Oxford Medical Publications

Oxford Textbook of

Public Health

Oxford Textbook of
Public Health

FIFTH EDITION

Roger Detels
Distinguished Professor of Epidemiology and Infectious Diseases, Schools of Public Health and Medicine, University of California, Los Angeles, Los Angeles, California, USA

Robert Beaglehole
Professor Emeritus, University of Auckland, Auckland, New Zealand

Mary Ann Lansang
Professor of Medicine and Clinical Epidemiology, College of Medicine, University of the Philippines, Manila, The Philippines

Martin Gulliford
Professor of Public Health, Department of Public Health Sciences, King's College London, London, United Kingdom

OXFORD
UNIVERSITY PRESS

OXFORD
UNIVERSITY PRESS

Great Clarendon Street, Oxford OX2 6DP

Oxford University Press is a department of the University of Oxford.
It furthers the University's objective of excellence in research, scholarship,
and education by publishing worldwide in

Oxford New York

Auckland Cape Town Dar es Salaam Hong Kong Karachi
Kuala Lumpur Madrid Melbourne Mexico City Nairobi
New Delhi Shanghai Taipei Toronto

With offices in

Argentina Austria Brazil Chile Czech Republic France Greece
Guatemala Hungary Italy Japan Poland Portugal Singapore
South Korea Switzerland Thailand Turkey Ukraine Vietnam

Published in the United States
by Oxford University Press Inc., New York

First edition 1984
Second edition 1991
Third edition 1997
Fourth edition 2002 (reprinted in paperback 2004, 2005 twice)
Fifth edition 2009
First published in paperback 2011

British Library Cataloguing in Publication Data

Data available

Library of Congress Cataloguing in Publication Data
Data available

Typeset by Cepha Imaging Pvt. Ltd., Bangalore, India
Printed in Great Britain on acid free paper by
Ashford Colour Press Ltd., Gosport, Hampshire

ISBN 978–0–19–921870–7 (Set)

ISBN 978–0–19–957943–3 (Vol. 1)

ISBN 978–0–19–957944–0 (Vol. 2)

ISBN 978–0–19–957945–7 (Vol. 3)

ISBN 978–0–19–969347–4 (Combined pbk.)

3 5 7 9 10 8 6 4

Available as a set only

Preface to the fifth edition

Much has happened in the world and in the field of public health since the publication of the 4th edition of the *Oxford Textbook of Public Health*. Sudden acute respiratory syndrome (SARS) has come and gone, H5N1, H1N1 and the probability of new variant influenzas are the emerging infectious diseases of greatest concern, the health gap between rich and poor countries and within many countries has widened, HIV continues to be a major problem despite the development of effective treatments and strategies to prevent mother-to-child transmission, wars continue to be waged causing massive loss and disruption of human life and displacement of people, violence and terrorism have increased, and the epidemics of obesity and asthma have intensified. Our inability to effectively meet disasters has been demonstrated with the tsunami devastating northern Indonesia, Sri Lanka, and southern Thailand (2004), although the rapid, effective response by the Chinese to the Sichuan earthquake (2008) gives evidence that our ability to respond to natural disasters is improving.

On the positive side, the World Health Organization and member states are in the process of developing international reporting systems for emerging diseases, we have made strides in preventing chronic diseases such as cancer and heart disease (although these diseases are already a major cause of morbidity and mortality in low- and middle-income countries), polio has been eliminated in much of the world through effective new immunization strategies, and environmental pollution and global warming are now recognized as major problems and have attracted political concern—a major step in implementing effective solutions. Further, the burgeoning field of genomics holds promise of transforming both medicine and public health, but we must be concerned that it is applied to the improvement of the health of individuals and society and not used to discriminate against genetically vulnerable persons. Although private organizations have long contributed to public health, there has been a recent surge in private support of public health, particularly in the field of HIV/AIDS. While these contributions have had very positive effects on the health of people, particularly in low- and middle-income countries, they have also had unexpected impacts.

Public health continues to be a dynamic, exciting field which challenges creative thinking and demands implementation of innovative strategies. For the 5th edition of the Textbook, we have outlined these continuing and new public health problems and have recruited authors who are leaders in recognizing and addressing them. Although we have continued dividing the basic structure of the Textbook into three major topic areas, the scope of public health, the methods of public health, and the practice of public health, we have added chapters to reflect the growth and changes in the field since 2002 and the emergence of new public health strategies. Thus, we have added new chapters on management of public health disasters, collective violence including war, applications of genomics to the field of public health, gene–environment interactions, clinical epidemiology, private support of public health, and the global health agenda for the twenty-first century, among others. All other chapters have been updated, most of them by new leaders in their respective fields. Further, we have recruited public health professionals from all the major regions of the world, reflecting the global scope of public health and the textbook.

We hope that this 5th edition will contribute to the advancement of the field of public health through its presentation of the scope, concerns, strategies, and applications of the field. The Textbook is intended for public health researchers, practitioners, students of the field, and other health professionals who wish to understand the field and their opportunities for contributing to the health and well-being of the people of the world.

Roger Detels
Robert Beaglehole
Mary Ann Lansang
Martin Gulliford

Introduction

The scope of public health

The scope of public health is vast and ever widening. The *Oxford Textbook of Public Health* provides a conceptual framework encompassing the scope of public health as it strives to cope with the enormous challenges of the twenty-first century.

Despite remarkable health gains achieved in the world over the past century, the increasing complexity of human interactions has considerably expanded public health concerns. Traditional public health approaches to epidemics have had to be redefined in the face of new global threats like severe acute respiratory syndrome (SARS) and avian influenza, as well as older microbial diseases with new biosecurity implications. The growing burden of noncommunicable diseases, the severe consequences of global warming, the repercussions of globalization, and the serious social dislocations resulting from rapid urbanization and armed conflicts have escalated the challenges to public health.

The persistence of HIV/AIDS, malaria, and tuberculosis, particularly among low- and middle-income countries, has spurred public health practitioners to utilize innovations in the fields of vaccinology, genomics, and proteomics to implement realistic solutions through sound health policies and systems strengthening, community engagement, and intersectoral partnerships. A major concern of public health is the growing recognition of the social determinants of health and the wide health disparities among nations, income groups, genders, and social classes. This concern for social justice and equity requires that public health professionals incorporate strategies from the social sciences, ethics, and human rights in the collective and organized pursuit of 'health for all'.

The Oxford Textbook of Public Health maps the breadth of public health through four updated sections: the history and development of public health, determinants of health and disease, public health policies, and public health law and ethics. Chapter 1.1 provides an overarching framework for public health and defines an expanded list of 13 functions covering the range of technology, social sciences, and politics. The next three chapters (Chapters 1.2–1.4) describe how public health has evolved in the context of rich and poor countries as well as those in economic transition, and the unique roles of the public and private sectors in addressing inequities in these different settings.

Critical to the development of interventions for public health problems is a thorough understanding of the structural and intermediary determinants of social inequities, coupled with a participative approach to address these determinants through intersectoral policies (Chapter 2.2). Globalization can potentially aggravate health inequities; hence, the economic, social, and political processes associated with these transnational interactions must be recognized and effectively managed (Chapter 2.1). The behavioural determinants, once viewed as the dominant factors for health and disease, are discussed within an ecological frame, thus providing a more integrated view of the complex interplay of behaviour with biologic, economic, political, and environmental factors (Chapter 2.3). In Chapters 2.4–2.7, important biologic determinants are elaborated. Genetic risks, which are increasingly being understood through the Human Genome Project, as well as genome-based technologies, have a growing potential to yield important public health interventions in the future, but there are also complex behavioural, economic, and ethical concerns that must be considered (Chapter 2.4). Almost taken for granted by the developed world, but still critically inadequate in many parts of the globe, are safe water, basic sanitation, food security, and good nutrition. Chapters 2.5 and 2.6 discuss the health risks and challenges associated with their absence, shortage, or—in the case of obesity—oversupply. Chapter 2.7 reviews the major infectious diseases, which remain significant causes of ill health globally and which present new threats with the emergence of new microbial pathogens and increasing antimicrobial resistance. The risks to human health and survival posed by a variety of environmental exposures, greenhouse gas accumulation, and ozone depletion, among others, are described in Chapter 2.8 and require urgent collaborative action.

There is ample evidence to demonstrate the value of providing essential packages through quality health services in reducing risks and improving health (Chapter 2.9). By assessing the burden of disease and underlying risk factors (Chapter 2.10), it is possible to prioritize the essential health care packages and interventions that will be most cost-effective and equitable in a given population.

An understanding of health determinants must translate into effective policies and strategies for action. Many countries have responded by addressing these root causes systemically and developing mechanisms to reduce health inequities (Chapter 3.1). With few exceptions, many high-income countries have used knowledge generated from biomedical and public health research to protect and improve public health (Chapter 3.2). In contrast, multiple factors such as poor governance, inadequate financing of health care, the distortion of national health priorities vis-à-vis global health initiatives, and an inadequate evidence base for decision-making are common features of the policy environment in low- and middle-income countries (Chapter 3.3). Of paramount importance to effective policy-making is strong public health leadership at all levels, characterized by strategic thinking in addressing public health problems and the ability to engage and mobilize multiple stakeholders in the process (Chapter 3.4).

Chapter 4.1 affirms the commitment of public health to achieve the 'highest attainable standard of health' and offers a rights-based approach to health (Chapter 4.1). This human right is elaborated in the context of public health legislation (Chapter 4.2) and international public health instruments (Chapter 4.3). Finally, the evolution of principles and guidelines of public health and research ethics are discussed in Chapter 4.4, with particular attention given to the principle of social justice as it relates to public health practice and research.

The extensive responsibilities and dynamic scope of public health described in this volume dictate that public health professionals employ a wide range of disciplines, seek and build intersectoral partnerships and international coalitions, and, most importantly, engage communities to achieve the goals of improving population health and promoting equity for all.

The methods of public health

The *Oxford Textbook of Public Health* remains central to the ambitions of the fifth edition. This volume presents the methods which form the basis of the scientific credibility of the public health endeavour. With a firm and broad grounding in the methods of public health, students and practitioners will ensure that their research and practice is based on robust evidence. In the absence of this grounding, we are vulnerable to charges of bias, and our efforts to improve the health of populations, and especially the health of the most disadvantaged populations, will inevitably be questioned by authorities with other aims and outlooks.

The range of health conditions facing populations is increasing, and so the scope of public health must widen to ensure an effective response. As the demographic, nutrition, and physical activity transitions spread to all parts of the world, the methods of public health must be adapted to meet the new challenges. Since the fourth edition appeared in 2002, global challenges to public health have become even more obvious, especially the effects of globalization on health and the increasing importance of global environmental changes, notably climate change. These new challenges are more difficult to study than the traditional concerns of infectious and non-infectious diseases and local environmental issues. The adaptation of old methods and the development of new methods will validate the ongoing relevance of public health research. Public health practitioners have always struggled to balance methodological rigor with the need to act expeditiously. This difficult balancing act will continue and will become even more difficult since the new challenges are much less amenable to direct observational study and not at all suitable for experimental study.

All chapters in this volume have been extensively revised, and new chapters added. This volume is organized around four sections: information systems and sources of intelligence; epidemiological and biostatistical approaches; social science and environmental techniques; and occupational sciences. Information systems are the foundation of all public health research and action. The lack of good information is still a barrier to effective action in much of the world. Basic information on births and deaths is not routinely available for most low-income and many middle-income countries. This gap remains a major impediment to tracking progress towards international development goals. Fortunately, a concerted effort is now being made to close the gap, especially for maternal and child statistics and with the support of philanthropic foundations. Three chapters in this section (Chapters 5.1–5.3) examine the contrasting challenges facing information systems in both high-income and low- and middle-income countries.

Epidemiology (Chapters 6.1–6.6) and biostatistics (Chapter 6.15) are the key sciences of public health. Public health practice requires a firm connection to the priority health needs of populations. Epidemiological research is almost always required to establish this connection, and exceptions are few; some major acute outbreaks or overwhelming catastrophes do not allow for serious epidemiological investigation before the response is mounted. However, epidemiological study is required to assess the scope of the problem and the effectiveness of the response. Public health methods are evolving to ensure the appropriateness of inferences (Chapter 6.13) drawn from public health investigations—perhaps the most difficult and certainly the most contentious aspect of public health science. This process often requires a systematic approach to ensuring that all data from all studies—published and unpublished—are synthesized into a useable summary assessment (Chapter 6.14). A critical and expanding methodological area deals with interventions and their effectiveness (Chapters 6.7–6.10). Technological advances—computers and the Internet—are changing the scope of public health and opening new possibilities, from data collection to the early identification of disease outbreaks and the modelling of disease transmission to predict future needs (Chapters 6.4 and 6.16). The methods and special issues facing clinical epidemiology are discussed in Chapter 6.11. The final chapter in this section stresses the continuing importance of surveillance to effective public health action (Chapter 6.17).

Social science techniques are assuming even greater importance to the practice of public health with the recognition that epidemiological information alone is not sufficient for the development and implementation of effective public health policies and programmes (Chapter 7.1). Demography is another underappreciated basic science of public health; the ageing of all populations, especially in low- and middle-income countries, will be a critical public health issue of this century (Chapter 7.2). Health economics and the use of cost-effectiveness analysis (Chapter 7.4) have expanded the audience for public health research to sectors outside health, especially the finance and development sectors, nationally and globally. Health promotion expands the focus of public health from a primary concern with disease prevention and control towards an understanding of the underlying determinants of health (Chapter 7.3).

These and other social science tools, including management of the health programmes (Chapter 7.5), are of equal relevance to the development and implementation of public health policy in all countries (Chapters 7.6 and 7.7).

Environmental and occupational health sciences cover traditional public health issues, as well as the even more difficult global health challenges that are discussed in The Scope of Public Health. This section deals with traditional environmental and occupational health hazards (Chapters 8.1–8.6). The increasingly important issues of risk assessment and management, and risk perception and communication are covered in Chapters 8.7 and 8.8.

The importance of methodological advances in public health is illustrated by the way in which many chapters in other volumes of this Textbook consider methodological issues in considerable detail—for example, the chapters on measuring the global burden of diseases and responding to global environmental challenges. The chapters in this section illustrate the evolution and breadth of public health methods as its scope continues to expand. No doubt, this process will continue well into the future.

The practice of public health

> *Public health is what we, as a society, do collectively to assure the conditions for people to be healthy. This requires that continuing and emerging threats to the health of the public be successfully countered . . . through effective, organised, and sustained efforts led by the public sector.* Institute of Medicine (1988)

The Textbook provides a state-of-the-art account of the practice of public health through forty-seven chapters written by leading experts. The contents of this volume continue the shift in thinking, already introduced in The Scope and Methods of Public Health, that considers public health not only as a matter of local and national concern and a key responsibility of governments and public agencies, but also as an international issue that must be addressed through optimal global governance. This change in thinking has led to the inclusion of new chapters that reassess priorities, recognize the evolving burden of disease, and recommend new strategies for intervention.

The Practice of Public Health begins with a discussion of the major groups of non-communicable disorders (Section 9). This section includes, for the first time, separate chapters on obesity and diabetes, reflecting the growing concern for the increasing impact of these conditions on global health. Current estimates suggest that there are about 1.1 billion overweight and obese adults in the world, with an estimated 10% of all children now being overweight. More than half of those affected are in middle- or low-income countries.

The series of chapters on communicable diseases has been similarly expanded, with new chapters on tuberculosis, malaria, hepatitis, and emerging diseases. Together, these conditions represent major priorities: tuberculosis accounts for an estimated 1.6 million deaths worldwide each year, with 8.8 million new cases; malaria accounts for 46.5 million disability-adjusted life years lost annually; while one out of every 40 deaths is attributed to liver cirrhosis or primary liver cancer. In addition to outlining problems and their causes, each of these chapters discusses potential solutions, including national and international strategies for disease control and prevention.

The emphasis on intervention for prevention of disease and promotion of health is continued in the volume's second section on public health hazards, including tobacco, alcohol, drug abuse, injuries, and violence (Section 10). The proposed intervention strategies encompass both population-based approaches—including, for example, regulation, the use of deterrents and incentives, and public education—and strategies targeted at individuals at high risk through health care services. It remains clear, however, that the greatest risks are generally found among those groups for whom interventions are least accessible.

In keeping with the equity orientation of public health, Section 11 considers the public health needs of different population groups, paying particular attention to groups that, for a range of reasons, are vulnerable to public health hazards and disease risks. Separate chapters outline the needs of families, women, children, adolescents, older people, ethnic minorities, people with disabilities, and forced migrants and displaced populations. Collectively, these chapters emphasize the importance of the public health role in analysing the health needs of these often marginalized populations and advocating for their rights to health.

Section 12 presents an analysis of the core public health skills required for improving population health and reducing inequalities in health. This section begins with a discussion of the concept of need, as a capacity to benefit from health intervention. This is accompanied by a practical guide to the assessment of need in public health practice. Needs must often be met through a combination of intervention strategies, and this is exemplified by chapters on current strategies for control of non-communicable and infectious diseases. A series of chapters then outlines opportunities for intervention through the health sector, including health care services, population screening, and environmental health practice. However, addressing the main determinants of health requires the development and implementation of public health interventions that extend well beyond the health sector. The difficulties of multisectoral intervention are illustrated by the complex problems of tackling health inequalities in either high-income or middle- and low-income countries. As Davidson Gwatkin observes, achieving change is critically dependent on political will.

In the final section of the book, Roger Detels and Sheena Sullivan question the assumption that intervention on public health problems must be led by the public sector. They describe a re-emerging role for powerful private sector advocates of public health intervention, while at the same time drawing attention to some of the difficulties of this approach and the importance of the stewardship role of governments. The final chapter by Margaret Chan and colleagues summarizes many of the key issues that have been raised in earlier chapters of the book. The authors conclude that technical skills will be insufficient to achieve the public health goals of improving population health and reducing inequalities. 'Efforts to provide good health for all' must be underscored by an ethical focus driven by recognition that 'the highest attainable standard of health is one of the fundamental rights of every human being'.

Institute of Medicine (1988). *The future of public health.* Washington DC. National Academies Press. Page 19.

Brief Contents

Contents

The scope of public health

SECTION 4
Public health law and ethics

The methods of public health

SECTION 5
Information systems and sources of intelligence

SECTION 6
Epidemiological and biostatistical approaches

SECTION 7
Social science techniques

SECTION 8
Environmental and occupational health sciences

The practice of public health

SECTION 9
Major health problems

List of contributors

Quarraisha Abdool Karim Columbia University (Department of Epidemiology), University of KwaZulu Natal (School of Family Medicine and Public Health) and CAPRISA (Centre for the AIDS Programme of Research in South Africa), South Africa.
Chapter 9.13 Acquired immunodeficiency syndrome

Salim S. Abdool Karim, Pro Vice Chancellor (Research), University of KwaZulu-Natal; Director, Centre for the AIDS Programme of Research in South Africa (CAPRISA); Professor in Clinical Epidemiology, Columbia University Adjunct; Professor in Medicine, Cornell University, South Africa.
Chapter 9.13 Acquired immunodeficiency syndrome

Maia Ambegaokar London School of Hygiene and Tropical Medicine, London, UK.
Chapter 3.4 Leadership in public health

Ian Anderson Professor for Indigenous Health, Centre for Health and Society & Onemda VicHealth Koori Health Unit, School of Population Health, University of Melbourne, Melbourne, Australia.
Chapter 11.5 Ethnic minorities and indigenous peoples

Roy M. Anderson Rector, Imperial College London, London, UK.
Chapter 6.16 Mathematical models of transmission and control

Samira Asma Associate Director, Global Tobacco Control, Centers for Disease Control and Prevention, USA.
Chapter 10.1 Tobacco

Gunilla Backman Senior Researcher, Human Rights Centre, University of Essex, UK.
Chapter 4.1 The right to the highest attainable standard of health

Rajiv Bahl Medical Officer, Department of Child and Adolescent Health and Development, World Health Organization, Geneva, Switzerland.
Chapter 11.3 Child health

Dean Baker Professor and Director, Center for Occupational and Environmental Health, University of California, Irvine, CA, USA.
Chapter 8.5 Occupational health

Hilary J. Bambrick Senior Lecturer, School of Medicine, University of Western Sydney, Campbelltown NSW Australia; Visiting Fellow, National Centre for Epidemiology and Population Health, The Australian National University, Canberra ACT, Australia.
Chapter 2.8 The global environment

Catherine R. Bateman School of Public Health and Community Medicine, University of New South Wales, Sydney, Australia.
Chapter 11.8 Forced migrants and other displaced populations

Robert Beaglehole Professor Emeritus, University of Auckland, Auckland, New Zealand.
Chapter 12.5 Prevention and control of chronic, non-communicable diseases

Ruth L. Berkelman Department of Epidemiology, Rollins School of Public Health, Emory University, Atlanta, GA, USA.
Chapter 6.17 Public health surveillance

Douglas Bettcher Director, Tobacco Free Initiative, World Health Organization, Geneva, Switzerland.
Chapter 4.3 International public health instruments
Chapter 10.1 Tobacco

Zulfiqar Ahmed Bhutta Husein Lalji Dewraj Professor of Pediatrics, and Chairman, Department of Pediatrics & Child Health, The Aga Khan University, Karachi, Pakistan.
Chapter 2.7 Infectious diseases

Stella Bialous President, Tobacco Policy International, San Francisco, USA.
Chapter 10.1 Tobacco

Fred Binka Dean School of Public Health, College of Health Sciences, University of Ghana, Legon, Ghana.
Chapter 5.2 Information systems and community diagnosis in low- and middle-income countries

Jennifer Bishop Department of Food Safety, Zoonoses and Foodborne Diseases, World Health Organization, Geneva, Switzerland.
Chapter 4.3 International public health instruments

Marike Boezen Unit Chronic Airway Diseases (head), Department of Epidemiology, University Medical Center Groningen, University of Groningen, Groningen, The Netherlands.
Chapter 9.4 Chronic obstructive pulmonary disease and asthma

Paolo Boffetta International Agency for Research on Cancer, Lyon, France.
Chapter 9.3 Neoplasms

Diana Bonta Vice President, Public Affairs, Kaiser Foundation Health Plans and Hospitals, Southern California Region, USA.
Chapter 7.5 Governance and management of public health programmes

Cynthia Boschi-Pinto Medical Officer, Department of Child and Adolescent Health and Development, World Health Organization, Geneva, Switzerland.
Chapter 11.3 Child health

James Bowen Center at Evergreen, Kirkland, WA, USA.
Chapter 9.10 Neurologic diseases, epidemiology, and public health

James W. Buehler Department of Epidemiology, Rollins School of Public Health, Emory University, Atlanta, GA, USA.
Chapter 6.17 Public health surveillance

Wylie Burke Professor and Chair, Department of Medical History and Ethics, University of Washington, Seattle, WA, USA.
Chapter 2.4 Genomics and public health

Jason W. Busse Assistant Professor, Department of Clinical Epidemiology & Biostatistics, McMaster University, Hamilton, Ontario, Canada; Scientist, Institute for Work & Health, Toronto, Ontario, Canada.
Chapter 6.11 Clinical epidemiology

Julie E. Byles Director, Research Centre for Gender, Health and Ageing Faculty of Health, University of Newcastle, NSW, Australia.
Chapter 11.7 Health of older people

Meredith Cagle Cagle Consulting Services.
Chapter 7.5 Governance and management of public health programmes

Simon Carroll Associate Director, Centre for Community Health Promotion Research, University of Victoria, Canada.
Chapter 7.3 Health promotion, health education, and the public's health

Margaret Chan Director General, World Health Organization, Geneva, Switzerland.
Chapter 12.14 Global health agenda for the twenty-first century

Venkatraman Chandra-Mouli Head, Adolescent Health and Development, Department of Child and Adolescent Health and Development (CAH), World Health Organization, Geneva, Switzerland.
Chapter 11.4 Adolescent health

Leda Chatzi Department of Social Medicine, Medical School, University of Crete, Heraklion, Greece.
Chapter 6.3 Cross-sectional studies

Chien-Jen Chen Academician and Distinguished Research Fellow, Genomics Research Center, Academic Sinica, National Taiwan University School of Medicine, Taipei, Taiwan.
Chapter 8.1 Environmental health issues in public health

Virasakdi Chongsuvivatwong Professor of Community Medicine, Epidemiology Unit, Faculty of Medicine, Prince of Songkla University, Hatyai, Thailand.
Chapter 12.5 Prevention and control of chronic, non-communicable diseases

Aileen Clarke Associate Clinical Professor in Public Health & Health Services Research, Health Sciences Research Institute, Warwick Medical School, University of Warwick, Coventry, UK.
Chapter 12.2 Needs assessment: A practical approach

Thomas Clasen Department of Infectious and Tropical Diseases, London School of Hygiene and Tropical Medicine, London, UK.
Chapter 2.5 Water and sanitation

Myles Cockburn Associate Professor, Department of Preventive Medicine, Keck School of Medicine; Department of Geography, College of Letters, Arts and Sciences, University of Southern California, USA.
Chapter 8.2 Radiation and public health

Bernadette Daelmans Department of Child and Adolescent Health and Development, World Health Organization, Geneva, Switzerland.
Chapter 11.3 Child health

Peter Davis Department of Sociology, University of Auckland, New Zealand.
Chapter 7.6 Public health sciences and policy in high-income countries

Manuel M. Dayrit Director, Human Resources for Health, World Health Organization, Geneva, Switzerland.
Chapter 3.4 Leadership in public health

Judith Bueno de Mesquita Senior Researcher, Human Rights Centre, University of Essex, UK.
Chapter 4.1 The right to the highest attainable standard of health

Katherine DeLand Senior Technical Officer, Tobacco Free Initiative, World Health Organization, Geneva, Switzerland.
Chapter 4.3 International public health instruments
Chapter 10.1 Tobacco

Rodolfo Dennis Head, Departments of Medicine and Research, Fundacion Cardioinfantil; Professor of Medicine, Pontificia Universidad Javeriana, Bogota, Colombia.
Chapter 6.11 Clinical epidemiology

Roger Detels Distinguished Professor of Epidemiology and Infectious Diseases, Schools of Public Health and Medicine, University of California, Los Angeles, Los Angeles, CA, USA.
Chapter 1.1 The scope and concerns of public health
Chapter 6.1 Epidemiology: The foundation of public health
Chapter 9.13 Acquired immunodeficiency syndrome
Chapter 12.13 Private support of public health

Ana V. Diez-Roux Department of Epidemiology, University of Michigan School of Public Health, Ann Arbor, MI, USA.
Chapter 6.2 Ecologic variables, ecologic studies, and multilevel studies in public health research

Allan Donner Department of Epidemiology and Biostatistics, Schulich School of Medicine and Dentistry, University of Western Ontario London, Ontario, Canada.
Chapter 6.8 Methodological issues in the design and analysis of community intervention trials

Manjit Dosanjh Advisor to the Director General, Life Sciences and International Organisations, CERN, Geneva.
Chapter 8.2 Radiation and public health

John M. Douglas, Jr Director, DSTDP, NCHHSTP, CDC, Atlanta, GA, USA.
Chapter 9.12 Sexually transmitted infections

Jeroen Douwes Associate Director, Centre for Public Health Research, Massey University Wellington Campus, Wellington, New Zealand.
Chapter 9.4 Chronic obstructive pulmonary disease and asthma

Lesley Doyal Professor of Gender and Health, School for Policy Studies, University of Bristol, Bristol, UK; Visiting Professor, University of Cape Town, South Africa.
Chapter 11.2 Women, men, and health

Shah Ebrahim Professor of Public Health, Department of Epidemiology & Population Health, London School of Hygiene and Tropical Medicine, London, UK.
Chapter 11.7 Health of older people

Matthias Egger Professor of Epidemiology and Public Health, Institute of Social & Preventive Medicine (ISPM), University of Bern, Switzerland.
Chapter 6.14 Systematic reviews and meta-analysis

Marcos Espinal Executive Secretary, Stop TB Partnership, Geneva, Switzerland.
Chapter 9.14 Tuberculosis

Daniel Ferrante World Health Organization, Geneva, Switzerland.
Chapter 10.1 Tobacco

Josep Figueras Director, European Observatory on Health Systems and Policies, Head, WHO Centre for Health Policy, Brussels.
Chapter 12.10 Strategies for health services

J. Peter Figueroa Chief, Epidemiology & AIDS, Ministry of Health, Kingston, Jamaica.
Chapter 7.7 Public health sciences and policy in low- and middle-income countries

Louise Finer Senior Researcher, Human Rights Centre, University of Essex, UK.
Chapter 4.1 The right to the highest attainable standard of health

Baruch Fischhoff Howard Heinz University Professor, Department of Social and Decision Sciences, Department of Engineering and Public Policy; Department of Social and Decision Sciences, Carnegie Mellon University, Pittsburgh, PA, USA.
Chapter 8.8 Risk perception and communication

Olivier Fontaine Department of Child and Adolescent Health and Development, World Health Organization, Geneva, Switzerland.
Chapter 11.3 Child health

Sven Francque Division of Gastroenterology and Hepatology, University Hospital Antwerp, Belgium.
Chapter 9.16 Chronic hepatitis and other liver disease

Melvyn Freeman Extraordinary Professor, University of Stellenbosch, South Africa.
Chapter 9.7 Public mental health

Julio Frenk Dean, Harvard School of Public Health, Boston, USA.
Chapter 3.3 Health policy in developing countries

Lawrence M. Friedman Independent Consultant, Rockville, MD, USA.
Chapter 6.7 Methodology of intervention trials in individuals

Fu Paul Fu, Jr. Associate Professor of Pediatrics and Public Health, David Geffen School of Medicine at UCLA, and UCLA School of Public Health, CA, USA.
Chapter 5.1 Information systems in support of public health in high-income countries

Michelle Funk Michelle Funk, Coordinator, Mental Health Policy and Service Development (MHP), Department of Mental Health and Substance Abuse, World Health Organization, Geneva, Switzerland.
Chapter 9.7 Public mental health

Gary Giovino Senior Research Scientist and Director, Tobacco Control Program, Roswell Park Cancer Institute, Buffalo, USA.
Chapter 10.1 Tobacco

Lynn R. Goldman Professor, Environmental Health Sciences, Johns Hopkins University, Bloomberg School of Public Health, Baltimore, MD, USA.
Chapter 12.8 Environmental health practice

Bernard D. Goldstein Professor, Department of Environmental and Occupational Health, University of Pittsburgh Graduate School of Public Health, Pittsburgh, PA, USA.
Chapter 8.7 Toxicology and risk assessment in the analysis and management of environmental risk

Octavio Gómez-Dantés Researcher, National Institute of Public Health, Mexico.
Chapter 3.3 Health policy in developing countries

Miguel Angel González-Block Executive Director of the Center for Health Systems Research, INSP—National Public Health Institute, Mexico.
Chapter 3.3 Health policy in developing countries

Fernando González-Martín International Health Regulations Secretariat, World Health Organization, Geneva, Switzerland.
Chapter 4.3 International public health instruments

Sherwood L. Gorbach Professor of Public Health, Medicine, and Molecular Biology/Microbiology, Tufts University School of Medicine, Boston, MA, USA.
Chapter 2.7 Infectious diseases

Lawrence W. Green Adjunct Professor, Department of Epidemiology and Biostatistics, School of Medicine, University of California at San Francisco, CA, USA.
Chapter 2.3 Behavioural determinants of health and disease

Manfred S. Green Center for the Study of Bioterrorism, Tel Aviv University, Israel Center for Disease Control, Ministry of Health, Israel.
Chapter 10.8 Public health aspects of bioterrorism

Sander Greenland Professor, Department of Epidemiology and Department of Statistics University of California, Los Angeles, CA, USA.
Chapter 6.12 Validity and bias in epidemiological research
Chapter 6.13 Causation and causal inference

Emily Grundy Centre for Population Studies, London School of Hygiene and Tropical Medicine, London, UK.
Chapter 7.2 Demography and public health

Martin Gulliford Department of Public Health Sciences, King's College London, London, UK.
Chapter 2.9 Health services as determinants of population health
Chapter 11.5 Ethnic minorities and indigenous peoples

Davidson R. Gwatkin The World Bank, Washington, DC, USA.
Chapter 12.4 Reducing health inequalities in developing countries

Davidson H. Hamer Associate Professor of International Health and Medicine, Department of International Health, Boston University School of Public Health, Department of Medicine, Boston University School of Medicine; Adjunct Associate Professor of Nutrition, Tufts University Friedman School of Nutrition Science and Policy, Boston, MA, USA.
Chapter 2.7 Infectious diseases

Christopher Hamlin Professor, Department of History, and in the Program of History and Philosophy of Science, University of Notre Dame, Notre Dame, IN, USA; Honorary Professor, Department of Public Health and Policy, London School of Hygiene and Tropical Medicine, London, UK.
Chapter 1.2 The history and development of public health in developed countries

Summer Hammide Student researcher, UCLA School of Public Health.
Chapter 4.3 International public health instruments

Marian T. Hannan Associate Professor of Medicine, Harvard Medical School, Co-Director of Musculoskeletal Research, Institute for Aging Research, Hebrew SeniorLife, Boston, MA, USA.
Chapter 9.9 Musculoskeletal diseases

Piya Hanvoravongchai Lecturer in Health Policy, Department of Public Health and Policy, London School of Hygiene and Tropical Medicine, London, UK.
Chapter 12.11 Public health workers

David Heymann Assistant Director General, Health Security and Environment, and Polio Eradication, World Health Organization, Geneva, Switzerland.
Chapter 9.17 Emerging and re-emerging infections

Robert A. Hiatt Co-Chair, Department of Epidemiology and Biostatistics, School of Medicine, University of California at San Francisco, CA, USA.
Chapter 2.3 Behavioural determinants of health and disease

Marcia Hills Professor, School of Nursing, Director, Centre for Community Health Promotion Research President, Canadian Consortium for Health Promotion Research University of Victoria, Canada.
Chapter 7.3 Health promotion, health education, and the public's health

Katherine J. Hoggatt Assistant Professor, Department of Epidemiology, University of Michigan, Ann Arbor, MI, USA.
Chapter 6.13 Causation and causal inference

Walter W. Holland Emeritus Professor of Public Health Medicine, Visiting Professor, LSE Health and Social Care, London School of Economics and Political Science, London, UK.
Chapter 3.1 Overview of policies and strategies
Chapter 12.7 Population screening and public health

T. Déirdre Hollingsworth Department of Infectious Disease Epidemiology, Faculty of Medicine, Imperial College London, London, UK.
Chapter 6.16 Mathematical models of transmission and control

Robert L. Hubbard Director, National Development and Research Institutes, Raleigh, NC, USA.
Chapter 10.2 Drug abuse

Paul Hunt UN Special Rapporteur on the right to the highest attainable standard of health (2002–2008); Professor, Human Rights Centre, University of Essex (England); Adjunct Professor, University of Waikato, New Zealand.
Chapter 4.1 The right to the highest attainable standard of health

Adnan A. Hyder Johns Hopkins University, Bloomberg School of Public Health, Department of International Health; Center for Injury Research & Policy, Baltimore, MD, USA.
Chapter 10.4 Injury prevention and control: The public health approach

Sopon Iamsirithaworn International Field Epidemiology Training Program, Bureau of Epidemiology, Department of Disease Control, Ministry of Public Health, Thailand.
Chapter 6.4 Principles of outbreak investigation

Alec Irwin Associate Director, François-Xavier Bagnoud Center for Health and Human Rights, Harvard School of Public Health, Boston, USA.
Chapter 2.2 Overview and framework

Philip James London School of Hygiene and Tropical Medicine, London, UK; International Obesity TaskForce, IASO, London, UK.
Chapter 9.5 Obesity

Dean T. Jamison Professor, Department of Global Health, University of Washington, Seattle, WA, USA.
Chapter 7.4 Cost-effectiveness analysis: Concepts and applications

Stephen Jan Senior Health Economist, The George Institute for International Health; Associate Professor, Faculty of Medicine, University of Sydney, NSW, Australia.
Chapter 12.1 Need: What is it and how do we measure it?

Don C. Des Jarlais Director of Research, Baron Edmond de Rothschild Chemical Dependency Institute, Beth Israel Medical Center, New York, NY, USA; Professor of Epidemiology and Population Health, Albert Einstein College of Medicine, Bronx, NY, USA.
Chapter 10.2 Drug abuse

Mary L. Kamb International Coordinator, Division of STD Prevention, Centers for Disease Control & Prevention (CDC), USA.
Chapter 9.12 Sexually transmitted infections

Nancy Kass Phoebe R. Berman Professor of Bioethics and Public Health, Berman Institute of Bioethics, Johns Hopkins Bloomberg School of Public Health, Baltimore, USA.
Chapter 4.4 Ethical principles and ethical issues in public health

Jennifer L. Kelsey Professor Emeritus, Stanford University School of Medicine, Department of Health Research and Policy, Stanford, CA, USA; Professor (part-time), University of Massachusetts Medical School, Departments of Medicine and of Family Medicine and Community Health, Worcester, MA, USA.
Chapter 9.9 Musculoskeletal diseases

Leeka Kheifets Professor, UCLA School of Public Health, Department of Epidemiology, Los Angeles, CA, USA.
Chapter 8.2 Radiation and public health

Rajat Khosla Senior Researcher, Human Rights Centre, University of Essex, UK.
Chapter 4.1 The right to the highest attainable standard of health

Muin J. Khoury Director, National Office of Public Health Genomics, Centers for Disease Control and Prevention, Atlanta, GA, USA.
Chapter 2.4 Genomics and public health

Robert J. Kim-Farley Professor, Departments of Epidemiology and Community Health Sciences, UCLA School of Public Health, Los Angeles, USA.
Chapter 12.6 Principles of infectious disease control

Mary Kindhauser Office of the Director General, World Health Organization, Geneva, Switzerland.
Chapter 12.14 Global health agenda for the twenty-first century

Richard S.G. Knight Professor of Clinical Neurology, National CJD Surveillance Unit, University of Edinburgh, Western General Hospital, Edinburgh, UK.
Chapter 9.11 The transmissible spongiform encephalopathies

Manolis Kogevinas Professor and co-Director, Centre for Research in Environmental Epidemiology (CREAL) Municipal Institute of Medical Research (IMIM), Barcelona, Spain.
Chapter 6.3 Cross-sectional studies

David Koh Head, Department of Community, Occupational and Family Medicine; Yong Loo Lin School of Medicine, National University of Singapore, Singapore.
Chapter 8.5 Occupational health

Dragana Korljan Human Rights Officer, Office of the High Commissioner for Human Rights.
Chapter 4.1 The right to the highest attainable standard of health

Walter A. Kukull Professor, Epidemiology, Director, Nat'l Alzheimer's Coord Ctr (NACC), Department of Epidemiology, University of Washington, Seattle, WA, USA.
Chapter 9.10 Neurologic diseases, epidemiology, and public health

Vipat Kuruchittham Lecturer, College of Public Health Sciences, Chulalongkorn University, Bangkok, Thailand.
Chapter 5.2 Information systems and community diagnosis in low- and middle-income countries

Kamakshi Lakshminarayan Assistant Professor, Department of Neurology, School of Medicine, University of Minnesota, Minneapolis, USA.
Chapter 9.2 Cardiovascular and cerebrovascular diseases

Mary Ann Lansang Professor of Medicine and Clinical Epidemiology, College of Medicine, University of the Philippines, Manila.
Chapter 7.7 Public health sciences and policy in low- and middle-income countries
Chapter 12.2 Needs assessment: A practical approach

Kelley Lee Head, Public and Environmental Health Research Unit, London School of Hygiene and Tropical Medicine, London, UK.
Chapter 2.1 Globalization

June Leung Intern, Hospital Authority, Hong Kong Special Administrative Region, People's Republic of China.
Chapter 10.1 Tobacco

Barry S. Levy Adjunct Professor of Public Health, Tufts University School of Medicine, Sherborn, MA, USA.
Chapter 10.6 Collective violence: War

Khanchit Limpakarnjanarat Communicable Disease Surveillance and Response (CSR), Department of Communicable Diseases (CDS), WHO SEARO.
Chapter 12.12 Planning for and responding to public health needs in emergencies and disasters

Annette Lin A candidate for a JD (juris doctorate) and MPH (masters of public health) joint degree at the University of California in Los Angeles, CA, USA.
Chapter 4.3 International public health instruments

Paul J. Lioy Professor and Vice Chair, Department of Environmental and Occupational Medicine, RWJMS, Deputy Director of Government Relations and Director of the Exposure Science Division of the Environmental and Occupational Health Sciences Institute (EOHSI), Robert Wood Johnson Medical School (RWJMS), UMDNJ and Rutgers University, Piscataway, NJ, USA.
Chapter 8.4 The science of human exposures to contaminants in the environment

Alexander Lo Dak Wai Solicitor, Hong Kong; Solicitor, England and Wales (non-practising); Chinese Medical Practitioner, Hong Kong; Professional Consultant, School of Law, The Chinese University of Hong Kong.
Chapter 4.2 Comparative national public health legislation

Donald Lollar Senior Research Scientist, National Center on Birth Defects and Developmental Disabilities, Centers for Disease Control and Prevention, United States Department of Health and Human Services, Atlanta, GA, USA.
Chapter 11.6 People with disabilities

A.D. Lopez School of Population Health, University of Queensland, Brisbane, Australia.
Chapter 2.10 Assessing health needs: The global burden of disease approach

Adetokunbo Lucas Adjunct Professor, Harvard University, Cambridge, MA, USA.
Chapter 3.3 Health policy in developing countries

Jeff Luck Department of Health Services, UCLA School of Public Health, CA, USA.
Chapter 5.1 Information systems in support of public health in high-income countries

Russell V. Luepker Mayo Professor, Division of Epidemiology and Community Health School of Public Health University of Minnesota, Minneapolis, USA.
Chapter 9.2 Cardiovascular and cerebrovascular diseases

Johan P. Mackenbach Department of Public Health, Erasmus MC, University Medical Centre Rotterdam, Rotterdam, The Netherlands.
Chapter 12.3 Socioeconomic inequalities in health in high-income countries: The facts and the options

Dermot Maher Senior Clinical Epidemiologist, Medical Research Council/ Uganda Virus Research Institute, Entebbe, Uganda.
Chapter 9.14 Tuberculosis

Lindiwe Makubalo Chief Director, Health Information, Epidemiology, Evaluation & Research, Department of Health, South Africa.
Chapter 7.7 Public health sciences and policy in low- and middle-income countries

Zoe Marshman Clinical Lecturer in Dental Public Health School of Clinical Dentistry, Claremont Crescent, Sheffield, UK.
Chapter 9.8 Dental public health

Robyn Martin Professor of Public Health Law, Centre for Research in Primary and Community Care, University of Hertfordshire, Hatfield, UK; Visiting Professor, The Chinese University of Hong Kong; Honorary Professor, London School of Hygiene and Tropical Medicine, London, UK; Director, European Public Health Law Network.
Chapter 4.2 Comparative national public health legislation

Jose Martines Department of Child and Adolescent Health and Development, World Health Organization, Geneva, Switzerland.
Chapter 11.3 Child health

Elizabeth Mason Director Department of Child and Adolescent Health and Development (CAH), World Health Organization, Geneva, Switzerland.
Chapter 11.3 Child health

Colin Douglas Mathers Coordinator, Mortality and Burden of Disease, Department of Health Statistics and Informatics, World Health Organization, Geneva, Switzerland.
Chapter 2.10 Assessing health needs: The global burden of disease approach

Di McIntyre Professor and South African Research Chair in 'Health and Wealth', Health Economics Unit, School of Public Health and Family Medicine, University of Cape Town.
Chapter 12.1 Need: What is it and how do we measure it?

Martin McKee European Centre on Health of Societies in Transition, London School of Hygiene and Tropical Medicine, London, UK.
Chapter 12.10 Strategies for health services

Anthony J. McMichael NHMRC Australia Fellow, National Centre for Epidemiology and Population Health, The Australian National University, Canberra ACT Australia.
Chapter 2.8 The global environment

Pierre-André Michaud, Médecin chef, Unité multidisciplinaire de santé des adolescents, Lausanne, Switzerland.
Chapter 11.4 Adolescent health

Peter Michielsen, Division of Gastroenterology and Hepatology, University Hospital Antwerp, Belgium.
Chapter 9.16 Chronic hepatitis and other liver disease

Edward Mills Canada Research Chair, Global Health, Faculty of Health Sciences, University of Ottawa, Ottawa, Ontario, Canada.
Chapter 6.11 Clinical epidemiology

Mark R. Montgomery Professor of Economics, Stony Brook University; and Senior Associate, Population Council, NY, USA.
Chapter 10.7 Urban health in low- and middle-income countries

Gavin Mooney Professor of Health Economics, Department of Public Health, University of Sydney, Australia and Health Economics Unit, University of Cape Town, South Africa.
Chapter 12.1 Need: What is it and how do we measure it?

Myfanwy Morgan Professor of Sociology and Health, Department of Public Health Sciences, King's College London, London, UK.
Chapter 7.1 Sociology and psychology in public health
Chapter 11.5 Ethnic minorities and indigenous peoples

Richard Morrow Professor of International Health, Johns Hopkins Bloomberg School of Public Health, Baltimore, MD, USA.
Chapter 9.15 Malaria

William Moss Associate Professor of Epidemiology, Johns Hopkins Bloomberg School of Public Health, Baltimore, MD, USA.
Chapter 9.15 Malaria

Alvaro Muñoz Professor of Epidemiology, Johns Hopkins Bloomberg School of Public Health, Baltimore, MD, USA.
Chapter 6.6 Cohort studies

C.J.L. Murray Institute for Health Metrics and Evaluation, University of Washington, Seattle, USA.
Chapter 2.10 Assessing health needs: The global burden of disease approach

F. Javier Nieto Professor and Chair, Department of Population Health Sciences, University of Wisconsin School of Medicine and Public Health, Madison, WI, USA.
Chapter 6.6 Cohort studies

D. James Nokes KEMRI-Wellcome Trust Programme, Kilifi, Kenya; Reader, Department of Biological Sciences, University of Warwick, Coventry, UK.
Chapter 6.16 Mathematical models of transmission and control

Ellen Nolte Senior Lecturer, European Centre on Health of Societies in Transition, London School of Hygiene and Tropical Medicine, London, UK.
Chapter 12.10 Strategies for health services

Don Nutbeam Provost and Deputy Vice Chancellor, University of Sydney, NSW, Australia.
Chapter 12.9 Structures and strategies for public health intervention

Roderico H. Ofrin Technical Officer, Emergency and Humanitarian Action, WHO SEARO.
Chapter 12.12 Planning for and responding to public health needs in emergencies and disasters

Jane Ogden Professor of Health Psychology, Department of Psychology, University of Surrey, Guildford, UK.
Chapter 7.1 Sociology and psychology in public health

Lisa Oldring Special Advisor to Mary Robinson, GAVI Fund Board of Directors.
Chapter 4.1 The right to the highest attainable standard of health

Jørn Olsen Professor and Chair, Department of Epidemiology, School of Public Health, UCLA, CA, USA.
Chapter 12.5 Prevention and control of chronic, non-communicable diseases

Adrian Ong Office of the Director General, World Health Organization, Geneva, Switzerland.
Chapter 12.14 Global health agenda for the twenty-first century

Krishna M. Palipudi Senior Survey Statistician, Office on Smoking and Health, Centers for Disease Control and Prevention (CDC), Atlanta, Georgia, USA.
Chapter 10.1 Tobacco

George C. Patton VicHealth Professor of Adolescent Health, Centre for Adolescent Health, Murdoch Children's Research Institute, Melbourne, Australia.
Chapter 11.4 Adolescent health

Sarah Payne Reader in Social Policy, School for Policy Studies, University of Bristol, Bristol, UK.
Chapter 11.2 Women, men, and health

Neil Pearce Director, Centre for Public Health Research, Massey University Wellington Campus, Wellington, New Zealand.
Chapter 9.4 Chronic obstructive pulmonary disease and asthma

Corinne Peek-Asa Professor, University of Iowa, Occupational and Environmental Health, Injury Prevention Research Center, Iowa City, IA, USA.
Chapter 10.4 Injury prevention and control: The public health approach

John Powell Associate Clinical Professor of Epidemiology and Public Health, Health Sciences Research Institute, Warwick Medical School, University of Warwick, Coventry, UK.
Chapter 12.2 Needs assessment: A practical approach

John Powles Senior Lecturer in Public Health Medicine, Department of Public Health and Primary Care, Institute of Public Health, Robinson Way, Cambridge, UK.
Chapter 3.2 Public health policy in developed countries

Deborah Prothrow-Stith Professor, Harvard University School of Public Health, Boston, Mass, USA.
Chapter 10.5 Interpersonal violence prevention: A recent public health mandate

Denis J. Protti Professor, Health Information Science, Human & Social Development Building, University of Victoria, Victoria, Canada; Visiting Professor, Health Informatics, City University, London, UK.
Chapter 5.1 Information systems in support of public health in high-income countries

Laura Punnett Professor, Department of Work Environment; Director, Center to Promote Health in the New England Workplace (CPH-NEW); Senior Associate, Center for Women and Work (CWW), University of Massachusetts Lowell, MA, USA.
Chapter 8.6 Ergonomics and public health

Pekka Puska Director General, National Public Health Institute (KTL), Helsinki, Finland.
Chapter 6.9 Community-based intervention studies in high-income countries

Mario Raviglione Director, Stop TB Department, World Health Organization, Geneva, Switzerland.
Chapter 9.14 Tuberculosis

K. Srinath Reddy President, Public Health Foundation of India, New Delhi, India.
Chapter 1.4 The development of the discipline of public health in countries in economic transition: India, Brazil, China

Margaret Reid Professor of Women's Health, Public Health and Health Policy, Community Based Sciences, University of Glasgow, Glasgow, UK.
Chapter 7.1 Sociology and psychology in public health

Peter G. Robinson School of Clinical Dentistry, University of Sheffield, UK.
Chapter 9.8 Dental public health

Robin Room Professor, School of Population Health, University of Melbourne; and Director, AER Centre for Alcohol Policy Research, Turning Point Alcohol & Drug Centre, Fitzroy, Victoria, Australia.
Chapter 10.3 Alcohol

Julia Royall Chief, Office of International Programs, US National Library of Medicine, USA.
Chapter 5.3 Web-based public health information dissemination and evaluation

Jonathan Samet Professor, University of Southern California, Los Angeles, California, USA.
Chapter 10.1 Tobacco

Rodolfo Saracci Director of Research in Epidemiology, IFC-National Research Council, Pisa Italy.
Chapter 9.1 Gene–environment interactions and public health

Benedetto Saraceno Director, Department of Mental Health and Substance Abuse, Acting Director, Department of Chronic Diseases and Health Promotion, World Health Organization, Geneva, Switzerland.
Chapter 9.7 Public mental health

Jorgen Schlundt Director, Department of Food Safety, Zoonoses and Foodborne Diseases, World Health Organization, Geneva, Switzerland.
Chapter 4.3 International public health instruments

Eleanor B. Schron Program Director, National Heart, Lung, and Blood Institute, National Institutes of Health ,Bethesda, MD, USA.
Chapter 6.7 Methodology of intervention trials in individuals

John C. Scott President, Center for Public Service Communications, Arlington, Virginia, USA.
Chapter 5.3 Web-based public health information dissemination and evaluation

Than Sein Director, Noncommunicable Diseases and Mental Health, World Health Organization, Regional Office for Southeast Asia, New Delhi, India.
Chapter 1.3 The history and development of public health in low- and middle-income countries

Shira Shafir Department of Epidemiology, School of Public Health, UCLA, CA, USA.
Chapter 8.3 Control of microbial threats: Population surveillance, vaccine studies, and the microbiological laboratory

Prakash S. Shetty Professor of Public Health Nutrition, Institute of Human Nutrition, School of Medicine, University of Southampton, Southampton, UK.
Chapter 2.6 Food and nutrition

Daniel Shouval Liver Unit, Hadassah-Hebrew University Hospital, Jerusalem, Israel.
Chapter 9.16 Chronic hepatitis and other liver disease

Victor W. Sidel Distinguished University Professor of Social Medicine, Montefiore Medical Center and the Albert Einstein College of Medicine, Bronx, NY, USA; Adjunct Professor of Public Health at Weill Medical College of Cornell University in New York City, NY, USA.
Chapter 10.6 Collective violence: War

Elliot R. Siegel Associate Director for Health Information Programs Development, US National Library of Medicine, US National Institutes of Health, US Department of Health and Human Services, Bethesda, MD, USA.
Chapter 5.3 Web-based public health information dissemination and evaluation

Chitr Sitthi-Amorn Professor and Senior Consultant, College of Public Health Sciences, Chulalongkorn University, Bangkok, Thailand.
Chapter 5.2 Information systems and community diagnosis in low- and middle-income countries

George Davey Smith Professor of Clinical Epidemiology, Department of Social Medicine, University of Bristol, UK.
Chapter 6.14 Systematic reviews and meta-analysis

Ian Smith Office of the Director General, World Health Organization, Geneva, Switzerland.
Chapter 12.14 Global health agenda for the twenty-first century

Orielle Solar Ministry of Health, Chile; and World Health Organization, Geneva, Switzerland.
Chapter 2.2 Overview and framework

Frank Sorvillo Department of Epidemiology, School of Public Health, UCLA, CA, USA.
Chapter 8.3 Control of microbial threats: Population surveillance, vaccine studies, and the microbiological laboratory

Jonathan Sterne Professor of Medical Statistics and Epidemiology, Department of Social Medicine, University of Bristol, UK.
Chapter 6.14 Systematic reviews and meta-analysis

Alison Stewart Principal Associate, Foundation for Genomics and Population Health, Cambridge, UK.
Chapter 2.4 Genomics and public health

Allison Streetly Programme Director, NHS Sickle Cell and Thalassaemia Screening Programme, Department of Public Health Sciences, King's College London, London, UK.
Chapter 12.7 Population screening and public health

Steven Sugden The Hygiene Centre, Department of Infectious and Tropical Diseases, London School of Hygiene and Tropical Medicine, London, UK.
Chapter 2.5 Water and sanitation

Patrick S. Sullivan Department of Epidemiology, Rollins School of Public Health, Emory University, Atlanta, GA, USA.
Chapter 6.17 Public health surveillance

Sheena G. Sullivan National Center for AIDS/STD Control and Prevention, Chinese Center for Disease Control and Prevention, Beijing China; Edith Cowan University, Perth, Australia.
Chapter 6.10 Community-based intervention trials in low- and middle-income countries
Chapter 12.13 Private support of public health

Julien O. Teitler Associate Professor of Social Work and Sociology, Columbia University, New York, NY, USA.
Chapter 11.1 The changing family

Tim Tenbensel School of Population Health, University of Auckland, New Zealand.
Chapter 7.6 Public health sciences and policy in high-income countries

Puja Thakker Research Associate, Public Health Foundation of India, New Delhi, India.
Chapter 1.4 The development of the discipline of public health in countries in economic transition: India, Brazil, China

Elma B. Torres Director, Health Safety and Environmental Management Consultancy Services, Inc., Philippines.
Chapter 12.8 Environmental health practice

Peter Tugwell Canada Research Chair in Health Equity; Director, Centre for Global health, Institute of Population Health, University of Ottawa, Canada.
Chapter 6.11 Clinical epidemiology

Kumnuan Ungchusak Director, Bureau of Epidemiology and International Health Regulation (IHR) Focal point Department of Diseases Control, Ministry of Public Health, Thailand.
Chapter 6.4 Principles of outbreak investigation

Nigel Unwin Professor of Epidemiology, Institute of Health and Society, Newcastle University, UK.
Chapter 9.6 The epidemiology and prevention of diabetes mellitus

Pierre van Damme Centre for the Evaluation of Vaccination, Vaccine & Infectious Disease Institute, University of Antwerp, Belgium.
Chapter 9.16 Chronic hepatitis and other liver disease

Koen Van Herck Centre for the Evaluation of Vaccination, Vaccine & Infectious Disease Institute, University of Antwerp, Belgium.
Chapter 9.16 Chronic hepatitis and other liver disease

Erkki Vartiainen Director, Department of Health Promotion and Chronic Disease Prevention, Helsinki, Finland.
Chapter 6.9 Community-based intervention studies in high-income countries

Carlo La Vecchia Head, Laboratory of General Epidemiology, Istituto di Ricerche Farmacologiche 'Mario Negri', Milano, Italy.
Chapter 9.3 Neoplasms

Jeanette Vega Vice Minister of Health, Chile.
Chapter 2.2 Overview and framework

Gemma Vestal World Health Organization, Geneva, Switzerland.
Chapter 10.1 Tobacco

Paolo Vineis Chair in Environmental Epidemiology, Imperial College London, UK.
Chapter 9.1 Gene–environment interactions and public health

Hester J.T. Ward Consultant in Epidemiology and Public Health, National CJD Surveillance Unit, University of Edinburgh, Western General Hospital, Edinburgh, UK.
Chapter 9.11 The transmissible spongiform encephalopathies

Noel S. Weiss School of Public Health and Community Medicine, University of Washington, WA, USA.
Chapter 6.5 Case–control studies

Vivian Welch Institute of Population Health, University of Ottawa, Ottawa, Canada.
Chapter 6.11 Clinical epidemiology

Suwit Wibulpolprasert Senior Advisor on Disease Control, Ministry of Public Health, Thailand.
Chapter 12.11 Public health workers

Gail Williams School of Population Health, Faculty of Health Sciences, University of Queensland, Australia.
Chapter 6.15 Statistical methods

Marilyn Wise School of Public Health, University of Sydney, NSW, Australia.
Chapter 12.9 Structures and strategies for public health intervention

Fred B. Wood Office of Health Information Programs Development, US National Library of Medicine, US National Institutes of Health, Bethesda, MD, USA.
Chapter 5.3 Web-based public health information dissemination and evaluation

Zunyou Wu Director, National Center for AIDS/STD Control and Prevention, Chinese Center for Disease Control and Prevention, Beijing, China.
Chapter 6.10 Community-based intervention trials in low- and middle-income countries

Derek Yach Vice-President, Global Health Policy, PepsiCo Foundation, USA.
Chapter 10.1 Tobacco

Gonghuan Yang Deputy Director, China Center for Disease Prevention and Control, Beijing, China.
Chapter 10.1 Tobacco

Ron Zimmern Executive Director, Foundation for Genomics and Population Health, Cambridge, UK.
Chapter 2.4 Genomics and public health

Paul Zimmet Director Emeritus and Director of International Research, Baker IDI Heart and Diabetes Institute, Melbourne Australia.
Chapter 9.6 The epidemiology and prevention of diabetes mellitus

Anthony B. Zwi School of Public Health and Community Medicine, University of New South Wales, Sydney, Australia.
Chapter 11.8 Forced migrants and other displaced populations

SECTION 1

The development of the discipline of public health

1.1

The scope and concerns of public health

Roger Detels

Abstract

Public health is the art and science of preventing disease, prolonging life, and promoting health through the organized efforts of society. The goal of public health is the biologic, physical, and mental well-being of all members of society. Thus, unlike medicine, which focuses on the health of the individual patient, public health focuses on the health of the public in the aggregate. To achieve this broad, challenging goal, public health professionals engage in a wide range of functions involving technology, social sciences, and politics. Public health professionals utilize these functions to anticipate and prevent future problems, identify current problems, identify appropriate strategies to resolve these problems, implement these strategies, and finally, evaluate their effectiveness.

In this chapter, we introduce the reader to the scope and current major concerns of public health as we enter the twenty-first century, giving examples of each. It is the goal of the chapter to assist the readers in understanding the conceptual framework of the field, which will help them in placing the subsequent more detailed chapters in the context of the entire field of public health.

Introduction

There have been many definitions and explanations of public health. The definition offered by the Acheson Report (Acheson 1988) has been widely accepted:

> *Public health is the science and art of preventing disease, prolonging life, and promoting health through the organized efforts of society.*

This definition underscores the broad scope of public health and the fact that public health is the result of society's efforts as a whole, rather than that of single individuals.

In 2003, Detels defined the goal of public health as:

> *The biologic, physical, and mental well-being of all members of society regardless of gender, wealth, ethnicity, sexual orientation, country, or political views.*

This definition or goal emphasizes equity and the range of public health interests as encompassing not just the physical and biologic, but also the mental well-being of society. Both the World Health Organization (WHO) and Detels' goals or definitions depict public health as being concerned with more than merely the elimination of disease.

To achieve the WHO goal of 'health for all', it is essential to bring to bear many diverse disciplines to the attainment of optimal health, including the physical, biologic, and social sciences. The field of public health has adapted and applied these disciplines for the elimination and control of disease, and the promotion of health.

Functions of public health

To accomplish its task of ensuring the well-being of the population, public health must perform a wide range of functions, which are listed in Table 1.1.1. The primary functions are to prevent disease and injuries and to promote healthy lifestyles and good health habits; but in order to succeed in these two objectives, public health must perform additional functions.

Public health *identifies*, *measures*, and *monitors* community health needs through surveillance of disease and risk factors (e.g. smoking) trends. Analysis of these trends and the existence of a functioning health information system provides the essential information for predicting or anticipating future community health needs.

In order to ensure the health of the population, it is necessary to *formulate*, *promote*, and *enforce* sound health policies to prevent and control disease and to reduce the prevalence of factors impairing the health of the community. These include policies requiring reporting of highly transmissible diseases and health threats to the community and control of environmental threats through the regulation of environmental hazards (e.g. water and air quality standards and smoking). It is important to recognize that influencing politics, particularly in a democracy, is an essential function of public health.

There are limited resources that can be devoted to public health and the assurance of high-quality health services. Thus, an essential function of public health is to effectively *plan*, *manage*, and *administer cost-effective health services*, and to ensure their availability to all segments of society.

In every society, there are *health inequalities* that limit the ability of some members to achieve their maximum ability to function.

Table 1.1.1 Functions of public health

1.	Prevent disease and injuries.
2.	Promote healthy lifestyles and good health habits.
3.	Identify, measure, monitor, and anticipate community health needs.
4.	Formulate, promote, and enforce essential health policies.
5.	Organize and ensure high-quality, cost-effective public health and health-care services.
6.	Reduce health disparities and ensure access to health care for all.
7.	Promote and protect a healthy environment.
8.	Disseminate health information and mobilize communities to take appropriate action.
9.	Plan and prepare for natural and man-made disasters.
10.	Reduce interpersonal violence and aggressive war.
11.	Conduct research and evaluate health-promoting/disease-preventing strategies.
12.	Develop new methodologies for research and evaluation.
13.	Train and ensure a competent public health workforce.

Source: Adapted from Office of the Director, National Public Health Performance Standards Program. *10 essential public health services.* [Online]. Centers for Disease Control; 1994. (Available from: http://www.cdc.gov/od/ocphp/nphpsp/EssentialPHServices.htm) and Pan American Health Organization. *Essential public health services.* [Online]. 2002. (Available from: http://www.sopha.cpha.ca/english/ephf_e.html)

Although these disparities primarily affect the poor, minority, rural, and remote populations and the vulnerable, they also impact on society as a whole, particularly in regard to infectious and/or transmissible diseases. Thus, there is not only an ethical imperative to reduce health disparities, but also a pragmatic rationale.

Technological advances and increasing commerce have done much to improve the quality of life, but these advances have come at a high cost to the environment. In many cities of both the developed and developing world, the poor quality of air—contaminated by industry and commerce—has affected the respiratory health of the population, and has threatened to change the climate, with disastrous consequences. We have only one world. If we do not take care of it, we will ultimately have difficulty living in it. Through education of the public, formulation of sound regulations, and influencing policy, public health must restore and monitor the environment to *ensure that the population can live in a healthy environment.*

To ensure that each individual in the population functions to his or her maximum capacity, public health needs to *educate the public and stimulate the community* to take appropriate actions towards the optimal conditions for the health of the public. Ultimately, public health cannot succeed without the support and active involvement of the community.

We cannot predict, and rarely can we prevent, the occurrence of natural and man-made disasters, but we can prepare for them to ensure that the resulting damage is minimized. Thus, *disaster preparedness* is an essential component of public health, whether the disaster is an epidemic such as influenza or the occurrence of typhoons.

Unfortunately, in the modern world, interpersonal *violence and war* have become common. In some segments of society (particularly among adolescent and young adult minority males), violence has become the leading cause of death and productive years of life lost. Public health cannot ignore that violence and wars are major factors dramatically reducing the quality of life for millions.

Many of the advances in public health have become possible through *research*. Research will continue to be essential for identifying health problems and the optimal strategies for confronting public health problems. Strategies that seem very logical may, in fact, not succeed for a variety of unforeseen reasons. Therefore, public health systems and programmes cannot be assumed to function cost-effectively without continuous monitoring and evaluation. Thus, it is essential that new public health strategies undergo rigorous evaluation before being scaled up, and once scaled up, periodically reviewed to ensure their continuing effectiveness.

Over the last century, the quality of research has been enhanced by the *development of new methodologies*, particularly in the fields of epidemiology, biostatistics, and laboratory sciences. The development of the computer has increased our ability to analyse massive amounts of data, and to use multiple strategies to aid in the interpretation of data. As new technologies continue to be developed, it is essential that public health continues to use these new technologies to develop more sophisticated research strategies in order to address public health issues.

The quality of public health is dependent on the competence and vision of the public health *workforce*. Thus, it is an essential function of public health to *ensure the continuing availability of a well-trained, competent workforce* at all levels, including leaders with the vision essential to ensure the continued well-being of society and the implementation of innovative, effective public health measures.

Contemporary health issues

Underlying almost all the pubic health problems of the world is the issue of poverty. More than half of the world's population lives below the internationally defined poverty line. Although the majority of the world's poor live in developing countries, there are many poor living in the wealthiest countries of the world—underscoring the disparity of wealth between developed and developing countries as well as between the poor and the rich in all countries. Unfortunately, the disparity between the rich and the poor is increasing, not only within countries, but also between rich and poor countries. It is incumbent on public health to reduce these disparities to ensure that all members of the global society share in a healthy quality of life.

The twentieth century witnessed the transition of major disease burdens, defined by death, from infectious and/or communicable diseases to chronic diseases (Table 1.1.2). In 1900, the leading cause of death in the United States and other developed countries was reported to be pneumonia and influenza. By the end of the century, diseases of the heart were the leading cause of death, and pneumonia and influenza dropped to the seventh place, primarily affecting the elderly. Commensurately, the average lifespan increased significantly, compounding the problems introduced by population growth. The reduction in communicable diseases was not primarily due to the development of better treatments, although vaccines played an important role in the second half of the twentieth century, but through public efforts to reduce crowding and improve housing, improve nutrition, and provide clean water and safe disposal of wastes.

By 1980, many leading public health figures felt that infectious diseases had been eliminated as a primary concern for public

Table 1.1.2 Leading causes of death in the United States (1900, 1950, 1990, 1997, 2001)

	1900	1950	1990	1997	2001
Diseases of the heart	167	307	152	131	248
Malignant neoplasms	81	125	135	126	196
Cerebrovascular disease	134	89	28	26	58
Chronic obstructive lung diseases	—	4	20	13	44
Motor vehicle injuries	—	23	19	16	15
Diabetes mellitus	13	14	12	13	25
Pneumonia and influenza	210	26	14	13	22
HIV infection	—	—	10	6	5
Suicide	11	11	12	11	10
Homicide and legal intervention	1	5	10	8	7

Values expressed as rates per 100 000, age-adjusted.
Source: Updated from McGinnis JM, Foege WH. Actual causes of death in the United States. *Journal of the American Medical Association* 1993; **270**:2007–12 and Department of Health and Human Services, National Center for Health Statistics *Health, United States, 1999*. Washington (DC): US Government Printing Office; 1999.

health; however, the discovery and expanding pandemic of acquired immunodeficiency syndrome (AIDS) caused by the human immunodeficiency virus (HIV) in the early 1980s, and subsequently, sudden acute respiratory syndrome (SARS) outbreaks in the late 1990s demonstrated the fallacy of their thinking. Although infectious and/or communicable diseases persist as a major public health concern, globally, even in poor, developing countries, chronic diseases have become a major health problem. In fact, 74 per cent of the deaths due to non-communicable or chronic diseases at the beginning of the twenty-first century occurred in developing countries. This, of course, reflects that the majority of the world's population lives in developing countries with limited resources and incomes. Communicable diseases, however, still accounted for 30 per cent of the deaths worldwide in 2005 (Fig. 1.1.1). This statistic is particularly disturbing, as the majority of the communicable diseases are now preventable through vaccines, improved sanitation, behavioural interventions, and better standards of living.

An essential step in defining health is to identify appropriate methods for measuring it. Traditionally, public health has defined disease in terms of mortality rates because they are relatively easy to obtain and death is indisputable. The use of mortality rates, however, places the greatest emphasis on diseases that end life, and tends to ignore those which compromise function and quality of life without causing death. Thus, the problems of mental illnesses, accidents, and disabling conditions are seriously underestimated if one uses only mortality to define health.

Two other strategies to measure health that evolved in the last half of the twentieth century have been 'years of productive life lost' (YPLL) (Lopez *et al.* 2006) and 'disability-adjusted life years' (DALYs) (Murray & Lopez 1995). The former emphasizes those diseases that reduce the productive lifespan (currently arbitrarily defined as 75 years), whereas the latter emphasizes those diseases that compromise function but also includes a measure of premature mortality. Using either of these alternatives to define health results in very different orderings of diseases and/or health problems as public health priorities (Fig. 1.1.1).

Using death to identify disease priorities, the leading cause is chronic diseases, which account for 61 per cent of the diseases worldwide (Fig. 1.1.1). Among the chronic diseases, cardiovascular diseases account for almost half (49 per cent) of the deaths.

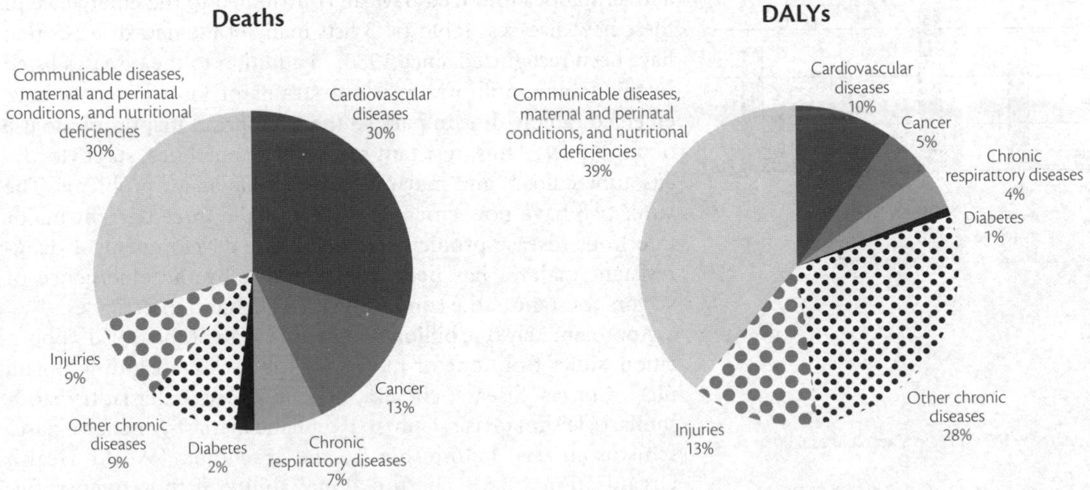

Fig. 1.1.1 Main causes of death and global burden of disease (DALYs) in the world for all ages, projections for 2005.
Source: World Health Organization. *Preventing chronic diseases: A vital investment.* [Online]. 2005. Available from: http://whqlibdoc.who.int/publications/2005/9241563001_eng.pdf.

The proportion, however, varies markedly by regions of the world and level of affluence of the countries. Communicable diseases remain the major cause of death only in Africa, although they account for a significant proportion of deaths in Southeast Asia and the eastern Mediterranean (Figs 1.1.2 A and B). The major victims of these communicable diseases are infants and children under five. The persistence of communicable diseases in these areas represents a major public health challenge.

DALYs and YPLL may be considered as better measures of the quality of life and functioning capacity of a country than mortality. Using DALYs to establish global disease priorities emphasizes communicable diseases and injuries, which tend to disproportionately affect the young, and reduces the relative importance of cardiovascular diseases and other chronic diseases that primarily affect the elderly (Fig. 1.1.1). The WHO has projected that the ranking of total DALYs for neuropsychiatric disorders, injuries, and non-communicable and/or chronic diseases will increase by 2020, whereas the ranking for communicable diseases other than HIV/AIDS will decline (Figs 1.1.3A–D) (Mathers & Loncar 2006). Communicable diseases, which currently account for 40 per cent of the DALYS, are expected to decline to 30 per cent by 2030 (Mathers & Loncar 2006).

On the other hand, according to projections by the WHO, HIV, tuberculosis, and malaria (currently major communicable disease problems globally) will account for an even greater number of YPLL per 1000 population by 2030, whereas other communicable diseases will yield to intervention efforts and account for progressively fewer YPLL (Fig. 1.1.4). The YPLL per 1000 population due to chronic diseases that tend to affect older people, however, is projected to remain constant, perhaps reflecting the optimism regarding the development of strategies for earlier diagnosis and better drugs to sustain life with these conditions.

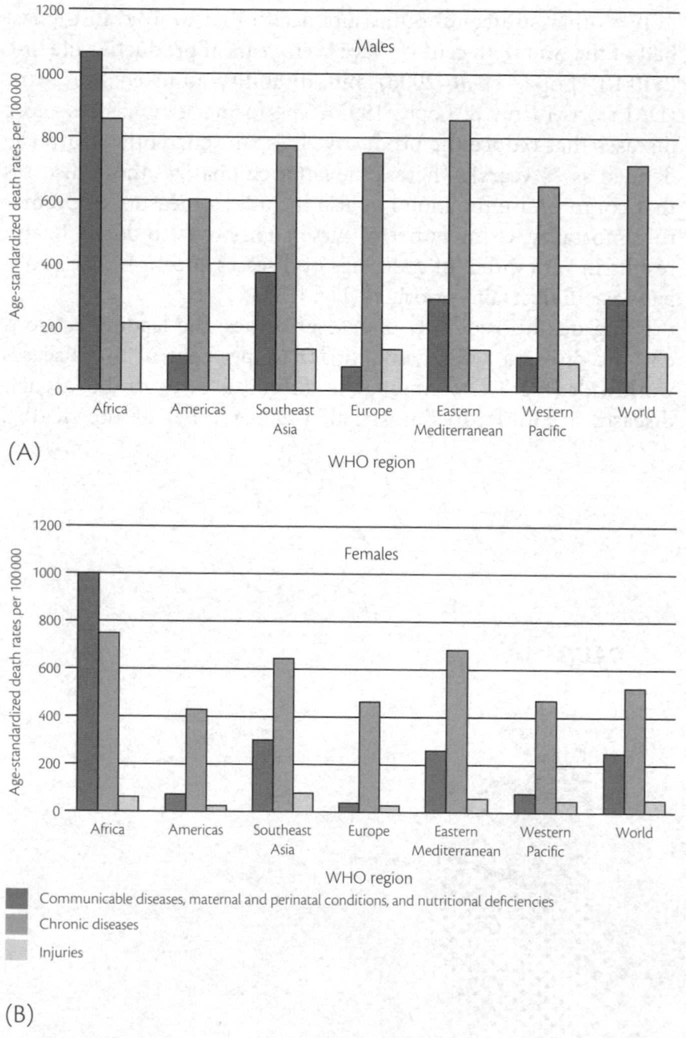

Fig. 1.1.2 Projected main caused of death by WHO region for all ages, 2005: (A) males and (B) females.
Source: World Health Organization. Main causes of death and global burden of disease (DALYs), world, all ages, projections for 2005. [Online]. Available from: http://www.who.int/chp/chronic_disease_report/contents/part2.pdf [accessed 2007 May].

Communicable diseases

The WHO's regional offices working with individual countries have conducted intensive immunization programmes against the major preventable infectious diseases of childhood, but there are significant barriers to complete coverage, including poverty, geographic obstacles, low levels of education, civil unrest and wars, and mistrust of governments. Poverty, weak governments, and misuse of funds have also prevented the control of disease vectors, provision of clean water, and safe disposal of sanitation, all essential for the control of communicable diseases. Another major factor in the rapid spread of communicable diseases has been the rapid growth in transportation. It is now possible for an individual with a communicable disease to circumnavigate the globe while still infectious and asymptomatic. Thus, cases of SARS were reported throughout Southeast Asia and as far as Canada within weeks of the recognition of the first cases in Hong Kong (Lee 2003).

Another source of communicable diseases is the continuing emergence of new infectious agents, many of them adapting to humans from animal sources. Figure 1.1.5 identifies new disease outbreaks from 1981 to 2003, including newly drug-resistant variants of new diseases occurring worldwide. Changes in food production, crowding of animals, mixing of live animal species in 'wet markets' in Asia and elsewhere, and the introduction of hormones and antibiotics into feed have all contributed to the emergence of these new diseases. Table 1.1.3 lists many of the new diseases that have been recognized since 1980. In addition to the diseases listed in this table, antibiotic-resistant strains of known agents have emerged rapidly due, in part, to the widespread inappropriate use of antibiotics. Thus, resistant strains of gonorrhoea, staphylococcus, tuberculosis, and malaria have become major problems. The latter two have now emerged as two of the three current major infectious disease problems globally. The development of drug-resistant malaria has been compounded by the emergence of vectors resistant to the commonly used chemical insecticides.

Approximately one billion people, one sixth of the world's population, suffer from one or more tropical disease, including Buruli ulcer, Chagas' disease, cholera, dengue, dracunculiasis, trypanosomiasis, leishmaniasis, leprosy, lymphatic filariasis, onchocerciasis, schistosomiasis, helminthiasis, and trachoma (World Health Organization 2006). The functional ability of those who suffer from one or more of these diseases is severely compromised, in turn affecting the ability of the poorest countries, which suffer the greatest burden of these tropical diseases, to compete in the

Income group	Rank	Disease or injury	Per cent of total deaths
Worldwide	1	Ischaemic heart disease	13.4
	2	Cerebrovascular disease	10.6
	3	HIV/AIDS	8.9
	4	COPD	7.8
	5	Lower respiratory infections	3.5
	6	Trachea, bronchus, lung cancers	3.1
	7	Diabetes mettitus	3.0
	8	Road traffic accidents	2.9
	9	Perinatal conditions	2.2
	10	Stomach cancer	1.9
High-income countries	1	Ischaemic heart disease	15.8
	2	Cerebrovascular disease	9.0
	3	Trachea, bronchus, lung cancers	5.1
	4	Diabetes mellitus	4.8
	5	COPD	4.1
	6	Lower respiratory infections	3.6
	7	Alzheimer's and other dementias	3.6
	8	Colon and rectum cancers	3.3
	9	Stomach cancer	1.9
	10	Prostate cancer	1.8
Middle-income countries	1	Cerebrovascular disease	14.4
	2	Ischaemic heart disease	12.7
	3	COPD	12.0
	4	HIV/AIDS	6.2
	5	Trachea, bronchus, lung cancers	4.3
	6	Diabetes mellitus	3.7
	7	Stomach cancer	3.4
	8	Hypertensive heart disease	2.7
	9	Road traffic accidents	2.5
	10	Liver cancers	2.2
Low-income countries	1	Ischaemic heart disease	13.4
	2	HIV/AIDS	13.2
	3	Cerebrovascular disease	8.2
	4	COPD	5.5
	5	Lower respiratory infections	5.1
	6	Perinatal conditions	3.9
	7	Road traffic accidents	3.7
	8	Diarrhoeal diseases	2.3
	9	Diabetes mellitus	2.2
	10	Malaria	1.8

Fig. 1.1.3A Ten leading causes of death by income group (baseline scenario), 2030.
Source: Mathers CD, Loncar D. Projections of global mortality and burden of disease from 2002 to 2030. *PLoS Medicine* 2006;**3**(11):e442. Available from: http://medicine.plosjournals.org/perlserv/?request=slideshow&type=table&doi=10.1371/journal.pmed.0030442&id=9665 [accessed 2007 May].

world marketplace. However, major strides have been achieved in reducing the burden of diseases such as leprosy, guinea worm disease, and lymphatic filariasis. Continuing efforts are needed to further reduce the burden of these and other tropical diseases.

We now recognize that we will continue to see new human pathogens emerging in the future, and need to be prepared to contain them. Table 1.1.4 lists the factors that contribute to the emergence of these new agents and disease threats. Unless the world faces the consequences of changing the environment in which we live, newly emerging diseases will continue to plague us.

Chronic diseases

With the increasing control of communicable diseases and the increasing lifespan, chronic diseases have emerged as the major global health problem in both developed and developing countries. Even in developing countries, chronic diseases have assumed greater importance. The prevalence of type 2 diabetes in rural India is 13.2 per cent (Chow & Raju 2006). Cardiovascular diseases have become a major cause of death in China. Eighty-seven per cent of stroke deaths occur in low- and/or middle-income countries (Lopez *et al.* 2007).

The causes of chronic diseases are many and complex (Fig. 1.1.6). Although the immediate causes are factors such as increasing blood pressure, increasing blood glucose, abnormal lipids and fat deposition, and diabetes, the underlying causes are behavioural and social. These behavioural factors include unhealthy diets that substitute pre-packaged and fast foods high in fats for a balanced diet, physical inactivity, and tobacco use; these in turn are the products of social change, including globalization, urbanization, and aging. Some chronic diseases have been associated with infectious disease agents. For example, *Chlamydia pneumoniae* has been implicated in the development of atherosclerosis (Kuo & Campbell 2000), and hepatitis C as a leading cause of hepatocellular (liver) cancer.

Another aspect of chronic diseases is the increasing survival of compromised individuals who would not otherwise have survived, many of whom are handicapped. These individuals require modified environments to experience a reasonable quality of life and to realize their full potential in order to contribute to society.

Most chronic diseases can be reduced by a combination of healthy behaviours, including not smoking, moderate alcohol use, and exercise (Breslow & Breslow 1993). Many developed countries have been promoting healthy lifestyles, but there is need for greater

Group	Cause	Average annual change (per cent) in age-standardized death rate	
		Males	Females
All causes		−0.8	−1.1
Group I		−1.4	−1.9
	Tuberculosis	−5.4	−5.3
	HIV/AIDS	3.0	2.1
	Malaria	−1.3	−1.5
	Other infectious diseases	−3.4	−3.3
	Respiratory infections	−2.7	−3.4
	Perinatal conditions[a]	−1.7	−1.9
	Other Group I	−3.0	−3.6
Group II		0.0	−0.8
	Cancer	−0.2	−0.4
	Lung cancer	0.1	0.3
	Diabetes mellitus	1.1	1.3
	Cardiovascular diseases	−1.1	−1.2
	Respiratory diseases	0.3	−0.1
	Digestive diseases	−1.3	−1.7
	Other Group II	−0.7	−1.1
Group III		0.0	−0.2
	Unintentional injuries	−0.2	−0.2
	Road traffic accidents	1.1	1.1
	Intentional injuries	0.2	−0.2
	Self-inflicted injuries	−0.3	−0.4
	Violence	0.4	0.2

[a]Causes arising in the perinatal period as defined in the ICD, principally prematurity and birth asphyxiz, and does not include all deaths occurring in the neonatal period (under 1 mo).
DOI: 10.1371/journal.pmed.0030442.t001

Fig. 1.1.3B Projected global tobacco-caused deaths (baseline scenario), by cause, 2015.
Source: Mathers C.D., Loncar D. Projections of global mortality and burden of disease from 2002 to 2030. *PLoS Medicine* 2006;**3**(11):e442. Available from: http://medicine.plosjournals.org/perlserv/?request=slideshow&type=table&doi=10.1371/journal.pmed.0030442&id=9667 [accessed May 2007].

Category	Disease or injury	2002 rank	2030 ranks	Change in rank
Within top 15	Perinatal conditions	1	5	−4
	Lower respiratory infections	2	8	−6
	HIV/AIDS	3	1	+2
	Unipolar depressive disorders	4	2	+2
	Diarrhoeal diseases	5	12	−7
	Ischaemic heart disease	6	3	+3
	Cerebrovascular disease	7	6	+1
	Road traffic accidents	8	4	+4
	Malaria	9	15	−6
	Tuberculosis	10	25	−15
	COPD	11	7	+4
	Congenital anomalies	12	20	−8
	Hearing loss, adult onset	13	9	+4
	Cataracts	14	10	+4
	Violence	15	13	+2
Outside top 15	Self-inflected injuries	17	14	+3
	Diabetes mellitus	20	11	+9

Fig. 1.1.3C Changes in rankings for 15 leading causes of DALYs (baseline scenario), 2002 and 2030.
Source: Mathers C.D., Loncar D. Projections of global mortality and burden of disease from 2002 to 2030. *PLoS Medicine* 2006;**3**(11):e442. Available from: http://medicine.plosjournals.org/perlserv/?request=slideshow&type=table&doi=10.1371/journal.pmed.0030442&id=9669.

emphasis and development of these programmes in developing countries, where the major global burden of chronic diseases occurs.

Mental illness

Public health professionals have only relatively recently recognized the need to address the mental health needs of society on a global scale, partly due to the difficulties in defining it. It is now estimated that 10 per cent of the world's population suffers from mental illness at any given time, and that mental illness represents 12 per cent of the global burden of disease. Mortality rates seriously underestimate the burden of mental health on society. Mental illness accounts for 31 per cent of DALYs, a better measure of its impact on society (Murray & Lopez 1995). However, the true extent of mental illness is probably greater—only 73 per cent of the countries have a formal mental health reporting system, and only 57 per cent have done epidemiologic studies or have data collection systems for documenting mental illness (World Health Organization 2001).

Income group	Rank	Disease or injury	Per cent of total DALYs
Worldwide	1	HIV/AIDS	12.1
	2	Unipolar depressive disorders	5.7
	3	Ischaemic heart disease	4.7
	4	Road traffic accidents	4.2
	5	Perinatal conditions	4.0
	6	Cerebrovascular disease	3.9
	7	COPD	3.1
	8	Lower respiratory infections	3.0
	9	Hearing loss, adult onset	2.5
	10	Cataracts	2.5
High-income countries	1	Unipolar depressive disorders	9.8
	2	Ischaemic heart disease	5.9
	3	Alzheimer and other dementias	5.8
	4	Alcohol use disorders	4.7
	5	Diabetes mellitus	4.5
	6	Cerebrovascular disease	4.5
	7	Hearing loss, adult onset	4.1
	8	Trachea, bronchus, lung cancers	3.0
	9	Osteoarthritis	2.9
	10	COPD	2.5
Middle-income countries	1	HIV/AIDS	9.8
	2	Unipolar depressive disorders	6.7
	3	Cerebrovascular disease	6.0
	4	Ischaemic heart disease	4.7
	5	COPD	4.7
	6	Road traffic accidents	4.0
	7	Violence	2.9
	8	Vision disorders, age-related	2.9
	9	Hearing loss, adult onset	2.9
	10	Diabetes mellitus	2.6
Low-income countries	1	HIV/AIDS	14.6
	2	Perinatal conditions	5.8
	3	Unipolar depressive disorders	4.7
	4	Road traffic accidents	4.6
	5	Ischaemic heart disease	4.5
	6	Lower respiratory infections	4.4
	7	Diarrhoeal diseases	2.8
	8	Cerebrovascular disease	2.8
	9	Diabetes mellitus	2.8
	10	Malaria	2.5

Fig. 1.1.3D Ten leading causes of DALYs by income group and sex (baseline scenario), 2030.
Source: Mathers C.D., Loncar D. Projections of global mortality and burden of disease from 2002 to 2030. *PLoS Medicine* 2006;**3**(11):e442. Available from: http://medicine.plosjournals.org/perlserv/?request=slideshow&type=table&doi=10.1371/journal.pmed.0030442&id=9671 [accessed 2007 May].

Global provisions for treatment of mental illness are still significantly below what is necessary to adequately address the problem. Although 87 per cent of the world's governments offer some mental health services at the primary-care level, 30 per cent of them have no relevant programme and 28 per cent have no budget specifically identified for mental health. Mental illness robs society of a significant number of potentially productive persons. With the diminishing proportion of productive people of working age and the increasing proportion of elderly dependants, it is important to assist those who are not productive because of mental illness to become healthy, productive members of society.

Population changes

Although the rate of growth of the world's population has slowed in the latter half of the twentieth century, the world's population, currently over 6.5 billion people, is estimated to grow to 9 billion by 2050 (Fig. 1.1.7) (United States Census Bureau 2006). The growth in the population will be mostly among the elderly and the old elderly (those over 80 years of age). By 2050, at least 30 per cent of the population in most developed countries and in China will be over 65 years of age (Fig. 1.1.8). In the United States, the number of elderly is expected to double over the next 30 years. Because women survive longer, the majority of the elderly will be women. The gender ratio (M:F) for the world's population was 101.4 in 2007, but is estimated to be 101.3 by 2010. However, among those 80 years and over, the ratio was 56.3 in 2007 and is estimated to be 57.3 by 2010.

Currently, one of the major problems facing the world is the deterioration of the environment caused by the increasing numbers of people and the accumulation of wastes produced by them, their vehicles, and the industries they support. Thus, the quality of the air that we breathe has declined, especially in developing countries, where increased economic output has come at the expense of the environment. The most polluted cities of the world are concentrated in developing countries, which have the least capacity and political will to reduce pollutants. Pollution of the world's oceans, which receive massive amounts of biological and chemical wastes annually, affects not only the quality of the water but also the ability of the ocean to sustain marine life, an important source of food.

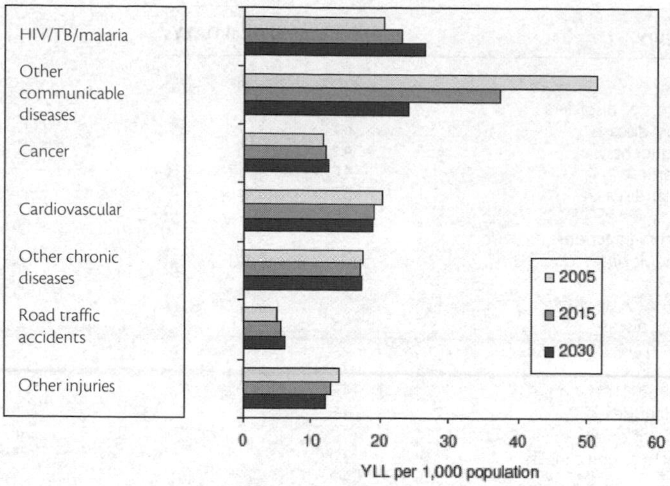

Fig. 1.1.4 Trends in global years of life lost (YLL) per 1000 population, by broad cause group and income group, 2002–2030 (2005).
Source: Mathers C.D., Loncar D. *Updated projections of global mortality and burden of disease, 2002–2030: data sources, methods and results*. Geneva: World Health Organization; 2005. Available from: http://www.who.int/healthinfo/statistics/bodprojections2030/en/index.html [accessed 2007 May].

As the population grows, there is increasing pressure to provide food, water, and other necessities to maintain a high quality of life. Fertile farmlands are increasingly being converted to residential areas. Thus, more people need to be supported on less land. Will agricultural efficiency grow at a rate commensurate with population growth? Will we be able to find alternative fuel sources when oil and other natural resources are depleted? Will we be able to provide sufficient water to sustain populations and agriculture, currently a major global problem?

The well-being of society is dependent on the ratio of those who produce to those who are dependent. The fact that the majority of the population growth in the coming decades will be among the old and old elderly, not through increasing birth rates, will result in a diminishing proportion of producers and an increasing proportion of dependants. In 2000, the proportion of the world's population who were 60 years and over was 10 per cent; by 2050, it will be 50 per cent. This will be further exacerbated because the majority of the oldest elderly will be single women who traditionally have more limited resources and lower levels of education, particularly in developing countries. Thus, the productivity and efficiency of those who produce must increase if we are to sustain or improve the quality of life for all. Improved technology and strategies will be required to increase worker productivity.

The occurrence of disease in old age is directly correlated with unhealthy behaviours developed in early life. Unfortunately, concurrent with population growth, there has been a worldwide epidemic of obesity and decreased physical activity, which has increased the proportion of elderly who suffer from chronic debilitating diseases in both the developed and developing world. Thus, unless efforts to promote health lifestyles are successful, not only will there be an increase in the proportion of elderly, but also an increasing proportion of them will require supportive care, placing a further economic burden on society.

Other public health issues

Oral health

Good dental health is essential for maintaining adequate nutrition and a healthy quality of life. However, it was estimated that in 2004 there was an average of 1.6 decayed, missing, or filled teeth (DMFT) among children 12 years old globally (WHO Oral Health Program 2004). The number of DMFT ranged from a low of 0.3 in Togo and Rwanda to 6.3 per 12-year-old in Martinique. The percentage of

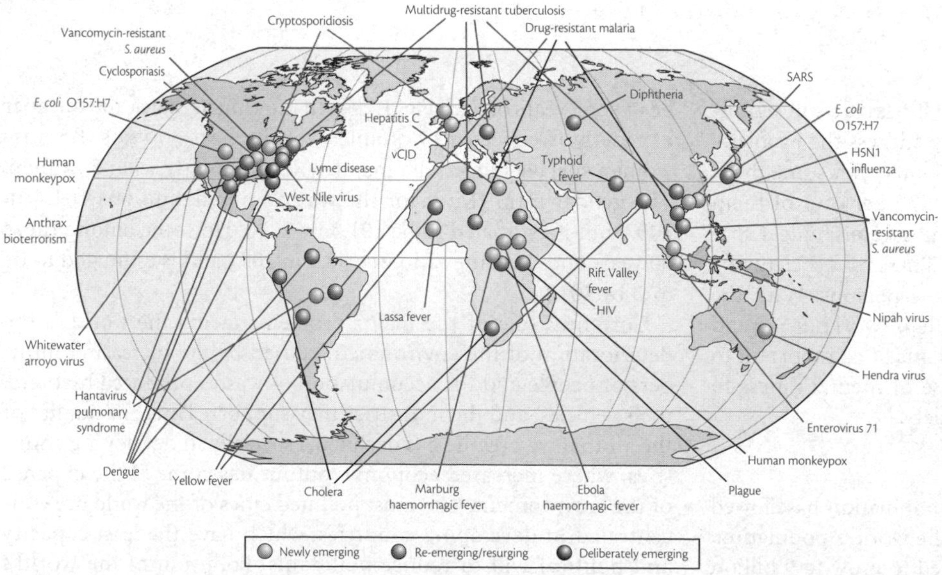

Fig. 1.1.5 Emerging and re-emerging disease worldwide, 1981–2003.
Source: Morens D.M., Folkers G.K., Fauci A.S. *Nature* 2004; **430**:242–9. Updated and reproduced with permission of A. Fauci [2007 June].

Table 1.1.3 Newly identified infectious diseases and pathogens

Year	Disease/pathogen
2004	Avian influenza (human cases)
2003	SARS
1999	Nipah virus
1997	H5N1 (avian influenza A virus)
1996	New variant Creutzfelt-Jacob disease; Australian bat lyssavirus
1995	Human herpes virus 8 (Kaposi's sarcoma virus)
1994	Savia virus; Hendra virus
1993	Hanta virus pulmonary syndrome (Sin Nombre virus)
1992	*Vibrio cholerae* O139
1991	Guanarito virus
1989	Hepatitis C
1988	Hepatitis E; human herpes virus 6
1983	HIV
1982	*Escherichia coli* O157:H7; Lyme borreliosis; human T-lymphotropic virus type 2
1980	Human T-lymphotropic virus

Source: World Health Organization. Workshop presentation by David Heymann. Geneva: World Health Organization; 1999.

adults in the United Kingdom with total tooth loss in 1998 was 13 per cent, and increased with decreasing social class (Table 1.1.5) and education (Fig. 1.1.9). These high rates of DMFT and tooth loss reflect poor dental hygiene and preventive care (Pine & Harris 2007). Unfortunately, many people believe that dental care is an expendable luxury, and that visits to dentists are only necessary when there is a problem. Poor dental hygiene is probably a major reason for the 119 730 cases of oral cancer worldwide in 2000, and why the five-year prevalence of oral cancer is estimated to be 6.8 per cent globally (WHO Oral Health Program 2004). Even in Western Europe, the five-year prevalence of oral cancer was estimated at almost 50 000 cases (WHO Oral Health Program 2004). Clearly the public health message regarding the importance of good dental hygiene, regular tooth brushing, and regular dental check ups is not reaching the majority of the people.

Injuries

Injuries and violence caused 9 per cent of all deaths and 12 per cent of the global burden of diseases in 2002, accounting for 5.2 million deaths (World Health Organization 2004). Deaths due to injuries are almost three times greater in developing than in developed countries. However, most of the injuries do not cause death, but may result in disability. Furthermore, they occur more commonly among younger persons and children.

Injuries can be broadly categorized in the following groups: motor vehicle accidents, suicide, homicide, and other unintentional injuries, including occupational injuries and falls. Motor vehicle accidents account for the largest proportion of deaths due to injury (Fig. 1.1.10); globally, they were the sixth leading cause of death in 2001, and the third leading cause of YPLL lost in the United States in 2000. The WHO projects that motor vehicle accidents will become the third highest cause of DALYs globally by 2020. Falls, particularly among the elderly, are a major cause of DALYs, and ranked thirteenth globally in 1999 according to the WHO.

Occupational injuries are another major cause of death and DALYs. Globally, over 350 000 deaths and 270 million injuries are currently attributable to occupation-related factors annually. The burden is greater in developing countries, where the drive to produce goods cheaply has been given greater importance than providing a safe work environment.

Homicide, violence, and suicide

Homicide, violence, and suicide represent a growing problem, particularly among the young. Homicide and suicide are among the top ten leading causes of death in the United States. In some minority groups in the United States, homicide and violence are the leading cause of death of youth, followed by suicide. In China, suicide remains the leading cause of death among women in rural areas. Globally, the WHO predicts that homicide and suicide will account for an increasing proportion of deaths. Unfortunately, the WHO predicts that by 2020, war will become the sixth leading cause of DALYs, violence the twelfth, and self-inflicted injuries the fourteenth.

Unintentional injuries are largely preventable through community and governmental intervention. Thus, improved roads, separation of different modes of transportation, enactment, and enforcement of seat belt and helmet laws, and improved designs of ladders and other equipment and tools have all been shown to significantly reduce injuries and deaths due to accidents. Stronger emphasis on a safer work environment, especially in developing countries, will significantly reduce both injuries and the severity of injuries that occur in the workplace.

Vulnerable populations

Public health has always been concerned with the health and well-being of vulnerable groups who require special attention. The definition of a vulnerable population and who constitute a vulnerable population varies by time, situation, and culture, but the common characteristic across all vulnerable groups is their susceptibility to adverse health and poor quality of life. Often, they live at the margins of society and have difficulty accomplishing the basic functions of living and accessing healthcare. Thus, they require assistance. In many societies, particularly in developing countries, the family acts as the safety net for these groups; but if the family itself is vulnerable, this safety net is absent. Societies with resources have developed social support programmes that assist the vulnerable, but these programmes seldom cover the full range of vulnerable groups, and may not adequately support those whom they target. Universal healthcare is one component of assisting the vulnerable, but presently, even in rich, developed countries such as the United States, healthcare is not available to all, and strategies to fund universal healthcare are difficult to implement.

The list of vulnerable groups includes the poor, minorities, women, children, the elderly, the handicapped, the illiterate, orphans and street children, immigrants, refugees and displaced people, the homeless, and the mentally ill. In certain situations, other groups may be considered vulnerable. For example, in the face of epidemics such as HIV/AIDS, one could also consider adolescents to be a vulnerable group.

Table 1.1.4 Factors contributing to the emergence or re-emergence of infectious diseases

1.	Human 'demographic change' by which persons begin to live in previously uninhabited remote areas of the world and are exposed to new environmental sources of infectious agents, insects, and animals.
2.	Breakdowns of sanitary and other public health measures in overcrowded cities and in situations of civil unrest and war.
3.	Economic development and changes in the use of land, including deforestation, reforestation, and urbanization.
4.	Climate changes cause changes in geography of agents and vectors.
5.	Changing human behaviours, such as increased use of child-care facilities, sexual and drug-use behaviours, and patterns of outdoor recreation.
6.	Social inequality.
7.	International travel and commerce that quickly transport people and goods vast distances.
8.	Changes in food processing and handling, including foods prepared from many different animals and transported great distances.
9.	Evolution of pathogenic infectious agents by which they may infect new hosts, produce toxins, or adapt by responding to changes in the host immunity (e.g. influenza, HIV).
10.	Development of resistance of infectious agents such as *Mycobacterium tuberculosis* and *Neisseria gonorrhoeae* to chemoprophylactic or chemotherapeutic medicines.
11.	Resistance of the vectors of vector-borne infectious diseases to pesticides.
12.	Immunosuppression of persons due to medical treatments or new diseases that result in infectious diseases caused by agents not usually pathogenic in healthy hosts (e.g. leukaemia patients).
13.	Deterioration in surveillance systems for infectious diseases, including laboratory support, to detect new or emerging disease problems at an early stage.
14.	Illiteracy limits knowledge of prevention strategies.
15.	Lack of political will—corruption, other priorities.
16.	Biowarfare/bioterrorism—an unfortunate potential source of new or emerging disease threats (e.g. anthrax and letters).
17.	War, civil unrest—creates refugees, food and housing shortages, increased density of living, etc.
18.	Famine.

In almost every country, developed or developing, there are homeless people, many of whom suffer from multiple problems, including mental illness. Complicating the ability of many vulnerable groups, including the homeless, mentally ill, alcoholics, and drug addicts, to achieve good health and to function adequately are poverty, prejudice, and stigmatization by society. Thus, we not only need programmes to assist the vulnerable, but also to encourage society to take action to assist them in realizing their maximum potential.

Complicating the issue of vulnerable groups is the fact that the specific problems and needs of each of these groups are different, and thus require differing specific public health action. For some of these groups, such as mothers and children and the handicapped, there are well-established programmes, although coverage is far from complete and the quality of these programmes varies widely. For others, such as the illiterate and migrants, there are fewer established programmes. If we are to meet the public health goal of 'Health for All', we need to identify and assist the vulnerable groups within societies to achieve their maximum possible health and function.

The environment

> *Environmental health comprises those aspects of human health, including quality of life, that are determined by physical, chemical, biological, social, and psychosocial processes in the environment.* (WHO)

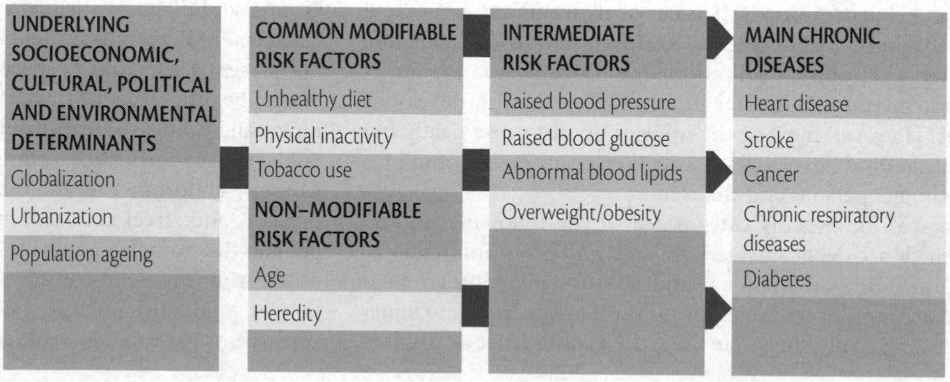

Fig. 1.1.6 Causes of chronic diseases. *Source*: World Health Organization. Main causes of death and global burden of disease (DALYs), world, all ages, projections for 2005. [Online]. Available from: http://www.who.int/chp/chronic_disease_report/contents/part2.pdf [accessed 2007 May].

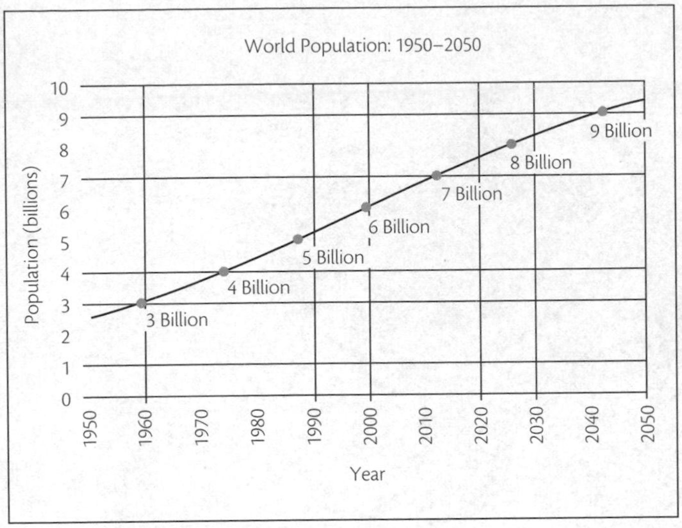

Fig. 1.1.7 World population, 1950–2050.
Source: United States Census Bureau. *International database.* [Online]. 2006 Aug. Available from: http://www.census.gov/ipc/www/idbnew.html [accessed 2007 May].

The number of known chemicals globally exceeds 14 million, of which over 60 000 are commonly used. All of these ultimately end up in the environment. They are the result of the huge proliferation of industry, technology, and automobiles in the twentieth century. Murray and Lopez (1996) have estimated that 1 379 238 DALYs are caused annually by environmental exposures. As we enter the twenty-first century, the number of pollutants will continue to increase.

Problems of the environment occur at the personal level (at home and the workplace), the community level (air and water pollution), and globally (global warming, hazardous and radioactive waste). Although these problems may be viewed separately, they are in fact all global issues affecting both local and remote populations. Thus, air pollution caused by slash-and-burn cultures in Sumatra severely affects the health of residents of Singapore and Malaysia. Industrial pollutants released in the industrial states of Northeastern United States cause acid rain, which adversely affects crops and people in the Midwestern United States and southern Canada. Pollution of rivers upstream can adversely affect communities and countries downstream, as happened in 2005 when nitrobenzene was released into the Songhua River in Heilongjiang, China, contaminating drinking water downriver in both China and Siberia, Russia.

Air pollution

The rapid increase in automobiles and industry has caused widespread air pollution in most urban areas of the world, the worst occurring in the developing countries, which have rapidly industrialized at the expense of their environment. Now, in the early part of the twenty-first century, many of these countries are realizing the need to protect the environment. Unfortunately, reversal of decades of pollution is far more difficult and costly than prevention.

The harmful effects of air pollution extend beyond the environment. Many members of society, including asthmatics and persons with chronic respiratory disease, are vulnerable to even relatively low levels of pollutants. Studies of the urban air in Southern California have demonstrated that children chronically exposed to high levels of both primary pollutants and photochemical oxidants have decreased lung function (Detels *et al.* 1979). Recent studies have demonstrated that children living near freeways in Southern California also suffer long-term lung damage (Gauderman *et al.* 2007). Levels of pollutants observed in many developing countries, especially in China and India, are considerably higher than in developed countries, but few studies have documented the cost of these high levels of pollutants to the health of children, as well as adults, in these countries. Thus, the true cost of uncontrolled industrialization in these countries is not known.

Water pollution

Those who live in developed countries take the provision of safe drinking water for granted, but 40 per cent of the world's population does not have access to clean drinking water, a basic necessity of life. As the world population expands, the production of waste increases, and the problem of protecting water supplies also increases. Approximately 60 per cent of the world does not have adequate facilities for waste disposal. Even in leading cities in developed countries, pollution of the water supply occurs, as happened in Milwaukee, Wisconsin, when cryptosporidia contaminated the water supply, causing severe illness and death, especially in vulnerable populations compromised by immune deficiency disorders (MacKenzie *et al.* 1994). The increased rate of upper respiratory infections and gastrointestinal disorders among surfers and others using the ocean for recreational purposes has been well documented. Beaches in most urban areas are frequently closed when the sewage disposal systems become overwhelmed. Acid rain from industrialization has caused acidification of lakes, making them inhospitable for fish and other marine life, thus compromising the food supply. Recently there has been discussion about whether the benefits of omega-3 fatty acids found in fish outweigh the risk of mercury poisoning among those who eat large quantities of fish. Ensuring a safe, adequate water supply for people in both developed and developing countries must become a public health priority.

Other pollutants

As the population of the world rapidly increases and technology produces new substances and processes, not only the amount of pollutants, but also the varieties of pollutants increases. As new substances are developed, their use should not be permitted until plans and provisions have been developed and implemented for their safe disposal. This seldom happens!

Biodegradable pollutants have a limited lifespan in the environment, but we are increasingly producing non-biodegradable substances such as plastics, which are now ubiquitous, and hazardous materials such as radioactive wastes that persist for generations. It is likely that the amount of these hazardous substances will increase as natural energy sources are exhausted by the burgeoning and increasingly affluent population. The problem of discarding these waste products safely has become a major public health issue. Developed countries are now paying developing countries to accept their hazardous waste products. This strategy does not solve the problem, but shifts it to those countries that have fewer resources with which to deal with the problem, thus solving a local problem but creating a global problem! A major public health issue of the twenty-first century will be global warming due to the release of carbon dioxide and other 'greenhouse gases'.

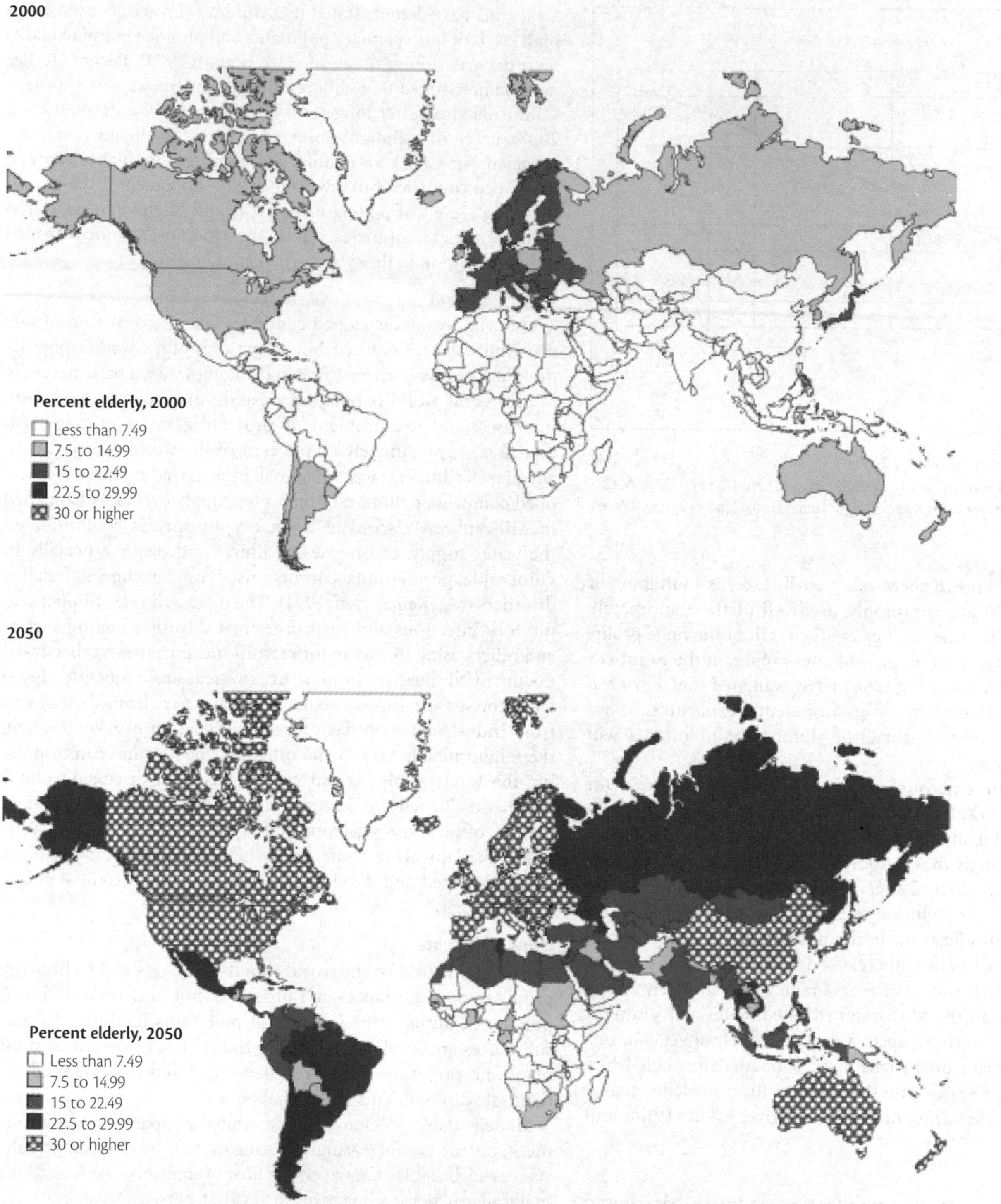

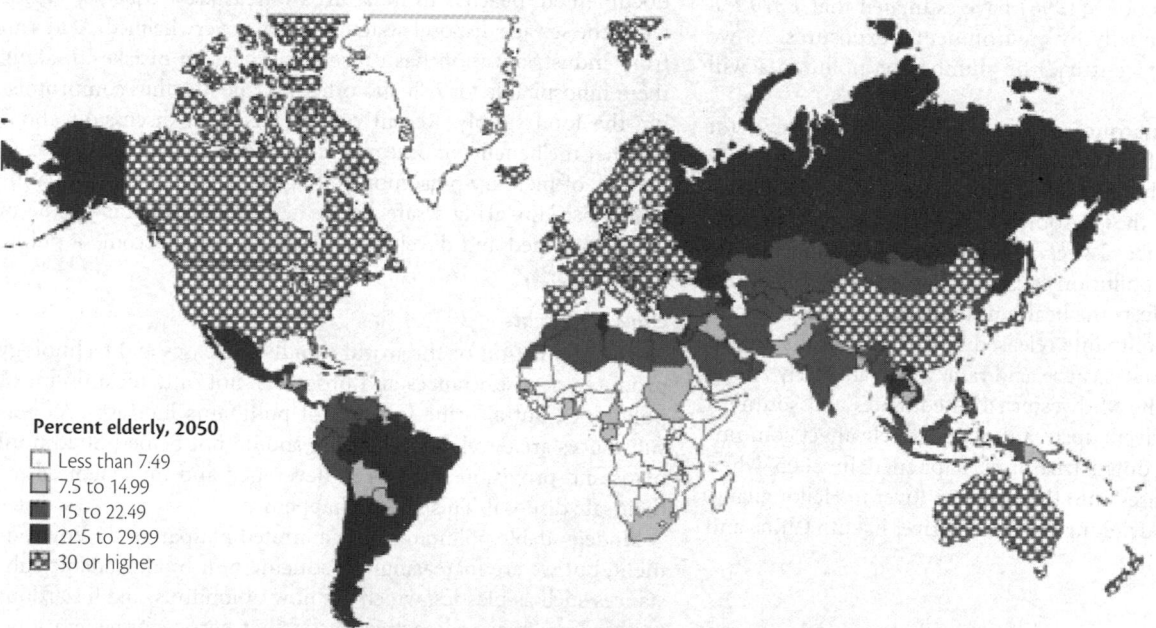

Fig. 1.1.8 Percentage of elderly (age 65 and over) by country, 2000 and 2050.
Source: Kaneda T. Percentage of elderly (ages 65 and over) by country, 2000 and 2050. [Online]. Population Reference Bureau. Available from: http://www.prb.org/Articles/2006/iticalWindowforPolicymakingonPopulationAginginDevelopingCountries.aspx [accessed 2007 May].
United Nations Population Division, *World Population Prospects: The 2004 Revision* (New York: United Nations, 2005).

Rescuing the environment

The key to rescuing the environment is to induce the political will of the countries of the world to take steps towards reversing and preventing further degradation of the environment. Global warming represents an example of these problems. The United States is the major producer of carbon dioxide and other greenhouse gases responsible for global warming, yet it is one of the few countries unwilling to sign the treaty on global warming! In order to induce the political will to protect the environment and public health globally, political leaders will need to collaborate with other countries

Table 1.1.5 Percentages of adults with total tooth loss in the United Kingdom for different age, gender, and social class groups in 1978, 1988, and 1998

	1978	1988	1998
Age (years)			
25–34	4	1	0
35–44	13	4	1
45–54	32	17	6
55–64	50	37	20
65 and over	79	67	45
All ages	30	21	13
Gender			
Male	25	16	10
Female	33	25	15
Both	30	21	13
Social class of head of household			
I, II, III NM (skilled non-manual)	22	15	8
III M (skilled manual)	29	24	15
IV, V (unskilled)	38	32	22
All	30	21	13

Source: Walker and Cooper (eds), 2000; Todd and Lader, 1991
Petersen PE. Inequalities in oral health: the social context for oral health. In: *Community oral health*. 2nd ed. London: Quintessence Publishing; 2007. p. 38.

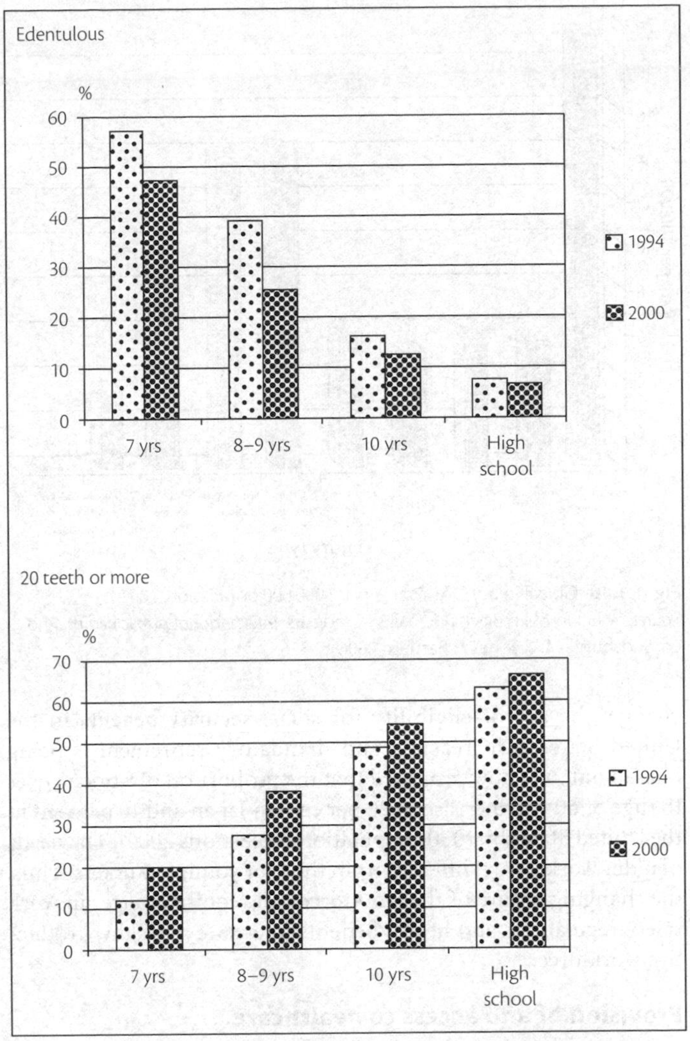

Fig. 1.1.9 Percentages of interviewed elderly (65 years or more) who reported being edentulous or having at least 20 teeth present in relation to number of years having attended school and year of study.
Source: Petersen PE. Inequalities in oral health: the social context for oral health. In: *Community oral health*. 2nd ed. London: Quintessence Publishing; 2007. p. 39.

to confront cultural norms, strong economic interests (e.g. industry), and current attitudes of much of the world's population. Regulations will need to be promulgated and implemented, which, out of necessity, will compromise the current lifestyle of much of the world's population. It is unlikely that risk from environmental pollution and hazardous waste can be reduced to zero. Thus, the concept of 'acceptable risk' will be a part of the process. Determining the level of acceptable risk might not be a scientific process, but a political one in which public health must play a strong role.

Occupational health

Occupational diseases are different from other diseases, not biologically, but socially. (Henry Sigerist 1958)

In 1999, Dr. Jukke Takala, Chief of the International Labour Organization's Health and Safety Programme, estimated that there were 1.1 million work-related deaths, 250 million work-related injuries, and 160 million cases of occupational disease annually worldwide (International Labour Organization 1999). Twelve million of these serious injuries occurred among young workers. This is more people than those who have myocardial infarcts (heart attacks), strokes, or newly diagnosed malignancies annually. A significant proportion of these deaths and injuries are preventable by improving safety in the workplace. However, safeguarding the worker is often given less priority than the need to produce cheap goods, especially in developing countries.

The nature of the workplace is constantly changing, with increasing proportions of workers being involved in communications and services rather than production of goods. Increasingly, the production of goods is moving from developed countries to developing countries, where labour costs are cheaper and safety regulations are fewer. Increasingly, women are entering the workforce and must juggle work and family. Because the costs of healthcare are rising more rapidly than the cost of living, industry is seeking relief from providing healthcare benefits, and healthcare is increasingly not provided as part of the employment package. Shifting from a formal full-time workforce to an informal part-time workforce is one strategy for reducing labour costs. Thus, the informal part-time workforce, not usually able to receive work-related benefits, now represents 50 per cent or more of the workforce globally. This segment of the workforce is particularly vulnerable to injury and limited access to healthcare.

As noted earlier, the population is aging, and the proportion of the population that produces is diminishing. In response to this

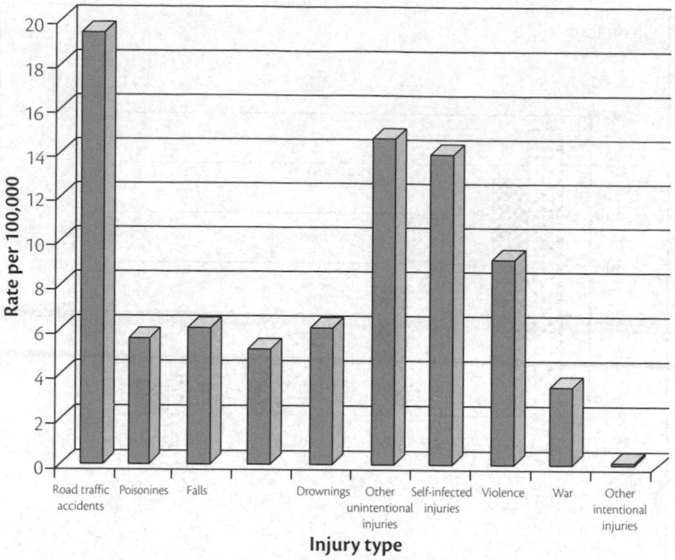

Fig. 1.1.10 Global injury DALY rates per 1 000 000 population, 2001.
Source: Merson M.H., Black R.E., Mills J.E., editors. *International public health*. 2nd ed. Sudsbury [MA]: Jones & Bartlett; 2006. p. 326.

change, the age of eligibility for social security benefits in the United States is increasing, and mandatory retirement is being phased out. It is now projected that the proportion of workers over the age of 60 will increase to 20 per cent in Japan and 10 per cent in the United States by 2030 (Population Projections 2000). The needs of older workers are different from those of younger workers. Thus, the changing nature of the workforce will require changes in work safety regulations and health benefits to ensure a healthy, productive workforce.

Provision of and access to healthcare

Access to preventive and curative care is a requirement for health in every society, whether rich or poor. Access to healthcare has long been a problem for the poor and for rural residents, especially in developing countries. However, in the United States, access to healthcare is even a problem for the middle class. Health insurance is prohibitively expensive and beyond the reach of many in the middle class, unless it is subsidized by the employers. Increasingly, employers are attempting to free themselves from the cost of health insurance for their employees through a variety of strategies. Thus, the proportion of those without healthcare is likely to increase. The elderly also have problems with healthcare; because healthcare costs increase with age, insurance companies are less willing to cover the elderly, and many governments, even in developed countries, do not provide adequate support for the elderly. In developing countries, the rural poor are particularly at risk. Few health professionals are willing to work in rural areas, and the cost of providing care in less populated areas is greater than in urban areas. Innovative strategies are needed to ensure that the rural poor and elderly have access to reasonable healthcare.

Bioterrorism and war

Biotererrorism has been used as a weapon for hundreds of years. In the middle ages, corpses of plague victims were catapulted into castles under siege. Recently, anthrax was used to contaminate the US postal system, resulting in several deaths. There has been a sharp increase in terrorist activities in this century. The WHO and public health agencies of individual countries have developed plans to quickly diagnose and control bioterrorist incidents. These threats to the health of the public will continue until we address the underlying causes of terrorism and bioterrorism.

Few actions can have the magnitude of negative impact on the health of the public that war has. Men, women, and children are killed, homes are destroyed, major segments of the population become displaced refugees, and the social and/or economic fabric of the countries involved is destroyed. Recovery usually takes years to decades. The outside world, particularly those countries adjacent to warring nations, must cope with the huge influx of displaced persons, and action needs to be implemented to help those still in the country suffering from the impact of the war. In many cases, the so-called rationale for the aggressive action is spurious. One suspects that had the billions of dollars that were spent on the wars in Iraq, Vietnam, and Afghanistan been put into humanitarian and public health support, it would probably have achieved a greater goal and more goodwill, not only on the part of the nations involved, but globally. The world must find a better way to resolve international conflicts.

Ethics in public health

Although ethics is implicit in the delivery of public health, it was only after the Second World War and the recognition that 'scientific experiments' in Nazi Germany violated human rights that an emphasis was placed on recognizing the ethics of public health actions, particularly research. The Declaration of Helsinki (World Medical Association 2002), the Belmont Report (US National Commission for the Protection of Human Subjects of Biomedical and Behavioral Research 1978), and the Council for International Organizations of Medical Science (CIOMS 2002) have promulgated ethical guidelines for research and the establishment of institutional review boards worldwide to ensure that medical and/or public health research is conducted ethically and does not violate human rights. However, there are inherent ethical conflicts in many public health actions. For example, the human rights of 'typhoid Mary', a typhoid carrier who insisted on working as a cook, were violated when she was incarcerated to prevent her from preparing food that initiated epidemics. Protecting the human rights of a man to refuse testing for HIV may result in his unknowingly infecting his wife, yet-to-be-born children, and other sexual contacts. By protecting his human rights, the human rights of his wife or partner and future family will be violated.

Implementing public health programmes and research often results in ethical conflicts and the need to balance the good of society against potential harm to the individual. It is usually necessary to inform society, particularly those who will be involved in the public programme or research, about the nature of the ethical conflicts inherent in action. For example, a trial evaluating the effectiveness of prophylactic treatment to prevent HIV infection in sex workers in Cambodia was stopped by the prime minister, who felt that the prevention trial exploited Cambodian sex workers. A more intense effort on the part of the researchers to inform the public and politicians about the nature of the study and the potential benefit to sex workers, not only in Cambodia but everywhere, might have averted this unfortunate outcome.

Public health interventions

One important task of public health professionals is to raise the level of anxiety of the public about public health problems to the level at which they will be willing to take an appropriate action. Raising the level of anxiety efficiently will result in inadequate or no action. On the other hand, raising the level too high will promote a fatalistic attitude and, as in the case of the recent HIV/AIDS epidemic, may promote stigmatization and isolation of affected individuals, seriously complicating the task of intervention. The difficulty for the public health professional is creating the level of anxiety that results in the required action.

Public health interventions can be divided into four categories: social/biologic/environmental, behavioural, political, and structural. The public health professional must use strategies in all four categories to achieve the maximum health of the public.

Social, biologic, and/or environmental interventions

The strategy that has had the greatest impact on improving the health of the public has been an improved standard of living, including provision of clean water and safe disposal of wastes. Unfortunately, these interventions have not reached much of the world where crowding, unsafe and insufficient water, and accumulation of wastes, and a lack of economic development persist.

The most cost-effective biologic intervention strategy is immunization, in part because it requires minimal behavioural change and usually only a single action. The WHO has taken the lead in promoting vaccine coverage worldwide through its Expanded Programme on Immunization. The appropriate use of vaccines has virtually eliminated the majority of childhood infections from the developed countries and significantly reduced them in most developing countries. Smallpox, a major infectious disease problem until the latter half of the twentieth century, has now been eliminated. We are well on our way to eliminating polio, but more challenges, such as hepatitis and tuberculosis, remain. Next may be measles. However, it is important to realize that development and production of a vaccine is only the first step. An effective vaccine against smallpox was available for over 150 years before smallpox was eliminated. The key was the strategy of vaccine coverage, 'search and contain', that permitted global elimination of the disease. Thus, the strategy for utilizing the vaccine is perhaps equally important as the efficacy of the vaccine itself.

Another biologic strategy is to eliminate the vectors of disease, the major approach currently in use for the control of dengue, arboviral diseases, and many of the parasitic diseases. However, overzealous use of pesticides can also create problems. For example, dichloro-diphenyl-trichloroethane (DDT), used widely in the twentieth century as an insecticide, still contaminates the food supply, creating other health problems, including the risk of malignancy.

Treatment can also be considered a biologic intervention strategy. To confront tuberculosis, one of the major infectious diseases of the twenty-first century, directly observed treatment short course (DOTS) has been successfully implemented in countries where the disease persists. Treatment of sexually transmitted infections and contacts is a major strategy for control of transmission, but has yet to prove effective in stopping the current epidemic.

Behavioural interventions

Most public health interventions depend ultimately on behaviour, whether it is personal or community behaviour. At the personal or individual level, promotion of good health habits and avoidance of smoking, excess alcohol use, and other dependency disorders are important interventions that have a major impact on health. At the community level, attitudes towards acceptable sexual behaviour and persons with dependency disorders and stigmatizing diseases are key to establishing community 'norms' that promote a healthy lifestyle and include all segments of society. However, modifying individual behaviour and community norms is difficult; it is even more difficult to ensure persistence of the modified behaviour. Yet, the majority of the public health interventions will not be successful unless they are embraced and sustained by the community at the local, national, and international levels. The success of the antismoking campaigns in the United States and Britain and population control in China (the one-child policy) affirm that it is possible to change community norms.

Many theories identifying strategies to modify behaviour have been proposed. One of the most interesting is the Popular Opinion Leader model proposed by Jeffrey Kelly (2004), which utilizes the natural leaders found in any social group as agents of change. In the United States, this strategy has been demonstrated to change behaviour in groups of men who have sex with men, and is now being evaluated in other populations worldwide.

Political interventions

Public health *is* politics. Any process that involves obtaining the support of the public will involve politics and differing points of view. For example, the campaign to stop smoking was strongly opposed by the tobacco industry, which spent millions of dollars trying to counter the many reports on the adverse health effects of smoking. Countering the efforts of the tobacco industry required obtaining the political support of the public in order to pass laws and regulations limiting smoking, placing health warnings on cigarette packages, and raising taxes on cigarettes.

If we are to succeed in safeguarding the oceans, inland waters, and the air we breathe, it will be through the political process. This process has already begun in many of the developed countries, which have passed strong laws regulating the emissions from automobiles and factories. Now this process must be expanded to the developing countries, where the worst pollution is currently occurring.

One of the most urgent issues before the public today is the battle over emission of 'greenhouse gases', which are causing a rise in temperatures globally. This temperature rise will adversely affect the quality of life of our children, grandchildren, and their grandchildren. Unfortunately, we have not yet achieved the political will to take the necessary steps to reverse this detrimental warming trend. The United States, the richest, most politically powerful nation in the world, even refuses to sign an international treaty signed by many other nations to address this problem.

It is important that the political process to improve the health of the public be based on sound scientific evidence. Pushing agendas not based on sound scientific evidence will undermine the credibility of public health professionals and our ability to accomplish our legitimate goals. Obtaining this evidence is not always easy. For example, accumulating evidence on the long-term (induction period of years to decades) impact of adverse exposures is not easily established, and often requires extrapolation from data on the impact of acute high-dose exposures to lower doses. This often requires relying on models, which are difficult for the public to understand, and are often subject to debate within the scientific community.

Structural interventions

The end result of the political process is the passage of laws and regulations. This action, if implemented, can have a very significant impact on the improvement of the health of the public. For example, the law reducing the maximum speed in California from 65 to 55 miles per hour had a significant impact on lowering the automobile fatality rate; unfortunately, this lower speed limit has been reversed. The passage and enforcement of helmet laws for motorcycles in Indonesia has reduced the incidence of associated brain injuries and deaths. The incidence of lung cancer and heart disease among men in California has been significantly reduced, probably due to the laws regulating smoking and the high taxes imposed on cigarettes. Many of the current public health problems of the world, particularly those involving protection of the environment, can be addressed through structural changes requiring passage and implementation of laws and regulations. To accomplish this will require changing the attitudes and behaviour of the public.

Private support of public health

Private support has played an important role in the development of public health, especially in the twentieth century. The Rockefeller Foundation supported the first school of public health in the United States at Johns Hopkins University; set up the International Health Commission in 1913; established the China Medical Board in 1914, which established the first public health university in China, the Peking Union Medical College, in 1921; and has continued to contribute to global health since its founding in 1913 (Berman 1983; Brown 1979). Other foundations, including the Ford Foundation, the Carnegie Foundation, and the Robert Wood Johnson Foundation, have made similar significant contributions to public health.

Private support of public health has been implemented through three strategies: establishment of charitable foundations by industry; development of international, national, and local non-governmental organizations (NGOs); and direct contributions by industry. Each makes and can continue to make a significant contribution to the health of the public.

Foundations have contributed enormously to the advancement of public health, but most often identify their own priorities for funding. Usually they provide support for important public health needs, but foundations and public health leaders do not always agree on what the most important priorities are. Thus, massive infusions of money into public health by organizations such as the Gates Foundation, which makes contributions to fight HIV, malaria, and tuberculosis, can have a significant positive impact, but they also tend to influence public health priorities. Some argue that developing strong public health infrastructures in developing countries will have a much greater impact on improving health than focusing funds on specific health issues (Garrett 2007).

NGOs tend to focus on specific health problems (e.g. American Cancer Society), specific health issues such as refugee health or medical care for the underserved (e.g. Doctors without Borders), and specific populations (e.g. drug users and sex workers). Often they can be more effective in reaching vulnerable populations and specific health problems and issues because they are closer to the problem than health professionals who must confront a broad range of concerns. Public health programmes can increase their cost-effectiveness by cooperating with NGOs in addressing specific issues, health problems, and populations.

Industry is often viewed as part of the problem. Certainly, industry is frequently the source of public health problems (e.g. air and water pollution). On the other hand, economic development can lead to an improved economic situation that reduces poverty and benefits all of society. However, industry, particularly the advertising industry, has clearly demonstrated that they are better at creating demand and influencing lifestyles than public health. Thus, it would behoove public health to learn from industry and to work with industry to develop and implement healthy economic growth, while safeguarding the environment and benefiting the public.

Private support has greatly benefited public health in the twentieth century. The challenge for the twenty-first century is for public health and private support to agree on the most effective use of private funds for achieving public health goals.

The future of public health

Public health does not lack challenges requiring solutions: emerging infections will continue to present new problems. Public health professionals recognize the threat that H5N1 influenza may mutate to cause human-to-human transmission, but given a virus as labile as influenza, other pandemics are also likely to occur. Early recognition of new strains by genetic monitoring of circulating influenza viruses will help.

An increasing proportion of the world's population will live to be old. We have been successful at adding 'years to life', but chronic diseases such as Alzheimer's have reduced the quality of life of the years of life added. We must now concentrate on adding 'life to years', helping older people to continue to be productive.

We cannot afford to continue to ignore the quality of the environment. Continuing contamination of the air and water will not only cause and/or exacerbate chronic and infectious diseases, but will rob us of important sources of food. Addressing these problems will require eliciting the political will and commitment of the public and changes in lifestyle. Unchecked population growth will further exacerbate the problem of protecting the environment.

Despite the economic and health advances of the past century, disparities between the rich and the poor are widening. This gap must be narrowed if not eliminated, not at the expense of those who are better-off, but by improving the economic situation and health of the poor and disadvantaged.

Injuries and violence are robbing an increasing number of people of their ability to function and to enjoy a reasonable quality of life. Injuries can be easily prevented through a variety of preventive strategies, including better design of the workplace and tools such as ladders, but also include implementing behavioural and structural strategies. Violence and war represent greater challenges, and will most likely require new strategies not hitherto widely used in public health.

We in public health know what needs to be done to significantly reduce chronic diseases such as cardiovascular diseases, stroke, and cancer, but we need to develop more effective ways to change behaviour and promote healthy lifestyles.

We have made tremendous strides to improve the health of the public, but the challenge to do better remains. In subsequent chapters, public health experts discuss the challenges and potential solutions in detail.

References

Acheson E.D. On the state of the public health [the fourth Duncan lecture]. *Public Health* 1988;**102**(5):431–437.

Berman E.H. *The ideology of philanthropy: the influence of the Carnegie, Ford, and Rockefeller foundations on American foreign policy*. New York (NY): University of New York Press; 1983.

Breslow L., Breslow N. Health practices and disability: some evidence from Alameda County. *Preventive Medicine* 1993;**22**:86–95.

Brown E.R. *Rockefeller medicine men: medicine and capitalism in America*. Berkeley (CA): University of California Press; 1979.

Chow C.K, Raju R. The prevalence and management of type 2 diabetes in India. *Diabetes Care* 2006;**29**:1717–1718.

Council for International Organization of Medical Sciences (CIOMS). *International ethical guidelines for biomedical research involving human subjects*. Geneva: World Health Organization; 2002.

Department of Health and Human Services, National Center for Health Statistics, *Health, United States, 1999*. Washington (DC): US Government Printing Office; 1999.

Detels R., Rokaw S.N., Coulson A.H. *et al.* The UCLA population studies of chronic obstructive respiratory disease: I. Methodology and comparison of lung function in areas of high and low pollution. *American Journal of Epidemiology* 1979;**109**(1):33–58.

Garrett L. The challenge of public health. *Foreign Affairs;* 2007 Jan/Feb.

Gauderman W.J., Vora H., McConnell K. *et al.* Effect of exposure to traffic on lung development from 10 to 18 years of age: a cohort study. *Lancet* 2007;**369**:571–577.

Sigerist H.E. *A History of Medicine.* Oxford and New York: Oxford University Press, 1958–1961.

International Labour Organization. Report of the 15th World Congress on Occupational Safety and Health. [Online]. 1999. Available from: http://www.ilo.org/public/english/bureau/inf/pr/1999/9.htm [accessed 2007 May].

Kaneda T. Percentage of elderly (ages 65 and over) by country, 2000 and 2050. [Online]. Population Reference Bureau. Available from: http://www.prb.org/Articles/2006/ACriticalWindowforPolicymakingonPopulationAginginDevelopingCountries.aspx [accessed 2007 May].

Kelly J.A. Popular opinion leaders and HIV prevention peer education: resolving discrepant findings, and implications for the development of effective community programmes. *AIDS Care* 2004;**16**(2):139–50.

Kuo C.C, Campbell L.A. Detection of Chlamydia pneumoniae in arterial tissues. *Journal of Infectious Diseases* 2000;**181**:S432–S436.

Lopez A., Mathers C., Ezzati M., Jamison D., Murray C. Global and regional burden of disease and risk factors, 2001: a systematic analysis of population health data. *Lancet* **367**(9524):1747–1757, 2007.

Lee S.H. The SARS epidemic in Hong Kong. *Journal of Epidemiology and Community Health* 2003;**57**(9):652–4.

Lopez A.D, Mathers C.D, Ezzati M. *et al.* Global burden of disease and risk factors. In: *Disease control priorities project*. Oxford: Oxford University Press; 2006.

MacKenzie W.R., Hoxie N.J., Proctor M.E. *et al.* A massive outbreak in Milwaukee of cryptosporidium infection transmitted through the public water supply. *New England Journal of Medicine* 1994;**331**:161–7.

Mathers C.D., Loncar D. Projections of global mortality and burden of disease from 2002 to 2030. [Online]. *PLoS Medicine* 2006;**3**(11):e442.

McGinnis J.M., Foege W.H. Actual causes of death in the United States. *Journal of the American Medical Association* 1993;**270**:2007–2012.

Merson M.H., Black R.E., Mills J.E., eds. *International public health*. 2nd edn. Sudsbury (MA): Jones & Bartlett; 2006. p. 326.

Murray C.J.L., Lopez A.D. A comprehensive assessment of mortality and disability from diseases, injuries, and risk factors in 1990, and projected to 2020. In: *The global burden of disease*. Cambridge (MA): Harvard University Press; 1995. vol 1.

Murray C.J.L., Lopez A.D. (eds). The global burden of disease. In: *The global burden of disease*. Cambridge (MA): Harvard University Press; 1996. (Global burden of disease and injury series; vol 1).

Office of the Director, National Public Health Performance Standards Program. *10 essential public health services*. [Online]. Centers for Disease Control; 1994. Available from: http://www.cdc.gov/od/ocphp/nphpsp/EssentialPHServices.htm

Pan American Health Organization. *Essential public health services*. [Online]. 2002. Available from: http://www.sopha.cpha.ca/english/ephf_e.html

Petersen P.E. Inequalities in oral health: the social context for oral health. In: *Community oral health*. 2nd edn. London: Quintessence Publishing; 2007. p. 38–39.

Pine C., Harris R. *Community oral health*. London: Quintessence Books; 2007.

Population Projections. *Health Affairs;* 2000 May/June.

United States Census Bureau. *International database*. [Online]. 2006. Available from: http://www.census.gov/ipc/www/idbnew.html [accessed 2007 May].

US National Commission for the Protection of Human Subjects of Biomedical and Behavioral Research. *The Belmont report*. Washington (DC): US National Commission for the Protection of Human Subjects of Biomedical and Behavioral Research; 1978.

WHO Oral Health Program. [Online]. Sweden: Malmo University; 2004. Available from: http://www.whocollab.od.mah.se/index.html [accessed 2007 May].

World Health Organization. *Atlas mental health resources in the world, 2001*. [Online]. 2001. Available from: http://whqlibdoc.who.int/whr/2001/WHR_2001.pdf [accessed 2007 May].

World Health Organization. Causes of chronic diseases. [Online]. 2005. Available from: http://www.who.int/chp/chronic_disease_report/contents/part2.pdf [accessed 2007 May].

World Health Organization. Indicators for Policy and Decision Making in Environmental Health. Geneva, Switzerland: WHO; 1997.

World Health Organization. *Injury Report*. [Online]. 2004. Available from: http://www.wpro.who.int/internet/templates/HLT_Topic.aspx?NRMODE=Published&NRORIGINALURL=%2Fhealth_topics%2Finjuries_and_violence_prevention%2F&NRNODEGUID=%7BF17BB93C-267E-49F1-B089-F4C4710AED39%7D&NRCACHEHINT=NoModifyGuest [accessed 2007 May].

World Health Organization. Main causes of death and global burden of disease (DALYs), world, all ages, projections for 2005. [Online]. Available from: http://www.who.int/chp/chronic_disease_report/contents/part2.pdf [accessed 2007 May].

World Health Organization. Neglected tropical diseases—hidden successes, emerging opportunities. [Online]. 2006. Available from: http://whqlibdoc.who.int/hq/2006/WHO_CDS_NTD_2006.2_eng.pdf [accessed 2007 May].

World Health Organization. Trends in global years of life lost (YLL) per 1,000 population, by broad cause group and income group, 2002–2030. [Online]. 2005. Available from: http://www.who.int/healthinfo/statistics/bodprojectionspaper.pdf [accessed 2007 May].

World Health Organization. *World Health Report, 2001*. Geneva: World Health Organization; 2001.

World Medical Association. *Declaration of Helsinki*. 5th revision. Washington (DC): World Medical Association; 2002.

1.2

The history and development of public health in developed countries

Christopher Hamlin

Abstract

This chapter explores the problem of defining the proper domain of public health as a science and department of public action. It examines three elements of public health, which have been important in its past in the developed world: The response to epidemics, the policing of towns (and states) in ordinary times, and efforts to produce a systematic betterment of population health. The chapter also argues that a 'golden age' from 1880 to 1970, when public health rationales were relatively unquestioned, has given way to a new era of complexity: The agenda of public health is less clear and there has been renewed fundamental debate on such ancient issues as how to understand cause as well as on what kinds of changes are possible and warranted.

Introduction

Much more than is usually realized, public health is both a central and a problematic element of the history of the developed world—here conceived as Europe and the 'Neo Europes'; that is, the set of nations in broad latitude bands of the northern and southern hemispheres in which European institutions and biota have been particularly successful (Crosby 1986).

Over the last three centuries, health status has changed profoundly in these regions; arguably, it is in terms of health that our lives differ most strikingly from those of our ancestors. We live longer. Rarely do parents experience the death of their young children; rarely do young adults experience the gradual 'consumption' of pulmonary tuberculosis. Affluence and transportation mean most of us are no longer subject to periodic famines, and much less subject to epidemics of deadly infectious diseases, although we are less confident about that than we were two decades ago. Nor are most of us wracked with chronic pain, with abscesses, or with induced deformities. Most of us do not see life as a continuously painful experience and death as a merciful release, a view that is rather commonly found in books of theology from three centuries ago (Browne 1964).

Our health is adversely affected by aspects of the world we have built and the ways we choose to live individually and communally. A good deal is known about how to prevent those effects even if we do not always do so. Nonetheless, an expectation of health and a preoccupation with it are hallmarks of modernity. The freedom of action that ideally characterizes the lives of individuals in the developed world is predicated on health; so much of the agenda of development concerns health, that this transformation has some claim to be seen as one of the monumental changes in human history. It might be argued that economic and political progress are subordinate to securing health—they are means; health, which surely translates into life, liberty, and the pursuit of happiness, is the end.

Surprisingly, the history of public health is under-studied. Few general texts give it much attention (but see McNeill 1976); there remain vast gaps in empirical knowledge, and relatively little comparative work (but see Baldwin 1999; Porter 1999; Kunitz 2007). Compared with the grand dramas of history, public health has sometimes seemed to historians a marginal and uncontroversial function of modern society. After all, we provide medicine, collect and evaluate demographic data, test water, and keep cities clean in roughly similar ways, according to the conventions of science, technology, and public administration that developed mainly in the nineteenth century. This view partly reflects a distortion of the history of public health by the modern professions and institutions of public health, which have often found it prudent to reduce the significance of the fact that they are necessarily political, even if their business is politics by medical means.

Public health is treated more broadly in this chapter. It is concerned with the general questions of how, why, and in what manners states came to take an interest in the peoples' health. The questions of what 'health' is, of what we mean by 'public', and of what we understand to be the proper domain of 'public health' are, and have always been, contested matters. To define public health as that part of health that is the responsibility of the state does not help: What constitutes the state, and what are presumed to be state responsibilities vary in time and place. However broadly or narrowly we define 'health', it will be clear that many public actions affect the public's health, yet will not necessarily be seen to belong to the domain of 'public health' or its predecessors.

An examination of actions taken in the name of the public to protect or improve the health of the public will illuminate the enigmatic relationship between that universal goal, the health of the public, and public health as an institution—as a profession, science, component of public administration, and theme of moral and political philosophy (Porter 1999; Fee 1993; Rosen 1958). Within that framework, there will be more diversity, contingency, complexity, and controversy in its history than is usually apparent. Ultimately, however, there can be no single narrative. A history of public health is necessarily part of an ongoing conversation about a programme of social change that is both rational and moral. The story we tell about it will depend on what we think public health should be, just as our notions of it will themselves reflect the evolution of the professions and institutions we have inherited, and of the myths, memories, and sensibilities that sustain them.

Themes and problems in the history of public health

It will help at the outset to recognize several of the most troublesome issues that face any historian of public health. Among these are the following:

I. The units of public health: States and publics

- *The public and the state:* 'State' and 'public' are not always interchangeable terms. The state, concerned with population, may arrive at different health-related policies from a public sphere of groups of citizens, carrying out a rational and critical dialogue among equals (Sturdy 2002).
- *The diversity of states:* Even when widely accepted reasons of the state and agendas of state responsibility arose, not every state was in the position to act on them. The focus of public health was quite often at the level of local states, whose responsibility and jurisdiction were often unclear or overlapping. But the state itself was an artificial unit for addressing problems, like many epidemic diseases, which were global in nature.
- *Goals of the state:* Although health is now thought of in terms of the biological autonomy of individuals, this has rarely, and only recently, been the goal of programmes of public health. Health sometimes has meant a good supply of labour or of soldiers, control of excess population, protection of élites, enhancement of the genetic stock of a population, or environmental stability.

II. The condition that is truly health

- *The definition of health:* The combating of epidemic infectious diseases has often seemed to be the core of public health. When we go beyond these diseases, questions arise of what level and kind of physical and mental well-being the state should guarantee or require of its citizens, and of the status of health as a source of imperatives vis-à-vis other sources of imperatives such as the market, the environment, or individual liberty. What sort of normality will a society demand?
- *The problem of causation of disease:* In a broad sense, diseases have many causes—personal, social, cultural, political, and economic, as well as biological. Among the multiple antecedents that converge in the production of an epidemic or endemic disease, there are numerous opportunities to intervene (MacMahon & Pugh 1970: Chapter 2). Notions of rights that must be respected, or of political or technical practicality, narrow that list. Discussion of cause has often included notions of responsibility or preventability—of where in a social system there is flexibility, of who or what must change to prevent disease.
- *Equality and rights—race, class, gender:* The idea of 'health for all' disguises the fact that the interests of the so-called public have not always been the interests of all of its members. Public health actions have often reflected, and sometimes exacerbated, a view of the world in which some groups were seen primarily as a threat to others. Often, views of the standards of health that were properly matters for the state varied with respect to different groups: Key divisions were by sex, by age (infants, working adults, and the aged all had a different status), by wealth, and by race, religion, or historical heritage (indigenous people had a different status from colonial rulers). Whether the public's response to disease was to advise, aid, or condemn, or to imprison, banish, or kill, reflected the allocation of rights and the distribution of power more than the status of the biological threat.

III. The health that is truly public

- *Health and public health:* Most modern states have in principle distinguished aspects of health that are the business of the public from those that are for the individual to pursue in the medical marketplace, although the borders have been drawn in many different ways.
- *Medical and non-medical public health:* Although public health has evolved into an ancillary medical science, with occasional involvement of relevant areas of engineering and the social sciences, the fact that health has been improved by many non-medical factors—prosperity, town planning, architecture, religious and humanitarian charity, the power of organized labour, and even the enlargement of political or economic rights—suggests that any comprehensive account of improved health must include these factors.
- *Health as authority:* Given the amorphous nature of the concept of health and its status as the supreme good of human existence, it has been attractive as an imperative for political action. If other 'reasons of state' carry more immediacy, public health has better claim to the moral high ground because it is seen to be universal and apolitical, exactly the qualities that make it attractive to act politically in the name of health.

These issues are too many to address fully, but they inform what follows. The history of public health in the developed world can be conceived in terms of three relatively distinct missions: Public health as a reaction to epidemics, as a form of police, and as a means of human betterment. Public health was initially reactive; faced with epidemic disease, early modern European states closed borders and ports, instituted fumigation, shut down dangerous (smelly) trades, and isolated victims. Second, public health acted as a form of police. It is probably the case that wherever humans live in communities, customs arise for the regulation of behaviour and the maintenance of the communal environment. Gradually, much of the enforcement of community standards became medical. The control of food adulteration or prostitution, of the indigent and the transient, or concern over dung or smoke overlapped with the control of epidemics, but went well beyond it, and occurred in normal as well as in epidemic times.

Finally, public health became a proactive political vision for improvement of the health of all. Well into the nineteenth century, the view remained common that high urban or infant death rates were inevitable. A proactive public health involved the determination that normal conditions of health, if they could be improved, were not acceptable conditions of health. This shift was partly due to technical achievements—such as smallpox inoculation, and later, vaccination—and to better demographic information, but it rested on changed conceptions of human rights coupled with greater technical and economic optimism. Such visions sustained the building of comprehensive urban water and sewerage systems before there was wide acceptance that these needed to be universal features of cities; such visions have periodically led public health to venture beyond traditional medical bounds, to recognize, for example, nuclear warfare or gun violence as public health problems.

The public health of epidemic crisis: Reaction

Regardless of their virulence and pervasiveness, epidemic and, even more so, endemic diseases do not necessarily warrant comment or action—they may simply be acknowledged as part of life. For the public to decide to fight an epidemic, it must believe it can do something to mitigate the problem, and it must be just sufficiently concerned. It is true that a belief in *the possibility of effective action* is a prerequisite for public health; one of the most intriguing problems in its history is the emergence of this belief. It does not coincide with the replacement of the supernatural by naturalistic explanations of disease causation. 'Will-of-God' explanations of disease have sometimes incited public action, but on other occasions implied abject resignation.

Similarly, naturalistic explanations—attributing epidemics to a mysterious element in the atmosphere or, as in the case of classical conceptions of smallpox, to a normal process of fermentation in the growing body—have on some occasions been taken as proof that we can do nothing beyond giving supportive care and on other occasions have sanctioned preventive public action. In each case, assessments of technical and political practicality are mixed with assessments of propriety: Is taking such action part of our cultural destiny?

These issues are already evident in the first European account of a widely fatal epidemic, the unidentified plague that struck Athens in 430 BC. Athenians both recognized contagion and acknowledged a duty to aid the afflicted, as Thucydides informs us, but these recognitions did not translate into expectations of prevention, mitigation, or escape (Carmichael 1993; Longrig 1992; Nutton 2000; Thucydides 1950). Few fled; on the contrary, the epidemic was exacerbated by an influx from the countryside. Although it was appreciated that those who survived the disease were unlikely to be affected again, and some hoped it would bring permanent immunity from all afflictions, the main response was to accept one's fate. The disease was attributed to the seasons, as well as to the gods, and was said to have be prophesied. Such resignation would be central to the moral philosophies of the Roman world, Stoicism and Epicureanism, both of which taught one to accept what was fated or necessary (Veyne 1987). Later writers in the Christian world attributed the failure of Islam to take active steps against plague to such an outlook. Although classical Islamic doctors developed a science of hygiene to a remarkable degree (Gori 2002), it did not follow that one should apply this knowledge in an epidemic: If plague came, that was Allah's will. To fight it would be futile and impious; one's duty was to trust (Conrad 1992; Dols 1977).

In contrast, the response to epidemic disease in the medieval Christian Latin countries was activism. One could prevent disease from taking hold in a community, or extinguish it if it did, or at least avoid it personally. This activism had many avenues, indicative of the syncretism of Medieval Latin culture. In the Old and New Testaments alone, disease had a multiplicity of significations. It represented the dispensation of God to an individual, perhaps as punishment or a test. To act against disease by intervening to help others stricken by a dangerous epidemic was an act of devotion. If one died in such a situation, it was a sign of grace; if one did not die, and helped to save others, this was equally a sign of grace. The laws of hygiene in the Pentateuch permitted a naturalistic interpretation of disease. Unclean acts or other transgressions, such as failing to isolate lepers from society, generated the retribution of disease, perhaps through God's appointed secondary or natural causes. Disease might even be naturally communicative; in such a case, communal decisions to maintain the Levitical laws were means not only of acting against potential epidemics but also of policing the community, and perhaps, of augmenting its welfare (Amundsen & Ferngren 1986; Dorff 1986; Douglas 1966; Lieber 2000; Winslow 1980). Such views would become widespread among nineteenth-century sanitarians.

The two diseases that did spur medieval Europeans to comment and react were leprosy and the plague. Although it is difficult to assess the number of lepers in medieval Europe, the common view is that there was a vast overreaction, in terms of both investment in institutions to house victims of the disease—there were said to be several thousand leprosaria—and the detection and isolation of cases to prevent transmission. In keeping with the prominence of leprosy in the Bible, the professionals who diagnosed it were churchmen, not medical men. The diagnosis was a loose one; it might be based on skin blemishes alone.

Often it involved an accusation. It led to the expulsion of the victim from ecclesiastical and civil society, symbolized in a ceremony resembling a funeral. Subsequently, no one was to touch or come near the leper or to touch what the leper touched. The theory of contagion provided the rationale for such action, but Skisnes (1973) has argued that the clinical characteristics of the disease itself—for example, its slow development, the visible disfigurement it produced—triggered such a reaction (Brody 1974; Carmichael 1997; Richards 1977; Touati 2000). Even if leprosy precautions did embody empirical knowledge of contagion, it, like most other diseases, belonged to the sphere of providence. While leprosy was sometimes seen as a punishment of sin, it might also reflect grace: God's singling out of an individual to bear a particular burden of suffering.

The prototypical institutional responses to epidemic disease, however, were those that arose in response to plague. The first wave of plague, the Black Death, spread across Europe from 1347 to 1353, and thereafter the disease returned to most areas about once every two decades for the next three centuries. This was a catastrophic disease, with case-fatality rates ranging from 30 to nearly 100 per cent depending on the strain of 'plague' (the identity of the microbe has recently been questioned; for a review, see Carmichael 2003), the means of transmission, and the immunological state of the population. Plague and accompanying diseases reduced the

European population by roughly a third or more in the fourteenth century and were responsible for only a very slow population growth during the following two centuries. As in the case of leprosy, the aetiology of plague and the associated means of prevention and mitigation of the disease were conceived in terms of divine will and natural processes, although even more clearly than with leprosy the distinction is misleading: Nature, whether in the courses of the stars, in meteorological phenomena, or in the process of contagion, was God's instrument (Nohl 1926; Ziegler 1969).

It is clear that in many communities the coming of plague was unacceptable. It could not be reconciled with the usual course of events, but indicated some fundamental violation of the cosmos, of an order which included human society. Boccaccio (1955), whose *Decameron* is a document on the Black Death, testifies to one form of activism—a discarding of social convention and religious duty, a devil-may-care indulgence in the present founded on the recognition that life was short and the future uncertain. Those with the means often fled plague-ridden places. Others, taking the view that the plague reflected God's just anger with hopelessly corrupt civil and ecclesiastical authority, saw a clear need to take charge of matters temporal and spiritual, to cleanse themselves, the state, and the church. Righteousness would end the plague.

Thus, the plague precipitated a social crisis, as would epidemics of other diseases in subsequent centuries. Beyond the massive disruption caused by high mortality and morbidity and an interruption of commerce and industry, the loss of faith in the conventions and institutions of society was a critical blow. Why respect property, family, or communal obligations, pay taxes, invest money, or tolerate rivals and others? Latent tensions within society had an excuse to become active.

When people acted precipitately and independently, civil and ecclesiastical institutions were threatened, and it is in their responses that we clearly see the emergence of public health as a form of public authority. For a state, to act in a crisis was to keep the state going; one maintained authority by acting authoritatively. If some state actions were rational in terms of the naturalistic aspects of theories of the plague, the viability of civic authority itself was probably more crucial than any lives they might save.

All these issues are evident in the manifold responses to plague from the mid-fourteenth to the early eighteenth century. Particularly in Germany, the response to the Black Death was to challenge civil and ecclesiastical authority. In 1349, lay flagellant groups paraded from town to town, giving public penitential performances to end the plague. Although they were usually well received, and their practices were unorthodox, the movement did draw attention to what the Church had failed to do, and Pope Clement VI condemned it.

However, the state response to such actions could not have been uniform, for medieval and early states were not monoliths but fragile alliances of multiple levels and kinds of authority, existing in continual tension with one another. In Basel, the majority Christian population blamed the plague on Jews—either it came by direct divine action because Jews had been allowed to live in the town, or through a natural agent with which the Jews had presumably poisoned the town's water. The town's Jews were rounded up, sequestered on an island, and burned. Here it was a local state, the town council, which took the action. Its credibility was at stake; it needed to be seen to act boldly in order to secure an end to the epidemic, its action built on pre-existing anti-Semitism. To the central state, the Holy Roman Empire, such actions against one group of its subjects verged on anarchy. Emperor Charles IV condemned the persecution and asserted on the basis of medical and religious authority that the Jews were not responsible for the plague (Ziegler 1969).

In contrast, the approaches to plague prevention and control developed in the next two centuries in the Italian city-states were humane, focused mainly on naturalistic intervention, and probably relatively successful. Plague control measures emerged out of a tradition of close municipal management, and in a cosmopolitan intellectual environment. Italy, after all, was the main European centre for receiving Galenic and Islamic medical knowledge; included were concepts of hygiene, disease causation, and the purification of enclosed spaces. The preventive measures taken in Italian city-states were eclectic. They included the development of the forty-day hold on ships or other traffic coming from potentially infected places (the quarantine), the isolation of victims (and families of victims), and numerous means of purifying the air and/or destroying contamination: Bonfires, burning sulphur, burning clothes and bedding, washing surfaces with lime or vinegar, and killing or removing urban animals. Such actions were predicated on an understanding that the disease moved from place to place through some medium or media, possibly involving, although probably not limited to, person-to-person contact.

Although the eclecticism of this response is certainly indicative of uncertainty about how plague spread, the actions do show a responsive civil authority (Carmichael 1986; Cipolla 1979, 1992). Indeed, in some ways plague prevention initiatives were themselves a means of state growth. Plague control required officials to oversee quarantine or isolation procedures. It required a staff to disinfect, and a structure to gather information on health conditions at remote ends of the state. An embassy, which in the high Middle Ages signified an official visit by one state to another, became the permanent presence of one state in the territory of another in the Italian city-states. Its initial purpose was to monitor the public health in the host country and to send word home if plague broke out (Cipolla 1981; Slack 1985).

Plague set the template for responses to epidemics of other diseases (often generically called plague)—flight, exacerbation of social tensions leading to scapegoating, a heightening of religious seriousness (often combined with a collapse of normal customs and obligations), and a mix of pragmatic efforts to disinfect people, places, goods, or the environment, and to isolate victims or potentially contagious strangers, and somehow to control the poor (Carmichael 1986; Briggs 1961). The particular mix of these actions reflected the current state of debate between proponents of atmospheric theories, including miasmatic theories, which located the origins of the epidemic in some unusual state of air, and of contagionist theories, which emphasized various forms of interpersonal transmission, and presumed that epidemics could spread only as far as infected humans (or human products) carried them. Only rarely were contagionist and environmental explanations mutually exclusive, as a wide range of factors were implicated in disease (Kinzelbach 2006; Pelling 2001).

Thus, in the nineteenth century, the series of cholera pandemics which arrived in Europe in the early 1830s brought forth accusations by the poor that the rich were poisoning them (particularly the doctors who wanted their bodies for teaching and research), and by the rich that the poor wantonly persisted in living in disease-nurturing squalor. It also engendered calls for public fasts, pure living, and declamations against sinful society, and a variety of attempts to disinfect, quarantine, and isolate (Briggs 1961; Delaporte 1986; Durey 1979; Evans 1990; McGrew 1965; Richardson 1988; Rosenberg 1962; Snowden 1995). In nineteenth-century America, the response to yellow fever and malaria was regular flight and the abandonment of cities during the summer by those who could afford to do so (Ellis 1992; Humphreys 1992). The summer home, in cooler, cleaner, and higher ground, became a mark of upper-middle-class life.

Significant alterations of that pattern came through efforts to control three other diseases: Venereal diseases (particularly syphilis), smallpox, and a mix of diseases including typhus, typhoid, relapsing fever, and a mix of ill-defined conditions known as continued fever (or just 'fever').

Whether syphilis came to Europe from America or Africa, or had been present in Europe in a milder form (perhaps labelled as leprosy), has been much debated. What is clear is that a virulent epidemic often known as the French disease or pox began to spread quickly in the last years of the fifteenth century, and can be traced to the intercourse between Italian prostitutes and French and Spanish soldiers during the siege of Naples in 1494. The connection between the disease and sex was made quickly, partly because of the initial symptoms on the external genitalia—the more expressive German term *lustseuche* had been adopted by 1510. As had not been the case with plague or leprosy, syphilis represented a serious epidemic disease that constituted a state problem (surely, plague was a state problem?), particularly because it affected military strength, but which was not susceptible to large-scale public action. It was further complicated by having variable symptoms and effects, having a long course during parts of which it was not clearly manifest, and varying in contagiousness and virulence.

If syphilis was to be controlled, states must prevail on individuals to avoid behaviours that spread the disease. One might expect the moral opprobrium related to contracting a disease usually acquired through illicit sexual contact to have had some role in discouraging such practices, but it did not. For an adventurous young man, a case of pox was a cost of doing business, even a badge of achievement. The disease was deemed curable, chiefly through mercurial treatments. Although there are suggestions that by the eighteenth century syphilis had become something to hide (though not necessarily for moral reasons), such was not the case during the sixteenth century, when the disease was spreading rapidly (Arrizabalaga 1993; Arrizabalaga *et al.* 1997).

State attention shifted from cure to prevention only in the eighteenth century, partly because syphilis was becoming more clearly distinguished from other venereal conditions and as the varied phenomena of tertiary syphilis were becoming more evident. Whereas the European states varied significantly in the priority they put on syphilis as a public problem, their approaches did not vary greatly: The disease was to be controlled by regulating prostitutes, who were regarded as the reservoir that maintained the contagion. Such approaches may well have had a significant effect in controlling the disease, but they exposed tensions between state and individual rights that have since become common in public health.

Such conflicts developed first in the United Kingdom following the first Contagious Diseases Act of 1862, even though its programme against venereal disease was much smaller than that of France, where regulation of prostitution was a central feature of public hygiene (Baldwin 1999). The British Act allowed the police in designated garrison towns to arrest and inspect women presumed to be prostitutes and to confine infected women in hospital. It led to a sustained campaign for repeal, which was ultimately successful in 1885. The repealers represented a broad coalition: Some objected that the legislation was morally indefensible because it acquiesced in the immoral industry of prostitution, others that it singled out women as responsible for a problem that was as much the responsibility of the men who used the services of prostitutes, while still others objected that the practice of arresting women was arbitrary (except with respect to class) and stigmatized working-class women who were not prostitutes (McHugh 1982; Walkowitz 1980).

The problem that the British parliament faced stemmed from liberal principles of human rights. Ironically, the Contagious Diseases Act had been touted as respecting rights—the rights of men: The state would inspect women because male soldiers and sailors would not put up with genital inspection. Nor should they be expected to in a state in which the male franchise was broadening and the public was becoming increasingly uneasy with declarations that part of its population existed as cannon fodder. But recognizing the rights of men simply made it all the more clear that they were not accorded to women.

The issues that arose in combating venereal diseases arose in a more general way with regard to smallpox. While the ninth-century doctor Al-Razi had viewed smallpox as a normal childhood condition, a particularly dangerous stage of growth, it had become more virulent in fifteenth- and sixteenth-century Europe (Clendening 1942)—why the change? By the eighteenth century, it had accounted for 10–15 per cent of the deaths. It was then widely recognized as a contagious disease of childhood. Many parents intentionally exposed their young children to it: Sooner or later, one would be exposed, and the older child who died from it was a multi-year investment lost; the younger one who survived was subsequently immune.

Small pox induction had arisen in many parts of the world. Independently of medical statistics, it was recognized that some means of inducing the disease made it significantly less virulent. Mortality rates of 25 per cent or more might drop to a few per cent. Notwithstanding assertions that such practice defied providence, and its inherently counter-intuitive character, such logic and experience had much to do with the relatively rapid acceptance of inoculation after 1721, when it was introduced into Western Europe by Lady Mary Wortley Montagu, a well-connected aristocrat who had observed the process in Turkey. It was first taken up in the British Isles; its subsequent spread depended on the patronage of royalty and nobility, on increases in the safety of the procedure, especially when carried out by the most highly skilled practitioners, and the acquiescence of at least a segment of the medical profession (Hopkins 2002; Miller 1957; Razzell 1977).

In 1798, the English practitioner Edward Jenner made immunization significantly safer by introducing the practice of vaccination with cowpox. Increasingly, smallpox prevention, hitherto a personal matter, became a state concern. Presumably, the institutions that orchestrated quarantines could also ensure universal vaccination. But here too there was ambiguity: In whose interests were vaccination programmes to be undertaken? England began offering free vaccination in 1840, made it compulsory in 1853, and instituted fines for non-compliance in 1873. The initial assumption that all would take advantage of this free medical service proved unfounded; as the authorities sought to give the vaccination laws more teeth, they encountered growing opposition and decreasing rates of compliance.

In 1898, anti-vaccinationists gained permission for conscientious objectors to forgo having their children vaccinated. The opposition was able to show that the dangerous procedure was not carried out everywhere with sufficient skill or care, and a real decline in smallpox meant decreasing risk to the unvaccinated. But mandatory vaccination also exposed underlying tension between the state and the public: In an atmosphere of distrust of the state, the more insistent the state became, the more convinced the public became that the state's actions were not in their interests (Baldwin 1999; Brunton, in press; Durbach 2005; Porter & Porter 1988). Yet anti-vaccination movements were sporadic and often isolated: Certainly, lack of opposition did not necessarily signify trust in the state?

It is important to emphasize that for most of the history of the West, efforts to combat epidemic disease had not reflected any sense of obligation to the health of individuals. At stake was the military, commercial, and cultural welfare of the state, and often, the protection of élites: The welfare of individual subjects (a better term than 'citizens' for much of the period) was incidental. Although states devoted substantial resources to enforcing quarantines and other health regulations (and absorbed considerable costs in lost commerce), it would be misleading to think of them acting in some quasi-contractual way as agents for groups of individuals who had recognized that public actions were necessary to secure their own health. Although many places had town or parish doctors, and there was often an expectation that the state take steps to protect the welfare of its subjects (such as making food affordable in times of dearth), early modern political theorists recognized no obligation of the state to protect the health of individuals. What was at risk in an epidemic was the state itself: The collection of taxes, the maintenance of defence, the continuance of commerce, and even the orderly transfer of property at a time of high mortality.

Perhaps, nowhere was the tension between individual and state so great as in the combating of what was called 'continued fever'. Typhus, typhoid, relapsing fever, and yellow fever were among the several epidemic diseases that appeared or became increasingly prominent in the aftermath of the Black Death. This continued fever (malaria was generally distinguished as 'remittent' or 'intermittent' fever) was endemic as well as epidemic, and amidst vast disagreement about classification and cause, there was general agreement about its frequent association with social catastrophe and squalor—with war, jails, pestilence, famine, and overcrowded slums (Geary 1995; Hamlin 1998, 2006; Smith 1981; Wilson 1978). Although it was often associated with class, it did not limit itself to the poor. Many theorists believed the fever could spread from poor to rich, whether by person-to-person contact or by diffusion through some environmental medium from hovels and slums to mansions. But, as would later be the case with tuberculous diseases, it was not clear whether one could disentangle any single factor from the many conditions of poverty, nor did medical men necessarily think it made sense to try.

The public action that might have been taken was the comprehensive improvement of living conditions—the prevention of overcrowded dwellings; the insurance of sufficient food, fuel, and clothing; the provision of personal and environmental cleanliness, a safe work place, and a non-exhausting work day—in short, all the physical and social changes that would produce a sound human being. Yet, such far-reaching actions to defend the state also threatened to transform it, and in essential ways—in its social distinctions, its institutions of property, even in the political rights it recognized. When the young Prussian radical doctors Rudolph Virchow and Sebastian Neumann investigated a typhus outbreak in Silesia in 1848, they argued that liberal political and economic reforms were the antidote to the squalor which caused the epidemic (Rosen 1947). Irish physicians made similar diagnoses in the pre-famine years—perhaps a little more on the Irish contribution because it is not as well-known as Virchow *et al.*

The public health of communal life: Police

Beyond the response to epidemic outbreaks of specific diseases, Western societies had from early times taken steps to regulate their communities for the common good or the public peace. By the eighteenth century, the term generally used for such efforts was 'police', but the control of crime was only a small part of it. It generally referred to matters of internal public order; that is, to all aspects of government other than military and diplomatic affairs, the raising of funds, import and export duties, matters of land tenure, and civil litigation. Common police functions included:

- The enforcement of basic rules of public behaviour
- The enforcement of standards of building construction and use, with regard to noxious trades and basic sanitation
- The care for the poor, the disabled, and for abandoned children or orphans
- The regulation of hours and modes of work
- The conduct of markets and the quality of the commodities sold in them
- The regulation of marriage and midwifery
- The supply of water to people and the treatment of cattle and other animals
- The inspection and regulation of transients and prostitutes
- The appropriate disposal of the dead, both human and animal
- The prevention of fire and injury
- The investigation of accidental deaths and other forensic matters
- The maintenance of population statistics
- The regulation of medical practice

Sometimes, town or public doctors were involved in this enforcement, and some of these matters—such forensic diagnosis—were overtly medical, at least as often doctors were part of the domain to be regulated.

The issues under the heading of police constituted problems at various levels: For individuals as town dwellers, or adjoining property owners within a neighbourhood, for towns as corporate entities, and for regional or national states. Public health, in the sense of a recognized obligation to protect the health of the people through public regulation, was only rarely the rationale for police, although improvement in the public's health was likely often a consequence of police action. Some matters of police represented public means for the resolution of disputes between individuals as property owners, such as those that arose when the drainage, smoke, or dung of one person's premises encroached on another's.

At a municipal level, a widespread concern with the policing of commerce and manufacture reflected the town's dependence on its markets. The privileges of trade and industry within a town were rarely free; the concern with the quality of foods and drugs was less a matter of consumers' health than of fair competition, consumer satisfaction, and maintenance of the market's good reputation. And it was in the interest of guilds, such as the medical guilds, to keep out outsiders—the regulation of medical practice was in the self-interest of established practitioners, even if done under the auspices of maintaining the quality of public medical care. Finally, at the state level, concern with midwifery, nutrition, or demographic statistics did not necessarily reflect concern with individuals' health. Early modern statecraft equated state strength with population. In the crudest forms of that equation that population was understood as cannon fodder.

The character of institutions of police varied considerably, although most medieval (and ancient) European towns had some kind of institution(s) to carry out the tasks listed earlier (Hope & Marshall 2000). Typically, these mirrored the political structure of the state. In medieval Islamic towns, a *muhtasib*, an appointee of the caliph (or in early modern Spain, a *mutasaf*) oversaw public morals and commerce, but also regulated medical and veterinary practice, refuse disposal, water supply, the cleansing of the public baths, and the licensing of prostitutes (Karmi 1981; López-Piñero 1981; Palmer 1981). In England, where the state was weak and towns strong, police institutions were more community-based; this bottom-up character of dispute resolution would evolve into common law. Among medieval English institutions of local government were the *leet* juries (groups of citizens who biannually perambulated through the town and 'presented' the nuisances they found to the magistrates, who would order abatement), and the courts of sewers, which acted similarly in trying to resolve conflicts about drainage. Whenever a landowner altered drainage patterns, others were affected, often deleteriously. The sewers court was a means of minimizing those adverse effects and compensating for the damage when they were unavoidable. In a similar way, London's Assize of Nuisances managed disputes between neighbours about the location and cleansing of privies (Chew & Kellaway 1973; Leongard 1989; Novak 1996; Redlich & Hirst 1970; Webb & Webb 1922).

The concept of 'nuisance', if not the term, underlay much of the work of public police. In the Anglo-French tradition, a 'nuisance' was an accusation, subsequently backed by a legal determination, that actions on one person's property or in the public domain annoyed and/or interfered with the enjoyment of another's rights (Novak 1996; Blackstone 1892; Hamlin 2002). Common forms of 'nuisance' included conditions offensive to health and sensibility, such as concentrations of pig manure or butchers' waste, as well as antisocial forms of behaviour.

It is clear that the business of the public police did affect health in many ways and also that it covered much of what would later belong to the domain of public health. The priority, however, was usually with amenity, morality, and conflict resolution. However, although the motives and contexts of police initiatives were broader than public health matters, there were overlaps in both practice and theory. The police institutions in late medieval Italian city-states evolved from means of plague response (Carmichael 1986), and almost always, a poorly administered town was looked upon as ripe for an epidemic. Moreover, within Hippocratic and Galenic frameworks, amenity was not clearly distinct from health: To feel well was to be well; unpleasant sights or smells, noises or incidents, even if they led to nothing we would recognize as disease, constituted both a form of trespass and an assault on health (Carlin 2005). Concepts of specific diseases and vectors were far in the future. Notwithstanding the occasional speculation, such as that of the sixteenth-century Italian doctor Girolamo Fracastoro that each disease might be the product of an invisible living seed, most medical men were not thinking about individual diseases in a way that would encourage them to look for discrete distinguishing causes. Because amenity, order, and health were so closely linked, a medical rationale could provide a basis for social action on behalf of a community.

Too little is known about the operation of these police institutions. What is known suggests that their performance varied enormously. It also suggests that the popular image of the pre-modern town as filthy and ungoverned is misleading. There may well have been filth on the streets, but clearly in some cases it was put there at prescribed hours prior to the rounds of the municipal street sweepers, who would collect it for manure or otherwise dispose of it. Many urban cottage industries—dyeing, soap making, the treating of leather or textiles—did use unpleasant animal products; complaints about them often reflect the struggle between classes for control of the urban environment, with wealthy merchants or professionals appealing to supposedly universal standards of sensibility and health to enhance their status over those who worked in what Guillerme calls the fermentation industries (Guillerme 1988; Kearns 1988).

Two examples of the ongoing legacy of such institutions of police can be seen in the regulation of the food supply and the evolution of the concept of 'nuisances' in Anglo-American public health. The fight for pure food and drugs that developed in the later nineteenth century is often seen as an early manifestation of consumerism, and equally, the product of advances in chemistry, microscopy, and bacteriology as applied to foods. Currently, regulation of the food supply is one of the most common duties of public health departments—efficient inspection of meat- and milk-processing plants and institutional kitchens is seen as an essential component of a civilized society. There were changes in the late nineteenth century in the recognition of a wider range of food contaminants, and due to the need to grapple with a more ingenious group of food adulterers, whose doings were better hidden by an increasingly complicated system of food production and distribution.

But, the concerns of consumers with food safety and their view that food inspection was a duty of government was old and widely shared. The concern of many medieval food inspection officers was with honest weights and measures, but quality was always implicit—the just measure did not satisfy if the ale was diluted. Although there might not have always been objective ways of determining food quality, consumers knew and enforced a moral economy on transgressing vendors: The records of civil discord are packed with the trashing of shops and the thrashing of vendors (Thompson 1971).

Traditions of market regulation affected public health more broadly. Concern about water quality in metropolitan London, for example, reflected consumer outrage at high prices and poor quality and quantity of the water well before there was any epidemiological evidence of it causing cholera. Equally, public willingness to accept that epidemiological evidence was tied to anger at paying too much for an irregular and visibly dirty water supply

(Hamlin 1990; Taylor & Trentmann 2005). It is also likely, although difficult to show, that the ready acceptance of the new scientific forms of food inspection in the late nineteenth century reflected consumer expectations that the service was necessary and appropriate for government to undertake (Waddington 2006).

In the case of environmental nuisances too, institutions of public health took over from long-standing institutions for settling civil disputes. Whereas in earlier centuries the concept had been very broad—including excessive noise, disturbances of the peace, the blocking of customary light—by the mid-nineteenth century, the quintessential nuisance had become urban dung, human and animal, and action against nuisances acquired a basis in statute law that supplemented its status in civil law. Beginning with the first English Nuisances Removal Act of 1847, passed in an expectation of the return of cholera, doctors, and later a new functionary called an inspector of nuisances (later a sanitary inspector), were charged with identifying nuisances and taking steps to have them removed (Hamlin 2005; Wilson 1881). The change from civil to criminal law reflects a recognition that a legal tradition built upon the power of property was ill-suited to a situation in which most property was not occupied by its owners, and which depended upon an outrage to sensibility was ill-suited to a situation in which most peoples' sensibilities were insufficiently attuned to the particular states of environment presumed to be associated with cholera.

Although this change was an emergency response, its effects were more far reaching. It represented the investing of community standards for health in a permanent institution with enforcement powers, rather than leaving them to be worked out incident-by-incident, through common law.

The inspectors of nuisances did not restrict themselves to documented causes of disease, but continued to respond to community complaints, which sometimes were primarily aesthetic. They became the defenders of the ever-rising standards of middle-class life, and however far their activities might stray from any direct relation to disease control, they carried with them the authority of public health imperative (Hamlin 1988, 2005; Kearns 1991).

Towards the end of the nineteenth century, some epidemiologists, recognizing that the tracing of cases and contacts informed by the new science of bacteriology provided a more exact means of disease control, suggested that concern with general environmental quality was an unjustified expense that deflected the attention of public health departments from what really mattered (Cassedy 1962; Rosenkrantz 1974). In some cases, they were effective in severing sanitation and public works from public health, but often they found that the public, who tended to support clean streets and pleasant neighbourhoods, continued (and continues) to appeal to public health as justification for their concern. More common than the wholesale replacement of sanitation by bacteriology was the emergence of what has been called a 'sanitary–bacteriological synthesis' (Barnes 2006). Here too, scientific medicine, however distantly it might be linked to the environmental condition under scrutiny, gave public action a legitimacy that would otherwise have been difficult to create.

The medicalization of public police that these examples suggest was clearly underway by the mid-eighteenth century. The concept of medical police first arose in Germany and Austria, later in Scotland, Scandinavia, Italy, and Spain; in France the rough equivalent was *hygiene publique*. In America and in England, the term and concept never really caught on (Carroll 2002). Medicine's rise to prominence reflected an alliance between medical practitioners who sought state patronage and the 'enlightened despots'—rulers who, such as Austria's Joseph II, sought a science of good government that would significantly strengthen their states. Increasingly, rulers like Joseph felt obliged to test their policies against some tenets of rationality; health seemed to offer a well-defined arena of rational government, a set of means to improve the state and to measure the progress of that improvement (Rosen 1974a,b). How much the regulation of personal behaviour could improve the health of soldiers and sailors was becoming recognized; why not practice the same techniques on the rest of society? The effect of this medicalization was to move matters of police further from the realm of local social relations and towards an all-encompassing scientific rationality.

The classic text of eighteenth-century medical police is Johann Peter Frank's six volume *System einer Vollständingen Medicinischen Polizey*, or *A System of Complete Medical Police*, which appeared between 1779 and 1819 (Frank 1976). Frank (1745–1821) had a distinguished career as a medical professor and a public health and hospital administrator, mainly in Vienna. He began his giant work with a discussion of reproductive health (two volumes), including suggestions for the regulation (and encouragement) of marriage, prenatal care, obstetrical matters, and infant feeding and care. He turned then to diet, personal habits, public amusements, and healthy buildings. The fourth volume covered public safety, which involved everything from accident prevention to the injuries supposedly inflicted by witches, the fifth volume dealt with safe means of interment, and the sixth with the regulation of the medical profession. In Frank's cameralist view, anything that adversely affected health was a matter for public policy and an appropriate subject for regulation—rights, traditions, property, and freedom had no status if they interfered with the welfare of the population.

In its most far-reaching definitions, modern public health approaches the domain of a comprehensive police. It also recognizes that a wide range of factors are implicated in health conditions—current public health concerns include the effects of violent entertainment, the prevention of gun violence, and the conditions of the work place. But in modern liberal democracies, much of what Frank saw as the obvious business of the state is deeply problematic. For, in the nineteenth century, public health shifted radically in mission and constituency. It became less a means of maintaining the state, and more a means by which the state served its sovereign citizens with an (increasing) standard of health that they (increasingly) took as a right of citizenship.

The public health of human potential

We often think that health is a service that governments owe their citizens, that what separates past from present is not intent but simply sufficient knowledge of the means to provide that service—this is not so. A public health that is not merely reactive or regulative but which takes as its goal the reduction of rates of preventable mortality and morbidity, and sees this as its duty to its populace, is a product of the eighteenth century. It is also one of the most remarkable changes of sensibility in human history. Its causes are complex but poorly understood; it clearly did require the development both of knowledge of the problem and of the means to solve it. The concepts of preventable mortality and excess morbidity required being able to show that both death and illness existed at much higher rates in some places than in others.

Although there were a few attempts in seventeenth and eighteenth century Europe to determine local bills of mortality, they were too few to provide a basis for comparison. In contrast, by the late nineteenth century, annual mortality rates were an important focus of competition among English towns. The central government's public health officials, notably John Simon, chief medical officer of the Privy Council from 1857 to 1874, badgered towns with poor showings. Simon and his successors urged them to analyse the reasons for their excess mortality and to take appropriate action (Brand 1965; Eyler 1979; Lambert 1965; Wohl 1983). By the end of the century, and during the twentieth century, reliable morbidity statistics were available to provide a better understanding of the remediable causes of disease. The gathering of such data, and after about 1920 their analysis by means of statistical inference, has become a central part of modern public health (Desrosières 1998; Magnello 2002).

The mission of prevention was also tied to a very real growth in knowledge of the means of prevention. The widespread adoption of inoculation, and after 1800, of vaccination for smallpox was the first clearly effective means to intervene decisively to prevent a deadly disease. Initially through the development of the numerical method and the cultivation of pathological anatomy in the Parisian hospitals in the first decades of the nineteenth century, and subsequently through bacteriological and later serological methods, infectious diseases were distinguished and their discrete causes and vectors identified (Ackerknecht 1967; Bynum 1994). Such recognition ultimately led not only to the 'magic bullet' thinking of vaccine development, but also underwrote campaigns to improve water quality and provide other means of sanitation, and sometimes, as with tuberculosis and typhoid, programmes to identify, monitor, and regulate carriers.

Yet these factors alone cannot account for the widespread conviction that human health could, and must be, significantly improved—they are means, not ends. Whatever the symbolic significance of effective action against smallpox in boosting confidence, vaccination successes did not imply that all infectious diseases were amenable to a similar strategy. In most cases, the new medical knowledge did not precede the determination to improve the health of all but was developed in the process of achieving that goal. A great deal of success was achieved despite quite erroneous conceptions of the nature of the diseases and their causes. The great sanitary campaign against urban filth (based on a vague and flexible concept of pathogenic miasms) is the best-known example (Barnes 2006).

Recognition of differential mortality was not new in the early 1800s, but it did not necessarily convey a need for action. That there was a mortality penalty associated with poverty, infancy, and urban living was clear; but some regarded the town as a necessary corrective to the overfecundity of the countryside, and characterized the poor peasant as occupying a fixed station in life, one whose chief attributes were higher mortality than the virtuous middle classes (though not necessarily than the profligate aristocracy) as well as compensating benefits, such as lowered anxiety (Sadler 1830; Weyland 1968). And even humane and optimistic writers saw infant mortality rates of 25 per cent or more as providential (Roberton 1827). To the influential eighteenth-century Lutheran clergyman Christoph Christian Sturm, God's providence was evident in the symmetry of the curve of mortality by age: Mortality rates were high among the very young and very old, and low in between (Strum 1832).

This is in contrast with the modern sensibility which admits no justifiable reason (beyond, perhaps, the climatic factors that determine the range of some disease vectors) for differential mortality or morbidity. These changes in sensibilities towards state provision can be divided into three periods: An age of liberalism from 1790 to 1880; a golden age of public health to 1970; and a more confusing post-modern period in the last four decades, which may, at least in its most positive aspects, be seen as a return to liberalism.

The age of liberalism: Health in the name of the people, 1790–1880

The social and intellectual movement known as liberalism, which began to prevail in the second half of the eighteenth century, included a wide range of philosophical, political, economic, and religious ideas, but at its heart were notions of individual freedom and responsibility, and usually, of equality in some form. In 1890, when John Simon, England's first chief medical officer and a pioneer of state medicine, surveyed progress in public health during the past two centuries in his *English Sanitary Institutions*, he included a lengthy chapter on the 'New Humanity'. In it, he covered the antislavery movement, the rise of Methodism, growing concern about cruelty to criminals and animals, legislation promoting religious freedom, the replacement of patronage by principle as the motor of parliamentary democracy, the introduction of free markets, the rationalization of criminal and civil law, and efforts towards international peace. Simon saw little need to explain how this concerned public health; he was sketching a fundamental change in 'feeling' that underlay changes in public health policy.

> *Society had become readier than before to hear individual voices which told of pain or asked for redress of wrong; abler . . . to admit that justice does not weight her balances in relation to the ranks, creeds, colours, or nationalities of men.*

No longer were humans so much cannon fodder; the best policies were those which maximized 'human worth and welfare' (Simon 1890; compare with Pettenkofer 1941; Coleman 1974; Haskell 1985).

What Simon recognized was that with the granting of equal political and economic rights and responsibilities, it had become impossible to see health status as appropriately constrained by class, race, or sex. Nineteenth-century French and English liberals recognized that some—particularly women, children, and the poor—still suffered ill health disproportionately, but they saw such consequences as incidental, accidental, and increasingly, as unnecessary and objectionable: In principle, all had an equal claim to whatever version of human and health rights a society was prepared to recognize. As Simon also recognized, this change in feeling was both the cause and effect of the widening distribution of political power.

And yet liberalism was no clear and compact doctrine, and its implications for public health were, and still are, by no means clear. Few of the pioneers of liberal political theory bothered to translate human rights into terms of health. They wrote mainly with middle-class men in mind, and saw the threats to life, liberty, and property as political rather than biosocial. The expansion (or translation) of political rights into rights to health was gradual, piecemeal (it has never been the rallying cry of revolution), complicated, and even fundamentally conflictual—it was, and is, not always the case that the choices free individuals make will protect the public's health, or even their own. Concern with public health arose accidentally, and in different ways and at different times in the developed nations. At the beginning of the twenty-first century, an obligation to maintain and/or improve the health of all citizens exists only in varying degrees.

Many early liberals found health rights hard to recognize because so much of public health had been closely associated with the medical police functions of an overbearing state. In revolutionary France, the first instinct was to free the market in medical practice by abolishing medical licensing, a policy quickly recognized as disastrous for maintaining the armies of citizen–soldiers who were protecting the nation (Foucault 1975; Riley 1987; Weiner 1993; Brockliss & Jones 1997). Even after new, meritocratic, and science-based medical institutions had been established, the cadre of public health researchers that it fostered—at the time, the world's leaders in epidemiology is this France?—found it difficult to conceive how their findings of the preventable causes of disease could be translated into proposals for preventive legislation. Poverty, and to some degree, working and living conditions were dictated by the market; government mandates would induce dependence or simply shift the problem elsewhere. Thus, France was the scientific leader in public health for the first half of the nineteenth century without finding a viable political formula for translating that knowledge into prevention (LaBerge 1992; Coleman 1982).

In early-nineteenth-century Britain, the ideas of T.R. Malthus led a broad range of learned public opinion, both liberal and conservative, to similar conclusions. Disease was among the natural checks that kept population within the margins of survival. Successful prevention of disease would be temporary only; it would postpone an inevitable equilibration of the food–population balance that would occur through some other form of human catastrophe (Hamlin 1998; Dean 1991). Malthusian sentiment blocked attempts to establish foundling hospitals. Notwithstanding the fact that such institutions were notoriously deadly to their inmates, it was felt that their existence encouraged irresponsible procreation—faced with full economic responsibility for their actions, men (or women, depending on how one viewed the prevailing legal arrangements for child support) would stifle their urges (McClure 1981). Malthusian views were prominent in British policy with regard to Ireland, Scotland, and India.

By 1850, in both France and England, it was no longer possible to maintain what for many was a complacent and convenient faith in the welfare-maximizing actions of a completely free society. A number of factors shattered this faith. First, no government ever adopted the programme of the early nineteenth-century liberals in full. In Central, Eastern, and Southern Europe, the old concerns of state security continued to govern their public health. In Sweden and later France, concern about a state was weakened by depopulation-fostered attention to the health and welfare of individuals.

Second, working-class parties, although often generally sympathetic with political liberalism, saw no advantage in economic liberalism. Often, they demanded adherence to the moral economy of the old order, in which governments damped fluctuations in grain prices and enforced the working conditions that craft guilds had established. Most important is that many liberals themselves arrived at what is properly called a biosocial vision, a concept of society which recognized that it was impractical, inhumane, and injudicious to impose economic and political responsibilities on people who were biologically incapable of meeting those responsibilities: Liberty had biological prerequisites.

These considerations were central to debates in France and Britain in the 1830s and 1840s. Governments in both countries were apprehensive of revolution and wary of an alienated underclass, urban and rural, of people who could not be trusted with political rights and seemed immune to the incentives of the market. Such people represented a reservoir of disease, both literal physical disease and metaphorical social disease, that could infect those clinging precariously to the lower rungs of respectability. Reformers proposed to somehow transform these dangerous classes, usually with Bibles, schools, or experimental colonies. Such was the political background against which Edwin Chadwick (1800–1884), secretary of the English bureau charged with overseeing the administration of local poor relief, developed 'the sanitary idea' in the late 1830s (Finer 1952; Hamlin 1998; Lewis 1952; Richards 1980; Chadwick 1965).

Chadwick justified public investment in comprehensive systems of water and sewerage on the grounds that saving lives—particularly of male breadwinners—would be recompensed in lowered costs for the support of widows and orphans. But he also suggested that sanitation would remoralize the underclass, and for many supporters, this was its most important feature. Politically, sanitation was a brilliant idea, as every other general reform was deeply controversial: Proposals for religion and education were plagued by sectarianism, calls to improve welfare by allowing free trade in grain (leading to lower food prices) ran afoul of powerful agricultural interests, proposals for regulating working conditions were unacceptable to powerful industrial interests. Notwithstanding complaints that towns should be allowed to reform in their own ways and their own good time rather than being forced to adopt Chadwick's technologies and deadlines, sanitation achieved remarkable popularity in nineteenth-century Britain. It was the locus of hope not just for improved health, but in general, for a prettier, happier, and better world.

In treating insanitation as the universal cause of disease, Chadwick hoped to establish a public health that was truly liberal. He sought to deflect attention from other causes of disease, such as malnutrition and overwork, for these were areas of great potential conflict between public health and liberal policy. For many, the liberty of the free (or more properly in the case of women, the unmarried) adult to bargain in the market for labour without state intervention to limit hours or kinds of work was axiomatic. And the need for food was to be the spur for work and self-improvement. Interventions by what has recently been called a 'nanny state' seemed to imply an obligation to the state and to affirm the desirability of dependence and subjugation. There were grounds for such concern: The relations of political status to health were fraught with ambiguity. Frank had written passionately of misery as a cause of disease amongst the serfs of Austrian Italy, but had not advocated the elimination of serfdom. Virchow argued, in 1848, that liberal political rights were the answer to typhus in Silesia, and in Scotland, WP Alison argued on the contrary that too rigorous a liberal regime was the cause of poverty-induced typhus (Frank 1941; Rosen 1947; Weindling 1984; Hamlin 2006).

For about a generation, from 1850 to 1880, sanitation was unchallenged in Britain (and in much of its empire) as the keystone of improved health. Chadwick's campaigns led to a series of legislative acts—beginning with the Public Health Act of 1848 and culminating with a comprehensive act in 1875—that established state standards for urban sanitation and a bureau of state medicine, staffed by medical officers in central and local units of government and charged with detecting, responding to, and preventing outbreaks of disease (Wohl 1983).

Outside Britain, although the ideals of sanitation might have had similar appeal, they did not warrant the same conclusions about state responsibility or sanitary technology. The English paradigm of a water-centred sanitary system was adopted only in the twentieth century (Simson 1978; Göckjan 1985; Goubert 1989; Labisch 1992; Münch 1993; Ramsey 1994; Melosi 2000; Hennock 2000). Often, the heritage of medical police was more prominent than that of sanitary engineering. Networks of local medical officers to control contagious disease transmission through the regulation of travel and prostitution were important.

Through the 1880s, the United States remained an exceptional case, coming closest to following a policy that an individual's health was a private matter alone. The national government maintained a system of marine hospitals along the coasts and navigable rivers, less for controlling the spread of epidemics than for relieving ports of the burden of caring for sick seamen. In the early 1880s, it established a National Board of Health to advance knowledge on public health issues of common import, but despite a superb research performance, the Board was scrapped within a few years on the grounds that public health was the business of individual states and cities (Duffy 1990).

Often dominated by rural interests, many state legislatures had little enthusiasm for public health. Louisiana, which established a state board of health to combat yellow fever, was an exception (Ellis 1992). Towns and cities were more active, but often only sporadically, taking steps when faced with epidemics. States that did establish boards of health usually focused on specific problems rather than on public health in general: In Massachusetts, the allotment of pure water resources was a key issue; elsewhere, it was food quality, care for the insane, vital statistics, or the threat of immigrants (Rosenkrantz 1972; Shattuck 1972; Kraut 1994). In Michigan, concern about kerosene quality (it was being adulterated with volatile and explosive petroleum fractions) and arsenical wallpaper dyes spurred the establishment of a state board of health in 1873 (Duffy 1990).

1880–1970: The golden age of public health?

By the 1880s, the classic liberalism of the first half of the nineteenth century was giving way to a resurgent statism. The European nations, the United States, and later, Japan competed for colonies and international influence. If the newly liberated or the newly enfranchised had some claim to a right to health, they also had a duty to the state to be healthy. In most of the industrialized nations, there was renewed interest in monitoring social conditions.

Although the emerging techniques of empirical social research gave this inquiry the aura of quantitative precision, the surveys disclosed little that was distinctly new about the lives or health of the mysterious poor, the usual targets of public health and social reform. Much of it seemed new, however, because it now registered as problematic (Turner 2001). For example, the enormous contribution of infant deaths to total mortality had long been clear, but only towards the end of the century did infant mortality, persistently high even in relatively well-sanitized Britain, become a problem in itself as distinct from an indicator of sanitary conditions in general. The health conditions of women too, and of workers, began to command attention in a way that they had not done previously (Sellars 1997).

Although these newly recognized public health problems partly reflected the changing distribution of political power, they also reflected anxiety about the nation's vulnerability, and even the decadence of its population. Worried about the strengths of their armies, states such as Britain discovered in the 1890s that too few of those they would call up were competent to be mobilized, and they attributed the problem to a vast range of causes: Poor nutrition (coupled with lack of sunlight in smoky cities), bad sanitation, bad mothering, and bad heredity (Soloway 1982; Pick 1989; Porter 1991a, 1999; Stradling & Thorsheim 1999). Epidemics of smallpox following the Franco-Prussian War of 1870 and again in the 1890s disclosed the gaps in vaccination programmes (Baldwin 1999; Brunton in press). The usual response was to redouble the state's efforts to take responsibility for the immune status of its population. The persistence of syphilis registered at a new level of unacceptability (Brandt 1985; Baldwin 1999).

This led to an expanded public health, one highly successful in terms of reduced mortality and morbidity. It was undertaken jointly in the name of the state and the people, but it involved the regulation of an individual's life—home, work, family relations, recreation, sex—that went beyond the medical police of the previous century. From a later standpoint, such intimate regulation of the individual by the state may seem overbearing, but, with some notable exceptions, the populations of developed countries accepted it as an appropriate and even desirable role for the state.

New diseases, or old diseases that were (or seemed) more prevalent or virulent, new institutions for the practice of public health medicine, and advances in medical and social science contributed to this new relation between states and people. During the 1860s, a long-standing analogy of disease with fermentation matured into the germ theory of disease as the research of Louis Pasteur and John Tyndall made clear the dependence of fermentation on some microscopic living ferment (Pelling 1978; Worboys 2000).

During the 1880s, primarily through the work of emerging German and French schools of determinative bacteriologists, it became possible to distinguish many microbe species from one another, to ascertain the presence of particular species with some degree of confidence, and therefore, to link individual species with particular diseases (Bulloch 1938). Through serological tests developed in the succeeding decades, the presence of a prior infection could be determined, regardless of whether anyone had noticed symptoms.

Notwithstanding the increasing recognition of the many ways by which microbial agents of disease were transmitted from person to person, the effect of the rise of the germ theory was to focus attention on the body that housed and reproduced the germ—for example, the well-digger working through a mild case of typhoid—even when there were alternative strategies (water filtration or, by the second decade of the twentieth century, chlorination) that protected the public reasonably well most of the time (Hamlin 1990; Melosi 2000). The general interest in the human as germ-bearer and culture medium brought with it an emphasis on the labour-intensive business of case-tracing, of keeping track not only of those who showed symptoms of the disease but also those with whom they had contact.

In the key diseases of typhoid fever, syphilis, and tuberculosis, concern with the inspection and regulation of people was exacerbated by the recognition that not all who were infected were symptomatic. The case of 'Typhoid Mary' Mallon, the asymptomatic typhoid carrier who lived for 26 years as an island-bound 'guest' of the City of New York, is notorious, but it was also important in the working out of both legal limits and cultural sensibilities with regard to the trade-off between civil rights and public health (Leavitt 1996). Newly virulent forms of diphtheria and scarlet fever, deadly childhood diseases transmitted person to person or by common domestic media, also gave immediacy to decisive public health intervention.

Such monitoring could not have occurred without a large rank and file of local public health officers. It was during the late nineteenth century that public health was identified as a distinct division of medicine and when most of the developed countries solidified a reasonably complete network of municipal and regional public health officers: In Germany, the *Kreisartz*; in France, the *Officier de Santé*; and in Britain, the Medical Officer of Health, assisted by the sanitary inspector. Increasingly, these officers worked as part of hierarchical national health establishments to which they reported local health conditions and from which they received expert guidance.

Whereas preceding generations of public doctors had often been drawn from the ranks of undercapitalized young doctors, beginning in the mid-1870s, many were specially trained and certified for public health work (Novak 1973; Watkin 1984; Acheson 1991; Porter 1991b). A commitment to public health was increasingly incompatible with ordinary medical practice, not wholly because of its specialized knowledge, but because it was built upon a quite different ethic. There had long been economic tension between public and private medicine in areas of practice such as vaccination, in which public authorities either took over entirely or inadequately compensated private practitioners for services that had traditionally been part of the ordinary medical marketplace (Brunton, in press; White 1991).

But monitoring healthy carriers and those who might be susceptible to disease introduced a new regime of medicine—one which responded to an ethic of public good, even if there were no client-defined complaints. Effectively, bacteriology, epidemiology, and associated measures of immunological status redefined disease away from the patient complaint. The healthy carrier might see no need to seek medical care, but to the public health doctor that person was a social problem. On occasion, private doctors were appealed to for a diagnosis (bronchitis, pneumonia) that would protect one from the health officer's diagnosis of tuberculosis, which would bring loss of employment and social stigma (Smith 1988).

Rivalling the germ theory as the major motif of public health thinking from the 1890s to the 1950s was the application of the emerging science of heredity to the improvement of human populations—the science and practice of eugenics (Paul 1995; Kevles 1995). Whether or not eugenic concerns were the source of the greatest anxiety about the public's health is debatable, but they were the locus of the greatest hope for health progress, the home of a residue of utopianism that had coloured the medical police and sanitary literature. Even more than other forms of public health, eugenics exposed a class, and sometimes a racial, division that had long been a part of public health: Much public health practice was predicated on a distinction between those, usually the poor, who were seen as the objects of public health efforts and those, often the well-to-do, who authorized intervention, whether to improve the lot of the poor, to protect 'society', or perhaps even to block the physical or moral contagia that might infect their own class (Kraut 1994; Anderson 1995; Bashford & Hooker 2001; Carlin 2005). Eugenics appealed mainly to those with wealth and power: Those others who were to be improved rarely identified heredity as the source of their problems.

Such an attitude is reflected in the most infamous application of the eugenic viewpoint, the attempt by Nazi Germany to exterminate Jews and other 'races' regarded as inferior and unfit not only to intermarry with so-called 'true Aryans', but even to exist. Although historians' views of the origins of the Holocaust differ, some of the immediate precedents for a state policy of negative eugenics—the prevention of the reproduction of those regarded as unfit—came from the sterilization laws that American states had begun to pass in the first decade of the century. The American laws focused on persistent immorality or criminality, and on what was called 'feeble-mindedness'.

In Germany, the acceptance of sterilization translated rather easily into the acceptance of euthanasia of the permanently institutionalized, and on to the extreme measures of the death camps, which were conceived of as facilities of state medicine. Even during the Holocaust, the prevailing rationality remained that of public health: The trade-off between individual rights and the welfare of the state was a part of the working moral world of the public health officer. Just as an excision of corrupt or cancerous matter might be necessarily to maintain the body of the individual, so too an excision of a part of society might be necessary to maintain the health of the nation (Lifton 1986).

The horrors of the extreme version of eugenics practised in Nazi Germany have discredited eugenics to such a degree that it is difficult to recapture how central it seemed to reformers of the left as well as of the far right. It appealed for a number of reasons. First, it explained the failure of prior reforms, particularly sanitation, which was to have effected the thorough physical and moral renewal of the lower classes.

Second, it seemed to be implied by Darwin's discoveries, which were themselves founded on deep familiarity with the remarkable transformations achieved by scientific agriculturalists in animal breeding. Those discoveries seemed particularly applicable within the utilitarian framework of the new statism: The task of governments was to reverse the trend towards decadence and produce uniform, reliable humans. Such concerns became powerful especially for nations that perceived themselves to be in demographic crisis, such as Sweden, which was experiencing depopulation and persistent tuberculosis, and the United States, where successive groups of immigrants found reasons to deplore the effects on the nation of the next immigrant group (Johannisson 1994; Kraut 1994; Broberg & Roll-Hansen 1996).

Finally, it flattered those who held power and prominence by assuring them that this was no accident. It offered a simple explanation, one resistant to empirical falsification, of all that was wrong, and a simple remedy for improvement based on an attractive sociological formula: More sex for those who should breed (sometimes with new partners) and less for those regarded as inferior.

Eugenics sanctioned an enormous range of practices. Although eugenists focused attention on the human genotype and urged the inadequacy of public health programmes that ignored heredity, they were by no means uniformly dismissive of social and environmental reforms. These were needed to allow the better stock to fulfil its potential and because many believed that nurture *could* affect nature: Heredity might be a limiting factor, but significant reforms were needed to fulfil hereditary potential. In almost every country in which eugenics was prominent—the United States, Britain, Japan, Germany, Russia, Brazil, and Argentina—it fitted into a comprehensive concept of social hygiene, albeit one that translated rather easily into racial hygiene (Schneider 1990; Stepan 1991; Porter 1991a; Gallagher 1999).

A third element of this phase of the development of public health was the rise of nutritional science. Although the effects of food on health had broadly been central to Western medicine throughout its history, and it was no mystery that poor food led to poor health, with the exception of the linkage between scurvy and a lack of fresh vegetables, matters of malnutrition and famine had remained outside public health. Remarkably, a science of nutrition that discriminated the particular effects of particular foods only began to take shape in the second half of the nineteenth century, chiefly in the new institutes of agricultural science where animal diets were being studied (Carpenter 1994). Most important was the link of several clinically distinct conditions with a deficit in trace substances in the diet. Particularly remarkable were Goldberger's association of pellagra in the American south with a too heavy reliance on maize, and the recognition of the roles of vitamin D and sunlight in the emergence of rickets. By the 1930s, public health included attention to a varied diet which ensured adequate vitamins (Etheridge 1972; Apple 1996; Marks 2003; Kunitz 2007). Diet, like genes, loomed in the public imagination as the cause of all troubles, and a universal source of hope.

Thus, during this golden age of public health, people in the developed world learned to fear three malign entities: The invisible germs of disease, which might come through the most casual contact; the mysterious genes in their gonads; and the peculiar set of trace nutrients that their food might not contain. Their health and survival depended on all these, yet governments could control them only partially; successful control depended on their behaviour. Hence, a significant role of public health was to educate, advise, and admonish. The citizen, particularly the female citizen, was now being asked to uphold a new standard of cleanliness and to clean things that were not visibly dirty with new kinds of disinfectants. It became important to exercise new prudence in choosing a mate and controlling sexuality. A doctor was required to see whether the baby was being properly fed (Apple 1987; Hoy 1995; Tomes 1998).

Ignorance heightened these hygienic demands. It was clear from tuberculin tests, for example, that exposure to tuberculosis was widespread, in some places nearly universal, but far from clear what was required for exposure to evolve into pulmonary consumption: Whether it was a matter of concentrated exposure, the victim's own constitution, or the diet and environment. All seemed plausible; the advice of public health authorities (who were concerned with infected cases and with their potential for infecting others) involved every aspect of life. It was not simply a matter of not spitting, but of disinfecting eating utensils, clothes, and bedclothes; transforming relations with a spouse, family, and co-workers; and changing diet, leisure activities, and the climate of dwellings (Newsholme 1935; Dubos & Dubos 1987; Smith 1988; Barnes 1995).

Some modern historians have been surprised that these long lists of seemingly exhausting and impossible hygienic expectations, each with no guarantee of health, did not trigger widespread resentment, victim-blaming, and excessive violations of rights (Armstrong 1983). Four factors are important: First, this was an age stunned by scientific and technical achievement and lacking for the most part a critical vocabulary for mediating expert advice. Second, it was an age of mass aspiration to middle-class standards of living, which were manifested in health, behaviour, and cleanliness. Third, all this was taking place against the backdrop of falling mortality and morbidity, and increasing domestic comfort. Fourth, these efforts were redolent with the ethos of progressive development of the community and the state (Lewis 1986).

The return of liberalism, 1970 to the present day: Lifestyle, environment, and welfare

The decades following the Second World War brought a marked shift in the focus of public health and the expectations of the public. In the developed world, the infectious diseases that had so long been the chief focus of public health receded, with polio being the last of the shock epidemics to fall victim to immunizations, antibiotics, or epidemiological or environmental control (Rogers 1990). With the conquest of fascism and the subsequent decline of communism, liberalism re-emerged. This was symbolized in the mission statement of the World Health Organization (WHO) that health and welfare were the birthright of all (WHO 1968). It was the obligation of states to deliver that right to their populations, who now, at least in the developed world, were made up of those who saw themselves as individual free agents, diverse perhaps in culture but equal in rights. In such a situation, the conflict between the imperatives of public health and civil rights re-emerged. It remains the most formidable issue that public health faces.

The retreat of infectious disease made clearer the failure of the developed nations to grapple with chronic diseases, some of which were the price of longer lifespans (Fox 1993). Some of these were clearly conditions that could be prevented by changes in behaviour: Epidemiological studies in the 1950s and 1960s showed the deadly effects of good living—of smoking and a rich diet (Susser 1985; Marks 1997; Porter 1999). A new set of personal disciplines emerged to control lifestyle diseases and prevent accidents—as well as not smoking, avoiding fats, recreational drugs, and alcohol, exercising one's heart and shedding weight, and using condoms (not to mention flossing and straightening one's teeth), one was to use seat belts and child harnesses, cope with childproof caps on medicine bottles, and accept a fluoridated water supply. All these measures met with objections in terms of their intrusion into personal liberty or on culture, or because they were found to be irksome or unpleasant.

Another feature of post-war public health concern was the shift from individual hygiene back to the environment (Hays 1987; Gottlieb 1993). To many, these heart diseases and cancers, along with other diseases and pathological conditions that seemed even more serious—for example, other forms of cancer, birth defects, lowered sperm counts—had broader structural causes and could be prevented only by comprehensive changes in the physical and social environment (Epstein 1979; McNeill 2000). Thus, part of the liberal resistance to public health imposition was the argument that a focus on disciplining lifestyles came at the cost of attention to grander and more serious political issues (Tesh 1987; Turshen 1987; Levins & Lopez 1999).

Although this new environmentalism had links with the nineteenth-century view of public health as environmental improvement, there were greater differences. The fear of insidious invisible radiation or the toxic chemicals that might lurk in numerous consumer products reflects the terror of germs or of the invisible odourless miasmas which germs replaced; however, the blame was quite differently directed. The new problems of environmental public health were those in which individuals were victimized by corporate oligopolies and by the governments they influence.

Although Chadwick and his associates had warned of vested interests, such as those that perpetuated slum housing, nineteenth-century environmental health problems had a communal character that was missing from the twentieth. Everyone in a nineteenth-century town produced excrement, smoke, ash, and rubbish; the great problem was to find within the community the will and means to act collectively (Wohl 1977; Kearns 1988). Few in a twentieth-century community produced radiation or toxic chemical waste, and the reasons why nothing was done about these seemed all too clear. Public health had failed in its police function; an institution that had evolved to stop the selling of spoiled food by the individual grocer or restaurateur could not cope with the conglomerate or the vast industry that sold goods whose harmful effects were less obvious and slower to appear but which might be much more widely distributed.

The result was an increasingly adversarial relationship between the people and the public health institutions that were supposedly safeguarding their health. To the degree that governments were seen as colluding with the proliferation of these dangerous materials, institutions of public health, as departments of government, were implicated too (Steneck 1984; Brown & Mikkelsen 1990; Edelstein 2004). An epidemiology that spoke the language of 'risk factors' could seem a way to dodge the blame (Rothstein 2003). Even the establishment of new departments of environmental protection, although it might be a means to apply new kinds of expertise to problems of environmental health, did not fundamentally alter the climate of distrust. Public health again became a matter for grassroots political agitation with the emergence of neopopulist Green parties, whose platforms gave prominent attention to health as part of environmental good, and who put their marginality to established governments at the centre of their appeal to the electorate. Public participation became an increasingly important concern (Jasanoff 2005). Nor could victims be confident that the government's epidemiologists would even recognize their disease unless a community of sufferers took it upon themselves to agitate for attention (Packard *et al.* 2004).

Such a focus on bad environmental policy even informed the response to AIDS and to other new infectious diseases, such as Ebola fever, that appeared in the 1980s and 1990s. Although it became clear that these diseases could be largely controlled through the traditional means of changes in personal behaviour and isolation or restriction of the activities of victims, these recognitions were not fully reassuring. They did little to deflect demand for a vaccine, or the investment of hope in curative medicine. They too could be seen as environmental diseases, caused by environmental changes that had allowed animal viruses to acquire secondary human hosts for whom they were highly virulent. Chief among these changes was the unwise exploitation of tropical forests by a globalizing oligopoly that put profit ahead of prudence (Garrett 1995).

Even those diseases most closely linked to lifestyle choice could be attributed to the broader social environment. People smoked, drank, used drugs, ate too much or vastly too little, practised unsafe sex, spent hours immobilized before televisions absorbing images of violence, hit their spouses and children, or shot their co-workers or themselves because they could no longer cope. To expect disciplined personal behaviour from alienated people living in a stressful world was unrealistic, and the institutions of public health should recognize this.

But the critics were ambivalent as to what such an analysis implied. For some, the obvious response was to remake a society whose support structures were more consistent with the health behaviours it wished to promote. How absurd, for example, for a state to subsidize the production of tobacco and the addiction to it of people in other nations, while blaming its own citizens for smoking (Brandt 2006). For others, such a response sounded like an even more invidiously intrusive state, bent on removing not only the means by which we satisfied unhealthful temptations, but also the temptations themselves. In this 'critical public health' view, the lifestyle agenda was suspicious. It was the public health agenda of an untrustworthy state, not that its people would have chosen. It was not clear that the personal benefits of delayed or denied gratification were worth it: Perhaps one should just enjoy life and rely on the miracles of modern medicine for redemption (Petersen & Lupton 1996).

This view, together with the emergence of widespread cancers and other chronic illnesses for which there was no clear preventive strategy, including the debilitating conditions of ageing, raised the question of why supportive and curative medical care did not form a part or priority in public health. It also raised the question of how far-reaching were the health obligations of the liberal state to its citizens. This issue had vexed public health practitioners throughout the liberal era, although it had often been suppressed because it was seen as too politically volatile.

In socialist or social democratic politics, or where the legacy of medical police remained strong (even when adopted, as in Sweden, by a democratic polity), there was often no clear boundary between public health and the public medical care most people demanded and received (Porter 1999). But elsewhere, the recognition that public health was bound up in the larger issue of human welfare, which in turn included the rest of medical care, was problematic. Many of the newly prominent diseases were not infectious; they could be experienced privately without disturbing community or state, hence the reactive and police rationales for public health did not apply. But they did disrupt the fulfilment of human potential, exacted great costs on productivity, and hence could justly take their place among the demands citizens could make of their governments.

In France, Germany, and Russia, public health services had emerged from, and had remained closely linked to, medical services for the poor (Labisch 1992; Solomon 1994; Ramsey 1994). In mid-nineteenth-century England, Edwin Chadwick, notwithstanding his own post as chief administrator of relief to the poor and the existence of a comprehensive national network of poor law medical officers, had deliberately severed public health (which he equated with sanitary engineering and saw as exclusively preventive) from medical care for the poor. Such medical care was second-rate, grudgingly made available because it was seen as a constitutional right. Expectations of effectiveness were low, however: It was hoped that the poor quality of public medical relief would spur the poor to pay for something better. While moderating the focus on sanitary engineering, Chadwick's English successors retained a distinction between public health medicine and social welfare, which seemed to them only marginally medical and to have more to do with the moral chastisement of the feckless or the warehousing of the incompetent or neglected (Hamlin 1998).

In Ireland, by contrast, an integrated system of public health, welfare, and medical care did emerge during the late nineteenth century, but more by accident than design (Cassell 1997). At the end of the nineteenth century, the Fabian socialists presented British parliament with a clear choice. The Fabians (mainly Beatrice Webb) proposed a much expanded scheme of prevention, although one which made even greater demands on personal and social behaviour as the price the citizen must pay for greater guarantees from the state. The liberals, whose view prevailed, would not discipline personal hygiene, but offered instead an insurance plan to pay for the medical care needed by stricken working men (Fox 1986; Eyler 1997). It was a policy acceptable to the rank and file of the medical profession and that retained and reinforced the split between public health and medicine.

Subsequent efforts to expand state responsibility for health into matters of care and cure have generally worked when medical professions have seen them as advantageous, yet the relationship between even this expanded public medicine and the broader questions of social welfare remain problematic (Starr 1982; Fox 1986; Levins & Lopez 1999; Epstein 2003). The kinds of objections that were made to Webb's scheme still arise: However laudable prevention as a goal, ironically, as we have seen with the concerns about lifestyles and the environment, the strategies and priorities of the preventive public health of the last two centuries have not always been those most desired by the masses of people. To many it has seemed that if the state was going to discipline behaviour for its own purposes, those who suffered that imposition deserved compensation for their trouble when things still went wrong.

Such logic was clearest in compensating veterans of wars. It underwrote the post-war establishment of Britain's National Health Service, which would provide 'health for heroes' and sustains the Veterans Administration medical system in the United States as it lurches from scandal to reform. Thus, what some have complained of as an unrealistic demand for risk-free living, in which people demand a political right to complete freedom of action without accepting responsibility for the consequences (as if one could somehow live free of one's biological self), may be better understood as a complaint about the fairness of the basic social contract of modern societies.

This problem of the relationship between the institutions of public health and the citizenry on whose behalf they claim to act is the greatest challenge currently facing public health in the developed world. That the problems that confront both public health and regular medical practice often stem from a wide range of social causes is plain. That it is so difficult to develop political will to respond to these problems is not chiefly a matter of epidemiological uncertainty. Such pathological phenomena are clearly the product of many causes on many levels, and accordingly, there are numerous points of access where defensible preventive measures might be taken. But almost all of them are likely to intrude on what are claimed as personal or cultural rights, and almost always attempts to act will be met with the response that it is fairer to act elsewhere. In such cases, epidemiology necessarily requires a large supplement, not from ethics so much as from a moral and political philosophy, that must be acceptable to an increasingly diverse community. Without such a foundation, public health is forced to take refuge in science that is frequently challenged; but simultaneously, it is not clear whether the professional and educational institutions of public health, or the legal, political, and administrative structures that create and maintain it, will be able to initiate and implement a satisfactory enquiry about how these conflicting rights are to be adjudicated.

Key points

- Economic and political progress are subordinate to securing health—they are the means; health is the end.
- Most modern states have distinguished aspects of health that are the business of the public from those that are for the individual to pursue.
- Public health, in the sense of a recognized obligation to protect the health of the people, was only rarely the rationale for policy.
- In the nineteenth century, public health shifted radically in mission and constituency. It became less a means of maintaining the state and more a means by which the state served its citizens.
- A new set of personal disciplines emerged to control lifestyle diseases and prevent accidents.
- Efforts to expand state responsibility for health into matters of care and cure have generally worked when medical professions have seen them as advantageous.

References

Acheson R. The British diploma in public health: birth and adolescence. In: Fee E, Acheson R, editors. *A history of education in public health: health that mocks the doctors rules*. Oxford University Press; 1991. pp. 44–82.

Ackerknecht E. *Medicine at the Paris hospital, 1794–1848*. Baltimore: Johns Hopkins University Press; 1967.

Bynum W.F. *Science and the practice of medicine in the nineteenth century*. Cambridge University Press; 1994.

Amundsen D., Ferngren G. The early Christian tradition. In: Numbers R., Amundusen D., editors. *Caring and curing: health and medicine in the Western religious traditions*. New York (NY): Macmillan; 1986. pp. 40–64.

Anderson W. Excremental colonialism: public health and the poetics of pollution. *Critical Inquiry* 1995;**21**:640–69.

Apple R. *Mothers and medicine: a social history of infant feeding, 1890–1950*. Madison (WI): University of Wisconsin Press; 1987.

Apple R.D. *Vitamania: vitamins in American culture*. New Brunswick (NJ): Rutgers University Press; 1996.

Armstrong D. *The political economy of the body*. Cambridge University Press; 1983.

Arrizabalaga J., Henderson J., French R. *et al. The great pox: the French disease in Renaissance Europe*. New Haven (CT): Yale University Press;1997.

Arrizabalaga J. Syphilis. In: Kiple K, editor. *Cambridge world history of human disease*. Cambridge: Cambridge University Press; 1993. pp. 1025–33.

Baldwin P. *Contagion and the state in Europe, 1830–1930*. New York (NY): Cambridge University Press; 1999.

Barnes D. *The great stink of Paris and the nineteenth-century struggle against filth and germs*. Baltimore (MD): Johns Hopkins University Press; 2006.

Barnes D. *The making of a social disease: tuberculosis in nineteenth-century France*. Berkeley (CA): University of California Press; 1995.

Bashford, A., Hooker, C., editors, *Contagion: Historical and Cultural Studies*. London, New York: Routledge; 2001.

Blackstone W. *Commentaries on the laws of England*. New York (NY): Strouse; 1892.

Boccaccio, G. *The Decameron*. London: Dutton; 1955.

Brand J.L. *Doctors and the state: the British medical profession and government action in public health, 1870–1912*. Baltimore (MD): Johns Hopkins University Press; 1965.

Brandt A. *No magic bullet: a social history of venereal disease in the United States since 1880*. New York (NY): Oxford University Press; 1985.

Brandt A. *The cigarette century: the rise, fall and deadly persistence of the product that defined America*. New York (NY): Basic Books; 2006.

Briggs A. Cholera and society in the nineteenth century. *Past and Present* 1961;**19**:76–96.

Broberg G., Roll-Hansen N., editors. *Eugenics and the welfare state: sterilization policy in Denmark, Sweden, Norway and Finland*. East Lansing (MI): Michigan State University Press; 1996.

Brockliss L., Jones C. *The medical world of early modern France*. Oxford: Clarendon Press; 1997.

Brody S. *The disease of the soul; leprosy in medieval literature*. Ithaca (NY): Cornell University Press; 1974.

Brown P., Mikkelsen E. *No safe place: toxic waste, leukemia, and community action*. Berkeley (CA): University of California Press; 1990.

Browne T. Religio medici. In: *Religio medici and other works*. Oxford: Clarendon Press; 1964.

Brunton D. *Political medicine: the construction of vaccination policy across Britain, 1800–1871*. University of Rochester Press; in press.

Bulloch W. *The history of bacteriology*. New York (NY): Oxford University Press; 1938.

Carlin C., editor. *Imagining contagion in early modern Europe*. New York (NY): Macmillan Palgrave; 2005.

Carmichael A. Leprosy: larger than life. In: Kiple K, editor. *Plague, pox, and pestilence*. New York (NY): Barnes and Noble; 1997. pp. 50–7.

Carmichael A. Plague and more plagues. *Early Science and Medicine* 2003;**8**:253--66.

Carmichael A. *Plague and the poor in Renaissance Florence*. Cambridge: Cambridge University Press; 1986.

Carmichael A. Plague of Athens. In: Kiple K, editor. *Cambridge world history of human disease*. Cambridge: Cambridge University Press; 1993. pp. 934–7.

Carpenter K. Protein and energy: a study of changing ideas in nutrition. Cambridge University Press; 1994.

Carroll P. Medical police and the history of public health. *Medical History* 2002;**46**:461–94.

Cassedy J. *Charles V: Chapin and the public health movement*. Cambridge (MA): Harvard University Press; 1962.

Cassell R.D. *Medical charities, medical politics: the Irish dispensary system and the poor law, 1836–1872*. Woodbridge, Suffolk: Royal Historical Society/Boydell Press; 1997.

Chadwick E. Report on the sanitary condition of the labouring population of Great Britain. Edinburgh University Press; 1965.

Chew H., Kellaway W.E., editors. *London assize of nuisance, 1301–141: a calendar*. London: London Record Society; 1973.

Cipolla C. Faith, reason, and the plague in seventeenth century Tuscany. New York (NY): Norton; 1979.

Cipolla C. *Fighting the plague in seventeenth-century Italy*. Madison (WI): University of Wisconsin Press; 1981.

Cipolla C. *Miasmas and disease: public health and the environment in the pre-industrial age*. Potter E, translator. New Haven (CT): Yale University Press; 1992.

Clendening L. *Source book of medical history*. New York (NY): Dover Publications; 1942.

Coleman W. *Death is a social disease: public health and political economy in early industrial France*. Madison (WI): University of Wisconsin Press; 1982.

Coleman W. Health and hygiene in the *Encyclopedie*: A medical doctrine for the bourgeoisie. *Journal of the History of Medicine* 1974;**29**:399–421.

Coleman W. *Yellow fever in the North: the methods of early epidemiology*. Madison (WI); University of Wisconsin Press; 1987.

Conrad L. Epidemic disease in formal and popular thought in early Islamic society. In: Ranger T, Slack P, editors. *Epidemics and ideas: essays on the historical perception of pestilence*. Cambridge University Press; 1992. pp. 77–99.

Crosby A. *Ecological imperialism: the biological expansion of Europe, 900–1900*. Cambridge University Press; 1986.

Dean M. *The constitution of poverty: toward a genealogy of liberal governance*. London: Routledge; 1991.

Delaporte F. *Disease and civilization, the cholera in Paris, 1832*. Cambridge (MA): MIT Press; 1986.

Desrosières A. The politics of large numbers: A history of statistical reasoning. Naish C, translator. Cambridge (MA): Harvard University Press; 1998.

Dols M. *The Black Death in the Middle East*. Princeton (NJ): Princeton University Press; 1977.

Dorff E. The Jewish tradition. In: Numbers R, Amundusen D, editors. *Caring and curing: health and medicine in the Western religious traditions*. New York (NY): Macmillan; 1986. pp. 5–39.

Douglas M. Purity and danger: an analysis of the concepts of pollution and taboo. London: Routledge; 1966.

Dubos R., Dubos J. *The white plague: tuberculosis, man and society*. New Brunswick (NJ): Rutgers University Press; 1987.

Duffy J. *The sanitarians: a history of American public health*. Urbana (IL): University of Illinois Press; 1990.

Durbach N. *Bodily Matters: The Anti-vaccination Movement in England, 1853–1907*. Durham: Duke University Press; 2005.

Durey M. *The return of the plague: British society and cholera, 1831–32*. Dublin: Gill and MacMillan; 1979.

Edelstein M. *Contaminated communities: social and psychological impacts of residential toxic exposure*. 2nd ed. Boulder (CO): Westview; 2004.

Ellis J.H. *Yellow fever and public health in the New South*. Lexington (KY): University Press of Kentucky; 1992.

Epstein R. Let the shoemaker stick to his last: a defense of the 'old' public health. *Perspectives in Biology and Medicine* 2003;**46**:s138–s159.

Epstein S. *The politics of cancer*. Revised edition. New York (NY): Anchor; 1979.

Etheridge E. *The butterfly caste: a social history of pellagra in the South*. Westport (CT): Greenwood Press; 1972.

Evans R.J. *Death in Hamburg: society and politics in the cholera years, 1830–1910*. London: Penguin Books; 1990.

Eyler J. *Sir Arthur Newsholme and state medicine, 1885–1935*. Cambridge University Press; 1997.

Eyler J.M. *Victorian social medicine: the ideas and methods of William Farr*. Baltimore (MD): Johns Hopkins University Press; 1979.

Fee E. Public health, past and present: a shared social vision. In: Rosen G, editor. *A history of public health*. Expanded edition. Baltimore (MD): Johns Hopkins University Press; 1993. pp. ix–lxvii.

Finer S.E. *The life and times of Sir Edwin Chadwick*. London: Methuen; 1952.

Foucault M. *The birth of the clinic*. New York (NY): Vintage; 1975.

Fox D. *Health policies, health politics: British and American experience, 1911–1965*. Princeton (NJ): Princeton University Press; 1986.

Fox D. *Power and illness: the failure and future of American health policy*. Berkeley (CA): University of California Press; 1993.

Frank J.P. *A system of complete medical police; selections from Johann Peter Frank*. Baltimore (MD): Johns Hopkins University Press; 1976.

Frank J.P. Academic address on the people's misery. *Bulletin of the History of Medicine* 1941;**9**:88–100.

Gallagher N. *Breeding better Vermonters*. Hanover (NH): University Press of New England; 1999.

Garrett L. *The coming plague: newly emerging diseases in a our world of balance*. New York (NY): Penguin; 1995.

Geary L. Famine, fever, and the bloody flux. In: Poirteir C, editor. *The Great Irish Famine*. Dublin: Mercier Press; 1995. pp. 74–85.

Göckjan G. Kurieren und Staat Machen: Gesundheit und Medizin in der burgerlichen welt. Frankfurt am Main: Suhrkamp; 1985. pp. 19.

Gori L. Arabic treatises on environmental pollution upto the end of the thirteenth century. *Environment and History* 2002.**8**:475–88.

Gottlieb R. *Forcing the spring: the transformation of the American environmental movement*. Washington (DC): Island Press; 1993.

Goubert J.P. *The conquest of water*. Wilson A, translator. London: Polity Press; 1989.

Guillerme A. *The age of water: the urban environment in the north of France, AD 300–1800*. College Station (TX): Texas A & M University Press; 1988.

Hamlin C. *A science of impurity: water analysis in nineteenth century Britain*. Adam Hilger/University of California Press; 1990.

Hamlin C. Environmental sensibility in Edinburgh, 1839–1840: the 'fetid irrigation' controversy. *Journal of Urban History* 1994;**20**:311–39.

Hamlin C. Muddling in bumbledom: local governments and large sanitary improvements: the cases of four British towns, 1855–1885. *Victorian Studies* 1988;**32**:55–83.

Hamlin C. Predisposing causes and public health in the early nineteenth century public health movement. *Social History of Medicine* 1992;**5**: 43–70.

Hamlin C. *Public health and social justice in the age of Chadwick: Britain 1800–1854*. Cambridge University Press; 1998.

Hamlin C. Public sphere to public health: the transformation of 'nuisance'. In: Sturdy S, editor. *Medicine, health, and the public sphere in Britain, 1600–2000*. London: Routledge; 2002. pp. 190–204.

Hamlin C. Sanitary policing and the local state, 1873–74: a Statistical study of English and Welsh towns. *Social History of Medicine* 2005; **18**:39–61.

Hamlin C. William Pulteney Alison, the Scottish philosophy, and the making of a political medicine. *Journal of the History of Medicine and Allied Sciences* 2006:547–66.

Haskell T. Capitalism and the origins of the humanitarian sensibility. *American Historical Review* 1985;**90**:339–61.

Hays S. *Beauty, health, and permanence: environmental politics in the United States, 1955–1985*. Cambridge University Press; 1987.

Hennock E.P. The urban sanitary movement in England and Germany, 1838–1914: a comparison. *Continuity and Change* 2000;**15**:269–96.

Hope V., Marshall E., editors. *Death and disease in the ancient city*. London: Routledge; 2000.

Hopkins D. *Princes and peasants: smallpox in history*. New edition. Chicago (IL): University of Chicago Press; 2002.

Hoy S. *Chasing dirt: the American pursuit of cleanliness*. New York (NY): Oxford University Press; 1995.

Humphreys M. *Yellow fever and the South*. New Brunswick (NJ): Rutgers University Press; 1992.

Jasanoff S. *Designs on nature: science and democracy in Europe and the United States*. Princeton (NJ): Princeton University Press; 2005.

Johannisson K. The people's health: public health policies in Sweden. In: Porter D, editor. *The history of public health and the modern state*. Amsterdam: Rudopi; 1994. pp. 165–82.

Karmi G. State control of the physician in the Middle Ages: an Islamic model. In: Russell A, editor. *The town and state physician in Europe from the Middle Ages to the Enlightenment*. Wolfenbüttel, Germany: Herzog August Bibliothek; 1981. pp. 63–84.

Kearns G. Cholera, nuisances, environmental management in Islington, 1830–1855. In: Bynum WF, Porter R, editors. *Living and dying in London*. London: Wellcome Institute for the History of Medicine; 1991. pp. 94–125.

Kearns G. Private property and public health reform in England, 1830–1870. *Social Science and Medicine* 1988;**26**:187–99.

Kevles D. *In the name of eugenics: genetics and the uses of human heredity*. Cambridge (MA): Harvard University Press; 1995.

Kinzelbach A. Infection, contagion, and public health in late Medieval and early Modern German imperial towns. *Journal of the History of Medicine* 2006;**61**:369–89.

Kraut A. *Silent travelers: germs, genes, and the 'immigrant menace'*. New York (NY): Basic Books; 1994.

Kunitz S. *The Health of Populations: General Theories and Particular Realities*. New York: Oxford University Press; 2007.

LaBerge A. *Mission and method: the early-nineteenth-century French public health movement*. Cambridge University Press; 1992.

Labisch A. *Homo hygienicus: Gesundheit und Medizin in der Neuzeit*. New York (NY): Campus; 1992.

Lambert R. *Sir John Simon and English social administration*. London: McGibbon and Kee; 1965.

Leavitt J. *Typhoid Mary: captive to the public's health*. Boston (MA): Beacon Press; 1996.

Leongard J., editor. *London viewers and their certificates, 1508–1558: certificates of the sworn viewers of the City of London*. London: London Record Society; 1989.

Levins R., Lopez C. Toward an ecosocial view of health. *International Journal of Health Services* 1999;**29**:261–93.

Lewis J. *What price community medicine? The philosophy, practice, and politics of public health since 1919*. Brighton: Wheatsheaf Books; 1986.

Lewis R.A. *Edwin Chadwick and the public health movement, 1832–1854*. London: Longmans Green; 1952.

Lieber E. Old Testament 'leprosy', contagion and sin. In: Conrad LI, Wujastyk K, editors. *Contagion: perspectives from pre-Modern societies*. Aldershot, UK: Ashgate; 2000. pp. 99–136.

Lifton R. *The Nazi doctors: medical killing and the psychology of genocide*. New York (NY): Basic Books; 1986.

Longrig J. Epidemic, ideas and classical Athenian society. In: Ranger T, Slack P, editors. *Epidemics and ideas: essays on the historical perception of pestilence*. Cambridge University Press; 1992. pp. 21–44

López-Piñero J.M. The medical profession in sixteenth-century Spain. In: Russell A, editor. *The town and state physician in Europe from the Middle ages to the Enlightenment*. Wolfenbüttel, Germany: Herzog August Bibliothek; 1981. pp. 85–98.

MacMahon B., Pugh T. *Epidemiology: pinciples and methods*. Boston (MA): Little, Brown; 1970.

Magnello E. The introduction of mathematical statistics into medical research: the roles of Karl Pearson, Major Greenwood, and Austin Bradford Hill. In: Magnello E, Hardy A, editors. *The road to medical statistics*. Amsterdam: Rodopi; 2002. pp. 95–123.

Marks H. Epidemiologists explain pellagra: gender, race, and political economy in the work of Edgar Sydenstricker. *Journal of the History of Medicine and Allied Sciences* 2003;**58**:34–55.

Marks H. *The progress of experiment: science and therapeutic reforming the United States, 1900–1990*. Cambridge University Press; 1997.

McClure R. *Coram's children: the London Foundling Hospital in the eighteenth century*. New Haven (CT): Yale University Press; 1981.

McGrew R. *Russia and the cholera, 1823–1832*. Madison (WI): University of Wisconsin Press; 1965.

McHugh P. *Prostitution and Victorian social reform*. London: Croom Helm; 1982.

McNeill J.R. *An environmental history of the twentieth-century world*. New York (NY): Norton; 2000.

McNeill W. *Plagues and peoples*. New York (NY): Anchor Doubleday; 1976.

Melosi M. *The sanitary city: urban infrastructure in America from colonial times to the present*. Baltimore (MD): Johns Hopkins University Press; 2000.

Miller G. *The adoption of inoculation for smallpox in England and France*. Philadelphia (PA): University of Pennsylvania Press; 1957.

Münch P. *Stadthygiene im 19 und 20 jahrhundert*. Göttingen, Germany: Vandenhoeck und Ruprecht; 1993.

Newsholme A. *Fifty years in public health: a personal narrative with comments*. Vol 1: *The years preceding 1909*. London: George Allen and Unwin; 1935.

Nohl J. *The Black Death*. London: George Allen and Unwin; 1926.

Novak SJ. Professionalism and bureaucracy: English doctors and the Victorian public health administration. *Journal of Social History* 1973;**6**:440–62.

Novak WJ. The people's welfare: law and regulation in nineteenth-century America. Chapel Hill (NC): University of North Carolina Press; 1996.

Nutton V. Did the Greeks have a name for it? Contagion and contagion theory in classical antiquity. In: Conrad LI, Wujastyk K, editors. *Contagion: perspectives from pre-Modern societies*. Aldershot, UK: Ashgate; 2000. pp. 137–62.

Packard RM, Brown PJ, Berkelman RL *et al.*, editors. Introduction: emerging illnesses as social process. In: *Emerging illnesses and society: negotiating the agenda of public health*. Baltimore (MD): Johns Hopkins University Press; 2004.

Palmer R. Physicians and the state in post-medieval Italy. In: Russell A, editor. *The town and state physician in Europe from the Middle Ages to the Enlightenment*. Wolfenbüttel, Germany: Herzog August Bibliothek; 1981. pp. 47–62.

Paul DB. *Controlling human heredity: 1865 to the present*. Atlantic Highlands (NJ): Humanities Press; 1995.

Pelling M. *Cholera, fever, and English medicine, 1825–1865*. Oxford University Press; 1978.

Pelling M. The meaning of contagion: reproduction, medicine and metaphor. In: Bashford A, Hooker C, editors. *Contagion: historical and cultural studies*. London: Routledge; 2001. pp. 15–38.

Petersen A., Lupton D. *The new public health: health and self in the age of risk*. London: Sage; 1996.

Pettenkofer M. *The value of health to a city* [translation, with an introduction by HE Sigerist]. Baltimore (MD): Johns Hopkins University Press; 1941.

Pick D. *Faces of degeneration: a European disorder, c. 1848–1918*. Cambridge University Press; 1989.

Pickstone JV. Dearth, dirt, and fever epidemics: rewriting the history of British 'public health', 1780–1850. In: Ranger T, Slack P, editors. *Epidemics and ideas: essays on the historical perception of pestilence*. Cambridge University Press; 1992. pp. 125–48.

Porter D., Porter R. The politics of prevention: anti-vaccinationism and public health in nineteenth century England. *Medical History* 1988;**32**:231–52.

Porter D. 'Enemies of the race': biologism, environmentalism, and public health in Edwardian England. *Victorian Studies* 1991a;**34**:159–78.

Porter D. *Health, civilization and the state*. London: Routledge; 1999.

Porter D. Stratification and its discontents: professionalization and conflict in the British public health service, 1848–1914. In: Fee E, Acheson R, editors. *A history of education in public health: health that mocks the doctor's rules*. Oxford University Press; 1991b. pp. 83–113.

Ramsey M. Public health in France. In: Porter D, editor. *The history of public health and the modern state*. Amsterdam: Rudopi; 1994. pp. 45–118.

Razzell P. *The conquest of smallpox: the impact of inoculation on smallpox mortality in eighteenth century England*. Firle, Sussex: Caliban; 1977.

Redlich J., Hirst F. *The history of local government in England* [reissue of Book I of *Local government in England*]. 2nd ed. New York (NY): Augustus Kelley; 1970.

Richards P. State formation and class struggle. In: Corrigan P, editor. *Capitalism, state formation, and Marxist theory*. London: Quartet; 1980. pp. 49–78.

Richards P. *The medieval leper and his northern heirs*. Totowa (NJ): Rowman and Littlefield; 1977.

Richardson R. *Death, dissection, and the destitute*. London: Penguin; 1988.

Riley JC. *The eighteenth century campaign to avoid disease*. London: Macmillan; 1987.

Roberton J. *Observations on the mortality and physical management of children*. London: Longman, Rees, Orme, Brown; 1827.

Rogers N. *Dirt and disease: polio before FDR*. New Brunswick (NJ): Rutgers University Press; 1990.

Rosen G, editor. Cameralism and the concept of medical police. In: *From medical police to social medicine: essays on the history of health care*. New York (NY): Science History; 1974a. pp. 120–41.

Rosen G, editor. The fate of the concept of medical police, 1780–1890. In: *From medical police to social medicine: essays on the history of health care*. New York (NY): Science History; 1974b. pp. 142–58.

Rosen G. *A history of public health*. New York (NY): MD Publications; 1958.

Rosen, G. What is social medicine: a genetic analysis of the concept. *Bulletin of the History of Medicine* 1947;**21**:674–733.

Rosenberg C: *The cholera years: the United States in 1832, 1849, and 1866*. Chicago (IL): University of Chicago Press; 1962.

Rosenkrantz B. *Public health and the state: changing views in Massachusetts, 1842–1936*. Cambridge (MA): Harvard University Press; 1972.

Rosenkrantz BG. Cart before horse: theory, practice and professional image in American public health, 1870–1920. *Journal of the History of Medicine* 1974;**29**:55–73.

Rothstein W. *Public health and the risk factor: a history of an uneven medical revolution*. Rochester (NY): University of Rochester Press; 2003.

Sadler M. *The law of population*. A treatise in six books, in disproof of the superfecundity of human beings, and developing the real principle of their increase. London: John Murray; 1830.

Schneider WH. *Quality and quantity: the quest for biological regeneration in 20th century France*. Cambridge University Press; 1990.

Sellars C. *Hazards of the job: from industrial disease to environmental health science*. Chapel Hill (NC): University of North Carolina Press; 1997.

Shattuck L. *Report of a general plan for the promotion of public and personal health, devised, prepared, and recommended by the commissioners … relating to a sanitary survey of the state*. New York: Arno; 1972.

Simon J. *English sanitary institutions, reviewed in their course of development, and in some of their political and social relations*. London: Cassell; 1890.

Simson JV. Die Flussverungsreinigungsfrage im Jahrhundert. *Vierteljahrschirft für sozial-und wirtschaftgeschichte* 1978;**65**:370–90.

Skisnes O. Notes from the history of leprosy. *International Journal of Leprosy* 1973;**41**:220–37.

Slack P. *The impact of the plague in Tudor and Stuart England*. London: Routledge and Kegan Paul; 1985.

Smith DC. Medical science, medical practice, and the emerging concept of typhus. In: Bynum WF, Nutton V, editors. *Theories of fever from Antiquity to the Enlightenment*. London: Wellcome Institute for the History of Medicine; 1981. pp. 121–34.

Smith FB. *The retreat of tuberculosis, 1850–1950*. London: Croom Helm 1988.

Snowden F. *Naples in the time of cholera 1884–1911*. Cambridge University Press; 1995.

Solomon SG. The expert and the state in Russian public health: continuities and changes across the revolutionary divide. In: Porter D, editor. *The history of public health and the modern state*. Amsterdam: Rudopi; 1994. pp. 183–223.

Soloway RA. *Birth control and the population question in England, 1877–1930*. Chapel Hill (NC): University of North Carolina Press; 1982.

Starr P. The social transformation of American medicine. New York (NY): Basic Books; 1982.

Steneck N. *The microwave debate*. Cambridge (MA): MIT Press; 1984.

Stepan N. *The hour of eugenics: race, gender, and nation in Latin America*. Ithaca (NY): Cornell University Press; 1991.

Stradling D., Thorsheim P. The smoke of great cities: British and American efforts to control air pollution, 1860–1914. *Environmental History* 1999;**4**:6–31.

Sturdy S., editor. Introduction: medicine, health, and the public sphere. *Medicine, health, and the public sphere in Britain, 1600–2000*. London: Routledge; 2002. pp. 190–204.

Sturm C.C. *Sturm's reflections on the works of God, and his providence throughout all nature*. Philadelphia (PA): Woodward; 1832.

Susser M. 'Epidemiology in the United States after World War II: the evolution of technique.'. *Epidemiologic Reviews* 1985;7:147–77.

Taylor V., Trentmann F. From users to consumers: water politics in nineteenth-century London. In: Trentmann F, editor. *The making of the consumer: knowledge, power and identity in the modern world*. Oxford: Berg; 2005.

Tesh S.N. *Hidden arguments: political ideology and disease prevention*. New Brunswick (NJ): Rutgers University Press; 1987.

Thompson E.P. The moral economy of the English crowd in the eighteenth century. *Past and Present* 1971;**50**:76–136.

Thucydides. *The history of the Peloponnesian War*. Crawley R, translator. New York (NY): EP Dutton; 1950.

Tomes N. *The gospel of germs: men, women, and the microbe in American life*. Cambridge (MA): Harvard University Press; 1998.

Touati F-O. Contagion and leprosy: myth, ideas and evolution in medieval minds and societies. In: Conrad LI, Wujastyk K, editors. *Contagion: perspectives from pre-Modern societies*. Aldershot, UK: Ashgate; 2000. pp. 179–201.

Turner S. What is the problem with experts?. *Social Studies of Science* 2001;**31**:123–49.

Turshen M. *The politics of public health*. New Brunswick (NJ): Rutgers University Press; 1987.

Veyne P., editor. The Roman empire. In: *A history of private life. Vol I: From pagan Rome to Byzantium*. Goldhammer A, translator. Cambridge (MA): Belknap Press of Harvard University Press; 1987. pp. 222–32.

Waddington K. *The bovine scourge: meat, tuberculosis and public health, 1850–1914*. Woodbridge, UK: Boydell; 2006.

Walkowitz J. *Prostitution and Victorian society: women, class and the state*. Cambridge University Press; 1980.

Watkin D. The English revolution in social medicine, 1889–1911. Unpublished PhD thesis. University of London; 1984.

Webb S., Webb B. *English local government from the Revolution to the Municipal Corporations Act: statutory authorities for special purposes*. London: Longmans Green; 1922.

Weindling P. Was social medicine revolutionary? Rudolph Virchow and the Revolution of 1848. *Bulletin of the Society for the Social History of Medicine* 1984;**34**:13–8.

Weiner D. *The citizen-patient in revolutionary and imperial Paris*. Baltimore (MD): Johns Hopkins University Press; 1993.

Weyland J. *The principles of population and production as they are affected by the progress of society with view to moral and political consequences* [original, 1816]. New York (NY): Augustus Kelley; 1968.

White K. *Healing the schism: epidemiology, medicine and the public's health*. New York (NY): Springer; 1991.

Wilson F.R. *A practical guide for inspectors of nuisances*. London: Knight; 1881.

Wilson L. Fevers and science in early nineteenth century medicine. *Journal of the History of Medicine* 1978;**33**:386–407.

Winslow C.A. *The conquest of epidemic disease: a chapter in the history of ideas* [original ed 1943]. Madison (WI): University of Wisconsin Press; 1980.

Wohl A. *The eternal slum: housing and social policy in Victorian London*. London: Edward Arnold; 1977.

Wohl A.S. *Endangered lives: public health in Victorian Britain*. Cambridge (MA): Harvard University Press; 1983.

Worboys M. *Spreading germs: disease theories and medical practice in Britain, 1865–1900*. Cambridge University Press; 2000.

World Health Organization. *Constitution of the World Health Organization in WHO Basic Documents*. 19th ed. Geneva: World Health Organization; 1968.

Ziegler P. *The Black Death*. New York (NY): Harper Torchbooks; 1969.

1.3

The history and development of public health in low- and middle-income countries

Than Sein

Introduction

Public health broadly deals with identification of health problems that affect the entire population with mechanisms to address these problems effectively. Historically, public health interventions are those that promote and protect people's health, and are chiefly undertaken by the governments. Ko Ko (1986) charted the progress of public health development over five eras—empirical health, basic science, clinical science, public health, and political science. Detels and Breslow (2000) described public health as a process of mobilizing local, state, national, and international resources to ensure the conditions in which people can be healthy. Beaglehole and Bonita (2004) referred to it as a collective action for sustained population-wide health improvement, emphasizing the hallmarks of sustained health actions and interventions addressing the health of the whole population. The notion of public within the term, public health, encompasses the interventions for health development by the people themselves individually and collectively, in addition to those carried out by the government or its agents. In general, public health is a comprehensive measure by the government and the people, covering promotive, preventive, curative, and rehabilitative aspects. Public health actions, for many centuries and even today, mainly focus on prevention and control of diseases or conditions that particularly affect a large number of people. Public health interventions not only deal with control and management of diseases, but also address the prevention or reduction of risks and root causes of these problems. Since fundamental characteristics of public health actions lie primarily on the social and other determinants of health, that are outside the domain of the health sector and also beyond the individual's action, these actions are not only the responsibility of the government, but also that of the people themselves.

The socioeconomic health and other development status of the world have changed rapidly and radically in recent years. Spectacular scientific advancement has led humans into outer space and also to apply such advanced knowledge and skill to health sciences, with which millions of lives have been saved. Yet, majority of people in over 150 countries around the world had a per-capita Gross National Income (GNI) of below US$10 725 in 2005, which are known generally, as the low- and middle-income (LMI) countries as classified by the World Bank (World Bank 2006a). People in many LMI countries live in poverty with inadequate healthcare and low health status. The present chapter reviews the history and development of public health in LMI countries of which about one-third are classified as least-developed nations. It provides an insight that could contribute to the solution of present and future challenges and opportunities for health development which actually influence the health of the world. Learning from the experience of past developments in public health is an essential element in modern public health education. Some examples of public health development in LMI countries of Asia and the Pacific are highlighted.

The chapter firstly traces health systems development from the colonial period to the present century. It documents the post-independent efforts of LMI countries in their health development, within the context of socioeconomic and political development, including collaborative work at inter-country and international levels. In the next section, it briefly touches upon disease prevention and control, especially how LMI countries cope with the prevailing high morbidity and mortality conditions, and the major public health achievements and failures. The lessons in eradication and elimination efforts for preventing and controlling priority diseases provide a clear perception on the application of principles and practice of public health. It also highlights the links between the epidemiological, political, and financing aspects of disease control. The next section covers why and how there is a shift in major causes of deaths and diseases in LMI countries with an increasing burden of chronic non-communicable diseases. This has led to adoption of measures and interventions beyond the usual health-sector functions for reducing risks, such as legislative, environment, and educative actions. These include the reduction of tobacco and alcohol use, avoiding unhealthy diets and promoting physical activity, or adopting multisectoral measures for road safety and injury prevention.

At the turn of the twentieth century, many LMI countries moved towards another era of public health development, with new thinking from a narrow view of vertical disease control interventions to a wider perspective of multisectoral interventions. Besides the usual public health measures undertaken by governments, an increasing number of non-governmental organizations and the private sector agencies, both at the local and global levels, were involved in public health development. In addition to the international agencies dealing with health under the UN system, many intergovernmental and international bodies and philanthropic organizations, foundations, and alliances are supporting and complementing the global public health functions. In summary, public health essentially deals with the health of the population in its totality. The success of public health measures depends on adhering to the basic principles of equity, social justice, and partnerships.

Protecting people's health

Public health practices during the colonial period

From time immemorial, human beings have dealt with the spread of dreadful diseases like diarrhoeal diseases, smallpox, plague, or syphilis, through various aspects of personal hygiene and other public health practices, including civic duties on sanitation measures, which were enforced by royal decrees. Since those ancient periods, measures to promote and protect the health of the people remained as the dedicated actions of the statehood in many countries in Asia, Africa, the Americas, and Europe. Modern public health principles and practices were further developed during the so-called Victorian period of the eighteenth–nineteenth centuries. With increasing ability to identify the causal factors of the diseases and conditions, knowledge on the social, environmental, and political dimensions of the diseases and their prevention grew tremendously. In addition to the establishment of medical care facilities, a series of legislative measures similar to that of colonial countries were initiated in order to protect the health of their own people. Such legislative measures on public health matters—such as improved sanitation facilities and practices, installation of safe water supply systems, and the preventive and control responses to epidemics—might have varied according to the origin of the colonial powers, but were effective in reducing the outbreaks of communicable diseases. The definite imprints of these legislative measures—such as the Public Health Acts, Local Government and Municipality Acts, Vital Registration Act, Factory Act, Food Adulteration Act, Vaccination Act, Contagious Diseases Act, etc.—are still in existence in many LMI countries. Only a few years ago, some laws and acts were updated or replaced with newer legislation. Some health systems' practices like hospital care, maternity homes, sanatoria, and quarantine places are still functioning as they did for centuries. The European model of a national social health insurance scheme also spread to other countries, especially to those in East Asia.

Many missionaries with western education and an allopathic medical background had established education, medial care, and research institutions, the so-called western institutions. The introduction of western medicine by missionaries resulted in first exposure and increasing access by the local populace to the western way of allopathic medical practices. The infectious diseases were identified as tropical diseases, since they mainly existed in the tropical countries. The prevention, control, and management of tropical diseases became priority teaching subjects for medical professionals and public health workers who liked to work in the colonies (Uragoda 1987; Harrison 1994). Many researchers and public health professionals in Europe and America became well known after they did their practices and research studies on the epidemiology and control of infectious diseases in the tropical countries. During the late eighteenth century, education in public health and tropical diseases flourished in Europe and North America with new institutions for undergraduate and postgraduate training. Many pioneer public health schools and tropical disease research institutions were established in the colonial home countries starting from the eighteenth century. These were institutions like Johns Hopkins School of Public Health in the United States, the London and Liverpool Schools of Tropical Medicine in Britain, and the School of Public Health in Spain. These institutions acted as home-based training institutions for research and development to spread the knowledge and information on the prevention and control of tropical diseases, and to train people who would like to serve in the tropical countries. Discoveries of causative organisms and ways of stopping transmission of malaria, sleeping sickness, and worm infestations, and also identification of nutritional disorders through clinical and public health research studies were initiated by these schools. These education and research practices were later spread to the people and institutions in the colonies and other countries. With technical and financial support of the Rockefeller Foundation and the technical support of the Johns Hopkins School of Public Health, the London School of Tropical Medicine was transformed into the London School of Hygiene and Tropical Medicine in 1920, expanding the scope of research and teaching in tropical medicine, public health administration, medical statistics, and epidemiology (Wilkinson & Power 1998). Spain established its National School of Public Health in 1924 and introduced a public health component into its comprehensive rural medical care network. The British authorities also established similar public health educational and research institutions in India starting from the early 1920s, such as the Institute of Tropical Medicine and the All-India Institute of Hygiene and Public Health in Kolkata (Calcutta) to undertake research in tropical diseases and to train local people on hygiene and public health. After that, a series of research and training institutions and laboratories were established for undertaking basic and applied research and training on specific diseases in India, which later became the exemplary institutions serving India and its neighbours for several decades (Jaggi 1979). Other colonial rulers also established similar medical and public health educational and research institutions in their respective colonies. Independent countries like Poland, China, Thailand, and Japan also followed similar developments. These educational institutions worked closely with their colonial counterparts to strengthen the skill, knowledge, and expertise on control of tropical diseases.

Actually, the development of public health and medical care services for the general public or natives in the colonies remained rudimentary. Local people were suffering from epidemic outbreaks not only from indigenous infectious sources but also from diseases imported through trade and migration routes. Moving millions of people to totally unfamiliar areas made them vulnerable to new diseases. Thousands of people died in new territories due to smallpox, malaria, yellow fever, typhus, typhoid, and cholera, or were disabled due to yaws, leprosy, and syphilis. Similarly, people who went for trade and commodities brought back infectious diseases to their homes in Europe and America. While the Americans initially launched the control of malaria and yellow fever campaigns in the eighteenth century, the British, French, and Dutch colonials initiated major international public health initiative for control of smallpox through vaccination, first among the people within the colonial administration and the workers employed, and later the general public. The colonials later launched community-based health interventions and research-cum-action projects for malaria control and worm infestation in some tropical countries, to have a better knowledge for the prevention and control that could be replicated in other parts of the world (Foster & Anderson 1978).

Foundation for international public health

Efforts in international public health were intensified in the mid-1800s, when the United States of America and the European nations started applying protective legislative measures to prevent the importation of diseases from trading ships and their cargo. An international sanitary conference, organized by a group of European nations in Paris in 1851, looking for solutions for protecting epidemic diseases coming from the tropics, drafted the international quarantine regulations, which was the precursor of today's International Health Regulations. Over the next 50 years, a series of international conferences held in Europe and America covered health and social issues including trafficking in liquor and opium. A major milestone at the eleventh international sanitary conference held in Paris in 1903 was the adoption of the first international sanitary convention for prevention and control of three tropical diseases, viz. plague, cholera, and yellow fever. Based on the recommendation of this convention, the French Government established in Paris in 1907 the first international health office—*L'Office International d'Hygiene Publique* (OIHP), whose main objective was to protect Europe from three tropical diseases (Howard-Jones 1974). Similar international health institutions were established in different parts of the world, mainly as regional bodies, responsible for reporting and controlling the outbreaks of diseases for cross-border transmission. One of the earliest institutions was the *L'Conseil Sanitaire Maritime et Quarantenaire d'Egypte*, situated in Alexandria since 1881. Following the decision of the 2nd international conference of American States, the International Sanitary Bureau for Americas was established in 1902, to facilitate the exchange of information on infectious diseases among the countries in the American continent. When the OIHP was established, this American sanitary bureau changed its name to the Pan American Sanitary Bureau (PASB), which later became the executive bureau of the Pan American Sanitary Organization (PASO). The PASO, under the agreement in 1949 as per WHO Constitution, acted as the Regional Organization of WHO for the Americas. The PASO was renamed as the Pan American Health Organization (PAHO) in 1957, with its headquarters in Washington, in the United States.

By 1911, just a few years before the outbreak of World War I, the task of OIHP in Paris was expanded, to become the first truly international health agency with the main responsibility of monitoring and reporting the outbreaks of the three tropical diseases occurring around the world, and providing information through a monthly bulletin to the general public, on health measures undertaken to combat these diseases (McNeill 1977). Around 1910–1920, major epidemics of infectious diseases due to plague, typhus, cholera, and the great influenza pandemic were rampant in many countries. After World War I, the countries formed an alliance for peace by establishing the League of Nations. Since the OIHP with its small staff and funding could not cope with major international public health crisis, the League of Nations in 1920 agreed to establish a new international health organization under its auspices. After intensive negotiations between the countries in the League and other independent nations, the League of Nations Health Organization (LNHO) was established in 1923, while the OIHP continued its function (Howard-Jones 1977). The LNHO was assigned to handle international health matters including organization of conferences and symposia, provision of technical assistance to countries, and the clearing-house function. The Weekly Epidemiological Records published since then by the OIHP was continued to date by its successor, the World Health Organization. The LNHO also initiated a series of basic, clinical, and field research studies on medicine and public health. It organized a series of international conferences and meetings of various experts in a wide range of subjects, such as malaria, tuberculosis, leprosy, maternal and child health, health systems, and medical education. It also promoted international medical education, including post-graduate education in public health (WHO 1967).

As early as the 1930s, senior public health administrators from the colonies expressed their concerns at the health status of the population, especially those from rural areas, at the international health conferences organized by the LNHO. The Conference of Far-Eastern Countries on Rural Hygiene organized by the LNHO in 1937 at Bandung, the Netherlands East Indies (present-day Indonesia) was a cornerstone in public health and rural health development in Asia. At this Conference, while noting the rampant condition of communicable diseases and nutritional deficiency disorders in the rural areas, the senior health administrators had identified health as central to development and emphasized the need for integrating health and intersectoral actions. They also recognized that adoption of basic health service approaches by bringing maternal and child healthcare and basic medical care through hospitals and dispensaries nearer to the people could reduce the morbidity and mortality (LNHO 1937).

Many LMI countries became the battlefields and victims of the devastating war for about 6 years during World War II. They had experienced the destruction, destitution, and diseases as well as human misery and suffering with very heavy death tolls. The virtual non-existence of the basic health infrastructure or public utility distribution system had resulted in miserable conditions. The spirit of international peace, solidarity, security, and tranquillity was transcended immediately after the War. The original draft of the UN Charter did not include health. The UN General Assembly (UNGA) in June, 1946 approved to include health in its Charter, and also called for an international conference whose main purpose was to foster consensus in the establishment of a new international health organization in place of the OIHP and LNHO. On 22 July 1946, at the New York conference, a total of 61 nations, many of which were still under colonial rule, approved the Constitution of the World Health Organization (WHO). After ratification by the twenty-sixth Member State, the WHO Constitution came into force on 7 April 1948, the date being celebrated as World Health Day every year. The main functions assigned to WHO were: To direct and coordinate international health work and to cooperate with Member States and partners in international health development (WHO 1992). WHO is collaborating closely, with its Member States, for over 60 years, through its six regional organizations and its headquarters, as a leading international health organization.

Health systems in post-independence period

With the people's movements, democratic reforms, and international pressure, many LMI countries gained independence one after another within a few years from the end of World War II, and some only in the mid-1950s. These countries started reconstruction and rehabilitation activities in various sectors to achieve the rapid economic growth and social development, while catching up with the technological advances in the colonials. Only a few fortunate countries in Asia, the Pacific, and Africa entered the post-World War II period in a relatively calm and favourable condition that helped them in rapid growth and reconstruction. Some countries were challenged by their own internal ethnic conflicts, thereby delaying the development efforts. Even after a few decades of independence, healthcare facilities were very few, rudimentary, and mainly concentrated in urban areas. A number of paramedical training institutes, public health training and research institutions, and health development centres were established in the rural areas, with technical assistance from bilateral and UN agencies. The *Kalutara* rural health training unit in Sri Lanka, the *Aung San* health demonstration unit in Myanmar, and the *Singur* rural health centre in India were a few of them. Exactly two decades after the Bandung Rural Health Conference, another international rural health conference was held at New Delhi in India in 1957, at which the concept and functioning of basic health services in the rural areas in Asia were reviewed including the training and use of multipurpose health workers, enhancement in prevention and control of infectious diseases, promoting intersectoral action, and participation of the local community, including formation of village health committees. The conference highlighted the importance and the need for strengthening rural health centres which were the basic units where comprehensive healthcare was provided (WHO 1957).

Many LMI countries till the 1960s had weak health infrastructure in providing maternal and child health (MCH) care. While a few of them had the technical and managerial authoritative bodies for MCH matters at the central level, the MCH services were mainly provided by the briefly trained nurse-aids, midwives, or nurse-midwives at the hospitals and hospital-based clinics which existed mostly in the urban areas. After a few decades, it was realized that the vertical approach of opening MCH centres and deploying MCH workers alone did not serve the purpose of expanding MCH care. Various strategies were adopted to integrate and expand the MCH as part of the essential basic healthcare packages. In the 1960s, many LMI countries started adopting comprehensive population policies, which included family planning as part of MCH care, to address both demographic and maternal health problems. Even though simple and effective technology for the family planning services was available during the 1960s, only 9 per cent of women in LMI countries had access to contraceptive services.

According to the United Nations Millennium Development Goal (UN-MDG) Report in 2006, an estimated 824 million people in the developing countries were affected by chronic hunger as measured by the proportion of people lacking the food needed to meet their daily needs. The countries in sub-Saharan Africa and South Asia were the worst hit, with 20–30 per cent of the people living with insufficient food (UN 2006). Protein-energy malnutrition (PEM) is a major nutritional deficiency disease due to inadequate energy intake leading to wasting and stunting. The research studies in LMI countries especially in Asia in 1980s showed that PEM was in fact due to calorie deficiency (Gopalan 1992; WHO 1986). The highest levels were found in South Asia (46 per cent) and the lowest in Latin America (7 per cent) and the Caribbean (5 per cent). More than 20 million children were born with low birth weight in the developing world, and more than half of these children were in South Asia. The risk of being malnourished as measured by weight was 1.2 times higher in Asia than in Africa, and 3 times higher in Africa than in Latin America. There has been little progress (from 20 per cent in 1990 to 17 per cent in 2000) of the prevalence of malnutrition among LMI countries. The percentage of children under 5 years with stunted growth or underweight in low income countries remained at 43 per cent; and the proportion of low birth weight babies was also around 20 per cent (World Bank 2005).

The hidden-hunger or micronutrient deficiency disease was more widespread than PEM. Around 1999, an estimated 5 billion people suffered from iron deficiency anaemia (IDA) alone, which had profound effects on overall health and development of the people. The IDA actually enhanced the morbidity and mortality of mothers and young children, and limiting the learning capacity, impairing the immune function, and reducing productive capacity. The vitamin A deficiency (VAD) is another micronutrient deficiency responsible for blindness among children. After extensive clinical trials in LMI countries, nutrition supplementation programme with vitamin A was introduced as part of activities for promotion of breastfeeding and dietary improvement, with the support of UN and bilateral agencies. Although there was an increase in coverage of vitamin A supplementation from 50 per cent in 1999 to 70 per cent in 2004, the VAD remains a public health problem of today (UNICEF 2006). The iodine deficiency disorders (IDD) is another important micronutrient deficiency disorder, which is widespread in Asia and Africa. While the universal iodization of salt and diversification of dietary intakes had successfully reduced the prevalence of IDD in the western and some Asian countries by 1980s, there were over 200 million people worldwide with goitre and 26 million people suffered from brain damage, associated with IDD, including 6 million children being identified as cretins. The IDD elimination policy and programme actions were proposed at the thirty-eighth World Health Assembly (WHA) in 1986 and later endorsed as an ambitious target in 1990 at the Global Summit for Children. By 1995, it was estimated that IDD was still a significant public health problem in 118 countries, affecting around 43 million people. Fortification of iodine in the widely consumed food and salt, and the advice on diversification of iodine-rich dietary intakes were promoted as main public health strategies in combating IDD. Bhutan, a land-locked Himalayan country, witnessed a remarkable reduction in the prevalence of IDD from 65 per cent in 1990 to 14 per cent in 2000, using a multisectoral approach including extensive availability and use of iodized salt to the whole population, monitoring by health staff on the iodine content of salt at various points of distribution and at the consumers' homes, and promoting social mobilization (WHO 1999a). A similar pattern of reduction in Myanmar, from 33 per cent of goitre rate among school children (6–11 years of age) in 1994 to less than 5.5 per cent (almost reaching the elimination target of 5 per cent) in 2004, was achieved through extensive publicity campaigns and rapidly expanded coverage of more than 90 per cent with universal iodization of salt (Ko Ko *et al.* 2005). By 2005, only 67 per cent of all types of salt consumed in LMI countries were fortified with iodine (World Bank 2005). The success with IDD elimination would depend upon the political commitment for sustained provision of iodine fortified salt for daily household use, promotion of diversified iodine-rich dietary intakes, and effective public education.

One of the key factors contributing to health development is having competent human resources for health or health workforce, i.e. the right numbers and mix of health professionals with the right knowledge, skills, and attitude at the right location and at the right time. As human resources for health consume as much as 60–70 per cent of the health budget, it is essential that they are fully developed and optimally utilized. Very often, health professionals have found it difficult to keep pace with new knowledge and skills. Hence, education and training of health personnel, whether pre-service, in-service, or continuing education, requires to equip them with the requisite knowledge, skills, and attitude, to effectively keep up with the rapid advancement in health and other technologies, as well as to keep responding to the changes in health needs. Almost all LMI countries have pre-service educational programmes for various health personnel to be deployed in their own national health systems. Each country is striving towards ensuring the quality and relevance of health personnel education. In the area of medical education, countries have established useful linkages for conducting collaborative training programmes among different institutions. The World Health Report 2006 provided a global situation analysis of the health work force in 2006 and identified effective strategies to strengthen allied health services and education (WHO 2006a).

Countries are still confronted with issues such as lack of clear national policies for health personnel development; inadequate norms and standards for health professionals resulting in an inappropriate mix of health personnel; lack of mechanisms for the exchange of information on health professionals' education and training; lack of common standards for health professionals' education and training; and absence of quality control mechanisms in health professionals' practices. Numerous strategies had been identified to strengthen the health workforce's services and education, which included among others: Development of comprehensive human resources for health; ensuring curriculum to meet changing service needs and technology and to provide evidence-based and cost-effective care; uniformity in education quality and products; establishing/strengthening national and regional centres of excellence that would address the changing health workers' needs.

Access to essential medicines continues to be the core element of healthcare. With technical advancement, more and more medicines and vaccines would be available and LMI countries need to strengthen their national medicines policies, including food and drugs quality control in order to improve access, promote rational use, and ensure quality, quantity, safety, and efficacy. Most LMI countries have developed national lists of essential medicines and vaccines, and enhanced the work of their Drug Regulatory Authorities to ensure safe, effective, and quality medicines. With the expansion of the private sector in healthcare, access to essential medicines has become an important issue. Most countries have long-standing price control mechanisms for essential medicines, but it is difficult to keep the medicines affordable and provide a sufficient return to the manufacturers. An information exchange mechanism between countries and evaluation of drug pricing systems has been established. The public health impact of the Trade Related Intellectual Property Rights (TRIPs) is being debated to find ways and means to solve the problems of countries, having been prevented from obtaining new medicines and vaccines essential for their public health needs in future. Intellectual property rights are important for innovation relevant to public health and are a factor in determining access to medicines. But neither innovation nor access depend on just intellectual property rights. The work of the commission on intellectual property rights, innovation, and public health, established by WHO in 2005, focused on the interactions between intellectual property rights, innovation, and public health. Based upon the commission's report, further debate is continuing to identify possible policy interventions for innovations useful for public health development (WHO 2007a).

Environmental health promotion

The promotion of environmental health including personal hygiene and public sanitation has always been part of healthy public and personal practices since the early days of health development in Asia. The nineteenth century experience of the high-income and some LMI countries showed that improvement in personal hygiene, provision of adequate and safe water supply, and enhancement of environmental health had prevented and controlled many infectious diseases. The incidence of water- and food-borne diseases including cholera in these countries had reduced dramatically through improvement in the water supply and sanitation, even when effective medicines were not yet available. Environmental health promotion is a part of civic duties and a main function of public bodies such as municipalities and local administrative bodies. Despite these legislative measures supplemented by education campaigns and subsidy support, progress in environmental health promotion in the LMI countries was not satisfactory. By 2000, about 2.4 billion people around the world still lacked access to improved sanitation facilities. Figure 1.3.1 showed the proportion of population having access to improved sanitation facilities in the countries of Asia, an average of the least-developed countries and the world in 2004, comparing with those in 1990. More than 50 per cent of the vast population of China, India, and many other Asian countries and many of the least-developed countries have no access yet to improved sanitation facilities (UNDP 2006), which had actually aroused to call for at the UN Millennium Summit at 2000, to halve the proportion of people without sustainable access to safe drinking water and sanitation by 2015. It was a formidable challenge for LMI countries especially in Asia and Africa, with more than half of their population not having access to safe water supply and sanitation.

The provision of improved sanitation facilities is often regarded as the responsibility of individuals and family members rather than public bodies. It would not be possible for a rural community to build and run a community-based sewerage system (for a whole village of 1000 households), which would be an equivalent of a public water-supply system for urban population, due to the heavy investment and maintenance costs. Many national sanitation programmes thus promoted the use of an on-site sanitation facility at the household level. For many poor families, the benefit of having clean water from a single common water supply source with a little cost incurred by them seemed to have more visible impact than the long-term benefit of having improved latrine for each household with a similar small investment. A study in a few least-developed countries in Asia showed that it would take 20 days' wages to build a simple pit latrine. Asian Development Bank had estimated in 2005 that the annual value of time saved by having better access to clean, safe, and reliable water supply, and sanitation facilities would amount to US$54 billion for achieving the UN MDG target, and US$109 billion to improve water supply and sanitation for all in Asia alone (ADB 2005). Community involvement in local decision-making is also a key to success. People will demand more if they

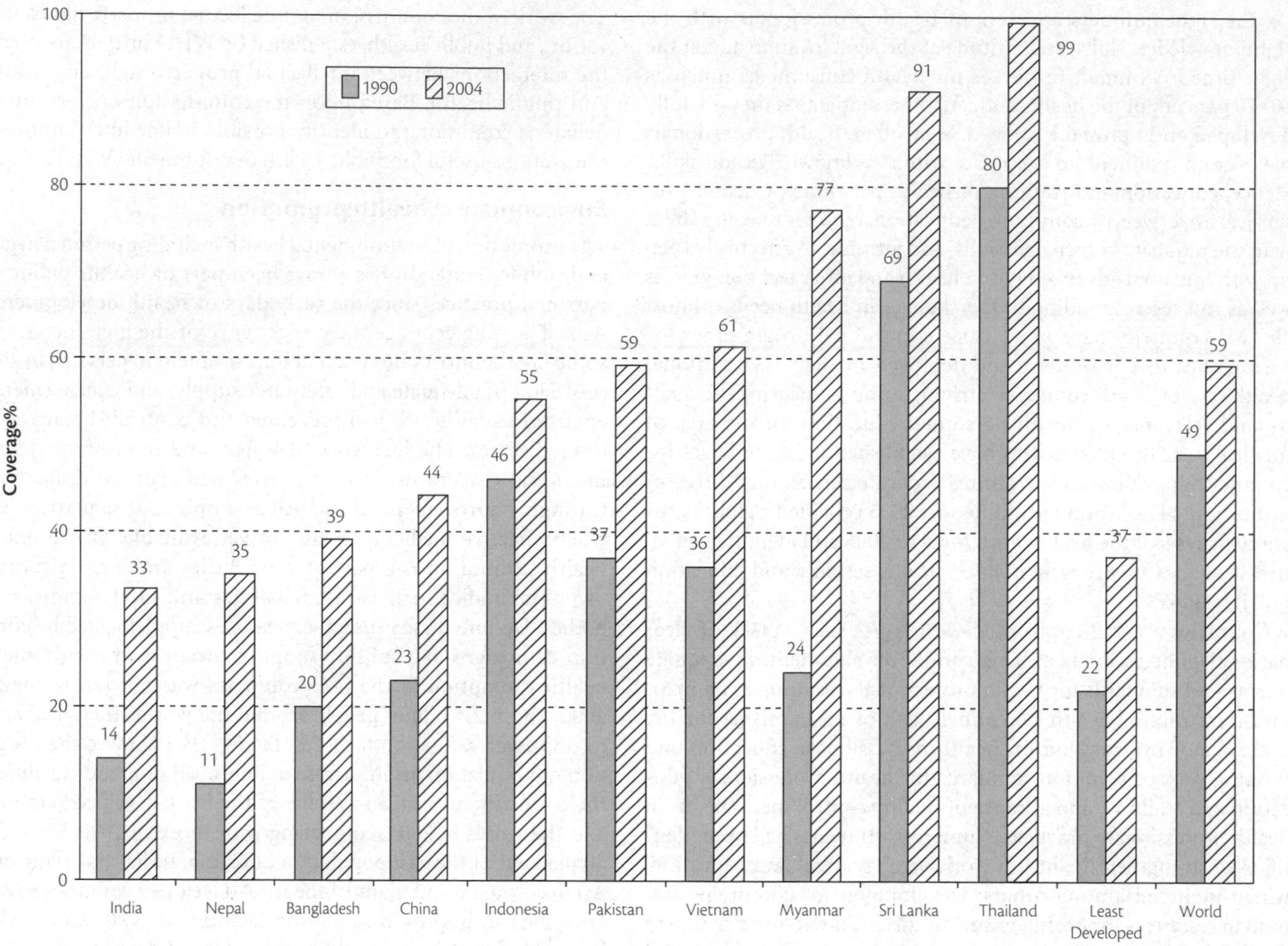

Fig. 1.3.1 Proportion of population with sustainable access to improved sanitation of the World, the least-developed countries and selected Asian nations, 1990 and 2004. *Source*: UNDP Human Development Report (2006).

know the benefits of having improved sanitary facilities. The use of public and private electronic and print media and the organization of national and sub-national sanitation campaigns are important strategies for promoting environmental sanitation, in addition to educating school children and mothers. With the existing economic growth, most middle-income countries could afford to invest a proportion of the national budget for initiating mass sanitation campaigns within the next decade to attain the UN MDG goal in this area. However, low-income countries may need additional financial support for achieving the target.

Reforming public health systems

Health-for-all movement

During 1950–60s, the LMI countries with the support of international agencies had made tremendous efforts to reduce the burden of communicable diseases with the establishment of nation-wide medical care and public health systems. Actually, the organized public health systems in the modern sense intended to benefit the whole population barely existed a century ago in these countries. Some countries adopted the so-called modern (allopathic-based) health systems as recently as the 1960–70s. Till date, the major works of the health systems in some LMI countries were run by the charitable or non-governmental organizations (NGOs). Some forms of a social insurance system as part of the welfare schemes for employed workers were introduced in a few middle-income countries, copying the social welfare model from western countries. After 30 odd-years, countries started realizing that healthcare systems based on hospitals and health centres were a burden on the public due to the high costs of medicines, technological equipment, and staff, as well as other facilities. Rapid expansion of basic health centres without properly trained human resources could not provide essential healthcare to the vast majority of rural people. The integration of specialized disease control programmes into general health services also moved slowly, with many vertical disease control programmes continuing as autonomous bodies for more than 4–5 decades. There was little coordination in planning and management between various sections of the health ministry itself and between the health and health-related sectors. Much of the health planning was done at the central level without the close involvement of the people responsible for implementation (Djukanovic & Mach 1975; WHO 1978a).

By mid-1970s, there were glaring contrasts in health status between high-income and LMI countries as well as among LMI countries. The average life expectancy at birth in LMI countries was around 55 years, with many countries having infant and child mortality above 100 per 1000 live births. Most infant and young children's deaths were due to infectious diseases that were easily preventable and controlled. Despite these drawbacks, a few LMI countries showed significant improvement in health status with little investment in health. Examples of Cuba, Chile, Sri Lanka, Tanzania, Kerala state of India, and rural health in China were used as the best policies and practices for successful health achievements. The underlying factors of successes in many LMI countries were the national policies and programmes addressing equity, social justice, community involvement, appropriate technology, and multisectoral approaches. The need for closing the gaps between those who achieved good health and those who were not able to do so led to the adoption of a historic resolution at the World Health Assembly in 1977 which set the main social target of Member States and WHO, of the attainment by all the citizens of the world by the year 2000 of a level of health that would permit them to lead a socially and economically productive life. This universal social target was termed as—Health for All by the year 2000 or HFA2000. It was meant to be a political and social aspiration that people would use better approaches than they had before, individually and by the community as a whole, for preventing and controlling diseases and alleviating unavoidable illness and disability. It was conceived as a process leading to progressive improvement in the health of the people and not as a single finite target. Essential healthcare would be accessible to individuals and families in acceptable and affordable ways with their full involvement. These principles were further clarified at the International Conference on Primary Health Care (PHC) jointly organized by WHO and UNICEF at Alma-Ata in the then USSR in 1978 which adopted the path-breaking Declaration of Alma-Ata (WHO 1978b). This Declaration and the accompanying report of the Conference called for urgent action by all governments, health and development workers, and the world community to protect and promote the health of all the people of the world using primary healthcare as the key approach. LMI countries saw the outcome and recommendations of the Alma-Ata Conference as well as the principles of the Declaration as an opportunity for restructuring their health systems, using the PHC approach as a practical, scientifically sound, and socially acceptable public health measure. They had formulated new health policies and strategies, as well as plans of action to launch and sustain their healthcare systems within the common framework of global HFA strategies. The adoption of the universal goal helped many countries to recognize new ways of reaching a higher level of health status, and to place greater emphasis on adherence to health goals. Some countries concentrated on vertical types of healthcare interventions like immunization, family planning, and maternal care, while others tried to be as comprehensive as possible in their public health development. For example, UNICEF and many other development agencies initially introduced the vertical programmes like MCH and family planning, growth monitoring, oral rehydration, breast-feeding, and immunization. The accessibility of essential healthcare, in fact, improved in most countries, with over 80 per cent of population covered with basic healthcare by 1980s. However, the progress on some aspects of healthcare, like essential care for pregnant mothers and safe delivery, immunization to infants and children, or provision of adequate water supply and sanitation, remained very slow in some LMI countries, particularly the least-developed ones. Healthcare for pregnant mothers as measured by the coverage of attendance by trained health personnel during pregnancy and childbirth was less than 25 per cent in many countries. Despite widespread acceptance by national health authorities of the idea of integrated health systems since the early days of health system developments in the 1950s, there were practical operational constraints in transforming semi-autonomous vertical or selective health development programmes into the general health services. One of the main factors that slowed implementation of HFA strategies using primary healthcare as the key approach was lack of a full understanding of the fundamental policies and principles of PHC and HFA that were applicable to national health systems development. This led to achieving an insufficient level of universal access to essential healthcare. There was inadequate coordination and collaboration between specific health intervention campaigns and the development of basic health infrastructure (district health systems development). This further led to difficulties in involving communities in health action, and slowed the pace of integration of vertical disease control campaigns into the general health infrastructure. It was further compounded by weak planning and management of health development, especially at the operational levels, and the imbalance and irrelevance of human resources for health (Tarimo & Webster 1994).

The late 1990s saw an intense democratization process in many LMI countries, which, in turn, led to a certain amount of devolution/decentralization of power and responsibility to the people, thereby increasing their involvement in the planning and management of development programmes including health. The World Bank, IMF, and many other multilateral and bilateral donors used these changes in devolution as a condition for extending external assistance. Thus, many reforms for health systems initiated in LMI countries in the last few decades included devolution of authority to local bodies on health matters as an important strategy. The approach varied among countries depending on the extent of devolution and decentralization, division of responsibility and resources, and the management capacity at each level of the health systems. Most nationwide health development programmes promoted community awareness and the creation of active and effective mechanisms for community involvement. A few successful programmes in various parts of the world showed that the conventional approach of merely expanding basic health services had proved inadequate. It was proving impossible economically to bear the cost of expansion of basic healthcare services by the public sector to the entire population in the face of the existing resource constraints. Thus, many countries adopted to deploy a large number of community-level health volunteers, trained for short periods, who constituted as a third force of human resources for health. This proved to be a success for expanding essential healthcare coverage in many countries. With their involvement in health action, many essential public health interventions especially in disease prevention and control including epidemic control and immunization, health promotion, maternal and child healthcare including nutrition promotion, information gathering and surveillance, treatment of minor ailments, and environmental health promotion were undertaken. Such public health initiatives received international attention as well as recognition, and their movements had been promoted by instituting the Sasakawa Health Prize, the Health for All medals, and other forms of recognition.

A series of new health reforms, such as improving the content of essential packages for health and the way these were financed, were undertaken as the third generation of health reforms. Many models of health financing either at national scale or local level were developed in LMI countries, including reforms in expanding social health insurance. Another global trend in health development is the increasing role of the private sector both for profit and non-profit. The issue of an appropriate public and private mix in health systems had been extensively debated, that stemmed from the fact that the larger proportion of health expenditure came out of private sources mainly from out-of-pocket (OOP) payment, while the governments could not increase their expenditure on health. Fewer agencies of non-profit were involved in public health development and medical care to the unserved populations. It is not a simple solution of either private or not, but a balanced mix of both that can fit within the existing socioeconomic, political, and health situation of the country and also how far the national health plans would ensure that wider reforms would address the gaps in healthcare and create a pro-poor health system.

Health development in the twenty-first century could be achieved through a dynamic yet harmonious balance between health in terms of consumption and health as an investment. Bringing in theory and practices of economic and social sciences, health development programmes had been designed by introducing the cost-effective health intervention packages tailored to economic and social realities of each country. New generations of health reforms were undertaken within the framework of health for all policy for the twenty-first century, as adopted in the World Health Declaration in May 1998 (WHO 1998a). Many LMI countries, especially those receiving substantial external investments in health from multilateral financial institutions like the World Bank, had used essential healthcare packages as part of their national health sector-wide programmes.

Health policy and planning

After WHO had introduced the country health planning (CHP) process for health sector development in the 1980s as part of capacity strengthening for policy-making and health development planning, planning and budgeting in the health sector became the norm for national development in many LMI countries. The centrally directed planning framework using CHP process had moved many LMI countries to a higher level of health attainment. It was highly successful in the era when selective healthcare interventions like immunization, malaria or leprosy control, and MCH/Family Planning were promoted through federally or centrally controlled development projects. The development assistance by bilateral and multilateral financing institutions in the 1990s had enhanced the financing of vertical programmes and later that of integrated health sector programmes. Attempts were made from a wider socioeconomic perspective by fostering greater involvement of national and international stakeholders in sectoral policy development and planning, both for short- and long-term periods.

With the initiatives of the World Bank and other external donors, the national poverty reduction strategy papers had included health as an integral part of development efforts. The long- and medium-term national health sector development plans in line with the global goals, such as HFA goals, Child-Summit goals and UN-MDG were developed, using the Sector Wide Approach (SWAp). SWAp is a wider consultative process involving the civil society groups, public and private sectors, and external donors. A shared policy framework using SWAp and a common or pooled programme budget has allowed less duplication, better resource allocation, and more opportunity for working in partnership (Cassels 1997). The health development plans were much more results-oriented and outcomes focused, and the development activities and efforts are geared toward achieving health impacts. By pulling all health development plans together into one framework using SWAp, the national health planners and programme managers could better identify the strategies and activities needed to achieve national and global objectives with estimated resources. There was growing experience in using SWAp for health development in LMI countries, which suggested that SWAp represented an effective investment in health systems capacity and government ownership. The evidence also showed that the successes would depend upon how far specific and high priority objectives were embedded for targeting the poor in the health sector plans (WHO 2000a). The recent initiative in one team, one programme, and one budget, for the country's development as part of UN reforms also fits in this perspective.

Health financing

While the high-income countries continued to increase spending on health in response to growing expectations, LMI countries were struggling with major problems in managing and financing their health systems. In the poorer LMI countries, the health sector financing had stagnated or even contracted over the last 25 years, whilst the demands for health had grown exponentially. The investment in health in terms of the proportion of GNP spent on health ranged from 1 to 6 per cent in many LMI countries as compared to more than 10 per cent in the developed world. Due to relatively low public investment in health, people had to spend more from out-of-pocket for appropriate access to essential healthcare. In most of LMI countries especially least developed nations, the OOP payment constituted a major source of financing. For example, according to the World Health Report 2006, the OOP payment for Nepal accounted for 73 per cent of total health expenditure, while it was 75 per cent in Bangladesh and 66 per cent in China (WHO 2006a).

Many LMI countries in the mid-1980s had introduced user charges, with a view to cover some part of the public health expenditure. While some might support that the user fees would increase revenue that could be used to improve the quality of public health services and expand coverage, but the amount of revenue recovered was not high enough to recover the increasing amount of health expenditure. Moreover, the poor would not be able to afford the fee, and access the most essential necessary healthcare services. In some LMI countries, community financing is organized and managed by the community, with some form of Government subsidy or technical support. The main aim of universal coverage of health financing is to develop health systems that guarantee universal access to effective health services regardless of a person's income or social status (Kutzin 1998). While the coverage of social health insurance (SHI) was high in the Americas, it was very low in many LMI countries of Asia and Africa, and almost non-existent in some LMI countries. Those who had such social health insurance usually had the coverage for formally employed workers as part of social welfare schemes usually managed by the Ministry of Labour. The major challenge in all these countries was how to extend the coverage of social health protection from the formal sector to the non-formal sector of employment, to non-working spouses, or to the child dependants and other family members (Than Sein 2002). A health system predominately funded by public sources including general taxation and social health insurance provides more equitable access by all members to a wide range of health services. These types of prepayment-based financing arrangements reduce the undue financial burdens from medical care costs and contain costs of health services (WHO 2006b).

Health research and development

Health research and development have been progressive with advancements in science and technology, and health systems development. In the past, LMI countries relied on the results of research and development from the high-income countries. In practical terms, many scientific breakthroughs in health actually came from the experiences gained in LMI countries such as identification of causal organisms for communicable diseases and the way they are transmitted, immunization against smallpox and other infectious diseases, development and use of contraceptives, and multidrug therapy. Promotion of research capability in LMI countries was high on the development agenda for many years. With the support and strengthening of WHO Collaborating Centres and networks of national centres of excellence around the world, and with the establishment of regional and global advisory committees on health research by WHO during the 1960–70s, the scientific communities from LMI countries played significant roles in international research promotion and development. A series of research and development efforts were initiated in the area of prevention and control of tropical diseases including vaccines, promotion of human health and reproduction including contraception and other fertility control measures, strengthening of health systems, protection of environmental health, control of non-communicable diseases, and development of essential healthcare technologies.

In order to promote innovation and intensification of health reforms during the post Alma-Ata era, people realized that health systems research (HSR) was an important tool for innovation and programme development for strengthening health systems based on PHC and HFA principles, especially in setting priorities for health research (Nuyens 2007). Many countries established and strengthened their HSR units/sections within the ministries of health or as separate autonomous national institutes to conduct health systems and health policy research, and to provide appropriate scientific, evidence-based information to decision-makers. Considerable progress was made in capacity building and capability strengthening in promoting health systems research. The development works further pave the way for developing an effective national health research system. International exchanges of experiences of the countries on health research system development had been promoted through various forums and networks of institutions and expertise had been established in recent years such as Asia-Pacific Health Research System Network and African Health Research System Network. When compared with investment in basic science research, the budget allocation for HSR remained relatively small both at national or international levels. There has been an attempt to recommend that the developing countries need to invest at least 2 per cent of national health expenditures in health research and research capacity strengthening, and at least 5 per cent of the development aid for the health sector from external agencies has to be earmarked for the same purpose (WHO and World Bank 1990). The Ad Hoc Committee on Health Research established by WHO in 1996 concluded that the central problem in health research promotion and development was the '10/90' disequilibrium of investing in health research and development (WHO 1996). An estimated US$56 billion was invested globally for health research, yet only 5–10 per cent was spent on health research on issues that affected the large majority of the world's population. This concern became even more acute in the context of the public health challenges of the twenty-first century.

Improving performance

For over half a century, economic performance indicators, such as Gross Domestic Product (GDP), Gross National Product (GNP) or Gross National Income (GNI), and inflation rates, have been available to policy makers and political leaders accountable for economic management. Using the scientific development and evidence, WHO had attempted to introduce a framework for *health system performance assessment*, with relevant concepts, possible indicators, and an initial report on measuring performance for improving health systems for its 190 Member States in its World Health Report 2000 (WHO 2000b). The original purpose of the framework for measuring health system performance was to establish a foundation for a solid body of evidence on the relationship between the organization and outcomes of health systems, with a view to provide governments with information for health policy development and to enable users to understand better the functions of health systems, and to access information about the extent to which health system outcomes attained. The World Health Report 2000 had created an unprecedented level of interest and debate all over the world, though not necessarily with positive reactions. While some experts, researchers, and governments made formal protests and questioned the underlying theoretical basis, the statistical techniques selected, the reliability of the data, and the reliability of ranking the social outcomes using a composite index, others had expressed their support for further improving the methodology. WHO had attracted extensive media attention and contributed a much-needed debate, but such high visibility could run the risk of a counterproductive effect if technical mistakes remained uncorrected and resultant rankings unsupportable (WHO 2001; Jamaison & Sandhu 2001). A series of technical publications were brought out on various aspects of summary measures of health including development of a composite index for health development (WHO 2002a). A few countries have even attempted the application of such analytical tools either at national or sub-national levels with a view to identifying policy gaps in improving health system performance of respective countries (IIPS/WHO 2006; WHO 2007d). Although several countries expressed strong views on the methodology especially the ranking, the experts highlighted the need for a critical analysis with scientific rigour on the assessment of health system performance in individual countries. Further development and wider consultation would be required to develop acceptable, effective tools and methods for assessment of health system performance.

Disease eradication and elimination

Disease control campaigns

With the advancement and expansion in the application of science, technology, and knowledge immediately after World War II, a number of vaccines, pharmaceuticals, and diagnostic tools were developed and used for public health interventions. Vaccination campaigns against infectious diseases such as smallpox, tuberculosis, and poliomyelitis were started from early 1950s as nation-wide campaigns. Similarly, some tropical diseases were put under control through mass use of chemotherapy. High-income countries had assisted LMI ones to contain the spread of infectious diseases at their source.

Campaign for control of yaws was initiated in Africa, Asia, the Pacific, and Latin America almost immediately after World War II, since antibiotics became available. As early as 1948, WHO and UNICEF had initiated a campaign for global control of yaws by introducing mass treatment with long-acting penicillin. At that time, there were an estimated 20 million cases of yaws worldwide, half of them in Asia. Although yaws was almost eliminated in many LMI countries by the early 1970s, scattered foci of infection still persisted in some parts of Latin America, the Pacific and South and Southeast Asia. A resurgence of yaws cases occurred in India in the mid-1980s. Due to concerted efforts, the annual incidence of yaws in India steadily declined from a peak of 3500 in 1996 to 46 cases in 2003, and no more reported cases since 2004. The spectacular success of yaws control, using the early case identification and mass treatment strategy, provided a boost to the control of other diseases through campaign approach.

Malaria was a tropical disease aimed for control and later eradication since millions of people died during the 1940s. Assured of massive support from international and bilateral agencies, many governments launched large-scale malaria control campaigns in 1950s that expanded progressively in scope and coverage in later decades. Many LMI countries established national malaria research/vector control institutes to provide technical direction, research development and training related to malaria and vector control. Initiated by the World Health Assembly in May 1955, nearly all newly independent LMI countries around the world started launching national malaria eradication programmes, utilizing the strategies such as active case finding with treatment and controlling mosquitoes with DDT insecticide. The malaria eradication in its earlier years saw dramatic successes. The reduction in malaria caseload during 1950–60s was spectacular, as seen from the experience of the countries of WHO Southeast Asia. The malaria caseload in these countries declined from over 100 million cases in 1950 to as low as 230000 in 1965. Through this global funding of Malaria Special Account in the 1960s, the insecticide—DDT and the antimalarial medicines, being produced in the western countries, were supplied to the needy countries in Asia and Africa. This helped to solve to some extent, the deficit in national programmes in LMI countries especially in Asia. Substantial stocks for DDT insecticide and necessary spraying equipment, personnel, and transport for large-scale operations was beyond the means of LMI countries. The inadequate supply and irrational use of medicines for malaria also led to drug resistance. This situation was followed in many countries by reverting programmes for the eradication of malaria to those for control during the mid-1970s. Despite this drawback, there was the beneficial effect of the use of DDT spraying on the control of another infectious disease called kala-azar which was highly endemic in the same groups of countries, and the disease almost completely disappeared by the 1960s (WHO 1992). Many countries also tried to integrate the control programmes for all vector-borne diseases under one national programme. Conceptually as well as managerially, it might be possible to have all vector-borne diseases under one consolidated national programme, practically it had been difficult to implement successfully and effectively. Many vector-borne diseases are still prevailing in many LMI countries.

LMI countries recognized leprosy as a priority communicable disease for centuries. In the absence of effective control methods earlier, people with leprosy and their families were isolated from others and this is still practised in some parts of the world. The discovery of dapsone (DDS) in 1943 and its immediate availability in the early 1950s for treatment of leprosy provided a major boost to leprosy control. The main strategies for leprosy control were mass screening, early detection and treatment with long-term dapsone therapy, case holding and release from control along with health education. Millions of leprosy cases were identified and registered and put under long-term treatment with dapsone. For numerous leprosy patients, dapsone therapy brought the long-denied hope and promise (Than Sein & Kyaw Lwin 2003).

During the eighteenth century, syphilis was usually regarded as the disease of the foreigners, and some Asians used to call it as *Farangi Roga*. Actually, limited information showed that syphilis had already been rampant among the populace in Asia earlier than those periods. Many LMI countries in the 1950s introduced national prevention and control programme for sexually-transmitted disease (STD) including syphilis, using strategies like early case detection, treatment with long-acting penicillin, and health education. Availability of treatment with penicillin actually conveyed a false sense of security, and the STD programmes totally ignored the increasing prevalence of prostitution, promiscuity, and homosexuality, which are the main social determinants. Since these main issues could not be addressed properly, newer STDs like HIV/AIDS, HBV infection, etc. are coming up and flourishing till date.

Cholera is one of the most feared infectious diseases in public health. The public health experience during the nineteenth century in Europe, the Middle-East, and Asia showed that adequate sanitation and safe water supply, as well as adequate personal and food hygiene practices could contain many local epidemics and the six global pandemics of cholera effectively in the past 10 decades. The use of new therapeutics and adequate rehydration therapy with early case detection demonstrated that many deaths from cholera could be averted. A series of cholera epidemics that occurred since 1991 due to the new O139 strain had affected more than 120 countries around the world. One of the serious concerns is that it would become the eighth cholera pandemic (Lee 2001). For LMI countries with more than 1 billion people without access to safe water supply and improved sanitation, it would be a major challenge to address the potential pandemic of cholera in the years to come.

Smallpox control—a public health success

Control of smallpox is to be recorded as the most successful public health intervention. Using the traditional technique of variolation—inoculation of pus taken from smallpox cases to healthy persons in Asia for many centuries—Edward Jenner in 1796 introduced a modified technique, not from human smallpox but from cowpox cases. The wider application of this method—vaccination—to the general population in Europe and the Americas had resulted in controlling smallpox within a shorter period (Henderson 1997). The spread of smallpox could not be controlled widely in other parts of the world, due to the variable purity and potency of the vaccine, poor vaccination techniques, and low coverage among the general population. In the early 1950s, nearly a million cases were reported in more than 100 countries/territories, with 58 per cent of cases being reported from British India alone. Lack of commitment and lack of broad humanitarian objectives by the colonial administration, limitation of technical and human resources, and lack of confidence in vaccination by the local populace were hindering the progress for control of smallpox through vaccination (Ko Ko *et al.* 2002). Thus, even more than a century after the discovery of smallpox vaccination, the disease continued to rage throughout the world. With the assurance of continued supply of freeze-dried smallpox vaccine, WHO, in 1958, advocated for worldwide smallpox control, through mass vaccination campaigns aiming at eradication. Initially, many LMI countries were sceptical on global campaign, since there was an inadequate supply of smallpox vaccine as well as inaccessibility of health facilities by a large segment of population. With intensive advocacy and support by international agencies, they later adopted smallpox control, organized through mass campaigns using basic health staff and institutions backed by legislation.

By the middle of the 1960s, several LMI countries achieved the smallpox eradication status (WHO 1964). However, smallpox still killed 2–3 million people annually worldwide as recently as 1967 and till the mid-1970s; and some countries in Asia and Africa had experienced sporadic outbreaks. Intensive case-detection and mass vaccination in affected areas successfully contained the disease, even in those countries where the incidence was high and relatively few people were vaccinated (Foege *et al.* 1971; Fenner *et al.* 1988). India launched a massive public health campaign called Operation Smallpox Zero in the early 1970s which led to the last case in May 1975 (Basu *et al.* 1979). Other neighbouring countries also followed suit leading to no more smallpox cases by 1975. The last naturally-acquired human smallpox case in the world was reported in Somalia in October 1977. After considering the final report of the global international commission on smallpox eradication, the 33rd World Health Assembly in May 1980 made a declaration that the world was free from natural transmission of smallpox. This was certainly the most spectacular public health achievement of the twentieth century. However, the final extinction of the smallpox virus itself has remained controversial from the scientific point of view. Especially after anthrax was used as a biological weapon in USA in 2001 and the occurrence of pandemic avian influenza in recent years, a consensus has not been reached on the timing for destruction of existing variola virus stocks. Currently, the decision for destruction of the variola virus has been deferred to 2010 (WHO 2006c).

The possibility of eradicating disease was mentioned by Thomas Jefferson in 1800 referring to the discovery of smallpox vaccine by Jenner. Eradication and elimination of infectious diseases such as the eradication of smallpox, yellow fever, and yaws or the elimination of soil-transmitted helminthes had been attempted for decades as public health goals. Achieving the eradication of smallpox by 1980 provided an impetus to develop acceptable public health strategies for eradication and elimination of many infectious and non-infectious diseases. A number of such diseases have been examined and identified as candidate diseases for possible global and local eradication or elimination. Accelerated development and rapid application of scientific and other technological knowledge in public health with increased access to healthcare in all corners of the world, has made a tremendous impact on disease prevention and control, especially prevention and control of immunizable diseases.

Expanded programme of immunization

By 1970, many safe, effective, and affordable vaccines, medicines and other chemicals, and diagnostic means were available to expand activities related to the prevention and control of both infectious and non-infectious diseases. While some diseases were aimed for elimination (to have zero cases, but the risk of disease remains), some were targeted for eradication (to have zero cases with zero risk) (Goodman & Foster 1998). With improved availability of vaccines for infectious diseases such as measles, poliomyelitis, diphtheria, tetanus, and others, many LMI countries initiated the Expanded Programme of Immunization (EPI) in the mid-1970s, in collaboration with WHO, UNICEF, and other partners, with the aim of controlling these diseases through the expansion of coverage of universal child immunization (immunizing at least 80 per cent of all 2-year-old children with essential vaccines). It took more than two decades for many LMI countries to improve the immunization coverage to the desired levels for elimination or eradication of vaccine-preventable diseases. Many LMI countries initially felt that the goal of universal child immunization might not be achievable, since they lacked human and financial resources to effectively deliver vaccines. Bilateral and multilateral donors, regional financial institutions, and UN system agencies provided large-scale assistance to LMI countries to improve immunization coverage through support of national EPI programmes. Within 10 years, nearly 80 per cent of all 2-year-old children globally were immunized against six major vaccine-preventable diseases. As an outcome, the lives of approximately 2 million children were saved from disability and deaths from six diseases. It is actually a concerted global effort with input of large financial and human resources to achieve and maintain a higher level of coverage. The EPI initiative was termed by many public health professionals as a silent revolution in public health in the twentieth century.

Figure 1.3.2 shows the immunization coverage of major childhood vaccines from 1980 to 2005, from the available data from the WHO Southeast Asia (SEA) Region. New vaccine for HepB was introduced as part of vaccines to be covered under routine EPI programme in late 1990s in several endemic countries, but the coverage does not yet reach to a higher level. GAVI initiative has provided necessary financial and material support to enhance this immunization programme. There was a parallel improvement in the production, transport, and storage of the EPI vaccines. Extensive training of health staff at various levels of the national health systems for programme management and epidemiology was undertaken. Similarly, the extended social mobilization efforts had boosted the increase in coverage of immunization (WHO 1993). Countries in the Americas, Europe, and some parts of Asia were able to achieve effective control of poliomyelitis by higher immunization coverage from 1980 onwards. This experience had led to a strong belief by many health policy makers and planners and public health professionals that the world might be ready to adopt plausible eradication and elimination strategies for prevention and control of diseases especially through effective immunization, both locally, nationally, regionally, and later globally. Community involvement in such extensive public health measures emerged as a significant strategy, together with improved mechanisms for bringing together the private and public sector agencies (WHO 1998b).

In 1988, the world community resolved to achieve global eradication of poliomyelitis by 2000 within the existing global EPI initiative, and also within the context of strengthening health systems and disease surveillance. This global call for poliomyelitis eradication provided LMI countries with challenges as well as opportunities, since they had to improve and sustain the expanded coverage

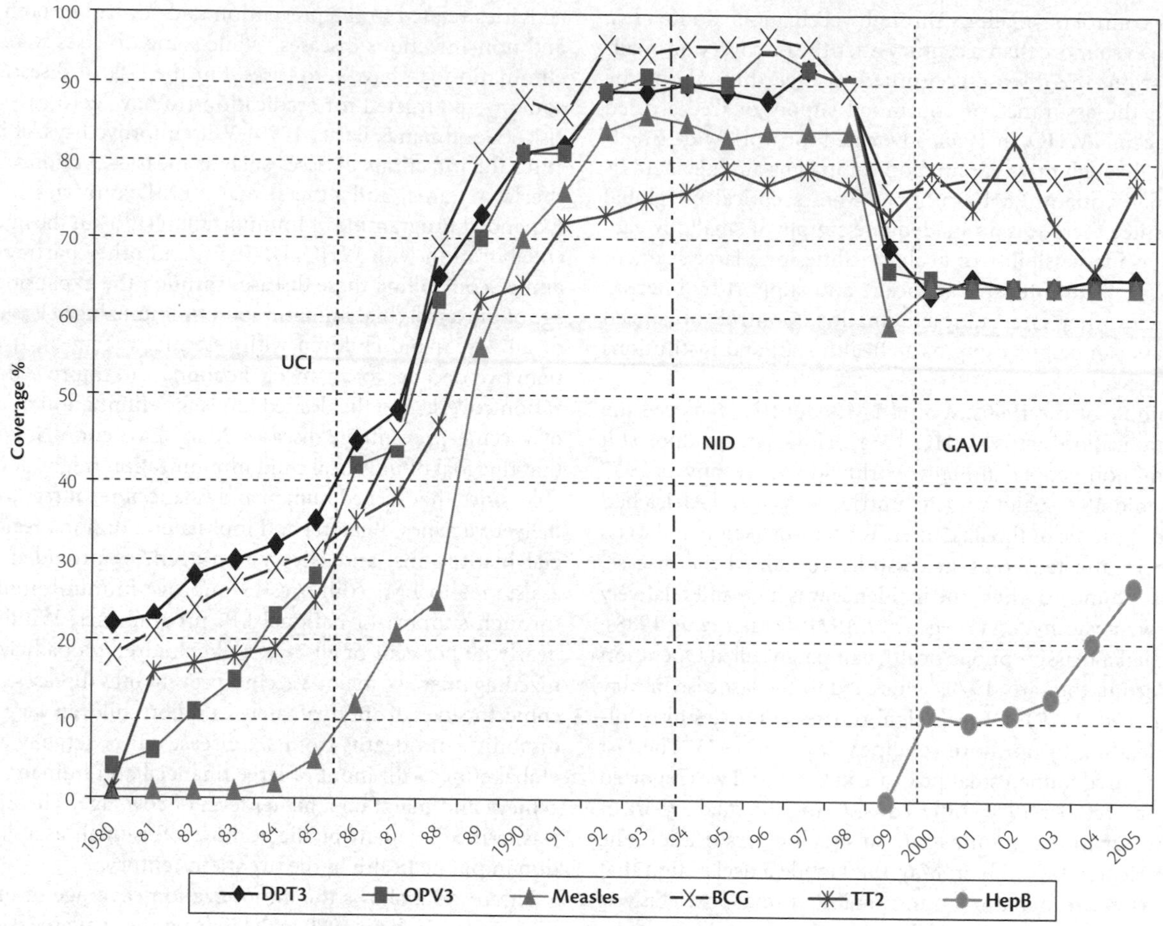

Fig. 1.3.2 Immunization coverage, WHO SEA Region, 1980–2005.
Source: WHO/SEARO, IVD Unit (UCI-Universal Child Immunization; NID-National Immunization Days).

of immunization, while they were improving their health infrastructure. At the start of the global poliomyelitis eradication campaign, the wild poliomyelitis virus was circulating in more than 125 countries in five continents, disabling more than 1000 children every day. While the average global coverage of poliomyelitis immunization had remained over 80 per cent since 1990, some LMI countries were not able to achieve that level and some were even less than 50 per cent. In order to improve this situation and also with the possibility of the interruption of transmission of wild virus by high coverage, an additional strategy was piloted in the Philippines and China, then followed as nation-wide campaigns in other polio-endemic countries. This new strategy was the adoption of a national immunization day (NID) by assigning a fixed date of a year as a special day for immunization. By the end of 1997, more than 450 million children under-5 years of age (almost half of the world's children) in at least 80 LMI countries were immunized with oral polio vaccine through NID campaigns, in addition to over 500 million children immunized through routine EPI programme. Surveillance of acute flaccid paralysis (AFP) in these countries was also intensified with additional human resources, proper case investigations, and prompt laboratory support.

Figure 1.3.3 shows the trends of polio immunization coverage by WHO regions in 1980, 1990, and 1996 to 2005, where the coverage of polio vaccine for infants is the lowest in the countries of Africa. With GAVI support, there was some improvement in coverage in other regions, compared with Africa. By 2003, around 415 million children under-5 years in the 55 LMI countries were immunized with over 2.2 billion doses of oral polio-vaccine. Similarly, 14 previously polio-free countries in Africa and Asia were able to stop the epidemics of poliomyelitis that had occurred by importation of wild poliovirus from other countries in 2005. Egypt with indigenous polio transmission existed for more than 5000 years from the time of Pharaohs and was declared a polio-free status by January 2005. China, after two rounds of NID in 1993 and 1994, showed the reduction of poliomyelitis from 5000 cases in 1990 to almost zero in 1995. India has been implementing the NID campaigns for poliomyelitis elimination as part of its national EPI programme from 1993; however, the wild poliovirus is still circulating in certain parts of the country even in 2007.

By early 2007, only four countries—India, Afghanistan, Pakistan, and Nigeria—remain endemic with indigenous transmission of wild poliovirus. They accounted for 92 per cent of all new cases of poliomyelitis. The remaining 8 per cent of cases occurred in a few countries where local wild poliovirus transmission is controlled but being reintroduced. Surveillance on new polio cases and acute flaccid paralysis cases with timely and prompt response for control is crucial in these countries. A concerted effort to intensify the polio eradication by interrupting transmission of wild poliovirus is required by implementing the multiple rounds of supplementary immunization activities, and by limiting the risk of reintroducing

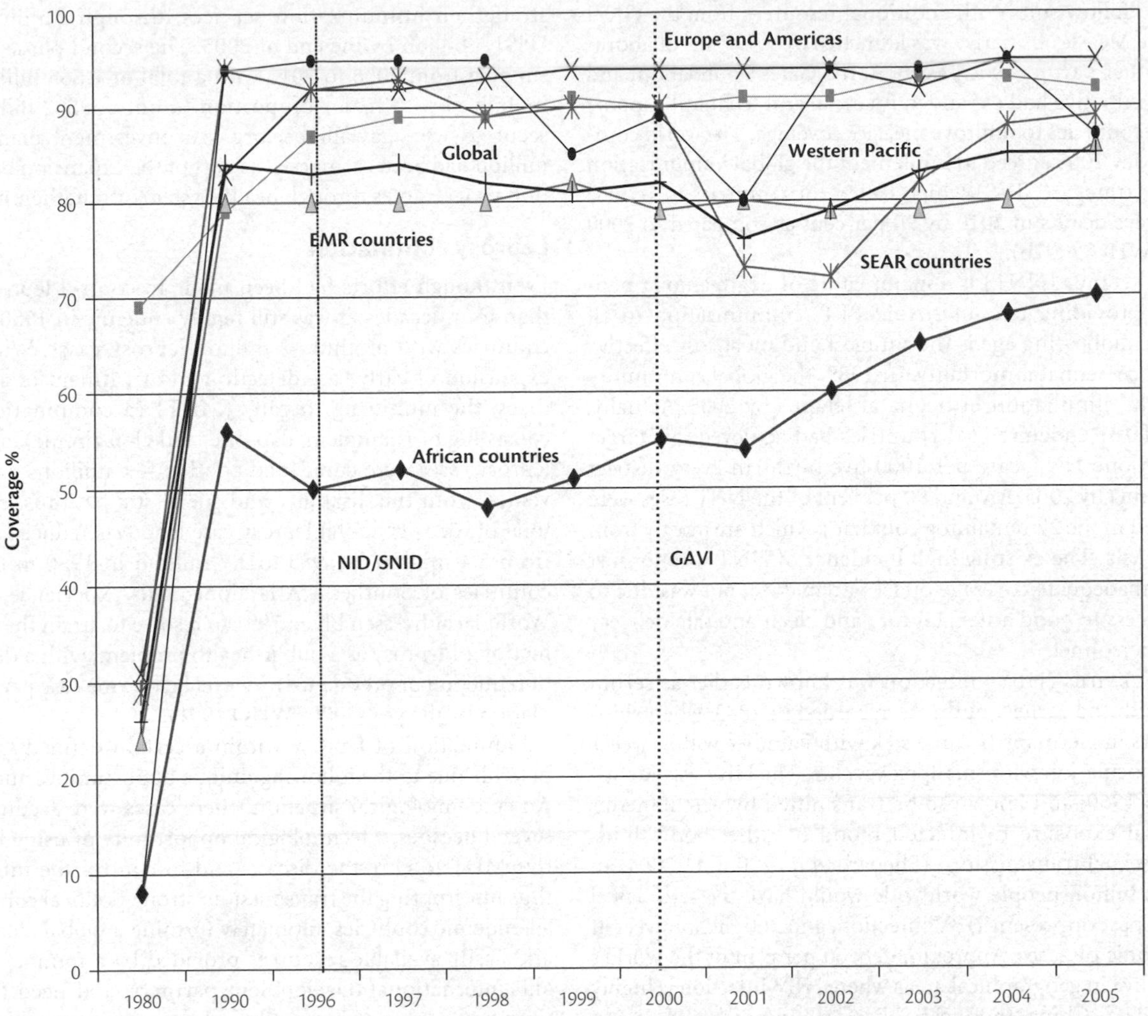

Fig. 1.3.3 Polio Immunization Coverage for < 1 year of age by WHO Regions, 1980, 1990, and 1996–2005.
Source: WHO/IVD Unit 2007.

wild poliovirus into poliomyelitis-free areas with stronger political will and support with national and international resources. An unprecedented level of financial support to the global polio eradication effort by the bilateral and multilateral donors, Rotary International and the Bill and Melinda Gates Foundation has ensured the intensification of polio elimination campaigns. By 2010, it is expected that all the countries around the world will be free from indigenous transmission of wild poliovirus (WHO 2006d). If and when, efforts to eradicate wild poliovirus from the world succeed by 2010, this would represent a major landmark in public health in this new Millennium.

Other immunizable diseases

While success on a global scale for polio elimination is imminent, there were disturbing declining trends in routine immunization during the last few years, especially among LMI countries. The donor-driven EPI programmes organized solely for the purpose of improved immunization coverage in the 1990s were short-lived and collapsed after the withdrawal of external inputs. Immunization coverage of women of child-bearing age with anti-tetanus vaccination had never reached the expected level of more than 80 per cent in most countries, and similar patterns were also seen for other vaccinations. By 2003, more than 27 million children worldwide were still missed for immunization in their first year of life, and each year, around 1.4 million children under 5 years of age died from vaccine-preventable diseases. Intensified efforts for sustaining coverage through routine immunization services were necessary to achieve the desired reduction in mortality and morbidity.

Measles is an easily transmitted viral infection responsible for around 10 per cent of deaths from all causes among under-5 children globally. While more than 20 million children are affected by measles and nearly 800 000 children were dying annually, the routine measles coverage during the last decades globally was around 70–80 per cent. A majority (>95 per cent) of these deaths occurred in the low-income countries with GNP per capita less than US$1000. The main reason for high measles morbidity and mortality was the failure to deliver at least a single dose of measles vaccine to more than 90 per cent of infants. A concerted effort to boost the coverage of measles vaccination from around 70 per cent to a higher and sustained level of over 90 per cent of every birth cohort was required to interrupt transmission of measles especially among the children in these countries. Maintaining a high level of coverage over 90 per cent and the ultimate elimination of measles in the Americas in 2000 had prompted other developed and developing countries to follow suit. With additional resources from the GAVI Alliance, the Measles Initiative was launched by WHO in collaboration with other partners such as JICA, the Gates Foundation, and CIDA. The initiative had expanded financial and technical support to endemic countries to improve measles coverage. The world community in May 2005 agreed to implement the global immunization and vision strategy (GIVS) which called for countries to reduce global measles deaths in 2010 by 90 per cent as compared to 2000 estimates (WHO 2007b).

Neonatal tetanus (NNT) is a major cause of death among neonates, and providing tetanus toxoid (TT) immunization to all women of childbearing age is the simplest and most cost-effective way to reduce neonatal mortality. In 1989, the global community called for the elimination of neonatal tetanus by 2005. Actually, only 104 of 161 endemic LMI countries had achieved this target of less than one NNT case per 1000 live births in every district (www.who.int) by 2005. Around 90 per cent of the NNT cases were concentrated in the 27 remaining countries, which are mostly from Africa and Asia. The existing high incidence of NNT was not just because of inadequate coverage of TT vaccination, but was due to the poor access to good antenatal care and clean and safe delivery by trained personnel.

Hepatitis B virus (HBV) infection was known earlier as serum hepatitis, with the earliest outbreak recorded in 1883, when shipyard workers in Germany became sick with jaundice within weeks following inoculation with smallpox vaccine. The HBV was identified only in 1960, and known to be transmitted by percutaneous and mucosal exposure to infected blood or other body fluids (including sexual transmission) (Shepard *et al.* 2006). In 2004, an estimated 2 billion people worldwide would have the serological evidence of past or present HBV infection, and 360 million were at risk for chronic diseases. Approximately 60 per cent of the world's population live in geographical areas where HBV infection is highly endemic such as China, Indonesia, Nigeria, and much of Asia and Africa (WHO 2004a). More than 150 countries worldwide had adopted the immunization against Hepatitis B as part of national EPI programmes. With the recommendation of WHO for utilizing the plasma-derived Hepatitis B (HepB) vaccine, many endemic countries had introduced it since 1992. The plasma-derived vaccine was later replaced by the recombinant HepB vaccine. Countries that started HepB vaccination since mid-1980s showed that the sero-prevalence among children was reduced from 10 per cent to less than 1 per cent, and the annual incidence rate of hepatocellular carcinoma among children of 6–14 years had reduced by half after a decade. If properly managed, HepB infection would be eliminated within the next 20 years.

Since the early 1990s, some LMI countries started introducing new vaccines against mumps, meningitis, rubella, HepB and HepC infections, and haemophilus influenza. Acknowledging the decreasing trends of routine immunization coverage and also the non-availability of vaccines against major diseases that are still prevalent in LMI countries, the Global Alliance for Vaccines and Immunization (GAVI) was launched in 2000 as a public–private partnership, comprised of partners such as WHO, UNICEF, the Bill and Melinda Gates Foundation, the World Bank, the Rockefeller Foundation, the governments of the developing and developed countries, vaccine manufacturers, civil society groups, as well as the research and technical institutes. The GAVI provided 74 LMI countries with new vaccines and related equipment, technical and financial support to strengthen immunization services, through funding of nearly US$1.5 billion by the end of 2005. The second phase of the GAVI support from 2006 to 2010 with a total of US$5 billion has been mobilized with major proportion (around US$2 billion) already secured (www.gavialliance.org). An investment plan of US$500 million had been earmarked as part of the expansion of immunization programmes through health systems strengthening.

Leprosy elimination

Even though efforts had been made to control leprosy for more than four decades, it was still highly endemic in 1980 in over 120 countries with around 12 million leprosy cases. With the rapid expansion of early case detection and treatment of all registered cases, the multidrug therapy (MDT) (a combination of drugs consisting of rifampicin, dapsone, and clofazimine), a few million leprosy cases were cured, and another few millions had been prevented from the disability and social stigma, thus, reducing the total burden. The total leprosy case load was reduced significantly from 5.4 million in 1985 to 3.7 million in 1990 in the endemic countries of Southeast Asia alone. This experience had led the World Health Assembly in 1991 to resolve to attain the global elimination of leprosy as a public health problem, with a defined target of reduction of prevalence to a level below one case per 10 000 population by the year 2000 (WHO 1991).

Elimination of leprosy within a certain defined target date is possible due to the following unique opportunities and principles: An epidemiological situation where cases were accumulated over several decades; a technological opportunity of using highly effective MDT to cure the disease, and to control the infective cases, thus interrupting the transmission; strong political commitment in all endemic countries, ultimately forming a global alliance; readily and easily available resources provided by a number of national and international development partners; and need for setting a time-bound target since such a situation or opportunity may not last for long. WHO together with the Nippon Foundation of Japan, the International Federation of Anti-Leprosy Associations (ILEP), the Novartis Foundation for Sustainable Development, the UN and its specialized agencies, multilateral and bilateral donors and other philanthropic societies, and the endemic countries themselves, formed a Global Alliance on leprosy and the alliance had provided generous and sustained contributions, in terms of financial, material, and human resources to the global effort for leprosy elimination. As a result of joint national and international efforts within a decade or more, the coverage of MDT in endemic countries had improved tremendously, and the case load had decreased significantly. By 2001, 107 out of 122 endemic countries had achieved the global target of leprosy elimination, i.e. reducing the prevalence of leprosy to a level below one case per 10 000 population (WHO 2002b). While China achieved the global elimination target by 1981, Myanmar could achieve it in early 2003. India could reach that target only in 2005.

Globally, a total of 296 500 new cases were detected in 2005, which was almost half of the level in 2000. By early 2007, 117 endemic countries had achieved the global elimination target, with around 200 000 leprosy cases being still registered for treatment with MDT. There are five endemic countries (Brazil, Nepal, DR Congo, Mozambique, and Tanzania), which have yet to achieve the elimination target. Sustained efforts on early case detection, treatment with MDT, and strengthened routine and referral services still remain the cornerstone of leprosy control. The Global Alliance had intensified necessary financial and human resources and logistic support to make leprosy control services sustainable and to ensure quality care easily available to the population through an integrated approach (WHO 2005a). If the current trend in disease reduction is well sustained with the full support from global alliance, the global leprosy elimination goal could be achieved and the burden of the disease further reduced in all endemic countries in the near future. Leprosy elimination would be another case of a successful public health initiative in the twenty-first century.

Neglected tropical diseases

While efforts are made to prevent and control many tropical diseases around the world, some countries felt that there are some neglected tropical diseases (NTD), such as visceral leishmaniasis or kala-azar, onchocerciasis, dracunculiasis, soil-transmitted helminthic infections, lymphatic filariasis, trachoma, schistosomiasis, the Chagas' disease, African trypanosomiasis, and leprosy, because they are localized conditions or of low morbidity or mortality, or interventions may not yet be available or may be too expensive.

For example, visceral leishmaniasis first came to the attention of Western doctors in 1824 in India where it was initially thought to be a variant form of malaria. Local people gave the name 'kala-azar' to the disease, meaning a disease with high temperature and darkening of the skin on abdomen and extremities. Visceral leishmaniasis is a parasitic disease transmitted by infected sand flies. It is highly prevalent in various localities in Asia, Africa, and southern Europe. Due to the extensive use of residual insecticide DDT for the malaria campaigns during the 1960–70s, the prevalence of visceral leishmaniasis has reduced to a large extent. The new medicine *Miltefosine* as an oral medicine is currently available in India and in neighbouring countries. The Institute for OneWorld Health, an international public–private partnership charity organization, is piloting the visceral leishmaniasis control programme using paromomycin, which was originally identified as the drug of choice in the 1960s and abandoned because of non-profitability for production. Until newer drugs are available at affordable price and accessible means to the mass population in these endemic countries, the misery and suffering due to visceral leishmaniasis would continue.

Onchocerciasis also known as river blindness is another parasitic infection caused by the filarial worm (*Onchocerca volvulus*) and transmitted by female black flies (*Simulium*). Even after the launching of Global Onchocerciasis Control Programme launched in 1974 in partnership with WHO, FAO, UNDP, the World Bank, and a coalition of more than 20 donors and agencies, some 86 million people were at risk and about 18 million were infected, 99 per cent of whom were in Africa, by 1990. A million people were visually impaired and over 350 000 were blind as a consequence of infection. The onchocerciasis programme in the Americas was converted into an elimination campaign in 1991. Similar changes occurred in Africa in 1996. The renewed initiative for elimination of river blindness with additional support from Carter Center, the Bill and Melinda Gates Foundation, Merck & Co., Inc., Lions Clubs, and US-CDC was launched again in the early 2000s, to reduce severe pathological manifestations of the disease through wider use of case management with an effective microfilarial drug (*ivermectin*) (WHO 2006e).

Before 1980, more than 10 million cases of dracunculiasis also known as guinea worm disease, were reported in Africa and South Asia annually. A global campaign to eradicate dracunculiasis was initiated in 1980 by the Centres for Disease Control and Prevention (CDC), USA, taking into account the implementation of International Drinking Water Supply and Sanitation Decade (IWSSD), 1981–1990. Although no medicine was available for this disease, the world community in 1986 called for its elimination by disruption of transmission through improvement of water supply and sanitation as well as promoting personal hygiene. African ministers of health resolved in 1988 to eradicate dracunculiasis by the end of 1995. The endemic countries in Africa and Asia launched elimination campaigns using combined strategies such as clean and safe drinking water supply and sanitation as part of IWSSD activities, improved community awareness and involvement in personal hygiene, surveillance and case containment, and larval control, and also with some cash incentives to identify cases. With concerted effort, the number of cases had been reduced from 3.2 million in 1986 to less than a million in 1989, and subsequently, to around 10 000 cases by 2005 with almost 90 per cent of these remaining cases in Ghana and Sudan. Main reasons of failure to control in the latter two countries were inadequate human resources, poor sanitation and water supply, and the continuing civil war that hampered the implementation of eradication campaigns (WHO 2006f).

Trachoma was an infectious chronic eye disease affecting around 400 million people in 1980, of which more than six million people became blind. Trachoma affected more in poor people and children due to inadequate water supply and unhygienic personal practices. People living in the dry and un-arid zones of the endemic tropical countries were being affected most. Many endemic countries implemented the SAFE strategy (surgery, antibiotics, facial cleaning, and environmental health) under the integrated trachoma control programme, within the Vision 2020 strategy, and with the ultimate aim of elimination of the disease. WHO estimated that in 2002 there were 3.6 million cases of blinding trachoma worldwide, and the majority is in LMI countries. A Global Alliance called GET 2020 (Alliance for Global Elimination of Blinding Trachoma by 2020) was established in 1996 with the partnership of endemic countries, WHO, Helen Keller Worldwide, the Carter Center, the Conrad N. Hilton Foundation, *Christoffel Blinden Mission* (CBM), Pfizer's International Trachoma Initiative (ITI) among others. During the last 7 years, nearly 41 million antibiotic treatments have been administered, approximately 240 000 people have received sight-saving surgery, and a few million people in endemic countries have benefited from health education and improved access to water and sanitation. If the constraints on the availability of antibiotics and specialized surgical sets could be overcome through the efforts of international alliances, the elimination of trachoma could even be achieved by 2010, 10 years ahead of the target set under the GET 2020 campaign (Tun Aung Kyaw 2005).

Lymphatic filariasis (LF) is another parasitic disease aimed for elimination, which is a blood-borne infection by microscopic, thread-like parasitic worms—microfilariae. By 2005, an estimated 1.3 billion people in 83 endemic countries were at risk. Of these, around 80–100 million people are having the disease but no symptoms. Another 15–20 million people would suffer from elephantiasis (swelling of the legs, hands, and genital organs). An improvement in the environmental health could interrupt the transmission and reduce the parasitic levels. Since the 1960s, national LF control programmes were introduced in many countries by adopting mass blood surveys and treatment of cases with appropriate medicine, in combination with appropriate vector control. Despite these efforts for decades, the disease continues to be highly prevalent in many countries mainly in Asia, the Pacific, and Africa. The 50th World Health Assembly in 1998 called for the elimination of lymphatic filariasis as a public health problem (WHO 2000c). Later, endemic countries developed national LF elimination programmes, with an aim of reducing it to a cumulative incidence rate over 5 years of less-than one new case per 1000 susceptible individuals. All endemic countries joined WHO and the development partners, including multinational pharmaceutical corporations like SmithKline Beecham and Merck & Co., by launching a global programme for eliminating lymphatic filariasis (GPELF) with the main goals of interrupting the transmission of infection by providing appropriate mass drug administration (MDA), and alleviating and preventing both the suffering and disability caused by the disease by providing appropriate healthcare (Molyneux *et al.* 2000). By 2006, 42 of the 82 endemic countries were implementing the MDA programmes with over 250 million people being treated with multidrug therapy for mass population. Most of these countries had completed five rounds of mass treatment in the endemic districts and were assessing withdrawing the MDA (WHO 2006g). There is hope that it may be possible to eliminate LF in the near future in some LMI countries through sustained and concerted strategies.

The Global Network for Neglected Tropical Diseases Control (GNNTDC) was a public–private partnership launched in 2006 to raise the profile of neglected tropical diseases and to stimulate a paradigm shift in disease control efforts. This partnership will concentrate on the control of a single tropical disease, and will work in collaboration with WHO to design an integrated drug administration platform that would address the seven neglected tropical diseases such as trachoma, soil-transmitted helminthic infections, and other parasitic diseases. The aim of the global network was to contribute toward the achievement of the UN MDG by eliminating and controlling the neglected diseases through an integrated mass drug delivery approach. A synergistic approach will streamline operational activities, improve efficiencies, and ensure that the priority health needs of impoverished communities in LMI countries are met (www.gnntdc.org).

Since the idea for eradication was started with the efforts to eradicate yellow fever in the eighteenth century, the terms—eradication and elimination—were used extensively and loosely for prevention and control of communicable diseases and later even for non-communicable diseases. This led to a misunderstanding of the purposes and sometimes inappropriate adoption of public health strategies. As far back as 1988, when the global eradication and elimination campaigns against many infectious diseases were launched, the International Taskforce for Disease Eradication had clarified various terms: Control as reduction of disease morbidity or mortality to an acceptable level with continued control measures; elimination as reduction to zero of an incidence of a specified disease in a defined geographical area with concerted and continued control measures; and eradication as a permanent reduction to zero of the worldwide incidence of infection caused by a specified agent, such that control measures could stop (www.cartercenter.org). With the rapid advancement of science and technology, there is a possibility of eliminating or eradicating some of the existing candidate diseases. Newer candidates might also be added in the near future.

Enhancing healthy lives

Burden of chronic non-communicable diseases

In recent years, many public health experts are debating on the proxy indicators for measuring health status in addition to the usual morbidity and mortality statistics. No measure is still perfect for the purpose of summing up the health of a population. The introduction of a new measure in health science being much debated as advocated in the World Health Report 1999 was the disability-adjusted life expectancy-DALE or healthy life expectancy-HALE. In simple terms, it is most easily calculable and well understood, reflecting all states of health. It is the expected years of life at birth with the adjustment of time spent in poor health, and easily understood as the number of years in full health that a newborn can expect to live, based on current rates of ill-health and mortality. The Global HALE at birth for women in 1999 was 57.8 years, which was 2 years higher than that for men. While infectious diseases continue to be a major public health problem, there were ominous signs that chronic non-communicable diseases (NCD) became increasingly prevalent in LMI countries. Recent estimates of global burden of disease and risk factors showed that over 26 million people died (almost 53 per cent of all deaths) in 2001 in LMI countries, due to chronic non-communicable diseases, such as cardiovascular diseases, diabetes, cancer, mental disorders, injuries, and other disabled diseases and conditions (World Bank 2006a).

Cardiovascular diseases, diabetes, and cancers

Cardiovascular disease (CVD) is a group of disorders of the heart and blood vessels, consisting of hypertension (high blood pressure), coronary heart disease, cerebrovascular disease, rheumatic heart disease, congenital heart disease, cardiomyopathies, deep vein thrombosis, and other heart and blood vessel disorders. More than 60 per cent of the global burden of coronary heart disease occurred in LMI countries (WHO 2004b). With increasing adoption of the lifestyle of the high-income countries by the people in LMI countries, there is likely to be greater exposure to various risk factors such as increased use of tobacco and alcohol, high blood pressure, unhealthy diets with high saturated fat leading to elevated serum cholesterol level and physical inactivity (Reddy & Yusuf 1999). Many large-scale, well-designed clinical trials on reducing risk factors primarily conducted in the established market economies had shown that lowering common risk factors could reduce illness and death from CVD. The dual approach of screening and intervening in cases of relatively high risk of CVD and of fostering population-wide preventive activities is as appropriate in LMI countries as in the high-income countries (Lenfant 2001). Over the past 30 years, mortality from cardiovascular diseases has decreased considerably in the high-income countries due to concerted and sustained efforts of a combination of health promotion, legislative and policy action, prevention of risks, and better case management (NIH 2000). Necessary policy steps could easily be introduced in LMI countries to adopt population-based health promotion and prevention, in combination with management of high-risk cases with proven therapeutic agents. The promotion of healthy diets that limit the intake of saturated fats and sodium, effort to prevent people from use of tobacco and alcohol, and effort to encourage life-long physical activity could be done as a population-wide, large-scale, public health intervention programme for prevention and control of CVD.

Diabetes mellitus is another chronic non-communicable disease, either insulin dependent (Type 1) or non-insulin dependent (Type 2), affecting around 170 million people of over 20 years of age worldwide in 2000. Even though insulin was discovered in 1921 for the treatment of diabetes, many people suffering from insulin-dependent diabetes in LMI countries are not yet accessing it adequately. The people affected by diabetes may increase to 370 million by 2030 if a proper prevention and control strategy is not in place (Wild *et al.* 2004). LMI countries such as India, China, Indonesia, Brazil, and Bangladesh would have a majority of diabetic cases. Maintaining a balanced body weight by height, being physically active for at least 30 min of moderately intense exercise, and taking low sugar and high consumption of vegetables and fruits are the simple and effective strategies for preventing and controlling diabetes. With early screening, diagnosis, and effective management with diet, exercise, and essential medicines, diabetes and its complications can easily be controlled.

Cancer has been a well-known chronic non-communicable disease for many decades, and a leading cause of deaths worldwide with more than 70 per cent of all cancer deaths occurring in LMI countries. Cancer is absent or low on the health agendas of LMI countries. Cancer is actually a generic term used for a group of more than 100 diseases and conditions that affect mainly the liver, lungs, breast, colorectum, cervix, prostate, and stomach. Liver cancer affects approximately 5.5 million people, predominantly caused by the viral hepatitis. In countries of low endemic viral hepatitis, chronic alcoholism and high content of aflatoxins in food are major risk for liver cancer. Stomach cancer is another common cancer caused by *Helicobacter pylori* infection. High consumption of salt, and salted, smoked, pickled, and preserved food is also the common risk for stomach cancer. Introduction of refrigerators and adoption of better methods for food preservation have considerably brought down the incidence of stomach cancer in many countries. Cancer of the breast is another common disease among women which is intimately related to a high-calorie diet, lack of exercise, and reproductive factors. While early detection with proper screening and increasing improvement in therapy has reduced the mortality associated with breast cancer, it is unfortunately not accessible to large segments of the population in LMI countries. Early diagnosis and treatment could reduce mortality of breast cancer by 45 per cent in women above the age of 50 years. Cancer of the uterine cervix is another cancer prevalent among women of childbearing age, which is mainly due to sexually transmitted human papillomavirus (HPV) infection. Pap smear screening has significantly reduced mortality from cervical cancer, and it could bring down the incidence of cervical cancer to less than 5 per 100 000 population in some countries of Europe and North America. Broad implementation of this approach in LMI countries could be hindered by the financial constraints and poor health infrastructure. The introduction of HPV vaccine, especially in low-resource settings could be hindered by its high cost and other challenges in implementing vaccination programmes. All people with incurable cancers could also obtain appropriate palliative care. Most of the population in LMI countries has little access to radiotherapy or other modern oncological services. The rational use of medicines would improve affordability of cancer chemotherapy. Specialists and radiotherapy facilities are few and tend to be located in the metropolitan areas. In the absence of appropriate financial mechanisms and protection, out-of-pocket payment for the diagnosis and treatment of cancer could devastate the affected families and individuals. The installation and maintenance of high-technology equipment stand in the way of equitable radiotherapy service. Cancer control plans should be developed in all LMI countries starting from now, in order to tackle effectively the silent epidemics.

Reducing tobacco and alcohol use

There was a major increase in tobacco-related illnesses and deaths worldwide during the last decades, with four million people killed every year, and if no proper control measures are instituted, the deaths may go up to 10 million. After the United States, four LMI countries, viz. China, Brazil, India, and Indonesia, are the highest producers of tobacco, and total production by these four countries is more than two-third of the tobacco produced globally in 2004 (Mackay *et al.* 2006). Among the various forms of tobacco used, cigarettes account for the largest share of manufactured tobacco products in the world. In addition, people used tobacco in various forms. Tobacco consumption among the youth is also increasing. With an intensive global campaign, WHO launched its global tobacco free initiative in 1998 to galvanize global political support for evidence-based tobacco policies, build and strengthen new and existing partnerships for action, accelerate national, regional, and global strategies for tobacco control, and mobilize resources. The initial focus was on developing the WHO Framework Convention on Tobacco Control (FCTC), the first health treaty initiated by WHO using its constitutional mandate. The WHO FCTC was approved by the World Health Assembly in May 2003, and became an international legal instrument by February 2005 after a mandated number of countries had ratified it. As of February 2007, a total of 168 countries are signatory to the Convention and 146 countries are parties to the Convention (www.who.int/tobacco). The WHO FCTC asserts the importance of national policies and strategies for reducing demand and addressing supply issues for tobacco use. The main provisions of the WHO FCTC includes the regulation of contents, packaging, and labelling of tobacco products, prohibition of sales to and by minors, illicit trade in tobacco products, and smoking in work and public places. It also called for a reduction in consumer demand by price and tax measures, a comprehensive ban on tobacco advertising, promotion and sponsorship, education, training, raising awareness and assistance with quitting, protection of the environment, and the health of tobacco workers. The Convention will help promote the economies that are not dependent on tobacco products, strengthening the women's roles in tobacco control, and supporting the countries by making people aware about the dangers of tobacco, and protecting most vulnerable communities. Several countries in the world now have comprehensive national tobacco control legislation, conforming to the provisions of the WHO FCTC. Under the leadership of the Conference of the Parties, the challenge is to build on the experience of the Convention and to develop strong national and international protocols on specific issues, as well as to support the countries, especially the least-developed nations, in implementing their obligations.

The World Health Report 2002 indicated that there were about 2 billion people worldwide who consume alcoholic beverages, and 76.3 million suffered from alcohol use disorders. A WHO sponsored study conducted in India that showed the financial losses to the state in the long-term were far greater than the immediate revenue (WHO 2006h). A wide range of policy options and interventions for reducing public health problems caused by harmful use of alcohol was advocated. One policy option proposed was to allocate part of the taxes generated from the sales of alcohol to support health promotion, including community education, sports, and recreational activities. Thailand has adopted, under its health promotion act, the use of sin tax on tobacco and alcohol, the proceeds being used for health promotion activities including reducing alcohol consumption and related problems. Other legislative measures adopted by many LMI countries included various measures on the limitation of physical availability of alcohol, by setting a minimum legal age limit, restricting the number, density and locations of sale outlets, or limiting hours and days of sale, and imposing some other restrictions on sale. In recent decades, community-level efforts to control harmful use of alcohol in some countries have been successful through enhanced partnerships and networks, involving public agencies and NGOs.

Other diseases and conditions

An estimated 400 million people worldwide suffer from mental and neurological disorders and other psychosocial problems including substance abuse. According to the World Health Report 2001, an estimated 12.3 per cent of all DALYs were attributable to mental and neurological disorders in 2000. Mental health disorders such as dementia, depression, and schizophrenia, generally affect the elderly. While many LMI countries have established national mental health policies, legislative measures, or mental health promotion programmes, some national policies, legislation, and programmes are based on outdated knowledge, concepts, and approaches (Rafei 2004). A major problem with the community-based approach was the lack of awareness among the community and lack of trained personnel, particularly community-level health workers who would be able to carry out basic essential mental healthcare services. Currently, many LMI countries are particularly affected by the problem of substance dependence. Most countries have developed policies to control substance abuse, with the focus on demand reduction and prevention of harm to substance abusers.

Injuries have emerged as a major public health problem worldwide, as estimated in World Health Report 2004, with almost 16 000 people dying from all types of injuries everyday worldwide. About 50 per cent of these deaths occurred in the countries of Asia and the Pacific. In LMI countries, 34 per cent of all deaths due to injuries are road traffic related. Road traffic injuries are the second leading cause of deaths among both children 5–14 years and young adults aged 15–29 years worldwide. The rapidly rising number of motor vehicles and motorcycles in the world and especially in LMI countries has seen an equally rapid increase in the number of injuries and deaths. Many countries have made progress in implementing national programmes to prevent and control injuries. Some have not yet put injury prevention on the public health agenda, since they considered injury as the problem to be tackled by sectors other than health such as the police, transport, education, and legal authorities. In a few LMI countries, injury prevention and control started with improving medical care services such as the establishment of accident and trauma centres, strengthening emergency ambulance services, and promoting the training on injury care and management. The first step of a public health approach to injury prevention and control is to have appropriate information in order to ascertain the magnitude and characteristics of injuries and their basic causes. An injury surveillance system provides relevant information on the kind of injuries suffered, on those affected, on places and time how people are injured, etc.

Healthy ageing

Many LMI countries have started giving attention to promoting the health of the elderly, focusing on partnerships and promotion of social welfare and healthcare at home and in the community, promotion of traditional family ties, making optimal use of existing healthcare delivery systems, and establishment of old-age homes. Some countries have formulated national policies on ageing and health. A few have started collection and analysis of related information for advocacy, policy and programme development, decision-making, dissemination to the general public, pensioners, healthcare professionals, and policy-makers to promote appropriate services, advice, and practice on healthy ageing. Efforts are also being made to develop an advocacy strategy in close collaboration with government agencies, NGOs, and the media, aiming at influencing public opinion and encouraging support for community-based programmes for healthy ageing. A few countries have also organized research studies related to epidemiology, patterns of the ageing population, and determinants of healthy ageing and improved the capacity of healthcare providers in the area of care of the elderly. The economic, social, and health status of the fast-growing elderly population poses a great challenge to all sectors. The major difficulties in developing appropriate healthcare for the elderly include the lack of reliable data for programme planning, a virtual absence of national policies and strategies for the care of the elderly, and an inadequate infrastructure to cope with their rapidly increasing health needs. The joint family system and family values are gradually being eroded in many countries. With regard to health status, around 6 per cent of the aged are immobile due to various disabling conditions. Approximately 50 per cent of the elderly suffer from chronic diseases. At the same time, health services for the elderly are inadequate. Knowledge among health workers on the specific needs of the elderly is also minimal.

Addressing risks

Since human behaviour occurs in a specific milieu, comprehensive policy interventions that improve the physical, social, and economic environments and modify the social norms of the population have proven to be far more effective in reducing the NCD burden and improving health, rather than a sole focus on behaviour change at the individual level. It is also uneconomical to promote unregulated growth of expensive specialized healthcare services focused on addressing individual patients, usually who come and seek services in an advanced stage of diseases. Healthy public policies are needed to change the physical and socioeconomic environment. Population-wide interventions aimed at reduction of tobacco and alcohol consumption, and promoting physical activity and healthy eating habits coupled with interventions targeting high-risk groups and individuals could greatly reduce the burden of NCD and improve public health outcomes with the potential to prevent at least 80 per cent of cardiovascular disease and diabetes, and 40 per cent of cancers (WHO 2005d). The costs of care and treatment of individual NCD cases are increasingly overstretching the public health systems, as well as the budgets of affected families. It could be considerably reduced by application of cost-effective interventions at the primary prevention level so that people may not even suffer from the diseases. Establishment of basic health facilities and community-based treatment, rehabilitative and palliative services no doubt contributed significantly in improving the quality of life of people with disabilities and those in the terminal stages of chronic diseases. A majority of effective public health interventions for prevention and control of NCD are primarily beyond the direct control of the health ministry.

Comprehensive NCD policies and programmes would require addressing the NCD prevention holistically. The measures include: Development and modification of healthy public policies and appropriate health legislation, regulations and financing mechanisms, modification of physical environment, and resource-sensitive organization and delivery of health services. National programmes need to select the interventions potentially feasible for implementation within existing resources and realistically increased resources in the short and medium term. The ministry of health should take a leadership role in coordinating and promoting partnerships that would involve stakeholders beyond government sectors such as the private sector, civil society groups, individual philanthropists, and international agencies. Governments also have a central role to play in establishing appropriate health financing mechanisms and models.

Health promotion as a core function of public health is effective in reducing the burden of both communicable and non-communicable diseases and in mitigating the social and economic impact of such diseases. It contributes to positive social and behavioural changes among individuals and communities resulting in the reduction of risks, premature deaths, and illness. The goal in promoting health is to mitigate the impact of risk factors associated with broad determinants of health leading to premature death and illness, and ultimately to improve the quality of lives of individuals and communities. To effectively address the identifiable determinants of health, health promotion requires strategic directions and policies to be formulated in addition to political commitment. The Bangkok Charter for Health Promotion in a Globalized World, 2006, confirmed the need to focus on health promotion actions to address the determinants of health. It encouraged stakeholders in all sectors and settings to advocate for health based on human rights and solidarity, to invest in sustainable policies, actions and infrastructure to address the determinants of health, to build capacity for policy development, leadership, health promotion practice, knowledge transfer and research, and health literacy, to regulate and legislate to ensure a high level of protection from harm and enable equal opportunity for health and well-being for all people; and to build alliances with public, private, non-governmental and international organizations, and civil society to create sustainable actions.

New paradigm of public health

Globalization of public health

The transformation of local societies to a global society resulted in the blurring of territories. An analysis on the impact of globalization and health is available in many health and development literature (Chen *et al.* 1999; Society for International Development 1999; Drager & Beaglehole 2001). It is accepted that globalization actually enhanced the opportunities for human advancement as well as economic and cultural growth of all peoples, through sharing of resources. Global markets, global finances, global technology, global knowledge, global solidarity, global governance, and global security—all of these entities have the ability to improve the health of people everywhere and achieve the target of health-for-all. The threats to and opportunities in public health were also analysed extensively within the context of globalization (Yach & Bettchnner 1998; Berlinguer 1999; Navarro 1999; UN 2003). Berlinguer used the term 'microbial unification of the world' as the phenomenon of the transmission of disease epidemics across countries and continents as part of globalization.

Today, the occurrence of a local epidemic of a disease has become a global issue. The rapidly increasing numbers of people travelling and migrating to neighbouring countries or across the world would pose the threat of spreading diseases. As disease agents could pass over any physical boundaries among nations and territories, transmission of disease could take place at any time anywhere in the world. A revised International Health Regulations had been adopted at the 58th World Health Assembly in 2005, in order to prevent, protect against, control, and provide a public health response to the international spread of disease, in ways that are commensurate with and restricted to public health risks, and avoid unnecessary interference with international traffic and trade (WHO 2005b).

The new measures adopted under IHR (2005) included among others: Immediate notification and verification of a public health emergency of international concern; internationally coordinated public health response; and provision of public health measures, including strengthening global surveillance. Certain infectious diseases could also be transmitted through food exports and tourism. If the preparations of food and food products are not carried out in accordance with good manufacturing practices, there are possible threats of spreading infectious diseases associated with the consignments. If proper manufacturing and export practices are followed, the export products could be consumed safely. Yet, there are many trade-related cases from Asia, the Americas, and Africa where exports from LMI countries are restricted or sanctioned by high-income nations, for the purpose of protecting from infectious diseases. Peru lost over US$770 million during the cholera outbreak in 1991, due to trade sanctions by several high-income countries by trade sanction on imports of Peruvian fishes and fishery products. Similarly, India lost around US$4000 million from export earnings due to the plague outbreak in 1994. Several African countries lost millions of dollars due to an embargo on certain fishery products during the cholera outbreaks in 1998 (Kinnon 1998; Miyagishima & Kaferstein 1998).

Emerging and re-emerging diseases

While many old scourges like tuberculosis, malaria, human plague, and leprosy remained or re-emerged as high burden diseases, a few new or previously unrecognized infections such as HIV-AIDS, ebola and other haemorrhagic diseases, SARS, and avian influenza are being reported both in the high-income and LMI countries. Main factors that aggravate this situation include: The change in human demography and job opportunities leading to mass migration; change of human behaviour, especially sexual relations; advancement in technology and industrial development such as air-conditioning, food processing, and preservation; environmental degradation; microbial adaptation and resistance; and the breakdown of public health infrastructure especially surveillance.

Acquired immunodeficiency disease syndrome (AIDS) was unknown before 1981 and its causal organism—the Human

Immunodeficiency virus (HIV) was discovered only in 1983. After a decade of a Global Programme on AIDS (GPA) launched by WHO, UNDP, the World Bank, and other partners, its work was consolidated into a UN AIDS Control Programme (UNAIDS). In the absence of an effective vaccine, the main strategies of prevention and control of HIV/AIDS were political advocacy, mass education on disease including sex education, behavioural intervention and social mobilization, and integrated social development. In industrialized countries, the number of deaths due to AIDS has dropped rapidly due to increasing accessibility of proper care and appropriate therapy. The impact on human development had gone beyond mortality as the epidemic had affected the sustainability of households and the socioeconomic resources of communities (UNDP 1998). An overwhelming majority of people with HIV infection or AIDS are living in LMI countries. The progress in improving life expectancy in the 1970–80s in many LMI countries, especially those in Africa, were reversed by the high burden of HIV/AIDS (WHO 1999b). An effective vaccine is still a long way off. With WHO advocacy in 2005 and support from the Global Fund, access to antiretroviral drugs (ARV) has improved tremendously in many endemic countries.

Tuberculosis (TB), an age-old scourge continues as a globally dangerous infection that led to adoption of a global Stop TB programme in 1991. The problem of TB is more complex than before since drug-resistant TB cases have increased and there is an increasing incidence of co-infection of TB and HIV. Effective case management and the vaccination of infants with BCG, and health education were the main control strategies. Improving socioeconomic conditions, access to good housing and reducing in-door and out-door pollution, and good personal hygienic practices played an important public health role in reducing TB morbidity and mortality. High-burden countries have been compelled to use the directly observed treatment, short-course (DOTS) strategy for effective management of infectious TB cases, thus reducing the infectious case load in a short period. A total of 183 countries and territories were implementing the DOTS strategy during 2004. More than 26 million TB patients were treated under the DOTS programmes over 11 years from 1995 to 2005 (WHO 2006i). The global prevalence of tuberculosis fell from 297 per 100 000 population in 1990 to 229 in 2004, partly as a consequence of DOTS expansion. This enhancement of coverage of TB treatment was accomplished with the support of the Stop TB partnership and the arrangement of the Global Drug Facility.

Even after initiating eradication campaigns during 1950–60s and implementing extensive control programmes in 1970–80s, malaria remains a major public health threat worldwide. Every year, over 3 billion people are at risk of contracting malaria and more than 500 million people suffer from acute disease resulting in more than 1 million deaths. Countries along the Mekong river in Asia and other high-malaria endemic countries in Africa joined together to fight the drug-resistant malaria. Many countries had introduced multidrug therapy as the first- and second-line therapy for malaria. Rapid deterioration in the malaria situation in many countries calls for greater efforts by governments of endemic countries and the full support of the international agencies. The global malaria control strategy was adopted at the Ministerial Conference on Malaria held at Amsterdam in 1992 and subsequently endorsed by the World Health Assembly and the UN General Assembly in 1993. In 1998, another global movement—Roll Back Malaria (RBM), was initiated as a global partnership between WHO, UNDP, UNICEF, and the World Bank, to combat malaria by using the strategies already adopted at the Ministerial Malaria Summit. The programme anticipated a 50 per cent reduction in the number of deaths from malaria within a decade through better access by all people in malaria-affected areas to a range of effective interventions (WHO 1999b). Development partners worked together with the malaria-affected countries to achieve this new goal. In recent years, through various funding mechanisms such as the Medicines for Malaria Venture, the Global Fund to Fight AIDS, Tuberculosis and Malaria, the malaria initiative of the President of USA, the World Bank Booster programme for malaria control and the Bill & Melinda Gates Foundation, many national programmes have enhanced their malaria prevention and control activities, especially in improving access to multidrug therapy including adoption of Artemisinin-based combination therapy (ACT), increasing coverage of selected indoor residual spraying and use of effective insecticide-treated bednets (ITN), and increasing availability of rapid diagnostic tests. Funds in millions of dollars were poured into malaria endemic countries to expand the coverage of treatment and use of ITN. Many countries had adopted revised malaria control strategies by scaling up coverage and proper use of ITN, expanding the coverage of diagnosis and treatment coverage with multidrug therapy, and promoting rapid diagnosis tests (RDT), revamping surveillance, and strengthening monitoring and evaluation, organizing advocacy, and launching malaria campaign weeks (WHO 2006j).

The Global Fund to Fight AIDS, Tuberculosis and Malaria (Global Fund) is a partnership between the governments, civil society, the private sector, and the affected communities to operate as a financial instrument to dramatically increase resources to fight three of the world's most devastating diseases. At the sixth round of proposal reviews in 2006, a total of US$846 million worth of proposals from 63 countries around the world had been approved, of which US$453 million was for HIV in 34 countries, US$202 million for malaria in 19 countries, and US$190 million for tuberculosis in 34 countries. Since 2001, the Global Fund has attracted US$4.7 billion for financing, through 2008. During its first two rounds of approving grants, it has committed US$1.5 billion in funding support for 154 programmes in 93 countries worldwide (www.globalfund.org). With this large-scale investment by the Global Fund, millions of people infected with HIV and suffering from AIDS, millions of tuberculosis cases especially multidrug-resistant cases, and millions of malaria cases had been identified and treated, and millions have been prevented from getting such diseases.

Human plague cases have dramatically declined in many LMI countries due to improvement in sanitary measures, use of antibiotics and insecticides, and proper handling of dead rats (rat falls). The total number of people who suffered from human plague during 1989–2003 was 38 310, with 2845 deaths, as reported in 25 countries. Sporadic cases of rat falls and annual reported human plague cases of about 1000–3000 occurred in many parts of Asia, Africa, and the Americas. After silent periods of about 30–50 years, human plague was reported in three geographical areas: India in 1994 and 2002, Indonesia in 1997, and Algeria in 2003 (WHO 2004c). The outbreak of plague in India in 1994 somehow created a wave of public panic, both within and outside the country. Inadequate sharing of information with the general population caused the country to lose billions of dollars in export earnings. Since pneumonic plague can kill a person in 3–4 days after infection, the potential for using the plague bacilli as a biological weapon is a threat. Current research is going on to address the preventive action against possible terrorist-caused plague disease outbreaks (www.niaiad.nih.gov/factsheets/plague.html).

About 90 per cent of an estimated 200 000 yellow fever (YF) cases occurred annually in Africa, where both the urban and jungle type of transmission existed (WHO 2003). The disease is still endemic in 34 African countries with several in Western and Eastern Africa reporting sporadic outbreaks every year since 1994. Some countries in South America are still at risk, predominated by the jungle type of YF. Even though the disease can be efficiently and effectively prevented and controlled through immunization, it is still persisted as a threat for international spread. Thousands of lives could easily be lost, unless a good surveillance system and higher immunization coverage in the countries at risk are sustained.

There is an annual worldwide incidence of 1.5 million cases of clinical viral hepatitis due to hepatitis A (HepA) virus, and if seroprevalence data were used, this annual incidence might be as high as tens of millions of people (WHO 2000d). The disease is most endemic in LMI countries where poor environmental conditions and inadequate hygienic practices facilitate the transmission especially among children with predominant asymptomatic infection. Essentially the entire population would have been infected before reaching adolescence. The disease is more serious in high-income and some LMI countries with a better standard of living and good hygiene, where the majority of population may not have any immunity to the HepA infection and could lead to sporadic community-wide outbreaks. Immunization against HepA has been an effective tool for protection of persons who travel to high-endemic countries and also in reducing incidence among the population in communities where annual incidence is rather high (Wasley 2006).

The advent of inexpensive and effective oral rehydration therapy (ORT) for diarrhoea and simplified case management for ARI and other childhood illnesses in the early 1970s resulted in conceivable progress in implementing effective clinical interventions as part of promoting the integrated management of childhood illness (IMCI). Poor sanitation and housing conditions including unclean and smoky kitchens, inadequate supply of safe water, and improper personal hygiene resulted in a high incidence of diarrhoeal diseases and ARI. The total number of ARI episodes in young children throughout the world has been estimated to be around 2000 million a year. The action to impart the knowledge and skill to basic health workers on IMCI has required a lot of professional and financial resources. Greater efforts are required to ensure that 80 per cent of the families in LMI countries have access to IMCI, in order to reduce the burden of diarrhoeal diseases and ARI. Not just developing more and more expensive medicines, research efforts need to be made on development of appropriate vaccines in the short-time span (e.g. expediting the development of rotavirus vaccination). Similarly political and financial investments have to be made in improving the water supply and sanitation, housing, reducing indoor and outdoor pollution, and also improving hygienic practices. These would ultimately lead to reducing the total burden of diarrhoeal diseases and ARI in the long run.

Dengue and dengue-haemorrhagic fever (D-DHF) have been major vector-borne diseases affecting the high mortality and morbidity among children in urban areas of Asia and the Pacific for many decades. Except in the improvement in management of the cases which had saved a lot of lives of children, the prevention and control of D-DHF concentrated only on active surveillance of the disease which is more of seasonal and cyclical in nature and effective reduction of mosquitoes in the immediate vicinity of where the epidemics occurred. The disease is further spreading in rural areas and also other continents such as Africa, Middle-East, and the Americas. Now, the disease is endemic in more than 100 countries with more than 2.5 billion people being at risk. Development of Dengue vaccine has been initiated since a few decades ago, but not yet been successful for wider use. Ebola is another haemorrhagic fever transmitted to humans by direct contact with the blood or body fluids of infected persons, mainly reported in a few countries of Africa since 1974. Except supportive intensive care being provided to the patient and precautionary infection control measures for health personnel who attended patients, there is no specific treatment or vaccine available for ebola (WHO 2004d). Another emerging viral haemorrhagic fever similar to ebola caused by Marburg virus infection mainly affected infants and young children in Africa reported as early as 1967 (www.itg.be/ebola). Japanese encephalitis (JE) is a vector-borne viral infection occurring in rural and peri-urban areas of Asia and the Pacific. There is no specific treatment, but JE vaccine is available now and a few countries have started including it as part of routine EPI programme.

Another seriously emerging disease is the avian influenza, caused by a highly pathogenic H5N1 virus which primarily causes diseases to domestic and migratory birds. It became a global alert in 2003 due to its potential rapid transmission around the globe. Only a little over 100 human cases with 70 per cent case-fatality rate were reported since December 2003 till January 2007 from nine countries. But, several countries around the world, mainly from Asia, Africa, Middle-East, and Europe, had confirmed existence of H5N1 virus in wild and domestic birds. Some countries have effectively controlled poultry outbreaks, but the virus may have been entrenched in domestic birds as shown by reported H5N1 outbreaks which re-emerged in these countries. Some countries in East Asia have introduced the poultry immunization on a large scale since 2004, and curtailed the poultry outbreaks significantly. Local preparedness and response to the epidemic control of both animal and human outbreaks of H5N1 infection are most crucial in determining the outcome, when the countries are challenged by the dreadful virus (WHO 2006k). There is a strong need to have global collaborative research to combat the avian influenza, since the H5N1 virus is a significant threat to animal and human health globally.

Health emergencies and health security

WHO's Constitution clearly states that the health of all peoples is fundamental to the attainment of peace and security. The terrorist attacks on the USA in September 2001, and countless terrorist acts against civilian populations in many parts of the world including use of biological weapons are in themselves threats to the health of the people. Communal violence and armed conflicts of long duration in many parts of the world have also caused psychosocial and other illnesses to the people and compounded by needlessly prolonged destruction of their health services. During the last 15 years, more than 10 000 events of natural and human-made disasters, including armed conflicts and complex emergencies occurred around the world, affecting around 4 billion people with nearly 2 million deaths, which cost more than US$1 trillion.

The most devastating disaster was the Asian Tsunami and earthquakes, which occurred on one single day on 26 December 2004, and affected several millions and took thousands of lives of the people around the countries of Southeast Asia (WHO 2005c). Since then, a series of natural disasters, like earthquakes, tsunami, and hurricanes, etc. had happened in various parts of the world with millions people dying or becoming homeless. Many actors at local, intercountry, and international levels are necessary to have quick responses to such catastrophic incidences, since health systems and other infrastructure in most cases also collapsed at the same time. A global system for surveillance and control of health and human security is required to protect the world public from any attack of infectious and other contagious threats, irrespective of national boundaries. Priorities include: Improving access to essential healthcare for vulnerable people; strengthening coordination among health partners; establishing and strengthening disease surveillance, early warning and response systems; supporting systems to reduce maternal, infant, and under-5 mortality and morbidity; and strengthening health and psychosocial support to victims. A global vision of health for all had instigated a climate of trust and improved the international relations. Governments of affected countries, majority of which are of LMI countries, in collaboration with multilateral financial institutions, international NGOs and foundations, donor agencies of high income countries, and WHO and other UN agencies had to respond to the death menace and saved countless lives and helped millions of victims.

Social medicine and public health

The initial ideas of social medicine or social dimension of public health had emerged around the early twentieth century (Ko Ko 1996). Professor Winslow defined public health as the science and art of preventing disease, prolonging life, and promoting physical health and efficiency through organized community efforts. This definition was debated for long as to whether it should fall in the area of preventive medicine or public health or beyond. The expansion of the concept of social medicine had emerged since the late 1940s as a new public health discipline. The leaders of both clinical medicine and public health questioned the polarization of curative and preventive medicine and specialization in each field, as if they were in water-tight compartments. Although new knowledge about causal factors, risks, and prevention and control of chronic non-communicable diseases were available since 1950–60s, the application for development of healthy public policy and public health interventions were done in the 1980s. The social and behavioural aspects that influenced illness and well-being became recognized. and many social interventions were proposed as part of health promotion. Without in-depth consideration of the basic concept of social medicine, many medical universities and faculties converted their departments or schools of public health into those of preventive and social medicine. Instead of teaching social medicine or new public health, educational institutions considered public health equating with preventive and social medicine and teaching more of conventional public health. Most of the associated changes are more of a change in designation than in the evolving concept of public health.

Because of the political needs and demands of the community, the widening gaps between health needs and available resources, and the rising pressure of societal factors, many health planners come out strongly that the tasks before them required fitting clinical medicine into a social context. Socialized healthcare had become the most reasonable, workable, and acceptable approach. The relationships between health and poverty were highlighted in an effort to find appropriate solutions. People themselves became more aware of the social and economic determinants impacting health. Empirical evidences were studied from both parts of the world. The value of health as a fundamental human right and its attainment as an essential social goal were firmly recognized. Mahler, WHO Director-General Emeritus, said that without health, life had little quality, for even if health was not everything, without it, the rest was nothing (WHO 1992). As a result of debates on the linkages of health with social, environmental, economic, and political factors, there are more discussions now to give a political dimension to international public health.

Policy makers are increasingly becoming concerned about finding equitable, realistic, and sustainable approaches for improving health. Meanwhile, experience has shown that many governments in LMI countries regarded the health expenditure by the public sector as purely a commodity of consumption. The total spending on health as a percentage to GDP in these countries is still around or even below 5 per cent. International agencies have encouraged these LMI countries to set priorities and improve resource allocation. A new paradigm for public health emerged in the early 1990s that health was central to development and to the quality of life. After three decades since the Alma-Ata Conference, the analysis of global health situation revealed that sustained progress in health development using PHC as the main approach towards achieving universal goal of health for all was a complex and difficult task for many LMI countries. Despite these draw backs, a few countries in Asia, Latin America, and Africa could display to the world that they could achieve major improvements in health outcomes while keeping the total public health spending at the lowest or modest levels (Rannan-Eliya 2006). Governments in these countries have adopted consistent multi-sectoral policies and programmes reaching the poor and the vulnerable, with the most effective preventive, promotive, and curative health interventions, in addition to other social and economic development programmes. Extensive use of health volunteers in providing essential primary healthcare and also expanding health knowledge through mass media and school education were the success factors.

In spite of the rapid expansion and improvement in health systems development over three decades, not all citizens in LMI countries have access to minimum essential healthcare. Many children in some LMI countries have missed basic services like polio, measles, and tetanus immunization. A majority of TB, malaria, HIV/AIDS, or leprosy patients do not have access to multidrug therapy. The challenge during the next century is what kind of public health policies are needed to ensure universal access to healthcare by all citizens. WHO has advocated the new universalism in health meaning that universal coverage is aimed for all, but not of everything (WHO 1999a). Essential public health interventions could be efficient and effective with quality, and should not be dependent on who is providing. These essential interventions for each country may need to be defined based upon the health financing mechanisms, health systems infrastructure, social behaviour, and other aspects of socioeconomic development. Public health development in the last couple of centuries had explicitly shown the need for increasing interdependence between high-income and LMI countries, in order to promote the health of the citizens of the world. The health risks are shared by every citizen of the world and could also be seen as opportunities for improvement. Debates in recent years have been intensified on the issues of global public health development and global governance of health (Dodgson *et al.* 2002; Kickbusch & Payne 2004). During the last 50 years, many intercountry, intergovernmental, international, bilateral, and multilateral development agencies and organizations, as well as alliances have emerged out of necessity to deal increasingly with international developmental issues, both in policy and programme terms including health and other social development.

In November 2006, Chan, the newly-elected WHO Director-General, defined a new role for the World Health Organization that could be a step towards becoming a truly international as well as a global health organization (WHO 2006l). While the main mission of WHO continues to be attaining for all people the highest possible level of health, it further adopts a corporate strategic framework that will result in achieving greatest possible contribution to world health (WHO 2007c). LMI countries need to work in close collaboration with WHO and other partners by focusing the global efforts to build healthy populations and communities in addressing the excess burden of sickness and suffering resulting from both communicable and non-communicable diseases especially in poor and marginalized populations. Partnerships could be established to sustain and support health system development so that equitable health outcomes are achieved and peoples' demands are met.

Looking ahead

The final decades of the twentieth century witnessed a rapidly changing political situation and severe economic upheavals, especially towards the end of the Cold War in the 1990s. Strong demands were made for pluralistic democracy, good governance, social justice, and respect for human rights for a clearly defined role of the State and for economic globalization. Social expectations and awareness of social and economic development linked with health improvement were infused in many LMI countries. There was a dramatic change in international public health development, especially the global health governance and international health cooperation. The centrality of health to human development was charted in a wide range of national and international agreements and affirmed in action by a wide-ranging set of stakeholders. A multiplicity of new actors in national and international health had redefined the boundaries of health sector, each with its own unique expertise and vision. Groups of individuals united in a particular cause, such as patient groups or civil society groups, become major players for policies and programme development, by creating powerful lobbies and raising public awareness. Increased access to the Internet and other new communication tools has revolutionized the people's reach for information with a certain degree of freedom of choice. Growing involvement of more non-governmental organizations in direct delivery of healthcare had complemented the efforts of national health systems. They become influential players in policy development and decision-making in socioeconomic and health-related issues.

New mechanisms for health financing with public–private partnerships and the scale of resources brought in by new partners are changing the way health is externally funded in many countries. This new paradigm in public health development, especially in low-income countries who had to rely heavily on external aids, has led to a complex relationship among traditional and new players in international health and health-related development, planning and use for resources, and the need for delineation and harmonization of responsibilities. Partnerships could enhance the value of public health interventions that were previously dominated by the public sector. Partnerships offer opportunities for involving the private sector and civil society groups, in scaling up the response to global health issues. There were however some concerns that the partnerships might widen the gaps by increasing fragmentation of international cooperation in health, overwhelming the national capacity, distorting the national priorities, diverting the scarce human resources, and also marginalizing the UN system agencies.

Conclusion

Health is a cause rather than an effect of economic development. The history of public health development among the high-income and LMI countries showed that important breakthroughs in public health have led to great improvements in economic development, as witnessed by the rapid growth of Britain and Japan during the industrial revolution in the late eighteenth century, and some countries in Asia and Middle-East during 1960–70s. Health actually determines economic productivity, intellectual prosperity, physical and emotional well-being of the people. Disease burden slows economic growth that is presumed to solve the health problems. For example, more than half of Africa's growth shortfall relative to the high-growth countries of East Asia could be explained statistically by disease burden, demography, and geography, rather than by more traditional variables of macroeconomic policy and political governance (Bloom & Sachs 1998).

The population afflicted with a high infant mortality rate usually lacks the secure knowledge of its children's longevity, witnesses higher rates of fertility, and experiences the quality–quantity tradeoff in child rearing. The efforts of national and international communities should be aimed at promoting healthy living, reducing the double burden of disease, and making essential healthcare accessible to all. Ever since the HFA movement initiated over three decades ago, health, equity, and social justice remain the main themes of social and health policy. These values and principles of solidarity, social justice, and ethics for primary healthcare and health for all continue to be relevant and will continue in the future. It is essential for all public health professionals and the international community to sustain these values.

References

Asian Development Bank (ADB) (2005). *Asia Water Watch 2025: Are countries in Asia on track to meet target 10 of the Millennium Development Goals*? ADB, Manila.

Basu, Z. *et al.* (1979). *Eradication of smallpox from India*, Regional Publication Series No. 5, WHO, New Delhi.

Beaglehole, R. and Bonita, R. (1997). *Public health at the crossroads*. Cambridge University Press, Cambridge.

Berlinguer, G. (1999). Globalization and global health. *International Journal of Health Services*, **29**, 579–95.

Bloom, D.E. and Sachs, J. (1998). *Geography, demography, and economic growth in Africa*. Revised October 1998, pp. 36–8. (www.clas.ufl.edu/users/bbsmith/Sachs_Geography.pdf)

Cassels, A. (1997). *A guide to health sector-wide approach: Concepts, issues and working arrangement*. WHO, Geneva (WHO/ARA97.12).

Chen, L.C. *et al.* (1999). Health as a global public good. In (eds. I. Kaul *et al.*) *Global public goods.* Oxford University Press, New York.

Dodgson, R. *et al.* (2002). *Global health governance: A conceptual review.* WHO, Geneva and London School of Hygiene and Tropical Medicine.

Detels, R. and Breslow, L. (2000). Current scope and concerns in public health. In (eds. Detels *et al.*) *Oxford textbook of public health*, 4th edition, Vol. 1. p. 3, Oxford University Press, New York.

Drager, N. and Beaglehole, R. (2001). Globalization: Changing the public health landscape. *Bulletin of World Health Organization*, **79** (9), 803.

Djukanovic, V. and Mach, E.P. (eds.) (1975). *Alternative approaches to meeting basic health needs in developing countries.* A joint UNICEF/WHO study. WHO, Geneva.

Fenner, F. *et al.* (1988). *Smallpox and its eradication*, pp. 473–516. WHO, Geneva.

Foege, W.H. *et al.* (1971). Selective epidemiologic control in smallpox eradication. *American Journal of Epidemiology*, **94**, 311–5.

Foster, G.M. and Anderson, B.G. (1978). *Medical anthropology*, pp. 224–5. John Wiley & Sons, New York.

Goodman, R.A. and Foster, K.L. (eds.) (1998). Global disease elimination and eradication as public health strategies, Proceedings of a conference held in Atlanta, Georgia, USA, February 1998, pp. 23–25, *Bulletin of the World Health Organization*, 1998, **76** (Suppl 2), 5–162.

Gopalan, C. (1992). *Nutrition in developmental transition in South-East Asia.* Regional Health Paper No. 21, pp. 9–11, WHO, New Delhi.

Harrison, M. (1994). *Public health in British India: Anglo-Indian preventive medicine 1859–1914*, Cambridge University Press, Cambridge.

Henderson, D.A. (1997). Edward Jenner's vaccine. *Public Health Reports*, **112**, 116–21.

Henderson, D.A. (1998). Smallpox eradication—a cold war victory, *World Health Forum*, **19**, 113–9.

Howard-Jones, N. (1974). The scientific background of the international sanitary conferences 1851–1938. *WHO Chronicle*, **28**, 159–71 and 455–70.

Howard-Jones, N. (1977). International public health: The organizational problems between the two World Wars (2). *WHO Chronicle*, **31**, 449–60.

International Institute for Population Sciences (IIPS) and World Health Organization (WHO) (2006). *Health system performance assessment: World health survey, 2003: India*, WHO-India, New Delhi.

Jaggi, O.P. (1979). *History of science, technology and medicine in India*, Volume XIII, Western Medicine in India: Medical Education and Research, Atma Ram & Sons, Delhi.

Jamaison, D.T. and Sandhu, M.E. (2001). WHO Ranking of health system performance. *Science*, August, **293**, 1595–6.

Kickbusch, I. and Payne, L. (2004). *Constructing global public health in the 21st century.* Lecture delivered at the meeting on global health governance and accountability, 2–3 June 2004, Harvard University, USA.

Kinnon, C.M. (1998). World trade: bringing health into the picture, *World Health Forum*, **19**, 397–406.

Ko Ko (1986). *Public health: Myth, mysticism and reality.* WHO, New Delhi.

Ko Ko (1996). *Closing the gaps in health care—A holistic approach to medical education.* In SEA Regional Conference on Medical Education, February 7–9, pp. 152–67, Bangkok.

Ko Ko *et al.* (2002). *Conquest of scourges in Myanmar*, pp. 51–2. Myanmar Academy of Medical Science, Yangon.

Ko Ko *et al.* (2005). *Conquest of scourges in Myanmar: An update*, p. 238, 309. Myanmar Academy of Medical Science, Yangon.

Kutzin, J. (1998). Enhancing the insurance function of health systems: A proposed conceptual framework. In (eds. S. Nitayarumphong and A. Mills) *Achieving universal coverage of health care.* Office of Health Care Reform, Ministry of Public Health, Nonthaburi, Thailand.

Lee, K. (2001). The global dimensions of cholera. *Global change and human health*, Vol. 2, No. 1, pp. 6–17.

Lenfant, C. (2001). Can we prevent cardiovascular diseases in low and middle income countries? *Bulletin of the World Health Organization*, **79** (10), 980–2.

League of Nations Health Organization-LNHO (1937). *Report of the intergovernmental Conference of Far-Eastern countries on rural hygiene*, held at Bandoeng (Java), August 3–13, Geneva.

Mackay, J. *et al.* (2006). *The tobacco atlas*, 2nd edition. American Cancer Society.

McNeill, W.H. (1977). *Plagues and peoples.* Basil Blackwell, Oxford.

Miyagishima, K. and Kaferstein, F.K. (1998). Food safety in international trade. *World Health Forum*, **19**, 407–11.

Molyneux, D.H. *et al.* (2000). Elimination of lymphatic filariasis as public health problem- lymphatic filariasis: Setting the scene for elimination. *Transactions of the Royal Society of Tropical Medicine and Hygiene*, **94**, 589–91.

National Institutes of Health (NIH) (2000). *Morbidity & mortality: 2000 chart book on cardiovascular, lung and blood diseases.* National Heart, Lung, and Blood Institute, Bethesda, MD, USA.

Navarro, V. (1999). Health and equity in the world in the era of globalization, *International Journal of Health Services*, **29**, 215–26.

Nuyens, Y. (2007). Setting priorities for health research: Lessons from low- and middle-income countries. *Bulletin of the World Health Organization*, April, **85** (4), 319–21.

Rafei, U.M. (2004). *Health development in the South-East Asia Region: An overview*, (SEARO Regional Publications No. 44) pp. 34–6, WHO, New Delhi.

Rannan-Eilya, R. (2006). Sri Lanka's health miracle, *South Asia Journal*, October–November, No. 14: pp. 63–73.

Reddy, K.S. and Yusuf, S. (1998). Emerging epidemic of cardiovascular disease in developing countries. *Circulation*, **97**, 596–601.

Society for International Development (1999). Responses to globalization: Rethinking health and equity. *Development*, **42** (4), 1–158.

Shepard, C. *et al.* (2006). Hepatitis B virus infection: Epidemiology and vaccination, *Epidemiology Reviews*, **28**, 112–25.

Tarimo, E. and Webster, E.G. (1994). *Primary health care concepts and challenges in a changing world: Alma-Ata revisited.* Current Concerns: SHS Paper No. 7 (WHO/SHS/CC/94.2), WHO, Geneva.

Than Sein (2002). A *policy brief on health care financing reforms in WHO South-East Asia Region*, (unpublished internal document). WHO, New Delhi.

Than Sein and Kyaw Lwin (2003). A million smiles: Elimination of leprosy in South-East Asia. *Regional Health Forum*, Vol. 7, No. 1. pp. 11–25. WHO, New Delhi.

Tun Aung Kyaw (2005). Control of trachoma in Myanmar. In (eds. Ko Ko *et al.*) *Conquest of scourges in Myanmar: An update*, p. 187. Myanmar Academy of Medical Sciences, Yangon.

UN (United Nations) (2003). *Human security now: Commission on human security*, pp. 95–112. New York.

UN (United Nations) (2006). *The UN report on millennium development goals 2006*, pp. 4–5, New York (http://mdgs.un.org/).

UNDP (United Nations Development Programme) (1998). *Human development report 1998.* UNDP, New York.

UNDP (United Nations Development Programme) (2006). *Human development report (HDR) 2006; Beyond scarcity: Power, poverty and the global water crisis.* UNDP, pp. 119–20.

UNICEF (United Nations Children's Fund) (2006). *States of the world's children 2006.* Oxford University Press, New York.

Uragoda, C.G. (1987). *A history of medicine in Sri Lanka–from the earliest times to 1948.* Sri Lanka Medical Association, Colombo.

Wasley, A. *et al.* (2006). Hepatitis A in the era of vaccination. *Epidemiological Review 2006*, **28**, 101–11.

Wilkinson, L. and Power, H. (1998). The London and Liverpool Schools of tropical medicine 1898–1998. *British Medical Bulletin*, **54**, 281–92.

Wild, S. *et al.* (2004). Global prevalence of diabetes: Estimates for the year 2000 and projections for 2030, *Diabetes Care*, **27** (5), May, 1047–53.

WHO (World Health Organization) (1957). *Report on rural health conference*, held during 14–26 October 1957. Document SEA/RH/9, WHO, New Delhi.

WHO (World Health Organization) (1964). *WHO expert committee on smallpox: First report*. WHO Technical Report Series No. 283, pp. 7, 9–11, 15, 24, 31.

WHO (World Health Organization) (1967). *Twenty years in South-East Asia: 1948–1967*. WHO, New Delhi.

WHO (World Health Organization) (1978a). *A decade of health development in South-East Asia 1968-1977*. WHO, New Delhi.

WHO (World Health Organization) (1978b). *WHO Alma-Ata 1978: Primary health care*. HFA Series No.1, WHO, Geneva.

WHO (World Health Organization) (1986). *Regional advisory committee on medical research for South-East Asia: Proceeding of the special session commemorating the tenth anniversary*. Held on 12 April 1985, Regional Publications Series No.15, WHO, New Delhi.

WHO (World Health Organization) (1991). *Resolution WHA44.9 on leprosy elimination*. WHO, Geneva.

WHO (World Health Organization) (1992). *WHO Collaboration in Health Development in South-East Asia: 1948–1988, Fortieth Anniversary publication (updated)*. WHO, New Delhi.

WHO (World Health Organization) (1993). *Implementation of global strategy for health for all by the year 2000: Eight report on the world situation*. Volume 1, WHO, Geneva.

WHO (World Health Organization) (1996). *Investing in health research and development: Report of the Ad hoc committee on health research relating to future intervention options*. WHO, Geneva (TDR/Gen/96.1).

WHO (World Health Organization) (1998a). *Health for all in the 21st century* (Document A51/5) and *World Health Declaration annexed to Resolution WHA51.7*, WHO Geneva.

WHO (World Health Organization) (1998b). *The World health report 1998: Life in the 21st century: A vision for all*. WHO, Geneva.

WHO (World Health Organization) (1998c). *Evaluation of the implementation of the global strategy for health for all by the year 2000, 1979–1996*. WHO, Geneva (Document WHO/HST/98.2).

WHO (World Health Organization) (1999a). *Health situation in the South-East Asia Region 1994–1997*, p. 155. WHO, New Delhi.

WHO (World Health Organization) (1999b). *The World health report 1999: Making a difference*. WHO, Geneva.

WHO (World Health Organization) (1999c). *Nutrition for health and development: Progress and prospects on the eve of the 21st century*. (WHO/NHD/99.9), WHO, Geneva,

WHO (World Health Organization) (2000a). *Sector-wide approaches for health development, a review of experience*, by Mike Foster *et al.* (WHO/GPE/00.1), WHO, Geneva.

WHO (World Health Organization) (2000b). *The World Health Report 2000, Health systems: Improving performance*. WHO, Geneva.

WHO (World Health Organization) (2000c). *Eliminate filariasis: Attack poverty. Proceedings of the First Meeting of The Global Alliance to eliminate lymphatic filariasis*, Spain, 4–5 May 2000 (CDS/CEE/200.5). WHO, Geneva (http://www.filariasis.org/) and International Filaria Journal (http://www.filariajournal.com/).

WHO (World Health Organization) (2000d). Hepatitis A Vaccines, *Weekly Epidemiology Record*, February, **75** (5): pp. 38–44, WHO: Geneva.

WHO (World Health Organization) (2001). *Assessment of health systems performance*, (EB107/9 and Resolution EB107.R8), WHO, Geneva.

WHO (World Health Organization) (2002a). *Summary measures of population health: Concepts, ethics, measurements and applications*, by Murray *et al.* (eds.). WHO, Geneva.

WHO (World Health Organization) (2002b) Leprosy control. *Weekly Epidemiology Record*, **77**, pp. 1–8, WHO, Geneva.

WHO (World Health Organization) (2003). Yellow fever vaccine, *Weekly Epidemiology Record*, October, **78** (40): pp. 349–360, WHO: Geneva.

WHO (World Health Organization) (2004a). Hepatitis B vaccines. *Weekly Epidemiology Record*, July, **79** (28), pp. 255–63. WHO, Geneva.

WHO (World Health Organization) (2004b). *The atlas of heart disease and stroke*. pp. 18–19, WHO Geneva.

WHO (World Health Organization) (2004c). Human plague. *Weekly Epidemiology Record*, August, **79** (33), pp. 301–8, WHO, Geneva.

WHO (World Health Organization) (2004d). Ebola haemorrhagic fever. *Fact Sheet No. 103*, May. WHO, Geneva (http://www.who.int/).

WHO (World Health Organization) (2005a). *Global strategy for further reducing the leprosy burden and sustaining leprosy control activities (2006–2010)*, (WHO/CDS/CPE/CEE/2005.53). WHO, Geneva.

WHO (World Health Organization) (2005b). *Resolution WHA58.3 revision of international health regulations*. WHO, Geneva.

WHO (World Health Organization) (2005c). *Moving beyond the tsunami: The WHO story*. WHO, New Delhi.

WHO (World Health Organization) (2005d). *Global report: Preventing chronic diseases: A vital investment*. WHO, Geneva.

WHO (World Health Organization) (2006a). *World health report 2006: Health workforce*. WHO, Geneva.

WHO (World Health Organization) (2006b). *Strategy on health care financing for countries of the Western Pacific and South-East Asia Regions (2006–2010)*. WHO, New Delhi.

WHO (World Health Organization) (2006c). *Smallpox eradication: Destruction of variola virus stocks*. (EB120/11 and Resolution EB120. R8), WHO, Geneva.

WHO (World Health Organization) (2006d). *Poliomyelitis eradication*. (EB120/4 Rev.1), WHO, Geneva.

WHO (World Health Organization) (2006e). Onchocerciasis Control. *Weekly Epidemiology Record*, July, No. **30**, pp. 293–6, WHO, Geneva.

WHO (World Health Organization) (2006f). Dracunculiasis. *Weekly Epidemiology Record*, May, **18**, pp. 173–188. WHO, Geneva.

WHO (World Health Organization) (2006g). Global programme to eliminate lymphatic filariasis, *Weekly Epidemiology Record*, June, **81** (22): pp. 221–232, WHO: Geneva.

WHO (World Health Organization) (2006h). *Public health problems caused by harmful use of alcohol in South-East Asia: Gaining less or losing more?* WHO, New Delhi (Alcohol Series No. 4).

WHO (World Health Organization) (2006i). *Global tuberculosis control: Surveillance, planning and financing: WHO report 2006*, p. 27, WHO, Geneva.

WHO (World Health Organization) (2006j), *The revised Malaria Control Strategy: South-East Asia Region 2006–2010*, (SEA-MAL 243) pp. 8–11, WHO, New Delhi.

WHO (World Health Organization) (2006k). *Report by the Secretariat on avian and pandemic influenza: developments, response and follow-up, and application of IHR (2005)*. (EB120/15), WHO, Geneva.

WHO (World Health Organization) (2006l). *Speech to the special session of World Health Assembly by the Director-General Elect Dr Margaret Chan on 9 November 2006*. WHO, Geneva, accessed at (http://www.who.int/dg/speeches/) on 12 February 2007.

WHO (World Health Organization) (2007a). *Public health, innovation and intellectual property: Towards a global strategy and plan of action*, (EB120/Inf.Doc./1), and *Public health, innovation and intellectual property: towards a global strategy and plan of action: Follow-up to the first session of the Intergovernmental Working Group*, (EB120/Inf.Doc/5), WHO, Geneva.

WHO (World Health Organization) (2007b). *Fact Sheet No. 286 on Measles*, January 2007. (http://www.who.int/).

WHO (World Health Organization) (2007c) *Medium Term Strategic Plan for 2008-2013 and Programme Budget for 2008–2009*. WHO, Geneva.

WHO (World Health Organization) (2007d). *Sub-national Health System Performance Assessment, Country Report on Indonesia*, WHO, Jakarta, Indonesia, April 2007. (http://www.who.or.id/eng/products/ow6/sub2/indexsub.asp?id=5).

WHO and UNICEF (2000). *Report on the global water supply and sanitation assessment*, WHO, Geneva and UNICEF, New York.

WHO and World Bank (1990). *Commission on health research for development: Essential link to equity in development*. Oxford University Press, New York.

World Bank (2005). *World development indicator 2005*. p. 114, Table 2.17.

World Bank (2006a). *The World development report 2007: Development and the Next Generation*, Washington, p. 285.

World Bank (2006b). *Global burden of disease and risk factors: Disease Control Priorities Project*, Lopez et al. (eds.), Oxford University Press, New York.

Yach, D. and Bettcher, D. (1998). The globalization of public health: Threats and opportunities. *American Journal of Public Health*, **88**, 735–43.

1.4

The development of the discipline of public health in countries in economic transition: India, Brazil, China

Puja Thakker and K. Srinath Reddy

Abstract

The three low- and middle-income countries (LMICs) profiled in this chapter are countries which together constitute nearly 45 per cent of the global population. These countries represent societies wherein the economies are on the upswing and are accompanied by demographic and epidemiological transitions profoundly influencing the agenda of public health as well as the level of resources available to address it. The dominant ideologies of both the state and society of the time, as can be seen in the social, political, and economic histories of these countries, have significantly influenced the development of public health.

As these countries focus on establishing strong systems for the delivery of health care, the role of the state has undergone substantial changes over time. The increasing dominance of market economics even in the health-care sector has substantially shaped the role of the private sector, and thus, the health-seeking behaviour of the population. Although a progressing economy has significantly increased national income per capita, the transition has varying impacts on the health system, especially raising concern over the quality of care delivered and the widening inequities in access to care.

Public health in LMICs has not succeeded in drawing upon interdisciplinary research and multisectoral action to the extent needed. Presently, the capacity for developing and implementing intersectoral policies is missing, and the active engagement of public health academia and health workers with the health system and policymakers is suboptimal. Although promising signs of a change are visible in some of these countries, the extent to which the discipline will advance further over the next two decades will be a critical determinant of health and development in the high-velocity transitional period that lies ahead.

Introduction

An overwhelming majority of the world's population presently resides in low- and middle-income countries (LMICs). The three LMICs profiled in this chapter are countries that together have a population size of 2.6 billion and constitute nearly 40 per cent of the global population. Hence, the development of public health in these countries, both as an academic discipline and as a delivery system, is of great importance to the state of global health. Key health indicators of these countries are summarized in Table 1.4.1.

The evolution of public health as a discipline in populous LMICs, such China, India, and Brazil, has been influenced by multiple interactive factors. These include the following:

1. Changing global and national perceptions, over time, of the ambit of public health as an academic discipline and its contribution as an application pathway for improving the health of the population.
2. Growing recognition of the multiple determinants of health, demanding interdisciplinary amalgamation of academic learning and directing public health practice into multisectoral action channels.

Table 1.4.1 Key health indicators for India, China, and Brazil (2007)

	Under-5 mortality (per 1000 live births)	MMR (per 100 000 live births)	Underweight children under 5 years of age (%)	Vaccination coverage* (%)
India	74	301	44	55–78
China	27	48	6	91–94
Brazil	33	260	3.7	92–99

* Estimates for BCG, DPT1, DPT3, polio, tetanus, MCV vaccines.

Source: CIA World Factbook: https://www.cia.gov/library/publications/the-world-factbook/ (accessed on 3 November, 2007); WHO/UNICEF: Immunization Profile, India. Website: http://www.who.int/vaccines/globalsummary/immunization/countryprofileresult.cfm?C='IND' (accessed on 31 October, 2007); Immunization Profile, China. Website: http://www.who.int/vaccines/globalsummary/immunization/countryprofileresult.cfm?C='CHI' (accessed on 31 October, 2007); Immunization Profile, Brazil. Website: http://www.who.int/vaccines/globalsummary/immunization/countryprofileresult.cfm?C='BRA' (accessed on 31 October, 2007).

3. The relative balance between preventive- and clinical-care components of public health services, as reflected in policymaker priorities and fiscal allocations.
4. The composition and characteristics of the health system, including the public–private–voluntary mix, the roles and responsibilities of different categories of health-service personnel, the size of the public health workforce, and the nature and strength of linkages between health services and educational/training institutions, which are charged with the task of creating the capacity of public health professionals and functionaries.
5. Economic transitions influencing the growth patterns and distributional dynamics of income and opportunity within the global and national settings.
6. Demographic and social transitions propelled by relatively late industrialization, recent but rapid urbanization, and fast-paced globalization.
7. Epidemiological and health transitions which are reordering the principal public health challenges, in terms of disease burdens, and rearranging priorities for public health action
8. The levels of access to the enlarging pool of global knowledge and expanding array of technological innovations which advance the precept and practice of public health.
9. National capacity for knowledge creation and knowledge management as well as the ability to identify and overcome barriers in knowledge translation.
10. National and international partnerships that are available to strengthen the intellectual as well as institutional resources needed for advancing public health.
11. Collaborative agreements with international agencies, such as the World Health Organization (WHO) and the World Bank as well as bilateral and multilateral development partners, which influence the overall agenda of public health programmes as well as determine the level of technical and financial resources available for specific programmes.

This chapter profiles some of these determinants, as generally applicable to these selected LMICs, and briefly describes the evolution of public health in each of them.

Defining public health

The debate on what defines the discipline of public health and what delineates the ambit of public health policies and programmes has witnessed several paradigm shifts over the past century. From an initially restricted mandate of ensuring public sanitation, safe water supply, and food safety, public health expanded to include services aimed at individual protection (such as immunization and contraception) and health promotion (mainly through health education). In recent years, recognition of the need to influence the upstream social determinants (which impact on group and individual behaviours, and thereby alter the biology of individuals to produce disease or promote health) has led to public health also adopting social legislation and regulation in areas such as tobacco control and nutrition.

The disciplinary mandate of public health has, therefore, expanded from providing essential hygienic services and disease-preventive personal protection to broader social-engineering efforts, which combine public education and policy interventions that have a population-wide effect, for health promotion. This global trend has also influenced the evolution of the discipline in LMICs, although the speed and scale of change have varied across countries.

Determinants of health

The course of public health has also been influenced by a growing understanding of the multiple determinants of health, their independent and interactive contributions to the health of societies and their constituent individuals, as well as the need for planned interventions to influence these determinants. The initial preoccupation with factors operating at the individual level (an interplay of beliefs, behaviours, and biology) gave way to greater recognition of determinants that operate at family and community levels (perceptions, priorities, and pathways). In recent years, awareness of the social and economic determinants that operate at national levels has increased, along with the recognition that these upstream factors are increasingly becoming dominant in the wake of globalization and economic liberalization rapidly rewriting social and trade policies. The factors that operate at the national and global levels, such as development, distribution, and demand–supply levers of trade, now impact profoundly on the health of the community, the family, and the individual. The evolution of public health as a discipline needs to integrate an understanding of all of these determinants (Fig. 1.4.1) as well as the underpinnings in society in order to influence each of them through appropriate interventions.

In LMICs, non-personal policy interventions, which have a population-wide impact (e.g. tobacco taxes and food prices), are likely to have a greater impact than education, in a short time frame, in promoting individual behaviour change. Public health leaders in LMICs have not yet realized the full potential of such policy interventions, and consequently, transdisciplinary research, multisectoral action, and multi-stakeholder advocacy have so far remained slow and subdued in their response to the rapid changes to the social determinants of health. Even as scientific advances in molecular genetics tend to swing the pendulum of causation discourse to individual susceptibility, the profound impact of social and environmental determinants remains inadequately addressed. This imbalance needs to be corrected if public health has to evolve to its full potential.

Determining the balance between preventive and clinical medicine

Even as definitional debates on the scope of public health have continued, the key factor influencing the evolution of public health in

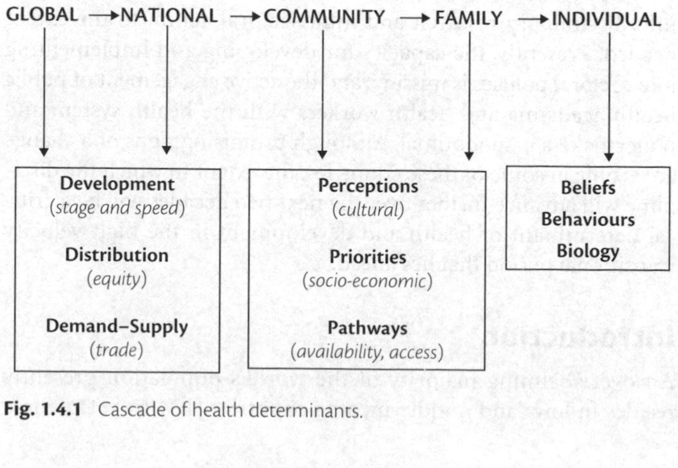

Fig. 1.4.1 Cascade of health determinants.

LMICs has been the level of resource allocation for preventive and promotive public health programmes, in comparison with that provided for public-sector clinical services. In resource-constrained economies, the emphasis was initially on providing essential clinical services, especially in primary health care. Public health programmes were resourced at lower levels and mainly involved immunization, disease control for major infectious diseases, and in the case of India, population control. Public health was more often viewed as the vehicle for extending the outreach of personalized clinical interventions across the population rather than as a pathway for promoting the health of the population. Even in terms of individual health protection, public health systems were used to deliver sporadic interventions at select points in an individual's life, in staccato style, rather than adopt a lifespan approach to the protection, preservation, and promotion of health at all stages of life. It is only in recent years, with a spurt in the growth of national economies, that public health is being better supported through increased financial allocation and is beginning to adopt a broader agenda of action. As public spending on health increases, public health is beginning to get greater attention within the health sector, even though clinical care is likely to continue as the major area of health expenditure.

Designing of health systems

Because the design and operation of efficient health systems which provide a mix of health-promotive, disease-preventive, diagnostic, and clinical services to all sections of the population is considered to be within the mandate of public health, the individual and collective contributions of public, private, and voluntary sectors become relevant to the evolution of this field. In many LMICs, the public sector was the principal provider of health services, at all levels, in the early stages of health-system development. Later, the role of the private sector grew, covering not only a large segment of tertiary care but also extending into secondary care. Private health care now also caters to much of urban primary health care in countries such as India. The not-for-profit voluntary sector has become actively engaged in health care at various levels in India, but the extent of its coverage remains limited.

The size of the workforce in the health sector overall, and in public health services in particular, has determined the level of efficiency of the health system. The misdistribution of health personnel, with urban preponderance and rural paucity, as well as chronic shortages of qualified health personnel, aggravated by migration to richer nations, have affected the performance of the health systems in India and Brazil. The lack of medical personnel also spurred on the creation of other categories of health-service personnel, such as 'barefoot doctors', community health workers, and volunteers (with varied nomenclature), and sustained the presence of traditional health-system practitioners as care givers to large segments of the population. The evolution of health systems in LMICs has yet to fully assimilate and accommodate these varied contributors into an integrated framework.

Disconnect between public health education and health-system operations

Ideally, institutions engaged in public health education and research should have been closely connected to the health systems. This would have been mutually beneficial, with the needs of the health systems and learnings from the reality of 'field' experiences influencing the curriculum and pedagogical methods of public health educational programmes and the academic institutions. This, in turn, could have invigorated the health systems through policy- and programme-relevant research as well as contributed to training programmes. However, public health training institutions, whether located in medical colleges or in university settings, remained largely distanced from the general health system. They also played a limited role in influencing the organization and performance of the health systems. This disconnect is especially visible in countries such as India, where the lack of such engagement has adversely affected the evolution of public health.

Development and rights perspectives

Against this background, the economic transitions of the past two decades have rapidly changed the way in which health is perceived by countries and the manner in which health services are provided. In resource-constrained economies, social-sector spending was initially considered a lower priority than 'growth' and infrastructure spending, and it was assumed that health would passively benefit from economic development. It became clear during the 1990s that investments in health are essential for accelerated economic growth. This 'human capital' approach, wherein the productivity of the workforce was linked to their health status, was complemented by a 'rights' approach, whereby the right to health became ably articulated as an essential right by increasingly assertive civil-society groups. The setting up of the National Commission on Macroeconomics and Health and the growth of the People's Health Movement (with public hearings on the 'right to health' organized by it in concert with the National Human Rights Commission), in the past decade in India, are illustrative of this convergent advocacy for health both as a developmental imperative and an inalienable human right.

Dangerous fallout of structural reforms

At the same time, the integration of LMIC economies into the global market posed several challenges. While promising increased growth opportunities, it also made them more vulnerable to the vagaries of the global market. The influence of international agencies promoting economic liberalization led to 'structural reforms' in the health system, wherein the role of the public sector became diminished, and several public health services such as water and sanitation were labelled as not being cost-effective (World Bank 1993). As a result, public health services suffered a setback in several LMICs. For example, the rapid shift from state-provided health care to limited availability of insured health care or private purchased health care has had an adverse impact on rural health services in China, in the post-liberalization phase, and correctives are now being applied. In India too, out-of-pocket (OOP) health expenditure has reached a level of 77 per cent, despite the state's commitment to the public sector as the primary provider of free health services.

Disparities

The economic growth of China, India, and Brazil has brought about an increase in per-capita incomes. Although this increase is expected to have a favourable impact on health states, the skewed distributional patterns of the wealth created during this growth phase have aggravated socioeconomic inequalities within these societies, resulting in major disparities in health outcomes. To illustrate, Table 1.4.2 showcases the urban–rural inequality that exists

Table 1.4.2 Socioeconomic inequalities exacerbate risk factors

	Access to improved drinking water sources (%)		Access to improved sanitation (%)	
	Urban	Rural	Urban	Rural
India	89	48	59	22
China	93	67	69	28
Brazil	96	57	83	37

Source: World Health Organization. World health statistics 2007. Geneva: World Health Organization; 2007 and National Council of Applied Economic Research (2000). *Rural Households Survey.*

in access to improved sanitation and clean drinking water within these three countries.

Health expenditure

The evolution of public health in LMICs has to be understood against the backdrop of these profound changes accruing in their economies and the resultant impact on health financing, health services, and health indicators. Figures 1.4.2.1–1.4.2.3 show the recent changes in the government's share (as a percentage) of the total health spending against the increase in gross national product (GNP) per capita.

Governmental contributions to total health expenditures are indicative of the political will and commitment towards health. A higher commitment from the government, in general, reduces out-of-pocket expenditures, and protects the poor from the financial risk associated with a health accident. Although several studies have shown that government spending on health benefits the middle and affluent class the most, it nevertheless serves as an essential safety net for the poorest segment of the population. Brazil (Fig. 1.4.2.3) has shown consistently upward trends in government spending on health as the GNP per capita has increased over the last decade. Government health expenditure in China (Fig. 1.4.2.2) has continually declined in recent years, despite its rapid economic growth. In India (Fig. 1.4.2.1), government health spending has been more erratic, and is currently at 17.3 per cent of the total health spending (Government of India 2005). With recent schemes such as the National Rural Health Mission, launched in 2005, and the National Urban Health Mission, launched in April 2008 , the government aims to increase this spending to 25 per cent of the total health spending by 2010.

A positive relationship between national income and health trends has long been observed across the globe. The lower national incomes of LMICs leave their populations disadvantaged in terms of their health states. Developing countries account for 84 per cent of the global population but 90 per cent of the global disease burden. Due to severe budget constraints, they also tend to spend much less on health. Developing countries account for 20 per cent of global gross domestic product (GDP) but only 12 per cent of all health spending. Even after adjusting for differences in the cost of living, high-income countries spend 30 times more on health per capita than low-income countries (Gottret & Schieber 2006). Further, a large percentage of health expenditure in LMICs tends to be OOP, as a consequence of missing safety-net policies within the health system and low overall public spending on health, leaving the poorest segment unprotected from catastrophic health spending.

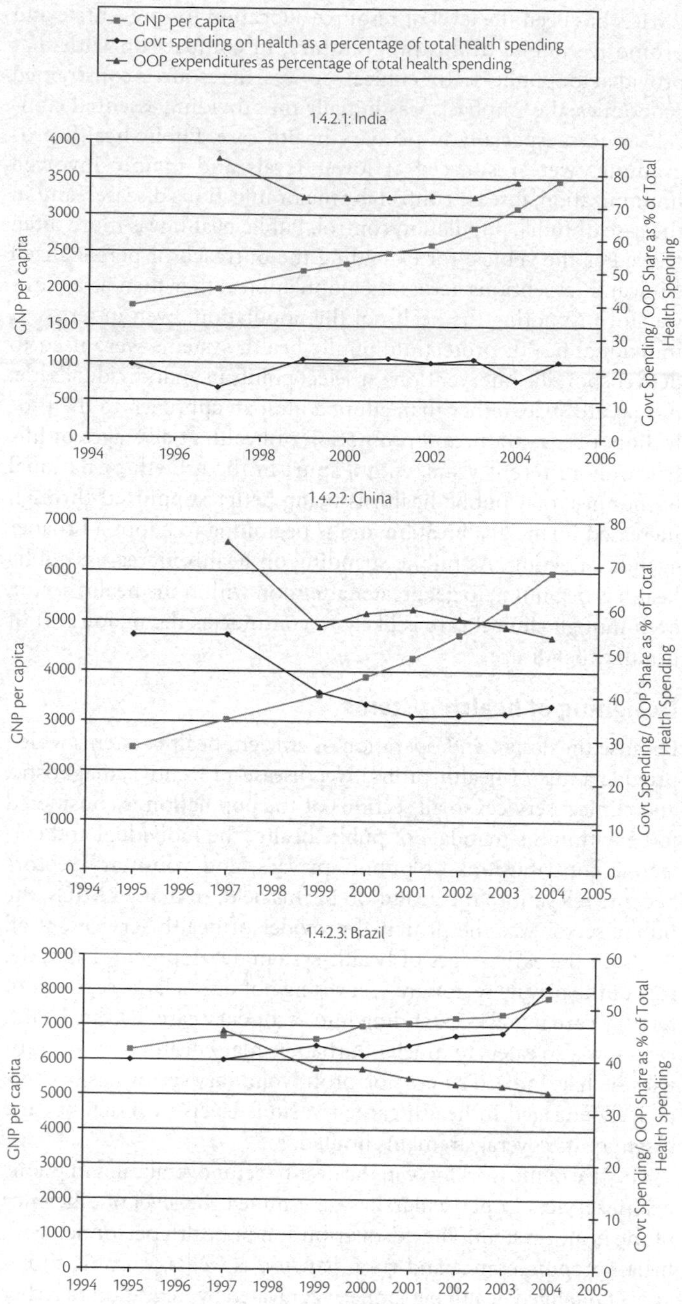

Fig. 1.4.2 Government spending on health as a percentage of the total health spending compared with changes in gross national product (GNP) per capita: (1.4.2.1) India, (1.4.2.2) China, and (1.4.2.3) Brazil.

Garg and Karan (2006) estimated that 32.5 million people fall below the national poverty line due to OOP payments in India each year.

The percentage of OOP expenditure is indicative of how equitably health services are being financed within a state. The general trend shows that greater government spending on health decreases OOP spending. OOP spending trends in India and China have remained virtually unchanged since 1999, still high at 77 per cent and 53 per cent in 2004, respectively (World Health Organization 2007). OOP expenditures in Brazil have declined marginally since 1999, to 34 per cent in 2004 (World Health Organization 2007). Rising OOP spending in recent years also reflects a shift in emphasis towards

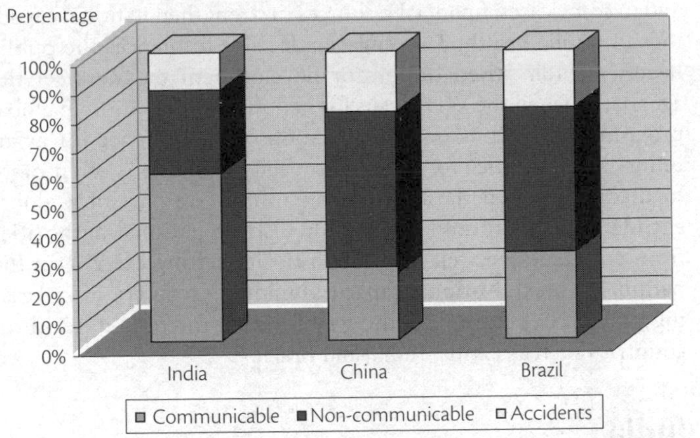

Fig. 1.4.3 Years of life lost (YLL), by cause.

curative care, with the declining role of the state in the provision of health-protecting and health-promoting activities.

The relationship between economic reform and public health has been salient from the time of the Great Depression in the 1930s. In the preceding decades, most spending by the state was limited to sectors which were direct drivers of economy, such as industry, agriculture, and infrastructure. It was only after World War II that the role of the state became significant for the delivery of several social functions such as health, education, etc. To execute such an undertaking, taxation was increasingly used and the concept of social welfare became more clearly defined among governments.

Historically, economic or political crises have often been the drivers behind economic reform. As a consequence of budget cuts during economic crises, government expenditures on health, education, and other 'soft sectors' are usually compromised first. Countries with low incomes have thus been unable to prioritize health as a critical investment. Confronted with changing disease burdens and socio-demographics as part of the development process, health systems are faced with new challenges that they are not adequately equipped to handle.

As countries progress across the development spectrum from low-income to middle-income, or from middle-income to high-income, they are escorted by large demographic and epidemiological changes that are reflected in the health of the population absorbing the economic growth. Economic growth of a country brings about several changes in the health states of its population. Juxtaposed with globalization, this recent economic growth has lead to rapid urbanization in countries in transition. Urbanization has brought about profound changes in living habits. Exposure to risk factors of non-communicable diseases such as obesogenic foods, alcohol, and tobacco in addition to reduced physical activity and augmented stresses associated with modern-day living have become increasingly prevalent. Urbanization itself has also brought about a greater number of deaths due to injuries (including homicide, suicide, and traffic accidents).

As population segments within LMICs witness morbidity and mortality shifts towards non-communicable diseases, as predicted with the advancement of the epidemiological transition, they continue to carry a high burden of infectious and other poverty-related diseases as well. As a consequence, countries in economic transition battle a dual burden: The rising share of non-communicable diseases such as cardiovascular illnesses, cancer, diabetes, and depression, and the traditional problems of infectious disease and malnutrition. Figure 1.4.3 shows the growing trend of non-communicable diseases in the three countries. While communicable diseases such as malaria, tuberculosis, cholera, and AIDS still persist in these countries, non-communicable diseases account for 56 per cent and 50 per cent, respectively, of the years of life lost (YLL) in China and Brazil today (World Health Organization 2007). Escalating at rates parallel to economic growth, non-communicable diseases have grown to become major contributors to premature death and disability. In India, 29 per cent of the YLL are to non-communicable causes.

The evolution of public health in LMICs has also to be understood in the context of the epidemiological transition that accompanies economic and demographic transitions.

In 1971, Omran (2005) broadly explained epidemiological transition as occurring mainly in three stages:

- Era of *pestilence* and *famine*, characterized by high mortality rates, short life expectancy, and no population growth.
- Era of *receding pandemics*, characterized by declining mortality due to large epidemics and stable population growth.
- Era of *degenerative* and *man-made diseases*, characterized by a sharp decline in mortality, a higher life expectancy and demographic growth as determined by fertility, and a shift to chronic (non-communicable) diseases as the major cause of mortality.

In 1985, Olshansky and Ault (1985) proposed a fourth era:

- The era of *delayed degenerative disease*, in which degenerative and man-made diseases are still the major killers, but whose distinguishing characteristic is the delayed *age* at which most of the deaths due to them occur.

Based on the experience of Russia and other post-Soviet republics in Eastern Europe, Yusuf *et al.* in 2001 proposed a fifth era:

- The era of *health regression* and *social upheaval*, in which war or other causes of social upheaval lead to increases in alcoholism and violence, increased ischaemic and hypertensive diseases in the young, as well as increased infectious disease caused by the breakdown of social and health structures. This regressive stage is marked by decreased life expectancy due to the resurgence of diseases from the first two eras, while diseases from the third and fourth stages continue to persist.

The onset of globalization in the twenty-first century has presented LMICs with new health challenges brought on by economic development. Increased rates of urbanization and industrialization marked by rapid deforestation, exponential vehicular growth, and loss of biodiversity have led to a sharp increase in ambient levels of air pollution. Further, the effects of climate change have compromised agricultural yields, thus contributing further to the risk of poor nutrition. The Food and Agricultural Organization (2007) has estimated that, in sub-Saharan Africa, climate change could reduce yields of major crops by 40 per cent over the next 25 years.

The increasing use of agricultural products in the quest for newer sources of energy has also raised concerns about food security and its consequences on nutrition levels. The expanding demand for biofuels such as biodiesel and ethanol, produced from crops such as maize and sugarcane, has also hiked the price of these crops, making them unavailable to the poor. For example, only 10 per cent of the global sugar harvest going into the production of ethanol has caused the price of sugar to double (Integrated Regional Information Network 2007). Brazil, the world's largest sugar producer and exporter, is now converting half of its sugar harvest into ethanol fuel. Such commercial farming is also leading to increased deforestation. Thus, both direct and indirect outcomes of changes in the environment have direct implications for the health of the population.

Characterized by the early onset of respiratory-related conditions in the short term and rising mortality due to several cancers and natural disasters in the long run, worsened by direct risks to nutritional status, a sixth era has presented itself as a new phase of the epidemiological transition:

- The era of *environmental degradation*, which is marked by acute deaths from natural calamities and infectious diseases from their aftermath, as well as chronic conditions such as cancers, emphysema, and asthma due to changes in the surrounding environment. Indirect effects of climate change on health also present issues such as the lack of food security and increased risks of malnutrition. The effects of degradation of the ambient and global natural environment may cause regression into any of the previous five eras, bringing about declines in life expectancy for all age groups.

Epidemiological transitions do not necessarily occur in a linear or unidirectional manner. Countries in economic transition continuously face the risk of regression due to resurgence of a condition that persisted in a previous phase of the epidemiological transition. The sequence of these phases may vary greatly, depending upon the developmental cycle of a country. The rate at which it transitions from one phase to another also depends upon the rate at which it develops economically, and is unique from other countries. In fact, due to persistent regional inequalities, the rate of transition, and the prevalent phase of transition, may even vary within different parts of the same country, as is seen in the case of urban and rural China.

The mid-phase of the epidemiological transition marks an overall shift in the leading causes of mortality from communicable to non-communicable diseases. This shift, juxtaposed with substantial gains in life expectancy, now pose a serious challenge to the health systems in economies in transition, which are still to be reconfigured to respond to these new threats.

Knowledge generation and management

In an increasingly globalizing world, not only are the agents of disease transmitted across nations (be they microbes or tobacco) but also knowledge and technologies integral to the advancement of public health become disseminated rapidly. The ability of LMICs to access these is also a factor that influences the speed at which public health can gain strength from science and technology for overcoming major challenges. Proprietary science and patent-restricted access to technologies become barriers to countries that are resource-constrained. Growth in national capacity for knowledge generation, through strengthening of academic institutions and networks engaged in research, and development of indigenous capacity for technological innovation are essential for LMICs to ensure that these barriers do not limit the growth of public health. Countries such as India, China, and Brazil are increasingly investing in building such capacity.

Partnerships

Partnerships with other countries and with international organizations such as the WHO are also useful in providing access to technical, and in some cases, financial resources to strengthen national capacities in public health. This engagement also influences the public health agenda, when donors or development partners set the agenda, or when the WHO calls for national participation in global programmes such as polio eradication or surveillance for avian influenza. Assistance for national capacity-building is often more forthcoming when the health programmes are part of a global agenda, but this should not unduly distract national authorities from conducting a well-informed priority-setting exercise in the national context. National capacity-building, in an era of increasing global cooperation, is the way forward for public health in countries such as China, India, and Brazil.

India

Public health in India has undergone several changes during its periods of political, social, and economic transition. From the time of British colonization, there has existed an organized framework for the delivery of public health services. The British first established their presence in India in the 1600s. In those times, much emphasis was placed on sanitation, waste management, and outbreak control, similar to the sanitary movements in England that had just occurred. However, these services and measures were in place largely to protect British civilians and their army cantonments, with an emphasis on the early detection of contagious diseases, such as cholera and plague, to prevent their spread to the ruling class (Das Gupta 2005).

The public health system established by the British had several strengths. They put into place the Indian Medical Service (IMS) in the 1760s, which despite its predominantly military orientation, laid the foundation for future health developments in years to come. The British also established medical colleges in Calcutta, Bombay, and Madras in 1835.

The continued interest of the British in the development of preventive health services was rooted in the high mortality of their soldiers during the uprising in 1857, which claimed hundreds of thousands of combatant and civilian lives. It is noted that as many as 69 out of every 1000 soldiers sent from Britain died during their first year of arrival (Harrison 1994), and became a huge cause for concern back in Britain. A commission was set up to investigate the high number of deaths of British soldiers and to evaluate hygiene standards within in its cantonments, the result of which was the setting up of separate establishments for British soldiers and civilians. It was ultimately recognized that the health of British civilians and soldiers could not be seen in isolation from that of the Indian people as they regularly interacted with Indian civilians, despite their deliberately distant habitations from them.

The plague outbreak in the early twentieth century reiterated the need for further investments and attention to public health. The British rulers undertook the establishment of several high-quality academic institutes for training and research, such as the Malaria Institute of India, the Haffkine Institute at Bombay, the Vaccine Research Laboratories at Kasauli, and the King Institute of Preventive Medicine at Madras (Banerji 1997). The School of Tropical Medicine and the All India Institute of Hygiene and Public Health in Calcutta were established shortly thereafter in the 1920s. These institutes of medical training and research were, however, symbols of elitist western civilization in India, and still did not serve the vast needs of the indigenous people.

During the decades preceding independence in 1947, health conditions of the masses were especially poor. Malnutrition and undernutrition rates were high, and communicable diseases were on a constant rise. According to the National Planning Committee (NPC) of 1948, malaria—the most predominant of all infectious diseases at the time—accounted for 100 million cases each year, of which a million proved to be fatal (Banerji 1997). Other infectious diseases such as tuberculosis, cholera, smallpox, dysentery, and diphtheria took a heavy toll of life, and cases of leprosy, filariasis, worm infestations, and venereal disease were also prevalent. Widespread disease and impoverishment were exacerbated by weak access to health care because western systems of medicine were mostly available only to the affluent class.

Further, as methods of western medicine gained popularity, the demand for indigenous medical practices also gradually diminished within the affluent class. Because the indigenous systems had historically thrived on their contributions, this decrease in demand undermined the financial sustainability of these systems. The underprivileged masses, who earlier relied almost exclusively on them, suffered the consequences of their withering. High taxation and exploitation by the colonial regime added substantially to the burden of indigenous families. These miserable conditions led to widespread discontentment and ultimately provided the impetus for a movement demanding health services for the people, and added fuel to the already existing fervour for independence from the British.

On the forefront of the public health movement were eminent medical professionals who were also prominent activists in the struggle for freedom. They were generous in envisioning a health system for India which was vast in scope. One of the main aspirations of the movement was to put in place a system that would serve the people of India, which was something the British rulers had notoriously neglected. The Indian National Congress (an organized opposition against the British empire, which later became the nation's dominant political party for several decades), played a significant role in this movement. Subhash Chandra Bose, President of the Congress in 1938, set up an NPC to be headed by Jawaharlal Nehru (soon to become the first prime minister of independent India). In order to evaluate the existing health conditions and systems, the NPC set up a national health subcommittee (also known as the Sokhey committee).

Concurrently, the British established a health survey and development committee chaired by Sir Joseph Bhore. Although colonial in origin, this committee—later known as the Bhore committee—was greatly influenced by the objectives of the national movement through the assessment and actions recommended by the Sokhey committee. The Bhore committee was eclectic in its constitution, drawing upon experts from various health-science institutions of India, officials such as the Minister of Health, the Director General of the Indian Medical Service, and the Director of the Medical Council of India; other experts from the United States, Britain, and the Soviet Union; and most importantly, representatives of the Indian civil society. The report of the Bhore committee is one of the founding doctrines of health policy in India even today.

Guided by principles that were remarkably similar in essense to the Alma Ata Declaration of 1972, the Bhore committee's recommendations strived for equity in access and health for all. First, the Bhore committee emphasized the need for improved access to primary health services through the setting up of primary health centres (PHCs) throughout rural areas. The establishment of five PHCs and one secondary health unit (SHU) per district in 1952, soon after independence, was perhaps the most direct outcome of this recommendation. It was also planned that these would be increased to 25 PHCs and two SHUs over a 10-year period (Banerji 1997). The Committee also emphasized that preventive and curative services must be well-integrated at all levels of administration. At the lowest level, it recommended the involvement of the community for the implementation of national health programmes. The setting up of a village health committee consisting of residents of the village, who would practice health promotion, was envisaged. Third, the Committee recognized the importance of addressing the social causes of disease, and therefore, recommended the social reorientation of physicians and medical graduates. Recognizing the lack of adequate educational institutes for public health, the Committee also recommended the setting up of centrally sponsored institutes for high-quality research and training programmes in the health sciences, at the graduate and postgraduate level. The All India Institute of Medical Sciences (AIIMS), set up in 1956, was a result of this recommendation. Even though some of the recommendations of the Committee were considered to be ambitious, they set the benchmark for policymakers in the decades to come.

One clear failure of the Bhore committee was that, despite its futuristic response to the public health challenges of the time, it overlooked the potential role of non-clinical researchers and professionals, and as a result excluded them completely from the formal practice of public health. Much emphasis was placed on the social reorientation of physicians by significant modification of the curriculum in medical colleges, as well as through an additional short three-month training course in public health, or preventive and social medicine (PSM) as it was then known. Doctors training doctors left little scope for the inclusion of non-medical personnel such as social scientists, economists, managers, and activists in training and research areas, and public health education remained this way for several decades. It was only in the 1990s that institutes such as the Sree Chitra Tirunal Institute for Medical Sciences and Technology in South India began to offer public health training programmes for the non-clinical community, but these have been few and far between, with only a small number of public health professionals being trained in multidisciplinary settings.

Even within the medical fraternity, PSM was limited in its scope and slow in its development. With a sudden surge in the number of medical colleges in the country post independence, quality control and standardization of education became a challenge. Authoritarian ways of curriculum development, and hierarchical administrations within these institutions did not exhibit any flexibility for change (Narayan 1984). The minimal requirements set by the Medical Council of India did little to promote excellence. Within medical colleges, PSM departments were often neglected and starved of resources. Often considered poor alternatives to clinical medicine, they suffered from low prestige and failed to attract the best talent into the PSM stream.

Fifteen years later, the Mudaliar committee (1961) was appointed to assess the performance of the health sector since the submission of the Bhore committee report. This Committee found the conditions in PHCs to be unsatisfactory and recommended the strengthening of already existing PHCs before the establishment of new ones. The Committee also pressed for the development of an Indian cadre of public health professionals along the lines of the

Indian Medical Service that existed during the British rule. In order to build capacity for the same, it recommended the establishment of a school of public health, in each state, that would grant degrees in public health and train both medical and non-medical personnel. Several other committees in later years also recommended the augmentation of trained public health workforce in the country.

Several of these recommendations, however, did not get the political attention they deserved. In fact, national plans in the initial years post independence have shown regressive policy trends, which have had serious repercussions on the development of the public health system and health policy, which would have potentially benefited from the operationalization of the Bhore and Mudaliar recommendations (Narayan 1984). It was not until the late 1990s that flaws of the public health education system, and the weak influence that it has had on practice, were beginning to be recognized. Poor health outcomes of public health programmes have attested to this neglect. Public health education in India has been too disease-oriented rather than determinants-oriented, and too programme-oriented rather than systems-oriented, lacking a multidisciplinary approach to public health analysis. This is perhaps a consequence of the exclusion of non-medical personnel during the early years of the development of public health training and services in India, as well as policy trends that prevented the convergence of clinical and non-clinical professionals on public health issues.

The paradigm of public health has essentially evolved according to the dominant ideology of both the state and society of the time. The period immediately following independence, namely from 1947 to 1970, was the era of centralized planning characterized by state-led growth of the economy. The state was socialist in its conceptualization, as was reflected in the setting up of its egalitarian health system. Public health developments were centred around the prioritization of primary health services, especially for the rural population, through the setting up of the PHCs. The state became the dominant provider of health at that time.

The first two decades post independence from 1947 to 1967 have been referred to as the golden decade of public health in India (Banerji 1997). Several disease-specific vertical programmes were created; PHCs were established; the state-sponsored Family Planning (later Family Welfare) programme was initiated; steps were taken to promote indigenous systems of medicine; water supply and sanitation was given emphasis in rural areas under the community development programme; and the Integrated Child Development Services (ICDS) was initiated to address malnutrition and undernutrition of children in the preschool years. Human resources for health also developed considerably: A large number of multipurpose workers (MPWs) were trained and recruited, through a scheme launched in 1971, and community health volunteers, later the village health workers, were also trained and recruited within the health system.

It was only a decade later that recommendations similar to the Bhore and Mudaliar committees were made once again in the Alma Ata Declaration of 1978. The declaration urged all governments and health workers to take urgent action to work towards achieving health for all by the year 2000. As one of the signatories, India seized the opportunity to deliberate upon its recent trends in health policy, and revisit the recommendations of the Bhore and Mudaliar committees. The western models of education, training, research, and practice of public health, which had been so predominant, were found 'inappropriate and irrelevant' to the needs of the population (Government of India 2002) . The Indian government also realized that the disease-oriented approach to health-care delivery was benefiting the upper class and urban populations the most. Several programmes, existing and new, attempted to augment the goals of the declaration thereafter.

During the first four decades after independence, the country adopted a 'mixed economy' model, consistent with the dominant political ideology of 'democratic socialism'. This allowed the private sector to flourish, along with state control of key infrastructure, industries, and major public services. In health too, private health-care providers were widely represented, from individual general practitioners to secondary-care hospitals. The indigenous systems of medicine continued to have a presence, especially in the rural areas.

The health sector was jolted by the economic reforms that began in 1991. These reforms led to extensive liberalization of the economy. After half a century of inward orientation, India's contribution to world trade and industry grew substantially. It witnessed a large increase in foreign direct investment and began its journey on the path to becoming one of the largest economies of the world. Unfortunately, the health sector benefited little from these economic developments. Government spending on health as a percentage of the GDP plummeted from 1.3 per cent in 1990 to 0.9 per cent by 2000. As central spending on health steadily declined, more of the financial responsibility was transferred to the states.

In recent years of the post-reform period, the role of the central government in the health sector has diminished greatly, under the influence of neoliberal economics, structural reform, and the spectacular liberalization of India's markets. The central government divested itself of a lot of social responsibility during its transition from a socialist to a capitalist economy. Such patterns of development have had a significant impact on the health sector. Since then, the private sector has grown phenomenally in the health-care delivery arena over the past two decades, mostly at the tertiary- and secondary-care levels. The public sector has begun to adopt practices such as 'user fees', making access more difficult for the poor, and has also begun to divest the management of public-sector health facilities to the private sector under ill-defined 'public–private partnerships'.

Public health systems, unlike most personal medical services, produce 'public goods', and are of high priority and assure good health outcomes for a nation. Although the government was expected to play a critical role in the effective planning and equitable delivery of central health agencies in a large federated union of states such as India, it has performed inadequately ever since India became independent. The nation has faced heavy economic costs for this neglect. For instance, the WHO estimated that the 1994 plague epidemic in Surat resulted in losses totalling US$1.7 billion due to the lack of an adequate public health system. The lack of timely public health action to prevent chronic (non-communicable) diseases has led to high costs of productivity losses and health-care expenditures caused by these neglected diseases. The WHO also estimated that India suffered a loss of US$9 billion in 2005 due to cardiovascular diseases, cancers, and diabetes. These losses are expected to cumulatively lead to US$237 billion by 2015 (World Health Organization 2005).

Due to demographic and epidemiologic transitions, the public health challenges of the country have expanded in recent decades, but have remained largely unmet by the weak response attempted by the national health system, the political leadership, and the academia at large. Unevenly distributed infrastructure, human resource constraints, and low budgetary allocations have significantly contributed to this failure. It is no surprise that efforts of the past have had little impact on health outcomes, despite having a well-developed administrative system, good technical skills in many fields, and an extensive network of medical institutions for research, training, and diagnostics. Although policy priorities have overlooked fundamental public health functions, the system also has deep management flaws that hinder effective use of resources (Das Gupta & Rani 2004).

The public health system as it exists today is an extensive network of district-level hospitals, block-level community health centres, cluster-level PHCs, and subcentres at the village level. Central to the rural public health system is the PHC. Each PHC covers approximately five to six villages, with a subcentre in each village to serve as the first point of access. Patients are referred to a higher tier when more elaborate treatment is required. Similar to a PHC, urban areas have urban health centres (UHCs) or urban family welfare centres and a general hospital (GH) serving a larger population.

The rural population is increasingly reliant on private health care or has no option but to resort to amateur 'doctors' and faith healers, even to treat deadly diseases such as tuberculosis (TB) and malaria. Often, because of the cost of travel and the fear of losing income while they are away, the rural sick tend to use the moderately better health-care services that are located in urban areas only when they are gravely ill. Conditions that could be easily treated, and at little expense, often prove fatal because they have reached an advanced stage by the time they can seek adequate treatment. Kala azar (black fever), for instance, is known by public health workers as an 'epidemic rooted in poverty'. Even though it is curable, it claimed the lives of 60 000 rural poor due to their lack of access to adequate health care (Parwini & Woreck 2004).

A dearth of critical health manpower has only exacerbated the problem of inequities in access to quality care. Despite the presence of over 250 medical colleges in the modern system of medicine and over 400 in traditional Indian system throughout the country, there is a serious shortage of trained health-care providers, particularly in rural areas, and a considerable drain of human resources due to migration of doctors and nurses to other countries.

To address the largely unmet needs of the rural population, the central government launched the National Rural Health Mission (NRHM) in April 2005 and proposed to increase its total health spending on health from 0.9 per cent of the GDP to 2–3 per cent of the GDP by 2012. Since its implementation, current health spending has increased to 1.13 per cent of the GDP (The Economist 2007). The focus of the NRHM is to improve rural health conditions, with a special focus on states with weak public health infrastructure and poor health indicators. The NRHM is improving access to the public health delivery system by the most marginalized segments of the population, including women and children, thereby reducing urban–rural disparities.

The NRHM was launched simultaneously with the Reproductive and Child Health (RCH) programme phase II. The NRHM is a larger and integrative health programme that encompasses all programmes in the area of family welfare, reproductive and child health, and others that are partially or entirely centrally funded, including vertical health programmes for specific diseases such as malaria, filariasis, blindness, etc.

Originally, the RCH-I was launched as a five-year project within the framework of fifty-year-old nationwide National Family Planning programme. Post-Alma-Ata, the Government of India, in its national health policy (NHP), envisaged Health for All by 2000. A mid-decade evaluation of the NHP revealed the need to restrategize in order to achieve certain reproductive health indicators. It was thought that the goals envisaged in the new RCH approach may coincide with the ninth five-year plan of the country. The RCH-I programme introduced a new approach of managing population growth by eliciting more community participation, especially the empowerment of women to take care of their own reproductive health. The RCH-II is now being implemented over the period of 2005–2010, and is a large component of the NRHM. Central to the NRHM is the positioning of at least one accredited social health activist (ASHA) in each village. The main task of this community health worker is to liaise between people of her village and the health facility. She serves as the primary contact of the public health system with the population. Not just a provider of basic curative medicines and first aid, an important part of her role is to facilitate preventive care via certain interventions as well as health education. The presence of the ASHA has caused a decline in fatalities due to unsafe motherhood in several states.

The central government also launched an urban analogue to this scheme, called the National Urban Health Mission (NUHM), in April 2008 (The Economist 2007). Urban social health activists (USHAs), urban counterparts of the ASHAs, will be trained and recruited to promote urban health, especially for homeless and street children, focusing on decreasing the levels of malnutrition and prevention of infectious disease through improved vaccination coverage.

Although financial allocations to the health sector are increasing and new national health programmes are being implemented to increase the outreach of health services, public health has not adequately engaged with policies that are traditionally considered outside the health sector but do exercise a profound impact on the health of the population, often more than policies in the health sector do. Policies related to agriculture, food processing, water resources, urban design, environment, trade, and education are among such policies, which need to become sensitive to and supportive of public health. Taxation and regulation too are measures that, when used judiciously, can influence the determinants of health. Tobacco control is a public health imperative requiring such multisectoral action. India's response to the growing epidemic of non-communicable diseases has now begun to evolve, commencing with a comprehensive legislation on tobacco control (2003) and now has extended to a new national programme for cardiovascular diseases, diabetes, and stroke (2008). This commitment must now extend to policies and actions outside the health sector. Public health must evolve to involve all of the government in policymaking for health and all of society in advancing health action.

In order to infuse greater public health expertise into the health system and broaden the scope of cross-cutting sectors such as public health to extend beyond the health sector, recent initiatives, such as the Public Health Foundation of India (PHFI), have come into existence. The mandate of this not-for-profit organization, created through a public–private partnership, includes the setting up of several institutes of education and training for public health programmes at the graduate and postgraduate level, the establishment of pathways for public health action that are truly multisectoral, and the advancement of a transdisciplinary research agenda which would inform policy and empower programmes. The attainment of such goals would necessitate that public health education be truly interdisciplinary in including subject areas such as epidemiology, biostatistics, behavioural sciences, health economics, health-services management, environmental health, health inequities and human rights, gender and health, health communication, and ethics of health care and research. Initiatives such as the PHFI are attempting to establish synergistic links between these diverse disciplines and the health system to improve the design and delivery of health care.

The Indian government needs to play a proactive role in developing a health policy that ensures equitable access of health resources to all strata of society. Although health is enlisted as a state subject under the Indian constitution, the central government needs to ensure good management of state health systems and oversight in addition to providing financial support, with checks and balances in place. Health financing is an area that needs to ensure equity and affordability while assuring the sustainability of health services. These policy challenges need to be addressed quickly to develop a robust framework for the further evolution and advancement of public health in India.

China

Public health practices in China date back several centuries into a rich history of traditional medicine. The formal practice of public health as a modern academic discipline can be traced back to the 1920s and 1930s, with the establishment of the Peking Union Medical College following the pneumonic plague outbreak in Manchuria in 1911. The college had a formal department of public health, which did some groundbreaking work in the establishment of a primary health-care network, and conducted studies to address the problems of insufficient drug supply in rural China. Guided by the principles of health for all, the university made recommendations for the provision of primary health care (Lee 2004). However, public health academics and health-systems development soon forked from each other, and it is only in recent years that convergence has been sought once again.

Public health in China has also been deeply influenced by its long social and political history over several centuries. These developments have been unique in that no other country (besides Russia) has undergone a political and economic transition so dramatic. The shift from autocratic to decentralized politics, from a closed economy to open markets, and from a predominantly agrarian to an increasingly industry-driven economy (Grant Thornton International Business Report 2008) have had a drastic impact on the health sector. The following paragraphs describe a brief history of China's social and political changes over the second half of the twentieth century and the influence of these changes on the development of the public health system in the decades that followed.

In 1949, Mao Zedong proclaimed the establishment of the People's Republic of China in a victory over imperialism and the Kuomintang (KMT), the opponent party of social democrats. Mao's regime marked a major era in Chinese history. He was one of the founding members of the Chinese Communist Party (CCP), formed in 1921. A revolutionary by conviction, Mao was a radical thinker. Even though his successors deviated from Mao's radical thoughts, 'Maoism', or Marxism as it was interpreted by Mao, is the guiding philosophy of the government even today. The political and socioeconomic changes brought about by the Mao regime had several implications for the health sector.

Before the founding of the People's Republic of China in 1949, very few health facilities existed apart from traditional Chinese medicine clinics and dispensaries, and preventive medicine was virtually non-existent. In the first National Health Congress of 1950, four basic guidelines for the health system were specified, stating that (i) medicine should serve the workers, peasants, and soldiers; (ii) preventive medicine should be emphasized over curative services; (iii) traditional medicine practices should be integrated with western medicine; and (iv) health-related work should be combined with mass movements (Beaglehole & Bonita 2004). Mass campaigns were launched several times a year, and were very effective in the control of infectious diseases. Another outcome of the Congress was the mandate of the Ministry of Health requiring all local governments to establish health centres in rural areas and assign health workers to them. Policies and guidelines such as this promoted the establishment and development of an institutional framework for public health across the nation, particularly benefiting rural China.

To understand the development of the Chinese public health system, it is pertinent to understand the social administration of the time. China was primarily agrarian, with 85 per cent of its population living in rural areas and employed in agriculture (Liu & Wang 1991). The CCP's attempt to speed up the socialization of China through a planned economy led to the practice of collectivization of agriculture in China. Mao implemented the organization of people into 'communes', and made them official state policy in 1958. Communes were essentially cooperatives comprising smaller agricultural units, and were integral to the social fabric of the nation. Communes were an effort to create a truly egalitarian society where everything was shared, and equality was sought in all aspects of life. The cooperatives controlled the prices and production of agricultural goods. Under the communal way of life, produce was merged and redistributed according to household size, and most public services were collectively financed. Health expenses in communes were met by the Cooperative Medical Scheme (CMS), a prepaid mechanism that would provide reimbursements for most medical expenses to its contributors. The CMS inherently increased equity within the system, by making health care affordable and accessible to all.

The period from 1949 to 1976 was an era of centrally planned and managed health services. A three-tier health-care network was established in 1957, which was constituted by village, town, and county in rural China, as part of its social welfare system. Village health clinics providing basic preventive and curative care at the local level served as the first point of access to health care, township health institutions served as the intermediary unit providing primary and secondary health services between the village clinics and the larger county hospitals, and county hospitals, in addition to providing tertiary care, also served as technical guidance centres for personnel and technical training to the lower-tier institutions. These institutions were well-coordinated at each level. They were mutually reliant and supported one another for the provision of comprehensive preventive and curative care through a bottom-up referral system.

There was also an elaborate system for the provision of preventive care through the setting up of epidemic prevention stations (EPSs) at each level of administration, which were closely knit with clinical services. In addition to the preventive services offered within the three-tier health system, there also existed maternal and child health centres, and specialized disease prevention and treatment centres for specific diseases such as TB, malaria, schistosomiasis, leprosy, and other endemic diseases. At the county and provincial level, there were as many as 3600 EPSs for epidemic control and disease prevention, which were responsible for several preventive services such as the early detection and control of infectious disease, inspections for environmental and food hygiene in industrial worksites and schools. All of these were united by the Academy of Preventive Medicine, the national-level institution responsible for research in preventive medicine, which provided technical support to all the other public health institutions at lower levels (Liu & Mills 2002).

Before the establishment of the People's Republic of China, most health expenditures were met by OOP spending of households. With the establishment of the three-tier network and the CMS, households were no longer burdened with health-care costs. However, inequalities still persisted because of an urban bias in the postings of physicians. The severe shortage of skilled medical personnel affected the quality of care delivered to rural areas the most. The unmet demand for providers resulted in the formation of a cadre of minimally trained health personnel, or 'barefoot doctors' in rural China. Barefoot doctors were typically agricultural workers themselves, and provided clinical care to their agricultural units and cooperatives (which later became villages) on a part-time basis. Plenty of resources were allocated by the central government towards the development of the CMS and for the training of barefoot doctors. Although they were only able to provide very basic health services to the peasant class, they existed in large numbers and were widely available (more than one per 1000 members of the population). By 1976, 96 per cent of the agricultural production teams were covered by the service of barefoot doctors (Guangpeng *et al.* 2007).

Although this was a period of relatively lower individual income, China witnessed stellar gains in the health of its people during this egalitarian period. The average life expectancy of the Chinese rose from 35 to 68 years, infant mortality decreased from 250 to 40 deaths per 1000 live births, and the prevalence of malaria was slashed from 5.5 per cent to 0.3 per cent of the population (Hsiao 1995). However, these remarkable gains in health outcomes could not be sustained because of the political and economic changes that took place with the advent of the Cultural Revolution in 1966.

The Revolution was a period of immense social upheaval with the dismissal of several civil rights—a tremendous setback to economic development. China fell even further behind industrialized powers of the world. It was only under the leadership of Deng Xiaoping, post 1978, that the party and the government relaxed control over people, and granted them certain civil rights in a new constitution that was adopted in 1975. In this new phase of reform and development, China went through a remarkable transition from an inward-looking closed economy to an open market-oriented economy, exhibiting immense growth. Global trade increased, diplomatic relations improved, and participation in international organizations was assumed. China became one of the fastest growing economies of the world.

With the end of the Cultural Revolution in the mid-1970s and the economic changes that followed, collective farming was abolished and individual household responsibility was introduced. This drastic change in agricultural policy led to the reorganization of the social structure, and therefore of the health system that was built around it. The breakdown of collective farming led to the collapse of the collectively financed CMS. Health centres sustained by contributions from the communes were now turned into self-financing township, county, and village health centres (Schuchend & Suzhen 2007). The effects of the economic reforms of the 1980s on the rural Chinese population and their health status were paradoxical. On one hand, as the rural economy developed, individual household incomes increased. Rural areas also witnessed the creation of a variety of institutes such as the county maternal and child health centres, county specialized disease prevention and treatment institutes , county centres for disease control, and county health supervision institutes (Gu & Tang 1995). Despite the increase in the number of institutions, the health of the population suffered and health gains from the previous decades started to erode. Inequities in affordability, accessibility, and availability of health services set in and rapidly escalated. There were three chief reasons for this:

1. Reduced government subsidies: The government cut subsidies to health institutions to an amount that accounted for just about 25 per cent of their revenue, covering only basic wages for their staff (Dummer & Cook 2007). In order to remain financially sustainable, health facilities were made to generate additional revenue from charging user fees and dispensing of drugs.
2. Fiscal decentralization: There was tremendous decentralization of the fiscal system to the provinces. Health spending was further decentralized from provincial to county and township governments. As a consequence of diminished government control, the vertical lines of communication within the health system became significantly weakened (Liu 2004).
3. Privatization: Liberalization of the public sector allowed private dispensaries to fill the unmet health needs of the population on the basis of their ability to pay. The increased availability of health services was offset by decreased affordability.

The consequences of these changes on health outcomes were profound:

1. User fees: Introduction of user fees into the health system, in addition to the collapse of the CMS, changed the health-seeking behaviour of those it was meant to serve. The unaffordable fees led to a reduction in the utilization of health services by the poorer segment of the population, creating greater disparities in health outcomes. OOP expenditures as a percentage of the total health spending increased dramatically, and remain high even today. In recent decades, OOP spending has risen from 38 per cent in 1991 to nearly 60 per cent in 2000. Although this number was 53 per cent in 2003, the decline has only been marginal (The Economist 2007).
2. Fragmentation of health system: When health centres were left to generate their own revenue, there was a loss of coordination within the three-tiered system. Health facilities started competing for patients rather than working together through referrals to provide comprehensive care.
3. Inequitable redistribution of health facilities: Centres that were located in poor neighbourhoods and were unable to generate sufficient revenue from user fees and drug prescriptions had to close down and merge with a neighbouring facility (Gao *et al.* 2002).

This redistribution exacerbated hardships in accessing health facilities for the poor.

4. Poor quality care: Health facilities in higher-income areas that generated sufficient revenues were able to pay higher wages to staff, thus attracting professionals of higher calibre. Health facilities in poor areas, if they managed to stay afloat, were unable to attract highly skilled physicians and health workers, as was reflected in the quality of care delivered.
5. Overprescription of drugs and services: There has been growing evidence that patients were prescribed unnecessary drugs and procedures such as X-rays (*The Economist* 2007) in an effort to generate higher revenue (Hsiao 1995; Akin *et al.* 2005; Collins *et al.* 2000), which has negatively impacted the health of the population. In some areas, drug resistance has risen as a dangerous consequence of the consumption of unnecessary drugs.
6. Marginalization of preventive services: EPSs were also adversely affected during the decades following the economic reforms and the consequent changes in government subsidies. The changed financing mechanisms led them to focus more on activities that were revenue-generating, rather than on preventive services, which were essentially free. Whereas in 1985, government subsidies accounted for nearly 80 per cent of their total income, this number was reduced to only 40 per cent in 1997 (Liu *et al.* 1999).

Government spending on health in China has since progressively declined (Fig. 1.4.2.2). More than 50 per cent of the total health spending came from government funds in 1991, but declined to 38 per cent by 2004, and OOP expenses rose from 38 per cent to 60 per cent during the same period (World Health Organization 2007).

There are multiple challenges that the health system must address, and adapt to the altered health needs due to changing disease patterns and demography. China's success in curtailing its fertility rate over the recent years, juxtaposed with major gains in life expectancy, presents it with the real problem of a large aging population. The unique and demanding health needs of this age group further burden a health system that is already pressed for resources.

The Chinese public health system has evolved into a vast establishment, with institutions at each level of the government involved with preventive care, curative care, and surveillance, and overseen by the Academy of Preventive Medicine at the centre. In recent years, the focus of the Academy has been primarily on activities that are hygiene-related and on other preventive services delivered through the EPSs, based on a biomedical model. China has since invested vast resources for the establishment of disease surveillance systems, especially after the recent SARS and avian flu epidemics. The establishment of the China Centre for Disease Control and Prevention (China CDC) in 2004 has been a milestone in the history of Chinese public health. Based on the Academy model, the China CDC's mandate extends to include a more broad-based approach to public health. Some of its main functions are disease surveillance and prevention, emergency response, health promotion and health education, training and applied research, and international cooperation (China Center for Disease Control 2008). It consists of an elaborate four-tiered network for disease control. It is also considered to be multisectoral in nature, through its partnerships with several ministries at the central level, universities, and research institutions. Collaborations with professional and non-governmental organizations make the China CDC a cross-cutting body with a key role in influencing policymaking.

Health-systems research has also been given increasing importance among policymakers, with the setting up of the Health Policy Advisory Board within the Ministry of Health in mid 1980s, and the founding of the China Health Economics Network shortly thereafter (Zhang & Zou 1998). After the SARS outbreak in 2003, research institutes and universities have been increasingly engaged in health policy and systems research, and their expertise for health-systems development has been sought at different levels of the government (Lei 2005). The establishment of the Health Policy and Regulation department within the Ministry of Health in 2004 is a result of such collaborations. While there is an increasing demand for public health researchers within the system, human resources are lacking and vacancies are plentiful. Although pathways for their close integration into the health sector are being paved, China has yet to see adequate investments in capacity-building for public health professionals.

Other challenges to the health sector

Uneven economic growth

China's growth rate of >9 per cent of the GDP for the last two decades has led to significant overall economic development of urban and rural populations. However, urban segment areas, especially in the 'Gold Coast' and the eastern provinces, have benefited much more. Rural areas such as the Yunnan, Guizhou, and Hunan provinces are still developing at a much slower pace than urban China, and will continue to lag behind for quite some time. The widening gap between urban and rural socioeconomic positions has only exacerbated disparities in health outcomes.

Technological barriers

China's open markets have brought in high-quality medical equipment, advanced biotechnological interventions, modern medical amenities, and the latest drugs. However, their availability depends largely on a persons ability to pay, and is concentrated in urban areas. With the diminishing role of the government in health-care delivery and increasing role of market forces, inequalities in access to health care and health status have continued to rise in recent years. Further, secondary translational barriers have prevented the health system from making technological advancements in health widely available to the masses. In the past, as resources for health have increased, government investment in public health has been skewed towards vaccination programmes and clinical care, with preventive and promotive care subsequently marginalized. Developing countries have realized in recent years that interventions need to be more evidence-based, context–specific, and resource-sensitive, and that following western models of public health need not lead to successful outcomes.

Human resources

After reforms in medical education, barefoot doctors were required to earn a certification and practice as a 'village doctor'. This deterred several barefoot doctors from practising, resulting in the loss of several trained health workers. Further, an urban bias in the preferences of medical graduates for employment has left the void created by the loss of several barefoot doctors unfilled. The lack of adequate public health personnel is also a lacuna that needs to be addressed.

Stark disparities in health outcomes

Disparities in maternal and infant mortality rates between urban and rural areas have been widening. Official data from the Ministry of Health and the WHO report that the infant mortality rate in urban areas is 10.1 per 1000 live births and in rural areas is 24.5 per 1000 live births. Maternal mortality indicates a similar disparity, with rates of 26.1 per 100 000 live births in urban areas and 63 per 100 000 live births in rural areas. Non-communicable diseases are simultaneously on the rise, affecting both rural and urban areas. Rural areas also face an increased risk of infectious diseases. According to Ministry of Health estimates, 80 per cent of the TB patients in China live in rural areas, particularly in the less-developed western regions, where the epidemiological transition is still in the early stages (Dummer & Cook 2007). Although levels of risk factors for chronic disease are higher in urban areas, the very low chances of detection and treatment of those with risk factors in rural areas leaves them highly vulnerable to adverse events such as stroke and heart disease.

Environmental degradation

Rapid industrialization and urbanization has increased the ambient air pollution in urban areas, which is an inherent risk factor for several respiratory illnesses. The lack of urban planning and unregulated vehicular growth further contribute to this. After the United States, China is the second largest contributor to environmental pollution in the world. Deforestation and decline in the number of open spaces in cities is damaging the biodiversity of these areas considerably, often beyond reversal. The short-term gains in health from the effects of globalization have long been replaced by the ill-effects of mass consumerism, such as depletion of natural reserves and deterioration of the natural environment. The World Bank estimates that by 2020, China will be paying US$390 billion (13 per cent of its projected GDP) to treat diseases indirectly caused by coal burning (Dummer & Cook 2007). Policymakers will have to proactively take measures to ensure the regulated and planned growth of new cities and intervene with environmental standards to protect, conserve, and restore China's natural resources, with active involvement of the public health community.

The Chinese experience shows that economic growth does not necessarily translate into better health outcomes. Progressive health-sector policies have often been left outside the purview of economic developments in transitional economies under the influence of neoliberal structural reforms. The Chinese experience also shows that the provision of health services cannot be left to the mercy of market economics. Meng *et al.* (2004) estimated that nearly 50 per cent of the village clinics in rural areas were privately owned. Excessive privatization without adequate government regulation and planning has compromised the quality of care. The role of the state in the assurance of, if not the provision of, health services has not been clearly defined. The resurgence of infectious diseases such as TB and schistosomiasis attests to the weak role of the state in the provision of preventive care.

Brazil

The development of public health, or *collective health*, as it is known in Brazil, has been markedly different from India and China, and any other country in Latin America. The development of the health system and the civil movement for political stability have played a mutually influential role in each other's development.

Development of the health system

State-provided health care in Brazil dates back to 1923, as a component of the social security system that was a promulgation of the Eloy Chavez law. Under this social welfare system, urban workers employed in the private sector received coverage for health care through compulsory contributions to pension and retirement funds (CAPS), later organized into institutes by professional category (IAPs), through payroll deductions and employer contributions. By default, workers in excluded professional categories, the unorganized sector, the unemployed, and the rural population were almost entirely devoid of health coverage from this system. These centrally regulated social security funds in turn provided reimbursements for health services provided by the private sector. For several decades, this system was financed by employers and employees, with very little involvement of the government in setting of health priorities. Government funds were used mainly to contract-out services to the private sector, or as subsidies for the construction of private hospitals and clinics. Further, most facilities that existed were concentrated in the more developed south and south-east, and further exacerbated issues off access to health-care facilities among poorer segments and those living in less developed areas.

The government during that period was known for its policies propagating rigid centralization and prioritization of economic development over social services (Cortes 2006). Until the 1960s, the social welfare system was centred on the provision of medical care to workers in the private sector, and the Ministry of Health, formed in 1953, was involved mainly with issues of community health and vaccine distribution through various campaigns and disease-specific vertical programmes. Although its mandate also included the provision of basic medical care to low-income populations where adequate services did not exist, it owned very few hospitals, which mainly specialized in contagious diseases and psychiatry (Medici 2007). Issues related to universal access to care were not prioritized on the agenda of policymakers. It has been estimated that barely 30 per cent of the country received coverage from an IAP by the end of the 1950s (Oliveira 2008).

However, significant changes occurred in this structure with the unification of these institutes to form the National Social Welfare Institute (INPS) in 1966, and brought about a growing trend towards expanding health-care coverage for categories not previously covered. The authoritarian government that came into power in 1964 recognized the lacunae existing within the fragmented health system and attempted to expand health-care delivery by contracting services to a larger network of private establishments in order to meet the greater demand for health care. A large portion of public funding was, thus, provided for the expansion of the private sector. Although several minor institutional and structural changes took place over the next couple of decades, the welfare system remained practically unchanged until the mid-1980s when a new constitution was adopted. This new constitution redefined social security to be inclusive of the rights to welfare, health, and social assistance, providing coverage to the entire population, independently of their professional job or any affiliation. A new unified national health-care system was established in 1988.

The public health reform movement

The development of public health in Brazil has been strongly influenced by the Latin American Social Medicine (LASM) movement which began in 1966. Inspired by similar historical social movements and political processes in France, Germany and England, led by Rudolf Virchow and others in mid-nineteenth century, the movement was deep-rooted in the economic and political changes that Brazil was witnessing. By the 1970s, what began as the struggle for democratization of health services had taken the shape of a much larger nationwide struggle against military rule. Drawing participation from across groups, professions, and communities such as health-services researchers, political party representatives, and health workers' organizations (Elias & Cohn 2003), the public health reform movement expressed itself through several symposia, conferences, and academic gatherings.

Although democracy was not established in Brazil till 1985, the Movement was able to exert an important influence over the post-dictatorial reforms (Collins *et al.* 2000). Many of the leaders of the Movement came from academic backgrounds. Its forerunners were protesting university students, especially those in health-related fields, who became involved in the political movement for democracy. As a result, they chose practices that promoted political change even after they had graduated. Given the heavy involvement of students and professionals in the political movement, their orientation towards social justice and politics in turn influenced curricula within educational institutes, which initially led to the introduction of social medicine in medical schools. Pioneered by the University of Rio de Janeiro in Brazil, separate graduate-level master's programmes in preventive and social medicine were offered across several countries in Latin America over the next decade (Waitzkin *et al.* 2001).

With the adoption of the new constitution in 1988 in democratic Brazil, health care was specified as a constitutional right and a responsibility of the state. During the same period, several Latin American countries were implementing neoliberal reforms, propagated by the World Bank, that encouraged privatization and the limiting of the state's involvement in the provision of health services to regulation only (Homedes & Ugalde 2005). Contrariwise, Brazilian health reforms aimed to increase the role of the state not only in health-service delivery but also in research and training, and largely curbed the dominance of the private sector. The role of the state was finally confirmed. Inspired by Italian health reforms of the 1960s and 1970s, Brazilian health reforms propagated decentralization, or *municipalization* as a means of de-concentrating power at the centre and strengthening the public sector. This was done through the establishment of the Unified Health System or the Sistema Único de Saúde (SUS) in 1988, which consisted of a three-tier network of primary health centres and hospitals owned by the central, state, and municipal governments (known as *municipios*). The SUS was to be nationally coordinated by the state and jointly implemented with local and state authorities. Health-care delivery by the private sector existed as a supplementary health network known as the SSAM, and was complementary to and coordinated with government services. The federal government would, through the Ministry of Health, play a larger regulatory role in the creation and implementation of the national health policy, and in national programmes for communicable diseases and nutrition. Public health activities such as disease surveillance, health promotion, and immunizations would also be delivered through the SUS (Buss & Carvalho 2007). Some of the key features of the democratization of the health sector were community participation, the decentralization of health services, and fiscal devolution at each level of the government (Medici 2007).

Before the establishment of the SUS, health-care delivery relied exclusively on centrally regulated social security funds, and the care delivered was largely dependent on the private sector. Now, it is almost entirely funded by local state and regional governments, and the role of the government in the provision of services has increased, but inequities still persist. Today, the SUS stretches nationwide and strives to provide a complete medical package, covering more than 70 per cent of Brazil's population (Schmidt & Duncan 2004). The complementary private system, or SSAM, provides care to the remaining population consisting of lower-risk individuals in the higher- and middle-income groups. As a result, expensive procedures not covered by the private SSAM network, and costs for high-risk individuals, are left entirely for the SUS to meet.

Through the 1990s, health services continued to be increasingly decentralized—both in terms of fiscal devolution and decision-making authority. Decentralization was facilitated through the transfer of power and funds to local municipalities to use on health services at their discretion. Fiscal devolution to the regional- and local-level authorities gave greater flexibility to the local governments to respond more appropriately to the needs of the population, as they were better informed about ground realities. This was managed by the members of two commissions—the Tripartite commission at the national level, consisting of representatives from all three levels of government, and the Bipartite commission at the state level, consisting only of state and municipal representatives. However, it also introduced competition between local and state governments for central government funding and further exacerbated inequities in access to quality health care.

Community participation, an important aspect of Brazil's health-reform policies, was mandated by law for state and local governments to be eligible for central funding. Civil society was involved by the creation of health councils at each level of the government. These were essentially advisory bodies that assisted with policy decisions regarding the implementation of the SUS. The councils were constituted such that they involved participation from several actors within the community, including members of civil society, the users as well as providers of health services. Although the actual distribution of power among the stakeholders within the councils has been skewed towards government representatives, the very existence of these councils made decision making a diverse and inclusive process (Tajer 2003). The establishment of a participatory forum helped the democratization of Brazilian institutions, empowering social sectors that were traditionally excluded from direct representation in the political system. Presently, under the PRO-SAUDE programme, Brazil's institutions providing training to the health workforce receive financial support for projects aimed at realigning the health system to the needs of the community.

Decentralization and devolution have been central to the debate on health-sector reform for decades, and Brazil duly illustrates its pros and cons. Although decentralization is meant to bring about greater equity and efficiency within the system, the varying levels of development and performance of local governments may also lead to greater disparities in health outcomes and fragmentation of the system. The attainment of equity and assured quality are challenges that Brazil's SUS faces today.

New developments

The Ministry of Health initiated the Family Health Programme (PSF) in 1992 in an effort to enhance the provision of basic health services including preventive services to underserved populations. The core of the PSF is the placement of a team of providers and specialists in a certain geographic area that serves roughly 1000 families. This programme currently serves 47 per cent of Brazil's population (Medici 2007). The PSF focuses on several health-promoting activities such as child development, vaccinations, prenatal examinations, promotion of personal hygiene, breastfeeding campaigns, and water and sanitation requirements within communities. It is currently one of the most effective programmes being carried out in the country (Buss & Carvalho 2007). In 2006, the National Commission on Social Determinants of Health (CNDSS) was also launched within the Ministry of Health. This commission consists of state and municipal health council representatives as well as ministers from cross-cutting sectors.

Several intersectoral programmes extending beyond the Ministry of Health have also been launched in recent years: The Family Grant Programme (PBF), managed by the Ministry of Social Development, offers financial support to families below the poverty line; the Family Agriculture Programme, managed by the Ministry of Agriculture, promotes family agriculture instead of industrial agriculture, thus improving nutritional levels and ensuring sustainable agriculture; the National Programme of Food and Nutrition (PNAN), tied closely to the PSF, sets nutritional guidelines for the Brazilian population and takes on several health-education campaigns to disseminate information on health-promoting dietary practices; the Healthy Cities/Communities initiative (CCS) is a network of municipal governments and universities and schools of public health, existing entirely at local levels, without the involvement of the central government; the Health Promoting Schools programme (EPS) is another intersectoral initiative between the Ministry of Health and the Ministry of Education to promote healthy practices within schools among teachers, students, and their families.

Brazil has been one of the most advanced countries for scientific theory and research generation in Latin America, with plenty of state support since the 1990s. An increasing number of graduate programmes in preventive and social medicine, extending beyond the medical community, have helped to shape the public health movement as a tool for political and social justice. The Brazilian health sector has significantly advanced due to thriving health-services research and the coming together of several professional and political organizations. The national health service now depends on academic support for various functions such as programme planning, implementation, monitoring, and evaluation (Schmidt & Duncan 2004). The CNDSS recommendations, in 2006, to the Ministry of Health resulted in the allocation of significant funding towards research on social determinants and inequity in health . A consortium of several public health education and research-based organizations such as FIOCRUZ, the Brazilian Association of Postgraduation in Collective Health (ABRASCO), and Canadian Public Health Association (CPHA) are currently carrying out the intersectoral Actions for Health project, which aims at capacity-building and knowledge exchange between different institutions across the country. Prizes for academic excellence and funding for health-systems research related to issues within the SUS are being increasingly awarded to researchers to build synergies between research outputs and the requirements of the health system. In 2007, 90 medical, nursing, and dental colleges received grants for making curricular changes that would promote engagement between different faculties of health-care professionals, primary care, and action learning (Global Health Workforce Alliance 2008). The case of Brazil exemplifies how academia and policymakers mutually benefited from one another and together contributed to the development of the national health system and strengthened the practice of public health.

Conclusion

The three countries profiled in this chapter (China, India, and Brazil) represent societies wherein the economies are on the upswing and are accompanied by demographic and epidemiological transitions, profoundly influencing the agenda of public health as well as the level of resources available to address it. Despite growth in their economies and increasing urbanization, they also have large segments of rural or otherwise disadvantaged populations, posing challenges not only to health equity but also presenting diversity in dominant disease burdens.

All of these countries have focused on developing health systems which will extend health care to all sections of the population. In doing so, clinical care was prioritized over preventive and promotive measures by all of them. It is only in recent years that countries such as China and India are paying greater attention to building broader public health capacity and looking at multisectoral interventions for promoting population health. In Brazil, the political discourse that shaped popular movements and governmental policies, over the past two decades, has accorded a high priority to public health. As the value of better health as an accelerator of economic development and its relevance to human rights gain greater recognition in each of these societies, public health is likely to grow in its influence and impact.

Even as the focus has been on establishing strong systems for delivery of health care, the role of the state has undergone substantial changes, over time, in these countries. China has dramatically shifted from universal state-supported and communitized models of health care to a mixed model of state-/employer-supported care and private purchased care. India, which always had a mixed model, has substantially reduced the role of the state in the supply of health services and has allowed an unregulated private sector to emerge as a major provider, increasing market distortions in the availability, quality, and pricing of health care. The rising out-of-pocket expenditures on health care in these countries are a cause for concern, because the poor may be deprived of affordable health care. Brazil, on the other hand, has emphasized the primary responsibility of the state in extending health care to all sections of the people and has clearly defined a small but supplementary role for the private sector.

Although decentralization has been accepted by each of these countries as essential for efficient operationalization of public health programmes, it has not been implemented with an equal measure of success everywhere. China's shift to decentralization has reduced state support for services. India's commitment to decentralization is becoming more manifest in new national programmes such as the National Rural Health Mission, but the serious gaps in the availability of health workforce, lack of public health expertise, and limited coordination among multiple vertical programmes raises concerns about the limited ability of local stakeholders in taking full advantage of a decentralized system. Brazil, on the other hand, has built a robust model of well-coordinated but adequately decentralized health-care system. As these countries develop further, they have to carefully balance local autonomy and central support so that the public health system is operationally unchained but not left rudderless. Even as democratic devolution and efficiency are promoted though decentralized systems, central coordination would be needed for ensuring commitment to goals, quality of services, and to provide for early recognition of and rapid response to emerging or exacerbated inequities.

In an era of rapid globalization, the pressures to free the markets will see these LMICs move towards greater privatization in all sectors, including health. However, the need for a strong role for the state in planning for universally available and affordable health care, and its predominant position in advancing policies and programmes for public health should not be overlooked. The state must act as the guarantor of services for the vulnerable sections of the people and a promoter of policies that protect the health of the entire population. Access to adequate and affordable health services must be fully assured by the state, even if not fully provided by it.

Even as the role of public health is enhanced in the priorities and programmes of these economically advancing countries, capacity-building for public health needs greater attention. Adequately trained and motivated human resources as well as strong institutional structures and networks for advancing public-health-related education and research are needed. As schools of medicine, nursing, and dentistry must upscale the public health components of their curriculum, schools of public health which provide interdisciplinary learning to medical as well as non-medical public health professionals must be developed. The limited biomedical model of health sciences must be replaced, through such education and research, with a trans-disciplinary model of applied public health sciences that integrates knowledge and perspectives from life sciences, social sciences, economics, quantitative sciences (such as epidemiology and biostatistics), and management sciences.

At the same time, public health education and research must become more closely connected to the development, evaluation, and strengthening of health systems. Public health will evolve into a stronger discipline with a greater ability to make a substantial societal contribution if it moves along these new directions of growth in the LMICs. Although promising signs of such a change are visible in some of these countries, the extent to which the discipline will advance further over the next two decades will be a critical determinant of health and development in the high-velocity transitional period that lies ahead.

Key points

- The disciplinary mandate of public health, globally and nationally, has expanded from providing essential hygienic services and disease-preventive personal protection to broader social-engineering efforts, which combine public education and policy interventions that have a population-wide effect, for health promotion.
- Health systems have been influenced by many of the economic and social changes that have occurred in LMICs, and have developed within that context.
- Economic transitions have been accompanied by profound demographic and epidemiological changes. The rapidly increasing burden of non-communicable (chronic) diseases juxtaposed with gains in life expectancy and lowered fertility rates are challenging present health systems in new ways.
- Skewed distributional patterns of the wealth created during this growth phase in the LMICs have aggravated socioeconomic inequalities, resulting in major disparities in health outcomes.
- A clearly defined role of the state in setting health priorities and assuring health services is key to improving health outcomes, especially among the poorer segments.
- Adequate engagement of public health researchers, policymakers, and practitioners is vital for the development of the discipline to its full potential.

References

Akin J.S., Dow W.H., Lance P.M. *et al.* Changes in access to health care in China, 1989–1997. *Health Policy and Planning* 2005;**20**(2):80–9.

Banerji D. *Landmarks in the development of health services in the countries of South Asia.* Delhi, India: Consul Press; 1997.

Beaglehole R., Bonita R. *Public health at a crossroads—achievements and prospects.* 2nd ed. London: Cambridge University Press; 2004. pp. 227–32.

Berman P., Ahuja R. (2008). Government Health Spending in India. *Economic and Political Weekly,* June–July. Vol. 43 (26, 27) pp. 209–216.

Buss P., Carvalho A. Health promotion in Brazil. *Promotion and Education* 2007;**14**(4):209.

China Center for Disease Control. People's Republic of China; 2008. Available from: http://www.chinacdc.net.cn

Collins C., Araujo J., Barbosa J. *et al.* Decentralising the health sector: issues in Brazil. *Health Policy* 2000;**52**:113–7.

Cortes S.M.V. Building up user participation: councils and conferences in the Brazilian health system. *Sociologias* 2006;**1**:1–23.

Das Gupta M., Rani M. India's public health system: how well does it function at the national level? Policy Research Working Paper 3447. Washington (DC): World Bank; 2004. p. 1–24.

Das Gupta M. Public health in India: an overview. Policy Research Working Paper 3787. Washington (DC): World Bank; 2005. p. 1–12.

Dummer B., Cook G. Exploring China's rural health crisis: processes and policy implications. *Health Policy* 2007;**83**(1):1–16.

Economic and Social Data Service. World Bank Data – China. Website: http://ddp.ext.worldbank.org (Accessed November 15th, 2007).

Elias P., Cohn A. Health reform in Brazil: lessons to consider. *American Journal of Public Health* 2003;**93**(1):44–8.

Food and Agricultural Organization. Paying farmers for environmental services. In: The state of food and agriculture. Rome, Italy: Food and Agricultural Organization; 2007.

Gao J., Qian J., Tang S. *et al.* Health equity in transition from planed to market economy in China. *Health Policy and Planning* 2002;**17** Suppl 1:20–9.

Global Health Workforce Alliance. *Scaling up, saving lives.* Geneva: World Health Organization; 2008.

Gottret P., Schieber G. Health transitions, disease burdens, and expenditure patterns. In: *Health financing revisited: a practitioner's guide.* Washington (DC): World Bank; 2006.

Government of India. National health accounts. Mumbai, India: Reserve Bank of India; 2005.

Government of India. *National health policy.* India: Ministry of Health; 2002.

Government of People's Republic of China. The Chinese statistical yearbook. People's Republic of China: Ministry of Health.

Grant Thornton International Business Report. Emerging markets: Brazil, Russia, India, China (BRIC). 2008.

Gu X., Tang S. Reform of the Chinese health care financing system. *Health policy* 1995;**32**:181–91.

Guangpeng Z., Xiaoyan L., Junhua Z. *et al.* The history and development of three-tier health care network in rural China. People's Republic of China: Health Human Resources Development Center (HHRDC), Ministry of Health; 2007.

Harrison M. *Public health in British India*. Cambridge: Cambridge University Press; 1994.

Homedes N., Ugalde A. Why neo-liberal health reforms have failed in Latin America. *Health Policy* 2005;**71**:83–96.

Hsiao W. The Chinese health care system: lessons for other nations. *Social Sciences and Medicine* 1995;**41**(8):1047–55.

Integrated Regional Information Network (IRIN). Combustion or consumption? Balancing food and biofuel production. UN Office for the Coordination of Humanitarian Affairs; 2007 Apr 25.

Lee L. The current state of public health in China. *Annual Review of Public Health* 2004;**25**:327–39.

Lei H. *Health systems research in China: macro situations*. Peoples Republic of China: Department of Health Policy and Regulation, Ministry of Health; 2005.

Liu X., Mills A. Financing reforms of public health services in China: lessons for other nations. *Social Science and Medicine* 2002; **54**:1691–8.

Liu X., Wang J. An introduction to China's health care system. *Journal of Public Health Policy* 1991 Spring:105–17.

Liu Y., Hsiao W.C., Eggleston K. *et al*. Equity in health and health care: the Chinese experience. *Social Science and Medicine* 1999; **49**:1349–56.

Liu Y. China's public health care system: facing the challenges. *Bulletin of the World Health Organisation* 2004;**82**:532–8.

Medici A. Structure of the health system. Brazil: Ministry of Foreign Affairs. Available from: http://www.mre.gov.br/cdbrasil/itamaraty/web/ingles/polsoc/saude/estsist/index.htm [accessed 2007 Dec].

Meng Q., Shi G., Yang H. *et al*. *Health policy and systems research in China*. Geneva: World Health Organization; 2004.

Narayan R. 150 years of medical education rhetoric and relevance. *Medico Friend Circle Bulletin* 1984;**97–98**:1–9.

O'Donnell O., Doorslaer E., Rannan-Eliya R. *et al*. Explaining the incidence of catastrophic expenditures on health care: comparative evidence from Asia. EQUITAP Project; 2005. Working paper 5.

Oliveira F. Social welfare. Brazil: Ministry of Foreign Affairs. Available from: http://www.mre.gov.br/CDBRASIL/ITAMARATY/WEB/ingles/polsoc/previd/apresent/index.htm [accessed 2008 Feb].

Olshansky S., Ault A. The fourth stage of the epidemiological transition: the age of delayed degenerative disease. In: *Should medical care be rationed by age?* Lanham (MD): Rowman and Littlefield; 1985.

Omran A. The epidemiologic transition: a theory of the epidemiology of population change. *The Milbank Quarterly* 2005; **83**(4):731–57.

Parwini Z., Woreck D. Black fever in India: an epidemic rooted in poverty 30th December, 2004. *The World Socialist Web* 2004.

Schmidt M., Duncan B. Academic medicine as a resource for global health: the case of Brazil—improving population health demands stronger academic input. *British Medical Journal* 2004;**329**(2):753–4.

Schuchend W., Suzhen F. The history, current status, and future prospects of barefoot doctors in China. People's Republic of China: Health Human Resources Development Centre, Ministry of Health; 2007.

Tajer D. Latin American social medicine: roots, development during the 1990s and current challenges. *American Journal of Public Health* 2003;**93**:2023–7.

The Economist (2007). Missing the barefoot doctors. October 2007. Website: http://www.economist.com/world/asia/displaystory.cfm?story_id=9944734 (accessed November 2, 2007).

Waitzkin H., Iriart C., Estrada A. *et al*. Public health then and now. *American Journal of Public Health* 2001;**91**:1952–1601.

World Bank. Investing in health: world development indicators. In: *World development report*. Washington (DC): World Bank; 1993.

World Health Organization. *WHO report 2006: working together for health*. Statistical Annexe; 2006.

World Health Organization. *World health report 1995: bridging the gaps*. Statistical Annexe; 1995.

World Health Organization. *World health report 1996: fighting disease, fostering development*. Statistical Annexe; 1996.

World Health Organization. *World health report 1997: conquering suffering, enriching humanity*. Statistical Annex; 1997.

World Health Organization. *World health report 1998: a life in the 21st century—a vision for all*. Statistical Annexe; 1998.

World Health Organization. *World health report 1999: making a difference*. Statistical Annexe; 1999.

World Health Organization. *World health report 2000: health systems—improving performance*. Statistical Annexe; 2000.

World Health Organization. *World health report 2001: mental health—new understanding, new hope*. Statistical Annexe; 2001.

World Health Organization. *World health report 2002: reducing risks, promoting healthy life*. Statistical Annexe; 2002.

World Health Organization. *World health report 2003: shaping the future*. Statistical Annexe; 2003.

World Health Organization. *World health report 2004: changing history*. Statistical Annexe; 2004.

World Health Organization. *World health report 2005: make every mother and child count*. Statistical Annexe; 2005.

World Health Organization. *World health report 2006: health workforce*. Statistical Annexe; 2006a

World Health Organization. *World health statistics 2007*. Geneva: World Health Organization; 2007.

Xinhua News Agency. TB tops list of China's killer diseases. 2006 May 10.

Yusuf S., Reddy K.S., Ounpuu S. *et al*. Global burden of cardiovascular diseases: Part I: general considerations, the epidemiologic transition, risk factors, and impact of urbanization. *Circulation* 2001;**104**:2746–53.

Zhang T., Zou H. Fiscal decentralization, public spending, and economic growth in China. *Journal of Public Economics* 1998;**67**:221–40.

SECTION 2

Determinants of health and disease

2.1

Globalization

Kelley Lee

Abstract

Globalization, defined as the closer integration or interconnectedness of human societies across national borders through spatial, temporal, and cognitive changes, is creating wide ranging impacts on public health. This interconnectedness is characterized by cross-border flows of people, other life forms, goods and services, capital, and knowledge to an unprecedented degree in terms of intensity and extensity (geographical reach). The emergence of a global economy, for example, has led to the restructuring of many health-related industries such as pharmaceuticals, food, and tobacco. Other global changes taking place, such as the increased movement of populations, environmental change, and financial transactions, have had indirect yet profound impacts on health determinants and outcomes.

To date, the public health community has played a limited role in influencing the nature of the changes taking place, which have been largely driven by powerful economic and political interests. Contemporary globalization, as a result, has been characterized by an inequitable distribution of costs and benefits within and across countries. For the public health community, there is a need to better understand the linkages between globalization and health, and the possible interventions available to protect and promote public health. A review of key activities in public health practice suggests the need for a 'global public health' approach which seeks to minimize the costs, and maximize the benefits, to public health arising from globalization. Recent developments in infectious disease outbreak control, environmental health, health promotion, and monitoring of health status provide examples of the challenges faced. These include opposition by powerful vested interests to stronger regulation, the need for effective collective action across all societies to tackle crossborder public health issues, and the current weaknesses of global health governance. Nonetheless, there are opportunities for the public health community to influence globalization by demonstrating the shared benefits to be gained. Greater attention to the public health impacts of globalization, through redistributive policies, greater attention to health equity, and appropriate social and environmental protections will, in turn, contribute to more sustainable forms of globalization.

Introduction

'Globalization' is a term associated with complex and varied changes to the world around us, and has received substantial research and policy attention in a wide range of fields. While scholars, policy makers, and practitioners continue to debate the benefits and drawbacks of these changes, there is agreement that better understanding of the nature of these changes, and their specific impacts on human societies, is much needed.

There is now a substantial body of scholarship on globalization and public health which seeks to explain how contemporary flows of people, other life forms, goods and services, capital, and knowledge are influencing the determinants of health and health outcomes (Lee 2003b; Lee & Collin 2005; Kawachi & Wamala 2006). The unprecedented scale of these flows, in some cases rendering the national borders of individual countries irrelevant, has posed three major challenges for the public health community: How can the evidence base on globalization and health be strengthened; what effective policy responses are needed to optimize the benefits, and minimize the costs to public health, arising from globalization; and how can these policy options be practically and effectively implemented?

This chapter is concerned with how globalization is influencing public health. It begins by defining globalization, and how it is a distinct and contemporary phenomenon. This includes the increasingly used concept of 'global public health'. The key drivers of globalization are described, alongside an understanding of the types of changes occurring as a result. The chapter then focuses on the implications raised by globalization for key functions of public health policy and practice. Many of the issues raised in this chapter are addressed in more detail elsewhere in this textbook, a reflection of the importance of global forces now at play in so many aspects of public health. The chapter concludes by considering the governance issues raised. While the public health community has found itself at the frontline of many of the impacts resulting from globalization, and needing to adapt to many of the changes taking place, it remains somewhat in the background when it comes to shaping and managing globalization. The public health community must increase its capacity to influence such decisions if globalization is to prove a positive force for human health.

What is globalization?

The popular and widespread use of the term 'globalization' has led to considerable variation, and at times lack of clarity, of what it actually means. In many cases, the term has been used to replace 'international', denoting subjects that concern two or more countries. Alternatively, the term is defined more narrowly to refer to increased international trade, the spread of Hollywood films or other relics of western culture, or the greater movement of people across borders. Alongside definitional vagueness lie marked differences in how globalization is normatively assessed. Some writers see globalization as a unifying and progressive force, bringing unprecedented economic growth and prosperity (Dollar & Kraay 2000; Feachem 2001). Others believe that globalization is a new form of colonialism which serves to reinforce inequalities of wealth and power, and consequently health and other social conditions, within and across countries (Cornea 2001; Labonte *et al.* 2005). These differences in perspective are reflected in the highly contested nature of scholarship in this field.

While it is beyond the scope of this chapter to review these debates in detail, including the substantial evidence now accumulating of the costs and benefits of globalization, it is an important starting point to approach the term critically. In the broadest sense, globalization has become widely understood as the closer integration or interconnectedness of human societies across national borders. Different societies have long interacted across vast distances (e.g. migration of the human species out of Africa in one million BC, the Silk Road trade route, and the Age of Discovery from the fifteenth century). Globalization can thus be recognized as an historical process. At the same time, we can see that there are contemporary forms of globalization in which there has been intensified flows of people, other life forms, goods and services, capital, and knowledge across borders to an unprecedented degree since the mid to late twentieth century. In recent decades, not only has there been a vast increase in the quantity of social interaction across populations, but the reach of those linkages to virtually all parts of the world is also new. Held *et al.* (1999) write that it is this greater intensity and extensity of linkages across human societies that define globalization today.

Three types of changes to human societies are occurring as a result of globalization (Lee 2003a). The *spatial dimension* refers to changes to how people organize and interact with physical or territorial space. The now clichéd image of globalization as a shrinking world or 'global village' refers to the extension of economic, political, and social linkages to a worldwide scale. E-mail, long-haul package holidays, cyberspace, and the global operations of transnational corporations are all examples of the restructuring of social space. For the most part, our experience of the world is that it is 'shrinking' because of a greater capacity to access distant locations. In other cases, novel ways of organizing social interactions are emerging, largely through new information and communication technologies. The creation of virtual communities, such as YouTube™ and Facebook®, for example, allow individuals to communicate, and form social connections and networks, irrespective of geographical location.

The *temporal dimension* concerns changes to how we think about and experience time. The contemporary world is largely characterized by an acceleration of the timeframe which things can be, and are expected to be, done. For instance, financial transactions involving currency trading, buying and selling of equities (stocks and shares), and the securing of credit can take place in a matter of seconds through global information and communication systems, even when involving parties located in different parts of the world. Similarly, advances in transportation technology have enabled larger numbers of people to travel greater distances in shorter amounts of time (e.g. bullet train, supersonic jets). Modern life has been one of time pressures to 'multi task', speed dial and 'drive through'.

Third, the *cognitive dimension* concerns changes to how we think about ourselves and the world around us. The dissemination and adoption of knowledge, ideas, values, and beliefs have become worldwide in scale through the global reach of the mass media (including the advertising industry), research and educational institutions, consultancy firms, religious groups, and political parties. The ascendance of English, as the leading language for diplomacy, science, air transportation systems, and entertainment is also a result of cognitive globalization. Some argue that this is leading to the marginalization of local cultures and languages, and corresponding domination by Western values and beliefs defined by individualism and consumerism (Barber 2003). Huntington (2002) warns of a potential 'clash of civilizations' as competing ideologies and value systems come together to cause religious or political conflict. However, others believe cognitive globalization is progressively spreading shared ideas and principles which support human rights, gender equity, environmental and labour standards, and democracy. In public health, Benatar *et al.* (2003) write of the development of global health ethics such as the human rights based approach. Overall, the three types of changes taking place as a result of globalization—spatial, temporal, and cognitive—are closely intertwined, and together are leading to a mixture of positive and negative impacts.

Another point of substantial debate surrounding globalization is an understanding of what is driving these change processes. Globalization is clearly enabled by technological advances which make flows across borders possible. As the capacity of these technologies expands, and the cost of using such technologies decline, they have become more accessible to larger numbers of people. For example, the industrial policies pursued by many governments since the 1970s has emphasized the achievement of increased economic competitiveness through promoting access to cheaper transport and fuel. This has led to a decline per ton of sea and air freight which, in turn, has encouraged the rapid growth of international trade (US Department of Transport 2000; Teitel 2005). Overlooking the environmental impacts, the advent of low cost air travel amid fierce competition has made holidays abroad accessible for the first time to millions of people (Swan 2007). Communication costs have declined even more rapidly. When desktop computers (microcomputers) became commercially available in the late 1970s, a desktop computer cost around US$5000, putting them out of reach of most private users. By 2007, the cost had declined to a few hundred dollars for many times the processing power of the original machines (Lee & Collin 2005). Not surprisingly, information and communication technologies have been frequently cited as the major force behind globalization (Hundley *et al.* 2003).

For some writers, however, technology is an enabler, but not the driver, of globalization. The real factors driving technological developments and their application are, it is argued, economic in nature. The global spread of capitalism has been driven, on the one hand, by untold thousands of producers seeking access to the cheapest inputs (i.e. raw materials, labour, research and development, transport and communications), most efficient (and greatest) economies of scale, and largest potential markets. Millions of consumers around the world, on the other hand, fuel this process by demanding the highest quality and quantity of goods and services at the lowest possible price. The millions of economic transactions that result, what eighteenth century economist Adam Smith called the 'invisible hand' of the market, is seen as the real force behind globalization (Dicken 1999).

A further perspective rejects globalization as an essentially technological or economically driven process which implies a degree of rationality and progress. Instead, some scholars point to current and dominant forms of globalization as driven by certain ideologically-based values and beliefs broadly referred to as neoliberalism. It has been the global spread of this ideology that has, for instance, defined the industrial policies facilitating the development of such technologies (e.g. the promotion of an information economy through deregulation and privatization of telecommunications sector), and their dissemination for particular purposes (e.g. deregulation of financial markets). It is argued that neoliberalism has also defined economic policies which encourage international trade (e.g. trade negotiations), market driven competition, and foreign investment (e.g. tax incentives, and a minimal role for the state at the expense of social welfare and environmental protections (Falk 1999).

Not surprisingly, differences in perspective about the drivers of globalization reflect variation in views about whether, on balance, such changes are beneficial or costly to human societies. So-called globalists (supporters of contemporary globalization) predict a world of closer integration, shared identities, greater efficiency and productivity, more rapid economic growth, and increased prosperity. While there may be bumps to negotiate along the way, such as temporary inequalities in wealth within and among countries, it is believed that the globalization path is progressive in the longer term, and will bring largely benefits for the greatest number of people. In sharp contrast, the opponents of contemporary globalization, who see its associated changes as largely driven by a neoliberal defined agenda, do not agree that the resultant changes taking place are mainly positive. A broad range of individuals and organizations, often referred to as the anti-globalization movement, see fundamental flaws inherent within the assumptions underpinning current globalization processes. Of particular note are stark imbalances in power and influence within the emerging global order, dividing the world into winners (those with access to technology, capital, knowledge and gainful employment) and losers (i.e. poor, unskilled), with the latter far greater in number. Although globalization may generate increased aggregate wealth, critics challenge the assumption that this wealth will eventually 'trickle down' to those at the bottom of the global pecking order. Rather, anti-globalists cite substantial evidence which is strongly suggestive that, without strong commitment to redistributive policies, along with appropriate social and environmental protections, neo-liberal globalization will lead to a widening gap between haves and have-nots including health inequities (Kim *et al.* 2000; Mittelman 2002). Moreover, if allowed to continue unabated, many critics argue that current forms of globalization are socially and environmental unsustainable in the longer term.

This chapter is broadly located within the latter perspective. From a public health perspective, globalization is leading to diverse and complex changes to health determinants, resulting in both positive and negative health outcomes. For the protection and promotion of public health, and to ensure the longer-term sustainability of globalization, these changes must be actively managed to ensure that the positive outweigh the negative impacts, and that any costs to health are equitably and fairly shared across societies. In order to develop effective responses to the public health implications raised by globalization, it is useful to consider in greater detail what changes are taking place.

Features of contemporary globalization

Current forms of globalization can be seen as dominated by the integration and convergence of systems of economic production, distribution and consumption on a worldwide scale. While economist have varied opinions on the precise timing of when these processes began to emerge, most agree that the creation of the Bretton Woods Institutions—the World Bank, International Monetary Fund (IMF) and General Agreement on Tariffs and Trade (GATT) after the Second World War laid its institutional and normative foundations. Each has played an important role in facilitating the emergence of a global economy defined by the liberalization of capital flows, and opening of national markets to trade and investment.

The first major pillar of the global economy, liberalization of capital flows, was introduced in the US from the mid 1970s which, in turn, precipitated a complete restructuring of financial markets across the world. Historically, banks, insurance companies, investment companies, and brokerage firms have been subject to heavy governmental regulation. Deregulation of financial markets, such as the removal of restrictions on the types of securities that financial institutions could trade, levels of interest that could be paid on specific types of securities and bank accounts, and types of institution entitled to act as financial intermediaries, was introduced to increase competitiveness within the market and encourage greater capital flows within and across countries. Information and communication technologies enabled high-speed electronic-based transactions which eventually linked financial markets across countries. The result has been the creation of a globally integrated financial market capable of 24-hour trading in foreign exchange and related money markets, the international capital markets, the commodity market, and the markets for forward contracts, options, swaps, and other derivatives (Valdez 2006). The scale of capital flows has correspondingly boomed. The world's financial assets totaled US$136 trillion in 2005, and will exceed US$228 trillion by 2010. Global crossborder capital flows reached a record US$6 trillion in 2006, more than double their level in 2002. Foreign exchange trading increased from US$17.5 trillion/year to US$1.5 trillion/day between 1979 and 2002 (OECD 2005; McKinsey & Company 2007).

A second key pillar of the global economy is the trade of goods and services. While trade has been the lifeblood of commerce for thousands of years, it is the restructuring and integration of production processes across the world, accompanied by the growth in scale and scope of trade, which characterizes the global economy of recent decades. Historically, trade among countries has been dominated by raw materials and natural resources (e.g. oil, timber), commodities (e.g. grains, metals) or manufactured products (e.g. textiles and clothing, food products). In 1948, the GATT was established as an agreement under which signatories could negotiate reductions in tariffs on traded goods. Originally, the GATT was to become an international organization like the World Bank or IMF. However, without consensus among member states, this could not be achieved. Instead, the GATT remained an agreement under which eight trade rounds were carried out between 1948 and 1994 through which thousands of concessions on tariff reductions were reached. During this period, membership grew from 23 countries in 1947 to 125 countries in 1994, thus establishing a worldwide trading system.

The boom in traded goods and services since 1945 led to renewed support for a permanent organization. In 1995, following the conclusion of the Uruguay Round of trade negotiations, the GATT was replaced by the World Trade Organization (WTO). Membership has since increase to 150 member states, with many more countries seeking accession. Moreover, the scope of the world trading system has broadened to embrace trade in services, agriculture, intellectual property rights, government procurement and other areas (Wilkinson 2006). The overall effect has seen a growth in the scale and range of international trade. Since 1948, world trade has consistently grown faster (6 per cent annually in real terms) than world output (3.9 per cent). In 2006, this trend continued with world merchandise exports increasing by 15 per cent to US$11.76 trillion, and commercial services exports growing by around 11 per cent (US$2.71 trillion) compared with global gross domestic production (GDP) growth of 3.7 per cent (WTO 2007).

The global restructuring of production and exchange processes has been an integral part of the boom in international trade over the past half century. In many sectors, transnational corporations (TNCs) have emerged which have geographically relocated components of their business to different parts of the world (Dicken 1999). Thus, resource extraction may take place in one country, manufacturing in another, and research and marketing in still others. The targeted consumers have also changed, with TNCs increasingly seeing the world as a single marketplace. According to the *Forbes Global 2000*, a ranking of the world's top corporations by sales, profit, assets and market value, the increase in so-called 'global brands' has been a key feature of a restructured world economy. In 2005, *BusinessWeek* ranked the top five global brands (measured as the 'most valuable') as Coca-Cola, Microsoft, IBM, General Electric and Intel (Anon 2005).

While global restructuring has not occurred in all industrial sectors, it can be observed in many sectors with direct or indirect impacts on public health. One important example is the pharmaceutical industry which, as a result of mergers and acquisitions, is today dominated by a small number of large companies. Pharmaceutical companies ranked among the largest 100 global corporations in 2006 led by Pfizer (35), Johnson and Johnson (57), Sanofi Aventis (58), GlaxoSmithKline (82), Novartis (83), Unilever (87), and Roche (97) (Forbes 2006). Table 2.1.1 describes the largest companies in 2004 by sales, growth and market share, all of which are headquartered in major industrialized countries. Table 2.1.2 lists the leading pharmaceutical trading countries, led by Switzerland with a trade surplus of £5561 million in 2004. The overall trend in the sector has been towards larger and fewer companies, controlling a growing share of the market. In 1992, the 10 largest companies accounted for one-third of world revenue (Tarabusi & Vickery 1998). By 2002, this share had increased to one-half (Busfield 2005). The trend towards larger pharmaceutical companies has been driven by global competition. The cost of

Table 2.1.1 Top world pharmaceutical corporations (2007)

	Country	Sales (£) million	Growth* (%)	Market share** (%)
Pfizer	USA	22 292	−2	6.7
GlaxoSmithKline	UK	18 847	1	5.6
Novartis	SWI	17 154	9	5.1
Sanofi Aventis	FRA	16 788	8	5.0
Astrazeneca	UK	15 010	9	4.5
Johnson & Johnson	USA	14 478	5	4.3
Roche	SWI	13 814	18	4.1
Merck & Co	USA	13 631	8	4.1
Abbott	USA	9570	8	2.9
Lilly	USA	8335	13	2.5
Leading 10		**149 920**	**6**	**44.9**
Amgen	USA	8188	1	2.5
Wyeth	USA	7949	8	2.4
Bayer	GER	7020	13	2.1
Bristol-Myers Squibb	USA	6519	6	2.0
Boehringer Ingelheim	GER	6277	11	1.9
Schering-Plough	USA	6181	10	1.9
Takeda	JAP	5479	9	1.6
Teva	ISR	5300	12	1.6
Novo Nordisk	DEN	3336	18	1.0
Daiichi Sankyo	JAP	2925	7	0.9
Leading 20		**209 093**	**7**	**62.6**

* Calculated in US$
** IMS audited markets
Source: Reprinted with permission by the Association of the British Pharmaceutical Industry (ABPI). Available at http://www.abpi.org.uk/statistics/section.asp?sect=1.

research and development (R&D), large-scale manufacturing, and worldwide marketing and distribution, means that successful companies need to be of a certain size with considerable resources. For example, the industry estimates that developing and launching a new drug product onto the world market costs around US$403 million in 2000 (DiMasi *et al.* 2002). The desire to gain access to overseas markets and 'pipeline' products has further encouraged mergers and acquisitions with local companies.

As industry ownership has become more concentrated, and so-called 'Big Pharma' has pursued the most profitable products to recover associated costs, concerns have been raised within the public health community about the neglect of certain diseases and populations deemed to offer insufficient financial returns. For conditions where there are a relatively small number of sufferers, or the potential market is a population unlikely to afford available treatment, companies have not invested resources (Trouiller *et al.* 2002). Another major concern is the assertion of intellectual property rights (IPRs) by pharmaceutical companies over new drugs. Patent protection entitles companies to exclusive marketing rights and to charge higher prices in order to recover R&D investment.

Table 2.1.2 World trade in pharmaceuticals, 2007

	Exports (£)	Imports (£)	Balance (£)
Switzerland	20 206	9336	10 870
Ireland	9664	1520	8144
Germany	24 395	18 810	5586
UK	14 567	10 291	4276
France	13 675	10 135	3540
Sweden	4726	1731	2995
Netherlands	7439	7276	163
Italy	7607	8466	−859
Spain	4142	5227	−1085
Japan	1736	4625	−2889
USA	17 491	35 801	−18 310

Source: Reprinted with permission by the Association of the British Pharmaceutical Industry (ABPI). Available at: http://www.abpi.org.uk/statistics/section.asp?sect=1.

Higher prices, however, has meant reduced access to new drugs by the poor. The need to improve access to essential medicines, such as second line anti-retroviral drugs, to treat major public health problems led to the Doha Declaration on IPRs and Public Health in 2003. Tensions between trade and public health policy, however, persist as practical implementation of the declaration's provisions in low-income countries remains a major challenge (Kerry & Lee 2007).

The food industry has undergone similar pressures to 'go large', with the ascendance of TNCs increasingly controlling food production from 'plow to plate'. The history of food production and consumption is closely linked to the migration of human populations, raising and exchange of food crops, and domestication of animals. The distinct feature of contemporary globalization is the industrialization of food production and consumption into a complex of global businesses (excluding subsistence farming). Among the Fortune Global 500 are food retailers Wal-Mart (2), Carrefour (25), Metro (55), and Tesco (59), and manufacturers Nestlé (53), Unilever (106), and PepsiCo (175), all of which command sizeable proportions of the world market. As global food brands have gained ground, local and small-scale producers have become increasingly marginalized in the name of economies of scale and efficiencies.

The globalization of the food industry raises a wide range of public health issues. The rapid rise in rates of obesity, as discussed further below, has led to concerns about the global trend towards diets high in fat, salt and sugar intake (Cassels 2006). In a follow-up to WHO's Global Strategy on Diet, Physical Activity and Health (WHO 2004), Lang *et al.* (2006) assessed compliance by 25 of the world's largest food manufacturers and retailers to recommendations concerning such factors as ingredients, advertising, portion size, and labelling. The report found only a small proportion of companies acting to reduce salt, sugar, and fats from their products, four (Cadbury Schweppes, Danone, Nestlé, and Unilever) had any policies on advertising, two (Kraft and McDonalds) were acting to reduce portion sizes, and 11 were improving labelling. While the public health community has pushed for stronger regulation of this hugely powerful industry, governments to date have largely resisted in favour of voluntary codes.

The tobacco industry offers a further example of the public health implications arising from the global restructuring of the world economy. As smoking prevalence has steadily declined in high-income countries, the tobacco industry has turned its efforts to so-called 'emerging markets' in Asia, Africa, Eastern Europe, and Latin America. Consequently, the industry has consolidated through numerous mergers and acquisitions into four transnational tobacco companies (TTCs) which control around 75 per cent of the world cigarette market: Philip Morris, British American Tobacco, Japan Tobacco International, and Imperial Tobacco. This excludes the Chinese National Tobacco Corporation, a state monopoly which supplies 98 per cent of the 300 million smokers in China, the world's largest tobacco market. Importantly, globalization has facilitated the tobacco industry's expansion into emerging markets through trade liberalization, overseas manufacturing, marketing and advertising, and economies of scale (Bettcher & Yach 2000; Callard *et al.* 2001). Consequently, based on current trends, it is predicted that deaths from tobacco use will rise from 5 million in 2006 to 8.4 million by 2020, with 70 per cent occurring in the developing world (WHO 2002b).

Finally, the global economy has a dark underbelly of illicit activity with important implications for public health. Of particular note is the growing problem of smuggled and counterfeit goods. The trade in illegal psychoactive drugs is a serious worldwide problem, with 200 million people (or 5 per cent of the global population age 15–64) having used illicit drugs at least once in the last 12 months. In recent decades, the trade has become global in the number of countries in which (producers and consumers are located), and the transnational network of criminal organizations involved. In 2003, the retail (street) value of the trade was estimated at US$322 billion (United Nations Office on Drugs and Crime 2006). The global nature of cigarette smuggling, representing around 20–25 per cent of total consumption, also poses a major problem by supplying the market with cheaper priced products and thus undermining national tobacco control policies. Counterfeit goods now comprise 5–7 per cent of world trade. Many counterfeits, notably medicines, food products and cigarettes, are of dubious quality and content, and can pose direct risks to public health. WHO estimates that counterfeit drugs account for 10 per cent of all pharmaceuticals, with the number rising to as high as 60 per cent in developing countries. For example, a survey in Nigeria found 80 per cent of drugs distributed in major pharmacies in Lagos to be counterfeit (WHO 2006a). Counterfeit baby milk powder in rural China caused the deaths of 50 children and acute malnutrition in hundreds of others (Watts 2004).

As well as the restructuring of economies, globalization has contributed to unprecedented levels of population mobility in terms of frequency and distance travelled. Population movements are not new—humankind has been on the move since *Homo erectus* migrated out of Africa in one million BC. Mass migrations, both voluntary and forced, have been prompted by the search for food, water, and arable land, and to escape hardship, conflict, and natural disasters. The migration of Europeans to the Americas from 1492 marked a period of large-scale movement of populations over the next 500 years. For example, 15 million slaves were transported from Africa to the Americas during the eighteenth and nineteenth centuries. More than 30 million people moved as indentured workers after the abolition of slavery in 1850. Around 59 million people migrated from Europe to the Americas, Australia, New Zealand, and South Africa between 1849 and 1939 in search of economic opportunities (ILO 2000). Global migration is thus part of an ongoing historical process.

What have characterized population movements since the mid twentieth century are the unprecedented volume, speed, and geographical reach of travel. All regions of the world have seen increasing numbers of people on the move. International migration now accounts for approximately 130 million people (2 per cent of the world's population) per year. Two million people cross international borders daily, and 500 million people cross borders on commercial airlines annually. Between 1995 and 2010, an increase of 80 per cent in long haul travel is predicted (Anon 2007). Total international tourist arrivals reached 842 million in 2006, growing by 20 per cent since 2002. International refugees receiving UN assistance increased from 1.4 million in 1961 to 9.2 million in 2004. It is estimated that 900 000 people were trafficked internationally in 2003. For all of these reasons above, by 2006 up to 200 million people (1 in 33 people) were living outside their country of birth, compared with 75 million in 1965 (UNFPA 2003). Furthermore, internal migration (movement within a single country) has occurred at an even greater magnitude. In the mid-1980s, one billion people, or about one-sixth of the world's population, moved within their own countries (Castles & Miller 2003).

The International Labour Organisation (ILO 2007) reports that, although more people globally are working than ever before, the number of unemployed remained at an all time high (195.2 million) in 2006. For the relatively educated, highly skilled, and mobile, globalization has created new employment opportunities. For the poorly educated and low skilled, globalization has brought employment insecurity. For healthcare, the most direct impact has been the accelerated migration of health workers. While the migration of health workers from poor countries, notably sub Saharan Africa, to the industrialized world has received much needed attention, migration patterns are recognized to be more widespread. The decision to migrate is an individual one, based on personal circumstances and employment prospects, but broader forces shaped by globalization, affecting work and living conditions are also at play (Bach 2003). The *World Health Report 2006* (WHO 2006c) estimates that there are 59.2 million full-time paid health workers worldwide, and an estimated shortage of almost 4.3 million doctors, midwives, nurses, and support workers. The shortage is most critical in 57 countries, especially in sub-Saharan Africa and parts of Southeast Asia. The African region has 24 per cent of the global health burden but only 3 per cent of health workers commanding less than 1 per cent of the world health expenditure. The so-called 'brain drain', caused by the flow of health workers from low- to high-income countries, has gravely worsened this problem. On average one in four doctors and 1 in 20 nurses trained in Africa is working in OECD countries.

The implications of globalization for public health

The Institute of Medicine (1997) defines 'global health' as 'health problems, issues, and concerns that transcend national boundaries, may be influenced by circumstances or experiences in other countries, and are best addressed by cooperative actions and solutions'. Public health is concerned with improving the health of whole populations, rather than the health of individuals (Walley *et al.* 2001: 19). The US Health and Human Services Public Health Service (1995) identifies 10 core activities of public health:

1. Preventing epidemics
2. Protecting the environment, workplace, food, and water
3. Promoting healthy behaviour
4. Monitoring the health status of the population
5. Mobilizing community action
6. Responding to disasters
7. Assuring the quality, accessibility, and accountability of medical care
8. Reaching out to link high-risk and hard-to-reach people to needed services
9. Researching to develop new insights and innovative solutions
10. Leading the development of sound health policy and planning

Global public health, in this sense, concerns how globalization is impacting on each of these core activity areas. Globalization is not only leading to public health issues transcending national boundaries, but to the need for collective efforts across countries to help shape more socially just and sustainable forms of globalization. The remainder of this chapter examines some of these key functions of public health, how globalization may impact on their practice, and how the public health community might effectively respond to these impacts.

Globalization and the control of infectious disease outbreaks

The prevention, control, and response to, infectious disease outbreaks are a core activity in public health. Historically, disease-causing microbes have travelled across vast distances for as long as mobile human populations have come into contact with each other and other animal species. For example, the shift from hunting-gathering to agrarian societies and the domestication of animals, between 8000 and 3500 BC, led to the emergence and spread of new zoonotic diseases (Swabe 1999). The so-called 'Columbian exchange', following the arrival of Christopher Columbus in the Americas, is noted by historians for the widespread exchange of plants, animals, foods, human populations (including slaves), and ideas that followed. Diseases, such as bubonic plague, cholera, influenza, measles, malaria, smallpox and tuberculosis, were also exchanged, resulting in the decimation of up to 90 per cent of the indigenous American population (Crosby 1972). Another notable example is the influenza pandemic of 1918–1919 at the end of the First World War, which killed around 25 million people. The pandemic similarly demonstrated the capacity of infectious disease to spread across the world amid large-scale human migration and weakened social structures.

Contemporary globalization, characterized by unprecedented volume, speed, and geographical reach of population mobility, is leading to growing evidence that infectious disease outbreaks have a greater capacity to emerge and spread more rapidly and further afield. This is because globalization, in its current forms, potentially influences a broad range of biological, environmental, and social factors that influence human infections.

First, globalization may alter what populations are at risk of certain infections. The Global Burden of Disease Study estimates that infectious diseases were responsible for 22 per cent of all deaths and 27 per cent of disability-adjusted life years worldwide in 2000 (Lopez *et al.* 2006). Many infections continue to disproportionately affect the poor within and across countries, and globalization can worsen their vulnerability by, for example, contributing to rapid urbanization without sufficient attention to basic needs such as water, sanitation, gainful employment, and healthcare. This lesson was gradually recognized in nineteenth-century Europe during the Industrial Revolution, which prompted social reforms that eventually led to a decline in infectious diseases, and vast improvements in health status, during the first half of the twentieth century. Today, it is no coincidence that infectious diseases still account for a large proportion of death and disability among those who have been excluded from, and in many cases bear a disproportionate share of the costs associated with, globalization processes.

At the same time, globalization can 'democratize' certain infectious diseases, making all populations vulnerable to them. While tuberculosis and cholera are diseases historically associated with poverty, because of the role of poor quality housing and sanitation in their spread, other infections do not discriminate by socioeconomic class. Some infections, such as measles, diphtheria, and tetanus, can be caught by any population, but vaccination reduces their reach. Where prevention is not possible, such as pandemic influenza, the consequences for whole populations, regardless of socioeconomic status, can be devastating. The rapid and extensive reaction to the outbreak of severe acute respiratory syndrome (SARS) in 2002–2003 was due to the perceived vulnerability of all populations, rich or poor (Woollacott 2003). Moreover, the rapid spread of SARS from China to around 25 countries within weeks, illustrated how quickly infectious diseases can spread within a globalized world. There are similar concerns about the potential for avian influenza to cause a human influenza pandemic of unprecedented proportions amid globalization.

Second, globalization may influence the *prevalence* (number of people with a disease within a given population) and *incidence* (number of new cases of a disease in a specified period of time per total population) of infectious diseases. De Vogli and Birbeck (2005) argue that vulnerability to HIV/AIDS, tuberculosis, and malaria is closely linked to poverty, gender inequality, development policy, and health sector reforms that involve user fees and reduced access to care. Dorling *et al.* (2006) similarly argue that 'global inequality in wealth will have compounded the effects of AIDS on Africa', notably caused by globalization-related policies such as structural adjustment programmes.

Third, globalization may influence the emergence of novel infections or re-emergence of diseases previously in decline. Environmental degradation, such as the felling of rainforests or dumping of toxic wastes, can increase contact with new sources of infection or lead to mutation of existing infectious agents (e.g. cholera Bengal). Perhaps the most worrying potential 'public health emergency of international concern' is an influenza pandemic involving a highly pathogenic strain such as H5N1. Intense animal rearing practices, alongside human populations, is believed to be contributing to an increased risk of antigenic shift of the influenza virus. The prospect of an influenza pandemic spreading across continents today has led to unprecedented efforts to prepare and coordinate across countries and regions (Lee & Fidler 2007). The SARS outbreak provided a worrying example, not only of the speed and reach of outbreaks, but the weak capacity by public health systems around the world to cope with a large-scale outbreak of this kind.

A cautionary note should be appended here. To prove that globalization is responsible for the increasing prevalence of a specific infection would require standardized monitoring of the exposure (the process of globalization being studied), the outcome (incidence of a particular infectious disease), and other determinants of disease (e.g. immunity, treatment, socioeconomic factors) over many years. The necessary studies would be extremely difficult to construct, and highly vulnerable to confounding due to new and unforeseen factors developing out of the enormous transformations occurring in most aspects of contemporary political, economic and cultural life. In addition, surveillance systems describing the incidence and prevalence of infectious diseases over time are very rare, particularly for populations in low-income countries, who are often the most likely to experience the adverse health effects of global transformations. Even if a causal association were detected, there would likely be considerable dispute over whether the relevant process, for instance global warming, was in fact caused by globalization. Thus, the assessment of health risks associated with globalization must accommodate much unavoidable uncertainty (Saker *et al.* 2006). This does not mean that no conclusions should be drawn on the influence of global processes on past, present and future disease patterns. Indeed, poor or absent supportive evidence of the benefits of globalization has not dissuaded proponents of unregulated economic globalization from arguing forcefully for its introduction. The need to respond in situations where we do not have full and incontrovertible evidence for our actions is well expressed by the precautionary principle: 'Where there are threats of serious or irreversible damage, lack of full scientific certainty shall not be used for postponing cost-effective measures' (UN Conference on the Environment and Development 1992).

The perceived heightening of infectious disease risks from a globalizing world has prompted actions to develop more effective public health responses. Alongside risks, globalization brings opportunities to improve the capacity of public health institutions to respond more effectively to infectious disease outbreaks. Foremost is the advent of new information and communication technologies which, in principle, enable faster, cheaper, and more efficient gathering and sharing of knowledge. ProMED-mail (see Box 2.1.1) and regional disease surveillance networks have sprung up to facilitate the collection and reporting of epidemiological data. The lessons learned from SARS led to renewed efforts to revise the International Health Regulations (IHR), which came into effect in 2007, to harness a broader range of information sources. Another change is the expansion of the scope of the IHR beyond named diseases, notably plague, yellow fever, and cholera, to the broader term 'public health emergencies of international concern'. This may include human or natural disasters. Beyond surveillance, technological advances are also permitting faster development, such as drugs, vaccines, because of the capacity for more rapid development and testing, and potential dissemination of new knowledge within the medical research community (WHO 2005).

Protecting environmental health in a global context

The discipline of environmental health concerns 'the theory and practice of assessing, correcting, controlling, and preventing those

Box 2.1.1 Programme for Monitoring Emerging Diseases (ProMED-mail)

The Programme for Monitoring Emerging Diseases (ProMED)—mail was established in 1994, with the support of the Federation of American Scientists and SatelLife, as an Internet-based reporting system dedicated to rapid global dissemination of information on outbreaks of infectious diseases and acute exposures to toxins that affect human health, including those in animals and in plants grown for food or animal feed. Electronic communications enable ProMED-mail to provide up-to-date and reliable news about threats to human, animal, and food plant health around the world, seven days a week.

By providing early warning of outbreaks of emerging and re-emerging diseases, public health precautions at all levels can be taken in a timely manner to prevent epidemic transmission and to save lives.

ProMED-mail is open to all sources and free of political constraints. Sources of information include media reports, official reports, online summaries, local observers, and others. Reports are often contributed by ProMED-mail subscribers. A team of expert human, plant, and animal disease moderators screen, review, and investigate reports before posting to the network. Reports are distributed by email to direct subscribers and posted immediately on the ProMED-mail Web site. ProMED-mail currently reaches over 30 000 subscribers in at least 150 countries.

A central purpose of ProMED-mail is to promote communication amongst the international infectious disease community, including scientists, physicians, epidemiologists, public health professionals, and others interested in infectious diseases on a global scale. ProMED-mail encourages subscribers to participate in discussions on infectious disease concerns, to respond to requests for information, and to collaborate together in outbreak investigations and prevention efforts. ProMED-mail also welcomes the participation of interested persons outside of the health and biomedical professions.

Source: International Society for Infectious Diseases. About ProMED-mail. http://www.promedmail.org/pls/promed/f?p=2400:1950:17654933971171386906 (accessed 12 March 2007)

factors in the environment that can potentially affect adversely the health of present and future generations' (Pencheon *et al.* 2001: 206–207). Environmental threats to public health range from local, small-scale factors (e.g. household exposures) to widespread exposures affecting whole populations. Protecting against a perceived environmental health threat involves identifying the hazard, determining the relationship between the hazard and the effect (dose-response assessment), exposure assessment, and risk characterization.

The possible impacts of globalization on environmental health are wide-ranging, going beyond global-scale threats to potentially affecting populations at the regional, community, occupational and household levels. Impacts from globalization can be direct, such as through the transport and dumping of hazard waste across borders, relocation of hazardous occupations (such as ship breaking in low-income countries), or damage caused by acid rain or a nuclear accident. Economic globalization, in which companies compete on a worldwide scale to increase returns, are raising concerns that there are incentives to undermine environmental health. Governments, seeking to attract foreign direct investment to fuel economic growth and employment, may engage in a so-called 'race to the bottom' by offering reduced taxation rates, low wages, or weak environmental, health and safety protections (Brecher & Costello 1994). As stated by the environmental organization, the Sierra Club (2000), 'By promoting economic growth without adequate environmental safeguards, trade increases the overall scale and pace of resource consumption; promotes adoption of high-consumption, high-polluting lifestyles; and prompts countries to seek international advantage by weakening, not raising, environmental protections'. China's rapid integration into the global economy, for example, has come at the cost of severe environmental degradation:

> *Scores of rivers have dried up in northern China over the past 20 years. More than 75 per cent of river waters are not suitable for drinking or fishing. China's cities are an environmental disaster, since urban infrastructure has not kept up with the influx of people. Many cities face serious sanitation problems, with sewage and wastewater going straight into rivers. Large cities, including Beijing, are smothered in smog. Old and weak people are often warned to stay indoors. Between 2001 and 2020 almost 600 000 people in China are expected to suffer premature death every year due to urban air pollution.* (Lovgren 2005)

The World Bank (2000) argues that '[e]very society has to decide for itself on the relative value it places on economic output and the environment'. Others argue, however, that there can be substantial inequity in who bears the environmental costs. In addition, many of the environmental impacts can affect more than one country and can even be global in scope. More commitment is thus needed to better balance the 'tradeoffs' between economic growth and environmental protection, including a fuller understanding of environmental health risks.

In managing this trade-off, the indirect effects of globalization on environmental health must also be recognized. A change in investment or lending policy by a global financial institution, such as the IMF, can have health consequences for local communities. For example, policy conditions set by the World Bank, or requirements to repay substantial sums of foreign debt, can restrict the public expenditure of borrowing countries on environmental protection or investment in basic infrastructure, such as water and sanitation. A cholera outbreak in South Africa in 2000–2001, which led to around 120 000 cases and 265 deaths, has been blamed on the introduction of user fees following the privatization of water utilities as part of the country's structural adjustment programme. As water supplies were cut to poor people unable to pay for the new charges, many resorted to using polluted river water (Anon 2006). Today, more than 2.6 billion people—over 40 per cent of the world's population—do not have access to basic sanitation, and more than one billion people still use unsafe sources of drinking water

(WHO/UNICEF 2006). Predictions of the growing scarcity of fresh water supplies globally, and the continued trend towards the privatization of water utilities with ownership dominated by large TNCs, is likely to worsen this situation.

The capacity of the public health community to correct, control, and prevent environmental health risks can be affected by globalization. For example, globalization poses additional challenges for identifying a hazard. In a more interconnected world, causal relations can become more extended and complex. The tasks associated with identifying a hazard must take account of factors that extend far beyond national borders, a greater range of stakeholders, and jurisdictions that lie beyond the reach of public health authorities. A good example is the increase in reported outbreaks of foodborne illnesses involving more than one country which has been linked, in part, to the globalization of the food industry (Kaferstein *et al.* 1997; Hall 2002). Tracing the source and cause of such an outbreak can be hindered by inadequate recordkeeping in some countries, lack of timely sharing of information, inconsistency in labelling, or lack of access to production facilities abroad. The work of environmental health workers can be made even more difficult by hazards arising from illicit activities such as dumping, counterfeiting or smuggling across borders (Kimball 2006).

The undertaking of risk assessment, defined as 'the process of estimating the potential impact of a chemical, physical, microbiological, or psycho-social hazard on a specified human population or ecological system under a specific set of conditions and for a certain timeframe' (Pencheon *et al.* 2001: 208), is also made more challenging by globalization. The population of interest may be widely dispersed, because of their mobility or transience, and identifying and measuring a suspected hazard requires large-scale analysis. Weiland *et al.* (2004) study 650 000 subjects as part of the International Study of Asthma and Allergies in Childhood. A collaboration with 155 participating centres worldwide, it is the first study 'to take a global view [of] . . . the relationship between asthma and eczema and climate' (Graham 2004).

Global health promotion

The rapid growth of the health burden from non-communicable diseases (NCDs) worldwide in recent decades, such as ischemic heart disease, cancer, and diabetes (Beaglehole & Yach 2003; Matthews & Pramming 2003) has led to growing attention to the need for global approaches to health promotion (Lee 2007). NCDs are the leading causes of death and disability worldwide. Disease rates from these conditions are accelerating globally, advancing across every region and pervading all socioeconomic classes. The *World Health Report 2002: Reducing risks, promoting healthy life*, indicates that the mortality, morbidity, and disability attributed to the major chronic diseases currently account for almost 60 per cent of all deaths and 43 per cent of the global burden of disease. By 2020, their contribution is expected to rise to 73 per cent of all deaths and 60 per cent of the global burden of disease. Moreover, 79 per cent of the deaths attributed to these diseases occur in the developing countries. Four of the most prominent chronic diseases—cardiovascular diseases (CVD), cancer, chronic obstructive pulmonary disease, and type 2 diabetes—are linked by common and preventable biological risk factors, notably high blood pressure, high blood cholesterol and overweight, and by related major behavioural risk factors: Unhealthy diet, physical inactivity, and tobacco use. Action to prevent these major chronic diseases should focus on controlling these and other key risk factors in a well-integrated manner.

Health promotion is the process of enabling people to increase control over, and to improve, their health (WHO 1986). Interventions address three areas of activity in order to prevent disease and promote the health of a community: Communication, service delivery, and structural (enabling factor) components (Walley *et al.* 2001: 147). A global approach to health promotion takes into account the ways in which globalization may be influencing the broad determinants of health, and health behaviours, as well as offering opportunities for providing appropriate interventions. The adoption of the Bangkok Charter for Health Promotion in a Globalized World in 2005 was in recognition of the major challenges, actions, and commitments needed to address the determinants of health in a globalized world by reaching out to people, groups, and organizations that are critical to the achievement of health. How this might be achieved can be understood in relation to two key issues—obesity and tobacco control.

The rapid increase in the incidence of overnutrition and obesity, among both adults and children, has attracted substantial public health concern in recent years (Taubes 1998). According to WHO and the International Obesity Taskforce (IOTF), around 300 million people worldwide are obese (BMI > 30), with levels continuing to rise rapidly in the early twenty-first century. At least 155 million school-age children are overweight or obese, with 30–45 million classified as obese. This accounts for 2–3 per cent of the world's children aged 5–17 years. In the EU, childhood obesity is described as 'out of control':

> *The number of children affected by overweight and obesity is now rising at more than 400 000 a year and already affects almost one in four across the entire EU, including accession countries in 2002. The new prevalence of 24 per cent in 2002 is five points higher than had been expected based on original trends in the 80s and is already higher than the predicted peak for 2010.* (IOTF 2004)

Also, the obesity epidemic is not limited to high-income countries. Changes in diet, levels of physical activity, and nutrition (known as the 'nutrition transition') have led to sharp increases in rates of obesity in such wide ranging countries as India, Thailand, Brazil, and China. As Drewnoski and Popkin (1997: 32) write:

> *Whereas high-fat diets and Western eating habits were once restricted to the rich industrialized nations . . . the nutrition transition now occurs in nations with much lower levels of gross national product (GNP) than previously. . . . First, fat consumption is less dependent on GNP than ever before. Second, rapid urbanization has a major influence in accelerating the nutrition transition.*

Similarly, Prentice (2006) links the trend to globalization of food production and lifestyles:

> *The pandemic is transmitted through the vectors of subsidized agriculture and multinational companies providing cheap, highly refined fats, oils, and carbohydrates, labour-saving mechanized devices, affordable motorized transport, and the seductions of sedentary pastimes such as television. This trend has been linked*

to the globalisation of sedentary lifestyles alongside changes in food production and consumption.

Many interventions to address the obesity epidemic have focused on the modification of individual behaviours, such as healthy eating initiatives and the promotion of physical activity. Global health promotion, however, must also seek to tackle the structural factors that constrain or enable lifestyle choices. This includes what and how food is produced and marketed by an increasingly globalized food industry. For example, the Institute of Medicine (2005) report, *Food Marketing to Children and Youth: Threat or Opportunity?* recognizes that dietary patterns begin in childhood and are shaped by an interplay of many factors—genetics and biology, culture and values, economics, physical and social environments, and commercial media environments. Importantly, the report provides the most comprehensive review to date of the scientific evidence on the influence of food marketing on diets and diet-related health of children and youth. It argues that environments supportive of good health require leadership and action from the food, beverage, and restaurant industries; food retailers and trade associations; the entertainment industry and the media; parents and caregivers; schools; and the government.

Global-level regulation of food-related industries, however, remains problematic. The process of adopting the WHO Global Strategy on Diet, Physical Activity and Health was fraught with efforts by the food industry to avoid the setting of explicit recommendations on healthy levels of salt, sugar, and fats intake, amid calls for binding regulation of marketing, labelling and other industry activities by public health advocates (Lang *et al.* 2006). In the US, the politically powerful food industry has instead succeeded in promoting self-regulation. As Kelly (2005) writes:

The global hegemony of the United States in the production and marketing of food, while a marvel of economic success, has contributed to the epidemic of obesity that is particularly afflicting children. So far the U.S. government has declined to regulate the aggressive ways in which food producers market high-energy, low-nutrition foods to young people. That public-health responsibility has been left to an industry-created scheme of self-regulation that is deeply flawed; there is a compelling need for government involvement.

Lessons for global health promotion can also be drawn from efforts to strengthen tobacco control worldwide. As described above, the globalization of the tobacco industry has led to a rise in tobacco consumption, facilitated by the industry's consolidation, greater economies of scale, and aggressive marketing strategies to gain entry to emerging markets (Bettcher & Yach 2000). WHO initiated negotiations for a Framework Convention on Tobacco Control (FCTC) in the mid 1990s in recognition of the need to globalize tobacco control policies (Reid 2005). Referring to the impact of globalization on the tobacco pandemic, then WHO Director-General Gro Harlem Brundtland stated:

[O]ver the past fifteen years, we have seen that modern technology, has limited the effectiveness of national action. Tobacco advertising is beamed into every country via satellite and cable. Developing countries are the subject of massive marketing campaigns by international tobacco companies. In the slipstream of increasing global trade, new markets are opened to international tobacco companies which see these emerging markets as their main opportunity to compensate for stagnant or dwindling markets in many industrialized countries. (Brundtland 2000)

As the first multilaterally negotiated public health treaty, the FCTC negotiation process encompassed regional consultations, public hearings, contributions by civil society organizations, and old-fashioned diplomacy among WHO's 192 member states. The process also faced extensive efforts by the powerful tobacco industry to undermine negotiations through seeking representation on some national delegations, lobbying of tobacco producing countries and farmers, orchestrated criticism of WHO for neglecting other public health priorities, and even challenges to long established science on tobacco and health (Lynn & Lerner 2002; Waxman 2002; Hammond & Assunta 2003).

Despite persistent industry opposition, public health advocates prevailed in successfully adopting a comprehensive treaty which sets out measures to address both the supply of and demand for tobacco. As of October 2008, 168 countries have signed, and 160 countries have fully ratified the treaty. Importantly, the FCTC represents a collective effort across WHO member states to address a clear global public health challenge. The involvement of a broad spectrum of stakeholders, notably civil society organizations, was critical to raising public awareness and support at the regional, national and local levels. The mobilization of public health advocates, led by the Framework Convention Alliance, was greatly facilitated by the use of the Internet (focused on the *Globalink* network) which allowed groups to keep abreast of negotiations, organize advocacy activities, and share experiences to an unprecedented degree (Collin *et al.* 2004). While weaker on some aspects of globalization, such as international trade, than initially hoped, the treaty will accommodate other transborder issues such as smuggling and marketing (e.g. sports sponsorship, satellite broadcasting) through the negotiation of additional protocols.

Initiating high-profile policies, such as the Global Strategy on Diet, Physical Activity and Health and the FCTC, can raise the profile of health promotion and be effective vehicles for addressing the global aspects of the challenges faced. The experiences of established campaigns, such as the WHO/UNICEF International Code on the Marketing of Breastmilk Substitutes and Health Cities Initiative, and more recently initiatives such as the Public–Private Partnership for Handwashing, shows that adoption of agreements is a starting point. Implementation requires longer term mobilization of political will, resources and technical capacity to translate commitments into effective action. In the context of globalization, trade flows, information and communication technologies, and marketing strategies are beginning to be harnessed for health promotion purposes. For example, the tobacco control community has developed countermarketing campaigns to challenge the use of advertising imagery associating cigarette smoking with glamour and excitement in emerging markets (Box 2.1.2). Worldwide consumer boycotts of TNCs, such as Nestlé and McDonalds, have been organized to pressure companies to change their marketing practices or unhealthy product ranges (Yach & Beaglehole 2003).

In summary, the global spread of unhealthy lifestyles and behaviours pose new challenges for health promotion. In many cases,

Box 2.1.2

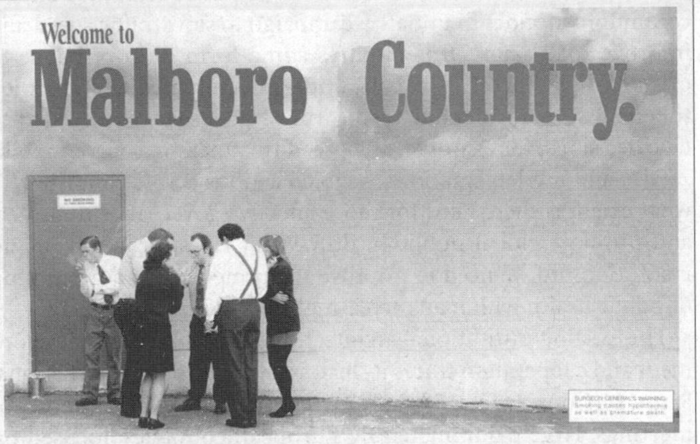

powerful vested interests within key sectors of the global economy have facilitated this process through foreign investment, production, trade and marketing practices. There is accumulating evidence that these practices are resulting in a sharp increase in NCDs. The public health community faces major challenges in influencing these practices, as well as opportunities to harness aspects of globalization to promote healthier lifestyles and behaviours. Collective efforts across countries to appropriately regulate harmful aspects of the global economy is clearly needed.

Monitoring the health status of the population

Assessing the health of a given population is the starting point for a wide range of public health activities such as policy reviews, programme development, goal setting and resource allocation. There are well recognized steps for assessing population health status:

- Define the purpose of the assessment
- Define the population concerned and any comparator population
- Define the aspects of health to be considered
- Identify and review existing data sources
- Select the most appropriate existing data (Gentle 2001)

In assessing the linkages between globalization and population health status, two challenges are presented. First, there is variable capacity across countries to collect and manage basic health data. Data remains of poor quality or limited in availability in many low- and middle-income countries. According to WHO (2006b):

> *A country health information system comprises the multiple sub-systems and data sources that together contribute to generating health information, including vital registration, censuses and surveys, disease surveillance and response, service statistics and health management information, financial data, and resource tracking. The absence of consensus on the relative strengths, usefulness, feasibility, and cost-efficiency of different data collection approaches has resulted in a plethora of separate and often overlapping systems. Too often, inappropriate use is made of particular data collection methods, for example, the use of household surveys to produce information on adult mortality.*

The WHO Health Metrics Network (HMN) is a global partnership working to strengthen and align health information systems around the world. The partnership is comprised of countries, multilateral and bilateral development agencies, foundations, global health initiatives, and technical experts that aim to increase the availability and use of timely, reliable health information by catalysing the funding and development of core health information systems in developing countries. As described by WHO:

> *HMN partners agree to align around a common framework that sets the standards for health information systems. The HMN framework will serve to define the systems needed at country and global levels, along with the standards, capacities and processes for generating, analysing, disseminating, and using health information. It links the normative framework for measurement in health with participatory assessment, planning, and implementation modalities that are objective, transparent, and include all stakeholders. Thus, it focuses the inputs of donors and technical agencies around a country-owned plan for health information development, thereby reducing the overlap and duplication. At both the country and global level, the HMN framework will enable access to and use of health information, thereby serving the needs of individual countries while also generating global public goods.*

In seeking to improve health information systems, a second challenge is the limitations of existing data sources in capturing health needs that cut across the national level (i.e. transnational). For each country, health data is collected and managed by a department of health and associated institutions. The WHO Statistical Information System (WHOSIS), in turn, collects and coordinates data on core health indicators, mortality and health status, disease statistics, health system statistics, risk factors and health service coverage, and inequities in health from its 192 member states. This is compiled in the *World Health Statistics*. By definition, globalization is eroding, and even transcending, national borders so that health and disease patterns may be emerging that do not conform to such delineations. As a result, national level data may need to be aggregated and disaggregated in novel ways to reveal these new patterns.

A good example is the above discussed increase in obesity rates. Improving data on trends in different countries reveal a complex picture. In high-income countries, obesity is rising rapidly across all social classes but is particularly associated with social deprivation. In the UK, for example:

> *Obesity is linked to social class, being more common among those in the routine or semi-routine occupational groups than the managerial and professional groups. The link is stronger among women. In 2001, 30 per cent of women in routine occupations were classified as obese compared with 16 per cent in higher managerial and professional occupations.* (UK Office of National Statistics Office)

In France, Romon *et al.* (2005) found that genetic predisposition influences the prevalence of obesity and changes in body mass index (BMI) among children from the higher social class. For children within the lowest social class, which has seen an increase in BMI across the whole population, environmental factors appear to have

Table 2.1.3 Per cent of population that is overweight, selected countries, 2002 and 2010 (Projected)

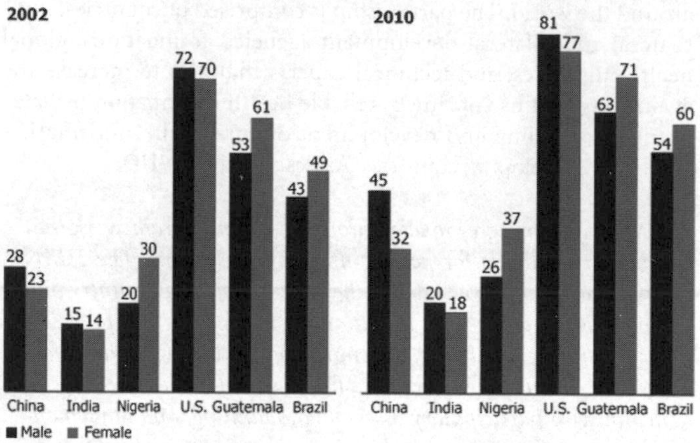

Note: 'Overweight' is defined as having a body mass index (weight in kilograms divided by height in metres squared) of between 25 and 30. 'Obese' is defined as having a body mass index of 30 or more.

Source: Reprinted with permission from the Population Reference Bureau.

played a more important role. In contrast, in low- and middle-income countries, the total number of obese or overweight people is projected to grow by 50 per cent by 2015 alongside the persistence of undernutrition (Table 2.1.3). Social class is one factor. In such diverse countries as Kenya, China, India, and Brazil, obesity among an increasingly affluent middle class has been observed (McLellan 2002). A high BMI may even be considered socially desirable as a sign of affluence. At the same time, some populations within the lower social classes are also experiencing rising rates of overweight and obesity. For example, Monteiro *et al.* (2004) find that a country's level of wealth is an important factor, with obesity starting to fuel health inequities in the developing world when the GNP reaches a value of about US$2500 per capita. Trends in over/undernutrition, in other words, are complex and changing over time, and require sufficiently detailed and comparable data across population groups defined along additional variables (e.g. gender, socioeconomic status, occupation).

The need to improve available data on the health of populations affected by globalization is illustrated by a wide range of other examples. The outsourcing of manufacturing to the developing world by TNCs, for example, has led to the employment of hundreds of thousands of workers. What public health needs to these workers have and are they addressed by local occupational health policies? Similarly, the greater movement of people across national borders may require increased attention to the health needs of different types of migrants. Alternatively, what public health issues arise for populations from global environmental change? All of these examples suggest the need to redefine new population groups within a global context, and to develop data sources that measure population health patterns which do not conform to national borders.

The governance of global public health

Governance broadly concerns the agreed actions and means adopted by a society to promote collective action and solutions in pursuit of common goals. Governance takes place whenever people seek to organize themselves to achieve a shared end through agreed rules, procedures, and institutions. This can take place at different levels of decision-making and action. In public health, if a local community decides to initiate a campaign to slow traffic speed and improve road safety, this requires some form of governance to organize the effort. If a global campaign is initiated to strengthen tuberculosis control, an agreed form of governance is needed to take decisions, for example, on agreed treatment, resource mobilization, and implementation of agreed actions across countries. To what extent is there need for more effective governance to protect and promote global public health? What rules, procedures, and institutions do we need to improve the protection and promotion of public health within an increasingly globalized context.

The existing institutional architecture for global health development and cooperation traces its historical roots to the International Sanitary Conferences of the nineteenth century. This series of meetings, largely dominated by European countries, focused on protecting trading interests from certain epidemic diseases such as cholera and plague. The institutions eventually created, such as the *Office International d'Hygiène Publique*, were primarily concerned with collecting and disseminating epidemiological data on these diseases (Fidler 2001). The creation of the WHO as a specialized agency of the United Nations in 1948 was intended to universalize the membership, and broaden the scope of, international health cooperation. Its objective, 'the attainment by all peoples of the highest possible level of health', was reflected in the vast array of programmes initiated under WHO's auspices.

Recent decades have seen challenges to WHO's designated role as 'the directing and co-ordinating authority on international health work' [WHO Constitution, Article 2(a)]. In part, this has arisen from differences in perspective on whether WHO should be biomedically (disease) focused, or whether the organization should address the broad determinants of 'health for all'. These debates have been accompanied by rapid changes in WHO's operating environment, with the ascendance of new institutional players and ideological perspectives. From the 1980s, the World Bank became a major influence as the biggest source of financing for health development (Buse 1994), while other UN bodies such as the UN Children's Fund and UN Development Programme (UNDP) expanded their health portfolios. The 1990s saw the creation of numerous global public-private partnerships for health which attracted additional resources, but rendered the policy environment far more complex and crowded (Buse & Walt 2000). In recent years, charitable foundations led by the Gates Foundation, have also become major players in the funding of health projects in the developing world (Birn 2005). This influx of institutions and resources has, on the one hand, reflected the higher priority to health development given by governments, corporations and civil society organizations. On the other hand, there is substantial evidence of overlapping mandates, duplication of effort, and, above all, a lack of collective strategic thinking about how to effectively tackle the public health challenges posed by globalization.

The governance of global public health can thus be presently seen as undergoing a period of transition. In principle, the formal institutions governing public health remain focused on governments. Public health authority lies within the ministries of health of each WHO member state, and collaboration across countries and regions takes place on a wide range of functions through governmental bodies. However, as described in this chapter, intensified flows of people, other life forms, goods and services, capital, and knowledge are influencing the determinants of health and health outcomes in diverse ways. Effective regulation of these flows can require collective action across governments and, in some cases, the participation of institutions beyond government. Many scholars of global governance point to the need for new institutional arrangements, a kind of political globalization, to enable more effective action. As Homedes and Ugalde (2003) write, 'If international health problems are to be solved, political, cultural, and social interdependence need to be built with the same impetus by which policymakers promote international trade'. Examples described in this chapter—such as tobacco control, food and nutrition, and infectious disease outbreaks—demonstrate the need for innovation.

What can the public health community do to foster such innovation? Globalization is now an established subject of discussion and debate at public health meetings around the world, and there has been no shortage of commitments to address its impacts. The Final Communiqué of the 13th Commonwealth Health Ministers Meeting (2001) included attention to the 'Impact of Globalisation on Health' as follows:

In discussing globalisation, Ministers identified poverty as the main obstacle to development. Poverty prevents countries from exploiting the potential benefits of globalisation, which has the effect of widening the gap between rich and poor countries. Ministers urged the Commonwealth to develop structured responses to globalisation that would promote positive impact on health. These responses should acknowledge the inextricable links between health and the wider socio-economic development agenda. They should take account of moral and ethical considerations relating to equity in resource distribution.

Ministers expressed strong views about the imposition of conditions linked to development assistance, such as the removal of public subsidies. This militates against the development efforts of poorer countries, and is unfair if not applied in the same way to the more developed countries. Ministers urged the Commonwealth to work for fairness in financing and ensure that the rules apply to developing and developed countries alike.

In 2001, the World Federation of Public Health Associations issued a Call to Action which commits itself to work with WHO 'to clarify areas of emerging public health risk associated with globalization, ranging from infectious and occupational diseases to diseases which are a product of the growing world-scale of anti-health forces' (World Federation of Public Health Associations 2001). The Mumbai Declaration of the People's Health Movement, agreed in 2004, calls for an end to 'corporate-led globalization' (People's Health Movement 2004). The Sixth Global Conference on Health Promotion in 2005 issued the Bangkok Charter which identifies actions, commitments and pledges required to address the determinants of health in a globalized world through health promotion.

Given widespread recognition of the need to address the impacts of globalization within the public health community, the essential next step is to seek influence within those policy communities which drive contemporary globalization. Public health representation within ongoing trade negotiations, for example, is critical. WHO and other public health institutions have so far remained marginal observers in the WTO and other key decision-making forums. The controversy surrounding intellectual property rights and access to medicines, the substantial concern by consumers about the social and environmental harms of globalization, and the potential costs to the global economy of a major infectious disease pandemic demonstrate the scope for greater collaboration across sectors. Lee *et al.* (2007) describe the potential role of health impact assessment for informing non-health-policy proposals. The global public goods for health approach addresses the growing globalization of health from an economic perspective. The concept identifies where a good or service (such as knowledge of an infectious disease outbreak), which would be of benefit globally, will not be produced or disseminated if left to the market because no one can be excluded from accessing the good, and thus no charge can be levied for its use and no costs recouped. At the national level, the production of these goods is usually ensured by government intervention, but at the global level there remains no 'global government' to undertake this role. Certain functions of public health may be classed as global public goods (e.g. immunization programmes, disease surveillance), which require collective action to overcome market failures (Smith *et al.* 2003). The concept might thus be an appealing rationale to non health policy makers shaping global change.

Conclusion

This chapter has described key ways in which globalization is relevant to the theory and practice of public health. There are both threats and opportunities arising from the complex and diverse changes created by globalization, although current forms of globalization is clearly characterized by an inequitable distribution of winners and losers. For the public health community, there is a need to understand and contribute to more effective management of the rapid changes taking place. Greater attention to these public health impacts will, in turn, contribute to more socially and environmentally sustainable forms of globalization.

References

Anon (2005). Global Brand Scorecard, The 100 Top Brands. *BusinessWeek*, 1 August.

Anon (2006). Report: Water problems remain in rural areas. *Guardian* and *Mail*, 12 July.

Anon (2007). World tourism marks another record year with 842 million arrivals, UN agency reports. *UN News Service*, 30 January. http://www.un.org/apps/news/story.asp?NewsID=21383&Cr=tourism&Cr1=# (accessed 26 March 2007).

Bach, S. (2003). International migration of health workers: labour and social issues. Working Paper, Sectoral Activities Programme, ILO, Geneva. http://www.ilo.org/public/english/dialogue/sector/papers/health/wp209.pdf (accessed 26 March 2007).

Barber, B. (2003). Jihad vs McWorld. In *The Globalization Reader* (eds. H. Lechner and J. Boli), pp. 21–26. Blackwell Publishing, London.

Beaglehole, R., and Yach, D. (2003). Globalisation and the prevention and control of non-communicable disease: the neglected chronic diseases of adults. *Lancet*, **362,** 903–6.

Benatar, S., Daar, A.S., and Singer, P.A. (2003). Global health ethics: the rationale for mutual caring. *International Affairs*, **79**(1), 107–38.

Bettcher, D.W., and Yach, D. (2000). Globalisation of tobacco industry influence and new global responses. *Tobacco Control*, **9**(2), *206–16.*

Birn, A.E. (2005). Gates's grandest challenge: transcending technology as public health ideology. *Lancet*, **366**(9484)**,** 514–9.

Brecher and Costello (1994), *Global Village or Global Pillage, Economic Reconstruction from the Bottom Up*, South End Press, Cambridge, MA.

Brundtland, G.H. (2000). Opening Statement. First Meeting of Intergovernmental Negotiating Body, Framework Convention on Tobacco Control, Geneva, 16 October. http://www.who.int/director-general/speeches/2000/english/20001016_tobacco_control.html (accessed 27 March 2007).

Buse, K. (1994). Spotlight on international organizations: The World Bank. *Health Policy and Planning*, **9**, 95–9.

Buse, K., and Walt, G. (2000). Global public-private partnerships: Part I – a new development in health? *Bulletin of the World Health Organisation*, **78**(4), 549–61.

Busfield, J. (2005). The globalization of the pharmaceutical industry. In *Global change and health* (eds. K. Lee and J. Collin), pp. 94–110. Open University Press, Maidenhead.

Callard, C., Chitanondh, H., and Weissman, R. (2001). Why trade and investment liberalisation may threaten effective tobacco control efforts. *Tobacco Control*, **10**, 68–70.

Castles, S., and Miller, M. (2003). *The Age of Migration, International Population Movements in the Modern World, 3rd edition*. Macmillan, London.

Collin, J., Lee, K., and Bissell, K. (2004). Negotiating the Framework Convention on Tobacco Control: The politics of global health governance. In *The Global Governance Reader* (eds. R. Wilkinson and C. Murphy), pp. 254–73, Routledge, London.

Commonwealth Health Ministers Meeting (2001). *13th Commonwealth Health Ministers Meeting Final Communiqué*, 25–29 November, Christchurch, New Zealand. http://www.thecommonwealth.org/document/34293/35232/35242/13th_commonwealth_health_ministers_meeting_final_c.htm (accessed 20 June 2007).

Cornea, G.A. (2001). Globalization and Health: results and options. *Bulletin of the World Health Organization*, **79**(9), 834–41.

Crosby, A. (1972). *The Columbian Exchange: Biological & Cultural Consequences of 1492*. Greenwood Press, Connecticut.

De Vogli, R., and Birbeck, G.L. (2005). Potential Impact of Adjustment Policies on Vulnerability of Women and Children to HIV/AIDS in Sub-Saharan Africa. *Journal of Health Population and Nutrition*, **23**, 105–20.

Dicken, P. (1999). *Global Shift, Transforming the World Economy*. Paul Chapman Publishing, London.

diMasi, J.A., Hansen, R.W., and Grabowski, H.G. (2002). The price of innovation: new estimates of drug development costs. *Journal of Health Economics*, **22**, 151–85.

Dollar, D., and Kraay, A. (2000). Growth is good for the poor. *Research Paper*, World Bank, Washington DC.

Dorling, D., Shaw, M., and Davey Smith, G. (2006). Global inequality of life expectancy due to AIDS. *BMJ*, **332**, 662–4.

Drewnoski, A., and Popkin, B. (1997). The Nutrition Transition: New Trends in the Global Diet. *Nutrition Reviews*, **55**(2), 31–43.

Falk, R. (1999). *Predatory globalization, a critique*. Polity Press, London.

Feachem, R. (2001). Globalisation is good for your health, mostly. *BMJ*, **323**, 504–6.

Fidler, D. (2001). The globalization of public health: the first 100 years of international health diplomacy. *Bulletin of the World Health Organization*, **79**(9), 842–9.

Forbes (2000). *The world's biggest public companies*. http://www.forbes.com/lists/2006/18/Rank_1.html (accessed 20 June 2007).

Gentle, P. (2001). Assessing health status. In *Oxford handbook of public health practice* (eds. D. Pencheon, C. Guest, D. Melzer and J.A. Muir Gray). Oxford University Press, Oxford.

Graham, S. (2004). Global Study Links Climate to Rates of Childhood Asthma. *Scientific American*, 21 June. http://scientificamerican.com/article.cfm?chanID=sa003&articleID=000624A7-66A2-10D3-A6A283414B7F0000 (accessed 27 March 2007).

Hall, G., D'Souza, R.M., and Kirk, M. (2002). Foodborne disease in the new millennium: out of the frying pan into the fire? *MJA*, **177**(11/12), 614–8.

Hammond, R., and Assunta, M. (2003). The Framework Convention on Tobacco Control: promising start, uncertain future. *Tobacco Control*, **12**(3), 241–2.

Held, D., McGrew, A., Goldblatt, D., and Perraton, J. (1999). *Global transformations*. Stanford University Press, Stanford.

Homedes, N., and Ugalde, A. (2003). Globalization and Health at the United States-Mexico Border. *American Journal of Public Health*, **93**(12), 2016–22.

Hundley, R.O., Anderson, R.H., Bikson, T.K., and Neu, C.R. (2003). *The Global Course of the Information Revolution, Recurring Themes and Regional Variations*. RAND National Defense Research Institute, Washington DC.

Huntington, S. (2002), *The Clash of Civilizations and the Remaking of World Order, 2nd edition*. Free Press, New York.

ILO (2007). *Global Employment Trends Brief 2007*. International Labour Organisation, Geneva. http://www.ilo.org/public/english/employment/strat/download/getb07en.pdf (accessed 20 June 2007).

ILO (2000), *Workers without Frontiers - The Impact of Globalization on International Migration*. International Labour Organization, Geneva.

IMF (2005). The IMF and the Fight against Money Laundering and the Financing Of Terrorism. *Fact Sheet*, September, Washington DC. http://www.imf.org/external/x10/changecss/changestyle.aspx (accessed 13 March 2007).

Institute of Medicine (1997). *America's Vital Interest in Global Health*. National Academy Press, Washington DC.

Institute of Medicine (2005). *Food Marketing to Children and Youth: Threat or Opportunity?* National Academy Press, Washington DC.

IOTF (2004). EU childhood obesity 'out of control'. *Press Release*, International Obesity Taskforce, Geneva. http://www.iotf.org/popout.asp?linkto=http://www.iotf.org/media/IOTFmay28.pdf (accessed 28 March 2007).

Kaferstein, F.K., Motarjemi, Y., and Bettcher, D.W. (1997). Foodborne disease control: A transnational challenge. *Emerging Infectious Diseases*, **3**(4), 503–10.

Kawachi, I., and Wamala, S. (eds.) (2006). *Globalization and Health*. Oxford University Press, Oxford.

Kelly, D. (2005). To quell obesity, who should regulate food marketing to children? *Globalization and Health*, 1(9). http://www.globalizationandhealth.com/content/1/1/9

Kerry, V.B., and Lee, K. (2007). TRIPS, the Doha declaration and paragraph 6 decision: what are the remaining steps for protecting access to medicines? *Globalization and Health*, **3**(3), 1–12.

Kim, J.Y., Irwin, A., Millen, J., and Gershman, J. (2000). *Dying for Growth: Global inequality and the health of the poor*. Common Courage Press, Monroe ME.

Korten. D. (1995) *When Corporations Ruled the World*. Kumerian Press and Berrett-Koehler, Bloomfield, Connecticut.

Kimball, A.M. (2006), *Risky Trade Infectious Disease in the Era of Global Trade*. Ashgate, London.

Labonte, R., Schrecker, T., and Sen Gupta, A. (2005). *Health for some: death, disease and disparity in a globalizing world*. Centre for Social Justice, Toronto.

Lang, T., Rayner, G., and Kaelin, E. (2006). *The Food Industry, Diet, Physical Activity and Health: a Review of Reported Commitments and Practice of 25 of the World's Largest Food Companies*. Centre for Food Policy, City University, London. http://www.city.ac.uk/news/press/The%20Food%20Industry%20Diet%20Physical%20Activity%20and%20Health.pdf (accessed 13 June 2007).

Lee, K. (2003a). *Globalization and health, an introduction*. Palgrave Macmillan, London.

Lee K. ed. (2003b). *Health impacts of globalization, towards global governance*. Palgrave Macmillan, London.

Lee, K. (2007). Global health promotion: How can we strengthen governance and build effective strategies? *Health Promotion International,* **21**(1), 42–50.

Lee, K., and Collin, J. (eds.) (2005). *Global change and health.* Open University Press, Maidenhead.

Lee, K., and Fidler, D. (2007). Avian and pandemic influenza: Progress and problems for global governance. *Global Public Health,* **2**(3), 215–34.

Lee, K., Ingram, A., Lock, K., and McInnes, C. (2007). Bridging health and foreign policy: The role of health impact assessment? *Bulletin of the World Health Organization,* **85**(3), 207–11.

Lopez, A., Mathers, C.D., Ezzati, M., Jamison, D.T., and Murray, C.J.L. (2006). *Global burden of disease and risk factors.* World Bank Publications, Washington DC.

Lovgren, G. (2005). China's Boom is Bust for Global Environment, Study Warns. *National Geographic,* 16 May. http://news.nationalgeographic.com/news/2005/05/0516_050516_chinaeco.html (accessed 23 March 2007).

Lynn, P., and Lerner, D. (2002). NGOs release new hard-hitting evidence of global tobacco industry tactics to subvert public policy. *Press Release,* 20 March, Corporate Accountability International, Boston. http://www.stopcorporateabuse.org/cms/page1294.cfm (accessed 15 June 2007).

Matthews, D., and Pramming, S. (2003). Diabetes and the global burden of non-communicable disease. *Lancet,* **362**(9397), 1763–4.

McKinsey Global Institute (2007). *Mapping the global capital markets, third annual report.* McKinsey & Company, San Francisco.

McLellan, F. (2002). Obesity rising to alarming levels around the world. *Lancet,* **359**(315), 1412.

Mittelman, J.H. (2002). Making globalization work for the have nots. *International Journal on World Peace,* **19**(2), 3–25.

Monteiro, C.A., Conde, W.L., Lu, B., and Popkin, B.M. (2004). Obesity and inequities in health in the developing world. *International Journal of Obesity,* **28**(9), 1181–6.

OECD (2005). *Measuring Globalisation, OECD Economic globalisation indicators.* Organisation for Economic Cooperation and Development, Paris.

Pencheon, D., Guest, C., Melzer, D., Muir Gray, J.A. (2001). *Oxford handbook of public health practice.* Oxford University Press, Oxford.

People's Health Movement (2004). *The Mumbai Declaration from the 3rd International Forum for the Defence of People's Health.* 14–15 January, Mumbai, India. http://www.phmovement.org/files/md-english.pdf (accessed 15 June 2007).

Prentice, A. (2006). The emerging epidemic of obesity in developing countries. *International Journal of Epidemiology,* **35**(1), 93–9.

Reid, R. (2005). *Globalizing Tobacco Control, Anti-smoking campaigns in California, France, and Japan.* Indiana University Press, Bloomington.

Romon, M., Duhamel, A., Collinet, N., and Weill, J. (2005). Influence of social class on time trends in BMI distribution in 5-year-old French children from 1989 to 1999. *International Journal of Obesity,* **29,** 54–59.

Saker, L., Lee, K., and Cannito, B. (2006). Globalization and infectious disease. In *Globalization and Health* (eds. I. Kawachi, I., and S. Wamala), pp. 19–38, Oxford University Press, Oxford.

Sierra Club (2000). *Comments to the Trade Policy Staff Committee, United States Trade Representative,* 20 May, Washington DC. http://www.sierraclub.org/trade/summit/testimony2.asp (accessed 20 June 2007).

Smith, R., Beaglehole, R., Woodward, D., and Drager, N. (eds.) (2005). *Global public goods for health, Health economic and public health perspectives.* Oxford University Press, Oxford.

Swabe, J. (1999). *Animals, disease, and human society: human-animal relations and the rise of veterinary medicine.* Routledge, London.

Swan, W. (2007). Misunderstandings about airline growth. *Journal of Air Transport Management,* **13**(1), 3–8.

Tarabusi, C., and Vickery, G. (1998). Globalization in the pharmaceutical industry. *International Journal of Health Services,* **28**(1), 67–105.

Taubes, G. (1998). As obesity rates rise, experts struggle to explain why. *Science,* **280**(5368), 1367–8.

Teitel, S. (2005). Globalization and its disconnects. *Journal of Socio-Economics,* **34**(4), 444–70.

Trouiller, P., Olliaro, P., Torreele, E., Orbinski, J., Laing, R., and Ford, N. (2002). Drug development for neglected diseases: a deficient market and a public-health policy failure. *Lancet,* **359**(9324): 2188–94.

UK Office for National Statistics (2001). *Obesity among adults: by sex and NS-SeC, 2001: Social Trends 34.* London. http://www.statistics.gov.uk/STATBASE/Product.asp?vlnk=11130&More=Y (accessed 15 June 2007).

UN Conference on the Environment and Development (1992). Rio Declaration on Environment and Development. Rio de Janiero, Brazil. http://www.un.org/documents/ga/conf151/aconf15126-1annex1.htm (accessed 20 June 2007).

UN Office on Drugs and Crime (2006). *2006 World Drug Report.* New York. http://www.unodc.org/pdf/WDR_2006/wdr2006_volume2.pdf (accessed 13 June 2007).

US Health and Human Services Public Health Service (1995). *For a healthy nation: returns on investment in public health.* US Government Printing Office, Washington DC.

Valdez, S. (2006). *An introduction to global financial markets.* Palgrave Macmillan, London.

Walley, J., Wright, J., and Hubley, J. (2001). *Public Health, an action guide to improving health in developing countries.* Oxford University Press, Oxford.

Watts, J. (2004). Chinese baby milk blamed for 50 deaths. The Guardian, 21 April. http://www.guardian.co.uk/china/story/0,7369,1196996,00.html (accessed 13 June 2007).

Waxman, H. (2002). The Future of the Global Tobacco Treaty Negotiations. *New England Journal of Medicine,* **346**(12), 21 March, 936–9.

Weiland, S.K., Hüsing, A., Strachan, Rzehak, P., Pearce, N., and the ISAAC Phase One Study Group (2004). Climate and the prevalence of symptoms of asthma, allergic rhinitis and atopic eczema in children. *Occupational and Environmental Medicine,* **61**(7), 609–15.

Wilkinson, R. (2006). *The WTO, Crisis and the governance of global trade.* Routledge, London.

World Bank (2000). Is Globalization Causing A 'Race To The Bottom' In Environmental Standards? *Briefing Papers,* April, PREM Economic Policy Group and Development Economics Group, Washington DC. http://www1.worldbank.org/economicpolicy/globalization/documents/AssessingGlobalizationP4.pdf (accessed 27 March 2007).

World Federation of Public Health Associations (2001). Public Health and Globalization. Proposed by the Resolutions Committee, WFPHA 35th Annual Meeting, 14 May, Washington DC. http://www.wfpha.org/pdf/01.23%20Public%20Health%20and%20Globalization.pdf (accessed 15 June 2007).

WHO (1986). *The Ottawa Charter for Health Promotion.* First International Conference on Health Promotion, Ottawa, 21 November 1986.

WHO (2002a). *Global Crises – Global Solutions, Managing public health emergencies of international concern through the revised International Health Regulations.* International Health Regulations Revision Project, Geneva.

WHO (2002b). WHO Atlas maps global tobacco epidemic. *Press Release,* 15 October, Tobacco Free Initiative, Geneva. http://www.who.int/mediacentre/news/releases/pr82/en/ (accessed 13 June 2007).

WHO (2004). *Global strategy on diet, physical activity and health.* WHA57.17, 57th World Health Assembly, Geneva.

WHO (2005). The World Health Assembly adopts resolution WHA59.2 on application of the International Health Regulations (2005). to strengthen pandemic preparedness and response. Epidemic and Pandemic Alert and Response, Geneva. http://www.who.int/csr/ihr/wharesolution2006/en/index.html (accessed 20 June 2007).

WHO (2006a). Counterfeit medicines. *Fact Sheet No. 275*, 14 November, Geneva. http://www.who.int/mediacentre/factsheets/fs275/en/print.html (accessed 13 June 2007).

WHO (2006b). *Health Metric Network (HMN) Workshop – better health information systems.* Health Metrics Network, Geneva. http://www.who.int/healthmetrics/news/20061027/en/index.html (accessed 20 June 2007).

WHO (2006c). *World Health Report 2006 – Working together for health.* Geneva.

WHO/International Obesity Taskforce (2000), *Obesity – Preventing and Managing the Global Epidemic.* WHO, Geneva.

WHO/UNICEF (2006). *Meeting the MDG drinking-water and sanitation target: the urban and rural challenge of the decade.* Water, Sanitation and Health, Geneva. http://www.who.int/water_sanitation_health/monitoring/jmpfinal.pdf (accessed 27 March 2007).

WHO/WTO (2002). The WTO Agreements relevant to health. In *WTO Agreements and Public Health* (Geneva: WHO/WTO).

Woollacott, M. (2003). The new killer threatening rich and poor alike. The Guardian, 25 April. http://www.guardian.co.uk/comment/story/0,,943179,00.html (accessed 20 June 2007).

WTO (2007). Risks lie ahead following stronger trade in 2006, WTO reports. *Press Release*, 472, Geneva. http://www.wto.org/english/news_e/pres07_e/pr472_e.htm (accessed 13 June 2007).

Yach, D., and Beaglehole, R. (2003). Globalization of Risks for Chronic Diseases Demands Global Solutions. *Perspectives on Global Development and Technology*, **3**(1–2), 1–21.

2.2

Overview and framework

Orielle Solar, Alec Irwin, and Jeanette Vega

Introduction

This chapter presents a conceptual framework within which to understand the multiple determinants that shape patterns of disease and well-being in populations. This provides a basis for evaluating where and how public health can intervene most effectively to improve health, particularly for vulnerable groups. This chapter starts from the premise that the central challenges for public health today include not just improving average health indicators, but reducing the unfair differences in health that currently exist among social groups, between and within countries. In other words, public health practice must be concerned with strengthening health equity. Getting to grips with this challenge requires finding answers to three fundamental problems:

1. Where do health differences among social groups originate, if we trace them back to their deepest roots?
2. What pathways lead from root causes to the stark differences in health status observed at the population level?
3. In light of the answers to the first two questions, where and how should we intervene to reduce health inequities?

This chapter seeks to provide a framework that can establish responses to the first two of these questions, in particular. Later chapters will investigate specific health determinant topics in greater detail. Our discussion here paints in the 'big picture' within which the more detailed analyses reveal their full meaning.

We begin by defining key concepts. We then review influential paradigms for understanding health determinants. Subsequent sections present a conceptual framework for analysis and action on the determinants of health, paying special attention to the determinants of health inequities. A final section sketches implications of this model for public health policy and practice. This chapter reflects work undertaken from 2004 to 2007 within the former Department of Equity, Poverty and Social Determinants of Health[1], World Health Organization, in connection with the WHO-sponsored Commission on the Social Determinants of Health (Solar & Irwin 2007).

Key concepts

Clarity on the meaning of a number of basic concepts is required for the arguments developed in this chapter, and for understanding how this discussion relates to later chapters in this volume and to ongoing debates in public health.

Health equity

Recent decades have seen broad gains in life expectancy and other average health indicators in most regions of the world. At the same time, however, gaps in health status between population groups are increasing, within and between countries. During the past two decades, some regions, in particular sub-Saharan Africa and parts of the former Soviet Union, have experienced stagnation or even reversals of earlier progress in population health indicators. In turn, the impact of these reversals has been unevenly distributed across social groups within the countries and regions concerned. In light of these trends, *health equity* has emerged as a defining challenge for public health practice in the early twenty-first century.

The WHO Department of Equity, Poverty and Social Determinants of Health defines health equity as 'the absence of unfair and avoidable or remediable differences in health among population groups defined socially, economically, demographically, or geographically' (WHO 2004). In essence, health inequities are health differences which are: Socially produced; systematic in their distribution across the population; and unfair (Dahlgren & Whitehead 2006). Identifying a health difference as inequitable is not an objective description, but necessarily implies an appeal to ethical norms (Braveman & Gruskin 2003).

Awareness of health inequities is hardly a new phenomenon. Historians have found evidence of lucid observation of the inequitable impacts of occupation and social status on health in Egyptian papyri written thousands of years before the Common Era (Sigerist 1943; Berlinguer 2006). In recent times, public health and political leaders' concern with inequities has tended to rise and fall somewhat cyclically. The Alma-Ata Declaration on Primary Health Care (1978) and the Ottawa Charter on Health Promotion (1986) were moments in which the special health needs of poor and vulnerable populations, and hence health equity as a policy goal, emerged strongly in international debates. The Alma-Ata Declaration laid out a vision of equitable health improvement based on 'development in the spirit of social justice' (WHO and UNICEF, 1978). Primary healthcare as defined at Alma-Ata included the creation of healthy living and working conditions through intersectoral programmes. It was expected that such programmes would favour rapid health gains among poor and vulnerable populations.

[1] Now the Department of Ethics, Equity, Trade and Human Rights.

During the later 1980s and 1990s, in contrast, equity as a guiding principle for health and social policy receded, arguably as the result of neoliberal economic models emphasizing market-based solutions in health and a reduced redistributive role for the state, within a geopolitical context marked by the collapse of communism and the ascendancy of corporate-driven globalization (see Chapter 2.1]).

Epidemiological research has clarified the nature and scope of health inequities through investigations revealing the existence of persistent *social gradients in health* for a wide variety of health indicators. The Whitehall Study of health outcomes among British civil servants was pioneering in this regard (Marmot *et al.* 1978). The Whitehall Study went beyond confirming the long-standing perception that the rich live longer, healthier lives than the very deprived. It showed that, even among relatively well-off members of society, a social gradient in health exists, with the most privileged category showing better outcomes than the group immediately below, which in turn enjoys better health than the category just beneath it, and so forth. Similar patterns have since been documented in numerous contexts around the world. The gradient effect is observed for practically all diseases and health status measures and across all segments of the socioeconomic spectrum. Action on health equity must grapple explicitly with the challenges posed by the social gradient (Graham & Kelly 2004).

During the late 1990s and early 2000s, evidence accumulated that existing global and national health policies had failed to reduce inequities, and indeed that substantial progress in average health indicators had been accompanied by widening health gaps between privileged and disadvantaged groups. Momentum for new, equity-focused approaches grew, at first primarily in wealthy countries. In recent years, public health's responsibility to confront health inequities at global, national, and local levels has been increasingly recognized (Evans *et al.* 2001).

Determinants of health

The determinants of health include all those factors that exert an influence on the health of individuals and populations. Classically, several major categories of health determinants have been identified, including: Genetic determinants; the impact of the natural environment; behavioural factors; and social, economic, cultural, and political arrangements. The many important factors that fall under the latter category are grouped together under the concept of 'social determinants of health'.

The concept of social determinants of health has been defined broadly to include the full set of social conditions in which people live and work, summarized in Tarlov's phrase as 'the social characteristics within which living takes place' (Tarlov 1996). Within the field encompassed by this concept, not all factors have equal importance. Causal hierarchies can be ascertained. The factors that directly determine individual health outcomes are not the same as the forces that shape the distribution of disease and well-being across populations. The conceptual framework elaborated in this chapter is fundamentally concerned with clarifying these distinctions and making explicit the relationships between underlying determinants of health inequities among social groups and the more immediate determinants of individual health.

Paradigms for understanding health determinants

In the contemporary context, several quite different paradigms coexist and inform public health policy and practice. These paradigms can be complementary. However, they may also lead to contradictory options. Here, we discuss three influential paradigms, which respectively emphasize biomedical interventions; individual lifestyle and behavioural factors; and a more comprehensive social approach to health.

The biomedical paradigm emerged in the late 1800s based on bacteriological discoveries and has been strengthened by advances in pharmacology and medical technology throughout the past century. This paradigm is essentially focused on deploying technological responses to disease at the level of the individual human body and its constituent organs. Primary emphasis tends to be on treating and when possible curing existing pathologies, rather than on preventive or promotive strategies. The current concern with genetic factors in disease processes is an outgrowth of the biomedical model, with distinctive long-term prospects for both curative and preventive techniques (see Chapter 2.4). The biomedical approach continues to constitute the dominant paradigm in health action today. The continued primacy of the biomedical model cannot be separated from economic motives and the high profits generated by the pharmaceutical industry and other components of the 'medical-industrial complex' (cf. Chapter 2.1).

An approach to health based on so-called 'lifestyle' and other behavioural determinants gained increased attention beginning in the 1970s. The 1974 Lalonde Report to the Canadian government acted as an important trigger. Lalonde argued that health for the majority of the population could not be attained through a concentration of public resources on personal medical services. The report described four major influences on the health field: Human biology, environment, lifestyle, and healthcare organization. In some respects, this analysis offered a welcome challenge to the biomedical model. Unfortunately, however, Lalonde's emphasis on health risks linked to individual lifestyle choices downplayed the differential impact of socioeconomic structures and political processes on people's opportunities for health. Instead, Lalonde's analysis lent itself to an interpretation of health as largely a matter of personal decision-making and hence private responsibility. In the international arena, this argument unintentionally played into the hands of neoliberal constituencies pressing for curtailment of state responsibility in the health sector, accompanied by aggressive privatization. While this was not Lalonde's intention, the report set precedents for a narrow, decontextualized understanding of 'lifestyle' and personal risk factors detached from social and political analysis (Colgrove 2002; Szreter 2002). This tendency has been dominant in many subsequent health promotion programmes.

In contrast to the narrow focus on individual behaviours and lifestyle choices, traditions in critical public health have developed more comprehensive paradigms that analyse the effects of a complex array of social and political factors on health outcomes. An understanding of the impact of structural social forces on health informed the work of some of the nineteenth century pioneers of modern public health. Rudolf Virchow (1985 [1848]), for example, wrote: 'Do we not always find the diseases of the populace traceable to defects in society?' This concept does not refer only to the direct impact on population health of the organization of the labour market and of social policy, including welfare state policies.

Rather, this structural perspective recognizes that a given model of social organization determines and shapes to a significant extent the options individuals have and their possibilities for changing their behaviour. During the twentieth century, traditions of social medicine developed in several global regions, from the Nordic countries to Latin America. These traditions have analysed the impact of socioeconomic structures on health and linked health progress for disadvantaged groups to community self-empowerment and movements for political and social change (Tajer 2003).

Different theories on the social patterning of disease

Epidemiological research has shown with increasing clarity that patterns of disease within populations are socially produced. This is already an important basic step towards answering the question of the origins of health differences among population groups. However, this insight leaves many questions still unanswered. Over recent years, various theoretical models have emerged to explain the processes through which social conditions and people's experience of life in society translate into differential health outcomes.

Among epidemiologists who acknowledge the primary shaping impact of social arrangements on health and illness, two major schools of thought have emerged. These can be labelled as: (1) Psychosocial approaches; (2) approaches that emphasize the social production of disease through the lens of what can be termed the political economy of health. These theoretical directions are not mutually exclusive. Both approaches seek to elucidate principles capable of explaining social inequalities in health, and both represent what Krieger has called theories of disease distribution, which presume but cannot be reduced to mechanism-oriented theories of disease causation. These approaches differ in their respective emphasis on particular social and biological factors that influence population health, how they integrate social and biological explanations, and thus in their recommendations for action (Krieger 2001, 2005).

The first school places primary emphasis on *psychosocial factors*, and is associated with the view that people's 'perception and experience of personal status in unequal societies lead to stress and poor health' (Raphael 2006; Raphael & Bryant 2006). This school traces its origins to a classic study by Cassel (1976), in which he argued that stress from the 'social environment' alters host susceptibility, affecting neuroendocrine function in ways that increase the organism's vulnerability to disease. More recent researchers, prominently including Richard Wilkinson, have sought to link altered neuroendocrine patterns and compromised health capability to people's perception and experience of their place in social hierarchies. According to these theorists, the experience of living in social settings of inequality forces people constantly to compare their status, possessions, and other life circumstances with those of others, engendering shame and anger in the disadvantaged, along with chronic stress that undermines health. At the level of society as a whole, meanwhile, steep hierarchies in income and social status weaken social cohesion, with this disintegration of social bonds also seen as negative for health. This research has inspired a substantial literature on the relationship between (perceptions of) social inequality, psychobiological mechanisms, and health status (e.g. Lynch *et al.* 2001; Marmot & Wilkinson 2001; Lobmayer & Wilkinson 2002; Marmot 2004; Wilkinson & Pickett 2006).

The contrasting *social production of disease/political economy of health* framework is sometimes also described as a materialist or neomaterialist position. Researchers adopting this approach do not deny negative psychosocial consequences of income inequality. However, they argue that interpretation of links between income inequality and health must begin with the structural causes of inequalities and emphasize inequality's material aspects, instead of focusing primarily on perceptions of inequality. Under this interpretation, the effect of income inequality on health reflects both lack of resources held by individuals, and systematic under-investments across a wide range of community infrastructure (Kaplan *et al.* 1996; Lynch *et al.* 1998). Economic processes and political decisions condition the private resources available to individuals and shape the nature of public infrastructure—education, health services, transportation, environmental controls, availability of food, quality of housing, occupational health regulations—that forms the 'neomaterial' matrix of contemporary life. Thus, income inequality per se is but one manifestation of a cluster of material conditions that affect population health (Davey Smith 2003).

Recently, some innovative theoretical approaches have opened new perspectives. Krieger's 'ecosocial' approach and other emerging multilevel frameworks have sought to integrate social and biological reasoning and a dynamic, historical, and ecological perspective to develop new insights into determinants of population distribution of disease (Krieger 2001, 2002, 2005). Krieger's notion of 'embodiment' is a suggestive concept 'referring to how we literally incorporate biologically influences from the material and social world in which we live, from conception to death; a corollary is that no aspect of our biology can be understood absent knowledge of history and individual and societal ways of living'. Armed with such constructs, Krieger (2001) argues, 'we can begin to elucidate population patterns of health, diseases, and well-being as biological expressions of social relations'.

These alternative theoretical directions in social epidemiology have given rise to strident polemics, but they can largely be reconciled. All contribute to an understanding of social differences in health. In order to draw full benefit from their respective insights, the contributions of these models must be situated within a comprehensive framework enabling us to visualize the complete causal chain of determinants that engender health inequities.

A framework for analysis and action on the determinants of health

Our goal is to present a framework that can provide clear answers to the first two questions that guide our discussion in this chapter: i.e. What causes health inequities, and what pathways lead from root causes to measured differences in health status among population groups. In addition, the framework described below defines levels of policy intervention on health determinants and helps suggest the potential scope and limits of policy action in each area. This aspect will be taken up more extensively in later sections. A comprehensive health determinants framework should achieve the following:

(a) Identify the determinants of health and the determinants of inequities in health

(b) Show how major determinants relate to each other

(c) Clarify the mechanisms by which social determinants generate health inequities

(d) Provide criteria for evaluating which determinants are the most important to address

The framework presented below draws substantially on the contributions of many previous researchers, prominently including Finn Diderichsen. Diderichsen's and Hallqvist's 1998 model of the social production of disease was subsequently adapted by Diderichsen, Evans, and Whitehead (2001). The concept of social position is at the centre of Diderichsen's interpretation of 'the mechanisms of health inequality' (Diderichsen 1998). In its initial formulation, Diderichsen's model emphasized the pathway from society through social position and specific exposures to health status. The framework was subsequently elaborated to give greater emphasis to 'mechanisms that play a role in stratifying health outcomes', including 'those central engines of society that generate and distribute power, wealth and risks' (Diderichsen *et al.* 2001) Diderichsen's model showed that these 'engines' give rise to social stratification that in turn engenders differential exposure to health-damaging conditions and differential vulnerability, depending on where people are placed within the social hierarchy. The concept of differential vulnerability includes both health conditions per se and people's ability to access material resources to respond to health problems. Social stratification likewise determines differential consequences of ill health for more and less advantaged groups. An injury or episode of illness is likely to have very different consequences for the life of a person living precariously at the bottom of the socioeconomic scale than for someone belonging to a more privileged category, with easier access to material resources and support options. The unequal results of ill health include economic and social consequences, as well as differential health outcomes as such.

Power as a factor in the social production of disease

Before examining in detail the proposed framework for the analysis of health determinants and health equity, it is important to discuss explicitly an underlying factor sometimes ignored in such discussions: Power. As a critical factor shaping social hierarchies and thus conditioning health differences among groups, power demands careful analysis from researchers concerned with health equity and the determinants of health. Understanding the causal processes that underlie health inequities, and assessing realistically what may be done to alter them, requires understanding how power operates in multiple dimensions of economic, social, and political relationships. On the other hand, while power is 'arguably the single most important organizing concept in social and political theory' (Ball 1992), this central concept remains contested and subject to diverse and often contradictory interpretations.

Recent social theory, particularly feminist theory, has shown the importance of distinguishing among several fundamental types of power: (1) 'Power over' (the ability to influence or coerce); (2) 'power to' (understood as the capacity to organize and change existing hierarchies in society); (3) 'power with' (power from collective action); and (4) 'power within' (power from individual consciousness) (Luttrell & Quiroz 2007). The coercive aspect of political, economic, and social power obviously has considerable relevance for analysing the forces undermining health opportunities for oppressed social groups. On the other hand, the dimension of power as collective action also carries promise for alternative models of public health action based on the empowerment of vulnerable communities.

An understanding of power as collective action connects suggestively with a model of social ethics based on human rights. As one commentary has argued: 'Throughout its history, the struggle for human rights . . . has consisted of one basic reality: A demand by oppressed and marginalized social groups and classes for the exercise of their social power' (Instituto de Estudios Politicos para America Latina y Africa 2005). Understood in this way, a human rights agenda means supporting the collective action of historically dominated communities to analyse, resist, and overcome oppression, asserting their shared power and altering social hierarchies in the direction of greater equity.

Theories of power remind us that any serious effort to reduce health inequities will involve changing the distribution of power within society to the benefit of disadvantaged groups. Changes in power relationships can take place at various levels, from the 'micro' level of interpersonal dynamics within individual households or workplaces to the 'macro' sphere of structural relations among social constituencies, mediated through economic, social, and political institutions. Power analysis makes clear, however, that micro-level modifications will be insufficient to reduce health inequities unless micro-level action is supported and reinforced through structural changes. By definition, then, action on the social determinants of health inequities is a political process that engages both the agency of disadvantaged communities and the responsibility of the state.

The emphasis on state action and the significance for marginalized groups of expressing their power politically takes on added importance, given the recent spread of largely de-politicized models of 'empowerment' in mainstream international development discourse and practice. Critics have observed how the idea of empowerment, originally generated in the context of grassroots movements pressing for redistribution of social, economic, and political power to marginalized groups, has been increasingly appropriated by mainstream development actors, such as the World Bank. In some contexts where these organizations have exerted influence, 'community empowerment' has arguably been reinterpreted as a substitute for substantial political and economic change, rather than a means to achieve it (Luttrell & Quiroz 2007). In practice, 'empowerment' of civil society and community groups often functions as a code word sanctioning government withdrawal from responsibility for service provision in health and social protection. Communities are 'empowered' to tackle their own health and underlying socioeconomic problems—meaning that they are given sole responsibility for doing so, but often without the financial and institutional resources needed to exercise this responsibility. For this reason, it is vital that those planning and implementing public health agendas be specific about what they mean by terms like 'empowerment', and about how public health policies will contribute to vulnerable people's capacity to control the factors that influence their health.

Introduction to the framework

The framework illustrated in Fig. 2.2.1 defines the major domains that must be differentiated and analysed in order to arrive at satisfactory answers to our guiding questions. This section offers an initial overview of the major components of the framework. Subsequent sections will analyse each specific component in detail.

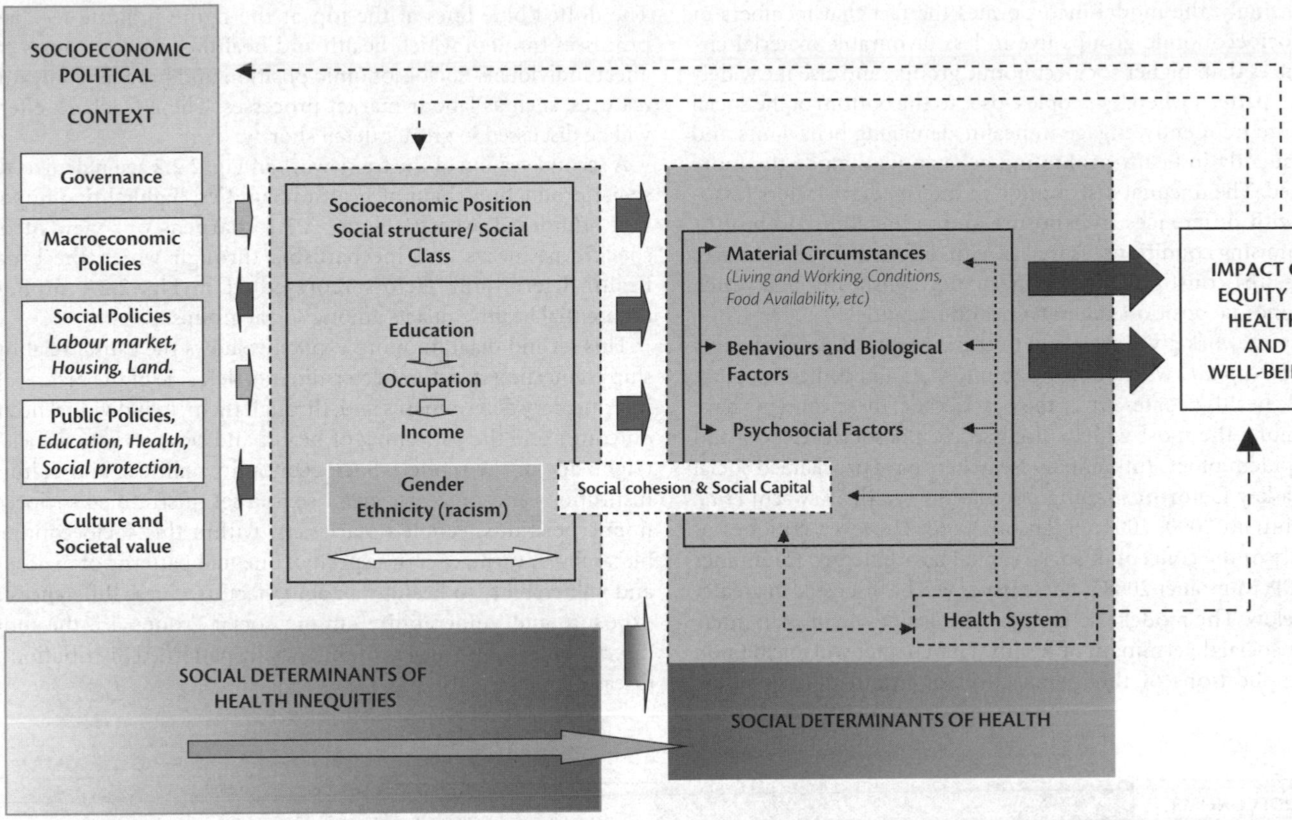

Fig. 2.2.1 Framework for understanding social determinants of health and health inequities.
Source: WHO Department of Equity, Poverty and Social Determinants of Health (Solar and Irwin 2007).

The framework defines two major domains. The first is that of *structural determinants*, which include people's socioeconomic position as well as relevant characteristics of the socioeconomic and political context. The second is that of *intermediary determinants*. This concept embraces what are often referred to as proximal determinants of health, and which at the individual level are termed risk factors, such as diet and exercise habits, smoking, or conditions of exposure to environmental pollutants in neighbourhoods, workplaces, and homes. A key aim of the framework is to clarify the relationship between structural and intermediary determinants.

In the far left column, the diagram shows the main *contextual factors that affect inequities in health*, e.g. governance, macroeconomic policies, social policies, public policies in other relevant areas, culture and societal values, and epidemiological conditions. 'Socioeconomic and political context' is a deliberately broad term that refers to the spectrum of factors in society that cannot be directly measured at the individual level. Context therefore encompasses a broad set of structural, cultural, and functional aspects of a social system whose impact on individuals tends to elude quantification but which exert a powerful formative influence on patterns of social stratification and thus on people's health opportunities. Within the context in this sense will be found those social and political mechanisms that generate, configure, and maintain social hierarchies.

Moving to the right, the next column of the diagram highlights the essential expression of social hierarchy, i.e. *socioeconomic position*, which reflects social structure and class relationships. People's socioeconomic position locates them with respect to the differential distribution of power, prestige, and resources in society. Since variables like 'power', 'prestige', and 'access to resources' may be difficult to measure, studies and evaluations of equity frequently use income, education, and occupation as proxies for these domains. When we refer to prestige and the related category of social discrimination, we find them strongly related to gender, ethnicity, sexuality, and education. Thus these latter factors are also included in the second column of the model, as factors linked to socioeconomic position.

Moving to the right once more, we reach the next stage in the social 'production chain' of health inequities (Diderichsen *et al.* 2001). Socioeconomic position influences people's health by acting through more specific, intermediary determinants. Those intermediary factors include: *Material circumstances*, such as neighbourhood, working and housing conditions; *psychosocial circumstances*, and also *behavioural, and biological factors*. Strenuous debates have characterized public health scientists' efforts to describe the interrelationships among these intermediary factors, with some groups giving relatively greater importance to psychosocial dynamics, others insisting on the primacy of the material dimension. The model presented here highlights material circumstances as the more fundamental area for action, while recognizing that material, psychosocial, and behavioural/biological factors influence each other through complex interactive patterns. Science has yet to understand the full set of mechanisms in play in these interactions. The fundamental point, however, is that all three categories of intermediary factors are shaped at a deeper level by the structural processes that assign individuals to different position in the socioeconomic hierarchy.

Accordingly, the model incorporates the fact that members of lower socioeconomic groups live in less favourable material circumstances than higher socioeconomic groups, and also the widely observed pattern whereby people closer to the bottom of the social scale more frequently engage in health-damaging behaviours and less frequently in heath-promoting behaviours than do the more privileged. The unequal distribution of intermediary factors (associated with differences in exposure and vulnerability to health-compromising conditions, as well as with differential consequences of ill-health) constitutes the primary mechanism through which socioeconomic position generates health inequities.

The framework gives attention to the concepts of *social cohesion* and '*social capital*', which occupy an unusual (and contested) place in public health debates. Over the past decade, these concepts have been among the most widely discussed in the social sciences and social epidemiology. Influential researchers have proclaimed social capital a key factor in shaping population health (Kawachi *et al.* 1997; Putnam 2000, 2001; Ferguson 2006). However, critiques of the utility of the concept of social capital have emerged (Muntaner *et al.* 1999; Muntaner 2004). These issues will be discussed in greater detail below. The model also includes the *health system* as an intermediary social determinant of health. This chapter will touch upon some implications of this perspective for health policymaking. The dotted blue lines at the top of the figure indicate feedback processes through which health and health equity outcomes can affect individuals' socioeconomic position and broader contextual features, such as labour market processes. These feedback effects will be discussed in greater detail shortly.

A second version of the framework in Fig. 2.2.2 again depicts the social production chain of health inequities, highlighting important additional aspects. Figure 2.2.2 sharpens our view of the specific pathways and mechanisms through which the broad health-determining factors represented in Fig. 2.2.1 produce differential health impacts among social groups.

This second diagram more explicitly shows the causal relationship connecting structural determinants (left side of the picture) to intermediary determinants and, through them, to individual health outcomes and the patterning of health and sickness across society (right side of the model). Socioeconomic, political, and cultural institutions and processes give rise to a set of stratified socioeconomic positions. People's placement within this socioeconomic hierarchy in turn generates specific, unequal patterns of exposure and vulnerability to health-damaging factors. These differences in exposure and vulnerability among social groups are the more directly observable triggers of the socially patterned distribution of disease.

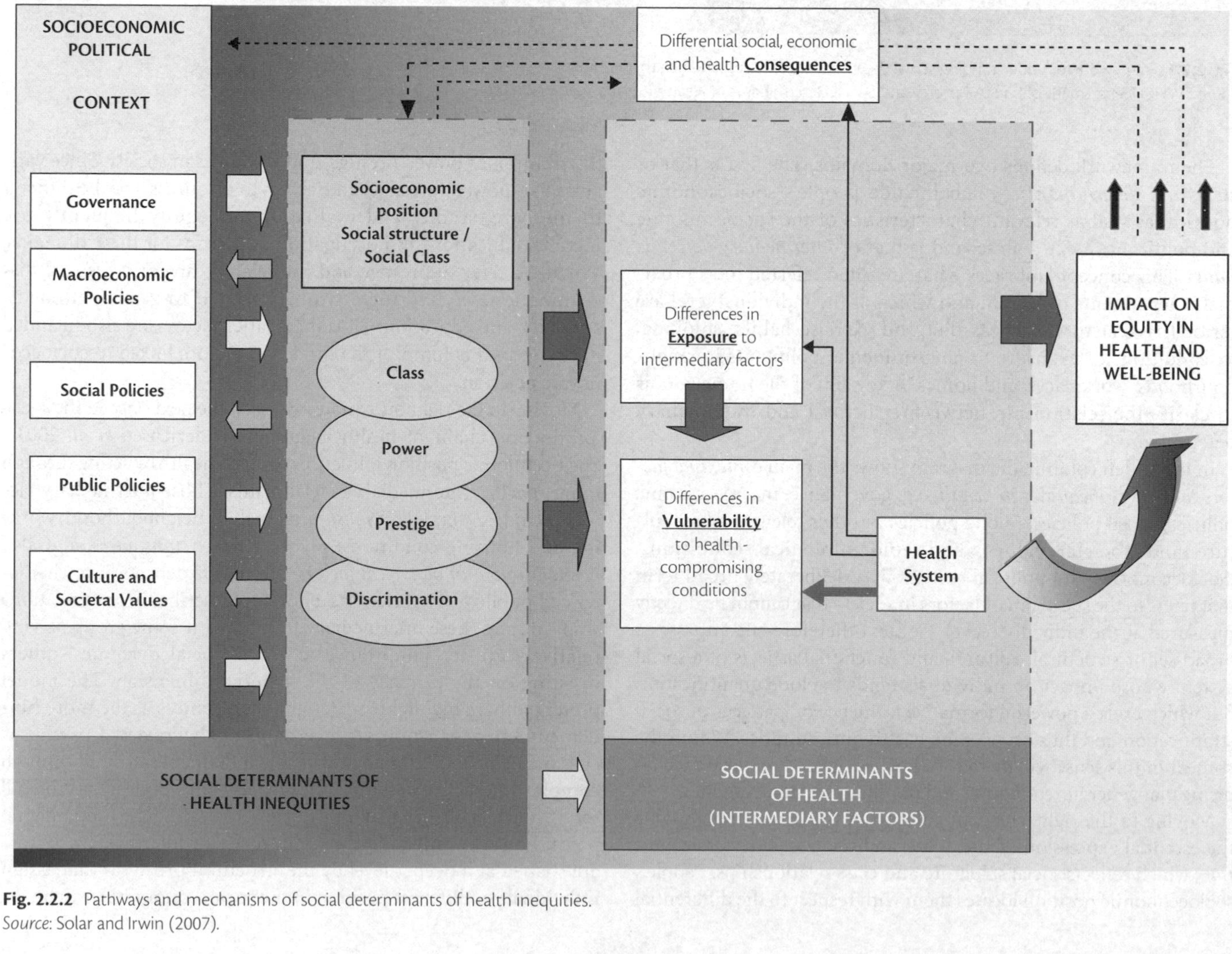

Fig. 2.2.2 Pathways and mechanisms of social determinants of health inequities.
Source: Solar and Irwin (2007).

Under the heading of 'socioeconomic position', Fig. 2.2.2 gives added emphasis to the concept of social class. As an inherently relational variable, class is able to shed particular light on the mechanisms associated with the social production of health inequities. By definition, class position is connected with the economic base and people's ability to access and control resources. Class is also linked with people's degree of power in society. The structures and mechanisms through which power is exercised, and the capacity of individuals and groups to wield power and exert control over decisions that affect their well-being, are in turn influenced by the political context (including functioning democratic institutions or their absence, corruption, access to media and information, etc.).

The inclusion of 'prestige' and 'discrimination' as facets of the social production of health/disease underscores that, in each society, the distribution of resources and power among groups is entwined with a hierarchical status system that assigns some groups higher social rank and greater respect than others. Though closely related to the unequal distribution of wealth and power, social status rankings are not identical with these other forms of hierarchy. Evidence suggests that forms of social prestige and/or systematic discrimination directed towards selected groups may exert health effects independent of wealth and material living conditions, as when studies show persistent differentials in life expectancy and other key health indicators between ethnic majority and minority groups, even when factors such as income and education are controlled for (Gee 2002).

The dotted lines at the top of Fig. 2.2.2, leading back from the right towards the left side of the diagram, illustrate significant 'feedback' effects that reveal an additional dimension of the dynamic interrelation between social conditions and health. Socioeconomic inequalities in health can in fact be partly explained by the impacts of health and sickness on socioeconomic position, e.g. when someone experiences a drop in income because of a work-induced disability or the medical costs associated with major illness. Persons who are in poor health less frequently move up and more frequently move down the social ladder than healthy persons. It may be noted, in addition, that some specific diseases can impact people's socioeconomic position not only by undermining their physical capacities, but also through associated stigma and discrimination, e.g. in the case of HIV/AIDS.

These observations help clarify why it is useful to view the health system itself as a social determinant of health. The model suggests the capacity of the heath sector to influence the social production of health/disease in at least three ways, by acting upon: Differences in exposures; differences in vulnerability; and differences in the consequences of illness for people's health and their social and economic standing. This is in addition to the health sector's key role in promoting and coordinating policy action across government sectors to address other social determinants of health.

Because of their magnitude, certain diseases, such as HIV/AIDS and malaria, can also impact key components of the socioeconomic and political context directly, e.g. the labour market and governance institutions. This effect is illustrated by the blue arrow in the diagram. The whole set of 'feedback' mechanisms just described is brought together under the heading of 'differential social, economic, and health consequences'. The framework includes the impact of existing social position on these mechanisms, indicating that path with a red arrow.

The following sections will discuss in greater detail each of the major components of the framework.

First element of the framework: Socioeconomic and political context

The model of health determinants developed in this chapter differs from some others in the importance attributed to the *socioeconomic and political context*. Political institutions and processes have been largely ignored in a substantial portion of the recent literature on health determinants. Population health researchers now routinely acknowledge that the health of individuals and populations is strongly influenced by social determinants. However, as Navarro and others have argued, it is much less common for public health scholars to recognize that the quality of determinants is in turn shaped by the policies that guide how societies (re)distribute material resources among their members (cf. Esping-Andersen 2002). In the growing area of determinants research, a subject rarely studied is the impact on social inequalities and health of political movements and parties and the policies they adopt when in government (Navarro & Shi 2001). Chung and Muntaner (2006) find similarly that few studies have explored the relationship between political variables and population health at the national level, and none has included a comprehensive number of political variables to understand their effect on population health, while simultaneously adjusting for economic determinants. As an illustration of the powerful impact of political variables on health outcomes, these researchers concluded in a recent study of 18 wealthy countries in Europe, North America, and the Asia-Pacific region that 20 per cent of the differences in infant mortality rate among countries could be explained by the type of welfare state they have adopted. Similarly, different welfare state models among the countries accounted for about 10 per cent of differences in the rate of low-birth-weight babies.

In general, the construction/mapping of context should include at least six points: (1) *Governance* in the broadest sense and its processes, including definition of needs, patterns of discrimination, civil society participation, and accountability/transparence in public administration; (2) *macroeconomic policy*, including fiscal, monetary, balance of payments and trade policies, and underlying labour market structures; (3) *social policies* affecting factors such as labour, social welfare, land and housing distribution; (4) *public policy* in other relevant areas such as education, medical care, water, and sanitation; (5) *epidemiological conditions*, particularly in the case of major epidemics such as HIV/AIDS, which exert a powerful influence on social structures and must be factored into global and national policy-setting; (6) *culture and societal values*.

While the category of culture and societal values includes a wide range of factors, one especially relevant aspect is the value placed on health and the degree to which health is seen as a collective social concern. This differs greatly across regional and national contexts. Elsewhere, following pioneering work undertaken by Kleczkowski *et al.* (1984), we have argued that the social value attributed to health in a country constitutes an important and often neglected aspect of the context in which health policies must be designed and implemented (Solar *et al.* 2004). In constructing a typology of health systems, Roemer and Kleczkowski have proposed three domains of analysis to indicate how health is valued in a given society:

- The extent to which health is a priority in the governmental/societal agenda, as reflected in the level of national resources allocated to health.
- The extent to which the society assumes collective responsibility for financing and organizing the provision of health services.

In maximum collectivism (also referred to as a state-based model), the system is almost entirely concerned with providing collective benefits, leaving little or no choice to the individual. In maximum individualism, ill health and its care are viewed as private concerns.

- The extent of societal distributional responsibility. This is a measure of the degree to which society assumes responsibility for the distribution of its health resources. Distributional responsibility is at its maximum when the society guarantees equal access to services for all.

Among many aspects of culture that operate as contextual determinants of health, the social value attributed to health may carry especially important consequences, not only by moulding individual and group behaviour, but also because this underlying valuation influences society's willingness to invest in public policies to address the determinants of health and health equity.

Second element of the framework: Socioeconomic position

The concept of 'socioeconomic position' locates people within complex, interpenetrating systems of social hierarchy. The two major variables used to operationalize socioeconomic position in studies of social inequities in health are *social stratification* and *social class*. The term stratification is used in sociology to refer to social hierarchies in which individuals or groups can be arranged along a ranked order of some attribute. Income or years of education provide familiar examples. Measures of social stratification are important predictors of patterns of mortality and morbidity. 'Social class', meanwhile, is defined by relations of ownership or control over productive resources (i.e. physical, financial, organizational) (Muntaner *et al.* 2003). Social class has important consequences for the lives of individuals. Class, in contrast to stratification, indicates the employment relations and conditions of each occupation. The task of class analysis is precisely to understand not only how macro structures (e.g. class relations at the national level) constrain micro processes (e.g. interpersonal behaviour) but also how micro processes can affect macro structures (for example, through collective action) (Muntaner *et al.* 1999).

Adler *et al.* (1994) observe that social class is among the strongest known predictors of illness and health and yet is, paradoxically, a variable about which very little systematic research has been conducted. Muntaner and colleagues have likewise noted that, while there is substantial scholarship on the psychology of racism and gender, little research has been done on the effects of class ideology (i.e. classism). This asymmetry could reflect that in most wealthy democratic capitalist countries, income inequalities are perceived as acceptable while gender and race inequalities are not (Muntaner *et al.* 1999). The concept of class adds significant value and should be included as a distinct component in discussions of socioeconomic position.

Historically, two central figures in the study of socioeconomic position were Karl Marx and Max Weber. For Marx, socioeconomic position was entirely determined by social class, whereby an individuals are defined by their relation to the 'means of production' (for example, factories, land). Social class and class relations are characterized by the conflict between exploited workers and the exploiting capitalists who control the means of production. This underscores that class is not an inherent property of individual human beings, but a relational characteristic generated by a social structure. Weber developed a different view of class and social location. Weber saw differential societal position as incorporating three dimensions: Class, status and party (or power). Class has an economic base. It implies ownership and control of resources and is indicated by measures of income. Status is considered to be prestige or honour in the community. Weber considers status to imply 'access to life chances' based on social and cultural factors such as family background, lifestyle and social networks. Finally, power is related to a political context (Liberatos *et al.* 1988). In this chapter, we use the term 'socioeconomic position', acknowledging the three separate but linked dimensions of social class reflected in the Weberian conceptualization.

More recently, Krieger, Williams, and Moss (1997) have treated socioeconomic position as an aggregate concept that includes both resource-based and prestige-based measures. Resource-based measures refer to material and social resources and assets, including income, wealth, and educational credentials; terms used to describe inadequate resources include 'poverty' and 'deprivation'. Prestige-based measures refer to individuals' rank or status in a social hierarchy. Given distinctions between resource-based and prestige-based aspects of socioeconomic position and the diverse pathways by which they affect health, epidemiological studies should state clearly how measures of socioeconomic position are conceptualized. Educational level creates differences between people in terms of access to information and the level of proficiency in benefiting from new knowledge, whereas income creates differences in access to scarce material goods. Occupational status includes both these aspects and adds to them benefits accruing from the exercise of specific jobs, such as prestige, privileges, power, and social and technical skills.

Socioeconomic position can be usefully measured at three complementary levels: Individual, household, and neighbourhood. Each level may independently contribute to distributions of exposure and outcomes. Also, socioeconomic position can be measured meaningfully at different points of the lifespan: e.g. infancy, childhood, adolescent, adult (current, past 5 years, etc.). Relevant time periods depend on presumed exposures, causal pathways, and associated aetiologic periods. Today it is also vital to recognize gender, ethnicity, and sexuality as social stratifiers linked to systematic forms of discrimination (Krieger *et al.* 1993).

A close relationship exists between the social–political context and what we term the structural determinants of health inequities. The framework posits that *structural determinants* are those that generate or reinforce social stratification in the society and that define individual socioeconomic position. These mechanisms configure the health opportunities of social groups based on their placement within hierarchies of power, prestige, and access to resources (economic status). We prefer to speak of *structural determinants*, rather than 'distal' factors, in order to capture and underscore the causal hierarchy of social determinants involved in producing health inequities. Structural social stratification mechanisms, joined to and influenced by institutions and processes embedded in the socioeconomic and political context (e.g. redistributive welfare state policies), can together be conceptualized as *the social determinants of health inequities*. In all cases, structural determinants present themselves in a specific political and historical context. At the same time, the context forms part of the origin and foundation of a given distribution of power, prestige, and access to material resources in a society and thus of the pattern of social stratification and social class relations existing in that society. The positive significance of this relationship is that it is possible to address the effects of the structural determinants of health inequities through purposive action on contextual features, for example through public policy measures addressing the education system, the labour market, land ownership, social protection and redistribution, and other mechanisms impacting stratification at a structural level.

Third element of the framework: Intermediary determinants

Structural determinants operate through a series of *intermediary social factors* or *social determinants of health*. The structural determinants or social determinants of health inequities are causally antecedent to these intermediary determinants, which are linked, on the other side, to a set of individual-level influences, including health-related behaviours and physiological factors. The intermediary factors flow from the configuration of underlying social stratification and, in turn, determine differences in exposure and vulnerability to health-compromising conditions. A recent revision of Diderichsen's model sheds additional light on the processes (Diderichsen 2004). Both *differential exposure* and *differential vulnerability* may contribute to the relation between social position and health outcomes, as can be tested empirically (Whitehead *et al.* 2000). Ill-health has serious social and economic consequences due to inability to work and the cost of healthcare. These consequences depend not only on the extent of disability but also on the individual's social position and on the society's environment and social policies. At the most proximal point in the models, genetic and biological processes are emphasized, mediating the health effects of social determinants (Graham 2004). The social and economical consequences of illness may feed back into the aetiological pathways and contribute to the further development of disease in the individual.

The main categories of intermediary determinants of health are: Material circumstances; psychosocial circumstances; behavioural and/or biological factors; the health system itself as a social determinant, and social cohesion. These elements are reviewed in turn.

Material circumstances

These include determinants linked to the physical environment, such as housing (relating both to the dwelling itself and its location), consumption potential, i.e. the financial means to buy healthy food, warm clothing, etc., and the physical working and neighbourhood environments. Depending on their quality, these circumstances both provide resources for health and contain health risks. In the model, material circumstances are highlighted as fundamental, exercising a strong causal influence on the other categories of intermediary determinants. Patterns of interaction among intermediary determinants are complex, however. Much remains to be understood about the interrelationships among material, psychosocial, and behavioural/biological factors in different contexts.

Social-environmental or psychosocial circumstances

These include psychosocial stressors (for example, negative life events, job strain), stressful living circumstances (e.g. high debt) and (lack of) social support, coping styles, etc. Different social groups are exposed to different degrees to experiences and life situations that are perceived as threatening, frightening, and difficult to deal with. This partly explains the long-term pattern of social inequalities in health. Stress may be a direct causal factor in triggering forms of illness. Additionally, a background condition of ongoing, long-term stress may be part of the causal complex behind other illnesses. A person's socioeconomic position may itself be a source of long-term stress, and will also affect the opportunities to deal with stressful and difficult situations.

Behavioural and biological factors

These include smoking, diet, alcohol consumption, and physical exercise. Such factors can be either health protecting and enhancing (like exercise) or health damaging (cigarette smoking and obesity). Biological factors, including genetic factors, are situated at this same level of analysis.

Social inequalities in health have also been associated with social differences in behaviours, or what are often referred to as 'lifestyle' factors. Such differences are found in nutrition, physical activity, tobacco, and alcohol consumption. This indicates that differences in behaviour could partially explain social inequalities in health, but researchers do not agree on their importance: Some regard differences in personal behaviour as a sufficient explanation without further elaboration; others regard them as contributory factors that in turn result from more fundamental causes. For example, Margolis *et al.* (1992) found that the prevalence of both acute and persistent respiratory symptoms in infants showed dose–response relationships with socioeconomic position. When risk factors such as crowding and exposure to smoking in the household were adjusted for, relative risk associated with socioeconomic position was reduced but still remained significant (cf. Marmot *et al.* 1984).

Cigarette smoking is strongly linked to socioeconomic position, including education, income, and employment status, and it is significantly associated with morbidity and mortality, particularly from cardiovascular disease and cancer (e.g. Marmot *et al.* 1991). A linear gradient between education and smoking prevalence was also shown in a community sample of middle-aged women: Additionally, among current smokers the number of cigarettes smoked was related to socioeconomic position. Significant employment grade differences in smoking were found in the Whitehall II study, which examined a new cohort of 10 314 subjects from the British Civil Service beginning in 1985 (Marmot *et al.* 1991). Moving from the lowest to the highest employment grades, the prevalence of current smoking among men was 33.6, 21.9, 18.4, 13.0, 10.2, and 8.3 per cent, respectively. For women, the comparable figures were 27.5, 22.7, 20.3, 15.2, 11.6, and 18.3 per cent, respectively. Social class differences in smoking are likely to continue because rates of smoking initiation are inversely related to socioeconomic position, while rates of cessation are positively related to people's socioeconomic rank (e.g. Escobedo *et al.* 1990; Kaprio & Koskenvuo 1988).

Behavioural factors are relatively accessible and measurable for research. Partially as a result, a large literature on behavioural or so-called 'lifestyle' influences on health has developed. The existence of a body of research in this area does not mean, however, that behavioural factors are the most important causes of social inequalities in health. Other, more fundamental factors may be at the root of variations in both personal behaviours and health—a crucial consideration when it comes to planning appropriate interventions (see Macintyre 2007). Some surveys indicate that differences in lifestyle can only explain a small proportion of social inequalities in health (Marmot *et al.* 1978). For instance, material factors may act as a source of psychosocial stress, and psychosocial stress may influence health-related behaviours. Each of them can influence health through specific biological factors. For example a diet rich in saturated fat will lead to atherosclerosis, which will increase the risk of a myocardial infarction. Stress will activate hormonal systems that may increase blood pressure and reduce the immune response. Adoption of health-threatening behaviours is a response to material deprivation and stress. Environments determine whether individuals take up tobacco, use alcohol, have poor diets, and engage in physical activity. Tobacco and excessive alcohol use, and carbohydrate-dense diets, are means of coping with difficult circumstances (Mackenbach & Bakker 2002).

The health system as a social determinant of health

Many models have paid insufficient attention to the health system as a social determinant. The health system can directly address socially conditioned differences in people's exposure and vulnerability to health damage not only by improving equitable access to care, but also in the promotion of intersectoral action to improve health status. Examples would include food supplementation through the health system and transport policies and intervention for tackling geographic barriers to healthcare access. A further aspect of great importance is the role the health system plays in mediating the differential consequences of illness in people's lives. The health system is capable of ensuring that health problems do not lead to a further deterioration of people's social status, and of facilitating sick people's social reintegration. Examples include programmes for the chronically ill to support their reinsertion in the workforce, as well as appropriate models of health financing that can prevent people from being forced into (deeper) poverty by the costs of medical care.

A crosscutting determinant: Social cohesion/social capital

Bernales (2006) has recently provided a review of debates on this topic. In the most influential recent discussions, three broad approaches to the characterization and analysis of social capital can be distinguished: Communitarian approaches, network approaches, and resource distribution approaches. The *communitarian approach* defines social capital as a psychosocial mechanism, corresponding to a neo-Durkheimian perspective on the relation between individual health and society (Popay 2000). The *network approach* considers social capital in terms of resources that flow and emerge through social networks. It begins with a systemic relational perspective; in other words, an ecological vision is taken that sees beyond individual resources and additive characteristics. This involves an analysis of the influence of social structure, power hierarchies and access to resources on population health (Moore *et al.* 2006). This approach implies that decisions that groups or individuals make, in relation to their lifestyle and behavioural habits, cannot be considered outside the social context where such choices take place. Finally, the *resource distribution approach,* adopting a materialistic perspective, suggests that there is a danger in promoting social capital as a substitute for structural change when facing health inequity. Some representatives of this group openly criticize psychosocial approaches that have suggested social capital and cohesion as the most important mediators of the association between income and health inequality (Lynch *et al.* 2000). The resource distribution approach insists that psychosocial aspects affecting population health are a consequence of material life conditions (Lynch 2000).

Recent work by Szreter and Woolcock (2004) has enriched the debates around social capital and its health impacts. These authors distinguish between bonding, bridging, and linking social capital. *Bonding social capital* refers to the trust and cooperative relationships between members of a network that are similar in terms of their social identity. *Bridging social capital*, on the other hand, refers to respectful relationships and mutuality between individuals and groups that are aware that they do not possess the same characteristics in socio-demographic terms. Finally, *linking social capital* corresponds with the norms of respect and trust relationships between individuals, groups, networks, and institutions that interact from different positions along explicit gradients of institutionalized power. Collaborative relationships between civil society or community-based organizations and state institutions provide one example.

Impact of determinants on equity in health and well-being

According to the analysis we have developed, the structural factors associated with the key components of socioeconomic position are at the root of health inequities measured at the population level. This relationship is confirmed by a substantial body of evidence.

Socioeconomic health differences are reflected in general measures of health, like life expectancy, all-cause mortality, and self-rated health (Kubzansky *et al.* 2001; Mackenbach *et al.* 2002). Differences correlated with people's socioeconomic position are found for rates of mortality and morbidity from almost every disease and condition (Antonovsky 1967; Illsley & Baker 1991). Socioeconomic position is also linked to prevalence and course of disease and self-rated health. Socioeconomic health inequalities are evident in specific causes of disease, disability, and premature death, including lung cancer, coronary heart disease, accidents, and suicide. Low birth weight provides an additional important example. This is a sensitive measure of child health and a major risk factor for impaired development through childhood, including intellectual development (Graham 2005). There are marked differences in national rates of low birth weight, with higher rates in the US and UK and lower rates in Nordic countries like Sweden, Norway, and the Netherlands. These rates vary in line with the proportion of the child population living in poverty (in households with incomes below 50 per cent of average income): At their lowest in low-poverty countries like Sweden and Norway, and at their highest in high-poverty countries like the UK and US (Emerson 2004).

Impact along the gradient

There is evidence that the association of socioeconomic position and health occurs at every level of the social hierarchy, not simply below the threshold of poverty. Not only do those in poverty have poorer health than those in more favoured circumstances, but those at the highest level enjoy better health than do those just below (e.g. Marmot *et al.* 1984, 1991). The effects of severe poverty on health may seem obvious through the impact of poor nutrition, crowded and insanitary living conditions, and inadequate medical care. Identifying factors that can account for the link to health all across the socioeconomic hierarchy may shed light on new mechanisms that have heretofore been ignored because of a focus on the more readily apparent correlates of poverty. The most notable of the studies demonstrating the SEP-health gradient is the Whitehall study of mortality (Marmot *et al.* 1984). Similar findings emerge from census data in the United Kingdom (Susser *et al.* 1985).

Despite the demonstrated important impact of socioeconomic position on health, disconcertingly little is known about how socioeconomic position operates to influence biological functions that determine health status. Part of the problem may be the way in which socioeconomic position is conceptualized and analysed. Socioeconomic position has been almost universally relegated to the status of a control variable and has not been systematically studied as an important aetiologic factor in its own right. It is usually treated as a main effect, operating independently of other variables to predict health.

Life course perspective

A life course approach explicitly recognizes the importance of time and timing in understanding causal links between exposures and outcomes within an individual life course, across generations, and in population-level diseases trends (e.g. Lynch & Smith 2005). Adopting a life course perspective directs attention to how social determinants of health operate at every level of development—early childhood, childhood, adolescence, and adulthood—both to immediately influence health and to provide the basis for health or illness later in life. The life course perspective attempts to understand how such temporal processes across the life course of one cohort are related to previous and subsequent cohorts and are manifested in disease trends observed over time at the population level. Time lags between exposure, disease initiation, and clinical recognition (latency period) suggest that exposures early in life are involved in initiating diseases processes prior to clinical manifestations. However, the recognition of early-life influences on chronic diseases does not imply deterministic processes that negate the utility of later-life intervention.

Two main mechanisms are identified. The '*critical periods*' model is when an exposure acting during a specific period has lasting or lifelong effects on the structure or function of organs, tissues, and body systems which are not modified in any dramatic way by later experiences. This is also known as biological programming, and is also sometimes referred to as a latency model. This conception is the basis of hypotheses on the foetal origins of adult diseases. This approach does recognize the importance of later life effect modifiers, for example in the linkage of coronary heart disease, high blood pressure, and insulin resistance with low birth weight (e.g. Frankel *et al.* 1996).

The '*accumulation of risk*' model suggests that factors that raise disease risk or promote good health may accumulate gradually over the life course, although there may be developmental periods when their effects have greater impact on later health than factors operating at other times. This idea is complementary to the notion that as the intensity, number, and/or duration of exposures increase, there is increasing cumulative damage to biological systems. Understanding the health effects of childhood social class by identifying specific aspects of the early physical or psychosocial environment (such as exposure to air pollution or family conflict) or possible mechanisms (such as nutrition, infection, or stress) that are associated with adult disease will provide further aetiological insights. Circumstances in early life are seen as the initial stage in the pathway to adult health but with an indirect effect, influencing adult health through social trajectories, such as restricting educational opportunities, thus influencing socioeconomic circumstances and health in later life. Risk factors tend to cluster in socially patterned ways, for example, those living in adverse childhood social circumstances are more likely to be of low birth weight, and be exposed to poor diet, childhood infections, and passive smoking. These exposures may raise the risk of adult respiratory disease, perhaps through chains of risk or pathways over time where one adverse (or protective) experience will tend to lead to another adverse (protective) experience in a cumulative way.

Ben-Shlomo and Kuh (2002) argue that the life course approach is not limited to individuals within a single generation but should intertwine biological and social transmission of risk across generations. It must contextualize any exposure both within a hierarchical structure as well as in relation to geographical and secular differences, which may be unique to that cohort of individuals. Recently the potential for a life course approach to aid understanding of variations in the health and disease of populations over time, across countries, and between social groups has been given more attention. Davey Smith (2003) suggests that explanations for social inequalities in cause-specific adult mortality lie in socially patterned exposures at different stages of the life course.

Children born into poorer circumstances are at greater risk of the forms of developmental delay associated with intellectual disability, including speech impairments, cognitive difficulties, and behavioural problems (Maughan *et al.* 1999; Power & Hertzman 2004). Some other conditions, like stroke and stomach cancer, appear to depend considerably on childhood circumstances, while for others, including deaths from lung cancer and accidents/violence, adult circumstances play the more important role. In another group are health outcomes where it is cumulative exposure that appears to be important. A number of studies suggest that this is the case for coronary heart disease and respiratory disease, for example (Davey Smith 2003).

Selection processes and health-related mobility

People with weaker health resources, allegedly, have a tendency to end up or remain low on the ladder of socioeconomic position. According to some analysts, the status of research on selection processes and health-related mobility within the socioeconomic structure can be summarized in three points: (1) variations in health in youth have some significance for educational paths and for the kind of job a person has at the beginning of his or her working career; (2) for those who are already established in working life, variations in health have little significance for the overall progress of a person's career; (3) people who develop serious health problems in adult life are often excluded from working life, and often long before the ordinary retirement age (see e.g. Manor *et al.* 2003). One might assume such effects to be inevitable. But they are in part due to discriminatory practices, in part also to failures to adapt educational institutions and working life to special needs. To the extent that this is the case, social selection is neither necessary, nor inevitable, nor fair. This phenomenon particularly affects persons with disabilities, persons from immigrant backgrounds and, to a certain extent, women (Graham 2004).

Impact on the socioeconomic and political context

From a population standpoint, we observe that the magnitude of certain diseases can translate into direct effects on features of the socioeconomic and political context, through high prevalence rates and levels of mortality and morbidity. The HIV/AIDS pandemic in sub-Saharan Africa can be seen in this light, with its associated plunge in life expectancy and stresses on agricultural productivity, economic growth, and sectoral capacities in areas such as health and education. The magnitude of the impact of epidemics and emergencies will depend on the historical, political, and social contexts in which they occur, as well as on the demographic composition of the societies affected. These are aspects that must be considered when analysing welfare state structures, in particular models of health system organization that may be considered to respond to such challenges.

Distinguishing determinants of health from determinants of inequities in health

Hilary Graham (2004) has rightly observed that the central concept of 'social determinants' remains ambiguous in much of the relevant public health literature. The term is used to refer simultaneously to the determinants of health and to the determinants of inequalities in health. Graham notes that: 'Using a single term to refer to both the social factors influencing health and the social processes shaping their social distribution would not be problematic if the main determinants of health—like living standards, environmental influences, and health behaviours—were equally distributed between socioeconomic groups'. But the evidence points to marked socioeconomic differences in access to material resources, health-promoting resources, and in exposure to risk factors. Furthermore, policies associated with positive trends in health determinants (e.g. a rise in living standards and a decline in smoking) have also been associated with persistent socioeconomic disparities in the distribution of these determinants (marked socioeconomic differences in living standards and smoking rates) (e.g. Howden-Chapman *et al.* 2000). We have attempted to resolve this linguistic ambiguity by introducing additional differentiations within the field of concepts conventionally included under the heading 'social determinants'.

We adopt the term *structural determinants* to refer specifically to the components of people's socioeconomic position. Structural determinants, combined with the main features of the socioeconomic and political context described above, together constitute what we call the *social determinants of health inequities.* This concept corresponds to Graham's notion of the 'social processes shaping the distribution' of downstream social determinants. Our term *intermediary determinants of health* refers to these more downstream factors. As noted, the vocabulary of 'structural' and 'intermediary' seeks to emphasize the causal linkage between the two categories and the priority of structural factors (Graham 2004).

Graham argues that what is obscured in many previous treatments of these topics 'is that tackling the determinants of health inequalities is about tackling the *unequal distribution of health determinants*'. Focusing on the unequal distribution of determinants is important for thinking about policy. This is because policies that have achieved overall improvements in key determinants such as living standards and smoking have not reduced inequalities in these major influences on health. When health equity is the goal, the priority of a determinants-oriented strategy is to reduce inequalities in the major influences on people's health. Tackling inequalities in social position is likely to be at the heart of such a strategy. For, according to Graham, social position is the pivotal point in the causal chain linking broad determinants to the risk factors that directly damage people's health. Graham emphasizes that policy objectives will be defined quite differently, depending on whether our aim is to address determinants of health or determinants of health inequities:

- *Objectives for health determinants* are likely to focus on reducing overall exposure to health-damaging factors along the causal pathway. The UK, for example, has focused on raising educational standards and living standards (important constituents of socioeconomic position) and reducing rates of smoking (a major intermediary risk factor).
- *Objectives for health inequity determinants* are likely to focus on levelling up the distribution of major health determinants. How these objectives are framed will depend on the health inequities goals that are being pursued. One example would be progressive tax structures to redistribute income (Graham 2004).

Implications for public health policies

Three key policy orientations can be derived from the framework presented in this chapter:

- Arguably the single most significant lesson of the framework is that interventions and policies to reduce health inequities must not limit themselves to intermediary determinants, but must include policies crafted to tackle structural determinants. Interventions addressing intermediary determinants can improve average health indicators while leaving health inequities unchanged. For this reason, policy action on structural determinants is necessary. To achieve solid results, determinants policies must be designed with attention to contextual specificities, which should be rigorously characterized using methodologies developed by social and political science.
- Cross-sectoral or intersectoral policymaking and implementation are crucial for progress on health equity. This is because structural determinants can only be tackled through strategies that reach beyond the health sector. The health sector's work with other sectors can involve different levels: From simple coordination of objectives and strategies among different sectors, through more substantive cooperation, up to genuine integration of policies. Policy integration is required to tackle the structural determinants of health.
- Participation of civil society and affected communities in the design and implementation of policies to address health determinants is essential to success. Social participation is an ethical obligation for governments. In addition, the empowerment of civil society and communities and their ownership of the determinants agenda could build a sustained global movement for health equity.

Figure 2.2.3 summarizes the policy implications of the determinants framework in a visual representation. It highlights the need to promote context-specific strategies to address structural as well as intermediary determinants. Such strategies will necessarily include cross-sector and intersectoral policies, through which structural determinants can be most effectively addressed, and will aim to ensure that policies are crafted so as to engage and ultimately empower civil society and affected communities. These broad directions for policy action can utilize various entry points or levels of engagement, represented in the image by the cross-cutting horizontal bars.

Moving from the lower to the higher bars (from more 'downstream' to more structural approaches), these entry points include: Seeking to palliate the differential consequences of illness; seeking to reduce differential vulnerabilities and exposures for disadvantaged social groups; and, ultimately, altering the patterns of social stratification. At the same time, policies and interventions can be targeted at the 'micro' level of individual interactions; at the 'meso'

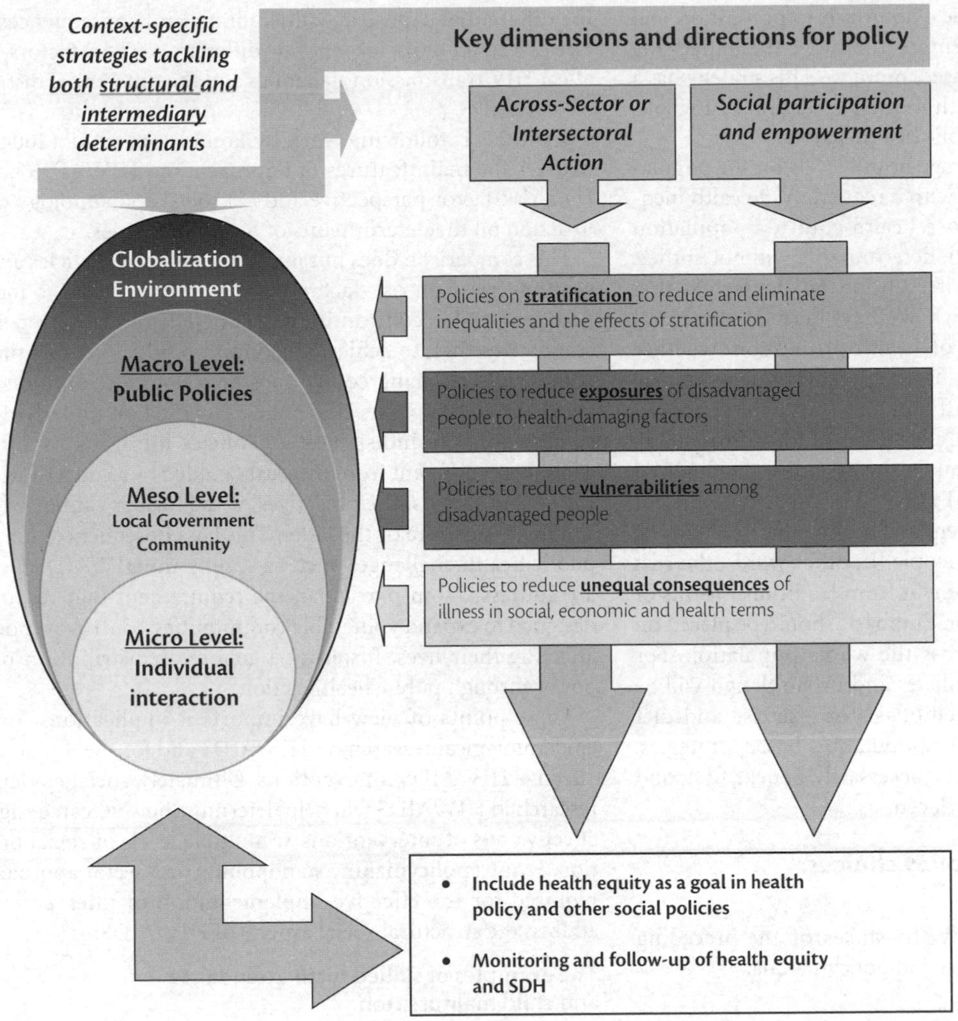

Fig. 2.2.3 Framework for policy action on social determinants of health and health equity.
Source: Solar and Irwin (2007).

level of community conditions or local government; or at the broadest 'macro' level of universal public policies and the global environment.

Individual vs. population approaches in epidemiology and public health policy

Modern epidemiology has been heavily oriented to the study of risk factors for chronic non-communicable and communicable emergent diseases (McMichael 1999). The primary concern has been to understand disease occurrence in individual terms, looking at aspects such as consumer behaviour, individual exposures, metabolic factors and genetic effects. Epidemiology has become adept at determining which individuals are at increased risk of disease, looking at factors that are measurable at the individual level, but it has not been as successful at understanding the distribution of diseases within and between populations. Factors that are important causes of diseases in an individual within a population may be very different from the factors that primarily determine disease rates in the whole population (Rose 2001).

Implicit in the focus on proximate risk factors is the assumption that the individual is the site of aetiologic actions and, therefore, the natural unit of epidemiological observation. Larger scale variables that affect whole groups or populations, such as poverty and cultural disruptions, are only viewed as important because and to the extent that they translate into individual-level risk factors. Poverty affects diet; cultural disruptions (such as economic transitions, rural-to-urban migration) spur increases in alcoholism, etc. However, this population vs. individual distinction needs careful examination, in light of the framework explored in this chapter. Are we distinguishing between structural and intermediary determinants and their proximate manifestations? Or is there a category of risk factor that, in some collective way, influences the health of the population at large via processes that do not have direct, proximate manifestations? Further, complex entities such a poverty, for example, can have very different meanings and can measure qualitatively different constructs at the individual and population levels (Schwartz 1994).

These distinctions are not only important for building appropriately comprehensive theoretical frameworks. They also have far-reaching implications for all aspects of public health policy. Individual and population-based approaches yield very different strategies for practice in both prevention and curative care. The individual approach seeks to identify high-risk, susceptible individuals and to offer them forms of personalized protection or treatment. In contrast, the population strategy seeks to control the determinants of incidence in the population as a whole. The 'high-risk individual' strategy is the traditional biomedical approach to prevention and cure. The population strategy attempts to remove the underlying causes that make the relevant diseases common. This strategy has a large potential for improving health in the population as a whole, but it raises new challenges for public health action.

Moreover, improvements in average health levels for the population are not necessarily associated with a reduction in health inequities. If the objective is to improve health equity, a population approach focused on intermediary determinants will not suffice. The strategy must also include intervention on the factors that determine health inequities, which we have termed structural determinants. Traditional forms of health promotion, whether adopting individual or population-based approaches, may actually widen health gaps between well-off and disadvantaged sectors of society, if policies do not incorporate measures to address structural factors. This is especially clear in the case of individualized interventions. As Macintyre (2000) notes: 'The capacity to benefit from individualized risk management and health education may be least among more disadvantaged people'. In other words, the rich are more likely to attend to and benefit from traditional forms of health promotion than are the poor. Emphasis should be placed on policies that can reduce risks across the whole population. For example, focusing on transport policies and urban design will be more useful that the traditional emphasis on exercise and diet alone. However, even in the case of population-based strategies, the groups in greatest need will not necessarily benefit first, and inequities will not necessarily be reduced.

Public health research and policy choices: Concrete examples

Specific examples will help clarify the stakes of the preceding discussion for public health research and policymaking.

The example of HIV/AIDS

Early studies of the human immunodeficiency virus/acquired immunodeficiency syndrome (HIV/AIDS) focused on individual characteristics and behaviours in determining HIV risk, a classic case of 'biomedical individualism' (Fee & Krieger 1993). Biomedical individualism is the basis of risk factor epidemiology; by contrast, social epidemiology emphasizes social conditions as fundamental causes of disease. Social epidemiologists examine how persons become exposed to risk or protective factors and under what social conditions individual risk factors are related to disease. Social factors are thus the focus of analysis and are not simply adjusted for as potentially confounding factors or used as proxies for unavailable individual-level data.

Social factors are critical to understanding non-uniform infectious disease patterns that emerge as a result of the dependent nature of disease transmission, incorporating the idea that an outcome in one person is dependent upon outcomes and exposures in others. Applying the vocabulary developed in this chapter, structural social determinants must be examined along with the intermediary determinants connected to individual factors—including biological, demographic, and behavioural risk factors—that may influence the risk of HIV acquisition and disease progression. Structural determinants are central to understanding the diffusion and differential distribution of HIV/AIDS in population subgroups. Structural determinants include people's socioeconomic position, as well as the legal and policy environment. Laws and policies can mitigate the differential exposure, vulnerability, and consequences people face as a result of socioeconomic differences. These factors, in turn, affect HIV transmission dynamics and the differential distribution of HIV/AIDS.

Table 2.2.1, following work by Poundstone *et al.* (2004), summarizes the main features of approaches to HIV/AIDS based on: (1) a risk-factor perspective and (2) social epidemiology oriented to action on the determinants of health inequities.

This comparison does not imply an 'either/or'. Policies and interventions based on risk-factor analysis and responsive to individual needs are vital in confronting a major epidemic. However, the table emphasizes that, to achieve maximum results in combating HIV/AIDS while reducing equity gaps between more and less advantaged social groups, specific policies focused on underlying structural factors are indispensable. Policies informed by this social analysis are different from measures guided by a concern with individual risk factors; the objectives of the former cannot be met by simply doing more of the latter. This has consequences for the way public health challenges such as scaling up HIV/AIDS treatment are addressed—in particular, the requirement that responses be designed to expand vulnerable communities' control over decisions affecting their lives, fostering a genuine redistribution of social power through public health action.

These points of view have important implications for future epidemiological research on HIV/AIDS and for the design of more effective HIV/AIDS interventions. Ultimately, social epidemiology research in HIV/AIDS will help determine how we can design more effective sets of interventions at multiple levels of social organization. From a policymaking standpoint, cross-sector approaches are required for the effective implementation of interventions that address the structural social aspects of HIV/AIDS.

The examples of skilled birth attendance and child malnutrition

Two additional examples analyse the comparative impacts of the conceptual framework's main components—including socioeconomic position and intermediary determinants—on specific forms of health inequity. The analysis highlights the powerful impact of socioeconomic position in determining inequities across a broad spectrum of health challenges. At the same time, these examples show that the effects of specific categories of intermediary determinants, such as health system factors, vary considerably when we consider different areas of health action. This has important implications for public health policymaking, as well as for the monitoring systems needed to provide evidence for policymaking and programme management.

The pervasive impact of socioeconomic position

Figure 2.2.4 shows the results of analyses carried out by the WHO Department of Equity, Poverty and Social Determinants of Health[2] in 2007, based on data from the Demographic and Health Surveys (DHS) in a group of countries in Africa. This work generated an equity analysis grounded in the determinants framework presented in this chapter. The researchers identified items on the DHS survey that could provide information on each of the main framework components: Structural determinants (including socioeconomic–political context and socioeconomic position) and intermediary

[2] Now the Department of Ethics, Equity, Trade and Human Rights.

Table 2.2.1 HIV/AIDS epidemiology and intervention strategies using different paradigms (adapted from Poundstone *et al.* 2004)

Research paradigm	Key research questions	Understanding of determinants of health	Intervention model and strategy
Risk factor epidemiology	What individual characteristics are associated with development of AIDS and disease progression?	1. Risk of HIV/AIDS is manifest at the individual level. 2. To change unhealthy or risky behaviours, individual responsibility and choice are sufficient.	1. Interventions focus on the individual a) Behaviour change to prevent HIV transmission b) Access to clinical AIDS care *Strategy based on tackling intermediary determinants*
Social epidemiology incorporating social determinants of health inequities	How do economic and political determinants help establish and perpetuate inequalities in HIV/AIDS distribution within and between populations? How do social factors influence psychology or behaviour to place persons at higher risk of HIV infection?	1. Limited access to resources places persons at risk of HIV infection and AIDS disease progression. 2. Psychosocial factors are conditioned and modified by the larger social context in which they occur. 3. Social determinants affect HIV/AIDS risk by shaping patterns of population susceptibility and vulnerability.	1. Interventions focus on policies and programmes to address structural social factors, enabling large reductions in HIV/AIDS at the population level and gains in equity 2. Interventions focus on creating space for vulnerable groups to gain greater control over their own lives: redistribution of social power *Strategy based on tackling structural determinants*

determinants (including behavioural factors and health system factors). An analysis was performed using a decomposable health concentration index. The purpose was to quantify the contributions of the different social determinants of health to the total wealth-related inequity in the area of skilled birth attendance. In all countries analysed, socioeconomic position plays a fundamental role, accounting for between 50.3 and 77.6 per cent of the observed inequities in skilled birth attendance. Intermediary factors, such as living and working conditions and behaviours, play a minor role, not more than 7 per cent in the countries studied. The health system itself was found to cause between 11.5 and 33.3 per cent of inequities. Across all countries and all public health indicators for which comparable analyses has been performed, socioeconomic position regularly emerges as the most powerful determinant of inequities in health among social groups. The arguments developed in this chapter suggest that this is because socioeconomic position reflects people's level of power in society.

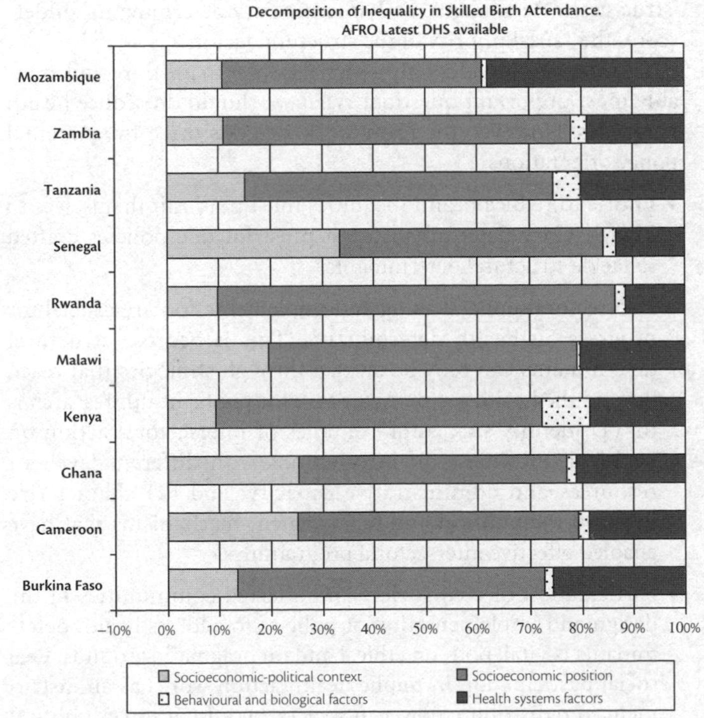

Fig. 2.2.4 Contributions of social determinants to inequities in skilled birth attendance in several African countries. Analysis performed by the former WHO Department of Equity, Poverty and Social Determinants of Health (Hosseinpoor et al. 2007).

Different health challenges show different profiles

Figure 2.2.5 compares the relative causal impact of determinants on equity in two different key health indicators in Mozambique: Skilled birth attendance and child malnutrition. The results confirm that socioeconomic position plays the major role in shaping inequities in both these areas, accounting for 51 per cent of the observed inequities in malnutrition and 48 per cent in skilled birth attendance. Intermediary factors, such as living and working conditions and behaviours, play a minor role in connection with skilled birth attendance, although they constitute a somewhat more important determinant of inequities in malnutrition.

Significant differences between malnutrition and skilled birth attendance emerge when the impact of health systems factors on inequities is considered. Public health policy to address these issues will look very different, as monitoring and evaluation processes are configured to provide information on a wide spectrum of social determinants of health—in this case, especially the respective impacts of health systems factors on inequities. In the case of child malnutrition, the health system accounts for only 9 per cent of observed inequities. In skilled birth attendance, the proportion of inequities directly linked to health system factors rises to almost 38 per cent.

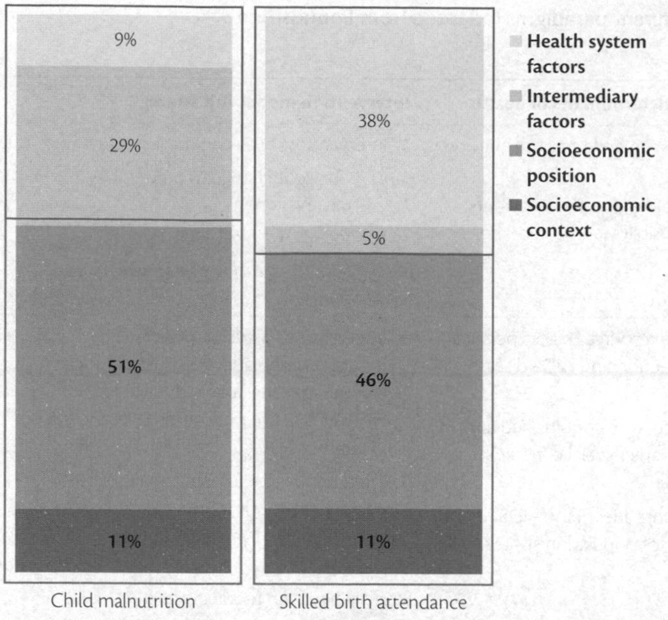

Fig. 2.2.5 Contribution of social determinants to health inequities in malnutrition and skilled birth attendance in Mozambique. Data source: DHS 2003. Analysis: WHO Department of Equity, Poverty and Social Determinants of Health (Hosseinpoor *et al.* 2007).

This suggests very different opportunities for the health sector to reduce inequities through direct action in these two areas.

At the same time, even in the case of skilled birth attendance, in the best case scenario, actions that can be undertaken directly by the health system still leave more than 60 per cent of health inequities untouched, given that the largest determinants of inequity lie beyond the reach of the health sector. This finding constitutes an argument that can be used to engage other sectors in work towards health equity. The bulk of inequities remain rooted in areas that must be addressed through coordination, cooperation, and integration of health policies and programmes with those of other sectors.

The picture emerging from these examples implies major differences in the nature of policy priorities to address equity challenges connected with different health problems, and in the degree of autonomy health officials enjoy to directly implement measures that can be expected to have a significant positive impact on health equity in these various areas. An approach sensitive to these differences is only possible when researchers and programme managers incorporate a social determinants perspective into their analyses, and when managers and policymakers recognize the causal hierarchy of determinants, as regards their origins, interrelationships, and respective impact. This highlights the need to develop health monitoring systems that provide information on social determinants of health, as a complement to more conventional population health indicators.

Conclusion

This chapter opened with three questions:

1. If we trace health differences among social groups back to their deepest roots, where do they originate?
2. What pathways lead from root causes to the stark differences in health status observed at the population level?
3. In light of the answers to the first two questions, where and how should we intervene to reduce health inequities?

The framework presented in these pages has been developed to provide responses to these problems. To the first question, on the origins of health inequities, we have answered as follows. The root causes of health inequities are to be found in the social, economic, and political mechanisms that give rise to a set of hierarchically ordered socioeconomic positions within society, whereby groups are stratified according to income, education, occupation, gender, race/ethnicity, and other factors. The fundamental mechanisms that produce and maintain (but that can also reduce or mitigate effect) this stratification include: Governance; the education system; labour market structures; and redistributive welfare state policies (or their absence). We have referred to the component factors of socioeconomic position as *structural determinants*. Structural determinants, together with the features of the socioeconomic and political context that shape their impact, constitute the *social determinants of health inequities*. The structural mechanisms that configure social hierarchies according to key stratifiers are the root cause of health inequities.

Our answer to the second question, about pathways from root causes to observed inequities in health, was elaborated by tracing how the underlying social determinants of health inequities operate through a set of what we call *intermediary determinants of health* to shape health outcomes. The main categories of intermediary determinants of health are: Material circumstances; psychosocial circumstances; behavioural and/or biological factors; and the health system itself as a social determinant. The vocabulary of 'structural determinants' and 'intermediary determinants' underscores the causal priority of the structural factors.

This chapter provides only a partial answer to the third and arguably most important question: What we should do reduce health inequities. However, the framework suggests three fundamental policy orientations:

- Efforts to reduce health inequities must not limit themselves to intermediary determinants, but must include policies crafted to tackle structural determinants.
- Intersectoral policymaking and implementation are crucial for progress on health determinants. This is because structural determinants can only be tackled through strategies that reach beyond the health sector. A key task for public health research is to: (1) identify successful examples of intersectoral action on health determinants in jurisdictions with different levels of resources and administrative capacity; and (2) characterize in detail the political and management mechanisms that have enabled effective intersectoral programmes.
- Participation of civil society and affected communities in the design and implementation of policies to address health determinants is vital, both on ethical and on pragmatic grounds. Real social participation in public health action works as an instrument to redistribute power in society, because it forces political authorities to listen to the voices and demands of excluded communities. In this sense, authentic participation can change the structural determinants of health inequities and give sustainability to these changes.

Subsequent chapters in this section will explore the role of specific determinants in greater detail. Chapters 3.2, 3.3, and 4.2, in particular, will delve further into the challenges of public health policy.

References

Adler, N.E., Boyce, T., Chesney, M.A. *et al.* (1994). Socioeconomic status and health: The challenge of the gradient. *American Psychologist*, **49**, 15–24.

Antonovsky, A. (1967). Social class life expectancy and overall mortality. *Milbank Memorial Fund Quarterly*, **45**, 31–73.

Ball, T. (1992). New faces of power. In (ed. T. Wartenberg) *Rethinking power*, pp. 11–24. SUNY Press, Albany.

Ben-Shlomo, Y. and Kuh, D. (2002). A life course approach to chronic disease epidemiology: Conceptual models, empirical challenges and interdisciplinary perspectives. *International Journal of Epidemiology*, **31**, 285–93.

Berlinguer, G. (2006). The social determinants of disease. Unpublished manuscript.

Bernales, P. (2006). Social capital review. Unpublished background study for the WHO conceptual framework on social determinants of health. WHO Department of Equity, Poverty and Social Determinants of Health, Geneva.

Braveman, P. and Gruskin, S. (2003). Defining equity in health. *Journal of Epidemiology and Community Health*, **57**, 254–58.

Cassel, J. (1976). The contribution of the social environment to host resistance. *American Journal of Epidemiology*, **104**, 107–23.

Chung, H. and Muntaner, C. (2006). Political and welfare state determinants of infant and child health indicators: An analysis of wealthy countries. *Social Science and Medicine*, **63**, 829–42.

Colgrove, J. (2002). The McKeown thesis: A historical controversy and its enduring influence. *American Journal of Public Health*, **92**, 725–9.

Dahlgren, G. and Whitehead, M. (2006). *Levelling up (part 1): A discussion paper on European strategies for tackling social inequities in health*. WHO EURO, Copenhagen.

Davey Smith, G. (2003). *Health inequalities: Lifecourse approaches*. Policy Press, Bristol.

Diderichsen, F. (1998). Towards a theory of health equity. Unpublished draft manuscript.

Diderichsen, F. (2004). *Resource allocation for health equity: Issues and methods*. The World Bank, Department of Health, Nutrition and Population (HNP), Washington.

Diderichsen, F., Evans, T., and Whitehead, M. (2001). The social basis of disparities in health. In *Challenging inequities in health* (eds. T. Evans, M. Whitehead, F. Diderichsen, A. Bhuiya and M. Wirth). Oxford University Press, New York.

Emerson, E. (2004). Poverty and children with intellectual disabilities in the world's richer countries. *Journal of Intellectual and Developmental Disability*, **29**, 319–37.

Escobedo, L.G., Anda, R.F., Smith, P.F. *et al.* (1990). Sociodemographic characteristics of cigarette smoking initiation in the United States: Implications for smoking prevention policy. *Journal of the American Medical Association*, **264**, 1550–5.

Esping-Andersen, G. (2002). *Why we need a new Welfare State*. Oxford University Press, New York.

Evans, T., Whitehead, M., Diderichsen, F. *et al.* (eds.)(2001). *Challenging inequities in health*. Oxford University Press, New York.

Fee, E. and Krieger, N. (1993). Understanding AIDS: Historical interpretations and the limits of biomedical individualism. *American Journal of Public Health*, **83**, 1477–86.

Ferguson, K. (2006). Social capital and children's wellbeing: A critical synthesis of the international social capital literature. *International Journal of Social Welfare*, **15**, 2–18.

Frankel, S., Elwood, P., Sweetnam, P. *et al.* (1996). Birthweight, body-mass index in middle age, and incident coronary heart disease. *Lancet*, **348**, 1478–80.

Gee, G.C. (2002). A multilevel analysis of the relationship between institutional and individual racial discrimination and health status. *American Journal of Public Health*, **92**, 615–23.

Graham, H. (2004). Social determinants and their unequal distribution. *Milbank Quarterly*, **82**, 101–24.

Graham, H. (2005). Intellectual disabilities and socieconomic inequalities in health: An overview of research. *Journal of Applied Research in Inequalities*, **18**, 101–11.

Graham, H. and Kelly, M.P. (2004). *Health inequalities: Concepts, frameworks and policy*. NHS Health Development Agency Briefing Paper. NHS Health Development Agency, London.

Hosseinpoor, A., Prasad, A., and Vega, J. (2007). *WHO report on inequities in maternal and child health in Mozambique*. Mission report, Department of Equity, Poverty and Social Determinants of Health, WHO, Geneva.

Howden-Chapman, P., Blakely, T., Blaiklock, A.J. *et al.* (2000). Closing the health gap. *New Zealand Medical Journal*, **113**, 301–2.

Illsley, R. and Baker, D. (1991). Contextual variations in the meaning of health inequality. *Social Science and Medicine*, **32**, 359–65.

Instituto de Estudios Politicos para America Latina y Africa (2005). Curso sistematico de derechos humanos. Online training course. Available at: <http://www.iepala.es/curso_ddhh/ddhh27.htm>. Accessed 8 December 2007.

Kaplan, G.A., Pamuk, E.R., Lynch, J.W. *et al.* (1996). Inequality in income and mortality in the United States: analysis of mortality and potential pathways. *British Medical Journal*, **312**, 999–1003.

Kaprio, J. and Koskenvuo, M. (1988). A prospective study of psychological and socioeconomic characteristics, health behavior and morbidity in cigarette smokers prior to quitting compared to persistent smokers and non-smokers. *Journal of Clinical Epidemiology*, **41**, 139–50.

Kawachi, I., Kennedy, B.P., Lochner, K. *et al.* (1997). Social capital, income inequality, and mortality. *American Journal of Public Health*, **87**, 1491–8.

Kleczkowki, B.M., Roemer, M., and Van Der Werff, A. (1984). *National health systems and their reorientation toward health for all: Guidance for policymaking*. WHO, Geneva.

Koopman, J.S. and Longini, I.M. (1994). The ecological effects of individual exposures and nonlinear disease dynamics in populations. *American Journal of Public Health*, **84**, 836–42.

Krieger, N. (2001). Theories for social epidemiology in the 21st century: An ecosocial perspective. *International Journal of Epidemiology*, **30**, 668–77.

Krieger, N. (2002). A glossary for social epidemiology. *Epidemiological Bulletin*, **23**, 7–11.

Krieger, N. (2005). Embodiment: A conceptual glossary for epidemiology. *Journal of Epidemiology and Community Health*, **59**, 350–5.

Krieger, N., Williams, D.R., and Moss, N.E. (1997). Measuring social class. *Annual Review of Public Health*, **18**, 341–78.

Krieger, N., Rowley, D.L., Herman, A.A. *et al.* (1993). Racism, sexism and social class, implications for studies of health, diseases and well being. *Annual Journal of Preventive Medicine*, **9**, 82–122.

Kubzansky, L.D., Sparrow, D., Vokonas, P. *et al.* (2001). Is the glass half empty or half full? A prospective study of optimism and coronary heart disease in the normative aging study. *Psychosomatic Medicine*, **63**, 910–16.

Lalonde, M. (1974). *A new perspective on the health of Canadians*. Ministry of Health and Welfare, Ottawa.

Liberatos, P., Link, B.G., and Kelsey, J.L. (1988). The measurement of social class in epidemiology. *Epidemiology Review*, **10**, 87–121.

Lobmayer, P. and Wilkinson, R.G. (2002). Inequality, residential segregation by income, and mortality in US cities. *Journal of Epidemiology and Community Health*, **56**, 183–7.

Luttrell, C. and Quiroz, S. (2007). *Understanding and operationalising empowerment*. Joint electronic publication by: poverty-wellbeing.net/ Swiss Agency for Development and Cooperation/Inter-Development/ Overseas Development Institute.

Lynch, J. (2000). Income inequality and health: expanding the debate. *Social Science and Medicine*, **51**, 1001–5.

Lynch, J., Due, P., Muntaner, C. *et al.* (2000). Social capital: Is it a good investment strategy for public health? *Journal of Epidemiology and Community Health*, **54**, 404–8.

Lynch, J.W., Kaplan, G.A., Pamuk, E.R. *et al.* (1998). Income inequality and mortality in metropolitan areas of the United States. *American Journal of Public Health*, **88**, 1074–80.

Lynch, J. and Smith, G.D. (2005). A life course approach to chronic disease epidemiology. *Annual Review of Public Health*, **26**, 1–35.

Lynch, J., Smith, G.D., Hillemeier, M. *et al.* (2001). Income inequality, the psychosocial environment, and health: Comparisons of wealthy nations. *Lancet*, **358**, 194–200.

Macintyre, S. (2000). Modernizing the NHS: Prevention and the reduction of health inequities. *British Medical Journal*, **320**, 1399–1400.

Macintyre, S. (2007). *Inequalities in health in Scotland: What are they and what can we do about them?* MRC Social and Public Health Sciences Unit Occasional Paper No. 17. Medical Research Council Social and Public Health Sciences Unit, Glasgow.

Mackenbach, J.P. and Bakker, M.J. (eds.) (2002). *Reducing inequalities in health: A European perspective*. Routledge, London and New York.

Mackenbach, J.P., Bakker, M.J., Kunst, A.E. *et al.*(2002). Socioeconomic inequalities in health in Europe: An overview. In *Reducing inequalities in health: A European perspective* (eds. J.P. Mackenbach and M.J. Bakker). Routledge, London and New York.

Manor, O., Matthews, S., and Power, C. (2003). Health selection: The role of inter- and intra-generational mobility on social inequalities in health. *Social Science and Medicine*, **57**, 2217–27.

Margolis, P.A., Greenberg, R.A., Keyes, L.L. *et al.* (1992). Lower respiratory illness in infants and low socioeconomic status. *American Journal of Public Health*, **82**, 1119–26.

Marmot, M. (2002). The influence of income on health: views of an epidemiologist. *Health Affairs* (Millwood), **21**, 31–46.

Marmot, M. (2004). *The status syndrome: How social standing affects our health and longevity*. Henry Holt, New York.

Marmot, M.G., Rose, G., Shipley, M. *et al.* (1978). Employment grade and coronary heart disease in British civil servants. *Journal of Epidemiology and Community Health*, **32**, 244–9.

Marmot, M.G., Shipley, M.J., and Rose, G. (1984). Inequalities in death—specific explanations of a general pattern? *Lancet*, May 5, **1**(8384), 1003–6.

Marmot, M.G., Smith, G.D., Stansfeld, S. *et al.* (1991). Health inequalities among British civil servants: the Whitehall II study. *Lancet*, **337**, 1387–93.

Marmot, M. and Wilkinson, R.G. (2001). Psychosocial and material pathways in the relation between income and health: A response to Lynch *et al. British Medical Journal*, **322**, 1233–6.

Maughan, B., Collishaw, S., and Pickles, A. (1999). Mild mental retardation: Psychosocial functioning in adulthood. *Psychological Medicine*, **29**, 351–66.

McMichael, A.J. (1999). Prisoners of the proximate: Loosening the constraints on epidemiology in an age of change. *American Journal of Epidemiology*, **149**, 887–97.

Moore, S., Haines, V., Hawe, P. *et al.* (2006). Lost in translation: a genealogy of the "social capital" concept in public health. *Journal of Epidemiology and Community Health*, **60**, 729–34.

Muntaner, C. (2004). Commentary: Social capital, social class, and the slow progress of psychosocial epidemiology. *International Journal of Epidemiology*, **33**, 674–80.

Muntaner, C., Borell, C., Benach, J. *et al.* (2003). The associations of social class and social stratification with patterns of general and mental health in a Spanish population. *International Journal of Epidemiology*, **32**, 950–8.

Muntaner, C., Lynch, J., and Oates, G.L. (1999). The social class determinants of income inequality and social cohesion. *International Journal of Health Services*, **20**, 699–732.

National Association of County and City Health Officials (NACCHO) (2002). *Creating Health Equity through Social Justice*. Draft Working paper. NACCHO, Washington.

Navarro, V. and Shi, L. (2001). The Political Context of Social Inequalities and Health. *International Journal of Health Services*, **31**, 1–21.

Popay, J. (2000). Social capital: the role of narrative and historical research. *Journal of Epidemiology and Community Health*, **54**, 401.

Poundstone, K.E., Strathdee, S.A., and Celentano, D.D. (2004). The social epidemiology of human immunodeficiency virus/acquired immunodeficiency syndrome. *Epidemiology Review*, **26**, 22–35.

Power, C. and Hertzman, C. (2004). Health and human development from life course research. In *Population Health:*
Policy dilemmas (eds. M. Barer, R. Evans, C. Hertzman and J. Heyman). Oxford University Press, Oxford.

Putnam, R. (2000). *Bowling alone: The collapse and revival of American community*. Simon & Schuster, New York.

Putnam, R. (2001). Foreword. In *Social capital and poor communities* (eds. S. Saegert, J.P. Thompson and M.R. Warren), pp. xv–xvi. Russell Sage Foundation, New York.

Raphael, D. (2006). Social determinants of health: Present status, unanswered questions, and future directions. *International Journal of Health Services*, **36**, 651–77.

Raphael, D. and Bryant, T. (2006). Maintaining population health in a period of welfare state decline: Political economy as the missing dimension in health promotion theory and practice. *Promotion & education*, **13**, 236–42.

Rose, G. (2001). Sick individuals and sick populations. *International Journal of Epidemiology*, **30**, 427–32.

Schwartz, S. (1994). The fallacy of the ecological fallacy: the potential misuse of a concept and the consequences. *American Journal of Public Health*, **84**, 819–24.

Sigerist, H. (1943). *Civilization and disease*. University of Chicago Press, Chicago.

Smith, G.D. and Egger, M. (1996). Commentary: understanding it all—health, meta-theories, and mortality trends. *British Medical Journal*, **313**, 1584–5.

Solar, O. and Irwin, A. (2007). *A conceptual framework for action on the social determinants of health*. Working paper of the WHO Department of Equity, Poverty and Social Determinants of Health and the Commission on Social Determinants of Health. WHO, Geneva.

Solar, O., Irwin, A., and Vega, J. (2004). Equity in health sector reform and reproductive health: Measurement issues and the health systems context. Unpublished working paper. WHO Health Equity Team, Geneva.

Susser, M., Watson, W., and Hopper, K. (1985). *Sociology in medicine*. Oxford University Press, New York.

Szreter, S. (2002). Rethinking McKeown: The relationship between public health and social change. *American Journal of Public Health*, **92**, 722–5.

Szreter, S. (2004). Industrialization and health. *British Medical Bulletin*, **69**, 75–86.

Szreter, S. and Woolcock, M. (2004). Health by association? Social capital, social theory, and the political economy of public health. *International Journal of Epidemiology*, **33**, 650–67.

Tajer, D. (2003). Latin American social medicine: Roots, development during the 1990s, and current challenges. *American Journal of Public Health*, **93**, 2023–7.

Tarlov, A. (1996). Social determinants of health: The sociobiological translation. In *Health and social organization* (eds. D. Blane, E. Brunner and R.Wilkinson), pp. 71–93. Routledge, London.

Virchow, R. (1985 [1848]). *Collected essays on public health and epidemiology*. Science History Publications, Cambridge.

Whitehead, M., Burström, B., and Diderichsen, F. (2000). Social policies and the pathways to inequalities in health: A comparative analysis of lone mothers in Britain and Sweden. *Social Science and Medicine*, **50**, 255–70.

WHO (2004). Glossary of equity, gender, human rights, poverty, social determinants and related issues in health. Unpublished working document. WHO Health Equity Team, Geneva.

WHO and UNICEF (1978). *Declaration of Alma Ata*. WHO, Geneva.

Wilkinson, R.G. (2000). Inequality and the social environment: A reply to Lynch *et al*. *Journal of Epidemiology and Community Health*, **54**, 411–3.

Wilkinson, R.G. and Pickett, K.E. (2006). Income inequality and population health: A review and explanation of the evidence. *Social Science and Medicine*, **62**, 1768–84.

2.3

Behavioural determinants of health and disease

Lawrence W. Green and Robert A. Hiatt

Introduction

That behaviour is associated with health and disease has never been in doubt. Indeed, the tendency to blame sinful, negligent, indulgent, ignorant, reckless, or selfish behaviour for health problems has too often placed undue emphasis on individual responsibility and culpability when the solution to health problems of populations demanded attention to the social and physical environment. But no matter how behaviour is framed or moralized in relation to its causes, it remains an inescapable variable in the pathway between ultimate upstream aetiologies and the incidence or prevalence of most diseases and health conditions downstream. Approaches to public health have sought throughout the history of civilization (1) to control or cajole the health-related behaviour of individuals, (2) to protect individuals from the behaviour of others, and (3) to mobilize the behaviour of groups to influence health-related social and physical environments.

This chapter reviews the ways in which behaviour relates to the spectrum of health and disease determinants, from environmental to genetic, in shaping health outcomes. It builds on the previous chapters in recognizing the powerful influence of socioeconomic factors, especially poverty, in influencing both behaviour and health. Many commentaries in the past two decades have attempted to correct the early overemphasis on behavioural determinants of health by discounting and sometimes disparaging any focus on individual behaviour in disease prevention and health promotion. This chapter seeks a middle ground, building on the growing understanding of the ecological context of the behaviour–health relationship. It seeks to integrate that knowledge in an approach to public health that acknowledges the reciprocal determinism of behavioural, environmental, and biologic determinants rather than minimizing the importance of behaviour in these complex interactions.

The shifting role of behaviour as a determinant of health and disease

Simple, discrete behaviours account for many of the infections and injuries of the past. Today's growing chronic disease burden relates more to complex behaviours. We use the term 'complex behaviour' to refer to combinations of interrelated practices and their environmental contexts, reflecting patterns of living influenced by the family and social history of individuals and communities, their environmental and socioeconomic circumstances, and their exposure to cultures and communications. We know that discrete behaviours can be influenced directly by health education targeted at individuals and groups. Complex behaviour changes more slowly and usually requires some combination of educational, organizational, economic, and environmental interventions in support of changes in both behaviour and conditions of living. This combination of strategies has defined health promotion and public health programmes addressing complex behaviour change (Green & Kreuter 2005; Smith *et al.* 2006).

Obesity and HIV/AIDS present the obvious contemporary examples of health-related conditions and diseases awaiting technological solutions, for which behaviour, in the meantime, is a necessary route of intervention and change. Virtually every public health breakthrough has had a behavioural change process that served the public until the technology was at hand. Then, behavioural change processes were needed to diffuse, adapt, and apply the new technology to varying cultural and social circumstances. Unless and until an obesity prevention vaccine or HIV vaccine is developed, society must depend on behavioural preventive measures to curb the spread of obesity and AIDS. These include, of course, policies, environmental changes, and health educational programmes that support behavioural changes.

Much of the early success in controlling HIV infections through change in sexual practices (especially use of condoms) among men in urban gay communities appear to have been in response to health education programmes (Petrow 1990). Reviews also show increases in the use of clean needles for at least 15 years among intravenous drug users (e.g. Wodak 2006), which has required a combination of policy and educational interventions to make clean needles accessible and more acceptable than the culture of needle-sharing. Evidence that health education leads to the regular use of condoms among sexually active adolescents, however, has not held up consistently (James *et al.* 2006; Koniak-Griffin & Stein 2006; Walker *et al.* 2006). The parallel lessons from the success of tobacco control programmes also point to the need for combined policy, regulatory, organizational, environmental, and educational interventions to influence population changes in tobacco consumption (Eriksen *et al.* 2007) and many of the same types of interventions are under consideration for obesity control (Mercer *et al.* 2005).

Specific behaviours and health—the causal links

Some behaviour clearly increases the risk of developing disease and can be considered a proximal cause of disease, such as hygienic practices that expose one to infections. Other behaviours correlate with and precede better health, increased longevity, and decreased disease risk, but their causal link is more tenuous, warranting their inclusion with more distal determinants, such as general dietary and physical activity patterns. Examining the relationships between specific behavioural patterns and indicators of health and disease status provides the foundation for assessing behavioural factors as population health determinants. Examining the covariation of these relationships with other characteristics of the populations and their environmental circumstances helps put behaviour into its ecological, social, and cultural context.

The causal link is relatively easy to establish for single-agent communicable or infectious diseases. Evidence from observational epidemiological studies, human experimental trials, and animal models, together with clear mechanisms of biological action, lead one to conclude that many behaviours are, in fact, contributing causes (causal risk factors) of specific diseases. Again, the easiest examples of clear causal linkages are those established for single-action behaviours such as ingesting a contaminated food, getting an immunization that confers lifetime immunity, or taking a one-dose medication that leads to rapidly improved symptoms, or even a cure. As the number of booster shots required for immunization or doses required for cure increase, the behaviour becomes more complex, requiring repetition or timing, and the causal linkage more difficult to unravel among the biomedical agent, the behaviour, and all the other events and circumstances that might have intervened and influenced the outcome along the way.

Complex behaviours and health—the causal pathways and synergies

More difficult still are causal attributions and allocations for long-term behavioural patterns that are not under medical supervision and relate to multiple-cause chronic diseases and conditions (Krieger 1984; Glass & McAtee 2006). We present three examples of evidence supporting causal links between behaviours and coronary heart disease: Smoking, diet, and physical activity. These three examples illustrate that even in the absence of direct experimental evidence in human beings, strong evidence of other types can be combined for the steps in a causal chain from behaviour through physiological effects to disease or health. In addition, the synergistic effects of two or more behaviours on health outcomes have been established.

A plausible biological model of the relationship between smoking behaviour and coronary heart disease has been available for decades (Dawber 1960). Observational epidemiological studies—including within- and between-population designs, case-control, and prospective designs—produced strong and consistent measures of association, the hypothesized temporal sequence, and dose–response relationships in subsequent decades (Stamler 1992). Additional randomized trials have included smoking cessation programmes that provide experimental evidence for smoking as a cause of coronary heart disease. Although the overall results of the Multiple Risk Factor Intervention Trial (MRFIT) in the United States were disappointing, in both MRFIT (Okene *et al.* 1990) and the British trial on the effect of smoking reduction (Rose & Colwell 1992), cessation interventions showed decreases in coronary heart disease mortality respectively of 13 per cent after 20 years and 12 per cent after 10.5 years. In addition, when smokers at baseline from the experimental and control groups were pooled, quitters had a significant decrease in their risk of mortality from coronary heart disease compared with non-quitters (Okene *et al.* 1990).

On the dietary front, evidence that saturated fat and cholesterol consumption behaviour contributes to coronary heart disease came first from ecological studies showing a correlation between dietary patterns and serum cholesterol levels (Keys *et al.* 1958), and later dietary fat consumption levels, and the corresponding geographical coronary heart disease incidence rates and mortality (Keys 1970). A 30-year follow-up of the Framingham cohort samples showed that high levels of serum cholesterol predicted the risk of coronary heart disease development (Anderson *et al.* 1987). In a meta-analysis of 27 trials, Mensink and Katan (1992) found that changes in dietary saturated fat and cholesterol led to changes in serum cholesterol. In the Helsinki Heart Study, Frick *et al.* (1987) showed that interventions to lower serum cholesterol levels decreased the occurrence of coronary heart disease. A definitive demonstration of the diet–heart hypothesis by a true experimental study might never occur because of the large sample size required, the sustained differential changes needed between intervention and control groups, and the long-term follow-up required for such a trial. The strong evidence for each step in a causal chain from diet to coronary heart disease and mortality, however, led to major national and international recommendations that diet be a first-line approach to reduce blood cholesterol to prevent disease, and more urgently today in the face of the global obesity epidemic (e.g. Health Canada 2003; NHLBI 1993; US Department of Health and Human Services 2001; WHO 1990, 2000).

Physical inactivity as a risk factor for coronary heart disease is the third example. Evidence that physical inactivity contributes to coronary heart disease came from studies of the biological effects of exercise on cardiovascular physiology, observational epidemiological studies, and randomized controlled trials of physical activity and physiological coronary heart disease risk factors, such as high blood pressure, obesity, and diabetes. The biological effects of exercise training to enhance cardiovascular health were well established by the 1980s (McArdle *et al.* 1986). Epidemiological evidence continues to show consistent and relatively strong associations, the hypothesized temporal sequence, and a dose–response relationship between physical activity and coronary heart disease (Blair *et al.* 1993). Observational epidemiological and randomized controlled trials demonstrated the beneficial effects of physical activity on blood pressure (Arroll & Beaglehole 1992) and on blood lipids and lipoproteins (Lokey & Tran 1989), which have, in turn, been causally linked with subsequent coronary heart disease. The combination of these sources of evidence for each of the steps in a causal chain provides a plausible model for the sequence.

Some of the immediate causal risk factors are not themselves behaviours, but have determinants that are behaviours. In these cases, the behavioural determinants can be regarded as indirect risk factors that act earlier in the causal pathway. For example, a combination of overeating and sedentary behaviour produce high caloric intake and low energy output, which together mediate the behavioural determinants of obesity. Obesity, in turn, is a physiological risk factor for cardiovascular diseases and type 2 diabetes (Stern 1991).

Behaviour also contributes to the prognosis of diseases at each stage where the screening, diagnosis, or the compliance with prescribed regimens of treatment or self-care affects outcomes. For example, the prognosis of breast cancer depends on the stage of disease at which the woman obtains screening, diagnosis, and medical care. The prognosis for type 1 (insulin dependent) diabetes depends on the patient's compliance with his or her insulin prescriptions. Because behaviour is so central to disease outcomes, a large literature on patient education and patient compliance with medical regimens has been catalogued and subjected to meta-analyses with regularity (e.g. Mullen *et al.* 1985; D.G. Simons-Morton *et al.* 1992; Malik & Hu 2007).

Behavioural risk factors in population health

The causal pathways by which behaviour can influence health (or its negative manifestations) can be broadly classified as direct (as shown by arrow 1 in Fig. 2.3.1) and indirect, where the indirect pathways (arrows 2 and 3 in Fig. 2.3.1) are largely mediated through the environment or through healthcare organization and personnel. These three determinants of health—behaviour, environment, and healthcare organization—in addition to human biology, were cast as the 'Health Field Concept' as part of the Lalonde Report on the Health of Canadians (Canada 1974), which many credit with having launched the health promotion and population health movements in public health. The third indirect pathway could be drawn through genetics, the main pathway by which individuals can make some reproductive decisions independent of the medical care system, but such non-medically mediated decisions are largely mediated by the social environment. Figure 2.3.1 is hardly a full representation of the three sets of variables (behaviour, environment, healthcare organization), much less the genetic interactions, insofar as there is much reciprocal determinism between behaviour and each of the various environments, as well as with genetics. These environmental influences on behaviour will be examined in the next section, and behaviour's influence on the environment in a later section.

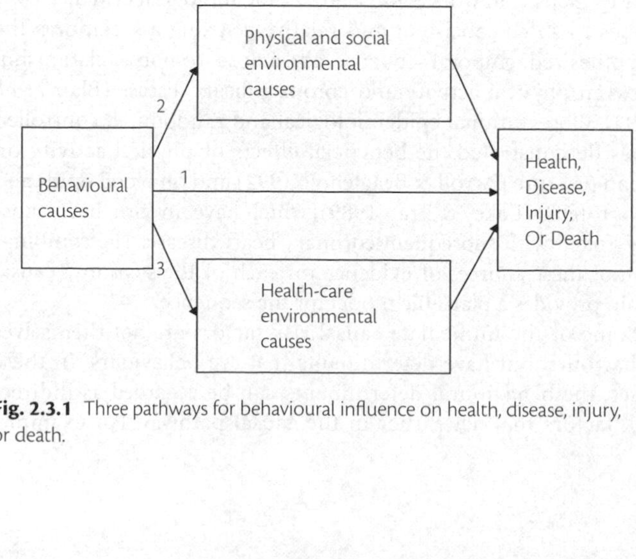

Fig. 2.3.1 Three pathways for behavioural influence on health, disease, injury, or death.

Behaviour itself as a risk factor for disease

The direct pathway suggested by Fig. 2.3.1 includes the broad array of actions people take, consciously or unconsciously, that can have an immediate or cumulative effect on their health status. The effect on health may be intended (health-directed) or unintended (health-related), but the behaviour is nevertheless direct in its effect. The most dramatic of these are the violent injury-causing actions people may take behind the wheel of an automobile, with weapons, or unintentionally with the careless use of tools or toxic substances or merely walking absent-mindlessly on a slippery or cluttered surface. Less dramatic, but no less lethal, are the cumulative little actions people take each time they light a cigarette, imbibe or inject an addictive or mind-altering substance, or abide by neglect of physical activity or healthful foods.

Table 2.3.1 lists the nine leading causes of death in most of the more developed countries, as reflected here by the United States, and relates those to the risk factors for each in column 2, which McGinnis and Foege (1993, 2004) and Mokdad *et al.* (2004) refer to as the 'actual causes of death'. Colditz (2001) has noted that more than half of all cancer is a consequence of behaviour, much of which is embedded in culture. Most of the risk factors in Table 2.3.1 are themselves behaviours. Those that are not behaviours themselves—such as high serum cholesterol, obesity, hypertension, and diabetes mellitus—are the consequence, in large part, of behaviours. The behavioural determinants of physiological risk factors in column 3 present some of the most challenging targets for public health intervention, because they require decreasing behaviours that are perceived as pleasurable (e.g. types of food, sedentary entertainment, spontaneous sexual encounters) and increasing behaviours perceived as boring, painful, or inconvenient (e.g. less sugary or salty foods, more strenuous or frequent physical activity, use of condoms). Their challenges are compounded by the fact that most of the instances of these behavioural determinants of risk can be carried out very privately with limited opportunity for monitoring or social influence.

Tobacco consumption alone accounts for a large proportion of deaths in developed countries, implicated as a direct risk factor in all five of the leading causes of death shown in Table 2.3.1. At least one of the three main behavioural risk factors—smoking, dietary practices, and alcohol use—is causally related to each of the 10 leading causes of death shown in Table 2.3.1. Active smoking has been established as a risk factor for coronary heart disease, diabetes, stroke, and adverse pregnancy outcomes, such as low birth weight, premature rupture of membranes, and abruption placentae (USDHHS 2004). As examples of how the behaviour of some individuals can influence the health of others, passive smoking (i.e. exposure to environmental tobacco smoke) has been related to lung cancer and other respiratory diseases, as an independent risk factor for coronary heart disease, and exposure to environmental tobacco smoke in the home has been associated with asthma, other respiratory conditions, and with ear infections in infants and children (US Department of Health and Human Services 2006). Although still controversial, the California Environmental Protection Agency (2005) has concluded from its reviews that passive smoking is also a risk factor for breast cancer.

As noted in previous chapters, the causes of death in developing countries differ markedly from the patterns reflected in Table 2.3.1, although the demographic profiles are converging. WHO estimates of the four leading causes of death for the developing countries have been respiratory diseases, infectious and parasitic diseases,

Table 2.3.1 The nine leading causes of death in the United States (2003), their generally accepted behavioural (in italics) and physiological risk factors, and the behavioural determinants of the physiological risk factors

Causes of death (age-adjusted death rates in the United States per 100 000 population)	Selected risk factors	Behavioural determinants of physiological risk factors
Diseases of the heart (232.3)	*Smoking* *Physical inactivity* High serum cholesterol Obesity Hypertension Diabetes mellitus	 High-fat diet High-calorie diet, physical inactivity High-salt diet High-calorie diet (obesity)
Malignant neoplasms (190.1)	*Smoking* *High-fat diet* *Low-fibre diet* *Physical inactivity* Sexually transmitted diseases	 *Sexual behaviours*
Cerebrovascular diseases (53.5)	Hypertension Atherosclerosis *Smoking*	*High-salt diet* *High-fat diet*
Chronic obstructive pulmonary disease (43.3)	*Smoking*	
Unintentional injuries (37.3)	*Alcohol abuse* *Unsafe driving* *Seat-belt non-use* *Smoking* *Drug use*	
Diabetes mellitus (25.3)	*Physical inactivity* Obesity	*High-calorie diet+*
Pneumonia and influenza (22.0)	*Drug use* Immunization Status Malnutrition	 *Failure to receive immunization* Diet
Suicide (10.8)	*Alcohol use* *Hand gun use* *Drug use*	
Chronic liver disease and cirrhosis (9.3)	*Alcohol abuse*	

Source: Adapted from National Center for Health Statistics, CDC (2006), p. 179. Death: Final data from 2003. *National Vital Statistics Reports*, **54**, 1–120; Mokdad et al. (2004).

cardiovascular diseases, and perinatal mortality. As tobacco use has increased and problems of macro-nutrients have replaced some of the micro-nutrient problems in those countries, other chronic diseases, in addition to cardiovascular diseases, have increased. By 2020, according to WHO (1998) estimates, the tobacco epidemic is expected to kill more people than any single disease. Because it is a known probable determinant of at least 25 diseases, and the most important determinant of some of the leading causes of death, tobacco use will cause nearly 18 per cent of all deaths in developed countries and 11 per cent in developing countries. This alone warrants the concerted global attention to this behaviour that has been proposed by the Framework Convention on Tobacco Control.

Behaviour as a determinant of other risk factors

Besides the cumulative effect of behaviours on physiological risk factors, such as the energy balance mentioned earlier between calorie intake and physical activity producing weight gain, obesity, and hypertension, many of the health consequences of behaviour are secondary to their impact on the immediate environment. Individuals are not merely the passive victims of the environments they inhabit or traverse. They are agents of change in those environments, and their ability to alter or control environmental threats to their own health increases with technological innovations. The growing capacity of individuals and groups to alter their environments through technological means, such as transport, also produces negative consequences for their health. Hence, health promotion and health protection have emphasized mobilizing individuals and groups to undertake personal conservation behaviours and collective actions to support policy changes and regulatory initiatives in support of more healthful environments.

Among the most striking differences in health between the developed and the developing countries are the perinatal-juvenile mortality rates. In their analysis of 66 countries, Hertz *et al.* (1994) found the three most important predictors of infant mortality rates to be percentage of households with sanitation, total literacy rate, and the percentage of households without safe water. The major public health goals in developing nations have related to the provision of immunization, access to a sufficient supply of clean water, and the installation of proper sanitation facilities (WHO 1981). But the more recent Millennium Development Goals (MDG) aim to cut global poverty by half by the year 2015, with three goals focused directly on health, covering maternal mortality, infant mortality, HIV/AIDS, malaria, and tuberculosis.

These environmental and age-specific or disease-specific health measures, however, achieve their intended health goals only to the extent that an informed population accepts and uses them properly. A report by the World Bank (1993) suggested that the single most important public health policy for developing countries lies in the improvement of the education of young girls. Better educated women have fewer children, who tend to be healthier and, in turn, better educated and able to respond to the technological advances offered by such environmental measures. They also become a better informed electorate to demand and support healthful policies for the installation of such facilities. In short, behaviour remains a critical mediator of the relationships between environmental measures and health outcomes, as well as the relationship between the health needs and the political actions to create the environmental changes.

The behaviour–policy link in the causal chains becomes more important as the chronic diseases creep into the developing countries. Inspection of the recent trends in the richest of the developing countries provides evidence that improvement of the socioeconomic condition is accompanied by a shift in mortality towards the chronic diseases and their behavioural risk factors reviewed earlier. In Mexico, for example, as early as 1991, infectious and parasitic diseases were only the fourth leading cause of death, following diseases of the heart, malignant neoplasms, and accidents. Developing countries are now the primary target for market expansion for the multinational tobacco companies, with convenience food companies close behind them. Behaviour will be an issue both in personally resisting the temptations offered by these industries and in collective action to restrain their advertising, promotion, ingredients, and location.

Behaviour as a consequence of cognitions, environments, and genetics

Notwithstanding the implied simplicity of identifying a few behaviours that account for the majority of deaths in developed countries, those and other behaviours are highly complex, value-laden, and over-determined. Most behavioural risk factors and healthcare behaviours as well, are the product of a variety of component behaviours, tasks, or actions. For example, food consumption confronts most people with a chain of related behaviours that includes procuring and selecting food, planning menus or selecting from a menu, preparing or ordering foods, and eating with literally hundreds of food-related choices, including where to shop or eat, what to purchase or prepare, how to season food, and with whom to eat (B.G. Simons-Morton *et al.* 1986). One can identify similar chains of component behavioural choices for each of the other health behaviours identified in Table 2.3.1.

Not only are the behaviours complex, but each behaviour has numerous influences or determinants. Factors that influence behaviours can be grouped into three major categories (Green & Kreuter 2005, with adaptation from Andersen, 1969): Predisposing, enabling, and reinforcing, as shown in Fig. 2.3.2. Both positive and negative behaviours are predisposed, enabled, and reinforced by forces in the culture and the environment. This broad categorization has proved useful in public health programme planning (with more than 970 published applications, see www.lgreen.net for bibliography) because it groups the determinants of behaviour according to the major strategies used in public health to influence them. *Direct communications* through mass media, schools, worksites, other organizations, and through patient counselling in health clinics are used to influence the predisposing factors. *Indirect communications* through parents, teachers, clergy, community leaders, employers, peers, and others are used to strengthen the reinforcing factors with organizational rewards or social-normative influence. *Community organization, political activation, and training* strengthen the enabling factors by mobilizing and moving resources, policies, and building skills and capacities.

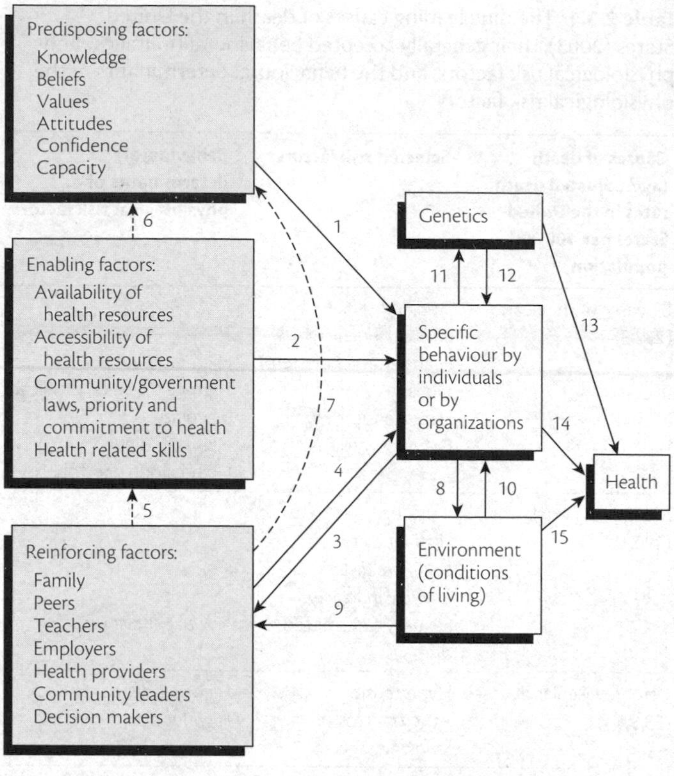

Fig. 2.3.2 This portion of the Precede–Proceed Model includes additional lines and arrows to outline a theory of causal relationships and order of causation and feedback loops for the three sets of factors influencing behaviour. In addition to the lines shown, an arrow from 'enabling factors' to 'environment' would elaborate the ecological aspect of factors that influence behaviour indirectly through changes in the environment. (Kreen & Kreater, 2005, p. 149, with permission.)

Predisposing factors

Predisposing factors reside in the individual and include attitudes, values, beliefs, and perceptions of need, but these are shaped over time by cultural and social exposures, which produce reinforcing factors (see below). Predisposing factors are those antecedents to behaviour that provide the rationale, motivation, or drive for an individual's or group's behaviour. They mostly fall in the psychological domain of determinants, though genetics and environment shape them across the life span. They include the cognitive and affective dimensions of knowing, feeling, believing, valuing, and having self-confidence or a sense of self-efficacy.

Because these determinants of behaviour reside in individuals, public health must seek to influence behaviour by assessing the prevalence and distribution of key predisposing factors and look for opportunities to communicate differentially with various segments of the populations, according to an educational diagnosis or 'social marketing' assessment of their knowledge, attitudes, values, beliefs, and perceptions. The behavioural science literature, especially in health psychology, is replete with competing theories of the relative importance of particular predisposing factors and how they interact with each other (e.g. Glanz *et al.* 2002). Some of these theories, such as the Health Belief Model (Becker 1974), Social Cognitive Theory (Bandura 2004), and the Transtheoretical Model of Stages of Change (Prochaska *et al.* 2002), have become mainstays of the intervention literature on health education and behaviour change. These frequent uses of selected models have produced sufficient numbers of comparable studies or programme evaluations to permit meta-analyses of their applications across different health behaviours (e.g. Harrison *et al.* 1992; Netz *et al.* 2005; Spencer *et al.* 2005).

Enabling factors

Underplayed in most psychological studies of health behaviour, but critical to the role of public health as a complement to the roles of parents, schools, and mass media in the development of a healthy population, are the enabling factors influencing behaviour. These are often conditions of the environment that facilitate (or impede) the performance of a predisposition or motivated action by individuals or groups. Included are the availability, accessibility, and affordability of healthcare and community resources. Also included are conditions of living that act as facilitators or barriers to action, such as availability of transportation or child care to release a parent from that responsibility long enough to participate in a health programme, clinic, or service. It also includes features of the built environment, such as bicycle lanes, sidewalks, proximity of housing to workplaces, and other physical conditions of the environment that make physical activity more or less convenient and inviting (e.g. Taylor *et al.* 2007). Enabling factors also include new skills that a person needs—or new capacities that a group, organization, or community needs—to be able to accomplish health goals.

Public health addresses the enabling factors for behavioural change through policy changes and resource allocations at the national, regional, and local level, community organization for such policy and resource allocation at the local level when government programmes and services are insufficient or inappropriate to local perceptions of need. Training in the skills needed to take certain complicated actions is the other behavioural intervention used by public health to address the enabling factors.

In an era of constrained public health resources, many communities have resorted to more intensive community organization to build coalitions of multiple agencies including government and NGOs, and intersectoral collaboration between the health agencies and the community's schools, worksites, transportation, and other such sectors. Public–private collaboration on issues of enabling a more healthful food supply in school lunches, for example, or less accessibility of children to vending machines with cigarettes or 'junk food', have become increasingly common strategies for addressing the behaviour–environment interaction issues at the heart of most enabling factors.

Reinforcing factors

Before chronic diseases became the prevailing concern of public health in developed countries, behaviour was perceived as less important than today. The types of behaviour required to implement many of the most important public health interventions such as immunization and fluoridation were less complex. Immunizations, for example, could confer long-term immunity for an individual with a single act. Fluoridation or chlorination of water supplies could be implemented in many communities with no engagement of the public, although when fluoridation did become a local political issue requiring a local vote, the behaviour in question for most people was, again, a single action. As chronic diseases became more prevalent, the behaviours in question were largely ones that had to be repeated frequently, some for a lifetime, such as dietary practices, hypertension medication regimens, smoking cessation, and physical activity. For these behaviours, the predisposing and enabling factors remain important, but reinforcing factors take on increased importance because maintaining a behaviour requires reinforcement.

Reinforcing factors are those consequences of action that determine whether the actor receives positive (or negative) feedback and is supported socially or financially after it occurs. Reinforcing factors thus include social support, peer influences, and advice and feedback by healthcare providers, as well as a sense that the benefits of the action outweigh the costs. In consideration of the benefits (and costs), they also include physical consequences of behaviour, which may be separate from the social context. Examples include the feeling of well-being (or pain) caused by physical exercise and the alleviation of respiratory symptoms (or the experience of side effects) following the use of asthma medication, or gaining weight while quitting cigarettes.

Public health uses reinforcing factors such as denormalizing smoking in public places, social reinforcement with encouraging words in personal counselling, small-group health education sessions in which behaviour is publicly endorsed and praised, or mass media images of attractive role models with whom people wish to be associated by their own behaviour. No matter how effective these extrinsic reinforcements might be in the short term in strengthening a behavioural tendency, they must be internalized over time to become intrinsic motivation. Token rewards lead to token behaviour if the individuals do not replace them over time with the belief that the behaviour is intrinsically valuable because it accords with their own personal values (Green *et al.* 1986).

Table 2.3.2 gives examples of the more commonly identified influences on each of four most important behavioural risk factors. These behaviours interact with each other, such that changes in one influence predisposing, enabling, and reinforcing factors for others. Young women, for example, may take up smoking in the belief that it will help them control their appetite and thereby their weight. Other examples are athletes quitting smoking and limiting alcohol intake to improve their physical activity or sport performance; and contraceptive use leading to fewer, more spaced births, which lead in turn to women seeking other opportunities to improve their health and that of their families.

Public health strategies to influence determinants of behaviour

Another chapter in this volume will deal with the full range of health promotion and health education strategies (Kickbusch 2008). The focus of this section is specifically on how the aspects of the environment discussed above that shape health-related behaviour can be targeted for strategic intervention for public health purposes. Three types of strategies are used in public health to accomplish health promotion and disease prevention goals through behaviour change:

- *Educational strategies* inform and educate the public about issues of concern, such as the dangers of drug misuse, the benefits of automobile restraints, or the relationship of maternal alcohol consumption to foetal alcohol syndrome.
- *Automatic-protective strategies* are directed at controlling environmental variables, that minimize the need for individual decisions in structuring each behaviour, such as public health measures providing for milk pasteurization, fluoridation, infant immunizations, and the burning or chemical killing of marijuana crops, but these often involve individual and group decisions and actions about which policies to support, since they limit degrees of freedom in choice of behavioural options.
- *Coercive strategies* employ legal and other formal sanctions to control individual behaviour, such as required immunizations for school entry, mandatory tuberculosis testing of hospital employees, compulsory use of automobile restraints, and arrests for drug possession or use.

Table 2.3.2 Some known and suspected influences on four major behavioural risk factors

Cigarette smoking	Dietary practices	Alcohol use/abuse	Physical inactivity
Knowledge of adverse health effects of smoking	Personal food preferences	Expectations of alcohol effects	Beliefs in physical activity benefits
Attitudes about smoking	Cultural food preferences	Child of alcoholic	Attitudes toward physical activity
Skills in smoking cessation/prevention	Perceived social acceptance of foods	Alternatives to alcohol	Self-motivation
Cigarette cost	Social context of eating	Psychological stress	Self-efficacy
Availability of cigarettes	Availability and convenience of foods	Low self-esteem	Accessibility of exercise facilities
Cigarette advertising	Skills in menu planning	Early drinking experience	Skills in relapse prevention
Peer influences to smoke	Skills in food preparation	Heavy social drinking	Skills in goal setting
Social support for non-smoking	Skills in food selection	Parent and peer influences	Enjoyability of physical activity
	Food advertising	Alcohol advertising	Family support
		Cost of alcohol	Design of the built environment
		Availability of alcohol	
		Supervision of drinking	

Illustrative of successful public health measures reflecting this range of strategies directed at influencing health-related behaviours are the efforts to control tobacco consumption. Influencing tobacco-related knowledge and attitudes has been declared one of the great public health achievements of the twentieth century, at least in the United States (Centers for Disease Control 1999) and several other countries. Considering that these successes, as measured by the reductions in tobacco consumption behaviour, were achieved largely in the last third of the century, they represent both a remarkable turn-around of an epidemic of smoking behaviour that had increased inexorably through the first two-thirds of the century, and an inspiration for public health approaches to other health-related behaviours that now show similar epidemic trends. The application of the lessons from tobacco control to reversing, for example, the obesity epidemic through similar influences on dietary and physical activity behaviours has become a point of major public health debate in the early years of the new millennium (Eriksen *et al.* 2007; Green *et al.* 2006; Mercer *et al.* 2005).

Influences on smoking initiation and cessation are numerous, and many of them are also intertwined with diet, alcohol, and physical activity. Predisposing factors include attitudes about smoking and beliefs about and knowledge of the health effects of smoking. Enabling factors of access to tobacco products and price are influential. The price elasticity has been documented at a 3 per cent decrease in tobacco consumption for every 10 per cent increase in the price, and a greater relative decrease in youth, for whom disposable income is less (Jha & Chaloupka 2000; Ranson *et al.* 2002). The influence of raising taxes on cigarettes, then, has been a major public health strategy with known effects on consumption. With the dedication of part of the tax revenues to the funding of comprehensive tobacco control programmes, some jurisdictions have achieved a doubling and even tripling of the rate of decline in per capita consumption compared with other jurisdictions in the same country (Mercer *et al.* 2005). But more powerful still are the cumulative reinforcing factors of growing social support and pressure for smoke-free environments as smoking becomes denormalized with the decline in prevalence rates and the legal restrictions on smoking in public places (Eriksen *et al.* 2007).

Cigarette advertising and promotions by the tobacco industry have proved to be powerful negative predisposing and reinforcing influences on smoking behaviour that are highly adaptable to changing regulatory attempts to control their content and channels. Initial restrictions on US tobacco advertising in the broadcast media in the mid-1960s, for example, resulted in the tobacco industry voluntarily withdrawing from radio and television advertising, but adroitly using those resources from mass media to expand its advertising vastly on more targeted print media in magazines, billboards, and youth-oriented outlets. Sponsorship of sports and arts events and clubs, for example, provided a more targeted venue for reaching youth and other susceptible markets. Response of some jurisdictions in restricting these sponsorships has produced reductions in youth uptake of tobacco products (Hagmann 2002). Diversification of advertising to youth-oriented media and point-of-purchase settings such as stores near schools has resulted in increased restrictions in many jurisdictions. The results have been largely disappointing, which is attributed to the agility of the industry in finding loopholes and ways to circumvent the new legal restrictions.

Attempts to control the determinants of tobacco consumption also illustrate an essential public health lesson in the importance of comprehensive programmes to affect the complex behaviours associated with chronic diseases (CDC 1999). Comprehensive approaches have proved critical because:

- No single intervention reaches all segments of susceptible people in a population (Green & Glasgow 2006).
- No single intervention reaches different segments with the same degree of effectiveness (e.g. Contento *et al.* 1993).
- Different interventions are differentially effective in the different phases of change (Prochaska *et al.* 2002).
- Different interventions variously influence the predisposing, enabling, and reinforcing determinants of behaviour in a population (Green & Kreuter 2005).

This comprehensiveness lesson has been carried forward to public health efforts in diet, alcohol, and physical activity insofar as they have increasingly engaged multiple organizations in community coalitions and multiple sectors and national programmes to address the various determinants that extend beyond the purview of the medical and public health sectors at the local level.

The promotion of physical activity or active living illustrates the lessons of comprehensiveness and multi-sector involvement in public health strategies to influence a complex behaviour. The numerous influences on sedentary behaviour or physical activity include predisposing beliefs about the importance of physical activity and attitudes about physical activity, enabling accessibility of exercise facilities, walking lanes or paths, skills in relapse prevention and in goal setting, and reinforcing factors of discomfort or inconvenience of exercise, and family support (Frankish *et al.* 1998). Increasing attention has been given in recent years to the built environment, including the density of housing, mixed-use neighbourhoods, and sidewalks that encourage walking to and from home for shopping, work, and recreation; provision of mass transit that also supports walking the distance to and from transit stops rather than driving to work and other destinations (Frank 2000).

The recent growth of the active living field is an extension and integration of traditional public health approaches with more collaborative approaches involving sectors such as housing, parks and recreation, and transportation. It responds to the increasing recognition of the complexity of health-risk behaviours related to chronic diseases and their numerous determinants. The performance of each behaviour is interwoven with or ecologically embedded in other behaviours and their mutual genetic determinants and their social, cultural, and physical environments.

Behaviour as determinant of environmental and genetic predispositions

Population behavioural and educational diagnoses enable public health to intervene strategically on the behaviour of populations. But health problems have other determinants in the environment and in genetics. Behaviour also can play a role in influencing those determinants.

The reciprocal influence of individual behaviour on environments

A fundamental precept of human ecology is the reciprocal determinism of behaviour and the environment (Green *et al.* 1996). The literature on health promotion took a sharp turn away from behaviour in the 1980s to give attention to the policy and environmental determinants of health. This was partly in response to a period in which public health was perceived to have taken too much of a psychological approach to the determinants of health (Green 2006). As early as 1968, Edward S. Rogers had appealed to sociology for the assistance of public health needed from the social sciences to address the ecological issues (Rogers 1968). Psychologists, however, were more available, at least in the US, to step into the perceived social science void of public health and to take up the new professorships in public health. They brought an emphasis on testing theories of individual behavioural change. As the ecological imperative of multi-level interventions (individual, family, organizational, community, regional, national, and global) gained growing emphasis in public health (e.g. Green *et al.* 1996; Kickbusch 1989), a gradual turn to the study of behaviour-in-context gave reciprocal determinism a new lease on life in public health (Institute of Medicine 2001, 2003; Stoto *et al.* 1997) in the decade bridging the millennium. One theory of behavioural change that gained particular public health prominence in this era was Albert Bandura's social cognitive theory, with its emphasis on self-efficacy and individual agency in changing one's environment at the same time that it gave prominence to the social environment in shaping behaviour (Bandura 2004).

Some of the environmental determinants of health beyond the behavioural control of individuals nevertheless lend themselves to group political behaviour or collective action through community intervention. Communities, neighbourhoods, or special-interest (self-help) groups can organize, vote, lobby, boycott, and otherwise support or prevent some environmental changes. To varying degrees, individuals can avoid or limit their exposure to environmental risks such as solar radiation, lead paint, and ambient smoke. In short, individual behaviour can be mobilized to influence the environment, so that individuals need not be seen only as passive objects of environmental influence.

The projected but still limited influence of behaviour on genetics

The Human Genome Project and the explosion of research on human genetics have raised very hopeful scenarios of 'personalized medicine', in which individuals could know more precisely their genetic risk of certain diseases or causes of death. The usual assumptions are that such information could be made readily available to individuals, and that having such information would be considerably more compelling in motivating behaviour than the usual statistical risk of groups of people without the personalized association with the individual in question.

The first assumption remains to be supported by true evidence of effectiveness. For example, in about 30 per cent of women with breast cancer, over-expression of a protein called HER2/neu is associated with a worse prognosis and in such women the drug trastuzumab is especially effective. The FDA approved the drug and a test for HER2/neu for use in women with metastatic breast cancer in 1998 and more recently for women with early stage breast cancer (Braga *et al.* 2006; Hortobagyi 2005; Piccart-Gebhart *et al.* 2005). The co-development and approval of the drug and test is considered one of the real successes of the application of genetics to modern medical practice and among the best examples of 'personalized medicine'. One might think the story is complete. However, although this information about the efficacy and availability of the test and the drug was published and promulgated by commercial backers, the behaviour of clinicians and their patients has been a more complicated matter. There is little known about how many women have access to testing and treatment. The costs of both are high and cost-effectiveness issues have not been resolved. Also how best to administer the test has not been resolved (e.g. timing) and there are reports of an increased risk of heart failure, the effect of which on acceptance is not known.

The second assumption, that having such information would motivate more concerted effort to change one's behaviour, is only partially supported by: (1) the logic and evidence from other areas of health counselling and communications that more personally tailored health information based on the individual's own family history or biological risk information adds motivational value to the experience with health advice that is based on more generic information (Kreuter & Wray 2003; Kreuter *et al.* 2003, 2004, 2005);

(2) limited direct evidence from the few instances in which such genetic information has been used to counsel individual behavioural choices of action. The latter is illustrated by the examples in the previous paragraph and those from prenatal testing and counselling for birth defects. However, a meta-analysis of 21 controlled trials showed that while genetic counselling improved knowledge of cancer genetics, it did not increase the level of perceived risk and few studies examined cancer surveillance behaviours (Braithwaite *et al.* 2006).

Public health faces two major limiting factors in pursuing this pathway of behaviour influencing health through genetic determinants: (1) the limited influence of the genes so far implicated in specific mortality or morbidity outcomes, and their interactions with the environment, (2) the ethics of offering such information to the individual with anything more than a cautionary note of possible relevance to their reproductive decisions or their behavioural choices. The first is a limit that could be partially overcome with further breakthroughs in the human genomics research. But apart from some prenatal tests for genetic defects in the fetus, most of the other genetic markers associated with predispositions to illnesses or premature mortality are highly interactive with other genes and the environment. Therefore, any course of action recommended to the individual remains probabilistic in its assurance of a health benefit. In combination with the other risk factors that can be more readily identified, the addition of personalized genetic information might raise the probabilities sufficiently to help the individual reach a tipping point in motivation to take action on complex health-related behaviours. But whether it really adds motivational value to what could be similarly known from a good family history has yet to be demonstrated.

The other limiting factors for this behaviour–genetic pathway as a public health consideration are the ethical complications that arise with the technology and the information. The concern, as in other screening technologies, with false-positive results can be multiplied in their ethical considerations for genetic information on individuals. The usual issues of protecting the privacy of such information and the potential discrimination in hiring, placement, retention, and promotion of individuals with known genetic predispositions will continue to be debated before the 'personalized medicine' potential of expanding the behaviour–genetic pathway can be pursued as public health policy. Meanwhile, private medicine is opening opportunities for individuals to explore this option in structuring their behavioural response to personal genetic information. Another chapter in this volume addresses human genetics more thoroughly.

The interaction of socioeconomic status (SES), environments, and behaviour

Of all the interactions in the association of behaviour and health, none is more pervasive, consistent, and robust than that of socioeconomic status. The relationship between SES and measures of health or mortality is shown in previous chapters to be a gradient rather than a threshold effect, though threshold effects are sometimes found beyond which income or other SES indicators have no further beneficial effects (e.g. Finch 2003). Those at the top of the SES hierarchy usually have better health and lower mortality rates than those just below them who are themselves better off than the others, and so on down to those in poverty at the very bottom. The gradient adheres whether the SES measure is education, income, occupational status, or place of residence. The gradient globally is anchored at the lowest end by the poorest developing countries. Some one billion people globally live in extreme poverty on an income of just US$1 a day, of whom 70 per cent live in Asian and Pacific countries. Many of the poor lack access to basic health services and are at exaggerated risks for many of the leading causes of death in those countries.

The question here is how the mortality and morbidity gradients with socioeconomic status might operate through health-related behaviours and environments to suggest mechanisms by which the pervasive SES gradient influences health.

SES as a predisposing determinant of behaviour

The ecological perspective on SES as a determinant of behaviour related to health would suggest first that environments shape behaviour from early childhood onward. Shaping behaviour in the first instance (rather than enabling it in the second or reinforcing it in the third) qualifies this environmental influence as a predisposing factor. Homes, neighbourhoods, towns, cities, regions, and whole countries with their variable physical, social, economic, and cultural environments differ in relation to SES measured at individual, family, neighbourhood, and other geographic levels. Once the measures of SES and health or mortality are aggregated above the individual level, their relationships constitute ecological correlations. Studies have examined the ecological relationship between mortality rates and various indicators of social inequalities in geographical areas varying in size from metropolitan areas (Lynch *et al.* 1998) to whole countries (Wilkinson & Marmot 1998). These studies showed that those areas where inequalities between those at the top of the hierarchy and those at the bottom were the largest were also those in which the mortality gradient was the strongest (Wilkinson 1996). Similar findings were found with other indicators of social inequities such as differences in social capital (Kawachi *et al.* 1997). Health disparities between socioeconomic groups appear from Canadian data to increase with age across the lifespan, which supports the notion of a cumulative effect over time of the health- and mortality-SES gradient (e.g. Prus 2007).

One implication of this relative deprivation dimension of the SES-health gradient is that perception of one's status relative to others de-motivates or discourages one's efforts to take greater control over the behavioural and environmental determinants of one's health. Whether consciously discouraged or unconsciously conditioned by repeated confrontations with inequalities and inequities that conspire against one's efforts, the hypothesis is that disparities make those exposed to relative deprivation less predisposed or motivated to take preventive and healthcare actions. Two specific mechanisms have been suggested for this de-motivation or lack of predisposition to undertake behaviour. One is a chronic pessimism that has been found in adolescent children of lower SES parents, and that pessimism was associated with stress (Finkelstein *et al.* 2007). The other possibly related mechanism is the theoretical construct of 'self-efficacy', widely measured in association with social cognitive theory applications in health behaviour research (Bandura 2004).

SES as an enabling determinant of behaviour

Socioeconomic standing also confers capabilities and resources that enable the predisposed behaviours to be carried out, for better or for worse. With higher standing come more resources and the associated education and training that endow individuals, families, groups, and communities with enabling judgements, resources, and skills. No matter how motivated people may be by their predisposing factors, they may not have the income and other resources, including accessible and affordable services within reach of their residences or workplaces, to be able to carry out the behaviour without great sacrifice and inconvenience. But environmental variables of accessible fruit and vegetable outlets in local neighbourhoods, for example, only partially explain or mediate the relationship between SES and fruit or vegetable consumption (Ball *et al.* 2006).

The educational enabling influence of SES on behaviour

Among the SES indicators, education has for decades demonstrated the strongest association with most health-behaviour measures (Green 1970a,b; Metcalf *et al.* 2007). It also stands out among the indicators of inequities in confirming the relative deprivation hypothesis above (Kunst & Mackenbach 1994). Education can be viewed as a proxy for a variety of predisposing and enabling factors in explaining the causes of behavioural determinants as mediators of at least part of the SES-health gradient. Prominent among these are optimism (a predisposing factor) and education as an enabling or coping resource (Finkelstein *et al.* 2007), with the knowledge, attitudes, and skills that come with years of schooling.

The Canadian Health Promotion Survey (Adams 1993) showed that men and women with a higher level of education self-rated their health as excellent or good in a much higher proportion than individuals with lower education. The proportion of people in Canada who are smokers is double in people with elementary or lower education, compared with people with university degrees (Health and Welfare Canada *et al.* 1993). This spread in proportions of smokers was greater for the highest and lowest education categories than for the highest and lowest income or occupational status categories (Pederson 1993). Data from the major US community trials in cardiovascular disease prevention showed that the dramatic drop in smoking prevalence over the 1980s was more pronounced for people with higher education compared with peoples with less education (Winkleby *et al.* 1992 b; Luepker *et al.* 1993). The same trend was observed in Canada for the period 1985–1991 (Millar & Stephens 1993).

These historical associations between health behaviours and SES have been confounded in the more recent tracking of obesity, physical activity, and food consumption. The more sedentary work and modes of travel of a majority of white collar workers blurs the educational, income, and occupational correlations with physical activity (e.g. Canadian Institute for Health Information 2006; Tjepkema 2005). In Canada, for example, 'of the demographic variables examined, income, occupation, and employment status were unrelated to obesity, while education was negatively associated with the prevalence of obesity' (Raine 2004, p. 6.).

The cultural–environmental predisposing influence of SES

The strong relationships between education and smoking and other health behaviours are only slightly less so when adjusted for age, sex, and ethnicity (Winkleby *et al.* 1992; Shea *et al.* 1991). Culture and gender do appear to play important roles, but these are highly intertwined with education and acculturation. The early ecological studies remain some of the most compelling in establishing and explaining the role of culture in health. The studies of Japanese men who had lived in Japan and emigrated to California showed clear dietary changes and increased heart disease and stroke rates only in their offspring, i.e. the second generation. Those who emigrated to Hawaii had intermediate rates of dietary change and coronary and stroke rates (Keys *et al.* 1970; Kato *et al.* 1973). As the Japanese became acculturated, they assumed both the dietary and cardiovascular patterns of their new country.

Another classic study providing evidence of the effects of culture on health was the series on the Roseto community. Early observations showed that this ethnically homogeneous Pennsylvania community experienced a significantly lower mortality from myocardial infarction than the nearby community of Bangor despite a higher prevalence of hypertension and obesity and a similar proportion of smokers (Lynn *et al.* 1967). These results were attributed to the apparent protective effect of a unique social, ethnic, and family cohesion in the community (Bruhn *et al.* 1982). More recent analyses show that Rosetans lost that relative protection over subsequent decades (Egolf *et al.* 1992). This loss was accompanied by an increase in the number of intermarriages of Rosetans with people of non-Italian decent, a decrease in social participation in Roseto, and an increase in the general wealth of the community, as the original Italian-born generation was gradually replaced by their ageing American-born offspring (Lasker *et al.* 1994).

In short, to the extent that minority cultures can remain sheltered from the pervasive influences of the majority culture, they can have powerful predisposing influences on health-related behaviour. With acculturation, however, comes the displacement of minority cultural influence with the majority culture. Culture, nevertheless, remains a conceptually useful construct for understanding both the minority and majority processes of socially transmitted beliefs and values that predispose people to one choice of behaviour over another.

SES as a reinforcing determinant of behaviour

A behaviour that is predisposed and enabled might still fail to persist beyond a trial stage of development if it fails to produce satisfying results. Satisfaction comes from various sources that can have the effect of reinforcing behaviour. SES can contribute to the availability of reinforcements by putting people into association with other people and environments that are more likely to produce satisfaction with behaviours. Two examples follow.

The 'status identity factor' and social norms

The social-normative theory underlying the notion of SES functioning like a reinforcing factor would predict that people will identify with a place in the social hierarchy that they can justify on the basis of their highest achievement. Unlike the usual measure of SES produced by averaging standardized or weighted measures of education, income, and occupation, one hypothesis derived from social reinforcement theory was that people will aspire to and adhere to that norm of a particular behaviour associated with their highest measure on the gradient of SES. For example, a person who is relatively high on education, but of moderate income and occupational status, would tend to adhere to the behavioural norms of the highest, rather than the average, of the three status scores. The hypothesis was tested in a California state-wide sample of mothers of children under 5, demonstrating that the immunization status of the children and five other measures of early childhood care followed a gradient with SES, but that the best predictor of the mother's behaviour on these five measures was her highest standardized SES among income, education, and occupation, not the average. This inferred 'status identity' of the mothers provided a basis for linking the psychological phenomena of identification and role modelling with the sociological concept of normative influence (Green 1970a).

Denormalizing behaviour

In retrospect, one of the most important elements of the tobacco control success of the last third of the twentieth century in the US and Canada was the 'denormalization' of smoking behaviour in public places (Eriksen *et al.* 2007). What had been a normative behaviour of smoking in the workplace and in restaurants, meeting rooms, and other public places became increasingly unacceptable, first by legal restrictions, then by social norms, by which the growing majority of non-smokers expected and even insisted on smoke-free environments. The combination of new smoke-free or 'clean air' ordinances and by-laws with mass media emphasizing the carcinogenic properties of second-hand smoke and the rights of non-smokers to be spared the exposure to this carcinogen resulted in a dramatic drop in this public behaviour. It was during this period of the 30-year decline in smoking that the rate of decline accelerated most dramatically. One reason for the importance of this element of the tobacco control campaigns was that the passage and enforcement of policies restricting a personal behaviour faced strong opposition as long as it was perceived by the public to be a matter of individual rights and the threat to be only to the person's own health. When the threat is seen to be to other people's health, especially to the health of children, the support of passage and enforcement of the laws and regulations grows. Other public health campaigns are attempting to model this experience, which builds on the social responsibility notions associated with communicable diseases of the past, but with most of the chronic disease-related behaviours, such as overeating and sedentary living, it has been more complicated to relate the normative behaviour of individuals to the health of others.

The interaction of socioeconomic status, gender, and behaviour

Men's and women's relative risk of disease or death in relation to specific behavioural risk factors such as smoking are generally similar (e.g. Oliveira *et al.* 2007), but their experiences with health differ markedly (Chapman Walsh *et al.* 1995). These differences cannot be attributed solely to biological determinants related to sexual differentiation (Krieger *et al.* 1993). The social construct of gender, as opposed to the biological categories of sex, was conceptualized to refer to cultural and social conventions, roles and behaviours assigned to men and women (Krieger 1996). These in turn shape the social, political, cultural, and economic circumstances experienced by men and women. Gender thus attempts to capture this differential experience that men and women have with their environment and the possibilities and constraints associated with these differences (Potvin & Frohlich 1998). A growing body of research is showing that some of these constraints and possibilities are interacting with the living conditions associated with SES to shape the health of people.

The correlation of SES with health appears stronger for men than for women; the SES-health gradient is steeper for men (Arber & Cooper 1999), except in their twenties and thirties when the gradients are similar (Matthews *et al.* 1999). The gender interactions with SES and health have been variously attributed to differential occupational experiences (e.g. Ross & Bird 1994), marital experiences (Koskinen & Martelin 1994), and degree of emancipation of women (Kawachi *et al.* 1999). These and other possible explanations generally require assumptions of behavioural mediators. Such mediators are more likely to be 'health-related' behaviour (e.g. sedentary living or food consumption patterns) rather than 'health-directed' behaviour (e.g. exercise or high-fibre diet). This distinction (Green & Kreuter 2005) recognizes the centrality of behaviour in the causal chains even when (perhaps especially when) it is not consciously health-*directed* behaviour.

Relationships among health-related behaviours

The interplay among habitual behavioural patterns and the socioeconomic and cultural conditions reviewed in the last half of this chapter leads one to put into a broader context the reductionist examinations, presented in the first half, of specific behaviours as they relate to health, disease, and mortality. The dynamic relationships among the specific measures creates a complex system of social, economic, cultural, and behavioural factors, interwoven with disease risk factors and health status, and influenced by the healthcare and physical environments.

Early studies of the relationships among health behaviours showed weak correlations, typically below r=0.20 (Green 1970b; Steele & McBroom, 1972). Those in subsequent studies that maintained correlations in the 0.20 range were smoking with alcohol use, alcohol use and exercise (Calnan 1989), and smoking and diet (Blaxter 1990). With the decline in smoking, less variation in smoking produces less co-variation with other behavioural variables. Given these low correlations, there is little evidence supporting a one-dimensional concept of health-related behaviours (Calnan 1994).

Conclusion

Behaviour is an inescapable link in the chain of causation between most environmental and genetic determinants and the health outcomes in which they are implicated. Some toxins and infectious environmental agents can affect health directly without behaviour as a mediator, but even these *can* be mediated by individual action to avoid exposures, and collective behaviour of groups or communities to protect themselves.

The *social* environment presents a further complexity in the mediating and moderating of behaviour and environment in their determination of population health. Most health-related behaviour occurs in the context of the social environment, so it involves the behaviour of other people as well as that of the person whose health is in question. The individuals are acting upon, and in reaction to, each other as their health outcomes are being shaped by their actions. This reciprocal determinism of behaviour and the social environment applies as well to the physical environment and the genetic determinants of health. These interactions make up the ecology of health, and call upon public health to take an ecological approach to the management of population health.

One way to structure the ecological approach to the planning of public health programmes in which behaviour change has a role is to examine the factors that influence behaviour in three categories of determinants: Predisposing factors, enabling factors, and reinforcing factors. These roughly correspond to strategies, respectively, that would use (1) direct communications to influence the knowledge, attitudes beliefs, and perceptions of the population concerning the behaviour–health relationship; (2) legal, engineering, financial, organizational levers and resource development that would enable or prohibit the behaviour; and (3) indirect communications through social organizations, parents, peers, employers, and others who control rewards and approval that would reinforce behaviour. By combining public health strategies directed at these three categories of determinants (predisposing, enabling, and reinforcing factors) the strategies will be comprehensive in their coverage and impact.

All of what has been understood as determinants of the health behaviour of individuals applies with some variation to the behaviour of health professionals, other practitioners and policy-makers who could serve as channels through which to reach individuals, groups, and whole populations to influence their health behaviour. The actions of all of these categories of individuals, as well as their organizations, can be analysed in relation to the factors that predispose, enable, and reinforce their actions, and these analyses can point, in turn, to the development of strategies to change those behaviours.

Acknowledgements

We are indebted to Denise Simons-Morton, MD, PhD, and Louise Potvin, PhD, co-authors of this chapter in the previous editions, for significant remnants of their earlier contributions that remain in this edition. We also thank Julie Miller for bibliographic assistance.

References

Adams, O. (1993). Health status. In *Health and welfare Canada. Canada's health promotion survey 1990: Technical report* (eds. T. Stephens and D. Fowler Graham), p. 23. Ministry of Supply and Services, Ottawa.

Adler, N.E., Boyce, T., Chesney, M.A. *et al.* (1994). Socioeconomic status and health: The challenge of gradient. *American Psychologist*, **49**, 15.

Andersen, R.M., Mullner, R.M., and Cornelius, L.J. (1987b). Black-white differences in health status: Method or substance. *Milbank Memorial Fund Quarterly*, **65** (Suppl 1), 71.

Anderson, K.M., Castelli, W.P., and Levy, D. (1987a). Cholesterol and mortality: 30 years of follow-up from the Framingham Study. *Journal of the American Medical Association*, **257**, 2176–80.

Anderson, P., Cremona, A., Paton, A. *et al.* (1993). The risk of alcohol. *Addiction*, **88**, 1493.

Anderson, R.M. (1969). *A behavioral model of families' use of health services*. University of Chicago Center for Health Administration Studies, Research Series No. 25, University of Chicago Press, Chicago.

Andersen, R.M., Mullner, R.M., and Cornelius, L.J. (1987). Black-white differences in health status: Method or substance. *Milbank Memorial Fund Quarterly*, **65** (Suppl 1), 71.

Antonovsky, A. (1967). Social class, life expectancy and overall mortality. *Milbank Memorial Fund Quarterly*, **45**, 31.

Arber, S. and Cooper, H. (1999). Gender differences in health in later life: The new paradox? *Social Science and Medicine*, **48**, 61.

Arroll, B. and Beaglehole, R. (1992). Does physical activity lower blood pressure: A critical review of the clinical trials. *Journal of Clinical Epidemiology*, **45**, 439–47.

Austoker, J. (1994a). Cancer prevention in primary care: Diet and cancer. *British Medical Journal*, **308**, 1610–14.

Austoker, J. (1994b). Cancer prevention in primary care: Reducing alcohol intake. *British Medical Journal*, **308**, 1549–52.

Ball, K., Crawford, D. and Mishra, G. (2006). Socio-economic inequalities in women's fruit and vegetable intakes: a multilevel study of individual, social and environmental mediators. *Public Health Nutrition*, **9**, 623–30.

Bartecchi, C.E., MacKenzie, T.D. and Schrier, R.W. (1994). The human cost of tobacco use, Part 1. *New England Journal of Medicine*, **330**, 907.

Basta, N.E. (2007). Community-level socio-economic status and cognitive and functional impairment in the older population. *European Journal of Public Health*, **18** (1): 48–54.

Becker, M.H. (1974). The Health Belief Model and personal health behaviour. *Health Education Monographs*, **2**, 324.

Berkman, L.F. and Syme, S.L. (1979). Social networks, host resistance, and mortality: A nine year follow-up of Alameda county residents. *American Journal of Epidemiology*, **109**, 186.

Berlin, J.A. and Colditz, G.A. (1990). A meta-analysis of physical activity in the prevention of coronary heart disease. *American Journal of Epidemiology*, **132**, 12–28.

Blair, S., Powell, K., Bazzarre, T. *et al.* (1993). Physical activity. American Heart Association Prevention Conference III: Behaviour change and compliance, keys to improving cardiovascular health. *Circulation*, **88**, 1402.

Blaxter, M. (1990). *Health and lifestyles*. Routledge, London.

Bor, W., Naiman, J.M., Anderson, M. *et al.* (1993). Socioeconomic disadvantage and child morbidity: An Australian longitudinal study. *Social Science and Medicine*, **36**, 1053.

Braga, S., dal Lago, L., Bernard, C. *et al.* (2006). Use of trastuzumab for the treatment of early stage breast cancer. *Expert Review of Anticancer Therapy*, **6**, 1153–64.

Braithwaite, D., Emery, J., Walter, F. *et al.* (2006). Psychological impact of genetic counseling for familial cancer: A systematic review and meta-analysis. *Familial Cancer*, **5**, 66–75.

Bruhn, J.G., Philips, B.U., and Wolf, S. (1982). Lessons from Roseto 20 years later: A community study of heart disease. *Southern Medical Journal*, **75**, 575.

Brunner, E. and Marmot, M. (1999). Social organization, stress and health. In *Social determinants of health* (eds. M. Marmot and R.G. Wilkinson), p. 17. Oxford University Press.

Bandura, A. (2004). Health promotion by social cognitive means. *Health Education and Behavior*, **31**, 143.

California Environmental Protection Agency (2005). *Proposed identification of environmental tobacco smoke as a toxic air contaminant*. California Environmental Protection Agency, Sacramento.

Calnan, M. (1989). Control over health and patterns of health-related behavior. *Social Science Medicine*, **26**, 435.

Calnan, M. (1994). Lifestyle and its social meaning. *Advances in Medical Sociology*, **4**, 69.

Canada (1974). *A new perspective on the health of Canadians (Lalonde Report)*. Department of National Health and Welfare, Ottawa.

Canadian Institute for Health Information (2006). *Improving the health of Canadians: Promoting healthy weights*. Canadian Institute for Health Information, Ottawa.

Carmelli, D., Swan, G.E., and Rosenman, R.H. (1986). The relationship between wives' social and psychologic status and their husbands' coronary heart disease. *American Journal of Epidemiology*, **122**, 90.

Cavelaars, A.E.J.M., Kunst, A.E., and Mackenbach, J.P. (1997). Socioeconomic differences in risk factors for morbidity and mortality in the European Community. *Journal of Health Psychology*, **2**, 90.

Centers for Disease Control and Prevention (1999). Achievements in public health 1900–1999: Tobacco use—United States, 1900–1999. *Morbidity and Mortality Weekly Reports*, **48**, 986–93.

Chapman Walsh, D., Sorensen, G., and Leanord, L. (1995). Gender, health and cigarette smoking. In *Society and health* (eds. B.C. Amick III, S. Levine, A.R. Tarlov, and D. Chapman Walsh), p. 131. Oxford University Press, New York.

Colditz, G.A. (2001). Cancer culture: epidemics, human behavior, and the dubious search for new risk factors. *American Journal of Public Health*, **91**, 357.

Colditz, G.A., Willett, W.C., Stampfer, M.J. *et al.* (1990). Weight as a risk factor for clinical diabetes in women. *American Journal of Epidemiology*, **132**, 501.

Connelly, S., O'Reilly, D., and Rosato, M. (2007). Increasing inequalities in health. Is it an artifact caused by the selective movement of people? *Social Science and Medicine*, **64**, 2008–15.

Contento, I.R., Basch, C., and Sheaa, S. (1993). Relationship of mothers' food choice criteria to food intake of preschool children: Identification of family subgroups. *Health Education Quarterly*, **20**, 227.

Corin, E. (1994). The social and cultural matrix of health and disease. In *Why are some people healthy and others not? The determinants of health populations* (eds. R.G. Evans, M.L. Barer, and T.R. Marmor), pp. 93–132. Aldine de Gruyter, New York.

Cotrell, L.S. (1976). The competent community. In *Further explorations in social psychiatry* (eds. B.H. Kaplan, R.N. Wilson, and A.H. Leighton), p. 195. Basic Books, New York.

Crawford, D., Ball, K., Mishra, G. *et al.* (2007). Which food-related behaviours are associated with healthier intakes of fruits and vegetables among women? *Public Health Nutrition*, **10**, 256–65. Erratum in *Public Health Nutrition*, **10**, 536.

Custer, S.J. and Doty, C.R. (1992). Assessment of self-motivation and selected physiological characteristics as predictors of adherence to exercise in a corporate setting. *Journal of Health Education*, **23**, 232.

Davis, N.J. and Robinson, R.V. (1988). Class identification of men and women in the 1970s and 1980s. *American Sociological Review*, **53**, 103.

Dawber, T.R. (1960). Summary of recent literature regarding cigarette smoking and coronary heart disease. *Circulation*, **22**, 164.

Egolf, B., Lasker, J., Wolf, S. *et al.* (1992). The Roseto effect: A 50-year comparison of mortality rates. *American Journal of Public Health*, **82**, 1089.

Emery, C.F. and Blumenthal, J.A. (1991). Effects of physical exercise on psychological and cognitive functioning of older adults. *Annals of Behavioral Medicine*, **13**, 99.

Epp, J. (1986). Achieveing health for all: A framework for health promotion. *Health Promotion International*, **1**, 419.

Eriksen, M.P., Green, L.W., Husten, C.G. *et al.* (2007). Thank you for not smoking: The public response to tobacco-related mortality in the United States. In *Silent victories: The history and practice of public health in twentieth-century America.* (eds. J.W. Ward and C. Warren). New York: Oxford University Press.

Eriksen, M. P., Green, L. W., Huston, C. *et al.* (2007). Tobacco control in the United States: After the great public health triumphs of the Twentieth Century, what must we emphasize in the Twenty-First? In *A safer and healthier America: Public health in the 20th century* (eds. J.W. Ward and C.S. Warren), in press.

Ewart, C.K., Taylor, C.B., Reese, L.B. *et al.*(1983). The effects of early myocardial infarction exercise testing on self-perception and subsequent physical activity. *American Journal of Cardiology*, **51**, 1076.

Finch, B.K. (2003). Socioeconomic gradients and low birth-weight: Empirical and policy considerations. *Health Services Research*, **38**, 1819.

Finkelstein, D.M., Kubzansky, D.M., Capitman, J. *et al.*(2007). Socioeconomic differences in adolescent stress: The role of psychological resources. *Journal of Adolescent Health*, **40**, 127–34.

Fox, A.J., Goldblatt, P.O., and Jones, D.R. (1986). Social class mortality differentials: artifact, selection, or life circumstances. In *Class and health: Research and longitudinal data* (ed. R.G. Wilkinson), p. 35. Tavistock Publications, London.

Fox, S.H., Koepsell, T.D., and Daling, J.R. (1994). Birth weight and smoking during pregnancy – effect modification by maternal age. *American Journal of Epidemiology*, **139**, 1008.

Frank, L.D. (2000). Land use and transportation interaction: Implications on the public health and quality of life. *Journal of Planning Education and Research*, **20**, 6–22.

Frankish, C.J., Milligan, C.D., and Reid, C. (1998). A review of relationships between active living and determinants of health. *Social Sciences and Medicine*, **47**, 287–301.

Frick, M.H., Elo, M.O., Happa, K. *et al.* (1987). Helsinki Heart Study: Primary-prevention trial with gemfibrozil in middle-aged men with dyslipidemia. Safety of treatment, changes in risk factors, and incidence of coronary heart disease. *New England Journal of Medicine*, **137**, 1237–45.

Glanz, K., Rimer, B.K., and Lewis, F.M. (eds.) (2002). *Health behavior and health education: Theory, research, and practice*, 3rd edition. Jossey Bass, San Francisco.

Glass, T. A. and McAtee, M. J. (2006). Behavioral science at the crossroads in public health: Extending horizons, envisioning the future. *Social Science & Medicine*, **62**, 1650.

Goeppinger, J. and Baglioni, A.J., Jr (1985). Community competence: A positive approach to needs assessment. *American Journal of Community Psychology*, **13**, 507.

Gottlieb, N.H. and Green, L.W. (1987). Ethnicity and lifestyle health risk: Some possible mechanisms. *American Journal of Health Promotion*, **2**, 37.

Green, L.W. (1970a). Manual for scoring socioeconomic status for research on health behavior. *Public Health Reports* **85**, 185.

Green, L.W. (1970b). *Status identity and preventive health behaviour*. Pacific Health Education Reports, No. 1. University of California School of Public Health. Berkeley, CA.

Green, L.W. (1986). The theory of participation: A qualitative analysis of its expression in national and international policies. In *Advances in health education and promotion* (eds. W.B. Ward, Z.T. Salisbury, S.B. Kar, and J.G. Zapka), Vol. 1, Part A, p. 211. JAI Press, Greenwich, CT.

Green, L.W. (2006). Public health asks of systems science: To advance our evidence-based practice, can you help us get more practice-based evidence? *American Journal of Public Health*, **96**, 406.

Green, L.W. and Glasgow, R. (2006). Evaluating the relevance, generalization, and applicability of research: Issues in external validation and translation methodology. *Evaluation & the Health Professions*, **29**, 126.

Green, L.W. and Kreuter, M. (2005). *Health program planning: An educational and ecological approach*, 4th edition. New York, McGraw-Hill Higher Education.

Green, L.W. and McAlister, A.L. (1984). Macro-intervention to support health behavior: Some theoretical perspectives and practical reflections. *Health Education Quarterly*, **11**, 322.

Green, L.W., Orleans, C.T., Ottoson, J.M. *et al.* (2006). Inferring strategies for disseminating physical activity policies, programs, and practices from the successes of tobacco control. *American Journal of Preventive Medicine*, **31**(Suppl 4), S66.

Green, L.W., Richard, L., and Potvin, L. (1996). Ecological foundations of health promotion. *American Journal of Health Promotion*, **10**, 270.

Green, L.W., Wilson, A., and Lovato, C.Y. (1986). What changes can health promotion produce and how long will they last? Trade-offs between expediency and durability. *Preventive Medicine*, **15**, 508.

Haan, I., Kaplan, G.A., and Camacho, T. (1987). Poverty and health. Prospective evidence from the Alameda County Study. *American Journal of Epidemiology*, **125**, 989.

Hagmann, M. (2002). WHO attacks tobacco sponsorship of sports. *Bulletin of the World Health Organization*, **80**, 80.

Hancock, T. (1986). Lalonde and beyond: looking back at 'A new perspective on the health of Canadians'. *Health Promotion: An International Journal*, **1**, 93.

Harrison, J.A., Mullen, P.D., and Green, L.W. (1992). A meta-analysis of studies of the Health Belief Model. *Health Education Research*, **7**, 107.

Health and Welfare, Canada, Stephens, T., and Fowler Graham, D. (eds.) (1993). *Canada's health promotion survey 1990: Technical report.* Minister of Supply and Services, Ottawa.

Health Canada (2003). *Canadian Guidelines for Body Weight Classification in Adults*. Health Canada, Ottawa.

Hertz, E., Hebert, J.R., and Landon, J. (1994). Social and environmental factors and life expectancy, infant mortality, and maternal mortality rates: Results of a cross-national comparison. *Social Science and Medicine*, **39**, 105.

Hortobagyi, G.N. (2005). Trastuzumab in the treatment of breast cancer. *New England Journal of Medicine*, **353**, 1734.

House, J.S., Kessler, R.C., and Herzog, A.R. (1990). Age, socioeconomic status, and health. *Milbank Quarterly*, **68**, 383.

Hunninghake, D.B., Stein, E.A., Dujovne, C.A. *et al.* (1993). The efficacy of intensive therapy alone or combined with lovastatin in outpatients with hypercholesterolemia. *New England Journal of Medicine*, **328**, 1213.

Hunt, K. and Annandale, E. (1999). Relocating gender and morbidity: Examining men's and women's health in contemporary Western societies. Introduction to special issue on gender and health. *Social Science and Medicine*, **48**, 1.

Institute of Medicine (2001). *Health and behavior: The interplay of biological, behavioral, and societal influences*. National Academies Press, Washington, DC.

Institute of Medicine (2003). *The future of public health in the 21st century*. National Academies Press, Washington, DC.

James, S., Reddy, P., Ruiter, R. A. *et al.* (2006). The impact of an HIV and AIDS life skills program on secondary school students in Kaw Zulu-Natal, South Africa. *AIDS Education and Prevention*, **18**, 281.

Jha, P. and Chaloupka, F. J. (eds). (2000). *Tobacco control in developing countries*. Oxford University Press, New York.

Kaplan, R.M., Atkins, C.J., and Reinsch, S. (1984). Specify efficacy expectations medicate compliance in patients with COPD. *Health Psychology*, **3,** 223.

Kato, H., Tillotson, J., Nichaman, M.Z. *et al.* (1973). Epidemiological studies of coronary heart disease and stroke in Japanese men living in Japan, Hawaii, and California. Serum lipids and diet. *American Journal of Epidemiology*, **97**, 372.

Kawachi, I., Kennedy, B.P., Gupta, V. *et al.* (1999). Women's status and the health of women and men: A view from the States. *Social Science and Medicine*, **48**, 21.

Kawachi, I., Kennedy, B.P., Lochner, K. *et al.* (1997). Social capital, income inequality, and mortality. *American Journal of Public Health*, **87**, 1491.

Keil, J.E., Sutherland, S.E., Mapp, R.G. *et al.* (1992). Does equal socio-economic status in black and white men mean equal risk of mortality. *American Journal of Public Health*, **82**, 1133–6.

Keys, A. (1970). Coronary heart disease in seven countries. *Circulation*, **41** (Suppl 1), 1.

Keys, A., Kimura, N., Kusukawa, A. *et al.* (1958). Lessons from serum cholesterol studies in Japan, Hawaii, and Los Angeles. *Annals of Internal Medicine*, **48**, 83.

Kickbusch, I. (1989). Approaches to an ecological base for public health. *Health Promotion*, **4**, 265–68.

Koniak-Griffin, D. and Stein, J. A. (2006). Predictors of sexual risk behaviours among adolescent mothers in a human immunodeficiency virus prevention program. *Journal of Adolescent Health*, **38**, 297.e111.

Koskinen, S. and Martelin, T. (1994). Why are socioeconomic mortality differences smaller among women than among men? *Social Science and Medicine*, **38,** 1385–96.

Kreuter, M.W. and Wray R.J. (2003). Tailored and targeted health communication: strategies for enhancing information relevance. *American Journal of Health Behavior*, **27** (Suppl 3), S227–32.

Kreuter M.W., Steger-May K., Bobra S. *et al.* (2003). Sociocultural characteristics and responses to cancer education materials among African American women. *Cancer Control*, **10** (5 Suppl), 69–80.

Kreuter, M.W., Skinner, C.S., Steger-May, K. *et al.* (2004). Responses to behaviorally vs culturally tailored cancer communication among African American women. *American Journal of Health Behavior*, **28,** 195–207.

Kreuter, M.W., Sugg-Skinner, C., Holt, C.L. *et al.* (2005). Cultural tailoring for mammography and fruit and vegetable intake among low-income African-American women in urban public health centers. *Preventive Medicine*, **41**, 53–62.

Krieger, N. (1984). Epidemiology and the web of causation. Has anyone seen the spider? *Social Science and Medicine*, **39**, 887.

Krieger, N. (1996). Inequality, diversity, and health: thoughts on 'race/ethnicity' and 'gender'. *Journal of American Medical Women's Association*, **51**, 133.

Krieger, N., Rowley, D.L., Herman, A.A. *et al.* (1993). Racism, sexism, and social class: Implications for study of health, disease, and well being. *American Journal of Preventive Medicine*, **9** (Suppl), 82.

Kuller, L.H., Ockene, J.K., Meilahn, E. *et al.* (1991). Cigarette smoking and mortality, MRFIT Research Group. *Preventive Medicine*, **29**, 638.

Kunst, A.E. and Mackenbach, J.P. (1994). The size of mortality differences associated with educational level in nine industrialized countries. *American Journal of Public Health*, **84**, 932.

Lahelma, E., Manderbaka, K., Rahkonen, O. *et al.* (1994). Comparison of inequalities in health: Evidence from national surveys in Finland, Norway, Sweden. *Social Science and Medicine*, **38**, 517.

Lahelma E., Martikainen, P., Rahkonen, O. *et al.* (1999). Gender differences in health in Finland: Patterns, magnitude and change. *Social Science and Medicine*, **48**, 7.

Lasker, J.N., Egolf, B.P., and Wolf, S. (1994). Community social change and mortality. *Social Science and Medicine*, **39**, 53.

Lokey, E.A. and Tran, Z.V. (1989). Effects of exercise training on serum lipid and lipoprotein concentrations in women: a meta-analysis. *International Journal of Sports Medicine*, **10**, 424.

Lorig, K. and Laurin, J. (1985). Some notions about assumptions underlying health education. *Health Education Quarterly*, **12**, 231.

Link, B.G. and Phelan, J. (1995). Social conditions as fundamental causes of disease. *Journal of Health and Social Behavior*, (special issue) 80.

Luepker, R.V., Rosamond, W.D., Murphy, R. *et al.* (1993). Socioeconomic status and coronary heart disease risk factor trends: The Minnesota Heart Health Survey. *Circulation*, **88**, 2172.

Lynch, J.W., Kaplan, G.A., Pamuk, E.R. *et al.* (1998). Income inequality and mortality in metropolitan areas of the United States. *American Journal of Public Health*, **88**, 1074.

Lynn, T.N., Duncan, R., Naughton, J.P. *et al.* (1967). Prevalence of evidence of prior myocardial infarction, hypertension, diabetes, and obesity in three neighboring communities in Pennsylvania. *American Journal of Medical Services*, **254**, 385.

McArdle, W.D., Katch, F.L., and Katch, V.L. (1986). *Exercise physiology: Energy, nutrition, and human performance*, 2nd edition. Lea and Febiger, Philadephia, PA.

McGinnis, J.M. and Foege, W.H. (1993). Actual causes of death in the United States. *Journal of the American Medical Association*, **270**, 2270.

McGinnis, J.M., and Foege, W. (2004). The immediate vs the important. *Journal of the American Medical Association*. **10**;291(10): 1263–4.

Macintyre, S. (1993). Gender differences in longevity and health in Eastern and Western Europe. In *Locating health: Sociological and historical explanations* (eds. S. Platt, T.H. Scott, and G. Williams), p. 57. Avebury UK, Aldershot.

Macintyre, S. (1997). The Black Report and beyond: What are the issues. *Social Science and Medicine*, **44**, 723.

Macintyre, S., Hunt, K., and Sweeting, H. (1996). Gender differences in health: Are things really as simple as they seem? *Social Science and Medicine*, **42**, 617.

Malik, V.S. and Hu, F.B. (2007). Popular weight-loss diets: from evidence to practice. *Nature, Clinical Practice, Cardiovascular Medicine*, **4**, 34–41.

Marmot, M.G., Rose, G., Shipley, M.J. *et al.* (1978). Employment grade and coronary heart disease in British civil servants. *Journal of Epidemiology and Community Health*, **32**, 244.

Marmot, M.G., Shipley, M.J., and Rose, G.A. (1984). Inequalities in death. Specific explanations of a general pattern? *Lancet*, **i**, 1003.

Marmot, M.G., Smith, G.D., Stansfeld, S. *et al.* (1991). Health inequalities among British civil servants: The Whitehall II study. *Lancet*, **337**, 1387.

Marmot, M.G., and Wilkinson, R.G. (eds.) (1999). *The social determinants of health*. Oxford University Press, Oxford.

Matthews, S., Manor, O., and Power, C. (1999). Social inequalities in health: Are there gender differences? *Social Science and Medicine*, **48**, 49.

McKinley, J.B. and Marceau, L.D. (2000). To boldly go . . . *American Journal of Public Health*, **90**, 25.

Mechanic, D. (1979). The stability of health and illness behavior: Results from a 16-year follow-up. *American Journal of Public Health*, **69**, 1142.

Mensink, R.P. and Katan, M.G. (1992). Effect of dietary fatty acids on serum lipids and lipoproteins: A meta-analysis of 27 trials. *Arteriosclerosis and Thrombosis*, **12**, 911.

Mercer, S. L. Kahn, L. K., Green, L.W. *et al.* (2005). Drawing possible lessons for obesity prevention and control from the tobacco control experience. Chapter 11 In *Obesity prevention and public health* (eds. D. Crawford and R.W. Jeffrey), pp. 231–64. New York and London: Oxford University Press, New York.

Metcalf, P., Scragg, R., and Davis, P. (2007). Relationship of different measures of socioeconomic status with cardiovascular disease risk factors and lifestyle in a New Zealand workforce survey. *New Zealand Medical Journal*, **120**(1248), U2392.

Millar, W.T. and Stephens, T. (1993). Social status and health risk in Canadian adults: 1985–1991. *Health Reports*, **5**, 143.

Mittendorf, R., Herschel, M. Williams, M.A. *et al.* (1994). Reducing the frequency of low birth weight in the United States. *Obstetrics and Gynecology*, **83**, 1056.

Mokdad, A.H., Marks, J.S., Stroup, D.F. *et al.*(2004). Actual causes of death in the United States, 2000. *Journal of the American Medical Association*, **291**, 1238. Erratum, *Journal of the American Medical Association*, **293**, 293.

Mullen, P.D., Green, L.W., and Persinger, G.S. (1985). Clinical trials of patient education for chronic conditions: A comparative meta-analysis of intervention types. *Preventive Medicine*, **14**, 753.

National Center for Health Statistics (2006). *Health, United States, 2006*. U.S. Department of Health and Human Services, Centers for Disease Control, p. 179, Hiattsville, MD.

Netz, Y., Wu, M.J., Becker, B.J. *et al.* (2005). Physical activity and psychological well-being in advanced age: A meta-analysis of intervention studies. *Psychology and Aging*, **20**, 272.

NHLBI (National Heart, Lung, and Blood Institute) (1993). *Detection, evaluation and treatment of high blood cholesterol in adults*, NIH Publication 93, p. 3095. National Institutes of Health, Bethesda, MD.

North, F, Syme, S.L., Feeney, A. *et al.* (1993). Explaining socioeconomic differences in sickness absence: The Whitehall II Study. *British Medical Journal*, **306**, 361.

Nuckolls, K.B., Cassels, J., and Kaplan, B.H. (1972). Psychosocial assets, life crisis and the prognosis of pregnancy. *American Journal of Epidemiology*, **95**, 431.

Ockene, J.K., Kuller, L.H., Svendsen, K.H., and Meilahn, E. (1990). The relationship of smoking cessation to coronary heart disease and lung cancer in the Multiple Risk Factor Intervention Trial (MRFIT). *American Journal of Public Health*, **80**, 954–8.

Office of Environmental Health Hazard Assessment (OEHHA), California Environmental Protection Agency (1997). *Health effects of exposure to environmental tobacco smoke*. Final report. Sacramento, CA.

Office of Health and Environmental Assessment (1992). *Respiratory, health effects of passive smoking: lung cancer and other disorders*. EPA/600/(6-90/0006F), US Environmental Protection Agency, Cincinnati, OH.

Ogston, S.A. and Parry, G.J. (1992). EUROMAC. A European concerted action: maternal alcohol consumption and its relation to the outcome of pregnancy and child development at 18 months. Results-strategy of analysis and analysis of pregnancy outcome. *International Journal of Epidemiology*, **21** (Suppl 1), S45.

Oliveira, A., Buros, H., Maciel, M. J. *et al.* (2007). Tobacco smoking and acute myocardial infarction in young adults: A population-based case-control study. *Preventive Medicine*, **44**, 311.

Peck, M.N. (1994). The importance of childhood socio-economic group for adult health. *Social Science and Medicine*, **39**, 553–6.

Pederson, L. (1993). *Tobacco use. Canada's health promotion survey 1990: Technical report* (eds. Health and Welfare Canada, T. Stephens and D. Fowler Graham), pp. 97–108. Minister of Supply and Services Canada, Ottawa.

Petrow, S. (1990). *Ending the HIV epidemic*. Network Publications, Santa Cruz, CA.

Piccart-Gebhart, M.J., Procter, M., Leyland-Jones, B. *et al.* Herceptin Adjuvant (HERA) Trial Study Team (2005). Trastuzumab after adjuvant chemotherapy in HER2-positive breast cancer. *New England Journal of Medicine*, **353**, 1659–72.

Poland, B., Green, L.W., and Rootman, I.R. (2000). *Settings for health promotion: Linking theory and practice*. Sage, Thousand Oaks, CA.

Pooling Project Research Group (1978). Relationship of blood pressure, serum cholesterol, smoking habit, relative weight and ECG abnormalities to incidence of major coronary events: Final report of the Pooling Project. *Journal of Chronic Disease*, **31**, 201.

Potvin, L. and Frohlich, K.L. (1998). L'utilité de la notion de genre pour comprendre les inégalités de santé entre les homes et les femmes. *Ruptures, Revue Transdisciplinaire en Santé*, **5**, 142.

Prattala, R. Kaaaristo, A., and Berg, M.A. (1994). Consistency and variation in unhealthy behaviour among Finnish men 1982–1990. *Social Science and Medicine*, **39**, 115.

Prochaska, J. O., Redding, C. A., and Evers, K. E. (2002). The Transtheoretical model and stages of change. In *Health behavior and health education: Theory, research, and practice*, 3rd edition (eds. K. Glanz, B. K. Rimer, and F. M. Lewis), pp. 99–120. Jossey-Bass, San Francisco.

Prus, S. G. (2007). Age, SES, and health: A population level analysis of health inequalities over the life course. *Sociology, Health and Illness*, **29**, 275–96.

Raine, K. D. (2004). *Overweight and obesity in Canada: A population health perspective*. Canadian Institute for Health Information, Ottawa.

Ranson, M.K., Jha, P., Chaloupka, F.J. *et al.* (2002). Global and regional estimates of the effectiveness and cost-effectiveness of price increases and other tobacco control policies. *Nicotine and Tobacco Research*, **4**, 311–19.

Richard, L., Potvin, L., Kishuck, N. *et al.* (1996). Assessment of the integration of the ecological approach in health promotion programs. *American Journal of Health Promotion*, **10**, 318.

Rimm, E.B., Manson, J.E., Stampfer, M.J. *et al.* (1993). Cigarette smoking and the risk of diabetes in women. *American Journal of Public Health*, **83**, 211.

Robbins, A.S. Manson, J.E., Lee, I.M. *et al.* (1994). Cigarette smoking and stroke in a cohort of US male physicians. *Annals of Internal Medicine*, **120**, 458.

Rogers, E.S. (1968). Public health asks of sociology . . . Can the health sciences resolve society's problems in the absence of a science of human values and goals. *Science*, **159**, 506.

Rose, G. and Colwell, L. (1992). Randomized controlled trial of anti-smoking advice: Final (20-year) results. *Journal of Epidemiology and Community Health*, **46**, 75.

Ross, C.E. and Bird, C.E. (1994). Sex stratification and health lifestyle: Consequences for men's and women's perceived health. *Journal of Health and Social Behavior*, **35**, 161.

Rozin, P. (1984). The acquisition of food habits and preferences. In *Behavior health: A handbook of health enhancements and disease prevention* (eds. J.D. Matarzzo, S.M. Weiss, J.A. Herd *et al.*), p. 590. Wiley, New York.

Rutten, A. (1995). The implementation of health promotion: A new structural perspective. *Social Science and Medicine*, **41**, 1627.

Shea, S., Stein, A.D., Basch, C.E. *et al.* (1991). Independent associations of educational attainment and ethnicity with behavioral risk factors for cardiovascular disease. *American Journal of Epidemiology*, **134**, 567.

Simons-Morton, B.G., O'Hara, N.M., and Simons-Morton, D.G. (1986). Promoting healthful diet and exercise behaviors in communities, schools, and families. *Family and Community Health*, **9**, 1.

Simons-Morton, B.G., Brink, S.G., Parcel, G.S. *et al.* (1990). *Preventing acute alcohol-related health problems in adolescents and young adults.* Centers for Disease Control, Atlanta, GA.

Simons-Morton, B.G., Greene, W.H., and Gottlieb, N.H. (1995). Social change. In *Introduction to health education and health promotion*, 2nd edition. p. 193. Waveland Press, Prospect Heights, IL.

Simons-Morton, D.G., Simons-Morton, B.G., Parcel, G.S. *et al.* (1988a). Influencing personal and environmental conditions for community health: A multilevel intervention model. *Family and Community Health*, **11**, 25.

Simons-Morton, D.G., Brink, S.G., Parcel, G.S. *et al.* (1988b). *Promoting physical activity among adults: A CDC community intervention handbook.* Center for Disease Control, Atlanta, GA.

Simons-Morton, D.G., Mullen, P.D., Mains, D.A. *et al.* (1992). Characteristics of controlled studies of patient education and counseling for prevention behaviors. *Patient Education and Counseling*, **19**, 175.

Smith, B.J., Tang, K. C., and Nutbeam, D. (2006). WHO Health Promotion Glossary: new terms. *Health Promotion International*, **21**, 340–5.

Spencer, L., Pagell, F., and Adams, T. (2005). Applying the transtheoretical model to cancer screening behavior. *American Journal of Health Behavior*, **29**, 36–56.

Stamler, J. (1992). Established major coronary risk factors. In *Coronary heart disease epidemiology: From aetiology to public health* (eds. M. Marmot and P. Elliott), pp. 35–66. Oxford University Press, Oxford.

Stamler, J., Wentworth, D., and Neaton, J.D., for MRFIT Research Group (1986). Is the relationship between serum cholesterol and risk of premature death from coronary heart disease continuous and graded. Findings in 356,222 primary screenees of the Multiple Risk Factor Intervention Trial (MRFIT). *Journal of American Medical Association*, **256**, 2823–8.

Steele, J. and McBroom, W. (1972). Conceptual and empirical dimensions of health behavior. *Journal of Health and Social Behavior*, **13**, 382.

Stern, M.P. (1991). Primary prevention of type II diabetes mellitus. *Diabetes Care*, **14**, 399.

Steuart, G.W. (1965). Health, behavior, and planned change. *Health Education Monographs*, **20**, 3.

Stoto, M. A., Green, L. W., and Bailey, L. A. (eds.) (1997). *Linking research and public health practice: A review of CDC's program of Centers for Research and Demonstration of Health Promotion and Disease Prevention.* National Academy Press, Washington, DC. http://books.nap.edu/catalog/5564.html

Stout, C., Morrow, J., Brandt, E.N. *et al.* (1964). Unusually low incidence of death from myocardial infarction in an Italian-American community in Pennsylvania. *Journal of American Medical Association*, **188**, 845.

Stronks, K., Van de Mheen, D., Loomanm C.W.N. *et al.* (1996). Behavioural and structural factors in the explanation of socio-economic inequalities in health: An empirical analysis. *Sociology of Health and Illness*, **18**, 653.

Taylor, W.C., Sallis, J.F., Lees, E. *et al.* (2007). Changing social and built environments to promote physical activity: Recommendations from low income, urban women. *Journal of Physical Activity and Health*, **4**, 54–65.

Tjepkema, M. (2005). *Nutrition: Findings from the Canadian Community Health Survey. Issue No. 1 measured obesity: Adult obesity in Canada.* Statistics Canada, Ottawa.

Townsend, P., Davison, N., and Whitehead, M. (1988). *Inequalities in health.* Penguin, Harmondsworth.

UNICEF (1993). *The state of the world's children 1993.* Oxford University Press, New York.

U.S. CDC (US Centers for Disease control). (1993). Cigarette smoking attributable mortality and years of potential life lost United States, 1990. *Morbidity and Mortality Weekly Reports*, **42**, 645.

U.S. Department of Health and Human Services (2001). *Healthy people 2001: National health promotion and disease prevention objectives.* UC Government Printing Office, Washington, DC.

U.S. Department of Health and Human Services (2004). *The health consequences of smoking: A report of the Surgeon General.* U.S. Department of Health and Human Services, Centers for Disease Control and Prevention, Coordinating Center for Health Promotion, National Center for Chronic Disease Prevention and Health Promotion, Office on Smoking and Health, Atlanta. US Government Printing Office, Washington, DC.

U.S. Department of Health and Human Services (2006). *The health consequences of involuntary exposure to tobacco smoke: A report of the Surgeon General—executive summary.* U.S. Department of Health and Human Services, Centers for Disease Control and Prevention, Coordinating Center for Health Promotion, National Center for Chronic Disease Prevention and Health Promotion, Office on Smoking and Health, Atlanta.

Verbrugge, L.M. (1989). The twain meet: Empirical explanations of sex differences in health and mortality. *Journal of Health and Social Behavior*, **30**, 282.

Villas, P., Cardenas, M., and Jameson, C. (1993). Instrument development using the PRECEDE model to distinguish users/triers from non-users of alcoholic beverages. *Wellness Perspectives: Research, Theory and Practice*, **10**, 46.

Walker, D., Gutierrez, J. P., Torres, P. *et al.* (2006). HIV prevention in Mexican schools: Prospective randomized evaluation of intervention. *British Medical Journal*, **332**, 1189.

Ward, J. W. and Warren, C. S. (eds.) (2007). *A safer and healthier America: Public health in the 20th century.* Oxford University Press, New York.

WHO (World Health Organization) (1981). *Global strategy for health for all by the year 2000.* WHO, Geneva.

WHO (World Health Organization) (1990). *Prevention in childhood and youth adult cardiovascular diseases: Time for action.* WHO technical report 792. WHO, Geneva.

WHO (World Health Organization) (1998). *Tobacco epidemic: Health dimensions.* Fact Sheet No. 154, revised. WHO, Geneva.

WHO (World Health Organization) (2000). *Obesity: Preventing and managing the global epidemic.* WHO technical report series no. 894. World Health Organization, Geneva.

Wilkinson, R.G. (1992a). Income distribution and life expectancy. *British Medical Journal*, **304**, 165.

Wilkinson, R.G. (1992b). National mortality rates: The impact of inequality. *American Journal of Public Health*, **82**, 1082.

Wilkinson, R.G. (1996). *Unhealthy society. The afflictions of inequality.* Routledge, London.

Wilkinson, R.G. (1999). Income inequality, social cohesion, and health: Clarifying the theory—A reply to Muntaner and Lynch. *International Journal of Health Services*, **29**, 525.

Wilkinson, R.G. and Marmot, M. (1998). *The solid facts.* World Health Organization, Geneva.

Wilkinson, R.G. and Pickett, K.E. (2008). Income inequality and socioeconomic gradients in mortality. *American Journal of Public Health*, **98**, 699–704.

Winkleby, M.A., Jatulis, D.E., Franck, E. *et al.* (1992a). Socio-economic status and health: how education, income, and occupation contribute to risk factors for cardiovascular disease. *American Journal of Public Health*, **82**, 816.

Winkleby, M.A., Fortman, S.P., and Rockhill, B. (1992*b*). Trends in cardiovascular risk factors by educational level: The Stanford Five City Project. *Preventive Medicine*, **21**, 592.

Wodak, A. (2006). Controlling HIV among injecting drug users: The current status of harm reduction. *HIV AIDS Policy and Law Review*, **11**, 77–80.

World Bank (1991). *World development report. Special population issues.* World Bank, Washington, DC.

World Bank (1993). *World development report 1993. Investing in health.* Oxford University Press, New York.

2.4

Genomics and public health

Alison Stewart, Wylie Burke,
Muin J. Khoury, and Ron Zimmerns

Introduction and historical perspectives

Public health has not traditionally been concerned with genomics. Practitioners of public health have regarded populations as essentially homogeneous, differing only in their exposures to environmental and social determinants of health such as poverty, poor housing, or toxic or infectious agents. Until recently, genomics and public health rarely came together except in the context of population screening programmes for certain genetic conditions. The first of these was newborn screening for the inherited metabolic disease phenylketonuria (PKU), for which biochemical screening and diagnostic tests became available during the 1960s (Botkin 2005). Although this genetic disease was rare, screening was recognized as a public health responsibility because early diagnosis and treatment of affected infants could prevent serious mental and physical disability in the population.

At around the same time, the speciality of medical genetics began to be recognized in some countries as a clinical discipline in its own right. As new interventions such as antenatal diagnosis for some genetic disorders were developed during the next few decades, geneticists and some public health professionals became involved in assessing population needs for services offering these interventions (Royal College of Physicians 1991) and, in countries such as the United Kingdom where public health has a role in healthcare service organization and delivery, in commissioning and allocating resources for them.

In some countries, enthusiasm for population screening broadened after the success of the early newborn screening programmes to include screening of sections of the adult population for some genetic conditions. In the United States, for example, mandatory screening of the African American population for sickle cell disease was introduced in the early 1970s. However the programme was ill-conceived: No clinical or public health benefits were identified, and there was evidence of stigmatization and discrimination against unaffected carriers of the condition (Markel 1997). Some other programmes met with more success, notably a carrier screening programme for Tay Sachs disease in the Ashkenazi Jewish community (Markel 1997) and screening for β-thalassaemia in Sardinia and Cyprus (Cao *et al.* 2002). Although newborn screening programmes continued, a general distrust of public health motives for population screening, together with the malign legacy of the eugenics movement of the early to mid-twentieth century, resulted during the late 1970s and 1980s in a general distancing of medical genetics from mainstream public health.

The impact of the 'new' genetics

In 1990, the Human Genome Project began. This ambitious enterprise aimed to sequence the entire 3 billion DNA base pairs of the human genome within a 15-year time frame, providing the raw material for discovering the sequences of the complete set of human genes and, eventually, finding out their functions and how they participate both in normal physiology and during the initiation and progression of disease. As it turned out, the sequencing project was finished ahead of schedule: A 'reference sequence' for the genome, including the almost complete sequences for its complement of around 25 000 genes, was published in 2003 (Collins *et al.* 2003).

The Human Genome Project accelerated progress in finding the genes that, when mutated, cause heritable diseases such as cystic fibrosis, Duchenne muscular dystrophy, and Huntington's disease. By the early years of the twenty-first century, the genes implicated in some 1800 of these genetic diseases (most of them very rare) had been identified and catalogued in the Online Mendelian Inheritance in Man database (http://www.ncbi.nlm.nih.gov/entrez/query.fcgi?db=OMIM). The availability of molecular diagnosis for many of these conditions began to transform the practice of medical genetics and spurred attempts to find better treatments.

During the same period, attention was also turning towards the subject of 'normal' human genetic variation and the opportunity of using the information and technology generated by the Human Genome Project to identify common genetic variants (or alleles) associated with disease in human populations (Willard *et al.* 2005). Many genetic epidemiology projects were initiated to search for gene–disease associations. In an effort to provide tools for such studies, the Human Genome Project consortia instigated first the single nucleotide polymorphism (SNP) project and then the HapMap project (Guttmacher & Collins 2005). The SNP and HapMap initiatives aimed to provide a map of common variation at the single-base level across the genome and to identify 'tagging' SNPs that characterized particular clusters of variants, or haplotypes, in different populations. These resources are beginning to bear fruit in successful whole-genome association studies, where markers distributed across the entire genome are scanned for possible association with a disease or other condition (Hirschhorn &

Daly 2005). These studies, often carried out by large international consortia and involving many thousands of study participants, have successfully identified common genomic variants associated with conditions including type II diabetes, coronary artery disease, and breast cancer (see, for example, The Wellcome Trust Case Control Consortium 2007).

The aim of all these studies is to achieve a better understanding of the molecular basis of human health and disease and to use this knowledge to develop a more accurate categorization of disease and susceptibility, together with new diagnostic technologies and more effective interventions, both preventive and therapeutic (Guttmacher *et al.* 2001; Collins & McKusick 2001). Alongside these aims is the hope of harnessing an understanding of human genomic variation to develop interventions that are targeted at those most likely to benefit.

Public health genomics

The population-level goals of the Human Genome Project, and the expectation that its achievements will in time bring profound changes both to clinical health services and to disease prevention, pose clear challenges and opportunities for public health practice (Khoury 1996). It may no longer be tenable for public health practitioners to regard populations as homogeneous, with 'one size fits all' answers to the problems posed by common, chronic conditions such as coronary heart disease, diabetes, or dementia. Genomic factors will also have to be incorporated into the assessment and control of important public health issues such as environmental health, nutrition, and infectious disease.

Nevertheless, doubts have been raised about the timing and occurrence of the widely touted 'genomics revolution' in medicine, and there are concerns that an over-emphasis on genomic contributors to disease may result in neglect of other factors such as environmental exposures, social structure, and lifestyle. Along with clear advances, genome-based research will almost certainly generate many promising ideas that do not ultimately yield health benefits.

As with other emerging technologies, the challenge is to devise an efficient strategy to distinguish between innovative advances and false leads. The potential benefits offered by the Human Genome Project need to be weighed against the resources required to implement them and against the potential harms.

The recognition of these challenges and opportunities and the need for a strategy to address them have led over the last decade to the emergence of the new field of public health genomics (Khoury 2003; Khoury *et al.* 2000; Stewart *et al.* 2007). The use of the term 'genomics' rather than 'genetics' signals that the subject matter is not confined to rare heritable diseases. The scientific basis for public health genomics is all the information stemming from the Human Genome Project and related '-omics' initiatives: Not only gene sequences and gene–disease associations, but also information about the spectrum of gene expression activity, gene products and metabolites in different tissue types, and in normal and disease states (functional genomics, proteomics, and metabolomics). Diagnostic and predictive biomarkers developed as a result of research in molecular and cell biology will increasingly be applied in clinical and preventive medicine, bringing opportunities to realize benefits for population health.

In this chapter, we will first outline the theoretical underpinnings of public health genomics: The recognition of genes as determinants of health, the importance of gene–environment interactions, and the relationships between genomic factors and disease. We will then look in more detail at some important areas where public health and genomics intersect: The use and evaluation of genetic and genomic tests, the criteria for population screening programmes involving genomic factors, and the use of genomics in disease prevention. This analysis will be followed by consideration of the ethical principles for the application of genomics in public health practice and, finally, by discussion of the challenges and prospects for public health genomics both immediately and in the coming decades.

We assume that readers have an understanding of the basic principles of genetics. For those needing background information or revision, there are many excellent Web-based tutorials such as *DNA from the Beginning*, produced by the Cold Spring Harbor Laboratory (http://www.dnaftb.org/dnaftb). A glossary of important terms and their definitions is provided in Box 2.4.1.

Genes as determinants of health

It has been known for many years that individuals differ in their susceptibility to environmental agents such as diet, housing, air and water quality, sanitation, and infectious agents. For example, in the nineteenth century when tuberculosis was rife in western European populations, physicians knew that individuals varied in their susceptibility to infection and attributed this variation to differences in individual 'constitution'. However, nothing was known about the 'constitutional' (essentially, genetic) factors involved, and so for all practical purposes they were ignored.

The new era of genomics mandates a change from this way of thinking, to one that explicitly recognizes genes as determinants of health (Fig. 2.4.1). An important feature of this model is that it emphasizes the interplay between genomic and environmental factors (an 'environmental' factor in this context is anything that is not genomic). Obesity presents a classic example. Genomic factors are known to influence an individual's appetite and sensation of satiation after a meal. Individuals with impaired mechanisms of appetite and satiation will seek more food and, if food is in abundant supply, will put on weight, sometimes to the point of obesity. Environmental factors can also influence genes: For example, ionizing radiation may cause DNA mutations that lead to cancer; if mutations affect germ-line cells, they may be transmitted to future generations.

Whether a disease appears to be primarily 'genetic' or 'environmental' depends on the relative prevalence of the causative factors. Once again, history provides an example. Vitamin D deficiency is known to cause the disease rickets, a discovery made during an era when the disease was relatively common due to the prevalence of childhood malnutrition. Today, however, childhood malnutrition is rare in the developed world, and the few cases of rickets that are seen are more likely to be caused by rare genetic disorders of vitamin D metabolism.

Rothman (1986) observed that any disease can be shown to be both 100 per cent inherited and 100 per cent environmental. The classic example is PKU. We refer to PKU as a genetic disease because the dietary factor, phenylalanine, is ubiquitous whereas the genetic

Box 2.4.1 Glossary of basic terms in genetics and genomics

Alleles	Variant forms of the same gene
Autosomes	Chromosomes that are not concerned with sex determination. Humans have 22 pairs of autosomes and two sex chromosomes
Biomarker	A factor used to indicate or measure a biological process (for example, a specific protein or genetic polymorphism)
Carrier	Usually refers to an individual who is heterozygous for a recessive disease-causing allele
Chromosomes	The structures within cells that carry the genetic information in the form of DNA
Dominant	A characteristic that is expressed even when the relevant gene is present in only one copy
Epigenetic	A factor or mechanism that changes the expression of a gene without affecting its DNA sequence, and is stably transmitted during cell division
Genome	The complete set of genetic information of an organism
Genotype	The specific genetic constitution of an individual
Germ-line	Relating to the sex cells, which transmit genetic information from one generation to the next
Haplotype	A specific set of alleles located on the same chromosome
Heterozygous	Carrying two different alleles of a gene
Homozygous	Carrying two identical alleles of a gene
Karyotype	A description of the number and structure of chromosomes in an individual
Locus	The location of a gene or DNA marker on a chromosome
Marker	A gene or other segment of DNA whose chromosomal position is known
Mendelian	Relating to the laws of inheritance discovered by Gregor Mendel
Meiosis	The specialized cell division that takes place when sex cells (sperm or eggs) are produced. The members of each chromosome pair separate so each sex cell receives only one copy of each gene
Mutation	A change in the sequence of DNA
Nucleotide	The molecular units that make up DNA and RNA. A nucleotide of DNA consists of a base (A, C, G, or T) linked to the sugar deoxyribose and a phosphate group
Penetrance	The likelihood that an individual carrying a specific genetic variant will show the characteristic determined by that variant
Phenotype	The observable traits of an organism
Polymorphism	A common genetic variant or allele (present in at least 1–2 per cent of the population)
Recessive	A characteristic that is only expressed when two copies of the relevant gene are present
SNP	Single nucleotide polymorphism: A DNA sequence variation that involves a change in a single nucleotide
Somatic	Relating to the cells of the body other than the germ-line (sex) cells and their precursors

defect is rare, occurring in around 1 in 10 000 births. If, in an alternative world, a population all had the genetic abnormality that we associate with PKU but phenylalanine was not found in the diet of that population, the few cases of PKU observed in that world would be deemed to be toxic or nutritional in origin.

It is clear, then, that the well-known 'nature versus nurture' debate in disease causation is meaningless, as are attempts to classify diseases as '*x* per cent genetic and *y* per cent environmental': All disease results from the combined effects of genes and environment. Box 2.4.2 presents some examples of effects of genetic and environmental exposures on disease risk.

The role of genes in disease

'Genetic' diseases

Although both genes and environment contribute to all diseases, in some cases a single alteration to the genetic code—a mutation—appears to be sufficient to cause disease. Examples of such classical 'genetic diseases' include cystic fibrosis, Huntington's disease, and sickle cell disease. Genetic diseases of this type are also sometimes known as Mendelian diseases because they show patterns of transmission from one generation to the next that conform to Mendel's laws of inheritance.

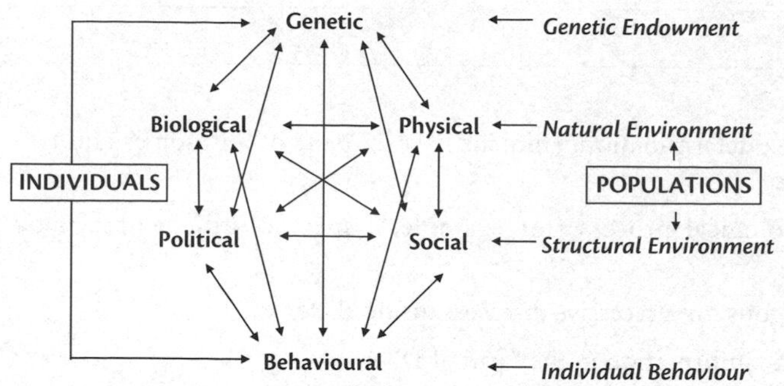

Fig. 2.4.1 Determinants of health.

Chromosomal disorders—caused by deletions, duplications, translocations, or inversions of whole chromosomes or chromosome segments—are also generally classed as genetic diseases because they are clearly correlated with an observable genetic lesion. An example of a chromosomal disorder is Down syndrome, which is caused by an extra copy of chromosome 21.

Although *potentially* heritable, genetic diseases are not always inherited. Almost all cases of Down syndrome arise as a result of a sporadic genetic lesion, usually during maternal meiosis. Some other genetic diseases show a similarly high proportion of sporadic cases. For example, approximately one-third of cases of the genetic disease tuberous sclerosis are inherited, whereas the remaining two-thirds arise from new mutations. In most cases, the cause of the new mutation is unknown.

In many countries of the developed world, specialist clinical genetics services care for individuals and families affected by genetic diseases. A recent book by Read and Donnai (2007) provides an excellent, practical background to all aspects of medical genetics and its clinical practice.

Mendelian diseases and chromosomal disorders are individually rare. However, collectively they represent a substantial burden of morbidity and mortality: Around 4000 Mendelian diseases have been recognized, with a combined birth frequency of approximately 1–2 per cent in populations in the developed world (Royal College of Physicians of London 1991).

The prevalence of genetic diseases may vary substantially in different populations, probably reflecting selective factors operating on the genes involved. For example, the birth prevalence of sickle cell disease, a recessive disorder, is very low in populations of Northern European origin, but as high as 1 in 80 in some black African populations (World Health Organization 1996). The reason is thought to be that, in the heterozygous state, sickle cell alleles confer resistance to malaria and so have been maintained by evolutionary pressures in populations exposed to malaria, despite the severe disadvantage they cause for homozygous individuals.

In some cases a 'founder effect' may be implicated: Particular alleles that arose in a small, isolated founder population may persist in the population through many generations if it remains relatively genetically isolated from other population groups. A probable example of a founder effect is the relatively high prevalence, in Ashkenazi Jews, of alleles causing the recessive disorder Tay Sachs disease.

The role of genes in common disease

Genes also play a role in susceptibility to the common diseases of later life such as coronary heart disease, type II diabetes, Alzheimer's dementia, and cancers. An indication that genomic factors are at work comes from the observation that in many cases such diseases show a tendency to 'run in families', though shared environment also contributes to familial effects. It is thought that genetic susceptibility to common disease is attributable to the combined action of many different common genomic variants that are individually of weak effect.

Box 2.4.2 Some patterns of relative risk in gene–environment interactions

The table shows three examples of different patterns of risk for three classical genetic diseases that have an environmental component, assuming dichotomous genetic susceptibility and environmental exposure.

In the first example, xeroderma pigmentosum (XP), exposure to ultraviolet light increases the risk of developing skin cancer in non-carriers of XP mutations, but the combination of these mutations and exposure to ultraviolet light vastly increases the risk. In theory, if individuals with XP mutations completely avoid ultraviolet light their risk of skin cancer becomes close to the background risk.

In the second example, phenylketonuria (PKU), only individuals with recessive mutations in the causative gene who are exposed to phenylalanine in the diet are susceptible to PKU.

In the third example, deficiency in the alpha-1-antitrypsin gene, both non-smokers who are at genetic risk and smokers who are not at genetic risk have an increased risk of developing emphysema, and the combination (smokers who are at genetic risk) is associated with the highest risk.

Gene variant	Environmental exposure	Relative risk (XP)	Relative risk (PKU)	Relative risk (emphysema)
Absent	Absent	1.0	1.0	1.0
Present	Absent	~1.0	1.0	Modest
Absent	Present	Modest	1.0	Modest
Present	Present	Very high	Very high	High

Reprinted with permission from Macmillan Publishers Ltd: Hunter, DJ. *Nature Reviews Genetics* **6**, 287–98, copyright 2005.

The genomic variants that affect susceptibility to common disease are so far mostly unknown. Many reported genotype–disease associations have not yet been independently validated though, as discussed previously, large-scale whole-genome association studies are now beginning to yield replicable associations. An example of an association that is supported by good evidence concerns alleles of the gene encoding the protein component of a blood lipoprotein, apolipoprotein E (APOE). Individuals with one copy of the *APOE4* allele have a risk of Alzheimer's dementia that is 2.5–3 times the risk of individuals with two copies of the more common *APOE3* allele. Homozygosity for the *APOE4* allele increases the relative risk still further, to 10–15 times the risk of *APOE3* homozygotes. Table 2.4.1 lists some other examples of validated gene–disease associations.

For some common diseases, including common cancers such as breast/ovarian cancer and colorectal cancer, there are families in which several family members are affected by the same disease, often at an early age, and the disease shows a Mendelian inheritance pattern through the family, suggesting the existence of a single mutation that confers a high risk of disease. In these Mendelian (single gene) subsets of common disease, genotype can be used with a fairly high degree of certainty to predict the development of disease.

An example is familial hypercholesterolaemia, a dominantly inherited condition that is characterized by a build-up of cholesterol and a high risk of premature cardiovascular disease. The disease is caused by mutations in a gene encoding a cell-surface receptor for a blood lipoprotein. About 1 in 500 people are thought to carry the mutant gene, and virtually all will develop symptoms of the disease at some stage of their life. In the population as a whole, only about 1 in 20 people who develop hypercholesterolaemia carry a strongly predisposing single-gene mutation; in general, single-gene subsets of common diseases account for a maximum of 5–10 per cent of the total burden of disease.

Complexities of gene–disease relationships

In Mendelian diseases and chromosomal disorders, a single genetic defect can be sufficient to cause disease. Such diseases are said to be completely or highly penetrant. The penetrance of a genotype is the probability that an individual with that genotype will be affected by the disease. Penetrance is always associated with a time frame; for example, lifetime penetrance, or penetrance by age 60, and so on. Cystic fibrosis is generally fully penetrant during early childhood, while Huntington's disease is fully penetrant by late middle age. Not all Mendelian diseases are fully penetrant, though in most cases penetrance is high; essentially, it is high penetrance that causes the disease to be recognized as Mendelian. For example, breast cancer associated with mutations in the *BRCA1* gene has a lifetime penetrance of 40–85 per cent (Antoniou *et al.* 2003; the higher estimates come from families with multiple cases of the disease, and the lower estimates from population-based studies).

Table 2.4.1 Selected genetic associations validated through meta-analysis

Gene	Variant (contrast)	Disease	OR	95% CI
ACE	DD (DI/II)	Myocardial infarction	1.28	1.09–1.50
KCNJ11	E23K KK (EK/EE)	Diabetes type 2	1.92	1.29–2.97
TGFA	Taq1 (allele2 vs 1)	Nonsyndromic cleft lip	1.58	1.13–2.21
MTHFR	677 (TT vs CC/CT)	Neural tube defects	1.70	1.31–2.21
MAPT	Allele AD vs others	Parkinson disease	1.52	1.22–1.90
GSTM1	null/null vs others	Bladder cancer	1.54	1.27–1.86
F5	Leiden vs others	Preeclampsia	2.22	1.46–3.38
DRD2	Ser311Cys Cys vs ser	Schizophrenia	1.43	1.16–1.76

Noncomprehensive list from 50 genetic associations validated through meta-analysis as reported by Ioannidis *et al.* (2006).

Incomplete penetrance is an indication that other factors are involved in determining whether an individual will be affected: These other factors may be other genes and/or environmental factors. Even for diseases whose penetrance is high, other genetic and/or environmental factors are likely to affect the expressivity of the disease: For example, characteristics such as the range and severity of symptoms, or the age of onset.

Complexity is also evident in the spectrum of mutations that may be associated with the 'same' disease. This phenomenon, known as genetic heterogeneity, is a complicating factor in the development and clinical application of genetic tests. Genetic heterogeneity may be allelic (different alleles of the same gene associated with the same disease) or non-allelic (alleles of different genes associated with the same disease; also called locus heterogeneity).

Genetic heterogeneity is extremely common. For example, more than 1000 different pathogenic mutations have been found in the *CFTR* gene associated with cystic fibrosis. Similarly, familial breast cancer may be caused by any of hundreds of different mutations in the *BRCA1* or *BRCA2* genes. Sometimes, particular mutations may be more common in a specific population. For example, in cystic fibrosis patients of Northern European origin the frequency of the ΔF508 mutation in the *CFTR* gene is about 70 per cent, whereas in African American cystic fibrosis patients it is only about 40 per cent. For this reason, clinical genetic testing protocols may need to be modified depending on the racial or ethnic origin of the person being tested.

DNA sequence variation is not the only source of variation in gene function. In multicellular organisms, different types of cells acquire their functional characteristics by expressing different subsets of their genome in a specific temporal pattern. Differential gene expression is associated with chemical modifications to the DNA (such as methylation) that do not change the primary DNA sequence and are termed epigenetic. As cells of a specific type multiply, they stably transmit these epigenetic modifications to the cells they give rise to. Epigenetic mechanisms are likely to play a role in mediating changes in gene expression in response to environmental signals (Jaenisch & Bird 2003). Disruption in epigenetic processes is known to play a role in some diseases, including cancer. Epigenetic changes are not generally thought to be heritable by the organism's offspring but there is some emerging evidence that trans-generational effects may occur (Richards 2006).

Because biological systems are so complex, it is almost always an over-simplification to speak in terms of a 'gene for' a particular characteristic or disease: No gene acts in isolation.

Genetic and genomic tests

Virtually all medical tests are to some degree 'genetic', because genetic factors have played a part in the development of the characteristics (for example blood pressure, eyesight, or bone density) that are tested.

A US Task Force on Genetic Testing defined a genetic test as 'the analysis of human DNA, RNA, chromosomes, proteins, and certain metabolites in order to detect heritable disease-related genotypes, mutations, phenotypes, or karyotypes for clinical purposes' (Holtzman & Watson 1997). This definition implies that a genetic test is a test that enables a direct inference about the state of the germ-line genetic material. Any diagnostic test for a Mendelian disease or chromosomal disorder qualifies as a genetic test because it allows such an inference. For example, a renal ultrasound test for autosomal dominant polycystic kidney disease may be considered a genetic test because it enables the inference that there is or is not a lesion in one of the genes causally implicated in this disease. A biochemical analysis to detect haemoglobin variants causing sickle cell disease is also a genetic test. Any direct DNA test is a genetic test, whether it relates to a single-gene or chromosomal disorder, or to a low-penetrance genetic factor implicated in a common disease. However, a blood pressure test, for example, is not a genetic test by this definition because it does not enable any direct inference about the sequence or properties of a specific gene or genes.

The nature and implications of a genetic test can vary widely, depending largely on the penetrance of the condition or the genotype in question. It is important, when using the term genetic test, to be clear about whether it is being used to denote a test for a genetic (highly penetrant heritable) disease, or simply to mean a test of the genetic material (Zimmern 2001). A test for a genetic condition may have serious implications both for the person tested and for his or her blood relatives. In contrast, a test for a common DNA polymorphism associated with susceptibility to, say, coronary heart disease will probably have no more serious implications for health than analysis of blood lipids, and no greater consequences for other family members.

The US Task Force's definition specifically excludes somatic genetic tests, such as tests of the genetic material in tumour cells or gene expression profiles in different tissues or organs. However, the development, use, and evaluation of somatic genetic tests—perhaps better termed 'genomic tests'—also pose both opportunities and challenges for public health. Somatic genomic tests may also include tests for other complex genomic biomarkers such as proteomic or metabolomic profiles.

Uses of genetic and genomic tests

Genetic and genomic tests may be used in:

- Diagnosis of a disease.
- Prediction of risk for a disease.
- Prediction of response to a therapeutic or preventive intervention. The most familiar scenario is prediction of response to a therapeutic drug. This use of genetic test information is known as *pharmacogenetics*.

It has recently been suggested that this categorization in fact misses the point, and that diagnosis and prediction are only means to various ends. The ultimate purpose of carrying out a genetic test is (a) to reduce morbidity or mortality, (b) to provide salient health information that will benefit the clinical care of the patient, or (c) to enable reproductive choice; and the effectiveness of the test should be evaluated with regard to the stated purpose (Burke *et al.* 2007).

Diagnostic genetic tests

Diagnostic genetic tests may be used at any stage of life (preimplantation, prenatal, newborn, childhood, adolescence, or middle age) to detect a DNA or chromosomal variant (or variants) associated with a disease. At present they are only in routine clinical use for highly penetrant single-gene (Mendelian) diseases and chromosomal disorders (see Table 2.4.2 for some examples). In the future, DNA tests may be used to clarify the diagnosis of specific molecular subtypes of common disease.

Diagnostic DNA tests carried out before birth (preimplantation or prenatal genetic diagnosis) may be used by couples at risk of transmitting a specific genetic disease to determine whether the embryo or foetus is affected by the disease. The purpose of testing is to enable the couple to exercise reproductive choice by either preparing for the birth of an affected child or opting to terminate the pregnancy. In the case of preimplantation diagnosis, only unaffected embryos are used to establish a pregnancy.

Diagnostic genetic tests in the postnatal period may be used to provide a definitive diagnosis in cases where genetic disease is suspected. For example, in an infant affected by severe muscle wasting, a DNA test may confirm a diagnosis of Duchenne muscular dystrophy.

A special category of diagnostic test is a carrier test, which is used to detect a carrier of a Mendelian autosomal recessive or sex-linked disease. Individuals in families or populations affected by such diseases may wish to know whether they are carriers and therefore, although not themselves affected, at risk of transmitting the disease to their children.

Diagnostic genomic biomarkers

Genomic biomarkers such as gene expression, proteomic or metabolomic profiles convey information about the molecular-genetic characteristics of somatic cells that may be correlated with clinical parameters such as disease staging, prognosis, and response to therapy. Gene expression and proteomic profiling is an active area of clinical research, particularly in oncology. For example, gene expression profiling, using microarrays, has been used to distinguish different tumour subtypes in diffuse large B-cell lymphomas (Staudt & Dave 2005). Serum proteomic profiling has been investigated as a screening test for early diagnosis of ovarian cancer (Petricoin *et al.* 2002).

However, although one Phase III clinical trial of gene expression profiling in breast cancer is underway, and some commercial 'kits' for gene expression and proteomic profiling are available, these technologies are not yet ready for mainstream clinical implementation (Quackenbush 2006). Difficulties that need to be overcome include inadequate reproducibility, lack of standardization, failure to demonstrate improved outcomes as compared with current clinical practice, and poor positive predictive values, especially when used as screening tests in a population setting.

Predictive genetic tests

Because an individual's germ-line DNA remains largely unchanged throughout life, DNA testing can in some circumstances be used in

Table 2.4.2 Examples of molecular genetic tests

Condition	Genes	Reported uses of testing
Neurological		
Spinocerebellar ataxia	*SCA1, SCA2, SCA3, SCA6, SCA7, SCA10, DRPLA*	Diagnostic, predictive
Fragile X syndrome	*FMR1*	Diagnostic, antenatal
Huntington's disease	*HD*	Diagnostic, predictive, antenatal
Connective tissue		
Ehlers–Danos syndrome, vascular type	*COL3A1*	Diagnostic, antenatal
Marfan syndrome	*FBN1*	Diagnostic, antenatal
Oncological		
Familial adenomatous polyposis	*APC*	Diagnostic, predictive
Hereditary non-polyposis colorectal cancer	*MLH1, MSH2, PMS2, MSH3, MSH6*	Diagnostic, predictive
Familial breast/ovarian cancer	*BRCA1, BRCA2*	Diagnostic, predictive
Haematological		
Beta-thalassaemia	Beta-globin (*HbB*)	Carrier detection, antenatal
Haemophilia A	*F8C*	Prognostic, carrier detection, antenatal
Haemophilia B	*F9C*	Carrier detection, antenatal
Renal		
Polycystic kidney disease (autosomal dominant and autosomal recessive)	*PKD1, PKD2, PKHD1*	Predictive, antenatal
Multisystem		
Achondroplasia	*FGFR3*	Antenatal
Alpha1-antitrypsin deficiency	*AAT*	Diagnostic, predictive
Galactosaemia	*GALT*	Newborn screening, carrier detection, antenatal
Neurofibromatosis type 1	*NF1*	Antenatal
Neurofibromatosis type 2	*NF2*	Predictive, antenatal

Source: Adapted from Burke, W. *New England Journal of Medicine* **347**, 1867–75.

an asymptomatic individual to predict the risk of a specific disease occurring in the future. The classic example is Huntington's disease, which may be predicted with almost 100 per cent certainty by a DNA test even before birth. A positive test result for a pathogenic mutation in the *APC* gene associated with familial adenomatous polyposis, an inherited form of bowel cancer, predicts future disease with 90–100 per cent certainty. In the context of highly penetrant Mendelian conditions, predictive testing is sometimes termed *presymptomatic testing*.

However, this high degree of predictive value is rare. Huntington's disease has a population prevalence of about 1 in 20 000–40 000, and fewer than 0.5 per cent of bowel cancer cases are thought to be due to inherited mutations in the *APC* gene. In relation to common disease, the predictive value of DNA test information is much lower; such tests may be better described as susceptibility or predispositional tests.

Pharmacogenetic tests

Heritable genetic factors are known to affect responses to many classes of therapeutic drugs. Variable responses may include increased or decreased sensitivity to the drug, as well as adverse or toxic drug reactions. For example, variants of genes encoding members of the cytochrome P450 family of enzymes affect dosage requirements for a wide range of drugs including warfarin, codeine, clozapine, and timolol (Wolf *et al.* 2000). Certain polymorphisms in the gene encoding the enzyme thiopurine *S*-methyltransferase (TPMT) are associated with serious adverse reactions to thiopurine immunosuppressive drugs, such as azathioprine, used in oncology and other fields of medicine (Gardiner & Begg 2006).

The concept underlying pharmacogenetics is that it may be possible to use DNA testing to tailor drug prescribing to an individual's genetic make-up, thereby optimizing response and minimizing adverse reactions. The path from discovery of a validated polymorphism influencing drug response to a clinically useful pharmacogenetic test is a complex one. The anti-coagulant drug warfarin provides an instructive example. Warfarin dose requirement is affected by variation in the *CYP2C9* gene (Sanderson *et al.* 2005). However, other factors such as age, sex, other genes, and drug interactions also affect warfarin response (and response to most other drugs); the predictive value of *CYP2C9* testing is not known accurately but may be only about 20 per cent (Sconce *et al.* 2005). It is not clear whether *CYP2C9* testing would offer appreciable advantages over current best practice in warfarin prescribing, which includes careful clinical evaluation of the patient and post-prescription monitoring.

Proposed pharmacogenetic tests need careful consideration on a case-by-case basis, including determination of sensitivity, specificity, positive and negative predictive values, and cost-effectiveness. The optimal parameters for a pharmacogenetic test will vary for different test indications.

Pharmacogenetic tests for heritable variants remain mostly at the research stage but some somatic pharmacogenetic tests are already in clinical use, particularly in oncology. An example is the typing of *HER2* gene expression in breast tumours to test for responsiveness to the drug Herceptin® (trastuzumab), an antibody drug that targets the HER2 protein on the surface of tumour cells.

Gene expression profiling is also under investigation as a tool to guide optimal treatment. For example, patients whose tumour gene expression profile, together with standard clinical criteria, indicates a good prognosis and a low probability of metastasis may be spared debilitating aggressive treatment with adjuvant chemotherapy. As discussed previously, gene expression profiling needs further evaluation before adoption for mainstream clinical use.

Evaluation of genetic and genomic tests

Public health professionals have a role in ensuring that any diagnostic, predictive, or pharmacogenetic tests used in clinical or public health practice are properly evaluated in order to protect patients and health services. A genetic test (or any other clinical test) encompasses more than a laboratory assay. Rather, it is a complex process that is part of an overall regime of disease prevention or management for a specific individual (Kroese *et al.* 2004). A test is best conceived of as the application of an assay for a particular disease, in a particular population, and for a particular purpose (Kroese *et al.* 2004). An assay may be deemed highly effective in one set of circumstances but not in another.

The first attempt to devise an evaluation framework for genetic tests was the ACCE project (Haddow & Palomaki 2004), using criteria originally proposed by the 1997 Task Force on Genetic Testing (Holtzman and Watson 1997). ACCE is an acronym standing for **A**nalytical validity, **C**linical validity, **C**linical utility, and **E**thical, legal, and social implications. Recently, it has been acknowledged that ethical, legal, and social implications such as potential discrimination, stigmatization, and psychosocial consequences form part of the assessment of the overall utility of a test (Grosse & Khoury 2006), and there has been a trend away from regarding them as a separable set of issues.

Analytical validity

The analytical validity is the means by which an assay is evaluated. It is defined as the assay's ability to measure accurately (in the case of a genetic test) the genotype of interest. It is important to define the genotype precisely. A test to detect 24 specific mutations in the *CFTR* gene is not the same test as one designed to detect only 4 mutations, for example. The test characteristics will differ in these two circumstances because the reference standard will be different. A distinction can also be made between open-ended assays such as karyotyping (microscopic examination of the chromosomes) or mutation scanning across a gene, in which any abnormality is sought, and closed assays, which specify in advance the spectrum of mutations or abnormalities the assay is designed to test (Burke & Zimmern 2007).

Clinical validity

Clinical validity is the ability of a test to diagnose or predict a specific phenotype (usually, a specific disease); here, the reference standard is a clinical one. The clinical validity of a test encompasses more than a demonstration of good epidemiological association between a test result (the presence of a genetic variant) and the disease. There must additionally be a formal evaluation of test performance in practice.

For closed assays, parameters such as sensitivity, specificity, positive and negative predictive values, likelihood ratios, and the receiver operating characteristic (ROC) curve can be measured. Even if there is a strong association between a genetic variant and a disease, as has been shown for the *TCF7L2* polymorphism and type II diabetes, a clinical test for this polymorphism may have very limited predictive value and thus poor clinical validity (Janssens *et al.* 2006).

Assessment of clinical validity is more difficult for open-ended assays. As a result, proxies must be used to estimate the clinical performance of an open-ended test. Microarray comparative genomic hybridization (CGH) offers an example (Subramonia-Iyer *et al.* 2007). CGH is a new technique for detecting submicroscopic chromosomal abnormalities, including some never detected before and some that are unlikely to be of clinical significance. In this setting, measures based on biological plausibility can be used to estimate the likelihood that a detected abnormality is clinically significant (e.g. nature and location of the abnormality; whether similar chromosomal abnormalities have been described in normal populations). With the use of these parameters, the test can be evaluated for its estimated diagnostic yield (proportion of those tested with a positive result) and false positive yield.

Clinical utility

Clinical utility refers to the likelihood that a test will lead to an improved health outcome, whether in terms of the clinical course of the disease by way of reduced mortality or morbidity, or in terms of reduced impact of the disease on the individual or his or her family. Factors that may be considered include the clinical risks and benefits of testing, such as the availability of an effective intervention and the risks associated with any interventions (Burke 2002; Burke *et al.* 2002), and health economic assessment.

Clinical utility may be poor if, for example, available interventions are not genotype-specific. Carriers of the Factor V Leiden or *G20210A* prothrombin variants have an increased risk for venous thromboembolism (VT). However, genetic testing of VT patients does not aid clinical management, as current evidence suggests that these genetic variants do not significantly increase the recurrence risk for VT.

Clinical utility has proved very difficult to assess in practice. Burke and Zimmern (2007), using criteria based on Donabedian's work on the quality of medical care, suggest that the main dimensions of clinical utility relate to the purpose for which a test is used (legitimacy, efficacy, effectiveness, and appropriateness), and the feasibility of test delivery (acceptability, efficiency, and the economic dimensions of optimality and equity) (Table 2.4.3).

The full evaluation of a genetic test is a complex process that requires significant resources. Because it is not possible to apply the full process to all tests, different levels of evaluation may be applied, depending on the nature of the test, its purpose, and the population in which it is to be carried out. For example, most tests for rare disorders require a less stringent programme of evaluation than tests for common disorders or population screening. This is because, when penetrance is high, the association between a positive test and ultimate outcome is more predictable, and the rarity of the condition means that the number of tests will be small.

In the United States, an ongoing model initiative of the Centers for Disease Control and Prevention, called the Evaluation of Genomic Applications in Practice and Prevention (EGAPP, http://www.egappreviews.org/default.htm), is attempting to integrate various models of genetic test evaluations including in-depth assessments and fast-track evaluation.

Genomics in disease prevention

All disease results from the combined effects of genetic and non-genetic factors. It follows that there may be opportunities to prevent disease by modifying either the genetic or the non-genetic component, or both. Juengst (1995) has distinguished these two theoretical modes of prevention as genotypic and phenotypic prevention, respectively.

Preventive strategies may be primary (preventing or delaying disease onset), secondary (encompassing early detection and treatment), or tertiary (delaying or preventing complications and deterioration).

Table 2.4.3 Key questions in genetic test evaluation

Domain	Questions
Assay	**How accurate is the assay?**
Analytical validity	What are the analytical sensitivity, specificity, PPV, and NPV of the assay, as compared to a gold standard?
Reliability and reproducibility	How reproducible are the test results under normal laboratory conditions?
Clinical validity	**What is the predictive value of the test in a defined population, for the specified disease?**
Gene–disease association	What is the strength of the association between genotype and disease?
	Is the genotype a minimally sufficient cause of disease?
	Is the genotype necessary for disease to occur?
Clinical test performance	What are the sensitivity, specificity, PPV, NPV, LR+, LR-, and ROC of the test, compared to a gold standard?
	If these measurements are not possible, what is the basis for proposing clinical validity for the test?
Clinical utility	
Test purpose	**What is the purpose of the test?**
Legitimacy	Is the proposed test in keeping with societal values, norms, and ethical principles?
	Is test delivery in compliance with laws and regulations?
Efficacy	Can the test and associated services achieve the intended purpose under ideal circumstances?
Appropriateness	What are the benefits and negative consequences of testing?
	Do the benefits sufficiently outweigh the negative consequences?
Feasibility of test delivery	**Can the test and associated services be delivered equitably, and in an acceptable manner, for a reasonable cost?**
Acceptability	Is the test delivered in conformity to the wishes, desires, and expectations of patients and their families?
Efficiency	Can the cost of the test and associated services be lowered without diminishing benefits? If there is an alternative for achieving the same purpose, is the test more or less efficient?
Optimality	What are the costs of the test relative to the benefits? Is a formal analysis of cost-effectiveness needed?
Equity	Can the test and associated services be provided equitably among different members of the population?

Source: Burke and Zimmern (2007).

Genotypic prevention

Genotypic prevention is a mode of primary genetic prevention. Examples include the use of antenatal genetic diagnosis and termination of pregnancy by couples wishing to avoid the birth of a child affected by a serious genetic disease. Genotypic prevention must always be a matter for personal choice by the individuals concerned, not a public health goal. Couples who know they are at risk of transmitting a genetic disease to their child should receive specialist advice and counselling by clinical genetics professionals before they make their choice.

Preimplantation genetic diagnosis (PGD) is considered by some to be a more acceptable form of genotypic prevention as it involves embryo selection rather than abortion, but there may still be ethical objections on the grounds that those embryos that are not selected for implantation are destroyed. Purchasers and commissioners of health services may also place restrictions on the use of PGD because of the high costs of the procedure, which involves *in vitro* fertilization as well as complex processes of embryo biopsy and molecular genetic testing.

In some countries, there are explicit programmes of antenatal genetic screening for some genetic diseases. Under such programmes, a whole population or population subgroup, who may not be aware that they are at risk, is offered a screening test to determine if the risk of their having an affected child is sufficiently high for them to be offered a definitive diagnostic test for the condition in question. For example, the United Kingdom has a national antenatal screening programme for Down syndrome (National Collaborating Centre for Women's and Children's Health 2003) and antenatal carrier screening programmes for sickle cell disease and the thalassaemias (NHS Sickle Cell and Thalassaemia Screening Programme). All pregnant women are offered screening as part of routine antenatal care. In countries such as the United Kingdom (but not in all countries) such programmes are considered ethically acceptable as long as informed choice by individuals determines who takes up the offer of screening.

Using genomics in secondary prevention: Newborn screening

Unfortunately most highly penetrant genetic diseases are incurable, but clinical management of many of these conditions has improved in recent years, and for some conditions life expectancy has increased significantly. In some cases, early detection of the disease, and early initiation of treatment, can significantly reduce mortality and morbidity. The classic example is the disease PKU, which is caused by deficiency of the enzyme phenylalanine hydroxylase (Kaye *et al.* 2006). If the disease is untreated, build-up of phenylalanine causes irreversible brain damage soon after birth. Early detection and initiation of a phenylalanine-free diet enables near-normal development. Sickle cell disease and cystic fibrosis also respond to early diagnosis and initiation of treatment in the newborn period, though the benefits are less dramatic than for PKU (Kaye *et al.* 2006). Newborn screening programmes may have other less direct benefits, such as in sparing parents of an affected child the often prolonged process of obtaining a diagnosis and in counselling parents about the risk to subsequent pregnancies.

Newborn screening programmes for various conditions are in place in many western countries (see Table 2.4.4 for examples). In some jurisdictions, including the United States, newborn screening programmes are state-mandated. In others, for example the United Kingdom, parental consent is sought.

The apparent success of newborn screening for PKU, the development of new diagnostic technologies such as tandem mass spectrometry, and powerful advocacy by some patient groups have led to pressure for widening newborn-screening programmes to include an increasing number of conditions [see, for example, the recent recommendations of the American College of Medical Genetics (Watson *et al.* 2006)].

However, serious concerns have been expressed about pressure to expand newborn screening panels (Botkin *et al.* 2006; Grosse *et al.* 2006). A major criticism is that many of the additional conditions depart from the key criteria identified by Wilson and Jungner (1968) for ensuring that population screening programmes deliver public health benefits. These criteria include the need to demonstrate that the natural history of the disorder is understood, that the characteristics of the screening test have been thoroughly evaluated, that an effective preventive intervention is available, and that screening is necessary to prevent death or serious disability.

For many of the conditions represented in the American College of Medical Genetics screening recommendations, evidence is not available to fulfil these criteria. Moreover, screening has the potential to cause harm (Grosse *et al.* 2006). Problems may include unnecessary or even harmful therapies given either to children who are incorrectly identified as having a disease or to children with mild or asymptomatic disease. False positive results may cause acute parental anxiety and damage family well-being. Insufficient thought has been given to the implications of identifying unaffected carriers of recessive conditions. Screening programmes have resource implications and opportunity costs that have not been sufficiently considered.

A further consideration is the need to ensure that health-service capacity, structures, and resources are in place to enable effective long-term follow-up of individuals identified by newborn screening programmes, so that the health benefits of early identification are not subsequently lost. There is evidence for a lack of effective long-term management of some individuals identified by newborn screening programmes for PKU and sickle cell disease (Botkin *et al.* 2006). For all these reasons, it has been suggested that new screening programmes should initially be introduced only within a research paradigm, so that their risks and benefits can be carefully assessed before widespread implementation (Botkin 2005).

Table 2.4.4 Examples of genetic disorders included in newborn screening programmes

Disorder	Screening method	US states offering screening	Offered in the UK?	Treatment
Phenylketonuria	Guthrie bacterial inhibition assay Fluorescence assay Amino-acid analyser Tandem mass spectrometry	All	Yes	Diet restricting phenylalanine
Congenital hypothyroidism	Measurement of thyroxine and thyrotropin	All	Yes	Oral levothyroxine
Sickle cell disease	Haemoglobin electrophoresis Isoelectric focusing High-performance liquid chromatography Follow-up DNA analysis	All	Yes	Prophylactic antibiotics Immunization against *Diplococcus pneumoniae* and *Haemophilus influenzae*
Galactosaemia	Beutler test Paigen test	All	No	Galactose-free diet
Maple syrup urine disease	Guthrie bacterial inhibition assay	Most	No	Diet restricting intake of branched-chain amino acids
Congenital adrenal hyperplasia	Radioimmunoassay	Most	No	Glucocorticoids Mineralocorticoids Salt
Cystic fibrosis	Immunoreactive trypsinogen followed by DNA testing	Some	Yes	Improved nutrition Management of pulmonary symptoms
Medium-chain acyl CoA dehydrogenase deficiency (MCADD)	Tandem mass spectrometry	Most	Planned	Avoidance of fasting Aggressive medical management during illness

Source: Khoury, MJ McCabe, and McCabe, E.R.B. (2003). *New England Journal of Medicine* **348**, 50–8.

The approach to the assessment of potential population screening programmes varies in different countries. In the United Kingdom, a National Screening Committee considers the evidence base for all proposed screening programmes, including those for genetic conditions. The Health Technology Assessment programme has carried out reviews of newborn screening for some conditions (see, for example, Pandor *et al.* 2004), and most proposed programmes are piloted on a regional basis before being rolled out nationally. For example, a national newborn screening programme for medium chain acyl CoA dehydrogenase deficiency (MCADD) is being introduced following a successful pilot study (National Screening Committee 2007). Critics of this cautious approach claim that lives are lost and children harmed by long delays before programmes are introduced. Ideally, research and clinical trials of new screening technologies should be funded promptly and adequately so that evidence to inform decisions about proposed screening programmes can be obtained as efficiently as possible.

Using genomics in primary phenotypic prevention of disease

The Holy Grail for those wishing to apply genomics in public health would be the ability to use genotypic information to identify individuals who are at increased risk of disease and who could be offered opportunities to reduce their risk by means of interventions aimed at modifiable environmental factors such as diet. However, this is by no means a simple goal to attain.

The predictive value of genotypic information

The first problem in using genotypic information for prevention is the low penetrance of most of the alleles implicated in susceptibility to common disease. Individually, such alleles are typically associated with odds ratios of around 1.1–2, though rarer alleles may confer higher risks (see Table 2.4.1 and Janssens *et al.* 2004). For this reason, the positive and negative predictive values of tests for single alleles are likely to be low (see Fig. 2.4.2): Most individuals who tested positive would gain no benefit from a preventive intervention because they would not have developed the disease in any case. Those who tested negative might be falsely reassured.

Some applications of the use of genotypic information in prevention have already been suggested. For example, since the discovery of the *HFE* gene, which is mutated in the iron-overload disease hereditary haemochromatosis, population screening for hereditary haemochromatosis has been proposed, based on *HFE* genotype. The rationale is that serious disease (liver cirrhosis, fibrosis, or diabetes) may be prevented by the simple procedure of frequent phlebotomy. However, although about 25–50 per cent of people with a predisposing *HFE* genotype have evidence of iron overload, it is not known how many of these people would, if untreated, progress to symptomatic disease; the penetrance of overt liver disease may be as low as 1–10 per cent. Public health has played an important role in the evidence-based evaluation of population screening for hereditary haemochromatosis. (Box 2.4.3)

It has been suggested that the predictive power of genotypic information would be increased if more alleles were considered together. This approach is sometimes called genomic profiling (Yang *et al.* 2003). Although individuals who carry multiple risk alleles will have a very high risk of disease, these individuals constitute a very small percentage of the population (Janssens *et al.* 2004). For the bulk of the population, genomic profiling will be extremely complex, depending on the number of risk genotypes tested for, the spectrum of risk alleles an individual carries, and the odds ratios associated with each of them (Janssens & Khoury 2006).

Pleiotropic effects of susceptibility genes must also be taken into account. For example, the *APOE4* variant increases risk for both Alzheimer's dementia and coronary heart disease but reduces risk for macular degeneration. Interventions aimed at preventing the negative effects of a gene variant might increase risk for another disease.

Behavioural responses to genomic risk information

A second question is whether risk information based on genetic factors is likely be effective in motivating the sustained behavioural change that would be needed to achieve health benefits. Current evidence on this issue is limited and more research is needed. Research to date suggests that risk information alone plays only a small part in people's ability to change their behaviour (Marteau & Lerman 2001). The availability of an effective intervention is important, as is the individual's assessment of his or her ability to achieve behavioural change; this assessment, in turn, is strongly dependent on the person's familial and social environment.

There is some evidence that reactions to genetic risk information may differ from those to other types of risk information. For example, one study compared attitudes about risk-reducing interventions in people with a clinical diagnosis of familial hypercholesterolaemia, with and without a mutation-positive DNA test result (Marteau *et al.* 2004). Although there was no difference in people's belief that cholesterol-lowering interventions were important for their health, those with a DNA-based diagnosis were less likely to believe that dietary intervention would be effective and more likely to believe that cholesterol-lowering medication would be required. This reaction suggests some degree of fatalism in attitudes about genetic information and the need to present genetic risk information in such a way that it does not undermine the individual's belief in the efficacy of behavioural change.

There could also be a danger that information indicating an average or reduced genetic risk might be falsely reassuring, leading people to underestimate their risk and ignore advice about a healthy lifestyle. To date there is little evidence that false reassurance is a significant concern, though some more subtle effects of negative genetic test results have been observed. For example, among people with a family history of Alzheimer's disease (and therefore at increased risk), those whose risk estimate included a negative test result for the *APOE4* polymorphism perceived their risk as lower than those with the same risk estimate based only on family history information (LaRusse *et al.* 2005).

A further relevant factor is the likelihood that people will take up an offer of genetic testing to indicate their risk. The public health impact of genetic susceptibility testing is likely to be low if few are motivated to take advantage of it. Those who have poor motivation to improve their health through behavioural and lifestyle change, or perceive a test result as a threat to their well-being rather than an opportunity to improve their health, are unlikely to perceive benefits from genetic susceptibility testing.

High-risk versus population approaches to prevention

The fundamental rationale for using genomics in the primary prevention of common diseases with environmental causes has also been questioned (see, for example, Merikangas & Risch 2003).

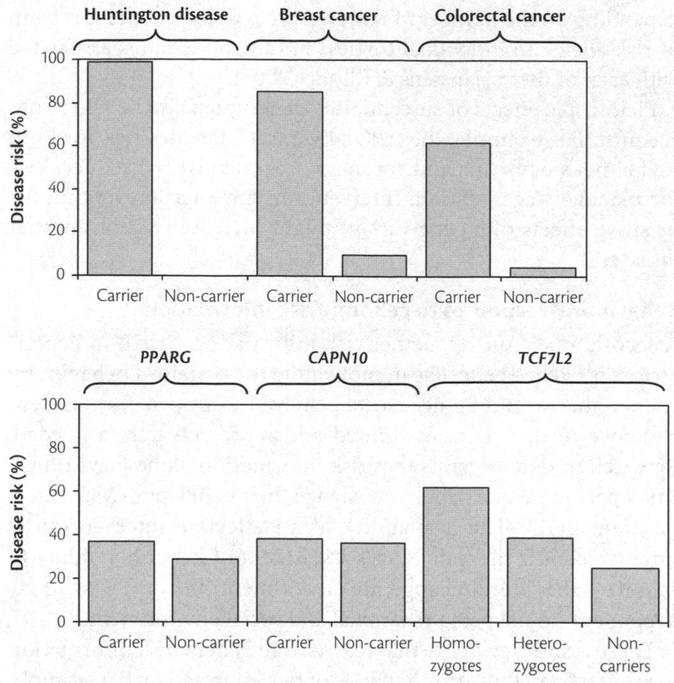

Fig. 2.4.2 Disease risks of carriers and non-carriers in genetic testing. In monogenic (Mendelian) disorders (top panel), carriers have a substantially increased risk of disease; non-carriers have a disease risk that approximates the population average. In the case of common disease (bottom panel), because risk alleles are generally common (population frequency >1 per cent), carriers and non-carriers have disease risks that are only slightly higher or slightly lower, respectively, than the population average. Reproduced from Janssens and Khoury (2006).

One argument is based on Rose's (1985) observation that a greater reduction in overall disease incidence can be achieved by a small reduction in disease risk over a whole population, whereas targeting an intervention at a high-risk group results in a larger absolute reduction in risk for those individuals. However, the example of obesity, discussed at the beginning of this chapter, suggests that population-level interventions may not be successful if they fail to take individual differences into account: Advice about healthy and moderate eating may have little effect on individuals whose genomic make-up predisposes them to a constant craving for high-calorie food. Moreover, Rose also pointed out that the population and high-risk approaches to prevention are complementary: Both have a role to play in prevention.

A further issue is the need for caution in applying population-derived risk estimates to decisions about individual patients (Rockhill *et al.* 2000). For example, Elmore and Fletcher (2006) have calculated that, although the Gail model for breast cancer risk prediction performs well at a population level, with a concordance of 0.96 between the expected and actual number of women in a population who develop breast cancer, at an individual level the concordance is only about 0.6. This problem is, of course, not unique to risk estimates based on genetics. Population-based risk estimates may best be used to stratify risk (so that, for example, an individual falls into a specific quintile) rather than to attempt to pinpoint individual risk. Population-based data will generate hypotheses about preventive action but these hypotheses must be tested rigorously in prospective outcome studies.

In summary, there is currently insufficient evidence to support the use of genetic testing or genomic profiling in the primary prevention of common diseases (Haga *et al.* 2003). In the future,

Box 2.4.3 Public health action to evaluate a proposed population screening programme: Hereditary haemochromatosis

With discovery of the *HFE* gene in 1996 and the identification of *HFE* mutations as the primary cause of hereditary haemochromatosis, many experts identified *HFE* mutation testing as a model for genetic screening of adult populations. Public health leadership has played an important role in evaluating this potential intervention.

1997 Meeting convened in the United States by National Human Genome Research Institute (NHGRI) and Centers for Disease Control and Prevention (CDC) to evaluate state of knowledge about *HFE* and hereditary haemochromatosis, resulting in:

- Consensus statement calling for more research on *HFE* mutation penetrance before screening
- Series of articles defining current knowledge and practice standards

1999 International jury convened to develop evidence-based recommendations regarding screening for haemochromatosis, under auspices of CDC and European Association for the Study of the Liver

- Jury recommended against population screening in absence of research documenting outcome benefit
- Jury recommended that diagnosis of hereditary haemochromatosis be reserved for symptomatic patients (as opposed to asymptomatic patients identified by biochemical or DNA-based testing)

2000–04 Population-based study of screening for hereditary haemochromatosis in 100 000 subjects funded by National Heart Lung and Blood Institute and NHGRI

- Penetrance of HFE mutations low (consistent with smaller studies from USA, Australia, and Europe)
- Symptomatic hereditary haemochromatosis rare

2004 Launch of CDC Web site (http://www.cdc.gov/genomics/training/perspectives/hemo.htm) providing education about hereditary haemochromatosis for healthcare providers and the general public.
Emphasis on identification of early symptoms of hereditary haemochromatosis by healthcare providers and a family tracing approach rather than population-based screening.

scientifically validated genotypic risk information may be best used to enhance the predictive value of a 'package' of risk information that also incorporates measures of lifestyle and behavioural factors as well as relevant phenotypic biomarkers. Further research is needed to determine the best way to communicate genetic risk information in order to achieve beneficial health outcomes.

Using family history in disease prevention

It is likely to be many years, perhaps decades, before it will be possible to use genotypic information routinely in the assessment of risk for common chronic diseases. It has been suggested that, in the meantime, family history information represents a useful surrogate that could be used more effectively and systematically in preventive healthcare than is currently the case (Yoon *et al.* 2002).

Family history is a risk factor for almost all diseases of public health significance, including most chronic diseases. Family history reflects the consequences of shared genetic variation at multiple loci (first-degree relatives such as siblings share 50 per cent of their genes), shared exposures to environmental factors, and shared behaviours.

Methods have been proposed for quantifying the risk associated with family history based on the number of family members affected, the degree of closeness of their biological relationship to the individual under consideration, and their ages at onset of disease (Yoon *et al.* 2002). From this information about their relatives, it is suggested that people can be stratified into average risk, moderate risk, and high risk groups and given appropriate preventive advice (Khoury *et al.* 2005). Those at average risk would be encouraged to adhere to standard public health prevention recommendations. Those at moderate or high risk would be given personalized recommendations including, for example, assessment and modification of risk factors, lifestyle changes, alternative early detection strategies, and perhaps chemoprevention. Those at high risk would also be referred to the specialist clinical genetics service to investigate the possibility of a high-penetrance genetic disorder. Although only a few people are expected to fall into the high risk group, a much larger number will be assessed as being at moderate risk, offering the possibility of augmenting and improving the standard population approach to prevention.

Risk stratification based on family history is already in clinical practice as a form of triage for individuals concerned about a family history of some common cancers, such as breast/ovarian and colorectal cancer [see, for example, guidelines of the United Kingdom's National Institute for Health and Clinical Excellence (2006) for management of women with a family history of breast cancer]. This approach is not, however, used proactively as a screening programme.

The added value of the proactive use of family history risk-stratification as an adjunct to population-level prevention activities needs rigorous evaluation (Khoury *et al.* 2005). Issues that must be addressed include the degree of accuracy of family history reporting, the optimum algorithm for stratifying risk, and the value of family history as a motivator for behavioural change. Particularly rigorous evaluation will be needed if a positive family history is used as an indication for any preventive intervention that carries risk, such as chemoprevention. Health service providers, particularly family practitioners, will need education and training in taking and assessing family histories, and provision must be in place for effective follow-up of individuals who fall into higher-risk groups. Health economic analysis should also form part of the overall assessment of the family history approach.

Genomics and public health ethics

The combination of genetics and public health has had an uneasy history, largely because of the legacy of the eugenics movement. Even today, there are still concerns about the potential tension between the population-level objectives of public health and the sensitive and personal nature of genomic information. It is important to allay these fears, which in many cases arise from an exaggerated perception of the 'power' of genomic information and from a misunderstanding of the motives of public health professionals who become involved with genomics.

The legacy of eugenics

The term 'eugenics', literally meaning 'well born', was coined by Francis Galton in 1883. Its central philosophy was that the human gene pool could be 'improved' by selective breeding (Kevles 1995). Individuals judged to have a 'good' genetic constitution would be encouraged to have children, while those with 'poor' genes would be discouraged. The idea gained ground both in a number of European countries (including the United Kingdom and Sweden) and in the United States. Some eugenic programmes involved the involuntary sterilization of large numbers of people deemed genetically 'unfit' because they were poor, homeless, or 'morally degenerate'. In Nazi Germany, eugenic principles were invoked to justify the murder of millions of people.

The application of eugenics to humans is problematic on two key counts: First, that eugenic programmes violate human rights; and second, that 'good' and 'poor' human characteristics are complex traits that have no objective definition and result from multiple genetic, environmental, and social influences. Even if 'good' and 'bad' traits could be defined, it would be impossible to select simultaneously for multiple 'good' traits and against multiple 'bad' traits. The eugenics movement has been rightly condemned, and repudiated in most countries of the world.

Use of genomic information: Balancing the rights of individuals and society

Revulsion against eugenics has led to an insistence that genomic information is the property of the individual and his or her family. Individual autonomy, informed consent, and the privacy and confidentiality of genomic information have been paramount concerns. Numerous authors have warned about the dangers of stigmatization and discrimination against individuals on the basis of genetic characteristics.

Recently there have been attempts to re-balance the ethical debate and to move away from the concept that genetic information necessarily has a power and significance beyond that of other types of personal medical information—a concept known as 'genetic exceptionalism' (Murray 1997). The serious issues faced by families affected by highly penetrant genetic diseases do not generally apply to the luckier majority whose genetic risk of disease is much lower (Janssens & Khoury 2006).

The focus of public health is the population rather than the individual. The development of applications for genomics in population health will depend on the willingness of individuals to allow their genomic information to be used in population-based research projects designed to investigate low-penetrance genomic variants and gene–environment interactions that affect disease susceptibility.

Concerns have been raised about the privacy and confidentiality of the genetic information of individuals participating in such projects. For example, full anonymization of samples and data may not be possible because the research may depend on the ability to link data to individuals. Moreover, the prospective nature of some epidemiological projects can mean that informed consent is difficult to implement fully: Individuals may be asked to consent now to future uses of their samples and data that are currently unknown.

However, the ethical problems of large population studies may have been over-played. Population-based research involving genetics will have meaningful public health implications but these studies will not generally reveal clinically relevant information about individual participants and consequently will entail few physical, psychological, or social risks for those individuals or their families (Beskow *et al.* 2001). Although individual rights must be upheld, and genetic information must be protected just like any other personal data, community-centred ethical values such solidarity, altruism, and citizenry must also be given due weight (Knoppers & Chadwick 2005). In this view, biobanks and population genomic research are seen as global public goods to be used for the benefit of current society and future generations (Knoppers 2005).

These arguments do not deny the importance of high ethical standards for population-based projects and biobanking initiatives, in order to maintain the degree of public confidence that will be essential for the success of these long-term projects. Iceland's deCODE project attracted criticism as a result of the Icelandic Government's decision to assume that every individual in the country would be a participant in the project unless they specifically opted out, and to grant a commercial monopoly on any results from the project to the deCODE company. Other large-scale population biobanking projects (see Table 2.4.5, later in this chapter) have been more careful to avoid ethical controversy, for example by establishing mechanisms for independent ethical oversight, paying careful regard to procedures for seeking informed consent from participants, and carrying out public consultations on project plans. Such measures appear to command broad approval although some disquiet persists, for example over issues such as feedback of results to individuals, and terms for commercial access to samples and data. The international Public Population Project in Genomics (P3G) (http://www.p3gconsortium.org) is providing a platform for sharing best practice in ethical standards for biobanking initiatives.

Integrating genomics into public health practice

We are moving from an era in which genetics has been a small specialist clinical service dealing with patients and families affected by rare heritable diseases, to one in which genomic information and technologies may become a normal part of mainstream clinical and public health practice (Guttmacher *et al.* 2001). During the past 10 years, public health professionals have begun to realize that this transformation must be rationally managed and to put in place organizations and strategies for achieving this aim.

The emergence of public health genomics

During the 1990s, some public health professionals in the United States and the United Kingdom began to realize that public health practice must take account of developments in genomics. In the United States, the report of a Task Force on Genetics and Disease Prevention convened by the Centers for Disease Control and Prevention (CDC) led to the establishment of the Office of Genetics and Disease Prevention (now the National Office of Public Health Genomics, NOPHG, http://www.cdc.gov/genomics) at CDC in Atlanta in 1997 (Centers for Disease Control and Prevention 1997). At around the same time, the idea of public health genomics as a new subdiscipline of public health began to emerge and multidisciplinary academic programmes in public health genomics were developed at the Universities of Michigan and Washington (Austin *et al.* 2000).

In the United Kingdom, two reports to Government by expert advisory groups signalled the first awareness, on the part of the country's National Health Service, that genomics would in time evolve beyond the confines of a small specialized service for rare genetic disorders (NHS Central Research and Development Committee 1995, 1996). The first public health organization with an explicit interest in genomics was the Public Health Genetics Unit (now the Foundation for Genomics and Population Health, http://www.phgfoundation.org), established in Cambridge in 1997.

In the decade since 1997, public health genomics has increased in strength and influence. A growing body of academic literature has established the intellectual foundations of the discipline. Projects and activities undertaken at the NOPHG, the Foundation for Genomics and Population Health and elsewhere have made important contributions in areas such as genetic test evaluation, human genome epidemiology, and public policy for the use of human tissue and genomic information. Other groups focused on public health genomics have been set up within both government organizations (for example, the Office of Population Health Genomics in the Western Australian Department of Health) and academia (for example, Centers of Genomics and Public Health at the Universities of Washington and Michigan).

The Bellagio model for public health genomics

In 2005, a multidisciplinary workshop attended by 18 experts from the United States, United Kingdom, France, Germany, and Canada was convened in Bellagio, Italy, with the aim of seeking a consensus on the definition, scope, and goals of public health genomics (Bellagio group 2005; Burke *et al.* 2006). The group arrived at the following definition:

Public health genomics is the responsible and effective translation of genome-based knowledge and technologies for the benefit of population health.

Building on this consensus definition, the workshop developed a visual representation of the 'enterprise' of public health genomics (Fig. 2.4.3). The functions and activities shown in dark grey define the scope of the field. Several key features emerge from this representation:

1. The input to the enterprise is knowledge generated by genome-based science and technology, together with knowledge derived from academic research in the population sciences, as well as the humanities and social sciences.
2. The driving force of public health genomics is knowledge integration. This term encompasses the activity of selecting, storing, collating, analysing, integrating, and disseminating knowledge,

both within and across disciplines. It is the means by which information is transformed into knowledge.

3. The integrated and interdisciplinary knowledge base is used to underpin four core sets of activities:
   (a) Communication and stakeholder engagement (including, for example, public dialogue and involvement, and engagement with industry)
   (b) Informing public policy (including applied legal and policy analysis, engagement in the policy-making process, seeking international comparisons, and working with government)
   (c) Developing and evaluating health services (including strategic planning, manpower planning, and capacity building; service review and evaluation; and development of new programmes and services)
   (d) Education and training (including programmes of genetic literacy for health professionals and generally within society, specific training for public health genomics specialists, and development of courses and materials).
4. The mode of working of public health genomics is described by the cycle of analysis—strategy—action—evaluation, which is a widely recognized representation of public health practice.
5. Public health genomics does include a research component, shown at the bottom of the diagram. This component is not generally basic research; rather, it is programmes of applied and translational research that contribute directly to the goal of improving population health and also identify gaps in the knowledge base that need to be addressed by further basic research.
6. Public health genomics does not operate in a vacuum. It is embedded within a social and political context and is informed by societal priorities.
7. Double-headed arrows throughout the diagram indicate the dynamic and interactive nature of the enterprise: It generates knowledge as well as using it, and it is modulated by the effects of its own outputs and activities.

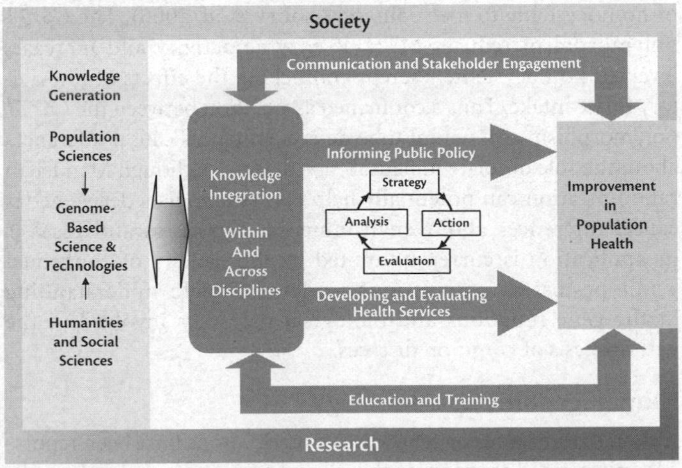

Fig. 2.4.3 The 'enterprise' of public health genomics. The scope of public health genomics is defined by the areas shown in dark grey.

An international network, the Genome-based Research and Population Health International Network (GRaPH *Int*, http://www.graphint.org) has been established to support the development of public health genomics and the sharing of resources worldwide (Stewart *et al.* 2006). The administrative hub of the network is based in Montreal and funded by the Public Health Agency of Canada.

Challenges and prospects for public health genomics

Integrating genomics into public health and behavioural research

Research is needed to strengthen the evidence base for applications of genomics in public health, particularly with respect to major public health problems such as obesity, outbreaks of infectious disease, or effects of exposure to environmental toxins and pollutants (Khoury *et al.* 2004, 2005).

Toxicogenomics and nutrigenomics

Toxicogenomics (sometimes referred to as 'ecogenomics') and nutrigenomics are important evolving areas of research that are attempting to unravel interactions between genomic variants and responses to toxic environmental agents and dietary constituents, respectively. There is good evidence that genomic variants do affect responses to these exposures but, as with alleles associated with susceptibility to common disease, the predictive value of the individual risk alleles is generally low. For example, a polymorphism in the *DPB1* gene (part of the major histocompatibility complex, which encodes components of the immune system) increases risk of sensitization to inhaled beryllium dust, encountered by workers in the nuclear industry. However, although the relative risk conferred by the sensitizing *DPB1* allele is high (odds ratio ~10), the specificity of the *DPB1* marker is low, thus limiting its utility.

Many reported associations and gene–environment interactions in toxicogenomics and nutrigenomics have not been independently confirmed. For example, different studies have found opposite effects of the Pro12Ala variant of the PPAR-γ gene on the association between the dietary P:S (polyunsaturated:saturated fat) ratio and body mass index. Although non-replication can be due to poor study design, under-powered studies, and type 1 errors, these differences could also reflect true differences between the populations studied, as well as the known biological complexity of the role of PPAR-γ.

The fields of toxicogenomics and nutrigenomics are in their infancy, and it is likely that many years of research will be needed before validated evidence will be available to inform public health action. It is also important to ensure that this evidence, when it does become available, is used responsibly. Genetic effects on responses to environmental toxins or dietary components may identify some individuals or populations at high risk for whom specific preventive advice may be appropriate. Toxicogenomic and nutrigenomic research will also reveal important aspects of the biological mechanisms of interaction between environmental exposures and the human body. Such information could lead, for example, to better definition of the lowest tolerable dose for a toxin, based on the most susceptible genotype.

In terms of prevention, however, genomics is unlikely to supersede the value of standard public health advice for the bulk of the population. Public health practitioners must ensure that the benefits and risks of any proposed interventions or programmes based on toxicogenomics or nutrigenomics are carefully weighed, and that people are not misled by unsupported claims made by companies selling direct-to-consumer genetic test kits.

Infectious disease

The complete genomes of many important human pathogens have been sequenced, including those of the organisms implicated in tuberculosis, malaria, plague, leprosy, diphtheria, cholera, and typhoid. Genomic information is being used to develop new diagnostics, vaccines, and drug treatments. For example, genomic technology has improved diagnosis of leishmaniasis and dengue fever in some Latin American countries (Singer & Daar 2001). Research on the genome of the malaria parasite *Plasmodium falciparum* identified an unusual biochemical pathway for steroid synthesis and suggested that a drug known to inhibit a crucial step in a similar pathway operating in bacteria and plants might be useful in treating malaria. The drug, fosmidomycin, has shown promise in several clinical studies.

The process of infection involves not just the pathogen genome but also that of the host organism. The genomes of human populations have co-evolved with those of the pathogens that infect them, and resistance or susceptibility to infection has been a strong selective pressure in human evolution. A wide range of human genes, including the highly polymorphic genes of the immune system, are involved in human responses to pathogens. In some cases a single genetic variant appears to be significantly associated with susceptibility or resistance to a disease. For example, a specific polymorphism in the gene encoding the cell-surface receptor molecule CCR5 is associated with resistance to infection by human immunodeficiency virus (HIV). This gene was chosen for analysis because the receptor was known to be involved in entry of the virus into specific cells of the immune system. Analysis of genomic variants in resistant individuals may suggest new mechanisms and targets for drug development, or strategies for enhancing protective immunity in exposed populations.

Behavioural research

Public health programmes of disease prevention depend to a large extent on promoting behavioural change, but genomics has so far had little impact on behavioural research. As discussed earlier in this chapter, there is a need for better understanding of the effect of genotypic risk information on human behaviour (Marteau & Lerman 2001). It is particularly important, for example, that individuals who believe genetic testing has revealed they are at reduced risk from, for example, bladder cancer due to smoking, or coronary heart disease due to a high-fat diet, do not interpret 'reduced risk' as 'no risk'.

In addition, the role of genomic factors in health-related behaviours must be more fully explored. For example, genomic factors are known to affect the likelihood that smokers will develop lung cancer, but the picture is incomplete without an understanding of the genomic factors that affect risk-taking behaviour and nicotine addiction. A fuller understanding of the role of genomics in human behaviour may suggest new strategies to promote public health and prevent avoidable death and disease.

The impact of genomics on epidemiology

Genomics offers new opportunities for epidemiological research. In time, the familiar 2×2 table correlating disease status (for example, in a case-control study) with the presence or absence of an exposure or risk factor may routinely be replaced by a 2×4 table in which the underlying genotype at a particular locus or groups of loci will be measured and evidence sought for interaction with the risk factor.

New tools and resources are being developed for epidemiological studies involving genomics. For example, as mentioned earlier in this chapter, genomics is inspiring the establishment of large population cohorts and 'biobanks' to provide resources for the discovery and characterization of genes associated with common diseases (Table 2.4.5). In addition to promoting gene discovery, biobanks will help epidemiologists to quantify the occurrence of diseases in different populations and to understand their natural histories and risk factors, including gene–environment interactions. Large cohorts may also be used for nested case-control studies or case-only studies as an initial screening method. These studies will produce a large amount of data on disease risk factors, lifestyles, and environmental exposures, and they will provide opportunities for data standardization, data sharing, and joint analyses (Khoury *et al.* 2004; Davey Smith *et al.* 2005).

Genomic research may also help to identify unknown environmental risk factors for disease or confirm suspected environmental risk factors, through the approach of Mendelian randomization (Davey Smith *et al.* 2005). The reasoning behind this approach is that if a genetic polymorphism affects the level of a biological intermediate in a way that mirrors the effect of an environmental exposure on the same intermediate, and if the biological intermediate in turn affects disease risk, then an association between the polymorphism and disease risk can act as a proxy for the relationship between the environmental exposure and disease risk. Mendel's law of random assortment of traits during transmission from parents to offspring means that this proxy relationship can be viewed as protected from the various confounding factors that affect observational studies of exposures.

The concept of Mendelian randomization can be illustrated by the example of the *C677T* polymorphism of the methylenetetrahydrofolate reductase (*MTHFR*) gene, which is needed for conversion of homocysteine to methionine (Khoury *et al.* 2005). The *C677T* polymorphism reduces MTHFR enzyme activity and increases levels of homocysteine, thereby mimicking the effects of low dietary folate intake. Thus a confirmed association between the *C677T* polymorphism and neural tube defects enhances causal inferences about the role of folate in neural tube defects. Although Mendelian randomization can potentially help epidemiologists derive better causal inferences about environmental exposures and disease, its application is currently limited by the paucity of confirmed genotype-disease associations, and incomplete understanding of the gene functions and biological pathways involved in the pathogenesis of common diseases.

Human genome epidemiology

Although thousands of gene–disease associations have been reported, only a small fraction of these have been independently replicated and fewer still can be considered fully validated (Khoury *et al.* 2007). Problems include publication bias, confounding by

Table 2.4.5 Examples of large population-based research biobanks (planned and current)

	Sample size (*n*)	Participating countries	Recruitment	Age at recruitment	URL
Cohort studies					
EPIC Europe	>500 000	Ten European countries	1993–97	45–74	http://www.iarc.fr/epic/Sup-default.html
CARTaGENE	50 000 (in two phases)	Quebec	2007–09 (Phase 1)	25–69	http://www.cartagene.qc.ca
Generation Scotland	50 000 family members	Scotland	Ongoing	35–55	http://129.215.140.49/gs/
UK Biobank	500 000	England	Ongoing	40–69	http://www.ukbiobank.ac.uk
Twin cohorts					
GenomEUtwin	>600 000 twin pairs	Six European countries	Varies among the eight different twin cohorts	Various	http://www.genomeutwin.org
Total populations					
DeCode Genetics	>100 000	Iceland	Ongoing	Various	http://www.decode.com
Esonian Genome Project	>100 000	Estonia	Ongoing	Various	http://www.geenivaramu.ee
Western Australian Genome Project	~2 000 000	Western Australia	Awaits funding	Various	http://www.genepi.org.au

Source: Adapted (and updated) from Davey Smith Ebrahim, S. Lewis, S. (2005). *Lancet* **366**, 1484–98.

population stratification, faulty selection of control subjects, genotyping errors, deviations from Hardy–Weinberg equilibrium, linkage disequilibrium issues, misclassification of exposures and outcomes, inadequate statistical power, and type 1 errors (false positive associations). These problems point to a need for systematic evaluation and meta-analysis of studies to identify validated associations, question unsubstantiated claims, and flag promising candidates for further investigation.

The Human Genome Epidemiology Network, HuGENet, is a global collaboration of individuals and organizations that develops methods and guidance for integrating and disseminating knowledge on the prevalence of genomic variants in different populations, genotype–disease associations, gene–gene and gene–environment interactions, as well as evaluating genetic tests for screening and prevention (Khoury 1999; Little *et al.* 2003).

HuGENet's Web-accessible knowledge base captures ongoing publications in human genome epidemiology and is searchable by disease, gene, and disease risk factors. In collaboration with several journals, HuGENet also sponsors systematic reviews of the evidence on genotype–disease associations, using specific published guidelines for this work (the HuGENet handbook) as well as applying quantitative methods for evidence synthesis. Over 50 HuGENet reviews have been published on various diseases ranging from single-gene conditions to common complex diseases.

In 2005, HuGENet formed a network of investigator networks; these are mostly disease-specific research consortia that share knowledge, experience, and resources for human genome epidemiology investigations. The HuGENet Network of Networks has published a 'road map' for using consortia-driven pooled data and meta-analyses to augment the knowledge base on gene–disease associations (Ioannidis *et al.* 2006) and guidelines on the assessment of cumulative evidence on genetic associations (Ioannidis *et al.* 2008). HuGENet is also working on ways of integrating genetic epidemiological evidence on gene–disease associations with biological evidence.

Genomics in the developing world

Genomics and genomic technology will not replace traditional public health measures such as combatting malnutrition, providing clean water and access to sanitation, alleviating poverty, and promoting sexual health. However, genomics offers potential benefits to the developing world, for example in more rapid and accurate diagnosis of infectious disease (as discussed earlier in this chapter), enhancing the nutritional value of staple foods, bioremediation to reverse environmental degradation, and prevention of widespread human suffering by better recognition and management of genetic disease (Daar *et al.* 2002; Genomics Working Group of the Science and Technology Task Force of the United Nations Millennium Project 2004).

It will be appropriate for different countries to adopt different strategies depending on the nature of their health problems, their economic situation, their social and political climate, their clinical and public health infrastructure, and the availability of trained medical and public health personnel. It is important to ensure that applications of genetics and genomic technology are thoroughly evaluated in pilot studies; that local expertise is fully engaged at all stages of the research, development and implementation pathway; and that international aid is focused appropriately on developing local capacity, networks, and partnerships to cascade expertise and promote best practice.

Management and prevention of genetic disease

As mentioned earlier in this chapter, the developing world carries the heaviest burden of genetic disease, contributing to a birth defects prevalence that is 50–100 per cent higher than in the developed world (Christianson *et al.* 2006). The most prevalent genetic disorders in the developing world are the haemoglobin disorders (sickle cell disease and thalassaemia) and glucose-6-phosphate deficiency. Approximately 7 per cent of the world's population are carriers of a haemoglobin disorder, and 300 000–400 000 babies with severe forms of these diseases are born every year, mostly in tropical regions (Weatherall & Clegg 2001). The public health impact of haemoglobin disorders is substantial and in some regions is increasing, as falling rates of childhood mortality due to malnutrition and infection mean that more individuals survive to present for diagnosis and treatment. Demographic changes such as migration are also increasing the prevalence of haemoglobin disorders in the developed world.

Chromosomal disorders and multifactorial conditions with a strong genetic component also have a significant impact on the developing world. For example, lack of effective family planning, leading to high birth rates for older mothers, contributes to a significant birth prevalence for Down syndrome. Congenital heart defects and neural tube defects make a substantial contribution to childhood mortality and morbidity. High rates of consanguineous marriages in some societies may increase the birth frequency of rare recessive diseases.

As a first step towards improving management and prevention of genetic conditions, both low-income and middle-income countries should seek to educate their communities and health professionals about these conditions, promote family planning, improve maternal health and nutrition, and establish child health services (Christianson *et al.* 2006). If economic and political circumstances allow, it may be possible to establish a medical genetics service, including training appropriate health professionals in clinical diagnosis of genetic conditions and basic genetic counselling, and considering implementation of appropriate neonatal and antenatal screening programmes.

Cultural, religious, and economic factors dictate different strategies in different countries, but all countries with a significant prevalence of haemoglobin disorders need good diagnostic facilities and provision for treatment. For sickle cell disease, the most cost-effective approach is likely to be the development of national centres with expertise in screening, DNA diagnosis, education, counselling, and management of the conditions (World Health Organization Advisory Committee on Health Research 2002). Ideally, such centres would support and train personnel for a network of peripheral screening clinics focusing on neonatal screening and administration of oral antibiotic prophylaxis in childhood, and taking the lead in programmes of public education.

The thalassaemias present a different range of problems. Simple and cheap diagnostic techniques are available to diagnose the condition and detect carriers. However, disease management is more complex and costly than for sickle cell disease because the severe forms require lifelong blood transfusion (using blood that has been screened to prevent transmission of pathogens) and expensive drug treatment to remove the excess iron introduced by multiple transfusions. In some countries, programmes of antenatal carrier screening are considered acceptable to reduce the birth prevalence of disease. Once again, the model of centralized diagnostic laboratories and a network of peripheral screening clinics (in this case, for antenatal screening) may be appropriate. Antenatal carrier screening programmes have been in operation for many years in some Mediterranean countries, where as a result the birth frequency of β thalassaemia has fallen by over 80 per cent (Cao *et al.* 2002).

In some middle-income, developing countries, such as the countries of Southeast Asia, changing lifestyles are leading to an increasing burden of disease from multifactorial conditions such as heart disease and diabetes, which may before long overtake communicable diseases as the major public health scourge in these countries. Although, as in the developed world, preventive strategies will be aimed at altering diet and lifestyle, some of the genetic variants underlying susceptibility to these conditions are likely to be population-specific. Genomic research in developing-world populations will be needed for a full understanding of the aetiology of disease and may point to a need for therapies and preventive interventions that are tailored for different population groups.

Genomic technologies in the developing world

In the wider sphere of genomic biotechnology, too, different strategies are appropriate for different countries (Genomics Working Group of the Science and Technology Task Force of the United Nations Millennium Project 2004). For some of the poorest countries, cheap genomics-based diagnostics may be cost-effective in programmes of infectious disease monitoring and control. International collaborations between the developed and developing world can help scientists in developing countries to gain access to appropriate technology, and to adapt this technology to a low-resource setting and a specific set of local conditions. Ongoing evaluation of any applications is also essential.

Some middle-income countries such as Cuba, Brazil, and Thailand are in a position to be able to develop their own biotechnology capacity. Governments in such countries need to create a favourable policy environment for genomic technology by investing in appropriate research, instituting transparent legal and regulatory frameworks and protection for intellectual property rights, stimulating their own biotechnology and pharmaceutical industries, and fostering public–private partnerships that are accountable to the public interest (World Health Organization Advisory Committee on Health Research, 2002). Policies for applications of genomics and genetics must be sensitive to the ethical and cultural values of the country.

Training partnerships between industrialized and developing countries can help to develop human resources, and in some cases joint academic or clinical appointments can prevent the 'brain drain' of highly trained scientists and clinicians to more lucrative jobs in the developed world. Innovative industrial partnerships between the developed and developing world can, if carefully managed, help to provide both resources and expertise for the development of local industry.

Education and training

In both the developed and the developing world, public health professionals must be prepared for the impact genomics will have on their practice (Austin *et al.* 2000; Burton 2003). As well as a working knowledge of basic genetics, they will need an understanding of human genome epidemiology and the criteria for evaluation of genetic tests, and an appreciation of the ethical, legal, psychosocial, and policy dimensions of applications of genomics and genomic technologies.

A set of competencies in genomics for the US public health workforce has been developed by the US National Office of Public Health Genomics (2001). Competencies are documented for the workforce as a whole and for specific groups including leaders/administrators, clinicians, epidemiologists, health educationalists, laboratory staff, and environmental health workers.

In addition, some individuals will require an in-depth knowledge of public health genomics, for example, those involved in screening and other preventive programmes, health service development and evaluation, public health education, and policy analysis and development. Educational programmes in public health genomics are already underway at some centres.

Conclusion

The full benefits of genomics for clinical medicine and public health are likely to take many years to materialize; public health genomics must play a long game (Halliday *et al.* 2004; Davey Smith *et al.* 2005). However, there is a need now to establish capacity and infrastructure for the decades ahead. Leadership, sharing of resources (Box 2.4.4), and knowledge through international networks such as GRaPH *Int* and the Public Health Genomics European Network (PHGEN, http://www.phgen.nrw.de/typo3/index.php), programmes of professional education and training, and engagement with public policy development for genomics will all contribute to timely progress.

Several challenges must be addressed. A concerted interdisciplinary effort will be required to understand interactions between genetic, environmental, and social contributors to health. Genome-based technologies and interventions need to be critically evaluated through prospective study of health outcomes. Effective implementation of genome-based advances will require new policy and educational initiatives.

Genomic research offers great promise for population health benefit. However, potential uses of genomic information must be critically scrutinized. Some seemingly promising technologies or interventions may yield little benefit or pose unexpected harms; others may provide unique opportunities to improve health.

Box 2.4.4 Examples of some current initiatives in public health genomics

Centres

National Office of Public Health Genomics, US Centers for Disease Control and Prevention

http://www.cdc.gov/genomics

Carries out research on how human genomic discoveries can be used to improve health and prevent disease. Established and coordinates the HuGE Net (Human Genome Epidemiology Network) initiative.

Foundation for Genomics and Population Health (formerly the Public Health Genetics Unit)

http://www.phgfoundation.org

Multidisciplinary group that assesses advances in genetic science and their impact on health services and healthcare policy.

Centers for Genomics and Public Health

http://www.sph.umich.edu/genomics/
http://depts.washington.edu/cgph/

Established by collaboration between the US Centers for Disease Control and Prevention and the Association of Schools of Public Health, and located at the Universities of Michigan and Washington. The Centers contribute to the knowledge base, provide technical assistance to local, state, and regional public health organizations and develop and deliver training to the public health work force.

Genomics, Health, and Society

http://genopole-toulouse.prd.fr/index.php?id=57

A multidisciplinary research centre located at the Toulouse Genopole, University of Toulouse, France, and including biologists, clinicians, geneticists, lawyers, sociologists, and economists.

Office of Population Health Genomics, Western Australian Department of Health

http://www.genomics.health.wa.gov.au/home/index.cfm

Aims to facilitate the integration of genomics into all aspects of public health, policy, and programmes.

Resources

HumGen

http://www.humgen.umontreal.ca

An international database on the legal, ethical, and social aspects of human genetics, developed as a collaboration between academia, government, and industry by the Centre de recherche en droit public at the University of Montreal.

Box 2.4.4 Examples of some current initiatives in public health genomics *(Continued)*

GDPinfo

http://apps.nccd.cdc.gov/genomics/GDPQueryTool/default.asp

A searchable database of all the documents available on the Office of Genomics and Disease Prevention Website, including the HuGE Net database.

PHGU Genomics Policy Database

http://www.phgfoundation.org/policydb

A searchable web-based database of literature on policy development for genomics in health services and healthcare.

Projects

Evaluation of Genomic Applications in Practice and Prevention (EGAPP)

http://www.cdc.gov/genomics/gtesting/egapp.htm

The project aims to develop a coordinate process for evaluating genetic tests and other genomic applications that are in transition from research to clinical and public health practice.

P3G Consortium—Public Population Project in Genomics

http://www.p3gconsortium.org/

An international consortium to provide the international population genomics community with the resources, tools, and know-how to facilitate data management for improved methods of knowledge transfer and sharing.

Canadian Programme on Genomics and Global Health

http://www.utoronto.ca/jcb/genomics/index.html

Promotes the use of genomics and biotechnologies to improve health in developing countries.

HuGE Net

http://www.cdc.gov/genomics/hugenet/default.htm

A global collaboration of individuals and organizations committed to the assessment of the impact of human genome variation on population health and how genetic information can be used to improve health and prevent disease.

Cross-disciplinary partnerships, research infrastructures, and effective communication among stakeholders will promote an efficient and beneficial translation process.

References

Antoniou, A. *et al.* (2003). Average risks of breast and ovarian cancer associated with BRCA1 or BRCA2 mutations detected in case series unselected for family history: A combined analysis of 22 studies. *American Journal of Human Genetics*, **72**, 1117–30.

Austin, M.A., Peyser, P.J., and Khoury, M.J. (2000). The interface of genetics and public health: Research and educational challenges. *Annual Review of Public Health*, **21**, 81–9.

Bellagio group (2005). *Genome-based research and population health.* Report of an international workshop held at the Rockefeller Foundation Study and Conference Center, Bellagio, Italy, 14–20 April 2005. http://www.graphint.org/docs/BellagioReport230106.pdf.

Beskow, L.M. *et al.* (2001). Informed consent for population-based research involving genetics. *JAMA*, **286**, 2315–21.

Botkin, J.R. (2005). Research for newborn screening: Developing a national framework. *Pediatrics*, **116**, 862–71.

Botkin, J. *et al.* (2006). Newborn screening technology: Proceed with caution. *Pediatrics*, **117**, 1800–5.

Burke, W. (2002). Genetic testing. *New England Journal of Medicine*, **347**, 1867–75.

Burke, W. and Zimmern, R. (2007). *Moving beyond ACCE: An expanded framework for genetic test evaluation.* Paper prepared for the UK Genetic Testing Network.

Burke, W. *et al.* (2002). Genetic test evaluation: information needs of clinicians, policy makers, and the public. *American Journal of Epidemiology*, **256**, 311–8.

Burke, W., Khoury, M.J., Stewart, A. *et al.* for the Bellagio group (2006). The path from genome-based research to population health: Development of an international public health genomics network. *Genetics in Medicine*, **8**, 451–8.

Burke, W., Zimmern, R.L., and Kroese, M. (2007). Defining purpose: A key step in genetic test evaluation. *Genetics in Medicine*, **9**, 675–81.

Burton, H. (2003). *Addressing genetics, delivering health.* Public Health Genetics Unit, Cambridge, UK.

Cao, A., Rosatelli, M.C., Monni, G. *et al.* (2002). Screening for thalassaemia: A model of success. *Obstetrics and Gynecology Clinics of North America*, **29**, 305–28.

Centers for Disease Control and Prevention (1997). *Translating advances in human genetics into public health: A strategic plan.* http://www.cdc.gov/genomics/about/strategic.htm

Christianson, A., Howson, C.P., and Modell, B. (2006). *March of Dimes global report on birth defects. The hidden toll of dying and disabled children.* March of Dimes Birth Defects Foundation. White Plains, New York.

Collins, F.S. and McKusick, V.A. (2001). Implications of the human genome project for medical science. *JAMA*, **285**, 540–4.

Collins, F.S., Morgan, M., and Patrinos, A. (2003). The human genome project: Lessons from large-scale biology. *Science*, **300**, 286–90.

Daar, A., Thorsteindottir, H., Martin, D.K. *et al.* (2002). Top ten biotechnologies for improving health in developing countries. *Nature Genetics*, **32**, 229–32.

Davey Smith, G., Ebrahim, S., Lewis, S. *et al.* (2005). Genetic epidemiology and public health: Hope, hype, and future prospects. *Lancet*, **366**, 1484–98.

Elmore, J.G. and Fletcher, S.W. (2006). The risk of cancer risk prediction: "What is my risk of getting breast cancer?" *Journal of the National Cancer Institute*, **98**, 1673–5.

Gardiner, S.H. and Begg, E.J. (2006). Pharmacogenetics, drug metabolising enzymes and clinical practice. *Pharmacological Reviews*, **58**, 529–90.

Genomics Working Group of the Science and Technology Task Force of the United Nations Millennium Project (2004). *Genomics and global health*. University of Toronto Joint Centre for Bioethics, Toronto.

Grosse, S.D. and Khoury, M.J. (2006). What is the clinical utility of genetic testing? *Genetics in Medicine*, **8**, 448–50.

Grosse, S.D., Boyle, C.A., Kenneson, A. *et al.* (2006). From public health emergency to public health service: The implications of evolving criteria for newborn screening panels. *Pediatrics*, **117**, 923–9.

Guttmacher, A.E. and Collins, F.S. (2005). Realizing the promise of genomics in biomedical research. *JAMA*, **294**, 1399–402.

Guttmacher, A.E., Jenkins, J., and Uhlmann, W.R. (2001). Genomic medicine: Who will practice it? A call to open arms. *American Journal of Medical Genetics*, **106**, 216–22.

Haddow, J. and Palomaki, G. (2004). ACCE: A model process for evaluating data on emerging genetic tests. In *Human genome epidemiology* (eds. M. Khoury, J. Little, and W. Burke), pp. 217–33. Oxford University Press, Oxford.

Haga, S.B., Khoury, M.J., and Burke, W. (2003). Genomic profiling to promote a healthy lifestyle: Not ready for prime time. *Nature Genetics*, **34**, 347–50.

Halliday, J.L., Collins, V.R., Aitken, M.A. *et al.* (2004). Genetics and public health – evolution, or revolution? *Journal of Epidemiology and Community Health*, **58**, 894–9.

Hirschhorn, J.N. and Daly, M.J. (2005). Genome-wide association studies for common diseases and complex traits. *Nature Reviews Genetics*, **6**, 95–107.

Holtzman, N.A. and Watson, M.S. (eds.) (1997). *Promoting safe and effective genetic testing in the United States*. Final report of the Task Force on Genetic Testing. http://www.genome.gov/10001733

Hunter, D.J. (2005). Gene-environment interactions in human disease. *Nature Reviews Genetics*, **6**, 287–97.

Ioannidis, J.P.A., Trikalinos, T.A., and Khoury, M.J. (2006). Implications of small effect sizes of individual genetic variants on the design and interpretation of genetic association studies of complex diseases. *American Journal of Epidemiology*, **164**, 609–14.

Ioannidis, J.P.A. *et al.* (2006). A road map for efficient and reliable human genome epidemiology. *Nature Genetics*, **38**, 3–5.

Ioannidis, J.P.A. *et al.* (2008). Assessment of cumulative evidence on genetic associations: interim guidelines. *International Journal of Epidemiology* **37**, 120–32.

Jaenisch, R. and Bird, A. (2003). Epigenetic regulation of gene expression: How the genome integrates intrinsic and environmental signals. *Nature Genetics*, **33**(Suppl.), 245–54.

Janssens, A.C.J.W. and Khoury, M.J. (2006). Predictive value of testing for multiple genetic variants in multifactorial diseases: Implications for the discourse on ethical, legal and social issues. *Italian Journal of Public Health*, **4**, 35–41.

Janssens, A.C., Gwinn, M., Valdez, R. *et al.* (2006). Predictive genetic testing for type 2 diabetes. *BMJ*, **333**, 509–10.

Janssens, A.C.J.W., Pardo, M.C., Steyerberg, E.W. *et al.* (2004). Revisiting the clinical validity of multiplex genetic testing in complex disease. *American Journal of Human Genetics*, **74**, 585–8.

Juengst, E.T. (1995). 'Prevention' and the goals of genetic medicine. *Human Gene Therapy*, **6**, 1595–605.

Kaye, C.I. *et al.* (2006). Newborn screening fact sheets. *Pediatrics* **118**, e934–63.

Kevles, D.J. (1995). *In the name of eugenics: Genetics and the uses of human heredity*. Harvard University Press, Cambridge, USA.

Khoury, M.J. (1996). From genes to public health: The applications of genetic technology in disease prevention. *American Journal of Public Health*, **86**, 1717–22.

Khoury, M.J. (1999). Human genome epidemiology (HuGE): Translating advances in human genetics into population-based data for medicine and public health. *Genetics in Medicine*, **1**, 71–3.

Khoury, M.J. (2003). Genetics and genomics in practice: The continuum from genetic disease to genetic information in health and disease. *Genetics in Medicine*, **5**, 261–8.

Khoury, M.J., Burke, W., and Thomson, E.J. (2000). *Genetics and public health in the 21st century*. Oxford University Press, New York.

Khoury, M.J., Davis, R., Gwinn, M. *et al.* (2005). Do we need genomic research for the prevention of common diseases with environmental causes? *American Journal of Epidemiology*, **161**, 799–805.

Khoury, M.J., Little, J., Gwinn, M. *et al.* (2007). On the synthesis and interpretation of consistent but weak gene-disease associations in the era of genome-wide association studies. *International Journal of Epidemiology*, **36**, 439–45.

Khoury, M.J., McCabe, L.L., and McCabe, E.R.B. (2003). Population screening in the age of genomic medicine. *New England Journal of Medicine*, **348**, 50–8.

Khoury, M.J., Millikan, R., Little, J. *et al.* (2004). The emergence of epidemiology in the genomics age. *International Journal of Epidemiology*, **33**, 936–44.

Knoppers, B.M. (2005). Of genomics and public health: Building public 'goods'. *Canadian Medical Association Journal*, **173**, 1185–6.

Knoppers, B.M. and Chadwick, R. (2005). Human genetic research: Emerging trends in ethics. *Nature Reviews Genetics*, **6**,75–9.

Kroese, M., Zimmern, R.L., and Sanderson, S. (2004). Genetic tests and their evaluation: Can we answer the key questions? *Genetics in Medicine*, **6**, 475–80.

LaRusse, S. *et al.* (2005). Genetic susceptibility testing versus family history-based risk assessment: Impact on perceived risk of Alzheimer disease. *Genetics in Medicine*, **7**, 48–53.

Little, J. *et al.* (2003). The human genome project is complete. How do we develop a handle for the pump? *American Journal of Epidemiology*, **157**, 667–73.

Markel, H. (1997). Scientific advances and social risks: Historical perspectives of genetic screening programs for sickle cell disease, Tay Sachs Disease, neural tube defects and Down Syndrome, 1970–1997. Appendix 6 in *Promoting safe and effective genetic testing in the United States. Final report of the Task Force on Genetic Testing* (eds. N.A. Holtzman and M.S. Watson). http://www.genome.gov/10001733

Marteau, T. and Lerman, C. (2001). Genetic risk and behavioural change. *BMJ*, **322**, 105–6.

Marteau, T. *et al.* (2004). Psychological impact of genetic testing for familial hypercholesterolaemia within a previously aware population: A randomized controlled trial. *American Journal of Medical Genetics*, **128**, 285–93.

Merikangas, K.R. and Risch, N. (2003). Genomic priorities and public health. *Science*, **302**, 599–601.

Murray, T. (1997). Genetic exceptionalism and 'future diaries': Is genetic information different from other medical information? In *Genetic secrets: Protecting privacy and confidentiality in the genetic era* (ed. M.A. Rothstein), pp. 60–73. Yale University Press, New Haven.

National Collaborating Centre for Women's and Children's Health (2003). *Antenatal care: Routine care for the healthy pregnant woman*. http://www.rcog.org.uk/resources/Public/pdf/Antenatal_Care.pdf

National Institute for Health and Clinical Excellence (2006). *Familial breast cancer: The classification and care of women at risk of familial breast cancer in primary, secondary and tertiary care.* http://www.nice.org.uk/guidance/CG41

National Office of Public Health Genomics (2001). *Genomic competencies for the public health workforce.* http://www.cdc.gov/genomics/training/competencies/default.htm

National Screening Committee (2007). *National Screening Committee policy – medium chain acyl CoA dehydrogenase deficiency screening.* http://www.library.nhs.uk/guidelinesfinder/ViewResource.aspx?resID=57173

NHS Central Research and Development Committee (1995). *Genetics of common disease.* Department of Health, London.

NHS Central Research and Development Committee (1995). *Report of the Genetics Research Advisory Group.* Department of Health, London.

NHS Sickle Cell and Thalassaemia Screening Programme. *Policy framework for antenatal screening programme for England.* http://www.kcl-phs.org.uk/haemscreening/Documents/AnScreenPolicy.pdf

Pandor, A., Eastham, J., Beverley, C. *et al.* (2004). Clinical effectiveness and cost effectiveness of neonatal screening for inborn errors of metabolism using tandem mass spectrometry. *Health Technology Assessment*, **8** (12).

Petricoin, E.F. *et al.* (2002). Use of proteomic patterns in serum to identify ovarian cancer. *Lancet*, **16**, 572–7.

Quackenbush, J. (2006). Microarray analysis and tumour classification. *New England Journal of Medicine*, **354**, 2463–72.

Read, A. and Donnai, D. (2007). *New clinical genetics.* Scion, Bloxham.

Richards, E.J. (2006). Inherited epigenetic variation – revisiting soft inheritance. *Nature Reviews Genetics*, **7**, 395–401.

Rockhill, B., Kawachi, I., and Colditz, G.A. (2000). Individual risk prediction and population-wide disease prevention. *Epidemiological Reviews*, **22**, 176–80.

Rose, G. (1985). Sick individuals and sick populations. *International Journal of Epidemiology*, **14**, 32–8.

Rothman, K.J. (1986). *Modern epidemiology.* Little, Brown and Company, Boston.

Royal College of Physicians of London (1991). *Purchasers' guide to genetic services in the NHS.* Royal College of Physicians, London.

Sanderson, S., Emery, J., and Higgins, J. (2005). CYP2C9 variants, drug dose, and bleeding risk in warfarin-treated patients: A HuGENet systematic review and meta-analysis. *Genetics in Medicine*, **7**, 97–104.

Sconce, E.A. *et al.* (2005). The impact of *CYP2C9* and *VKORC1* genetic polymorphism and patient characteristics upon warfarin dose requirements: Proposal for a new dosing regimen. *Blood*, **106**, 2329–33.

Singer, P.A. and Daar, A.S. (2001). Harnessing genomics and biotechnology to improve global health equity. *Science*, **294**, 87–9.

Staudt, L.M. and Dave, S. (2005). The biology of human lymphoid malignancies revealed by gene expression profiling. *Advances in Immunology*, **87**, 163–208.

Stewart, A., Brice, P., Burton, H. *et al.* (2007). *Genetics, health care and public policy.* Cambridge University Press, Cambridge.

Stewart, A., Karmali, M., and Zimmern, R. (2006). GRaPH Int: An international network for public health genomics. In *Genomics and public health. Legal and socio-economic perspectives* (ed. B.M. Knoppers), pp. 257–71. Martinus Nijhoff Publishers, The Netherlands.

Subramonia-Iyer, S. *et al.* (2007). Array-based comparative genomic hybridization for investigating chromosomal abnormalities in patients with learning disability: Systematic review and meta-analysis of diagnostic and false-positive yield. *Genetics in Medicine*, **9**, 74–9.

The Wellcome Trust Case Control Consortium (2007). Genome-wide association study of 14,000 cases of seven common diseases and 3,000 shared controls. *Nature*, **447**, 661–78.

Watson, M.S. *et al.* (eds.) (2006). Newborn screening: Toward a uniform screening panel and system. Executive summary. *Genetics in Medicine*, **8** (Suppl), 1S–11S.

Weatherall, D.J. and Clegg, J.B. (2001). Inherited haemoglobin disorders: An increasing global health problem. *Bulletin of the World Health Organization*, **79**, 704–12.

Willard, H.F., Angrist, M., and Ginsburg, G.S. (2005). Genomic medicine: Genetic variation and its impact on the future of health care. *Philosophical Transactions of the Royal Society Series B*, **360**, 1543–50.

Wilson, J.M.G. and Jungner, G. (1968). *Principles and practice of screening for disease.* Public health paper no. 34. World Health Organization, Geneva.

Wolf, C.R., Smith, G., and Smith, R.L. (2000). Science, medicine and the future: Pharmacogenetics. *BMJ*, **320**, 987–90.

World Health Organization (1996). *Control of hereditary diseases.* WHO, Geneva. http://whqlibdoc.who.int/trs/WHO_TRS_865.pdf

World Health Organization Advisory Committee on Health Research (2002). *Genomics and world health.* World Health Organization, Geneva.

Yang, Q. *et al.* (2003). Improving the prediction of complex diseases by testing for multiple disease susceptibility genes. *American Journal of Human Genetics*, **72**, 636–49.

Yoon, P.W., Scheuner, M.T., Peterson-Oehlke, K.L. *et al.* (2002). Can family history be used as a tool for public health and preventive medicine? *Genetics in Medicine*, **4**, 304–10.

Zimmern, R. (2001). What is genetic information: Whose hands on your genes? *Genetics Law Monitor*, **1**, 9–13.

2.5

Water and sanitation

Thomas Clasen and Steven Sugden

Abstract

The lack of safe drinking water and basic sanitation impose a heavy health burden, especially on young children and the poor; it also aggravates poverty, poor school attendance, and overall development. Unlike many of the other challenges in public health, the water and sanitation solutions are well-known. However, despite strong evidence of the effectiveness and cost-effectiveness of improved water and sanitation against diarrhoea and certain other diseases and support for the intervention at the highest international levels, coverage still lags behind the MDG targets, especially for sanitation. This chapter describes the aetiological agents of the leading water- and sanitation-related diseases, presents the evidence concerning the effectiveness of water and sanitation interventions to prevent such diseases, and summarizes the economic implications of such interventions and some of the other non-health benefits associated therewith. Recent and emerging developments in water, sanitation, and health are discussed, including new methods for assessing and measuring the risks associated with unsafe water and sanitation, technologies, programmatic approaches, and implementation strategies. The chapter closes with a discussion of some of the continuing challenges in water and sanitation, including efforts to scale up interventions among the most vulnerable populations in an effort to secure the benefits of water and sanitation for all.

Introduction

Background

Safe drinking water and sanitary waste disposal are among the most fundamental of public health interventions. When readers of the *British Medical Journal* were asked in 2006 to name the 'greatest medical advance' since 1840, their top choice was clean drinking water and waste disposal, beating antibiotics, anaesthesia, vaccines, and germ theory (Ferriman 2007). Deaths from diarrhoeal diseases and typhoid fever showed dramatic declines in Europe and North America when cities and towns began filtering and chlorinating their water and safely disposing of human and animal excreta (Cutler & Miller 2005). The field of epidemiology arguably has its origins in John Snow's nineteenth century mapping of cholera cases and the eventual intervention at London's Broad Street pump that demonstrated waterborne transmission of the disease.

While diseases associated with poor water and sanitation are now comparatively unknown in higher income countries, they still impose a heavy burden elsewhere, especially among young children, the poor, the immuno-compromised, and the displaced. Diarrhoeal diseases alone kill an estimated 1.7 million people each year, and account for 17 per cent of deaths in children under five in developing countries (WHO 2005). According to the World Health Organization (WHO), 94 per cent of such deaths could be averted by improvements in water, sanitation, and hygiene (Prüss-Üstün & Corvalán 2007). Because they interfere with normal adsorption of nutrients, the diseases associated with poor water and sanitation are also a major cause of malnutrition, a separate source of significant morbidity and mortality (Fewtrell *et al.* 2007).

Water and sanitation are not only a matter of public health, but also of poverty, equity, and justice (UNDP 2006). Because they are less likely to have access to safe water and sanitation, the poor bear most of the burden of water-related diseases, driving them further into poverty through lost productivity and expenditure on treatment (Blakley *et al.* 2006). Time spent in collecting water from distant sources and the inability to procure sufficient quantities of water for irrigating crops, watering animals, and carrying out other productive activities aggravates poverty. Inadequate water and sanitation are also associated with poor school attendance (Hutton *et al.* 2007). For these and other reasons, water and sanitation have been recognized as a fundamental human right (UNICEF 1999; United Nations 2002).

Nevertheless, basic water security and sanitation still elude much of the world's population living in low-income countries. An estimated 1.1 billion people lack improved access to water supplies; 2.6 billion people—40 per cent of the world's population—lack access to improved sanitation. Coverage is lowest in developing regions, where people are most vulnerable to infection and disease. In Africa, improved water and sanitation coverage is just 56 per cent and 37 per cent, respectively (WHO/UNICEF 2005). Rural areas also lag behind their urban counterparts, with three times as many rural dwellers lacking improved sanitation as urban dwellers; improved water reaches less than 50 per cent of rural populations in 27 developing countries. If current trends continue, more than half of the rural population will still be without sanitation coverage in 2015, and more than 700 million mainly poor rural dwellers will still lack improved water (WHO/UNICEF 2006).

The shortfall in water and sanitation coverage is not the result of a failure to recognize the need or declare goals at the highest international levels. The 1977 Mar del Plata Declaration by the United Nations expressed the goal of providing safe water and sanitation for all by 1990, launching the Water and Sanitation Decade (1981–1990) (Cairncross 1992). In 1990, the UN renewed the call and extended the deadline to the end of the century. The United Nations Millennium Development Goals (MDGs) call for halving, by 2015, the portion of the population without sustainable access to safe drinking water or basic sanitation (United Nations 2000). As the research described in this chapter suggests, such coverage would not only advance the environmental security targets under MDG Goal 7, but also make contributions to reducing poverty (Goal 1), increasing primary education (Goal 2), promoting gender equality (Goal 3), reducing child mortality (Goal 4), and combating major diseases (Goal 6). In a further effort to attract attention to this deficit and additional priority to the sector, the United Nations General Assembly declared 2005–15 as the Decade for Action, Water for Life (WHO/UNICEF 2005), and 2008 as the International Year of Sanitation.

Traditionally, much of the work in water and sanitation has been undertaken by engineers and has consisted of infrastructural improvements. Low-cost community- and household-based interventions, such as protected wells, boreholes, and communal stand pipes for improved water supplies, and various types of latrines, septic tanks, and composting systems for improved sanitation, have been largely conceived by and constructed with the assistance of engineers. There are numerous books, manuals, and other resources that describe these systems in detail, including Cairncross and Feachem (1993), DFID (1998), Davis and Lambert (2002), the quarterly *Waterlines*, and the World Bank Water and Sanitation Programme (WSP) *Field Notes* (www.wps.org). Readers are encouraged to refer to such sources for details on the design, installation, and operation of such systems, technology innovations, and the programmatic challenges associated with achieving widespread use on a sustained basis.

This chapter focuses solely on the public health issues concerning water and sanitation. After introducing some basic terminology, it begins by describing the diseases associated with inadequate water and sanitation and their contribution to the overall burden of disease. It then presents evidence of the effectiveness of water and sanitation interventions to prevent such diseases, the economic implications (especially cost-effectiveness and cost–benefits) of such interventions, and some of the other non-health benefits associated therewith. Recent and emerging developments in water, sanitation, and health are then discussed, along with some issues relevant to designing water and sanitation interventions. The chapter closes with a discussion of some of the continuing challenges in water and sanitation, including efforts to scale up interventions among the most vulnerable populations in an effort to secure the benefits of water and sanitation for all.

Terminology

At the outset, it is useful to understand some of the terminology used in describing the diseases, transmission routes, and interventions associated with the water and sanitation sectors. Water-related diseases are sometimes classified according to their disease transmission routes as *waterborne* (ingested in drinking water), *water-washed* (associated with inadequate supplies of water for proper personal hygiene), *water-based* (transmitted through an aquatic invertebrate host), or linked to a *water-related vector* (involving an insect vector breeding in or near water) (White *et al.* 1972). Most waterborne organisms that are human pathogens colonize the gut of humans and certain other mammals and are transmitted through the *faecal–oral* route. The transmission of common waterborne diseases can thus be interrupted by improvements in sanitation (*excreta disposal*), personal hygiene (especially *hand washing*), and microbiological *water quality*, while those that are water-washed are impacted by improvements in *water supplies* (quantity and access) for personal hygiene. Improving water supplies can also help prevent water-based diseases (such as schistosomiasis and dracunculiasis) by reducing the need to enter infected water bodies.

The term 'sanitation' is vague with multiple meanings. Within the sanitation sector two definitions are used. Under the broader definition, sanitation extends to the process whereby people demand, effect, and sustain a hygienic and healthy environment for themselves. This definition could include safe food production, solid waste management, industrial waste, hygiene behaviour change, hand washing, control of chemicals, environmental pollution, storm water drainage, wastewater disposal, human settlements, prevention and control of communicable diseases, HIV/AIDS, vector and vermin control, occupational health and safety, mining and quarrying, port health, and disposal of the dead. A second definition is more specific, extending only to the process of separating humans from their excreta. This chapter uses this second, more specific definition and regards sanitation as a system in which excreta is (i) collected safely and with dignity, (ii) transported to a suitable location, (iii) treated or contained for some period of time, and (iv) reused and/or discharged to the environment.

The MDG targets for water and sanitation are expressed in terms of *sustainable access to safe drinking water* and of *basic sanitation*. The water target has been interpreted as 'sufficient drinking water of acceptable quality as well as sufficient quantity of water for hygienic purposes' (UN Millennium Project 2005). Basic sanitation, in turn, has been defined as 'the lowest-cost option for securing sustainable access to safe, hygienic, and convenient facilities and services for excreta and sewage disposal that provide privacy and dignity, while at the same time ensuring a clean and healthy living environment both at home and in the neighbourhood of users (UN Millennium Project 2005). Progress toward the MDGs, however, is measured with reference to the Joint Monitoring Programme (JMP) which adopts an indicator approach based on facilities or level of service. For water supplies, the JMP distinguishes only between *improved water supplies* (piped-in tap water, public tap/standpipe, borehole/tubewell, protected well/spring, rainwater harvesting), and *unimproved water supplies* (surface water, unprotected well/spring, tankered water, bottled water). *Improved sanitation* includes a private flush or pour-flush toilet or latrine connected to a piped sewer system or septic system, simple pit latrine with slab, ventilated improved pit (VIP) latrine, or composting toilet; *unimproved sanitation* includes any other flush or pour-flush latrine, open pit latrine, bucket latrine, hanging latrine, any public or shared facility, or open defecation (WHO/UNICEF 2002).

Burden of disease

General

Poor water and sanitation are associated with a variety of infectious diseases transmitted through various pathways by helminths, protozoa, bacteria, and viruses. Table 2.5.1 summarizes the most important of these diseases, their transmission routes, aetiological agents, and epidemiological significance. Further details are provided in Sections 'General' *et seq.* Some of these diseases also contribute to malnutrition, a separate cause of substantial morbidity and mortality that is not reflected in the direct burden of disease figures cited below (Black *et al.* 2003).

Certain diseases associated with water are not addressed in this chapter. First, in addition to microbial agents, water is a medium for the transmission of chemical pathogens, including arsenic and other metals, fluoride, nitrates, and volatile organic compounds (including pesticides and herbicides). Accordingly, WHO guidelines and many national water standards establish maximum allowable limits for such chemicals (WHO 2004). However, except for arsenicosis and fluoridosis, which are especially serious in focal areas in Asia and parts of Africa, most of these contaminants represent hazards to health only over the longer term. Second, although improvements in water supplies (to discourage contact with water) and point-of-use water treatment (with filters) are important interventions in preventing dracunculiasis (Cairncross *et al.* 2002), efforts to control Guinea worm infection have been largely successful and the disease is now of public health interest in limited areas. Finally, this chapter does not address a variety of diseases associated with waterborne pathogens, such as poliomyelitis and hepatitis A & E, which are controlled mainly by vaccines and other non-environmental measures (Leclerc *et al.* 2002).

Diarrhoeal diseases

Diarrhoeal diseases kill an estimated 1.8 million people each year (WHO 2005). Among infectious diseases, diarrhoea ranks as the third leading cause of both mortality and morbidity (after respiratory infections and HIV/AIDS), placing it above tuberculosis and malaria. Young children are especially vulnerable, bearing 68 per cent

Table 2.5.1 Principal infectious diseases, disease agents, transmission routes, and annual morbidity and mortality related to poor water and sanitation

Disease	Aetiological agent	Transmission	Morbidity*	Mortality*
Diarrhoea (dysentery, cholera)	**Viruses** *Rotavirus*	Faecal–oral	4 billion (annual)	1.8 million
	Bacteria *E.coli (ETEC)* *Shiguella* sp. *Salmonella* sp. *Vibrio* sp. *Campylobacter* sp.	Faecal–oral		
	Protozoa *Giardia lambia* *Cryptosporidium parvum* *Emtamoeba histolytic*	Faecal–oral		
Schistosomiasis	*S. haematobium* *S. mansoni* *S. japonicum*	Penetration through skin exposed to contaminated freshwater	187 million	27 000–280 000
Ascariasis	*Ascaris lumbricoides*	Faecal–oral	1.2 billion	
Trichuriasis	*Trichuris trichuria*	Faecal–oral	795 million	
Hookworm infection	*Necator americanus*	Penetration through skin exposed to faecally-contaminated soil	740 million	
	Ancylostoma duodenale	Faecal–oral		
Typhoid and paratyphoid fever	*Salmonella* sp.	Faecal–oral	26 million	216 000
Trachoma	*Chlamydia trachomatis*	Fingers Clothing Eye-seeking flies (*M. sorbens*) Coughing/sneezing	6 million blind 150 million with active trachoma	

* Estimates vary according to method. Morbidity and mortality estimates for diarrhoeal disease are from WHO (2005); those for soil-transmitted helminth infections (STH) (ascariasis, trichuriasis, hookworm) and schistosomiasis are from deSilva *et al.* (2003) and Hotez *et al.* (2006). Mortality estimates for STH and schistosomiasis vary significantly, depending on the method used for estimation (Hotez *et al.* 2006). Typhoid and paratyphoid estimates are from Crump *et al.* (2004). Trachoma figures are from Kumaresan and Mecaskey (2003).

of the total burden of diarrhoeal disease (Bartram 2003). Among children younger than 5 years, diarrhoea accounts for 17 per cent of all deaths (United Nations 2005). For those infected with the human immunodeficiency virus (HIV) or who have developed acquired immunodeficiency syndrome (AIDS), diarrhoea can be prolonged, severe, and life-threatening (Hayes *et al.* 2003).

Diarrhoea is characterized by stools of decreased consistency and increased number. The clinical symptoms and course of the disease vary greatly with the age, nutritional and immune status, and the pathogen (Black & Lanata 1995). Most cases resolve within a week, though a small percentage continue for 2 weeks or more and are characterized as 'persistent' diarrhoea. Dysentery is a diarrhoeal disease defined by the presence of blood in the liquid stools. Though epidemic diarrhoea such as cholera and shigellosis (bacillary dysentery) are well-known risks, particularly in emergency settings, their global health significance is small compared to endemic diarrhoea (Hunter 1997).

The immediate threat from diarrhoea is dehydration, a loss of fluids and electrolytes. Thus, the widespread promotion of oral rehydration therapy (ORT) has significantly reduced the case-fatality rate associated with the disease. Such improvements in case management, however, have not reduced morbidity, which is estimated at four billion cases annually (Kosek *et al.* 2003). And since diarrhoeal diseases inhibit normal ingestion of foods and adsorption of nutrients, continued high morbidity is an important cause of malnutrition, leading to impaired physical growth and cognitive function, reduced resistance to infection, and potentially long-term gastrointestinal disorders.

The infectious agents associated with diarrhoeal disease are transmitted chiefly through the faecal–oral route (Leclerc *et al.* 2001). Safe excreta disposal thus represents a primary barrier that should contribute to the prevention of indirect transmission via food, water, hands, fomites, and mechanical vectors (flies) (Fig. 2.5.1). A wide variety of bacterial, viral, and protozoan pathogens excreted in the faeces of humans and animals are known to cause diarrhoea. The importance of individual pathogens varies among settings, seasons, and conditions. Although diarrhoea is also associated with the ingestion of metals, nitrates, organics, and other chemicals, the burden of disease arising from such exposure is small relative to infectious diarrhoea (Hunter 1997).

Schistosomiasis

Schistosomiasis affects 187 million people all over the world, with *S. haematobium* and *S. mansoni* being the most common species. The schistosomiasis life cycle involves contamination of freshwater by eggs-carrying excreta and urine and an intermediate host, a freshwater snail. Larvae released in the water infect humans by penetrating through the skin. Parasites develop and migrate to the intestines and bladder where thousands of eggs are produced. Like other intestinal helminths, schistosomes are associated with impaired physical and mental development and anaemia. Furthermore, schistosomiasis may cause serious damage to the bladder and intestine walls as a result of parasite egg entrapment within tissues. Chronic infection with *S. haematobium* has been associated with increased risk of bladder cancer in adulthood (Gryssels *et al.* 2006).

Soil-transmitted helminth infection

More than two billion of the world's population, mostly in developing countries, are infected with soil-transmitted helminths. About 300 million people suffer from heavy worm load and related severe morbidity (deSilva *et al.* 2003). *Ascaris lumbricoides, Trichuris trichuria*, and hookworm (*Ancylostoma duodenale* and *Necator americanus*) are the most prevalent intestinal helminths. Transmission occurs via ingestion of eggs present in faecally-contaminated soil, or via penetration of the larvae through the skin. Children are particularly vulnerable to chronic and heavy infections which result in malnutrition, stunted growth, reduced physical fitness, and impaired cognitive development (Stephenson *et al.* 2000). Hookworm infection is an important cause of anaemia, not only in children, but also among women of reproductive age and pregnant women leading to premature birth and low birthweight (Hotez *et al.* 2004).

Typhoid and paratyphoid fevers

While enteric fevers such as typhoid and paratyphoid were leading causes of waterborne disease in previous centuries, morbidity and mortality diminished dramatically with the provisions of disinfected water supplies and improved sanitary facilities (Cutler & Miller 2005). The aetiological agents for typhoid and paratyphoid fevers

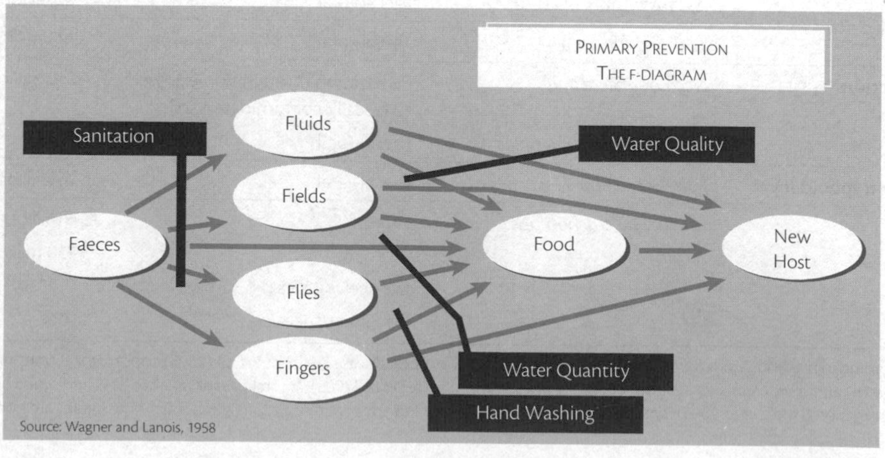

Fig. 2.5.1 The F-diagram (from Wagner & Lanois 1958).

are *Salmonella typhi* and *Salmonella paratyphi*; a proposed new nomenclature would change the *S. typhi* to *S. enterica* serovar Typhi and *S. paratyphi* to *S. enterica* serovar Paratyphi A and B. A recent review estimates 21 million cases of typhoid annually, causing 216 000 deaths (Crump *et al.* 2004). The milder paratyphoid accounts for an additional 5 million cases each year.

Trachoma

Trachoma accounts for 15 per cent of world blindness, with 6 million people affected and 150 million at risk of visual impairment (Kumaresan & Mecaskey 2003). Trachoma is caused by repeated eye infection with *Chlamydia trachomatis*. Children are the main reservoir for infection, with high prevalence of active trachoma (Mabey *et al.* 2003). Repeated infections result in deformation of the upper eye lid, abrasion of the cornea, and progressive loss of vision in later life. *C. trachomatis* is transmitted from the discharge of an infected eye via contaminated fingers, clothing, and eye-seeking flies (*M. sorbens.*) Although the role of flies in the transmission of infection remains unclear, studies have shown that *M. sorbens* breed mainly in solid human faeces present in the environment and not in latrines (Emerson *et al.* 2000). Thus, safe excreta disposal may play an important role in reducing trachoma transmission. Improving water supplies and sanitationis part of the WHO-backed SAFE (surgery, antibiotics, facial hygiene, environmental improvement) strategy for controlling and preventing the disease.

Effectiveness of water and sanitation in preventing disease

Barriers to transmission of faecal–oral diseases

As illustrated by the so-called 'F-diagram' (Fig. 2.5.1), the safe disposal of human faeces is the primary barrier in preventing faecal–oral transmitted diseases. Without removing excreta from potential contact with humans, animals, and insects, pathogens may be carried on unwashed hands, in contaminated water or food, or via flies and other insects on to further human hosts. Whether or not sanitation is adequate, hands can become contaminated with faeces, especially during anal cleansing following defecation or in cleaning a child after defecation. This may result in further transmission, either directly or indirectly through food, water, or other beverages, or fomites. Accordingly, hand washing is an important secondary barrier to faecal–oral disease transmission (Curtis & Cairncross 2003). Other secondary barriers include (i) water quality interventions to prevent contamination (e.g. safe distribution and storage or use of a residual disinfectant to prevent recontamination), (ii) water supply interventions to increase the quantity and availability of water for personal and domestic hygiene, (iii) proper cooking and food handling, and (iv) control of mechanical vectors such as flies.

Rigorously assessing the impact of water and sanitation interventions on human health presents a number of methodological problems (Blum & Feachem 1983; Esrey *et al.* 1986). Blinded, randomized, controlled trials (RCTs), the gold standard of epidemiological evidence (Chapter 6.8), are impossible for most water and sanitation interventions, as it is impractical or politically inexpedient to randomly deliver the intervention to large numbers of a study population while leaving others as controls, and often impossible to blind infrastructural interventions. Studies that purport to achieve sufficient sample size by randomly allocating the intervention to the population of one village while using a second village serve as controls are, in fact, a one-to-one comparison, yielding a sample size of just two and limiting the statistical significance of any observed differences (Blum & Feachem 1983). Most interventional studies of water and sanitation follow a quasi-randomized (quasi-experimental) design where the intervention has not been allocated randomly, but the investigators otherwise treat as a controlled trial. Blinded RCTs have been used to assess certain water quality interventions of household-based interventions (Colford *et al.* 2002). Recent studies of sanitation interventions have followed cluster-randomized (Emerson *et al.* 2004) and step-wedge approaches (Smith & Morrow 1996) to address some of the challenges of RCTs to assess water and sanitation interventions.

Most studies of the water and sanitation thus follow observational designs (cross-sectional, case-control, and cohort studies). While these studies can yield valuable information in developing hypotheses and seeking associations between the intervention and outcome of interest, they must measure and control for numerous known confounders. Age is particularly important: Diarrhoeal disease morbidity and mortality is highest among children after weaning and before development of immune systems; other enteric infections also tend to follow demographic patterns consistent with their exposure. Faecal–oral diseases such as diarrhoea are characterized by significant seasonal variations that make it difficult to make before–after comparisons (as opposed to comparisons with a contemporaneous control group) and challenging to estimate sample sizes (Schmidt *et al.* 2007). Other important confounders include quantity and quality of water available, distance and other barriers to access, collection and storage practices, sanitation facilities, and use, and hygiene practices. Households who take special steps to improve their water supplies or build latrines are self-selected and, as they also tend to be wealthier, better educated, and more conscious of hygiene, are more likely to adopt other behaviour that protect their families from faecal–oral disease.

Regardless of the study design, there are significant challenges in assessing the effectiveness of water and sanitation interventions to prevent diarrhoeal disease. First, there are different ways of defining the disease itself. While many studies use the standard WHO definition for diarrhoea (3 or more loose stools in 24 h) (WHO 1993), others use local definitions (Moy *et al.* 1991). Although some studies use clinical assays or serology to confirm infection, most assessments of diarrhoeal diseases rely on self-reporting which can be biased by recall errors (especially for periods longer than the previous 48 h) and potential reporting since diarrhoea is private or embarrassing and often regarded as more of an annoyance than a disease. Comparing results between studies is also complicated by different measures of disease frequency (incidence, period prevalence, longitudinal prevalence) and measures of effect of the intervention (risk ratios, rate ratios, odds ratios, longitudinal prevalence ratios). While collecting information on incidence may be necessary for assessing risk, longitudinal prevalence may be a more efficient means of measuring the effectiveness of an intervention while minimizing Hawthorne effect and courtesy bias and the challenge of distinguishing separate episodes of diarrhoea (Morris *et al.* 1996; Schmidt *et al.* 2007). Another common error in the analysis of results is the failure to adjust the data for lack of independent observations (e.g. repeated observations of the same subject and for intra-cluster correlations, such as among subjects living within the same household). Owing to the challenges of measuring actual use of a latrine or improved water supply, many studies fail to report on compliance with the intervention even though this has been shown to be an important aspect of the effectiveness of the intervention.

It is important for those engaged in research involving water and sanitation interventions to consider these methodological issues when designing studies and assessments. These issues should also be borne in mind in evaluating the evidence of the effectiveness of water and sanitation interventions described in the next section.

Evidence of effectiveness

Scores of studies have been conducted and published on the effectiveness of water, sanitation, and hygiene interventions to prevent infection and disease. By one estimate, more than 285 studies were published between 1980 and 2003 solely on water quality interventions to prevent diarrhoea (Clasen *et al.* 2006). Systematic reviews (Chapter 6.14) are a means of identifying, summarizing, synthesizing, explaining, and assessing the methodological quality of evidence of the effectiveness of health interventions with a variety of studies relating to a particular health intervention. In some cases, such reviews also employ meta-analysis or other statistical methods to estimate the pooled effect of the intervention across the studies included in the review. A number of such reviews have examined the evidence of effectiveness of water, sanitation, and hygiene interventions to prevent disease and infection.

Diarrhoeal diseases

Table 2.5.2 summarizes the results of five different systematic reviews of water and sanitation interventions to prevent diarrhoeal diseases published over the last 25 years. They demonstrate that improvements in water quantity, water quantity and quality, water quality and availability, and sanitation all make substantial contributions to the prevention of diarrhoeal diseases.

In the past, Esrey's conclusions have been oversimplified to suggest that improving water quantity and sanitation may be more effective in preventing diarrhoea than improving water quality. An analysis of the actual review, however, suggests that only when the water supply is delivered on plot are the health gains realized (Cairncross & Valdmanis 2006). This is consistent with the more recent reviews. Clasen *et al.* (2006) suggest that household-based interventions are about twice as effective in preventing diarrhoeal diseases than conventional interventions at the source or point of distribution (e.g. protected wells, boreholes, and communal tap stands), and are roughly comparable to the impact of hand washing and sanitation. The biological basis for the added protection offered from point-of-use interventions has been shown in dozens of studies that demonstrate how water that is safe at the source becomes contaminated during collection, storage, and use in the home (Wright *et al.* 2004). Among household-based interventions, filtration was associated with the largest reductions in diarrhoeal disease, perhaps because it also improves water aesthetics which may increase use (compliance) with the intervention.

Recent reviews also challenge three other widely-held notions in public health engineering. First, the evidence does not suggest that an improved supply of water is essential for water quality interventions to prevent diarrhoea (Clasen *et al.* 2006). This finding confirms the WHO's recent strategy to pursue household water treatment and safe storage as a means of accelerating the health gains of safe drinking water, even though it may not reduce the 1.1 billion currently without access to improved water supplies. Second, water quality interventions appear to be effective in preventing diarrhoea regardless of whether they are deployed in settings where sanitation

Table 2.5.2 Estimate of effect* (and number of studies) of systematic reviews of water and sanitation interventions to prevent diarrhoeal diseases

Intervention (Improvement)	Esrey *et al.* (1985) (range)	Esrey *et al.* (1991)	Fewtrell *et al.* (2005) (95% CI)	Clasen *et al.* (2006) (95% CI)	Clasen *et al.* (2008) (95% CI)
Water quantity	25% (0–100%) (17)	27% (7)			
Water quality			0.69 (0.53–0.89) (15)	0.57 (0.46–0.70) (38)	
Source	16% (0–90%) (9)	17% (7)	0.89 (0.42–1.90) (3)	0.73 (0.53–1.01) (6)	
Household			0.65 (0.48–0.88) (12)	0.53 (0.39–0.73) (32)	
Chlorination				0.63 (0.52–0.75) (16)	
Filtration				0.37 (0.28–0.49) (6)	
Solar disinfection				0.69 (0.63–0.74) (2)	
Floc-disinfection				0.69 (0.58–0.82) (6)	
Water quality and availability	37% (0–82%) (8)	16% (22)	0.75 (0.62–0.91) (6)		
Water and sanitation		20% (7)			
Sanitation	22% (0–48%) (10)	22% (11)	0.68 (0.53–0.87) (2)		0.67 (0.50–0.82) (7)

*For studies by Esrey and colleages, estimate of effect is the median reduction in diarrhoeal disease from the reported studies; for other studies, estimate of effect is the pooled risk ratio from meta-analysis using random effects model. To compare results, the percentage reduction is 1−RR (e.g. RR of 0.69 implies a 31% reduction in risk).

is improved or unimproved (Clasen *et al.* 2006). This is in contrast to conclusions that interventions to improve water quality are effective only where sanitation has already been addressed (Esrey 1986; VanDerslice & Briscoe 1995). Finally, contrary to conventional wisdom and results from disease-transmission modelling (Eisenberg *et al.* 2007), sub-group analysis does not demonstrate that the effectiveness of a water quality intervention to prevent diarrhoea is enhanced by adding hygiene instruction, a separate vessel to treat or store water, or by improving sanitation or water supply (Fewtrell *et al.* 2005; Clasen *et al.* 2006). This is consistent with the finding that the effectiveness of a water quality intervention does not depend on the baseline conditions in regard to other environmental parameters that are associated with diarrhoea. At the same time, it implies that the cost and effort of combining the water quality intervention with improved hygiene, water storage, water supply, or sanitation may not be justified on the basis of an incremental effect on diarrhoeal disease.

With respect to sanitation interventions, Esrey and colleagues reported median reductions in diarrhoea of 22 per cent (range of 0–48 per cent) from 10 studies of interventions that included excreta disposal (Esrey *et al.* 1985). A subsequent review that also included sanitation interventions reported a medium reduction in diarrhoea morbidity of 22 per cent from 11 studies (36 per cent from five studies the investigators deemed rigorous) (Esrey *et al.* 1991). An update of the Esrey reviews which was limited to interventional research designs identified just four such studies of improved sanitation, only two of which provided data that they could use in a meta-analysis (Fewtrell *et al.* 2005). Fewtrell and colleagues reported the interventions to be protective, with a pooled relative risk of 0.68 (95 per cen CI: 0.53–0.87)—a 32 per cent reduction in diarrhoea that would appear consistent with Esrey's findings. More recently, Clasen and colleagues reported a pool risk ratio from seven randomized and quasi-randomized controlled studies of 0.67 (95 per cent CI: 0.50–0.88), corresponding to a 33 per cent reduction in risk (Clasen *et al.* 2008). All of the interventional studies included in the Fewtrell and Clasen reviews combined the sanitation intervention with a water supply (and in some cases, hygiene) intervention, making it impossible to tease out the effect attributable solely to the improvement in excreta disposal facilities. Nevertheless, the consistency of results among these reviews and the underlying studies does provide some confidence that sanitation interventions are protective against diarrhoeal disease. And observational studies—such as a recent cohort study in Brazil in which increased sewer connections was associated with a 26 per cent reduction in diarrhoea (95 per cent CI: 15–37 per cent) (Barretto 2007)—provide additional support.

Soil-transmitted helminth infection

Esrey and colleagues (1991) reported a 4 per cent median reduction in hookworm (*Ancylostoma*) infection from nine studies of combined sanitation and water interventions; the reduction was also 4 per cent in the only included study they deemed rigorous. Esrey also reported a 4 per cent reduction in hookworm in the single study reporting on a sanitation intervention alone. Combined improvements in water supplies and sanitation were associated with a 28 per cent reduction in ascariasis morbidity from 11 studies (29 per cent from four rigorous studies).

In their review of randomized and quasi-randomized controlled trials of interventions to improve excreta disposal, Clasen and colleagues (2008) found consistent evidence that the interventions were protective, even though the limited number of clusters in each study made it impossible to calculate confidence intervals around the point estimates or to pool estimates using meta-analysis. The three studies that reported *Ascaris* infection as an outcome found the intervention group had reductions of 34 per cent (Chandler *et al.* 1954), 73 per cent (Messou *et al.* 1997), and 39 per cent (Zhang *et al.* 2000) compared to controls. The two studies that reported hookworm infection also found the intervention to be protective, with reductions of 87 per cent (Messou *et al.* 1997) and 66 per cent (Chandler *et al.* 1954). Two studies also reported the intervention to be effective against intestinal parasites that they did not specify: Chen *et al.* (2004) recorded a 77 per cent reduction in the intervention group compared with controls, while Zhang *et al.* (2005) found a 56 per cent reduction.

Schistosomiasis

Esrey and colleagues (1991) reported a median reduction in the prevalence of schistosomiasis of 73 per cent (range 59–87 per cent) from four water and sanitation interventions; the reduction was 77 per cent among the three studies they deemed rigorous. Piped-in water supplies and community washing and bathing facilities that reduced contact with surface waters were especially protective, leading to reductions in both prevalence and severity (Esrey *et al.* 1991). The reviewers noted that in Kenya, the installation of boreholes without laundry or shower facilities failed to reduce infection.

Two recent quasi-randomized, controlled interventional studies from China also suggest that improved excreta disposal is protective against schistosomiasis. In a 3-year quasi-RCT, Chen *et al.* (2004) recorded a 43 per cent reduction from combined water, sanitation, and hygiene interventions that also included a snail control component. Zhang *et al.* (2005) reported a 45 per cent reduction in a 2-year quasi-RCT that included water, sanitation, and hygiene. Once again, these trials did not include sufficient clusters to reliably calculate confidence intervals around the point estimates of effect.

Typhoid and paratyphoid

No studies of water or sanitation interventions to prevent typhoid or paratyphoid have been reported. Nevertheless, there is evidence suggesting the effectiveness of water quality interventions. Cutler and Miller (2005) have shown the historical evidence on reductions in mortality associated with the introduction of clean water and sanitation in the United States. Recent case-control studies do suggest that the diseases are still associated with unsafe water and sanitation. In a recent study in Uzbekistan where typhoid remains endemic, cases were more likely to drink unboiled surface water outside the home (OR 3.0, 95 per cent CI: 1.1–8.20) (Srikantiah *et al.* 2007). In a similar case-control study in Bangladesh, drinking unboiled water at home was a significant risk factor (OR 12.1, 95 per cent CI: 2.2–65.6) (Ram *et al.* 2007). Among the risk factors for typhoid and paratyphoid in an urban setting in Indonesia were lack of a toilet in the household (OR 2.20, 95 per cent CI: 1.06–4.55) and use of ice cubes (OR 2.27; 95 per cent CI: 1.31–3.93).

Trachoma

The evidence of the effectiveness of environmental interventions (including water and sanitation) alone to prevent active trachoma is not clear (Rabiu *et al.* 2007). Reviews of the WHO-backed SAFE strategy for trachoma control conclude that there is comparatively weak evidence of the effectiveness of the 'F' (facial cleanliness) and

'E' (environmental improvement) components that encompass improved access to water and better sanitation (Emerson *et al.* 2000a; Kuper *et al.* 2003). In a 6-month cluster RCT of 21 villages in the Gambia, Emerson and colleagues (2004) reported a reduction in fly catches among study clusters receiving latrines. However, the prevalence of active trachoma associated with the intervention was not statistically lower than among seven control clusters (RR 0.81, 95 per cent CI: 0.54–1.22). While trachoma is a water-washed disease that may be impacted by increased access to water, there is also a paucity of evidence that face washing alone is protective against active trachoma (Ejere *et al.* 2004) despite consistent evidence that improved facial hygiene was associated with lower prevalence of disease (Emerson 2000).

Economic implications of water and sanitation interventions

Economic evaluation

Although the evidence suggests that water and sanitation interventions are effective in preventing diarrhoea and certain other faecal–oral diseases, the extent to which interventions are ultimately deployed will not be determined on their effectiveness alone. With limited resources, particularly in developing countries, governments are forced to allocate health expenditures to an array of public health challenges. While public sector decisions on health expenditures are often based on political commitments or other expediencies, economic efficiency, by definition, requires that resources be directed to their most productive use. In the health context, such allocative efficiency means identifying and focusing on the intervention that will produce the greatest health gains for a given investment of resources (Witter *et al.* 2000). This implies more than cost; the lowest cost intervention is seldom the most effective. Economic evaluation is normally a function of both the cost of the intervention and the return on that cost, measured either in terms of overall economic benefits (a *cost–benefit analysis* or CBA) or in the realization of a social objective, such as the prevention of disease (a *cost-effectiveness analysis* or CEA). In a CBA, all of the outcomes of the investment are valued in economic terms, and the output is expressed as a return on the investment or the cost–benefit ratio. The output of a CEA is a ratio (the cost-effectiveness ratio) between the cost of the intervention and an operational outcome measured in its own units. For health interventions, a common unit of measurement is disability adjusted life years (DALYs) averted as a result of the intervention.

Cost-effectiveness analysis

In its *2002 World Health Report*, the WHO assessed the cost-effectiveness of interventions to increase coverage of water and sanitation services in accordance with the MDGs (WHO 2002). It concluded that achieving the MDG for improved water supplies would be the least costly to implement in each region, at a global cost of approximately I$37.5 billion over 10 years. It estimated health gains of approximately 30 million DALYs worldwide. A more recent CEA of water quality interventions to prevent diarrhoeal disease reached a similar conclusion when comparing source-based improvements to household-based interventions (Clasen *et al.* 2007). Among household-based interventions, point-of-use chlorination using sodium hypochlorite was the most cost-effective; additional health gains could be achieved at higher costs with household-based filters. In the lowest-income parts of Africa, for example, the cost per DALY averted was US$53 for household chlorination, US$61 for household solar disinfection, US$123 for source-based interventions, and US$142 for household filters. Direct cost saving, even if limited to the WHO estimates of those corresponding to health-related expenditures, more than offset the costs of implementing most water quality interventions. This means that governments, who are chiefly incurring such costs, would reduce their overall outlays by investing in the implementation of such interventions rather than in the treatment of cases of diarrhoeal disease.

In a recent CEA of improvements in water supplies and sanitation that included the value of time savings from improving the access as well as health benefits, Cairncross and Valdmanis (2006) reported a cost-effectiveness ratio of US$94 per DALY averted for installation of hand pumps or standposts, US$223 for household connections, US$47 for water sector regulation and advocacy, more than US$270 for latrine construction and promotion, and US$11 for promotion of basic sanitation.

Cost–benefit analysis

In another WHO-funded study, Hutton and colleagues (2007) assessed the cost–benefit ratios in 17 WHO epidemiological sub-regions of five categories of water and sanitation interventions based on the MDG water and sanitation targets and additional steps to minimize environmental exposure. The interventions included (1) improvements required to meet the MDGs for water supply, (2) interventions to meet the water and sanitation MDG, (3) increasing access to improved water and sanitation for everyone, (4) providing disinfection at point-of-use over and above increasing access to improved water supply and sanitation, and (5) providing regulated piped water supply in house and sewage connection with partial sewerage for everyone. Costs of the interventions were based on WHO estimates and included the full economic cost of construction and maintenance. Predicted reductions in the incidence of diarrhoeal disease were calculated for each intervention based on the expected population receiving these interventions. Benefits were based on such reductions in disease, and included time savings associated with better access to water and sanitation facilities, the gain in productive time due to less time spent ill, health sector and patient costs saved due to less treatment of diarrhoeal diseases, and the value of prevented deaths.

The analysis yielded a vast amount of valuable data on the cost of each intervention and on each of the categories of benefits. Table 2.5.3 summarizes the results of the analysis for the epidemiological sub-regions that comprise the continent of Africa. Significantly, most of the overall economic benefit is derived from time savings from improved access to water and sanitation. The cost–benefit ratio in Africa is 11, meaning a return of US$11 for every dollar invested in water and sanitation. In all regions and for all five interventions, the cost–benefit ratio is greater than 1, with values in developing regions of between 5 and 28 for Intervention 1, between 3 and 34 for Intervention 2, between 6 and 42 for Intervention 3, and between 5 and 60 for Intervention 4; returns were lowest (between 1.27 and 4.84) for Intervention 5. Significantly, the main contributor to benefits was the saving of time associated with better access to water supply and sanitation services; health benefits were a

Table 2.5.3 Economic benefits from investments in improved water and sanitation in Africa (based on Hutton 2007)

	Meeting MDG target	**Full coverage of safe water and basic sanitation**
Cases of diarrhoea avoided annually	173 million cases	245 million cases
Productive days gained annually	456 million	647 million
Value of productive days gained annually	US$116 million	US$168 million
Health sector treatment costs averted annually	US$1695 million	US$2410 million
Value of time saved	US$15 877 million	US$33 972 million
School days gained annually	99 million	140 million
Cost of interventions per year	US$2020 million	US$4040 million
Total economic benefits per year	US$22 910 million	US$44 040 million
Dollar benefits return per dollar invested (Cost Benefit Ratio)	11	11

comparatively minor part of the overall. While the authors review possible sources of financing- based benefits, they conclude that the health sector budget, which is often meagre anyway, cannot and should not be expected to fund improvements in water and sanitation.

Providing services and allocating costs

Cost-effectiveness analyses and cost–benefit analyses suggest that improvements in water and sanitation yield both health and other valuable benefits, not only to those who receive the intervention but also to the public sector. Inadequate water and sanitation services also have significant externalities (costs imposed on others), such as the costs of over-extraction from water supplies, pollution of water sources, and environmental degradation. Even those who promote water as a basic right accept that some value must be attached to water to reduce waste, encourage conservation and promote higher value uses. Infrastructural improvements in water and sanitation often fail to be initiated or sustained because of a reluctance to charge fully for the cost of delivering the services, inefficiency in collecting such charges or diversion of the fees away from operation and maintenance. Understanding who benefits from improvements in water and sanitation can help justify the allocation of costs and secure financing.

While water and sanitation services are traditionally provided by the public sector, private entrepreneurs, ranging from individual water vendors to large-scale concessionaires of water supply and sewer systems, also play a role. Studies that assess willingness to pay and ability to pay regularly show that people of even modest means can and will contribute to the cost of improving water and sanitation services in many cases (Whittington and Briscoe 1990; Whittington *et al.* 2002). For water, interventions that increase the convenience, reliability, quantity, and quality of water are especially attractive. Urban sanitation is particularly well-suited to the service sector, though even rural latrines are often constructed by specialized masons. Careful planning to assess and match the demand for improvements with the target population's willingness-to-pay help guide decisions on the appropriate level of services and ensure their financial sustainability.

Other benefits of water and sanitation interventions

Improving water availability (quantity and access)

As the Section 'Evidence of effectiveness' makes clear, improving water availability—even without a corresponding improvement in water quality—is associated with reductions of diseases transmitted through waterborne, water-washed, and water-based routes. This is partly due to the well-established relationship between the amount of water that people use and the time required to collect it (Cairncross & Feachem 1993). Figure 2.5.2 shows the plateau-shaped curve that characterizes water consumption patterns based on service levels. While significant quantities of water are used if delivered directly to the home, the quantity used is fairly constant when the collection time is 5–30 min and further diminishes for longer collection times. In lower-income settings, average daily per capita consumption is about 150 l for those with household

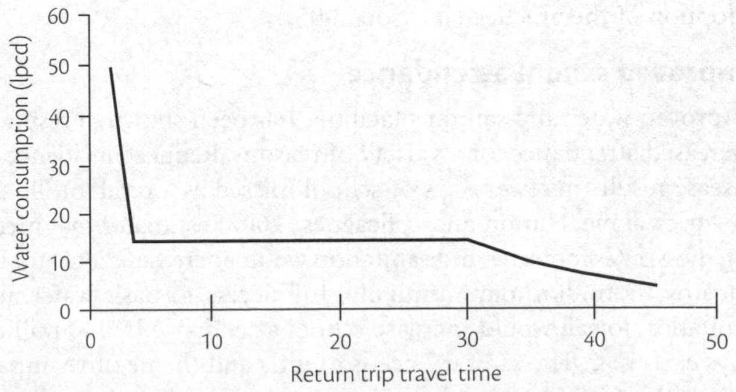

Fig. 2.5.2 Time travel (in min) versus consumption (in litres per capita per day) (from Cairncross & Feachem 1993).

connections, 50 l for yard taps, and just 15 l for communal sources such as stand posts, wells, and springs. Thus, assessments of water availability are expressed in terms of distance: Normally 1 km or round trip collection time (normally 30 min) (WHO/UNICEF 2000) but 0.5 km in disaster response (Sphere Project 2004).

Examining the evidence, a recent WHO report concludes that a minimum quantity of water for basic health protection is 20 l/person/day (Hutton & Bartram 2003). Of this, 7.5 l is for consumption (hydration and food preparation) and therefore must be of a quality to present minimal health risk; the balance is for basic personal and domestic hygiene. The report recognizes, however, that in addition to the direct health benefits associated with improving water supplies, there are indirect health and other benefits. Indirect health benefits may accrue from reducing the amount of time collecting water which can then be used more effectively at home caring for children or engaging in other productive activities (Cairncross 1987). Services at clinics, medical posts, and other healthcare facilities also benefit from improved water supplies. Sufficient water for irrigating gardens and crops can improve nutrition and generate income (Thompson *et al.* 2001). Vending water and making and selling beverages can also impact poverty. Finally, to the extent that people are paying for water, improved water supplies may result in savings that can be used for food and other necessities that may impact health outcomes.

Ecological sanitation

Within the sanitation sector there is an active group of advocates who promote the use of ecological sanitation (Winblad & Simpson-Hébert 2004). Ecological sanitation (EcoSan) works on the principle that urine and faeces are not just waste products, but assets that if properly managed, can contribute to better health and food production and reduce pollution. Managing such assets includes reducing pathogen loading to a safe level which is achieved by a combination of drying the faeces, increasing the pH, and storage for at least 12 months. Without good latrine management, pathogens can survive and create a risk to public health. The pathogen which causes greatest concern is *Ascarisis,* which has a long persistence in the environment and a low infective dose (Cairncross & Feachem 1993). Public health risks need to be balanced against the potential benefits. In areas where land fertility is low, artificial fertilizer is expensive, and livelihoods are dependent on subsistence farming, the benefits of using excreta as a fertilizer/soil improver could be considerable. Even when potential benefits can be demonstrated, local beliefs and taboos may limit acceptability or prevent adoption of the practice (Jackson 2005).

Improved school attendance

Improved water and sanitary facilities has been shown to result in increased attendance for a variety of reasons. Reduced incidence of disease results in fewer days of school missed as a result of illness. In Africa alone, Hutton and colleagues (2007) estimated that meeting the MDGs for water and sanitation would increase school attendance by 99 million days annually; full access to basic water and sanitation for all would increase school attendance by 140 million days each year. The sanitary needs of girls and the negative impact that lack of sanitation adversely impact their attendance levels. A UNICEF sanitation project in Bangladesh led to an 11 per cent increase in female enrolment by building appropriate school sanitation (UNICEF 1999). In Uganda, 94 per cent of girls reported problems at school during menstruation and 61 per cent reported staying away from school (IRC 2006). Cultural and religious constraints in many settings make menstruation a taboo. If menstruation lasts over a week, there is a tendency for girls to skip the entire school year (Bharadwaj & Patkar 2004). Sanitation pays an important role in improving educational access for children with disabilities, through the improvement of paths, latrine floors, and installation of handrails (Bannister *et al.* 2005).

Security and gender equality

Improved sanitation and water supplies improve security and gender equality for women and girls. Household sanitation can increase their safety by avoiding the dangers of sexual assault and harassment faced when practising open defecation or using latrines away from their homes. Safe, private, and proximate latrines are a particular issue for women in emergencies and conflicts (Sphere Project 2004). Research in Kenya revealed that women would defecate into plastic bags and throw them into streets ('flying toilets') because they feared being raped when using latrines shared with men (Maili Saba 2005). They were also afraid of being seen to be using latrines too regularly and preferred to bathe within their own homes after dark where they felt safer. Young children often prefer open defecation due to fear of falling into pits in poorly-designed or unsuitably-adapted latrines.

Advancing the fight against HIV/AIDS

It is well known that access to safe drinking water and sanitation prolongs the lives of people living with HIV/AIDS (PLWHA) by reducing the risk of opportunistic infections, including diarrhoeal diseases (Hayes 2003). Household-based water treatment has been shown to be an effective intervention in preventing mortality and morbidity in a population with one or more persons infected with HIV (Colford *et al.* 2005; Lule *et al.* 2006). Point-of-use water treatment products are now included in health kits for PLWHA (Colindres *et al.* 2007). Efforts are also underway to ensure that mothers infected with HIV have safe drinking water (or point-of-use water treatment products) to prepare infant formula for use as an alternative to breastfeeding in order to minimize mother–child transmission.

Recent and emerging developments in water and sanitation

Water safety plans and microbial risk assessment

Traditionally, the water sector relied on compliance with end-product standards to ensure the safety of drinking water. Most drinking water standards are based on WHO guidelines that establish maximum limits for known or suspected microbial and chemical pathogens as well as physical/aesthetic characteristics. Under this approach, drinking water is to be free of pathogens at the point of delivery as demonstrated by the absence of a prescribed indicator of faecal contamination, such as *E. coli* or thermotolerant coliforms (TTC). However, in the third edition of the WHO *Guidelines for Drinking-Water Quality* (GDWQ), the WHO adopted a risk assessment and risk management approach for improving drinking water quality (WHO 2004). The approach calls on water providers to develop and implement water safety plans similar to the hazard assessment critical control point (HACCP) approach used in the food industry to identify and control potential threats to safety.

This latest rolling revision to the GDWQ also encourages greater surveillance to verify compliance.

This risk-based approach uses health-based targets for water quality. This is based on quantitative microbial risk assessment (QMRA), an approach developed for calculating the burden of disease from potential pathogens. QMRA sets pathogen limits based on the evidence concerning exposure assessment, dose–response analysis, and risk characterization (Haas *et al.* 1999). Risk assessment and acceptable levels of risk are expressed in terms of DALYs. Reference pathogens are defined for each category of microbes. Significantly, these do not necessarily coincide with long-standing indicator organisms and may require capacity building in new laboratory techniques. Limited country-specific data and other resources may also delay full implementation of this approach in many countries.

Wastewater reuse

QMRA is also used in the recently-published second edition of the WHO's *Guidelines for the Safe Use of Wastewater, Excreta and Greywater* for agriculture and aquaculture (WHO 2006). As an estimated 70 per cent of water withdrawals from surface and subsurface sources are used for agricultural purposes (WRI 2007), the agricultural sector is particularly eager to develop safe, economical, and effective water sources for crop irrigation. Wastewater can be high in plant nutrients (nitrogen, phosphorus, and potassium), minimizing the need for chemical fertilizers and producing higher incomes for farmers (Ensink & van der Hoek 2007). As municipalities in lower-income settings struggle to treat even drinking water, however, few are able to remove potential pathogens from wastewater, leaving an estimated 80 per cent of sewage untreated. The WHO *Guidelines* attempt to balance the benefits of wastewater reuse with the need for food security. As treated wastewater is also being increasingly viewed as a potential source of drinking water in water stressed regions, additional guidance based on public health evidence will be necessary.

Household-based water treatment

For the hundreds of millions who lack household water connections that provide drinking water on a 24–7 basis, water is often collected and stored in the home until needed. It is well known that even water that is safe at the point of collection undergoes frequent and extensive re-contamination during collection (or compromised distribution), storage, and use in the home (Wright *et al.* 2004). While providing safe, piped in, disinfected water to each household is an important goal, even meeting the MDG targets for 50 per cent coverage would entail an investment of tens of billions of dollars each year to connect households at the rate of 300 000 per day (WHO/UNICEF 2005). Accordingly, the WHO and others have called for other approaches that will accelerate the heath and economic gains associated with safe water while progress is made in improving infrastructure.

Interventions to treat and maintain the microbial quality of water at the point of use are among the most promising of these alternatives (Sobsey 2002). In many settings, both rural and urban, populations have access to sufficient quantities of water, but that water is unsafe. Because point-of-use interventions ensure the microbiological integrity of the water at the point of ingestion, they are more likely to deliver health benefits. Recent systematic reviews have shown household-based interventions (home-based boiling, chlorination, filtration, solar disinfection, and flocculation/disinfection) to be significantly more effective than traditional, non-reticulated source-based interventions (protected wells and springs, boreholes, communal tap stands) in improving microbiological water quality and reducing diarrhoeal disease (Fewtrell *et al.* 2005; Clasen *et al.* 2006). The up-front cost of treating such water at the point-of-use can be dramatically less than the cost of conventional water treatment and distribution systems. Point-of-use water treatment, such as household-based chlorination, is the most cost-effective intervention to prevent diarrhoeal disease across a wide range of countries and settings (WHO 2002; Clasen *et al.* 2007). It is also among the most cost-beneficial (Hutton *et al.* 2007). In 2003, the WHO helped organize the International Network for the Promotion of Safe Household Water Treatment and Storage, a global collaboration of UN and bilateral agencies, NGOs, research institutions, and the private sector committed to improved household water management as a component in water, sanitation, and hygiene programmes. The Network's Website contains a considerable amount of information on household water management (http://www.who.int/household_water/en).

Technologic and programmatic innovations

Efforts to improve water supplies and sanitation, particularly in rural and remote locations, have proved especially challenging. Despite concerted efforts over past decades, the situation for many has not improved dramatically (Thompson *et al.* 2001). While a variety of communal and household-level options have been promoted as alternatives to customary approaches in order to improve water quality, quantity, and proximity, some of these have been found wanting in terms of technological suitability, cost, and sustainability. New challenges include natural or man-made chemical contamination, saline intrusion, increasing urbanization, falling water tables, threats associated with climate change, and increasing demand for agricultural and industrial uses of water (Chapter 2.10). High upfront costs, lack of financing, uncertain land tenure, inadequate skilled masons for construction, pit-emptying, longer-term waste disposal, and urbanization are major challenges in sanitation.

Public health professionals, programme implementers, social entrepreneurs, and the private sector have responded to these challenges by developing and promoting a variety of technological and programmatic innovations for improving water supplies and sanitation, especially among low-income populations. In water, these include developments in rainwater harvesting, water locating, borehole drilling, well digging, locally-fabricated pumps and other water lifting devices, self-supply strategies, chemical filters, and adsorption technologies. In sanitation, communal private latrines have been promoted widely in India and elsewhere, and technologies include cheaper, lightweight squatting slabs, composting toilets, digestion chemicals, multi-chamber pits, pit-emptying, and improved separation of liquid and solid excreta. Many of these innovations are accompanied by entrepreneurial initiatives, microfinance, and base-of-the-pyramid (BOP) marketing. While some of these innovations appear promising, lessons from the past suggest that understanding and responding to the particular circumstances present in a given setting—and especially what the target population itself wants and is willing to pay for—are especially important in achieving large-scale sustainable improvements that will also impact public health.

Water and wastewater testing and microbiology

American Public Health Association (APHA), the American Water Works Association (AWWA), and the Water Environment Federation (WEF) jointly publish *Standard Methods for the Examination of Water and Wastewater*, the definitive guide for water quality testing. The twenty-first edition published in 2005 contains methods for assessing physical properties, metals, inorganic non-metallic constituents, aggregate organic constituents, individual organic compounds, radioactivity, toxicity, microbiological examination, and biological examination (APHA *et al.* 2005). Nevertheless, there are continuing debates about even fundamental issues, such as the use of indicators of faecal contamination such as coliforms, thermotolerant coliforms (TTC), and *Escherichia coli* (Gleeson & Gray 1997). The International Water Association's Health Related Water Microbiology Specialist Group is a rich source of research and new developments in the microbiology of water and waste, including water and wastewater treatment and its effects on health and the environment (including chlorinated by-products), methods in microbiology, microbe tracking and behaviour in water systems and the environment, rapid testing and monitoring, issues presented by bioterrorism, epidemiology and microbial risk assessment, and treatment processes.

Total sanitation

First developed in Bangladesh in 1999 and now expanding elsewhere, Community-Led Total Sanitation (CLTS) is an approach that empowers local communities to stop open defecation and to build and use latrines without the support of external hardware subsidies. Through the use of participatory techniques, community members analyse their own sanitation situation, including the extent of open defecation and the possibilities of faecal–oral contamination. This is designed to ignite a personal sense of disgust and shame that translates into collective action to reduce the impact of open defecation (Kar 2003). By triggering collective behaviour change, CLTS places the community, rather than the household, at the centre of the decision-making process. Peer pressure and civic pride are important motivating factors. The particular design of a latrine is secondary to the emphasis on 100 per cent coverage. The results can be impressive, with whole communities changing from open defecation to latrine use in a matter of months (Kar 2003). The approach has since been rolled out in Africa and Asia, and there is some evidence of its sustainability (Kar & Bongartz 2006).

Sanitation marketing

Sanitation marketing uses a commercial approach to the production and delivery of sanitation technologies and engages the private sector for production and delivery in a financially and institutionally sustainable manner (Jenkins & Sugden 2006). Such a marketing approach has been recommended over typical public-sector promotion of sanitation since it helps ensure that people choose to receive what they want and are willing to pay for, is financially sustainable, is cost-effective, and can be taken to scale (Cairncross 2004). Sanitation marketing adopts a consumer perspective, starting with an understanding of which products and services the target population wants, will pay for, will maintain, and are appropriate to the local context. It seeks to develop a sustainable sanitation industry which is not dependent on external donors for hardware subsidies or long-term support for its continuation. It recognizes the household as the key decision maker regarding their defecation practice and the importance of effective public private partnerships. The extent to which the approach is capable of reaching the base of the economic pyramid has not yet been shown.

Scaling up sanitation; subsidies

Recent research has begun to explore the drivers and constraints toward latrine adoption (Jenkins & Curtis 2005; Jenkins & Scott 2007). Results demonstrate that while public health and economic benefits are the main societal reasons for investing in sanitation, householders have different reasons for wanting a latrine (Table 2.5.4). Research has shown that the rate of uptake of sanitation interventions increases as information spreads from one household to another, much like the adoption curves that characterize many new innovations (Cairncross 2004; Jenkins and Curtis 2004). Householder-perceived advantages of using a latrine become apparent as housing density starts to increase and when the need for privacy, convenience, and maintaining dignity become more important.

Subsidizing latrine construction is a controversial issue within the sanitation sector. Public incentives to private individuals are justified in an economic sense when there are externalities—social benefits that go beyond the private benefits associated with a given private action (Gregersen 1984; Pardo 1990). As the public health benefits of limiting open defecation are greater than the private benefits an individual gains by choosing use of latrines over open defecation, sanitation may constitute a public good, thus justifying subsidies. However, for scaling up of sanitation to be successful, subsidies must be used to encourage householders to build and use latrines and help them overcome the constraints rather than to cover the actual costs of construction. Moreover, the public service priority needs to focus on safely and efficiently managing excreta within the larger community, especially in dense urban slums, after it has left the private domain of households (Methra & Knapp 2005; Evans *et al.* 2004). Inappropriately-applied subsidies also have the negative effects of creating dependency, distorting the behaviour of the private supply market, and perhaps most importantly, not reaching the poor.

Challenges in water and sanitation

Failure to treat diarrhoea as a serious disease

One of the threshold constraints to scaling up water and sanitation is the belief that diarrhoea—the main health threat associated with poor water and sanitation coverage—is not a disease. Figueroa and Kinkaid (2008) cite numerous studies from various countries in which participants reported diarrhoea to be a natural and even desirable condition, especially in young children, not worthy of special preventative measures. Although health benefits often lack significant motivational impetus for driving preventative measures, the fact that diarrhoea is not even considered a disease by many of the most vulnerable populations further limits this strategy. Among policy makers and health officials faced with a variety of life-threatening diseases, diarrhoea may not receive the commitment of resources that its status as the third leading cause of morbidity and mortality from infectious disease would suggest it deserves.

Despite UN and other initiatives to draw attention to the need to expand water and sanitation coverage, there is no corresponding

Table 2.5.4 Inventory of stated benefits of improved sanitation from the private vs. public perspectives

Household perspective *	Society-public perspective **
◆ Increased comfort	◆ Reduced excreta-related disease burden (morbidity and mortality) leading to:
◆ Increased privacy	◇ Reduced public healthcare costs
◆ Increased convenience	◇ Increased economic productivity
◆ Increased safety, for women, especially at night, and for children	◆ Increased attendance by girls at school (for school sanitation) leading to broad development gains associated with female education
◆ Dignity and social status	◆ Reduced contamination of ground water and surface water resources
◆ Being modern or more urbanized	◆ Reduced environmental damage to ecosystems
◆ Cleanliness	◆ Increased safety of agricultural and food products leading to more exports
◆ Lack of smell and flies	◆ Increased nutrient recovery and reduced waste generation and disposal costs (for ecological sanitation)
◆ Less embarrassment with visitors	◆ Cleaner neighbourhoods
◆ Reduced illness and accidents	◆ Less smell and flies in public places
◆ Reduced conflict with neighbours	◆ More tourism
◆ Good health in a very broad cultural sense, often linked to disgust and avoidance of faeces	◆ National or community pride
◆ Increased property value	
◆ Increased rental income	
◆ Eased restricted mobility due to illness, old age	
◆ Reduced fertilizer costs (ecological sanitation)	
◆ Manure for crop production (ecological sanitation)	

*Compiled from the following case studies and project reports based on household interviews, surveys, and group discussions in many different settings: Jenkins (1999, 2004); Jenkins and Curtis (2005); Obika *et al.* (2002); Mukherjee (2000); Allen (2003); Ellmendorf and Buckles (1980); D'Souza (2005); WSP-EAP (2002); WSP (2004).
** Reasons for public action stated in studies and documents but rarely quantified or ranked (Evans *et al.* (2004); Jenkins and Sugden (2006)).

source of funds to meet the challenge. Roll Back Malaria, the Global Fund to Fight HIV/AIDS, Tuberculosis and Malaria, and the Presidents Emergency Plan for AIDS Relief (PEPFAR) are examples of high profile, well-financed, international campaigns against important infectious diseases. Though diarrhoea accounts for more mortality and morbidity than tuberculosis or malaria, there is no global fund or presidential initiative to address it even though it is largely preventable as evidenced by the minimal disease in middle- and high-income countries. Unless and until diarrhoea is recognized as a significant health threat rather than an embarrassing annoyance, it is not likely to attract its share of health resources.

Lack of public-sector coordination

In most countries, a variety of agencies and authorities are responsible for some part of water and sanitation. These typically include the ministries of water, health, water resources, environment, local government, rural development, and education. In many cases, there are also federal, regional, district, and local levels of government. Rarely do any of these ministries take full responsibility for all aspects of water or of sanitation. The result is often a patchwork effort that lacks funding and coordination. There are important examples of successful coordinated public sector efforts. In South Africa, strides in sanitation are occurring because of a national decision and plan which set out targets, clear strategies, significant resources, and accountability (Muller 2002). Ethiopia has also achieved considerable success in improving water and sanitation coverage, particularly in the Southern Nations, Nationalities and Peoples Region, where a commitment at the senior levels translated into coordinated and sustained action (Bibby & Knapp 2007).

Bias toward large, infrastructural solutions

Public-sector advocacy, funding, and support has been shown to be an important factor in the successful scaling up of oral rehydration salts, insecticide-treated nets, and other interventions directed at environmental health. To date, however, governmental support for community and household-based water and sanitation interventions programmes has not been extensive in most countries. This is due in part to the engineering orientation of the applicable ministries, and their emphasis on larger-scale, infrastructural improvements, especially in urban and peri-urban settings. Nearly all populations who do not enjoy piped-in water on a 24–7 basis express priority for increasing the quantity and access to water over improving its quality. Governments respond accordingly, aware not only of the political value from these popular projects (and the particularly photogenic value of water emerging from massive new pipes), but also the economic gains that are available from reducing the time people spend collecting and transporting water to their homes and from the productive use of water in agricultural activities. Multilateral and bilateral funding also tends to focus on such infrastructural water projects, despite compelling evidence that HWTS is more cost beneficial and highly cost-effective (Hutton *et al.* 2007; Clasen *et al.* 2007).

The term 'sanitation' is not only vague; it is often used interchangeably with the term 'sewerage'. Sewerage refers to a system of sewers that convey wastewater to a treatment plant and as such is depended on the provision, operation, and maintenance of an infrastructure of pipes, pumps, and screens. If working correctly, sewerage systems separate humans from their faeces, and is therefore a form of sanitation. But sewers are not the only form, and arguably not the most important with regard to increasing sanitation coverage in Africa. In Dar es Salaam, Kampala, and other African cities, 70 per cent of the population are served by pit latrines and only 10–12 per cent by the sewer system, despite heavy investment in the latter. This proportion is unlikely to increase over the coming years as cities are rapidly growing and sewerage systems are very expensive. Even so, Ministries of Water are often mainly interested in sewer systems and ignore on-site solutions. As the poor often cannot afford to connect to sewer systems, and the households served by the rehabilitated sewers already had access to sanitation, the net impact of the investment on the MDGs, health, and poverty reduction is limited. The funding allocated to low-cost, low-technology excreta management solutions used by the vast majority of the world's poor is comparatively low. The consequence of the bias towards sewer solutions is to direct resources away from the poor.

Uncertainty about the role of the private sector

Water and sanitation have traditionally been supplied by the public sector, particularly in Europe and North America where coverage, service levels, and costs are optimal. As governments, particularly in lower-income settings, have been unable to deliver services such as power, transportation, and even health and education to much of the population, they are increasingly relying on the private sector to provide such services. There are some apparent success stories where the private sector, through concessions, public–private partnerships, or other vehicles, enhance the coverage and service level of water and sanitation though increased investment and improved management of fee collection and delivery. At the same time, there are at least some notorious cases, such as Cochabamba, Bolivia, where a concession was opposed due to the perception at least that the private sector partners were putting profits ahead of performance. There is certainly a need for regulation, as these services are usually a natural monopoly and market forces, if left unchecked, will favour delivery to higher-density and higher income areas where paybacks are faster and costs/risks lower. The United Nations Development Programme (UNDP), World Bank, and others have examined the constructive role that the private sector can play in helping scale up the delivery of water and sanitation services (UNDP 2007). Balancing the potential contribution of the private sector against the needs of the target population will continue to represent a significant challenge for policy makers.

Decoupling sanitation from water

Since the 1990s, there has been an effort to always integrate water supply, sanitation, and hygiene promotion in developing countries within the same project. As a result, sanitation and hygiene have piggy backed on the political and community demand for improved water supplies. However, many effective interventions to improve excreta disposal do not require improvements in water supplies. While the water supply sector is dominated by engineers who lean towards technical solutions, sanitation and hygiene promotion rely more heavily on understanding and changing behaviour, a different set of skills. As a result, staff in integrated projects naturally concentrate on water supplies, whilst excreta disposal fails to receive the resources it requires. The sanitation element is usually built around the process of providing the water supply; in fact, sanitation differs in that it requires a household rather than a community decision, requires more time, and is more complex from a behaviour change perspective. By decoupling sanitation from water, it may be possible to increase coverage more rapidly, particularly in remote areas in which water interventions are unlikely to reach in the near future.

Excreta disposal in urban unplanned areas

While urban areas generally have higher rates of sanitation than rural areas, the rapid growth of informal settlements and urban slums presents a particular challenge for sanitation (WHO/UNICEF 2006). The lack of planning controls can result in ever increasing housing densities as plots are divided and subdivided either to house expanding extended families or to increase rental income. Eventually the area becomes saturated. This complicates excreta management in two ways: (i) streets and passages become very narrow making it impassable for latrine- and septic-emptying vehicles, and (ii) the space available in each compound is insufficient to build initial or replacement latrines.

Another important and sensitive question with urban sanitation is the divide between public and private responsibility. Public funds are used to install, manage, and maintain public sewers and tariffs or taxation used to recover costs. No such publicly funded services are provided for the poor living in the unplanned high density areas, and excreta disposal is regarded as being the sole responsibility of the household. It is arguable that the public health benefits from providing an appropriate pit emptying service could be so great that it warrants total public funding and provided free of charge to the poor.

Conflicting objectives in sanitation

Sanitation projects usually aim for a combination of four often-conflicting objectives. The first is to build a large number of latrines in a relatively short time, driven in part by the MDGs or national targets. In such cases, projects often use a supply-driven approach that coerces, entices, or persuades householders to build latrines by providing a generous subsidy, normally in the form of free hardware and/or labour. But when funding ends, the delivery and support mechanisms dissolve and the community members are left, as they started, with a lack of latrine component supply chains and nowhere to turn to for support. The second objective is to develop a sustainable sanitation industry that can continue providing latrines for many generations to come. This requires a good understanding of demand, the motivations and constraints of households in building and using latrines and the use of marketing techniques to develop, promote and supply better latrine components. This is a longer-term process which will not result in large number of latrines being built in a short period of time and is therefore not attractive to politicians, donors, government officials, and implementers wanting instant MDG-driven solutions and to be seen to be doing something. The third objective driving sanitation is to enhance sustainable livelihoods and environmental improvements. This can be achieved by taking an ecological sanitation approach to latrine building which ensures that the nutrients in the excreta are reused to grow crops. The fourth objective is organizational insistence that their work must be targeted at the poorest of the poor. These are the most risk adverse, hardest to reach, price sensitive members of the population who are also likely to be the least well educated and socially or politically connected. This makes them the least likely people to benefit from either a supply- or a demand-driven approach. While a targeted, sustainable, demand-driven, livelihood-enhancing latrine building programme that builds a large number of latrines in a short period of time is the ideal, decision makers need to understand the weaknesses of each approach and prioritize their expectations accordingly.

Conclusion

Unlike many of the other challenges in public health, the solutions for eliminating most of the disease burden associated with poor water and sanitation are well known. All but the poor have enjoyed the health, economic, and other benefits associated with safe drinking water and basic sanitation for decades. The fact that hundreds of millions still lack access to these fundamental resources is a scandal that generations have allowed to persist simply as a matter of misguided priorities. And as the 'haves' continue to make rapid gains, they are not only increasing the gap over the 'have-nots' but also using up larger amounts of the world's limited water supplies and capacity for waste disposal, making it more difficult and costly for others to join their privileged club.

The need to extend water and sanitation coverage is acknowledged at the highest international levels, and progress is being made. Whether these efforts will be any more successful than those expressed in previous international declarations and goals is not yet clear. As the poor continue to wait for the piped-in water supplies and sanitary disposal that they deserve, however, it is incumbent on the public health community to develop, assess, and promote effective, low-cost, and sustainable alternatives and creative delivery strategies in order to accelerate access to the health gains associated with safe drinking water and basic sanitation.

Key points

- While safe drinking water and sanitation are widely recognized as fundamental public health interventions, more than a sixth of the world's population still lack improved water supplies and 40 per cent lack basic sanitation.
- The infectious diseases associated with unsafe drinking water and poor sanitation impose a heavy burden, especially on the poor, the very young and the immuno-compromised; they also aggravate poverty, education, and economic development.
- There is strong evidence that interventions to improve water supplies or sanitation can be effective in preventing diarrhoea, soil-transmitted helminth infections, schistosomiasis, and typhoid fevers.
- Water and sanitation interventions have also been shown to be cost-effective and cost-beneficial, with significant savings to the public sector from reduced healthcare costs; there is also evidence of other economic and developmental benefits from improved access to water and sanitation.
- A variety of recent and emerging developments, including new methods for assessing and monitoring the risk of diseases associated with water and sanitation as well as alternative technologies, programmatic approaches, and implementation strategies, may contribute to improved targeting, coverage, uptake, and sustainability.
- Nevertheless, significant political, social, economic, and developmental challenges must be addressed in order to successfully scale up some of these interventions on a sustainable basis and thus provide the most vulnerable populations with the health and other benefits of safe drinking water and sanitation.

References

Allan, S.C. (2003). *The WaterAid Bangladesh / VERC 100% sanitation approach: Bangladesh*. IDS Working Paper 194. Institute of Development Studies, Brighton, Sussex.

APHA (2005). *Standard methods for the examination of water and wastewater*, 21st edition. American Public Health Association, the American Water Works Association (AWWA) and the Water Environment Federation (WEF), Washington, DC.

Bannister, M., Hannan, M.D., Jones, H. *et al.* (2005). *Water and sanitation for all: Practical ways to improve accessibility for disabled people*. 31st WEDC Conference, Maximising the benefits from water and environmental sanitation. Kampala, Uganda.

Barreto, M.L., Genser, B., Strina, A. *et al.* (2007). Effect of city-wide sanitation programme on reduction in rate of childhood diarrhoea in northeast Brazil: Assessment by two cohort studies. Lancet, **370**(9599), 1622–8.

Bartram, J. (2003). New water forum will repeat old message. *Bulletin of the World Health Organization*, **83**, 158.

Bharadwaj, S. and Patkar, A. (2004). *Menstrual hygiene and management in developing countries: Taking stock*. Junction Social, Social Development Consultants.

Bibby, S. and Knapp, A. (2007). *From burden to communal responsibility: A sanitation success story from southern region in Ethiopia*. Field Note. Washington: World Bank Water and Sanitation Programme.

Black, R.E. and Lanata, C.F. (1995). Epidemiology of diarrhoeal diseases in developing countries. In (eds. M.J. Blaser, P.D. Smith, J.I. Ravdin, H.B. Greenberg, and R.L. Guerrant) *Infections of the gastrointestinal tract*. Raven Press, New York.

Black, R.E., Morris, S.S. and Bryce, J. (2003). Where and why are 10 million children dying every year? *Lancet*, **361**, 2226–34.

Blakely, T., Hales, S., Kieft, C. *et al.* (2005). The global distribution of risk factors by poverty level. *Bulletin of the World Health Organization*, **83**, 118–126.

Blum, D. and Feachem, R.G. (1983). Measuring the impact of water supply and sanitation investments on diarrhoeal diseases: Problems in methodology. *International Journal of Epidemiology*, **12**, 357–65.

Cairncross, S. (1987). The benefits of water supply, In (ed. J. Pickford) *Developing world water*. Grosvenor Press, London.

Cairncross, S. (1992). *Sanitation and water supply: Practical lessons from the decade*. The World Bank, Washington DC.

Cairncross, S. (2004). *The case for marketing sanitation*. Field Note. Nairobi: Water and Sanitation Programme Africa.

Cairncross, S. and Feachem, R. (1993). *Environmental health engineering in the tropics: An introductory text*, 2nd edition). John Wiley & Sons Ltd., Chichester, West Sussex.

Cairncross, S., Muller, R., and Zagaria, N. (2002). Dracunculiasis (Guinea Worm Disease) and the eradication initiative. *Clinical Microbiology Reviews*, **15**, 223–46.

Cairncross, S. and Valdmanis, V. (2006). Water supply, sanitation and hygiene promotion. In (eds. D.T. Jamison, J.G. Breman, A.R. Measham *et al.*) *Disease control priorities in developing countries*, pp. 771–92, The World Bank, Washington DC.

Chandler (1954). A comparison of helminthic and protozoan infections in two Egyptian villages two years after the installation of sanitary improvements in one of them. *The American Journal of Tropical Medicine and Hygiene*, **3**, 59–73.

Chen, G., Wang, M.H.S., Ou, N. *et al.* (2004). Observation on the effect of the comprehensive measures of replacing cattle with machine and reconstructing water supply and lavatory to control the transmission of schistosomiasis. *Journal of Tropical Disease & Parasitology*, **2**, 219–22.

Clasen, T., Bostoen, K., Boisson, S. *et al.* (2008). *Improved excreta disposal for the prevention of diarrhoea, helminth infections and trachoma: A systematic review* (submitted).

Clasen, T., Do Hoang, T., Boisson, S. *et al.* (2008). Lessons in household water treatment from a cross-sectional study in rural Vietnam. *Environmental science & technology* (in press).

Clasen. T., Haller, L., Walker, D. *et al.* (2007). Cost-effectiveness analysis of water quality interventions for preventing diarrhoeal disease in developing countries. *Journal of Water and Health*, **5** (4), 599–608.

Clasen, T., Roberts, I., Rabie, T. *et al.* (2006). *Interventions to improve water quality for preventing diarrhoea (Cochrane Review)*. In The Cochrane Library, Issue 3, 2006. Update Software, Oxford.

Colford, J.M. Jr, Saha, S.R., Wade, T.J. *et al.* (2005). A pilot randomized, controlled trial of an in-home drinking water intervention among HIV + persons. *Journal of Water and Health*, **3** (2), 173–84.

Colford, J.M., Rees, J.R., Wade, T.J. *et al.* (2002). Participant blinding and gastrointestinal illness in a randomized, controlled trial of an in-home drinking water intervention. *Emerging Infectious Diseases*, **8**, 29–36.

Colindres, R., Mermin, J., Ezati, E. *et al.* (2007). Utilization of a basic care and prevention package by HIV-infected persons in Uganda. *AIDS Care*, **24**, 1–7.

Crump, J.A., Luby, S.P., and Mintz, E.D. (2004). The global burden of typhoid fever. *Bulletin of the World Health Organization*, **82**, 346–53.

Curtis, V. and Cairncross, S. (2003). Effect of washing hands with soap on diarrhoea risk in the community: A systematic review. The *Lancet Infectious Diseases*, **3**, 275–81.

Cutler, D. and Miller, G. (2005). The role of public health improvements in health advances: The twentieth-century United States. *Demography*, **42** (1), 1–22.

Davis, J. and Lambert, R. (2002). *Engineering in emergencies*. Intermediate Technology Publications, Ltd., London.

DFID (1998). *Guidance manual on water supply and sanitation programmes*. UK Department of International Development, London.

deSilva, N.R., Brooker, S., Hotez, P.J. *et al.* (2003). Soil-transmitted helminth infections: Updating the global picture. *Trends in Parasitology*, **19**, 547–51.

Eisenberg, J.N., Scott, J.C., and Porco, T. (2007). Integrating disease control strategies: Balancing water sanitation and hygiene interventions to reduce diarrheal disease burden. *American journal of Public Health*, **97** (5), 846–52.

Ejere, H., Alhassan, M.B., and Rabiu, M. (2004). *Face washing promotion for preventing active trachoma*. The Cochrane Database of System Reviews 2004, Issue 3.

Emerson, P.M., Bailey, R.L., and Mahdi, O.S. (2000). Transmission ecology of the fly *Musoca sorbens*, a putative vector of trachoma. *Transactions of the Royal Society of Tropical Medicine and Hygiene*, **94**, 1–5.

Emerson, P.M., Cairncross, S., Bailey, R.L. *et al.* (2000a). Review of the eidenc ebase fo the 'F' and 'E' component of the SAFE strategy for trachoma control. *Tropical medicine & international health*, **5** (8), 515–27.

Emerson, P.M., Lindsay, S.W., Alexander, N. *et al.* (2004). Role of flies and provision of latrines in trachoma control: Cluster-randomised controlled trial. *Lancet*, **363** (9415), 1093–8.

Ensink, J.H. and van der Hoek, W. (2007). New international guidelines for wastewater use in agriculture. *Tropical Medicine & International Health*, **12** (5), 575–7.

Esrey, S.A. and Habicht, J-P. (1986). Epidemiologic evidence for health benefits from improved water and sanitation in developing countries. *Epidemiologic Reviews*, **8**, 117–28.

Esrey, S.A., Feachem, R.G., and Hughes, J.M. (1985). Interventions for the control of diarrhoeal diseases among young children: Improving water supplies and excreta disposal facilities. *Bulletin of the World Health Organization*, **64**, 776–72.

Esrey, S.A., Potash, J.B., Roberts, L. *et al.* (1991). Effects of improved water supply and sanitation on ascariasis, diarrhoea, dracunculiasis, hookworm infection, schistosomiasis, and tracoma. *Bulletin of the World Health Organization*, **69**, 609–21.

Evans, B., Hutton, G., and Haller, L. (2004). *Closing the sanitation gap—the case for better public funding of sanitation and hygiene*. Commission on Sustainable Development, Oslo.

Ferriman, A. (2007). BMJ readers choose the "sanitary revolution" as greatest medical advance since 1840. *British Medical Journal*, **334**, 111.

Fewtrell, L., Kaufmann, R., Kay, D. *et al.* (2005). Water, sanitation, and hygiene interventions to reduce diarrhoea in less developed countries: a systematic review and meta-analysis. *The Lancet Infectious Diseases*, **5**, 42–52.

Fewtrell, L., Pruss-Ustun, A. Bos, R. *et al.* (2007). *Water, sanitation and hygiene—quantifying the health impact at national and local levels in countries with incomplete water supply and sanitation coverage*. Environmental Burden of Disease series No. 15. World Health Organization, Geneva.

Figueroa, M.E. and Kincaid, D.L. (2008). Social, cultural and behavioral correlates of household water treatment and storage. World Health Organisation Geneva (in press).

Gleeson, C. and Gray, N. (1997). *The Coliform Index and waterborne disease*. E & FN Spon, London.

Gryssels, B., Polman, K., Clerinx, J. *et al.* (2006). Human schistosomiasis. *Lancet*, **368**, 1106–18.

Guerrant, D.I., Moore, S.R., Lima, A.A.M. *et al.* (1999). Association of early childhood diarrhoea and cryptosporidiosis with impaired physical fitness and cognitive function four-seven years later in a poor urban community in Northeast Brazil. *The American Journal of Tropical Medicine and Hygience*, **61**, 707–13.

Gundry, S., Wright, J., and Conroy, R. (2003). A systematic review of the health outcomes related to household water quality in developing countries. *Journal of Water and Health*, **2** (1), 1–13.

Haas, C.N., Rose, J.B., and Gerba, C.P. (1999). *Quantitative microbial risk assessment*. John Wiley & Sons, New York.

Hayes, C., Elliot, E., Krales, E. *et al.* (2003). Food and water safety for persons infected with human immunodeficiency virus. *Clinical Infectious Diseases*, **36**(Suppl 2), S106–9.

Hotez, P., Brooker, S., Bethony, J. *et al.* (2004). Hookworm infection. *The New England Journal of Medicine*, **351**, 799–807.

Hotez, P.J., Bundy, D.A.P., Beegle, K. *et al.* (2006). Helminth infections: Soil-transmitted helminth infections and schistosomiasis. In (eds. B.D.T. Jamison, A.R. Measham, C *et al.*) *Disease control priorities in developing countries*, 2nd edition, pp. 467–97. Oxford University Press.

Hunter, P.R. (1997). *Waterborne disease epidemiology and ecology*. John Wiley & Sons, Chichester.

Hutton, G. and Bartram, J. (2003). *Domestic water quantity, service level and health*. World Health Organization, Geneva.

Hutton, G., Haller, L., and Bartram, J. (2007). Global cost-benefit analysis of water supply and sanitation interventions. *Journal of Water and Health*, **5** (4), 481–502.

IRC Water and Sanitation Centre (2006). Girl friendly toilets for school girls. (downloaded from http://www.schools.watsan.net/page/319).

Jackson, B. (2005). *A review of EcoSan experience in Eastern and Southern Africa*. Field Note. Washington: World Bank Water and Sanitation Programme.

Jenkins, M.W. and Curtis, V. (2005). Achieving the "good life"; why some people want latrines in rural Benin. *Social Science & Medicine*, **61**, 2446–59.

Jenkins, M.W. and Scott, B. (2007). Behavioral indicators of household decision-making and demand for sanitation and potential gains from social marketing in Ghana. *Social Science & Medicine*, **64** (12), 2427–42.

Jenkins, M.W. and Sugden, S. (2006). *Rethinking sanitation—Lessons and innovation for sustainability and success in the New Millennium*. UNDP HDR2006, Sanitation Thematic Paper, London School of Hygiene and Tropical Medicine.

Kosek, M., Bern, C., and Guerrant, R.L. (2003). The global burden of diarrhoeal disease, as estimated from studies published between 1992 and 2000. *Bulletin of the World Health Organization*, **81**, 197–204.

Kar, K. (2003). *Subsidy or self-respect? Participatory total community sanitation in Bangladesh*. IDS Working Paper 194. Institute of Development Studies, Brighton, Sussex, UK.

Kar, K. and Bongartz, J. (2006). Update on some recent developments in community-led total sanitation. Institute of Development Studies, Brighton, Sussex, UK.

Kuper, H., Solomon, A.W., Buchan, J. *et al.* (2003). A critical review of the SAFE strategy for the prevention of blinding trachoma. *The Lancet Infectious Diseases*, **3**(6), 372–81.

Kumaresan, J. and Mecaskey, J. (2003). The global elimination of blinding trachoma: Progress and promise. *The American Journal of Tropical Medicine and Hygiene*, **69**, 24–28.

Leclerc, H., Schwartzbrod, L., and Dei-Cas, E. (2002). Microbial agents associated with waterborne diseases. *Critical Reviews in Microbiology*, **28** (4), 371–409.

Lule, J.R., Mermin, J., Ekwaru, J.P. *et al.* (2005). Effect of home-based chlorination and safe storage on diarrhea among person with HIV in Uganda. *Tropical Medicine and International Health*, **73**, 926–33.

Mabey, D.C., Solomon, A.W., and Foster, A. (2003). Trachoma. *Lancet*, **362**(9379), 223–9.

Mackenbach, J. (2007). Sanitation: Pragmatism works. *British Medical Journal*, **6334** (Suppl 1), s17.

Maili Saba Research Report (2005). Livelihood and gender in sanitation and hygiene water services among urban poor.

Maybe, D., Solomon, A.W., and Foster, A. (2003). Trachoma. *Lancet*, **362**, 223–9.

Methra, M. and Knapp, A. (2005). *The challenge of financing sanitation for meeting the millennium development goals*. Commissioned by the Norwegien Ministry of the Environment for the Commission on Sustainable Development. Water and Sanitation Program—Africa. The World Bank, Nairobi, Kenya.

Messou, E., Sangare, S.V., Josseran, R. *et al.* (1997). Effect of hygiene measures, water sanitation and oral rehydration therapy on diarrhea in children less than five years old in the south of Ivory Coast. *Bulletin de la Société de pathologie exotique*, **90** (1), 44–7.

Morris, S.S., Cousens, S.N., Kirkwood, B.R. *et al.* (1996). Is prevalence of diarrhoea a better predictor of subsequent mortality and weight gain than diarrhea incidence? *American Journal of Epidemiology*, **144**, 582–8.

Moy, R.J.D., Booth, I.W., McNeish, A.S. *et al.* (1991). Definitions of diarrhoea. *Journal of Diarrhoeal Diseases*, **9** (4), 335.

Mukherjee, N. (2000). *Myth vs. reality in sanitation and hygiene promotion*. Field Note, Jakarta: World Bank Water and Sanitation Programme—East Asia and the Pacific.

Muller, M. (2002). *The National Water and Sanitation Programme in South Africa*. Field Note, Water and Sanitation Program—Africa: The World Bank, Nairobi, Kenya.

Obika, A., Jenkins, M., Howard, G. *et al.* (2002). *Social marketing for urban sanitation, Inception Report*. DFID KAR Project R7982. WEDC, Loughborough, UK.

Prüss-Üstün, A. and Corvalán, C. (2007). *Preventing disease through healthy environments: Towards an estimate of the environmental burden of disease*. World Health Organization, Geneva.

Rabiu, M., Alhassan, M., and Ejere, H. (2007). *Environmental sanitary interventions for preventing active trachoma*. Cochrane Database of Systematic Reviews 2007, Issue 4.

Ram, P.K., Naheed, A., Brooks, W.A. *et al.* (2007). Risk factors for typhoid fever in a slum in Dhaka, Bangladesh. *Epidemiology and Infection*, **135** (3), 458–65.

Rubenstein, A., Boyle, J., Odoroff, C.L. *et al.* (1969). "Effect of improved sanitary facilities on infant diarrhea in a Hopi village." *Public Health Reports*, **84** (12), 1093–7.

Schmidt, W.P., Luby, S.P., Genser, B. *et al.* (2007). Estimating the longitudinal prevalence of diarrhea and other episodic diseases: continuous versus intermittent surveillance. *Epidemiology*, **18** (5), 537–43.

Smith, P.G. and Morrow, R.H. (1996). *Field trials of health interventions in developing dountries: A Toolbox*. (2nd edition) Macmillan Education Ltd., London.

Sobsey, M.D. (2002). *Managing water in the home: Accelerated health gains from improved water supply*. The World Health Organization (WHO/SDE/WSH/02.07), Geneva.

Sphere Project (2004). *Humanitarian Charter and minimum standards in disaster response*. The Sphere Project, Geneva.

Srikantiah, P., Vafokulov, S., Luby, S.P. *et al.* (2007). Epidemiology and risk factors for endemic typhoid fever in Uzbekistan. *Tropical Medicine and International Health*, **12** (7), 838–47.

Stephenson, L.S., Latham, M.S., and Ottensen, E.A. (2000). Malnutrition and parasitic helminth infections. *Parasitology*, **121**, S23–38.

Thompson, J., Porras, I.T., Tumwine, J.K. *et al.* (2001). *Drawers of Water II: 30 years of change in domestic water use and environmental health in East Africa*. IIED, London.

Thylefors, B., Negrel, A.D., and Dadzie, K.Y. (1995). Global data on blindness. *Bulletin of the World Health Organization*, **73**, 115–21.

UN Millennium Project (2005). *UN millennium project task force on water and sanitation—Health, dignity and development: what will it take?* Earthscan, London.

UNDP (2007). *Beyond scarcity: Power, poverty and the global water crisis*. United Nations Development Programme: Human Development Report 2006.

United Nations (2000). United Nations Millennial Declaration. General Assembly Res. 55/2 (18 September 2000).

United Nations (2002). United Nations Committee on Economic, Cultural and Social Rights, General Comment 15, 27 November 2002.

Van Derslice, J. and Briscoe, J. (1995). Environmental interventions in developing countries: Interactions and their implications. *American Journal of Epidemiology*, **141**, 135–44.

Wagner, E.G. and Lanois, J.N.(1958). *Excreta disposal for rural areas and small communities*. WHO monograph series NO.39. WHO, Geneva.

White, G.F., Bradley, D.J., and White, A.U. (1972). *Drawers of water: Domestic water use in East Africa*. University of Chicago Press, Chicago.

Whittington, D. and Briscoe, J. (1990). Estimating the willingness to pay for water services in developing countries: A case study of the use of contingent valuation surveys in Southern Haiti. *Economic Development. & Cultural Change*, **38** (2), 293–311.

Whittington, D., Pattanayak, S., Yang, J-C. *et al.* (2002). Household demand for improved piped water services in Kathmandu, Nepal. *Water Policy*. **4** (6), 531–56.

WHO (1993). *The management and prevention of diarrhoea: Practical guidelines*, 3rd edition. World Health Organization, Geneva.

WHO (2004). *Guidelines for drinking-water quality*, Vol. 1, 3rd edition. World Health Organization, Geneva.

WHO (2005). *Progress towards the millennium development goals, 1990–2005*. World Health Organization, Geneva.

WHO (2006). *Guidelines for the safe use of wastewater, excreta and greywater*, Vols. 1–4. World Health Organization, Geneva.

WHO/UNICEF (2002). *Global water supply and sanitation assessment*. The World Health Organization and the United Nations Children's Fund, Geneva.

WHO/UNICEF (2005). *Water for life: Decade for action 2005–2015*. World Health Organization and United Nations Children's Fund Joint Monitoring Program, Geneva.

WHO/UNICEF (2006). *Meeting the MDG drinking water and sanitation target: The urban and rural challenge of the decade*. The World Health Organization and the United Nations Children's Fund, Geneva.

Winblad, U. and Simpson-Hébert, M. (eds.), (2004): *Ecological sanitation*. Stockholm Environmental Institute.

Witter, S., Ensor, T., Jowett, M. *et al.* (2000). *Health economics for developing countries*. Macmillan Education Ltd., London.

WRI (2007). Water Resources Institute. EarthTrends Environmental Resource Portal (downloaded from http://earthtrends.wri.org/text/water-resources/variable-10.html).

Wright, J., Gundry, S., Conroy (2003). Household drinking water in developing countries: A systematic review of microbiological contamination between source and point-of-use. *Tropical Medicine and International Health*, **9** (1), 106–17.

WSP-EAP (2002). *Selling sanitation in Vietnam: What works?* Jakarta: World Bank Water and Sanitation Program—East Asia and the Pacific.

Zhang, S-Q, Wang, T-P, Tao, C-G *et al.* (2005). Observation on comprehensive measures of safe treatment of night-soil and water supply, replacement of bovine with machine for schistosomiasis control. *Zhongguo Xue Xi Chong Bing Fang Ji Za Zhi* [*Chinese Journal of Schistosomiasis Control*], **17** (6), 437–42.

Zhang, W-P, Liu, M-X., Yin, W-H. *et al.* (2000). Evaluation of a long-term effect on improving drinking water and lavatories in rural areas for prevention of diseases. *Ji Bing Kong Ji Za Zhi* [*Chinese Journal of Disease Control & Prevention*], **4** (1), 76–8.

2.6

Food and nutrition

Prakash S. Shetty

Introduction

Food and nutrition are important determinants of a wide range of diseases of public health importance worldwide. Nutrition is a broad and complex subject which includes nutrient–gene interactions and the induction of such diseases as diabetes mellitus, coronary heart disease, and cancer and to conditions like impaired brain development. Nutrition also deals with the social, economic, and cultural issues related to making the right food choices, purchasing and eating the 'correct' types of food and in the 'appropriate' quantities as well as the factors that determine daily human activity and behaviour related to food. Thus, just as our gradual acquisition of the knowledge of microbiology influenced our understanding of infectious diseases, which in turn led to preventive measures for the population, so the historical advances in the field of nutrition have led to a more coherent understanding of the patterns of and the prevention of diet-related diseases of public health importance throughout the world.

Fluctuations in disease rates depend on environmental factors which include food and nutrition as one of the primary determinants. In the developing world, numerous deficiency diseases persist, which are the result of nutrient deficiencies in the daily diet. These now coexist with the increasing incidence of diet-related chronic diseases, which are typical of industrialized and economically developed countries. Thus developing societies now bear the 'double burden' of malnutrition with the emergence of the so called 'diseases of affluence' amidst persisting under-nutrition in their populations.

Significant changes in the patterns of disease and the causes of premature death within a population have little to do with advances in curative medicine and therapeutics. The changes in health depend largely on the environmental changes which include changes in social and economic conditions, the implementation of immunization programmes, improvements in women's social and educational status within the society, and changes in agriculture and food systems and in the availability of food. These changes have, in turn, been influenced in recent times by globalization and the increasing global trade and the social and cultural interactions that affect agricultural practices, the food systems, and the industrial and manufacturing sector and affect individual diets and lifestyles. National policies that seek to promote principally economic activity and international trade to boost foreign exchange earnings ignore the impact of these measures on the health of the populations. Most of the beneficial environmental influences on the other hand, operate through changes in the provision and access to hygienic and nutritious food; the availability of potable water, clean housing, sanitary surroundings, and lack of exposure to environmental toxins. Economic development is normally accompanied by improvements in the quantity and quality of a nation's food supply and improvements in the immediate environment and living standards of the community. These changes contribute to a nutritionally mediated improvement in the body's resistance to infections and the mutual interdependence of the immune and nutritional state of the population probably explains at least some of the gains in public health in Britain in the last century (McKeown 1976).

The quantitative and qualitative changes in our food patterns that lead to such dramatic changes in life expectancy also result in the problems of diet-related chronic diseases, but these are not inevitable. Diet-related chronic diseases occur typically in middle and later adult life and can by increasing the incidence of premature mortality undermine the gains in life expectancy. More importantly they lead to morbidity and the resultant disability adjusted life years lost as well as contributing to economic losses and reducing the quality of life. These diet-related chronic diseases are traditionally regarded as manifestations of overconsumption and self-indulgence in an affluent society. In practice, some of these chronic diseases may be compounded by relatively deficient intakes of some nutrients thus emphasizing the need for a diversified and balanced daily diet for good health.

Nutrition has re-emerged as of fundamental importance in public health. Nutritional issues were seen in industrialized and developed societies as relating to deficiency diseases which were conquered in the early part of the twentieth century while continuing to persist in the relatively poor, developing countries. Now, however, food and nutrition are recognized as one of the principal environmental determinants of a wide range of diseases of public health importance throughout the world. These diseases reflect the cumulative impact of a variety of pathophysiological processes over a lifetime and the interactions are often seen as reflecting individual genetic susceptibility, but the different disease patterns of groups living on different diets being manifestly a societal reflection of the impact of dietary factors. The display of nutrient–gene interactions is evident, for example, in obesity, alcoholism, cardiovascular disease, non-insulin dependent diabetes mellitus, many gastrointestinal disorders, neural tube defects, and the most prevalent cancers.

As molecular epidemiology unravels the basis for genetic susceptibility to these disorders, physicians interested in metabolic medicine eventually look for the gene inducers or repressors which then prove to be of dietary or environmental origin. Societal features which determine human behaviour and economic well-being as well as climate, tradition, culture, and the role of women, all affect food patterns and dietary practices. These are the features which need to be recognized when considering public health rather than simply the epidemiological aspects of dietary disease. This chapter seeks to take a global view of food and nutrition in public health terms and so nutritional deficiency disorders as well as other diet related diseases of public health importance would be considered. This is particularly important because deficiency diseases are widespread in several parts of the world and yet coexist in the same country with chronic adult diseases usually found in affluent, developed societies. Vitamin deficiencies, both clinical and subclinical continue to manifest in poor communities as well as in apparently healthy populations. Threat of hunger and starvation and severe dietary inadequacy resulting in malnutrition often emerges during conflict and other man-made emergencies. The chapter is structured in such a way that it deals with both sides of the 'mal' nutrition in humans.

Hunger and malnutrition

The pre-eminent determinant of hunger or household food insecurity is poverty in societies. The recognition that poverty and hunger go hand in hand is manifest in the UN's Millennium Development Goal 1 (MDG 1), which specifies targets for the reduction of both global poverty and hunger by the year 2015. Improving household food security is one of the stated objectives of all democratic societies and constitutes an important element of the human right to adequate food. *Food security* is defined as the access by all people at all times to the food they need for an active and healthy life. The inclusion of the term household ensures that the dietary needs of all the members of the household are met throughout the year. The achievement of household food security requires an adequate supply of food to all members of the household, ensuring stability of supply all year round, and the access, both physical and economic, which underlines the importance of the entitlement to produce and procure food. Food insecurity exists when individuals lack access to sufficient amounts of safe and nutritious food and, therefore, are not consuming enough for an active and healthy life. This situation may be a result of the unavailability of food, inadequate purchasing power, or inappropriate utilization of food at the household or individual level. Thus food security at the household level is a complex phenomenon attributable to a range of factors that vary in importance across regions, countries, and social groups, as well as over time (Shetty 2006). It is described in terms of the availability and stability of good quality, safe and nutritious food supplies, and the access to, and utilization of, this food. All these criteria must be met for the consumption of a healthy diet and the achievement of nutritional well-being.

Availability relates to the adequacy of a varied and nutritious food supply and is influenced principally by factors that promote agricultural production and trade. Issues that influence these factors include policies and incentives, access to natural resources, and the availability of agricultural inputs, skills, and technologies including biotechnology. Stability of the level and types of foods available for consumption is subject to seasonality and by the sustainability of the production and farming systems in practice. These factors, in turn, depend on the efficiency of market systems, including pricing mechanisms and infrastructure such as transport and warehousing, which influences the distribution and flow of food. While reduction of food losses through improvements in food storage and processing also affect stability, the nature of the farming system adopted and its effect on the environment and on sustainability is also a key determinant of the stability of food supplies in the medium- to long term.

Access that a community, household, or individual has to food is a reflection of the ability to either grow and retain the food grown for consumption, to purchase the food from the market, or to acquire it by a combination of strategies that Amartya Sen (1981) has described as representing 'entitlements' to food. This system depends on a range of factors such as: Access to resources such as land, water, agricultural inputs, and improved technologies; the nature of the food marketing system and the infrastructure to support it; purchasing power and food prices; consumer perceptions, behaviour, and preferences. Utilization is more concerned with the biological availability of the food after it has been ingested. While age, body size, and physical activity levels influence food utilization, the absence of disease and parasitic infestations also influences the utilization of nutrients by the body. As a consequence, utilization of food is largely influenced by factors such as health, clean water, and good sanitation.

The causes of malnutrition on the other hand are multi-dimensional and its determinants include both food and non-food related factors, which often interact to form a complex web of biological, socioeconomic, cultural, and environmental deprivations. Although establishing a relationship between these variables, and the indicators of malnutrition do not necessarily imply causality, they do demonstrate that in addition to food availability many social, cultural, health, and environmental factors influence the prevalence of malnutrition. Although, in general, people suffering from inadequacy of food are poor, not all the poor are undernourished. Even in households that are food secure, some members may be undernourished. Income fluctuations, seasonal disparities in food availability, and demand for high levels of physical activity, and proximity and access to marketing facilities may singly or in combination influence the nutritional status of an individual or a household. For example, the transition from subsistence farming to commercial agriculture and cash crops may help improve nutrition in the long run, however, they may result in negative impacts over the short term unless accompanied by improvements in access to health services, environmental sanitation, and other social investments. Rapid urbanization and rural to urban migration may lead to nutritional deprivation of segments of society. Cultural attitudes reflected in food preferences and food preparation practices, and women's time constraints including that available for child-rearing practices, influence the nutrition of the most vulnerable in societies. Inadequate housing and overcrowding, poor sanitation, and lack of access to a protected water supply, through their links with infectious diseases and infestations, are potent environmental factors that influence biological food utilization and nutrition. Inadequate access to food, limited access to healthcare, and a clean environment and insufficient access to educational opportunities are in turn determined by the economic and institutional structures as well as the political and ideological superstructures within society. The links between food security and malnutrition are evident as nutritional status is the outcome indicator. The presence of undernutrition is not only causally related to food insecurity at the household or individual level, but is also determined by other health-related factors such as access to safe water, good sanitation, and healthcare as well as the care practices that include proper breastfeeding and complementary feeding and ensuring fair and appropriate intra-household food distribution.

Poor nutritional status of populations affects physical growth, intelligence, behaviour, and learning abilities of children and adolescents. It impacts on their physical and work performance and has been linked to impaired economic work productivity during adulthood. Inadequate nutrition predisposes them to infections and contributes to the negative downward spiral of malnutrition and infection. Good nutritional status, on the other hand, promotes optimal growth and development of children and adolescents. It contributes to better physiological work performance, enhances adult economic productivity, increases levels of socially desirable activities, and promotes better maternal birth outcomes. Good nutrition of a population manifested in the nutritional status of the individual in the community contributes to an upward positive spiral and reflects the improvement in the resources and human capital of society.

Low birth weight

Intrauterine growth retardation resulting in low birth weights constitutes a major public health problem in developing countries. A WHO Technical Report (1995) recommended that the 10th percentile of a sex-specific, birth-weight-for-gestational-age distribution be designated for the classification of small-for-gestational-age infants. It is difficult to establish with certainty in all cases whether the reduced weight at birth is the result of *in utero* growth restriction. However, in populations in developing countries with high incidence of small for gestational age infants, the likelihood is that this is largely the result of intra-uterine growth retardation. The definition of intra-uterine growth retardation (IUGR) is an infant born at term (i.e. >37 weeks of gestation) with a low birth weight (i.e. <2500 g). The causes of IUGR are multiple and involve many different factors. The most important determinant of infant weight at birth is the maternal environment of which nutrition is the single most important factor. Poor maternal nutritional status at conception and inadequate maternal nutrition during pregnancy can result in IUGR. Short maternal stature, low maternal body weight and body mass index at conception, and inadequate weight gain during pregnancy are factors that are associated with IUGR. In developing countries IUGR is closely related to conditions of poverty and chronic undernutrition of economically disadvantaged mothers.

More than 96 per cent of low-birth-weight infants are born in the developing world and 20 million children are born each year weighing <2500 g, accounting for 16 per cent of all births in the developing world—a rate more than double the level in the developed world (7 per cent) (UNICEF 2007). The incidence of low birth weight varies across regions, but South Asia has the highest incidence, at 31 per cent with India being home to 40 per cent of all low-birth-weight babies in the developing world.

Low birth weights due to IUGR are associated with increased morbidity and mortality in infancy. It is estimated that term infants weighing less than 2500 g at birth have a four-times increased risk of neonatal death as compared to infants weighing between 2500 and 3000 g and 10 times higher than those weighing between 3000 and 3500 g. The risk of morbidity and mortality in later infancy is also considerably high in these low-birth-weight infants. In developing countries this is largely due to increased risk of diarrhoeal disease and respiratory infections. Barker's studies have consistently demonstrated a relationship between low birth and later adult disease and provide an important aetiological role for foetal undernutrition in amplifying the effect of risk factors in later life in the development of chronic diseases like heart disease and diabetes mellitus in adult life (Barker 2004).

Childhood undernutrition

The clinical conditions of childhood undernutrition or malnutrition are widely recognized as kwashiorkor, marasmus, and the mixed condition of marasmic kwashiorkor. These severe forms of malnutrition are, however, the tip of an iceberg of widespread mild and moderate childhood undernutrition within the community. It is this form of undernutrition in infants and children that is relevant from a public health nutrition perspective.

Poor diet and nutrition are not the only causes of childhood undernutrition. The determinants of child undernutrition can be considered as operating at three levels of causality: Immediate, underlying, and basic (Smith & Haddad 2000). The immediate determinants are dietary intakes and health status which are in turn influenced by three underlying determinants—household food insecurity, the concept of care for children and their mothers, and the health environment which includes access to safe water and to sanitation. Care encompasses such variables as breast-feeding and proper complementary feeding practices, the education of women—the caregiver, their status, their autonomy, and their access to resources. A poor health environment can result in frequent episodes of infection such as diarrhoeal diseases and even respiratory infections. A vicious cycle may be established with an intestinal infection in a young child leading to anorexia, intestinal damage with malabsorption, and secretory diarrhoea which then does not remit because the poor nutritional state of the child maintains the immunological deficit and this impairs the recovery of the intestine. Traditionally children in poor communities, fail to thrive once they have succumbed to an infectious disease and they then languish, responding poorly to standard therapy and failing to grow even when presented with apparently adequate amounts of food.

Undernutrition in childhood is characterized by growth failure, resulting in a body weight that is less than ideal for the child's age. Hence, in children, assessment of growth has been the single most important measurement that best defines their health and nutritional status. Measures of height and weight are therefore the commonly used indicators of the nutritional status of the child. Classification of childhood malnutrition based on height, weight, and age continues to be the backbone of nutritional assessment methods for both population and individual assessments (WHO 1995). Hitherto the standard reference for comparison has been the National Center for Health Statistics and WHO international reference population; however WHO has recently developed international growth standards for children, which will replace them (WHO 2006).

Children throughout the world when well fed and free of infection tend to grow at similar rates whatever their ethnic or racial origin and healthy children everywhere can, when fed appropriately, be expected to grow on average along the 50th centile of a reference population's weight and height for age. By expressing both height and weight as standard deviations or Z-scores from the median reference value for the child's age the normal range will correspond to the 3rd and 97th centile (i.e. ±2 SDs or ±2 Z-scores). By expressing data in this way, it is possible to express the weight and height data for all children across a wide age range in similar Z-score units and thereby produce a readily understandable comparison of the extent of growth retardation at different ages and in different countries.

A deficit in height is referred to as 'stunting', whereas a deficit in weight-for-height is considered as 'wasting'. These two measures are subsumed in the original designation of a child's failure to grow in terms of weight-for-age. Clearly this measure includes both the wasting and stunting features but fails to distinguish the important differences between the two. Wasting can occur on a short-term basis in response to illness with anorexia or malabsorption or because the child goes hungry for several weeks. Changes in weight-for-height therefore reflect the impact of short-term changes in nutritional status. Growth in height, however, is much more a cumulative index of long-term health because growth in length or height stops when a child develops an infection and the subsequent growth may be slow during the recovery period. Children normally grow in spurts and intermittently. Energy intake is not a crucial determinant of height and the energy cost of growth and weight gain is only 2–5 per cent of total energy intake once the child is 1 year of age. Impairment or slowing of growth in height occurs in many communities at the time of weaning and up to about 2 years of age and affects a fair proportion of children in many developing countries. Once the children have failed to maintain their proper growth trajectory for stature they tend to remain on the lower centiles and 'track' at this low level for many years.

Global estimates of the main forms of child undernutrition *viz* underweight and stunting as well as their prevalence in individual countries is compiled on a regular basis by WHO (de Onis *et al.* 2004) and the most recent available data is summarized in Table 2.6.1. Comparisons from earlier estimates indicate that the prevalence of underweight and stunting remain high despite substantial progress in most regions in the 1990s. In most parts of Africa the numbers of underweight and stunting increased during this period while the dramatic progress in Asia is outweighed by the persisting high prevalence and numbers of children affected. Stunting is a serious problem in both these regions and reflects poor nutrition during the early growth period; often the result of frequent infectious episodes during this period. Physical stunting is associated with poor mental development and socioeconomic deprivation resulting from reduced physical abilities and employment opportunities in adult life. Stunting in South Asia seems also to be related to the high incidence in low birth weight in this region.

Underweight in children is being used as an indicator for monitoring progress towards the Millennium Development Goals (MDG). Overall current analyses demonstrates some progress in reducing child undernutrition; but is uneven and in some countries has even deteriorated. To achieve the MDG more concerted effort is needed, especially in those regions with stagnating or increasing trends in child undernutrition. Well-nourished children have a better chance of surviving and growing into healthy adults. Improving child nutrition requires attention to all three components, i.e. access to adequate and safe food, freedom from illness, and appropriate care. Ensuring optimal child health and growth can contribute to a healthy adult population and accelerate economic growth of countries.

Table 2.6.1 Current estimates and progress since 1990 in the prevalence and numbers of child undernutrition globally and in developing countries of Africa, Asia, and Latin America

	Underweight		Stunting	
	1990	**2005**	**1990**	**2005**
Global				
Prevalence (%)	26.5	20.6	33.5	24.1
Numbers (× 10^6)	163.4	127.2	206.5	149.1
Africa				
Prevalence (%)	23.6	24.5	36.9	34.5
Numbers (× 10^6)	25.3	34.5	39.6	48.5
Asia				
Prevalence (%)	35.1	24.8	41.1	25.7
Numbers (× 10^6)	131.9	89.2	154.6	92.4
Latin America				
Prevalence (%)	8.7	5.0	18.3	11.8
Numbers (× 10^6)	4.8	2.8	10.0	6.5

Prevalence expressed as percentage below -2 SD of NCHS/WHO international reference value.
Global estimates are predominantly developing countries in the three regions.
Latin America includes the Caribbean.
Estimates reported by de Onis *et al.* (2004).

Adult undernutrition

For the last 50 years, nutritionists have focused on vulnerable groups in society, i.e. children, pregnant and nursing mothers, and the elderly, because they were considered to be particularly susceptible to nutritional deficiencies. It is now becoming apparent that undernutrition among the young adults has been neglected and this may have profound significance for the economic growth of developing countries. One simple measure of undernutrition in adults is adult weight in relation to height and *body mass index* (BMI) (i.e. body weight in kilograms divided by the square of the height in metres) is considered the most suitable index for both under- and overnutrition in adults (Shetty & James 1994). The choice of BMI for the assessment of nutritional status of adults was based on the observation that BMI was consistently highly correlated with body weight (a proxy for the available energy stores within the body) and was relatively independent of the stature of the individual. Adults with a BMI <18.5 are considered to be chronically undernourished while those with BMI >25 and >30 are considered overweight and obese, respectively (WHO 2000); and the same BMI cut-offs apply to both males and females. BMI is not only a sensitive index of adult undernutrition but also allows variations in relation to socioeconomic status, and seasonal fluctuations in the availability of food in the community to be detected. Undernourished adults show considerable impairment of physical well-being and exercise capacity and susceptibility to illness. The ability to promote and sustain effective agricultural productivity, particularly in rural societies, may therefore be limited by the vigour and well-being of the adults on whom the vulnerable in society depend. Thus, it is important to consider adult undernutrition alongside other vulnerable segments in a community.

Anthropometric measures of adult undernutrition provides an opportunity for objective estimates of the prevalence of undernutrition worldwide, hitherto dependent on estimates of food availability in countries and the numbers of people food insecure. In practice, children and adults may adapt to a shortage of food by reducing their physical activity without changing their body weight. Thus, measures of the prevalence of low weight-for-height provide only a limited index of food insecurity as physical activity is fundamental to children's play and exploration and therefore to their mental development. Similarly, in adults physical activity is desirable not only for physiological well-being and for limiting the development of chronic disease but also to allow societies to prosper through physically demanding economic activity and those sound developments which rely on an energetic and enterprising population.

For many years, the Food and Agriculture Organization of the UN (FAO) has attempted to assess the global prevalence of undernutrition by relating complex measures of food supply and its variable distribution between households with estimates of the population's energy needs (Naiken 2003). The number of undernourished estimated most recently by FAO, based on their method, is 854 million, of which 820 million are in developing countries (FAO 2006). Since reducing by half the proportion of the hungry or food insecure by 2015 is one of the targets set in MDG1, monitoring progress using this method has considerable importance. It is apparent that there has been progress in this direction although it has been recognized that progress has been slow in the last decade as compared to the previous decade. While the prospect of meeting the MDG1 target are good, progress has been variable with some regions such as Central Africa and East Asia having shown a worsening of the situation with increase in numbers of undernourished. Reliable global estimates of adult undernutrition based on BMI are not available since nutritional surveys rarely include adult men and the issue of adult undernutrition has also largely been ignored. With awareness of the increasing problem of overweight and obesity, it is likely that more information based on anthropometric surveys of adults will be generated which will also provide for data on adult undernutrition.

Public health initiatives that deal with this problem worldwide have to recognize that the basic causes of malnutrition are clearly political and socioeconomic. Agricultural revolutions such as the green revolution have increased food availability and helped meet the food needs of the population. Agricultural productivity has increased worldwide and developing countries are increasingly producing more food even when expressed on a per capita basis. Food prices for most commodities, particularly for cereals, have also fallen and been at their lowest until recently. However, poverty is often the basis of a failure to have access to food even when it is available and even when the prices are low as they are currently. Accelerated food production will alleviate hunger only to the extent that the resources used in the process reduce poverty more than they would if used in other ways. Thus food entitlement decline is a more important force in sustaining poverty and undernutrition than a decline in the availability of food in developing societies.

Micronutrient malnutrition

Micronutrient malnutrition, also referred to as 'hidden hunger' is caused by lack of adequate micronutrients such as vitamins and minerals in the habitual diet. Diets deficient in micronutrients are characterized by high intakes of staple food and cereal crops, but low consumption of foods rich in bioavailable micronutrients such as fruits, vegetables, and animal and marine products. Micronutrient deficiencies are important from a public health perspective as they affect several billion people worldwide (Table 2.6.2) and can impair cognitive development and lower resistance to disease in children and adults. They increase the risk to both mothers and infants during childbirth and impair the physical ability and economic productivity of men. The costs of these deficiencies in terms of lives lost and reduced quality of life are enormous not to mention the economic costs to society. Strategies to combat micronutrient deficiencies in communities have included: (i) *Supplementation* of specific nutrients to meet the immediate deficits. (ii) *Fortification* of staple food items in the daily diet—another successful strategy that has been adopted to deal with specific nutrient deficiencies—a good example is the fortification of common salt with iodine to tackle iodine deficiency and goitres. (iii) *Food-based approaches* which include promoting kitchen gardens to enable families to produce and consume a diversified diet rich in vitamins and improve the nutrition of households—promoted extensively to reduce vitamin A deficiency in developing countries. (iv) A potential strategy under investigation is to improve the nutrient quality of commonly consumed staples by agricultural biotechnology such as genetically modified crops—a process referred to as *biofortification*. The micronutrient deficiencies that will be addressed below in this chapter include only the significant ones from a public health viewpoint.

Iron deficiency

Iron deficiency is probably the most common nutritional deficiency disorder in the world and affects over 2 billion people with anaemia. Hence it is a major public health problem with adverse consequences especially for women of reproductive age and for young children. The predominant cause of iron deficiency worldwide is

Table 2.6.2 Estimated global impact of micronutrient malnutrition

Micronutrient malnutrition	Estimated impact
Vitamin A deficiency	140 million pre-school children affected with VAD[1]
	Contributes to 1.15 million deaths in children every year[2]
	4.4 million children suffer from xeropthalmia[1]
	6.2 million women suffer from xerophthalmia[1]
Iron deficiency	2.0 billion women (96 million of them pregnant)[2]
	67 500 maternal deaths per year from severe anaemia[2]
Iodine deficiency	1.98 billion at risk with insufficient or low iodine intakes[3]
	15.8% of population worldwide have goitre[3]
	17.6 million infants born mentally impaired every year[2]
Folate deficiency	Responsible for 200 000 severe birth defects every year[2]

[1] SCN (2004) *Fifth report on the world nutrition situation: Nutrition for improved development*

[2] UNICEF/Micronutrient Initiative (2004) *Vitamin and mineral deficiency: A World progress report*

[3] WHO (2004) *Iodine status worldwide*

nutritional, the diet failing to provide for the body's requirements of iron. In tropical countries, intestinal parasitosis exacerbates iron deficiency by increasing the loss of blood from the gastrointestinal tract. The increase in malaria in these countries also contributes to the anaemia. A low intake of iron and/or its poor absorption then fails to meet the enhanced demands for iron and anaemia results.

The consequences of iron deficiency are numerous as iron plays a central role in the transport of oxygen in the body and is also essential in many enzyme systems. Iron deficiency leads to changes in behaviour, such as attention, memory, and learning in infants and small children, and also negatively influences the normal defence systems against infection. T-lymphocyte function, phagocytosis, and the killing of bacteria by neutrophilic leucocytes are affected. In pregnant women iron deficiency contributes to maternal morbidity and mortality, and increases risk of foetal morbidity, mortality, and low birth weight (Viteri 1997). Iron deficiency results in a reduction in physical working capacity and productivity of adults both in agricultural and industrial work situations. These functional impairments are economically important as it is estimated that median value of productivity losses is about 0.9 per cent GDP and the economic impact of iron deficiency can vary from 2 per cent GDP in the case of Honduras to 7.9 per cent in Bangladesh (Horton & Ross 2003).

Iron deficiency disorders encompass a range of body iron depletion states. The least severe is *diminished iron stores* diagnosed by decreased serum ferritin levels and not usually associated with adverse physiological consequences. The intermediate, *iron deficiency without anaemia* on the other hand, is severe enough to affect production of haemoglobin without haemoglobin levels falling below clinical criteria indicative of anaemia and is characterized by decreased transferrin saturation levels and increased erythrocyte protoporphyrin. The severe form with clinical manifestation is *Iron Deficiency Anaemia*.

Iron deficiency anaemia (IDA) is a serious problem worldwide and the dominant cause in all cases is nutritional iron deficiency (Table 2.6.3). The highest prevalence figures for IDA are seen in developing countries: In infants and pre-school children (39 per cent), school-age children aged 5–14 years (48.1 per cent), and women aged between 15 and 59 years (52 per cent) (WHO 2001). Even in industrialized, developed countries the prevalence of IDA is significant and the estimated prevalence is 20.1 per cent among infants and pre-school children aged 0–4 years, 22.7 per cent among pregnant women, and 12 per cent in the elderly aged 60+ years. Based on the estimates of IDA as a risk factor for mortality, the total attributed global burden is estimated at 841 000 deaths and over 35 million DALYs (Stolzfus *et al.* 2004).

In Africa, Asia, and South America, the availability of iron in the diets has been deteriorating and IDA continues to be a massive public health problem. The availability of iron in the diet for absorption is affected by both the forms of iron and the nature of foods concurrently ingested. Iron exists in the diet in two forms: (i) as 'haem iron' it is found only in animal sources and is readily available for absorption and is not influenced by other constituents of the diet; and (ii) as 'inorganic iron' it is not readily available and is strongly influenced by factors present in foods ingested at the same time. Both animal foods and ascorbic acid (vitamin C) promote the absorption of inorganic iron. Diets, which are primarily cereal and legume-based, may contain much iron but, in the absence of cofactors such as ascorbic acid or presence of phytates, they provide only low levels of bioavailable iron. Concern about iron deficiency is an important nutritional reason for recommending the consumption of at least some meat as well as foods with ascorbic acid for populations who rely predominantly on a cereal-based diet.

The strategies to combat iron deficiency include: (1) iron *supplementation*; (2) iron *fortification* of certain foods; (3) *dietary modification* to improve the bioavailability of dietary iron by modifying the composition of meals; and (4) *parasitic disease control*. Iron and folate supplementation programmes for pregnant women are currently widely implemented in several countries; many countries have a universal preventive supplementation policy during pregnancy. Iron supplementations aimed at pre-school or school-aged children are being carried out in several countries. Fortification of foods with iron is a preventive measure aimed at improving and sustaining adequate iron nutrition over a longer term. Many industrialized countries like Canada and the United States have fortified foods with iron and studies in developing countries have demonstrated the

Table 2.6.3 Numbers of people (in millions) affected with iron deficiency anaemia based on blood haemoglobin concentration in different regions of the world

	Children		*Women (15–49 years)*		*Men*
	0–4 years	**5–14 years**	**Pregnant**	**All women**	***(15–59 years)***
	(millions)	(millions)	(millions)	(millions)	(millions)
WHO Regions					
Africa	45.2	85.2	10.8	57.8	41.9
Americas	14.2	40.6	4.5	53.8	19.4
Southeast Asia	111.4	207.8	24.8	215.0	184.8
Europe	12.5	12.9	2.4	27.1	13.3
Eastern Mediterranean	33.3	37.9	7.7	60.2	41.5
Western Pacific	29.8	156.8	9.7	158.7	174.4
Total All Regions	**246.4**	**541.2**	**59.9**	**572.6**	**475.3**

Source: Compiled from WHO (2001): *Iron Deficiency Anemia: Assessment, prevention and control.*

effectiveness of iron fortification of foods provided these programmes are based on careful planning and follow well-established guidelines (Viteri 1997). Improvement in the supply, consumption, and the bioavailability of iron in food is an important strategy to improve iron status of populations. The bioavailability of iron in foods is influenced by the composition of the meal and food preparation methods. The consumption of ascorbate-rich foods enhances iron absorption while limiting the content of phytate which inhibits iron absorption, will improve iron bioavailability. Malaria and intestinal parasites (especially hookworm) are important contributors to IDA in endemic areas. In populations where hookworm is prevalent, effective treatment of this helminth infection has reduced IDA in school-aged children (Stoltzfus *et al.* 1997). Thus, strategies that address iron nutrition, whether food based, or by supplementation or fortification, must be integrated with programmes such as malaria prophylaxis, helminth control, environmental health, and control of other micronutrient deficiencies to maximize effectiveness (WHO 2001).

Iodine deficiency

The term 'iodine deficiency disorder' (IDD) refers to a complex of effects arising from deficient intakes of iodine. The mountainous areas of the world are likely to be iodine deficient because the rain leaches the iodine from the rocks and soils. The most severely deficient areas are the Himalayas, the Andes, the European Alps, and the vast mountainous regions of China, i.e. elevated regions subject to glaciation and high rainfall which run off into rivers. It also occurs in flooded river valleys of Eastern India, Bangladesh, and Burma. The Great Lake basins of North America are also iodine deficient. Excessive intakes of goitrogens in food, (due to the excessive consumption of *cassava* or the *brassica* group of vegetables) and in water (water-borne goitrogens in Latin America) as well as the deficiency of certain trace elements in the soil or food chain (such as selenium) may interfere with the uptake and metabolism of iodine in the body and can thus cause or amplify the effects of iodine deficiency.

The prevalence of manifest IDD in the form of goitre varies globally and at present is confined to developing countries, largely because public health initiatives such as iodization of salt have been introduced in the developed world, and most have mandated or permitted salt iodization. Iodine deficiency and goitre is still prevalent in Central and Eastern Europe. According to recent estimates the goitre prevalence in developing countries is 15.8 per cent (WHO 2004). However, this figure masks the enormous numbers who are at risk of IDD based on urinary iodine status which reflects the insufficiency of iodine intake in the diet (Table 2.6.4). Iodine deficiency is also responsible for over 200 000 severe birth defects worldwide while also contributing to lower the intellectual capacity of almost all nations reviewed, by as much as 10–15 percentage points (UNICEF/Micronutrient Initiative 2004).

IDD in humans is predominantly the result of a primary deficiency of iodine in the diet. Both water and foods are sources of iodine, with marine fish being the richest source of iodine. Milk and meat are also rich sources of iodine. Fruits, legumes, vegetables, and fresh water fish are also important additional sources. Plant foods are likely to show a reduced content of iodine if the iodine content of the soils in which they are grown is low. Goitrogens in the diet are of secondary importance as aetiological factors in IDD. It has been shown that staple foods consumed largely by poor rural populations, such as cassava, maize, sweet potatoes, lima beans contain cyanogenic glucosides which release a goitrogen thiocyanate. Cassava is now implicated as an important contributor to the endemic goitre and cretinism in non-mountainous Zaire and in Sarawak in Malaysia. Selenium deficiency in the soil can result in manifestations of IDD in the presence of modest iodine deficiency since selenium is essential for thyroid metabolism. Selenium deficiency is now recognized as an aetiologic factor in the IDD in several regions of China.

Iodine is readily absorbed from the diet and forms a very important element in the synthesis of thyroid hormones in the body. Thyroid hormones are essential for normal growth and development. Just prior to birth, the levels of the biologically active triiodothyronine (T_3) increase and prepare the organism for the transition from intra-uterine to extra-uterine life. Failure to synthesize sufficient T_3 as a result of iodine deficiency may be a factor in the stillbirths that occur as a part of the spectrum of IDD. Thyroid hormone deficiency leads to severe retardation of growth and maturation of all organs. The brain is particularly susceptible to damage during the foetal and early postnatal periods. It is now confirmed that the thyroidal control of neonatal brain development is more important than foetal brain development since early and optimal thyroid hormone treatment after birth can lead to substantial improvement in thyroid function. The spectrum of IDDs in humans, from the foetus to the adult, have been outlined by Hetzel (1987).

Table 2.6.4 Proportion of population and number of individuals with insufficient iodine intake in school-age children (6–12 years) and the general population and total goitre prevalence in the same UN regions

UN Region	Insufficient iodine intake (urinary iodine <100 μg/l)		Total goitre prevalence
	School age children	General population	
Africa	42.7% (59.7 million)	43.0% (324.2 million)	26.8%
Asia	38.3% (187.0 million)	35.6% (1239.3 million)	14.5%
Europe	53.1% (26.7 million)	52.7% (330.8 million)	16.3%
Latin America and the Caribbean	10.3% (7.1 million)	10.0% (47.4 million)	4.7%
North America	9.5% (2.1 million)	64.5% (19.2 million)	–
Oceania	59.4% (2.1 million)	64.5% (19.2 million)	12.9%
Total	**36.5% (285.4 million)**	**35.2% (1988.7 million)**	**15.8%**

Summarized from *Iodine Status Worldwide*; WHO (2004).
Figures in parenthesis are numbers of individuals at risk estimated from UN population estimates for 2002.

The public health initiatives for correcting iodine deficiency require the provision of adequate iodine to the individual. This has been achieved by one of several methods: *Iodization* of salt has been the most favoured method and has greatly reduced the prevalence of IDDs in Switzerland, the United States, and New Zealand. Since its first successful introduction in the 1920s in Switzerland (Burgi *et al.* 1990) successful programmes have been reported in Central and South America, in Europe (Finland), and in Asia (China and Taiwan). However, several developing countries have encountered problems with their salt iodization programmes because it is difficult to produce and maintain enough high-quality iodized salt for large populations such as in India and Bangladesh. The extra costs of iodized salt and its availability and distribution in remote regions can also be a problem. These issues may be compounded by cultural prejudices about the use of iodized salt and the loss of iodine with cooking if salt is not added after cooking. *Iodized oil* injections have been used to prevent goitre and cretinism in New Guinea (Pharoah & Connolly 1987). Iodized oil is suitable for mass programmes and can be carried out alongside mass immunization programmes. These methods have been successful in China, Indonesia, and Nepal. The major problems with iodized oil are the cost, the initial discomfort, and the likely potential disadvantage associated with the transmission of Hepatitis B and HIV with the use of needles. The need for a primary healthcare team to inject the iodized oil can be a further disadvantage. Iodized oil by mouth may be an alternative and primarily health centres can readily administer this scheme. Oral iodized oil has been shown to be as effective in a single oral dose as an intramuscular injection (Phillips *et al.* 1988). However, the effects of oral iodized oil seem to last for only half as long as a similar dose of injected iodized oil. They do not, however, suffer from the disadvantages of iodized oil injections so it is a preferred method for use in remote areas. The IDDs are excellent examples of nutritional deficiency disorders of public health importance which can readily be abolished if mass community programmes are undertaken.

Vitamin A deficiency

Vitamin A deficiency leads to night blindness and xerosis (dryness) of the conjunctiva and cornea and disrupts the integrity of their surface and causes corneal clouding and ulceration and may lead to blindness in children. Xerophthalmia continues to be a major cause of childhood blindness despite the intensive prevention programmes of the last two decades. It is a widespread problem and the parts of the world most seriously affected include South and Southeast Asia, and many countries in Africa, Central America, and the Near East. Extrapolations from the best available data suggest that 140 million children under 5 and more than 7 million pregnant women suffer from vitamin A deficiency every year (SCN 2004). This report also states that another 4.4 million children and 6.2 million women suffer from xerophthalmia. Nearly half of the cases of VAD and xerophthalmia occur in South and Southeast Asia.

An additional 20–40 million suffer from mild or sub-clinical deficiency of vitamin A, which we now recognize as having serious consequences for survival since vitamin A deficiency (VAD) is now known to decrease the child's resistance to infections and increase mortality. Even before eye signs of VAD are detectable, changes in the surface linings of the gastrointestinal and respiratory tracts occur along with changes in cell-mediated immunity and these can increase the risk of morbidity and even mortality associated with infections in children. Recent evidence suggests that VAD may be associated with increased maternal morbidity and even mortality. The estimates are that between 1.2 and 3 million children and significant numbers of mothers die associated with vitamin A deficiency. Vitamin A is also now known to be involved in foetal development, haematopiesis, spermatogenesis, appetite, and physical growth.

Vitamin A is the parent of a class of compounds called retinoids. Pro-vitamin A carotenoids, chiefly β-carotene, is also included in the vitamin A family. Preformed vitamin A is chiefly found in dairy products such as milk, butter, cheese, egg yolk, in some fatty fish, and in the livers of farm animals and fish. Carotenes are generally abundant in yellow fruits (papayas, mangoes, apricots, peaches) and vegetables (carrots). Absorption of vitamin A is about 80 per cent complete in the presence of an adequate fat intake, while the absorption of carotenoids is highly bile salt dependent. Vitamin A (retinol and retinoic acid) plays a very important role in the body in cellular development and differentiation. Retinol also has a vital role in normal vision, particularly by the rods in the retina. Thus, one of the earliest manifestations of vitamin A deficiency is night blindness.

There is now increasing evidence that vitamin A supplements in deficient populations can reduce morbidity, mortality, and blindness. Xerophthalmia has become less prevalent in recent years in hyperendemic areas such as Indonesia and India. Intervention strategies that may have contributed to this include periodic megadose vitamin A supplementation either in the form of capsules, syrup, or as an injected dose. It is now the practice to provide vitamin supplements along with immunization programmes in many countries with the objective of providing at least one dose of vitamin A per year for all children aged 6 months to 5 years. The fortification of dietary items which are universally consumed, e.g. sugar, in Central America (Arroyave *et al.* 1981) and monosodium glutamate in Indonesia (Muhilal *et al.* 1988) have had a favourable impact on the vitamin A status of the whole population. Following on the success of sugar fortification in Central America it has been successfully tried in Zambia and South Africa and the Philippines have successfully implemented fortification of cereals (wheat and maize flour) with vitamin A (UNICEF/Micronutrient Initiative 2004). The problems with food fortification are essentially logistical and technological and many developing countries are beginning the process of fortifying staple foods and condiments with vitamins (and minerals) including margarine, cooking oil, and soya sauce. Food supplies from different regions of the world show limited vitamin A availability, but the problem is exacerbated by a tendency to withhold vegetables and fruits from children and from pregnant and lactating women for cultural and other reasons in some parts of the world. Nutrition education is the only answer when vitamin A deficiency develops despite fruit and vegetable sources of the vitamin being in plentiful supply. These foods are not incorporated into the diets of young children and mothers, due either to lack of knowledge or cultural biases. Nutrition education together with practical advice and help with growing cheap, nutritious vegetables in home kitchen gardens may help eradicate vitamin A deficiency. Horticultural approaches are increasingly recognized for their effectiveness and potential sustainability in improving not only vitamin A status, but also micronutrient status generally. The importance of combining increased vitamin A levels in the food supply with nutrition education and appropriate social marketing that promotes consumption by vulnerable groups within populations cannot be underestimated. Economic development and poverty reduction programmes are likely to improve the socioeconomic status and may indirectly contribute to reducing the problem of VAD.

Folate deficiency

Folate enables cell division and tissue growth. Adequate folate in the diet helps prevent malformations that affect the neural tube and spinal cord such as anencephaly and spina bifida as well as other birth defects like cleft lip and palate. Without adequate folate in the diet, 2 in every 1000 pregnancies may end up with a serious birth defect. Folate deficiency is also associated with increased risk of pre-term delivery and low birth weight (Scholl & Johnson 2000) and may also contribute to anaemia especially in pregnant and lactating mothers (Dugdale 2001). It may thus contribute indirectly to increased maternal illness and mortality. With the increasing awareness of the role folate plays in reducing the risk of heart disease and stroke, a case is being made for folate fortification of flour, a strategy already adopted in the United States and Canada.

It is important to acknowledge the contribution of several Non Government Organizations (NGOs), many of them specialized in addressing specific micronutrient deficiencies (e.g. International Council for the Control of Iodine Deficiency Disorders (ICCIDD) with the objective of the sustainable elimination of IDD) while many others such as Micronutrient Initiative (MI) tackle all major micronutrient deficiencies of public health significance. It would be futile to mention all of them, apart from emphasizing the important role they play in numerous ways to deal with the problem of 'hidden hunger' worldwide. They closely work in partnership with governments, AID agencies, and with the UN agencies and the community to further this laudable objective.

This section has hitherto dealt with only some of the more important nutritionally determined deficiency disorders of public health importance. It is important to recognize that segments of populations in the world suffer from other nutritional disorders such as those due to the deficiency of fluoride, zinc, selenium, B group vitamins, and ascorbic acid. Some of these seem to occur during seasonal deficiencies in their availability and accompany famine and conflict situations when they are seen in refugee camps. It is important to recognize that in all regions of the world there are still some populations affected by one or more of these deficiencies despite the significant advances that have been made in controlling nutritional deficiency disorders. In some regions of the world, largely the result of increasing population size, the numbers of undernourished are increasing even if the population prevalence is declining. In many there is shift in the severity of the deficiency diseases with decreasing numbers with severe deficiency and increasing numbers with mild to moderate deficiencies. For a majority of these countries there is still the need to pursue vigorous policies and targeted action to combat the various nutritional deficiency disorders as a part of the comprehensive health-oriented national food and nutrition policies.

Consequences of undernutrition and micronutrient deficiencies

An issue that deserves attention is to ask the question whether humanitarian considerations apart, does widespread undernutrition and micronutrient malnutrition matter? And is there a case for investing in better nutrition? According to UNICEF, approximately half the economic growth achieved by developed countries of Western Europe since 1790 until 1980 can be attributed to better nutrition and improved health and sanitation (UNICEF 1997). The social and economic costs, apart from costs to the individual due to poor nutrition, are huge. Improving nutrition of communities reduces healthcare costs. More than half of child mortality in developing countries is attributable to underweight and the consequent increased risk of infectious diseases. Underweight is the leading risk factor in the global burden of disease and, among developing countries with high mortality, it contributes to nearly 15 per cent of the attributable disability adjusted life years (DALYs) (WHO 2002). Preventing low birth weight and stunting also reduces childhood mortality and morbidity. The intimate links between undernutrition in early life including low birth weight and the increasing risk of chronic disease in later adult life is well established. Diagnosis and treatment of chronic diseases like heart disease, diabetes, and cancer is expensive and will distort the limited public health budgets of developing countries.

Undernourished children become smaller adults and demonstrate lower physiological performance and reduced physical and work capacity. Employment prospects and productivity of short-statured and undernourished individuals is impaired (Spurr 1987). It shortens productive lives and increases absence due to illness; impacting in turn on economic productivity of countries. Micronutrient deficiencies such as iron deficiency in adults also impairs physical capacity and work productivity and contributes to economic losses.

Poor nutrition impairs cognitive development and learning in undernourished children in developing societies. Grantham-McGregor (1995) has demonstrated that children who are stunted and live in deprived circumstances have major deficits in intellectual and cognitive development and social behaviour. Children's scholastic ability in their teens can be strongly influenced by interventions in the second and third year of life. Iodine deficiency and the syndrome of cretinism is another example of the role of nutrition in brain development and function. Even postnatal iodine deficiency can lead to slowing of mental processing that results in permanent impairment of mental development because of the need for adequate nutrition during critical periods of brain development. Similarly, Pollitt (1991a,b) has demonstrated that iron deficiency anaemia can permanently handicap children at a crucial time in their development even though iron deficiency per se is not enough to produce demonstrable clinical deficiency. Grantham-McGregor's (1995) studies show that food that stimulates longitudinal bone growth also stimulates brain development, thus implying a more generic demand for a range of nutrients if mental function is to improve. All of these have significant relevance to the fact that childrens' education is the cornerstone to social and economic development of nations and is now an important component of the MDGs (MDG2). The benefits of sustained mental and physical development from childhood into adult life ensures that healthy adults with the physical capacity to maintain high work outputs and with the intellectual ability to flexibly adapt to new technologies in this rapidly globalizing world will be a national asset. The importance of food and nutrition in the development of human capital in developing societies can never be underestimated.

Strategies to address the problem of undernutrition in developing societies

Reduction of poverty and hunger are high up among the MDG since achieving MDG 1—halving poverty and hunger by 2015 is central to achieving the other health-related MDGs. Economic growth and development should reduce the burden of undernutrition, but the reduction is slow and many people continue to suffer needlessly. There is thus a need for well-conceived policies for sustainable economic growth and social development that will benefit the poor and the undernourished. Given the complexity of factors that determine malnutrition of all forms, it is important that appropriate food and agricultural policies are developed to ensure household food security and that nutritional objectives are incorporated into development policies and programmes at national and local levels in developing countries. The deleterious consequences of rapid growth and development need to be guarded against and policies need to be in place to prevent one problem of malnutrition replacing another in these societies.

The pre-eminent determinant of household food insecurity is poverty in societies. Several policy measures undertaken by governments in developing countries are aimed at ensuring food supply and household food security. These include:

- Macroeconomic policies and economic development strategies that ensure both public-sector and private-sector investment in agriculture and food production.
- Appropriate policies to promote expansion and diversification of food availability and agricultural production in a stable and sustainable manner, and to regulate the import or export of foods and agricultural products to ensure food security.
- Policies that help create adequate employment opportunities for the rural poor and improving market efficiencies and opportunities.
- Policies that improve distribution and access to land, and to other resources such as credit, as well as other agricultural inputs.
- Legislating for policies that deter discrimination and ensure equal status for women, and ensuring their effective implementation.
- Identification of good and culturally appropriate caring practices and policies that protect, support, and promote good care and nutrition practices for children.
- Policies that enable public health measures to reduce the burden of infectious diseases and to ensure access to primary healthcare.

It is hoped that with good governance and democracy and with well-targeted aid from developed countries the implementation of these policies and the relevant programmes will reduce the burden of hunger and undernutrition in developing countries of the world.

Diet, nutrition, and chronic non-communicable diseases

The evidence relating food and nutrition to chronic non-communicable diseases such as non-insulin-dependent diabetes mellitus, and cancers comes from population-based epidemiological investigations and from controlled trials. Descriptive population-based epidemiological investigations yield valuable data which lead to important hypotheses, but they cannot be used alone to establish the causal links between diet and disease. The most consistent correlation between diet and chronic diseases has emerged from comparisons of populations or segments of population with substantially different dietary habits. Analytical epidemiological studies, such as cohort studies and case control studies that compare information from groups of individuals within a population usually provide more accurate estimates of such associations. It is important to recognize when examining population-based epidemiological data relating diet to disease that every population consists of individuals who vary in their susceptibility to each disease. Part of this difference in susceptibility is genetic. As the diet within a population changes in the direction that measures the risk of the specific disease, an increasing proportion of individuals, particularly those most susceptible to the risk, develop the disease. As a result of this inter-individual variability in the interaction of diet with an individual's genetic make-up and therefore the individual's susceptibility to disease, some diet–disease relationships are difficult to identify within a single population. In experimental clinical studies and randomized and controlled trials, long exposures may be required for the effect of the diet as a risk factor to be manifest. Strict inclusion criteria for participants need to be adopted to show the effect with small numbers in a reasonable length of time. These in turn may restrict the study to homogenous samples and thus limit the applicability of results to the population at large. Despite these limitations, when carefully designed studies show consistent findings of an association between specific dietary factors and a chronic disease, they generally indicate a cause and effect relationship.

Diet, nutrition, and cardiovascular diseases

The commonest cardiovascular diseases that are diet-related are coronary heart disease and hypertension.

Coronary heart disease (CHD)

CHD emerged as a burgeoning public health problem in Europe and North America after World War II and by the end of the 1950s had become the single major cause of adult death. The rates of CHD show marked international differences with overall rates being higher among men than women. Mortality rates are sevenfold higher in some Eastern European countries while three-fold differences are evident between Scotland and Spain or Portugal. Migration can contribute to either an increase as in the case of Japanese moving to the United States or decrease when Finns move to Sweden—migrants tending to approach the rates in their host countries. In the case of migrants from South Asia to the United Kingdom, however the rates exceed the hosts implying some genetic susceptibility increasing risk in the host environment.

Several prospective studies have documented the relationship between habitual diets and the risk of CHD in a given population. These longitudinal studies have shown that several foods and nutrients in the diet are protective and reduce risk of CHD—they include whole grain cereals, fish, fruits and vegetables, nuts, and moderate intakes of red wine while others such as dietary cholesterol, trans fatty acids, and increased consumption of coffee may increase the risk of CHD.

The nearly five-fold difference in CHD rates among different countries and the intra-population variations in rates, by socioeconomic class, ethnicity, and geographical location, have brought to our attention the dietary basis of CHD. The marked changes in CHD rates in migrant populations that moved across a geographical gradient in CHD risk provided further evidence of the environmental nature of the causative factor. The WHO Expert Committee on Prevention of CHD (1982) concluded, after reviewing the data on the relationship between blood cholesterol and the risk of CHD, that the relationship of lipids in the diet and blood met the criteria for an epidemiological association to be termed causal. These data were backed by several intervention trials in volunteers, clinical studies, and a wide range of animal experiments demonstrating the effects of diet on coronary artery atherosclerosis.

This relationship between dietary factors and CHD was supported by the results of the Seven Country Study (Keys 1980). The *saturated fat intake* varied between 3 per cent total energy in Japan and 22 per cent in Eastern Finland while the 15-year CHD incidence rates varied between 144 per 10 000 in Japan and 1202 per 10 000 in Eastern Finland. The annual incidence of CHD among 40–59-year-old men initially free of CHD was 15 per 100 000 in Japan and 198 per 100 000 in Finland. Measurement of food consumption by the people in 16 well-defined cohorts in seven countries and its correlation to 10-year incidence rate of CHD deaths provided further support for this causal association. The strongest correlation was noted between CHD and percentage of energy derived from saturated fat, while total fat was not significantly correlated with CHD.

In the Seven Country Study, the *serum total cholesterol* values were 165 mg dl in Japan and 270 mg dl in Eastern Finland, and suggested that the variation in serum total cholesterol levels between populations could be largely explained by differences in saturated fat intake and CHD incidence. On a population basis, the risk of CHD seems to rise progressively within the same population with increases in plasma total cholesterol. Observational studies suggest that one population with an average total cholesterol level 10 per cent lower than another will have one-third less CHD and a 30 per cent difference in total cholesterol predicts a four-fold difference in CHD (WHO 1990). The Seven Country Study showed a strong positive relationship between saturated fat intake and total cholesterol level; populations with an average saturated fat intake between 3 and 10 per cent of the energy intake were characterized by serum total cholesterol levels below 200 mg dl and by low mortality rates from CHD. As saturated fat intakes increased to greater than 10 per cent of energy intake a marked and progressive increase in CHD mortality was noticed. Saturated fats raise total and *low-density lipoprotein* (LDL) cholesterol; and of these fatty acids myristic and palmitic acids abundant in diets rich in dairy and meat products have the greatest effects (Table 2.6.5).

Several prospective studies have shown an inverse relation between *high-density lipoprotein* (HDL) cholesterol and CHD incidence. However, HDL cholesterol levels are influenced by several non-dietary factors and HDL levels do not contribute to explain differences in CHD mortality between populations. HDL levels are increased by alcohol, weight loss, and by physical activity. Populations who have high intakes of mono-unsaturated fatty acids (from olive oil) or have diets rich in n-3 polyunsaturates of marine origin (like Eskimos) also have low CHD rates. Both *mono-unsaturated* and n-3 and n-6 *polyunsaturated fatty acids* (PUFAs) lower plasma total and LDL cholesterol; PUFAs more effective than mono-unsaturates (Kris-Etherton 1999; Mori & Beilin 2001). There is good evidence that some isomers of fatty acids, such as *trans fatty acids* increase the incidence of CHD by increasing LDL cholesterol levels and decreasing the HDL levels, by interfering with essential fatty acid metabolism, and by enhancing the concentrations of the lipoprotein Lp(a) which, in genetically susceptible people, seems to be an additional risk factor through mechanisms which include an anti-plasminogen effect to limit fibrinolysis.

Table 2.6.5 Summary of strength of evidence of dietary and lifestyle factors and risk of developing cardiovascular disease

Evidence	Decreased risk	No relationship	Increased risk
Convincing	Regular physical activity	Vitamin E supplements	Myristic and palmitic acids
	Linoleic acid		Trans fatty acids
	Fish and fish oils[1]		High sodium intake
	Vegetables and fruits		Overweight
	Potassium		High alcohol intake[4]
	Alcohol intake (low to moderate)[2]		
Probable	α Linolenic acid	Stearic acid	Dietary cholesterol
	Oleic acid		Unfiltered boiled coffee
	NSP[3]		
	Whole grain cereals		
	Nuts (unsalted)		
	Plant sterols/stanols		
	Folate		

Adapted from WHO/FAO (2003) *Diet, nutrition and the prevention of chronic diseases*
[1] Eicosapentaenoic acid and docosapentaenoic acid
[2] For CHD risk
[3] NSP= non starch polysaccharide
[4] For risk of stroke

Other dietary components, e.g. *dietary fibre or complex carbohydrates* in the diet seem to influence serum cholesterol levels and the incidence of CHD. Population sub-groups consuming diets rich in plant foods with a high content of complex carbohydrates have lower rates of CHD; vegetarians have a 30 per cent lower rate of CHD mortality than non-vegetarians and their serum cholesterol levels are significantly lower than that of lacto-ovo-vegetarians and non-vegetarians. *Alcohol* consumption also reduces the incidence of CHD. A number of observational studies suggest that light-to-moderate drinkers have a slightly lower risk of CHD than abstainers. However, the relationship between alcohol intake and CHD is complicated by changes in blood pressure and also the nature of the alcoholic drink. The presence of phenolic compounds in red wine may contribute to the benefits of drinking red wine as compared to alcohol consumption *per se* in reducing the incidence of CHD.

The risk of CHD in individuals is dominated by three major factors: (i) High serum total cholesterol, (ii) high blood pressure, and (iii) cigarette smoking (WHO 1982). There is also a synergism between risk factors, with the Japanese notable for their high smoking rates and hypertension but very low cholesterol levels: Smoking and hypertension are particularly harmful to individuals with high cholesterol levels. Body weight changes induced by diet and levels of physical activity, are strongly related to changes in serum total cholesterol, blood pressure, and obesity. Obesity in turn, particularly when associated with high waist circumference or waist/hip ratio, is strongly related to diabetes mellitus, both of which are risk factors for CHD.

Hypertension and stroke

The risk of CHD and that of cerebrovascular disease presenting clinically as stroke, increases progressively throughout the observed range of blood pressure, in a number of different countries (MacMohan *et al.* 1990). From the combined data it appears that there is a five-fold difference in CHD and a ten-fold risk of stroke over a range of diastolic blood pressure of only 40 mm Hg. Analysis indicates that a sustained difference of only 7.5 mm Hg in diastolic blood pressure confers a 28 per cent difference in risk of CHD and a 44 per cent difference in risk of stroke.

Nutritional determinants of hypertension are contributory factors and are causally linked to stroke. Obesity and alcohol intake are related to hypertension since weight reduction and restricting alcohol intake can lower blood pressures. The dietary factors that are implicated (in addition to alcohol and caffeine intakes) are excessive sodium and saturated fat intake and low potassium and calcium intake. The role of dietary sodium in hypertension has been a subject of considerable debate. A critical review concluded that there was the relationship between intakes of salt and the prevalence of hypertension (Glieberman 1973). However, in a majority of the studies the methods for assessing both dietary sodium and blood pressure were inadequate. The Intersalt Study (1988) compared standardized blood pressure measurements with 24 h urinary sodium excretion in 10 000 individuals aged 20–59 years in 32 countries and showed that populations with very low sodium excretion (implying low sodium intakes) had low median blood pressures, a low prevalence of hypertension, and no increase in blood pressure with age. Although sodium intake was related to blood pressure levels and also influenced the extent to which blood pressures increased with age, the overall association between sodium, median blood pressure, and the prevalence of hypertension was less than significant.

A number of explanations have been put forward to explain why meticulous studies such as the Intersalt Study underestimate the relationship between dietary sodium and blood pressure. These include among others: Unreliability of assessing dietary intake of sodium accurately; genetic variability; and the contribution of other factors such as obesity or alcohol intake. Recent meta-analysis has correlated blood pressure recordings in individuals with measurements of their 24 h sodium intake (Law *et al.* 1991); an association which increases with age and with the initial blood pressure. The results of intervention trials of sodium restriction support this relationship. Aggregation of the results of 68 cross-over trials and 10 randomized control trials of dietary salt reduction have shown that moderate dietary salt reduction over a few weeks lowers systolic and diastolic blood pressure in those individuals with high blood pressure (Law *et al.* 1991). It was estimated that such reductions in salt intake by population would reduce the incidence of stroke by 26 per cent and that of CHD by 15 per cent in Western countries. Reduction of salt in processed food would lower blood pressure even further and would prevent as many as 70 000 deaths per year in the United Kingdom. Results of therapeutic trials of drug therapy also support the fact that the incidence of stroke can be reduced if blood pressure is lowered, although the beneficial effect of lowering the incidence of CHD is lower than expected.

The other dietary component that has been investigated by the Intersalt Study (1988) is potassium. Urinary potassium excretion, an assumed indicator of intake, was negatively related to blood pressure as was the urinary sodium/potassium concentration ratio. It has also been observed that potassium supplementation reduces blood pressure in both normotensive and hypertensive subjects (Cappucio & MacGregor 1991). Some, but not all, cross-sectional and intervention studies suggest a beneficial effect of calcium intake on blood pressure. Epidemiological studies also consistently suggest lower blood pressures among vegetarians than non-vegetarians independent of age and body weight. These studies may also support the role of other dietary components because vegetarian diets rich in complex carbohydrates are also rich in potassium and other minerals.

Nutritional intervention is likely to reduce the occurrence of hypertension and the consequent complications of stroke and CHD in the community, as demonstrated in Finland where the average blood pressure has fallen by nearly 10 mm Hg and the prevalence of hypertension is only a quarter of what it was prior to the intervention. Along with the falls in average cholesterol levels, CHD and stroke rates in Finland have fallen dramatically as the population's diet was transformed to change its fat content and to more than double the average vegetable and fruit intakes. The decline in CHD and stroke rates was predominantly dependent on the fall in cholesterol and blood pressure levels respectively and these changes occurred despite increasing obesity rates (Puska *et al.* 1995).

A summary of the strength of evidence (convincing and probable) on diet and lifestyle factors and risk of developing cardiovascular diseases (CHD and stroke) based on the recent Joint WHO/FAO Expert Consultation is provided in Table 2.6.5 (WHO/FAO 2003). There is now general agreement on the population strategies that need to be adopted to reduce both the frequency and extent of the risk factors of cardiovascular disease based on this report. The nutritional approach including increasing physical activity is aimed at reducing obesity, lowering blood pressure, lowering total and LDL cholesterol and increasing HDL cholesterol, and lowering sodium intakes. Current recommendations take into consideration both the entire spectrum of cardiovascular risks including effects on thrombosis as well as providing a holistic approach to recommending a healthy diet which will reduce all chronic non-communicable diseases including cancers. These recommendations include lowering total fat intake to between 30 and 35 per cent of total calories, restricting saturated fat intake to a maximum of 10 per cent of total calories, increasing contribution from monounsaturated and polyunsaturated fatty acids (n-3 and n-6 PUFAs), and to increase intakes of complex carbohydrates or dietary fibre. Translated into food components this would mean reducing in particular intake from animal fat, hydrogenated and hardened vegetable oils, and increasing the consumption of cereals, vegetables, and fruits.

Diet, nutrition, and cancers

It is now widely accepted that one-third of human cancers could relate directly to some dietary component (Doll & Peto 1981) and it is probable that diet plays an important role in influencing the permissive role of carcinogens on the development of many cancers. Thus up to 80 per cent of all cancers may have a link with nutrition.

Evidence that diet is a determinant of cancer risk comes from several sources. These include correlation between national and regional food consumption data and the incidence of cancers in the population. Studies on the changing rates of cancer in populations as they migrate from a region or country of one dietary culture to another have contributed to many important hypotheses. Case control studies of the dietary habits of individuals with and without a cancer and prospective studies as well as intervention trials have provided evidence for the effects of diet on cancer. The section below discusses only those human cancers where the role of diet or a nutrient is reasonably well established (summarized in Table 2.6.6). Many other cancers in which aspects of the diet may have a possible role have not been discussed since the aim is not to make this section exhaustive and all inclusive.

Cancers of the gastrointestinal tract may be influenced by the diet. The intake of alcohol appears to be an independent risk factor for oral, laryngeal, and pharyngeal cancers as well as for oesophagus, liver, and breast cancers. Consumption of salted fish (Cantonese style), preserved and fermented foods containing nitrosamines as weaning foods or from early childhood may introduce a substantial risk of *nasopharyngeal cancer*. *Stomach cancer* is also associated with diets comprising large amounts of salted and salty foods and low levels of fresh fruit and vegetables which may contain nutrients that possibly inhibit the formation of nitrosamines. Non-starchy vegetables, allium vegetables (onion, garlic, etc.), and fruits probably decrease risk of stomach cancer.

Cancers of the colon and rectum are the third commonest form of cancer and the incidence rates are high in Western Europe and North America while they are low in sub-Saharan Africa (Boyle *et al.* 1985). Almost all the specific risk factors of colon cancer are of dietary origin. International comparisons indicate that diets low in dietary fibre or complex carbohydrates and high in animal fat and animal protein increase the risk of colon cancer. The epidemiological data relating foods containing dietary fibre to colorectal cancer generally support the existence of an inverse relationship between the intake of foods which are rich in dietary fibre and colon cancer risk and meta analysis indicates a 10 per cent decreased risk per 10 g fibre per day. Diets rich in fibre are also rich sources of nutrients such as antioxidant vitamins and minerals with potential cancer inhibiting properties. Vegetarian diets seem to provide a protective effect from the risk of colon cancer. There is now convincing evidence that red meat and processed meat in the diet increases the risk of colon and colorectal cancers while physical activity decreases risk. Alcohol intake in men and women as well as obesity and abdominal fatness increase risk of this cancer (WCRF/AICR 2007).

Primary *liver cancers* have been correlated with mycotoxin (aflatoxin) contamination of foodstuffs. The primary causal factor for *lung cancer*, a leading cause of death among men, is cigarette smoking. Several studies have shown an interactive effect between cigarette smoking and low frequency of intake of green and yellow vegetables rich in β-carotene. In prospective studies, the frequency of the consumption of foods rich in β-carotene has been inversely associated with lung cancer risk. However, high intakes of β-carotene as supplements increases risk significantly; and so does arsenic in drinking water.

Breast cancer is a common cause of death among women both in the United States and in the United Kingdom. The most convincing evidence is that lactation protects against risk of breast cancer in both pre- and post-menopausal women. Physical activity probably also decreases risk while increase in body fatness after menopause increases risk. While other nutritional factors related to life events such as greater birth weight, attained adult stature, and weight gain increase risk, consumption of alcoholic drinks also convincingly increases risk of breast cancer both pre- and post-menopause.

Dietary factors thus seem to be important in the causation of cancers of many sites and dietary modifications may reduce cancer risk. In general diets high in plant foods, especially vegetables and fruits, are strongly associated with a lower incidence of a wide range of cancers. Such diets tend to be low in saturated fat, high in complex carbohydrate and fibre, and rich in several antioxidant vitamins. Sustained and consistent intake of alcohol, physical inactivity, and obesity and body fatness are also associated with several cancers. On the basis of the evidence, a recent report (WCRF/AICR 2007) makes the following recommendations: (i) be as lean as possible within the normal range of body weight for height and be physically active. (ii) Eat mostly foods of plant origin and limit intake of red meat and avoid processed meat. (iii) Limit consumption of energy dense foods and avoid sugary drinks. (iv) Limit alcohol intake. (v) Limit consumption of salt, and avoid mouldy food. (vi) Mothers must be encouraged and supported to breastfeed their children.

Table 2.6.6 Associations between nutritional factors and some common cancers

Cancer	Decreasing risk of cancer	Increasing risk of cancer
Breast	Lactation Physical activity	Alcohol Obesity
Colorectal	Physical activity NSP/dietary fibre Milk, calcium	Processed red meat Alcohol Obesity
Endometrium and kidney	Physical activity	Obesity
Liver		Aflatoxin Alcohol
Lung	Fruits Physical activity	High-dose supplements of β-carotene
Mouth, larynx, pharynx	Vegetables and fruits	Alcohol
Nasopharynx		Salted fish*
Oesophagus	Fruits and vegetables	Alcohol Obesity
Pancreas	Folate rich foods	Obesity
Prostate	Lycopene and selenium-rich foods	High-calcium diets
Stomach	Fruits and vegetables	High salt intake

Compiled from WCRF/AICR, (2007): *Food, nutrition, physical activity and the prevention of cancer: A global perspective.*
Both convincing and probable evidence for decreasing and increasing risk combined
NSP= non starch polysaccharide/dietary fibre
* Specifically Cantonese style salted fish

Diet, lifestyles, and obesity

Obesity is one of the most important public health problems and the prevalence of obesity is increasing in the developed, industrialized world. Even in developing countries, relatively affluent and urbanized communities in countries undergoing rapid economic growth and transition are showing an increasing prevalence of obesity among adults and children.

Overweight and obesity is normally assumed to indicate an excess of body fat. Like adult undernutrition, body mass index (BMI) is used as an indicator of choice to diagnose obesity in adults and Table 2.6.7 outlines the diagnostic criteria for overweight and obesity in infants and children, adolescents, and adults (WHO 1995; WHO 2000). Recent recommendations include the suggestion that a BMI of between 18.5 and 24.9 in adults be considered appropriate weight for height. A BMI between 25 and 29.9 is indicative of overweight and possibly a pre-obese state, while obesity is diagnosed at a BMI >30. The main health risk of obesity is premature death due to heart disease and hypertension and other chronic diseases. In the presence of other risk factors, (both dietary and non-dietary), obesity increases the risk of CHD, hypertension, and stroke. In women, obesity seems to be one of the best predictors of cardiovascular disease. Longitudinal studies have demonstrated that weight gain, both in men and women, is significantly related to increases in cardiovascular risk factors. Weight gain was strongly associated with increased blood pressure, elevated plasma cholesterol, and triglycerides and hyperglycaemia (fasting and post-prandial). The distribution of fat in the body in obesity may also contribute to increased risk; high waist–hip ratios (i.e. fat predominantly in abdomen and not subcutaneous) increase the risk of heart disease and type 2 diabetes. The coexistence of diabetes is also an important contributor to morbidity and mortality in obese individuals. Obesity also carries increased risk of gall bladder stones, breast and uterine cancer in females, and possibly of prostate and renal cancer in males as well as osteoarthritis of weight bearing joints and obstructive sleep apnoea. While obesity contributes to social problems such as low self-esteem and reduced employability it is also associated with increasing mortality both in smokers and non-smokers.

Several environmental factors, both dietary and lifestyle related, contribute to increase in obesity in communities. Social and environmental factors that either increase energy intake and/or reduce physical activity are of primary interest. Changes in the environment that affect the levels of physical activity among children and adults and changes both in the food consumed and in the patterns of eating behaviour may contribute to increase energy intakes beyond one's requirement, thus causing obesity. Increased intake of dietary fat as energy dense food may result in poor regulation of appetite and food intake while fibre-rich complex carbohydrates tend to bulk the meal and limit intakes. International comparisons reveal that obesity increases as the fat percentage of calories in the diet increases (Lissner & Heitmann 1995). Patterns of eating, particularly snacking between meals, may contribute to increased intakes. However, evidence supports the view that much of the energy imbalance which is responsible for the epidemic of obesity in modern societies is largely the result of dramatic reductions in physical activity levels (both occupational and leisure time) when food availability is more than adequate.

Tackling overweight and obesity that is approaching epidemic proportions worldwide is of crucial importance since it is associated with several co-morbidities and the consequent increased healthcare costs. It has been estimated that the direct costs of obesity for healthcare in the United States in 1995 was US$70 billion and that of physical inactivity another US$24 billion (Colditz 1999). These are enormous costs and a huge drain on healthcare budgets of countries.

Table 2.6.7 Diagnostic criteria for overweight and obesity in infants and children, adolescents, and adults

Infants and children		
(all ages)	Weight-for-height	>+2 Z scores
Adolescents		
Overweight	BMI-for-age	>85th percentile
Obese	BMI-for-age	>85th percentile of BMI plus
	Triceps-for-age	>90th percentile of TSkf
	Subscapular-for-age	>90th percentile of SSSkf
Adults		
Normal weight range	BMI	18.5–24.9
Overweight or pre-obese	BMI	25–29.9
Obese-Grade I	BMI	30–39.9
Grade II	BMI	35–39.9
Grade III	BMI	>40

Adapted from WHO (1995). *Physical status: the use and interpretation of anthropometry* and WHO (2000). *Obesity: Preventing and managing the global epidemic.*

Preventive measures to tackle the increasing obesity worldwide are reliant on the strength of evidence related to the factors that increase or reduce the risk of weight gain. The WHO report (WHO 2003) provides a summary of the evidence, but a more recent and critical review of the evidence is provided in Table 2.6.8 (WCRF/AICR 2007). Preventive measures have to start very early and primary prevention may have to be aimed at young children. This includes nutrition education of children and parents and dealing with problems of school meals, snacking, levels of physical activity, and other related issues. Public health initiatives need to address all social and environmental issues that contribute to the increasing energy and fat intakes and reduce physical activity levels. Since the issues are complex, attempts have to be made to interact with a wide range of stakeholders related to agriculture and trade, education, sport, transportation, etc., and address issues relevant to work sites, schools, supermarkets and deal with marketing, advertising, and promoting activity, etc., and not merely expect the health sector to provide solutions. A recent high-level exercise in the United Kingdom is a good example of such an integrated approach to the problem (Foresight 2007).

Non-insulin dependent diabetes mellitus (NIDDM)

NIDDM is a chronic metabolic disorder which occurs in middle adulthood and is strongly associated with an increased risk of CHD. NIDDM has to be distinguished from insulin dependent diabetes as well as from gestational diabetes of pregnancy. Obesity is a major risk factor for the occurrence of NIDDM; the risk being related both to the duration and the degree of obesity. The occurrence of

Table 2.6.8 Summary of factors that decrease risk (i.e. promote appropriate energy intake relative to energy expenditure) and those that increase risk (i.e. promote excess energy intake relative to energy expenditure) of weight gain and obesity

Evidence	Decreased risk	Increased risk
Convincing	Physical activity	Sedentary living
Probable	Low-energy-dense foods	Energy-dense foods
	Being breastfed	Sugary drinks
		'Fast foods'
		Television viewing

Source: Adapted from WCRF/AICR (2007): *Food, nutrition, physical activity and the prevention of cancer: A global perspective.*

1. Low-energy-dense food whole grain cereals, cereal products, non-starchy vegetables, and dietary fibre.
2. Energy-dense foods are mostly from animal fat and fast foods.
3. Sugary drinks have sucrose or high-fructose corn syrup.

NIDDM in a community appears to be triggered by a number of environmental factors such as sedentary lifestyle, dietary factors, stress, urbanization, and socioeconomic factors. Certain ethnic or racial groups seem to have a higher incidence of NIDDM, these include Pima Indians, Nauruans, and South Asians (i.e. Indians, Pakistanis, and Bangladeshis). NIDDM also seems to occur when the food ecosystem rapidly changes, e.g. urbanization of Australian aborigines or adoption of Western dietary patterns by Pima Indians.

The cause of NIDDM is unclear, but it seems to involve both an impaired pancreatic secretion of insulin and the development of tissue resistance to insulin. Overweight and obesity, particularly the central or truncal distribution of fat accompanied by a high waist/hip ratio and a high waist circumference seems to be invariably present with NIDDM. Hence the most rational approach to preventing NIDDM is to prevent obesity. Weight control and increasing physical activity levels is fundamental both as a population strategy for the primary prevention of this disorder and also to tackle high-risk individuals. Physical activity improves glucose tolerance by weight reduction and by its beneficial effects on insulin resistance. Diets high in plant foods are associated with a lower incidence of NIDDM, and vegetarians have a lower risk than non-vegetarians.

Expert groups have provided dietary recommendations for both the primary prevention of NIDDM, the management of diabetes, and the reduction of secondary complications which include CHD risk and the renal, ocular, and neurological complications of diabetes. Prevention of weight gain and reduction of obesity is the key, as is increasing levels of physical activity. The specific dietary recommendations include providing diets with carbohydrates providing 55–60 per cent of energy, maximizing content of complex carbohydrates and dietary fibre (non starch polysaccharide intake of 20 g per day) and reduction of simple sugar intakes. In addition the general recommendations for fat (saturated fat to <10 per cent of calories) is emphasized due to the associated high risk of CHD. Maintaining a desirable body weight and preventing weight gain is most important.

Diet and osteoporosis

The increase in numbers of elderly in the developed world has seen an increase in health problems of the elderly, which affects their quality of life. Fracture of the hip is an important health problem, particularly among post-menopausal women. Fractures occur in the elderly following what appears as relatively trivial falls when there is osteoporosis and the density of the bone is reduced. Bone density increases in childhood and adolescence and reaches a peak at about 20 years of age. Bone density falls from menopause in women and from about the age of 55 years in men. The variation in bone density between individuals and different racial groups is large and of the order of ±20 per cent. Since bone density declines with increasing age, those that attain high levels of peak bone mass at the end of adolescence and retain higher levels of bone density during adulthood become osteoporotic with advancing age much more slowly than those with lower bone densities to start with. Hence the range of factors that influence the attainment of peak bone density may play a crucial role in the development of osteoporosis and the occurrence of fractures as age advances.

Several factors determine the onset of osteoporosis and include the lack of oestrogen in post-menopausal women, degree of mobility, smoking, and alcohol intake. Calcium intake is a likely dietary determinant that may contribute to the onset and degree of osteoporosis. Evidence from some countries tends to indicate that the osteoporosis may be diet related since the fracture rate is halved among individuals in the higher calcium intake range compared to those on low calcium diets. However, there are regions where the lower rates of fracture due to osteoporosis are associated with lower calcium intakes. For example, the rates are lower in Singapore as compared with the United States, although the calcium intakes are lower than in the United States. The traditional emphasis on calcium intakes possibly reflects the recognition of its importance in contributing to the density of bone during growth and the need for attaining dense bones at the peak of adult life. High-protein and high-salt diets are known to increase bone loss while calcium supplements, well above what may be considered physiological, in post-menopausal women, may help to reduce the rate of bone loss and slow down the development of osteoporosis. Adequate levels of vitamin D either from the diet or by synthesis in the skin on exposure to sunlight are important factors that diminish risk of osteoporosis. Poor vitamin D status in the elderly have been linked with age-related bone loss and osteoporotic fractures. Many other nutrients may be important for long-term bone health and the prevention of osteoporosis. High intakes of alcohol increase risk of osteoporosis. Above all, the evidence is convincing that physical activity is an important determinant of good bone health.

It is generally believed that populations in developing countries are at less risk of developing osteoporosis in spite of low calcium intakes. This may be related to the fact that they do more physical work, smoke less, drink less alcohol, and have diets which are generally not high in protein or salt content. However, osteoporosis is seen in developing countries in regions where low intakes of dietary calcium are associated with high fluoride intakes. No osteoporosis occurs if high intakes of fluoride are accompanied by dietary intakes of calcium which are also high.

Diet and dental caries

Dental caries is a common disease of the teeth, which results in decay of the tooth surface, usually beginning in the enamel.

An essential feature in the causation of dental caries is dental plaque which is largely made up of microorganisms. Dietary sugars diffuse into the dental plaque where they are metabolized by the microorganisms to acids which can dissolve the mineral phase of the enamel causing dental decay. The process is, however, much more complex and is related to the quantity and quality of saliva produced in the mouth among other factors.

The evidence relating diet to dental caries is vast and has been well reviewed (Rugg-Gunn 1993). The overwhelming evidence indicates that sugars are cariogenic. There is good correlation between the sugar supply (in g per person per day) and the occurrence of dental caries in children and adults (WHO/FAO 2003). The consumption of refined sugar is a recent phenomenon in many parts of the world and seems to have been accompanied by an increase in dental caries in communities which were hitherto free of the problem. Cross-sectional studies correlating an individual's sugar consumption with the incidence of dental caries has demonstrated significant correlations between the two, particularly among young children. It also appears that the consumption of sugars between meals is associated with a marked increase in caries while consumption of sugars with meals is associated only with a small increase. Sucrose seems to be the predominant dietary agent that is cariogenic, although the current emphasis is on the consumption of all free sugars, particularly between meals. Despite suggestions that starch is also cariogenic, careful analysis of epidemiological data from several countries suggests that a much closer relationship exists between dental caries and free sugars than between caries and starchy cereal foods. Fresh fruit, although it contains intrinsic sugars, has a lower cariogenic potential while fruit juices are cariogenic, which may be related to the added sugars in fruit juices or from the lack of adequate salivary stimulation. Food may also contain protective factors that may prevent the occurrence of dental caries. This includes a sufficient daily ingestion of fluoride. Inorganic phosphates in the diet also seem to protect against dental caries.

Prevention of dental caries can be achieved by health education aimed at the individual beginning in infancy. Avoidance of the addition of free sugars to bottle feeds and milk and fruit drinks are a must. An adequate intake of fluoride is desirable quite early in life. During childhood and adolescence, the restriction of the three major sources that contribute to two-thirds of our intake of sugars, i.e. confectionery, table sugar, and soft drinks, will help reduce the increment of caries in childhood. At local and national level, the main interventions should include fluoridation of water supply, labelling of foods, and possible changes in policies that promote the production and marketing of free sugars.

Population nutrient intake goals in the prevention of chronic diseases

The distribution and determinants of risk factors in a population have direct implications for population-based prevention strategies. The foremost attribute that needs recognition is that risk typically increases across the spectrum of the risk factor and is a continuum. Thus those individuals at increased risk are not a distinct group or deviant minority, but a part of the risk continuum. Hence, population-based strategies must seek to shift the whole distribution of risk factors downwards and thus help reduce population incidence of the disease.

Population nutrient intake goals represents the mean population intake of the nutrient that is judged to be consistent with the maintenance of good health; health in this context implies a low prevalence of diet-related diseases in the population. There is usually no single best value and the safe range of intakes that constitute the nutrient goals would be consistent with maintenance of health. If the existing population averages move outside the recommended ranges, health concerns are likely to arise. Thus population nutrient intake goals are useful signposts for population-based strategies to help shift the risk distribution in a population downwards and thus reduce risk of the disease within the population. The recommended population nutrient goals based on critical examination of the available evidence from a recent Expert Consultation (WHO/FAO 2003) are summarized in Table 2.6.9.

Emerging food and nutrition issues of public health concern

Over the last decade several issues of public health concern related to food and nutrition have emerged both in the developed, industrialized countries, and in developing societies of the world. These include the problems related to the microbiological safety of foods, the frightening prospect of an epidemic of spongiform encephalopathies, concerns related to genetically modified foods, issues related to labelling of processed foods, and the emerging epidemic of diet-related chronic diseases and obesity in developing societies. Some of these issues will be dealt with briefly under this section.

Food safety

Food safety refers to whether food is safe for human consumption and hence lacking in biological and chemical contaminants that have the potential to cause illness. The increasing concern over the safety of foods in the developed world is a paradox in that the epidemiological evidence on the safety of foods is quite contrary to

Table 2.6.9 Ranges of the population nutrient intake goals

Dietary factor/nutrient	PNI goal*
Total fat	15–30%
Saturated fat	<10%
Polyunsaturated fatty acids (PUFAs)	6–10%
n-6 PUFAs	5–8%
n-3 PUFAs	1–2%
Trans fatty acids	<1%
Monounsaturated fats (MUFAs)	By difference
Total carbohydrate	55–75%
Free sugars	<10%
Protein	10–15%
Cholesterol	<300 mg per day
Sodium chloride	<5 g per day
Fruits and vegetables	>400 g per day

Source: Summarized from WHO/FAO (2003)
* Expressed as per cent of energy

the perceptions of the public and the media that the food available now is less safe than it used to be. The improvements in public health have virtually eradicated primarily food-borne infections that were until recently associated with considerable morbidity and mortality. The common food-borne diseases currently encountered are usually associated with mild self-limiting gastroenteritis. Studies of risk perception suggest that the public becomes alarmed by health threats which are disproportionate to the actual risk associated with the disease and that this public concern is fuelled by the media which make health issues into media health scares depending on the newsworthiness of the incidents.

There have been several food-borne epidemics in the developed world that have raised concerns about food safety in recent years. These include for instance the *Salmonella enteritidis pt4 (Se4)* epidemic. This was attributed to the ability of *Se4* to invade the oviduct of poultry and get deposited in the albumin of the egg. At the consumer level the outbreak of the infection was linked to the use of raw egg in recipes or cross-contamination from raw to cooked foods. *Campylobacter* infection is the commonest food-borne disease in the United Kingdom and the increase in its incidence may partly be explained by the better ascertainment and reporting of cases associated with this infection. The more recent food scare was the emergence of *E. coli 0157* in Scotland. The emergence of this food-borne infection which caused several deaths include changes in husbandry and the movement of livestock as well as the rapid growth of the fast food industry and poor food hygiene in these environments. *Listeria* is another cause of food-borne disease which is a good example of the role of international trade and globalization in the spread of food-borne diseases.

In the developing world the issues of food safety are related to microbiological agents that contaminate food and water and spread disease rapidly in the warm humid environments of these countries aided by the improper or poor food hygiene practices, poor environmental sanitation, and inadequate regulation of food-related commerce. The safety of foods in the developing world is also compromised by the presence of toxins such as aflatoxins which result from contamination with mycotoxins due to poor food storage practices or due to cyanogens in the diet due to inadequate preparation of staple foods such as cassava. In addition, the food chain in these poor countries is contaminated by pesticide and chemical residues thus compromising the safety of the food consumed by the populations in these countries.

Genetically modified (GM) foods

Another issue that has emerged over recent years and has created a considerable degree of controversy is the use of biotechnology to produce genetically modified foods. Genetic modification of food crops can be used to reduce food losses by increasing resistance to drought, frost, diseases and pests, and help control weeds and reduce post-harvest losses. Biotechnology can improve the nutritional value of foods, for example by increasing protein or micronutrient content or by reducing saturated fat content. They could help slow down ripening so that foods retain their quality much longer. Biotechnology can increase both the yield and the quality of crops grown on existing farmland and thereby reduce pressure on wildlife habitats. In the developed world, particularly in the United Kingdom and Europe, the opposition to GM foods is based largely on ecological arguments that raise concerns regarding the ecological damage that may follow large-scale use of GM crops. In the poor, developing countries the concerns are more related to the use of the 'terminator gene' technology and the dependence on the large multinationals for seeds and chemicals that the small farmers will inherit. At the heart of this controversy and the raging debate is the gulf between plant breeders, seed and agrochemical industries who promote biotechnology, and the campaigners who argue that GM technology may have hazardous consequences on the environment. This is a debate replete with numerous paradoxes and the climate of mistrust, some of it associated with the not too recent BSE and nvCJD scare, is obscuring the real issues and clouding objective decisions from being made with regard to the production and consumption of GM foods (Dixon 1999). Agricultural biotechnology is essential to increase food production to an increasing global population that is increasingly diverting food from human use to biofuels and animal feed; the latter the consequence of increased meat consumption with economic growth, as seen in China. It has the potential to improve the quality of the food to address both nutritional needs as well as consumer demands. It is interesting to note that the perception and acceptance of GM foods in developing societies, once the terminator gene threat has passed, is widely at variance to the concerns in developed countries (FAO 2004).

Food labelling

An important source of information for the consumer about the food on the supermarket shelf is the label on a food product. Food labels provide information that may be of interest to the consumer, especially with regard to the added chemicals (additives, pesticide residues, colouring and flavouring agents, and preservatives), fats, sugars, and energy content. Although, about two-thirds of shoppers claim to read the information on the labels of new or unfamiliar food products to check their contents, this interest in labels does not mean that consumers always understand the information in the labels. Consumers are even more confused by the nutrition information panel which appears on many food labels.

Food label information is usually designed by experts. A prototype label is produced by the *Codex Alimentarius Commission* of the FAO and WHO which is the Organization charged with advising on international food standards, and this prototype is followed by Food Standards Committees around the world. According to this prototype the nutrients—energy, carbohydrate, protein, and fats are listed according to their amounts per serving and per 100 g. Most consumers however, have hardly any idea of what a 100 g serving is, or for that matter what a normal or average serving is. A further problem is that these labels designed by experts is also beset with problems with terminology. One example is the term 'carbohydrate', which covers a wide range of compounds including sugars and starches, which have quite different health-related properties. Health benefits or nutritional claims are also not meant to be part of the food labels and they also do not provide information to cover ecological and ethical issues which may be of concern for some consumers. More recently the need to highlight the source or origin of foods and in particular the labelling of GM sources of the food product has been a serious concern of consumers. In January 2007, the Food Standards Agency in the United Kingdom agreed on the nutritional criteria for a 'traffic light' labelling of food products to identify products high in fat, sugar, and salt. While consumer organizations supported this move some of the major food companies and super markets have opposed the scheme. Food labelling is an important issue of public health concern and despite the considerable progress made so far there is much to be achieved.

Functional foods

New food products are being marketed as health-enhancing or illness-preventing foods. These are called functional foods or otherwise as 'pharmafoods' or 'nutriceuticals' or novel foods. Functional foods are generally defined as food products that deliver a health benefit beyond providing nutrients. The health benefits of functional foods may be conferred by a variety of production and processing techniques which include: Fortification of certain food products with specific nutrients, using phytochemicals and active microorganisms, and by genetic modification of foods. The topic of functional foods is complex and controversial. An assumption implicit in the functional foods and health benefit claims is that the food supply needs to be fixed or doctored (or medicalized) on public health grounds. The assumption therefore is that the current food supply is in some way deficient, that the habitual diets are inadequate and a technological fix will solve the problem. Thus the emerging debate viewed from the perspective of the proponents of functional foods is that these novel foods may reduce healthcare expenditure by promoting good health and that functional foods are a legitimate nutrition education tool, which will help inform consumers of the health benefits of certain food products. The opponents on the other hand rightly state that it is the total diet that is important for health. They believe that the functional foods are a 'magic bullet' approach which enables manufacturers to indulge in marketing hyperbole, exploit consumer anxiety, and essentially blur the distinction between food and drugs. Ironically the production and marketing of functional foods is on the rise in most developed countries.

Emerging epidemic of obesity and diet-related chronic diseases and the 'double burden' of malnutrition in developing societies

A critical examination of the principal causes of mortality and morbidity worldwide indicates that malnutrition and infectious diseases continue to be significant contributors to the health burden in the developing world. Although reductions in the prevalence of undernutrition is evident in most parts of the developing world, the numbers of individuals affected remain much the same or have even increased, largely the result of increases in the population in these countries. What is striking, however, is that the health burden due to non-communicable diseases (NCDs) such as heart disease and cancer is dramatically increasing in some of these developing countries with modest per capita GNPs, particularly among those that are in some stage of rapid developmental transition. Even the modest increases in prosperity that accompany economic development seems to be associated with marked increases in the mortality and morbidity attributable to these diet-related NCDs. These transitions in the disease burden of the population are mediated by changes in the dietary patterns and lifestyles which typify the acquisition of urbanized lifestyles.

Most developing countries, particularly those in rapid developmental transition, are in the midst of a demographic and epidemiologic transition. Economic development, industrialization, and globalization are accompanied by rapid urbanization. These developmental forces are bringing about changes in the social capital of these societies as well as increasing availability of food and changing lifestyles. The changes in food and nutrition are both quantitative and qualitative; there is not only access to more than adequate food among some sections of the population, but also a qualitative change in the habitual diet. Lifestyle changes contribute to a reduction in physical activity levels (occupational and leisure time) which promote obesity. The essence of these changes is captured by the term 'nutrition transition' (Popkin 1994), which accompanies the demographic and epidemiologic transition in these countries. The poor consumer resistance and inadequate regulation compromises food safety and increases contaminants in the food chain. In addition the deterioration of the physical environment, particularly the increase in levels of environmental pollution, contributes to the health burden. These developing societies suffer a 'double burden'—an unfinished agenda of pre-existing widespread undernutrition superimposed by the emerging burden of obesity and chronic diseases.

Food and nutrition in the prevention of diseases of public health importance

The public health approach to the prevention of nutrition and diet-related diseases requires the adoption of health-oriented nutrition and food policies for the whole population. In most developing countries, the first priority must be ensuring the production or procurement of adequate food supply and its equitable distribution and availability to the whole population along with the elimination of the various forms of nutritional deficiencies which include protein-energy malnutrition, vitamin, mineral, and trace element deficiencies. Efforts must also be made to improve the quality of the food which includes ensuring food safety while reducing spoilage and contamination of foods as well as diversifying the availability and use of foods. In agrarian societies, consideration must be given to the short- and long-term effects of agricultural policies that affect the income and buying power of the small producers. Particular attention needs to be paid to the impact the promotion of cash and export crops has on the availability and ability to procure the principal staples in the diet. Special attention needs to be paid to the feasibility of fortification of foods to deal with localized or widespread deficiencies of iodine, iron, and vitamin A as a mass intervention measure.

In developed countries, the burgeoning costs of tertiary healthcare related to the diagnosis and management of the increasing burden of obesity and diet-related NCDs has had an impact. There is increasing recognition of the need for prevention-oriented health and nutrition policies, and changes in behaviour and lifestyle to reduce the occurrence of these diseases. Some developed countries have been active in the field of public education using national dietary guidelines as a major stimulus. It is important to remember that nutrition education of the public operates in the area where advice is given on a balance of probabilities, rather than irrefutable evidence or any degree of certainty. There is bound to be information that does not fit in with the consensus view since the consensus is based on the balance of the available evidence. It is important to recognize that the causes of these chronic diseases are complex and dietary factors are only a part of the explanation. Individuals differ in their susceptibility to the adverse health effects of specific dietary factors or deficiencies of others. Within the context of public health the focus is the health of the whole population and interventions are aimed at lowering the average level of risk to the health of the whole population.

Changes in consumer preferences have emerged, initially among the upper socioeconomic and educated masses. The media attention, along with the behavioural changes in food preferences and food choices are in turn influencing the industry to modify the systems for food production and processing. However, progress in changing consumer behaviour and preferences is by its nature intrinsically rather slow and has until recently largely occurred without support from public policies in any but the health sector. The process of changing unsatisfactory dietary practices and thus promoting health is not easy to achieve both socially and politically. Despite these limitations the occurrence of and mortality associated with some diet-related NCDs such as heart disease have declined reflecting possible changes in lifestyles of the population.

The dynamic relationship between changes in a population's diet and changes in its health is reflected well in two critical situations. One is the changes in disease and mortality profiles of migrant populations moving from a low risk to a high risk environment. An example of this is the change in disease pattern of the Japanese migrants to the United States. The other is the rapid change seen within a country as rural to urban migration occurs or more frequently as a developing country undergoes rapid industrialization and economic development, and in the process acquires a dietary change and the consequent morbidity and premature mortality profile characteristic of a developed country. Several developing countries have urban pockets of affluent diet and lifestyles and related disease burdens in the midst of problems typical of a poor, developing country. Such countries in transition, like India and Brazil, bear the dual burdens of diseases of affluence and the widespread health problems of a poor country. Developing countries can hence benefit by learning from the experience of dietary change and adverse health effects of the developed world and the aim should be to avoid the diseases and premature deaths related to the changes in diets and lifestyles. By recognizing this problem, governments of developing countries can gain for their people the health benefits of avoiding nutritional deficiencies without encouraging at the same time the development of diet-related NCDs that invariably accompany economic and technological development.

It is thus possible for a country to achieve a reduction in infant and childhood mortality and an increase in life expectancy by the pursuance of health and nutrition policies that aim to provide adequate and equitable access to safe and nutritious food and to minimize at the same time the occurrence of diet-related chronic diseases. This in turn will help avoid the social and economic costs of morbidity and premature death in middle age—a period of highest economic activity and productivity to the nation and to society at large. If such a socially and economically desirable goal is to be achieved, then national governments in both developing and developed countries must aim towards achieving a population-based dietary change (WHO 1990). In the pursuance of this objective, FAO and WHO jointly established the scientific basis for developing and using Food-Based Dietary Guidelines (FAO/WHO 1996).

The development of Food-Based Dietary Guidelines (FBDGs)

FBDGs are developed and used in order to improve the food consumption patterns and nutritional well-being of individuals and populations. Guidelines would be needed by all countries given the important role that food and dietary practices play in nutrition-related disorders; both due to deficiencies or excesses. FBDGs can address specific health issues without the need to fully understand the biological mechanisms that may link constituents of food and diet with disease. However, FBDGs do take into account the considerable epidemiological data linking specific food consumption patterns with a low or high incidence of certain diet-related diseases.

Disseminating information and educating the public through the FBDGs is a 'user friendly' approach since consumers think in terms of foods rather than nutrients. They provide a means for nutrition education mostly as foods for the public. They are intended for use by individual members of the general public, are written in ordinary language, and as far as possible avoid the use of technical terms in nutritional science. FBDGs will vary with the population group and has to take into account the local or regional dietary patterns, practices, and culture. It is important to recognize that more than one dietary pattern is consistent with good health. This will enable the development of food-based strategies that are appropriate for the local region and take into consideration the local dietary practices.

FBDGs can serve as an instrument of nutrition policies and programmes. Since they are based directly on diet and health relationships of particular relevance to the individual country or region, they can help address those issues of public health concern, whether they relate to dietary insufficiency or dietary excess. Food and diet are not the only components of a healthy lifestyle and it is important that other relevant messages related to health promotion are integrated into dietary guidelines.

Global strategies to reduce the burden of nutritional disorders

The prevalence of chronic diseases is increasing dramatically, with the majority occurring in developing countries. WHO proposed an integrated global strategy for the prevention and control of non-communicable diseases entitled, 'Diet, physical activity and health' in 2003. More recently WHO has highlighted the fact that chronic diseases are the leading cause of disease and disability, but are neglected elements of the global health agenda (Beaglehole *et al.* 2007). WHO has proposed a global goal for the prevention and control of chronic diseases to complement the MDG. The goal is to reduce by 2 per cent per year the age-specific rates of death attributable to chronic diseases, achievement of which would avert 36 million deaths by 2015. Because most of the deaths averted would be in low- and middle-income countries and would mainly affect people less than 70 years, it would bring major economic benefits and reduce the health burden of these nations. Strategies that are developed to tackle nutritional problems need to be joined up to deal simultaneously with both ends of the spectrum of nutritional disorders and need to encompass a wide range of stake holders in a joined up and integrated manner to be effective.

References

Arroyave, G., Mejia, L.A., and Aguilar, J.R. (1981). The effect of vitamin A fortification of sugar on serum vitamin A levels of pre-school Guatemalan children: A longitudinal evaluation. *American Journal of Clinical Nutrition*, **34**, 41–9.

Barker, D.J.P. (2004). The developmental origins of adult disease. In *Fetal and neonatal physiology* (eds. R.A. Polin, W.W. Fox and S.H. Abman), Third edition. W.B. Saunders, Philadelphia.

Beaglehole, R., Ebrahim, S., Reddy, S. (2007) *et al.* Prevention of chronic diseases: A call to action. *Lancet*, **370**, 2152–7

Boyle, P., Earidze, D.G., and Simans, M. (1985). Descriptive epidemiology of colo-rectal cancer. *International Journal of Cancer*, **36**, 9–18.

Cappucio, F.P. and MacGregor, G.A. (1991). Does potassium supplementation lower blood pressure? A meta-analysis of published trials. *Journal of Hypertension*, **9**, 465–73.

Colditz, G. (1999). Economic costs of obesity and inactivity. *Medicine and Science in Sport and Exercise*, **31**, S663–7.

de Onis, M., Blossner, M., Borghi, E. *et al.* (2004). Estimates of global prevalence of childhood underweight in 1990 and 2015. *Journal of the American Medical Association*, **291**, 2600–6.

Dixon, B. (1999). The paradoxes of genetically modified foods. *British Medical Journal* **318**, 547–8.

Doll, R. and Peto, R. (1981). *The Causes of Cancer*. Oxford University Press, Oxford.

Dugdale, M. (2001). Anemia. *Obstetrics & Gynaecology Clinics of North America*, **28**, 363–81.

FAO (2004). *Agricultural biotechnology: Meeting the needs of the poor?* Food and Agricultural Organization, Rome.

FAO (2006). *State of food insecurity in the world*. Food and Agricultural Organization, Rome.

FAO/WHO (1996). *Preparation and use of food-based dietary guidelines*. World Health Organization, Geneva.

Foresight (2007). *Tackling obesity: Future choices-project report*. The Stationery Office, London.

Glieberman, L. (1973). Blood pressure and dietary salt in human populations. *Ecology of Food and Nutrition*, **2**, 143–56.

Grantham-McGregor, S. (1995). A review of the studies of the effect of severe malnutrition on mental development. *Journal of Nutrition*, **125**, 2232S–8S.

Hetzel, B.S. (1987). An overview of the prevention and control of iodine deficiency disorders. In *The prevention and control of iodine deficiency disorders* (eds. B.S. Hetzel, J.T. Dunn and J.B. Stanbury). Elsevier, Amsterdam.

Horton, S. and Ross, J. (2003). The economics of iron deficiency. *Food Policy*, **28**, 51–75.

Intersalt Cooperative Research Group (1988). Intersalt: An international study of electrolyte excretion and blood pressure. *British Medical Journal*, **298**, 920–4.

Keys, A. (1980). *Seven countries: A multivariate analysis of death and coronary heart disease*. Howard University Press, Cambridge, Massachusetts.

Kris-Etherton, P.M. (1999). Monounsaturated fatty acids and risk of cardiovascular disease. *Circulation*, **100**, 1253–8.

Law, M.R. Frost, C.D., and Wald, N.J. (1991). By how much does dietary salt reduction lower blood pressure? *British Medical Journal*, **302**, 811–24.

Lissner, L. and Heitmann, B.L. (1995). Dietary fat and obesity: Evidence from epidemiology. *European Journal of Clinical Nutrition*. **49**, 969–81.

MacMohan, S., Peto, R., Cutler, J. *et al.* (1990). Blood pressure, stroke and coronary heart disease. *Lancet*, **335**, 765–74.

McKeown, T. (1976). *The modern rise of population*. Edward Arnold, London.

Muhilal, P.D., Idjrodinata, Y.R., and Karyadi, D. (1988). Vitamin A fortified monosodium glutamate and health, growth and survival of children: A controlled field trial. *American Journal of Clinical Nutrition*, **48**, 1271–6.

Martin M.J, Hulley, S.B., Browner, W.S. *et al.* (1986). Serum cholesterol, blood pressure and mortality: Implications from a cohort of 361 662 men. Lancet, **ii**, 933–6.

Mori, T.A. and Beilin, L.J. (2001). Long-chain omega 3 fatty acids, blood lipids and cardiovascular risk reduction. *Current Opinion in Lipidology*, **12**, 11–17.

Naiken, L. (2003). Keynote Paper: FAO methodology for estimating the prevalence of undernourishment. *Proceedings of the International Scientific Symposium on Measurement and Assessment of Food Deprivation and Undernutrition*. Food and Agricultural Organization, Rome.

Pharoah, P.O.D. and Connolly, D.C. (1987). A controlled trial of iodinated oil for the prevention of endemic cretinism: A long-term follow-up. *International Journal of Epidemiology*, **16**, 68–73.

Phillips, D.I.W., Lusty, T.D., Osmond, C. *et al.* (1988). Iodine supplementation: Comparison of oral or intramuscular iodized oil with potassiumiodide. A controlled trial in Zaire. *International Journal of Epidemiology*, **17**, 142–7.

Pollitt, E. (1991a). Effects of diet deficient in iron on the growth and development of preschool children. *Food and Nutrition Bulletin*, **13**, 521–37.

Pollitt, E. (199b). Iron deficiency and cognitive function. *Annual Review of Nutrition*, **13**, 521–37.

Popkin, B. (1994). The nutrition transition in low-income countries: An emerging crisis. *Nutrition Reviews*, **52**, 285–98.

Puska, P., Tuomilehto, J., Nissinen, A. *et al.* (1995). *The North Karelia Project. 20 year results and experiences*. University Press, Helsinki.

Rugg-Gunn, A.J. (1993). *Nutrition and dental health*. Oxford University Press, Oxford.

Scholl, T.O. and Johnson, W.G. (2000). Folic acid: Influence on the outcome of pregnancy. *American Journal of Clinical Nutrition*, **71**, 1295S–303S.

SCN (2004). *Fifth report on the world nutrition situation: Nutrition for improved development*. Standing Committee on Nutrition, WHO, Geneva.

Scottish Office Home and Health Department (1993). *The Scottish diet: Report of a working party to the Chief Medical Officer in Scotland*. The Scottish Office, Edinburgh.

Sen, A. (1981). *Poverty and famines: An essay on entitlement and deprivation*. Clarendon Press, Oxford.

Shetty, P. (2006). The Boyd Orr Lecture: Achieving the goal of halving global hunger by 2015. *Proceedings of the Nutrition Society*, **65**, 7–18.

Shetty, P.S. and James, W.P.T. (1994). *Body mass index: An objective measure for the estimation of chronic energy deficiency in adults*. FAO Food and Nutrition Paper, Food and Agricultural Organization, Rome.

Smith, L.C. and Haddad, L. (2000). *Explaining child malnutrition in developing countries: A cross-country analysis*. International Food Policy Research Institute, Washington.

Spurr, G.B. (1987). The effects of chronic energy deficiency on stature, work capacity and productivity. *Chronic energy deficiency: Causes and consequences*. IDECG, Lausanne.

Stoltzfus, R.J., Chwaya, H.M., Tielsch, J.M. *et al.* (1997). Epidemiology of iron deficiency anaemia in Zanzibari schoolchildren: The importance of hookworms. *American Journal of Clinical Nutrition*, **65**, 153–9.

Stolzfus, R.J., Mullany, L., and Black, R.E. (2004). Iron deficiency anemia. In *Comparative quantification of health risks: The global and regional burden of disease attributable to selected major risk factors*(eds. M. Ezzati, A. Rodgers and C.J.L. Murray). World Health Organization, Geneva.

UNICEF (1997). *The state of the world's children 1997*. Oxford University Press, Oxford.

UNICEF (2006). *The state of the world's children 2007: Women and children*. UNICEF, New York.

UNICEF/Micronutrient Initiative (2004). *Vitamin and mineral deficiency: A World progress report*. Micronutrient Initiative, Canada.

Viteri, F.E. (1997). Prevention of iron deficiency. *Prevention of micronutrient deficiencies. Tools for policy-makers and public health workers.* Institute of Medicine. National Academy Press, Washington.

WHO (1982). *Prevention of coronary heart disease.* Technical Report Series. World Health Organization, Geneva.

WHO (1990). *Diet, nutrition and the prevention of chronic disease.* WHO Technical Report Series 797. World Health Organisation, Geneva.

WHO (1995). *Physical status: The use and interpretation of anthropometry.* World Health Organization, Geneva.

WHO (2000). *Obesity: Preventing and managing the global epidemic.* World Health Organization, Geneva.

WHO (2002). *The World Health Report: Reducing risks, promoting healthy life.* World Health Organization, Geneva.

WHO (2004). *Iodine status worldwide.* World Health Organization, Geneva.

WHO (2006). *WHO child growth standards.* World Health Organization, Geneva.

WHO/FAO (2003). *Diet, nutrition and the prevention of chronic diseases.* Technical Report series 916. World Health Organization, Geneva.

WHO/UNICEF/UNU (2001). *Iron deficiency anemia: Assessment, prevention and control.* World Health Organization, Geneva.

World Cancer Research Fund/American Institute for Cancer Research (2007). *Food, nutrition, physical activity and the prevention of cancer: A global perspective.* American Institute for Cancer Research, Washington.

2.7

Infectious diseases

Davidson H. Hamer, Zulfiqar Ahmed Bhutta, and Sherwood L. Gorbach

Introduction

Infectious diseases are a major cause of morbidity, disability, and mortality worldwide. During the last century, substantial gains have been made in public health interventions for the treatment, prevention, and control of infectious diseases. Nevertheless, recent decades have seen a worldwide pandemic of the human immunodeficiency virus (HIV), increasing antimicrobial resistance, and the emergence of many new viral, bacterial, fungal, and parasitic pathogens.

As a result of changes in a variety of different environmental, social, economic, and public health factors, morbidity and mortality due to infectious diseases have declined in industrialized countries during the last 150 years with the result being a gradual transition to chronic diseases including cardiovascular disease, diabetes mellitus, and cancer as major causes of mortality in these countries today. However, in contrast, in less developed countries, infectious diseases continue to contribute substantially to the overall burden of disease.

Detailed information on the definitions of infectious diseases, modes of transmission, and their control are provided in Chapter 12.6, by Robert J. Kim-Farley. An overview of issues related to emerging and re-emerging infections is provided in Chapter 9.17. Similarly, detailed information on diseases caused by prions, sexually transmitted infections, human immunodeficiency virus/acquired immunodeficiency syndrome (HIV/AIDS), tuberculosis, and malaria can be found in Chapters 9.11–9.15. This chapter will review the global burden of common infectious diseases in children and adults, determinants of the high infectious disease burden in resource-poor countries, and important aspects of the clinical manifestations, diagnosis, and treatment of the handful of infectious diseases that account for the major share of morbidity and mortality in children and adults worldwide.

Burden of infectious diseases

At the beginning of the twentieth century, infectious diseases were the leading cause of death throughout the world. At that time, three diseases—pneumonia, diarrhoea, and tuberculosis—were responsible for about 30 per cent of deaths in the United States. During the last century, there has been a decline in infectious diseases mortality in the United States from 797 deaths per 100 000 in 1900 to 36 per 100 000 in 1980. Despite substantial reductions in all-cause mortality due to diarrhoeal disease and tuberculosis, pneumonia and influenza have continued to be major causes of mortality (Armstrong *et al.* 1999). Concurrent with the growth of the AIDS pandemic worldwide, there was a rise in mortality rates among persons aged 25 years and older in developed and less developed areas of the world.

In the late twentieth century, substantial reduction in child mortality occurred in low- and middle-income countries. The fall in the number of child deaths during the period of time from 1960–90 averaged 2.5 per cent per year and the risk of dying in the first 5 years of life halved—a major achievement in child survival. In the period 1990–2001, mortality rates dropped an average of 1.1 per cent annually, mostly after the neonatal period. Most neonatal deaths are unrecorded in formal registration systems and communities with the greatest number of neonatal deaths have the least information related to mortality rates and interventions. Not surprisingly therefore current global burden figures of newborn and young infant deaths are largely estimates. These figures suggest that 10.6 million children under the age of 5 years die annually and, of the 130 million births, 3.8 million die in the first 4 weeks of life—the neonatal period, with some three quarters of neonatal deaths occurring in the first week after birth. In the period 2000–2003, four communicable diseases categories accounted for 54 per cent of childhood deaths; these included pneumonia (19 per cent), diarrhoea (18 per cent), malaria (8 per cent), and neonatal sepsis or pneumonia (10 per cent) (Bryce *et al.* 2005) (Fig. 2.7.1). The distribution of these causes of mortality was similar in World Health Organization (WHO) regions with the exception of malaria, which was concentrated in sub-Saharan Africa.

The Southeast Asian region accounts for the highest number of child deaths, over 3 million, whereas the highest mortality rates are generally seen in sub-Saharan Africa. Annually, sub-Saharan Africa and South Asia share 41 and 34 per cent of child deaths respectively (Table 2.7.1) (Black *et al.* 2003). Only six countries account for half of worldwide deaths and 42 for 90 per cent of child deaths with the predominant causes being pneumonia, diarrhoea, and neonatal disorders, with surprisingly little contribution from malaria and AIDS. In all, 99 per cent of neonatal deaths occur in poor countries (estimated average neonatal mortality rate (NMR) of 33/1000 live births) and the remaining are divided among 39 high-income countries (estimated average NMR of 4/1000 live births) (Table 2.7.2).

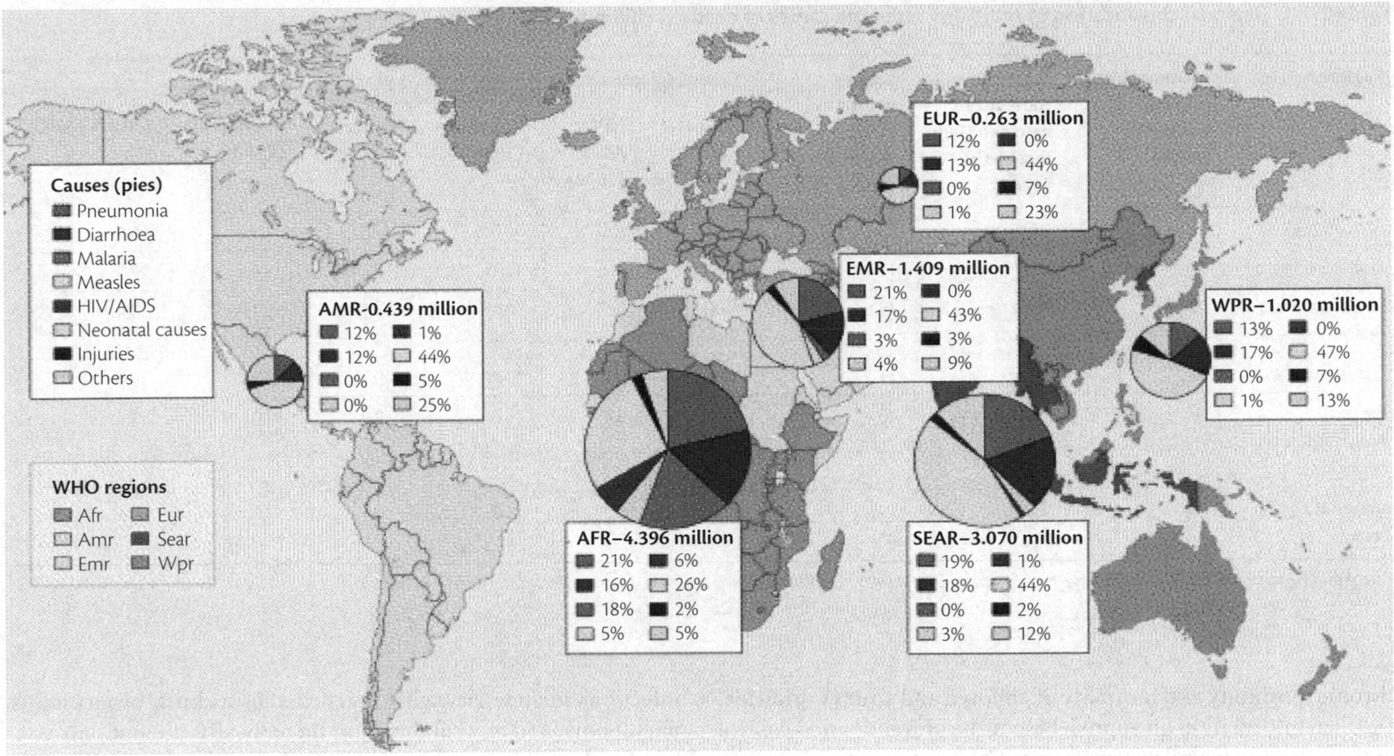

Fig. 2.7.1 Distribution of causes of child mortality worldwide; from: Bryce *et al.* (2005). WHO estimates of the causes of death in children. *The Lancet*, **365**, 1147–52.

As of the end of 2006, the Joint United Nations Programme on HIV/AIDS (UNAIDS) estimated that there were 39.5 million people living with HIV infection and that 4 million new infections occurred during 2006 along with 3 million deaths. The greatest increases in prevalence were in Central Asia and Eastern Europe while sub-Saharan Africa continued to account for nearly two-thirds of cases. In contrast to the continuing growth of the HIV/AIDS pandemic, global growth of tuberculosis slowed in the last few years. By 2004, the WHO estimated that there were 8.9 million new cases worldwide and that the incidence of tuberculosis was stable or declining in five of six WHO regions, the only exception being Africa (Nunn *et al.* 2007). Sadly, tuberculosis is responsible for approximately 10 per cent of HIV-associated deaths of children and adults in sub-Saharan Africa, despite substantial increases in the numbers of HIV-infected people receiving antiretroviral therapy in resource-poor countries.

Lower respiratory tract infections are the leading cause of DALYs worldwide, accounting for 6.4 per cent of the total. HIV/AIDS is third on the list accounting for 6.1 per cent, while diarrhoeal diseases and malaria rank fifth and ninth, accounting for 4.2 and 2.7 per cent of DALYs, respectively. In high-income countries, lower respiratory infections are the fourth leading cause of death. No communicable disease is among the top ten leading causes of DALYs in high-income countries. In contrast, pneumonia, HIV/AIDS, diarrhoea, tuberculosis, and malaria rank among the top ten causes of death and DALYs in low- and middle-income countries.

A number of factors are responsible for the decline in infectious diseases in industrialized nations during the last century. These include improved nutrition, safer food and water supplies, improved hygiene and sanitation, the introduction of antimicrobial agents, and immunizations, all of which resulted in decreased host susceptibility and reductions in disease transmission (Cohen 2000). While there have been substantial reductions in morbidity and mortality due to communicable diseases in the last century, there remain significant gaps in child and adult mortality between rich and poor countries.

Apart from the immediate causes of infections in childhood, a number of determinants contribute to the high burden of infectious diseases in developing countries. These include several distal determinants such as income, social status, and education, which work through an intermediate level of environmental and behavioural risk factors (Fig. 2.7.2). These risk factors, in turn, lead to the proximal causes of death (nearer in time to the terminal event), such as undernutrition, infectious diseases, and injury (Rice *et al.* 2000). The major social determinants affecting the mortality and morbidity of young children include poverty, crowding, poor housing conditions, malnutrition, inequity, lack of education, failure to implement breastfeeding and complementary feeding programmes, the presence of debilitating disease in addition to infections, complications of labour and LBW, inadequate health-related social behaviours and practices, and other social and cultural determinants of health.

Specific disease categories

As described above, a limited number of infectious diseases are responsible for a large proportion of the total global burden of morbidity and mortality, especially in resource-limited areas of the world. The following section will provide an overview of the major types of infectious diseases responsible for the bulk of acute and

Table 2.7.1 Regional classification of mortality rates and causes of death in children under 5 years

Region	<5 mortality rate per 1000 live births (2004)	Infant mortality rate per 1000 live births (2004)	Neonatal mortality rate per 1000 live births (2000)	Cause of death among children under 5 years					
				Neonatal Causes (2000)	HIV/ AIDS (2000)	Diarrhoea (2000)	Malaria (2000)	Pneumonia (2000)	Others (2000)
African region	167	100	43	26.2	6.8	16.6	17.5	21.1	5.6
American region	25	21	12	43.7	1.4	10.1	0.4	11.6	27.9
Southeast Asia region	77	56	38	44.4	0.6	20.1	1.1	18.1	9.9
European region	22	18	11	44.3	0.2	10.2	0.5	13.1	25.4
Eastern Mediterranean region	94	69	40	43.4	0.4	14.6	2.9	19.0	13.5
Western Pacific region	31	25	19	47.0	0.3	12.0	0.4	13.8	18.4

The World Health Report 2006: Working together for health. Geneva, World Health Organization, 2006 (http://www.who.int/whr/2006/annex/en).

chronic morbidity and mortality of children and adults worldwide. Detailed information on approaches for the prevention and control of these diseases is available in Chapter 12.6.

Acute respiratory infections (ARIs)

ARIs are classified as upper or lower respiratory tract infections. Upper respiratory tract infections include the common cold, otitis media, sinusitis, and pharyngitis while lower respiratory tract infections include laryngitis, tracheitis, bronchitis, bronchiolitis, pneumonia, and any combination thereof. ARIs are not only confined to the respiratory tract, but may also have systemic effects due to extension of infection into the bloodstream, the production of microbial toxins, inflammation, and reduced lung function.

ARIs, especially bronchiolitis and pneumonia, are the most common causes of both illness and mortality in children under 5 years with. In adults, pneumonia and influenza are major causes

Table 2.7.2 Global burden of diseases: Deaths and disability adjusted life years (DALYs), 2001

	Low and middle-income		High-income		World	
	Deaths	DALYs (3, 0)[a]	Deaths	DALYs (3, 0)[a]	Deaths	DALYs (3, 0)[a]
Total for all causes (thousands)	48 351	1 386 709	7891	149 161	56 242	1 535 871
Rate per 1000 population	9.3	265.7	8.5	160.6	9.1	249.8
Age-standardized rate per 1000[b]	11.4	281.7	5.0	128.2	10.0	256.5
Selected cause groups	Number in thousands (per cent)					
Communicable diseases[c]	17 613 (36.4)	552 376 (39.8)	552 (7.0)	8561 (5.7)	18 166 (32.3)	560 937 (36.5)
HIV/AIDS	2552 (5.3)	70 796 (5.1)	22 (0.3)	665 (0.4)	2574 (4.6)	71 461 (4.7)
Diarrhoea	1777 (3.7)	58 697 (4.2)	6 (<.1)	444 (0.3)	1783 (3.2)	59 141 (3.9)
Malaria	1207 (2.5)	39 961 (2.9)	0 (0.0)	9 (<0.1)	1208 (2.1)	39 970 (2.6)
Lower respiratory infections	3408 (7.0)	83 606 (6.0)	345 (4.4)	2314 (1.6)	3753 (6.7)	85 920 (5.6)
Perinatal conditions	2489 (5.1)	89 068 (6.4)	32 (0.4)	1408 (0.9)	2522 (4.5)	90 477 (5.9)
Protein-energy malnutrition	241 (0.5)	15 449 (1.1)	9 (0.1)	130 (<0.1)	250 (0.4)	15 578 (1.0)

Notes: Numbers in parentheses indicate percentage of column total. Broad group totals in bold are additive but should not be summed with all other conditions listed in table. *Source*: World Health Organization. Global burden of disease estimates 2001 (www.who.int/healthinfo/bodgbd2001/en/index.html).

[a] DALYs (3, 0) refer to the version of the DALY based on a 3 per cent annual discount rate and uniform age weights.

[b] Age-standardized using the WHO World Standard Population.

[c] Includes only causes responsible for more than 1 per cent of global deaths or DALYs in 2001.

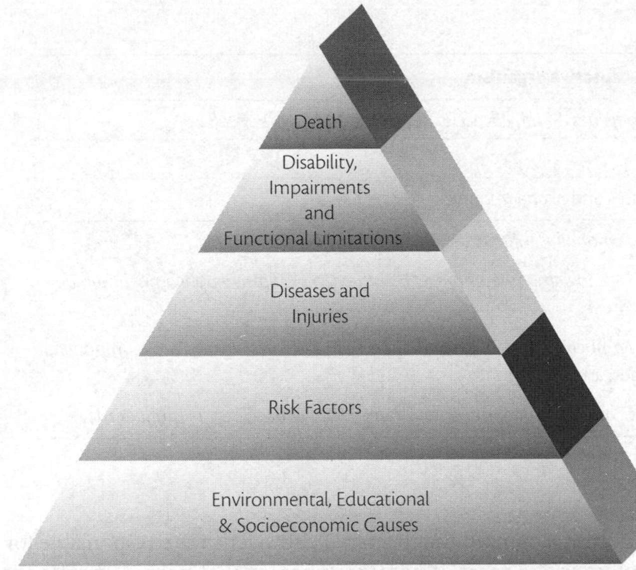

Fig. 2.7.2 Overview of the burden of disease framework. This diagram is intended for a broader scale since environmental factors can be proximate causes of death but injuries can directly cause disability or death.

of morbidity and mortality in developed as well as less-developed nations.

Global and regional epidemiology

The annual incidence in children in Europe and North America is 34–40 cases per 1000, higher than at any other time of life, except perhaps in adults older than 75 or 80 years of age. Pneumonia is the most severe and largest killer of children, causing almost 20 per cent of all child deaths globally. Recent estimates indicate that there are approximately 1.9 million pneumonia deaths annually (95 per cent confidence interval, 1.6–2.2 million), with 75 per cent of all childhood pneumonia cases occurring in just 15 countries.

Most of the deaths from ARIs are due to pneumonia. The annual incidence of pneumonia is estimated at 151 million new cases per year, of which 11–20 million (7–13 per cent) cases are severe enough to require hospitalization. Serious neonatal infections account for 30–50 per cent of neonatal mortality in different regions, and it is difficult to disentangle sepsis and deaths from pneumonia. With the inclusion of neonatal pneumonia, recent estimates indicate that pneumonia is the single largest contributor to child mortality, accounting for almost 28–34 per cent of all under-5 deaths globally. It is also important to note that in contrast to diarrhoeal deaths where mortality rates have reduced dramatically, despite the introduction of a global programme for the control of ARIs almost 15 years ago, there has been little change in overall burden of deaths from pneumonia.

There are about 4 million adults who develop pneumonia in the United States each year, of whom greater than 1 million are hospitalized. In terms of the overall burden of disease, upper and lower ARIs account for a major proportion of outpatient visits, antibiotic prescriptions, and healthcare costs in the United States and Western Europe. Despite gains in the availability and quality of healthcare in industrialized countries, ARIs, especially lower respiratory tract infections, remain a major cause of morbidity and mortality for adults and children. In fact, even today pneumonia and influenza together are the sixth most common cause for death among adults in the United States. Recovery from pneumonia in the elderly takes longer and complications and mortality are also more frequent than in younger populations. Pneumonia is one of the most common causes of hospitalization and decreased activities of daily living among the elderly. Risk factors for death from pneumonia in adults include advanced age, alcohol consumption, leucopenia, bacteraemia, hypoxemia, co-morbid conditions such as diabetes mellitus, congestive heart failure, active malignancies, and immunosuppression, and certain signs and symptoms including hypothermia, hyperthermia, tachypnoea, hypotension, and altered mental status. In addition, post-obstructive pneumonia, aspiration pneumonia, and infections due to *Staphylococcus aureus* and gram-negative bacilli are independently associated with increased mortality risk.

Many factors such as the presence of certain co-morbid medical conditions, use of certain drugs, changes in physiochemical characteristics of the non-specific host defence system such as cilia and mucus of the respiratory tract, malnutrition, and mechanical devices contribute to an increased incidence of pneumonia among the elderly. However, an important predisposing factor to the increased incidence of infections is the age-associated decline in immune responsiveness. Changes in immune response not only decrease resistance to pathogens but also contribute to increased morbidity and mortality due to respiratory infections.

Aetiology

A wide range of different bacterial and viral pathogens are responsible for community-acquired pneumonia in children and adults. Foremost among them is *Streptococcus pneumoniae*, which accounts for up to half of all cases. Other commonly encountered bacterial pathogens include *Haemophilus influenzae*, *Chlamydia pneumoniae*, *Moraxella catarrhalis*, *Legionella pneumophila*, *Mycoplasma pneumoniae*, *S. aureus*, and Gram-negative rods such as *Klebsiella pneumoniae* and *Escherichia coli* (Table 2.7.3). During recent years, the role of viral pathogens in the aetiology of acute lower respiratory tract infections has been increasingly described. While influenza is well recognized as a cause of viral pneumonia, several studies have demonstrated the importance of parainfluenza virus, respiratory syncytial virus (RSV), adenovirus, and human metapneumovirus.

Issues in presentation and diagnosis

Currently, the standard WHO algorithm for ARIs defines non-severe pneumonia as cough or difficult and fast breathing (respiratory rate of 50 breaths per minute or more for children aged 2–11 months; or respiratory rate of 40 breaths per minute or more for children aged 12–59 months) and either documented fever of above 101°F or chest in-drawing. Severe pneumonia has been defined as having cough or difficult breathing, with tachypnoea and in-drawing of the lower chest wall (with or without fast breathing); and very severe pneumonia/disease—cough or difficult breathing with one or more danger signs (central cyanosis, inability to drink, or unusually sleepy). The WHO has defined pneumonia solely on the basis of clinical findings obtained by visual inspection and setting respiratory rate cut-offs. It is recognized that mortality in children due to ARIs could be reduced by one-half if early detection and appropriate treatment could be provided.

In contrast to the simple, clinical definition of pneumonia recommended by the WHO for use in developing countries, pneumonia

Table 2.7.3 Pathogen-specific causes of childhood and adult pneumonia

Age range	Most common causative organism
Neonates (from birth to 30 days after birth)	*Streptococcus pyogenes*, *Staphylococcus aureus*, and *Escherichia coli*
Infants (from 3 weeks to 4 months)	*S. pneumoniae*
Infants older than 4 months and preschool-aged children	Respiratory viruses and *S. pneumoniae*
Children in developing countries	*S. aureus* and *Haemophilus influenzae* including non-typable strains
Adults—outpatient	*S. pneumoniae*, *Mycoplasma pneumoniae*, *H. influenzae*, *Chlamydiophila pneumoniae*, and respiratory viruses
Adults—inpatient	*S. pneumoniae*, *M. pneumoniae*, *C. pneumoniae*, *H. influenzae*, *Legionella pneumophila*, respiratory viruses, and aspiration
Adults—intensive care unit	*S. pneumoniae*, *S. aureus*, *L. pneumophila*, Gram-negative bacilli, and *H. influenzae*

in resource-rich countries is usually based on the presence of characteristic signs and symptoms (e.g. dry or productive cough, tachypnoea, fever, focal findings on respiratory examination), hypoxaemia, and the presence of infiltrates on chest radiograph. In general, the elderly tend to present with fewer or atypical symptoms of pneumonia than younger patients and therefore non-specific features such as fever or mental status change may be indicators of an underlying lower respiratory tract infection.

Microbiological studies can be pursued to support the diagnosis of pneumonia due to specific infectious agents and to facilitate decision making for antibiotic management. While broad spectrum empirical antimicrobial coverage is recommended in various guidelines, there is a potential risk for clinical failure and increased mortality if inappropriate antibiotic therapy is initiated. If available and adequate quality specimens can be obtained, blood cultures and sputum gram stain and culture should be performed. Rapid diagnostic tests may be useful when specific diagnoses are being considered such as RSV, influenza, or *L. pneumophila*.

Clinical approaches for the management of childhood pneumonia are significantly hampered by the lack of a gold standard, as classic microbiological methods have poor sensitivity and current algorithms lack sufficient specificity. It is therefore likely that community strategies for the recognition and management of pneumonia by ancillary health workers that rely on simple clinical criteria, other than auscultation, will overdiagnose bacterial pneumonia. There are legitimate concerns that widespread use of first-line antibiotics for all acute respiratory infections will lead to loss of effectiveness.

Evidence-based interventions

Only in the early 1980s, long after immunization and diarrhoea control programmes were launched, did the international community become aware of the epidemiological magnitude of pneumonia in children. This need for action led the WHO and UNICEF to decide that reduction of mortality from pneumonia should be the main objective of the initial ARI programme. Only about half of children with pneumonia receive appropriate medical care, and, according to limited data from the early 1990s, less than 20 per cent of children with pneumonia received antibiotics. Since early microbiological studies of lung aspirates taken from hospitalized, untreated children with pneumonia in developing countries showed that bacteria were present in more than 50 per cent of cases and it was recognized that bacterial pathogens were responsible for the most severe cases, it became apparent that prompt treatment with a full course of effective antibiotics could be life-saving.

Antibiotic treatment of pneumonia

Although recommendations for antibiotic therapy for pneumonia are based on aetiological diagnosis, identification of the causative organism in routine clinical care is very difficult and empirical antibiotic therapy is often instituted. Guidelines for the treatment of pneumonia in immunocompetent adults in industrialized nations generally recommend a macrolide or doxycycline for outpatients; an advanced macrolide such as azithromycin or clarithromycin plus a beta-lactam or a respiratory fluoroquinolone alone for less acutely ill inpatients; and a beta-lactam plus either an advanced macrolide or respiratory fluoroquinolone for adults requiring intensive care (Mandell *et al.* 2007). The preferred treatment options must be modified for certain high-risk groups and in patients who have had recent antimicrobial therapy.

Since *S. pneumoniae* and *H. influenzae* are the most common causes of childhood pneumonia in developing countries, the WHO recommends using oral cotrimoxazole or amoxicillin as first-line drugs for the treatment of non-severe pneumonia at first level health facilities. Cloxacillin or other anti-staphylococcal antibiotics should be available to treat cases in which the initial combination fails within 48 h. Young infants with signs of pneumonia, sepsis, or meningitis should be referred to hospital for parenteral treatment. Similarly children with pneumonia and malnutrition should be referred to hospital for differential diagnosis of tuberculosis and for parenteral antimicrobial treatment for bacterial pneumonia.

The various modalities for antibiotic treatment in children according to disease severity are shown in Table 2.7.4. However, the emergence of resistance to first-line antimicrobial drugs recommended for home treatment of non-severe pneumonia has been associated with treatment failure rates as high as 22 per cent. Recent data on the failure of standard antimicrobial treatment with parenteral penicillin or amoxicillin in 24 per cent of cases for severe pneumonia among HIV-infected children in Africa are even more alarming.

The current WHO treatment guidelines for ARIs were designed before the rise of HIV infection in sub-Saharan Africa, and they do not include empiric treatment for *Pneumocystis carinii* pneumonia. Daily administration of cotrimoxazole is advocated since it reduces

Table 2.7.4 Treatment of paediatric pneumonia according to disease severity

Signs/symptoms	Classification	Treatment
Fast breathing: ≥60 breaths/min in child aged <2 months ≥50 breaths/min in child aged 2–11 months ≥40 breaths/min in child aged 1–5 years	Pneumonia	Home care
		Give appropriate antibiotics for 5 days
Definite crackles on auscultations		Soothe the throat and relieve the cough with a safe remedy
		Advise the mother when to return immediately
		Follow up in 2 days
Signs of pneumonia plus chest wall in-drawing	Severe pneumonia	Admit to hospital
		Give recommended antibiotics
		Manage airway
		Treat high fever if present
Signs of severe pneumonia plus central cyanosis, severe respiratory distress, and inability to drink	Very severe pneumonia	Admit to hospital
		Give the recommended antibiotics
		Give oxygen
		Manage airway
		Antipyretics

deaths from opportunistic infections in symptomatic HIV-infected children, including pneumonia caused by *P. carinii*. A multi-centre randomized control trial, by the APPIS Group, showed that standard empiric therapy for severe pneumonia with injectable penicillin or oral amoxicillin in severe pneumonia in infants is inadequate where HIV prevalence is high (Addo-yabo *et al.* 2004). The benefits of these guidelines would be enhanced if they could also be applied (with modification) throughout areas with high rates of HIV infection and where the pneumonia burden is high, even in HIV-negative children.

Integrated management of childhood infections (IMCI)

In the mid-1980s, WHO initiated a control programme for ARIs that focused on cases managed by health workers. The current case management of ARIs has been incorporated into the global IMCI which train health workers to recognize fast breathing, lower chest wall in-drawing, or danger signs in children with respiratory symptoms (such as cyanosis or inability to drink).

Preventive measures

Poverty, overcrowding, air pollution, malnutrition, harmful traditional practices, and delayed and inappropriate case management are important underlying determinants for high ARI case fatality rates. Preventive strategies for pneumonia include immunizing children with the pneumococcal, measles, and *H. influenzae* type b (Hib) vaccines, hand washing, reduction of the incidence of LBW, ensuring warmth after birth and appropriate feeding, promoting adequate nutrition (including exclusive breastfeeding and zinc intake), and reducing indoor air pollution (Bhutta 2007; WHO Collaborative Group on Breastfeeding 2000).

Three vaccines have the potential to substantially reduce deaths in children <5 years of age—(the Hib, measles, and pneumococcal vaccines). Two kinds of vaccines are currently available against pneumococci: A 23-valent polysaccharide vaccine (23-PSV), which is more appropriate for adults than children, and a 7-valent protein-conjugated polysaccharide vaccine (7-PCV). The rate of invasive pneumococcal disease (IPD) has decreased among both immunized children and non-immunized adults since the introduction of heptavalent pneumococcal conjugate vaccine (PCV7) for use in infants in the United States in 2000. Moreover, newer versions of the pneumococcal conjugate vaccine might become available as early as 2008, and have the potential to significantly reduce pneumonia deaths in developing countries.

Controlled trials of hand washing promotion in child-care centres in developed countries have reported significant reduction (12–32 per cent) in rates of upper respiratory-tract infections. A community-based cluster randomized trial of hand washing promotion from Pakistan also reported that frequent hand washing (with or without soap) led to a 50 per cent reduction in pneumonia incidence and a 36 per cent lower incidence of impetigo.

About 3 billion people still rely on solid fuels, 2.4 billion on biomass, and the rest on coal, mostly in China. Globally, there is marked regional variation in solid fuel use in relation to poverty with use rates of <20 per cent in Europe and Central Asia and >80 per cent in sub-Saharan Africa and South Asia, intricately linking to poverty. More than half of all the deaths and 83 per cent of DALYs lost attributable to solid fuel use occur as a result of lower respiratory tract infection (pneumonia) in children under 5 years of age and a systematic review of the evidence for the impact of indoor air pollution on a wide range of health outcomes including pneumonia indicates substantial benefits on pneumonia prevention.

Previously, a meta-analysis of trials of daily preventive zinc supplementation showed a significant impact on pneumonia incidence (Zinc Investigators' Collaborative Group 1999). A recent update of this meta-analysis reaffirms the impact on reduction in the risk of respiratory tract infections (by 8 per cent, respectively) but not on duration of disease (Aggarwal 2007).

Public health implications

Despite the introduction of a global programme for the control of ARIs almost 15 years ago, there has been little change in overall burden of deaths from pneumonia. The bulk of deaths from childhood pneumonia disproportionately affect the poor who have higher exposure rates to risk factors for developing ARIs, such as overcrowding, poor environmental conditions, malnutrition, and also limited access to curative health services. The importance of reaching the poor with pneumonia in community settings must be underscored. Such strategies involve recognizing and ambulatory management of pneumonia in community settings through community health workers, assuring transportation and access to facilities for severe pneumonia and availability of antibiotics.

Neonatal sepsis

Sepsis and meningitis are significant causes of morbidity and mortality in newborns, particularly in preterm, LBW infants. Serious infections among newborns are estimated to cause 30–40 per cent of neonatal deaths, especially in rural populations and are associated with several risk factors.

Neonatal sepsis may be defined using clinical criteria (Table 2.7.5) and/or microbiological testing, by positive blood and/or cerebrospinal fluid (CSF) cultures. It may also be classified according to the time of onset of the disease: Early onset (EOS) and late onset (LOS). Meningitis can occur as a part of sepsis in both the early and late onset time periods or as focal infection with late-onset disease. The distinction has clinical relevance, as EOS disease is mainly due to bacteria acquired before and during delivery, and LOS disease to bacteria acquired after delivery (nosocomial or community sources). In the literature, however, there is little consensus as to what age limits apply, with EOS ranging from 48 h to 6 days after delivery.

Global and regional epidemiology

Severe bacterial infections are responsible for 460 000 deaths annually, apart from 300 000 fatalities from tetanus, many of which are due to neonatal tetanus. The reported incidence of neonatal sepsis varies from 7.1 to 38 per 1000 live births in Asia, from 6.5 to 23 per 1000 live births in Africa, and from 3.5 to 8.9 per 1000 live births in South America and the Caribbean, 6–9 per 1000 in the United States and Australia. The incidence of neonatal meningitis is 0.1–0.4/1000 live births and is higher in developing countries. Despite major advancement in neonatal care, overall case-fatality rates from sepsis range from 2 to as high as 50 per cent.

Unfortunately, hospitals in developing countries are also hot beds of infection transmission, especially multi-drug-resistant nosocomial infections. Reported rates of neonatal sepsis vary from 6.5 to 38 per 1000 live hospital-born babies and the rates of bloodstream infection range from 1.7 to 33 per 1000 live births, with rates in Africa clustering around 20 and in South Asia around 15 per 1000 live births. Factors responsible for hospital-acquired neonatal sepsis include lack of aseptic technique for procedures, inadequate hand hygiene and glove use, deficient sterilization and disinfection practices, overuse of invasive devices, re-use of disposable supplies without adequate sterilization, re-use of single-use vials, overcrowded and understaffed labour and delivery rooms, unhygienic bathing and skin care, contaminated bottle feedings, inappropriate and prolonged use of antibiotics, and lack of effective infection control practices.

Table 2.7.5 World Health Organization clinical criteria for diagnosis of neonatal sepsis and meningitis*

Sepsis	Meningitis
Symptoms	*General signs*
Convulsions	Drowsiness
Inability to feed	Reduced feeding
Unconsciousness	Unconsciousness
Lethargy	Lethargy
Fever (>37.7°C or feels hot)	High-pitched cry
Hypothermia (<35.5°C or feels cold)	Apnea
Signs	*Specific signs*
Severe chest in-drawing	Convulsions
Reduced movement	Bulging fontanelle
Crepitations	
Cyanosis	

**The more symptoms a neonate has, the higher the probability of the disease.*

Aetiology

In general, Gram-negative pathogens are responsible for a substantial proportion of EOS. In contrast to industrialized countries where group B streptococci are common causes of neonatal sepsis, *Klebsiella pneumoniae* is an important aetiology in developing countries. LOS is most commonly due to *E. coli*, *S. aureus*, *S. pyogenes*, *S. pneumoniae*, and *Salmonella* spp. The organisms causing neonatal sepsis and meningitis in developing and developed countries are listed in Table 2.7.6.

Evidence-based interventions to address neonatal infections

Child survival and safe motherhood strategies have yet to adequately address mortality in the neonatal period. The fourth Millenium Development Goal (MDG-4) commits the international community to reducing mortality in children aged <5 years by two-thirds from 1990 base figures by 2015. Real progress in saving newborns will depend upon provision of a good mix of preventive and therapeutic services.

Medical treatment

Reaching and treating sick newborn infants promptly is critical to survival. Normally, a combination of ampicillin and gentamicin is used by health staff for suspected cases of neonatal sepsis (Table 2.7.7). However, increasing antibiotic resistance among common organisms causing neonatal sepsis in both community and hospital settings presents a challenge to the selection of appropriate antibiotics. Case management of neonatal infections is mainly provided through child-health services, both in facilities and through family-community care. Scaling up of emergency

Table 2.7.6 Major bacterial causes of neonatal sepsis and meningitis

Neonatal sepsis		Neonatal meningitis	
Developing countries	**Developed countries**	**Developing countries**	**Developed countries**
Gram-negative bacilli (more common)	Gram-negative bacilli	Gram-negative bacilli (more common in neonates <1 week old)	Gram-negative bacilli
Klebsiella spp.	*Escherichia coli* (more common)	*Klebsiella* spp.	*E. coli*
E. coli		*E. coli*	
Pseudomonas aeruginosa		*Serratia marscesens*	
Salmonella spp.		*P. aeruginosa*	
		Salmonella spp.	
Gram-positive cocci (less common)	Gram-positive cocci	Gram-positive organisms	Gram-positive organisms
Staphylococcus aureus	*Streptococcus agalactiae* (Group B streptococci) (GBS) (more common)	*Listeria monocytogenes*	GBS
Coagulase-negative staphylococci (CONS)	CONS	*Streptococcus pneumoniae* (more common in neonates <1 week old)	*S. pneumoniae*
S. pneumoniae	*S. aureus*	CONS	*L. monocytogenes*
S. pyogenes		*S. aureus*	

obstetric care and sick neonatal care can be combined. Guidelines for integrated management of pregnancy and childbirth identify opportunities for assimilating maternal and neonatal care. Similarly Integrated Management of Childhood Illness (IMCI) has been widely implemented as the main approach for addressing child health in health systems. However, IMCI management guidelines do not as yet include the first week of life—the period of highest risk for child mortality, and also rely on the sick child being brought to a health facility. The recent modification of IMCI to include the neonatal period (IMNCI) and expand to community settings has now been included as a public health strategy in many countries including India. The ideal strategy would be to provide a linked

Table 2.7.7 Antimicrobial therapy of neonatal meningitis and sepsis

Patient group	Likely aetiology	Antimicrobial choice	
		Developed countries	**Developing countries**
Sepsis			
Immunocompetent children	Developed countries Group B streptococci *E. coli* Developing countries *Klebsiella* spp. *Pseudomonas* spp. *Salmonella* spp.	Ampicillin or penicillin plus an aminoglycoside	Ampicillin or penicillin plus gentamicin Or co-trimoxazole plus gentamicin
Meningitis			
Immunocompetent children (age <3 months)	Developed countries Group B streptococci *E. coli* *L. monocytogenes** Developing countries *S. pneumoniae* *E. coli*	Ampicillin plus ceftriaxone or cefotaxime	Ampicillin plus gentamicin
Immunodeficient	Gram-negative bacilli *L. monocytogenes*	Ampicillin plus ceftazidime	

strategy of care in community settings with referral to facilities in case of need.

Following the demonstration of significant reduction in neonatal mortality with the use of oral co-trimoxazole and injectable gentamicin by community health workers, this strategy could be employed in circumstances where referral is difficult. Currently in some health systems, outreach health workers, community nutrition, and child development workers are being trained to visit all mothers and neonates at home two to three times within the first 10 days, starting soon after birth, to provide home-based preventive care/health promotion and to detect neonates with sickness requiring referral. Extra contacts are proposed for LBW babies. With slight modifications, these visits can also be used to provide postpartum care to the mother as well.

Preventive measures

Preventive interventions need to bridge the continuum of care from pregnancy, through childbirth and the neonatal period, and beyond. Lack of positive health-related behaviour, education, and poverty are underlying causes of many neonatal deaths, either through increasing the prevalence of risk factors such as maternal infection or by reducing access to effective care.

Attempts to reduce the proportion of LBW births at the population level, have had limited success. Many deaths in preterm babies and in those born at term with LBW can be prevented with extra attention to warmth, feeding, and prevention or early treatment of infections. In developing countries, 90 per cent of mothers deliver babies at home without skilled health professional present. Simple low-cost interventions, notably tetanus toxoid vaccination, exclusive breastfeeding, counselling for birth preparedness, breastfeeding promotion through peer counsellors and women's groups, have been shown to reduce newborn morbidity and mortality (Darmstadt *et al.* 2005). Postnatally, kangaroo mother care for LBW infants, hand washing and decreased congestion in facilities, attention to environmental hygiene and sterilization, antibiotics for neonatal infections, are additional health system measures. Alcohol-based antiseptics for hand hygiene are an appealing innovation because of their efficacy in reducing hand contamination and their ease of use, especially when sinks and supplies for hand-washing are limited. Creation of a 'step-down' neonatal care unit for very LBW babies with mothers providing primary care also led to early discharge and reduction in hospital-acquired infection rates in another nursery in Pakistan. These interventions can be delivered through facility-based services, population outreach, and family-community strategies.

Early initiation of breastfeeding affects neonatal health outcomes through several mechanisms. Mothers who suckle their offspring shortly after birth have a greater chance of successfully establishing and sustaining breastfeeding throughout infancy, and also provide a variety of immune and non-immune components that accelerate intestinal maturation, resistance to infection, and epithelial recovery from infection. Prelacteal feeding with non-human milk antigens may disrupt normal physiologic gut priming. Although WHO currently recommends dry cord care for newborns, application of antiseptics such as chlorhexidine has been shown to be effective against both gram positive and gram negative bacteria and, in community studies, to reduce rates of cord infection and sepsis in newborns. A closely related issue is the need for general skin care. A randomized controlled trial of topical application of sunflower seed oil to preterm infants in an Egyptian NICU showed that treated infants had substantially improved skin condition and half the risk of late-onset infection.

At least two doses of tetanus toxoid should be given during pregnancy so that protective antibodies can be transferred to the foetus, to protect it from neonatal tetanus. Women with a history of prolonged rupture of membranes, especially if preterm, should be given prophylactic antibiotics. This approach improves neonatal outcome by increasing the latency of pregnancy. Maternal antibiotic therapy in this situation is effective in prolonging pregnancy and reducing maternal and neonatal infection-related morbidities. A multi-country study (ORACLE I) from urban centres suggested that administration of erythromycin to women with preterm premature rupture of membranes (PPROM) was associated with significant health benefits for the newborn. A domiciliary cadre of trained birth attendants potentially can be trained to recognize PPROM and provide referral and, possibly, initial antimicrobial therapy.

An important aspect of prevention of neonatal infection in developed countries relates to group B streptococcal (GBS) disease. The joint guidelines developed and implemented in the United States have led to a significant reduction in the burden of disease. The majority of newborns born to mothers with risk of GBS colonization undergo a full diagnostic evaluation and empiric therapy.

In recent years, the importance of hospital-acquired infections in newborn infants, frequently with multi-resistant organisms has been recognized. It is imperative that preventive strategies such as hand washing, reducing overcrowding and congestion, and environmental control are strictly enforced.

Meningitis in neonates, children, and adults

Acute meningitis is a potentially fatal infection caused by several microorganisms including bacteria, viruses, parasites, and fungi (Sáez-Llorens & McCracken 2003). In addition, meningitis is associated with a risk of chronic morbidity and developmental disability. Although the exact incidence of meningitis in developing countries is uncertain, case fatality rates range from 10 to 30 per cent. Even if effective treatment is provided, between 20 and 50 per cent of survivors still develop neurological sequelae. Successful outcome of neonatal meningitis relates to several factors including age, time, and clinical stability before effective antibiotic treatment, species of microorganism, number of bacteria or quantity of active bacterial products in the CSF at the time of diagnosis, intensity of the host's inflammatory response, and time elapsed to sterilize CSF cultures. The highest rates of mortality and morbidity occur following meningitis in the neonatal period.

Aetiology

The three most common bacterial pathogens, *S. pneumoniae*, *H. influenzae*, and *N. meningitidis*, account for more than 80 per cent of cases of bacterial meningitis in the United States overall, although *Listeria monocytogenes* is a greater problem for the elderly, immunocompromised, and pregnant women (Table 2.7.8). There is a relative paucity of microbiological information from developing countries, but beyond the neonatal period, the main agents of meningitis include Hib, *S. pneumoniae*, and *Neisseria meningitidis* with reported CFRs of 7.7, 10, and 3.5 per cent, respectively. Table 2.7.9 shows the common bacteria causing meningitis in developing and developed countries.

Table 2.7.8 Aetiology and treatment of bacterial meningitis

Patient group	Common organisms	Antimicrobial therapy
Immunocompetent children (age ≥3 months–18 years)	*H. influenzae* *S. pneumoniae* *N. meningitidis*	Developing countries: Ampicillin plus chloramphenicol Developed countries: Cefotaxime or ceftriaxone*
Immunodeficient, pregnant, and elderly (>50 years)	*L. monocytogenes* *S. pneumoniae* *N. meningitides* Aerobic Gram-negative bacilli	Ampicillin plus ceftazidime
Neurosurgical problems and head trauma	*S. aureus* *S. pneumoniae*	Vancomycin + third-generation cephalosporin

*For resistant *S. pneumoniae*, the American Academy of Pediatrics recommends vancomycin plus cefotaxime or ceftriaxone as empiric therapy.

Issues in presentation and diagnosis

The clinical features that may help in diagnosing meningitis are summarized in Table 2.7.10. In general, clinicians should have a low threshold for investigating and excluding meningitis in children as features may be non-specific. The clinical diagnosis can be confirmed by lumbar puncture and the examination of CSF. The CSF will have a cloudy appearance, elevated protein, increased leucocyte counts with a predominance of neutrophils, and the presence of pathogens on gram stain and/or culture provide a definitive diagnosis of bacterial meningitis. The use of latex agglutination or the *S. pneumoniae* C-polysaccharide antigen test (Binax NOW) may serve to confirm the diagnosis, especially if the child has been pre-treated with antibiotics (Saha *et al.*). A bacterial meningitis score has been shown to have an excellent negative predictive value for the presence of bacterial meningitis. If patients do not have one of the following factors—positive CSF Gram stain, CSF absolute neutrophil count ≥1000 cells/μl, CSF protein ≥80 mg/dl, peripheral blood absolute neutrophil count ≥10 000 cells/μl, or history of seizure before or at the time of presentation, they are very unlikely to have bacterial meningitis (negative predictive value = 99.9 per cent) (Nigrovic *et al.* 2007).

Medical treatment

The mainstay of treatment is prompt antibiotic therapy for suspected bacterial meningitis. Antibiotics need to be started before the results of CSF culture and sensitivity are available. This requires selection of an appropriate antibiotic, known to be effective against the common bacterial pathogens prevalent locally. An increasing number of β-lactamase-producing strains of Hib are resistant to ampicillin, and a smaller number of chloramphenicol acetyltransferase-producing strains are resistant to chloramphenicol. Additionally, the proportion of CSF isolates of *S. pneumoniae* that is non-susceptible to penicillin, ceftriaxone, and cefotaxime has also increased. Currently, the drugs for suspected or confirmed bacterial meningitis include cefotaxime (or ceftriaxone) alone or with ampicillin (preferred). If this is not available, then ampicillin + either gentamicin or chloramphenicol may be used. If sepsis is suspected, then cases should be treated with ampicillin or penicillin plus an aminoglycoside, until meningitis is confirmed. Antimicrobial therapy is described further in Table 2.7.8.

Table 2.7.9 Comparison of bacterial meningitis aetiology in children in the developing and developed world (prior to the widespread introduction of the Hib vaccine)

	Developing countries	Developed countries
H. influenzae	30%	65%
S. pneumoniae	23%	13%
N. meningitidis	28%	18%
Other organisms	19%	4%

Very early parenteral administration of corticosteroids (before or with initiation of antibiotics) significantly reduces severe adverse outcomes and case fatality rates. Similarly, there is evidence to suggest that restriction of fluids in the first 48 h may improve outcomes. While a meta-analysis of randomized, controlled trials

Table 2.7.10 Signs and symptoms of pediatric meningitis

Symptoms or presenting history	Signs
Vomiting	Stiff neck
Inability to feed and drink	Repeated convulsions
A headache or pain in back of neck	Fontanelle bulging
Convulsions	Petechiae or purpura
Irritability	Irritability
History of recent head trauma	Lethargy Evidence of head trauma
Signs of raised intracranial pressure	
Unequal pupils	
Rigid posture or posturing	
Focal paralysis in any limbs or trunk	
Irregular breathing	

has shown the benefit of steroids in all-cause bacterial meningitis, predominantly Hib meningitis, a recent study restricted to their use in pneumococcal meningitis found no significant benefits. However, there was a significantly lower rate of hearing loss in the treatment group at 3 months post-discharge. A recent Cochrane systematic review found that corticosteroids protect against severe hearing loss and neurological sequelae, and reduce mortality among adults with community-acquired bacterial meningitis in high-income countries (van de Beek *et al.* 2007). While this review found evidence of a benefit for children from resource-rich countries, there was no beneficial effect of corticosteroids for children in low-income countries.

Preventive measures

Although poverty, malnutrition, overcrowding are important risk factors for disease, delayed and inappropriate case management is a common determinant of adverse outcomes, the development of effective vaccines has been a major factor in the reduction of the burden of meningitis in the developed world. These include the Hib, pneumococcal conjugate, and meningococcal vaccines.

Haemophilus influenzae type b (Hib) vaccine

Currently three Hib conjugate vaccines are available for use in infants and young children with comparable efficacy (protective efficacy of Hib against development of laboratory confirmed invasive disease >90 per cent). All industrialized countries now include Hib vaccine in their national immunization programmes, resulting in the virtual elimination of invasive Hib disease. There is comparable impressive evidence of benefit from several developing countries following introduction of Hib vaccine and many countries are beginning to include Hib vaccine in their repertoire with GAVI support.

Pneumococcal vaccine

The older 23-valent pneumococcal polysaccharide vaccine is unsuitable for use in young children. The recent development of the 7-valent protein-conjugate polysaccharide vaccine, 9-valent and 11-valent vaccines is a major advance in the control of invasive pneumococcal disease. In the United States, the 7-PCV was included in routine vaccinations of infants and children under 2 years in 2000 and by 2001 the incidence of all invasive pneumococcal disease in this age group had declined by 69 per cent. Currently several Latin American countries are beginning to introduce pneumococcal conjugate vaccine as part of their EPI programmes.

Meningococcal vaccine

Meningococcal polysaccharide vaccine is available for A, C, W-135, and Y strains. This quadrivalent vaccine is being introduced in several developed countries as part of routine vaccine schedules, especially for adolescents who will be rooming in crowded dormitories while attending university. In many developed countries this vaccine has been replaced by the quadrivalent meningococcal conjugate vaccine, which is more immunogenic and, because it induces memory cells, is likely to lead to a longer lasting protective immune response.

Gastrointestinal tract infections

Diarrhoea, the most common manifestation of intestinal tract infections, is a leading cause of preventable death in most developing countries where its greatest impact is seen in infants and children. Infectious diarrhoea may be accompanied by numerous complications (Table 2.7.11). The financial burden associated with medical care and lost productivity due to infectious diarrhoea amounts to more than US$20 billion a year in the United States alone.

Invasive diarrhoea refers to diarrhoea caused by bacterial pathogens that invade the bowel mucosa, causing inflammation and tissue damage and may cause blood in stools (bloody diarrhoea). Invasive diarrhoea accounts for approximately 10 per cent of diarrhoeal episodes in children under 5 years of age and approximately 15 per cent of diarrhoea-associated deaths in this age group worldwide. Although less frequent, bloody diarrhoea generally lasts longer, is associated with higher risk of complications and case fatality rates, and is more likely to adversely affect a child's growth.

Global and regional epidemiology

The aetiology and severity of gastrointestinal infections are determined by several epidemiological factors. Young children and the elderly are at greatest risk for more severe disease and complications. The presence of underlying medical conditions, especially those that compromise immunity, greatly enhances the risk of acquiring an infection and its ultimate severity. Poor sanitation,

Table 2.7.11 Complications of gastrointestinal infections

Complication	Causative pathogens
Dehydration	*Vibrio cholerae, Cryptosporidium parvum* (especially in immunocompromised hosts), enterotoxigenic *Escherichia coli* (ETEC), rotavirus
Severe vomiting	Staphylococcal food poisoning, norovirus, rotavirus
Haemorrhagic colitis	*Campylobacter jejuni*, enterohemorrhagic *E. coli* (EHEC), *Salmonella, Shigella, V. parahaemolyticus*
Toxic megacolon, intestinal perforation	EHEC, *Shigella, C. jejuni* (rare), *Clostridium difficile* (rare), *Salmonella* (rare), *Yersinia* (rare)
Haemolytic uremic syndrome (HUS), thrombotic thrombocytopenic purpura (TTP)	EHEC, *Shigella, C. jejuni* (rare)
Reactive arthritis	*C. jejuni, Shigella, Salmonella, Yersinia*
Malabsorption/malnutrition	*Cyclospora cayetanensis, Giardia lamblia, C. parvum* (especially immunocompromised hosts)
Distant metastatic infection	*Salmonella, C. jejuni* (rare), *Yersinia* (rare)
Guillain–Barré syndrome	*C. jejuni* (rare)

inadequate water supplies, and increasing globalization of food transport systems all predispose to the development of large epidemics of food- and water-borne outbreaks of gastrointestinal disease. Seasonal or cyclic weather variations also influence the epidemiology of diarrhoeal disease and food poisoning.

Several recent reviews have evaluated diarrhoea burden and mortality rates. A review carried out two decades ago estimated that 4.6 million children died annually from diarrhoea. Kosek *et al.* have recently updated these estimates by reviewing 60 studies of diarrhoea morbidity and mortality published between 1990 and 2000 (Kosek *et al.* 2003). They concluded that diarrhoea accounts for 21 per cent of all deaths at <5 years of age and causes 2.5 million deaths per year, although morbidity rates remain relatively unchanged. Despite the different methods and sources of information, each successive review of the diarrhoea burden over the past three decades has demonstrated declining mortality but relatively stable morbidity rates. Persistent high rates of diarrhoea morbidity may have significant long-term effects on linear growth and physical and cognitive function in children. Figure 2.7.3 shows specific trends for diarrhoea in the world from 1954–2000.

Aetiology

Common aetiologies of non-inflammatory diarrhoea include enterotoxigenic *E. coli* (ETEC) and other strains such as enteroaggregative (EAEC), diffusely adhering, and enteropathogenic *E. coli*, *Vibrio cholerae*; non-01 choleras such as *V. vulnificus*; parasites including *Giardia lamblia*, *Cryptosporidium parvum*, and microsporidia; and several different virus species including rotavirus, noroviruses, and astroviruses (Hamer and Gorbach, in press). Acute inflammatory diarrhoea is the result of infection with bacterial enteropathogens such as *Shigella*, *Campylobacter*, *Salmonella* spp., enterohaemorrhagic *E. coli* (EHEC), *V. parahaemolyticus*, and *Clostridium difficile*. Among the parasites, *Entamoeba histolytica* is the most common cause of dysenteric illness although *Balantidium coli*, *Schistosoma mansoni*, *S. japonicum*, *Trichuris trichiura*, hookworms, and *Trichinella spiralis* can all cause bloody, mucoid diarrhoea.

Infectious microorganisms in contaminated food and drink are the main source of travellers' diarrhoea. High-risk foods include uncooked vegetables, salsa, meat, and seafood. Tap water, ice, unpasteurized milk and dairy products, salads, and unpeeled fruits are also associated with an increased risk. Although many different pathogens may be responsible, the leading culprits are various forms of *E. coli*, particularly ETEC and EAEC. *C. jejuni* is encountered in a significant proportion of cases, particularly during cooler seasons. Viruses, *Shigella*, *Salmonella*, *Giardia*, *Cryptosporidium*, and *Cyclospora* spp. are responsible for a minority of travellers' diarrhoea cases.

Food poisoning is most commonly caused by the consumption of food contaminated with bacteria or bacterial toxins. Food poisoning can also be due to parasites (for example, trichinosis), viruses (e.g. hepatitis A), and other toxins (e.g. *Amanita* mushrooms). The most well-recognized causes of bacterial food poisoning are the following: *Clostridium perfringens*, *S. aureus*, *Vibrio* spp. (including *V. cholerae* and *V. parahaemolyticus*), *Bacillus cereus*, *Salmonella* spp., *C. botulinum*, *Shigella* spp., toxigenic *E. coli* (ETEC and EHEC), and certain species of *Campylobacter*, *Yersinia*, *Listeria*, and *Aeromonas*.

Issues in presentation and diagnosis

Gastrointestinal infections usually result in three principal syndromes: Non-inflammatory diarrhoea, inflammatory diarrhoea, and systemic disease. Non-inflammatory diarrhoea primarily involves the small intestine, whereas inflammatory diarrhoea predominantly affects the colon. The location of infection influences the clinical characteristics and certain diagnostic features of the diarrhoeal disease (Table 2.7.12). Thus, organisms that target the small intestine tend to produce watery, potentially dehydrating diarrhoea, while those infecting the large intestine cause bloody mucoid diarrhoea associated with tenesmus.

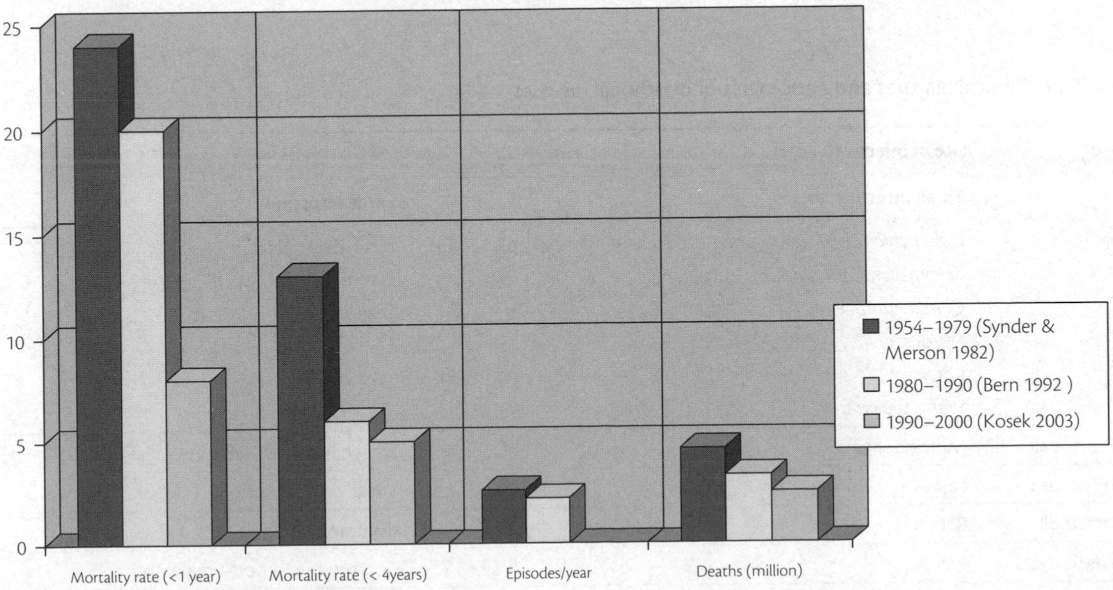

Fig. 2.7.3 Trends in worldwide diarrhoea mortality and morbidity rates.

Acute watery diarrhoea can be rapidly dehydrating, with stool losses of 250 ml/kg/day or more, a quantity that quickly exceeds total plasma and interstitial fluid volumes, and is incompatible with life unless aggressive fluid therapy can be provided. Such dramatic dehydration is usually due to rotavirus, ETEC, or *V. cholerae*, and it is most dangerous in the very young.

Persistent diarrhoea is defined as diarrhoea lasting 14 days or longer, is manifested by malabsorption, nutrient losses, and wasting, and is typically associated with malnutrition. Although persistent diarrhoea accounts for 8–20 per cent of diarrhoea episodes, it is associated with a disproportionately increased risk of death. Persistent diarrhoea more commonly follows an episode of bloody diarrhoea and is associated with a 10-fold higher risk of mortality. HIV infection is another risk factor for persistent diarrhoea in both adults and children.

Inflammatory diarrhoea is a manifestation of invasive intestinal infection that is associated with intestinal damage and nutritional deterioration, often with systemic manifestations including fever. Although clinicians often use the term bloody diarrhoea interchangeably with dysentery, the latter is a syndrome consisting of the frequent passage of characteristic, small-volume, bloody mucoid stools, abdominal cramps, and tenesmus. Agents that cause bloody diarrhoea or dysentery can also provoke a form of diarrhoea that does not present clinically with visible blood in the stool, although mucosal damage and inflammation are present and faecal blood and white blood cells are usually detectable by microscopy.

Because of the significant morbidity and costs associated with infectious diarrhoea, making a specific laboratory diagnosis can be useful epidemiologically, diagnostically, and therapeutically. A definitive diagnosis is achieved mainly through study of faecal specimens, using bacteriological culture, viral culture, or direct electron microscopy for viral particles, and identification of microbial antigens (viruses, bacteria, parasites, or toxins). DNA probes, PCR, and immunodiagnostic tests can now be used to identify several pathogens in stool specimens. Although some diseases can be diagnosed by elevations of serum antibody titres, this method is usually retrospective and often inaccurate.

Evidence-based interventions

Increased use of oral rehydration therapy, improved nutrition, increased breastfeeding, better supplemental feeding, female education, measles immunization, and improvement in hygiene and sanitation are believed to have contributed to the decline in morbidity and mortality of diarrhoea. Syndromic diagnosis provides important clues to optimal management and is both programmatically and epidemiologically relevant. The correct treatment of diarrhoea requires mothers to recognize the problem and seek medical care promptly, and that health workers give oral rehydration solution (ORS) or other fluids to prevent or treat dehydration, dispense an appropriate antibiotic when needed, provide advice on appropriate feeding, and provide follow-up, especially for children at increased risk of serious morbidity or death. In recent years, low osmolarity ORS and zinc supplementation (10–20 mg/day) have led to significantly improved diarrhea outcomes (Aggarwal 2007).

Medical treatment

Since the most devastating consequences of acute infectious diarrhoea result from fluid losses, the major goal of treatment is the replacement of fluid and electrolytes. While the intravenous route of administration has been traditionally used, ORS have been shown to be equally effective physiologically and logistically more practical and less costly to administer, especially in developing countries. ORS is the treatment of choice for mild-to-moderate diarrhoea in both children and adults, as long as vomiting is not a major feature of the gastrointestinal infection. ORS can also be used in severely dehydrated patients after initial parenteral rehydration.

Although there is no doubt about the value of ORS in treating dehydrating diarrhoea, the optimal sodium concentration of the solution remains in dispute, particularly in regard to the treatment of mild-to-moderate diarrhoea in well-nourished children in industrialized countries. The high concentration of sodium (90 mmol) in the standard WHO ORS formulation may cause hypernatraemia and even seizures in children with non-cholera watery diarrhoea. Consequently, lower concentrations of sodium and a reduced osmolarity solution have been found to be effective

Table 2.7.12 Clinical features and aetiologies of diarrhoeal diseases

Feature	Site of infection	
	Small intestine	**Large intestine**
Pathogens	*Escherichia coli* (enteropathogenic *E. coli*, enterotoxigenic *E. coli*) *Cryptosporidium parvum* *Giardia lamblia* Norovirus Rotavirus *Vibrio cholerae*	*E. coli* (EIEC, EHEC) *Entamoeba histolytica* *Shigella* spp.
Location of pain	Mid abdomen	Lower abdomen, rectum
Volume of stool	Large	Small
Blood in stool	Rare	Common
Faecal leukocytes	Rare	Common (except in amebiasis)
Sigmoidoscopy	Normal	Mucosal ulcers, haemorrhagic foci, friable mucosa

for rehydration and not to be associated with any serious adverse clinical events (Hanh *et al.* 2001). The substitution of starch derived from rice or cereals for glucose in ORS has been another approach. Rice-based salt solutions produce lower stool losses, a shorter duration of diarrhoea, and greater fluid and electrolyte absorption than do glucose-based solutions in treating childhood and adult diarrhoea.

The provision of zinc supplements in conjunction with oral rehydration therapy serves to shorten the duration of diarrhoea and reduce the risk of subsequent episodes among children in resource-poor settings. This approach is now advocated by the WHO for the routine treatment of childhood diarrhoea in developing countries.

Dietary abstinence, the traditional approach to an acute diarrhoeal illness, restricts the intake of necessary calories, fluids, and electrolytes. During an acute attack, the patient often finds it more comfortable to avoid spicy, high-fat, and high-fibre foods, all of which can increase stool volume and intestinal motility. Although giving the bowel a rest provides symptomatic relief, continued oral intake of fluids and foods is critical for both rehydration and the prevention of malnutrition. In children, it is particularly important to restart feeding as soon as the child is willing to accept oral intake.

Because certain foods and fluids can increase intestinal motility, it is wise to avoid fluids such as coffee, tea, cocoa, and alcoholic beverages. Ingestion of milk and dairy products can potentiate fluid secretion and increase stool volume. Besides the oral rehydration therapy outlined above, acceptable beverages for mildly dehydrated adults include fruit juices and various bottled soft drinks. Carbonated drinks should be allowed to 'de-fizz' by letting them stand in a glass before ingestion. Soft, easily digestible foods are generally acceptable to the patient with acute diarrhoea.

Since most patients with infectious diarrhoea, even those with a recognized pathogen, have a mild, self-limited course, neither a stool culture nor specific treatment is required for such cases. For more severe cases, however, empirical antimicrobial therapy should be instituted, pending the results of stool and blood cultures. Gastrointestinal infections likely to respond to antibiotic treatment include cholera, giardiasis, cyclosporiasis, shigellosis, *E. coli* diarrhoea in infants, symptomatic travellers' diarrhoea, and *C. difficile* diarrhea (Table 2.7.13). The choice of antimicrobial drug should be based on *in vitro* sensitivity patterns, which vary from region to region. A fluoroquinolone antibiotic is a good choice for empirical therapy, since these agents have broad-spectrum activity against virtually all bacterial pathogens responsible for acute infectious diarrhoea (except *C. difficile*). Resistance to fluoroquinolones in South and Southeast Asia is an increasing problem.

In patients with severe community-acquired diarrhoea—characterized by more than four stools per day lasting for at least 3 days or more with at least one associated symptom such as fever, abdominal pain, or vomiting—there is a high likelihood of isolating a bacterial pathogen. In this setting, a short course of a fluoroquinolone, namely 1–3 days duration, will generally provide prompt relief with a low risk of adverse effects. Fluoroquinolones will not be effective for parasitic infections—specific antiparasitic drugs should be prescribed after identification of the offending pathogen in stool smears.

Self-treatment with an effective antimicrobial agent is advised for traveller's diarrhoea. While a fluoroquinolone is the treatment of choice, travellers to countries in Asia where resistance has become widespread should be provided with azithromycin for standby therapy. Rifaximin may also be used but this non-absorbable antibiotic is not recommended for treatment of invasive diarrhoea, which is common among travellers to Asia, especially Thailand.

There are conflicting reports regarding the efficacy of antimicrobial drugs in several important infections, such as those caused by *Campylobacter* spp., and insufficient data for infections caused by *Yersinia and Aeromonas* spp., vibrios, and several forms of *E. coli.* In cases of EHEC, there is evidence that antibiotics are not helpful and may even be harmful.

The duration of antimicrobial therapy has not been clearly defined. While courses of anywhere from 3 to 10 days of treatment have been recommended, there are several studies that included severe forms of diarrhoea which suggested that a single dose is as effective as more prolonged therapy. For example, single-dose fluoroquinolone therapy is highly effective for infections due to *V. cholerae*, *V. parahaemolyticus*, and most *Shigella* species. On the other hand, short-course treatment of salmonella gastroenteritis with fleroxacin has not been found to be clinically beneficial. When treatment is indicated, a number of studies have shown that the combination of an antimicrobial drug and an antimotility drug provides the most rapid relief of diarrhoea.

Antimotility drugs are particularly useful in controlling moderate-to-severe diarrhoea. These agents disrupt propulsive motility by decreasing jejunal motor activity. Opiates may decrease fluid secretion, enhance mucosal absorption, and increase rectal sphincter tone. The overall effect is to normalize fluid transport, slow transit time, reduce fluid losses, and ameliorate abdominal cramping. In contrast to the potential utility of antimotility drugs, adsorbents such as kaolin, pectin, and activated charcoal are not useful for treatment of acute diarrhoea.

Loperamide is the best agent because it does not carry a risk of habituation or depression of the respiratory centre. Treatment with loperamide produces rapid improvement, often within the first day of therapy. Although there has been a long-standing concern that antimotility agents might exacerbate cases of dysentery, this has largely been dispelled by clinical experience. Patients with shigellosis, even *S. dysenteriae* type 1, have been treated with loperamide alone and have had a normal resolution of symptoms without evidence of prolonging the illness or delaying excretion of the pathogen. However, as a general rule, antimotility drugs should not be used in young children or in patients with acute severe colitis, whether infectious or non-infectious in origin.

Preventive measures

Diarrhoeal disease affects rich and poor, old and young, and those in developed and developing countries alike, yet a strong relationship exists between poverty, an unhygienic environment, and the number and severity of diarrhoeal episodes—especially for children under 5 years. Poverty also restricts the ability to provide age-appropriate, nutritionally balanced diets, or to modify diets when diarrhoea develops so as to mitigate and repair nutrient losses. The impact is exacerbated by the lack of adequate, available, and affordable medical care. Thus preventive and management strategies for diarrhoea must have an equity focus.

Malnutrition is an independent predictor of the frequency and severity of diarrhoeal illness and can lead to a vicious cycle in which sequential diarrhoeal disease leads to increasing nutritional deterioration, impaired immune function, and greater susceptibility to infection.

Table 2.7.13 Therapy of bacterial infectious diarrhoea*

	Antibiotic of choice	Dose, route, and duration	Alternative drugs
Recommended in symptomatic cases			
Shigella	Ampicillin Ampicillin-resistant strains: Trimethoprim-sulphamethaxazole (TMP–SMX)	500 mg PO q.i.d. or 1 g IV q.6h. × 3 days 50–100 mg/kg/day for children One double-strength tablet PO b.i.d. or, for children, 10 mg/kg/day TMP and 50 mg/kg/day SMX × 3 days (maximum of 320 mg/1600 mg per day)	Fluoroquinolones, nalidixic acid, azithromycin
Traveller's diarrhoea	Ciprofloxacin	500 mg PO bid × 3 days	TMP–SMX, other fluoroquinolones, azithromycin
Enteropathogenic *E. coli*, Enteroaggregative *E. coli*, and diffusely adherent *E. coli* in infants; enteroinvasive *E. coli*	TMP–SMX	As for shigellosis	Fluoroquinolones, azithromycin
Typhoid fever	Ciprofloxacin	500 mg PO b.i.d. × 7 days	Amoxicillin 1 g PO q.i.d. × 14 days; TMP–SMX; chloramphenicol 500 mg PO or IV q.i.d. × 14 days azithromycin; third-generation cephalosporins
Cholera	Tetracycline[1] Doxycycline[1]	500 mg PO q.i.d. or, for children, 40 mg/kg/day in 4 doses (max. 4g/day) × 3 days 100 mg PO b.i.d. × 3 days	Ciprofloxacin, TMP–SMX, furazolidinone, azithromycin
Salmonella (unusual cases)	Ampicillin Ampicillin-resistant strains: TMP–SMX	50–100 mg/kg/day in 4 doses × 10–14 days One double-strength tablet PO b.i.d. or, for children, 8 mg/kg/day TMP and 40 mg/kg/day SMX (max. of 320 mg/1600 mg per day) × 14 days	Ciprofloxacin 500 mg PO b.i.d. × 14 days
Not generally recommended due to lack of conclusive findings or no studies			
Campylobacter jejuni	Erythromycin	500 mg PO b.i.d. × 5 days	Ciprofloxacin 500 mg PO b.i.d. × 5 days Azithromycin 500 mg PO on day 1, 250 mg PO qd days 2–5
Yersinia enterocolitica	Fluoroquinolones, TMP–SMX, chloramphenicol		Aminoglycosides, tetracycline
Aeromonas species	TMP–SMX, third-generation cephalosporins, fluoroquinolones		Tetracycline, chloramphenicol
Vibrio, noncholera species	Tetracycline		
EPEC, EAggEC, or DAEC in adults, EHEC	TMP–SMX		
Not recommended (except in unusual cases)			
Nontyphoidal *Salmonella*			
ETEC			

*Since resistance to commonly used drugs (penicillins, TMP/SMX, and fluoroquinolones) is so widespread, it is difficult to make recommendations without knowing local susceptibility patterns of enteropathogens.

[1]Should not be administered to children less than 8 years of age.

Family knowledge about diarrhoea must be reinforced in areas such as prevention, nutrition, hand washing and hygiene, measles vaccination, preventive zinc supplements, and when and where to seek care. It is estimated that, in the 1990s, more than 1 million deaths related to diarrhoea may have been prevented each year, largely attributable to the promotion and use of these therapies.

A meta-analysis of three observational studies in developing countries shows that breastfed children under age 6 months are 6.1 times less likely to die of diarrhoea than infants who are not breastfed. Continued breast feeding during the diarrhoea episode provides nutrients the child, prevents weight loss, and improves recovery from diarrhoea. Contaminated and poor-quality complementary foods are associated with increased diarrhoea burden and stunting (Huttly 1997). Ideally, complementary foods should be introduced at age 6 months, and breastfeeding should continue for up to 2 years or even longer. Appropriate, safe, and aptly initiated complementary feeding has been shown to significantly reduce mortality in young children. Diarrhoea frequently causes fever, altering host metabolism and leading to the depletion of body stores of nutrients. These losses must be replenished during convalescence, which takes much longer than the illness does to develop. For these reasons, appropriate feeding strategies during diarrhoea episodes are a corner stone of treatment.

Probiotics, especially *Lactobacillus rhamnosus* GG, effectively reduce the frequency and duration of diarrhoea in children and adults. Probiotics are also useful for the prevention of antibiotic-associated diarrhoea.

Various studies suggest that zinc-deficient populations are at increased risk of developing diarrhoeal diseases, respiratory tract infections, and growth retardation. A meta-analysis published in 1999 showed that continuous zinc supplementation was associated with decreased rates of childhood diarrhoea (Zinc Investigator's Collaborative Group 1999), and a recent meta-analysis confirms the previous findings and indicates that zinc supplementation for young children leads to reduction in the risk of diarrhoea (by 14 per cent), serious forms of diarrhoea, and the number of days of diarrhoea per child (Aggarwal 2007).

Human faeces and contamination are the primary source of diarrhoeal pathogens. Poor sanitation, lack of access to clean water, and inadequate personal hygiene are responsible for an estimated 90 per cent of childhood diarrhoea. Promotion of hand washing reduces diarrhoea incidence by an average of 33 per cent and rigorous observational studies demonstrated a median reduction of 55 per cent in all-cause child mortality associated with improved access to sanitation facilities. Hand washing promotion strategies have also been shown to reduce diarrhoea burden with ancillary benefits in community settings.

Strict adherence to food and water precautions as outlined above will help those who travel to less developed areas of the world to decrease their risk of acquiring gastrointestinal infections. Parasitic infections, such as strongyloidiasis and hookworms, can be avoided by the use of footwear. Avoiding contact with freshwater such as rivers and lakes in endemic areas serves to prevent schistosomiasis.

Immunization represents an ideal way to prevent certain bacterial and viral diseases, but has not yet proved successful for combating many gastrointestinal pathogens. The cholera vaccine that has been available for decades suffers from low efficacy, a moderate risk of side-effects, and a short duration of action. Newer oral cholera vaccines, such as the inactivated B subunit vaccine, are highly effective for prevention of severe cholera. New rotavirus vaccines, now available for the prevention of rotaviral diarrhoea in children, have not been associated with intussusception. Measles is known to predispose to diarrhoeal disease secondary to measles-induced immunodeficiency, and it is estimated that measles vaccine at varying levels of coverage (45–90 per cent) could prevent 44–64 per cent of measles cases, 0.6–3.8 per cent of diarrhoeal episodes, and 6–26 per cent of diarrhoeal deaths among children under 5 years. Global measles immunization coverage is now approaching 80 per cent, and the disease has been eliminated from the Americas, raising hopes for global elimination in the near future, with a predictable reduction in diarrhoea as well.

Typhoid fever

Typhoid fever, a systemic disease caused by *Salmonella enterica* serovar Typhi, is an acute illness characterized by protean and non-specific symptoms, including fever and gastrointestinal infection. The systemic disease caused by *S. paratyphi* (A, B, or C) is also clinically similar; both typhoid and paratyphoid are collectively labelled as enteric fevers. The emergence of drug-resistant strains, especially multi-drug-resistant (MDR) *S. typhi*, resistant to ampicillin, chloramphenicol, trimethoprim-sulphamethoxazole, and, more recently, fluoroquinolones, is a growing problem.

Global and regional epidemiology

The global incidence of typhoid fever in 2000 was estimated to be 21.6 million cases, with more than 200 000 deaths (Crump *et al.* 2004). Approximately 12.5 million cases of typhoid fever occur annually in the developing world (excluding China), with 7.7 million cases in Asia alone. In South Asia, recent community-based studies indicate that a large proportion of cases occur in children under 5, with significant morbidity and mortality. The global case fatality rate of 1 per cent is based on conservative estimates from hospital-based fever studies; actual mortality figures may be higher in areas where referral is difficult and health services dysfunctional. Table 2.7.14 shows the regional distribution of crude typhoid incidence rates.

There have been dramatic point-source outbreaks of typhoid related to contamination of food sources or water supply. The use of contaminated ground water, consumption of street foods, and poor personal hygiene are common risk factors for infection.

Issues in presentation and diagnosis

After ingestion in contaminated food or water, *S. typhi* penetrates the small bowel mucosa and makes its way rapidly to the lymphatics, the mesenteric nodes, and finally the bloodstream. Following an initial bacteraemia, the organism is sequestered in cells of the reticuloendothelial system where it multiplies and re-emerges several days later in recurrent waves of bacteraemia, an event that initiates the symptomatic phase of infection. The incubation period ranges from 5 to 14 days.

Typhoid fever is a febrile illness of prolonged duration, characterized by hectic fever, delirium, persistent bacteraemia, splenomegaly, and a variety of systemic manifestations. Most children present with fever, headache, and abdominal discomfort, diarrhoea, sore throat, anorexia, dry cough, or myalgia and constipation. In the later phase of illness, more specific physical signs including hepatomegaly and splenomegaly may be observed. Rose spots may be seen in an early stage of the illness in fair-skinned children and large proportions have a centrally coated tongue (Bhan *et al.* 2005).

Table 2.7.14 Crude typhoid incidence rates by region, 2000

Area/region	Crude incidence*	Typhoid cases	Incidence classification
Global	178	10 825 487	High
Africa	50	408 837	Medium
Asia	274	10 118 879	High
Europe	3	19 144	Low
Latin America/ Caribbean	53	273 518	Medium
Northern America	< 1	453	Low
Oceania	15	4656	Medium

Source: Data summarized from Crump *et al.* (2004).
*Per 100 000 persons per year.

Pulse–temperature dissociation is present in some patients. In approximately 50 per cent of patients, there is no change in bowel habits; in fact, constipation is more common than diarrhoea in children with typhoid fever. As a result of recurrent waves of bacteraemia, patients with typhoid fever can develop pneumonia, pyelonephritis, osteomyelitis, septic arthritis, and meningitis. Intestinal haemorrhage and perforation, the most common complications, often occur in the third week of infection or during convalescence. The most serious complication, intestinal perforation, occurs in 0.5–3 per cent of the patients with typhoid, and because they occur most commonly in areas where optimal medical care is not readily available, it may be associated with case fatality rates ranging from 4.8 to 30.5 per cent.

Diagnosis of typhoid and paratyphoid fever requires culture of blood, bone marrow, stools, or urine to confirm growth of *S. typhi*. Laboratory findings commonly include leucopenia, thrombocytopenia, proteinurea, and elevated transaminases, but these are relatively non-specific and uncommon. In developing countries, culture facilities are expensive and mostly confined to hospitals, while most typhoid patients are diagnosed clinically and treated in outpatient settings. In other instances, serological diagnosis may be made with the Widal test. The latter, though useful, is insufficiently sensitive in endemic areas. Newer diagnostic tests have been developed, such as the Typhidot and Tubex, which detect IgM antibodies against specific *S. typhi* antigens (Bhutta 2006). Since these newer assays have not proven to have adequate sensitivity and specificity for routine use in community settings, there is a need for further refinement in serological or molecular diagnosis of the disease.

Medical treatment

In the pre-antibiotic era, typhoid fever case fatality rates approached 20 per cent. Treatment with effective antimicrobial agents—ampicillin, chloramphenicol, cotrimoxazole, and later ciprofloxacin—has progressively reduced case fatality rates to <1 per cent, except for MDR isolates. Fluoroquinolones and third-generation cephalosporins are effective in MDR typhoid but over the last few years there have been increasing reports in Asia of *S. typhi* strains with reduced fluoroquinolone susceptibility. The presence of nalidixic acid resistance *in vitro* is associated with clinical treatment failures with fluoroquinolones. Alternative therapies including azithromycin or third-generation cephalosporins are recommended in these circumstances. Given the considerable morbidity and higher mortality rates reported with MDR typhoid in children, it is imperative that appropriate antibiotic therapy be instituted promptly and, when the appropriate facilities are available, treatment choices should be guided by susceptibility testing.

Preventive measures

Detection of sources of infection related to recent typhoid fever in household contacts, commercial food handlers, or contaminated drinking water sources is essential to design effective preventive measures for disease containment.

Although the old whole-cell-inactivated typhoid vaccine has been withdrawn because of side effects, there are two licensed vaccines for prevention of disease: Ty21a (an attenuated strain of *S. typhi* administered orally) and Vi (the purified bacterial polysaccharide vaccine, given parenterally). These two vaccines have comparable protective efficacy and while they have been largely used for travellers, recently the Vi vaccine has been used for school vaccination programmes in large public health settings in Asia. For younger children and infants the Vi conjugate vaccine has been shown to provide a high degree of protection in a series of studies in Vietnam. However, the conjugate vaccine has as yet not been produced for public health use.

Dengue fever

In recent years, dengue fever, a mosquito-borne arboviral disease, has become one of the most common and rapidly spreading vector-borne diseases (after malaria) and thus now represents a major international public health concern. The dengue virus belongs to the genus *Flavivirus* (single-stranded, non-segmented RNA viruses), which includes four serologically distinct serotypes (DEN-1, DEN-2, DEN-3, and DEN-4). Variations in virus strains within and between the four serotypes influence disease severity. There is limited protection across serotypes. Secondary infections (particularly with serotype 2) are more likely to result in severe disease and dengue haemorrhagic fever.

Global and regional epidemiology

Humans and mosquitoes are the principal hosts of dengue virus. although some non-human primates can also be infected. Dengue epidemics occur during the warm, humid, rainy seasons, which favour breeding conditions for the mosquito vector, *Aedes aegypti*. More than two-fifths of the world's population (~2.5 billion) lives in areas potentially at risk for dengue, which is endemic in more than 100 countries across the globe, with tropical areas of Asia, the Western Pacific, Latin America, and the Caribbean being the most seriously affected regions.

In some case series, dengue fever has been reported as the second most frequent cause of hospitalization (after malaria) among travellers returning from the tropics. It causes an estimated 100 million illnesses annually, including 250 000–500 000 cases of dengue haemorrhagic fever—a severe manifestation of dengue—and 24 000 deaths (Deen *et al.* 2006). Around 95 per cent of cases occur in children less than 15 years of age, with infants representing 5 per cent of the cases.

Issues in presentation and diagnosis

The incubation period can vary from 3 to 14 days (typically between 5 and 7 days) and viraemia can persist up to 12 days (typically 4–5 days). Fever usually lasts for 5–7 days; fevers persisting beyond 10–14 days suggest another diagnosis. The clinical features of dengue vary with patient age. Most dengue infections, especially in children, are minimally symptomatic or asymptomatic (Fig. 2.7.4). Children may also present with atypical syndromes such as encephalopathy and fulminant liver failure.

Classic dengue fever is characterized by a high fever of abrupt onset, sometimes with two peaks (saddle back fevers), severe myalgias, arthralgia, retro-orbital pain, headaches, and any of the three types of rashes, including a petechial rash, diffuse erythematous rash with isolated patches of normal skin, and a morbilliform rash, haemorrhagic manifestations, and leucopenia. Other manifestations include flushed facies, sore throat, cough, cutaneous hyperesthesia, and taste aberrations. Convalescence may be prolonged and complicated by profound fatigue and depression.

When the only haemorrhagic manifestation is provoked (by a tourniquet test), the case is categorized as Grade I dengue haemorrhagic fever, but a spontaneous haemorrhage, even if mild, indicates Grade II illness. Grades III and IV dengue haemorrhagic fever (incipient and frank circulatory failure, respectively) represent dengue shock syndrome which is characterized by sustained abdominal pain, persistent vomiting, sudden change from fever to hypothermia, alteration of consciousness, and a sudden drop in platelet count. Around 40 per cent of patients also have enlargement and tenderness of the liver. Rare presentations of infection include severe haemorrhage, severe hepatitis, rhabdomyolysis, jaundice, parotitis, cardiomyopathy, and variable neurological syndromes.

Infection with one serotype is thought to produce lifelong immunity to that serotype but only partial immunity to the others. Previous infection with a specific serotype followed by infection with a new serotype greatly increases the risk of dengue haemorrhagic fever.

Dengue virus serotypes are distinguishable by complement-fixation and neutralization test. Other diagnostic tests for patients with dengue include packed cell volume, platelet count, liver function tests, prothrombin time, partial thromboplastin time, electrolytes, and blood gas analysis. Laboratory findings commonly associated with dengue include leucopenia, lymphocytosis, increased concentration of liver enzymes, and thrombocytopenia. Diagnosis can be confirmed with several laboratory tests, especially the haemagglutination inhibition test and IgG or IgM enzyme immunoassays. Platelet counts and haematocrit determinations should be repeated at least every 24 h to allow prompt recognition of the development of dengue haemorrhagic fever and institution of fluid replacement. Diagnostic criteria for dengue fever are provided in Table 2.7.15.

Evidence-based interventions

Rapid urbanization has led to an increase in the environmental factors that contribute to the proliferation of *Aedes* mosquitoes. These include uncontrolled urban development, inadequate management of water and waste, presence of a range of large water stores, and disposable, non-biodegradable containers that become habitats for the larvae. These factors can change a region from non-endemic (no virus present) to hypoendemic (one serotype present) to hyperendemic (multiple serotypes present).

Medical treatment

No specific therapeutic agents exist for dengue fever apart from analgesics and medications to reduce fever. Treatment is supportive; steroids, antivirals, or carbazochrome (which decreases capillary permeability) have no proven role. In contrast, ribavirin, interferon alpha, and 6-azauridine have shown some antiviral activity *in vitro*. Mild or classic dengue is treated with antipyretic agents such as acetaminophen, bed rest, and fluid replacement (usually administered orally and only rarely parenterally); most cases can be managed on an outpatient basis.

The management of dengue haemorrhagic fever and the dengue shock syndrome is purely supportive. Aspirin and other non-steroidal anti-inflammatory drugs should be avoided owing to the increased risk for Reye's syndrome and haemorrhage.

Preventive measures

In the absence of a vaccine, control of the vector mosquito, *Aedes aegypti*, is the only effective preventive measure. At a personal level, the risk of mosquito bites may be reduced by the use of protective clothing and repellents. The single most effective preventive measure for travellers in areas where dengue is endemic is to avoid mosquito bites by using insect repellents containing *N*,

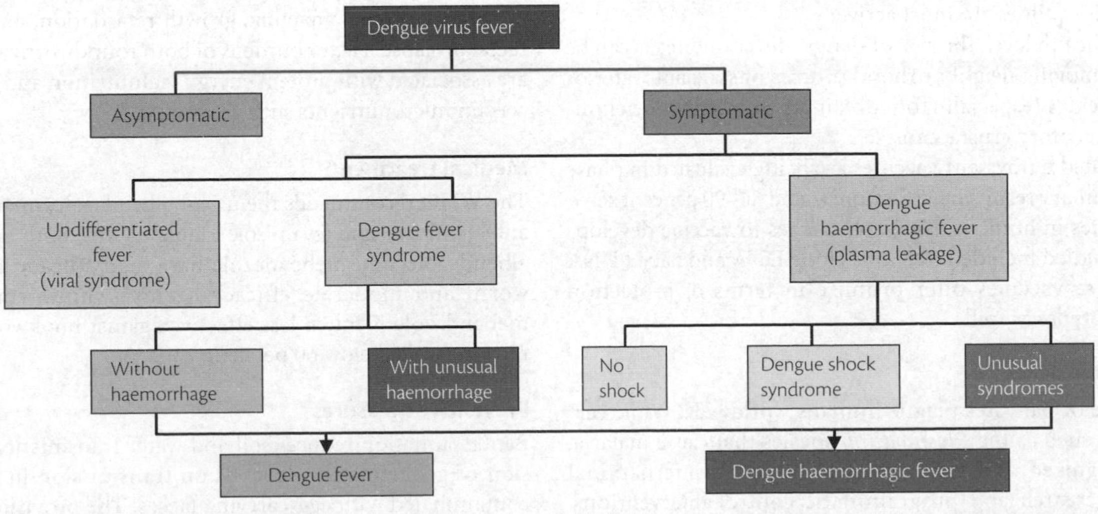

Fig. 2.7.4 WHO classification of symptomatic dengue infection.

Table 2.7.15 Diagnostic criteria for dengue fever

Dengue fever

Acute illness with two or more of:

Headache, retro orbital pain, myalgia, arthralgia, rash, haemorrhagic manifestations, and leucopenia

WHO definition for dengue haemorrhagic fever (WHO 2006)

- Fever
- Platelet count ≤100 000/mm^3
- Haemorrhagic manifestations
- Evidence of plasma: Leakage caused by increased vascular permeability manifested by at least one of the following:
  - Elevated haematocrit (≥20 per cent over baseline or a similar drop after intravenous fluid replacement),
  - Pleural or other effusion (e.g. ascites)
  - Low protein

Dengue shock syndrome

Criteria for dengue haemorrhagic fever:

- Pulse pressure <20 mm Hg or
- Hypotension (defined as systolic pressure <80 mm Hg for those aged <5 years or <90 mm Hg for those >5)

Probable diagnosis

At least one of following:

- Supportive serology
- Occurrence at same location and time as confirmed cases of dengue fever

Confirmed diagnosis

At least one of following:

- Isolation of dengue virus
- Four-fold or greater increase in serum IgG or increase in IgM antibody
- Detection of dengue virus or its genomic sequences by reverse transcription.

N-diethyl-3-methyl-benzamide (DEET) or picaridin. The insect repellents should be used in the early morning and late afternoon, when *Aedes* mosquitoes are most active.

At a public health level, the risk of dengue fever outbreaks can be reduced by removing neighbourhood sources of stagnant water or by using larvicides (especially for containers that cannot be eliminated), and predatory crustaceans.

Live attenuated tetravalent vaccines are being evaluated in phase 2 trials. Preliminary results have demonstrated 80–90 per cent seroconversion rates in humans. New approaches to vaccine development being studied include infectious clone DNA and naked DNA vaccines. These vaccines offer promise in terms of protection against all serotypes as well.

Parasitic infections

A broad range of parasites plague humans worldwide. While certain parasites, such as the *Plasmodium* species that cause malaria, are well recognized and have received intensive international support for research and programmatic control interventions, others are considered among the world's most neglected diseases. Some of the main neglected tropical parasitic diseases include the protozoan infections: Human African trypanosomiasis, visceral leishmaniasis, and American trypanosomiasis (Chagas disease) and helminthic infections such as the soil-transmitted nematodes (ascariasis, hookworms, trichuriasis), schistosomiasis, lymphatic filariasis, onchocerciasis, and dracunculiasis.

Of the 20 major helminth infections of humans, the commonest are the geo-helminths. Roundworms, members of the phylum Nematoda, are responsible for an estimated 1 billion or more human infections. In many low-income countries, it is more common to be infected than not. Indeed, a child growing up in an endemic community can be infected soon after weaning, and continue to be infected and constantly re-infected for life.

Global and regional epidemiology

Recent global estimates indicate that more than a quarter of the world's population is infected with one or more helminths. The geographic distribution of roundworms in many tropical and subtropical regions closely parallels socioeconomic and sanitary conditions. In locales where several species of intestinal parasites are found, coinfection with *Ascaris lumbricoides, Trichuris trichiura,* and hookworms is common. In low- and middle-income countries, about 1.2 billion people are infected with the roundworm, *Ascaris lumbricoides*, while more than 700 million are infected with hookworm (*Necator americanus* or *Ancylostoma duodenale*) or whipworm (*Trichuris trichiura*) (Hotez *et al.* 2004). In 2002, the WHO estimated that 27 000 people die annually from geo-helminthic infections. Many investigators, however, believe that this figure is an underestimate. It has been estimated that 155 000 deaths annually occur from these infections (CFR 0.08 per cent).

Issues in presentation

Children of school age are at greatest risk from the clinical manifestations of disease. Studies have shown associations between helminth infection and undernutrition, iron deficiency anaemia, stunted growth, poor school attendance, and poor performance in cognition tests. Some 44 million pregnancies are currently complicated by maternal hookworm infection, placing both mothers and children at higher risk of anaemia and death during pregnancy and delivery. Intense whipworm infection in children may result in trichuris dysentery syndrome, the classic signs of which include bloody diarrhoea, anaemia, growth retardation, and occasionally rectal prolapse. Heavy burdens of both roundworm and whipworm are associated with protein energy malnutrition and deficiencies of certain micronutrients such as vitamin A.

Medical treatment

The WHO recommends the use of albendazole, mebendazole, pyrantel pamoate, and levamisole (Table 2.7.16). Both benzimidazoles, albendazole, and mebendazole have high efficacy against roundworm and moderate efficacy against whipworm. Single-dose mebendazole is much less effective against hookworm, with cure rates typically below 60 per cent.

Preventive measures

Better sanitation reduces soil and water transmission as transmission of geohelminths depends on transmission in environments contaminated with egg-carrying faeces. The provision of adequate sanitation is the only definitive intervention to eliminate helminthic

Table 2.7.16 Diagnosis and treatment of major intestinal nematode infections

Organism	Type of specimen	Specimen preparation	Size of eggs or larvae (μm)	Drug of choice	Alternative therapies
Trichuris trichiura	Stool	Direct smear or concentration	50–54 × 23	Mebendazole, 100 mg orally (PO) twice daily (bid) × 3 days	Albendazole, 400 mg PO once
Ascaris lumbricoides	Stool	Direct smear or concentration	45–70 × 35–50	Mebendazole, 100 mg PO bid × 3 days or Albendazole, 400 mg PO once or Pyrantel pamoate, 11 mg/kg PO once (max 1 g)	Piperazine citrate, 75 mg/kg bid (max 1 g) by nasogastric tube × 2–3 days until resolution of obstruction
Ancylostoma duodenale *Necator americanus*	Stool	Direct smear or concentration	55–70 × 35–45	Mebendazole, 100 mg PO bid × 3 days	Albendazole, 400 mg PO once or Pyrantel pamoate, 11 mg/kg PO × 3 days (max 1 g)
Enterobius vermicularis	Adhesive tape preparation	Direct microscopy	50–60 × 20–30	Mebendazole, 100 mg PO once or Pyrantel pamoate, 11 mg/kg PO once Repeat in 2 weeks	Albendazole, 400 mg PO once Repeat in 2 weeks
Strongyloides stercoralis	Stool, duodenal aspirate	Concentration or Baermann method	400–500 × 15	Ivermectin, 150–200 μg/kg PO × 1–2 days*	Thiabendazole, 25 mg/kg PO bid × 2 days (max 3 g/day)

*Intrarectal ivermectin is an option for treatment of high-grade strongyloidiasis.

infections, but to be effective it should cover a high percentage of the population. With high costs involved, implementing this strategy is difficult where resources are limited. Both the World Bank and WHO promote helminth control programmes and considers it as one of the most cost effective strategies to improve health in developing countries. These programmes emphasize mass drug administration as a major component of control.

Recommended drugs for use in public health settings include albendazole (single dose: 400 mg, reduced to 200 mg for children between 12 and 24 months), or mebendazole (single dose: 500 mg), as well as levamisole or pyrantel palmoate. Programmes aim for mass treatment of all children in high-risk groups (communities where worms are endemic) with antihelmintic drugs every 3–6 months. A recent systematic review of randomized controlled trials found that deworming increases haemoglobin by 1.71 g/l (95 per cent confidence interval 0.70–2.73), which could translate into a small (5–10 per cent) reduction in the prevalence of anaemia (Gulani *et al.* 2007).

Home delivery of antihelminthics is problematic for several reasons and thus school-based deworming programmes are preferred. These have been showed to boost school participation and are practical as schools offer a readily available, extensive, and sustained infrastructure with a skilled workforce that can be readily trained. In Kenya, such a programme reduced school absenteeism by a quarter, with the largest gains among the youngest children. Perhaps even more importantly, this study showed that those children who had not been treated benefited from the generally lowered transmission rate in the schools. These school-based programmes have resulted in improvements in overall nutritional status, growth, physical fitness, appetite, anaemia, and cognitive development. The above measures must be coupled with community behaviour change strategies with the aim of reducing contamination of soil and water by promoting the use of latrines and hygienic behaviour. Without a change in defecation habits, periodic deworming cannot attain a stable reduction in transmission.

Table 2.7.17 Public health interventions and their effect on diseases

Major intervention	Disease prevented or treated
Effective antenatal care	Neonatal sepsis and meningitis, pneumonia
Skilled maternal and neonatal care	Neonatal sepsis and meningitis, neonatal tetanus
Maintenance of good personal hygiene	Neonatal sepsis and meningitis, diarrhoea, typhoid fever
Antimicrobial therapy	Neonatal sepsis, meningitis, bacteraemia, diarrhoea, pneumonia, typhoid fever, malaria, helminths
Vaccines	Pneumonia, typhoid fever, meningitis, bacteraemia
Oral rehydration therapy	Diarrhoea
Vitamin A	Diarrhoea, measles, malaria
Zinc	Diarrhoea, pneumonia, malaria
Provision of safe water, sanitation, and hygiene	Neonatal sepsis and meningitis, diarrhoea, pneumonia, typhoid fever, helminths
Breast feeding	Neonatal sepsis and meningitis, diarrhoea, pneumonia
Complementary feeding	Neonatal sepsis, diarrhoea, pneumonia
Intermittent preventive therapy in pregnancy	Malaria
Insecticide-treated nets	Malaria
Integrated vector control	Malaria, dengue, other vector-borne diseases

Conclusion

The global burden of infectious diseases contributing to childhood and adult mortality is considerable. The situation is further compounded by increasing antimicrobial resistance and the emergence of newer infections with viruses such as avian influenza (H5N1) and the coronavirus responsible for the severe acute respiratory syndrome (SARS). Although the contribution of neonatal infections to overall child mortality has only recently been recognized, the persistent global burden of deaths due to diarrhoea and pneumonia underscore the need for improved public health strategies for change. There are interventions that can make a difference to childhood and adult infectious diseases (Table 2.7.17). What is needed is their implementation at scale to populations at greatest risk. This will require not only biomedical approaches but measures to address the social determinants of disease.

References

Addo-Yobo, E., Chisaka, N., Hassan, M. *et al.* (2004). Oral amoxicillin versus injectable penicillin for severe pneumonia in children aged 3 to 59 months: A randomised multicentre equivalency study. *The Lancet*, **364**, 1141–1148.

Aggarwal, R., Sentz, J., and Miller, M.A. (2007). Role of zinc administration in prevention of childhood diarrhea and respiratory illnesses: A meta-analysis. *Pediatrics* **119**, 1120–30.

Armstrong, G.L., Conn, L.A., and Pinner, R.W. (1999). Trends in infectious disease mortality in the United States during the 20th century. *Journal of the American Medical Association*, **281**, 61–6.

Bhan, M.K., Bahl, R., and Bhatnagar, S. (2005). Typhoid and paratyphoid fever. *The Lancet*, **366**, 749–62.

Bhutta, Z.A. (2006). Current concepts in the diagnosis and treatment of typhoid fever. *British Medical Journal*, **333**, 78–82.

Bhutta, Z.A. (2007). Dealing with childhood pneumonia in developing countries: How can we make a difference? *Archives of Diseases of Childhood*, **92**, 286–8.

Black, R.E., Morris, S.S., and Bryce, J. (2003). Where and why are 10 million children dying every year? *The Lancet*, **361**, 2226–34.

Bryce, J., Boschi-Pinto, C., Shibuya K. *et al.* (2005). WHO estimates of the causes of death in children. *The Lancet*, **365**, 1147–52.

Cohen, M.L. (2000). Changing patterns of infectious disease. *Nature*, **406**, 762–7.

Crump, J.A., Luby, S.P., and Mintz, E.D. (2004). The global burden of typhoid fever. *Bulletin of the World Health Organization*, **82**, 346–53.

Darmstadt, G.L., Bhutta, Z.A., Cousens, S. *et al.* (2005). Lancet Neonatal Survival Steering Team. Evidence based cost-effective interventions: how many newborn babies can we save? *The Lancet*, **365**, 977–88.

Deen, J.L., Harris, E., Wills, B. *et al.* (2006) The WHO dengue classification and case definitions: time for a reassessment. *The Lancet*, **368**, 170–173.

Gulani, A., Nagpal, J., Osmond, C. *et al.* (2007). Effect of administration of intestinal anthelminthic drugs on haemoglobin: Systematic review of randomised controlled trials. *British Medical Journal*, **doi: 10.1136**, 1–6.

Hamer, D.H. and Gorbach, S.L. Gastrointestinal infections. In (eds. D.A. Warrell, T.M. Cox, and J.D. Firth). *The Oxford textbook of medicine*, 5th edition. Oxford University Press, Oxford, England; in press.

Hanh, S.K., Kim, Y.J., and Garner, P. (2001). Reduced osmolarity oral rehydration solution for treating dehydration due to diarrhoea in children: A systematic review. *British Medical Journal*, **323**, 81–5.

Hotez. P.J., Brooker, S., Bethony, J.M. *et al.* (2004). Hookworm infection. *New England Journal of Medicine*, **351**, 799–807.

Huttly, S.R., Morris, S.S., and Pisani, V. (1997). Prevention of diarrhoea in young children in developing countries. *Bulletin of the World Health Organization*, **75**, 163–74.

Kosek, M., Bern, C., and Guerrant, R.L. (2003). The magnitude of the global burden of diarrheal disease from studies published 1992–2000. *Bulletin of the World Health Organization*, **81**, 197–204.

Mandell, L.A., Wunderink, R.G., Anzueto, A. *et al.* (2007). Infectious Diseases Society of America/American Thoracic Society consensus guidelines on the management of community-acquired pneumonia in adults. *Clinical Infectious Diseases*, **44**, S27–S72.

Nigrovic, L.E., Kupperman, N., Macias, C.G. *et al.* (2007). Clinical prediction rule for identifying children with cerebrospinal fluid pleocytosis at very low risk of bacterial meningitis. *Journal of the American Medical Association*, **297**, 52–60.

Nunn, P., Reid, A., and De Cock, K.M. (1997). Tuberculosis and HIV infection: The global setting. *Journal of Infectious Diseases*, **196** (Suppl 1), S5–S14.

Rice, A.L., Sacco, L., Hyder, A. *et al.* (2000). Malnutrition as an underlying cause of childhood deaths associated with infectious diseases in developing countries. *Bulletin of the World Health Organization*, **278**, 1207–21.

Sáez-Llorens, X. and McCracken, G.H. (2003). Bacterial meningitis in children. *The Lancet*, **361**, 2139–48.

Saha, S.K., Darmstadt, G.L., Yamanaka, N. *et al.* (2005). Rapid diagnosis of pneumococcal meningitis: Implications for treatment and measuring disease burden. *Pediatric Infectious Disease Journal*, **24**, 1093–8.

Van de Beek, D., de Gans, J., McIntyre, P. *et al.* (2007). Corticosteroids for acute bacterial meningitis. *Cochrane Database of Systematic Reviews*, CD004405.

WHO Collaborative Study Team on the Role of Breastfeeding on the Prevention of Infant Mortality (2000). Effect of breastfeeding on infant and child mortality due to infectious diseases in less developed countries: A pooled analysis. *The Lancet*, **355**, 451–5.

Zinc Investigators' Collaborative Group (1999). Prevention of diarrhea and pneumonia by zinc supplementation in children in developing countries: Pooled analysis of randomized controlled trials. *Journal of Pediatrics*, **135**, 689–97.

2.8

The global environment

Anthony J. McMichael and Hilary J. Bambrick

Introduction

We, the human species, have reached an unfamiliar crossroads with respect to the health risks posed by the external environment. We not only continue to face the health risks posed by long-familiar forms of environmental contamination, but now also face an emerging range of larger-scale and more systemic environmental hazards. As the sheer size and economic intensity of human endeavour, globally, has escalated in recent decades, its impact on the natural systems and processes of the global environment has increased—and, in consequence, environmental changes at that larger scale are becoming evident (Kennedy 2006).

These changes, such as global climate change, freshwater depletion, soil erosion, and the loss of species, are occurring on an unprecedented scale. They represent a weakening of Earth's life-support systems, a weakening of the foundations of biological health and life upon which human health ultimately depends. They therefore pose current and future risks to human health. Meanwhile, the ongoing increases in interconnectedness and 'globalization' of economic systems, trade, food systems, cultural diffusion, human mobility, electronic communication, and the spread of infectious agents are adding further to the contemporary emergence and strengthening of macroscopic influences on population health and disease.

These human-induced 'global environmental changes' are thus expanding the topic scope of 'environment and health'. Contamination by additives (chemicals, radiation, microbes) has long been the main source of environmental risks, and it remains so in many of the world's poorer and more vulnerable communities and populations. Meanwhile, populations everywhere are beginning to encounter this further dimension of health risk from larger-scale disruptions of environmental and ecosystem processes. Food yields, for example, are becoming less secure, and infectious disease occurrence is becoming more varied and volatile.

In essence, whereas traditional environmental hazards to human health mostly arise from the unintended *addition* of contaminants to air, water, soil, or food—or from excessive exposure to naturally occurring environmental factors (e.g. solar radiation)—these emerging larger-scale hazards arise from the *loss* of environmental attributes such as stability, productivity, regenerative and absorptive capacity. This added depth, indeed qualitative extension, to the category 'environmental health' necessitates some new and modified research strategies. It also requires a shift in how we think about and apply preventive strategies.

Implications for research concepts and methods

During the past half-century, the environment has mostly been treated by public health researchers and practitioners in a reductionist, itemized fashion. The health risks associated with specific physical, chemical, or microbiological agents have been characterized and quantified, one by one, and targeted interventions to reduce those risks have then been formulated and evaluated. This has been an important and fruitful strategy for the detection, characterization, and quantification of the health risk of each new contaminant and other agents entering the environment—and for the subsequent risk management strategy, often by setting exposure standards. This 'classical' type of environmental epidemiological study has often assumed the risk to be mediated by a straightforward causal relation between the specified exposure and health outcome, exhibiting either linear or curvilinear risk function. From such modelled relationships, the health risks at different doses can be estimated.

That focus and strategy of research (risk identification and assessment) and risk management remains important. As industrialization, agricultural production, and overall economic development have spread and intensified around the world, many new and often localized exposures to specific chemical and physical agents have resulted. New technologies—such as the use of mobile phones—can entail specific new exposure hazards. Vigilance is necessary on the research and policy fronts in relation to all such specific physical, chemical, and microbiological hazards to human health.

For all environmental exposures, old and new, there is the opportunity to study the relations with health outcomes at one or several levels of aggregation. Where widely-acting environmental exposures (e.g. urban air pollution and the post-Chernobyl ionizing radiation exposure) impinge on whole communities fairly evenly, it is appropriate for whole communities or populations to be the unit of analysis. Similarly, many epidemiological studies have estimated the percentage change in the study population's death rate associated with each unit increase in level of ambient air pollution. Other environmental exposures may impinge unevenly between individuals, with considerable difference in the 'dose' received. In such situations it is desirable to compare sets of individuals for whom estimates of individual-level exposure are possible. Conveniently, some such exposures are measurable at the individual level (via concentrations in blood, urine, saliva, or hair; or with molecular biomarkers), and this allows their associated health risks to be estimated at varied levels of received dose.

It is likely that much of the research on the health risks posed by global environmental changes will be conducted at the level of population or community. If climate change affects the altitude of transmission of malaria within a highland region, the primary research question is whether there has been an observable change in the physical range of malaria occurrence. Subsequent questions about which age-groups, families, or communities have been most affected are of interest, but are not specific to the climate change issue. Similarly, if heat-waves become more frequent and more severe under climate change conditions, there is need for research to assess how the exposure of populations to unusually high temperatures or unusually long heat-waves affects the immediate rates of death—overall, by specified cause, and for relevant identifiable sub-populations (age, sex, socioeconomic position, urban versus rural, etc.).

This type of research question refers to indices of the exposure and vulnerability of whole communities in relation to an environmental change entailing the disturbance of a natural system (e.g. the world's climate) that reflects the pressures exerted by human societies as a consequence of their way of living. The research and risk assessment question has a clear 'ecological' character. This has fundamental implications for how we could, indeed should, think about reducing or averting the risk to health.

Thinking 'ecologically'

The advent of a range of larger-scale environmental influences on human health is requiring researchers as public health practitioners to think in ecological terms. (The word 'ecological', here, refers to understanding relations within and between communities of living organisms, and between them and their physical environment. It does *not* refer to the regrettably mislabelled 'ecological studies', as classified by epidemiology textbook orthodoxy.) This need to think more ecologically will require an enhanced understanding of how these complex environmental systems are changed by human actions, and by what pathways, both direct and indirect, these changes then affect health.

To estimate the current and, importantly, the future health consequences of these systemic changes will require advances in many of our research methods. This would include developments in the following: Spatial analysis; time-series analysis; and techniques of modelling (both statistical and process-based) to estimate future health risks, handle uncertainties inherent in future scenarios, define the parameters of future 'health risk', and explore how the combined impact of concurrent environmental and social changes affects health risks.

An appropriate response to this challenge will also enrich research and policy thinking in other domains. For example, if in considering the health impacts of the urban environment we view cities as no more than an aggregation of specific 'toxic' exposures (lead from petrol, air pollutants, noise levels, road trauma, etc.), then we only address part of the health impact agenda. By viewing the city as a system that reflects and affects human ecology, the urban environmental health calculus then also includes consideration of how city design and transport systems affect physical activity (and obesity); access to, and type of, food retail outlets; mental health stresses in suburbia; infectious disease contact networks; and the release of greenhouse gases with their subsequent climate-changing and, hence, health consequences.

In summary, human-induced changes in the environment at large—the human-built environment, the globalizing geopolitical and economic environment, and the natural systems of the biosphere—pose major new challenges for epidemiologists and public health practitioners. The environmental health agenda of the twenty-first century will encompass much more than it did during the preceding two centuries. During those centuries, industrialization and urban living gathered momentum and affected local environments. Contemporary China provides a compelling reminder of how extensively such activities can contaminate environments and endanger health. Today, the scale of those human activities and their resultant pressures on the environment are affecting the environment and its natural systems at global and regional levels.

The 'environment'—local and global

History of evolution of ideas about environment and health

Concern over environmental conditions substantially shaped the historical evolution of public health and its core research discipline, epidemiology. In nineteenth-century Britain, there was a need to understand and remedy, for example: Toxic hazards in locally-brewed alcoholic drinks, the cholera outbreaks in London, mortality differentials between contrasting geographic and socioeconomic groups, and various specific occupational exposure hazards.

During earlier centuries, there persisted the age-old belief that disease reflected God's retributory judgement on the human condition. Then, in the seventeenth century, new philosophical perspectives emerged as the foundations of modern empirical science were laid in Western Europe. Francis Bacon argued for scientific enquiry based on empirical observation and comparison. René Descartes propounded a reductionist framework for studying the external 'machine-like' world.

This Enlightenment thinking about the role of scientific enquiry, the rise of inductive logic (drawing generalized inferences about relationships and physical laws from specific sets of observations), and a utilitarian approach to the fruits of scientific enquiry nurtured a more activist approach to managing the environment. Consequently, the 'social hygiene' movement arose in late seventeenth-century Europe, seeking to improve and cleanse the environment. Major social expenditures were required, ranging from draining marshes, removing urban refuse, and improving roadways.

In the wake of the French Revolution, social ideologies gave greater emphasis to egalitarianism. There was recognition that the widespread damaging environmental impacts of intensified mechanized production methods, crowding, and the disposal of wastes and excreta impinged heavily on the health of urban-industrial populations. In Britain, for more pragmatic and utilitarian reasons, the Sanitary Idea emerged in the 1840s in response to the perceived chronic poverty, illness, and debilitation of the urban workforce. The sanitary engineering idea also became linked with early notions of urban sustainability—including the recycling of sewage, attaining local self-sufficiency in food production, and achieving full employment. Later that century, in England, Ebenezer Howard's ideal of smaller decentralized 'garden cities', with green-belts and with residential areas separated from work zones, became popular as a means of countering the health-endangering miasmas emanating from dank, dirty, and crowded urban-industrial environments.

Meanwhile, improvements in nutrition, the urban environment and general social progress were ushering in the first public health revolution (McKeown *et al.* 1972). Other health gains arose via changes in human social organization and economic practices. For example, the mechanization of European agriculture from the mid-eighteenth century, with increased fodder production, stimulated a growth in cattle herds. This caused a reduction in human malaria, since the malaria-transmitting anopheline mosquitoes much prefer their blood-meals from cattle than from humans.

The spectacular rise of bacteriology in the 1880s caused a frame-shift in perspective. Microbes were now deemed to be the primary cause of disease. This influential 'Germ Theory', along with new theories of cell biology and heredity, of micronutrient deficiencies, and the medicalization of child-bearing and child-rearing, all refocused the health sciences on the individual. Ideas of shared environmental exposures and the resultant shared health risks receded.

The model of specific causation—and hence prevention and treatment—of disease inherent in the Germ Theory prevailed early in the twentieth century. However, some counterbalancing of ideas arose from new knowledge about the vector-based transmission (by mosquitoes, ticks, biting flies, etc.) of major diseases such as malaria, schistosomiasis, dengue fever, yellow fever, and leishmaniasis. This underscored the important influences of wider environmental and ecological conditions. It led to new environmental management strategies in tropical and subtropical regions, including the spraying of mosquito breeding sites with DDT, control of surface water, and the control of alternative mammalian host species.

By the mid-twentieth century, the spread of industry and motorized transport had greatly increased local environmental exposures. Major urban air pollution episodes occurred, and these helped stimulate new environmental legislation in Western countries during the 1960s and beyond. Meanwhile, in her iconic book *Silent Spring*, Rachel Carson (1962) focused attention on a new concern—the apparently pervasive ecological damage caused by the bioaccumulation of pesticides, such as DDT and other chlorinated hydrocarbons. Concentrations of these human-made chemicals increased up the food chain. Humans, she argued, were on notice that such human-made chemicals, rippling through the natural world, would eventually damage human biology.

In the 1970s, the recognition of 'acid rain' heightened awareness that some types of environmental health hazards were transcending landscapes and national boundaries. As the increasing fire power of modern epidemiology began to yield information about health risks from long-term follow-up studies of occupational cohorts, new concerns also arose about the health hazards posed by cumulative exposure to various industrial and agricultural environmental contaminants. These included, especially, the environmentally persistent chlorinated hydrocarbons and several heavy metals (especially lead and cadmium). Exposures to these agents can, variously, impair the immune system, reproductive system, and neurological system—along with liver and kidney functioning and bone architecture.

During the 1970s and 1980s, concerns about chemical pollution of the environment and other forms of environmental damage assumed more of a 'life of their own' in public discourse. This is evident in much of the language of the UN's famous 1972 Stockholm Conference on the Environment, and in the orientation of the report *Our Common Future*, in 1987, from the UN's World Commission on Environment and Development (the 'Brundtland Commission') (World Commission on Environment and Development 1987). Both were particularly concerned to explore how environmental conservation and quality could be achieved in concert with the anticipated, and desired, increases in economic development.

In high-income countries, epidemiologists and the health sector at large became preoccupied with new insights and new ways of studying the health risks arising from specific individual-level behaviours and exposures, including cigarette smoking, alcohol consumption, aspects of the 'Western' diet, oral contraceptive use, sexual behaviours, personal solar exposure, and domestic chemical exposures. There was a partial eclipse of research interest in understanding how aspects of the ambient environment affect rates of disease.

Acting as a modern Isle of Iona, air pollution epidemiology largely kept alive an interest in understanding how changes in types and levels of ambient environmental exposure affected health outcomes in whole communities. Then, in the late 1980s and the 1990s, it began to emerge that there was yet another—different and larger—category of environmental hazard looming over human health. That is the major focus of this chapter.

Current burden of disease due to environmental exposures

The World Health Organization estimates that one-quarter of the global burden of disease is due to modifiable environmental factors in air, water, soil, and food (Prüss-Üstün & Corvalán 2006). The figure in children is higher, over one-third—and predominantly from diarrhoeal disease, lower respiratory infections, unintentional injuries, and malaria. This environment-related burden is much greater in low-income than high-income countries: An estimated 25 per cent of deaths in developing regions versus 17 per cent in developed. Comparing low-income to high-income countries, healthy life-years lost to environmentally caused disease are 25 times higher for road crashes, 140 times higher for diarrhoeal diseases, and 800 times higher for respiratory infections. Children in developing countries lose an estimated eight times more healthy life-years from environmental diseases than do their developed country counterparts.

These environmental hazards remain enormously important in lower income countries, especially in socioeconomically and politically disadvantaged communities. Technically, many of them can be managed or eliminated on a local basis. But this requires political will and resources, and a moral or ideological responsiveness to the existence of health inequalities.

Meanwhile, these ongoing environmental health hazards are being supplemented, increasingly, by the emergence of health risks due to changes in the 'global environment'. Those changes are occurring at a much larger scale, and involve various systemic disturbances and shifts that have direct and indirect consequences for human health. The best-known, and the most important with respect to the future sustainability of health-supporting conditions for human populations, are the 'global environmental changes' (GEC) such as climate change, biodiversity loss, and degradation of food-producing ecosystems on land and in the oceans.

These GECs can be thought of as a major component of a wider set of 'global changes' that typify the growing scale, speed, and intensity of changes in environmental, social, economic processes and conditions in the world at large. That larger set is shown schematically in Fig. 2.8.1.

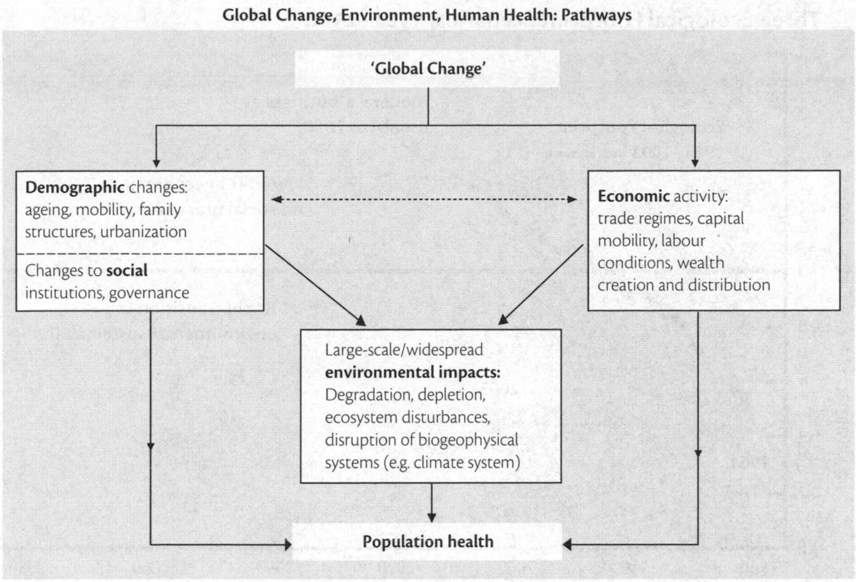

Fig. 2.8.1 Schematic diagram of major domains of 'global change'. Demographic, social, and economic variables generate and influence the pressures on the natural environment. Those variables and associated large-scale environmental changes affect human health.

Global environmental changes: Larger and systemic influences on population health

There is an urgent need for a fuller understanding of how human-induced global environmental changes pose risks to human health. These large-scale hazards to health have arisen from the disruption or depletion of complex biophysical and ecological systems that is now occurring on an increasing scale as a result of expanded and intensified human economic activity.

These emerging global environmental changes entail the *loss* of natural environmental capital and *disruption* of ecosystems. That type of human impact on the environment is qualitatively distinct from the more familiar process of (mostly time-limited and reversible) local environmental *contamination*. The elucidation of these hazards to health requires more than the mono-disciplinary and single-factor approaches that have generally served epidemiologists, toxicologists, and environmental scientists well in the past.

It is important, here, to clarify the nature and the dimensions of this recent development in the ways in which human activities are now altering many aspects of the structure and functioning of the natural world.

The 'ecological footprint'

A widely used measure of human impact on the environment is the 'ecological footprint'. This relates directly to the more familiar concept of environmental 'carrying capacity'—i.e. how many individuals can be sustained over time by a specified unit of land area. The 'footprint' reverses the arithmetic: It asks how many units of environment are required to meet the needs (or wants) of a specified unit of human population—an individual, community, city, or population.

Several recent assessments have been made of the global human population's aggregated 'footprint' on Earth's environment. The consistent conclusion is that humanity is collectively consuming more materials and generating more waste than the natural environment can supply and absorb, respectively, on a recurrent basis. That is, we are operating in 'ecological deficit', depleting Earth's stocks of natural environmental 'capital'—in order to meet our now excessive demands on the environment.

The World Wide Fund for Nature (WWF) has estimated the world population's ecological footprint by analysing trends in stocks and flows at national level over recent decades, focusing particularly on major categories of ecological systems, including freshwater, marine, and forest ecosystems. Figure 2.8.2 shows the WWF's estimation for the period 1961–2003. The size of the human footprint is expressed as the number of Planet Earths needed to meet the total environmental demands. Beyond the year 2003, the figure comprises three scenario-based estimates of future aggregate environmental demands, assuming that the specified economic development, policy, and technology trajectories will apply.

A separate recent analysis, comparing national indices (Dietz *et al.* 2007), concludes that population size and rising affluence (with its associated patterns of production and consumption) are the principal drivers of humanity's pressures on the natural environment. Other commonly postulated determinants such as the extent of urbanization, type of economic structure, and population age distribution were found to have relatively little effect. The analysis also found that higher levels of education and life expectancy were not associated with elevated environmental pressures. This finding suggests that some important aspects of human well-being can be improved without significant risk to the environment.

Of course, a prime purpose for seeking to understand the health consequences of human-induced changes to the global environment is to enrich the evidence base for policy-making. Big decisions need to be made about the choice of technologies and the form of physical and social development. How should we generate energy? How can our cities be made sustainable and socially congenial? What forms of transport should we use? What aspects of trade should be encouraged, and what aspects discouraged?

That last question leads to consideration of one of the major other 'global' developments in today's world that is exerting increasing influence on human health—international trade. This, in concert, with an increasing international cultural diffusion that is influencing patterns of consumer preference and behaviours, is a good illustration of the category of emerging large-scale influences on human health that are not primarily mediated by changes in the natural environment.

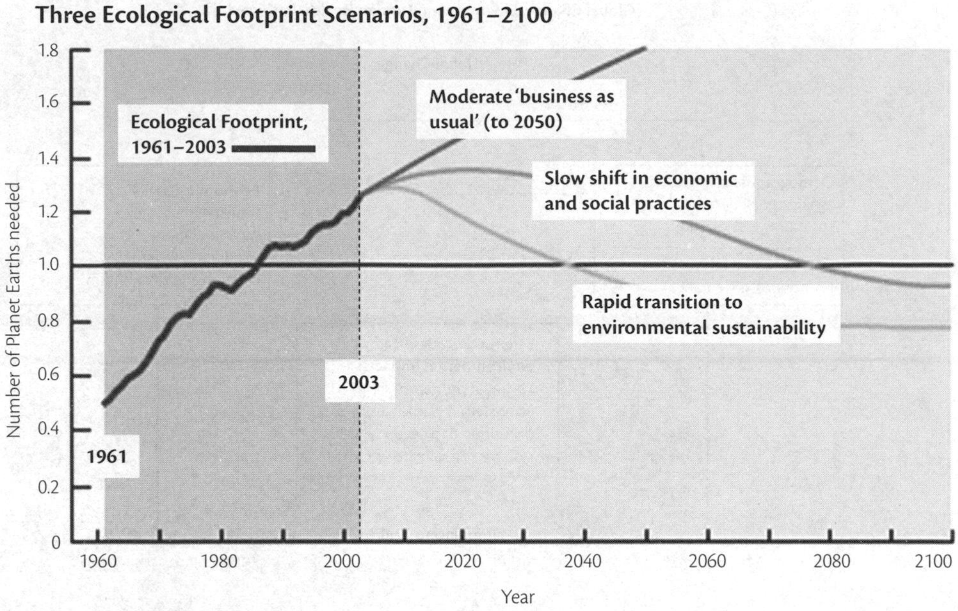

Fig. 2.8.2 Estimated time-trends in the total human ecological footprint, expressed as the changing number of Planet Earths needed for 1961–2003 (data-based) and 2003–2100 (scenario-based) (WWF International 2006).

International trade, globalization, and health

Historically, various environmental health hazards have arisen from rapid urban immigration (where crowding and poor sanitation can amplify infectious disease transmission, for example) and from localized pollution due to the rapid expansion of poorly regulated industry. Many of these hazards have been of a relatively simple, direct-acting, kind. Today, increasingly, intensive international trade, especially in food and therapeutic goods, presents new and complex challenges to global environmental health.

Food producers are under increasing pressure to be economically competitive—usually to produce the most food for the least cost. Increasingly mechanized production may be economically cheap in conventional market terms, but it often requires more energy to produce the food than is available from the food produced. The environmental consequences, many of which pose health risks, include a growing contribution to global greenhouse gas emissions (FAO 2006). Other intensive farming practices, such as the use of hormones and antibiotics to promote animal growth, can both damage the environment and produce food that is potentially unsafe.

Today's 'factory farmed' meat has a very different lipid profile from the wild-animal meat that was consumed during much of our species' evolutionary history. The latter type of meat has much lower saturated fat content and is higher in omega-3 fatty acids (the so-called 'fish oils') (McMichael 2005). Further, people in many countries are now consuming considerably more meat (currently 125 kg annually per capita in the United States) (Brown 2005) than would have been available in earlier times, and they expend less energy to get it. This systemic energy imbalance in our modern way of life further underpins the global obesity epidemic.

Industrial agriculture, now spreading worldwide with ever increasing pressure to become more and more economically 'efficient' poses additional health risks via the extensive use of fertilizers and pesticides, feed formulations that include animal tissues, arsenic and antibiotics, and the consequent environmental pollution (Bambrick 2004). Complex and 'unnatural' food chains—whereby herbivores such as cattle are fed the remains of other animals—continues in some countries (and indeed is deemed to be acceptable practice under international standards applied by the World Trade Organization). Such practices continue despite the UK 'mad cow' (bovine spongiform encephalopathy) epidemic disaster of the 1990s. That economic and public health disaster was caused by feeding mammalian (cattle and sheep) offal to cattle—and it resulted in the transmission of the novel infectious agent, or prion, to human consumers, causing the neurodegenerative disorder 'variant Creutzfeldt–Jakob disease' (Nathanson *et al.* 1997).

Chickens are commonly fed fish-meal from unintended by-catch, much of which is shark that is so high in mercury content that it is unfit for human consumption (Bambrick & Kjellström 2004). Insufficient research attention has been paid to studying the human health risks that might result from eating such chickens, or their eggs. Similarly intensive practices are being applied, increasingly, to various forms of aquaculture, with the same potential for contamination of the human food supply. Where aquaculture employs netted enclosures in the open ocean, antibiotics, pesticides, and disease can spread freely to non-farmed areas.

Food, as an increasingly global commodity, often has such complex and multidirectional pathways that it obscures the origins of individual ingredients in manufactured items. This poses difficulties of four main kinds: (i) Identifying an outbreak (which may occur in disseminated fashion) of a food-borne disease; (ii) responding to it by recalling all affected items; (iii) determining where in the supply chain the contamination occurred; and (iv) implementing prevention, since legislation at the place of origin may be inadequate or not enforceable.

Even as these various economic pressures and practices in an increasingly competitive global marketplace are jeopardizing various aspects of foods safety, the international trade rules applied by the World Trade Organization seriously limit the capacity of individual countries to employ domestic legislation to protect public health (such as by restricting imports) (Bambrick 2004). Such trade agreements seek primarily to limit non-tariff barriers to trade. However, they may also erode food safety, because nations importing food are discouraged from setting regulatory standards higher than the often low standards of the exporting nation.

Similar problems—complexity in origin, multidirectional trade, and pressures to reduce regulatory standards—exist in the international trading of therapeutic goods, including human blood and plasma products. For example, some rich countries rely on blood and plasma purchased from the poor in developing countries, both to shore up their national supply and to manufacture blood-derived therapeutic products for subsequent export (Bambrick *et al.* 2006).

Global environmental change: Definition, context, significance

Human pressures on the Earth System

The various above-mentioned human-induced changes to natural environmental (biophysical and ecological) systems are a consequence of the aggregated regional and global pressures exerted by the continuing growth in human population size and economic activity. They accompany, and to some extent are caused by, aspects of 'globalization', as social, economic, cultural, technological, and political connectedness increases among human societies around the world. The total environmental impact of humankind is now so great that it is inducing changes in components of the Earth System (Millennium Ecosystem Assessment 2005). For key environmental parameters, the Earth System has recently moved well outside the range of natural variability that applied over the last half million years or so. This is unprecedented in human experience.

The Earth System is now becoming a major focus of interdisciplinary study. It is a self-regulating system that comprises physical, chemical, biological, and human components. The interactions and feedbacks between component parts of the geosphere and biosphere are complex and exhibit multi-scale temporal and spatial variability. Recently, and for the first time, human activities have begun significantly to alter Earth's atmosphere, land surface, oceans, coasts, biological diversity, hydrological and biogeochemical cycles. These anthropogenic changes are now equalling some of Nature's great forces in extent and impact. Human activities have, for example, approximately doubled the amount of activated nitrogen (ammonia and other nitrogen compounds) that is produced each year. Many of these global environmental changes (GEC), including global climate change (Rahmstorf *et al.* 2007)—appear to be accelerating.

The manifestations of these changes are many. Forest cover is declining in many tropical regions. There is a widespread and continuing loss of productive agricultural and pastoral soil on all continents. With industrialized fishing fleets, we have over-fished most of the large ocean fisheries. Farming and industrial activities have severely depleted many of the great aquifers upon which the future of irrigated agriculture and urban sustainability depends. The widespread use of nitrogenous fertilizer, along with fossil fuel combustion, has doubled the rate at which activated nitrogenous compounds enter the global environment. Most irreversible of all, human pressures are extinguishing whole species and many local populations at an historically unprecedented overall rate. Indeed, we are, in reality, perpetrating the Sixth Great Extinction to have occurred since vertebrate life emerged on Earth around a half billion years ago (Leakey & Lewin 1995).

These GECs represent a reduction in the capacity of the natural environment to supply and replenish resources, absorb, and recycle the wastes products of the activities of humans and other animals (e.g. cattle, pigs), and to provide climatic–environmental stability and physical buffering processes. This diminution of capacity results from changes to the structure, composition, and function of Earth's biophysical and ecological systems (i.e. 'life-support systems').

Box 2.8.1 the main types of global environmental changes

- Changes to atmospheric composition and, therefore, function:
  - Greenhouse gas accumulation, leading to climate change
  - Stratospheric ozone depletion
- Changes to food-producing ecosystems:
  - Land cover, soil fertility
  - Coastal and marine ecosystem stocks
- Biodiversity changes:
  - Loss/extinction
  - Redistribution (invasion)
- Internal rearrangements (balance)
- Changes to cycles of elements (especially N, P, S)—in addition to the carbon cycle (climate change)
- Changes to the hydrological cycle, and depletion of freshwater supplies
- World-wide dissemination of persistent organic pollutants (POPs)
- Urbanization
- Desertification

Global environmental changes: Types, inter-relations

The various GECs that are symptoms of this human overloading of the Earth System are listed in Box 2.8.1. They are 'global' in one or other of two senses. Some, such as climate change and stratospheric ozone destruction, are spatially integrated at world scale. Others such as species extinctions and land degradation occur via the worldwide aggregation of local changes.

Figure 2.8.3 illustrates the main pathways by which GECs can affect human health (Earth System Science Partnership 2006). Neither the set of pathways nor the categories of health impacts shown are exhaustive. For example, many of the impacts shown would also be associated with mental health problems (e.g. post-traumatic stress disorders, suicides), while other environmental changes would result in conflicts or refugee flows in response to depleted resources. In the complex real world of human politics and culture there are also, of course, many important modulating 'non-environmental' influences on these GEC-related health risks.

The area with particular need for research is shown within the grey-shaded rectangle. Much research remains to be done on the health consequences of stratospheric ozone depletion and global climate change. However, that research domain needs less 'affirmative action' than do the relationships shown in the grey area—many of which are intrinsically complex, entailing perturbations of ecosystems and feedbacks between concurrent environmental change processes. Some of the complexity inherent in tackling the health impacts of global environmental change is discussed in Box 2.8.2.

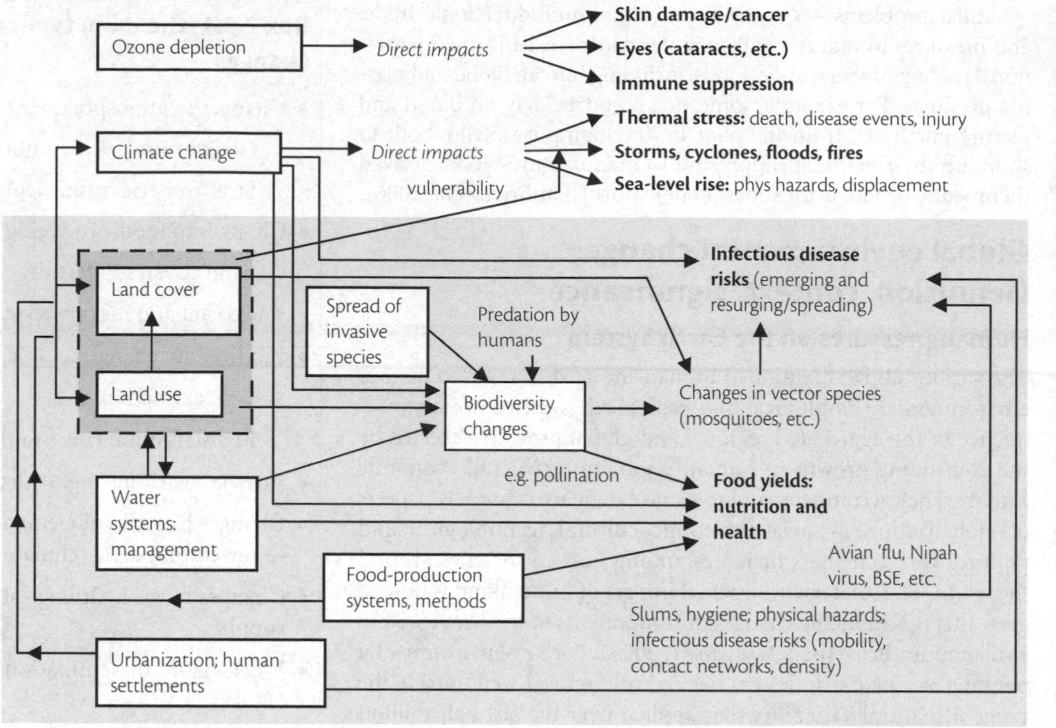

Fig. 2.8.3 Schematic diagram of the main types of biogeophysical pathways by which Global Environmental Changes (shown in red) can affect human health. From Earth System Science Partnership: Global Environmental Change and Human Health project (2006).

Box 2.8.2 Millennium Development Goals: The nexus between GECs, sustainability, human well-being, and health

At the turn of the century, the United Nations embraced a set of eight Millennium Development Goals (United Nations 2000). The first six of these seek reductions in poverty, illiteracy, gender inequality, malnutrition, child deaths, maternal mortality, and major infectious diseases. The seventh goal seeks 'environmental sustainability'. While highlighting several areas of major challenge to human health, this itemization of goals creates a disconnect that all-too-easily separates environmental considerations from health considerations.

Poverty, for example, cannot be eliminated against a counter-current of degraded and non-productive environments, especially when the environmental deficits impinge primarily on the poor and exacerbate the risks of disease. Likewise, adequate food and freshwater supplies require soil fertility, climatic stability, river flows, and various ecological functions (e.g. pollination). Infectious diseases cannot be contained in conditions of climatic instability, land disturbance, environmental refugee flows, and environment-related poverty.

Further, the goal of 'environmental sustainability' must extend well beyond addressing traditional, long-standing, physical, chemical, and microbiological hazards in local environments—even though those exposures remain important, particularly as accompaniments to industrialization and urbanization in lower income countries, and have the greatest impact on poor and vulnerable communities (Butler & McMichael 2005). Lower income groups have been most affected by air pollution in Sao Paulo, leaded house paint in inner-urban USA, and isocyanate poisoning in Bhopal, for example (McMichael 2002). These localized hazards, while serious, are remediable; they do not entail an enduring, perhaps permanent, loss of natural environmental capital.

The health risks from *global* environmental changes also impinge unequally, both within and between populations. Further, the health risk disparities due to climate change, agroecosystem degradation, freshwater shortages, and other GECs may well increase in coming decades, reflecting differences in location, economic conditions, social and human resources, political power, and the extent of direct dependency on local environments (Prüss-Üstün & Corvalán 2006). Most arable land has now been privatized, and access to stocks of wild species (fish, land-animals, wild plants) is declining as population pressures and commercial activities intensify. Freshwater is increasingly being privatized as natural sources become depleted or degraded.

Health risks from global environmental changes

Climate change

Global climate change is the most widely recognized of the GECs. It is becoming generally understood that our prevailing pattern of energy generation and use, and of agricultural (including livestock) production, is increasing the concentration of energy-trapping (greenhouse) gases in the lower atmosphere. That additional trapped energy manifests as heat, which then warms the Earth's surface. This human-driven increment in the atmosphere's natural 'greenhouse' capacity (which achieves a warming of around 33°C) keeps the planet comfortably above freezing point. The human-generated greenhouse gases comprise, principally, carbon dioxide, methane, nitrous oxide, and industrial halocarbons.

The reality of human-induced climate change is now largely agreed by climate scientists around the world. Nevertheless, many details remain in relation to process, timing, and the uncertainty of critical thresholds that may be reached. The Fourth Assessment Report of the Intergovernmental Panel on Climate Change (IPCC 2007) concludes that there is at least 90 per cent certainty that the unusual warming in recent decades has been mostly due to human actions.

During the last century, the world's average surface temperature increased by approximately 0.6°C; two-thirds of that warming occurred after 1975. Other evidence shows that climate variability has increased in various regions. Further warming of 1.8–4.0°C (including another 0.6°C rise already in the pipeline) is forecast for this century (Fig. 2.8.4). The actual outcome will depend largely on how human societies adjust their energy metabolism and agricultural practices over coming decades. Rainfall patterns will also change. Importantly, there will also be a generalized increase in variability of weather patterns, although this will itself vary by geographic region. Indeed, all these anticipated changes in climatic conditions will vary by region.

The IPCC's Fourth Assessment Report is, a year or two further on, widely viewed as being rather conservative in its projections. In large part this reflects the fact that it had necessarily had a 'cut-off' date for admissible published evidence in early 2006. Subsequent evidence during 2006–2007 has pointed to an apparent acceleration in emissions, warming, glacier melting, and sea level rise (Rahmstorf *et al.* 2007).

This ongoing warming is affecting physical and biotic systems. More than 90 per cent of the significant changes to physical and biological systems observed since 1970 are consistent with warming (IPCC 2007b). Ice-sheets are melting faster than foreshadowed in the previous assessment; long-term drying is already emerging in southern and western Africa, southern Europe, India, and Australia (IPCC 2007a). The seasonal cycles of birds, bugs, butterflies, bears, and buds are changing, and are getting out of kilter with one another: Many finely tuned ecological systems are becoming uncoupled (IPCC 2007b).

Much early public discussion about climate change focused on risks to economic growth, physical infrastructure, and recreational amenities. The real risk is more profound. Climate change is a serious threat to the physical and ecological systems upon which biological function and health depend. That is, it endangers health and life on Earth. From an anthropocentric view, the public health task is to address prevention at two distinct levels. The essential primary prevention task, by definition, is to reduce global greenhouse gas emissions. However, since climate change is already occurring and more change is inevitable ('committed'), we must also develop strategies to lessen the adverse impacts on health.

Health effects of climate change

The health effects of global climate change are, in small part, with us already—but are difficult to identify and attribute at this early stage. Now and, increasingly, in the future, they will occur via various direct and indirect pathways (see Fig. 2.8.5, and also Fig. 2.8.3) (McMichael 2006). Some effects would be immediate, some would be delayed. The impacts will vary between regions and populations,

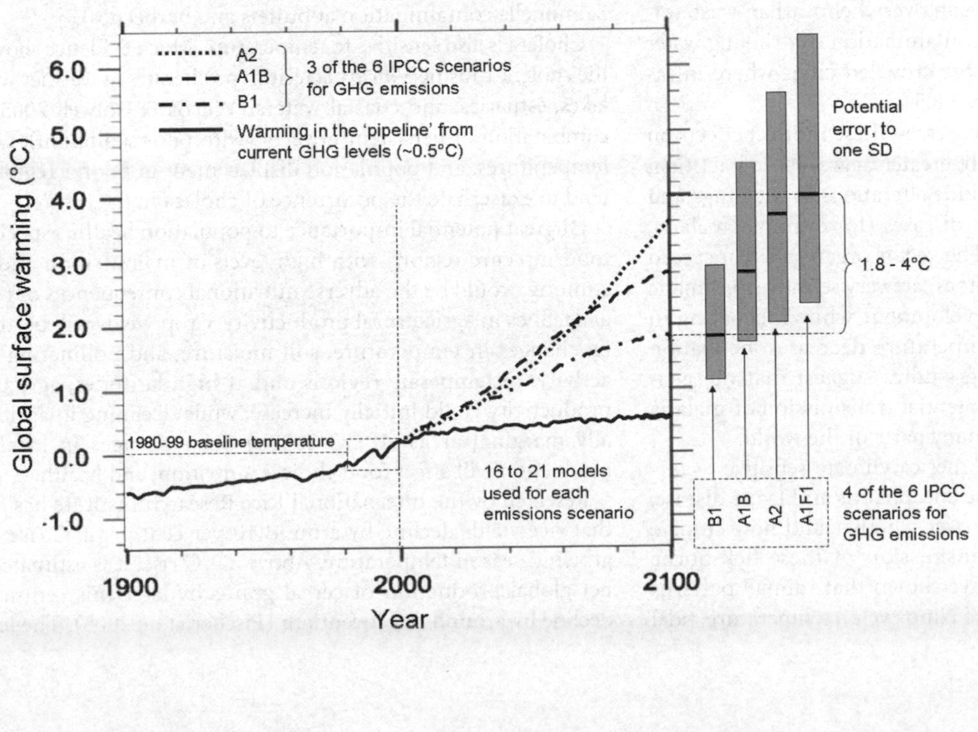

Fig. 2.8.4 Recent and projected (modelled) future change in average Earth-surface temperature.
Source: modified from IPCC Fourth Assessment Report (Meehl *et al.* 2007). The four scenarios included here span the full range (1.8–4.0°C) between the best (central) estimates of the six scenarios used in the original modelling.

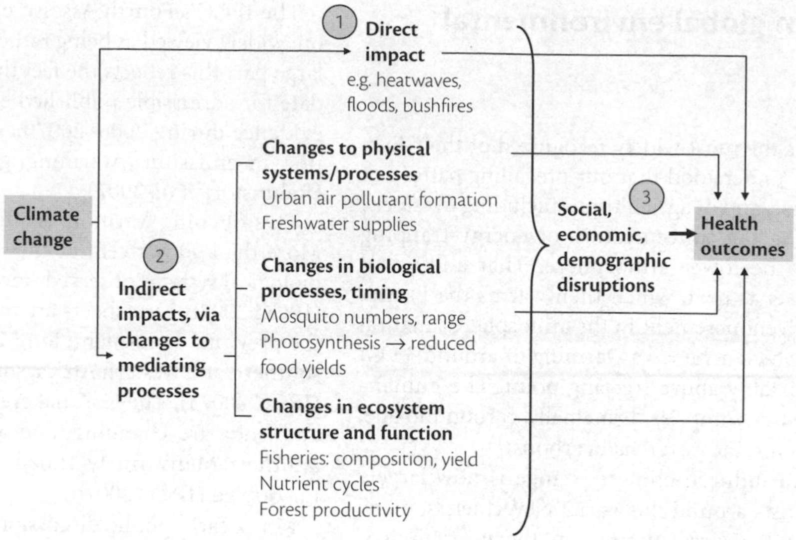

Fig. 2.8.5 Schema of main pathways by which climate change can affect human health.

in particular as a function of the geographic pattern of climatic trends and events and the vulnerability of the local population, which would be affected by, for example, the underlying burden of chronic disease, poverty levels, and the capacity of local infrastructure to respond to environmental change.

Some health outcomes in some populations would be beneficial. For example, some low-latitude regions may become too hot for mosquitoes, and winter cold periods would become milder in various temperate-zone countries where death rates currently tend to peak in wintertime. However, there is a broad consensus that most of the anticipated health effects of climate change would be adverse (McMichael 2006; IPCC 2007b). The direct health effects would include changes in mortality and morbidity from altered exposures to thermal extremes; the respiratory health (including asthma) consequences of increased exposures to photochemical pollutants and aeroallergens; and the physical hazards of the increased occurrence of storms, floods, or droughts, in at least some regions. Intensified rainfall, with flooding, can overwhelm urban wastewater and sewer systems, leading to contamination of drinking water supplies. This is most likely in large crowded cities where infrastructure is old or inadequate (Box 2.8.3).

Over time, as climate change progresses, these indirect effects on health are likely to have a relatively greater aggregate impact than the direct effects. These would include alterations in the range and activity of vector-borne infectious diseases (for example, malaria, dengue fever, and leishmaniasis). The vector organisms that spread these diseases (for example, mosquitoes) are very sensitive to climatic conditions, as is the parasite's development while incubating in the vector: Increased ambient temperature decreases incubation period. Scenario-based modelling studies suggest that the geographic zone and seasonality of potential transmission of malaria and dengue fever will increase in many parts of the world.

In temperate Europe and North America, climate-sensitive vector-borne infections include tick-borne encephalitis and Lyme disease. There is uncertainty, and debate, over whether and how climate change will affect patterns of transmission of these tick-borne infections. In Australia, studies have shown that rainfall patterns (especially in association with the El Niño cycle), temperature, tidal movements, and the ecology of vertebrate host species influence outbreaks of mosquito-borne Ross River virus disease, the major Australian arboviral infection.

Changes in climatic conditions will also affect the rates of transmission of many person-to-person infections, especially food- and water-borne pathogens. *Salmonella*, and various other bacteria that cause food poisoning, proliferate more rapidly at higher temperatures. A weaker seasonal relationship exists for infection by *Campylobacter*. Diverse studies have shown that short-term temperature increases are followed by increased notifications of non-specific food-poisoning in the United Kingdom (Bentham & Langford 2001) and of diarrhoeal diseases in Peru and Fiji (Checkley *et al.* 2000; Singh *et al.* 2001). Simple monotonic associations exist between temperature and salmonellosis notifications in European countries (Kovats *et al.* 2004) and Australia (D'Souza *et al.* 2004). Outdoor temperatures might also affect exposures via seasonal changes in eating patterns (e.g. eating foods more prone to Salmonella contamination at buffets and barbecues).

Cholera is also sensitive to temperature. Much evidence shows that the cholera-causing *Vibrio* bacterium proliferates in warmer water in lakes, estuaries, and coastal waters (Wilcox & Colwell 2005). The combination of persistent poverty (with poor sanitation), warmer temperatures, and population displacement in poorer regions will tend to exacerbate the occurrence of cholera in the future.

Of great potential importance to population health, especially in food-insecure regions with high levels of malnutrition and child stunting, would be the adverse nutritional consequences of regional declines in agricultural productivity. Crop yields will be affected by changes in temperature, soil moisture, and pollinating insect activity. In temperate regions and at high latitudes, agricultural productivity could initially increase, while declining in agriculturally marginal areas (IPCC 2007b) Such changes in local food production will affect food choices, nutrition, and health.

Research by the International Rice Research Institute has shown that rice yields decline by around 10 per cent per 1°C rise in the growing-season temperature. Above a 3°C rise, it is estimated that net global production of cereal grains by later this century will decline by around one-twentieth (Fischer *et al.* 2005). The level of

Box 2.8.3 Climate change will exacerbate existing health inequalities

The impact of climate change will differ between rich and poor countries. It will disproportionately affect diseases which already place major health burdens on poorer countries. Many of the 30 most significant causes of premature death around the world are closely linked with the environment and will be substantially and directly affected by climate change (Fig. 2.8.6). Poor countries already suffer many times the burden than richer countries.

Malaria, for example, leads to more than 10 000 times as many years of life lost in the poorest 20 per cent of countries than in the richest 20 per cent. Deaths among young children from diarrhoeal disease and from malnutrition—both closely related to climate—are likely to increase with further stress on water supplies and reduced crop yields. Many other important causes could be affected indirectly; increased depression and suicide among rural populations and farmers with prolonged drought, or more deaths resulting from wars over scarcer resources. Other mosquito-borne diseases and diarrhoeal diseases are responsible for between one and three thousand times more years of life lost in the poorest compared to the richest countries and, being directly dependent on climate, are predicted to increase with climate change.

The poorest countries will not only be exposed to heightened disease risks from climate change, but will have least capacity to adapt technologically, and their health systems will be least able to respond.

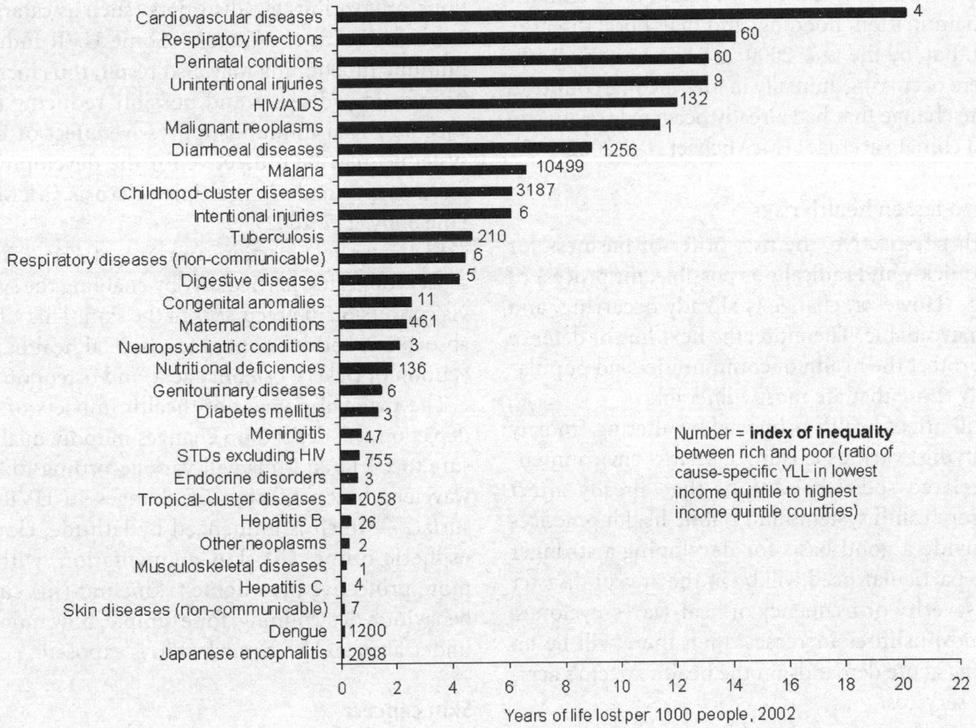

Fig. 2.8.6 The 30 most significant causes of permature death worldwide (years of life lost: YLL), and also showing an index of inequality between rich and poor countries. YLL data from WHO (2007).

decline in many already food-insecure populations in low-latitude regions is estimated at around 10–20 per cent (Lobell & Field 2007). Droughts and floods could further impair local production. Declines are also projected for wild fisheries and, perhaps, aquaculture production (IPCC 2007b).

There is a potentially very large, but more diffuse and harder-to-quantify, category of risk to health. Climate change will inevitably adversely affect physical and psychological health in the wake of loss of livelihoods, displacement of population, and economic disruption. This will occur particularly because of rising sea levels (for example, small island states, coastal Bangladesh, and the Nile Delta), agroecosystem decline, and freshwater shortages.

Detecting health impacts

Initially, most climate-induced health impacts will be difficult to detect. If an ice-sheet melts it must be because its environment is warmer. If plants flower early, that almost certainly reflects changed climatic conditions. However, evidence that malaria is moving higher in East African highlands (Patz *et al.* 2002) could reflect the associated warming—or it could reflect changes in land use, population movements, mosquito spray programmes, antimalarial drug resistance, or all of the above.

Further, human health is often well buffered by culture, behaviour, and healthcare. The signal is thus hidden. For example, if climate change affects local grain yields, then (unlike polar bears no longer able to catch prey because of the receding ice floes) humans can trade or switch to other crops. Either the evidence or the actual occurrence of health impact can thus be masked or deferred, making detection more difficult.

Various infectious diseases are quite probably now responding to climatic changes. Viewed together, the recent shifts in physical range of malaria (sub-Saharan Africa), tick-borne encephalitis (Sweden), and the schistosomiasis water-snail (eastern China)—all associated with warming—and the changing seasonal and inter-annual pattern of some enteric bacterial infections (cholera, other vibrios, salmonellosis) suggest that climate change is now affecting at least some infectious diseases (McMichael *et al.* 2006; McMichael & Woodruff 2007).

Meanwhile, using a rather conservative statistical formula confined to four causes of death with known relations to climatic variables (malaria, malnutrition, flooding, and diarrhoeal disease), WHO has estimated that, by the year 2000, around 150 000 deaths from those causes were occurring annually in low-income countries because of the climate change that had already occurred (relative to the 1961–1990 global climate average) (McMichael *et al.* 2002).

Adaptive strategies to lessen health risks

From a public health perspective, the first order of business for society is to curb, as quickly and radically as possible, the process of global climate change. However, change is already occurring, and some more is now unavoidable. Therefore, the next line of defence is to take actions to protect the health of communities and populations, and particularly those that are most vulnerable.

Climate change will affect health primarily by altering (mostly increasing or intensifying) various existing climatic–environmental exposures and related social conditions that already affect human health. Existing health systems and public health practices should therefore provide a good basis for developing a stronger coping capacity. One particular need will be in the area of disaster preparedness. If the severity or frequency of heat-waves, cyclones, floods, landslides, and bushfires increases, then there will be an increase in the episodic acute demands on the health system's accident-and-emergency services.

To achieve long-term effectiveness of health protection, however, adaptive strategies will be needed that extend across sectors. These would include:

- Public education about the health risks of climate change;
- Early-alert systems for impending weather extremes;
- Community-based neighbourhood support/watch schemes;
- Better (i.e. climate-proofed) housing design and urban planning;
- Disaster preparedness, and an enhanced health-system 'surge' capacity;
- Expanded infectious disease control programmes (vaccines, vector control, rapid case treatment);
- Improved surveillance of risk-indicators and health outcomes; and
- Appropriate workforce training and career development.

Stratospheric ozone depletion

Stratospheric ozone depletion is a separate phenomenon from greenhouse gas accumulation in the lower atmosphere (troposphere). It results in an increase in ultraviolet irradiation (UVR) at the Earth's surface. The major ozone-destroying chemicals, chlorofluorocarbons (CFCs), have been used as refrigerants and propellants since the 1920s. They were first suspected of damaging atmospheric ozone in the 1970s. Rapid international response ensued, with the signing of the Vienna Convention for Protection of the Ozone Layer in 1985, followed by the Montreal Protocol in 1987 mandating a global phasing out of CFCs. Compliance has been good, though not complete.

Because of their long atmospheric lifetimes, the increase in UVR exposure is yet to peak, sometime within the next decade, and then decline slowly back to normal levels by around mid-century. Meanwhile, the increased exposure to the ultraviolet B radiation (UBV) is expected to cause slight increases in the severity of sunburn and the incidence of skin cancers in fair-skinned populations, and various eye disorders (such as cataracts) are expected to increase (Lucas *et al.* 2006). Some UVR-induced suppression of immune functioning may also result, thus increasing susceptibility to infectious diseases and possibly reducing the efficacy of some vaccines. That immunosuppressive effect of UVR, both local and systemic, may be protective for the development of autoimmune diseases, particularly multiple sclerosis (McMichael & Hall 1997; Ponsonby *et al.* 2002).

Exposure to a certain amount of UVR is beneficial to other aspects of health, particularly by enabling the synthesis of vitamin D via conversion of precursors in the skin. This vitamin assists calcium absorption and is essential for skeletal health, particularly the prevention of rickets, osteomalacia, and osteoporosis.

The regional population health impacts of stratospheric ozone depletion will depend on changes in individual-level received exposure to UVR, and this will vary according to: (i) the amount and wavelength constitution of changes in UVR flux at the Earth's surface—which is influenced by latitude, cloud cover, and stratospheric ozone; (ii) skin pigmentation, with darker skin being more protective than lighter skin; and (iii) cultural practices and behaviour, determining, for example, how much outdoor activity is undertaken and how much skin is exposed.

Skin cancers

Estimates made in the 1990s indicated that the increased exposure to UBV would cause basal cell carcinoma incidence to increase, temporarily, by around 15–20 per cent at mid–high latitudes, but to increase very much less at intermediate latitudes. The estimated percentage increases in incidence of squamous cell carcinoma would be twice as great as for basal cell carcinoma. One widely cited study, using integrated mathematical modelling, estimated that non-melanoma skin cancer rates would rise to a peak excess incidence of approximately 10 per cent in the United States and Europe around the middle of the twenty-first century (Slaper *et al.* 1996).

Eye health

Acute exposure to a high dose of UVB results in acute inflammation of the cornea and conjunctiva (photokeratitis and photoconjunctivitis or snow blindness). Chronic exposure is one risk factor for the development of pterygium (a fleshy, wing-shaped growth on the eye's medial surface).

Cataracts are extremely common among older age groups in some populations and cause visual impairment, ranging up to complete blindness. They are associated with an increased risk of mortality in both developed and developing countries. Chronic UVR exposure, especially to UVB, appears to be an important cause of cortical and posterior subcapsular cataract, whereas intense exposure in childhood and young adulthood may cause nuclear cataracts (Neale *et al.* 2003). Even a marginal impact of increased UVB exposure on the incidence of already-common cataract would significantly affect population health.

Indirect and ecological effects

A potentially important, although indirect, health detriment could arise from UVB-induced impairment of photosynthesis on land (terrestrial plants) and at sea (phytoplankton, as the base of the marine food web). Although such effects could reduce the world's food yields, few relevant data are yet available.

Biodiversity: Losses and invasions

Through humankind's spectacular reproductive and technological 'success', the natural habitats of many other species have been occupied, damaged, or eliminated. Biologists estimate that this ongoing human-induced mass extinction may cause extinction of around one-third of all species alive in the 1800s by the end of this century (Pimm *et al.* 1995). The rate of species loss in today's world is three to four orders of magnitude faster than the natural background rate of extinction.

The loss of various key species would weaken whole ecosystems. This would have consequences that would often be adverse to human interests, such as changing the ecology of vector-borne infections and of food-producing systems that depend on pollinators and the predation of pests, and impairing the cleansing of water and the circulation of nutrients that normally cycle through ecosystems. Much genetic and phenotypic material would also be lost. To maintain the hybrid vigour and environmental resilience of 'food' species, a diversity of wild species is needed as a source of genetic additives. Further, a high proportion of modern medicinal drugs in Western medicine has natural origins, and many defy synthesis in the laboratory. Scientists test thousands of novel natural chemicals each year, seeking new drugs to treat HIV, malaria, drug-resistant tuberculosis, and cancers.

The obverse of this problem of species losses is the accelerating spread of 'invasive' species. This is occurring particularly in response to environmental disturbance and change and to the increased intensity of long-distance trade, tourism, and migration. These are discussed further, below. Another example comes from the vast proliferation of water hyacinth (a decorative plant from Brazil) in Lake Victoria, eastern Africa, which has reportedly extended the breeding grounds for the water snail that transmits schistosomiasis.

Field studies have shown how depletion of certain mammalian species within complex ecological communities boosts the intensity of replication and transmission of certain microbes that can infect humans (e.g. the spirochaete *Borrelia burgdorferi* that causes Lyme Disease), or leads to a greater exposure of humans, no longer protected by other biteable targets, to disease-transmitting mosquitoes (Dobson *et al.* 2006).

Land-use and sea-use changes: Consequences for food and malnutrition

The increase in land degradation has great implications for food supplies and therefore for nutrition, child growth and (physical and neurocognitive) development, and health. During recent decades the combination of erosion, desiccation, and nutrient exhaustion, plus irrigation-induced water-logging and salinization, has seriously degraded up to around one-third of the world's 1.5 billion hectares of readily arable farmland (Millennium Ecosystem Assessment 2005).

The 'Green Revolution', which fed much of the expanding human population during the 1960s to the 1980s, depended on laboratory-bred, high-yield cereal grains, fertilizers, groundwater, and arable soils. In retrospect, those productivity gains appear to have come substantially at the expense of using up environmental and ecological 'capital'—especially topsoil and groundwater. Today, as greater food yields are pursued to feed an increasing population, an estimated 850 million people are malnourished (FAO 2005).

Meanwhile, at sea, many of the world's great fisheries are now on the brink of being overexploited. The United Nations' Food and Agriculture Organization (FAO) estimates that the sustainable fish-catch limit has been neared—around 100 million tonnes per year (FAO 2002).

Changes to global element cycles (e.g. nitrogen and phosphorus)

An under-remarked category of global environmental change is the changing and intensification of cycling of elements and associated compounds through the biosphere. There is an emerging view among expert scientists that the build-up of activated nitrogen (ammonia and other nitrogen compounds) is beginning to pose a substantial threat to the composition and functioning of aspects of the natural world around us. The agricultural (including livestock) sector is a major source of disturbance to these global and regional cycles.

Intensive agriculture affects water quality not only by increasing the sediment load, but by leaching nutrients and agricultural chemicals and toxic chemicals into streams and rivers. Since 1960, there has been a sevenfold increase, globally, in fertilizer application and a 70 per cent increase in irrigated cropland area (Millennium Ecosystem Assessment 2005; Earth System Science Partnership 2006). Agricultural fertilizer use and livestock excreta comprise the largest source of excess nitrogen and phosphorus entering waterways and coastal zones. Indeed, humans now generate as much biologically activated nitrogen as do all of Nature's pathways—volcanoes, lightning, vegetation, and others. Indeed, the human contribution, especially from nitrogenous fertilizers, is on track to increase by a further 65 per cent by 2050. We are thereby changing the chemistry of soils and waterways widely around the world.

This poses various risks to human health, both direct and indirect, including:

- Diminished crop yields (soil nitrification and acidity), posing risks to nutritional sufficiency
- Eutrophication (nitrates and phosphates) of waterways, potentiating cholera outbreaks (via planktonic blooms, the natural reservoir for the cholera vibrio)
- Stomach cancer (nitrate ingestion)—long hypothesized, but not clearly resolved

- Nitrogen oxides as ambient (and domestic) air pollutants
- Methaemoglobinaemia ('blue babies')

Depletion of freshwater supplies

The issue of large-scale changes in the supply and quality of freshwater is fundamental to the health of the environment, and it has intersections with various other global environmental changes (Millennium Ecosystem Assessment 2005). The basic problem, of course, is that the growth in human numbers and the intensification of industrial and food production processes (irrigation, livestock production, etc.) means that the renewable supply of freshwater in many parts of the world is now being exceeded. Hence the diminution of flows in many great rivers, and the decline in aquifers (including 'fossil water' from the previous glaciations).

As the world's climate changes, mountain glaciers are shrinking on all continents, and some river flows are, therefore, being diminished. Further, in a warmer world, run-off from rain is affected, both because evaporation is more rapid and soil surfaces have undergone change.

Freshwater is critical to many aspects of health: Domestic hygiene, food production, food processing and cooking, and sanitation systems. The storage of freshwater has consequences for mosquito populations and, hence, diseases such as malaria and dengue fever. The building of canals (e.g. in China) affects the probabilities of spread of water-snails and, hence, schistosomiasis.

The Millennium Assessment (2005) concludes that:

> *Current patterns of human use of water are unsustainable. From 5% to possibly 25% of global freshwater use exceeds long-term accessible supplies and is met through engineered water transfers or the overdraft of groundwater supplies. More than one billion people live in areas without appreciable supplies of renewable freshwater and meet their water needs in this way.*

Persistent organic pollutants

Various chemical pollutants, particularly the chlorinated organic chemicals such as the polychlorinated biphenyls (PCBs), persist within the environment and have become globally pervasive. They are referred to as persistent organic pollutants, or 'POPs'. The semi-volatile members of this class of chemicals undergo a type of serial distillation process in the atmosphere, as they pass from 'cell' to 'cell', moving from low to high latitudes. Via this intriguing process, they ultimately emerge at higher concentrations in living creatures at the circumpolar regions than in their counterpart at lower latitudes where the chemicals are produced, used, and released.

Some of these environmentally persistent chemicals are likely to affect neurological, immune, and reproductive systems in humans, who obtain their food at the top of the increasingly contaminated food chain. Weakening of ecosystems—as perhaps foreseen by Rachel Carson in *Silent Spring* in 1962—may also occur, resulting in various flow-on environmental health effects in human populations.

GECs and infectious disease: A global transition in human–microbe relations?

There has been a recent and continuing increase in tempo in the emergence and spread of infectious diseases in human populations. This has occurred since the mid-1970s, across all continents. Approximately 40 previously unknown or unrecognized infectious diseases in humans have been identified (Institute of Medicine 2003).

In the decade between 1994 and 2003, the following human infectious diseases have emerged:

2003	Severe acute respiratory syndrome (SARS)
1999	Nipah virus
1997	H5N1 flu virus (avian influenza) Variant Creutzfeldt–Jakob disease (human 'mad cow disease')
	Australian bat lyssavirus
1995	Human herpes virus 8 (Kaposi sarcoma virus)
1994	Sabia virus (Brazil) Hendra virus

This development suggests that, today, a critical combination of social and technological change, intensity of human action, and disruption of environments is creating a new round of ecological opportunities for many previously unknown or unrecognized infectious agents (see also Box 2.8.4). That combination includes: Increased human mobility, more long-distance trade, intensification of food production, more large dam and irrigation projects, accelerating urbanization, extended sexual contact networks, antibiotic over-use, expanding numbers of refugees, and the exacerbation of poverty in inner-urban ghettos, shanty towns, and in poor undernourished populations everywhere. All these trends have great consequences for the emergence and spread of infectious diseases (Weiss & McMichael 2004).

The intensification of livestock production provides an important example. We have seen the emergence in recent decades of various new infectious agents that have crossed from 'food' animals to humans—such as mad cow disease (bovine spongiform encephalopathy) and its human variant Creutzfeldt–Jakob disease, Nipah virus disease (from pig farming in Malaysia), severe acute respiratory syndrome (SARS) apparently from animals brought into the wet food markets of East Asia, and highly pathogenic H5N1 avian influenza apparently from poultry production processes in southern China and Southeast Asia.

These outbreaks reflect, more generally, the transformation and intensification of agriculture and livestock production, especially 'factory farming' on a large scale. Industrialized crop and animal production is increasing rapidly near the urban centres of Asia, Africa, and Latin America. In this way the traditional relations between small farmers, their animals, and the local environment are being broken, disrupting environments, livelihoods and community structures, and mobilizing 'new' human-infecting microbes—and often in socioeconomic and political environments that are slow to detect and respond to a new threat.

As humans encroach further into pristine environments, new contacts between wild fauna, insect vectors, domesticated livestock, and humans occur. This increases the risk of cross-species infection. An example of such contact followed the establishment of large commercial piggeries close to the tropical forest in Perak, northern Malaysia. There, in 1997–98, the Nipah virus first crossed over from fruit bats (flying foxes, *Pteropus* species) to pigs and thence to pig farmers (Daszak *et al.* 2006). That zoonotic infection illustrates how the conjunction of intensified animal husbandry in association with large-scale environmental change and ecosystem disruption can potentiate a new zoonotic infection. In that case, forest-clearing and, perhaps, El Niño regional drying reduced the natural forest fruit supplies for bats, the natural reservoir of the virus. The presence of pig-farming, in cleared forest settings with associated fruit orchards, acted as an alternative food source for the bats, which then infected the pigs and, thence, the pig farmers.

More generally, the clearance and fragmentation of forest has increased the exposure of rural populations in low-income countries to a number of infectious diseases, such as various newly encountered arenaviruses that cause haemorrhagic fevers in South American populations. Other research in the Peruvian Amazon has shown that the abundance of *Anopheles darlingi* mosquitoes, the major local malaria vector, increases by several orders of magnitude over locations with progressively intensive levels of forest clearance (Patz *et al.* 2000).

On the social–behavioural front, especially in the urban environment, relaxation of traditional cultural norms has yielded newer, freer, patterns of human behaviour, including in relation to sexual activities and illicit drug use. Modern medical manoeuvres, including blood transfusion and organ transplantation, also create new opportunities for viruses to pass from person to person.

Long-distance trade amplifies the dissemination of various infectious diseases. Outbreaks of the potentially lethal toxin-producing *E. coli* O157 in North America and Europe in the 1990s were caused by contaminated beef imported from infected cattle in Latin America. Large development projects, particularly dams, irrigation schemes, and road construction, often potentiate the spread of infectious diseases spread by vectors or intermediate hosts, such as malaria, dengue fever, and schistosomiasis.

Meanwhile, as discussed above, a new and longer shadow is now falling over future infectious disease risks by human-induced changes in the world's climate (Dobson *et al.* 2006).

Box 2.8.4 Major factors affecting the emergence and spread of infectious diseases in humans

- Population growth and density (often accompanied by peri-urban poverty)
- Urbanization: Changes in social and sexual relations
- Globalization of travel and trade (distance and speed)
- Intensified livestock production
- Live animal food markets: Longer, faster, supply lines
- Changes to ecosystems (deforestation, biodiversity loss, etc.)
- Global climate change
- Biomedical exchange of human tissues (transfusion, transplantation)
- Misuse of antibiotics (humans and domestic animals)
- Increased human susceptibility to infection: Due to population ageing, HIV infection, intravenous drug use, increased UVR exposure from ozone depletion

Research: Scope, methods, policy role

Categories of research question

From the preceding text it is clear that this is a complex and challenging domain in which to conduct research to identify causal relations, assess health risks, and develop and evaluate interventions. With complexity comes uncertainty, and this, in turn, requires some new ways of thinking about and communicating research results. It has implications, of course, for policy development. When uncertainties are considerable, and risks to health are potentially great, what is the role of precaution?

There are three broad categories of epidemiological research task—which can be thought of as inspection, detection, and projection. Much of that research needs to be conducted in collaboration with other disciplines. The research tasks are:

1. Study the 'baseline' relations between a specified health outcome and natural variations in climatic–environmental conditions. This research extends the information base, which, in turn, is needed for each of the next two categories of research.
2. Seek early evidence of changes in rates of occurrence of disease or disease risk factors (e.g. mosquito population range or altered allergy seasons) that are reasonably attributable to recent local environmental or climatic change.
3. Use the baseline information to estimate how future scenarios of climatic–environmental change (generated from scenarios of future human pressures on the environment) will affect the rate and/or range of occurrence of specified health outcomes.

The third of these research areas is complex, and relatively unfamiliar to mainstream epidemiology and population health research. It will often require high-level integrated mathematical modelling. That integration can be of two main types—vertical integration (along the central causal chain), and horizontal integration (which brings into the calculus other non-climate variables and processes that may modify steps in the central causal chain).

Integrated assessment of health impacts

The impacts of environmental change on human health and survival are a long way 'to the right' in the causal chain. Most of the research done to date in this 'global environmental' domain has been in relation to climate change. The following discussion therefore uses climate change-related research as the template for thinking more generically about the risk assessment challenges.

Most research energy in the realm of integrated assessment has been (understandably) expended further to the left of the causal chain. This has sought to enhance the capacity of climate models to provide valid and more precise estimates of the impact of plausible scenarios of future global greenhouse gas emissions on future climate projections. Once this step is deemed satisfactory, those modelled climate change 'output' scenarios can be used to model future changes in health-determinant variables: Mosquito populations, flood patterns, local food production, the likely duration and frequency of heat-waves, and so on. These 'exposures' are then applied to the existing, known, exposure–effect (dose–response) relationships, to estimate changes in probabilities of health outcomes.

A more sophisticated approach incorporates into the model, via 'horizontal integration', information about ongoing trends in other determinants of health outcomes for which reasonable extrapolation of future trends is possible. Examples would be demographic trends in age structures, likely future uptake of domestic air-conditioning by 2050; advent of relevant vaccines and likely consequent population immunity, and the introduction and extension of deliberate and specific 'adaptive' changes such as mosquito control programmes, heat-wave warning systems, and flood protection measures.

Integrated assessment, as currently practised, is (mostly) inherently conservative in that it assumes future smooth changes in both climatic mean conditions and variability. Step-changes and the consequences of passing critical thresholds are much less easy to foresee and model. This can be illustrated by considering the integrated-assessment modelling of climate change impacts on regional cereal grain yields. This modelling has been based on physiological models of how temperature and soil moisture affect plant growth, and has not been able to take account of, for example, a change in the pattern of outbreaks of plant pests and diseases or a change in patterns of extreme weather events (floods, storms, etc.)—events that would be rather stochastic. Further, it is also not possible to include projections of those types of social and technological changes that are not reasonably foreseeable.

Adaptations to reduce health risks: Further dimension for integrated modelling

Human-induced climate change is occurring this decade, and more change is unavoidable because of the time-lags in this complex process. Hence, beyond steps taken to curtail greenhouse gas emissions, there is need for societies to take health protecting 'adaptive' actions.

There are two main categories of adaptation. These are: (i) spontaneous (e.g. physiological adaptation to higher temperature; ongoing improvements in housing; unscheduled discovery of effective vaccines); and (ii) planned (e.g. heat-wave warnings; improved mosquito control programmes; public education about hazards).

Research on climate change impacts has, to date, mostly used rather simple assumptions about possible adaptive responses (behavioural, technological, health, and economic). Little attention has been paid to considering how health systems and other social institutions might respond to climate change, or how these might interact to reduce exposure and enhance adaptive capacity.

Enriching mitigation and adaptation policy decisions

Elucidating the risks to population health from GEC will enable better informed social policy responses. Policy decisions must encompass the following:

1. Mitigation policies aimed at stopping detrimental environmental change. (Concern over health risks motivates many people to address the issue of climate change and other environmental changes. Research that enriches the evidence of health risks should therefore add further rationale and stimulus to the policy discussion of mitigation strategies.)
2. Adaptive strategies, policies, and measures to reduce current and future adverse health impacts of global environmental changes.
3. 'Portfolio' solutions that combine mitigation and adaptation (such as solar power for home, clinics, schools, agriculture, and small businesses; water purification; pumping and crop irrigation; desalination, public transport).

While GECs occur at global/worldwide scale, many of the health impacts will be site-specific and path-dependent; that is, they will depend on local circumstances. For example, malaria epidemics occur following rainy seasons in some regions, but during droughts (with local stasis of water) in others. Therefore, as ever, public health interventions must be designed at a scale and of a kind that is appropriate to the health outcome of local concern.

Interventions will be required at local, national, regional, and global scales. Research will therefore have maximum translational impact if, in aggregate, it spans all of these levels.

Implications for public health policy and practice

It is evident from this chapter that there are very many, often complex and interacting, ways in which human-induced changes to the environment-at-large affect—and will increasingly affect—risks to health. Beyond slowing, ceasing, or reversing the environmental change itself, the main task for the health sector is to take actions to minimize the translation of those risks into actual adverse health outcomes. A central consideration, and one that should help guide the priorities for action, is the differential vulnerability of sub-populations and groups.

Population vulnerability

The vulnerability of a particular population, sub-population, or local group to the potential health impacts of GEC depends is a function of: (i) the extent of the external exposure; (ii) the 'constitutional' sensitivity of the population/group and its support structures; and (iii) the level of adaptive resources and capacity. In more detail:

1. Magnitude of exposure to environmental change: This includes changes in both average environmental conditions and in the extent of their variability. Repeated weather extremes (e.g. repeated heavy rains) or sequential extremes (such as prolonged drought followed by heavy rains and flooding) can deplete a community's coping mechanisms and resources thereby increasing vulnerability to stresses.
2. Extent to which health status, or the natural or social systems on which health outcomes depend, are sensitive to ('susceptible' to) the environmental change: This refers, in essence, to the form of the exposure–response relationship for that 'target' entity. The sensitivity of ecosystems (e.g. agroecosytems) may also be important if the environmental stresses are likely to alter essential health-supporting functions such as water supplies, food production, carbon sinks, and stabilization of infectious disease transmission.
3. Adaptive capacity: This reflects resources and actions, both potential and those already in place, to reduce the extent of incurred adverse health outcome. A simple example is that the prevalence of air-conditioning within an urban area will help to reduce the impacts of heat extremes. The effectiveness of any existing adaptive interventions partially determines the above-mentioned exposure–response relationship.

In general, the vulnerability of a population depends on the level of material resources, effectiveness of governance and civil institutions, quality of public health infrastructure, access to relevant local information, and pre-existing burden of disease (Woodward *et al.* 2001). Indeed, a mix of individual, community, political, social, economic, cultural, and geographical factors determine vulnerability. These factors are not uniform across a region or nation; rather, there are geographic, demographic, and socioeconomic differences. Hence, the effective targeting of prevention or adaptation strategies requires understanding which demographic or geographic subpopulations may be most at risk.

One particular challenge in developing adaptation strategies is the issue of scale. The drivers of, and hence the potential for response to, GEC can operate at international, national, and local levels. Ozone depletion is a global issue, with chlorofluorocarbons (CFCs) produced locally affecting global stratospheric concentrations. Deforestation, international trade, and travel have local, national, regional, and international environmental and social impacts. These can influence the emergence of infectious diseases across these scales. Infectious diseases emerging in one part of the world can affect nations throughout the world. Clearly, the choice of effective interventions requires understanding of the scale at which the drivers of change and health outcomes occur.

Preventive strategies: Examples in relation to climate change

Many local actions can be taken to reduce the vulnerability of communities and whole populations to the health hazards of climate change. Climate change will act primarily by intensifying many of the existing climatic–environmental exposures and associated social and ecological conditions that affect human health. Hence, existing health systems and public health practices ought to provide a good base for adaptive strategies to reduce health impacts.

Major components of the health sector task—which will vary considerably between regions and countries—are as follows:

1. Preventive programmes, such as vaccines, mosquito control, food hygiene and inspection, nutritional supplementation
2. Public education (including via doctors' waiting rooms and hospital clinics)
3. Surveillance of disease occurrence and disease risk factors
4. Forecasting of likely future health risks, from:
   a. Projected climate change
   b. Mitigation and adaptation strategies
5. Health sector workforce training and in-career development
6. Minimization of greenhouse gas emissions from health system infrastructure

To achieve long-term effectiveness, adaptive strategies must extend well beyond the formal health sector, to include:

1. General public education about the health risks of climate change
2. Early-alert systems for impending weather extremes
3. Community-based neighbourhood support/watch schemes, to protect the most vulnerable
4. Better (climate-proofed) housing design, urban planning, water catchment, agricultural extension services (improved farming practices)
5. Disaster preparedness, including health-system 'surge' capacity

Beyond these adaptive strategies lies the greater preventive challenge of slowing, then averting, climate change via radical and far-sighted policy decisions at national and international levels. Health professionals everywhere have both the opportunity (via their knowledge, community engagement, and policy influence) and the responsibility to help make this happen.

Conclusion

The relations between human population health and the conditions of the social and natural environments is a profound and long-term one—and is at the core of the quest for sustainability. This fundamental ecological relationship is buffered by culture, and it therefore often lacks the immediacy that is apparent elsewhere in nature. However, viewed in ecological and population-level terms, the limits to, and the characteristics of, a population's health profile are determined in the medium-to-longer term by environmental conditions.

Over the past half-century there has been a growing awareness of the health risks that arise from environmental exposures, including from modern industrial and agricultural practices. This spectrum of health hazards encompasses toxicological, physical, and microbiological exposures, all usually confined within a localized setting. Local air pollution, environmental tobacco smoke, and pesticide residues in local food produce are familiar examples. Such localized environmental hazards remain important public health issues, particularly in many developing countries.

Today, however, as the scale of human impact on the world's environment increases, larger scale and more complex changes in ecological and biogeophysical systems portend potentially greater, and longer lasting, risks to human health and survival. The aggregate pressures of human societies, regionally and globally, are now disrupting and depleting various of the planet's large-scale natural environmental systems—as evidenced by greenhouse gas accumulation and climate change, stratospheric ozone depletion, depletion of freshwater supplies, degradation of fertile land, depletion of ocean fisheries, marked changes to the cycling of several elements (especially nitrogen and its biologically activated forms), loss of biodiversity and associated disruptions of ecosystems, and, via biophysical processes, the global dispersion of persistent organic pollutants.

These global environmental changes are unprecedented in human experience, at least at this scale, and some of them (such as climate change, stratospheric ozone depletion, and the global amplification of activated nitrogen) are new at any scale. The increasingly urgent challenge for public health researchers and practitioners is to understand how today's remarkable human-induced changes to larger-scale environmental systems are influencing—and are likely to influence increasingly—the health of populations around the world.

The modern 'environmental health' agenda therefore must address these larger, increasingly prominent, systemic influences on human health. This requires broad, collaborative, engagement across disciplines and across cultures and economies. The need for global research capacity-building in this domain is both urgent and crucial. The need for public and policy receptivity to these dimensions, with their often longer time horizons, is equally critical.

References

Bambrick, H. (2004). *Trading in food safety: The impact of trade agreements on quarantine in Australia*. The Australia Institute, Canberra.

Bambrick, H. and Kjellström, T. (2004). Good for your heart but bad for your baby? Revised guidelines for fish consumption in pregnancy. *The Medical Journal of Australia*, **181**(2), 61–62.

Bambrick, H., Faunce, T., and Johnston, K. (2006). Potential impact of the AUSFTA on Australia's blood supply. *The Medical Journal of Australia*, **185**(6), 320–3.

Bentham, G. and Langford, I.H. (2001). Environmental temperatures and the incidence of food poisoning in England and Wales. *International Journal of Biometeorology*, **45**(1), 22–6.

Brown, L. (2005). *Learning from China: Why the Western Economic Model will not work for the world [online]*, Earth Policy Institute. www.earth-policy.org/Updates/2005/Update46.htm.

Butler, C. and McMichael, A. (2005). Environmental Health. In (eds. B. Levy and V. Sidel) *Social injustice and public health*, pp. 318–36. Oxford University Press, Oxford.

Carson, R. (1962). *Silent spring*. Houghton Mifflin, Boston.

Checkley, W., Epstein, L.D., Gilman, R.H. *et al.* (2000). Effects of El Niño and ambient temperature on hospital admissions for diarrhoeal diseases in Peruvian children. *Lancet*, **355**, 442–50.

D'Souza, R.M., Becker, N.G., Hall, G. *et al.* (2004). Does ambient temperature affect foodborne disease? *Epidemiology*, **15**(1), 86–92.

Daszak, P., Plowright, R., Epstein, J.H. *et al.* (2006). The emergence of Nipah and Hendra virus: pathogen dynamics across a wildlife-livestock-human continuum. In *Disease ecology: Community structure and pathogen dynamics* (eds. S.K. Collinge and C. Ray), pp. 186–201 Oxford University Press, New York.

Dietz, T., Rosa, E., and York, R. (2007). Driving the human ecological footprint. *Frontiers in Ecology and the Environment*, **5**, 13–18.

Dobson, A., Cattadori, I., Holt, R. *et al.* (2006). Sacred cows and sympathetic squirrels: The importance of biological diversity to human health. *PLoS Medicine*, **3**, e231–45.

Earth System Science Partnership (2006). *Global environmental change and human health (GEC&HH)*. http://www.essp.org/en/joint-projects/health.html.

FAO (2005). *The state of food and agriculture*, United Nations.

FAO (2006). *Livestock's long shadow. Environmental issues and options*, 414 pages. FAO, Rome.

Fischer, G., Shah, M., Tubiello, F.N. *et al.* (2005). Socio-economic and climate change impacts on agriculture: An integrated assessment, 1990–2080. *Philosophical transactions of the Royal Society of London. Series B, Biological sciences*, **360**(1463), 2067–83.

Institute of Medicine (2003). *Microbial threats to health: Emergence, detection, and response*, Institute of Medicine of the National Academies. http://www.iom.edu/CMS/3783/3919/5381.aspx.

IPCC (2007a). *Climate change 2006, Vols. I, II, and III. IPCC Third Assessment Report*. Cambridge University Press. New York.

IPCC (2007b). *Climate change 2007: Climate change impacts, adaptation and vulnerability. IPCC WGII Fourth Assessment Report*, Intergovernmental Panel on Climate Change. http://www.ipcc-wg2.org/index.html.

Kennedy, D. (ed.) (2006). *The state of the planet 2006–2007*. Island Press, Washington DC.

Kovats, R.S., Edwards, S.J., Hajat, S. *et al.* (2004). The effect of temperature on food poisoning: a time-series analysis of salmonellosis in ten European countries. *Epidemiology and Infection*, **132**, 443–53.

Leakey, R. and Lewin, R. (1995). *The Sixth Extinction: Pattern of life and the future of mankind*. Doubleday, New York.

Lobell, D.B. and Field, C.B. (2007). Global scale climate-crop yield relationships and the impacts of recent warming. *Environmental Research Letters*, **2**(014002).

Lucas, R., Repacholi, M., and McMichael, A. (2006). Is the current public health message on UV exposure correct? *Bulletin of the World Health Organization*, **84**(6), 485–91.

McKeown, T., Brown, R.G. and Record, R.G. (1972). An interpretation of the modern rise of population in Europe. *Population Studies*, **26**(3), 345–82.

McMichael, A. (2002). The urban environment and health in a globalising world: Issues for developing countries. In *Urban health in the third world* (ed. R. Akhtar), pp. 423–46. APH Publishing, New Delhi.

McMichael, A. (2005). Integrating nutrition and ecology: Balancing the health of humans and biosphere. *Public Health Nutrition*, **8**, 706–15.

McMichael, A. and Hall, A. (1997). Does immunosuppressive ultraviolet radiation explain the latitude gradient for multiple sclerosis? *Epidemiology*, **8**, 642–5.

McMichael, A. and Woodruff, R. (2007). Climate change and infectious disease. In *Social ecology of infectious disease* (eds. K. Mayer and H. Pizer). Academic Press, New York.

McMichael A.J., Campbell-Lendrum D., Kovats S. *et al.* Climate Change. In: Ezzati M, Lopez AD, Rodgers A, Mathers C (eds.) *Comparative Quantification of Health Risks: Global and Regional Burden of Disease due to Selected Major Risk Factors.* Geneva: World Health Organization; 2004. pp. 1543–1650.

McMichael, A.J., Woodruff, R.E., and Hales, S. (2006). Climate change and human health: Present and future risks. *Lancet*, **367**(9513), 859–69.

McMichael, T., Campbell-Lendrum, D., Kovats, S. *et al.* (2002). *Comparative risk assessment for climate change.*

Meehl, G.A., Stocker, T.F., Collins, W.D. *et al.* (2007). Global climate projections. In *Climate change 2007: The physical science basis. Contribution of working Group I to the fourth assessment report of the Intergovernmental Panel on Climate Change* (eds. S. Solomon, D. Qin, M. Mannin, Z. Chen, M. Marquis, K.B. Averyt *et al.*). Cambridge University Press, Cambridge, United Kingdom and New York, NY, USA.

Millennium Ecosystem Assessment (2005). *Ecosystems and human wellbeing: Synthesis*. Island Press, Washington, DC.

Nathanson, N., Wilesmith, J., and Griot, C. (1997). Bovine spongiform encephalopathy (BSE): Causes and consequences of a common source epidemic. *American Journal of Epidemiology*, **145**(11), 959–69.

Neale, R.E., Purdie, J.L. *et al.* (2003). Sun exposure as a risk factor for nuclear cataract. *Epidemiology*, **14**(6), 707–12.

Patz, J.A., Graczyk, T.K., Geller, N. *et al.* (2000). Effects of environmental change on emerging parasitic diseases. *International Journal for Parasitology*, **30**(12–13), 1395–405.

Patz, J.A., Hulme, M., Rosenzweig, C. *et al.* (2002). Climate change - regional warming and malaria resurgence. *Nature*, **420**(6916), 627–8.

Pimm, S., Russell, G., Gittleman, J. *et al.* (1995). The future of biodiversity. *Science*, **269**, 347–50.

Ponsonby, A.L., McMichael, A., and van der Mei, I. (2002). Ultraviolet radiation and autoimmune disease: insights from epidemiological research. *Toxicology*, **181–182**, 71–8.

Prüss-Üstün, A. and Corvalán, C. (2006). *Preventing disease through healthy environments. Towards an estimate of the environmental burden of disease.* World Health Organization, Geneva.

Rahmstorf, S., Cazenave, A., Church, J. *et al.* (2007). Recent climate observations compared to projections. *Science*, **316** (5825), 709.

Singh, R.B., Hales, S., de Wet, N. *et al.* (2001). The influence of climate variation and change on diarrheal disease in the Pacific Islands. *Environmental Health Perspectives*, **109**(2), 155–9.

Slaper, H., Velders, G.J.M., Daniel, J.S. *et al.* (1996). Estimates of ozone depletion and skin cancer incidence to examine the Vienna Convention achievements. *Nature*, **384**(6606), 256–8.

United Nations (2000). *Millennium development goals*. New York.

Weiss, R.A. and McMichael, A.J. (2004). Social and environmental risk factors in the emergence of infectious diseases. *Nature Medicine*, **10**(12 Suppl), S70–6.

WHO (2007). *Global burden of disease statistics*. Last updated, date accessed 30 April 2007. http://www.who.int/healthinfo/bod/en/index.html.

Wilcox, B.A. and Colwell, R. (2005). Emerging and re-emerging infectious diseases: biocomplexity as an interdisciplinary paradigm. *Ecosystem Health*, **2**, 244–57.

Woodward, A., Hales, S., and de Wet, N. (2001). *Climate change: Potential effects on human Health in New Zealand*. Report prepared for the Ministry for the Environment as part of the NZ Climate Change Programme. Wellington. pp. 1–22. http://www.mfe.govt.nz/publications/climate/effect-health-sep01/effect-health-sep01.pdf.

World Commission on Environment and Development (1987). *Our common future: Report of the World Commission on environment and development*, United Nations, 317 pages, Oxford University Press, Oxford.

WWF International (2006). Living planet report 2006. World Wildlife Fund International, Gland, Switzerland. http://assets.panda.org/downloads/living_planet_report.pdf.

2.9

Health services as determinants of population health

Martin Gulliford

Abstract

This chapter evaluates the relationship between health services and public health and asks 'what is the role of health services in improving population health?'. Traditional thinking in public health has been sceptical of the value of health services at improving health. This stems from recognition of the importance of wider determinants of health, the limited effectiveness of healthcare interventions, and the importance of iatrogenic illness. A number of efficiency-oriented strategies have been developed to increase the health gains from healthcare including needs assessment, health technology assessment and cost-effectiveness analysis, implementation research to promote the uptake of research findings, and strategies to improve the organization and delivery of healthcare. Estimates suggest that healthcare now adds about 5 years to life expectancy at birth in high-income countries. Application of similar techniques to the health problems of middle- and low-income countries suggests that about a quarter of the overall burden of disease in these countries could be prevented through implementation of packages of low-cost but highly effective interventions. Investment in these health interventions would be justified by the economic benefits associated with improved population health. Implementation of the essential package of care approach is hampered by the relative or absolute lack of health services for poor populations in middle- and low-income countries. The distribution of health services in middle- and low-income countries generally shows substantial pro-rich inequity and the financial costs of accessing healthcare may further impoverish poor households. Primary care, with its emphasis on universality and affordability, has been successfully implemented in some countries with favourable health outcomes. In high-income countries, where universal coverage and equitable access to primary care have been more widely achieved, pro-rich inequity exists in accessing preventive medical interventions and specialist care for more serious illnesses. These inequities may contribute to some adverse health outcomes in lower socioeconomic groups. Public health specialists should advocate principles of efficiency and equity and contribute to realizing these through participation in processes of needs assessment, health technology assessment, quality improvement, and facilitating access to needed healthcare for all groups.

Introduction

Healthcare represents one of the largest investments that societies make in the health needs of the population but the role of health services in improving population health is disputed. According to one argument, healthcare should not be regarded as one of the determinants of population health because it is largely ineffective at prolonging life and even causes premature mortality through iatrogenic disease (Illich 1976). A more mainstream view is that health services play an important role in delivering clinical interventions for the treatment and cure of disease, as well as population interventions for the prevention of disease and promotion of health. Health services represent one of three key areas of public health activity alongside health protection and health improvement (Faculty of Public Health 2007). Public health specialists often play an important role in planning and managing health services. This chapter evaluates the relationship between healthcare and public health; it asks 'What is the role of health services in improving population health?'

Definition of healthcare

The boundaries of health services and health systems are difficult to define (Box 2.9.1). Broader definitions encompass 'all the activities whose primary purpose is to improve or maintain health' (Murray & Frenk 2000). This includes interventions that are not implemented through healthcare services including, for example, improvements to road and vehicle safety. In this chapter, multi-sectoral interventions are considered to contribute to health improvement and not healthcare (Box 2.9.2). The objective of this chapter is to evaluate whether healthcare contributes to population health independent of intervention on wider determinants of health.

Health services at different levels of economic development

In order to set the chapter in context, Table 2.9.1 provides illustrative data for health services indicators for several countries at different levels of economic development (World Bank 2006). It is clear that the countries with the lowest-incomes and worst health

Box 2.9.1 Definitions of health systems, healthcare, and health services

- **Health systems:** (i) All the activities whose primary purpose is to improve or maintain health (Murray and Frenk 2000); (ii) the economic, fiscal, and political management method that nations use to run the national healthcare services (Last 2007) (iii) a local or regional group of organized health services (Last 2007)
- **Healthcare:** Services provided to individuals or communities by agents of the health services or professions to promote, maintain, monitor, or restore health. Healthcare is not limited to medical care, which implies therapeutic action by or under the supervision of a physician. The term is sometimes extended to include self-care (Last 2001)
- **Health services:** Services that are performed by healthcare professionals, or by others under their direction, for the purpose of promoting, maintaining, or restoring health. In addition to personal healthcare, health services include measures for health protection, health promotion, and disease prevention (Last 2001)

also have the smallest share of resources committed to health services. In the high-income countries, per capita expenditure on health is some 200 times greater than in the low-income countries and health conditions, measured in terms of life expectancy at birth, are substantially better. These variations among countries illustrate enormous inequality in distribution of healthcare resources at the global level.

Table 2.9.1 also illustrates considerable variation among countries in the same income category. There is variation in the overall level of resources devoted to the health sector; in the relative proportions of public and private sector spending; as well as variation among countries in health outcomes at a given level of expenditure on health. Among middle-income countries, Costa Rica has been successful at mobilizing resources for health and life expectancy is higher than expected. Among the high-income countries, the United States is unusual in having exceptionally high health expenditure but life expectancy is lower than expected. These variations reflect, to a greater or lesser extent, the prevailing philosophies that shape societal views of the purpose of health services as well as the policies, institutions, and community responses to questions of health and healthcare.

Box 2.9.2 Aspects of health

Healthcare need	Capacity to benefit from health care (Stevens *et al.* 2004)
Health improvement	Population health benefit associated with intervention on the determinants of health
Health gain	Individual or population health benefit associated with healthcare intervention
Health outcome	Change in individual or population health status associated with utilization of needed healthcare

Concepts and values in healthcare

Purpose and value of health services

Health services serve several objectives. Health services can improve health by preventing or delaying the onset of disability or death; they contribute to relieving pain and suffering; healthcare is also valued for providing information concerning diagnosis and prognosis. Healthcare is concerned more generally with how individuals' lives will begin and end and with what opportunities they will have in between. The US Presidents' Commission (President's Commission for the Study of Ethical Problems in Medicine and Biomedical and Behavioural Research 1983) observed that healthcare is valued beyond its immediate benefits 'touching on countless important and in some ways mysterious aspects of personal life investing it with significant value as a thing in itself'. Healthcare represents a tangible expression of the value placed on life and health.

For individuals, as well as for private providers and commercial interests, healthcare is valued as a private good that can be utilized to preserve or improve health. Despite this, markets generally fail to provide a satisfactory distribution of healthcare. The risk of illness is unpredictable, the costs of healthcare can be extremely high, and consumers may have limited information on which to base choices. For these reasons, communities and national governments are usually involved in arrangements for the delivery of healthcare in order to pool risks and regulate healthcare markets. However, healthcare often yields benefits that extend beyond individual recipients. For example, the treatment of pulmonary tuberculosis has value in controlling the spread of disease to others. Such positive externalities may be valued more by communities than by individuals. Societies therefore value healthcare as a merit good, which is typically under-utilized when distributed by market forces that allow individuals to value only the personal benefits they obtain. Extending this argument, healthcare may contribute to generating public goods that benefit all. Thus, the eradication of smallpox, or the control of antimicrobial drug resistance, offer benefits that are freely accessible to the global population with a value extending beyond national boundaries (Smith *et al.* 2003).

Dimensions for evaluation

The diverse objectives, and the complex organization and delivery of healthcare, require evaluation on several different conceptual dimensions. Maxwell's (1984) framework of six dimensions is frequently used (Box 2.9.3). Each of Maxwell's dimensions represents a complex, multi-faceted concept that is not easily defined. The dimensions can be broadly grouped into those associated with efficiency, including efficiency and effectiveness; and those associated with equity, including equity and access. Relevance to need, and social acceptability, contribute to the definition of both efficiency and equity. The relative importance assigned to the concepts of efficiency and equity is important in shaping health services and is the subject of significant ideological debate concerning how the inputs and outputs of health services should be organized and valued.

Table 2.9.1 Health expenditures and health services indicators at different levels of economic development around 2003–2004

	Gross national income per capita (2004 US$)	Health expenditure (per cent GDP)	Public expenditure (per cent total)	Health expenditure per capita (US$)	Doctors per 1000 population	Hospital beds per 1000 population	Life expectancy at birth years)
Low-income							
Kenya	480	4.3	38.7	20	0.1	1.6	48
Pakistan	600	2.4	27.7	13	0.7	0.7	65
Middle-income							
Albania	2120	6.5	41.7	118	1.3	3.1	74
Costa Rica	4470	7.3	78.8	305	1.3	1.4	79
Indonesia	1140	3.1	35.9	30	0.1	0.7	67
High-income							
Japan	37 050	7.9	81.0	2662	2.0	14.3	82
United Kingdom	33 630	8.0	85.7	2428	2.2	4.2	79
United States	41 440	15.2	44.6	5711	2.3	3.3	77

Source: World Bank (2006).

Ideological and philosophical drivers

On the input side, obtaining needed healthcare is regarded at one extreme as the responsibility of individuals and families. This is often the case in low-income countries where government or externally funded health services may not be available and families necessarily make out-of-pocket payments to private providers or do not obtain healthcare (van Doorslaer *et al.* 2006b). In high-income countries, obtaining needed care is sometimes also viewed primarily as an individual responsibility with the government, representing the organized efforts of society, having a minimal role in the regulation of the healthcare market. This libertarian view is most evident in the organization of healthcare in the United States (Blake *et al.* 2003). One proposed justification is that taxation to provide healthcare for others infringes against individuals' freedom of choice. From this perspective, fairness only concerns basic opportunities to compete for health resources and does not require that a fair distribution of healthcare be realized. As greater income and wealth are generally associated with better access to healthcare but with fewer health needs, this libertarian approach will not usually lead to an equitable distribution of healthcare. This is in contrast to the more egalitarian approach that has prevailed in most high-income countries with the ideal of universal eligibility to comprehensive services and the objective of equity of access to healthcare (Mossialos *et al.* 2003).

Box 2.9.3 Dimensions for evaluation of health services

Effectiveness	Extent to which a healthcare intervention achieves the intended outcome (Last 2007)
Efficiency	Outcome achieved in relation to expenditure of resources (Last 2007)
Equity	Fairness, or justice, in respect of treatment of different individuals or groups (Last 2007)
Access	Extent to which services are available, can be utilized, deliver needed services, and achieve appropriate outcomes (Gulliford *et al.* 2002)
Appropriateness	Relevance to need (Maxwell 1984)
Responsiveness	Social acceptability (Maxwell 1984)

Source: Maxwell (1984).

A separate set of tensions concerns how the outputs of healthcare should be distributed. According to utilitarian doctrine, society in general and health services in particular should aim to maximize the health gains obtained across all individuals. This idea is summed up by the slogan 'the greatest good for the greatest number'. This utilitarian approach is sometimes regarded as 'the guiding principle for many of the decisions and actions of public health professionals' (Last 2007, p. 385). The objective of maximizing the health gain to be achieved from the available resources is closely related to the economic principle of efficiency. Resources for health will be used most efficiently when health gain is maximized (Box 2.9.3).

The simple form of utilitarianism is problematic. This approach only requires that the sum of health gains in a population should be maximized, it does not require that all individuals receive a fair distribution of potential benefits from healthcare. This is in contrast to approaches based on concepts of human rights and social justice in which each individual is considered to have a right to health. According to this approach, all individuals are considered to be entitled to healthcare even when the contribution this makes to the aggregate benefit of the wider community does not require that they receive it (Dworkin 1977). The rights to health and medical care are recognized in the Universal Declaration of Human Rights (United Nations 2007). The International Covenant on Economic, Social and Cultural Rights goes further and requires that governments create 'conditions which would assure all medical services and medical attention in the event of sickness' (Office of the High Commissioner for Human Rights 2007). These international statements do not guarantee that access to needed services will be possible for all individuals but they are important in offering a degree of protection to marginalized and vulnerable groups. An approach based on human rights favours a just or equitable distribution of healthcare over the maximization of potential health gains across the population. The pursuit of equity is also justified in terms of Rawl's theory of justice as fairness which proposed that a just society will be arranged so as to achieve fair equality of opportunity, with inequalities only permitted if they are of the greatest benefit to the least-advantaged members of society (Daniels *et al.* 2004). Based on the concepts of human rights and social justice, equity may be regarded as a moral value which health services should strive to promote (Braveman *et al.* 2001). Efficiency will often be compromised through this approach, as for example, if equitable access to specialist services is to be provided in sparsely populated rural areas, or if insulin therapy for insulin-dependent diabetes is to be ensured in low-income country settings.

The conflicting principles underlying the financing and delivery of healthcare outlined in this section are apparent in the differing approaches to provision of health services in different countries. Existing health systems result from compromises that are made through the policy process. In the healthcare systems of high-income countries, collective healthcare provision based on universal eligibility is favoured but individuals may not be prevented from purchasing healthcare privately. Equity of access is an objective, but this is only to the extent to which it is considered acceptable to compromise efficiency. In other systems, such as the United States or in middle-income countries, private financing of healthcare through insurance or out-of-pocket payments may predominate, but governments may facilitate access to basic health services for vulnerable groups such as the poor and elderly.

In the following sections, approaches to the relationship between health services and population health are divided into those that are predominantly motivated by the pursuit of efficiency and those driven by the goal of greater equity. Two specific questions are addressed: 'How do health services aim to optimize health gains?' and 'How do health services ensure an optimal distribution of health gains?'

Efficiency-driven approaches

Underlying problems

Lack of effectiveness

A basic assumption underlying the efficiency-driven approach is that utilization of healthcare is associated with health gains. This assumption was challenged by Illich who claimed that 'a vast amount of contemporary clinical care is incidental to the curing of disease, but the damage done by medicine to the health of individuals and populations is very significant' (Illich 1976, p. 23). Illich acknowledged that medicine has some effect in preventing and curing infectious diseases through the use of vaccinations and antimicrobial drugs but he argued that the historical reductions in mortality from infectious diseases in high-income countries occurred before these technologies became available. In his opinion, treatment of non-communicable diseases such as cancer and cardiovascular disease was of negligible benefit and may cause considerable harm (Illich 1976).

Illich's interpretation was supported by McKeown's (1979) analysis of historical trends in mortality in Britain. This analysis was important in identifying the limited role of medicine as a determinant of health in the historical era. For example, relative reductions in mortality between 1881 and 1950 ranged from 30-fold for tuberculosis, 20-fold for digestive diseases, and 15-fold for respiratory disease (Office for National Statistics 1998). Most of these reductions occurred before widespread use of specific antimicrobial treatment after 1945. These trends support the interpretation that environmental influences, particularly improved nutrition, clean water supplies, and better housing and sanitation, were largely responsible for historical reductions in mortality from infectious diseases in high-income countries with limited gains from health service interventions (McKeown 1979).

Consistent with McKeown's analysis, the historian Wooton suggested that before the late nineteenth century medical practice had little capacity to improve health, and was generally only harmful (Wooton 2006). It was only through the development of the germ theory of infectious disease causation, and its practical application in antiseptic surgery from 1865 onwards, that medicine first began to implement procedures that gave greater benefit than harm. Wooton (2006) argued that in the historical era, progress in medicine was largely confined to the development of a body of scientific knowledge concerning health and disease. This knowledge was not translated into practical applications and consequently medicine did not develop as a technology for improving health until more recent decades.

A similar argument was developed earlier by Cochrane in his book *Effectiveness and Efficiency* (Cochrane 1972). Cochrane commented on the rising costs of medical care and the dominance of treatment of established disease over preventive medicine. He showed that in many instances there was little evidence available concerning whether medical interventions were beneficial, ineffective, or harmful. When randomized controlled trials were conducted, they often showed that benefits of intervention were smaller than anticipated and unexpected adverse effects of treatment were not uncommon. For example, one large clinical trial showed that routine use of corticosteroid drugs in patients with head injury was associated with a relative increase in mortality of 15 per cent (95 per cent confidence interval 7–24 per cent) (Roberts *et al.* 2004). Cochrane advocated a now generally accepted view that all healthcare interventions should be tested in randomized controlled trials, and the results of all such trials should be systematically collected, analysed, and implemented in clinical practice. He advocated greater emphasis on applied research, rather than pure scientific research with little potential for benefit to patients or the public.

The dissociation between the scientific prestige associated with different medical specialities and their potential for improving health was noted by McKeown in his Introduction to *The Role of Medicine* (McKeown 1979). Tradition and professional opinion were, for a long time, the main drivers of clinical practice and the organization and delivery of medical care. However, tradition came under attack through research from epidemiologists and social scientists that questioned the effectiveness of widely used procedures, demonstrated inexplicable variations in clinical practice, widespread problems with medical errors and poor quality of care, and showed that methods for organizing and delivering care were not consistent with patients' wants and needs.

Quality of care and variations in practice

'Quality of care' is a wide ranging concept that includes departures from optimal standards of healthcare judged on any of Maxwell's dimensions (Maxwell 1984). In Donabedian's framework (Donabedian 2003), quality may be assessed in terms of the organizational structures for care, the processes of care that are delivered, or the health outcomes of care.

Problems with quality of care are often revealed through variations in the organization and delivery of care. For example, in Brazil 72 per cent of women giving birth in private clinics had Caesarean sections, compared with 31 per cent in public hospitals; yet, 70–80 per cent of women in either setting expressed a preference for vaginal delivery (Potter *et al.* 2001). In Pakistan, 68 per cent of subjects in a household survey had received one or more injections for treatment of acute symptoms in the preceding 3 months, with an average of 13.6 injections per person per year. A new needle was reportedly used in only 53 per cent of instances (Janjua *et al.* 2005). In Trinidad in 1993, 59 per cent of diabetic patients with hypertension were treated with a combination of reserpine, clopamide, and dihydroergocristine; this combination was rarely used in neighbouring islands (Mahabir & Gulliford 2005). In England in 2000, 26 per cent of patients diagnosed with 'influenza' in primary care, and 13 per cent with 'common colds', were prescribed antibiotics (Ashworth *et al.* 2004). At different family practices the proportion prescribed antibiotics ranged from 0 to 97 per cent for influenza and 0 to 84 per cent for common colds (Ashworth *et al.* 2005).

Variations such as these may originate in uncertainty concerning the optimal use of specific medical interventions. This uncertainty permits the outcome of clinical decisions to be influenced by factors such as the supply of medical services, or practitioner and patient preferences, leading to wide and often idiosyncratic variations in practice. Variations in practice may result in health resources being used inefficiently; in patients being treated in ways that are contrary to their expressed preferences; in the widespread use of potentially harmful procedures; or patients being denied the potential benefits of effective therapy.

Iatrogenic illness and patient safety

Iatrogenic illness and problems with patient safety represent a particular set of concerns with quality of care. Errors in medical care have been shown to be common, especially in hospital settings. In the US Harvard Medical Practice Study of 30 121 subjects from 51 acute hospitals in 1984 (Brennan *et al.* 1991), injuries caused by medical management occurred in 3.7 per cent of hospital admissions. A quarter of these adverse events were judged to be caused by negligence; 2.6 per cent were permanently disabling, and 13.6 per cent led to death. Based on these results, it was estimated that there may be between 44 000 and 88 000 deaths in the United States annually from errors in medical care (Kohn *et al.* 2000). In primary care, there may be significant errors in 0.1–1 per 100 consultations (Bhasale *et al.* 1998). These include delays in diagnosis, wrong diagnoses, errors in prescribing, failure to prescribe needed treatment, and difficulties with communication and referral (Bhasale *et al.* 1998).

Healthcare-associated infections are an increasing problem. In England in 2006, there were 55 681 cases of *Clostridium difficile* infection in people aged 65 years and over, generally associated with broad-spectrum antibiotic use in hospitals (Health Protection Agency 2007). Over-utilization of antimicrobial drugs is leading to the emergence of organisms that show multiple resistance, leading to healthcare-acquired infections that are difficult to treat. In England and Wales, the number of methicillin-resistant Staphyloccus aureus (MRSA) related deaths increased from 669 in 2000 to 1168 in 2004 (Office for National Statistics 2006). Multi-drug-resistant tuberculosis has emerged as an important threat with an estimated 450 000 cases worldwide in 2006 (World Health Organization 2007a).

Misallocation of resources and problems in service organization and delivery

The World Health Report for 2000 characterized health services as often 'poorly structured, badly led, inefficiently organized, and inadequately funded' (World Health Organization 2000) (p. xiv). A common problem is over-allocation of resources to hospitals. In high-income countries about 70 per cent of health services expenditure is on hospital services. This pattern of expenditure has been exported to middle- and low-income countries, often in the form of development projects that provide hospital infrastructure, not always accompanied by the required running costs. Hospital-based services generally deliver interventions of low cost-effectiveness compared with those delivered in primary care (World Bank 1993). Other problems concern the relationship between public and private sectors with doctors employed in the public sector often 'moonlighting' in private clinics, or charging for services provided in public clinics (World Health Organization 2000). The private sector may be inadequately regulated. There is often a lack of respect for the comfort, dignity, and concerns of patients (Phillips 1996).

Proposed solutions

Clinical effectiveness and health technology assessment

Cochrane's book *Effectiveness and Efficiency* was influential in leading to the development of strategies for improving clinical effectiveness, including the promotion of 'evidence-based medicine' grounded in the belief that clinical decision-making should be informed as far as possible by the results of well-conducted randomized controlled trials (RCTs) that provide evidence for the effectiveness of interventions (Sehon & Stanley 2003). This requires that the results of all available RCTs should be summarized in the results of systematic reviews and meta-analyses such as those produced by the Cochrane collaboration. This approach has been extended to cover not just therapeutic interventions but diagnostic techniques, screening strategies, and methods for delivering care under the more general heading of health technology assessment.

Health technology 'includes any method used to promote health, prevent and treat disease and improve rehabilitation or long-term care' (The NHS Health Technology Assessment Programme 2007). Health technology assessment includes evaluation of both the effectiveness and resource use associated with new medical technologies. Cost-effectiveness analysis is now commonly integrated into the implementation of randomized controlled trials so that the cost per unit benefit from an intervention may be estimated. Cost-utility analysis allows the health benefits from different interventions to be compared using a common metric such as the quality-adjusted life year (QALY). This permits more explicit comparison of the benefits obtained, and the resources used by different interventions, thus informing choices made in resource allocation decisions. Processes for assessing population health needs have also been made more explicit, based on the incidence and prevalence of disease and the effectiveness of interventions, so that health services can be designed to deliver services that are relevant to the population's health problems (Stevens *et al.* 2004).

Quality improvement, implementation research, and patient safety

The increasing availability of objective evidence concerning effective treatment for different conditions has been associated with increased evaluation of medical care against agreed standards. It is clear that there is widespread failure to achieve standards of good clinical practice or to implement fully interventions that have been shown to be effective in randomized controlled trials. For example, the technique of cumulative meta-analysis showed a delay of many years between evidence of efficacy and implementation of thrombolytic therapy in myocardial infarction (Lau *et al.* 1992). These problems have given rise to a new area of research known as 'implementation research' that aims to evaluate and identify methods to encourage health professionals to practice in accordance with evidence-based guidelines (Eccles *et al.* 2005). Studies in implementation research typically combine a range of interventions such as the provision of guidelines, invitations to educational meetings, provision of advice from respected peers, or the inclusion of prompts in the medical record. Such combinations of interventions commonly offer modest benefits in terms of promoting evidence-based practice (Oxman *et al.* 1995). In the United Kingdom, the government recently introduced a system of contractual financial incentives to encourage family doctors to deliver specified processes of care and designated intermediate outcome targets in their patients, with a main emphasis on chronic illness management (Roland 2004). Initial results appear to be impressive (Doran *et al.* 2006).

Alongside quality improvement initiatives, and requiring similar techniques for implementation, there have been specific initiatives to increase patient safety. In some countries, special organizations have been set up with the brief of improving patient safety through surveillance of critical events, identifying risks, and feeding back information to improve services. In 2004, the World Health Organization launched a World Alliance for Patient Safety with a headline campaign of 'Clean Care is Safer Care' focusing on safe blood transfusion, injection and immunization, safer clinical procedures, clean water, sanitation, and hand hygiene (World Alliance for Patient Safety 2007).

Systems redesign and service organization and delivery research

The focus of health technology assessment is primarily at the micro-level of the interaction between individual patients and health professionals. Increasingly, the organizational context in which care is delivered is viewed as important in influencing the effectiveness and efficiency of care (Sheldon 2001). Whether services are delivered in primary or secondary care, by physicians or nurses, by specialist teams or generalists may be important in influencing the costs and outcomes. The size and workload of an organization, its staffing levels, the management strategies, and organizational culture may also influence the quality and safety of services (Mannion *et al.* 2005). Consequently, there has been an expansion of social-science-based research into organization and delivery of health services. This includes investigation of the nature of patient and carer interactions with the health system, the roles of the healthcare workforce, or the impact of organizational change on the various dimensions of quality of care (Fulop *et al.* 2003). At the same time, there has been a much greater interest in experimentation with different models of organizing care including transferring care from hospital to primary and community settings, utilizing staff with different types of training, or integrating specialist skills into primary care service delivery. Such changes have sometimes been facilitated by health sector reforms that remove commissioning and service planning functions from the hands of service providers.

Redesign and modernization of service delivery have been particularly important in the management of chronic conditions. Health services have been designed traditionally to deal with acute episodes of illness but most contacts with health services are now for chronic conditions (Bodenheimer *et al.* 2002). More than two-thirds of adults in high-income countries have one or more chronic conditions, and chronic conditions account for 80 per cent of primary care consultations and 60 per cent of hospital bed days. The management of chronic conditions requires ongoing surveillance of patients' condition, management of risk factors, early detection of complications, and education of patients so that they can actively manage their own illness and reduce risk through appropriate lifestyle and behavioural changes. Traditionally designed health services are often very ineffective at delivering services that can achieve these outcomes. The US Institute of Medicine referred to a 'quality chasm' representing the discrepancy between the potential for delivering effective care and the reality of chronic illness management (Institute of Medicine 2005). This has led to the development of new models of service delivery in chronic illness care with a focus on developing care in primary settings, linking appropriately trained staff skilled in education and promoting self-care, with easy access to specialist advice, supported by reliable and easy to use clinical information systems (Bodenheimer *et al.* 2002).

Healthcare and population health

Perceptions of the role of health services as determinants of population health have evolved. Historically, medical care was of limited importance as a determinant of health; medical care was often ineffective and had a considerable capacity for causing harm. In the twentieth century however, the pace of technological innovation accelerated and from 1948 onwards the application of randomized controlled trials to evaluate the effectiveness of health technologies was increasingly accepted. Effective interventions came to be widely used. These included vaccination and immunization against infectious disease, screening for early stages of cancer, treatment of risk factors for cardiovascular disease, or treatment services for the major causes of mortality. The impact of the widespread implementation of such interventions on population health is difficult to evaluate because of the contribution of wider and more powerful determinants of population health cannot be readily controlled as they might be in a randomized trial. Three main approaches have been used to evaluate the impact of healthcare on population health indicators.

'Avoidable' mortality

The 'avoidable' mortality argument is that if a given condition is amenable to medical intervention, then there should be few or no deaths from the condition. Mortality rates may be used as sentinel indicators of the effectiveness of healthcare services. For example, if surgical services are effective then there should be few deaths from acute appendicitis, cholecystitis or abdominal hernia. This approach was developed and implemented most extensively by Holland and co-workers (Holland 1991) who mapped the distribution of 'avoidable' deaths in Europe. The approach has been extended to monitoring of morbidity and health service utilization in routinely published indicator datasets. However, the approach suffers from the limitations that definition of 'avoidability' may often be grounded in low level evidence, and there are few health conditions for which the wider determinants of health are not important in determining the distribution of mortality.

Time-series analysis

If a health service intervention is implemented across a population over a short space of time, changes in trends in mortality or morbidity may be used to evaluate the effectiveness of the intervention. There have been well-documented reductions in the incidence of infectious diseases following the implementation of new vaccination programmes. There have also been changes in mortality from cancer following the implementation of screening programmes. This approach is complicated by underlying secular trends in disease incidence as well as by changes over time in the effectiveness of case management.

Modelling

Modelling approaches to the evaluation of health service effectiveness vary in their sophistication but all utilize evidence concerning the incidence and prevalence of disease, the effectiveness of clinical interventions, and the expected coverage and quality of services in the population at risk. This information is used to estimate the contribution of medical care to real or projected changes in mortality or other health outcomes in populations of interest.

Healthcare and population health: High-income countries

Bunker and colleagues (Bunker *et al.* 1994) modelled the contribution of medical care to life expectancy in the US population. Examples of their estimates are shown in Table 2.9.2. Their report concluded that medical care, including preventive and treatment services, contributed about 5 years additional life expectancy in the United States with potential for gain of an additional 1.5–2 years if effective interventions were implemented more completely, with improved population coverage and higher standards of care. In a more recent study, Cutler *et al.* (2006) estimated changes in life expectancy at birth in the United States between 1960 and 2000. The cumulative increase in life expectancy during this period was 6.97 years with reduced mortality from cardiovascular disease accounting for 4.88 years (70 per cent) and reduced rates of infant deaths accounting for 1.35 years (19 per cent). Based on Bunker's estimates, as well as analyses of the decline in mortality from cardiovascular disease (Unal *et al.* 2004), Cutler *et al.* (2006) attributed half of this increased life expectancy to more effective medical intervention. Several examples illustrate the substantial benefits to be obtained from effective medical care.

Survival with human immunodeficiency virus (HIV)

The first illustration concerns the survival of people who are infected with HIV. Lohse *et al.* (Lohse *et al.* 2007) compared the survival of HIV-infected individuals in Denmark with that of controls matched for age, sex, and place of residence drawn from the general population. The estimated median survival of incident HIV cases after 25 years of age was 7.6 years in 1995–6, 22.5 years in 1997–1999, and 32.5 years in the period 2000–2005. This dramatic improvement in survival following diagnosis was attributed to the introduction of highly active antiretroviral therapy (HAART). This improvement is all the more remarkable when it is remembered that HIV was first identified in 1984. This example illustrates the capability of medical care to change the clinical course of a condition. In this case HIV became a chronic disease requiring active medical therapy over many years, with a prognosis similar to that of a diagnosis of insulin-treated type 1 diabetes mellitus. Indeed, before insulin treatment became available, the prognosis of type 1 diabetes was similar to, or worse than that of HIV infection in the pre-HAART era.

Breast cancer mortality

Another example concerns mortality from breast cancer, the most frequent cancer among women in high-income countries. In the United Kingdom, population-based mammographic screening was introduced for women aged 50–64 years after 1988. The decision to introduce screening was based on strong, but disputed, evidence from randomized controlled trials (Gotzsche & Olsen 2000; Nystrom *et al.* 2002). Around this time, there was also accumulating evidence for increasing survival following clinical diagnosis through more effective use of specific therapies, including the oestrogen receptor antagonist tamoxifen. An analysis of breast cancer mortality for women aged 55–69 years in England and Wales, showed an estimated 21.3 per cent reduction in breast cancer mortality between 1990 and 1998 compared with the predicted trend (Blanks *et al.* 2000). The authors estimated that approximately one-third of this decrease could be attributed to breast cancer screening with two-thirds of the reduction attributed to improved treatment.

Table 2.9.2 Measuring the effects of medical care. Estimated increases in life expectancy for the population from clinical preventive and curative services

Examples: Condition treated	Relevant population	Estimated gain in life years in those receiving the service	Estimated gain in life expectancy distributed across the US population	
			Current	Potential
Cervical cancer screening	Adult women	96 days	2 weeks	1 week
Immunization for diphtheria	All children	10 months	10 months	0
Cervical cancer treatment	Affected women	21 years	2 weeks	1 week
Ischaemic heart disease	Affected adults	14 years	1.2 years	6–8 months
Appendicitis	Affected individuals	50 years	4 months	0
Trauma	Affected individuals	24–38 years	1.5–2 months	3–4 months
Estimated overall gain from preventive and curative services			5 years	1.5–2 years

Source: Bunker *et al.* (1994).

Allgood *et al.* (2008) compared women who died of breast cancer with control women who did not die and found that attending for breast screening was associated with between a 35 and 65 per cent reduction in odds of mortality depending on assumptions. Cancer Research UK (2008) reported that 5-year survival of women diagnosed with breast cancer increased from 52 per cent in 1971–3 to 80 per cent in 2001–3. The example of breast cancer, illustrates the difficulty of analysing longer term outcomes of health service interventions. Analysis required estimation of the secular trend, in this case increasing, as well as separate effects of a population screening intervention and the outcomes of improved clinical treatment.

Coronary heart disease (CHD) mortality

These same difficulties are also evident in the third example, which concerns the impact of healthcare on declining mortality from coronary heart disease. In Finland, as in a number of other high-income countries, coronary heart disease mortality has been declining since the 1960s. During the 1980s and 1990s, a number of new therapies were introduced, whose effectiveness had been demonstrated in large randomized controlled trials. These included more effective drug therapy for patients with myocardial infarction, angina or heart failure as well as coronary artery bypass surgery for patients with angina. There were also declining trends in the major risk factors for CHD including elevated cholesterol and blood pressure levels and cigarette smoking. Based on observed trends in risk factors and uptake of specific therapies, Laatikainen and colleagues (Laatikainen *et al.* 2005) estimated that about 53 per cent of the reduction in CHD mortality in Finland between 1982 and 1997 could be attributed to changes in risk factor levels, while 23 per cent could be attributed to more effective medical care, including secondary prevention, in those affected by the condition. In England and Wales, coronary heart disease mortality declined by 62 per cent in men and 45 per cent in women between 1981 and 2000, and about 42 per cent of the decline was attributed to medical intervention (Unal *et al.* 2004).

These analyses of CHD trends and their determinants raise important questions concerning the priority to be given to prevention efforts through population strategies as compared to healthcare intervention, contributing 'high risk' approaches to primary prevention and to secondary and tertiary prevention in those with established disease. Comparison of the potential costs and outcomes of population strategies for primary prevention, as compared to medical care intervention, should generally favour the former. However, the dominant epidemiological approach to evaluation, the randomized controlled trial, lends itself most readily to the evaluation of medical care interventions. The application of epidemiological designs to the evaluation of population-wide prevention strategies has generally given disappointing results (Ebrahim & Smith 2001). This may have encouraged epidemiologists to give undue priority to medical care interventions with less attention given to the implementation and evaluation of population strategies. For example, Wald and Law (Wald & Law 2003) used the results of meta-analyses of clinical trials to support the concept that a 'polypill' containing a number of effective but low-cost pharmaceuticals (a statin, three blood pressure-lowering drugs, as well as aspirin and folic acid) may have the potential to prevent up to 80 per cent of stroke and coronary heart disease deaths. However, a pill is not a panacea for a lifetime of exposure to unhealthy risks and a strategy grounded in the high-risk approach may not be appropriate for population-wide implementation.

Healthcare and population health: Middle- and low-income countries

Immunization

In high-income countries, environmental changes associated with economic development mostly occurred before effective medical interventions became available. This was not true for the low-income countries and did not always apply to the poor in middle-income countries. The health gains from clinical and public health interventions that were provided through health services in these countries were more obvious than in the high-income countries, and this was especially so for the effects of immunization programmes.

Between 1967 and 1977, the World Health Organization organized a programme to eradicate smallpox, based on systematic delivery of smallpox vaccination to populations at risk. In 1967, there were up to 2 million deaths from smallpox annually, but there have been no naturally occurring cases since 1977. The additional cost of the smallpox eradication programme was modest (Fenner *et al.* 1988). The success of this programme showed that the widespread use of a highly effective but low-cost intervention had the potential to have a major impact on mortality. Following on from the smallpox eradication programme, the WHO established the Expanded Programme on Immunisation (EPI). This aimed to deliver immunization against polio, diphtheria, pertussis, measles, tetanus, and BCG against tuberculosis to children as well as tetanus immunization for pregnant women, achieving 80 per cent coverage for the main vaccines in children since 1990 (World Health Organization 2007b). The EPI programme was estimated to reduce the overall burden of disease among children under 5 by 20–25 per cent (World Bank 1993). The Global Polio Eradication Initiative has been successful in further reducing the spread of polio, with only four countries (Afghanistan, Pakistan, India, and Nigeria) still experiencing indigenous polio transmission in 2006. Between 1988 and 2005 an estimated 5 million people avoided long-term disability from Polio as a result (Global Polio Eradication Initiative 2006). Immunization programmes are now being extended to include additional vaccines including hepatitis B and *Haemophilus influenzae* type B (World Health Organization 2007b). For example, a decrease in *Haemophilus influenzae* type B disease burden was recorded in South Africa following the introduction of the new vaccine (von Gottberg *et al.* 2006).

Investing in Health

Building on the success of immunization programmes, the World Bank's World Development Report for 1993 (World Bank 1993) applied the tools of needs assessment, health technology assessment, and cost-effectiveness analysis to modelling potential solutions to a wider range of health problems in middle- and low-income countries. The motivation behind the report was summarized in its title, *Investing in Health*. A healthy population is a major resource that can contribute to stronger economic growth and improving standards of living (Bloom *et al.* 2004). On average, each 10 per cent increase in life expectancy at birth in a country is associated with an increase in economic growth of 0.3–0.4 per cent per year (Commission on Macroeconomics and Health 2001). Improved health can lead to greater productivity because there are more economically active adults, fewer dependent adults affected by illness, children who are better able to participate in education enhancing their productivity as adults, and rising expectations of longevity providing a motivation to save for later life.

The 1993 World Bank Report argued that existing resources for healthcare were utilized extremely inefficiently and that major health gains could be achieved through focused investment in limited packages of highly effective but low-cost clinical interventions and public health measures delivered through health and other services. This investment could be justified in economic terms through the benefits it could bring to productivity and economic growth.

The Global Burden of Disease study and the Disease Control Priorities project were influential in identifying, quantifying, and prioritizing needs for healthcare intervention in countries at different levels of development (Lopez *et al.* 2006). Using information about the burden of disease and the cost-effectiveness of different interventions it was possible to model the health gain, measured in terms of disability adjusted life years (DALYs), that could result from different interventions and identify priorities for investment. The World Development Report estimated that a gain of DALYs equivalent to about 25 per cent of the burden of disease in middle- and low-income countries could be achieved through implementation of programmes of low-cost public health interventions, partly delivered through health services, as well as essential cost-effective clinical services (Table 2.9.3) (World Bank 1993). A recommended package of essential measures included extended and increased uptake of immunization, improved nutrition education and micronutrient supplementation, treatment of sick children, and reproductive health interventions including prevention and treatment of sexually transmitted diseases and safe motherhood. It was estimated that significant health gains could be achieved with little additional overall cost to governments, through disinvestment from public spending on what it termed 'discretionary clinical services', including interventions of low cost-effectiveness delivered in hospital settings.

Developments from *Investing in Health*

The 1993 World Development Report contributed to an important shift in thinking in several respects. Providing health services to the poor in middle- and low-income countries was no longer to be regarded as a weak form of buffering against the consequences of poverty. Instead, delivering health interventions to the poor was viewed as attacking the causes of poverty and contributing towards establishing conditions that could lead to economic growth, providing households with a route out of a continuing cycle of poverty and illness. Following on the publication of the Report, the World Health Organization established a Commission on Macroeconomics and Health (2001) whose report endorsed the importance of preventing and treating disease as a means of promoting wealth as well as health. This facilitated the mobilization of resources for health in middle- and low-income countries. A Global Fund was established to attract funds to be directed towards programmes for the prevention and treatment of AIDS, TB, and malaria (The Global Fund 2007). The Global Alliance on Vaccines and Immunisation (GAVI) was set up to promote immunization programmes in the poorest countries through both public and private sector funding (GAVI Alliance 2007).

The 1993 Report was also important in encouraging a more explicit approach to rationing of services and priority setting for health investment, justified by the extent of health gains that could be achieved through this approach. For example, it is estimated that for a cost of US$1 million the loss of 50 000 to 500 000 DALYs could be averted through extended vaccine coverage, the loss of 50 000 to 125 000 DALYs could be averted through improved malaria treatment programmes (Jamison *et al.* 2006). Estimates such as these encouraged governments to retreat from the ideal of universal access to comprehensive services and to promote instead

Table 2.9.3 Actual and proposed allocation of public expenditure on health in developing countries and potential health gains, 1990

Package component	Proposed spending on package ($ per capita)	Estimated actual spending 1990	Reduction in disease burden: Per cent	Reduction in disease burden: Millions of DALYs
Public health	5	1	6	77
Immunization (EPI plus[a]), school health interventions, HIV/AIDS prevention, tobacco and alcohol control, nutrition and family planning education, STD[b] control, malaria (selected prevention measures)				
'Essential' clinical services	10	4–6	19	225
Treatment of TB, maternal health and safe motherhood, family planning, integrated management of childhood illness, treatment of sexually transmitted diseases, malaria treatment, non-communicable diseases and injuries (selected early screening and secondary prevention)				
'Discretionary' clinical services	6	13–15		
All other services including low-cost-effectiveness treatment of cancer, cardiovascular disease, major trauma, neurological and mental health conditions				
Total	21	21	25	302

[a] EPI plus, Expanded Programme on Immunisation with additions (see text for explanation)
[b] STD, sexually transmitted disease
Sources: World Bank (1993) and World Health Organization (2000).

the notion of universal access to essential services (World Health Organization 2000). Updated estimates were published for the global burden of disease and risk factors (Lopez *et al.* 2006) and revised estimates for the costs and effectiveness of different packages of intervention were published (Jamison 2007; Laxminarayan *et al.* 2006). These included a growing appreciation of the present and likely future impact of chronic non-communicable diseases affecting adults in middle- and low-income countries, together with a recognition that selected interventions for these conditions could be very cost-effective.

The thinking of *Investing in Health* was also influential in high-income countries. For these countries, a major implication is that appropriate healthcare as well as population strategies to promote health are an increasingly important investment in order to contain the costs associated with an ageing population affected by a high prevalence of chronic illness. In the United Kingdom, the Treasury commissioned a former chief executive of a leading bank to examine the case for increasing investment in health services (Wanless 2004). His report recognized the increasing costs associated with chronic conditions and argued for the need 'to invest in reducing demand by enhancing the promotion of good health and disease prevention' (p. 3) with 'health services evolving from dealing with acute problems through more effective control of chronic conditions to promoting the maintenance of good health' (p. 10) (Wanless 2004).

Criticisms of *Investing in Health*

The approach of *Investing in Health* was grounded in modelling the potential health gains that might be achieved through optimal use of specific interventions. This approach was endorsed by the later World Health Report 2000 (World Health Organization 2000) and by the report of the Commission on Macroeconomics and Health (Commission on Macroeconomics and Health 2001). Nevertheless, there is a concern that anticipated benefits from essential packages of care have not been fully realized, leading to two main types of criticism of the approach. First, there are technical criticisms of the methods used in estimating the costs and outcomes of intervention in different conditions. Several important assumptions are disputed. The estimation of DALYs in the 1993 report utilized weights that assigned greater value to life years of economically active adults than infants or older people. The same discount rate was used across different countries, but low-income countries would generally value present benefits more highly than high-income countries. Costs of intervention were estimated as average rather than marginal costs (Williams 1999). The balance of costs and benefits may vary in different settings. This is illustrated by the observation that there have been no cases of wild-type poliomyelitis in the United States since 1979, but polio control costs US$230 million annually, and there are an average of nine polio cases per year linked to oral polio vaccine (Taylor *et al.* 1997). While these methodological criticisms are important at the margin, they do little to vitiate the general conclusion that if effective low-cost interventions were employed more efficiently there would be considerable health gains.

A second type of criticism concerns the lack of a well-developed strategy for implementation of essential packages of care. Proposed disinvestment from regressive, specialist services of low-cost effectiveness is unlikely to prove politically acceptable in most countries (Gwatkin *et al.* 2004). Investment in essential packages of intervention requires appropriate policies and structures that will support the financing and delivery of services, especially for the poor. Cost-effectiveness analysis is useful in defining the set of interventions that should be delivered by health services but has a more limited role in defining the systems that should be developed to implement them. This is illustrated by the debate concerning the appropriateness of the strategy for polio eradication (Taylor *et al.* 1997). The resources allocated to short-term intensification of polio vaccination activity may have been better invested in long-term efforts to strengthen health systems that can deliver interventions for a range of priority conditions (Taylor *et al.* 1997). The counter-argument is that the Polio Eradication strategy is implemented with a subsidiary aim of strengthening heath systems, and some empirical evidence from a range of low-income countries suggests that this has been achieved, although possibly to a more limited extent than was possible (Loevinsohn *et al.* 2002). Both arguments point to the need for the development of health systems that offer access to affordable care to everyone.

Equity-driven approaches

Equity-driven approaches to health services are primarily motivated by a concern for social justice. Equity requires that all individuals or groups in the population should be treated fairly, with a just distribution of the costs of providing services, as well as a fair distribution of the benefits obtained through utilization of health services. The data shown in Table 2.9.1 illustrate substantial inequity in the distribution of health resources between rich and poor countries. This global inequity is sometimes addressed through the concept of the right to health. For example, facilitating access to essential medicines, such as antiretroviral therapy, represents a practical means of approaching the realization of the right to health (Hogerzeil 2006).

More than 150 countries recognize the right to the highest attainable level of health; yet, most societies tolerate inequalities in the determinants of health to a varying extent. The unequal distribution of determinants, especially income and education, fosters the development of inequalities in health. Inequality in the distribution of income between groups in a country may be summarized using the Gini coefficient, which provides a numerical index of inequality ranging in value from zero, indicating perfect equality in income, to one indicating maximal inequality in income distribution. Gini coefficients for countries generally fall in the range 0.2–0.6. There is evidence that more unequal societies have worse health (Wilkinson & Pickett 2006).

Health and normal functioning are necessary prerequisites of the fair equality of opportunity that is required in a just society (Daniels *et al.* 2004). Therefore, health systems should be organized so as to minimize inequalities in health and improve the health status of all groups in a population (Daniels *et al.* 2004). Universal access to healthcare is the objective, but 'What is access to healthcare?' and 'How can we judge whether a just distribution of access to care has been realized?'

Access to healthcare

In general terms, 'access to healthcare' is said to exist when individuals or families can mobilize the resources they need to preserve or improve their health (Gulliford *et al.* 2002). At the simplest level, having access to healthcare may be judged in terms of the availability of services (Box 2.9.4). This may include the geographical proximity or physical accessibility of services. Availability may also

Box 2.9.4 Dimensions of access to healthcare

Dimension of access	Meaning	Potential indicators
Availability	Whether there is an adequate supply of health services in an area	◆ Number of physicians or nurses per 1000 population ◆ Number of hospital beds per 1000 population ◆ Distance to nearest primary care provider ◆ Distance to nearest hospital
Utilization	Whether health services are utilized	◆ Primary care consultations for 1000 population ◆ Hospital admissions per 1000 population
Relevance to need	Whether appropriate services are received by people who need them	◆ Proportion of births attended by trained healthcare professional ◆ Proportion of subjects with elevated blood pressure who receive antihypertensive therapy
Outcomes	Whether achievable health outcomes are realized	◆ Maternal mortality rate ◆ Mortality rate from appendicitis

encompass the supply of services in terms of the numbers of doctors, nurses, or hospital beds per 1000 population (Table 2.9.1). At the next level, gaining access to healthcare means that services are utilized when they are needed. There may be considerable barriers to the uptake of services even when these are available. Obstacles to utilization include financial barriers, such as the costs to individuals or households of utilizing care; physical barriers, including distance or difficulties of travel; personal barriers, as when services are not viewed as culturally appropriate, socially acceptable or consistent with personal beliefs; or organizational barriers, as when there are difficulties obtaining a consultation, or delays in receiving needed treatment, because of waiting lists or limited capacity of services (Aday & Anderson 1981; Pechansky & Thomas 1981). Utilization of services only offers benefit when care provided is relevant to need and is effective in addressing people's health problems (Box 2.9.4). Finally, access to healthcare should deliver effective care that meets people's health needs and achieves the intended health outcome.

Equity in access to healthcare

Equity in healthcare can be evaluated in several different ways (Box 2.9.5). An important distinction, which is attributed to Aristotle, is the one between horizontal as compared to vertical equity (Gillon 2005). Horizontal equity requires that equals should be treated in proportion to their equality, while vertical equity requires that unequals should be treated in proportion to their inequality. It is generally easier to evaluate horizontal equity, as this requires that all people with the same needs have access to the same services, 'equal access for equal need'. Horizontal inequity in access to healthcare, like inequality in income or health, is often measured using Gini-like metrics known as concentration indices (Wagstaff *et al.* 1991; Mackenbach & Kunst 1997).

In reality, different groups in a population often have different needs and require appropriately differentiated services. This is evident, for example, in the healthcare needs of indigenous peoples in Australia whose life expectancy at birth is some 17 years shorter than that of the general population. Mooney posed the question,

Box 2.9.5 Aspects of equity in health and healthcare

Equity	Fairness, or justice, in respect of treatment of different individuals or groups (Last 2007)
Horizontal equity	The extent to which equals are treated in proportion to their equality
Vertical equity	The extent to which unequals are treated in proportion to their inequality
Equity in financial contribution	The extent to which individual or household contributions are consistent with their capacity to pay
Equity in access to healthcare	The extent to which there is a fair distribution of access to healthcare in relation to need, including equal access for equal need (horizontal) and unequal access for unequal need (vertical)
Equity in health	The extent to which there is a fair or just distribution of health among individuals and groups in a population
Effective coverage	The proportion of the population in need of an intervention that has received an effective intervention (Shengelia *et al.* 2005)

'what would amount to a fair distribution of health resources, given this large difference in health status?' (Mooney 1996). There is little consensus, on how questions concerning this vertical dimension of equity should be answered (Mooney 2000). Marginalized groups such as indigenous populations, new migrants, homeless people, or prisoners may be regarded as 'hard to reach' or at least 'underserved' by standard services and there may sometimes be a case for developing targeted services. There is a concern that such targeted services may become 'poor services for poor people'. More generally, there is increasing emphasis on designing local services to meet locally expressed needs, leading to greater variation in the organization and delivery of services, in contrast to the uniform approach implied by the pursuit of horizontal equity. In the United Kingdom, the tension between these two dimensions of equity has been addressed by introducing national level service specifications, while accommodating local discretion in organizing their implementation.

Equity of access: Availability of services

There are generally substantial inequities in healthcare access among different groups in the populations of middle- and low-income countries. Gwatkin characterized health systems in middle- and low-income countries as 'consistently inequitable, providing more and higher quality services to the well-off, who need them less, than to the poor, who are unable to obtain them'. (Gwatkin *et al.* 2004) (p. 1273).

Health services in middle- and low-income countries do not usually provide full population coverage. In some of the more affluent middle-income countries, such as the small islands of the Caribbean, government services offer access to primary care services that are mainly used by the poor, while private practitioners' services are utilized by the better off. However, as national income decreases, government expenditure on healthcare as a per cent of GDP declines and population coverage by government services diminishes (Table 2.9.1). Services tend to be concentrated close to urban areas, where they may be more readily utilized by better off groups leading to a markedly pro-rich distribution of expenditure on government health services. The distribution of expenditure on primary healthcare services generally shows a lesser degree of inequity than all healthcare spending (Fig. 2.9.1). In rural areas, access to government health services may be extremely limited, with non-governmental organizations such as religious bodies and charities sometimes offering alternative sources of provision. Thus, not only is the overall supply of services in middle- and low-income countries generally limited, but also the geographical distribution of services disadvantages the poor. Geographical barriers to accessing services are important not only in terms of distance but also in terms of the difficulty and costs of travelling long distances to access services.

In China, the lack of availability of rural health services was addressed between 1965 and the early 1980s by the development of 'barefoot doctors'. These were rural farm workers who were given basic health training over several months in order to provide a combination of traditional Chinese and Western medicines to rural communities. The success of this strategy is debated. However, the barefoot doctor approach was regarded as a model for the development of community health workers in other countries and provided an important inspiration for the 1978 Alma Ata Declaration that initiated the 'Health for All' strategy. The Alma Ata Declaration promoted access to primary care, with an emphasis on community participation and universality, as a means of facilitating equity in health.

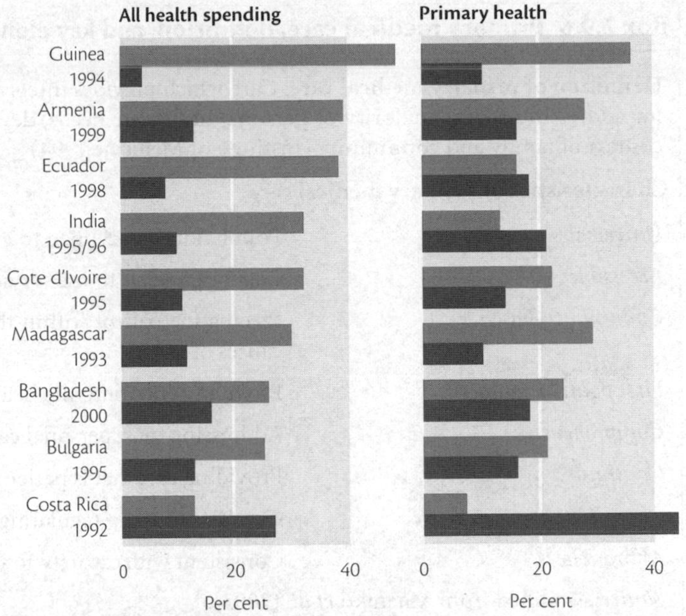

Fig. 2.9.1 Share of public spending that accrues to the richest (top bar) and poorest fifths (bottom bar) of the population.
Source: World Bank (2004).

The importance of the concept of primary healthcare was restated recently by Margaret Chan in her speech to the World Health Assembly following her election as Director General of WHO in 2006 when she said 'When we talk about capacity, we absolutely must talk about the importance of primary healthcare. It is the cornerstone of building the capacity of health systems' (Chan 2006).

Definition of primary healthcare

There are several definitions of primary healthcare. The WHO makes a distinction between primary healthcare, which encompasses public health activities directed at environmental determinants of health, and primary medical care, including first point of contact care in the community. The UK Departments of Health define primary healthcare simply as care provided outside hospitals by family health services (including family physicians, dentists, pharmacists, and opticians) and community health services (including community doctors, dentists, nurses, midwives, and health visitors and other allied professions). Other definitions characterize primary healthcare according to key attributes (Box 2.9.6). Primary care providers are community-based, easily accessible, and offer population coverage. Primary care provides the first point of contact with the health system and is comprehensive in its scope, addressing all potential health problems. Primary care also provides ongoing care over time with continuity or longitudinality representing a key element in most definitions. Primary care services are generally less costly and more affordable than specialist services. In high-income countries, primary medical care practitioners generally have a gatekeeper role in which they regulate and coordinate access to specialist care (Starfield 1992). However, specialist expertise is increasingly being embedded in primary care teams in order to improve the quality of chronic illness management (Bodenheimer *et al.* 2002).

Through its emphasis on universality, accessibility, and affordability, primary medical care generally promotes equity of access to healthcare. Through its community orientation and emphasis on

Box 2.9.6 Primary medical care, definition, and key elements

Definition of primary medical care: Care which provides integrated, accessible healthcare services by clinicians who are accountable for addressing a large majority of personal healthcare needs, developing a sustained partnership with patients, and practising in the context of family and community (Institute of Medicine 1994)

Characteristics of primary medical care

Universal	Population-based, open to everyone
Accessible	Enabling people to use services when they are needed
Community-based	Placing the patient within the wider familial or social context necessary for addressing multiple causes of illness
First point of contact	Providing entry into the health system
Comprehensive	Addressing most personal care needs including preventive, curative, and rehabilitative
Continuity	Providing care that is patient-focused over time
Coordination	Coordinating and regulating use of other levels of care
Affordable	Consistent with capacity to pay

Source: Modified from Macinko *et al.* (2003).

out-of-hospital care, primary medical care generally enhances efficiency through the application of more cost-effective and appropriate health technologies. The gatekeeper role of the primary care practitioner generally has the consequence of promoting more efficient utilization of resources compared with systems where individual patients can gain direct access to specialists.

Primary care and population health

Does the availability of primary healthcare contribute to improved population health? In general, those countries that have followed policies emphasizing universal primary healthcare coverage have achieved more favourable health outcomes. The Cuban health system is frequently cited as one that has successfully adopted the primary care approach. In 2001, life expectancy at birth in Cuba was 76.3 years compared with 77.4 years in the United States, and the infant mortality rate was 7.2 per 1000 in both countries in spite of the great disparity in economic conditions (Pan American Health Organization 2007). In Costa Rica, commitment to the development of public health services and primary care has been associated with favourable health outcomes and the second highest life expectancy in the Americas (Table 2.9.1) (Unger *et al.* 2007).

Evidence is also provided by ecological analyses from high-income countries. In the United States, states with a greater supply of family physicians have lower mortality rates after adjusting for income inequality and smoking (Shi *et al.* 1999). In the United Kingdom, districts with higher supply of family physicians have lower mortality from all causes but while this association is sensitive to adjustment for several measures of healthcare needs. Hospital utilization shows a strong negative association with the supply of primary care physicians (Gulliford 2002). In an analysis of data for eighteen Organisation for Economic Cooperation and Development (OECD) countries, Macinko and colleagues (Macinko *et al.* 2003) suggested that the strength of a country's primary healthcare system is associated with lower all-cause mortality and reduced premature years of life lost from all-causes and from respiratory and cardiac disease.

These studies provide preliminary information about the relationship between systems of organizing the delivery of healthcare and population health outcomes. Given the ecological nature of the data, and the imprecise and incomplete measurement of confounding variables, there is a risk of bias. Illich observed that 'the fact that the doctor population is higher where certain diseases have become rare has little to do with the doctors' ability to control or eliminate them. It simply means that doctors deploy themselves as they like, more so than other professionals, and that they tend to gather where the climate is healthy, water is clean and where people are employed and can pay for their services' (Illich 1976, p. 30).

Inverse care law

Inequality in the availability of health services is a concern for all countries for the reasons outlined by Illich (1976); without regulation, the supply of healthcare resources is distributed towards more affluent areas with fewer health needs. This situation was described by the British general practitioner Julian Tudor Hart as an 'inverse care law' with 'the availability of good medical care tending to vary inversely with the need for it in the population served' (Tudor Hart 1971) (p. 405).

In countries which, like the United Kingdom, have a dominant national health service funded from general taxation, this situation has been addressed through the development and application of explicit formulae linking the allocation of resources for hospital and community services in different areas to measures of population size and health needs (Smith *et al.* 1994). The number of primary care doctors in an area is also regulated. Nevertheless, historical patterns of the supply of services have been resistant to change and socioeconomically deprived areas continue to have fewer doctors and less well-developed primary care facilities (Gulliford *et al.* 2004). Similar resource allocation methods have been recommended for application to public services in some middle- and low-income countries (Laxminarayan *et al.* 2006). In countries with more pluralistic systems of providing care, or where fee-for-service payment is dominant, greater inequities in the supply of services develop. For example, in US cities, the poor are significantly 'underserved' by health services, both because of inequalities of supply and because of financial barriers to accessing care (Institute of Medicine 2003). In most countries, the rural poor are significantly disadvantaged by relative or absolute lack of availability of services.

Equity of access: Utilization of services

The availability of services does not ensure that those who need them will use them, and there may be important personal, financial, or organizational barriers to the uptake of services. The probability of an individual utilizing services depends on their perceptions of their needs, on social and cultural norms and expectations, and on previous experiences of utilizing care. Patterns of utilization may not be consistent with medically defined need, as when people do not take up preventive services, delay in presenting with serious conditions, or utilize services for apparently trivial conditions. In many health systems, the financial cost of utilizing healthcare may present a very significant barrier to utilization.

Financial barriers to access

Out-of-pocket expenditure is an important method of funding healthcare in middle- and low-income countries (Table 2.9.1) and the impact of these financial contributions is usually disproportionate for poorer groups (Pannarunothai & Mills 1997). This has the consequence that poor people may be unable to obtain needed healthcare, or may find it necessary to utilize less costly and less appropriate forms of care such as private drug vendors (Whitehead *et al.* 2001). People may delay accessing care until their illness becomes more severe, requiring more costly treatment (Whitehead *et al.* 2001). Health expenditures for serious illness may then be catastrophic leading to impoverishment of households. In Asia, illness is one of the principal reasons for households falling into poverty. Across eleven Asian countries, if household expenditures on healthcare are taken into account, then an estimated additional 2.7 per cent of the population (78 million people) live in absolute poverty with household incomes of less than US$1 per person per day when compared with conventional estimates (van Doorslaer *et al.* 2006b). Xu and colleagues (Xu *et al.* 2003) reported a multi-country study of catastrophic health expenditures, which they defined as health expenditure exceeding 40 per cent of household income after subsistence needs were met. In household survey data, more than 2 per cent of households in 17 out of 59 countries experienced catastrophic expenditures. Based on between-country comparisons, high healthcare expenditures were more likely if health services require direct payment, if households have limited capacity to pay, and if methods to pool risks are lacking. This leads to a paradox observed by Frenk (2006) that while healthcare should be an important factor in reducing poverty, expenditure on healthcare is itself a cause of poverty. This paradox was addressed in Mexican health reforms through the introduction of a new form of health insurance (Seguro Popular) that extends coverage of the poor and provides access to a set of basic medical interventions (Frenk *et al.* 2006). Bleich *et al.* (2007) found that hypertensive subjects who were insured through Seguro Popular were more likely to have their hypertension treated and controlled, compared with sociodemographically matched but uninsured controls. However, the achievement of better hypertension treatment was also dependent on an adequate supply of health professionals in an area (Bleich *et al.* 2007). More generally, there is a lack of evidence concerning the costs, outcomes, and consequences for equity of such models of financing care (Palmer *et al.* 2004; Gwatkin *et al.* 2004).

Equity of healthcare utilization in high-income countries

Many studies have evaluated the overall impact of barriers to the utilization of medical care in high-income countries that, with the exception of the United States, offer universal healthcare coverage. In a recent study, the utilization of physician services was evaluated in relation to respondents' self-rated needs for care (van Doorslaer *et al.* 2006a). Gini-like indices of horizontal inequity were estimated to summarize the utilization of care in relation to household income level. The results showed that utilization of primary care visits was generally either equitably distributed among income groups, or showed a pro-poor distribution (Fig. 2.9.2). However, utilization of specialists' services generally showed some degree of pro-rich inequity, that is higher-income groups utilized more specialist care than lower-income groups at a given level of need. This is a consistent finding from a number of studies and suggests that higher socioeconomic position, including higher income or education, may facilitate access to specialist care through increased ability to negotiate financial or organizational barriers. These results from a range of

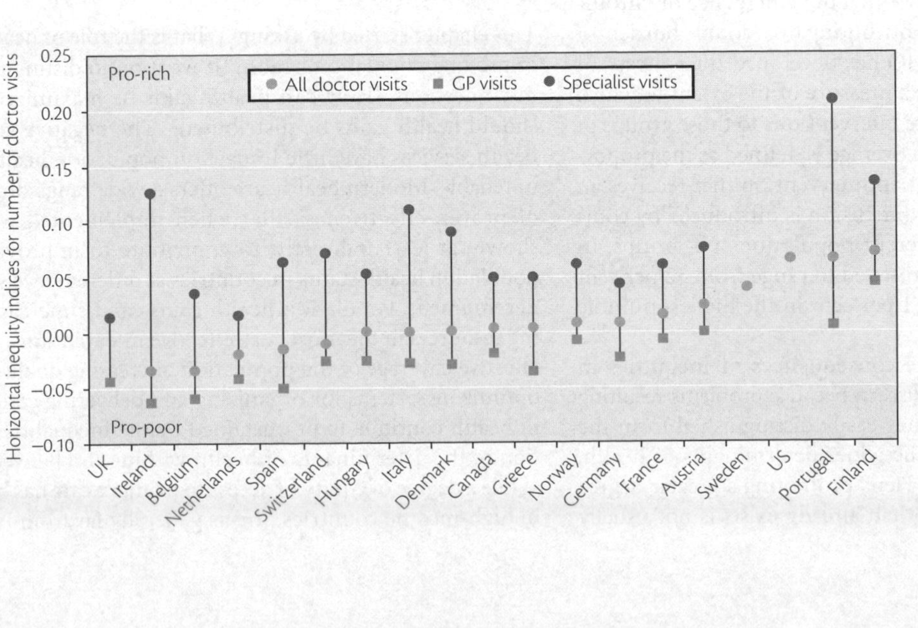

Fig. 2.9.2 Horizontal inequity (HI) indices in relation to household income for the annual mean number of visits to a doctor in 19 OECD countries.
Source: van Doorslaer *et al.* (2006a).

countries suggest that in many instances a degree of equity of access to primary care has been achieved, but inequity persists in the utilization of specialist care.

Equity of access: Relevance and effectiveness

Socio-economic groups differ not only with respect to the volume of care consumed but also with respect to the type of care utilized. There is a considerable body of evidence to show that preventive medical interventions are taken up less by lower socioeconomic groups, with a risk of increasing inequalities in health. In Belgium, for example, overall utilization of family physician services showed substantial pro-poor inequity, but there was marked pro-rich inequity in the uptake of influenza vaccination, cholesterol testing, mammography, and cervical cancer screening (Lorant *et al.* 2002). Problems of poor quality care typically vary between socioeconomic groups with disadvantaged groups receiving lower quality care. The US Institute of Medicine has reviewed a large and consistent body of evidence to show that US black and ethnic minority populations are less likely to receive needed care even after allowing for socioeconomic variables including insurance status, income, age, and severity of condition (Institute of Medicine 2003). For example, there are lower rates of utilization of appropriate cardiac treatment including coronary artery bypass surgery, lower rates of renal dialysis or transplantation, but higher rates of unfavourable events such as diabetes-related lower limb amputations.

Access to care and equity in health

In low-income countries, it is clear that lack of access to healthcare contributes to unfavourable population health outcomes. The 1993 World Development Report estimated that 32 per cent of the burden of disease in low-income countries could be avoided by extending coverage of low-cost interventions (World Bank 1993). This is recognized in the Millennium Development Goals that aim to improve the status of the world's poorest populations with specific health-related objectives of reducing child mortality, improving maternal health and combating HIV/AIDS, malaria, and other diseases. There have now been significant increases in life expectancy, leading to reduced between-country inequalities, but preventable mortality and morbidity from malaria, TB, diarrhoea, and pneumonia remain important in the poor populations of many countries (Jamison 2007). At the same time, the emergence of chronic non-communicable diseases is contributing to a 'double burden' of disease (Jamison 2007). The WHO has developed the concept of 'effective coverage' (Box 2.9.5) as a measure of the extent to which health services deliver appropriate interventions to those groups of people who need them. Effective coverage is defined as the proportion of the population in need of an intervention that receives an effective intervention. An equity dimension is introduced by comparing effective coverage in different population sub-groups. In Mexico, effective coverage was estimated to range from 52 per cent in the lowest wealth quintile to 61 per cent in the highest quintile (Lozano *et al.* 2006).

In high-income countries, the consequences of inequities in healthcare access are less easy to discern because problems resulting from inadequate healthcare are not easily distinguished from the consequences of inequalities in the wider determinants of health, often sustained over generations. Here, promoting a greater degree of equity of access to healthcare than already exists is not usually viewed as a major strategy for reducing inequalities in health. Instead, inequalities in the wider determinants must be addressed more directly (Acheson 1998). In England, among ten headline indicators on inequalities in health requiring action by local health bodies, only one, the number of primary care professionals per 10 000 population, refers to the provision of healthcare. This does not mean, however, that it is not important to ensure that all groups have equal access to the benefits offered by effective healthcare interventions.

Some indirect evidence suggests that inequity in access to specialist care may contribute to inequalities in health in high-income countries. In England and Wales, there are substantial socioeconomic inequalities in survival with cancer that have been increasing over time and are greater for treatable cancers (Coleman *et al.* 2004). For example, the difference in 5-year survival between the highest and lowest quintiles of deprivation in women is 5.8 per cent for breast cancer, 8.3 per cent for rectal cancer, and 7.3 per cent for colon cancer, compared with 0.2 per cent for oesophageal cancer, a less treatable condition. Evidence such as this has been used to advocate the routine implementation of 'equity audit' as part of routine service evaluation. In the United States, there are significant black–white inequalities in mortality, with life expectancy for black men being 6.3 years lower, and for women 4.5 years less, than for whites. Cardiovascular disease and diabetes account for 35 per cent of this difference in men and 52 per cent in women (Harper *et al.* 2007). Differential access to healthcare may contribute to these differences (Institute of Medicine 2003).

In order to promote equity in health, new policies and services have sometimes been implemented on the basis of their potential to reduce inequalities in health. In England, following a White Paper on cigarette smoking, smoking cessation services were developed in deprived areas, providing nicotine replacement therapy free of charge (Chambers 1999). Universal antenatal and newborn screening programmes for sickle cell disease and thalassaemia were implemented with specific recognition of their potential to reduce health inequalities associated with black and ethnic minority status (Sassi *et al.* 2001). At local level, outreach services have been developed to target specific groups such as homeless people with serious mental illness.

Conclusion

This chapter started by asking 'What is the role of health services in improving population health?' It went on to distinguish two separate questions: 'How can health gains be maximized?' and 'How should health gains be distributed?' The negative argument that health services have little impact on population health now seems untenable. Modern healthcare offers a wide range of interventions of proven effectiveness that when implemented widely can be shown, at least indirectly, to contribute to improving trends in population health status in countries at different levels of economic development. Population health gains can be increased by investing resources in the most cost-effective interventions, by increasing effective coverage of the population, increasing quality of care, and optimizing systems for organizing and delivering care. Inequalities in health continue to be sustained by the inequalities in distribution of the determinants of health within- and between-countries. While a degree of equity of access to primary care has been achieved in high-income countries, this is generally far from being the case in middle- and low-income countries. The challenge now is to ensure that all groups obtain a fair share of the benefits of healthcare intervention. Public health specialists should advocate principles of efficiency and equity and contribute to realizing these through participation in processes of needs assessment, health technology assessment, quality improvement, and facilitating access to needed healthcare for all groups.

References

Acheson, E.D. (1998). *Independent inquiry into inequalities in health*. The Stationery Office, London.

Allgood, P.C., Warwick, J., Warren, R.M.L. *et al.* (2008). A case-control study of the impact of the East Anglian breast cancer screening programme on breast cancer mortality. *British Journal of Cancer*, **98**, 206–9.

Ashworth, M., Charlton, J., Ballard, K. *et al.* (2005). Variations in antibiotic prescribing and consultation rates for acute respiratory infection in UK general practices 1995–2000. *British Journal of General Practice*, **55**, 603–8.

Ashworth, M., Latinovic, R., Charlton, J. *et al.* (2004). Why has antibiotic prescribing for respiratory illness declined in primary care? A longitudinal study using the General Practice Research Database. *Journal of Public Health*, **26**, 268–74.

Bhasale, A.L., Miller, G.C., Reid, S.E. *et al.* (1998). Analysing potential harm in Australian general practice: An incident-monitoring study. *The Medical Journal of Australia*, **169**, 73–6.

Blake, S.C., Thorpe, K.E., and Howell, K.G. (2003). Access to healthcare in the United States. In *Access to healthcare* (eds. M.C. Gulliford and M. Morgan), Routledge, London.

Blanks, R.G., Moss, S.M., McGahan, C.E. *et al.* (2000). Effect of NHS breast cancer screening programme on mortality from breast cancer in England and Wales, 1990–8: comparison of observed with predicted mortality. *British Medical Journal*, **321**, 665–9.

Bleich, S.N., Cutler, D.M., Adams, A.S. *et al.* (2007). Impact of insurance and supply of health professionals on coverage of treatment for hypertension in Mexico: Popualtion-based study. *British Medical Journal*, doi:10.1136/bmj.39350.617616.BE (published 22 October 2007).

Bloom, D.E., Canning, D., and Jamison, D.T. (2004). Health, wealth and welfare. *Finance and Development*, 10–15.

Bodenheimer, T., Wagner, E.H., and Grumbach, K. (2002). Improving primary care for patients with chronic illness. *Journal of the American Medical Association*, **288**, 1775–9.

Braveman, P., Starfield, B., Geiger, H.J. *et al.* (2001). World Health Report 2000: How it removes equity from the agenda for public health monitoring and policy Commentary: Comprehensive approaches are needed for full understanding. *British Medical Journal*, **323**, 678–81.

Brennan, T.A., Leape, L.L., Laird, N.M. *et al.* (1991). Incidence of adverse events and negligence in hospitalized patients. Results of the Harvard Medical Practice Study I. *New England Journal of Medicine*, **324**, 370–6.

Bunker, J.P., Frazier, H.S., and Mosteller, F. (1994). Improving health: Measuring effects of medical care. *Milbank Quarterly*, **72**, 225–58.

Cancer Research UK (2008). *Breast cancer survival statistics.* Cancer Research UK, London. Source: http://info.cancerresearchuk.org/cancerstats/types/breast/survival/ accessed 25th January 2008.

Chambers, J. (1999). Being strategic about smoking. *British Medical Journal*, **318**, 1–2.

Chan, M. (2006). *Speech to the World Health Assembly*. World Health Organization, Geneva. Available at http://www.who.int/dg/chan/speeches/2006/wha/en/index.html accessed 21st June 2007.

Cochrane, A.L. (1972). *Effectiveness and efficiency. Random reflections on health services*. Nuffield Provincial Hospitals Trust, London.

Coleman, M.P., Rachet, B., Woods, L.M. *et al.* (2004). Trends and socioeconomic inequalities in cancer survival in England and Wales up to 2001. *British Journal of Cancer*, **90**, 1367–73.

Commission on Macroeconomics and Health (2001). *Macroeconomics and health: Investing in health for economic development*. Report of the Commission on Macroeconomics and Health. World Health Organization, Geneva.

Cutler, D.M., Rosen, A.B., and Vijan, S. (2006). The Value of Medical Spending in the United States, 1960–2000. *New England Journal of Medicine*, **355**, 920–7.

Daniels, N., Kennedy, B., and Kawachi, I. (2004). Health and inequality, or why justics is good for our health. *Public health, ethics and equity*. Oxford University Press, Oxford.

Donabedian, A. (2003). *An Introduction to quality assurance in healthcare*. Oxford University Press, Oxford, New York.

Doran, T., Fullwood, C., Gravelle, H. *et al.* (2006). Pay-for-Performance Programs in Family Practices in the United Kingdom. *New England Journal of Medicine*, **355**, 375–84.

Dworkin, R. (1977). *Taking rights seriously*. Duckworth, London.

Ebrahim,S. and Smith,G.D. (2001). Exporting failure? Coronary heart disease and stroke in developing countries. *International Journal of Epidemiology*, **30**, 201–5.

Eccles, M., Grimshaw, J., Walker, A. *et al.* (2005). Changing the behavior of healthcare professionals: The use of theory in promoting the uptake of research findings. *Journal of Clinical Epidemiology*, **58**, 107–12.

Faculty of Public Health (2007). *Three key domains of public health practice*. Faculty of Public Health, London. Available at http://www.fphm.org.uk/about_faculty/what_public_health/3key_areas_health_practice.asp accessed 21st June 2007.

Fenner, F., Henderson, D.A., Arita, I. *et al.* (1988). *Smallpox and its eradication*. World Health Organization, Geneva.

Frenk, J., Gonzalez-Pier, E., Gomez-Dantes, O. *et al.* (2006). Comprehensive reform to improve health system performance in Mexico. *Lancet*, **368**, 1524–34.

Fulop, N., Allen, P., Clarke, A. *et al.* (2003). From health technology assessment to research on the organisation and delivery of health services: Addressing the balance. *Health Policy*, **63**, 155–65.

GAVI Alliance (2007). *Global alliance on vaccines and immunisation*. Available at http://www.gavialliance.org/ accessed 21st June 2007.

Gillon, R. (2005). *Philosophical medical ethics*. John Wiley, Chichester.

Global Polio Eradication Initiative (2006). *Global Polio Eradication Initiative. 2005 Annual Report*. World Health Organization, Geneva.

Gotzsche,P.C. and Olsen, O. (2000). Is screening for breast cancer with mammography justifiable? *Lancet*, **355**, 129–34.

Gulliford,M., Figueroa-Munoz,J., Morgan,M. *et al.*(2002). What does 'access to healthcare' mean? *Journal of Health Services Research and Policy*, **7**, 186–8.

Gulliford, M.C., Jack, R.H., Adams, G. *et al.* (2004). Availability and structure of primary medical care services and population health and healthcare indicators in England. *BMC Health Services Research*, **4**, 12.

Gulliford, M.C. (2002). Availability of primary care doctors and population health in England: is there an association? *Journal of Public Health Medicine*, **24**, 252–4.

Gwatkin, D.R., Bhuiya, A., and Victora, C.G. (2004). Making health systems more equitable. *Lancet*, **364**, 1273–80.

Harper, S., Lynch, J., Burris, S. *et al.* (2007). Trends in the Black-White Life Expectancy Gap in the United States, 1983-2003. *Journal of the American Medical Association*, **297**, 1224–32.

Health Protection Agency (2007). *Health Protection Agency publishes quarterly Clostridium difficile and MRSA figures*. Available at http://www.hpa.org.uk/infections/topics_az/hai/Mandatory_Results.htm accessed 21st June 2007.

Hogerzeil, H.V. (2006). Essential medicines and human rights: What can they learn from each other? *Bulletin of the World Health Organisation*, **84**, 371–5.

Holland, W.W. (1991) *European community atlas of 'Avoidable Death'.* Second Edition. Oxford Medical Publications, Oxford.

Institute of Medicine (1994). *Defining primary care. An interim report.* National Academies Press, Washington DC. Available at http://books.nap.edu/openbook.php?record_id=9153andpage=1 accessed 21st June 2007.

Institute of Medicine (2005). *Crossing the quality chasm. A new health system for the 21st Century.* National Academy Press, Washington, DC.

Institute of Medicine (2003). *Unequal treatment: Confronting racial and ethnic disparities in healthcare.* National Academies Press, Washington DC.

Ivan Illich (1976). *Limits to medicine. Medical nemesis: The expropriation of health.* Penguin Books, Harmondsworth.

Jamison, D.T. (2006). *Investing in health.* In *Disease control priorities in developing countries.* Chapter 1 (*eds.* D.T. Jamison *et al.*). World Bank Group, Washington DC. Available at http://files.dcp2.org/pdf/DCP/DCP01.pdf accessed 21st June 2007.

Janjua, N.Z., Akhtar, S., and Hutin, Y.J.F. (2005). Injection use in two districts of Pakistan: Implications for disease prevention. *International Journal for Quality in Healthcare*, **17**, 401–8.

Kohn, L,T., Corrigan, J.M., and Donaldson, M.S. (2000). *To err is human; building a safer health system.* National Academy Press, Washington DC.

Laatikainen, T., Critchley, J., Vartiainen, E. *et al.* (2005). Explaining the decline in coronary heart disease mortality in Finland between 1982 and 1997. *American Journal of Epidemiology*, **162**, 764–73.

Last, J.M. (2007). *A dictionary of public health.* Oxford University Press, Oxford.

Last, J.M. (2001). *Dictionary of epidemiology.* Oxford University Press, Oxford.

Lau, J., Antman, E.M., Jimenez-Silva, J. *et al.* (1992). Cumulative meta-analysis of therapeutic trials for myocardial infarction. *New England Journal of Medicine*, **327**, 248–54.

Laxminarayan, R., Mills, A.J., Breman, J.G. *et al.* (2006) Advancement of global health: Key messages from the Disease Control Priorities Project. *Lancet*, **367**, 1193–208.

Loevinsohn, B., Aylward, B., Steinglass, R. *et al.* (2002). Impact of targeted programs on health systems: A case study of the polio eradication initiative. *American Journal of Public Health*, **92**, 19–23.

Lohse, N., Hansen, A.B.E., Pedersen, G. *et al.* (2007). Survival of persons with and without HIV infection in Denmark, 1995 to 2005. *Annals of Internal Medicine*, **146**, 87–95.

Lopez, A.D., Mathers, C.D., Ezzati, M. *et al.* (2006). Global and regional burden of disease and risk factors, 2001: Systematic analysis of population health data. *Lancet*, **367**, 1747–57.

Lorant, V., Boland, B., Humblet, P. *et al.* (2002). Equity in prevention and healthcare. *Journal of Epidemiology and Community Health*, **56**, 510–16.

Lozano, R., Soliz, P., Gakidou, E. *et al.* (2006) Benchmarking of performance of Mexican states with effective coverage. *Lancet*, **368**, 1729–41.

Macinko, J., Starfield, B., and Shi, L. (2003). The contribution of primary care systems to health outcomes within Organization for Economic Cooperation and Development (OECD) countries, 1970–1998. *Health Services Research*, **38**, 831–65.

Mackenbach, J.P. and Kunst, A.E. (1997). Measuring the magnitude of socio-economic inequalities in health: An overview of available measures illustrated with two examples from Europe. *Social Science and Medicine*, **44**, 757–71.

Mahabir, D. and Gulliford, M.C. (2005). Changing patterns of primary care for diabetes in Trinidad and Tobago over 10 years. *Diabetic Medicine*, **22**, 619–24.

Mannion, R., Davies, H.T., and Marshall, M.N. (2005). Cultural characteristics of 'high' and 'low' performing hospitals. *Journal of Health Organisation and Management*, **19**, 431–9.

Maxwell, R.J. (1984). Quality assessment in health. *British Medical Journal*, **288**, 1470–2.

Mckeown, T. (1979). *The role of medicine.* Blackwell, Oxford.

Mooney, G. (2000). Vertical equity in healthcare resource allocation. *Healthcare Analysis*, **8**, 203–15.

Mooney, G.H. (1996). And now for vertical equity? Some concerns arising from aboriginal health in Australia. *Health Economics*, **5**, 99–103.

Mossialos, E., and Thomson, S. (2003). Access to healthcare in the European Union: the impact of user charges and voluntary health insurance. In *Access to Healthcare* (eds. M.C. Gulliford and M. Morgan). Routlegde, London.

Murray, C.J. and Frenk, J. (2000). A framework for assessing the performance of health systems. *Bulletin of the World Health Organisation*, **78**, 717–31.

Nystrom, L., Andersson, I., Bjurstam, N. *et al.* (2002). Long-term effects of mammography screening: Updated overview of the Swedish randomised trials. *Lancet*, **359**, 909–19.

Office for National Statistics (1998). *DH2. Number 25.* Office for National Statistics, London.

Office of the High Commissioner for Human Rights (2007). *International covenant on economic, social and cultural rights.* Office of the High Commissioner for Human Rights, Geneva. Available at http://www.unhchr.ch/html/menu3/b/a_cescr.htm accessed 21st June 2007.

Office for National Statistics (2006). Report: Deaths involving MRSA: England and Wales, 2000-2004. *Health Statistics Quarterly*, **29**, 63–8.

Oxman, A.D., Thomson, M.A., Davis, D.A. *et al.* (1995). No magic bullets: A systematic review of 102 trials of interventions to improve professional practice. *Canadian Medical Association Journal*, **153**, 1423–31.

Palmer, N., Mueller, D.H., Gilson, L. *et al.* (2004) Health financing to promote access in low income settings—how much do we know? *Lancet*, **364**, 1365–70.

Pan American Health Organization (2007). Regional Core Health Data System. Country Profile: Cuba. Data updated for 2001.

Pannarunothai, S., and Mills, A. (1997). The poor pay more: Health-related inequality in Thailand. *Social Science and Medicine*, **44**, 1781–90.

Phillips, D. (1996). Medical professional dominance and client dissatisfaction: A study of doctor-patient interaction and reported dissatisfaction with medical care among female patients at four hospitals in Trinidad and Tobago. *Social Science and Medicine*, **42**, 1419–25.

Potter, J.E., Berquo, E., Perpetuo, I.H.O. *et al.* (2001). Unwanted caesarean sections among public and private patients in Brazil: Prospective study. *British Medical Journal*, **323**, 1155–8.

President's Commission for the Study of Ethical Problems in Medicine and Biomedical and Behavioural Research (1983). *Securing access to healthcare.* US Government Printing Office, Washington DC.

Roberts, I., Yates, D., Sandercock, P. *et al.* for CRASH trial collaborators. (2004). Effect of intravenous corticosteroids on death within 14 days in 10008 adults with clinically significant head injury (MRC CRASH trial): Randomised placebo-controlled trial. Lancet, **364**, 1321–8.

Roland, M. (2004). Linking Physicians' Pay to the Quality of Care—A Major Experiment in the United Kingdom. *New England Journal of Medicine*, **351**, 1448–54.

Sassi, F., Le Grand, J., and Archard, L. (2001). Equity versus efficiency: A dilemma for the NHS. *British Medical Journal*, **323**, 762.

Sehon, S.R. and Stanley, D.E. (2003). A philosophical analysis of the evidence-based medicine debate. *BMC Health Services Research*, **3**, 14.

Sheldon, T.A. (2001). It ain't what you do but the way that you do it. *Journal of Health Services Research and Policy*, **6**, 3–5.

Shengelia, B., Tandon, A., Adams, O.B. *et al.* (2005). Access, utilization, quality, and effective coverage: An integrated conceptual framework and measurement strategy. *Social Science and Medicine*, **61**, 97–109.

Shi, L., Starfield, B., Kennedy, B. *et al.* (1999). Income inequality, primary care, and health indicators. *Journal of Family Practice*, **48**, 275–84.

Smith, R., Beaglehole, R., Woodward, D. *et al.* (2003). *Global public goods for health. Health economic and public health perspectives.* Oxford University Press, Oxford.

Smith, P., Sheldon, T.A., Carr Hill, R.A. *et al.* (1994). Allocating resources to health authorities: Results and policy implications of analysis of use of inpatient services. *British Medical Journal*, **309**, 1050–4.

Starfield, B. (1992). *Primary care: Concept, evaluation and policy*. Oxford University Press, New York.

Starfield, B. (2000). Is US health really the best in the world? *Journal of the American Medical Association*, **284**, 483–5.

Stevens, A., Raftery, J., and Mant, J. (2004). The epidemiological approach to healthcare needs assessment. In (Eds.), *Healthcare needs assessment: the epidemiologically based needs assessment reviews* (eds. A. Stevens, J. Raftery, J. Mant, and S. Simpson), pp. 1–15. Radcliffe Medical Press, Oxford.

Taylor, C.E., Cutts, F., and Taylor, M.E. (1997). Ethical dilemmas in current planning for polio eradication. *American Journal of Public Health*, **87**, 922–5.

The Global Fund (2007). *The Global Fund to fight AIDS, Tuberculosis and Malaria*. Available at http://www.theglobalfund.org/en/ accessed 21st June 2007.

The NHS Health Technology Assessment Programme (2007). Health Technology Assessment.

Tudor Hart, J. (1971). The inverse care law. *Lancet*, **297**, 405–12.

Unal, B., Critchley, J.A., and Capewell, S. (2004). Explaining the decline in coronary heart disease mortality in England and Wales between 1981 and 2000. *Circulation*, **109**, 1101–7.

Unger, J.P., De Paepe, P., Buitron, R. *et al.* (2008). Costa Rica: Achievements of a heterodox health policy. *American Journal of Public Health*, **98**, 636–43.

United Nations (2007). Universal Declaration of Human Rights. United Nations, New York. Available at http://www.un.org/Overview/rights.html accessed 21st June 2007.

van Doorslaer, E., Masseria, C., Koolman, X. and for the OECD Health Equity Research Group (2006a). Inequalities in access to medical care by income in developed countries. *Canadian Medical Association Journal*, **174**, 177–83.

van Doorslaer, E., O'Donnell, O., Rannan-Eliya, R.P. *et al.* (2006b). Effect of payments for healthcare on poverty estimates in 11 countries in Asia: An analysis of household survey data. *Lancet*, **368**, 1357–64.

von Gottberg, A., de Gouveia. L., Madhi, S.A. *et al.* (2006). Impact of conjugate Haemophilus influenzae type b (Hib) vaccine introduction in South Africa. *Bulletin of the World Health Organisation*, **84**, 811–18.

Wagstaff, A., van Doorslaer, E., and Paci, P. (1991). On the measurement of horizontal inequity in the delivery of healthcare. *Journal of Health Economics*, **10**, 169–205.

Wald, N.J. and Law, M.R. (2003). A strategy to reduce cardiovascular disease by more than 80%. *British Medical Journal*, **326**, 1419.

Wanless, D. (2004). *Securing good health for the whole population. Final report*. HMSO, London.

Whitehead, M., Dahlgren, G., and Evans, T. (2001). Equity and health sector reforms: can low-income countries escape the medical poverty trap? *Lancet*, **358**, 833–6.

Wilkinson, R.G. and Pickett, K.E. (2006). Income inequality and population health: A review and explanation of the evidence. *Social Science and Medicine*, **62**, 1768–84.

Williams, A. (1999). Calculating the global burden of disease: Time for a strategic reappraisal? *Health Economics*, **8**, 1–8.

Wooton, D. (2006). *Bad medicine: Doctors doing harm since Hippocrates*. Oxford University Press, Oxford.

World Alliance for Patient Safety (2007). *Clean care is safer care*. World Health Organization, Geneva.

World Bank (2004). *World Development Report 2004. Making services work for poor people*. World Bank, Washington DC, Oxford University Press.

World Bank (2006). *World Development Indicators 2006*. World Bank, Washington DC.

World Bank (1993). *World Development Report 1993*. World Bank, New York, Oxford University Press.

World Health Organization (2007a). *2006 Tuberculosis facts*. Geneva, World Health Organization.

World Health Organization (2000). *The World Health Report 2000*. Geneva, World Health Organization.

World Health Organization (2007b). *WHO vaccine preventable diseases: monitoring system. 2006 global summary*. World Health Organization, Geneva.

Xu, K., Evans, D.B., Kawabata, K. *et al.* (2003). Household catastrophic health expenditure: A multicountry analysis. *Lancet*, **362**, 111–17.

2.10

Assessing health needs: The global burden of disease approach

C.J.L. Murray, A.D. Lopez, and Colin Douglas Mathers

Introduction

The epidemiological transition and rapid changes in disease patterns have posed serious challenges to health-care systems and forced difficult decisions about the allocation of scarce resources. Epidemiological information is often required at all levels of health systems, and compilations of mortality and morbidity statistics at the national and subnational levels have been published by many countries for several decades. However, prior to the first global burden of disease (GBD) study, which began in 1992, there had been no comprehensive efforts to provide comparable regional and global estimates and projections of disease and injury burden based on a common methodology and denominated in a common metric.

The first GBD study was commissioned by the World Bank in 1991 to provide a comprehensive assessment of the disease burden in 1990 for 107 diseases and injuries and 10 selected risk factors for the world and 8 major regions (Murray & Lopez 1996b, 1996c; World Bank 1993). One of the major goals of the GBD 1990 study was to facilitate the inclusion of non-fatal health outcomes into debates on international health policy, which had largely drawn on the mortality data available in countries, much of it referring to children. Second, there was a need to decouple epidemiological assessment from advocacy so that estimates of the mortality or disability from a condition are developed as objectively as possible. In addition, there was a need to quantify the burden of disease using a measure that could then be used for cost-effectiveness analysis.

The basic philosophy guiding the burden of disease approach is that best-estimates of incidence, prevalence, duration, and death can be generated through the careful analysis and correction for bias of all available sources of information in a country or region. To assess the burden of disease, a time-based metric that combined years of life lost due to premature mortality and years of life lost due to time lived in health states less than ideal health, the DALY, was developed (Murray 1996). The GBD 1990 study represented a quantum step in the global and regional quantification of the impacts of diseases, injuries, and risk factors on population health. Its results have been widely used by government and non-government agencies alike to inform debates on priorities for research, development, and policy response.

In 2000, the World Health Organization (WHO) began publishing annual updates of the GBD for the world and 14 WHO subregions as annex tables to the World Health Reports (World Health Organization 2000, 2004). These were based on an extensive analysis of mortality data for all regions of the world together with systematic reviews of epidemiological studies and population health surveys for selected causes, as well as incorporating a range of methodological improvements. Additionally, a major and expanded research programme, the Comparative Risk Assessment project, was undertaken to quantify the global and regional attributable mortality and burden for 26 major risk factors (World Health Organization 2002).

The WHO GBD analysis for the year 2001 was used as the framework for cost effectiveness and priority-setting analyses carried out for the Disease Control Priorities Project, a joint project of the World Bank, WHO, and the National Institutes of Health, funded by the Gates Foundation (Jamison *et al.* 2006). The GBD results were documented in detail, with information on data sources and methods as well as uncertainty and sensitivity analyses, in a book published as part of the Disease Control Priorities Project (Lopez *et al.* 2006).

Despite these considerable efforts to quantify the burden of disease, the WHO updates were incremental updates that did not achieve a complete systematic reassessment of the data on all diseases and injuries. Additionally, changes in methods and data with successive updates meant that results were not comparable with earlier estimates, particularly those for 1990 from the first study. The WHO revisions have continued to largely rely on the original GBD weights, although better population-based methods and data are now available to develop improved disability weights included in the GBD. For these reasons, the Bill and Melinda Gates Foundation has funded a consortium lead by the Institute for Health Metrics and Evaluation involving the WHO, University of Queensland, Johns Hopkins University, and Harvard University to undertake a complete revision of the GBD for 1990 and 2005 (known as the GBD 2005 study). This 3-year project intends to publish results in 2010.

Measuring disease burden

The incorporation of the burden of premature mortality and disability into one summary measure requires a common metric. Since the late 1940s, researchers have generally agreed that time is an appropriate currency: Time (in years) lost through premature death and time (in years) lived with a disability. A range of such time-based measures has been used in different countries, many of them variants of the so-called quality-adjusted life year. For the GBD study, an internationally standardized form of the quality-adjusted life year was developed, called the disability-adjusted life year or DALY. The DALY expresses years of life lost to premature death and years lived with a disability of specified severity and duration. Here, a premature death is defined as one that occurs before the age to which a person could have expected to survive if he or she were a member of a model population with a life expectancy at birth approximately equal to that of the world's longest-surviving population—Japan. One lost DALY can be thought of as one lost year of 'healthy' life (either through death or illness/disability), and total DALYs (the burden of disease) as a measurement of the gap between the current health of a population and an ideal situation where everyone in the population lives into old age in full health.

To calculate total DALYs for a given condition in a population, years of life lost (YLL) and years lived with disability (YLD) for that condition must each be estimated, and then summed. The YLL for deaths at a given age *x* are calculated from the number of deaths, d_x, at that age multiplied by a global standard life expectancy, L_x, which is a function of age *x*. The GBD 1990 study chose not to use an arbitrary age cut-off such as 65 or 70 years in the calculation of YLL, but rather specified the loss function L_x in terms of the life expectancies at various ages in standard life tables with life expectancy at birth fixed at 82.5 years for females and 80 years for males. YLD for a particular condition in a particular time period are calculated by multiplying the number of incident cases, i_x, at each age *x* in that period by the average duration of the condition for each age of incidence, l_x, and a weight factor, dw_x, that reflects the severity of the condition on a scale from 0 (full health) to 1 (dead). YLD are generally calculated either for the average incident case of a given disease, or for one or more disabling sequelae of the disease. For example, YLD for onchocerciasis are calculated by adding the YLD for the sequelae of low vision, blindness, and itchy dermatitis.

The first GBD study chose to apply a 3 per cent time discount rate to the YLL in the future to estimate the net present value of YLL in calculating DALYs, and also incorporated non-uniform age weights that gave less weight to years of healthy life lost in early childhood or at older ages. When discounting and age weighting are both applied, a death in infancy corresponds to 33 DALYs, whereas deaths at ages 5–20 equate to around 36 DALYs. A more complete account of the DALY, and the value choices it incorporates, is given elsewhere (Murray 1996; Murray *et al.* 2002). All DALY results discussed here use age-weighted and discounted DALYs, although results have also been published elsewhere using other value choices.

Summary measures of population health

Over the past thirty or so years, several indicators have been developed to adjust mortality in order to reflect the impact of morbidity or disability. These summary measures of population health fall into two basic categories: Health expectancy and health gap (Fig. 2.10.1) (Murray *et al.* 2000). Within the former category, Sullivan (1971) first suggested weighting life expectancy to measure the health of a population using a single indicator, disability-free life expectancy. Disability-free life expectancy incorporates a dichotomous weighting scheme; that is, it does not account for varying levels of severity. Wilkins and Adams (1983) suggested a more sensitive weighting scheme based on functional limitations, leading to the disability-adjusted life expectancy approach.

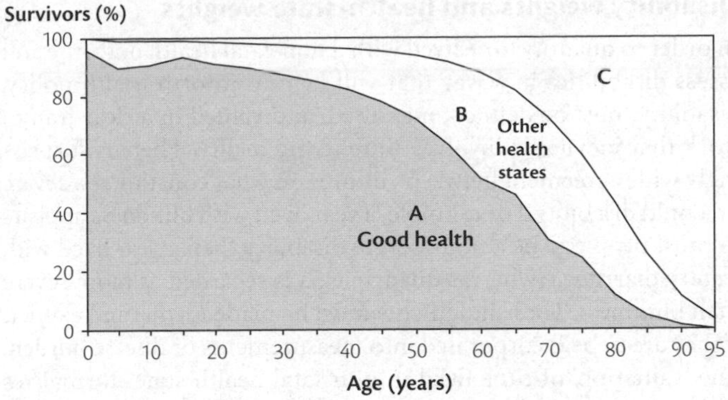

Fig. 2.10.1 The relationship between health expectancies and health gaps in a stationary population.
The health gap is area C + *f*(B), where *f*(B) is a function of B in the range 0 to area B representing the lost equivalent years of full health lived in states B. The health expectancy is the area A + *g*(B), where *g*(B) = B – *f*(B) represents the equivalent years of full health lived in states B.

As a summary measure of the burden of disability from all causes in a population, disability-adjusted life expectancy has two advantages over other summary measures (Murray & Lopez 1996c). The first is that it is relatively easy to explain the concept of a lifespan without disability to a non-technical audience. The increasing popularity of health expectancy indicators among policy makers has been documented (Robine *et al.* 2003). The second is that it is easy to calculate disability-adjusted life expectancy using the Sullivan method, which relies on prevalence data.

The DALY is an example of a particular type of health gap summary measure that allows the disaggregation of overall disease burden into the burden attributed to specific diseases, injuries, or exposures. In the GBD study, the aim was to develop a summary measure based on explicit and transparent value choices that may be readily debated and modified. Overall, the DALY used in the GBD study is an egalitarian measure, in that it is built on the principle that only two characteristics of individuals that are not directly related to their health, their age and their sex, should be taken into consideration when calculating the burden of a given health outcome in that individual. Other characteristics, such as socioeconomic status, race, or level of education are not considered.

Along with ongoing efforts to improve the analysis of mortality and epidemiological data for the estimation of DALYs, the WHO explored the use of health-adjusted life expectancies (HALEs) as a single summary indicator of population health (Mathers *et al.* 2004), and also extensively explored the ethical, conceptual, and philosophical underpinnings for quantifying population health as part of the overall effort to foster summary measures of population health (Murray *et al.* 2002).

Disability weights and health-state weights

In order to quantify time lived with a non-fatal health outcome and assess disabilities in a way that will help to inform health policy, disability must be defined, measured, and valued in a clear framework that inevitably involves simplifying reality. There is surprisingly wide agreement between cultures on what constitutes a severe or a mild disability. For example, a year lived with blindness appears to most people to be a more severe disability than a year lived with watery diarrhoea, whereas quadriplegia is regarded as more severe than blindness. These judgments must be made formal and explicit if they are to be incorporated into measurements of disease burden. The 'valuation' of time lived in non-fatal health states formalizes and quantifies social preferences for different states of health as disability weights (dw_x). Depending on how these weights are derived, they are variously referred to as disability weights, quality-adjusted life year (QALY) weights, health-state valuations, or health-state preferences. Because the DALY measures loss of health (unlike the QALY, which measures equivalent healthy years lived), the disability weights for DALYs are inverted, running from 0 (ideal health) to 1 (state comparable to death).

A number of methods have been developed to formalize social preferences for different states of health. Most involve asking people to make judgments about the trade-off between quantity and quality of life. This can be expressed as a trade-off in time (how many years lived with a given disability would a person trade for a fixed period of perfect health), a trade-off between persons (whether the person would prefer to save 1 life-year for 1000 perfectly healthy individuals or 1 life-year for perhaps 2000 individuals in a worse health state), or a 'standard gamble' between remaining in a certain health state or accepting a given risk of death in order to return to a state of perfect health.

The original GBD study used two forms of the person trade-off method to value health states and asked participants in weighting exercises to make a composite judgment about the severity distribution of the condition and the preference for time spent in each severity level. This was largely necessitated by the lack of population information on the severity distribution of most conditions at the global and regional levels. In a formal deliberative exercise involving small groups of health workers from all regions of the world, health-state valuations were derived for a set of 22-indicator disabling conditions—such as blindness, depression, and conditions that cause pain. Disability weights for other GBD sequelae were then derived by ranking against these conditions. Subsequent valuation exercises carried out in various cultures have closely matched the results of the original GBD exercise and suggest that cross-cultural variation in health-state preferences is less important than has been argued by some commentators (Salomon & Murray 2002a).

A Dutch disability weight study also attempted to address concerns that valuations by health professionals may differ from those of the general population (Stouthard *et al.* 1997). Using similar methodology to the original GBD study with three panels of public health physicians and one lay panel, this study concluded that it makes little difference whether the valuation panels comprise medical experts or lay people, as long as accurate functional health-state profiles are provided. In this study, the distribution of health states associated with each sequela was defined using the EuroQol health profile to describe the health states.

The valuation methods used in the original GBD have been criticized on the grounds that the groups used to elicit weights were not representative of the general global population, that the person trade-off method used in the GBD is unethical, in that it involves hypothetical scenarios trading off saving the lives of people in full health versus saving the lives of people with specified health conditions (Arnesen & Nord 1999), and that the inclusion of disability in the DALY implies that people with disability are less valued than people in full health (Mont 2007). In response, the conceptual basis of the DALY has been further developed to clarify that the DALY is quantifying loss of health, not broader valuations of the 'quality of life', 'wellbeing', or 'utility' associated with health states (Salomon *et al.* 2003). As used in the DALY, the term 'disability' is essentially a synonym for health states of less than full health. Subsequent GBD work on eliciting health-state valuations has moved away from reliance on the person trade-off method, and has also made use of large representative population surveys (Salomon *et al.* 2004), although a full revision of the disability weights used in the GBD is only now being undertaken as part of the GBD 2005 study.

Other social value choices incorporated in the DALY

To assess premature mortality, the GBD studies have utilized a standard life table for all populations, with life expectancies at birth fixed at 82.5 years for women and 80 years for men. A standard life expectancy allows deaths at the same age to contribute equally to the burden of disease irrespective of where the death occurs. Alternatives, such as using different life expectancies for different populations that more closely match their actual life expectancies, violate this egalitarian principle. As life expectancy is rarely equal for men and women, the GBD assigned men a lower reference life expectancy than women. However, because much of the difference between men and women is determined by men's higher exposure to various risks such as alcohol, tobacco, and occupational injury rather than purely biological differences, this choice could be modified in future revisions of the Study (Waldron 1993; Wong *et al.* 2006).

If individuals are forced to choose between saving a year of life for a 2-year-old and saving it for a 22-year-old, most prefer to save the 22-year-old. A range of studies confirms this broad social preference to weight the value of a year lived by a young adult more heavily than one lived by a very young child or an older adult. Adults are widely perceived to play a critical role in the family, community, and society. It was for these reasons that the GBD study incorporated age-weighting into the DALY. It was assumed that the relative value of a year of life rises rapidly from birth to a peak in the early twenties, after which it steadily declines.

Individuals commonly discount future benefits against current benefits similarly to the way that they may discount future dollars against current dollars. Whether a year of healthy life, like a dollar, is also deemed preferable now rather than later is a matter of debate among economists, medical ethicists, and public health planners, as discounting future health affects both measurements of disease burden and estimates of the cost-effectiveness of an intervention. There are arguments for and against discounting. In the GBD studies to date, future life years have been discounted by 3 per cent per year. This means that a year of healthy life bought for 10 years hence is worth around 24 per cent less than one bought for now, as discounting is represented as an exponential decay function.

As the impact of discounting is significant, GBD findings have been published for DALYs with and without discounting and age weights. Discounting future health reduces the relative impact of a child death compared with an adult death. Another effect is that it reduces the value of interventions that provide benefits largely in the future, such as vaccinating against hepatitis B, which may prevent thousands of cases of liver cancer, but some decades later. The Disease Control Priorities Project chose to use DALYs with discounting but not age weights, as have some national burden of disease studies. With the increased emphasis on DALYs as quantifying loss of health rather than the social value of health, it is likely that future revisions of the GBD will revisit the choices for discounting and age-weighting.

Sensitivity analyses

To gauge the impact of changing these social choices on the final measures of disease burden, both the GBD 1990 and the GBD 2001 assessments were recalculated with alternative age-weighting and discount rates, and with alternative methods for weighting the severity of disabilities (Murray & Lopez 1996c; Mathers *et al.* 2006).

Weighting the years of healthy life lost uniformly at all ages, compared to non-uniform age weights, resulted in somewhat more weight being given to the chronic diseases of older ages and somewhat less weight being given to mental disorders and injuries, which affect younger adults disproportionately. In low- and middle-income countries, people aged 60 years and older suffered 21 per cent of the total burden of disease and injury. This declined to 13 per cent when non-uniform age weights were used, increasing the weight placed on young and middle-aged life years. The rates of discounting the future stream of life have important effects on the proportion of the burden due to non-fatal outcomes (YLD), on the age distribution of disease burden, and on the distribution of the burden by broad cause group. Discounting future years of lost healthy life at 3 per cent resulted in 36–38 per cent of the burden being due to YLD, depending on whether or not age weights were also applied, compared to just over one quarter when the discount rate was set to zero. Because, for most causes, the 'duration' associated with the years lost due to premature death is longer than the duration with disability for an incident case, discounting has a greater effect on reducing YLL than on YLD. Different choices of discount rates and age weights do not cause any large changes in the rank ordering of diseases and injuries.

In addition to these sensitivity analyses, Mathers *et al.* (2006) attempted to estimate uncertainty ranges for the GBD results at regional level arising from data limitations. Uncertainty in estimated all-cause mortality ranged from ±1 per cent for high-income countries to ±15–20 per cent for sub-Saharan Africa, reflecting differential data availability. Uncertainty ranges were even larger for deaths from specific diseases. Uncertainty ranges for YLD assessments varied considerably, ranging from relatively certain estimates for diseases such as polio, for which intensive surveillance systems are in place, to highly uncertain estimates for those such as osteoarthritis, for which in some regions no usable data source was found, and for others the latest available data were decades old. Typical uncertainty for regional prevalence estimates ranged from ±10 per cent to ±90 per cent, with a median value of ±41 per cent, among a subset of diseases for which uncertainty analysis was carried out (Mathers *et al.* 2006).

The conclusion drawn from both sets of sensitivity analyses was that, in general, the accuracy of the underlying basic epidemiological data from which disease burden is calculated will influence the final results much more than the discount rate, the age weight, or the disability weighting method. If, for example, estimates of the incidence of blindness are off by a factor of 2, then the results, whatever the social value choices used in the metric, will be substantially incorrect. Thus, much more effort needs to be invested in improving the basic epidemiological data than in analysing the effects of what are eventually minor adjustments to the particular summary measure of population health employed.

Estimating mortality and disability

Classification

As many developing countries still have only limited information about the distribution of causes of death in their populations, a primary objective of the GBD study has been to develop comprehensive internally consistent mortality estimates worldwide for each major cause. Diseases and injuries that cause death and burden of disease were classified using a tree structure based on the International Classification of Diseases (Murray & Lopez 1996c). The highest level of aggregation consists of three broad cause groups: Group I (communicable, maternal, perinatal, and nutritional conditions), Group II (non-communicable diseases), and Group III (injuries). Group I causes are those conditions that occur largely in poorer populations and typically decline at a faster pace than all-cause mortality during the epidemiological transition.

Each group was then subdivided into categories; for example, cardiovascular diseases and malignant neoplasms are two subcategories of Group II. Beyond this level, there are two further disaggregation levels such that over 120 individual causes can be listed separately. The GBD cause list was slightly expanded for the WHO revisions, resulting in 135 disease and injury categories.

The basic units of analysis for the first GBD study were the eight World Bank regions defined for the 1993 World Development Report. The heterogeneity of these large regions limited their value for comparative epidemiological assessments. For the WHO updates, a more refined approach was followed. Mortality estimates by disease and injury cause, age, and sex were first developed for each of the 192 WHO member states using different methods for countries with different sources of information on mortality. Epidemiological estimates for incidence, prevalence, and YLD were developed for 17 groupings of countries, and then imputed to country populations using available country-level information and methods to ensure consistency with the country-specific mortality estimates. The resulting country-level estimates were made available by WHO at a summarized level for 14 subregions of the six WHO regions, and also facilitated the production of regional estimates for any desired regional groupings of countries (World Health Organization 2008).

Estimating regional mortality patterns

The GBD 1990 study and the WHO updates drew on four broad sources of mortality data: Death registration systems with medically certified cause-of-death information, sample death registration systems for India and China relying predominantly on verbal autopsy-based information, epidemiological assessments for specific causes, and cause-of-death models. We summarize the approach used for the GBD 2002 estimates; more detail is provided by Mathers *et al.* (2006).

Life tables specifying mortality rates by age and sex for 192 WHO Member States were developed for 2002 from available death registration data (112 member states), sample registration systems

(India, China) and data on child and adult mortality from censuses and surveys such as the Demographic and Health Surveys (DHSs) and UNICEF's Multiple Indicator Cluster Surveys (MICSs). For countries without useable death registration data, estimated levels of child and adult mortality were applied to a modified logit life table model, using a global standard, to estimate the full life table for 2001 (Murray *et al.* 2003). For 55 countries, 42 of them in sub-Saharan Africa, no information was available on levels of adult mortality. Based on the predicted level of child mortality in 2001, the most likely corresponding level of adult mortality (excluding HIV/AIDS deaths where necessary) was selected, along with uncertainty ranges, based on regression models of child versus adult mortality as observed in a set of almost 2000 life tables judged to be of good quality.

Death registration data containing useable information on cause-of-death distributions were available for 107 countries, the majority of these in the high-income group, Latin America and the Caribbean, and Europe and Central Asia. Population-based epidemiological studies, disease registers, and notifications systems (in excess of 2700 data sets) also contributed to the estimation of mortality due to 21 specific communicable causes of death, including HIV/AIDS, malaria, tuberculosis, childhood immunizable diseases, schistosomiasis, trypanosomiasis, and Chagas disease. Almost one third of these data sets related to sub-Saharan Africa.

In order to address information gaps relating to other causes of death for populations without useable death registration data, models for estimating broad cause-of-death patterns based on GDP and overall mortality levels were used. These are based on the fact that the broad cause structure of mortality is closely related to the level of mortality in a population. Such models estimate the distribution of deaths by cause in a population from historical studies of mortality patterns in countries with vital registration. The models developed for the initial GBD study drew on a data set of 103 observations from 67 countries between 1950 and 1991, and were used primarily to provide plausibility bounds on estimates derived from epidemiological assessments. The approach to cause-of-death modelling for the GBD 2000–2002 estimates was revised and enhanced, drawing on a substantially larger data set of 1613 country–year observations (Salomon & Murray 2002b).

Assessing disability

A disease or injury may have multiple disabling effects, or sequelae. For example, diabetes may result in diabetic vascular disease, retinopathy, or amputation. To estimate the total burden of disability, the GBD measured the amount of time lived with each of the various disabling sequelae of diseases and injuries, in both treated and untreated states, and weighted for their severity in each population. In all, 271 disabling sequelae of disease and injuries were analysed for GBD 2000–2002, for all regions and age groups, and for both sexes.

Calculating the number of years lived with a disabling condition requires information about its incidence, the average age of onset, the average duration of the disability, and the severity weight for the condition. Epidemiological experts were requested to estimate each of these variables for each condition based on an in-depth review of published and unpublished studies. For each sequela, prevalence, case-fatality, remission, and mortality were estimated. This information allowed correction of the preliminary estimates for internal consistency; that is, ensuring that the estimated prevalence was consistent with estimated incidence and vice versa. Consistency was validated using DISMOD software specifically developed for the GBD (Fig. 2.10.2). DISMOD is a computer model (DISease MODel) that allows simultaneous estimation of age patterns of basic epidemiological parameters, such as incidence, prevalence, case-fatality, and duration, based on knowledge of a limited set of these variables (Barendregt *et al.* 2003). When inconsistencies were detected, epidemiological experts were asked to revise their initial estimates.

The number of years lived with a given disability for each individual were calculated from the incidence of the disability, with the 'stream' of disability arising from it measured from the age of onset, for the estimated duration of the disability, multiplied by the condition's severity weight. To calculate the years lived with disability due to a condition in any given population, the number of years lived with disability lost per incident case must be multiplied by the number of incident cases. A case of asthma, for example, carries a disability weight of 0.1 if untreated and 0.06 if treated. If the annual incidence of asthma in males aged 15–44 years is 1 million cases, the untreated proportion is 35 per cent, and the average duration is 7 years, then this sequela alone is estimated to cause 664 000 years lived with disability for that demographic group. Unlike the estimates of YLL, not all sequelae of all conditions could be explicitly assessed for years lived with disability. Estimates for conditions not explicitly considered were made based on information about the ratio of total premature mortality to disability for each broad cause group.

While the GBD 2000–2002 updates drew on substantially more data for both mortality and epidemiological estimates, an incremental revision strategy was followed and new systematic reviews and estimates were not completed for all causes; some such as dengue and Japanese encephalitis continued to rely on the original GBD assessments of the mid 1990s. Additionally, YLD estimates for most causes continued to be based on the disability weights estimated for the original GBD study (Murray 1996).

Data sources for YLD estimation included disease registers, epidemiological studies, health surveys, and health-facility data (where relevant). Mathers *et al.* (2006) estimated that around 8700 data sets were used to quantify the YLD estimates for GBD 2000–2002, of which more than 7000 related to Group I causes. One quarter of the data sets related to populations in sub-Saharan Africa, and around one fifth to populations in high-income countries. Together with the more than 1370 additional data sets used for the estimation of YLL, the 2000–2002 GBD study incorporated information from over 10 000 data sets relating to population health and mortality.

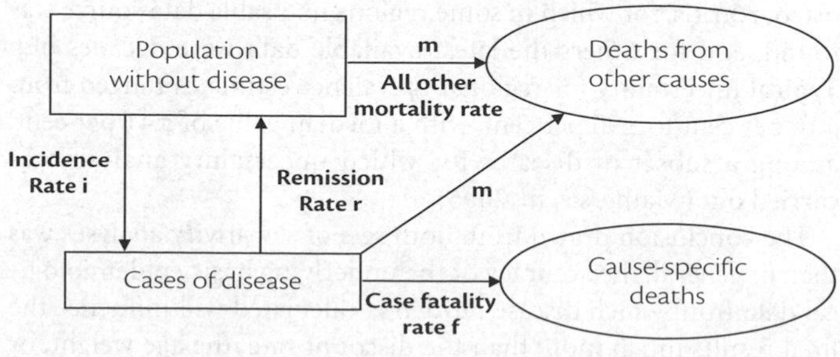

Fig. 2.10.2 The basic disease model underlying DISMOD (DISease MODel).

Global burden of disease 1990 study

Initial results of the GBD 1990 study were published in the 1993 World Development Report (World Bank 1993) and in WHO publications (Murray & Lopez 1994; Murray *et al.* 1994). After further revisions of epidemiological assessments and disability weights, the final results were published in 1996 (Murray & Lopez 1996a, 1996b, 1996c). The results of the Study demonstrated clearly that disability plays a central role in determining the overall health status of a population. Yet that role had previously been almost invisible to public health. The leading causes of disability were shown to be substantially different from the leading causes of death, which has considerable implications for the practice of judging a population's health from its mortality statistics alone.

The leading causes of disease burden in 1990 were childhood diseases (lower respiratory diseases, diarrhoeal diseases, and perinatal causes such as birth asphyxia, birth traumas, and low birth weight), in part because of the greater weight given to deaths at younger ages by the DALY. Depression ranked fourth globally, ahead of ischaemic heart disease, cerebrovascular disease, tuberculosis, and measles. Road traffic accidents also ranked in the top 10 causes of DALYs worldwide. The results of the original GBD study were surprising to many health policy makers, more familiar with the pattern of causes represented in mortality statistics. Neuropsychiatric disorders and injuries were major causes of lost years of healthy life as measured by DALYs, and were greatly undervalued when measured by mortality alone (Murray & Lopez 1996a, 1997). More broadly, non-communicable diseases, including neuropsychiatric disorders, were estimated to have caused 41 per cent of the global burden of disease in 1990, only slightly less than communicable, maternal, perinatal, and nutritional conditions combined (44 per cent), with 15 per cent due to injuries.

The methods and findings of the original (1990) GBD study were widely published, and the GBD approach was widely adopted by countries and health-development agencies alike as the standard for health accounting. The methods and findings of the original GBD study stimulated quite a number of national disease burden studies of varying scope and methodological rigour during the 1990s. The earliest comprehensive studies were for Mexico (Lozano *et al.* 1995) and Mauritius (Vos *et al.* 1995), followed by studies in the late 1990s in the Netherlands (Stouthard *et al.* 1997; Melse & Kramers 1998; Ruwaard & Kramers 1998) and Australia (Mathers *et al.* 1999). Since 2000, comprehensive national burden of disease studies have also been carried out in countries such as Brazil, Iran, Malaysia, Turkey, South Africa, Zimbabwe, Thailand, and the United States, and recently, follow-up analyses of burden of disease have been carried out for Australia (Begg *et al.* 2008) and Mexico (Mexican Ministry of Health, National Institute of Public Health, Harvard Initiative for Global Health 2008). New or follow-up studies are now underway in a number of other countries.

Disease and injury burden in 2002: An overview

A key aim of the GBD studies has been to quantify the burden of fatal and non-fatal health outcomes in a single measure, the disability-adjusted life year (DALY). This section gives an overview of the main results of the GBD update for 2002 in terms of mortality and DALYs. More details on the age–sex–cause and sequelae patterns can be found elsewhere (World Health Organization 2008; Mathers *et al.* 2006). Results are presented here in terms of World Bank geographic regions, with high-income countries aggregated as a separate group.

Global and regional mortality in 2002

Slightly over 56 million people died in 2002, 10.5 million (or nearly 20 per cent) of whom were children younger than 5 years of age. Of these child deaths, 99 per cent occurred in low- and middle-income countries. Additionally, there are a comparatively high number of deaths in low- and middle-income countries at young and middle-adult ages. In these regions, 30 per cent of all deaths occur at ages 15–59 years, compared to 15 per cent in high-income countries (Fig. 2.10.3). The causes of death at these ages, as well as in childhood, are thus important in assessing public health priorities.

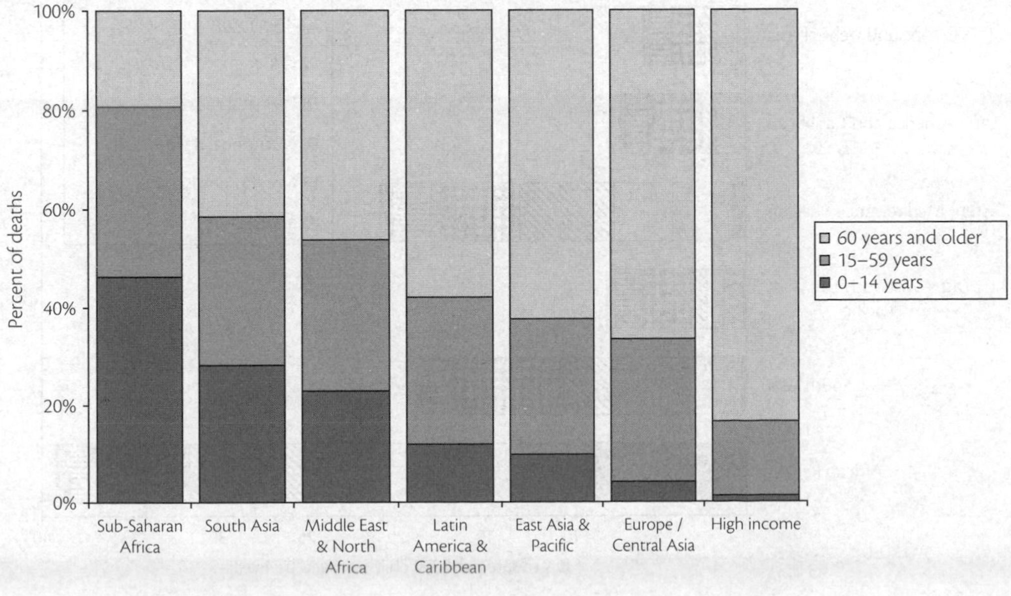

Fig. 2.10.3 Per cent distribution of deaths by age group and region, 2002.

Worldwide, one death in every three is from a Group I cause (communicable, maternal, and perinatal conditions, and nutritional deficiencies). This proportion remains almost unchanged from 1990, with one major difference: Whereas HIV/AIDS accounted for only 2 per cent of Group I deaths in 1990, it accounted for an estimated 15 per cent in 2002. This latter figure has subsequently been revised downward to around 11 per cent, as described in the following paragraphs.

The risk of a child dying before age five ranged from 17 per cent in sub-Saharan Africa to 0.7 per cent in high-income countries in 2002. Low- and middle-income countries accounted for 99 per cent of global deaths among children under the age of 5 years, and 85 per cent of these were in the low-income countries. Just five preventable conditions—pneumonia, diarrhoeal diseases, malaria, measles, and perinatal causes—are responsible for 70 per cent of all child deaths (see Fig. 2.10.4). If all countries had the Japanese rates for child mortality, the lowest in the world, the annual number of child deaths would fall by 90 per cent, to around 1 million.

In developing countries, Group II causes (non-communicable diseases) were responsible for more than 50 per cent of deaths in adults aged 15–59 in all regions except South Asia and sub-Saharan Africa, where Group I causes including HIV/AIDS remained responsible for one third and two thirds of the deaths, respectively (Fig. 2.10.5). In other words, the epidemiologic transition is already well established in most developing countries.

The leading causes of death in 2002 are shown in Table 2.10.1. The extent of epidemiological transition worldwide is reflected in the dominant role of ischaemic heart disease and stroke (cerebrovascular disease) as the leading killers, together accounting for more than 1 in 5 deaths. Major communicable diseases such as lower respiratory infections, diarrhoeal diseases, and tuberculosis are among the top ten causes of death as are road traffic accidents and lung cancer. It should be noted that since the GBD estimates for 2002 were published in the World Health Report 2004 (World Health Organization 2004), WHO and UNAIDS estimates of incidence, prevalence, and mortality for HIV have been substantially revised to take into account advances in methodology and increased data availability (UNAIDS, World Health Organization 2007). The estimated global prevalence of HIV for 2002 was revised downwards by around 16 per cent and the estimated global deaths due to HIV were revised from 2.7 to 2 million, making it the sixth rather than fourth leading cause of death globally. The single biggest reason for this reduction was the intensive exercise to assess India's HIV epidemic, which resulted in a major revision to the country's estimates, almost halving the estimated prevalence. Around 70 per cent of the reduction in HIV estimates is due to changes in India and five African countries: Angola, Kenya, Mozambique, Nigeria, and Zimbabwe.

Leading causes of disability

The original GBD study brought to the attention of health policy makers the previously largely ignored burden of non-fatal illnesses, particularly mental disorders. The findings of the GBD for 2002, based on updated data and analyses, confirm that disability and states of less than full health, caused by diseases and injuries, play a central role in determining the overall health status of populations in all regions of the world.

The overall burden of non-fatal disabling conditions is dominated by a relatively short list of causes. In all regions, neuropsychiatric conditions are the most important causes of disability, accounting for 35 per cent of YLDs among adults aged 15 years and over. The disabling burden of neuropsychiatric conditions is almost the same for males and females, but the major contributing causes are different. Whereas depression is the leading cause of disability for both males and females, the burden of depression is 50 per cent higher for females than males, and females also have higher burden

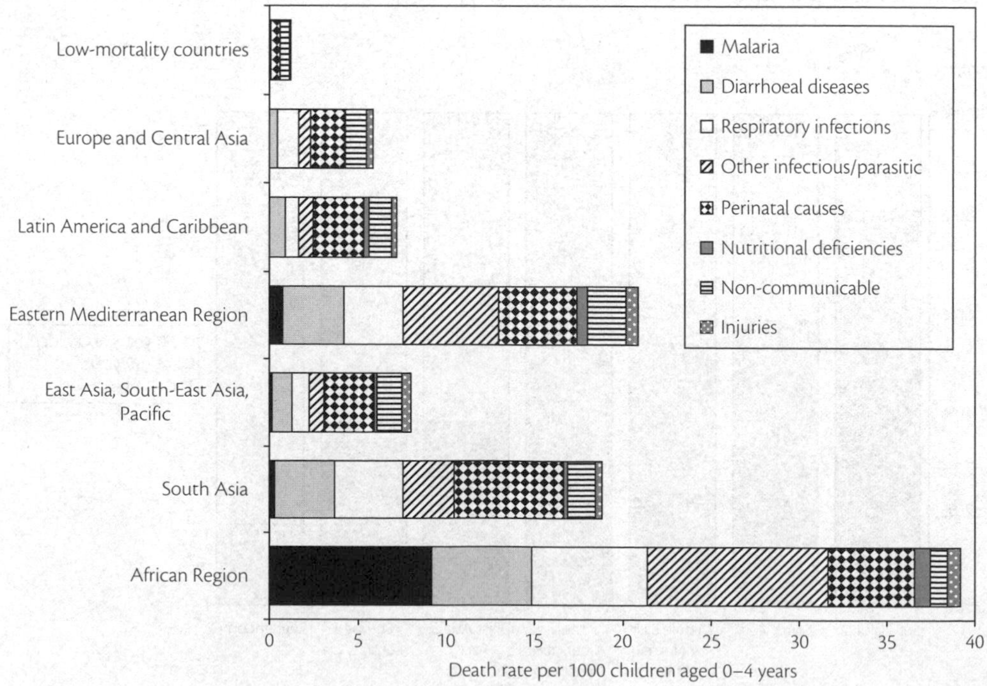

Fig. 2.10.4 Death rates by broad cause group and region, children aged 0–4, 2002.

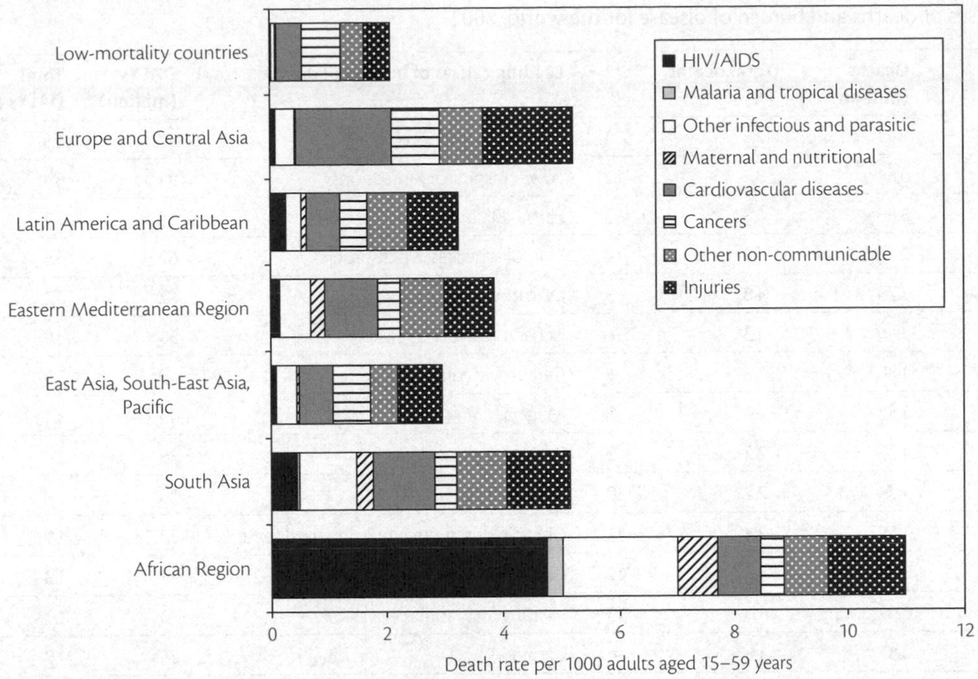

Fig. 2.10.5 Death rates by broad cause group and region, adults aged 15–59, 2002.

from anxiety disorders, migraine, and senile dementias. In contrast, the male burden for alcohol and drug use disorders is nearly six times higher than that for females, and accounts for one quarter of the male neuropsychiatric burden.

Surprisingly, more than 80 per cent of global non-fatal health outcomes occur in middle- and low-income countries. Nearly half of all YLDs arise due to diseases and injuries in the low-income countries. Although the prevalence of disabling conditions such as dementia and musculoskeletal disease is higher in countries with long life expectancies, this is offset by lower contributions to disability from conditions such as cardiovascular disease, chronic respiratory diseases, and the long-term sequelae of communicable diseases and nutritional deficiencies. In other words, people living in low-income countries not only have lower life expectancies (higher risk of premature death) than those in high-income countries, but also live a higher proportion of their lives in poor health.

The burden of diseases and injuries

The analyses presented here reinforce the conclusions of the original GBD study about the importance of including non-fatal outcomes in a comprehensive assessment of global population health. They have also confirmed the growing importance of non-communicable diseases in low- and middle-income countries. The results also highlight important changes in population health in some regions since 1990, as discussed in the following paragraphs.

The epidemiological transition in low- and middle-income countries has resulted in a 20 per cent reduction since 1990 in the per-capita disease burden due to Group I causes (communicable, maternal, perinatal, and nutritional conditions). Without the HIV/AIDS epidemic and the associated lack of decline in tuberculosis burden, this reduction would have been substantially greater, closer to 27 per cent over the period. HIV/AIDS is now among the leading cause of burden of disease globally, and the leading cause in sub-Saharan Africa, followed by malaria. Seven other Group I causes also appear in the top ten causes for this region (see Fig. 2.10.5).

The burden of non-communicable diseases is increasing, accounting for nearly half of the global burden of disease (all ages), a 10 per cent increase from estimated levels in 1990. Indeed, more than 40 per cent of the adult disease burden in low- and middle-income countries of the world is now attributable to non-communicable disease. Implementation of effective interventions for Group I diseases, coupled with population ageing and the dynamics of risk for non-communicable disease, in many developing countries are the likely causes of this shift. The burden of disease in Europe and Central Asia is dominated by ischaemic heart disease and stroke, which together account for more than 20 per cent of total disease burden. In contrast, in Latin America and Caribbean countries, these diseases account for only 6 per cent of disease burden. However, there are very high levels of diabetes and endocrine disorders in this region, compared to others.

The per-capita disease burden in Europe and Central Asia increased by nearly 20 per cent over the period since 1990, so that this region now has worse health than all other regions of the world apart from South Asia and sub-Saharan Africa. This largely reflects the substantial increases in adult male mortality and disability in the 1990s, leading to the highest male–female differential in disease burden in the world. A significant factor in this trend is thought to be increasing alcohol abuse, particularly among males, which led to high rates of accidents, violence, and cardiovascular disease (McKee & Shkolnikov 2001; Men *et al.* 2003; Shkolnikov *et al.* 2001). From 1991 to 1994, the risk of adult (15–59 years) premature death increased by 50 per cent for Russian males. It improved somewhat between 1994 and 1998, but has increased significantly again in the first few years of the twenty-first century.

Violence is the sixth leading cause of burden in Latin America and Caribbean countries: Although it is not ranked in the top ten in any other region, it is nonetheless significant. Injuries primarily affect young adults, often resulting in severe disabling sequelae. All forms of injury accounted for 14 per cent of adult burden in the world in 2002. Road traffic accidents, falls, violence, and self-inflicted

Table 2.10.1 The twenty leading causes of deaths and burden of disease for the world, 2002

	Leading causes of death	Deaths (million)	Total deaths (%)		Leading causes of burden of disease	DALYs (million)	Total DALYs (%)
1	Ischaemic heart disease	7.21	12.6	1	Perinatal conditions	97	6.5
2	Cerebrovascular disease	5.51	9.7	2	Lower respiratory infections	91	6.1
3	Lower respiratory infections	3.88	6.8	3	HIV/AIDS	84	5.7
4	HIV/AIDS	2.78	4.9	4	Unipolar depressive disorders	67	4.5
5	Chronic obstructive pulmonary disease	2.75	4.8	5	Diarrhoeal diseases	62	4.2
6	Perinatal conditions	2.46	4.3	6	Ischaemic heart disease	59	3.9
7	Diarrhoeal diseases	1.80	3.2	7	Cerebrovascular disease	49	3.3
8	Tuberculosis	1.57	2.7	8	Malaria	46	3.1
9	Malaria	1.27	2.2	9	Road traffic accidents	39	2.6
10	Trachea, bronchus, lung cancers	1.24	2.2	10	Tuberculosis	35	2.3
11	Road traffic accidents	1.19	2.1	11	Chronic obstructive pulmonary disease	28	1.9
12	Diabetes mellitus	0.99	1.7	12	Congenital anomalies	27	1.8
13	Hypertensive heart disease	0.91	1.6	13	Hearing loss, adult onset	26	1.7
14	Self-inflicted injuries	0.87	1.5	14	Cataracts	25	1.7
15	Stomach cancer	0.85	1.5	15	Measles	21	1.4
16	Cirrhosis of the liver	0.79	1.4	16	Violence	21	1.4
17	Nephritis and nephrosis	0.68	1.2	17	Self-inflicted injuries	21	1.4
18	Colon and rectum cancers	0.62	1.1	18	Alcohol use disorders	20	1.4
19	Liver cancer	0.62	1.1	19	Protein-energy malnutrition	17	1.1
20	Measles	0.61	1.1	20	Falls	16	1.1

injuries are all among the top 20 leading causes of burden. The former Soviet Union and other low- and middle-income countries of Europe have rates of injury death and disability among males similar to those in sub-Saharan Africa. In Latin America and the Caribbean, as well as the Europe and Central Asian region, and the Middle East and North Africa, more than 30 per cent of the entire disease and injury burden among male adults aged 15–44 is attributable to injuries, including road traffic accidents, violence, and self-inflicted injuries. Additionally, injury deaths are noticeably higher for women in some parts of Asia and the Middle East and North Africa, in part due to high levels of suicide and violence.

The GBD results clearly illustrate the 'double burden' of disease faced by the poorer developing countries of South Asia and Africa. Countries that are still struggling with 'old' and 'new' infectious disease epidemics must now also deal with the emerging epidemics of chronic non-communicable disease such as heart disease, stroke, diabetes, and cancer.

Regional imbalances in the burden of disease

Sub-Saharan Africa and South Asia (which includes India) together accounted for more than 53 per cent of the total global burden of disease in 2002, although they made up only 34 per cent of the world's population. In contrast, the high-income countries, with about 15 per cent of the world's population, together bore less than 8 per cent of the total disease burden. China emerged as substantially the most 'healthy' of the low- and middle-income countries, with 15 per cent of the global disease burden and a fifth of the world's population. This means that about 546 years of healthy life were lost for every 1000 people living in sub-Saharan Africa, compared with just 127 for every 1000 people in the high-income countries, a more than fourfold differential (Fig. 2.10.6).

The global burden of risk factors in the 2000s

Perhaps the most important methodological progress since the GBD 1990 study has been with respect to quantification of disease burden caused by risk factors. In the initial study, the population health effects of ten risk factors were quantified, but there was limited emphasis on the comparability of the estimates. Different risk factors have very different epidemiological traditions, particularly with regard to defining 'hazardous' exposure, the strength of evidence on causality, and the availability of epidemiological research on exposure and outcomes. Moreover, classical risk-factor research has treated exposures as dichotomous, with individuals either exposed or non-exposed, with exposure defined according to some, often arbitrary, threshold value. Recent evidence for such continuous exposures as cholesterol, blood pressure, and body mass index (BMI) suggests that such arbitrarily defined thresholds are inappropriate, because hazard functions for these risks rise (or decline)

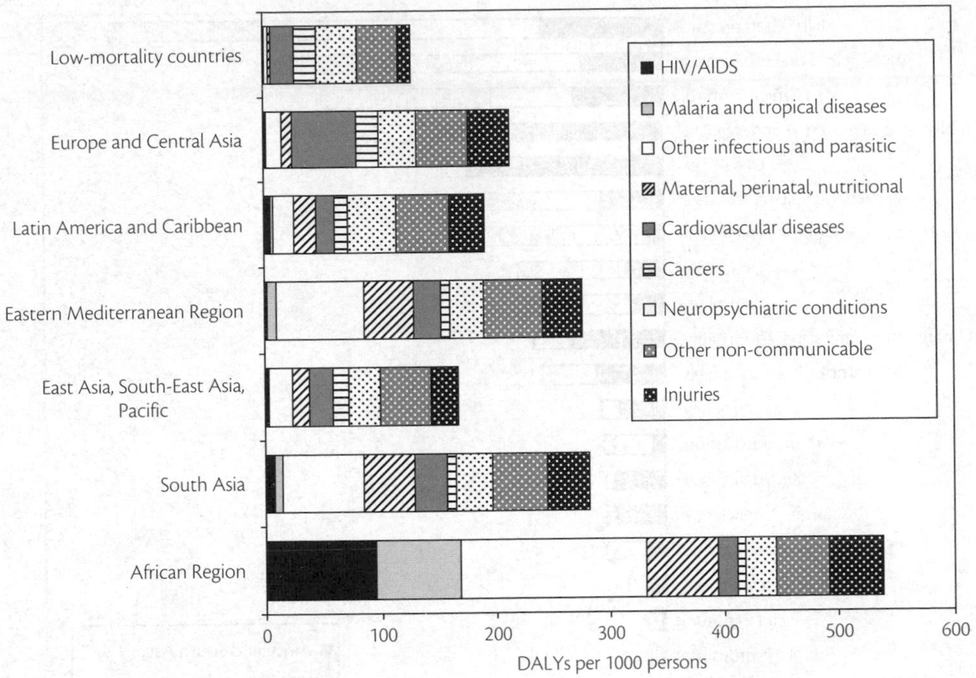

Fig. 2.10.6 The burden of disease, by broad cause group and region, 2002.

continuously across the entire range of measured exposure levels, with no obvious threshold (Eastern Stroke and Coronary Heart Disease Collaborative Research Group 1998).

For the GBD 2000 study, a new framework for quantifying risk-factor burden was defined, which measured changes in disease burden that would be expected under different population distributions of exposure (Murray & Lopez 1999). Fractions of disease burden attributable to a risk factor were then calculated based on a comparison of disease burden expected under the current (i.e. 2000) estimated distribution of exposure, by age, sex, and region, with that expected if a 'counterfactual' distribution of exposure had applied. To improve comparability across risk factors, a counterfactual distribution was defined for each risk factor as the population distribution of exposure that would lead to the lowest levels of disease burden. Thus, for example, in the case of tobacco, this theoretical-minimum-risk (counterfactual) exposure distribution would be 100 per cent of the population being life-long non-smokers; for overweight and obesity, it would be a narrow distribution of BMI centred around an optimal level (e.g. 21 [SD 1] kg/m^2), and so on. The theoretical-minimum-risk exposure distributions for the risk factors quantified in the WHO Comparative Risk Assessment (CRA) study (the risk-factor arm of the GBD 2000 study) were developed by expert groups for each risk factor, together with systematic reviews and analyses of extant sources on risk-factor exposure and hazard, using an iterative process that increased comparability across risk factors (Ezzati *et al.* 2002, 2004).

The comparative risk assessment for 26 global risk factors, carried out as part of the GBD 2000 study are summarized in Figs 2.10.7 and 2.10.8, and in Table 2.10.2. The analysis was carried out for 14 subregions of the six WHO regions; these subregions were further grouped into 'developed', 'low-mortality developing' including China and much of Latin America, and 'high-mortality developing' including sub-Saharan Africa, and many countries in Western and Southern Asia, including India, Bangladesh, and Myanmar. These results show that risk factors for communicable, maternal, perinatal, and nutritional conditions (e.g. unsafe sex, child and maternal undernutrition, indoor air pollution from household use of solid fuels, and poor water, sanitation, and hygiene)—whose burden is primarily concentrated in the low-income regions of sub-Saharan Africa and South Asia—and risk factors for non-communicable diseases (e.g. smoking, alcohol, high blood pressure and cholesterol, and overweight and obesity) are leading causes of global disease burden, the latter being globally widespread.

These results suggest that the world is currently experiencing a 'risk-factor' transition, in developed countries characterized by high disease burden from tobacco, suboptimal blood pressure, alcohol, cholesterol, and overweight. Disease burden in the poorest countries, on the other hand, is primarily caused by underweight, unsafe sex, unsafe water and sanitation, indoor air pollution, and micronutrient deficiencies (zinc, iron, vitamin A). Interestingly, the risk factors causing, on average, the greatest disease burden among the 2.4 billion people living in low-mortality, developing countries are a mixture of both, led by alcohol, suboptimal blood pressure, and tobacco, followed by underweight and overweight. This juxtaposition of what might be termed 'new' and 'old' risk factors strongly suggests that health policy in developing countries must increasingly address risks such as tobacco and blood pressure that have often mistakenly been labelled, and treated, as conditions of affluence.

Undernutrition was the leading global cause of health loss in 2000, as it was in 1990 (the 2000 results disaggregate undernutrition into underweight and micronutrient deficiencies). Undernutrition was responsible for a lesser proportion of the global burden of disease in 2000 as compared to an estimated 15.6 per cent in 1990. Part of this reduction is due to a real decrease in levels of undernutrition, and part to the improved methods of the GBD 2000 study. Similarly, due to a mix of reduced exposure and methodological improvements, the estimated burden attributable

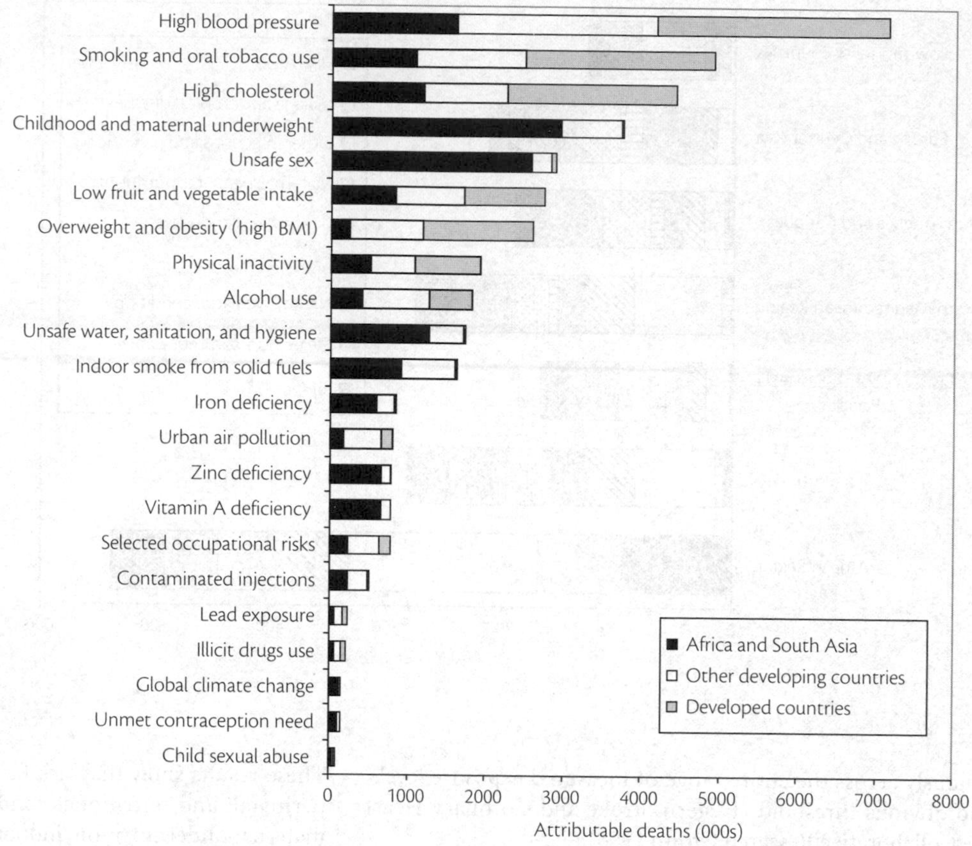

Fig. 2.10.7 Attributable mortality, by selected major risk factors and region, 2000.

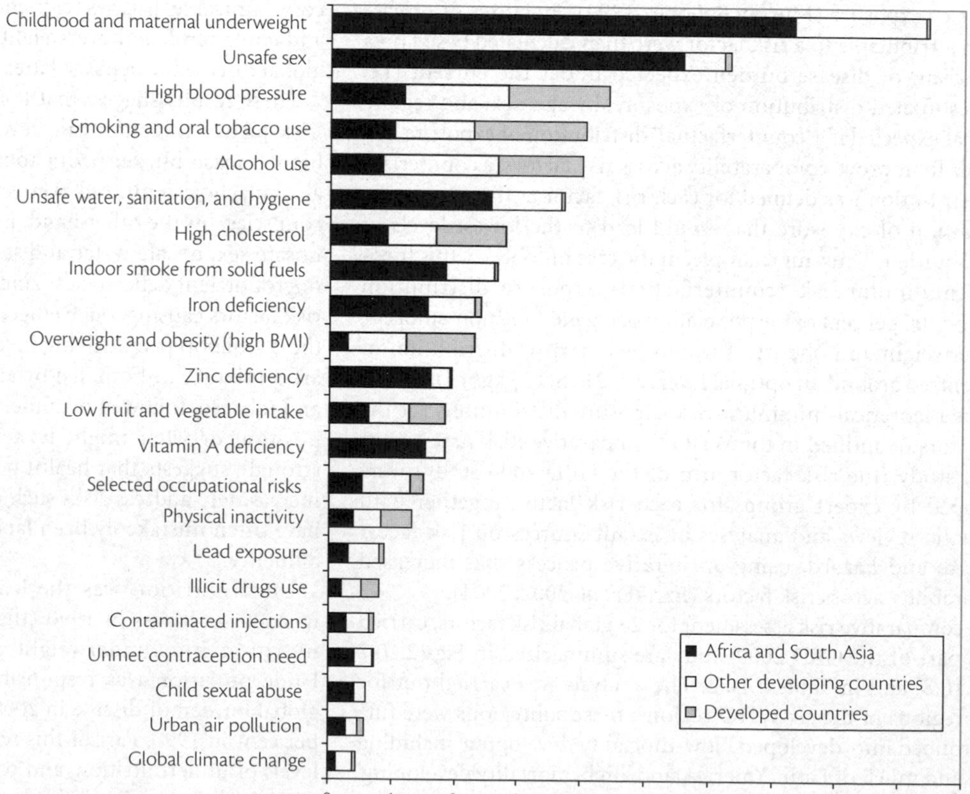

Fig. 2.10.8 The burden of disease, by selected major risk factors and region, 2000.

Table 2.10.2 The twenty leading risk factors for deaths and burden of disease, for the world, 2000

Attributable mortality				**Attributable burden of disease**			
	Risk factor	**Deaths (million)**	**Total deaths (%)**		**Risk factor**	**DALYs (million)**	**Total DALYs (%)**
1	High blood pressure	7.1	12.8	1	Childhood and maternal underweight	137.4	9.4
2	Smoking and oral tobacco use	4.9	8.8	2	Unsafe sex	91.9	6.3
3	High cholesterol	4.4	7.9	3	High blood pressure	64.3	4.4
4	Childhood and maternal underweight	3.7	6.7	4	Smoking and oral tobacco use	59.1	4.1
5	Unsafe sex	2.9	5.2	5	Alcohol use	58.3	4.0
6	Low fruit and vegetable intake	2.7	4.9	6	Unsafe water, sanitation and hygiene	54.2	3.7
7	Overweight and obesity (high BMI)	2.6	4.6	7	High cholesterol	40.4	2.8
8	Physical inactivity	1.9	3.4	8	Indoor smoke from household use of solid fuels	38.5	2.6
9	Alcohol use	1.8	3.2	9	Iron deficiency	35.1	2.4
10	Unsafe water, sanitation and hygiene	1.7	3.1	10	Overweight and obesity (high BMI)	33.4	2.3
11	Indoor smoke from household use of solid fuels	1.6	2.9	11	Zinc deficiency	28.0	1.9
12	Iron deficiency	0.8	1.5	12	Low fruit and vegetable intake	26.7	1.8
13	Urban air pollution	0.8	1.4	13	Vitamin A deficiency	26.6	1.8
14	Zinc deficiency	0.8	1.4	14	Selected occupational risks[a]	21.9	1.5
15	Vitamin A deficiency	0.8	1.4	15	Physical inactivity	19.1	1.3
16	Selected occupational risks[a]	0.8	1.4	16	Lead exposure	12.9	0.9
17	Contaminated injections in healthcare settings	0.5	0.9	17	Illicit drugs use	11.5	0.8
18	Lead exposure	0.2	0.4	18	Contaminated injections in healthcare settings	10.5	0.7
19	Illicit drugs use	0.2	0.4	19	Non-use and use of ineffective methods of contraception	8.8	0.6
20	Global climate change	0.2	0.3	20	Child sexual abuse	8.2	0.6

[a] Includes occupational risk factors for injuries, occupational carcinogens and airborne particulates, ergonomic stressors, and occupational noise.

to unsafe water and sanitation declined from 6.8 per cent in 1990 to 3.7 per cent in 2000.

The 2000 study attributed 4.4 per cent of the global burden of disease to higher than optimal blood pressure, taking into account all increased cardiovascular disease risk for systolic blood pressure distributions relative to a counterfactual distribution with mean 110 mmHg and SD 10 mmHg; on the other hand, the 1990 study attributed only 1.4 per cent of the global burden of disease to hypertension (also using a reference level of 110 mmHg). The GBD 2000 results for smoking and unsafe sex were also much higher than those estimated for 1990—4.1 per cent in 2000 versus 2.6 per cent in 1990 for smoking and 6.3 per cent in 2000 versus 3.5 per cent in 1990 for unsafe sex. Work carried out since the GBD 2000 has examined risk factors for cancers and cardiovascular disease in more detail, and has also updated the analyses of the attributable burden of child and maternal undernutrition (Danaei 2005, 2006; Black 2008).

Despite substantially improved comparability in GBD 2000, the quantification of risk-factor burden needs to expand to include a larger number of risk factors for tropical diseases, injuries, and mental health. The GBD 2005 study will examine the feasibility of including additional important public health risks.

Projections of the global burden of disease

To plan health services effectively, policy makers need to know how health needs might change in the future. To meet this need, the GBD 1990 study included projections of mortality and disability from 1990 to 2020, by cause, for all regions and both sexes. A set of relatively simple models was used to project future health trends for baseline, optimistic, and pessimistic scenarios, based largely on projections of economic and social development, and using the historically observed relationships of these with cause-specific mortality rates (Murray 1997). Updated projections of future trends for mortality and burden of disease between 2002 and 2030 have been prepared by WHO using similar methods to the GBD 1990 study and updated inputs (Mathers & Loncar 2006).

Projection methods

Rather than attempt to model the effects of the many separate direct, or proximal, determinants of disease from the limited data that are available, mortality change was modelled as a function of a limited number of socioeconomic variables: (a) income per capita; (b) the average number of years of schooling among adults, termed 'human capital'; and (c) time, a proxy measure for the secular improvement in health in the twentieth century that partly resulted from accumulating knowledge and technological development. These socioeconomic variables show clear historical relationships with mortality rates; for example, income growth is closely related to the improvement in life expectancy that many countries achieved in the twentieth century. Because of their relationships with death rates, these socioeconomic variables may be regarded as indirect, or distal, determinants of health. In addition, a fourth variable, tobacco use, was included because of its overwhelming impact on health, using information from more than four decades of research on the time lag between persistent tobacco use—measured in terms of 'smoking intensity'—and its effects on health (Peto *et al.* 1992).

Separate projection models were used for HIV and tuberculosis, with various scenarios for scale up of treatment, and with modifications for the interaction between HIV and tuberculosis. In addition to baseline projection scenarios, optimistic and pessimistic scenarios were also developed using different projections of the independent variables.

The data inputs for the projections models were updated by Mathers and Loncar (2006) to take account of the greater number of countries reporting death registration data to the WHO, particularly from developing regions, and to use the latest projections for HIV/AIDS, tuberculosis, tobacco smoking, and overweight and obesity.

Mortality projections

According to both sets of projections, overall (age-standardized) mortality rates worldwide are expected to decline by around 0.5–1 per cent per year over the next 30 years, but at two to three times this rate for most major communicable diseases. While the proportion of deaths from non-communicable diseases is expected to rise everywhere, rates of mortality from these diseases collectively are expected to decline at somewhat less than 1 per cent per year. Major failures with tobacco and obesity control efforts could dramatically alter this prediction, as was seen in several Western countries in the 1950s and 1960s.

Among young children and adolescents under the age of 15 years, the risk of death is projected to decline dramatically in all regions, falling by about two thirds in sub-Saharan Africa and India. Deaths from communicable, maternal, and perinatal conditions, and nutritional deficiencies (Group I) are expected to fall substantially in developing regions, and this projected overall reduction runs counter to the now widely accepted belief that infectious diseases are making a comeback worldwide. It partly reflects the relative contraction of the world's 'young' population, and the growth of the older adult populations. In addition, the projection reflects the observed overall decline in Group I conditions over the past four decades owing to increased income, education, and technological progress in the development of antimicrobials and vaccines.

Clearly, it should not be taken for granted that the progress of the past four decades against infectious diseases will be maintained. It is possible, for example, that antibiotic development and other control technologies will not keep pace with the emergence of drug-resistant strains of important microbes such as *Mycobacterium tuberculosis*. If such a scenario were to prove correct, and in addition, if case-fatality rates were to rise because of such drug-resistant strains, the gains of the present century could be halted or even reversed. The evidence to date nonetheless suggests that, as long as current efforts are maintained, Group I causes are likely to continue to decline.

Deaths from non-communicable diseases are projected to climb from 33 million deaths in 2002 to 51 million in 2030, a 50 per cent increase in absolute numbers. In proportionate terms, Group II deaths are expected to increase their share of the total from 59 per cent in 2002 to 69 per cent in 2030. Mortality attributable to tobacco is expected to rise from its 2002 level of 8 per cent of deaths worldwide to more than 11 per cent of deaths in 2030. Many governments have yet to confront this global health emergency.

Non-communicable diseases are projected to dominate the burden in 2030

When disability is taken into account as well as death, a different view of the future emerges—one that emphasizes adult health problems still further. By 2030, the disease burden due to communicable diseases, maternal, and perinatal conditions, and nutritional deficiencies (excluding HIV/AIDS) is expected to fall to one fifth of the total. The burden attributable to non-communicable diseases, accordingly, is expected to rise sharply, and the burden from injuries is also expected to rise to around 75 per cent of that of Group I conditions, largely from increased traffic accidents. In low- and middle-income countries as a group, deaths from non-communicable diseases are expected to rise from 47 per cent of the burden to almost 70 per cent.

The steep projected increase in the burden of non-communicable diseases worldwide is largely driven by population ageing, augmented by the large numbers of people in developing regions who are now exposed to tobacco. The projected small decrease in the age-specific rates of these diseases in low-income countries is far outweighed by the large and demographically driven increase in the absolute numbers of adults at risk for these diseases, augmented by the tobacco epidemic.

In 2002, the three leading causes of disease burden were, in descending order, conditions arising in the perinatal period, pneumonia, and HIV/AIDS. The three conditions projected to take their place by 2030 are depression, ischaemic heart disease, and road traffic accidents. Perinatal conditions is expected to fall to fourth place and pneumonia to seventh. According to latest UNAIDS projections, HIV would fall to around eleventh place by 2030. Not surprisingly, these changes are not expected to be evenly dispersed worldwide. The total number of lost years of healthy life in the high-income countries is likely to fall slightly, whereas it will increase in sub-Saharan Africa, partly due to a substantial rise in the projected burden of injuries from road accidents.

Limitations of the GBD projections

The 1990 GBD study's HIV/AIDS projections severely underestimated the spread of the epidemic in sub-Saharan Africa, particularly southern Africa; by 2000, HIV/AIDS was estimated to have killed several times more people than projected. On the other hand, the projections published by Mathers and Loncar (2006) probably severely overestimated the projected deaths due to HIV in future years.

In late 2007, UNAIDS and WHO revised estimates and projections of HIV deaths downwards from around 3 million deaths annually to 2 million deaths annually and also concluded that the epidemic had already peaked in sub-Saharan Africa. Rather than continuing to increase to 6 million deaths per annum globally in 2030, the latest projections of HIV mortality suggest that it could decline to around 1 million deaths in 2030.

Apart from the inherent difficulties in predicting the future course of epidemic diseases such as HIV, there can be considerably more confidence in the general picture provided by the projections for the future course of non-communicable disease mortality, based on the historical evidence on the epidemiological transition and on the strong influence of population ageing. However, by their very nature, projections of the future are highly uncertain and need to be interpreted with caution. The burden and mortality projections are not intended as forecasts of what will happen in the future but as projections of current and past trends, based on certain explicit assumptions and on observed historical relationships between development and mortality levels and patterns. The results also depend strongly on the assumption that future mortality trends in low-income countries will have the same relationship to economic and social development as has occurred in the higher-income countries in the recent past.

The GBD projections have not taken explicit account of trends in major risk factors apart from tobacco smoking, and in the recent update, to a limited extent overweight and obesity. If broad trends in risk factors are for worsening of risk exposures with development, rather than the improvements observed in recent decades in many high-income countries, then the GBD projections for low-income countries may be optimistic. There is a need to develop more comprehensive projection models that take explicit account of available information on trends in a wide range of risk factors.

The GBD 2005: Priorities for a new and comprehensive assessment

The Bill and Melinda Gates Foundation has provided funding for a new GBD 2005 study, to be carried out over 3 years, commencing in 2007. The study will be led by the new Health Metrics and Evaluation Institute, hosted by the University of Washington (Moszynski 2007), with key collaborating institutions including Harvard University, the WHO, Johns Hopkins University, and the University of Queensland. This study will also draw on the world's cumulative descriptive epidemiology expertise through a network of around 40 expert working groups. As well as developing new and improved methods to make full use of the increasing amount of health data, particularly from developing countries, the GBD 2005 study will include a comprehensive and consistent revision of disability weights, and assess trends from 1990 to 2005, with projections to 2010.

Several hundred collaborating experts in approximately 40 scientific working groups will conduct systematic reviews of the incidence and prevalence of disease and disabling sequelae, and of exposure and effects of risk factors. The new GBD study will attempt to make full use of new sources of primary data that have recently become available including the WHO World Health Surveys and a number of national health interview and examination surveys. New methods are under development for estimating adult mortality, analysing verbal autopsy data, modelling cause-of-death composition, computing attributable fractions for multiple risk factors, correcting for differential item functioning in health surveys, and imposing internal consistency constraint. Responding to critiques and improvements in the field, the new study will aim to make major progress in disability assessment, using new survey instruments to update disability weights and gather data on health states.

Discussion and conclusions

The GBD study has provided a bold and much needed strategy to estimate current and projected health needs. In particular, it has shown that non-communicable diseases are rapidly becoming the dominant causes of ill health in all developing regions except sub-Saharan Africa, has revealed the extent to which mental health problems have been underestimated worldwide, and has shown the significance of injuries as a problem for the health sector in all regions.

The development and widespread application of a single summary measure of population health (DALYs) has greatly facilitated scientific and political assessments of the comparative importance of various diseases, injuries, and risk factors, particularly for priority-setting in the health sector. Comparative rankings of DALYs have led to strategic decisions by some agencies, such as the WHO, to invest greater effort in programme developments in order to address priority health concerns such as tobacco control and injury prevention. The subsequent GBD 2000–2002 updates, and a plethora of country applications, have led to substantial improvements in both methods and data availability, as well as in the comparability of results. Such global comparative assessments have identified dramatic changes in global health conditions, including impressive reductions in child and adult mortality in many middle-income countries, and some low-income countries, the explosion of the HIV/AIDS epidemic during the 1990s in sub-Saharan Africa, and the dramatic adult health reversal in the former Soviet countries in the 1990s.

The comparable analyses of the GBD/CRA 2000 frameworks have confirmed the advanced epidemiological transition in most regions for both diseases and their risk factors, with the possible exception of South Asia and Africa. To the unfinished agendas of the neglected tropical diseases, malaria, tuberculosis, HIV/AIDS, child and maternal mortality have been added new agendas of non-communicable disease prevention and control, injury prevention and control, and new health threats associated with globalization and trade, particularly tobacco.

The burden of disease methodology and the DALY measure have stimulated considerable debate, particularly in the international and national health policy arenas, among the health economics and epidemiological research communities, and among disability interest groups (Fox-Rushby 2002). Criticisms of the GBD approach fall into two main groups. First, there are concerns about the desirability and implications of extrapolation of population health estimates where data are limited, uncertain, or missing (Cooper *et al.* 1998). Second, there has been a lively debate in the literature about the way that the DALY summarizes fatal and non-fatal health outcomes (Mont 2007; Anand & Hanson 1997; Williams 1999).

Murray and colleagues have argued that health planning, including that based on uncertain assessments of the available evidence which synthesizes the available data and information while ensuring consistency and adjustment for known biases, will almost always be more informed than planning based on ideology, special interests, or crude statistics that are often biased and inconsistent (Murray *et al.* 2003). Murray has recently clarified the roles of crude, corrected, and predicted health statistics (Murray 2007). Although we strongly advocate that corrected and predicted health statistics should be used to produce a comprehensive and unbiased picture of the global burden of disease for health policy and planning, evaluation and monitoring of health systems and interventions, on the other hand, should be based on corrected, but not predicted, statistics.

One of the major innovations of the GBD study was the attempt to measure and value states of health worse than perfect health in a comparable fashion across various societies. Self-report instruments currently in use lack cross-cultural comparability, with the result that the measurement of health in various populations is largely not comparable. The development and operation of a conceptual framework to measure and describe health in a way that improves comparability across populations is a key challenge for burden of disease research (King *et al.* 2003). The GBD 2005 study will also explicitly approach the quantification of health-state preferences as quantifying loss of health, not of broader valuations of 'quality of life' or 'well-being'.

The issue of co-morbidity is another measurement problem to emerge from the GBD which requires further methodological work. In the GBD work to date, co-morbid conditions have been valued separately and time spent in these combined states valued as the sum of the individual state valuations. This additive model is clearly problematic and more sophisticated approaches have been developed in some national studies and for the calculation of overall levels of disability in populations (Mathers *et al.* 2006; Begg *et al.* 2007). More data are required on the prevalence of major co-morbidities in order to avoid multiple attributions in health-state valuations.

Widespread use of published summary measures provides clear evidence that there is a demand for the simplification of epidemiological complexity that summary measures provide. Of course, the provision of summary measures does not preclude the full dissemination of the underlying internally consistent incidence, prevalence, and mortality estimates. In particular, there is considerable demand for a revised GBD study that reliably measures changes in global health and disease patterns over the past 15 years or so. More money is being spent on global health than ever before—by governments, private foundations, and non-governmental organizations. Donors and others in the global health community are increasingly demanding a better understanding of trends in health in order to better allocate their resources and make real progress in improving health. Critical policy questions depend upon understanding trends. The new GBD study will also revise 1990 estimates using consistent data and methods to assess trends in the global burden of diseases and injuries from 1990 to 2005.

As international programmes and policies to improve health worldwide become more widespread, so too will the need for more comprehensive, credible, and critical assessments to periodically monitor population health and the success, or otherwise, of these policies and programmes. Repeated one-off assessments of the global burden of disease do not provide comparability over time due to improvements in data and methods. There is a need to move beyond these, towards truly consistent and comparable monitoring of the world population's health over time.

References

Anand S., Hanson K. Disability-adjusted life years: a critical review. *Journal of Health Economics* 1997;**16**(6):685–702.

Arnesen T., Nord E. The value of DALY life: problems with ethics and validity of disability adjusted life years. *British Medical Journal* 1999;**319**(7222):1423–5.

Barendregt J., van Oortmarssen G.J., Vos T. *et al.* A generic model for the assessment of disease epidemiology: the computational basis of DisMod II. *Population Health Metrics* 2003;**1**:4.

Begg S.J., Vos T., Barker B. *et al.* Burden of disease and injury in Australia in the new millennium: measuring health loss from diseases, injuries and risk factors. *Medical Journal of Australia* 2008;**188**(1):36–40.

Begg S., Vos T., Barker B., Stevenson C., Stanley L., Lopez A. *The burden of disease and injury in Australia 2003.* Canberra, Australian Institute of Health and Welfare; 2007.

Cooper R.S., Osotimehin B., Kaufman J.S. *et al.* Disease burden in sub-Saharan Africa: what should we conclude in the absence of data?. *Lancet* 1998;**351**(9097):208–10.

Eastern Stroke and Coronary Heart Disease Collaborative Research Group. Blood pressure, cholesterol, and stroke in Eastern Asia. *Lancet* 1998;**352**:1801–7.

Ezzati M. *et al.*, Comparative Risk Assessment Collaborative Group. Selected major risk factors and global and regional burden of disease. *Lancet* 2002;**360**(9343):1347–60.

Ezzati M., Lopez A.D., Rodgers A. *et al. Comparative quantification of health risks: global and regional burden of disease attributable to selected major risk factors.* Geneva: World Health Organization; 2004.

Fox-Rushby J.A. *Disability adjusted life years (DALYS) for decision-making? An overview of the literature.* London: Office of Health Economics; 2002.

Jamison D.T., Breman J.G., Measham A.R. *et al. Disease control priorities in developing countries.* 2nd ed. New York (NY): Oxford University Press; 2006.

King G., Murray C.J.L., Salomon J.A. *et al.* Enhancing the validity and cross-cultural comparability of measurement in survey research. *American Political Science Review* 2003;**93**(4):567–83.

Lopez A.D., Mathers C.D., Ezzati M. *et al. Global burden of disease and risk factors.* New York (NY): Oxford University Press; 2006.

Lozano R., Murray C.J.L., Frenk J. *et al.* Burden of disease assessment and health system reform: results of a study in Mexico. *Journal for International Development* 1995;**7**(3):555–64.

Mathers C.D., Iburg K.M., Begg S. Adjusting for dependent comorbidity in the calculation of healthy life expectancy. *Population Health Metrics* 2006;**4**:4.

Mathers C.D., Iburg K., Salomon J. *et al.* Global patterns of healthy life expectancy in the year 2002. *BMC Public Health* 2004;**4**(1):66.

Mathers C.D., Loncar D. Projections of global mortality and burden of disease from 2002 to 2030. *PLoS Medicine* 2006;**3**(11):e442.

Mathers C.D., Lopez A.D., Murray C.J.L.. The burden of disease and mortality by condition: data, methods and results for 2001. In: Lopez AD *et al.*, editors. *Global burden of disease and risk factors.* New York (NY): Oxford University Press; 2006. p. 45–240.

Mathers C.D., Salomon J.A., Ezzati M. *et al.* Sensitivity and uncertainty analyses for burden of disease and risk factor estimates. In: Lopez A.D. *et al.*, editors. *Global burden of disease and risk factors.* New York (NY): Oxford University Press; 2006. p. 399–426.

Mathers C.D., Vos T., Stevenson C. *The burden of disease and injury in Australia.* Canberra: Australian Institute of Health and Welfare; 1999.

McKee M., Shkolnikov V. Understanding the toll of premature death among men in eastern Europe. *British Medical Journal* 2001;**323**(7320):1051–5.

Melse J.M., Kramers P.G.N. Berekening van de ziektelast in Nederland. Achtergronddokument bij VTV-1997; deel III, hoofdstuk 7 [Calculation of the burden of disease in the Netherlands. Background document to VTV-1997: III; chapter 7]. Bilthoven, the Netherlands: Rijksinstituut voor Volkgezondheit en Milieu [National Institute of Public Health and the Environment]; 1998.

Men T., Brennan P., Boffetta P. *et al.* Russian mortality trends for 1991–2001: analysis by cause and region. *British Medical Journal* 2003;**327**(7421):964.

Mexican Ministry of Health, National Institute of Public Health, Harvard Initiative for Global Health. *Mexico health metrics 2005 report: section 1—comparative risk assessment*. Mexico: Systema Nacional de Informacion en Salud (SINAIS); 2005. Available from: http://sinais.salud.gob.mx/metrica/areas/mcr.html [accessed 2008 Jan 15].

Mont D. Measuring health and disability. *Lancet* 2007;**369**(9573): 1658–63.

Moszynski P. Gates Foundation funds new institute to evaluate global health data. *British Medical Journal* 2007;**334**(7606):1238.

Murray C.J.L., Ferguson B.D., Lopez A.D. *et al.* Modified logit life table system: principles, empirical validation and application. *Population Studies* 2003;**57**(2):1–18.

Murray C.J.L., Lopez A.D., Jamison D.T. The global burden of disease in 1990: summary results, sensitivity analysis and future directions. *Bulletin of the World Health Organization* 1994;**72**(3):495–509.

Murray C.J.L., Lopez A.D. Evidence-based health policy—lessons from the Global Burden of Disease Study. *Science* 1996a;**274**(5288):740–3.

Murray C.J.L., Lopez A.D. *Global comparative assessments in the health sector: disease burden, expenditures and intervention packages: collected reprints from the Bulletin of the World Health Organization*. Geneva: World Health Organization; 1994.

Murray C.J.L., Lopez A.D. *Global health statistics*. Cambridge (MA): Harvard University Press; 1996b.

Murray C.J.L., Lopez A.D. Global mortality, disability and the contribution of risk factors: global burden of disease study. *Lancet* 1997;**349**(9063):1436–42.

Murray C.J.L., Lopez A.D. On the comparable quantification of health risks: lessons from the global burden of disease study. *Epidemiology* 1999;**10**(5):594–605.

Murray C.J.L., Lopez A.D. *The global burden of disease: a comprehensive assessment of mortality and disability from diseases, injuries and risk factors in 1990 and projected to 2020*. Cambridge (MA): Harvard University Press; 1996c.

Murray C.J.L., Mathers C.D., Salomon J.A. Towards evidence-based public health. In: Murray C.J.L., Evans D, editors. *Health systems performance assessment: debates, methods and empiricism*. Geneva: World Health Organization: 2003. p. 715–26.

Murray C.J.L., Salomon J.A., Mathers C.D. *et al. Summary measures of population health: concepts, ethics, measurement and applications*. Geneva: World Health Organization; 2002.

Murray C.J.L., Salomon J.A., Mathers C.D. A critical examination of summary measures of population health. *Bulletin of the World Health Organization* 2000;**78**(8):981–94.

Murray C.J.L. Rethinking DALYs. In: Murray C.J.L., Lopez A.D., editors. *The global burden of disease*. Cambridge (MA): Harvard University Press; 1996. p. 1–98. vol 1.

Murray C.J.L. Towards good practice for health statistics: lessons from the Millennium Development Goal health indicators. *Lancet* 2007;**369**(9564):862–73.

Peto R., Lopez A.D., Boreham J. *et al.* Mortality from tobacco in developed countries: indirect estimation from National Vital Statistics. *Lancet* 1992;**339**(8804):1268–78.

Robine J.M., Jagger C., Mathers C.D. *et al. Determining health expectancies*. Chichester: John Wiley & Sons; 2003.

Ruwaard D., Kramers P.G.N. Public health status and forecasts. Health prevention and health care in the Netherlands until 2015. Elsevier, the Netherlands: National Institute of Public Health and Environmental Protection; 1998.

Salomon J., Mathers C.D., Chatterji S. *et al.* Quantifying individual levels of health: definitions, concepts and measurement issues. In: Murray C.J.L., Evans D., editors. *Health systems performance assessment: debate, methods and empiricism*. Geneva: World Health Organization; 2003. p. 301–18.

Salomon J.A., Murray C.J.L. Estimating health state valuations using a multiple-method protocol. In: Murray C.J.L. *et al.*, editors. *Summary measures of population health: concepts, ethics, measurement and applications*. Geneva: World Health Organization; 2002a.

Salomon J.A., Murray C.J.L. The epidemiologic transition revisited: compositional models for causes of death by age and sex. *Population and Development Review* 2002b;**28**(2):205–28.

Salomon J.A., Tandon A., Murray C.J.L., World Health Survey Pilot Collaborating Group. Unpacking health perceptions: multi-country survey study using anchoring vignettes to enhance comparisons of self-rated health. *British Medical Journal* 2004;**328**(7434):258–61.

Shkolnikov V., McKee M., Leon D. Changes in life expectancy in Russia in the mid-1990s. *Lancet* 2001;**357**(9260):917–21.

Stouthard M., Essink-Bot M., Bonsel G. *et al. Disability weights for diseases in the Netherlands* Rotterdam, the Netherlands: Department of Public Health, Erasmus University; 1997.

Sullivan D.F. A single index of mortality and morbidity. *HSMHA Health Reports* 1971;**86**(4):347–54.

UNAIDS, World Health Organization. *AIDS epidemic update: December 2007*. Geneva: UNAIDS; 2007.

Vos T., Tobias M., Gareeboo H. *et al. Mauritius health sector reform, national burden of disease study*. Mauritius: Ministry of Health and Ministry of Economic Planning and Development; 1995.

Waldron I. Recent trends in sex mortality ratios for adults in developed countries. *Social Science and Medicine* 1993;**36**(4):451–62.

Wilkins R., Adams O.B. Health expectancy in Canada, late 1970s: demographic, regional and social dimensions. *American Journal of Public Health* 1983;**73**(9):1073–80.

Williams A. Calculating the global burden of disease: time for a strategic reappraisal?. *Health Economics* 1999;**8**:1–8.

Wong M.D., Chung A.K., Boscardin W.J. *et al.* The contribution of specific causes of death to sex differences in mortality. *Public Health Reports* 2006;**121**(6):746–54.

World Bank. *World development report 1993. Investing in health*. New York (NY): Oxford University Press for the World Bank; 1993.

World Health Organization. *Global burden of disease estimates*. Geneva: World Health Organization; 2008. Available from: http://www.who.int/healthinfo/bodestimates/en/index.html [accessed 2008 Feb 27].

World Health Organization. *World health report 2000. Health systems: improving performance*. Geneva: World Health Organization; 2000.

World Health Organization. *World health report 2002. Reducing risks, promoting healthy life*. Geneva: World Health Organization; 2002.

World Health Organization. *World health report 2004: changing history*. Geneva: World Health Organization; 2004.

SECTION 3

Public health policies

3.1

Overview of policies and strategies

Walter W. Holland

Introduction

The prime aim of health policies worldwide has been the maintenance and improvement of the health status of populations. This implies an understanding of human health and disease in order to determine the major biological, political, social, environmental, and lifestyle factors influencing health status and the burden of disease. The risk factors which influence health differ between countries, and the examples in this book illustrate their investigation, influence on health, and methods of control. Thus, policies for health will be influenced by different factors in each country and region. Although it may appear that the problems addressed in this chapter are mainly concerned with developed countries, it is important to emphasize that the issues are the same in all countries at all stages of development. Public health problems in the developing world may appear different and greater, but the principles are the same.

Health status

Knowledge of the health status of a population is essential in the formulation of any public health strategy. Although, in general, health has improved, variations in health status both between countries, within countries, and between different gender, social, and ethnic groups remain and, in some instances, have become more pronounced. This chapter deals with some of the changes and differences in health in different parts of the world. In developed countries the most important causes of mortality are from the chronic diseases. Infective diseases have become less important as a major cause of mortality, although with the appearance of AIDS, SARS etc. are still important. In the developing countries infectious diseases such as malaria, tuberculosis, acute respiratory infections, gastrointestinal conditions are still of great importance, although in many chronic diseases have already overtaken the toll of death from infectious diseases.

With the increase in the chronic diseases and ageing of the population the measurement of mortality has become a less important measure of the health status of any population. Morbidity and disability are an important measure of health status. The difficulty is, however, in the acceptability of measures which have been proposed. Mathers (2007) provides a succinct review and analysis of the various measures which have been proposed and are being used. For most purposes, the combination of mortality with disability would provide a good measure to describe the health status of any population group. Sullivan (1966), Sanders (1964), and Robine *et al.* (2003) devised a method combining such data to estimate disability-free life expectancy. However it was found that this required information based on community surveys. The problem with this is the impossibility of comparing results cross-nationally (or even within a country) because of different expectations and norms for health in different groups.

In view of these difficulties a number of other measures have been tried, such as healthy-life expectancies, potential years of life lost, and disability adjusted life years (DALY). The latter is a summary measure which combines time lost through premature death and time lived in states of less than optimal health, referred to as 'disability'. The DALY is, essentially, a measure of the potential years of life lost (PYLL) but includes lost good health. It is thus, theoretically, a better measure of the burden of disease of any population group. Mathers (2007) describes how these measures have been developed and are used. The health state measures do reflect the severity of a disease dependent on the social preference for different states of health—they can thus be used as a 'common currency' for combining mortality and non-fatal health events in the comparison of health status of different groups. They can thus also be thought of as quality adjusted life years (QALY) widely used in economic evaluations. However, it must be emphasized that all these measures depend on assessment of 'disability' by individuals responding to interviews or questionnaires. Mortality, by contrast, depends on the measurement of an event.

WHO, in its analysis of the burden of disease comparisons between communities and regions, uses the DALY approach (Murray 1996). The summary measures are thus based on a mixture of reasonably accurate, comparable data (mortality) and level and frequency of 'disability' on responses to enquiries. Although there is reasonably reproducible and comprehensive data available on the latter in many developed countries, information on this are less adequate for developing countries as they often rely on proxy replies rather than responses of individuals. Nonetheless, they may provide a rough guide to the importance of different conditions and their burden, which should assist those responsible for the development of proper public health strategies. Mathers (2007) describes the criticisms of the WHO measures and provides tables for the 'burden of disease' as measured by mortality and DALYs in both low- and middle-income versus high-income countries and the world as a whole. For both groups, ischaemic heart disease, cerebrovascular disease, and lower respiratory infections, in that order, have the highest death rates; high blood pressure, smoking, and high cholesterol are the global risk factors with the highest death rates. If DALYs are used, the order for death rates is perinatal conditions, lower respiratory infections, and ischaemic heart disease, while childhood underweight, high blood pressure, and unsafe sex are the most important risk factors. This illustrates the importance of using a variety of measures for the determination of the health status of any population, the need for public health to define precisely the method used in the description of health status, and to be clear as to the reason for which the health status measurement will be used.

Health services

As the health of most of the populations of the developed world has improved, complaints and concerns with the health services have risen. All health systems face the challenges of demographic change (ageing of the population), increasing population mobility, growing social exclusion, costly new therapeutic techniques, and rising public demands and expectations. While all these place mounting pressure on service provision at a time that public spending is under tight constraints, there are new opportunities for prevention and treatment, there is growing interest in prevention and health promotion, and the quality, as well as quantity, of life is generally improving.

The public has widely different views on the quality of health services, ranging from 95 per cent considering that health services are good in France to only 25 per cent in Greece (Ferrara 1993). All countries face similar problems as follows:

(1) Inequalities in both health status and health service provision between different geographic areas and social groups.

(2) Variations in the utilization of services for similar conditions (e.g. hysterectomy).

(3) Difficulties in the apportionment of limited resources to different strategies (e.g. prevention versus cure, or cure versus care) or between services (e.g. cardiac services versus renal services).

(4) Many of the problems are related to lifestyle behaviour and political/economic issues (e.g. cigarette smoking).

These issues have been described in detail for the countries of the European Union (Abel-Smith *et al.* 1995; Holland & Mossialos 1999).

The following chapters all illustrate the approaches adopted in individual countries to cope with these dilemmas. Most people accept that difficult choices need to be made. Most concentrate on the provision of health services, but health services in themselves do relatively little to bring about an improvement in the health status of populations. Environmental factors, such as housing, traffic, and employment, and behavioural factors, such as smoking, diet, and alcohol consumption, probably make greater contributions. Nonetheless, health services have an essential role in improving quality of life and can produce specific valuable improvements in other aspects of health status.

In its World Health Report (2000), WHO attempted to assess the performance of health systems. It considers that the key functions of health systems are 'providing services, generating the human and physical resources that make service delivery possible; raising and pooling the resources used to pay for healthcare and setting and enforcing the rules of the game and providing strategic direction for all the actors involved'. The Report assesses the performance of a country's health system on the 'basis of three overall goals: Good health, responsiveness to the expectations of the population, and fairness of financial contribution'.

The Report gives details of the measures used in its assessments. Population health, the defining objective of any health system, was assessed on the basis of the measures described above in the section on health status—mortality and DALYs. Responsiveness was assessed on the basis of responses by key informants on respect for persons, which included respect for dignity, confidentiality, and autonomy as well as client orientation which included prompt attention, quality of amenities, access to social support networks, and choice of provider.

Fair financing means 'that the risks each household faces due to the costs of the health system are distributed according to ability to pay rather than to the risk of illness: A fairly financed system ensures financial protection for everyone'. Thus, 'the way healthcare is financed is perfectly fair if the ratio of total health contributions to total non-food spending is identical for all households independently of their income, their health status or their use of the health system'. A great deal of effort was expended on developing information on expenditure on health and constructing national health accounts.

The final score on the performance of an individual country's health performance based on the above criteria was weighted as follows: Health (DALYs)—total 50 per cent, overall or average 25 per cent, distribution or equality, 25 per cent; responsiveness—total 25 per cent, overall or average 12.5 per cent, distribution or equality 12.5 per cent; fair financial contribution—distribution or equality 25 per cent.

The World Health Report (2000) gives details of the variation of each of these measures between countries as well as the total score achieved by a country on the above scale. Full statistical details are given for each of the above measures, as well as for the main causes of mortality in each country. The Report concludes by making the overall health attainment, according to the WHO index. Japan has rank 1, followed by Switzerland, Norway, and Sweden. France comes in at Number 6, the United Kingdom ninth, the United States fifteenth. Niger, Somalia, Central African Republic, and Sierra Leone are last at 188–191. In general, African countries have the lowest scores.

Not unexpectedly, this analysis has given rise to a great deal of discussion. Individual countries objected to the order in which they were placed. However for public health purposes the publication of the Report has encouraged analysis of the components of an 'ideal' health system. The individual measures included are open to a great deal of criticism—the report is transparent that many of the judgements made were subjective, based on selected respondents and not tested for reliability. But, at the very least, it opened the debate on both the adequacy of an individual country's system as well as the measures required by assessment.

Organization and financing

The promotion of services to improve health by those working in public health and the influence that can be brought to bear on the management and administration of all services are important contributions to health service planning. Most health systems in developed countries have well-developed mechanisms for funding and provision. The problems in developing and developed countries may differ widely. In the former, health services are usually well organized in the urban areas, with deficits in the rural areas. But there are also problems in the former. In many developing countries most doctors are paid by the state, and are not well paid. However, opportunities usually exist for doctors in urban areas to supplement their income by private practice, which leads to great difficulties and disparities both between different groups of practitioners as well as between different areas in a country. There are also problems relating to the distribution of health workers caused by migration to developed countries. This may have grave implications for the supply and quality of health services. Different solutions are being developed; one suggestion is that all doctors who provide clinical services should be in private practice, and only those in public health and/or health planning should be employed by the state at a reasonable salary.

Although this problem also exists in developed countries, it does not have such an impact on the delivery of basic health services. Countries differ, however, in their ability to use these structures to initiate broad policies to maximize the population's health. All health systems operate within a framework of national law. In some countries, such as the United Kingdom, the state is clearly visible as a regulator and provider of services. In others, legislation creates an environment in which doctors, hospitals, and insurance agencies operate with less visible state intervention. The ability of health services to co-operate with other agencies varies but it is less where there is little formal control beyond legislation of the health system itself. Most countries have endorsed the World Health Organization (WHO) *Health for All* charter but there is great variation in implementation in national and local policies. The state is involved in all health systems in varying degrees:

(1) As legal regulator of the arrangements for patients to receive medical care and doctors to receive remuneration

(2) As a contributor to healthcare financing, either through formal taxes or through quasi-taxes such as compulsory social insurance

(3) As a guardian, to ensure that the correct balance of resources is used to achieve optimum population health

Healthcare may be conceived in an economic framework as an exchange of goods. Patients seeking medical care are making demands while doctors are supplying services. However, there are ways other than medical treatment of using resources to improve population health and the priorities of medical practice emphasizing technical over social models of care do not always provide optimal health benefits. There is a role in all healthcare systems for an overview of resource allocation, health policy, and population health outcomes; this is the task of health commissioning. The latter is the means to secure the best value by specifying and procuring services for the population to deliver the best possible health and well-being outcomes within the best use of available resources. For example, in an area with many childhood accidents, it may be better to commission services which help to reduce road and home accidents than to improve accident and emergency services.

The problems of organization and financing are particularly great in the low- and middle-income countries. As the World Health Report demonstrates, it is in these countries that mortality and disability rates are particularly high. Not only do these countries suffer from a high burden of acute infective diseases, but also from increasing incidence of chronic diseases. It is these countries that suffer from poor environmental conditions, inadequate transport, and above all poor, inadequate education.

Many of these poor countries are the successors to a past colonial regime. In some instances, this has left a deficient system of governance and great turmoil. Hence, not only are these countries poor and unhealthy, they also have great extremes of poverty and wealth. Thus, their ability to develop fair, equitable systems of organization and financing are grossly impaired. It is these, the poorer countries and areas, that have the most health problems—and the worst health systems. This circle of inadequacy is compounded by the emigration of the educated health service workers to the wealthier nations which have needs for such trained personnel. The problem in low-income countries is compounded by their aspirations. The need in these areas is mainly for the development of public health and primary healthcare facilities. Unfortunately, few have the willingness (or ability) to restrict the development of secondary and tertiary healthcare, much more expensive in both monetary terms as well as skills required by personnel. Thus, the reduction of levels of ill-health is impeded by the desire to develop (unnecessary) secondary and tertiary facilities.

Health commissioning (in the past, the term 'health administration' subsumed 'commissioning')

Health commissioning needs to take into account the following factors:

(1) Improvement in health status (e.g. targeting smokers to reduce smoking should result in fewer cases of ischaemic heart disease)

(2) Risk reduction (e.g. as above, reducing the number of smokers in a population)

(3) Services and protection needed to achieve improvements in health and reduction of risks (e.g. product labelling)

(4) Data needs for monitoring the achievement of the tasks identified (discussed in detail by Holland (1995))

The prerequisites for achieving these goals need to be clear. The best model for this is that developed in the Netherlands (Ministry of Health, Welfare and Cultural Affairs 1993) which considers that health is seen as 'the possibility for every member of society to function normally and to participate in social life'. Thus, the need for healthcare is 'to enable an individual to share, maintain, and if possible improve his or her life together with other members of the community'. This implies that necessary healthcare is that which allows the individual to be a full participant in society. This societal perspective is a little different from the individual perspective, where health is seen as the balance between what the individual wants to do and what the individual can do, or the professional approach where health is the absence of disease. The Dutch model is the best one to follow in the arena of public health choices. It should be noted that although this is an excellent model, even in the Netherlands, changes in the structure and financing of services for health have been difficult to achieve. A recent publication,

Exter *et al.* (2004), gives an interesting chronological account of the various changes and emphasizes that there are many interested groups and powerful lobbies which slow down progress in implementing changes. Government in Holland cannot impose changes without consent. Since 1993 there have been at least 15 major reports concerned with change. Within that framework it is necessary to consider the place of public health. For that the current British definition is helpful as discussed below.

It is often considered that health commissioning is particularly suited for wealthy countries. But it is just as applicable in countries with few resources. The crucial prerequisite is for those responsible for the administration of services for health are committed to improving health status rather than only the provision of clinical (health) services. If it is accepted that a country's goal is to improve health status then, by having a robust system of health commissioning, priorities can be set to favour the development of appropriate measures to reduce risks, e.g. by smoking policies or immunization, rather than the provision of 'rescue' services such as the treatment of lung cancer or pneumonia. This is addressed in greater detail under priorities.

Role of public health

> *Public Health is the science and art of preventing disease, prolonging life, promoting health through the organised efforts of society. Public Health Medicine is that branch of medicine which specialises in public health. Its chief responsibilities are the surveillance of the health of the population, the identification of its health needs, the fostering of policies which promote health and the evaluation of health services.* (Acheson 1988)

For the proper application of these principles it is essential to appreciate the methods to be used. Epidemiology, which is the science fundamental to the study and practice of public health, increases the understanding of the determinants of health and disease and the knowledge of their occurrence in populations and groups. Such information indicates the action that can be taken to prevent disease and promote health by health education or social policies which aim to modify behaviour, prophylactic procedures like immunization, screening for identification of those at special risk or in need of special care, and protection against specific environmental hazards. Preventive programmes also need to be monitored to determine whether they are achieving their objectives, at what cost, and how they may need to be modified.

A further function is the study of the nature and extent of disease and disability in the population and how this varies with age, sex, economic, and social circumstances, occupation, and environment. Information on the patterns of disease is essential in defining health needs and tasks for health services and in setting priorities. It also allows the review of the services as they now are and the identification of those who do and do not use them so that the need for new services or the modification of the present ones can be judged. In addition, it is necessary to evaluate how effective the services are in helping the community in cure and care, in the relief of suffering, the maintenance of working capacity, rehabilitation of the disabled, and lowering of death rates. It also needs to assess how efficient the services are in using the community's resources. Both aspects are critical in ensuring value for money, and are an integral part of health service management and resource planning—the more so since technology is always offering expensive new options.

Thus, the problems for which public health action is required include:

(1) Outbreaks of disease caused by infectious or toxic agents, e.g. smallpox, typhoid, food poisoning, bovine spongiform encephalopathy, radiation, and so on;

(2) Problems arising from social and environmental issues such as inadequate housing, unemployment, poverty, abortion, fluoridation of water, and global environmental and population issues (McMichael & Powles 1999; Raleigh 1999);

(3) Behavioural concerns such as smoking, excessive consumption of alcohol, drug abuse, and insufficient exercise;

(4) Health service issues including assessment of healthcare needs and outcomes, and the effectiveness and efficiency of particular services.

Public health, as a discipline, should not become involved in the direct management of clinical services in the community or within institutions—it lacks the expertise essential for these tasks. Its prime responsibilities are to promote health and to prevent and control disease. It thus has responsibility for surveillance and for the planning and co-ordination of measures that promote and maintain health. It must be involved in the planning and distribution of clinical services in accordance with measures of need and demands and the assessment of effectiveness.

The UK Faculty of Public Health considers that public health practitioners need to have skills in nine key areas:

(1) Surveillance and assessment of the populations' health and well-being

(2) Assessing the evidence of the effectiveness of health and healthcare interventions, programmes, and services

(3) Policy and strategy development and implementation

(4) Strategic leadership and collaborative working for health

(5) Health improvement

(6) Health protection

(7) Health and social service quality

(8) Public health intelligence

(9) Academic public health

These are considered to be the main skills needed for the three main domains of public health practice—health protection, health improvement, and service quality. A number of chapters in this Textbook address these issues in much greater detail.

Assurance of appropriateness

Few countries, at present, appear to have developed an organizational framework whereby the principles and methods of determining appropriateness are systematically applied.

In considering the provision of services for health, it is important to be clear about what is to be achieved. In most countries, it is now accepted that everyone who needs healthcare must be able to obtain it. However, that is not always the rule, as is shown in the following chapters.

The form and content of the right to healthcare are the result of a series of political and social compromises. As the Dutch *Report on Choices in Health Care* emphasizes, responsibility for others, the ideal of equality, and the social benefits of good public health have encouraged the belief that people are responsible for their own health, and are free to choose how to use healthcare and which risks they are willing to take (Ministry of Health, Welfare and Cultural Affairs 1993). The fusion of such different starting points has always brought strain to the design of healthcare systems That these strains are limited in the determination of rights is partly due to a pragmatic coupling between equality and freedom of choice so that, in principle, everyone has equal rights to virtually all of the facilities of healthcare. People do not need everything they want and not all needs for healthcare are equally important. There is a need for healthcare services to maintain or restore health, for care and nursing of impaired health, or to relieve suffering. The concept of health is therefore the most appropriate standard to determine as to when there is a need for healthcare. A definition of 'health' is that it is the ability to function normally. In this definition, there will be a need for healthcare when people are restricted in their normal functioning or when there is a threat of such restriction. Such a need is more essential when the restrictions are greater or threaten to be greater. From a community-oriented view of health, this is an incomplete statement. Health has a value in itself because it allows a people to participate in social life and to develop themselves. The more the health problems restrict a person's possibilities in society, the more the need for healthcare.

As stated above, there are a variety of approaches to health. From the perspective of the individual, health is linked to self-determination or autonomy. To be healthy is to be able, as an individual, to achieve in society what one has chosen to aim for. Whether that is possible depends not only on one's physical, material, and psychological resources, but also on what one wishes to achieve. Health can be described as a balance between what people want and what they can achieve. Thus, there will be differences in how individuals express a desire for healthcare.

From the medical professional perspective, health is the absence of disease, and is seen as a deviation from normal biological function. In this definition, there is a clear distinction between healthcare for the sick and social services for people who are not sick, where healthcare must be seen as professionally given care, provided on the basis of indications defined objectively by the provider.

The effectiveness of care is also defined objectively with the most important criteria being danger to life and the extent of normal biological function. Biological functions seem ultimately to be directed at survival and reproduction. From that perspective, demands can be sorted according to gravity, and it is possible to distinguish necessary from less necessary care.

From the community-oriented approach, health is seen as the possibility of every member of the society to function normally. The choices are made at the level of society because individual health is linked to the possibility of participation in social life. Care is thus necessary when it enables an individual to share, maintain, and if possible improve his or her life together with other members of the community. Of course this question is not answered in the same way by all communities. There are three points of departure: The fundamental equality of people, the fundamental need for the protection of human life, and the principle of solidarity. Thus, the major aim of any such system is the improvement of health and the ability to participate within society. If one accepts this Dutch model, then it is possible to define the different types of care that need to be provided in a variety of ways.

The WHO (Europe) has discussed the key areas specifically for public health (WHO 1999). These can be summarized as understanding health and disease, measuring health status, appropriate disease surveillance and control, promoting health and well-being, evaluating and improving health outcomes, intersectoral and collaborative working, and advocacy and communications. These define the role of public health within a health system which includes healthcare and ensures that appropriate decisions are made.

Criteria, access, and utilization

The first criterion that needs to be established is whether care is necessary or not. The second criterion is the effectiveness of the services provided, the efficiency with which they are provided, and whether the individual could take responsibility for providing them.

These principles are established in some way or another in most health systems. They are thus concerned with improvement of health status, risk factor reduction, and improvement of services and protection.

In most developed countries, there is now a split between provision and purchasing for healthcare. The relative role of those who purchase healthcare varies between countries. In most private insurance systems, what is insured constitutes what is bought; however, in those that have managed care, or purchasing authorities, these decide what care should be purchased and where it should be obtained. It is thus feasible to introduce healthcare systems that consider the improvement of health on a societal basis. The characteristic that prevents medical care becoming an ordinary market, from an economic viewpoint, is that the receivers of services are often unable to make informed choices about care. However, it should be noted that patients do make many of the key choices over healthcare, whether their feelings and symptoms indicate that they are ill, and whether to consult a doctor.

There are wide variations between the different methods of organization and responses of individuals to healthcare. Similarly, doctors do not perform uniformly. Individual doctors vary in their action when faced with similar conditions. In both the National Health Services and social insurance systems, doctors are gate keepers to resources. They legitimize a patient's claim for services. Health systems seek to influence doctors' decisions broadly, e.g. in the level of remuneration given to a particular service.

As indicated, in all systems it is crucial that there is interaction between the different sectors of society. Health can only be improved through changes in the environment, through occupation, including agriculture as well as health services and education, and unless there is some degree of co-ordination between these activities the optimal distribution of resource will be lacking. This also has an important impact on the improvement of health which is the aim of most national health systems. Most systems have now come to terms with the fact that they cannot only treat established disease but also have to be considered with the improvements of health and the prevention of disease.

International trends in healthcare

Abel-Smith *et al.* (1995) reviewed trends in healthcare. They note that there is a worldwide trend towards giving every citizen in a country the same rights to healthcare, but not in the United States. President Clinton made proposals so that would also have been the case in America. Although there seems to be little chance of this right being available for all the citizens of the country with the largest healthcare expenditure, some US states, e.g. Massachusetts, are experimenting in providing this. There has been an increase in public financing of healthcare quantitatively whether by compulsory insurance contribution or taxation in most countries. There is some trend towards consumers making a contribution in the forms of co-payments, e.g. prescription charges. Some countries are following the trend set by the United Kingdom in 1978 (Department of Health and Social Security 1976) of distributing resources on a geographical per head of population basis.

Recent developments in the United Kingdom, as well as in some other European countries, e.g. Sweden, have been to develop quasi-markets with an increase in consumer-choice. This has been achieved by the development of privately financed healthcare facilities, mainly for simple elective procedures, e.g. cataract and hip replacement. Patients choosing these providers have the costs met by the NHS.

Some countries are encouraging people to take out private insurance or even to contract out of the public system.

Most countries are attempting to improve efficiency and effectiveness by introducing charters for waiting times. These indicated the right to be treated within a given time and reduce travel times by locating services in individual practices or locations rather than concentrated in a few large centres; however, some specialist services (e.g. cancer) are only provided in a limited number of institutions. All countries and political regions have become concerned with quality and effectiveness and a few, e.g. the European Union, have developed indices of outcome (Holland 1997).

Unfortunately, in most developed and many developing countries, the trend has been to increase expenditure on clinical services while simultaneously diminishing, or slowing the rate of growth, for public health and preventive services.

Politicians and electorates in most countries demand the development of clinical services which can demonstrate their benefit rapidly, but are much less concerned with promoting or developing public health preventive services where the benefit is far more long-term, in spite of many academic studies demonstrating the cost effectiveness of the latter.

Provider–purchaser model for both public health and personal health services

The separation of commissioning and providing services discussed above theoretically enables better decisions to be made over which services are to be provided within a limited budget. Theoretically, it should also be possible to balance preventive, curative, and rehabilitative services. For this to be effective an adequate knowledge of the epidemiology, including the natural history, of conditions is necessary. However, this is not possible for more than a small number of conditions, although a few, such as coronary heart disease, chronic obstructive lung disease, and lung cancer, may represent a large proportion of the disease burden in a particular population.

Coronary heart disease may be used as an example. The prevalence of the various stages of the disease can be ascertained in a defined population by appropriate epidemiological studies or estimated by extrapolation from studies in equivalent populations. Incidence figures for each stage of the condition are obtained in the same way. Many of the factors responsible for the development of coronary heart disease, e.g. smoking cigarettes, blood pressure, and poor diet are known. Evidence of the effectiveness of various approaches to prevention, e.g. advise school children not to start smoking, counselling adults smokers to stop when they attend the doctor, banning cigarette advertising, and so on, is known (or required). Evidence of the effectiveness and procedures to be used for the treatment of the early stages of diseases such as angina is available.

It is thus possible to devise an appropriate model of the requirement for different treatment strategies like the use of aspirin, thrombolytics, and anticoagulants, and the need for efficient ambulance services, coronary care beds, and so on. Finally, knowledge is available of the appropriate rehabilitative services that are effective after a myocardial infarction.

From this complex model, it is thus possible to consider the balance of resources to be devoted to, or invested in, the development of effective methods to both reduce the burden of coronary heart disease as well as to improve the outcome of those who develop the condition.

Obviously, this scheme is idealistic so far, but it remains the underlying rationale for the separation of purchasing and providing health services. Managed care, now so popular in the United States, is an example of this type of separation. All these models rely on the development of knowledge of the effective methods of treatment or prevention of a condition.

The problem in all countries is that, although the effectiveness of many procedures or treatments is known, understanding of many common ailments, e.g. arthritis, is still poor. Thus, all countries are involved in a variety of schemes to identify cost-effective methods of investigation, prevention, treatment, and rehabilitation (Holland & Mossialos 1999).

It is encouraging that many countries, e.g. Ireland, England, France, and some cities in the United States, e.g. New York, have, by 2007, introduced a ban on smoking in public places—recognizing that this public health measure will have a major impact on the incidence of smoking-related diseases as it has already led to a reduction in the prevalence of smoking.

The role of public health in the determination of priorities

The role of public health is in the determination of priorities among these possibilities for improving health. Theoretically, the role of public health is clear in almost all the systems described here. It has the necessary tools to describe the problems and to devise appropriate mechanisms for their solution. In all the systems, however, the ability for public health to influence health policy is limited. Few of the countries described have effective mechanisms to influence individual health behaviours (e.g. the smoking of cigarettes) or to consider investment in non-health activities (e.g. education or employment) which are known to have more profound effects on health status than the use of medical care services (Black 1980; Acheson 1998). Nonetheless, the framework and structures currently being devised, coupled with concerns about the environment and demography, as well as increasing fiscal constraints in all systems, is forcing all countries to begin to confront these issues.

Previously, decisions on expenditure and treatment were largely controlled by those who were providing services. The treatment or service delivered to an individual or community was rarely questioned. With improvements in educational attainments and rising costs of medical procedures all societies have begun to question health expenditure. Thus, decisions on priorities have become more explicit and democratic. Most countries have begun to debate how and what should be done; e.g. should preventive services be provided to all the population or should heart transplants be available on demand (dependent on a sufficient supply). As a result, most countries have also begun to spend resources more effectively and to examine ethical issues involved in the setting of priorities and supply of services.

To address these issues, countries have developed a variety of mechanisms to involve the public more in such issues, e.g. citizen juries, opinion surveys, focus groups, and including patients or consumers in the groups which advise on priorities in an area or country. The problem is that, although the inclusion of 'consumers' is welcome, it also gives rise to problems. In public health priority setting, an attempt is made to rank the priorities by their importance in terms of impact on the health of a population. Thus, in developed western countries the most important risk factor is smoking as a cause of disease. Thus, it should rank as first priority. In a developing country, e.g. in Africa, smoking is uncommon, so the first priority might be the containment/eradication of malaria or a safe water supply. This illustrates the importance of knowledge of local conditions and is equally true for all parts of the world. Priorities for health services must be concerned with local needs.

The setting of priorities is a political process. Several chapters in this book discuss priorities in different areas of the world and for different conditions. These take into account the importance and severity of the condition and should also be concerned with the effectiveness and possibilities for intervention, such as available trained manpower, facilities, drugs, etc. All of this is fine in theory, but practice often is more murky. In many developed areas the consumer—who elects the politicians who are ultimately responsible—will be interested in the priorities for interventions likely to be of benefit to him/her. The immediate return from a clinical/curative intervention is usually more attractive than the long-term investment for a public health intervention. It must not be forgotten that, in addition, most politicians and senior administrators at the government level are not usually qualified but are no different to the average consumer. Thus, to develop and implement public health intervention priorities requires a great deal of skill by individual public health practitioners including the ability to communicate. We may have excellent technical schemes—as described above—but the main public health skill of ability to communicate is crucial. The other main contributor to the setting of priorities is also the occurrence of a scandal—e.g. an outbreak of typhoid will have/has had a dramatic effect on concern with water and food safety. All these issues are addressed in this book. But, a word of caution: In spite of the appreciation by most practitioners that alleviation of poverty is crucial for the achievement of most public health priorities, few countries have developed adequate interventions.

Conclusion

The chapters describing the policies and strategies of various countries demonstrate the progress that has been made not only in the control of disease but also in the delivery of services. Most countries demonstrate a willingness to consider a wider perspective in the provision of health services than purely concern with treatment activities. Most countries, with the notable exception of the United States, have developed mechanisms for beginning to address the problem of inequalities and deprivation. Most are facing the problem of increasing costs of medical care by rational deliberations and are beginning to consider alternative approaches, including an increased investment in public health research, in order to be able to introduce appropriate and effective preventive strategies.

References

Abel-Smith, B., Figueras, J., Holland, W. *et al.* (1995). *Choices in health policy; an agenda for the European Union*. Darmouth, Aldershot.

Acheson, E.D. (Chairman) (1988). *Public health in England. Report of the Committee of Inquiry into the Future Development of the Public Health Function*. HMSO, London.

Acheson, E.D. (1998). *Independent inquiry into inequalities in health*. HMSO, London.

Black, D. (1980). *Inequalities in health*. Department of Health and Social Security, London.

Department of Health and Social Security (1976). *Sharing resources for health in England. Report of the Resource Allocation Working Party*. HMSO, London

Exter, A., Hermans H., Dosljak M. *et al.* (2004). *Health care systems in transition: Netherlands, Copenhagen*. WHO Regional Office for Europe on behalf of the European Observatory on Health Systems and Policies.

Ferrera, M. (1993). *EC citizens and social protection: main results from a Eurobarometer survey*. Commission of the European Communities, Brussels.

Holland, W.W. (1995). Achieving an ethical health service: the need for information. *Journal of the Royal College of Physicians, London*, **29**, 325–34.

Holland, W.W. (Project Director) (1997). *EC atlas of 'avoidable death'* (3rd edn), pp. 1–2, Oxford Medical Publications.

Holland, W. and Mossialos, E. (Ed.) (1999). *Public health policies in the European Union*. Ashgate, Aldershot.

Mathers, C. (2007). Epidemiology and world health. In: *The Development of Modern Epidemiology*, Ed. W.W. Holland, J. Olsen, C. Florey, Oxford Union Press, Chapter 5 pp. 41–60.

McMichael, A.J. and Powles, J.W. (1999). Human numbers, environment, sustainability and health. *British Medical Journal*, **ii**, 977–80.

Ministry of Health, Welfare and Cultural Affairs (1993). *Report on choices in health care*. Ministry of Health, Welfare and Cultural Affairs, The Hague. MUG.

Murray, C.J.L. (1996). Rethinking DALY's. In: *The Global Burden of Disease*, Ed. C.J.L. Murray and A.D. Lopez, Global Burden of Disease and Injury Series, Volume 1, Harvard University Press, Cambridge, MA.

Raleigh, V.S. (1999) World population and health in transition. *British Medical Journal*, **2**, 981–4.

Robine, J.M., Jagger C., Mathers C.D. *et al.* (2003). *Determining Health Expectancies*. John Wiley & Sons, Chichester.

Sanders, B.S. (1964). Measuring community health levels. *American Journal of Public Health*, **54**, 1063–70.

Sullivan, D.F. (1966). *Conceptual problems in developing an index of health*. National Centre for Health Statistics, Rockville, MD. (available at http://www.cdc.gov/nchs/data/series/sr_02/sr02_017.pdf).

WHO (World Health Organization) (1999). *The changing role of public health in the European region*. EUR/RC 49/10 and EUR/RC 49/Conf. Doc./6 Appendix 1. WHO, Geneva.

World Health Organization (2000). *The World Health Report 2000. Health systems: improving performance*. WHO, Geneva.

3.2

Public health policy in developed countries

John Powles

Persuasion requires shared standards of evidence, chains of authority, networks of trust, and accepted rules of logic and evidence. Changes in the rules of discourse and communication, no less than the knowledge unearthed by science, are the background to the changes in health and longevity that are the mark of the 'modern' age. (Mokyr 2002 p. 180)

Abstract

In the developed market economy (OECD) countries, adult mortality risks halved in the second half of the twentieth century. Trends were less favourable in Eastern Europe and were actually adverse in the Slavic and Baltic republics of the former Soviet Union.

These variable health gains cannot easily be related to explicit health policies or to organizational forms within health ministries. An alternative approach is to explore ways in which knowledge has been developed and used in response to leading adult health risks. In the last half century, there were historically unprecedented levels of investment in medical research, especially in the Scandinavian and English-speaking countries.

New knowledge has been used to protect and enhance health in a variety of ways according to the nature of the health risks being addressed. In general, knowing what to do has been powerfully permissive of it (ultimately) being done.

Linkages between the development and successful use of knowledge have not, however, been tight—in part, because openly published science is a global public good. The United States, in particular, has been more successful as a generator than as a successful user of knowledge, suggesting that health protection and enhancement are being impeded by distinctive features of its political economy.

The diverse ways in which knowledge has been used extend well beyond processes appropriately described as 'interventions'. Decentralized, informal, and 'spontaneous' uses have also played important roles.

Investments in medical research by government, civil, and commercial organizations should be sustained at high levels in expectation of continuing favourable returns to human well-being. Difficult unsolved problems—such as those related to excess adiposity and ecological disruption—are likely to require a wide repertoire of inventive responses, suggesting a need to leave space for decentralized activity and institutional creativity.

Introduction: The nature and scope of public health policy

The scope and purpose of public health policy may be seen as implicit in widely used definitions of public health. Winslow's definition, as adapted by the Acheson Report in England, is:

The science and art of preventing disease, prolonging life and promoting health through organised efforts of society (Secretary of State for Social Services 1988).

Public health policies might thus be thought of as the policies that guide these 'organized efforts' to protect and improve health. The scope of such policies depends a good deal, however, on what is considered to be entailed by 'organized efforts', and on how these 'organized efforts' are understood to be related to efforts that are less organized, more informal, more decentralized, or perhaps even 'spontaneous'.

Approaches that favour restricting the scope of public health to the more formal actions of state organizations may do so with a more or less positive attitude towards the benefits of such state action. Either way, these interpretations have the merit of identifiability and concreteness: It is not too difficult to identify the proclaimed public health policies of governments or to trace the actions of official bodies that follow their adoption.

Interpretations which emphasize the beneficent effects of state action are common in the public health literature. But the political tide in most developed countries has recently been flowing in a contrary—liberal conservative—direction and the case for governmental or other collective action now needs to be made in a more sceptical environment. Liberal opinion, both classical and 'neo', is sceptical both of the legitimacy and of the effectiveness of actions to improve well-being that are mediated by state institutions. Exponents of a strong (or 'hard') liberal viewpoint—for example, Friedrich von Hayek—emphasize that it is individuals who understand best what is needed for their own good. The knowledge needed to optimize well-being is thus essentially decentralized and it is best put to use through the mediation of institutions that facilitate the exchange of decentralized knowledge, that is, by markets. It is simply not possible, in Hayek's view, for officials in centralized institutions, even when enlightened and well-intentioned, to possess the detailed knowledge needed to act in the best interests of large, highly diverse publics. Hayek's censure fell not only on public officials but also on scientific intellectuals who dreamt of bringing social practices more in line with scientific discoveries—a tendency he called 'scientism' (Hayek 1942, 1943, 1944; Gamble 2006). In Hayek's view, this 'visible hand of human reason . . . lacked the all-important sanction of [social] evolutionary experience, and therefore risked claiming a knowledge which humans could not possess' (Gamble 2006, p. 126).

Hayek played an important role in the revival of 'hard' liberalism in the second half of the twentieth century, with politicians such as Margaret Thatcher acknowledging their debt to him (Gamble 1996, p. 151). Hayek preferred the liberal (though undemocratic) political economy of nineteenth-century Britain and regretted the expanding role of state institutions from that century's end. From a public health perspective this is rather unfortunate as this was the period when child mortality risks declined rapidly from the high levels that had persisted throughout the Victorian age. Historical analyses reveal that much of the improvement in health through the late nineteenth and early twentieth centuries was not market-mediated (Easterlin 1999; Szreter 1988; Mokyr 2002). If, counterfactually, the political economy of Hayek's golden age had been maintained, the price in child health gains foregone, may have been considerable.

Looking back from the first decade of the twenty-first century, the transformations of health during the second half of the twentieth century are more salient than the transformation of child health at its beginning. Figure 3.2.1 summarizes the reductions between 1950 and 2000 in the risks of dying before age 15 and between ages 15 and 60.

Between 1950 and 2000, the downward trajectory in the risks of dying in childhood tended, if anything, to accelerate, with those countries starting with the highest levels showing the biggest absolute gains by century's end. These may be identified by reading from the right on the X axis of Fig. 3.2.1 (A): The points are, respectively, for Portugal, Bulgaria, Slovakia, Spain, Hungary, and Japan. Reductions in the risk of dying in childhood in Japan, Portugal, Spain, Italy, Austria, the Czech and Slovak republics, and Finland, all exceeded 90 per cent. In England and Wales, childhood mortality risks fell by 81 per cent, and in the United States, they declined by 76 per cent. Although proportional differences remained substantial by century's end, the absolute range was small: From 0.5 per cent in Sweden to 2.4 per cent in Russia, exceeding 1 per cent only in the ex-Soviet states, Hungary, Slovakia, and Bulgaria. (Among the ex-Soviet states, only the Slavic republics—Russia, Ukraine, and Belarus—and the Baltic republics—Estonia, Latvia, and Lithuania—are included in these analyses.)

Achievements in reducing mortality risks between ages 15 and 60 were much more variable, with all the ex-Soviet states included here actually experiencing higher risks in 2000 than in 1959 (when their data series commence). Risks were roughly halved in the OECD countries, with Japan, Spain, Italy, Finland, and Australia achieving the biggest proportional reductions (all above 55 per cent), and with reductions of around 50 per cent in England and Wales and 45 per cent in the United States. At the turn of the century, absolute risks in the OECD countries included here were concentrated in a narrow range, being lowest in Sweden, Japan, Italy, Switzerland, and Australia (all below 8 per cent) and highest in the United States (11.3 per cent).

Some US economists have assessed the value of that country's reductions in adult mortality risks during the second half of the twentieth century to be very substantial—bearing comparison with the value of the total increase in economic product during this period (Nordhaus 2002).

How one traces these divergent recent gains and losses in adult health via their social and institutional causes to the policies that may have helped make them possible will colour one's interpretation

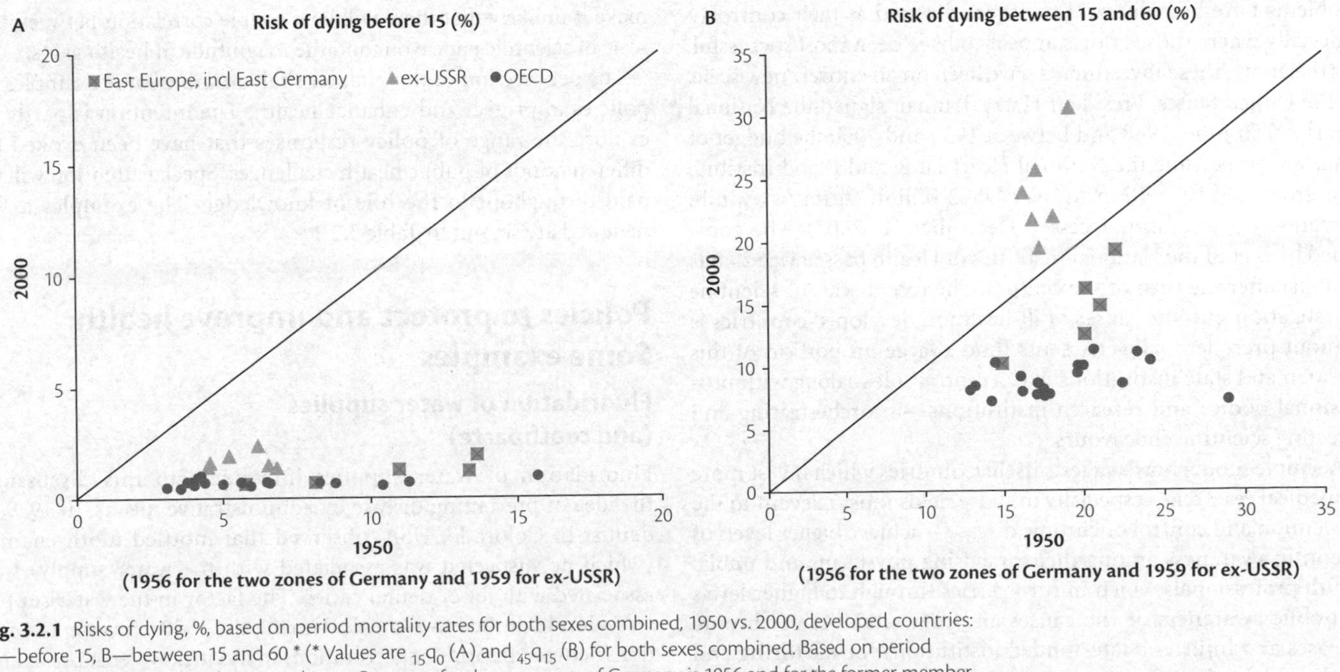

Fig. 3.2.1 Risks of dying, %, based on period mortality rates for both sexes combined, 1950 vs. 2000, developed countries: A—before 15, B—between 15 and 60 * (* Values are ${}_{15}q_0$ (A) and ${}_{45}q_{15}$ (B) for both sexes combined. Based on period mortality rates. Diagonals indicate no change. Base year for the two zones of Germany is 1956 and for the former member states of the USSR is 1959, not 1950. Data for the two zones of Germany are kept separate to 2000.
Source: Human Mortality Database (www.mortality.org).

of the role of public health policy in today's developed societies. The dramatic deterioration in the performance of the ex-Soviet states—which had been relatively impressive up to around 1960 but turned disastrous afterwards—suggests a failure of institutional adaptation as the composition of adult mortality risks came to be dominated by vascular disease and injury.

The reason for singling Hayek out above is because of the central role he accords, in his analytic approach, to the way in which societies use knowledge. This emphasis on the use (and we may add, generation) of knowledge offers a potentially fruitful approach to understanding how public policy in developed countries has served to protect and enhance health—or, alternatively, has failed to do so. Valuing Hayek's emphasis on the role of knowledge does not require agreement with his other views on political economy. We can provisionally agree that how knowledge is mobilized and used to enhance well-being is a fundamental characteristic of a country's political economy and leave open, for further consideration, the extent to which these processes are actually and properly sensitive to public policy. We have already noted how successes in reducing child mortality in the early twentieth century raise serious difficulties for those wishing to follow Hayek in deprecating 'scientism'.

The scope of this chapter can now be reconsidered. When Winslow was drawing lessons from the dramatic reduction in child mortality in the early decades of the twentieth century, he was reflecting on a period in which the scientific advances of preceding decades were put to work only after some delay. Application of the new bacteriological knowledge to control infectious disease in urban and domestic settings had been delayed by the reluctance of physicians to accept it. Time was also needed to build the institutional means for its propagation among the public (principally among mothers) (Ewbank & Preston 1989). The situation with the control of chronic disease (paradigmatically ischaemic heart disease) and injury (paradigmatically road traffic injury) in the second half of the twentieth century has been essentially different: Investments in the development of new knowledge to deal with these problems have been integral to efforts directed at their control—especially where those efforts appear to have been most successful. Furthermore, these investments have been on an entirely new scale. In the United States, President Harry Truman signed the National Heart Act in June, 1948 and between 1950 and 2000 the budget of what was to become the National Heart Lung and Blood Institute rose from US$10 million to over US$2 billion (http://www.nih.gov/about/history.htm, accessed December 18, 2007). The combined budget of the National Institutes of Health passed US$20 billion just after the turn of the century. The recent scale of scientific investigation into the causes of ill-health in developed countries is without precedent. Governments fund a large proportion of this research and state institutions play a central role—along with professional bodies and research institutions—in orchestrating and directing scientific endeavours.

A simple model now suggests itself: Countries which invest more in medical research—especially in those fields most relevant to the prevention and control of chronic disease—achieve higher levels of scientific awareness among their practising physicians and public health professionals which in turn carries through to higher levels of public awareness of the causes and preventability of chronic diseases and injuries. State-funded institutions for nurturing and guiding the scientific quest to understand and control disease have developed strongly in many OECD countries. By contrast, the corresponding Soviet institutional response was very weak. The authoritarian political culture inhibited the use of science to address problems with a potential social or political dimension (McKee 2007; Krementsov 1997). The Soviet State may have seemed strong in its ability to control many parameters of citizens' lives, but as a collective problem-solving agency it was a timid shadow of its Western counterparts.

Figure 3.2.2 provides a convenient bibliometric index of research publications on cardiovascular disease during the 1990s. Although there may be some bias against Cyrillic language publications in this source, this is unlikely to account for the overall pattern which shows higher publication rates in the OECD countries, and extremely low publication rates in the ex-USSR countries, with the Eastern European countries generally in between. Identifying a society's mobilization of scientific endeavour towards the solution of its health problems as an important part of its public health policy response seems reasonable. But a closer look at differences between countries suggests that it is, indeed only part of the picture. The United States, for example, appears to have been much more proficient as a contributor to the advancement of knowledge relevant to disease prevention than it has been as a successful user of such knowledge. Portugal, on the other hand, has shown dramatic reductions in adult mortality risks despite its low publication rate. To the extent that gains in countries such as Portugal have been built on the advancing global stock of knowledge they will have benefited from the character of openly published scientific knowledge as a 'global public good': No one may be excluded from using it and use by one party does not diminish the opportunity for others to use it (technically, goods are 'public' when 'consumption' is 'non-excludable' and 'non-rival').

It is also clear that there are important determinants of adult mortality levels and trends that are independent of deliberate efforts to control disease—countries with Mediterranean or East Asian food cultures, for example, have enjoyed some protection against the epidemic waves of ischaemic heart disease, that was independent of deliberate efforts to achieve this result. Observations such as this also make it unlikely that there will be a simple correlation between the scale of scientific endeavour and the magnitude of health gains.

The next section of this chapter shall examine some examples of policies to protect and enhance health. The intention is partly to explore the range of policy responses that have been evoked by different kinds of public health challenges. Special attention will be paid throughout to the role of knowledge. The examples to be reviewed are set out in Table 3.2.1.

Policies to protect and improve health: Some examples

Fluoridation of water supplies (and toothpaste)

Fluoridation of water supplies introduces to this discussion the idea of preventing disease by administrative means. In 1929, a dentist in Colorado, USA, observed that mottled tooth enamel (which he suspected was associated with the water supply) was associated with fewer dental caries. The factor in the water supply was soon identified as fluoride. During the 1930s, inverse associations between fluoride concentrations in 21 cities' water supplies and a newly developed quantitative index of dental caries (DMFT, decayed, missing, and filled teeth) were reported. Caries prevalence

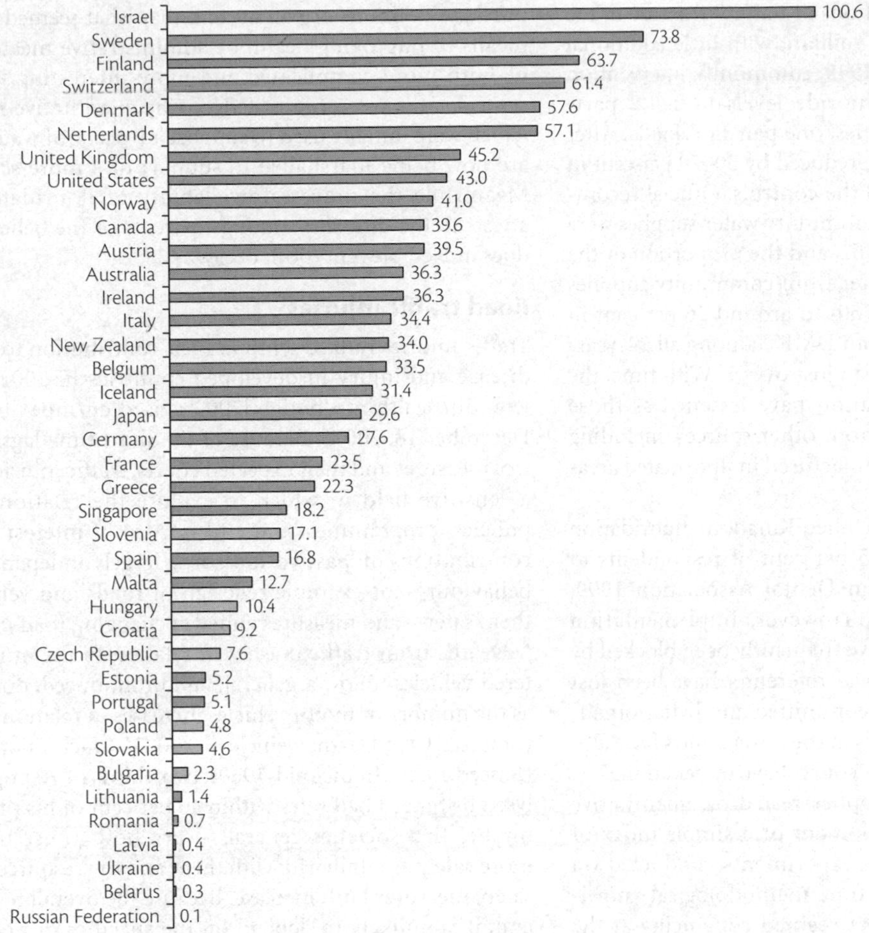

Fig. 3.2.2 Publications on cardiovascular disease indexed in Medline, 1991–2001, per million population.
Source: MacKay and Mensah 2004.

Table 3.2.1 Some types of public health policy responses with illustrative examples

Type of policy response	Nature of problem addressed	Examples (those in italics are discussed further in the text)
Administrative measures applied to whole populations	Problems amenable to specific measures administered by public agencies and requiring little public involvement for their effect	Regulation of the sale and of use of hazardous chemicals; Regulation of occupational hazards. (Discussed elsewhere in this textbook.)
Combinations of administrative measures and mass behaviour change	Problems addressed by combinations of regulation and mass behaviour change	*Fluoridation (of water supplies and of toothpaste (1));* *Control of road traffic injury* (including changes in the design of roads and of motor vehicles) (2).
Large-scale change in behaviour	Problems whose solution requires large-scale behavioural change, typically requiring supporting institutional changes	*HIV infection and sudden infant death syndrome (3);* *Disease attributable to smoking (4);* Disease attributable to non-optimal dietary composition
Enhanced use of clinical procedures applied to individuals (for prevention)	Problems where 'organized efforts' are used to enhance population coverage by clinical procedures of defined efficacy and feasibility	Immunization; *Enhanced clinical management of vascular risk (especially from raised blood pressure) (5)* Cancer screening
Unsolved	Problems without clearly defined solutions with current knowledge and within current institutional arrangements	*Disease attributable to declining physical activity and excess adiposity (6);* Asthma and allergic diseases; *Effects of large-scale ecological disruption (7).*

was reported to decline as concentrations of natural fluoride in the water supply approached 1 part per million, with little additional benefit at higher concentrations. In 1945, community intervention trials of the effects of adjusting fluoride levels to 1–1.2 parts per million began in four pairs of cities, one pair in Canada. After 13–15 years caries was reported to be reduced by 50–70 per cent in the experimental cities compared to the controls. Official recommendations for the fluoridation of community water supplies were formalized in the United States in 1962, and the proportion of the population receiving fluoridated water from community supplies rose from 40 per cent in the mid-1960s to around 56 per cent in 1992. Over this same period, the mean DMFT among all 12-year-olds fell dramatically from around 4 to just over 1. With time, the potential benefits of water fluoridation have lessened as those without such supplies get fluoride from other sources, including toothpaste and drinks and foods manufactured in fluoridated areas (Division of Oral Health 1999).

In both the United States and the United Kingdom, fluoridation enjoys the support of around 70–75 per cent of respondents to national opinion surveys (American Dental Association 1999; British Dental Association 1999). However, implementation requires local decisions, and these have frequently been blocked by opponents. In the United States, local referenda have been lost because opponents have been more committed and better organized than proponents. Legal challenges in the lower courts have also blocked adoption, though the highest courts have upheld none.

Proposals to flouridate water supplies rested on quantitative research in populations. The development of a simple index of tooth decay was important as were experiments conducted on whole communities. However, with time methodological knowledge has advanced and evidence that seemed convincing at the time may seem less robust when set against today's standards. Scientific reviewers in the United Kingdom have recently 'been surprised by the poor quality of the evidence and the uncertainty surrounding the beneficial and adverse effects of flouridation' (Cheng *et al.* 2007 p. 699). The best estimate (by these reviewers) of the increase, in flouridated areas, in the proportion of children free of caries, was a median of 15 per cent with an interquartile range of 5–22 per cent. Even this wide range understated the uncertainty because 'potential confounders were poorly adjusted for' (NHS Centre for Reviews and Dissemination 2000). Evidence for the effectiveness of flouridated toothpastes is much more certain, being based on some 70 randomized controlled trials (preventive fraction 24 per cent, 95 per cent confidence interval 21–28 per cent) (Marinho *et al.* 2003).

Opponents of flouridation have claimed harmful effects. There is now a much more adequate understanding of how difficult it is to exclude harms of potential public health importance—say increases of 20 per cent for non-trivial conditions with relatively low background risks. It is now understood that studies of sufficient size and duration to detect such effects have not been done.

One of the most interesting observations from the recent reviews has been the marked secular declines in caries prevalence in EU member states, reflecting the declines, noted above, in the United States. These declines bear little obvious relationship to the prevalence of water flouridation (Cheng *et al.* 2007). It is plausible that the widespread use of flouridated toothpastes deserves a substantial part of the credit. If true it could mean that the main benefits of the flouride hypothesis are being realized through the decentralized purchase decisions of parents and that what seemed at first to be a means of improving health by administrative means turns out to be both more complicated and more interesting. What remains central is the role of knowledge—the quantitative methodologies which were initially used to support advocacy of water fluoridation are now being marshalled in support of a more sceptical stance. Meanwhile the universal availability of flouridated toothpaste attests to the diffusion amongst parents of the belief that flouride does indeed prevent tooth decay.

Road traffic injuries

Traffic injuries ranked tenth in their contribution to the burden of disease and injury in developed countries in 2002 (http://www.who.int/healthinfo/bodgbd2002revised/en/index.html, accessed December 18, 2007). Because of the short time lags between control measures and their expected effects, traffic injuries also provide a sensitive field in which to explore the relationship between policies, programmes, and effects. Also of interest is the relative contributions of 'passive' measures, largely independent of driver behaviour—for example redesign of roads and vehicles to make them safer—and measures aimed at changing road user behaviour.

Deaths from traffic crashes in relation to the number of registered vehicles follow a general, and pronounced, downward trend as the number of motor vehicles increases in relation to population (Smeed's Law: Deaths/vehicle = $0.0003(\text{vehicles/population})^{-0.66}$) (Smeed 1972). In the mid-1960s, two-thirds of 70 populations analysed by Smeed had rates within 40 per cent of his prediction. This implies that societies generally learn how to use motor vehicles more safely as familiarity with them and the resources available for safety measures both increase. Because the overall tendency is general, it is unlikely to depend on the specifics of policies variably adopted—although it may be contributed to by the 'public good' character of enhanced vehicle crashworthiness (all tend to benefit from design changes introduced in large demanding markets). But it is also the case, that around the general trends, some societies have performed better than others.

Figure 3.2.3 shows the decline in Victoria, Australia, in deaths per 10 000 vehicles as the number of vehicles increased in relation to population. Over 80 per cent of the reduction in fatalities per 10 000 vehicles that occurred between 1920 and 2005 happened before 1970. During these five early decades, Victoria generally had ratios in excess of Smeed's prediction. Then, in a little more than two decades from 1970, it changed from being a relatively poor performer in this domain to being one of the best (Fig. 3.2.4).

During the 1960s, there had been a growing political consensus in Victoria that the loss of so many lives on the roads was no longer tolerable. In December 1970, it became the first jurisdiction in the world to make the wearing of seat belts compulsory. A string of legislative measures followed, including random testing of the breath alcohol concentrations of drivers in 1977. After the decline in fatality rates faltered in the late 1980s, a very strong 'social marketing' campaign was launched in combination with intensive policing (Powles & Gifford 1993). The number of speed camera checks per year rose to 8 per licensed driver and the proportion of vehicles recorded as speeding fell from 20 to 3 per cent. In 1994, 1.6 million random breath tests were performed, a number equal to about half of the driving age population (Hendrie & Ryan 1995, p. xi–xii). Fatality rates fell sharply and have stayed down. Since the early 1990s, the Transport Accident Commission (TAC), which carries all

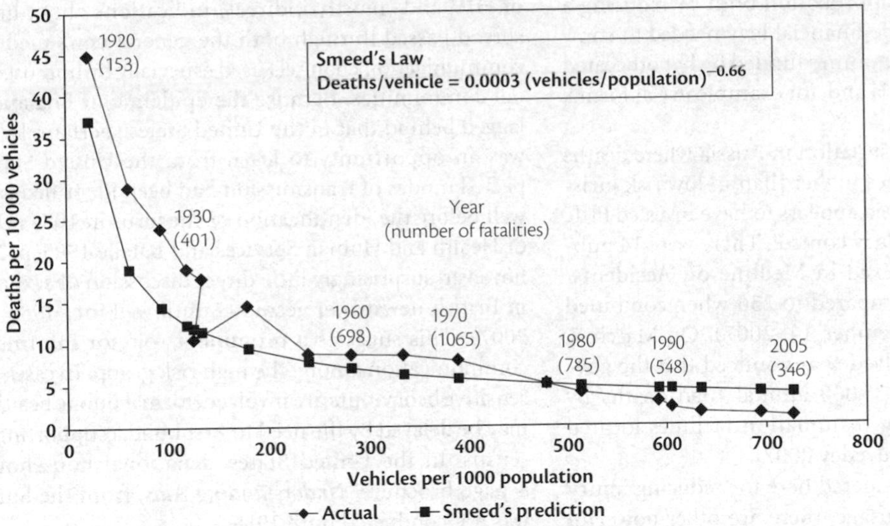

Fig. 3.2.3 The actual versus predicted decline in traffic fatalities per 10 000 vehicles with increasing motorization, State of Victoria, Australia, 1920–2005.
Sources: Hawthorne (1991); Smeed (1972); Australian Transport Safety Bureau (2007).

compulsory traffic injury insurance and makes 'no-fault' compensation payments to victims, has spent significantly on traffic accident prevention programmes, including intensive use of paid television advertising. Ten per cent of the spend has been allocated to evaluation, from which the TAC has been able to conclude that its benefits-to-costs ratio, from reduced injury claims, has been very favourable (Cameron & Newstead 1996). By 2005, the fall in deaths per 10 000 vehicles relative to the level in 1960 was around tenfold.

Several points can be made about this spectacular public health success: (1) Most of the very large secular declines in traffic injury deaths per unit vehicles (or distance travelled) observed around the world are likely to have occurred with a substantial degree of independence from the specific policies and programmes adopted in different political jurisdictions; (2) Against this broad background trend, a second order, but never-the-less important degree of variation seems attributable to the intensity and nature of the specific control measures taken locally; (3) In the relatively compact political environment of an Australian state, it was possible to build support for the escalation of control measures as less forceful measures proved inadequate to achieve widely desired goals—notwithstanding a political culture that valued personal independence; (4) The comparative trend line for Britain (in Fig. 3.2.4), ending with rates among the lowest in Europe, shows that Victoria does not differ so much in the level it has attained as in the distance it has travelled (so to speak) over four decades of intensive political attention; (5) Success has depended on knowing what to do—guided by research bodies such as the Monash University Accident Research Centre (in Victoria), the Insurance Institute for Highway Safety (in the United States), and the Transport Research Laboratory (in the United Kingdom); (6) Although not easy to identify in the illustrated data for Victoria, improved vehicle crashworthiness is likely to have also been a major contributor to mortality decline. Robertson (2001) allocates 90 per cent of US vehicle occupant mortality decline between 1964 and 1990 to this source.

This example also illustrates the powerful social benefits of having single, substantial 'pots of gold' for dealing with leading sources of disease or injury. By linking the size of the 'pot' to the scale of the problem—in this case by the level of compensation payments for traffic injuries—a resource is created that bears some commensurability with the public health challenge faced. The custodians

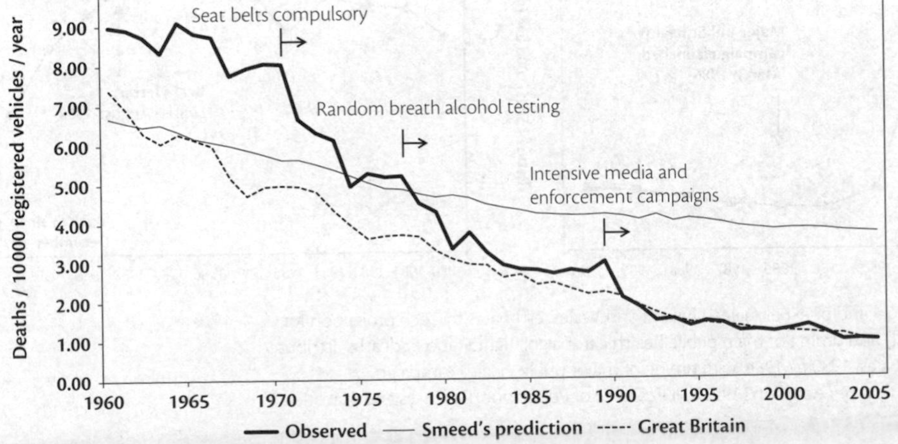

Fig. 3.2.4 Decline in traffic fatalities per 10 000 vehicles, 1960–2005, State of Victoria, Australia and Great Britain (with predicted trend using Smeed's Law).
Source: Smeed (1972); Australian Transport Safety Bureau (2007); Department for Transport (2007).

of this fund can then gain social approbation both by reducing a recognized evil and by reducing the financial levy needed to compensate for it. (Anti-smoking programmes funded by hypothecated tobacco taxes, as also exist in Victoria and, for example in California, exploit an analogous linkage.)

As a contrast, one may note the situation in Russia where deaths per 10 000 vehicles are over 10 times higher than in low risk jurisdictions (OECD 2007, p. 236). Russia appears to have invested little in the science needed for traffic injury control. There were 14 publications in the last 10 years indexed in Medline on 'Accidents/traffic' combined with 'Russia', compared to 236 when combined with 'Australia' (searched on December 14, 2007). On March 7, 2007, Deputy Prime Minister Medvedev announced that the government was responding to the 35 000 annual road deaths by 'examining the issue of equipping reanimation facilities located throughout the road network' (Medvedev 2007).

In addition to the measures considered here for reducing injury risks per unit of exposure to car usage, there are other powerful health and environmental considerations favouring a reduction in car use itself (Woodcock *et al.* 2007).

Human immunodeficiency virus (HIV) and sudden infant death syndrome (SIDS)

The epidemic of HIV infection in Europe followed that of the United States. The time course of the epidemic through the population of homosexual and bisexual males in England and Wales has been reconstructed by 'back projection' from the subsequent epidemic of AIDS (de Angelis *et al.* 1998). The incidence of HIV infection appears to have peaked in 1983 and then to have fallen sharply (Fig. 3.2.5).

Against the time course of the infection rate can be set the timing of the formal control measures. Intensive 'social marketing' campaigns to promote changes to safer sexual practices were not launched by the UK government until March 1986 (Acheson 1993). It is thus likely that most of the change in sexual practices responsible for the sudden turnaround and decline in HIV incidence after 1983 had occurred before the formal programme began. How is this to be explained? New knowledge about the dire consequences of HIV and (mostly indirect) indications about how it might be spread passed through both the general news media and through communication channels used especially by homosexual and bisexual communities. Because the epidemic in England substantially lagged behind that in the United States (perhaps by 3 years), there was an opportunity to learn from the United States where suspected modes of transmission had been identified as early as 1982, well before the identification of the virus in 1984 (US Department of Health and Human Services and Batelle 1995, p. 29). There was, however, surprisingly little direct discussion of sexual transmission in British newspaper accounts until well into 1983 (Hilliard *et al.* 2007). This suggests a prominent role for informal, 'horizontal' communication among the high risk group. In cases like this where sensitive behaviours are involved, formal public health programmes may be delayed by the need to first build a supporting political consensus. In the United States, a national household drop of an 8-page brochure, *Understanding Aids*, from the Surgeon General was not conducted until 1988.

The decline in Sudden Infant Death Syndrome (SIDS) in England (also shown in Fig. 3.2.5) illustrates apparently similar communication processes. In August 1988, a letter from an Adelaide paediatrician was published in *The Lancet* in which results from several small studies were pooled. It showed that front sleeping had a statistically significant association with increased risk (Beal 1988). Death rates from SIDS fell by more than a third in the next 3 years before the UK government's formal public health programme ('Back to sleep') began in December 1991 (OPCS 1988 and 1995; Hiley & Morley 1994), suggesting that mass behaviour change began well in advance of the formal programme. Why it did so is something of a mystery. Coverage of SIDs in British newspapers during this period increasingly emphasized that scientists were busy on the case and that a wide range of hypotheses was under investigation. No special salience was given to the role of sleeping position (Hilliard *et al.* 2007). The rate of decline in SIDS did, however, accelerate sharply after the national 'Back to sleep' programme began, with incidence halving in the subsequent 12 months. Official advice on sleeping position changed in the Netherlands before it did in the United Kingdom, and in the United Kingdom before the

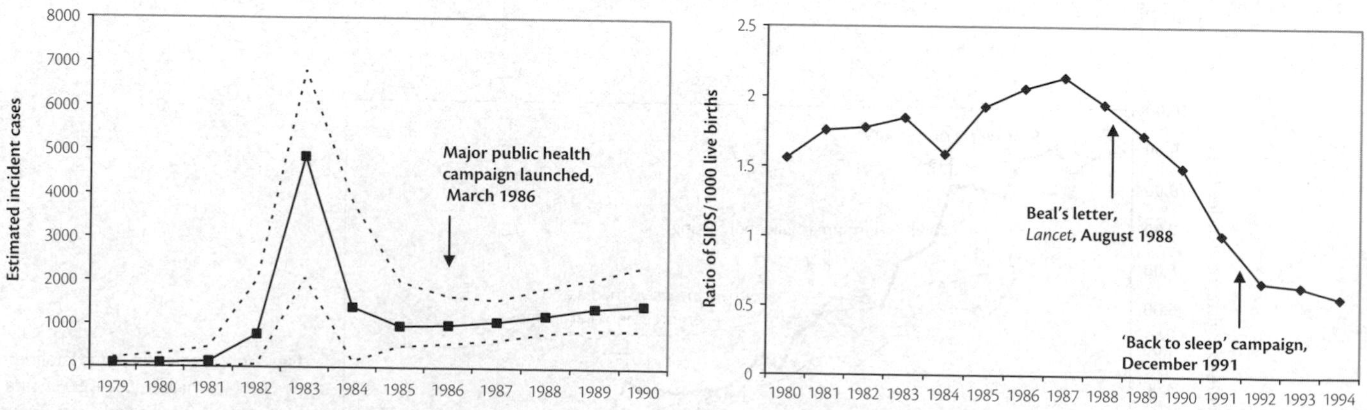

Fig. 3.2.5 Left: HIV incidence in homosexual and bisexual males, England and Wales, estimates by back-projection for 1979–90 (with 95 per cent credible interval) and timing of main public health campaign; Right: Ratio of deaths attributed to SIDS per 1000 live births, England and Wales, 1980 to 1984, with timing of major public health campaign.
Sources: HIV: De Angelis, personal communication, Acheson (1993); SIDS: Office of Population, Censuses and Statistics (1988, 1995).

United States. Gilbert and colleagues have gathered evidence on the sleeping positions of control infants in epidemiological studies showing that the prevalence of the hazardous front sleeping position fell first in the Netherlands, then in the United Kingdom, and finally in the United States (Gilbert *et al.* 2005, Fig. 3.2.4). The national declines in SIDS occurred in the same sequence.

These two examples—of HIV and of SIDS—show how, in highly literate and health-conscious populations, much of the benefit from new knowledge may flow more or less automatically from its dissemination through channels other than formal public health programmes. In these circumstances, it is the advance of science, perhaps even more than the strength of public health programmes, that sets the pace for health improvement (Dwyer & Ponsonby 1996). This is not to claim that the incremental gain from formal programmes is typically negligible; it may still be very worthwhile relative to their typically modest resource requirements.

In these two examples, informed publics seem to have made their own good use of new knowledge, without the necessity of professional or administrative mediation. This casts doubt on the helpfulness of the widespread practice of equating of 'medicine' with the knowledge held by and acted on by physicians. On the basis of this equation, one might conclude that the decline in the HIV epidemic in England in the early 1980s (for example) was due to 'non-medical measures'. A semantic sleight of hand of this kind led Thomas McKeown astray in his attempts to explain earlier falls in mortality. (McKeown 1976) The reality is that the lay public and physicians draw on the same stocks of knowledge: Conflating medicine as a social institution with its professional practice is an avoidable source of confusion.

In relation to the decline in SIDS, Gilbert and colleagues' demonstration that if, counterfactually, current methods of evidence synthesis had been available in 1970 and used to pool data from the two case control studies published by then, the cumulated odds ratio for front versus back sleeping would have been determined to be 2.9 (95 per cent CI 1.15–7.47). They estimate that over 50 000 excess infant deaths occurred in North America, Europe, and Australasia because of the delay in advocating back sleeping (Gilbert *et al.* 2005, p. 883). This example shows how capacities to protect and improve health may owe as much to advances in methodological knowledge (in this case, knowing how to make the best use of what is known) as to advances in substantive knowledge.

Tobacco smoking

It is ironic that medicine provided a 'cultural bridge' across which tobacco was transferred from the exotic rituals of the Amerindian cultures to the everyday life of seventeenth-century Europe. By explaining tobacco's properties within the contemporary humoral theories of well-being, physicians such as the Sevillian Nicolas Monades provided what was to be the main, medical, justification for tobacco use until into the nineteenth century, when 'recreational' justifications came to the fore (Goodman 1993). With the advent of manufactured cigarettes in the late nineteenth century, tobacco use was made more convenient and more deadly. In the twentieth century, increased purchasing power resulting from economic development has been almost universally accompanied by widespread adoption of cigarette smoking (Tobacco Advisory Group 2000). These epidemics of nicotine addiction can, on the experience of 'early adopters' such as England, be expected to last at least a century (Lopez *et al.* 1994). As a public health problem, cigarette smoking is thus distinguished not only by the great quantity of disease attributable to it—accounting at its peak, in the United Kingdom, for almost a half of male and a quarter of female deaths between 35 and 69 (Peto & Lopez 1994, p. 206)—but also by the protracted time scale over which it evolves. It will, for example, be half a century before the full health effects of onsets of nicotine addiction in today's adolescents become fully manifest. Tobacco smoking is, in addition, a form of addiction that is both legal and extremely profitable.

Although earlier studies were published in Nazi Germany, for readers of the English-language literature the health effects of cigarette smoking were mostly revealed to by epidemiological studies conducted between the late 1940s and the mid-1960s. A question of interest is how this new knowledge (since much strengthened) has influenced the course of the smoking 'epidemic' and the epidemics of disease that have followed in its train.

From around 1950 to the mid-1960s, it was the general news media that conveyed new knowledge of the health effects of smoking to the public. The Royal College of Physicians report in the United Kingdom in 1962 (Royal College of Physicians 1962) and the Surgeon General's report in the United States in 1964 (which it stimulated) (United States Public Health Service 1964) were 'organized efforts' that, nevertheless depended for their effects on such news coverage. A study of this process in the United States showed that the intensity of print media discussion of the risks of smoking was closely mirrored in adult smoking cessation rates through the 1950s and 1960s (Pierce & Gilpin 2001).

The intensification of 'organized efforts' to discourage tobacco smoking dates mainly from the 1970s. The main measures have included price increases (by specific taxes), bans on advertising and other forms of promotion, requirements for warning labels on tobacco products and on advertisements, restrictions on smoking in public places, health education in schools, mass education and persuasion, enhanced advice, and assistance with cessation.

Attempts to assess the contribution of these measures to national trends in smoking prevalence (and with appropriate lags, to national trends in attributable mortality) needs to take account of the variation in the time of onset of the smoking epidemics, before its health effects were understood. In Europe, UK males and females and Finnish males (but not females) were 'early adopters' of cigarette smoking (Lopez 1996). A general pattern of 'first in, first out' of the smoking epidemic might have been expected, to some extent independently of the timing and strength of national counter measures. Lung cancer mortality in early middle-aged males (ages 35–54) peaked in the 1950s in United Kingdom, in the 1960s in Finland, and in the 1970s in the United States. Falls since these peaks have exceeded 70 per cent in the United Kingdom and Finland and been around 50 per cent in the United States. Rates in 2000 were respectively: 15.4, 13, and 23 per 100 000 person-years (age standardized using equal weights, Peto *et al.* 1994, 2003).

It also happens that Finland (which banned tobacco advertising in 1978) (Harkin *et al.* 1997, p. 29) and the United Kingdom have been among the leaders in efforts to reduce smoking. Finnish females, whose delayed smoking epidemic came to maturity during a period of tobacco control activity, have experienced a lung cancer mortality peak (at about 7/100 000 for 45–54-year-olds in 1990) less than one-third as great as that experienced by UK females (about 27/100 000 for 45–54-year-olds in 1975) (Peto & Lopez 1994): The size of the smoking epidemic in UK females was largely determined in the pre-control period (Lopez 1996). This pattern—of smoking epidemics having lower amplitudes when maturing in an environment of tobacco control activity—suggests that control measures are effective.

Although trends in adult smoking prevalences in developed countries have generally been favourable, trends since the early 1990s in smoking uptake by adolescents have been mixed. In many European countries 30-day smoking prevalences in 15–16-year-olds have been in the range of between 20 and 40 per cent between 1995 and 2003 (Hibbel *et al.* 2003). In the United States, the remarkable California Tobacco Control Program appears to have succeeded with adolescents where many others have failed. In 2004, 30-day smoking prevalences for 9th–12th graders (roughly 15–17-year-olds) were only 13 per cent, compared to a US national average of 22 per cent (California Department of Health Services 2007).

To summarize: Cigarette smoking remains the leading public health problem in developed countries. As a specific behaviour it is without rival in the disease burden it generates. It illustrates well how the evolution of some public health problems may need to be viewed within a very prolonged time frame. Peak smoking prevalences appear to have been lower in the higher educated strata in 'late uptake' countries—where knowledge of health effects has had more opportunity to influence behaviour—there are notable exceptions, such as the high smoking prevalences among Spanish physicians as recently as the 1990s (Harkin 1997, p. 10). Reductions in attributable mortality within the next half century will need to mainly come from encouraging and supporting cessation in current smokers. But if the course of the epidemic of nicotine addiction is to be curtailed, inter-generational transmission must also be minimized. This will be helped if there are declines in parental smoking whilst their children are at the ages most sensitive to their influence. The relevant parental ages will presumptively be before 40 or so. This keeps the reduction of smoking uptake in adolescence, and an increase in quitting in the early adult years both in the frame as important objectives.

The history of efforts to reduce health losses from tobacco also illustrates how the development of quantitative methods has supported appropriate policy responses. It is striking that high level policy debates in the United Kingdom during the 1950s and 1960s revolved around a largely illusory search for 'proof of causation' rather than quantifying how much was at stake (Pollock 1999). Artificial stimulation of this controversy over causation was also a deliberate strategy of commercially powerful tobacco companies. With increased acceptance of epidemiological reasoning and its transmission to political and wider publics (for example Peto & Lopez 1994), quantitative assessments have become much more central to policy deliberations. Changes, like this, in the rules of discourse, have enhanced the propensity to act on new knowledge (as noted by Mokyr in quote at start of chapter).

Enhanced clinical management of vascular risk

Half a century of epidemiological research on ischaemic heart disease and stroke has progressively clarified the quantitative relationships between the three main risk factors—usual blood pressure, usual blood cholesterol concentration, and smoking—and the risk of heart attack and stroke. Even measurements made on a single occasion—which capture usual values only with some error—are sufficient to stratify individuals into groups at vastly differing levels of vascular risk (Stamler *et al.* 1986).

For persons in their 60s, risk of heart attack is lower by 25 per cent and risk of stroke by 35 per cent for each 10 mmHg reduction in usual systolic blood pressure (Lawes *et al.* 2004a, p. 325, 326) and the risk of heart attack is lower by 30 per cent for each 1 mmol/l reduction in usual cholesterol concentration (Lawes *et al.* 2004b, p. 428). All of the excess stroke risk appears to be reversible if blood pressure is lowered to target levels by medication and about two-thirds of the excess risk of heart attack may be reversible.

This predictability and demonstrated reversibility of vascular risk in individuals has provided the basis for the prevention of heart attack and stroke by the clinical management of risk factors—especially blood pressure and blood cholesterol concentration. The United States has national programmes for each—The National High Blood Pressure Education Program (NHBPEP), established in 1972 and the National Cholesterol Education Program, established in 1985. The former has been running for longer, and it will be explored a little further here.

The NHBPEP has aimed to make case-finding more complete and control more effective. National progress in blood pressure control is monitored through the National Health and Nutrition Examination Survey (NHANES) (Table 3.2.2). Despite the limitations of these data on the proportions of 'hypertensives' 'aware, treated, and controlled', they suggest a substantial improvement in case-finding and control between the late 1970s and the turn of the century. The proportion of those defined as hypertensive who were taking medication doubled from 31 per cent in 1976–80 to 61 per cent in 1999–2004. Proportions controlled rose from 10 to 35 per cent over the same period (National Heart Lung and Blood Institute 2007).

The Framingham Study cohorts have provided the opportunity to track changes over a longer time span, though in a population that is likely to be more health conscious than average. The proportion of those aged 45–74 who reported antihypertensive medication increased from 2 per cent in the 1950s to 25 per cent in the 1980s in males and from 6 to 28 per cent in females. Those with blood pressures above 160/100 measured on a single occasion (and irrespective of treatment status) fell from 19 to 9 per cent in the case of males and from 28 to 8 per cent in the case of females. Bigger proportionate declines occurred in progressively higher blood

Table 3.2.2 United States: Trends in awareness, treatment, and control of high blood pressure in persons 18–74, 1976 to 1994

	Per cent of those either above 140/90 at time of survey or reporting antihypertensive medication			
	1976–80	**1988–91***	**1991–1994***	**1999–2004**
Aware that they have high blood pressure	51	73	68	72
Report taking anti-hyptertensive medication	31	55	53	61
Controlled (below 140/90 at time of survey)	10	29	27	35

* These estimates are based on NHANES III in which blood pressure was measured on 2 occasions.

Source: Joint National Committee 1997, p. 3; National Heart Lung and Blood Institute 2007.

pressure strata and the prevalence of left ventricular hypertrophy fell markedly. These findings are consistent with other data pointing to substantial secular declines, especially in severe hypertension (Mosterd *et al.* 1999).

In assessing the National High Blood Pressure Education Program and other formal public health programmes seeking to enhance control of blood pressure, three questions need to be addressed: (1) To what extent has the improvement in case-finding and management for high blood pressure been attributable to the 'organized effort' of programmes such as the NHBPEP? (2) How much effect has improved treatment had on the numbers at risk because of raised blood pressures? And (3) How much of the observed decline in vascular risk is likely to be attributable to the reduction of blood pressures by clinical means?

Studies designed to answer the first two questions appear to have been very limited. In rural Kentucky a community high blood pressure control programme was run in two counties between 1979 and 1984, with a third county serving as control. In the intervention counties, the percentage of 'hypertensives' whose blood pressure was controlled to below 140/90 rose from 37 to 53 per cent, with no change in the control county. Cardiovascular mortality fell in the intervention counties, while remaining constant in the control (Kotchen *et al.* 1986).

Some US observers believed, in the early 1980s, that '... the documented improvements in hypertension control since the beginning of the NHBPEP must be considered a major contribution ...' to the decline in cardiovascular mortality rates' (Lenfant & Roccella 1984). Over the longer period from 1963 to 2004 in the United States, age-adjusted death certification rates for heart attack and stroke each fell by around 70 per cent (National Heart Lung and Blood Institute 2007). There is a good deal of credit waiting to be attributed somewhere.

For persons aged 60–74, data from the US national health surveys show a substantial shift downwards in blood pressure distributions from the early 1960s to the most recent survey period around 2000. Because nearly all treated persons stay above the median, reductions in the median provides a more robust measure of shifts in the central tendency due to causes other than treatment. Median systolic pressures at ages 60–74 fell over this period by about 16 mmHg, from 148 to 132 mmHg. The fall had actually occurred by the early 1990s and there is little evidence of further reduction since. The reduction in the upper tail of the distribution was more marked, with 90th centiles falling by about 30 mmHg—from around 191 mmHg to 160 mmHg (estimates from smoothed distributions in Fig. 3.2.1 of Burt *et al.* 1995 and analyses of data from NHANES IV (http://www.cdc.gov/nchs/nhanes.htm)). Some of the credit for these improvements should go to enhanced clinical control of blood pressure.

Rose coined the term 'prevention paradox' to describe how, when risk is related monotonically to a quantitative attribute such as blood pressure, the interventions which offer most to the individuals at high risk contribute less to reducing the population burden of the disease than do small downward shifts in the whole distribution (Rose 1985). Strachan and Rose reworked these analyses taking account of the misclassification of risk status when blood pressure is only measured on a single occasion. Assuming a reliability coefficient of 0.5, over 50 per cent of the population risk of fatal stroke attributable to true (usual) blood pressures higher than those in the lowest decile, was to be found in those whose true pressures were in the top decile. Yet, even in these apparently promising circumstances, a 'high risk' case-finding strategy that correctly identified all in the true top decile and that achieved an average reduction of 7.5 mmHg diastolic in all those offered treatment, would reduce stroke mortality only by about the same amount as would result from a 3 mmHg reduction in diastolic blood pressures across the whole distribution (Strachan & Rose 1991). Thus, although classification on the basis of usual blood pressures enhances the relative effectiveness of the 'high risk' strategy in relation to stroke, it still remains modest when compared to downward shifts in the whole distribution of blood pressures. Earlier analyses of the contribution of hypertension treatment to the decline in stroke mortality between 1970 and 1980 placed it in the range of 6–25 per cent (Bonita & Beaglehole 1989).

Rose expounded his 'prevention paradox' by considering one risk factor at a time. Optimal strategies for risk reduction in multicausal diseases like ischaemic heart disease have since been further clarified. Law and Wald showed that the important thing was to identify persons whose absolute vascular risk was high—whether from modifiable or non-modifiable causes—because the absolute benefit from risk lowering therapy is directly proportional to the absolute risk. Preventive efforts should therefore be calibrated against absolute risk and not against the levels of individual modifiable risk factors (Law & Wald 2002). This approach is now incorporated in guidelines for prescribing expensive statin drugs in the UK National Health Service.

To conclude this example: The 'organized efforts' of the NHBPEP and other similar programmes will account for part of the improved case-finding and management for persons with usual blood pressures above treatment thresholds. This improved management will account for part of the decline in the prevalence of persons above treatment thresholds. The decline in the prevalence of persons above treatment thresholds will account for part of the decline in stroke and ischaemic heart disease mortality attributable to raised blood pressures.

Despite this cumulative diminution of the contribution of the NHBPEP that contribution is still likely to have been very worthwhile because even small reductions in the heavy burdens imposed by heart attack and stroke will add up to a big benefit in absolute terms. Furthermore, the gains attributable to the NHBPEP are notable for having been achieved within a pluralistic and organizationally diverse system of medical care.

The relatively limited likely contributions of clinical control to substantial secular declines in blood pressure and blood cholesterol concentrations leaves open the attribution of much of the credit for large declines in death from vascular causes attributable to favourable shifts in risk factor distributions. Between 1970 and 2000, the death certification rates for coronary heart disease at ages 35–74 fell by about two-thirds in the United States and by almost four-fifths in Australia (National Heart Lung and Blood Institute 2007). For the United States, it has been estimated that risk factor changes contributed about half the fall in deaths from coronary disease 'prevented or deferred' between 1980 and 2000 (Ford *et al.* 2007). The proportional contribution of risk factor change to life years gained will have been greater because deaths averted by risk factor changes, yield, on average, longer streams of life. The diffusion of knowledge about risk factors to the general public is likely to have made a substantial contribution to these declines. In societies that have been less successful in reducing vascular risk, popular knowledge of risk factors may be very much lower (Dokova *et al.* 2005).

> *Unless Prudence be a constant attendant on Opulence . . . tis better living on a slender fortune.* Richard Mead (1673–1754)

Unsolved problems: Physical inactivity and adiposity

The material basis of modernization lies in the replacement of muscle, wind, and water power by energy carried by steam, electricity, and liquid hydrocarbons. Of the main adverse consequences for health, two—air pollution and transport injuries—have been largely brought under control. The third—the physiological consequences of declining energy expenditure—remains unsolved.

Data, of known validity, on time trends in energy expenditure is generally unavailable for developed populations. Because of the technical difficulties involved, the measurement of total energy turnover in representative free-living individuals is a major challenge for contemporary public health surveillance. The 'doubly labelled water' technique provides a gold standard but is too expensive for large-scale use. Individually calibrated heart rate monitoring is the next best but so far only one study has reported findings from a broadly representative study population (Wareham *et al.* 1997).

In the absence of data on trends in energy expenditure over time, data on recorded energy consumption may be used as a proxy, bearing in mind that such records tend to underestimate true intake and that an assumption of a roughly constant under-reporting bias over time is required. Data for English adults show substantial declines since the first 7-day-weighed dietary intakes of the 1930s (Widdowson 1936; Widdowson & McCance 1936; Bingham *et al.* 1981; Prentice & Jebb 1995). Data abstracted from a large series of dietary studies in the United States show falls of around 17 per cent in recorded energy consumption of US adults (without adjustment for increasing body weight) between the 1940s and the early 1980s (Stephen & Wald 1990).

The Physical Activity Level (PAL) is the ratio of total energy expenditure to basal metabolic rate (James & Schofield 1990). It is an important determinant of public health via two types of effects. First, activity is directly protective of health (independently of its effects on body composition and of its contribution to aerobic fitness) (US Department of Health and Human Services 1996, Wareham *et al.* 2000). Second, as activity levels decline, the prevalence of obesity increases (Prentice & Jebb 1995).

Tentative suggestions are that mean PALs of the order of 1.75 may be needed to help prevent mass obesity. This compares with current average values for developed countries of around 1.55–1.60. To close the gap would require the addition of around 1 h of moderately intensive activity to the average citizen's daily routine (Saris *et al.* 2003). The effect of the decline in physical activity levels over past decades is compounded by the increased availability and declining real prices of energy dense foods, which some analysts see as the more important contributor to the rise in adiposity (Bleich *et al.* 2008).

The widespread rise of obesity in developed countries is visible to all. Recent declines in adult mortality in rich countries have, in most cases, been occurring in spite of adverse trends in two related health determinants—physical activity and adiposity. What might be required to reverse these trends?

The difficulty faced may be compared with that of changing the composition of the diet in order to favour health. Although there are hedonic attractions in unhealthy dietary compositions—chocolate, ice cream!—attractive alternatives that favour health are also available—for example, Mediterranean diets. But exertion is, alas, not as attractive as indolence. During our evolutionary past, there was unlikely to have been a survival advantage in exertion in the absence of hunger or other immediate need. In this light, the origins of our problems with obesity and inactivity are profoundly social: They are a consequence not so much of individual misbehaviour as of our collective transformation of the way we provision society and the resulting marked reduction in the need for muscular exertion.

Investment in new knowledge is a clear priority. Strategic importance, and the indications that solutions will not be easy, both point to the need to establish physical activity and energy balance as high priorities in public health research. Given the rapid advances in identifying genetic susceptibility, preventive strategies will be needed at all levels—universal (for the whole population), selective (for the susceptible), and targeted (for those already affected) (World Health Organization 1998, p. 168). Assuming further research confirms the fundamental importance of low physical activity levels, the most feasible and attractive ways of increasing such activity will need to be found. These are likely to entail significant and pervasive institutional change.

Unsolved problems: Sustainability

Averting harm to health from the disruption of the ecological systems on which human well-being depends is unlike other public health challenges. The need for action cannot be inferred from empirical observations of previous harm from this source, but rather is to be inferred from highly uncertain models of what may happen in the future. Those averse to 'speculation' might be inclined to defer judgement until there has been time for the relevant models to be more thoroughly challenged, and the contributory evidence better marshalled. The argument against delay is that the interacting momenta of population increase and economic development are likely to result in 'overshoot and collapse' unless corrective action begins now. If attempts to extend the current pattern of energy and resource-intensive industrialism to the whole of an increasing human population are likely to come seriously unstuck, then the sooner the transition to more sustainable material culture is begun the better. This topic is too vast to be properly addressed here—beyond noting that transitions to durable solutions (if made in time) are likely to require fundamental institutional changes. Many of the needed changes could also bring 'health dividends', for example via increased energy expenditure in moving around and reduced consumption of red meat (McMichael *et al.* 2007).

Some reflections on the examples considered

The topic of public health policy in developed countries is a vast one. I have sought to approach it by asking first whether knowledge plays a more important role than is implied by its relative neglect in commonly invoked models of the 'wider determinants of health'.

Several conclusions can be drawn from the examples considered.

1. Knowing what to do—to protect and enhance health—is powerfully permissive of it (ultimately) being done. This emerges clearly from all the examples where substantial gains in health

have been achieved (1 to 5 above). The relationship is not one to one. Health protective changes may occur for other reasons and knowing may not lead to doing because of the difficulties involved (adiposity provides the obvious example).

2. Because openly published science is a global public good, the proximity between the generation of new knowledge and the capacity to use it need not be close. The United States, for example, ranks more highly as a generator of knowledge than it does as a successful user. Generation and use are not too disjoint however, because a high investment in research relevant to public health is associated with a diffusion of the relevant 'rules of discourse'. Publics familiar with 'risk' and 'risk factors' will more readily assimilate new knowledge expressed in this way.
3. New knowledge may flow to its ultimate users through a variety of channels, ranging from formal health education programmes (sleeping position and SIDS in the United Kingdom, from December 1991) to highly informal, horizontal channels (sexual practices and HIV).
4. Advances in methodological knowledge—knowing better how we can know and how to make the best use of what we do know—have in some cases been as important as advances in substantive knowledge.
5. 'Interventions' that tell people what to do have often been found to be ineffective. These null results have often occurred against a background of favourable, and presumptively knowledge-based, changes in the relevant behaviours in the host population. This apparent paradox—of interventions without success against a background of success without interventions—is discussed further below.

Restoring knowledge to a central role in recent health trends in developed countries has an additional merit: It provides a common theme with explanations of trends in other times and in other populations. In the early twentieth century, the decline of childhood mortality was powerfully determined by the propagation to parents of new bacteriological knowledge (Ewbank & Preston 1989). For last decades of the twentieth century in low- and middle-income countries, Jamison and colleagues have concluded that:

> *Increased access to knowledge and technology has accounted for perhaps as much as two-thirds of the impressive 2 per cent per year rate of decline in under five mortality rates* (Jamison 2006, p. 4).

Liberalism and knowledge: Standing Hayek on his head

Liberalism tends to view politics as artificial (Zvesper 1987) and emphasizes the decentralized use of knowledge. Hayek's 'hard liberalism' sees the way knowledge is used as a central characteristic of political economy and deprecates centralized uses of knowledge.

The examples I have reviewed reinforce the central role of knowledge in the protection and enhancement of health in developed countries over the last half century. Some also demonstrate the importance of diffuse and decentralized processes in the successful use of knowledge. But the centrality of politics (think of the protracted tobacco wars) and the role of state and other centralized institutions—professions, scientific institutions, research 'charities'—in these processes, can neither be denied as a reality nor valued negatively. Massive state investments in medical research—most notable, ironically, in countries espousing economic liberalism and most deficient in the former communist states make the case. We can therefore accept Hayek's proposition that how knowledge is used is a fundamental characteristic of a society then turn him on his head and view positively rather than negatively the political and often centralized processes that have made the generation and diffusion of knowledge about how to protect and enhance health so fruitful of human well-being over the last half century.

Interventions without success and success without interventions

The idea of an intervention—defined by the *Oxford English Dictionary* as 'The action of intervening, "stepping in", or interfering in any affair, so as to affect its course or issue' (http://dictionary.oed.com)—has become pervasive in medicine and public health. Interventions clearly need intervenors: Professionals, programme administrators, or others. Recent medical usage links the idea to actions that can be subject to tests of effectiveness by a randomized control trial (RCT)—the most potent known salve for cognitive insecurity. Being testable in an RCT in turn implies actions that can be objectively pre-specified. This would seem to rule out actions that are informal, spontaneous, contingent, or 'one off'.

We have seen above how many of the processes leading to the turnaround in the HIV epidemic and to the reduction in SIDS (up to the formal programme at the end of 1991) appear to have been of an informal kind, making them, to a large degree 'successes without interventions'. There is only space here to add a couple of examples from the field of tobacco control, namely 'George Godber's lunch' and The California Tobacco Control Program.

In the late 1950s, George Godber was Deputy Chief Medical Officer in Britain and was very keen to act on the increasing knowledge of the harmful effects of smoking. But the Chief Medical Officer did not want to take the matter forward with the Minister of Health. Godber visited Charles Fletcher, a respiratory physician, at a London teaching hospital and invited him to his club for lunch so that they could discuss strategies. They decided on working through the Royal College of Physicians in order to by-pass the Chief Medical Officer. The College took up the matter energetically and decided to produce a report aimed at a large audience. In 1962, *Smoking and Health* appeared and quickly sold out (Pollock 1999; Lock *et al.* 1998). The United States was stimulated to follow suit and in 1964 the Surgeon General's report on *The Health Effects of Smoking* appeared. News media coverage of smoking and health was responsive to these reports and Pierce and colleagues have shown that smoking cessation rates in US middle-aged adults were, in turn, responsive to the extent of news coverage. (Pierce & Gilpin 2001) The point of this story is that all these processes are knowledge-based without qualifying as interventions.

Only a compulsive sceptic could doubt that the California Tobacco Control Program has contributed importantly to the reduction of tobacco smoking in that state. Since it achieved dedicated funding it has included many activities that would qualify as interventions. But the programme itself was created and sustained by a protracted political process—beginning with an 'indoor air ordinance' in Berkeley in April 1977 and reaching a decisive step with the passage of Proposition 99 in a statewide referendum in November 1988. This placed a tax of 25 cents on each pack of cigarettes that was hypothecated to the Program. The first city to make its restaurants 100 per cent smoke-free was Lodi in June 1990, and in January 1998 bars were made smoke free statewide. (Glantz & Balbach 2000). The proportion of households reporting themselves smoke free rose from 51 per cent in 1993 to 77 per cent in 2002. 'It is likely that the emphasis placed on the dangers of secondhand smoke by the California Tobacco Control Program media campaign, led to the adoption of home smoking restrictions'. (California Department of Health Services 2003, pp. 6–9.) (Such restrictions were not initially promoted by the Program.) Complex dynamics of this kind, including protracted political contests and 'spontaneous' household behaviour changes are not well captured in the idea of 'interventions'. But these elements are very likely to have contributed to the success of the Program.

Knowledge may thus be acted on in many ways in order to protect and enhance health, only some of which are appropriately described as 'interventions'.

Public health problems and public health investments

One reason why it is not always easy to see in health levels the short- to medium-term effects of public health programmes is that the causal path may go in the opposite direction: The nature and magnitude of health problems experienced may determine the strength of the public health response. Finland and Australia provide cases in point.

In the late 1960s, mortality from vascular disease in middle-aged males in the Finnish province of North Karelia was far above levels in other developed countries and the risk of dying before 65 approached 50 per cent. These risks were perceived, by the local people, as unacceptable and so they petitioned the national government to mount a preventive programme. From this the North Karelia Project was born and it in turn, stimulated investment in public health institutions (Vartiainen *et al.* 1994). Despite its modest population, Finland now has over 1000 staff in its National Institute of Public Health, and it ranks at the top in its rate of publication in leading international epidemiological journals (Fig. 3.2.6). Proportional mortality reductions in Finland have been amongst the biggest in the developed countries. Evaluative studies of the North Karelia project itself suggest it was effective. Lung cancer mortality fell sooner and further there consistent with early results for changes in smoking prevalence (Puska *et al.* 1993).

Australia, like Finland, faced adverse mortality trends in the sixth and seventh decades of the twentieth century with male life expectancy at birth falling during the seventh decade. Rising death rates from coronary heart disease, car crashes, and suicide were responsible. A country which had been notable for its favourable mortality levels at the beginning of the century, that had experienced a long post-war economic boom and that thought of its way of life as being especially favourable to health had to come to terms with a serious loss of rank in international health comparisons. Strong institutional responses evolved in relation to traffic injuries, heart disease, and tobacco control (Powles & Gifford 1993). These institutional developments have plausibly contributed to Australia's recent ranking as a relatively good performer in reducing overall mortality.

The strong development of public health institutions oriented towards chronic disease control in countries such as Finland and Australia may be contrasted with experience in countries such as France, Italy, and Spain where the evolving nature of public health challenges has been different. Vascular mortality in these countries did not persist at high levels, but tended to fall, often rapidly: This brought down all-cause mortality rates and made the case for re-invigorating public health institutions to prevent chronic disease less pressing. In these countries, traffic injuries, HIV, tobacco control, and the reduction of harm from alcohol use are among the most salient challenges.

The challenge of inequality

Recent favourable trends in overall adult mortality have been accompanied by growing inequalities in countries across Western

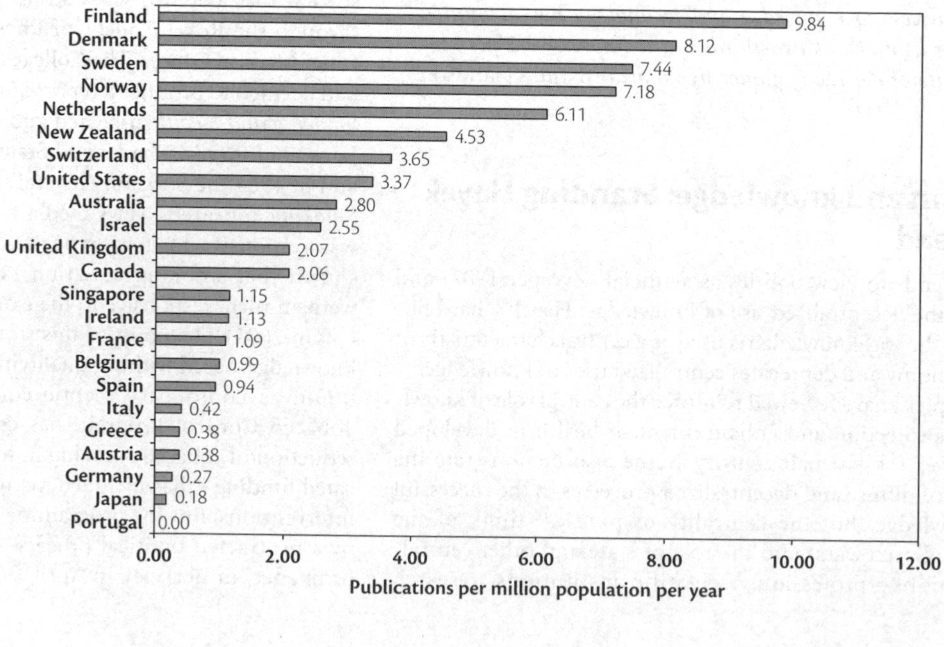

Fig. 3.2.6 Publications in the *American Journal of Epidemiology* plus the *International Journal of Epidemiology* classified by country of author's address, per million population, average for 1995–98. *Source*: Author's calculations using Medline records.

Europe because mortality declines have been proportionally greater in more favoured strata. Increasing inequalities in vascular mortality has been an important contributor (Mackenbach 2003). The causes of, and appropriate remedies for, these inequalities in health have been a major pre-occupation in policy discussions in the United Kingdom (Black *et al.* 1980; Acheson 1998). There is no tendency for mortality inequalities to be lesser in countries with higher income equality. The causes of death contributing most to these differences do, however, vary markedly between countries: '. . . mortality from ischaemic heart disease was strongly related to occupational class in England and Wales, Ireland, Finland, Sweden, Norway, and Denmark, but not in France, Switzerland, and Mediterranean countries. In the latter countries, cancers other than lung cancer and gastrointestinal diseases made a large contribution to class differences in total mortality. Inequalities in lung cancer, cerebrovascular disease, and external causes of death also varied greatly between countries' (Kunst *et al.* 1998b).

Black and colleagues have articulated a 'materialist' interpretation of the cause of inequalities in the United Kingdom. This gives primacy to 'material deprivation' (both absolute and relative) and draws attention to the marked increase in income inequalities there between 1979 and 1995/96—for example, over this period, the number of persons living in households with less than half the national average income increased from 4.5 to 12.2 million persons (Black *et al.* 1999). However, the finding of Kunst and colleagues that relative mortality inequalities are not less in countries with more equal income distributions does not support this interpretation. Furthermore, constrained consumption opportunities are not everywhere associated with high mortality levels: Cretan villagers observed in the 1960s and 1970s in the Seven Countries study had favourable mortality levels, despite their extremely frugal circumstances (Keys 1980). Thus, within some material cultures (all of which seem to have warm-ish climates!), it has become possible to attain low mortality on low incomes. The health effects of limited consumption opportunities therefore appear to depend strongly on the context in which consumption choices are made. Materialist explanations, if they are to be persuasive, need either to acknowledge their limited sphere of applicability ('northern commodity-intensive cultures'?) or, more informatively, to incorporate explicit reference to the kinds of differences between life in a Cretan village in the 1960s and life on housing estate in a British industrial city in the 1990s that are likely to be most important for health: Dietary traditions (related also to local food producing possibilities), norms governing alcohol and tobacco use (and purchasing power for cigarettes), and obligatory daily energy expenditure might be starters. Given that the relative importance of causes contributing to mortality inequalities varies by country, responses should also differ. In France, where inequalities in males appear to be amongst the largest within Western Europe, chronic diseases related to the volume of alcohol consumed make a major contribution; policies to reduce consumption will therefore be important. In Finland, injuries related to drunkenness are more salient, pointing to the need both for 'harm reduction' policies (such as control of drunk driving), and for programmes to encourage a change away from the traditional 'peak drinking' pattern. Measures to counter smoking are of primary importance in countries where a mature smoking epidemic is combined with a high background risk of vascular disease (roughly the 'northern' countries). (In countries at earlier stages in their smoking epidemics, programmes to encourage quitting may have the effect of increasing mortality inequalities. This does not, of course, mean that they should not be implemented.)

Jarvis and colleagues have shown for the United Kingdom that the current social gradient in smoking prevalence has been mainly created by greater rates of smoking cessation in the upper social strata: 'What we need to explain above all is not so much why poor people start smoking, but why they do not give it up' (Jarvis & Wardle 1999). Plasma cotinine levels among smokers show that nicotine dependence increases systematically with deprivation and that poor smokers obtain more nicotine per cigarette smoked. Using the indirect method of Peto, Lopez, and others (1992) (in which lung cancer mortality is used as a measure of tobacco exposure to estimate the proportion of other deaths attributable to smoking), it is estimated that, in the United Kingdom, smoking attributable deaths contribute about two-thirds of the excess mortality in the less favoured groups. The most obvious short-term policy response is to greatly strengthen assistance for quitting. In the long term, all measures that contribute to making tobacco use uncommon will have helped to reduce a major actual or potential cause of health inequality.

Making progress safe

Material progress—understood as the intensification of commodity production—both favours and harms health. One of the continuing challenges for public health institutions is to help resolve this ambivalence by countering the manifest and potential harms to health arising from material progress. This enables the net effect of affluence on health to approximate more closely towards those effects which are intrinsically beneficial. In nineteenth century Britain, industrialism did not impress as 'progress' until ways had been found to control the increase of fatal infection in the new industrial towns (Szreter 1997). In the twentieth century, the increased consumption opportunities generated by economic development has permitted a global epidemic of nicotine addiction which, especially when combined, in susceptible food cultures, with 'early dietary affluence' resulted in epidemic waves of tobacco-caused cancer and tobacco-amplified vascular disease. These epidemics were sometimes big enough, at least in males, to substantially nullify beneficial effects of economic development on traditional infective killers of adults such as tuberculosis and pneumonia. Now, as we have noted these two related epidemics are generally in retreat in developed countries. But history has not ended. Challenges and unsolved problems are ever renewed. As noted above, the uptake of tobacco smoking by young people has ceased declining in many developed countries and there is no plausible solution to the rising prevalence of obesity in sight. Industrialism in its current form is now known not to be generalizable to the whole human population without serious damage to planetary systems. Although we cannot predict the exact ways in which the cumulative disruption of major ecological processes will rebound on our health, the likelihood of serious harm from this source is now substantial. Public health endeavour will continue to be an important determinant of what we are able to mean by 'progress' and of whether we shall be able to make it safe.

Acknowledgements

I am grateful to Nick Day for the examples relating to HIV transmission and the decline in SIDS, to Daniela de Angelis for the model data on HIV in England, and to Christine Lim for help with Fig. 3.2.1.

Key points

- Adult mortality risks in established market economies and in European communist countries diverged markedly during the last four decades of the twentieth century.
- A fruitful approach to understanding these processes is to examine how knowledge has been developed and used in response to leading adult health risks.
- Knowing what to do has been powerfully permissive of it (ultimately) being done.
- The ways in which knowledge is used to protect and enhance health extend beyond formal 'interventions' to informal, decentralized, and 'spontaneous' processes.
- Creative institutional responses in areas such as heart disease prevention, tobacco control, and traffic injury control have extended the boundaries of what is achievable with given stocks of knowledge.
- So far, there has been little success in preventing the rise of excess adiposity, or in achieving transitions to sustainable productive systems. These provide current tests for the capacity of states to act as stewards over society's problem-solving capacities.

References

Acheson, E.D. (1993). Behold a pale horse: A view from Whitehall. *PHLS Microbiology Digest*, **10**, 133–40.

Acheson, E.D. (1998). *Independent inquiry into inequalities in health*. The Stationery Office, London.

American Dental Association (1999). *Fluoridation facts (revised)*. American Dental Association, Chicago (http://www.ada.org/consumer/facts/ff-menu.html, accessed November 12, 1999).

Australian Transport Safety Bureau (2007). *Road deaths Australia 2006 Statistical summary*. Australian Transport Safety Bureau, Canberra.

Beal, S. (1988). Sleeping position and SIDS [letter]. *Lancet*, **2**, 512.

Berry, C.J. (1994). *The idea of luxury: A conceptual and historical investigation*. Cambridge University Press, Cambridge.

Bingham, S.A., McNeil, N.I., and Cummings, J. H. (1981). The diet of individuals: A study of a randomly chosen cross section of British adults. *British Journal of Nutrition*, **45**, 23–35.

Black, D., Morris, J.N., Smith, C., and Townsend, P. (1980). *Inequalities in health: Report of a research working group*. Department of Health and Social Security, London.

Black, D., Morris, J.N., Smith, C. *et al.* (1999). Better benefits for health: Plan to implement the central recommendation of the Acheson report. *British Medical Journal*, **318**, 724–7.

Bleich, S., Cutler, D., Murray, C. *et al.* (2008). Why is the developed world obese? *Annual Review of Public Health*, **29**, 273–95.

Bonita, R. and Beaglehole, R. (1989). Increased treatment of hypertension does not explain the decline in stroke mortality in the United States, 1970–1980. *Hypertension*, **13**, I69–73.

Breslow, L. (1996). Social ecological strategies for promoting healthy lifestyles. *American Journal of Health Promotion*, **10**, 253–7.

British Dental Association (1996). *Oral health, tooth decay and the need for water fluoridation (Parliamentary Briefing)*. British Dental Association, London (http://www.derweb.ac.uk/bfs/bdaparli.html, accessed November 12, 1999).

Bunker, J.P. (2000). Medicine matters after all. *Journal of the Royal College of Physicians of London*, **29**, 105–12.

Burt, V.L., Culter, J.A., Higgins, M. *et al.* (1995). Trends in the prevalence, awareness, treatment, and control of hypertension in the adult US population. Data from the health examination surveys, 1960 to 1991 [published erratum appears in Hypertension 1996 May; **27**(5):1192]. *Hypertension*, **26**, 60–9.

California Department of Health Services, Tobacco Control Section (2003). Tobacco control successes in California: A focus on young people, results from the California Tobacco Surveys, 1990–2002 (http://www.dhs.ca.gov/tobacco, accessed December 18, 2007).

California Department of Health Services, Tobacco Control Section. (2007) Prevalence: Youth smoking (http://www.dhs.ca.gov/tobacco, accessed December 18, 2007).

Cameron, M. and Newstead, S. (1996). *Mass media publicity supporting police enforcement and its economic value*. Monash University Accident Research Centre, Melbourne (www.general.monash.edu.au/muarc/media/media.htm, accessed October 20, 1999).

Cheng, K.K., Chalmers, I., and Sheldon, T.A. (2007). Adding fluoride to water supplies. *BMJ*, **335**, 699–702.

De Angelis, D., Gilks, W.R., and Day, N.E. (1998). Bayesian projection of the acquired immune deficiency syndrome epidemic. *Applied Statistics*, **47**, 449–98.

Department for Transport (2007). *Road casualties Great Britain: 2006*. Department for Transport, London.

Division of Oral Health, Centers for Disease Control (1999). Fluoridation of drinking water to prevent dental caries. *Morbidity and Mortality Weekly Report*, **48**, 933–40.

Dokova, K.G., Stoeva, K.J., Kirov, P.I. *et al.*(2005). Public understanding of the causes of high stroke risk in northeast Bulgaria. *The European Journal of Public Health*, **15**, 313–16.

Dwyer, T. and Ponsonby, A.L. (1996). The decline of SIDS - a success story for epidemiology. *Epidemiology*, **7**, 323–5.

Easterlin, R.A. (1999). How beneficent is the market? A look at the modern history of mortality. *European Review of Economic History*, **3**, 257–94.

Ewbank, D.C. and Preston, S.H. (1989). Personal health behaviour and the decline in infant and child mortality: the United States, 1900–1930. In *What we know about health transition; The cultural, social and behavioural determinants of health: Proceedings of an international workshop,Canberra, May 1989* (ed. J.C. Caldwell *et al.*), pp. 116–49. Australian National University, Canberra.

Ford, E.S., Ajani, U.A., Croft, J.B. *et al.* (2007). Explaining the decrease in U.S. deaths from coronary disease, 1980–2000. *The New England Journal of Medicine*, **356**, 2388–98.

Gamble, A. (1996). *Hayek: The iron cage of liberty*. Polity Press, Cambridge.

Gamble, A. (2006). Hayek on knowledge, economics, and society. In *The Cambridge companion to Hayek* (ed. E. Feser), pp. 111–31. Cambridge University Press, Cambridge.

Gilbert, R., Salanti, G., Harden, M. *et al.* (2005). Infant sleeping position and the sudden infant death syndrome: systematic review of observational studies and historical review of recommendations from 1940 to 2002. *International Journal of Epidemiology*, **34**, 874–87.

Glantz, S.A. and Balbach, E.D. (2000). *Tobacco war: Inside the California battles*. University of California Press, Berkeley.

Goodman, J. (1993). *Tobacco in history: The cultures of dependence*. Routledge, London and New York.

Harkin, A.M., Anderson, P., and Goos, C. (1997). *Smoking, drinking and drug taking in the European Region*. WHO Regional Office for Europe, Copenhagen.

Hawthorne, G. (1991). *Pre-driver education: An evaluation of a traffic safety education program for senior students in Victorian post-primary schools*. PhD thesis submitted to Monash University 1991. Monash University, Melbourne, Australia.

Hayek, F.A. (1942). Scientism and the Study of Society, Part I. *Economica*, **9**, 267–91.

Hayek, F.A. (1943). Scientism and the Study of Society, Part II. *Economica*, **10**, 34–63.

Hayek, F.A. (1944). Scientism and the Study of Society, Part III. *Economica*, **11**, 27–39.

Hendrie, D. and Ryan, G.A. (1995). *Review of road safety practices in Australia and recommendations for Western Australia*. Road Accident Prevention Research Unit, Department of Public Health, University of Western Australia, Perth.

Hibell, B., Andersson, B., Bjarnason, T. *et al.* (2003). *The ESPAD Report: Alcohol and other drug use among students in 35 European countries*. The Swedish Council for Information on Alcohol and Other Drugs, Stockholm.

Hiley, C.M.H. and Morley, C.J. (1994). Evaluation of government's campaign to reduce risk of cot death. *British Medical Journal*, **309**, 703–4.

Hilliard, N., Jenkins, R., Pashayan, N. *et al.* (2007). Informal knowledge transfer in the period before formal health education programmes: Case studies of mass media coverage of HIV and SIDs in England and Wales. *BMC Public Health*, **7**, 293.

James, W.P.T. and Schofield, C. (1990). *Human energy requirements*. Oxford University Press, Oxford.

Jamison, D.T. (2006). Investing in Health. In *Disease control priorities in developing countries* (2nd edn.), (ed. D.T. Jamison *et al.*), pp. 3–36.

Jarvis, L. (1997). *Smoking among secondary school children in 1996: England*. The Stationery Office, London.

Jarvis, M.J. and Wardle, J. (1999). Social patterning of individual health behaviours: The case of cigarette smoking. In *Social determinants of health* (eds. M.G. Marmot and R.G. Wilkinson), pp. 240–55. Oxford University Press, Oxford.

Joint National Committee (1997). The sixth report of the Joint National Committee on prevention, detection, evaluation, and treatment of high blood pressure [published erratum appears in Arch Intern Med 1998 Mar 23;**158**(6):573]. *Archives of Internal Medicine*, **157**, 2413–46.

Keys, A. (1980). *Seven countries: A multivariate analysis of death and coronary heart disease*. Harvard University Press, Cambridge.

Kotchen, J.M., McKean, H.E., Jackson-Thayer, S. *et al.* (1986). Impact of a rural high blood pressure control program on hypertension control and cardiovascular disease mortality. *Journal of the American Medical Association*, **255**, 2177–82.

Krementsov, N.L. (1997). *Stalinist science*. Princeton University Press, Princeton, NJ.

Kunst, A.E., Groenhof, F., and Mackenbach, J.P. (1998a). Mortality by occupational class among men 30–64 years in 11 European countries. EU Working Group on socioeconomic inequalities in health. *Social Science and Medicine*, **46**, 1459–76.

Kunst, A.E., Groenhof, F., Mackenbach, J.P., and EU working group on socioeconomic inequalities in health (1998b). Occupational class and cause specific mortality in middle aged men in 11 European countries: Comparison of population based studies. *British Medical Journal*, **316**, 1636–42.

Law, M.R. and Wald, N.J. (2002). Risk factor thresholds: Their existence under scrutiny. *BMJ*, **324**, 1570–6.

Lawes, C.M.M., Vander Hoorn, S., Law, M.R. *et al.* (2004a). High blood pressure. In *Comparative quantification of health risks: Global and regional burden of diseases attributable to selected major risk factors*, Vol. 1 (eds. M. Ezzati *et al.*), pp. 281–390. World Health Organization, Geneva.

Lawes, C.M.M., Vander Hoorn, S., Law, M.R. *et al.* (2004b). High cholesterol. In *Comparative quantification of health risks: Global and regional burden of diseases attributable to selected major risk factors* (eds. M. Ezzati *et al.*), pp. 391–496. World Health Organization, Geneva.

Lenfant, C. and Roccella, E.J. (1984). Trends in hypertension control in the United States. *Chest*, **86**, 459–62.

Lock, S., Reynolds, L.A., and Tansey, E.M. (1998). *Ashes to ashes: The history of smoking and health*. Rodopi, Amsterdam.

Lopez, A. (1996). The lung cancer epidemic in developed countries. In *Adult mortality in developed countries* (ed. A. Lopez), pp. 111–34. Oxford University Press, Oxford.

Lopez, A.D., Collishaw, N.E., and Piha, T. (1994). A descriptive model of the cigarette epidemic in developed countries. *Tobacco Control*, **3**, 242–7.

Mackay, J. and Mensah, G. (eds.) (2004). *The atlas of heart disease and stroke*. World Health Organization, Geneva.

Mackenbach, J.P., Bos, V., Andersen, O. *et al.* (2003). Widening socioeconomic inequalities in mortality in six Western European countries. *International Journal of Epidemiology*, **32**, 830–7.

Marinho, V.C., Higgins, J.P., Sheiham, A. *et al.* (2003). Fluoride toothpastes for preventing dental caries in children and adolescents. *Cochrane Database of Systematic Reviews*, CD002278.

McKee, M. (2007). Cochrane on Communism: The influence of ideology on the search for evidence. *International Journal of Epidemiology*, **36**, 269–73.

McKeown, T. (1976). *The modern rise of population*. Arnold, London.

McMichael, A.J., Powles, J.W., Butler, C.D. *et al.* (2007). Food, livestock production, energy, climate change, and health. *Lancet*, **370**, 1253–63.

Mead, R. (1775). *The medical works of Richard Mead, M.D.* Alexander Donaldson & Charles Elliot, Edinburgh (reprint by AMS Press, New York, 1978), p. 438.

Medvedev, D. (2007). Excerpts from the transcript of the session of the Presidential Council for Implementing Priority National Projects and Demographic Policy. Kremlin, Moscow (http://www.kremlin.ru/eng/text/speeches/2007/03/07/1944_type82913type82917_119295.shtml, accessed December 18, 2007).

Mokyr, J. (2002). *The gifts of Athena: Historical origins of the knowledge economy*. Princeton University Press, Princeton, N.J.

Mosterd, A., D'Agostino, R.B., Silbershatz, H. *et al.* (1999). Trends in the prevalence of hypertension, antihypertensive therapy, and left ventricular hypertrophy from 1950 to 1989. *New England Journal of Medicine*, **340**, 1221–7.

National Heart Lung and Blood Institute (2007). Factbook. (http://www.nhlbi.nih.gov/about/factbook/chapter4data, accessed December 18, 2007)

NHS Centre for Reviews and Dissemination (2000). *A systematic review of public water fluoridation*. NHS CRD, York.

Nordhaus, W. D. (2002). *The health of nations: The contribution of improved health to living standards*. Working Paper 8818. National Bureau of Economic Research, Boston.

OECD (2007). *Factbook 2007*. OECD, Paris.

Office of Population, Censuses and Statistics (1988, 1995). *OPCS Monitor, Series* DH3 Sudden Infant Deaths. OPCS, London.

Peto, R., Lopez, A.D., Boreham, J. *et al.*(1994). *Mortality from smoking in developed countries, 1950–2000: Indirect estimates from national vital statistics*. Oxford University Press, Oxford.

Peto, R., Lopez, A.D., Boreham, J. *et al.* (1992). Mortality from tobacco in developed countries: Indirect estimation from national vital statistics. *Lancet*, **339**, 1268–78.

Peto, R., Lopez, A.D., Boreham, J. *et al.* (2003). *Mortality from smoking in developed countries, 1950–2000* (2nd edn.). Clinical Trials Service Unit, Oxford University (web based update of first edition), Oxford. (http://www.ctsu.ox.ac.uk/~tobacco, accessed December 18, 2007).

Pierce, J.P. and Gilpin, E.A. (2001). News media coverage of smoking and health is associated with changes in population rates of smoking cessation but not initiation. *Tobacco Control*, **10**, 145–53.

Pollock, D. (1999). *Denial and delay: The political history of smoking and health, 1951–1964*. Action on Smoking and Health, London.

Powles, J.W. and Gifford, S. (1993). Health of nations: Lessons from Victoria, Australia. *British Medical Journal*, **306**, 125–7.

Prentice, A.M. and Jebb, S.A. (1995). Obesity in Britain: Gluttony or sloth? *British Medical Journal*, **311**, 437–9 (and response to correspondence in **311**, 1568–9).

Puska, P., Korhonen, H.J., Torppa, J. *et al.* (1993). Does community-wide prevention of cardiovascular diseases influence cancer mortality? *European Journal of Cancer Prevention*, **2**, 457–60.

Robertson, L.S. (2001). Groundless attack on an uncommon man: William Haddon, Jr, MD. *Injury Prevention*, **7**, 260–2.

Rose, G. (1985). Sick individuals and sick populations. *International Journal of Epidemiology*, **14**, 32–8.

Royal College of Physicians (1962). *Smoking and health*. Pitman Medical, London.

Saris, W.H., Blair, S.N., van Baak, M.A. *et al.* (2003). How much physical activity is enough to prevent unhealthy weight gain? Outcome of the IASO 1st Stock Conference and consensus statement. *Obesity Reviews*, **4**, 101–14.

Secretary of State for Social Services (1988). *Public health in England: The report of the Committee of Inquiry into the future development of the Public Health Function* (D. Acheson, Chairman). HMSO, London.

Smeed, R.J. (1972). The usefulness of formulae in traffic engineering and road safety. *Accident Analysis and Prevention*, **4**, 303–12.

Stamler, J., Wentworth, D., and Neaton, J.D. (1986). Is relationship between serum cholesterol and risk of premature death from coronary heart disease continuous and graded? Findings in 356,222 primary screenees of the Multiple Risk Factor Intervention Trial (MRFIT). *JAMA*, **256**, 2823–8.

Stephen, A.M. and Wald, N.J. (1990). Trends in individual consumption of dietary fat in the United States, 1920–1984. *American Journal of Clinical Nutrition*, **52**, 457–69.

Strachan, D. and Rose, G. (1991). Strategies of prevention revisited: effects of imprecise measurement of risk factors on the evaluation of "high-risk" and "population-based" approaches to prevention of cardiovascular disease. *Journal of Clinical Epidemiology*, **44**, 1187–96.

Szreter, S. (1988). The importance of social intervention in Britain's mortality decline c.1850–1914: A re-interpretation of the role of public health. *Journal of the Society for the Social History of Medicine*, **1**, 1–37.

Szreter, S. (1997). Economic growth, disruption, deprivation, disease, and death: on the importance of the politics of public health for development. *Population and Development Review*, **23**, 693–728, 929,931.

Tobacco Advisory Group, Royal College of Physicians (2000). *Nicotine addiction in Britain*. Royal College of Physicians, London.

United States Public Health Service (1964). *Smoking and health: Report of the advisory committee to the Surgeon General of the Public Health Service*. US Department of Health, Education and Welfare, Washington.

US Department of Health and Human Services and Batelle (1995). *For a healthy nation: Returns on investment in public health*. US Government Printing Office, Washington.

US Department of Health and Human Services (1996). *Physical activity and health: A report of the Surgeon General*. US Department of Health and Human Services, Centers for Disease Control and Prevention, Atlanta, GA.

Vartiainen, E., Puska, P., Jousilahti, P. *et al.* (1994). Twenty-year trends in coronary risk factors in North Karelia and in other areas of Finland. *International Journal of Epidemiology*, **23**, 495–504.

Wareham, N.J., Hennings, S J., Prentice, A.M. *et al.* (1997). Feasibility of heart-rate monitoring to estimate total level and pattern of energy expenditure in a population-based epidemiological study: the Ely Young Cohort Feasibility Study 1994–5. *British Journal of Nutrition*, **78**, 889–900.

Wareham, N.J., Wong, M.Y., and Day, N.E. (2000). Glucose intolerance and physical inactivity: The relative importance of low habitual energy expenditure and cardiorespiratory fitness. *American Journal of Epidemiology*, **152**, 132–9.

Widdowson, E.M. (1936). A study of English diets by the individual method, part I. Men. *Journal of Hygiene*, **36**, 269–92.

Widdowson, E.M. and McCance, R.A. (1936). A study of English diets by the individual method, part II. Women. *Journal of Hygiene*, **36**, 293–309.

Woodcock, J., Banister, D., Edwards, P. *et al.* (2007). Energy and transport. *Lancet*, **370**, 1078–88.

World Health Organization (1998). *Obesity: Preventing and managing the global epidemic. Report of a WHO Consultation on obesity, Geneva 2–5 June 1997*. World Health Organization, Geneva.

Zvesper, J. (1987). Liberalism. In *The Blackwell encyclopaedia of political thought* (ed. D. Miller), pp. 285–89. Blackwell, Oxford.

3.3

Health policy in developing countries

Miguel Angel González-Block, Adetokunbo Lucas, Octavio Gómez-Dantés, and Julio Frenk

Abstract

Health policy making in developing countries is increasingly being envisaged as a stewardship process concerned with attaining trust and legitimacy between a government and its people towards the improvement of the welfare of populations. Health policy today involves multiple actors and an increased role by global and international agencies. Increased investment in the context of the Millennium Development Goals is also placing greater attention on good national and international governance. Particular attention is being paid to governance of the new breed of vertical programmes. This approach has demonstrated benefits for the specific diseases being tackled, yet it threatens other programmes and the capacity of local authorities to meet broad health needs. Developing country governments should set clear priorities on the basis of health needs and infrastructure capacity as well as on sound ethical guidance that help achieve maximum improvement in health in return for minimum expenditure.

Comprehensive national health accounts is an important policy tool to track health spending from all sources. Performance assessment can support policy making in monitoring and evaluating attainment of critical outcomes and the efficiency of the health system in a way that allows comparison over time and across systems. Particular attention is being given to financing healthcare for the more than 1.3 billion rural poor and informal sector workers in developing countries without financial protection against the catastrophic costs of healthcare. Success with these and other innovations will depend on solving the multiple challenges facing the health workforce. Relying on public–private mix of services to address health infrastructure faces the question of the capacity by government to develop contracts, set prices, and monitor and supervise private providers.

It is not always easy to reconcile efficiency and equity in health policy. Equity should be a primary concern for sustainable policy making, and tools are available to trace the extent to which investments at national levels benefit the poor and needy. In many respects, health policy in developing countries is all about the encouragement of innovation and the scaling-up of life-saving technologies and systems. Access to knowledge and technology has accounted for a high proportion in the decline in mortality rates. New strategies for organizing health research systems can contribute to make evidence-based policy a reality in developing countries.

Introduction

Most developing nations are making important strides towards better health and universal health service coverage through policies that are increasingly influenced by international experience. The flow of financial resources is also rapidly increasing thanks to the role that health investments are playing in the wider strategy towards democracy, economic growth, and global security (Frenk & Gómez-Dantés 2007; Hecht & Shah 2006; Brown *et al.* 2001). Health policy in the South is thus increasingly being influenced by globalization, both by responding to global threats and by doing so through extensive use of the pool of global experiences.

Health policy has been critical for the diffusion of life-saving technologies and knowledge that are behind the drop in disparities in life expectancy across rich and poor countries at least since the middle of the last century. Taken as a group, the poorer countries have seen gains of about 5 years on average per decade since 1960, against half this much by the better-off. Critically, the pace of technology diffusion has been more influential for health than changes in the levels of income. Increased access to knowledge and technology thanks to appropriate health policies has accounted for perhaps as much as two-thirds of the 2 per cent per year rate of decline in under-5 mortality rates (Jamison 2006).

However, health policy still has important challenges in a world saddled with conflict, poverty, and the pandemic of HIV/AIDS. In some African countries, the trend in the mortality rate for children under 5 has been reversed. While, between 1960 and 1990, African countries made substantial progress in reducing this rate, in many countries this effort was slowed down considerably, and in some others mortality even rose between 1990 and 2002 (UNICEF 2004).

In this chapter, we review the context in which health policies are being developed in low- and middle-income countries. We discuss several key concepts associated with health policy; and we describe some of the tools available for policy making. In the first part, we discuss the role of health policy as a stewardship instrument and the general context in which health policies are being designed and implemented in developing nations. In the second part, we describe some of the novel tools available for policy making, including burden of disease, national health accounts, and health system performance assessment. We discuss the increasing international financing for healthcare and the alternatives for providing financial protection against catastrophic costs of healthcare to the rural and urban poor. We then analyse the search for equity in health and discuss the role of international agencies and health research in the design and implementation of health policies. The main messages of the chapter are the following:

1. Health policy is being called not only to address the pressing needs of infectious diseases and malnutrition and the emerging problems of non-communicable diseases and injuries, but also the new challenges related to globalization.
2. Sound health policy making can contribute to the consolidation of democracy, to economic growth, and to global security. The broad consensus generated around this issue has helped to mobilize **more money for health** in developing nations.
3. Policy-making should be evidence-based, and also results-oriented. Careful planning and skilled management can achieve good results and allow developing countries to deliver **more health for the money**.

Health policy as stewardship

Health policy making in developing countries is seeking a new model of action to increase health and welfare, largely based on the separation of health system stewardship from service delivery through various forms of decentralization (Murray & Frenk 2000; Bossert 1998). Policy making is increasingly being envisaged as a stewardship process concerned with attaining trust and legitimacy between a government and its people towards the improvement of the welfare of populations (Londoño & Frenk 1997; Gilson 2003; Bankauskaite *et al.* 2007; Garret 2007). The *World Health Report 2000* defined stewardship of the health system by national governments as a critical function to realign incentives and to mobilize and allocate resources to achieve the final goals of health gain, financial protection, and responsiveness. Stewardship has also been defined as a function of international agencies to enable co-ordination of health systems at the global level (WHO 2000).

Stewardship is an ethically based, outcome-oriented policy approach and as such it is more interventionist than the economically driven agency approach to state regulation (Fig. 3.3.1). The notion of stewardship, if properly developed, is also consistent with an evidence-based health policy framework (Saltman 2000). A national health strategy based on stewardship can marshal the available evidence to support population-based measures that can improve overall health status. Stewardship capacity is synonymous with the quality of governing institutions within countries, and with the trust that societies place in their governments. In a global climate of increased support for public investments in health, increasing attention is being paid to differentiate countries with 'good' and 'stressed' governance in order to marshal international aid support for policy making.

The process of policy making for the health sector has become increasingly intricate. Health practitioners, policy makers, and planners have to contend with three main issues: **Diversity, complexity, and change.**

There is often great **diversity** within developing countries, as well as between and within different geographical areas. Ecological and geographical factors are recognized as important determinants of health conditions. Economic, social, and cultural determinants also contribute to diversity. The association of poverty, exclusion, and discrimination with poor health status is a consistent finding in both developed and developing countries and has a long research tradition (Evans *et al.* 1994). In general, policy making fails to systematically recognize and act on these determinants. The WHO Commission on Social Determinants of Health is attempting to redress this shortcoming by creating awareness of such determinants among political leaders and stakeholders, and helping countries adopt comprehensive health and development policies oriented towards them (Irwin *et al.* 2006).

Complexity in health needs of populations is another challenge. In contrast with rich countries that experienced a substitution of old for new patterns of disease, developing nations are facing

Characteristic	Agency theory	Stewardship theory
1. Model of man	Economic man	Self-actualizing man
Behaviour	Self-serving	collective serving
2. Psychological mechanisms		
Motivation	Lower order/econimic needs (physiological, security, economic)	Higher order needs (growth, achievement, self-actualization)
	Extrinsic	Intrinsic
Social comparison	Other managers	Stakeholders
Identification	Low value commitment	High value commitment
Power	Institutional (legitimate, coercive, reward)	Personal (expert, referent)
3. Situation mechanisms		
4. Management philosophy	Control-oriented	Involvement-oriented
Risk orientation	Control mechanisms	Trust
Time frame	Short-term	Long-term
Objective	Cost control	Performance enhancement
	Individualism	Collectivism
5. Cultural differences	High-power distance	Low-power distance

Fig. 3.3.1 Comparison of agency theory and stewardship theory. *Source*: Armstrong (1997), adapted from Davis *et al.* (1997).

a triple burden of ill health: First, the unfinished agenda of infections, malnutrition, and reproductive health problems; second, the emerging challenges represented by non-communicable diseases and injuries, which already comprise half the disease burden in low- and middle-income countries; third, the health risks associated with globalization, including the threat of pandemics like AIDS and influenza, the trade in harmful products like tobacco, and other drugs, the health consequences of climate change, and the dissemination of harmful lifestyles.

Annual changes in mortality projections between 2002 and 2020 suggest decreases in tuberculosis of over 5 per cent yet increases of between 2.1 and 3 per cent for HIV/AIDS. Diabetes mellitus and road traffic mortality are projected to increase over 1 per cent per year, an alarming rate (Table 3.3.1). In projections to 2030 (Table 3.3.2), cardiovascular disease will account for 13.4 per cent of the total world mortality and will rank as the first or second cause of mortality in all income regions. Tobacco consumption is largely responsible for many disease trends, and particularly ischaemic heart disease. This is a product of relentless push of industry into new, unregulated contexts susceptible to lifestyle changes.

While knowledge and innovative health technologies have been critical in healthcare in developing countries, the explosion of new technologies designed for rich countries as well as innovations of critical importance to the South such as ARV and IMCI have markedly increased the **complexity of healthcare**. The expanding scope of prophylactic, diagnostic, and therapeutic options demands an increasing range of specific programmes with the associated need for specialist personnel, new categories of support staff, high-technology equipment, and infrastructure. Figure 3.3.2 illustrates the complex interaction of medical and non-medical factors that are involved in perpetuating the high maternal mortality rates occurring in the developing world. It also offers clues as to the package of interventions that are required to reduce maternal mortality (McCarthy & Maine 1992). A particular challenge is a renewed tendency to deliver new technologies through vertical programmes that may fail to support the health system while weakening existing programmes (WHO 1996; Molineaux & Nantulya 2004; Unger *et al.* 2003; Garret 2006).

The interaction of medical and non-medical factors in the dynamics of health and disease calls for a critical analysis of needs and opportunities as a basis of designing and managing health programmes. Rather than blindly attempting to deliver standardized, pre-packaged, stereotyped interventions, policy makers should try to match the services to suit local needs. Because of the important influence of non-medical factors on health, it is necessary to mobilize inter-sectoral action to complement strictly medical inputs from the health sector. However, policy makers in developing countries should measure their capacity and ensure they first reap their benefits of interventions they can directly control within their health systems (Jamison 2006).

Policy making in developing countries also has to be fluid and dynamic to adapt strategies and programmes to the many **changes** that are occurring in the environment. Two critical changes are accountability and socioeconomic change.

Global as well as national influences are leading towards greater **accountability** of policy makers to parliaments, provincial stakeholders, as well as to donors, clients, and populations. Decentralization has continued its pace giving provincial authorities and local officials greater autonomy for innovations but also increased responsibility (Hutton 2002; Bossert 1998). Policy making in the health sector is thus moving from a technical and highly hierarchical approach towards recognizing the role of new actors and processes set in a political and participatory environment.

Table 3.3.1 Projected average annual rates of change in age-standardized death rates for selected causes: World 2002–2020

Group	Cause	Average annual change (per cent) in age-standardized death rate	
		Males	**Females**
All Causes		−0.8	−1.1
Group I		−1.4	−5.3
	Tuberculosis	−5.4	−5.3
	HIV/AIDS	3.0	2.1
	Malaria	−1.3	−1.5
	Other infectious diseases	−3.4	−3.3
	Respiratory infections	−2.7	−3.4
	Perinatal conditions*	−1.7	−1.9
	Other Group I	−3.0	−3.6
Group II		0.0	−0.8
	Cancer	−0.2	−0.4
	Lung cancer	0.1	0.3
	Diabetes mellitus	1.1	−1.3
	Cardiovascular diseases	−1.1	−1.2
	Respiratory diseases	0.3	−0.1
	Digestive diseases	−1.3	−1.7
	Other Group II	−0.7	−1.1
Group III		0.0	−0.2
	Unintentional injuries	−0.2	−0.2
	Road traffic accidents	1.1	1.1
	Intentional injuries	0.2	−0.2
	Self-inflicted injuries	−0.3	−0.4
	Violence	0.4	0.2

[a] Causes adding in the perinatal period as defined in the ICD, principally prematurity and birth asphyxia, and does not include all deaths occurring in the neonatal period (under 1 mol)

Source: Mathers & Loncar (2006).

Changes in the economic and social situation in the country may have a profound effect on the health sector. Health policies have had to be modified in the light of rapid development in some countries and economic recession in others. In the immediate post-World War II era, macroeconomic policies emphasizing central planning and welfare programmes gained popularity. During the 1980s and 1990s, this trend was reversed, with national policies increasingly favouring free market economy in place of welfare programmes and central control. These changes brought about a slow-down in public health sector investments and the introduction of user fees, without visible improvements (Alliance HPSR 2004). Today, international agencies such as the IMF and the World Bank have reversed their policies (WB IMF Development Committee 2003), and funding has been substantially increased aiming to double the level of international aid to support the

Table 3.3.2 Mortality rate rank and percentage of total deaths projected to 2030. World and income regions

Income group	Rank	Disease or injury	Per cent of total deaths
World	1	Ischaemic heart disease	13.4
	2	Cerebrovascular disease	10.6
	3	HIV/AIDS	8.9
	4	COPD	7.8
	5	Lower respiratory infections	3.5
	6	Trachea bronchus, lung cancers	3.1
	7	Diabetes mellitus	3.0
	8	Road traffic accidents	2.9
	9	Perinatal conditions	2.2
	10	Stomach cancer	1.9
High-income countries	1	Ischaemic heart diseases	15.8
	2	Cerebrovascular disease	9.0
	3	Trachea, bronchus, lung cancers	5.1
	4	Diabetes mellitus	4.8
	5	COPD	4.1
	6	Lower respiratory infections	3.6
	7	Alzheimer and other dementias	3.6
	8	Colon and rectum cancers	3.3
	9	Stomach cancer	1.9
	10	Prostate cancer	1.8
Middle-income countries	1	Cerebrovascular disease	14.4
	2	Ischaemic heart disease	12.7
	3	COPD	12.0
	4	HIV/AIDS	6.2
	5	Trachea, bronchus, lung cancers	4.3
	6	Diabetes mellitus	3.7
	7	Stomach cancer	3.4
	8	Hypertensive heart disease	2.7
	9	Road traffic accidents	2.5
	10	Liver cancer	2.2
Low-income countries	1	Ischaemic heart disease	13.4
	2	HIV/AIDS	13.2
	3	Cerebrovascular disease	8.2
	4	COPD	5.5
	5	Lower respiratory infections	5.1
	6	Perinatal conditions	3.9
	7	Road traffic accidents	3.7
	8	Diarrhoeal disease	2.3
	9	Diabetes mellitus	2.1
	10	Malaria	1.8

Source: Mathers & Loncar (2006).

Millennium Development Goals. Government capacity is being revamped to ensure efficiency and equity in investments.

Countries face different degrees of resource development, of government control, and of public and private investment. These dimensions define a spectrum of country situations that goes from the accumulated conditions of poverty and underdevelopment seen in low-income countries, to the emerging conditions most notably seen in middle-income countries (Fig. 3.3.3). This chapter focuses on eight critical issues along this spectrum:

1. Health reform with special emphasis on structural reform and decentralization
2. Tools for policy making—burden of disease, national health accounts, and performance assessment
3. Financing healthcare—SWAPs and health insurance
4. Human resources for health
5. Public–private contracting
6. Equity in health
7. International agencies and public–private partnerships
8. Health research

Health reform

The rapid advances in health technologies, the increasing demands and expectations of populations, and the escalating costs of healthcare are challenging governments both in developed and developing countries. Governments are responding to these changes and the associated challenges by undertaking reforms of the health sector.

Structural reform

Health sector reform has been defined as the sustained and purposeful change to improve efficiency, equity, and effectiveness of the health sector (Berman & Bossert 2000; Roberts *et al.* 2003). Reforms have also been equated with comprehensive and integral change at the structural, programmatic, organizational, and instrumental levels of the health system (Frenk 1994; Gonzalez Block 1997).

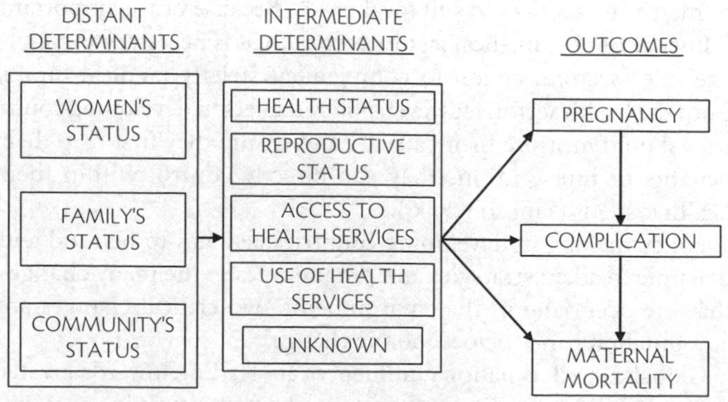

Fig. 3.3.2 Interaction of factors involved in the epidemiology of maternal mortality.
Source: McCarthy & Maine (1992).

COMPONENT	TYPE OF CHALLENGE	
	Accumulated	Emerging
Population	• **Epidemiological backlog** • Common infections • Malnutrition • Reproductive health problems • **Health gap** • **Inequity**	• **New pressure** • Non-communicable diseases • Injuries • Emerging infections • **Changes in demand patterns** • **Political pressures**
Institutions	• **Insufficient coverage** • **Poor technical quality** • **Allocational inefficiency** • **Inadequate patient referral** • **Deficient management of institutions**	• **Cost escalation** • **Inadequate incentives** • **Financial insecurity** • **Patient dissatisfaction** • **Technological expansion** • **Deficient management of the system**

Fig. 3.3.3 Challenges facing health systems in developing countries, by population and institutional components.
Source: Londoño & Frenk (1997).

At the **structural** level, changes such as the universalization of access to services, new financing arrangements and the separation of stewardship and delivery functions have been critical. In turn, reforms at the **programmatic** level may include the definition of specific service rights and predefined packages of interventions through explicit choices based on a calculus of benefits and costs. Changes at the **organizational** level may involve increasing provider choice and introducing provider payment mechanisms to promote quality and efficiency. At the **instrumental** level, reforms may imply increasing reliance on research, evaluation, and monitoring mechanisms, as well as incentives for human resource and technology development.

Health reforms require the development of monitoring mechanisms to ensure the attainment of objectives in the mid to long term. Such mechanisms should pay attention both to the technical and the ethical components of health reforms. A number of technical areas for monitoring and decision making have been identified. These areas include effective coverage; general level and distribution of health conditions; general level and distribution of responsiveness; and fair financing (see below under Performance Assessment) (WHO 2000). This framework was successfully used for monitoring and evaluation purposes at the subnational level in the recent reform experience of the Mexican health system (Frenk *et al.* 2006).

The ethical monitoring of health sector reforms has been enabled through a set of benchmarks of fairness (Daniels *et al.* 1996). These benchmarks identify and measure the degree of fairness of health systems and of the different objectives pursued by health reforms. While this approach was developed to assess reforms brought about by managed care in the United States, it has been tested in several developing countries with some success (Daniels *et al.* 2005).

Decentralization

The decentralization of the planning and management of health services from national authorities to provincial governments is a common feature of structural reforms. However, we are witnessing new trends towards recentralizing services, due both to an assessment of past strategies but more importantly as a result of scaling-up efforts for disease control.

Especially in large countries with dispersed populations, governments cannot efficiently manage the delivery of healthcare from their central offices. In a decentralized system, the central Ministry of Health can set national goals and targets, whilst devolving the responsibility for detailed management of the services to local authorities. Such arrangements promise improved allocative and technical efficiency, organizational innovation to meet local needs, improved service quality as well as greater equity together with transparency, accountability, and legitimacy for the health sector as a whole. Three questions are critical to assess the effectiveness of decentralization: (a) The amount of choice that is transferred from central institutions to institutions at the periphery of health systems, (b) what choices local officials make with their increased discretion, and (c) what effect these choices have on the performance of the health system; see Fig. 3.3.4 and Table 3.3.3 (Bossert 1998).

Beyond the administrative form that decentralization takes (deconcentration, delegation, or devolution), policy making depends on the relationships established between diverse actors and on the various influences they can exert on each other.

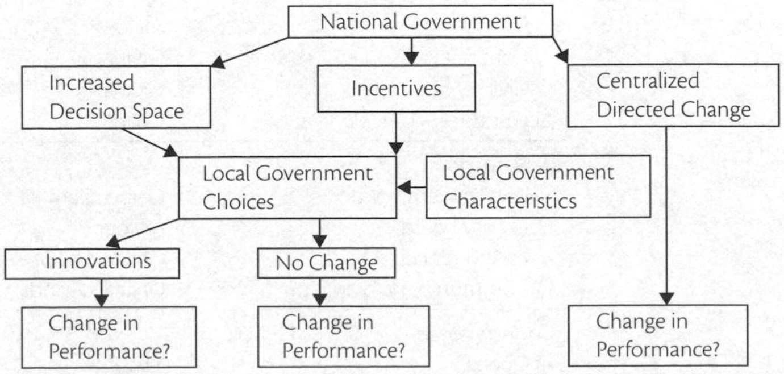

Fig. 3.3.4 Decision space and changes in performance in a decentralized healthcare system.
Source: Bossert (1998).

Decentralization entails the establishment of principal–agent relationships, whereby the principal transfers responsibilities but tries to maintain overall control, for example, on the kind of services provided, their quality and the equity attained (Bossert 1998). Information, assessment, and monitoring instruments are therefore critical for the success of decentralization reforms. Economic theories based on the choice that consumers have on the consumption of public resources have been useful to understand decentralization in developed countries. However, under conditions of meagre resources there is less local political and economic competition. More importantly perhaps is the reliance on trusted institutions at the local level and the strengthening of their capacity to ensure common interests across the multiple actors and often multiple principals that exert influence on health service providers (Gilson 2003).

Decentralization has not been without its critics, arguing that it has been often imposed upon local governments as a means of reducing central government obligations (Ugalde & Homedes 2006). The assessment of the effects of decentralization is now leading to recentralize a number of health functions in both rich and poor countries. This is the case of hospital administration in Norway (Bankauskite *et al.* 2007) and of public health surveillance in Mexico. Of greater significance for recentralization, however, is the increased funding by global health initiatives for disease control programmes such as malaria and HIV/AIDS. A new breed of vertical programmes is thus emerging, with forceful central funding, planning, and supervision yet relying on often decentralized primary healthcare services for their implementation. This approach has demonstrated benefits for the specific diseases being tackled, yet it threatens other programmes and the capacity of local authorities to meet broad health needs (Garrett 2007).

Tools for policy making

Policy making in developing countries has not always been guided by the best available evidence. In the immediate post-independence period, some developing countries copied models of health services in developed countries with particular emphasis on specialized curative care and the construction of large tertiary hospitals. The high cost of maintaining such establishments often distorted the national health budget, leaving very little resources for supporting less expensive but highly effective community-based services. Because of severe resource constraints, developing countries should set clear priorities and adopt policies that help achieve maximum improvement in health in return for minimum expenditure.

The establishment of priority lists of disease conditions and interventions was relatively easy in the traditional epidemiological situation where a few major conditions, mainly acute infectious diseases, accounted for a high proportion of deaths. In such situations one could rank priorities by considering the mortality rates from specific acute infectious diseases or the prevalence of chronic disabling diseases like onchocerciasis, a blinding disease. The process of priority setting has become more complex with the epidemiological transition and the increasing differentiation of health systems.

Efficient decision making for the allocation of scarce resources for health interventions requires setting priorities in terms of a

Table 3.3.3 Comparing the decision space in Ghana, Philippines, Uganda, and Zambia

	Range of choice		
Functions	**Narrow**	**Moderate**	**Wide**
Financing			
Source of revenue	Zambia	Ghana, Uganda	Philippines
Expenditures		All four	
Income from fees		Ghana, Zambia, Uganda	Philippines
Service organization			
Hospital autonomy	Ghana, Zambia	Uganda	Philippines
Insurance plans	Ghana, Uganda		Zambia, Philippines
Payment mechanisms	Ghana, Uganda	Philippines	Zambia
Contracts with private providers		Ghana, Zambia, Philippines	Uganda
Human resources			
Salaries	All four		
Contracts	Ghana,	Philippines	Zambia, Uganda
Civil service	Ghana	Zambia, Uganda, Philippines	
Access rules	Ghana	Zambia, Uganda, Philippines	
Governance			
Local government	Ghana, Zambia		Uganda, Philippines
Facility boards	All four		
Health offices	Ghana, Philippines	Zambia, Uganda	
Community participation	Ghana, Uganda	Zambia Philippines	
Country totals			
Ghana	11	4	0
Zambia	5	7	3
Uganda	5	7	3
Philippines	3	7	5

Source: Bosser & Buveais (2000).

wide range of considerations (Musgrove 1999, Gericke *et al.* 2005), to include: (i) The potential health impact and cost of interventions; (ii) the 'public good' character of interventions as well as their externalities and their consequence for catastrophic expenditure in the absence of public interventions; (iii) anti-poverty and equity considerations; and (iv) the capacity of health systems to implement new interventions

Burden of disease and priority setting

Health measures are critical for policy making, in general, and for priority setting, in particular. One of the most widely applied indexes used to measure health needs is disability adjusted life years (DALYs), which combines losses from premature death and from disability (Murray 1994 a,c).

The most common use of the DALY is simply to rank diseases and conditions by the burden of disease that they contribute, thus highlighting their relative importance for population health. The DALY is also being used to measure the burden of disease attributable to specific risk factors such as tobacco and obesity. On the basis of such measures, DALYs have been used to assess the impact of major control programmes and to estimate cost-effectiveness of interventions by comparing the cost of averting a DALY across them. In its 2000 World Health Report, WHO published data on Healthy Life Expectancy (HALE), which is defined as the average number of years that a person can expect to live in 'full health' by taking into account years lived in less than full health due to disease and/or injury.

The DALY approach has been critiqued by several authors with respect to technical, methodological and conceptual issues (Schneider 2001). The data required to estimate the DALY is extensive and is not always available to the extent necessary or with the required quality in developing countries. This has led to the use of questionable assumptions, such as the use of data for non-representative population segments. Another difficulty with the DALY is the combination of death and disability measures under the assumption that these phenomena lie on the same continuum along time (Anand & Hanson 1997).

Most critique of the DALY has centred on the large number of value-based judgements necessary to assign unequal age weights, to estimate the discounting of future health years, as well as to establish the disability weights (Anand & Hanson 1997). Furthermore, disability is quantified with respect to the limitation that diseases impose on individual functionality and does not consider pain and suffering.

The DALY is proving a useful tool but more work is required to refine and simplify it. Under the guidance of WHO, low- and middle-income countries are striving to improve the quality of data collection so as to improve the accuracy of national estimates of burden of disease. Some middle-income countries like Sri Lanka, Mexico, and Brazil are already making effective use of these tools (Morrow & Bryant 1995; Hyder *et al.* 1998). In Tanzania, the burden disease approach was adapted to prioritize interventions in the rural districts of Morogoro and Rufiji. After a 5-year period of offering a package of essential health services, under-5 mortality rates had declined by 40 per cent, to less than 100 deaths per 1000 live births, in contrast with the child mortality rate for the country as a whole which remained in 160 deaths during the period of the intervention (deSavigny *et al.* 2004).

The public good character of interventions offers another criterion for priority setting. Public investment will be justified if the interventions do not have sufficient supply or demand. Such is the case for vector control or environmental risk surveillance. However, even if there is some private supply and demand, the public intervention would be justified if it can be demonstrated that enlarging services would benefit an even wider population beyond that which is consuming the service directly. Such is the case of immunizations, where individual consumption offers herd immunity to populations at large.

The risk by the poor or the near-poor of incurring catastrophic expenditures when seeking healthcare or as a result of disability to work is in itself a reason to invest public resources. Indeed, in Mexico, around 3 million households suffer impoverishing or catastrophic health expenditures annually, a situation that led the government to implement the programme Seguro Popular de Salud (Popular Health Insurance) as a means of universalizing public insurance (Knaul & Frenk 2005).

The condition of poverty of specific population groups is in itself an important criterion to consider for allocating resources on a priority basis. However, poverty in itself is not a reason to provide services indiscriminately, as scarce resources would not be used efficiently in the fight against poverty. This is why it is ethically acceptable to provide a package of highly cost-effective services for the poor, so long as the package is also acceptable to the poor themselves.

The criteria thus far considered for prioritizing public investments in health interventions can be summarized in Fig. 3.3.5, which suggests that investments should be spent on public goods only when they are cost-effective and when they have inadequate private supply and demand. Interventions that particularly benefit the poor should also be prioritized, as are those threatening with catastrophic health expenditure. Vertical and horizontal equity will not always be compatible with cost-effectiveness, leaving decision making open to political criteria (Musgrove 1999).

The setting of priorities to invest in specific interventions should also consider the capacity of the health systems to formulate appropriate programmes and to deliver on the ground. Assessing health system capacity is today paramount, as new interventions are being scaled-up for the control of malaria, TB, and HIV/AIDS, among other diseases. These interventions require human, technical, and material resources that are often lacking. Four dimensions have been proposed for the assessment of the organizational and economic context (Gericke *et al.* 2005): (i) Technical characteristics of interventions; (ii) the logistical and delivery requirements; (iii) the requirements stemming from governmental regulation; and (iv) the characteristics of demand and utilization.

Technical characteristics of interventions include the basic design of products and technologies, such as stability and shelf-life. Product standardization is critical as similar interventions will be more easily implemented. Costs that are incurred during implementation but that may not have been considered in cost-effectiveness analysis include safety monitoring, supervision, storage and regular, on-time delivery. Regulatory costs can be considerable, such as accreditation of health providers and facilities to ensure service quality as well as measures to curb corruption. Often the costs necessary to ensure compliance and coercion are not considered when formulating new programmes, leading to low enforcement of measures to increase quality and efficiency. Finally, priority setting should consider the ease of use of technologies by the population at large, including the extent to which health education is required to ensure demand and compliance. Ease of use may also be related

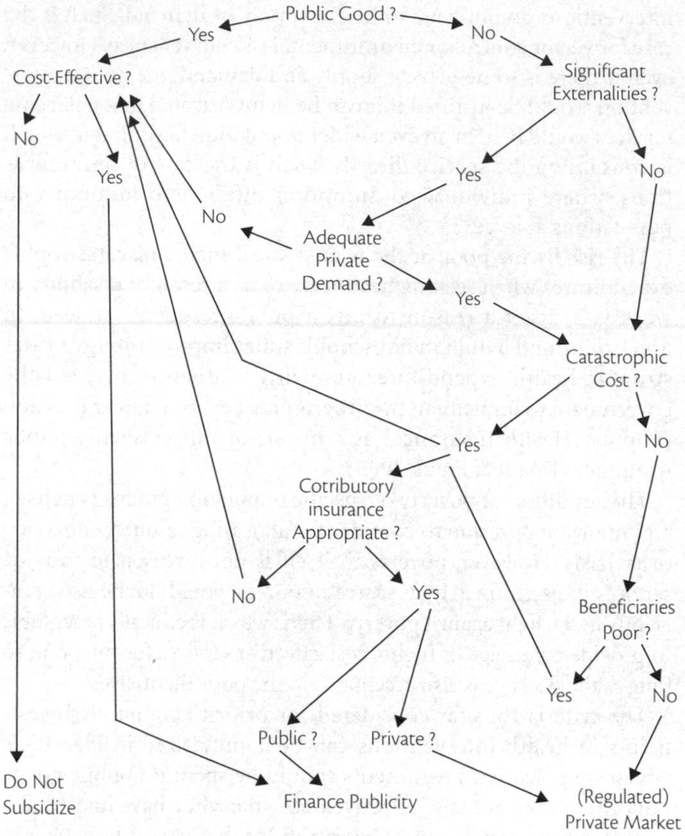

Fig. 3.3.5 Decision tree for assessing public investments in health.
Source: Musgrove (1999).

to the proliferation of black markets and forgery for which countermeasures should be implemented.

National health accounts

In the past, policy makers concentrated mainly on spending within the public sector, ignoring private spending through insurance, corporate arrangements, and employees' schemes, and out-of-pocket spending. Furthermore, spending within the public sector lacked clear indicators on resource flows, thus contributing to growing inequity and inefficiency. Policy makers now obtain a more comprehensive view of health expenditures thanks to the use of national health accounts developed through a uniform methodology. These analyses integrate health spending from all sources—public and private, corporate, and personal—within comprehensive accounts. National health accounts can affect the choices made within the public sector but also influence the role of public agencies in providing guidelines to the private sector and to communities regarding the most cost-effective uses of their investments and expenditures.

Health accounts consist of a basic matrix, where the columns list all sources of health spending—public (taxation and national social insurance), and private sources including employment-based schemes, privately financed insurance, and out-of-pocket expenditure. The rows of the matrix show the distribution of expenditure for personal healthcare, public health, and environmental sanitation services, and administration. Disaggregating the items in the columns and rows generates more elaborate analyses, providing more detailed information about sources and spending. Thus, the analyses could show variations over time, by geography, by population sub-groups, or any other variable that is relevant to policy making (Berman 1997; WHO 2003). Today, health accounts are being prepared not only at the national level but also by specific programmes such as HIV/AIDS and reproductive health.

Health system performance assessment

The *World Health Report 2000* offered a comprehensive methodology and reported results to assess the overall performance of health systems in terms of health gain, responsiveness to the legitimate expectations of the population, and fairness of financing (WHO 2000). These outcomes are conceived as the direct consequence of the health system functions of stewardship, financing, resource generation, and service provision (Fig. 3.3.6). The three health system outcomes were assessed in terms of equity and efficiency, except financial fairness for which only equity is appropriate. Health gain was measured through healthy life expectancy, already described under the priority setting section above. The methodology enabled the measurement of each health system goal separately as well as through a combined indicator. All WHO member countries were then ranked as a means of highlighting the benefits and limitations of health system designs as well as to promote analysis and improvements.

Performance assessment can support policy making in monitoring and evaluating attainment of critical outcomes and the efficiency of the health system in a way that allows comparison overtime and across systems. Performance assessment enables to measure the relationship between design of health systems and outcomes and to disseminate evidence on the benefits of diverse health system designs and reforms. The use of a widely accepted, comparative method was intended to feedback the policy debate as well as to empower the public with information relevant to their well-being (Murray & Evans 2003).

The methodology for performance assessment was widely debated by academics and governments. It was argued that intersectoral action for health was not subject to monitoring, focusing only on those functions and outcomes that are more directly under the control of ministries of health. Given that health sector policy making may be the result of actions taken in an indefinite past, it will not be clear whose actions are being assessed at any given point in time.

Perhaps most controversial was the lack of consensus on the weighting that was given to each of the three separate dimensions of performance, where following a Web survey, health gain was assigned 50 per cent and responsiveness and financial protection 25 per cent each. Data used for the 2000 report was also faulted for excessive use and lack of clarity of the estimations that were necessary, given poor data quality and availability in many countries.

Performance assessment has been widely endorsed as a tool for policy making for developing countries and, as mentioned above, was the basis for the monitoring of health sector reform in Mexico. However, improvements need to be made. Greater attention should be placed to the broader health system as well as to the relationship between measured outcomes and health system functions. Inequality should be more broadly measured, to include both health as well as socioeconomic inequality. Sub-national analyses should be carried out to identify success and limitations that can be more easily disseminated at the national level. Furthermore, national health information systems need to be strengthened as tools for performance assessment through the development of a broad range of health metrics (WHO 2007).

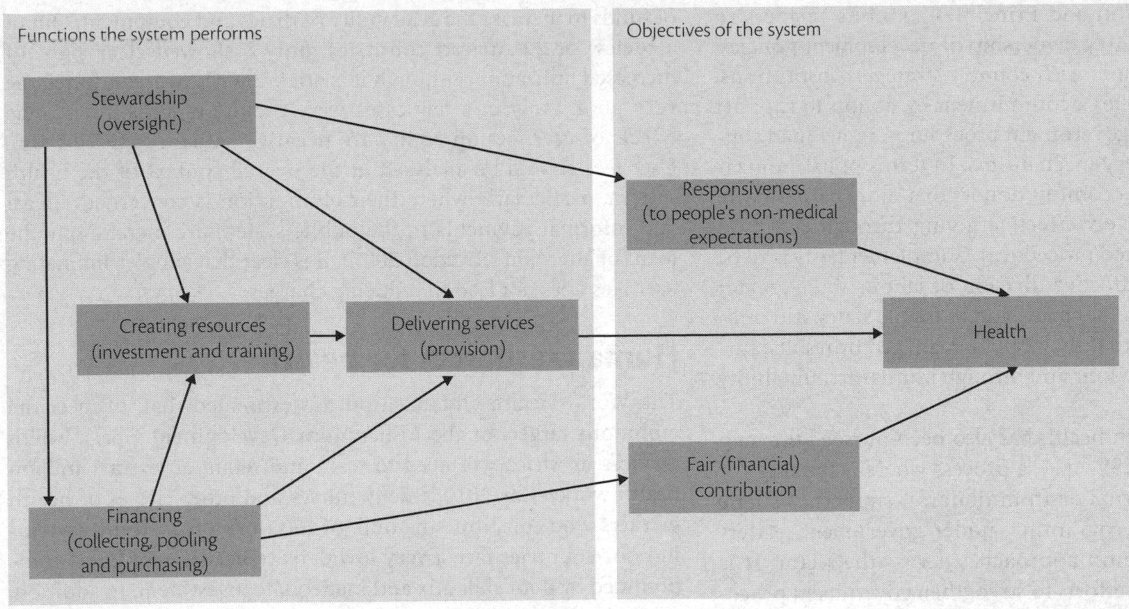

Fig. 3.3.6 Functions and objectives for the measurement of health system performance.
Source: WHO (2000), Fig. 2.1.

Mexico demonstrates how middle-income countries with reasonably developed information systems can make use of data for health system performance assessment. From 2000 to 2006, a set of health conditions and service benchmarks were systematically measured at state level and disseminated at yearly intervals. Evidence indicates that state authorities agreed on the quality and relevance of these measures and have accepted on this basis to be systematically monitored by federal health authorities and interested actors. Systematic monitoring has also led to the development of effective coverage measures, defined as the proportion of potential health gain that could be delivered by the health system to that which is actually delivered (Lozano *et al.* 2006). A total of 14 health interventions have been monitored and overall effective coverage assessed through a comprehensive indicator. Overall coverage ranged from 54 per cent in Chiapas, a poor state, to 65.1 per cent in Mexico's capital. These findings suggest that basic health interventions are much more equitably distributed in Mexico with respect to other health indicators.

Financing and contracting for healthcare

During the 1980s, international financing agencies restrained public investments in health as part of structural adjustment programmes with negative consequences for health systems. These policies have now been reversed as the UN enshrined the Millennium Development Goals (MDGs) with important health targets for maternal and child health as well as HIV/AIDS, TB, and malaria among other epidemic diseases. MDGs served as a basis on which to mobilize national and international resources (WB IMF Development Committee 2003). Also, the Commission on Macroeconomics and Health, convened by WHO under the leadership of Jeffrey Sachs, produced analytical data advocating massive investments in health as a means of spurring economic growth (Commission on Macroeconomics and Health 2001). The Monterrey Consensus agreed at the 2002 UN Financing for Development Conference intends to double the level of international aid through an additional US$20 billion per annum to enable poor countries to achieve the MDGs (Sachs 2004).

Scaling up health financing in poor countries

Government capacity is now being revamped in many countries to ensure that massive scaling-up of health interventions can be undertaken under conditions of efficiency and equity. However, before interventions can be scaled up, low-income countries under stress—essentially countries with low governance—will have to strengthen their institutional capacity to ensure efficient and equitable resource allocation. It has also been recommended that resources be allocated to interventions whose delivery is least covered by the market so as to increase the impact of government services (Filmer *et al.* 2000).

The IMF and World Bank estimate that large increases in aid (a doubling or more of current flows) could be used effectively in countries with good governance such as Bangladesh, India, Indonesia, Pakistan, and Vietnam, and in some sub-Saharan African countries, such as Ethiopia. These countries have a combination of good policies and prospects for further improvement, large unmet needs relative to the MDG targets, and relatively low levels of aid dependence. Sub-Saharan African countries considered to have good governance such as Burkina Faso, Mozambique, Tanzania, and Uganda could also use additional aid productively to supplement the sizable flows they already receive—an increase of about 60 per cent on average in the medium-term.

Evidence suggests that international short-term health aid is indeed supporting economic growth, regardless of the strength of governments (Clemens *et al.* 2004). Effective low-cost health interventions have also been effectively put in place and sustained in countries with weak governments or even under conflict situations (Medlin *et al.* 2006; Center for Global Development 2007).

Aid harmonization and sector-wide approaches

Donors and recipient countries have achieved a high degree of consensus regarding the provision of international aid. The Paris Aid

Harmonization Declaration and Principles commits partners to recognize developing country ownership of development policies, and the alignment of donors with country strategies, institutions, and procedures. This implies a commitment by donors to support capacity strengthening of government procedures, rather than supporting specific aid delivery mechanisms. In terms of harmonization, the Paris declarations commit donors to a more harmonized, transparent, and collectively effective giving through common arrangements and simplified procedures. Complementarity is to be sought through a more effective division of labour while greater attention should be paid to aid provision in fragile states. Aid policies should be devised so that they can be managed by results, furthering collaborative behaviour and through mutual accountability (Paris Declaration 2005).

Donor harmonization in health has also been pursued through Sector Wide Approaches (SWAps), a process whereby funding for the sector—whether internal or from donors—supports a single policy and expenditure programme, under government leadership, and adopting common approaches across the sector. It is generally accompanied by efforts to strengthen government procedures for disbursement and accountability. A SWAp should ideally involve broad stakeholder consultation in the design of a coherent sector programme at micro, meso, and macro levels, and strong co-ordination among donors and between donors and government. (Brown *et al.* 2001).

Health insurance and financial protection

Attention is increasingly being paid on how to finance healthcare for the more than 1.3 billion rural poor and informal sector workers in low- and middle-income countries without financial protection against the catastrophic costs of healthcare. Community health insurance has been proposed to improve access by rural and informal sector workers to needed heath care. Macro-level cross-country analyses give empirical support to the hypothesis that risk-sharing in health financing matters in terms of its impact on both the level and distribution of health, financial fairness, and responsiveness indicators (Preker *et al.* 2003; Alliance HPSR 2004).

Five key policies are available to governments to improve the effectiveness and sustainability of community financing schemes:

- Increased and well-targeted subsidies to pay for the premiums of low-income populations
- Insurance to protect against expenditure fluctuations and re-insurance to enlarge the effective size of small risk pools
- Effective prevention and case management techniques to limit expenditure fluctuations
- Technical support to strengthen the management capacity of local schemes
- Establishment and strengthening of links with the formal financing and provider networks

Middle-income countries with segmented health systems face particular challenges to extend insurance coverage to a rising population employed in the informal sector. New schemes have been implemented aiming at universal access to care through voluntary, government-subsidized schemes. Short-term assessments point to success (Gaikidou *et al.* 2006).

It is clear now that where user fees are established, critical factors for success in utilization are exemptions for the poor and the retention of funds to increase the availability of drugs and equipment. Out of a review of 22 African countries, only 8 showed clear signs of increased utilization, although it is not known how fees affected the very poor. Only in a few cases were exemptions instituted. The effects of user fees on equity are negative (Alliance HPSR 2004). User fees should be analysed in the overall context of the health system, particularly where their elimination is concerned. Illegal and informal payments in the public system are increasingly the focus of attention (Savedoff 2007). It is clear that simply eliminating user fees does not lead to reducing charges.

Human resources for health

The World Health Organization has estimated that, to meet the ambitious targets of the Millennium Development Goals, health services in Africa will need to train and retain an extra 1 million health workers by 2010, chiefly nurses and other classes of health workers who constitute the bulk of the workforce. Health systems in poor countries face a very low density health workforce, compounded by poor skill mix and inadequate investment. In addition, migration of trained human resources to more developed countries is becoming an ever more important issue.

Mass migration of health personnel is often a symptom of the 'sick system syndrome', in which many essential components of healthcare services are malfunctioning and mismanaged. Policies on migration must tackle the 'pull factors', which induce trained personnel to seek better living conditions abroad, as well as the 'push factors', which make disaffected and frustrated health workers seek employment elsewhere. Health challenges, such as the HIV/AIDS epidemic, impose additional pressures on health workers in their workplaces and at home, exposing them to contagious hazards, which adversely affect the morbidity and mortality of the workforce. The 'anchor factors' which encourage workers to remain in public service are important too. These should include financial incentives as well as well designed training programmes, that increase workers' skill and competence, boost their morale, increase their job satisfaction, and improve the performance of services (Lucas 2005).

Effective policy making for human resources has to overcome the low attention that is given by both national governments and international agencies. Fiscal discipline depends on restriction of staff numbers and compensation levels, with staff salaries now consuming 60–80 per cent of diminished public budgets in the health sector. There is also a lack of coherent and integrated investment strategies to strengthen the workforce, resulting in an overemphasis on workshops and training sessions that have an unclear effect. Such constraints operate in a context of health-sector and civil-service reforms that have altered the work environment through expansion of the private sector, downsizing, and decentralization in the public sector. Public–private contracting has thus been increasingly sought after as a means of addressing multiple constraints.

An informal global network of health leaders supported by the Rockefeller Foundation's Joint Learning Initiative has proposed four immediate steps towards a reinvigorated human resources for health policy (Joint Learning Initiative 2004):

- Large-scale advocacy to achieve heightened political awareness within countries and globally, leading to a social mobilization to respond to the crisis in the short term.

- Improve information and develop a commonly accepted framework of ideas, terms, and relations to guide analysis for policy formulation, particularly on the mobility of health professionals and the relations between health equity and human resources.
- Learn from history and identify success stories demonstrating the goodwill and commitment of health workers in spite of adverse conditions. Lessons from BRAC in Bangladesh are highlighted, employing over 30 000 village health workers to raise awareness of health issues among the rural poor.
- Address the supply, demand, and mobility of personnel, linking across training and education, health systems, and labour markets to develop a system that ensures continuity of policies over time. This includes a process of addressing low wages, as well as creating an incentive structure that supports providers over the course of their working lives.

International debate around the responsibilities of all actors has also produced an interesting range of proposals, including ethical recruitment guidelines and financial compensation for exporting countries. (Brush *et al.* 2004). Diagnostic approaches are required to inform evidence-based action: Identify signs and causes of the 'sick system syndrome'. These should lead to develop and adopt policies on human resources which are relevant, affordable, and sustainable, and are realistic about migration of trained staff (Lucas 2005).

Policy making and the public–private mix

The private health sector may be defined as comprising all providers who exist outside the public sector, whether their orientation is philanthropic or commercial, and whose aim is to treat illness or prevent disease (Mills *et al.* 2002). However, the public and private sectors are highly related as public sector workers often have a private practice and many public facilities offer private wards or services or operate in such a manner that they are indistinguishable from profit-seeking private providers (Meng *et al.* 2004).

As stated previously, even in developing countries with a widespread public system such as Mexico, catastrophic or impoverishing out-of-pocket health expenditures, which imply an extensive use of private medical services, affect a large proportion of the population (Knaul & Frenk 2005). In these contexts, it is vital to support consumers in their use of health services. Such efforts could stimulate appropriate demand through improving consumer information or could make services or products more affordable. Efforts can also influence the supply of services through creating institutions that give consumers greater authority to challenge care of poor quality (Mills *et al.* 2002, Soderlund *et al.* 2003).

Social marketing is an approach to stimulate demand of cost-effective interventions by increasing consumer information and subsidizing access to services. This approach has been particularly used to demand services within the private sector for reproductive health and basic sanitation. Limitations have been identified with regard to the extent to which social marketing stimulates or rather limits the private sector, the targeting of the poor, and leakage of benefits to the better-off who could afford to pay full-price for health services and commodities.

The use of vouchers has been tested on a limited scale as a means of targeting the poor without having to provide a generic subsidy. Protection of patients has also been pursued through the establishment of specialized government agencies to facilitate the settlement of malpractice and negligence, attempting to reduce the costs and negative consequences of litigation (Tena & Sotelo 2005).

Efforts on the supply side to improve the quality and value of private providers have included the promotion of professional training and accreditation as well as giving access to their patients to a limited range of public goods or services as for the treatment of TB (Marek *et al.* 1999). However, the most important efforts have been in the area of purchasing or contracting of a full range of primary or hospital services for specific population groups. These functions involve the separation of purchasing and provision at the government level and exercising stewardship functions, as already noted at the beginning of this chapter. The main challenge with these approaches lies in the capacity by government to develop contracts, set prices, and monitor and supervise private providers (Slack & Savedoff 2001; Palmer *et al.* 2003).

Equity in health

Policy makers in most developing countries are aware that poverty and ill health are intertwined and that important differences in health exist both across countries and provinces and across socio-economic groups (Figs 3.3.7 and 3.3.8). It is now accepted that poverty breeds ill health and that ill health keeps poor people poor (Fig. 3.3.7). The concept of equity in health is based on a fundamental principle: That differences in health that are the result either of the exposure to unhealthy life or working conditions or limited access to essential health services are morally unacceptable (Whitehead 1990; Dahlgren & Whitehead 1991).

Inequality in the health status of individuals and communities is a global phenomenon. Such disparities have been observed even in the most affluent countries but are most striking in developing countries where the poorest citizens often lack access to the most basic healthcare. Efforts to reduce such disparities have only been partially successful and too little is known on the reasons behind failure (Wagstaff 2002).

Equity can be assessed in three complementary dimensions: In health status of families, communities, and population groups; in allocation of financial, technical, and material resources and, in access to and utilization of high-quality services. Attention must be paid to political commitment towards equity and to equitable policy formulation To this end, information, monitoring, and evaluation for equity should be in place. Each of these dimensions of equity and of their political and policy dimensions are now considered.

The basic dimensions of health equity

Gross inequality in health status is regarded as prima facie evidence of inequities in the healthcare system. Significant inequalities in health status are found even in the most affluent developed countries, with long traditions of national health services that are designed to provide universal coverage (Black *et al.* 1998; Pollock 1999). A consistent finding is the strong association between poverty and poor health as defined by such indicators as the expectation of life, the incidence of acute diseases and injuries, the prevalence of chronic diseases and disabilities, and low access to services (Gwatkin 2000; Wagstaff 2002).

This consistent association of poverty with ill health makes it necessary for health systems to address the needs of the poor, and it strengthens the case in favour of programmes for the alleviation of poverty as important strategies for health promotion. It also draws

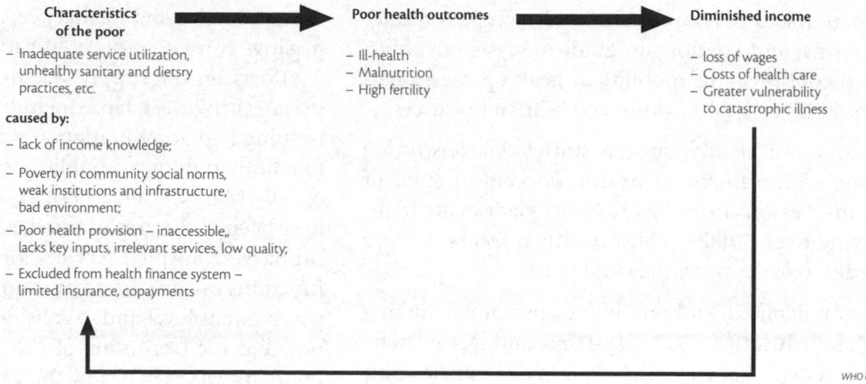

Fig. 3.3.7 The cycle of health and poverty.
Source: Wagstaff (2002).

attention to the influence of factors outside the health sector on health development: Education especially of girls, access to adequate quantity of safe water, environmental sanitation; as well as food and nutrition. Lifestyle and human behaviour, including such personal choices like smoking, use of alcohol, sexual behaviour, and physical exercise, also have important effects on health outcomes (Gwatkin 2003).

Equity is also examined in terms of the allocation of resources to different sections of the population. On moral and ethical grounds, the objective of allocative equity is for public resources to be shared out in a fair manner (Taipale 1999). The simplest formula would be a uniform per capita allocation. However, if large differences in health status already exist, an equal allocation would tend to perpetuate the inequalities. It can be argued that it is the responsibility of governments to perform a re-distributive function by allocating resources from the more affluent sector of society to meet the needs of lower-income individuals and families, the so-called vertical equity already mentioned when addressing priority setting, above.

Another view of equity is that everyone should have an equal opportunity of receiving care. This so-called horizontal equity proposes that individuals in like situations should be treated in like manner. Access is often defined in terms of the availability of services and its geographical coverage but experience has shown that the potential access, i.e. the services are within geographical range, does not necessarily correspond to real access as measured by the utilization of services (Jacobs & Price 2006).

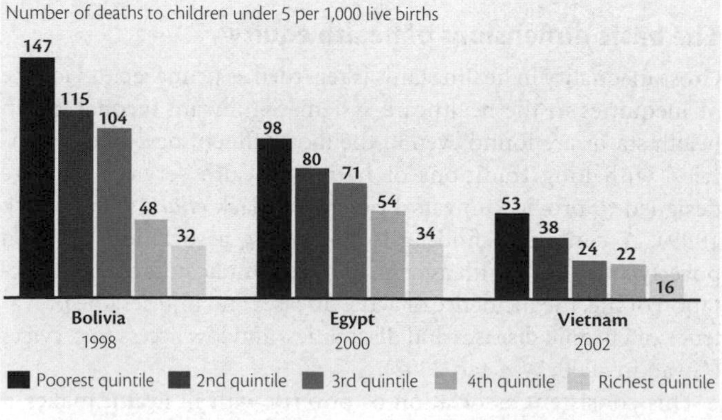

Fig. 3.3.8 Inequalities in under-5 mortality rates within socioeconomic groups of selected developing countries. 1998–2002.
Source: Gwatkin *et al.* (2003).

Marked disparities are often found in the geographical distribution of health facilities: Between regions, between urban and rural areas, between rural areas and within urban areas. (Phillips 1990). The differential ratios of persons per facility—hospital beds, nurses, and doctors—are used to measure the disparities. The distribution of health centres and other institutions in relation to the population—how far people have to travel to reach such facilities—are also used to indicate the uneven distribution of resources.

Political commitment for equity and equitable policy formulation

The political commitment of the government is the essential basis for promoting equity in health (Feacham 2000). The objective of equity in health fits well with the political philosophy in welfare states that have the clear goal of providing universal coverage of comprehensive healthcare for the entire population 'from the womb to the tomb'. In such countries, the question is not whether the State should embrace equity in health but how to achieve this goal in practice. Many developing countries have adopted more limited but realistic goals of providing universal access to a cost-effective package of services, together with universal financial protection through social health insurance (Frenk *et al.* 2006). In Mexico, a package of essential health services was devised using cost-effectiveness criteria as a priority-setting tool. However, the package was also a means to ensure that all citizens, regardless of their labour or socioeconomic status, have the right to universal access to healthcare. The Mexican model may be seen as reconciling two extremes: The selective, technocratic approach to the distribution of healthcare, which provides practical alternatives but is usually morally neutral, and the rights-based approach, which has a strong value foundation but has lacked operational support (Frenk & Gómez-Dantés 2007).

Political commitment for equity is also required to correct the inequities that result from discrimination on the basis of gender, race, ethnic group, and religion. Often, inequalities in health status reflect the marginalization of disadvantaged groups (Brockerhoff & Hewett 2000). The plight of indigenous populations in the Americas and Australasia is a special case.

In weighing policy options, a good guideline would be to examine critically the expected impact of the selected option on equity. The formulation of health policies has to contend with a variety of pressures including the increasing demands of populations for more services, the desire to achieve maximal improvement in health of the populations served, and the need to contain costs. Reforms of the health sector aim at improving efficiency, effectiveness, cost-effectiveness, and equity. It is not always easy to reconcile these goals. For example, the delivery of care to the populations in remote areas is relatively expensive and less cost-effective than services to dense urban areas. However, in the interest of equity, health services should reach the underserved populations even in remote settings.

The impact of macroeconomic policies on health also deserves attention. For example, under pressure from the international finance agencies, some developing countries undertook Structural Adjustment Programmes (SAP) and markedly reduced public investment in health and other social sectors. UNICEF (2004) and other agencies drew attention to negative impact of SAP on the health of children. In future, careful analysis and relevant research would be used to design macroeconomic policies that would not harm the health of vulnerable groups. The international community has responded to this problem by adopting policies for alleviating poverty. Debt relief for the poorest nations has been one of the major mechanisms for alleviating poverty.

One aspect of equity is that the government should allocate financial resources fairly to the entire population. A simple demographic formula that allocates funds simply on population size may need to be adjusted to take note of special needs of particular regions; otherwise, the uniform allocation may tend to perpetuate inequalities. Another source of inequity is the degree to which local authorities can raise additional funds through taxation and by retaining user fees (Brikci & Phillips 2007). Again, the fact that the more affluent areas are able to raise much larger funds than the poorer areas may tend to widen the gap in the quantity and quality of healthcare.

Within the health budget, there is the difficult task of allocating resources to the needs of the various groups within the community. (Castro-Leal *et al.* 2000; Makinen *et al.* 2000) With finite resources, even the most affluent nations have to accept limits to the services that the public sector can provide. Hence, rationing is an inevitable feature of health planning. In the interests of equity and social justice, if economies have to be made, the burden should be fairly shared among various sectors of the community. Quantitative estimates of burden of disease and of the cost-effectiveness of various interventions help to rationalize the selection of priorities (Murray 1994a,b,c; Hyder 1998). But a point is reached at which hard choices cannot be made solely on the basis of objective measurements. At this stage, the debate must include philosophical and ethical considerations about the value of human life (Morrow & Bryant 1995).

The Poverty Reduction Strategy Papers (PRSPs) are a promising avenue to focus policy making on the poor, although much needs to be done to influence health policy making through this strategy (Laterveer *et al.* 2003). The majority of PRSPs lack country-specific data on the distribution and composition of the burden of disease, a clear identification of health system constraints and an assessment of the impact of health services on the population. More importantly, they make little effort to analyse these issues in relation to the poor. Furthermore, only a small group explicitly includes the interests of the poor in health policy design. Attention to policies aiming at enhancing equity in public health spending is even more limited. Few papers that include expenditure proposals also show pro-poor focused health budgets.

Tools are available to trace the extent to which investments at national levels benefit the poor and needy, taking into consideration the effects on income and health and considering the relative size of benefits given the levels of health and income (Gwatkin 2000, 2003). The better-off in Africa and in India benefit far more than the poor from public spending (Castro Leal *et al.* 2000). Recent analyses in Mexico suggest that the incidence of health benefits is improving for the poor thanks to financial reforms, although still inequitable (Frenk *et al.* 2006). However, analysis of a wide range of evidence suggests that tax-based funding distributes health benefits more evenly and targets the poor more effectively than social health insurance (Wagstaff 2007).

New tools are also being developed to forecast demand for global health funding of programmes benefiting the poor (Sekhri 2006). These efforts stem from the realization that the lack of accurate and credible information about the demand for essential health products costs lives. Gaps and weaknesses in demand forecasting result in a mismatch between supply and demand—which in turn leads to both unnecessarily high prices and supply shortages.

Equity information, monitoring, and evaluation

In order to design services that are equitable and to monitor performance of health services, each health authority needs an appropriate management information system which must include measuring inequalities in health status and inequities in access to healthcare. The data collecting instruments must be designed to take note of groups and sub-groups especially vulnerable groups whose access to services is restricted by geographical, economic, social, and cultural factors. It should include the usual demographic indicators—age, sex, and marital status, as well as socioeconomic indicators—race, ethnic origin, occupation, residence, and other social variables (Rosen 1999).

The health system should include mechanisms for monitoring equity objectively. Interest in measuring equity has generated some useful tools and some valuable experience is accumulating. In the first instance, monitoring equity is the responsibility of health authorities at each level of care. They must build into their service, sensitive indicators that would inform them of their performance with regard to equity and access to care.

In addition to such internal processes, it would be valuable to commission independent reviews of equity within the health system by groups outside the health departments. Another option would be to assign responsibility for a national equity watch to a local non-governmental organization.

International organizations

International organizations are influential in developing country policy in many conditions. A new breed of agencies, the Global Health Programs and the Public–Private Partnerships (PPPs) are also increasing their influence, particularly through financing health interventions.

UN agencies

The World Health Organization is the lead agency for health within the United Nations system. In recent years, other international agencies have increased their involvement in the health sector. The United Nations Children's Fund (UNICEF) through its child survival programme, provides massive input into the health sector often in collaboration with WHO. Other UN agencies like the United Nations Fund for Population Action (UNFPA), the International Labour

Organisation (ILO), and the Food and Agricultural Organisation (FAO) have relevant programmes involving specific aspects of the health sector. Through its lending programme, the World Bank represents an important source of external finance for the health sector and has stimulated countries to develop more efficient and cost-effective health programmes.

Generally, these external agencies operate independently of each other at country level but there have been some attempts at co-ordination and collaboration. UNICEF and WHO have established mechanisms of collaboration including such formal mechanism as the Task Force for Child Survival. WHO also sometimes executes health programmes on behalf of other external agencies. A more ambitious attempt at inter-agency collaboration is the UNAIDS programme; six UN agencies jointly manage this programme for the global control of HIV/AIDS epidemic.

Global Health Programmes and public–private partnerships

There has been a proliferation of Global Health Programmes (GHPs) and public–private partnerships, with more than 70 in existence. They account for close to 20 per cent of international aid for health. Examples include Roll Back Malaria (RBM); the Global Alliance on Vaccines and Immunization (GAVI), the International AIDS Vaccine Initiative. (IAVI) and the Global Fund for AIDS, TB and Malaria (GFATM). The vast majority focus on communicable diseases—60 per cent of identified GHPs target the big three diseases—HIV/AIDS, TB, and malaria—with HIV/AIDS attracting the most GHPs by some margin. However, almost all the 'most neglected' diseases (such as lymphatic filariasis and leishmaniasis) are now supported by at least one GHP, many of which have been established in recent years. No GHPs address non-communicable diseases, or health systems per se.

Africa has the highest number of GHPs per country, followed by Asia (East, Southeast, and Central). GHPs vary substantially in scale, cost, operational structure, and impact on systems at country level, including research and development as well as technical assistance and service support. GHPs which support improved service access may provide discounted or donated drugs, and give technical assistance. Some GHPs are dedicated to advocacy for increased international and/or national response and resource mobilization. The Global Fund is dedicated to financing for specific disease programmes.

GHPs are generally considered to deliver positive results in the following areas: Leverage of additional funds (including from private sector); promotion of global public goods; raising profile of neglected issues; more inclusive governance; enhanced aid effectiveness through pooling of resources, and reduced commodity prices. On the other hand, common criticisms levelled at GHPs are the creation of additional complexity in an international aid system that is already overloaded. For certain GHPs, poorer countries do not meet eligibility criteria or have the capacity to frame successful proposals. Other limitations include the distortion of national priorities; the provision of international aid made ad hoc and less predictable; dysfunctional national coordination mechanisms; the establishment of parallel structures or additional burden on existing national systems; displacement of existing government services; disproportionate demands on time of Ministers and senior officials; national strategic planning and budgeting processes undermined, and diminished political accountability (Buse & Wasxman 2001; Widdus 2003).

Health research

In many respects, health policy in developing countries is all about the encouragement of innovation and the scaling-up of life-saving technologies and system processes. As highlighted previously, increased access to knowledge and technology has accounted for perhaps as much as two-thirds of the 2 per cent per year rate of decline in under-5 mortality rate (Jamison 2006). Furthermore, there is increasing realization that research and evaluation can play a valuable role for shared learning from health sector reforms (González Block 1997).

The case has been made that it is as unethical to introduce health reforms that have not been previously validated or thoroughly analysed as it is to introduce untested medical technology into healthcare. Indeed, both can have important health consequences, even more so population interventions that are adopted on a massive scale (Daniels 2006). WHO has recognized that 'Ignoring research evidence is harmful to individuals and populations, and wastes resources' (WHO 2004).

Health research—including health policy and systems research—thus plays a double role in policy making. As a core function of health systems, research contributes knowledge as one of the most critical resources for healthcare. Formulating and implementing health research policy is therefore a key component of health policy overall. On the other hand, research on health policy and systems contributes knowledge and applications to improve the way that societies organize themselves to respond to health problems and challenges (Alliance HPSR 2004). Such knowledge is today one of the scarce resources limiting health system performance.

Health research systems and policy

WHO together with the Council on Health Research for Development and the Global Forum for Health Research advocating health research policy through the development of health research systems at national level and through a well- structured international architecture (Pang *et al.* 2003). Health research systems should be strengthened by building relevant capacity, developing capable leadership, providing essential monitoring and evaluation tools, improving capacity for ethical review of research, and putting in place necessary ethical standards and regulations for population health, health services, and clinical research. Health systems should further promote access to reliable, relevant, and up-to-date evidence on the effects of interventions, based on systematic reviews of the totality of available research findings (WHO 2004).

Health research systems provide a promising opportunity to link knowledge generation with practical concerns to improve health and health equity. Pioneer health research systems from Canada and the UK show that academic centres and service agencies can be related in ways that encourage the utilization of research (Lomas 2000; Henkel *et al.* 2006), such as networking between existing stakeholders (Department of Health 2006). A key issue is the balance between funding research through independent research councils that have science-led priorities and funding research in response to the priorities of healthcare systems.

New science frameworks are solving these dilemmas through positing a move from the traditional discipline-centred mode of knowledge production (characterized as Mode 1), towards a broader conception (Mode 2) where knowledge is generated through a context of application and thus addresses problems identified through continual negotiation between actors from a variety of settings (Gibbons *et al.* 1994). Another conceptualization, Pasteur's Quadrant, suggests how types of research can be considered according to two dimensions, a quest for understanding and considerations of use. This gives rise to three categories of research depending on the extent to which general understanding arises in the process of solving specific problems, or whether only pure knowledge or pure application is generated (Stokes 1997).

Evidence-based policy making

The new science frameworks are being applied to policy making though novel strategies such as the interfaces and receptor model (Hanney *et al.* 2003) or the 'linkage and exchange' model proposed by the Canadian Health Services Research Foundation (Lomas 2000). Such strategies are promoting collaborative approaches to organizing health research systems. It has also promoted the use of knowledge brokers between researchers and policy makers. In the end, demonstrating the benefits or research for policy making and for population health and national well-being will be critical (Hanney & Gonzalez Block 2006).

Evidence-based policy making can be made a reality if research and analysis is carefully introduced along the critical steps of issue identification, policy development, implementation, monitoring, evaluation, and feedback. Evidence can provide the rationale for an initial policy direction; it can set out the nature and extent of the problem, suggest possible solutions, look to the likely impacts in the future, and evidence from piloting and evaluation can provide motivation for adjustments to a policy or the way it is to be implemented (Campbell *et al.* 2007).

Conclusion

Policy making for the design, implementation, and management of effective, efficient, and equitable health systems is today more critical than ever to address the developing country health challenges. Health policy is being called not only to address the pressing needs of infectious diseases and malnutrition and the emerging problems of violence, lesions, tobacco, and obesity. New challenges are being addressed, including the fight against poverty and the increasing global threats. The belief that sound health policy making can contribute to democracy, economic growth, and global security has influenced the availability of greater financial resources for health. However, relaxing this constraint has now brought much greater awareness to needs in key areas such as human resources and health system strengthening and research.

The information now being produced can provide valuable guidance to policy makers, although it also threatens to overpower capacities in poor countries. Not only must policy making be knowledge-based—it must also be result-oriented. Careful planning and skilled management can achieve good results even where financial resources are limited. The countries that have achieved good health at low cost challenge other countries to adapt and adopt relevant aspects of their policies.

Policy makers must give high priority to strategies that will eliminate the major items of the unfinished agenda that still plague many developing countries. Many lives can be saved and much disability prevented by measures like boosting immunization programmes, ensuring access to adequate supplies of safe water and good sanitation, by providing effective treatment for common childhood ailments, and ensuring skilled care during childbirth including emergency obstetric care (Center for Global Development 2007). More daunting tasks include the pandemic of HIV/AIDS and the emerging non-communicable challenges, which may require complex and expensive care. Experience has shown that some progress can be made through the application of social and behavioural interventions, that can act on those risks that are responsible for the increasing burden of disease associated to chronic ailments and injuries in the developing world.

Key points

- Health policy making in developing countries is intricately related to global health policies and actors.
- Health financing is increasing, thanks to policy advocacy, but more resources and improved governance are required to meet the Millennium Development Goals.
- Policy tools are available to support decision making at national and global levels.
- Equity and efficiency trade-offs should be addressed on the basis of sound research and health research systems.

References

Alliance AHPSR (2004). *Strengthening health systems: The role and promise of policy and systems research*. Alliance AHPSR, Geneva, Switzerland.

Ameratunga, S., Hijar, M., and Norton, R. (2006). Road-traffic injuries: Confronting disparities to address a global-health problem. *Lancet*, **367**, 1533–40.

Armstrong, J.L. (1997) Stewardship and public service. Ottawa, Canadian Public Service Commission, (discussion paper).

Anand, S. and Hanson. K. (1997). Disability-adjusted life years: A critical review. *Journal of Health Economics*. Dec; **16**(6), 685–702.

Bankauskaite, V., Dubois, H.F.W., and Saltman, R. (2007). Patterns of decentralization across European health systems. In *Decentralization in health care* (eds. R. Saltman *et al.*), pp. 22–43. WHO, UK.

Berman, P.A. (1997). National health accounts in developing countries: Appropriate methods and recent applications. *Health Economics*, **6**, 11–30.

Berman, T.J. and Bossert, T. (2000). *A decade of health sector reform in developing countries: What have we learned?* Data for Decision Making Project. IHSG. Harvard School of Public Health.

Black, D., Morris, J.N., Smith, C. *et al.* (1998). Better benefits for health: plan to implement the central recommendation of the Acheson report. *British Medical Journal*, **318**, 724–7.

Bossert, T. and Beauvais, J.C. (2002). Decentralization of health systems in Ghana, Zambia, Uganda and the Philippines: A comparative analysis of decision space. *Health Policy and Planning*, **17**, 14–31.

Bossert, T., Larrañaga, O., Giedion, U. *et al.* (2003). Decentralization and equity of resource allocation: Evidence from Colombia and Chile. *Bulletin of the World Health Organization*, **91**, 95–100.

Bossert, T. (1998). Analyzing the decentralization of health systems in developing countries: Decision space, innovation and performance. *Social science & medicine*, **47**, 1513–27.

Brikci, N., Philips, M. (2007). User fees or equity funds in low-income countries. *Lancet*, **369**(9555), 10–11.

Brockerhoff, M. and Hewett, P.C. (2000). Inequality of child mortality among ethnic groups in sub-Saharan Africa. *Bulletin of the World Health Organization*, **78**, 30–41.

Brown, A.M. Foster, A., Norton, A. *et al.* (2001). *The status of sector-wide approaches.* Working Paper 142. ODI, London.

Brush, B., Sochalski, J., and Berger, A. (2004). Imported care: Recruiting foreign nurses to US health care facilities. *Health Affairs*, **23**(5).

Buse, K. and Waxman, A. (2001). Public–private health partnerships: A strategy for WHO. *Bulletin of the World Health Organization*, **79**(8).

Campbell, S., Benita, S., Coates, E. *et al.* (2007). *Analysis for policy: Evidence-based policy in practice.* Government Social Research Unit, HM Treasury, London.

Castro-Leal, F., Dayton, J., Demery, L. *et al.* (2000). Public spending on health care in Africa: Do the poor benefit? *Bulletin of the World Health Organization*, **78**(1), 66–74.

Centre for Global Development (2007). *Millions saved: Proven successes in global health.* 2007 Edition. CGD, Washington.

Cleland, J. and Van Ginneken, J. (1989). Maternal schooling and childhood mortality. *Journal of biosocial science*, **10**(Suppl.), 13–34.

Clements, M., Radelet, S., and Bhavnani, R. (2004). *Counting chickens when they hatch: The short-term effect of aid on growth.* Working Paper 44, Center for Global Development, Washington DC.

Commission on Macroeconomics and Health (2001). *Macroeconomics and Health: Investing in Health for Economic Development—Report of the Commission on Macroeconomics and Health.* December 20, World Health Organization, Geneva.

Dahlgren, G. and Whitehead, M. (1991). *Policies and strategies to promote equity in health.* WHO Regional Office, Copenhagen.

Daniels, N. (2006). Toward ethical review of health system transformations. *American Journal of Public Health*, **96**, 3.

Daniels, N., Flores, W., Pannarunotha, S. *et al.* (2005). An evidence-based approach to benchmarking the fairness of health-sector reform in developing countries. *Bulletin of the World Health Organization*, **83**(7), 534–539.

Daniels, N., Light, D.W., and Caplan, R.L. (1996). *Benchmarks of fairness for health care reform.* Oxford University Press, New York.

Dare, L. and Reeler, A. (2005). Health systems financing: Putting together the 'back office'. *British Medical Journal*, **331**, 759–62.

De Savigny, D., Kasale, H., Mbuya, C. *et al.* (2004). *Fixing health systems.* IDRC, Ottawa.

Denis, J. and Lomas, J. (2003). Convergent evolution: The academic and policy roots of collaborative research. *Journal of Health Services Research & Policy*, **8**, 1–6.

Department of Health (2006). *Best research for best health: A new national health research strategy.* London.

Davis, J., Donaldson, L., Schoorman, D. (1997) Towards a stewardship theory of management. Academy of Management Review, **22**(1), 20–47.

Evans, R., Barer, M., and Marmor, T. (1994). Why are some people healthy and others not? The determinants of health of populations. Aldine de Gruyter, Hawthome (NY).

Feacham, R.G.A. (2000). Poverty and inequity: A proper focus for the new century. *Bulletin of World Health Organization*, **78**(1), 1.

Filmer, D., Hammer, J.S., and Pritchett, L.S. (2000). Weak links in the chain: A diagnosis of health policy in poor countries. *World Bank Research Observer*, **15**(2), 199–224.

Frenk, J. and Gómez-Dantés, O. (2007). La globalización y la nueva salud pública. *Salud publica de Mexico*, **49**(2), 156–164.

Frenk, J. (1994). Dimensions of health system reform. *Health Policy*, **27**(1), 19–34.

Frenk, J., Bobadilla, J., Sepúlveda, J. *et al.* (1989). Health transition in middle-income countries: New challenges for health care. *Health Policy and Planning*, **4**(1), 29–39.

Frenk, J., Gonzalez-Pier, E., Gómez-Dantes, O. *et al.*(2006). Comprehensive reform to improve health system performance in Mexico. *Lancet*, **368**, 1524–34.

Frenk, J., Lozano, R., and Gonzalez Block, M.A. (1994). *Economía y salud: propuestas para el avance del sistema de salud en México.* Fundación Mexicana para la Salud, 1994, Mexico, DF.

Gakidou, E., Lozano, R., González-Pier, E. *et al.*(2006). Assessing the effect of the 2001–06 Mexican health reform: An interim report card. *The Lancet*, **368**(9550), 1920–35 E.

Garret, L. (2007). The challenge of global health. *Foreign Affairs*, **86**, 14–38.

Gericke, C.A., Kurowski, C., Ranson, M.K. *et al.* (2005). Intervention complexity – a conceptual framework to inform priority-setting in health. *Bulletin of the World Health Organization*, **83**, 285–293.

Gibbons, M., Limoges, C., Nowotny, H. *et al.* (1994). *The new production of knowledge: The dynamics of science and research in contemporary societies.* Sage, London.

Gilson, L. (2003). Trust and the development of health care as a social institution. *Social Science & Medicine*, **56**, 1453–68.

Gonzalez-Block, M.A. (1997). Comparative research and analysis methods for shared learning from health system reforms. *Health Policy*, **42**, 187–209.

Gwatkin, D.R. (2000). Critical reflection: Health inequalities and the health of the poor: What do we know? What can we do? *Bulletin of the World Health Organization*, **78**(1), 3–18.

Gwatkin, D.R. (2003). How well do health programmes reach the poor? *Lancet*, **361**, 540–1.

Hanney, S. and González-Block, M.A. (2006). Building health research systems to achieve better health. *Health Research Policy and Systems*, **4**, 1–6. www.health-policy-systems.com/content/4/1/10

Hanney, S.R., Gonzalez-Block, M.A., Buxton, M.J. *et al.* (2003). The utilisation of health research in policy-making: Concepts, examples and methods of assessment. *Health Research Policy and Systems*, **1**: 2.

Harrison, K. (1997). The importance of the educated healthy woman in Africa. *Lancet*, **349**, 588.

Hecht, R.M. and Shah, R. (2006). Recent trends and innovations in development assistance for health. In *Disease Control Priorities in Developing Countries* (eds. D.T. Jamison, J.G. Breman, A.R. Measham, G. Alleyne, M. Claeson, D.B. Evans *et al.*), 2nd edition, pp. 3–34. Oxford University Press for The World Bank, 2006, Washington, DC.

Hutton, G. (2002). *Decentralization and the sector-wide approach in the health sector.* SDS, Basel.

Hyder, A.A., Rotllant, G., and Morrow, R.H. (1998). Measuring the burden of disease: Healthy life-years. *American Journal of Public Health*, **88**, 196–202.

Irwin, A., Valentine, N., Brown, C. *et al.* (2006). The Commission on social determinants of health: Tackling the social roots of health inequities. *PLoS medicine*, **3**(6), e106. doi:10.1371/journal.pmed.0030106.

Jacobs, B. and Price, N. (2006). Improving access for the poorest to public sector health services: Insights from Kirivong Operational Health District in Cambodia. *Health Policy Plan*, Jan, **21**(1), 27–39.

Jamison, D.T. (2006). Investing in Health. In *Disease control priorities in developing countries* (eds. D.T. Jamison, J.G. Breman, A.R. Measham, G. Alleyne, M. Claeson, D.B. Evans *et al.*), 2nd edition, pp. 3–34. Oxford University Press for The World Bank, 2006, Washington, DC.

Joint Learning Initiative (2004). *Human resources for health. Overcoming the crisis.* Harvard University Press, Cambridge.

Knaul and Frenk (2005). Health insurance in Mexico: Achieving universal coverage through structural reform. *Health Affairs*, **24**, 1467–76.

Kogan, M., Henkel, M., and Hanney, S. (2006). *Government and research: Thirty Years of evolution*, 2nd edition. Springer, Dordrecht.

Laterveer, L., Niessen, L.W., and Yazbeck, A.S. (2003). Pro-poor health policies in poverty reduction strategies. *Health Policy Plan*, **18**, 138–45.

Lavorack, G. and Labonte, R. (2000). A planning framework for community empowerment goals within health promotion. *Health Policy and Planning*, **15**(3), 255–62.

Lomas, J. (2000). Using 'linkage and exchange' to move research into policy at a Canadian Foundation. *Health Affairs*, **19**, 236–40.

Londono, J. and Frenk, J. (1997). Structured pluralism: Towards an innovative model for health system reform in Latin America. *Health Policy*, **41**(1), 1–36.

Lopez, A.D., Mathers, C.D., Ezzati, M. *et al.* (2006). Global and regional burden of disease and risk factors, 2001: Systematic analysis of population health data. *Lancet*. Jul 29; **368**(9533), 365.

Lozano, R., Soliz, P., Gakidou, E. *et al.* (2006). Benchmarking of performance of Mexican states with effective coverage. *The Lancet*, **368** (9548), 1729–41.

Lucas, A.O. (2005). Human resources for health in Africa. Better training and firm national policies might manage the brain drain. *British Medical Journal*, 5 November, **331**, 1037–8.

Lucas, A.O. (1992). Public access to health information as a human right. *Proceedings of the International Symposium on Public Health Surveillance. Morbidity & Mortality Weekly Report*, **41**, 77–8.

Makinen, M., Waters, H., Rauch, M. *et al.* (2000). Inequalities in health care use and expenditures: Empirical data from eight developing countries and countries in transition. *Bulletin of the World Health Organization*, **78**, 55–65.

Marek, T., Diallo, I., Ndiaye, B. *et al.* (1999). Successful contracting of prevention services: Fighting malnutrition in Senegal and Madagascar. *Health Policy and Planning*, **14**(4), 382–9.

Mathers, C.D. and Loncar, D. (2006). Projections of global mortality and burden of disease from 2002 to 2030. *PLoS Medicine*, **3**(11), e442. doi:10.1371/journal.pmed.0030442

McCarthy, J. and Maine, D. (1992). A framework for analyzing the determinants of maternal mortality. *Studies in family planning*, **23**, 23–33.

Medlin, C.A., Chowdhury, M., Jamison, D.T. *et al.* (2006). Improving the health of populations: Lessons of experience. In *Disease control priorities in developing countries* (eds. D. Jamison *et al.*), The World Bank, Washington DC.

Meessen, B., Van Damme, W., Kirunga Tashobya, C. *et al.* (2006). Poverty and user fees for public health care in low-income countries: lessons from Uganda and Cambodia. *The Lancet*, **368**, 2253–7.

Meng, Q., Shi, G., Yang, H. *et al.* (2004). *Health policy and systems research in China*. UNICEF/UNDP/World Bank/WHO. Special Programme for Research and Training in Tropical Diseases (TDR), Geneva.

Mills, A., Brugha, R., Hanson, K. *et al.* (2002). What can be done about the private health sector in low-income countries? *Bulletin of the World Health Organization*, **80**, 325–30.

Molineux, D. and Nantulya, V. (2004). Linking disease control programmes in rural Africa: A pro-poor strategy to reach Abuja targets and Millennium Development Goals. *British Medical Journal*, **328**(7448), 1129–32.

Morrow, R.H. and Bryant, J. (1995). Health policy approaches to measuring and valuing human life: Conceptual and ethical issues. *American journal of public health*, **85**, 1356–60.

Murray, C.J. (1994a). Quantifying the burden of disease: The technical basis for disability-adjusted life years. *Bulletin of the World Health Organization*, **72**, 429–45.

Murray, C.J. (1994b). National health expenditures: A global analysis. *Bulletin of the World Health Organization*, **72**, 623–37.

Murray, C.J. (1994c). Cost-effectiveness analysis and policy choices: Investing in health systems. *Bulletin of the World Health Organization*, **72**, 663–74.

Murray, C.J.L. and Evans, D.B. (eds.)(2003). *Health systems performance assessment: Debates, methods and empiricism*. WHO, Geneva.

Musgrove, P. (1999). Public spending on health care: How are different criteria related? *Health Policy*, 47.

Narasimhan, V., Brown, H., Pablos-Mendez, A. *et al.* (2004). Responding to the global human resources crisis. *Lancet*, **363**(9419), 1469–72.

Palmer, N., Mills, A., Wadee, H. *et al.* (2003). A new face for private providers in developing countries: What implications for public health? *Bulletin of the World Health Organization*, **81**(4), 292–7.

Pang, T., Sadana, R., Hanney, S. *et al.* (2003). Knowledge for better health—a conceptual framework and foundation for health research systems. *Bulletin of the World Health Organization*, **81**(11).

Paris declaration on AID effectiveness Ownership, Harmonisation Alignment Results and Mutual Accountability Paris, 2 March 2005.

Phillips, D.R. (1990) '*Health and health care in the third world*. Chapter 4. Longmans, UK.

Population Reference Bureau (2004). *Improving the health of the world's poorest people*. Population Reference Bureau, Washington.

Pollock, A.M. (1999). '*Devolution and health: challenges to Scotland and Wales*'. *British Medical Journal*, **319**, 94–8.

Preker, A.S., Carrin, G., Dror, D. *et al.* (2002). Effectiveness of community health financing in meeting the cost of illness. *Bulletin of the World Heaflth Organization*, **80**(2), 143–50.

Preker, A.S., Suzuki, E., Bustero, F. *et al.* (2003). *Costing the Millennium Development Goals*. Background paper to The Millennium Development Goals for Health: Rising to the Challenges, World Bank, Washington, DC.

Roberts, M.J., Hsiao, W., Berman, P., Reich, M.R. (2004). Getting Health Reform Right: A guide to Improving Performance and Equity. Oxford University Press, New York.

Rosen, M. (1999). Data needs in studies on equity in health and access to care—ethical considerations. *Acta Oncologica*, **38**, 71–5.

Sachs, J. (2004). Health in the developing world: Achieving the Millennium Development Goals. *Bulletin of the World Health Organization*, Dec; **82**(12) 947–952.

Saltman, B. and Ferroussier-Davis, O. (2000). On the concept of stewardship in health policy. *Bulletin of the World Health Organization*, **78**(6), 732–9.

Savedoff, W.D. (2007). *Transparency and corruption in the health sector: A conceptual framework and ideas for action in Latin America and the Caribbean*. Inter-American Development Bank, Health Technical Note 03/2007, Washington, DC.

Schneider, M. (2001). *The setting of health research priorities in South Africa*. South African Medical Research Council, Burden of Disease Research Unit, Johannesburg.

Sekhri, N. (2006). *Forecasting for global health: New money, new products & new markets*. Background Paper for the Forecasting Working Group. Center for Global Development, Washington.

Slack, K., Savedoff, W.D. (2001). '*Public purchaser-private provider contracting for health services: Examples from Latin America and the Caribbean*'. Sustainable Development Department Technical Paper 111, Inter-American Development Bank, Washington, DC.

Söderlund, N., Mendoza-Arana, P., and Goudge, J. (2003). *The new public/private mix in health: Exploring the changing landscape*. Alliance for Health policy and Systems Research, Geneva.

Spiegel, J.M. and Yassi, A. (2004). Lessons from the margins of globalization: Appreciating the Cuban health paradox. *Journal of public health policy*, **25**(1), 85–110(26).

Stokes, D.E. (1997). *Pasteur's quadrant: Basic science and technological innovation*. Brookings Institute, Washington DC.

Taipale, V. (1999). 'Ethics and allocation of health resources—the influence of poverty on health'. *Acta Oncologica*, **38**(1), 51–5.

Tena–Tamayo, C. and Sotelo, J. (2005). Malpractice in Mexico: Arbitration not litigation. *British Medical Journal*, 20 August; **331**, 448–51.

Unger, J.P., De Paepe, P., and Green, A. (2003). A code of best practice for disease control Programmes to avoid damaging health care services in developing countries. International *Journal of Health Planning and Management*, **18**, S27–S39.

Ugalde, A. and Homedes, N. (2006). Decentralization: The long road from theory to practice. In *Health services decentralization in Mexico. A case study in state reform* (eds. A. Ugalde and N. Homedes). Center for US-Mexico Studies, La Jolla.

UNICEF (2004). *Progress for children. A child survival report card: Number 1.*

Whitehead, M. (1990). The concepts and principles of equity and health. WHO Regional Office, Copenhagen.

Wagstaff, A. (2002). Poverty and health sector inequalities. *Bulletin of the World Health Organization*, **80**(2), 97–105.

Wagstaff, A. (2007). *Social health insurance reexamined*. World Bank Policy Research Working Paper 4111, January.

WHO (2000). *'Health systems: Improving performance'*. World Health Report 2000, WHO, Geneva.

WHO (2003). *Guide to producing national health accounts with special applications for low-income and middle-income countries*. WHO, 2003, Geneva.

WHO (2004). *Knowledge for better health: Strengthening health systems*. The Mexico Statement on Health Research from the Ministerial Summit on Health Research. Mexico City, November 16–20.

WHO (2004). Ministerial Summit (Web). World Health Organization. World Health Report 2004. *Changing history*. WHO, 2004, Ginebra.

WHO (2005). *Preventing chronic diseases: A vital investment*. WHO, Geneva.

WHO (2006) Human resources for health: The World Health Report 2006, Working Together for Health. WHO, 2006, Geneva.

WHO (2006) *Investing in Health Research and Development. Report of the Ad Hoc Committee on Health Research Relating to Future Intervention Options.* WHO, Geneva.

WHO (2007). Health Metrics Network Biennial Report 2005/2006. WHO, Geneva.Widdus, R. (2003). Public–private partnerships for health require thoughtful evaluation. *Bulletin of the World Health Organization*, **81**(4), 235.

World Bank–IMF Development Committee (2003). *Supporting sound policies with adequate and appropriate financing'*. Discussion paper, World Bank, Washington DC.

3.4

Leadership in public health

Manuel M. Dayrit and Maia Ambegaokar

Introduction

Imagine that tomorrow you were suddenly appointed into a prominent health leader position in your country—as a Director of Department or perhaps even Minister of Health. Upon taking office, you are presented with the following urgent dilemmas by your chief advisers:

- We are suffering perennial outbreaks of water-borne diarrhoea in the urban slums of our largest city, caused by the illegal tapping of water lines. How can we prevent this in both the short and long terms?
- Other departments are preventing us enacting any measures to stop smoking in public places. How can we convince them to collaborate on this critical health issue?
- How can we take steps to provide anti-retrovirals for the tens of thousands of our citizens suffering from HIV/AIDS?
- Our government is in moral opposition to abortion, despite scientific evidence showing that decriminalizing abortion prevents maternal deaths from sepsis. Illegal abortion is high in our country. What action should we take?

How would you proceed to address these issues? Would you be able to think on your feet and respond promptly and effectively to the health needs of your populace? In other words, are you capable of being a public health leader?

These questions are examined below as we explore the nature of leadership and the possibility of learning it.

Chapter overview

There is growing recognition of the importance of leadership in public health. This is reflected in recent domestic and international initiatives to train or 'develop' leaders in the health sector (Cardenas *et al.* 2002; Saleh *et al.* 2004; Umble *et al.* 2005; Wright *et al.* 2001), to identify the skills and personal qualities of leaders (NHS Leadership Centre 2006; Wright *et al.* 2000), and to assess the effect of different types of leadership on outcomes (Firth-Cozens & Mowbray 2001; Xirasagar *et al.* 2005). In this chapter, we examine what is involved in public health leadership and illustrate our themes with experiences from the working lives of some contemporary health sector leaders. We set four tasks: To define the difference between management and leadership; to describe the core competencies and personal characteristics of leaders; to discuss whether leadership can be taught; and to demonstrate why leadership is so important in public health. We argue that it is the complex, multi-organizational, and team-based nature of health work that necessitates leadership at many levels in order to result in success.

The broader goal in this chapter is to present the reader with the information required to forge a personal 'path to leadership'. There is an urgent need around the world for strong public health leaders to promote the health of populations, particularly the poor and vulnerable. Unfortunately, calls for stronger and better leadership are often taken as imprecise and unachievable demands. In this chapter, we attempt to circumvent that accusation by demonstrating that effective leaders have existed and continue to exist in health, and that strong leadership can be encouraged and developed. In addition, we have built the chapter on findings from interviews with individual health sector leaders.

We look in detail at the way in which the perception of leadership has evolved over the years. Having established the important distinction between 'management' and 'leadership', we explore three different aspects of leadership: the competencies of leadership; the personal characteristics of recognized leaders; and the broad division of leadership styles into either transactional or transformational. We then look to the question of whether leadership can be taught, examining existing methods and frameworks for leadership instruction and development, and we investigate how to measure leadership ability and assess the impact made by individual leaders. Finally, we compare the more theoretical findings of our chapter with public health leadership in practice, discovering the complex nature of the reality faced by public health leaders today.

At the end of the chapter, we turn to the targeted reader of this book—an early-to-mid-career public health worker—and suggest ways to develop his or her own 'path to leadership'. We urge the aspiring health leader not to forget the inseparable link between what is needed for leadership to occur and the kind of principled leadership most required in global health today.

Among the chapter's most important points:

- There is a distinction between leadership and management. Leadership has to do with the visionary activities of setting direction, while management has to do with the controlling tasks associated with implementation.

- Public health leaders need to be able to imagine and create evidence-based change. They need to be able to influence and lobby key actors for support of their public health agenda. They must operate across disciplinary and organizational boundaries, and they must be skilled at developing and working through diverse teams.
- Leaders are not simply born. Public health leaders can be developed by means of team-based training, mentoring and repeated practice of leadership skills at all levels and all types of public health organization. The aspiring health leader can create her or his path to leadership.
- Public health challenges are often politically and procedurally complex and do not lend themselves to simple medical or technical solutions. A set of guiding principles will help the leader to define appropriate actions.

Evolution of thinking about leadership

A century or so ago, thinking about leadership focused on the inherent personality of the individual and 'his or her characteristics and traits . . . were thought to be hereditary' (*Turning Point* 2001, p. 14).

> *This 'Great Man Theory' approached leadership capacities as innate, fixed and cross-contextual. Skills and competencies as learned activities were disregarded. Instead, they were thought to be anchored in some internal personality or genetic set with which one was born. . . .[T]his earlier understanding of leadership [also] focused on the leader as solitary actor, as if the followers or context had no role in the leadership situation.* (*Turning Point* 2001, p. 14)

This 'great leader' theory has certainly been invoked in the health sector. For example, Halfdan Mahler, a former head of the World Health Organization, and James Grant, a former head of UNICEF, were widely thought to have innate leadership qualities that largely explained the success of their agendas. It is true, as the experiences described in our interviews demonstrate, that leaders are often people who are willing to take risks and to do things that defy convention. However, research and thinking on the question of leadership moved on in the middle of the twentieth century to consider the skills and competencies that anyone in a leadership position, regardless of personality, might develop in order to influence followers to take desired actions.

More recently, the focus has been on leaders as those who can see the way forward in the context of complexity and constant change. For a leader, achieving results in such a context requires not just the use of skills that will enable individuals to get things done, but also the ability to facilitate disparate group efforts by collaborating and sharing the leadership task:

> *. . . [W]e have shifted from a view of leader as sole or unitary actor to a team or community centred view of leadership, . . .[and] the social and economic times of most organizations have produced a demand for skills and abilities that are as complex as the situations in which they are found. The rapid change has moved leadership from a hierarchical model of leadership into collaborative models.* (*Turning Point* 2001, p. 15)

In public health, the collaborative approach may be a necessity, as discussed in a later section of this chapter dealing with the complexity inherent in public health practice. This shift in the way of thinking about leadership—from a top-down model to a participatory one—has been similar to that in the way of thinking about organizational management. So what is the relationship between management and leadership?

Leadership is not the same as management

Much literature and research conflate leadership and management, but the two are not identical.

> *'Management' derives from the Latin word* 'manus' *(meaning hand) and the subsequent Italian word* 'maneggiare' *(to control, often horses). In effect, the origin of 'management' is manifest in Ben Hur's epic chariot races—it concerns the control of unruly beasts. 'Leadership', however, is from the Old German word* 'Lidan' *and the Old English derivation* 'lithan' *(to travel, to show the way, to guide).* (Grint 2002, p. 248)

This distinction between the controlling tasks associated with implementation and the visionary activities associated with setting a direction is a useful, if simplified, way of defining management as compared to leadership. In practice, the two are often linked, in a single individual or in a particular job description. As a result, separating the characteristics of good leadership from those of good management is not straightforward.

To a certain extent, the confusion arises because historical reviews of research on leadership often begin with the early research on what makes a good manager. For example, Stone and Patterson (2005) begin with Max Weber's interest in bureaucratic hierarchies as an efficient solution to getting things done in the workplace. This led to Classical Management Theory, with its emphasis on using the bureaucracy to achieve objectives, and Scientific Management theories with their focus on 'control, ruthless efficiency, quantification, predictability, and de-skilled jobs' (Stone & Patterson 2005, p. 2). In this context, managers who could organize and direct workers below them in the hierarchy were crucial. There was little emphasis, during this period in the early part of the twentieth century, on the behavioural aspects of organizations. Instead, workers were seen as machine-like, and managers needed only to establish and oversee the correct procedures. By the middle of the twentieth century, management theorists shifted their focus to the factors that motivate people at work and the ways in which managers could harness motivation to achieve results. 'A new theory of organizations and leadership began to emerge based on the idea that individuals operate most effectively when their needs are satisfied' (Stone & Patterson 2005, p. 3). In this context, good managers were perceived as those who could do more than structure the work and give orders. They also needed to inspire their workers to lead them.

The tendency to link the characteristics of good managers with those of leaders is thus partly the result of changes in the understanding of the role of a manager. Still, the distinction between the leadership role and the managerial role is widely perceived as the difference between vision and implementation. Table 3.4.1, for example, shows one typical set of divisions.

These distinctions between leaders and managers apply as well in the health sector. For example, the director of a health district might choose to have an operations director who manages the finances and daily implementation, thus allowing her/himself the freedom

Table 3.4.1 Leadership vs. management functions

	Leadership functions	Management functions
Creating an agenda	*Establishing direction*: Vision of the future, develop strategies for change to achieve goals	*Plans and budgets*: Decide actions and timetable, allocate resources
Developing people	*Aligning people*: Communicate vision and strategy, influence creation of teams which accept validity of goals	*Organizing and staffing*: Decide structure and allocate staff, develop policies, procedures, and monitoring
Execution	*Motivating and inspiring*: Energize people to overcome obstacles, satisfy human needs	*Controlling, problem solving*: Monitor results against plan and take corrective action
Outcomes	Produces positive and sometimes dramatic change	Produces order, consistency, and predictability

Source: Huczynski & Buchanan, 2007, p. 698; based on John P. Kotter (1990) *A Force for Change: How Leadership Differs from Management*, Free Press, New York.

to develop strategies and engage diverse actors in a shared vision of the district's health goals. A hospital, to give another example, needs a manager who with limited finances can organize and implement a detailed schedule of surgeries involving people, equipment, and other resources. However, a hospital also needs a leader who can motivate staff to provide high-quality work in the context of budget restrictions. Sometimes these skills and job responsibilities may exist in the same person, but the nature of management tasks differ from leadership tasks.

In this chapter, we are particularly interested in leadership, rather than management. We do not mean to imply that competent management is not important. On the contrary, the ability to take care of the controlling tasks associated with implementation is crucial to the delivery of programmes and services in public health, and there is a great deal of research and funding targeting the improvement of management in order to strengthen the functioning of health systems (see, for example, Egger *et al.* 2005). However, the current interest in public health leadership is in itself worth exploring. Public health requires people who can move the agenda in a world dominated by the politics of vested interest groups. It requires individuals who can take scientific evidence and use it to change the direction of policy. This calls for 'big picture' skills and the ability to influence people both inside and outside the public health field.

What do these leaders do, exactly? We consider this question next, looking at critical competencies, personal characteristics, and the difference between transactional and transformational leadership.

Leadership competencies and personal qualities

The literature on leadership is replete with definitions and lists of leadership characteristics. In this section, we present two that are particularly thorough and intuitively useful in public health. However, we do so with a couple of caveats. First, research on leadership has not yet presented definitive descriptions, much less definitive prescriptions. As Grint (2002, p. 249) says: 'a science of leadership . . . has proved incredibly elusive . . . [and yet] there are indeed plenty of leadership recipes on the market'. In the health sector, this is as true as in other sectors.

Second, there is reason to be concerned that some of the elements of these lists may be 'culture-bound' and thus more accurate in the North American and European settings in which they were developed. Some research has identified culture-specific differences in observed leadership traits. For example, 'participatory' working behaviour may be more relevant in some cultural contexts than others (Flahault & Roemer 1986). Having said this, there is no harm in advocating the leadership behaviours presented in the two lists below—such as acting with high ethical integrity, developing an evidence-based vision of the future, and empowering others to work towards public health goals—whatever the cultural context.

Competencies of leaders in health

What do we expect leaders in public health to be able to do? One comprehensive list (Wright *et al.* 2000) defines the following core competencies of public health leaders:

1. Transformation—Public health needs and priorities require leaders to engage in systems thinking, including analytical and critical thinking processes, envisioning of potential futures, strategic and tactical assessment, and communication and change dynamics.
2. Legislation and politics—The field of public health requires leaders to have the competence to facilitate, negotiate, and collaborate in an increasingly competitive and contentious political environment.
3. Transorganization—The complexity of major public health problems extends beyond the scope of any single stakeholder group, community unit, profession or discipline, organization or government unit, thus requiring leaders with the skills to be effective beyond their organizational boundaries.
4. Team and group dynamics—Effective communication and practice are accomplished by leaders through building team and work group capacity and capability (Wright *et al.* 2000, p. 1204).

In other words, public health leaders need to be able to imagine and create evidence-based change; they need to be able to influence and lobby politicians for support of their public health agenda; they must operate across disciplinary and organizational boundaries; and they must be skilled at developing and working through diverse teams. The authors go on to give more detail about each competency area (Wright *et al.* 2000). We present a summary in Table 3.4.2. In a practical way, the information in this table answers the question: What do public health leaders do?

Interviews with public health leaders suggest that this is an appropriate list of the types of skills public health leaders need and use in varying degrees. All the leaders interviewed for this chapter had some vision of an alternate future to which they are committed. Whether it was to improve the health services in a remote location of Uganda, strengthen the performance of an international public health bureaucracy, or lead research towards better understanding of breast cancer, each had a vision of contributing towards improving

Table 3.4.2 Competencies needed by leaders in public health

Creating change	Influencing politics	Working trans-organizationally	Building teams
Visionary leadership Be able to articulate an evidence-based vision of the future and incorporate it into strategy. *Sense of mission* Facilitate the development of a mission, communicate it, and 'model' it through personal behaviour. *Effective change agent* Think creatively and analytically about systems and change strategies, and facilitate dialogue and empowerment of others to take action.	*Political processes* Determine appropriate actions on policy and political issues, organize key actors to cooperate for regulatory and legislative changes, and translate policies into programmes and services. *Negotiation* Mediate potential crises, bargain, and coordinate with key stakeholders. *Ethics and power* Identify and use alliances based on ethical principles. *Marketing and education* Use social marketing and health education to influence key audiences.	*Understanding of organizational dynamics* Assess and develop systems structures based on an understanding of culture and organizational behaviour. *Inter-organizational collaborating mechanisms* Involve key actors and networks across a broad range of organizations and groups in collaborative coalitions. *Social forecasting* Analyse trends and communicate predictions to consortium partners.	*Develop team-oriented structures and systems* Change system infrastructure to encourage innovative, learning teams. *Facilitate development of teams* Empower, motivate, and reward teams. *Serve in facilitation and mediation roles* Negotiate and intervene to help teams function. *Serve as an effective team member* Through own behaviour, 'model' the key characteristics of listening, encouraging and motivating while displaying integrity, commitment, and honesty.

Source: Adapted from Wright *et al.* 2000.

the people's health and well-being. Interviewees acknowledged the necessity of working in the political arena, although the extent of political engagement much depended on whether their job allowed them the opportunity to do so. The frustration of not being able to effectively exert influence beyond the health sector was a frequent observation. This confirmed the importance of working trans-organizationally as well as trans-sectorally. Working with ministries of finance was a frequently cited example of doing so. The interviewees acknowledged the critical importance of collaborative work, of building and working in teams. However, it was also suggested by some interviewees that the conventional way in which medical doctors were trained did not necessarily provide them with the skills to work collaboratively in public health teams.

Personal characteristics of leaders

The ability to conduct the change-related, trans-organizational, political, and team-building activities associated with public health leadership seems to rely on a core set of personal qualities. One particularly useful summary argues for a framework of 15 qualities important in a public health leader, broken down into three groups: Personal, cognitive, and social qualities (NHS Leadership Centre 2006).

As Fig. 3.4.1 demonstrates, at the core are the five personal qualities of self-belief, self-awareness, self-management, drive for improvement, and personal integrity. The five cognitive qualities at the top make possible the necessary analytical and procedural skills: Seizing the future, intellectual flexibility, broad scanning, political astuteness, and drive for results. These are then rounded off by five social qualities at the bottom: Leading change through people, holding to account, empowering others, effective and strategic influencing, and collaborative working.

The ten qualities associated with 'setting the direction' and 'delivering the service' shown as the outer ring of the doughnut in Fig. 3.4.1 can be viewed as another way of presenting the same basic material we have illustrated in Table 3.4.2. But the core personal qualities presented at the centre of the doughnut are worth emphasizing because they represent the personal behaviour

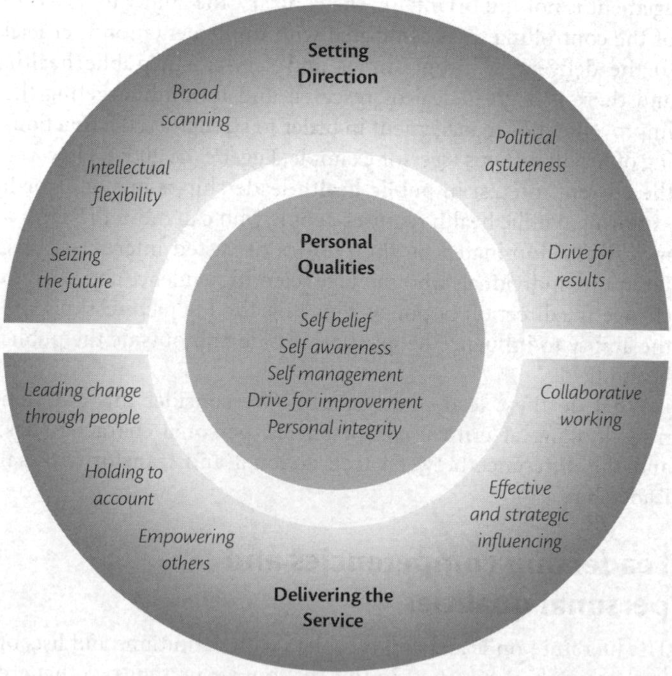

Fig. 3.4.1 NHS Leadership qualities framework.

of a leader. These core personal characteristics explain *how* leaders are able to do what they do. Self-belief, for example, is a 'positive "can do" sense of confidence which enables [outstanding leaders] to be shapers rather than followers, even in the face of opposition' (NHS Leadership Centre 2006, p. 4). Leaders are also self-aware. They know their own emotions and learn from mistakes (NHS Leadership Centre 2006, p. 13). Leaders demonstrate self-management. They are 'tenacious and resilient' in complex and difficult working environments (NHS Leadership Centre 2006, p. 5). They do not lose control, but manage their emotions (NHS Leadership Centre 2006, p. 14). Public health leaders have a vocation that feeds a 'drive for improvement': 'Outstanding leaders are motivated by wanting to make a real difference to people's health . . . [by] investing their energy in bringing about health improvements—even to the extent of wanting to leave a legacy which is about effective partnerships, inter-agency working and community involvement [rather than their own reputation]. . .' (NHS Leadership Centre 2006, p. 5). And finally, leaders demonstrate personal integrity: 'a strongly held sense of commitment to openness, honesty, inclusiveness and high [ethical and performance] standards . . .' (NHS Leadership Centre 2006, p. 16).

Transactional versus transformational leadership

In addition to their personal qualities, leaders tend to behave in one of two ways when seeking to accomplish something: They may be 'transactional' or 'transformational' in their approach (Avolio & Bass 1999). Transactional leaders are explicitly instrumental, for example by complimenting a junior for work well done or by arranging a *quid pro quo* ('you do something for me and I will do something for you'). Transactional leaders use rewards and punishments deliberately. In contrast, transformational leaders are more likely to present a co-worker with a vision of how things could be done differently. Transformational leaders give lots of personal attention to the people they work with, providing stimulation and inspiration to those around them.

Research on leaders in the public sector (including health workers) suggests they are more likely to be transformational in their approach (Alban-Metcalfe & Alimo-Metcalfe 2000). Research on the leadership styles of doctors also indicates that those with transformational behaviours are perceived as more effective leaders and are able to deliver better healthcare results (Xirasagar *et al.* 2005). Some may argue that this is likely to be true generally of health sector leaders, but the importance of the distinction could depend on context. Perhaps transactional leaders are needed in certain urgent settings (such as emergency epidemic responses or operating theatres) while transformational leaders are needed in the more operationally complex domains (such as influencing changes in health policy). However, it is worth noting that '[T]ransformational leadership has been documented to enable superior organizational performance in almost all settings that it has been tested' (Xirasagar *et al.* 2006, p. 105).

That said, a cautionary view has also been expressed by other researchers that the notion of transformational leadership must not trap the leader into thinking that he/she must have all the answers, that 'they have to do it all on their own, standing apart and moulding their organizations into shape'. The leader must be able to find the right balance that works for the specific situation at hand and must be aware of his/her personal limitations so that they can seek and receive help from colleagues (Binney *et al.* 2005, p. 104–5).

Emphasizing the special qualities of public health leaders, as we have done in this section, seems to imply that leaders are somehow born exceptional. As Firth-Cozens and Mowbray (2001) say:

> *It seems clear that certain traits such as arrogance, authoritarianism, and strong competitiveness may be prejudicial to good leadership, and that sociable, confident people who work well under stress have a head start in making good leaders.*

Nonetheless, the personal qualities and competencies cited above, such as self-knowledge and political skill, might also result from a maturity of experience. Similarly, transformational or transactional behaviour might be picked up by people as they progress through their careers. Thus, it seems likely that leadership can be learned, at least in part. But can it be taught? We turn next to that question.

Training and assessing leaders

Training leaders

Around the world, initiatives to train health sector leaders are being developed and implemented. Some training efforts are focused on the traditional attempt to ensure that public health leaders have the epidemiological and statistical skills to understand—if not necessarily to implement—research and evaluation of interventions and outcomes. For example, the Training Programmes in Epidemiology and Public Health Interventions Network (TEPHINET), in association with the World Health Organization, has been part of training public health personnel around the world.

> *There is a growing interest among ministries of health in establishing new TEPHINET programmes. These programmes are becoming increasingly recognized as catalysts for strengthening the scientific basis of policy-making through the continuous examination of data. . . .* (Cardenas *et al.* 2002, p. 196)

In order to be able to analyse trends and articulate a vision of the future, public health leaders clearly need to be able to assess and use the available research evidence. This skill is conventionally believed to be one that can be taught. What about skills like trans-organizational work and team-building? Can these be conferred on a potential leader by means of a training programme? Some recent, interesting evaluations suggest they can.

Saleh *et al.* (2004) evaluated training provided by the Northeast Public Health Leadership Institute (NEPHLI) in the US. Issues covered in the year-long programme include such slightly nebulous topics as building collaborative relationships, group problem solving, and dealing with cultural diversity. The evaluation results show that the participants clearly believe their abilities were enhanced in the 15 competency areas assessed. In addition, those who had reason to use certain particular skills as part of their work were more likely to perceive an improvement in their competence as a result of training. A key aspect of this training was, thus, the relevance of the topics to the participants' daily work. There may be, of course, a distinction between the participants' perception that the training improved their skills and the reality when they apply these skills. Nevertheless, it seems reasonable that those (such as doctors and nurses) whose basic training and earlier work skills are technical medical ones would benefit from training that emphasizes a very different set of procedural skills. For example, in this case, the '[t]opics covered included influencing others, measuring and improving public health performance, developing collaborative relationships and partnerships, risk communication, team building, group problem solving, responding to the needs for cultural diversity and competence, and emergency preparedness training' (Saleh *et al.* 2004, p. 1245).

Another training programme evaluation sheds some light on the mechanism by which these behavioural skills are transferred to the participants. Umble *et al.* (2005) assessed a leadership training programme in which all the members of a public health team participated together in the training. In addition, the training was based on the participants' real work and on typical projects. The results showed improved outcomes with regard to collaborating and networking, key aspects of leadership.

As Fig. 3.4.2 illustrates, the training approach seems to have improved the participants' confidence to work collaboratively and to lead a team, as well as improving their practice of these behaviours. The authors conclude from this evaluation that 'networks and collaborative leaders can be developed through education, and that groups thus created can improve services and programmes' (Umble *et al.* 2005, p. 642). This approach to bringing together, as a team, leaders who will have to work together to solve public health problems, has the potential to work elsewhere. See, for example, a story from the Philippines presented in Box 3.4.1.

In addition to formal training programmes, the development of leaders has also been promoted by means of 'mentoring', 'shadowing', or 'coaching' (*Turning Point* 2001, p. 51). Mentoring is the process by which a more experienced person guides a more junior person with regard to various work- and career-related decisions. It may involve helping the junior person solve problems at work by empathetic listening and feedback. Mentoring may also involve the experienced person giving career advice to the junior.

Shadowing can work with a more senior person either being shadowed or doing the shadowing. In the former approach, a more junior person follows the senior one in his or her job over several months. In this way, learning takes place by observing and participating in the work of an established leader. The latter approach involves a more experienced person shadowing a junior over a shorter period of a day or few days, and then giving constructive feedback on the junior's behaviour and activities at work.

Coaching does not necessarily involve a senior and junior person. A coach can provide assessment and feedback of skills and

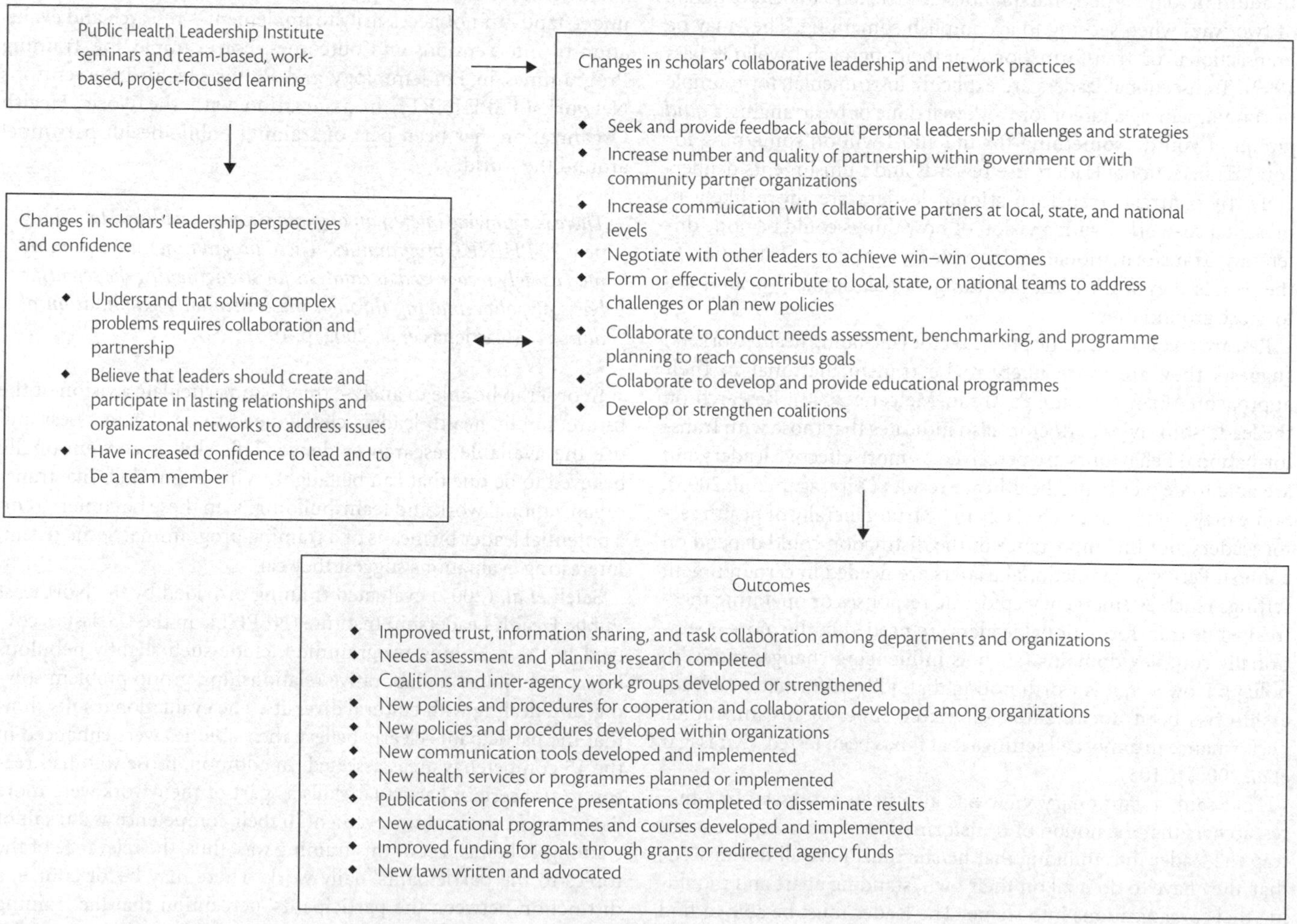

Fig. 3.4.2 Changing leadership practices through collaborative team training.
Source: Umble *et al.* (2005).

Box 3.4.1 Training local teams to be health leaders in poor communities: A case from the Philippines

The Philippines provides the story of an innovative approach to the need for leadership to address the health needs of the most deprived and vulnerable populations. Begun in 2002, the Leaders for Health Program (LHP) was predicated on the understanding that health professionals must work in concert with political and community actors if basic health problems are to be addressed in low-income communities. This 'Tri-Leader' approach brought together the community doctor, the mayor, and a local community leader and trained them, both individually and as a team.

To address the need that medical leaders understand and are able to use evidence to inform policy, doctors received post-graduate training resulting in a Master in Community Health Management. Recognizing that the local political and community leaders often did not have an advanced level of education, the programme created a certificate course in community health management tailored to them, but paralleling the master's training provided to doctors. Joint workshops and training sessions were also held for the tri-leaders together. In addition, all three benefited from coaching and mentoring from a more experienced leader of their own category in another part of the country. Once this team began to identify priorities in its locality, the LHP provided assistance in identifying donors for specific interventions. For example, some communities invested in sanitation and clean water systems. One community established a local pharmacy; another invested in a boat for emergency transport of patients.

By taking this innovative approach to leadership—one that recognizes the importance of joint leadership in the medical, political, and local communities in order to address public health needs—the LHP has been able to demonstrate greater success than other initiatives that focus only on placing trained doctors in low-income areas. Its success would seem to be due to the programme's understanding of the complexity of health systems. For example, addressing water-borne diseases properly requires sanitation systems, and sanitation systems cannot be built without political support. In addition, the programme's training of doctors together with mayors and community leaders helps doctors to see beyond the narrowly bio-medical domain to the broader political and sociological setting in which public health problems must be tackled. One mayor reported that earlier attempts to post doctors to his village were unsuccessful because the doctor was perceived to be making demands arrogantly of a resource-poor community, rather than working with the community to reach a common understanding.

Similar team-based approaches to training public health leaders have shown success elsewhere. (For an example from the United States, see our discussion in Umble *et al.* [2005].) Training medical, political, and community leaders together fosters the networking skills and builds the very communication links needed to address public health priorities. The evidence suggests that this is an approach that might reasonably be tried elsewhere.

Source: Baquiran *et al.* 2006; Leaders for Health Program 2005.

practice with a leader or someone wishing to develop leadership skills. Coaches may set goals and tasks for the subject, followed by discussion sessions designed to help him or her learn from the experience. Peers may sometimes coach one another, although this may be more successful when the peers not in direct competition with one another (*Turning Point* 2001, p. 52).

Among the leaders we interviewed, mentoring and shadowing experiences occupied a prominent place in their development. Many cited their mentors with great fondness and appreciation. And there were instances when more than one mentor was acknowledged by a leader.

It appears, then, that the training and development of leaders is possible. The former assumption that leaders are born with innate skills that cannot be taught, no longer seems true. Waiting for great leaders to emerge is not necessary. Instead, the health sector can seek to train, develop, and promote leaders. But, how do we discern which individuals exhibit leadership traits and which ones are performing well as leaders? There must be some mechanism for assessing leaders, and we turn next to that problem.

Measuring leadership ability

There are many leadership assessment tools, but three are based on empirical research. The Leadership Practices Inventory (Kouzes & Posner 1997) measures leaders on five dimensions: Challenging the process; inspiring a shared vision; enabling others to act; modelling the way; and encouraging the heart. The Multifactor Leadership Questionnaire (Avolio & Bass 1999) measures characteristics associated with transformational leadership, transactional leadership, and the absence of leadership (*laissez-faire* way of working in a leadership position). The Transformational Leadership Questionnaire (Alban-Metcalfe & Alimo-Metcalfe 2000) measures nine factors:

- Genuine concern for others
- Political sensitivity and skills
- Decisiveness, determination, self-confidence
- Integrity, trustworthy, honest, and open
- Empowers, develops potential
- Inspirational networker and promoter
- Accessible, approachable
- Clarifies boundaries, involves others in decisions
- Encourages critical and strategic thinking.

All three of these leadership tools are applied by asking someone other than the leader (sometimes a superior, sometimes a subordinate) to assess the leader's performance on each element along a scale. Each of the three has been applied in various settings and found to be useful in distinguishing high-performing leaders from those who demonstrate weaker leadership skills despite being in a job requiring leadership.

There are two uses for these types of tests. The first is to help individuals identify their own areas of strength and weakness in order to develop as leaders. The second is to select people for leadership positions. Neither of these is being implemented to any great extent in health sectors around the world, although richer countries probably do so more. The use of such tools could help health-sector managers to improve the leadership profile of their workforce. However, as has been noted about all attempts to list leadership characteristics, more work needs to be done to identify tools that work well across different cultures.

In this chapter so far, we have looked at the theory and thought behind leadership studies and research. We have also seen how various approaches to train and develop leaders have been implemented. But, beyond this, how does leadership work in the gritty, very real world of day-to-day public health work?

Leadership in health today

Acknowledging and addressing complexity—putting theory into practice

Health systems are complex. In all countries, health systems are broad and multi-sectoral. They involve complicated interactions among politics and policy-making, financing, training and education, and public and private organizations. It is not easy to define where public health activities end: A large manufacturing company may employ someone to conduct health education with its staff, just as the government might engage outreach workers to do the same with villagers. In the context of a very complex system that extends far beyond the boundaries of any one organization, it is not possible to 'manage' things in a mechanical way (Plsek & Wilson 2001). It is not possible to impose simple managerial or technical solutions to a public health problem and thus solve it.

Indeed, if technical and mechanistic solutions were all that were needed to address public health problems, we would not need leaders. Instead, the complex, multi-organizational, and team-based nature of public health work requires people who can inspire others to achieve results working through the complexity. And leaders are not needed just at the top of the pyramid. Increasingly, as solutions require collective action, leadership in public health is needed at all levels (Grint 2002). The 'command and control' approach will not serve to address the myriad and varied issues faced in national health sectors around the world, not to mention internationally.

Public health leaders must exercise their leadership in a complex environment. What does this mean, exactly? The leaders we interviewed voiced both enthusiasm and frustration with the work they were engaged in. While they spoke of positive gains in their work, they also spoke of conditions beyond their sphere of influence, and of existing economic and political forces far beyond their personal or their organization's capacities to change. Despite these difficulties, hardly any interviewee suggested that they should give up. The following quote from *Living Leadership: A Practical Guide for Ordinary Heroes* may be helpful in providing perspective on how leaders might conduct themselves in the face of complexity:

> *Coming alive is when leaders are able to use all their intelligence, senses and experience to connect with others and make sense of the context. They don't forget their life experience. They are able to acknowledge when a situation is different from ones they have experienced before and they need to pause and think again. They are able to tolerate the complexity of events and people and not rush to simple-minded solutions that don't make sense. Their focus is on both long- and short-term issues. They can ask for and receive help.* (Binney *et al.* 2005, p. 93)

We observed that the fundamental premise that keeps public health leaders going despite the difficulties is this: That a public health leader is there to serve people. And the goal of service is to improve the quality of life of people by preventing, treating, and even eliminating disease wherever possible.

This imperative to serve has to be expressed concretely. The public health leader quickly finds that his or her mission of service will lead to problems and dilemmas inherent to this complex world. Let us look at some examples of how this complexity manifests itself in the challenges that leaders face.

Consider the relationship between disease and poverty manifest in epidemics. In Manila, there are perennial outbreaks of diarrhoea in the urban slums because residents illegally tap water lines causing contamination of water. When such a water-borne outbreak occurs, the water company needs to step in. It removes the illegal connections, repairs leaks, flushes out the contamination, and increases the chlorination levels in the affected water lines. Public health authorities undertake epidemic investigations and related measures to treat the sick and prevent the infection from spreading in households.

While appearing to be a local issue, this phenomenon is a microcosm of a global problem described in the text of a WHO poster that reads: 'For the first time in history, more than half of the world's population lives in urban settings. Three billion people live in cities. One billion people live without access to safe drinking water'.

What can be done to prevent perennial outbreaks of water-borne diarrhoea in the urban slums of Manila caused by the illegal tapping of water lines? How would the public health leader deal with this situation in order to find a longer term answer to it?

The relationship between disease and people's lifestyles presents many interesting challenges. The association between smoking cigarettes and cancer is now well established. In 2003, the World Health Assembly ratified the Framework Convention on Tobacco Control, which urged member states to undertake a variety of actions in order to reduce smoking among their populations. Despite scientific advances leading to a better understanding of the ill effects of smoking and the aforementioned landmark global agreement, the prevalence of smoking among youth and women is on the rise in many countries. And while some countries have set forth legislation to ban smoking in public places, governments in many countries seem not to be doing enough to discourage and reduce smoking among their constituents.

How would the public health leader, such as a city health officer, deal with a situation where the city mayor or the city council have not enacted any measures to stop smoking in public places?

Consider the relationship between a disease, the necessary medicines for its treatment, and the commercial interests involved in making those medicines accessible to the people who need them. HIV/AIDS has become a determinant of social and economic development. Life expectancies have been shortened drastically in many African countries because thousands of people succumb to AIDS at an early age. Large numbers of AIDS orphans are overwhelming the capacities of families and societies to provide and care for them. Anti-retrovirals exist, but they are expensive and still inaccessible to millions of infected people.

How would a public health leader, such as a Minister of Health in a country with a large burden of HIV/AIDS, take steps to provide anti-retrovirals for thousands of citizens with the disease?

And what does a public health leader do when people's choices come into direct confrontation with tradition, and prevailing moral views and teachings of religious institutions? It is now commonplace for women to seek abortions in order to terminate unwanted pregnancies. Often, these abortions are conducted under surreptitious and illegal conditions, placing women at high risk of life-threatening bleeding and infection. There is ongoing debate that legalizing abortions will result in better regulation of the practice of abortion, thereby making the procedure less risky.

How does a public health leader deal with a situation where the scientific evidence shows that decriminalizing abortion prevents maternal deaths from sepsis, but where his moral beliefs run counter to implementing such a change?

The above examples are only a few of the many complex issues that public health leaders face. As they bring themselves to lead under these challenging circumstances, their aforementioned personal qualities, technical and social competencies will be tested. It can be overwhelming to lead in such complex situations, and leaders must be realistic about what they and their organizations can accomplish.

Principled leadership

In the face of such challenges, leaders need more than the attributes described above to help them succeed. Also vitally important is a set of principles that can serve as a guide to thought and action. Where would public health leaders derive such a set of principles? We offer five principles derived from the WHO Constitution (see Box 3.4.2):

1. Commitment to the vision of total human development
2. Commitment to empowering the poor and the vulnerable with knowledge and opportunity
3. Pursuit of evidence and truth
4. Commitment to fairness and equity in the provision of adequate health and social measures
5. Trustworthiness and public accountability

Applied singly or in varying combinations, we submit that these principles provide the foundation and inspiration to public healthwork.

In the first challenge discussed above, public health leaders are asked to find a longer-term solution to control water-borne outbreaks of diarrhoea in the urban slums of Manila. Principle 1, which calls for commitment to total human development, urges these leaders to think beyond epidemic control. It challenges them to address the problem of urban slums to tackle the social determinants of water-borne outbreaks. This is exceedingly complex and difficult. However, where Principle 1 is combined with Principle 2, more durable solutions have been found. The experience of Gawad Kalinga in the Philippines demonstrates how a movement to eradicate urban slums has improved the health of people in such communities and in the process has prevented the perennial occurrence of outbreaks there (see Box 3.4.3). By addressing the land and housing issues at the root of urban slum communities, Gawad Kalinga was able to build low-cost houses and proper water supplies for the families previously dwelling in slums.

Principle 5, trustworthiness and public accountability, is applicable to the second challenge. The campaign against smoking is another complex issue. There are big business interests that protect and promote the sale of cigarettes. Some of these business interests may even have philanthropic projects which benefit the public, such as grants to educational institutions or youth scholarships.

Box 3.4.2 WHO constitution

THE STATES Parties to this Constitution declare, in conformity with the Charter of the United Nations, that the following principles are basic to the happiness, harmonious relations and security of all peoples:

- Health is a state of complete physical, mental, and social well-being and not merely the absence of disease or infirmity.
- The enjoyment of the highest attainable standard of health is one of the fundamental rights of every human being without distinction of race, religion, political belief, economic or social condition.
- The health of all peoples is fundamental to the attainment of peace and security and is dependent upon the fullest co-operation of individuals and States.
- The achievement of any State in the promotion and protection of health is of value to all.
- Unequal development in different countries in the promotion of health and control of disease, especially communicable disease, is a common danger.
- Healthy development of the child is of basic importance; the ability to live harmoniously in a changing total environment is essential to such development.
- The extension to all peoples of the benefits of medical, psychological and related knowledge is essential to the fullest attainment of health.
- Informed opinion and active co-operation on the part of the public are of the utmost importance in the improvement of the health of the people.
- Governments have a responsibility for the health of their peoples, which can be fulfilled only by the provision of adequate health and social measures.

ACCEPTING THESE PRINCIPLES, and for the purpose of co-operation among themselves and with others to promote and protect the health of all peoples, the Contracting Parties agree to the present Constitution and hereby establish the World Health Organization as a specialized agency within the terms of Article 57 of the Charter of the United Nations.

Source: WHO Constitution was adopted by the International Health Conference held in New York from 19 June to 22 July 1946 (Reference: WHO Basic Documents, 2007).

It can be convenient for public health leaders to take the path of least resistance and not call for a ban of cigarettes in public places. Principle 5 calls on public health leaders to be faithful to their calling of safeguarding public health despite the odds against them. In this respect, they are trustworthy and accountable to the public for their actions, even if some of their actions may be politically unpopular. There are public health leaders who have unstintingly used the built-up scientific evidence on the ill effects of smoking to persist in the campaign to ban smoking in public places. To them, the public owes a debt of gratitude for their courage and persistence.

Box 3.4.3 Gawad Kalinga: Improving well-being by empowering the poor

Gawad Kalinga (GK) translated in English means to Guardian of care. GK is a non-profit foundation whose vision for the Philippines is a slum-free, squatter-free nation through a simple strategy of providing land for the landless, homes for the homeless, and food for the hungry in order to attain dignity and peace in poor Filipino communities.

What started in 1995 as a daring initiative by a faith-based organization to rehabilitate juvenile gang members and help out-of-school youth in a large squatters' relocation area in Metro Manila, has now evolved into a movement for nation-building. Local and multinational corporations have engaged with GK as part of their programmes for corporate social responsibility. Together with its partners, Gawad Kalinga is now in the process of transforming slum communities with the goal of building 700 000 homes in 7000 communities in 7 years (2003–2010). At the time of writing, Gawad Kalinga is in over 900 communities all over the Philippines. GK villages have also been recently introduced in Papua New Guinea, East Timor, Cambodia, and Indonesia.

As a growing multi-sectoral movement, GK works actively in the poorest urban areas and aims to improve the quality of life of its residents by providing decent homes and the resources necessary for self-sufficiency. It seeks a holistic approach to poverty alleviation which includes various components: The provision of basic healthcare, community organization, livelihood programmes, and values formation. GK has extended its activities to include poor Muslim communities in its Highway of Peace campaign where Muslim and Christians together build GK homes. In some outstanding cases of inter-community bridge building, long-standing family feuds have been reversed by one community building a house for a rival community

Even before a GK house is built in a slum community, issues of land ownership, capital for house materials, participation of the residents in the construction of the houses, eventual ownership of the built houses, and community building are considered and dealt with. Complex social dynamics are involved in dealing with these varied issues.

In 2006, GK launched its 'One Million Heroes' campaign, designed to encourage intensified volunteerism in the GK communities. Part of the current success of GK is attributed to this stewardship component which integrates leadership building into the GK communities. Every GK village has a Caretaker Team comprised mainly of resident volunteers who undertake specific responsibilities like assisting in resolving conflicts, ensuring the proper management of the resources for constructing the houses, and seeing to it that the GK standards for a well-organized community are maintained.

Principle 4, commitment to fairness and equity, may be applicable in the third challenge. In the face of the complex issues concerning the way in which pharmaceuticals are produced, sold, and distributed, answers must be found to address the lack of access to medicines by millions of people. The solutions to these imbalances are not straightforward. They involve the dynamics of the domestic and international market for medicines. Where patent issues for new medicines are involved, there are international agreements that govern the production and marketing of generic copies during the patent term. Notwithstanding these complexities, public health leaders, seeking to broaden their populations' access to medicines, have persevered to find ways to accomplish this goal. At the Sixtieth World Health Assembly in May 2007, public health leaders from around the world tackled this very issue and produced resolution WHA60.30, initially proposed by Brazil. The way this resolution was debated and eventually passed by the World Health Assembly is an example of how public health leaders from different countries can come together to agree on an exceedingly complex public health issue.

The final example focuses on the issue of abortion. The application of Principle 3—the pursuit of evidence and truth—may guide an advocate for the legalization of abortion to argue that this policy significantly decreases maternal deaths. But those against abortion will resist this evidence, taking the view that no law can justify terminating the foetus in early pregnancy. People's beliefs and values vary. In the Philippines, while there are data showing that septic abortions happen in the thousands, legalization of abortion would be unacceptable as public policy. In contrast, in Iran, abortion was made legal to address mothers' health risk in certain pregnancies (Reproductive Health Matters 2005). So, even as public health leaders pursue the evidence to justify health interventions, there may be other, historical and social considerations that override it. Public health leaders, whatever their moral beliefs, will have to respect those realities.

It is indeed exciting and challenging for the public health leader to bring together personal qualities, technical and social competencies, and principles to the job at hand.

Effective leadership

There are a variety of public health sector jobs that will allow leaders to exercise their full range of talents. At the national level, leading a public health organization (or certain programmes within the organization) is one such job. Ensuring that the bureaucracy delivers the services that the public expects of it will require the leader to exercise competencies such as empowering others, driving for results, and being held to account. Providing immunization services to millions of children every year in order to protect them from vaccine-immunizable disease is a good example of this. The leader has to keep the programme on track in the face of many competing priorities, ensuring that the right people are in place to run the programme. The leader must see to it that funds are available to procure the vaccines, and that the vaccines are delivered and used properly at the points of service throughout the country. The leader relies on a well-functioning organization to do this. Immunization targets have to be set and results achieved; and the leader must hold his/her people to account for their performance, even as he/she is held to account by his/her superiors and the public.

Where one sees an immunization programme with high immunization coverage rates, one can find examples of successful public health leadership. While the immunization example above discusses leadership at the national level, there are additional levels of leadership necessary to the programme. At the international level, global immunization strategies and targets are set in consultation with experts and various stakeholders, including Member States, international development agencies, and non-governmental organizations. At a sub-national level, leadership undertakes the planning and implementation of all the details of the programme.

This includes ensuring that the staff members are properly trained, motivated, and supervised, that vaccines and supplies are available, and that the health facilities are organized and well-prepared to deliver the service. Furthermore, there is leadership at the various levels of the service delivery chain to see to it that the children in the communities and households actually get immunized. Even at the community level, village health-workers and volunteers may play leadership roles in providing information to parents, encouraging them to ensure their children are vaccinated.

The results of effective leadership in a national immunization programme are profound in terms of preventing life-threatening illnesses in children. High-coverage rates of measles immunization have significantly reduced illness and deaths among children from pneumonia, diarrhoea, and malnutrition that are the sequelae of severe measles infection.

In times of organizational change, public health leaders will need to exercise other competencies such as seizing the future, intellectual flexibility, and broad scanning. For example, when the Philippine Department of Health decentralized its services in 1992, it devolved all provincial hospitals and municipal health centres to local governments. More than 500 hospitals, 1000 health centres, and 35 000 staff were devolved. It was a huge change, and public health leaders at all levels faced the challenge of continuing to provide services, while adapting to new organizational relationships.

The onus on the top leadership of the Department of Health was tremendous in terms of managing the transition. The devolved parts of the organization resisted the change and while they were legally bound to implement, performance dipped. The non-devolved half of the organization found itself having to implement programmes through lower levels of the organization, which were no longer under their direct administrative control.

What was once an unbroken chain of command from national to municipal level was cut in two places: The provincial and municipal levels now reported to their respective local executives.

The devolution of health services was part of an administrative re-structuring of government. It was driven by the principle of increasing the powers and responsibilities of local government, particularly in the administration of public services. Public health leaders had to manage this change as best as they could and work with local governments, many of which were unready to take over the responsibility of managing health services. During such a critical transition, public health leaders needed to provide visionary guidance and practical savvy to calm the organizational turmoil, deal with the anger of devolved staff, and the haplessness of local governments, and provide a steady and reassuring presence in what was a very trying time.

Public health leaders are not immune to political battles and on many occasions they will have to decide whether or not to engage in the fight. It is not an easy decision to take. Engagement is costly in terms of personal time and energy, as well as organizational resources. Some of the fiercest political battles involve the business sector. Regulating the sales and marketing of infant formulas in developing countries is one example of a thorny issue. Government regulates the aggressive marketing practices of the milk companies, which are known to run counter to breastfeeding promotion among mothers. In the Philippines, milk companies have filed suits against the Department of Health to challenge government regulation of these marketing practices. In instances like this, public health leaders must stand firm in the face of litigation.

Public health leaders are found not just in the state or government sector. They also work in non-governmental organizations, academia, and the private commercial sector. Activities of non-state-sector organizations do affect public health. For instance, the marketing behaviour of pharmaceutical companies affects patterns of public consumption. Non-governmental organizations' activities during disasters and natural calamities contribute to public health. The research done in academic institutions helps inform public health policy. Health leadership can thus be considered a shared responsibility. It is, therefore, critical for the leaders of the various sectors to engage in honest and effective dialogue to attain synergy of purpose and action.

Have public health leaders made a difference in this complex world? Where is the evidence that they have changed the lives of their constituents for the better? Assessing leadership is by nature a retrospective activity. It is, therefore, always difficult to know for sure whether in any particular context another leader in the same position would have acted differently, and more important, whether there would have been a different outcome had someone else been making the decisions. Furthermore, would a leader who was successful in dilemma 'X' have shone equally had he/she instead been placed into dilemma 'Y'? It is evident that in a complex reality, a leader and his/her context are in fact inseparable: Put the right person in the right place at the right time, and leadership happens. Beyond this, instinct and personal experience tells us that public health leaders *do* make a difference, and they can be responsible for collective success or failure. We can look to historical examples as further evidence.

We can look first to the 1854 cholera outbreak in Soho, London, and the famous demonstration of leadership that in many ways marked the beginning of modern epidemiological public health as a discipline. Supported by his exceptional technical, medical, and scientific skills, John Snow exhibited several of the characteristics of leadership covered in this chapter. In particular, his self-belief and confidence, and vision and belief in a better state of affairs were all monumentally demonstrated.

The historical context must especially be appreciated: Snow was active prior to the formulation of the germ theory—the theory that proposes that microorganisms are the cause of many diseases—a cornerstone of modern medicine and medical microbiology. At the time, the predominant scientific belief concerning the mechanism of spreading disease was that expounded in the Miasma theory: That diseases such as cholera and the plague were spread by poisonous air. For some years, Snow argued that this theory was mistaken, and he became convinced from his research upon various outbreaks in London that cholera was in fact spread by water.

Battling scientific convention was only a part of the struggle for what Snow thought would save lives. Implementing his theory led to another difficult conflict. When Snow postulated that the source outbreak at the time appeared to be a water pump and consequently recommended that it be blocked, there was understandable resistance from the inhabitants of the area who depended on the pump for their daily drinking water. With both science and the affected population against him, it is an extraordinary feat of negotiation that Snow eventually succeeded in convincing the local authorities to remove the handle from the pump, bringing an end to the incidence of infection and no doubt saving many lives. Snow's actions also led directly to a new understanding of how disease can spread.

Snow's leadership continued after the outbreak was under control, when he demonstrated the utmost integrity in doubting his own conclusion—pondering whether the fact that the outbreak was already on decline prior to the handle removal meant that he had been mistaken. Hence, he persevered in mapping out each cholera case in the context of its proximity to the well. In doing so, he not only consolidated the correctness of his decision, but also gave birth to what we now call epidemiology.

John Snow did not seek to be a leader. Neither was he appointed into his position as local health hero and scientific pioneer. It is clear from the story that his technical skills were secondary to his leadership qualities. His knowledge of himself, belief and vision in an improved understanding of health, personal integrity, perseverance, and a desire to serve people regardless of their social class, pushed him to succeed in the situation he found himself in the middle of.

In contrast to this first evidential example of public health leadership—historical, local, and focused on an individual—as a second example we can examine a case typical of the complex modern reality and necessary leadership of today. The successful containment of SARS in 2003 involved multi-level, multidisciplinary, collective international leadership and would not have been possible without it. One might be tempted to point to WHO and other coordinating bodies at the time as the self-appointed 'leader', but in reality a 'network of leadership' was crucial to the urgent halting of the new disease.

Originating in a Hong Kong hotel, but rapidly spreading globally via the fast-moving web of international transport, SARS proved the cliché that disease recognizes no national boundaries and does not discriminate between types of people. With such a highly contagious, little-understood, deadly respiratory disease, every human life was under threat. On the other hand, human reality *does* recognize national boundaries and so a successful public health response to SARS relied on strong leadership at the national and local levels, which simultaneously cooperated internationally. Furthermore, the impact of SARS reached far beyond the health sphere: Mass hysteria surrounding the emerging disease damaged tourism and economies, costing Asian businesses alone around US$60 billion in lost revenue (Dayrit 2004). All sectors needed to work together to minimize the human cost incurred by SARS. Given these facts, what exactly was required of national public health leadership—particularly in the more affected countries?

A typical national public health strategy to fight the disease can be considered as having rested upon five pillars:

- Minimizing the entry of imported cases through monitoring and screening of passengers in seaports and airports
- Averting local transmission of cases through contact tracing, quarantining of suspected carriers, and isolation of cases
- Preventing SARS deaths with supportive hospital treatment
- Disseminating information and health advisories to the public to control fear and panic
- Mitigating the non-health consequences of SARS

It is worth noting that of these public health responsibilities, only the third point—hospital treatment—is a purely health-oriented task. The other pillars all required public health leadership in multisector responses to a health threat. In many cases, national leaders had to make brave and controversial decisions in the interest of the health of their people, such as implementing new quarantine laws necessary for the protection of the population but risked being seen as limitations on civil liberties or human rights. Leaders needed to be communicative and bold, demonstrating integrity and acting with the best interests of the people at heart. Underlying their actions were not only their own guiding principles, but globalized principles of human well-being and equity, which are increasingly shared across all boundaries.

All considered, and given the immediacy and gravity of the situation, this was a massive responsibility for national health leaders and their colleagues. With the support of international bodies such as WHO, however, in winning the fight against SARS the multi-country leadership set a precedent for dealing with future international health threats, strengthening global preparedness in the process. Without that collaborative leadership, SARS would almost definitely have taken countless more lives, cost billions more to the global economy, and could still be very much at large.

We have seen a classic example of individual, localized, public health leadership in the exceptional efforts of John Snow and a contemporary, complex, international, collaborative leadership example in the multi-leader response to SARS. Both undoubtedly made an impermeable difference to the health and well-being of the world today.

Examples of leadership are multiple and varied, and yet there are common elements that can be found in them all. It is by embracing these elements that, regardless of the plethora of leadership examples, a personal 'path to leadership' can be forged.

The path to leadership

You too can become a public health leader—but how can you develop the personal qualities and competencies needed to do so?

The public health leaders we interviewed first entered the profession with a strong desire to serve. Through the course of their careers, they were exposed to circumstances that deepened their commitment. Frequently, they sought out challenging circumstances in which to gain much needed experience. They travelled, engaged in development work, often involving poor countries and communities. In the course of this exposure, they took up more advanced public health studies, perhaps did some research, wrote articles in scientific journals, or managed a healthcare facility. Some had long periods of service in their own country before being exposed to international work. For others, international exposure came early, usually through some clinical- or public health training abroad.

There are several paths to leadership. Some moved into public health after years of working in the clinics, practising a speciality like paediatrics, obstetrics, or surgery. Others came into positions of leadership through the field services, rising through a public health organization, or a non-governmental organization. Others were involved in academia, teaching and research, consulting, or working with a development agency. Public health leaders could also have been involved in politics. Or they could once have been cause-oriented activists, involved in issues such as HIV prevention and primary healthcare.

Mentors play a significant role in the development of the public health leader. Nearly everyone we interviewed cited people significant to their career at various stages.

One public health leader we spoke to for this chapter put it this way: 'A leader creates a path for others to succeed'. Another interviewee mentioned how his boss and mentor encouraged him and other young people in the organization to think up and explore new ideas. These contemporary nuggets of advice are reminiscent of a gem of wisdom found in the ancient text of the *Tao Te Ching*:

> *Go to the people. Live with them. Learn from them. Love them. Start with what they know. Build with what they have. But with the best leaders, when the work is done, the task accomplished, the people will say 'We have done this ourselves'.*

Many public health leaders of the last generation lived by this maxim. Similar expressions paraphrasing this attitude were made by several of the leaders we interviewed.

Central to the growth and development of the public health leader are the years when he/she developed the personal qualities of self-awareness, self-belief, and self-management. In many, there was the strong conviction that their involvement in public health was imbued with higher purpose and that they were instruments of a higher power to do good work. Certainly, the sense of 'other-orientedness' was quite a major motivation infusing the leaders' sense of service. Among those interviewed, none said that money was a strong motivating factor for the choice of a public health career. A desire to continue learning new things was often mentioned as a source of great satisfaction. One public health leader emphasized the necessity to listen and learn from others before making decisions.

Personal integrity is another of the personal qualities greatly valued by public health leaders. It is the inner core of public credibility. Trustworthiness, transparency on the job, and incorruptibility are among the attributes that they strive to maintain in themselves and look for in their colleagues. When leaders lose personal integrity—as when they fall into the trap of self-serving personal agendas, unethical conflicts of interest, or even bribe-taking—their loss of public credibility will eventually occur, just as death follows disease. Since we do not live in a perfect world, it is not unknown for public health leaders to fall from grace and lose their integrity and credibility. It is a sad day when a person in a position of public health leadership is found to have betrayed the public trust one way or the other. The path to public health leadership must strengthen and ennoble both mind and heart.

When does one know that one is ready to lead? The opportunity to lead may be sought, but very often it is given, when the higher authority deems that the individual is ready to exercise leadership. The opportunity to lead is a gift. But just as the public health leader has been selected to lead, so too is it his/her job to select others to take up positions of leadership. Leaders should nurture future leaders. Selecting a person for a leadership position is often one of the biggest decisions that a public health leader can make.

The potential health leaders of tomorrow are encouraged to forge their 'path to leadership' on three fronts:

1. Know your guiding principles.
2. Seek mentors and aim to learn from every situation you face.
3. Pursue leadership, not the leadership position.

Know your guiding principles

The WHO constitution—drawn up in a fertile climate of unprecedented hope by international leaders in every field—can be distilled into fundamental guiding principles that are central to a public health leader's work. In reality, individual context, culture, and background dictate that each leader will interpret these principles slightly differently and will complement them with principles derived from additional underlying foundations that constitute their personal philosophy of life. Together, this collection of principles will serve to give focus and meaning to the health leader's work.

Nonetheless, these principles must be embedded firmly in the mind. Leaders need to think and act on their feet. Unless one is sure of one's principles, in a time of crisis—with perhaps many lives at stake—panic and uncertainty might take over. There will not be time to think—about remembering your principles when the need to make a decision is immediate. For this reason, taking the time to understand what guides you—to 'know thyself'—is invaluable. Take time to think about what it is that guides you, or what you would like to guide you. Find your principles. Write them down. Read them out aloud. Explain and discuss them with a close friend or mentor. Take regular moments to revisit them so that they are forever under your skin, in your subconscious, never far from the surface. Together, they will serve as your guiding beacon during times that test your leadership.

Seek mentors and aim to learn from every situation you face

Both the literature on leadership and the practical experience of today's health leaders underline the crucial importance of mentorship in the development of the complete public health leader. To achieve self-improvement, being prepared to learn from superiors, fellow colleagues, friends, and public figures is essential. But how does one 'obtain' a mentor?

There is no fixed prescription for mentorship. By its very nature, it is a personal arrangement between two parties, and sometimes one of the parties (the mentor) does not even need to be aware of the fact. Some programmes encourage their participants to go out and seek a mentor other than their direct supervisor—someone they admire, probably working in their vicinity—and to invite them to act as a mentor. Following this, an arrangement can be struck that is convenient and suitable to the mentor and the mentee. The mentoring relationship could be formal and structured, with regular meetings and log book entries; or it could be more informal and sporadic, with the occasional chat over coffee or e-mail correspondence.

In whatever case best suits the people involved, the opportunity should be taken for the mentor to impart advice, the mentee to report on recent events, and for both to share thoughts on work and even wider aspects of life, particularly if relevant to a career in health and leadership. Ideally, a mentoring relationship should be mutually beneficial, with both parties learning from one another, enriching their understanding of their work and purpose.

For of course, a mentor can gain much from a mentee. One can learn as much from subordinates or peers as one learns from superiors. In this sense, mentors surround us, wherever we are. Rarely is one person not able to learn something from another. A mentor does not need to (and rarely does) exhibit all the aspects of leadership covered in this chapter. More often, elements of leadership can be found in part in various people met in the course of a career. The challenge is to identify the skills and to attempt to understand how to integrate them into one's own work and behaviour. This form of fragmented menteeship does not need to take the form of the more contractual approach mentioned above. It is up to the mentees to observe and learn by themselves—a kind of secret mentorship.

Pursue leadership, not the leadership position

Looking back to the beginning of this chapter, at the distinction between leadership and management (Tables 3.4.1 and 3.4.2 and Fig. 3.4.1), it is clear that whereas to exercise management it is necessary to be in a management position, the skills, characteristics, and competencies of leadership can more or less be practised regardless of one's position in a hierarchy. One pursues leadership by steadily inculcating in oneself the personal qualities, competencies, and principles that make up a true leader. One does not acquire these necessary attributes and skills simply by ascending to a leadership position, often via political patronage, especially if one lacks adequate preparation. Study, training, reflection, exposure, and experience are all elements of this preparation. Thus, as one's leadership traits flourish, the time will come when one is ready to assume a leadership position. Leadership should be sought in this way from day one of any career and hence, any strong public health organization should encourage leadership development at all levels.

When does one know that he/she is ready to take up a position of leadership?

The trajectory of an individual's path to leadership can rise steeply or gently. It is one's willingness to step forward, given one's self-awareness and knowledge of the prospective job, however incomplete, which might mark a person's readiness to lead. A potential leader will almost always be selected by having already demonstrated leadership and by showing readiness to lead. In deciding if one is ready to assume the responsibility of a public health leader, it of course helps to discuss the opportunity with mentors, co-workers, and family members.

Once in a leadership position, the leader must keep learning. Mistakes will be made, disappointments and conflicts will occur. The strong face of leadership is well-observed, but how do top health leaders deal with themselves during the dark hours, when the tasks seem overwhelming and when results fall short of expectations? It is often said that in these situations, leaders dig deep into themselves to find internal resources of strength. The capacity to affirm self-belief and overcome self-doubt is an important ingredient in surviving the difficult times; but it is also true that the leader turns outward to others for strength. One leader from Kenya whom we interviewed emphasized that she turned to her community for rejuvenation and inspiration. 'We hold on to each other', she said. Others turn to family members or colleagues for support. And there are many who through prayer and meditation, turn to their faith or guiding principles to find inner strength.

It is hoped that the above will help to direct the interested and motivated reader in tracing his/her own 'path to leadership'—imparting some of the information and advice needed to one day lead within the area of public health. Before bringing this chapter to a close, and as a final pointer for those wishing to serve the needy through public health leadership, we might want look at things from another perspective. Instead of asking 'What do I need in order to become a health leader?' perhaps we should ask 'What kind of leader does the world need?'

Getting the public health leaders the world needs

We need public health leaders everywhere and at every level of the health system. However, good leaders are most needed in places where people are poor and suffering simply because there is such a scarcity of them there. Committed and effective leaders often provide the vision and impetus to mobilize people and resources in needy areas (see Box 3.4.3).

How can the international health community help developing countries develop the needed leaders? A good starting point is to aim at strengthening educational institutions, which can provide relevant, team-based training, and at providing support towards helping governments and their partners to improve workplace conditions, including financial and non-financial incentives. From an international perspective we can work towards empowering nations to do this self-sufficiently, strengthening their own frameworks for leadership. Health leaders have used the term 'capacity release' in reference to this kind of endeavour (Chan 2007). It must be stressed that training programmes are only one component of a comprehensive approach that should include strategies to retain promising public health workers and sustain the idealism of leaders who are prepared to venture forth to places of hardship. We must encourage and support them to stay where they are most needed. Examples of work being done on this include the WHO framework on training leaders and managers (Egger *et al.* 2005) and related work to strengthen leadership at all levels of the health system.

Conclusion

As we come to the end of this chapter, let us summarize its most important points:

- The literature makes an academic distinction between leadership and management. Leadership has more to do with the visionary activities of setting direction, while management leans towards the controlling tasks associated with implementation. In practice, the two are often linked in the job description and work of an individual;
- Leaders possess certain personal qualities, skills, and principles that enable them to do what they need to do. These attributes are acquired through a variety of ways. The constant manifestation and practice of these attributes, skills, and principles is a continuing challenge in a leader's job and career;
- In the face of ever-increasing complexity in the world around us, public health leadership is needed to prevent, treat, and eliminate disease and promote the health of people. This capability to lead should be developed and nurtured in prospective individuals in varying social and cultural contexts and at all levels and types of public health organizations;
- Each 'path to leadership' is unique and very personal. However, exposure, training, mentors, and guiding principles all help in the development of leadership qualities in individuals who aspire to lead. They should be sought by anyone interested in serving as a public health leader.

In closing, the pursuit of leadership must ennoble the mind and the heart of those who aspire to it. It is a noble and never-ending quest. We bid the reader all success.

Notes

1 Leaders we spoke to were chosen from among current and former work colleagues. Information was derived from direct interviews or informal conversations. In some instances, speeches and curriculum vitae were referred to. Where interviews were made, there was no standard structure. Informants were told in advance that the purpose of the interview was to learn about their experiences as a leader in public health. They were asked simply to talk about their background and to tell stories from their experience. Follow-up questions focused on some of the broad themes arising from the literature.

Acknowledgements

The authors would like to thank Amimo Agola, Anand Kurup, Chadia Wannous, Christine Lamoureux, Claudia Vivas, Delanyo Dovlo, Dick Chamla, Francis Omaswa, Guangyuan Liu, Helen Robinson, Lealou Reballos, Maria Eufemia Yap, and Miriam Were, among others, for their insights into the issues of leadership in public health.

We would also like to acknowledge the contributions of Daniel Shaw for editing the text and providing useful material for the text and boxes. Thanks also to Carmen Dolea for her valuable comments on the manuscript and to Joanne McManus for polishing the final draft.

References

Alban-Metcalfe, Robert, J., and Alimo-Metcalfe, B. (2000). An analysis of the convergent and discriminant validity of the transformational leadership questionnaire. *International Journal of Selection and Assessment*, **8**(3), 158–75.

Avolio, B.J. and Bass, B.M. (1999). Re-examining the components of transformational and transactional leadership using the multifactor leadership questionnaire. *Journal of Occupational & Organizational Psychology*, **72**(4), 441–62.

Baquiran, R., Yap, M.E., and Bengzon, A.R.A. (2006). *Terminal grant report: Leaders for Health Program 2002–2006*. Pfizer Philippines Foundation Inc., Manila.

Binney, G., Wilke G., and Williams, C. (2005). *Living leadership, a practical guide for ordinary heroes*. Pearson Education Limited, England.

Bonita, R., Beaglehole, R., and Kjellström, T. (1993). *Basic Epidemiology*. WHO, Geneva.

Cardenas, V.M., Roces, M.C., Wattanasri, S. *et al.* (2002). Improving global public health leadership through training in epidemiology and public health: The experience of TEPHINET. Training Programs in Epidemiology and Public Health Interventions Network. *American Journal of Public Health*, **92**(2), 196–7.

Chan, M. (2007). Address to WHO staff. 4 Jan 2007. World Health Organization, Geneva.

Dayrit, M.M. (2004). *Health and population. The Macapagal–Arroyo presidency and administration – Record and legacy (2001–2004)*. University of the Philippines Press, Quezon City, Philippines.

Dickinson, H., Peck, E., and Smith, J. (2006). *Leadership in organisational transition – what can we learn from research evidence?* March 2006. National Health Service Institute for Innovation and Improvement Health Services Management Centre, United Kingdom.

Dweggah, M. (2007). *Managment of Staff*. Interview with Dr Margaret Chan, Director-General, WHO; May 2007 UN Special, Geneva.

Egger, D., Travis, P., Dovlo, D. *et al.* (2005). *Strengthening management in low-income countries*. Making Health Systems Work: Working Paper Series Number 1. World Health Organization, Geneva.

Firth-Cozens, J. and Mowbray, D. (2001). Leadership and the quality of care. *Quality in Health Care*, **10** (Suppl 2), ii3–7.

Flahault, D. and Roemer, M.I. (1986). *Leadership for primary health care*. World Health Organization, Geneva.

Gawad Kalinga. Main site. http://www.gawadkalinga.org/. Accessed 10 July 2007.

Grint, K. (2002). Management or leadership? *Journal of Health Services Research & Policy*, **7**(4), 248–51.

Huczynski A.A. and Buchanan D.A. (2007). *Organizational Behaviour, an Introductory Text*, 6th edition. Pearson Education Limited, England.

Kouzes, J.M. and Posner, B.Z. (1997). *Leadership practices inventory (LPI): Facilitators Guide*, 2nd edition. Jossey-Bass, San Francisco.

Leaders for Health Program (2005). *The LHP experience: 5 stories of hope and transformation in municipal health practices (Program Document)*. Ateneo Professional Schools, Makati, Philippines. www.leadersforhealth.ph.

McGrew, R.E. (1985). *Encyclopedia of Medical History*. The MacMillan Press, London.

NHS Leadership Centre (2006). *NHS leadership qualities framework*. National Health Service Institute for Innovation and Improvement, United Kingdom.

Plsek, P.E. and Wilson, T. (2001). Complexity, leadership, and management in healthcare organisations. *British Medical Journal*, **323**(7315), 746–9.

Reproductive Health Matters (2005). 'Round Up – law and Policy'. *Reproductive Health Matters*, **13**(6), 180–6.

Saleh, S. S., Williams, D., and Balougan, M. (2004). Evaluating the effectiveness of public health leadership training: The NEPHLI experience. *American Journal of Public Health*, **94**(7), 1245–9.

Stone, A.G. and Patterson, K. (2005). *The history of leadership focus*. Servant Leadership Research Roundtable – August 2005. School of Leadership Studies, Regent University.

Thomas, J.C. (2005). Ethics in public health: Skills for the ethical practice of public health. *Journal of Public Health Management Practice*, **11**(3), 260–1.

Turning Point Program. (2001). *Collaborative leadership and health: A review of the literature*, 80 pages. Leadership Development National Excellence Collaborative, Turning Point Program, Seattle, WA.

Umble, K., Steffen, D., Porter, J. *et al.* (2005). The National Public Health Leadership Institute: Evaluation of a team-based approach to developing collaborative public health leaders. *American Journal of Public Health*, **95**(4), 641–4.

Wikipedia contributors, 'Gawad Kalinga', *Wikipedia, The Free Encyclopedia*. http://en.wikipedia.org/wiki/Gawad_Kalinga_777. Accessed 10 July 2007.

World Health Organization. *Knowledge network on urban settings* (Poster). WHO Commission on Social Determinants of Health, WHO Centre for Health Development, Kobe, Japan.

World Health Organization. *The health leadership service*. World Health Organization, Geneva, Switzerland. http://www.who.int/health_leadership/en/. Accessed on 11 July 2007.

World Health Organization (2003). *WHO Framework Convention on Tobacco Control*. World Health Organization, Geneva, Switzerland. http://www.who.int/tobacco/framework/WHO_FCTC_english.pdf. Accessed on 9 July 2007.

World Health Organization (2007). *Managing the health millennium development goals – the challenge of management strengthening: Lessons from three countries*. World Health Organization, Geneva, Switzerland.

World Health Organization. (2007). *Public health, innovation and intellectual property. 60th World Health Assembly Resolution WHA60.30*, May 2007.World Health Organization, Geneva, Switzerland. http://www.who.int/gb/ebwha/pdf_files/WHA60/A60_R30-en.pdf. Accessed on 9 July 2007.

Wright, K., Rowitz, L., and Merkle, A. (2001). A conceptual model for leadership development. *Journal of Public Health Management and Practice*, **7**(4), 60–6.

Wright, K., Rowitz, L., Merkle, A. *et al.* (2000). Competency development in public health leadership. *American Journal of Public Health*, **90**(8), 1202–7.

Xirasagar, S., Samuels, M.E., and Curtin, T.F. (2006). Management training of physician executives, their leadership style, and care management performance: An empirical study. *The American Journal of Managed Care*, **12**(2), 101–8.

Xirasagar, S., Samuels, M.E., and Stoskopf, C.H. (2005). Physician leadership styles and effectiveness: An empirical study. *Medical Care Research & Review*, **62**(6), 720–40

SECTION 4

Public health law and ethics

4.1

The right to the highest attainable standard of health[1]

Paul Hunt, Gunilla Backman, Judith Bueno de Mesquita, Louise Finer, Rajat Khosla, Dragana Korljan, and Lisa Oldring

Abstract

This chapter introduces the right to the highest attainable standard of health, which is enshrined in several legally binding international treaties, as well as numerous national constitutions. It outlines the complementary relationship between public health and the right to the highest attainable standard of health, and provides a framework for analysing this human right. This analytical framework is then applied, by way of illustration, to neglected diseases, mental disability, sexual and reproductive health, and water and sanitation. The conclusion identifies the key features of a health system from the perspective of the right to the highest attainable standard of health.

Human rights

What are human rights?

Human rights are freedoms and entitlements concerned with the protection of the inherent dignity and equality of every human being. They include civil, political, economic, social, and cultural rights. The international community has accepted the position that all human rights are universal, indivisible, interdependent, and interrelated (UN 1993).

Although inspired by moral values, such as dignity and equality, human rights are more than moral entitlements: They are legally guaranteed through national and international legal obligations on duty bearers. They are enshrined, for example, in various international treaties and declarations.

International human rights treaties (often called covenants or conventions), such as the International Covenant on Economic, Social and Cultural Rights (ICESCR), are legally binding on the States that ratify them ('States parties'). In contrast, human rights declarations, such as the Universal Declaration of Human Rights, are non-binding, although many of them do include norms and principles that reflect obligations that are binding under customary international law.

Human rights have traditionally been concerned with the relationship between the State, on one hand, and individuals and groups on the other. By ratifying international human rights treaties, States assume binding legal obligations to give effect to the human rights enumerated within them.

Additionally, all States have national laws that protect some human rights. Moreover, some States have enshrined human rights—civil, political, economic, social, and cultural—in their constitutions.

Historic neglect of economic, social, and cultural rights, such as the rights to health and shelter, is gradually being overcome, thanks in part to civil society organizations across the world that have campaigned for their equal representation and advocated for specific mechanisms for their enforcement.

Who has human rights duties?

Although only States are parties to international and regional human rights treaties, and are thus fully accountable for compliance with their provisions, all members of society have responsibilities regarding the realization of human rights, including the right to the highest attainable standard of health (UN 1948, preamble; UNCESCR 2000, para. 42). This includes health workers,[2] families, communities, inter- and non-governmental organizations, civil society groups, as well as the private business sector: These so-called 'non-State actors' all have responsibilities regarding the realization of the right to health. States, as parties to international treaties, have a duty to provide an environment in which all of these individuals and groups can discharge their human rights responsibilities.

[1] The 'right to health' or the 'right to the highest attainable standard of health' are used as shorthand for 'the right of everyone to the enjoyment of the highest attainable standard of physical and mental health', the full title envisaged in Article 12 of the International Covenant on Economic, Social and Cultural Rights (ICESCR).

[2] A generic term encompassing doctors, nurses, midwives, public health professionals, managers/administrators, traditional health workers, as well as those working in particular contexts or specializations, such as prison health or obstetrics and gynaecology. According to the WHO definition, health workers are 'all people engaged in actions whose primary intent is to enhance health' (WHO 2006a).

Approaches to human rights

One approach to the vindication of human rights is via the courts, tribunals, and other judicial and quasi-judicial processes (the 'judicial' approach). Another approach, however, brings human rights to bear upon policy-making processes so that policies and programmes that promote and protect human rights are put in place (the 'policy' approach). Although the two approaches are intimately related and mutually reinforcing, the distinction between them is important because the 'policy' approach opens up challenging new interdisciplinary possibilities for the operationalization of human rights.

Lawyers have played an indispensable role in developing the norms and standards that today constitute international human rights law. Naturally, when it comes to the 'judicial' and 'policy' approaches, some lawyers are professionally drawn to the former. Indeed, in the context of the right to health, despite some suggestions to the contrary, this approach has a vital role to play and many courts have demonstrated that they have a crucial contribution to make.[3] It is important that this judicial contribution deepens and becomes more widespread.

In addition to this approach, however, it is vital that the right to health is brought to bear upon all relevant local, national and international policy-making processes This 'policy' approach depends upon techniques and tools—indicators, benchmarks, impact assessments, and so on—that demand close cooperation across a range of disciplines. Given its historic role and traditional expertise, public health has an indispensable contribution to make to the 'policy' approach. The Section 'New tools and techniques' below briefly introduces some of these techniques and tools in the specific context of the right to the highest attainable standard of health.

What is the right to health?

Sources of the right to health[4]

The origins of the international right to the highest attainable standard of health can be traced back over 50 years. Adopted in 1946, the World Health Organization's Constitution States: 'The enjoyment of the highest attainable standard of health is one of the fundamental rights of every human being without distinction of race, religion, political belief, economic or social condition'. Two years later, article 25(1) of the Universal Declaration of Human Rights laid the foundations for the international legal framework for the right to health. Since then, the right to health has been codified in numerous legally binding international and regional human rights treaties, and enshrined in many national laws, some of which are signalled in the following paragraphs. This gives rise to one of the most important and distinctive characteristics of human rights, including the right to the highest attainable standard of health. Human rights place legally binding obligations on States.

International human rights law

Concrete legal duties are conferred upon States when they ratify international treaties; they must ensure that all individuals within their jurisdiction can enjoy the rights envisaged within them. The cornerstone protection of the right to health in international law is found in Article 12 of ICESCR. Over 155 States have legally bound themselves, through ratification of this treaty, to its implementation.

Additional right to health protections are contained in international treaties that address issues specific to marginalized groups, such as the International Convention for the Elimination of All Forms of Racial Discrimination (ICERD);[5] the International Convention on the Elimination of All Forms of Discrimination Against Women (CEDAW);[6] and the Convention on the Rights of the Child (CRC).[7]

Authoritative and interpretive guiding principles of several of these treaty provisions on the right to health—called General Comments or General Recommendations—shed further light on the parameters and content of the right to health generally, and in relation to the application of the right to specific groups. In 2000, for example, the United Nations (UN) treaty-body responsible for monitoring ICESCR adopted General Comment 14 on the right to the highest attainable standard of health.

Moreover, some UN treaty-bodies have decided cases that shed light on the scope of health-related rights. Recently, for example, the Human Rights Committee considered the case of a 17-year old Peruvian who was denied a therapeutic abortion. When K.L was 14 weeks pregnant, doctors at a public hospital in Lima diagnosed the foetus with an abnormality that would endanger K.L's health if pregnancy continued. However, K.L. was denied a therapeutic abortion by the hospital's director. In *K.L. v Peru*, the Human Rights Committee decided that by denying the young woman's request to undergo an abortion in accordance with Peruvian law, the Government was in breach of its right-to-life obligations under the International Covenant on Civil and Political Rights (UNHRCttee 2003).

Further standards relating to specific groups are set out in non-binding legal instruments, such as the Declaration on the Elimination of Violence against Women. Additional international human rights instruments contain protections relevant to the right to health in various situations, environments and processes, including armed conflict, development, the workplace, and detention (UNCHR 2003a, Annex I).

Significantly, resolutions of the UN Commission on Human Rights, including those on disabilities and access to medication (UNCHR 2002a, b), have articulated the right to the highest attainable standard of health; while other important resolutions contain provisions that bear closely upon the right (UNCHR 2003a, Annex II).

Far-reaching commitments relating to the right to health have been made in the outcome documents of numerous UN world conferences, such as the International Conference on Population and Development (UN 1994), the Fourth World Conference on Women (UN 1995), and the Millennium Declaration (UNGA 2000). These conferences have helped to place international problems, including health issues such as HIV/AIDS, at the top of the global agenda and their outcome documents influence international and national

[3] For an overview of jurisprudence on the right to health, see UNHRC (2007, paras 55–89).

[4] The 'right to health' or the 'right to the highest attainable standard of health' is employed as shorthand for the full title which is 'the right of everyone to the enjoyment of the highest attainable standard of physical and mental health'.

[5] ICERD provides protection for racial and ethnic groups in relation to 'the right to public health (and) medical care' (Article 5 (e) (iv)).

[6] CEDAW provides several provisions for the protection of women's right to health (Articles 11 (1) f, 12 and 14 (2) b).

[7] CRC contains extensive and elaborate provisions on the child's right to health, including one which is fully dedicated to the right to the health of the child (Article 24), and others containing protections for especially vulnerable groups of children (articles 3 (3), 17, 23, 25, 32, and 28).

policy-making. Several refer to the right to health and health-related rights.

Regional human rights law

The right to health is recognized in human rights treaties drafted and monitored by the different regional human rights systems. These have effect only in their respective regions and include: The African Charter on Human and Peoples' Rights (Article 16); the African Charter on the Rights and Welfare of the Child (Article 14); the Additional Protocol to the American Convention on Human Rights in the Area of Economic, Social and Cultural Rights, known as the 'Protocol of San Salvador' (Article 10); and the European Social Charter (Article 11). Other regional instruments provide, through health-related rights, indirect protection of the right to health.[8]

At regional level there are also judicial and other mechanisms that adjudicate cases involving the right to health. A notable case in 2002 was the finding by the African Commission on Human and Peoples' Rights of a violation of the right to health by the Federal Republic of Nigeria, on account of violations against the Ogoni people in relation to the activities of oil companies in the Niger Delta (ACHPR 2001).

Significantly, regional mechanisms have also found breaches of other health-related rights, including the violation of the right to a home and family and private life, arising from environmental harm to human health in *López Ostra v. Spain* (ECtHR 1994), as well as the negative consequences on children's health stemming from the occurrence of child labour in *ICJ v. Portugal* (ECSR 1998).

Another important development has come from the Inter-American Commission on Human Rights, which expressed its willingness to 'take into account' provisions of the regional treaty (the Protocol of San Salvador) related to the right to health when analysing the merits of a case, even though it lacked competence to determine violations under them (IACHR 2000).

National law

A study has shown that 67.5 per cent of the constitutions of all nations have provisions regarding health and healthcare (Kinney & Clark 2004). In addition, a large number of constitutions set out States' duties in relation to health, such as the duty to develop health services, from which it is possible to infer health entitlements.

In some jurisdictions these constitutional provisions have generated significant jurisprudence, such as the decision of the Constitutional Court of South Africa in *Minister for Health v. Treatment Action Campaign*. In this case, the Court held that the Constitution required the Government 'to devise and implement a comprehensive and coordinated programme to realize progressively the right of pregnant women and their newborn children to have access to health services to combat mother-to-child transmission of HIV' (CCSA 2002, para. 135 (2) (a)). This case—and numerous other laws and decisions at the international, regional, and national levels—confirms that the courts have an important role to play in the protection of the right to the highest attainable standard of health.

Right to health in the context of other human rights

As already indicated, the right to health is closely related to and dependent upon the realization of other fundamental human rights contained within international law. These include the rights to life, food, housing, work, and education, as well as rights based on the freedom not to be tortured or discriminated against. Similarly, the rights to privacy, equality, access to information, and freedom of association, as well as other rights and freedoms, relate to and address integral components of the right to health.

The right to health—like other economic, social, and cultural rights—does not escape controversy and ideological objections. Some States are still reluctant to see it as a right of similar weight to others, such as the right to a fair trial. However, under international law, the right to the highest attainable standard of health is an integral part of the international code of human rights and must be given equal treatment and attention. Importantly, the interdependence and equal footing of all human rights was reaffirmed in the Vienna Declaration (UN 1993, para. 5). Furthermore, jurisprudence and international standards are gradually clarifying the mutually reinforcing relationship between the right to health and other health-related rights, such as the right to life (UNCESCR 2000, para. 3).

The complementary relationship between public health and the right to health

With a few exceptions, the relationship between health and human rights was not subject to close examination until the 1990s. Of course, the Constitution of WHO (WHO 1946) affirms the right to health and so does the Declaration of Alma-Ata (WHO 1978a). Also, some of those who were struggling against HIV/AIDS in the 1980s recognized the crucial importance of human rights. But, for the most part, these important developments were not accompanied by a detailed examination of the substantive relationship between health and human rights. That had to wait until the early 1990s. A great debt is owed to the late Jonathan Mann and his colleagues at the Harvard School of Public Health and the Francois-Xavier Bagnoud Center for Health and Human Rights for their pioneering work on the relationship between health and human rights, especially in the context of HIV/AIDS.

In the 1990s, however, Dr. Mann and others suffered from a serious limitation that does not apply today. At that time, although there was a widespread and detailed understanding of many human rights, there was no comparable understanding of the right to the highest attainable standard of health, even though this human right is the cornerstone of the relationship between health and human rights.

Today, however, the situation is significantly different. In 2000, an authoritative understanding of the right to health emerged when the UN Committee on Economic, Social and Cultural Rights, working in close collaboration with WHO and many others, adopted General Comment 14 (UNCESCR 2000). Also, some international bodies like WHO, UNFPA, UNICEF, and UNAIDS, as well as civil society organizations, have begun to give more careful attention to health-related rights, including the right to the highest attainable standard of health. These and other developments have deepened understanding of the right to health, enabling linkages to be made between public health and human rights, a process that continues to accelerate through good practice, the academic literature and widening jurisprudence.

8 These include the American Declaration on the Rights and Duties of Man, the American Convention on Human Rights, the Inter-American Convention on the Prevention, Punishment and Eradication of Violence against Women, and the European Convention for the Protection of Human Rights and Fundamental Freedoms and its protocols.

Although in some quarters there is a presumption that the right to health relates to medical care, such a narrow definition is in fact inconsistent with international human rights law, which encompasses both medicine and public health, as confirmed by Article 12 of ICESCR and Article 24 of CRC. As well as access to medical care, the right to health encompasses the social, cultural, economic, political, and other conditions that make people need medical care in the first place (WHO 1948, preamble; Beaglehole 2002), as well as other determinants of health such as access to water, sanitation, nutrition, housing, and education. This wider perspective underscores the very extensive common ground between public health and the right to the highest attainable standard of health.

The right to the highest attainable standard of health depends upon public health measures, such as immunization programmes, the provision of adequate sanitation systems and clean drinking water, health promotion (e.g. regarding domestic violence, healthy eating, and taking exercise), road safety campaigns, nutrition programmes, the promotion of indoor stoves that reduce respiratory diseases, and so on. Also, however, the classic, long-established public health objectives can benefit from the newer, dynamic discipline of human rights. In other words, just as public health programmes are essential to the realization of the right to health, so too can human rights help to reinforce existing, good, health programmes and identify new, equitable, health policies. This chapter focuses on the relevance of the right to the highest attainable standard of health to public health. However, the indispensable contribution of public health to the right to the highest attainable standard of health also deserves careful study.

Both public health and human rights advocates wish to establish effective, integrated, responsive health systems that are accessible to all. Both stress the importance not only of access to healthcare, but also to water, sanitation, health information, and education. Both understand that good health is not the sole responsibility of the Ministry of Health, but belongs to a wide range of public and private actors. Both prioritize the struggle against discrimination and disadvantage, and both stress cultural respect. At root, those working in health and human rights are both animated by a similar concern: The well-being of individuals and populations.

Health workers—defined in the World Health Report of 2006 (WHO 2006a) as 'all people engaged in actions whose primary intent is to enhance health'—can use health-related rights to help them devise more equitable policies and programmes; to place important health issues higher up national and international agendas; to secure better coordination across health-related sectors, as well as between services within the health sector; to raise more funds from the treasury; to leverage more funds from developed countries to developing countries; in some countries, to improve the terms and conditions of those working in the health sector; and so on. The right to the highest attainable standard of health is not just a rhetorical device, but also a tool that can save lives and reduce suffering, especially among the most disadvantaged.

The following sections provide examples that illustrate the resonance between public health and the right to the highest attainable standard of health.

Although these two disciplines are, in many ways, complementary, in practice public health has been used by some States as a ground for limiting the exercise of some human rights. Indeed, under international law, States are allowed to impose some limitations on human rights, in some circumstances, for the protection of public health, an issue briefly revisited in the following section.

The contours and content of the right to health

The right to health is not a right to be healthy. It is a right to facilities, goods, services, and conditions that are conducive to the realization of the highest attainable standard of physical and mental health. Understanding of the content of the right has evolved considerably over the last 50 years, with jurisprudence, international standards, and practical implementation of the right all contributing to this process.

As we have seen, an inclusive approach to implementing the right to the highest attainable standard of health calls for its reach to extend not only to timely and appropriate medical care, but also to the underlying determinants of health, such as access to safe and potable water and adequate sanitation, healthy occupational and environmental conditions, and access to health-related education and information (UNCESCR 2000, para. 8).

The right to health can also be broken down into more specific entitlements, such as the rights to: Maternal, child, and reproductive health; healthy workplace and natural environments; the prevention, treatment and control of diseases, including access to essential medicines; and access to safe and potable water.

In times of emergency, States have a joint and individual responsibility to cooperate in providing disaster relief and humanitarian assistance, including medical aid and potable water as well as assistance to refugees and internally displaced persons (UNCESCR 2000, para. 40).

Certain limitations on the right to health do exist, as issues of public health are sometimes used by States as grounds for limiting the exercise of other fundamental rights. For such limitations to be implemented legitimately, they must be in accordance with the law and international human rights standards. In particular, they should be strictly necessary for the promotion of the general welfare in a democratic society, proportional, subject to review, and of limited duration (UNCESCR 2000, paras. 28–9; UN ECOSOC 1985, Annex).

The right to health analytical framework

In recent years, the Committee on Economic, Social and Cultural Rights, WHO, the Special Rapporteur on the right of everyone to the enjoyment of the highest attainable standard of physical and mental health, civil society organizations, academics, and many others, have developed a way of 'unpacking' or analysing the right to health with a view to making it easier to understand and apply to health-related policies, programmes, and projects in practice. The analytical framework that has been developed is made up of 10 key elements and has general application to all aspects of the right to health, including the underlying determinants of health: This has been demonstrated by the Special Rapporteur in his use of the framework throughout his work.

- *National and international human rights laws, norms and standards*

The relevant laws, norms, and standards relevant to the particular issue, programme, or policy must be identified. These will include both general provisions and standards relating to the right to health, in addition to international instruments that relate to specific groups and contexts (see the Section 'What is the right to health?' above) (UNCHR 2003a, Annex 1).

◆ *Resource constraints and progressive realization*

International human rights law recognizes that the realization of the right to health is subject to resource availability. Thus, what is required of a developed State today is of a higher standard than what is required of a developing State. However, a State is obliged—whatever its resource constraints and level of economic development—to realize progressively the right to the highest attainable standard of health (UN 1966b, Art. 2(1)). In essence, this means that a State is required to be doing better in 2 years time than it is doing today. In order to measure progress (or the lack of it) over time, indicators and benchmarks must be identified (see the Section 'New tools and techniques').

◆ *Obligations of immediate effect*

Despite resource constraints and progressive realization, the right to health also gives rise to some obligations of immediate effect, such as the duty to avoid discrimination (UNCESCR 2000, para. 43). These are obligations without which the right would be deprived of its raison d'être and as such they are not subject to progressive realization, even in the presence of resource constraints. (UNCESCR 1990, para.10). The precise scope of these immediate obligations has not yet been clearly defined; for the health and human rights communities, this remains important work-in-progress.

◆ *Freedoms and entitlements*

The right to health includes both freedoms (for example, the freedom from discrimination or non-consensual medical treatment and experimentation) and entitlements (for example, the provision of a system of health protection that includes minimum essential levels of water and sanitation). For the most part, freedoms do not have budgetary implications, while entitlements do.

◆ *Available, accessible, acceptable and good quality*

All health services, goods, and facilities should comply with each of these four requirements. An essential medicine, for example, should be *available* within the country. Additionally, the medicine should be *accessible*. Accessibility has four dimensions: Accessible without discrimination, physically accessible, economically accessible (i.e. affordable), and accessible health-related information. As well as being available and accessible, health services should be provided in a culturally *acceptable* manner. This requires, for example, effective coordination and referral with traditional health systems. Lastly, all health services, goods, and services should be of *good quality*; a medicine, for example, must not be beyond its expiry date. These four requirements are further explored and applied in Section 'Right to health issues through the analytical framework'.

Note the similarity between these requirements and the four 'As' of public healthcare envisaged since the 1978 Alma Ata Declaration: Geographical accessibility; financial accessibility; cultural accessibility; and functional accessibility (WHO 1978b).

◆ *Respect, protect, fulfil*

This subsidiary framework relates to the tripartite obligations of States to respect, protect, and fulfil the right to the highest attainable standard of health, as explained and used by CESCR, the Committee on the Elimination of Discrimination Against Women (CEDAW) and the Sub-Commission on the Promotion and Protection of Human Rights. A version of this subsidiary framework is also enshrined in the Constitution of South Africa.

For example, the obligation to *respect* places a duty on States to refrain from interfering directly or indirectly with the enjoyment of the right to health. The obligation to *protect* means that States must prevent third parties from interfering with the enjoyment of the right to health. The obligation to *fulfil* requires States to adopt necessary measures, including legislative, administrative and budgetary measures, to ensure the full realization of human rights, including the right to the highest attainable standard of health.

◆ *Non-discrimination, equality and vulnerability*

Because of their crucial importance, the analytical framework demands that special attention be given to issues of non-discrimination, equality, and vulnerability in relation to all elements of the right to the highest attainable standard of health.

◆ *Active and informed participation*

Participation is grounded in internationally recognized human rights, such as the rights to participate in the formulation and implementation of government policy, to take part in the conduct of public affairs, and to freedom of expression and association.[9] The right to health requires that there be an opportunity for individuals and groups to participate actively and in an informed manner in health policy-making processes that affect them (UNCESCR 2000, para. 54).

◆ *International assistance and cooperation*

In line with obligations envisaged in the UN Charter and some human rights treaties,[10] developing countries have a responsibility to seek international assistance and cooperation, while developed States have some responsibilities towards the realization of the right to health in developing countries.

◆ *Monitoring and accountability*

The right to health introduces globally legitimized norms or standards from which obligations or responsibilities arise. These obligations have to be monitored and those responsible held to account. Without monitoring and accountability, the norms and obligations are likely to become empty promises. Accountability mechanisms provide rights-holders (e.g. individuals and groups) with an opportunity to understand how duty-bearers have discharged their obligations, and it also provides duty-bearers (e.g. ministers and officials) with an opportunity to explain their conduct. In this way, accountability mechanisms help to identify when—and what—policy adjustments are necessary. Accountability tends to encourage the most effective use of limited resources, as well as a shared responsibility among all parties. Transparent, effective, and accessible accountability mechanisms are among the most crucial characteristics of the right to the highest attainable standard of health.

These 10 key elements of the right-to-health analytical framework underscore what the right to health contributes to public health. For example, the pre-occupation with non-discrimination, equality, and vulnerability requires a State to take effective measures to address the health inequities that characterize some populations. The focus on active and informed participation requires a State to adopt, so far

[9] For example, *International Covenant on Civil and Political Rights* (ICCPR), articles 19, 22, 25; *International Covenant on Economic, Social and Cultural Rights* (ICESCR), article 13; *Convention on the Elimination of All Forms of Discrimination Against Women* (CEDAW): articles 7, 8.

[10] UN Charter; ICESCR (Article 2); CRC (Article 4).

as possible, a 'bottom-up' participatory approach in health-related sectors. The requirement of monitoring and accountability can help to ensure that health policies, programmes, and practices are meaningful to those living in poverty.

Crucially, the key elements of the right-to-health analytical framework are not merely to be followed because they accord with sound management, ethics, social justice, or humanitarianism. States are required to conform to the key features *as a matter of binding law*. Moreover, they are to be held to account for the discharge of their right-to-health responsibilities arising from these legal obligations.

Right to health issues through the analytical framework

In this section, elements of the analytical framework signalled in Section 'The contours and content of the right to health' are applied to a selection of health issues. While space does not permit all of the elements to be applied to all of the selected issues, each element is applied to at least one of them.

The selected health issues are: Neglected diseases; mental disability; sexual and reproductive health, including maternal mortality; and water and sanitation. The right to health is among the most extensive and complex in the international lexicon of human rights. As already signalled, it extends much further than these four issues which are simply provided as an illustration of how the right-to-health analytical framework applies to this selection of important health issues.

Neglected diseases[11]

Although there is no standard global definition of 'neglected diseases', nor are they homogenous, they tend to share some common features. For example, they typically affect neglected populations, those least able to demand services. They are a symptom of poverty and disadvantage. Fear and stigma are attached to some neglected diseases, leading to delays in seeking treatment and to discrimination against those afflicted.

Neglected diseases include lymphatic filariasis, schistosomiasis, onchoocerciasis (river blindness), trachoma, buruli ulcer, soil-transmitted helminths, leishmaniasis, leprosy, and human African trypanosomiasis (sleeping sickness). According to WHO, 'the health impact of . . . neglected diseases is measured by severe and permanent disabilities and deformities in almost 1 billion people' (WHO 2002).

Where curative interventions for neglected diseases exist, they have generally failed to reach populations early enough to prevent impairment. Furthermore, the development of new tools to diagnose and treat them has been underfunded, largely because there has been little or no market incentive (WHO 2004a, p. 22).

◆ *Non-discrimination, equality and vulnerability*

Discrimination and social stigma can be both causes and consequences of certain neglected diseases. As non-discrimination and equal treatment are cornerstone principles in international human rights law, a rights-based approach to neglected diseases pays particular attention to policies, programmes, and projects that impair the equal enjoyment of the human rights of people suffering from these diseases.

Stigmatization and discrimination heighten people's vulnerability to ill health. Often, stigmatization is based on myths, misconceptions, and fears, including those related to certain diseases or health conditions. In turn, fear of stigmatization can lead people living with neglected diseases to avoid diagnosis, delay seeking treatment and hide the diseases from family, employers, and the community at large.

Discrimination involves acts or omissions which may be directed towards stigmatized individuals on account of their health status and/or related disabilities. For example, leprosy, lymphatic filariasis and leishmaniasis may cause severe physical disabilities, including deformities and scarring, giving rise to discrimination in the workplace, and access to healthcare and education.

The socioeconomic consequences of stigmatization and discrimination associated with neglected diseases can have devastating consequences for individuals and groups that are already marginalized, leading to further vulnerability to neglected diseases. For example, stigma related to tuberculosis can be greater for women: It may lead to ostracism, rejection, and abandonment by family and friends, as well as loss of social and economic support and other problems (WHO 2001, p. 12). Social and behavioural research on stigma and neglected diseases suggests that women also may experience more social disadvantages than men, in particular from physically disfiguring conditions like lymphatic filariasis (Coreil *et al.* 2003, p. 42).

The guarantee of non-discrimination and equal treatment enshrined under national and international human rights law requires the government to adopt wide-ranging measures, including through the implementation of health-related laws and policies, which confront discrimination in the public and private sector.

◆ *Active and informed participation*

A human rights approach not only attaches importance to reducing the incidence and burden of neglected diseases, but also to the democratic and inclusive processes by which these objectives are achieved. Such processes require the active, informed, and meaningful participation of communities affected by neglected diseases.

Affected communities have sometimes participated in aspects of prevention, treatment, and control of neglected diseases. For example, they are sometimes involved in vector control programmes, such as bed net impregnation to combat malaria, or housing improvements to combat Chagas disease, which is caused by parasites living in cracks in housing. Communities have also been involved in treatment strategies, for example, through community health workers who have been selected and trained to administer vaccinations and treatment (Espino *et al.* 2004).

However, the human rights approach means that affected communities should participate in a range of contexts, not just in implementing programmes. They should be actively involved in setting local, national, and international public health agendas; decision-making processes; identifying disease control strategies and other relevant policies; and holding duty bearers to account. While it is not suggested that affected communities should participate in all the technical deliberations that underlie policy formulation, their participation can help to avoid some of the top-down, technocratic tendencies often associated with old-style development plans and policy implementation.

Although effective participation is not straightforward, and takes time to generate, it is nonetheless an important means by which to empower and build capacity in affected communities, enhance accountability, and improve the effectiveness of interventions.

[11] See WHO and TDR (2007).

Therefore, as demonstrated in the following examples, participation has a positive impact on the enjoyment of the right to health.

In Peru in the 1980s, patients' associations, spontaneously set up in response to the government's failure to provide drugs and financial compensation for people who had suffered from leishmaniasis, were eventually successful in securing support from the regional and national health authorities. They became forums for discussions of wide-ranging social and political issues. This movement, which became more structured and organized over time, provided local institutions with detailed knowledge and made links with local populations so that it became possible to determine the best control and intervention strategies, and implement them successfully (Guthman *et al.* 1997).

In Uganda, Village Health Teams are able to help dispel the neglect that characterizes certain diseases and populations, ensuring that local needs are clearly identified, understood, and addressed. Moreover, the Teams can provide the crucial grassroots delivery mechanisms for community interventions in relation to neglected diseases, and health protection generally.

Vehicles for community participation such as these require adequate resources, training, and support. They must be listened to and used strategically as delivery mechanisms in relation to neglected diseases, with smooth and effective coordination, cooperation, and collaboration between them and the local political structure and health centres. For this reason, government, development actors, and others should sustain and foster vital community-based initiatives to ensure that full and effective participation can support the realization of the right to health.

◆ *Monitoring and accountability*

In practice, few accountability mechanisms give sufficient attention to neglected diseases, and often prove inaccessible to impoverished members of neglected communities. Within a national jurisdiction, parliamentarians might hold the Minister of Health to account in relation to the discharge of his or her responsibilities, yet the ability of these and other general mechanisms (such as judicial processes) to provide adequate accountability in relation to neglected diseases and the right to health is doubtful.

The right to the highest attainable standard of health demands accessible, transparent, and effective monitoring and accountability mechanisms that are meaningful to neglected communities. These could include independent national human rights institutions that monitor the incidence of neglected diseases and the initiatives taken to address them. Adopting an evidence-based approach, the institution could scrutinize who is doing what and whether or not they are doing all that can reasonably be expected of them to realize the right to health of those concerned. Whenever possible, the institution should identify realistic and practical recommendations for all those involved.

International human rights machinery can also draw attention to the issue of neglected diseases and neglected populations. For example, when a relevant State presents its periodic reports to CESCR, both the Government's reports and the human rights body's examination of them, should give careful attention to the issue of neglected diseases and neglected populations, in accordance with the national and international right to health standards to which the Government is bound.

◆ *International assistance and cooperation*

This feature of the right to health requires that donors and the international community pay particular attention to the health problems of the most vulnerable and disadvantaged individuals and communities in developing countries. For example, donors and the international community have a duty to help developing countries enhance their capacity so they can determine their own national and local health research and development priorities, such as neglected diseases.

Mental disabilities[12]

Too often, disability issues do not attract the attention they demand and deserve. This is especially true in the context of mental disabilities. The right to the highest attainable standard of health demands that due attention is given to both physical and mental disabilities.

A significant development in the field of disability was achieved with the adoption of a new international human rights treaty in 2006, the Convention on the Rights of Persons with Disabilities. Alongside this important new treaty, which will enter into force once ratified by 20 States, there are many important provisions contained in non-binding principles that have profound connections to the right to health, even if some elements are inadequate and need revisiting.[13] Where appropriate, these specialized instruments should be used as interpretive guides in relation to the right to health as it is enshrined in international law.

International human rights treaties and specialized international instruments relating to mental disabilities are mutually reinforcing, even if, as the UN Secretary General recently put it, 'a more detailed analysis of the implementation of State human rights obligations in the context of mental health institutions would be desirable' (UNGA 2003, para. 43). Inadequate attention has been given to the implementation of these obligations to date. In this context it is heartening that the new UN Convention received the highest number of signatories of any such Convention on its opening day.[14]

◆ *Freedoms and entitlements*

Freedoms

Freedoms of particular relevance to the experience of individuals with mental disabilities include the right to control one's health and body. Forced sterilizations, rape, and other forms of sexual violence, to which women with mental disabilities are particularly vulnerable, are inherently inconsistent with their sexual and reproductive health rights and freedoms, are psychologically and physically traumatic, and thus jeopardize mental health even further.

Several international human rights instruments allow for exceptional circumstances in which persons with mental disabilities can be involuntarily admitted to a hospital or another designated

[12] Noting the wide range of terminology available, the generic term 'mental disability' has been adopted for efficiency as an umbrella term, though it is recognized that it encompasses many profoundly different conditions. These include all major and minor mental illness and psychiatric disorders, as well as intellectual disabilities. 'Disability' refers to a range of impairments, activity limitations, and participation restrictions, whether permanent or transitory.

[13] See, for example, the *UN Principles for the protection of persons with mental illness and the improvement of mental health care*, ('UN Mental Illness Principles') (1991) (UNGA 1991).

[14] 82 countries signed the Convention on the day it opened to signature, 30 March 2007.

institution (ECHR, Article 5 (1) (e); UN Mental Illness Principles, Principle 16). However, because involuntary detention is an extremely serious interference with the freedom of persons with disabilities, in particular their right to liberty and security, international and national human rights law attaches numerous procedural safeguards to involuntary detention cases. Moreover, these safeguards are generating a significant jurisprudence, most notably in regional human rights commissions and courts (ECtHR 1979; Gostin & Gable 2004; Gostin 2000; Lewis 2002).

Entitlements

The right to health includes an entitlement to a system of health protection which provides equality of opportunity for all people to enjoy the highest attainable standard of health through access to both healthcare and the underlying determinants of health, all of which play a vital role in ensuring the health and dignity of persons with mental disabilities (UNGA 1993, Rules 2–4).

States are required to take steps to ensure a full package of community-based mental healthcare and support services conducive to health, dignity, and inclusion. These should include medication, psychotherapy, ambulatory services, hospital care for acute admissions, residential facilities, rehabilitation for persons with psychiatric disabilities, programmes to maximize the independence and skills of persons with intellectual disabilities, supported housing and employment, income support, inclusive and appropriate education for children with intellectual disabilities, and respite care for families looking after a person with a mental disability 24 h a day. In this way, unnecessary institutionalization can be avoided.

Scaling up interventions to ensure equality of opportunity for the enjoyment of the right to health requires that adequate numbers of appropriate professionals be trained. Similarly, primary care providers should be provided with essential mental healthcare and disability sensitization training to enable them to provide front-line mental and physical healthcare to persons with mental disabilities.

Underlying determinants of health that are particularly relevant to persons with mental disabilities, who are disproportionately affected by poverty and as such often deprived of important entitlements, include adequate sanitation, safe water, and adequate food and shelter (UNCESCR 2000, para. 4). The conditions in psychiatric hospitals, as well as other institutions used by persons with mental disabilities, are often grossly inadequate from this point of view.

◆ *Obligations of immediate effect and progressive realization*

It is reasonable to expect that countries, even those with very limited resources, undertake to implement certain measures towards realization of the right to health for people with disabilities. For example they can be expected to: Include the recognition, care, and treatment of mental disabilities in training curricula of all health personnel; promote public campaigns against stigma and discrimination of persons with mental disabilities; support the formation of civil society groups that are representative of mental healthcare users and their families; formulate modern policies and programmes on mental disabilities; downsize psychiatric hospitals and, as far as possible, extend community care; in relation to persons with mental disabilities, actively seek assistance and cooperation from donors and international organizations (WHO 2001b, pp. 112–15).

◆ *Respect, protect, fulfil*

Specifically in relation to mental disabilities, the obligation to *respect* requires States to refrain from denying or limiting equal access to healthcare services and underlying determinants of health, for persons with mental disabilities. They are also required to ensure that persons with mental disabilities in public institutions are not denied access to healthcare and related support services, or underlying determinants of health, including water and sanitation (IACHR 1997).

The obligation to *protect* means that States are required to take actions to ensure that third parties do not harm the right to health of persons with mental disabilities. For example, States should take measures to protect persons with mental disabilities from violence and other right to health-related abuses occurring in private healthcare or support services.

The obligation to *fulfil* requires States to recognize the right to health, including the right to health of persons with mental disabilities, in national political and legal systems, with a view to ensuring its implementation. States should adopt appropriate legislative, administrative, budgetary, judicial, promotional, and other measures towards this end (ICESCR Article 2(1); UNCESCR 2000, para. 36). For example, States should ensure that the right to health of persons with mental disabilities is adequately reflected in their national health strategy and plan of action, as well as other relevant policies, such as national poverty reduction strategies, and the national budget (WHO 2004c). Mental health laws, policies, programmes, and projects should embody human rights and empower people with mental disabilities to make choices about their lives; give legal protections relating to the establishment of (and access to) quality mental health facilities, as well as care and support services; establish robust procedural mechanisms for the protection of those with mental disabilities; ensure the integration of persons with mental disabilities into the community; and promote mental health throughout society (WHO 2005a). Patients' rights charters should encompass the human rights of persons with mental disabilities. States should also ensure that access to information about their human rights is provided to persons with mental disabilities and their guardians, as well as others who may be institutionalized in psychiatric hospitals.

◆ *International assistance and cooperation*

The record shows that mental healthcare and support services are not a priority health area for donors. Furthermore, donors have sometimes supported inappropriate programmes, such as the rebuilding of a damaged psychiatric institution constructed many years ago on the basis of conceptions of mental disability that have since been discredited. In so doing, the donor inadvertently prolongs, for many years, seriously inappropriate approaches to mental disability.

It is unacceptable for a donor to fund a programme that, in moving a psychiatric institution to an isolated location, makes it impossible for its users to sustain or develop their links with the community (MDRI 2002). If a donor wishes to assist children with intellectual disabilities, it might wish to fund community-based services to support children and their parents, enabling the children to remain at home, instead of funding new facilities in a remote institution that the parents can only afford to visit once a month, if at all (Rosenthal 2000).

Donors have a right to health duty to consider more—and better quality—support in the area of mental disability. In accordance with their responsibility of international assistance and cooperation, they are required to consider adopting measures such as: Supporting the development of appropriate community-based care and support services; supporting advocacy by persons with mental disabilities, their families and representative organizations; and providing policy and technical expertise. Furthermore, donors should ensure that all their programmes promote equality and non-discrimination for persons with mental disabilities, while international agencies fulfil the role that corresponds to them by providing technical support.

◆ *Monitoring and accountability*

The right to health requires that States have in place effective, transparent, and accessible monitoring and accountability mechanisms in relation to the health of persons with mental disabilities.

In many countries, there is an absence of sustained and independent monitoring of mental healthcare, resulting in frequent abuses in large psychiatric hospitals and community-based settings going unnoticed. The Mental Illness Principles emphasize the importance of inspecting mental health facilities, as well as investigating and resolving complaints where an alleged violation of the rights of a patient is concerned (UN Mental Illness Principle 22).

Lack of surveillance is doubly problematic because persons with mental disabilities, especially those who are institutionalized, are often unable to access independent and effective accountability mechanisms when their human rights have been violated. Where accountability mechanisms do exist, the severity of their condition may render them unable to protect their interests independently through legal proceedings, to demand effective procedural safeguards where these may be lacking, or to access legal aid.

For example, the right to health requires that an independent review body must be made accessible to persons with mental disabilities, or other appropriate persons, to review cases of involuntary admission and treatment periodically (UN Mental Illness Principle 17).

Although there is a range of detailed international standards concerning the human rights of persons with mental disabilities, and procedural safeguards to protect them (UN Mental Illness Principles 11, 18), their lack of implementation poses a real challenge. The new Convention on the Rights of Persons with Disabilities will be crucial to international monitoring and accountability, especially if its Optional Protocol, which introduces a procedure under which individuals and groups can lodge complaints, were to come into force. Significantly, this mechanism strengthens the existing standards relating to the right to health of persons with mental disabilities that do not establish specific monitoring or accountability mechanisms.

Alongside this Convention, other international human rights treaties (including ICESCR, CRC, CEDAW and CERD, and ICCPR,) extend protections to persons with mental disabilities. For this reason, States should pay greater attention to them in their State party reports, and examination of these reports by the human rights treaty bodies should, in turn, give a greater focus to these issues through their discussions with States parties, concluding observations, and general comments or recommendations. Relevant civil society organizations, including representatives of persons with mental disabilities, play an important role by engaging with UN treaty bodies and special procedures.

Sexual and reproductive health, including maternal mortality

The Commission on Human Rights confirmed in 2003 that 'sexual and reproductive health are integral elements of the right of everyone to the enjoyment of the highest attainable standard of physical and mental health' (UNCHR 2003b, preamble and para. 6). The outcomes of world conferences, in particular the International Conference on Population and Development (UN 1994), the Fourth World Conference on Women (UN 1995), and their respective 5-year reviews, confirm that human rights have an indispensable role to play in relation to sexual and reproductive health issues.

More recently, there has been a deepening conceptual understanding of maternal mortality as a human rights issue (Cook *et al.* 2006; Freedman 2003). Although the issue is connected to a number of human rights, the right to the highest attainable standard of health is of particular relevance, and is the focus of the following remarks.

◆ *Freedoms and entitlements*

Freedoms

In the context of sexual and reproductive health, freedoms include a right to control one's health and body. Rape and other forms of sexual violence, including forced pregnancy, non-consensual contraceptive methods (e.g. forced sterilization and forced abortion), female genital mutilation/cutting (FGM/C), and forced marriage all represent serious breaches of sexual and reproductive freedoms, and are therefore fundamentally and inherently inconsistent with the right to health. In the specific context of maternal mortality, relevant freedoms include freedom from discrimination; harmful traditional practices, such as early marriage and violence.

For example, some cultural practices, including FGM/C, carry a high risk of disability and death. This means that where the practice exists, States should take appropriate and effective measures to eradicate it, in accordance with their obligations under the Convention on the Rights of the Child. Early marriage, which disproportionately affects girls, is predominantly found in South Asia and sub-Saharan Africa, where over 50 per cent of girls are married by the age of 18. Among other problems, early marriage is linked to health risks including those arising from premature pregnancy. Finally, in the context of adolescent health, States are obliged to set minimum ages for sexual consent and marriage (UNCRC 2003, paras. 9, 19).

Entitlements

Entitlements that form part of the rights to reproductive and sexual health include equal access, in law and fact, to reproductive and child health services, as well as information about sexual and reproductive health issues.

Specifically, States are required to provide a wide range of appropriate and, where necessary, free sexual and reproductive health services, including access to family planning, pre- and post-natal care, emergency obstetric services, and access to information. They should also ensure access to such essential health services as voluntary testing, counselling, and treatment for sexually transmitted infections, including HIV/AIDS, and breast and reproductive system cancers, as well as infertility treatment.

Unsafe abortions kill some 68 000 women each year, and thus constitute a right to life and right to health issue of enormous proportions. They also give rise to high rates of morbidity.

Women with unwanted pregnancies should be offered reliable information and compassionate counselling, including information on where and when a pregnancy may be terminated legally. Where abortions are legal, they must be safe: Public health systems should train and equip health service providers and take other measures to ensure that such abortions are not only safe but accessible (WHO 2003). In all cases, women should have access to quality services for the management of complications arising from abortion. Punitive provisions against women who undergo abortions are inconsistent with the right to the highest attainable standard of health.

Certain entitlements envisaged in international law are directly relevant to reducing maternal mortality (CEDAW Article 12 (2); UNCESCR 2000, para. 14) and, if fulfilled, would reduce its incidence. For example, an equitable, well-resourced, accessible, and integrated health system—a crucial entitlement arising from the right to health—is widely accepted as a vital pre-condition for guaranteeing women's access to the interventions that can prevent or treat the causes of maternal deaths (Freedman 2005). Other entitlements include education and information on sexual and reproductive health (UNCEDAW 1999a, para.18), safe abortion services where not against the law,[15] and primary healthcare services (UNCESCR 2000, paras. 14, 21; UNCEDAW 1999a para. 27; UN 1994, para. 8.25) especially universal access to reproductive healthcare (UNMP 2005b).

The entitlement to specific underlying determinants of health relevant to maternal mortality must also be guaranteed. The failure to safeguard women's rights is often manifested in low status of women, poor access to information and care, early age of marriage, and restricted mobility, among other problems (DFID 2005). Specifically, gender equality[16] has an important role to play in preventing maternal mortality as alongside empowerment it can lead to greater demand by women for family planning services, antenatal care, and safe delivery. Another relevant determinant of health and element of the right to health that must be ensured in order to address problems of maternal mortality is water and sanitation, which are vital to the provision of prenatal care and emergency obstetric care.

◆ *Available, accessible, acceptable and good quality*

In many countries, information on sexual and reproductive health is not readily available and, if it is, it is not accessible to all, in particular women and adolescents. Sexual and reproductive health services are often geographically inaccessible to communities living in rural areas, or provided in a form that is not culturally acceptable to indigenous peoples and other non-dominant groups. Similarly, services, and relevant underlying determinants of health, such as education, are often of substandard quality.

In order to address the problem of maternal mortality, the concept of availability calls for collective action to enhance care and improve human resource strategies, including increasing the number and quality of health professionals and improving terms and conditions (UNMP 2005c). Accessibility considers whether physical access and the cost of health services influence women's ability to seek care (UNMP 2005c). Furthermore, discriminatory laws, policies, practices, and gender inequalities prevent women and adolescents from accessing good quality services or information on sexual and reproductive health, and have a direct impact on maternal mortality (Cook *et al.* 2006). To prevent maternal mortality, scaling up technical interventions, or making the interventions affordable is insufficient: Strategies ensuring the *acceptability* of services through their sensitivity to the rights, cultures and needs of pregnant women, including those from indigenous peoples and other minority groups, are also vital (Shiffman 2006). Quality of care will influence both a woman's decision whether or not to seek care, as well as the outcome of interventions, and so is key to tackling maternal mortality through the provision of maternal healthcare services.

◆ *Discrimination, vulnerability and stigma*

Discrimination and stigma continue to pose a serious threat to sexual and reproductive health for many groups, including women, sexual minorities, refugees, people with disabilities, rural communities, indigenous persons, people living with HIV/AIDS, sex workers, and people held in detention. Some individuals suffer discrimination on several grounds, e.g. gender, race, poverty, and health status (UNCHR 2003a, para. 62).

Discrimination based on gender hinders the ability of many women to protect themselves from HIV infection and to respond to the consequences of HIV infection. Women and girls' vulnerability to HIV and AIDS is compounded by other human rights issues including inadequate access to information, education, and services necessary to ensure sexual health; sexual violence; harmful traditional or customary practices affecting the health of women and children (such as early and forced marriage); and lack of legal capacity and equality in areas such as marriage and divorce.

Stigma and discrimination associated with HIV/AIDS may also reinforce other prejudices, discrimination, and inequalities related to gender and sexuality. The result is that those affected may be reluctant to seek health and social services, information, education, and counselling, even when those services are available. This, in turn, will contribute to the vulnerability of others to HIV infection.

Vulnerability in the context of sexual and reproductive health is particularly relevant to adolescents and young people, who find themselves lacking access to relevant information and services during a period characterized by sexual and reproductive maturation. Important protections for adolescents are enshrined in CRC, which includes a number of cross-cutting principles which have an important bearing on adolescent's sexual and reproductive health, namely: The survival and development of the child, the best interests

[15] UN human rights bodies have also held that absolute legal prohibitions on abortion can violate the rights to life and health where they contribute to maternal mortality. For example, in its Concluding Observations on Colombia, CEDAW noted, with great concern: 'That abortion, which is the second cause of maternal deaths in Colombia, is punishable as an illegal act. No exceptions are made to that prohibition, including where the mother's life is in danger or to safeguard her physical or mental health or in cases where the mother has been raped. . . . The Committee believes that legal provisions on abortion constitute a violation of the rights of women to health and life and of article 12 of the Convention' (UN CEDAW 1999b, para. 393).

[16] States should 'take all appropriate measures to eliminate discrimination against women in the field of healthcare in order to ensure, on a basis of equality of men and women, access to healthcare services, including those related to family planning' (CEDAW, article 12.1).

of the child, non-discrimination, and respect for the views of the child (CRC Articles 2,3,5,6,12; UNCRC 2003, para.12).

Discrimination on the grounds of sexual orientation is impermissible under international human rights law. The legal prohibition of same-sex relations in many countries, in conjunction with a widespread lack of support or protection for sexual minorities against violence and discrimination, impedes the enjoyment of sexual and reproductive health by many people with lesbian, gay, bisexual, and transgender identities or conduct.[17] Similarly, criminalization can impede programmes which are essential to promoting the right to health and other human rights.[18]

Arising from their obligations to combat discrimination, States have a duty to ensure that health information and services are made available to vulnerable groups. For example, they must take steps to empower women to make decisions in relation to their sexual and reproductive health, free of coercion, violence and discrimination. They must take action to redress gender-based violence and ensure that there are sensitive and compassionate services available for the survivors of gender-based violence, including rape and incest. States should ensure that adolescents are able to receive information, including on family planning and contraceptives, the dangers of early pregnancy, and the prevention of sexually transmitted infections including HIV/AIDS, as well as appropriate services for sexual and reproductive health. Consistent with *Toonen v. Australia* and numerous other international and national decisions, they should ensure that sexual and other health services are available for men who have sex with men, lesbians, and transsexual and bisexual people. It is also important to ensure that voluntary counselling, testing, and treatment of sexually transmitted infections are available for sex workers (UNHRCttee 1994).

Finally, in the context of sexual and reproductive health, breaches of medical confidentiality may occur. Sometimes these breaches, when accompanied by stigmatization, lead to unlawful dismissal from employment, expulsion from families and communities, physical assault, and other abuse. Also, a lack of confidentiality may deter individuals from seeking advice and treatment, thereby jeopardizing their health and well-being. States are obliged to take effective measures to ensure medical confidentiality and privacy.

Water and sanitation

Healthcare attracts a disproportionate amount of attention and resources. Yet access to water and sanitation, as well as other underlying determinants of health, are integral features of the right to the highest attainable standard of health.

- *Available, accessible, acceptable and quality*

Available

The right to health requires a State to do all it can to ensure that safe water and adequate sanitation is available to everyone in its jurisdiction. The quantity of water available for each person should correspond to the quantity specified by WHO (Howard & Bartram 2002), though some individuals and groups may require additional water due to health, climate, and work conditions, and the State should therefore ensure that this is also available. The right to health stipulates that States must ensure the availability of safe water for personal and domestic uses such as 'drinking, personal sanitation, washing of clothes, food preparation, personal and household hygiene' (UNCESCR 2003 para 12 (a)).

Accessible

The right to health also requires that water and sanitation be accessible to everyone without discrimination. In this context, accessibility has four dimensions:

First, water and sanitation must be within safe physical reach for all sections of the population, in all parts of the country. Water and sanitation therefore should be *physically accessible* within, or in the immediate vicinity of, the household, educational institution, workplace, and health or other institution (UN 2005, guideline 1.3). The inaccessibility of water within safe physical reach can seriously impair health, including the health of women and children responsible for carrying water. Carrying heavy water containers for long distances can cause fatigue, pain, and spinal and pelvic injuries, which may lead to problems during pregnancy and childbirth. Similarly, the absence of safe, private sanitation facilities subjects women to a humiliating, stressful, and uncomfortable daily routine that can damage their health (UNMP 2005a, pp. 23–5). When designing water and sanitation facilities in camps for refugees and internally displaced persons, special attention should be given to prevent gender-based violence. For example, facilities should be provided in safe areas near dwellings (UNHCR 2005).

Second, water and sanitation should be *economically accessible*, including to those living in poverty. Poverty is associated with inequitable access to health services, safe water, and sanitation. If those living in poverty are not enjoying access to safe water and adequate sanitation, the State has a duty to take reasonable measures that ensure access to all.

Third, water and sanitation should be *accessible* to all *without discrimination* on any of the grounds prohibited under human rights law, such as sex, race, ethnicity, disability, and socioeconomic status.

Finally, reliable *information* about water and sanitation must be *accessible* to all so that they can make well-informed decisions.

Acceptable

The right to health requires that water and sanitation facilities be respectful of gender and life-cycle requirements and be culturally *acceptable*. For example, measures should ensure that sanitation facilities are mindful of the privacy of women, men, and children.

Quality

Both water services and sanitation facilities must be of good *quality*: This reduces susceptibility to anaemia, diarrhoea, and other conditions that cause maternal and infant mortality and morbidity (UNMP 2005a, p. 18). Water required for personal and domestic use should be safe and free from 'micro-organisms, chemical substances and radiological hazards which constitute a threat to a person's health' (UNCESCR 2003, para. 12(b)). States should establish water quality regulations and standards on the basis of the *WHO Guidelines for Drinking Water Quality* (WHO 2006c).

17 Other Special Rapporteurs have documented violence and discrimination based on sexual orientation (UNCHR 2001, paras. 48–50; UNGA 2001, paras 17–25).

18 For example, 'criminalization of homosexual activity . . . would appear to run counter to the implementation of effective education programmes in respect of HIV/AIDS prevention' (UNHRCttee 1994, para 8.5).

Similarly, each person should have affordable access to sanitation services, facilities, and installations adequate for the promotion and protection of their human health and dignity. Good health requires the protection of the environment from human waste; this can only be achieved if everyone has access to, and utilizes, adequate sanitation (UNCHR 2004, para. 44).

New tools and techniques

The 'Human rights' section introduced the idea, which is increasingly recognized, that one way of vindicating the right to the highest attainable standard of health is by way of the 'policy approach' i.e. the integration of the right to health in national and international policy-making approaches. For this approach to prosper, the traditional human rights techniques—taking test cases in the courts, 'naming and shaming', letter-writing campaigns, slogans, and so on—will not be sufficient. The 'policy approach' demands the development of new right-to-health skills and tools, such as budgetary analysis, indicators, benchmarks, and impact assessments. In recent years, the health and human rights community has made significant progress towards the development of these new methodologies. Here, by way of illustration, indicators, benchmarks, and impact assessments are briefly introduced in the context of the right to the highest attainable standard of health.

A human rights-based approach to health indicators

The international right to the highest attainable standard of health is subject to progressive realization. Inescapably, this means that what is expected of a State will vary over time. With a view to monitoring its progress, a State needs a device to measure this variable dimension of the right to health. The most appropriate device is the combined application of indicators and benchmarks. Thus, a State selects appropriate indicators that will help it monitor different dimensions of the right to health. These indicators might include, for example, maternal mortality ratios and child mortality rates. Most indicators will require disaggregation, such as on the grounds of sex, race, ethnicity, rural/urban, and socioeconomic status. Then the State sets appropriate national targets or benchmarks in relation to each disaggregated indicator.

In this way, indicators and benchmarks fulfil two important functions. *First*, they can help the State to monitor its progress over time, enabling the authorities to recognize when policy adjustments are required. *Second*, they can help to hold the State to account in relation to the discharge of its responsibilities arising from the right to health, although deteriorating indicators do not necessarily mean that the State is in breach of its international right to health obligations (UNCHR 2006, para. 35). Of course, indicators also have other important roles. For example, by highlighting issues such as disaggregation, participation, and accountability, indicators can enhance the effectiveness of policies and programmes.

Health professionals and policy makers constantly use a very large number of health indicators, such as the HIV prevalence rate. Is it possible to simply appropriate these health indicators and call them 'human rights indicators' or 'right to health indicators'? Or do indicators that are to be used for monitoring human rights and the right to health require some special features? If so, what are these special attributes?

The considered view is that some of these health indictors may be used to monitor aspects of the progressive realization of the right to health, provided the following conditions are met (UNGA 2004):

1. They correspond, with some precision, to a right to health norm.
2. They are disaggregated by at least sex, race, ethnicity, rural/urban, and socioeconomic status.
3. They are supplemented by additional indicators—rarely found among classic health indicators—that monitor five essential and inter-related features of the right to health:
    - A national strategy and plan of action that includes the right to health
    - The participation of individuals and groups, especially the most vulnerable and disadvantaged, in relation to the formulation of health policies and programmes
    - Access to health information, as well as confidentiality of personal health data
    - International assistance and cooperation of donors in relation to the enjoyment of the right to health in developing countries
    - Accessible and effective monitoring and accountability mechanisms

In this way, many existing health indicators, such as the maternal mortality ratio and HIV prevalence rate, have an important potential role to play in measuring and monitoring the progressive realization of the right to health, provided that they conform to these conditions.

Impact assessments and the right to the highest attainable standard of health

A further tool that can be employed to monitor the fulfilment of the right to health and hold duty-bearers to account is through impact assessments. They are an aid to equitable, inclusive, robust, and sustainable policy making, and have the objective of informing decision-makers and the people likely to be affected by a new policy, programme, or project so that the proposal can be improved to reduce potential negative effects and increase positive ones. They are one way of ensuring that the right to health—especially of marginalized groups, including the poor—is given due weight in all national and international policy-making processes. From the right to health perspective, an impact assessment methodology is a key feature of a health system and an essential means by which a government can gauge whether or not it is on target to realize progressively the right to health.

At least two distinct methodological approaches are available: To develop a self-standing methodology for human rights impact assessments such as has been done in other fields, such as environmental and social policy; or to integrate human rights into *existing* types of impact assessments. The second approach is consistent with the call on governments to mainstream human rights into all government processes and requires interdisciplinary collaboration (UNGA 2007, para. 39).

In order that an impact assessment uphold rights-based principles, it must: (1) Use an explicit human rights framework, (2) aim for progressive realization of human rights, (3) promote equality and non-discrimination in process and policy, (4) ensure meaningful participation by all stakeholders, (5) provide information and protect the right to freely express ideas, (6) establish mechanisms to hold the State accountable, and (7) recognize the interdependence of all human rights (Hunt and MacNaughton 2006, p. 32).

If the second approach above is adopted, there are six steps that should be followed to ensure that the right to health is integrated into existing impact assessments: (1) Perform a preliminary check on the proposed policy to determine whether or not a full-scale right-to-health impact assessment is necessary; (2) prepare an assessment plan and distribute information on the policy and the plan to all stakeholders; (3) collect information on potential right-to-health impacts of the proposed policy; (4) prepare a draft report comparing the potential impacts with the State's legal obligations arising from the right to health; (5) distribute the draft report and engage stakeholders in evaluating the options; and (6) prepare the final report detailing the final decision, the rationale for the choices made and a framework for implementation and evaluation.

Overall, the human rights framework for impact assessment adds value because human rights (1) are based on legal obligations to which governments have agreed to abide, (2) apply to all parts of the government encouraging coherence to policy-making and ensuring that policies reinforce each other; (3) require participation in policy making by the people affected, enhancing legitimacy and ownership of policy choices; (4) enhance effectiveness by demanding data disaggregation, participation and transparency; and (5) demand mechanisms through which policy makers can be held accountable.

Conclusion: Key features of a health system from a right to health perspective

The right to the highest attainable standard of health can be understood as a right to an effective and integrated health system, encompassing healthcare and the underlying determinants of health, which is responsive to national and local priorities, and accessible to all.

At the heart of this understanding of the right to health is a package of health services, facilities, and goods, extending to healthcare and the underlying determinants of health, such as access to safe water, adequate sanitation, and health-related information. This package must be available, accessible, and of good quality. Also, it must be sensitive to different cultures. While this package will have many features that are common to all countries, there will also be differences between one country and another, reflective of different disease burdens, cultural contexts, resource availability, and so on. This chapter has signalled some elements of this package in relation to neglected diseases, mental disability, sexual and reproductive health, and water and sanitation.

However, besides this essential package of health services, facilities, and goods, a health system must have some additional features if it is to reflect the right to the highest attainable standard of health. These additional features derive from international norms, including CESCR's General Comment 14 on the right to the highest attainable standard of health. While some of these additional features have been described in the preceding paragraphs, they include the following:

1. Formal legal recognition of the right to health in either a national Constitution, or bill of rights, or other statute.
2. An elaboration of what the right to health means, for both the public and private sectors, for example by way of regulations, guidelines and codes of conduct.
3. Research and development for national and local health priorities.
4. A comprehensive situational analysis identifying, inter alia, the health needs of the population, upon which (5) is based.
5. A comprehensive national health plan, including objectives, timeframes, who is responsible for what, reporting procedures, indicators and benchmarks (to measure progressive realization), and a detailed budget.
6. A health financing system that is equitable and evidence-informed.
7. An ex-ante right to health impact assessment methodology that permits the Government to foreshadow the likely impact of a draft law, policy, or programme on the enjoyment of the right to the highest attainable standard of health, thereby enabling it, when necessary, to revise the projected initiative.
8. As much 'bottom up' participation as possible, in relation to policy-making, implementation, and accountability.
9. Access to health-related information and data; data will have to be disaggregated so that the health situation of disadvantaged populations is properly understood, enabling the authorities to devise measures that address health inequities and disadvantage; at the same time, however, arrangements must be in place to ensure that personal medical data remains confidential.
10. As well as effective mechanisms for co-ordination within the health sector, there must also be effective mechanisms for intersectoral coordination in health, because the right to health extends beyond the health sector; moreover, where relevant, there must be effective coordination and referral with traditional health systems.
11. A sufficient number of domestically trained health workers enjoying good terms and conditions of employment; they should be reflective of the country's cultural diversity, including language, and strike a balance between men and women; health workers' training should include human rights.
12. An international dimension, for example, low-income countries should seek international assistance and cooperation in health and high-income countries should provide it.
13. Educational campaigns and other arrangements so that the public knows about its right to health entitlements and how to vindicate them.
14. Effective, transparent, and accessible monitoring and accountability mechanisms, including redress, for both the public and private health sectors.

States have a legal obligation to ensure that their health systems not only include an appropriate package of health services, facilities, and goods, but also the additional features briefly summarized in points 1–14.

Key points

- The right to the highest attainable standard of health is enshrined in several international treaties and numerous national constitutions.
- It gives rise to legally binding obligations on States.

- There is a complementary relationship between public health and the right to the highest attainable standard of health.
- The right to health analytical framework deepens understanding of contemporary public health issues and can help to identify appropriate responses to them.
- The right to the highest attainable standard of health can be understood as a right to an effective and integrated health system, encompassing healthcare and the underlying determinants of health, which is responsive to national and local priorities, and accessible to all.

References

ACHPR (African Commission on Human and Peoples' Rights) (2001). *Communication No. 155/96: The Social and Economic Rights Action Center for Economic and Social Rights v. Nigeria*. Fifteenth Annual Activity Report of ACHPR, 2001–2002, Annex V.

Annan, K. (2001). *Speech to the National Urban League Conference.* 30 July 2001, Washington DC.

Bartram, J. *et al.* (2005). Focusing on improved water for sanitation and health. *Lancet*, **365**, 810–12.

Beaglehole, R. (2002). Overview and framework. In *Oxford Textbook of Public Health* (ed. R. Detels), 4th edition. OUP, Oxford.

Chapman and Russel (eds.) (2002). *Core obligations: Building a framework for economic, social and cultural rights*, Intersentia, 2002.

CCSA (Constitutional Court of South Africa) (2002). *Minister of Health et al v. Treatment Action Campaign et al.* Case CCT 8/02, decided on 5 July 2002.

Cook, R., Dickens, B. *et al.* (2006). *International policy on sexual and reproductive health and rights*. Swedish International Development Cooperation Agency.

Coreil, J., Mayard, G., and Addiss, D. (2003). *Support groups for women with lymphatic filariasis in Haiti*. Report Series No. 2, Social, Economic and Behavioural Research, Special Programme for Research and Training in Tropical Diseases (TDR), 2003, p. 42.

Council of Europe (1950). *Convention for the protection of human rights and fundamental freedoms*. ETS No. 5.

DFID (Department for International Development) (2005). *How to reduce maternal deaths: Rights and responsibilities*. DFID, London.

ECSR (European Committee on Social Rights) (1998). *International Commission of Jurists v. Portugal*. Case No. 1/1998.

ECtHR (European Court of Human Rights) (1979). *Winterwerp v. The Netherlands, Judgement 24 October 1979*. Application No. 6301/73. Reported at 2 EHRR 387.

ECtHR (European Court of Human Rights) (1990). *E. v. Norway, Judgement of 29 August 1990*. Application No. 11701/85, Series A, No. 181–A.

ECtHR (European Court of Human Rights) (1994). *Lopez Ostra v. Spain, Judgement of December 9, 1994*. Case No. 41/1993/436/515.

Espino, F., Coops, V., and Manderson, L. (2004). *Community participation and tropical disease control in resource-poor settings*. UNICEF/UNDP/World Bank/WHO Special Programme for Research and Training in Tropical Diseases, Geneva.

Evans, B. *et al.* (2004). *Closing the sanitation gap: The case for better public funding of sanitation and hygiene behaviour change*. Organization for Economic Co-operation and Development (OECD) 13th Round Table on Sustainable Development. OECD, Paris.

Freedman, L. (2003). Human rights, constructive accountability and maternal mortality in the Dominican Republic: A Commentary. *International Journal of Gynecology and Obstetrics*, **82**.

Freedman, L. (2005). Achieving the MDGs: Health systems as core social institutions. *Development*, **48**(1).

Gostin, L.O. (2000). Human rights of persons with mental disabilities: The ECHR, *International Journal of Law and Psychiatry*, **23**.

Gostin, L.O. and Gable, L. (2004). The human rights of persons with mental disabilities: A global perspective on the application of human rights principles to mental health. *Maryland Law Review*, **63**.

Guthman, J. *et al.* (1997). Patients' associations and the control of leishmaniasis in Peru. *Bulletin of the World Health Organization*, **75**: 6–13. p.17.

Howard, G. and Bartram, J. (2002). *Domestic water quantity: Service level and health*. World Health Organization (WHO) 2002. WHO, Geneva.

Hunt, P. and MacNaughton, G. (2006). *Impact assessments, poverty and human rights: A case study using the right to the highest attainable standard of health*. UNESCO. http://www2.essex.ac.uk/human_rights_centre/rth/docs/Impact%20Assessments%209Dec06[1].doc

IACHR (Inter-American Commission on Human Rights) (1997). *Victor Rosario Congo v. Ecuador*. Case 11.427, Report No. 12/97, OEA/Ser.L/V/II.95 Doc. 7 rev at 257 (1997)

IACHR (Inter-American Commission on Human Rights) (2000). *Jorge Odir Miranda Cortez et al v. El Salvador*. Case 12.249, Report No. 29/01, OEA/Ser.L/V/II.111 Doc. 20 rev. at 282 (2000).

ICJ (International Court of Justice) (1996). *Advisory opinion: Legality of the threat or use of nuclear weapons*, ICJ Reports 1996. Vol. I. ICJ, The Hague.

Kinney, E. (2001). The international human right to health: What does this mean for our nation and world? *Indiana Law Review*, **34**.

Kinney, E. and Clark, B.A. (2004). Provisions for health and health care in the constitutions of the countries of the world, 37 *Cornell international law journal*, 285.

Lewis, O. (2002). Protecting the rights of people with mental disabilities: The ECHR. *European journal of health law*, **9**(4).

MDRI (Mental Disability Rights International) (2002). *Not on the agenda: Human rights of people with mental disabilities in Kosovo*. MDRI, Washington.

OAS (Organization of American States) (1948). *American declaration of the rights and duties of man*. OAS Res. XXX, adopted by the Ninth International Conference of American States (1948). OAS, Washington DC.

OAS (Organization of American States) (1969). *American convention on human rights*. OAS Treaty Series No. 36, 1144 U.N.T.S. 123. Adopted at the Inter-American Specialized Conference on Human Rights, San Jose, Costa Rica, 22 November 1969. OAS, Washington DC.

OAS (Organization of American States) (1994). *Inter-American convention on the prevention, punishment and eradication of violence against women, "Convention of Belém do Pará"*. Adopted at the 24th Regular Session of the General Assembly, 9 June 1994. OAS, Washington.

Rosenthal, E. *et al.* (2000). Implementing the right to community integration for children with disabilities in Russia: A human rights framework for international action. *Health and Human Rights: An International Journal*, **4**.

Shiffman, J. and Garces del Valle, A. (2006). Political histories and disparities in safe motherhood between Guatemala and Honduras. *Population and Development Review*, **32**(1).

Skogly, S. (2006). *Beyond national borders: States' HR obligations in their international cooperation*, Intersentia.

UN (1945). *UN Charter*, adopted 26 June 1945, entered into force 24 October 1945, as amended by GA Res. 1991 (XVIII) 17 December 1963, entered into force 31 August 1966 (557 UNTS 143); 2101 of 20 December 1965, entered into force 12 June 1968 (638 UNTS 308); and 2847 (XXVI) of 20 December 1971, entered into force 24 September 1973 (892 UNTS 119). UN, New York.

UN (1948). *Universal declaration of human rights*. GA Resolution 217A (III), UN GAOR, Resolution 71, UN Document A/810. UN, New York.

UN (United Nations) (1965). *Convention on the elimination of all forms of racial discrimination*, (ICERD). UN GA Resolution 2106A (XX). UN, New York.

UN (1966a). *International Covenant on Civil and Political Rights*, (ICCPR). UN GA Resolution 2200A (XXI), 16 December 1966. UN, New York.

UN (1966b). *International Covenant on Economic, Social and Cultural Rights*, (ICESCR). UN GA Resolution 2200A (XXI), 16 December 1966. UN, New York.

UN (1979). *Convention on the elimination of all forms of discrimination against women* (CERD). GA Resolution 34/180, UN GAOR, 34th Session, Supplement No.46 at 193, UN Document A/34/46. UN, New York.

UN (1989). *Convention on the rights of the child*, (CRC). UN GA Resolution 44/25, 20 November 1989. UN, New York.

UN (1990). *International convention on the protection of the rights of all migrant workers and members of their families*, (ICRMW). GA Resolution 45/158, 18 December 1990. UN, New York.

UN (1991). *Principles for the protection of persons with mental illness and the improvement of mental health care*, GA Resolution 46/119, 17 December 1991. UN, New York.

UN (1993). United Nations General Assembly. *Vienna declaration and programme of action. World conference on human rights*, Vienna 14–25 June 1993, UN Document A/CONF.157/23. UN, New York.

UN (1994). *International conference on population and development*. 5–13 September 1994, Cairo, Egypt.

UN (1995). *Report of the fourth world conference on women*. Beijing, China 4–15 September 1995. UN Document A/CONF.177.20.

UN (2002). *Johannesburg plan for the implementation of the world summit on sustainable development*. 26 August–4 September 2002, Johannesburg, South Africa.

UN (2005). *Sub-Commission draft guidelines for the realisation of the right to drinking water and sanitation*. Adopted by the Sub-Commission in Resolution 2006/10. UN Document A/HRC/Sub.1/58/L11.

UNCEDAW (United Nations Committee on the Elimination of Discrimination Against Women) (1999a). *General Recommendation No. 24 on Women and Health*, EDAW/C/1999/1/WGII/WP2/Rev.1. UN, Geneva.

UNCEDAW (United Nations Committee on the Elimination of Discrimination Against Women) (1999b). *Concluding Observations on Colombia*. 5 February 1999. UN Document A/54/38, paras. 337–401. UN, Geneva. para. 393.

UNCESCR (United Nations Committee on Economic, Social and Cultural Rights) (1990). *General Comment No. 3 (Fifth Session). The nature of States parties obligations (Art.2, par.1)*. UN Document E/1991/23. UN, Geneva.

UNCESCR (United Nations Committee on Economic, Social and Cultural Rights) (1994). *General Comment No. 5 (Eleventh Session). Persons with disabilities*. UN Document E/C.12/1194/13. UN, Geneva.

UNCESCR (United Nations Committee on Economic, Social and Cultural Rights) (2000). *General Comment No. 14 (Twenty Second Session). The right to the highest attainable standard of health*. UN Document E/C.12/2000/4. UN, Geneva.

UNCESCR (United Nations Committee on Economic, Social and Cultural Rights) (2003). *General Comment No. 15 (Twenty Ninth Session). The right to water*. UN Document E/C.12/2002/11. UN, Geneva.

UNCHR (United Nations Commission on Human Rights) (1991). *Second progress report of Mr Danilo Turk, special rapporteur on the realization of economic, social and cultural rights*, 18 July 1991, UN Document E/CN.4/Sub.2/1991/17. UN, Geneva. paras. 6–48.

UNCHR (United Nations Commission on Human Rights) (2001). *Civil and political rights, including the question of disappearances and summary executions: Report of the special rapporteur*, 11 January 2001, UN Document E/CN.4/2001/9). UN, Geneva.

UNCHR (United Nations Commission on Human Rights) (2002a). *Access to medication in the context of pandemics such as HIV/AIDS*, Resolution 2002/32, 22 April 2002. UN, Geneva.

UNCHR (United Nations Commission on Human Rights) (2002b). *Human rights of persons with disabilities*, Resolution 2002/61, 25 April 2002. UN, Geneva.

UNCHR (United Nations Commission on Human Rights) (2003a). *The right of everyone to the enjoyment of the highest attainable standard of physical and mental health, Report of the Special Rapporteur*, 13 February 2003, UN Document E/CN.4/2003/58). UN, Geneva.

UNCHR (United Nations Commission on Human Rights) (2003b). *The right of everyone to the enjoyment of the highest attainable standard of physical and mental health*. 22 April 2003, Resolution 2003/28. UN, Geneva. Preamble and para 6.

UNCHR (United Nations Commission on Human Rights) (2003). Extrajudicial, summary or arbitrary executions, *Report of the Special Rapporteur*, 11 January 2001, UN Document E/CN.4/2001/9). UN, Geneva. paras 48–50.

UNCHR (United Nations Commission on Human Rights) (2004). *Relationship between the enjoyment of economic, social and cultural rights and the promotion of the realization of the right to drinking water supply and sanitation: Final report of the UN sub-commission Special Rapporteur*. 14 July 2004. UN Document E/CN.4/Sub.2/2004/20. UN, Geneva, para 44.

UNCHR (United Nations Commission on Human Rights) (2006). *The right of everyone to the enjoyment of the highest attainable standard of physical and mental health, report of the Special Rapporteur*, 3 March 2006, UN Document E/CN.4/2006/48). UN, Geneva.

UNCRC (United Nations Committee on the Rights of the Child) (2003). *General Comment No. 4. Adolescent health and development in the context of the Convention on the Rights of the Child*. UN Document CRC/GC/2003/4. UN, Geneva. paras 9 and 19.

UNDP (United Nations Development Programme) (2006). *Human development report: Beyond scarcity: Power, poverty and the Global Water Crisis*. UN, Geneva.

UN ECOSOC (United Nations Economic and Social Council) (1985). *Siracusa principles on the limitation and derogation provisions in the international covenant on civil and political rights*. UN Document E/CN.4/1985/4, Annex.

UNGA (United Nations General Assembly) (1993). *Standard rules on the equalization of opportunities for persons with disabilities*. Adopted by Resolution 48/96, 20 December 1993. UN, New York.

UNGA (United Nations General Assembly) (2000). *United Nations Millennium Declaration*. Adopted by Resolution 55/2, 8 September 2000.

UNGA (United Nations General Assembly) (2001). *Question of torture and other cruel, inhuman or degrading treatment or punishment, Note by the Secretary-General*. 3 July 2001, UN Document A/56/156. paras 17–25.

UNGA (United Nations General Assembly) (2003). *Progress of efforts to ensure the full recognition and enjoyment of the human rights of persons with disabilities: Report of the Secretary General*. 24 July 2003, UN Document A/58/181. UN, New York. para 43.

UNGA (United Nations General Assembly) (2004). *Report of the Special Rapporteur on the right of everyone to the enjoyment of the highest attainable standard of physical and mental health*, 8 October 2004, UN Document A/59/422. UN, New York.

UNGA (United Nations General Assembly) (2007). *Report of the Special Rapporteur on the right of everyone to the enjoyment of the highest attainable standard of physical and mental health*, 8 August 2007, UN Document A/62/214. UN, New York.

UNHCR (United Nations High Commissioner for Refugees) (2005). *Access to water in refugee situations: Survival, health and dignity for refugees*. UNHCR, Geneva.

UNHRCttee (UN Human Rights Committee) (1994). *Toonen v. Australia*, 4 April 1994, UN Document CCPR/C/50/D/488/1992. UN, New York. para 8.5.

UNHRCttee (UN Human Rights Committee) (2003). *Karen Noelia Llantoy Huaman v. Peru (K.L. v. Peru)*. UN Document CPR/C/85/D/1153/2003. UN, New York.

UNHRC (United Nations Human Rights Council) (2007). *Report of the Special Rapporteur on the right of everyone to the enjoyment of the highest attainable standard of physical and mental health*,

Paul Hunt, 17 January 2007, UN Document A/HRC/4/28. UN, New York.

UNMP (United Nations Millennium Project) (2005a). *Health, Dignity and Development: What Will it Take?* Report of the Task Force on Water and Sanitation. UN, New York. pp. 23–25.

UNMP (United Nations Millennium Project) (2005b). *Taking action: Achieving gender equality and empowering women.* Report of the Taskforce on Education and Gender Equality. Earthscan, London.

UNMP (United Nations Millennium Project) (2005c). *Who's got the power?* Report of the Task Force on Child Health and Maternal Health. UN, New York.

UNOHCHR (United Nations Office of the High Commissioner for Human Rights) (2006). *Frequently asked questions on a human rights based approach to development cooperation*, 2006, UN Document HR/PUB/06/8. UN, New York and Geneva.

UNOHCHR (United Nations Office of the High Commissioner for Human Rights) (2006). *Principles and guidelines for a human rights approach to poverty reduction strategies.* UN, Geneva. para 77.

WHO (World Health Organization) (1946). *Constitution of the World Health Organization*, adopted by the International Health Conference, New York, 19 June-22 July 1946, and signed on 22 July 1946. WHO, Geneva.

WHO (World Health Organization) (1978a). *Declaration of Alma-Ata: International conference on primary health care.* 6–12 September, USSR.

WHO (World Health Organization) (1978b). *A joint report by the Director-General of the WHO and the Executive Director of UNICEF presented at the international conference on primary health care*, 1978, Alma-Ata. WHO, Geneva.

WHO (World Health Organization) (2001). *A human rights approach to tuberculosis.* WHO, Geneva. p.12.

WHO (World Health Organization) (2001). *World Health Report 2001. Mental health: New understanding, new hope.* WHO, Geneva. pp. 112–15.

WHO (World Health Organization) (2002). *Global defence against the infectious disease threat.* WHO, Geneva.

WHO (World Health Organization) (2003). *Safe abortion: Technical and policy guidance for health dystems.* WHO, Geneva.

WHO (World Health Organization) (2004a).*Intensified control of neglected diseases: Report of an international workshop, Berlin, 10–12 December 2003.* WHO/CDS/CPE/CEE/2004.45. WHO, Geneva. p22.

WHO (World Health Organization) (2004b). *Water, sanitation and hygiene links to health: Facts and figures*, 2004. WHO, Geneva.

WHO (World Health Organization) (2004c). *Mental health policy, plans and programmes.* WHO, Geneva.

WHO (World Health Organization) (2005a). *Resource book on mental health, human rights and legislation.* WHO, Geneva.

WHO (World Health Organization) (2005b). *World Health Report 2005, make every mother and child count.* WHO, Geneva.

WHO (World Health Organization) (2006a). *World Health Report 2006, Working together for health.* WHO, Geneva.

WHO/UNICEF (World Health Organization/United Nations Children's Fund) (2006b). *Joint monitoring programme, meeting the MDG global water and sanitation target, the urban and rural challenge of the decade.* WHO, Geneva.

WHO (World Health Organization) (2006c). *Guidelines for drinking water quality.* WHO, Geneva.

WHO (World Health Organization) and TDR (Special Programme for Research and Training in Tropical Diseases) (2007). *Neglected diseases: A human rights analysis.* Document reference TDR/SDR/SEB/ST/07.2. WHO, Geneva.

4.2

Comparative national public health legislation

Robyn Martin and Alexandra Lo Dak Wai

Abstract

Law is an important tool in containment of communicable and non-communicable disease. International instruments require states to undertake measures which require legal underpinning. However, the meaning of 'law', and understandings of the extent to which the state can intervene in private life for the benefit of public health, differ across states. In some legal cultures, law is to be found in a form other than legislation, making difficult a comparison of state legislation. This chapter will examine limitations to a world comparison of public health legislation, and consider representative national laws from Western and Asian legal cultures in relation to three public health threats—communicable disease, tobacco harms, and obesity—to analyse ways in which law can play a part in global public health. The legislation discussed in the course of this chapter is that in force in December 2007.

Introduction

Early public health practice focused on poor sanitation and hygiene as sources of disease transmission. Law played an important role in underpinning public health interventions by providing surveillance duties together with powers of compulsory detention, quarantine, and in some instances, powers of compulsory vaccination or treatment. Improvements in scientific medicine throughout the twentieth century enabled the focus of public health to shift from sanitation to medical prevention and cure of disease. Non-medical interventions were considered less important, and by the mid-twentieth century, the role of law in public health had declined. Law came to be considered a redundant mechanism for disease control.

More recently, faced with new and re-emerging infectious diseases, we have been forced to recognize that science alone cannot contain threats posed by communicable disease. While science has made enormous strides in developing medical means of protection and containment, disease has consistently kept one step ahead of medicine. A legal framework for disease control measures is essential to public health disease containment strategy, and it is now also clear that a legal framework is equally important for effective containment of non-communicable diseases. Law is an essential tool in the armoury of contemporary public health, yet states the world over have looked to their public health legislation only to find that it is based on outdated science, and premised on outdated notions of the balance between public good and private right.

Since 2003 and the threat of SARS, many states have begun the process of rethinking and reforming their public health laws. This process has been made more urgent by the requirements of the revised WHO International Health Regulations (IHR) (Fidler & Gostin 2006). While some states have simply amended their laws to bring new disease threats within traditional legal disease frameworks, other states have taken the view that nineteenth-century legislative approaches are no longer valid, and have begun the process of designing entirely new laws to fit new public health environments. Much public health law across the world is in the process of reform, and the legislation discussed in this chapter is that in force in December 2007.

Comparing national public health legislation

The importance of political and social context to the content of public health law means that there is little to be gained in a simple comparison of legal rules or a compilation of state legislation. We must place any comparative analysis within its legal culture, the 'way in which values, practices, and concepts are integrated into the operation of legal institutions and the interpretation of legal texts' (Bell 1995). One way of going about this would be to locate legal systems in the context of world legal 'cultural families' (Van Hoecke & Warrington 1998). Any detailed comparison of laws across cultural families is of limited value as these cultures differ fundamentally in their approach to what constitutes law, and the role of law in society. We can, however, examine legal systems within a legal culture in order to identify the different ways in which public health laws are used to solve particular public health problems (Zweigert & Kötz 1998).

There is no universal understanding of the meaning of 'law' or 'regulation'. Some legal cultures recognize law only as the content of a written statutory act, code, or regulation, or the decision of a court. The WHO in the context of food law defines 'regulation' more widely to include 'any law, statute, guideline or code of practice issued by any level of government or self-regulatory organization' (WHO 1996). Other cultures have an even wider understanding of law which would include administrative orders, guidelines, local edicts and customary law. Legal pluralism, whereby traditional, religious, kinship, tribal, local, and community laws coexist alongside state laws, is common in many parts of the world. Public health is an issue which will in some states be governed not only by 'hard' law but also by 'soft' law which cannot be found in any formal document. It would be misleading then to assume that because a state has no public health legislation, then it has no public health laws. The requirement of compliance with the revised IHR, and the globalization of disease information and exchange, have prompted many states to formalize their primary public health laws, such that increasingly states are enshrining laws in publicly accessible legislation. However, it remains the case that in many states, particularly those not influenced by Western approaches to law, public health powers and duties fall within the domain of 'soft law', complicating any comparison of laws across states.

Much comparative law literature has been devoted to the identification of world legal cultures or families. Any such categorization will inevitably be simplistic and, if applied uncritically, potentially biased towards Western concepts of law because in Western legal philosophy the sources of law are more easily identifiable. Contemporary comparative legal theory has taken a social anthropological approach to defining legal systems which share fundamental characteristics, identifying four distinct legal cultures: Western, Asian, Islamic, and African (Van Hoecke & Warrington 1998). Grouping legal cultures in this way permits some macro-comparison of underlying concepts and underpinning theories, and enables us to take example states from legal families to make more manageable a world comparison. More importantly, some, even if superficial, understanding of the meaning and purpose of law in different legal cultures is essential to any examination or comparison of national laws in order to avoid drawing misleading conclusions about comparative public health legal regimes and in order to avoid examining national public health laws through a filter of Eurocentric legal theory.

The ideal approach in this chapter would have been to examine legislation in states from these four legal cultures. Such an ideal is, however, confounded by the fact that many states have no dedicated public health laws in the sense of published 'hard' law, although there may be conventional powers of quarantine, exclusion, or even compulsory treatment contained within traditional or 'soft' laws. This is particularly the case in states within Islamic or African legal cultures. Sources of public health law such as the WHO International Digest of Health Legislation focus primarily on states that have addressed public health by means of a parliamentary process and that have published laws in the Western tradition, and contain little information about public health laws and practices in states within Islamic and African legal cultures.

It is inevitable then that this comparison of public health legislation will focus on public health law within Western and Asian legal cultures, where states have chosen to enact dedicated public health legislation. This chapter will consider selected legal systems within these two legal families in order to compare approaches to public health law. It is important, however, not to forget that other legal cultures take different approaches to the use of law as a public health tool, and where possible reference will be made to approaches in other legal cultures.

The analysis will be undertaken on the premise that only laws which perform the same function are susceptible to comparison. This approach complies with the 'principle of functionality' (Mechlem 2000) whereby a comparative analysis should start with a legal question rather than with a legal norm. The discussion will focus on three public health questions: How can law support infectious disease control, how can law help to reduce the harms caused by tobacco, and the potential role of law in tackling obesity. In the course of comparison, issues of compliance of national laws with human rights and with the revised IHR will be addressed.

Defining public health law

What is public health law?

While communicable diseases still pose a catastrophic threat to health in many parts of the world, mortality and morbidity in the developed world are primarily the consequence of non-communicable diseases such as heart disease, stroke, and cancer, and their common risk factors such as diet, tobacco, and alcohol. This requires new public health strategies and new public health interventions. Defining public health law is not an easy task when it is realized that public health responsibility now extends to matters such as road traffic safety, domestic violence, lifestyle choice, media freedom, and taxation. The most commonly accepted definition is that by Gostin (2000):

> *Public health law is the study of the legal powers and duties of the state to assure the conditions for people to be healthy (e.g. to identify, prevent, and ameliorate risks to health in the populations) and the limitations on the powers of the state to constrain the autonomy, privacy, liberty, proprietary or other legally protected interests of individuals for the protection or promotion of community health.*

This definition makes clear that public health law is about the relationship between the state and its populations rather than between health practitioners and patients. Public health law governs the organized efforts of the state for population health on the assumption that a state has responsibility for the health, and the conditions for health, of its citizens. Law may be needed to authorize interventions to address foreseeable risks of harm even where those interventions infringe the rights of individuals. At the same time, a public health end does not justify all possible means, and public health law will operate to set appropriate limits to infringement of individual rights and freedoms.

Law also has a wider role to play in the protection of public health. Laws might operate initially by means of direct provision of powers and duties, but will also serve to make a public statement of acceptability of behaviour which will indirectly alter public attitudes and actions. Laws against pollution or smoking in public places are effective only in part because of enforcement provisions. They are effective also because they have created minimum acceptable standards of protection. Laws, regardless of the legal system in which they operate, can change socio-cultural norms.

The absence of law also serves to send messages about acceptable behaviours. Where there is no law to regulate tobacco use, this implies that there is nothing socially unacceptable about cigarette advertising or smoking in proximity to others. Increasingly where individuals have little control over their living environments, even within Western individualistic societies, populations expect the state to intervene to reduce health risks and to set health standards.

Hence the content of public law has a value which is greater than the sum of its parts. Public health law reflects the importance that a government attributes to addressing threats to health, and reflects the standards that the state expects of its citizens in relation to health behaviours. Unreformed public health laws, based on outdated science and cultural values, create a dissonance between law and contemporary public health practice. Law reform must reflect social context, and it can prove counterproductive to transplant laws from another jurisdiction with a different social culture. Where law conflicts with contemporary understandings of the balance between individual right and public benefit, and where law fails to accommodate advancements in public health science, then law undermines the work of the state to protect its citizens from harm by eroding respect for public officials charged with implementing law.

Public health law in context

Gostin's definition presents a universal framework for the scope of public health law, but does not dictate the content of law. Public health law in each state will depend on the political and social context of that state. The recognition of health risk which might justify the application of law will vary according to understandings of medical science, public appreciation of risk, and public belief in the possibility of the control of risk. Where Western medical science is only one health belief system alongside others such as traditional medicine or religion, then law will play a different role in risk reduction. Public health operates within an ethical framework of communitarianism and utilitarianism, presupposing both that there are circumstances in which the greater good of the community justifies the overriding of autonomy of the individual, and that the intervention which results in the greatest health benefit for the greatest number is the most appropriate. However, the balance between communitarianism, utilitarianism, and autonomy is dependant on acceptance of state intervention in private life in pursuance of public health goals. The relationship between citizen and state, and the acceptability of intervention into individual rights for the public good, will be different, for example, in an authoritarian state than in a democracy. While Western health and legal systems prioritize autonomy as an underpinning health principle, other states, where the organization of society is based on religious or communitarian norms, may support more intrusive state activity to achieve public health goods.

Because of the importance of social and political context to the content of public health law, it will be useful, before examining legislation, to consider a brief overview of differing approaches to law within Western and Asian legal cultures.

Western legal culture

Western legal culture accommodates both common law and civil law states. Britain, Australia, Canada, New Zealand, and the United States, for example, have common law systems based on the English tradition in which law is embodied both in judicial decisions and in statutory form. So also do states and territories such as Cyprus, Malta, India, Hong Kong, Singapore, and Malaysia, although in these states the British system has been adapted to accommodate aspects of other cultures such as Asian or, in the case of Malaysia, Islamic legal culture. Former African colonies also apply English common law. Kenya has a basis of common law overlain with Islamic customary and tribal law, and the legal system of Nigeria is substantially common law combined with customary law.

France, Germany, Spain, Portugal, Italy, Turkey, along with South American and North African states with European colonial histories, have adopted the civil law tradition in which authoritative law has been codified, deriving from Justinian (Roman) law and developed by the French Code Civile or the German BGB. Other states such as the Philippines, South Africa, and Sri Lanka have legal systems containing both the common law and civil law traditions as a consequence of their history of colonialism, in each case overlain with values derived from Asian or African social traditions.

Legal systems within Western legal culture are secular, and independent of religion and morality. Law in a Western culture provides the main method of conflict resolution amongst individuals and between individuals and the state. One consequence of secularism is that of rationalism, whereby the legal system is organized according to principles and rules which must be justified by logic or reason rather than by religious or moral belief. A primary feature of Western legal culture is its presumption of autonomy of the individual. Western legal philosophy has given rise to an emphasis on human rights in both the civil and political, and social and economic spheres. While many of these human rights are universal and embedded in international treaties and conventions, the origin of much human rights doctrine in Western political philosophy has resulted in some distrust of human rights arguments in non-Western societies. In Western legal cultures, human rights focus on the relationship between the individual and the state and provide remedies for individuals in dispute with the state, and as such they constrain interference with private life even when that interference might be justified on the basis of a wider community or public benefit. Other legal cultures place more value on family and collective relationships, and hence individual human rights play a more significant role in Western legal culture than elsewhere.

Asian legal culture

The family of Asian legal systems includes China, Japan, the Republic of Korea, and Thailand. Other Asian states and territories such as Singapore, Malaysia, and Hong Kong, which inherited a common law system; Vietnam, which has a legal system based on Marxist–Leninist ideology; Macau, which inherited the Portuguese civil law legal system; and the Philippines, which has a mixed common law and civil law system, interpret law through a filter of Asian and/or Islamic values. In many respects, the legal systems of Asian states have little in common. Their political contexts vary widely and they have all introduced some Western law superimposed over traditional laws giving rise to pluralist systems. Nevertheless, there are aspects of Asian legal systems which contrast them from other legal cultures, most notably the influence of Confucianism and Buddhism which impose duties of loyalty to family and society. Additionally, most Asian governments are characterized by a strong bureaucracy and the absence of a doctrine of separation of powers.

Asian legal culture differs from Western culture in relation to the role of law in the regulation of private or social life. Whereas Western legal systems presuppose that the private life of citizens falls within the remit of objective state law, and that the limits of law are imposed by a philosophy of liberalism which guarantees personal freedoms, in Asian legal tradition it is not rational thought but rather an accepted natural order of things, derived from religious and moral belief, which underpins law. In this tradition, each individual has a status in the societal hierarchy. The duty of the individual is not to question, challenge, or debate, but rather to accept and obey the natural order. Individuals are characterized by duty rather than by autonomy. There is no consensus as to whether and to what extent modern Asian systems maintain this traditional approach, but there is nevertheless an accepted view that Asian legal culture shuns the adversarial style of Western dispute resolution in favour of a system of conciliation and compromise, whereby the end goal is not a vindication of rights but rather a result which restores harmony or creates the least disturbance to the natural order. This can still be seen in the reliance on mediation rather than litigation in the redress of rights in many Asian cultures.

The most significant consequence of respect for the natural order has been the approach to the balance between public good and private right. In Asian legal culture, rights are inseparable from duties (Diokno 2000), and there is in consequence a greater willingness on the part of individuals to suffer sacrifice for the benefit of the family or community. Government authority and some curtailment of rights are considered necessary to state welfare and social and political order. There has developed some resistance in Asia to Western approaches to human rights on the basis that human rights are values which derive from history and culture, giving rise to the claim for recognition of 'Asian values' (Bell 1996). Attempts to impose Western human rights on Asian legal systems have led to accusations of cultural imperialism (Svennson 2000). It has been argued that in developing Asian states, economic and social rights need to be constrained in pursuance of economic growth (Neary 2002), although some critics dispute that rights do in fact hamper economic growth (Sen 1997). Chinese scholars defend Asian interpretations of human rights (De Bary & Tu 2001), arguing that rights are communitarian and dependant on context. The view that Asian legal philosophy accepts wider government responsibility and greater intrusion into private life is still prevalent (Brems 2001). The Chairman of China's National People's Congress notes that Asian civilizations have developed through mutual influences based on a tradition that values harmony, and this should continue so as to allow Asian countries to develop their own cultural and foreign policies (South China Morning Post 2007).

Public health legislation in Western legal culture

Legislation supporting communicable disease control in Western legal culture

Public health legislation across much of Western legal culture has undergone little updating since the mid-twentieth century. Hence law is based on outdated science and fails to recognize human rights and ethics. Within Western legal culture, there is a range of approaches to legal public health powers and duties addressing communicable disease control. A study of legislation governing tuberculosis in 14 European states (Coker *et al.* 2007) demonstrates that approaches to public health law fall into four broad typologies, authoritarian (Russia, Estonia, Switzerland, and Norway), moderate (England, Germany, Israel, the Czech Republic, Hungary, Poland, and Finland), preventive (France and the Netherlands), and *laissez faire* (Spain). Differences of approach can be explained in part by the social and political histories of each state.

Nevertheless there are some common features to Western approaches to public health law. Most Western public health law focuses on protection of the healthy from sources of disease, including from human sources of disease, rather than on treatment and care of the ill. Most Western law provides penalties for persons who expose others to risk of disease by their health behaviours. It is now accepted in most Western states that human rights doctrine must provide limits to the power of the state to intervene for the public good, and human rights arguments have been used to challenge state public health powers. In *Enhorn v Sweden*, the European Court of Human Rights upheld a claim against the state of Sweden by an HIV-positive man detained under Swedish public health legislation, on the grounds that detention breached the claimant's right to liberty and to private and family life by being disproportionate to the public health risk (Martin 2006a).

Legislation supporting communicable disease control in England and Wales

The legal system in England and Wales is the English common law system. Authoritative law can be found both in the form of legislation (statutes and regulations) and of judicial decisions binding on lower courts by means of the doctrine of precedent. The main source of English public health law is in statutory form.

England led the world in developing legal powers and duties for population health. In the early nineteenth century, Britain faced environmental health threats from developing industrialization and urban populations well before other states. After the influenza and typhoid epidemics in 1837 and 1838, the lawyer Edwin Chadwick conducted an enquiry which concluded that much spread of disease resulted from living conditions. The first Public Health Act was passed in 1848 and the revised Public Health Acts became a model for legal regulation of public health across the world. British colonies from Hong Kong to Australia inherited British legislation, and states such as Japan, with very different legal systems, borrowed the British public health legal framework as a starting point for developing their own public health law (Tatara 2002).

The principles of public health law in England and Wales remain little changed since this early legislation. Disease control is governed by the Public Health (Control of Disease) Act 1984 and the Public Health (Infectious Disease) Regulations 1988. The other UK countries, Scotland and Northern Ireland, have similar legislation. Public health powers can only be invoked in relation to diseases classified as notifiable, as listed in the Act and in the Schedule to the Regulations. SARS and H5N1 influenza, for example, are currently not notifiable diseases and so there are no powers in relation to these diseases. The Act imposes a duty on medical practitioners to report notifiable diseases, and provides to the local authority powers of compulsory medical examination, powers of removal, and powers of detention in a hospital of persons with specified diseases. There are no powers of quarantine of persons exposed to disease, and no powers of isolation of persons with disease other than in a hospital. The Act imposes penalties on persons who expose others to risk of disease, although as the legislation is based on outdated science, some provisions provide penalties for behaviour that creates no public health risk. It is an offence, for example, for a person suffering from disease to return books to the library, although there is no known disease risk associated with library books (Atenstaedt 2006).

The 1984 Public Health Act is a consolidation of old public health laws, and powers were formulated at a time when it was accepted that private rights could be infringed for the benefit of a public good. There is concern that some powers provided by the Act may now be vulnerable to challenge under the Human Rights Act 1998 which brought into domestic law provisions of the European Convention for the Protection of Human Rights and Fundamental Freedoms. The decision of the European Court of Human Rights in *Enhorn v Sweden* (above) suggests that the exercise of public health powers which infringe liberty and private life can only be justified in circumstances where detention is proportional to the public health risk, and where detention is a last resort measure. As English public health legislation does not authorize measures less intrusive than hospital detention, some exercises of detention powers will not be a last resort (Martin 2006a). The absence of review and appeal procedures, and the fact that applications for detention can be made *ex parte* (such that the subject of the application cannot oppose it), make the legislation vulnerable to challenge under Article 6 of the European Convention which protects the right to a fair trial (Harris & Martin 2004).

Consistent with Western approaches to the public/private balance, only minor infringements of the rights to privacy and to private life will be tolerated even where the health of the population is threatened. English law does not, for example, authorize compulsory treatment or compulsory vaccination, whatever the public health risk, as consent to treatment is a fundamental principle of English jurisprudence.

English public health law is currently undergoing a process of amendment to ensure compliance with the revised IHR. There have long been calls for reform of the legal framework of public health (Coker & Martin 2006). In March 2007, a Consultation Paper was published (Department of Health 2007) proposing that revised legislation take an 'all hazards' approach rather than be based on notifiable diseases, and so cover new diseases as well as chemical or radiation contamination. The proposals recommend recognition within the legislation that powers be subject to principles of human rights. New powers of quarantine and compulsory counselling are proposed, powers of detention and medical examination are refined, and consistent with the principle of autonomy, powers of compulsory medical treatment are rejected. The paper argues against the requirement that subjects of public health powers be notified of applications to exercise powers so as to enable them to mount a defence, but does propose that there be opportunity for an order for exercise of compulsory powers to be reviewed. Statutory surveillance procedures are to be simplified and brought up to date in line with IHR requirements.

Legislation supporting communicable disease control in France

France is a republic with a centralist government structure. Despite the strong powers of central government, French philosophy favours individual over collective rights and there is reluctance in France to impinge on personal freedoms, what is known as the 'French paradox' (Morella 1996). The French legal system is a civil law system, in which authoritative law is codified. Law (*loi*) in the French legal system has a somewhat broader meaning than in English law, and covers the constitution, codes, statutes, *ordonnances* (which are time limited and lapse without later statutory ratification), regulations (*décrets* issued by the president or prime minister and *arrêtes* issued by a minister or mayor), orders, and circulars. There is no doctrine of precedent as in the English legal system, although court decisions are influential in the interpretation of law.

The *Code de la Santé Publique* recognizes the fundamental right to protection against health threats, guarantees equal access to the best possible health security, and protects the right to respect for dignity and freedom from discrimination.

The history of public health in France is very different from that in Britain. The association between hygiene, morality, and disease meant that the church for a long time played a role in public health initiatives. Indeed, there was suspicion around the involvement of the state in the private matter of health (Da Lomba & Martin 2004). Early public hygiene measures instituted by the church included detention, exclusion, and coercive treatment, but these measures were unsupported by legislation.

The first significant state intervention into public health came with the 1916 *Lois Bourgeois* and the 1919 *Honnorat* which created dispensaries for the purpose of detecting incidences of tuberculosis, and provided medicines to the poor and public sanitoriums. The 1994 *Loi relative á la santé publique et á la protection sociale* simplified the disease control framework. As a result, disease control in France relies primarily on notification of specified diseases and compulsory vaccination, including compulsory vaccination of both school children (vaccination is a precondition to public benefits such as schooling) and of persons working in specified activities (*Code de la Santé Publique*). There are also some powers of exclusion from activities (*Code de la Santé Publique*), but there are now no statutory powers of detention, quarantine, compulsory medical examination, or compulsory treatment, favouring instead voluntary and non-statutory measures and respect for the primacy of the patient/doctor relationship of trust. However, specific groups such as prisoners (*Code de Procédure Pénale* 1999) and foreigners (*Décret* no 46-1574 of 1946) may be subject to powers of compulsory medical examination and isolation in relation to diseases such as tuberculosis, and there are powers of containment of persons suffering from smallpox (*Décret* no 2003-313 of 2003). The Prefect of each *département* has the power to issue laws (*arrêtés*) in the short term in case of emergency, and central government has emergency powers, so law could provide powers in a public health emergency. Overall, however, France has few legislated public health powers compared to England or other Western states (Coker *et al.* 2007). France is considering the introduction of statutory powers of compulsory medical examination (where there is suspicion of disease), quarantine, and isolation in response to the SARS epidemic and in the light of the revised IHR (Sommade 2004).

Public health law reform for communicable disease in Western legal culture

The threat of SARS and pandemic influenza, and the requirement of compliance with the revised IHR, have provided an incentive to all states to revisit the role of law in public health. Public health legislation in Western legal culture has tended to be reactive, responding to existing public health concerns and consisting of precise duties and powers with little room for exercise of discretion (Martin 2006b). Law reform proposals tend to be more open-textured, more flexible, and more focused on rapid response to public health risk than traditional legislation.

Another feature of law reform proposals is an overt examination of the underpinning rights and values which provide the framework of public health activity, and in particular recognition that in Western jurisprudence, individual rights such as autonomy and privacy can only in exceptional circumstances be sacrificed to the public good. Whereas traditional public health legislation made no reference to the constraints of public health ethics or human rights, law reform proposals tend to make clear the balance between public good and private right in the context of the particular culture of the state.

An early example of law reform is the Australian Capital Territory's Public Health Act 1997. The ACT has a common law legal system. The Act introduced an approach to public health law driven by the notion of risk, with the objectives of providing tools for rapid response to public health risk and ensuring protection of individual liberty and privacy. The Health Minister may declare at any time a particular activity that might give rise to transmission of disease or that might otherwise affect the health of individuals, to be a public health risk activity. Any person carrying out a public health risk activity is obliged to comply with a code of practice, enforced by registration and licensing procedures. Duties of disease notification apply only where notification is necessary to protect public health, and powers of confinement of individuals apply only where confinement is necessary to avert an imminent and serious risk to public health.

Quebec, Canada, which has a civil law legal system, introduced its new Public Health Act in 2001. The legislation establishes a public health ethics committee with responsibility for overseeing public health surveillance so as to ensure ethics compliance, and notification is based on risk to public health. The Act allows for compulsory exclusion, isolation of both persons with disease and persons exposed to disease, medical examination, and, more unusually, for the compulsory medical treatment of persons with disease with the objective of reducing contagion. In a case of public health emergency, the Act provides compulsory vaccination powers. There is recognition of responsibility to sufferers of disease as well as to the healthy in the form of a general duty to see that all persons with disease are provided with access to medical care and treatment.

Scotland, which has a legal system based on Roman Dutch and common law, has published a consultation paper on public health law reform (Scottish Executive 2006). A focus of the paper is the determination of rights and values which are to provide a framework for public health practice in Scotland, suggesting that those primary values might be personal autonomy and privacy, along with care for others. Responsibility for the public's health lies with the individual as well as with the state. The Scottish proposals recognize that public health responsibilities and powers should reflect the objective of risk reduction. Proposed duties of notification are predicated on the requirement that the disease or condition pose an appreciable risk to the public's health. Duties of notification would consider moral and cultural sensitivities and comply with ethical and legal guidance. Powers of medical examination, exclusion, quarantine, or detention would need to be consistent with human rights principles of least restrictive alternative, proportionality, and individual rights. The Scottish proposals, like the English proposals, do not entertain the possibility of compulsory medical treatment in recognition of the primacy of the autonomy of the individual.

Legislation to address tobacco harms in Western legal culture

The use of law in the control of non-communicable disease is comparatively recent. Law is particularly important in this area because much non-communicable disease is a product of lifestyle choices and environmental influences on choices. Law has the power both directly and indirectly to change lifestyle environments, to ensure informed lifestyle choices, and to control commercial exploitation.

While the effectiveness of legal intervention into smoking behaviours is still subject to research, preliminary studies suggest that voluntary codes of behaviour do not work (Jones 1999), and that enforced smoking prohibitions serve both to improve the health environment of non-smokers, and to assist in discouraging smoking behaviours (Euromonitor International 2006a; Allwright 2005; Fichtenberg 2002). Within Europe, a number of states, including Ireland, the United Kingdom, Italy, Malta, Spain, the Netherlands, Norway, and France, have introduced laws restricting or prohibiting smoking in public places. Germany, the largest consumer of tobacco in Europe, is planning laws to ban smoking in restaurants, bars, and transport facilities. More widely in the Western world, laws have been introduced in Canada, the United States, New Zealand, and Australia providing smoke-free environments and regulating tobacco advertising, tobacco packaging and warnings, taxation on tobacco products, and restrictions on the sale of tobacco. Other laws such as occupational health and discrimination laws also provide protection from tobacco harms. In Australia, an asthmatic successfully sued a hotel under the Disability Discrimination Act 1992 because failure to provide a smoke-free environment prevented her, as a sufferer of asthma, from using hotel premises (*Francey and Meeuwissen v. Hilton Hotels of Australia* 2000).

The importance of law as a tool in the control of tobacco harms was recognized in the first ever global public health treaty, the WHO Framework Convention on Tobacco Control, adopted in 2003. In February 2005, the Convention became international law, and set international standards on tobacco price and tax increases, tobacco advertising and sponsorship, labelling, trade, and second hand smoke. The Convention requires signatory states to impose restrictions on tobacco sale, advertising, sponsorship and promotion, to regulate tobacco labelling, to protect indoor places from smoke polluted air, and to criminalize tobacco smuggling. Indeed legal interventions constitute the backbone of the Convention strategies.

Legislation to address tobacco harms in England and Wales

The United Kingdom ratified the Framework Convention on Tobacco Control in 2004, and subsequently individual UK countries produced legislation in compliance with the framework. The Health Act 2006 provides generally for designation of smoke-free areas, for possible exemptions from smoking prohibitions, and for signage to make clear where smoking is permitted. In England smoking prohibitions are contained in the Smoke Free (Premises and Enforcement) Regulations 2006 and the Smoke Free (Exemptions and Vehicles) Regulations 2007 has similar regulations. Any enclosed or substantially enclosed area or vehicle which is open to the public, or where people work, must now be smoke-free and must display signs making this clear. This includes restaurants, cafes, pubs, cinemas, clubs, public transport, company cars, offices, and factories. Exemptions from the prohibitions include prisons, adult residential care homes, residential mental healthcare centres, and designated hotel rooms. Significant warnings on tobacco packaging are required by the Tobacco Products Labelling (Safety) Regulations 1991 as updated, and the Tobacco Products (Manufacture, Presentation and Sale) Regulations 2002.

The 2005 European Union Tobacco Advertising Directive applies to tobacco advertising and sponsorship with a cross-border dimension but is limited to merchandizing and sports sponsorship. In England and Wales, the Tobacco Advertising and Promotion Act 2002 and regulations prohibit national advertising, promotion and sponsorship of tobacco products, including brandshare products (Tobacco Advertising and Promotion (Brandshare) Regulations 2004), with limited exceptions such as advertising near the till where cigarettes are to be sold in shops. The Children and Young Persons (Sale of Tobacco etc.) Order 2007 amends the Children and Young Persons (Protection from Tobacco) Act 1991 to raise the age at which young persons can be sold tobacco products from 16 to 18. Further laws are planned to prohibit the display of cigarettes in shops and supermarkets, requiring tobacco products to be kept under the counter. Similar laws are being considered in Scotland, Norway, New Zealand, and Scotland. The government also hopes to pass laws to prohibit vending machines in pubs, to fine persons who drop cigarette butts, and to restrict the sale of packs of 10 cigarettes as smaller packets are more attractive to children. Small packs of cigarettes are already prohibited in Australia, New Zealand, Canada, France, and some US states.

Legislation to address tobacco harms in France

Cigarette smoking has long been a feature of French café culture. France is also a producer of tobacco. Attempts to prohibit smoking in public places have been strongly resisted on both economic and cultural grounds. In 1991, France passed law to ban direct tobacco advertising, to require health warnings on tobacco packs, and to require all restaurants and bars to provide no-smoking areas. The restrictions on smoking in public places were in practice rarely enforced. In 1999, the French government issued a circular restricting smoking in healthcare establishments (Circular DGS/DH/SP 3 No 99-330 of 8 June 1999). France ratified the WHO Framework Convention on Tobacco Control in 2003 and in 2007 a smoking ban came into effect to include schools, shops, transport facilities, offices, public buildings, and other enclosed spaces. The smoking bans were not promulgated in legislative form but rather by government decree following a parliamentary committee recommendation (*Décret* no 2006-1386 of 15 November 2006). Smoking prohibitions in restaurants, bars, and nightclubs were delayed until 2008. Prohibition on tobacco advertising was introduced in France in 1993 (*Loi Evin*). These laws were amended to allow televised sports events from states where tobacco advertising is not prohibited. Sale of tobacco products to persons under 16 is prohibited by *Loi* no *2003-715 of 2003*, and the sale of cigarettes in packets of 10 is prohibited.

The potential role of law in tackling obesity in Western legal culture

WHO recognizes obesity to be one of the greatest public health challenges of the twenty-first century and a disease in its own right (WHO 2003). Law has long had a role in controlling toxic food content but until recently played no part in constraining and influencing lifestyle choices. Law has traditionally been predicated on the understanding that humans are rational actors, but theories of behaviouralism, which propose that external events and circumstances can bias the ability to make rational judgements, have paved the way for law's involvement in countering market manipulation of preferences (Harvard Law Review Note 2003). Research on the influence of advertising on food choices (Borzekowski *et al.* 2001) and on misleading food labelling has provided an evidence base for law. This 'new frontier of public health law' (Mello *et al.* 2006) has not been free of controversy. Legal intervention has prompted civil liberties arguments of freedom of choice and freedom of speech. Ethics literature has raised concerns of the 'nanny state' and of paternalism in relation to issues of personal responsibility (Holm 2007). While tobacco can be classified as a dangerous substance, much food at the centre of obesity arguments is not in itself dangerous, only becoming so as part of an overall unhealthy diet. One food manufacturer commented in relation to a chocolate bar, '. . . health warnings are for dangerous things. Whilst we recognise the problem I do not think that a Curly Wurly is a dangerous thing' (House of Commons UK 2004). However, it is now accepted that some foods can be classified as healthy or unhealthy, and the food industry itself has begun to promote what it terms 'healthy eating' ranges of food.

The role of law in the relationship between food and public health has become more important in the changing dynamic of food systems (Lang 2006). Governments, concerned about the rising costs of obesity, are looking to law not only as a means of controlling market practices but also as a means of shaping consumers' knowledge and understanding of health risks, their purchasing patterns, and their eating habits.

The role of law in tackling obesity in England and Wales

Obesity is one of the most pressing public health concerns in Britain. Public health interventions to prevent increasing levels of obesity are a government priority (Department of Health 2004, 2006). The government has recognized the health problems posed by obesity in a series of papers which reflect changing approaches to the role of the state in obesity (Martin 2008). Obesity is categorized as a medical problem (National Audit office 2001), an economic problem (Wanless 2002, 2004), a societal problem (House of Commons 2004), and a public health problem (Department of Health 2004) in which the role of government is to:

> *. . . support consumers, providing them with easier access to a wide range of healthier foods and, crucially, the information and knowledge needed to make informed choices about their diets. And this may mean targeting action to meet the needs of particular groups and tackle inequalities.*

More recently obesity has been classed as a personal problem whereby 'Our problems are not, strictly speaking, public health questions at all. They are questions of individual lifestyle. . . . They are not epidemics in the epidemiological sense. They are the result of millions of individual decisions' (former prime minister Tony Blair 2006a). In this context, the government has on the whole favoured voluntary industry regulation.

However, industry has been slow to achieve the levels of protection demanded by the public health community, and gradually the government is turning to law to enforce food health standards. The Education (Nutrition Standards for School Lunches) (England) Regulations 2006 set minimum nutritional requirements in the provision of school lunches. The Food Labelling Regulations 1996 have been amended to require clearer labelling of food content, although labelling of the nutritional content of food is currently only required where the manufacturer makes particular nutritional claims for its product. The Food Standards Agency recommend a 'traffic lights' system of food labelling to allow easy identification of healthy foods, but some major supermarkets have rejected this approach in favour of a system based on percentage of guideline daily amount (GDA) of a nutrient, resulting in inconsistent labelling across the industry. In recognition of the relationship between breastfeeding and childhood obesity, the English government is considering the introduction of laws to protect breastfeeding in public along the lines of the Breastfeeding (Scotland) Act 2005.

The most contested area of legal intervention in obesity control is the proposal to prohibit the advertising of unhealthy foods targeted at children. The foods most commonly advertised to children in the United Kingdom (Hastings 2003), as elsewhere (Caraher 2006), are those which have high levels of fat, salt, and sugar. The House of Commons Health Committee acknowledges '. . . the food industry's relentless targeting of children through intense advertising and promotion campaigns, some of which explicitly aim to circumvent parental control by exploiting "pester power"' (House of Common Health Committee 2004). The Food Standard Agency accepts the '. . . causal link between promotional activity and children's food knowledge, preference and behaviours' (Food Standards Agency 2003).

In 2006, Ofcom, the independent regulator of television, radio, telecommunications, and wireless communications services in the United Kingdom, published a consultation document in which it concluded that self-regulation alone would not be sufficient to deal with the problem of advertising to children. Ofcom recommended that advertising of food and drink products be prohibited during programmes aimed at children or which will be of interest to children aged between 4 and 9 years, extended to cover programmes for children aged 4 to 15 in 2008 (Ofcom 2007). The public health community argued that these restrictions were insufficient to protect children and proposed that all food and drink advertising should be prohibited before 9 pm. As a result the 2007 Private Members Television (Food Advertising) Bill, proposed prohibiting advertising between 5 am and 9 pm of foods which fail to meet specified nutritional standards. It must be borne in mind that national legislation regulating television content in Europe is weakened by the European Television without Frontiers Directive which specifies that broadcasting is governed by the laws of the country in which it originates. This allows British viewers to access television programmes from other European states where there is no regulation of food advertising. The Directive on Audiovisual Media Services proposed in 2008–09 will attempt to limit advertising of food, tobacco, and alcohol products across Europe.

The role of law in tackling obesity elsewhere in Western legal culture

Obesity is a health concern across the Western world, and states are increasingly considering legal interventions. In Europe, in 2006, the WHO Ministerial Conference adopted a European Charter on Counteracting Obesity (WHO Regional Office for Europe 2006) which acknowledged that obesity posed a serious problem not only for health but also for economics and social development in Europe. The Charter recommends that governments and national parliaments ensure consistency and sustainability of approach to obesity through regulatory action, including legislation. A report by the International Association of Consumer Food Organizations for the World Health Organization consultation on a global strategy for diet and health has recommended international controls on food advertising including cross-border controls (IACFO 2003).

In Australia, obesity levels are particularly high. Laws in relation to health are devolved to state governments and so differ from state to state despite there being no real borders between states. Approaches in Australia to issues such as food content, food labelling, and the placement of food vending machines tend to favour voluntary industry regulation. Food labelling, for example, is governed by the Australian Food Standards Code which provides uniform food standards and outlines food labelling requirements. It is planned to amend the Code to introduce a 'traffic' light system of food labelling along the lines of the proposed British system, but this will continue to be embodied in a code of practice rather than in law. Some Australian states have begun to introduce legislation in recognition that voluntary industry compliance has not been successful.

Elsewhere, Laws in Sweden and Norway prohibit advertising of junk food aimed at children under 12, but programmes for older children are often accompanied by advertisements for crisps and soft drinks (WHO 2006). Viewers have access to television programmes from other European states with no restrictions. In Canada, Quebec has legislated to restrict all marketing of food and beverage products to children under 13, but as with European legislation, protection is weakened by access to viewers in Quebec to programmes from other Canadian states and from the United States. New Zealand has introduced a food classification scheme which will restrict food advertising on terrestrial television in designated time bands. France now requires advertising of unhealthy food to carry a health warning. Spain has a Code of Self Regulation of the Advertising of Food Products Directed at Minors which requires that there be caution on advertisements aimed at children under 12, and prohibits use of celebrities in advertisement of unhealthy foods. Ireland has prohibited television advertising of fast foods and sweets, as well as the use of celebrities in the promotion of junk food to children.

Some states, Canada and the United States, for example, have legislated to require that the trans fat content of all pre-packaged foods be displayed on labels, and the New York City Health Code prohibits restaurants in New York from serving foods that contain more than 0.5 g of trans fat per serving (Gostin 2007). The Australia New Zealand Food Standards Code 2002 introduced mandatory nutrition labelling of packaged foods for Australia and New Zealand. Germany and Norway are planning on raising taxes on foods high in fats, sugars, and salt. School vending machines are prohibited in some jurisdictions, for example, in Latvia, California, and France, and are restricted in what they can sell in other places, such as Chicago. In New Zealand, the National Administration Guidelines were amended in 2007 to require schools to limit the sale of unhealthy food and drink in vending machines.

States across Western legal culture are actively exploring ways in which law might be used to control production, sale, advertising, and access to unhealthy foodstuffs. Objections by the food industry have carried little weight since voluntary industry codes have been unsuccessful, and food manufacturers are now changing approach. Many major food suppliers have introduced sugar-, salt-, and fat-reduced products, along with 'healthy' food ranges. Much food advertising now focuses on the health value of products, and many manufacturers have begun to improve food labelling, although not always in a manner consistent across the industry. Industry objections to television advertising have so far proved more successful based on freedom of speech arguments, but again the failure of voluntary codes has led many states to consider legislation. As the full health and economic consequences of obesity become more apparent, there is willingness across the Western world to use legislative tools to intervene in lifestyle choices, especially where children are at risk. Western consumers are generally in support of stronger controls. While protection of privacy and freedom of speech are fundamental Western rights, there is sufficient public concern about obesity to accept that laws are needed to ensure informed consumer choice in relation to diet and lifestyle.

Public health legislation in Asian legal culture

Legislation supporting communicable disease control in Asian legal culture

Legislation supporting communicable disease control in China

The revised IHR (2005) give member states new mandates and responsibilities to prevent, protect against, and control the international spread of disease. This development constituted the most far-reaching change in international public health regulation since the nineteenth century (Fidler 2005), and was the outcome of a shift from a 'Westphalian' (reliance on state sovereignty) to a 'post-Westphalian' (global health governance and international co-operation) regulatory model (Fidler 2004). China was at the epicentre of the 2003 SARS epidemic, and learned first hand the importance of law in support of public health. Since then China has enacted much needed public health legislation.

Public health programmes and interventions must be planned and delivered in the context of national health and political systems (Merson 2006). Under the Constitution of the People's Republic of China, the National People's Congress (NPC) is the highest organ of state power. The NPC and its Standing Committee are empowered with rights of legislation, decision, supervision, election, and removal. The State administration is collectively known as the Central People's Government and is responsible for carrying out the principles and policies of the Communist Party of China. In practice much of the detail of contemporary Chinese law has its origins in Japanese law, the civil law systems of Germany and France, and the common law of England and the United States. However, it remains the case that cultural influences have survived in the practice and enforcement of laws.

The primary legislation is the Communicable Diseases Law, promulgated at national level in 1989 and substantially revised in 2004. The Ministry of Health acknowledged in the promulgation notice that the law was amended in the light of experience gained from the SARS epidemic, and that its revision aimed to enhance the overall standard of disease prevention (*zheng ti shui ping*) and to achieve perfection (*jian li, wan shan*) of the public health system. Article 1 states the purpose of the law, to prevent, control, and eliminate the occurrence and spread of communicable diseases in order to protect the health of individuals and the public. Article 1 also clarifies the legislation's policy focus (*zhi dao si xiang*) on prevention (*yu fang wei zhu*), to include a combination of preventive and therapeutic measures (*fang zhi jie he*), and the adoption of 'diverse control measures' (*fen lei guan li*) based on scientific knowledge and the needs of the people. The infectious diseases (*chuan ran bing*) covered by the legislation fall into three categories. Type A includes plague and cholera, Type B includes SARS, avian influenza, anthrax, pulmonary tuberculosis, viral hepatitis, dysentery, typhoid, AIDS, syphilis, and measles, and Type C contains a long list of infectious diseases. Other diseases may be added to Types B and C on the decision of the national health authority attached to the State Council, as necessitated by outbreaks, the epidemiological situation or disease seriousness. SARS, anthrax, and avian influenza, which are highly pathogenic to humans and classified as Type B, may at times be subject to more rigorous preventive and control measures as if they were Type A diseases.

Article 8(1) entrenches the role of traditional medicine such as Chinese medicine (TCM) as a complementary partner to modern medicine in the prevention and treatment of communicable disease. While the role of TCM is protected by the Chinese Constitution, the reiteration here is a reflection of the belief that the use of TCM in China contributed significantly to the control and abatement of the spread of SARS, particular in the Guangdong region. The role of international co-operation is expressly encouraged (Article 8(2)). Individuals and units (*dan wei*) within the PRC are now required under Article 12 to comply with measures such as investigation, inspection, sample collection, isolation (*ge li*), and supply of accurate information as required by the health authorities, subject to the duty to respect privacy and the right of appeal. A new surveillance system (Article 17), warning system (Article 18), and pathogen databank (Article 26) are to be established. The 'diverse control measures' (*fen lei guan li*) focus on health promotion activities (Article 13), vaccination programmes with emphasis on free vaccination for children (Articles 14–16), enforcement through medical institutions (*yi liao ji gou*) (Article 21), laboratories (Article 22), blood collection, supply, and research institutions (Article 23), and agricultural ministries with responsibility for zoonosis (Article 25). Article 24 envisages that further regulations will be enacted with regard to AIDS, while provinces are expressly required to take more active steps to contain HIV/AIDS.

The Frontier Health and Quarantine Law 1986, Food Hygiene Law 1995, Law on Practising Doctors 1998, and Law on the Prevention and Treatment of Occupational Diseases 2001 are other examples of national law relevant to disease prevention. In 2003, Regulations on the Urgent Handling of Public Health Emergencies were promulgated by State Council. State Council also has the power to enact national administrative legislation under the Chinese Constitution, and through its ministries and bureaux, industry-specific administrative regulations. Such regulations must comply with national law to be valid. The Implementing Rules of the Frontier Law 1989 and the Regulations on the Handling of Major Animal Epidemic Emergencies 2005 are examples. At a further level, administrative bureaux such as the Ministry of Health and the State Administration of Quality Supervision, Inspection and Quarantine are vested with authority to enact measures such as the Measures for the Handling of Food Poisoning Incidents 2000, the Measures for the Administration of Information Reporting on Monitoring Public Health Emergencies and Epidemic Situation of Infectious Diseases 2003 and the Regulation on the Urgent Handling of the Entry-Exit Inspection and Quarantine of Frontier and Port Public Health Emergencies 2003.

Provincial national people's congresses and governments have legislative power to enact law governing their territories that are consistent with national law, which may further regulate activities in accordance with regional needs. Article 4 of the Communicable Diseases Law gives provincial governments the power to bring within the legislation locally prevalent diseases as Type B or C diseases without prior central government approval, though the notice of publication has to be filed with the central government. Article 10 of the Public Health Emergency Regulations empowers provincial governments to formulate regional plans for handling emergencies taking into consideration local circumstances, to supplement the national plan.

Border control issues are dealt with under the Frontier Law of 1986. Diseases are classified either as quarantinable (*jian yi chuan ran bing*) or monitored diseases (*jian ce chuan ran bing*). These provisions reflect the international obligations undertaken by China under the IHR 1969. The key obligation is set out in Article 7, which provides that all persons (*ren yuan*) and conveyances (*jiao tong gong ju*) are subject to quarantine inspection at the first frontier port of their arrival. Article 24 of the Frontier Law provides that where the provisions of the law differ from those of international treaties on health and quarantine to which China is a party, the provisions of such international treaties shall prevail with the exception of treaty clauses in relation to which the PRC has declared reservations.

An overview of Chinese public health law is not complete without reference to the stringent legal liability regime introduced by the Public Health Emergency Regulations in the wake of the SARS epidemic. Officials can be sanctioned, demoted, or removed from office if they fail to perform their reporting or other duties, or delay or cause false reports to be made directly or by enabling others to conceal information. Criminal sanctions may apply if such behaviour results in disease spread. While China was criticized for initially withholding information in relation to the SARS outbreak, China was quick to demonstrate that the delay was caused by decisions of recalcitrant officials who were subsequently removed from office, rather than state policy. Administrative or criminal sanctions will also apply to persons who propagate rumour, artificially push up prices, or defraud consumers during a public health emergency period (Articles 45–52).

Legislation supporting communicable disease control in Japan

Under the Japanese Constitution of 1947, the National Diet is the highest organ of state power. The Japanese legal system was modelled on the feudal Chinese legal system, but after the Meiji reformation, the legal system has largely followed the German model. As in China, laws are supplemented by administrative directions and suggestions (*gyôsei shidô*). Article 25 of the Constitution provides that all people shall have the right to maintain the minimum standards of wholesome and cultured living, and the State shall use its endeavours for the promotion and extension of social welfare and security, and of public health, in all spheres of life.

The main legislation on communicable diseases control in Japan is the 1999 Law Concerning the Prevention of Infectious Diseases and Medical Care for Patients of Infections, under which doctors are required to report 86 infectious diseases classified in 5 categories. In 1997 the epidemiology arm of The National Institute of Infectious Diseases was reformed as an independent Infectious Disease Surveillance Centre, with power to monitor and collect reports of infectious agents from prefectures, ordinance designated cities, and special wards (prefectures). The NIID also has power to conduct investigations in the event of an infectious disease outbreak and to exchange information with overseas agencies.

Pursuant to a requirement that the legislature review the law after 5 years, substantial amendments were introduced in 2004, with emphasis on tackling problems brought about by bioterrorism (anthrax and smallpox), the threat of terrorist attacks, and SARS. These amendments relate principally to strengthening the role of government in infectious disease control in an emergency, reviewing the control strategy of zoonosis, and reviewing the list of categorized diseases, especially Category IV. Article 15 empowers the national government to conduct epidemiological investigations in addition to those carried out by regional governments, and to provide suggestions for handling an outbreak. In a threatened breakout, the national government may require prefectures to establish concrete preparedness plans (Articles 9 and 10) and may issue directives to the local governors of the prefectures (Articles 51(2) and 63(2)).

Supplementary decisions made by the Diet provide that examination of patients with suspected SARS infection must take place only at specified hospitals. There is to be education at places of work and schools to ensure against discrimination and prejudice in relation to patients with infectious diseases and their families. Education is to be provided to ensure consideration of disease patients' human rights. Finally, international medical cooperation is to be promoted through WHO and through bilateral deliberations between countries.

The Quarantine Law was amended simultaneously to provide powers to expand the range of medical examinations and inspections at quarantine stations and to oblige persons suspected of suffering from an infectious disease to report their health conditions for a period after entry into Japan. In 2005, the Tuberculosis Control Law was revised with particular emphasis on medical screening in line with a further amendment to the Infectious Diseases Control Law in 2006, and the two laws are expected to improve control of infectious diseases.

Legislation supporting communicable disease control in Hong Kong

The Quarantine and Prevention of Disease Ordinance (Cap. 141) and the Prevention of the Spread of Infectious Diseases Regulations (Cap. 141B) constitute the legislative framework for the prevention and control of infectious diseases in Hong Kong. This legislation is based on early English public health laws. The primary legislation applies mainly to the 1969 IHR quarantinable diseases (cholera, plague, and yellow fever) and the regulations apply to other infectious diseases as listed in the First Schedule to the primary legislation. The legislation needs to be amended every time a new disease is added, and in 2003 there were delays in control measures in relation to SARS while the amendment procedures were undertaken (LegCo Select Committee Hong Kong 2004).

Under the regulations medical practitioners have a duty to report disease where they have reasonable grounds to suspect the existence of disease, and others such as police officers, relatives, occupiers, and hotel keepers have a duty to report when they have knowledge of disease. There is a presumption of knowledge such that the burden lies on the person with reporting responsibility to show that he had no knowledge. The regulations provide powers of entry onto premises, powers of forcible removal of persons from premises, powers of quarantine of persons exposed to disease, and powers of detention of a person with disease until he is no longer infectious. Statutory public health offences include exposure of others to risk of disease and failure to comply with a public health order. Certain extraordinary amendments were made during SARS. The Prevention of the Spread of Infectious Diseases (Amendment) Regulations 2003 inserted into the main legislation a new Part VIA with powers to restrict persons from leaving Hong Kong, to stop and detain, and to conduct medical examination of persons arriving in or leaving Hong Kong.

Hong Kong also has the Public Health and Municipal Services Ordinance (Cap. 132), which focuses on sanitary sources of disease, and the Emergency Regulations Ordinance (Cap. 241) which enables the Chief Executive in Council to make any regulations in a circumstance of public emergency and danger which he considers to be in the public interest. There are currently no regulations in pursuance of this Ordinance. The Hong Kong Bill of Rights Ordinance (Cap. 838) protects the right to life, liberty, freedom from torture, and rights to privacy, honour, and equality before the law. There are some exceptions to these rights on grounds such as public health, and measures may be taken in derogation of human rights in a situation of emergency.

In February 2007, proposals were introduced to the Panel on Health Services of Hong Kong's legislature to enable Hong Kong to comply with the revised IHR. The paper proposes amendments to strengthen the ability to respond to outbreaks and to provide for preventive and control measures by requiring travellers to produce proof of vaccination, prophylaxis, or declarations, to submit to medical examination, tests, and isolation measures. There will be powers to refuse entry or exit of travellers. It is also proposed to provide legal powers for combating and controlling the effect of public health emergencies and to ensure the territory's preparedness for public health emergencies. Proposed amendments include updating and expanding the list of notifiable diseases, requiring notification of any release of dangerous infectious agents, surrender or submission of specimens, requiring doctors to provide information, and placing sick persons under medical surveillance.

Legislation supporting communicable disease control in other Asian states

Asian states have high incidences of many infectious diseases and are particularly vulnerable to H5N1 strain influenza attributable in part to unhygienic poultry husbandry and lax biosecurity (Melville and Shortridge 2004). One of the common difficulties encountered in Asian states is that while the legal framework may be in place, resources and political will can be lacking.

Malaysia has a legal system based on English common law, but Islamic law also constitutes a significant source of law particularly in relation to private relationships. Malaysia has a large population of migrant workers from Vietnam, China, and Nepal suffering high incidences of tuberculosis, syphilis, and hepatitis B. All semi-skilled and unskilled foreign workers are screened before visas are issued and are required to undergo regular medical examination. Foreign travellers entering Malaysia from specified countries are required to show proof of vaccination against diseases such as yellow fever. The 1988 Prevention and Control of Infectious Diseases Act provides a wider range of duties and powers than equivalent legislation in Western cultures. As well as powers of isolation, medical examination, and quarantine, there are powers to enter into any vehicle arriving in Malaysia, to examine any person or property on board, and to take necessary samples. The Minister has the power to order any area of Malaysia to be designated an infected area, and in relation to an infected area there are powers to put persons under surveillance and powers of compulsory treatment and immunization. Malaysian legislation is currently undergoing reform to enhance surveillance capacity in compliance with the IHR 2005.

The legal system of the Philippines is a mixture of common and civil law. The 1987 Constitution of the Republic of the Philippines provides that the state shall protect and promote the right to health of the people and shall instil health consciousness. Principal law-making powers lie with the Congress of the Philippines, but there is considerable decentralized law-making power. Law may take the form of a presidential decree, a statute of the republic, an executive order, a local government ordinance, or a barangay (community) ordinance. Under Executive Order 102 of 1999, health services are devolved to local governments. The central Department of Health continues to provide services in relation to specific programmes such as tuberculosis and malaria eradication, to manage disease and surveillance systems, and to articulate national policy. The Local Government Code 1991 gives responsibility to local government for health promotion and prevention in relation to communicable and non-communicable diseases, and local health boards carry out this work. In case of widespread public health threats or epidemics, the Secretary of Health can be directed by the President of the Republic to take temporary control of health operations in a local government area for the duration of the emergency.

The prevalence of communicable diseases in the Philippines is high. Philippines has one of the highest incidences of TB in Asia, and non-completion of treatment is common. The Philippine Department of Health Web site attributes TB prevalence to the low priority given to anti-tuberculosis activities, poor availability of anti-TB drugs, insufficient laboratory networking, poor health infrastructures, and lack of trained personnel. These problems are now being addressed, and Directly Observed Therapy has been introduced to ensure completion of treatment. Childhood vaccination against diseases such as tuberculosis and hepatitis B is compulsory (Republic Act No. 7846 of 1994).

The Quarantine Act 2004 gives to the Bureau of Quarantine within the Department of Health powers of examination at ports of entry in relation to both domestic and international vessels, powers and duties of surveillance, and power to enforce rules and regulations necessary to prevent introduction, transmission or spread of 'public health emergencies of international concern'. The Director of the Bureau has power to exercise, in relation to port entry, intervention strategies such as health education, compulsory vaccination of persons entering the Philippines, medical examination of travellers, apprehension, detention, quarantine, and surveillance. Regulations under the Act enable, in an outbreak of a public health emergency, the Bureau Director to recommend to the Secretary for Health a range of disease control measures including apprehension, detention/isolation, and surveillance of suspect cases, surveillance of persons exposed to disease and the power to declare an area or community under quarantine.

Legislation to address tobacco harms in Asian legal culture

Legislation addressing tobacco harms in China

When China ratified the WHO Framework Convention on Tobacco Control in 2005, the Regional Director for the WHO Western Pacific Region stated in a press release that it was 'perhaps the clearest indication yet that the world is increasingly committed to addressing the global tobacco epidemic' (WHO 2005). Studies had predicted a significant increase in tobacco-related mortality in China (Liu 1998; Lam 2001). Current Ministry of Health figures suggest that in China there are 350 million smokers and 450 million passive smokers, and despite the fact that 100 000 die annually from passive smoking, only a third of the population is aware of the dangers of passive smoking (Reuters 2007a).

In 2000, at the National Conference on Policy Development on Tobacco Control in China in the twenty-first Century, participants from the Chinese Academy of Preventive Medicine, Ministry of Health, the WHO, and from other states proposed comprehensive legislation on tobacco control to include increases in tobacco tax, advertising, promotion and sponsorship bans, and package warnings, together with measures to reduce second-hand smoke and strengthen national mass-media campaigns (John Hopkins 2000). In ratifying the Framework Convention, the Chinese government declared that it was committed to strong tobacco control policy in order to fulfil its treaty obligations, and the Standing Committee of the National Peoples Congress took the opportunity to ban cigarette automatic vending machines (National People's Congress 2005). In 2007 eight ministries were established to co-ordinate treaty compliance operations. The 2007 China Tobacco Control Report was released in May 2007 to coincide with the Global Smoke Free Day (Ministry of Health China 2007).

Tobacco harms, particularly those to children, were already covered by the Law on the Protection of Minors 1991, the Law on the Prevention of Juvenile Crime 1999 which imposed duties on parents and teachers to educate minors not to smoke, Tentative Measures on the Administration of Tobacco Advertisements, the Implementing Measures on the Designation of Smoke Free Cities within China 2003, and the Measures on the Prohibition of Smoking in Public Transport and Waiting Rooms 1997. In 2006 substantial amendments were made to the Law on the Protection of Minors to introduce a ban on sale of cigarettes to persons under 18, and a complete ban on smoking in schools, nurseries, and youth activity centres. However, such policies were not implemented without dissent. It was reported (Reuters 2007b) that an official of the State Tobacco Monopoly Association told NPC delegates that while 'smoking harms people's health, restraining smoking threatens social stability', based on the estimate that the tobacco industry contributed 80 billion yuan per day in tax.

China continues to face tension between tobacco ownership interests and public health arguments. The 2007 Tobacco Control Report painted an alarming picture (Ministry of Health China 2007). For example, 180 million passive smokers in China are children under 15. It was recognized that '. . . our country is still considerably far from fulfilling the goals set down by the treaty'. The Report acknowledged that legislation prohibiting smoking in public places is an effective way of tobacco control, citing laws in other countries as well as survey results suggesting that the smoking bans would not be detrimental to businesses. Coupled with China's treaty obligation to prevent passive smoking under Article 8, the Report provides an incentive for the government to take tougher control measures. At the same time, China is the world's largest producer of tobacco with the Chinese government controlling monopoly interests in tobacco production (Peng 1997). Tobacco sales contribute significantly to tax revenues and the tobacco market in China is predicted to continue to expand (Euromonitor International 2006B).

China gave directions to health authorities, universities, and NGOs to promote the 20th Global Smoke Free Day on 31 May 2007, stating that China would be the first nation to host an Olympic games after the implementation of the Tobacco Framework. With international commitment and national pride in favour of tobacco control, China's policy to implement the Framework seems to have gained the upper hand. However, determination and concern for the health and well-being of its population are crucial if China is to counter economic objections and enforce laws in accordance with the requirements of the Tobacco Framework.

Legislation addressing tobacco harms in Japan

As recently as 2004, Japan was still home to over 31 million smokers, with high rates of smoking in young men and women (Omi 2004). Smoking prevalence among physicians and nurses was also high (WHO 2004). After ratifying the Tobacco Framework Convention in 2004, the Japanese government through the National Institute of Public Health began to strengthen its national programmes to control the use of tobacco. It was recognized that tobacco control might be a uniquely different issue in Japan because the Japanese tobacco industry was administered by the government. Indeed the Tobacco Industry Law of 1984 called for activities that promoted tobacco, and tobacco sales constituted a substantial source of revenue (Mochizuki-Kobayashi 2004). This is also reflected in the fact that the Ministry of Finance holds a nearly 50 per cent share in Japan Tobacco, and upon retirement from political life, officials of the Ministry often assume high positions in the company, so powerful individuals have an interest in maximizing tobacco profits (Mochizuki-Kobayashi 2004). The Ministry of Finance and the Ministry of Health, Labour and Welfare presented opposing views during the Framework deliberations. The Health Minister proposed a focus on ways to reduce tobacco consumption so as to promote health, but the Finance Minister argued that the role of government should be to provide information to enable individuals to decide for themselves and that no measures should be taken to reduce or ban tobacco use (Hanai 2003).

Much early tobacco legislation in Japan is contained in local ordinances. In 2001, a municipal ordinance in Aomori Prefecture prohibited the placement of vending machines for cigarettes. In 2002, Chiyoda Ward in Tokyo introduced an ordinance which prohibited smoking and discarding cigarette butts in designated areas. The first national legislation was the 2003 Health Promotion Law containing a provision on the responsibility of administrators for the prevention of passive smoking in public places, and so prompting large enterprises such as Japan Railway to adopt smoke-free policies in railway stations. Government buildings, schools, department stores, hospitals, cinemas, and theatres became smoke-free, but smoking in workplaces and other public places has yet to be prohibited. It remains to be seen what restrictions Japan will implement with regard to the obligation to undertake a comprehensive ban of all tobacco advertising, promotion, and sponsorship as required by the Framework Convention.

Legislation addressing tobacco control in Hong Kong

The Smoking (Public Health) (Amendment) Ordinance (Cap.371) was enacted in Hong Kong in 1982 providing prohibitions against smoking in areas such as banks and shopping malls, and stipulating that restaurants providing seating for over 200 people must designate not less than one-third of such area as smoke-free. However, the public was still subjected to considerable second-hand smoke. The bodies with responsibility for regulation are the Hong Kong Council on Smoking and Health established in 1987 under the Hong Kong Council on Smoking and Health Ordinance (Cap. 389) and the Tobacco Control Office within the Department of Health. To comply with the Framework Convention, the Smoking Ordinance was substantially revised in 2006. Changes pertained to expansion of statutory no smoking areas to cover most indoor areas in workplaces and public places, tightening of restrictions on advertisement, promotion and sponsorship of tobacco products, and requiring tobacco packages to bear health warnings with pictorial or graphic content. During the early days of application of the Ordinance there was confusion as to the meaning of terms such as 'indoor' areas, leading to a large number of exemptions being granted. Despite these unresolved issues, the amendments have resulted not only in cleaner air in indoor settings, but also a cultural shift whereby inconsiderate smokers are no longer condoned.

Legislation addressing smoking harms in other Asian states

Most Asian states are signatories to the Framework Convention on Tobacco Control including India, Pakistan, Republic of Korea, and People's Democratic Republic of Korea, Myanmar, Thailand, and Vietnam. Many states are introducing tobacco control legislation but as in Japan, smoking is an ingrained part of Asian culture and there is much resistance.

Singapore, a Convention signatory, began legislating against tobacco use in 1970. The Smoking (Prohibition in Certain Places) (Amendment) Notifications 1997 extended the ban so that it covered schools, universities, cinemas, air-conditioned restaurants, and air-conditioned shops. Further amendments in 2006 extended the smoking ban to cover outdoor food outlets, karaoke bars, and nightclubs. The 1998 amendments to the Smoking (Control of Advertising and Sale of Tobacco) (Licensing) Regulations regulate sale of tobacco to minors and tobacco advertising. Singapore now has one of the strongest anti-smoking regimes in the world.

Malaysia, also a signatory to the Convention, has one of the highest rates of smoking in the region. Malaysia passed the Control of Tobacco Products Regulation in 1993 but tobacco industry pressures resulted in limited prohibition (Assunta & Chapman 2004). Amendment regulations in 1997 prohibited the sale of tobacco products to persons under the age of 18 and increased the number of places where smoking is prohibited. Smoking is now prohibited in most public places including schools, government buildings, public waiting areas, air-conditioned restaurants, shopping malls, and sports complexes. However, indirect advertising of tobacco products still takes place and much needs to be done to comply with the Framework Convention.

Smoking incidence is high in the Philippines but appears to be declining among adolescents (CDC 2005). Tobacco is a major source of revenue for the Philippines. The 2003 Tobacco Regulation Act attempts a compromise between health and revenue, stating that it is the policy of the state both to protect the right to health, and to protect workers and other stakeholders in the tobacco industry. The result is that the emphasis of the tobacco control movement is on education and warnings of health risks. Smoking is prohibited in schools and recreational facilities for persons under 18, hospitals, and transport facilities. Other public areas such as covered areas open to the public, private workplaces and restaurants are required to provide designated smoking areas. No tobacco product can be sold within 100 m of a school. Tobacco advertising is allowed but must not be aimed at minors, must not feature celebrities, must not use cartoons, must not be placed in printed media where more than 25 per cent of readers are under 18, and must not be placed on a billboard or mural near a school. Parallel to these measures are compensation measures for farmers who voluntarily cease to grow tobacco to support them in the change to other crops, and provisions to assist displaced cigarette factory workers.

The potential role of law in tackling obesity in Asian legal culture

Obesity may once have been primarily a Western problem, but no longer. One-fifth of the population in China is now overweight, and China has seen an alarming increase in childhood obesity (Wu 2006). The health risks associated with obesity tend to occur at lower body mass index (BMI) in Asian populations, and the Western Pacific Region of WHO have proposed new definitions of overweight and obesity based on lower levels of BMI for Asia (Regional Office for the Western Pacific 2000).

Obesity in Asia has been attributed to changing Asian diets and the adoption of Western food practices, together with low levels of exercise (Tee 2002). Asian culture has traditionally regarded excess weight as evidence of wealth and prosperity, and parents are proud of fat babies (Ip 1999). The result is that while obesity in the Western world is associated with poverty, in Asia it is associated with affluence (China Daily 2006). The opening up of Asian markets, particularly the enormous and lucrative Chinese market, to foreign foods and media advertising has resulted in the targeting of Asian populations by major food and drink manufacturers.

While there have been some restrictions on advertising in China, restrictions have tended to focus on cultural impact rather than on health (Ha 1996). However, evidence suggests that parents in China perceive that food advertising to children encourages poor quality, and expensive, eating habits and there is increasing pressure on government to regulate aggressive and deceptive advertising (Chan & McNeal 2003). Elsewhere in Asia, in 2007, South Korea announced restrictions on the advertising of 'fast' food from 2008, to be extended in 2010 to all foods containing high levels of sugar or fat. In June 2007, the government of Malaysia announced that fast-food companies were banned from sponsoring children's television programmes. In Thailand, all food advertisements must be approved by a national government body.

In South Korea, from 2007, the Korean Food and Drug Administration will require all foods to be labelled to make clear the levels of trans fat, and by 2010 no packaged food will be allowed to contain more than 1 per cent of trans fat. From 2007, in Malaysia, all fast-food chains will be required to label their food with cholesterol, fat, and sugar content. In Singapore, labelling of trans fats is voluntary but the largest supermarket chain, FairPrice, declares trans fats on its own brand labels and plans to reduce the number of its products containing trans fats. Thailand, the Philippines, Brunei Darussalam, Indonesia, and Singapore all restrict false advertising of the nutritional content of products (Tee 2002). The Philippine Food Fortification Act 2000 goes further and in recognition that the Filipino diet is deficient in nutrients, legislates for food fortification for locally processed products and food products for sale and distribution in the Philippines. For example, rice is to be fortified with iron; and wheat, sugar, and cooking oil, with vitamin A.

In South Korea, from 2007, no fast foods can be sold within 200 m of a school. Following a report by the Delhi Diabetics research centre, the Delhi government has proposed a ban on all junk food in schools.

China and Malaysia also regulate the content of school foods. Vietnam prohibits marketing of food and beverage products in schools.

Concern about the rapid increase in obesity and obesity-related health problems in Asian states has prompted consideration of government intervention in content, labelling, and marketing of processed foodstuffs. Because there is in general greater acceptance in Asian culture of state intervention in private life, particularly in states with some Islamic laws, civil liberties arguments have carried little weight. Concern has been more for economic consequences of restrictions, but unlike in the tobacco context where governments have a vested financial interest in tobacco production, these have not been sufficient to counter public health concerns for the health and economic consequence of obesity. Asian states are keen to learn from the problems faced by Western countries and to preempt the development of Western levels of obesity, and this has resulted in increasing regulation of food products with high levels of fat, salt, and sugar. Such measures are in accord with the concern of Asian states to protect cultural traditions, including traditional food practices, from Western influences, making food control laws more popular and less controversial than in Western states. However, WHO notes that most self-regulatory codes of practice on issues of food have developed in Europe, Australasia, and North America rather than in Asia, and that there has been relatively little activity to restrict marketing in low- to middle-income countries where promotional activities are growing faster and have the greatest impact (WHO 2006).

Conclusion

Increasingly states are resorting to law to provide a sound framework for non-medical interventions in public health. Increasingly also, international legal instruments are being developed to provide some coherence and consistency in approach to global public health problems.

In the context of communicable disease the revised IHR 2005 have the objective of achieving global public health security by strengthening national disease surveillance, prevention, control and response systems, and by strengthening WHO global alert and response systems. While the IHR 1969 focused on disease control at borders, the IHR 2005 address not only strengthening of border controls but also disease prevention and control at disease source, requiring states to introduce national measures to prevent the spread of disease. The IHR 1969 applied only to three diseases (cholera, plague, and yellow fever), but the IHR 2005 apply to all public health threats of international concern. The IHR also introduce into state and global disease responses respect for internationally recognized human rights. State parties to the Regulations are obliged to implement the core capacity requirements of the IHR by 2009. Law in statutory form, at least in a non-authoritarian state, must result from a parliamentary process which is inevitably slow. Hence many states are, at the time of writing, either in the process of reforming their public health legislation, or designing new legislation to strengthen 'soft' law public health powers.

In the context of tobacco control the 2003 WHO Framework Convention on Tobacco Control, developed in recognition of the global nature of the tobacco epidemic, requires signatory states to provide protection against tobacco smoke, regulation of tobacco product content, sale and traffic, regulation of tobacco labelling and warnings, regulation of tobacco advertising, promotion and sponsorship, and health education and promotion. The greater part of these requirements requires legal underpinning because the requirements involve interference with commercial activity and constraint on individual lifestyle behaviours. Again many states have begun to frame law to implement the framework, requiring new legislation aimed specifically at the control of public health tobacco harms.

The WHO has not yet used its law-making powers for obesity, but has initiated a Global Strategy on Diet, Physical Activity and Health to support policies that promote accessibility to foods low in fat, salt, and sugar. In 2006 WHO published reports on Reducing Salt Intake in Populations, on The Extent, Nature and Effects of Food Promotion to Children: A Review of the Evidence, and on Marketing of Food and Non-alcoholic Beverages to Children, for the purpose of developing an evidence base on mechanisms for reducing obesity levels. The reports recognize that self- regulation has not proved sufficient, particularly in reducing the volume of food and drink marketing to children and in minimizing the effects of marketing. The reports recommend that self-regulation operate in a legal framework in which there are incentives for compliance (WHO 2006).

These global instruments provide a common framework of legislative public health tools, but the content of law in response to the IHR and the Framework Convention will differ widely across states. Unlike science, which purports to be neutral, objective, and universally applicable, law is the formalization of social contracts between the state and its citizens and will reflect the social relationships ingrained in the culture of the state. National history, politics, geography, and economics will have forged very different understandings of what law is, who has the power to exercise it, and how it operates. Cultural and political circumstances and public awareness will influence the nature of restrictions appropriate to particular health threats (WHO 2006).

Over time it may be that these differences in understanding will be eroded by the effects of globalization. Global media reports, global recognition of the need for intervention for the protection of public health, and global agreement to international health and human rights instruments may eventually lead to some harmonization, or at least convergence, of public health laws. We have not yet reached that point, and for now approaches to law as a tool for public health vary widely.

It has not therefore been possible to identify world themes of public health law. It has not even been possible to collate a representative sample of national public health legislation across the world, given that the term 'legislation' already imposes a Western approach to control of populations and population behaviour. Much public health intervention is operated, particularly in African and Islamic legal cultures, on the basis of customary law or authority of the state without the need for legislation. The agreement of such states to international instruments such as the IHR or the Framework Convention has prompted some legislative activity, and there has been some minimal commonality of content of national legislation across signatory states. But as can be seen by the response of Japan and the Philippines to the Framework Convention, local conditions and local culture have led to very different commitments to tobacco prohibition.

This chapter has focused on Western and Asian legal cultures because legislation plays a more significant role in the meaning of law in these cultures. Approaches to law in the Western states we have examined demonstrate that autonomy and private rights are fundamental to the framing of law, and only rarely does law in Western legal culture envisage measures such as treatment and vaccination without consent, even when it might be in the public interest to treat or vaccinate. Recognition of human rights documents also plays a significant role in the extent to which Western states are prepared to interfere with privacy and autonomy, particularly in relation to communicable disease where public health measures might call for infringement of physical liberties. However, Western states have generally been rigorous in legislating restrictions on tobacco use, even where restrictions impinge on commercial interests and constrain lifestyle choices. Similarly Western states have been ready to use law in relation to other 'lifestyle' diseases such as obesity, regulating food content, food advertising, and food labelling.

States which have elements of Asian legal culture, prioritizing community and state interests over individual interests, have been prepared to adopt more stringent legal measures for communicable disease control than Western states. Hence Asian states are more likely to legislate for powers that potentially infringe autonomy such as compulsory treatment and vaccination. This is not because Asian states are prepared to override human rights, but rather because recognition of Asian values results in different interpretations of the meaning of rights. At the same time, Asian states have been less prepared to interfere with cultural lifestyle choices where to do so would impinge on state commercial interests, public revenue, employment rights of workers in the tobacco industry, and cultural smoking behaviours. Tobacco laws in Asian states have emphasized health education and health warnings over interference with smoking practices. There are signs, however, that Asian states are prepared to intervene in dietary choices, particularly in relation to imported Western food practices which threaten not only health of populations and the economy of the state but are also harmful to cultural food practices and traditions.

Globalization inevitably leads to some measure of cultural imperialism, and over time the predominance of Western approaches to regulation, rights, and legislative expression of law is filtering into approaches in other legal cultures. The significant presence of persons from Western cultures in international organizations, and their representation in the framing of international instruments, has meant that Western approaches to public health and to rights have influenced the content of international public health frameworks. International frameworks presuppose that national laws are formalized, with the result that all states will over time enshrine their public health laws in statutory form.

We are a long way from a common international stance on the use of law as a public health tool, but the renewed willingness of the WHO to use its treaty and law-making powers in the interests of global health will slowly lead to some convergence of national public health legislation. Only when all states choose to use statutory powers, published in legislative form and publicly available, to endorse public health interventions, will we able to undertake a comprehensive worldwide analysis of national public health legislation.

Key points

- Law is an important tool for containment of both communicable and non-communicable disease.
- Law is not a neutral instrument, and the meaning and process of 'law' differ widely across legal cultures.
- Any comparison of national public health legislation is made difficult by absence of legislation addressing public health in many states. States within Western and Asian legal cultures are more likely to enshrine law in legislative form.
- Many states within Western and Asian legal cultures have legislated to control communicable disease and to control tobacco harms, and are beginning to consider legislation to address obesity.
- International legal instruments such as the revised International Health Regulations and the Framework Convention for Tobacco Control will require many more states to consider legislation to comply with international requirements.

References

Allwright, S., Paul, G., and Bernie, J. (2005). Legislation for smoke-free workplaces and health of bar work before and after study. *British Medical Journal*, **331**, 1117–26.

Assunta, M. and Chapman, S. (2004). Industry sponsored youth smoking prevention programme in Malaysia: A case study in duplicity. *Tobacco Control*, **13**, ii37–42.

Atenstaedt, R. (2006). Does danger lurk in the library? *Public Health*, **120**(8), 776–7.

Bell, D. (1996). The East Asian challenge to human rights: Reflections on an East West dialogue. *Human Rights Quarterly*, **18.3**, 641–67.

Bell, J. (1995). Comparative law and legal theory. In *Prescriptive formality and normative rationality in modern legal systems* (eds. W. Krawietz, N. MacCormick, and G. von Wright). Duncker and Humblot, Berlin.

Borzekowski, D. and Robinson, T. (2001). The 30-second effect: An experiment revealing the impact of television commercials on food preferences of preschoolers. *Journal of the American Diet Association*, **101**, 42–6.

Brems, E. (2001). *Human rights: Universality and diversity*. Martinus Nijhoff, The Hague.

Caraher, M. (2006). Television advertising and children: Lessons from policy development. *Public Health Nutrition*, **9**(5), 596–605.

CDC (2005). Tobacco use among students aged 13 to 15 years – Philippines, 2001 and 2003. *MMWR*, February 4, 2005.

Chadwick, E. (1842). *Report on the sanitary conditions of the labouring population of Great Britain*, London.

Chan, K. and McNeal, J. (2003). Parental concern about television viewing and children's advertising in China. *International Journal for Public Opinion Research*, **15**(2), 151–66.

China Daily (2006). Hong Kong parents must take lead in obesity battle. *China Daily*, 3 October 2006.

Coker, R. and Martin, R. (2006). Introduction: The importance of law for public health policy and practice. *Public Health*, **120**(Suppl.) 2–8.

Coker, R., Mounier-Jack, S., and Martin, R. (2007). Public health law and tuberculosis control in Europe. *Public Health*, **121**(4), 266–73.

Dalacoura, K. (2003). *Islam, liberalism and human rights*. L.B.Tauris, London.

Da Lomba, S. and Martin, R. (2004). Public health powers in relation to infectious tuberculosis in England and France: A comparison of approaches. *Medical Law International*, **6**, 117–47.

De Bary, Tu. (2001). *Confucianism and human rights*. Columbia University Press, Columbia.

Department of Health (2004). *Choosing health: Making healthy choices easier*. Department of Health White Paper, 16 Nov 2004.

Department of Health Western Australia (2005). *A new public health Act for WA*. Department of Health, Perth.

Department of Health (2006). *Forecasting obesity to 2010*. Department of Health July 2006.

Department of Health (2007). Review of Parts II, V and VI of the Public Health (Control of Disease) Act 1984: a Consultation. Department of Health, London.

Diokno, M. (2000). Once again, the Asian values debate: The case of the Philippines. In *Human rights and Asian values* (eds. M. Jacobsen and O. Bruun). Curzon Press, Richmond.

Durand de Bousingen, D. (2001). French court enforces Formula 1 tobacco advertising ban. *Lancet*, **9273**, 2036.

Enhorn v Sweden [2005] E.C.H.R. 56529/00.

Euromonitor International (2006a). *NRT smoking cessation aids in Ireland.*

Euromonitor International (2006b). *Tobacco in China*. December 2006.

Fidler, D. (2004). SARS, governance and the globalization of disease. Palgrave, McMillan, UK.

Fidler, D. (2005). From international sanitary conventions to global health security: The new international health regulations. *Chinese Journal of International Law*, **4**(2), 325–92.

Fidler, D. and Gostin, L. (2006). The new international health regulations: An historic development for international law and public health. *Journal of Law and Medical Ethics*, 85–94.

Fichtenberg, C. and Glantz, S. (2002). Effect of smoke-free workplaces on smoking behaviour: systematic review. *British Medical Journal*, **325**, 188–94.

Food Standards Agency (2003). Academic panel examines food promotion and children reviews. 26 November 2003.

Francey and Meeuwissen v Hilton Hotels of Australia H 97/50, 10 March 2000.

Gostin, L. (2000). *Public Health Law: Power, duty, restraint*, p. 4. University of California Press, Berkeley.

Gostin, L. (2007). Law as a tool to facilitate healthier lifestyles and prevent obesity. *JAMA*, **298**, 87–90.

Hanai (2003). Reported in Mochizuki-Kobayashi Y *et al.* (2004). Tobacco Free*Japan. Recommendations for Tobacco Control. Tobacco Free*Japan, Tokyo and Institute for Global Tobacco Control, Department of Epidemiology, Johns Hopkins Bloomberg School of Public Health, at 268.

Ha, L. (1996). Concerns about advertising practices in a developing country: An examination of China's new advertising regulations. *International Journal of Advertising*, **15**, 91–102.

Harris, A. and Martin, R. (2004). The exercise of public health powers in an era of human rights: The particular problem of tuberculosis. *Public Health*, **118**(5), 312–22.

Harvard Law Review Note (2003). The elephant in the room: Evolution, behaviouralism and counteradvertising in the coming war against obesity. *Harvard Law Review*, **116**(4), 1161–84.

Hastings, G. *et al.* (2003). *Review of the research on the effects of food promotion to children*. Centre for Social Marketing, Glasgow.

Holm, S. (2007). Obesity interventions and ethics. *Obesity Reviews*, **8**(1), 207–10.

House of Commons UK (2004). *Response to consultation by the select committee on health, Third Report.* House of Commons, London.

House of Commons Health Committee (2004). Press Notice, 'Obesity Report Published'. 26 May 2004.

IAFCO (2003). *Broadcasting bad health*. July 2003.

Ip, H. (1999). Comment by Dr Henrietta Ip, Chair, Hong Kong Child Health Foundation, to the BBC. May 23 1999.

Jacobsen, M. and Bruun, O. (eds.) (2000). *Human rights and Asian values.* Curzon Press, Richmond.

Johns Hopkins (2000). *National conference on policy development on tobacco control in China in the 21st century*, reported at http://www.jhsph.edu./global_tobacco/policy_development/china_national_plan/.

Jones, K., Wakefield, M., and Turnbull, D. (1999). Attitudes and experiences of restaurateurs regarding smoking bans in Adelaide, South Australia. *Tobacco Control*, **8**, 62–6.

Lam, T., Ho, S., Mak, K. *et al.* (2000) Mortality and smoking in Hong Kong: Case-control study of all adult deaths in 1998. *British Medical Journal*, **323**, 361.

Lang, T. (2006). 'Food, the law and public health'. *Public Health*, Special edition edited by Coker, R. and Martin, R., **120**, 30–41.

LegCo Select Committee Hong Kong (2004). *Report of the Select Committee to inquire into the handling of the severe acute respiratory syndrome outbreak by the government and the hospital authority*. Legislative Council, Hong Kong.

Liu, B-Q., Peto, R., Chen, Z-M. *et al.* (1998). Emerging tobacco hazards in China: 1. Retrospective proportional mortality study of one million deaths. *British Medical Journal*, **317**, 1311–1422.

Maffeis, C. and Tatò, L. (2001). Long term effects of childhood obesity on morbidity and mortality. *Hormone Research*, **55**(1), 42–5.

Martin, R. (2006a). The exercise of public health powers in cases of infectious disease: Human rights implications. *Medical Law Review*, **14**(1), 132–43.

Martin, R. (2006b). The limits of law in the protection of public health and the role of public health ethics. *Public Health*, Special edition edited by Coker, R. and Martin, R., **120**, 71–80.

Martin, R. (2008). The role of law in the control of obesity in England: looking at the contribution of law to a healthy food culture. *Australia and New Zealand Health Policy*. In press.

Mbeke, T. (2000). *HIV=AIDS controversy: What's all this then?* Thabo Mbeke's letter to world leaders on AIDS in Africa.

Mechlem, K. (2000). Legal reform in developing countries: The use of comparative law and law and economics. In *Governance, decentralization and reform in China, India and Russia* (ed. J. Dethier). Kluwer Academic Press, Dordrecht/London/Boston.

Mello, M., Studdert, D., and Brennan, T. (2006). Obesity—the new frontier of public health law. *New England Journal of Medicine*, **354**(24), 2601–10.

Melville, D. and Shortridge, K. (2004). Influenza: Time to come to grips with the avian dimension. *Lancet Infectious Diseases*, **4**(5), 261–2.

Merson, M., Black, R., and Mills, A. (2006). *International public health: Diseases, programs, systems, and policies.* Jones and Bartlett, Sudbury, Mass.

Mill, J. (1869). *On Liberty*. Longman, Roberts and Green, London.

Ministry of Health China (2007). *China tobacco control report 2007*. Office of the Team of Leaders for Conforming to the FCTC, Ministry of Health, Beijing, May 2007 (Chinese only).

Ministry of Health New Zealand (2002). *Public health legislation: Promoting public health, preventing ill health, and managing communicable diseases.* Ministry of Health, Wellington.

Mochizuki-Kobayashi, Y. *et al.* (2004). *Tobacco Free * Japan. Recommendations for Tobacco Control*. Tobacco Free*Japan, Tokyo and Institute for Global Tobacco Control, Department of Epidemiology, Johns Hopkins Bloomberg School of Public Health.

Morella, A. (1996). *La Défaite de la Santé Publique*, pp. 266–9. Flammarion, France.

National Audit Office (2001). *Tackling obesity in England*. National Audit Office, 15 February 2001.

National People's Congress (2005). Decision of the standing committee of the tenth national people's congress about ratifying the framework convention on Tobacco Control promulgated on 28 August 2005, reported at http://www.lawinfochina.com.

Neary, I. (2002). *Human rights in Japan, South Korea and Taiwan*. Routledge, London.

Ofcom (2006). *Television advertising of food and drink to children: Options for new restrictions*. 28 March 2006.

Ofcom (2007). *Television advertising of food and drink to children: Final statement*. 22 February 2007.

Omi, S. (2004). *Message for tobacco free Japan. Forward to recommendations for tobacco control policy*. WHO Western Pacific Region Office.

Parliament of South Australia (2007). *Fast food and obesity inquiry*. Adelaide, 27 March 2007.

Peng, Y. (1997). *Smoke and power: The political economy of Chinese tobacco*, University of Oregon PhD thesis, referenced in de Bayer, J. *et al.* (2004), *Research on tobacco in China*, Health, Nutrition and Population Discussion Paper, World Bank.

Pickett, K., Kelly, S., Brunner, E. *et al.* (2005). Wider income gaps, wider waistbands? An ecological study of obesity and income inequality. *Journal of Epidemiology and Community Health*, **59**, 670–4.

Prime Minister Tony Blair (2006a). Healthy living. July 2006.

Prime Minister Tony Blair (2006b). How do we lead healthier lives? 26 July 2006.

Regional Office for the Western Pacific (2000). *The Asia-Pacific perspective: Redefining obesity and its treatment*. WHO, February 2000.

Reuters (2007a). '100,000 Chinese die annually from passive smoking'. 29 May 2007.

Reuters (2007Bb). 'Smoking curb could "upset China stability"'. 7 March 2007.

Scottish Executive (2006). *Public health legislation in Scotland*. Scottish Executive, Edinburgh.

Sen, A. (1997). Human rights and Asian values: What Lee Kuan Yew and Le Peng don't understand about Asia. *The New Republic*, July 14.

Sommade, C., Haut Comité Français pour la Défense Civile (2004). Quarantine Conference, Wilton Park, 22 January 2004.

South China Morning Post (2007). The debate on Asian values gets a revival. April 23. Hong Kong.

Stanton, R., Mehta, A., Morton, H. *et al.* (2005). Food advertising and broadcasting legislation – a case of system failure? *Nutrition and Dietetics*, **62**(1), 26–32.

Svennson, M. (2000). The Chinese debate on Asian values and human rights: Some reflections on relativism, nationalism and orientalism. In *Human rights and Asian values* (eds. M. Jacobsen and O. Bruun). Curzon Press, Richmond.

Tan Poh-ling (1997). *Asian legal systems*. Butterworths, Australia.

Tatara, K. (2002). Philosophy of public health: Lessons from its history in England. *Journal of Public Health Medicine*, **24**(1), 11–15.

Tee, E-S. (2002). Nutritional labelling and claims: Concerns and challenges; experiences from the Asia Pacific Region. *Asia Pacific Journal of Clinical Nutrition*, **11**, S215–S223.

Van Hoecke, M. and Warrington, M. (1998). Legal cultures, legal paradigms and legal doctrine: Towards a new model for comparative law. *International and Comparative Law Quarterly*, **47**, 495–536.

Wanless, D. (2002). *Securing our future health: Taking a long-term view*. HM Treasury, London.

Wanless, D. (2004). *Securing good health for the whole population*. HM Treasury, London.

WHO (2000). WHO Western Pacific region tobacco-free initiative country specific database, quoted in *Tobacco Free * Japan. Recommendations for Tobacco Control*. Tobacco Free*Japan, Tokyo and Institute for Global Tobacco Control, Department of Epidemiology, Johns Hopkins Bloomberg School of Public Health, at 270.

WHO (2003). Factsheet: *Obesity and overweight,* http://www.who.int/hpr/NPH/docs/gs_obesity.pdf.

WHO (2005). *'China joins the global war on smoking'*. Press release 30 August 2005.

WHO (2006). *Marketing of food and non-alcoholic beverages to children*. WHO, Geneva.

WHO Regional Office for Europe (2006*). European charter on counteracting obesity*. Istanbul 16 November 2006.

Wu, Y. (2006). Overweight and obesity in China. *British Medical Journal*, **333**, 362–3.

Zweigert, K. and Kötz, H. (1998). *Introduction to comparative law*. Clarendon Press, Oxford.

4.3

International public health instruments

Douglas Bettcher[1], Katherine DeLand[1], Jorgen Schlundt[1], Fernando González-Martín[1], Jennifer Bishop, Summer Hamide, and Annette Lin

Abstract

Norms, standards, agreements, and regulations have been used, since the nineteenth-century International Sanitary Conferences, as governance tools in public health diplomacy. With globalization attaining an unprecedented level at the end of the twentieth century, it appeared that some public goods were increasingly difficult to provide efficiently at the state level. The reason for this is that as states increased their interconnectedness, the interrelation between domestic public goods common to the interacting states also increased. Correlatively, the singular nature of some of what were once solely domestic public goods progressively declined and the creation and maintenance of those public goods became shared enterprises. This led to the emergence of the concept of the global public good (GPG). This chapter examines the ideas of health as a GPG and international law in general, and international health instruments in particular, as intermediate GPGs utilized to protect and promote health. As intermediate GPGs for health, international legal instruments take on an additional layer of importance in global health governance. In providing a robust framework for improving and occasionally even creating health, these instruments are important not only for what they are already doing, but for the potential new instruments that may be developed. Through the presentation of case studies examining three international instruments that the World Health Organization (WHO) has been involved in developing, the chapter focuses on the evolution and implementation of emerging, salient international health-specific legal agreements. As WHO continues to grow into its normative role, it is likely that additional opportunities to exercise its constitutional quasi-legislative powers will present themselves. The three examples of intermediate GPGs examined in this chapter have laid a solid foundation on which WHO and its Member States may build, to continue working toward achieving the GPG of health.

Notwithstanding over 150 years of the use of regulatory approaches to public health protection and promotion, their relevance is still intensely debated. In today's world characterized by the phenomenon of globalization, what is the relevance of norms, standards, agreements, and regulations in multilateral disease control initiatives? In what ways could the usefulness and utility of regulatory and normative mechanisms be enhanced to diminish the morbidity and mortality burdens of communicable and non-communicable diseases on vulnerable groups in developing countries? Can normative and regulatory mechanisms play any meaningful role in financing global health, and the distribution of health dividends as GPGs in a sharply divided world?

This chapter will first present the economic concept of GPGs and examine the idea of health as a GPG and international health instruments as intermediate GPGs utilized to protect and promote health (Kaul *et al.* 1999; Taylor & Bettcher 2000; Fidler 2003). Next, through the presentation of case studies examining three international instruments that the WHO has been involved in developing, the chapter will focus on the evolution and implementation of emerging, salient international health-specific legal agreements. Finally, the chapter will provide a brief discussion of the 'soft law' and 'hard law' international legal paradigms, and WHO's role in creating these instruments.

As the WHO Constitution provides, health is not merely the absence of disease or infirmity, but is also 'a state of complete physical, mental, and social well being' (WHO 2007a). Because of the broad nature of health, concerted multinational action on all levels is required to provide health. This chapter aims to provide some insight and overview into the relationship between international law and the improvement of public health using the concept of GPGs.

[1] The author is a staff member of the World Health Organization. The author alone is responsible for the views expressed in this publication, and they do not necessarily represent the decisions or the stated policy of the World Health Organization.

Section I: Global public goods—health and international health instruments

Health as a global public good

The concept of public goods form a core economic tool used since the eighteenth century to think about and analyse national governance. A public good is a good that has two characteristics: (1) It is non-rival in consumption; that is, its consumption by an individual does not impede someone else from consuming it, and (2) it is non-excludable, which means that one cannot prevent someone from consuming it. For instance, a public park can be considered a public good. The fact that someone is spending some time in a public park does not, under normal circumstances, impede someone else from coming into the park. Furthermore, in a normal situation, a public park is open to anyone and no one is allowed to prevent someone else from accessing it. It should be noted, however, that public goods do not necessarily have to be tangible. For instance, security or education can also be considered public goods. Since public goods tend to be underprovided in the absence of government intervention, due to the 'free-rider problem' (i.e. taking advantage of a public good without providing for its existence or maintenance), governments often focus on activities dedicated to providing public goods.

With globalization attaining an unprecedented level at the end of the twentieth century, it appeared that some public goods were increasingly difficult to provide efficiently at the state level. The reason for this is that as states increased their interconnectedness, the interrelation between domestic public goods common to the interacting states also increased. Correlatively, the singular nature of some of what were once solely domestic public goods progressively declined and the creation and maintenance of those public goods became shared enterprises. This led to the emergence of the concept of the GPG. Kaul *et al.* (1999) define GPG as a public good having three characteristics:

1. It covers more than one group of countries.
2. Its benefits [...] reach [...] a broad spectrum of the global population (which means that access to them must not be limited to certain economic classes, gender, religious groups, or any other discrete community).
3. It meets the needs of present generations without jeopardizing those of future generations.

Based on these criteria, health is arguably a GPG. As a public good, health is a positive sum: One person's good health does not detract from another's. Indeed, better individual health usually has positive effects on entire populations—for example, through reduced disease transmission. As health is not only an end in itself, but is also inseparable from social and economic welfare, health is also a key element for economic and social growth. An improvement in individual health can improve the community-level economy and social fabric.

Furthermore, although the onus of providing health remains primarily on national governments, globalization means that the determinants of health, as well as the requisite means to deliver health, are increasingly global (Jamison *et al.* 1998). Countries are more and more interdependent with regard to health issues. This is clearly true for those matters related to communicable disease, as illustrated by the 2002 SARS outbreak, which required concerted, multilateral action to contain. Though less obvious, this is no less true for non-communicable diseases (Beaglehole & Yach 2003). In fact, a range of non-infectious transnational health threats have emerged in recent years, including *inter alia* the marketing of tobacco, environmental degradation, alcohol and illicit drug use, anti-microbial resistance, hunger and food insecurity, and diet and obesity, all of which now constitute globalized threats to health and human security. As these threats demonstrate, globalization is not limited to the movement of people and goods across borders, but also can affect individual and collective behavioural patterns which can, in turn, have dramatic impact on health.

Two forces are moving health progressively toward the centre of the stage in the discussion of GPGs. First, as already noted, enhanced international linkages in trade, migration, and information flows have accelerated the cross-border transmission of disease and the international transfer of behavioural health risks. Second, intensified pressure on common-pool global resources, such as air and water, has generated shared, transnational environmental threats. The result is that diseases, and other threats harmful to health, present enormous international (and often global) challenges that are beyond the governance capabilities of individual nation states. Accordingly, efficiently addressing these issues requires coordination and action at a supranational level.

It should be noted, however, that the notion of health as a GPG is not uncontested. It has been argued that an individual's health—or even an entire county's health status—primarily benefits only the individual or country and that the resources necessary to provide better health are indeed 'predominantly rival and exclusive' (Woodward & Smith 2003). This school agrees that some aspects of health may be GPGs, including control of globally threatening communicable disease, like HIV/AIDS and tuberculosis, but there is some concern that 'relaxing' the interpretation of GPG to include health may dilute the usefulness of GPGs as means to secure funding (Smith & Woodward 2003). Perhaps most importantly, if health as a GPG is limited to very prescribed circumstances, like control of certain infectious disease, then it loses its capacity as an organizing principal for global health priorities (Smith *et al.* 2004).

Nonetheless, even among those who maintain that health is not a GPG, there is a strong sense that collective action and coordination, as the core notion of GPGs, can be used to great and measurable effect to promote and improve global health. While this chapter argues that heath is, in and of itself, a GPG, it does so in the same spirit as those who contest this first, basic notion. Namely, the idea of health as a GPG is a useful tool, both to an intellectual examination of global health status, progress and possibilities, and to the development of practical, applicable health interventions. Insofar as this chapter focuses on international instruments, developed via collective global action, its premise finds the common ground between the health as a GPG camp and the opposing view.

As well as being the means to a GPG end (in this case, health), the coordination and actions themselves could also be considered GPGs, insofar as they provide a shared platform for the process of improving social and economic welfare. The agreements to coordinate and to act in concert, while critical for reaching a GPG, are part of the process rather than an outcome in and of themselves. This conceptualization allows us to introduce a typology that distinguishes two different types of GPGs—final GPGs and intermediate GPGs:

1. Final GPGs are outcomes rather than 'goods' in the standard sense. They may be tangible (such as the environment or the

common heritage of mankind) or intangible (such as peace or financial stability).

2. Intermediate GPGs, such as international regimes, contribute towards the provision of final GPGs (Kaul *et al.* 1999).

The WHO Framework Convention on Tobacco Control (WHO FCTC) provides an example of an intermediate GPG. As an intermediate GPG, the WHO FCTC establishes a rubric of coordinated action among states, which will bring about a significant health improvement not otherwise efficiently obtainable by states acting on their own (Taylor *et al.* 2003).

Health-related international instruments as intermediate GPGs

The evolution of normative and regulatory approaches to the transnational spread of disease dates back to the European-led International Sanitary Conferences in the mid-nineteenth century. The European cholera epidemics of 1830 and 1847 catalysed the earliest regulatory and normative approaches to cross-border disease control. From 1851 to the end of the nineteenth century, ten International Sanitary Conferences were convened, and eight sanitary conventions were negotiated on the cross-border spread of cholera, plague, and yellow fever in Europe.

Insofar as these instruments were negotiated long before any of the European countries had experienced an epidemiologic transition from infectious to chronic disease burdens (Omran 1971), these normative, regulatory frameworks were narrowly focused on infectious disease control, the primary threat to health and a substantial cross-border concern. The agreements were a prominent feature of the European-led international sanitary conferences and the emphasis on infectious disease was mirrored in the disease surveillance-oriented mandates of pioneer multilateral health organizations, including the Pan American Sanitary Bureau, Office International d'Hygiene Publique, Health Office of the League of Nations, and Office International des Epizooties.

The globalization of public health provides a context in which the continued development and implementation of public health-related global norms and standards is becoming increasingly relevant. As there is no supranational authority that can ensure the provision of GPGs, the implications of globalization include the need for increased transnational cooperation and partnerships, as well as greater intersectoral action. Intermediate GPGs, like international norms, agreements, and regulations, play an important role in this dynamic (Kaul *et al.* 2003; Taylor *et al.* 2003; Fidler 2002). The globalization of public health has catalysed global health governance, involving states, international organizations, and non-state actors in the process of designing multinational health interventions and agreements (Kickbusch 2003; Dodgson *et al.* 2002; Taylor & Bettcher 2000).

Although WHO has made limited use of its constitutional powers to adopt agreements under Article 19, regulations under Article 21 and recommendations under Article 23, during the 1990s, the Organization launched two initiatives suggesting that international law may be seen as a more important instrument of global public health policy in the future. The first involved the revision of the International Health Regulations (IHR) to make them more relevant to the global problems caused by emerging and re-emerging infectious diseases. The second was the decision to develop the WHO FCTC. Additionally, although not exclusively about health, many multilateral instruments negotiated by states, intergovernmental organizations (IGOs), and non-governmental organizations (NGOs) in areas like international environmental law, international trade law, international human rights law, international humanitarian law, international law on arms control, international law on narcotic drugs and international labour law have included the protection of human health as an embedded objective (Taylor *et al.* 2002).

Using the intermediate GPG international law to achieve the GPG for health

The use of international law in the production of health as a GPG comprises four essential aspects. First, states use international law to establish formal institutions empowered to work on global public health problems. The modern classic example of this is, of course, the WHO, but it is reasonable also to see certain others, including the United Nations Environment Program (UNEP) and the International Labor Organization (ILO), that also, if somewhat indirectly, promote and foster health.

Second, states use international law to establish procedures through which states and non-state actors can tackle specific global public health problems. For example, in order to effectively address the transnationalization of health risks and diseases, instruments like the WHO FCTC and the International Health Regulations (IHR) provide frameworks for efficient multilateral information and surveillance systems. Implementation and ongoing evolution and improvement of these systems are critical and the complexity inherent in this kind of information gathering is exemplified by WHO's strengthening global monitoring and alert systems, which link together, *inter alia*, specialized laboratories, disease surveillance systems, sources of relevant expertise, and state governments via electronic and printed media.

Third, states use international law to craft substantive duties in connection with particular global public health challenges. The IHR, for example, obligates WHO Member States to notify the Organization of specific public health events. The WHO FCTC requires Parties to implement specific obligations, like adhering to a discrete tobacco product labeling and warning regime, as well as to incorporate the general obligations and objectives of the Convention into their approaches to providing health.

Fourth, states use international law to create mechanisms to enforce substantive legal duties undertaken by states that have agreed to be bound by international instruments. Enforcement mechanisms come in many forms, from states self-reporting on progress made in connection with certain goals articulated in a treaty, as is common in multilateral environmental agreements like the Basel Convention (1992), to formal adjudication of state-to-state disputes by an international tribunal, as seen in the WTO's dispute-settlement mechanism.

While various instruments can be intermediate GPGs for health, international legal agreements are among the most important. International legal agreements provide a foundation for many other intermediate products with global public benefits, including institutionalized forums for global cooperation, research, surveillance, technical assistance programmes, and information clearing-houses. Global agreements like the WHO FCTC, the IHR, and the Codex Alimentarius are negotiated to secure global cooperation and that cooperation, in turn, leads to the sustained creation and promotion of health and related GPGs.

Section II: Case studies

The intermediate GPGs that comprise health-related international normative agreements, strategies, and instruments, will improve public health, reduce the burden of disease, and lead to reductions in poverty and increases in economic development. Globalization has been a cardinal factor triggering the expansion of international health law, which is recognized as inextricably interrelated to other areas of international normative concern, including international environmental law, labour law, and arms control. The WHO FCTC signalled a turning point in WHO's approach to international health lawmaking, and its entry into force heralded a new era in international health cooperation. As demonstrated by the WHO FCTC and the revision of the IHR, the forces of globalization at work in international health are compelling the international community to think creatively and to develop new models of cooperation, including the expanded use of international health law, to protect and promote the health of populations worldwide.

The three case studies that follow illustrate the relevance of norms, standards, agreements, and regulations in transnational disease control and discuss the impact of such instruments now and in the future. First we will examine the WHO FCTC, the first global health treaty negotiated under the auspices of WHO. The Convention is an evidence-based treaty that represents a paradigm shift in developing a regulatory strategy to address addictive substances; in contrast to previous drug control treaties, the WHO FCTC asserts the importance of demand reduction strategies as well as supply reduction issues. Second, we will present the IHR, WHO's legally binding regulations designed to address the spread of general and specific infectious disease. States Parties to the IHR are required to develop, strengthen, and maintain core surveillance and response capacities to detect, assess, notify, and report public health events to WHO and respond to public health risks and public health emergencies. Third, we will discuss the International Food Safety Authorities Network (INFOSAN) and the Codex Alimentarius, which has become the global reference point for consumers, food producers and processors, national food control agencies, and the international food trade as the benchmark against which national food measures and regulations are evaluated within the legal parameters of the WTO Agreements.

Case study: The WHO Framework Convention on Tobacco Control

The WHO FCTC is a carefully balanced legal instrument, adopted following vigorous negotiations, which took into account scientific, economic, social, and political considerations. The launch of WHO's first treaty negotiation was catalysed by a unique convergence of a number of factors:

- The accumulation of solid scientific evidence over a 50-year period, demonstrating the causal links between tobacco use and more than 20 major categories of disease (Doll 1998), and evidence pointing to the global toll of tobacco-related diseases;
- The strengthening of the evidence pointing to the adverse economic implications of the tobacco epidemic (World Bank 1999)
- The strengthening of the evidence that cost-effective tobacco control measures exist (World Bank 1999)
- The release as a result of litigation in the United States of over 35 million pages of previously secret tobacco industry documents, which provided a unique opportunity to better understand the strategies and tactics of the tobacco industry and, in doing so, to advance the public health agenda (Yach & Bettcher 2000)
- The establishment of a WHO cabinet project, the Tobacco Free Initiative, to focus international attention, resources, and action on the global tobacco epidemic
- The examples of different countries with successful tobacco control experiences
- The support of civil society in the form of public pressure on governments for strengthened tobacco regulations as the public became more aware of the dangers of tobacco (Da Costa e Silva & Nikogosian 2003)

The WHO FCTC focuses on the global implementation of evidence-based strategies to decrease demand rather than focusing solely on the supply side of the equation (Yach & Bettcher 2000). It is designed to act as a global complement to, not a replacement for, national and local tobacco control programmes and activities.

This case study explores the economic and public health evidence that provides the foundation for the WHO FCTC, demonstrates how the provisions of the Convention promote evidence-based interventions that have been proven to effectively reduce the demand for tobacco, and finally discusses how the WHO FCTC is an intermediate GPG for health.

The globalization of the tobacco epidemic

The WHO FCTC was developed in response to the ongoing globalization of the tobacco epidemic, which was amplified by a variety of complex factors with cross-border effects, including trade liberalization, foreign direct investment, global marketing, transnational tobacco advertising, promotion and sponsorship, and the international movement of contraband and counterfeit cigarettes. To strengthen and coordinate global responses to the tobacco epidemic, the World Health Assembly adopted, on 24 May 1999, a resolution to pave the way for accelerated multilateral negotiations on a framework convention on tobacco control and possible related protocols. This represented the first time that WHO Member States had exercised their treaty-making powers under Article 19 of the WHO Constitution (WHO 2007a).

Tobacco use is the second leading cause of death worldwide (WHO 2002c). Annually, 5.4 million people die prematurely from tobacco-related disease and it is expected that the developing countries' share of total tobacco-related deaths will reach 84 per cent in 2030 (Mathers & Loncar 2006). Indeed, while the number of tobacco consumers in developed countries is now quite stable (and even decreasing in a few countries), it has been rapidly increasing in developing countries. As a result, 84 per cent of tobacco users are in developing countries and this share is expected to reach 88 per cent by 2025, even if we assume a decrease of 1per cent in prevalence annually (Guindon & Boisclair 2003). The consequences will be dramatic: By 2030, the number of deaths per year attributable to tobacco globally will be 8.3 million (Mathers & Loncar 2006).

Besides the harm that tobacco causes its users, it is now well established that second-hand smoke also considerably increases the risk of contracting tobacco-related illnesses, both for adults and children. The health consequences for them can be dramatic and immediate. Finally, a well-known impact of tobacco use on others is the effects it can have on unborn babies, particularly when mothers smoke or are exposed to second-hand smoke.

Economic consequences of the tobacco epidemic

In recent years, the adverse impact of tobacco consumption on economic development has been confirmed by an increasing number of studies. The European Commission has stated that it 'clearly recognizes the importance of tobacco control as a development issue' (European Commission 2003).

There are a number of ways in which tobacco consumption can have negative economic impact. National revenue is directly reduced because tobacco kills about a quarter of its consumers in their middle age, depriving families of essential financial resources. This in turn reduces the level of education and health which are 'critical input[s] into poverty reduction, economic growth, and long-term economic development at the scale of whole societies' (WHO 2001). The fact that purchasing tobacco products requires a greater proportion of income the poorer a consumer is also detracts from the basic needs of families with tobacco users. For instance, it is estimated that, in Bangladesh, 'over 350 young children per day could be saved from death by malnutrition, if their parents redirected some of their tobacco money to food' (Efroymson *et al.* 2001).

The healthcare costs attributable to smoking are particularly high in developed countries and are increasing in developing countries. When these costs are borne by the government, they decrease the ability of the government to provide other services and the kinds of infrastructure that are essential for economic growth. When borne by individuals, these costs represent a heavy financial burden on the smokers and their families.

Another crucial economic issue related to tobacco use is the effect that it can have on employment. The tobacco industry has abundantly used the argument that tobacco growing and manufacturing provide jobs in communities and are therefore important for many economies. However, this argument is misleading. First, in high-income countries, tobacco manufacturing is highly capital intensive and provides for only a very few jobs (World Bank 1999). In these countries, if tobacco consumption were to decrease, the money previously spent on tobacco products would shift to other, probably more labour intensive goods, thereby creating more jobs. In low- and middle-income countries, while the tobacco industry employs a large number of people, these jobs often represent a 'poverty trap' for an important proportion of those employed. The *bidi* factories in India and Bangladesh, for example, employ mostly women and children, many of whom work 11–16 h per day, without enough pay to cover their basic needs (Blanchet 2002; Raghavan 2002). The employment of children by the tobacco industry prevents them from receiving a proper education, as well as putting them at risk for the severe health problems associated with tobacco cultivation, including 'green tobacco sickness' and pesticide exposure (Blanchet 2002; Raghavan 2002). Additionally, imported raw tobacco, heavy dependence on government subsidies, trade barriers, and prohibitive loans that reinforce the global tobacco oligopsony all make tobacco farming unprofitable for farmers and governments (World Bank 1999).

Finally, international tobacco smuggling presents both serious public health and economic problems. As documented in the World Bank Report *Curbing the Epidemic*, it is estimated that some 30 per cent of internationally traded cigarettes, which amounts to about 355 billion pieces, are lost to smuggling each year (World Bank 1999). Tobacco smuggling undermines the legal tobacco market, thereby needlessly causing governments to lose substantial tax revenue. Moreover, young people, who are most sensitive to the prices of tobacco products (World Bank 1999), are most at risk from smuggled cigarettes, which often are sold more cheaply than legal cigarettes and often do not contain the legally mandated product warnings and information that legal cigarettes do.

Demand-side measures: Evidence-based interventions to reduce tobacco use

It has been clearly demonstrated that cost-effective demand reduction interventions for tobacco use can be useful in reducing tobacco consumption in both developing and developed country settings (World Bank 1999; WHO 2002). The WHO FCTC incorporates evidence-based provisions that reaffirm the right of all people to the highest standard of health. The Convention's objective provides a solid foundation for the treaty to reduce the public health and economic damage inflicted on individuals, communities, and countries by tobacco use.

This section maps out the evidence-based interventions that have been proven to reduce tobacco consumption and outlines the main provision of the WHO FCTC that correspond to these interventions; the WHO FCTC provides a global roadmap for comprehensive tobacco control.

Price measures

Price and tax measures are an important and effective means of reducing tobacco consumption, especially among young people (World Bank 1999)—a fact specifically recognized in the WHO FCTC in Article 6. Many countries have experienced important reductions in tobacco consumption after having increased their tax level. South Africa increased its taxes on tobacco, making the price of cigarettes go up by nearly 85 per cent between 1993 and 1999 and its estimated smoking prevalence decreased by 14.4 per cent (Van Walbeek 2002). Generally, it is estimated that a 10 per cent increase in the price of cigarettes will reduce consumption by approximately 4 per cent in a high-income country and by approximately 8 per cent in a low- or middle-income country (World Bank 1999). Furthermore, it has been shown that tax increases have a stronger impact on young people, which is particularly important, as the risk of lung cancer increases exponentially with the duration of smoking. Lastly, increases in tobacco taxes increase government revenue.

Non-price measures

Protection from exposure to tobacco smoke. Article 8 of the WHO FCTC requires Parties to provide 'for protection from exposure to tobacco smoke in indoor workplaces, public transport, indoor public places and, as appropriate, other places' (WHO 2003c). Where a Party lacks legal jurisdiction to do this at the national level, it is to 'actively promote' equivalent measures at the subnational level. For the United States, where the workplace is covered by this provision, it is estimated that consumption was reduced 4 to 10 per cent when these kinds of restrictions were implemented (World Bank 1999). Recognizing the importance of protection from tobacco smoke, the second session of the Conference of the Parties to the WHO FCTC (the governing body for the Convention) adopted guidelines for the implementation of Article 8 that include a ban on smoking in public and work places.

Packaging and labeling of tobacco products. When warning labels contain large, graphic, thought provoking, and factual information, they are effective in deterring tobacco use. This is recognized in Article 11 of the WHO FCTC, which contains obligations for Parties to appropriately label packages of tobacco products.

Tobacco product label warnings are unique in prevention because the consumer receives the warning at the time of use. When new and graphic cigarette labels were introduced in Canada in 2000, 41.2 per cent of those surveyed in one study had intentions to quit smoking within 6 months (Hammond 2003). In Poland, new warning labels occupying 30 per cent of the largest sides of cigarette packs greatly influenced smokers' decisions to halt or reduce their smoking (World Bank 1999).

Communication, media, and dissemination of scientific information. In the area of education, communication, training, and public awareness, addressed in Article 12 of the WHO FCTC, Parties are required to adopt legislative, executive, administrative, or other measures that promote public awareness and access to information on the dangers of tobacco.

As more people become educated regarding the effects of tobacco, fewer choose to use it. In the United States, tobacco consumption declined 30 per cent from the 1930s to the end of the 1970s (World Bank 1999), a period during which there were three tobacco information shocks, including the groundbreaking tobacco control report issued by the Surgeon General in 1964 (United States 1964). In areas where funds are limited, including developing countries, an inexpensive method that has been used to achieve similar information shocks is to record smoking behaviour on individuals' death certificates and then publicly disseminate the resulting data.

The use of counter-advertising in various media has channeled negative images of smoking to the public. A study conducted between 1954 and 1981 in Switzerland revealed that counter-advertising in the media dramatically reduced smoking by 11 per cent (World Bank 1999). Finland and Turkey have had similar success with anti-smoking campaigns.

Tobacco advertising, promotion, and sponsorship. Bans on cigarette promotion can also reduce smoking. A comparison of 100 countries, some with complete bans on advertising and others with no such bans, showed that countries that banned advertisements had a significant decrease in consumption (World Bank 1999).

Article 13 of the WHO FCTC requires each Party to undertake comprehensive bans of all tobacco advertising, promotion, and sponsorship, as far as constitutionally possible for each Party. This is a centrepiece of an evidence-based approach for reducing the demand for tobacco products. Parties whose constitution or constitutional principles do not allow them to undertake a comprehensive ban must apply a series of restrictions on all advertising, promotion, and sponsorship of tobacco products.

Cessation interventions

Cessation interventions include individual training, hospital treatment, counselling, and numerous pharmacological products known as nicotine replacement therapy (NRT) that have the benefit of being self-administered. Patches, gums, sprays, and inhalators are types of NRT that deliver small doses of nicotine free of harmful tobacco smoke. They are considered safe and effective and have been shown to help double the success rate of other cessation efforts (World Bank 1999). Models based on data from the United States suggest that if NRT were made available over the counter, rather than just by prescription, significantly more people would quit smoking (World Bank 1999). Furthermore, there is evidence that smokers want this type of help: In the United States, sales of NRT products increased by 150 per cent between 1996 and 1998 (World Bank 1999). The roles of policy-makers, health professionals, researchers, and the international community are important in the cessation movement (WHO 2003a).

In the area of cessation, Article 14 of the WHO FCTC requires Parties to endeavour to:

- Create cessation programmes, not only in healthcare facilities, but also in workplaces, educational institutions, and other settings
- Include diagnosis and treatment of nicotine dependence in national health programmes
- Establish programmes for diagnosis, counselling, and treatment in healthcare facilities and rehabilitation centres
- Collaborate with other Parties to the Convention to increase the availability of cessation therapies, including pharmaceutical products

Supply side measures: Elimination of illicit trade in tobacco products

The World Bank has concluded that the only supply side measure that leads to effective demand reduction is the elimination of illicit trade (World Bank 1999). The causes of illicit trade in tobacco products are multi-factorial, requiring concerted multilateral action by all countries. Contrary to assertions by tobacco companies that price differentials between countries are the only significant cause of illicit trade, World Bank research has also identified corruption as an equally important cause of illicit trade in tobacco (World Bank 1999).

The WHO FCTC in Article 15 recognizes that the elimination of smuggling and all forms of illicit trade in tobacco products is an essential component of tobacco control. Moreover, the WHO FCTC includes a detailed provision on the illicit trade in tobacco products which incorporates provisions on tracking and tracing of such products. At the second session of the Conference of the Parties to the WHO FCTC, the Parties recognized that the elimination of smuggling and counterfeiting is an essential component of global tobacco control and, as such, it established a subsidiary body to negotiate the Convention's first protocol, which will address illicit trade in tobacco products.

Comprehensive multisectoral intervention

The best results in the reduction of tobacco use within a country are achieved when several interventions are combined. India experienced success with this approach, as noted by the tobacco industry and reflected in a report in the Tobacco Journal International, a tobacco industry publication. The report states that India's tobacco industry suffered a 4 per cent decline during the 1999–2000 period, due to excise duty on cigarettes, smoke-free workplaces, bans on tobacco sales at railway stations, and cigarette advertising bans (Tobacco Journal International 2000). In this regard, the WHO FCTC in one of its core guiding principles acknowledges that 'comprehensive multisectoral measures and responses to reduce consumption of all tobacco products at the national, regional and international levels are essential' (WHO 2003c).

Impact of WHO FCTC

All of the WHO FCTC's methods have already proven their impact over time. The most obvious of these impacts have been in the economic and public health areas, but ground has been gained on the political and multisectoral fronts as well.

Empirically, increasing the price of tobacco products is the primary method of curbing consumption. The potency of this measure is clear in economic terms: A 33 per cent increase in the price of tobacco would yield a cost-effectiveness ratio of US$3 to US$42 for every disability adjusted life year (DALY) averted in low- and middle-income countries, and US$85 to US$1773 for every DALY averted in high-income countries (Jamison *et al.* 2006). Levels of taxation currently avert about 15 million DALYs annually; further increases can avert even more DALYs (Shibuya *et al.* 2003). An averted DALY has sizable financial implications, with less public and private expenditure on healthcare for tobacco-attributed illnesses. And contrary to critics' fears, taxation on tobacco products actually raises government revenues because consumption usually falls at a slower rate than price increases (Frank *et al.* 2000).

These financial gains are linked with public health and broader economic gains. A healthy and long-living workforce, with incentives to invest in human capital, has positive implications for long-term development. Increasing tobacco prices by 70 per cent could avert 10–26 per cent of all smoking-related deaths globally, an outcome that would particularly affect low- and middle-income countries, young people, and men (Jamison *et al.* 2006). But tax increases can be more effective if implemented with other measures—in developed countries, the demand is price-inelastic, and additional methods, such as comprehensive bans on tobacco advertising, bans of smoking in public and work places, and strong counter-marketing measures must be utilized (Shibuya *et al.* 2003). Non-price methods, such as nicotine replacement therapies, can be more expensive than raising cigarette prices, but are still cost effective, if also 'extremely sensitive to context'—where public health messages are readily absorbed, such costs could be low (Jamison *et al.* 2006). Promoting cessation among current smokers will have its impact during the next 50 years, and prevention efforts will have their impact afterwards (Jamison *et al.* 2006).

Less apparent than the economic and health impact of the WHO FCTC's methods is its political and multisectoral impact. Cooperation and political resolve have become essential as more sectors become involved with the battle against the tobacco epidemic. There is a growing awareness of the effectiveness of the multisectoral approach's synergistic core; as Dr Margaret Chan, Director-General of WHO, stated: 'multiple sectors influence health, and should pay attention to the health impact of their policies' (Chan 2007). Each of the WHO FCTC's measures enhances the efficacy of the others—thus the whole of the WHO FCTC is greater than the sum of its parts.

The WHO FCTC provides the context for a substantial scale up of WHO's efforts at country-level to reduce the non-communicable burden of disease by implementing a core package of cost-effective, demand reduction measures. The treaty itself has catalysed Organizational and national programmatic movement to address the effects of non-communicable disease and its determinants.

The WHO FCTC as an intermediate global public good for health

The WHO FCTC and the process of negotiating the WHO FCTC both have important intermediate GPG characteristics. The Convention and its negotiation are intermediate GPGs in that both have facilitated the development of tobacco control policies globally (Taylor *et al.* 2003). Having entered into force, the WHO FCTC provides a mechanism to respond to the GPG aspects of tobacco control. The WHO FCTC will facilitate the flow of information about tobacco control and serve as a mechanism to coordinate various transnational aspects of tobacco control, including smuggling, advertising, packaging, and labelling. It will enhance global surveillance, information exchange, and international technical, legal, and financial cooperation in support of the GPGs of tobacco control. Even now, the WHO FCTC process continues to provide a global instrument for public health professionals to distribute their evidence to governments and to get this evidence incorporated into binding agreements (Wipfli *et al.* 2002), including future protocols to the Convention.

Conclusion

The strength of the WHO FCTC resides primarily in three elements. First, it is an evidence-based treaty. All the tobacco control measures required by the WHO FCTC have been proven to be effective and are based on numerous experiences and facts. Second, it is a comprehensive tool that addresses all the effective tobacco control policies that can be implemented to reduce tobacco consumption; its effect will exceed the sum of the results of each measure taken separately because some measures increase the effectiveness of others. Third, the global aspect of the convention will enhance its effectiveness far beyond action implemented at the national or even regional level. The burden of disease induced by the tobacco epidemic is huge and increasing. The number of smokers in the world is estimated to be about 1.3 billion and it is expected that, if the current trend continues, this number will increase to 1.7 billion in 2025 (WHO 2003a; Guindon & Boisclair 2003). Half of these people will eventually die from tobacco-related illnesses.

It has been estimated that reduction of consumption and initiation of tobacco use by 50 per cent by 2050 has the potential to avert up to 200 000 000 deaths from tobacco use (Peto & Lopez 2000). As a powerful intermediate GPG designed to reduce tobacco consumption, the WHO FCTC will significantly decrease this burden, which will in turn lead to improved overall health and economic conditions.

Case study: The international health regulations

While the WHO FCTC was the WHO Member States' first exercise of the WHO Constitutional powers to adopt conventions or agreements within the purview of the Organization's mandate, the power to adopt regulations found in Article 21 of the WHO Constitution was tapped into decades ago, in response to the threat of infectious disease. The result was the International Health Regulations (IHR), legally binding regulations adopted by most countries to contain the threats from diseases that may rapidly spread from one country to another (WHO 2007b). The current IHR are designed to address not only emerging infectious diseases like SARS, but also those cross-border threats that arise as a result of public health risks and emergencies like chemical spills or waste that has been dumped.

The version of the IHR that was in place through the end of the twentieth century, the 1969 IHR, included only three diseases: Cholera, plague, and yellow fever. The measures were oriented to border control and the notification and control measures were relatively passive, reflecting a strong sense of independent, domestically oriented disease control. When the WHO Member States called for a revision of the 1969 IHR, it was based on the need for stronger, more collaborative measures to adequately respond to the globalized nature of infectious disease. Its revision in 2005 demonstrates a global commitment to contain public health risks and emergencies at the source, not only at national borders. The revised IHR, the 2005 IHR, was adopted by the World Health Assembly in May 2005, and came into force, generally, on 15 June 2007.

The compelling question of whether or not the IHR constitutes an intermediate GPG for health was addressed by Giesecke prior to the 2005 adoption by the World Health Assembly of the 2005 IHR (Giesecke 2003). Giesecke accurately projected what a revised IHR would need to contain to be considered an intermediate GPG for health. Indeed, his vision of the revised IHR as an intermediate GPG for epidemic control mirrors, to a great extent, what was ultimately adopted by the 192 WHO Member States at the close of the decade-long process of revising the 1969 IHR.

This case study describes the relevant new provisions in the Regulations and seeks, in part, to illustrate how the 2005 IHR, or aspects thereof, may be considered an intermediate GPG for health.

Strengthening of the IHR through increased roles and responsibilities for WHO and Parties

The 2005 IHR increased the rights and obligations of WHO and Parties both substantially and substantively. This expansion of roles is analysed below in the context of the Regulations as an intermediate GPG for health.

New mandates for WHO

Five key changes to the 1969 IHR found a place in the final text of the 2005 IHR. These changes strengthen WHO's role and contribute to establishing the Regulations as an effective tool to attain the ultimate GPG for epidemic control. These include (1) use of other information sources by WHO; (2) informal and confidential notification to WHO; (3) a wider remit (scope); (4) guaranteed assistance by WHO to control outbreaks; and (5) a rapid, transparent decision mechanism to make recommendations on any necessary health measures.

The use of information from sources other than official governmental notifications or consultations and provisional confidentiality of notified information. For the past decade, WHO's alert and response operations team has been using information from non-official sources to detect public health events of international importance and to conduct timely risk assessment with countries. With the advent of the 2005 IHR this mechanism has been further refined and formalized. Article 9.1 of the 2005 IHR firmly establishes WHO's mandate to 'take into account reports from sources other than notifications and consultations' with the proviso that these reports must be assessed on the basis of sound epidemiological principles and communicated to the country where the event is occurring (WHO 2005). Before taking action on these reports, WHO is required to seek verification thereof from the Party in which the event is allegedly occurring (WHO 2005).

Consultation. WHO is no stranger to consultations with its Member States' public health officials and has engaged in countless discussions on public health events of national and potentially international concern with key personnel in ministries of health. Article 8 of the 2005 IHR provides a legal framework for this consultation process, including consultation under circumstances where the information available may be insufficient to perform the assessment required for notification to the Organization. Critically, the information communicated to WHO under this provision is subject to the provisional restrictions placed on its dissemination to other Parties as set out in Article 11 of the 2005 IHR. According to the text of Article 11, WHO must, as a general matter, consult with the Party in whose territory the event is occurring as to its intent to make this information available to other States.

A broader purpose and scope. As has been discussed earlier, the purpose and scope of the 2005 IHR are far broader than those of the 1969 IHR, which was limited to Parties being required to notify WHO only when one of three diseases (cholera, plague, and yellow fever) became apparent in their jurisdictions. By contrast, one of the cornerstones of the 2005 IHR is notification to WHO of public health events on the basis of contextual criteria without restriction to a limited list of diseases. While not intended to detract from this broad language, for a number of political and policy reasons, WHO Member States were in favour of including a short list of diseases for mandatory notification, although the value of including a list of notifiable diseases in the Regulations is debatable.

WHO support to States Parties in their response to public health risks and emergencies of international concern. The Organization has been supporting countries in their response to national and international public health emergencies for many years, including through the Global Outbreak Alert and Response Network, managed by the WHO alert and response operations group. The 2005 IHR further institutionalizes and harmonizes these processes for both Parties and WHO. Articles 10 (Verification) and 13 (Public health response) of the 2005 IHR carve out a specific role for WHO in terms of when and how the Organization is required to support Parties. The verification procedure established in Article 10 requires that WHO, when it receives information of an event that may constitute a public health emergency of international concern (PHEIC), offers to collaborate with the Party concerned to assess the potential for international disease spread, possible interference with international traffic, and the adequacy of control measures. Although a Party is not necessarily obliged to accept such an offer, a refusal on its part does not prevent WHO from sharing available public health information with other Parties should this be warranted by the 'magnitude of the public health risk' involved, while taking into account the views of the Party (World Health Organization 2005). With regard to public health response, in Article 13 WHO is required generally to collaborate with Parties 'in the response to public health risks and other events by providing technical guidance and assistance and by assessing the effectiveness of the control measures in place, including the mobilization of international teams of experts for on-site assistance, when necessary' (World Health Organization 2005).

A transparent decision-making process within WHO. A number of countries raised concerns regarding the decision-making procedure at WHO during the 2003 SARS crisis, which in turn had a profound impact on the IHR negotiations in 2004 and 2005. Indeed, World Health Assembly resolution WHA56.28 expressly requested the Director-General of WHO 'to take into account evidence, experiences, knowledge and lessons acquired during the SARS response when revising the International Health Regulations' (WHO 2003b). This request was accommodated in the 2005 IHR, which, for example, establishes a specific procedure for the *determination* of a PHEIC by the Director-General and the issuance of any corresponding health measures (WHO 2005). Although it remains the duty of the Director-General to determine whether a particular public health event constitutes a PHEIC, s/he is required to first seek the view of an Emergency Committee of relevant independent experts before informing other countries of his/her decision, unless the affected Party agrees with the determination. With regard to the adoption of specific control measures following such a determination, the Director-General must invariably take into account the views of the Committee. It should be noted that the views of the Committee are not binding on the Director-General, who may decide to reject them.

New rights and obligations for States Parties

With regard to Parties' obligations, the need to strengthen national surveillance was central to creating a successful IHR. From the perspective of promoting a GPG for health, epidemiology training and capacity building, including improved communications and laboratory facilities, are prerequisite to the successful control of epidemics. Annex 1A of the 2005 IHR establishes a set of minimum core public health capacities for surveillance and response that all Parties to the Regulations must meet within a pre-defined time period set out in Articles 5 (Surveillance) and 13 (Public health response). These new provisions stipulate that each Party 'shall develop, strengthen and maintain, as soon as possible, but no later than five years from the entry into force of these Regulations, the capacity:

(1) To detect, assess, notify and report events

(2) To respond promptly and effectively to public health risks and public health emergencies of international concern

It should be noted that this 5-year period may be extended 'on the basis of a justified need and an implementation plan' for an additional 2-year period. Finally, on an exceptional basis, the Director-General may grant a Party an additional 2-year extension to meet its obligations under Articles 5 and 13 of the 2005 IHR. The Director-General's decision, however, is contingent on first consulting the Review Committee.

The 2005 IHR as an intermediate global public good for health

The concept of public goods and what make them global have been defined and discussed elsewhere in this chapter and will, therefore, be dealt with only briefly here. Relevant to the examination of the IHR, disease control at the national level through the adoption of regulatory measures can be seen as a public good for health. That is, such a public good is non-excludable because it benefits those who are not even aware that there is a risk (of disease) and non-rivalrous due to the fact that one person benefiting from disease control does not prevent another from also benefiting. With regard to the global nature of the public good of infectious disease control it is clearly the intent of the 2005 IHR to be a transboundary, globally inclusive instrument. Article 3 (Principles) of the 2005 IHR provides that the implementation of the new rules 'shall be guided by the goal of their universal application for the protection of all people of the world from the international spread of disease' (WHO 2005).

In terms of the IHR as an intermediate GPG for health, the freedom from epidemics (or epidemic control) is a final GPG for health, while the surveillance and control mechanisms required to attain this goal are an intermediate GPG for health. A functioning IHR provide the set of rules that establish administrative and legislative structures in support of these intermediate GPGs for health. Therefore, inasmuch as they deal with epidemic control, the 2005 IHR may constitute an intermediate GPG for health. The conditional is employed here because, as the Regulations entered into force only on 7 August 2007 for all WHO Member States that adopted them in May 2005, it is too early to tell what the level of compliance with the new rules will be and whether the 2005 IHR are being successfully implemented. Indeed, for the fate of the 2005 IHR to be different than that of the 1969 Regulations, which had become largely ineffective, full implementation and respect for its provisions are pre-requisite to play this enabling role as an intermediate GPG for health. The ineffectiveness of the 1969 IHR resulted, in part, from their scope being limited to three diseases; the failure by WHO Member States to notify WHO of outbreaks in a timely fashion, in accordance with the Regulations; and the application by Member States of excessive measures affecting traffic and trade.

Although it is premature to assess the extent to which the 2005 IHR will be an effective tool to curb epidemics, it is clear that its purpose and scope make it a firm candidate as an intermediate GPG for health. This is shown by the broad scope of the IHR as set out in Article 2 of the Regulations which provides that:

> *The purpose and scope of these Regulations are to prevent, protect against, control and provide a public health response to the international spread of* disease *in ways that are commensurate with and restricted to* public health risks, *and which avoid unnecessary interference with international traffic and trade.* (emphasis added) (WHO 2005)

The scope is further delineated through the definitions of key terms such as PHEIC, disease, international traffic, and public health risk. Given the far-reaching scope of the 2005 IHR and, with 194 Parties and its quasi-universal geographical coverage, it could easily be argued that the 2005 IHR has the potential to become an intermediate GPG for health, as described above. Although the scope of the proposed revised Regulations was somewhat controversial during the revision negotiations in 2004 and 2005 (Plotkin *et al.* 2007), and the text itself is not explicit on this point, the coverage of the 2005 IHR is considered broad enough to encompass relevant public health risks involving biological, chemical, or radiological agents (WHO 2007), including those that are naturally occurring, accidental, or intentional in nature (Fidler & Gostin 2006). It is also important to highlight that, as was the case with the 1969 version of the Regulations, the 2005 IHR is designed to contain the international spread of disease while at the same time ensuring that the international movement of people and goods is not unnecessarily restricted. This nexus between public health and international traffic, as well as between the law of infectious disease and trade law, is an important and defining aspect of the Regulations, both today and historically.

Conclusion

The 2005 IHR clearly has the potential to become an intermediate GPG for health, as discussed in this case study. Their purpose of preventing and protecting against the international spread of disease, including epidemic control, while avoiding unnecessary interference with world traffic, falls squarely within the definition of a public good. Moreover, the global nature of this public good is clear, given the Regulations' textual intent of universal application. Whether or not the 2005 IHR actually plays this enabling role as an intermediate GPG for health, however, will largely depend on its effective implementation. The most important challenge is, therefore, to create incentives for States Parties to comply with the 2005 IHR (Aginam 2005) and rally support for their implementation. This will require substantial human and financial resources and a strong commitment from a broad array of partners and stakeholders, including the donor community. Without this, the 2005 IHR role as an intermediate GPG for health will remain purely aspirational. Every effort must be made to ensure that governments and international organizations, including WHO, prioritize their effective implementation.

Case study: Food safety—the Codex Alimentarius Commission (CAC) and the International Food Safety Authorities Network (INFOSAN)

Food safety and food control have been recognized as important issues in many countries for decades. Many major initiatives both in safe food production and in control philosophy have contributed to systems perceived by many to be efficient in the prevention of foodborne disease in most developed countries. The recent outbreaks of foodborne disease have, however, shaken the consumers' trust in these food safety systems. BSE, dioxin, *Escherichia coli* O157, *Salmonella*—all foodborne hazards that were virtually unknown 10–15 years ago are now household names in most families.

Many countries now realize that foodborne disease continues to be a major public health issue. Foodborne diseases are some of the most widespread health problems in the world and they have implications on both the health of individuals and the development of societies. Deeply concerned by this, the Fifty-third World Health Assembly adopted a resolution in May 2000 calling upon WHO and its Member States to recognize food safety as an essential public health function (WHO 2000). The resolution also called for the development of systems to enable a reduction of the burden of foodborne disease.

One of the primary multilateral responses to the need for food safety management is the Codex Alimentarius Commission (CAC), an intergovernmental body operated under the auspices of the Food and Agriculture Organization of the United Nations (FAO) and WHO. The objective of the CAC is to protect the health of consumers and to ensure fair practices in the food trade, while promoting coordination of all food standards work undertaken by intergovernmental and non-governmental organizations (FAO and WHO 2007). The international food standards and related texts adopted by CAC constitute the *Codex Alimentarius*. All food standards and related texts in the Codex Alimentarius are of voluntary nature and may become binding only when they are converted into national legislation or regulation. The membership of CAC is open to all member nations and associate member nations of FAO and WHO, and currently covers more than 99 per cent of the world population. To complement the CAC standard setting, and in response to two World Health Assembly resolutions and a CAC request (CAC 2004), WHO established a list of primary official contact points in each of its Member States for the exchange of information in food safety emergency situations. This network, the International Food Safety Authorities Network (INFOSAN), also provides tools and support to increase Member State capacity to develop their national food safety systems and respond to health emergencies posed by natural, accidental, and intentional contamination of food.

This case study examines the global burden of foodborne disease and provides overviews of CAC and INFOSAN, the most salient international responses to food safety concerns. As part of the review of these mechanisms, the question of CAC and INFOSAN providing intermediate GPGs for health is considered.

Foodborne disease burden

It is estimated that up to 2 million people die each year from diarrhoeal diseases, mostly attributed to contaminated food and drinking water. Studies estimate that each year in the United States, foodborne diseases result in 76 million illnesses, 325 000 hospitalizations, and 5000 deaths (Mead *et al.* 1999). It is estimated that foodborne diseases in the United States caused by *Campylobacter*, *Salmonella*, *E. coli O157*, and *Listeria monocytogenes* cost almost US$7 billion annually.

Extrapolations such as this one from the United States, are scarce at the global level. In addition, data collected through surveillance systems for foodborne disease do not provide the real incidence of such diseases. Available data often pertain mostly to outbreaks, which are only the tip of the iceberg. Data on sporadic diarrhoeal illness (of which most are caused by food) is largely obtained through passive surveillance systems whose quality varies greatly between countries and diseases. For example, underreporting of *Salmonella* diarrhoea, including both sporadic and outbreak cases, differs from country to country and has recently been estimated at from 3.2 to 3.9 per cent in the United Kingdom (Adak *et al.* 2002; Wheeler *et al.* 1999) to 38 per cent in the United States (Mead *et al.* 1999). No information on under notification of diarrhoea is presently available for developing countries, but it could be assumed the underreporting is even more prevalent and therefore more important in areas with poorer general health coverage.

The additional contribution of foodborne disease to the vicious circle of malnutrition and diarrhoea should not be forgotten. The FAO estimates that malnutrition affects about 800 million people. Malnutrition increases host susceptibility to foodborne infections through a number of mechanisms. Diarrhoea caused by *E. coli*, which is probably the most important cause of children's diarrhoea in developing countries, has a longer duration and a greater potential for long-term nutritional consequences in malnourished children. In general malnutrition can result in a 30-fold increase in the risk for diarrhoea-associated death (Morris & Potter 1997).

It is important to reiterate that diarrhoeal diseases only constitute a fraction of disease caused by food. Microorganisms transmitted through food can cause many other types of disease, including very serious long-term infections. Even more important, the disease burden caused by chemical hazards in food is largely unknown, with estimation of a very serious fraction of all cancers caused by such hazards. Therefore, it is generally recognized that determinations of the impact of foodborne disease have always relied heavily on estimates and assumptions. We do not have the full picture yet.

Foodborne diseases not only significantly affect people's health and well-being; they also have economic consequences for individuals, families, communities, businesses and countries. These diseases impose a substantial burden on healthcare systems and markedly reduce economic productivity. The loss of income due to foodborne disease perpetuates the cycle of poverty. Estimating direct as well as indirect costs of foodborne disease is difficult. An estimate in the United States places the medical costs and productivity losses in a population of approximately 250 million in the range of US$6.6–37.1 billion (Butzby & Roberts 1997).

Global food trade is increasing with feed, food ingredients, partially processed food, and final food products being bought and sold around the world. Food is also sent abroad for processing and then returned to the country of origin for sale. According to FAO trade statistics, the value of trade in agricultural products was estimated at US$552 billion in 2005. International travel also represents a significant source of foodborne disease for some countries. For example, in 2005, Sweden reported that 80.2 per cent and The Netherlands reported 87 per cent of their salmonellosis cases acquired their infection while overseas (EFSA 2007).

Thus, it has become imperative to address the matters related to food safety at the international level—to complement and assist in the actions taken by national governments that carry the primary responsibility to ensure food safety for their population.

The Codex Alimentarius Commission (CAC)

Legal basis and organizational structure

The CAC was established as a joint commission on the basis of Article VI.1 of the FAO Constitution (FAO 1961) and under Article 18 of the WHO Constitution (WHO 1963), as the executive organ of the Joint FAO/WHO Food Standards Programme. CAC enjoys certain autonomy on procedural and programmatic matters, whereas the strategic direction of the Joint Programme is laid out by the Member States in the respective governing bodies of the two parent organizations. The highest governing body of Codex Alimentarius is the CAC. It meets annually in Rome and in Geneva on an alternate basis. The CAC is assisted by an Executive Committee. The Secretary of the CAC is jointly appointed by the Directors-General of FAO and WHO from the staffs of these organizations.

The preparatory work of the Codex Alimentarius (i.e. development of draft international standards and related texts), is undertaken by the subsidiary bodies of CAC—Codex committees and task forces. They are classified into two categories. The general subject committees address horizontal aspects of food standards (additives, contaminants, labelling, methods of analysis, and sampling, etc.); the commodity committees address specific groups of commodities (fish and fishery products, milk and milk products, etc.).

The provision of scientific advice, based on risk analysis principles, by FAO and WHO to Codex and to member states, occurs through expert committees, such as: Joint FAO/WHO Expert Committee on Food Additives (JECFA), Joint FAO/WHO Meetings on Pesticide Residues (JMPR), and Joint FAO/WHO Expert Meetings on Microbiological Risk Assessment (JEMRA).

Operations and procedure

The operation of the CAC system is guided by the Rules of Procedure, adopted by CAC and endorsed by the Directors-General of FAO and WHO. The process of elaboration and adoption of international standards and related texts follows a procedure consisting of eight steps:

Step 1: A proposal for new work is reviewed and a decision on whether or not to undertake new work is taken by the Commission.

Steps 2–4: A draft text is prepared and circulated to governments and all interested parties for comment, followed by review by the relevant Committee.

Step 5: The Commission reviews the progress made and agrees that the draft should go to finalization.

Steps 6 and 7: The approved draft is sent again to governments and interested parties for comment and is finalized by the relevant Committee.

Step 8: Following a final round of comments, the Commission adopts the draft as a formal Codex text.

An accelerated procedure whereby the elaboration of a text is concluded by adoption at Step 5 can be used, thereby skipping steps six through eight.

International importance

The Codex Alimentarius has become the global reference point for consumers, food producers and processors, national food control agencies, and the international food trade. The status of Codex Alimentarius standards recognized in the World Trade Organization's (WTO) Agreement on the Application of Sanitary and Phytosanitary Measures (WTO/SPS Agreement) and the Agreement on Technical Barriers to Trade (WTO/TBT Agreement) both encourage the international harmonization of food standards. As a result, Codex Alimentarius standards have become the benchmarks against which national food measures and regulations are evaluated within the legal parameters of the WTO Agreements.

In particular, the SPS Agreement specifically designates Codex Alimentarius standards, guidelines, and recommendations as the international standards in food safety, with which WTO members are encouraged to harmonize their sanitary measures. The SPS Agreement acknowledges that governments have the right to take sanitary measures necessary for the protection of human health. WTO members applying measures that are more stringent than Codex standards are allowed to do so but are required to provide scientific justification for those measures.

The International Food Safety Authorities Network (INFOSAN)

In collaboration with FAO, WHO initiated INFOSAN in 2004. The mandate to establish INFOSAN lies in two World Health Assembly Resolutions. World Health Assembly Resolution 53.15, adopted in 2000, called for improved communication among WHO and its Member States on matters of food safety (WHO 2000). World Health Assembly Resolution 55.16, adopted in 2002, expressed serious concern about natural, accidental, and intentional contamination of food that can lead to health emergencies (WHO 2002a). Member States requested that WHO provide tools and support to increase their capacity to respond to such emergencies. The INFOSAN mandate was also based on recommendations from a series of international conferences which called for a coordinated approach for the effective management of public health emergencies, including those caused by contaminated food. In 2004, the CAC requested that WHO establish a list of primary official contact points in each of its Member States for the exchange of information in food safety emergency situations.

Based on these mandates, and recognizing the continuous increase in global food trade and travel, INFOSAN was developed to share food safety information and experience, as well as to promote collaboration between food safety authorities at national and international levels. An integral part of the INFOSAN network is the rapid exchange of emergency information between such authorities relative to food safety events or emergencies. This is known as INFOSAN Emergency.

As of February 2009, INFOSAN has 172 member countries and is advised on its strategic functions by an external advisory group. To facilitate the sharing of food safety experience, INFOSAN Information Notes, describing the latest food safety knowledge, are developed 6–12 times per year. Multilateral communication is also encouraged as a means of countries learning from each others' experiences.

INFOSAN Emergency operates within the International Health Regulations (2005) (WHO 2005) and oversees all food safety related events, inclusive of food contamination and foodborne disease. On average, 200 food safety events per month are investigated to determine their public health impact, including events of unusual or unexpected natures, distribution, and possible trade restrictions. The network actively shares information about 1 or 2 such events per month deemed of international public health significance. For example, when two shigellosis outbreaks occurred in two countries both implicating baby corn from a third country, INFOSAN Emergency sought information from the exporting country. Through this process it was determined that a further three countries were at risk since they had imported the affected baby corn. INFOSAN Emergency alerted all three countries, enabling a process where these countries could determine the risk for their population and implement their own appropriate risk management options. In the baby milk powder event in China, involving the export of different products contaminated with melamine, the Chinese authorities actively used INFOSAN to communicate information on needed recalls to a number of other countries.

Membership in INFOSAN is voluntary. However, the legal obligation with regard to INFOSAN Emergency is a mix of both hard and soft law: The 2005 IHR (hard law) and the instruction to WHO to maintain a list of primary contacts from the CAC (soft law). Codex Alimentarius encourages the rapid notification of food safety events or emergencies associated with imported foods to international bodies and to the exporting country.

CAC and INFOSAN as intermediate GPGs for health

Both CAC and INFOSAN have proven capacity to improve health and health systems, the predicate for an intermediate GPG for health. The success of the CAC as the multilateral framework for global food safety is the result of the global scale and scope of over 180 commodity standards, 1112 food additives provisions, covering 292 food additives and 2930 Maximum limits for pesticide residues, covering 218 pesticides (FAO and WHO 2006). In addition, many consider Codex Alimentarius and CAC a successful United Nations initiative because of a high level of transparency ensured by the participation of a number of governmental and non-governmental observer organizations in the 8-step rule-based standards-setting process.

Contributing to the success of the Codex Alimentarius is the Codex Trust fund. The trust fund was established to provide financial support to developing countries, so that their officials can participate directly in CAC meetings. The Codex Alimentarius contributes significantly to a general public health improvement in many countries, where the expertise and food safety system necessary to obtain the most recent scientific information and knowledge of food safety advice and regulation is not available. As developing nations and regions move to comply with WTO trade and SPS obligations and monitor the impact of agri-food industry globalization and global food trade liberalization on food safety, the work of the CAC in establishing a basis for standards harmonization continues to grow in importance.

INFOSAN has demonstrated its function as an intermediate GPG for health, strengthening international as well as national food safety systems and providing a platform for the development of the GPG of health, itself. The provision of INFOSAN Information Notes provides technical support for national food regulators when considering the impact and management of evolving food safety issues. INFOSAN Emergency activities enable rapid alerts to countries about food safety events or emergencies that may impact both the health and the economy of these countries. INFOSAN also assists national governments with the necessary public health response as required.

Conclusion

The ability of national governments to regulate food safety as they simultaneously move to increase food security presents many challenges. The necessary changes in food production systems should be matched with the food safety lessons learned throughout the developments in the industrialized food producing countries. There is no need to repeat the food safety mistakes in these countries in other parts of the world. At the present time, national governments are forced to acknowledge the inability of nations to unilaterally regulate domestic food systems. When confronted with growing levels of international food trade, cross-border competition, increasing corporate and supplier power, and rapid consolidation of global agri-food markets and industries, governments increasingly engage in collective policy action at the multilateral level to protect citizens and to achieve the collective good.

The high level of foodborne disease, together with the globalization of the food trade and international travel, signify that foodborne disease is an issue of international public health concern. In recognition of this, WHO has developed, in collaboration with other United Nation and international agencies, the Codex and INFOSAN–both strong examples of intermediate GPGs for health.

Section III: International legal paradigms, enforcement, and intermediate global public goods for health

As noted earlier in this chapter, the production of GPGs for health is most effective when states create international legal instruments that contain four essential aspects:

1. The establishment of formal institutions empowered to work on global public health problems
2. The establishment of procedures through which states and non-state actors can tackle specific global public health problems
3. The enumeration of substantive duties in connection with particular global public health challenges
4. The creation of mechanisms to enforce substantive legal duties undertaken by states that have agreed to be bound by international instruments

The WHO FCTC and the 2005 IHR both integrate all four aspects, as they address institutional, procedural, substantive, and enforcement aspects of the regulation of tobacco products and disease spread, respectively. As binding instruments, these instruments are often called 'hard law'. However, as demonstrated by the non-binding Codex Alimentarius and the voluntary INFOSAN, it is not only binding multilateral legal instruments that make up the landscape of intermediate GPGs for health. Those agreements and arrangements that are non-binding, and sometimes identified as 'soft law', can play a critical role in establishing the foundations required to produce the ultimate GPG—in this case, health.

This section provides a brief review of health as a GPG in the context of international law and the spectrum of agreements between nations. The contrasts and similarities between hard and soft international law are presented and the institutional capacity, responsibility, and role of WHO in the creation of intermediate GPGs for health is examined.

Law and non-law: Binding and non-binding international instruments and GPGs for health

The ideas and characteristics of soft law and hard law, and their relationship and usefulness, are common themes among international legal scholars and practitioners. With regard to the GPG of health, a very cogent and useful set of articles on this area was presented in the Bulletin of the WHO in December 2002, a special edition focusing on international law and public health (WHO 2002b).

As exemplified by the case studies in this chapter, public health concerns are becoming increasingly complex as globalization progresses; so, too then, must and have the international responses been. In overcoming the Westphalian notion of single nation solutions, 'the complex network of global health governance structures that are emerging . . . indicates the need for an inclusive approach to engagement with new global health actors', including civil society, private actors, and public organizations (Taylor & Bettcher 2002; Taylor 2002). It is perhaps reasonable, then, to assert that the first step to producing the GPG of health is to examine the entire spectrum of stakeholders and create processes that are inclusive, to ensure that the intermediate GPG international legal instruments are as effective and efficient as possible.

Among the intermediate GPG legal instruments, traditional legal instruments—namely, treaties—provide the strongest, most effective tools for improving health (Taylor 2002), though they are commensurately difficult to negotiate because they bind parties to discrete, identifiable obligations. Although treaties have variable success in being implemented and enforced, the gestalt created by a negotiation, adoption, and entry into force can be tremendous (Taylor 2002). This certainly was the case for the WHO FCTC process, during which 'the power of the process' was often noted as one of the key ingredients to its success. In this way, not only the instrument, but also the attendant process and investment by interested entities, becomes an intermediate GPG for health.

Perhaps because of the substantial challenges inherent in successfully negotiating a treaty on a topic as multifaceted as health, non-binding instruments have become increasingly utilized as nations seek to reach agreement and move a number of multilateral agendas forward (Chopra *et al.* 2002). The force behind this is likely that non-binding agreements provide the kind of flexibility that allows nations to act cooperatively and in concert without limiting their own autonomy (Chopra *et al.* 2002). In their article, Taylor and Bettcher note, however, that the position and essential nature of non-binding instruments like resolutions and codes, sometimes called soft law and sometimes called 'non-law', remain unsettled in the rubric of international law (Taylor & Bettcher 2002). In terms of intermediate GPGs for health, non-binding arrangements like the Codex and INFOSAN certainly have demonstrated their usefulness, even in the face of not having the more robust implementation and enforcement opportunities that come with traditional international legal instruments.

Global health and global health governance is a dynamic, exciting arena with an increasingly complex landscape being painted with each new transboundary health challenge that emerges or is identified. The relationship between hard and soft law has and will continue to adapt to best respond to the needs of global communities, which will in turn look to the WHO FCTC, 2005 IHR and the Codex as models of intermediate GPGs on which to build.

WHO and institutional roles and responsibilities in the creation of intermediate GPGs for health

In a review of the nature and usefulness of international instruments for health, it would be remiss not to consider the role of WHO, as the United Nations specialized agency for health, in the creation of these intermediate GPGs for health. As the institutional umbrella home of all the instruments considered in this chapter, it plays a key and central role in fostering and providing a forum for its Member States to create agreements. Notwithstanding this, though, the question of what it can do and what it should do remain topics worth considering.

According to its Constitution, WHO is not simply an institutional home for multilateral health programmes and technical expertise; WHO is vested with substantial normative functions as well, including the Articles 19 and 21 powers to adopt conventions and regulations on matters within its competence (WHO 2007a). Though, with the exception of regulations, these powers are only 'quasi-legislative' in that Member States are not automatically bound to provisions of a given negotiated text, this is nonetheless one of the Organization's most important functions (Burci & Vignes 2004). As Taylor notes, 'WHO's leadership in coordinating codification and implementation efforts among the diverse global actors actively engaged in health lawmaking could, in theory, foster the development of a more effective, integrated and rational legal regime and, consequently, better collective management of global health concerns' (Taylor 2002). The Organization has, essentially, a bully pulpit and, if exercised with care, political acumen, and vision, there is tremendous opportunity to promote international law as a primary tool for the GPG of health.

By design of its founding Member States, WHO does not, and perhaps should not, have full legislative capacity (Burci & Vignes 2004). It does have substantial comparative advantage, though, in being the agent for actualizing international agreements on health. The Organization has the capacity to coordinate its Member States, promote dialogue, and set the global health agenda and provide a platform for negotiations (Taylor 2002), provided it maintains adequate supporting political will and consensus among its constituency (Burci & Vignes 2004; Taylor 2002). WHO is one of, if not *the*, most potent sources of intermediate GPGs for health.

Conclusion

As intermediate GPGs for health, international legal instruments take on an additional layer of importance in global health governance.

In providing a robust framework for improving and occasionally even creating health, these instruments are important not only for what they are already doing, but for the potential good new instruments might be able to deliver. As WHO continues to grow into its normative role, it is likely that additional opportunities to exercise its Constitutional quasi-legislative powers will present themselves. The three examples of intermediate GPGs examined in this chapter, the WHO FCTC, the 2005 IHR, and the Codex and INFOSAN, have laid a solid foundation on which WHO and its Member States may build to continue to work toward achieving the GPG of health.

Acknowledgement

The authors would like to acknowledge Obijiofor Aginam and Kazuaki Miyagishima for their contributions towards this chapter.

Key points

- Health is arguably a GPG: One person's good health does not detract from another's and an improvement in individual health can improve the community-level economy and social fabric. Furthermore, although the onus of providing health remains primarily on national governments, globalization means that the determinants of health, as well as the requisite means to deliver health, are increasingly global.
- Insofar as international health instruments provide an infrastructure critical for reaching GPGs, but are part of the process rather than an outcome in and of themselves, they can be considered intermediate GPGs.
- The WHO Framework Convention on Tobacco Control (WHO FCTC), with its foundations in economic and public health, promotes evidence-based interventions that have been shown to improve health by effectively reducing the demand for tobacco, is an intermediate GPG for health.
- Intended to prevent and protect against the international spread of disease, including epidemic control, while avoiding unnecessary interference with world traffic the 2005 International Health Regulations (IHR) clearly have the potential to become an intermediate GPG for health, if effectively implemented.
- Insofar as both the Codex Alimentarius and INFOSAN strengthen international as well as national food safety systems and provide a platform for the development of the GPG of health, they are also both intermediate GPGs for health.
- WHO is one of, if not *the*, most potent sources of intermediate GPGs for health; the Organization has the capacity to coordinate its Member States, promote dialogue and set the global health agenda and provide a platform for negotiations, provided it maintains adequate supporting political will and consensus among its constituency.

References

Aginam, O. (2005). *Global health governance: International law and public health in a divided world*, p. 82. University of Toronto Press, Toronto.

Adak, G.K., Long, S.M., and O'Brien, S.J. (2002). Trends in indigenous foodborne disease and deaths, England and Wales: 1992 to 2000. *Gut*, **51**, 832–41.

Beaglehole, R. and Yach, D. (2003). Globalization and the prevention and control of noncommunicable disease: The neglected chronic diseases of adults. *The Lancet*, **362**, 903–8.

Blanchet, T. (2002). Child work in the bidi industry – Bangladesh. In *Tobacco and poverty: Observations from India and Bangladesh* (ed. D. Efroymson), pp. 37–43. PATH Canada, Dhaka.

Burci, G.L. and Vignes, C-H (2004). Normative functions. In *World Health Organization*, pp.124–53. Kluwer Law International, The Hague.

Butzby, J.C. and Roberts, T. (1997). Guillain-Barré syndrome increases foodborne diseases costs. *Food Review*, **20**, 36–42.

CAC (2004) Principles and guidelines for the exchange of information in food safety emergency situations. CAC/GL 19-1995, Rev.1-2004. www.codexalimentarius.net/download/standards/36/CXG_019e.pdf

Chan, M. (2007). Speech to interns. 24 August 2007, World Health Organization, Geneva.

Da Costa e Silva, V.L. and Nikogosian, H. (2003). Convenio marco de la OMS para el control del tabaco: la globalizacion de la salud publica.[WHO Framework Convention on Tobacco Control: the globalization of public health.] *Prevencion del Tabaquismo* [Prevention of tobacco addiction], **5**, 71–5.

Dodgson, R., Lee, K., and Drager, N. (2002). Global health governance: A conceptual review *Key Issues in Global Health Governance Discussion Paper No. 1* Centre on Global Change & Health and World Health Organization, Geneva. Available from: http://whqlibdoc.who.int/publications/2002/a85727_eng.pdf

Doll, R. (1998). Uncovering the effects of smoking: historical perspective. *Statistical Methods in Medical Research*, **7**, 87–117.

Efroymson, D., Saifuddin, A., Townsend, J. *et al.* (2001). Hungry for tobacco: An analysis of the economic impact of tobacco consumption on the poor in Bangladesh. *Tobacco Control*, **10**, 212–17.

European Commission (2003). *Tobacco control in EC development policy: A background paper for the high level round table on tobacco control and development policy*, p. 2. European Commission, Brussels.

European Food Safety Authority (EFSA) (2007). *The Community Summary Report on trends and sources of zoonoses, zoonotic agents, antimicrobial resistance and foodborne outbreaks in the European Union in 2005.* EFSA, Brussels.

FAO/WHO (2006) Understanding the Codex Alimentarius. Third Edition. Rome. ftp://ftp.fao.org/codex/Publications/understanding/Understanding_EN.pdf

FAO/WHO (2007) Codex Alimentarius Commission. Procedural Manual. Seventeenth Edition, Rome. ftp://ftp.fao.org/codex/Publications/ProcManuals/Manual_17e.pdf

Fidler, D. (2002). *Global health governance: Overview of the role of international law in protecting and promoting global public health* (*Key issues in Global Health Governance Discussion Paper 3*). World Health Organization and London School of Hygiene and Tropical Medicine. Available from: http://www.lshtm.ac.uk/cgch/ghg3.pdf

Fidler, D. and Gostin, L. (2006). The new International Health Regulations: An historic development for international law and public health. *Journal of Law, Medicine and Ethics*, **34**, 85–94.

The Food and Agriculture Organization (FAO) (1961). 11th FAO Conference Resolution No. 12/61, FAO, Rome.

Frank, J., Chaloupka, F.J., Hu, T. *et al.* (2000). The taxation of tobacco products. In *Tobacco control in developing countries* (eds. P. Jha and F. Chaloupka), pp. 237–72. Oxford University Press, Oxford.

Giesecke, J. (2003). International health regulations and epidemic control. In *Global public goods for health*: *Health economic and public health perspectives* (eds. R. Smith, R. Beaglehole, D. Woodward and N. Drager), pp. 196–211. Oxford University Press, Oxford.

Guindon, G.E. and Boisclair, D. (2003). Past, current and future trends in tobacco use *HNP Discussion Paper No.6, Economics of Tobacco Control Paper No. 6*. The World Bank, Washington, DC.

Hammond, D., Fong, G.T., McDonald, P.W. *et al.* (2003). Impact of the graphic Canadian warning labels on adult smoking behaviour. *Tobacco Control*, **12**, 391–5.

Jamison, D.T., Frenk, J., and Knaul, F.I. (1998). International collective action in health: Objectives, functions, and rationale. *The Lancet*, **351**, 514–7.

Jamison, D.T., Breman, J.G., Measham, A.R. *et al.* (2006) Cost-effective strategies for noncommunicable diseases, risk factors, and behaviors. *Prioroties in health*, pp. 97–128. Oxford University Press, New York.

Kaul, I., Grunberg, I., and Stern, M.A. (1999). Defining global public goods. In *Global public goods, international cooperation in the 21st century* (eds. I. Kaul, I. Grunberg, and M.A. Stern), pp. 2–19. Oxford University Press, Oxford.

Kickbush, I (2003). Global health governance: Some theoretical considerations on the new political space. In *Health impacts of globalisation: Towards global governance* (ed. K.), pp. 192–203. Palgrave, Macmillan, London.

Mathers, C. and Loncar, D. (2006). Projections of global mortality and burden of disease from 2002 to 2030. *PLoS Medicine*, **3**, 2011–30.

Mead, P.S., Slutsker, L., Dietz, V. *et al.* (1999). Food-related illness and death in the United States. *Emerging Infectious Disease*, **5**, 607–25.

Morris, J.G. Jr. and Potter, M. (1997). Emergence of new pathogens as a function of changes in host susceptibility. *Emerging Infectious Diseases*, **3**, 435–41.

Omran, A. (1971). The epidemiologic transition: A theory of the epidemiology of population change. *Milbank Quarterly*, **49**, 509–38.

Plotkin, B., Hardiman, M., González-Martin, F. *et al.* (2007). Infectious diseases surveillance and the international health regulations. In *International Disease Surveillance* (eds. N.M. M'Ikanatha, R. Lynfield, C.A. Van Beneden, and de Valk, eds.), pp. 18–31. Blackwell Publishing, Oxford.

Raghavan, P. (2002). Bidi workers in Ahmedabad, India: Monotonous work, low pay. In *Tobacco and poverty: Observations from India and Bangladesh* (ed. D. Efroymson), pp. 31–6. PATH Canada, Dhaka.

Report of the Commission on Macroeconomics and Health (2001). *Macroeconomics and health: Investing in health for economic development*, chaired by Jeffrey D. Sachs, World Health Organization, p.21.

Shelton, D. (2000). Law, non-law and the problem of "soft law" In *Commitment and compliance: The role of non-binding norms in the international system* (ed. D. Shelton), pp. 1–20. Oxford University Press, Oxford.

Shibuya, K., Ciecierski, C., Guindon, E. *et al.* (2003). WHO framework convention on tobacco control: Development of an evidence based global public health treaty. *British Medical Journal*, **327**, 154–7.

Smith, R.D. and Woodward, D. (2003). Global public goods for health: Use and limitations. In *Global public goods for health: A reading companion*. World Health Organization, Geneva. Available at http://www.who.int/trade/distance_learning/gpgh/gpgh9/en/index.html

Smith, R., Woodward, D., Acharya, A. *et al.* (2004) Communicable disease control: A 'Global Public Good' perspective. *Health Policy and Planning*, **19**, 271–8.

Taylor, A.L. (2002). International health law and the WHO. *Bulletin of the World Health Organization*, **80**, 975–80.

Taylor, A.L., Bettcher, D.W., and Peck, R. (2003). International law and the international legislative process: The WHO Framework Convention on Tobacco Control. In *Global public goods for health: Health economic and public health perspectives* (eds. R. Smith, R. Beaglehole, D. Woodward, and N. Drager), pp. 212–32. Oxford University Press, Oxford.

Taylor, A.L. and Bettcher, D.W. (2002). WHO framework convention on tobacco control: A global 'good' for public health. *Bulletin of the World Health Organization*, **78,** 920–9.

Taylor, A.L., Bettcher, D.W., Fluss, S.S. *et al.* (2002). International health instruments: An overview. In *Oxford Textbook of Public Health: The scope of public health*(eds. R. Detels, J. McEwen, R. Beaglehole, and H. Tanaka), pp. 359–86. Oxford University Press, Oxford.

United States (1964). Smoking and health: Report of the advisory committee to the Surgeon General of the public health service. *Public Health Service Publication No. 1103* Public Health Service, Office of the Surgeon General.

Van Walbeek, C. (2002). Recent trends in smoking prevalence in South Africa: Some evidence from AMPS data. *South African Medical Journal*, **92**, 468–72.

World Bank (1999). *Curbing the epidemic: Governments and the economics of tobacco control*. World Bank, Washington, DC.

World Health Organization (WHO) (1963). Article 18 of the WHO Constitution, the 16th World Health Assembly Resolution WHA16.42, WHO, Geneva, Switzerland.

WHO (1983) *International Health Regulations, 3rd annotated edition*. WHO Press, Geneva.

WHO (2000). Food Safety. *World Health Assembly Resolution WHA53.15*. Available from http://ftp.who.int/gb/archive/pdf_files/WHA53/ResWHA53/15.pdf.

WHO (2002a). Global public health response to natural occurrence, accidental release or deliberate use of biological and chemical agents or radionuclear material that affect health. *World Health Assembly resolution WHA55.16*. Available from: http://www.who.int/gb/ebwha/pdf_files/WHA55/ewha5516.pdf.

WHO (2002b). Special theme issue: Global public health and international law. *Bulletin of the World Health Organization*, **80**, 923–1000.

WHO (2002c). *The World Health Report 2002: Reducing risk, promoting health life*, p. 8. WHO Press, Geneva.

WHO (2003a). *Policy recommendations for smoking cessation and treatment of tobacco dependence*. WHO Press, Geneva.

WHO (2003b). *Revision of the International Health Regulations*. World Health Assembly resolution WHA56.28. Available from: http://www.who.int/gb/ebwha/pdf_files/WHA56/ea56r28.pdf.

WHO (2003c). *WHO framework convention on tobacco control*. WHO Press, Geneva.

WHO (2005). *Revision of the International Health Regulations*. World Health Assembly resolution WHA58.3. Available from: http://www.who.int/gb/ebwha/pdf_files/WHA58/WHA58_3-en.pdf.

WHO (2007a). *Basic Documents*, 46th edition, pp.1–18. WHO Press, Geneva.

WHO (2007b). *The World Health Report 2007: A safer future: Global public health security in the 21st century*, p. 5. WHO Press, Geneva.

Wheeler, J.G., Sethi, D., Cowden, J.M. *et al.* on behalf of the Infectious Intestinal Disease Study Executive (1999). Study of infectious intestinal disease in England: Rates in the community, presenting to general practice, and reported to national surveillance *British Medical Journal*, **318**, 1046–50.

Wipfli, H., Bettcher, D., Subramaniam, C. *et al.* (2001). Confronting the global tobacco epidemic: Emerging mechanisms of global governance. In *International co-operation in health* (eds. M. McKee, P. Garner, and R. Stott), pp. 189–231. Oxford University Press, Oxford.

Woodward, D. and Smith, R.D. (2003). Global public goods and health: Concepts and issues. In *Global public goods for health: A reading companion*. World Health Organization, Geneva. Available at http://www.who.int/trade/distance_learning/gpgh/gpgh1/en/index.html

Yach, D. and Bettcher, D. (2000). Globalisation of tobacco industry influence and new global responses. *Tobacco Control*, **9**, 206–16.

Tobacco Journal International (2000). Taxation structure hits Indian cigarette market: Country Special, India. *Tobacco Journal International*.

4.4

Ethical principles and ethical issues in public health[1]

Nancy Kass

Abstract

Public health ethics examine and consider the moral dimensions of public health practice and public health research. While the field of medical ethics dates back hundreds of years, and writings on bioethics began to emerge in the 1960s and 1970s, the field of 'public health ethics', articulated as such by name, did not appear significantly in the literature for several more decades. More recently, there has been an explosion of interest in defining public health ethics, examining how it resembles or differs from medical ethics or bioethics, laying out frameworks and codes, and trying to provide both conceptual and practical guidance on how ethics plays a role in public health practice and research. This chapter will describe briefly the history of medical ethics and bioethics; work in bioethics with direct relevance for public health; the principles, codes, and frameworks recently articulated to provide guidance on public health ethics; and discuss the recent and growing literature on ethics and public health *research*, including whether and how public health research ethics might differ from the ethical guidance and regulations that have been created to more broadly oversee the ethics of research with human participants.

History of medical ethics and bioethics

Medical ethics has a long and important history. While some cite the Hippocratic Oath as the first articulation of the moral duties of physicians, and others cite nineteenth century writers such as John Gregory and Thomas Percival as giving birth to medical ethics, clear codes and teachings about the moral duties of the physician as a professional and as a caretaker have existed for hundreds, if not thousands, of years (Percival 1985; McCullough 1998). The depth of this work has grown: It is the focus of significant scholarship both in philosophy and other disciplines, the American Medical Association has longstanding professional codes of medical ethics, and instruction on medical professionalism is currently required by 99 per cent of US and Canadian medical schools (Kao *et al.* 2003). The American Association of Medical Colleges insists that principles related to medical ethics should be taught as part of the Graduate Medical Education (GME) Core Curriculum (Allen 2007). Medical history, understandably, remains focused predominantly on the individual interactions between a physician and his or her patient.

Bioethics, in contrast, emerged within the last 50 years, bringing with it an explicitly broader focus. Emerging out of questions of resource allocation, moral questions raised by new reproductive and genetic technologies, a growing patients' rights movement, and a lack of oversight in human subject research, bioethics focused significantly on the societal and public policy implications of healthcare, research, and new medical and/or scientific discovery. The name 'bioethics' began to appear in the 1960s and 1970s. Early issues animating this new field of bioethics included whether social 'worth' should be relevant in allocating early kidney dialysis, whether Karen Ann Quinlan, a young woman in a persistent vegetative state, ought to be removed from a respirator when she had no meaningful cognition, and how to respond to a series of US-government-funded research studies viewed as potentially exploitive and inappropriate. Important scholarship grew in all of these areas and, in the early 1970s, a national commission was convened at the request of the US Congress to examine questions of ethics and human research. The National Commission drafted the *Belmont Report* (National Commission for the Protection of Human Subjects of Biomedical and Behavioral Research 1979) that delineated three ethics principles to be followed in conducting human research—beneficence, respect for persons, and justice.

Bioethics as a field took off. Centres were created, journals were started, meetings were convened, and professionals from a variety of disciplines began to call themselves 'bioethicists'. The three 'Belmont principles' became the foundation for one of the preeminent texts in bioethics (Beauchamp & Childress 1979) and, while some suggested alternative approaches to navigate through tough situations of bioethics, they remain widely cited both by scholars and as a practical framework through which to reason moral problems in healthcare and research (Clouser 1995; Jonsen 1995; Pellegrino 1995).

The early framers of these three principles suggested that no principle, a priori, ought to have moral superiority over any other. Nonetheless, the issues that animated bioethics in the early

[1] The first half of this chapter (until the section heading Public Health Research) is drawn significantly from two previously published articles by the author: 1. Kass, N., Public health ethics: From foundations and frameworks to justice and global public health, *The Journal of Law, Medicine, and Ethics*, 2004, **32**(2), 232–42; 2. Kass, N. An ethics framework for public health, *American Journal of Public Health*, 2001, **91**(11), 1776–82.

years—the need to tell patients and research subjects the truth and the right to refuse medical care or research participation—were ones where the principle of respect for autonomy, perhaps given too little moral attention previously, was now given pre-eminent moral status (Callahan 1984; Pellegrino & Thomasma 1988; Steinbock 1996). Informed consent, a practical application of the autonomy principle, became a hallmark of the new bioethics. Codes of ethics for clinical practice, which had focused for a century on not harming patients and upholding professional decorum, now added clauses requiring physicians to 'best protect the dignity of man in patients or research subjects' (Ramsey 1973).

The sub-field of *public health ethics*, articulated as such, did not appear significantly in the literature until approximately 10 years ago. An important exception, however, was a chapter, 'Ethics and Public Health', in the 1986 edition of the Maxcy-Rosenau text *Public Health and Preventive Medicine* (Lappe 1986).[2] This chapter outlined some of the core challenges in public health ethics: Fair distribution of resources, rights of individuals vs. those of groups, and promoting efficiency while recognizing the 'special standing of those in greatest need of health protection and services'. Moreover, Lappe compared medical ethics to public health ethics. Medical ethics is more concerned with individual autonomy and the duties of single health professionals, whereas public health ethics focuses more on equity and efficiency in the distribution of health resources as well as on the community in having its health protected. Lappe suggested that individual rights can be compromised for the sake of community interests, but only when there is proportionality. That is, the benefit must be larger than the sacrifice, and the absolute level of infringement on individual rights must be minimal. Related, since many public health programmes do not grant individuals the right of refusal, there must be evidence that the programmes will provide the good on which they are premised. At least as much as community good vs. individual rights being at stake, he suggested, there is an inevitable tension between utilitarianism and justice or, stated differently, between efficiency and equity. An ethic of public health captures the urgency for efficiency, while recognizing the special standing of those in greatest need of health protection and health services.

An additional exception worth noting is the work of Dan E. Beauchamp. Beauchamp suggested that social justice and communitarian traditions are and ought to be the driving forces behind public health practice and that these might define a somewhat separate 'ethic' (Beauchamp 1976). While public health practitioners had recognized, importantly, for more than a century, the relationship between social conditions and health (Fee 1977),[3] Beauchamp's work was striking in laying out as a new idea *within bioethics* that exclusive attention to individual interests, particularly through a notion of market justice, 'plague attempts to protect the public's health . . . This new ethical paradigm will require thinking about and reacting to the problems of disability and premature death as primarily collective problems of the entire society' (Beauchamp 1976).

Furthermore, Beauchamp challenged bioethics to realize that much of the work of public health is to further the interests of community. Community, Beauchamp asserted, does not mean simply that the government ensures that individuals' interests are not offended by the actions of others. Rather, community means that we have shared commitments to one another, and that through collective actions related to health and safety, for example, we share a commitment to the common life, 'a central practice by which the body politic defines itself and affirms its values' (Beauchamp 1985). While Beauchamp did not literally use the words 'public health ethics', his work is foundational in describing how public health has its own set of moral priorities, and that these are critical to the functioning of a civil society.

Similarly, some of the issues that animated bioethics discourse in the 1960s and 1970s produced a literature that now, arguably, would be categorized as centrally relevant to questions of public health ethics despite not using the language, 'public health ethics'. In the next section, three of these ethics issues will be described: Ethics and health promotion, resource allocation, and the civil liberties vs. public health questions precipitated by the HIV/AIDS epidemic.

Ethics and health promotion

The degree to which governments should become involved in regulating personal behaviour became a matter of heated debate, and several scholars began to address the ethics issues inherent to health promotion, government involvement, and public health. At the core of the debates was whether it was acceptable to intervene only when behaviour change was relevant to protecting the health of others, as traditionally had been the norm in public health, or whether, now, paternalistic justifications, allowing intervention to improve the health of the person who would be the object of an intervention, also would be considered morally acceptable. Daniel Wikler, an important scholar for this body of literature, further suggested that promoting certain lifestyles or modes of behaviour itself conveyed a certain set of moral values about what constitutes right behaviour: 'It is not self-evident that this vision of a safe society, with its lack of immoderation, stress, and risk-taking, is to be favoured over others whose constitutive elements have incidental adverse effects upon health' (Wikler 1978).

Edmund Pellegrino, considered as one of the 'fathers of bioethics', wrote about an ethics of prevention (Pellegrino 1981). Preventive interventions, he suggested, ranged in how voluntary the intervention was, citing approaches like health education, opinion manipulation through mass media, tax and insurance incentives and disincentives, legal prohibitions. Pellegrino reminded us that health education and promotion include at the very least persuasion and, at times, coercion in the name of what some consider to be 'the good life'. And yet, he rightly explains, there 'is unlikely to be universal consensus on these matters in a democratic society that promises a maximal degree of personal choice'. Nonetheless, as a society, we inevitably are forced to make decisions about what constraints we will accept to further the common good.

[2] Note that the 11th edition of the same text book (1980) had a chapter entitled 'Legal and Ethical Issues in Public Health' by Sidney Shindell. The bulk of this chapter is devoted to legal issues in public health, however, rather than ethics issues, and thus is not discussed here.

[3] Note that this article describes the work of Edward Chadwick in England in the early 1800s demonstrating that differences in social conditions led to a more than twofold difference in life expectancy between upper and lower classes. Also in the 1800s, governments began conducting investigations of housing conditions and garbage heaps and mapping them in relation to outbreaks of disease, and by the end of the nineteenth century, state and local boards of health were being created to enforce sanitary regulations.

Faden and Faden, similarly, described a spectrum of interventions from facilitation to persuasion to manipulation to coercion, and argued that the acceptability of such approaches ultimately rests on how rational they are, and how resistible they are (Faden & Faden 1978). Described here, to be cited frequently throughout future public health ethics writings, was the concept of *proportionality:* The burden posed by interventions (particularly non-voluntary interventions) should be low and the benefit high. As such, incentives should be favoured over disincentives, true education should be favoured over manipulative messages, and government intervention ought not occur unless there is considerable evidence about the effectiveness of the proposed intervention.

Scholars of this period agree that voluntary approaches are ethically preferable to compulsory ones. The Society of Public Health Educators' code of professional ethics goes further, however, calling voluntariness as the *only* acceptable approach. According to the Code, health educators must 'support change by choice, not by coercion' (Society for Public Health Education 1976).

Purely voluntary interventions do not always work, however (Glanz *et al.* 1997; Roter *et al.* 1998). The operative question for ethics scholars, then, became whether or under what conditions more directive or controlling interventions could be implemented. Furthermore, since it would be governments implementing stricter measures, how could one ensure that the agenda was related to public health rather than to politics (Faden 1987)? Involuntary measures also assume 'a benign, wise, and responsive government, something history finds singularly rare' (Pellegrino 1981).

Shifting in focus from what governments can impose on individuals was Dan Beauchamp. Beauchamp suggested that the legal authority of public health should be used to regulate the behaviour of those who market and distribute harmful products rather than regulating the behaviour of individuals (Beauchamp 1976). If outside influences allow an individual unknowingly to alter his or her preferences, this diminishes the autonomy with which those choices are made (Wikler 1978). Coercive measures may be needed to control the facilitation, persuasion, and manipulation of messages that run counter to the interests of public health.

Resource allocation (Faden & Kass 1991)

In the 1970s and 1980s, a significant body of literature emerged regarding the fair distribution of healthcare resources. Articles examined access to healthcare and whether there was a moral 'right' to healthcare (Fried 1975; Fried 1976; Beauchamp & Faden 1979; Daniels 1981; Menzel 1983; Engelhardt 1986). The President's Commission for the Study of Ethical Problems in Medicine and Biomedical and Behavioral Research commissioned papers on this topic (President's Commission for the Study of Ethical Problems in Medicine and Biomedical and Behavioral Research 1983), and other scholars built on this work.

Since many political figures and advocates were calling for a right to healthcare, philosophical examinations of rights theory emerged during this period. A right to healthcare differs from healthcare being a privilege, or being provided out of charity (Beauchamp & Faden 1979). Given that there is no legal right to healthcare in this country, scholars have examined whether morally there is the obligation to provide citizens with healthcare. During this period, contrasting views of justice were put forward (Brody 1981; Gibbard 1982; Green 1983; Walzer 1983; Buchanan 1984; Daniels 1985), yet all scholars agreed that healthcare access must be improved. Furthermore, despite differences about how to achieve it, there was agreement that individuals should be guaranteed some minimum of healthcare services.

Inevitably, questions of increasing access to healthcare led to questions of how to most fairly allocate limited resources (Winslow 1986; Churchill 1987; Blank 1988; Callahan 1988; Pellegrino 1988). There were calls to recognize both the implicit rationing inherent in the American healthcare system and the need for a morally acceptable and explicit rationing policy. One of the more controversial proposals was to ration by age. Both Daniel Callahan and Norman Daniels wrote books suggesting it is morally defensible to use age in resource allocation decisions (Callahan 1988; Daniels 1992). Pellegrino and Thomasma, in contrast, stated that most of the hard rationing decisions could be avoided if we shifted spending from less valuable goods, such as the US$65 billion spent on cosmetics or the US$30 billion spent on alcohol (Pellegrino & Thomasma 1988).

While the allocation and rationing literature of this period did not explicitly discuss public health or invoke the language of public health ethics, scholars ultimately argued that preventive and primary care services should be privileged in resource allocation decisions. Mainstays of public healthcare delivery—prenatal care and immunizations—often were cited as among the least controversial services to be included in a basic, minimum package of services (President's Commission for the Study of Ethical Problems in Medicine and Biomedical Behavioral Research 1983; Churchill 1987).

HIV and bioethics

Few public health challenges have forced the examination of ethics issues as often as HIV/AIDS. Essentially all of the classic public health ethics tensions emerged, from societal rights vs. individual liberties to justice and healthcare access, and issues emerged in range of core functions of public health: Surveillance, disease reporting, containment, and resource allocation. As policy makers contended with tough decisions, a large body of bioethics literature emerged, much in what might now be called public health ethics. Indeed, arguably, it was the HIV epidemic that introduced much of the bioethics world to the world of public health, its priorities, tools, and responses.

In 1983, the Public Health Service recommended that gay men be discouraged from donating blood (CDC 1983). Ronald Bayer, among the founders of public health ethics, responded with one of the earliest pieces on ethics and HIV (Bayer 1983). Two major US public policy documents, *Confronting AIDS* from the quasi-public Institute of Medicine (IOM 1986) and the *Report of the Presidential Commission on the Human Immunodeficiency Virus Epidemic* (Presidential Commission on the Human Immunodeficiency Virus Epidemic 1988) included significant sections on the ethical issues raised by the epidemic. Fear and uncertainty precipitated calls for restrictive proposals, from tattooing infected persons to full quarantine. While there was almost uniform rejection from the bioethics and legal communities of isolation of this sort (Gostin & Curran 1986; Koop 1986; Macklin 1986; Musto 1986; Porter 1986), policy proposals continued that advocated for the exclusion of HIV-infected persons from specific opportunities, such as employment, housing, insurance, and school. The bathhouses of San Francisco and the case of Ryan White—a child with haemophilia and HIV barred from his school—became symbols of the fear and discrimination that prompted questions about how to respond to the new public health crisis. Bioethics could not help but jump into the fray to help articulate an appropriate public health response.

Bridging clinical and public health ethics were examinations of the moral responsibilities of physicians to the wives of bisexual men, particularly HIV-infected bisexual men. Public health traditionally has protected unknowing contacts from risks of infection, while clinical medicine has enforced a tradition of patient confidentiality. Could bioethics help navigate the right response when these duties conflicted? Arguably, the area in which bioethics most engaged with the HIV epidemic and traditional public health was in debates about how best to design HIV screening programmes. Screening is a mainstay of public health. Back in the 1920s, criteria were established that needed to be satisfied before screening programmes could be implemented (Wilson & Jungner 1968; Cochrane & Holand 1971; Whitby 1974). In response to HIV, bioethicists, for the first time, put forward ethical requirements that must be in place before a public health screening programme can be imposed (Bayer 1989; Bayer *et al.* 1986; Gostin & Curran 1987; Gostin *et al.* 1987; Hunter 1987; Childress 1987). What types of screening programmes should be implemented was particularly vexing in the mid 1980s, a time when the screening tool had been licensed, but no treatments were yet available. Thus, those screened would not be helped, and they would be subject to discrimination. HIV screening was put forward so that infected persons might learn their status and, theoretically, would take precautions to prevent the spread to unknowing others. Little empirical evidence was available to demonstrate whether this assumption was true, however. Indeed, the limited research available provided somewhat contradictory findings (Doll *et al.* 1987; Coates *et al.* 1988; McCusker *et al.* 1988; Van Griesven *et al.* 1988). One study found that, while HIV-infected persons decrease their risky sexual practices once learning their status, uninfected persons engage in riskier behaviour once they are told they are uninfected (Fox *et al.* 1987). Such findings have tremendous implications given that, even in the highest prevalence communities, screening is likely to identify more uninfected persons than infected ones.

HIV also renewed interest in the ethics of other traditional tools of public health. Calls were made for mandatory reporting of HIV, contact tracing, and partner notification. Advocates of reporting suggested that more accurate understanding of the disease could be achieved with mandatory reporting and that education and potential treatments could be targeted to those found to be infected. Critics argued that education and potential treatments can be provided with or without reporting, while reporting was an unjustified invasion of privacy, particularly when strong antidiscrimination laws did not exist. As a result, they feared, at risk individuals would be driven from testing out of fear of the consequences. Not surprising, the momentum for mandatory reporting increased when treatments became available.

HIV also prompted ethics analysis regarding health education, duty to treat, resource allocation, access to care, and healthcare financing. Indeed, HIV stimulated public policy debate in almost every existing area of public health. As HIV gripped the United States, so did it grip the community of bioethicists, who became introduced to public health, why it exists, and how it operates. Through this more intimate knowledge of public health, bioethics began to ponder when, ethically, public health should use particular response tools, and what criteria must be satisfied before the more invasive tools of public health can be dispatched. The phrase 'public health ethics', again, was not yet used, but the foundation of the field had been laid.

Public health ethics

After the important work of Beauchamp and Lappe, there was somewhat of a hiatus in thinking about public health ethics, formally, for another 15 years. Much more recently, however, there was a ground swell within bioethics recognizing that the ethics issues that emerged through public health were somewhat different in nature from ethics issues raised through medicine or other areas of bioethics and/or that similar ethics challenges emerged, but deserved to be *resolved* differently when encountered through public health. Several commentators offered frameworks, definitions, and analyses of public health ethics, claiming public health ethics to be its own subfield of bioethics, with its own priorities and approaches. In 2001 and 2002, four articles were published that defined public health ethics, its territory, and/or offered tools to use in its analysis (Kass 2001; Callahan & Jennings 2002; Childress *et al.* 2002; Roberts & Reich 2002), and in 2002, for the first time, the American Public Health Association, an organization that had existed since 1832, published its first code of ethics (APHA Code of Ethics 2002).

One article called for a framework of analysis for public health ethics that might differ from the existing frames for medical and research ethics (Kass 2001). Such a framework would give priority to certain public health interests while keeping in moral check the legally sanctioned police powers of public health. Another article sought to 'map the terrain' of public health ethics and identified particular ethics considerations that arise predictably in public health, from maximizing utility to preventing harm to distributing benefits fairly (Childress *et al.* 2002). Both of these contributions provide frameworks for analysis that include identifying programme goals, determining effectiveness, minimizing burdens, proportionality, and procedural justice.

Callahan and Jennings pointed out that public health has been concerned with social and economic inequality since nineteenth century, while bioethics, in its first decades, was more visibly concerned with the good of the individual. They identified four areas of public health that typically raise ethics issues: Health promotion, risk reduction, epidemiologic research, and interventions to reduce structural and economic disparities (Roberts & Reich 2002). Notably, they call for bioethics as a community to become more aware of the ethics issues that arise in public health.

Not coincidentally, all three of these articles also devote attention to social justice. Social justice is highly correlated with better health outcomes, and social justice is a recurring theme of public health (Powers & Faden 2006). Indeed, as will be described subsequently, public health practitioners rarely go far in examining epidemiologic correlations without finding important associations between poor health outcomes and social class and/or social position. An important question for public health ethics, then, is to what extent do public health professionals have an affirmative obligation to better *social* rather than, narrowly, health-related, conditions, in the name of public health? Such 'positive duties' remain more controversial than do the 'negative duties' of ensuring that citizens' health, rights, and opportunities are not interfered with by others, and yet there is growing literature within public health and public health ethics that such affirmative duties, at least to ensure the conditions under which individuals can be healthy, is indeed an obligation of public health.

Public health research

Literature related to ethics and public health research fall into two categories. First, there are articles that try to examine how public health research can be distinguished, both conceptually and operationally, from public health practice (CDC 1999; Casarett *et al.* 2000; Bellin & Dubler 2001; Amoroso & Middaugh 2003). This body of literature tries to lay out criteria defining when an activity is 'simply' quality assurance or evaluation vs. when it crosses the line to become research with humans. At stake in such a distinction is not simply intellectual precision; activities deemed to be research with humans cannot be conducted until they have been approved by an Institutional Review Committee, in accordance with the Code of Federal Regulations pertaining to human research, and individuals cannot be asked to participate or contribute their data until they have provided written consent or until those in charge obtain a waiver.

Second, there is a body of literature related to public health research and ethics that focuses more specifically on activities that unquestionably are research, but that ask whether public health research is different, again, from clinical research. As such, ought it to be exempt from certain types of review or requirements, and, in addition, do different ethics challenges emerge when one targets populations rather than individuals to be the subject of research intervention and inquiry. Both of these bodies of literature will be summarized briefly here.

Distinguishing public health research from non-research activities of public health

An early and widely cited document that sought to distinguish public health research from non-research was put forward by the Centers for Disease Control and Prevention (CDC) in 1999 (CDC 1999). This document built on an earlier published report from two CDC staff members (Snider & Stroup 1997). The CDC guidelines were written in response to queries from outsiders that certain activities conducted by CDC in the name of public health practice perhaps ought to have been categorized as research (Burris, Buehler & Lazzarini 2003). While the CDC guidelines were written primarily for CDC employees to help guide them in their own work, the distinctions raised are relevant to others in public health as well. The document acknowledges that federal regulations, when drafted, did not address whether or how they would apply to the mandatory data collection requirements of health departments. Specifically, all health departments have statutory authority to collect systematic data from individuals, using methods similar to those used in formal research investigations. And while federal regulations provide a definition of human research, the definition does not adequately distinguish public health research from 'non-research'. The 1999 CDC guidelines outline three public health activities—surveillance, emergency response, and evaluation—that are particularly susceptible to the quandary over whether the activity is research or non-research (CDC 1999). According to the CDC document, distinctions rest on what was the primary intent of the activity. If, primarily, the activity is designed to help a public health department do its job furthering the health interests of a particular community, even if it *also* produces data of more generalizable interest, the activity can and should be called non-research. Research, in contrast, always is intended to produce generalizable data, and the activity is designed from the beginning to have relevance beyond the population or programme from which data were collected. Surveillance activities, for example, are likely to be considered non-research when they are in response to 'lawful state disease reporting or monitoring' activities. When they are collected to learn information more broadly about similar populations or settings or more broadly about a given health condition, then activities are more likely to be considered as research. Sometimes, a state health department could be engaged in both. That is, they may be collecting data for purposes of statutorily authorized surveillance and reporting. However, they may also be collecting additional data on etiological causes of disease that would be of broader interest. This latter component may then be considered a research activity, but the data collected more narrowly for surveillance purposes would retain its categorization as a non-research activity. Conducting an evaluation is viewed by the CDC guidelines similarly. If the evaluation is conducted to examine how well a particular programme achieved its own objectives within a given setting or population, it likely would be considered non-research. If, instead, the evaluation were conducted to see if programmes *of this sort* generally worked with populations *of this sort*, then the activity likely would be considered research. Moreover, to the extent that environments are manipulated (e.g. one group receives a programme and the other does not, and outcomes are compared), activities are more likely to be considered research.

The CDC states that outbreak investigations and other emergency responses are and must be considered non-research. Indeed, state and local health departments arguably could not conduct their state-mandated functions if they were not classified in this way.

Academic scholars also have taken on this question of when an activity is research vs. non-research. Casarett *et al.* proposed two criteria for distinguishing quality improvement from research activities. While not focusing on the public health context *per se*, these authors set forward criteria that are quite different from those urged by the CDC. Rather than focusing on the purpose or intent of the activity, these authors are perhaps more consequentialist. Activities should be regulated as research, they say, if (1) the majority of patients involved are not expected to benefit directly from the knowledge to be gained and (2) additional risks and burdens exist as a result of wanting findings to be generalizable. That is, rather than asking if the activity is designed to gather generalizable knowledge, they ask, does creating generalizable knowledge change the risk/benefit ratio. They further suggest that their approach is more practical, contending that it may be difficult to determine intent and also that the results of most QI activities are generalizable to some degree. When lines are blurry, they say, it is appropriate to consider risk. This recommendation is corroborated, to some extent, by the recommendations from a CDC workshop on the topic of practice vs. research (MacQueen 2004). MacQueen and Buehler describe participants at this workshop debating two particular cases and recommending that the need for research oversight be determined on level of risk, while also stressing the need to ensure ethical and professional conduct, rather than making distinctions based on primary intent.

Bellin and Dubler, in contrast, say that an activity can be considered QI (rather than research) if there is a commitment, in advance of data collection, 'to a corrective action plan given any one of a number of possible outcomes. The sponsor of this review must have both clinical supervisory responsibility and the authority to impose change' (Bellin & Dubler 2001). That is, an activity should be considered quality improvement if there is a direct and clear commitment from someone with the power to make changes that evaluation results will lead to modifications, as necessary, in how the programme is structured or run. Otherwise, they say, the activity must be considered research. Amoroso and Middaugh continue the theme, suggesting that practice refers to interventions designed solely to enhance the well being of *specific* individuals, whereas research creates generalizable results (Amoroso & Middaugh 2003). They acknowledge, however, that in actual cases, categorizing particular activities can be challenging and they emphasize that such decisions should be made in advance and not left to journals to decide whether submitted manuscripts need to have had their work reviewed by an IRB.

Burris *et al.*, however, take on a more conceptual question. They contend that, while many of the tools and activities of public health practice resemble the tools and activities of research, a fundamental moral difference exists between public health departments performing these activities and others doing so. Public health departments are government agencies, 'carrying out a statutory mission to protect and promote collective health'. As such, when *they* collect data, they are doing so as a means of fulfilling their government-mandated *practice functions*. Burris, then, believes that the work of public health departments systematically should be exempt from the federal regulations and posits that those who suggest otherwise simply do not understand what public health agencies do. Under such a view, even those activities conducted by public health departments that others would put in the 'research' category—activities designed to gather generalizable knowledge—would be exempt from oversight by the Common Rule, expressly *because* they are conducted by public health departments. Importantly, however, an alternative, internal system would need be created to ensure that the 'human beings who become involved in activities that increase our knowledge (whether defined as research or not) should be protected'. Having internal review rather than using the preexisting Common Rule system is suggested not only out of efficiency (so that critical public health data collection activities can occur in a timely manner), it also is suggested because of a view that the usual balancing IRBs are asked to perform when they review research is misplaced if applied to public health departments. That is, most human research reviewed by IRBs ultimately is discretionary while the research of public health departments, in these authors' view, is less so since it is conducted as a means of fulfilling their public mandate. They propose that systems be put in place to ensure that data collection activities are conducted in the least harmful, least restrictive, and most respectful way possible, but should be judged less on whether or not they should be conducted (Burris *et al.* 2003).

The National Bioethics Advisory Commission (NBAC) suggested that, just as the physician performs clinical activities on behalf of the individual patient, public health professionals act on behalf of the population as a whole (National Bioethics Advisory Commission 2001). Furthermore, public health practice professionals are bound by a variety of laws that provide comparable ethics protections to the safeguards offered by IRBs. Specifically, public health laws 'address the requirements for informed consent, protections for privacy and confidentiality, procedures for collecting and handling information . . . and penalties for public health professionals when they do not comply with legal requirements' (National Bioethics Advisory Commission 2001). NBAC, however, takes a different position from Burris and, echoing CDC guidelines, suggests that projects *intended* to produce generalizable knowledge must be subject to the oversight provided by the Common Rule.

Perhaps the strongest voices in the literature for continued and ongoing oversight of public health data collection activities come from Fairchild and Bayer. Their view is that *all* data collection activities conducted by federal or state governments should be subject to ethical review, whether classified as practice or research. While not suggesting that IRBs necessarily perform this review, they advocate for universal review of these activities. Indeed, they argue, it is expressly because of the statutory requirement for data collection in public health that someone must ensure that public health does not overstep its reach: 'The invocation to act, especially when the individual rights of privacy and liberty may be impinged, must be subject to limits' (Fairchild & Bayer 2004). They provide as a hypothetical example that public health might try to link HIV registries with school registries, a proposal that might be denied if reviewed by an ethical board. Ethical review, they suggest, would help to keep public health authorities' power to collect identifiable data in check.

Ethical issues raised by public health research

The second body of literature summarized here examines activities clearly labelled as research. At stake, however, is whether ethics issues in *public health research* might differ somewhat from those of clinical research. Related, this literature asks whether the review considerations of IRBs should change to some degree when evaluating investigations labelled as public health research.

A series of papers, drafted mostly by epidemiologists, began to appear in the literature in the 1970s that suggested the need for certain types of epidemiological studies to maintain identifiers and, importantly, to waive the usual requirement for individual informed consent (Gordis *et al.* 1977; Kelsey 1981; Waters 1985). Gordis *et al.* contended that epidemiologists have important responsibilities in maintaining confidentiality, but also maintained that requiring patients' consent for researchers accessing patients' medical records would make retrospective record review studies essentially impossible to conduct (Gordis *et al.* 1977). They provide dozens of examples, from identifying the link between cigarette smoking and lung cancer, to the link between high concentrations of oxygen for premature infants and blindness, to the link between oral contraceptives and stroke, illustrating that epidemiologic record review studies have contributed enormously to our clinical and public health knowledge. Kelsey went further and suggested that, in some cases, written consent also should be waived for interview studies conducted in person, suggesting that the spirit of consent is important, but the act of signing may discourage some individuals from enrolment and simply may not be necessary for lower risk research

(Kelsey 1981). As a whole, these papers point out that epidemiologic research is less likely than clinical research to include patients and associated drug risks and more likely to be analysing records with associated privacy risks. Thus, they begin to suggest that there might be ways in which public health research is 'different' from clinical research. More specifically, they suggest that risks generally are low in epidemiologic research, leading them to make procedural recommendations for research review and oversight.

More recently, a conceptual literature has begun to explore whether and how population-based research and/or prevention research differ in ethically relevant ways from clinical research. Taylor and Johnson suggest that the research ethics literature generally has focused on the important ethics challenges from clinical research (generally with individuals) but has given little attention to issues raised by population-based research (Taylor & Johnson 2007). For example, population-based research may not allow individual participants the opportunity to refuse participation, something generally considered fundamental to ethical research with humans. Providing interventions at the level of the community rather than the level of the individual, by definition, means that everyone in that community automatically is exposed to the intervention. Studies, for example, have evaluated community-wide interventions, such as measuring the effect of fortifying flour or cereals in some but not all communities' rations, or determining the impact of health promotion media campaigns provided in some communities and not in others. When individuals cannot refuse their participation in a study, IRBs must determine that the level of risk for individuals is minimal and that the public health benefit resulting from the research outweighs the compromise to autonomy imposed by individuals' inability to refuse. Almost always in such cases, data are collected at the population level and without any individual identifiers. In some cases, there are mechanisms to inform the population as a whole that the research is being conducted, allowing for some level of disclosure or 'informing' to occur, even absent the ability to individually agree or decline participation.

Another ethics risk that may be more likely to exist in population-based research is social stigma or stereotyping of identifiable groups. Population-based research sometimes will target specific geographic, religious, or ethnic communities, or may target groups defined by a risk behaviour such as injection drug use or sexual orientation. As such, it has the potential to create social harms seen less often in clinical research that targets individuals. Specifically, not only might individuals enrolled in studies that target particular groups be at social risk by virtue of being associated with the study; moreover, the research study's results may be used to label or stereotype the population as a whole. Thus, even if researchers rigorously follow usual measures to safeguard confidentiality of individual identities, population-based research carries the risk that outsiders might think differently about an entire social group due to the research having been conducted. Consequently, it is from population-based research that community advisory boards (Strauss *et al.* 2001; Morin *et al.* 2003; Quinn 2004) and community-based participatory methods (Israel *et al.* 1998; Macaulay *et al.* 1999) have emerged as a means to get community input into planned designs as well as into how findings will be disseminated and described afterward. When communities potentially are put at risk by research, it is important, ethically, to get the views of groups best able to represent community-wide interests, just as individuals must provide input for clinical research. Communities can give voice to, and respond to how rights and interests of communities will be protected in proposed research and how benefits that might offset any existing risks will be realized.

Finally, in the same way that traditional clinical trials have faced the question of whether successful interventions needed to be provided to research subjects—or at least to those who had been in the placebo group—after the trial is over, population-based trials increasingly are needing to consider what, if anything, will be made available to study communities when the research is completed. Particularly for research conducted in resource-poor communities, this new question has become quite contentious and has been the subject of significant bioethics attention. This has been the focus of some literature on Community Based Participatory Research. Also, guidelines of the Council for International Organization of Medical Sciences (CIOMS), drafted to advise researchers on ethical conduct for research in resource-poor settings, delineate that successful research interventions should be made 'reasonably available for the benefit of that population or community', although this is qualified in the CIOMS commentary by saying that decisions about what should be provided and in what manner must be decided on a case-by-case basis (CIOMS 2002). The World Health Organization's guide for developing countries on creating research ethics committees similarly says that 'a description of the availability and affordability of any successful study product to the concerned communities following the research' is a reasonable piece of ethics committee review but does not suggest that research should be approved only when future access can be guaranteed (WHO 2000). The National Bioethics Advisory Commission went further, suggesting that 'prior agreements'—that is, 'arrangements made before a trial begins that address the post-trial availability of effective interventions to the host community and/or country after the study has been completed'—should be made among 'producers, sponsors, and users' of research products; such agreements likely would lay out what will be available, to whom, for how long, and who will pay (National Bioethics Advisory Commission 2001). While clearly an attractive idea in principle, some have criticized this recommendation, saying that many policy commitments from donors and/or governments for translating important research findings into public health practice never could have been secured until the dramatic study results were in hand. Requiring agreements in advance, they say, would stifle important research from going forward. An empirical study with a variety of stakeholders, however, showed that 83 per cent of participants, 29 per cent of IRB chairs, and 42 per cent of researchers thought that an HIV-related intervention, if shown to be effective in a study, should be made available to all HIV-infected persons globally either for free or at a level they could personally afford (Pace *et al.* 2006). Another study showed that 37 per cent of US investigators working on intervention studies in developing countries believed it was 'true or sometimes true' that 'the intervention being tested is unlikely to be available to most citizens of the developing country in the foreseeable future' (Kass *et al.* 2003).

Finally, important in the evolution of thinking about public health research and ethics was a controversial legal case of 2001 related to a lead abatement trial conducted in the 1990s in Baltimore (Ericka Grimes vs. Kennedy Krieger Institute, Inc. 2001). This trial targeted low income housing units in old neighbourhoods that had both significant lead paint in units and where units often were in disrepair; that is, where children would be at risk of lead poisoning due to the existing poor conditions (Farfel & Chisolm 1990; Farfel & Chisolm 1991; Farfel & Chisolm 1994; Pollak 2002). Despite evidence for decades of the danger of lead paint, particularly to children, and despite continued high rates of lead poisoning among children in Baltimore, no laws existed requiring that houses be safe or abated before they could be rented to families. Thus, in the trial, households were randomized to one of several different lead abatement strategies in order to see the effect on both household lead dust and children's own blood lead levels of the varying abatement strategies. Two families later brought lawsuits, charging that researchers failed to warn them in a timely manner of children's continued risk of exposure and that families had not been fully informed of the risks of the research. The judge's ruling in the case garnered significant public attention for many reasons, including that he stated that this research was analogous to the Tuskegee syphilis study of 1932–1972 where poor, African-American men were deliberately denied penicillin for their syphilis. The judge further stated that families were 'enticed . . . into living in potentially lead-tainted housing', while researchers claimed that families benefited from having houses at least partially abated, given that public policy otherwise allowed landlords to rent completely unabated housing units to low-income families in these neighbourhoods.

This case was paradigmatic of certain types of public health research, in that it targeted a particular community, it dealt with prevention of a major public health problem and, significantly, it was designed to respond to a series of baseline conditions that were harmful to public health. Thus, debate ensued focused on what research ethics requires when public health research interventions are being evaluated in *settings of neglect*. Are public health researchers responsible for eliminating all of the neglect in order to be able to work in such environments? Or can public health researchers test interventions meant to ameliorate the harmful effects of such environments? Related, a panel was convened by the National Academy of Sciences to investigate ethics and prevention research in response to the issues raised by this case (Lo and O'Connell 2005).

To date, there continues to be no consensus regarding whether research is exploitive when situated in settings of neglect and when testing interventions that may improve conditions, but will not improve them as much as other, existing, currently unavailable interventions. Scholars have raised whether conducting research on 'partial solutions' condones the idea that partial solutions are adequate for the disadvantaged (Spriggs 2004; Farmer and Campos 2004; Buchanan and Miller 2006; Kass [under review]).

A few key ethics questions arise with this type of research. First, do the preexisting, risky background conditions (in this case, of lead paint poisoning) count as a risk of the study, or the condition being studied (Spriggs 2005)? Second, how likely, actually, is it that the partial solutions being tested through the research will have a better chance of being translated into practice, if shown to be effective, than 'full solutions' had been previously? That is, what justifies conducting research on partial abatement, or short course AZT for pregnant HIV-infected women in poor countries, or a number of other 'partial solutions' is that they might be simpler, more affordable, or otherwise generally more realistic as a policy option for governments, health departments, and individuals to consider using on a widespread basis. Presumably, studies of this sort only are considered where the 'full solution', existing interventions (like full lead abatement, or longer courses of AZT for pregnant women) simply are not required or not otherwise being provided to communities at risk.

Miller and Buchanan suggest that rejecting all research on partial solutions out of a 'presumption that a particular conception of justice will eventually prevail'—that is, that the disadvantaged eventually will get access to existing, better interventions they have previously been unable to access—sacrifices the welfare of 'literally millions' of (in this case) children who could benefit from the results of the partial solutions tested through public health prevention research. Related, they assert that it is inappropriate to blame researchers for 'the lack of social consensus' on the right to better social conditions and that doing so is 'misplaced indignation' (Buchanan & Miller 2006).

Others, however, suggest that even the perception of exploitation raised through this case is harmful for the research enterprise and suggests a need for 'true partnership in the research enterprise, particularly when proposed research involves vulnerable communities' (Mastroianni & Kahn 2002).

Conclusion

Public health has only recently been given significant attention in the bioethics literature, both in terms of public health practice and public health research. However, the population focus of public health means that its duties are to safeguard the wellbeing of communities and populations as a whole rather than, primarily, the rights and well being of individuals. As such, public health practice must balance furthering the health of communities through education, surveillance, interventions, and regulations with needing to restrict the freedoms or privacy of individuals affected to the minimum degree possible. Public health is granted statutory authority to protect the public's health and, indeed extraordinary public health improvement has been achieved through sanitary measures, restaurant inspections, immunizations, and health education. At the same time, it is expressly because of this authority that ethics has such a critical role to play. Clear frameworks of ethics that lay out a need for data, minimizing of harms, and fair procedures, and clear principles to follow, including transparency, reciprocity, and equity, can help public health to do its duty to improve health on behalf of all of us, while allowing individuals who comprise 'the public' to feel confident that any restrictions are appropriate and fairly defined. Public health research requires some new considerations for research ethics. Research ethics will continue to require prior review by ethics committees—or IRBs—and will continue to require that benefits and risks be balanced and study populations be chosen fairly. Within public health research, however, new considerations will allow IRBs to be more mindful of the implications of research for populations as a whole, for finding creative ways to seek community-wide input, and to begin to consider how to ensure that communities, as well as individuals, realize research benefit.

References

Allen, R. (2007) Fostering professionalism during medical school and residency training. CME Report 3-A-01. *Report of the Council on Medical Education.* American Medical Association, Chicago.

American Public Health Association (2002). *APHA Code of Ethics.* Washington, DC.

Amoroso, P. and Middaugh, J. (2003). Research vs. public health practice: when does a study require IRB review? *Preventive Medicine*, **36**, 250–3.

Bayer, R. (1983). Gays and the stigma of bad blood. *Hastings Center Report*, **13**, 5–7.

Bayer, R. (1989). Ethical and social policy issues raised by HIV screening: the epidemic evolves and so do the challenges. *AIDS*, **3**, 119–24.

Bayer, R., Levine, C., Wolf, S.M. (1986). HIV antibody screening: an ethical framework for evaluating proposed programs. *Journal of the American Medical Association*, **256**, 1768–74.

Beauchamp, D.E. (1976). Alcoholism as blaming the alcoholic. *International Journal of Addiction*, **11**, 41–52.

Beauchamp, D.E. (1985). Community: the neglected tradition of public health. *The Hastings Center Report*, **15**, 28–36.

Beauchamp, D.E. (1985). Public health as social justice. *Inquiry*, **13**, 1–14.

Beauchamp, T.L. and Childress, J.L. (1979). *Principles of Biomedical Ethics*. Oxford University Press, Oxford.

Beauchamp, T.L. and Faden, R.R. (1979). The Right to Health and the Right to Health Care. *Journal of Medicine and Philosophy*, **4**, 118–131.

Bellin, E. and Dubler, N.N. (2001). The Quality Improvement-Research Divide and the Need for External Oversight. *American Journal of Public Health*, **91**, 1512–1517.

Blank, R.H. (1988). *Rationing Medicine*. Columbia University Press, New York.

Brody, B. (1981). Health Care for the haves and have nots. Toward a just basis of distribution. Shelp E.E., ed. In *Justice and Health Care*. Reidel, Boston, 151–159.

Buchanan, A.E.(1984). The right to a decent minimum of health care. *Philosophy and Public Affairs*, **13**, 55–78.

Buchanan, D.R. and Miller, F.G. (2006). Justice and Fairness in the Kennedy Krieger Institute Lead Paint Study: the Ethics of Public Health Research on Less Expensive, Less Effective Interventions. *American Journal of Public Health*, **96**, 781–787.

Burris, S, Buehler, J, Lazzarini, Z (2003). Applying the Common Rule to Public Health Agencies: Questions and Tentative Answers about a Separate Regulatory Regime. *J Law Med Ethics*, **31**, 638–653.

Callahan, D. (1984). Autonomy: A Moral Good, Not a Moral Obsession. *The Hastings Center Report*, **14**, 40–42.

Callahan, D. (1988). Meeting Needs and Rationing Care. *Law, Medicine and Health Care*, **16**, 261–66.

Callahan, D. (1988). *Setting Limits: Medical Goals in an Aging Society*. Touchstone Books, New York.

Callahan, D. and Jennings, B. (2002). Ethics and Public Health: Forging a Strong Relationship. *American Journal of Public Health*, **92**, 169–176.

Casarett, D., Karlawish, J.H.T., Sugarman, J. (2000). Determining When Quality Improvement Initiatives Should Be Considered Research: Proposed Criteria and Potential Implications. *Journal of the American Medical Association*, **283**, 2275–2280.

Centers for Disease Control (1983). Current Trends Prevention of Acquired Immune Deficiency Syndrome: Report of Inter-Agency Recommendations. *Morbidity and Mortality Weekly Report*, **32**, 101–3.

Centers for Disease Control (1999). *Guidelines for Defining Public Health Research and Public Health Non-Research*. Atlanta.

Childress, J.F. (1987). An Ethical Framework for Assessing Policies to Screen for Antibodies for HIV. *AIDS Public Policy Journal*, **2**, 28–31.

Childress, J.F. *et al.* (2002). Public Health Ethics: Mapping the Terrain. *Journal of Law, Medicine, and Ethics*, **30**, 170–178.

Churchill, L. (1987). *Rationing Health Care in America*. University of Notre Dame Press, Notre Dame.

Clouser, K.D. (1995). Common Morality as an Alternative to Principlism. *Kennedy Institute of Ethics Journal*, **5**, 219–236.

Coates, T.J., Stall, R.D., Kegeles, S.M., Lo, B., Morin, S.F., McKusic, L (1988). AIDS antibody testing. *American Psychology*, **43**, 859–64.

Cochrane, A.L. and Holland, W.W. (1971). Validation of Screening Procedures. *British Medical Bulletin*, **27**, 3–8.

Council for International Organizations of Medical Sciences (2002). *International Ethical Guidelines for Biomedical Research Involving Human Subjects*, World Health Organization, Geneva.

Daniels, N. (1981). Health-care needs and distributive justice. *Philosophy and Public Affairs*, **10**, 146–79.

Daniels, N. (1985). *Just Health Care*. Cambridge, New York. 245.

Daniels, N. (1992). *Am I My Parent's Keeper? An Essay on Justice Between the Young and Old*. Oxford University Press, New York.

Doll, L.S., Darrow, W., O'Malley, P., Bodecker, T., Jaffe, H. (1987). *Self-reported Behavioral Change in Homosexual Men in the San Francisco City Clinic Cohort*. Presented at 3rd International AIDS Conference, Washington, DC.

Engelhardt, H.T. (1986). Rights to Health Care, Social Justice, and Fairness in Healthcare Allocations. In *Foundation of Bioethics*. Oxford University Press, New York.

Ericka Grimes, v. Kennedy Krieger Institute, Inc. (2001). West's Atl Report. 2001, **782**, 807–62. Baltimore, MD.

Faden, R.R. (1987). Ethical issues in government sponsored public health campaigns. *Health Education Quarterly*, **14**, 27–37.

Faden, R.R. and Faden, A.I. (1978). the ethics of health education as public policy. *Health Education Monographs*, **6**, 180–197.

Faden, R.R. and Kass, N.E. (1991). Bioethics and public health in the 1980s: resource allocation and AIDS. *Annual Reviews of Public Health*, **12**, 335–360.

Fairchild, A.L., Bayer, R. (2004). Public health: ethics and the conduct of public health surveillance. *Science*, **303**, 631–632.

Farfel, M.R. and Chisolm, J.J. (1990). Health and environmental outcomes of traditional and modified practices for abatement of residential lead-based paint. *American Journal of Public Health*, **80**, 1240–1245.

Farfel, M.R. and Chisolm, J.J. (1991). An evaluation of experimental practices for abatement of residential lead-based paint: report on a pilot project. *Environmental Research*, **55**, 199–212.

Farfel, M.R. and Chisolm, J.J. (1994). The longer-term effectiveness of residential lead paint abatement. *Environmental Research*, **66**, 217–221.

Farmer, P. and Campos, N.G. (2004). New malaise: bioethics and human rights in the global era. *Journal of Law and Medical Ethics*, **32**, 243–251.

Fee, E. (1977). History and development of public health. In *Principles of Public Health Practice* (Scutchfield F.D., Keck C.W., eds.). Delmar Publishers, Boston, 10–30.

Fox, R., Odaka, N.J., Brookmeyer, R., and Polk, B.F. (1987). Effect of HIV antibody disclosure on subsequent sexual activity in homosexual men. *AIDS*, **1**, 241–46.

Fried, C. (1975). Rights in health care—beyond equity and efficiency. *New England Journal of Medicine*, **293**, 241–245.

Fried, C. (1976). Equality and rights in medical care. *Hastings Center Report*, **6**, 29–34.

Gibbard, A. (1982). The prospective Pareto principle and equity of access to health care. *Milbank Memorial Fund Quarterly*, **60**, 399–428.

Glanz, K., Lewis, F.M., and Rimer, B.K. (1997) *Health Behavior and Health Education: Theory, Research and Practice (2nd Ed.)* Jossey-Bass, San Francisco.

Gordis, L., Gold, E., and Seltser, R. (1977). Privacy protection in epidemiologic and medical research: a challenge and a responsibility. *American Journal of Epidemiology*, **105**, 163–168.

Gostin, L. and Curran, W.J. (1986). The limit of compulsion on controlling AIDS. *Hastings Center Report*, **16**, 24–29.

Gostin, L. and Curran, W.J. (1987). Legal control measures for AIDS: reporting requirements, surveillance, quarantine, and regulation of public meeting places. *American Journal of Public Health*, **77**, 214–218.

Gostin, L., Curran, W.J., and Clark, M.E. (1987). The case against compulsory casefinding in controlling AIDS—testing, screening and reporting. *American Journal of Law and Medicine*, **12**, 7–53.

Green, R.M. (1983). The priority of health care. *Journal of Medical Philosophy*, **8**, 373–380.

Hunter, N.D. (1987). AIDS prevention and civil liberties: the false security of mandatory testing. *AIDS Public Policy Journal*, **2**, 1–10.

Institute of Medicine (1986). *Confronting AIDS: Directions for Public Health, Health Care, and Research*. National Academies Press, Washington, DC.

Israel, B.A., Schulz, A.J., Parker, E.A., Becker, A.B. (1998). Review of community-based research: assessing partnership approaches to improve public health. *Annu Rev Public Health,* **19**, 173–202.

Jonsen, A.R. (1995). Casuistry: an alternative or complement to principles? *Kennedy Institute of Ethics Journal,* **5**, 237–251.

Kao, A., Lim, M., Spevick, J., Barzansky, B. (2003). Teaching and evaluating students' professionalism in US Medical Schools, 2002–2003. *JAMA,* **290**, 1151–1152.

Kass, N.E. Just research in an unjust world [manuscript under review].

Kass, N.E. (2001). An Ethics Framework for Public Health. *American Journal of Public Health,* **91**, 1776–1782.

Kass, N., Dawson, L., Loyo-Berrios, N.I. (2003). Ethical oversight of research in developing countries. *IRB Ethics & Human Research,* **25**, 1–10.

Kelsey, J.L. (1981). Privacy and confidentiality in epidemiological research involving patients. *IRB,* **3**, 1–4.

Koop, C.E. (1986). Surgeon generals report on acquired immune deficiency syndrome. *Journal of the American Medical Association,* **256**, 278–89.

Lappe, M. (1986). Ethics and public health. In *Maxcy-Rosenau Public Health and Preventive Medicine, Twelfth Edition* (Last J.M., ed.), Appleton-Century-Crofts, Norwalk, Connecticut, 1867–77.

Lo, B. and O'Connell, M.E. (2005). Ethical considerations for research on housing-related health hazards involving children. *Committee on Ethical Issues in Housing-Related Health Hazard Research Involving Children, Youth and Families,* National Academies Press, Washington DC.

Macaulay, A.C. *et al.* (1999). Participatory research maximizes community and lay involvement. *British Medical Journal,* **319**, 774–778.

Macklin, R. (1986). Predicting dangerousness and public health response to AIDS. *Hastings Center Report,* **16**, 16–23.

MacQueen, K.M. and Buehler, J.W. (2004). Ethics, practice, and research in public health. *American Journal of Public Health,* **94**, 928–931.

Mastroianni, A.C. and Kahn, J.P. (2002). Risk and responsibility: ethics, Grimes v Kennedy Krieger, and public health research involving children. *American Journal of Public Health,* **92**, 1073–1076.

McCullough, L.B., ed. (1998). *John Gregory's Writings on Medical Ethics & Philosophy of Medicine*, Kluwer Academic Publishers, Dordrecht.

McCusker, J, Stoddard, A.M., Mayer, K.H., Zapka, J, Morrison, C, Salzman, S.P. (1988). Effects of HIV antibody test knowledge on subsequent sexual behaviors in a cohort of homosexually active men. *American Journal of Public Health,* **78**, 462–67.

Menzel, P.T. (1983). *Medical Costs, Moral Choices: A Philosophy of Health Care Economics in America*. Yale University Press, New Haven.

Morin, S.F., Maiorana, A., Koester, K.A., Sheon, N.M., Richards, T.A. (2003). Community consultation in HIV prevention research: a study of community advisory boards at 6 research sites. *JAIDS,* **33**, 513–520.

Musto, D.F. (1986). Quarantine and the problem of AIDS. *Milbank Memorial Fund Quarterly,* **64**, 113.

National Bioethics Advisory Commission (2001). *Ethical and Policy Issues in Research Involving Human Participants: Volume I: Report and Recommendations of the National Bioethics Advisory Commission.* Bethesda, MD.

National Commission for the Protection of Human Subjects of Biomedical and Behavioral Research (1979). *The Belmont Report: Ethical Principles and Guidelines for the Protection of Human Subjects of Research.*

Pace, C. *et al.* (2006). Post-trial access to tested interventions: the views of IRB/REC chair, investigators, and research participants in a multinational HIV/AIDS study. *AIDS Research and Human Retroviruses,* **22**, 837–841.

Pellegrino, E.D. (1981). Health promotion as public policy: the need for moral groundings. *Preventive Medicine,* **10**, 371–378.

Pellegrino, E.D. (1988). Rationing health care: the ethics of medical gatekeeping. In *Medical Ethics: A Guide for Health Professionals* (Monagle J.F., Thomasma D.C., eds), Aspen, Rockville, MD, 261–70.

Pellegrino, E.D. (1995). Toward a virtue-based normative ethics for health professions. *Kennedy Institute of Ethics Journal,* **5**, 253–277.

Pellegrino, E. and Thomasma, D.C. (1988). *For the Patient's Good: The Restoration of Beneficence in Health Care.* Oxford University Press, New York.

Percival, T. (1985). Medical Ethics; or a Code of Institutes and Precepts, adapted to the Professional Conduct of Physicians and Surgeons . . . together with an Introduction by Edmund D. Pellegrino. Classics of Medicine Library, Birmingham.

Pollak, J. (2002). The lead-based paint abatement repair and maintenance study in Baltimore: historic framework and study design. *Journal of Health Care Law and Policy,* **6**, 89–108.

Porter, R. (1986). History says no to the policeman's response to AIDS. *British Medical Journal,* **293**, 1589–90.

Powers, M. and Faden, R. (2006). *Social Justice: The Moral Foundations of Public Health and Health Policy*. Oxford University Press, New York.

Presidential Commission on the Human Immunodeficiency Virus Epidemic (1988). *Final Report*. Government Printing Office, Washington DC.

President's Commission for the Study of Ethical Problems in Medicine and Biomedical and Behavioral Research (1983). *Securing Access to Health Care: The Ethical Implications of Differences in the Availability of Health Services.* Volume One: Report, 1983. Government Printing Office, Washington DC, 201.

Quinn, S.C. (2004). Ethics in public health research: protecting human subjects: the role of Community Advisory Boards. *American Journal of Public Health,* **94**, 918–22.

Ramsey, P. (1973). The nature of medical ethics. In Veatch R.M., Gaylin W., Morgan, eds, *National Conference on the Teaching of Medical Ethics*, pp. 14–28. New York: Hastings Center.

Roberts, M.J. and Reich, M.R. (2002). Ethical analysis in public health. *The Lancet,* **359**, 1055–9.

Roter, D.L., Hall, J.A., Merisca, R., Ruehle, B., Cretin, D., Svarstad, B. (1998). Effectiveness of interventions to improve patient compliance: a meta-analysis. *Medical Care,* **36**, 1138–61.

Snider, D.E. and Stroup, D.F. (1997). Defining research when it comes to public health. *Public Health Reports,* **112**, 29–112.

Society for Public Health Education (1992). *Code of Ethics for the Health Education Profession*. Section 4. http://www.sophe.org/ Accessed 11/4/03.

Spriggs, M. (2004). Canaries in the mines: children, risk, non-therapeutic research, and justice. *Journal of Medical Ethics,* **30**, 176–81.

Steinbock, B. (1996). Liberty, responsibility, and the common good. *The Hastings Center Report,* **26**, 45–47.

Strauss, R.P. *et al.* (2001). The role of Community Advisory Boards: involving communities in the informed consent process. *American Journal of Public Health,* **91**, 1938–43.

Taylor, H.A. and Johnson, S. (2007). Ethics of population-based research. *Journal of Law, Medicine & Ethics,* **35**, 295–9.

Van Griesven, G.J.P. *et al.* (1988). Impact of HIV antibody testing on changes in sexual behavior among homosexual men in the Netherlands. *American Journal of Public Health,* **79**, 1575–77.

Walzer, M. (1983). *Spheres of Justice.* Basic Books, New York.

Waters, W.E. (1985). Ethics and epidemiological research. *International Journal of Epidemiology,* **14**, 48–51.

Wikler, D.I. (1978). Coercive measures in health promotion: can they be justified? *Health Education Monographs,* **6**, 223–41.

Wikler, D.I. (1978). Persuasion and coercion for health. *Milbank Memorial Fund Quarterly/Health and Society,* **56**, 303–33.

Whitby, L.G. (1974). Screening for disease: definitions and criteria. *Lancet,* **819**.

Wilson, J.M.G. and Jungner, F. (1968). *Principles and Practice of Screening for Disease.* Public Health Papers, No 34. World Health Organization, Geneva.

Winslow, G.R. (1986). Rationing and publicity. In *The Price of Health* (eds Agich, G.J. and Begley, C.E.) Reidel, Boston, 199–215.

World Health Organization (2000). *Operational Guidelines for Ethics Committees That Review Biomedical Research.* WHO, Geneva.

SECTION 5

Information systems and sources of intelligence

5.1

Information systems in support of public health in high-income countries

Paul Fu, Jr., Jeff Luck, and Denis J. Protti

Abstract

The field of public health has greatly benefited from the effective application of the principles of information science and information management, and the effective implementation of information technology. Information systems are at the core of all modern public health activities in high-income countries. This chapter will review how information systems, especially those that employ electronic information technology, are applied in public health, and how those applications are changing as information technology evolves.

It discusses the emergence of the fields of biomedical informatics and health information science in the context of the changes in health care and the information revolution. Biomedical informatics focuses on health-related data, information, and knowledge and the storage, retrieval, and optimal use for problem-solving and decision-making activities. Health information science is the study of the nature of information and its processing, application, and impact within a health-care system. Individuals with skills and training in these areas can more effectively manage organizations, people, and processes, as well as information systems. Effective management of information will enable the organizational transformation necessary to stay competitive in the modern era.

Information technology advances are creating new opportunities to collect, analyse, and share information more rapidly, cheaply, and effectively. This chapter describes successful examples in which information technology has been used effectively for public health operations, including data collection (vital statistics, population surveys, disease surveillance, facility-based data collection, and data from providers and payers); data analysis and policy development (computerized statistical and epidemiologic analyses, health indicators, geographic information systems, linked databases and data warehousing); and data access and dissemination (public health and medical literature, downloadable data sets, online query systems, information sharing, and providing health data to community members).

There are many challenges for future public health information systems in high-income countries, many of which focus upon how to make existing solutions more cost-effective in an era of limited funding and high-cost technology-based solutions. Rapid developments in information technology and network communications make data collection and analysis available to a far greater number of users, including untethered or mobile individuals. At the same time, greater availability means greater need to stringently safeguard the confidentiality and privacy of data that is collected.

Information technology, management, and systems support a wide range of public health activities, and broader application of information systems will improve our ability to achieve the goals of public health.

Introduction

The field of public health has greatly benefited in the past and will benefit even more from the effective application of the principles of information science and information management, and the effective implementation of information technology. Public health practitioners have at times been required to avail themselves of technology and systems designed to meet the requirements of the private sector or the acute-care medical sector. As Friede *et al.* (1994) point out, public health information requirements are different and their needs unique. In the traditional clinical setting, the focus is on a single patient; in the public health setting, the focus is on the population.

Clinical information systems developed for patient care or the clinical laboratory are typically oriented towards facilitating the entry and review of a single record or of several hundred records of subjects in a study. By contrast, public health practitioners often need to examine thousands of records, although they may only require summary information about the population and not need detailed information of each individual. In addition, holders of data are often eager to share selections of their data with others, and to engage in collaborative studies, whereas sharing is explicitly restricted with patient-care systems in order to safeguard patient privacy.

A *health information system* in the broadest sense comprises data as well as procedures to collect, store, analyse, transfer, and retrieve that data. The data may be stored in paper and/or electronic form, and the collection, analysis, transfer, and retrieval may be performed by human beings or electronic information technology, but usually by some combination of both. *Information technology* consists of computers, the networks and telecommunications systems that connect them, and the software that operates the computers and networks. Dramatic advances in all aspects of information technology are driving profound changes in organizations and societies.

Information systems are at the core of all public health activities. The ultimate purpose of a public health information system is to convert raw data into information that can be used for decision making. One major challenge in developing information systems for public health is the great diversity of data that must be captured (demographic, clinical, geographic, administrative, and financial) and the diversity of sources from which it originates (patients, health providers, laboratories, hospitals, restaurants, etc.). A second challenge is the number and diversity of users of public health information, including policymakers, public health professionals, managers, community-based organizations (CBOs), and the population at large.

Information science

Information science investigates how systems, humans, and/or machines retrieve information rather than just receive it. The science focuses on the meaningfulness of information and the usefulness of information to the user. Humans are active rather than passive; they search for information for a specific purpose and do not just wait to process it, should it happen to pass by (Radford 1978).

The field of information science is perhaps best defined by Meadow (1979), who views it as a study concerned with the following:

1. Nature of information and information processes
2. Measurement of information (including its value) and information processes
3. Communication of information between humans and information machines
4. Organization of information and its effect on the design of machines, algorithms, and human perception of information
5. Human behaviour with respect to the generation, communication, and use of information
6. Principles of design and measurement of the performance of algorithms for information processing
7. Artificial intelligence applied to information processing

Biomedical informatics

There has been significant evolution of the descriptors used to describe the interface of information technology and health and public health. The literal translation of the French term *informatique* and the German term *informatik* is 'the rational scientific treatment, notably by computer, needed to support knowledge and communications in technical, economic, and social domains'.

Over the past 35 years, many have published their opinions as to what constitutes the field of biomedical informatics. Reichertz (1973) defined medical informatics as 'the science of analysis, documentation, steering, control, and synthesis of information processes within the health-care delivery system', especially in the classical environment of hospitals and medical practice. Levy (1977) defined medical informatics as 'the acquisition, analysis, and dissemination of information in health-care delivery processes', concluding that on the grounds of relevance and direct appropriateness to modern medicine, informatics is a basic medical science. Expressing a similar view, Van Bemmel (1984) wrote that medical informatics comprises the theoretical and practical aspects of information processing and communication, based on knowledge and experience derived from processes in medicine and health care.

Shortliffe (2002) took the broader view, as informed by progress in the field over time, writing that biomedical informatics can be defined as 'the scientific field that deals with biomedical information, data, and knowledge—their storage, retrieval, and optimal use for problem solving and decision making'. Spanning both basic and applied research, specific subdomains within biomedical informatics focus research and application at differing levels of focus (see Fig. 5.1.1). Building upon this framework, Yasnoff *et al.* (2000) defined public health informatics as 'the systematic application of information and computer science and technology to public health practice, research, and learning'.

Health information science

Protti (1982) defined health information science as 'the study of the nature of information and its processing, application, and impact within a health-care system'. This definition was not intended to be unique and mutually exclusive of the work of others. It was rather an attempt to broaden the Reichertz domain of hospitals and medical practice to encompass all of health care.

A health information scientist or health informaticist should therefore be concerned with:

1. The nature of information and information processes in all aspects of health promotion, detection, and delivery of care
2. The measurement of information and information processes
3. The organization of information and its effect on the performance of health practitioners, researchers, planners, and managers
4. The communication of information between patients, health-care providers, administrators, evaluators, planners, and legislators
5. The behaviour of patients, health-care providers, administrators, planners, and legislators, with respect to the generation and use of information

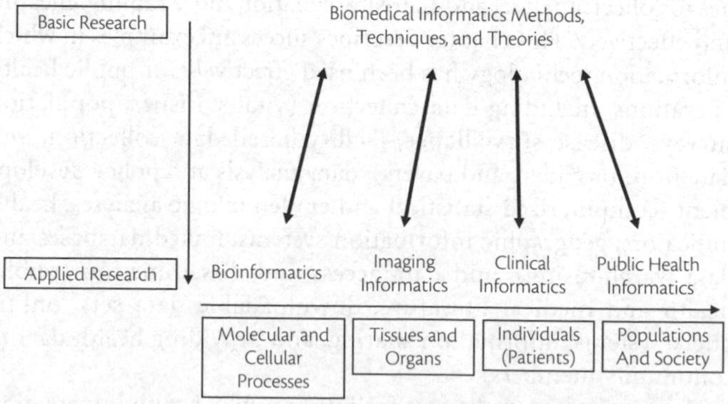

Fig. 5.1.1 Biomedical informatics. (From Shortliffe E.H. JBI status report. *Journal of Biomedical Informatics* 2002;**35**:279–80. *With permission.*)

Many of the conceptual foundations of health information science are borrowed from other fields such as mathematics, economics, psychology, engineering, sociology, and biology. It is a discipline that is not distinctively different from these in subject content, but is different in outlook. Information science in health is concerned with the individual and group behaviour of health-care personnel in their interaction with information and with the technology, which processes information.

Information technology

Evolution of information technology

Information technology is not a new phenomenon; it has been around since the beginning of time. It entails people communicating with one another, and recording their thoughts, ideas, and actions for others to read or hear. The broad definition of contemporary information technology includes:

- Computers (mainframes to workstations, desktop personal computers, and multimedia)
- Telecommunications (switching systems to faxes to digital communications systems)
- Networks (local area and wide area)
- Document reproduction
- Artificial intelligence and speech recognition expert systems

To understand information technology in a modern context, it is important to realize that the electronic computer is only one component in an elaborate and highly differentiated infrastructure. This infrastructure has grown through a succession of technology generations, each of which represents one or more major advances. The concept of technology generations captures important aspects of computing technology such as cost decrease, size decrease, and computational power increase. However, it fails to account for the qualitative changes that have given computing its distinct character in each generation.

The change from mechanical to electronic devices made it possible to store programmes as data and enabled the use of computers as a general-purpose tool, and then, the development of programming language compilers. The transistor made reliable operation possible and enables routine electronic data processing, and then, interactive time-sharing. Integrated circuits reduced costs to the level where computers became commonplace and made possible the personal computer dedicated to the single user. Each generation represents a revolution in technology with a qualitatively different impact. Each generation subsumes the capabilities of that preceding it, providing much better facilities at much lower cost, and adding new capabilities not possessed by the previous generations.

Computer hardware

Computer hardware is becoming continuously more powerful. Moore's Law is an observation that the number of transistors that can be packed onto a semiconductor chip doubles every 18 months, with corresponding increases in computing power. As manufacturing costs do not rise nearly as fast, the price per unit of computing power continues to plummet. The capacity of disk storage devices has risen by more than 50 per cent per year for several years, yielding more dramatic reductions in the price per unit of electronic data storage. These trends have resulted in affordable shared server computers, powerful desktop computers costing less than US$500, portable computers of equivalent power but higher cost, and a growing range of small hand-held computers.

Networks and telecommunications

Computers are increasingly being connected to each other via *networks*: Local area networks (LANs) within buildings, wide area networks (WANs) within organizations with multiple locations, and the Internet worldwide. WANs and the Internet use the publicly available *telecommunications* infrastructure. The benefits of this increasing interconnection are summarized by Metcalfe's Law: The observation that the value of a computer network grows exponentially by the number of computers connected to it, as every new computer can access, and be accessed by, every other computer on the network.

The transmission capacity of a computer network, measured by amount of data transferred per unit time, is referred to as the network's bandwidth. Due to rapid construction and development of more powerful computerized network switching devices and technologies such as fibre optics, the available bandwidth of networks is growing at a dramatic rate, with concomitant drops in price. The result is that persons connected to the robust computer networks found in universities and large corporations take for granted practically instant access to information from computers around the world. Technologies such as cable modems and digital subscriber line (DSL) telephone service are now making this high bandwidth and low cost available to homes.

Within a decade, most of the population of many industrialized countries will have routine, low-cost access to bandwidth sufficient for real-time video and audio communication. Portable and hand-held computers will be able to access networks via wireless connections, albeit at lower bandwidth. Bandwidth availability in developing countries will vary widely, both across countries and between urban and rural areas. However, the dropping price of wired, fixed wireless, and satellite telecommunications will provide more and more locations in low- and middle-income countries with bandwidth sufficient to support important information systems applications.

Software

Computers require elaborate, specialized instructions to store, process, display, and share data. These instructions or programmes are known as *software*. As software is only a type of information, the marginal cost of duplicating it is nearly zero. However, the writing and testing of software is a very labour-intensive process conducted by skilled programmers. Therefore, advances in individual software programmes are less dramatic than the increases in hardware and network capabilities, but a new programme can be distributed to millions of users within weeks at minimal cost. For example, easy-to-use browser software distributed for free enabled the explosion of network and Internet use in the last half of the 1990s.

Software now exists for thousands of applications, including database creation and maintenance, quantitative analyses (e.g. scientific, statistical, epidemiologic, and financial), communications, management, and entertainment. New software is being written and disseminated continuously throughout the world to take advantage of advances in computer hardware and telecommunications.

Technology and society

Society is experiencing its second major revolution in less than two hundred years. The first was the Industrial Revolution of the nineteenth century, which saw the substitution of mechanical processes for human muscles. It changed the nature and types of work, although not the size of the required workforce, as well as society's view of human values. It provided untold opportunities for the individual to hold a job at some level. The steam engine pushed us out of the field, into huge crowds in darkened halls; television returned us to our own darkened living rooms. The compass and chronometer made intercontinental travel possible; the aeroplane made it simple; and advances in communications technology may make some travel unnecessary.

The second major revolution is the information revolution. Technology is changing everyone's job. What is both exciting and frightening is that the rate of change does not appear to be diminishing. As Kaiser (1999) put it:

> *We are at the cusp of a new century, but the alteration we are about to undergo is much more than a change in digits. It is far greater than the incremental steps—in science, art, or engineering—that each century has so far brought us. It will be a quantum leap in consciousness, a dramatic step forward. The Internet, the electronic global brain, is behind this revolution. It will bring us to a new consciousness because it will allow us to share all the information we are able to gather from cultures past and present. And this sharing of information, this global conversation, will change the consciousness of the planet.*

The fundamental economic activities of our society—agriculture, manufacturing, and service industries—continue, but a new decision-making process increasingly influences them. Vastly more information (on markets, costs, techniques, other options) is being made available to decision makers because of the information technology now available. This information is being eagerly sought because more informed decisions are likely to produce better results, be they in politics, operating factories, hospitals, public health agencies, or any organization.

A popular way of looking at information technology is in terms of its utility. The most frequently used reasoning to justify purchases of information technology goes as follows: Labour expenses are increasing and labour-saving computer costs are decreasing; it then logically follows that one should always trade an expensive commodity, such as labour, for an inexpensive commodity, such as computers. One of the resulting dilemmas is that value has become less personal and more social or group-oriented. In a technological society, the individual has the potential of becoming insulated against ethical and moral decisions as these responsibilities are projected onto society itself. For people whose identities have been embedded in their jobs, traditional culture provides no guidelines to help them value themselves after they have been more or less excluded from the productive parts of society.

Evolution of the health-care industry

The future of the health-care industry is not the same globally. In many parts of the world, the health-care industry is struggling to satisfy the most basic and fundamental of needs; in other parts of the world, the rapid advances in medical science are putting strains on governments to provide the best possible care, given the limited resources available. In the United States and the United Kingdom, the future of the health-care industry is a competitive one, where competition is being redefined to include price and marketing as important factors, and the key to being competitive is how well information is provided and used.

The increasing emphasis on competition has spurred the movement for the delivery of health-care services away from traditional, and costly, hospital settings. Tests that were once run in the hospital or in large clinical laboratories are now being performed in doctors' offices in minutes and at a fraction of the previous cost. An increasing number of surgical procedures are performed routinely in outpatient day surgery units and in private surgicentres. Technological advances, such as the lithotripter, replace complex and costly inpatient surgeries.

Medical costs are also being reduced by treatments that can be performed at home, such as in-home intravenous medication administration, telemedicine-assisted self-care for chronic conditions such as diabetes, and hospice care. The benefits extend well beyond lower costs. Recovery or remission rates for many patients are dramatically reduced in the familiar and comfortable home environment. A lens implant in the eyes of a 75-year-old person allows a patient to continue to live independently in the home and community; the quality of life is infinitely 'better' than moving to a home for the blind in a nearby town or city. Neonatal intensive-care units are allowing life to be continued where death would have been a certainty 25 years ago. Microprocessor technology provides artificial voices for the mute, reading workstations for the blind, and communication for those paralysed by stroke.

Information management

Given the 'information revolution' our society is experiencing, it is not uncommon to assume that 'information' implies only the involvement of computers and communication technology. In organizational settings, one often further assumes that the major issue involved is the introduction of information technology within the organization. What is often overlooked is that the introduction of information technology in an organization is much more of a social process than a technical one. If the people involved in information management are to coordinate the acquisition and provision of information effectively, they must understand how people process information, both as individuals and as members of organized groups or units.

Organizations and information

An organization is an administrative and functional structure of human resources, material, and resources coordinated in some manner to achieve a purpose. Organizations are held together by the methodologies of acquiring, processing, retaining, transmitting, and utilizing information.

The purpose of an information system is to support managerial activities of all types at all levels of an organization. It connects, classifies, processes, and stores data and retrieves, distributes, and communicates data to decision makers. This processed data may or may not then be transformed into information by the human decision maker.

In an organizational setting, such systems are often called *management information systems*. Davis (1983) defined a management information system as 'an integrated, man–machine system for providing information to support the operations, management, and decision-making functions in any organization'. The system uses computer hardware, software, manual procedures, management and decision models, and a database. In many ways, information systems are an extension of the study of organizations, organizational systems, organizational behaviour, organizational functions, and management.

An organizationally based information system acquires, processes, stores, and transmits raw material, which is usually a mixture of (1) factual data; (2) material that has been subjected to interpretation in its passage through the system (information); and (3) other content that is openly acknowledged to be the opinions, judgments, and observations of individuals both within the organization and outside it (wisdom). The value of this material, that is information, depends upon the use to which it can be put. Measuring information, decision making, and productivity in information processing is an unresolved problem. Information is an essential commodity and a unique resource. It is often not depreciable and a 'purchaser' may not be able to determine the value of an information item without examining it. Information is not a 'free good'; it is a resource no less essential to the survival of an organization than are personnel, material, and natural resources. As with any other resource, data and information are resources that must be conserved, recycled, protected, and managed.

Managing information

In health-care settings, information is needed to support decisions that relate to:

1. Promoting wellness, preventing illness, and curing or ameliorating disease;
2. Monitoring, evaluating, controlling, and planning health-care resources;
3. Formulating health and social services policy; and
4. Advancing knowledge through research and disseminating knowledge through education.

Information exchange between health-care facilities, governments, and other constituencies is becoming more prevalent, and the need for individuals within an organization to share and use the same information is becoming much more common. Information systems are often pursued as a solution to this need for information collaboration. However, the real challenge in implementing successful information systems is that of managing people and their perceptions. Understanding how people process information both as individuals and as members of organized groups or units is the critical factor for success.

A new field of professionals has emerged to manage information and information systems projects: Informaticists and information scientists focus on the people and the nature of data, information, and information processes within the organization. They are more likely to assess the value of information and its effect on the performance of the decision makers within the organization. Active in planning, designing, implementing, managing change, developing, and deploying information systems to meet the needs of rapidly changing health-care systems, informaticists and information scientists are change agents—a bridge between older systems and models, and newer technologies and techniques—individuals who must be aware of how and why information is communicated between patients, clients, health-care providers, epidemiologists, administrators, evaluators, and planners. The use to which end-users put information is, in the end, the most critical measure of success of an information system that vary greatly in complexity.

The information management challenge is also addressed from an architectural perspective. With the rapid proliferation of data stores and information systems, it is important that organizations align their information systems to the strategic direction, objectives, and structure of the organization. Determining the investment to be made in information systems and providing a rigorous and disciplined framework for evaluating benefits versus costs help to ensure that all data and information assets are coordinated and help to support operations in the most cost-effective, least data- and system-redundant manner. Once acquired, specific standards and guidelines for the definition, measurement, use, and disposition of information help with interoperability, or communication and exchange of data, between differing systems.

Individuals charged with leading change through information systems should possess excellent interpersonal, written, and verbal communication skills such that they are effective at working with end-users at multiple levels of the organization. Effective information managers understand the organization's mission and the business that it is in. They also understand the complexity and dynamics of health-care delivery and are able to function in multidisciplinary teams and environments. System implementation is challenging because, frequently, short-term success must be demonstrated while making progress on the long-range information systems implementation. To do so, they must understand the present and future capabilities of information technology and must be technologically credible to their peers and staff.

Effective information managers demonstrate leadership through effective listening, team building, and consensus building. They are creative, innovative, and have a vision of the future. Most of all, they have an honest concern for the organization's most critical resource—its people.

Organizational transformation

Information technology presents new strategic opportunities for organizations that reassess their mission and objectives. Organizations go through three distinctive stages as they respond to changing environments:

1. Automate—reduce the cost of production, usually by reducing the number of workers. As an example, scanners, bar codes, and universal product codes are being introduced for more than identifying goods.
2. Inform—what happens when automated processes yield information as a by-product. This necessitates that knowledge workers develop new skills to work with new information tools; it often entails new ways of thinking.
3. Transform—a stage characterized by leadership, vision, and a sustained process of organization empowerment. It includes the broad view of quality but goes beyond this to address the unique opportunities presented by the environment and enabled by information technology.

Production workers will become analysers, a role offering a different level of conceptual skill from what was needed before as a doer or machine minder; it will require an ability to see patterns and understand the overall process rather than just looking at controlling information on a screen.

The ability of information technology to affect coordination by shrinking time and distance permits an organization to respond more quickly and accurately to the marketplace. Successful application will require changes in management and organizational structure. This not only reduces idle assets of the organization but also improves perceived output quality. The 'metabolic' rate of the organization—the rate at which information flows and decisions are made—is constantly accelerating. The measurements, rewards, incentives, and required skills all require rethinking in an information-technology-impacted world.

A major challenge for management in the next millennium will be to lead their organizations through the transformation necessary to prosper in the globally competitive environment. Management must ensure that the forces influencing change move through time to accomplish the organization's objectives. Evidence to date is that, at the aggregate level, information technology has not improved profitability or productivity. Some of the reasons are as follows:

- Benefits are there, but simply not visible.
- Improvement is in lower prices or better quality.
- Investment in information technology is necessary to stay in business.
- The external world is demanding more.
- Use of information technology in low pay-off areas.
- Information technology is laid on top of existing services.
- No cost reduction, just cost replacement.

To go successfully through the transformation process, organizations must have a clear business purpose and a vision of what the organization is to become; a large amount of time and effort must be invested to enable the organization to understand where it is going and why. The organization must have a robust information technology infrastructure in place, including electronic networks and understood standards; it must invest heavily and early enough in human resources—all employees must have a sense of empowerment. Last, but by no means least, understanding one's organizational culture and knowing what it means to have an innovative culture is the first key step in a move towards an adaptive organization.

Applying information systems in public health

Public health is a data-intensive field. Paper-based information systems can be found in public health programmes in any country. In industrialized countries, information technology has been applied in public health programmes for decades. Initially, centralized computers were used to aggregate and analyse data collected in the field. Desktop computers made it possible for more and more sophisticated analyses to be performed on a distributed basis, and telecommunications links allowed the electronic transmission of data. Management and some clinical functions in laboratories, clinics, and hospitals were also computerized. Nevertheless, the actual collection of data in the field and in most facilities is still accomplished with paper records.

Mutually reinforcing advances in all aspects of information technology are creating huge new opportunities to collect, analyse, and share information more rapidly, cheaply, and effectively. Other industries have completely re-engineered their processes to take advantage of these information technology capabilities (Hammer 1990). Although many public health organizations and some health departments have begun using the Internet for information dissemination, most have not yet taken full advantage of information technology to fundamentally transform how they accomplish their missions.

In other industries, re-engineering processes to take advantage of information technology capabilities have resulted in dramatic efficiency and performance improvements, better customer service, and more effective analyses of company-wide data to formulate management strategy. Public health agencies can use information technology to improve operations in several ways. First, core public health activities, ranging from data collection in the field through transmission, analysis, and dissemination, can be fully computerized. Personal health services providers are moving in this direction, with an electronic medical record (EMR) as the ultimate goal (Dick *et al.* 1997). Such automation ensures that data is shared more quickly, analysed more easily, and is available to multiple users simultaneously. Second, information systems can be implemented to more efficiently manage administrative activities such as procurement, contracting, human resources, and financial management. These systems can be modelled closely on successful similar systems in other industries. Third, data from information systems in different programmes can be aggregated and linked together in centralized databases to facilitate population-level analyses, policy development, and dissemination to a wide range of users.

The fundamental goals of public health agencies will not be changed by information technology, nor will basic activities such as disease surveillance, treatment, education, facility inspection, and epidemiologic analysis be eliminated. However, innovative agencies will likely transform how those activities are performed. For example, geographic analyses of disease patterns have been essential to public health since John Snow's work. Geographic information systems (GIS) software makes it possible to combine and display geographically coded data more effectively to make public health workers more efficient.

Public health programmes

Local health departments in industrialized countries establish programmes to carry out their legally mandated functions, such as communicable disease control, environmental health, substance abuse prevention/treatment, and the public health laboratory. Each of these programmes may have its own information system, built upon a database containing information about persons, facilities, and service providers with whom the programme interacts. These information systems are essential to the effective functioning of the programmes, and provide essential data on the health of the underlying population. For example:

- Information systems that support communicable disease investigation and treatment are *person-oriented*; that is, their major data elements are demographics of infected persons and contacts, disease characteristics, provider IDs, and treatment status. Other person-oriented information systems support nutrition and maternal and child health promotion programmes.
- Information systems that support environmental health programmes which carry out inspections of facilities that prepare food as well as other facilities that serve the population, such as

public swimming pools, are *facility-oriented*. Los Angeles County (CA) has an Environmental Health Management Information System database of records of inspections carried out at facilities, including facility characteristics, violations found, sanctions applied, and dates of correction.

- Information systems that support substance abuse prevention and treatment programmes in the United States, which accomplish their mission by funding contractors that provide services to persons with substance abuse problems, are *provider-oriented* as well as *person-oriented*. That is, the database must contain contractor characteristics, number of clients served, funding, and contract status, as well as data describing the persons under treatment.
- Information systems that support public health laboratories which process hundreds of thousands of specimens per year for community providers and other public health agencies are *transaction-oriented*. That is, they electronically capture data from instruments and store the results in a database. Public health laboratories can purchase and install these commercially developed systems with minimal customization.

The ability to use information collected by paper-based field data collection processes, such as for communicable disease outbreaks, is limited by the timely input of data into a supporting information system. To improve the responsiveness of this process, more data collection is likely to become electronic. For example, reporting of adverse health events by the public, such as foodborne illnesses contracted at restaurants, can easily be accomplished over the Internet. Public health field staff who collect large amounts of data, such as public health nurses administering directly observed therapy to tuberculosis patients or food preparation facility inspectors, can input data to portable or hand-held computers in the field, with wireless or network uploading to the central database.

Health departments also perform many tasks generic to any large organization, including accounting and finance, human resource management, procurement, contracting, and equipment inventories. Information systems to perform these functions can be purchased from commercial vendors to other industries or government agencies, or developed by suppliers to those industries. In small health departments or in low- and middle-income countries, desktop computer spreadsheets and database programmes can be adequate to accomplish these functions.

Data collection

All public health activities rely on accurate population health data. This includes data on events such as mortality, population health status and behaviour, communicable disease case and treatment reports, and utilization of health-care services. Each of these major types of data is usually collected by a specialized public health programme, using its own customized information systems.

Vital statistics

Because the US Census Bureau conducts a complete census only every 10 years, the Census Bureau, as well as many state and county governments, use vital statistics data to make inter-censal population projections. Natality and mortality are the main categories of vital statistics information. Each birth and death event is recorded, so that vital statistics registries are an ongoing census of these events in the population. Additional data items about each event, such as race or ethnicity of a newborn's parents or causes of deaths, are also recorded in standardized fashion. For example, the California death record has over 100 data items.

Vital statistics activities lend themselves to computerization and the collection of vital statistics data is highly computerized in industrialized countries. For example, the Automated Vital Statistics System (AVSS) is used to input birth and death data in all 58 counties in California. These records are aggregated at the state level. The National Center for Health Statistics (NCHS) compiles national-level natality and mortality data files in its National Vital Statistics System (NVSS). Summary and detail files from NVSS allow analyses of deaths by factors such as location, age group, race, gender, year, and cause of death (Centers for Disease Control and Prevention 2008).

Vital statistics can be used for planning public health services. For example, the number, location, and characteristics of births can help project the need for children's health services. Mortality data is essential for planning disease prevention programmes.

Population surveys

Although vital statistics are collected as a census, many other important types of information necessary for public and health services research analyses are collected from surveys of representative samples of the population of a nation or region. This includes information on the determinants of health, the health status and needs of communities, health services access and insurance coverage, and health behaviours.

Given the diverse types of information to be gathered, industrialized countries conduct a broad spectrum of health surveys, each designed to collect specific data from a defined population. Some of the major national health surveys in the United States are briefly described in the following text as examples of the data collection methods employed and the resulting information resources available for public health analyses:

- The National Health Interview Survey (NHIS) is conducted by the NCHS. This in-person survey, conducted annually, targets a nationally representative cluster sample of 40 000 households. In addition to underlying demographic data on each household, NHIS collects data on health status and health services utilization, including acute and chronic conditions, activity limitations due to health problems, insurance coverage, and utilization of outpatient and inpatient health services. Specialized modules, covering topics such as cancer prevention and control, are added periodically (Centers for Disease Control and Prevention 2008).
- The National Health and Nutrition Examination Survey (NHANES), also conducted by the NCHS, is a much more intensive survey of 5000 randomly sampled persons annually. Respondents complete interviews and in-depth physical examinations and testing. The data collected include diet, nutrition, health behaviours, and risk factors. This combination of behavioural and biomedical data from a nationally representative population allows prevalence estimates of diseases and risk factors, as well as analyses of the links between health behaviours and health status (Centers for Disease Control and Prevention 2008).
- The National Health Care Survey (NHCS) is composed of several surveys drawing data on patient characteristics and services utilization at a wide range of health-provider organizations: Hospitals, ambulatory surgery facilities, ambulatory-care clinics, nursing homes, and hospices. These surveys are also conducted

by the NCHS and they draw data from medical records at nationally representative samples of facilities; tens of thousands of records are reviewed in each survey. Some of the surveys are annual, others periodic (Centers for Disease Control and Prevention 2008).

- The Medical Expenditure Panel Survey (MEPS) is conducted by the US Agency for Healthcare Research and Quality (AHRQ). This in-person household survey details data on insurance coverage and utilization of and payment for health services, as well as personal health information, allowing these data to be linked longitudinally. The household survey is supplemented by data collection from health providers and employers to provide a more complete picture of health insurance and health expenditures (Agency for Healthcare Research and Quality 2008).
- The Behavioral Risk Factor Surveillance System (BRFSS) is a telephone survey conducted by the CDC. BRFSS is a concatenation of surveys conducted in each state, comprising over 150 000 interviews annually. Data is collected on a variety of health risk and behaviours, including tobacco and alcohol use, exercise and diet, chronic disease prevention and screening, and injury prevention. Individual states can add questions tailored to their public health needs (Centers for Disease Control and Prevention 2008).
- Private foundations often conduct surveys that provide data useful for public health analyses. An example is the National Survey of America's Families (NSAF). Designed to assess the effect of policy changes such as welfare reform, NSAF oversampled low-income households and collected a range of data on family demographics and welfare, including health. Primarily a telephone survey, it collected data from a nationally representative sample of over 44 000 households (Urban Institute 2008).

Information systems are used to support all phases of survey design and execution in industrialized countries. In-person survey interviewers often use laptop computers to collect data, and computer-assisted self-interview (CASI) software may be used to collect data on particularly sensitive topics. Telephone survey interviewers use automated questionnaires on computer-assisted telephone interview (CATI) software (Aday 1996). Specialized software is used for other aspects of survey design, analysis, and management, including sample design, random-digit dialling, call centre management, data cleaning and imputation, and calculation of weights (e.g. for non-response and adjustment to population proportions).

Ideally, computerized data collection systems feed data directly into a computerized database of results. This includes the use of the Internet for data collection. For local health assessment and planning, rapid surveys with samples sizes of a few hundred can be conducted rapidly and inexpensively, especially if utilizing the Internet for participant response (Husein *et al.* 1993; Kipp *et al.* 1994; Satia *et al.* 1994). Copies of survey instruments and documentation can also be made available on the Internet, enabling users to correctly analyse and interpret survey results. However, Internet data collection will probably not supplant in-person or telephone methods, as the response rate to Internet surveys is expected to mirror the relatively low response rates of mail surveys.

Disease surveillance

Surveillance of communicable diseases (CDs) is a fundamental public health activity (Drotman & Strassburg 2001). Surveillance techniques and information systems are further discussed in Chapter 6.17 (Berkelman *et al.* 2009).

In industrialized countries, laws require that several dozen communicable diseases be reported to local health departments by physicians, clinics, hospitals, and laboratories. Reports are aggregated for state or provincial health departments, and then to national government health agencies. Sentinel sites, or facilities that provide services to a large enough population to capture significant numbers of patients with the target diseases and have the resources for ongoing data collection, may be the focus of communicable disease reporting (Woodall 1988). Sampling from a network of carefully chosen locations can provide reporting representative of the population, as is done in China (Chunning 1992).

Most communicable disease reporting is still accomplished through paper forms submitted to the local health department. There, the data from the form is inputted to computerized databases, and reporting to state and national levels is often electronic. Paper forms are less reliable and can be too slow for rapid response to outbreaks of emerging infectious diseases, such as West Nile virus.

Laboratories and hospitals that use sophisticated computerized information systems are beginning to use electronic reporting in some jurisdictions. Internet-based reporting is increasing as more physician offices are connected to the Internet, and capabilities for secure Internet transmission of confidential information expand.

The CDC have developed the National Electronic Disease Surveillance System (NEDSS), which is a comprehensive electronic communicable disease reporting system (Centers for Disease Control and Prevention 2008). Components include the following:

- Data standards for uniform generation, transmission, and aggregation of communicable disease reports
- Record-matching software to eliminate duplicate reports of the same case of a communicable disease
- A common user interface for all computerized CDC reporting systems
- Standardized Internet-based, secure transmission links from health departments to the CDC
- Standardized data definitions to facilitate data sharing and analysis

Facility-based data collection

Facility-based data collection occurs when data that can be very useful in describing patterns of disease and treatment, as well as the underlying demographic data on patients, is compiled from clinical information systems. Data sets are submitted on electronic media or as electronic data files. A major shortcoming of this data is that patients using the reporting facilities may not be representative of the overall population. This is especially a problem in low- and middle-income countries, where access to health care is very limited and many people with diseases do not present to facilities for treatment. Nevertheless, in many countries, this data is the best available (Cibulskis & Izard 1996).

An example is the standardized reporting of procedures that are almost always performed at large facilities, or of diseases almost always diagnosed or treated there. For example, in the United States, hospitals in 35 states are required to report data on inpatient discharges (Love 2000). Required data on each discharge includes length of stay, diagnosis, mortality, patient demographics, and payer. A state government department aggregates the data and removes personally identifiable data so that complete files can be made public. These data are then made available for use in a range of management, health services research, and policy analyses.

Inpatient discharge reporting does not capture all data on procedures, however, because ambulatory surgeries are becoming more common, and are performed in free-standing centres as well as in hospitals. Therefore, some states have now begun to require that ambulatory surgeries be reported as well, whether performed at hospital or at centres certified by Medicare (Love 2000).

Cancer registries are another facility-based system that provides data of great value for cancer epidemiology, health services research, and environmental health analyses. For example, California requires that all diagnosed neoplasms be reported, along with treatment data and underlying patient demographics (California Cancer Registry 2008). All hospital and facilities that treat cancer are required to file reports, as are physicians who treat cancer. Reported data are aggregated at the state level, personally identifiable data are removed, and complete files made available for public use.

Data collection from payers and providers

Data on disease patterns and health services utilization can be collected from payers, such as health insurers, or directly from providers when they are reimbursed by government health agencies. Payers who reimburse physicians and hospitals on a fee-for-service (FFS) basis receive claims data for each outpatient encounter or inpatient stay. This data is limited in clinical and demographic detail due to being collected for billing purposes, but can cover very large segments of the population. Data collection from providers can also be effective when a government payer requires encounter or discharge data to be submitted as a condition for receiving capitation or global budget allocations. Because a claim for each encounter need not be submitted under a capitated payment system, getting providers to submit complete and timely data is a major challenge, and so the resulting data sets may not be fully complete. No matter how encounter data is collected, privacy concerns must be addressed by removing personally identifiable fields from data files.

The Centers for Medicare and Medicaid Services (CMS) gathers and formats data to support its operations. Medicare is a health insurance programme for all US residents older than 65 years of age or with a disabling condition or end-stage renal disease. It reimburses fee-for-service for over 80 per cent of its beneficiaries, and so the resulting claims data is quite comprehensive. Medicaid is the US health insurance programme covering persons in poverty. It is operated and financed jointly by state governments and CMS. The CMS makes limited data sets available for health services research and policy analyses (Centers for Medicare and Medicaid Services 2008).

In the long term, EMRs will facilitate the capture and sharing of data by health providers. Ideally, data captured at the bedside or in a clinic can be electronically transmitted to central payer or government data repositories, and then aggregated across the entire population.

Data analysis and policy development

Specialized software has been developed to provide data that can be analysed to provide information for planning and policy development, including epidemiologic studies, resource allocation decisions, programme design and evaluation, and quality assessment, in a format usable by decision makers and communities.

Computerized statistical and epidemiologic analyses

Almost all statistical and epidemiologic analyses in industrialized countries are now performed using computerized analysis software. The increase in memory storage capacity and processing power of desktop and portable computers enables even very large data sets to be analysed on inexpensive computers using powerful statistical programmes such as SAS (SAS Institute 2008), Stata (STATA Corporation 2008), and SPSS (SPSS 2008).

Analysis of survey data requires special statistical procedures to properly account for the sample design, but survey data analysis programmes such as SUDAAN also run on microcomputers (RTI International 2008). Epidemiology software is also available, such as the widely used Epi Info™ programme, available as a free download from the CDC (Centers for Disease Control and Prevention 2008). This software performs a full range of epidemiologic functions, including basic mapping.

Geographic information systems

A geographic information system (GIS) takes data from one or more databases of different types of information, such as population characteristics and census area boundaries or health-facility locations and street maps, links the data using a common geographical coordinate system, and then presents the data using maps to convey the various dimensions and information perspectives (United States Geographic Survey 2008). Locations of events or facilities can be presented, or areas of the map can be colour-coded to indicate differing levels of a population characteristic. GIS are applicable to numerous aspects of public health (Yasnoff & Sondik 1999).

Specialized software is used to compile the database and generate the maps. The two most common commercial GIS systems are ESRI ArcView (www.esri.com) and PitneyBowes MapInfo (www.mapinfo.com). Although very powerful, these systems are relatively costly and require substantial user training to be used most effectively. The CDC EpiMap module of Epi Info is freely available (www.cdc.gov/epiinfo/index.htm). GIS capabilities are also built into many Internet sites. The US Census Bureau's TIGER mapping system allows users to generate maps of population characteristics derived from Census data (United States Census Bureau 2008).

A GIS analysis consists of several steps. The first is to obtain basic geographic data *layers*, such as street grids, political or census boundaries, or pollution source locations. The next step is to *geocode* the health events of interest, such as deaths or reported communicable disease cases. In geocoding, each event is assigned a latitude and/or longitude coordinate, by which it will be related to other data layers. Geocoding is not a perfect process, however, because address data collected in surveys may be incorrect or garbled. After geocoding, maps displaying the desired data layers can be produced and refined. Individual events may be displayed as points on the map. Average values for defined areas, such as census tracts within a county or states within a nation, can also be used to colour-code map regions. Maps can be modified interactively by the user to address particular health questions, by adding or subtracting layers, zooming in and out, or changing colour-coding schemes. GIS databases can perform other analyses in addition to producing descriptive statistical maps, such comparing rates over time, calculating optimal locations for new facilities, or correlating disease patterns to pollution sources.

Statistical and epidemiologic methods must be properly incorporated into GIS analyses for public health. For example, disease rates in small geographic areas may be based on small numbers of cases, and therefore may be highly variable from year to year. Spatial statistical techniques, such as *kriging* (University of Iowa 2008), have been developed to interpolate rates from observed data to locations between observations.

Health indicators

Health indicators are useful for comparing health status across populations, examining analyses of health trends over time, and developing policies to address a community's most important health problems. An indicator that combines measures of both morbidity and mortality is very useful for broad comparisons across communities defined by geography, race or ethnicity, or income. The disability-adjusted life years (DALY) is a health gap measure or indicator weighting for diseases and health conditions and is described in detail in Chapter 2.10 (Murray *et al.* 2009).

Indicator sets describe the health of a population in a summary fashion, including features such as the socio-economic environment, disease patterns, access to health services, and mortality. They can highlight health disparities, as well as health-system strengths and weaknesses that can be the targets of policy initiatives. Indicator sets do not provide a single measure of the population's health status.

One example set is the core health indicators developed by the Pan American Health Organization (PAHO), which it publishes for its member countries (see Table 5.1.1 for some of these indicators). Developing an indicator report for a community is a multi-step process (Durch *et al.* 1997) (also see Chapter 5.2; Kuruchittham *et al.* 2009) . The first step is collaboration among stakeholders to choose the indicators to be measured, given the state of development and most pressing problems faced by the community. Many indicator sets are publicly available, and can be used to choose individual indicators for a community's own efforts. Example sets include:

- The PAHO Core Health Data indicators, which are appropriate for comparisons both in and across developing countries.
- The US government's Healthy People 2010 objectives, which establish goals for a broad range of public health objectives (United States Department of Health and Human Services 2008).
- The Institute of Medicine's book *Improving Health in the Community: A Role for Performance Monitoring*, which describes the process by which communities develop indicator sets, and contains extensive lists of potential indicators (Durch *et al.* 1997).
- The Health Plan Employer Data and Information Set (HEDIS), which was developed to assess the quality of health maintenance organizations (HMOs). Although it has substantial shortcomings, it is the most widely used indicator set for comparing the quality of health care delivered by these organizations (National Committee on Quality Assurance 2008).

The second step is to compile, from many different sources, data to calculate the indicators. Third, indicators must be calculated and published. Finally, policymakers and community-based organizations (CBOs) can use the results as a basis for discussion, policy decisions, and resource allocation. Once the process for collecting and analysing data is in place, future cycles are less labour-intensive, and the data can be compared to the baseline period in order to evaluate the implemented policies.

Linked databases and data warehousing

In-depth health policy and public health analyses often combine data on many different aspects of a population's health, such as those summarized by health indicator sets. However, compiling the raw data for these analyses is the most labour-intensive part of the effort, as the various data elements frequently reside in disparate information systems developed and maintained by separate public health programmes, other government agencies, hospitals and clinics. One method of aggregating data for analysis is to extract data from stand-alone databases through batch data files or real-time data messaging, transform the data so that the data elements are comparable and use the same units of measure or quantity, and finally load the transformed data into a data warehouse (Sanders & Protti 2008). Once data is consolidated into the data warehouse, it can be used for analysis of complex questions, such as investigating patterns of infant mortality by combining vital statistics and hospital discharge data, or assembling an overall picture of a population's health.

Despite this great promise, several technological and organizational challenges must be overcome before public health data warehouses can become widespread:

- Different information systems have different formats for data such as personal identifiers, geographic locations, and medical terminology. The uploading of data from operational systems to the data warehouse must therefore standardize data element formats, a time-consuming process.

Table 5.1.1 Selected PAHO core health indicators

National health expenditures as % GDP	Birth rate	Immunization coverage in infants
Total population	Death rates:	Communicable disease incidence
Population growth rate	◆ All causes	◆ Measles
% urban population	◆ Communicable diseases	◆ Cholera
Life expectancy	◆ Malignant neoplasms	◆ TB
Literacy rate	◆ Circulatory system	◆ Malaria
% with access to safe water	◆ External causes	◆ AIDS
% with access to sewerage	Infant mortality rate	
MDs, nurses, dentists per 10 000	◆ % under-5 deaths diarrhoeal	
Hospital beds per 1000	◆ % under-5 deaths acute respiratory	

Source: Pan American Health Organization. Regional core health data initiative. [Online]. Available from: http://www.paho.org/English/DD/AIS/coredata.htm [accessed 2008 May 1].

- Combining data from vital statistics registries, health surveys, and disease surveillance systems may require the use of different statistical analysis techniques for data from different sources. Recent, well-publicized disclosures of personal health information illustrate the importance of implementing practices and technologies that will assure the highest standard of privacy and confidentiality protection, and are continually re-evaluated to protect against new threats.
- Gaining community stakeholder cooperation for sharing data from sources outside the public health organization, such as hospitals or health plans, can be difficult (Multnomah County Health Department 1999).

Data access and dissemination

Once information has been collected or created, dissemination via the Internet is much faster and simpler than by print or physical digital media, such as CD-ROMs. Types of public health information available online include documents (e.g. books, papers, reports, brochures), downloadable data sets, and query systems. Internet data access tools vary in sophistication, from those intended for analysts with advanced training to ones targeted at the public.

Internet search engines facilitate the access of data or information that is available online, which are databases compiled by software that automatically accesses and catalogues all types of Web pages. Users can perform simple or complex keyword searches of all these Web pages simply by accessing the search engine's main Web page. For example, Google (www.google.com) and Yahoo! (www.yahoo.com) are considered the leading English-language search engines. Both claim to have indexed several billion Web pages and documents, and possess sophisticated algorithms to provide ranked search results by likely relevance to the user's query. Bibliographies of Internet resources in particular disciplines are often maintained by libraries or non-profit organizations, and can offer users very efficient access to relevant Web sites. Useful bibliographies of public health Internet resources are provided by the University of California, Berkeley (University of California 2008), the University of Washington (University of Washington 2008), and the University of Iowa (University of Iowa 2008).

Increased availability of these and similar tools, and of high bandwidth network connections will make Internet public health resources available to more users, and will allow access to larger and more interactive databases.

Public health and medical literature

More and more of the published academic and policy literature relevant to public health is becoming available online. The largest resource for accessing the biomedical, public health, and health services research literature online is PubMed, the US National Library of Medicine (NLM) bibliographic database (www.pubmed.gov), where full citations and abstracts can be downloaded as well as an increasing number of full-text articles.

Many government agencies make their reports and publications available online. The *Morbidity and Mortality Weekly Report* published by the US CDC, an essential tool for dissemination of public health data, is now fully available via the Internet (www.cdc.gov/mmwr). Some prominent medical journals, such as the *British Medical Journal* (bmj.bmjjournals.com), are freely accessible in full text for eligible low- and middle-income countries. Others, such as the *New England Journal of Medicine* (content.nejm.org), make abstracts and some articles available for free, but require a subscription fee for complete access. Universities and other organizations, such as the US Institute of Medicine (www.iom.edu), make reports and texts available online.

Downloadable data sets

Although some public-use versions of data sets from vital statistics registries or surveys are still available on magnetic tape or CD-ROM format, an increasing number of data resources are being made available for download via the Internet.

Demographic data for geographic regions is fundamental to public health analyses. For example, data on the age and gender of residents within specified geographic boundaries are necessary to calculate mortality or disease prevalence rates. The Data Extraction System at the US Census Bureau Internet site (www.census.gov) provides access to public-use versions of data from the decennial census as well as from other ongoing surveys of income and other population characteristics. Users define the parameters of the data they require (i.e. variables and geographic boundaries), and receive the data set by email. Other demographic data, such as vital statistics on births and deaths, can also be accessed online. One example is the US NCHS National Death Index (part of the NVSS).

Data obtained from many of the health surveys and disease surveillance systems described earlier are also available via the Internet. For example, public-use data sets from several US NCHS surveys and other national surveillance systems are available via a dedicated Internet data portal, called CDC WONDER (Centers for Disease Control and Prevention 2008). The USAID-funded Demographic and Health Surveys provide comparable, high-quality data for many low- and middle-income countries, and these data sets are also available for download (Macro International 2008). For users wishing to learn about downloadable data sources available on particular topics, the University of Michigan maintains a list of numerous such resources (University of Michigan 2008).

Online query systems

Online query systems can provide quantitative information about population health, including demographics, health indicators, and health services utilization, to users who need such data for decision-making activities, such as understanding rates of different diseases in order to rationally allocate limited resources. Often accessible via the Internet, these information systems are much more flexible than printed reports, which show only a few of the many potential ways to present large data sets.

The underlying databases are categorized along the dimensions that can be queried. This may be a data set composed of individual observations (such as vital statistics registries), or even multiple linked data sets. Statistical analyses are performed by calling pre-programmed routines. Therefore, to provide faster response to users and to ensure confidentiality, many query systems draw their responses from large, preformatted summary tables. Databases are constructed to protect confidentiality and patient privacy.

To effectively serve users who are not trained analysts, the user interface should be direct and simple. Cross-sectional output tables, time trends, and bar charts for comparisons over time and across groups are some of the standard results format. Maps can also be used, to select geographic regions as part of a query and to display results by colour-coding map regions.

Recent advances in Internet, database, and statistical analysis software allow online users to perform sophisticated analyses of

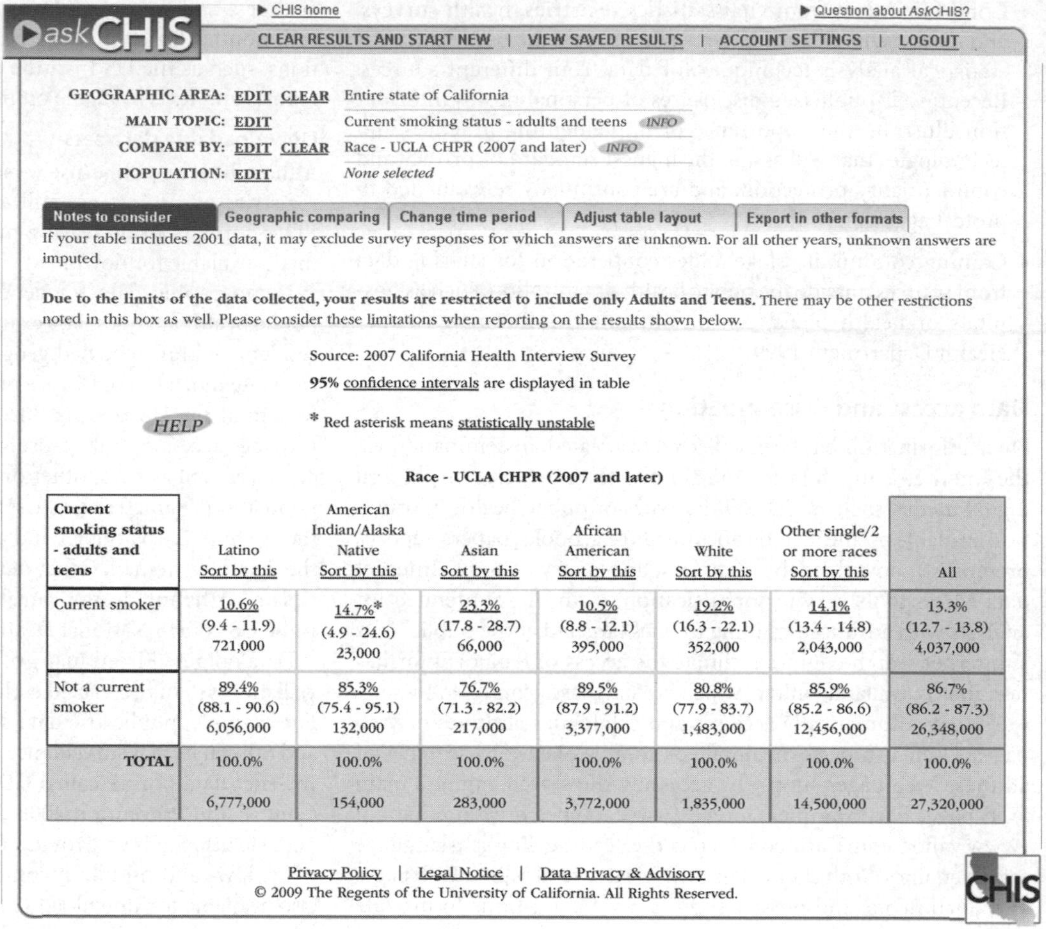
askCHIS

▶ CHIS home ▶ Question about AskCHIS?

CLEAR RESULTS AND START NEW | VIEW SAVED RESULTS | ACCOUNT SETTINGS | LOGOUT

GEOGRAPHIC AREA: EDIT CLEAR Entire state of California

MAIN TOPIC: EDIT Current smoking status - adults and teens INFO

COMPARE BY: EDIT CLEAR Race - UCLA CHPR (2007 and later) INFO

POPULATION: EDIT *None selected*

Notes to consider | Geographic comparing | Change time period | Adjust table layout | Export in other formats

If your table includes 2001 data, it may exclude survey responses for which answers are unknown. For all other years, unknown answers are imputed.

Due to the limits of the data collected, your results are restricted to include only Adults and Teens. There may be other restrictions noted in this box as well. Please consider these limitations when reporting on the results shown below.

Source: 2007 California Health Interview Survey

95% confidence intervals are displayed in table

HELP

* Red asterisk means statistically unstable

Race - UCLA CHPR (2007 and later)

Current smoking status - adults and teens	Latino Sort by this	American Indian/Alaska Native Sort by this	Asian Sort by this	African American Sort by this	White Sort by this	Other single/2 or more races Sort by this	All
Current smoker	10.6% (9.4 - 11.9) 721,000	14.7%* (4.9 - 24.6) 23,000	23.3% (17.8 - 28.7) 66,000	10.5% (8.8 - 12.1) 395,000	19.2% (16.3 - 22.1) 352,000	14.1% (13.4 - 14.8) 2,043,000	13.3% (12.7 - 13.8) 4,037,000
Not a current smoker	89.4% (88.1 - 90.6) 6,056,000	85.3% (75.4 - 95.1) 132,000	76.7% (71.3 - 82.2) 217,000	89.5% (87.9 - 91.2) 3,377,000	80.8% (77.9 - 83.7) 1,483,000	85.9% (85.2 - 86.6) 12,456,000	86.7% (86.2 - 87.3) 26,348,000
TOTAL	100.0% 6,777,000	100.0% 154,000	100.0% 283,000	100.0% 3,772,000	100.0% 1,835,000	100.0% 14,500,000	100.0% 27,320,000

Privacy Policy | Legal Notice | Data Privacy & Advisory

© 2009 The Regents of the University of California. All Rights Reserved.

CHIS

Fig. 5.1.2 *Ask*CHIS query system using the California Health Interview Survey (CHIS) results. (From University of California. California health interview survey (CHIS) [Online]. Available from: http://www.chis.ucla.edu/main/default.asp [accessed January 17, 2009]. With permission.)

population health data derived from surveys or vital statistics. For example, the *Ask*CHIS query system (Fig. 5.1.2) provides extensive data about the demographics and health of California's population, based on results from the biennial California Health Interview Survey (CHIS). Users can produce bivariate statistics, stratify by selected variables, combine levels of variables, and compare years simply by selecting from menus (University of California 2008).

The PAHO core health indicators described earlier in this chapter can be queried via the Internet (Pan American Health Organization 2008). An example output is shown in Fig. 5.1.3.

Information sharing among public health professionals

The Internet greatly improves the efficiency with which public health professionals can share information on best practices. Such sharing is especially important in public health, because development of new procedures and programmes is costly and time consuming and public health professionals in different cities, states, countries usually perform very similar functions and can borrow ideas from each other easily.

There are many ways to share information over the Internet. Email list servers simplify communications by allowing groups of users to exchange email using a single group list email address. All members of the list receive the questions, answers, and notices posted to the list by its members. Discussion forums are online tools that enable online interactive discussion in thematic subject 'threads'. Web logs (blogs) are Web pages where information is serially posted for public dissemination. Collaboration portals frequently provide all of these tools at a single location and are often sponsored by an organization or government entity.

More structured information sharing can be sponsored by government agencies or non-profit organizations. For example, several US government and non-profit organizations have formed the 'Partners in Information Access for the Public Health Workforce' programme (2008) to facilitate access to a variety of public health data sources.

Providing health data to community members

Individual members of the population are increasingly turning to the Internet as a source of health information on topics such as disease prevention, health promotion, and the appropriate utilization of health services, potentially leading to a beneficial impact on public health (Wellner 2000). However, sites that contain inaccurate information or information biased due to commercial sponsorship pose a risk to the health of online consumers.

The Internet is an ideal medium for publishing reference materials, and community resource guides are a reference that can assist those seeking health services. Government and non-profit organizations frequently offer health information over the Internet as a public service. The Cancer Information Service at the National Cancer Institute is an extremely useful resource for consumers faced with the need to learn about cancer diagnosis and treatment (National Cancer Institute 2008). Agencies and public health departments can post important information on their Web sites

Regional Core Health Data Initiative. Table Generator System

Instructions

You can to:

- Generate a new table maintaining the values for the rows and the and the columns, yet select a new value for the fixed dimension.
- Export the table, by clicking on *To export...* link. This will generate a table accessible in Microsoft Excel. For more information see: HELP.
- Print the table, by clicking on *To print...* link. This will generate a table with a layout appropriate for printing. Automatically divides the table in several narrower tables to facilitate easy printing.
- Access reference sources for each value or definition for any indicator, by click on the value or indicator name. A window will open containing this information.

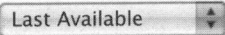

Last Available

Table for the Year: Last Available

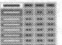

	Argentina	Bolivia	Brazil	Chile	Colombia	Ecuador	Paraguay	Peru	Uruguay	Venezuela
B.1.0.0-Calories availability [Kcal/day per capita]	2,959	2,219	3,146	2,872	2,567	2,641	2,524	2,579	2,883	2,272
B.2.0.0-Literacy rate [%]	97.6	90.3	90.5	96.5	93.6	92.6	93.7	90.5	98.0	93.0
B.3.0.0-Gross primary enrollment ratio [%]	113.1	108.9	140.3	103.7	116.0	116.7	111.7	116.4	113.1	104.3
B.4.0.0-Gross National Income (GNI), per capita, current US$ (Atlas Method) [$ per capita]	5,150	1,100	4,710	6,810	3,120	2,910	1,410	2,980	5,310	6,070
B.5.0.0-Gross National Income (GNI), per capita, international $ (PPP-adjusted) [US$]	11,670	3,810	8,700	11,300	6,130	6,810	4,040	6,490	9,940	10,970
B.6.0.0-Gross Domestic Product (GDP), per capita, international $ (PPP-adjusted) [US$]	11,984.53	3,937.24	8,949.44	13,029.52	6,377.91	7,145.15	4,033.81	7,091.85	10,203.00	11,060.39
B.7.0.0-Annual GDP growth rate [%]	8.5	4.6	3.7	4.0	6.8	3.9	4.3	7.7	7.0	10.3
B.8.0.0-Highest 20%/Lowest 20% income ratio [Ratio]	17.9	42.0	21.0	15.8	21.0	17.6	25.8	15.3	10.1	15.8
B.9.0.0-Proportion of population below the international poverty line [%]	6.6	23.2	7.5	2.0	7.0	17.7	13.6	10.5	2.0	18.5
B.10.0.0-Proportion of population below the national poverty line [%]	...	...	21.5	17.0	64.0	46.0	21.8	54.3	...	...
B.11.0.0-Unemployed proportion of the labor force [%]	10.2	5.4	8.9	6.9	9.5	7.7	7.9	11.4	12.2	15.0
B.12.0.0-Inflation: consumer prices index's annual growth rate [%]	10.9	4.3	4.2	3.4	4.3	3.0	9.6	2.0	6.4	13.7

Fig. 5.1.3 Pan American Health Organization Regional Core Health Data Initiative. (From Pan American Health Organization. Regional core health data initiative: table generator system. [Online]. Available from: http://www.paho.org/english/sha/coredata/tabulator/newTabulator.htm [accessed January 17, 2009].)

for easier access, such as advisories of health hazards or current environmental conditions—such as the cross-US government agency Web site AIRNow (United States Environmental Protection Agency 2008) that reports on air quality across the US (Fig. 5.1.4).

Many consumer-focused portal sites have been created to provide health information to consumers. WebMD® (www.webmd.com) and RevolutionHealth™ (www.revolutionhealth.com) are two of the better-known Web sites currently in this space. Other Web sites, such as Healia® (communities.healia.com) focus on using social networking tools to bring together groups of individuals with common health conditions. These sites offer a wide range of information on health promotion, specific conditions, and treatments.

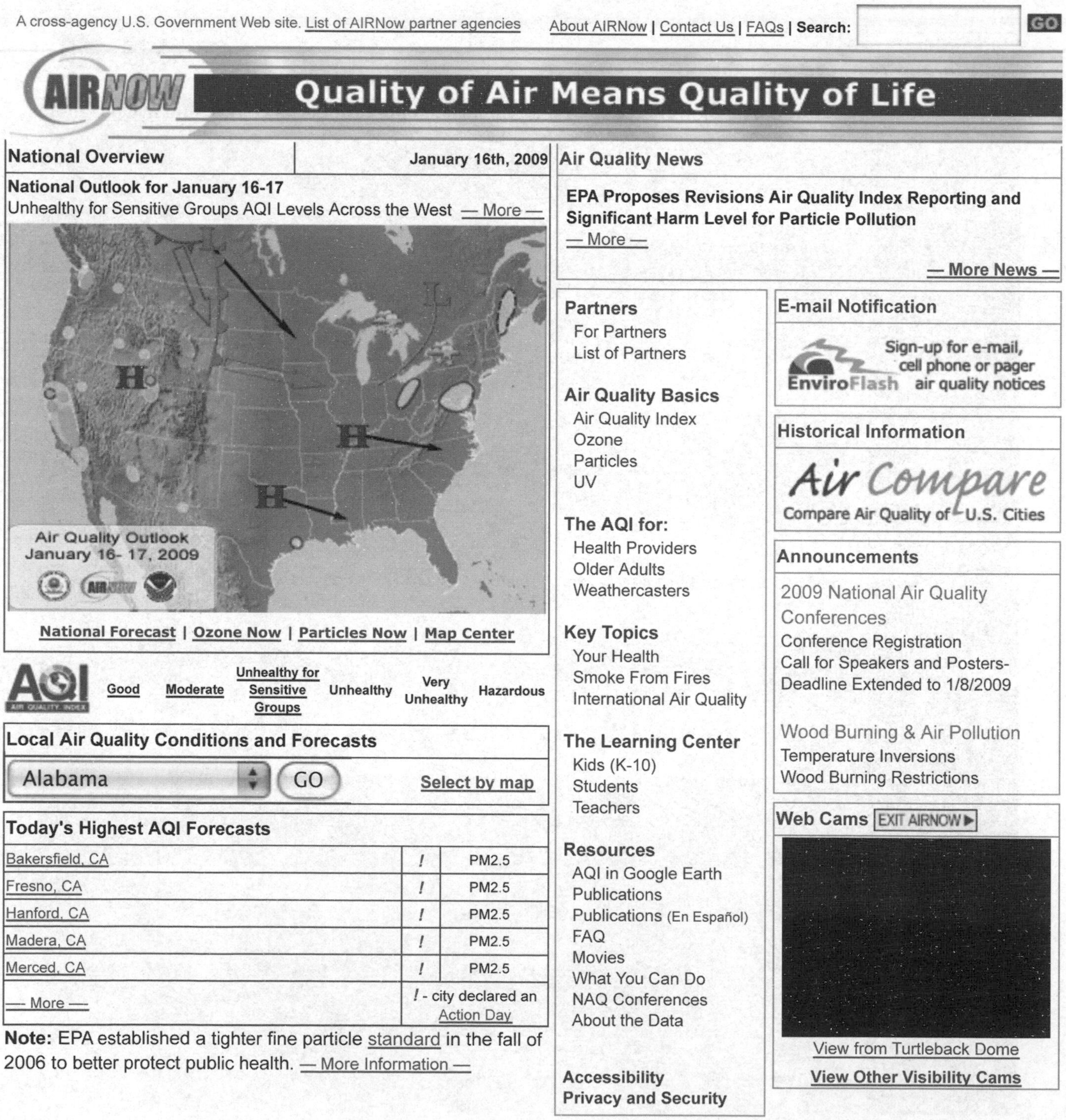

Fig. 5.1.4 US AIRNow Web site. (From United States Environmental Protection Agency. AIRNow homepage. [Online]. Available from: http://airnow.gov [accessed January 17, 2009].)

The best of these sites are easy to use, often containing well-researched and clearly written information.

Search engines also make it relatively easy for consumers to find information on the Internet about the health topics of interest to them. The largest search providers have created 'vertical' search engines that focus on health (Yahoo!®, health.yahoo.com; Google™, www.google.com/Top/Health; Microsoft™, health.live.com). However, the quality of search results is not guaranteed, and most consumers are not trained to evaluate the validity of the information they access. There are Web sites focused on educating consumers about Web sites that espouse ineffective or dangerous treatments (quackwatch.org). Health on the Net Foundation promotes and certifies Web sites that offer reliable and useful health and medical information (www.hon.ch), but it is not universally used.

Public reporting of quality of care measures

Improved quality in the delivery of health services contributes to public health by conserving resources and improving the health of patients. In industrialized countries, quality measurements focus on all types of potential problems: Underuse of efficacious procedures, overuse of procedures whose risks exceed their benefits, and misuse that leads to avoidable complications (Chassin 1998). Information systems will play a key role in improving the process of care.

Measurement of the quality of health care can be broken down into the measurement of three different aspects (Blumenthal 1996; Brook *et al.* 1996; Donabedian 1980):

- Structure: Institutional capabilities and qualifications
- Process: Technical and interpersonal aspects of the care provided to patients
- Outcome: Patients' morbidity, mortality, functional status, and quality of life

Structural aspects are the easiest to measure, but have only an indirect effect on outcomes.

Process measures can be derived from hospital or clinic information systems. When process criteria are clearly linked to outcome improvements, such as prescribing beta-blockers to post-myocardial infarction patients, process measurements that fall short of goals may directly indicate where quality improvement interventions should be targeted. Information systems can also be used for ongoing monitoring after interventions are implemented (McLaughlin & Kaluzny 1999). Clinical information systems, especially computerized order-entry systems or EMRs, can incorporate clinical practice guidelines. When properly designed and integrated in the organizational context of a clinic or hospital, such information systems can significantly improve the quality of care, for example, by reducing the incidence of medication errors (Evans *et al.* 1998).

Public reporting of many process measures is becoming widespread in the United States. For example, the CMS Hospital Compare Web site provides online access to process measures for several conditions such as heart attack, heart failure, and pneumonia, as well as patient satisfaction survey results, from hospitals nationwide (United States Department of Health and Human Services 2008).

Health outcomes are what patients and providers ultimately want to improve, but measurements of outcomes must adjust for confounding risk factors, such as the severity of patients' underlying illnesses and the presence of co-morbidities. Nevertheless, successful outcome measurements provide important policy and clinical data. For example, small area variation studies have shown that rates of common surgical procedures vary greatly over small geographic distances, without correlation to the disease patterns of the underlying populations (Wennberg 1999). New York has collected clinical data and applied sophisticated statistical risk adjustment models to compare mortality after coronary artery bypass graft (CABG) surgery at all hospitals in the state. Hospitals performing low volumes of the surgery were found to have higher risk-adjusted mortality. This measurement programme has been credited with improving outcomes by reducing the fraction of CABG surgeries performed at lower-volume hospitals (New York Department of Health 2008). Compiling data from facilities in sufficient clinical detail to construct risk-adjusted outcome measures requires sophisticated information systems.

Challenges to applying information systems in public health

The previous subsections have outlined many ways in which information systems can contribute to improving public health. Continued technological advancement and innovative applications of those technologies in organizations will certainly foster even more ideas in the years to come. However, three challenges must be overcome before this full potential can be realized.

Information technology and telecommunications infrastructure

The adoption of information systems and programmes that support the enhancement of public health, such as Web-based multimedia health education or fully electronic disease surveillance systems, depends on the widespread availability of high-bandwidth (broadband) telecommunications connections. However, the degree of Internet connectivity varies greatly across and within industrialized countries. While broadband connections are generally available in urban and most suburban areas, rural and underserved communities still have challenges in connectivity.

The next challenge is to push access to the mobile consumer or public health professional, so that information is available to be accessed or entered in the field or at the point of requirement. Next-generation cellular-based telephone networks and handsets will be required to achieve this goal. As described in Chapter 5.3 (Siegel *et al.* 2009), advances in wireless communications will allow important public health applications of information systems to proceed long before hardwired telecommunications services are universal.

Funding availability

In most industrialized countries, the core public health activities of disease prevention and health promotion, as well as primary health care, have historically been underfunded. Paradoxically, information systems development and implementation requires significant initial investments in hardware, software development, network infrastructure, and training before benefits can begin to accrue. This will remain a major hurdle to the broader application of information systems in public health. Public health leaders must therefore become more knowledgeable about information systems (Yasnoff *et al.* 2000) and argue vigorously with policymakers when the long-term benefits of such investments clearly exceed the short-term costs.

Privacy and confidentiality protection

Health data are among the most sensitive of personal information, and organizations that collect it from individuals are obligated to protect it from unauthorized use or disclosure. However, wider applications of information systems in health care mean that more and more personal health data are available in electronic form, and is therefore subject to new and worrisome disclosure risks. Public concerns over protecting the privacy of personal health data are especially strong in countries such as the United States, where the majority of the population is not covered by universal health insurance.

Organizations that collect personal health data, including public health agencies, health services providers, and health-financing organizations, must protect against three different types of confidentiality breaches:

1. Access to stored health information by unauthorized persons. This is accomplished by controlling access to information systems with tools such as passwords and restricted access to the most sensitive types of data.
2. Interception of information while it is being transmitted from the source to the collecting organization, or between organizations. This is accomplished using encryption technology.
3. Sharing of information among organizations without the originating person's full consent. The solution to this problem is not a technological one, but rather requires health organizations to adopt and enforce strict procedures with regard to sharing the information they have collected.

In the United States, federal legislation carrying significant penalties establishes the framework for the protection of consumer health information. The 'administrative simplification' provisions of the Health Insurance Portability and Accountability Act (HIPAA) of 1996 require that health organizations comply with national standards for the protection of health data and electronic sharing ('transactions') of that data.

Data collected through vital statistics systems, disease surveillance, and health surveys are often highly sensitive and personally identifiable. However, there are important public health reasons for making these data as widely available as possible. Agencies that collect such data must therefore strike a balance between easy access and necessary privacy protection. Several techniques are employed to accomplish this. Access to complete data files should be restricted to authorized users working under clear confidentiality procedures. Public-use data files are stripped of all personal identifying information, such as name or address. Because combinations of individual characteristics (e.g. age, race, income, and education) can allow salient individuals to be identified in small population divisions, geographic identifiers in public-use data sets may be very general (e.g. state only).

Conclusion

Information technology, management, and systems support a wide range of public health activities and broader application of information systems can improve our ability to achieve the goals of public health. Rapid technological evolution makes it impossible to predict future trends precisely, but what we can already realistically envision is remarkably exciting. In summary:

- Biomedical informatics and health information science are disciplines that have arisen in response to the flood of data that characterizes health and public health in this century.
- Because information technology allows for collaboration and information sharing beyond physical boundaries, organizations must transform in order to manage their data and information assets wisely and to use them in the most productive manner possible to fulfil their mission and vision.
- Effective information management is critical if organizations are to successfully re-engineer workflow processes to meet the challenges of the next decade.
- Public health organizations, although slower than organizations in other economic sectors, have embraced information technology at multiple levels and an increasing amount of data is collected and disseminated online.
- The Internet has transformed the ability for the public health worker to access multiple data sources and use them for very sophisticated analyses and comprehensive policy development.

References

Aday L.A. *Designing and conducting health surveys: a comprehensive guide*. San Francisco (CA): Jossey-Bass; 1996.

Agency for Healthcare Research and Quality. Medical Expenditure Panel Survey homepage. [Online]. Available from: www.meps.ahrq.gov/ [accessed 2008 Apr 30].

Berkelman R.L., Sullivan P.S., Buehler J.W. *et al.* Public health surveillance. In: Detels R, Beaglehole R, Lansang MA *et al.*, editors. *Oxford Textbook Of Public Health*. 5th ed. Oxford: Oxford University Press; 2009.

Blumenthal D. Part 1: Quality of care—what is it?. *New England Journal of Medicine* 1996;**335**:891–4.

Brook R.H., McGlynn E.A., Cleary P.D. *et al.* Quality of health care. Part 2: measuring quality of care. *New England Journal of Medicine* 1996;**335**:966–70.

California Cancer Registry. Welcome to California Cancer Registry. [Online]. Available from: www.ccrcal.org/[accessed 2008 May 9].

Centers for Disease Control and Prevention. Behavioral Risk Factor Surveillance System (BRFSS). [Online]. Available from: www.cdc.gov/brfss/[accessed 2008 Apr 30].

Centers for Disease Control and Prevention. National Electronic Disease Surveillance System (NEDSS). [Online]. Available from: www.cdc.gov/NEDSS/[accessed 2008 May 7].

Centers for Disease Control and Prevention. National Health and Nutrition Examination Survey (NHANES). [Online]. Available from: www.cdc.gov/nchs/nhanes.htm [accessed 2008 May 5].

Centers for Disease Control and Prevention. National Health Care Survey (NHCS). [Online]. Available from: www.cdc.gov/nchs/nhcs.htm [accessed 2008 Apr 30].

Centers for Disease Control and Prevention. NCHS: mortality data from the National Vital Statistics System (NVSS). [Online]. Available from: www.cdc.gov/nchs/deaths.htm [accessed 2008 May 4].

Centers for Disease Control and Prevention. NCHS: National Health Interview Survey (NHIS). [Online]. Available from: www.cdc.gov/nchs/nhis.htm [accessed 2008 Apr 30].

Centers for Disease Control and Prevention. What is Epi Info™? [Online]. Available from: www.cdc.gov/epiinfo/[accessed 2008 Apr 30].

Centers for Disease Control and Prevention. WONDER. [Online]. Available from: wonder.cdc.gov/[accessed 2008 May 9].

Centers for Medicare and Medicaid Services. Overview—limited data sets. [Online]. Available from: www.cms.hhs.gov/LimitedDataSets/[accessed 2008 May 8].

Chassin M.R. Is health care ready for Six Sigma quality? *Milbank Quarterly* 1998;**76**: 510,565–91.

Chunning C. Disease surveillance in China. *Morbidity and Mortality Weekly Report* 1992;**41**(Suppl):111–22.

Cibulskis R., Izard J. *Monitoring systems. Health policy and systems development: an agenda for research.* Kanovsky J, editor. Geneva: World Health Organization; 1996.

Cooke A. Quality of health and medical information on the Internet. *Clinical Performance and Quality Health Care* 1999;**7**:178–85.

Davidow W.H., Malone M.S. *The virtual corporation: lessons from the world's most advanced companies.* New York (NY): Harper Business; 1992.

Davis G. Evolution of information systems as an academic discipline. *Administrative Sciences Association of Canada conference proceedings.* Vancouver: WBC Press; 1983. p.185–9.

Dick R.S., Steen E.B., Detmer D.E. *et al.*, editors. *The computer-based patient record: an essential technology for health care.* Washington (DC): National Academy Press; 1997.

Donabedian A. *The definition of quality and approaches to its assessment.* Ann Arbor (MI): Health Administration Press; 1980.

Drotman D.P., Strassburg M.A. Infectious disease data: sources and management. In: Thomas J *et al.*, editors. *Epidemiologic methods for infectious diseases.* New York (NY): Oxford University Press; 2001.

Durch J.S., Bailey L.A., Stoto M. *et al.*, editors. *Improving health in the community: a role for performance monitoring.* Washington (DC): National Academy Press; 1997.

Evans R.S., Pestotnik S.L., Classen D.C. *et al.* A computer-assisted management program for antibiotics and other antiinfective agents [see comments]. *New England Journal of Medicine* 1998;**338**:232–8.

Friede A., Rosen D.H., Reid J.A. *et al.* CDC WONDER: A co-operative processing architecture for public health. *Journal of American Medical Informatics Association* 1994;**1**:303–12.

Hammer M. Reengineering work: don't automate, obliterate. *Harvard Business Review* 1990;**68**:104–12.

Hardin Library, University of Iowa. E-resources by subject. [Online]. Available from: www.lib.uiowa.edu/hardin/eresources.asp?subj=124 [accessed 2008 May 9].

Husein K., Adeyi O., Bryant J. *et al.* Developing a primary care information system that supports the pursuit of equity. *Social Science and Medicine* 1993;**36**:585–96.

Institute of Medicine. *The future of public health.* Washington (DC): National Academy Press; 1998.

Kaiser L. Quantum leaps in healing. *Health Forum Journal* 1999;**42**:50.

Kipp W., Kielman A.A., Kwered E. *et al.* Monitoring of primary health care services: an example from Western Uganda. *Health Policy and Planning* 1994;**9**:155–60.

Kuruchittham V., Binka F., Sitthi-Amorn C. *et al.* Information systems and community diagnosis in low- and middle-income countries. In: Detels R., Beaglehole R., Lansang M.A. *et al.*, editors. *Oxford textbook of public health.* 5th ed. Oxford: Oxford University Press; 2009.

Levy A.H. Is informatics a basic medical science? In: Shires D., Wolfe H., editors. Medinfo 1977. Proceedings of the 2nd World Congress on Medical Informatics. Amsterdam: North Holland; 1977. p. 979–81.

Lorenzi N.M., Riley R.T. *Organizational aspects of health informatics: managing technological change.* New York (NY): Springer Verlag; 1995.

Love D. *State data sources.* Los Angeles (CA): Association for Health Services Research Annual Meeting; 2000.

Macro International. MEASURE DHS homepage. [Online]. Available from: www.measuredhs.com/[accessed 2008 May 9].

Mathers C. Global burden of disease: determinants and assessment. In: Detels R, Beaglehole R, Lansang MA *et al.*, editors. *Oxford textbook of public health.* 5th ed. Oxford: Oxford University Press; 2009.

McLaughlin C.P., Kaluzny A.D. *Continuous quality improvement in health care: theory, implementation and applications.* Gaithersburg (MD): Aspen Publishers; 1999.

Meadow C.T. Information science and scientists in 2001. *Journal of Information Science* 1979;**1**:217–21.

Multnomah County Health Department. *Designing a public-private integrated health information system for use in local public health planning and policy development.* Portland (OR): Multnomah County Health Department; 1999.

National Cancer Institute. Cancer information service (CIS). [Online]. Available from: cis.nci.nih.gov [accessed 2008 May 9].

National Committee on Quality Assurance. Healthcare Effectiveness Data and Information Set (HEDIS) and quality measurement. [Online]. Available from: www.ncqa.org/tabid/59/Default.aspx [accessed 2008 May 9].

New York Department of Health. Cardiovascular disease data and statistics. [Online]. Available from: www.health.state.ny.us/statistics/diseases/cardiovascular/[accessed 2008 May 9].

O'Carroll P., Yasnoff W. *et al.*, editors. *Public health informatics and information systems.* Gaithersburg (MD): Aspen Publishers; 2000.

Pan American Health Organization. Regional core health data initiative: table generator system. [Online]. Available from: www.paho.org/english/sha/coredata/tabulator/newTabulator.htm

Pan American Health Organization. Regional core health data initiative. [Online]. Available from: www.paho.org/English/DD/AIS/coredata.htm [accessed 2008 May 1].

Partners in Information Access for the Public Health Workforce. Partners in information access for the public health workforce homepage. [Online]. Available from: phpartners.org/[accessed 2008 May 9].

Protti D.J., editor. A new under-graduate program in health informatics. Proceedings of the AMIA Congress. San Francisco (CA): Masson Publishing; 1982. p. 241–5.

Radford K.J. *Information for strategic decisions.* New York (NY): Reston Publishers; 1978.

Relchertz P. Protokollder Klausurtangung Ausbildungsziele, inhalte und *ethoden in der Medizinischen Informatik* 1973;2:18–21.

RTI International. SUDAAN 9. [Online]. Available from: www.rti.org/sudaan/[accessed 2008 May 9].

Sanders D., Protti D.J. Data warehouses in healthcare: Fundamental principles. *Electronic Healthcare* 2008;**6**(3). [Online]. Available from: www.longwoods.com/product.php?productid=19510&cat=524&page=1 [accessed 2008 May 14].

SAS Institute. SAS: business intelligence software and predictive analytics. [Online]. Available from: www.sas.com [accessed 2008 May 9].

Satia J.K., Mavalankar D.V., Sharma B. *et al.* Micro-level planning using rapid assessment for primary care health services. *Health Policy and Planning* 1994;**9**:318–30.

Sheldon Margin Public Health Library, University of California. Public health resources on the Internet. [Online]. Available from: www.lib.berkeley.edu/PUBL/internet.html [accessed 2008 May 9].

Shortliffe E.H. JBI status report. *Journal of Biomedical Informatics* 2002;**35**:279–80.

Siegel E.R, Wood F.B, Scott J.C. *et al.* Web-based public health information dissemination and evaluation. In: Detels R., Beaglehole R., Lansang M.A. *et al.*, editors. *Oxford textbook of public health.* 5th ed. Oxford: Oxford University Press; 2009.

SPSS. Data mining, statistical analysis software. [Online]. Available from: www.spss.com [accessed 2008 May 8].

STATA Corporation. Stata: data analysis and statistical software. [Online]. Available from: www.stata.com [accessed 2008 May 8].

United States Census Bureau. Mapping and cartographic resources. [Online]. Available from: tiger.census.gov [accessed 2008 May 7].

United States Department of Health and Human Services. Healthy People 2010 homepage. [Online]. Available from: www.healthypeople.gov [accessed 2008 May 9].

United States Department of Health and Human Services. Hospital compare. [Online]. Available from: www.hospitalcompare.hhs.gov [accessed 2008 May 13].

United States Environmental Protection Agency. AIRNow homepage. [Online]. Available from: airnow.gov [accessed 2008 May 9].

United States Geographic Survey. Geographic information systems (GIS) poster. [Online]. Available from: erg.usgs.gov/isb/pubs/gis_poster [accessed 2008 May 9].

University of California. California Health Interview Survey (CHIS). [Online]. Available from: www.chis.ucla.edu/main/default.asp [accessed 2008 May 13].

University of Iowa. Geographical information systems (GIS): improving public health. [Online]. Available from: www.uiowa.edu/~geog/health/ [accessed 2008 May 3].

University of Michigan. Statistical resources on the Web: health. [Online]. Available from: www.lib.umich.edu/libhome/Documents.center/ sthealth.html [accessed 2008 May 9].

University of Washington. Public health toolkit. [Online]. Available from: healthlinks.washington.edu/public_health [accessed 2008 May 9].

Urban Institute. Assessing the new Federalism. [Online]. Available from: www.urban.org/center/anf/nsaf.cfm [accessed 2008 May 8

Van Bemmel J.H. The structure of medical informatics. *Medical Informatics* 1984;**9**:175–80.

Wellner A.S. Casting the health net. *American Demographics* 2000; **22**:46–9.

Wennberg J.E. Understanding geographic variations in health care delivery. *New England Journal of Medicine* 1999;**340**:52–3.

Winker M.A., Flanagin A., Chi-Lum B. *et al.* Guidelines for medical and health information sites on the internet: principles governing AMA web sites. *Journal of the American Medical Association* 2000;**283**:1600–6.

Woodall J.P. Epidemiological approaches to health planning, management, and evaluation. *World Health Statistics Quarterly* 1988;**41**:2–10.

Yasnoff and Sondik 1999

Yasnoff W.A., O'Carroll P.W., Kou D. *et al.* Public health informatics: improving and transforming public health in the information age. *Journal of Public Health Management and Practice* 2000;**6**:67–75.

5.2

Information systems and community diagnosis in low- and middle-income countries

Vipat Kuruchittham, Fred Binka, and Chitr Sitthi-Amorn

Abstract

Effective information systems are the essence of public health planning to improve health status of communities by capturing key information and trends on health problems and their determinants. A frequently used medium to gather health information from several sources (e.g. vital registration and censuses, routine reporting, and surveillance) is information technology, which offers a better and faster mode for data collection, processing, analyses, retrieval, and dissemination. Investing in technology by no means guarantees the desired health outcomes. To successfully implement information systems, public health leaders must understand technology and commit to improve community health status, and involve those who provide health services early in the development of information systems. Effective information systems enhance the ability of public health policy-makers and healthcare providers to employ evidence-based interventions and also enhance their roles in setting priorities and solving problems of communities. Although information systems offer great benefits in improving health, developing and implementing the systems is costly and risky and therefore low- and middle-income countries must prudently consider which investments in technology will meet their needs and means.

Overview

Information is the basis for planning for a rational allocation of resources to address public health problems. Information should shed light on health situations, help to set priorities—among various public health problems, appraise options, develop and implement programmes, and monitor and evaluate actions to determine whether they adequately address the situations. Information is the essence of the planning process. Decision-makers balance evidence from information with their values and societal imperatives to arrive at the best choices. Information includes what is measured, what is not measured, and what is inherently immeasurable. Most information systems, which rely on information technology, collect measurable quantifiable information at the expense of less explicit soft and qualitative information. Therefore, an appropriate mix of quantitative and qualitative information will be needed. Although the information is rarely perfectly accurate, its accuracy can be enhanced through the development of clear operational definitions, training and motivating the personnel gathering information, and interactions with stakeholders to standardize interpretations.

The definition of a community can have many interpretations such as a neighbourhood or a collection of people in a given similar geographical area. A community also refers to a group of people who share the same stakes and common interests such as trade unions, those who are mobilized around a given activity, or the users of health services. Some have even expanded the definition of a community to include those employed in a workplace, the population of a nation, or a civil society. In this chapter, a community can encompass several interpretations such as a village, sub-district, district, province, or nation. A fundamental purpose of an information system is to enhance the ability of decision-makers to employ evidence-based actions and enhance their roles in solving problems of a community however defined. A community is not a static entity; therefore any meaningful information system for the diagnosis of community problems requires a dynamic interaction between the members of the community and the managers of information systems. It is important to make use of the best available information and interpret information into meaningful strategic options that reflect the reality of health and healthcare systems in a given community or society. Any information produced should then be fed back to the community members to enhance their future involvement. This feedback can then be the driving force in linking information to actions because the community will press for the kind of information they can use.

Public health policy-makers and healthcare managers need timely, useful, and balanced information (quantitative and qualitative) for the diagnosis of health needs, their determinants, and trends to achieve effective planning and monitoring of healthcare interventions. This chapter discusses the importance and role of information systems in the evaluation of health problems and their determinants, programme planning, monitoring, and the development and evaluation of intervention options.

The objectives of public health actions

An overall objective of public health actions is to estimate the magnitude of the health problems and their determinants as well as to analyse trends and changing paradigms of these problems and determinants. Because the community consists of heterogeneous groups, the overall objective needs to be expanded to include many value-laden issues such as health needs and determinants, equity, responsiveness to expectations, efficiency, protection of individuals, and fairness. The results of community diagnosis can then be used as evidence for discussion among the stakeholders in the community, balancing the values of the various stakeholders in setting priorities and making decisions for resource allocation acceptable to the community. The priorities and decisions for prevention and control strategies should take into account not only the current status of health but also the impact that controls may have on the health of future generations.

The priorities and decisions for prevention and control strategies depend not only on the indicators used for the diagnosis but also on the explicit or tacit values of a health system. The World Health Organization (WHO) suggested some possible value-laden objectives (Box 5.2.1) of a health system (WHO 2000). Indicators for these value-laden objectives are being developed to measure how well a health system has achieved its objectives.

Improving average health status and reducing the burden of disease

Improving average health status and reducing the burden of disease as measured by life expectancy, death rates by age groups, disease or morbidity rates, and the measurement of the burden of disease combining mortality and morbidity are important functions of public health professionals. The disability adjusted life year (DALY), combining both years of life lost (YLL) and years lost due to disability (YLD) into one measure, is the metric employed by WHO to estimate the global burden of disease. A systematic analysis of world population health data in 2001 showed that five of the ten leading causes of the burden of disease in low- and middle-income countries were communicable diseases including HIV/AIDS, which is the fourth leading cause among low- and middle-income countries and the leading cause in sub-Saharan Africa, whereas all the ten leading causes in high-income countries were non-communicable diseases (Lopez *et al.* 2006).

In addition to monitoring the global burden of disease, there has been an ongoing effort to monitor progress of the eight Millennium Development Goals (MDGs) for 2015 with 48 indicators, 17 of which are health indicators (WHO 2005). Examples of health indicators are prevalence of underweight children under 5 years of age, infant mortality rate, maternal mortality ratio, HIV prevalence among pregnant women aged 15–24 years, prevalence and death rates associated with malaria and tuberculosis, and proportion of population with access to affordable essential drugs on a sustainable basis. Some have suggested that, in their assessment, at least half of the health indicators cannot attract major international attention or investments and that in low- and middle-income countries data availability on these indicators is limited (Murray 2007). Therefore, good information systems are needed to help collect health information essential for health monitoring and planning in low- and middle-income countries.

Box 5.2.1 Possible value-laden objectives of a health system (WHO 2000)

- Improving average health status and reducing the burden of disease
- Reducing health inequity and inequality
- Responding to the legitimate expectations of individuals
- Improving the efficiency of health system
- Protecting individuals and enhancing fairness

Reducing health inequity and inequality

Equity is particularly important if planning involves allocation of resources for health from the public sector. The agencies implementing the plans can be the government or non-governmental organizations supported by the government. In contrast, the private health system does have more responsibility to satisfy individuals who pay for their services, rather than the responsibility for reducing inequities. Therefore, the reduction of health inequities as an indicator does not apply as much to the private sector as to the government system.

Health inequality is linked to the agenda of poverty and material deprivation. The WHO has developed a set of measures for health inequalities including social, household, and individual differences in health. Health inequalities differ in various continents with different stages of human development, as exemplified by the mean life expectancies of 48.8 years in Africa compared with that of 77.4 years in North America in 2000–2005 (Dorling *et al.* 2006). Not only does health inequality differ in different continents, but also differ within a country. For example, there were regional inequalities in life expectancy among administrative regions of Lithuania, where differences among males were up to 10.8 years and among females were up to 7.2 years (Kalediene & Petrauskiene 2000). Measuring inequalities gives health a central theme in the development agenda.

In terms of investment in research, a 10/90 disequilibrium exists between global health expenditures for research and the burden of disease (Global Forum for Health Research 2004). The '10/90 gap' refers to the estimate that less than 10 per cent of global health research funds are spent for research on diseases affecting 90 per cent of the global burden, occurring mainly in low- and middle-income countries. Thus the Global Forum keeps track of health research resource flows to inform decision-makers and funders and plan a more balanced allocation of resources, both globally and locally, according to needs.

Responding to the legitimate expectations of individuals

The legitimate expectations of individuals reflect an attempt to fulfil their right to health services because they are citizens of a country and a community. Legitimate expectations do not include expectations based on self-interest at the expense of the public. Examples of legitimate expectations include the provision of emergency services and services with high public health values such as immunization, preventive and promotive services, and the treatment of infectious diseases.

One measure of the response to the legitimate expectations of individuals is satisfaction with services. Satisfaction has multiple dimensions including access, cost, and quality of care. There are significant differences in the satisfaction with health systems among countries. Satisfaction with health services in the community can also be compared within regions in countries and between the public and private sectors.

Improving the efficiency of health systems

The efficiency of a health system depends on the allocation of resources to services with high public health values (allocative efficiency) and the provision of technically efficient services (technical efficiency) including clinical services. Technical efficiency involves the use of cost-effective services and some form of competition and market mechanism, and therefore can readily apply to the private sector. It is difficult to prescribe the optimal mix between equity, efficiency, and satisfaction with services. The challenges are to use the available resources to best achieve health system goals agreed upon by the society.

There are variations in healthcare expenditures with respect to the gross domestic product of countries. For example, Viet Nam spends more on health as a percentage of gross domestic product than Malaysia in 2003 but has the same life expectancy and higher child mortality than Malaysia (WHO 2007). Some information for planning healthcare has to involve centralized efforts to monitor service standards and to protect the public. Information is needed to monitor financing, to provide services at public and private facilities, and to enable the public to make appropriate choices.

Protecting individuals and enhancing fairness

Protecting individuals and enhancing fairness are two important goals of health. Citizens of a country have a right to a certain level of health regardless of whether they are rich or poor. Rights to health promotion services, disease prevention such as immunization, treatment of emergencies, and acute infections are some examples. Governments can involve the stakeholders to determine the level of health all citizens can have within the constraints of limited resources.

Each of the above five objectives can help direct the development of variables to measure the current health situation as well as to assess changes over time. A good variable has to be reliable, valid, sensitive to change, and credible to the stakeholders.

Although fulfilment of many of these objectives would lead to similar decisions, this may not be true for all cases. For example, coping with inequity by focusing on the health of the underprivileged groups to enhance social justice will require different decisions than improving the average health status of both the elite and the underprivileged groups of the society.

Clear objectives will identify the minimum information needed to make decisions. Clear objectives will help focus on the improvement of an information system to enhance its utility to meet the objectives of the health system. One important argument for not using information for planning is that information is not accurate and that basing a decision on incomplete information can do more harm than good. By having clear objectives, a minimum level of information useful for decision-making can be determined. In the case of inadequate information, efforts can be mounted to collect additional information through various methods, such as a rapid survey or focus group discussions.

Key components and sources of public health information systems

The major components and sources of health information that will need systematic information for planning include: (a) Vital registries and census, (b) morbidity data, (c) risk factor surveillance, (d) health outcomes, (e) health facilities and services, (f) healthcare utilization and costs, and (g) information infrastructure. The contributors and managers of health information for planning can be policy analysts, healthcare providers, epidemiologists, physicians, social scientists, and economists, among others. The gatherers and users of health information are often different people at different levels of the healthcare system. For policy decisions, policy analysts will need information to facilitate policy recommendations. Those who provide health services and have the task of being accountable for the services they provide should also be involved in the development of information system components.

Vital registries and census

Vital registries and census are major sources of public health information maintained by the national statistical offices. Vital registries provide information on births, deaths, and may also include information on marriages and divorces. In addition the registries may provide information on infant and child health by linking birth certificates and death reports. The registries also track population dynamics including information on life expectancy, fertility, and population growth rates.

There are examples in low- and middle-income counties where vital events are under-reported due to the lack of quality assurance of the reporting system, even to document all deaths and their causes. For example, a study comparing four data collection methods to detect deaths in Bavi District, a rural area of Vietnam, showed that the accuracy varied (Huy *et al.* 2003). Quarterly household follow-up was the most accurate method, detecting 99.8 per cent of all deaths, followed by re-census repeated every 2 years (96.0 per cent) and Commune Population Registration System (81.1 per cent), while neighbourhood survey over-reported deaths by 65.6 per cent.

The inaccuracy of death reports and inadequate medical certification of deaths limit the ability to infer the causes of death (e.g. communicable and non-communicable diseases, accidents, injuries, homicides, and suicides), particularly in those occurring outside hospital or clinical settings. When the causes of mortality cannot be defined in majority of cases, verbal autopsy may be used as a method to estimate the causes through data gathered from relatives and friends. Accurately determining the causes of deaths can assist public health professionals in monitoring and measuring the impact of interventions especially in identifying, tracking, and controlling epidemics of emerging infectious diseases.

In addition to vital registries, a census is done every decade to determine socio-demographic profiles, migration, and other population data for a given geographic area. Small area population data from census are essential to government offices such as the ministry of interior to draw boundaries of each administrative unit and the ministry of public health to predict future needs of the public and the resources required.

Morbidity data

Morbidity data are not only indicators of various disease conditions within the population but also indicators of accidents, injuries, homicides, and suicides. Prevalence and incidence are the key measures of morbidity data. Prevalence is defined as the number of persons having a disease at a specific period of time in the population, divided by the number of persons at risk of having a disease at a specific period of time in the population. The difference between prevalence and incidence is that incidence measures only new cases while prevalence includes both new and old cases of disease in the numerator. Problems arise on accurately determining both the numerator and denominator. With existing health systems in most low- and middle-income counties, patients may seek care in more than one place; and double counting is unavoidable as there is no nationwide information system to trace each patient.

Data sources used to calculate prevalence and incidence are most readily available from health facilities such as clinics and hospitals. The numbers or proportions of patients who seek care are commonly presented to indicate the burden of disease. This method has particular appeal because of its simplicity and low cost. If survey information is not available or gives incomplete information, routine reporting from hospitals and health facilities, elaborated in the section **'Routine reporting systems'**, can give information on the health status and burden of disease in a target catchment area that is useful for planning and monitoring health service.

How data sources get reported from the local to the national level is a key area for intervention and disease monitoring. This is especially true for communicable diseases like SARS where timeliness of data is crucial to react, control, and stop the spread of disease. When data come from several sources, a data collection method should be standardized and should provide the simplest way of recording and reporting since healthcare professionals at lower levels of the health system, especially in low- and middle-income countries, are already overloaded with routine work. Data should be reported at the greatest detail possible; for example, reporting of cancer should specify the stage of disease as this information will provide useful information for cancer treatment and prevention programmes.

Morbidity data is also used to track the effectiveness of campaigns such as reduction of accidents from a 'Don't drink and drive' campaign. Moreover having the whole spectrum of morbidity data is useful for health policy planning because the national burden of disease can be determined and healthcare resources can be allocated accordingly. In order to monitor changes over time on the health status of a nation, trend analyses may be performed including plotting trend in prevalence. Figure 5.2.1 shows that HIV prevalence rates have stabilized since 2000 in sub-Saharan Africa even though the actual number of infected individuals continues to increase due to population growth (UNAIDS 2006).

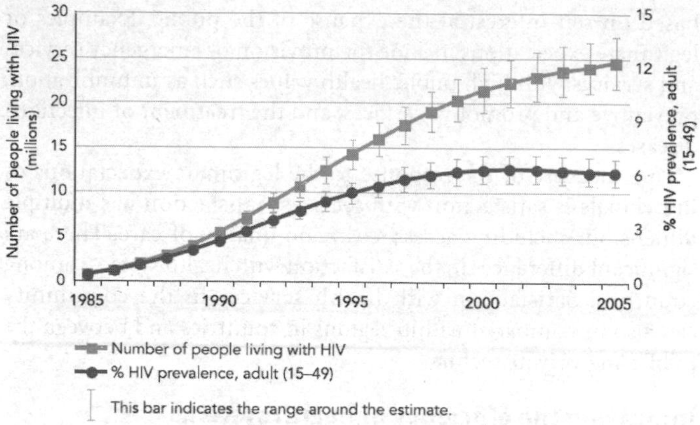

Fig. 5.2.1 HIV epidemic in sub-Saharan Africa, 1985–2005.
Source: UNAIDS 2006.

Risk factor surveillance

Governmental healthcare agencies are periodically encouraged to conduct a large-scale health risk factor survey, which records information on a large number of health-related variables including but not limited to tobacco use, drug use, alcohol intake, exercise or physical activities, diet, cancer screening (e.g. mammography, pap smear, and colonoscopy), healthcare utilization, and existing health conditions such as hypertension and hypercholesterolemia. Risk factor surveys offer useful information especially when combined with existing information being routinely reported by health facilities and collected by vital registries and census.

Information on various risk factors allow researchers to perform epidemiologic investigation to learn not only possible causes of illness and disease but also the effectiveness of intervention programmes (e.g. smoking cessation, cancer screening awareness) being implemented both in a community and nationwide. In addition information on risk factors can be applied to make predictions; for example, risk factors such as sex, age, hypertension, diabetes, and level of physical activity could be used to estimate the probability of developing coronary heart disease (Ma *et al.* 2005). Furthermore periodic information from risk factor surveillance over time can be analysed to track changes in epidemics, health conditions, and health risk behaviours.

Planning of health risk factor surveys is essential to obtain reliable and valid data that are representative of the entire population and to determine how these data can be linked with existing information such as morbidity and mortality rates. For example, data on frequencies of women having mammogram screening can be linked with breast cancer incidence and mortality rates to determine the effectiveness of screening and treatment programmes for early detection of breast cancer. In an effective programme, shifting incidence rates from late to early stages and a decline in mortality rate should be observed. Results from the analysis can be used as evidence to promote good heath behaviours and enact public health policy. Furthermore comparisons across geographic regions may yield new epidemiologic insights on geographic variations observed, and can inspire additional studies on these variations and how to reduce health gaps.

Health outcomes

Traditional outcomes of care are usually measured using mortality and morbidity rates. Although these are important indicators, they do not take into account the impact of diseases and deaths on the individuals and their families as well as on the economic and social well-being of the society. Deaths of young adults have more impact on the productivity of the society than deaths of the incapacitated elderly. Therefore the definition of outcome of care needs to take into consideration the lifetime consequences of diseases, impact of diseases and death, the well-being of society, and productivity.

Health outcomes should not be merely a measure of deaths and disabilities, but the outcomes should capture important domains of health-related quality of life in individuals, including physical and mental status, social networks, and environmental factors. The field of health outcome measurement has been increasingly receiving attention with the realization that there is much more to the overall satisfaction of individuals than what physicians are able to capture through traditional methods. Because individuals have their own values, belief, and preferences, two individuals with exactly the same condition and treatment may feel and rate their health differently. Hence overall health status should be measured by individuals rather than by physicians or others unless they are unable to rate their own health, in which case, relatives or family members may act as a proxy.

Health status measurements can be categorized into generic and disease-specific measurements. Generic measurements provide an overall measure of the individual's health status regardless of age, disease, or treatment over a wide range of the health continuum, whereas disease-specific measurements focus on measuring a particular range of health in detail. Many applications utilize a general health measure, supplemented with a disease-specific measure to capture the individual's health status and to compare this with other groups of diseases or populations. Examples of generic measures include the European Quality of Life Index (EQ-5D), Medical Outcome Study Short Forms (SF-36 and SF-12), World Health Organization Quality of Life (WHO-QOL), Quality of Well-Being scale (QWB), and Nottingham Health Profile (NHP), and some examples of disease-specific instruments are the Alzheimer's Disease Assessment Scale and the McGill Pain questionnaire (Skevington *et al.* 2004; McDowell 2006).

There are two types of measurement scales: Non-preference-based and preference-based. A non-preference-based scale, which utilizes psychometric methods, produces a separate summary score for each health dimension and also aggregates various health dimension scores into a summary score. A preference-based scale which is particularly useful for economic evaluation employs utility theories to produce a single score ranging from 0 (for death) to 1.0 (for full health).

Whenever possible, we should use existing valid and standardized measures and instruments and should avoid developing a new health status instrument because it takes time and resources to construct and validate a new instrument, and it is difficult to make comparisons with previous studies utilizing other instruments.

Health status applications may be applied in many areas including: (a) To monitor health status and establish norms of different disease conditions in the population; (b) to evaluate the effectiveness of treatments, new drugs, or devices by comparing baseline and post-intervention results; (c) to track improvement over time of chronically ill patients; and (d) to estimate the burden of disease in order to inform the health policy agenda.

An example of health status applications is that after tsunami disaster in Thailand, the SF-36, Harvard Trauma Questionnaire (HTQ), and Hopkins Checklist-25 (HSCL-25) were used to measure mental health problems among adults in tsunami-affected areas (van Griensven *et al.* 2006). Results indicated elevated rates of symptoms of post-traumatic stress disorder (PTSD), anxiety, and depression among survivors decreased over time between the period of 2 and 9 months after the tsunami. Another similar study was conducted in the same areas but in children using the UCLA PTSD Retraction Index, Birleson Depression Self-Rating Scale, and tsunami-modified version of the PsySTART Rapid Triage System; the study found a slight decrease in prevalence of PTSD symptoms (Thienkrua *et al.* 2006). These studies showed that health status measures may not only be used to track mental health improvement over time, but also to evaluate the effectiveness of mental health services provided to those affected by the disaster.

Health facilities and services

Health facilities and services play a major role in maintaining and improving the individual's health, which in turn reflects the overall health of a population. The services are provided by both the public and private sectors. While the public sector should provide services to all individuals regardless of their ability to pay, the private mainly targets middle- to high-income groups that are able to pay for faster and better services, even though these may not necessarily yield better outcomes.

Health facilities can be categorized into primary, secondary, and tertiary care units. Primary care units should be the place where everyone seeks the first level of care, but this is not always the case. Many would bypass this first level and go directly to secondary care units where services would be provided by physicians and nurses. With a shortage of health service providers in many low- and middle-income countries, primary care units may be staffed by a couple of nurses and health volunteers with no physicians.

The World Health Report (2006) showed a critical shortage of health service providers in several countries, mostly located in Africa and some parts of Asia. The report also demonstrated that more health workers help save more lives. There were huge gaps in total health workforce, as large as ten-fold, between African countries and countries in America, when comparing health service providers and health management and support workers of low- and middle-income countries with high-income countries. Thus much more trainings of healthcare professionals are needed especially in low- and middle-income countries.

In addition to providing curative care services at different levels, health facilities also provide information on various health indicators that are needed to estimate national burden of disease, and plan for prevention and control of diseases. National guidelines should be established on the kind of information to be reported from facilities, as well as the methods and frequency of reporting. The guidelines should also specify how often reported information will be compiled and analysed to depict the national health status. Moreover health facilities should also take part in promotive services to encourage good health behaviours, which ultimately would reduce burden of curative care.

Healthcare services provided at healthcare facilities may vary across regions in term of quality of care. Responsible offices such as the ministry of public health and accreditation agency should establish a framework for quality and performance assessments of these health facilities. These assessments should be used as key information for improving quality of care rather than as a basis for penalizing poor performing facilities.

Healthcare utilization and costs

In order to efficiently allocate limited healthcare resources, it is important to have information on healthcare utilization and costs. Healthcare utilization or variations in health services can be measured from the perspective of the provider or consumer.

Utilization includes issues of acquisition, diffusion, use, and control of access to health technology.

Variations in service provision can depend on the scheme used to pay healthcare providers (for example, fee-for-service or capitation scheme). The price of certain procedures might be inappropriately increased if the fee-for-service scheme is adapted to the point that the financing system cannot be sustained in the context of a greater emphasis on treatment rather than prevention.

If coverage refers to the degree to which effective provision is given to those who have a real need, it is not always true that more services lead to more coverage. Conversely, hospitals may avoid providing standard services if they are costly, or may not join the programme of healthcare financing schemes if capitation is in place. If the hospitals fail to provide proven efficacious and standard care because the services are too expensive, certain ethical issues may arise. By analysing healthcare utilization and costing information, such issues can be identified.

Individuals who are covered by private healthcare financing schemes might overutilize health resources because they perceive that it is their right to obtain services. Services that are overutilized might lead to inequitable access to services by other low-income groups. On the other hand, under certain healthcare financing schemes, individuals might underutilize services because they may perceive that they are receiving inferior care, or they might overutilize services due to a perception that healthcare is inexpensive with cost being subsidized.

Combining healthcare utilization throughout the nation is a daunting task unless standardization of coding like diagnosis related groups (DRGs) is applied. If healthcare financing schemes were to have health facilities claim their cost of services using standardized coding, abuse of the system may occur by reporting a code with higher remuneration while providing less expensive services.

In addition to healthcare utilization, tracking costs or medical expenditures should not be overlooked. Costs under the various healthcare financing schemes, their trends, the relative proportions of people covered under the various schemes, and the percentage of gross national product used for each scheme need to be assessed in order to monitor and determine the operative efficiency and effectiveness of the programme. Information on costs is also needed to estimate the unit cost of caring for various health conditions, which is important for the allocation of the healthcare budget.

Information infrastructure

Health information infrastructure is a major component of public health planning to improve the effectiveness, efficiency, and equity in health in the nation. Since planning for public health actions needs information, several healthcare organizations have developed their own information systems to serve these needs, but without considering the overall national information infrastructure. Hence information systems often lack inter-operability, which makes data sharing among systems and maintenance difficult. Redundancy of data entry is also unavoidable with independently developed systems because patients may receive care from more than one place. In addition busy healthcare professionals may be averse to the extra burden of filling out data into multiple surveillance report forms from different agencies. Having good information systems would free up time from duplicate paper work, and provide more accurate and timely information needed for health planning.

Due to inter-operability between systems, government agencies such as ministry of public health must play a leadership role in facilitating the participation of all stakeholders in both the public and private sectors in the development of the national health information infrastructure. These government agencies are the body that should specify the standards to be adopted for system inter-operability, and issue legislations and regulations on privacy, confidentiality, and security of information.

The national health information infrastructure is a collection of inter-operable systems linking public health, clinical, and individual health information, which would create a comprehensive evidence-based public health practices. The infrastructure would improve healthcare services as individuals are able to access their personal health information from anywhere, any place, and any time. Not only would the infrastructure provide personalized care, but also enable tracking of population health, including monitoring disease outbreaks.

In addition to inter-operability between systems, issues of privacy, confidentiality, and security of information must be considered when building health information infrastructure. Health information at the individual level must be protected as individuals have basic rights to privacy and informed consent must be obtained before disclosing such information to others. Laws must clearly state how health information at different levels should be handled in order to safeguard privacy, confidentiality, and security of health information. There may be exceptional instances when individual health information may be disclosed, for example, when there is an urgent need to contain pandemics like avian influenza.

All agencies handling health information should apply good practices to secure and protect individuals' information. Security policies include: Who can access and modify the information, how to access and modify the information including audit trails, and a place to securely store the information. The process of ensuring that only authorized users have access to the information is called authentication, which is composed of two major methods: (a) Password management or what users know, (b) physical security or what users have, which may be smart cards or biometrics (fingerprint, retinal scan, face recognition, and voice authentication). While all the information systems should have the basic minimum of password management as a method of authentication, higher security may be implemented using smart cards or biometrics of individuals when the information is highly sensitive.

Building a good infrastructure is not easy as information technology is costly and difficult to implement. It involves several parties including government agencies, healthcare providers, purchasers of healthcare plans, and industries developing information technology. Electronic connections must be established to link organizations and information flows have to be presented in interchangeable formats such as extensible markup language (XML), which supports sharing data across multiple information systems. Although Internet is such an essential medium to ease collection and rapid transfer of surveillance data, Internet access is still limited in low- and middle-income countries. In 2004 the average numbers of Internet users per 1000 people were only 24 and 92 in low- and middle-income countries, respectively, compared to 545 in high income countries (UNDP 2006). This digital divide may be reduced by establishing partnerships between local and international funding agencies as in the case of the Multilateral Initiative on Malaria

Communications Network (MIMCom) in Africa which was established with aims to improve access to the Internet, to facilitate research efforts, and to promote information sharing (Royall *et al.* 2005). The MIMCom network in Africa had grown from two sites in one country in 1997 to 19 sites in 12 countries in 2005.

Benefits of a good national health information infrastructure include: (a) Enhancement of inter-operability between systems due to standardization; (b) faster and more secure reporting of public health data, which reduces response time for public health actions; (c) data warehouse, which generates evidence-based public health information; and (d) reduced redundancy and burden of data entry among overworked health professionals. Although information systems provide numerous benefits, they are good only if health professionals appreciate these benefits and use the system properly. Training of health professionals needs to be given alongside with building the information system.

Information systems and public health in low- and middle-income countries

This section details how several components and sources of public health information can be integrated into systems that would help low- and middle-income countries to effectively identify health problems, plan and monitor health interventions to resolve those problems. The information systems include: (a) Demographic surveillance systems, (b) community key informants, (c) health information systems, and (d) geographic information systems. After describing all the information systems, an example of evidence-based public health is given to demonstrate how collected information can be utilized.

Demographic surveillance systems

Demographic surveillance systems (DSS) and sample registration systems with verbal autopsy offer reasonably good solutions to obtaining vital events such as births and deaths for health policy and planning. DSSs involve continuous longitudinal recording of demographic data usually within small geographically defined populations and on a regular basis. The periodicity of follow-up varies somewhere between monthly household visits (Matlab, Bangladesh) to about yearly visits (Agincourt, South Africa) (Razzaque & Streatfield 2002; Collinson *et al.* 2002). However, for most of the DSSs the average visitation cycle is about three times a year. DSSs start with an initial census to define the baseline denominator population and thereafter continuously monitor this population at well-defined periods of time in order to observe changes or events that occur to or within the initial population. During the routine visits, vital events such as births, deaths, migrations and, in some areas, pregnancies are registered and monitored. Since DSSs follow-up the population at very regular intervals, it is possible to have fairly accurate accounts of individual and household characteristics that allow for almost a near complete capture of vital events in the DSS area.

One major criticism of the DSS is that because it covers small geographical populations, the representativeness of the data may be questioned. However, with the increasing numbers of DSS sites in many countries, they may potentially become sentinel sites that can represent a broader part of the country (for example, in Tanzania, the government has constituted a sentinel system of about five DSS sites located in different parts of the country, which collects data for informing health policy at the national level (Mubyazi & Gonzalez-Block 2005).

A closely related viable solution to the provision of health information is sample vital registration (SVR) with verbal autopsy. Unlike DSSs, SVR involves nationally representative cluster samples with active continuous registration of vital events such as births, deaths, and migrations (Setel *et al.* 2005). Once a death is registered, this is followed by a verbal autopsy to establish the probable cause of death. The difference between SVR and the DSS is that while SVR is based on a nationally representative cluster sample, DSSs are usually based on small well-defined geographical areas such as a district or part of a district and often cover every individual in that geographical entity. SVR is now fully functional in China and India and represents the best source for generating nationally representative vital events such as births and deaths for planning purposes (Setel *et al.* 2005).

Verbal autopsies represent a source of collecting data on causes of death in settings where routine health facility data on causes of death are lacking, particularly in settings where most deaths occur outside of health facilities. The method involves interviewing relatives or caregivers of the deceased persons who were closely associated with the deceased during the period leading to death. In DSSs or in areas where there is a sample registration system, deaths recorded by field workers are followed with a verbal autopsy interview with the caregivers or relatives who were around at the time of death to ascertain the conditions that occurred prior to death. Interviews are based on standardized field-based protocols that seek to elicit information on the illness or health conditions observed or reported by the person prior to death. A panel of physicians reviews the forms and assigns a probable cause of death. A cause of death is assigned based on the concordance of at least two or more physicians. The use of verbal autopsies to ascertain cause of death has proven to be a useful tool to determine the cause of death structure in Africa (Greenwood *et al.* 1987; Snow *et al.* 1992; Ghana Vitamin A Supplementation Trials (VAST) Team 1993). Verbal autopsies have been used extensively in many parts of low- and middle-income countries, particularly in Africa and Asia, to ascertain information on causes of death especially among children and to evaluate the impact of health intervention programmes. The assumption guiding the use of verbal autopsies is that every cause of death has certain observable and distinguishable symptoms that can be recognized and recalled by relatives of deceased persons. Hence verbal autopsies are usually very specific for certain conditions such as accidents, injuries, measles, and stroke.

Community key informants

A major innovation that DSSs have introduced to improve data collection is the use of community key informants (CKI). CKIs are members selected by their communities to work with managers of DSS sites to report on birth and death events within their own communities. The CKIs are usually trusted and respected people and are often privy to events that occur in the community. With basic training on how to record births and deaths in simple notebooks, the CKIs are able to complement routine demographic data collection at the DSS sites. Because they reside in the communities, they are able to record an event first-hand as and when it occurs. This often reduces the time delay between the occurrence of the event and when it is reported, if at all. Thus, the CKIs help to reduce problems of misreporting and recall biases associated with delays in capture.

The novelty in the concept of the CKI is its relation with the routine data collection machinery at the DSS sites. The CKIs do not operate independently of the routine field operations at the sites. They work closely with the field team because field supervisors from the DSS sites visit the CKIs fortnightly to collate possible events recorded over the past 2 or 3 weeks and reconcile these events with those recorded by the routine field workers. Through this process the number of missed events is reduced considerably (Binka *et al.* 1999) and also forestalls falsification of data since the CKI and fieldworkers serve as checks on one another. Hence the quality and integrity of the data are assured.

Health information systems

Health information systems are interdependently connected systems of acquiring, processing, and disseminating of health information. Health information systems integrate several public health systems (e.g. census, surveillance, surveys, and vital registration systems) into a unified system so that information can be easily accessible from a single place and sound policy decision making and planning can be based on knowledge-based information rather than incomplete information from a particular system. For example, to design interventions for chronic diseases and to monitor the progress, morbidity data alone is insufficient and the data must be combined with behavioural risk factor data to allow effective programme to be designed according to the behaviour of the targeted population. In addition health information systems should not be only accessible to public health professionals but health consumers as well.

Health information systems have moved from traditionally paper-based to electronic-based systems utilizing information technology that enables information to be processed much faster and results to be disseminated and shared across our borderless world. Since health information systems integrate information from various sources, standards must be established to allow information sharing between systems. For comparability of information among countries, global health indicators must be established.

Health-related MDG indicators have been widely endorsed as global health indicators to track progress towards the goals by 2015. Low- and middle-income countries have been pressured to strengthen their health information systems to facilitate regular reporting of related indicators as data availability among these countries is very limited. For all health-related MDG indicators data availability was only 15 per cent in low- and middle-income countries during 1990–2005 (Murray 2007). Besides what have been suggested by MDGs, health indicators should include non-communicable diseases, injuries, and their associated risk factors (Boerma & Stansfield 2007).

Although health information systems pose benefits, building health information systems is expensive and low- and middle-income countries may not be willing to invest in them. However these expensive systems were shown to lead to cost savings due to improved system efficiencies and health outcomes; the estimated annual costs per capita for essential information systems ranged from US$0.53 in low-income countries to US$2.99 in high-income countries (Stansfield *et al.* 2006).

To assist low- and middle-income countries in developing their health information systems, the Health Metrics Network (HMN) has been established as a global partnership with the goal to 'increase availability, accessibility, quality and use of health information that are critical for decision making at global and country levels'. HMN also has provided a framework consisting of components, standards, and a road map for implementation to guide overall direction of health information systems (HMN 2006). With well-established health information systems public health policy makers will have reliable, timely, and accurate information to allocate resources, design health programmes, track their progress and impact, and make sound decisions to overall improve health in the nation.

Geographic information systems

Geographic information systems (GIS) are a combination of computer hardware and software used to store, manipulate, analyse, and display spatial or geographic data. GIS had been widely used in many disciplines such as agriculture, forestry, environmental engineering, and urban planning prior to its applications in public health. Today, more public health professionals are aware of the usefulness of GIS; spatial data in small areas are more readily available and technology is more easily accessible.

Years before a personal computer was even invented, mapping of information had been used by John Snow, an English physician who investigated the cause of cholera deaths in central London in 1854 by plotting each cholera death on a map of London neighbourhoods. The finding was that a large number of cases were clustered around a water pump on Broad Street, which Snow hypothesized might be the root of the outbreak. After having the pump removed, the epidemic stopped.

Geographic information systems handle both spatial (map) and non-spatial (attribute) data. Attribute data (e.g. country name, area, and population) are stored in a database and these attribute data are linked to spatial data, which are represented with points, lines, or polygons. Analyses of spatial data using spatial statistics can reveal if point data are randomly scattered or clustered in a specific area, as in the cholera epidemic investigated by Snow. Some examples of GIS applications in public health are: (a) Analysing spatial clustering of health events, e.g. investigation of cancer clusters around an industrial plant; (b) mapping general health information, e.g. display of mammography screening utilization in each province; and (c) analysing access to health services, e.g. finding the shortest path to the closest hospital.

Several GIS tools include choropleth mapping, which assigns different shades or colours to geographic areas according to their values, and geocoding, which automatically matches addresses on the map. For example, choropleth maps were used to display the HIV epidemic in Thailand over the decadal period as shown in Fig. 5.2.2 (Torugsa *et al.* 2003). Darker shading displayed higher prevalence of HIV in men. Figure 5.2.2 shows that initially most high-HIV-prevalence areas were in the upper northern region but prevalence has declined over time, which likely occurred due to effective public health interventions.

Evidence-based public health: An example of utilizing collected information

There are many evidence-based medicine products developed for busy clinicians but few evidence-based public health resources are available for public health practitioners. Evidence-based medicine is defined as 'the conscientious, explicit, judicious use of the current best evidence in making decisions about the care of individual patients' while evidence-based public health focuses on the current

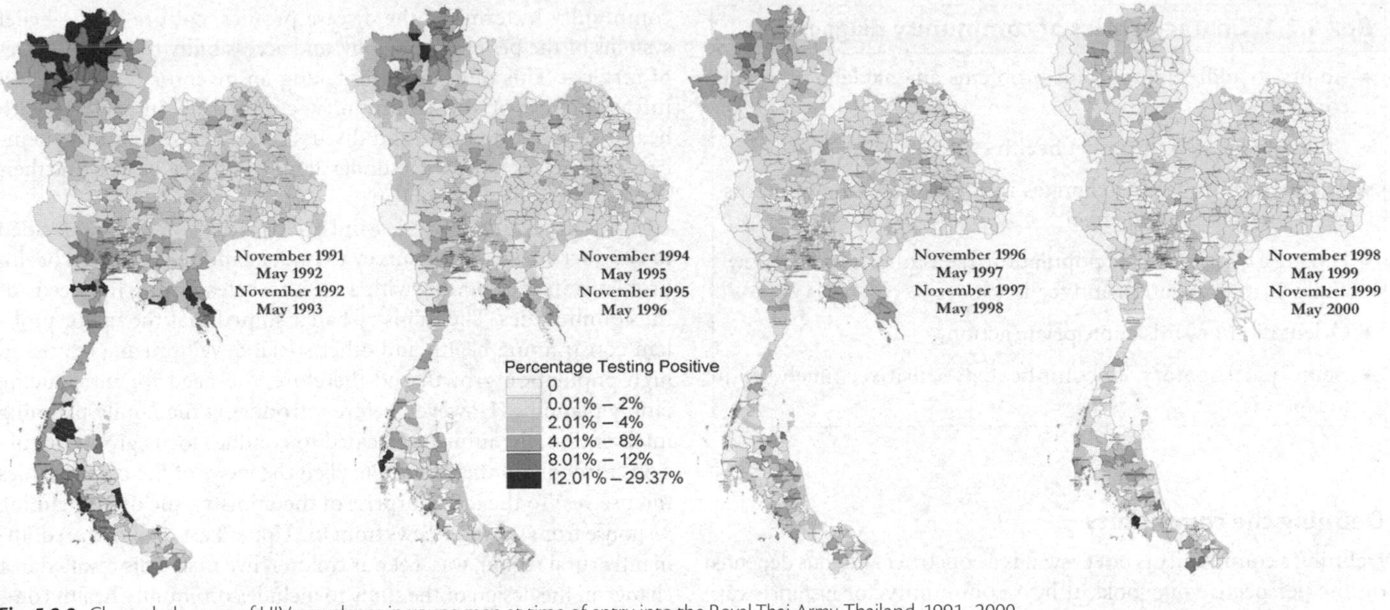

Fig. 5.2.2 Choropleth maps of HIV prevalence in young men at time of entry into the Royal Thai Army, Thailand, 1991–2000.
Source: Torugsa *et al.* 2003.

best evidence in making decisions in routine public health practice, and in developing public health policies and programmes (Sackett *et al.* 1996). Evidence-based public health practice requires integrating practitioner expertise, accumulated public health and basic science knowledge, and regulatory requirements, with the best evidence from systematic research.

Three types of public health evidence are: (a) Definitive clinical and epidemiologic studies of human subjects and populations; (b) consensus of experts based on historical observation and experience in human populations; and (c) findings from basic science research extrapolated to humans. Since the field of public health is very broad and diverse, there are multiple disciplines (knowledge domains) within the field of public health. Some examples of disciplines involved in public health are: Medicine, nursing, epidemiology, statistics, food and nutrition sciences, health economics, environmental engineering, and political science.

To develop evidence-based practice for public health, initial steps are to define the knowledge domains of public health and to identify and assess existing sources of relevant evidence. After having access to existing sources, the next steps are to examine, classify, evaluate existing models for synthesizing evidence and delivering evidence-based contents to public health practitioners, and to identify characteristics of evidence-based medicine synthesis and delivery methods potentially relevant to models for delivery of evidence-based public health contents. The last step is to propose models for synthesis and delivery of current evidence-based public health contents for selected knowledge domains and related practitioner groups. With the abundance of new information available daily, information systems should be implemented in a way that public health practitioners can easily learn and utilize current best practices from evidence-based public health.

With the limited resources that low- and middle-income countries have, public health policy makers should only invest in health promotion and public health strategies that prove to be effective. Although the Cochrane group has provided the most extensive systematic reviews, they have had a limited role in providing evidence-based public health in low- and middle-income countries because: (a) A majority of systematic reviews do not reflect the health priorities of these countries; (b) many effective interventions cannot be applied in resource-poor countries; and (c) a limited number of reviews were conducted in low- and middle-income countries compared to high-income countries (McMichael *et al.* 2005).

The general framework for community diagnosis

The importance of engaging the community in health management has long been recognized and indeed forms a central component of public health practice. After all health is about people and if we view people as part of a community however defined, then the need to understand that community becomes imperative. Public health is as much about facilitating a process whereby communities participate in defining their health needs as it is about providing prevention and treatment for common diseases and conditions. Thus the notion of community diagnosis is grounded in the practice of public health, particularly in relation to primary healthcare. An understanding of the general status of people requires knowledge of the socio-cultural conditions of the people, their belief systems and the social construction of disease, the health-seeking behaviour of the people, ecological and environmental conditions under which they live, and the types of health facilities available and accessible to them, among others. This process of understanding the community constitutes what is generally referred to as community diagnosis. The characteristics defining good community diagnosis include some observable or noticeable attributes in place (Box 5.2.2). The general framework for community diagnosis includes: (a) Defining the community, (b) health needs and situations, (c) health indicators, (d) environmental situation, (e) sources of information and the methods that can be used for community diagnosis, and (f) community involvement in healthcare.

Box 5.2.2 Characteristics of community diagnosis

- Ability to address important problems amenable to practical control
- Ability to identify the target health events
- Adequacy in reflecting changes in the distribution of events over time, place, and person
- Having a clearly defined population, data collection, data flow, analysis, interpretation and feedback
- Orientation towards appropriate action
- Being participatory, uncomplicated, sensitive, timely, and inexpensive

Defining the community

Defining a community is not easy; it is a construct and thus depends on the perspective one looks at it. A community, for instance, can be defined by physical boundaries or distance to a known point so that the people inhabiting that space are referred to as a community irrespective of whether they have shared interests or not. From the sociological perspective, however, a community may refer to a group of people with a common shared interest, characteristics, values, belief systems, or culture, without necessarily having a physical boundary.

However defined, a community usually refers to a target population that shares a common defining factor. In terms of healthcare or service provision, if a community is defined as a geographic entity, then decisions on provision of services require consideration of transient populations such as migrants, whose usual place of residence is different from that geographic entity. On the other hand, if the defining characteristic of a community is based on some criteria other than geography then that criterion becomes the basis for characterizing or mobilizing that community. For instance, we could have a community of gay people, people living with HIV/AIDS, people of a certain religious denomination or sect.

For purposes of health planning or implementation of interventions, one may need specific information about communities, the need to determine the most appropriate way to obtain that information. A large community may require selecting a sample from which the information is collected. However, if the target population or community is small, the researcher or public health practitioners may decide to collect information from the entire population. Depending on the issue of interest in community diagnosis, various measurements may have to be taken, for example: Demographic characteristics, educational infrastructure (schools) and educational attainment, markets, environmental conditions including waste disposal, housing conditions, vector control, nutritional status of the population, and the social environment (MacQueen *et al.* 2001).

Health needs and situations

The needs of a particular community depend on the disease burden of the community and the available health infrastructure (personnel, equipment, and other resources), as well as the socioeconomic configuration of the community. Therefore in defining the health needs of a community, it is imperative to understand the community in terms of the disease profiles, culture or the belief systems of the people, geography, and accessibility to major centres of services. This often requires taking an inventory of the health infrastructure of the community, conducting interviews with health service providers, and discussions with community members themselves in order to understand what they perceive as their most pressing health problems.

For example, in 1991, the Ministry of Health of Ghana decided to conduct a nationwide survey to understand the common health problems in the country with a view to determining the needs of the communities. The ministry had assumed that the major problem constraining health and other social developments related to high population growth and therefore, the need for introducing family planning. However, before introducing the family planning intervention, the ministry decided to conduct focus group discussions throughout the country to elicit the views of the communities themselves. To the utter surprise of the ministry, the overwhelming response from the interviews from the Upper East region, a predominantly rural region, was 'Let our children live first'. This resulted in a change in the design of the study to include community health component, which was not part of the original design of the study. This example illustrates the fact that in determining what the health needs of a community are, the communities themselves would have to be consulted (Binka *et al.* 1995).

Health indicators

Health indicators are standardized measures that are used to determine the health status of a population, and to support health authorities and providers to monitor and evaluate the performance level of the health system. In measuring the quality of a health system as well as the health of the population itself, one has to consider factors such as major non-medical determinants of health, the quality of health services received, and characteristics of the community or the health system.

Health indicators are usually expressed in crude or adjusted age-specific mortality rates as well as other indicators of well-being of a population. Common health indicators include age-specific mortality rates (e.g. infant mortality rates, mortality of children under 5 years of age, maternal mortality rates). Other mortality indicators include probabilities of dying at various adult ages, for example, the probability of dying between age 15 and 60, which is an indicator of adult mortality. One other important health indicator commonly used is life expectancy at birth for males and females. Non-mortality indicators include healthy years of life lived, years of life lost to specific diseases and to injuries.

Environmental situation

The environment has a direct impact on health. The three major components of the environment— physical, biological, and social— all affect and are affected by humans. The physical environment, which comprises the non-living part of the environment, includes things like the soil, air, water, minerals, and climate. The biological environment on the other hand is made up of the living aspects of the earth and includes things like plants, animals, and other micro-organisms while the social environment is entirely man-made and represents the case of man as a member of society. It does include things like social organization, the family, the community, cultural aspects such as the belief system, the laws, education, social services, healthcare, politics, and governance.

Understanding the environment is important in community diagnosis because community diagnosis seeks to understand the different facets of the community, including the environment and how these impact on the health of the people. To understand the community thus requires an understanding of the environment. To do that, public health practitioners need to collect data on the different facets of the environment such as climate and rainfall patterns, the vegetation, water sources and quality, waste disposal, construction sites, and animal reservoirs. In addition, there is a need to gather information on housing types, toilet facilities, pollutants, food hygiene, etc. An understanding of these environmental factors will help in the diagnosis of the community with respect to the provision of health.

Sources of information and the methods that can be used for community diagnosis

Information for public health policy and planning generates from several sources (Box 5.2.3). While each of these sources of data are important and complementary, they all have their strengths and shortcomings. For instance, while both censuses and nationally representative sample surveys tend to have a national character, censuses cover the entire population in the country while national sample surveys (e.g. demographic and health surveys) are usually made up of a representative sample of the population. However, both sources are often unable to adequately register vital events such as births and deaths. Details of these different information sources are discussed in the succeeding sections.

Routine reporting systems

Although it is widely recognized that accurate statistics on births and deaths are critical to rational policy formulation, data on such vital events are lacking in most low- and middle-income countries, particularly in Africa. The most widely available source of health statistics is from health facility records. Data are captured from patients presenting at health facilities for treatment. This information can provide a general picture of the burden of disease in the catchment area of the facility. Health managers can use this information for their planning in the absence of survey or other population level health information.

Analysis of data from routine reports can signal a disease outbreak in an area. For instance, an unexpected increase in the number of routinely reported cases of meningitis in one year to the next would signify an outbreak of meningitis. In this scenario, routine annual monitoring of cases reported is the key indicator of a potential outbreak.

Box 5.2.3 Sources of information and methods for community diagnosis

- Routine reporting systems
- Surveys
- Surveillance
- Routine screening
- Contact tracing
- Vital registration and censuses

Information from routine reports of a key facility for the treatment of drug-dependent patients in Thanyarak Hospital (Thailand) indicated that the spread of HIV seroprevalence among drug users occurred first in the central region of Thailand including Bangkok, followed by the north, the south, and the northeast.

On the other hand, routine reports are fraught with certain biases. Attendance at health facilities depends on several factors including geographic, financial, and cultural considerations. Thus there may be selection bias when only routine reports from facilities are used. In addition one cannot determine the population at risk from routine reports, hence rates cannot be calculated.

Surveys

Surveys are social and epidemiological tools that are used to capture specific information, either in one snapshot, or where there is need to monitor trends over time, in repeated waves at specified intervals. In public health or epidemiological studies, practitioners, health managers, or public health specialists may wish to have a deeper understanding of a particular health issue or a series of issues that may have emerged from either routine surveillance or findings from other settings. Surveys may also help elucidate the cultural context and the belief system relating to a particular health problem.

In designing surveys one may have to consider several factors. What is the question that the survey aims to answer? How do I design my survey instrument to capture information that will allow me to answer that question? Who is the target population? Is there a need to stratify the population? What is the sample size that is required to reach a scientifically sound conclusion? Is the sample representative? There is also a need to make plans for the dissemination of the survey results in order to affect policy.

In conducting surveys the community must be active participants and must be engaged very early in the process. Very often in disseminating survey results the community members are not involved. Community members must be seen as active participants in the entire process, especially when the attitude or behaviour of the community is the focus of health programmes. For example, public health practitioners and researchers in northern Ghana were interested in knowing whether lay counsellors could be used to promote voluntary counselling and testing (VCT) for HIV/AIDS in a rural setting where there was a shortage of health workers. A special survey was conducted to determine the feasibility of this concept. Results showed that it is possible to use lay counsellors to promote VCT services in settings where health personnel are in short supply (Baiden *et al.* 2007).

Surveillance

Surveillance involves the maintenance of an ongoing disease monitoring system in order to provide timely information on the occurrence or outbreak of a disease. Surveillance can be on a large scale involving whole communities or restricted to specific groups and can either be passive or active depending on the potential transmissibility of the disease in question. Surveillance can also be in the form of sentinel reporting. Diseases that are often put under routine surveillance include those that have the potential of exploding into epidemics and need to be monitored closely so that intervention mechanisms are put in place to forestall extensive spread. Active surveillance can be a costly endeavour, hence most countries usually have a passive system of surveillance.

Sentinel surveillance, which involves a selection of specific facilities where routine information is collected on specific disease conditions,

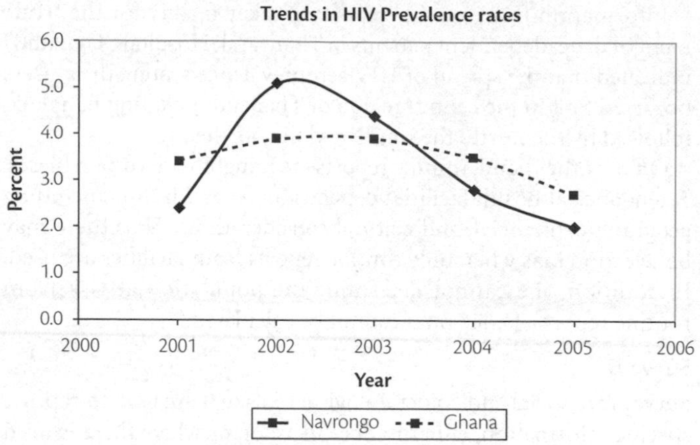

Fig. 5.2.3 Trends in HIV prevalence rates of selected sentinel sites in Ghana. *Source*: National AIDS/STI Control Programme Ghana Health Service 2004.

is one way of keeping costs down. For example, in Ghana 40, centres have been set up as sentinel points to monitor the prevalence of HIV in the country (Fig. 5.2.3). On the other hand, while surveillance traditionally was used mainly in the monitoring of disease epidemics, surveillance has now been extended to the monitoring of biological and chemical reactions, including the use of chemical toxins and other chemical effects on humans.

Routine screening

The objective of screening is to allow for early detection of health conditions or risk factors associated with disease conditions. Screening is important in chronic diseases such as hypertension, diabetes, cancers of the breast and cervix in women, and prostrate cancers in men. The target for screening can be the general population or specific high-risk groups. It is also useful in screening infected but asymptomatic individuals. For example, genital chlamydial infection is a common sexually transmitted infection that is often asymptomatic, but associated with long-term morbidity in many women. Early infection can be diagnosed reliably using non-invasive methods and treated effectively with antibiotics. Screening for genital chlamydial infection in high-risk settings, such as genitourinary medicine and abortion clinics has been documented to be effective (Stephenson 1998).

In deciding to undertake screening there must be obvious benefits to both the patients and the general public as a whole. For instance, if screening is mandatory for a particular disease then health authorities will have to provide treatment if a patient is found to have one of the conditions for which the screening is instituted. Also, screening has the potential to identify risk factors for certain disease conditions. Early detection can lead to appropriate interventions such as reduction in weight or appropriate dietary restrictions in high blood pressure patients, thereby reducing the burden of the disease.

Contact tracing

Contact tracing is particularly useful when information from routine systems and surveillance suggests the need for a clarification of the pattern of the disease spread. It is also useful to estimate acute illness episodes and disease problems among illegal migrants and mobile ill-defined populations such as tourists and migrant workers. The purposes of contact tracing (community visiting team) are: (a) To confirm diagnosis and determine aetiology; (b) to determine the pattern of risk behaviours; (c) to estimate the magnitude of health problems; (d) to identify possible control measures; (e) to identify where and to whom to apply control measures; and (f) to recommend control measures.

Contact tracing increases the validity of the estimate of the magnitude of a health problem by allowing cases who failed to receive health services from health facilities to be included. In addition contact tracing can enable better targeting of control measures, leading to increased efficiency of the health system.

Vital registration and censuses

Although it is widely recognized that accurate statistics on births and deaths are critical to rational policy formulation, data on such vital events are lacking in most low- and middle-income countries, particularly in Africa. Vital registration systems, which typically record many of these events, are non-existent in many countries. Even where they exist, they are fragmented, incomplete, and often limited in coverage. Health facility records are limited in coverage because many births and deaths occur outside health facilities, which means that for such individuals there is no record of either their birth or death, much less the cause of death. Thus for the limited cases captured through the health system, they are invariably fraught with selection bias because the health facilities are often only accessible to the well-to-do, certain segments of the population that have better geographic access, or those reached by specific projects that proactively encourage recording of specific events.

Vital registration systems are premised on the notion that all persons will voluntarily report vital events such as births or deaths to a central agency, in most cases the national statistical agencies or the birth and death registry, as is the case in some countries. Registration systems are often passive in nature, i.e. they rely on the goodwill of the population or the enlightened few who proactively seek to register events such as births and deaths. The laissez-faire attitude to registration results from the fact that there are no penalties for non-registration and no rewards for registration. Thus, to the extent that registration systems remain passive without penalties for non-compliance, vital events capture will remain low.

Community involvement in healthcare

One of the cardinal principles in public health is community involvement in healthcare delivery. If public health programmes are ever to make an impact, communities for which programmes are designed must be involved and brought to the forefront as active participants in the delivery of healthcare. Community involvement comes in different forms and levels. One form is actual involvement in control programmes. For instance, if there is an epidemic, the community must be actively mobilized, sensitized, and assigned roles so that they become part of the control strategy. The community has to understand its role in stemming further disease spread from infected members to uninfected members and in managing those already infected. Another level of community involvement is using community agents or representatives as part of the frontline staff in health promotion and delivery. For example, the Ghana Health Service (GHS) launched in 2004 a programme for transforming clinic-based primary healthcare and reproductive health services to community-based health services. Known as the Community-based Health Planning and Service (CHPS), the programme promotes the idea that communities can be active participants in the provision of their own healthcare. CHPS places community health officers (CHOs) and volunteers in all 138 districts of the country to provide basic health services to all communities in Ghana. The CHOs and volunteers live and work in the communities providing door-to-door services to individuals within households. The CHPS programme is the government of Ghana programme of action to get communities involved in the delivery of healthcare (Nyornator *et al.* 2005).

Conclusion

Low- and middle-income countries must invest in resources to capture essential information and trends on health problems. This will help to decide whether investments in the healthcare system will yield the desired health outcomes. These countries must not be trapped into investing in high technology for sophisticated information systems that are beyond their needs and means. We propose some guidelines for making decisions on information system projects. First, system users must be involved from the beginning in order to establish a clear and realistic goal. Second, a comprehensive review of existing solutions must be done before decisions on high-technology investments are made. Third, some assurance of adequate support and continuity from the vendor must be obtained since low- and middle-income countries will be very dependent on the support system. Finally, the reality of organizational constraints on the systems must be taken into account, for example, the adequacy of human resources to operate the system. Therefore, it is important to 'think big' (holistic manner), 'start small' (adopt an evolutionary not a 'big bang' approach), and 'act rationally' in order to advance the objectives of the healthcare system (Wyatt 1994).

References

Baiden, F., Akanlu, G., Hodgson, A. *et al.* (2007). Using lay counsellors to promote community-based voluntary counselling and HIV testing in rural northern Ghana: A baseline survey on community acceptance and stigma. *Journal of Biosocial Science*, **5**, 1–13.

Binka, F.N., Nazzar, A., and Phillips, J.F. (1995). The Navrongo community health and family planning project. *Studies in family Planning*, **26**, 121–39.

Binka, F.N., Ngom, P., Phillips, J.F. *et al.* (1999). Assessing population dynamics in a rural African society: The Navrongo Demographic Surveillance System. *Journal of Biosocial Science*, **31**, 373–91.

Boerma, J.T. and Stansfield, S.K. (2007). Health statistics now: Are we making the right investments? *Lancet*, **369**, 779–86.

Collinson, M., Mokoena, O., Mgiba, N. *et al.* (2002). Agincourt demographic surveillance system, South Africa. In *Population and health in developing countries*, INDEPTH Network.

Dorling, D., Shaw, M., and Smith, D.G. (2006). Global inequality of life expectancy due to AIDS. *British Medical Journal*, **332**, 662–64.

Ghana Vitamin A Supplementation Trials (VAST) Study Team (1993). Vitamin A supplementation in northern Ghana: Effects on clinical attendance, hospital admissions, and child mortality. *Lancet*, **342**, 7–12.

Global Forum for Health Research (2004). *The 10/90 report on health research 2003-2004*. Global Forum for Health Research, Geneva.

Greenwood, B.M., Greenwood, A.M., Bradley, A.K. *et al.* (1987). Deaths in infancy and early childhood in a well-vaccinated rural West African population. *Annals of Tropical Paediatrics*, **7**, 91–9.

Health Metrics Network (2006). *Health Metrics Network framework and standards for the development of country health information systems*. WHO, Geneva.

Huy, T.Q., Long, N.H., Hoa, D.P. *et al.* (2003). Validity and completeness of death reporting and registration in a rural district of Vietnam. *Scandinavian Journal of Public Health*, **31** (Suppl. 62), 12–18.

Kalediene, R. and Petrauskiene, J. (2000). Regional life expectancy patterns in Lithuania. *European Journal of Public Health*, **10**, 101–4.

Lopez, A.D., Mathers, C.D., Ezzati, M. *et al.* (2006). Global and regional burden of disease and risk factors, 2001: Systematic analysis of population health data. *Lancet*, **367**, 1747–57.

Ma, T., Jong, G.P., Ueng, K.C. *et al.*(2005). Establishing a prediction model for coronary angiography based on coronary risk factors. *International Heart Journal*, **46**, 57–68.

MacQueen, K.M., McLellan, E., Metzger, D.S. *et al.* (2001). What is community? An evidence-based definition for participatory public health. *American Journal of Public Health*, **91**, 1929–38.

McDowell, Ian (2006). *Measuring health: A guide to rating scales and questionnaires*. Oxford University Press, New York.

McMichael, C., Waters, E., and Volmink, J. (2005). Evidence-based public health: What does it offer developing countries? *Journal of Public Health*, **27**, 215–21.

Mubyazi, G. and Gonzalez-Block, M. (2005). Research influence on antimalarial drug policy change in Tanzania: Case study of replacing chloroquine with sulfadoxine-pyrimethamine as the first-line drug. *Malaria Journal*, **4**, 51.

Murray, C.J. (2007). Towards good practice for health statistics: Lessons from the Millennium Development Goal health indicators. *Lancet*, **369**, 862–73.

National AIDS/STI Control Programme Ghana Health Service (2004). *HIV Sentinel Survey Report 2003*. Ghana AIDS Commission, Ghana.

Nyonator, F.K., Awoonor-Williams, J.K., Phillips, J.F. *et al.* (2005). The Ghana community-based health planning and services initiative: Fostering evidence-based organizational change and development in a resource-constrained setting. *Health Policy Planning*, **20**, 25–34.

Razzaque, A. and Streatfield, K. (2002). Matlab demographic surveillance system, Bangladesh. In *Population and Health in Developing Countries*, INDEPTH Network.

Royall, J., van Schayk, I., Bennett, M. *et al.* (2005). Crossing the digital divide: The contribution of information technology to the professional performance of malaria researchers in Africa. *African Health Sciences*, **5**, 246–54.

Sackett, D.L., Rosenberg, W.M., Gray, J.A. *et al.* (1996). Evidence based medicine: What it is and what it isn't. *British Medical Journal*, **312**, 71–2.

Setel, P.W., Sankoh, O., Rao, C. *et al.* (2005). Sample registration of vital events with verbal autopsy: A renewed commitment to measuring and monitoring vital statistics. *Bulletin of the World Health Organization*, **83**, 561–640.

Skevington, S.M., Sartorius, N., and Amir, M. (2004). Developing methods for assessing quality of life in different cultural settings. The history of the WHOQOL instruments. *Social Psychiatry and Psychiatric Epidemiology*, **39**, 1–8.

Snow, R.W., Armstrong, J. R., Forster, D. *et al.* (1992). Childhood deaths in Africa: Uses and limitations of verbal autopsies. *Lancet*, **340**, 351–5.

Stansfield, S.K., Walsh, J., Prata, N. *et al.* (2006). Information to improve decision making for health. In *Disease control priorities in developing countries* (eds. D.T. Jamison, J.G. Breman, A.R. Measham *et al.*),2nd edItion. Oxford University Press and The World Bank, New York.

Stephenson, J.M. (1998). Screening for genital chlamydial infection. *British Medical Bulletin*, **54**, 891–902.

Thienkrua, W., Cardozo, B.L., Chakkraband, S. *et al.* (2006). Symptoms of posttraumatic stress disorder and depression among children in tsunami-affected areas in southern Thailand. *Journal of the American Medical Association*, **296**, 549–59.

Torugsa, K., Anderson, S., Thongsen, N. *et al.* (2003). HIV Epidemic among young Thai men, 1991–2000. *Emerging Infectious Diseases*, **9**, 881–3.

United Nations Development Programme (2006). *Human Development Report 2006*. UNDP, New York.

United Nations Programme on HIV/AIDS (2006). *2006 Report on the global AIDS epidemic*. UNAIDS, Geneva

van Griensven, F., Chakkraband, S., Thienkrua, W. *et al*. (2006). Mental health problems among adults in tsunami-affected areas in southern Thailand. *Journal of the American Medical Association*, **296**, 537–48.

World Health Organization (2000). *Health systems: Improving performance*. WHO, Geneva.

World Health Organization (2005). *Health and the Millennium Development Goals*. WHO, Geneva.

World Health Organization (2006). *World health statistics 2006*. WHO, Geneva.

World Health Organization (2006). *Working together for health*. WHO, Geneva.

World Health Organization (Accessed Feb 11, 2007). Countries: Statistics [Web Page]. Available at: http://www.who.int/countries/en/.

Wyatt, J.C. (1994). Clinical data systems, part 3: Development and evaluation. *Lancet*, **344**, 1682–8.

5.3

Web-based public health information dissemination and evaluation

Elliot R. Siegel, Fred B. Wood, John C. Scott, and Julia Royall

Abstract

This chapter focuses on the current status of what is called Web-based health information dissemination. The chapter highlights the proliferation of Web sites for public health organizations and institutions of all types that has occurred in recent years. The chapter next addresses the dramatic potential of Web-based applications for Emergency Preparedness and Disaster Management for all countries, whether high-, middle-, or low-income. This includes the use of Web-based networks of satellites, sensors, data mining, and analytics.

The chapter presents two case studies on emergency preparedness: Wireless Information System for Emergency Responders (WISER); and Central American Network for Disaster Health Information (CANDHI). The chapter then discusses a major Web-based health application in low-income countries—the Health InterNetwork Access to Research Initiative (HINARI); and provides an update on the Multinational Initiative on Malaria (MIM) and its use of Web-based dissemination of scientific research.

Finally, the chapter presents a multidimensional approach to Web evaluation that includes methods to determine: (1) How well the Web sites are meeting customer or citizen needs; and (2) what design, content, functionality, and performance improvements may be needed to better meet user needs.

The Web will continue to grow as an important part of the public health information infrastructure in many countries. The key role of the Web can exacerbate the digital divide, to the extent access and use are more heavily concentrated in urbanized and higher income areas. On the other hand, the Web can help improve access to public health information much more broadly than was possible in the pre-Web era. Given the growing role of the Web in public and consumer health, a robust approach to Web evaluation is important.

Introduction

In the last decade, the Internet and World Wide Web (Web) has revolutionized the process by which public and consumer health information is disseminated to users. The Internet has evolved from a niche technology in the early 1990s to a strong presence in the post-industrial nations by the late 1990s, to what is now a dominant global position in information networking and access of all sorts. The Internet is the technology pathway over which the information flows, and the Web is the key to accessing this information. The Web is a system of interlinked, hypertext documents accessed via the Internet. With a Web browser, a user views Web pages that may contain text, images, and other multimedia and navigates between them using hyperlinks for Web access.

The Web revolution is now spreading to the recently industrialized nations and most developing nations. Web traffic in the more mature user nations is growing more slowly due to the high levels of earlier growth and the beginning of market saturation. This is the familiar 'S curve' of technological innovation. The greatest rates of growth are now in countries such as the People's Republic of China and India.

In the post-industrial nations, the health sector is one of the largest user segments on the Web. In the United States, surveys estimate that 40–50 per cent or more (some estimate up to 80 per cent) of Web users search for health information: For themselves and their families and friends, and as professionals for scientific, research, healthcare provision, and administrative purposes (Abreu, M., Cybercitizen Health, 2006 survey results, Manhattan Research LLC; Fox 2005, 2006; Madden & Fox 2006).

Among the more advanced technological nations, almost all major public health departments at the Federal and many State (or Province) levels have Web sites, as do virtually all of the health and biomedical research and scientific institutions. Likewise, many of the major healthcare provider institutions also have Web sites, and increasingly are using Web sites to provide information in support of patient care. In the United States, a growing percentage of physician and other provider practices are using Web sites or referring patients to other Web sites (Abreu, M., Taking the Pulse, 2006 survey results, Manhattan Research LLC; Siegel *et al.* 2006).

The advent of Web-based dissemination of public and consumer health information for myriad purposes has generated a need to make sure that these information services are well designed and user friendly. While Web evaluation lags well behind Web applications, evaluation is a revolution in the making.

Much of the information in this chapter is based on the domestic and international experience of the US National Library of Medicine (NLM). The NLM is the largest biomedical library in the world, and operates some of the most heavily used US Government consumer health and biomedical Web sites, such as MedlinePlus and PubMed/MEDLINE. NLM is an operating unit of the US National Institutes of Health (NIH), which is part of the US Department of Health and Human Services (HHS).

The intent of the chapter is to provide an overview of major aspects of the revolution in Web-based public health information dissemination and evaluation. The material presented should be applicable to public health, consumer health, and biomedical research organizations in all parts of the world that make significant use of Web-based information dissemination.

Public health information on the Web

Globalization of Web usage

The last 5 years have witnessed the maturation of the Web, as Internet connectivity has spread from the major urban centres in high-income countries to widespread availability in those countries, including small towns and some rural areas, plus connectivity in the urban centres of many low- and middle-income countries. Rural and remote areas still have limited Internet connectivity in low- and middle-income countries and even to some extent in high-income countries including the United States.

The Internet World Stats organization tracks Internet use by global region and on a country-specific basis. As of June 2007, the data highlight that Africa is still far underrepresented in Internet usage, and to a lesser extent the Middle East and Asia. North America has by far the heaviest concentration of Internet usage, and, to a lesser extent, Europe (see Table 5.3.1).

Analysis of country-specific data indicates that there are many African, Middle Eastern, and Asian countries still with very low levels of Internet use. In this sense, the digital divide still exists for most low- and middle-income countries. Maps of global Internet bandwidth likewise show very large bandwidth available for the United States and Europe, and large bandwidth for East Asia. Comparatively, the rest of the world has limited bandwidth (see www.telegeography.com).

The digital divide is generally considered to be a function of several variables, including low per capita income and educational levels, a low-tech culture, and inadequate political support, as well as limited computer and Internet availability and bandwidth (Peters 2001).

Notwithstanding digital divide issues, NLM's usage data on its own Web sites document the inevitable trend toward globalization of Web users. NLM's two most heavily used Web sites are PubMed (www.pubmed.gov, for accessing MEDLINE, the bibliographic database of the biomedical and health research literature), and MedlinePlus, a consumer health information portal (www.medlineplus.gov). Non-US users now account for over one-half of PubMed unique visitors per month and about one-third of MedlinePlus unique visitors.

comScore/MediaMetrix, a major Internet audience measurement company, estimates that as of early 2007, about 80 per cent of total global Web usage for home users (users accessing the Web from a home computer) was non-US, and about 20 per cent was US. Thus overall Web usage is already heavily dominated by countries other than the United States (Fisher, L., comScore Health Information Usage Reports, 2007; Wood *et al.* 2005).

Within the health information sector for home users, the US versus non-US usage split is less dramatic, with about 60 per cent non-US and 40 per cent US, averaged across numerous Web sites. To some extent, US Web site usage is magnified so long as a disproportionately large percentage of leading Web sites in a given topic area are based in the United States. Non-US users account for over 90 per cent of *MedlinePlus en espanol* usage (http://medlineplus.gov/spanish), apparently because thus far *MedlinePlus en espanol* is perceived as a leading health information Web site within the Spanish-speaking user community regardless of country. Typically, for *MedlinePlus en espanol*, about one-fifth of the users are from Mexico and one-fifth from Spain, one-tenth from Peru, and one-twentieth from Chile and Colombia.

As of 2007, US National Institutes of Health Web sites, including NLM's, as a group constitute the most heavily used international source of health information on the Web. This is presumed to be because of the highly regarded and non-commercial nature of NIH and its Web sites, and the widespread use of English as a common language in the health sector. It may also reflect the concerted effort that some NIH Web sites have made to implement Web evaluation, including user feedback, to improve their Web presence. (See the last section of this chapter for a discussion of Web evaluation.)

Going forward, it is likely that health sector usage of the Web will continue to increase globally, and that the relative non-US share will also increase, as low- and middle-income countries get better connected to the Internet infrastructure and develop their own health Web sites. At present, less than one-sixth of the world population uses the Web, and the vast majority of the non-using population lives in sub-Saharan Africa, the Middle East, Eastern Europe, Central and South Asia, and parts of East and Southeast Asia. Many of the countries in these regions speak English as a second or third language, if at all. These countries with developing or transitional economies can be expected to eventually develop more health Web sites in their native languages.

Table 5.3.1 Distribution of Internet usage and penetration by global region (as of June 2007)

World Region	% World population	% World Internet usage	% Internet penetration
Africa	14.2	2.9	3.6
Asia	56.5	36.0	11.0
Europe	12.3	28.2	39.4
Middle East	2.9	1.7	10.0
North America	5.1	20.4	69.0
Latin America/ Caribbean	8.5	9.0	18.4
Ocean/Australia	0.5	1.7	54.4

Source: Internet World Stats, 2007, http://www.internetworldstats.com/stats.htm

% World Internet usage = Percentage of total world Internet usage accounted for by use from the specified world region.

% Internet penetration = Percentage or regional population that used the Internet.

A health Web overview

The US Food and Drug Administration (FDA) has compiled a list of nations with one or more publicly accessible Web sites for health departments or ministries, and also Web sites related to food and drugs.

The length of the list is yet another indicator of how pervasive the Web has become in the health arena (see http://www.fda.gov/oia/agencies.htm):

- Asia and the Pacific—19 countries with 55 health department or similar Web sites
- Europe—38 countries with 126 Web sites
- Middle East—8 countries with 16 Web sites
- Africa—16 countries with 32 Web sites
- Americas—25 countries with 55 Web sites (not including the United States)

Based on the FDA list, it would appear that about 95 countries have Web sites for their main health department or ministry. Most are in English or have an English option. Some are in the native language only (e.g. Russian, Chinese). In addition, most international health organizations have a major Web presence. Examples include the: World Health Organization (http://www.who.int/en); Pan American Health Organization (http://www.paho.org); and European Commission on Health and Human Protection (http://ec.europa.eu/dgs/health_consumer/index_en.htm).

In addition to national and international health-related Web sites, in some countries such as the United States, many state or provincial level health departments or the equivalent have their own Web sites. The US Centers for Disease Control and Prevention has compiled the Web sites for all US state-level departments of health and makes that information available via a Web-based clickable map (see http://www.cdc.gov/mmwr/international/relres.html).

In addition, the NLM in the United States coordinates a National Network of Libraries of Medicine that includes about 6000 medical libraries at medical schools, hospitals, health clinics, and health information centres in all regions of the country (http://www.nlm.nih.gov/network.html). Most of these US medical libraries and the larger medical facilities have one or more Web sites. NLM also coordinates a GoLocal Network that links information on local healthcare facilities and health provider services in 18 States, and some of these local facilities and providers have Web sites as well (http://www.nlm.nih.gov/medlineplus/golocal/index.html). In general, the smaller facilities and small practice providers are less likely to have Web sites, although the percentage is increasing.

Likewise, in the United States and many other nations, the universities make extensive use of the Web, and this includes the schools of public health and related fields. The Association of Schools of Public Health has prepared a list of the Web sites of all 38 accredited and 7 associate member Schools of Public Health in the United States (see http://www.asph.org/document.cfm?page=200).

The World Federation of Public Health Associations has 65 national public health association members and five regional association members. The World Federation membership list includes Web links to a majority of its members (http://www.wfpha.org/pg_mbr_overview.htm). Many of these organizations in turn link to various in-country academic and research organizations.

At least two other regions of the world (besides the United States) have public health academic associations with Web links to member institutions, including universities and affiliated research centres. These are the Latin American and Caribbean Association of Education in Public Health (http://www.alaesp.sld.cu/html/informe.htm), and the Asia-Pacific Academic Consortium for Public Health (http://apacph.org/site). The Association of Schools of Public Health in the European Region has many links (http://www.aspher.org/index.php?auto=aspher_membership), including in most cases the individual school Web sites.

The Web has penetrated and become an integral part of the public health research infrastructure, and is vital to all aspects of the health research enterprise. This is one of the basic premises of the HINARI discussed in a later section of this chapter. HINARI helps health researchers in sub-Saharan Africa and other low-income countries gain access to the Web-based journal literature.

As another example, NLM maintains a National Information Center on Health Services Research and Healthcare Technology (NICHSR) with comprehensive Web-based information on all aspects of the health research enterprise, with hundreds of Web links (see http://www.nlm.nih.gov/nichsr/nichsr.html). The NICHSR Web site well illustrates the complexity and power of the Web information resources available to US and global health researchers. Those researchers and regions of the world without effective Web access are at a disadvantage in this arena.

The wide prevalence of Web sites extends to the volunteer health sector as well. The International Medical Volunteers Association has compiled a list of many dozens of volunteer medical and health organizations, including their Web sites (see http://www.imva.org/Pages/orgdb/wblstfrm.htm) and provides an overview of the governmental and non-governmental organizations (NGOs) in the health sector along with their Web sites (http://www.imva.org/Pages/orgfrm.htm).

Last but not least, the Web has enabled the development and vibrancy of widespread consumer health information dissemination, something that was much more difficult in the pre-Web era. NLM is one of the leaders in providing information intended to be useful to the general public, as well as for health providers, researchers, and librarians. In addition to MedlinePlus (in English and *en espanol*), PubMed (and PubMedCentral, http://www.pubmedcentral.nih.gov), and the NICHSR, NLM offers other Web sites that focus on:

- Special populations (e.g. NIHSeniorHealth, http://nihseniorhealth.gov; Arctic Health, http://www.arctichealth.org; Native American Health, http://americanindianhealth.nlm.nih.gov; Asian American Health, http://asianamericanheatlh.nlm.nih.gov)
- Special topics, with some overlap with special populations (e.g. Environmental Health and Toxicology, http://toxnet.nlm.nih.gov; Chemical Information, http://sis.nlm.nih.gov/chemical.html; HIV/AIDS Information, http://sis.nlm.nih.gov/hiv.html, and AIDSInfo, http://www.aidsinfo.nih.gov)

In sum, at NLM and throughout the public health sector in the United States and around the world, the Web has become a key tool for the organization and dissemination of public health information at all levels—from the international health organizations and public health departments of nations and states, to health researchers and academics, to health providers, to medical and health volunteers, and to health consumers.

In less than a decade, the Web has transitioned from an experimental information technology to a key part of basic information infrastructure for the health sector, as with most other major sectors of society. Thus the need to pay much more attention to Web evaluation to help assure that health Web sites are effective in meeting the needs of their sponsors and, equally (or some would say more) important, their clients and users.

Web evaluation is the topic of the last section of this chapter. But first, a look in greater depth at two areas of Web application: Disaster management and emergency preparedness; and health information in low- and middle-income countries.

Disaster management and monitoring on the Web

The confluence of a mature World Wide Web and its underlying Internet infrastructure, combined with a growing list of major natural and man-made disasters, has focused attention on the use of the Web for disaster management and emergency preparedness. The public health sector has historically been a key player in this arena, and recent events have intensified the need and perceived priority in the supporting library community.

NLM's Long Range Plan for 2006–2016 (NLM, 2006) gives special attention to disaster management and the role of libraries and librarians when disasters strike. NLM's emphasis is on the role of medical libraries that directly serve the public health, consumer health, biomedical research, and emergency responder communities. But medical libraries could also serve the public at large, and the emergency preparedness role of libraries could extend to public and academic research libraries as well as medical libraries.

In the aftermath of Hurricanes Katrina and Rita in 2005, NLM's national network of libraries was highly effective in obtaining useful information from affected communities, rerouting requests for services, and getting equipment and personnel to locations serving evacuees and temporary health facilities. Many public libraries served as communication and social service centres for evacuees.

There is ample evidence of the enormous communication and information dissemination problems that arise in large-scale disasters. The area is ripe for additional research that builds on NLM's existing strengths and research portfolio.

Work already undertaken by NLM has produced:

- Portable devices with toxic chemical information used by emergency responders after Hurricane Katrina
- Software tools for robust DNA identification of victims of the September 11, 2001, terrorist attacks and of Hurricane Katrina
- Prototype self-healing wireless networks to restore connectivity
- Smart tags to track patients during triage, transportation, and treatment; new insights into the evolution of flu viruses derived from the analysis of genomic data, which suggest more effective strategies for vaccine development
- Identification of key resources for disaster recovery (http://sis.nlm.nih.gov/enviro/hurricane.html), including digital libraries or repositories of important literature (e.g. CANDHI project and PHpreparedness.info)

Going forward, the use of Web-based systems and technologies offers numerous opportunities to create and strengthen disaster management and emergency response capabilities. The Web is a natural platform for the collection, structuring, and dissemination of information on the entire cycle of emergency planning, scenario building, training, preparedness, response, and remediation. The Web can be used to implement complex information systems in user-friendly ways, including use of Wikis, blogs, and Web-based conferencing and collaboration software, as well as a wide range of general and special purpose Web sites (Palen *et al.* 2007; Currion *et al.* 2007; Turoff *et al.* 2006; Turoff *et al.* 2004).

The overall concept of Web-based emergency information management seems broadly applicable to and needed by all countries that have to deal with the possibility of a natural or man-made disaster. And the role of medical and associated libraries in disaster response likewise seems appropriate for those countries that have a reasonably well-developed library infrastructure.

The following sections present some examples of information technology applications to disaster management and emergency response. These are drawn from the experience of NLM and other US Government agencies, and have broad relevance to all nations facing a disaster management challenge.

In the United States, a large amount of disaster management and emergency preparedness information is already on the Web. For example, the Centers for Disease Control and Prevention (CDC) provides key health information for individuals, emergency responders, disaster workers, and health professionals on behalf of all federal agencies. CDC is a primary resource for electronically available up-to-the-minute disease, injury, prevention, and treatment information for disasters. The CDC home page on Natural Disasters & Severe Weather (http://www.cdc.gov/nceh/hsb/extreme/) links to information on earthquakes, tornadoes, wildfires, and other natural disasters. The Emergency Preparedness and Response home page (http://www.bt.cdc.gov/) includes information on and links to man-made disasters: Bioterrorism, Chemical Emergencies, Radiation Emergencies, Mass Casualties, and Recent Outbreaks and Incidents.

These and other Web sites increasingly are linking emergency and disaster-relevant information from multiple sources, including, as discussed below, networks of ground, air, and satellite-based sensors and information collection sources.

Remote sensing of health disasters

Early warning or early detection systems started in the physical sciences, and typically consist of telemetry between remote sensing or detection devices, and the scientists involved with the specific phenomenon, e.g. seismologists for earthquakes, meteorologists and oceanographers for severe storms and tsunamis. The telecommunications component of these applications provides data, usually via dedicated telecommunications systems, making scientists and public health workers aware of the occurrence of a disaster and its parameters, or its potential characteristics. Many communities and countries are putting in place disaster preparedness plans that are supported by remote sensing technologies that go beyond disaster response, to disease prevention and control following disaster. The Web is increasingly used for dissemination of this information.

Remote sensing technologies can help to assess and communicate the areas and extent of damage when disasters strike. An accurate description of the location, estimated number of people and types of facilities affected, and infrastructure damage all enables a coherent response and planning for the implementation of appropriate public health measures. Remote sensing data can also help public health officials and responders better distribute emergency resources throughout an area, and help to inform health and medical facilities of the likelihood of injuries, diseases, epidemics, and other adverse public health consequences of a disaster.

Remote sensing and surveillance are already being used by health sector disaster managers for health monitoring and disease forecasting and control. Baseline surveillance data on endemic disease distribution in an area provided by Geographic Information Systems (GIS) can be used to assess the nature of disease threats to displaced people and enable public health action, such as immunization, to be taken to protect groups at risk. These types of data may also be used to evaluate the evolution of eventual outbreaks or epidemics, and to adapt disease control strategies.

The 1990 Baguio City earthquake in the Philippines is an early example. In the wake of the earthquake, the Philippines Department of Health issued a warning of the potential spread of typhoid fever, diarrhoea, amoebiasis, and cholera that had developed in refugee encampments in the area. By employing public warning systems, health authorities appealed to the public to cooperate with measures designed to check the incidence of these deadly diseases (Scott 1998; Rantucci 1994).

Another disease-based example is influenza, also known as the flu, which is a contagious respiratory disease caused by a virus. Most people who get flu recover in a week or two, but some people develop life-threatening complications (such as pneumonia). In the United States, the number of state-based influenza surveillance programmes is growing rapidly. North Carolina is a good example. In 2004, 1686 people in North Carolina died of pneumonia and influenza. Fortunately, since the 2000–2001 flu season, North Carolina's General Communicable Disease Control Branch and the State Laboratory of Public Health have continuously participated in the US Influenza Sentinel Physicians Surveillance Network (Sloane *et al.* 2006; North Carolina Department of Health and Human Services 2007).

By watching for outbreaks of flu and testing for different strains of flu, public health agencies can help control outbreaks, determine appropriate treatments, and determine the effectiveness of vaccines. In the Sentinel Physicians Surveillance Network, each week, sentinel physicians, university health centres, hospitals/medical centres, and public health agencies across the state report 'influenza-like illness' (ILI) to the US Centers for Disease Control and Prevention (CDC) and collect representative samples for virus strain identification. The reports include the total number of patient visits to each practice or agency for that week and the number of those patients with symptoms of influenza-like illness (ILI), broken down into four age groups. For purposes of this surveillance programme, the ILI case definition is a fever of 100°F or higher, along with a cough or sore throat.

For the 2006–2007 flu season, 74 health providers in 45 counties throughout the state agreed to participate in the sentinel programme and to regularly report ILI to CDC. This group of sentinels includes a wide variety of physician practice types (paediatrics, family practice, and internal medicine) in 19 local health departments, 15 college and university student health centres, 34 private practices, and 6 hospital clinics. In addition to tracking flu cases among North Carolina residents, this system enables North Carolina and CDC to monitor influenza in a very diverse student population that includes students from other states and countries.

The larger goal for individual States and the United States as a whole, and by extension for other countries and regions, is the use of real-time data collection and analysis to strengthen public health surveillance at both regional and national levels. The intent is to strengthen surveillance systems by using readily available information in real-time, thereby increasing the power of these systems to detect disease outbreaks sooner.

Although symptom and diagnostic data have long since been stored in a variety of administrative healthcare databases, the challenge is developing automated systems for integrating these data so that abnormal patterns of disease can be detected in a timely manner. The 2001 and 2002 bioterrorist anthrax attacks in the United States highlighted deficiencies in detection and warning systems.

A 2003 pilot project at the Children's Hospital of Boston, MA, supported by NLM, demonstrated how an enhanced data acquisition infrastructure, combined with appropriate analytic tools, could be used to recognize disease clusters as soon as possible once patients begin appearing at healthcare sites (Que *et al.* 2006; Reis & Mundl 2004; Bourgeois *et al.* 2006; Wagner *et al.* 2004). Researchers established a surveillance network by virtually integrating multiple hospital emergency department (ED) databases in real-time. This provided a picture of regional population patterns of disease. Furthermore, at one of these hospitals, retrospective databases with many years of historical data were created that were critical for establishing normal and abnormal ('alert') ranges for the analytic models. The project first established normal patterns of disease and then built models that enabled the detection of deviations from these patterns with a minimum of false alarms ('false positives').

Another example of electronic disease monitoring and reporting is WHO's GOARN—the Global Outbreak Alert & Response Network. GOARN electronically connects member countries and warns them of disease outbreaks (see http://www.who.int/csr/outbreaknetwork/en/ and http://www.who.int/csr/alertresponse/realtimealert/en/index.html). Applications like these, and especially when using a Web-based platform, offer the prospect of increasing several fold the power of health disaster surveillance systems to detect disease outbreaks sooner and more accurately.

Electronic information tools for emergencies: Case study on WISER

A recent electronic information tool that is being incorporated into regular use by emergency responders in the United States is WISER (Wireless Information System for Emergency Responders, http://wiser.nlm.nih.gov), a National Library of Medicine-designed programme to assist emergency responders in hazardous material incidents. WISER provides a wide range of information on hazardous substances, including substance identification support, physical characteristics, human health information, and containment and suppression guidance. Its features include:

- Mobile support, providing Emergency Responders with critical information
- Comprehensive decision support, including assistance in identification of an unknown substance and, once the substance is identified, providing guidance on immediate actions necessary to save lives and protect the environment
- Access to 400+ substances derived from NLM's Hazardous Substances Data Bank (HSDB), which contains detailed information on over 5000 critical hazardous substances

- Rapid access to the most important information about a hazardous substance

WISER data comes from the Hazardous Substances Data Bank (HSDB) and contains information on human exposure, industrial hygiene, emergency handling procedures, environmental impacts and risks, regulatory requirements, and related areas. All data are referenced and derived from a core set of books, government documents, technical reports, and selected primary journal literature.

Many of the sources of data available via WISER are used by first responders already and include guidebooks, databases, hazardous materials specifications, and other information prepared by governmental and non-profit agencies.

While WISER currently focuses on substances of interest to the United States, the basic concept is applicable to other nations and to multinational and international organizations.

Regional disaster health information networks: Case study on CANDHI

In October 1998, Hurricane Mitch hit Central America, leaving more than 18 000 dead and 12 000 injured (Centre for Research on the Epidemiology of Disasters 2007; United Nations Commission of Latin America and the Caribbean 1998). Major public health, economic, and social lifelines were crippled, including health facilities and communications services. Within a year of this tragedy, NLM, together with the Pan American Health Organization (PAHO), began a special project to support the rebuilding and improvement of local and national health information infrastructure, first in Honduras and Nicaragua, and then in El Salvador. The result of this initiative is the Central American Network for Disaster Health Information (CANDHI).

The principal goal of the project is to contribute to disaster reduction in the region. This is being achieved through capacity building activities in the area of disaster-related information management. Through participation in the project, participating countries have improved their capacities to collect, index, manage, store, disseminate, and share public health, medical, and other information related to disasters (Arneson *et al.* 2007, 2005, 2003). The project strategy provides health sciences libraries and information centres with the knowledge, training, and technology resources needed to have sufficient capacities to act as reliable information providers to a host of other users in these countries. In the longer term, the establishment of disaster information centres should also facilitate the development of improved disaster prevention and mitigation policy and planning in participating countries.

Before the CANDHI initiative, the Regional Disaster Information Center for Latin America and the Caribbean (Spanish acronym known as CRID) counted its regular users worldwide at approximately 6500. These were mainly professionals from the health and environment, academic, humanitarian, grass roots, and civil defence sectors. Information provided by CRID was frequently used for planning and decision-making purposes, as well as for training. CRID is the coordinator of the CANDHI project.

CRID's collection is comprised primarily of non-conventional or grey (unpublished, non-peer reviewed) literature resulting from expert meetings; case studies and evaluations; university research and assessments; guidelines and technical reports issued by governmental authorities; and publications, resolutions, journals or bulletins, and technical proceedings. Many of these materials were prepared by United Nations and other specialized organizations (for example, PAHO, the World Meteorological Organization, and the Economic Commission for Latin America and the Caribbean). All documents are available from CRID in full text.

Before CANDHI, CRID maintained a bibliographic database of documents, but the documents were not available full-text online. One of CRID's major efforts was fulfilling requests for these documents. The majority of requests (80 per cent) came via the Internet, with the balance received via fax and post. Most of the email requests came from people using CRID's Web site, and most of these were from outside of the region. Even though there were a significant number of 'clients' using the Internet, many of CRID's principal users, particularly those who might have used CRID-derived information for operational purposes, such as Civil Defense and Ministries of Health, were not using the Internet. The primary users of Internet were academics.

Despite increased use of CRID's Web site and email, the documents were only available in print and fulfillment of a request for a document at CRID took on the average of from 1 to 3 weeks. The documents were physically scanned or photocopied and then mailed via regular post or, for short documents, sent by fax.

CANDHI provided the opportunity for CRID to develop a digital library of its collection, and now nearly 70 per cent of the collection is available online. This greatly reduces the need to mail or fax documents and provides almost instantaneous access to the literature on disasters and health.

Not only has CANDHI proven to be a good emergency preparedness and disaster management tool, the project also has served as a catalyst for the modernization of the medical school libraries in the region. The CANDHI centres in Honduras, Nicaragua, El Salvador, Panama, and Guatemala have all developed their own local CANDHI Web sites. Although each Web site has its unique features, all of the affiliated Web sites provide access to the CRID bibliographic database on disasters, the CRID digital library, a digital library of local documents, as well as other local resources and contacts. Costa Rica is the next country that will make its Web site publicly available. Although Web site statistics are not yet available from all CANDHI centres, in 2005, over 25 000 unique visitors accessed five of the CANDHI Web sites and over 170 000 unique visitors accessed the CRID Web site. In addition, over 9500 people visited the CANDHI centres to obtain information.

A CANDHI portal Web site is operational (see http://www.candhi.org/). This Web site lists and links the participating centres and CRID and uses the CANDHI meta-search engine for enhanced retrieval of disaster information across Central America. The portal also serves to describe the CANDHI programme, links to the Disaster Information Center Toolkit, and provides a framework for identifying and retrieving local and regional information on disasters. The Web site is also used to share software tools developed for CANDHI, and as a forum for discussion and collaboration among the participants. CRID was responsible for the initial development of the portal, and it is anticipated that several CANDHI centres will rotate responsibility for the maintenance of the site.

The CANDHI concept and use of Web-based information dissemination have been successful thus far, and provide a model that could be replicated in other countries and regions of the world.

Public health research information dissemination in low- and middle-income countries: The case of HINARI

Since the early years of the World Wide Web, most low- and middle-income countries have had very limited Internet connectivity and little benefit from Web-based health information. Most of these nations and their medical libraries are faced with limited financial and staff resources. Biomedical and health researchers, administrators, and providers in these nations are often unable to gain access to the world's biomedical and public health literature.

In recent years, several special programmes were established to improve literature access as Internet connectivity improved. Perhaps the most well known of these programmes is the Health InterNetwork Access to Research Initiative (HINARI), a partnership led by the World Health Organization (WHO). The HINARI programme is supported by international publishers of research journals in biomedicine and related subjects that offer access to the full text of more than 2800 journals to medical researchers, clinicians, economists, and policy makers in 113 countries. Access to the entire collection is free, for qualifying institutions in 69 of the countries where the annual per capita GNP was US$1000 or less in December 2000. An annual fee of US$1000 is collected for institutions in 44 countries where the GNP was between US$1001 and US$3000. HINARI users of NLM's PubMed Web site also benefit from direct links to full-text articles from HINARI journals.

Previous investigations by the WHO concluded that access to key biomedical literature by researchers in low- and middle-income countries was their single biggest information need. HINARI was launched in January 2002 with the content of the six largest medical journal publishers, and now offers full content from 75 of the world's leading publishers for the last 8–10 years of volumes. HINARI receives support from Yale University and the US National Library of Medicine, as well as WHO, and others. As of mid-2006, over 2000 institutions in over 100 countries had registered for the HINARI.

A sister programme, Access to Global Online Research in Agriculture (AGORA) was launched in October 2003. AGORA is a partnership led by the United National Food and Agriculture Organization (FAO).

Research and policy benefits

A recent evaluation (Scott, J., Usage review of HINARI and AGORA, Center for Public Service Communications, June 2006) has concluded that HINARI and AGORA were making dramatic contributions to scientific research in the fields of biomedicine and health in the developing world. HINARI and AGORA have enabled students to pursue health and agricultural studies in ways inconceivable before. Students engaged in writing theses or dissertations reportedly use HINARI/AGORA as their principal research tool. HINARI and AGORA also are instrumental in enabling academic and research institutions to interact on a more equal footing with their counterparts in high-income countries. As just one example, a Ugandan research institute presented 10 papers at an international AIDS Congress in Toronto in 2006, made possible through HINARI research. And the first evidence-based guidelines in Vietnam for medical treatment in paediatrics were based on HINARI research.

Teachers and researchers are not the only ones benefiting from Web-based access to medical and health literature. Web-based HINARI information is also used to inform public policy makers of national governments. The following examples from Tanzania suggest the likelihood of similar applications in other countries that have access to HINARI and use the Web as a research tool.

The Tanzanian National Institute for Medical Research has a mandate to advise the Government of Tanzania on health policy issues of national significance, and the Institute uses HINARI to inform the policy-making process. The institute's director, who is also chair of the National Advisory Committee for Malaria and an adviser to Tanzania's Anti Malarial Drug Research Network, reported an example of using HINARI for this purpose. He uses HINARI to search for research findings of experts as well as experiences of other national policies with respect to drug-resistant malaria. HINARI was also used extensively to search for research findings that demonstrate results for insecticide-treated bed nets and experience with implementing successful bed net programmes.

This use of HINARI went beyond benefit to the health sector by providing access to research that suggested a reduction or removal of a tax on importing bed nets might stimulate the national bed net market (an effective malaria prevention measure) and encourage more suppliers in Tanzania to develop and market products. Further HINARI-enabled literature searches led Tanzanian researchers to experiences with bed net programmes reported in China, India, and Vietnam. The results of these experiences encouraged them to recommend local production of bed nets as an alternative to the government's earlier focus on reducing or removing import taxes on foreign-made bed nets as a way to increase the availability of bed nets in Tanzania. As a result, not only is Tanzania realizing the medical benefits of increased use of bed nets, they have also found a way to provide job opportunities and stimulate the national and local economies of the country.

Another significant public policy issue in Tanzania that has benefited from HINARI-enabled research is the current discussion of whether or not to re-introduce the use of DDT to eradicate mosquitoes. With the increase of malaria in Tanzania public health officials debated the decision whether or not to re-introduce widespread use of DDT to control the spread of the disease. HINARI was a principal tool used by health policy makers of the Tanzanian government to research the pros and cons of the argument.

HINARI was also cited for its role in enabling accreditation for the Master of Science in Nursing (MSN) programme at the Aga Khan University in Uganda. The Aga Khan University (AKU) in Uganda currently offers two major programmes. Over the past 5 years, Aga Khan University has developed a part-time study programme that allows practicing nurses to learn and apply new skills. At the most basic level nurses completing the programme are upgraded to the position of a Registered Nurse. The second programme enables nurses at the diploma level to move on to receive a BSN degree. The Aga Khan University would like to offer the MSN, which is offered nowhere else in the country. The librarian of the advanced nursing studies programme trains his students to use HINARI and believes that access to nursing and other journals through HINARI will help to ensure that the appropriate ministries and other bodies regulating nursing programmes in Uganda will accredit the university programme.

Continuing barriers to access

Prior research on HINARI has indicated that while access to the biomedical journal literature has increased markedly due to HINARI, there are continuing serious issues that pose barriers to effective access (Smith *et al.* 2007). In a study of five African countries, the majority of respondents (at four medical schools in Cameroon, Nigeria, Tanzania, and Uganda and one medical research organization in Gambia) had recently used the Internet for health information. However many respondents reported problematic Internet connectivity, limited bandwidth that slows download speeds, intermittent power outages, problems with passwords, and in general a relatively low awareness of HINARI and its services, and limited training in using HINARI. Few respondents reported having access to an Internet-enabled computer at home or in their private offices. Many depended on computers in common areas or in Cyber cafes (Smith *et al.* 2007). These five-country results were similar to a study of medical staff at a major teaching hospital in Nigeria (Ajuwan 2006).

A multi-regional evaluation (Scott J, Usage review of HINARI and AGORA, Center for Public Service Communications, June 2006) extended to a dozen countries—including Senegal, Ghana, Cameroon, Ethiopia, Tanzania, and Uganda in sub-Saharan Africa; Ecuador, Costa Rica, and Honduras in Central America; and Vietnam, Bangladesh, and Cambodia in Southeast Asia. The results were similar.

In Cameroon, for example, most Internet users have limited bandwidth. Downloading a four-page journal article can take as long as 10–15 min during business hours. A creative approach to dealing with this problem was attempting to download articles after work hours, but this met with new frustrations. Because of the instability of electric power in Yaoundé, the capital city, computers would shut down in the middle of downloads. When the power returned, it was often with a surge that would blow out the computer system, resulting in the loss of the searched material as well as the computers themselves.

But where there's a will there's a way, and the example of the Ghana Agricultural Information Network System (GAINS), part of the Institute for Scientific and Technological Information (INSTI) headquartered in Accra, is a good one. The INSTI solution to providing access to Web-based research is creative, but time-consuming. In the absence of good Internet access, and until access is improved throughout the country, the INSTI coordinator asked researchers in stations outside of Accra to choose the five journals that are most relevant to their work. By 'snail mail', the GAINS coordinator sends the abstracts of those journals to the researchers who then can identify the full-text articles of interest. The GAINS office in Accra then conducts the Internet search, downloads the full-text articles, and sends them, again via snail mail, to the remote researchers.

There are physical challenges too. In other cases, for example in Dhaka, Bangladesh, researchers and other users of HINARI and AGORA who are not fortunate enough to be located at institutions that have computers and Internet access must travel, sometimes great distances, through very congested traffic, in order to use the system. In addition to the challenges of travel, they must take time off from work to do their HINARI/AGORA searches. It is not uncommon to take a half-day or even a day off from work in order to get to publicly available HINARI/AGORA workstations.

After poor Internet connectivity, language may be the principal obstacle in many countries to efficient use of journal articles and other medical literature. The Dean of the Faculty of Medicine of the Universidad Central del Ecuador reported that only about 20 per cent of the students at Ecuador's principal medical school speak English. Similarly, it is estimated that, at best, 40 per cent of doctors in Vietnam speak English and only 20–30 per cent students are sufficiently conversant with English (Tran Thanh Xuan, Director of the library at the University of Medicine and Pharmacy in Ho Chi Minh City, personal communication). The percentage of professors using English was only slightly higher. Because of their limited English proficiency, most medical students in Vietnam tend to rely more on Vietnamese journals. Post-graduate students tend to have better English literacy than younger students and use literature, usually acquired through HINARI searches, for thesis research. At this time, most HINARI users in Vietnam are professors or researchers.

Many libraries in HINARI countries have limited collections, and therefore put even more emphasis on Internet access for downloading full text. For example, the university libraries in Cameroon, among them Yaoundé 1, which is reputed to be the best in Cameroon, have poor collections of books and journals measured in numbers of volumes, currency of their collections and condition. Even what looked to be a reasonable volume of literature at Yaoundé 1 University in practical terms was not particularly useful; many of the books, side-by-side on the shelves, were in several languages (French, English, Dutch, Spanish, German, and others) thereby limiting their likely value to students, most of whom read only French or English.

Other barriers identified included: Confusion over passwords and log-in procedures; excessive error messages; shortages of librarians and trained information technology professionals at participating institutions; and a general lack of awareness of and training on HINARI and AGORA.

The multi-regional evaluation concluded that HINARI and AGORA offer significant realized value added. But the contribution falls short of potential due to the barriers identified. The evaluation made several recommendations:

- Promote awareness of the availability of HINARI/AGORA to current non-users in participating countries
- Increase training opportunities on use of HINARI/AGORA (and of the Internet generally for research and information sharing) for end users and for staff
- Clarify and streamline policies for access to and sharing of user names and pass- words for HINARI/AGORA
- Increase funding and technical support to HINARI/AGORA and participating institutions, so that Internet connectivity and performance continues to improve (perhaps by broadening the financial support base to include other agencies of the United Nations, development agencies of donor agencies, and private foundations)

Update on the Multinational Initiative of Malaria Communications Network (MIMCom): A case study of Web access in Africa

While there has been an improvement in communications at the global level, access to the benefits of information technology has been difficult for researchers in much of sub-Saharan Africa due to limited telecommunications infrastructure. For example, in 1997, the US National Library of Medicine (NLM) made MEDLINE, its premier database of the world's medical literature, available free to the networked world through PubMed, which has over 15 million records for biomedical articles. For scientists with access to the Web, this service made it possible to search MEDLINE, read abstracts, and carry out research. However, most researchers in developing countries, especially those in Africa, have not been able to take full advantage of PubMed due to very limited, or nonexistent, and expensive Internet access.

From its creation in 1997, the Multilateral Initiative on Malaria Communications Network (MIMCom) started reversing this state of affairs and has provided an ideal application for PubMed to be used by researchers in underserved areas of Africa. MIMCom was conceived by African malaria researchers and has been designed, implemented, and overseen by the US National Library of Medicine (NLM) in collaboration with over 30 partners in Africa, the United States, and the United Kingdom. MIMCom has grown as a research network, the first of its kind in Africa, from two sites in one country to 19 sites in 13 countries. The map in Fig. 5.3.1 identifies the locations of African health institutes whose access to email and the Internet has been enabled or enhanced with initial assistance from MIMCom. Phase I sites were assisted, for the most part, by their own funding agencies. Phase II sites applied for and were funded by a grant from a development agency in Europe. The reach of MIMCom News, with nearly 2,000 subscribers, is indicated in Fig. 5.3.1.

MIMCom also comprises a Web site, training programmes, monitoring and evaluation activities, document delivery service, and support of specific malaria research agendas. Most importantly, since this initial start-up effort that MIMCom provided, sites are now able to choose from an array of technologies currently available, making their own decisions about how access can best support their scientific research and build the research capacity so desperately needed on the continent.

NLM examined the use of information technology (IT) by scientists, students, and administrative personnel at MIMCom sites, focusing on the use of IT as a tool to facilitate communication, retrieve information, obtain documents, write proposals, and prepare papers for publication (Royall *et al.* 2005).

The study showed that MIMCom has become a dynamic tool in the research process. For researchers, the Internet connection to colleagues and to current information has gone a long way toward addressing the distances of time and space. Electronic communication has enabled research teams to engage in discussions with colleagues in other parts of the world and participate in real-time problem-solving; coordinate research activities; store information; share information; search for literature; submit manuscripts for publication; and send research proposals to funding agencies. Electronic communication also has made possible long distance

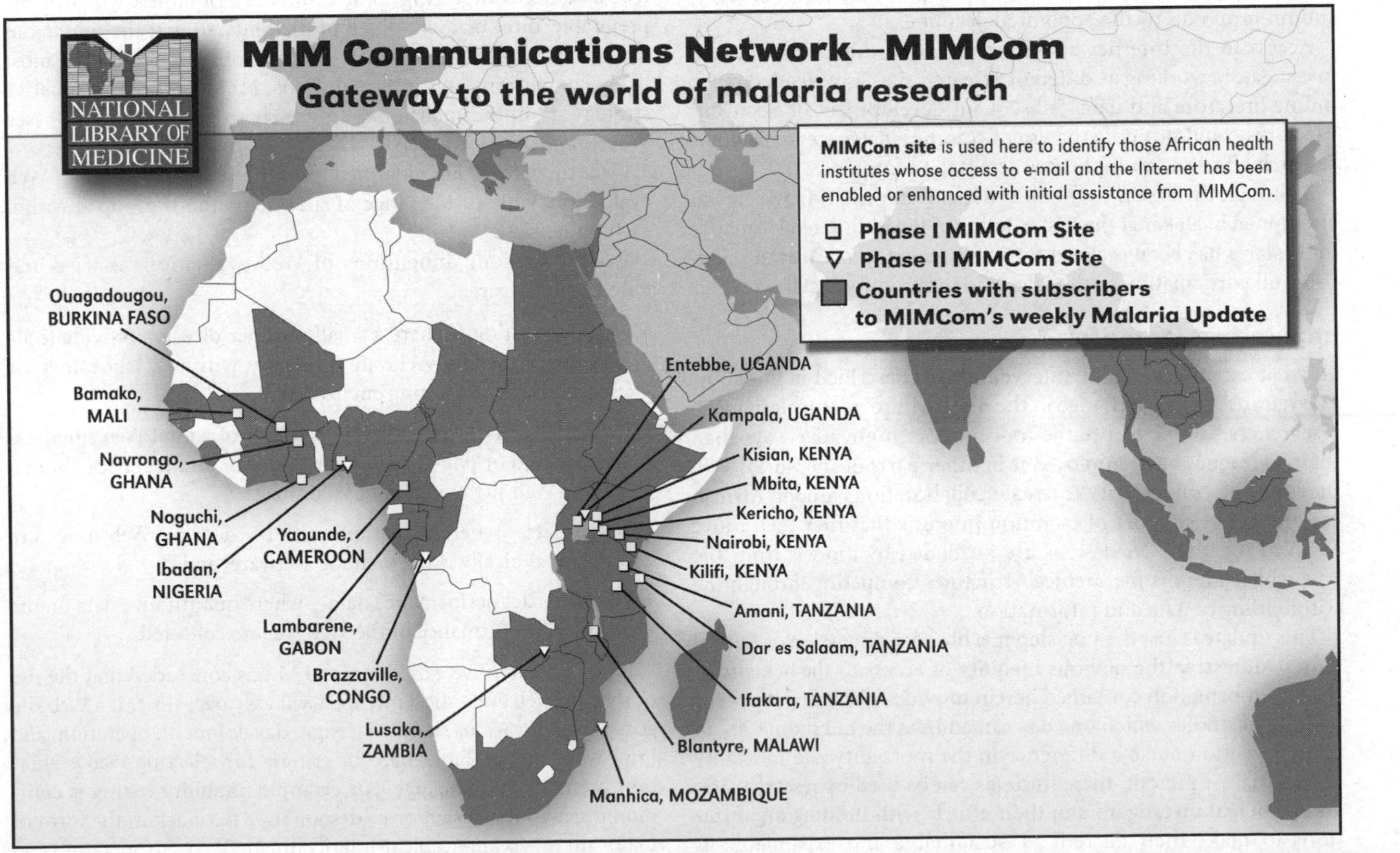

Fig. 5.3.1 MIM Communications Network—MIMCom—Gateway to the world of malaria research.
Source: Julia Royall.

educational/training activities and improved communication between students and supervisors. MIMCom has helped remove geographic as well as intellectual isolation—among the greatest challenges faced by researchers in the sites reviewed.

Overall, MIMCom has provided researchers in the sites reviewed with four key opportunities: (1) Researchers can now download PDF files of journal articles, making the Internet link a lifeline for many. Large files are sent through email, saving money and time; (2) the scientists in these centres are now capable of competing favourably with their colleagues in other parts of the world in proposal writing, acquisition of literature, and submission of papers for publication; (3) users no longer waste large amounts of time looking for Internet cafés; and (4) for some junior scientists, MIMCom facilities are the only means by which they can access the information they need for their training.

The speed with which IT enables researchers to carry out simple tasks, thus saving time, energy, and money, appears to be the most important result of enhanced connectivity at the participating sites. The new facility has, within limits, made a positive contribution to researchers' productivity and efficiency and, subsequently, to each site's research agenda. Further, enhanced connectivity and access to information have affected each site's financial bottom line through savings in areas such as transportation related to communication, telephone and facsimile transmissions, and ordering supplies; and by supporting development and submission of research grant applications. Respondents mentioned the importance of being able to communicate with donors in a timely fashion, of being able to collaborate effectively with others on proposals, and finally, to submit proposals by the appointed deadline.

Access to the Internet enables rapid communication between investigators working at different research sites as well as access to online literature and data. Subsequent development of electronic networks could promote the use of common databases to facilitate research efforts at multiple sites across the continent.

Although the access to the Internet and information which was envisioned in Dakar at the first meeting of the Multilateral Initiative on Malaria has been realized for many researchers, African scientists' full participation in the scientific community is still evolving.

Implications for the future

To what extent does an IT intervention, as described in this summary, translate into a change in the disease burden of malaria? Will researchers be able to use the tool in more innovative ways than their colleagues have employed it in other parts of the world? Will they use the connectivity to create collaborations among African researchers in support of common interests that they then move forward together? Next steps are burdened by models from the past which support hierarchical structures competing through the withholding of data and information.

This update is just the first step in a broader discussion of critical issues addressing the obvious inequity of access to the benefits of IT. The information contained herein provides a building block for additional studies which one day can address the question: Can an IT intervention make a difference in the morbidity and mortality of malaria? At present, these findings can be used by research sites and principal investigators in their efforts with funding organizations to make their current IT sustainable and expandable as required. The findings also can be used by consortia such as the Multilateral Initiative on Malaria as they work proactively to promote interaction among information technology, research, and better health. Their target audiences may include governments in Africa (i.e. regulatory bodies, telephone company monopolies, ministries of health, and policy makers), foundations, corporations, and international aid organizations. IT is critical to widening the circle to include African researchers as part of the international scientific community (Royal *et al.* 2004).

Evaluation of public health Web sites

During the last 5 years, the use of Web sites in the public health sector has become commonplace, almost universally in high-income countries, and selectively in low- and middle-income countries. Improvements in Internet connectivity in developing regions have opened the door to a wide range of special projects intended to make public health-related information more broadly accessible. Web sites have become indispensable to public health professionals around the world, and, increasingly, to emergency responders, health researchers and providers, and the general citizenry.

The more critical the role of Web sites in disseminating health information, the more important it is to evaluate public health Web sites to assure that mission and user needs are being met and resources are being effectively applied.

NLM now has over a decade of experience with Web evaluation. NLM has tried out numerous evaluation methods and approaches. One of the major findings is that no one evaluation method will suffice when it comes to Web evaluation. No single method is perfect or all encompassing. Best results are obtained when using, preferably, three or more different methods, so that the results can be compared and 'triangulated' to find convergence on the most likely conclusions and interpretations. NLM calls this evaluative strategy a 'multidimensional approach to Web evaluation' (see Wood *et al.* 2003).

Over time, NLM has identified four different dimensions of Web evaluation, with a wide range of specific methods grouped within each dimension.

Briefly, the four dimensions of Web evaluation, as tried and tested by NLM, are:

- Usability testing—where a small number of users provide feedback on a specific Web site, typically within a laboratory or specially designed testing environment;
- User feedback—where a larger number of actual Web site users are surveyed or polled as to their opinions and feedback about a specific Web site or group of Web sites;
- Usage data—where actual quantitative data on Web usage are collected typically using Web log software; and
- Web/Internet performance data—where quantitative data on the technical performance of the Web site are collected.

Based on extensive experience, NLM has concluded that the use of specific Web evaluation methods will vary over time, as a Web site goes through various stages of design, development, operation, and improvement. See Table 5.3.2 for criteria for selecting Web evaluation methods at each stage. For example, usability testing is common during Web design or re-design; user feedback in the form of major surveys is applicable primarily during Web site operation and improvement; Web usage data and Web/Internet performance data are key tools for monitoring Web site operations.

Table 5.3.2 Criteria for selecting Web evaluation methods Stages in Web Site Life Cycle

Evaluation method	Web development	Web operations	Web improvement	Web use/impact
USABILITY TESTING				
Heuristic/Expert review	√√		√√	
Usability lab testing	√√√		√√	√
Informal usability feedback	√		√	
USER FEEDBACK				
Online internal user survey		√√√	√√√	√√√
Online external user survey		√	√	
Focus group	√√	√√	√√√	√√√
Nationwide syndicated survey	√	√√	√√	√√
Unsolicited user feedback		√√	√√	√
USAGE DATA				
Web log data analysis		√√√	√√√	√√
Internet audience measurement	√	√√	√√	√√
WEB/NET PERFORMANCE DATA	√	√√	√√	
SPECIAL OUTREACH PROJECTS	√	√√	√√√	√√√

Key: √√√ = very important; √√ = moderately important; √ = less important; no check mark = generally not applicable or not important.

Source: Fred B. Wood and Elliot R. Siegel (1998).

The major Web evaluation methods are discussed below, including a brief history of NLM's experience with the method and some examples.

For context, Web site design, development, and improvement elements include (based in part on the American Customer Satisfaction Index framework, see Wood *et al.* 2007):

- Content—completeness, accuracy, quality, organization, and freshness of information on the Web site
- Look and feel—user-friendliness of the site, such as ease of reading, clarity of the site organization, and simplicity of the site layout
- Navigation—ability of the user to find desired information on the site and in a minimum number of steps or clicks
- Search—utility and effectiveness of the search function on the Web site to help the user find desired information, and present search results in an understandable way
- Site performance—technical performance of the site such as speed of downloading pages and reliability of downloading
- Privacy—ability of the site to limit collection of personal information and protect from unauthorized disclosure of any privacy information that is collected
- Functionality—overall ability of the site to provide useful information in an easy, convenient way that helps the user meet his or her needs
- Satisfaction—extent to which the site meets the overall expectations of the user

This framework should be kept in mind throughout the following discussion of specific methods.

Where possible, we provide cost estimates for various evaluation methods. The estimated dollar cost range can be considered representative of costs for Western high-income countries (when converted to local currencies). Costs in low- and middle-income countries would be expected to be somewhat to significantly lower, depending on the local economy and competitive marketplace.

Usability testing

The usability testing group of Web evaluation methods includes: Heuristic/Expert review; Formal usability testing; and Informal usability testing.

Heuristic/expert review

One of the most straightforward Web evaluation methods is to have one or a small group of Web evaluation experts review and evaluate one's Web site. This method is used almost exclusively during the original Web site design stage, to get some outside, independent feedback on the design elements and site functionality, and secondarily during site re-design and improvement.

The term 'heuristic' is sometimes used interchangeably with 'expert,' and refers to the application of principles and standards of Web design. In the early years of the Web, there were no generally accepted design principles. But that has changed in recent times, and Web design is now the subject of numerous papers, books, and Web sites (see, for example, Wikipedia 2007; Koyani *et al.* 2003; Cato 2001; Nielsen 2000; Sklar 2000).

The NIH and DHHS have made significant efforts to develop Web design frameworks, and some of these are publicly available for use by anyone (US Department of Health and Human Service 2007a,b; 2006).

Arranging for an expert review of a Web site is basically paying someone who makes a profession out of mastering and applying Web site design standards, and who keeps up on and assimilates varied Web design standards-development initiatives. The expert review also usually has the advantage of bringing in an outside perspective, independent of the person or organization developing the Web site.

NLM's experience has been that expert review can be helpful when a Web site design is far enough along that there is something concrete to review, but not so far along that significant changes or rethinking would be too costly or disruptive. So the timing of an expert review is important—not too late, not too early in the Web design (or re-design) process.

Web design experts can also be involved from square one in the Web design process, when the basic site concept is being formulated, and before there is even a test site suitable for review. This is more likely to be in the context of contracting out for some or all of a Web site design process. And when outsourcing is used, it is important as well that someone with expert review capabilities be involved in the effort.

Expert reviews can typically be conducted quickly, in a few weeks to a month or two, and at modest cost (US$10 000 range).

Notwithstanding the value of expert reviews at specific points in the Web design and re-design, it is incumbent on all Web managers to be familiar with relevant Web design standards, and particularly those of the Web manager's organization (if applicable). And furthermore, the astute Web manager needs to be able to view expert review input with a degree of detachment and expertise. Experts can be helpful, but their advice is not always correct or appropriate.

Usability testing

Expert review means just that, involvement by experts. Usability testing means getting feedback on a Web site from actual users. Feedback can be informal, for example, by asking a small group of users to conduct searches and answer questions about a specific Web site.

NLM made use of informal usability testing primarily in the early years of the Web. For example, shortly after the launch of the MedlinePlus consumer health Web site (www.medlineplus.gov), NLM conducted several pilot tests that included informal usability testing with public librarians at various locations in the Eastern and Southern United States. Librarians were asked to access MedlinePlus and provide what amounted to structured feedback on the Web site, its content, and performance (Wood *et al.* 2000).

Informal usability testing can, for certain purposes, provide useful results. The cost is usually minimal, since frequently the participants are other employees or volunteers. But the informality means that results are less rigorous and likely to have less validity, due to the many factors that can affect results and are not controlled for in an informal setting.

For these reasons, over time, NLM has gravitated toward more intensive use of so-called formal usability testing for major Web sites. Formal usability testing is typically conducted by professional service organizations in a laboratory setting, with a technical set-up that allows monitoring of the participant's verbal and physical responses and movements, including keystrokes. A formal usability test usually includes at least six to eight persons, selected to represent a cross-section of the target user community for the Web site being tested.

Formal usability testing can be very good at simulating a real user environment with a small sample of real users. NLM does not have its own usability laboratory, and for the most part contracts with Web evaluation organizations that do usability testing. The usability testing industry pre-dated the Web, with its roots in industrial design and product testing in the commercial sector, and in aerospace and transportation engineering, as examples. Applied social scientists and industrial engineers have adapted usability testing to the Web environment. And the Web usability testing sector is now considered mature, with several companies well established in major US and overseas markets. In addition, in the United States, some governmental agencies and private companies have their own usability labs.

NLM's MedlinePlus consumer health Web site and NLM's home page (www.nlm.nih.gov) have both made extensive use of formal usability testing. The testing results have helped the Web managers and designers to identify changes in site layout, use of fonts and colours, navigation, and content. In general, usability testing is conducted periodically—at most annually or usually less often. Such testing is fairly closely tied to the Web site design or redesign schedules.

While the laboratory setting predominates in NLM's usability testing, on occasion testing is conducted with paper mock-ups and Web page prototypes. This approach would apply in the early design stages, prior to development of even a prototype working Web site.

The cost of formal usability testing is typically in the range of US$15 000 to US$35 000, for testing with a dozen or so individual users. This cost includes recruitment of participants, development of test protocols and questions, use of the testing lab, and analysis and reporting of testing results.

Overall, NLM has found formal usability testing to be one of the most valuable Web evaluation methods employed to date.

User feedback

The primary purpose of a public or consumer health Web site is to disseminate information to persons interested in public or consumer health topics. The relative success of a Web site typically is gauged by the degree of satisfaction expressed by users, and the extent to which users report that they are able to find the information they seek from that Web site. Success may also be defined in terms of user feedback on various specific aspects of Web site content and performance, and the extent to which users would return to the Web site again and consider the Web site as a primary resource.

Over the last decade, NLM has experimented with a wide range of methods for obtaining feedback from Web site users. These methods vary widely in the number of users sampled or included in the feedback process, and whether users are queried or measured directly by NLM or by third-party vendor organizations.

Many consumer health information Web sites have on the Web site a place for users to provide unsolicited feedback. This type of feedback can be quite helpful, but it is *ad hoc* and unscientific.

The four major and more systematic user feedback methods considered here are: Randomized online user surveys; 'external' online user panel surveys; in person or online focus groups; and syndicated nationwide surveys.

Randomized online user surveys

Background. NLM has used customer surveys since the advent of online health information, a couple of decades before the Web revolution began. Customer or user surveys are widely recognized as one of the best ways to get direct feedback from users of any service, and information services are no exception. NLM conducted its last pre-Web user survey in 1994–1995. Since that time, NLM has focused on surveying Web site users.

In the early years of the Web, NLM and other organizations running Web sites tried so-called 'bounce back' surveys where questions were posted on the Web site and anyone could respond. While the results of these surveys had some value-added, they were not statistically valid since the sample was not randomized.

Snapshot surveys. About the turn of the century, NLM migrated to what are known as 'snapshot' surveys of Web users. Basically, a randomized sample of Web users is given the opportunity to respond to a survey. The survey is typically offered on a pop-up basis, and the sampling period ideally is about 2–3 weeks—thus the 'snapshot' terminology. The sampling rate is a function of the overall usage or traffic level on the Web site, and is set so that about 1000–3000 responses are received during the 2–3 weeks the survey is in the field.

NLM had good success with the snap-shot surveys, which were conducted for MedlinePlus, the NLM home page, PubMed (www.pubmed.gov, the Web version of the MEDLINE biomedical journal database, and more), and ToxNet (http://toxnet.nlm.nih.gov/, an environmental toxicology Web site). These surveys set the original benchmark for NLM, and convincingly established that randomized online surveys can be effectively implemented, at least for Web sites with sufficient traffic. (When traffic is too low, it takes too long to obtain the minimum number of completed survey response for a statistically significant result.)

The snapshot surveys provided new insights into the demographics of Web site users, levels of customer satisfaction, and feedback on various site characteristics. Importantly, the snapshot surveys offered the ability to craft customized questions that asked users how they learned about the Web site, why they were coming to the Web site, and what they intended to do with the information they found on the Web site.

The limitations of the snapshot survey are that, first, by definition, the survey is taken for a limited period of time, and as a practical matter, NLM never ran such a survey more than once a year on any Web site, and more typically once every 2–3 years. Second, the cost per survey was US$20 000–30 000, which even for NLM precluded running a survey very often. Hence over time, the survey response data might become outdated. Third, the snapshot surveys offered only very limited ability to benchmark the results against similar survey results of other Web sites.

Continuous surveys. The next major advance in online user surveys for NLM came in 2004, when some NLM Web sites participated in a pilot project using the American Customer Satisfaction Index (ACSI) online user survey methodology.

The ACSI is a randomized survey methodology but with several added features. First, the survey is run continuously, for an entire year, with roughly 300–400 completed responses each month. Results are continuously updated. Second, the ACSI combines both standardized and customized questions. Third, the ACSI provides benchmarking of the standardized results, and in particular a measure of overall satisfaction, with numerous other US Government agencies and private sector companies participating. Fourth, and of special importance in the US Government context, the ACSI has been approved by the US Office of Management and Budget for use by Federal agencies. Fifth, the ACSI is offered by the Federal Consulting Group of the US Department of the Treasury at about the same price point as typical snapshot surveys. Based on favourable results of the 2004 pilot test, NLM led an NIH-wide initiative to obtain funding for an enterprise approach to using the ACSI online survey methodology. The trans-NIH project included over 60 NIH Web sites from 31 different NIH organizational units.

The trans-NIH ACSI project ran for 2 years, and the majority of participating Web site staffs found considerable value in both the survey results and the opportunities for sharing lessons learned (see Wood *et al.* 2008). The survey results helped many participating Web site staffs better understand their customers, why they were coming to the site, and what aspects of the Web site were found to be most useful or satisfying. The trans-NIH enterprise approach also allowed the use of customized questions to generate an NIH-wide profile of Web site users and their health information-seeking behaviour. Overall, the NIH Web sites fared well in customer satisfaction levels when benchmarked against other US Government Web sites and private sector sites. Non-response bias is still an issue for randomized online surveys in the Web environment. NLM has found that response rates are quite low (in the order of 5 per cent of those offered the survey actually complete the survey, typical of all such online surveys regardless of sponsor or specific method). With a low response rate, a concern is that the respondents are not representative of the total customer population. To address this issue, NLM compares survey results with other evaluative results, for example with Web log data (see later section), to look for consistency. Overall, NLM, and most online survey vendors, believe that randomized survey results are reasonably valid.

Based on about 6 years experience with online surveys, NLM has concluded that the randomized online user survey is one of the most valuable Web evaluation methods. The online survey is strongly recommended for any major public or consumer health Web site with moderate to high traffic levels (anything above 50 000–100 000 unique visitors per month should be sufficient to generate an adequate number of completed surveys in a reasonable period of time).

Online 'external' user panel surveys

As an alternative survey approach, various private companies maintain independent panels of users that can be tapped for various survey purposes. That is, rather than surveying users directly as they come to a Web site, a subset of an 'external' panel of users can be sampled for feedback on a specified Web site. These private sector panels typically include up to tens of thousands of members, or virtual members (who are available for participation in specific survey projects).

NLM has used this survey approach on two occasions in the last several years, both times for getting user feedback on MedlinePlus and several other consumer health information Web sites. These have been called Web site comparative analysis studies. In each case, the surveys were designed to obtain 100–200 completed forms from respondents familiar with each of, typically, five Web sites in the comparative analysis. The intent is that respondents from the panel have some familiarity with the Web sites about which they are being queried. Thus the panel responses are thought to be more valid because panelists have used the Web site(s) of interest over a period of time and/or are asked to use the Web site(s) prior to answering questions.

The comparative questions cover topics similar to those used in randomized direct surveys of Web site users. The results of the two comparative studies indicate that MedlinePlus is perceived by users to be on a par with WebMD, which is the leading private sector consumer health Web site in terms of overall usage levels. The implication of these studies is that WebMD's higher usage is due to marketing and promotional activities, not due to some significant advantage in site content, functionality, or performance. The combined study results indicate that online health information consumers perceive both MedlinePlus and WebMD as more useful than other sites such as Yahoo Health, MSN Health, AOL Health, Mayo Health, and InteliHealth.

NLM has concluded that the use of external panels for user surveys can meet specialized, niche needs, such as getting comparative feedback with other Web sites in the same market space. The cost of panel surveys is about US$30 000–45 000. Panel surveys are not, however, a substitute for surveying your own users directly when they visit your Web site.

Focus groups—in person or online

Focus groups are part of the standard repertoire of product and service development, and have been employed by NLM for decades with regard to health information services. The need for focus groups has continued as NLM's information services have evolved from paper to online electronic to Web-based.

The purpose of a focus group is to engage a small number of persons, presumably actual users or those who are representative of current or future users, in providing feedback on a specific Web site. Focus groups can potentially provide a deeper and more robust level of user feedback than can randomized online surveys. But focus group results are not generalizable to a larger user population in a statistical sense.

Traditionally, focus groups have been held in person. But in-person focus groups can be difficult to schedule, and incur travel costs—for the participants and/or the facilitators.

Over the last 5 years, NLM has experimented with the use of online focus groups for several Web sites, including: MedlinePlus in English and en Espanol (http://medlineplus.gov/spanish/); Environmental Health and Toxicology (http://sis.nlm.nih.gov/enviro.html); and ToxTown (http://toxtown.nlm.nih.gov/). The online focus groups are less expensive, by perhaps a factor of two (US$5000 online compared to US$10 000 in-person), and eliminate any geographic barriers and the need for travel. But the online discussion is more constrained than when meeting face-to-face. Also, online focus groups by definition exclude the less Web-savvy users.

NLM believes that focus groups should be included as part of the Web evaluation strategy for any major public or consumer health information Web site.

Nationwide syndicated survey

Another way to get general user feedback is through subscription to nationwide surveys that are conducted by public or private polling organizations. In the United States, a leading example of a public organization is the Pew Internet & American Life Project, which for several years has conducted public opinion surveys on various Internet and Web-related topics. The results of Pew surveys are mostly free to anyone and available for download from the Pew Web site (http://www.pewinternet.org/). Pew has conducted several studies on the topic of online health information-seeking (see, e.g. Fox 2006; Madden & Fox 2006).

NLM has subscribed to several syndicated health sector surveys. Like all syndicated surveys, the costs of the survey recruitment, design, fielding, data collection, analysis, and reporting are spread over multiple clients. This makes access to the survey results much more affordable than having to cover the entire cost alone. An annual subscription cost for a survey with 2000 respondents might typically be in the range of US$25 000– 50 000.

NLM has found such surveys very helpful in understanding overall and health sector trends in Internet and Web usage, what kinds of information users seek on health Web sites, the reasons they seek such information, and what they do with the information they find. Additionally, these surveys provide important information on levels of public awareness of various health organizations and Web sites, and the ways that users gain access to such Web sites and related health information, including use of search engines, wireless technologies, and the like. Finally, some surveys cover the physician or provider perspective regarding online health information, and provide a helpful complement to the consumer perspective.

The annual price for a syndicated survey usually includes several monthly or quarterly 'hot topic' deliverables, access to an online portal for download of detailed survey results, assistance from a survey analyst for a set level of effort, and input to the formulation of each year's survey instruments.

Usage data

User feedback data, discussed above, are largely qualitative, which are sometimes converted to quantitative form (for example, by scaling or quantizing qualitative responses to questions). User feedback data are based on perceptions of the Web site customers. These data are very important but do not provide a true quantitative indicator of actual levels of Web site usage.

Usage data are defined as quantitative measurements of various metrics of Web site usage. These metrics and the data collected on them are not water tight, and are subject to various uncertainties. But usage data are an essential component to an overall Web evaluation strategy.

NLM has collected Web usage data for over a decade, since the launch of its first major Web sites—PubMed and MedlinePlus. NLM has studied the evolution of Web metrics in recent years and in 2001, and after considerable deliberation, settled on three core measures of Web usage and one optional measure. These include:

- Unique visitors—the number of different persons who visit a specific Web site in one month's period of time, correcting for repeat visitors;
- Total visits—the number of total visits by all persons visiting a specific Web site in one month's period of time, counting multiple visits per person equally;
- Pages downloaded—the total number of pages downloaded (also called page views) from a specific Web site in one month's time;
- Searches conducted (optional for NLM)—the total number of searches conducted on a specific Web-based database in a given

month (this metric applies only to Web sites that have searchable, structured databases, such as PubMed in the case of NLM).

These definitions have stood the test of time. The two primary ways NLM collects data on these metrics are: Web log analysis software loaded on NLM's own internal Web servers; and Internet Audience Measurement services based on external user panels. The main difference is that Web log software measures users by collecting data on the number of Internet Protocol (IP) addresses that visit the Web site being monitored, whereas Internet user panels measure the actual number of persons on the panel using specific Web sites and then extrapolate that data to national averages.

Web log data analysis

All major Web sites should have Web log software loaded on the main server. This has long since become standard operating procedure. The software in most situations will be readily available Commercial off the Shelf (COTS), and in some cases custom written for addressing unique or specialized needs. NLM currently uses commercial software on several sites, along with freeware on smaller sites and custom software for some of the very large sites.

Most Web log software collects data on the core metrics—unique visitors, total visitors, pages downloaded—plus data on several other supplemental metrics, such as: Country breakdown; top pages downloaded; top referral sites; site loyalty (frequency of visits); time online (per visit or session); browsers used; operating systems used; and search engines used.

Web log data are typically reported monthly, and in time series, and made available on a protected access Web site. NLM has found that Web log data are useful to Web managers and top-level management for tracking overall usage trends, and for comparing Web log data with other usage information (e.g. external Internet Audience measurements, see below).

However, data users need to keep in mind the limitations—the data are numbers of IP addresses, and tend to under-count institutional users such as libraries where many people may use the same computer and IP address in a given period of time. On the other hand, individual users from computers with dynamic IP addresses may be over-counted.

Nonetheless, Web log data are considered a mainstay of an overall Web evaluation strategy.

Internet audience measurement

Web log data are frequently used to estimate the number of Web site users, and trends in growth or decline of the volume of usage over time. However, as noted, Web log data are an approximation, due to several possible error factors. Further, many Web managers desire to understand the relative positioning of their Web site compared to other Web sites in the same market space. Web log data are generally considered proprietary, and are very difficult to obtain for Web sites outside of one's own organization.

The use of external panels of users to estimate media usage levels pre-dates the Internet and Web. For several decades, estimates of prime time television viewing audiences have been based on extrapolations of the viewing habits of a relatively small number of people. The same concept has been applied to the Internet and Web over the last decade, first to the US market and in recent years increasingly to international markets.

This service is formally called 'Internet Audience Measurement' in the United States. However, panels and other techniques are actually used to estimate usage of various Web sites, and thus really should be called Web Site Audience Measurement, or similar. Since the late 1990s, NLM has used various US measurement services (Wood *et al.* 2005).

NLM currently uses comScore Networks/MediaMetrix, which has the largest panel size—about one million US domestic panel members, and about one million combined panelists for non-US countries (mostly concentrated in Western Europe, but with some coverage in over 150 countries).

comScore's greatest strength in the health sector is the home consumer health market, that is, estimating usage of individuals who search for health information from home. The comScore panel also includes some college student panelists (in residence halls) and some office workers. However, comScore under-represents the scientific, research, and library users of health information. All comScore panelists agree to have their Web usage monitored and recorded, in terms of number of visits to each Web site, number of pages downloaded, the number of minutes per visit, and similar metrics. Data are collected and aggregated by month, and then extrapolated to national and global averages by using demographic, census, and other polling data.

NLM uses comScore data to monitor Web usage levels in the health information and government information market spaces. The comScore data are a useful complement to Web log data in order to cross-verify usage data and better understand national and global health information usage trends.

NLM has found that Internet audience measurement services are a practical and cost-effective way to comprehensively understand broader Web site usage trends and the competitive landscape relevant to specific Web sits. A 1-year subscription to comScore or Neilsen/NetRatings costs US$40 000–50 000.

Web/Internet performance data

An important component of Web site performance is the speed of downloading pages. Even if the Web content is excellent, and the Web site well-designed, a poor Internet connection could mean long download times and a frustrated user. Some unhappy customers will log off or move on to another Web site, and never come back.

While somewhat esoteric, it behooves all Web managers to pay attention to the technical performance of their Web sites. This is somewhat challenging because there are so many factors that can affect Internet performance and Web download times.

NLM has found that, besides designing Web sites for optimal download, the most important step is to have an Internet performance monitoring capability. For the last decade, NLM has experimented with a variety of approaches to measuring Internet performance, both home-grown and commercial (Wood *et al.* 1998). At present, NLM uses a combination of: (1) An NLM-centric network of medical libraries whose Internet pathways to (and from NLM) are monitored, measured, and reported on an hourly basis 24/7; and (2) a commercial service known as Keynote that maintains a virtual network of Points of Presence (POPs) in the United States and overseas for measuring average and Web site-specific download times.

These performance measurements allow NLM to isolate and trouble-shoot slow download times reported by users or partner institutions. Even if the problem is out of NLM's direct control, the performance data allow NLM to advise others as to what to do or who to talk with to help solve the problem.

The state-of-the-art of Web/Internet performance software and services has advanced markedly in recent years. Useful measurement services and data can be obtained for as little as US$2000 per Web site per year.

Planning for Web evaluation

The Web has become an integral part of the public health infrastructure in the United States and other high-income countries, and trends are moving in that direction in other countries as well. The Web can support many of the informational, research, epidemiologic, health promotion, disease prevention, and care support and advocacy goals of public and consumer health, nationally and globally.

The central role of the Web argues strongly that Web evaluation be a key part of the Web design, development, operation, improvement, and re-design cycle. And a multidimensional approach to Web evaluation is likely to be most effective in optimizing Web site performance and meeting user needs.

NLM's decade of work with Web evaluation suggests that some combination of usability testing, online surveys, and focus groups, Web usage data from log files and external user panels, and monitoring download speed will meet the need for most Web sites. The exact combination and deployment of Web evaluation methods will depend on the size and traffic level of the Web site, and on available staff and financial resources.

In NLM's experience, an investment in Web evaluation helps significantly increase the return on investment in the biomedical, research, and consumer health information Web sites.

Conclusions

The last 5 years have witnessed a revolution in the use of the World Wide Web in the public health sector. The number of Web sites used by national and provincial health departments, public health associations, schools of public health, and public health-related volunteer and advocacy organizations has proliferated.

Some overarching conclusions:

1. The Web revolution in the public health arena will continue, as the Web matures and the user community increases in sophistication and expectations. This is especially true for public and consumer health information dissemination.
2. There is still a digital divide between the developed and developing nations, as reflected in differential levels of Internet usage and bandwidth availability.
3. The Web presents opportunities to help further bridge the divide, such as with the HINARI programme, for accessible health and biomedical journal literature in low- and middle-income countries.
4. The Web offers exciting new opportunities for Disaster Management and Emergency Preparedness globally. Natural and human disasters do not respect national boundaries.
5. Given the key role of Web sites in public and consumer health information dissemination, evaluation of Web sites warrants greater attention and a more sophisticated approach—a multidimensional approach to Web evaluation.
6. All Web developers and Web masters, and their respective management teams, need to be sensitive to the universal need for Web evaluation. The major public and consumer health Web sites would benefit greatly from a substantial evaluative activity.

Acknowledgements

The authors acknowledge helpful reviews of all or parts of this chapter and/or useful suggestions from Stacey Arneson, Victor Cid, Martha Fishel, Dennis Benson, and Ione Auston of the NLM.

References

Abreu, M. (2006). Cybercitizen Health: 2006 Survey Results. Unpublished report prepared by Manhattan Research LLC for the National Library of Medicine, Bethesda MD, USA.

Abreu, M. (2006). Taking the Pulse: 2006 Survey Results. Unpublished report prepared by Manhattan Research LLC for the National Library of Medicine, Bethesda MD, USA.

Aguwon, G. (2006). Use of the Internet for health information by physicians for patient care in a teaching hosopital in Ibadan, Nigeria. *Biomedical Digital Libraries,* **3**, 12–21.

Arnesen, S., Scott, J., Perez, R. *et al.* (2003). Prevention pays: NLM/PAHO partnership helps health professionals get information before disasters strike in Central America. In *Proceedings of the 103rd Annual Meeting of the Medical Library Association.* San Diego CA, USA.

Arnesen, S., Cid, V., Scott, J. *et al.* (2005). Central American Network for Disaster and Health Information (CANDHI): Enhancing information management capacities at health sciences libraries promotes disaster preparedness. In *Proceedings of the 9th World Congress on Information and Libraries.* Salvador-Bahia, Brazil.

Arnesen, S.J., Cid, V.H. Scott, J.C. *et al.* (2007). The Central American Network for Disaster Health Information. *Journal of the Medical Library Association,* **95**, 316–22.

Bourgeois, F.T., Olson, K.L., Brownstein, J.S. *et al.* (2006). Validation of syndromic surveillance for respiratory infections. *Annals of Emergency Medicine,* **47**, p. 265e1, Epub.

Cato, J. (2001). *User-centered Web design.* Addison-Wesley, London, UK.

Centre for Research on the Epidemiology of Disasters (2007). *The OFDA/CRED international disaster database.* US Agency for International Development/Office of Foreign Disaster Assistance and Universite Catholiqu de Louvain, Brussels, Belgium.

Currion, P., de Silva, C., and Van de Walle, B. (2007). Open source software for disaster management. *Communications of the ACM,* **50**, 61–5.

Fox, S. (2006). *Online health search 2006.* Pew Internet & American Life Project, Washington DC, USA.

Fox, S. (2005). *Health information online.* Pew Internet & American Life Project, Washington DC, USA.

Fisher, L. (2007). comScore Health Information Usage Report. Unpublished report prepare by comScore Networks Inc. for the National Library of Medicine, Bethesda MD, USA.

Koyani, S., Bailey, R., and Nall, J. (2003). *Research-based Web design & usability guidelines.* National Institutes of Health, National Cancer Institute, Bethesda MD, USA.

Madden, M. and Fox, S. (2006). *Finding answers online in sickness and in health.* Pew Internet & American Life Project, Washington DC, USA.

National Library of Medicine (2006). *Charting a course for the 21st century: NLM's long range plan 2006-2016.* US Dept. of Health and Human Services, Public Health Service, National Institutes of Health, National Library of Medicine, Bethesda MD, USA.

Nielsen, J. (2000). *Designing Web usability.* New Riders Publishing, Indianapolis, IN, USA.

North Carolina Department of Health and Human Services, Division of Public Health (2007). EpiNotes. Available at: http://www.epi.state.nc.us/epi/gcdc/flu.html (accessed 23 May 2007).

Palen, L., Hiltz, S., and Liu, S. (2007). Online forms supporting grassroots participation in emergency response. *Communications of the ACM*, **50**, 54–8.

Peters, T. (2001). *Spanning the digital divide: Understanding and tackling the issues*. Bridges.org, Durbanville, South Africa, and Washington DC, USA.

Que, J., Tsui, F.C., and Wagner, M.M. (2006). Timeliness study of radiology and microbiology reports in a healthcare system for biosurveillance. *American Medical Informatics Association Symposium Proceedings*, p. 1068.

Rantucci, G. (1994). *Geological disasters in the Phillipines: July'90 earthquake and June'91 eruption of Mt. Pinatubo, description, effects, lessons learned*. Diane Publishing, Darby, PA, USA.

Reis, B.Y. and Mandl, K.D. (2004). Syndromic surveillance: The effects of syndrome grouping on model accuracy and outbreak detection. *Annals of Emergency Medicine*, **44**, 235–41.

Royall, J., Schayk, I., Bennett, M. *et al.* (2005). Crossing the digital divide: The contribution of information technology to the professional performance of malaria researchers in Africa. *African Health Sciences*, **5**, 246–54.

Royall, J., Bennett, M., van Schayk, I. *et al.* (2004). Tying up lions: Multilateral Initiative on Malaria Communications: The first chapter of a malaria research network in Africa. *American Journal of Tropical Medicine and Hygiene*, **71**(Suppl 2), 259–67.

Scott, J. (1998). Applications of telecommunications and information technology for humanitarian health initiatives. In *Proceedings of the Pacific Medical Technology Symposium—PACMEDTek* (eds. R. Nelson, A. Gelish, and S. Mun). IEEE Computer Society, Los Alamitos CA, USA.

Scott, J. (1997). *Earth observation, hazard analysis, and communications technology for early warning*. United Nations International Decade for Natural Disaster Reduction, Early Warning Programme, New York, NY, USA.

Scott, J. (2006). Health InterNetwork Access to Research Initiative (HINARI)/Access to Global Online Research in Agriculture (AGORA) Usage Review. Unpublished report prepared for the World Health Organization, Food and Agriculture Organization, and United Kingdom Department for International Development.

Siegel, E., Logan, R., Harnsberger, R. *et al.* (2006). Information Rx: Evaluation of a new informatics tool for physicians, patients, and libraries. *Information Services & Use*, **26**, 1–10.

Sklar, J. (2000). *Principles of Web design*. Thompson Learning, Cambridge, MA, USA.

Sloane, P., MacFarquhar, J., Sickbert-Bennett, E. *et al.* (2006). Syndromic surveillance for emerging infections in office practice using billing data. *Annals of Family Medicine*, **4**, 351–8.

Smith, H., Bukirwa, H., Mukasa, O. *et al.* (2007). Access to electronic health knowledge in five countries in Africa: A descriptive study. *MBJ Health Services Research*, **7**, 72–7.

Turoff, M., Chumer, M. and Hitlz, S. (2006). Emergency planning as a continuous game. In *Proceedings of the International ISCRAM Conference* (eds. M Turoff and B. Van de Walle). Newark, NJ, USA.

Turoff, M., Chumer, M., Van de Walle, B. *et al.* (2004). The design of a dynamic emergency response management information system (DERMIS). *The Journal of Information Technology Theory and Application*, **5**, 1–35.

United Nations Economic Commission of Latin America and the Caribbean (1998). *Central America: Assessment of the damage caused by Hurricane Mitch: Implications for economic and social development and for the environment*. The Commission, Santiago, Chile.

United States Department of Health and Human Services (2007a). *HHS Web standards*, final version January 5, 2007. Available at: http://www.samhsa.gov/IT/Docs/HHSWebStandardsFinal010507.pdf (accessed 9 September 2007).

United States Department of Health and Human Services, Assistant Secretary for Public Affairs (2007b). *Usability.gov: Your guide for developing usable and useful Web sites*. Available at: http://www.usability.gov/ (accessed 9 September 2007).

United States Department of Health and Human Services (2006). *Research-based Web design & usability guidelines*. Available at: http://usability.gov/pdfs/guidelines_book.pdf (accessed 9 September 2007).

Wagner, M.M., Espino, J., Tsui, F.C. *et al.* (2004). Syndrome and outbreak detection using chief-complaint data—experience of the Real-Time Outbreak and Disease Surveillance project. *Morbidity and Mortality Weekly Report*, **53**(Suppl), 28–31.

Wikipedia (2007). *Web design*. Available at: http://en.wikipedia.org/wiki/Web_design (accessed 9 September 2007).

Wood, F., Siegel, E., Feldman, S. *et al.* (2008). Web evaluation experiment at the US National Institutes of Health: Use of the American Customer Satisfaction Index online customer survey. *Journal of Medical Internet Research*, Jan–Mar; 10(1): e4. Published online 2008 February 15. doi: 10.2196/jmir.944.

Wood, F., Benson, D., LaCroix, E-M. *et al.* (2005). Use of Internet audience measurement data to gauge market share for online health information services. *Journal of Medical Internet Research*, **7**, e31.

Wood, F., Siegel, E., LaCroix, E-M *et al.* (2003). A practical approach to E-government web evaluation. *IT Pro (Information Technology Professional)*, **5**, 22–8.

Wood, F., Lyon, B., Schell, M.B. *et al.* (2000). Public library consumer health information pilot project: Results of a National Library of Medicine evaluation. *Bulletin of the Medical Library Association*, **88**, 314–22.

Wood, F., Cid, V., and Siegel, E. (1998). Evaluating Internet end-to-end performance: Overview of test methodology and results. *Journal of the American Medical Informatics Association*, **5**, 528–45.

World Health Organization (2003). Forty new countries given low cost access to health journals [press release, 17 Jan 2003]. Available at: www.who.int/mediacentre/releases/2003/pr3/en/print.html (accessed 9 September 2007).

SECTION 6

Epidemiological and biostatistical approaches

6.1

Epidemiology: The foundation of public health

Roger Detels

Abstract

Epidemiology is the basic science of public health, because it is the science that describes the relationship of health or disease with other health-related factors in human populations, such as human pathogens. Furthermore, epidemiology has been used to generate much of the information required by public health professionals to develop, implement, and evaluate effective intervention programmes for the prevention of disease and promotion of health, such as the eradication of smallpox, the anticipated eradication of polio and guinea worm disease, and the prevention of heart disease and cancer. Unlike pathology, which constitutes a basic area of knowledge, and cardiology, which is the study of a specific organ, epidemiology is a philosophy and methodology that can be applied to learning about and resolving a very broad range of health problems. The 'art' of epidemiology is knowing when and how to apply the various epidemiological strategies creatively to answer specific health questions; it is not enough to know what the various study designs and statistical methodologies are.

The uses and limitations of the various epidemiological study designs are presented to illustrate and underscore the fact that the successful application of epidemiology requires more than a knowledge of study designs and epidemiological methods. These designs and methods must be applied appropriately, creatively, and innovatively if they are to yield the desired information. The field of epidemiology has been expanding dramatically over the last three decades, as epidemiologists have demonstrated new uses and variations of traditional study designs and methods. We can anticipate that the scope of epidemiology will expand even more in the future as increasing numbers of creative epidemiologists develop innovative new strategies and techniques.

The chapters in this section present detailed discussions of the principles and methods of epidemiology. In this introductory chapter, I will attempt to define epidemiology, to present ways in which epidemiology is used in the advancement of public health, and finally, to discuss the range of applications of epidemiological methodologies.

What is epidemiology?

There are many definitions of epidemiology, but every epidemiologist will know exactly what it is that he or she does. Defining epidemiology is difficult primarily because it does not represent a body of knowledge, as does, for example, anatomy, nor does it target a specific organ system, as does cardiology. Epidemiology represents a method of studying a health problem and can be applied to a wide range of problems, from transmission of an infectious disease agent to the design of a new strategy for healthcare delivery. Furthermore, this methodology is continually changing as it is adapted to a greater range of health problems and more techniques are borrowed and adapted from other disciplines such as mathematics and statistics.

Maxcy, one of the pioneer epidemiologists of the past century, offered the following definition:

> *Epidemiology is that field of medical science which is concerned with the relationship of various factors and conditions which determine the frequencies and distributions of an infectious process, a disease, or a physiologic state in a human community* (Lilienfeld 1978).

The word itself comes from the Greek *epi*, *demos*, and *logos*; literally translated, it means the study (*logos*) of what is upon (*epi*) the people (*demos*). John Last, in the *Dictionary of Epidemiology*, has defined epidemiology as follows:

> *The study of the distribution and determinants of health-related states or events in specified populations, and the application of this study to the control of health problems.*

Last's definition underscores that epidemiologists are concerned not only with disease but also with 'health-related events', and that ultimately epidemiology is committed to control of disease. All epidemiologists, however, will agree that epidemiology concerns itself with populations rather than individuals, thereby separating it from the rest of medicine and constituting the basic science of public health. Following from this, therefore, is the need to describe health and disease in terms of frequencies and distributions in the population. The epidemiologist relates these frequencies and distributions of specific health parameters to the frequencies of other factors to which populations are exposed in order to identify those that may be causes of ill health or promoters of good health. Inherent in the philosophy of epidemiology is the idea that ill health is not randomly distributed in populations, and that elucidating the reasons for this non-random distribution will provide clues regarding the risk factors for disease and the biological mechanisms that result in loss of health.

Because epidemiology usually focuses on health in *human* populations, it is rarely able to provide experimental proof in the sense of Koch's postulates, as can often be done in the laboratory sciences. Epidemiology more often provides an accumulation of increasingly convincing indirect evidence of a relationship between health or disease and other factors. This process, referred to as causal inference (see Chapter 6.13, by Hoggatt and Greenland), includes considering an observed relationship in terms of its strength, consistency, specificity, temporality, biologic gradient, plausibility, coherence, and experimental evidence (Hill 1965).

Although they will differ on the exact definitions of epidemiology, most epidemiologists will agree that they try to characterize the relationships among the *agent*, the *environment*, and the *host* (usually human). The epidemiologist considers health to represent a balance among these three forces, as shown in Fig. 6.1.1.

Changes in any one of these three factors may result in loss of health. For example, the host may be compromised as a result of treatment with steroids, making him or her more susceptible to agents that do not ordinarily cause disease. On the other hand, a breakdown in the water supply system may result in an increased exposure of people to agents such as cryptosporidium, as happened in 1993 in Milwaukee, WI (MacKenzie *et al.* 1994). Finally, some agents may become more or less virulent over time—often because of the promiscuous use of antibiotics—thereby disturbing the dynamic balance among agent, host, and environment. Two examples are the cases of acute necrotizing fasciitis caused by group A streptococcus (Communicable Disease Surveillance Centre 1994) and the development of multi-drug-resistant tuberculosis (Chapman & Henderson 1994).

The epidemiologist uses another triad to study the relationship of agent, host, and environment: *time–place–person*. Using various epidemiological techniques, described in subsequent chapters, the epidemiologist describes disease or disease factors occurring in the population in terms of the characteristics of time (e.g. trends, outbreaks, etc.), place (the geographic area in which the disease is occurring), and person (the characteristics of the affected individuals; e.g. age, gender, etc.) to elucidate the causative agent, the natural history of the disease, and the environmental factors that increase the likelihood of the host acquiring the disease. With this information, the epidemiologist is able to suggest ways to intervene in the disease process to prevent either disease or death.

Epidemiology has been described as the 'art of the possible'. Because epidemiologists work with human populations, they are

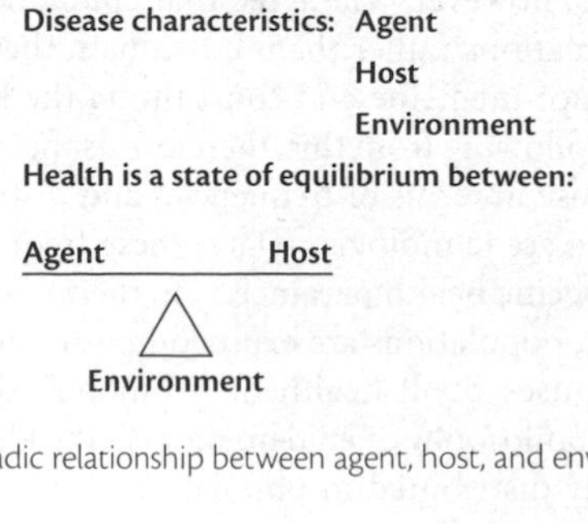

Fig. 6.1.1 The triadic relationship between agent, host, and environment in epidemiology.

rarely able to manipulate events or the environment as can the laboratory scientist. They must, therefore, exploit situations as they exist naturally to advance knowledge. They must be both pragmatic and realistic; they must realize both the capabilities and limitations of the discipline. Morris has said that the 'epidemiologic method is the only way to ask some questions . . ., one way of asking others and no way at all to ask many' (Morris 1975). The art of epidemiology is to know both when epidemiology is the method of choice and when it is not, and how to use it to answer the question.

Applying the epidemiological method to resolve a health question successfully can be compared to constructing a memorable Chinese banquet. It is not enough to have the best ingredients and to know the various Chinese cooking methods. The truly great chefs must be able to select the appropriate ingredients and cooking methods to bring out the flavours of each dish, and further, must know how to construct the correct sequence of dishes to excite the palate without overwhelming it. They create a memorable banquet by adding their creative genius to the raw ingredients and the established cooking methods. Similarly, it is not enough for the epidemiologist to know the various strategies and methods of epidemiology; the innovative epidemiologist must be able to apply them creatively to obtain the information needed to understand the natural history of the disease. It is not enough to know what a cohort study is; the epidemiologist must know when the cohort design is the appropriate design for the question at hand, and then must apply that design appropriately and creatively. These skills make epidemiology more than a methodology. It is this opportunity for creativity and innovation that provides excitement for the practitioner and makes the successful practice of epidemiology an art.

For example, Imagawa *et al.* (1989) identified probable transient HIV-1 infection in men, implying clearance of the virus by the immune system of the men, by focusing their viral isolation studies on the relatively few HIV-1-antibody-negative homosexual men who had many different sexual partners; a simple cohort study of antibody-negative individuals would have required a cohort of thousands of men rather than the 133 studied. The effects of passive smoking were demonstrated by cohort studies of non-smoking family members of smokers and in nursing students by comparing the reported symptoms in room-mates of smokers and non-smokers who kept diaries of their symptoms: The room-mates of the smokers had a 1.8 greater risk of episodes of phlegm than room-mates of non-smokers (Schwartz & Zeger 1990). Colley *et al.* (1974), Tager *et al.* (1979), and Tashkin *et al.* (1984) demonstrated that children of smokers had lower levels of lung function than children of non-smokers. All of these investigators used traditional study designs, but demonstrated their creativity by applying that design to those specific populations which were most likely to reveal a relationship if it existed.

Epidemiologic studies rarely provide 'proof' of a causal relationship. Thus, there is continuing debate among epidemiologists about what constitutes adequate criteria for inferring a causal relationship from epidemiological studies (Rothman 1988). Hill (1965) suggested the following criteria for establishing a causal relationship: Strength of association (statistical probability and risk ratio), consistency of findings across multiple studies, specificity of the relationship, temporality (outcome follows causation), biologic gradient (a dose–response relationship), plausibility, coherence (consistency with prior knowledge), experimental evidence, and analogy (relationship hypothesized is similar to that in known relationships).

Susser has added to these criteria the ability of the observed relationship to correctly predict other relationships (Rothman 1988). The debate goes on, but the principle is the same: Epidemiologic studies seldom provide 'proof' of a causal relationship in the sense of Koch's postulates, but may be used to reveal a possible relationship and build a convincing case that this relationship is causal.

Uses of epidemiology in support of public health

Epidemiology is the basic science of public health because it is the health science that describes health and disease in *populations* rather than in individuals, information essential for the formulation of effective public health initiatives to prevent disease and promote health in the community. I have taken the liberty of updating the 'Functions of Epidemiology', first expounded by Morris (1957) and Holland *et al.* (2007). They are as follows:

1. *Describe the spectrum of the disease*: Disease represents the end point of a process of alteration of the host's biological systems. Although many disease agents are limited in the range of alterations they can initiate, others, such as measles, can cause a variety of disease end points. For example, the majority of infections with rubeola (measles) virus result in the classical febrile, blotchy-rash disease, but the rubeola virus can also cause generalized haemorrhagic rash and acute encephalitis. Years after initial infection, rubeola can also cause subacute sclerosing panencephalitis (SSPE), a fatal disease of the central nervous system.

   Various types of epidemiological studies have been used to elucidate the spectrum of disease resulting from many agents and conditions; for example, cohort studies have been used to document the role of high blood pressure as a major cause of stroke, myocardial infarct, and chronic kidney disease. For rare diseases such as SSPE and multiple sclerosis, case–control studies have been useful to identify the role of the rubeola virus (Alter 1976; Detels *et al.* 1973). Knowing the spectrum of disease that can result from specific infections and conditions allows the public health professional to design more effective intervention strategies; for example, education, screening, and treatment programmes to reduce the prevalence of high blood pressure will also reduce the incidence of myocardial infarct, stroke, and chronic kidney disease (Hypertension Detection and Follow-up Program Cooperative Group 1979).

2. *Describe the natural history of disease*: Epidemiological studies can be used to describe the natural history of disease, to elucidate the specific alterations in the biological system in the host, and to improve diagnostic accuracy. For example, cohort studies of individuals who were infected with HIV, the 'AIDS virus', revealed that a drop in the level of T-lymphocytes having the CD4 marker was associated with being infected with HIV (Polk *et al.* 1987), and that a further decline in CD4 cells was associated with developing clinical symptoms and AIDS (Detels *et al.* 1987). This observation stimulated immunologists to focus their research on the interaction of the immune system and HIV. From a clinical perspective, clinicians can target HIV-antibody-positive individuals who have declining CD4 cells for prophylactic treatment when it is most likely to be effective. Epidemiology can also be used to describe the impact of treatment on the natural history of disease. For example, a cohort study design was used to demonstrate the public health effectiveness of combined highly active antiretroviral therapy on reducing the incidence of AIDS and extending survival of those who already had the disease (Detels *et al.* 1998). Thus, describing the natural history of AIDS among both treated and untreated individuals has assisted researchers to focus their studies and clinicians to use the limited treatment modalities available more effectively (Phair *et al.* 1992). The field of 'clinical epidemiology' applies research on the natural history of disease to improving the diagnostic accuracy of physicians in their clinical practice (Sackett *et al.* 1991).

3. *Community diagnosis*: Epidemiological surveys are often used to establish the morbidity and mortality from specific diseases, allowing efficient use of limited public health funds for control of those diseases having the greatest negative impact on the health of the community. For example, an epidemiological survey in one area of China identified the epidemic of HIV due to plasma donations in villages (Ji *et al.* 2006; Wu & Detels 1995; Wu *et al.* 2001). The use of disability-adjusted years (DALYs) has allowed quantification of the importance of non-lethal conditions on the public's health (Murray 1994).

4. *Describe the clinical picture of a disease*: Epidemiological strategies can identify who is likely to get a disease such as capillariasis, the characteristic symptoms and signs, the extent of the epidemic, the risk factors, and the causative agent, and can help to determine the effectiveness of treatment and control efforts (Detels *et al.* 1969b).

5. *Identify factors that increase or decrease the risk of acquiring disease*: Having specific characteristics increases the probability that individuals will or will not develop disease. These 'risk factors' may be social (smoking, drinking), genetic (ethnicity), dietary (saturated fats, vitamin deficiencies), and so on. Knowing these risk factors can often provide public health professionals with the necessary tools to design effective programmes to intervene before disease occurs. For example, descriptive, cross-sectional, case–control, cohort, and intervention studies have all shown that smoking is the biggest single risk factor for ill health, because it is a major risk factor for cardiovascular disease, chronic respiratory disease, and many cancers (e.g. of the lung, nasopharynx, and bladder). Thus, smoking is the leading cause of disability and death in developed countries, if not the world. Health education campaigns and other strategies to stop or reduce smoking, based on these epidemiologic studies, are now a major public health activity in most countries of the world.

6. *Identify precursors of disease and syndromes*: High blood pressure, a treatable condition, has been identified through case–control and cohort studies as a precursor to heart disease, stroke, and kidney disease (Joint National Committee on Prevention, Detection, Evaluation, and Treatment of High Blood Pressure 1997).

7. *Test the efficacy of intervention strategies*: A primary objective of public health is to prevent disease through intervention in the disease process. But a vaccine or other intervention programme must be proved effective before it is used in the community. Double-blind placebo-controlled trials are a necessary step in developing an intervention programme, whether that programme is administration of a new vaccine, a behavioural intervention strategy to stop smoking, or a community intervention

study to lower heart disease. Although it may be argued that injection of a saline placebo is no longer considered ethical, a proven vaccine, such as polio, can often be used as a placebo for a trial of a new vaccine for a different disease, as was used for trials of rubella vaccines in Taiwan (Detels *et al.* 1969a). Widespread use of an intervention not subjected to epidemiological studies of efficacy may result in implementation of an ineffective intervention programme at great public expense, and may actually result in greater morbidity and mortality because of an increased reliance on the favoured but unproven intervention and a reduced use of other strategies that are thought to be less effective but which are actually more effective.

Although an intervention such as a vaccine may have been demonstrated to have efficacy in double-blind trials, it may fail to provide protection when used in the community. Double-blind trials may demonstrate the 'biological efficacy' of the vaccine; but if the vaccine is not acceptable to the majority of the public, they will refuse to be vaccinated, and the 'public health effectiveness' of the vaccine will be very low. For example, the typhoid vaccine provided some protection against small infecting inocula, but the frequency of unpleasant side effects with the whole cell vaccines and the need for multiple injections in the past influenced many people against being vaccinated (Chin 2000).

Another problem of inferring public health efficacy from small vaccine trials is that volunteers for these trials may not be representative of the general public, which needs to be protected against a specific disease. Thus, broad-based intervention trials also need to be carried out, to demonstrate the acceptability and public health effectiveness of a vaccine or other intervention to the population in need of protection.

As there are adverse effects associated with any vaccine, ongoing evaluations of the cost–benefit relationship of specific vaccines are important. By comparing the incidence of smallpox with the incidence of adverse effects from the smallpox vaccine, Lane *et al.* (1969) demonstrated that more disease resulted from routine use of the vaccine in the United States than by transmission from imported cases.

There are several epidemiological strategies that can be used for ongoing evaluation of intervention programmes. Serial cross-sectional studies can be used to determine if there has been a change in the prevalence of disease or of indicators of health status over time. The cohort design can be used to compare incidence of disease in comparable populations receiving and not receiving the prevention programme. The case–control design can be used to determine if there are differences in the proportion of cases and non-cases who had the intervention programme.

8. *Investigate epidemics of unknown aetiology*: Epidemiological strategies were used to establish the extent, cause, modes of transmission, and risk factors for Ebola haemorrhagic fever, which first occurred in the Congo in 1976 (King 2003; Feldmann *et al.* 1996), and capillariasis in the Philippines in the mid-1960s (Detels *et al.* 1969b).
9. *Evaluate public health programmes*: Departments of health are engaged in a variety of activities to promote the health of the community, ranging from vaccination programmes to clinics for the treatment of specific diseases. Ongoing evaluation of such programmes is necessary to ensure that they continue to be cost-effective. Periodic review of routinely collected health statistics can provide information about the effectiveness of many programmes. For programmes for which relevant statistics are not routinely available, cohort studies and serial cross-sectional studies of the incidence and changing prevalence of the targeted disease in the populations which are the intended recipients of these programmes can measure whether the programmes have had an impact and are cost-effective. For example, most countries have established STD clinics, but studies in Thailand (Prempree *et al.* 2007) and Beijing (Zhao *et al.* 2007) have demonstrated that the majority of the patients with STDs do not attend the government STD clinics.
10. *Elucidate mechanisms of disease transmission*: Understanding the mechanisms of disease transmission can suggest ways in which public health professionals can protect the public by stopping transmission of the disease agent. Epidemiological studies of the various arboviral encephalitides have incriminated certain species of mosquitoes as the vectors of disease and specific animals as the reservoirs for the viruses. For example, public health efforts in California to prevent western equine encephalitis have concentrated on control of the mosquito vector and vaccination of horses, which are a reservoir of the virus. Although an effective vaccine for smallpox had been available for almost two hundred years, eradication of the disease was not achieved until the recognition that the low infectivity of varicella virus and the relatively long incubation for development of smallpox could be used to develop a strategy of surveillance for cases, with identification and immediate vaccination of all susceptible contacts (containment). Using this containment strategy based on epidemiologic principles, smallpox was eradicated through a worldwide effort in less than ten years (Fenner *et al.* 1988).
11. *Elucidate the molecular and genetic determinants of disease progression*: Epidemiological strategies helped to elucidate the changes in the human immune response by CD4 and CD8 cells that accompany infection by disease agents (Detels *et al.* 1983; Fahey *et al.* 1984; Ho *et al.* 1995), and genetic factors (such as CCR5 absence or heterozygosity) that prevent HIV infection and slow progression of HIV disease (Liu *et al.* 2004).

From the examples given in the preceding list, it should be clear that epidemiology functions as the backbone or core of evidence-based public health practices, as well as a key strategy for evaluating the effectiveness of both clinical and public health interventions.

Applications of epidemiology

Specific epidemiological study designs are used to achieve specific public health goals. These goals range from identifying a suspected exposure–disease relationship to establishing that relationship, to designing an intervention to prevent it, and finally, to assessing the effectiveness of that intervention. The usual sequence of study designs in the identification and resolution of a disease problem are as follows:

- Ecologic studies
- Cross-sectional (prevalence) surveys
- Case–control studies
- Cohort studies
- Experimental studies

There are, however, many exceptions to the application of this sequence of study designs, depending on such things as the prevalence and virulence of the agent and the nature of the human response to the agent.

The earliest suspicion that a relationship exists between a disease and a possible causative factor is frequently obtained by observing correlations between exposure and disease from existing data such as mortality statistics and surveys of personal or national characteristics. These can be correlations observed across geographical areas (ecological studies) or over time, or a combination of both. Many of the initial epidemiological investigations on chronic bronchitis used vital statistics data, particularly data on mortality. Case–control studies identified smoking as a possible causal factor for chronic bronchitis. Subsequent prevalence studies confirmed the relationship, as have cohort studies. Finally, a decline in respiratory symptoms of chronic bronchitis and a concurrent but slower decline in lung function has been observed in individuals who cease smoking (Colley 1991).

Although this is the usual sequence in which the various epidemiological study designs are applied, there are exceptions to this sequence. Furthermore, all study designs are not appropriate to answer all health questions. The usual applications of each of the epidemiological study designs and their limitations are, therefore, presented briefly in this subsection and in greater depth in subsequent chapters.

Ecologic studies (see Volume 2, Chapter 6.2)

The use of existing statistics to correlate the prevalence or incidence of disease in groups or populations to the frequency or trends over time of suspected causal factors in specific localities has often provided the first clues that a particular factor may cause a specific disease. These epidemiological strategies, however, document only the co-occurrence of disease and other factors in a population; the risk factors and the disease may not be occurring in the same people within the population. These types of descriptive studies are inexpensive and relatively easy to perform, but the co-occurrence observed may be merely due to chance. For example, the incidence of both heart disease and lung cancer has increased concurrently with the increased use of automatic washing machines in the United States. Few people, however, would attribute the increase in these two diseases to the use of automatic washing machines. Thus, ecologic studies must be interpreted with caution. Nonetheless, they often reveal important relationships and can provide a strong rationale for undertaking more expensive analytic studies.

Cross-sectional/prevalence surveys (see Volume 2, Chapters 6.3, 6.4, 6.17)

Cross-sectional/prevalence surveys establish the frequency of disease and other factors in a community. Because they require the collection of data, however, they can be expensive. They are useful to estimate the number of people in a population who have disease and can also identify the difference in frequency of disease in different subpopulations. This descriptive information is particularly useful to health administrators who are responsible for developing appropriate and effective public health programmes.

Cross-sectional studies can also be used to document the co-occurrence of disease and suspected risk factors not only in the population but also in specific individuals within the population. The cross-sectional study design is useful to study chronic diseases such as multiple sclerosis, which has a reasonably high prevalence, but an incidence that is too low to make a cohort study feasible (Detels *et al.* 1978). On the other hand, they are not useful for studying diseases that have a very low prevalence, such as subacute sclerosing panencephalitis or variant Creutzfeldt-Jakob disease. Cross-sectional studies are subject to problems of respondent bias, recall bias, and undocumented confounders. Further, unless historical information is obtained from all the individuals surveyed, the time-relationship between the factor and the disease is not known. Also, prevalence surveys identify people who have survived to that time point with disease, and thus, under-represent people with a short course of disease.

The cross-sectional study design is used in two special types of studies: Field studies and surveillance. Field studies are usually investigations of acute outbreaks, which require immediate identification of the causative factors if effective public health interventions are to be implemented in a timely fashion. Surveillance is the monitoring of disease or health-related factors over time and uses serial cross-sectional surveys to observe trends. Surveillance is important to identify diseases that are becoming an increasing public health problem, to assure that diseases already brought under control remain under control, and to evaluate the impact of public health intervention strategies.

Case–control studies (see Volume 2, Chapter 6.5)

The case–control study compares the prevalence of suspected causal factors between individuals with disease and controls. If the prevalence of the factor is significantly different in cases than it is in controls, this factor may be associated with the disease. Although case–control studies can identify associations, they do not measure risk. An estimate of relative risk, however, can be derived by calculating the odds ratio. Case–control studies are often the analytic study design used initially to investigate a suspected association. Compared to cohort and experimental studies, they are usually relatively cheap and easy to perform. Cases can often be selected from hospital patients and controls either from hospitalized patients with other diseases or by using algorithms or formulas for selecting community (neighbourhood) or other types of controls. Selection bias, however, is often a problem, especially when using either hospitalized cases or controls. The participants are seen only once, and no follow-up is necessary. Although time sequences can often be established retrospectively for factors elicited by interview, they usually cannot be for laboratory test results. For example, an elevation in factor B may either be causally related, or it may be a result of the disease process and not a cause. Furthermore, factors elicited from interview are subject to recall bias; for example, patients are often better motivated to recall events than controls because they are concerned about their disease.

The case–control study is particularly useful for exploring relationships noted in observational studies. A hypothesis, however, is necessary for case–control studies. Relationships will be observed only for those factors studied. Case–control studies are not useful for determining the spectrum of health outcomes resulting from specific exposures, because a definition of a case is required in order to do a case–control study. On the other hand, these studies are the method of choice for studying rare diseases, and are often indicated when a specific health question needs to be answered quickly.

Cohort studies (see Volume 2, Chapter 6.6)

Cohort studies follow defined groups of people without disease to identify risk factors associated with disease occurrence. They have the advantage of establishing the temporal relationship between an exposure and a health outcome, and thus measure risk directly. Because the population studied is often defined on the basis of its known likelihood of exposure to suspected factors, cohort studies are particularly suitable for investigating health hazards associated with environmental or occupational exposures. Further, these studies will measure more than one outcome of a given exposure, and therefore, are useful for defining the spectrum of disease resulting from exposure to a given factor. Occasionally, a cohort study is done to elucidate the natural history of a disease when a group that has a high incidence of disease but in which specific risk factors which are not known can be identified. Although this cohort is not defined based on a known exposure, questions are asked and biological specimens are collected from which exposure variables can be identified concurrently or in the future.

Unfortunately, cohort studies are both expensive and time consuming. Unless the investigator can define a cohort in which risk factors were measured at some time in the past and has the assurance that the cohort has been completely followed up for disease outcomes in the interim (historical cohort), this design can take years to decades to yield information about the risks of disease resulting from exposure to specific factors. Ensuring that participants remain in a cohort study for such long periods of time is both difficult and expensive. Further, the impact of those who drop out of follow-up must be taken into account in the analysis and interpretation of these studies. Finally, exposures may vary over time, complicating the analysis of their impact.

Because of the cost and complexity of cohort studies, they are usually done only after descriptive, cross-sectional, and/or case–control studies have suggested a causal relationship. The size of the cohort to be studied is dependent, in part, on the anticipated incidence of the disease resulting from the exposure. For diseases with a very low incidence, population-based cohort studies are usually not feasible, either in terms of the logistics or of the expense of following very large numbers of people, or both. Cohort studies establish the risk of disease associated with exposure to a factor, but do not 'prove' that the factor is causal; the observed factor may merely be very closely correlated with the real causative factor or may even be related to the participants' choice to be exposed.

A variant of the cohort study that has become popular is the 'nested case–control study' (Gange *et al.* 1997). Cases arising from a cohort study are compared with individuals followed in the cohort who have not developed disease using the usual case–control analytic strategies. The advantage of this type of study is that the exposure variables are collected before knowledge of the outcome, and therefore, are unlikely to be tainted by recall bias.

Experimental studies (see Volume 2, Chapters 6.7–6.10)

Experimental studies differ from cohort studies because it is the investigator who makes the decision about who will be exposed to the factor based on the specific design factors to be employed (e.g. randomization, matching, etc.). Therefore, confounding factors such as choice that may have led to the subjects being exposed in the cohort studies are usually not a problem in experimental studies. Because epidemiologists usually study human populations, there are few opportunities for an investigator to deliberately expose participants to a suspected factor. On the other hand, intervention studies of randomly assigned individuals (Chapter 6.7) or communities (Chapters 6.7–6.10) to receive or not receive an intervention programme that demonstrates a subsequent reduction in a specific health outcome in the intervention group do provide strong evidence, if not proof, of a causal relationship. Because of the serious implications of applying an intervention that may alter the biological status of an individual or the socio-political behaviour of a community, intervention studies should not be undertaken until the probability of a causal or risk relationship has been well established using the other types of study designs.

Meta-analysis (see Volume 2, Chapter 6.14)

Because individual epidemiologic studies rarely provide proof of causation and results of different studies can vary for a number of reasons, including small sample size, a recent trend has been to combine similar studies to increase the power of the analysis. This strategy for data synthesis is known as *meta-analysis*. It has been especially helpful in studying diseases with a low incidence or where similar studies have given conflicting results.

Methodological issues (see Volume 2, Chapters 6.12, 6.13)

Epidemiologic studies, because they deal with humans, are subject to problems such as bias (deviation of results from truth), due to the strategies of recruiting participants or to differential recall among persons with and without disease, and confounding, due to factors which are associated with both the exposure variables and outcome variable under study. In the last several decades, many new techniques have been developed to reduce the effect of these factors, which can influence the outcome of a study and, in some instances, can cause apparent relationships to be observed which are in fact false.

Summary

Epidemiology is the core science of public health because it defines health and disease in human populations, describes disease aetiology, and evaluates public health control efforts. It achieves these goals through a variety of strategies and methods. Epidemiology is a dynamic science, and is continually evolving new strategies and methods in support of public health goals.

References

Alter M. Is multiple sclerosis an age-dependent host response to measles? *Lancet* 1976;1(7957):456–7.

Chapman S.W. and Henderson H.M. New and emerging pathogens multiply resistant *Mycobacterium tuberculosis. Current Opinion in Infectious Diseases* 1994;7:231–7.

Chin J. *Control of communicable diseases manual.* Washington (DC): American Public Health Association; 2000.

Colley J.R.T., Holland W.W., Corkhill R.T. *et al.* Influence of passive smoking and parental phlegm on pneumonia and bronchitis in early childhood. *Lancet* 1974;2(7888):1031–4.

Colley J.R.T. Major public health problems: respiratory system. In: Holland WW, Detels R *et al.*, editors. *Oxford textbook of public health.* 2nd ed. Oxford University Press; 1991. p. 227–48. vol. 3.

Communicable Disease Surveillance Centre. Invasive group A streptococcal infections in Gloucestershire (England/Wales). *Communicable Disease Report* 1994;**4**:97–100.

Detels R., Fahey J.L., Schwartz K. *et al.* Relation between sexual practices and T-cell subsets in homosexually active men. *Lancet* 1983;**1**(8325):609–11.

Detels R., Grayston J.T., Kim K.S. *et al.* Prevention of clinical and subclinical rubella infection: efficacy of three HPV-77 derivative vaccines. *American Journal of Diseases of Children* 1969a;**118**:295–300.

Detels R., Gutman L., Jaramillo J. *et al.* An epidemic of intestinal capillariasis in man: a study in a barrio in northern Luzon. *American Journal of Tropical Medicine and Hygiene* 1969b;**18**(**5**):676–82.

Detels R., McNew J., Brody J.A. *et al.* Further epidemiological studies of subacute sclerosing panencephalitis. *Lancet* 1973;**819**:11–4.

Detels R., Muñoz A., McFarlane G. *et al.* Effectiveness of potent antiretroviral therapy on time to AIDS and death in men with known HIV infection duration. *Journal of the American Medical Association* 1998;**280**(**17**):1497–503.

Detels R., Visscher B.R., Fahey J.L. *et al.* Predictors of clinical AIDS in young homosexual men in a high-risk area. *International Journal of Epidemiology* 1987;**16**:271–6.

Detels R., Visscher B.R., Haile R.W. *et al.* Multiple sclerosis and age at migration. *American Journal of Epidemiology* 1978;**108**:386–93.

Fahey J., Prince H., Weaver M. *et al.* Quantitative changes in T-helper or T-suppressor/cytotoxic lymphocyte subsets that distinguish acquired immune deficiency syndrome from other immune subset disorders. *American Journal of Medicine* 1984;**76**:95–100.

Feldmann H., Slenczka W., Klenk H.D. Emerging and reemerging of filoviruses. *Archives of Virology* 1996;**11** Suppl:77–100.

Fenner F., Henderson D.A., Arita I. et al. *Smallpox and its eradication*. Geneva: World Health Organization; 1988.

Gange S., Munoz A., Schrager L.K. *et al.* Design of nested studies to identify factors related to late progression of HIV infection. *Journal of Acquired Immune Deficiency Syndromes and Human Retroviruses* 1997;15 Suppl: S5-S9.

Hill A.B. The environment and disease: association or causation? *Proceedings of the Royal Society of Medicine* 1965;**58**:295–300.

Ho D.D, Neumann A.U., Perelson A.S. *et al.* Rapid turnover of plasma virion and CD4 lymphocytes in HIV-1 infection. *Nature*; 1995;**373**:123–126.

Hoggatt K. and Greenland S., Causation and causal inference. *Oxford Textbook of Public Health*. 5th ed. Oxford: Oxford University Press; 2008.

Holland W.W., Olsen J., Florey C.D.V. *et al.*, editors. *The development of modern epidemiology: personal reports from those who were there*. Oxford: Oxford University Press; 2007. p. 177–8.

Hypertension Detection and Follow-up Program Cooperative Group. Five-year findings of the hypertension detection and follow-up program. I: Reduction in mortality of persons with high blood pressure, including mild hypertension. *Journal of the American Medical Association* 1979;**242**:2562–71.

Imagawa D.T., Lee M.H., Wolinsky S.M. *et al.* Human immunodeficiency virus type 1 infection in homosexual men who remain seronegative for prolonged periods. *New England Journal of Medicine* 1989;**320**:1458–62.

Ji G., Detels R., Wu Z. *et al.* Correlates of HIV infection among former blood/plasma donors in rural China. *AIDS* 2006;**20**(**4**):585–91.

Joint National Committee on Prevention, Detection, Evaluation, and Treatment of High Blood Pressure. The sixth report of the Joint National Committee on Prevention, Detection, Evaluation, and Treatment of High Blood Pressure. *Archives of Internal Medicine* 1997;**157**:2413–46.

King J.W. Ebola virus. [Online]. Emedicine.com, Inc; 2003 Nov [last updated 2008 Apr 2]. Available from: http://www.emedicine.com/MED/topic626.htm

Lane J.M., Ruben F.L., Neff J.M. *et al.* Complications of smallpox vaccination, 1968: national surveillance in the United States. *New England Journal of Medicine* 1969;**281**:1201–8.

Lilienfeld D.E. Definitions of epidemiology. *American Journal of Epidemiology* 1978;**107**:87–90.

Liu C., Carrington M., Kaslow R.A. *et al.* Lack of associations between HLA class II alleles and resistance to HIV-1 infection among white, non-Hispanic homosexual men. *Journal of Acquired Immune Deficiency Syndromes* 2004; **37**(**2**):1313–7.

MacKenzie W.R., Hoxie N.J., Proctor M.E. *et al.* A massive outbreak in Milwaukee of cryptosporidium infection transmitted through the public water supply. *New England Journal of Medicine* 1994;**331**:161–7.

Morris J.N. *Uses of epidemiology*. 3rd ed. London: Churchill Livingstone; 1975.

Morris J.N. *Uses of epidemiology*. London: Churchill Livingstone; 1957.

Murray C.J. Quantifying the burden of disease: the technical basis for disability-adjusted life years. *Bulletin of the World Health Organization* 1994;**72**:429–45.

Phair J., Jacobson L., Detels R. *et al.* Acquired immune deficiency syndrome occurring within 5 years of infection with human immunodeficiency virus type-1: the Multicenter AIDS Cohort Study. *Journal of Acquired Immune Deficiency Syndromes* 1992;**5**:490–6.

Polk B.F., Fox R., Brookmeyer R. *et al.* Predictors of the acquired immunodeficiency syndrome developing in a cohort of seropositive homosexual men. *New England Journal of Medicine* 1987;**316**:61–6.

Prempree P., Detels R., Ungkasrithongkul M. *et al.* The sources of treatment of sexually transmissible infections in a rural community in central Thailand. *Sex Health* 2007;**4**(1):17–9.

Rothman K.J., editor. *Causal inference.* Chestnut Hill (MA): Epidemiology Resources; 1988.

Rotman K.J., Greenland S., Pool C., Lash T.L. Validity and bias in epidemiologic research. *Oxford textbook of public health*. 5th ed. Oxford: Oxford University Press; 2008.

Sackett D.L., Haynes R.B., Buyatt G.H. *et al. Clinical Epidemiology, a basic science for clinical medicine*. London: Little, Brown; 1991.

Schwartz J., Zeger S. Passive smoking, air pollution, and acute respiratory symptoms in a diary of student nurses. *American Review of Respiratory Disease* 1990;**141**:62–7.

Tager I.B., Weiss S.T., Rosner B. *et al.* Effect of parental cigarette smoking on the pulmonary function of children. *American Journal of Epidemiology* 1979;**110**:15–26.

Tashkin D.P., Clark V.A., Simmons M. *et al.* The UCLA Population Studies of Chronic Obstructive Respiratory Disease: VII. Relationship between parental smoking and children's lung function. *American Review of Respiratory Disease* 1984;**129**:891–7.

Wu Z., Detels R. HIV-1 infection in commercial plasma donors in China. *Lancet* 1995;**346**:61–2.

Wu Z., Rou K., Detels R. *et al.* Prevalence of HIV infection among former commercial plasma donors in rural Eastern China. *Health Policy and Planning* 2001;**16**(**2**):41–6.

Zhao G., Detels R., Gu F. *et al.* The distribution of people seeking STD services in the various types of healthcare facilities in Chao Yang District, Beijing, China. *Sexually Transmitted Diseases* 2007;**35**:65–7.

6.2

Ecologic variables, ecologic studies, and multilevel studies in public health research

Ana V. Diez-Roux

Abstract

This chapter reviews the use of ecologic variables, ecologic studies, and multilevel studies in epidemiology and public health. It begins with a discussion of the ecologic fallacy and the sources of the ecologic fallacy, placing it in the context of other fallacies related to the presence of multiple levels of organization. Other fallacies including the atomistic fallacy, psychologistic (or individualistic) fallacy and sociologistic fallacy are also reviewed. This is followed by a discussion of the uses of ecologic or group-level variables in epidemiology, distinguishing the use of these variables as proxies for individual-level data and as measures of true group-level constructs. The final sections contrast the advantages and disadvantages of individual-level studies, ecologic studies, and multilevel studies. Multilevel analysis is briefly reviewed. The chapter concludes with a discussion of the challenges inherent in multilevel studies and multilevel analysis. The importance of conceptualizing the multiple levels of organization relevant to a particular research question is emphasized throughout the chapter.

Introduction

There has been much discussion in epidemiology about the utility of ecologic variables and ecologic studies; most of these centre on the limitations of ecologic studies in drawing inferences regarding the relationship between individual-level variables. These limitations are due to the presence of the ecologic fallacy; that is, the well-established logical fallacy inherent in making inferences regarding individual-level associations based on group-level data (Piantadosi *et al.* 1988; Greenland 1992; Morgenstern 1995). Because of these limitations, it is often argued that ecologic studies should be limited to 'hypothesis generation', leaving the more esteemed process of 'hypothesis testing' to individual-level data.

A key notion that has received much attention in epidemiology over the past few years is that not all disease determinants can be conceptualized as individual-level attributes, hence the need to consider features of the groups to which individuals belong when studying the causes of ill health. This has led epidemiologists and public health researchers to rethink the ideas on ecologic studies and ecologic variables traditionally espoused in epidemiology (Von Korff *et al.* 1992; Schwartz 1994; Susser 1994; Susser 1994; Diez-Roux *et al.* 1998; Blakely & Woodward 2000; Macintyre & Ellaway 2000; Diez-Roux 2004b) More generally, there has been renewed interest in the idea that group-level (or ecologic)[1] variables may provide information that is not always captured by individual-level data, and in rethinking the ways in which these group-level constructs can be examined in epidemiologic analyses. This reconceptualization of ecologic or group-level variables has been manifested, for example, in research and debate on the possible health effects of group-level constructs such as income inequality (Lynch *et al.* 2003; Subramanian & Kawachi 2003) social capital (Kawachi *et al.* 1999; Lynch *et al.* 2000), and neighbourhood characteristics (Pickett & Pearl 2001; Diez-Roux 2004a; Oakes 2004; Subramanian 2004; Diez-Roux 2007). The renewed interest in 'ecologic', 'macro', or 'group-level' determinants of health has occurred within a broader recognition of the need to consider multiple levels of organization (e.g. from molecules to society) in studying the determinants of health and disease.

Many of the conceptual and analytical issues that arise when considering the uses of ecologic studies and ecologic variables are derived from the presence of multiple levels of organization and nested data structures more generally. For example, many problems that arise when dealing with individuals nested within groups (e.g. persons nested within geographical areas) are also present when dealing with groups nested within larger groups (e.g. states nested within countries), persons nested within families, or multiple measurements on individuals over time (in this case, the 'group' is the individual and the 'individuals' are the measurement occasions). The need to deal with multiple levels of organization is the norm rather than the exception in epidemiology.

The presence of multiple levels has two important implications. First, the units of analysis (or observations for which independent and dependent variables are measured) can be defined at different levels.

[1] In this chapter, the terms 'group-level' or 'ecologic' will be used interchangeably to refer to variables that characterize groups.

The unit of analysis determines the level at which variability is examined. For example, a study with individuals as the units of analysis (in which each observation is an individual) can investigate the causes of inter-individual variation in the outcome. A study with groups as the units of analysis (in which observations are groups) can investigate the causes of inter-group variation in the outcome. A study involving repeated measurements on individuals over time (in which measures at different points in time are the units of analysis) can investigate the causes of variability across measures. As will be seen, the use of units of analysis at one level to make inferences about the causes of variability at a different level leads to a series of methodological problems.

The second implication is that constructs relevant to health can be conceptualized (and measured) at different levels. Constructs pertaining to a higher level may be important in understanding variability at a lower level, and conversely, constructs defined at a lower level may be important in understanding variability at a higher level. For example, characteristics of the groups to which individuals belong may be important in explaining inter-individual variability, and characteristics of individuals constituting the groups may be important in explaining inter-group variability. Analogously, when looking at multiple measures on individuals over time, individual characteristics may be important in understanding variability across measures, and factors specific to measurement occasions may be important in understanding inter-individual variability.

This chapter discusses the use of ecologic variables and ecologic, individual-level, and multilevel studies in epidemiology within the broader context of the implications of multiple levels of organization for understanding disease aetiology. Although the discussion will focus on the simple case of individuals nested within groups, it is generalizable to many other situations involving nested data structures, as noted earlier. The first subsection reviews the classic distinction between ecologic and individual-level studies made in epidemiology, and provides historical examples of the use of ecologic studies in public health. The next subsection summarizes the sources of the 'ecologic fallacy', placing this fallacy within the context of other fallacies, which may arise when the presence of multiple levels is ignored. The third subsection revisits the full range of study designs available to investigators, based on the units of analysis (and the level at which variability is examined) and the levels at which relevant constructs are defined and measured. The final subsection highlights some challenges faced by epidemiology as it attempts to investigate the multilevel determinants of health.

Ecologic studies and their use in public health

Epidemiology has traditionally distinguished two types of studies based on the units of analysis: Ecologic studies and studies of individuals. Ecologic studies are studies in which groups are the units of analysis: Both the dependent and the independent variables are measured for groups, and inter-group variations (and associations between independent and dependent variables across groups) are examined. For example, common ecologic studies in public health involve measuring rates of disease for different geographic areas and relating these rates to area social or physical characteristics (e.g. measures of area median income, levels of air pollution, water hardness, and radiation). Ecologic studies are often cross-sectional with independent and dependent variables measured at the same point in time. However, ecologic studies can also involve repeated measures on a group, or several groups, over time, as in time-trend studies (Susser 1994; Morgenstern 1995). For example, an ecologic study could examine yearly incidence rates of disease for different regions over a ten-year period and investigate the relation of these incidence rates to area characteristics that do and do not change over time. Ecologic studies could also involve the analysis of groups randomized to receive or not receive an intervention. In many ecologic studies, the predominant analytic approach involves the estimation of correlation coefficients between the group-level exposure and the group-level outcome. However, many other analytic approaches are also possible, including the estimation of other measures of association (such as rate differences or rate ratios) using linear or log-linear models (Morgenstern 1995).

In contrast, in individual-level studies, the units of analysis are individuals: Both independent and dependent variables are measured for individuals, and inter-individual variations (and associations between independent and dependent variables across individuals) are investigated. Based on their design, individual-level studies can be cross-sectional (when both independent and dependent variables are measured at the same point in time), cohort (when individuals free of the outcome at baseline are followed over time to compare risk of the outcome in the exposed and unexposed), or case–control (when a sample of persons with the outcome is compared with a sample of controls with regard to the presence of certain exposures).

Because the units of analysis differ in ecologic and individual-level studies, the information they provide (and the information they lack) also differs. Ecologic studies include information on group characteristics (which may sometimes be simply summaries of the characteristics of individuals in the group), but lack information on the cross-classification of individual-level characteristics within groups. For example, an ecologic study may relate the percentage of smokers in different groups to mortality rates, but has no information on whether within groups smokers were actually the ones more likely to die. On the other hand, individual-level studies focus on inter-individual variations and have information on individual-level characteristics, but often lack information on characteristics of the groups to which individuals belong. Although the omission of relevant group-level characteristics in individual-level studies is rarely recognized as a problem, it also can lead to incorrect inferences, as will be discussed in more detail in the subsections that follow.

Uses of ecologic studies in public health

Descriptive ecologic studies in which rates of disease or death are compared over time or across geographic areas have been a staple of epidemiology for centuries. Chadwick (Chadwick 1965) used an ecologic approach in his famous *Report on an Inquiry into the Sanitary Condition of the Labouring Population of Great Britain* in 1842. Table 6.2.1 shows a portion of Chadwick's report, in which mortality for a drained area is compared to mortality for an undrained area at three parallel points in time. By comparing mortality rates over time in both communities (one drained and the other undrained), he was able to draw inferences regarding the relationship between drainage and ill health. Drainage was the exposure, mortality the outcome, and communities the units of analysis.

Table 6.2.1 Death rates compared in three successive decades in a drained and an undrained town

The following has been the proportion of deaths in the population in the two towns:

	Beccles	Bungay
Between 1811 and 1821	1 in 67	1 in 69
Between 1821 and 1831	1 in 72	1 in 67
Between 1831 and 1841	1 in 71	1 in 59

You will therefore see that the rate of mortality has gradually diminished in Beccles since it has been drained, whilst in Bungay, notwithstanding its larger proportion of rural population, it has considerably increased.

Source: Chadwick E. *Report on the sanitary conditions of the labouring population of Great Britain*. Edinburgh, UK: Edinburgh University Press; 1965. p. 103. Reproduced from Susser M. *Causal thinking in the health sciences*. New York (NY): Oxford University Press; 1973. With permission. Copyright © 1973 Oxford University Press.

With these findings, Chadwick had grounds to institute a system of sanitation nationwide. Although the miasmatic theory of disease causation which Chadwick espoused (and which he believed was supported by his data) was later proved false, the method of sanitation that Chadwick introduced was probably as important as any other single measure in modern times (Susser 1973).

Early in his studies, John Snow (1855) also used an ecologic approach in comparing cholera rates for London districts, and examining whether differences in these rates were related to differences in the sources of water (Susser 1973, Table 2). The units of analyses were districts, and both the independent variable (source of water) and the dependent variable (cholera rates) were measured at the district level. At the beginning of this century, Goldberger *et al.* (Goldberger *et al.* 1920; Terris 1964) used an ecologic approach to compare incidence rates of pellagra across villages. Their findings linking food availability at the village level to village pellagra rates contributed to the demonstration that pellagra was not an infectious disease, as was believed by many at the time.

More recently, ecologic studies relating rates of cardiovascular disease across countries to risk factor prevalences (Keys's Seven Countries Study) laid the foundation for future work on the epidemiology and causes of cardiovascular disease (Keys 1980). For example, data from the Seven Countries Study showed a relationship between the average proportion of calories derived from saturated fat and coronary heart disease mortality. Another recent example is provided by psychiatric epidemiology; ecologic studies have demonstrated that the incidence of acute transient psychoses varies dramatically across sociocultural settings. In the WHO Ten Country Study, for instance, the incidence of non-affective acute remitting psychosis was tenfold higher in developing than in developed country settings (Susser & Wanderling 1994). These studies have led to testing of specific hypotheses about causation, including antecedent fever and culturally normative life events.

Much useful public health information has been obtained from ecologic studies. However, as will be illustrated throughout this chapter, both studies of individuals and studies with groups as the units of analysis have their limitations. The degree to which a given study design is appropriate depends on the particular research problem. Snow's research provides an illustrative example. Four years after Snow's initial investigation (Table 6.2.2), one of the companies, the Lambeth Company, had moved its waterworks to a point higher up on the Thames, thus obtaining a supply of water free from the sewage of London. This meant that within a single district, some houses were receiving water drawn from one place on the Thames and others were receiving water drawn from a different point. Thus, the district as the unit of analysis was no longer appropriate. In Snow's words: 'To turn this grand experiment into account, all that was required was to learn the supply of water to each individual house where a fatal attack of cholera might occur' (cited in Susser, 1973, p. 59). Snow subsequently confirmed the conclusions drawn from his prior ecologic analysis by examining the relationship between source of water and cholera risk with households, rather than districts, as the units of analysis (Table 6.2.3).

The following section, which focuses on 'fallacies' related to the existence of multiple levels of organization, discuss some of the limitations and potentialities of ecologic studies and studies of individuals. The section begins with a discussion of the ecologic fallacy because it is the fallacy most commonly mentioned in epidemiology. We then discuss how the presence of multiple levels may also lead to related fallacies in studies of individuals.

The ecologic fallacy and other fallacies related to the presence of multiple levels of organization

The ecologic fallacy is the fallacy of drawing inferences at the individual level (i.e. regarding variability across individuals) based on group-level data. The most common example of the ecologic fallacy involves situations in which group-level variables are used as proxies for unavailable individual-level exposures. For example, to study the relation between exposure to substance X and cancer in the absence of individual-level data, the prevalence of exposure to X in different areas is related to cancer rates in those areas. In this case, we do not have information on exactly who is exposed to X and who is not, so the area prevalence of X is used as a rough approximation for the exposure of each area resident. Because we lack information on the joint distribution of exposure and outcome at the individual level (i.e. we do not know if persons who developed cancer were actually exposed to X), we cannot conclude that individuals exposed to X have a higher risk of lung cancer even if we find that areas with a higher per cent exposed to X have higher cancer rates.

Another example is provided by the relation between mean country income and obesity when mean income is used as a proxy for individual-level income. Suppose a researcher finds that, at the country level, higher mean income is associated with higher prevalence of obesity (or increasing body mass index [BMI]). If he or she infers that within countries higher income is associated with higher BMI, he or she may be committing the ecologic fallacy, because BMI may always be higher for low-income than high-income persons within countries.

Sources of the ecologic fallacy

The ecologic fallacy arises when associations between two variables at the group level (or ecologic level) differ from associations between analogous variables measured at the individual level. The typical ecologic fallacy applies when aggregate measures for the group (e.g. the percentage of persons with a certain attribute or the mean attribute across persons) are used as proxies for individual-level data.

Table 6.2.2 Mortality from cholera, and the water supply, in the districts of London in 1849

District	Population	Deaths from cholera	Deaths from cholera per 10 000	Annual value of house and shop room per person (in #)	Water supply (waterworks)
Rotherhithe	17 208	352	205	4.238	Southwark and Vauxhall, Kent, tidal ditches
St. Olave, Southwark	19 278	349	181	4.559	Southwark and Vauxhall
St. George, Southwark	50 900	836	164	3.518	Southwark and Vauxhall, Lambeth
Bermondsey	45 500	734	161	3.077	Southwark and Vauxhall
St. Saviour, Southwark	35 227	539	153	5.291	Southwark and Vauxhall
Newington	63 074	907	144	3.788	Southwark and Vauxhall, Lambeth
Lambeth	134 768	1618	120	4.389	Southwark and Vauxhall, Lambeth
Wandsworth	48 446	484	100	4.839	Pump-wells, Southwark and Vauxhall, Wandle River
Camberwell	51 714	504	97	4.508	Southwark and Vauxhall, Lambeth,
West London	28 829	429	96	7.454	New River
Bethnal Green	87 263	789	90	1.480	East London
Shoreditch	104 122	789	76	3.103	New River, East London
Greenwich	95 954	718	75	3.379	Kent
Poplar	44 103	313	71	7.360	East London
Westminster	64 109	437	68	4.189	Chelsea
Whitechapel	78 590	506	64	3.388	East London
St. Giles	54 062	285	53	5.635	New River
Stepney	106 988	501	47	3.319	East London
Chelsea	53 379	247	46	4.210	Chelsea
East London	43 495	182	45	4.823	New River
St. George's, East	47 334	199	42	4.753	East London
London City	55 816	207	38	17.676	New River
St. Martin	24 557	91	37	11.844	New River
Strand	44 254	156	35	7.374	New River
Holborn	46 134	161	35	5.883	New River
St. Luke Kensington (expect Paddington)	110 491	260	33	5.070	West Middlesex, Chelsea, Grand Junction
Lewisham	32 299	96	30	4.824	Kent
Belgrave	37 918	105	28	8.875	Chelsea
Hackney	55 152	139	25	4.397	New River, East London
Islington	87 761	187	22	5.494	New River
St. Pancras	160 122	360	22	4.871	New River, Hampstead, West Middlesex
Clerkenwell	63 499	121	19	4.138	New River
Marylebone	153 960	261	17	7.586	West Middlesex
St. James, Westminster	36 426	57	16	12.669	Grand Junction, New River
Paddington	41 267	35	8	9.349	Grand Junction
Hampstead	11 572	9	8	5.804	Hampstead, West Middlesex
Hanover Square and May Fair	33 196	26	8	16.754	Grand Junction
London	2 280 282	14 137	62	—	—

The districts are arranged in the order of their mortality from cholera.

Source: Snow J. On the mode of communication of cholera. In: *Snow on cholera.* (2nd ed 1936). New York (NY): The Commonwealth Fund; 1855. p. 62–3. Reproduced from Susser M. *Causal thinking in the health sciences.* New York (NY): Oxford University Press; 1973. With permission. Copyright © 1973 Oxford University Press.

Table 6.2.3 Cholera death rates by company supplying household water

Company	Number of houses	Deaths from cholera	Deaths per 10 000 houses
Southwark and Vauxhall Company	40 046	1263	315
Lambeth Company	26 107	98	37
Rest of London	256 423	1422	59

Source: Snow J. On the mode of communication of cholera. In: *Snow on cholera.* (2nd ed 1936). New York (NY): The Commonwealth Fund; 1855. p. 86. Reproduced from Susser M. *Causal thinking in the health sciences.* New York (NY): Oxford University Press; 1973. With permission. Copyright © 1973 Oxford University Press.

These differences between individual-level and group-level associations for apparently analogous variables were first described for correlation coefficients (Robinson 1950) but may also be present for other measures of associations such as linear regression coefficients (Morgenstern 1982). Because the use of correlation coefficients raises additional complexities (and because of its limitations as a measure of association), the following discussion will focus on regression coefficients as the main measure of association estimated at both the group and the individual level.

The example on income and obesity mentioned earlier is illustrated in Fig. 6.2.1. At the group or country level, mean BMI increases with increasing mean income. At the same time, for individuals within countries, BMI decreases with increasing individual-level income. This situation arises because group-level mean income is related to BMI independently of individual-level income (or in other words, because there is a group effect). Persons living in countries with higher mean income have generally higher BMIs than those living in countries with lower mean income, regardless of their individual-level income.

Another situation is depicted in Fig. 6.2.2, where the relation between individual-level income and BMI differs by mean country income: In countries with higher mean income, individual-level income is strongly and inversely related to BMI, whereas this relation is non-existent, or perhaps exists in the opposite direction, in countries with lower mean income. Here, the group-level variable (average income of the country in which a person lives) modifies the effect of individual-level income on the outcome. In this case, group-level associations (the relationship between mean country income and mean country BMI) will also differ from individual-level associations (the relationship between individual-level income and individual-level BMI). In addition, individual-level associations will differ from country to country, according to levels of mean country income. Thus, when a group-level variable is related to the outcome independently of the analogous variable measured at the individual level, or when the group-level variable modifies the effects of its individual-level analogue on the outcome, ecologic associations (which express the relationship between group-level variables and group-level outcomes) will differ from the corresponding individual-level associations (which express the relationship between individual-level variables and individual-level outcomes) (Hammond 1973; Firebaugh 1978; Greenland & Morgenstern 1989; Levin 1995).

The concepts summarized here can also be expressed mathematically. Suppose the 'true' relationship between country mean income, individual-level income, and individual-level BMI is reflected in the following equation:

$$Y_{ij} = \beta_0 + \beta_1 X_{ij} + \beta_2 \bar{X}_j + U_j + e_{ij} \qquad (6.2.1)$$

where,

Y_{ij} = BMI for *i*th individual in *j*th country

X_{ij} = income for *i*th individual in *j*th country

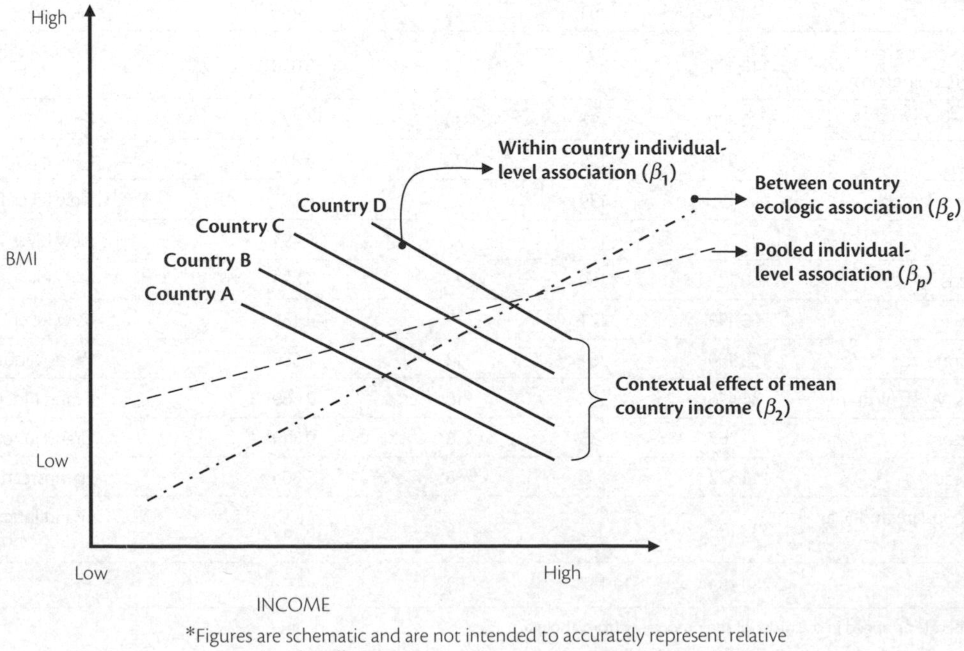

Fig. 6.2.1 Hypothetical associations of income with body mass index (BMI) within and between countries. Mean country income does not modify the effect of individual-level income.*

*Figures are schematic and are not intended to accurately represent relative magnitudes of coefficients.

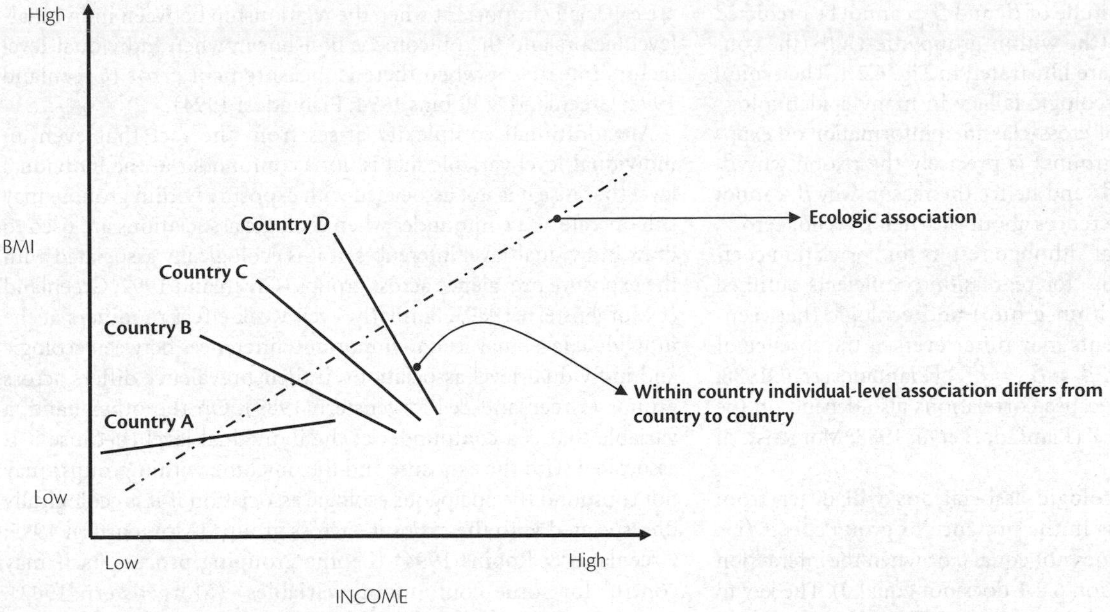

Fig. 6.2.2 Hypothetical associations of income with body mass index (BMI) within and between countries. Mean country income modifies the effect of individual-level income.

$\bar{X}_j$ = mean X_{ij} in country j

e_{ij} and U_j are individual-and country-level errors, respectively
β_1 = mean difference in individual-level BMI per unit difference in individual-level income
β_2 = mean difference in individual-level BMI per unit difference in mean country income

Thus, BMI for each individual is related not only to his or her own income, but also to the mean income for the country in which he or she lives. In Equation 6.2.1, β_1 reflects the individual-level relation between X_{ij} and Y_{ij}. As it is 'adjusted' for the group effect (to the extent that between-group differences are entirely captured by β_2 and the group-level error U_j), it is equivalent to the within-group effect of individual-level income (or the average within-group effect if this varies across groups). β_1 is what we would like to estimate in order to quantify the individual-level effect of X_{ij} on Y_{ij}. β_2 reflects the relationship between mean country income ($\bar{X}_j$) and Y_{ij}, after controlling for X_{ij} (i.e. the effect of mean country income on individual-level BMI after controlling for individual-level income). (Equation 6.2.1 can also be modified to allow interactions between X_{ij} and $\bar{X}_j$, as shown in Fig. 6.2.2. For reasons of simplicity, this situation will not be illustrated, but the discussion that follows applies as well.)

Suppose that instead of this full equation showing the relationship between BMI and individual level income and mean country income, we fit the ecologic equation shown in the following:

$$\bar{Y}_j = \beta_{e0} + \beta_{e1}\bar{X}_j + e_j \qquad (6.2.2)$$

where,
$\bar{Y}_j$ = mean BMI in country j
$\bar{X}_j$ = mean income in country j

β_{e1} = mean difference in mean country BMI per unit change in mean country income
(The subscript e is used in this case because regression coefficients refer to ecologic or group-level associations.)

In this case, β_{e1} reflects the ecologic relation between mean country income ($\bar{X}_j$) and mean country BMI ($\bar{Y}_j$). It is sometimes referred to as the between-group effect. Clearly, β_{e1} (the between-group effect) is not equivalent to β_1 (the within-group effect of X_{ij}) or β_2 (the effect of $\bar{X}_j$) of Equation 6.2.1. In fact, both the individual-level within-group effect (β_1) and the effect of mean $\bar{X}_j$ (β_2) are confounded in the ecologic regression coefficient (β_{e1}): β_e in Equation 6.2.2 is the sum of β_1 and β_2 of Equation 6.2.1 (Raudenbush & Bryk 2002).

Yet another alternative is to fit a purely individual-level equation ignoring group membership, as in Equation 6.2.3:

$$Y_{ij} = \beta_{p0} + \beta_{p1}X_{ij} + e_{ij} \qquad (6.2.3)$$

The subscript p is used in this case because regression coefficients refer to associations between individual-level variables pooled across groups. β_{p1} reflects the effect of X_{ij} on Y_{ij} pooling across groups and ignoring group membership (it is unadjusted for any potential group effects). When group effects are present, β_{p1} will differ from β_1 (the within-group effect) of Equation 6.2.1, and will also differ from β_{e1} (the ecologic effect of $\bar{X}_j$) of Equation 6.2.2. Both the within-group effects of X_{ij} and the effect of $\bar{X}_j$ on Y_{ij} are confounded in β_{p1}.

In the absence of group effects (e.g. when β_2 of Equation 6.2.1 equals 0) and when there is no interaction between $\bar{X}_j$ and X_{ij} (the group- and individual-level variables), β_1 (within-group effect), β_{e1} (ecologic effect), and β_{p1} (pooled individual effect) are all equivalent. However, in the presence of group effects, β_e does not equal β_1 or β_{p1} (source of the ecologic fallacy). In addition, β_{p1} does not equal β_{e1} or β_2. When group effects are present, β_{p1} will be a weighted average of β_1 and β_{e1}, and will lie between them, although the order of magnitude of β_1 and β_{e1} cannot be predicted (Piantadosi *et al.* 1988). β_1 (the within-group effect), β_2 (the contextual effect), β_{e1}, and β_{p1} are illustrated in Fig. 6.2.1. The typical explanation given for the ecologic fallacy in many epidemiology textbooks (i.e. the absence of cross-classified information on exposure and outcome within groups) is precisely the reason why β_2 and β_1 are confounded in β_e, and hence the reason why β_e cannot reliably be used to make inferences about β_1 when β_2 is not zero.

It is important to note that although results for correlation coefficients generally follow those for regression coefficients outlined earlier, individual-level (within-group) and ecologic (between-group) correlation coefficients may differ even in the absence of group effects (i.e. even when $\beta_1 = \beta_{e1} = \beta_{p1}$) (Piantadosi *et al.* 1988; Hammond 1973). This is because correlations also depend on the relative dispersion of X and Y (Piantadosi *et al.* 1988; Morgenstern 1982).

As illustrated earlier, ecologic associations will differ from individual-level associations in the presence of group effects (i.e. when β_2 in Equation 6.2.1 does not equal 0 or when the interaction between X_{ij} and $\bar{X}_j$ in Equation 6.2.1 does not equal 0). The key to understanding the sources of the ecologic fallacy therefore lies in specifying the conditions under which β_2 (the independent effect of $\bar{X}_j$) or the interaction between $\bar{X}_j$ and X_{ij} will differ from 0. Several different situations may result in non-zero values for β_2 or for the interaction term between X_{ij} and $\bar{X}_j$. These include (a) situations where group mean X_{ij} ($\bar{X}_j$) is a marker for omitted individual-level variables which individuals in a group tend to share; and (b) situations where mean X_{ij} at the group level measures a different construct than X at the individual level. Both situations will be discussed in more detail in the following subsection.

$\bar{X}_j$ is a marker for omitted individual-level variables that individuals in a group tend to share

It is possible that $\bar{X}_j$ is a marker for omitted individual-level variables which individuals in a group tend to share; that is, groups differ in the distribution of individual-level variables causally related to the outcome. In the BMI example, unmeasured individual-level factors (e.g. diet, exercise, genetic factors) may vary from country to country, and their prevalence may be associated with mean country income. These individual-level factors may affect the risk of the outcome independently of individual-level income or may modify the association of individual-level income with the outcome. If these factors are unmeasured in the analyses, their effects will be reflected in the coefficient for mean income in Equation 6.2.1 (β_2), or in the mean income by individual-level income interaction, and in the ecologic regression coefficient relating mean income to mean BMI (β_{e1} in Equation 6.2.2). Thus, differences in the distribution of these individual-level confounders or effect modifiers across groups may lead to discordances between the group-level and individual-level associations of income and BMI. Summary ecologic measures of these individual-level factors for each group are sometimes available (e.g. per-cent sedentary or mean dietary fat). However, controlling for these summary measures in ecologic analyses is often insufficient to account for the confounding effects of individual-level variables (although in some cases controlling for multiple summary measures of the same variable may reduce confounding to some extent) (Morgenstern 1995; Greenland & Morgenstern 1989; Greenland & Robins 1994). It is even possible for this ecologic adjustment to actually increase bias (Greenland & Morgenstern 1989). The limitations of the use of summary measures are especially important when the relationship between individual-level factors and the outcome is non-linear, when individual-level factors interact or when there is measurement error (Greenland 1992; Greenland & Robins 1994; Piantadosi 1994).

An additional complexity arises from the fact that even an individual-level variable that is not a confounder at the individual level (because it is not associated with exposure within groups) may still operate as a confounder when ecologic associations are used to draw individual-level inferences, if it is ecologically associated with the exposure prevalence across groups (Greenland 1992; Greenland & Morgenstern 1989). Similarly, even weak effect modifiers at the individual level may lead to important differences between ecologic and individual-level associations, if their prevalence differs across groups (Greenland & Morgenstern 1989). On the other hand, a variable that is a confounder at the individual level (because it is associated with the exposure and the outcome within groups) may not confound the analogous ecologic association if it is ecologically unassociated with the exposure across groups (Morgenstern 1995; Greenland & Robins 1994) (i.e. the grouping process itself may control for some confounding variables) (Morgenstern 1982). Brenner *et al.* (1992) have also shown that although non-differential misclassification of a binary variable seriously hinders the ability to control for that variable in individual-level studies, it does not always reduce the ability to control for that variable in ecologic studies. Thus, in some cases, the ecologic analysis may avoid the confounding present in individual-level analyses.

The absence of information on individual-level confounders (which may differ from group to group) and the limitations inherent in using ecologic summaries (and interactions between ecologic summaries) to control for individual-level confounders or non-linearities in the individual-level effects is the most common critique of ecologic studies in epidemiology. A key underlying assumption of this critique (which often goes unstated) is that the ecologic measures (e.g. mean country income) and the individual-level measures (individual-level income) are indicators of the same construct; that is, if it were somehow possible to control for the unavailable individual-level information on other confounders and to fully capture non-linearities, it would be perfectly legitimate to infer things about how individual-level income is related to the outcome based on how mean country income is associated with it. But this assumption is not always true. Even if all possible individual-level confounders are controlled, ecologic associations may differ from individual-level associations because the ecologic measure of exposure and its individual-level namesake may be tapping into different constructs. This brings us to another important source of the ecologic fallacy, discussed as follows.

$\bar{X}_j$ and X_{ij} measure different constructs

An alternative interpretation of Fig. 6.2.1 (or Fig. 6.2.2) is that country mean income and individual level income are measuring different constructs ($\bar{X}_j$ measures a group-level construct and X_{ij} measures a distinct individual-level construct), and the group-level construct is related to BMI independently of individual-level income. Firebaugh (Firebaugh 1978, p. 560) has noted that 'The demystification of cross-level bias begins with the recognition that an aggregate variable often measures a different construct than its namesake at the individual level'. In this case, country mean income is a measure of a truly group-level attribute and not a proxy for individual-level data. Living in countries with high mean income places individuals at greater risk of having high BMI regardless of their individual-level income (or modifies the relation between individual-level income and BMI, as in Fig. 6.2.2). Thus, mean country income is said to exert a contextual effect on BMI. Both country-level and individual-level income provide distinct information, and both are needed to completely understand the distribution of BMI. In this case, the origin of the ecologic fallacy lies in assuming that the group-level measure is tapping into the same construct as the individual-level measure, when in fact it is not. Mean country income is associated with increased BMI, after controlling for individual-level income, but within countries individual-level income is negatively associated with BMI. In this situation, the ecologic fallacy can be thought of as a problem of construct validity: It arises because the aggregate measure is assumed to be measuring an individual-level construct when in fact it is measuring a group-level construct (Schwartz 1994).

The contextual effect of mean income may be mediated through a variety of different mechanisms. For example, countries with higher levels of mean income may rely to a greater extent on mass food production and this may in turn be associated with higher fat contents, and higher fat in the diets of individuals. In addition, the higher standard of living may be related to more sedentary occupations, higher frequency of food consumption outside the home, exposure to food advertisements, dieting behaviours, etc. Of course, because disease is defined at the level of individuals, in order to affect health, contextual effects must ultimately be mediated through individual-level processes (i.e. through processes defined at a lower level of organization), just as the effects of individual-level behaviours, for example, are mediated through biological mechanisms. Mediators of a contextual effect do not necessarily involve the individual-level namesake of the group-level variable. In our BMI income example, for instance, the contextual effect of mean income may work through individual-level variables other than income. As in any epidemiologic analysis, the extent to which contextual effects should be estimated before or after adjustment for individual-level factors depends on whether the latter are conceptualized as confounders or mediators. The key point here is that β_2 differs from 0 not because individual-level confounders that vary across groups are ignored, but because mean country income and individual-level income are measuring different constructs.

A variant of the preceding example is when the ecologic variable investigated is actually associated with another group-level attribute, which exerts a contextual effect on the outcome. Thus, the ecologic effect is actually the result of confounding by another group-level or ecologic variable. For example, mean income may be a proxy for level of industrialization; that is, it is not mean income rather level of industrialization that exerts a contextual effect on BMI. In this case, the observed contextual effect of mean income is the result of confounding by level of industrialization. The discordance between the group and individual effects of income arises because mean income is a proxy for level of industrialization, which is related to BMI independently of individual-level income.

Grouping on the dependent variable

Hammond (Hammond 1973) notes another (related) reason for differences between ecologic and individual-level regression coefficients: Grouping by the dependent variable. For example, if persons are grouped into neighbourhoods based on their income (due to social processes driving economic residential segregation) and we are interested in estimating the relationship between race and income at the individual-level, the ecologic regression coefficient between per-cent Black and mean neighbourhood income would differ from the individual-level coefficient relating race to individual-level income because of the grouping process involved. Similarly, if persons were grouped into neighbourhoods based on the presence of disease, and we are interested in the relationship between a certain risk factor and disease, the ecologic relation between the percentage of persons in the neighbourhood with the risk factor and the disease rate would be a biased estimate of the individual-level association between the risk factor and the probability of having the disease. Essentially, the grouping process generates a 'group effect' analogous to the contextual effects of mean group X described earlier.

Relationship between sources of the ecologic fallacy

The three sources of the ecologic fallacy described earlier all pertain to situations in which there is some form of 'group effect'. This includes situations where there is a failure to distinguish constructs at different levels (e.g. mean group X is assumed to measure the same thing as individual-level X), where something about the groups is associated with individual-level predictors of the outcomes (mean group X is associated with other individual-level factors related to Y), or when some process results in grouping of persons by the dependent variable. It is important to emphasize that the simple presence of differences in the distribution of 'confounders' of individual-level variables (e.g. diet and exercise in the BMI example) across groups (countries in the example) may be an indication that group-level constructs play a causal role in the development of these individual-level factors. In common epidemiologic discussions of the ecologic fallacy, these group effects are viewed as a nuisance that makes it difficult for epidemiologists to draw inferences regarding individual-level associations based on group-level data. However, more recently, epidemiologists have become increasingly interested in investigating these group effects, and in understanding their implications for epidemiologic analyses more broadly.

The previous discussion (similar to typical discussions of the ecologic fallacy) focuses on the situation in which the independent variable at the group level is an aggregate of characteristics of individuals in the group. Thus, the group-level variable (mean income) has an individual-level namesake (individual-level income). However, other ecologic variables do not involve aggregates of individual-level data (e.g. the existence of a certain law) and the problem of separating-out contextual effects from individual-level effects of the variable (e.g. the effects of mean country income from that of individual-level income) is not an issue. In this situation, it is clear that the ecologic variable is measuring a group-level construct. However, ecologic studies relating these types of predictors to outcomes may still be limited in their ability to draw individual-level inferences because of the absence of information on individual-level confounders or effect modifiers which may differ from group to group.

Other reasons for differences between ecologic and individual-level regression coefficients

In addition to the conceptual issues discussed earlier, there are statistical considerations which may lead to a discrepancy between estimates from ecologic and individual-level studies. The example used throughout this subsection (country mean income, individual-level income, and BMI) is based on a continuous individual-level dependent variable, and on the limitations inherent in using a linear ecologic model as a proxy for a linear individual-level model. Additional complexities arise when the individual-level outcome is binary. The use of a linear regression ecologic model as a proxy for a non-linear individual-level regression model (e.g. a log-linear or multiplicative model) may not always be appropriate. Fitting the aggregate or ecologic regression model that directly corresponds to a non-linear individual-level regression model is not always simple or possible with available ecologic data (see Greenland, 1992, for details). Failure to correctly specify the ecologic model to be used as a proxy for the individual-level model may be yet another source of differences between individual-level and aggregate-level regression coefficients. However, all the sources of the ecologic fallacy described in the preceding subsections may still be present even if the form of the ecologic model is appropriate for the individual-level model it is attempting to proxy.

It is important to emphasize that the degree to which ecologic and individual-level coefficients differ may vary from situation to situation. The logical possibility of the ecologic fallacy should not be taken as evidence that the fallacy necessarily occurs in all cases (Greenland & Robins 1994) or that when it occurs it has a critical impact. Some researchers have proposed strategies which may sometimes help reduce the ecologic fallacy, particularly when the group-level aggregate exposure is simply a proxy for unavailable individual-level data. These strategies include selecting regions so as to minimize within-region variability and maximize between-region variability in individual-level exposure, comparing groups with similar covariate distributions, conducting sensitivity analyses, and comparing results based on different specifications of the ecologic model (Greenland 1992), as well as other statistical approaches (King 1997). Many of these approaches assume that no other group-level effects are present or that the aggregate proxy is not serving as a proxy for group-level constructs. Despite these approaches, and for all the reasons outlined here, the use of ecologic studies to estimate individual-level relationships is often problematic.

Other fallacies related to the existence of multiple levels

The ecologic fallacy is only one of a set of possible 'fallacies' that are derived from the existence of multiple levels of organization (Diez-Roux *et al.* 1998). Because, at least recently, epidemiologists have been mostly concerned with drawing inferences regarding the causes of inter-individual variability, the ecologic fallacy has received much more attention than its counterpart, the atomistic fallacy. The atomistic fallacy is the fallacy of drawing inferences regarding variability across groups based on individual-level data. The effect of an individual-level predictor on an outcome in a study of individuals is not necessarily the same as the effect of its group-level namesake on group-level outcomes. Thus, the use of individual-level associations to draw inferences regarding group-level associations may also lead to incorrect inferences. In the BMI example, β_{p1} (the relation between individual-level income and BMI pooling individuals across groups) does not equal β_{e1} (the ecologic relation between country mean income and country mean BMI). In addition, β_1 (the within-group effect of individual-level income) does not equal β_{e1} either. Moreover, the BMI example includes multiple groups (countries) and individuals within them, but many individual-level studies only include individuals from a single group. Factors that explain variability across individuals within groups are not necessarily the same as those that explain variability across groups. For example, if stress levels are relatively invariant within groups (e.g. communities or countries), stress may not be important in explaining variability in coronary heart disease within groups, but may be strongly associated with differences in coronary heart disease rates across groups. This is another reason why the use of individual-level data to infer group-level effects may lead to incorrect inferences.

Both the ecologic and atomistic fallacies can be thought of as methodological problems inherent in drawing inferences at one level when the data are collected at another level. These fallacies arise when the conceptual model being tested corresponds to one level, but the data are collected at another level, or in Riley's (Riley 1963) words, when 'the methods fail to fit the model'. We have seen that the sources of these problems lie in (a) the lack of information on constructs pertaining to another level of organization; and (b) the failure to realize that a variable defined and measured at one level of organization may tap into a different construct than its namesake at another level, and that constructs at both levels may be relevant to the outcome studied. Both of these issues point to a more general problem, which is that even when making inferences about a given level other levels of organization may need to be taken into account. For example, the failure to consider group characteristics in drawing inferences regarding the causes of variability across individuals, and the failure to consider individuals in drawing inferences regarding the causes of variability across groups, gives rise to another set of fallacies, which are closely related to the ecologic and atomistic fallacies described earlier. In these fallacies (which have been termed the psychologistic, or individualistic, and sociologistic fallacies), although the level at which data are collected may fit the conceptual model being investigated, important facts pertaining to other levels have been ignored; in Riley's (Riley 1963) words, 'The methods may fail to fit the facts'.

Ignoring relevant group-level variables in a study of individual-level associations may lead to what Riley has termed the psychologistic fallacy; that is, assuming that individual-level outcomes can be explained exclusively in terms of individual-level characteristics. For example, a study based on individuals might find that immigrants are more likely to develop depression than natives. But suppose this is only true for immigrants living in communities where they are a small minority. A researcher ignoring the contextual effect of community composition might attribute the higher overall rate in immigrants to the psychological effects of immigration per se or even to genetic factors, ignoring the importance of community-level factors and thus committing the psychologistic fallacy (Riley 1963; Valkonen 1969). (The term 'psychologistic fallacy' is not the most appropriate because the individual-level factors used to explain the outcome are not always exclusively psychological. Other authors have used the term individualistic fallacy (Valkonen 1969), but because the term has also been used as a synonym of the atomistic fallacy (Alker 1969; Scheuch 1969), it will be avoided here.)

Analogously, ignoring the role of individual-level factors in a study of groups may lead to what has been termed the sociologistic fallacy (Riley 1963). Suppose a researcher finds that communities with higher rates of transient population have higher rates of schizophrenia, and he or she concludes that higher rates of transient population lead to social disorganization, breakdown of social networks, and increased risk of schizophrenia among all community inhabitants. But suppose that schizophrenia rates are only elevated for transient residents (because transient residents tend to have fewer social ties, and individuals with few social ties are at greater risk of developing schizophrenia); that is, rates of schizophrenia are high for transient residents and low for non-transient residents, regardless of whether they live in communities with a high or a low proportion of transient residents. If this is the case, the researcher would be committing the sociologistic fallacy in attributing the higher schizophrenia rates to social disorganization affecting all community members rather than to differences across communities in the percentage of transient residents.

Both the psychologistic and the sociologistic fallacies arise because relevant variables pertaining to other levels have been excluded from the model which led to an inappropriate explanation for the association. Although it is didactically useful to distinguish both sets of fallacies (ecologic and atomistic versus psychologistic and sociologistic), they are closely interrelated and are essentially different manifestations of the same phenomenon: The failure to recognize that constructs defined at different levels may be important in understanding the causes of variability within a given level, and the failure to adequately distinguish constructs defined at different levels.

The types of fallacies are summarized in Table 6.2.4.

The full range of epidemiologic studies

In considering the most appropriate study design to answer a given research question, investigators need to consider two issues. The first issue is the level of organization about which inferences are to be made; for example, are we interested in drawing inferences regarding causes of variation in the outcome among groups or among individuals? The answer to this question will determine the most appropriate unit of analysis. The second issue is the level of organization at which the constructs of interest in explaining the outcome are conceptualized. The answer to this second question will determine the predictors to be investigated and the level at which they are conceptualized. Constructs relevant to health may be conceptualized, and measured, at different levels of organization (e.g. countries, states, neighbourhoods, peer groups, families, couples, persons, and measurement occasions). Factors defined at a higher level may be important in understanding variability at a lower level, and vice versa, factors defined at a lower level may be important in understanding variability at a higher level. Decoupling the unit of analysis from the level of organization of the constructs investigated may be helpful in discussing the full range of studies available to epidemiologists and the advantages and disadvantages of each for a particular research question.

Clearly specifying the constructs of interest is an important requirement of any study. Lack of clarity on exactly which constructs group-level or ecologic variables are measuring underlies an important part of the confusion generated by the use of ecologic studies and the interpretation of group-level or ecologic effects. In the following subsection, we review the use of group-level variables in epidemiology based on the constructs which they are intended to be measuring. We then consider study designs with different units of analysis in terms of the types of inferences that can be drawn from them and the types of constructs they are best suited to investigating.

Table 6.2.4 Types of fallacies

Unit of analysis	Level of inference	Type of fallacy
Group	Individuals	Ecologic
Individual	Groups	Atomistic
Individual (relevant group-level variables excluded)	Individuals	Psychologistic[a]
Group (relevant individual-level variables excluded)	Groups	Sociologistic

[a] Also called *individualistic* by some authors.

Source: Diez-Roux AV *et al*. Bringing context back into epidemiology: variables and fallacies in multilevel analysis. *American Journal of Public Health* 1998;**88**(2):216–22.

Group-level variables in epidemiology

Group-level variables as proxies for individual-level variables

One of the most common uses of ecologic variables in epidemiologic studies is as proxies for individual-level variables, either because individual-level data are unavailable or because individual-level measurements are prone to measurement error. For example, in the absence of detailed information on smoking among individuals, median smoking levels in the area in which an individual lives may be used as a proxy. Of course, the use of these group-level proxies implies loss of information: We do not know whether a given person smokes or not, and we use mean smoking levels in the area as an approximation. In this case, the group-level measure is a second-class alternative to the ideal individual-level measurement. The relevant construct (smoking) is defined at the individual-level, but a group-level measurement is used as a proxy for it because direct individual-level measurements are unavailable. If a valid and reliable measure of individual-level exposure were available, it would be used instead.

Group-level variables are also used as proxies for individual-level data in cases in which individual-level measures are subject to a lot of measurement error, or when intra-individual variability makes a single measure a poor marker for the person's true exposure. For example, the mean yearly hours of sunlight in an area may be used as a proxy for individual-level exposure to sunlight and average per capita fat consumption in a group may be used as a proxy for the fat consumption of each member (due to limitations in characterizing an individual's fat intake based on a single, one-day measurement). In these situations, the ecologic measure is believed to be a better indicator of the 'true' individual-level exposure than the individual-level measure itself, because the ecologic measure reduces the 'noise' associated with measurement error or intra-individual variation.

Group-level proxies for individual-level variables can be used in studies with individuals or groups as the units of analysis. Regardless of the study design in which they are used, the key assumption in the use of these variables is that the group-level measure is an adequate proxy for the individual-level construct; that is, even if there is a measurement error, the construct being tapped into by the measure is an individual-level property rather than a group-level property.

But this may not always be true: It is possible that the group-level measure is capturing information about a group-level attribute rather than about the individual-level characteristics of persons comprising the group. For example, it is theoretically possible that areas with a higher percentage of smokers have higher cancer rates not because smokers develop cancer but because there is something about these areas (e.g. per-cent smokers may exert a contextual effect on cancer risk mediated, for example, through exposure to second-hand smoke), which places everyone in the area at higher risk regardless of whether they smoke or not. Unless individual-level data are available, it may not be possible to differentiate the effects of individual-level smoking from the contextual effect of per-cent smoking in the area (or other group-level properties associated with it). Thus, in considering the use of group-level variables as proxies of individual-level data, researchers may wish to consider two issues: (1) the degree of measurement error in the individual-level construct inherent in using the group-level variable (e.g. misclassification of smokers as non-smokers); and (2) the degree to which the group-level measure is tapping into a group-level construct rather than the individual-level construct it purports to proxy.

Group-level variables as measures of group-level constructs

Another application of ecologic variables is to measure group-level constructs. Variables that reflect the characteristics of groups have been classified into two basic types (Morgenstern 1995; Von Korff *et al.* 1992; Valkonen 1969; Lazarsfeld & Menzel 1971; Blalock 1984): Derived variables and integral variables. *Derived variables* (also termed *analytical* or *aggregate variables*) summarize the characteristics of individuals in the group (means, proportions; e.g. percentage of persons with incomplete high school education, median household income, *etc.*) Although created through the aggregation of information from the individual members of a group, derived variables are often used as measures of group-level properties and often provide information distinct from their individual-level analogue. For example, mean neighbourhood income and individual-level income are indicators of two distinct constructs, each of which may be important to health. Mean neighbourhood income may be a marker for neighbourhood-level factors potentially related to health (such a recreational facilities, school quality, road conditions, environmental conditions, types of foods available and their cost), and these factors may affect everyone in the community regardless of their individual-level income. Similarly, community unemployment level is a community-level property that may affect everyone in the community regardless of whether they are unemployed or not.

A special subset within derived variables is the average of the dependent variable within the group (Susser 1994). As noted by Ross (1916) in his theory of happenings, for some types of events, the frequency of occurrence may depend on the number of individuals already affected. The prevalence of a given infection in the group to which a person belongs will affect his or her risk of infection, or may modify the relationship between individual-level risk factors and the risk of disease (Halloran & Struchiner 1991; Koopman *et al.* 1991; Koopman & Longini 1994). The classic concept of herd immunity is a variant of this notion: The prevalence of immunity in a community will determine whether an epidemic of disease does or does not occur, and will therefore influence a non-immune individual's risk of acquiring disease. The contextual effect of the dependent variable's prevalence within a group may also be important in understanding other health outcomes. For example, the prevalence of obesity in a community may influence the likelihood that an individual is obese. This effect may operate through several different mechanisms. The prevalence of obesity may itself generate societal norms regarding acceptability and desirability of obesity, which may influence an individual's risk of being obese. In addition, the probability of adopting behaviours conducive to obesity (e.g. certain types of diet or physical activity patterns) may be higher in situations in which the behaviour is highly prevalent in the community. Although infrequently considered, these types of contextual effects may be important in understanding the distribution (and causes) of health-related behaviours (smoking and alcoholism are two common examples).

Integral variables (also termed *primary* or *global variables*) describe group characteristics that are not derived from characteristics of its members (e.g. the existence of certain types of laws, availability of health care, political system, or population density). Integral variables do not have analogues at the individual level. They may be discrete and dichotomous (e.g. an intervention or a disaster, presence of a certain law), scaled and polychotomous (e.g. social disorganization, intensity of newborn care), or continuous (e.g. physicians per capita). A special type of integral variable refers to patterns and networks of contacts or interactions between individuals within groups. These patterns are derived from how individuals are connected to each other, and yet they are more than aggregates of individual characteristics. Lazarsfeld and Menzel (1971) have referred to these variables as *structural variables*, although the term *structural effects* has also been used to refer to the effects of group-level properties more generally (Blau 1960). Patterns of interconnections among individuals may be important determinants of individual risk, particularly for infectious diseases, but possibly for many other health outcomes as well (Koopman *et al.* 1991; Koopman & Longini 1994; Koopman & Lynch 1999). In addition, these patterns may modify the relationship between certain individual-level attributes and risk of disease (Koopman *et al.* 1991). These patterns of interactions can be summarized in the form of group-level attributes such as network size or structure (Lazarsfeld & Menzel 1971; van den Eeden & Huttner 1982). Just as other 'group-level' variables can refer to groups of various sizes, these patterns may characterize a whole continuum of groups depending on the particular research problem: Large groups, smaller groups within larger groups, or even pairs of individuals.

When group-level variables are used to characterize group-level properties, there is no ambiguity in defining whether individuals are or are not exposed (as there is when group-level variables are used as proxies for individual-level exposure data). The group-level variable (whether derived or integral) applies equally to all individuals within the group; for example, all are 'exposed' to living in a neighbourhood with high unemployment regardless of whether they themselves are employed, all are 'exposed' to existing laws regarding seat belt use. Thus, the measurement error problem which may be present when group-level measures are used as proxies for measures of individual-level constructs is not present (although there may be measurement error in the measure of the group-level construct itself, as there may be for any measure). As we discuss in the following, such group-level constructs can be investigated in studies with either individuals or groups as the units of analysis.

Study designs based on the units of analysis

Studies with groups as units of analysis

Studies with groups as the units of analysis (ecologic studies) are most appropriate when investigators are interested in explaining variation between groups and the constructs of interest can be conceptualized as group-level properties. These group-level properties may be either derived or integral variables. Numerous studies have examined the relationship between area measures of deprivation or socio-environmental characteristics (derived variables) and area disease or mortality rates with geographic regions as the units of analysis (see, for example, Townsend *et al.* 1988; Wing, Barnett *et al.* 1992; Benach, Yasui *et al.* 2001; Janghorbani, Jones *et al.* 2006). This analytical approach is most appropriate if the research question is formulated at the area (group) level and the main construct investigated (deprivation or socio-environmental characteristics) is conceptualized as an area or group-level attribute. In these cases, area socio-environmental characteristics are conceptualized as group attributes that affect all individuals living within the community and the interest lies in drawing inferences regarding differences between areas.

An example involving integral group-level variables is provided by studies that relate national legislation restricting tobacco advertising in different countries to country smoking rates: A country-level construct is examined and the interest lies in drawing country-level inferences. Ecologic designs may also be appropriate for the evaluation of the effects of group-level interventions on group-level outcomes (Morgenstern 1982). For example, a study may want to investigate the relationship between the introduction of a mass media campaign to prevent teenage smoking (an integral variable) and the prevalence of teenage smoking in the area. Because the mass media campaign may affect all community inhabitants (regardless of whether they actually saw the ads or not) through mechanisms involving diffusion, peer pressure, and so on, the intervention can be conceptualized as a group-level attribute.

As discussed in the subsection on the ecologic fallacy, these studies are limited in their examination of the role of individual-level constructs—as confounders, mediators, or effect modifiers of the group-level associations. In the previous example, differences in the effects of the mass media campaign by individual-level characteristics (effect modification) could not be investigated. Neither could the impact of differences in individual exposures to the mass media campaign. In addition, in the case of ecologic variables with individual-level analogues (e.g. area unemployment and individual-level unemployment), studies with groups as the units of analysis cannot differentiate the contextual effect of the variable from its individual-level effect. For example, an ecologic study showing that area unemployment is related to higher rates of adverse mental health outcomes could not differentiate whether the increased rate of mental illness is seen only for the unemployed or is present for all area inhabitants regardless of whether they are unemployed or not. However, from a public health perspective, the group-level association may itself be of great interest. If the association observed is causal, decreasing the unemployment rate would decrease the rate of mental illness regardless of whether the effect was due to the group or individual effect of unemployment. Similarly, the country-level relationship between income inequality and health may have important policy implications regardless of whether it is due to a contextual effect of income inequality itself, or to the fact that more unequal countries tend to have more people in the lower-income categories.

It is often argued that ecologic studies may be particularly useful when investigating the health effects of individual-level attributes with little within-group variation but large between-group variation. For example, if dietary fat is homogeneous within countries but varies greatly from country to country, an individual-level study restricted to individuals from a single country may find no association between dietary fat and cardiovascular disease, but an ecological study comparing country rates to country average fat intake may find a strong relationship. From this perspective, the advantage of the ecological study results purely from the fact that it is able to include more variability in the exposure of interest. The same research question could be addressed in a study of individuals that included individuals from different countries and thus ensured sufficient variation in the exposure. But often this option is not feasible, whereas country-level measures may be available from standard sources. Of course, the presence of significant between-country differences in diet raises the important question of why countries differ in diet to begin with, and suggests that the diet of individuals has important country-level determinants. Despite the potential advantage of increasing variability in the exposure of interest, ecologic studies of diet and health outcomes are subject to the limitations of ecologic studies outlined earlier in terms of the presence of group effects and the inability to control for individual-level variables which may vary from group to group. Both of these may limit the utility of these studies in drawing inferences regarding the individual-level relationship between diet and health.

Although they will not be discussed here in detail, studies with groups as the units of analysis are subject to many of the same analytical issues as individual-level studies with respect to confounding, establishment of temporality, selection biases, and so on. In addition, these types of analyses raise additional methodological issues, such as the need to have adequate numbers of groups as well as enough individuals per group, the need to account for differences in the variability of outcomes (i.e. estimated rates) for the different groups due to the fact that they may be based on different numbers of observations, and the possibility of multicollinearity between the predictors examined (which is often more of a problem in ecologic studies than in individual-level studies) (Morgenstern 1982). Further, studies in which the units of analysis are geographic areas may need to use statistical methods to account for the fact that areas geographically closer to each other may tend to be more similar (in outcomes) than those more distant from each other (due to unmeasured factors that cluster in space), which leads to violation of the assumption of independence of observations (e.g. Clayton, Bernardinelli *et al.* 1993; Zhu, Gorman *et al.* 2006). Time-trend studies also raise additional methodological issues related to time-series analyses generally (Morgenstern 1995).

Studies with individuals as units of analysis

Individual-level studies are most appropriate when investigators are interested in drawing inferences regarding variability across individuals, and all potential constructs of interest can be conceptualized as individual-level properties. The most common epidemiologic studies are of this type. The assumption is that all constructs relevant to the outcome being studied are individual-level constructs.

Studies with individuals as the units of analysis and with information limited to individual-level constructs cannot examine the role of group-level constructs as antecedents of individual-level variables, as independent predictors of outcomes, or as confounders of individual-level associations. They cannot determine whether the effect of a given individual-level variable is only present in certain group contexts, or varies from group to group, as a function of group characteristics. In order to answer these questions, other types of studies are needed.

Studies limited to individuals from a single group are clearly unable to examine the role of group-level constructs in causing the outcome (or in interacting with individual-level variables), because group-level properties are invariant within groups (Schwartz & Carpenter 1999). If group-level factors are important in causing the outcome, studies focused on a single group may fail to detect important disease determinants. In the dietary fat example, we noted that a study based on individuals from a single country would not detect dietary fat as a risk factor if it were invariant within countries. More fundamentally, the country-level factors that influence large variations in fat intake across countries is the salient variable that the individual-level study could not capture.

If the study involves individuals from many different groups, relevant group-level properties may be included in individual-level analyses. For example, group-level variables can be included in regression equations with individuals as the units of analysis. These types of analyses have been called *contextual analyses* (Blalock 1984; Iversen 1991). Susser (1994) has referred to studies which investigate the effects of group-level variables on individual-level outcomes as mixed studies. A simple example of the type of regression models fitted in contextual analysis is shown in Equation 6.2.4:

$$Y_{ij} = \beta_0 + \beta_1 C_j + \beta_2 X_{ij} + e_{ij} \quad (6.2.4)$$

where,

Y_{ij} = outcome for *i*th individual in *j*th group
C_j = group-level variable
X_{ij} = individual-level variable
e_{ij} = error for *i*th individual in *j*th group

Contextual models can include multiple group-level and individual-level variables as well as their interactions. In Equation 6.2.4, β_1 estimates the effect of the group-level characteristic on the individual-level outcome (after adjustment for X_{ij}) and β_2 estimates the effect of the individual-level variable on the outcome (after adjustment for C_j). Contextual models can be used, for example, to investigate the effects of neighbourhood context on fertility outcomes by including characteristics of the neighbourhoods where individuals live (derived or integral variables) together with individual-level characteristics in individual-level regression models.

In these models, special methods may be necessary to account for residual within-group correlations in individual-level outcomes. Ignoring this correlation may lead to incorrect estimates of standard errors (Diggle *et al.* 2002). Efficiency of estimation may also be reduced (Diggle *et al.* 2002) One common approach to account for within-group correlations is to use marginal models (Zeger *et al.* 1988), also referred to as population-average models (Diggle *et al.* 2002) or covariance pattern models (Brown & Prescott 1999). Marginal or population-average models use the population-average response as a function of covariates without explicitly accounting for heterogeneity across groups (Zeger *et al.* 1988). In contrast to the multilevel models described in the next subsection, marginal models do not allow examination of group-to-group variability per se, or of the factors associated with it. Neither do they allow decomposition of total variability in the individual-level outcome into within- and between-group components. Although contextual analysis can be used to simultaneously investigate the effects of group-level and individual-level constructs in shaping individual-level outcomes, it does not allow examination of group-to-group variability per se, or of the factors associated with it. The unit of analysis remains the individual and only inter-individual variation is examined.

Studies with both groups and individuals as the units of analysis (multilevel studies)

Over the past few years, multilevel studies and multilevel analysis have emerged as promising approaches in several fields including education, sociology, and public health (Raudenbush & Bryk 2002; Mason *et al.* 1983; Hermalin 1986; Paterson & Goldstein 1991; Diprete & Forristal 1994; Duncan & Jones 1998; Kreft & deLeeuw 1998; Diez-Roux 2000; Diez-Roux 2002; Subramanian 2003; Bingenheimer & Raudenbush 2004). Multilevel studies simultaneously examine groups (or samples of groups) and individuals within them (or samples of individuals within them). Variability at both the group level and the individual level can be simultaneously examined, and the role of group-level and individual-level constructs in explaining variation between individuals and between groups can be investigated. For example, a study may have information on a series of country-level characteristics (e.g. GNP, inequality in the distribution of income) and on the individual-level characteristics of a sample of individuals within each country (including health outcomes). Researchers may be interested in investigating how country-level and individual-level factors are related to health outcomes, as well as the extent to which between-country and between-individual variability in the outcomes are explained by variables defined at both levels. Thus, multilevel analysis allows researchers to deal with the micro-level of individuals and the macro-level of groups or contexts simultaneously (Duncan & Jones 1998). Multilevel models can be used to draw inferences regarding the causes of inter-individual variation and the extent to which it is explained by individual-level or group-level variables, but inferences can also be made regarding inter-group variation, whether it exists in the data, and to what extent it is accounted for by group- and individual-level characteristics.

In the case of multilevel analysis involving two levels (e.g. individuals nested within groups), the model can be conceptualized as a two-stage system of equations. The case for a normally distributed dependent variable is illustrated in Equation 6.2.5. For reasons of simplicity, the illustration will focus on the case of only one independent variable at the individual and one independent variable at the group level (although models can be extended to include as many independent variables as needed).

In the first stage, a separate individual-level regression is defined for each group.

$$Y_{ij} = \beta_{0j} + \beta_{1j} I_{ij} + \varepsilon_{ij} \qquad \varepsilon_{ij} \sim N(0, \sigma^2) \quad (6.2.5)$$

where,

Y_{ij} = outcome variable for *i*th individual in *j*th group (or context)

I_{ij} = individual-level variable for ith individual in jth group (or context)
β_{0j} is the group-specific intercept
β_{1j} is the group-specific effect of the individual-level variable

Individual-level errors (e_{ij}) within each group are assumed to be independent and identically distributed with a mean of 0 and a variance of σ^2. Regression coefficients (β_{0j} and β_{1j}) are allowed to vary from one group to another.

In a second stage, each of the group- or context-specific regression coefficients defined in Equation 6.2.1 (β_{0j} and β_{1j} in this example) are modelled as a function of group-level variables.

$$\beta_{0j} = \gamma_{00} + \gamma_{01} C_j + U_{0j} \qquad U_{0j} \sim N(0, \tau_{00}) \qquad (6.2.6)$$

$$\beta_{1j} = \gamma_{10} + \gamma_{11} C_j + U_{1j} \qquad U_{1j} \sim N(0, \tau_{11}) \qquad (6.2.7)$$
$$\text{cov}(U_{0j}, U_{1j}) = \tau_{10}$$

where,
C_j = group-level or contextual variable
γ_{00} is the common intercept across groups (where C_j is 0)
γ_{01} is the effect of the group-level predictor on the group-specific intercepts
γ_{10} is the common slope associated with the individual-level variable across groups (where C_j is 0)
γ_{11} is the effect of the group-level predictor on the group-specific slopes

The errors in the group-level equations (U_{0j} and U_{1j}), sometimes called 'macro errors', are assumed to be normally distributed with mean 0 and variances τ_{00} and τ_{11} respectively. τ_{01} represents the covariance between intercepts and slopes; for example, if τ_{01} is positive, as the intercept increases the slope increases. Thus, multilevel analysis summarizes the distribution of the group-specific coefficients in terms of two parts: A 'fixed' part, which is unchanging across groups (γ_{00} and γ_{01} for the intercept, and γ_{10} and γ_{11} for the slope), and a 'random' part (U_{0j} for the intercept and U_{1j} for the slope), which is allowed to vary from group to group.

By including an error term in the group-level equations (Equations 6.2.6 and 6.2.7), these models allow for sampling variability in the group-specific coefficients (β_{0j} and β_{1j}) and also for the fact that the group-level equations are not deterministic (i.e. the possibility that not all relevant macro-level variables have been included in the model) (Wong & Mason 1985). The underlying assumption is that group-specific intercepts and slopes are random samples from a normally distributed population of group-specific intercepts and slopes (or equivalently, that the groups or macro errors are 'exchangeable') (Diprete & Forristal 1994).

An alternative way to present the model fitted in multilevel analysis is to substitute Equations 6.2.6 and 6.2.7 in Equation 6.2.5 to obtain:

$$Y_{ij} = \gamma_{00} + \gamma_{01} C_j + \gamma_{10} I_{ij} + U_{0j} + U_{1j} I_{ij} + e_{ij} \qquad (6.2.8)$$

The model includes the effects of group-level variables (γ_{01}), individual-level variables (γ_{10}), and their interaction (γ_{11}) on the individual-level outcome Y_{ij}. It also includes a random intercept component (U_{0j}) and a random slope component (U_{1j}), which together with the individual-level errors e_{ij} constitute a complex error structure. Because of the presence of this complex error structure, special estimation methods must be used. Although multilevel or random effects models were first developed for continuous dependent variables, analogous methods have been developed or are under development for other types of outcomes (Raudenbush & Bryk 2002; Wong & Mason 1985; Goldstein 1995).

By simultaneously including information on both groups and individuals, multilevel models avoid the limitations of ecologic studies and individual-level studies outlined in the subsection on fallacies. Both individuals and groups are units of analysis, and both inter-group and inter-individual variability can be examined. Multilevel studies thus provide an opportunity to link traditional ecologic and individual-level studies. Multilevel models allow investigation of a variety of interrelated research questions. They allow separation of the effects of context (i.e. group characteristics) and of composition (characteristics of the individuals in groups): Do groups differ in average outcomes after controlling for the characteristics of individuals within them? Are group-level variables related to outcomes after controlling for individual-level variables? Multilevel models can also be used to examine the effects of individual-level variables: Are individual-level variables related to the

Table 6.2.5 Types of study designs used in public health based on unit of analysis, level at which variability is examined, and constructs most appropriately investigated

Type of study	Unit of analysis	Level at which variability is examined	Constructs investigated as potential 'causes' of variability	
			Group-level	**Individual-level**
Ecologic	Groups	Groups (utility for inter-individual variability limited)	Yes	Only group-level proxies
Individual level	Individuals	Individuals (utility for inter-group variability limited)	No (yes in contextual)	Yes
Multilevel	Groups and individuals	Groups and individuals	Yes	Yes

outcome after controlling for group-level variables? Do individual-level associations vary from group to group, and is this partly a function of group-level variables? Multilevel models also allow quantification of variation at different levels (e.g. within group and between group) and the degrees to which these sources of variation are 'statistically explained' by individual-level and group-level variables. For example, is there significant variation in group-specific intercepts or slopes (do τ_{00} and τ_{11} differ significantly from 0)? How does this variability change as individual-level or group-level variables are added? What per cent of the variability in individual-level outcomes in between and within groups?

The types of studies, the levels at which variability is examined, and the types of constructs which they are more suited to investigate are summarized in Table 6.2.5.

Challenges in multilevel studies and multilevel analysis

The recognition of the need to examine constructs defined at multiple levels in understanding the causes of ill health has stimulated discussions of the many challenges in conducting and analysing multilevel studies. A key requirement is to begin with a clearly articulated conceptual model of the levels and constructs most relevant to the health outcome being investigated. A multiplicity of different nested (or non-nested) groups or levels may be relevant for a particular research question. Specifying the relevant levels is part of the development of the theory that should precede the data collection and statistical analysis. An important methodological complexity is that the variance apportioned to a given level in multilevel models may be over- or underestimated if a relevant level is ignored in the analysis (Subramanian 2003). In addition, misspecification of the relevant level may result in incorrectly concluding that groups (or higher-level) effects are absent. For example, if the research question pertains to the impact of availability of healthy foods on diet, and neighbourhoods are specified as the higher-level unit for which food availability is measured, the absence of an effect of neighbourhood food availability could be entirely consistent with a large effect of country-level food availability. In this case, the absence of the neighbourhood effect could result from low variability in healthy food availability across neighbourhoods within the country. If this is so, neighbourhood food availability would not be detected as an important predictor of individual-level diet. The failure to include the country level in the analyses would lead the researcher to miss the country-level food availability effect (this situation is directly analogous to the inability of studies restricted to individuals from a single group to detect group effects (Schwartz & Carpenter 1999).

The 'groups' relevant to a specific health outcome may be difficult to define (e.g. neighbourhoods) or have fuzzy and changing boundaries (e.g. friendship groups). Data are often unavailable for the theoretically relevant group of interest, so a crude proxy is used (e.g. census tracts for neighbourhoods) (Diez-Roux 2007; Diez-Roux 2001; O'Campo 2003). This results in substantial misspecification of the group and the group-level construct of interest. Whereas epidemiology has become very sophisticated at measuring individual-level attributes, the measurement of group-level attributes remains in its infancy. In some cases, the measurement of group-level constructs may be very simple (e.g. the presence of a certain law), but in others (e.g. social capital, the structure of social networks, or features of neighbourhoods related physical activity or stress) it is not. Recent work has illustrated the measurement of group-level constructs using aggregated survey data (Raudenbush & Sampson 1999; Mujahid *et al.* 2007). This approach allows assessment of the agreement between respondents within a group, the reliability of the group-level measure for discriminating between groups, and the construct validity of the group-level measure (by relating the measure obtained to other sources of data) (Mujahid *et al.* 2007; Raudenbush 2003). Other measures of group-level constructs may involve approaches that do not necessarily involve aggregation of individual measures (e.g. the structure of connections between individuals within a group or the use of geographic information systems to develop measures of neighbourhood availability and accessibility of resources). As the study of group-level factors becomes more common, other approaches to measuring attributes of groups are likely to emerge.

Because group-level factors must ultimately affect individuals in order to influence health, their effects must necessarily be mediated through more proximate individual-level processes. At the same time, some individual-level factors may be confounders of group-level effects either because individuals are selected into groups based on their individual-level attributes (e.g. persons with low income are selected into disadvantaged neighbourhoods) or because individual-level factors and group-level factors are associated for other reasons (e.g. persons living in countries characterized by mass production of processed foods may also be less physically active). Indeed, much of the effort in the estimation of group-level effects in multilevel studies goes into controlling appropriately for individual-level confounders of group effects (Pickett & Pearl 2001; Duncan & Jones 1998). Residual confounding by mismeasured or unmeasured individual-level variables has long been a critique of studies of group effects (Oakes 2004; Diez-Roux 2001; Hauser 1970). On the other hand, many of these individual-level factors may be mediators of group effects, raising questions regarding whether of not group-level effects should be adjusted for these factors (Macintyre & Ellaway 2003). Even more complex situations may arise when a factor is both a mediator and a confounder of the higher-level effect.

It has been noted that the use of multiple regression approaches to partition indirect and direct effects (e.g. the portion of a group effect that is mediated through a given variable and the portion that is not) may lead to incorrect conclusions regarding the presence and strength of direct effects (Robins & Greenland 1992; Cole & Hernan 2002). The extent to which the approach of estimating a direct effect by comparing a group-level effect before and after adjusting for a mediator results in substantial bias in real-life situations (as opposed to hypothetical examples) remains to be fully determined (Blakely 2002). It is likely to vary from research problem to research problem depending on the extent to which adjustment for the mediator actually introduces substantial confounding by other unmeasured variables related to the mediator and the outcome. When individual-level variables may be both confounders and mediators of the effect of interest, special estimation procedures may be necessary to correctly estimate the effect (Robins 1989; Robins *et al.* 2000). The extension of these emerging methods to a multilevel data structure is likely to be quite complex.

Observational multilevel studies face the same problems as other observational studies in estimating causal effects from observational data. The ability to draw causal inferences is based on the extent to which the methods used approximate the counterfactual comparison of interest. One important limitation of past work in this regard especially prevalent in research on neighbourhood health effects has been the reliance on group-level derived variables (e.g. neighbourhood mean income) as proxies for the relevant integral group-level variable of interest (Pickett & Pearl 2001; Diez-Roux 2001; Macintyre & Ellaway 2002). This has limited the extent to which the data available allow researchers to approximate the counterfactual contrast of interest, even within the limitations of observational studies. Better specification of the group-level factors of interest (e.g. moving from crude proxies to measures of the specific constructs of interest) and the testing of specific hypotheses will improve the ability to draw causal inferences.

The extent to which group-level effects can be validly estimated through the use of multiple regression methods (including multilevel models) to control for individual-level confounders has been questioned (Oakes 2004). The adjusted comparison requires assumptions regarding the effects of the individual-level variable on the outcome across groups, and may involve extrapolations beyond the support in the data if there is little overlap in the distribution of the individual-level variable across groups (e.g. individual-level income across levels of neighbourhood disadvantage). The extent to which this is a problem is an empirical question and may vary from research problem to research problem (Diez-Roux 2004b). This is no different from similar situations involved in adjusted comparisons in individual-level studies. The use of propensity score (Rubin 1997) matching has recently been proposed as an alternative to traditional regression approaches in estimating some types of group effects (Harding 2003).

Another complexity of observational studies of group effects is that certain group-level properties may be at least partly endogenous to the characteristics of the individuals that make up the group (Oakes 2004; Subramanian 2003). This makes the identification of these group-level effects from observational data problematic. The extent to which group-level properties are endogenous to individual-level properties is likely to vary for different group-level constructs and different research questions (Diez-Roux 2004b; Subramanian 2004). Endogeneity may appear more of a problem in the case of derived group-level variables (e.g. mean neighbourhood income) that are constructed by aggregating the characteristics of individuals within a group. However, as noted earlier, these variables are often used as proxies for a more clearly exogenous integral group-level property. Endogeneity is also a possibility for some integral group-level variables (e.g. dietary habits of residents may influence neighbourhood availability of healthy foods). However, it is unlikely that all group-level attributes are fully endogenous to the individual characteristics of persons of which the group is composed. Strategies to at least partly deal with the problem of endogeneity in the multilevel context have been proposed (Subramanian 2004), but in situations where endogeneity is a major concern other analytical strategies more appropriate for the analysis of dynamic systems may be more appropriate (Auchincloss and Diez Roux 2008).

Finally, sample size and power calculations in multilevel studies are complex and remain an area of active research (Raudenbush & Bryk 2002; Snijders & Bosker 1999; Raudenbush & Liu 2000; Hox 2002). In general, the power for estimating the individual-level regression coefficients depends on the total sample size (Hox 2002). The power for higher-level (group-level) effects and cross-level interactions (interactions between group- and individual-level variables) depends more strongly on the number of groups than on the total sample size (Hox 2002). However, the power to estimate the ratio of between group to total variability (the intra-class correlation coefficient) is affected by the number of groups and the number of persons per group in a different manner than the power to detect associations of group-level variables with individual-level outcomes (the fixed effects of group properties) (Snijders & Bosker 1999). Power and sample size calculations need to specify the key multilevel parameters of interest, and tradeoffs may be involved.

Conclusion

In public health research, both predictors and outcomes may be conceptualized at different levels of organization, and understanding outcomes at a given level may require taking into account information pertaining to levels above or below it. Also, each system can be thought of as nested within another level, and dynamically interrelated with the levels above and below it. In addition, each level may acquire 'emergent' properties, unique characteristics confined to that level, which are different from the properties of its components. The selection of the appropriate study design should be based on the specific research question investigated, including the level of organization about which inferences are to be made, as well as the levels of organizations of the constructs of interest (including the main independent variables and potential confounders or effect modifiers of the association).

Problems related to the use of ecologic studies and ecologic variables in epidemiology often result from confusion regarding the level of organization to which the research question pertains, the level of organization at which the constructs of interest are defined and measured, and the sometimes inappropriate use of variables defined and measured at one level to proxy constructs defined at another level. Of course, researchers must necessarily focus on certain aspects of the continuum of levels of organization and not all studies need (or can) span all levels. Rather than defending or critiquing one study design in favour of another, it is more useful to evaluate whether the level of analysis investigated and the constructs examined are appropriate for the specific question being asked. Because 'ideal' study designs are often not possible, the key lies in determining whether the particular design employed is 'good enough' for the question being asked. The issues reviewed in this chapter may be helpful in making this judgment.

References

Alker H. A typology of ecological fallacies. In: Dogan M, Rokkam S, editors. *Social ecology*. Boston (MA): MIT Press; 1969. p. 69–86.

Auchincloss A.H. and Diez Roux A.V. A new tool for epidemiology? The usefulness of dynamic agent models in understanding place effects on health. *American Journal of Epidemiology*, 2008;**168**(1):1–8.

Benach J., Yasui Y. *et al.* Material deprivation and leading causes of death by gender: evidence from a nationwide small area study. *Journal of Epidemiology and Community Health* 2000;**55**(4):239–45.

Bingenheimer J.B. and Raudenbush S.W. Statistical and substantive inferences in public health: issues in the application of multilevel models. *Annual Review of Public Health* 2004;**25**:53–77.

Blakely T. Commentary: estimating direct and indirect effects—fallible in theory, but in the real world? *International Journal of Epidemiology* 2002;**31**(1):166–7.

Blakely T.A. and Woodward A.J. Ecological effects in multi-level studies. *Journal Epidemiology and Community Health* 2000;**54**(5):367–74.

Blalock H. Contextual-effects models: theoretical and methodological issues. *Annual Review of Sociology* 1984;**10**:353–72.

Blau P.M. Structural effects. *American Sociological Review* 1960;**25**:178–93.

Brenner *et al.* 1992.

Brown H. and Prescott R. *Applied mixed models in medicine*. New York (NY): Wiley; 1999.

Chadwick E. Report on the sanitary conditions of the labouring population of Great Britain. Edinburgh, UK: Edinburgh University Press; 1965.

Clayton D.G., Bernardinelli L. *et al.* Spatial correlation in ecological analysis. *International Journal of Epidemiology* 1993;**22**(6):1193–202.

Cole S.R. and Hernan M.A. Fallibility in estimating direct effects. *International Journal Epidemiology* 2002;**1**(1):163–5.

Diez-Roux A.V. *et al.* Bringing context back into epidemiology: variables and fallacies in multilevel analysis. *American Journal of Public Health* 1998;**88**(2):216–22.

Diez-Roux A.V. A glossary for multilevel analysis. *Journal of Epidemiology and Community Health* 2002;**56**(8):588–94.

Diez-Roux A.V. Estimating neighborhood health effects: the challenges of causal inference in a complex world. *Social Science and Medicine* 2004a;**58**(10):1953–60.

Diez-Roux A.V. Investigating neighborhood and area effects on health. *American Journal of Public Health* 2001;**91**(11):1783–9.

Diez-Roux A.V. Multilevel analysis in public health research. *Annual Review of Public Health* 2000;**21**:171–92.

Diez-Roux A.V. Neighborhoods and health: where are we and where do we go from here? *Revue d'Epidemiologie et Sante Publique* 2007.

Diez-Roux A.V. The study of group-level factors in epidemiology: rethinking variables, study designs and analytical approaches. *Revue d'Epidemiologie* 2004b;**26**:104–11.

Diggle P.J., Liang K.Y. *et al. Analysis of longitudinal data*. New York (NY): Oxford University Press; 2002.

Diprete T.A. and Forristal J.D. Multilevel models: methods and substance. *Annual Review of Sociology* 1994;**20**:331–57.

Duncan C. and Jones K. Context, composition and heterogeneity: using multilevel models in health research. *Social Science and Medicine* 1998;**46**(1):97–117.

Firebaugh G. A rule for inferring individual-level relationships from aggregate data. *American Sociological Review* 1978;**43**:557–72.

Goldberger J., Wheeler G.A. *et al.* A study of the relation of factors of a sanitary character to pellagra incidence in seven cotton-mill villages of South Carolina in 1916. *Public Health Report* 1920;**35**:1701–24.

Goldstein H. *Multilevel statistical models*. New York (NY): Halsted Press; 1995.

Greenland S. and Morgenstern H. Ecological bias, confounding, and effect modification. *International Journal of Epidemiology* 1989;**18**(1):269–74.

Greenland S. and Robins J. Ecologic studies—biases, misconceptions, and counter-examples. *American Journal of Epidemiology* 1994;**139**:747–60.

Greenland S. Divergent biases in ecologic and individual-level studies. *Statistics in Medicine* 1992;**1511**:1209–23.

Halloran M.E. and Struchiner C.J. Study designs for dependent happenings. *Epidemiology* 1991;**2**(5):331–8.

Hammond J. Two sources of error in ecological correlations. *American Sociological Review* 1973;**38**:764–77.

Harding D. Counterfactual models of neighborhood effects: the effect of neighborhood poverty on high school dropout and teenage pregnancy. *American Journal of Sociology* 2003;**109**:676–719.

Hauser R. Context and consex: a cautionary tale. *American Journal of Sociology* 1970;**75**:645–64.

Hermalin A. The multilevel approach: theory and concepts. *Population Studies Addendum Manual IX* 1986;**66**:15–31.

Hox J.P. Multilevel analysis: techniques and applications. Manwah (NJ): Lawrence Erlbaum; 2002.

Iversen G. *Contextual analysis*. Newbury Park (CA): Sage Publications; 1991.

Janghorbani M., Jones R.B. *et al.* Neighbourhood deprivation and excess coronary heart disease mortality and hospital admissions in Plymouth, UK: an ecological study. *Acta Cardiologica* 2006;**61**(3):313–20.

Kawachi I., Kennedy B.P. *et al.* Social capital and self-rated health: a contextual analysis. *American Journal of Public Health* 1999;**89**(8):1187–93.

Keys A. Seven countries: a multivariate analysis of death and coronary heart disease. Cambridge (MA): Harvard University Press; 1980.

King G. A solution to the ecological inference problem. Reconstructing individual behavior from aggregate data. Princeton (NJ): Princeton University Press; 1997.

Koopman J.S., Longini I.M., Jr. *et al. Assessing risk factors for transmission of infection. American Journal of Epidemiology* 1991;**133**(12):1199–209.

Koopman J.S., Longini I.M., Jr. The ecological effects of individual exposures and nonlinear disease dynamics in populations. *American Journal of Public Health* 1994;**84**(5):836–42.

Koopman J.S. and Lynch J.W. Individual causal models and population system models in epidemiology. *American Journal of Public Health* 1999;**89**(8):1170–4.

Koopman J.S., Prevots D.R. *et al.* Determinants and predictors of dengue infection in Mexico. *American Journal of Epidemiology* 1991;**133**(11):1168–78.

Kreft I., deLeeuw J. *Introducing multilevel modeling*. London: Sage; 1998.

Lazarsfeld P. and Menzel H. On the relation between individual and collective properties. In: Etzioni A, editor. *A sociological reader on complex organizations*. New York (NY): Holt, Rinehart, and Winston; 1971. p. 499–516.

Levin B. Annotation: accounting for the effects of both group- and individual-level variables in community-level studies. *American Journal of Public Health* 1995;**85**:163–4.

Lynch J., Due P. *et al.* Social capital—is it a good investment strategy for public health? *Journal of Epidemiology and Community Health* 2000;**54**(6):404–8.

Lynch J., Harper S. *et al.* Commentary: plugging leaks and repelling boarders—where to next for the SS income inequality? *International Journal of Epidemiology* 2003;**32**(6):1029–36;discussion 1037–40.

Macintyre S. and Ellaway A. Ecological approaches: rediscovering the role of the physical and social environment. In: Berkman L, Kawachi I, editors. *Social epidemiology*. New York (NY): Oxford University Press; 2000.

Macintyre S. and Ellaway A. Neighborhoods and health: an overview. In: Kawachi I, Berkman L, editors. *Neighborhoods and health*. New York (NY): Oxford University Press; 2003. p. 20–44.

Macintyre S. and Ellaway A. Place effects on health: how can we conceptualise, operationalise and measure them? *Social Science and Medicine* 2002;**55**(1):125–39.

Mason W., Wong G. *et al.* Contextual analysis through the multilevel linear model. In: Leinhardt S, editor. *Sociological methodology*. San Francisco (CA): Josey Bass; 1983. p. 72–103.

Morgenstern H. Ecologic studies in epidemiology: concepts, principles, and methods. *Annual Review of Public Health* 1995;**16**:61–81.

Morgenstern H. Uses of ecologic analysis in epidemiologic research. *American Journal of Public Health* 1982;**72**(12):1336–44.

Mujahid M.S., Diez Roux A.V. *et al.* Assessing the measurement properties of neighborhood scales: from psychometrics to ecometrics. *American Journal of Epidemiology* 2007.

O'Campo P. Invited commentary: advancing theory and methods for multilevel models of residential neighborhoods and health. *American Journal of Epidemiology* 2003;**157**(1):9–13.

Oakes J.M. The (mis)estimation of neighborhood effects: causal inference for a practicable Social Epidemiology. *Social Science and Medicine* 2004;**58**(10):1929–52.

Paterson L. and Goldstein H. New statistical methods for analysing social structures: an introduction to multilevel models. *British Educational Research Journal* 1991;**17**:387–93.

Piantadosi S., Byar D.P. *et al.* The ecological fallacy. *American Journal of Epidemiology* 1988;**127**(5):893–904.

Piantadosi S. Invited commentary: ecologic biases. *American Journal of Epidemiology* 1994;**139**(8):761–4; discussion 769–71.

Pickett K.E. and Pearl M. Multilevel analyses of neighbourhood socio-economic context and health outcomes: a critical review. *Journal of Epidemiology Community Health* 2001;**55**(2):111–22.

Raudenbush S. and Bryk A.S. Applications in organizational research. In: *Hierarchical linear models: applications and data analysis methods*. Thousand Oaks (CA): Sage; 2002. p. 99–159.

Raudenbush S. The quantitative assessment of neighborhood social environments. In: Kawachi I, Berkman L, editors. *Neighborhoods and health*. New York (NY): Oxford University Press; 2003. p. 112–31.

Raudenbush S.W., Liu X. Statistical power and optimal design for multisite randomized trials. *Psychological Methods* 2000;**5**(2):199–213.

Raudenbush S.W., Sampson R.J. Ecometrics: Toward a science of assessing ecological settings, with application to the systematic social observation of neighborhoods. *Sociological Methodology* 1999;**29**:1–41.

Riley M. Special problems of sociological analysis. In: *Sociological research I: a case approach*. New York (NY): Harcourt, Brace and World; 1963. p. 700–25.

Robins J. The control of confounding by intermediate variables. *Statistics in Medicine* 1989;**8**(6):679–701.

Robins J.M., Greenland S. Identifiability and exchangeability for direct and indirect effects. *Epidemiology* 1992;**3**(2):143–55.

Robins J.M., Hernan M.A. *et al.* Marginal structural models and causal inference in epidemiology. *Epidemiology* 2000;**11**(5):550–60.

Robinson W. Ecological correlations and the behavior of individuals. *American Sociological Review* 1950;**15**:351–7.

Ross R. An application of the theory of probabilities to the study of a priori pathometry: Part I. *Proceedings of the Royal Society Series A* 1916;**92**: 204–30.

Rubin D.B. Estimating causal effects from large data sets using propensity scores. *Annals of Internal Medicine* 1997;**127**(8 Pt 2):757–63.

Scheuch E. Social context and individual behavior. In: Dogan M., Rokkam S., editors. *Social ecology*. Boston (MA): MIT Press; 1969. p. 133–55.

Schwartz S. and Carpenter K.M. The right answer for the wrong question: consequences of type III error for public health research. *American Journal of Public Health* 1999;**89**(8):1175–80.

Schwartz S. The fallacy of the ecological fallacy: the potential misuse of a concept and its consequences. *American Journal of Public Health* 1994;**84**:819–24.

Snijders T.A.B. and Bosker R. Multilevel analysis: an introduction to basic and advanced multilevel modeling. London: Sage; 1999.

Snow J. On the mode of communication of cholera. In: *Snow on cholera*. [2nd ed 1936]. New York (NY): The Commonwealth Fund; 1855. p. 62–3.

Subramanian S.V. and Kawachi I. Response: in defence of the income inequality hypothesis. *International Journal of Epidemiology* 2003;**32**(6):1037–40.

Subramanian S.V. Multilevel methods for public health research. In: Kawachi I, Berkman L, editors. *Neighborhoods and health*. New York (NY): Oxford University Press; 2003.

Subramanian S.V. The relevance of multilevel statistical methods for identifying causal neighborhood effects. *Social Science and Medicine* 2004;**58**(10):1961–7.

Susser E. and Wanderling J. Epidemiology of nonaffective acute remitting psychosis versus schizophrenia: sex and sociocultural setting. *Archives of General Psychiatry* 1994;**51**:294–301.

Susser M. *Causal thinking in the health sciences*. New York (NY): Oxford University Press; 1973.

Susser M. The logic in ecological: I. *The logic of analysis. American Journal of Public Health* 1994;**84**:825–9.

Susser M. The logic in ecological: II. *The logic of design. American Journal of Public Health* 1994;**84**(5):830–5.

Terris M. *Goldberger on pellagra*. Baton Rouge: Louisiana State University Press; 1964.

Townsend P. *et al.* Health and deprivation, inequality and the North. London: Routledge; 1998.

Valkonen T. Individual and structural effects in ecological research. In: Dogan M., Rokkam S., editors. *Social ecology*. Boston (MA): MIT Press; 1969. p. 53–68.

van den Eeden P. and Huttner H.J. Multi-level research. *Current Sociology* 1982;**30**:1–178.

Von Korff M., Koepsell T. *et al.* Multi-level research in epidemiologic research on health behaviors and outcomes. *American Journal of Epidemiology* 1992;**135**:1077–82.

Wing S., Barnett E. *et al.* Geographic and socioeconomic variation in the onset of decline of coronary heart disease mortality in white women. *American Journal of Public Health* 1992;**82**(2):204–9.

Wong G. and Mason W. The hierarchical logistic regression model for multilevel analysis. *Journal of the American Statistical Association* 1985;**80**:513–24.

Zeger S.L., Liang K.Y. *et al.* Models for longitudinal data: a generalized estimating equation approach. *Biometrics* 1988;**44**(4):1049–60.

Zhu L., Gorman D.M. *et al.* Hierarchical Bayesian spatial models for alcohol availability, drug 'hot spots' and violent crime. *International Journal of Health Geographics* 2006;**5**:54.

6.3

Cross-sectional studies

Manolis Kogevinas and Leda Chatzi

Introduction

Cross-sectional studies examine the relationship between diseases (or other health-related characteristics) and other variables of interest as they exist in a defined population at a particular point in time (Last 2001). They could be defined as 'studies taking a snapshot of a society'. Synonyms used for cross-sectional include prevalence and disease-frequency studies.

The principal characteristic of cross-sectional studies is that they provide information on the *prevalence* of disease; that is, they include prevalent cases. In these studies, exposure and disease are measured at the same point in time, but this characteristic is shared by other epidemiologic designs; for example, case–control studies. In many cross-sectional studies, information on past exposures is not collected, but this should not be regarded as a characteristic defining these studies. The outcome measured in cross-sectional studies can be a continuous variable such as blood pressure or FEV1, as compared to a dichotomous outcome measured in case–control studies and, on most occasions, in cohort studies.

As is frequently the case in epidemiology, studies may use mixed designs; for example, a cross-sectional study may measure a biomarker referring to current exposure (e.g. vitamin E), may request information for the past (e.g. use of health services in the last year), may identify older and recent cases (e.g. subjects who had asthma in childhood or those who had their first attack of asthma in the last few months), and may convert into a cohort study if subjects included in the cross-sectional studies are followed up. The statistical analysis of cross-sectional studies depends on their hybrid design, and is frequently similar to that of a case–control study using logistic regression and calculating (prevalence)-odds ratios. Cross-sectional studies are extensively used to measure the prevalence of disease and exposures or other health-related variables. On these occasions, the representativeness of the studied sample is a prerequisite.

In this chapter, we will first describe the uses of cross-sectional studies in epidemiological and public health research, then discuss methodological issues concerning the design, the main biases of these studies, including response rates, and how to improve participation in the studies. We will finally discuss issues related to the statistical analysis of cross-sectional studies. Many of these issues are also relevant to other epidemiological designs.

Uses of cross-sectional studies

Cross-sectional studies have been used to evaluate the prevalence of diseases and of health-related variables, as well as to evaluate the aetiology of diseases. Large multipurpose national cross-sectional studies are conducted in several countries for administrative reasons, and to provide background documentation on the health status of a population.

National multipurpose surveys

National (or regional) multipurpose surveys are carried out routinely or ad hoc in several countries. The purpose and themes of these surveys are multiple, and they may cover different health problems in successive years. A description of the aims of the Health Survey in England is shown in Table 6.3.1.

The National Health and Nutrition Examination Survey (NHANES) is the largest national multipurpose survey, and is conducted on a routine basis (www.cdc.gov/nhanes): It is a programme of studies designed to assess the health and nutritional status of the civilian, non-institutionalized population of the United States. The survey is unique in that it combines interviews and physical examination.

Results of national health surveys can be used for several purposes, such as the study of time trends in risk factors or health symptoms, identification of causes of disease, and evaluation of health needs. Changes of health problems and risk factors in the population over time can be identified through repeated surveys. This type of information may allow health planning through the identification of the needs and effectiveness of existing policies and interventions. Time trends in obesity and in levels of toxic substances, such as lead in blood, are examples of the use of these types of surveys. Increases in overweight among children have been observed in many countries and are a public health concern, particularly because overweight children are at greater risk of becoming overweight adults. Trends in overweight children from the 1960s to the 1990s were examined in the United States, using data from consecutive NHANES surveys. Using age- and sex-specific reference data, children at the 95th percentile and above were classified as overweight. The percentage of overweight children and adolescents increased over three decades from the 1960s to the 1990s (Fig. 6.3.1). As shown in the figure, the percentage of

Table 6.3.1 Health Survey for England: description and aims

The Health Survey for England is a series of annual surveys about the health of people in England. The survey has been carried out since 1991 and was proposed to improve information on morbidity of the population by the (then) newly created Central Health Monitoring Unit within the Department of Health. This information is used to underpin and improve targeting of nationwide health policies.
The survey aims
◆ To provide annual data about the nation's health
◆ To estimate the proportion of the population with specific health conditions
◆ To estimate the prevalence of risk factors associated with those conditions
◆ To assess the frequency with which combinations of risk factors occur
◆ To examine differences between population subgroups
◆ To monitor targets in the health strategy
◆ To measure the height of children at different ages, replacing the national study of health and growth (from 1995)

overweight boys and girls aged 6–11 years increased from 4 per cent in 1965 to 13 per cent in 1999, and the percentage of overweight adolescents increased from 5 per cent in 1970 to 14 per cent in 1999.

The existence of a large national database has several advantages for the identification or confirmation of risk factors of a disease. Problems of cross-sectional studies that evaluate risk factors of diseases are discussed in the next subsection, particularly potential biases from the inclusion of prevalent cases and from frequent lack of information on past exposures. However, evaluation of a national representative population sample, as is the case in several multi-purpose surveys, has the advantage of capturing a global image of the society, including population groups that may be omitted in other types of design. Information on the population distribution of health problems and risk factors provide important clues to researchers on the causes of disease, and may also confirm previous hypotheses in large population samples.

An example provided here is of a study on cleaners, based on the NHANES. The importance of this study lies, among others, in the fact that domestic cleaners are a population group that is very hard to identify through the usual designs applied; identifying industry-based cohorts is an easier, more usual strategy. Arif *et al.* (2003) used data from the third National Health and Nutrition Examination

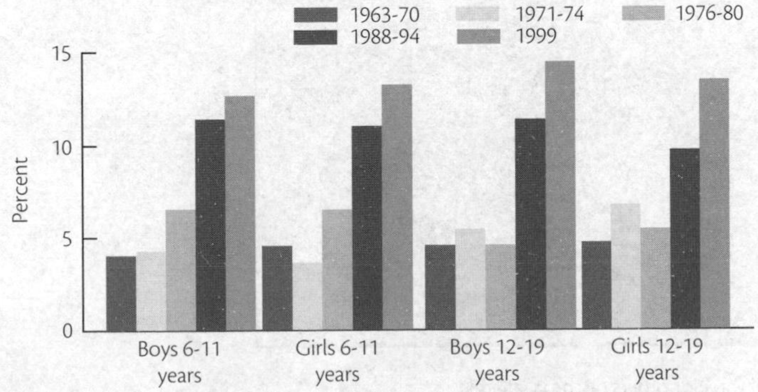

Fig. 6.3.1 Trends in overweight (BMI ≥ 95th percentile): United States.
Source: CDC/NCHS; NHES II/III (1963–70), NHANES I (1971–74), NHANES II (1976–80), NHANES III (1988–94). NHANES 1999.

Survey (NHANES III), 1988–94, to evaluate associations between occupation and work-related asthma and wheezing among US workers. They identified several occupations that were at risk of developing work-related asthma, with cleaners and equipment cleaners showing the highest risks: The population-attributable risk for work-related asthma was 26 per cent. The study confirmed a previous hypothesis on asthma in cleaners (Kogevinas *et al.* 1999), provided an evaluation of asthma risk in other occupations in the US population, and also gave an estimate of the burden of occupational asthma.

By identifying the health-care needs of the population, government agencies and private-sector organizations can establish policies and plan research, education, and health-promotion programmes that will help improve present health status and prevent future health problems.

Studies examining the prevalence of disease

Cross-sectional studies are, by definition, the appropriate design to evaluate the prevalence of diseases, which may be done for administrative purposes or for reasons related to the evaluation of aetiological factors. The main issues regarding the conduct of these studies include the representativeness of the sample, the size of the sample, and the measurement of outcomes and exposures. The International Study of Asthma and Allergies in Childhood (ISAAC) is among the largest of the cross-sectional studies ever done.

The ISAAC was designed to allow comparisons of the prevalence of allergic disorders in childhood between populations in different countries and their trends over time (Asher *et al.* 1995). In the early 1990s, although it was generally perceived that asthma prevalence was increasing, there existed very limited population-based estimates. The study included simple 'core' instruments for measuring the prevalence of allergic disorders suitable for different geographical locations and languages: (a) written questionnaires on the prevalence and severity of asthma, rhinitis, and eczema for self-completion by 13–14-year-olds or for completion by parents of 6- to 7-year-olds and (b) video questionnaires on the prevalence and severity of asthma for self-completion by 13–14-year-old children. In phase I, children aged 13–14 years were studied in 155 centres in 56 countries (n = 463 801) and children aged 6–7 years were studied in 91 centres in 38 countries (n = 257 800)

(The International Study of Asthma and Allergies in Childhood (ISAAC) Steering Committee 1998). Up to 20-fold variations in the prevalence of 'current wheeze' (in the last 12 months) were observed between centres worldwide (range 1.8–36.7 per cent), with a seven-fold variation observed between the 10th and 90th percentiles (4.4 per cent; 30.9 per cent). The highest 12-month-period prevalences were from centres in the United Kingdom, Australia, New Zealand, and the Republic of Ireland; the lowest prevalences were from centres in Eastern Europe, Albania, Greece, China, Taiwan, Uzbekistan, India, Indonesia, and Ethiopia (Fig. 6.3.2).

Aetiological research

Cross-sectional studies are particularly valuable for the investigation of the aetiology of non-fatal diseases, degenerative diseases, diseases with no clear point of onset (e.g. chronic bronchitis), and effects on physiologic variables (e.g. forced vital capacity [FVC] or liver enzyme levels). In diseases with no clear point of onset, it is difficult to identify incident cases and conduct cohort or incident case–control studies. The prevalence of a disease will be highest if it occurs relatively frequently and if the disease persists in time. A disease could be described as persistent if it is not rapidly fatal and if it does not manifest usually as a transitory condition. Diseases such as asthma and osteoarthritis, which have a relatively high prevalence, have frequently been examined in cross-sectional studies.

The European Community Respiratory Health Survey (ECRHS) is, in many aspects, similar in design to the ISAAC: It is an international cross-sectional study that was conducted on adults (20–44 years), mainly from European centres, to evaluate the prevalence and aetiology of asthma and related diseases (Burney *et al.* 1994). In an initial screening short questionnaire, the ECRHS included information from approximately 140 000 individuals of 22 countries. A subsample of the study incorporated extensive questionnaires, measurement of atopic markers, spirometry, and methacholine challenge. The key findings of the study are the large geographical differences in the prevalence of asthma, atopy, and bronchial responsiveness in adults, with high prevalence rates in English-speaking countries and low prevalence rates in the Mediterranean region and Eastern Europe. Analyses of risk factors have highlighted the importance of occupational exposure for asthma in adulthood (Kogevinas *et al.* 1999). The association between sensitization to individual allergens and bronchial responsiveness was strongest for indoor allergens (mites and cats). Analysis of treatment practices has confirmed that treatment of asthma varies widely between countries, and that asthma is often under-treated (Janson *et al.* 2001).

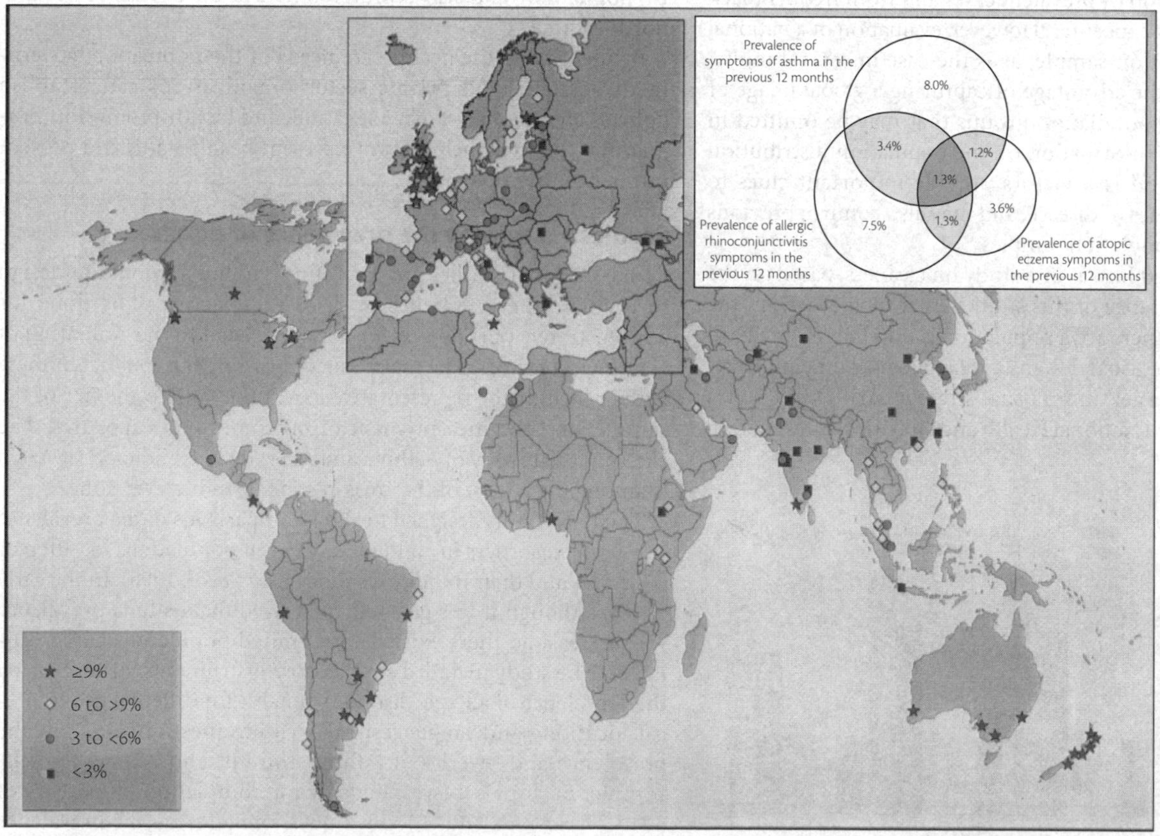

Fig. 6.3.2 ISAAC I: World map of 12-month prevalence of symptoms of at least two of three disorders (asthma, allergic conjunctivitis, atopic eczema). (From the International Study of Asthma and Allergies in Childhood [ISAAC] Steering Committee. Worldwide variation in prevalence of symptoms of asthma, allergic rhinoconjunctivitis, and atopic eczema. *Lancet* 1998;**351**[9111]:1225–32. With permission of Elsevier.)

Design of cross-sectional studies

Main design issues

The simplest form of a survey in a population is a one-time measurement of the prevalence of a disease (Checkoway *et al.* 2004). On some occasions, repeated surveys (panel studies) are conducted on the same or different individuals (Fig. 6.3.3).

When evaluating the prevalence of a disease, the sample studied should be representative of the base population from which subjects are recruited (internal validity). The random error of an estimate depends directly on the size of the study, and standard techniques exist to calculate this error (see, for example, free software such as EpiInfo™ [www.cdc.gov/epiinfo]). Measurement of outcomes may be particularly complicated because, frequently, prevalence studies are conducted for diseases that have a gradual onset and are not fatal. In addition, problems may occur when comparisons of prevalence are made between countries that may have different systems for the identification of the disease or even different perceptions and oral descriptions of a disease. For example, refer to the large prevalence studies conducted for the evaluation of prevalence of children's asthma, such as the ISAAC study mentioned earlier. Wheezing is a key symptom defining asthma in childhood. However, the perception of what is wheezing is not necessarily the same in different countries, and further, some languages do not have a single word to describe what in English is called 'wheezing'.

Generalizability is another aspect of representativeness, and refers to whether the findings in one population can be extrapolated to other populations (external validity). It is less of a problem when examining risk factors of disease, because biological mechanisms through which an agent may provoke disease tend to be similar between populations; it may, however, be more difficult to ensure when examining prevalence, because this may vary considerably within and between populations.

Panel studies use a modified longitudinal design that combines cross-sectional and cohort study methods: They are series of cross-sectional studies performed over time, usually on the same group of individuals or study sample, but also on different groups of a population in subsequent time periods. The objective is to evaluate change in health status in relation to changes in exposure. Small groups, or panels, of individuals are followed over short time intervals, and health outcomes, exposure, and potential confounders are ascertained for each subject on one or more occasions. This design is especially useful for the study of physiologic variables (such as pulmonary function, blood pressure) for which changes over several years may indicate early stages of disease processes. It is also useful to evaluate time trends in a disease.

The third phase of the ISAAC (ISAAC III) could be regarded as a panel study. ISAAC III was a repetition of the phase-I survey after 5–10 years to examine time trends in the prevalence of allergic disorders in centres and countries that had participated in the first phase.

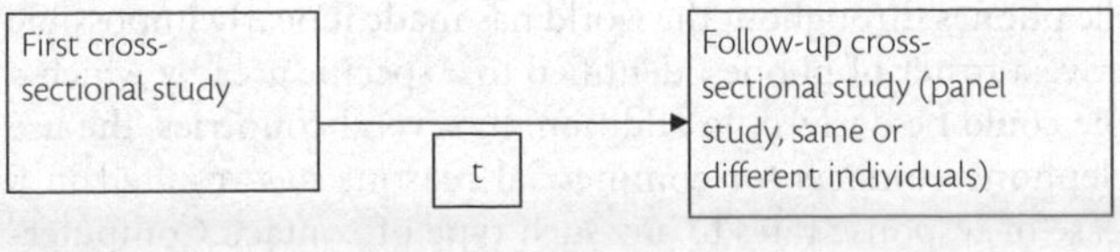

Fig. 6.3.3 Basic design of one-time or repeated cross-sectional studies.

The findings from ISAAC III indicate that international differences in asthma symptom prevalence have reduced, with decreases in prevalence in English-speaking countries and Western Europe, and increases in prevalence in regions where prevalence was previously low (Fig. 6.3.4). Although there was little change in the overall prevalence of current wheezing, the percentage of children reported to have had asthma increased significantly, possibly reflecting greater awareness of this condition and/or changes in diagnostic practices. The increases in asthma symptom prevalence in Africa, Latin America, and parts of Asia indicate that the global burden of asthma is continuing to rise, but the global prevalence differences are diminishing (Pearce *et al.* 2007).

Panel studies may also evaluate the same individuals before and after an intervention or an exposure. These types of studies have been extensively used in occupational and environmental epidemiology to evaluate changes in symptoms or physiological parameters following an intervention in a workplace or in the general environment, such as air pollution. An example is a study that examined the effects of short-term exposure to diesel traffic in 60 adults with asthma (McCreanor *et al.* 2007). Each participant walked for two hours along Oxford Street in London, and on a separate occasion, through Hyde Park. Physiological and immunologic measurements were performed after each occasion. It was found that walking for two hours on Oxford Street induced consistent reductions of up to 6.1 per cent in the forced expiratory volume in 1 s (FEV1) and up to 5.4 per cent in the forced vital capacity (FVC), which were significantly larger than the reductions in FEV1 and FVC after exposure in Hyde Park. Similar changes were also observed for markers of inflammation in the lungs.

Panel studies, particularly when examining the same individuals, could be regarded as prospective studies, and frequently this distinction between study designs is blurred. The study on Oxford Street is a cross-over study that includes aspects of both a prospective experimental design and a cross-sectional study. The main difference of cross-sectional panel studies with prospective designs is that panel studies examine the prevalence of a disease or a physiologic parameter rather than incidence.

Sampling and response rates

Cross-sectional studies aiming to identify the prevalence of a specific factor in a community should select a representative sample of that community. The same is, in principle, desirable in cohort and case–control studies, but in these studies the main issue is internal validity rather than external validity (generalizability). In cohort studies, the most important issue concerning subject selection and validity of results is the completeness of follow-up. In case–control studies, the crucial issue concerning selection of subjects is that cases and controls should be selected from the same study base; whether cases are representative of the general population is, by contrast, not crucial for the internal validity of a case–control study.

In a cross-sectional study, however, representative sampling is the only procedure that allows selection of subjects form a population that can be used as the basis of generalization. A sampling frame should be identified that allows identification of any subject in a population who could be included in a sample. Different methods can then be applied to select the subjects. Sampling error estimation has been exhaustively addressed in statistics. This depends on the number of subjects included in a study and can be estimated. Non-sampling error refers to bias, and may be of considerably

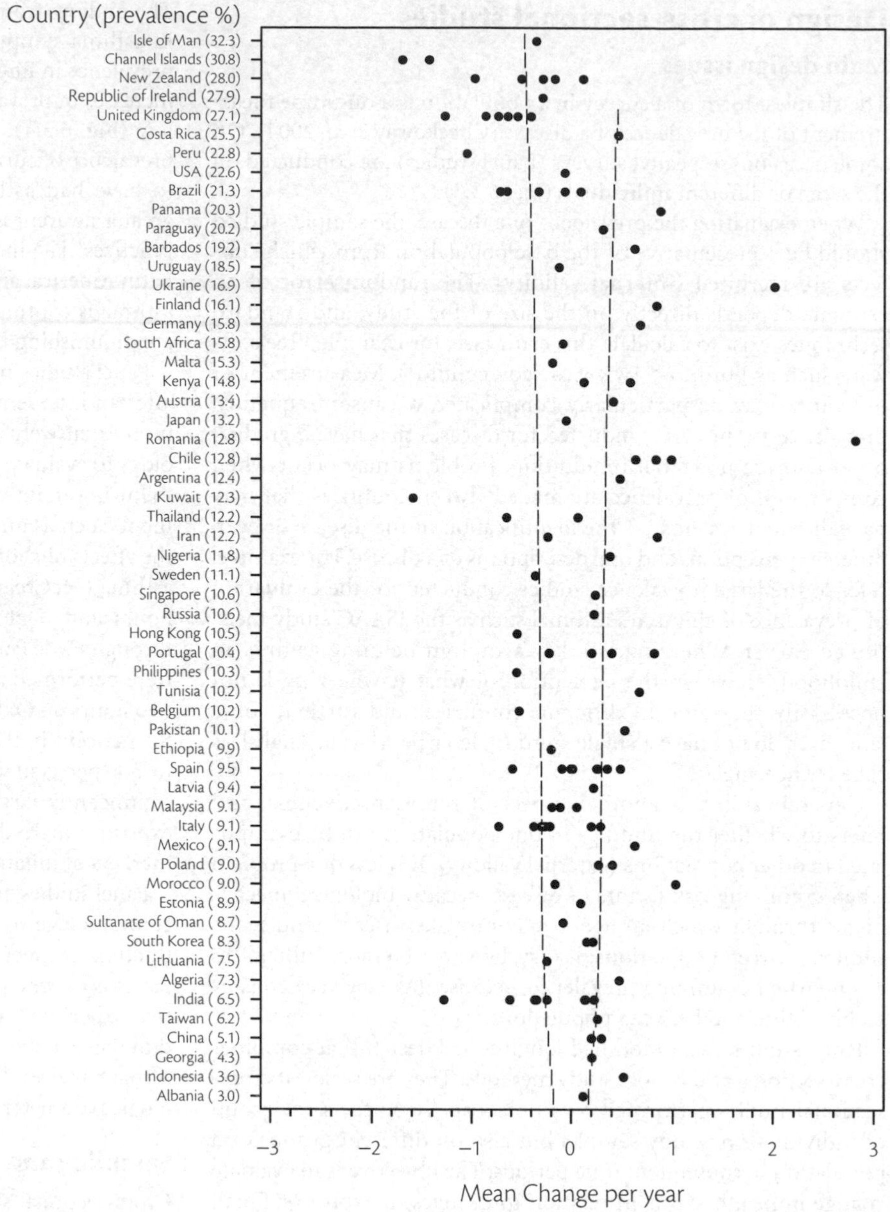

Fig. 6.3.4 Ranking plot showing the change per year in prevalence of current wheeze (wheeze in the past 12 months) in children aged 13–14 years for each centre by country; the ISAAC III. (*Source*: Pearce N., Ait-Khaled N., Beasley R. *et al.* Worldwide trends in the prevalence of asthma symptoms: phase III of the International Study of Asthma and Allergies in Childhood [ISAAC]. *Thorax* 2007;**62**:758–66. With permission of BMJ Publishing Group.)

greater importance than sampling error. Enlarging the sample does not reduce non-sampling error. Non-response may be non-random, and may therefore be related to factors of interest for a study such as education, ethnicity, or obesity.

Response rates and dealing with non-response

There is a general perception, not only among epidemiologists, that it is becoming increasingly difficult in many industrialized countries to achieve high response rates in surveys (Hartge 2006). In an evaluation of 355 original epidemiological papers published in ten high-impact journals, it was found that average participation in epidemiological studies has fallen in the last 30 years, and this has particularly affected controls in population-based studies (Morton *et al.* 2006). At least some information regarding participation was provided in 59 per cent of the cross-sectional studies, 44 per cent of the case–control studies, and 32 per cent of the cohort studies. In 51 of the 86 cross-sectional studies that reported response rates, the mean participation was 74 per cent, and ranged from 28 per cent to 100 per cent. In recent years, response rates of about 50 per cent among population controls are not uncommon. Participation in cross-sectional studies decreased by approximately 1 per cent per year from 1970 to 2003 (Morton *et al.* 2006).

The use of telephones as a means for defining a sampling frame has been rapidly decreasing. The main assumption for the use of random digit dialling (RDD) was that there would be one working residential phone number per household; this assumption is no longer valid because of rapid changes in telecommunications, particularly the use of mobile phones. The rapid increase in the use of mobile phones throughout the world has made it nearly impossible to derive a roster of phones identified to a specific area by which a sample could be derived. In addition, in several countries, the use of telephone contacts for commercial reasons has resulted in a decrease of response rates to any such type of contact. Computer-assisted telephone interviews are, however, an equally valid and efficient means of collecting information from subjects who have been contacted and have agreed to participate.

Studies collecting biological samples

In recent years, an increasing proportion of epidemiological studies collect biological samples, following the advances in molecular and genetic techniques and their application in large-scale studies. In the review of 355 studies mentioned earlier, very high participation rates (above 90 per cent) were identified in cohort and cross-sectional studies collecting biospecimens; however, only about a third of the studies reporting collection of biospecimens also reported response rates for the biological samples. A total of 134 of the 355 (38 per cent) articles reported collection of biologic specimens to measure exposure or disease, and the proportion of cohort and case–control studies that collected biologic specimens increased over time, while that of cross-sectional studies remained fairly constant (Morton *et al.* 2006). Large cross-sectional studies such as the NHANES regularly collect biological samples, and the inclusion of collection of biospecimens does not appear to influence the representativeness of the sample.

An increasing number of studies are collecting saliva or other biospecimens by mail. Several studies that have collected saliva samples by mail have obtained response rates that are not very different from those observed for paper-and-pencil questionnaires. In a study of 2994 subjects at Geneva University, Switzerland, the response rate for subjects requested to provide a mail questionnaire and saliva was 52 per cent, while for those requested to complete only the mail questionnaire was 63 per cent; using financial incentives increased the response rates by 6–11 per cent (Etter *et al.* 2005). Sociodemographic factors may affect response rates in such type of sampling. Self-collection of saliva was evaluated, concerning both the response and the quality of DNA retrieved, for a random sample of 611 men (ages 53–87 years) in Sweden (Rylander-Rudqvist *et al.* 2006). The response rate was 80 per cent, and varied from 89 per cent for those aged 67–71 years to 71 per cent for those aged 77–87 years. Similar to other studies, the DNA extracted was of high quality, and could be used as an alternative to blood DNA in molecular epidemiologic studies. There is little empirical evidence in several cultures to evaluate general tendencies regarding participation when biospecimens are collected. Whether non-response may differentially affect the analysis of biomarkers is unknown. One study examined a series of genetic data (polymorphisms, haplotypes, and short tandem repeats) from 2955 individuals of three studies and found no evidence of differential results by participation (Bhatti *et al.* 2005). A note of caution, however, has been made against assuming that willingness to participate should not vary with a particular polymorphism or other forms of genetic variation (Hartge 2006).

Improving non-response

The difficulties in achieving high response rates and the potential biases resulting from self-selection make indispensable the understanding of the reasons for non-response and the application of methods for limiting it. Numerous studies have evaluated factors affecting non-response in epidemiological and other types of studies. Most of the factors frequently identified, such as age, sex, education, exposure status, method of recruitment, and type of questionnaire used, may also be culture-specific. This indicates that, in addition to some general guidelines, there is a need to verify main approaches to increase responses in different sociocultural settings, and these may change in different time periods. Nevertheless, some general guidelines can be drawn based on numerous observational and randomized trials.

A comprehensive systematic review of available randomized trials from any relevant discipline (not restricted to medicine or epidemiology) evaluated factors that influence response to postal questionnaires (Edwards *et al.* 2002). Information from 292 randomized controlled trials was reviewed, which included 258 315 participants. A total of 75 strategies that could influence response to postal questionnaires were studied. The review identified questionnaire length, use of monetary incentives (particularly when not conditional on response), appearance of the package, layout of the questionnaire, type of follow-up, and registered delivery as the most influential factors in terms of participation rates. Figure 6.3.5 shows effect

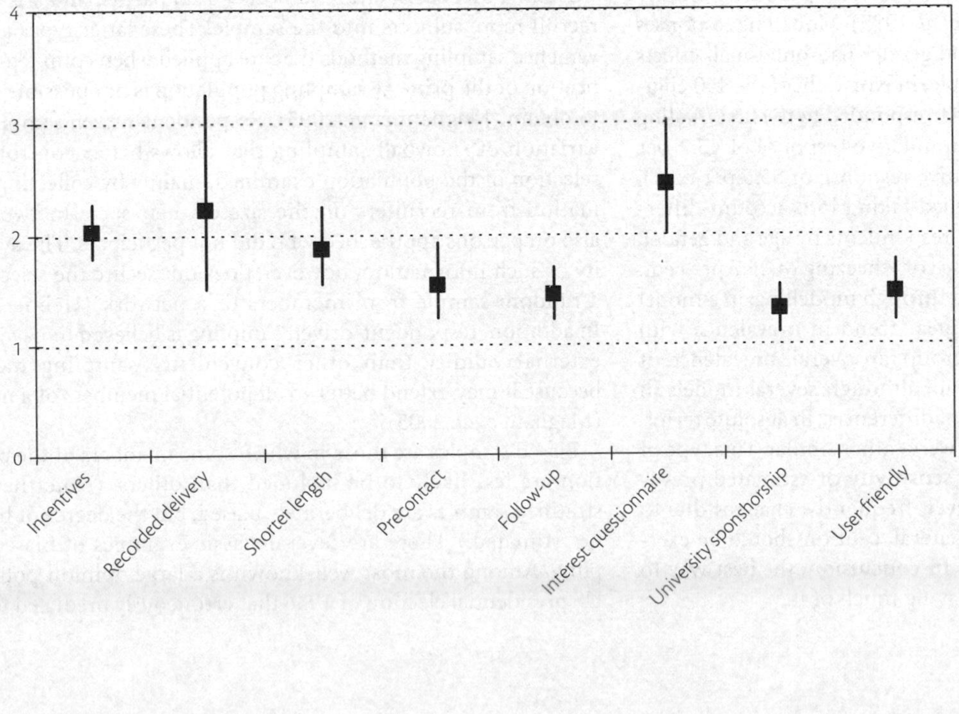

Fig. 6.3.5 Effects on questionnaire response (odds ratios and 95 per cent confidence intervals) of eight strategies where combined trials included over 1000 participants. (Adapted from Edwards P., Roberts I., Clarke M. *et al.* Increasing response rates to postal questionnaires: systematic review. *British Medical Journal* 2002;**324**:1183. With permission of BMJ Publishing Group.)

estimates for the most influential factors. Contacting participants before sending questionnaires increased response, as did follow-up contact. Questionnaires designed to be of more interest to participants were more likely to be returned, whereas those containing sensitive questions were less likely to be returned. Questionnaires originating from universities were more likely to be returned than those from other sources, such as commercial organizations. Overall, response to postal questionnaires can be improved by following strategies shown to be effective in other research.

Adjusting for non-response

The most important measure to deal with potential biases from non-response is to minimize, as much as possible, the number of non-responders. As already discussed, this is done by selecting adequate means of contact and through repeated contact with subjects. Several approaches have been described to evaluate and adjust estimates of prevalence, taking into account non-response.

An evaluation of the basic characteristics of non-responders is important and may offer clues concerning the representativeness of the sample. Such characteristics may be derived from information about the target population of other surveys; for example, the percentage of smokers. They can also be derived from a subsample of non-responders followed up intensively. Estimates of prevalence can then be weighed, using the data on respondents, but taking into account information on variables known for responders and non-responders, such as age, sex, residence, etc.

A typical procedure in prevalence surveys is to make repeated contact with subjects to increase response rates; the final estimates are derived from the total number of responders. Alternatively, it can be assumed that responders from different mailings or other contact are not representative of the population. Under this assumption, the overall prevalence estimates are modelled, using the prevalence of each mailing. A cumulative response at the time of each mailing can be calculated, taking into account different covariates (e.g. age, sex) of the samples responding in each mailing, and estimates of the prevalence of non-responders derived through extrapolation.

Such modelling was conducted by analysing responses of 13 007 subjects in the three English centres of the European Community Respiratory Health Survey (Chinn *et al.* 1995). Modelling responses to take into account centre, age, and gender had only small effects on estimated prevalence. For example, in Norwich, of the 440 eligible individuals aged 20–24 years, 141 responded to the first mailing (32 per cent), 58 to the second (cumulative response of 45.2 per cent), and 45 to the third (cumulative response of 55.5 per cent). Prevalence of wheezing was modelled taking into account differences among respondents and non-respondents by age and gender, and this gave an estimated prevalence of wheezing of 25.7 per cent. This estimate was further examined through modelling; in a model that included a parameter for a linear trend in prevalence with each mailing by age and gender group, an overall prevalence of 23.9 per cent was estimated. Overall, although several models in this study gave statistically significant differences, in absolute terms, the estimates of prevalence derived were rather similar. This type of modelling is useful to explore the sensitivity of estimated prevalence to non-response bias. However, frequently, changes due to such modelling are small, and in general, caution should be exercised when applying such models. In conclusion, the best way to adjust for non-response is by not having much of it.

Item non-response

Apart from the overall response rate, the quality of the respondents' answers deserves attention. The issue of item non-response has been little discussed and is usually not reported. What is usually discussed and reported as 'non-response' refers to non-contact with a selected person or the refusal of this person to participate (unit non-response). Failure of a respondent to answer an individual question or provide a sample (item non-response) should also be considered, and can equally affect the representativeness of specific analyses in a study. In a study of bladder cancer in Spain, the overall response rate to the main questionnaire was 85 per cent; however, the response to specific items was lower. For example, the answers on lifetime consumption of water and water quality in the subjects' residences were available for 1479 of the 2490 subjects (59.39 per cent) (Villanueva *et al.* 2007). An evaluation of differences in sociodemographic characteristics of subjects included or excluded from the water analyses, and also differences in the prevalence of known risk factors such as smoking, indicated that item non-response was not likely to bias results on this occasion. However, exclusion of subjects reduced the statistical power of the study.

Sampling methods

Different types of sampling may be applied in cross-sectional studies, depending on the aims of the study, characteristics of the population to be studied, available background information, and means available in each study.

In a simple random sample, all subsets of the sampling frame have an equal probability of being selected. Most frequently, large surveys use stratified sampling, which involves a first-stage selection of different categories of the population and subsequent selections at random within each stratum. The main reason for performing stratified sampling is efficiency, so as to secure adequate sampling of small population groups and avoid oversampling of larger groups. Several other probabilistic and non-probabilistic types of sampling have been applied—such as *cluster sampling*, in which the unit selected is a group of persons (e.g. a city block) rather than individuals; *snowball sampling*; and *respondent-driven sampling*, wherein a first set of study subjects ('seed participants') is used to recruit more subjects into the sample. These latter types are convenience sampling methods that are applied when complete identification of the primary sampling population is not possible or hard to obtain (Magnani *et al.* 2005). Respondent-driven sampling is a variation of snowball sampling that allows better control of the selection of the population examined, mainly by collecting information from recruiters on the size of their social network and also on persons approached who did not participate. The availability of such information, however, does not secure the selection of a random sample from members of a network (Heimer 2005). In addition, respondent-driven sampling is believed to have higher external validity than other convenience sampling methods, because it may extend better to all potential members of a network (Magnani *et al.* 2005).

Biased samples are those in which some members of the population are less likely to be included than others. (Note that some stratified samples are deliberately biased, but the degree of bias can be estimated.) There are several classic examples of biased sampling. Among the most well-known is a large opinion poll in the US presidential election of 1936 that erroneously predicted that the incumbent president, Franklin Roosevelt, would lose by a large margin. This poll of approximately two-million persons was based on people who were readers of a magazine, supplemented by records of registered automobile owners and telephone users. The error was generated because the sample overrepresented more affluent people who were less likely to vote for the Democratic candidate.

Examples of different sampling procedures are as follows: Sampling in a large multipurpose survey (NHANES) in the United States, a large international prevalence survey (ISAAC), and a local survey of a difficult-to-identify population of drug addicts in Spain.

The NHANES applies multistage (four stages) probability sampling to select participants representative of the civilian, non-institutionalized US population. In stage 1, primary sampling units (mostly single counties) are selected. In the second stage, these units are divided into segments (generally city blocks) and sample segments are selected, taking into account size. In stage 3, households within each segment are listed, and a sample is randomly drawn. In the final stage, individuals are randomly chosen from a list of all persons residing in the selected households within the designated age–gender–race strata. The NHANES is designed to sample larger numbers of certain subgroups of particular public health interest, including African Americans, adolescents, etc.

For the ISAAC, a combination of non-random and random methods was used. The areas participating within each country were not selected at random; instead, qualitative criteria and convenience sampling were used. Stratified random sampling was then used within a given geographical area to select school children. All schools in each geographical centre were listed and a random sample was selected. The sampling unit was the school and non-participating schools were replaced. All children in a selected school within the two specified age groups (6–7 years and 13–14 years) were included.

Snowball sampling was applied in a study of heroin users in three cities in Spain (de la Fuente de Hoz *et al.* 2005). This sampling is especially useful when the objective is to reach populations that are inaccessible or hard to find. The participants were 991 young, community-recruited heroin users in Barcelona, Madrid, and Seville. Most subjects were identified by other participants (40 per cent), or by non-participating drug users or ex-users (45 per cent). Because there was no sampling frame to select drug addicts from, non-probabilistic type sampling was used. In each of the three cities, social workers directly enrolled subjects who were drug consumers in different settings (targeted sampling). Selected subjects were then asked to nominate other drug users (snowball sampling), who were encouraged by providing incentives. To increase representativeness, the initial places and ways of capturing subjects were diversified, with an intention to capture different types of drugs users (very young, short-term users, etc).

Web-based research

Web-based research has been expanding in recent years. The Internet has been used in research and clinical settings to enhance contact with participants. Prevalence surveys have traditionally been based on self-administered paper questionnaires and face-to-face or telephone interviews. Internet surveys are said to have advantages compared to face-to-face or telephone interviews, including reduced turn-a-round time and lower expenses. These surveys, similar to computer-assisted personal or telephone interviews, have advantages over paper-and-pencil questionnaires with regard to data management.

The two main issues regarding the validity of Internet surveys are response rates and quality of the data collected. Several studies that focused on specific population groups with high indexes of Internet use have found comparable response rates between Internet-based questionnaires and more traditional approaches (Pealer *et al.* 2001). However, many of these studies reported response rates for persons recruited through the Internet rather than for population-based samples. These results are, therefore, difficult to generalize, although they indicate that in specific populations Internet-based surveys provide high-quality data.

There are few studies comparing population-based data using both the Internet and traditional approaches. Results differ and depend crucially on the level of education and computer literacy in different cultures, age, and sociodemographic groups. Women younger than 67 years and without a history of breast cancer who were referred for mammography at a Danish public hospital were randomized to receive either a paper questionnaire with a prepaid return envelope or the Internet-based (online) version of the same (Kongsved *et al.* 2007). The response rate was 18 per cent for the Internet group, compared with 73 per cent for the paper questionnaire. The quality of the information, however, was better in the Internet version, with 98 per cent having no missing data, compared with 63 per cent completing the paper questionnaire. An interesting aspect of this study was that after sending a reminder and with the possibility to use the alternative questionnaire form (i.e. paper questionnaire for the Internet group), the response rate for the Internet group became comparable with that of the group assigned the paper questionnaire. In the Millennium Cohort Study (Smith *et al.* 2007) of military personnel in the United States, a similar proportion of the approximately 70 000 respondents chose to reply via the Internet. Web responders were more likely to be male, younger, obese, smoke more cigarettes, have higher education, and work in technical occupations; they were less likely to be problem alcoholics and to report occupational exposures.

On the basis of existing evidence, it appears that Internet-based surveys may provide high response rates in select populations. For most general populations, however, Internet-based surveys do not yet seem to provide adequate response rates, and this may lead to selected sampling. Several studies indicate that these surveys may be efficiently combined with traditional techniques to save resources and perhaps provide more complete answers. Clearly, more research is needed in the future on population-based surveys to evaluate changes in response to Internet-based research.

Bias in cross-sectional studies

Cross-sectional studies may suffer from the same potential biases as other epidemiologic designs: Misclassification, selection bias, and confounders. Issues of particular concern for cross-sectional studies are the potential biases from the mixing of incident and prevalent cases, the frequent lack of information on past exposures, and consequently, the time sequence of events, and the lack of representativeness in studies evaluating the prevalence of disease or other health-related variables. Because of these difficulties, it has been recommended that cross-sectional studies examining the risk factors of disease are appropriate for diseases that produce little disability, and are also appropriate for the pre-symptomatic phases of more serious disorders (Coggon *et al.* 1997).

Incidence–prevalence bias

Incidence–prevalence bias (Neyman's bias; also, length-bias) is a type of selection bias due to the mix of incident and prevalent cases in cross-sectional studies. This bias refers specifically to the selection of a case group that is not representative of cases in the community. Figure 6.3.6 shows the hypothetical time of occurrence of disease and the duration of disease. The lines on these graphs represent the duration of disease, with the left endpoint representing the date that the disease was first diagnosed and the right endpoint representing the date that the patient died. In Fig. 6.3.6a, subjects are ordered by time of initial diagnosis. A cross-sectional study in January 2002 selected those patients who were alive at that time; this would include a disproportionately high percentage of cases with long duration, while those with more aggressive disease, and hence short duration, would have a lower probability of being sampled. The latter is exemplified in Fig. 6.3.6b: Patients with the shortest survival times appear at the bottom of the graph and those with the longest survival times appear at the top. Rarely do patients with short survival times appear among the prevalent cases. A bias would occur if survivors of a condition studied are atypical with respect to the exposure evaluated. If the exposure examined is not directly or indirectly related to survival, inclusion of prevalent cases would not bias any association. In addition, as noted by Hill *et al.* (2003), for diseases with extremely low case fatality (e.g. rheumatoid arthritis), studies based on prevalent cases are not subject to Neyman's bias, even if the risk factor under study produces increased mortality from other causes.

The association of smoking with Alzheimer's disease has been discussed as a potential outcome of incidence–prevalence bias. Several cross-sectional studies have suggested that smoking exerts a protective effect against Alzheimer's disease; however, evidence from a few cohort studies is controversial. A cross-sectional study that included a prospective component suggested that part of the protective effect could be attributed to Neyman's bias, specifically because smokers with dementia would have worse survival than smokers without dementia. The study was a population-based cohort of 668 people aged 75–101 years in Sweden (Wang *et al.* 1999). Smoking was negatively associated with prevalent Alzheimer's disease (adjusted odds ratio = 0.6, 95 per cent CI 0.4–1.1). Over the three-year follow-up (1989–92), the hazard ratios of incident Alzheimer's disease due to smoking was 1.1 (95 per cent CI 0.5–2.4). In addition, mortality in the follow-up was greater for smokers among the demented (hazard ratio = 3.4) than non-demented subjects (hazard ratio = 0.8). The authors concluded that smoking does not protect against Alzheimer's disease, and that the cross-sectional association might be due to differential mortality.

When examining prevalent cases, an additional problem may occur if the diseased persons modify their exposure; treatment of diabetes mellitus type 1 with insulin is an example. Before insulin was available, patients had a very poor survival of less than one year. At that time, a cross-sectional study simply would not identify many diabetics. With insulin treatment, survival has spectacularly increased to more than 20 years. A cross-sectional study evaluating diabetes and use of insulin would therefore find an association, simply because diabetics take insulin whereas non-diabetics do not. This bias has also been described as a type of Neyman's bias (incidence–prevalence bias), but in reality is a case of reverse causation provoked by misclassification due to an erroneous evaluation of the timing of exposure.

Other types of selection bias and misclassification

The study by Morris and Dale (1955) on the incidence and prevalence of cardiovascular disease among London bus drivers and conductors is an example of selection bias in a cross-sectional study. Bus drivers in London were shown to have very different lipid profiles, blood pressure patterns, and eventually, cardiovascular disease risk compared with bus conductors. Bus drivers were less physically active on the job than conductors, but could the difference in cardiovascular disease risk be ascribed to physical activity? One alternative explanation was that some characteristic, such as obesity, could have led to self-selection in a job that was more (bus conductors) or less active (bus drivers). The studies of London busmen were eventually the first to convincingly demonstrate the importance of physical activity for health.

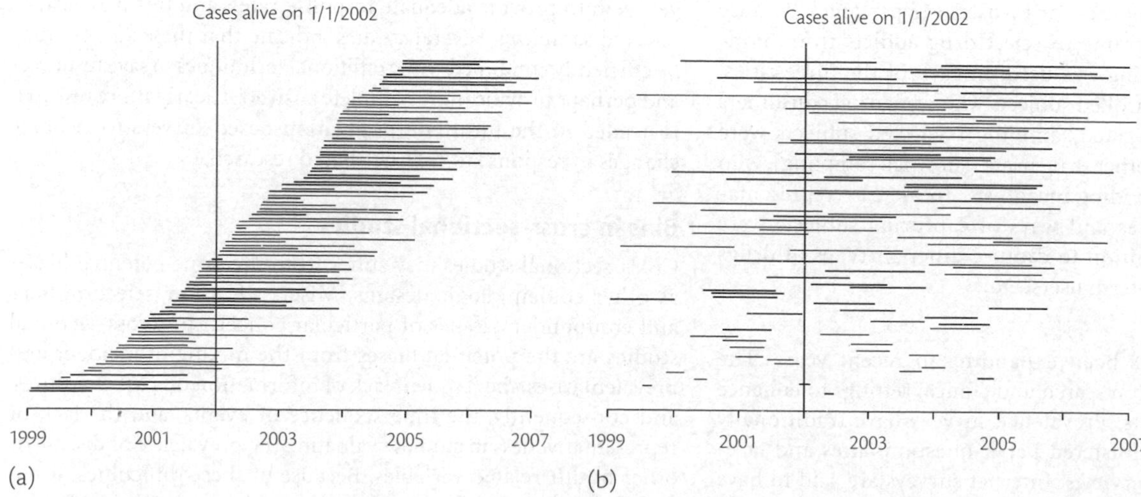

Fig. 6.3.6 Incidence–prevalence bias in cross-sectional studies. (Adapted from Simon S. Neyman bias. [Online]. Children's Mercy Hospitals and Clinics; 2004. Available from: http://www.childrens-mercy.org/stats/weblog2004/NeymanBias.asp)

The healthy worker effect may lead to an underestimation of an association in case–control studies that evaluate occupation and disease at a specific point in time (Checkoway *et al.* 2004). This happens because workers with health problems at work are more likely to change jobs than subjects without symptoms. In this case, the selection is not dropping out of the job, contrary to what was a potential problem in busmen. Any cross-sectional evaluation will therefore not capture cases that have occurred in the past, and will over-represent healthy individuals who have stayed on the job. An example of this was observed in a cross-sectional study on occupational asthma in Spain (Kogevinas *et al.* 1996). Subjects were asked about their current occupation and about current respiratory symptoms. The prevalence odds ratio (POR) for asthma in subjects employed in high-risk occupations was 1.4 (95 per cent CI of 0.6–3.3). Subjects were also asked whether they had suffered respiratory symptoms in the past, and if so, the type of job they were employed in: The POR for employment in a high-risk occupation at the time of respiratory problems was 2.8 (95 per cent CI 1.5–5.2), indicating that the cross-sectional analysis failed to identify health risks, because of the selective migration of subjects with respiratory symptoms out of high-risk jobs.

This type of bias is less of a problem if current exposure is a reliable surrogate for past exposure and is not a problem for non-changeable characteristics such as race, gender, and genetic variability. Case–control or cross-sectional studies are currently the most widely applied designs for evaluating the effects of genetic susceptibility, such as the effects of single nucleotide polymorphisms (SNPs) on disease risk.

Social desirability bias has long been recognized, and falls within the wider category of misclassification (Armstrong *et al.* 1994). Requesting information on behaviours that are regarded as sensitive by respondents may lead to refusal to participate or to a tendency to over-report behaviours regarded as socially desirable (or under-report what is regarded as socially undesirable). This has become particularly evident in recent years in large surveys that inquire into health-related behaviours such as sexual activity and drug use.

Extensive research has shown that self-administered questionnaires obtain more valid information on socially sensitive issues than do face-to-face interviews (Armstrong *et al.* 1994; Schuman & Presser 1981). In recent years, the use of computers in soliciting information has considerably expanded. In addition to computer-assisted personal interviews (CAPIs), the technique of audio computer-assisted self-interviewing (ACASI) has been proposed as an efficient method to enhance validity when evaluating behaviours than could be perceived as socially undesirable (Turner *et al.* 1998). In the ACASI (also known as audio-CASI), respondents hear the questions through headphones and enter their responses directly into a computer. An experimental comparison of sexual behaviours in adolescent males, using either a paper-and-pencil self-administered questionnaire or ACASI, identified an almost fourfold increase in the number of respondents reporting male–male sexual contact in the ACASI (5.5 per cent), compared with 1.5 per cent in the paper-and-pencil questionnaire (Turner *et al.* 1998). Among the reported advantages of ACASI is that it reduces the literacy requirements of respondents compared to other forms of self-administered questionnaires (paper and pencil or computer-assisted). The ACASI technique has been tested in multiple settings, and has generally been shown to provide higher estimates of the prevalence of socially undesirable behaviours than face-to-face interviews (Ghanem *et al.* 2005); results are less consistent when comparing it with self-administered questionnaires (Morrison-Beedy *et al.* 2006). Different computer-assisted methods (audio or text) may have little impact on reported socially undesirable behaviours, and the choice of one method over another should be based on an evaluation of wider considerations of the study settings.

Analysis of cross-sectional studies

Prevalence is the ratio of the number of cases of a disease in a population at a particular time to the size of the population at that time.

$$\text{Prevalence} = \frac{\text{Number of existing cases of disease}}{\text{Total population at that point in time}}$$

Point prevalence is estimated at one point in time, whereas period prevalence denotes the number of cases in a time interval (e.g. one year).

For example, in a given state in June 2007, there were 14 000 women diagnosed with breast cancer. The total female population in the same period was 1 558 000. So, the prevalence of breast cancer in this population on a specific date in this period would be 14 000/1 558 000, which equals 0.009 (or 0.9 per cent). This means that nearly 1 per cent of the women in June 2007 had breast cancer, a figure that corresponds to the actual prevalence of this disease in several industrialized countries. This estimate does not show how many new cases of breast cancer occurred each year or when the disease was diagnosed. In these types of estimates, it is usually assumed that none of the persons diagnosed with a chronic disease are entirely cured, although such calculations could be incorporated in the estimation of prevalence.

Strictly speaking, prevalence is a proportion, although it is sometimes indicated erroneously as a rate. Thus, the term *prevalence rate* should be regarded theoretically as an impossible concept (Elandt-Johnson 1975).

Prevalence reflects determinants of incidence as well as survival (duration of a disease). The prevalence of bladder cancer in the United States in January 2004 (377 523 persons alive with a history of bladder cancer) was higher than that of lung cancer (174 880 persons), even though the incidence of lung cancer (81.2 per 100) is clearly higher than that of bladder cancer (37.3/100). This reflects the much better prognosis for bladder cancer (5-year relative survival rate of 79.5 per cent) compared with the 15 per cent for lung cancer.)

Figure 6.3.7 shows the flow of subjects in and out of the pool of disease (Pearce 2004). In its simplest expression, the prevalence odds is equal to incidence rate times the duration of the disease:

$$\frac{P}{1-P} = I \times D$$

where P is prevalence, I is incidence, and D is duration (survival). This, however, is only true under stable conditions; that is, unchanging rates and population structure, which are unlikely on most occasions in true populations. If two populations are compared,

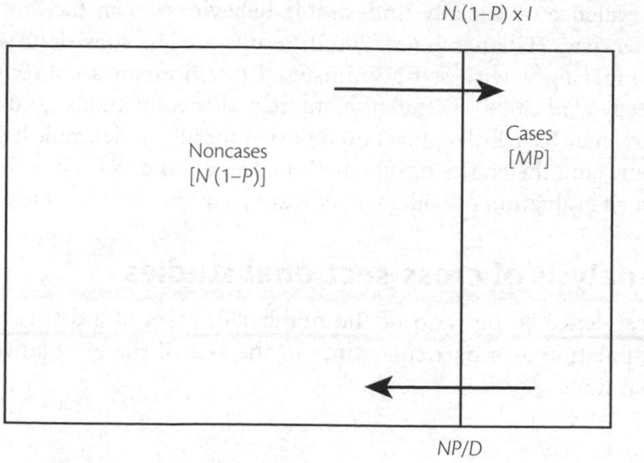

Fig. 6.3.7 The relationship between prevalence and incidence in a steady-state population. D, duration; I, incidence; N, population; P, prevalence. (From Pearce N. Effect measures in prevalence studies. *Environmental Health Perspectives* 2004;**112**:1047-50. With permission of Environmental Health Perspectives.)

and say 1 indicates the exposed and 0 the unexposed, the prevalence odds ratio (POR) can be calculated as

$$POR = \frac{P_1/(1-P_1)}{P_0/(1-P_0)} = \frac{I_1 D_1}{I_0 D_0}$$

If the duration of the disease is expected to be equal in the exposed and unexposed, the POR is equal to the incidence rate ratio (under steady conditions in the population). Under the same conditions, the ratio of prevalence (compared to the ratio of prevalence odds) will only estimate the incidence rate ratio if the prevalence of the disease is low. If so, 1−P would be roughly equal to 1.

There has been some controversy as to whether cross-sectional studies should calculate POR or prevalence ratios (PR) (Pearce 2004; Thomson *et al.* 1998). The choice of one or the other depends essentially on the purposes of the research, with POR having advantages compared to PR if aetiological research is conducted. However, the prevalence ratio, or probably, the absolute difference in prevalence may be preferred if two populations are compared regarding the prevalence of disease.

Statistical analysis in cross-sectional studies is frequently limited to descriptive statistics through the use of standard statistical measures for proportions or a comparison of distributions (e.g. blood pressure) between an exposed and an unexposed group. Standard statistical tests comparing means of a distribution, such as Student's *t*-test, can be used. For the evaluation of multiple variables, standard techniques such as multiple linear regression can be used. For dichotomous outcomes, POR is the most common effect measure estimated in cross-sectional studies comparing groups, with the application of logistic regression or equivalent techniques. A wide range of other analytical regression techniques is readily available for the modelling of prevalence ratios (Thomson *et al.* 1998; Barros & Hirakata 2003). Selection of the effect measure (i.e. POR versus PR) as the preferred effect measure should, therefore, not depend on the availability of statistical tools (Pearce 2004), rather on the objectives of the research.

Summary

Cross-sectional studies are among the most commonly applied designs. The principal characteristic of these studies is that they provide information on the prevalence of disease. In many cross-sectional studies, information on past exposures is not collected, but this should not be regarded as a characteristic defining these studies. On many occasions, cross-sectional studies tend to follow a hybrid design, an analysis incorporating aspects of cohort and case–control studies. Repeated cross-sectional studies (panel studies) offer the possibility of assessing short- and long-term physiologic changes. Large cross-sectional studies are conducted in several countries to provide background information on health-related variables, including health-service use. In recent years, these surveys have also incorporated collection of biospecimens. In aetiological research, cross-sectional studies are suitable epidemiological means for studying non-fatal diseases and effects on physiologic variables that do not have a clear time of onset. However, the design of these studies makes them less appropriate than other study designs for investigating causal associations. Among the major limitations of cross-sectional studies are the inclusion of prevalent rather than incident cases and the frequent lack of information on past exposures and the time sequence of events. The representativeness of the sample is crucial when evaluating prevalence of a disease, and several policies have been developed to increase participation in studies, reduce non-response, and improve the quality of the recorded information.

References

Arif A.A., Delclos G.L., Whitehead L.W. *et al.* Occupational exposures associated with work-related asthma and work-related wheezing among U.S. workers. *American Journal of Industrial Medicine* 2003;**44**:368–76.

Armstrong B.K., White E., and Saracci R. *Principles of exposure measurement in epidemiology*. New York (NY): Oxford University Press; 1994.

Asher M.I., Keil U., Anderson H.R. *et al.* International Study of Asthma and Allergies in Childhood (ISAAC): rationale and methods. *European Respiratory Journal* 1995;**8**:483–91.

Barros A.J. and Hirakata V.N. Alternatives for logistic regression in cross-sectional studies: An empirical comparison of models that directly estimate the prevalence ratio. *BMC Medical Research Methodology* 2003;**3**:21.

Bhatti P., Sigurdson A.J., Wang S.S. *et al.* Genetic variation and willingness to participate in epidemiologic research: data from three studies. *Cancer Epidemiology, Biomarkers, and Prevention* 2005;**14**:2449–53.

Burney P.G., Luczynska C., Chinn S. *et al.* The European Community Respiratory Health Survey. *European Respiratory Journal* 1994;**7**:954–60.

Checkoway H., Pearce N., Kriebel D. *Research methods in occupational epidemiology*. New York (NY): Oxford University Press; 2004.

Chinn S., Zanolin E., Lai E. *et al.* Adjustment of reported prevalence of respiratory symptoms for non-response in a multicentre health survey. *International Journal of Epidemiology* 1995;**24**:603–11.

Coggon D., Rose G., and Barker D.J.P. *Epidemiology for the unitiated*. London: BMJ Publishing Group; 1997.

de la Fuente de Hoz L., Brugal Puig M.T., Ballesta Gomez R. *et al.* Cohort study methodology of the ITINERE Project on heroin users in three Spanish cities and main characteristics of the participants. *Revista Espanola de Salud Publica* 2005;**79**:475–91.

Edwards P., Roberts I., Clarke M. *et al.* Increasing response rates to postal questionnaires: systematic review. *British Medical Journal* 2002;**324**:1183.

Elandt-Johnson R.C. Definition of rates: some remarks on their use and misuse. *American Journal of Epidemiology* 1975;**102**:267–71.

Etter J.F., Neidhart E., Bertrand S. *et al.* Collecting saliva by mail for genetic and cotinine analyses in participants recruited through the Internet. *European Journal of Epidemiology* 2005;**20**:833–8.

Ghanem K.G., Hutton H.E., Zenilman J.M. *et al.* Audio computer-assisted self-interview and face-to-face interview modes in assessing response bias among STD clinic patients. *Sexually Transmitted Infections* 2005;**81**:421–5.

Hartge P. Participation in population studies. *Epidemiology* 2006;**17**:252–4.

Heimer R. Critical issues and further questions about respondent-driven sampling: comment on Ramirez-Valles *et al.* 2005. AIDS and Behavior 2005;**9**:403–8.

Hill G., Connelly J., Hebert R. *et al.* Neyman's bias revisited. *Journal of Clinical Epidemiology* 2003;**56**:293–6.

Janson C., Anto J., Burney P. *et al.* The European Community Respiratory Health Survey: what are the main results so far? European Community Respiratory Health Survey II. *European Respiratory Journal* 2001;**18**: 598–611.

Kogevinas M., Anto J.M., Soriano J.B. *et al.* The risk of asthma attributable to occupational exposures: a population-based study in Spain. Spanish Group of the European Asthma Study. *American Journal of Respiratory and Critical Care Medicine* 1996;**154**:137–43.

Kogevinas M., Anto J.M., Sunyer J. *et al.* Occupational asthma in Europe and other industrialised areas: a population-based study. European Community Respiratory Health Survey Study Group. Lancet 1999;**353**:1750–4.

Kongsved S.M., Basnov M., Holm-Christensen K. *et al.* Response rate and completeness of questionnaires: a randomized study of Internet versus paper-and-pencil versions. *Journal of Medical Internet Research* 2007;**9**;e25.

Last J.M., Spashoff R.A., Harris S.G. *A Dictionary of Epidemiology*, 4th edition, New York, Oxford University Press.

Magnani R., Sabin K., Saidel T. *et al.* Review of sampling hard-to-reach and hidden populations for HIV surveillance. *AIDS* 2005;**19** Suppl **2**: S67–72.

McCreanor J., Cullinan P., Nieuwenhuijsen M.J. *et al.* Respiratory effects of exposure to diesel traffic in persons with asthma. *New England Journal of Medicine* 2007;**357**:2348–58.

Morris J.N. and Dale R.A. Epidemiology of coronary atherosclerosis. *Proceedings of the Royal Society of Medicine* 1955;**48**:667–72.

Morrison-Beedy D., Carey M.P., and Tu T. Accuracy of audio computer-assisted self-interviewing (ACASI) and self-administered questionnaires for the assessment of sexual behavior. *AIDS and Behavior* 2006;**10**:541–52.

Morton L.M., Cahill J., and Hartge P. Reporting participation in epidemiologic studies: a survey of practice. American Journal of Epidemiology 2006;**163**:197–203.

National Cancer Institute. SEER Cancer Stat Fact Sheets. [Online]. Available from: http://seer.cancer.gov/statfacts/

Pealer L.N., Weiler R.M., Pigg R.M., Jr. *et al.* The feasibility of a Web-based surveillance system to collect health risk behavior data from college students. *Health Education and Behavior* 2001;**28**:547–59.

Pearce N., Ait-Khaled N., Beasley R. *et al.* Worldwide trends in the prevalence of asthma symptoms: phase III of the International Study of Asthma and Allergies in Childhood (ISAAC). *Thorax* 2007;**62**:758–66.

Pearce N. Effect measures in prevalence studies. Environmental Health Perspectives 2004;**112**:1047–50.

Rylander-Rudqvist T., Hakansson N., Tybring G. *et al.* Quality and quantity of saliva DNA obtained from the self-administrated oragene method—a pilot study on the cohort of Swedish men. *Cancer Epidemiology, Biomarkers, and Prevention* 2006;**15**:1742–5.

Schuman H. and Presser S. Questions and answers in attitude surveys: experiments on question form, wording, and context. San Diego(CA): Academic Press; 1981.

Simon S. Neyman bias. [Online]. Children's Mercy Hospitals and Clinics; 2004. Available from: http://www.childrens-mercy.org/stats/weblog2004/NeymanBias.asp

Smith B., Smith T.C., Gray G.C. *et al.* When epidemiology meets the Internet: Web-based surveys in the Millennium Cohort Study. *American Journal of Epidemiology* 2007;**166**:1345–54.

The International Study of Asthma and Allergies in Childhood (ISAAC) Steering Committee. Worldwide variation in prevalence of symptoms of asthma, allergic rhinoconjunctivitis, and atopic eczema. *Lancet* 1998;**351**:1225–32.

Thomson M.L., Myers J.E., Kriebel D. Prevalence odds ratio or prevalence ratio in the analysis of cross-sectional data: what is to be done? *Occupational and Environmental Medicine* 1998;55:272–7.

Turner C.F., Ku L., Rogers S.M. *et al.* Adolescent sexual behavior, drug use and violence: increased reporting with computer survey technology. *Science* 1998;**280**:867–73.

Villanueva C.M., Cantor K.P., Grimalt J.O. *et al.* Bladder cancer and exposure to water disinfection by-products through ingestion, bathing, showering, and swimming in pools. *Am J Epidemiol* 2007;**165**:148–56.

Wang H.X., Fratiglioni L., Frisoni G.B. *et al.* Smoking and the occurrence of Alzheimer's disease: cross-sectional and longitudinal data in a population-based study. *American Journal of Epidemiology* 1999;**149**:640–4.

6.4

Principles of outbreak investigation

Kumnuan Ungchusak and Sopon Iamsirithaworn

Introduction

Knowledge of medicine and diseases has increased enormously over the last few decades. With the advance of knowledge, public health services in many countries can implement effective prevention programmes, and are able to protect people from many avoidable illnesses and death. However, people around the world still suffer and die from various known and unknown outbreaks of disease. Some outbreaks are old diseases that have re-emerged, some are newly identified or emerging, and some have been deliberately started (Fig. 6.4.1). Outbreaks can occur anywhere, from a very remote area where no health facility exists to nosocomial outbreaks in a very sophisticated hospital where hundreds of health personnel are employed. It is a challenge for the government and public health professionals of all countries to detect and control these outbreaks as early as possible. Outbreak investigations also provide the opportunity to discover new aetiological agents, to understand factors that promote the spread of the diseases, and to identify the weaknesses of existing prevention and health programmes. For these reasons, all public health professionals should have the ability to detect, conduct, or play essential roles in supporting outbreak investigations.

This chapter provides a definition and describes the objectives of outbreak investigation, the methods for planning and conducting an investigation, and what needs to be done after the investigation has been completed. For simplicity, mainly examples of communicable disease investigations have been discussed; however, the concepts and principles can be applied to non-communicable diseases as well.

What is an outbreak?

The terms *outbreak* and *epidemic* can be used interchangeably. However, most people understand the term *outbreak*, which coveys a greater sense of urgency. Some epidemiologists prefer to use the term *epidemic* only in a situation that covers a very wide geographical area and involves large populations. For example, it is possible to use the term 'outbreak of HIV' to describe a sharply increasing HIV prevalence rate among commercial sex workers in a city where the normal rate was low in the previous year. However, the term 'HIV epidemic' can be used when an abnormally high HIV prevalence is found among sex workers in many cities of the country.

In general, *outbreak* is used for a situation when diseases or health events occur at a greater frequency than normally expected within a specified period and place. There is often a misunderstanding that only communicable diseases can cause outbreaks. Non-communicable outbreaks such as mass sociogenic illnesses are sometimes reported as acute outbreaks of unexplained illness, especially in school settings (Centers for Disease Control and Prevention 1990, 1996).

Because the criteria for judging an outbreak can be very subjective, it is useful to define the term in a more measurable manner. The criteria for judging that an outbreak has occurred can be one of the following:

1. The occurrence of a greater number of cases or events than normally occurs in the same place and during the same period as in past years. An example is the detection of influenza outbreaks in the United States. The surveillance data from the 122 sentinel cities provides the seasonal baseline mortality attributed to influenza and pneumonia on a weekly basis, and an influenza outbreak is signalled by a rise of the mortality rates above the epidemic threshold (Fig. 6.4.2). Another example is the epidemic of Kaposi's sarcoma, a manifestation of AIDS, confirmed in New York when almost 30 cases were reported in 1981, whereas only two or three cases had been reported in previous years (Biggar *et al.* 1988).

2. A cluster of cases of the same disease occurs that can be linked to the same exposure. The term *cluster* means an aggregation of two or more cases, which is not necessarily more than expected. For example, three athletes were admitted to hospital with an acute febrile illness, and all of them had participated in a triathlon in Springfield, Illinois (Centers for Disease Control and Prevention 1998a). After receiving this report, the responsible unit started to suspect that an outbreak of febrile illness might be occurring among athletes who participated in the triathlon. The investigation revealed that *Leptospira* was the cause of the illness.

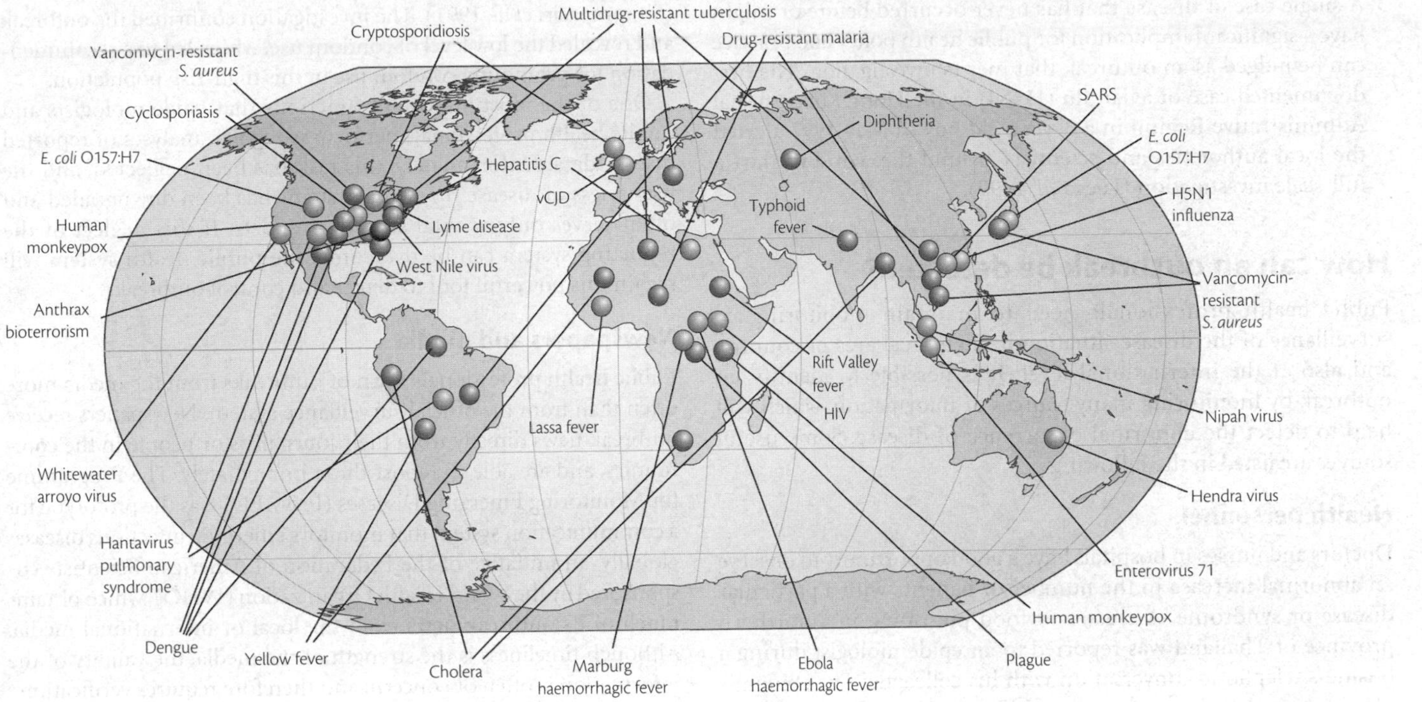

Fig. 6.4.1 Emerging and re-emerging disease worldwide, 1981–2003. (From Morens D.M., Folkers G.K., Fauci A.S. The challenge of emerging and re-emerging infectious diseases. *Nature* 2004;**430**:242–9. With permission of the author.)

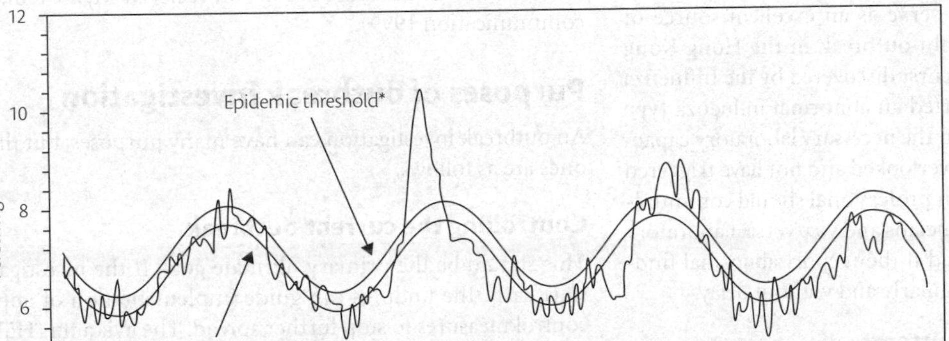

* The epidemic threshold is 1.645 standard deviations above the seasonal baseline.
† The seasonal baseline is projected using a robust regression procedure that applies a periodic regression model to the observed percentage of deaths from P&I during the preceding 5 years.

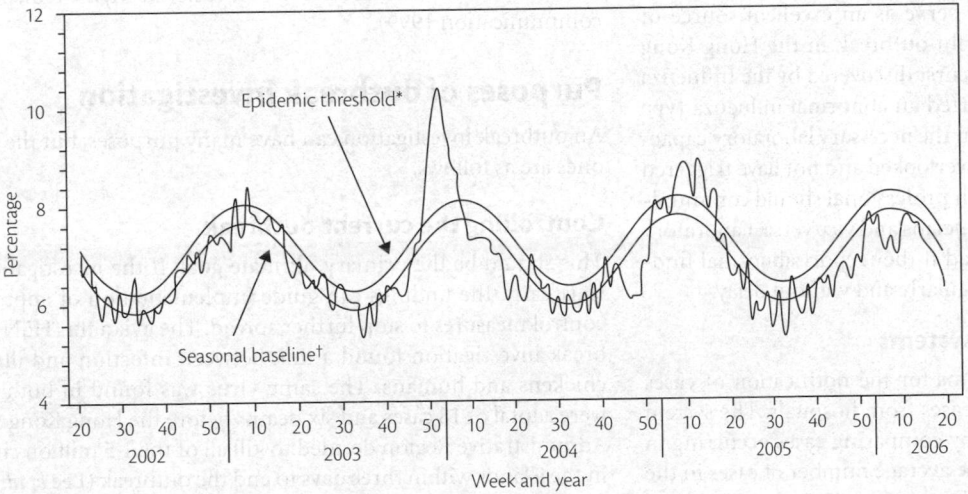

Fig. 6.4.2 Percentage of deaths attributed to pneumonia and influenza reported by the 122 Cities Mortality Reporting System, by week and year—United States, 2002–06. (Blanton L., Brammer L., Wang S. *et al.* Update: influenza activity—United States and worldwide, 2005–06 season, and composition of the 2006–07 influenza vaccine. *Morbidity and Mortality Weekly Report* 2006; **55**[23]:648–53.)

3. A single case of disease that has never occurred before or might have a significant implication for public health policy and practice can be judged as an outbreak that merits investigation. The first documented case of avian flu (H5Nl) in the Hong Kong Special Administrative Region in a 3-year-old boy in May 1997 alerted the local authorities and scientists around the world to start a full-scale investigation (Lee *et al.* 1999).

How can an outbreak be detected?

Public health professionals need to maintain monitoring or surveillance of the disease situation in their local area or country, and also at the international level. It is possible to identify an outbreak by monitoring many sources of information, which will help to detect the abnormal occurrence of disease. Some useful sources are listed in the following.

Health personnel

Doctors and nurses in hospitals have a good opportunity to observe an abnormal increase in the number of patients with a particular disease or syndrome. A cluster of food poisoning in a northern province of Thailand was reported to an epidemiologist during a business telephone conversation with his colleague. The epidemiologist started an investigation and identified the first confirmed outbreak of *Clostridium botulinum* food poisoning associated with home-canned bamboo shoots in the country (Centers for Disease Control and Prevention 1999a). Without this personal contact, the outbreak would not have been investigated. Thus, public health authorities should maintain a cordial relationship with doctors and hospital staff, both in the governmental and private sectors. Conversely, doctors should report all suspected outbreaks to local public health authorities.

Laboratory

Every laboratory or network can serve as an excellent source of outbreak notification. The avian flu outbreak in the Hong Kong Special Administrative Region was first discovered by the Influenza Surveillance Network, which reported an abnormal influenza type A (H5N1) (Lee *et al.* 1999). Without the necessary laboratory capacity, the avian flu might have been overlooked and not have triggered a field investigation. A public health professional should communicate regularly with laboratory technicians and vice versa. Laboratory scientists can prevent further spread if they report abnormal findings to public health authorities regularly and without delay.

Official disease notification systems

Most countries have official systems for the notification of cases and deaths of epidemic-prone diseases from hospitals. The system was designed to detect outbreaks by comparing cases occurring in the current week or month with the average number of cases in the same area during the same period in past years.

For some diseases such as HIV/AIDS, a sentinel surveillance system was designed to monitor and detect abnormal trends in particular sentinel populations and sites. The first HIV sentinel serosurveillance in Thailand, which started in June 1989, detected that the HIV prevalence among commercial sex workers in a popular northern tourist province was 44 per cent. This finding was very alarming, and prompted a field investigation to confirm the high prevalence and to look for risk factors of HIV infection among sex workers (Siraprapasiri *et al.* 1991). The investigation confirmed the outbreak and revealed the low level of condom use, which led to a recommendation for promoting condom use in this high-risk population.

One of the most important functions that epidemiologists and public health professionals perform is regular analyses of reported disease data. Unfortunately, this task has been neglected, and the usefulness of disease reporting systems has been downgraded and often serves only as vital statistics reports. If this neglect of the reporting system can be overcome, the public health system will regain this powerful tool to detect and control outbreaks.

Newspapers and media

Public health professionals learn of outbreaks from the media more often than from the official surveillance system. Newspapers receive outbreak news directly from their journalists or people in the community, and are able to report them immediately. The Programme for Monitoring Emerging Diseases (ProMED) was the prototype for a communication system that monitors emerging infectious diseases globally, an initiative of the Federation of American Scientists co-sponsored by the World Health Organization (WHO), which obtains much of its outbreak news from the local or international media. Although timeliness is the strength of the media, the validity of the information is often of concern, and therefore requires verification.

Village health volunteers

In rural areas where there are no health facilities and communication is limited, village leaders or village health volunteers can often help to recognize an abnormal increase in the numbers of some clinical diseases such as diarrhoea, dysentery, measles, fever, deaths from unknown aetiology, etc. For example, the headman in a village of Kachin state in the Union of Myanmar informed the health authorities that seven villagers had died from febrile illness. This information triggered a field investigation, which revealed that malaria was the cause of the outbreak (Dr Myint Win, personal communication 1999).

Purposes of outbreak investigation

An outbreak investigation can have many purposes, but the critical ones are as follows.

Controlling the current outbreak

This should be the primary ultimate goal. If the investigation can start early, the findings can guide implementation of appropriate control measures to stop further spread. The avian flu (H5N1) outbreak investigation found a link between infection and illness in chickens and humans: The same virus was found in both. There were a total of 18 cases and six deaths before the Hong Kong Special Administrative Region decided to kill all of the 1.5 million chickens in the islands within three days to end the outbreak (Lee *et al.* 1999). There has been no human case in Hong Kong since then. However, the outbreak of H5N1 in poultry has re-emerged in several countries in Asia and other continents, with increasing numbers of human cases since 2003. Up to 16 December 2008, there were 391 human cases with 247 deaths reported in 15 countries. To achieve the goal of controlling the current outbreak, it is necessary to eliminate the delay in detecting the outbreak, to start the investigation as soon as possible, and to immediately implement appropriate preventive measures indicated by the investigation results.

Prevention of future outbreaks

Not all investigations start at the beginning or before the peak of the outbreak. The findings or lessons learned from the investigation may be too late to help fully control the current outbreak, but they can still contribute to the prevention of future outbreaks. Through sound investigations, the weaknesses of the prevention programmes can be identified. If recommendations are taken seriously, the chance of recurrence of the same outbreak or other diseases that share common risk factors can be reduced.

Research to provide knowledge of the disease

Information about new diseases and their natural history, clinical spectrums, incubation periods, etc. can often be best learned during an outbreak investigation. The outbreak of encephalitis in Malaysia, which continued until the end of April 1999 and resulted in 257 cases and 100 deaths, prompted an international outbreak investigation, resulting in the discovery of a new Nipah virus (Centers for Disease Control and Prevention 1999b; 1999c). The mode of transmission was close contact with infected pigs through blood and secretions.

Evaluation of the effectiveness of prevention programmes

Investigation of an outbreak of disease, which is the target of a public health programme, may reveal weaknesses in that programme. Investigation of an outbreak of vaccine-preventable diseases often identifies populations that have not received the vaccine. For example, the investigation of a measles outbreak that occurred in 1993 in Espindola, a rural community in the Peruvian Andes, revealed that more than a quarter of the 553 residents were affected, and that more than 3 per cent of those with measles had died. One year before the outbreak, a national measles campaign targeting children less than 15 years of age had been conducted. Although national data reported the coverage to be 78 per cent, the investigation found that only 4 per cent of the children in Espindola had actually been vaccinated (Sniadack *et al.* 1999).

Evaluation of the effectiveness of the existing surveillance system

Some aspects of the surveillance system can be evaluated during an outbreak, such as the timeliness, validity, sensitivity, appropriateness of case definitions, and utilization of the surveillance information.

Training of health professionals

The Epidemic Intelligence Service of the US Centers for Diseases Control and Prevention (CDC) and over 30 Field Epidemiology Training Programs (FETP) around the world use real outbreaks as an opportunity for training health professionals, as well as to provide services by investigating the causes and determinants of outbreaks.

Responding to public, political, and legal concerns

In many situations, an investigation must be conducted because the media has publicized the complaints of people to politicians, or even rumours. The main objective for this kind of investigation is to verify the outbreak and diagnosis. If it is groundless, the investigator can supply the media with new information that can end the rumours. Conversely, if it is a true outbreak, investigators must decide on what steps need to be taken.

In general, for a real outbreak, many objectives can be achieved fully or at least partially. However, the ultimate goal is to control the current outbreak and to prevent future ones. It is unethical for investigators to compromise this ultimate goal with other goals such as training or non-essential research that does not directly contribute to control activities.

Components of an investigation team

In this chapter, the term 'investigators' will represent people who are directly involved in planning and conducting outbreak investigations from start to finish. In principle, local health professionals at the district or provincial level should assume the role of investigators and start work as soon as possible. For complicated or difficult field investigations, additional disciplines or international experts can provide assistance. It is best to form an investigation team with a single principal investigator in charge of the operation. A good investigation team should include the following:

1. A field epidemiologist who is technically competent to conduct field investigations systematically. The field epidemiologist usually serves as one of the primary investigators, and should be involved in all the investigative steps.
2. Disease control people who are experienced in implementing basic disease control measures such as food and environmental sanitation, vector control, and vaccination. If available, an educator who can provide essential knowledge to villagers in clear terms is also very useful for disease control implementation.
3. Laboratory technicians who are able to provide basic and advanced laboratory support to the investigation team. They might not need to travel to the field and collect the specimens themselves, except when a special collection procedure is required.
4. Specialists in particular areas (e.g. a veterinarian) would be very helpful for an outbreak investigation of zoonotic diseases. An entomologist is a key team member for an outbreak investigation of vector-borne diseases. A social scientist with expertise in qualitative methods will help identify risk behaviours among affected populations and assess the acceptability of the recommended interventions.
5. Public health administrators who are good at providing logistic support, mobilizing resources, and providing administrative expertise for the team.
6. In certain situations, when the outbreak has caused panic or has gained the intense attention of the public, the investigation team should recruit or appoint a person to be in charge of public relations and press releases. This person should appropriately reassure and not unduly alarm the public.

In practice, all of these team members are not always available at the subdistrict or district level, due to limited human resources. Public health professionals and field epidemiologists need to have basic knowledge of all these relevant disciplines and be able to assume these tasks if needed.

Due to the sudden nature of a field investigation, it is best to establish in advance a list of people who will be on call and ready to join an investigation team once an outbreak has occurred. The Thai Ministry of Public Health established 1030 surveillance and rapid respond teams (SRRTs) to serve as investigation and control teams at all districts nationwide when the avian influenza outbreak occurred in early 2004. Public health officers received practical epidemiology training, and subsequently became frontline armies tracking outbreaks in their local area.

Issues to be considered before implementing an investigation

The principal investigator should consider all of the following issues before initiating a field investigation.

Assessing the existence of the outbreak

No matter how outbreak news is obtained, an investigator should confirm the validity of the information. The best way is to have direct communication with the responsible local health authority or field staff. It is not unusual for the information to be groundless. Sometimes, the outbreak had in fact occurred, but the media incorrectly quoted the name of the location. The investigator should carefully check with all other possible local health authorities in order not to overlook the outbreak.

Gathering available basic information

If the local health authority or field staff confirms the existence of the outbreak, the investigator should ask for additional information related to the situation and control measures being implemented.

Information related to the disease situation

1. What are the main symptoms and signs of the patients?
2. By whom and how was the diagnosis made; for example, using only clinical or also laboratory evidence?
3. How many patients were seen and how many died?
4. What was the average age of the patients and were there any differences in gender distribution?
5. Where did the patients come from? Are they clustered or scattered?
6. When was the increased number first observed and what is the trend at the moment?

Information related to control and response activities

1. What has already been done in terms of the field investigation and implementation of control activities?
2. Are there any serious constraints that compromise the field investigation and/or implementing control measures?
3. Who are the key people responsible for the investigation and control activities?

It is not necessary to gather all of this information before leaving for the field, but having it will help investigators to plan an effective investigation.

Ensuring that clinical specimens and suspected materials are collected

It is absolutely critical to contact the doctors who saw the cases and made the diagnosis to obtain relevant clinical specimens such as serum and blood for future laboratory tests. The items to which the cases were exposed, such as food and water, should be collected immediately before anything is unintentionally destroyed. The investigator should contact the local and reference laboratories so that the necessary supplies and equipment can be obtained immediately.

Obtaining permission and adequate support from local and national authorities

The investigation team should ask the permission of the local health authorities, which will create a sense of shared responsibility and partnership. Usually, local authorities are pleased to receive assistance. In a few situations, the local authority might be unhappy about having outsiders conduct the field investigation because of the sensitive nature of the problem. The investigator needs to convince local authorities that a thorough and sound investigation will produce more benefits than cause harm. The investigator should also request field support from the key authorities, such as field staff who will facilitate the fieldwork and provide transportation, medication, etc. In some situations, if the outbreak is possibly of national and international concern, the principal investigator should inform national authorities so they are aware and can plan further necessary steps to deal with the media and international communities.

Planning the field operation

The investigator needs to have a short meeting with team members to summarize the situation, set up the objectives of the investigations, divide responsibility among team members, and check the readiness of laboratory and logistical support.

It is also important to plan the duration of the field investigation. The investigation team should stay in the field until all investigation processes such as data collection, analysis, interpretation, and the executive summary have been completed. Leaving the field without accomplishing all these objectives could delay the implementation of control measures. Most outbreak investigations should plan to obtain preliminary results and recommendations within a week of the investigation beginning to ensure that the findings will be timely enough for control of the current outbreak. Additional studies and subsequent investigations can be conducted later.

The investigation team should not spend too much time preparing a perfect plan, because of the urgency of the outbreak, rather should obtain what is most necessary and start the investigation as soon as possible.

Steps of outbreak investigation

An outbreak investigation is an observational study in nature, because the events have already occurred. Every outbreak investigation needs to start with a good descriptive study, followed by analytical studies whenever possible and necessary. Conclusions about the causes, mechanisms, and determinants of the outbreak need to be drawn, based on sound epidemiological, clinical, laboratory, and environmental evidence.

A descriptive study can help to identify the risk population and risk area so that immediate interventions can be directed to those who need the most attention. A good descriptive study can also generate hypotheses about how the outbreak has spread and what factors contributed to the abnormal occurrence of the disease. In theory, hypotheses derived from a descriptive study should be confirmed by further analytical study; in reality, this is not always possible, due to many constraints.

It is preferable to translate the methodology for outbreak investigation into steps of action. Gregg (1996) has divided the outbreak investigation process into 10 steps; with a slight modification, this 10-step investigation process has been summarized in Box 6.4.1. Steps 1–4 use descriptive epidemiology to generate basic facts and hypotheses, Steps 5–7 are processes to test the hypotheses and draw conclusions, and Steps 8–10 emphasize the importance of communication of the results and follow-up of the recommendations.

This outline does not imply a strict course of action. In real outbreak investigations, many steps may be undertaken concurrently, depending on the situation.

Box 6.4.1 Ten steps to take in an outbreak investigation

1. Confirm the existence of the outbreak.
2. Verify the diagnosis and determine the aetiology of the disease.
3. Develop a case definition, start case-finding, and collect information on cases.
4. Describe persons, places, and times, and generate hypotheses.
5. Test the hypotheses using an analytic study.
6. Carry out necessary environmental or other studies to supplement the epidemiological study.
7. Draw conclusions to explain the causes or the determinants of the outbreak, based on clinical, laboratory, epidemiological, and environmental studies.
8. Report and recommend appropriate control measures to concerned authorities at the local, national, and if appropriate, international levels.
9. Communicate the findings to educate other public health professionals and the general public.
10. Follow up the recommendations to ensure implementation of control measures.

Step 1: Confirm the existence of an outbreak

The main question is: 'Is this a true outbreak?' Applying the definition of an outbreak outlined in this chapter, the investigator should be able to establish or refute the existence of the outbreak. Investigators should review the number of cases with the local health officers or hospital staff and compare it with the number found during the same period recorded in past years.

For example, the outbreak of trichinosis in North Rhine-Westphalia, Germany, was confirmed because there were 52 cases in a 3-month period between November 1998 and January 1999, compared with no more than 10 cases annually during the same time period in the past 10 years (Centers for Disease Control and Prevention 1999d).

Step 2: Verify the diagnosis and aetiology of the disease

If the number of cases fit the case criteria for the outbreak, the next related questions are

- What is the correct diagnosis and aetiology of the disease?
- What can be done immediately to prevent new cases from occurring?

Knowing the exact diagnosis and aetiology of the disease will help to establish appropriate preventive measures immediately. This will protect susceptible people and allow the team to start educating villagers to avoid the risk factors. For example, many adults in a remote village were sick with fever, muscle and joint pain, rashes over the body, etc. If the diagnosis and aetiology of the disease is unknown, the local public health officials will find it very difficult to educate the public or implement effective preventive programmes. Until the serology of some patients showed sharply rising immunoglobulin M (IgM) antibodies to dengue virus, control measures to destroy the larvae of the *Aedes* mosquito, the vector of dengue which breeds in water containers, could not be started.

In many situations, an unknown or unclear diagnosis can cause panic due to rumours. This was demonstrated by an outbreak of pneumonic plague in Surat, India, in 1994, and of encephalitis in Malaysia in 1999, which resulted in severe panic among local people and foreign tourists. Thus, it is very important to obtain the exact diagnosis as rapidly as possible.

Investigators should have basic knowledge of the clinical diagnosis and of how to confirm the aetiology of suspected disease by using well-established laboratory techniques. It is recommended that investigators visit and talk with some patients, review and visualize the signs and symptoms, and hold discussions with the attending doctors. The information from this step will help to develop a case definition to facilitate active case-finding. The information on aetiology will also help to interpret the findings from the later descriptive study and establish a causal association.

The investigators should also visit the laboratory facilities and ask for either positive or negative results of the testing of specimens. It is not necessary that all cases be laboratory confirmed, but at least some of the apparent clinical cases or deaths should be confirmed. Once there are some laboratory-confirmed cases, the investigator will find it more reasonable to assume that other cases with the same clinical manifestations in the same period and location are the same disease.

It is unfortunate that specimens from patients are often thrown away when the primary results (either positive or negative) are obtained. The investigators should plan with the doctors and laboratory technicians to perform further investigations on the specific strain, and to establish drug sensitivities, genetic markers, etc. Many new laboratory technologies, such as serological testing, culture and isolation, and molecular techniques, are very powerful for diagnosing and tracking the connections between cases.

Step 3: Develop an appropriate case definition, start case-finding, and collect information on Cases

At this stage, the investigator needs to answer at least three questions:

- Who should be counted as a case?
- Are there more undetected cases in the hospitals and in the community?
- What are the characteristics of cases?

To answer these three questions, the investigators must follow three steps.

Develop an appropriate case definition

It is important that the investigator develop a case definition, which will be applied consistently during the investigation. The definition should be sensitive or adequate at the beginning, in order to capture actual cases. A good case definition for investigative purposes should be specific to time and location. The case definition should not include any specific suspected exposure that the investigator plans to verify. This would create selection bias when the investigator generates the hypothesis or tests the hypothesis in the subsequent steps. Using the information from the previous steps, the investigator can divide the case definition into different levels. For example, in an investigation of leptospirosis among athletes participating in a triathlon in Illinois and Wisconsin in 1998, the following definitions were used (Centers for Disease Control and Prevention 1998b):

1. A suspected case is a triathlon participant who manifests at least two of the following symptoms or signs during the period of 21 June to 13 August, 1999: chills, headache, myalgia, diarrhoea, eye pain, or red eyes. These criteria were based solely on a set of clinical signs and symptoms, and were rather loose.
2. A confirmed case is a suspected case who has laboratory confirmation by serology (IgM ELISA and microagglutination test titre ≥ 1:400), by positive tissue immunohistochemical test, or by a positive culture of *Leptospira*.

In some instances, the investigator might need to apply a definition of 'probable case'. A probable case is not fully confirmed by specific laboratory testing, but has unique clinical or preliminary laboratory test results or is epidemiologically linked to a confirmed case. The definition of the same disease in different investigations can be slightly different, based on the availability of laboratory support.

Active case-finding

In places where there is good surveillance, cases from all hospitals can be reported to the epidemiology unit at the district or provincial level. Investigators can apply the case definition and count the number of cases, and review data that are collected on the reporting form. If enough cases and basic information on cases have already been gathered, investigators can start descriptive epidemiology.

Conversely, if only a few cases have been seen at the health facility, the investigators should plan to search for cases in the community. The investigator must start a process called *active case-finding*. The objective of active case-finding is to have enough cases to analyse. At the same time, this case-finding will give a better picture of the magnitude of the outbreak. For example, in the outbreak of leptospirosis among triathlon athletes in Wisconsin and Illinois in 1998, only three cases were reported by the hospital at the beginning. The investigators cooperated with many state health departments by making a telephone call survey; in the end, they succeeded in interviewing 1194 athletes. Among them, 110 (9 per cent) had an illness that met the suspected case definition of leptospirosis. The investigators also obtained acute serum from 70 cases, 24 of whom were confirmed as having leptospirosis by both IgM and microagglutination tests (Centers for Disease Control and Prevention 1998b).

In the preceding example, it appeared that active case-finding by telephone interviews was not difficult. However, investigators need to try their best to do active case-finding whenever it is necessary, no matter how difficult it is. Investigators must frequently visit many hospitals in the outbreak area and review medical records themselves. Sometimes, they must search for cases in each village by interviewing from house to house, which is the true nature of outbreak field investigations and the way people learn epidemiology. This active case-finding in the community also provides two more benefits:

1. Control measures can be implemented if the aetiology of the disease is known and treatable. During an investigation, using active case-searching in a village that reported seven deaths from malaria in Kachin state in the Union of Myanmar, the investigator found 94 probable cases and 53 microscopically confirmed malaria infections. All of the probable and confirmed cases found by this active process were treated. Without this measure, there might be more deaths later on (Dr Myint Win, personal communication 1999).
2. Rapid environmental assessment can be started during the visit to the affected families or villages. From the direct interview with the cases, the investigators can develop hypotheses and implement necessary interventions immediately, such as sanitation improvement among food handlers and treatment of water to prevent a waterborne outbreak.

In situations in which the outbreak is not localized but widespread, the investigator might need to use the media to alert the public about the outbreak. People can then avoid suspected exposures and see a health-care provider if they have developed symptoms compatible with the case definition.

Collecting information on cases

For each case, the investigator should collect at least four types of information:

1. Identifying information: Name, hospital number, contact person, and address of contact. This additional information will help to avoid duplication of enumerated cases. The investigator can also maintain communication with these cases when more information is needed.
2. Demographic information: Age, gender, occupation, religion, ethnicity, area of residence, place of work, etc. This important information may help to determine the characteristics and distribution of cases.
3. Clinical information: Symptoms and signs, date of onset, duration of illness, and results of diagnostic procedures. These data will help to confirm that it is a true case, provide the pattern of clinical manifestations, and also, the distribution of cases by time.
4. Suspected risk factors: Investigators can ask for a history of exposure to factors before the disease developed. The timing of interest is usually one incubation period if the aetiology is known or suspected. Questions about contact with other patients who have similar clinical symptoms are also very helpful. If the diagnosis is not known, the investigator might collect this information in a qualitative manner.

The investigator should develop a questionnaire as a tool to collect the relevant information from the hospital or during active case-searching in the community. In practice, some of the information will not be available or not of good quality. The investigators should validate all data that are in doubt.

Step 4: Describe the outbreak in person, place, and time, and hypotheses formation

In this step, investigators need to answer the following questions:

- What are the main clinical features?
- What is the population at risk?

- What are the risk factors?
- What are the most likely explanations of how the outbreak began?

A simple approach is to analyse clinical information from each case and see the distribution of cases in terms of person, place, and time. The analysis should be done using rates rather than absolute numbers; the investigator needs to obtain the denominators from an available source or to estimate them. Using rates, the investigator can compare and determine the populations and areas of highest risk. With the advent of computers, many software programs are available to analyse these data. A popular one is EpiInfo™, which is public domain software from the US CDC that is designed specifically for field investigations. In the absence of a computer, investigators can still analyse the data manually. Individual questionnaires can be compiled into a line listing, which includes important variables of all cases. With this line listing, simple counts can be made. In this way, investigators will gain knowledge about populations and areas of risk. Resource and control measures can then be directed to the risk populations and risk areas. Enumeration will also produce information for hypothesis formation to explain how and why the outbreak occurred.

Clinical manifestations of cases

Signs and symptoms of cases can be analysed in percentages and shown in a summary table. In an outbreak of unknown aetiology, clinical information will help to differentiate the diagnosis. For an outbreak in which the aetiology is already known, the investigators still need to compare the clinical information found in the investigation with previous knowledge. Any discrepancy between the investigation and previous knowledge such as the attack rate, mortality rate, severity, etc. should be carefully examined, because this might indicate that a new strain or different specific host response is occurring. The high mortality rate of approximately 40 per cent in the Nipah encephalitis outbreak in Malaysia 1999 (Centers for Disease Control and Prevention 1999c) indicated that this outbreak might not be due to the usual endemic encephalitis.

Population at risk

Investigators should analyse the characteristics of cases by gender, age, occupation, ethnicity, etc. Initially this can be carried out by examining the proportion of all cases, but the specific attack rate by age and gender will be more useful for comparisons and hypothesis formation. The rates will provide useful indicators of the possible aetiology of the outbreak. In the Ebola hemorrhagic fever outbreak in Zaire in 1976, all ages and both genders were affected, but females slightly predominated. Age- and gender-specific attack rates indicated that adult females had the highest attack rate. This finding suggested that parenteral injection with unsterilized syringes and needles given during antenatal care in the local hospital was the means of transmission (World Health Organization 1978).

The outbreak of Nipah encephalitis in Malaysia in early 1999 was initially thought to be due to Japanese encephalitis alone. However, after careful analysis of the descriptive information, it was clear that the cases were mainly male, adult, involved in pig farming, and of Chinese ethnicity. This descriptive information did not fit the pattern for Japanese encephalitis, which mainly affects children of both genders, with no preference for a particular ethnicity. The investigator then began to suspect other organisms and to hypothesize that pig farming increased the risk of becoming ill.

Index and outlier cases: In infectious diseases, the first case on the epidemic curve or the index case is important, because of the possibility that he and/or she brought the disease into the community either from the local area or from other locales. Cases that appear at the very beginning or at the end of the epidemic should also be given careful attention. These cases are called *outlier cases*, and can provide important information about the source and the way in which the disease is spread.

Normally, the very first and very last cases in the epidemic curve should be critically appraised. The first case may not be the true index case because of misdiagnosis, a case unrelated to the epidemic, etc. The late cases may be due to misdiagnosis, a case unrelated to the epidemic, or a secondary case that had a different exposure than the majority of the cases in the epidemic.

During the outbreak of severe acute respiratory syndrome (SARS) in February 2003, the index case was identified as a 65-year-old medical doctor from Guangdong, mainland China, who stayed on the 9th floor of a hotel in Hong Kong (Fig. 6.4.3). He had treated patients with atypical pneumonia prior to his departure, and he was symptomatic upon arrival in Hong Kong. He had infected over a dozen guests and international visitors. During the outbreak investigation, the investigators aimed to identify contacts of this index case to prevent further transmission. A history and information of this index case obtained by the investigation team traced back to the previous atypical pneumonia outbreaks or undiagnosed SARS since late 2002 (World Health Organization Regional Office for the Western Pacific 2006).

Location

Investigators can calculate attack rates of cases in different locations. These can be places of residence, places of work, sites of exposure, etc. Locations with high attack rates often indicate the sources of infection or contamination. A spot map showing the locations of cases can give a very good idea of the source, as demonstrated by Snow in his classical investigation of a cholera outbreak in the Golden Square area of London between August and September 1854 (Frost 1936). In that investigation, Snow found most cases clustered around the Broad Street pump. From this information, Snow deduced that the Broad Street pump was probably the primary source of the outbreak.

If cases are scattered in many locations, investigators should explore the secular pattern of the cases over time, which will indicate whether the outbreak started in one area and spread to other areas, or whether people living in different places had a common exposure. The SARS outbreak is good example of when cases are distributed worldwide originally from a single source of infection.

Time

The aim is to show the occurrence of cases over time and look for a pattern of occurrence. In general, there are two major types of outbreaks: A common source and a propagated source. The way to differentiate between these two patterns of outbreak is to draw an epidemic curve that shows the number of cases (on the y-axis) over time of onset (on the x-axis). The epidemic curve of each outbreak will suggest whether the mode of spread is by a common source or from person to person.

Common source outbreak

This kind of outbreak occurs when people are infected by exposure to the same source of infection. For example, a group of people contract viral hepatitis A because they ate the same contaminated food served during a wedding party. A common source outbreak

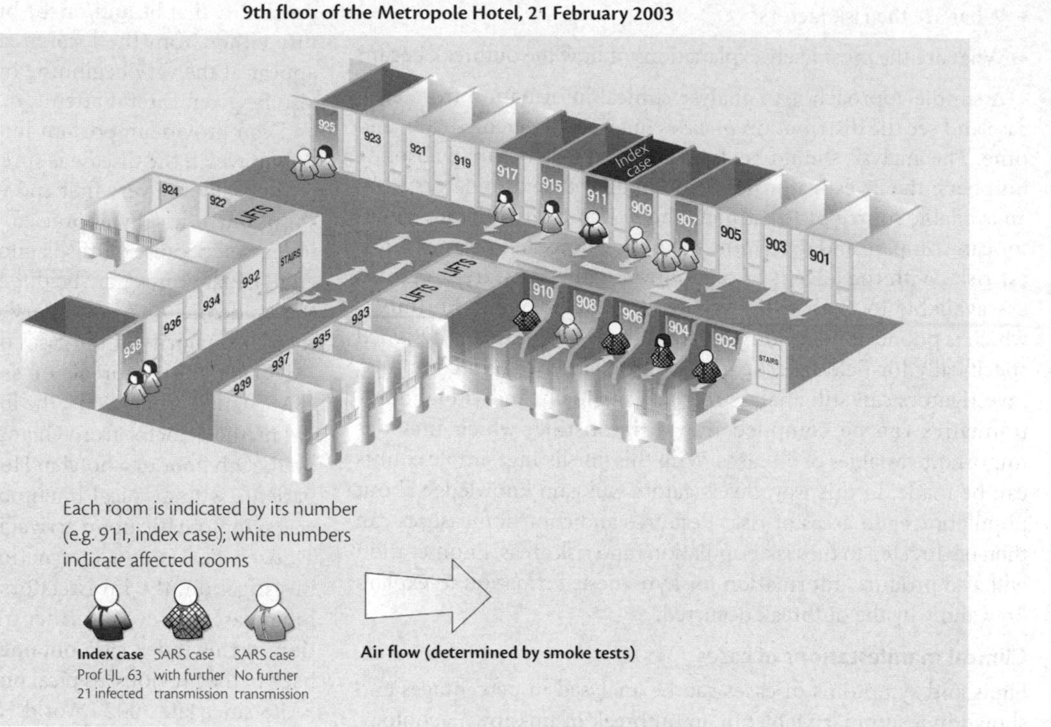

Fig. 6.4.3 Index case of SARS—Hong Kong, 2003.
Source: World Health Organization Regional Office for the Western Pacific. *SARS: how a global epidemic was stopped.* Manila, Philippines: World Health Organization, Western Pacific Region; 2006. With permission.

can be divided into a point common source and a continuous common source:

1. A point common source outbreak occurs when there is a single source that exists for a very short time and all cases have common exposure to it at that particular time.

2. A continuous common source outbreak occurs when there is only one source that provides continuous or intermittent exposure over a longer period of time.

Epidemic curve of a point common source outbreak: The epidemic curve shows a sharp increase of many cases suddenly followed by a rapid decline, although not as rapid as at the beginning of the epidemic. Another criterion to judge a point common source is that the first case and the last case usually occur within one incubation period.

If the aetiology and the data of the incubation period of the disease are known, the investigators can then roughly estimate the probable time of the initial exposure. This can be done by identifying the peak of the epidemic from the curve and counting back on the *x*-axis the equivalent of the incubation period. The investigator can also use the first case and count back on the *x*-axis the duration of the minimum incubation period, which will also give a rough estimate of the time of exposure.

If the aetiology of the disease is not known, but the epidemic curve fits well with a point common source outbreak, the investigator can estimate the average incubation period if he or she knows the times of common exposure.

In the outbreak of food poisoning caused by *Salmonella enteritidis* in Riga, Latvia, 2006, the peak of the outbreak was observed four days after the onset date of the index case (Fig. 6.4.4). All of the cases had a history of having a meal at the same restaurant. The implicated food items included tuna, beans, and Caesar salads with mayonnaise prepared from raw eggs, which were subsequently identified as the source of infection (Brila *et al.* 2006).

Epidemic curve for a continuous common source outbreak: The epidemic curve shows an abrupt increase in the number of cases, but instead of having a peak and a decline within one incubation period, new cases persist for a longer time, with a plateau shape instead of a peak before decreasing. However, if there are many peaks or irregular jagged curves, it suggests an intermittent common source.

Propagated outbreak

A propagated outbreak is caused by transmission from one person to another, and requires direct contact such as touching, biting, kissing, or sexual activity.

Epidemic curve of propagated source outbreak: The epidemic curve shows a slow increase in the number of cases, with progressive peaks approximately one incubation period apart. The investigators might observe an abrupt decrease in new cases, because everyone has already been infected. The span from the first to the last cases will also last longer than several incubation periods (Fig. 6.4.5).

The outbreaks of SARS in Singapore demonstrated the propagated source of transmission beginning from a young female who returned home from Hong Kong. This patient had stayed on the same hotel floor as the index case. She had initially infected many hospital staff before the disease spread for further generations (Kamps & Hoffmann 2003). The outbreak resulted in 238 cases and 33 deaths in a few months.

Step 5: Testing the hypotheses by analysis

In an outbreak of infectious disease, the investigator needs to answer the following questions:

- What is the aetiology of the disease?
- What is the source of infection?

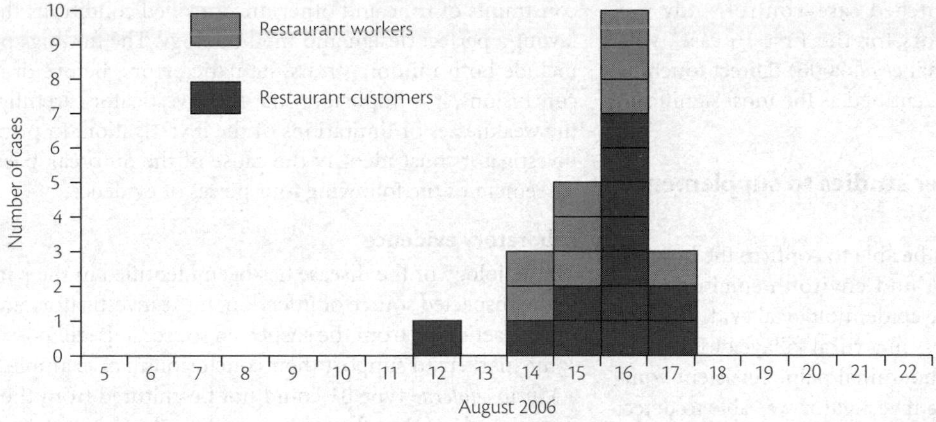

Fig. 6.4.4 Dates of illness onset for 23 cases in an outbreak of *Salmonella enteritidis* infection linked to a restaurant in Riga, Latvia, August 2006. (From Brila A, Innuse M, Perevoscikovs J *et al*. An outbreak of *Salmonella enteritidis* infections linked to a restaurant in Riga, August 2006. *EuroSurveillance* 2006;**26**:11. With permission of *Eurosurveillance*.)

- What is the pattern of spread?
- What are the risks factors for an individual to get the disease?
- What are the determinants of the outbreak or the factors which, when combined together, result in the outbreak?

The aetiology of the disease should be derived from the laboratory study. The pattern of spread can be identified by a careful descriptive study. Sometimes it is not as simple as expected, and a descriptive study does not give enough clues. The investigator must patiently re-examine the descriptive information, carry out more active case-finding, and re-analyse the data. The investigator also needs to directly observe the location, lifestyle, and/or behaviour of the cases. These additional investigations usually help the investigator to generate some reasonable hypotheses. For example, a cholera outbreak in a home for mentally disabled children in Nonthaburi, Thailand, persisted over a one-month period, and the epidemic curve showed a pattern of person-to-person spread. After looking into the attack rate in different buildings in the home, the investigator found that some buildings had a very high attack rate. When the investigator visited the home, he discovered that the building with the highest attack rate was very crowded. Two or three children shared a single bed. The children also bathed in a small room, where they were exposed to feces from other children. With this direct observation, the hypothesis was formulated that crowding promoted the spread of the disease. In this example, the hypothesis was very reasonable, and might not need to be tested. Improving the crowded conditions was recommended, and action was taken immediately.

In another example, the hypothesis needed to be tested by an analytical study design. The most common is a case–control study. The investigator needed to define the cases and measure the odds of suspected exposed factors found among cases in comparison to the odds of exposure found among appropriately selected controls. The case definition for the analytical study may be more specific than that used for a descriptive study in order to reduce misclassifying non-cases as cases. Conversely, the controls may also need to be tested to avoid classifying non-apparent cases as controls. An example is the analytic study for identifying risk factors for highly pathogenic avian influenza H5N1 among human cases, an emerging infectious disease in South-East Asia. On 23 January 2004, the Ministry of Public Health in Thailand reported the first confirmed human case of H5N1 infection following the outbreak in poultry. During February–November 2004, epidemiologists and health officials worked together to investigate the

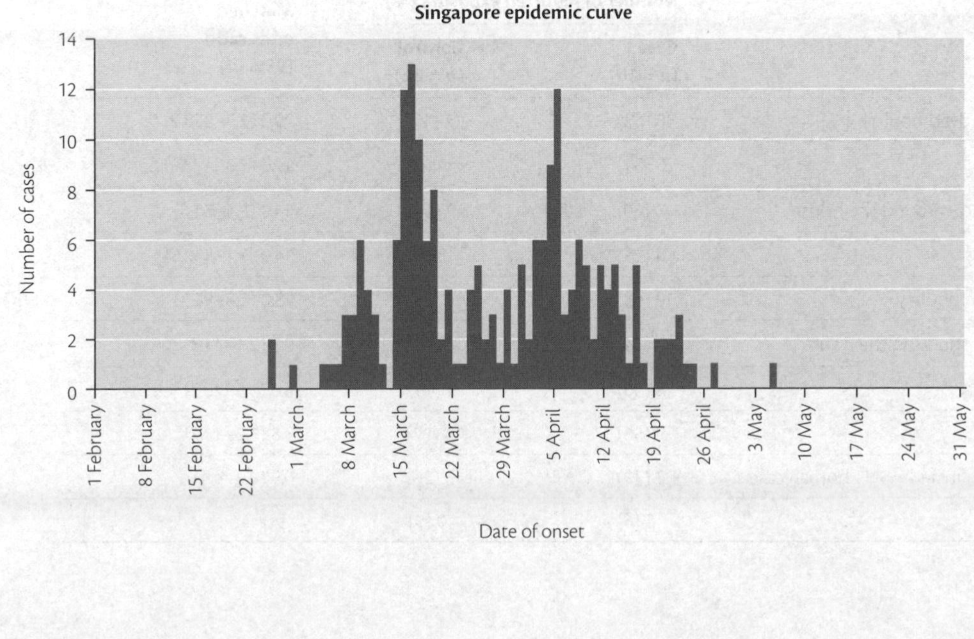

Fig. 6.4.5 SARS cases by date of onset—Singapore, 2003. (From World Health Organization Regional Office for the Western Pacific. *SARS: how a global epidemic was stopped.* Manila, Philippines: World Health Organization, Western Pacific Region; 2006. With permission.)

H5N1 outbreak in humans. A matched case–control study was conducted to determine risk factors for the first 16 cases who became ill with H5N1 (Areechokchai *et al.* 2006). Direct touching of unexpectedly dead poultry was identified as the most significant risk factor (Table 6.4.1).

Step 6: Environmental or other studies to supplement epidemiological findings

Although an analytical study might be able to confirm the hypothesis, the investigator still needs to find environmental or other evidence to support and explain the epidemiological evidence.

In an outbreak of unknown illness in a rural village of Egypt, in which the cases developed severe abdominal pain, persistent vomiting, and generalized weakness, the investigator was able to detect abnormally high blood lead levels among the cases. The analytical study revealed an association between high blood levels and eating flour from one mill factory. The mill implicated in the outbreak was visited. Upon arrival at the mill, the investigators noted a lead smelting pot in the corner of the mill. Lead was used by the miller to attach the crosspiece to the grinding stone. Occasionally, the lead would break off and contaminate the flour. The miller reported using about 2 kg of lead per year. Analysis of grain from the mill showed no lead; however, lead was found in flour from the surface of the mill stone and in samples of flour after grinding was complete (Abdel-Nasser 1996).

Step 7: Establishing the causes of the outbreak

Once the hypothesis has been tested and other necessary studies have been carried out, the investigators can draw their conclusions about the causes of the outbreak. This conclusion is very important, because action should follow. Many restaurants or factories have been closed because they were implicated as the source of the outbreak. Outbreak investigations are naturally faced with constraints of time and other uncontrolled conditions that do not favour a perfect design and methodology. The findings potentially include both random and systematic errors. Before drawing any conclusions, it is important that the investigator carefully examine the weaknesses or limitations of the investigation. In principle, the investigator must identify the cause of the outbreak based on the agreement of the following four pieces of evidence.

Laboratory evidence

The aetiology of the disease has been identified in the patients and in the suspected source of infection. If the investigator cannot identify the aetiology from the suspected source, it is still possible to use some markers to support their conclusions. For example, although a *Vibrio cholerae* type 01 could not be cultured from the drinking water supply of the affected community, the observation of human faecal coliform bacteria in the water helped to indicate that human faeces had contaminated the water.

Clinical evidence

It is necessary to verify that the incubation period and clinical manifestations of cases are compatible with the aetiological agents reported from the laboratory. In the SARS outbreak, most patients developed atypical pneumonia with rapid progression to respiratory failure and a fraction of them also had diarrhea which was explainable by the findings of SARS coronavirus both in the respiratory tract and stool of patients.

Environmental evidence

Careful investigation of the environment should reveal clues that the causative agent can pass from the source to the cases or the index case to subsequent cases. The investigation of early SARS cases revealed that the index case passed the virus to several people who stayed in the same floor and used the same elevator (CDC 2003).

Table 6.4.1 Numbers and percentages of reported exposures associated with influenza A (H5N1) disease by type of exposure—Thailand, 2004

Exposure (*n* = 80)	Number of reported exposure (%)		Matched odds ratio (95% CI)
	Case (*n* = 16)	Control (*n* = 64)	
Directly touching abnormal dead poultry	10 (63)	12 (19)	29.0 (2.7–308.2)
Dressing poultry	5 (31)	4 (6)	17.0 (1.6–177.0)
Having abnormal dead poultry around the house	8 (50)	9 (14)	14.0 (2.4–81.6)
Plucking dead poultry	4 (25)	3 (5)	14.0 (1.3–152.5)
Being within 1 metre of dead poultry	10 (63)	16 (25)	13.0 (1.8–96.3)
Storing sick/dead poultry products in the house	7 (44)	3 (5)	9.3 (2.1–41.3)
Directly touching sick poultry	8 (50)	9 (14)	5.6 (1.5–20.7)
Being within 1 m of sick poultry	9 (56)	14 (22)	3.8 (1.2–11.7)
Contact with suspected/confirmed H5N1 human case	3 (19)	13 (20)	0.9 (0.2–4.4)
Visiting live poultry market	1 (6)	0 (0)	very large

For an outbreak of food poisoning, a cooking environment that is dirty or located close to the toilet is convincing evidence of food being contaminated by faeces. Crowding in bedrooms is very convincing evidence for a respiratory tract disease outbreak.

Epidemiological evidence

Epidemiological evidence found in the descriptive and analytical studies should clearly explain the following aspects:

- Pattern of spread, as described by an epidemic curve
- Statistical strength of association between exposure and developing the disease
- Dose–response relationship, which demonstrates a higher strength of association when the exposure is increasing
- Exposure should precede an illness

It is not uncommon to see some disagreement in the evidence from different sources. In this event, the investigator needs to verify the validity of each piece of evidence and discuss the data with people who have expertise in that particular area in order to obtain more information and draw a valid conclusion.

Step 8: On-site reporting to and recommendations for concerned authorities

The most important step leading to a timely response is to report the findings to the responsible individuals both at the local and national levels so that they can take appropriate action. Keeping this in mind, the investigators need to complete two tasks before leaving the outbreak area:

1. Complete analysis and data interpretation: Leaving the field without completing these tasks will reduce the sense of urgency necessary to finish the work. Data are easier to retrieve when staying in the field rather than instructing field people to send them to the investigation team later.
2. Present the main findings with recommendations: Some findings may be very sensitive because they reflect the weaknesses or mistakes of the health or other authorities. The investigator needs to select the appropriate approach, either formal or informal, with those responsible. Leaving the field without providing the information that the team obtains from the investigation will be detrimental to other people who could be prevented from becoming ill if the information were known. In many urgent situations, the findings and recommendations might be regularly given to the people responsible during the outbreak investigation process instead of waiting until the end. The investigators also need to present or communicate the findings and recommendations to the national authorities as soon as possible. The recommendations for action should be based on the findings of the investigation. These might include the following aspects.

What can be done to control the outbreak

With timely investigation, some interventions can be implemented to stop further spread. In the outbreak of measles in a rural community in Peru, measles vaccines were given to children aged between 6 months and 15 years who were not measles cases, regardless of their previous immunization status. Using knowledge about the complication of measles in previous studies, the investigators estimated that the action prevented 87 cases of diarrhoea and 46 cases of pneumonia, and averted five deaths (Sniadack *et al.* 1999).

How to prevent future outbreaks

In many instances, interventions cannot be implemented for the current outbreak, but the findings can be used to set up new practices or policies. These recommendations can help prevent future outbreaks. In Thailand, the recommendation was made to change practices of chicken farming and avoiding direct contact with sick poultry, which was recommended through the results of the investigation of human H5N1 cases. The Egyptian government, after reviewing the results of the investigation of lead contamination in flour mills, agreed to ban the use of lead in privately owned flour mills (Abdel-Nasser 1996).

How to improve the investigation

The investigator should review the performance of the investigation and identify the weaknesses of the methodology or the field operation so that improvements can be made. These might include a more appropriate case definition, a better investigative design, improved laboratory support, a different team composition, lower costs, a shorter time course, etc.

How to improve surveillance

The best time to evaluate the surveillance system is during an outbreak investigation. In most outbreaks, the investigator must review data from existing surveillance systems. With this direct involvement, the investigator will be able to evaluate the timeliness, completeness, validity of diagnosis, sensitivity of the system, and utilization of the surveillance information. The investigation of human avian H5N1 influenza cases in Thailand led to an improved definition of a human case in the areas experiencing an H5N1 virus outbreak in poultry.

Step 9: Dissemination of information

In addition to on-site reporting, the investigator should disseminate the information to educate the public health community and the general public. There may be many other communities that are also prone to a similar outbreak. The information will raise the awareness of health and government authorities to assess their own situation and implement measures to prevent possible outbreaks. Dissemination of information should occur in a timely manner through weekly or monthly reports. Release of important findings through the mass media is also very useful for educating the public. Before releasing the investigation results through the media, the investigator must ensure that all the facts are delivered in a constructive manner and do not result in blame of any organization. The investigator should also report the investigation results in an international journal or bulletin such as the *Weekly Epidemiological Record* of the WHO or the *Morbidity and Mortality Weekly Report* of the CDC. This practice is necessary to alert health professionals in other countries and keep them informed of the problem.

In recent years, sharing of information for outbreak detection and control through the Internet and email has been increasingly utilized for timely responses. Telecommunications played an important role in the outbreaks of SARS when the disease was spread rapidly by air transportation to countries on the other side of the world. The teleconference on the clinical features and management of SARS was held by the WHO, which united 80 clinicians from 13 countries worldwide (World Health Organization Regional Office for the Western Pacific 2006).

Step 10: Follow-up to ensure implementation of control measures

Finally, the investigator should follow up the investigation by maintaining close communication with local health authorities. An absence of new cases for at least two incubation periods of the infectious disease under investigation could suggest that the outbreak is subsiding. A good investigator should follow up on the recommendations. An outbreak investigation is a waste of time if sound recommendations have not been implemented. The investigator should learn the reasons why the recommendations were or were not implemented. If the recommendations were implemented, the investigator can also learn the impact by observing the trend of the disease.

Cooperation for international outbreak investigation and preparedness

The world today is especially prone to outbreaks because of frequent cross-border movement, civil war and migration, rapid transportation, international trading, tourism, etc. An outbreak in one country can spread to other countries very easily. For example, in the multi-country SARS outbreak, international travelers were at risk of disease spreading from a single infectious case in a hotel (Centers for Disease Control and Prevention 2003). Ultimately, there were over 8000 cases reported in 26 countries worldwide. The world's experience with the SARS outbreak led to the commitment of countries around the world to improve surveillance and international joint investigation of emerging infectious diseases through the new International Health Regulation, which was adopted by the World Health Assembly in 2005.

A massive outbreak of botulism in northern Thailand in March 2006 tested the international capacity to respond to a public health emergency. Botulism poisoning due to contaminated home-canned bamboo shoots caused illness in 209 villagers, of whom 134 persons were hospitalized and 42 required mechanical ventilation. A global search for botulinal antitoxin began, involving international agencies, embassies, national laboratories, airlines, and commercial organizations in seven countries. Sufficient antitoxin was obtained from four sources for treatment of 90 patients, with a delay in treatment of five to nine days from time of exposure. Rapid local outbreak detection and an effective international response likely prevented mortality and additional morbidity (World Health Organization 2007).

An outbreak anywhere in the world must, therefore, be treated as a threat to all countries. It is important for each country to build up its capacity for surveillance, outbreak preparedness, and investigation. In addition to the US CDC Epidemic Intelligence Services, many countries have started training programmes and established a medical detective unit that is ready to investigate all kinds of outbreaks. These training programmes are known by different names, such as the Field Epidemiology Training Program (FETP) in over 30 countries, the Epidemiology European Training Program in the European Community, etc. The WHO has set up an outbreak verification network, a worldwide network of laboratories and reporting sites that collects information on reported and rumoured outbreaks nationally and worldwide. It is a wise investment, and a commitment that is needed by the international communities for information exchange and collaborative investigation of outbreaks.

Conclusion

Outbreak investigation is an essential function of public health professionals who care for the well-being of the community. It is an opportunity to gain new knowledge of diseases and to discover the weaknesses of current public health practices and systems. A good public health professional must always be alert to the possibility of outbreaks. Normal surveillance systems or unofficial sources, such as the mass media, can be a good source for detection of an outbreak. Before starting field investigations, investigators should organize the team, review previous knowledge, prepare the technical and management aspects, and start the investigation as soon as possible. The investigation can be conducted by following the 10 steps outlined earlier. The investigation usually starts by confirming the existence of the outbreak, verifying the diagnosis, gathering case information, descriptive epidemiology, formulating and testing the hypothesis when necessary, environmental surveys to supplement epidemiological evidence, and providing timely onsite reporting of the findings, with practical recommendations to local and national responsible authorities. Competent outbreak investigators combine sound scientific knowledge and good management skills. Direct participation in conducting the investigation is needed to gain the necessary skills. A good investigator should be a field-oriented person with strong levels of perseverance, skepticism, and common sense. The investigator should not end his or her work with the report, but should follow up on the recommendations and continue vigorous surveillance of the problem. In the future, increasing joint international investigations will be needed. Rich countries and resource-limited countries need to collaborate to detect and stop outbreaks before they get out of control. Through this cooperation, the world will be a safer place amidst the threat of old and emerging disease outbreaks.

References

Abdel-Nasser M.A. Outbreak investigation of an unknown illness in a rural village, Egypt, 1996. Cairo, Egypt: Field Epidemiology Training Programs; 1996.

Areechokchai D., Jiraphongsa C., Laosiritaworn Y. *et al.* Investigation of avian influenza (H5N1) outbreak in humans—Thailand, 2004. *Morbidity and Mortality Weekly Report* 2006;**55** Suppl 1:3–6.

Biggar R.J., Nasca P.C., Burnett W.S. AIDS-related Kaposi's sarcoma in New York City in 1977. *New England Journal of Medicine* 1988;**318**:252.

Blanton L., Brammer L., Wang S. *et al.* Update: influenza activity—United States and worldwide, 2005–06 season, and composition of the 2006–07 influenza vaccine. *Morbidity and Mortality Weekly Report* 2006;55(23):648–53

Brila A., Innuse M., Perevoscikovs J. *et al.* An outbreak of Salmonella enteritidis infections linked to a restaurant in Riga, August 2006. *Eurosurveillance* 2006;**26**:11.

Centers for Disease Control and Prevention. Food-borne botulism associated with home-canned bamboo shoots—Thailand, 1998. *Morbidity and Mortality Weekly Report* 1999a;**48**:437–9.

Centers for Disease Control and Prevention. Mass sociogenic illness in a day-care center, Florida. *Morbidity and Mortality Weekly Report* 1990;**39**:301–4.

Centers for Disease Control and Prevention. Outbreak of acute febrile illness among athletes participating in triathlons—Wisconsin and Illinois, 1998. *Morbidity and Mortality Weekly Report* 1998a;**47**:585–8.

Centers for Disease Control and Prevention. Outbreak of Hendra-like virus—Malaysia and Singapore, 1998–1999. *Morbidity and Mortality Weekly Report* 1999b;**48**:265–9.

Centers for Disease Control and Prevention. Outbreak of Nipah virus—Malaysia and Singapore, 1999. *Morbidity and Mortality Weekly Report* 1999c;**48**:335–7.

Centers for Disease Control and Prevention. Outbreak of unexplained illness in a middle school—Washington, April 1994. *Morbidity and Mortality Weekly Report* 1996;**45**:6–9.

Centers for Disease Control and Prevention. Trichinellosis outbreaks—North Rhine-Westphalia, Germany, 1998–1999. *Morbidity and Mortality Weekly Report* 1999d;**48**:488–92.

Centers for Disease Control and Prevention. Update: leptospirosis and unexplained acute febrile illness among athletes participating in triathlons—Illinois and Wisconsin, 1998. *Morbidity and Mortality Weekly Report* 1998b;**47**:673–6.

Centers for Disease Control and Prevention. Update: Outbreak of severe acute respiratory syndrome—worldwide, 2003. *Morbidity and Mortality Weekly Report* 2003;**52**:241–8.

Frost W.H. *Introduction to Snow on Cholera*. London: Oxford University Press and Commonwealth Fund; 1936.

Gregg M.B., editor. Conducting a field investigation. In: *Field epidemiology*. New York (NY): Oxford University Press; 1996. p. 44–59.

Kamps B.S. and Hoffmann C. Epidemiology. In: Kamps B.S., Hoffmann C., editors. *SARS reference*. 3rd ed. Flying Publisher; 2003. p. 71.

Lee S.Y., Mak K.H., Saw T.A. The avian flu (H5N1): one year on. *Public Health and Epidemiology Bulletin* 1999;**8**:1–8.

Siraprapasiri T., Thanprasertsuk S., Rodklay A. *et al*. Risk factors for HIV among prostitutes in Chiangmai, Thailand. *AIDS* 1991;**5**: 579–82.

Sniadack D.H., Moscoso B., Aguilar R. *et al*. Measles epidemiology and outbreak response immunization in a rural community in Peru. *Bulletin of the World Health Organization* 1999;**77**:545–52.

World Health Organization Regional Office for the Western Pacific. *SARS: how a global epidemic was stopped*. Manila, Philippines: World Health Organization, Western Pacific Region; 2006.

World Health Organization. Report of the International Commission. Ebola hemorrhagic fever in Zaire, 1976. *Bulletin of the World Health Organization* 1978;**56**:271–90.

World Health Organization. The need for global planned mobilization of essential medicine: lessons from a massive Thai botulism outbreak. *Bulletin of the World Health Organization* 2007;**85**(**3**):238–40.

6.5

Case–control studies*

Noel S. Weiss

Summary

Case–control studies compare ill or injured individuals (cases) with those at risk of the illness or injury (controls) with regard to prior exposures or characteristics, and so appear to proceed backwards, from consequence to potential cause. However, if a case–control study is able to enrol cases and controls from the same underlying population at risk of the outcome, and can measure exposure status of these persons in a valid manner, the results obtained will closely resemble those of a properly performed cohort study.

Introduction

In 1971, Herbst *et al.* (1971) reported that mothers of seven of the eight teenage girls diagnosed with clear cell adenocarcinoma of the vagina in Boston during 1966–1969 claimed to have taken a synthetic hormone, diethylstilboesterol, while pregnant. None of the mothers of the 32 girls without vaginal adenocarcinoma, matched to the cases mothers with regard to hospital and date of birth, had taken diethylstilboesterol during their pregnancy. Within a year, a New York study of five girls with and eight girls without vaginal cancer obtained similar results (Greenwald *et al.* 1971). The introduction of prenatal diethylstilboesterol use into obstetric practice in the United States during the 1940s and 1950s followed by the appearance of this hitherto unseen form of cancer some 20 years later supported a causal connection between *in utero* exposure to diethylstilboesterol and vaginal adenocarcinoma. The means by which *in utero* diethylstilboesterol exposure might predispose to the occurrence of clear cell vaginal adenocarcinoma was unknown in 1971. (It is now believed that diethylstilboesterol acts by interfering with normal development of the female genital tract, resulting in the persistence into puberty of vaginal adenosis in which adenocarcinoma can arise.) Nonetheless, a causal inference was made at that time by the Food and Drug Administration, which specified pregnancy as a contraindication for diethylstilboesterol use.

The investigation by Herbst *et al.* was a case–control study: A comparison of prior exposures or characteristics of ill people (cases) with those of people at risk for the illness in the population from which the cases arose. Generally, the prior experience of people at risk is estimated from observations of a sample of that population (controls). A difference in the frequency or levels of exposure between cases and control—that is, an association—may reflect a causal link.

A case–control, cohort, or any other form of non-randomized study has the potential to identify associations that are not causal, either because of chance or because of the influence of some other factor associated with both the exposure and outcome. Even so, the evidence that is provided by well-performed case–control studies can carry great weight when evaluating the validity of a causal hypothesis. Indeed, a number of causal inferences have been based largely on the result of case–control studies. These include, in addition to the diethylstilboesterol–vaginal adenocarcinoma relationship, the connection between aspirin use in children and the development of Reye's syndrome, and the use of absorbent tampons and the incidence of toxic shock syndrome.

One of the criteria used to assess the validity of a causal hypothesis is the strength of the association between exposure and disease, usually as measured by the ratio of the incidence rate in exposed and non-exposed people. In most case–control studies, it is not possible to measure incidence rates in either of these groups. Nonetheless, from the frequency of exposure observed in cases and controls, it is usually possible to estimate closely the ratio of the incidence rates.

To understand how this can be done, consider a cohort study in which exposed and non-exposed people are followed for a certain period of time. The table below summarizes their experience with regard to a particular disease:

	Diseased	Non-diseased	Total
Exposed	a	b	$a + b$
Non-exposed	c	d	$c + d$

The cumulative incidence of the disease in exposed and non-exposed people over a given period of follow-up is $a/(a + b)$ and $c/(c + d)$, respectively. The relative risk (RR) is the ratio of these:

$$\mathrm{RR} = \frac{a/(a+b)}{c/(c+d)}$$

* This chapter is an excerpt from *Epidemiologic Methods* by T.D. Koepsell and N.S. Weiss (2003).

If the incidence of the disease is relatively low during the follow-up period in both exposed and non-exposed people, then *a* will be small relative to *b* and *c* will be small relative to *d*. Therefore,

$$RR = \frac{a/(a+b)}{c/(c+d)} \approx \frac{a/b}{c/d} = \frac{a/c}{b/d}$$

In this expression, the numerator (*a/c*) is the odds of exposure in people who develop the disease and the denominator (*b/d*) is the odds exposure in people who remain well. Therefore,

$$\textit{Odds ratio}\ \ (OR) = \frac{a/c}{b/d}$$

The numerator can be estimated from a sample of cases, and the denominator can be estimated from a sample of non-cases. Neither estimate is influenced by the proportion of cases among the subjects actually chosen for study.

In the following hypothetical example, assume that 100 of 10 000 people exposed to a particular substance or organism developed a disease, compared with 300 of 90 000 non-exposed people:

	Diseased	Non-diseased	Total
Exposed	100	9 900	10 000
Non-exposed	300	89 700	90 000

Therefore,

$$RR = \frac{100/10\,000}{300/90\,000} = 3.00$$

If a case–control study had been carried out in this population, in which 50 per cent of the cases were included but only 1 per cent of the non-cases, then the following results would have been obtained:

	Diseased	Non-diseased
Exposed	100 × 0.5 = 50	9 900 × 0.01 = 99
Non-exposed	300 × 0.5 = 150	89 700 × 0.01 = 897

$$RR \approx OR = \frac{50/150}{99/897} = 3.02$$

In many studies, controls are chosen as they were in this example; that is, from people who have not developed the disease by the end of the same time period during which other people (the cases) have become ill. In such studies, the less common the disease in both the exposed and non-exposed people during the period, the better the odds ratio will estimate the ratio of cumulative incidence. In the example, only 0.1 per cent and 0.33 per cent of exposed and non-exposed people, respectively, developed the illness: So, the relative cumulative incidence and odds ratio are closely related (3 versus 3.02). However, it is also possible to choose controls from people free of disease only until the corresponding cases have been diagnosed; a person can appear in the study first as a control and later as a case. If this approach is used, the odds ratio will be a valid estimate of the ratio of incidence rates (i.e. cases divided by person–time at risk) irrespective of the disease frequency (Greenland & Thomas 1982; Pearce 1993).

Retrospective ascertainment of exposure status in cases and controls

Epidemiological studies seek to obtain information on exposures present during an aetiologically relevant period of time; that period varies across aetiological relationships. For example, although excess consumption of alcohol predisposes to both motor vehicle injuries and cirrhosis of the liver, it does so during considerably different time intervals before the occurrence of the injury or the onset of the illness, respectively.

Some case–control studies are nested within cohort studies in which specimens (e.g. blood or urine) have been obtained before diagnosis on all cohort members, but have not yet been analysed for the exposure(s) in question. When these analyses are carried out on cohort members who developed a particular illness and on controls selected from the cohort, the results obtained are not influenced by the events occurring after the diagnosis of the illness. (To avoid the possibility of occult illness in cases influencing levels of a suspected aetiological factor, many studies of this type exclude from the analyses specimens obtained in the period before diagnosis that might correspond to the preclinical stage of disease.) Also, among the large majority of case–control studies in which exposure status is not measured until the illness or injury has been diagnosed, some are concerned only with an exposure or characteristic that would have been the same at all times in a person's life. This is true for a genetically determined characteristic such as ABO blood type or the absence of glutathione transferase M_1 activity (an enzyme that metabolizes several potentially carcinogenic constituents of cigarette smoke). Clearly, these studies are no less valid for having had to measure exposure in retrospect.

However, most case–control studies are required to consider explicitly how best to assess in retrospect the subjects' exposure status during one or more possible aetiologically relevant time periods. Possible sources of exposure data include interviews or questionnaires, available records, and physical or laboratory measurements.

Interviews or questionnaires

For many exposures, a subject's memory is an excellent window to the past. A number of important aetiological relationships have been identified through interview-based case–control studies. Generally, study participants will report longer-term and more recent experiences with greater accuracy than shorter-term and more distant ones. Attention to the ways in which questions are asked (Armstrong *et al.* 1992), along with the use of visual aids when appropriate (e.g. pictures of medicines, or containers of household products, and calendars for important life events to enhance recall of the timing of other exposures), will maximize the accuracy of the information received. These efforts, along with the use of the same questions for cases and controls asked in the same way, will also minimize the potential for bias that could result from the subject's or interviewer's awareness of case or control status.

One advantage of exposure ascertainment via interview or questionnaire is that information can be sought for multiple points in the past. It is possible that a given exposure plays an aetiological role only if present at a certain age, for certain duration, or at a certain time in the past. Because there is often little guidance before a study starts that suggests the most relevant age, length, or recency, key exposures are often elicited throughout much of the subject's lifetime. However, care must be taken not to include exposures that took place after the illness began. An instructive example is provided by Victora *et al.* (1989) in a case–control study of infant death from diarrhoea as related to the type of feeding. These investigators asked mothers whether their child was or was not being breastfed immediately before the onset of the fatal illness (mothers of controls were queried about type of feeding prior to a comparable point in time). Mothers were also asked if subsequent to the onset of the illness there had been any changes in the type of feeding; following the development of diarrhoea, many children were switched to formula and cow's milk. Relative to infants who were solely breastfed, those who were supplemented with powdered or cow's milk prior to their illness had about four times the risk of diarrhoeal death. However, the authors showed that if one inappropriately considered the feeding method that was present during the illness, about a 13-fold increase in risk associated with supplementation would have been estimated.

Records

Case–control studies have exploited the presence of vital, registry, employment, medical, and pharmacy records, to name a few, as a means of obtaining information on exposures. However, because the information contained in the records is usually assembled for purposes other than epidemiological research, they may not provide precisely the information desired by the epidemiologist. For example, a death certificate or an occupational record may state an individual's job, but often not his or her actual exposure to the substance(s) of interest to the study. A pharmacy record will indicate a prescription having been filled, but not necessarily whether the patient took the medication on a given day, or took it at all. This sort of imprecision will impair a study's ability to discern a true association between an exposure and a disease—the greater the imprecision, the greater the impairment.

Nonetheless, some very strong associations have been identified through record-based case–control studies. For example, Daling *et al.* (1987) conducted a tumour-registry-based case–control study to test the hypothesis that homosexual men have a relatively high incidence of anal cancer. Although registry data do not specify a man's sexual preference, they do contain information regarding his marital status. The investigators found that three times more men with anal cancer than controls (men with colon or rectal cancer) had never been married. Being single is far from a perfect predictor of homosexuality, of course. Nonetheless, the presence of such a large case–control difference, given the very poor means of gauging the relevant exposure, was a stimulus to conduct interview-based studies that could elicit information regarding sexual history with greater precision. The latter studies showed an exceedingly strong association between anal cancer in men and a history of sexual intercourse with another man (Daling *et al.* 1987).

In case–control studies in which medical records are used to characterize exposure status, care must be taken to restrict the information obtained to that which precedes the case's diagnosis (and the presence of symptoms, if any, that led to the diagnosis). The records of controls must be truncated at similar points in time. Without this safeguard, it is possible that bias will arise because there are systematically more records available to review on cases than controls; the case's illness may have stimulated an enquiry by medical personnel into his or her past, whereas no corresponding enquiry would necessarily have occurred for control subjects.

Physical and laboratory measurements

The recognized limitations of interviews and records in characterizing a variety of potentially relevant exposures have stimulated the conduct of epidemiological studies that use laboratory and other methods of measurement. A woman cannot tell an investigator the level of her reproductive hormones, the concentration of various micronutrients in her blood, or whether her cervix is infected with human papillomavirus, but laboratory tests can. Unfortunately, such tests tell us what these things are only at the time that the specimens have been obtained. For some exposures, there will be a high correlation between the measured level following case and control identification, and that which was present during the aetiologically relevant time period. For example, lead enters and does not leave the dentine of teeth. Therefore, in young school-age children, lead dentine levels are an indicator of cumulative lead exposure, a good portion of which could be relevant to the development of intellectual impairment and other adverse neurological outcomes. In contrast, one would not rely on serum levels of reproductive hormones of postmenopausal cases of breast cancer and controls to indicate what their premenopausal levels were, much less their hormonal status during their very early reproductive years (at which time the hormones may be exerting their greatest impact on future risk of breast cancer).

Case definition

Ideally, the cases in a case–control study would comprise all (or a representative sample of) members of a defined population who develop a given health outcome during a given period of time. For studies of disease aetiology, that outcome is the disease incidence. For studies that seek to determine the efficacy of early disease detection or treatment, the outcome generally is the occurrence of complications of the disease or mortality; such studies have been described in detail elsewhere (Selby 1994; Weiss 1994), and will not be covered any further here.

The population from which cases are to be drawn may be defined geographically or on the basis of other characteristics such as membership in a prepaid health-care plan or an occupational group. The identification of all newly ill people in a defined population can be facilitated by the presence of a reporting system such as a cancer or malformation registry that seeks to accomplish this identification for other purposes. Occasionally, care for the condition being studied may be centralized, so that it will be necessary to review the records of only one or a few institutions to identify all cases in the population in which those institutions are located. However, in many instances, it is not feasible to identify all cases that occur in a given population; therefore, case–control studies are often based on cases identified from hospital records, or from the records of selected providers from whom patients had sought health care. The study by Herbst *et al.* (1971) on vaginal adenocarcinoma was of this type. Whether or not the cases are derived from a defined population, it is necessary that they be drawn in an unselected manner with regard to exposure status; for example, by including in the study all otherwise eligible cases diagnosed or receiving care during a defined time period.

Although the goal of a case–control study of aetiology is to enrol incident cases, under some circumstances it may be necessary to enrol prevalent cases at a particular point in time, irrespective of when each one's illness had begun. For some conditions, the date of occurrence may simply not be known; for example, in the absence of very close sero-monitoring, one generally cannot determine when a person acquired an HIV infection. Furthermore, for uncommon diseases of long duration, an incidence series may yield too few cases for meaningful analysis. The disadvantages of using prevalent cases in a case–control study relate in part to the added problems of accurate exposure ascertainment. For prevalent conditions whose date of diagnosis is known, pre-illness exposure information on study subjects must be obtained for more distant points in the past, on average, than would be necessary for an incident series. For prevalent conditions whose date of occurrence is unknown (e.g. HIV infection), there will be uncertainty as to the best point in time before which one should elicit exposure information. Also, by studying people remaining alive with a given condition, one is simultaneously studying not only aetiological factors but also those that influence survival from the condition.

Ideally, the criteria used to identify and select individual cases for study should be objective with high sensitivity and specificity for the disease. Specificity is of particular concern, because the inadvertent inclusion of people without disease into the case group will generally obscure any true association with the exposure. With this in mind, in the case–control study of Reye's syndrome and antecedent analgesic use conducted by the Centers for Disease Control (Hurwitz *et al.* 1985), only cases with a substantial degree of neurological impairment (stage 2 or higher) were included. The use of this criterion minimized the chances that children with a disease other than Reye's syndrome, which generally would have a lesser degree of severity, would be included in the case group. It also was intended to serve as protection against selective misclassification of Reye's syndrome based on knowledge of exposure status, because the hypothesis of the association of aspirin with Reye's syndrome was well-known by the time the study took place. Conceivably, the knowledge that the child had consumed aspirin could have led some doctors to diagnose Reye's syndrome in cases with an atypical illness.

Control definition

Occasionally, the proportion of ill people who have had a specific exposure is so high, unequivocally more than would be expected in the population from which they were derived, that the presence of an association (although not its magnitude) can be surmised from a case series alone (Cummings & Weiss 1998). For example, when it was learned that all cases of a form of pneumonia that was epidemic in Spain in 1981 had ingested adulterated rapeseed oil, a causal inference was drawn, leading to efforts to eliminate further use of this oil. This action was taken before any formal comparison of cases with controls was made (Tabuenca 1981).

However, in the vast majority of instances, an explicit control group is needed to estimate the frequency and degree of exposure that would have taken place among cases in the absence of an exposure–disease association. An ideal control group would be one that comprises individuals:

1. Selected from a population whose distribution of exposure is that of the population from which the cases arose
2. Who are identical to the cases with respect to their distribution of all characteristics (a) that influence the likelihood and/or degree of exposure, and (b) that, independent of their relation to the exposure, are also related to the occurrence of the illness under study or to its recognition
3. In whom the presence of the exposure can be measured accurately and in a manner that is identical to that used for the cases

If these criteria are not met in a particular study, then selection bias, confounding, or information bias, respectively, will be present.

Minimizing selection bias

If the cases identified in the study are all or a sample of those that occurred in a defined population, one can seek to achieve comparability by choosing as controls people sampled from that same population. For geographically defined populations, a number of different sampling methods have been used, including random digit dialling (RDD) of telephone numbers, area sampling, neighbourhood sampling, voters' lists, population registers, motor vehicle licences, and birth certificates, among others. When cases are members of a prepaid health-care plan who develop an illness or injury, a sample of people who were members of the health plan when the illness or injury occurred can serve as controls. When cases are ill or injured members of an employed population, controls can be selected from this same population.

If cases have not been selected from a definable population at risk for the disease, but from people treated for a particular illness at one or a few hospitals or clinics, then selection bias may be introduced if controls are not chosen from people who, had they developed the illness under study, would have received care at these hospitals or clinics, and if people who do and do not receive care from these sources differ with regard to the frequency or level of exposure.

Therefore, when cases are chosen from a narrow range of health-care providers, controls are often chosen from other ill people treated by these providers. Such ill controls may also be used if, irrespective of the source of the cases, there is no feasible way to sample from the population at large, or if sampling from the general population would result in a substantial level of non-response or information bias. For these reasons, in some studies of fatal illness, exposures in people with a given cause of death are compared with exposures in a sample of people who died from other causes.

However, the choice of ill or deceased controls can itself give rise to selection bias if the illnesses (causes of death) represented in the control group are in some way associated with the exposure of interest. For example, ill or recently deceased people tend to have been smokers of cigarettes more often than other people (McLaughlin *et al.* 1985), because smoking is associated with a variety of causes of illness and death. Because smoking histories of ill people overstate the use of cigarettes in the population from which the cases arose (even if that population cannot be defined), the odds ratio associated with smoking based on the choice of ill people as controls will be spuriously low.

To minimize selection bias related to having chosen ill or deceased controls, an attempt can be made to omit potential controls with conditions known to be related (positively or negatively) to the exposure. For example, in the analysis of a hospital-based case–control study of bladder cancer and earlier use of artificial sweeteners, the investigators excluded from their control group people who were admitted to hospital for obesity-related diseases (Silverman *et al.* 1983). They showed that without this restriction, the control group would have a spuriously high proportion of users of artificial sweeteners relative to the population from which their cases had actually come. This approach will succeed to the extent that one judges correctly which conditions are truly exposure-related, and how accurately the presence of those conditions can be determined. For many exposures, this may pose little problem, and judicious exclusion will yield a control group capable of providing an unbiased result. For others, such as cigarette smoking or alcohol consumption, it has been shown that admitting diagnoses or statements of cause of death are incapable of identifying all people with illnesses related to these exposures (McLaughlin *et al.* 1985).

Some case–control studies simply compare exposure status among subgroups of patients with the same outcome. For example, Laumon *et al.* (2005) obtained blood samples of 10 748 drivers involved in fatal road accidents in France during 2001–2003, and had these analysed for a metabolite of cannabis. The investigators contrasted the proportion testing positive between drivers judged to have been at fault for the crash ('cases') and drivers judged not to have been at fault ('controls'). The results of such a study will be valid when each of these accidents has a single driver at fault, and when it is possible to identify which driver that was. To the extent that these conditions do not hold, the misclassification that ensues will tend to make the size of the observed association smaller than the true one.

Occasionally, controls are chosen from individuals who are tested for the presence of the disease under study and are found not to have it. For example, people demonstrated to have coronary artery occlusion on coronary angiography have been compared with angiography patients without occlusion with regard to potential risk factors (Thom *et al.* 1992). As another example, the prior use of oral contraceptives was compared between women diagnosed with venous thromboembolism and women seen at the same institution for suspected venous thromboembolism who were diagnosed as not having this condition (Bloemenkamp *et al.* 1999). It may be relatively inexpensive to select controls from people who receive the same diagnostic evaluation as do cases, and it is also possible to achieve case–control comparability with regard to the choice of a health-care provider (and the correlates of that choice). This approach can have an impact on the study's validity if the frequency or degree of exposure differs between otherwise comparable members of a population who do and do not receive the test. It will increase the validity if the disease being investigated is generally asymptomatic, and so would not be detected in the absence of testing. Thus, the relation of the use of oral contraceptives with the incidence of *in situ* cancer of the cervix is best studied in women who have undergone cervical screening, by comparing oral contraceptive use between cases of *in situ* cancer and women with a negative screen. This is because:

- In most societies, women who use oral contraceptives are screened more commonly than women who do not.
- *In situ* cancers are asymptomatic and will not be identified in the absence of cervical screening.

Therefore, if controls are chosen from women in general, who may or may not have received cervical screening, an apparent excess of oral contraceptive users would be present among cases of *in situ* cancer even if no true association were present.

However, the choice of test-negative controls can detract from a study's validity if the large majority of the people who develop the disease would soon be diagnosed whether or not the test was administered. There was a controversy in the late 1970s regarding the suitability, in case–control studies of postmenopausal oestrogen use and endometrial cancer, of a control group restricted to women with no evidence of cancer on endometrial biopsy. Among women without endometrial cancer, oestrogen use differs greatly between those who have and have not undergone biopsy, because oestrogen use predisposes to uterine bleeding of non-malignant causes, which often leads to endometrial biopsy. Those investigators who believed that there was a great prevalence of occult endometrial cancer in the population suggested that the optimal control group ought to be women undergoing endometrial biopsy and found not to have cancer (Horwitz & Feinstein 1978). However, the majority of the investigators believed that no such large pool of prevalent, occult disease existed, and that choosing biopsy-negative controls would lead to a spuriously high estimate of oestrogen use in the population at risk, and thus, a spuriously low odds ratio (Shapiro *et al.* 1985).

No matter how controls are defined in a case–control study, selection bias may be introduced to the extent that exposure information is not obtained on all who have been selected to participate. The magnitude of this bias will increase in relation to the frequency of missing data and the degree to which exposure frequencies or levels differ between study subjects on whom exposure status is and is not known. The problem of incomplete ascertainment of exposure on study subjects is particularly common in interview- or questionnaire-based case–control studies. Strategies for minimizing the degree of non-response in case–control studies are discussed in detail elsewhere (Armstrong *et al.* 1992).

Minimizing confounding

Characteristics of confounding variables in case–control studies

Confounding occurs when the estimate of the relationship between an exposure and a disease is distorted by the influence of another factor. In any study design, confounding will occur to the extent that the other factor is associated with both the exposure (although not as a result of the exposure) and the disease or its recognition. In case–control studies alone, a factor may confound even if it is not associated with an altered risk of disease, if the proportions of cases and controls vary across levels or categories of the factor. For example, in a collaborative study of ovarian cancer and use of oral contraceptives (Weiss *et al.* 1981), an attempt was made to identify and interview all incident cases over several years in two American populations. In one of the populations (western Washington State), several controls per case were interviewed, whereas the control-to-case ratio in the other (Utah) was 1:1. Because oral contraceptive use was more common among women in Washington than in Utah, failure to take into account the state of residence in the analysis (e.g. by adjustment) would have led to a spuriously high estimate of the frequency of oral contraceptive use by controls relative to that by the cases.

Means of controlling for confounding

One straightforward way of preventing confounding is to restrict cases and controls to a single category or level of the potentially confounding variable. For example, in their study on physical activity and primary cardiac arrest, Siscovick *et al.* (1982) excluded people with conditions, such as clinically recognized heart disease, that could both predispose to cardiac arrest and might be expected to alter level of activity. A second way is to obtain information on exposures or characteristics that may differ between cases and controls, and then make statistical adjustments for those that are also found to be related to the exposure or characteristic under investigation (Rothman & Greenland 1998).

Finally, it is possible to match one or more controls to each case's category or level of a potentially confounding factor. It is appropriate to match if:

1. The variable is expected to be strongly related to both the exposure and disease. Thus, in a case–control study of breast cancer and use of hair dye, it would make sense to match on gender (if the study has not already been restricted to women) because use of dye is more common among women than men in most cultures. Although confounding by gender could be prevented even without matching by adjustment in the analysis, the statistical precision of the unmatched study would be substantially reduced relative to that of a case–control study having a more similar proportion of female cases and controls.
2. Information on possible matching variables can be obtained inexpensively. There are some means of control selection in which information regarding some confounders can be obtained at no cost. For example, from voters' lists or prepaid health-plan membership records, it would generally be possible to choose directly one or more controls who were identical to a given case's age. Conversely, if a population sampling scheme such as random digit dialling were being employed, the age of the respondent would not be known in advance of approaching him or her. Rather than omitting already contacted controls who did not match a particular case's age, the matching can be done much more broadly; additional control for finer categories of age can be accomplished in the data analysis.
3. Information on exposure status cannot be obtained inexpensively. The higher the cost of exposure ascertainment, the greater the incentive to limit the number of control subjects to the number of cases. Case–control differences regarding confounding factors particularly will reduce the statistical power of a study that does not have a surplus of controls. Enriching the group of controls selected with people more similar to the cases with regard to confounding factors (i.e. matching) can prevent this loss of statistical power.

In case–control studies of genetic characteristics as possible aetiological factors, some investigators have used a matched design in which a specific type of relative (e.g. parent, sibling, or cousin) is chosen as a control for each case (Yang & Khoury 1997; Witte *et al.* 1999). This approach has the advantage of minimizing potential confounding by other genetic characteristics with which the one of interest is associated. However, it has the disadvantage of excluding a possibly large fraction of cases for whom there is no relative available of the type needed to provide a sample for genetic analysis.

It should be remembered that matching alone is not sufficient to eliminate a variable's confounding influence: Failure to consider a matching variable in the analysis of the study can lead to a biased result (Rothman & Greenland 1998). Analyses of studies that have matched controls to cases on a given characteristic can adjust for that characteristic as if no matching had taken place. Alternatively, these analyses can explicitly consider cases and controls as matched sets. In the instance of matched case–control pairs and a dichotomous exposure variable, the following table could be constructed.

	Contents	
Cases	Exposed	Non-exposed
Exposed	*a*	*b*
Non-exposed	c	d

Only the *b* pairs in which the case was exposed but not the matched control, and the *c* pairs in which the reverse was true, would enter the analysis. The odds ratio would be calculated as *b/c*. When there is more than one control per case, the matched odds ratio can be calculated as well (Breslow & Day 1980).

Minimizing information bias

For case–control studies in which information on exposure status is sought via an interview or questionnaire, the chief safeguards against information bias entail asking questions about events that are salient to the respondent, that are framed in an unambiguous way, and that are presented identically to both cases and controls. Employment of these safeguards, however, will not prevent differential accuracy of reporting between cases and controls in all circumstances. Some past exposures or events will simply be more salient to people with an illness, who might have dwelled on possible reasons for its occurrence, than to people without that illness. Other exposures may be viewed as socially undesirable, and there may be a difference between cases and healthy controls in their willingness to admit to them. If the anticipated difference in the quality of information between cases and otherwise appropriate controls is too great, a control group that is less than ideal in other respects may be selected instead so as to minimize the potential for information bias. For example, some studies of prenatal risk factors for a particular congenital malformation that utilize maternal interviews as the source of exposure data have selected as controls infants with other malformations (Rosenberg *et al.* 1983). This control group will provide a more valid result than a control group that consists of infants in general if mothers of malformed and mothers of normal infants report prenatal exposures to a different degree even in the absence of an association, and the exposure in question is not associated with the occurrence of the malformations present in control infants.

Similar reasoning led Daling *et al.* (1987), when conducting their case–control study on anal cancer and a history of anal intercourse, to eschew the geographic population from which their cases had arisen as a sampling frame for controls. They feared that interviews that sought information about prior anal intercourse might be more complete among men with cancer than men in the population at large. Thus, they chose as controls men with a cancer of a different site (colon), which they believed was unlikely to have been aetiologically related to prior anal intercourse.

When the exposure under consideration is sufficiently imprecise or is open to subjective interpretation, there may not be any control group that will provide information comparable to that provided by cases. An instructive example comes from a case–control study on Down's syndrome (Stott 1958), conducted shortly before the chromosomal basis for the aetiology of this condition had been learned. The study sought to determine whether emotional 'shocks' during pregnancy might be a risk factor. The author interviewed mothers of children with Down's syndrome with regard to the occurrence of a 'situation or event [that would be] stress- or shock-producing if this would have been its expected effect on an emotionally stable woman'. Identical interviews were administered to mothers of normal children, and also to mothers of children with mental retardation who did not have Down's syndrome. Even though it is not possible that an emotional shock in pregnancy could play any aetiological role in a condition already determined at conception, a far higher proportion of mothers of cases of Down's syndrome reported an emotional shock than did mothers of normal controls (RR estimated from the data, 17.0). The use of other children with mental retardation as controls only partially reduced the spuriously high relative risk, to a value of 4.3.

When conducting an interview-based study of a rapidly fatal disease, or a disease that impairs a person's ability to provide valid interview data, it is necessary to obtain information from at least some surrogate respondents; typically, these respondents are close relatives of the cases. In general, for purposes of comparability, similar information ought to be obtained from surrogates of controls, even though the control would be expected to provide more accurate data. Results of case–control studies based on exposure information provided by surrogate respondents need to be interpreted with particular caution. Although by no means present in every instance (Nelson *et al.* 1990), there can be a large difference in the validity of the responses given by case and control surrogates. For example, Greenberg *et al.* (1985) investigated the basis for an apparent strong association between cancer mortality and 'nuclear' work among employees of a naval shipyard, which had been found during a comparison of work histories provided by surrogates of men who died from cancer and of those who died of other conditions. They observed that, regarding work in the nuclear part of the industry, surrogates of the cases generally provided information similar to that contained in employment records of the shipyard; in contrast, the surrogates of controls substantially misclassified the nature of their relatives' jobs as not involving radiation. Using the data provided by employment records, which included individual radiation dosimetry, little or no association was found between cancer mortality and radiation exposure received at the shipyard (Rinsky *et al.* 1981).

What was undoubtedly a spuriously negative association was found in a case–control study of lung cancer and passive cigarette smoking that used, for one analysis, information obtained from surrogate respondents (Janerich *et al.* 1985). In this analysis, the relative risk of lung cancer among non-smokers associated with a spouse's having smoked—0.33 (i.e. a 67 per cent reduction in risk)—would seem almost certainly due to a spurious minimization or the denial of smoking by spouses of cases, who may have feared their habit caused their spouse to develop lung cancer.

In most interview-based case–control studies, information is not sought from cases until days to months have elapsed following the diagnosis of their condition. These persons are queried regarding exposures that occurred during what is presumed to be the aetiologically relevant period prior to diagnosis. For controls, for whom there is no 'diagnosis' date, what is the appropriate time frame in which to focus the questions that are asked of them? If exposures that occurred some time in the past, or that occurred over an extended period, are most likely to be relevant, controls are generally asked about events during the same calendar time as the cases. However, when studying exposures that could act acutely to lead to illness, having the case recall events immediately prior to illness and the control do the same for the corresponding time in the past may lead to bias: Only the cases will have the onset of their illness to help in recalling events that took place shortly prior to that time. This difference could lead to relatively more complete ascertainment of exposure among cases.

In response to this concern, some case–control studies investigating potentially rapidly acting exposures query controls about the time period prior to the date of interview instead of the date of their case's diagnosis (or, in an unmatched study, the date of a typical case's diagnosis). So, in a study of risk factors for meningococcal disease in adolescents (Tully *et al.* 2006), cases were asked about events during the two weeks prior to diagnosis (which occurred, on average, 53 days before the interview) and controls about events during the two weeks just prior to the interview itself. The investigators felt that the plausibility of case–control comparability on recall of exposures involved in transmission (e.g. 'intimate kissing with multiple partners') would be greater using this approach than one in which the controls were asked about a two-week period ending 53 days prior to the interview. However, although a sound approach when trying to estimate the short-term influence of many exposures, this strategy can backfire if recall of an exposure diminishes over time to the same degree in cases and controls. For example, in the study of meningococcal disease, a far smaller proportion of cases than controls reported attending religious observances during their respective two-week intervals (adjusted odds ratio = 0.1, 95% confidence interval = 0.02–0.6). Almost certainly, this difference had more to do with relatively poorer recall of churchgoing among cases (who had to think back some two months) than to a genuine salutary effect of church attendance on the incidence of meningococcal disease.

Incomparable assessment of exposure status between cases and controls is not confined to interview- or questionnaire-based studies. Most laboratory-based studies seek to prevent this by testing samples blind to case and control status. If feasible, it is desirable to also carry out this blinding for studies in which exposure is to be determined from medical or other records. However, there are instances in which the nature of the information available in records has already been influenced by whether the subject is a case or a control. For example, it was found that among 100 infertile women who underwent laparoscopy (Stratby *et al.* 1982), 21 had endometriosis. Only 2 per cent of the 200 women who underwent laparoscopy for another indication, tubal ligation, were noted in the procedural records as having endometriosis. However, the interpretation of this association is unclear, because the identification and/or recording of endometriosis in cases and controls (women undergoing tubal ligation) may well have been incomparable—only in the infertile women was the laparoscopy expressly done as a diagnostic tool to investigate the possible presence of conditions such as endometriosis.

Estimating attributable risk from results of case–control studies

Occasionally, a case–control study identifies a large odds ratio relating an exposure to a disease, and for this and other reasons, a causal influence of the exposure may be suspected. The decision to seek to limit or eliminate that exposure requires weighing its negative and positive consequences. This weighing must be done in absolute, rather than in relative terms, because the same relative increase (or decrease) in risk is of far greater consequence for common than for rare outcomes. The absolute increase in the risk of disease believed to be due to a dichotomous exposure, sometimes referred to as the 'attributable risk' (AR), can be estimated directly from data gathered in cohort studies or randomized trials as the difference between the incidence among exposed (I_e) and non-exposed people (I_n). The formula $I_e - I_n$ can be rewritten as $RR(I_n) - I_n$, or as $I_n(RR - 1)$. Because the relative risk can be estimated from the results of a case–control study by means of the odds ratio, the only additional piece of information needed to estimate the attributable risk is an estimate of I_n. For the population in which the study has been conducted, I_n can be estimated if:

1. The overall incidence (I) of the disease in that population is known or can be approximated.
2. The frequency of exposure (P_e) in the controls selected for study reasonably reflects that of the population that gave rise to the cases.

Given (1) and (2),

$$\begin{aligned} I &= I_e(P_e) + I_n(1-P_e) \\ &= I_n RR(P_e) + I_n(1-P_e) \\ &= I_n(P_e[RR-1]+1) \end{aligned}$$

So,

$$I_n = \frac{I}{P_e(RR-1)+1}$$

Therefore,

$$AR = \frac{I(RR-1)}{P_e+(RR-1)} = \frac{I}{P_e+1/(RR-1)}$$

For example, consider a disease with an incidence rate of 10 per 100 000 per year in a population in which 5 per cent of people have been exposed during a relevant period of time. The following table summarizes data from a case–control study conducted in that population:

Exposed	Cases (%)	Controls (%)	OR
Yes	15	5	3.35
No	85	95	1

The attributable risk that corresponds to the estimated 3.35-fold increase in risk is

$$\frac{10}{0.05+1/(3.35-1)} = 21.0 \text{ Per } 100\,000 \text{ Per year}$$

From the results of case–control studies that suggest a causal relation, it is also possible to estimate the percentage of exposed people with the disease who developed it because of their exposure, rather than through one or more causal pathways not involving the exposure. This measure, often termed the 'attributable risk per cent' (AR%) among exposed people, is defined as

$$\frac{I_e - I_n}{I_e} \times 100$$

It can be described in terms of the relative risk alone:

$$AR\% = \frac{I_e}{I_e} - \frac{I_n}{I_e} = 1 - \frac{1}{RR} = \frac{RR-1}{RR} \times 100$$

Therefore, the results of a case–control study that provide a valid estimate of the relative risk (via the odds ratio) can provide the attributable risk per cent as well, with no additional assumptions or sources of data. It is also possible to estimate the percentage of a disease's occurrence in the population as a whole that resulted from the actions of given exposure. This measure, the 'population attributable risk per cent' (PAR%) or 'aetiological fraction', is simply the attributable risk per cent multiplied by the proportion of cases in that population who were exposed (P_e):

$$PAR\% = AR\%\ P_e$$

In the present example,

$$AR\% = \frac{3.35-1}{3.35} = 70.1\%$$

And

$$PAR\% = 70.1\%\ (0.15) = 10.5\%$$

The role of case–control studies in understanding disease aetiology

Randomized trials will not be able to answer all questions regarding the reasons for disease occurrence. Many potential disease-causing or disease-preventing exposures cannot be manipulated, either at all—for example, most genetic characteristics—or in any practical way for purposes of a study. For many exposure–disease relationships, either the disease is too uncommon or the induction period is too long to conduct a randomized trial that is not unfeasibly large in size or long in duration. Finally, it generally will not be possible to conduct separate randomized trials to measure the impact of all potential types, amounts, and durations of a class of exposure.

Also, it is not possible to rely solely on cohort studies for answers. Just as with randomized trials, the disease outcome being studied may be too rare to allow a cohort approach to be useful. This explains why the aetiologies of vaginal adenocarcinoma and Reye's syndrome, for example, have been evaluated exclusively by case–control studies—these diseases are simply too uncommon for most cohort studies to generate any cases, even in 'exposed' individuals. Prospective cohort studies are also of limited use when the induction period for the exposure–disease relationship is either very short or very long. If the induction period is very short and the exposure status of an individual varies over time, a cohort study would need to assess exposure status repeatedly among cohort members. For this reason, studies of alcohol consumption and the occurrence of injuries typically are case–control in nature (Holcomb 1938). Similarly, unless information on exposure status can be ascertained retrospectively, it would not be feasible to initiate a cohort study of a suspected aetiologic relation that requires a very long time (perhaps several decades) to manifest itself.

Although case–control studies may be of particular value in the evaluation of the aetiology of uncommon disease, they may have difficulty in obtaining statistically precise results if the frequency of the exposure in the population under study is either extremely common or extremely uncommon (Crombie 1981). Thus, only an association as strong as the one between cigarette smoking and lung cancer could have emerged reliably from case–control studies of several hundred British men conducted in the late 1940s (Doll & Hill 1950), given that well over 90 per cent of that population were cigarette smokers. For very uncommon exposures—for example, occupational exposure to a specific substance suspected of posing a risk to health, or an infrequently prescribed drug—barring a strong observed association based on a large number of subjects, even the best-designed case–control study will usually offer no more than a suggestion of the presence or absence of a relation with regard to the occurrence of a given illness.

Conclusion

- Case–control studies compare ill or injured persons (cases) with those at risk of the illness or injury (controls) in terms of prior exposures or characteristics.
- From most case–control studies of a given condition it is possible to obtain an estimate of the relative risk associated with an exposure by dividing the odds of exposure in cases by the odds of exposure in controls (odds ratio).
- The validity of the results of a case–control study can be compromised by differences between cases and controls with regard to exposures or characteristics that are also correlated with the likelihood or degree of the exposure in question.
- In most case–control studies, ascertainment of exposure status is undertaken after the cases have sustained their illness or injury. These studies will produce an unbiased estimate of an exposure–disease association to the extent that exposure status prior to disease onset can be ascertained with a high degree of sensitivity and specificity.
- In a setting in which (a) randomization of potential study participants is unethical or infeasible and (b) the outcome under study is an uncommon one, data from case–control studies may be the best available by which to judge a potential cause–effect relationship between the exposure and outcome.

References

Armstrong B.K., White E., and Saracci R. *Principles of exposure measurement in epidemiology*. New York (NY): Oxford University Press; 1992.

Bloemenkamp K.W.M., Rosendaal F.R., Buller H.R. *et al.* Risk of venous thrombosis with use of current low-dose oral contraceptives is not explained by diagnostic suspicion and referral bias. *Archives of Internal Medicine* 1999;**159**:65–70.

Breslow N.E. and Day N.E. *Statistical methods in cancer research*. Vol. 1: the analysis of case-control studies. Lyon, France: IARC Press; 1980. IARC Scientific Publication No. 32.

Crombie I.K. The limitations of case-control studies in the detection of environmental carcinogens. *Journal of Epidemiology and Community Health* 1981;**35**:281–7.

Cummings P. and Weiss N.S. Case series and exposure series: the role of studies without controls in providing information about the etiology of injury or disease. *Injury Prevention* 1998;**4**:34–57.

Daling J.R., Weiss N.S., Hislop T.G. *et al.* Sexual practices, sexually transmitted disease, and the incidence of anal cancer. *New England Journal of Medicine* 1987;**317**:973–7.

Doll R. and Hill A.B. Smoking and carcinoma of the lung. *British Medical Journal* 1950;**2**:739–48.

Greenberg E.R., Rosner B., Hennekens C. *et al.* An investigation of bias in a study of nuclear shipyard workers. *American Journal of Epidemiology* 1985;**121**:301–8.

Greenland S. and Thomas D.C. On the need for the rare disease assumption in case-control studies. *American Journal of Epidemiology* 1982;**116**: 547–53.

Greenwald P., Barlow J.J., Nasca P. *et al.* Vaginal cancer after maternal treatment with synthetic estrogens. *New England Journal of Medicine* 1971;**285**:390–3.

Herbst A.L., Ulfelder H., and Poskanzer D.C. Adenocarcinoma of the vagina: association of maternal stilbestrol therapy with tumor appearance in young women. *New England Journal of Medicine* 1971;**284**:878–81.

Holcomb R.L. Alcohol in relation to traffic accidents. *Journal of the American Medical Association* 1938;**111**:1076–85.

Horwitz R.I. and Feinstein A.R. Alternative analytic methods for case-control studies of estrogens and endometrial cancer. *New England Journal of Medicine* 1978;**299**:1089–94.

Hurwitz E.S., Barren M.J., Bregman D. *et al.* Public Health Service Study on Reye's syndrome and medications. Report of the pilot phase. *New England Journal of Medicine* 1985;**313**:849–57.

Janerich D.T., Thompson W.D., Varela L.R. *et al.* Lung cancer and exposure to tobacco smoke in the household. *New England Journal of Medicine* 1985;**323**:632–6.

Laumon B., Godegbeku B., Martin J.L. *et al.* Cannabis intoxication and fatal road crashes in France: population-based case-control study. *British Medical Journal* 2005;**331**:1371–4.

McLaughlin J.K., Blot W.J., Mehl E.S. *et al.* Problems in the use of dead controls in case-control studies. II. Effect of excluding certain causes of death. *American Journal of Epidemiology* 1985;**122**:485–94.

Nelson L.M., Longstreth W.T., Koepsell T.D. *et al.* Proxy respondents in epidemiologic research. *Epidemiologic Reviews* 1990;**12**:71–86.

Pearce N. What does the odds ratio estimate in a case-control study? International Journal of Epidemiology 1993;22:1189–92.

Rinsky R.A., Zumwolde R.D., Waxweiller R.J. *et al.* Cancer mortality at a naval nuclear shipyard. *Lancet* 1981;**1**:231–5.

Rosenberg L., Mitchell A.A., Parsells J.L. *et al.* Lack of relation of oral clefts to diazepam use during pregnancy. *New England Journal of Medicine* 1983;**309**:1282–5.

Rothman K.J. and Greenland S. *Modern epidemiology*. 2nd ed. Philadelphia (PA): Lippincott-Raven; 1998.

Selby J.V. Case-control evaluations of treatment and program efficacy. *Epidemiologic Reviews* 1994;**46**:91–101.

Shapiro S., Kelly J.P., Rosenberg L. *et al.* Risk of localized and widespread endometrial cancer in relation to recent and discontinued use of conjugated estrogens. *New England Journal of Medicine* 1985; **313**:969–72.

Silverman D.T., Hoover R.N., and Swanson G.M. Artificial sweeteners and lower urinary tract cancer: hospital vs. population controls. *American Journal of Epidemiology* 1983;**117**:326–34.

Siscovick D.S., Weiss N.S., Hallstrom A.P. *et al.* Physical activity and primary cardiac arrest. *Journal of the American Medical Association* 1982;**248**:3113–7.

Stott D.H. Some psychosomatic aspects of casualty in reproduction. *Journal of Psychosomatic Research* 1958;**3**:42–55.

Stratby J.H., Molgaard C.A., Coulam C.B. *et al.* Endometriosis and infertility: a laparoscopic study of endometriosis among fertile and infertile women. *Fertility and Sterility* 1982;**38**:667–72.

Tabuenca J.M. Toxic-allergic syndrome caused by ingestion of rapseed oil denatured with aniline. *Lancet* 1981;**2**:567–8.

Thom D.H., Grayston J.T., Siscovick D.S. *et al.* Association of prior infection with Chlamydia pneumoniae and angiographically demonstrated coronary artery disease. *Journal of the American Medical Association* 1992;**268**:68–72.

Tully J., Viner R.M., Coen P.G. *et al.* Risks and protective factors for meningococcal disease in adolescents. *British Medical Journal* 2006;**332**:445–50.

Ulfelder H. and Robboy S.J. The embryologic development of the human vagina. *American Journal of Obstetrics and Gynecology* 1976;**126**:769–76.

Victora C.G., Smith P.G., Vaughan J.P. *et al.* Infant feeding and deaths due to diarrhea. *American Journal of Epidemiology* 1989;**129**:1032–41.

Weiss N.S., Lyon J.L., Liff J.M. *et al.* Incidence of ovarian cancer in relation to the use of oral contraceptives. *International Journal of Cancer* 1981;**28**:669–71.

Weiss N.S. Application of the case-control method in the evaluation of screening. *Epidemiologic Reviews* 1994;**16**:102–8.

Witte J.S., Gauderman W.J., and Thomas D.C. Asymptotic bias and efficiency in case-control studies of candidate genes and gene-environment interactions: basic family designs. *American Journal of Epidemiology* 1999;**149**:693–705.

Yang Q. and Khoury M.J. Evolving methods in genetic epidemiology. III. Gene-environment interaction in epidemiologic research. *Epidemiologic Reviews* 1997;**19**:33–43.

6.6

Cohort studies

Alvaro Muñoz and F. Javier Nieto

Introduction

Cohort studies constitute one of the basic types of designs in epidemiologic research. The key element of cohort studies is time. Specifically, a cohort (i.e. group of individuals) who at enrolment is free from the disease (i.e. outcome) whose natural history is of interest and who have heterogeneous profiles of putative risk factors (whose simplest form is as exposed or unexposed) is followed over time. The central aim of this type of study is to determine the occurrence of an event of interest (e.g. disease, death) and to characterize its heterogeneity according to constellations of risk factors.

Following exposed and unexposed individuals over time, cohort studies are uniquely equipped to describe the processes and mechanisms by which exposures relate to the development of disease. Cohort studies are the primary tool to describe '*time* and *medicine*' as characterized by Samet (Samet 2000). They provide the data to describe *when* diseases occur and to track their consequences over time. Factors that cause disease or early signs of disease can be monitored over time as well. The diversity of the individuals followed in a cohort study provides the data to identify the risk factors that make certain individuals more susceptible to developing disease. Data collected in cohort studies are useful to describe the prognostic value of markers of exposures. This is described by providing estimates of the distribution of disease-free times in individuals with different values of exposures over time. Multisite cohort studies may serve the additional role of characterizing *where* diseases occur and to what extent diseases are spread in different geographical locations.

A cohort study with an adequate sample and follow-up period provides a means to determine how the exposure factors influence the natural history of the disease of interest, making this design the paradigm of epidemiologic research. Once a measure of the frequency of disease occurrence (e.g. incident cases in person-years, which is the number of cases expected among 100 person-years) is adopted, cohort studies allow the direct comparison of the risk of becoming ill in several groups; for instance, exposed and non-exposed to a specific factor. The comparison can be *relative*, that is, how many times higher (or lower) is the risk in the exposed compared with the unexposed (*relative risk*), or *absolute*, that is, how much difference in risk is there between the exposed and non-exposed (*attributable risk*). Briefly, the relative risk gives an idea of the strength of the association, which has considerable relevance if the aim is to investigate the causal relationship between exposure and disease; on the other hand, the attributable risk measures the change of incidence due to the exposure in question, which has great importance from the public health perspective because it quantifies the burden of disease that an exposure exerts in a population (Levin 1953; Uter *et al.* 2001).

The identification of exposures and risk factors for disease provides a basis for prevention. There are numerous examples of cohort-based exposure–disease associations that have resulted in beneficial prevention strategies: For instance, to prevent lung cancer, cigarette smoking should be avoided; to prevent infection with human immunodeficiency virus (HIV), high-risk sexual practices (e.g. unprotected anal receptive intercourse) and injection with unsterile needles should be avoided; to prevent the development of acquired immunodeficiency syndrome (AIDS) and death among individuals infected with HIV, high levels of HIV-RNA in plasma should be avoided (by treatment); to prevent heart disease, low levels of high-density and high levels of low-density lipids should be avoided (by diet, exercise, and/or medications which lower low-density lipids); to prevent cervical cancer, infection with human papilloma virus (HPV) should be avoided. Needless to say, there are instances in which the design of solid prevention strategies faces the complexity of multifactorial aetiology and of exposures that cluster so that exposures have to be taken into account jointly, and the lack of such recognition may lead to ascribing to a particular exposure an effect that is not appropriate. When an exposure of interest clusters with others, acting only on that exposure may not result in successful prevention strategies; for example, based on data from cohort studies, high levels of beta-carotene markers (purportedly resulting from appropriate diets) have been associated with protection against cancer (Willett *et al.* 1984), but supplementation with beta carotene only has not resulted in a lower incidence of cancer in clinical trials (ATBC Cancer Prevention Study Group 1994; Virtamo *et al.* 2003).

Types of cohort studies

This chapter refers to observational cohort studies, in which the investigator documents when the disease occurs and what exposures (including possible interventions available to individuals being followed) are present at different time points. The cohort design shares with the experimental design or controlled clinical trial the temporal relationship between exposure and disease, of the putative cause with the supposed effect. The clinical trial design is a special type of cohort study in which the study subjects are randomly assigned to the different experimental groups. The difference between these study designs lies on the weight or validity of the conclusions regarding the potential causal relationships between exposure and disease, given the inherent limitation of observational designs to control the problem of the potential confounding variables not identified by the investigator. The role of randomization in clinical trials is to make the two groups comparable so that the effect of the therapy can be determined.

Depending on when the data not fixed by the investigators are collected, other terms are used to refer to epidemiological study designs (Vandenbroucke 1991). In cohort studies and clinical trials, the investigator selects (fixes) study participants according to the exposure and conducts the studies to obtain data on the event of interest. In contrast, in case–control studies, the investigator selects the participants according to the occurrence of the event of interest and the study is conducted to obtain data on exposures deemed to have caused the event. Cohort studies and clinical trials are also called *prospective studies*, which contrast with *retrospective studies*, a term typically utilized for case–control studies.

In some studies, the investigator collects the data *concurrently* with the study being conducted, and in others, the data are available before the study is designed and the study is conducted to obtain that data (i.e. the data for the study precedes its conduct or the study is *non-concurrent*). This type of design is called 'retrospective study' by some authors (Vandenbroucke 1991; Kelsey *et al.* 1986), a term that can cause confusion because, as mentioned, it is also used for case–control studies. It is possible that studies collect data concurrently for some participants and non-concurrently (*historically*) for the remainder of the study population.

The simplest cohort design is to obtain exposure data at baseline and follow up individuals to only obtain data for when the event of interest occurs. A richer design includes regularly scheduled visits at which data on exposures are updated, and in many cases, biological samples are collected for testing to assess those exposures. Cohort studies with regularly scheduled visits for updating exposure information and/or determining outcomes are referred to as *panel studies* (Kelsey *et al.* 1986). If, in addition, the outcome of interest is not an event but the profile of a biomarker over time (e.g. change in kidney function measured by filtration rate), panel studies are referred to as *longitudinal studies*.

Design issues in cohort studies

The nature of a cohort study provides the temporal structure necessary to associate a particular exposure with a subsequent event of interest. Documentation of the time sequences of exposures and events generates data upon which the course of event development can be modelled. Such data provide flexibility to define the study outcome based on to the length of time elapsed between exposure and event. The time at which an exposure first occurs, placing individuals at risk for event development, is referred to as the *origin* (e.g. birth in population-level epidemiology, infection with a virus or bacteria in infectious disease epidemiology). Ideally, a cohort study will have complete data of the time elapsed between the origin and the event of interest for as many participants as possible. However, in most studies, not all individuals are followed up from the origin: Some will have been at risk for some time since the origin when enrolled into the cohort study. Those followed up from the origin are called the *incident* cohort and those entering the study after certain duration from the origin are called the *prevalent* cohort. Implementation of the appropriate statistical methods to combine incident and prevalent cohorts may not only yield more efficient estimates but also provide the means for appropriately describing the timing of events beyond the study duration (Muñoz *et al.* 1997).

For some diseases, the origin is well defined and observable, such as employment into an occupation deemed to place workers at risk for health events. For others, the origin is well-defined but difficult to observe, such as infection with a virus (e.g. sexual transmission of HPV, whose occurrence can be determined in a cohort study by following uninfected sexually active individuals with regularly scheduled visits at which the participants are tested for presence of antibodies to HPV). Still others do not have a well-defined origin, as in the case of end-stage renal disease in which the origin may be the time when a physiological defect is identified but may also be the time at which high blood pressure occurs and evolves into a chain of events conducive to renal disease. When the origin is not well-defined, data from cohort studies are typically assembled to describe the incidence of the event of interest (e.g. events per 100 person-years at risk) according to strata based on demographic attributes such as age and gender as well as biomarkers of disease progression (e.g. low-density lipoprotein cholesterol for cardiovascular disease, amount of a virus in infected individuals for infectious diseases). Cohort studies with data on individuals from origin to the event of interest as well as with baseline information and updated information on predictors at regular intervals between the origin and event provide the most complete data to describe the natural history of a disease (Muñoz *et al.* 1992, 1997; Muñoz & Xu 1996).

Study population

In a cohort design, the study population comprises individuals who are exposed or unexposed to the suspected risk factors and who are at risk for the disease of interest. In other words, all cohort members need to be *susceptible* to the disease under study. Thus, for example, if the aim is to investigate risk factors for uterine cancer, the basal examination is usually used to detect the persons at risk, which in this case are women who have not undergone surgical removal of the uterus (hysterectomy) and who have no clinical evidence of uterine cancer. If the risk for an infectious disease is investigated, it is of interest to exclude from the beginning individuals who are not susceptible to infection by the organism of interest (e.g. CCR5 homozygous individuals are not susceptible to HIV infection) and individuals who in spite of being infected are immune to disease progression. In the case of chronic diseases (e.g. cardiovascular diseases, cancer, hypertension, diabetes), the common practice is to exclude from the cohort individuals who already have clinical manifestations of the disease, which is determined at the baseline examination.

Once the study population has been deemed to be free of the event whose occurrence is to be documented during the proposed follow-up, it should be ensured that the participants have enough variability in the presence and/or magnitude of exposure to the risk factor or factors of interest. Logically, if the exposure were to be distributed homogeneously in a large part of the cohort, it would be practically impossible to detect an association between that exposure and the disease. Thus, for example, if certain components of drinking water were to be cardiovascular risk factors, it would be difficult to detect this association in a study limited to a locality in which the characteristics of the water supply are uniform (Rose 1985). After being selected, participants of a cohort study are classified according to the exposure factors at the baseline (initial) examination; exposure status can be updated throughout the follow-up if the participants are re-examined at regular intervals subsequent to the baseline examination.

The cohort can be the totality (or almost the totality) of a geographically and temporally defined population. For example, Hoffmans *et al.* (1988) constructed a non-concurrent study of mortality among Dutch males born in 1932. This cohort included the totality of the 84349 Dutch males who were 18 years old in 1950, when they were examined for eligibility to military service; the investigators used the data collected at baseline (when the individuals were 18 years old) to describe the relationship between obesity at 18 years and subsequent cause-specific mortality (Hoffmans *et al.* 1989).

Instead of the totality of a population, it is more common to include only a fraction or a sample of a population defined temporally and geographically. For instance, as outlined in Table 6.6.1, the Framingham study was initiated at the beginning of the 1950s in Framingham, Massachusetts (USA), with the goal of studying the incidence of and risk factors for cardiovascular diseases (Dawber 1980). From a list of residents aged 35–59 years (18000 persons in total), 6507 adults were randomly selected, among whom only 4469 agreed to participate in the initial examination. In order to compensate for the unexpectedly high rate of refusal, the investigators decided to include 734 individuals who, although not part of the random sample, had expressed interest in being part of the cohort. Of the resulting 5203 participants in the baseline examination, 76 persons were excluded for having clinical manifestations of cardiovascular disease, leaving a total of 5127 participants in the Framingham Heart Study cohort. The follow-up consisted of physical examinations every 2 years with comprehensive data collection particularly emphasizing on diet, physical activity, and stress.

The generalization of results obtained from a cohort study whose participants are a sample from a sole population may have serious limitations, which are overcome by other studies that enrol participants from diverse populations. Indeed, the tradition initiated by the Framingham cohort study was complemented by three large cohort studies of cardiovascular disease conducted in the 1980s, which covered practically the whole spectrum of adults (≥ 18 years) as well as diverse ethnic and socioeconomic groups in the United States. Specifically, the CARDIA study (Friedman *et al.* 1988) recruited a total of 5115 persons between 18 and 30 years of age in four states; the ARIC study (ARIC Investigators 1989) cohort comprised 15800 persons aged 45–64 years at the beginning of the study and residents of four states; and the CHS (Fried *et al.* 1991)

Table 6.6.1 Examples of cohorts in prospective studies

	Framingham	MACS	Norwegian electricians
Study aims	Incidence and risk factors for cardiovascular diseases and hypertension	Natural history of HIV infection and AIDS	Relationship between electromagnetic radiation and cancer incidence
Type of study	Concurrent	Concurrent	Non-concurrent
Date	1949–current	1984–current	1960–1991
Study population	Adult residents in Framingham (MA, USA)	Homosexual men in four metropolitan areas of the United States	Electricians in the 1960 Norwegian census
Simple size	5127	6972	37945
Sex	Males and females	Male	Males
Age at baseline (years)	30–62	18–70	20–70
Active follow-up	Study visits every 2 years including physical exam, electrocardiogram, and laboratory exams	Study visits every 6 months with extensive interviews including behaviour and medical care, physical exam, laboratory exams, and collection of blood samples for national repository	—
Passive follow-up	◆ Clinical records (in case of hospitalization) ◆ Death certificates	◆ Clinical records ◆ Death certificates ◆ National Death Index	◆ Cancer registries ◆ Death certificates

Sources: Dawber T.R. *The Framingham study. The epidemiology of atherosclerotic disease.* Cambridge (MA): Harvard University Press; 1980; Kaslow R.A., Ostrow D.G., Detels R. *et al.* The Multicenter AIDS Cohort Study: rationale, organization, and selected characteristics of the participants. *American Journal of Epidemiology* 1987;**126**:310–8 and Dudley J., Jin S., Hoover D. *et al.* The Multicenter AIDS Cohort Study: retention after 9-1/2 years. *American Journal of Epidemiology* 1995;**142**:323–30; Tynes T., Andersen A., Langmark F. Incidence of cancer in Norwegian workers potentially exposed to electromagnetic fields. *American Journal of Epidemiology* 1992;**136**:81–8.

followed up 2955 participants 65 years or older in another four communities of the United States.

In addition to strict temporal and geographic criteria, a cohort can also be defined by a group of individuals sharing common characteristics, which facilitates the follow-up and/or the accuracy and precision of the data to be collected. For example, the Multicenter AIDS Cohort Study (MACS) (Kaslow *et al.* 1987; Dudley *et al.* 1995) comprised homosexual men in four metropolitan areas of the United States with the overall aim of describing the natural history of HIV infection and AIDS, from the risk factors of infection with HIV to the hazard of death among those developing AIDS (see Table 6.6.1). Participants were recruited by close communication with community members and by active recruitment at gathering places. The cohort had been assembled before the virus (HIV) was identified as the causative agent of AIDS in 1985. The investigators had the foresight to collect blood samples at enrolment in 1984, which proved to be extremely valuable in 1987 when the test developed to identify antibodies against HIV was used to determine not only who were already infected at enrolment but also those among the HIV negative at baseline who subsequently seroconverted, based on the testing of blood samples collected every six months. The subcohort with antibodies to HIV at baseline is a classical example of a prevalent cohort, and those among the HIV negative at baseline who subsequently tested positive are an example of an incident cohort.

From April 1984 through March 1985, a cohort of 4954 men was recruited into the MACS in four metropolitan areas of the United States (Baltimore, Chicago, Los Angeles, and Pittsburgh). To increase minority enrolment, an additional 625 men, 69.3 per cent of whom were non-Caucasian, were recruited in 1987–91. To address issues of long-term effectiveness of therapies and their putative adverse effects, 1393 men were additionally enrolled in 2001–2003. The entire MACS cohort, therefore, consisted of 6972 men, 2883 (41 per cent) of whom were seroprevalent for HIV at entry into the study. All men were followed up every six months with repeat interviews, physical examinations, and collection of blood. Serologic tests for HIV antibody were routinely carried out at each visit. Up to September 2006, the dates of last negative and first positive visits (i.e. seroconverters) were known for 614 men. Using blood samples collected at each semi-annual visit in order to characterize the level of HIV-induced immunosuppression, mononuclear cells were analysed by two-colour flow cytometry with antibodies specific for CD3, CD4, and CD8. Confirmation of AIDS diagnoses were made by obtaining physician and hospital summaries and by reviewing medical records; 1877 AIDS cases were observed up to September 2006. Deaths were monitored by follow-up and through an ongoing search of death records. A total of 1956 participants died before September 2006. One of the principal investigators of the MACS (B. Frank Polk) led efforts in 1987–8 using similar methods to assemble a parallel cohort of injecting drug users (Vlahov *et al.* 1991). In 1994, the Women's Interagency HIV Cohort Study (Barkan *et al.* 1988) assembled a cohort of approximately 4000 high-risk or HIV-infected women to parallel and complement the MACS, which has resulted in mutually beneficial collaborations under a common data-coordinating centre.

When a specific registry with baseline data is available, it provides the opportunity to conduct a non-concurrent cohort study. For example, Nieto *et al.* (1992) used a registry of physical examinations carried out on schoolchildren between 1933 and 1945 in Hagerstown (MD, USA) to assemble a non-concurrent cohort of about 13 000 children in order to study the relationship between childhood obesity and adult mortality; the baseline information obtained between 1933 and 1945 was linked to the mortality experience of the cohort up to 1985. In other historical cohorts, the study population is defined from the beginning as a function of the exposure factors to be investigated. Thus, participants are selected explicitly according to the presence or absence of the characteristics considered to be possible risk factors, such as a cohort of Norwegian electricians. As summarized in Table 6.6.1, this historical cohort of 37 945 workers was defined from the registry of occupations of the working population in Norway according to the 1960 census (Tynes *et al.* 1992).

Baseline visit

The objective of the baseline visit in a concurrent cohort study is generally the classification of the study participants according to the exposure factor or factors under investigation. Furthermore, as discussed earlier, it is important to determine that the participants to be followed are indeed at risk for developing the event of interest. For example, Furth *et al.* (2006) designed a cohort of children with chronic kidney disease to determine the risk factors for progression towards end-stage renal disease; for this, they recruited 540 children aged 1–16 years with an estimated glomerular filtration rate of between 30 and 90 ml/min/1.73 m^2, indicating a level of insufficiency in their kidney function that put them at risk of end-stage renal disease.

The most important component of a cohort study is time: Specifically, the follow-up of participants in the study to properly characterize the temporal evolution of exposures and outcomes. At the time of recruitment, it is essential to convey to the participants the need to be retained in the study over time. Hence, potential participants who are unable or unwilling to return for subsequent examinations or to be followed up for the development of events of interest should not be recruited.

In the baseline and follow-up visits, information is collected about the evolution of the exposure of interest as well as about potential confounding variables and effect modifiers. Equally important is to collect information that facilitates the subsequent tracking of study participants for the follow-up visits. For example, in the initial visit of the ARIC study (ARIC Investigators 1989), the phone numbers and addresses of the primary physician and at least three relatives or friends of each participant were obtained. In addition, it is essential to obtain personal identifiers that will allow linkages with morbidity and mortality registries (such as cancer registries, national death indexes). These personal identifiers should be kept strictly confidential and be used only for the purposes authorized by the participants when they signed the consent to participate in the study.

In its simplest form, the baseline visit can take place over a single continuous time period until the desired sample size is reached. In many cases, however, additional participants are recruited (i) to replace those who have developed the event of interest or who have been lost to follow-up; (ii) to include groups of individuals who were under-represented in the original recruitment; and/or (iii) to respond to new scientific challenges due to the changing nature of the epidemiology of the disease of interest (e.g. new therapies introduced in 1995 changed a lethal infectious disease [AIDS] into a chronic condition highly controlled by effective suppression of viral replication in HIV-infected individuals [Schneider *et al.* 2005]).

Follow-up

The follow-up can be active, by repeated contacts via successive visits to a health centre, mailed questionnaires, or phone calls. Sometimes, the different forms of contacting participants are alternated. For example, in the follow-up of the ARIC study, participants were invited every three years to return to the clinic for a new physical examination and complementary assessments (ARIC Investigators 1989); in addition, each participant was called every year and asked about illnesses and hospitalizations occurring in the interim period since the last clinic visit. In the MACS, the visits are scheduled every six months and take place in dedicated settings instead of in a clinic. This is in contrast to clinic cohort studies in which visits take place according to the health needs of the participants.

For certain diseases and events (e.g. cancer), external sources (i.e. registries) can be used to record events occurring among the individuals enrolled in the study. The task of searching or recording *linkages* of each participant in these registries may be simpler if the registry is automated (stored in a computer accessible database), and a common identification number is used in the registry and the cohort study database. When a numerical identifier is not available, it is necessary to use the participant's name, birth date, and other identifiers to perform the linkage. The type and automation of the record linkage system is determined in each case by the availability of data and the characteristics of each particular registry (Oshima *et al.* 1979; Hole *et al.* 1981; Smith & Newcombe 1982; Newcombe 1984). When linking, it is important to rule out duplication because this could result in mismatches.

The quality of the information about the occurrence of events is fundamental for correct estimation of the incidence and its determinants. Therefore, in many cohort studies, a special effort is made to ensure that the information about disease occurrence or death is accurate. Generally, events recorded in interviews with study participants are verified by requesting documents such as the clinical records or death certificate of the subject, not only to verify the occurrence of the event but also to improve the information regarding diagnosis (e.g. to obtain the histological type in a study of lung cancer; to distinguish between thrombotic and haemorrhagic episodes in a study of cerebrovascular events, etc.). A major challenge in cohort studies with cause-specific mortality as the event of interest is the determination of the cause of death, which may require confirmation by inspecting clinical records or by interviewing the physician who attended to the participant before his or her death.

Incomplete observation of event of interest

Observations in a cohort study are incomplete because it is unfeasible for the investigator to observe the event in all participating individuals. This type of incompleteness in the data is called *censoring* and can be due to any of the following: Individuals being observed as event-free on the date of analysis, sometimes called *administrative* censoring; individuals being lost to follow-up (prior to the date of analysis) before developing the event; or deaths due to unrelated causes, precluding the observation of the event of interest.

When the follow-up is ended by the investigators (or the source of funding for the study is exhausted), the participants still under follow-up without having experienced the event of interest are considered administrative losses. When participants emigrate during the course of the follow-up, change addresses or telephone numbers making them untraceable, or refuse to continue participating, they are considered censored observations due to follow-up losses. When death is the reason for censoring an event of interest, it is more appropriate to use methods of analysis based on competing risk models, which consider the deaths as exits or removals from the risk set as opposed to treating the deaths as observations that could have been observed had the participants not died before the event of interest occurred.

For the most part, subjects who are lost to follow-up are *right-censored*, which means that their exit from observation is the last possible time they contributed information to the study (i.e. on the timeline of their participation represented by a scale running from left to right, no data are available to the right of the time of censoring.) Occasionally, information from sources external to the study (e.g. death certificates) are used to identify the interval of time during which individuals lost to follow-up and free of the event of interest are documented to have had the event because they died of the event of interest at some time point after the censoring. This interval is defined as the time between the date the individual was lost to follow-up and the date of death. Given that the individual died of the event of interest, the event must have occurred during this interval. These observations are called *interval-censored* observations.

In the subsection on survival analysis, we will discuss the issues regarding the relationships between the censoring mechanisms and the disease process, as well as the need for properly incorporating these issues into the data analysis.

Types and measures of exposures

The classification of study participants according to exposure factors is one of the most complex challenges in a cohort study. *Exposure factor* means any attribute of the subject or any external agent that can influence his or her health (Armstrong *et al.* 1992).

Types of exposures

Exposure factors include host factors (such as age, sex, race, genetic factors, metabolic factors, and immune function) and environmental factors (such as viruses and bacteria, environmental pollutants, diet, alcohol, and/or tobacco consumption). Sometimes, an exposure factor represents a set of factors that are difficult to separate. For example, social class encompasses external environmental factors, related to individual behaviour, access to health-care services, socioeconomic status, and others.

The exposures can be either fixed over time (e.g. sex), change directly with time (e.g. age and calendar), or not change directly with time (e.g. cigarettes smoked per day, biological marker levels, diet). When exposures not only change over time but do so heterogeneously (i.e. change differently over time in different individuals), they are referred to as *internal* (i.e. at the individual level) time-dependent exposures. Examples of internal time-dependent exposures include the following: The number of cigarettes smoked per day, body mass index (defined as weight/height^2 in kg/m^2), total serum cholesterol level and level of low- and high-density lipoproteins, CD4 cell count, viral load of an infectious organism, presence or absence of a symptom or a clinical condition, and use of medications. In contrast, exposures that change over time but affect groups or populations who are subject to the exposure in a similar way are referred to as *external* (i.e. at the population level) time-dependent exposures (i.e. they change equally over time for different individuals comprising a given population). The most common example of an external variable is a calendar, which is the same for the whole population. Other examples of external time-dependent exposures include the following: Levels of air pollution in a given region, supplements in the food and water supply, medical procedures used in different calendar periods, and types of therapies available in different calendar periods.

Follow-up visits in the setting of a cohort study provide the opportunity for collecting data to update internal time-dependent exposures. External time-dependent exposures may be obtained from external sources, but data obtained at the individual level can sometimes be used to define eras (i.e. calendar periods) when there are changes at the population level. For example, as described earlier, the MACS started in 1984 and has since been conducted concurrently with major advances in therapies effective against viral replication in HIV-infected individuals. In 1998, Detels *et al.* (Detels *et al.* 1998) determined the effectiveness of the potent antiretroviral therapies introduced in 1995 by showing a doubling of the AIDS-free times under the conditions of the first two years (Jul 1995–Jul 1997) of the highly effective antiretroviral therapy (HAART) era. In 2005, Schneider *et al.* (Schneider *et al.* 2005) determined the population effectiveness of prolonged use of HAART by showing that in the era when HAART was well established (i.e. Jul 2001–Dec 2005, six to ten years after its introduction in July 1995), the median survival time after AIDS diagnosis increased 10-fold from the 1.5 years in the era when no therapies were available.

In cohort studies, two types of effects of interventions can be measured. The first can be termed 'individual effectiveness', which mimics clinical trials by using treatment data at the individual level. These analyses must, via stratification and regression, overcome the lack of randomization and the confounding by indication, whereby those individuals at more advanced disease stages are the ones more likely to receive the therapies (Ahdieh *et al.* 2000). Measures of individual effectiveness *supplement* (and typically support and extend) the results of clinical trials, but are usually subject to an unknown amount of residual confounding (Phillips *et al.* 1999). Data-analysis methods for individual effectiveness require the use of multivariate methods of survival analysis, including the use of therapy as an internal time-dependent covariate; however, the complexity of the selection of individuals receiving therapies may require the use of more elaborate methods for causal inferences (Robins & Finkelstein 2000; Cole *et al.* 2003).

The second type of effect that can be measured in a cohort study can be termed 'population effectiveness', which compares the occurrence of disease in the population when the most ill are treated to the occurrence of disease in the population when none or only few are treated with a given therapy. Because the introduction and use of therapies are closely linked to calendar time, the primary comparison may be characterized by time periods. To control for survival bias and overall disease progression, this approach requires the comparison of groups reaching similar time at risk (e.g. duration of infection or time since disease diagnosis) in different eras defined by calendar periods (Schneider *et al.* 2005; Detels *et al.* 1998; Muñoz & Hoover 1995). Measures of population effectiveness *complement* the efficacy measured in clinical trials and provide a key public health index: The amount of disease burden that is reduced when only some (typically the most ill) receive the therapy of interest (Muñoz *et al.* 2000). Comprehensive data collected by cohort studies are essential to eliminate possible ecological fallaciousness (i.e. effectiveness due to changes over time other than changes in the therapies of interest). This includes not only prospectively collected data on therapy use, but also information on access, health-care utilization and practices, and adherence at the population level.

Measures of exposures

The exposure can be defined as a quantitative (continuous) variable (e.g. blood pressure) or qualitative (categorical) variable (e.g. non-smoker, ex-smoker, current smoker). To avoid imposing linear relationships for quantitative variables, the investigator could categorize them. For example, quantitative variables (such as blood pressure) can be categorized as dichotomous (hypertensive or normotensive), ordinal (with values 1–4), or polytomous (systolic blood pressure ≥180 mmHg, 160–179 mmHg, 130–159 mmHg, <130 mmHg). A variable such as tobacco consumption can be categorized as dichotomous (smoker or non-smoker), nominal, categorical (cigarettes, cigars, pipe), or continuous (mean number of cigarettes per day). The decision of defining a variable in one way or another has implications for the interpretation and inferences from analyses using multivariable regression methods.

When exposures are assessed repeatedly over time, the investigators can take into account not only the amount (dose) but also the duration of the exposure (Armstrong *et al.* 1992). There are several ways of quantifying dose and duration: (i) cumulative exposure (e.g. number of cigarette-years, number of rad-years of exposure to a radioactive compound at work); (ii) the average exposure during the latest years (e.g. average number of cigarettes per day, average number of rads in the work environment); or (iii) maximum exposure (e.g. maximum number of cigarettes per day, maximum level of radioactivity registered in the industry).

The most typical data-collection instruments in epidemiologic practice are questionnaires, physical examination, and registries. Questionnaires allow not only the obtaining of information on demographic data, personal and family history, and symptoms but also the recording of self-reported physical characteristics such as weight and height. They can be administered through personal or telephone interviews, they can be completed by the participants themselves, or they can be administered by a computer-assisted method, which is particularly useful for the collection of sensitive data (e.g. sexual behaviour, drug abuse). Physical examination includes the collection of data from the physical exploration as well as anthropometric, radiographic, electrocardiographic, and blood samples. Sometimes, the examination is made in the context of routine health care of patients in the hospital or health centre; at other times, it is performed during a visit specifically designed for the study. Registries are external sources that can be used to complement the active follow-up and are particularly useful to obtain vital status events or diagnosis of a condition of interest (e.g. cancer registries). In the non-concurrent or historical designs, the information collected in registries form the basis for classifying and quantifying the exposure of interest.

Types of outcomes

The scientific aims of a cohort study should dictate the type of outcome or measure of disease occurrence that should be collected during follow-up. The most common measure of disease in cohort studies is the time individuals at risk take to develop an end point. To properly describe this time, the following need to be defined: (1) the origin, which marks the time at which individuals are placed at risk for the development of the particular event of interest; (2) the end point, which typically is the onset of a clinical condition or the date an individual dies; and (3) the scale of time, which is typically measured in years or months, but could be days for events that take a short time to occur.

In most cases, even for groups of individuals with a persistent (e.g. fixed) exposure, the pattern of incidence of disease over the follow-up time is not the same at different durations at risk. An exposure whose deleterious effect monotonically accumulates over time will result in an incidence rate that increases with time (e.g. death after AIDS diagnosis in the absence of treatment). An exposure that first affects susceptible individuals so that those remaining free of the event over time represent resistance (i.e. some degree of immunity to the effects of exposure) will result in an increasing incidence followed by a decreasing incidence rate (e.g. a viral infection to which a subset of individuals are immune). An exposure that initially carries risk that ameliorates over time will result in a decreasing incidence rate (e.g. death after transplantation).

Events in person-time

In chronic diseases (e.g. cancer and cardiovascular disease) the origin at which individuals are placed at risk is often not well defined, or it is very difficult to measure. Furthermore, it is often the case that in the context of chronic diseases the primary interest is not to characterize the nature of the incidence rate at different times from the origin. Instead, the primary epidemiologic objective is to identify the exposures that describe heterogeneities in the incidence of disease. To identify such exposures, the relevant data from a cohort study are the number of events occurring in the total of person-years when individuals at risk had certain characteristics (e.g. age between 50 and 60 years, smoking 1–2 packs of cigarettes per day, having a particular genetic mutation). When employing these methods, it is expected that the incidence rate will be constant within each subgroup of the population. Therefore, it is desirable that the exposures that define the subgroups of individuals, including calendar and age, yield an approximately constant incidence rate. Under that assumption, whether one individual is contributing person-years from, say, 5 to 7 years from the origin or 9 to 11 years, they are considered to contribute 2 person-years equally.

In a cohort study that recruits individuals free of the event of interest at baseline and on whom data are collected to determine who develops the event of interest and after how many person-years, the outcome for the analysis of incidence rates is defined as the number of d events in n person-years. The investigators need to determine the cells defined by different exposures in which person-years from a cohort study will be accumulated (i.e. n person-years), and the number of events of interest will be enumerated (d events). The primary aim is to characterize the putative heterogeneity of the incidence rates between different cells defined by specific exposures.

Time to event

The nature of a cohort study provides the temporal structure necessary to associate a particular exposure with a subsequent event of interest. Documentation of the time sequences of exposures and events generates data upon which the course of event development can be modelled. Such data provide flexibility to define the study outcome according to the amount of time elapsed between exposure and event. The time at which an exposure first occurs, placing an individual at risk for event development, is referred to as the *origin*. The use of time-to-event outcomes requires that the *time* variable be anchored at the origin, resulting in the characterization of the event incidence across the time since origin. In other words, the incidence of the event from 5 to 7 years past the origin will be handled differently in the analysis than the incidence from 9 to 11 years, even though both time periods equally span 2 person-years.

Examples of time-to-event outcomes used in epidemiological research include the following: (1) in clinical epidemiology, the classic time from diagnosis of a clinical condition to death or the time from initiating therapy to response; (2) in infectious disease epidemiology, the time from infection to overt disease (i.e. the incubation period); (3) in cancer epidemiology, the time from remission to relapse; (4) in behavioural epidemiology, the time from enrolment into a smoking cessation programme to the time the individual quits smoking; and (5) in occupational epidemiology, the time from employment to the occurrence of an occupationally related health outcome.

Change of biomarkers

In some cohort studies, the primary event is not an event but whether a marker of disease changes over time differently in individuals exposed to different risk factors. For example, in the cohort study of children with moderate kidney function insufficiency, conducted by Furth *et al.* (2006), the primary objective was to identify the factors that predicted fast decline of kidney function. Another example is the cohort study conducted by Tager *et al.* (1983) in East Boston in the 1970s, showing the effect of maternal smoking on slowing the expected increase of pulmonary function in growing children. The study was seminal to the subsequent mounting evidence that second-hand (involuntary) smoking had detrimental health effects and guided the issuing of policies to ban smoking from work and public places as fundamental prevention measures for the health of the public. Furthermore, cohort studies have not only contributed substantially to the elucidation of disease aetiology but have also spurred the development of statistical methods to properly analyse data. For example, Rosner *et al.* (1985) developed methods for the analyses of data presented in their work in collaboration with Tager *et al.* (1983).

In the studies in which the participants are examined or interviewed repeatedly during follow-up in addition to the baseline examination, the successive study visits are generally used to update or complement the information about biomarkers that measure factors of outcomes and exposures. These cohort studies offer the opportunity to describe how exposures preceding changes of an outcome of interest may serve to describe the heterogeneity of the changes of the outcome. From a cross-sectional perspective, this design can be conceived as a series of cross-sectional studies repeated over the same cohort, which offers interesting methodological variations to the classic cohort design measuring the primary outcome as time to an event.

For cohort studies using change of a biomarker as the outcome, it is important to establish consistent and standardized methods across the sites of the study to measure the biomarker over time. The methods for the analyses of these data are those of longitudinal data analyses and, as discussed in the following subsection, they are of different nature than the methods of survival analyses or the analysis based on person-time.

Analysis

Comparison of the frequencies of disease occurrence in exposed and unexposed individuals is a primary objective of cohort studies. A fundamental condition for valid epidemiologic inferences is that for the disease to be (causally) linked to a given exposure, the exposed and unexposed groups should be comparable with respect to factors that are known to explain the heterogeneity of disease occurrence (i.e. no confounding). In clinical trials, randomization leads to this comparability. However, in cohort (observational) studies, comparability needs to be achieved by stratification and/or regression. The goal of regression methods is to mimic randomization so as to assess the effect of a given exposure in groups of individuals who differ in the exposure of interest, but who are otherwise comparable with respect to all variables known to be associated with disease.

Methods for the analysis of cohort studies have become increasingly sophisticated. It is widely recognized that the occurrence of most diseases is due to multiple factors and that disease progression usually involves the presence of several cofactors (effect modifiers). Therefore, simple methods of analysis involving only one factor are inadequate. Statistical methods for the analysis of multivariable data (i.e. several risk factors) have been developed and incorporated into readily available software supporting these applications. Multivariable methods are often of greater need when analysing data from observational cohort studies as compared to data collected from randomized trials. As such, the use of multivariable methods in the context of cohort study data has increased in parallel with the availability of these methods. This greater need for multivariable methods when analysing cohort data is largely due to the fact that the random assignment of an exposure (typically a treatment deemed to have potential health benefit) in clinical trials facilitates comparability among exposed and unexposed groups. If the randomization in a clinical trial is successful and assuming non-informative dropout with an appropriate sample size, univariate analysis of the (randomly assigned) exposure and outcome is sufficient (i.e. intent-to-treat analysis). Such is seldom the case in observational cohort studies. Univariate analysis is usually the first step, which typically evolves into multivariable regression models to adjust for confounders.

The type of outcome of interest determines the type of analytical technique most appropriate to yield a valid inference. Table 6.6.2 provides a succinct summary of the analytical methods for cohort studies reviewed here.

When the outcome data are collected as events in person-years, Poisson regression methods are the most appropriate for data analysis (I in Table 6.6.2). These methods are particularly useful for the analysis of trends and changes in incidence of disease over calendar time; they are of great utility for data in which an origin is not well defined or not of interest, which will be the case if the rate of disease occurrence is assumed to be constant within a defined interval or period.

When the outcome data are times to event from a well-defined origin (II in Table 6.6.2), the percentage of individuals remaining free of the event of interest at t units of time after the origin can be estimated by the Kaplan–Meier curve (Kaplan & Meier 1958) or by maximum-likelihood methods for the non-parametric and parametric (Cox *et al.* 2007) approaches, respectively. Two survival curves can be compared using the Mantel–Haenszel (Mantel & Haenszel 1959) test or the likelihood ratio test (Cox *et al.* 2007). Regression analysis can be accomplished under the semi-parametric assumption of proportional hazards (Cox 1972) or under richer parametric models (Cox *et al.* 2007) which lend themselves more directly to estimation of relative times quantifying not only how the hazard is modified by an exposure but also to what extent an exposure shortens (if deleterious) or extends (if beneficial) the event-free times.

When the outcome is a biomarker repeatedly measured at follow-up visits (III in Table 6.6.2), regression methods for correlated data need to be used. This is so because the biomarkers measured in the same individual over the follow-up visits are correlated so that the standard methods of regression methods for statistically independent outcomes are not appropriate.

Table 6.6.2 Main methods for the analysis of cohort studies

Outcome		Summary measure	Comparison		Measure of association
			Exposed/unexposed (two-sample)	**Multiple (regression)**	
I	Events in person-years	Incidence rate	$(O-E)^2$/variance	Poisson	Relative incidence
II	Time to event (exposure changing)	Kaplan–Meier; maximum likelihood estimates	Logrank or Mantel–Haenszel; likelihood ratio test	Proportional hazards; parametric (staggered entries)	Relative hazard; relative time
III	Biomarker repeatedly measured at follow-up visits	Change	t-test for simple measures of change between baseline and last visit	Regression for correlated data; marginal, conditional, random effects	Differences in change over time

Analysis based on person-time

Calculation of person-time and rates

The methods described in this subsection are useful for the analysis of the frequency of events in person-years in groups of individuals with different exposures and when anchoring at the origin is not important. The primary aim is to describe the heterogeneity of the incidence in subgroups of the population defined by exposures, often including age and calendar.

To illustrate the methods, we present data from the Precursors Cohort study. This cohort comprised 1337 medical students of the Johns Hopkins University who graduated between 1948 and 1964 (Klag *et al.* 1993). A total of 1271 students (95%) completed a questionnaire and were examined during their stay at the school. In order to study the determining factors ('precursors') of general mortality and the occurrence of cardiovascular diseases, this cohort was followed up through mailed questionnaires. When the participants reported that they have had a myocardial infarction or another cardiovascular event, the hospital records were requested in order to validate the diagnosis. The vital status of the participants who did not respond was systematically investigated through calls to relatives and friends and through matching with the National Death Index. Table 6.6.3 shows data obtained in the follow-up for each of the groups (smokers and non-smokers), the column named 'person-years' showing the totality of time units lived by the members of the cohort between the indicated years of age. Thus, for example, the non-smokers in the cohort lived a total of 862.5 years while being 20–24 years old and 1929.5 years while being 25–29 years of age.

In the data presented in Table 6.6.3, the axis of time was age. Time since the entrance to the school of medicine or calendar years could have also been used. In the Precursors study, the age of the students at the onset of follow-up was relatively uniform (around 22–25 years), with which the use of age is approximately equivalent to the use of years since admission. However, given that the recruitment of the students took place between 1948 and 1964, the possible existence of temporal trends can make it advisable to also control for the temporal scale of calendar years. One of the advantages of the person-time methodology is precisely its flexibility to utilize simultaneously several axes of time.

The person-time method also has great flexibility for the analysis of time-dependent exposures, as for example in longitudinal studies. Thus, for instance, from the data of the Framingham study (see Table 6.6.1), Sorlie *et al.* (1980) studied the mortality in the six-year periods that followed the visits numbered 1, 4, 7, and 10 in relation to body weight of the participants in the preceding visit. Therefore, the same participant could contribute to the denominator of the exposed (obese) in a period and to the non-exposed (non-obese) in another. The process of assignment of person-time in the case of time-dependent variables or in the case of multiple temporal scales can be very complicated and computer programs designed for this purpose can be useful (Pearce & Checkoway 1987; Macaluso 1992).

The method of calculation of rates based on person-time is commonly used in the case of events with low frequency of occurrence, for which a reasonable model is provided by the Poisson distribution (Armitage & Berry 1987; Breslow & Day 1987). Confidence intervals of the incidence rates can be easily calculated based on the Poisson distribution as the variance of the logarithm of the

Table 6.6.3 Internal comparison of the rates based on person-years. Cohort from the Precursors Study. Occurrence of mortality (all cause) until 1989, as a function of cigarette consumption at the baseline examination

Age (years)	Non-smokers			Smokers			
	Deaths	Person-years	Rate	Deaths	Person-years	Rate	Expected deaths*
20–24	1	862.5	0.00116	1	886.5	0.00113	1.0
25–29	2	1929.5	0.00104	2	2195.5	0.00091	2.3
30–34	0	2052	0	1	2360	0.00042	0
35–39	1	2064.5	0.00048	4	2354	0.00170	1.1
40–44	1	2029.5	0.00049	6	2280.5	0.00263	1.1
45–49	3	1940.5	0.00155	2	2182.5	0.00092	3.4
50–54	5	1501	0.00333	13	1819	0.00715	6.1
55–59	5	827	0.00605	11	1187	0.00927	7.2
60–64	4	370.5	0.01080	13	582	0.02234	6.3
65–69	0	103.5	0	4	106	0.03774	0
70–74	1	17.5	0.05714	0	23	0	1.3
75–79	0	1.5	0	0	0.5	0	0
Total	23			57			29.8

*Numbers of deaths that would occur in the group of smokers if they had the rate observed in the non-smokers.

incidence rate is simply the inverse of the number of events (Breslow & Day 1987).

Univariate analysis

Internal comparison: The comparison of exposed and unexposed within a cohort can be done through the calculation of the standardized mortality ratio (SMR). Using data from the Precursors study, the last column of Table 6.6.3 shows the deaths 'expected' in the smokers if they had had the rates of the non-smokers. For example, the number of deaths expected in smokers 45–49 years old would be 0.00155 (deaths/year) × 2182.5 (person-years) = 3.4 deaths. The ratio of total observed deaths to the total expected deaths in smokers (if the smokers had the same age-specific rates as the non-smokers) is the standardized mortality ratio (SMR), which in this case is 57/29.8 = 1.9.

External comparison: In other situations, it can be of interest to compare the mortality in the study group with the mortality of the total population that is used as reference. In this case, it is necessary to obtain the expected number of deaths using population-level rates from demographic statistics. Thus, in the Precursors study, the observed mortality can be compared with the mortality of the population of White males in the United States, as shown in Table 6.6.4. The total number of observed deaths (23 + 57 = 80) divided by the total number of expected deaths based on the demographic statistics provides the SMR of the cohort in comparison with the general population, which in case of data from Table 6.6.4 is 80/148.1 = 0.54. This result implies that the mortality is almost half of what would be expected if the cohort had the same rates as that of the general population of White males.

Table 6.6.4 External comparison of the rates based on person-years. Cohort of the Precursors Study. All-cause mortality until 1989, observed and expected according to national rates in 1980

Age (years)	National mortality rate*	Study cohort		
		Deaths	Person-years	Expected deaths†
20–24	0.001909	2	1749	3.3
25–29	0.001747	4	4125	7.2
30–34	0.001676	1	4412	7.4
35–39	0.002087	5	4418.5	9.2
40–44	0.003161	7	4310	13.6
45–49	0.005217	5	4123	21.5
50–54	0.008668	18	3320	28.8
55–59	0.013756	16	2014	27.7
60–64	0.021406	17	952.5	20.4
65–69	0.033121	4	209.5	6.9
70–74	0.050338	1	40.5	2.0
75–79	0.074685	0	2	0.1
Total		80	29676	148.1

*Mortality rates among white males, the United States, 1980.
†According to national rates.

Multivariable analysis

The aim of multivariable analysis is to identify the constellation of exposures that explain the variability of incidence of disease, allowing for random variation under a probability distribution model. The Poisson distribution provides a useful and reasonable model to carry out the multivariable analysis of incidence rates observed in cohort studies. Ideally, the final regression model from a multivariable analysis should have an appropriate goodness of fit and be optimally parsimonious (i.e. with all regression coefficients being statistically significant). The most appropriate method of multivariate analysis for data based on person-time is Poisson regression (Armitage & Berry 1987; Breslow & Day 1987).

Survival analysis

Time-to-event outcomes are used to accomplish the following epidemiologic objectives: Estimate the percentage of individuals that survive (i.e. remain event-free) for differing lengths of time from the origin, compare the survival of exposed and unexposed groups, and characterize the possibly multifactorial nature explaining observed heterogeneities in survival of different subgroups of individuals using multivariable analysis and regression methods.

Descriptors of the distribution of times to event

If T denotes the variable of time from origin to event, the simplest descriptor of the distribution of T is the *survival function* at time t (where t is a positive number), which is denoted by $S(t)$ and corresponds to the cumulative probability that an individual in the baseline cohort survives beyond time t. The survival function starts with a value of one and monotonically decreases towards zero. Its complement from one $1-S(t)$ is the cumulative probability that an individual in the baseline cohort has the event before or at time t. The *pth percentile*, which is denoted by $t(p)$, is the time by which p per cent develop the event of interest; that is, when $1-p=S\left[t(p)\right]$. A widely used descriptor of survival times is the median, which is simply the 50th percentile, or the time since origin by which half of the individuals develop the event of interest.

The *hazard function* at t, which is denoted by $h(t)$, corresponds to the proportion of individuals who develop the event in the next unit of time among those who survive event-free until time t. That is, $h(t)$ equals the rate of decline of S at t divided by $S(t)$. The rate of decline of S is the *density function*, which is denoted by $f(t)$ and fulfils the equation $f(t)=h(t)S(t)$. It is important to note that $h(t)$ is a conditional probability and refers only to the subset of the baseline cohort that survives event-free by time t. In addition, $h(t)$ is often called the instantaneous hazard or risk of the event at time t, given that as the unit of time approaches zero, $h(t)$ represents the hazard corresponding to a single instant in time. In contrast, $S(t)$ and $1-S(t)$ are cumulative probabilities that refer to the entire baseline cohort.

Figure 6.6.1 depicts the 25th percentile and hazard at $t=12$ years of a survival function. The 25th percentile is 6 years (i.e. $t(0.25)=$ 6 years), because it corresponds to the time by which 25 per cent of the individuals develop the event (i.e. 75 per cent survive). The hazard at $t=12$ years is 10 per cent and corresponds to the ratio of 0.04/0.40, which is the value of the rate of decline of the survival function at $t=12$ (i.e. the density $t=12$) divided by the value of S at $t=12$.

The accumulation of h from zero to t (i.e. the area under the curve described by h from zero to t) is defined as the *cumulative*

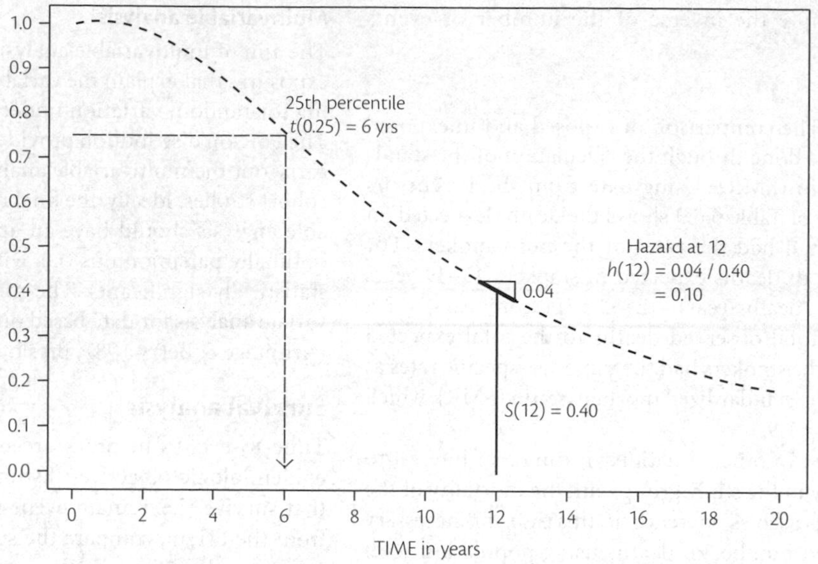

Fig. 6.6.1 Survival function ($S[12]$), the 25th percentile ($t[0.25]$), and hazard at t = 12 years ($h[12]$).

hazard at t, which is denoted by $H(t)$. In other words, $H(t)$ is the 'summation' of all instantaneous hazards ($h(t)$) between zero and t. There is a close and useful relationship between the survival function and the cumulative hazard at t: $S(t)=\exp[-H(t)]$, or equivalently, $H(t)=-\log[S(t)]$. Therefore, the cumulative hazard does not equate to the cumulative probability of events by time t because $-\log[S(t)]$ is not equal to $1-S(t)$.

Estimation of the survival function

The presence of censored observations is a case of missing data, and the fundamental role of the assumption that censored observations are not a selected subgroup is that, at any time during the study, individuals who remain under observation *represent* those subjects who were censored beforehand. The observation of events beyond the time an individual is censored provides the data to estimate when a censored individual is expected to develop the event had she or he remained in the study. Furthermore, because the individuals who are observed to develop the event are representative of the observations censored before their time of event, estimates of the hazard functions based on the observed individuals are unbiased, and thus are the hazards that the censored individuals would have experienced had they remained under observation in the study. Indeed, this forms the basis of the Kaplan–Meier method (Kaplan & Meier 1958), based on the calculation of the survival probability through the product of one minus the instantaneous hazards.

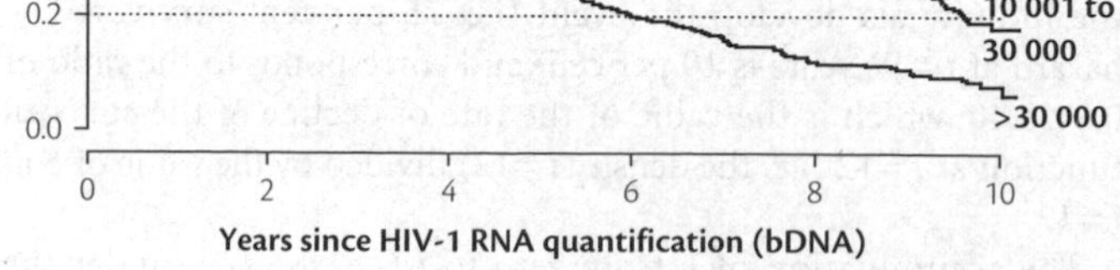

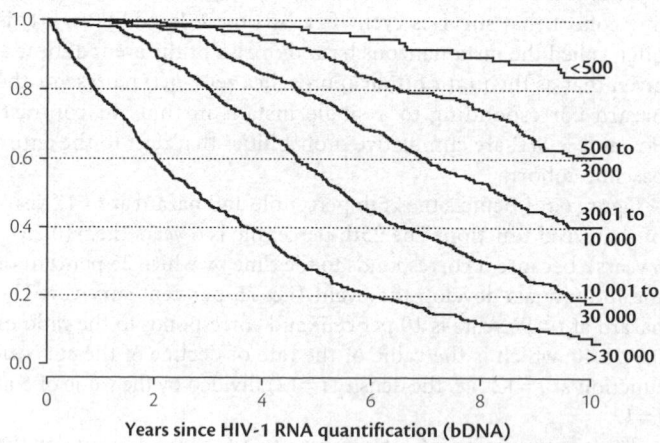

Fig. 6.6.2 Proportion AIDS-free, by plasma HIV-RNA (copies/ml).

Figure 6.6.2 shows five Kaplan–Meier curves according to the number of copies of HIV detected in 500 ml of plasma measured by bDNA in HIV-infected individuals followed up in the MACS cohort (Mellors *et al.* 1997). It clearly shows the great predictive value that viral load has for the development of AIDS. Indeed, investigators in the MACS have developed methods to quantify the variability of time to AIDS explained by viral load (Cox *et al.* 2007) and have shown that it alone explained approximately 50 per cent of the variability of time to AIDS (Mellors *et al.* 2007). The standard error of the estimators of the Kaplan–Meier survival function can be obtained from the formula proposed by Greenwood (Armitage & Berry 1987; Greenwood 1926).

Univariate analysis

Graphical display of the survival curves is generally quite useful to obtain an overall comparison of the experiences of groups subjected to different exposures (Fig. 6.6.2). There are two different ways to measure the association between exposure and survival, which correspond to horizontal (i.e. relative time) and vertical comparisons (i.e. relative hazard) of survival curves. The first one is the relative times defined as $t_1(p)/t_0(p)$, where $t_i(p)$ corresponds to the time taken by p per cent of group i to develop the event. The second one is the relative hazard, defined as $h_1(t)/h_0(t)$, where $h_i(t)$ is the hazard for the ith group at time t. If exposure shortens survival, the relative time will be less than 1 and the relative hazard will be greater than 1. If the relative times are independent of p and/or the relative hazard is independent of t, the times and/or the hazards are said to be proportional. In such cases, the relative times and/or hazards will be constant across all values of p and/or t, respectively. Methods based on parametric models (e.g. lognormal) are more amenable to estimation and testing of relative times (e.g. to compare, for instance, the median survival time in exposed and unexposed) and can also provide measures of relative hazards. Semi-parametric methods based on the proportionality of hazards focused attention to estimation and testing of relative hazards.

There are hypothesis-testing procedures to assess whether the difference between two or more survival curves is statistically significant. The most commonly used is the logrank test (Peto *et al.* 1977), which assumes that the hazards are proportional and tests whether the relative hazard is equal to 1. It is equivalent to the Mantel–Haenszel (Mantel & Haenszel 1959) statistic for the combination of tables constructed at each time an event occurs whereby the table describes how many individuals were at risk at that time and how many of them developed the event from each group being compared. The *p*-value is obtained from a χ^2 table with as many degrees of freedom as survival curves compared minus one.

Multivariable analysis

In the context of survival analysis, the most used method of multivariate analysis is the proportional hazards regression (Cox 1972). The semi-parametric proportional hazards regression model corresponds to the hazard of the group with covariates representing exposures and confounders $x_1 = x_2 = \ldots = x_K = 0$ (i.e. the reference group) being completely arbitrary, and the hazard of the group characterized by any other values of x_1 to x_K being a fixed multiple of the hazard of the reference group according to a linear combination of the covariates. Specifically, the hazard of the group with covariates $x_1, x_2, \ldots, x_K$ denoted by $h_x(t)$ is $h_0(t)\exp(\beta_1 x_1 + \beta_2 x_2 + \ldots + \beta_K x_K)$.

The interpretation of the parameters is directly linked to relative hazards. In particular, if we have two groups of individuals described by the constellation of covariates taking values *x* for one group and x^* for the other, the hazard at time *t* of the group described by x^* relative to the hazard at the same time of the group defined by *x* (i.e. the relative hazards) is given by $RH(t) = \exp\left[\sum_{k=1}^{K} \beta(x_k^* - x_k)\right]$. Because such an expression does not depend on *t*, the relative hazard is constant (i.e. the hazards are proportional). In particular, if *x* and x^* only differ in one unit in the k th covariate (i.e. $x^* = x_1, x_2, \ldots, x_k + 1, \ldots x_K$), then the relative hazard of the x^* group to the *x* group is simply $RH(t) = \exp(\beta_k)$.

When investigators from a cohort study are not only interested in relative hazards but also in describing the underlying hazard with the aim of characterizing mechanisms and the desire to quantify how exposures modify the magnitude of event-free times, parametric models are a more attractive option (Cox *et al.* 2007). To carry out parametric analyses of time-to-event data, the generalized gamma distribution offers a succinct yet flexible family of distributions. The generalized gamma distribution $GG(\beta, \sigma, \lambda)$ has three parameters whereby the location parameter β governs the value of the median for fixed values of σ and λ; the scale parameter σ determines the value of the interquartile ratio (i.e. IQr = 3rd quartile/1st quartile) for a fixed value of λ and independently of β; and the parameter λ determines the percentiles of the standard ($\beta = 0, \sigma = 1$) generalized gamma. The generalized gamma contains commonly used parametric models in the particular cases when λ is 0 and 1 corresponding to the lognormal and Weibull models, respectively. More importantly, the parameters λ and σ together determine the *type* of hazard function and yield a graphical taxonomy of the rich variety of hazards covered by the generalized gamma and described by Muñoz and colleagues for the first time in 2007 (Cox *et al.* 2007). Specifically, the taxonomy shows that the generalized gamma family includes all four of the common types of hazard functions: Increasing, decreasing, U or bathtub shape, and inverted U or arch shape.

The conventional generalized gamma regression model corresponds to $GG(\beta' x, \sigma, \lambda)$, describing the distribution of the times for the group of individuals with covariate vector *x*. In this case, the relative times of the group with covariates *x* to the group with covariates x^* are constant (i.e. proportional times) and are equal to $\exp[\beta'(x - x^*)]$. Lack of proportionality of times can be easily incorporated by allowing σ to depend on covariates *z* and full generalization of the model can be accomplished by further allowing λ to depend on covariates. Software is commonly available to implement generalized gamma regression in its full general form.

An example of the richness of parametric regression analyses for survival data is illustrated by Schneider *et al.* (2005), who used data from the MACS cohort of homosexual men and the WIHS cohort of women to characterize the changing pattern of survival after development of clinical AIDS from 1984 to 2004 when different antiretroviral therapies were introduced. Table 6.6.5 presents descriptive statistics, adjusted relative hazards, and relative times by therapy era. In the first three therapy eras, only those individuals with incident AIDS during the given period contributed data to the analysis; thus, the number of individuals seen is equivalent to the number with incident AIDS. Many individuals diagnosed with AIDS between January 1995 and June 1998 survived until after June 1998, and therefore potentially contributed person-time to each of the last two therapy eras. The primary purpose of the multivariate models was to attempt to put all subjects and eras under a 'common denominator'. Given the possible confounding effects of age, CD4 cell count at AIDS diagnosis, and type of AIDS diagnosis with therapy era, and to control for cohort study (i.e. sex), the bottom part of Table 6.6.5 presents the relative hazards obtained from a multivariable Cox proportional hazards regression model and the relative times obtained from a multivariable Weibull regression model. Substantial differences in survival were seen between the last two HAART eras and the no/monotherapy era, with the time from AIDS to death (adjusted by age, sex, type of AIDS diagnosis, and CD4 cell count at diagnosis) expanded by factors close to 8 and 11 in the periods July 1998–June 2001 and July 2001–December 2003, respectively. This analysis illustrates the role that cohort studies can play in providing measures of the effectiveness of interventions at the population level.

Longitudinal data analysis

The two analytical strategies explained in the preceding sections (person-time and survival analysis) are the tools regularly utilized for the analysis of the results of a typical epidemiologic cohort study when the dependent variable is the occurrence of an event such as disease or death. However, occasionally, the dependent variable of interest in a cohort study is not the occurrence of an event but the value of a determined biomarker such as blood pressure, weight, leukocyte count, viral load, glomerular filtration rate, pulmonary function, C reactive protein, or CD4 cell count.

To illustrate the power of longitudinal data in cohort studies collecting data at regularly scheduled visits, we used data collected at semi-annual visits by the Multicenter AIDS Cohort Study from 1984 to 2006. The person-visits of interest were those happening after the first time individuals tested positive for antibodies to HIV

Table 6.6.5 Descriptive statistics, adjusted relative hazards, and relative times for survival after an initial AIDS diagnosis in five calendar periods from July 1984 to December 2003. Data from the Multicenter AIDS Cohort Study and The Women Interagency HIV Study

	Calendar period				
Variable	**Jul 1984–Dec 1989**	**Jan 1990–Dec 1994**	**Jan 1995–Jun 1998**	**Jul 1998–Jun 2001**	**Jul 2001–Dec 2003**
Therapy era	No/monotherapy	Monotherapy/ combination therapy	HAART introduction	Short-term stable HAART	Moderate-term stable HAART
Number seen	633	660	472	496	464
% women	NA*	NA*	65%	72%	74%
Incident AIDS	633 (100%)	660 (100%)	472 (100%)	143 (29%)	57 (12%)
Median (IQR)† date of AIDS diagnosis	Oct 1987 (Apr 1986–Dec 1988)	Apr 1992 (Feb 1991–Jun 1993)	Jan 1996 (Jul 1995–Nov 1996)	Nov 1996 (Dec 1995–Sep 1998)	Mar 1997 (Jan 1996–Oct 1999)
Median (IQR)† age at AIDS diagnosis	36.5 (32.1–41.1)	39.7 (35.3–43.9)	39.7 (34.5–44.5)	39.8 (35.1–44.8)	40.1 (35.6–45.2)
Median (IQR)† CD4 cell count at AIDS diagnosis	141 (64–273)	90 (35–194)	196 (78–390)	241 (117–439)	268 (130–456)
Number of person-years	685	912	796	1156	992
Deaths (% of person-years)	388 (57%)	445 (49%)	109 (14%)	71 (6%)	44 (4%)
Relative hazard‡‖ (95% confidence interval)	1	0.65 (0.55, 0.77)	0.21 (0.15, 0.28)	0.08 (0.06, 0.13)	0.06 (0.03, 0.10)
Relative time§‖ (95% confidence interval)	1	1.42 (1.24, 1.62)	3.57 (2.77, 4.61)	7.82 (5.86, 10.45)	10.65 (7.66, 14.80)

*NA: not applicable since WIHS began in October 1994.
†IQR: inter-quartile range.
‡ Results of Cox proportional hazards regression.
§Results of Weibull regression under the assumption of proportional survival times.
‖ Adjusted by age at AIDS diagnosis, type of AIDS diagnosis, gender, and CD4 within one year prior to AIDS diagnosis.
Source: Reprinted with permission from Schneider M.F., Gange S.J., Williams C.M. *et al.* Patterns of the hazard of death after AIDS through the evolution of antiretroviral therapy: 1984–2004.
AIDS 2005;**19**:2009–18.

and with data on therapy received, CD4 cell count (a marker of immunosuppression), and HIV-RNA (copies of HIV per ml of plasma). The objective was to describe the distribution of HIV-RNA in four categories of CD4 cell count using 200, 350, and 500 cells/mm^3 as cut-off values and in four categories of therapy according to whether the participant at a given visit was not on any therapy, was just receiving antiretroviral therapy but not a triple combination, or was receiving triple combination therapy (HAART) and the visit occurred within three years or after three years from initiation. Two measures of HIV-RNA were used: (i) the median HIV-RNA and (ii) the percentage of person-visits in a given category of CD4 cell count and therapy with undetectable HIV-RNA (i.e. <50 copies/ml).

Figure 6.6.3 uses a diamond-shaped equiponderant graphical display of the effects of CD4 cell count and therapy on HIV-RNA whereby the shaded area on each square is proportional to the HIV-RNA (Li *et al.* 2003). Both panels show the great effectiveness of HAART in suppressing viral replication in all categories of CD4 cell count. It also shows that CD4 cell count and HIV-RNA are inversely correlated. Furthermore, non-HAART therapy had only a modest effect on viral replication. Finally, among those with CD4 cell count below 200 cells/mm^3, those who had initiated HAART more than 3 years before had a median viral load slightly higher than those who had initiated within three years, which is a possible indication of some individuals developing resistance.

Methods for the analysis of longitudinal data can be broadly classified in three categories: Marginal, conditional, and random-effects models. The primary aim of the marginal approach is to combine the multiple cross-sections corresponding to visits so as to provide the most efficient summary of the cross-sectional relationships between exposure and disease. In this approach, the longitudinal component is typically incorporated by including age or time since baseline as a covariate for the regression component of the model. Approaches for the incorporation of the correlation between repeated measurements within individuals include parametric (Jennrich & Schluchter 1986) and non-parametric methods, the latter handling the correlation as a nuisance (Zeger & Liang 1992). The primary aim of conditional models is to regress current outcome on past values of the outcome, and current and previous exposures. Classical Markovian models for binary data were introduced in 1979 (Korn & Whittemore 1979) and applied in 1980 to a study of air pollution and asthma (Whittemore & Korn 1980).

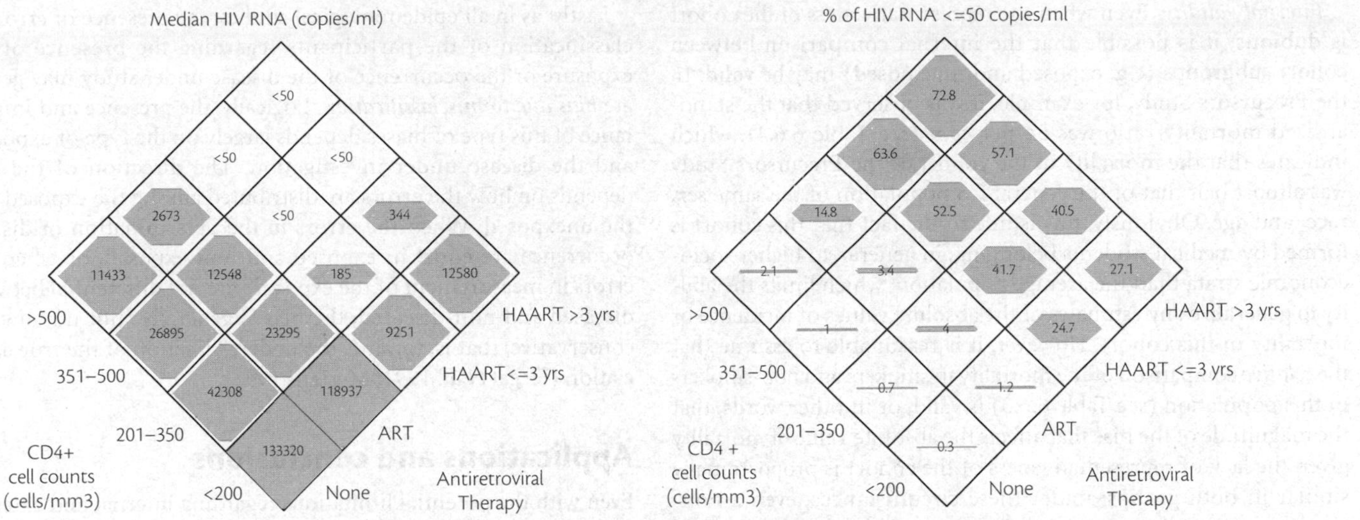

Fig. 6.6.3 Median HIV-RNA (copies/ml) and per cent with HIV-RNA ≤ 50 copies/ml in HIV-infected individuals according to CD4 cell count and antiretroviral therapy; the MultiCenter AIDS Cohort Study, 1984–2006.

Extensions for continuous outcomes were used for the study of the effect of cigarette smoking on respiratory function (Rosner *et al.* 1985). The primary aim of the random-effects models is to allow different individuals to have different intercepts and slopes according to components of variance and to provide direct averages of rates of change across individuals. Methods for random-effects models have been provided for Gaussian outcomes (Laird & Ware 1982), binary outcomes (Kupper & Haseman 1978), and for event-in-person-years outcomes (Breslow 1984).

When data are longitudinal assessments of a biomarker (e.g. pulmonary function, blood pressure, viral load of an infectious agent), linear models for normally distributed biomarkers allowing for both fixed and random effects (i.e. mixed effects) are apt to describe the probabilistic structure of the data. In the simplest case of two groups (i.e. an exposure taking the value 0 or 1) with linear trends over time, the fixed effects describe the two average lines for each group. That is, for the unexposed group, the average biomarker trajectory is given by $\beta_0 + \beta_1 t$, and for the exposed group, the average biomarker trajectory is given by $\left(\beta_0 + \beta_0^*\right) + \left(\beta_1 + \beta_1^*\right)t$. In this case, β_0^* represents the fixed effect of exposure on the levels at baseline and β_1^* represents the fixed effects of exposure on the rates of change of the biomarker over time. The random effects allow individuals in each of the two groups to vary randomly around the average lines of the fixed effects (i.e. each individual has his or her own line that varies randomly from the average line) (Laird & Ware 1982).

Validity and biases

The interpretation of the results of a cohort study is done in the context of its external and internal validity.

External validity: It refers to the extent to which the results of a cohort study can be extrapolated or generalized to the reference population. This concept is related to the 'representativeness' of the cohort and, thus, depends on the procedure of selection of its members. When the cohort is composed of volunteers, representativeness may be limited due to the fact that volunteers tend to be different than the general population. For example, in a cohort study of the American Cancer Society (Garfinkel 1985), it was observed that the members of the cohort (friends or relatives recruited by volunteers) included a larger proportion of subjects of White race as well as persons from the upper social class. Even when the study intends to attain a representative cohort following a probabilistic sampling selection procedure, representativeness may be limited by the fact that a number of the selected subjects refuse to participate in the study or decide to drop out before the follow-up is concluded. In the end, cohort studies almost always end up being composed of individuals who manifest certain degree of voluntariness.

For example, in a report from one of the first population-based cohort studies, the Framingham Heart Study (see Table 6.6.1), the investigators expressed their surprise for the low level of participation of the subjects invited to the study (69%). The investigators found among the non-participants a higher proportion of single men, heavy alcohol drinkers, and persons with low educational level. The fact that the participants or volunteers are on average people with higher educational level and healthier lifestyles makes the absolute values of incidence or mortality that are calculated in the cohorts biased (generally underestimated).

The representativeness or the lack of representativeness of the cohort in relation to the general population is also determined by the inherent characteristics of the sampling framework. Thus, for instance, even in the case that the members of the Framingham cohort were a representative sample of the population of this small town in New England, it is more than dubious that this population was representative of the general population. A sample from Framingham might be representative of the population of New England, but perhaps not so of the population of the United States. To address this latter issue, the cohorts in studies of cardiovascular epidemiology undertaken in the latest decade in the United States (CARDIA, ARIC, CHS) included participants from several regions of the country, trying to include populations with diverse social and ethnic composition. Even in this case, the representativeness of these cohorts can be questioned if one intends to obtain inferences applicable to the overall population of the continent or the world.

Internal validity: Even when the representativeness of the cohort is dubious, it is possible that the internal comparison between cohort subgroups (e.g. exposed and unexposed) may be valid. In the Precursors Study, for example, it was observed that the standardized mortality ratio was 54 per cent (see Table 6.6.4), which indicates that the mortality in the cohort of the Precursors Study was almost half that of the general US population of the same sex, race, and age. Obviously, this is due to the fact that this cohort is formed by medical students belonging, in general, to higher socio-economic strata than the average population, which limits the ability to generalize any estimates of the absolute values of incidence or mortality in this cohort. However, it is reasonable to assume that the *relative* comparison of the mortality in smokers and non-smokers in this population (see Table 6.6.3) is valid, or in other words, that the magnitude of the bias that affects the absolute value of mortality given the lack of representativeness of the cohort is proportionally similar in both groups; under these circumstances, even a non-representative cohort in the strict sense of the word, can yield unbiased estimates of the relative risk (or SMR in this case).

In cohort studies, the internal validity is based not only on the comparability of the selection process of exposed and unexposed when the cohort is established, but also on the comparability between the subjects who are lost to follow-up and those who continue under observation in the study. In other words, the losses to follow-up must be independent of the hypothesis under investigation. If the participants who are lost to follow-up have a different survival experience compared to those who remain under observation, the overall estimates of survival are biased (i.e. do not accurately represent the survival experience of the population in the original cohort).

In the evaluation of the possibility of biases due to the losses to follow-up, it is important to consider which type of losses have occurred. As was seen earlier, losses during follow-up can be produced by a refusal to continue in the study, by emigration, by death, or by 'administrative decision' of the investigator when ending the study. The latter have especial relevance in the studies in which participants are recruited during a long period of time. The biases due to differential losses to follow-up in a cohort study are conceptually analogous to the *selection biases* that affect case–control or other types of epidemiological studies.

There are other biases than can affect the internal validity of a cohort study. Among the information biases, one type of bias that could affect these types of studies is *surveillance bias*. This bias is present when the persons exposed to a determined risk factor are more carefully monitored or watched over than the persons without that factor. If the disease has a long subclinical phase, this can make the magnitude of the association between that factor and the disease exaggerated. Thus, for example, diabetics are generally subject to periodical checkups in which blood pressure is taken. Because in the natural history of hypertensive disease there exists a long asymptomatic phase and hypertension is much more likely to be diagnosed in diabetic persons given their periodical clinical assessment, it is possible that part of the strong association that exists between diabetes and hypertension is due in part to a surveillance bias. Even in cohort studies in which information is collected in a systematic form, if the observer knows the history of the participant, he can evaluate the presence of the disease in a biased form (*observer bias*). These biases are removed in large part in cohort studies in which a rigorous protocol for collection of information (preferably blinded) and well-trained observers exist.

Lastly, as in all epidemiological studies, the presence of errors in classification of the participants regarding the presence of the exposure or the occurrence of the disease under study may generate *bias due to misclassification*. Logically, the presence and importance of this type of biases depends largely on the type of exposure and the disease under investigation. The direction of the bias depends on how the errors are distributed among the exposed and the unexposed. When the errors in the determination of disease occurrence are equal in exposed and non-exposed, or when the errors in measurement of the exposure are not differential between diseased and non-diseased, the bias is generally (but not always) conservative; that is, towards the underestimation of the true association (Flegal *et al.* 1991; Mertens 1993).

Applications and conclusions

Even with the potential limitations regarding internal and external validity discussed in the previous subsection, the cohort study constitutes the design of reference for all other designs in observational epidemiology. Cohort studies are free from certain types of biases that complicate the interpretation of cross-sectional and case–control studies (Schlesselman 1982), as for example, recall bias (different recall of the exposure in cases and controls) and cross-sectional bias (due to different duration of disease in exposed and unexposed).

The essential characteristics of the cohort design, classifying the research subjects regarding the exposure and examining the occurrence of the event under study, reproduce the natural sequence of the causal phenomena that are investigated. The temporal relationship between the supposed cause (the exposure) and the supposed effect (the disease) is more clearly established than in a cross-sectional study or in a case–control study. Thus, for instance, the interpretation of an association between the presence of depression and an increased risk of myocardial infarction has very different implications depending on the design of the study. In a case–control study, it is practically impossible to discern how much of this association is due to the fact that depressed subjects have increased risk of coronary disease and how much to the fact that the patients who have experienced a myocardial infarction have a tendency to depression. However, in a cohort study it is possible to establish in a clear form if the presence of depression in individuals free of disease at the beginning of the study is associated with an increased incidence of infarction during follow-up.

The cohort design is more powerful for the establishment of the temporal relationship between cause and effect, one of the classical criteria for causality (Hill 1965). However, the design of a cohort study is not exempt from the problem of the potential confounding variables that determine the presence of an indirect, non-causal association; for example, an association between depression and coronary risk, even prospectively identified, might be due, not to that depression causes myocardial infarction but to that depression is more frequent in persons of low social class, who smoke more and have dietary habits that increase their cardiovascular risk.

From the logistic point of view, concurrent cohort studies have serious challenges inasmuch as the long time required for their implementation and the large numbers of participants required for diseases with low incidence (Lilienfeld & Lilienfeld 1980). It is for these reasons that, for many authors, concurrent cohort studies are indicated only when there exists enough evidence obtained from historical, case–control, or cross-sectional studies; when a new agent that can modify the risk of disease, as for example, oral contraceptives has been introduced (Kelsey *et al.* 1986); or when an outbreak of an unknown aetiology is identified (Fried *et al.* 1991).

Another advantage of cohort studies is the possibility of studying the occurrence of several events in addition to that initially planned. Thus, for instance, the Framingham cohort has been the basis for the investigation of several hypotheses in addition to those conceived in the initial aims of the study, as for example, the relationship between several factors and cancer (Kreger *et al.* 1991), senile dementia (Bachman *et al.* 1993), cognitive function (Elias *et al.* 1993), osteoporosis (Hannan *et al.* 1992), hearing defects (Gates *et al.* 1990), and others (Kannel 1990). Furthermore, cohort studies are a platform to expand the initial scientific scope of the studies as new knowledge is acquired and new questions arise. For example, when the MACS was established in 1983, not even the causative infectious agent (HIV) had been identified. It was only in 1985, two years into the conduct of the study, that HIV was identified and only then baseline samples kept in a repository were tested to find out who at enrolment was infected with HIV. The whole investigation focused on the infectious aetiology as opposed to other potential causes including an environmental exposure or a nutritional aetiology. Another example is provided by the neurological complications of HIV, as at the beginning, there were no neurological manifestations of HIV but, in the course of the epidemic, cases of dementia were recognized among HIV-infected individuals. Thus, a completely new battery of tests and procedures were implemented in the MACS to respond to the challenge of in whom and when cognitive decline ensued in HIV-infected individuals.

Cohort studies have proven to be extremely valuable in many areas of medical research including cardiovascular disease (Dawber 1980), cancer (Doll & Hill 1952; Doll *et al.* 2005), and infectious diseases (Samet & Muñoz 1998). Examples of contemporary studies demonstrate how the challenge of describing the effect of temporally varying exposures on disease risk can be met using modern epidemiologic approaches for the design and analysis of cohort studies (Willett & Colditz 1988; Muñoz & Gange 1998).

Cohort data may also be of great use for the development of public policy, such as treatment guidelines. Follow-up of cohorts before interventions are available provides the most appropriate data for the description of the natural history of disease. Furthermore, if these studies continue to collect data after interventions become available, three uses of these pre-intervention data are apparent: (i) as historical controls for assessing and/or confirming the effectiveness of interventions (Jacobson *et al.* 2002), (ii) as a reference point to establish the effectiveness of interventions at the population level once the interventions have been widely implemented (Schneider *et al.* 2005; Detels *et al.* 1998; Muñoz *et al.* 2000), (iii) as a mechanism to identify the subgroups who should receive treatment once an intervention has been proven efficacious in clinical trials (Phair *et al.* 2002; Cole *et al.* 2004).

Summary

The simplest cohort design is to obtain exposure data at baseline and follow up individuals to obtain data only from when the event of interest occurs. A richer design includes regularly scheduled visits at which data on exposures are updated. The exposures can be either fixed over time (e.g. sex), change directly with time (e.g. age and calendar), or not change directly with time (e.g. biological markers). According to the scientific aims of a cohort study, disease occurrence can be measured as an event in person-time, time to end point of interest, or change in a biomarker repeatedly measured at follow-up visits. Analytical methods include survival analyses to handle censored observations due to incomplete observation of the development of events and longitudinal data analyses for the trajectories of markers of disease progression. Stratification, multivariate regression, and causal inference methods are key tools to accomplish comparability among exposed and unexposed groups. Identification of exposures and risk factors for disease provides a basis for prevention strategies. Data from cohort studies can be used to assess the effects of interventions by using data at the individual level to determine individual effectiveness or by comparing occurrence of disease in the population when typically none or only a few are intervened to determine population effectiveness. From the public health perspective, population effectiveness quantifies the reduction of disease achieved by treating the subset of the population that needs therapies the most. In doing so, cohort studies are at the cornerstone of public health and policy.

References

Ahdieh L., Gange S., Greenblatt R. *et al.* Selection by indication of potent antiretroviral therapy use in a large cohort of women infected with human immunodeficiency virus. *American Journal of Epidemiology* 2000;**152**:923–33.

ARIC Investigators. The Atherosclerosis Risk In Communities (ARIC) Study: design and objectives. *American Journal of Epidemiology* 1989;**129**:687–702.

Armitage P., Berry G. *Statistical methods in medical research.* 2nd ed. Oxford: Blackwell Scientific Publications; 1987.

Armstrong B.K., White E., Saracci R. *Principles of exposure measurement in epidemiology.* Oxford: Oxford University Press; 1992.

ATBC Cancer Prevention Study Group. The effect of vitamin E and beta carotene on the incidence of lung cancer and other cancers in male smokers. *New England Journal of Medicine* 1994;**330**:1029–35.

Bachman D.L., Wolf P.A., Linn R.T. *et al.* Incidence of dementia and probable Alzheimer's disease in a general population: The Framingham Study. *Neurology* 1993;**43**:515–9.

Barkan S.E., Melnick S.L., Preston-Martin S. *et al.* The Women's Interagency HIV Study: WIHS Collaborative Study Group. *Epidemiology* 1988;**9**:117–25.

Breslow N. Extra-Poisson variation in log-linear models. *Applied Statistics* 1984;**33**:38–44.

Breslow N.E., Day N.E. *Statistical methods in cancer research.* Vol II: The design and analysis of cohort studies. Lyon, France: IARC Scientific Publications; 1987.

Cole S.R., Hernán M.A., Robins J.M. *et al.* Effect of highly active antiretroviral therapy on time to acquired immunodeficiency syndrome or death using marginal structural models. *American Journal of Epidemiology* 2003;**158**:687–94.

Cole S.R., Li R., Anastos K. *et al.* Accounting for lead time in cohort studies: evaluating when to initiate HIV therapies. *Statistics in Medicine* 2004;**23**:3351–63.

Cox C., Chu H., Schneider M. *et al.* Parametric survival analysis and taxonomy of hazard functions for the generalized gamma distribution. Statistics in Medicine 2007; **26**:4352–74.

Cox D. Regression models and life-tables. *Journal of the Royal Statistical Society* 1972;B**34**:187–202.

Dawber T.R. The Framingham study. The epidemiology of atherosclerotic disease. Cambridge (MA): Harvard University Press; 1980.

Detels R., Muñoz A., McFarlane G. *et al.* Effectiveness of potent antiretroviral therapy on time to AIDS and death in men with known HIV infection duration. *Journal of the American Medical Association* 1998;**280**:1497–503.

Doll R., Hill A.B. A study of the aetiology of carcinoma of the lung. *British Medical Journal* 1952;**2**:1271–86.

Doll R., Peto R., Boreham J. *et al.* Mortality in relation to smoking: 50 years observations on male British doctors. *British Journal of Cancer* 2005; **92**(**3**):426–9.

Dudley J., Jin S., Hoover D. *et al.* The Multicenter AIDS Cohort Study: retention after 9-1/2 years. *American Journal of Epidemiology* 1995;**142**:323–30.

Elias M.F., Wolf P.A., D'Agostino R.B. *et al.* Untreated blood pressure level is inversely related to cognitive functioning: the Framingham Study. *American Journal of Epidemiology* 1993;**138**:353–64.

Flegal K.M., Keyl P.M., Nieto F.J. Differential misclassification arising from non-differential errors in exposure measurement. *American Journal of Epidemiology* 1991;**134**:1233–44.

Fried L.P., Borhani N.O., Enright P. *et al.* The Cardiovascular Health Study: design and rationale. *Annals of Epidemiology* 1991;**1**:263–79.

Friedman G.D., Cutter G.R., Donahue R.P. *et al.* CARDIA: study design, recruitment, and some characteristics of the examined subjects. *Journal of Clinical Epidemiology* 1988;**41**:1105–16.

Furth S.L., Cole S.R., Maxey-Mims M. *et al.* Design and methods of the Chronic Kidney Disease in Children (CKID) prospective cohort study. *Clinical Journal of the American Society of Nephrology* 2006;**1**:1006–15.

Garfinkel L. Overweight and cancer. *Annals of Internal Medicine* 1985; **103**:1034–6.

Gates G.A., Cooper J.C., Kannel W.B. *et al.* Hearing in the elderly: the Framingham cohort, 1983–1985. *Part I. Basic audiometric test results. Ear and Hearing* 1990;**11**:247–56.

Greenwood M. The natural duration of cancer. In: *Reports on public health and medical subjects*. London: Her Majesty's Stationary Office; 1926. p. 1–26.

Hannan M.T., Felson D.T., Anderson J.J. Bone mineral density in elderly men and women: results from the Framingham Osteoporosis Study. *Journal of Bone and Mineral Research* 1992;**7**:547–53.

Hill A.B. The environment and disease: association or causation? Proceedings of the Royal Society of Medicine 1965;58:295–300.

Hoffmans M.D.A.F., Kromhout D., Lezenne C.C. Body mass index at the age of 18 and its effects on 32-year-mortality from coronary heart disease and cancer. *A nested case-control study among the entire 1932 Dutch male birth cohort. Journal of Clinical Epidemiology* 1989;**42**:513–20.

Hoffmans M.D.A.F., Kromhout D., Lezenne C.C. The impact of body mass index of 78,612 18-year-old Dutch men on 32-year mortality from all causes. *Journal of Clinical Epidemiology* 1988;**41**:749–56.

Hole D.J., Clarke J.A., Hawthorne V.M. *et al.* Cohort follow-up using computer linkage with routinely collected data. *Journal of Chronic Diseases* 1981;**34**:291–7.

Jacobson L.P., Li R., Phair J.P. *et al.* Evaluation of the effectiveness of highly active antiretroviral therapy in persons with human immunodeficiency virus using biomarker-based equivalence of disease progression. *American Journal of Epidemiology* 2002;**155**:760–70.

Jennrich R.I., Schluchter M.D. Unbalanced repeated-measure models with structured covariance matrices. *Biometrics* 1986;**42**:805–20.

Kannel W.B. Contribution of the Framingham Study to preventive cardiology. *Journal of the American College of Cardiology* 1990;**15**: 206–11.

Kaplan E.L., Meier P. Non-parametric estimation from incomplete observations. *Journal of the American Statistical Association* 1958;**53**:457–81.

Kaslow R.A., Ostrow D.G., Detels R. *et al.* The Multicenter AIDS Cohort Study: rationale, organization, and selected characteristics of the participants. *American Journal of Epidemiology* 1987;**126**:310–8.

Kelsey J.L., Thompson W.D., Evans A.S. *Methods in observational epidemiology*. New York (NY): Oxford University Press; 1986.

Klag M.J., Ford D.E., Mead L.A. *et al.* Serum cholesterol in young men and subsequent cardiovascular disease. *New England Jounal of Medicine* 1993;**328**:313–8.

Korn E.L., Whittemore A.S. Methods for analyzing panel studies of acute health effects of air pollution. *Biometrics* 1979;**35**:795–802.

Kreger B.E., Splansky G.L., Schatzkin A. The cancer experience in the Framingham Heart Study cohort. *Cancer* 1991;**67**:1–6.

Kupper L.L., Haseman J.K. The use of a correlated binomial model for the analysis of certain toxicological experiments. *Biometrics* 1978;**34**:69–76.

Laird N.M., Ware J.H. Random-effects models for longitudinal data. *Biometrics* 1982;**38**:963–74.

Levin M.L. The occurrence of lung cancer in man. *Acta Unio Internationalis Contra Cancrum* 1953;**9**:531–41.

Li X., Buechner J.M., Tarwater P.M. *et al.* A diamond-shaped equiponderant graphical display of the effects of two categorical predictors on continuous outcomes. *The American Statistician* 2003;**57**:193–99.

Lilienfeld A.M., Lilienfeld D.E. *Foundations of epidemiology*. 2nd ed. New York (NY): Oxford University Press; 1980.

Macaluso M. Exact stratification of person-years. *Epidemiology* 1992;**3**: 441–8.

Mantel N., Haenszel W. Statistical aspects of the analysis of data from retrospective studies of disease. *Journal of the National Cancer Institute* 1959;**22**:719–48.

Mellors J.W., Margolick J.B., Phair J.P. *et al.* Prediction of CD4 cell decline and predictive value of HIV-1 RNA, CD4 cell count and CD4 cell slope for progression to AIDS and death in untreated HIV-1 infection. *Journal of the American Medical Association* 2007;**297**:2349–50.

Mellors J.W., Muñoz A., Giorgi J.V. *et al.* Plasma viral load and CD4+ lymphocytes as prognostic markers of HIV-1 infection. *Annals of Internal Medicine* 1997;**126**:946–54.

Mertens T.E. Estimating the effect of misclassification. *Lancet* 1993;**342**: 418–21.

Muñoz A., Carey V., Taylor J.M.G. *et al.* Estimation of time since exposure for a prevalent cohort. *Statistics in Medicine* 1992;**11**:939–52.

Muñoz A., Gange S.J., Jacobson L.P. Distinguishing efficacy, individual effectiveness and population effectiveness of therapies. *AIDS* 2000;**14**:754–56.

Muñoz A., Gange S.J. Methodological issues for biomarkers and intermediate outcomes in cohort studies. *Epidemiological Reviews* 1998;**20**:29–42.

Muñoz A., Hoover D. Use of cohort studies for evaluating AIDS therapies. In: Finkelstein D., Schoenfeld D., editors. *AIDS clinical trials*. New York (NY): Wiley; 1995.

Muñoz A., Sabin C.A., Phillips A.N. The incubation period of AIDS. *AIDS* 1997;**11**:S69–S76.

Muñoz A., Xu J. Models for the incubation of AIDS and variations according to age and period. *Statistics in Medicine* 1996;**15**:2459–73.

Newcombe H.B. Strategy and art in automated death searches [editorial]. *American Journal of Public Health* 1984;**74**:1302–3.

Nieto F.J., Szklo M., Comstock G.W. Childhood weight and growth as predictors of adult mortality. *American Journal of Epidemiology* 1992;**136**:201–13.

Oshima A., Sakagami F., Hanai A. *et al.* A method of record linkage. *Environmental Health Perspectives* 1979;**32**:221–30.

Pearce N., Checkoway H. A simple computer program for generating person-time data in cohort studies involving time-related factors. *American Journal of Epidemiology* 1987;**125**:1085–91.

Peto R., Pike M.C., Armitage P. *et al.* Design and analysis of randomized clinical trials requiring prolonged observation of each patient. *II: analysis and examples. British Journal of Cancer* 1977;**351**:1–39.

Phair J.P., Mellors J.W., Detels R. *et al.* Virologic and immunologic values allowing safe deferral of antiretroviral therapy. *AIDS* 2002; **16**:2455–9.

Phillips A.N., Grabar S., Tassie J.M. *et al.* Use of observational databases to evaluate the effectiveness of antiretroviral therapy for HIV infection: comparison of cohort studies with randomized trials. *EUROSIDA, the French Hospital Database on HIV and the Swiss HIV Cohort Study Groups. AIDS* 1999;**13**:2075–82.

Robins J.M., Finkelstein D.M. Correcting for noncompliance and dependent censoring in an AIDS clinical trial with inverse probability of censoring weighted (IPCW) log-rank tests. *Biometrics* 2000;**56**:779–88.

Rose G. Sick individuals and sick populations. *International Journal of Epidemiology* 1985;**14**:32–8.

Rosner B., Muñoz A., Tager I.B. *et al.* The use of an autoregressive model for the analysis of longitudinal data in epidemiologic studies. *Statistics in Medicine* 1985;**4**:457–67.

Samet J.M., Muñoz A. Evolution of the cohort study. *Epidemiological Reviews* 1998;**20**:1–14.

Samet J.M. Concepts of time in clinical research. *Annals of Internal Medicine* 2000;**132**:37–44.

Schlesselman J.J. *Case-control studies.* New York (NY): Oxford University Press; 1982.

Schneider M.F., Gange S.J., Williams C.M. *et al.* Patterns of the hazard of death after AIDS through the evolution of antiretroviral therapy: 1984–2004. *AIDS* 2005;**19**:2009–18.

Smith M.E., Newcombe H.B. Use of the Canadian Mortality Database for epidemiological follow-up. *Canadian Journal of Public Health* 1982;**73**:39–46.

Sorlie P., Gordon T., Kannel W.B. Body build and mortality. *The Framingham Study. Journal of the American Medical Association* 1980;**243**:1828–31.

Tager I.B., Weiss S.T., Muñoz A. *et al.* Longitudinal study of the effects of maternal smoking on pulmonary function in children. *New England Journal of Medicine* 1983;**309**:699–703.

Tynes T., Andersen A., Langmark F. Incidence of cancer in Norwegian workers potentially exposed to electromagnetic fields. *American Journal of Epidemiology* 1992;**136**:81–8.

Uter W., Pfahlberg A. The application of methods to quantify attributable risk in medical practice. *Statistical Methods in Medical Research* 2001;**10**:231–7.

Vandenbroucke J.P. Prospective or retrospective: what's in a name? *British Medical Journal* 1991;302:249–50.

Virtamo J., Pietinen P., Huttunen J.K. *et al.* Incidence of cancer and mortality following alpha-tocopherol and beta-carotene supplementation: a post intervention follow-up. *Journal of the American Medical Association* 2003;**290**:476–85.

Vlahov D., Anthony J.C., Muñoz A. The ALIVE Study: a longitudinal study of HIV-1 infection in intravenous drug users—description of methods. *Journal of Drug Issues* 1991;**21**:759–76.

Whittemore A.S., Korn E.L. Asthma and air pollution in the Los Angeles area. *American Journal of Public Health* 1980;**70**:687–96.

Willett W.C., Colditz G.A. Approaches for conducting large cohort studies. *Epidemiological Reviews* 1988;**20**:91–9.

Willett W.C, Polk B.F., Underwood B.A. *et al.* Relation of serum vitamins A and E and arytenoids to the risk of cancer. *New England Journal of Medicine* 1984;**310**:430–4.

Zeger S.L., Liang K.Y. An overview of methods for the analysis of longitudinal data. *Statistics in Medicine* 1992;**11**:1825–39.

6.7

Methodology of intervention trials in individuals

Lawrence M. Friedman and Eleanor B. Schron

Introduction

An intervention trial, or a clinical trial, has been defined in various ways and may be of several kinds. The International Conference on Harmonisation defines a clinical trial as 'any investigation in human subjects intended to discover or verify the clinical, pharmacological, and/or other pharmacodynamic effects of an investigational product (s), and/or to identify any adverse reactions to an investigational product(s), and/or to study absorption, distribution, metabolism, and excretion of an investigational product(s) with the object of ascertaining its safety and/or efficacy' (International Conference on Harmonisation 1996). This definition has the advantage of applying to all phases of a clinical trial (I–IV), as traditionally defined (Friedman *et al.* 1998). The International Conference on Harmonisation definition has the disadvantage of not including trials of non-pharmacological or non-device interventions (for example, surgical procedures, diet, exercise). To encompass trials of all kinds of interventions, and given that even many trials of drugs, devices, and biologics do not neatly fit into the usual phases, it makes sense to think about early and late phase trials. Early phase trials generally address questions such as proper dose, physiologic response, tolerance, and toxicity in small number of subjects. The subjects are often healthy volunteers, but may also be people with disease who have not responded to other treatments. The early phase trials inform the design and conduct of subsequent late phase trials. This chapter will mainly address issues relating to late phase trials that use outcomes of clinical interest and are large enough to influence clinical practice. Such a clinical trial may be defined as 'a prospective study comparing the effects and value of intervention(s) against a control in human beings' (Friedman *et al.* 1998).

Clinical trials are needed because only rarely is the precise pattern or outcome of a disease or condition known. It is not yet possible to identify all of the genetic and environmental factors that lead to disease progression, recovery, and relapse. Also rare is the treatment that is so overwhelmingly successful that even with a vague understanding of the course of the disease, it is possible to say, in the absence of a control group, that the treatment is obviously beneficial and has few major adverse effects. More often, the treatment, while useful, is less than perfect. Therefore, in order to determine the true balance of potential benefit and harm from a new treatment or intervention, it is necessary to compare people who have received the treatment with those who have not. Ideally, this comparison will be made in an unbiased manner so that, at the end, any difference seen between those treated and those not treated is most likely due to the treatment.

This chapter can only cover some of the key issues in clinical trials. For more extensive discussions, the reader is referred to any of several textbooks (Friedman *et al.* 1998; Meinert & Tonascia 1986; Piantadosi 1997; Pocock 1983) as well as journals such as *Clinical Trials* and *Statistics in Medicine*.

Ethical issues in intervention studies

The issue of the ethics of conducting clinical trials has generated considerable discussion and debate. Because interventions may be harmful, as well as helpful, and participants are asked to undergo potential hazards, discomforts, and expenditure of time, the question being addressed in any clinical trial must be important. Knowledge of the answer to the question must be worth these possible harms. In addition, there must be what has been termed 'clinical equipoise' (Freedman 1987). That is, there must be uncertainty as to the usefulness of the intervention among those knowledgeable about the intervention. Individual investigators or doctors may have personal beliefs about the benefits of a new intervention. Those beliefs may prevent those investigators from participating in or entering participants into a clinical trial. The uncertainty in the medical community at large, however, is used to justify the conduct of the trial.

Informed consent of all study participants is essential. The nature of informed consent may differ in different countries and cultures, but the concept of individual choice to join or not join a trial must be universal (Council for International Organization of Medical Sciences (CIOMS) 2002; Nuremberg Code 1949; The National Commission for the Protection of Human Subjects of Biomedical and Behavioral Research 1979; World Medical Association 2000).

In addition to informed consent at the beginning of a trial, it is sometimes necessary either to modify the consent and/or to alert participants already in a trial to important new information. This can happen, for example, when an adverse effect that is important, but not so serious that a trial must be stopped, is noted. The Heart and Estrogen/Progestin Replacement Study (HERS), for example, observed an increase in thromboembolic events among the women taking the hormone therapy. This adverse outcome, which was not clearly stated in the consent form as a known risk, was uncommon, but serious. Rather than stop the trial, the investigators informed the participants of the findings and published the information in a 'Letter to the Editor' (Grady *et al.* 1997). It may also be necessary to reinform participants when one clinical trial of a similar nature or question or intervention is reported while another is ongoing (US Department of Health and Human Services 2005). The issue of conducting research in emergency settings or in other situations where informed consent is either not possible or must be delayed until after the intervention is started is a troublesome one. Such research can be extremely important, yet the imperative to only involve those who have understood the risks and volunteered to be subjects is considered by many to be unbreakable. The US FDA provides an exception from the informed consent requirement in limited settings, provided that certain policies are followed (US Food and Drug Administration 2006), as do Canadian authorities (Interagency Advisory Panel on Research Ethics 2001). The situation in other countries is less clear, though ICH guidance would appear to allow research in emergency settings (International Conference on Harmonisation 1996).

Selection of the comparison group raises ethical issues. Clinical trials may compare a new or unproven intervention against standard or usual therapy, against no therapy, against a placebo, or in combination with standard therapy against placebo in combination with standard or usual therapy. Whenever the comparison is against no therapy or placebo, the ethics of not treating someone in the best possible way are raised. If indeed there is no good treatment, then it is not a problem. But if a treatment known to be beneficial exists, then a control consisting of no therapy or placebo must be carefully justified. This might be possible if there is no appreciable risk to health or discomfort for the time that effective therapy is withheld (Ellenberg & Temple 2000; Temple & Ellenberg 2000). Often, placebo-controlled trials or trials that have no treatment as the control use both the new intervention and the control (placebo or no treatment) in addition to the best-known treatment or standard care. In such trials, the intent of evaluating the new intervention is not to replace an existing one, but to add to it. The ethics of this situation are similar to those where there is no known effective therapy. A more difficult issue exists when a treatment is commonly used in practice, but it is either of unproven benefit or is not the best-known therapy. This latter situation may occur when practitioners do not accept the evidence for the best therapy or there are practical (including financial) barriers to implementing it. Regardless of the reason for unproven or non-optimal treatment, some have advocated using usual therapy as a comparison, arguing that it provides the best test as to whether the new intervention is superior to what is being done (Eichacker *et al.* 2002). Investigators must consider the ethical issues of not using the best-known therapy as a control and the potential difficulties in interpretation of the results if the control group consists of a variety of interventions (some of which might be beneficial and others useless or even harmful).

Even when there is no known effective therapy, the ethics of using a placebo, and indeed of randomization, have been questioned (Hellman & Hellman 1991). The strictures of abiding by a study protocol reduce a clinician's freedom to do what he or she thinks is in the best interest of the patient. The interests of the individual patient cannot be sacrificed for those of society. Conversely, it has been pointed out that a clinician's views as to the best treatment are often misguided, that hunches about treatment are not particularly helpful to the patient, and that trials can be designed to take into account patient needs (Passamani 1991).

This last point is crucial. Trial design needs to incorporate the highest ethical standards. Whenever there is a potential conflict between the needs of the patient and those of the study, the interests of the patient must take precedence.

Study question

Primary and secondary questions

The most important factor in selection of the study design, population, and outcome measures is the question that is posed. Each intervention study has a primary question that is specified in advance and is used to determine the sample size. As implied by its name, in the usual two-armed study there is typically just one primary question. It is a question that is important to answer and feasible to address. By feasibility is meant the ability to identify and enrol adequate numbers of participants, to employ the intervention in an effective and presumably safe manner, to ensure that there is adequate adherence to the protocol, and to measure the outcome accurately and completely. In addition to the primary question, there may be a variety of secondary questions. Secondary questions may be less important or less feasible to answer. There may be fewer outcomes or the outcomes may be harder to measure. They may help the investigator to understand the mechanism of action of the intervention by examining biochemical or physiological processes.

Study outcomes (also termed endpoints or response variables) may be of several sorts. One way of categorizing them is as either discrete or continuous. That is, they may consist of the occurrence of an event, such as a myocardial infarction or survival from cancer, or of a measurement, such as level of blood pressure or number of CD4 lymphocytes. For late phase trials, these outcomes are usually clinically important. That is, they may be fatal or serious non-fatal events, or other clinically meaningful conditions such as alleviation of pain, increased functional status, or change in an important risk factor such as cigarette smoking.

Often, primary outcomes are composites of two or more kinds of events. For example, in studies seeking to reduce the incidence of coronary heart disease (CHD), the outcome might be a combination of death from CHD and non-fatal myocardial infarction. Sometimes, occurrence of coronary revascularization procedures might be included. The reasons for using a composite outcome are that it adds events, and therefore will reduce the required sample size, and that the individual events all represent the same underlying disease. Interpretation of the results, however, can be challenging, particularly if the outcomes are of different clinical importance. This is particularly true if the outcome perceived to be least important is most common, and dominates the analysis or if the comparisons between groups for the separate components trend in opposite directions (DeMets *et al.* 2006a).

Regardless of the primary outcome, several features pertain (Friedman *et al.* 1998). First, it must be specified in advance; written in a protocol. Second, it must be capable of being assessed in the same way in all participants. Third, it must be capable of unbiased assessment. Fourth, it must be assessed in all, or almost all, of the participants. As discussed below, significant amounts of missing data can seriously affect the interpretation of the trial.

Surrogate outcomes

Clinical trials can require large numbers of participants, last for years, and be expensive. Trials with a continuous variable as the outcome require fewer participants than do trials with dichotomous outcomes. Also, if the outcome can be assessed before a clinical event has occurred, the study may be shorter in duration. Therefore, there is considerable interest in the use of surrogate outcomes, which are often continuous. A surrogate outcome is one that substitutes for a clinical outcome; it may not, in itself, be important to the participant. An example is blood pressure. Elevated blood pressure is important primarily because it is a risk factor for stroke and heart disease, not because it is generally symptomatic. It has been shown in numerous clinical trials of both diastolic and isolated systolic hypertension that treatment reduces the occurrence of stroke and heart disease (Psaty 1997; SHEP Cooperative Research Group 1991; Staessen 1997). However, not all methods of reducing blood pressure are without risk or are equally effective in all people. Therefore, trials comparing different antihypertensive agents were conducted (ALLHAT Officers and Coordinators for the ALLHAT Collaborative Research Group 2002; Wing *et al.* 2003).

Similarly, we know that ventricular arrhythmias are associated with increased risk of sudden cardiac death (Bigger 1984). Therefore, for years it made sense to treat people with antiarrhythmic agents to reduce the occurrence of sudden death in those with heart disease and ventricular arrhythmias. Yet, when clinical trials of these agents were conducted, the results were sometimes unfavourable (The Cardiac Arrhythmia Suppression Trial (CAST) Investigators 1989; Waldo *et al.* 1995). Ventricular arrhythmia suppression is not a good surrogate for the clinical outcome of sudden cardiac death. Other examples of inadequate surrogate outcomes have been described (Fleming 1994; Fleming & DeMets 1996). Ideal characteristics of a surrogate outcome have been proposed (Prentice 1989) but these are unlikely to be fulfilled. Therefore, judgement as to the usefulness of a surrogate endpoint must be exercised. For early phase studies that do not attempt to address clinical questions, surrogate outcomes are entirely appropriate. For late phase trials, the kinds of issues that must be considered are the extent of correlation between the surrogate and the clinical event of interest, the ease or difficulty (and cost) of obtaining reliable surrogate outcome measurements on all of the participants, the feasibility of obtaining enough participants to conduct a clinical outcome study, the harm of a possibly wrong answer, and the urgency of obtaining an answer. With regard to the possibility of an incorrect answer if a surrogate outcome is used, this may be justified in certain circumstances. For example, if the disease or condition is life-threatening, doctors and patients may require less evidence of clinical benefit and may be less concerned with possible harm from an intervention. The results of a trial with a surrogate outcome may be sufficiently persuasive to allow use of the new intervention. Similarly, in truly life-threatening situations, getting an early answer using a surrogate outcome may outweigh the interest in getting a better, but delayed, answer using a clinical outcome. Early trials in AIDS used surrogate outcomes. At that time, unlike the situation today, no proven treatments were available.

Efficacy and effectiveness

Intervention studies are sometimes categorized as efficacy trials and effectiveness trials. An efficacy trial attempts to evaluate whether an intervention works under reasonably optimal circumstances. That is, if the active drug is taken as prescribed by essentially all in the intervention group, and if almost no one in the control group takes the active drug, will the drug alter some clinical outcome? An effectiveness trial allows for non-adherence to the assigned treatment; it resembles what is likely to happen in actual clinical practice. Most efficacy trials will be relatively short, as longer trials would have trouble maintaining optimal adherence (Friedman *et al.* 2004). The distinction between efficacy and effectiveness trials may sometimes be unclear as it is a continuum.

Studies of equivalency and non-inferiority

Studies of equivalency address whether the new intervention is similarly beneficial to an agent known to be worthwhile. Studies of non-inferiority look at whether the new intervention is at least as good as the standard therapy. Several factors need to be considered in the design and conduct of these kinds of trials. First, it is sometimes difficult to know that a comparison agent is worthwhile. Not all agents proven to be beneficial at some previous time will be so in all circumstances or to the same degree. This is the case with drugs such as antidepressants (Ellenberg & Temple 2000; Temple & Ellenberg 2000). Therefore, simply showing that a new intervention is no worse than the standard one may not truly prove that the new one is better than placebo. Second, 'equivalency' or 'non-inferiority' must be defined. It is not the same as failing to show a significant difference between the two agents. That could happen simply because the study has an insufficient number of participants, or because participants failed to adhere adequately to the treatments. Because the two agents cannot be shown to be identical (an infinite sample size would be needed), the new intervention must be shown to fall within some predefined boundary that is sufficiently close to the standard therapy. Defining how close will depend on the risks of inappropriately declaring the new agent to be effective and the feasibility of conducting a trial with a large enough sample size. Analysis and interpretation of equivalency and non-inferiority trials is somewhat different from interpretation in superiority trials. Failing to show a difference in a superiority trial does not necessarily entitle one to claim non-inferiority to the control or superiority to no treatment. The breadth of the confidence intervals, and the pre-specified hypothesis must be considered (Piaggio *et al.* 2006).

Clinical significance and statistical significance

An intervention study should have the ability to detect a clinically important difference between groups, if one exists. Conversely, simply showing that a statistically significant difference exists if the outcome is either not clinically meaningful or is so trivial in magnitude as to be unimportant is not worthwhile. Therefore, in determining the question to be posed, and the outcome to be measured, the issue of clinical significance needs to be considered. Factors that enter into the determination are the seriousness and prevalence of the condition or disease, the risks or cost of the intervention, and the usefulness of existing treatments (Friedman 2005).

Interventions versus intervention strategies

Not all interventions need to consist of single treatments. Sometimes, intervention strategies may be tested. In some trials of hypertension treatment, a stepped care approach was used (Hypertension Detection and Follow-up Program Cooperative Group 1979; SHEP Cooperative Research Group 1991). The intent was to see if successful lowering of elevated blood pressure resulted in reduction of stroke or heart disease. If the first antihypertensive agent did not adequately lower the blood pressure, another drug was used or added. At the end of this kind of study, it may not be possible to say that a particular drug is responsible for the observed benefits, but rather a strategy. Sometimes, the strategy may incorporate non-pharmacological as well as pharmacological approaches (for example, diet as well as drug in order to reduce blood pressure).

In trials that compared coronary artery bypass graft surgery against medical therapy (CASS [Coronary Artery Surgery Study] Principal Investigators and their Associates 1983), the comparison was not really coronary artery bypass graft versus medicine. Because, over the follow-up period, a large proportion of the participants in the medical arm received surgery, it was a strategy of early surgery versus surgery later if needed. Yusuf *et al.* (1994) reported 5-, 7-, and 10-year results from an overview of seven trials of coronary artery bypass graft surgery. At 5 years, 25 per cent of the participants assigned to the medical arms had received surgery; at 7 years 33 per cent had done so; at 10 years, 41 per cent had undergone surgery.

The Atrial Fibrillation Follow-up Investigation of Rhythm Management (AFFIRM) compared two strategies in patients with atrial fibrillation (AFFIRM Investigators 2002). One strategy attempted to correct the heart rhythm, using a variety of drugs; the other strategy was designed to control the heart rate. Despite the goal, only 62.6 per cent of the rhythm control group were actually in normal sinus rhythm at the end of 5 years, while 34.6 per cent of the rate control group were in sinus rhythm at the 5-year point. Nevertheless, the comparison of the two strategies addressed the appropriate and important clinical question of whether trying to convert those with atrial fibrillation to normal sinus rhythm was better than controlling the ventricular heart rate. At the end, the rate control group had mortality that was no worse than the rhythm control group, with fewer adverse effects.

These kinds of studies can be important and valid, but the objectives need to be clearly stated. Otherwise, the study may be criticized for not truly making the intended comparisons.

Quality of life and cost-effectiveness

Not all study outcomes need be mortality or major morbidity. Increasingly, clinical trials have evaluated outcomes such as quality of life (QOL) (sometimes referred to as health-related quality of life, well-being, or patient satisfaction) or the cost-effectiveness of administering a particular intervention as compared with another, either as primary or secondary outcomes.

There are many definitions of QOL. Essentially, QOL is a multidimensional concept that characterizes an individual's total well-being and includes psychological, social, and physical dimensions (Sartorius 1993). Many reliable and valid instruments have been developed for assessing QOL, both for a general population and for specific diseases and conditions (Ferrans & Powers 1985, 1992; McDowell 2006; Ware *et al.* 1995; Ware & Sherbourne 1992). Table 6.7.1 shows an example of a model that includes factors that may relate to QOL.

Assessment in clinical trials may be particularly valuable in cases when an intervention is not expected to alter survival but may affect a patient's perception of well-being. Cost-effectiveness evaluation may be important when interventions are expensive and where the difference between intervention and control on mortality or major morbidity is small. In a comparison of implantable cardiac defibrillators versus antiarrhythmic drugs, cost-effectiveness was a key secondary outcome. Patients with serious ventricular arrhythmias had a significant reduction in mortality from the defibrillator, but the costs were considerably greater (Larsen *et al.* 2002). Hlatky *et al.* (1997) compared quality of life, employment status, and medical care costs during 5 years of follow-up among patients treated with angioplasty or bypass graft surgery. Those in the surgical group had a better quality of life than those in the angioplasty group. Only in a subset of the participants was the cost lower in the angioplasty group.

There are ongoing improvements in methods of measuring and reporting these outcomes. The current status of QOL and cost-effectiveness assessment, however, is sufficiently robust that they can be appropriately used as clinical trial end-points.

Adverse events

As noted in the beginning of this chapter, clinical trials are designed to assess the balance of benefits and harms from a new intervention, as compared with another intervention. Incidence of adverse events comprises an important part of the harms. In the simplest case, adverse events are simply the reverse of the hoped for benefit in the primary outcome. But there are many other possible adverse events, some of which are expected; others are either unexpected

Table 6.7.1 Conceptual model for quality of life (Ferrans (1996))

Ferrans conceptual model for quality of life	
Health and functioning	**Social and economic**
Your health	Friends
Pain	Emotional support from friends
Energy (fatigue)	Home (house, apartment)
Ability to take care of yourself without help	Neighbourhood
	Job/unemployment
Ability to take care of family responsibilities	Ability to take care of financial needs
	Education
Usefulness to others	
Worries	
Control over life	
Chances of living as long as you would like	
Sex life	
Leisure time activities	
Healthcare	
Psychological/spiritual	**Family**
Satisfaction with life	Family happiness
Happiness in general	Spouse, lover, or partner
Achievement of personal goals	Children
Peace of mind	Emotional support from family
Faith in God	Family health
Personal appearance	
Satisfaction with self	

or, although expected, are more serious than anticipated. Assessment of adverse events is complicated by several factors. First, because many are looked at, it may not be easy to say which ones are truly significantly increased and which ones are due to chance. This is particularly the case with unexpected adverse events. Although it is reasonable to demand clear statistical significance when deciding that a new intervention is beneficial, investigators will generally be less statistically rigorous when assessing safety of study participants. Second, serious but uncommon adverse events may not occur often enough, even in large trials, to be properly evaluated. Furthermore, the trial may not last long enough for some kinds of adverse events to appear. These might only be discovered after a drug has been marketed, when many people have been on it for a long enough time. Sometimes, only when a drug is being evaluated for another indication, requiring a larger sample size and a longer follow-up, will an adverse event become clear. This occurred when COX 2 inhibitors, originally developed to treat inflammation due to arthritis, were studied for their effects on colon polyps (Bresalier *et al.* 2005; Solomon *et al.* 2006).

Study population

A key part of defining the question to be answered is specifying the kinds of people who will be enrolled in the clinical trial. That is done by means of eligibility criteria, of which there are various sorts (Friedman *et al.* 1998). First, eligible participants must have the potential to benefit from the intervention. That is, they must have the condition that the intervention might affect. Implicit in this is having the degree of severity at a time in the disease process that is modifiable. Also, any change in the condition must be detectable. That is, it cannot be so mild or slowly progressing that to detect a change, the study must be too large or last too long to be feasible. Second, participants cannot have known contraindications to the intervention. Third, they should not have other conditions which would make it difficult to detect changes in the condition of interest. An obvious example is someone who has both heart disease and cancer. If a 3-year study of an intervention for the heart disease is planned and the expected survival due to the cancer is less than that, it is unlikely that the person will contribute to answering the question about heart disease. Fourth, if the study requires participants to return for follow-up visits in order to assess the outcome, people who are unlikely to be able to do so should not be enrolled.

Figure 6.7.1 shows how the study participants are derived from the general population. People are excluded at various stages, based on the entry criteria. The final stage indicates that there are identified eligible participants who are not enrolled. This is because participating is strictly voluntary as a result of informed consent. Many people decide that they would prefer not to enrol in the trial.

The issue of who is and who is not enrolled in a trial raises the concepts of validity, generalization, and representativeness (Friedman *et al.* 1998). A properly designed and analysed trial will yield a valid result. That is, it will be possible to say whether or not the intervention is different from or better than the control, in the setting of the kinds of participants who were enrolled.

Depending upon how narrow or broad the study sample is will determine how much the results can be generalized. If the eligibility criteria are highly selective, then the results might only apply to that sort of participant. If the eligibility criteria are broad, with many identifiable kinds of participants, then the results would be more broadly applicable. The reasons for performing one or the other type of study will depend partly on how much is known about the mechanism of action of the intervention. Congestive heart failure may have several aetiologies. If it is known (or surmised) that the intervention only works in heart failure of a non-ischaemic origin, and therefore only such people are enrolled, then the results of the trial would only apply to people with non-ischaemic heart failure. Another reason for a narrowly defined study population might be concern over the risks versus benefits. For example, the first studies of blood pressure reduction were in people with quite elevated pressures (Hypertension Detection and Follow-up Program Cooperative Group 1979; Veterans Administration Cooperative Study Group on Antihypertensive Agents 1970; Veterans Administration Cooperative Study Group on Antihypertensive Agents 1967). Any benefit from treatment would be easier to find because of the greater likelihood of clinical events in this high-risk group. Also, any adverse effects of the intervention would be more likely to be balanced by the benefits. Not until other trials were conducted in people with lower levels of blood pressure was it possible to say with certainty that such people should be treated. The first studies could not be extrapolated to the lower risk population.

An example of a trial that successfully enrolled a broad population is the Heart Outcomes Prevention Evaluation Study (The Heart Outcomes Prevention Evaluation Study Investigators 2000). In that trial, an angiotensin-converting enzyme inhibitor was evaluated in over 9000 participants with either known vascular disease or diabetes plus a risk factor for cardiovascular disease, but without evidence of heart failure. Regardless of the type of patient, the

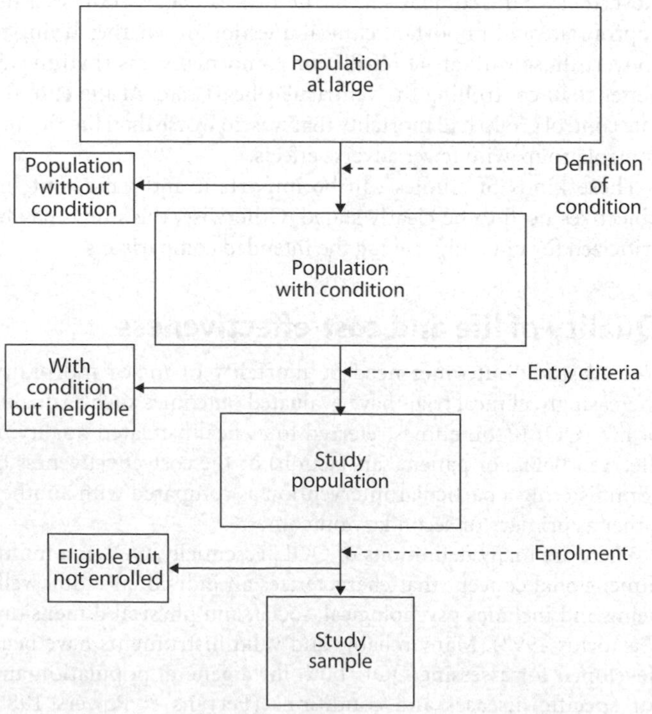

Fig. 6.7.1 Relationship of study sample to study population and population at large (those with and without the condition under study) (Friedman *et al.* 1998).

intervention was found to be highly effective in reducing mortality and morbidity.

No clinical trial is truly representative of the population with the condition being studied. Investigators conduct trials in people to whom they have ready access, rather than a random sample of the population. Eligibility criteria exclude some people for study design reasons and not because it is thought that they would not respond to the intervention in the same way as those enrolled. Additionally, there are always differences between volunteers and non-volunteers. If one is rigid, the results would be applied only to people who are identical in all relevant ways to those in the trial. The key word is 'relevant'. Judgement must be used in deciding to whom the results reasonably apply. Are the characteristics of the patient whom one wishes to treat different in respects likely to alter the effect of the intervention as observed in the trial?

One also needs to ask if the setting or way in which the trial was conducted were so special as to preclude wide generalization of the results. Particularly for trials of surgical procedures or that require other specialized expertise, the trial investigators are likely to be more experienced than the average clinician who will implement the intervention if proven to be beneficial. Therefore, translation of the results of these trials into general practice must be done cautiously, and with due consideration of the skills of the investigators (Flather *et al.* 2006).

Trial designs

Parallel design

In a parallel design study, participants are allocated to intervention or control and stay in that group until the end of the study. Although the typical study has two groups, one intervention and one control, many have more. Thus, there may be more than one intervention group and even more than one control group. When there are only two groups, the comparison is straightforward. When there are more than two groups, the comparisons can become complicated. For example, if there are three groups, two interventions and a control, there can be up to three main comparisons—each intervention against the control and one intervention against the other. This has implications for the overall type I error and therefore for the sample size. Conservatively, one would correct for the number of comparisons, in this case dividing the α level by 3. Instead of requiring a p value of, for instance, 0.05 for significance, each comparison might require a p value of 0.0167. To maintain adequate power to achieve this level of significance, the sample size will need to increase considerably. The possibly lower event rates in the two intervention groups (assuming benefit from the interventions) will also lead to the need for a larger sample size. If only the comparisons of the two interventions against the control are of interest, there is less penalty, and the three-arm design may be more efficient than initiating two individual studies, as the same control group can be used. Even here, as will be seen in the section on sample size, the control group may need to be larger than if there is only one intervention group.

Factorial design

If there is an interest in studying more than one intervention at a time, a factorial design study may be more efficient than a parallel design. The simplest factorial design is a two-by-two design. This design will have four groups: Treatment A plus treatment B, treatment A plus the control for treatment B, control for treatment A plus treatment B, and control for treatment A plus control for treatment B. The last is the only group that has no exposure to either of the interventions being tested. When this design is analysed, there are two primary analyses: The two groups with treatment A versus the two groups without treatment A and the two groups with treatment B versus the two groups without treatment B. It is unlikely that there will be adequate power to look at a single group against another single group. This would usually only happen if both interventions show differences, and are additive. An example where this happened is the Second International Study of Infarct Survival (ISIS-2 [Second International Study of Infarct Survival] Collaborative Group 1988). Factorial designs need not be just two by two. There can be more than two groups for each factor, or even more than two factors. In addition to efficiency, an advantage to the factorial design is that one might derive suggestions of differential effect of treatment in the presence or absence of the other treatment. However, this is also a weakness. If these so-called interactions are present, they may make it difficult to discern an overall effect, particularly if they go in opposite directions (Brittain & Wittes 1989). Examples of successful factorial designs, in addition to the ISIS trials (ISIS-2 [Second International Study of Infarct Survival] Collaborative Group 1988; ISIS-3 [Third International Study of Infarct Survival] Collaborative Group 1992), are the Physicians' Health Study (Hennekens & Buring 1989) and the Women's Health Initiative (The Women's Health Initiative Study Group 1998). Interestingly, for a three-arm parallel design, it is generally thought appropriate to adjust the α level for the number of comparisons. For factorial design, however, the usual practice is not to make such an adjustment.

Cross-over design

In the cross-over design, each participant serves as his or her own control (Friedman *et al.* 1998). In the simplest case, half of the participants would receive intervention followed by control, and the other half the reverse. The major advantage of this design is the smaller sample size. Because each participant is on both intervention and control, half the number of participants are needed. The sample may be even smaller, because the variability is less than in the standard parallel design. There are disadvantages, however. The most obvious one is that the outcomes must be reversible. A cross-over design is not possible if the primary outcome is mortality or a clinical event. A second disadvantage is that there is an assumption of no carry-over effect from one period to the next. If the effect of the intervention persists into the period when the control is being administered, then the apparent effect may be less than the real one. Often, to minimize the likelihood of carry-over, a washout period is inserted between the actual cross-over periods. Unfortunately, it is difficult to prove that a carry-over effect is absent and a participant has truly returned to baseline.

Randomization

The optimal way of allocating intervention or control to clinical trial participants is by means of randomization. Randomization does not guarantee balance in all factors between the groups, but the chances of balance are increased. Unknown as well as known and measured characteristics are likely to be comparable when there is randomization. A properly performed randomization procedure also reduces the opportunity for investigator bias in the allocation of intervention or control. Finally, randomization guarantees that statistical tests of significance will be valid.

Randomization does not require a one-to-one allocation to intervention or control, only that the allocation be unpredictable. Alternative assignment or assignment based on day of the month (for example, odd or even) is predictable, and is not equivalent to randomization. Matching on the basis of important characteristics is also not considered randomization. Flipping an unbiased coin to determine whether a participant is assigned to group A or B can be a valid way of randomizing. In practice, however, tables of random numbers or computer-produced random numbers are more often used.

Randomized studies can, by definition, only have a concurrent control group. That is, a historical control study cannot have randomized allocation. This yields another advantage of randomization, namely that the participants are enrolled in the same time period in both the intervention and control groups. Therefore, temporal trends in care or in the nature of the condition being studied are equal in the two groups.

Randomization procedures

Several procedures for randomly assigning treatments to participants have been developed. The simplest are the fixed allocation procedures. If, for example, 20 participants are needed for a study, a coin may be tossed when each participant is entered. However, the likelihood that the number of participants in the two groups will be different (for instance, 12 to 8 or even more extreme) is about 50 per cent. As the sample size increases, the likelihood of such a large uneven split is reduced. If 100 participants are enrolled, the chance of a 60 to 40 split is only about 5 per cent (Friedman *et al*. 1998).

Blocked randomization is commonly used because of this problem. In blocked randomization, equal numbers of participants in the groups is guaranteed after every several are enrolled. For example, if the block size is 4, and the sample size is 12, then after 4, 8, and 12 participants are enrolled, there would be equal numbers in treatments A and B. This would be accomplished by specifying that each block of four would have two participants assigned to A and two to B. The order within the block of four would be randomized. Thus, it could be ABAB, AABB, ABBA, BABA, and so on. The hazard with this approach is that if the block size is known to the investigator and the treatments are not completely blinded, the last one of the block (and sometimes the last two) can be predicted. Therefore, often, the block size, as well as the order within the block, is random, and the investigator entering the participants is kept ignorant of the block size.

Another advantage of blocked randomization would be if participant entry criteria are modified partway through a trial. In the absence of blocking, even if at the end of entering all participants there are more or less equal numbers in the groups, there may be imbalance in numbers when only some of the participants have been entered. If, because of lagging participant entry, the eligibility criteria are loosened, different sorts of participants may enrol later during recruitment than enrolled earlier. As a result, the characteristics of the participants in group A may differ from those in group B. With blocked randomization, equal numbers are ensured throughout the enrolment period, and changes in entry criteria would not lead to imbalances between the groups in type of participant.

Stratified randomization is a special kind of blocked randomization. Here, the investigator wishes to ensure that there is balance between group A and B, not only in numbers of participants, but in kind of participant. If, despite the randomization process, there is concern that there will be imbalance between groups for one or two key highly prognostic variables, randomization can be stratified on those variables. Thus, within decades of age, for example, blocked randomization would occur. If sex is also a key variable, there would be blocked randomization within each age–sex category. The problem is that even with only two or three characteristics, each one having two or more factors, the number of strata can rapidly increase (Friedman *et al*. 1998). This can lead to unfilled cells unless many participants are being enrolled. If the sample size is large, randomization will generally lead to good balance, making stratification unnecessary. Therefore, stratified randomization should be done judiciously. If, after the trial is over, it is found that there is a major imbalance in a key factor, an adjusted analysis can be performed. In multicentre trials, randomization is usually done by centre, making the centre one of the important strata. This minimizes the chance that different sorts of participants or different medical practices among centres will confound the results.

In addition to the above fixed randomization procedures, there are various adaptive randomization procedures. In baseline adaptive procedures (also termed adaptive stratification or covariate adaptive randomization), the likelihood of randomization to A or B changes in order to reduce imbalances in selected characteristics. In response adaptive procedures, the likelihood of randomization to one or another group changes based on the occurrence of study outcomes. Adaptive randomization procedures have not been used as frequently as fixed randomization. For more details of these procedures, see Friedman *et al*. (1998). and Rosenberger and Lachin (2002).

Blinding

Blinding, sometimes termed masking, is commonly used in clinical trials. In double-blind studies, neither the investigator nor the participant is aware of the intervention assignment. In single-blind trials, only the participant is not informed of the assignment. In unblinded, or open trials, all are aware of the assignment. Ideally, trials should be double-blind. This reduces the opportunity for bias in study management and outcome assessment. For most trials of procedures or life style change, it is not feasible to have anything other than an unblinded design. Here, special efforts to ensure unbiased outcome assessment should be employed.

Sample size

Clinical trials should be designed with adequate power to answer the question being posed. That is, by the end of the trial, there should be enough events or, in the case of continuous response variable, sufficient precision of the estimate to say with reasonable assurance that the intervention does or does not have the postulated effect. Several factors are considered in the calculation of sample size. For dichotomous outcome studies, these factors are event rate in the control group, expected benefit from the intervention, level of adherence to the intervention, level of adherence to the control regimen, α level, and power. For continuous outcome studies, the mean and variance of the control and intervention groups, plus the level of adherence, α level, and power, would be the relevant variables.

Various references provide formulas for calculating sample size; (Lachin 1981; Lakatos 1986; Wu 1988), as does Chapter 6.14. In essence, the factors that lead to the need for larger sample sizes in the dichotomous outcome situation are lower control group event rate, smaller benefit from the intervention (or lesser difference that one wants to detect), smaller α, greater power to detect a real difference (smaller β), and poorer adherence (or greater cross-over). Alpha is commonly selected to be 0.05 (two-sided); power is typically 0.8–0.9.

As discussed below, the preferred method of analysis is by 'intention to treat'. This means that, in general, participants remain in the randomization group to which they have been assigned, regardless of their future actions or the degree to which they adhere to the assigned regimen. To the extent that those assigned to the intervention group fail to comply with the intervention, for example by not taking their medication (often called 'drop-out'), the expected benefit from the intervention is reduced. Similarly, to the extent that those assigned to the control group begin taking the intervention (often called 'drop-in'), the control group event rate is altered. The net effect of this non-adherence is a narrowing of the difference between the groups. This, in turn, leads to a larger sample size in order to maintain the same power to detect a real difference. Non-adherence can have an appreciable effect on sample size. A correction factor proposed by Lachin multiplies the needed sample size by $1/(1 - R_0 - R_1)^2$, where R_0 is the drop-out rate and R_1 is the drop-in rate. Because the factor is squared, the sample size increases rapidly as soon as the combined non-adherence rate goes over 20 per cent. Even a combined non-adherence rate of only 10 per cent means a sample size increase of almost a quarter. More complicated sample size formulas take into account the fact that most non-adherence is not linear, but is often greater earlier in a trial than later (Lakatos 1986; Wu 1988). Another factor sometimes considered in sample size calculations is the estimated time for an intervention to make the postulated biological changes. For example, if cholesterol-lowering drugs act at least partly by affecting arterial plaque, then the time for that process to occur (so-called 'lag time') implies a larger sample size (and a longer study).

As noted in the section above on study question, studies of equivalency and non-inferiority may require large sample sizes, depending on what is meant by 'equivalence'. Because the sample size formula contains the difference to be detected in the denominator, if zero difference is planned, the sample size would be infinite. Therefore, one typically specifies a difference δ. If the two treatments show differences less than this, they are considered equal, or at least they have differences that are unimportant. Sample size formulas for such studies are available (Blackwelder & Chang 1984). It should be emphasized that, unlike studies where a difference is being sought, an underpowered study of equivalency or non-inferiority will lead to the 'desired' outcome. That is, it will confirm the null hypothesis of no difference. Even more, poor adherence will enhance the likelihood of seeing no difference for either the primary outcome or for adverse effects.

The needed sample size is an estimate because factors such as event rate and adherence are rarely known for certain. It may be prudent, therefore, to be conservative in the assumptions that enter into calculating sample size. The disadvantage of being conservative is that increased size or duration leads to increased cost. Also, entering more people into a trial than is necessary to answer the question may put more people at risk than is appropriate. Just as randomization can be adjusted, based on observed outcomes, so can sample size. This chapter is not the place to discuss adaptive sample size methods in detail. Those interested should see Proschan *et al.* (2006).

Recruitment of participants

A rule of thumb for all late phase clinical trials is that participant recruitment is always more difficult than expected. With medical records and other ways of identifying study participants now being increasingly available electronically, screening can be conducted more efficiently than in the past. At the same time, however, there is increased attention in many countries to privacy concerns (National Institutes of Health 2003; Peto *et al.* 2004; Trevena *et al.* 2006). Therefore, screening and contact of potential study participants must be conducted with proper consideration of privacy rights.

It is the uncommon clinical trial that finishes enrolment on schedule and the even rarer one that can do so without major recruitment strategy changes. Because recruitment is difficult, it is best to employ multiple strategies and to plan for back-up strategies in advance and to monitor progress closely throughout the enrolment period. Depending on the nature of the study population, back-up strategies would include adding sources of participants (for example, clinics, hospital units) or disseminating information about the trial more widely, to both medical personnel and potential participants. If sufficient resources are available, the strategies might include adding staff whose primary responsibilities involve enhancing enrolment or increasing incentives. The latter raises ethical questions if the incentives are inappropriate in amount or kind. Paying so-called 'finder's fees', for example, would not be acceptable.

If participant enrolment remains slow, several options are available. One approach is to extend the time of enrolment. This has the advantage of not changing other study design factors, but the disadvantages of additional cost and delay in answering the question. A second approach is to accept the smaller sample size. Depending upon how large the shortfall is, the reduced power may not be too great. If the power goes from 90 to 85 per cent or even 80 per cent, that can be acceptable. However, if it falls much below 80 per cent, the study is likely to be underpowered. Some have argued that conducting even underpowered trials is useful, as cumulative meta-analyses of similar trials will yield the answers (Antman *et al.* 1992), but that approach is not recommended here. A third option is to change the entry criteria, so that more people are eligible. Depending on the original criteria, this might be feasible. However, care needs to be taken to make sure that other design assumptions, such as the expected effect of the intervention and the event rate, are not materially changed. In addition, as noted above, a blocked randomization scheme needs to be used to ensure that there is no gross imbalance between groups in participants enrolled before and after the criteria change.

A fourth option is to change the study outcome, so that fewer participants are needed to obtain the same number of events. A study may be originally designed with the outcome of death due to heart disease or non-fatal myocardial infarction. Because of limited resources, other remedies for slow participant accrual may not be feasible. It may be decided that the intervention is as likely to affect other important outcomes, such as need for coronary revascularization, as it is to affect myocardial infarction. Adding that event to the primary outcome would increase the event rate considerably, and allow for an answer with fewer participants. In another example, incidence of hypertension may be the outcome in a study looking at prevention of hypertension with weight loss. Instead of using incidence of hypertension as the primary event, mean blood pressure might be used. Going from a dichotomous outcome study to a study using a continuous variable as the outcome will reduce the needed sample size. These sorts of design changes should not be made lightly. They require considerable thought and review. If, because of the changes, the results are not persuasive to the outside community of practising clinicians, there is little point in undertaking them.

Adherence

As discussed in the section above on sample size, adherence (or compliance) on the part of participants is a key factor in clinical trials. It can reduce the power of a trial, and, if truly bad, can make the study results uninterpretable. Therefore, most investigators take steps when planning a study to minimize poor participant adherence. One is to design the study so that the regimen is as simple as possible. For medications, once-daily dosing is preferable to more frequent doses. For lifestyle interventions such as diet or exercise, simpler, more easily remembered programmes are better. Shorter trials have better chances of maintaining good adherence than longer ones. A second method is to select participants who are more likely to adhere. One way is by means of a run-in phase prior to randomization. Unless study participants must be enrolled immediately, for example at the time of an acute event, a run-in period can be used to determine who adheres to the regimen. Potential participants might be given the active medication for several weeks. At the end of that time, only those who took at least 80 per cent (or some other reasonable amount) of the drug would be enrolled. The participants who could not adhere, even over the short term, would not be randomized. This approach has been successfully used in the Physicians' Health Study (Glynn *et al.* 1994; Steering Committee of the Physicians' Health Study Research Group 1989) and the Women's Health Study (Cook *et al.* 2005). Angiotensin-converting enzyme inhibitors may cause cough in some people. Therefore, to minimize the drop-out rate after randomization, studies of angiotensin-converting enzyme inhibitors have used a short run-in period to exclude those who might not tolerate the drug (Davis 1998). Excluding potential non-adherers on the basis of other demographic or psychosocial factors has been done, but the evidence that it successfully separates good from poor adherers is unclear (Dunbar-Jacob 1998). Educating potential participants about the trial is not only good practice from an informed consent standpoint, but is likely to lead to the enrolment of participants who are better adherers. Being unduly persuasive in enrolling participants may improve the recruitment figures, but it can lead to worse adherence statistics. Because the analysis is done on an intention-to-treat basis, the study is more harmed by someone who drops out after enrolment than by someone who does not enrol.

A variety of techniques to maintain good adherence have been tried. Those that appear to be useful are frequent contact and reminders, providing easy transportation and access to attractive facilities, providing continuity of care, providing special medication dispensers, such as calendar packs, and involving family members, particularly when the intervention is lifestyle change (Schron & Czajkowski 2001). Other techniques include attention to aspects of the trial regimen, such as single-dose formulation for medication, intervention schedules made similar to those in clinical practice, and the use of specially trained personnel.

Adherence monitoring has two purposes. One is to be able to advise participants who are not complying with their regimen on how they might improve. The second is to be able to interpret the results of the trial more accurately. The first requires knowledge of individual adherence; the latter only requires knowing how the groups are performing.

Monitoring individual adherence is important, but there is considerable debate about how accurately it can be done, except for interventions that take place entirely in clinics or hospitals (surgery, vaccine, periodic medication, food feeding studies). Self-reports are simple, but subject to considerable uncertainty. Participants may not remember accurately, and may have a desire to report better adherence than is truly the case. Assessment of activities such as nutritional intake and physical activity are particularly difficult. The use of diaries or other records may help, but still depend on accurate completion by the participant.

For studies involving medication, there are a variety of ways to assess adherence. Pill count is relatively simple, though there are studies that indicate that it over-reports adherence (Rand & Weeks 1998). Participants may forget to return the partially empty containers or may intentionally discard medication that was not taken. Laboratory measures of drug metabolites can be useful, but also may be misleading, as they do not reflect what was ingested long term or show the true pattern of medication usage. Use of special devices that register when a bottle cap is opened has been advocated (Rand & Weeks 1998). Electronic monitoring of this sort can provide a continuous record of dose taking. This probably provides a more accurate measure of adherence, but it is expensive. Even this technique does not prevent a participant from opening the bottle, removing a pill, and then discarding it.

Physiological or biochemical measures that reflect responses to the intervention can be used in some studies. For example, trials of cholesterol-lowering agents which have heart disease as the outcome would periodically measure lipid levels. These are not foolproof indicators of adherence, as individual responses vary, but they are particularly good at demonstrating that on average, after randomization, the intervention group has a different biochemical profile from the control group. One problem with using these sorts of measures as markers of individual adherence is that they may unmask the group to which a participant has been assigned.

Unless one is willing to go to considerable lengths and spend considerable resources, the simple measures of adherence are probably adequate for most purposes. They will certainly indicate gross problems overall, and allow the investigator to conclude, with reasonable assurance, that the intervention was or was not administered satisfactorily, and that there is or is not a difference between the groups in intermediate response variables or biomarkers. However, there is no single gold standard for measuring adherence. Furthermore in order to have a valid assessment of adherence, the use of more than one measure is recommended (DiMatteo 2004).

Data and safety monitoring

Data and safety monitoring is an essential part of any clinical trial. If the data become persuasive before the scheduled end of the trial, or if unexpected adverse events occur, the investigator is obligated either to stop the trial or to make necessary design changes. For many trials, the monitoring function is undertaken by a person or group external to the study investigator structure. For masked studies, this helps to keep the investigator blinded. But more importantly, for all trials, an outside group is less likely to have a bias and less likely to want the study to continue inappropriately because of financial or other reasons. The primary function of this group is to maximize participant safety. Secondarily, it helps ensure the integrity of the trial.

In the process of data and safety monitoring, several kinds of recommendations may be made. First, and most common, would be a recommendation to continue the trial without any change. Second would be a recommendation to modify the protocol in some way. Examples might be changing the participant entry criteria, changing the informed consent to take into consideration important new information, changing the frequency of certain tests to better ensure safety, or even dropping from the study certain types of participants for whom it may no longer be appropriate. Third, there might be reason to recommend extending the trial. This could occur if the participant accrual rate is slower than expected or if the overall event rate is much lower than expected. Fourth, there might be a recommendation to stop the trial early.

Data monitoring techniques

Regular data monitoring must be performed for ethical reasons. However, this carries a penalty:

> *If the null hypothesis, H_0, of no difference between two groups is, in fact, true, and repeated tests of that hypothesis are made at the same level of significance using accumulating data, the probability that, at some time, the test will be called significant by chance alone will be larger than the significance level selected. That is, the rate of incorrectly rejecting the null hypothesis will be larger than what is normally considered to be acceptable* (Friedman *et al.* 1998).

Therefore a variety of stopping boundaries or guidelines have been developed that maintain the overall prespecified α level. Biostatistics references can be consulted for the details of these methods. In essence, the methods fall into three categories: Classical sequential, group sequential, and curtailed sampling. In the classical sequential approach (Whitehead 1997), there is no fixed sample size. Participant enrolment and the study end when boundaries for benefit or harm are exceeded. A theoretical advantage of the classical sequential approach is that fewer participants might need to be enrolled than in a fixed sample size design. This design requires study outcomes to occur relatively soon after enrolment, however, so that decisions about enrolment of new participants can be made. As a result, it may have limited usefulness.

The most commonly used monitoring techniques are the group sequential methods. Here, after a group of participants have been enrolled, or after a length of time, the data are examined. In order to conserve the overall α level, the study is not stopped early even if the nominal p value (for example, 0.05) is exceeded. More extreme p values are required for early stopping. An example of such boundaries is that developed by O'Brien and Fleming (1979), which calls for very extreme results early in a study which gradually become less extreme towards the end. If the study goes to the expected end, the significance value is essentially what it would be without any interim monitoring. An approach proposed by Haybittle (1971) and Peto *et al.* (1976) uses a constant extreme value throughout the trial, with the usual p value for significance at the end. Both of these techniques allow the final significance value to be what would be used without monitoring because of the low likelihood of stopping early, given the extreme nature of the boundaries. A modification of these techniques uses what is termed an α spending function (Lan & DeMets 1989). This technique allows for more flexible selection of the times when the data will be monitored.

Another modification of the group sequential methods employs asymmetric boundaries. For many trials, even those that are not one-sided tests of the hypothesis, it would be inappropriate to continue a trial until the intervention is proven harmful, using the usual p value of 0.05. Therefore, instead of having the monitoring boundary for harm symmetric to the one for benefit, a less extreme monitoring boundary can be developed (DeMets & Ware 1982). Thus, if the one for benefit maintains the overall α at 0.05, the one for harm might maintain it at 0.1, or even less extreme. Even with one-sided tests of hypothesis, an advisory boundary for harm can be implemented, as was the case in the Cardiac Arrhythmia Suppression Trial (Pawitan & Hallstrom 1990).

Curtailed sampling addresses the probability of seeing a significant result if the trial were to continue to its end, given the data at the current time (that is, part way through the trial) (Lan & Wittes 1988). For example, if there is a strongly positive trend with three-quarters of the expected data in hand, one can examine the probabilities of having a statistically significant outcome under various assumptions regarding future data. A reasonable assumption might be that the control group event rate will continue, more or less, as it has been and that the null hypothesis is true. If, under those conditions, the outcome is still significant, there might be reason to stop the study. Conversely, if there is little or no benefit (or a trend towards harm) from the intervention, one might look at how large a benefit would be required from now on to see a significant benefit at the end. If there is little likelihood of that happening, the study might be stopped because continuation would be futile.

Descriptions of stopping decisions in clinical trials have been published (DeMets *et al.* 2006b). These include stopping early for overwhelming benefit, clear harm, or futility, as well as examples of complicated issues. A decision to stop a trial early is irrevocable; therefore, such a decision must be made carefully. Whenever a recommendation is made to stop a study early, factors other than whether or not the monitoring boundaries are crossed need to be considered (Friedman *et al.* 1998). Might the results be due to imbalance in baseline characteristics or to bias in ascertainment of the outcome? Might poor adherence or differential use of concomitant therapy be important? What might be the impact of outcomes other than the primary one on the interpretation of the conclusions? Are there major unexpected adverse effects that need to be considered? How might other ongoing research affect the results? Will the results be persuasive to others? The issues are not just statistical in nature. If they were, there would be little need for a monitoring committee. Instead, an algorithm could be created which would make the decision. But because the decisions depend on a complex interaction of statistics, understanding of the biological mechanism of action of the intervention, knowledge of other research findings, and judgement as to how the results will be received and interpreted, decisions to recommend continuation or stopping are rarely easy and often second-guessed.

Analysis issues

Whom to include

A purpose of assigning intervention or control by means of randomization is to ensure, as far as possible, that there is balance between the groups on both measured and unmeasured factors. Anything that alters that balance, such as removing from analysis some data from some participants, can induce bias. The reason is that it may be difficult to prove that the cause for the exclusion is unrelated to either a key baseline factor or to the intervention or control. Therefore, the general guideline for analysis is called 'intention to treat'. That is, once randomization has taken place, the data from all participants should be included and counted in the group to which they are assigned.

There are several reasons why one would want to withdraw participants or data from the analysis. First, it may be discovered, after enrolment, that a participant is not truly eligible for the trial. Therefore, that person would not contribute meaningfully to answering the question and, in fact, might confuse the issue by providing incorrect information. Also importantly, it might be hazardous for that person to be taking the intervention. Withdrawing such people from the study and the analysis might seem to be straightforward, but often it is not. If the decision that a person is ineligible is made after adverse effects or a clinical event has occurred, it might be viewed as an effort to manipulate the data. Eligibility criteria are commonly subjective and even in blinded trials there may be clues regarding the group to which the participant was assigned. Therefore, if participants are withdrawn from the trial because they are found to be ineligible, it must be done as soon as possible, before any events have occurred or follow-up measurements performed, and without knowledge of the treatment group. If that does not happen, then the best policy is to leave the participant in the study and analyse the data as if he or she is eligible. If it is possibly dangerous for the participant to be on the intervention, that can be discontinued without removing the person from the trial. If the percentage of ineligible people is small, that should not unduly affect the conclusions. If the percentage is large, such that the study integrity might be affected, then there is clearly a larger problem with the conduct of the trial.

A second reason for withdrawal of participants after randomization is poor adherence. As discussed in the sample size section, incomplete adherence to the protocol is best handled by increasing the number of people in the trial. Sometimes, however, it is decided to remove non-adherent participants from the analysis. The argument for doing this is that if they have not taken the intervention, there is no way that they can provide information as to its usefulness. The counter-argument is that lack of adherence may be a reflection of not being able to tolerate one or another of the treatments. Therefore, withdrawing poor adherers leads to an underestimate of the adverse effects. It also biases the analysis because those removed from one group are likely to be different from those removed from the other group. There have been attempts to adjust for non-adherence, but these approaches are questionable.

The classic example of how withdrawing poor adherers from analysis can lead to strange results is from the Coronary Drug Project, a trial of lipid lowering in heart disease patients. As expected, those assigned to the active medication group who did not take it fared worse than those who did. But those assigned to placebo who did not take the placebo also fared worse than those who did (Coronary Drug Project Research Group 1980). This outcome could not be accounted for by measured differences between the adherers and non-adherers. Therefore, unknown confounding factors must have been present, as the difference is not attributable to an inert substance. It is best to include the data from all participants, regardless of level of adherence, in the analysis. If, despite the best efforts of the investigator, adherence is so poor as to compromise the integrity of the trial, then that itself says something about the usefulness of the intervention.

Poor quality or, in the extreme case, missing data is a third reason for withdrawing participants from analysis. Every effort must be made to minimize these. If participants are lost to follow-up, or do not return for key outcome measurements, the data will be missing. To the extent that this constitutes more than a few per cent of the total data, the study is severely impaired. The reason, again, is that there is no assurance that the missing data are independent of the treatment. If participants do not return to the clinic because one of the treatments makes them feel unwell, the data in that group will only be from those who are healthier or better able to tolerate the treatment.

Various statistical methods have been proposed to take into account missing data, but none is perfect (Espeland *et al.* 1992; Proschan *et al.* 2001). In general, they make assumptions or a range of assumptions about the missing data (sensitivity analysis). They may use prior data from the individual or some average from the group to which that individual is assigned to impute the most likely values for the missing data. One assumption might be that all participants missing in one group had the most unfavourable results while all the other groups had the most favourable results, and vice versa. These techniques can be useful, but as with simply censoring missing data, are limited if the missing data are strongly related to treatment and there are large amounts of missing data. One hopes that regardless of the assumptions made, the overall conclusions are unchanged. If the amount of missing data is so great that, under reasonable assumptions, the conclusions vary, the investigator must question the validity of the study.

The same factors apply to poor-quality data or outliers. Ideally all analyses should be performed with and without including the outliers, as there may be important reasons for the apparently strange data that should not be ignored. One practice that is not encouraged is substituting data such as prior measurements from an individual for data that are thought to be incorrect or outlying.

Adjustment procedures

Despite best efforts, study groups may turn out to have imbalances in important factors at baseline. In such cases, it is tempting to adjust for these imbalances. Unless the imbalance is large and the factor is highly correlated with the outcome, however, adjustment is unlikely to make a major difference. Simply showing that there is a statistically significant difference in a baseline covariate is not sufficient reason to adjust on that factor. Conversely, large and potentially important differences may not be statistically significant because of small numbers. Furthermore, there may be several covariates that are imbalanced in a similar direction. Individually, they may not be important, but in the aggregate, they may lead to enough of an imbalance that adjustment is useful. In summary, adjustment for baseline imbalances is legitimate, and should be explored if there are apparent differences. Mostly, this is unnecessary. Certainly, if adjustment converts a non-significant result to a significant one, it needs to be interpreted cautiously.

Adjustment for post-randomization variables is strongly discouraged. Level of adherence is one example of such a variable. Others might be biomarkers or similar interim measures of the effect of the intervention, as well as concomitant therapy. Because such variables are, or may be related to, the intervention, unlike the baseline factors, adjustment for them can result in misleading interpretations. Response to an intervention can indicate better prognosis, even in the absence of the intervention (Anderson *et al.* 1983; Coronary Drug Project Research Group 1980). Adjustment on such a variable can make an intervention appear beneficial when it is not.

Subgroup analyses

In every clinical trial it is tempting to look at the effects of the intervention in subgroups of participants. This is particularly the case with trials that show no significant difference overall. Even without overall benefit, there might be some subsets that indeed benefit. The problem is that with enough creativity, one can almost always find a group that benefits (and a group that is harmed) from the intervention. Even in trials that have significant overall differences, there is a desire to find the types of participants who benefit the most.

It is generally the case that qualitative interactions are uncommon (Peto 1995). That is, an intervention is unlikely to be beneficial in one subgroup and harmful in another. Conversely, it is quite plausible that there are differential relative effects. Some kinds of people are indeed likely to be helped more than other kinds of people. The problem is that unless the subgroups of interest are specified in advance, it is likely that most of the observed differences are due to chance. The best way of confirming that subgroup differences are real is to examine an independent dataset, usually from another trial of the same question. Somewhat weaker is using independent data from the same trial. This can be done if, during data monitoring, a possible subgroup difference is identified. The data accrued during the remaining period of the trial on participants who have not yet had the event can be confirmatory. Other approaches, such as looking at trends in subgroups defined by continuous variables, especially where there is biological plausibility, can also be used.

As noted, with enough imagination, apparent subgroup differences can be uncovered. 'Fishing', or 'data-dredging' is a natural activity, as unexpected subgroup findings can be important sources of new information and new hypotheses. As opposed to raising new questions, however, conclusions should almost never be drawn from subgroups that are not prespecified. The examples of differences based on signs of the zodiac (ISIS-2 [Second International Study of Infarct Survival] Collaborative Group 1988) or similar characteristics are cautionary.

Meta-analyses

A separate chapter is devoted to meta-analyses (Chapter 6.13). Therefore, only a brief summary is provided here. Meta-analyses can be important ways of synthesizing data. They enable researchers to incorporate multiple studies of the same question. Because of the added numbers of participants, they provide better estimates of intervention effects in subgroups. They allow one to put together several small studies to see if a larger study should be conducted to address a question more clearly. They do have potential limitations, however. Most important is the effort expended in collecting all of the relevant studies and the judgement that must go into selection of the studies to be combined. Studies that show benefit from an intervention are more likely to be published (Dickerson *et al.* 1987). Therefore, if meta-analyses are not done carefully with clear criteria, biases can be introduced. Another limitation is that only some outcomes can be used. Typically, mortality or major morbidity is the outcome of interest. When deciding on whether or not an intervention is useful, other outcomes, such as adverse effects and quality of life, may be important, but are rarely incorporated into published meta-analyses. The ability to perform meta-analyses easily may lead to several inadequately powered studies yielding an overall statistically significant p value. Examples of probably misleading conclusions from these meta-analyses have been observed, once the single large trial was conducted (LeLorier *et al.* 1997). Any discouragement of the conduct of properly sized trials because of meta-analyses is unfortunate.

Reporting and interpretation

Several guidelines to the proper reporting of clinical trial results have been published (Moher *et al.* 2001; Piaggio *et al.* and for the CONSORT Group 2006). In essence, they call for objective recording of all pertinent aspects. It is recognized that space limitations restrict the amount of information that can be included in a publication. The advent of journal websites, however, allows for the dissemination of supplementary material. Ideally, all of the following should be included in a clinical trial report (Friedman *et al.* 1998).

1. Background and rationale.
2. Specification of the primary question and the response variables used to assess it.
3. Prespecified secondary questions.
4. Nature of the study population, including eligibility criteria, major reasons why people were not entered, and the fact that informed consent was obtained.
5. Sample size calculations and the assumptions used for that calculation.
6. Basic study design features and allocation procedures.
7. Data collection procedures, including efforts to minimize bias, quality control, and event classification.
8. Presentation of key baseline characteristics, by group.
9. Process measures, such as adherence, concomitant therapy usage, performance of procedures, amount of missing or poor quality data, and numbers of participants lost to follow-up.
10. Results for the primary outcome, secondary outcomes (prespecified and other), and adverse events. The statistics and tabulations should reflect the original intent and indicate whether the effects of repeated tests have been taken into account. Confidence intervals, relative risk reduction (or increase), and absolute risk reduction should be presented. Also noted should be where the data were analysed.

11. Adverse effects.
12. Special analyses, such as subgroups, covariate adjustment, and data-derived hypotheses.
13. Interpretation, implications, and conclusions in the context of both study data and information external to the trial.
14. A structured abstract that accurately reflects the body of the paper.

Conclusion

It is not easy to conduct well-designed clinical trials, and there are ethical issues that must be considered. Nevertheless, there is no substitute for good clinical trials in providing important information for clinical use and public health about the possible benefits of interventions. As a result of the development of clinical trial technologies over the past several decades, more clinical decisions are evidence based. Improvements in trial design and analysis are continuing and will have further impact, as will increasing knowledge about genetics, better understanding of disease aetiologies and processes, and pharmacology.

References

ALLHAT Officers and Coordinators for the ALLHAT Collaborative Research Group (2002). Major outcomes in high-risk hypertensive patients randomized to angiotensin-converting enzyme inhibitor or calcium channel blocker vs diuretic: The Antihypertensive and Lipid-Lowering Treatment to Prevent Heart Attack Trial (ALLHAT). *JAMA*, **288** (23), 2981–97.

Anderson, J.R., Cain, K.C., and Gelber, R.D. (1983). Analysis of survival by tumor response. *Journal of Clinical Oncology*, **1** (11), 710–19.

Antman, E.M., Lau, J., Kupelnick, B. *et al.* (1992). A comparison of results of meta-analyses of randomized control trials and recommendations of clinical experts. Treatments for myocardial infarction. *JAMA*, **268** (2), 240–8.

Bigger, J.T. (1984). Identification of patients at high risk for sudden cardiac death. *The American Journal of Cardiology*, **54** (9), 3–8D.

Blackwelder, W.C. and Chang, M.A. (1984). Sample size graphs for 'proving the null hypothesis'.*Controlled Clinical Trials*, **5** (2), 97–105.

Bresalier, R.S., Sandler, R.S., Quan, H. *et al.* and the Adenomatous Polyp Prevention on Vioxx (APPROVe) Trial Investigators (2005). Cardiovascular events associated with rofecoxib in a colorectal adenoma chemoprevention trial. *The New England Journal of Medicine*, **352** (11), 1092–1102.

Brittain, E. and Wittes, J. (1989). Factorial designs in clinical trials: the effects of non-compliance and subadditivity. *Statistics in Medicine*, **8** (2), 161–71.

CASS (Coronary Artery Surgery Study) Principal Investigators and their Associates (1983). Coronary artery surgery study (CASS): A randomized trial of coronary artery bypass surgery. Survival data. *Circulation*, **68**, 939–50.

Cook, N.R., Lee, I.M., Gaziano, J.M. *et al.* (2005). Low-dose aspirin in the primary prevention of cancer: The women's health study: A randomized controlled trial. *JAMA*, **294** (1), 47–55.

Coronary Drug Project Research Group (1980). Influence of adherence to treatment and response of cholesterol on mortality in the coronary drug project. *The New England Journal of Medicine*, **303** (18), 1038–41.

Council for International Organization of Medical Sciences (CIOMS) (2002). *International Ethical Guidelines for Biomedical Research Involving Human Subjects*. World Health Organization (WHO), Geneva.

Davis, C.E. (1998). Perandomization compliance screening: A statistician's views. In *The Handbook of Health Behavior Change* (eds. S.A. Shumaker *et al.*), 2nd edition, pp. 485–90. Springer, New York.

DeMets, D.L., Furberg, C.D., and Friedman, L.M. (2006a). Lessons learned. In *Data Monitoring in Clinical Trials: A Case Studies Approach* (eds. D.L. De Mets, C.D. Furberg, and L.M. Friedman), pp. 14–38. Springer, New York.

DeMets, D.L., Furberg, C., and Friedman, L.M. (2006b). *Data Monitoring in Clinical Trials: A Case Studies Approach*. Springer, New York.

DeMets, D.L. and Ware, J.H. (1982). Asymmetric group sequential boundries for monitoring clinical trials. *Biometrika*, **69**, 661–3.

Dickerson, K., Chan, S., Chalmers, T. C. *et al.* (1987). Publication bias and clinical trials. *Controlled Clinical Trials*, **8** (4), 343–53.

DiMatteo, M.R. (2004). Variations in patients' adherence to medical recommendations: A quantitative review of 50 years of research. *Medical Care*, **42** (3), 200–9.

Dunbar-Jacob, J. (1998). Predictors of patient adherence: Patient characteristics. In *The Handbook of Health Behavior Change* (eds. S.A. Shumaker *et al.*), 2nd edition, pp. 491–511. Springer, New York.

Eichacker, P.Q., Gersteinberger, E.P., Banks, S.M. *et al.* (2002). Meta-analysis of acute lung injury and acute respiratory distress syndrome trials testing low tidal volumes. *American Journal of Respiratory and Critical Care Medicine*, **166** (11), 1510–14.

Ellenberg, S.S. and Temple, R. (2000). Placebo-controlled trials and active-control trials in the evaluation of new treatments. Part 2: practical issues and specific cases. *Annals of Internal Medicine*, **133** (6), 464–70.

Espeland, M.A., Byington, R.P., Hire, D. *et al.* (1992). Analysis strategies for serial multivariate ultrasonographic data that are incomplete. *Statistics in Medicine*, **11** (8), 1041–56.

Ferrans, C.E. (1996). Development of a conceptual model of quality of life. *Scholarly Inquiry for Nursing Practice*, **10** (3), 293–304.

Ferrans, C.E. and Powers, M.J. (1992). Psychometric assessment of the quality of life index. *Research in Nursing & Health*, **15** (1), 29–38.

Ferrans, C.E. and Powers, M.J. (1985). Quality of life index: Development and psychometric properties. *Advances in Nursing Science*, **8** (1), 15–24.

Flather, M., Deahunty, N., and Collinson, J. (2006). Generalizing results of randomized trials to clinical practice: reliability and cautions. *Clinical Trials*, **3** (6), 508–12.

Fleming, T.R. (1994). Surrogate markers in AIDS and cancer trials. *Statistics in Medicine*, **13**, 1423–35.

Fleming, T.R. and DeMets, D.L. (1996). Surrogate end points in clinical trials: Are we being misled? *Annals of Internal Medicine*, **125** (7), 605–13.

Freedman, B. (1987). Equipoise and the ethics of clinical research. *The New England Journal of Medicine*, **317**, 141–5.

Friedman, L.M. (2005). Clinical significance vs. statistical significance. In *Encyclopedia of Biostatistics* (eds. P. Armitage and T. Colton), 2nd edition, pp. 847–8. Wiley, Chichester,.

Friedman, L.M., Furberg, C.D., and DeMets, D.L. (1998). *Fundamentals of Clinical Trials*, 3rd edition. Springer-Verlag, New York.

Friedman, L.M., Simons-Morton, D.G., and Cutler, J.A. (2004). Comparative features of primordial, primary, and secondary prevention trials. In *Clinical Trials in Cardiovascular Disease* (J.E. Manson *et al.*), 2nd edition, pp. 14–21. Elsevier Saunders, Philadelphia,.

Glynn, R.J., Buring, J.E., Manson, J.E. *et al.* (1994). Adherence to aspirin in the prevention of myocardial infarction. The physicians' health study. *Archives of Internal Medicine*, **154** (23), 2649–57.

Grady, D., Hulley, S.B., and Furberg, C. (1997). Venous thromboembolic events associated with hormone replacement therapy. *JAMA*, **278** (6), 477.

Haybittle, J.L. (1971). Repeated assessment of results in clinical trials of cancer treatment. *The British Journal of Radiology*, **44** (526), 793–7.

Hellman, S. and Hellman, D.S. (1991). Of mice but not men. Problems of the randomized clinical trial. *The New England Journal of Medicine*, **324** (22), 1585–9.

Hennekens, C.H. and Buring, J.E. (1989). Methodologic considerations in the design and conduct of randomized trials: The U.S. physicians' health study. *Controlled Clinical Trials*, **10**(Suppl 4), 142–50S.

Hlatky, M.A., Rogers, W.J., Johnstone, I. *et al*. and The Bypass Angioplasty Revascularization Investigation (BARI) Investigators (1997). Medical care costs and quality of life after randomization to coronary angioplasty or coronary bypass surgery. *The New England Journal of Medicine*, **336** (2), 92–9.

Hypertension Detection and Follow-up Program Cooperative Group (1979,). Five-year findings of the hypertension detection and follow-up program. I. Reduction in mortality of persons with high blood pressure, including mild hypertension. *JAMA*, **242** (23), 2562–71.

ICH (International Conference on Harmonisation). Guidance for industry. E6 good clinical practice: consolidated guidance. http://www.fda.gov/cder/guidance/959fnl.pdf. (1996). 4-12-0007. Ref Type: Electronic Citation

Interagency Advisory Panel on Research Ethics. Tri-Council Policy Statement (TCPS): Ethical conduct for research involving humans. http://www.pre.ethics.gc.ca/english/policystatement/section2.cfm#2F. 2001. Government of Canada. Ref Type: Electronic Citation

ISIS-2 (Second International Study of Infarct Survival) Collaborative Group (1988). Randomttd trial of intravenous streptokinase, oral aspirin, both, or neither among 17 187 cases of suspected acute myocardial infarction: ISIS-2. *The Lancet*, **332** (8607), 349–60.

ISIS-3 (Third International Study of Infarct Survival) Collaborative Group (1992). ISIS-3: A randomised comparison of streptokinase vs tissue plasminogen activator vs anistreplase and of aspirin plus heparin vs aspirin alone among 41 299 cases of suspected acute myocardial infarction. *The Lancet*, **339** (8796), 753–70.

Lachin, J.M. (1981). Introduction to sample size determination and power analysis for clinical trials. *Controlled Clinical Trials*, **2** (2), 93–113.

Lakatos, E. (1986). Sample size determination in clinical trials with time-dependent rates of losses and noncompliance. *Controlled Clinical Trials*, **7** (3), 189–99.

Lan, K.K.G. and DeMets, D.L. (1989). Changing frequency of interim analysis in sequential monitoring. *Biometrics*, **45** (3), 1017–20.

Lan, K.K.G. and Wittes, J. (1988). The B-value: A tool for monitoring data. *Biometrics*, **44** (2), 579–85.

Larsen, G., Hallstrom, A., McAnulty, J. *et al*. and AVID Investigators (2002). Cost-effectiveness of the implantable cardioverter-defibrillator versus antiarrhythmic drugs in survivors of serious ventricular tachyarrhythmias: results of the Antiarrhythmics Versus Implantable Defibrillators (AVID) economic analysis substudy. *Circulation*, **105** (17), 2049–57.

LeLorier, J., Gregoire, G., Benhaddad, A. *et al*. (1997). Discrepancies between meta-analyses and subsequent large randomized, controlled trials. *The New England Journal of Medicine*, **337** (8), 536–42.

McDowell, I. (2006). *Measuring Health a Guide to Rating Scales And Questionnaires*, 3rd edition. Oxford University Press, New York.

Meinert, C.L. and Tonascia, S. (1986). *Clinical Trials Design, Conduct, and Analysis*. Oxford University Press, New York.

Moher, D., Schulz, K. F., and Altman, D. (2001). The CONSORT statement: Revised recommendations for improving the quality of reports of parallel-group randomized trials.*JAMA*, **285** (15), 1987–91.

National Institutes of Health. Clinical Research and the HIPAA Privacy Rule. http://privacyruleandresearch.nih.gov/clin_research.rtf. (2003). 4-14-0007. Ref Type: Electronic Citation

Nuremberg Code (1949). *Trials of war criminals before the Nuremberg military tribunals under control council law no.10*. U.S. Government Printing Office, Washington, D.C., 2.

O'Brien, P.C. and Fleming, T.R. (1979). A multiple testing procedure for clinical trials. *Biometrics*, **35** (3), 549–56.

Passamani, E. (1991). Clinical trials—are they ethical? *The New England Journal of Medicine*, **324** (22), pp. 1589–92.

Pawitan, Y. and Hallstrom, A. (1990). Statistical interim monitoring of the cardiac arrhythmia suppression trial. *Statistics in Medicine*, **9** (9), 1081–90.

Peto, J., Fletcher, O., and Gilham, C. (2004). Data protection, informed consent, and research. *BMJ*, **328** (7447), 1029–30.

Peto, R. (1995). Clinical trials. In *Treatment of Cancer* (eds. P. Price and K. Sikora), 3rd edition, pp. 1039–43. Chapman and Hall, London.

Peto, R., Pike, M.C., Armitage, P. *et al*. (1976). Design and analysis of randomized clinical trials requiring prolonged observation of each patient. I. Introduction and design. *British Journal of Cancer*, **34** (6), 585–612.

Piaggio, G., Elbourne, D.R., Altman, D.G. *et al*. for the CONSORT Group (2006). Reporting of noninferiority and equivalence randomized trials: An extension of the CONSORT statement. *JAMA*, **295** (10), 1152–60.

Piantadosi, S. (1997). *Clinical Trials. A Methodologic Perspective*. Wiley, New York.

Pocock, S.J. (1983). *Clinical Trials. A Practical Approach*. Wiley, New York.

Prentice, R.L. (1989). Surrogate endpoints in clinical trials: Definition and operational criteria. *Statistics in Medicine*, **8**, 431–40.

Proschan M.A., Lan, K.K.G., and Wittes, J.T. (2006). Adaptive sample size methods. In *Statistical Monitoring of Clinical Trials: A Unified Approach*, pp. 185–211. Springer, New York.

Proschan, M.A., McMahon, R.P., Shih, J.H. *et al*. (2001). Sensitivity analysis using an imputation method for missing binary data in clinical trials. *Journal of Statistical Planning and Inference*, **96**, 155–65.

Psaty, B.M. (1997). Health outcomes associated with antihypertensive therapies used as first-line agents. A systematic review and meta-analysis. *JAMA*, **277** (9), 739–45.

Rand, C.S. and Weeks, K. (1998). Measuring adherence with medication regimens in clinical care and research. In *The Handbook of Health Behavior Change* (eds. S.A. Shumaker *et al*.), 2nd edition, pp. 114–32. Springer, New York,.

Rosenberger, W.F. and Lachin, J.M. (2002). *Randomization in Clinical Trials: Theory and Practice*. John Wiley and Sons, New York.

Sartorius, N. (1993). A WHO method for the assessment of health-related quality of life (WHOQOL). In *Quality of Life Assessment: Key Issues in the 1990s* (eds. S. Walker and R. Rosser), pp. 201–7. Kluwer Academic Publishers, Boston.

Schron, E.B. and Czajkowski, S.M. (2001). Clinical trials. In *Compliance in Health Care and Research* (eds. L.E. Burke and I.S. Ockene). Futura, New York.

SHEP Cooperative Research Group (1991). Prevention of stroke by antihypertensive drug treatment in older persons with isolated systolic hypertension. Final results of the Systolic Hypertension in the Elderly Program (SHEP).*JAMA*, **265** (24), 3255–64.

Solomon, S.D., Pfeffer, M.A., McMurray, J.J. *et al*. and APC and PreSAP Trial Investigators (2006). Effect of celecoxib on cardiovascular events and blood pressure in two trials for the prevention of colorectal adenomas. *Circulation*, **114** (10), 1028–35.

Staessen, J.A. (1997). Randomised double-blind comparison of placebo and active treatment for older patients with isolated systolic hypertension. The Systolic Hypertension in Europe (Syst-Eur) Trial Investigators. *The Lancet*, **350** (9080), 757–64.

Steering Committee of the Physicians' Health Study Research Group (1989). Final report on the aspirin component of the ongoing physicians' health study.*The New England Journal of Medicine*, **321** (3), 129–35.

Temple, R. and Ellenberg, S.S. (2000). Placebo-controlled trials and active-control trials in the evaluation of new treatments. Part 1: ethical and scientific issues. *Annals of Internal Medicine*, **133** (6), 455–63.

The Atrial Fibrillation Follow-up Investigation of Rhythm Management (AFFIRM) Investigators (2002). A comparison of rate control and rhythm control in patients with atrial fibrillation. *The New England Journal of Medicine*, **347** (23), 1825–33.

The Cardiac Arrhythmia Suppression Trial (CAST) Investigators (1989). Preliminary report: effect of encainide and flecainide on mortality in a randomized trial of arrhythmia suppression after myocardial infarction. *The New England Journal of Medicine*, **321** (6), 406–12.

The Heart Outcomes Prevention Evaluation Study Investigators (2000). Effects of an angiotensin-converting-enzyme inhibitor, Ramipril, on cardiovascular events in high-risk patients. *The New England Journal of Medicine*, **342** (3), 145–53.

The National Commission for the Protection of Human Subjects of Biomedical and Behavioral Research. The Belmont Report: Ethical Principles and Guidelines for the Protection of Human Subjects of Research. http://www.hhs.gov/ohrp/humansubjects/guidance/belmont.htm. (1979). Ref Type: Electronic Citation

The Women's Health Initiative Study Group (1998). Design of the women's health initiative clinical trial and observational study. *Controlled Clinical Trials*, **19** (1), 61–109.

Trevena, L., Irwig, L., and Barratt, A. (2006). Impact of privacy legislation on the number and characteristics of people who are recruited for research: A randomised controlled trial. *Journal of Medical Ethics*, **32** (8), 473–7.

U.S. Department of Health and Human Services. Protection of Human Subjects, Title 45 Code of Federal Regulations Part 46. http://www.hhs.gov/ohrp/humansubjects/guidance/45cfr46.htm#subparta. (2005). Ref Type: Electronic Citation

U.S. Food and Drug Administration. Exception from informed consent requirements for emergency research; Title 21 CFR Part 50. http://www.accessdata.fda.gov/scripts/cdrh/cfdocs/cfcfr/CFRSearch.cfm?fr=50.24. (2006). Ref Type: Electronic Citation

VA (Veterans Administration) Cooperative Study Group on Antihypertensive Agents (1970). Effects of treatment on morbidity in hypertension. II. Results in patients with diastolic blood pressure averaging 90 though 114 mm Hg. *JAMA*, **213**, 1143–52.

VA (Veterans Administration) Cooperative Study Group on Antihypertensive Agents (1967). Effects of treatment on mortality in hypertension. Results in patients with diastolic blood pressures averaging 115 through 129 mm Hg. *JAMA*, **202**, 1028–34.

Waldo, A.L., Camm, A.J., deRuyter, H. *et al.* (1995). Survival with oral d-sotalol in patients with left ventricular dysfunction after myocardial infarction: rationale, design, and methods (the SWORD trial). *The American Journal of Cardiology*, **75** (15), 1023–7.

Ware, J., Kosinski, M., Bayliss, M. *et al.* (1995). Comparison of methods for the scoring and statistical analysis of SF-36 health profile and summary measures: summary of results from the Medical Outcomes Study. *Medical Care*, **33**(Suppl 4), no. Apr, AS264–79.

Ware, J. and Sherbourne, C. (1992). The MOS 36-Item Short-Form Health Survey (SF-36). I. conceptual framework and item selection. *Medical Care*, **30**, 473–83.

Whitehead, J. (1997). *The Design and Analysis of Sequential Clinical Trials*. 2nd edition, Wiley, Chichester.

Wing, L.M., Reid, C.M., Ryan, P. *et al.* for the Second Australian National Blood Pressure Study Group (2003). A comparison of outcomes with angiotensin-converting—enzyme inhibitors and diuretics for hypertension in the elderly.*The New England Journal of Medicine*, **348** (7), 583–92.

World Medical Association. Declaration of Helsinki. http://www.wma.net/e/policy/b3.htm. (2000). World Medical Association. 4-12-0007. Ref Type: Electronic Citation

Wu, M.C. (1988). Sample size for comparison of changes in the presence of right censoring caused by death, withdrawal, and staggered entry. *Controlled Clinical Trials*, **9** (1), 32–46.

Yusuf, S., Zucker, D., Passamani, E. *et al.* (1994). Effect of coronary artery bypass graft surgery on survival: overview of 10-year results from randomised trials by the Coronary Artery Bypass Graft Surgery Trialists Collaboration. *The Lancet*, **344** (8922), 563–70.

6.8

Methodological issues in the design and analysis of community intervention trials

Allan Donner

Abstract

With the literature on community intervention trials showing rapid growth over the last two decades, there is an increasing need to better understand their methodological foundation. A key feature of such trials is the allocation of intact communities or clusters of individuals rather than individuals themselves to different intervention groups. Examples include trials evaluating a mass education intervention delivered through the media or alterations in the hygiene of villages located in low- and middle-income countries. Only recently, however, has it been recognized that the application of standard approaches to the design and analysis of such trials can lead to serious problems of interpretation. This is because methods that are extensively discussed in the clinical trial literature tend to assume that the outcomes on individuals within the same cluster are statistically independent, when in fact responses on individuals in the same community invariably tend to be more similar than responses on individuals in different communities. Moreover, the development of methods that take into account within-cluster dependencies becomes particularly challenging when a relatively small number of large communities are enrolled in the trial. This has led to the popularity of designs not frequently seen in large-scale clinical trials, such as pair-matching and repeated cross-sectional surveys.

In this chapter, we discuss a range of such issues, including the advantages and disadvantages of different study designs, methods of assuring adequate statistical power, and choice of analytic approach. Ethical issues arising from the need to obtain informed consent at both the cluster level and at the level of the individual are also discussed.

Introduction

The purpose of this chapter is to address methodological issues that arise in community-based intervention trials. Although the word 'community' is often now used in the literature to encompass a wide variety of social groupings, including, for example, schools, workplaces, and religious organizations, the focus here will be largely, but not exclusively, on geographical groupings, such as villages, towns, or entire cities. An intrinsic feature of such trials is that both implementation and randomization at the community level is either the most natural choice or a virtual necessity. For example, in mass education trials, it is difficult to provide advice concerning lifestyle modification to some people and not others in the same community without risking experimental contamination. Moreover, the interventions administered in such trials often have the potential to affect all or most individuals in a community even though they are actually delivered to only a fraction of residents.

This notion has been recognized explicitly by researchers evaluating the effect of vaccines through the concept of 'herd immunity', where immunization is expected to reduce the attack rate among all residents of a community, even though only some individuals have been vaccinated. However, it also may be a factor in other community-based trials that rely on a variety of mechanisms governing human interaction to help modify health risk behaviour. For example, cities were the unit of randomization in the Community Intervention Trial for Smoking Cessation (COMMIT Research Group 1995), a randomized, controlled multi-centre trial aimed at adult smokers, at least partly because it was expected that heavy smokers would find it easier to stop smoking in an environment where this practice was made less socially acceptable.

Methodological implications of community-based randomization

Trials that randomize communities or, more generally, 'clusters' of individuals to different intervention groups are almost always characterized by positive intracluster correlation, i.e. the tendency for responses among individuals in the same cluster to resemble each other more than the responses of individuals in different clusters. This concept can be equivalently viewed as 'between-cluster variation', which reflects the natural variation among clusters that exists even in the absence of an intervention effect. That is, the higher the degree of intracluster correlation, the greater the degree of between-cluster variation.

The reasons for between-cluster variation are diverse, usually cannot be disentangled without an extensive quantity of empirical information, and may be induced either externally or internally. As an example of externally induced clustering effects, differences in smoking by-laws across communities may affect the relative success of smoking cessation programmes. As a second example, differences in socioeconomic status may be related to variation in the success of community-based education programmes. However, clustering effects may also be internally induced, as when individuals with respiratory problems migrate to dry climates or elderly individuals migrate to warm climates. Such effects may also arise simply through the interaction of individuals living in close proximity.

Whatever the source of the clustering, it is now well-accepted that it must be accounted for at both the design and the analysis stages of the trial. Failure to account for the clustering in the estimation of trial power may lead to an elevated type 2 error (caused by a lower level of statistical power than planned for), while failure to account for it in the analysis stage may lead to an elevated type 1 error (higher rate of false significant differences than planned for). Thus, there are two potential pitfalls operating on parallel tracks—if an important intervention effect is present, the probability of detecting it is reduced, while if the effect of intervention is non-existent, the probability of falsely detecting it is increased. As Cornfield (1978) stated, 'Randomization by cluster accompanied by an analysis by individual (without adjustment for clustering) is an exercise in self-deception, however, and should be discouraged'. He might also have added a similar caution concerning the estimation of trial power.

A recent review of design and analysis strategies employed in cluster randomized trials was presented by Varnell *et al.* (2004), who surveyed 60 articles published in the *American Journal of Public Health and Preventive Medicine* from 1998 to 2002. Their review showed that only 15 per cent of these articles reported evidence of using appropriate methods of sample size estimation, while 54 per cent reported the use of appropriate analytic methods. These discouraging results are also fairly close to those found in a similar review published almost a decade earlier by Simpson *et al.* (1995).

Impact of the intracluster correlation

The intracluster correlation coefficient ρ may simply be defined as the standard Pearson product-moment correlation between any two observations in the same cluster. In community intervention trials, where negative values of ρ are usually regarded as implausible, ρ may be equivalently defined as the proportion of overall variance in the trial outcome that may be attributed to variation among clusters. More formally, we may define $\rho = \sigma_B^2/(\sigma_B^2 + \sigma_W^2)$, where σ_B^2 represents the variance component among clusters and σ_W^2 represents the variance component within clusters. Letting $\sigma^2 = \sigma_B^2 + \sigma_W^2$ denote the overall variance of the outcome measure, we may then write $\sigma_W^2 = \sigma^2(1-\rho)$, showing how the degree of resemblance among responses within a cluster increases with ρ. Equivalently, higher values of ρ lead to increased variation among clusters for a fixed value of σ^2.

It is also possible to interpret clustering effects in community-based trials in terms of 'effective sample size'. Consider a trial randomizing k communities of size m to each of two intervention groups. If $N = km$ denotes the total number of individuals per group, then the effective sample size per group is given by $N/[1+(m-1)\ \rho]$. Thus, when ρ achieves its maximum value of 1.0, the total amount of information available from each cluster is no more than that provided by a single individual, while at $\rho = 0$ each individual in the trial provides an independent piece of information.

The factor $\text{VIF} = [1+(m-1)\ \rho]$ is sometimes referred to as the 'variance inflation factor' or 'design effect', since it represents the factor by which the variance of a group mean or proportion must be multiplied by to appropriately account for the randomization by cluster. It is thus clear that the impact of clustering in any one trial depends not only on the value of ρ, but also on the size of the randomized clusters. Unfortunately this has sometimes been a source of misunderstanding on the part of investigators who have ignored clustering effects simply because the estimated value of ρ was close to zero. Note, for example, that values of ρ less than 0.01 are not uncommon in cluster randomized trials. If such a trial were to randomize clusters containing 100 subjects each, the variance inflation factor is seen to be almost 2.0, implying that the effective sample size is only half that of an individually randomized trial enrolling the same number of subjects.

The effect on type 1 error of ignoring the VIF in testing the equality of two means using an unpaired t-test has been quantified by Scariano and Davenport (1987). For example, their results show that at $m = 100$ and $\rho = 0.01$, the true type 1 error rate at a nominal significance level of 0.05 is given by 0.1658, a more than three-fold increase. Moreover, the inflation in type 1 error rate for given values of m and ρ becomes even greater when an analysis of variance F-test is used to compare three or more means.

The actual value of ρ in practice will depend on both the outcome measure of interest as well as the size of the clusters randomized. Although ρ is almost always small in size and positive, empirical evidence shows that it generally declines with cluster size, although relatively slowly. For example, in primary care settings ρ has been found to vary from about 0.01 to 0.05 (Campbell *et al.* 2000), while for very large communities values of ρ may be less than 0.001.

Some investigators may be tempted to perform a test of significance that attempts to rule out a positive value of ρ, interpreting a statistically nonsignificant result as an indication that clustering effects are absent. However, this strategy is not only conceptually flawed ('absence of evidence does not imply evidence of absence') but is particularly weak in this context given the low power of such tests for detecting small but influential values of ρ.

A detailed discussion as to how to account for the impact of clustering in performing standard statistical tests is presented in the Section 'Analysis strategies in community-based intervention trials'.

Specifying the unit of inference

The discussion above assumes that the unit of inference for the trial is at the individual level, while the unit of randomization is at the community (cluster) level. However, the literature shows that even for trials essentially evaluating the same intervention, there is considerable diversity in the choice of randomization unit. For example, West *et al.* (1991) report on a meta-analysis synthesizing the results of trials in which the allocation units included individuals, households, neighbourhoods and entire communities. However, in each case the choice of randomization unit has been largely a matter of practicality or convenience—the aim of each of these trials has been to investigate the biological effect of Vitamin A on child mortality. Therefore it is necessary in each of these trials to consider the impact of the variance inflation factor in both the design and the analysis.

However, in other trials, particularly those developed from a policy perspective, the units of randomization and of inference may be the same. For example, Diwan *et al.* (1995) evaluated a policy of 'group detailing' on the prescribing of lipid-lowering drugs in a trial randomizing community health centres. A primary endpoint in this study was the number of appropriately administered prescriptions per month, with the health centre serving as the unit of analysis. Therefore, standard methods of sample size and analysis were employed with no need to consider the role of the within-centre clustering effects. As a second example, the hospital-based rate of caesarian section was the primary endpoint in a trial designed to lower the rate of caesarian section at the hospital level in Latin America (Althabe *et al.* 2004). In trials such as these, where the observed results on any one subject are not of direct interest, the challenges that arise in design and analysis are essentially the same as those that which arise in individually randomized trials.

Failure of investigators to distinguish the primary unit of inference in the planning stages of a trial may lead to confusion in developing the trial protocol. Possibly related to this confusion is the terminology 'unit of analysis error', which implies that an analysis at the individual level is inevitably invalid when clusters are the unit of randomization. In fact, this is the case only if the clustering effects induced by the randomization are not appropriately accounted for.

The role of randomization

Randomized or non-randomized?

The discussion up to this point has assumed that communities will be assigned at random to different intervention groups. The advantages of randomization for community-based intervention trials are no different from those in any comparative trial, including the assurance that each eligible cluster has an equal chance of being assigned to a given intervention group, thus eliminating the risk of selection bias on the part of either the participants or the investigators. Randomization also tends to create groups that are comparable on factors (either known or unknown) that may influence response. Moreover, this protection extends not only to community-level characteristics, such as size and geographic location, but also to individual-level baseline characteristics, such as age and gender, provided the entire community (or a random subset of residents) is randomized. However, the probability of substantive imbalance on such characteristics is higher than in individually randomized trials allocating the same number of subjects. Therefore it is important in any one trial to confirm the effectiveness of the randomization by comparing the distribution of both community-level and individual-level characteristics across groups.

In the absence of randomization, it is almost impossible to rule out the possibility of selection bias in the allocation of communities to different intervention groups. As a result, the study findings run the risk of lacking credibility, particularly if they are unexpected. However, non-randomized community-based trials are still frequently implemented, usually for a variety of practical or ethical reasons. For example, if an intervention has already been implemented on a major scale, or if resources for implementing a new intervention are only available in certain communities, randomization may not be viewed as feasible. In other cases, it may be perceived that non-randomized designs would be easier to explain to public officials and to gain public acceptance, given the resistance to assignment by chance that some individuals have. This points to the importance of being able to communicate the purposes and advantages of randomization to key stakeholders, and to possibly offer incentives for their participation.

There are also some arguments against randomization that are less cogent. For example, it has sometimes been perceived that non-randomized designs may be preferable when the number of communities available for allocation is small. However, as pointed out by Koepsell *et al.* (1992), the availability of a limited number of clusters is not a strong reason to avoid randomization, since the increased probability of imbalance on important prognostic characteristics can be controlled by using stratification or pair-matching in the design. Moreover, the challenge of achieving balance when only a small number of communities in each group are available remains a problem whether randomization is employed or not.

In some studies, systematic allocation of geographically separated control and experimental communities has been seen as necessary to avoid experimental contamination, i.e. the spread of an intervention effect to individuals in the control group or vice-versa. However, if the eligible communities are fairly large, this concern can be at least partially dealt with by subsampling participants within the centre of a randomized community while keeping track of any changes of residence (e.g. see Hayes 1998). Another approach sometimes used to deal with this problem is to combine groups of similar clusters into larger randomization units so as to reduce the extent to which individuals in different intervention groups are likely to mingle. For example, Moulton *et al.* (2001) describe the design of a vaccine trial conducted among American Indian populations in which two to four geopolitical units were combined into larger units 'so as to minimize social interaction between the units'. Thus, the aim here was to sacrifice the potential gain in precision obtainable by choosing a smaller randomization unit in favour of reducing the possible bias due to cross-unit social interaction. Other practical methods of minimizing contamination while otherwise retaining strong internal validity in the context of randomization are discussed by Watson *et al.* (2004).

In spite of the lower quality of evidence usually obtained from non-randomized comparisons, it is clear that at the very least they may generate hypotheses that can be subsequently tested in a more rigorous experimental framework. Moreover, in the initial stages of an evaluation there is undoubtedly greater scope for more widespread use of relatively advanced approaches such as time-series experiments (e.g. Biglan *et al.* 2000) when it is felt to be premature to launch a full-scale randomized trial.

Subsampling and the risk of selection bias

In some trials, for example those randomizing worksites, all individuals in a cluster can be readily identified in advance and followed up. In this case, randomization by community will ensure that both cluster-level and individual-level characteristics will be well-balanced between groups, i.e. there will be no risk of selection bias at either of these levels. Such balance will also be preserved provided random subsamples of individuals are selected from communities after their initial randomization. However, for practical reasons or even out of necessity, subject recruitment is often done prospectively after randomization in an opportunistic manner, raising the possibility of intervention-related bias. For example, project staff who are responsible for recruiting participants to receive a new and promising intervention may be more enthusiastic or selective in their efforts than are individuals who are assigned to recruit participants into the control group. Torgerson (2001) has argued that such differential recruiting efforts could result in substantial imbalance between intervention groups with respect to both the number of the subjects recruited and their characteristics. Similar imbalances could result if willingness to participate differed by intervention group. In either case, much of the benefit of the original randomization may be lost, since then it is only the community-level characteristics that will not be subject to selection bias. In the context of trials randomizing medical practices, where it is routine to identify eligible patients after their practice has been randomized, this phenomenon may be referred to as 'detect and treat bias'.

If eligible subjects in a community cannot be identified before randomization, it may be possible to reduce this bias by ensuring that subject recruitment is done by an individual, ideally one who is independent of the study, who does not have prior knowledge of the group allocation. However, if it is the investigator who has responsibility for identifying the trial participants, he/she should be blinded to group membership until a potential subject is judged as eligible. Jordhøy *et al.* (2002) describe how serious problems of selection bias arose in a cluster randomized trial of palliative care that did not involve blinded group allocation.

Pair-matching and stratification

The attraction of pair-matching as a design strategy

In some community-based trials, it is desirable from both a methodological and logistical perspective not to impose any restrictions on the randomization scheme, i.e. to adopt a 'completely randomized' design. For example, Sommer *et al.* (1986) investigated the impact of vitamin A supplementation on childhood mortality in a trial randomizing over 200 villages in Indonesia to each of two intervention groups. With these many clusters, unrestricted randomization can be expected to offer reasonable assurance that the intervention and control groups are well balanced with respect to important prognostic characteristics. Furthermore, any remaining imbalance in either cluster-level or individual-level characteristics related to outcome can be controlled for in the analysis (see the section 'Adjusting for covariates').

However, in most community-based trials, budgetary and other resource-based limitations simply do not allow a large number of communities to be randomized. Moreover, the smaller effective sample size characterizing such trials implies that the probability of imbalance on any one such characteristic will be greater than in an individually randomized trial that recruits the same total of subjects. Thus, pair-matching, although not a common design choice for individually randomized trials, has an obvious attraction. With this strategy, communities are first matched with respect to selected baseline characteristics, such as geographic area and size, which are expected to be related to outcome. One member of a pair is then randomly assigned to the new intervention, with the other member serving as a control, thus providing assurance that the groups compared are similar at the outset with respect to important prognostic characteristics.

An example of a matched-pair design is provided by the COMMIT smoking cessation trial first discussed in the Section 'Introduction', in which the intervention programme was randomly assigned to one of two cities in each of 11 matched pairs, 10 in the US and one in Canada. Matching was done with respect to several baseline characteristics, including community size, population density, demographic profile, and geographical proximity. It is also interesting to note that COMMIT enrolled more than three times the number of pairs that were recruited in the first generation of community-based trials, and, perhaps not coincidentally, was the first to use formal power considerations at the design stage.

Although the matching factors selected in any given trial will naturally vary according to the selected endpoints, two factors very frequently selected are community size (e.g. small, medium, large) and geographic area (e.g. urban versus rural). Matching by size is particularly attractive since this factor may serve as a surrogate for other key prognostic factors that are more difficult to match on, such as socioeconomic status or access to healthcare resources (e.g. Lewsey 2004). For example, in trials conducted in developing countries larger communities may be advantaged with respect to certain outcomes simply because they are located closer to central health facilities than communities that are smaller in size. Matching by size is also an efficiency consideration since it provides assurance that the number of individuals assigned to each intervention group will be approximately the same.

Particularly large gains in efficiency may be achieved when it is possible to match on suitably categorized levels of the baseline version of the primary endpoint. For example, if this endpoint is an incidence rate, then the ability to match on the corresponding baseline incidence rate (or failing that, on a corresponding prevalence rate) can lead to considerable gains in precision. An interesting illustration of this effect is given by Todd *et al.* (2003) in the context of several HIV prevention studies conducted in East Africa.

A baseline survey that captures such information is also useful for other purposes, for example, in checking on some of the design assumptions that were used to estimate trial power, and in providing field experience to those staff who will be responsible for the final data collection. In making the decision as to whether it is worthwhile to conduct such a survey, Duffy *et al.* (1992) point out that pre-trial data may sometimes be obtained with a relatively minor increase in resources as compared to that required to secure the same amount of statistical power through increasing the study sample size. However, the decision as to how much baseline data should be collected should depend on how stable the outcome rates of interest have been in past years, as well as on the cost and ease of obtaining the required data retrospectively.

The efficiency of a matched-pair design is directly tied to the magnitude of the matching correlation ρ_m, which may be defined as the standard Pearson product-moment correlation coefficient between the members of a matched pair with respect to their observed endpoints. Since the actual gain in efficiency in reasonably large samples may be quantified by the factor $G = 1/(1-\rho_m)$, it is clear that high values of ρ_m may bring large gains in precision. For example, the HIV prevention trial reported by Grosskurth *et al.* (1995 generated a matching correlation of 0.94 as a consequence of effective pair-matching of communities on prior rate of sexually transmitted disease, location (roadside, lakeshore, or island), and geographic proximity. However, this degree of success in pair-matching is unusual, and indeed in some trials efficiency may even be lost relative to that of a completely randomized design. This is because many community-based trials can afford to randomize only a small number of units per group, in which case the available degrees of freedom associated with the test statistic used to evaluate the effect of intervention plays an influential role. For example, a trial with k matched pairs is typically analysed using a paired t-statistic with $k-1$ degrees of freedom, as compared to the $2(k-1)$ degrees of freedom available for an unmatched analysis. While this difference may not be important if $k>30$, Martin *et al.* (1993) have shown that it may have very tangible consequences in terms of power if $k<10$. In this case, they conclude that 'matching should be used only if the investigators are confident that the matching correlation is at least 0.20'.

Thus, the question may arise as to the efficiency of performing an unmatched analysis of data arising from a matched-pair design. Diehr *et al.* (1995) have investigated this question, showing that for $k<10$, breaking the matching and performing an unmatched analysis may in fact result in an increase in power for testing the effect of intervention. However, an important assumption here is that the decision to break the matches is made at the design stage of the trial. Thus, it would be inappropriate to base the decision to break the matches on the basis of the observed matching correlation, as this would lead to an elevated type 1 error.

Another limitation of the matched-pair design that arises even in the presence of effective matching results from its inability to directly estimate the intracluster correlation coefficient. This limitation arises because estimation of ρ requires, by definition, an estimate of the natural variation in response among clusters that are treated the same. However, it is clear that the effect of an intervention within a matched pair is confounded with such variation. Hence in the presence of a positive intervention effect, the usual estimator of between-cluster variation, and hence of the intracluster correlation coefficient, will be biased upwards.

Although the inability to directly estimate ρ in a matched-pair design does not affect the ability of investigators to perform a test of the intervention effect, which is inevitably based on between-stratum information, the lack of a valid estimator of between-cluster variation may serve as a handicap in appropriately powering future trials randomizing the same or similar units. Moreover, as discussed by Klar and Donner (1997) constraints will be placed on the nature of several secondary analyses that can be performed, including the ability to make inferences concerning individual-level covariates.

Given the analytic complexities associated with the pair-matched design, a preferable option under many circumstances may be the 'stratified design', as discussed in the next section.

The stratified design

Stratified designs can be viewed as a more general form of the matched-pair design that allocates several communities in each stratum to either intervention or control. For example, the Pathways intervention trial for the prevention of obesity in American Indian schoolchildren (Caballero *et al.* 2003) used this design to allocate 41 schools to either a multicomponent intervention or to a control. The investigators created primary strata based on four distinct field centres in the study catchment area followed by the construction of two secondary strata within these centres based on a school's median body fat percentage. Half the schools within each stratum were then randomized to either the intervention group or the control group, resulting in 41 schools distributed among a total of eight strata. As stated by the authors, the choice of a stratified versus a paired design was made 'under the assumption that stratification would provide adequate control for the difference in percentage body fat'.

Unlike the matched-pair design, the stratified design allows some degree of cluster-level replication in each combination of treatment and stratum. As pointed out by Klar and Donner (1997), this provides greater flexibility in the statistical analysis, since stratum effects may simply be represented by indicator variables in a regression analysis that appropriately adjusts for clustering effects. As discussed in the Section 'Statistical approaches to estimating trial power', such modelling is not possible in a pair-matched design without making special assumptions.

Although in theory the stratified design offers less control over the influence of key baseline characteristics than a pair-matched design that enrols the same number of clusters, the difficulty in practice of securing adequate pair-matches for all eligible clusters may mitigate this advantage. Moreover, there is reason to believe that 'over-matching' is not uncommon, given that trials enrolling more than 50 matched pairs have been frequently reported in the literature. Since matching can only be effective to the extent that the baseline risk of an event varies across strata, the question may arise as to whether such a large number of distinct matches can actually be constructed in advance. This suggests, for example, that a stratified design enrolling four communities in each of 26 strata or eight communities in each of 13 strata, may be as efficient as a matched-pair design enrolling two communities in each of 52 strata, while at the same time offering increased flexibility in the analysis and more degrees of freedom for the estimation of error. Although a completely randomized design without any stratification would provide even more degrees of freedom, this may not lead to a gain in power if the strata are wisely chosen.

Determining the required size of a trial

Statistical approaches to estimating trial power

The formal assessment of statistical power is now regarded as a fundamental step in the design of any comparative trial and is a staple of discussion in the clinical trial literature. Historically, however, many community-based intervention trials have been designed with little or no consideration of statistical power. This may be partly because any trial enrolling hundreds or even thousands of individuals may (erroneously) be perceived as obviously not lacking in power. However, even those investigators who recognized the issue of the smaller 'effective sample size' in cluster randomized trials did not have effective and easily accessible tools for dealing with this problem until the 1980s.

Appropriate sample size formulae are now easily available in both journals (e.g. Kerry & Bland 1998) and in textbooks (Donner & Klar 2000; Murray 1998). In their simplest form, they require that standard sample size formulae for comparing means or proportions be multiplied by an estimate of the likely variance inflation factor $\text{VIF}=1+(m-1)\rho$. Thus, for comparing either two means or two proportions, an investigator may use standard sample size formulas as would be applied in the design of individually randomized trials and multiply the result by an estimate of VIF.

As an example, let $Z_{\alpha/2}$ denote the two-sided critical value of the standard normal distribution corresponding to the desired type 1 error rate α, and Z_β denote the critical value corresponding to desired type 2 error rate β. Then, assuming the difference in sample means for the experimental and control groups can be regarded as approximately normally distributed, the number of subjects required per intervention group in a completely randomized design is given by $n = \frac{(Z_{\alpha/2} + Z_{\beta})^2 (2\sigma^2)[1+(m-1)\rho]}{(\mu_1 - \mu_2)^2}$, where $\mu_1 - \mu_2$ denotes the magnitude of the difference to be detected and m denotes the cluster size. Equivalently, the number of clusters required per group is given by $k = n/m$. For comparing two proportions P_1 and P_2, the required sample size may be obtained by replacing $2\sigma^2$ in the formula above by $P_1(1-P_1)+P_2(1-P_2)$.

For variable-sized clusters, Manatunga and Hudgens (2001) and Eldridge *et al.* (2006) have shown that this expression may be replaced by $VIF_A = 1 + [(cv^2+1)\overline{m} - 1]\ \rho$, where the coefficient of variation $cv = S_m/\overline{m}$, where $\overline{m}$ and S_m denote the mean and standard deviation, respectively, of the cluster sizes. Eldridge *et al.* (2006) also give some examples of the value of cv for sample sizes typically seen in cluster randomized trials.

In the presence of effective pair-matching or stratification, application of the formula above may be expected to be conservative. However, if prior information concerning the matching correlation ρ_m is available, a more precise estimate of the required size of sample for a matched-pair design may be obtained by multiplying n by $(1-\rho_m)$. Donner and Klar (2000) provide examples of sample size estimation for each of the completely randomized, matched-pair and stratified designs.

An alternative approach to estimate trial size is to formulate the problem directly in terms of the coefficient of variation between clusters rather than in terms of the intracluster correlation coefficient. A discussion of this approach is provided by Hayes and Bennett (1999), who also provide sample size formulae for trials in which outcomes are expressed as rates per person-year.

Ensuring the power is adequate

The requirement for an advance estimate of ρ in assessing the proper size of a cluster randomized trial is no different in principle than, for example, the need to have an advance estimate of the standard deviation of the primary outcome variable in an individually randomized trial. However, until the 1990s, values of ρ obtained from previous trial data have not been readily available to investigators. Fortunately this problem is now less serious, with many investigators now routinely reporting the estimated value of ρ for a variety of randomization units and outcome variables. Indeed some investigators have now reported such estimates for a range of study results obtained in a particular research area (e.g. Agarwal *et al.* 2005; Parker *et al.* 2005; Gulliford *et al.* 2005).

The review by Gulliford *et al.* (2005) is particularly notable in that it reveals an approximate linear relationship which holds on the log scale between the prevalence of a trait and the corresponding value of ρ. This suggests that the anticipated prevalence of an outcome variable may be used in some research contexts to make an informed assumption about the magnitude of clustering effects.

It is important to recognize that any particular value of ρ must be interpreted in the context of the trial design and analysis. For example, estimates may be obtained either taking into account the trial stratification factors and/or the individual level covariates adjusted for in the analysis. It is also useful to note that unadjusted values of the intracluster correlation coefficient, which are those most frequently presented, will generally be larger than their adjusted counterparts, implying their future use in sample size estimation will be conservative.

Even with the availability of an appropriate estimate of required trial size, it is useful to conduct a sensitivity analysis exploring the effect on sample size by varying the values of the intracluster correlation, the number of clusters per intervention group, and the cluster (or cluster subsample) size.

The increased attention that has been paid more recently to the formal assessment of the required sample size in the design of community-based intervention trials is particularly welcome given that many of these studies have historically been underpowered and thus found to be inconclusive (e.g. Susser 1995). This is not only because many investigators have not had ready access to the statistical tools needed for this purpose, but also because community-based trials may be particularly susceptible to problems of low power given the nature of the interventions evaluated and the heterogeneity of the populations to which they are administered. For example, many interventions are applied over a wide area on a group basis with relatively little attention given to individual study participants. Thus, the risk of both non-compliance and loss to follow-up is exacerbated, particularly since not only individuals but entire communities are subject to attrition. Moreover, many community-based trials are also prevention trials whose aim is to reduce event rates that may already be quite low in a relatively healthy population. The lengthy follow-up time typically required in these trials places a further burden not only on the ability of study participants to show reasonable levels of compliance but also on the efforts of project staff who are administering the intervention over large geographic areas, often with only limited resources at their disposal. Thus, it is perhaps not surprising, as stated by Susser (1995) that 'generally the size of effects has been meagre in relation to the effort expended'.

Some community intervention trials also have to contend with the immigration of new subjects after baseline, further complicating issues of ensuring that study power is adequate (Jooste *et al.* 1990). Additional discussion of this issue in the context of cancer prevention trials is given by Byar (1988).

Since the power available in a community-based trial is invariably limited by the degree of between-community heterogeneity, one strategy for increasing precision is to establish relatively narrow cluster-level eligibility criteria, for example, by randomizing communities of similar size and socio-economic status. For example, LaPrelle *et al.* (1992) enrolled communities in a smoking cessation trial that were known to be similar with respect to racial and educational make-up, while acknowledging the corresponding risk of some loss in generalizability. Similarly, clusters were deliberately selected to be homogeneous for the purpose of increasing statistical power in the HIV intervention trial described in Grosskurth *et al.* (1995).

For trials such as that described by LaPrelle *et al.* (1992), where there is some latitude in how the primary outcome variable can be defined, it is useful to recognize that continuous endpoints (e.g. number of cigarettes smoked per day) generally lead to much more statistical power than their dichotomous counterparts (e.g. quitting smoking or not), although issues of measurement error and ease of interpretability must also be considered here.

Some trials are also characterized by a degree of flexibility in the fundamental choice of the unit to be randomized. In this regard, Duan *et al.* (2000) have remarked that 'it is important to explore new conduits (such as churches) through which community-based interventions can be more effectively delivered to target subpopulations of heightened risk'. This argument recognizes that the choice of randomization unit may directly impact on statistical power through a variety of factors, both tangible and non-tangible.

A common rationale for avoiding individual randomization in the evaluation of a new intervention is to reduce the risk of experimental contamination. However, investigators have also recognized that power losses due to contamination may remain a problem even if intact social groups are randomized, particularly in the case of small adjacent clusters. Aside from its possible role in minimizing contamination, selective subsampling can also be used more directly to increase power. For example, a decision could be made to enrol only neighbourhoods within a larger community that are known to have higher levels of risk factors than the community as a whole. From a statistical perspective, this strategy would be consistent with the well-known effect on power of increasing the number of clusters in a trial versus increasing the sizes of these clusters. Thus, in a trial allocating k clusters of size m to each of two intervention groups, the variance of an estimated event rate $\hat{P}$ is given by $\text{Var}(\hat{P}) = (P(1-P)(1+[m-1]))/k$, where P is the value of the true event rate. It is therefore clear that increasing k for a fixed value of m steadily drives the value of this variance to zero, implying that the power of the trial can be increased indefinitely by increasing k. However, it is also clear that as m increases for a fixed number of clusters k, $\text{Var}(\hat{P})$ can only be reduced to a limiting threshold value given by $P(1-P)/k$, thus constraining the maximum power that can be obtained. In fact even when clusters are (hypothetically) infinite in size, the power of a trial may be held below 80 per cent if k is not sufficiently large.

A useful rule of thumb in this regard is that very little increase in power will be obtained for a fixed number of clusters after m exceeds the value $1/\rho$ (Donner & Klar 2004). For example, if $\rho = .01$, then the increased power obtained by enrolling more than 100 subjects per community will be small. Yet, as alluded to in the Section 'Introduction', investigators will often have practical reasons for enrolling very large numbers of subjects per community, even if not warranted from a strictly statistical perspective.

Torgerson (2001) and Farrin *et al.* (2005) have argued that the practice of randomizing intact social groups as a means of minimizing contamination effects may be overused. The argument made by these authors is that the loss of precision associated with cluster randomization often outweighs that which results from the contamination and subsequent dilution of intervention effect that can be expected under individual randomization. However, it must also be recognized that under individual randomization the presence of contamination will serve to bias the estimated intervention effect, a factor which must also be taken into account if the ultimate goal of the investigators is to estimate the magnitude of this effect when the intervention is applied in a non-experimental setting. Other factors to consider here include practical aspects involved in administering the intervention and the importance of reflecting 'real world' conditions while doing so.

If the correlation r between a baseline score and a follow-up score is fairly high, say 0.5 or larger, it would be more efficient to compare net changes in baseline between two intervention groups than it would be to compare the final scores alone. Moreover, empirical findings reported by Murray *et al.* (2000) suggest that the value of ρ estimated from a net change from baseline may be considerably smaller than that corresponding to the final score, adding further to the gain in efficiency. An extension of this strategy would be to take repeated measurements over time in each community. This was done in the REACT trial (Luepker *et al.* 2000), where the slope of the linear trend over time was defined as the primary endpoint.

Similar gains in precision may accrue from the incorporation of relevant covariates in the context of regression modelling. The gain in precision obtained by covariate adjustment can be estimated using the correlation coefficient between the outcome variable and the covariate in question. Again denoting this correlation by r, the error variance in a standard model for continuous outcome variables will be reduced by the factor $1-r^2$, a result also holding approximately for binary outcome variables. (For multiple covariates, r is replaced by the multiple correlation coefficient R.) It is thus seen that substantial gains in efficiency beyond that formally planned for can be secured if the appropriate covariates can be identified and measured in advance.

Trials allocating only one community to an intervention group and one to a control group are still occasionally reported in the literature. The flaw in these studies is not only one of low power but the questionable validity of the design itself. This is because any effect of intervention is totally confounded with intrinsic differences that are likely to exist between the two communities, even though on face value these communities may appear to be well matched. Thus, it is impossible to develop a valid significance test for evaluating the effect of intervention, similar to the difficulty that would be faced in a clinical drug trial randomizing one patient to each of two treatments. Nonetheless, this design might be helpful for pilot investigations whose main aim is to examine practical issues such as the acceptability of the intended intervention.

Once the appropriate sample size has been selected using statistical considerations, there remains the practical problem of ensuring that recruitment targets can actually be met. Shadish (2002) points out that this can be a particularly difficult challenge when researchers have had no previous experience with the communities to be enrolled, and cautions in this case that it is particularly important to conduct a pre-study survey that attempts to locate and count potential participants. This advice reflects continuing discussion in the literature that large-scale community-based intervention trials are sometimes launched without performing adequate feasibility studies of the complex intervention components and measurement instruments that tend to characterize these studies. An excellent example of how comprehensive feasibility studies can be used effectively in the planning stages of a large-scale community-based trial is given in a series of articles that describes the pilot phase of the Pathways obesity prevention study (Caballero *et al.* 2003).

Analysis strategies in community-based intervention trials

Basic methods of analysis

There are now many statistical procedures with an array of underlying assumptions that can be used to analyse data arising from cluster randomization trials. In this section, we provide a limited discussion of some of these procedures. This will be done separately for the completely randomized, matched pair, and stratified designs.

Underlying this discussion are some fundamental principles that apply to most comparative trials. The first of these is that the 'intent-to-treat' approach will be used for the primary analyses, implying that all subjects will be counted in the group to which they have been assigned and that outcome data on all subjects will be included in the analyses. In the context of community-based trials, this implies that once a cluster has been randomized, it must be retained in the allocated intervention group. Thus, the intent-to-treat principle provides a 'real-world' assessment of the effectiveness of an intervention rather than an 'efficacy' assessment reflecting optimal conditions. However, secondary analyses in which certain clusters or cluster members are not counted can be particularly useful for either strengthening the trial conclusions or suggesting that caution be used in their interpretation.

To ensure that the final evaluation of intervention effect is not subject to bias, every effort should be made to obtain outcome data on subjects who, because of refusal or other factors, become characterized as 'dropouts'. Since in spite of an investigator's best efforts outcomes on some subjects will inevitably remain missing, satisfactory methods must be used to handle this problem, as reviewed, for example, by Shadish (2002). These include relatively simple methods of imputation, where a missing data point is replaced by the mean of the remaining observations to more sophisticated methods of multiple imputation (Little & Schenker 1995). A difficulty unique to community randomized trials is that entire clusters may be lost, in which case imputation at the analysis stage is generally not an alternative. Instead every effort must be done in the planning stages of the trial to motivate key decision-makers in each community to undertake all reasonable efforts to prevent a community from suspending their participation.

In some trials, it has been the custom to perform a 'modified intent-to-treat analysis' in which certain subjects are removed on the grounds that treatment-related bias is highly unlikely, while statistical power will be improved. For example, in vaccine trials, it is common to remove subjects who fail to receive even a single injection of the vaccine assigned. In this case it is always prudent to perform a secondary analysis that includes all subjects randomized.

The completely randomized and stratified designs

If a completely randomized design is adopted, k clusters (communities) are randomized to each of two groups, usually with a binary or continuous variable chosen as the primary outcome measure. In this case the simplest and perhaps most intuitive approach to the analysis would be to adjust standard procedures such as the chi-square test (for comparing proportions) or the t-test (for comparing means) to account for clustering effects.

We illustrate this approach by considering the comparison of proportions in a completely randomized design. A detailed description of methods for comparing both means and proportions in cluster randomized trials, including examples of all procedures discussed in this section, is given by Donner and Klar (2000, Chapters 5–6).

Let m_{ij} denote the size of the jth community assigned to the ith group, $i=1, 2; j=1, 2 \ldots k$, with $M_i = \sum_{j=1}^{k_i} m_{ij}$ denoting the total number of subjects in group i, and $\hat{P}_i$ denoting the corresponding value of the overall event rate in this group. Then the standard Pearson chi-square statistic with one degree of freedom may be written as $x_p^2 = \sum_{i=1}^{2} M_i(\hat{P}_i - \hat{P})^2 / \hat{P}(1-\hat{P})$. However, application of this statistic to clustered data is invalid since the assumption of statistical independence required to insure the validity of this test will be violated. In particular, the effect of applying x_p^2 to data arising from a cluster randomized trial will, in general, lead to an elevated type 1 error, implying that an intervention effect declared as statistically significant may in fact not be significant if correctly evaluated.

Appropriate adjustment of x_p^2 for clustering effects requires an estimate of the underlying intracluster correlation coefficient ρ, which, under the null hypothesis of no intervention effect, may be assumed to be constant across intervention groups. The required estimate may be obtained by pooling the observations in both groups and then applying the 'analysis of variance approach' described by Donner and Klar (1994) and Donner and Klar (2000, Chapter 6). Let MSC and MSW denote the pooled mean square errors between and within groups, respectively. Then defining

$\bar{m}_{Ai} = \sum_{j=1}^{k_i} m_{ij}^2 / M_i$, we obtain

$\hat{\rho} = (MSC - MSW)/(MSC + [m_0 - 1]MSW)$, where

$$MSC = \sum_{i=1}^{2} \sum_{j=1}^{k} m_{ij} \left(\hat{P}_{ij} - \hat{P}_i\right)^2 / (k-2)$$

$$MSW = \sum_{i=1}^{2} \sum_{j=1}^{k} m_{ij} \left(1 - \hat{P}_{ij}\right) / (M-k)$$

and $m_0 \left[M - \sum_{i=1}^{2} \bar{m}_{Ai} \right] / (k-2)$

The value of x_p^2 is then adjusted by applying a correction factor which depends on both $\hat{\rho}$ and the values of the m_{ij}. Letting $C_i = 1 + (\bar{m}_{Ai})\hat{\rho}$ the adjusted chi-square statistic with one degree of freedom is given by $x_A^2 = \sum_{i=1}^{2} M_i \left(\hat{P}_i - \hat{P}\right)^2 / C_i \hat{P}(1-P)$.

At $\hat{\rho} = 0\,(C_1 = C_2 = 1)$ it is clear that x_A^2 reduces to x_p^2, while if all clusters are of the same size m, it reduces to $/[1+(m-1)\hat{\rho}]$.

As mentioned earlier, values of $\hat{\rho}$ computed as negative are usually truncated at zero, since truly negative clustering effects tend to be regarded as implausible in cluster randomization trials. It follows in this case that standard methods of statistical analysis may be applied to the trial data.

It is worth noting that the validity of this approach does not require the assumption that the correlation ρ between any two observations in the same cluster is constant (an assumption which in any case would be particularly dubious in the context of trials randomizing entire communities). Rather the only requirement in this regard is that the average value of ρ is reasonably constant from cluster to cluster.

However, application of the statistic x_A^2 does require that the total number of clusters is sufficiently large to allow ρ to be estimated to a reasonable degree of accuracy. Thus, for trials enrolling fewer than 10 clusters per group, as is the case in many community-based studies, it may be preferable to restrict analyses to the cluster level, for example by applying the standard two-sample t-test to comparing the mean event rates in the two groups. Although the required assumptions of normality and homogeneous variance for this procedure are clearly violated, particularly in the presence of variable cluster sizes, there is considerable evidence that the t-test is remarkably robust to such violations (e.g. Donner & Klar 1996).

An alternative is to apply nonparametric procedures such as the Wilcoxon rank sum test or Fisher's two-sample permutation procedure.

While the Wilcoxon procedure is computationally simpler, the permutation test uses the actual values of the observed event rates rather than their ranks and therefore tends to be more powerful. Exact statistical inferences for these procedures can be conducted using programmes such as Proc-StatXact (Mehta & Patel 1997). However, it is useful to note that both procedures require at least four clusters per group in order to achieve statistical significance at $p < 0.05$, reflecting their relatively weak power.

It is well-known that the interpretation of results from any comparative trial is enhanced by their presentation in terms of confidence limits. Following the approach above, an approximate two-sided 95 per cent confidence interval about a difference in proportions may be readily obtained as:

$$\left(\hat{P}_1 - \hat{P}_2\right) \pm 1.96\sqrt{\frac{C_1 P_1(1-P_1)}{M_1} + \frac{C_2 P_2(1-P_2)}{M_2}}.$$

At $\hat{\rho} = 0$, ($C_1 = C_2 = 1$), this expression reduces to the standard confidence interval about a difference between two proportions. However, the assumption of a common intracluster correlation coefficient, although guaranteed under the null hypothesis of no intervention effect, may not be appropriate for confidence interval construction. In this case separate estimates of ρ may be used in computing the variance inflation factors C_1 and C_2.

Since the stratified design may be viewed as a replication of the completely randomized design, straightforward extensions of the latter may be used to account for both stratification and clustering effects. For binary outcomes, Donner (1998) and Donner and Klar (2000, Chapter 6) have shown how the well-known Mantel-Haenszel test for combining several two-by-two contingency tables may be applied to a stratified cluster randomized design. For continuous outcome measures, a weighted *t*-test procedure may be used, as described by Donner and Klar (2000, Chapter 7).

As is the case for the completely randomized design, a stratified permutation test may be applied to this design when the number of clusters is small, such as that implemented using programs like Proc-StatXact. An example is given by Duan *et al.* (2000), who used this procedure to analyse data obtained from a church-based telephone-counselling trial, where the stratification factors were church characteristics thought to be strong predictors of the primary outcome variable.

In non-randomized community-based trials, the assumption of a common ρ may not be reasonable, although simulation studies performed by Jung *et al.* (2001) suggest that moderate differences in the value of ρ from group to group will only slightly disturb the properties of x^2_A. The ratio estimator approach, frequently used in the field of survey sampling (Rao & Scott 1992), requires no assumptions concerning the intracluster correlation coefficient and therefore may be preferred to x^2_A in trials that have not employed random allocation. However, a practical disadvantage of this procedure is that it requires many more clusters per group (at least 20) to ensure its validity (Donner *et al.* 1994).

The matched-pair design

In a matched-pair design the intervention of interest is randomly assigned to one community within a pair (stratum), with the remaining community acting as a control. Since a measure of between-cluster variation is not directly available from the communities within a pair, the test of intervention effect is typically performed using cluster-level procedures such as the paired (one-sample) *t*-test, in which the error variance is estimated using between-stratum information.

This procedure is natural for testing the effect of intervention on a continuous outcome measure, where it is applied to the differences d_j, $j = 1, 2, \ldots k$, between the two means in the *j*th stratum, $j = 1, 2, \ldots k$. However, it is also frequently used in the case of a binary outcome measure, since, as in the case of the two-sample *t*-test, research has shown (e.g. Gail *et al.* 1996) that the paired *t*-test is very robust to departures from the underlying assumption that the *dj* are normally distributed with constant variance.

Let d_j, $j = 1, 2, \ldots k$, denote the difference in means or proportions in the *j*th stratum, with mean $\bar{d} = \sum_{j=1}^{k} d_j / k$ and variance $S_d^2 = \sum_{j=1}^{k} (d_j - \bar{d})^2 / (k-1)$. Then the paired *t*-statistic is given by $tp = \left(\bar{d}\sqrt{k}\right) / S_d$ with (*k*-1) degrees of freedom.

This procedure was used to test for the effect of intervention in the community-based trial described in the Section 'The attraction of pair-matching as a design strategy' that was designed to reduce the rate of HIV (Grosskurth *et al.* 1995). After transforming the observed HIV rates to the logarithmic scale to improve normality, the precision of the analysis was further improved by defining the primary endpoint as the difference between the baseline rate and the observed two year rate.

Some investigators avoid the need to make modelling assumptions in the analysis of data obtained from a matched-pair design by alternatively applying either the Wilcoxon signed rank test or Fisher's one-sample permutation test. Exact inferences for these procedures may again be obtained using Proc-StatXact. However, both procedures require at least six pairs in order to achieve statistical significance at $p < 0.05$.

Adjusting for covariates

It was discussed in a previous section how design-based strategies can be used to control for the influence of cluster-level covariates. An alternative is to adjust for both cluster level and individual level covariates in the statistical analysis using regression modelling. Although adjustment for aggregated versions of individual level covariates can be achieved at the design stage (e.g. stratification by percentage of residents with high school education), statistical adjustment at the individual level for that covariate may bring greater efficiency as well as ease of interpretation due to the absence of the well-known 'ecological fallacy'. Moreover, since the likelihood of chance imbalance on any given covariate in a cluster randomized trial is greater than in an individually randomized trial enrolling the same number of individuals, regression modelling procedures may be essential for avoiding chance confounding. However, this is only possible if those covariates expected to have a strong relationship to outcome are measured at baseline. For example, Alexander *et al.* (1989) describe how failure to obtain baseline measures of socio-economic status in a community-based breast cancer screening trial led to severe problems of interpretation.

Although standard modelling procedures such as multiple linear regression (for continuous outcomes) and multiple logistic regression (for binary outcomes) will yield valid estimates of regression coefficients in the presence of clustering effects, their associated standard errors will be underestimated, possibly leading to spurious statistical significance. We now discuss extensions of these procedures that may be used to account for these effects.

The completely randomized and stratified designs

An approach that has now become standard for the control of either cluster level or individual level covariates in a completely randomized cluster randomized trial having a continuous outcome measure is mixed effects regression modelling, as discussed by Donner and Klar (2000, Chapter 7). The term 'mixed' in this expression arises because the model contains terms representing the fixed effect of intervention as well as random effects representing cluster effects and random error terms. Also referred to as either a two-stage nested or a repeated measures analysis of variance model, it may be written as

$$Y_{ijl} = \mu + G_i + V_{ij} + e_{ijl},\ i = 1, 2;\ j = 1, 2 \ldots, k;\ l = 1, 2, \ldots, m_{ij} \qquad (6.8.1)$$

The terms in this model include μ, the population mean response, and G_i, a constant representing the fixed effect of intervention group i ($i = 1, 2$). Two random effects are also included in the model. Random cluster effects, denoted by V_{ij} are assumed to be normally distributed with mean 0 and variance σ_A^2, i.e. $V_{ij} \sim N(0, \sigma_A^2)$, while the remaining random error variation is modelled by assuming $e_{ijl} \sim N(0, \sigma_w^2)$.

The assumption that the cluster effects can be modelled as random variables implies that communities are theoretically obtained as a random sample from a well-defined population. This assumption is sometimes formally realized, as it was in the HIV prevention trial discussed by Grosskurth *et al.* (1995). However, structured sampling schemes in which communities are selected at random are often not realistic. Indeed, as discussed in a previous section, they may be selected instead with the express purpose of reducing between-cluster variability. In this case, the generalizability of the results on a wider scale must rest largely on non-statistical factors, including judgment and past experience.

Maximum likelihood estimates of the intervention effect, adjusted for the influence of covariates, may be obtained in practice using the SAS procedure PROC MIXED. Stratification effects representing factors such as cluster size and geographic area can be easily added to the model given by Eq.(6.8.1) by suitably incorporating indicator variables.

A more complicated model is required if multiple outcome measurements are obtained after baseline and it is of interest to test if the time course of changes in the intervention communities differs from that in the control communities. Such an analysis may be of particular interest for examining the mechanism of action over time induced by an intervention. This approach was adopted by Resnicow *et al.* (2001), who evaluated a multicomponent intervention designed to increase fruit and vegetable consumption among African Americans as delivered through Black churches.

Further discussion of such models, which require treatment-by-interaction terms to be added to Eq.(6.8.1), is given by Koepsell *et al.* (1991).

For binary outcome measures, two main approaches tend to be used. The first is that of generalized estimating equations (GEE), developed by Liang and Zeger (1986), which leads to an extension of standard logistic regression that adjusts for clustering effects. The most common strategy used for this purpose is 'robust variance estimation', which implies that random sources of variability are estimated using between-cluster information, yielding what is often called the 'sandwich' estimator of variance. An attractive feature of this strategy is that although the within-cluster correlation structure must be specified in advance (the 'working correlation matrix'), subsequent statistical inferences will be valid even if this correlation structure is misspecified. The most common working correlation structure specified for cluster randomization trials is 'exchangeable', implying that the correlation between any two responses in the same cluster is identical.

As a consequence of this property, the validity of robust variance GEE is assured only if the number of clusters is fairly large. However, the minimum number of clusters required depends on many factors, including the cluster sizes and the number of covariates in the model, although research suggests that this figure ranges between 20 and 40 (e.g. Feng *et al.* 1996; Pan & Wall 2002). Although several small-sample adjustments to robust variance GEE have been proposed in the statistical literature (e.g. Mancl and DeRoune 2001; Pan & Wall 2002), further research is required to assess their effectiveness under a wide range of practical settings. Therefore, as discussed by Murray *et al.* (2004), this greatly hampers the application of GEE to all but the largest community-based intervention trials.

The use of a 'model-based' estimator of variance rather than a robust variance estimator will allow inferences using GEE to be valid in samples of much smaller size. This desirable property arises since the resulting standard errors are now based on an assumed within-cluster correlation structure rather than on between-cluster variation. However, it is clear that in a trial randomizing moderately sized communities, it would be very difficult to specify any particular correlation structure in advance, with the consequent risk of bias in the estimation of standard errors. Thus, robust variance estimators are much more widely applied than model-based estimators, in spite of their reduced efficiency and unreliability in small samples.

The GEE approach may be characterized as 'population-averaged' in that it measures the expected ('marginal') change in a response over all clusters as the value of the covariate increases by one unit. Thus, the regression coefficient estimating the effect of intervention estimates the difference in the expected response for subjects in the experimental communities as compared to subjects in the control communities, an interpretation similar to that for standard logistic regression. This is in contrast to an approach based on random effects or 'cluster-specific' models, which are characterized by the inclusion of parameters that are specific to each cluster, and which allows them to measure the expected change in response within a cluster as the value of a covariate increases by unit. Perhaps the most commonly used such model is the logistic-normal, which can be viewed as a standard logistic regression model with an added normally distributed random effect. The interpretation of the resulting regression coefficients is then conditional on these effects. Unlike GEE, implementation of this procedure requires data that provides more than one observation per cluster.

Both population-averaged and random effects approaches can now be implemented using the SAS procedures GENMOD and GLIMMIX, respectively, with analogous procedures available in STATA. Although these approaches estimate the same population parameters when the outcome variable is normally distributed, this equivalence disappears in the case of a binary outcome variable, and thus their interpretation is different. As pointed out by Neuhaus (1992), interpretation of estimated covariate effects obtained from random effects models may be difficult when the covariate is defined at the cluster level, i.e. takes on identical values within a cluster. This problem is most notable in cluster randomization trials, since the covariate of main interest tends to be the cluster level intervention effect. Interpretation of such an effect using a cluster-specific model must formally rely on the notion of a subject within a given cluster changing his or her intervention status, clearly a non-observable event. This inability to provide internal validation has led Neuhaus (1992) to remark that random effects models are most suitable for testing the effect of covariates that vary within clusters (e.g. subject age or gender), while population-averaged models such as GEE are preferable for testing the effect of cluster level covariates such as intervention status. However, it must also be noted that the differences between the two approaches disappear as the intracluster correlation coefficient approaches zero, and that more empirical work is needed to compare their advantages and disadvantages in practice. As pointed out by Omar and Thompson (2000), one advantage of the cluster-specific approach is that it provides direct estimates of variance components, and hence the intracluster correlation coefficient, quantities which are treated as nuisance parameters using the population-averaged approach. Moreover, it can also be extended to provide estimates of variance components at each of the multiple levels of clustering that arise in a natural hierarchy, such as villages selected from countries, or classrooms selected from schools that were in turn sampled from school districts. Some evidence also exists (e.g. Bellamy *et al.* 2000) that the logistic-normal procedure performs better than GEE when the number of clusters is relatively small. However, the basic problem remains that clustering effects cannot be accurately estimated in this case, and thus the application of either approach to the adjustment of covariates in community-based intervention trials enrolling only a few communities is unfortunately limited in scope. An excellent non-technical discussion of the distinction between population-averaged and random effects models is given by Hanley *et al.* (2003).

The matched-pair design

A fairly simple but very general method that can be applied to incorporate the effect of covariates in a matched-pair design with a binary outcome variable has been described in the context of the COMMIT trial by Gail *et al.* (1992). The first step is to fit a multiple logistic regression model to the trial outcome data that contains the cluster level and individual level covariates of interest but which omits the variable representing intervention status. For each cluster the difference between the observed success rate and the expected success rate based on this 'null' model can be calculated by summing expectations over all individuals in the cluster. Then one can perform a paired t-test or one-sample permutation test on these residuals to test the null hypothesis of no intervention effect that takes into account the covariates modelled at the first step. An analogous approach using multiple linear regression rather than multiple logistic regression may be used for the case of a continuous outcome variable.

While this approach may be used to control for the effect of both cluster level and continuous level covariates, it does not allow assessment of the independent effect of individual level covariates on outcome. Such an assessment may be of interest when a secondary objective of the trial is to test the effect of covariates such as age or baseline blood pressure on outcome. Although aggregated versions of such covariates, such as mean baseline blood pressure, may be easily modelled at the cluster level using standard methods, modelling at the individual level may be of more direct interest. However, owing to the difficulty in estimating ρ this objective cannot be accomplished in a matched-pair design without making special assumptions.

One option available to investigators in this case is to break the matches and then perform a mixed model regression analysis. However, a theoretical objection to this strategy may be raised when both the outcome variable and the covariate(s) of interest vary with the remaining stratum effects, since the effect of such residual confounding may lead to an elevated type 1 error. Donner *et al.* (2007) have shown that this problem may indeed arise when a large number of small clusters are randomized. However, when a relatively small number of large clusters are randomized, as is the case in most community-based trials, the resulting test of significance for the independent effect of an individual level covariate will in fact hold its significance level after the matches are broken. One caveat is that these results are restricted to the case of a continuous outcome variable and a single individual level covariate, with the case of binary and multiple covariates requiring further research.

Cohort versus cross-sectional designs

There has been considerable discussion in the literature as to the relative advantages of cohort versus cross-sectional designs for evaluating the effect of a community-based intervention. With the cohort approach, each individual is followed up over time, while for the cross-sectional design, different groups of individuals are independently sampled and assessed at each of several time periods. The former design is generally more powerful from a statistical perspective, since it permits an analysis that controls for individual baseline values, leading to a more precise estimate of the intervention effect. This is not possible in cross-sectional designs, where covariate adjustment is restricted to cluster level summary measures. However, this theoretical advantage of a cohort design must be weighed against the risk of loss to follow-up that arises in any longitudinal study. If the loss to follow-up is different across intervention groups, the final estimate of intervention effect may be subject to substantial bias. Moreover, there may be substantial losses of efficiency relative to a cross-sectional design even when the subject attrition is unrelated to treatment assignment. Other disadvantages of the cohort design, as reviewed by Atienza and King (2002), include a loss of representativeness of the target population related to the aging of the cohort, and 'learning effects' that may result from repeated assessments on the same individual.

From a conceptual perspective, the choice of design must also be considered in the light of how the primary question of scientific interest is posed. Thus, if interest focuses mainly on change at the broader community level, cross-sectional designs may be the more natural choice while cohort designs may be more natural if change at the individual level is of most interest. Further discussion may be found in Feldman and MacKinlay (1994).

Ethical issues in the design of community-based trials

Issues involving the need for informed consent

Guidelines for informed consent and other ethical issues are now well established for individually randomized clinical trials. Some of these guidelines apply to cluster randomized trials as well, such as the need for control group subjects to receive at least the current standard of local care and to be eligible to receive the new intervention on termination of the trial if it has been shown to be safe and effective. However, since the historical basis for such guidelines lies in the relationship between physician and patient, their direct application to cluster randomization trials, and community-based trials in particular, has proved to be controversial. As a result, ethical standards for such trials remain in the formative stage.

From this perspective, a distinctive feature of cluster randomized trials is that two levels of informed consent (and sometimes more) must be considered, one at the cluster level and one at the individual level. The first level of consent is generally provided by a key decision-maker such as a mayor or school principal on behalf of his/her constituents prior to randomization. In relatively small trials it also may be possible to obtain informed consent at the individual level prior to randomization. However, in many trials recruitment must instead be done prospectively after randomization due to an inability to identify all eligible subjects prior to randomization. In this case the development of appropriate consent procedures will be more complicated, since it involves consent to be followed up under a treatment regimen that has already been assigned. Post-randomization consent not only raises difficult ethical issues, but also the possibility of selection bias. Further complications arise when it is difficult or even impossible for a subject to withdraw from the study, as in the village-randomized trial described by Hutton (2001) that evaluated the efficacy of an insecticide spray.

Feasibility considerations alone will often present formidable obstacles to securing individual level informed consent in community-based trials, for example in trials that promote lifestyle changes through the media. In this case, where the intervention could be perceived as relatively benign, there may be little objection to the failure to secure informed consent at the individual level. Indeed the unawareness of the intervention programme on the part of community residents may in fact be perceived as a methodological strength of the study (Hutton 2001). However, more urgent challenges in securing informed consent may arise when relatively intrusive interventions are delivered, as in the case of trials delivering water fluoridation to all households in a community. In case of doubt, it seems reasonable to leave the decision to obtain informed consent to an independent committee, such as an Institutional Review Board (IRB). Unfortunately, this solution may not always be straightforward, as most IRB guidelines do not distinguish clearly between consent at different levels.

A distinction made by Edwards *et al.* (1999) may be useful in clarifying these issues. These authors classify cluster randomization trials as either 'cluster-cluster' or as 'individual-cluster', depending on how the intervention is delivered. Thus, in a cluster-cluster trial, the intervention is targeted at the entire community, as in the examples above, and it is difficult (although perhaps not impossible) for individuals to avoid. In this case, it may be argued that a decision-maker or 'guardian', such as a mayor or public health official, must not only provide permission for their cluster to be randomized, but should also sign a consent form clearly setting out the government's duties for safeguarding its constituents' interests. This approach can be seen to be consistent with guidelines for community-based research published by the World Health Organization and the Council for International Organizations of Medical Sciences (2002). However, other approaches have also been proposed, such as sampling the views of individuals selected from the community (Eldridge *et al.* 2005). This approach might be particularly attractive when the decision-maker will not necessarily be a recipient of the intervention and/or may have special interest in the trial results (Hutton 2001).

Cluster-cluster trials differ from individual-cluster trials in that for the latter it is possible to secure consent on an individual basis. As an example, a community-based prevention trial evaluating the effect of a new vaccine could allow any one individual the autonomy to accept or decline the intervention. Securing informed consent at the individual level should also be feasible in many health education trials and in trials administering supplementation by nutrients such as vitamin A, where the issues are very similar to those that arise in individually randomized trials. However, for trials conducted in developing countries, it is recognized that procedures for securing such consent may vary somewhat depending on norms peculiar to the local setting (Hayes 1998).

The need for trial monitoring

It is largely ethical concerns that motivate the need for trial monitoring and interim analyses in individually randomized clinical trials. Thus, data-dependent stopping plans, such as that proposed by O'Brien and Fleming (1979), have proved very helpful to researchers when termination of a study must be considered when one treatment shows unexpected early evidence of superior efficacy. The opportunity for early termination is particularly important for long-term trials having outcomes such as serious morbidity or mortality. However, it is interesting to note that cluster randomized trials in general, and community-based trials in particular, have not usually adopted formal procedures for trial monitoring. In some instances, this may be due to the belief that unexpected early harm or benefit is unlikely given the nature of the interventions compared. Although this may be the case for some interventions, such as those designed to influence behavioural change, there are clearly many exceptions, as in long-term trials evaluating the effect of nutritional supplements such as vitamin A on child mortality.

A second reason for the failure to adopt formal stopping rules in cluster randomized trials is that the theory underlying the most frequently adopted plans has invariably assumed individual randomization. However, Zou *et al.* (2005) have recently shown that the most commonly adopted plans may also be applied to cluster randomization trials with little difficulty. For trials that recruit communities prospectively, Lake *et al.* (2002) have also shown how an interim analysis of accumulating data can be used to re-estimate parameters such as the intracluster correlation coefficient, and hence insure that the final trial power is of adequate size.

Reporting of results

Many of the reporting guidelines for community-based randomized trials are similar to those for cluster randomized trials in general, as discussed by Donner and Klar (2000, Chapter 9) and by Campbell *et al.* (2004). A major contribution provided by the latter authors is an extension of the Consolidation of Standards for Reporting of Trials (CONSORT) Statement, developed over a decade ago as a template for reporting the results of individually randomized trials (Begg *et al.* 1996). A key element of CONSORT is a flow chart providing the number of subjects enrolled at each stage of randomization.

Some reporting guidelines have special relevance for community-based trials. For example, it was mentioned in the Section 'The completely randomized and stratified designs' that the communities participating in a trial are rarely selected at random from a larger population of communities, with the risk of questions arising as to the likely generalizability of the conclusions (external validity). However, some understanding of this issue may be obtained by listing the number and characteristics of those communities that met the trial eligibility criteria but declined to participate. Similar reporting guidelines apply at the individual level if a subsampling strategy has been used to select residents within a community

The interventions evaluated in many community-based trials are frequently complex, with many components. This has led to a debate in the literature as to whether it should be the 'function and process' of the intervention that should be standardized rather than its specific components, thus allowing flexibility in its tailoring to the prevailing local conditions (Hawe *et al.* 2004). However, in either case, it is incumbent on investigators to adequately describe the content of the intervention as it is actually delivered, whether administered directly to individual subjects or implemented solely at the community level. This again allows the reader to more easily generalize the results as well as facilitating its application by policy makers.

With respect to the randomization procedure, both the timing and the method used should be described in the context of the selected design. For stratified designs, the number of communities in each combination of intervention group and stratum should be reported.

The first table in a publication reporting the results of an individually randomized trial is usually a description of baseline characteristics in the two intervention groups. In cluster randomization trials, two such descriptions are required, one at the cluster level, for characteristics such as size, geographic location, etc. and the other at the individual level, with emphasis in both cases on those characteristics likely to be related to outcome.

The use of significance tests for comparing baseline characteristics in individually randomized trials is now widely discouraged, since under a properly executed randomization scheme the source of any observed baseline difference cannot be other than chance (e.g. Senn 1994). The problem will be compounded in community-based trials if these tests are performed without adjustment for clustering effects, since then the obtained p-values will be spuriously low. In any case, it should be the magnitude of such differences rather than their statistical significance that should be used to decide if covariate adjustment is required.

If experimental contamination can be regarded as a potential source of bias, a description of the steps taken to minimize this problem can allow a reader to judge its likely impact. For example, Grossskurth *et al.* (1995) describe how data on place of residence was used to track patterns of migration across communities in the HIV prevention trial described in the Section 'The attraction of pair-matching as a design strategy'.

Differential loss to follow-up across intervention groups can be a threat to the internal validity of any trial. Therefore, the reasons for such attrition, at both the cluster and individual level, should be provided. Reporting the overall individual loss to follow-up rate separately by cluster is also useful, since it allows the reader to understand if these losses are concentrated in communities having particular characteristics.

Since an assessment of between-cluster variation is crucial for sample size estimation, failure of investigators to report estimated values of the intracluster correlation coefficient handicaps the design of future trials in the same subject matter area. As mentioned previously, the magnitude of this problem has declined considerably in recent years. However, the review conducted by Varnell *et al.* (2004) indicates that there is still considerable room for improvement.

Campbell *et al.* (2007) have recently reviewed the rapidly growing methodology available for handling clustering effects in both the sample size calculations and the analysis. Given the relative unfamiliarity of these methods, it is incumbent on authors to provide a clear statement of the procedures adopted, and, where appropriate, to provide accessible references.

Final remarks

Despite the growing literature advising investigators on appropriate methodology, there is still considerable room for improvement at both the design and analysis stages of many community-based trials. From a statistical perspective, failure to account for clustering effects at either of these stages can lead to serious problems of interpretation. Thus, trials that fail to account for such effects in the design stage may fail to detect intervention effects having public health importance while those that fail to account for these effects in the analysis stage are prone to report spurious statistical significance.

Community-based trials also frequently adopt designs that are almost never used in large-scale individually randomized trials, such as the pairing of randomization units and repeated cross-sectional surveys. We have therefore discussed factors that should influence the choice of design in studies randomizing intact communities, as well as the unique analytical and ethical issues that may emanate from this choice. More generally, we have attempted to provide investigators with a better understanding of the many challenges involved in conducting a community-based trial and presented guidelines for meeting these challenges.

Key points

Clearly specify the unit of inference for the trial in terms of the stated objectives.

- Avoid the risk of selection bias if individuals are subsampled from communities.
- Be aware of the advantages and disadvantages of the completely randomized, matched-pair, and stratified designs.

- Ensure that the assessment of sample size and the approach to the statistical analysis adequately account for clustering effects.
- Use the CONSORT statement for cluster randomized trials as a guide to reporting trial results.

References

Alexander, F., Roberts, M.M., Lutz, W. *et al.* (1989). Randomization by cluster and the problem of social class bias. *Journal of Epidemiology and Community Health*, **43**, 29–36.

Althabe, F., Belizan, J.M., Villar, J. *et al.* (2004). The Latin-American cluster randomized controlled trial of mandatory second opinion for the reduction of unnecessary caesarean sections. *The Lancet*, **363**, 1934–40.

Agarwal, G.G., Awasthi, S., and Walter, S.D. (2005). Intra-class correlation estimates for assessment of vitamin A intake in children. *Journal of Health, Population and Nutrition*, **23**, 66–73.

Atienza, A.A. and King, A.C. (2002). Community-based health intervention trials: An overview of methodological issues. *Epidemiologic Reviews*, **24**, 72–9.

Begg, C.B. (1990). Significance tests of covariate imbalance in clinical trials. *Controlled Clinical Trials*, **11**, 223–5.

Begg, C., Cho, M., Eastwood, S. *et al.* (1996). Improving the quality of reporting of randomized controlled trials, The CONSORT statement. *Journal of the American Medical Association*, **276**, 637–9.

Bellamy, S.L., Gibberd, R., Hancock, L. *et al.* (2000). Analysis of dichotomous outcome data for community intervention studies. *Statistical Methods in Medical Research*, **9**, 135–59.

Biglan, A., Ary, D., and Wagenaar, A.C. (2000). The value of interrupted time-series experiments for community intervention research, *Prevention Science*, **1**, 31–49.

Buck, C. and Donner, A. (1982). The design of controlled experiments in the evaluation of non-therapeutic interventions. *Journal of Chronic Diseases*, **35**, 531–8.

Byar, D. (1988). The design of cancer prevention trials. *Recent Results in Cancer Research*, **111**, 34–48.

Caballero, B., Clay, T., Davis, S.M. *et al.* for the Pathways Study Research Group (2003). Pathways: A school-based, randomized controlled trial for the prevention of obesity in American Indian schoolchildren. *American Journal of Clinical Nutrition*, **78**, 1030–8.

Campbell, M.J., Donner, A., and Klar, N. (2007). Developments in cluster randomized trials and Statistics in Medicine. *Statistics in Medicine*, **26**, 2–19.

Campbell, M.K., Elbourne, D.R., and Altman DG for the CONSORT Group (2004). CONSORT statement: extension to cluster randomised trials. *British Medical Journal*, **328**, 702–8.

Campbell, M.K., Mollison, J., Steen, N. *et al.* (2000). Analysis of cluster randomized trials in primary care: A practical approach. *Family Practice*, **17**, 192–6.

COMMIT Research Group (1995). Community intervention trial for smoking cessation (COMMIT): I. Cohort results from a four-year community intervention. *American Journal of Public Health*, **85**, 183–92.

Cornfield, J. (1978). Randomization by group: A formal analysis. *American Journal of Epidemiology*, **108**, 100–2.

Council for International Organizations of Medical Sciences (CIOMS) (2002). *International ethical guidelines for biomedical research involving human subjects*. CIOMS, Geneva. Available at: http://www.cioms.ch/frame_guidelines_nov_2002.htm Accessed on 13 August 2007.

Diehr, P., Martin, D.C., Koepsell, T. *et al.* (1995). Breaking the matches in a paired *t*-test for community interventions when the number of pairs is small. *Statistics in Medicine*, **14**, 1491–1504.

Diwan, V.K., Wahlström, R., Tomson, G. *et al.* (1995). Effects of "Group Detailing" on the prescribing of lipid-lowering drugs: a randomized controlled trial in Swedish primary care. *Journal of Clinical Epidemiology*, **48**, 705–11.

Donner, A. (1998). Some aspects of the design and analysis of cluster randomization trials. *Applied Statistics*, **47**, 95–114.

Donner, A., Eliasziw, M. and Klar, N. (1994). A comparison of methods for testing homogeneity of proportions in teratologic studies. *Statistics in Medicine*, **13**, 1253–64.

Donner, A. and Klar, N. (1994). Methods for comparing event rates in intervention studies when the unity of allocation is a cluster. *American Journal of Epidemiology*, **140**, 279–89.

Donner, A. and Klar, N. (1996). Statistical considerations in the design and analysis of community intervention trials. *Journal of Clinical Epidemiology*, **49**, 435–9.

Donner, A. and Klar, N. (2000). *Design and analysis of cluster randomization trials in health research*. Oxford University Press, New York.

Donner, A. and Klar, N. (2004). Pitfalls of and controversies in cluster randomization trials. *American Journal of Public Health*, **94**, 416–21.

Donner, A., Taljaard, M., and Klar, N. (2007). The merits of breaking the matches: A cautionary tale. *Statistics in Medicine*, **26**, 2036–51.

Duan, N., Fox, S.A., Derose, K.P. *et al.* (2000). Maintaining mammography adherence through telephone counseling in a church-based trial. *American Journal of Public Health*, **90**, 1468–71.

Duffy, S.W., Rohan, T.E., and Day, N.E. (1992). Cluster randomization in large public health trials: The importance of antecedent data. *Statistics in Medicine*, **11**, 307–16.

Edwards, S.J.L., Braunholtz, D.A., Lilford, R.J. *et al.* (1999). Ethical issues in the design and conduct of cluster randomised controlled trials. *British Medical Journal*, **318**, 1407–9.

Eldridge, S.H., Ashby, D., and Feder, G.S. (2005). Informed patient consent to participation in cluster randomized trials: an empirical exploration of trials in primary care. *Clinical Trials*, **2**, 91–8.

Eldridge, S.H., Ashby, D., and Kerry, S. (2006). Sample size for cluster randomized trials: effect of coefficient of variation of cluster size and analysis method. *International Journal of Epidemiology*, **35**, 1292–300.

Esbensen, F.A., Deschenes, E.P., Vogel, R.E. *et al.* (1996). Active parental consent in school-based research. *Evaluation Review*, **20**, 737–53.

Farrin, A., Russell, I., Torgerson, D. *et al.* on behalf of the UK BEAM Trial Team (2005). Differential recruitment in a cluster randomized trial in primary care: The experience of the UK Back pain, Exercise, Active management and Manipulation (UK BEAM) feasibility study. *Clinical Trials*, **2**, 119–24.

Feldman, H.A. and McKinlay, S.M. (1994). Cohort versus cross-sectional design in large field trials: precision, sample size, and a unifying model. *Statistics in Medicine*, **13**, 61–78.

Feng, Z., McLerran, D., and Grizzle, J. (1996). A comparison of statistical methods for clustered data analysis with Gaussian error. *Statistics in Medicine*, **15**, 1793–806.

Feng, Z. and Thompson, B. (2002). Some design issues in a community intervention trial. *Controlled Clinical Trials*, **23**, 431–49.

Gail, M.H., Byar, D.P., Pechacek, T.F. *et al.* (1992). Aspects of statistical design for the community intervention trial for smoking cessation (COMMIT). *Controlled Clinical Trials*, **13**, 6–21.

Gail, M.H., Mark, S.D., Carroll, R.J. *et al.* (1996). On design considerations and randomization-based inference for community intervention trials. *Statistics in Medicine*, **15**, 1069–92.

Grosskurth, H., Mosha, F., Todd, J. *et al.* (1995). Impact of improved treatment of sexually transmitted diseases on HIV infection in rural Tanzania: Randomized controlled trial. *Lancet*, **346**, 530–6.

Gulliford, M.C., Adams, G., Ukoumunne, O.C. *et al.* (2005). Intraclass correlation coefficient and outcome prevalence are associated in clustered binary data. *Journal of Clinical Epidemiology*, **58**, 246–51.

Hawe, P., Shiell, A., and Riley, T. (2004). Complex interventions: How "out of control" can a randomised controlled trial be? *British Journal of Medicine*, **328**, 1561–3.

Hayes, R. (1998). Design of human immunodeficiency virus intervention trials in developing countries. *Journal of the Royal Statistical Society, Series A*, **161**, 251–63.

Hayes, R.J. and Bennett, S. (1999). Simple sample size calculation for cluster-randomized trials. *International Journal of Epidemiology*, **28**, 319–26.

Hutton, J.L. (2001). Are distinctive ethical principles required for cluster randomized controlled trials? *Statistics in Medicine*, **20**, 473–88.

Jooste, P.L., Yach, D., Steenkamp, H.J. *et al.* (1990). Drop-out and newcomer bias in a community cardiovascular follow-up study. *International Journal of Epidemiology*, **19**, 284–9.

Jordhøy, M.S., Fayers, P.M., Ahlner-Elmqvist, M. *et al.* (2002). Lack of concealment may lead to selection bias in cluster randomized trials of palliative care. *Palliative Medicine*, **16**, 43–9.

Jung, S., Ahn, C., and Donner, A. (2001). Evaluation of an adjusted chi-square statistic as applied to observational studies involving clustered binary data. *Statistics in Medicine*, **20**, 2149–62.

Kerry, S. and Bland, J.M. (1998). Analysis of a trial randomized in clusters. *British Medical Journal*, **316**, 549.

Kirkwood, B.R. and Morrow, R.H. (1989). Community-based intervention trials. *Journal of Biosocial Science*, **10 (Suppl)**, 79–86.

Kinmonth, A.L., Woodcock, A., Griffin, S. *et al.* on behalf of the Diabetes Care from Diagnosis Research Team (1998). Randomised controlled trial of patient centred care of diabetes in general practice: impact on current wellbeing and future disease risk. *British Medical Journal*, **317**, 1202–8.

Klar, N. and Donner, A. (1997). The merits of matching in community intervention trials. *Statistics in Medicine*, **16**, 1753–64.

Koepsell, T.D., Martin, D.C., Diehr, P.H. *et al.* (1991). Data analysis and sample size issues in evaluations of community-based health promotion and disease prevention programs; a mixed-model analysis of variance approach. *Journal of Clinical Epidemiology*, **44**, 701–13.

Koepsell, T.D., Wagner, E.H., Cheadle, A.C. *et al.* (1992). Selected methodological issues in evaluating community-based health promotion and disease prevention programs. *Annual Review of Public Health*, **13**, 31–57.

Lake, S., Kammann, E., Klar, N. *et al.* (2002). Sample size re-estimation in cluster randomized trials. *Statistics in Medicine*, **21**, 1337–50.

LaPrelle, J., Bauman, K.E., and Koch, G.C. (1992). High intercommunity variation in adolescent cigarette smoking in a 10-community field experiment. *Evaluation Review*, **16**, 115–30.

Lewsey, J.D. (2004). Comparing completely and stratified randomized designs in cluster randomized trials when the stratifying factor is cluster size: A simulation study. *Statistics in Medicine*, **23**, 897–905.

Liang, K-Y. and Zeger, S.L. (1986). Longitudinal data analysis using generalized linear models. *Biometrika*, **73**, 13–22.

Little, R.J. and Schenker, N. (1995). Missing data. In *Handbook of statistical modeling for the social and behavioral sciences* (eds. G. Arminger, C.C. Clogg and M.E. Sobel), pp. 39–75. Plemum Press, New York.

Luepker, R.V., Raczynski, J.M., Osganian, S. *et al.* (2000). Effect of a community intervention on patient delay and emergency medical service use in acute coronary heart disease: The Rapid Early Action for Coronary Treatment (REACT) Trial. *Journal of the American Medical Association*, **284**, 60–7.

Manatunga, A.K. and Hudgens, M.G. (2001). Sample size estimation in cluster randomized studies with varying cluster size. *Biometrical Journal*, **43**, 75–86.

Mancl, L. and De Rouen, T.A. (2001). A covariance estimator for GEE with improved small sample properties. *Statistics in Medicine*, **57**, 126–34.

Mantel, N. and Haenszel, W. (1959). Statistical aspects of the analysis of data from retrospective studies of disease. *Journal of the National Cancer Institute*, **22**, 719–48.

Martin, D.C., Diehr, P., Perrin, E.B. *et al.* (1993). The effect of matching on the power of randomized community intervention studies. *Statistics in Medicine*, **12**, 329–38.

Mehta, C. and Patel, N. (1997). *Proc-StatXact for SAS Users, statistical software for exact nonparametric inference user manual.* CYTEL Software Corporation, Cambridge, MA.

Moher, D., Schulz, K.F., and Altman, D.G. for the CONSORT Group (2001). The CONSORT statement: revised recommendations for improving the quality of reports of parallel group randomised trials. *Lancet*, **357**, 1191–4.

Moulton, L.H., O'Brien, K.L., Kohberger, R. *et al.* (2001). Design of a group-randomized Streptococcus pneumoniae vaccine trial. *Controlled Clinical Trials*, **22**, 438–52.

Murray, D.M. (1998). *Design and analysis of group-randomized trials*, pp.305–20. Oxford University Press, New York.

Murray, D.M., Clark, M.H., and Wagenaar, A.C. (2000). Intraclass correlations from a community-based alcohol prevention study: The effect of repeat observations on the same communities. *Journal of Studies on Alcohol*, **61**, 881–90.

Murray, D.M., Varnell, S.P., and Blitstein, J.L. (2004). Design and analysis of group-randomized trials: A review of recent methodological developments. *American Journal of Public Health*, **94**, 423–32.

Neuhaus, J.M. (1992). Statistical methods for longitudinal and clustered designs with binary responses. *Statistical Methods in Medical Research*, **1**, 249–73.

O'Brien, P.C. and Fleming, T.R. (1979). A multiple testing procedure for clinical trials. *Biometrics*, **34**, 549–56.

Omar, R.Z. and Thompson, S.G. (2000). Analysis of a cluster randomized trial with binary outcome data using a multi-level model. *Statistics in Medicine*, **19**, 2675–88.

Pan, W. and Wall, M.M. (2002). Small sample adjustments in using the sandwich variance estimator in generalizing estimating equations. *Statistics in Medicine*, **21**, 1429–41.

Parker, D.R., Evangelou, E., and Eaton, C.B. (2005). Intraclass correlation coefficients for cluster randomized trials in primary care: The cholesterol education and research trial (CEART). *Contemporary Clinical Trials*, **26**, 260–7.

Puffer, S., Torgerson, D.J., and Watson, J. (2003). Evidence for risk of bias in cluster randomised trials: review of recent trials published in three general medical journals. *British Medical Journal*, **327**, 785–8.

Rao, J.N.K. and Scott, A.J. (1992). A simple method for the analysis of clustered binary data. *Biometrics*, **48**, 577–85.

Resnicow, K., Jackson, A., Wang, T. *et al.* (2001). A motivational interviewing intervention to increase fruit and vegetable intake through black churches: Results of the Eat for Life trial. *American Journal of Public Health*, **91**, 1686–93.

Scariano, S.M. and Davenport, J.M. (1987). The effects of violations of independence assumptions in the one-way ANOVA. *The American Statistician*, **41**, 123–9.

Schellings, R., Kessels, A.G., Ter Riet, G. *et al.* (2006). Randomized consent designs in randomized controlled trials: Systematic literature search. *Contemporary Clinical Trials*, **27**, 320–32.

Shadish, W.R. (2002). Revisiting field experimentation: Field notes for the future. *Psychological Methods*, **1**, 3–18.

Siddiqui, O., Hedeker, D., Flay, B. *et al.* (1996). Intraclass correlation in a school-based smoking prevention study—outcome and mediating variables, by sex and ethnicity. *American Journal of Epidemiology*, **144**, 425–33.

Simpson, J.M., Klar, N., and Donner, A. (1995). Accounting for cluster randomization: a review of primary prevention trials, 1990 through 1993. *American Journal of Public Health*, **85**, 1378–82.

Sommer, A., Tarwotjo, I., Djunaedi, E. *et al.* and the ACEH Study Group (1986). Impact of vitamin A supplementation on childhood mortality. *Lancet*, **1**, 1169–73.

Susser, M. (ed.)(1995). Editorial: The tribulations of trials—Intervention in communities. *American Journal of Public Health*, **85**, 156–8.

Todd, J., Carpenter, L., Li, X. *et al.* (2003). The effects of alternative study designs on the power of community randomized trials: evidence from three studies of human immunodeficiency virus prevention in East Africa. *International Journal of Epidemiology*, **32**, 755–62.

Torgerson, D.J. (2001). Contamination in trials: Is cluster randomisation the answer? *British Medical Journal*, **322**, 355–7.

Varnell, S.P., Murray, D.M., Janega, J.B. *et al.* (2004). Design and analysis of group-randomized trials: A review of recent practices. *American Journal of Public Health*, **94**, 393–9.

Watson, L., Small, R., Brown, S. *et al.* (2004). Mounting a community-randomized trial: sample size, matching, selection, and randomization issues in PRISM. *Controlled Clinical Trials*, **25**, 235–50.

West, K.P., Pokhrel, R.P., Katz, J. *et al.* (1991). Efficacy of vitamin A in reducing preschool child mortality in Nepal. *Lancet*, **338**, 67–71.

Zou, G., Donner, A., and Klar, N. (2005). Group sequential methods for cluster randomization trials with binary outcomes. *Clinical Trials*, **2**, 479–85.

6.9

Community-based intervention studies in high-income countries

Pekka Puska and Erkki Vartiainen

Abstract

After World War II, with the emergence of cardiovascular and some other chronic disease epidemics and with increasing medical evidence on their risk factors, preventive efforts in many industrialized countries included community-based preventive programmes, projects, and studies. An important background was the notion that the strong risk factors relate closely to behaviours and lifestyles—especially to diet and smoking. It was also realized that in order to reduce the disease rates in the population, merely working with individuals with 'clinically high risk' is insufficient. Instead, to reduce the disease rates, a population-based approach is needed, i.e. changes in general lifestyle and reduction of general risk factor levels in the population.

The first major community-based project was the North Karelia Project in Finland, which was started in 1972 to plan, implement, and evaluate a comprehensive preventive cardiovascular preventive programme in this population with a very high mortality from cardiovascular diseases. Based on similar concepts, and later with the encouraging experiences from the North Karelia Project, many other community-based projects were started, with somewhat different background and approaches.

Today, many evaluation results and experiences are available about numerous community-based intervention studies in high-income countries. However, the results of the specific studies have not matched with the initial optimism. On the other hand, the results of the North Karelia Project and other community-based studies show the great potential of long-term, sustained, and comprehensive interventions.

The chapter describes some of the major community-based studies in high-income countries. It discusses further the many challenges of the design of such intervention studies and their evaluation. Despite many constraints, modern public health is very dependent on interventions on the main, well-established chronic disease risk factors in the community and in the national population. Community-based programmes have also helped to develop national policies and activities. At the same time further development in both our concepts, methods, and measurements with community-based interventions will be important to better serve public health.

Background

In high-income countries community-based intervention studies have mostly been used to assess the possibility and extent of chronic disease prevention in the population. Historically, community-based trials have been a logical follow-up from case-control and prospective studies that have identified likely causal risk factors, and from individual randomized trials. As early as the 1950s and 1960s, early cohort studies on cardiovascular diseases (Anderson *et al.* 1991) showed how three main risk factors (blood pressure, blood cholesterol, and smoking) were strongly associated with cardiovascular diseases both within and between populations.

To prove causality, randomized trials are generally needed. But very soon the many limitations of individual randomized trials in assessing the effectiveness of community-based interventions for cardiovascular diseases were realized. The proposed interventions should deal with a large number of people to introduce lifestyle changes that are, to a great extent, features of the community rather than individuals *per se*.

Epidemiological considerations further spurred the movement towards community-based intervention approaches. The risk of cardiovascular diseases increases continuously as the level of a risk factor increases, without any natural threshold limit. Most of the cardiovascular disease cases occur among individuals in the population with an average risk level, because they constitute the largest proportion of the population at risk. Although a very high risk factor level leads to a high disease risk for an individual, the number of cases from this risk group is relatively low because of the relatively low proportion of people in this population segment.

Following this, the discussion on prevention has focused on two major prevention strategies: The high-risk strategy and the population strategy. In the high-risk strategy people are screened for their risk factors (like high blood pressure, high LDL cholesterol), and preventive activities are directed to those at high risk. In the population strategy, preventive activities, such as health promotion and policy measures, are directed to all the people in the community, i.e. to the whole population.

The community-based approach is thus based on the observation that effective reduction of chronic disease rates in the population usually calls for changes in general risk-related behaviours or reduction in mean risk factor levels. Hence, the intervention predominantly involves general lifestyle changes. Another important feature of the community-based approach is that the intervention targets the community, aiming at modifying social and environmental determinants.

The relative merits of the two strategies in influencing blood cholesterol levels are illustrated by Finnish data derived from five independent risk factor surveys conducted between 1972 and 1992 at 5-year intervals (Jousilahti *et al.* 1998). About 30 per cent of the coronary heart disease (CHD) deaths came from the population group whose serum cholesterol level was ≥ 8 mmol/l. It was estimated that 20 per cent of the mortality could be prevented by reducing the cholesterol levels in the entire population by 10 per cent. In contrast, a 25 per cent reduction in cholesterol levels ≥ 8 mmol/l could reduce CHD mortality by only 5 per cent. (Fig. 6.9.1).

As early as the 1950s, it was observed that blood cholesterol level could be greatly influenced by a few dietary factors: Saturated fats increase blood cholesterol level; polyunsaturated fats decrease it. Also dietary cholesterol was found to increase blood cholesterol level (Keys *et al.* 1959). Since then, numerous studies have been carried out to further assess the role of diet on blood cholesterol level. Even in the most recent reviews the original findings have not changed very much. Only the effect of trans fatty acids on blood cholesterol in the 1980s is a new finding. Also, pectin, certain vegetables and plant sterols and stanols were found to have favourable effects on blood cholesterol. Blood pressure could be reduced by limiting sodium intake and obesity, in addition to the use of drugs (Lichtenstein *et al.* 2006). Based on these findings it became obvious that dietary habits of people in industrialized countries are key areas for intervention.

At the same time numerous studies had shown smoking to be a strong risk factor, both for cardiovascular diseases and for cancer. In addition, some other behavioural factors, especially physical inactivity and excess alcohol use, were shown to be important risk factors. These researches strengthened the evidence that most major chronic, noncommunicable diseases (NCD) are indeed strongly related to certain lifestyles, with individual, psychosocial

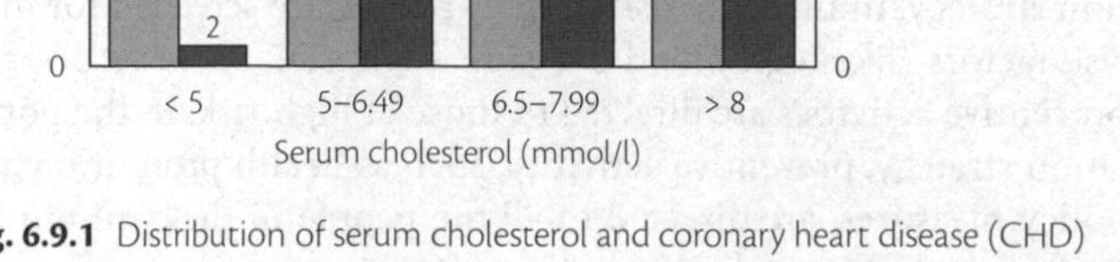

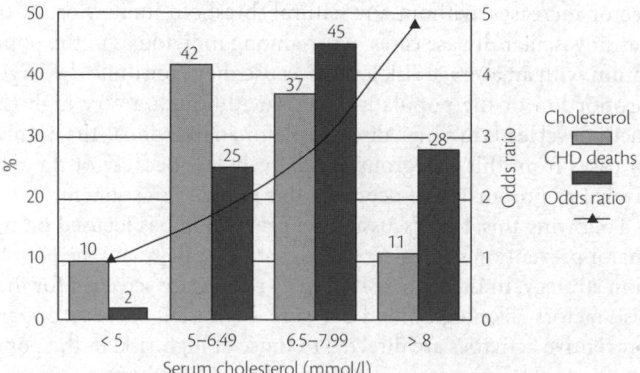

Fig. 6.9.1 Distribution of serum cholesterol and coronary heart disease (CHD) deaths of men aged 30–59 years (1972, 1977, and 1982 cohorts combined) and odds ratios of CHD mortality associated with serum cholesterol.
Source: Jousilahti *et al.* (1998).

and environmental determinants. Thus the World Health Organization (WHO) and others often refer to these diseases as 'lifestyle diseases'. The Global Strategy for NCD Prevention and Control targets smoking, unhealthy diet, and physical inactivity (WHO 2000).

Community-based programmes and studies were introduced to assess two questions: (1) can the mean risk factor level be reduced in an entire population, primarily through general lifestyle change; and (2) does such reduction lead to a decline in mortality and morbidity?

The first three cardiovascular prevention community programmes were started in the 1970s: The North Karelia Project in Finland (Puska *et al.* 1983), the Stanford Three Communities Study in the United States (Farquhar *et al.* 1977), and the CHAD (*C*ommunity syndrome of *H*ypertension, *A*therosclerosis, and *D*iabetes) programme in Israel (Abramson *et al.* 1981). In 1974, the European Office of WHO initiated the Comprehensive Cardiovascular Community Control Programme to help countries develop community-based cardiovascular disease prevention programmes and to facilitate learning from other experiences. Nine European countries participated in this programme (Puska *et al.* 1988).

In the 1980s, this programme evolved into the Countrywide Integrated Non-communicable Disease Prevention Program (CINDI), with the aim of enlarging the community programme to other chronic diseases sharing the same risk factors. These experiences were used in developing the WHO European strategy to prevent and control noncommunicable diseases (WHO 2006).

In the United States, three major demonstration programmes were started in the 1980s: The Stanford Five-City Project (Farquhar *et al.* 1990), the Minnesota Heart Health Program (Luepker *et al.* 1994), and the Pawtucket Heart Health Program (Carleton *et al.* 1995). In the United States, the latest development has been to use these experiences to carry out cardiovascular programmes with fewer resources (Goodman *et al.* 1995) and in hard-to-reach populations (Shea *et al.* 1992), and to develop the US national strategy to prevent coronary heart disease and stroke.

It should be noted that this chapter deals with studies where the 'community' has been defined in terms of geographical areas. A number of studies have used other type of 'communities', such as schools, work sites, or communities defined by profession. In the 1970s WHO coordinated a work site-based cardiovascular study, initially in England and Belgium, and later in Poland and Italy (WHO 1989).

Selectecd community-based intervention projects to reduce cardiovascular morbidity

The North Karelia Project was initiated in 1972 to reduce the extremely high cardiovascular mortality in the area (Puska *et al.* 1983). North Karelia is an Eastern province in Finland, consisting of a largely rural county with one main city, and with about 180 000 inhabitants. As a reference area a nearby province, similar to North Karelia, was chosen. The effect of the programme during the original 5-year period 1972–1977 was evaluated by examining independent random population samples at the outset (1972) and five years later (1977) both in the programme and in the reference area. Similar independent surveys were carried out in 1982 and thereafter also at 5-year intervals, but enlarged to a national risk factor monitoring system (Vartiainen *et al.* 2000).

At five years, statistically significant effects (net reduction in North Karelia) were noted in the programme among the middle-aged male population, namely: A 28 per cent reduction in smoking, a 3 per cent reduction in mean serum cholesterol, a 3 per cent fall in mean systolic blood pressure, and a 1 per cent fall in mean diastolic blood pressure. Among the females only the blood pressure was reduced significantly in North Karelia compared to the reference area. During the first five years of the project (1972–1977), the programme effectively reduced the population mean values of the major coronary risk factors. At 10 years the effects persisted for serum cholesterol concentrations and blood pressure and were increased for smoking.

After the original period, the project was continued for 25 years as a national demonstration programme. After 25 years a remarkable decline was seen in smoking among men, major dietary changes occurred, and serum cholesterol and blood pressure levels were markedly reduced. At the same time in North Karelia (among the male population of 35–64 years), CVD mortality declined by 68 per cent, CHD mortality by 73 per cent, cancer mortality by 44 per cent, lung cancer mortality by 71 per cent, and all-cause mortality by 49 per cent (Puska *et al.* 1998). During the original project period, 1972–1977, the reductions in target risk factors and in CHD mortality were significantly greater in North Karelia than in the reference area or nationally. Separate analyses have shown that most of this decline in CHD mortality could be explained by population level changes in the main risk factors (Vartiainen *et al.* 1994).

In the Stanford Three Community Study (Farquhar *et al.* 1977), three semi-rural communities with populations between 13 000 and 15 000 were chosen for the study. In two of these communities there were extensive mass media campaigns over a 2-year period, and in one of these, face-to face counselling was also provided to a small subset of high-risk individuals. A random sample of the same individuals was studied before and after the campaign over two years. In the control community the risk of cardiovascular disease increased over the 2-year study period, but in the treatment communities there was a substantial and sustained decrease in risk, specifically a greater reduction in plasma cholesterol, blood pressure, and smoking in the programme communities.

The CHAD programme was initiated in 1970, and the second screening was carried out in 1975 (Abramson *et al.* 1981). The CHAD programme serves adult residents aged 25 years and older in a housing project in Jerusalem. In the beginning 648 people were studied in the programme area, and 1995 served as the control neighbourhood. In 1975, 524 members from the same cohort in the intervention population and 1512 in the control population were examined. The programme depended primarily on face-to-face counselling of individuals and married couples in a local health centre providing primary healthcare services. Reductions in blood pressure, obesity, and smoking were greater in the programme area than in the control neighbourhood. No significant effect was observed on blood cholesterol levels.

The National Research Programme on Primary Prevention of Cardiovascular Diseases in Switzerland was conducted from 1977 to 1980 (Gutzwiller *et al.* 1985). Two towns (12 000 inhabitants each) in the French-speaking areas and two towns (16 000 inhabitants each) in the German-speaking part of the country were selected either for the intervention or the comparison group. The intervention involved different kinds of health education with various community involvements. In the intervention towns, 26.2 per cent of the regular smokers quit during the study period, compared to 18.1 per cent in the reference towns. A significant net increase in the proportion of hypertensive patients under effective control was observed in the intervention towns. The decline in serum cholesterol was similar in the intervention and comparator towns.

As a Mediterranean country Italy has had traditionally low coronary mortality rates, but during the 1970s the rates began to increase. The Martignacco community cardiovascular control project was started in 1977. The intervention community had 5259 inhabitants. A community of 7651 residents was selected as the control community (Feruglio *et al.* 1983). The programme included mass communication, and group and individual counselling. The mean serum cholesterol level decreased in the intervention community and increased in the control community over a 3-year follow-up of the same cohorts.

In the Stanford Five-City Project, two treatment cities ($N = 122\,800$) received a 5-year low-cost comprehensive programme that used a communication-behaviour change model, community organization principles, and social marketing methods. Two cities ($N = 197\,500$) served as controls. Risk factors were assessed both by cohort and independent cross-sectional surveys. After 30–64 months of education, significant net reductions in the intervention cities compared to the control cities were seen in plasma cholesterol (2 per cent), blood pressure (4 per cent), and smoking rate (13 per cent). Significant reductions were observed also in the cross-sectional surveys in cholesterol and blood pressure but not in smoking (Farquhar *et al.* 1990)

In the Minnesota Heart Health Program, three pairs of communities were matched in size and type. Each pair had one education site and one comparison site (Luepker *et al.* 1994). After a baseline survey, a 5–6-year programme involving mass media, community organization, and direct education for risk reduction was begun in the education communities. Against a background of strong secular trends with increasing health promotion and declining risk factors, the overall programme effect was modest in size and duration.

In the Pawtucket Heart Health Program, a random sample of residents aged 18–64 years were studied using cross-sectional and cohort surveys (Carleton *et al.* 1995). Pawtucket citizens of all ages participated in multi-level education, screening, and counselling programmes. The downward trend in smoking was slightly greater in the comparison city. The decline in blood pressure and cholesterol was similar in both cities. Achieving cardiovascular risk reduction at the community level was feasible, but maintaining statistically significant difference between the cities was not.

The Kilkenny Health Project was a community research and demonstration programme that aimed to reduce the risk of cardiovascular diseases in a county in the southeast of Ireland with total population of 70 000 (Shelley *et al.* 1995). Independent random samples were used to evaluate the effects of the programme from the intervention and reference counties. The health promotion programme was carried out in Kilkenny from 1985 to 1992. Blood pressure and cholesterol levels declined both in the intervention and reference area.

In former West Germany a community-oriented cardiovascular disease prevention programme was conducted in six regions over a 7-year period, starting in 1988 (Hoffmeister *et al.* 1996). The six intervention regions, comprising a total population of over one million, were scattered throughout the country. The national trend was used as reference. The prevention activities were aimed to promote healthy nutrition, increase physical activity, and reduce smoking, hypertension and hypercholesterolemia. In the pooled intervention area, the net reduction in mean systolic and diastolic blood pressure was 2 per cent, total serum cholesterol 1.8 per cent, and in smoking 6.7 per cent, as compared with the national trend.

The Hartslag Limburg community-based intervention project was started in 1998 in a general population of Maastricht region (population 185 000) in The Netherlands (Schuit *et al.* 2006). In the intervention area, two strategies were integrated: A population-wide strategy aimed at all inhabitants to change lifestyle to reduce risk factors, and a subgroup strategy focused on individuals with diagnosed cardiovascular disease or multiple physical risk factors. A random sample of 3000 individuals in the intervention area, and 758 in the reference area were studied in the beginning of the programme and after 5 years. Risk factors changed unfavourably in the reference group, whereas changes were less pronounced or absent in the intervention group. The programme had a significant effect on body mass index, waist circumference, systolic blood pressure; in women, the mean serum cholesterol and glucose level also decreased.

Community-based intervention projects for other major health problems

As stated earlier, in the field of prevention of chronic, noncommunicable diseases and health problems, much of the research activity and methodological discussions has concerned prevention of cardiovascular diseases. There have been many other activities and programmes to try to influence other health problems, like traffic and other accidents or just health-related lifestyles without any specific diseases and targets. Most of these have been programmes with varying degree of evaluation. Much less has there been systematic community-based intervention studies.

In the field of cancer, a major limitation is that the rates for specific outcomes, i.e. cancer rates, are usually smaller than cardiovascular rates and the time lag between the risk factor and disease changes are likely to be longer. In the 1990s, the COMMIT study (Community Intervention Trial for Smoking) was undertaken to reduce smoking rates in the intervention communities, with reduction in cancer as a goal. The results were modest and demonstrated the difficulties in assessing the effectiveness of multiple interventions with a larger number of intervention communities versus comparator communities (COMMIT Research Group 1995).

In the North Karelia Project, where there was a significant net reduction in smoking in the study areas, there was a significantly greater reduction in incidence and mortality from tobacco-related cancers in North Karelia compared to the rest of the country (Luostarinen *et al.* 1995; Puska *et al.* 1998).

With current international concern on the increasing problem of obesity and diabetes rates, many programmes and policy measures have been launched to help prevent diabetes. Although many of these have a community basis, there are few rigorous community-based studies. In Finland a community-based preventive programme for diabetes, FIND2D-project, was launched in 2003. It involves community-based prevention in five hospital districts, with baseline surveys in 2002/2003 and follow-up surveys in 2007 in the intervention areas and three reference areas (Saaristo *et al.* 2007).

In the field of injury prevention, Duperrex *et al.* (2002) conducted a study on safety education of pedestrians for injury prevention. In the field of environmental health, where communities are natural targets for health interventions, examples of community-based studies relate to water and sewage systems, traffic arrangements, and city planning. The introduction of congestion traffic charges has been studied as 'natural experiments' in London and Stockholm (Beevers *et al.* 2005; Hugosson *et al.* 2006).

Important methodological aspects of community studies

Study design

Most community-based studies have used a quasi-experimental design in which one or several communities are allocated to receive the experimental intensified intervention programme and one or several communities are selected to serve as reference areas which represent the development in the country. In the intervention community an innovative programme is implemented to apply the best possible approaches to change the population level of one or more risk factors in the whole community.

The reference community is not deprived of any new health developments that might occur other than those represented by the experimental programme. In fact the comparison between the communities is not a comparison of programme and no programme but is, in most cases, a comparison of two programmes. This is exemplified clearly in the US studies. In the Stanford Three Community Study, there was a clear effect on risk factors and some effect was seen in the Stanford Five-City Program but the effects in the Minnesota and Pawtucket Heart Health Programs were minimal or did not exist because of strong changes in risk factors at the national level. This secular trend is often thought to happen by itself, but this is unlikely to be correct. The more likely explanation is that strong national and local policies and activities were carried out at the same time.

The observation unit in community trials is a community. In cluster randomized trials, several communities should be used to allow use of the community as a unit in the statistical analyses. Communities can be matched by size and other characteristics of the population and randomly allocated to intervention and control conditions (for details, see Chapter 6.8, 'Methodological issues in the design and analysis of community intervention trials', by Allan Donner). However, in real life, it is usually not feasible to include a sufficient number of communities to use the community as a unit of statistical analysis. It is also difficult to run several community programmes at the same time. In addition, the use of the two or more communities creates interpretational complications in the event of a positive result in one community and a negative one in another.

In a truly experimental design with a sufficient number of communities randomly allocated into intervention and control communities, one other issue raised is how much this would comply with the basic idea of community interventions, that is, broad community participation and comprehensive community organization that benefit from a bottom-up approach.

In all quasi-experimental designs, where the assignment into experimental and control units is not random, there is the possibility of both biased selection of experimental and reference units and of biased sampling in the selection of study units. In the case of the North Karelia Project the experimental unit was already selected before sampling. The only choice for the evaluation was in the selection of a suitable reference unit. Another county in Eastern Finland was chosen as the reference area. Similarly, in the Israel CHAD programme the intervention area was first decided and the reference community was selected later.

Two designs in the evaluation of community programmes have been used. The main design for the assessment of the effect of an intervention on risk-factor levels is the 'separate-sampling pretest-post-test control group' design. Separate independent cross-sectional samples are drawn from the same populations, one in the intervention and another in the reference area, before and after the study period. The net reduction in disease and risk-factor levels in the intervention community (i.e. the reduction in the intervention area minus the reduction in the reference area) is considered to be the effect of the intervention. This design was used in the studies in North Karelia and Germany and in the three major cardiovascular risk studies in the United States, and is regarded to give the best estimates of the intervention effects from quasi-experimental studies.

A cohort design was used to evaluate the programmes in Israel, Italy, and the Netherlands. The same subjects were studied before and after the intervention. This was the only option in Italy and Israel because all the people were studied in the intervention and control areas. In the US studies where both designs were used, the results from the cohort design seemed to show more positive effects than those from the independent cross-sectional samples. This can be explained partly by the higher statistical power of the cohort studies or by the influence of the initial survey on those individuals, as explained in the subsection below on survey samples.

Whether cross-sectional, independent population samples, or a cohort design should be used in the assessment depends on the aims of the study. Independent samples are more likely to better assess the magnitude of changes in the population as a whole compared to follow-up of a single cohort. Thus this is the preferred method in assessing changes in the community. The cohort approach can give more information on the types of changes that have actually taken place at the individual level, and can thus give useful additional information.

Selection of intervention and reference communities

Ideally, the intervention community should be typical of the larger area to which the results are to be applied. Often, however, this choice is guided by historical or practical factors, as was the case in the decision to make North Karelia the setting for an intervention trial. In selecting a community it is particularly important that the area chosen does not have exceptionally good resources or other characteristics that will render the programme experience non-replicable in other parts of the country. North Karelia, for example, had the lowest level of service resources and was the least developed in socioeconomic terms among all the counties of Finland. If the intervention is successful in a community of average or below average resources, it is reasonable to conclude that the introduction of similar programmes would be feasible in other parts of the country.

Establishing an intervention programme in a small community is usually easier and makes the evaluation of the intervention process and risk factors simpler. Increasing the community size usually provides a setting more typical of the region or nation for which the intervention programme is ultimately to be applied. If the evaluation aims to assess the effects on disease rates, a large population is usually needed. Where it is only feasible to compare one intervention community against one reference community, each community should be large enough to provide a sufficient number of disease events of interest and to enable the use of relatively independent samples at subsequent time points and of sufficient size, so that the statistical significance of the net differences in the disease rates in the two communities can be tested. Depending on the disease rates and the length of follow-up, a community of 250 000–500 000 would be necessary for a community intervention study on CHD.

A reference community is essential because changes may occur 'spontaneously' as societies change their lifestyle, for example through increased popular awareness of the risk factors, technological or fashion changes, or increased or improved treatment of risk factors by health professionals. In order to separate the effect of the intervention from general trends of change, the intervention must be compared with a reference community. If risk-factor levels are decreasing nationally, then the 'net' reduction in the intervention community, i.e. the impact of the intervention programme, will be lowered.

Where the national trend is for risk-factor levels to increase, then there may not be sufficient time to reverse that trend although even a deceleration of the increase would suggest that the programme has some positive effect on lifestyles. If a cohort design is used, the ageing of the study subjects can increase some of the risk factors such as on blood pressure, cholesterol levels, and body mass index. This was observed in the Hartslag Limburg study (Schuit *et al.* 2006) and during long-term follow-up of participants in the Martignacco study (Feruglio *et al.* 1983).

Changes in an intervention area can be compared with national trends. This, however, may be misleading since often there is considerable within-country variation and the secular trends occurring in an area in the absence of intervention might not coincide with the national pattern. Thus it is preferable to select a reference community that is similar in all respects to the intervention community. In North Karelia, the decline in risk factors was faster during the first 5 and 10 years of the intervention than in the reference area, but subsequently the development was very similar to other areas of Finland (Vartiainen *et al.* 2000). It is difficult to determine whether these changes represent national trends independent of the intervention, whether the intervention programme contributed to national interest and lifestyle changes and risk-factor control, or whether there was direct 'spill-over' or contamination from North Karelia to the neighbouring county. In the 10-year follow-up of the CHAD programme in Israel the smoking prevalence continued to decline in the intervention population while the national survey did not show any decline in the age group studied (Gofin *et al.* 1986).

Study period

The length of time over which the intervention study continues is very important since a short study period may not provide sufficient time for permanent changes to occur, while a long study period may result in a levelling-off in the differences between areas. Furthermore, different end-points may have different optimum time periods. Changes in health behaviour, for example, can be detected quite quickly, changes in levels of risk factors somewhat

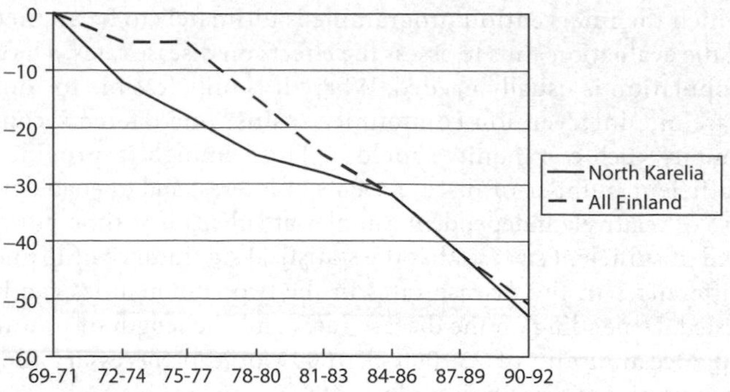

Fig. 6.9.2 Per cent decline in CHD mortality among men (35–64 years) in North Karelia and all Finland.
Source: Puska, P. *et al.* (1995).

later, while changes in disease incidence and finally mortality will be detected only after a considerably longer time period.

In first 5 years of the North Karelia project, for example, most of the reduction in cigarette smoking took place in the first year of the programme; most hypertensive individuals who brought their blood pressure under control achieved this by the end of the third year; dietary changes took place gradually over a 5-year period; and, as noted earlier, at the end of 5 years, a net reduction in risk-factor levels was observed. Concerning mortality, CHD incidence and mortality rates started to decline surprisingly quickly after the start of the intervention in North Karelia. In the rest of the country, a similar decline started several years later. Thus a significant net change in favour of North Karelia was observed, especially in 1974 to 1979 (Salonen *et al.* 1983). Thereafter, although the decline in North Karelia continued, the net decline was gradually reduced (Fig. 6.9.2). Thus maximal difference in favour of the intervention area was observed some 5–8 years after its start (Puska *et al.* 1995). For cancer mortality, a net reduction in favour of North Karelia could be observed much later, i.e. 5–10 years after the intervention commenced.

Survey samples

The aim of an intervention programme is to introduce changes in risk factors that will in turn lead to changes in disease rates. The success of a programme in achieving such changes is assessed by comparing risk-factor levels and disease rates in a cross-sectional sample at baseline with the findings from an independent cross-sectional sample at the end of the intervention.

Independent cross-sectional samples are used in preference to a longitudinal follow-up of a cohort because the latter severely limits its ability to estimate the impact of an intervention. Involvement in a survey may in itself affect the behaviour of the subjects, and those who participate in the survey preceding implementation of an intervention programme subsequently may be more sensitive to the programme activities. In this group, any observed change may be due in part to participation in the pre-test survey and not to the intervention. Thus the true magnitude of the effect in the intervention programme can be measured only by examining a new random sample of the population at the end of the trial period.

For these reasons, the main assessment of the impact of intervention is based on repeat cross-sectional samples. However, longitudinal follow-up of baseline survey samples can provide useful supplementary information, for example, about the characteristics of individuals who change their behaviour and lifestyles compared with those who do not. The cohort design also has certain analytical advantages such as higher statistical power, possibility for adjustment of differences in baseline levels of risk factors, and more efficient testing procedures.

The sample size usually depends on the magnitude of changes to be detected, the required level of confidence, and the cross-sectional intra- and interpersonal variation. Changes in the reference area must also be taken into consideration. The detection of risk factors does not usually need a very large sample size. However, detection of small net changes are important if these are in the same direction for all risk factors and will require a larger sample size. If several subgroups are to be analysed separately, a larger sample size is also needed.

The sample's age range is also an important issue. Obviously the whole population is the target of the intervention but often, as in North Karelia, the intervention programme, although comprehensive, emphasizes persons of certain ages because of the nature of the problem. Emphasis on lifestyle changes directs the age range towards younger age groups, while emphasis on disease end-points would be towards older age groups. With increased interest in 'healthy ageing' the tendency has been to include older age groups. On the other hand, children and youth are targeted in many studies that are not discussed here.

At the end of the intervention period either a second independent sample of the same age-groups is examined, or an independent cross-section of the same birth cohort. Use of the same birth cohort increases the comparability of the baseline and terminal measurements because it avoids any possible unrecognized birth cohort effects (e.g. due to wars or famines). However, this means that the sample at the end is, for example, 5 years older, which may bias the observed absolute changes (i.e. intervention-related changes in risk factors are countered by increases due to ageing). This effect is controlled for when the change in the intervention area is compared with the change in the reference area to describe the net change. Obviously, the analyses can, if necessary, be restricted to the same age-group at both time points.

Survey implementation

The pre- and post-test survey conducted in intervention and reference areas should be strictly comparable. The measurements should be well standardized and tested. Self-administered and pre-coded questionnaires are often used. The measurements are carried out by personnel (often nurses) who are carefully instructed and trained before the surveys to use standardized and often internationally accepted measurement techniques. Strenuous efforts must be made to use identical procedures in the study areas and in the two surveys. The time of the year should also be considered because of possible seasonal variation.

High participation rates are of vital importance to avoid bias in the results. In the North Karelia project, the data quality was strengthened by the high participation rates of both areas in the two surveys. The participation rate did vary between the two areas, although the variation was small. At the outset the participation was higher in the intervention area, presumably because people were interested in participating in the programme. At the end, however, the response rate was smaller in the intervention area, probably due to a waning of interest following exposure to the numerous intervention activities organized over the life of the programme.

Good laboratory standardization and standardization of survey measurements are important if results are to be comparable. Ideally samples should be sent to a central laboratory for analysis by technicians who do not know whether samples originated from the intervention or reference areas.

Disease and mortality surveillance

Monitoring disease and mortality rates at the community level has many problems. Examinations of cross-sectional representative samples do not give much information about the incidence of new cases.

A register, even with the most complete coverage and rigorous criteria, is dependent on individuals seeking health services or being identified in other ways. It is possible and even likely that an intensive community intervention stimulates people to seek medical aid more actively and with milder symptoms, which would tend to increase the incidence rates spuriously. In the North Karelia register it was found that incidence of 'definite' acute myocardial infarction decreased more than 'possible' acute myocardial infarction during the intervention. This might have been because, in response to the intervention, persons with milder symptoms were more eager to seek medical help. The actual decrease in the acute myocardial infarction incidence rate in North Karelia may thus have been greater than indicated by the register.

A further problem encountered with a community-based disease register is the maintenance of the same diagnostic criteria and coverage. A blind reclassification of cases may be done after the study period to confirm the consistency of the diagnostic criteria. To ensure the completeness of coverage, death certificates, hospital records, and other available sources of notification should be checked continuously.

The launching of a new permanent disease register in the reference area can represent a substantial intervention that may minimize the impact of the programme in the intervention area. And because a better health information system (including registers) can be part of the comprehensive intervention programme, its contribution cannot be assessed if a register is also established in the reference area. To avoid contamination due to the introduction of an *ad hoc* register, the ideal solution would be to monitor disease and mortality rates based on national routine statistics. This is adequate when a comprehensive centralized hospital data system is available. In some countries hospital discharge data achieve complete coverage although the reliability of the diagnostic data is less satisfactory. In other countries, where hospital discharge data are less complete and reliable, it is necessary to establish disease registers in both the intervention and reference areas.

The ultimate end-point is mortality, although there are limitations with regard to cause-specific mortality, especially in areas where autopsy rates are relatively low. The observed rates are dependent on physicians' practices in completing the death certificates and these may change over the course of the programme. Age- and sex-specific total mortality rates are, the more reliable indices; however, they lack sensitivity because mortality is the ultimate end-point in the course of the disease and, for example, only a portion of the total mortality is due to cardiovascular disease.

For most community intervention programmes, changes in risk factors are preferred as outcome measures instead of mortality or morbidity (Lindholm & Rosen 2000). This is only partly because of the above-mentioned difficulties in assessing the disease end-points. There are also other arguments: The medical evidence on effects of reduction of, for example, smoking rates, low-density lipoprotein cholesterol levels, and blood pressure levels on disease rates is overwhelming. Thus if we can convincingly show an effect on these indicators, we can be assured that useful prevention has been served. Obviously the use of surrogate end-points such as reduction of risk factors are acceptable only if there is shown to be a strong, independent, consistent association between the surrogate end-point and the 'hard end-points' such as morbidity or mortality reduction, particularly from prospective studies and randomized controlled trials. With a smaller community it is unrealistic to expect statistically significant effects on disease rates despite effective intervention.

Assessment of the intervention

A crucial but difficult question is how to actually evaluate the intervention. Obviously, the assessment of possible effects is meaningful only if we can be sure that a proper intervention has taken place. This relates both to appropriate theoretical frameworks and the intensity of the intervention. A common problem of most community programmes is the application of small 'doses' of these interventions, in contrast to their generally ambitious aims (Mittelmark *et al.* 1993).

The issue on the proper assessment of the input of intervention programmes is extremely important to understand public health implications. Negative or meagre results from some community-based interventions are often interpreted as proof that population-based interventions are not effective, while the actual reason may be that very little happened in the community.

In addition to the intensity or dose of the intervention, even more difficult is to assess the quality or type of the intervention. A population-based community intervention typically uses a whole range of intervention modalities ranging from media campaigns and health service interventions to community organization and environmental and policy changes. Some work has been done to assess factors like exposure to media or to preventive services (Flora *et al.* 1993), but assessment of factors such as community organization or environmental changes is even more difficult. Despite many efforts, there has been little progress concerning assessment of these complex interventions.

Evaluation priorities and components

Intervention programmes aim to prevent and control certain diseases in an area. The aims of the programme may have a different focus, which leads in turn to a different emphasis in the evaluation. Major long-term programmes in larger communities are interested in assessing, in epidemiological terms, whether the programme has influenced the level of risk factors in the target population and whether this in turn has resulted in decreased disease rates and improved health ('experimental' component). Other programmes are restricted only to demonstrating that certain activities lead to such changes in habits, risk factors, or environmental factors that are generally considered beneficial to prevention or control of certain chronic conditions ('demonstration' component). Still other programmes are primarily health service-oriented, i.e. the development of better ways to deliver the health services to control these diseases ('health service operational' component).

If the programme is health service-oriented (e.g. better detection and treatment), then the evaluation emphasizes health service-oriented research. But in intervention programmes to reduce chronic disease risk factors, much of the work goes far beyond the health services (e.g. various strategies in promoting lifestyles changes in the community) and evaluation focuses on other aspects, such as epidemiology and sociology. Even in a health service-oriented programme in a larger community it is advisable, in the long run, to evaluate performance also in terms of effects on mortality and morbidity.

Since in practice most programmes will combine different aims, the evaluation should accordingly be comprehensive, with the point of emphasis dependent upon the nature of the programme and upon local conditions. Generally the evaluation of community-based intervention programmes should consider the following evaluation components:

1. *Feasibility (or performance or input).* This is the assessment of whether the planned intervention activities could be implemented and to what extent, and what proportion of the target population was covered or reached by the programme. In feasibility evaluation, the final performance of the programme is compared with the initial list of planned activities, and this forms the basis for understanding the possible effects of the programme. If this part of the evaluation shows that the programme was not feasible under the local conditions, it is not necessary to conduct an effects evaluation.
2. *Effects.* This part of the evaluation is concerned with assessing whether the programme reached its stated objectives. Depending on the local programmes (as mentioned above), this may concern health-related habits, risk factors, and/or health service utilization, plus, possibly, mortality, morbidity, and/or disability rates (representing different levels of objectives).

   After defining the objectives, their respective indicators have to be defined and appropriate data sources and measurements (mortality statistics, disease registers, random sample surveys, health service utilization data, etc.) selected. A standardized system for comparing changes in these indicators will be required because the changes observed may be due to factors other than the programme ('spontaneous change', national development', etc.). For this purpose, a reference community is needed that is, ideally, matched with the programme community and selected by random sampling. The changes in the intervention community should also be compared with whatever statistics are available on a regional and national basis. This is important, especially in those cases where a specific reference area is not feasible.
3. *Process.* Process evaluation aims to assess how the different programme components in the local community (integrated with the local health services and social organization of the community) achieve the programme objectives over the life of the programme. This evaluation concerns detailed assessment of the different steps and measures in the intervention, changes in various intervening variables considered, and the occurrence of risk factors and disease changes with time. In the latter, the systems for monitoring these trends form the evaluation tool. In order to facilitate process evaluation, it is advisable at the planning stage to have a detailed flow-chart to illustrate the plan of action. Process evaluation is also related to the question of what kind of process leads or does not lead to the desired effects. This kind of evaluation calls for theoretical models of change that guide the process evaluation.
4. *Other consequences.* A major intervention in the community is likely to lead to consequences other than those specified in the objectives. These may include health- related, social, or psychological changes, and can be either positive or negative. Such consequences might be, for example, increased side effects or widespread medication, increased anxiety, or increased feelings of security, satisfaction about the services, and better quality of life. A major community-based pilot programme should pay attention to this part of evaluation because of its implications for nationwide application of the programme.
5. *Economic measures.* Assessment of programme costs in relation to the observed effects, i.e. the cost-effectiveness ratio of the programme (also termed efficiency), may be expressed, for instance, as costs per saved life. This information can be used to compare costs of different strategies leading to the same effect or to compare programmes leading to different effects but which cost a similar amount to run. On the other hand, a cost-benefit analysis quantifies and puts values on all benefits and costs associated with the programme and expresses them in a common denomination.

The first step in the evaluation of costs is to assess the direct costs of the project, i.e. the extra input (training, materials, co-ordination) that lead to the implementation of the integrated programme in the community. Thereafter, the direct community costs should be assessed, which include the costs of the health services and other activities in the community for the prevention and control of the diseases under study. It may, however, be advisable to differentiate between (the usually very large) costs that would have occurred in the absence of a specific programme and the extra costs (or savings) resulting from the intensified system. Comparison with the respective costs in the reference area may be used in such an evaluation.

The above discussion shows how community-based preventive studies can have different perspectives ranging from evaluation of a community-based programme (where the interest can often be in aspects of feasibility and observed risk factor changes) to a rigorous 'trial' (when the interest is in health effects and outcomes). Different kind of studies are needed, and an ideal trial may not be possible. Often the study has to balance between the different objectives.

Discussion of results

A number of publications have tried to summarize the results of major community-based preventive projects, particularly those concerning cardiovascular diseases prevention (Fortmann *et al.* 1995; Mittelmark *et al.* 1993; Ebrahim & Smith 1997; Sellers *et al.* 1997; Lindholm & Rosen 2000). So far practically all such studies have been carried out in high-income countries. Only during the last few years, with emergence of chronic diseases in low- and middle-income countries, have such studies been started in such countries with varying study designs and levels of evaluation.

A summary of the evaluation of the early European community-based cardiovascular preventive studies, linked to the WHO programme on Comprehensive Cardiovascular Community Control Programmes, showed that most of the nine European studies analysed showed a reduction in the risk factor levels in the intervention community, but a statistically significant net reduction was shown in three programmes for smoking, four for serum cholesterol, and five for blood pressure (Puska 1988).

Winkleby *et al.* (1997) made a review of the results of the Stanford Five City Project, Minnesota HHP, and the Pawtucket HHP. They showed that the joint estimates of intervention effect were in the expected direction in 9 of 12 gender-specific comparisons but were not statistically significant. It was concluded that the results illustrate the analytic challenges of evaluating community-based intervention trials and indicate smaller than expected net differences. Rigid evaluations of the projects showed only modest or no 'hard' effects on targeted risk factors or CVD rates in most of the projects. They also discussed the difficulties in assessing the true overall impact. This is because of the comprehensive nature of the intervention, caused by diffusion to other areas and linkage with national trends. A British review dealt with both community intervention trials and community studies and arrived at rather similar conclusions (Ebrahim & Smith 1997). It stated that for pooled effects on mortality, a small but potentially significant (about 10 per cent reduction) may have been missed.

Expectations for community-level interventions are often unrealistic, that is, based on overly high estimates of effect size and insufficient sample sizes to detect smaller effects. Commercial advertising campaigns, which generally have substantially more resources than community prevention trials, are typically satisfied with modest increases in market share. Mittelmark *et al.* (1993) called for 'realistic outcomes' in their review.

A very important aspect is thus the dose of the intervention, as discussed earlier. Because most of the projects in larger communities over a number of years have had only very limited resources, the dose of the intervention is small. Another important aspect is the nature of the intervention. Most of the projects carried out so far have, in spite of many efforts, been limited to educational and health service-based interventions. Among the projects, the North Karelia Project was perhaps the most 'community-based', i.e. influencing broadly the physical and social environment of the community.

It should also be noted that many community-based preventive projects have served as sites of training, advocacy raising, and demonstration for national programmes and policies. They have thus contributed to national preventive work in a way that has been very difficult to evaluate.

Perhaps the best example to illustrate the long-term experience and potential of sustained community-based and national heart health work is the experience in Finland. After the early success in the 1970s, and with significant net reductions in both risk factors and CHD mortality, intensive national work was started, to which the project actively contributed. During this latter period the decline in risk factors and disease rates accelerated in parallel between North Karelia and the whole of Finland.

Associated with the risk factor changes, a dramatic reduction was, indeed, seen in the cardiovascular mortality and a huge improvement in public health. This success has generally been attributed to a sustained, theory-based, and comprehensive intervention that was broadly integrated in the community of North Karelia and later on involved national policy and health promotion measures, all influencing the social and physical environments of the population.

Conclusions

Numerous community-based programmes have been implemented to change lifestyles for pilot, demonstration, and research purposes. Their evaluation and experiences have contributed greatly to national policy decisions and actions. Further development in our concepts, methods, and measurement with community-based interventions will be important to better serve public health. Despite many critical constraints, modern public health is very dependent on changes in the major, well-established risk factors in the community and in the national population.

Successful community-based programmes should do the right things and enough of them, that is, use sound theoretical frameworks and implement the interventions in the communities with a sufficient 'dose'. Usually environmental and policy decisions are key, but often they can be achieved only in conjunction with health promotion activities that influence the public agenda and people's intentions. At the same time, the human factor is crucial: Persistent and dedicated work is needed, combining enthusiastic and credible leadership with close involvement of, and ownership by, the population.

Key points

- Chronic disease risk factors are closely related to lifestyles that are strongly rooted in community features.
- The greatest potential in reducing cardiovascular and other chronic disease rates in the population are population-based strategies that reduce general risk factor levels in the community.
- Since the 1970s, many community-based studies in high-income countries have assessed the possibilities and effects of community-based prevention.
- While the direct effects of many studies have been less than expected, the great potential of long-term, sustained, and comprehensive population-based intervention is demonstrated by the long-term results of the North Karelia Project in Finland.
- Many community-based projects have greatly contributed to national activities and policies. At the same time, further work on concepts, methods and evaluation measurements is needed.

References

Abramson, J.H., Gofin, R., Hopp, C. *et al.* (1981). Evaluation of a community program for the control of cardiovascular risk factors: the CHAD program in Jerusalem. *Israel Journal of Medical Sciences*, **17**, 201–12.

Anderson, K.M., Wilson, P.W., Odell, P.M. *et al.* (1991). An updated coronary risk profile. A statement for health professionals. *Circulation*, **83**, 356–62.

Beevers, S.D. and Carslaw, D.C. (2005). The impact of congestion charging on vehicle emissions in London. *Atmospheric Environment*, **39**, 1–5.

Carleton, R.A., Lasater, T.M., Assaf, A.R. *et al.* (1995). The Pawtucket Heart Health Program: Community changes in cardiovascular risk factors and projected disease risk. *American Journal of Public Health*, **85**, 777–85.

COMMIT Research Group (1995). Community Intervention Trial for Smoking Cessation (COMMIT): I. Cohort results from a four-year communityiIntervention. *American Journal of Public Health*, **85**, 183–92.

Donner, A. (2009). Methodological issues in the design and analysis of community intervention trials. In *Oxford textbook of public health* (eds. R. Detels, R. Beaglehole, M.A. Lansang, and M.Gulliford), Oxford University Press, Oxford.

Duperrex, O., Roberts, I., and Bunn, F. (2002). Safe education of pedestrians for injury prevention. *BMJ*, **324**, 1129–33.

Ebrahim, S. and Smith, G.D. (1997). Systematic review of randomised controlled trials of multiple risk factor interventions for preventing coronary heart disease. *BMJ*, **314**, 1666–74.

Farquhar, J.W., Fortmann, S.P., Flora, J.A. *et al.* (1990). Effects of communitywide education on cardiovascular disease risk factors. The Stanford Five-City Project. *JAMA*, **264**, 359–65.

Farquhar, J.W., Maccoby, N., Wood, P.D. *et al.* (1977). Community education for cardiovascular health. *Lancet*, **1**, 1192–5.

Feruglio, G.A., Vanuzzo, D., Di Muro, G. *et al.* (1983). The Martignacco project: A community study. Outlines and preliminary results after four years. *Giornale di Arteriosclerosis*, **2**, 207–17.

Flora, J.A., Lefebvre, R.C., Murray, D.M. *et al.* (1993). A community education monitoring system: Methods from the Stanford Five-City Project, the Minnesota Heart Health Program, and the Pawtucket Heart Health Program. *Health Education Research*, **8**, 81–95.

Fortmann, S.P., Flora, J.A., Winkleby, M.A. *et al.* (1995). Community intervention trials: reflections on the Stanford Five-City Project Experience. *American Journal of Epidemiology*, **142**, 576–86.

Gofin, J., Gofin, R., Abramson, J.H.*et al.* (1986). Ten-year evaluation of hypertension, overweight, cholesterol, and smoking control: the CHAD program in Jerusalem. Community Syndrome of Hypertension, Atherosclerosis and Diabetes. *Preventive Medicine*, **15**, 304–12.

Goodman, R.M., Wheeler, F.C., and Lee, P.R. (1995). Evaluation of the Heart To Heart Project: lessons from a community-based chronic disease prevention project. *American Journal of Health Promotion*, **9**, 443–55.

Gutzwiller, F., Nater, B., and Martin, J. (1985). Community-based primary prevention of cardiovascular disease in Switzerland: methods and results of the National Research Program (NRP 1A). *Preventive Medicine*, **14**, 482–91.

Hoffmeister, H., Mensink, G.B., Stolzenberg, H. *et al.* (1996). Reduction of coronary heart disease risk factors in the German cardiovascular prevention study. *Preventive Medicine*, **25**, 135–45.

Hugosson, M.B., Sjöberg, A., and Byström, C. (2006). Facts and results from the Stockholm Trials - Final version - December 2006. Miljöavgiftskansliet/Congestion Charge Secretariat, City of Stockholm.

Jousilahti, P., Vartiainen, E., Pekkanen, J. *et al.* (1998). Serum cholesterol distribution and coronary heart disease risk: Observations and predictions among middle-aged population in eastern Finland. *Circulation*, **97**, 1087–94.

Keys, A., Anderson, J.T., and Grande, F. (1959). Serum cholesterol in man: diet fat and intrinsic responsiveness. *Circulation*, **19**, 201–14.

Lichtenstein, A.H., Appel, L.J., Brands, M. *et al.* (2006). Diet and lifestyle recommendations revision 2006: A scientific statement from the American Heart Association Nutrition Committee. *Circulation*, **114**, 82–96.

Lindholm, L. and Rosen, M. (2000). What is the "golden standard" for assessing population-based interventions?—problems of dilution bias. *Journal of Epidemiology and Community Health*, **54**, 617–22.

Luostarinen, T., Hakulinen, T., and Pukkala, E. (1995). Cancer risk following a community-based programme to prevent cardiovascular diseases. *International Journal of Epediomology*, **24**, 1094–9.

Luepker, R.V., Murray, D.M., Jacobs, D.R., Jr *et al.* (1994). Community education for cardiovascular disease prevention: risk factor changes in the Minnesota Heart Health Program. *American Journal of Public Health*, **84**, 1383–93.

Mittelmark, M.B., Hunt, M.K., Heath, G.W. *et al.* (1993). Realistic outcomes: Lessons from community-based research and demonstration programs for the prevention of cardiovascular diseases. *Journal of Public Health Policy*, **14**, 437–62.

Puska, P. (ed.) (1988). Comprehensive cardiovascular community control programmes in Europe. EURO Reports and Studies. World Health Organization. Regional Office for Europe. Copenhagen.

Puska, P. (2000). Do we learn our lessons from the population-based interventions? *Journal of Epidemiology and Community Health*, **54**, 562–3.

Puska, P., Tuomilehto, J., Nissinen, A. *et al.* (1995). The North Karelia Project. 20Year Results and Experiences. National Public Health Institute, Helsinki.

Puska, P., Salonen, J.T., Nissinen, A. *et al.* (1983). Change in risk factors for coronary heart disease during 10 years of a community intervention programme (North Karelia project). *British Medical Journal (Clinical Research Ed.)*, **287**, 1840–4.

Puska, P., Vartiainen, E., Tuomilehto, J. *et al.* (1998). Changes in premature deaths in Finland: successful long-term prevention of cardiovascular diseases. *Bulletin of the World Health Organization*, **76**, 419–25.

Saaristo, T., Peltonen, M., Keinänen-Kiukaanniemi, S. *et al.* for the FIN-D2D Study Group. (2007). *International Journal of Circumpolar Health*, **2**, 66–78.

Salonen, J.T., Puska, P., Kottke, T.E. *et al.*(1983). Decline in mortality from coronary heart disease in Finland from 1969 to 1979. *British Medical Journal (Clinical Research Ed.)*, **286**, 1857–60.

Schuit, A.J., Wendel-Vos, G.C., Verschuren, W.M. *et al.* (2006). Effect of 5-year community intervention Hartslag Limburg on cardiovascular risk factors. *American Journal of Preventive Medicine*, **30**, 237–42.

Sellers, D.E., Crawford, S.L., Bullock, K. *et al.* (1997). Understanding the variability in the effectiveness of community heart health programs: A meta-analysis. *Social Science and Medicine*, **44**, 1325–39.

Shea, S., Basch, C.E., Lantigua, R. *et al.* (1992). The Washington Heights-Inwood Healthy Heart Program: A third generation community-based cardiovascular disease prevention program in a disadvantaged urban setting. *Preventive Medicine*, **21**, 203–17.

Shelley, E., Daly, L., Collins, C. *et al.* (1995). Cardiovascular risk factor changes in the Kilkenny Health Project. A community health promotion programme. *European Heart Journal*, **16**, 752–60.

Vartiainen, E., Jousilahti, P., Alfthan, G. *et al.* (2000). Cardiovascular risk factor changes in Finland, 1972-1997. *International Journal of Epidemiology*, **29**, 49–56.

Vartiainen, E., Puska, P., Pekkanen, J. *et al.*(1994). Changes in risk factors explain changes in mortality from ischaemic heart disease in Finland. *BMJ*, **309**, 23–7.

Winkleby, M.A., Feldman, H.A., and Murray, D.M. (1997). Joint analysis of three U.S. community intervention trials for reduction of cardiovascular disease risk. *Journal of Clinical Epidemiology*, **50**, 645–58.

World Health Organization (2000). Global strategy for the prevention and control of noncommunicable disease. World Health Organization. WHA/A53/14.2000.

World Health Organization (2006). Gaining Health. The European Strategy for the Prevention and Control of Noncommunicable Diseases. World Health Organization. Copenhagen.

6.10

Community-based intervention trials in low- and middle-income countries

Zunyou Wu and Sheena G. Sullivan

Abstract

Community intervention trials began to be used in low- and middle-income countries about 20 years ago. Since then, they have been increasingly employed to test interventions that address urgent and preventable public health issues, particularly infectious disease control, neonatal mortality, malnutrition, and unhealthy behaviours. Various methodological considerations need to be considered in the planning, conduct, and analysis of community trials, especially when conducted in low- and middle-income countries. Selection of the study site needs to consider the baseline prevalence of the health problem of interest, the representativeness of the community chosen for the study, and the available resources. Background information is often absent before the trial and can be collected through qualitative research and community consultation. Engagement of the community at all stages of the trial is crucial for success and scale-up. Published trials have typically used pre/post or intervention/control comparisons to measure effectiveness. Where control groups are used and several communities are included in the study, the methodology should consider issues associated with conducting cluster-randomized trials which affect the sample size, statistical power, randomization, and statistical analyses. There are various ethical issues associated with conducting community trials, particularly with regard to obtaining informed consent from individuals versus community leaders, the use of control groups, and the distribution of incentives for participation. The type, intensity, and quality of the intervention must be considered acceptable and culturally sensitive to the communities. Simplicity, affordability, and sustainability of intervention strategies should always be emphasized. Success is often measured by morbidity and mortality rates associated with the disease of interest, but behavioural, psychosocial, environmental, and other indirect measures may also be used. Similarly cohort, cross-sectional or population-level data can be used for evaluation. Because they are often needs-driven, community-based intervention trials conducted in low- and middle-income countries have an enormous potential for scale-up. Scientific robustness of a trial should be maintained as much as possible while taking into account the limitations of working in low- or middle-income settings, including human resource and infrastructure limitations. Most of all, trials should prioritize the development of simple, cheap, effective, and sustainable solutions to health problems to facilitate uptake and use in routine public health work.

Introduction

In recent years, community-based intervention trials have been increasingly used to evaluate public health interventions to control disease and promote health. They can provide reliable data on the efficacy and cost effectiveness of disease control strategies to inform policy-makers in developing health policy and allocating resources. Typically, community-based interventions use lifestyle interventions that reflect community norms and are thus more readily integrated into current practices.

Community-based interventions were first used in high-income countries for reducing risk factors for cardiovascular and other chronic diseases. They began to be used in low- and middle-income countries in the late 1980s, initially to test programmes addressing maternal and child health. Early interventions targeted increasing immunization coverage (Desgrees du Lou *et al.* 1995; Brugha & Kevany 1996), decreasing general childhood mortality (Bang *et al.* 1990; Pandey *et al.* 1991; West *et al.* 1991), and maternal mortality (Fauveau *et al.* 1991). In the past 10–15 years, community-based intervention trials have been widely used in different settings targeting a broad range of public health issues in low- and middle-income countries. A community intervention trial was used to evaluate the impact of increased face-washing frequency on the prevalence of trachoma among children in Kongwa, Tanzania (West *et al.* 1995). Chavasse *et al.* (1999) used a community approach to evaluate whether fly control reduced the incidence of diarrhoea among children in Pakistan. Morrow *et al.* (1999) evaluated the impact of peer education on increasing exclusive breastfeeding to reduce diarrhoea among children. The effects of low-dose supplementation with vitamin A or β-carotene on mortality related to pregnancy were evaluated in villages in Nepal (West *et al.* 1999; Christian *et al.* 2000a). Community approaches have been used to trial interventions to control vector-borne diseases, such as dengue fever in Kenya (Wacira *et al.* 2007) and Vietnam (Vu *et al.* 2005).

Community trials have also played a major role in finding strategies to control the HIV epidemic, such as the STD treatment trials conducted in Uganda (Wawer *et al.* 1999; Kamali *et al.* 2003) and Tanzania (Grosskurth *et al.* 1995a), condom promotion among sex workers in Thailand (Wongkhomthong *et al.* 1995), and interventions to prevent the initiation of drug use in southern border areas of China (Wu *et al.* 2002). On a smaller scale they have been used to test programmes to reduce risk factors for chronic diseases, such as cardiovascular diseases (Dowse *et al.* 1995; Fang *et al.* 1999) and cancer (Ramadas *et al.* 2003).

Community-based intervention trials conducted in low- and middle-income countries have influenced clinical and public health practice not only in the countries in which they are conducted, but also in the industrialized world. For example, the STD treatment trials in Uganda and Tanzania demonstrated that improved control of STDs could reduce the incidence of HIV infection at the early stage of an HIV/AIDS epidemic (Hayes *et al.* 1997). This approach has been adopted as a best practices model, although more recently its efficacy has been called into question (Trollope-Kumar & Guyatt 2006).

Community-based intervention trials are often complicated and expensive. Due to the scarcity of resources available in middle-income and particularly in low-income countries, community-based intervention trials have design and methodological features that may be different from similar studies in high-income countries. This chapter reviews community-based intervention trials in low- and middle-income countries. The chapter will discuss study design, study population, intervention activities and quality of intervention, ethical issues, measurement issues, and interpretation and translation of results of community-based intervention trials conducted in low- and middle-income countries.

Design

Designing community-based intervention trials using a community as the study unit is more complicated than designing intervention trials at the individual level. Launching community-based intervention trials in low- and middle-income countries is even more difficult than doing them in high-income countries because background information is usually not available. In addition, the necessary infrastructure and competent personnel often do not exist, particularly in rural areas where public health interventions are most needed.

Defining communities

Communities are generally classified along geographical lines, which in low- and middle-income countries is often a village, urban district, or neighbourhood. In a study to examine the effect of vitamin A and β-carotene supplementation on postpartum illness in Nepal, randomization was by ward, a subunit of the study district consisting of several small subdistricts (Christian *et al.* 2000a; Christian *et al.* 2000b). Entire regions are also sometimes randomized, as was done in four regions of southern Guatemala for a study evaluating the effectiveness of information, education, and communication strategies to increase maternal awareness about pregnancy (Perreira *et al.* 2002). For interventions among children, schools often provide a suitable environment in which to conduct intervention activities. In South Africa, a drama-in-education programme, DramAide, was compared with information-only among high school students in 14 schools—seven randomized to the DramAide, seven to information-only (Harvey *et al.* 2000). Hospitals may also serve as the unit of randomization. In a study to reduce unnecessary blood transfusions in India, 12 hospitals were assigned to either intervention or control arms, where the intervention consisted of asking doctors to complete a transfusion request form that included a checklist to ascertain whether a transfusion was absolutely necessary (Bray *et al.* 2002). The reality, of course, is that in many low- and middle-income settings, interventions targeting only schools or hospitals will miss a sizeable portion of the target population. However, targeting a comprehensive range of sub-communities is a strategy that has been used to overcome this problem, such as in a Vietnamese trial to control dengue vectors, where local leaders, health volunteer teachers, and schoolchildren were all targeted (Kay *et al.* 2002).

Regardless of what unit of 'community' is chosen, having well-defined communities as a study unit or study venue is very important for successful community-based prevention trials. Ideally, the variations within and between communities should be low. However, in reality this is often not the case. The size of the communities selected and factors that can potentially interfere with the outcomes often vary between selected study venues. It is important to understand the maximum tolerance of heterogeneity among selected study venues.

Selection of study sites

The first stage of any study is to select an appropriate site for launching a trial. Several issues need to be considered. First, study sites must have a reasonably high prevalence of the events of interest, particularly sufficient high incidence. A high event rate is important to increase the cost-efficiency of the study and to reduce the duration of the trial. In low- and middle-income countries disease incidences are frequently high, particularly infectious diseases. In the STD treatment studies, high rates of key STDs were observed in study sites. In Mwanza, the average prevalence of syphilis was 15.6 per cent and the average prevalence of HIV antibody seropositivity was 4.1 per cent (Grosskurth *et al.* 1995a); in Rakai, the baseline prevalence was 10 per cent for syphilis and 15.9 per cent for HIV (Wawer *et al.* 1998); and in Mataka, baseline prevalence of active syphilis was 13.1 per cent and for HIV was 9.8 per cent (Kamali *et al.* 2003).

Second, existing resources, when available, should be used as much as possible; otherwise the intervention will be expensive and will not be sustainable when the trial is completed. Traditional birth attendants have long been used in interventions to reduce neonatal mortality (Bang *et al.* 1990; Jokhio *et al.* 2005). In the Tanzania study of the impact of face-washing on trachoma among children, neighbourhood meetings, followed by school plays, seminars with traditional healers, and meetings with other village groups were utilized (West *et al.* 1995). In the community drug prevention study in China, schools, families, communities, and health service infrastructures were all used (Wu *et al.* 2002). In Kenya, an intervention to increase the use of insecticide-treated bed nets used employers to promote the nets as one of the intervention components (Wacira *et al.* 2007).

Third, study sites should be representative of most communities affected by the diseases of interest. This is important because the intervention strategies and measures being tested in the trial should be expanded to other communities or even to the whole country or several countries if they are successful. In the stroke prevention study, Harbin, Changchun, Beijing, Zhenzhou, Shanghai, Changsha, and Yinchuan cities were chosen. The seven cities were representative of urban China in terms of geographic location, city size, and prevalence of risk factors and incidence of stroke (Fang *et al.* 1999).

Qualitative study of communities

Communities vary within regions and across regions. Usually little background information about study communities is available in low- and middle-income countries. It is essential to fully understand the community to assure the success of community-based intervention trials. Thus, collecting information about administrative structures and cultural characteristics is necessary before carrying out the trial.

Several methods can be used to collect existing and essential information. First, it is important to interview key informants in the community. Key informants include community administrative leaders, community religious leaders, opinion leaders, and, importantly, members of the target community. Information can also be sought from these people through focus group discussion. Wacira and colleagues (2007), in designing an intervention to increase the use of insecticide-treated bed nets in Kenya, conducted interviews and focus group discussions with representatives from government ministries, companies, and non-governmental organizations as well as employers and community members. Bhandari *et al.* (2003), in designing an intervention to improve perinatal and neonatal health outcomes, used qualitative methods to collect information about community characteristics, children's nutritional status, feeding practices, and reasons children may not be breastfed.

These qualitative methods may also be accompanied by on-site observation. This method was used in the NIMH Collaborative HIV/STD Prevention Trial study in five countries (NIMH Collaborative HIV/STD Prevention Trial Group 2007c). Anthropologists observed daily activity in food markets from 6 am when the markets opened to 6 pm when they closed. Their major objectives were to identify the most influential popular opinion leaders who could be selected and trained for delivery of the intervention and to identify existing social networks among food market vendors that could be used for diffusion of the intervention.

The amount of effort that should be put into a qualitative study prior to a trial varies from study to study and depends on how complex the proposed intervention is, how complex the communities involved in the trial are, how much background information already exists, the prior experience of the investigators, and how much money is available for the study. For the trial promoting exclusive breastfeeding, only a rapid ethnographic study of infant feeding was employed before the intervention trial was initiated (Morrow *et al.* 1999) but a comprehensive ethnographic study was conducted in the NIMH Collaborative HIV/STD Prevention Trial (NIMH Collaborative HIV/STD Prevention Trial Group 2007b).

Community consultation

Complementing the qualitative study should be a comprehensive consultation with the community. Different communities include different sub-groups of people. Each sub-group has its own characteristics, interests, and needs. Comprehensive consultation with different sub-groups is very important for developing effective interventions. In the drug prevention study in China, a wide range of people were consulted, including government leaders in different government sectors, such as education, health, public security, culture and entertainment, agriculture technology, ethnic group management, and poverty alleviation, as well as community leaders, youth leaders, women leaders, student leaders, teachers, village health workers, and drug users (Wu *et al.* 2002).

There is some debate about whether permission should be sought from communities before conducting community-based trials (Edwards *et al.* 1999). To a certain extent, community consultation with different stake holders goes some way towards seeking the consent of the community to conduct a trial. From a scientific point of view, seeking consent from every member of the community would compromise the results. But the approval, support, and involvement of key community stakeholders is an important part of project planning and design that can influence whether or not a project is in fact successful. In a review of 12 community-based intervention studies, 11 reported that community involvement had enhanced the quality of the intervention; two thought that it had improved the outcomes; eight believed it had improved enrolment; four noted better research methods and dissemination; and three described better descriptive measures (ARHQ 2003).

There is no rule to determine how much community consultation is needed. It depends on the complexity of the proposed intervention and the complexity of the community. The same targeted intervention may require different intensities of community consultation. In the study promoting consistent condom use among female sex workers in China, the extent of community consultation differed between study sites (Wu 1998). In Chengjiang County, comprehensive consultation was sought from officials from all government sectors involved in entertainment management as well as from establishment owners and the sex workers themselves. In Ruili and Longchuan counties, in which the investigators had had extensive prior experience, only local health officials, establishment owners, and sex workers themselves were consulted.

Consultation is not only important for developing appropriate and effective intervention strategies and work plans but also to provide the opportunity for local community members to learn skills, and to identify barriers for promoting changes in the community. Even more important, by being consulted, community leaders and members perceive that they are respected by the investigators, that they share the ownership of the project and, therefore, that they share the responsibility for the success of the project. To increase ownership, the process can be formalized through the establishment of a community advisory board (CAB). This board may include representatives of relevant local government units, such as the village leader, health workers, teachers, and law enforcement officers, influential members of the community, as well as members of the target community. The board typically reviews and advises investigators on a variety of intervention strategies.

Often people in the community think that they work for the investigators and not for themselves or for their community. This perception occurs because they are usually paid or partly paid by the project or its director, and they are told what the problems are and how to solve them. This perception is counterproductive, particularly for sustaining the changes after the trial is closed. It is important to promote the perception that the project is the community's project, that it will benefit the community, and that everyone has a responsibility to participate.

The control group

In principle, the control group is very important in community intervention trials to separate the impact of the intervention from other factors that might affect the trial. On the other hand, in quasi-experimental designs, rates before the intervention may instead serve as the baseline. In 1987, the Senegal government introduced immunization programmes into Bandafassi, an isolated area that previously had had no regular immunization programmes. Since immunizations were the only change introduced into the area during this period, it was possible to assess the impact of immunization on childhood mortality by comparing mortality rates before and after the immunization programme was introduced. Evaluation of the data indicated that after the introduction of immunizations, neonatal mortality declined by 31 per cent; the mortality rate for children between 1 and 8 months of age declined by 20 per cent; and the mortality rate for children between 9 and 59 months declined by 48 per cent (Desgrees du Lou *et al.* 1995).

In some cases, it is almost impossible to identify a robust control group and pre- and post-intervention comparisons are the only reasonable option. In the study promoting consistent condom use among female sex workers in China, high mobility among the sex workers precluded the researchers' ability to identify a suitable control group (Wu 1998). Sex workers would frequently work in several establishments at the same time or quickly move between establishments. Those sex workers coming from an intervention establishment to a control establishment who shared their new knowledge with coworkers would dilute the intervention effect and could incorrectly lead to the conclusion that condom promotion had had no effect.

Studies that use the mass media are particularly affected by contamination and preclude the use of a control group. In Burkina Faso, an intervention to distribute drugs against schistosomiasis was preceded by a nationwide information campaign utilizing television and radio to ensure high compliance with the treatment (Gabrielli *et al.* 2006). The campaign was nationwide, hence no control group was used and instead pre- and post-intervention comparisons were used.

In other cases, it is unethical to have a control group. In the early 1990s, the Thai government launched a national AIDS campaign promoting condom use and implemented a '100 per cent condom' policy in all brothels. It was not ethically acceptable to set up a parallel control group since condom use was already known to be effective in reducing sexual transmission of HIV. After condom promotion was implemented nationwide, the incidence and prevalence of STDs declined dramatically, accompanied by a decline in HIV infections (Wongkhomthong *et al.* 1995).

Where having a control group is unethical or impractical, it may be possible to compare two different interventions. This may also be the case if the researchers know that the methods being tested have both been successful in other communities, but they need to find the best intervention model for the community under study. In the study of trachoma in Tanzania, intervention villages received free treatment and health education while 'control' villages received the treatment only (West *et al.* 1995). The addition of health education carried an additional cost but the study showed it would be worth implementing on a wider scale since children in intervention communities were 60 per cent less likely to develop trachoma.

Trials to determine the best method of reducing a disease of interest may include more than two interventions as well as a control. In Honduras, a programme to increase the use of healthcare services compared four groups: (1) Money given directly to households; (2) resources to local health teams combined with a community-based nutrition intervention; (3) both packages; (4) neither package (Morris *et al.* 2004). In Mexico, two intervention groups with different counselling frequencies were compared with a control group to evaluate which had the greatest impact on increasing exclusive breastfeeding among mothers (Morrow *et al.* 1999).

Another way to obviate ethical concerns is to allocate enough funds in the project budget to have a waitlisted control—where the community receives the intervention once it has been shown to be effective. This was done in a programme that combined microfinance and gender/HIV training in South Africa (Pronyk *et al.* 2006). Communities were pair-matched, then randomized to receive the intervention at study onset or 3 years later.

The results of trials comparing pre- and post-intervention data or comparing two or more variations of an intervention can be difficult to interpret. Over long periods of time, many changes can occur in a community and can affect disease rates. Concurrent controls usually provide a more valid comparison and this design has been more commonly used in community-based intervention trials conducted in low- and middle-income countries. In the Mwanza study of the impact of improved STD treatment on the HIV epidemic, six pair-matched comparison communities were used. The baseline prevalence of HIV and syphilis, as well as most of the risk factors, were similar among the six comparison communities (Grosskurth *et al.* 1995a; Grosskurth *et al.* 1995b). In the Rakai STD study, ten comparable community clusters were randomized, with five assigned to intervention and five to control groups (Wawer *et al.* 1998).

In some studies, despite pre-baseline qualitative or quantitative data that suggested similarity between intervention and control communities, the baseline data indicate significant differences between communities for key outcomes. Thus, unlike the above studies where intervention and control communities were comparable at baseline, a simple comparison of the differences at follow-up between intervention and control is not statistically meaningful. In these cases, differences between pre- and post-intervention outcomes must be compared between intervention and control groups. To measure the impact of the World AIDS Campaign comparing the effectiveness of mass media alone with mass media plus small media (including leaflets, fliers, stickers, letters to families in the community, posters), both a parallel control group and a pre- and post-intervention control group were used and both confirmed changes within 2 months after the intervention was began (Du *et al.* 1999).

Communities may also switch between intervention and control arms of a study to gain better insight on the impact of the intervention. The randomized community trial to evaluate the impact of fly control on the incidence of childhood diarrhoea in Pakistan offered an unique example of different control groups (Chavasse *et al.* 1999). The study consisted of three areas: Area A, Area B, and a control area. Area A was sprayed in 1995, not sprayed in 1996, and traps were set in 1997. Area B was not sprayed in 1995, sprayed in 1996, and no traps were set in 1997. The control area was not sprayed from 1995 to 1997. Areas A and B were switched to control areas in 1995 and in 1996.

Sample size and statistical power

In community-based interventions, the unit of intervention is the community or cluster. Because of the dynamics that exist in communities, individuals within a community are more similar to each other than to individuals from another community and are therefore more likely to have the same outcome. This violates the assumption of independence between observations, which is essential in most statistical analyses. Thus, the correlation between individuals within and between communities needs to be considered in sample size calculations and analyses. The sum of these two components of variance, the variance between subjects in a cluster and the variance between clusters, is used to calculate the intracluster correlation (Kerry & Bland 1998b).

The intracluster correlation is used to estimate the design effect. This is the ratio of the total number of subjects required using cluster randomization to the number that would be required if individual randomization were used. The ratio obtained is used to estimate how much larger the sample size (of individuals) needs to be to achieve statistical power. For example, if the design effect is 1.17, then the number of participants needs to be increased by 17 per cent. Changes in the number of participants per cluster and in the intracluster correlation will change the design effect (Todd *et al.* 2003).

To a certain extent, increasing the number of individual observations in a cluster can reduce the variability within communities and increase statistical power, but at a certain point this effect plateaus and the number of clusters needs to be increased. In general, if communities are particularly heterogeneous, a larger number of small communities should be considered. However, the advantages of increasing the number of communities needs to be balanced with the feasibility and costs associated with targeting more communities. In the South African study to reduce intimate-partner violence, the number of clusters was limited to four in each study arm because of operational constraints, including the time required for recruitment and follow-up, the need to enrol all households in a village before expansion, and ethical concerns about withholding the intervention from control villages (Pronyk *et al.* 2006). Conversely, a smaller number of communities can be used if communities are relatively homogeneous. In either case, the number of individuals required in cluster-randomization is larger than would be needed for individual randomization.

Making estimates of intracluster variance in community-randomized trials is made difficult by the lack of existing data or previous studies that can be used to make estimates. Many researchers do not account for the cluster effect or have not published sufficient information to estimate the variance between groups (Kerry & Bland 1998a). In the community intervention trials discussed in this chapter, the number of communities involved varied; many did not account for the intra-cluster correlation and in certain study designs controls were not used; the study was not randomized; or only two communities were studied. In the Mauritius non-communicable disease prevention study, it was not feasible to use a control area in the small island, therefore only one unit was used, assessed by pre- and post-intervention cross-sectional surveys including 5080 and 5162 participants, respectively (Dowse *et al.* 1995). Emerson *et al.* (1999) used two pairs of villages (1124 children enrolled at baseline) to study control of trachoma and diarrhoea in Gambia (Emerson *et al.* 1999). In the study to promote exclusive breastfeeding in San Pedro Martir, 39 clusters with two to four city blocks each were randomized to one of two intervention conditions or a control. A total of 125 children were enrolled, which met the minimum required sample size of 120, based on $\alpha = 0{\cdot}05$ (one-sided), and giving 86 per cent power to detect a 20 per cent absolute difference in exclusive breastfeeding between intervention and control groups (24 per cent versus 4 per cent) if there was no design effect, or 76 per cent power if there was a design effect of 1.2. In Dhaka, 40 zones (20 intervention and 20 control) were randomly selected from 60 zones in a low socio-economic area to test an intervention to promote exclusive breastfeeding (Haider *et al.* 2000). The sample size was calculated based on achieving a 30 per cent difference in exclusive breastfeeding between intervention and control zones, at $\alpha = 0.05$, with 90 per cent power on a two-tailed test. The estimated required sample size, accounting for the design effect plus migration and loss to follow-up, was 312 mother–infant pairs in each arm, of which there were 288 intervention and 286 control participants remaining at the 6-month evaluation.

An alternative to increasing the sample size in an individual study or site is to pool data from different trials or run multi-site trials. The NIMH Collaborative HIV/STD Prevention Trial is a community-level study being conducted in five sites in five countries—China, India, Peru, Russia, and Zimbabwe—to assess the efficacy of an intervention involving popular-opinion leaders (NIMH Collaborative HIV/STD Prevention Trial Group 2007c). The trial uses comparable intervention strategies and data collection instruments that will allow the pooling of data to increase power, although individual sites have also been powered to observe an effect. Pooling data from trials that were not planned together requires that they have comparable outcome measures, which can be difficult to achieve. Even for the NIMH trial, this was a challenge (NIMH Collaborative HIV/STD Prevention Trial Group 2007a). In either case, site-specific sources of variance need to be taken into account when determining sample size and power and in analysing the results.

Further discussion on sample size calculations for cluster randomized trials can be found in Chapter 6.8, Methodological issues in the design and analysis of community-based intervention trials.

Randomization, matching, and stratification

Well-designed randomized community-based intervention trials are recognized as the gold standard for the evaluation of public health interventions. However, as noted above, randomization to intervention and control communities is not always feasible. In randomization, communities are assigned to the intervention or control condition on the basis of chance and unmeasured confounding factors are expected to be equally distributed in the intervention and comparison groups. Unbiased effect-estimates and valid confidence intervals can therefore be obtained.

When a randomized community intervention trial design is chosen, the unit of randomization is the community rather than the individual. This is known as group or cluster randomization. The number of units of randomization in community-randomized trials is usually smaller than in individually randomized trials, although the number of individuals may be large. In Nepal, the studies to improve postpartum outcomes randomized 270 wards in 30 village development committees to one of two intervention groups or a control but the total number of individuals enrolled in the study was more than 15 000 (Christian *et al.* 2000a; Christian *et al.* 2000b). Often, community trials have fewer communities available for randomization. When the number of communities is very small, randomization is less likely to achieve comparability between intervention and control groups (Rothman & Greenland 1996). If only a few communities are available for the study, then even with randomization, the intervention and control communities may not be comparable at baseline. If only two study communities are studied, no matter how well researchers do randomization, incomparability between intervention and control communities is likely to remain.

To overcome dissimilarity between intervention and control communities, researchers may consider matching, which involves matching communities on factors highly associated with the outcome variable, and then randomizing within the matched pair. The rationale for matching is to improve power in randomized studies. However, if matching variables are not strongly associated with the outcome, matching actually reduces study power through loss of degrees of freedom with a small number of experimental units (Martin *et al.* 1993). In the study of the effect of face-washing on trachoma, three paired villages were matched on the level of maternal education, baseline prevalence of clean faces in young children, and trachoma status. Within each pair, one village was randomized to the intervention and the other to the control group (West *et al.* 1995). In the Mwanza study, matching was used because there were variations in HIV prevalence and incidence in different parts of the study region (Hayes *et al.* 1995). Communities were matched on roadside, lakeshore, or rural location, geographic area, and preexisting level of STDs based on clinic records at the health centre. Randomization was performed within each matched pair.

An alternative to matching is stratification, where communities may be grouped rather than paired by variables associated with the outcome and later randomized within strata. In both matching and stratification, the degrees of freedom are reduced, but this can be offset by the decrease in the variance between communities, which in turn can reduce the design effect and improve power. The results of the three landmark HIV community-randomized trials conducted in Africa—the Mwanza trial (Grosskurth *et al.* 1995a), the Rakai study (Wawer *et al.* 1998), and the Masaka trial (Kamali *et al.* 2003)—were compared to examine the differential effects of stratification or matching (Todd *et al.* 2003). In Mwanza and Masaka, matching and stratification reduced between-community variance and improved the power of the study compared with an unmatched or unstratified design. In the Rakai trial, where communities had been selected to be relatively homogeneous, matching reduced the variance between communities but did not increase power.

Both stratification and matching require some background data prior to randomization upon which to base the matching or stratification. In the Indian study to promote breastfeeding, a baseline survey of all households with children younger than 2 years was first conducted, and a total score calculated based on socioeconomic indicators, child mortality, recent morbidity, and the prevalence of wasting and stunting. Communities were then paired to communities with similar scores and then randomized to intervention or control.

When study communities are similar in prevalence and incidence of events and related key risk factors, matching is not necessary. In this situation, randomization can be directly performed without matching. For example, in the Rakai STD prevention trial, matching was not used because of the homogeneous character of the study communities (Wawer *et al.* 1999).

Sometimes matching is not feasible either because data on the outcomes of interest and risk factors among study communities are not available, or the number of units is too small to permit effective matching. In the study to maximize immunization coverage through home visits in Ghana, only three towns were selected as study units. Neither randomization nor matching was performed (Brugha & Kevany 1996).

On the other hand, in certain circumstances, randomization of intervention units is not possible. This may occur, for example, when study villages are adjacent to one another and the risk of contamination is high. In a community-based intervention trial to reduce childhood mortality from pneumonia, random allocation was not performed (Bang *et al.* 1990). The intervention included mass education about childhood pneumonia and case management of pneumonia by village health workers and traditional birth attendants. A total of 102 villages in one contiguous area were studied, of which 58 villages were assigned to the intervention group and 44 villages were in the control group. The two groups were separated by a small 'buffer' zone of a few villages. In this example, given the geographic proximity of the intervention and control communities and the use of mass education, the other choices available to the researchers were randomization without using mass education, or using the mass media without a control area.

There are other issues with using randomization in settings based in low- and middle-income countries. Acceptability of research by the community sometimes is an issue. In some low- and middle-income countries, communities do not accept the concept of 'research' or 'study' nor do they understand the need for controls. They often only support community programmes or projects that they believe will be beneficial, or at least potentially beneficial to their communities. Randomization may give the community the impression that they are only being used as guinea pigs. Additionally, many poor countries believe that having control communities is not cost-effective because of the expenses involved in maintaining such communities. In these situations it is important to educate the government or communities about the need for controls and randomization in yielding scientifically valid findings.

Where randomization is chosen, investigators should follow the guidelines found in the CONSORT (consolidated standards of reporting trials) statement (Campbell *et al.* 2004). This statement was initially designed to guide the reporting of randomized clinical trials by providing a checklist and flow diagram. It has since been updated to provide guidance on the reporting of cluster-randomized trials and includes a 22-point checklist to remind researchers to include important information necessary for objective interpretation of the results, such as the intracluster correlation, design effect, and power and sample size calculations. Many medical journals now require adherence to the statement as a condition for publication (Campbell 2004).

Cohort versus repeated cross-sectional samples

Although community-based interventions are conducted at the community level, their assessment is at the individual level. Ideally, all individuals in the target population are sampled, but this is rarely feasible. In the two studies to reduce childhood mortality (Bang *et al.* 1990; Pandey *et al.* 1991), a cohort study design was used and all children in the communities were enumerated. In the India study (Bang *et al.* 1990), a census was carried out before the study. All births and deaths of children under 5 years were recorded by village health workers in each village. In the Nepal study (Pandey *et al.* 1991), a similar method was employed. A household census of children under 5 years was done at the start of the study, and all subsequent births and childhood deaths were registered throughout the subsequent 36 months.

Conducting either a census or a mixed design is expensive and often not logistically possible. Thus, researchers in low- and middle-income countries have generally needed to make a choice between one of two study designs: (1) A cohort study design, where a selected group of individuals is followed up for changes over the course of the study; or (2) a repeated cross-sectional survey design where different groups, usually randomly selected, are assessed at each time period. This decision depends on the characteristics of the outcome variable, the information-collecting system available at the study sites, the ability to follow the sample population, and the amount of funds available for the study.

Cohort studies are statistically more powerful than cross-sectional surveys, since individual baseline characteristics can be controlled for, which reduces sampling error. However, results based solely on a cohort may not be representative of the target population. Even if the population of interest were those who reside in the community continuously during the intervention, the cohort sample is usually a self-selected subset of that group who are willing to be followed up. Therefore, it probably is not representative of the entire target population. Attrition throughout the study may also decrease the external validity of the sample, particularly if the participants who leave the study are disproportionately reached by the intervention. Moreover, repeated measurement may act as a kind of intervention in itself, increasing participants' knowledge and confounding the results.

A cohort study design was used in the trachoma study (West *et al.* 1995). Children's trachoma status and facial cleanliness were observed at baseline and at 2, 6, and 12 months after intervention. In the study of peer counselling to promote exclusive breastfeeding in Mexico, the cohort study design was also used (Morrow *et al.* 1999). All study mothers were followed-up at 2, 4, and 6 weeks and at 2 and 3 months postpartum to record infant-feeding practices in the previous week and whether the infant had experienced diarrhoea since the last interview.

In South Africa, Pronyk and colleagues observed the effects of their intervention to reduce intimate-partner violence using three cohorts. Cohort 1 consisted of women enrolled in a microfinance programme; randomly selected household co-residents aged 14–35 years were included in Cohort 2; and randomly selected community members aged 14–25 years comprised Cohort 3 (Pronyk *et al.* 2006). Women in Cohorts 2 and 3 did not directly receive the intervention (microfinance plus HIV training curriculum) but were assessed to monitor the auxiliary benefits of the intervention.

Cross-sectional studies also have their own strengths and weaknesses. Given that the target population for community-based interventions is often the wider community, it has been argued that cross-sectional surveys are more appropriate to see changes in the communities targeted. They may include people who have had extensive or limited exposure to the intervention, thus giving a more representative picture of the intervention's reach. On the other hand, this may also be seen as a weakness, especially when limited exposure is associated with in-migration and a related short duration of exposure, rather than limited reach (Feldman & McKinlay 1994).

Cross-sectional surveys are often used to assess mass-media campaigns. In two HIV/AIDS-related education studies, repeated cross-sectional surveys were used to assess the impact of the intervention programme (Pauw *et al.* 1996; Du *et al.* 1999). Knowledge was assessed at baseline and after the education intervention programme had been implemented.

In some situations, the cohort study design is almost impossible to use, for example, in areas of high migration. In the trial to promote condom use among sex workers, repeated cross-sectional surveys were the only feasible choice given the high turn-over of sex workers in the study site (Wu 1998).

Sometimes a retrospective cohort can be reconstructed in repeated cross-sectional surveys. In the study of prevention of drug use in China (Wu *et al.* 2002), the incidence of drug use among adolescents and young adults was estimated based on a reconstructed retrospective cohort derived from repeated cross-sectional surveys. This was possible because there was very little migration in or out of the villages and the village leader was responsible for recording all in- and out-migrations.

In some cases, both a cohort and a cross-sectional survey have been used simultaneously. In Ghana, a study to improve the nutritional status of infants aged 6–12 months used both a cohort and cross-sectional design to evaluate the intervention (Lartey *et al.* 1999). Infants in the intervention group were individually randomized to receive either Weanimix (a cereal-legume blend jointly developed by UNICEF and the Ghanaian government) or one of three locally produced complementary foods. Infants were assessed at 6 and 12 months of age for iron, zinc, vitamin A, and riboflavin status. It was not possible to include a concurrent control group; hence a cross-sectional study conducted before and after the intervention collected anthropometric data on children not included in the intervention. All four foods improved nutritional status compared to the non-intervention group, and Weanimix showed the best overall improvements.

Ethical issues

We previously mentioned the debate over whether communities should be informed about the intervention and their consent obtained. Where an intervention is being directed to the community as a whole and does not involve individual recruitment of people into intervention activities, a Community Advisory Board has acted as guardians of the community under study. Whether this is sufficient is debatable (see *International Ethical Guidelines for Epidemiological Studies*, Discussion draft no. 3, CIOMS, WHO, April 2007. Available at: http://www.cioms.ch/080221feb_2008.pdf; accessed 13 August 2007).

Where individuals in a community are enrolled in the trial to receive specific intervention components, additional ethical issues arise, especially with regard to the control group. Unlike a drug trial, which can be double-blinded and where participants are aware that they may receive treatment or placebo, community trials often involve educational or other programmes and participants know whether they are receiving the intervention or not. By fully informing participants in the control group about the intervention during the informed consent process, contamination may be introduced by prompting the controls to seek out the information that their counterparts in the intervention group are receiving. If controls are receiving routine care, then it may be considered acceptable to withhold information regarding the intervention from them. In this way, individual consent to participate in intervention activities is sought only from those in the intervention communities, and consent for data collection and to be contacted for follow-up is taken from all parties (Edwards *et al.* 1999). If an intervention is shown to work, then the controls are sometimes treated as wait-listed controls and receive the intervention at a later time. As with a drug trial, if an intervention is shown to be overwhelmingly effective it could be stopped early and administered to all communities.

The problem of whether to fully inform controls about the intervention is further complicated when monetary incentives are introduced. In many low- and middle-income countries, financial or other incentives, such as free food, washing powder, or other household consumables, are provided for participation in a trial. Any financial or other incentive may be viewed as coercion given the poor financial situation of most eligible participants in low- and middle-income countries, but in many of these settings incentives are expected. The nature and amount of such incentives should be described in the study protocols submitted to ethics review committees, which will ultimately decide if the incentive implicates voluntary participation. Where controls are concerned, fairness and justice may be compromised. Both intervention and control participants would normally receive reimbursement for data collection activities, but controls that are not required to participate in any intervention activities, such as skills training, would not be eligible for any associated reimbursements. From a practical perspective, there is some risk that incentives increase the intervention effect by creating a motivation to participate that artificially increases exposure.

As researchers from high-income countries intensify their research activity in low- and middle-income countries, and as researchers from low- and middle-income countries increasingly bid for foreign funding, adherence to international ethical guidelines has become increasingly important. This includes the establishment of institutional structures, such as institutional review boards (IRB) or ethics committees that can monitor the progress of the research and protect the people enrolled in the trials.

Intervention activities

Types of interventions

The content of community interventions can include changes in public policy, the environment, community norms, or personal behaviours at both the individual and community levels. In broad terms, intervention programmes can be grouped into four types: (1) Individual-level programmes, such as self-study manuals, one-to-one communication or counselling, peer education programmes; (2) Mass media campaigns such as radio and television advertisements or newspaper stories; (3) Public policy changes, such as mandated non-smoking areas in public places and the use of seat belts; and (4) Group interventions such as educational programmes in schools or with informal groups such as support organizations of drug users or sex workers. Often community-wide interventions include programmes of each type. Choosing which types of interventions to use should be determined by the characteristics of the communities, the diseases of interest, cost, feasibility, and other factors.

Individually targeted intensive interventions may be of limited use in community trials because participation in these kinds of programmes is low, and thus the population-level impact will be small. Generally, a combined approach is more likely to be effective than one which uses only one approach because the combined approach will reach a wider audience. For example, the Indian intervention to promote exclusive breastfeeding employed a combination of interventions, namely: (1) Individual counselling by traditional birth attendants, immunization clinic nurses, and healthcare workers; (2) meetings between the healthcare workers and community representatives who in turn held neighbourhood meetings to promote breastfeeding among women in the community; and (3) printed educational materials including pamphlets, posters in clinics, flip books for health workers, and counselling guides to solve common breastfeeding problems (Bhandari *et al.* 2003). In Guatemala, an intervention to increase awareness of danger signs during pregnancy, delivery, and the postpartum period used: (1) A clinic-based programme which trained health providers on prenatal counselling and provided educational media to patients; (2) a community-based programme consisting of radio messages about obstetric complications; and (3) education sessions conducted through women's groups (Perreira *et al.* 2002).

Well-designed mass media campaigns are usually effective for increasing basic knowledge but may not be effective for correcting misconceptions (Du *et al.* 1999). Strategies that use the mass media are often unable to randomize communities and may also be unable to include a control group because it has such a wide reach that contamination is highly likely.

Public policy change is probably the most cost-efficient way to make an impact. For example, the '100 per cent condom' policy for brothel-based prostitutes in Thailand reduced the incidence and prevalence of STDs dramatically (Wongkhomthong *et al.* 1995). But even this approach was combined with mass education on the threat of HIV and the efficacy of condoms.

Appropriateness of intervention messages

Community interventions, particularly those that try to change people's behaviour, need to be carefully tailored to the target audience. Even those interventions that test treatments requiring only a minor change in behaviour encounter difficulties in ensuring compliance among patients. Thus the sensitivities of the target population should be integrated into intervention messages. For example, sex workers may be more receptive to HIV/STI prevention messages when they are put in the context of fertility (Liao *et al.* 2003). When the Thai government introduced the health warning, 'Smoking causes impotence', on packets of cigarettes, it was hoped that the message would strike a chord among young men who are typically resistant to health warnings (Chapman 1999).

However, in many cases knowledge and information is not enough to create change and structural interventions may be needed. A typical example is anti-smoking education among health professionals, which has largely failed on its own. New strategies that have included policy interventions, for example, regulations prohibiting smoking in hospital settings, have been more effective in stopping health professionals from smoking around clinical settings (Smith *et al.* 2005). Another example is knowledge education about drug injection-related harms among injecting drug users, who may be aware of the risks of sharing needles but will continue to practice risky injecting behaviours in the absence of readily available needles and syringes (Yap *et al.* 2002; Lin *et al.* 2004).

Difficulties in message framing are often exacerbated in low- and middle-income countries by limited education. For example, people may not understand how chronic behaviour, such as long-term smoking, can lead to adverse health consequences many years later (Chapman 1999). Thus the literacy levels of the population should also be taken into account.

Religion can also pose a barrier—the obvious example being condom use to prevent HIV/STD infection—although there are some examples where religion has successfully been incorporated into intervention activities. For example, harm reduction for drug users in Muslim communities has been advocated on the basis that an Islamic legal dictum provides that 'a lesser harm may be tolerated in order to eliminate a greater harm . . .' (IHRD 2006). Religious leaders in Xinjiang Autonomous Region in western China have been key players in harm reduction efforts there (XJHAPAC 2006).

Intensity of the interventions

The intensity of an intervention programme must reach a certain threshold in order to produce a change. For example, in the study to promote exclusive breastfeeding in San Pedro Martir, Mexico City, two intervention groups with different counselling frequencies, six visits and three visits, were compared with a control group that had no intervention (Morrow *et al.* 1999). Infants were followed up until 3 months of age to assess the effect of the peer education programme on promoting exclusive breastfeeding and on the incidence of diarrhoea among children. Exclusive breastfeeding was achieved in 67 per cent in the six-visit group, 50 per cent in the three-visit group, and 12 per cent in the control group.

In the study promoting condom use among female sex workers in China (Wu 1998), six on-site education and condom promotion programmes were given at all three study sites. However, one of the study sites was not able to provide sexual healthcare services, including STD diagnosis and treatment, to sex workers. Sex workers at that study site had a lower increase in knowledge and a lower increase in consistent condom use rate with clients, compared with the other two sites.

How much intervention is less than enough, how much is just enough, and how much is more than enough depends on such variables as the nature of the intervention, the characteristics of the target population, and the cultural characteristics of the society or community. Thus no guidelines can be formulated to cover all circumstances.

Often a community health intervention trial can be designed, funded, and implemented in a place where other health-related programmes may already be under way with public and/or private sponsorship in both experimental and control communities. Many community intervention trials may be testing only an incremental increase in the general level of health promotion in intervention communities, not the effectiveness of the intervention alone. Any community intervention programme must be sufficiently potent to be 'heard' beyond the background noise of ongoing health promotion activities. Thus an intervention programme should direct resources toward interventions that are relatively unique and not available in control communities.

Sustainability of interventions

The sustainability of an intervention is one of most important issues in conducting community-based interventions in low- and middle-income countries. Several factors affect sustainability. First, the cost-effectiveness of the intervention. The cheaper the intervention is, the more sustainable the programme is likely to be. In the Mwanza STD study, during the 2 years of follow-up, 11 632 cases of STDs were treated in the intervention health units; 252 HIV infections were averted each year in the intervention group compared with control group. The average per capita cost was US$0.39. It was estimated that the average cost per disability-adjusted life-year (DALY) saved was US$10 (range: US$2.51 to US$47.86). The estimated cost-effectiveness of the intervention, i.e. improved treatment services for STDs, compared favourably with the cost of childhood immunization programmes, US$12–US$17 per DALY (Gilson *et al.* 1997).

Second, the simpler the intervention is, the more sustainable the programme will be. In a study on reducing childhood mortality in Nepal (Pandey *et al.* 1991), the intervention programme focused on active case detection. Every day each health worker visited 10–15 households with children under 5 years of age, most within a half-hour walk from the worker's home. The worker completed a round of the target households (about 160) under his/her responsibility every 2 weeks. The intervention occupied about half his/her time and allowed him/her to continue his/her regular farming activities. In the Rakai STD study, because of the lack of a clinical infrastructure in the study areas and the high prevalence of STDs in the communities, a mass-treatment strategy was used and all consenting adults were given directly observed STD therapy in their home every 10 months, irrespective of laboratory test results or the presence of symptoms (Wawer *et al.* 1999). These strategies would be possible for many low- and middle-income countries.

Third, the higher the proportion of people in the community covered by the intervention, the more likely the programme will be sustained. In the Rakai STD study, all consenting adults were given treatment (Wawer *et al.* 1999); i.e. the STD rate in the community was reduced for the period of the trial and this would have at least a medium-term impact on keeping levels of infection low. However, without continued availability of free treatment to address new infections, the long-term sustainability is limited.

Fourth, the higher the intensity of the intervention, the less likely the programme will be sustained because maintaining high intensity is usually expensive, difficult, and often results in 'burn-out'. However, if the intensity is not high enough, the programme may not be able to produce changes.

If the programme itself can generate profits, the sustainability of the programme is likely. From July 1998 to August 1999, condom vending machines were installed in communities for condom social marketing in Shenzhen City, Guangdong Province, where many migrants live. The price of a single condom was 1 Chinese Yuan (then equivalent to US$0.12) and was thus affordable to everyone in the community. Taking into account the staff's salaries, the base price of condoms, and the cost of the vending machines for the 8-month period, the profits generated from condoms bought from the vending machines was estimated at 100 per cent (Wu 1999).

Measurement

While the unit of intervention in community-based trials is the community, the unit of measurement is often the individual. Since the overall aim of a community-based intervention programme is generally to reduce mortality and/or morbidity, these two types of rates are the most commonly used measures of the impact of the intervention.

In the childhood mortality studies in Nepal (Pandey *et al.* 1991), India (Bang *et al.* 1990), and Ethiopia (Ali *et al.* 2005) mortality was used as the outcome variable. Maternal mortality was an outcome in an antenatal care intervention in Bangladesh (Fauveau *et al.* 1991), in the night blindness study among postpartum women in Nepal (Christian *et al.* 2000a), and in the intervention to train traditional birth attendants in Pakistan (Jokhio *et al.* 2005).

In two diarrhoea control studies, the reported incidence of diarrhoea among children under 5 was used as the outcome measure to assess the effectiveness of the intervention (Chen and Liu 1991; Chavasse *et al.* 1999). In three STD studies conducted in Africa, the incidence rates of STDs and HIV infection were used to evaluate intervention effects (Grosskurth *et al.* 1995a; Wawer *et al.* 1999; Kamali *et al.* 2003).

Morbidity may also be measured not as disease incidence measured through biological methods, but also by using psychosocial measures. A number of these now exist to measure quality of life, addiction, depression, and other psychological symptoms, many of which have been translated and tested in the context of low- and middle-income countries. In India, the effectiveness of a day-care programme for the elderly was measured using standardized scales for assessing psychiatric morbidity and quality of life (Jacob *et al.* 2006).

Direct measures of outcome variables, such as disease incidence or mortality, provide valid data to assess the effectiveness of an intervention programme. However, determining them is often expensive. The high cost of individual-level measurements may limit the number of surveys that can be done and thus the statistical power of the evaluation. The high cost of measuring incidence often precludes long-term monitoring for latent effects, which can be important since the time lag between programme implementation and individual-level effects is often uncertain and may be long. Costs can be reduced to a certain extent by taking advantage of local health services records and using passive case detection, rather than surveying participants at specific times. In Ghana, an intervention to prevent malaria in children was measured by the incidence of malaria and anaemia as detected when children were hospitalized at any one of 11 health clinics in the study site (Chandramohan *et al.* 2005). In many low- and middle-income countries, however, health services may not be established well enough to make this feasible. Serial cross-sectional surveys may also reduce costs as they are usually less expensive than incidence studies.

Because of these problems, other measures are often used as surrogate markers for morbidity. Examples of surrogate or intermediate outcomes that are measured in a variety of behavioural intervention studies include knowledge, attitudes, beliefs, intentions, behavioural skills, and behaviours. In such studies, the assumption is that increasing knowledge and changing attitudes will lead to reduced risk behaviours and by reducing risk behaviours the likelihood of developing the disease is also reduced. In community-based HIV/AIDS education interventions, knowledge, sexual behaviours, and condom use behaviours are used as outcome variables to assess the impact of the interventions (Pauw *et al.* 1996; Bentley *et al.* 1998). Self-reported data are cheaper because they avoid costly clinical tests. Moreover, changes in behaviour may be expected to be seen to a larger extent than changes in the frequency of disease. Thus sample size calculations may become smaller, reducing overall study expenditure.

Data collected through self-report are less robust than objective measures such as biological testing because they may be affected by recall bias and social-desirability bias. Ideally, where funding is sufficient, self-reported behaviours are verified by more objective data, such as biological data, to verify that the changes in behaviour lead to the desired outcome, at least in the short term. Studies of condom use to prevent HIV infection will often ask participants about their risk behaviours but may verify this though biological assessments, such as testing for STDs (which generally have a higher incidence and infectivity than HIV, and hence are more likely to yield an observable change in prevalence), or observing whether participants can demonstrate correct condom use. In the Indian study to increase condom use among men, participants were asked about their risk behaviours and this was complemented with testing for HIV and STDs (Bentley *et al.* 1998). Men who reported that they always used a condom with a sex worker had lower HIV conversion rates and lower STD prevalence than those who reported having never used a condom.

Other general measures can include distribution of intervention materials or demand for services. In the nationwide schistosomiasis campaign launched in Burkina Faso, the number of immunizations was one outcome used to measure coverage (Gabrielli *et al.* 2006). In Brazil, STD/AIDS prevention was partially assessed by the demand for male and female condoms (Figueiredo & Ayres 2002).

Environmental factors can also act as objective measures of the success of an intervention. In the study to increase knowledge and modify behaviours related to dengue vectors in Vietnam, the main outcome was the prevalence of the *Aedes aegypti* mosquito larvae in water storage containers (Vu *et al.* 2005).

Interpretation

Interpretation of results is sometimes difficult. Cautious interpretation must be made especially when no control group is used. The Matlab study of maternal mortality in Bangladesh concluded that maternal mortality was significantly lower in areas with maternal and child healthcare programmes and family planning programmes (MCH-FP) than in the control area (Fauveau *et al.* 1991). However, continued observation indicated that there was no difference between the MCH-FP and comparison areas (Ronsmans *et al.* 1997). The authors thus concluded that the introduction of the maternity-care programme coincided with declining trends in direct obstetric mortality in the areas covered by the programme, although it is also possible that the effectiveness of the intervention declined.

Even with a control group, sometimes the relative benefits of an intervention are not observable. This may be because the investigators have failed to accommodate secular trends in the community under study. Conducting a pre-baseline survey before randomization can provide data to help interpret the influence of secular trends. Qualitative data can also help to interpret secular trends. In the South Africa study, qualitative data and analytic methods that could control for secular trends were used to detect reductions in intimate-partner violence (Pronyk *et al.* 2006).

Appropriate data analysis

A key issue in interpreting results from a community-based trial is using the correct data analysis, particularly when cluster-randomization has been used. The analysis of clustered data is by no means agreed upon by statisticians, and much less, there is no standardized notation. Moreover, because the analysis is complicated—requiring that both individual-level and group-level characteristics be accommodated—few researchers use the correct statistical analyses. A review of 56 papers in seven peer-reviewed journals identified few that had appropriate study designs or used the appropriate methods of analysis to allow for the intracluster correlation effect (Ukoumunne *et al.* 1999). In another review of cluster-randomized trials published between 1998 and 2002 in the *American Journal of Public Health* and *Preventive Medicine*, only nine of the 60 papers reviewed reported the correct analysis (Varnell *et al.* 2004). Among the community-randomized trials cited in this chapter many did not account for the design effect. In general, statisticians fail to take into account the group or design effect and data are analysed at the individual level. By ignoring the group effect, the relative benefits of the intervention are exaggerated and the intervention may seem more effective than it really is (Donner & Klar 2000) (see also Chapter 6.8, Methodological issues in the design and analysis of community intervention trials).

Accounting for the group and individual-level covariates can be achieved using a general or generalized linear model (GLM). This may also be referred to as random effects modelling, mixed modelling, random coefficient modelling, contextual modelling, hierarchical linear modelling, or multilevel analysis. Generalized estimating equations (GEE) are also used. Unfortunately, few statisticians in high-income countries, and even fewer in low- and middle-income countries, are experienced in the use of these models for cluster data. Detailed descriptions on the appropriate analyses for cluster-randomized data are provided by Donner and Klar (2000) and Ukoumunne *et al.* (1999).

Translating scientific studies to programme settings

Often, the scientific environment in which a study is conducted is quite different from programme settings. Investigators will often choose a study environment that will allow methodological robustness. For example, communities with low emigration are often used in scientific studies to maximize the likelihood of good follow-up of participants for the duration of the study. Scientific studies are also generally able to expend more resources (financial, human, and time) than would be feasible if the project were later institutionalized in the routine healthcare system in low- and middle-income countries. The capacity of health workers is a key issue in scaling up evidence-based interventions. In many low- and middle-income countries, health workers, particularly those in rural areas, have only had some high-school education, with additional training in first aid and preventive medicine. Intervention activities need to be within the capabilities of the health human resources that are reasonably available or that require a level of training that is realistic given local health budgets.

In low- and middle-income countries, trials are often done to determine their effectiveness, rather than their efficacy. The differences between these two objectives are important when considering whether or not to scale up an intervention. Efficacy measures the benefits of an intervention among those who take advantage of it or the benefits of an intervention given under fairly ideal conditions; effectiveness measures the benefits of an intervention among those offered or under programmatic or 'real-life' conditions. When scaling up a community intervention programme, the overall effectiveness of a programme is more important than knowing how good it could be if people were to use it, especially when trying to determine how best to use limited resources. This also extends to structural barriers that prevent people from using an intervention. In the study from Honduras that compared giving monetary incentives to women to use primary healthcare services with direct transfer of resources to local health teams, it was found that the household-level intervention had a large impact, but the transfer of resources could not be implemented properly because of legal complications (Morris *et al.* 2004). While the researchers acknowledged this limited interest in their findings, they stressed that their objective was to test effectiveness, rather than efficacy; the inability of the government to successfully transfer resources was therefore an important observation because of its implications for scale-up. Sometimes in community trials, particularly those conducted in low- and middle-income countries, feasibility is the most important study outcome.

Feasibilty is greatly aided by community consultation. As mentioned earlier, consultation with key community members in the design phase of a project can aid translation of research into policy by ensuring that the study asks questions which the community regard as important. Continued communication with these parties is essential for creating the sense of ownership required for politicians and government officials to support scale-up of an intervention. Strategies that facilitate the development of relationships among members in different, responsible sectors can facilitate this process of persuasion. They are especially important when recommending the scale up of interventions that benefit marginalized or stigmatized members of the population.

Conclusion

Community intervention trials are now used in low- and middle-income countries more than ever before and cover an increasing range of public health issues, including infectious diseases, neonatal mortality, malnutrition, and unhealthy behaviours, as well as chronic diseases. Their use is likely to continue to increase in coming years as concern grows over the evaluation of the delivery of health services, public education, and social policy. One advantage of conducting community intervention trials in low- and middle-income countries is that they often address urgent preventable health problems in these countries. However, it is often more challenging to implement community intervention trials in these countries because of the lack of background information, lack of infrastructure, and lack of trained and experienced resource personnel. Several criteria need to be considered before beginning community intervention trials in low- and middle-income countries:

- Study sites should have a reasonably high incidence of the health events of interest.
- A qualitative study of the social and cultural characteristics of the community may need to be conducted.
- Community consultation should be carried out before finalizing the intervention plan.
- Local resources should be used for the intervention to ensure sustainability.
- The type, intensity, and quality of the intervention must be considered acceptable and culturally sensitive to the communities.
- Simplicity, affordability, and sustainability of intervention strategies should always be emphasized.

Community interventions have been demonstrated to be effective in low- and middle-income countries but more trials are needed for the many public health problems still affecting these countries.

Acknowledgement

The authors are especially grateful to Professors Roger Detels and Mary Ann Lansang for their comments, suggestions, and helpful editing. The authors would also like to thank Ms Line Handlos-Neerup for her assistance with the literature review.

References

Ali, M., Asefaw, T., Byass, P. *et al.* (2005). Helping northern Ethiopian communities reduce childhood mortality: Population-based intervention trial. *Bulletin of the World Health Organization*, **83**, 27–33.

ARHQ (2003). Community-based participatory research: Assessing the evidence. Agency for Healthcare Research and Quality, US Department of Health and Human Services, Washington DC.

Bang, A.T., Bang, R.A., Tale, O. *et al.* (1990). Reduction in pneumonia mortality and total childhood mortality by means of community-based intervention trial in Gadchiroli, India. *Lancet*, **336**, 201–6.

Bentley, M.E., Spratt, K., Shepherd, M.E. *et al.* (1998). HIV testing and counseling among men attending sexually transmitted disease clinics in Pune, India: Changes in condom use and sexual behavior over time. *AIDS*, **12**, 1869–77.

Bhandari, N., Bahl, R., Mazumdar, S. *et al.* (2003). Effect of community-based promotion of exclusive breastfeeding on diarrhoeal illness and growth: A cluster randomised controlled trial. *Lancet*, **361**, 1418–23.

Bray, T.J., Salil, P., Weiss, H.A. *et al.* (2002). Intervention to promote appropriate blood use in India. *Transfusion Medicine*, **12**, 357–66.

Brugha, R.F. and Kevany, J.P. (1996). Maximizing immunization coverage through home visits: A controlled trial in an urban area of Ghana. *Bulletin of the World Health Organization*, **74**, 517–24.

Campbell, M.J. (2004). Extending CONSORT to include cluster trials. *British Medical Journal*, **328**, 654–5.

Campbell, M.K., Elbourne, D.R., and Altman, D.G. (2004). CONSORT statement: Extension to cluster randomised trials. *British Medical Journal*, **328**, 702–8.

Chandramohan, D., Owusu-Agyei, S., Carneiro, I. *et al.* (2005). Cluster randomised trial of intermittent preventive treatment for malaria in infants in area of high, seasonal transmission in Ghana. *British Medical Journal*, **331**, 727–33.

Chapman, S. (1999). Smoking and women: Beauty before age? *British Medical Journal*, **318**, 818.

Chavasse, D.C., Shier, R.P., Murphy, O.A. *et al.* (1999). Impact of fly control on childhood diarrhoea in Pakistan: community-randomised trial. *Lancet*, **353**, 22–5.

Chen, S. and Liu, X. (1991). Efficiency evaluation of combined intervention measures with improving drinking water first to prevent infantile acute diarrhea. *Chinese Journal of Epidemiology*, **12**, 289–91.

Christian, P., West, K.P. Jr., Khatry, S.K. *et al.* (2000a). Vitamin A or beta-carotene supplementation reduces symptoms of illness in pregnant and lactating Nepali women. *Journal of Nutrition*, **130**, 2675–82.

Christian, P., West, K.P. Jr., Khatry, S.K. *et al.* (2000b). Night blindness during pregnancy and subsequent mortality among women in Nepal: effects of vitamin A and beta-carotene supplementation. *American Journal of Epidemiology*, **152**, 542–7.

Desgrees du Lou, A., Pison, G., and Aaby, P. (1995). Role of immunizations in the recent decline in childhood mortality and the changes in the female/male mortality ratio in rural Senegal. *American Journal of Epidemiology*, **142**, 643–52.

Donner, A. and Klar, N. (2000). *Design and analysis of cluster randomization trials in health research*, London, Arnold Publishing Company.

Dowse, G.K., Gareeboo, H., Alberti, K.G. *et al.* (1995). Changes in population cholesterol concentrations and other cardiovascular risk factor levels after five years of the non-communicable disease intervention programme in Mauritius. Mauritius Non-communicable Disease Study Group. *British Medical Journal*, **311**, 1255–9.

Du, H., Wu, Z., Jia, P. *et al.* (1999). Comparison of effectiveness of mass media with small media and personal communication in the World AIDS Campaign in Beijing in 1997-1998. *Chinese Journal of STD & AIDS*, **5**, 113–116.

Edwards, S.J., Braunholtz, D.A., Lilford, R.J. *et al.* (1999). Ethical issues in the design and conduct of cluster randomised controlled trials. *British Medical Journal*, **318**, 1407–9.

Emerson, P.M., Lindsay, S.W., Walraven, G.E. *et al.* (1999). Effect of fly control on trachoma and diarrhoea. *Lancet*, **353**, 1401–3.

Fang, X.H., Kronmal, R.A., Li, S.C. *et al.* (1999). Prevention of stroke in urban China: A community-based intervention trial. *Stroke*, **30**, 495–501.

Fauveau, V., Stewart, K., Khan, S.A. *et al.* (1991). Effect on mortality of community-based maternity-care programme in rural Bangladesh. *Lancet*, **338**, 1183–6.

Feldman, H.A. and McKinlay, S.M. (1994). Cohort versus cross-sectional design in large field trials: Precision, sample size, and a unifying model. *Statistics in Medicine*, **13**, 61–78.

Figueiredo, R. and Ayres, J.R. (2002). Community based intervention and reduction of women's vulnerability to STD/AIDS in Brazil. *Revista de Saude Publica*, **36**, 96–107.

Gabrielli, A.F., Toure, S., Sellin, B. *et al.* (2006). A combined school- and community-based campaign targeting all school-age children of Burkina Faso against schistosomiasis and soil-transmitted helminthiasis: performance, financial costs and implications for sustainability. *Acta Tropica*, **99**, 234–42.

Gilson, L., Mkanje, R., Grosskurth, H. *et al.* (1997). Cost-effectiveness of improved treatment services for sexually transmitted diseases in preventing HIV-1 infection in Mwanza Region, Tanzania. *Lancet*, **350**, 1805–9.

Grosskurth, H., Mosha, F., Todd, J. *et al.* (1995a). Impact of improved treatment of sexually transmitted diseases on HIV infection in rural Tanzania: Randomised controlled trial. *Lancet*, **346**, 530–6.

Grosskurth, H., Mosha, F., Todd, J. *et al.* (1995b). A community trial of the impact of improved sexually transmitted disease treatment on the HIV epidemic in rural Tanzania: 2. Baseline survey results. *AIDS*, **9**, 927–34.

Haider, R., Ashworth, A., Kabir, I. *et al.* (2000). Effect of community-based peer counsellors on exclusive breastfeeding practices in Dhaka, Bangladesh: A randomised controlled trial. *Lancet*, **356**, 1643–7.

Harvey, B., Stuart, J., and Swan, T. (2000). Evaluation of a drama-in-education programme to increase AIDS awareness in South African high schools: A randomized community intervention trial. *International Journal of STD and AIDS*, **11**, 105–11.

Hayes, R., Mosha, F., Nicoll, A. *et al.* (1995). A community trial of the impact of improved sexually transmitted disease treatment on the HIV epidemic in rural Tanzania: 1. Design. *AIDS*, **9**, 919–26.

Hayes, R., Wawer, M., Gray, R. *et al.* (1997). Randomised trials of STD treatment for HIV prevention: report of an international workshop. HIV/STD Trials Workshop Group. *Genitourinary Medicine*, **73**, 432–43.

IHRD (2006). Is harm reduction "un-Muslim?" In *Harm reduction developments 2005: Countries with injection-driven HIV-epidemics*, p. 45. International Harm Reduction Program (IHRD) of the Open Society Institute, New York.

Jacob, M.E., Abraham, V.J., Abraham, S. *et al.* (2007). The effect of community based daycare on mental health and quality of life of elderly in rural south India: A community intervention study. *International Journal of Geriatric Psychiatry*, **22**(5), 445–7.

Jokhio, A.H., Winter, H.R., and Cheng, K.K. (2005). An intervention involving traditional birth attendants and perinatal and maternal mortality in Pakistan. *New England Journal of Medicine*, **352**, 2091–9.

Kamali, A., Quigley, M., Nakiyingi, J. *et al.* (2003). Syndromic management of sexually-transmitted infections and behaviour change interventions on transmission of HIV-1 in rural Uganda: A community randomised trial. *Lancet*, **361**, 645–52.

Kay, B.H., Nam, V.S., Tien, T.V. *et al.* (2002). Control of *aedes* vectors of dengue in three provinces of Vietnam by use of *Mesocyclops* (Copepoda) and community-based methods validated by entomologic, clinical, and serological surveillance. *American Journal of Tropical Medicine and Hygiene*, **66**, 40–8.

Kerry, S.M. and Bland, J.M. (1998a). The intracluster correlation coefficient in cluster randomisation. *British Medical Journal*, **316**, 1455.

Kerry, S.M. and Bland, J.M. (1998b). Sample size in cluster randomisation. *British Medical Journal*, **316**, 549.

Lartey, A., Manu, A., Brown, K.H. *et al.* (1999). A randomized, community-based trial of the effects of improved, centrally processed complementary foods on growth and micronutrient status of Ghanaian infants from 6 to 12 mo of age. *American Journal of Clinical Nutrition*, **70**, 391–404.

Liao, S.S., Schensul, J., and Wolffers, I. (2003). Sex-related health risks and implications for interventions with hospitality women in Hainan, China. *AIDS Education and Prevention*, **15**, 109–21.

Lin, P., Fan, Z.F., Yang, F. *et al.* (2004). Evaluation of a pilot study on needle and syringe exchange program among injecting drug users in a community in Guangdong, China. *Chinese Journal of Preventive Medicine*, **38**, 305–8.

Martin, D.C., Diehr, P., Perrin, E.B. *et al.* (1993). The effect of matching on the power of randomized community intervention studies. *Statistics in Medicine*, **12**, 329–38.

Morris, S.S., Flores, R., Olinto, P. *et al.* (2004). Monetary incentives in primary health care and effects on use and coverage of preventive health care interventions in rural Honduras: Cluster randomised trial. *Lancet*, **364**, 2030–7.

Morrow, A.L., Guerrero, M.L., Shults, J. *et al.* (1999). Efficacy of home-based peer counselling to promote exclusive breastfeeding: A randomised controlled trial. *Lancet*, **353**, 1226–31.

NIMH Collaborative HIV/STD Prevention Trial Group (2007a). Challenges and processes of selecting outcome measures for the NIMH Collaborative HIV/STD Prevention Trial. *AIDS*, **21** (Suppl 2), S29–36.

NIMH Collaborative HIV/STD Prevention Trial Group (2007b). Design and integration of ethnography within an international behavior change HIV/sexually transmitted disease prevention trial. *AIDS*, **21** (Suppl 2), S37–48.

NIMH Collaborative HIV/STD Prevention Trial Group (2007c). Methodological overview of a five-country community-level HIV/sexually transmitted disease prevention trial. *AIDS*, **21** (Suppl 2), S3–18.

Pandey, M.R., Daulaire, N.M., Starbuck, E.S. *et al.* (1991). Reduction in total under-five mortality in western Nepal through community-based antimicrobial treatment of pneumonia. *Lancet*, **338**, 993–7.

Pauw, J., Ferrie, J., Rivera Villegas, R. *et al.* (1996). A controlled HIV/AIDS-related health education programme in Managua, Nicaragua. *AIDS*, **10**, 537-44.

Perreira, K.M., Bailey, P.E., de Bocaletti, E. *et al.* (2002). Increasing awareness of danger signs in pregnancy through community- and clinic-based education in Guatemala. *Maternal and Child Health Journal*, **6**, 19–28.

Pronyk, P.M., Hargreaves, J.R., Kim, J.C. *et al.* (2006). Effect of a structural intervention for the prevention of intimate-partner violence and HIV in rural South Africa: A cluster randomised trial. *Lancet*, **368**, 1973–83.

Ramadas, K., Sankaranarayanan, R., Jacob, B.J. *et al.* (2003). Interim results from a cluster randomized controlled oral cancer screening trial in Kerala, India. *Oral Oncology*, **39**, 580–8.

Ronsmans, C., Vanneste, A.M., Chakraborty, J. *et al.* (1997). Decline in maternal mortality in Matlab, Bangladesh: A cautionary tale. *Lancet*, **350**, 1810–4.

Rothman, K. and Greenland, S. (1996). *Modern Epidemiology*, 2nd edition. Lippincott-Raven, Philadelphia.

Smith, D.R., Zhang, X., Zheng, Y. *et al.* (2005). Tobacco use among public health professionals in Beijing: the relationship between smoking and education level. *Australian and New Zealand Journal of Public Health*, **29**, 488–9.

Todd, J., Carpenter, L., Li, X. *et al.* (2003). The effects of alternative study designs on the power of community randomized trials: Evidence from three studies of human immunodeficiency virus prevention in East Africa. *International Journal of Epidemiology*, **32**, 755–62.

Trollope-Kumar, K. and Guyatt, G. (2006). Syndromic approach for treatment of STIs: Time for a change. *Lancet*, **367**, 1380–1.

Ukoumunne, O.C., Gulliford, M.C., Chinn, S. *et al.* (1999). Methods for evaluating area-wide and organisation-based interventions in health and health care: A systematic review. *Health Technology Assessment*, **3**, iii–92.

Varnell, S.P., Murray, D.M., Janega, J.B. *et al.* (2004). Design and analysis of group-randomized trials: a review of recent practices. *American Journal of Public Health*, **94**, 393–9.

Vu, S.N., Nguyen, T.Y., Tran, V.P. *et al.* (2005). Elimination of dengue by community programs using Mesocyclops(Copepoda) against Aedes aegypti in central Vietnam. *American Journal of Tropical Medicine and Hygiene*, **72**, 67–73.

Wacira, D.G., Hill, J., McCall, P.J. *et al.* (2007). Delivery of insecticide-treated net services through employer and community-based approaches in Kenya. *Trop Medicine & International Health*, **12**, 140–9.

Wawer, M.J., Gray, R.H., Sewankambo, N.K. *et al.* (1998). A randomized, community trial of intensive sexually transmitted disease control for AIDS prevention, Rakai, Uganda. *AIDS*, **12**, 1211–25.

Wawer, M.J., Sewankambo, N.K., Serwadda, D. *et al.* (1999). Control of sexually transmitted diseases for AIDS prevention in Uganda: a randomised community trial. Rakai Project Study Group. *Lancet*, **353**, 525–35.

West, K.P. Jr., Katz, J., Khatry, S.K. *et al.* (1999). Double blind, cluster randomised trial of low dose supplementation with vitamin A or beta carotene on mortality related to pregnancy in Nepal. The NNIPS-2 Study Group. *British Medical Journal*, **318**, 570–5.

West, K.P. Jr., Pokhrel, R.P., Katz, J. *et al.* (1991). Efficacy of vitamin A in reducing preschool child mortality in Nepal. *Lancet*, **338**, 67–71.

West, S., Munoz, B., Lynch, M. *et al.* (1995). Impact of face-washing on trachoma in Kongwa, Tanzania. *Lancet*, **345**, 155–8.

Wongkhomthong, S., Kaime-Atterhog, W., and Ono, K. (1995). *AIDS in the developing world: A case study of Thailand*. ASEAN Institute for Health Development, Mahidol University, Bangkok.

Wu, Z. (1998). *Promoting condom use among female prostitutes in natural settings in Yunnan, China*. 12th International AIDS Conference, Geneva.

Wu, Z. (1999). *Sustainability of condom vending machine in condom marketing in Shenzhen, Guangdong province*. Ministry of Health, Beijing.

Wu, Z., Detels, R., Zhang, J. *et al.* (2002). Community-based trial to prevent drug use among youths in Yunnan, China. *American Journal of Public Health*, **92**, 1952–7.

XJHAPAC (2006). *The Yining City injecting drug user harm reduction program experience gained, expansion achieved* [unpublished report]. Urumqi, Xinjiang HIV/AIDS Prevention and Care Project.

Yap, L., Wu, Z., Liu, W. *et al.* (2002). A rapid assessment and its implications for a needle social marketing intervention among injecting drug users in China. *The International Journal on Drug Policy*, **13**, 57–68.

6.11

Clinical epidemiology

Jason W. Busse, Edward Mills, Rodolfo Dennis, Vivian Welch, and Peter Tugwell

Abstract

Global society has reached a level of interdependence wherein there is a need to share healthcare knowledge and deploy resources in the best interests of people everywhere. Clinical and public health professionals can be united in this effort through their common reliance on epidemiology. Clinical epidemiology and its derivative—the evidence-based medicine movement—have many parallels with public health. Indeed, many clinicians with clinical epidemiology training develop research projects and subsequently research programmes that move beyond clinical decision-making to include a population focus.

In response to this global need, the International Clinical Epidemiology Network (INCLEN) programme has trained over 700 physicians and other health specialists at a Master's degree level in clinical epidemiology, social sciences, biostatistics, or clinical economics. INCLEN has established a global resource network to support fundamental changes in the way physicians, medical educators, and policy makers think about health and disease. INCLEN now has semi-autonomous regional networks in Africa, India, China, Southeast Asia, Latin America, Europe–Mediterranean, and Canada–United States.

A methods framework, the 'equity–effectiveness iterative loop', is used to demonstrate the interface between clinical epidemiology and public health, with special attention to ensuring that the disadvantaged are explicitly considered. The focus is on evidence-based, action-oriented epidemiology based upon the health needs of the relevant community. Various examples are used, such as circumcision to prevent male-acquired HIV infection.

The history and evolution of clinical epidemiology as related to public health

There is a growing concern that the costs of medical care may be exceeding the benefits, or at the very least that the same level of healthcare benefits could be achieved at lower costs (Cutler 2004). More importantly, there is clear consensus that inequitable distribution of these benefits abounds. It often seems that the majority of healthcare researchers and providers in the high-income countries have accorded public health a low priority (Tugwell *et al.* 2006a). According to the Institute of Medicine, the mission of public health is defined as 'fulfilling society's interest in assuring conditions in which people can be healthy' (Institute of Medicine 1988); public health emphasizes a collective action for the 'public good' over a 'private good'. Some of this disconnect can be explained by the separation of clinical medicine and public health, that began almost a century ago.

With the advent and remarkable successes of the germ theory in the nineteenth century, much of clinical medicine became focused on laboratory research—describing the pathophysiology of individual microorganisms—and little research was conducted on the host or environment. In 1916, the Rockefeller Foundation, endowed by John D. Rockefeller and chartered in 1913 for the well-being of people throughout the world, concluded that insufficient attention was being paid to environmental and social factors in disease, and that public health personnel were widely needed.

The Foundation's solution was to establish schools of public health apart from schools of medicine. The role of medicine was thus to provide care to individuals and investigate disease processes, and the role of public health was to research and impact the determinants of health and disease in populations. Epidemiology, the social sciences, and qualitative methods became the domain of public health, and medicine assumed dominance in clinical treatment advances.

In his 1938 president's address to the American Society for Clinical Investigation, John Paul introduced the term 'clinical epidemiology', which he defined as the application of epidemiological and related methods from a clinical perspective. The shift in the focus of clinical epidemiology from community ecology to individual patients and groups of patients took place in the 1960s. In 1964, Alvan Feinstein, who has been referred to as the father of clinical epidemiology (Fletcher 2001), published an influential series of papers on scientific methodology for clinical medicine in the Annals of Internal Medicine. When asked by an epidemiologist to provide a lecture on his work in epidemiology, Feinstein replied:

> *. . . I am not an epidemiologist. Epidemiologists are people who go around collecting useless statistics about the incidence and prevalence of syphilis in Tasmania. I don't do that.' A critic stated, 'Yes, you are; you study groups of people and apply statistics to them: That is what epidemiologists do.' And I said, 'Well, if I am, I am a clinical epidemiologist.* (Daly 2005)

Kerr White also felt the need to incorporate greater scientific rigour into medical practice. White's training included medicine and public health, and he felt that epidemiology—the basis of public health—had much to offer clinical medicine. In 1964, White was the founding chair of what became the Department of Health Policy and Management in the School of Public Health at John Hopkins University, where he attempted to bridge the gap between medicine and public health. However, many of his colleagues were threatened by what they perceived as efforts to usurp clinical authority. As noted by White: 'When proposing a population-based study of hospitals, for example, I was called before the local medical society and accused of trying to mount a communist plot!' (Daly 2005).

In 1966, David Sackett established the first Clinical Epidemiology Research Unit in the Department of Medicine at the State University of New York at Buffalo, United States. By 1967, he had moved to Canada and established the influential Department of Clinical Epidemiology and Biostatistics at the McMaster Medical School in Hamilton, Canada.

In 1972, Archibald (Archie) Cochrane compiled a series of lectures commissioned and published by the Nuffield Trust—Effectiveness and Efficiency: Random Reflections on Health—that compellingly articulated the need for rigorous scientific evaluation of diagnosis, treatment, and preventive medicine (Cochrane 1972).

The distinct field of public health was beginning to influence and challenge clinical medicine. The creation of these two parallel institutions with separate mandates resulted in what has been termed the schism between medicine and public health. This divide was not to the benefit of either group and in 1974 the Macy Conference reported:

> *. . . [T]he health professionals shut themselves up in their schools of public health, and the physicians stayed within the walls of the medical schools and hospitals. The latter felt that public health specialists 'were no longer doctors', while the health people believed themselves to be crusaders in a cause they had to win, imposing it if necessary on the community as well as on other physicians who did not understand them.* (Bowers 1974)

In 1977, John Knowles, then President of the Rockefeller Foundation, edited a collection of articles on American healthcare, and wrote:

> *Public health interests have been, and continue to be, isolated from American medical education and practice. Issues that influence health, such as nutrition, family size, population density, environmental mobility, poverty, racism, sexual practices, unemployment, housing, transportation, and the like, are rarely taken into account in any overall calculation of the health needs of the nation.* (Knowles 1977)

Seminal work by, in addition to the above individuals, Gene Glass, Richard Peto, Iain Chalmers, Gordon Guyatt, Brian Haynes, and Andrew Oxman developed methods by which to identify, appraise, select, and summarize healthcare literature to inform clinical questions (a systematic review) and, when appropriate, mathematically combine data to provide a more precise estimate of treatment effect (a meta-analysis). However, such efforts were initially not well-accepted within medicine.

In 1979, commenting on organized medicine's limited use of clinical epidemiology to inform best practices, Archie Cochrane wrote: 'It is surely a great criticism of our profession that we have not organized a critical summary, by specialty or subspecialty, adapted periodically, of all relevant randomized controlled trials' (Cochrane 1979).

Formal international dissemination of the principles of clinical epidemiology began in 1980 when Kerr White, who was Deputy Director for Health Sciences of the Rockefeller Foundation, initiated through the foundation, The International Clinical Epidemiology Network (INCLEN). This programme provided young clinicians from low- and middle-income countries with funding to pursue training in clinical epidemiology at Chapel Hill in the United States, McMaster University in Canada, University of Newcastle in Australia, or the University of Pennsylvania in the United States. As of January 2008, INCLEN included 81 clinical epidemiology units/centres in 33 countries (see Box 6.11.1).

In 1982, 44 years after the term was first coined, the first modern textbook in clinical epidemiology was published by Robert Fletcher, Suzanne Fletcher, and Edward Wagner at the University of North Carolina, United States (now in its 4th edition) (Fletcher & Fletcher 2005). Soon after, clinical epidemiology textbooks were published from McMaster University, Canada (now in its 3rd edition) (Haynes 2006) and Yale University, United States (Feinstein 1985) in 1985, from the University of Washington, United States in 1986 (now in its 3rd edition) Weiss 1996), and from McGill University, Canada in 1988 (Kramer 1988).

The United States government implemented a number of initiatives to improve collaboration between the US Public Health Service and the medical establishment, but in 1988 the Institute of Medicine drew attention to the ongoing 'poor relationships [of public health workers] with the medical profession' (Institute of Medicine 1988). Similar concerns were raised in Britain through The Report on the Committee of Inquiry into the Future Development of the Public Health Function (Acheson 1988).

In 1991, White advanced two main issues that he felt had limited the development of public health. First, the inability to attract and retain accomplished medical physicians. As an example he noted that the number of physicians employed in US state health departments had decreased by more than 34 per cent from 1979 to 1986. The second barrier he saw was the failure by most physicians to understand the public health perspective. White proposed that four root causes were to blame for this situation (White 1991):

1. The failed attempt to establish public health as a separate profession, apart from medicine
2. Failure to establish epidemiology as a fundamental science for medicine and public health
3. Failure to provide public health and epidemiological training to medical students
4. Failure of medicine and public health to cooperate and coordinate their efforts

Others have argued that the primary barrier to the development of public health was ideological; the belief of many physicians that their mandate was the application of basic science to improve health one individual and one treatment at a time. This ideology

Box 6.11.1 The International Clinical Epidemiology Network (INCLEN)

INCLEN (http://www.inclentrust.org) began as a strategy funded by the Rockefeller Foundation in 1980 to improve healthcare by providing health professionals, mostly physicians, with the necessary tools to plan, measure, and evaluate clinical care. Healthcare professionals, empowered in such a fashion, would provide an essential link to help develop functional health and health research systems in low- and middle-income countries. Currently with over 1500 members, the Network has trained physicians and other health specialists at a Master's degree level in clinical epidemiology, social sciences, biostatistics, or clinical economics. This strategy has built a global resource network to support fundamental changes in the way physicians, medical educators, and policy makers think about health and disease. INCLEN now has semi-autonomous regional networks in Africa, India, China, Southeast Asia, Latin America, Europe–Mediterranean, and Canada–United States. The natural result of this regionalization is a cultural and national tailoring of the programme to be more responsive to the local setting.

Vision

INCLEN's long-range goals are to strengthen national health systems and to improve healthcare practice globally by providing health professionals with the tools to analyse the efficacy, effectiveness, efficiency, and equity of health interventions and preventive measures.

Mission

INCLEN is dedicated to improving the health of disadvantaged populations, particularly in low- and middle-income countries, by promoting equitable healthcare based on the best evidence of effectiveness and the efficient use of resources. INCLEN achieves this by using the network to conduct collaborative, inter-disciplinary research on high-priority health problems, and to train future generations of leaders in healthcare research.

Examples of INCLEN outputs with public health implications

In the initiative, 'WorldSAFE and IndiaSAFE: Studying the Prevalence of Family Violence', the World Studies of Abuse in the Family Environment (WorldSAFE) teamed up with the family violence group from India (IndiaSAFE) in 1999 to examine the prevalence of physical and psychological maltreatment against adult women in the family and to review individual factors associated with family violence in India. The IndiaSAFE study was a population-based cross-sectional survey administered in seven sites (five of which were INCLEN centres). Through sampling, interviews, and focus groups, results were analysed and compared to the WorldSAFE model of family violence. Results from the IndiaSAFE study substantiated four of the six hypotheses generated by the WorldSAFE model of family violence, and were instrumental in the planning of strategies to support interventions worldwide (Peedicayil *et al.* 2004).

The study, 'Acceptability and cost-effectiveness of zinc supplementation in the treatment of acute, watery diarrhoea among children', launched in October 2002, was a randomized controlled trial to assess site-specific variations in the use of oral rehydration solutions (ORS), antimicrobials, and anti-diarrhoeal agents among children who received or did not receive zinc supplementation (Awasthi and INCLEN Childnet 2006a). Countries participating in the study were India, Brazil, the Philippines, Egypt, and Ethiopia. Recruited were 1020 and 992 children in the zinc and control groups, respectively. The study found that in the management of acute watery diarrhoea, an intervention package involving zinc plus ORS, along with culturally appropriate, site-specific messages in the local language, did not affect overall ORS use, decreased antibiotic/antidiarrhoeal use, and there was good patient adherence and no significant side effects from zinc. The zinc formative research guide produced in conjunction with this study was used by the United States Agency for International Development and other partner agencies for increasing the use of zinc worldwide.

The study, 'Danger signs of neonatal illnesses: Perceptions of caregivers and health workers', launched in July 2004, involved eight countries: Brazil, Cameroon, Colombia, Egypt, India, Indonesia, Mexico, and the Philippines (Awasthi *et al.* 2006b). This study targeted urban and rural healthcare givers and urban and rural community healthcare workers to understand their attitudes and practices regarding healthcare of neonates after birth in general and their perceptions regarding danger signs of illness in particular. This study had major implications on educational interventions to improve health-seeking behaviour and healthcare for neonatal illnesses. Results of this work directly fed into strategies for neonatal survival in the respective countries.

translated into financial benefit and increased authority for the clinical enterprise, resulting in the endorsement of what has now become known as 'eminence-based medicine' (Fox 1986).

In 1990, Gordon Guyatt approached the Department of Medicine at McMaster University (Canada) with the idea of incorporating a novel approach to educating physicians (Guyatt & Rennie 2002). In an effort to denote the importance that use of current scientific literature would have in this new curriculum, he proposed the term 'scientific medicine'. Some department members were incensed by the implication that what they were currently teaching was unscientific. This led to a modification of the term to 'evidence-based medicine', that relied heavily upon clinical epidemiology. In order to best define evidence-based medicine, it is helpful to quote the conclusions of Sackett *et al.* (1996), in their well-known article, 'Evidence-based medicine: What it is and what it isn't':

> *Good doctors use both individual clinical expertise and the best available external evidence, and neither alone is enough.*

Without clinical expertise, practice risks becoming tyrannized by evidence, for even excellent external evidence may be inapplicable to or inappropriate for an individual patient. Without current best evidence, practice risks becoming rapidly out of date, to the detriment of patients.

Prominent among the efforts to facilitate the implementation of evidence-based medicine in clinical practice is the Cochrane Collaboration—named in honour of Archie Cochrane—and formed under the leadership of Iain Chalmers in 1993. This collaboration is comprised of an international representation of patients (or professional consumers who claim to speak for patients), clinicians, and methodologists that aims to prepare systematic reviews of the effects of healthcare interventions. These reviews are targeted for updating every 2 years (although this is variable), and their results are available through paid subscription via the Internet (http://www.cochrane.org). Evidence-based medicine is not without its detractors (Straus *et al.* 2007; Feinstein 1997), but in 2006, the *British Medical Journal* designated evidence-based medicine one of the 15 greatest medical breakthroughs since 1840 (Ferriman 2007).

The separation of public health and medicine was the result of a deliberate attempt to create two professions. This divide was maintained, in part, due to social and political factors. It now seems evident that close collaboration between medicine and public health will serve society far better. The shift inherent in evidence-based medicine, from the authoritative approach of healthcare to one that attempts to use clinical epidemiology to incorporate the best evidence currently available, represents a challenge for all healthcare providers; however, the global society has reached a level of interdependence wherein there is a need to share healthcare knowledge and deploy resources in the best interests of people everywhere. Clinical and public health professionals and public health can be united in this effort through their common reliance on epidemiology (Institute of Medicine 2007).

The equity–effectiveness loop: A framework for the interface between clinical epidemiology and public health

Clinical epidemiology and its derivative—the evidence-based medicine movement—have many parallels with public health. Indeed many clinicians with clinical epidemiology training develop research projects and subsequently research programmes that move beyond clinical decision-making to include a population focus. This stimulated one of us (PT) and his colleagues to address this process systematically through an iterative measurement loop framework (Tugwell *et al.* 1985). The focus was on evidence-based, action-oriented epidemiology based upon the health needs of the relevant individuals and their community.

This has recently been updated with an 'equity lens' to ensure that the disadvantaged are explicitly considered (Tugwell *et al.* 2006a) (see Fig. 6.11.1). What was the stimulus to incorporate explicit attention by clinical epidemiologists to the disadvantaged? This was due to the realization that average improvement can hide important inequitably worse health effects amongst the disadvantaged. For example, impressive gains in health during the twentieth century, showing dramatic increases in average life expectancy in rich and poor countries (World Health Organization 1999), would meet the criteria we initially recommended in the 1985 paper, but there is a critical component missing. These averages obscure the fact that health in both high- and low- income settings is unevenly distributed according to socioeconomic position; health and longevity are highest for the richest, and decrease steadily with decreasing socioeconomic status (Wilkins & Adams 1983; Wilkinson 1996). Many of these inequalities are avoidable, and hence unfair.

These social gradients in health, or socioeconomic inequalities in health, are pervasive in all countries of the world (Diderichsen *et al.* 2001) and hold true for most diseases, injuries, and health behaviours. Modern health policy must increasingly be oriented not only to the production of health, but also the distribution of health (Gwatkin 2003). For example, the Millennium Development Goals state the need to include poor people in the benefits of development (United Nations 2001).

Therefore, the 'equity–effectiveness iterative loop', as its name implies, has been expanded to provide a logical way to apply an 'equity lens' as one moves from assessing needs through to assessing effectiveness, and cost-effectiveness, of interventions, leading to the development and evaluation of evidence-based health policy. This framework integrates the concepts of individual risk and socioeconomic status with intervention effectiveness from a population health perspective.

Step 1: Burden of illness

This step measures the burden of illness and its gradient by socioeconomic status. This includes downstream (individual), and upstream (societal) determinants of health (biological, cultural, political, psychosocial, and environmental).

Step 2: Differential equity–effectiveness

Controlled studies provide estimates of efficacy and effectiveness; efficacy measures how well an intervention can work in ideal circumstances (Sackett *et al.* 1985). Effectiveness measures how well an intervention works in real settings and systems at the community level. Community effectiveness is often substantially lower than efficacy because of a staircase effect with four 'steps': (1) the result of lower awareness, access, or coverage; (2) screening, diagnosis, or targeting; (3) compliance of providers; and (4) adherence of consumers. Poor people may have circumstances that reduce efficacy at all four steps and therefore a greater staircase effect may be observed compared to the least poor people. There is a need to assess equity issues across each step to identify barriers to implementation related to gradients in wealth.

Step 3: Economic evaluation

This step assesses the efficiency (health benefits such as number of disability-adjusted life years avoided for a specific cost that includes direct, indirect, and where possible intangible costs) of the intervention. Assessing the efficiency requires adequate evidence of efficacy and valid estimates of cost. Assessing the equity issues related to cost-effectiveness implies a trade-off between cost efficiency and population health equity. Priority funding of interventions with the best cost-effectiveness ratios might increase differences between the richest (or least poor) and poorest because the cost of reaching poor people may be higher and health benefits may be lower. Four approaches to this have been proposed (Drummond 2006). One promising method to assess equity issues related to cost-effectiveness

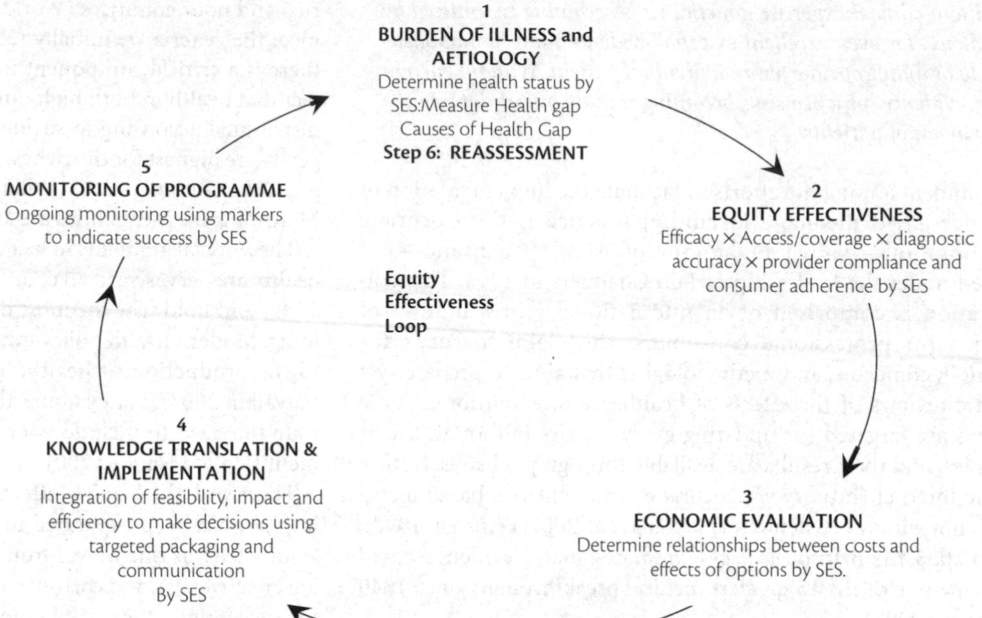

Fig. 6.11.1 Equity–effectiveness loop (SES: socioeconomic status).
Source: Tugwell (2006a).

is the development of an equity and quality-adjusted life year (EQ-QALY), as a complement to established measures of the difference between rich and poor, such as the concentration index (Wagstaff 2002).

Step 4: Knowledge translation and implementation

Translation of knowledge is defined as the process that transfers research results from producers of knowledge to its users, for the benefit of the population. Moving beyond the traditional domain of academic publication, it comprises three interlinked components of uptake and translation: Exchange, synthesis, and ethically sound application of knowledge (Birdsell *et al.* 2002). This step entails uptake and translation of knowledge into action (Birdsell 2002; Davis *et al.* 2003; Grimshaw *et al.* 2001).

There is therefore a need to develop new, effective means of packaging and communicating evidence on effectiveness across wealth gradients to the different policy, community, and practitioner groups or individuals responsible for each of the components of community effectiveness—access, diagnostic accuracy, compliance of providers, and adherence of consumers (Giuffrida 2000; Briggs *et al.* 2001; Mowatt *et al.* 2001; Zwarenstein & Bryant 2000). Evidence that interventions using knowledge translation are efficacious is currently lacking in most sectors. One exception is the work of INCLEN (see Box 6.11.1), which is developing methods explicitly to consider equity issues in developing and applying clinical guidelines (INCLEN 2004). By targeting the wealth gradient in knowledge translation strategies, we support the operational research agenda for optimizing the benefits to the poor of key interventions.

Steps 5 and 6: Monitoring and reassessment

Monitoring identifies the importance of process assessments and intermediate outcomes to assess success in affecting mortality and morbidity by socioeconomic group and deciding whether further remediable need exists; if so, an additional iteration of the equity–effectiveness loop is needed. The Whitehall cohort study, for example, showed that, even with equitable access to cardiac care, the social deprivation gradient still produces disparities in outcomes (Britton *et al.* 2004), indicating a need to tackle other causes, or 'steps', of disparities.

Step-by-step through the equity–effectiveness loop

We elaborate on the application of the equity–effectiveness loop using examples of interventions such as male circumcision to prevent transmission of HIV and other health challenges, particularly in low- and middle-income countries.

Male circumcision, the removal of the foreskin and thus removal of many of the Langerhans cells in the male genital area, has been examined as a prevention strategy since the early 1990s (Wawer *et al.* 2005). Given the rate that the HIV/AIDS pandemic is increasing, it is clear that we need to implement preventive strategies based on the highest quality evidence. Current strategies promoted for the prevention of HIV infection include education, condoms, sterile injection equipment, and abstinence. Other interventions, such as vaccines, pre-exposure prophylaxis, and microbicides are under study and their effectiveness is still unproven. Most recently, male circumcision has been promoted as a strategy to reduce infection (Wawer *et al.* 2005; Mills & Siegfried 2006). We will examine this issue in detail using the equity–effectiveness loop.

Step 1: Burden of illness

The HIV/AIDS pandemic now affects around 33 million people infected worldwide, with reason to believe that this will continue to increase unless effective interventions can be developed to slow the rate of transmission. Important gradients are present in HIV-affected populations across different social groups such as differing religions. Religion, even after adjusting for lifestyle risk factors across education and income, appears to predict HIV prevalence (Drain 2005). Higher income and higher education appear to present a paradoxical increase in HIV incidence in most African countries (Malawi National AIDS Commission, http://www.aidsmalawi.org.mw). The effect of HIV on the community impacts on the economy due to orphanhood, grandmothers caring for villages, a lack of health worker supply, and inadequate supplies of effective drugs.

Step 2: Efficacy, community effectiveness, and differential equity–effectiveness

In initial demographic analyses, investigators observed that populations in sub-Saharan Africa with large populations of the males circumcised had comparatively lower HIV/AIDS indices than populations that did not traditionally circumcise males (Drain *et al.* 2006).

Previous observational studies of males in HIV prevalent areas gave a relative risk of infection among circumcised men that ranged from 0.22 (95 per cent CI, 0.10–0.46) based on cohort studies to 0.41 (95 per cent CI, 0.35–0.49) based on cross-sectional studies. The biological rationale for circumcision as a preventative measure comes from the knowledge that the foreskin is highly susceptible to skin ruptures and possible permeability and has many Langerhans cells. These cells are believed to capture HIV-1 virions through site receptors that bind to antibody-coated virus, thus acting as reservoirs for the virus and serving as a site of replication.

Even with the high relative odds and a plausible biological explanation for a protective effect, observational studies sometimes provide unreliable estimates of the effectiveness of an intervention due to known and unknown confounding (Guyatt & Rennie 2002). In the HIV and circumcision example, an obvious confounding variable is that circumcision was predominantly practised in countries with large Islamic populations, and evidence from countries with lower Islamic populations demonstrated that Islamic populations tend to have lower prevalence of HIV/AIDS than their corresponding non-Islamic populations (Drain *et al.* 2006). With this conundrum, public health officials were, rightly, hesitant to recommend male circumcision on a population-wide level, given that the studies were observational and not randomized trials, (Siegfried *et al.* 2005). Figure 6.11.2 displays the widely accepted classification of evidence for implementing interventions in public health decision-making (Guyatt *et al.* 2000).

For a public health decision to be evidence-based, policy-makers should follow clear steps in: (1) formulating a question; (2) seeking the best available evidence; (3) determining the quality of that evidence; and (4) determining the applicability of the evidence to their settings.

Formulating a question: Any well-designed question should be composed of the following five criteria–PICOT:

1) Population
2) Intervention
3) Control
4) Outcome
5) Time-duration of the trial

To frame the scenario of male circumcision for HIV/AIDS prevention, we propose the following structured question:

In sexually active males (population) that have been circumcised (intervention), are rates of HIV infection (outcome) over 2 years (time–duration of the trial) importantly different from sexually active males that have not been circumcised (control)?

This structured question addresses all of the important components of an answerable question. Note that we state 'importantly different' rather than the more conventional 'statistically' different as there are examples where statistically significant results do not result in clinical or meaningful differences (Redelmeier *et al.* 1996; Wells *et al.* 2001).

As displayed in Fig. 6.11.2, the first choice for assessing a quantitative benefit of an intervention are systematic reviews or meta-analyses of randomized clinical trials (RCTs). Next are single well-conducted RCTs. Next are single observational studies, and so on. We are aware that the demographic and observational studies on male circumcision have existed since the 1990s and provide compelling rationale for considering the introduction of population-wide male circumcision, but we are also cautious that these observational studies may be vulnerable to confounding variables, such as religious behaviours (Drain *et al.* 2006). As a result, we would ideally like to find a meta-analysis of randomized trials or several well-conducted RCTs.

Seeking the best available evidence: For the purpose of this chapter, we searched the following electronic databases (from inception to 8 October 2007): MedLine (via PubMed); EMBASE; CINAHL; AMED; Cochrane CENTRAL; Cochrane Database of Systematic Reviews; and Relief Web (a database of freely accessible non-governmental organization reports and news reports).
Using the search terms 'HIV AND circumcision AND random*', we identified three RCTs published since 2005 in the biomedical literature (Auvert *et al.* 2005; Bailey *et al.* 2007; Gray *et al.* 2007). Next, we appraised the applicability and internal and external validity of each of these RCTs.

Critical appraisal: Three of the trials described RCTs were published in sub-Saharan Africa. All were conducted among sexually active males. All of the trials had a non-circumcised control group and all of the trials assessed HIV infection as their primary outcome. At this stage, all of the trials appear to provide us with

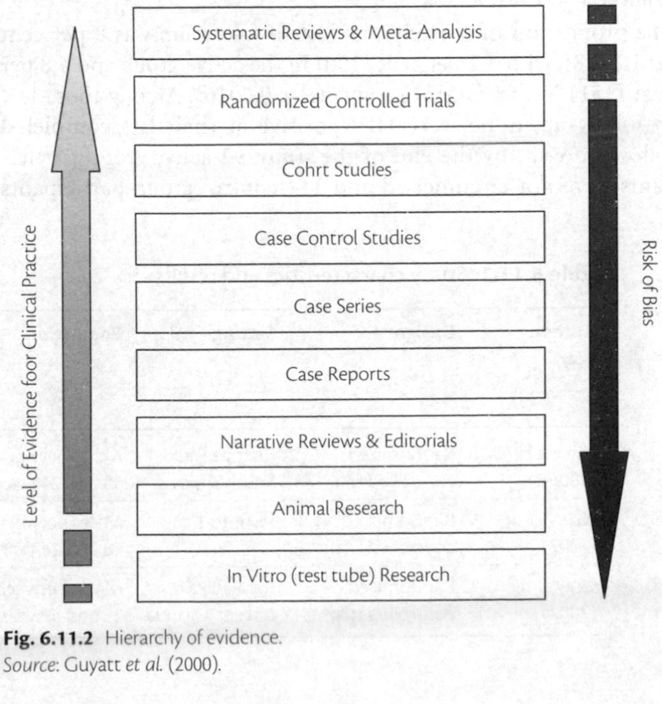

Fig. 6.11.2 Hierarchy of evidence.
Source: Guyatt *et al.* (2000).

information that addresses our initial question. Next, we determined if the trial quality was sufficient to provide strong inferences about the effectiveness of male circumcision for reducing HIV/AIDS.

In order to determine trial quality, we suggest using the users' guide, 'How to appraise an article about therapy', published by the McMaster EBM Working Group in 1994 (Guyatt *et al.* 1994). This tool has been modified for a variety of fields, but the utility of it remains (see Box 6.11.2).

Using the questions from the Users' Guide, we determined the quality and utility of each RCT (see Table 6.11.1).

Trial 1 (Auvert *et al.* 2005)

Primary guides on methods

In 2005, the first RCT of male circumcision was published to great media attention (Table 6.11.1) (Auvert *et al.* 2005). This study enrolled sexually active males between the ages of 18 and 24 years. The study randomly assigned the participants to receive surgical circumcision or remain uncircumcised. The study used urn randomization and allocation was concealed using opaque envelopes. Participants in the active arm were circumcised using the forceps guided method within a week of randomization. All data was analysed using an intent-to-treat approach, in addition to examining only those patients that underwent treatment according to the study arm they were randomized to (a per-protocol approach). The trial was stopped early due to benefit after the Data and Safety Monitoring Board's (DSMB) first interim analysis. The average duration of participants in the trial was 18.1 months (range 13–21).

Secondary guides on methods

Participants and health workers were not blinded to group allocation, although efforts were made to ensure confidentiality of the participant's circumcision status. Groups were largely similar at the start of the trial and almost all (~90 per cent) were sexually active at the start of the trial.

What were the results?

The proportion of participants lost to follow-up was 8 per cent (251/3128), with 3.2 per cent (100) in the active group and 4.8 per cent (151) in the control groups ($P = 0.0016$). Among those lost to follow-up, none were HIV-positive at their last completed follow-up visit. By the end of the study, 92 active group participants were not circumcised and 114 control group participants were circumcised. During the study, 20 active group participants and 49 control group participants acquired HIV infection, corresponding to incidence rates of 0.85 per 100 person-years (95 per cent CI, 0.55–1.32) and 2.1 per 100 person years (95 per cent CI, 1.6–2.8) in the intervention and control groups, respectively. The Relative Risk (RR) of HIV infection corresponds to 0.42

Box 6.11.2 Users' guides for an article about therapy

Adapted from: Guyatt *et al.* (1994)

I. Are the results of the study valid?

Primary guides

Was the assignment of study participants to the interventions randomized?

Were all patients who entered the trial properly accounted for and attributed at its conclusion?

Was follow-up complete?

Were study participants analysed in the groups to which they were randomized?

Secondary guides

Were study participants, health workers, and study personnel 'blind' to treatment?

Were the groups similar at the start of the trial?

Aside from the experimental intervention, were the groups treated equally?

II. What were the results?

How large was the treatment/intervention effect?

How precise was the estimate of the treatment/intervention effect?

III. Will the results help in caring for the target population?

Can the results be applied to the target population?

Were all population or group important outcomes considered?

Are the likely treatment benefits worth the potential harms and costs?

Table 6.11.1 Study characteristics and results

Author, year	Design	Setting	Population	*n*	Outcomes		Relative risk (95% confidence intervals)
					Intervention	Control	
Auvert *et al.* (2006)	Randomized controlled trial	Orange Farm, South Africa	Males between 18 and 24 years	3274	20/1546	49/1582	0.42 (0.25–0.70)
Bailey *et al.* (2007)	Randomized controlled trial	Kisumu, Kenya	Males between 18 and 24 years	2784	22/1391	47/1393	0.47 (0.28–0.77)
Gray *et al.* (2007)	Randomized controlled trial	Rural Rakai district, Uganda	Males between 15 and 49 years	4996	22/2387	45/2430	0.50 (0.30–0.83)

(95 per cent CI, 0.25–0.70) in favour of the intervention. Adverse events among the circumcised group were minor and included pain at the site (12/1495), excessive bleeding (9/1495), and haematoma (9/1495).

Will the results help in caring for a target population?

The participants enrolled in the trial likely represent males through sub-Saharan Africa, and there was a suitably broad set of inclusion criteria to represent males of different ethnic groups and religions. The trial reported adequately all important outcomes. We should be wary of the large effect size given that trials stopped early may inflate effect sizes (Montori *et al.* 2005). The question of whether the treatment benefits outweigh the harms and costs must be interpreted in a culturally specific manner. Will the broad population accept this intervention? Will perceived protection affect other established preventative measures such as condom use?

Trial 2 (Bailey *et al.* 2007)

Primary guides on methods

The next available trial (Bailey *et al.* 2007) was published simultaneously with the third RCT (Table 6.11.1) (Gray *et al.* 2007) in February 2007, although results had been available in the media since early January 2007. A total of 2784 men aged 18–24 years in Kisumu, Kenya, were randomly assigned to an intervention group (circumcision, $n=1391$) or a control group (delayed circumcision, $n=1393$). Most men identified themselves as unskilled workers, farm labourers, or fishermen ($n=1653$, 59 per cent); 632 (23 per cent) were students. Randomization employed stratification for established risk factors. Allocation concealment was ensured through the use of opaque envelopes. Circumcision generally occurred within 24 h of randomization, through the forceps guided method. Participants were counselled to refrain from sexual activity for at least 30 days after the procedure. The trial used an intent-to-treat analysis as well as per-protocol analyses. As with the first trial, this trial was stopped early by the DSMB due to benefit at the third interim analysis. The average duration of participants in the trial was 24 months (range: 18–24).

Secondary guides

Participants and medical staff were not blinded to group allocation. However, data analysts and HIV testers were blinded. Groups were similar at the beginning of the trial and were treated equally throughout, with the exception of the intervention.

What were the results?

Overall, follow-up for HIV status was incomplete for 240 (8.6 per cent) participants: 126 (4.5 per cent) in the circumcision group and 114 (4.1 per cent) in the control group. Circumcision provided a RR of 0.41 (95 per cent CI, 0.24–0.70) protective effect against HIV infection compared with the control group, and a Relative Risk Reduction (RRR) of 0.40 (95 per cent CI, 0.23–0.68) protective effect, after adjustments for non-adherence and for those individuals who were found to be HIV-positive at baseline. By the end of the trial, 18 participants were not circumcised in the active group and 12 participants from the control group were circumcised. Further, 4 participants were found to have been HIV-positive at baseline and so were excluded from the analysis. Adverse events among the circumcised group were minor and included bleeding (5/1391), infection (4/1391), and delayed healing (3/1391).

Will the results help in caring for the target population?

The participants in this trial are representative of the general Kenyan male population and were of mixed professional status and sexual history. It is likely that the results from this trial have applicability to populations throughout East Africa. Although stopped early, the trial largely completed its intended duration

Trial 3 (Gray *et al.* 2007)

Primary guides on methods

The final study (Gray *et al.* 2007) that met our eligibility criteria was published along with Bailey *et al.* (2007) in February 2007. The trial randomized 4996 uncircumcised, HIV-negative men aged 15–49 years in rural Rakai district, Uganda. Men were randomly assigned to receive immediate circumcision ($n=2474$) or delayed circumcision for 24 months ($n=2522$). Randomization occurred using urn randomization, with opaque envelopes to conceal allocation. Participants in the active group were circumcised within an average of 2 days post-randomization. Circumcision was done with the sleeve procedure, and patients were counselled to abstain from sexual intercourse until complete wound healing had occurred. The primary trial outcome, HIV infection, was assessed using intention-to-treat analysis for participants that provided a PCR-negative HIV test at study initiation. The trial was again terminated by the DSMB due to benefit at the second interim analysis, at which time 44 per cent of all participants had completed the entire trial.

Secondary guides

Participants and healthcare workers could not be blinded. Groups were similar at the beginning of the trial and were treated equally throughout, with the exception of the intervention.

What were the results?

A total of 114 (2.3 per cent) active group participants and 115 (2.3 per cent) control group participants were lost to follow-up over the trial duration. Further, 146 participants in the active group did not receive circumcision and 33 men in the control group were circumcised outside of the trial parameters. There were 22 HIV infections in the active group and 45 infections in the control group. This corresponds to an HIV incidence over 24 months of 0.66 cases per 100 person-years in the intervention group and 1.33 cases per 100 person-years in the control group. The rate of all adverse events related to surgery in the intervention group was 7.6 per cent (178 events in 2328 surgeries) and most were mild. The severe adverse events included one wound infection, two haematomas that required re-exploration and ligation of active bleeding vessels, one wound disruption due to external cause, and one case of severe postoperative herpetic ulceration not involving the surgical wound requiring hospitalization.

Will the results help me in caring for my population?

The population enrolled represents a relatively rural area of Uganda with broad inclusion criteria representing many different employment and sexual histories. It is likely that the results from this trial have applicability to other populations in East Africa and possibly throughout sub-Saharan Africa. The trial was stopped prior to completion and one should be cautious that the effects may be inflated (Montori *et al.* 2005).

Making sense of the study findings

The studies we included all reported that circumcision promoted important effects in preventing HIV infection. In general the studies were well reported and apparently well conducted. All three trials were stopped early due to benefit, prior to their intended completion. There is reason to believe that studies that stop early are at risk for yielding inflated effect sizes. In an analysis of 143 RCTs that stopped early, Montori *et al.* (2005) identified that studies that stopped prior to intended completion, and had small numbers of events, yielded much higher effect sizes. The fewer events that had accrued at the time investigators terminated their trial, the higher the risk of overestimation. In the study by Montori *et al.,* when comparing the trials with events fewer than the median number (66) to those above the median, they found the odds ratio for a magnitude of effect greater than the median (RRR of 47 per cent) was 28 (95 per cent CI, 11–73 per cent). Given the small number of events within each of our specific trials, we felt it was best to pool the studies to create a meta-analysis, thereby increasing the number of events available for interpretation.

Meta-analysis of included studies

We included data from all three RCTs in a meta-analysis to pool the effect size estimates in order to determine the likely effect size across all three trials.

In order to pool across studies, we need to be aware of the total sample size in each group, from each trial, that was exposed. We also need to determine the number of patients in each group that acquired the outcome (HIV infection). Table 6.11.1 displays these findings from our three included studies.

Meta-analysis is a statistical tool that can be relatively easy, as in this case where there are only three trials with clear outcomes, or more difficult (and may require the assistance of a statistician) when there is a more substantive number of trials and when differences across trials are examined using advanced methods such as sensitivity analyses, meta-regression, or sub-group analyses.

We pooled our data with Stats Direct, (StatsDirect Ltd. Manchester, UK, version 2.1), using a random effects model, namely the DerSimonian–Laird random effects method, which recognizes and anchors studies as a sample of all potential studies, and incorporates an additional between-study component to the estimate of variability (DerSimonian & Laird 1986). This method provides more conservative estimates than the fixed-effects model. We calculated the I^2 statistic and associated 95 per cent confidence interval for the pooled effect size, the percentage of between-study variability that is due to true differences between studies (heterogeneity) rather than sampling error (chance) (Higgins & Thompson 2002). We considered an I^2 value greater than 50 per cent to reflect substantial heterogeneity. The meta-analysis is plotted on a forest plot, with RR less than 1 indicating findings in favour of male circumcision (Fig. 6.11.3).

By combining data from the three RCTs, we found a pooled RR of 0.44 per cent (95 per cent CI, 0.33–0.60, $P = <0.0001$, $I^2 =$ 0 per cent, 95 per cent CI 0–35 per cent), corresponding to a RRR of 56 per cent (95 per cent CI, 40–67 per cent). There was no observable heterogeneity across the trials. Another way of interpreting results is the number needed to treat (Laupacis 1988). The number needed to treat to prevent one HIV infection was 58 (95 per cent CI: 48–81).

Applying the findings to the target populations

Our meta-analysis provides us with a strong inference that male circumcision may reduce HIV infection amongst men. We need to now determine whether it is practical and feasible to pursue male circumcision across the African population. When we consider that sexually active males in sub-Saharan Africa represent the group most responsible for infections in women and children, we recognize that reducing male likelihood of infection may protect partners and other groups exposed to sexual activity with the males. For that reason, the intervention is appealing.

We recognize, however, that implementing circumcision across a broad population is fraught with difficulties related to spiritual, religious, and other value-laden decisions (Ngalande *et al.* 2006). Even in North America, where circumcision was routine until the 1990s, there is now growing opposition to circumcision, and such arguments need to be considered in a compassionate and public health context (Auvert *et al.* 2006).

We also recognize that there are harms related to circumcision. Many males in sub-Saharan Africa are circumcised in traditional ceremonies and there is concern about a lack of sterility of the tools used and the potential for serious adverse events and potentially even HIV infection through exposure to unsterile equipment (Mills *et al.* 2006a). Further, in our analysis above, we found that minimizing adverse events in a sterile setting require considerable medical experience, which may not exist in settings with few healthcare workers, to ensure that the risk of infection and serious bleeding from the wound are minimized.

Differential effectiveness. Many controlled studies provide estimates of efficacy i.e. how well an intervention can work in ideal circumstances. The equity–effectiveness loop takes efficacy as the anchor point representing the maximum benefit that can be achieved. Community effectiveness is the measure of how well an intervention does work when delivered in real-life settings and systems at the community level. This 'community effectiveness' is

Study name	Statistics for each study			
	Risk ratio	Lower limit	Upper limit	*p*-Value
Auvert, RSA	0.42	0.25	0.70	0.001
Bailey, Kenya	0.41	0.24	0.70	0.001
Gray, Uganda	0.50	0.30	0.83	0.007
	0.44	0.33	0.60	0.000

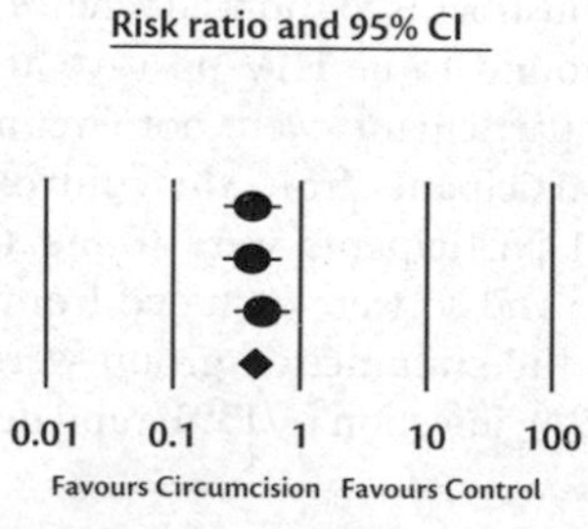

Fig. 6.11.3 Meta-analysis of circumcision trials (CI: confidence interval).

often substantially lower than the expected efficacy because of four systemic factors: Awareness/access/coverage, screening/diagnosis/targeting, provider compliance, and consumer adherence.

Circumcision is a very good example of this

Indeed, we are concerned that media and international agencies are sending out the wrong message—that circumcision reduces infection chances by 60 per cent (WHO/UNAIDS 2007). This is based on the efficacy data above. In support of the stability of the estimates is the fact that these efficacy trials were held in comparatively different economic conditions within the threshold of 'poverty-affected' populations (i.e. the poor populations of these countries are probably similar, even though GDPs may vary). Examining whether effect sizes within our meta-analysis may differ according to location (see Fig. 6.11.3), we can see that all trials displayed a similar rate of effectiveness. It is also remarkable that our pooled analysis is almost identical to the pooled cross-sectional estimate of 0.41 (95 per cent CI, 0.35–0.49) (Siegfried 2005).

However, in reality, the results should be presented as absolutes—which shows a much less impressive impact, i.e. the absolute risk reduction (ARR) is low, ARR 0.014 (95 per cent CI, 0.07–0.2), corresponding to a Number Needed to Treat of 72 (95 per cent CI, 50–143). This means that, contrary to media reports, 72 circumcisions will need to be conducted in order to prevent one infection over a period of 2 years. When stated in this stark contrast to the media reports, the individual protection is low, but the population effects are high.

The reasons for this dilution of the efficacy results from the trials are several. First, the trials we included in our meta-analysis were all held in settings with high levels of HIV infection, and patients were provided with education about HIV prevention and on reducing their number of sexual partners. Although such intensive education programmes may be included as ministries of health in Africa begin to roll out circumcision as a prevention tool, historically there has been a persistent, yet inadequate, response to prevention strategies in the past. Second, a potential difference between the trial settings and many settings in Africa is the age and specific practice of circumcision. In the included trials, young sexually active males were enrolled. Participants had to be uncircumcised prior to enrolment. In many settings in Africa, even those with high prevalence of HIV, circumcision is commonplace, and traditional healing practices and religion will either initiate circumcision at birth or as a coming of age ceremony. While circumcising at birth is arguably the safest surgical procedure for the patient, and reduces the likelihood of failing the intervention (i.e. having sexual intercourse before the scarring has healed), it would take a generation to determine its population effect. Rwanda, one country in Africa with a comparatively high HIV rate, has chosen to implement the widespread circumcision of adult males in an effort to bring about an immediate public health effect (Anon 2007). Circumcision will be available in ministry clinics free of charge. As a response to unprofessional circumcision strategies, such as traditional healers, many ministries of health have mandated that circumcision aspects of rituals be performed at clinic settings. The success of this mandate will be challenging, but appears to be accepted in some settings (Mills *et al.* 2006c).

We do not anticipate that consumer adherence will be a major challenge in circumcision given that the intervention requires only a one-time procedure. The immediate adherence challenges related to circumcision will be abstaining from sexual activity during the healing period.

Step 3: Economic evaluation

This step assesses the efficiency (health benefits [number of lives saved, number of quality]/disability-adjusted life years avoided) obtained for a specific cost (direct, indirect, and where possible the intangible costs expressed in monetary units such dollars, euros, or pounds) of the intervention. That is, whether the intervention is being delivered to those who would benefit from it with an optimal use of resources. Assessment of efficiency should not be done in the absence of adequate evidence of efficacy and valid estimates of cost. Application of an equity lens to this step implies a trade-off between cost-efficiency and population health equity. Priority funding of interventions with the best cost-effectiveness ratios might increase rich–poor differences because the cost of reaching the poor may be higher (e.g. distance to care) and health benefits may be lower. The concept of using equity-adjusted traditional utility metrics such as an Equity Adjusted Quality Adjusted Life Year (EQ-QALY) needs to be developed, as described above.

Applying this to the circumcision example, we need to recognize that there are costs related to any intervention and we need to determine if the cost of the intervention will make it inaccessible for some participant groups. In a cost-effectiveness analysis related to the Auvert *et al.* RCT, assuming full coverage of the male circumcision intervention in a South African province, with a 2005 adult male prevalence of 25.6 per cent, 1000 circumcisions would avert an estimated 308 (80 per cent CI, 189–428) infections over 20 years (Kahn *et al.* 2006; Williams *et al.* 2006). The estimated cost was US$181 (80 per cent CI, US$117–US$306) per HIV infection averted, and net savings were US$2.4 million (80 per cent CI, US$1.3 million–US$3.6 million). With a lower HIV prevalence of, say, 8.4 per cent, the estimated cost per HIV infection averted was US$551 (80 per cent CI, US$344–US$1071) and net savings were US$753 000 (80 per cent CI, US$0.3–US$1.2 million). This cost-effectiveness evaluation estimated that each circumcision costs US$47, a price that we would consider to be exceptionally high in sub-Saharan Africa, and that a widespread circumcision roll-out would substantially reduce those costs. The cost of lifetime clinical care in this assessment was US$11 948 with antiretroviral access and US$3793 without. Nonetheless, the cost of HIV/AIDS treatment in sub-Saharan Africa remains outside of the abilities of many nations, indicating that any costs saved through HIV infections averted would be an important saving for national health budgets.

Step 4: Implementation

The circumcision example emphasizes the importance of explicit consideration of the values and cultural acceptability. Individual rights overtook common public health strategies when, in the 1980s context of a lack of treatment, testing for HIV/AIDS was made voluntary, and disclosure of HIV status was viewed as an individual's right (Bayer & Fairchild 2006). Far be it for us to question the validity of this approach; we simply wish to display here that community values outweighed stricter public health strategies such as widespread testing or quarantine (Fairchild & Bayer 2004). As we see almost 30 years later, a greater emphasis is now being placed on community protection rather than individual rights and the United States as well as the World Health Organization now recommend routine testing of individuals using an opt-out approach (Mills & Chong 2006; Mills *et al.* 2006b).

The science of implementation overlaps substantially with the recently burgeoning 'knowledge translation' initiatives—see the section below.

Steps 5 and 6: Monitoring and reassessment

Monitoring identifies the importance of process assessments and intermediate outcomes (putting the human and physical resources in place, monitoring the identification, and treatment of those at risk/in need). The main purpose of these steps in the iterative loop is to assess success in affecting mortality and morbidity by socioeconomic group and deciding whether further remediable need exists; if so there needs to be an additional iteration of the loop.

Monitoring of any scaled up programme for circumcision to reduce HIV/AIDS is essential; just applying the evidence alone will be insufficient. There is compelling evidence that some strategies in sexual health have previously had negative outcomes when public health decision-makers were too eager to apply new interventions. The use of nonoxynol-9 spermicidal lubricant, for example, was widely marketed to prevent pregnancies during the 1980s and 1990s. It was also believed to potentially reduce HIV infection. However, when multiple trials were conducted, it became apparent that the intervention was harmful and may have contributed to increased infections (Wilkinson 2002). Recent microbicide trials to reduce HIV infection have had similarly disappointing results, despite the tremendous media attention and policy-maker promises of imminent effectiveness (WHO 2007). It is clear that if circumcision is to be implemented widely, there will be a need for intense monitoring and dealing with problems as they arise (Singh & Mills 2005).

An example of an approach to monitor HIV and other health programmes is the Equity Gauge of the Global Equity Gauge Alliance, funded by Rockefeller Foundation. This group has developed 'equity gauges' as a means of tracking gaps in health at the national or subnational levels (McCoy *et al.* 2003). This approach to equity includes three pillars: (1) measuring key indicators, (2) public participation, and (3) advocacy. Inclusion of all three pillars will ensure that information is acted upon. Equity Gauges have been or are being developed in Bangladesh, Chile, China, Ecuador, Kenya, South Africa, Thailand, Uganda, Zambia, and Zimbabwe (McCoy 2003).

WHO has developed a Health Metrics Network to enable performance-based monitoring of interventions and health systems. The Network will aim to build transparency and accountability, and ensure that policy decisions are based upon evidence. Equity is central to the proposed data indicators (AbouZahr & Boerma 2005).

Our stepwise illustration of the equity–effectiveness loop concludes here, showing the interface between clinical epidemiology and public health.

We will finish the chapter by describing a few other features of this interface.

Knowledge translation and innovation

This is an aspect of clinical epidemiology that has developed fairly recently, stimulated in part by being singled out for funding by agencies such as the Canadian Institutes of Health Research. This is highly relevant to public health and warrants discussion here.

We define knowledge translation as 'the synthesis, exchange, and application of knowledge by relevant stakeholders to accelerate the benefits of global and local innovation in strengthening health systems and improving people's health' (WHO 2006). Essentially, this involves uptake and translation of knowledge into action. To do this, tailored interventions are needed to reach a range of target groups, including researchers, local and national policy makers, professionals, affected communities, industry, media, and the general public.

However, one of the primary challenges facing these initiatives is to determine the most effective strategies to promote the use and application of research. A useful framework to provide direction for determining what strategies can work is the Ottawa Model of Research Use (OMRU), developed by Graham and Logan (2004).

This framework describes an evidence-based approach to selecting and tailoring strategies to promote the application of research. The framework consists of six key elements that should be assessed, monitored, and evaluated before, during, and after any knowledge translation effort (see Fig. 6.11.4). Three of the key elements relate to barriers and supports: (1) the structural, social, patients, and economic influences within the practice and policy environment; (2) the attitudes, knowledge, motivation, and skills of potential adopters or target audiences; and (3) the perceptions of the research evidence and innovation developed. The other three key elements are: (4) The implementation intervention strategies for diffusing, disseminating, or implementing research findings; (5) the adoption and use of the innovation; and (6) the impact or outcomes of research use.

Below, we illustrate the importance and the evidence available in knowledge translation in low- and middle-income countries, using each of the OMRU components (Santesso & Tugwell 2006). We propose that each step is assessed across the socioeconomic gradient using the equity-oriented knowledge translation cascade (Fig. 6.11.5), thus ensuring that interventions do indeed benefit the disadvantaged (Tugwell *et al.* 2006b).

1. *Perceptions of the research evidence and innovation*: Assessing and evaluating the external factors, such as the characteristics of the users and the environment they work in, is relatively straightforward. Assessing the perceptions of the research evidence, however, is less so. These latter characteristics relate primarily to how the evidence was created and the ease of application. For example, Logan and Graham (2004) explain that if the research evidence has been produced in a rigorous or transparent way or by credible developers, it may be more readily applied. But if the evidence is difficult to apply, not compatible with usual practice or not seen as advantageous, it may not be applied. Negative feelings about the evidence may also hinder its application. Haines *et al.* (2004) relate these concepts to knowledge transfer to the public. They found that the public is wary of evidence that is not congruent with existing cultural values.

   This emphasizes the importance of adapting innovations/interventions to potential users and the setting, and creating an innovation or intervention that is perceived positively. An example of a clinical initiative that gives a priority to local applicability is the INCLEN's Knowledge 'Plus' Program, which is based on the premise that developing, providing access to, and equipping healthcare professionals to use locally appropriate

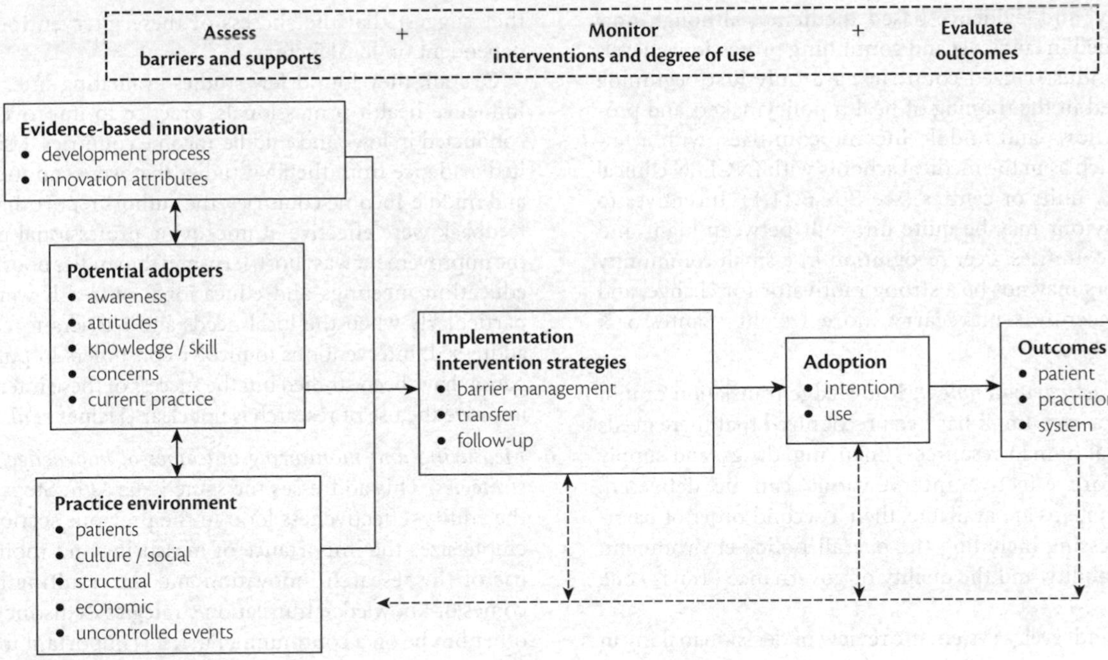

Fig. 6.11.4 The Ottawa Model of Research Use.
Source: Graham and Logan (2004).

and equitable guidelines enhances knowledge translation in low- and middle-income countries. The development of these guidelines, or Knowledge Plus Packages, is through a transparent and systematic process according to local health priorities and the healthcare environment, and involves healthcare professionals and stakeholders to capture local or 'tacit knowledge'. Knowledge Plus Packages for TB, acute respiratory infections, and hyperlipidaemia have been developed and are being applied in Colombia, India, and the Philippines. Tools to locally adapt the guidelines have also been developed for other settings (INCLEN 2004).

2. *Potential adopters*: Attitudes, knowledge, motivation, and skills. While many of the characteristics and barriers to research use in potential adopters may be similar between high- and low-income countries, some characteristics present unique challenges in low- and middle-income countries. 'Evidence-based

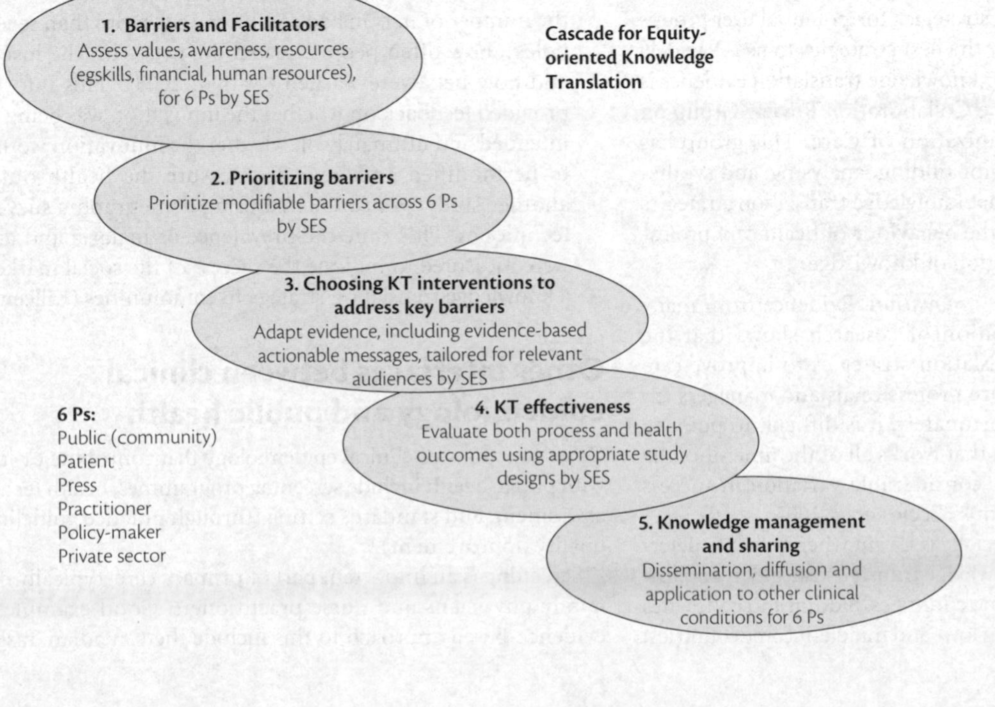

Fig. 6.11.5 Equity-oriented knowledge translation cascade.
Source: Tugwell (2006b).

health policy' and 'evidence-based medicine', although now widely included in curricula and continuing professional development in industrialized countries, are only just beginning to be included in the training of health policymakers and professionals in low- and middle-income countries, with a few exceptions such as in the medical schools with INCLEN clinical epidemiology units or centres (see Box 6.11.1). Incentives to change behaviour may be quite different between high- and low-income countries: Peer recognition in a small community with few peers may not be a strong motivator for change, and monetary incentives may carry more weight (Santesso & Tugwell 2003).

3. *Policy and practice environment*: Knowledge translation cannot take place in a vacuum. It has been recognized that there needs to be minimal human resources, financing, drugs, and supply systems before effective interventions can be delivered. Once these systems are available, then a second order of barriers need assessing including the overall policy environment, political instability, and the quality of governance (Travis *et al.* 2004).

   At this second level, a systematic review of decision making in healthcare management and policy making from Lavis *et al.* (2004) identifies that conflicts and rivalries between elected officials and civil servants may decrease the application of research evidence. Similarly, interviews with key informants in knowledge translation in low- and middle-income countries emphasize that the application of research may be hindered when the political environment is corrupt and unstable and when there is a lack of financial resources (Santesso & Tugwell 2003). At a clinical level, research evidence may be competing with institutionalized habits, superstitions, traditions, and cultures (Cutler 2004).

4. *Determining the implementation intervention strategies:* According to OMRU, once researchers have assessed the salient barriers and supports for knowledge translation, they can determine the best strategy to ensure the application of knowledge in their potential users. Research evidence and experiences evaluating knowledge translation strategies for potential user groups also informs decisions about the best strategies to use. A widely used evidentiary resource for knowledge translation evidence is available from The Cochrane Collaboration Review Group on Effective Practice and Organization of Care. This group has developed specific methods for finding, analysing, and synthesizing the evidence about what knowledge translation strategies work to change or improve the behaviour of healthcare professionals to ensure the application of knowledge.

5. *The adoption and use of the innovation*: Evidence from many reviews of the implementation of research shows that the majority of knowledge translation strategies to improve care that are targeted to healthcare professionals and managers are moderately successful. Unfortunately, it is difficult to point to any one type of intervention that works all of the time since the research shows that there is considerable variation in success within and across interventions (Eccles *et al.* 2005).

   This variation may be especially relevant when trying to determine if this research into knowledge transfer strategies is applicable to low- and middle-income countries. Siddiqi and colleagues (2005) reviewed the literature in low- and middle-income countries; they suggest that the success of these interventions is highly dependent on local factors.

   Overall, they found few studies evaluating interventions to influence health professionals' practice to improve healthcare conducted in low- and middle-income countries. Using the limited evidence from the few studies that were conducted in low- and middle-income countries, the authors report that audit and feedback were effective at improving professional practice but the improvement was short-term and the studies poorly designed; education meetings and educational outreach were effective, particularly when the local needs and barriers to change were addressed. Interventions to involve consumers in public participation have been studied but the success of these interventions to improve the use of research is not clear (Haines *et al.* 2004).

6. *Measuring and monitoring outcomes of knowledge translation strategies*: This addresses the same issue as in Steps 5 and 6 of the equity–effectiveness loop in the previous sections. OMRU emphasizes the importance of measuring and monitoring the use of the research/innovation and the resulting health outcomes of knowledge translation strategies as distinct from each other but lie on a continuum. First, it is important to determine whether the research is used or consulted by the target audience or is in place and reaching the target audience—outcomes to measure its use are necessary. If the research is used then the next question to ask is: Does it result in improved health outcomes—the primary objective of any knowledge translation activity?

   The distinction between the two is illustrated in the use of bed nets in Tanzania to prevent malaria. The Ifakara Health Research and Development Centre in Tanzania has developed social marketing strategies, which include intense promotion of the use of insecticide-treated mosquito nets in local communities, for example, through play skits performed in a community. The consistent use of, care of, and reapplication of insecticide to the bed nets are obviously key in whether the bed nets decrease malaria and mortality in those communities. Therefore, the researchers assessed the numbers of people who had bed nets, the number of nets in bad condition (e.g. more than seven large holes), how often people treated the nets with the insecticide, and how nets were washed (Nathan 2004). This information provided feedback on whether the innovation was being used as intended and ultimately on whether the innovation would need to be modified and how. To measure the health outcomes, another study was conducted using demographic surveillance techniques. This time the prevalence of malaria and anaemia were measured to indicate the success of the social marketing as a knowledge translation strategy to communities (Killeen 2007).

Other interfaces between clinical epidemiology and public health

Other functions of clinical epidemiology that contribute or interface with public health include screening programmes, health technology assessment, and standards setting (through practice guidelines and quality improvement).

Screening is an important part of primary care, typically done by family physicians and nurse practitioners. Good examples of an evidence-based approach to this include the Canadian Task Force on the Periodic Health Exam (Canadian Task Force on Preventive Healthcare (http://www.ctfphc.org), the US Preventive Services Task Force (http://www.ahrq.gov/clinic/uspstfix.htm), and guidelines for disease promotion in immigrants and refugees in Canada (Pottie *et al.* 2008). Many of these screening clinical actions need to be integrated with public health services.

Health Technology Assessment, defined by Battista as the bridge between science and policy, also bridges clinical epidemiology and public health. Indeed one of us (PT) has used the same stepwise iterative loop approach to systematizing the methods (Tugwell *et al.* 1995).

Standards setting through practice guidelines and quality assurance in clinical epidemiology also has many parallels with public health, especially public health units. Clinical guidelines are only as good as the evidence and judgements they are based on. For example, the international GRADE initiative has been developed for users of clinical practice guidelines and other recommendations to provide them with the information needed to know how much confidence they can place in the recommendations. Systematic and explicit methods of making judgements can reduce errors and improve communication. The GRADE system grades the quality of evidence and the strength of recommendations that can be applied across a wide range of interventions and contexts. Judgements about the strength of a recommendation require consideration of the balance between benefits and harms, the quality of the evidence, translation of the evidence into specific circumstances, and the certainty of the baseline risk. It is also important to consider costs (resource utilization) before making a recommendation. Inconsistencies among systems for grading the quality of evidence and the strength of recommendations reduce their potential to facilitate critical appraisal and improve communication of these judgements. This system for guiding these complex judgements balances the need for simplicity with the need for full and transparent consideration of all important issues. These are being used not only for clinical guidelines but also at the policy level, such as for the World Health Organization to assess the evidence for anti-virals for avian influenza (Schunemann *et al.* 2007).

Conclusion

In summary:

- The separation of clinical medicine and public health in the early twentieth century led to a schism between clinical care and the collective action for 'public good' over 'private good'. Epidemiology, the social sciences, and qualitative methods became the domain of public health, and medicine assumed dominance in clinical treatment advances.
- Clinical epidemiology has adopted many public health methods; conversely, it has contributed to methods for tackling public health problems.
- Clinical epidemiology training has led to many clinicians and other healthcare providers developing research programmes addressing public health problems.
- Equity, with a special focus on equity in effectiveness, has recently become a focus of clinical epidemiology, and complements the longstanding concern for this in public health.
- The equity–effectiveness framework is just one approach for systematically organizing the clinical epidemiological approach to public health problems.
- Clinical epidemiology has a contribution to make to public health.

References

AbouZahr, C. and Boerma, T. (2005). Health information systems: The foundations of public health. *Bulletin of World Health Organization*, **83**, 578–83.

Acheson, D. (1988). *Public Health in England: The report of the Committee of Inquiry into the future development of the public health function*. HMSO, London.

Anon. (2007). *Global challenges/Rwanda to launch mass male circumcision program to reduce spread of HIV/AIDS*. Available at: http://www.kaisernetwork.org/daily_reports/rep_index.cfm?DR_ID = 47626 (Accessed 22 September 2007).

Auvert, B., Sobngwi-Tambekou, J., Taljaard, D. *et al.* (2006). Corresponding Authors' reply to: The Potential Impact of Male Circumcision on HIV in Sub-Saharan Africa, *PLoS Medicine*, **3**, e67.

Auvert, B., Taljaard, D., Lagarde, E. *et al.* (2005). Randomized, controlled intervention trial of male circumcision for reduction of HIV infection risk: The ANRS 1265 Trial. *PLoS Medicine*, **2**, e298.

Awasthi, S. and INCLEN Childnet Zinc effectiveness for diarrhea group (2006a). Zinc supplementation in acute diarrhea is acceptable, does not interfere with oral rehydration, and reduces the use of other medications: a randomized trial in five countries. *Journal of Pediatric Gastroenterology and Nutrition*, **42**, 300–5.

Awasthi, S., Verma, T., and Agarwal, M. (2006b). Danger signs of neonatal illnesses. *Bulletin of World Health Organization*, **84**, 819–26.

Bailey, R.C., Moses, S., Parker, C.B. *et al.* (2007). Male circumcision for HIV prevention in young men in Kisumu, Kenya: A randomised controlled trial. *Lancet*, **369**, 643–56.

Bayer, R. and Fairchild, A.L. (2006). Changing the paradigm for HIV testing the end of exceptionalism. *The New England Journal of Medicine*, **355**, 647–9.

Birdsell, J.M., Atkinson-Grosjean, J., and Landry, R. (2002). *Knowledge translation in two new programs: Achieving "The Pasteur effect"*. Canadian Institutes of Health Research, Ottawa, Canada.

Briggs, C.J., Capdegelle P., and Garner, P. (2001). Strategies for integrating primary health services in middle- and low-income countries: effects on performance, costs and patient outcomes. *Cochrane Database Systematic Reviews*, 4, CD003318.

Britton, A., Shipley, M., Marmot, M. *et al.* (2004). Does access to cardiac investigation and treatment contribute to social and ethnic differences in coronary heart disease? Whitehall II prospective cohort study. *British Medical Journal*, **329**, 318–20.

Bowers, J. (1974). *Schools of Public Health in Latin America*. Report of a Macy Conference, Medellin, Colombia, November 17–19, 1974. *Josiah H. Macy, Jr. Foundation*, New York.

Cochrane, A.L. (1972). *Effectiveness and efficiency: Random reflections on Health Services*. Nuffield Provincial Hospitals Trust, London.

Cochrane, A.L. (1979). 1931–1971: A critical review, with particular reference to the medical profession. In *Medicines for the year 2000*, pp. 1–11. Office of Health Economics, London.

Cutler, D.M. (2004). *Your money or your life: Strong medicine for America's health care system*. Oxford University Press, New York.

Daly, J. (2005). Evidence-based medicine and the Search for a Science of Clinical Care. *University of California Press*, London.

Davis, D., Evans, M., Jadad, A. *et al.*(2003). The case for knowledge translation: shortening the journey from evidence to effect. *British Medical Journal*, **327**, 33–5.

DerSimonian, R. and Laird, N. (1986). Meta-analysis in clinical trials. *Controlled Clinical Trials*, **7**, 177–88.

Diderichsen, F., Evans, T., and Whitehead, M. (2001). The social basis of disparities in health. In *Challenging Inequities in Health. From Ethics to Action* (eds. T. Evans *et al.*), pp. 13–23. Oxford University Press, New York.

Drain, P.K., Halperin, D.T., Hughes, J.P. *et al.* (2006). Male circumcision, religion, and infectious diseases: An ecologic analysis of 118 developing countries. *BMC Infectious Diseases*, **6**, 172.

Drummond, M., Weatherly, H., Claxton, K. *et al.* (2006). *Assessing the challenges of applying standard methods of economic dvaluation to public health interventions.* Report prepared for the Department of Health by the Public Health Research Consortium, University of York. Available at: http://www.york.ac.uk/phrc/D1-05_FR.pdf Accessed 3 February 2008.

Eccles, M., Grimshaw, J., Walker, A. *et al.* (2005). Changing the behaviour of healthcare professionals: The use of theory in promoting the uptake of research findings. *Journal of Clinical Epidemiology*, **58**, 107–12.

Egger, M., Smith, G.D., and Altman, D.G. (eds.) (2001). *Systematic reviews in health care: Meta-analysis in context.* BMJ Publishing Group. London, (ISBN:0-7279-1488-X).

Fairchild, A.L. and Bayer, R. (2004). Public health. Ethics and the conduct of public health surveillance. *Science*, **303**, 631–2.

Feinstein, A.R. and Horwitz, R.I. (1997). Problems in the "evidence" of "evidence-based medicine". *The American Journal of Medicine*, **103**, 529–35.

Feinstein, A.R. (1985). *Clinical epidemiology; the architecture of clinical research.* WB Saunders, Philadelphia.

Ferriman, A. (2007). BMJ readers choose the "sanitary revolution" as greatest medical advance since 1840. *BMJ*, **334**, 111.

Fletcher, R. (2001). Alvan Feinstein, the father of clinical epidemiology, 1925–2001. *Journal of Clinical Epidemiology*, **54**, 1188–90.

Fletcher, R.W. and Fletcher, S.W. (2005). *Clinical epidemiology: The essentials* (4th edn.). Lippincott Williams & Wilkins, Philadelphia.

Fox, D.M. (1986). *Health policies, health politics: The British and American Experience, 1911–1965*, Princeton University Press, Princeton.

Giuffrida, A., Gosden, T., Forland, F. *et al.* (2000). Target payments in primary care: Effects on professional practice and health care outcomes. *Cochrane Database of Systematic Reviews*, 3, CD000531.

Graham, I. and Logan, J. (2004). Translating research: Innovations in knowledge transfer and continuity of care. *The Canadian Journal of Nursing Research*, **36** (2), 89–103.

Gray, R.H., Kigozi, G., Serwadda, D. *et al.* (2007). Male circumcision for HIV prevention in men in Rakai, Uganda: a randomised trial. *Lancet*, **369**, 657–66.

Grimshaw, J.M., Shirran, L., Thomas, R. *et al.* (2001). Changing provider behavior: An overview of systematic reviews of interventions. *Medical Care*, **39**(Suppl 2), I12–I45.

Guyatt, G.H. and Rennie, D. (2002). User guides to the medical literature. *A manual for evidence-based clinical practice.* AMA Press, Chicago.

Gwatkin, D. (2003). How well do health programmes reach the poor? *Lancet*, **361**, 540–1.

Haines, A., Kuruvilla, S., and Borchert, M. (2004). Bridging the implementation gap between knowledge and action for health. *Bulletin of the World Health Organization*, **82**, 724–31.

Haynes, R.B., Sacket, D., Guyatt, G. *et al.* (2006). *Clinical epidemiology: How to do clinical practice research.* Lippincott, Williams, Wilkins, Philadelphia.

Higgins, J.P. and Thompson, S.G. (2002). Quantifying heterogeneity in a meta-analysis, *Statistics in Medicine*, **21**, 1539–58.

INCLEN (2004). *Knowledge translation to policy and practice: INCLEN's Knowledge 'Plus' Program. INCLEN News.* Available at: http://www.inclentrust.org/pdf/inclennews/November%202004/INCLEN%27s%20Knowledge%20Plus%20Program.pdf Accessed on 28 October 2007.

Institute of Medicine (1988). *The future of public health.* National Academy of Health, Washington D.C.

Killeen, G.F., Tami, A., Kihonda, J. *et al.* (2007). Cost-sharing strategies combining targeted public subsidies with private-sector delivery achieve high bednet coverage and reduced malaria transmission in Kilombero Valley, southern Tanzania. *BMC Infectious Disease.* **7**, 121.

Knowles, J.H. (1977). *Doing better but feeling worse: Health in the United States.* Norton, New York.

Kramer, M.S. (1988). *Clinical epidemiology and biostatistics: A primer for clinical investigators and decision-makers.* Springer-Verlag, Berlin.

Laupacis, A., Sackett, D.L., and Roberts, R.S. (1988). An assessment of clinically useful measures of the consequences of treatment. *The New England Journal of Medicine*, **318**, 1728–33.

Lavis, J.N., Posada, F.B., Haines, A. *et al.* (2004). Use of research to inform public policymaking. *Lancet*, **364**, 1615–21.

Marmot, M. (2001). Inequalities in health. *The New England Journal of Medicine*, **345**, 134–6.

McCoy, D., Bambas, L., Acurio, D. *et al.* (2003). Global equity gauge alliance: Reflections on early experiences. *Journal of Health and Population Nutrition*, **21**, 273–87.

Mills, E.J. and Chong, S. (2006). Lesotho embarks on universal HIV testing. *HIV/AIDS policy & law review / Canadian HIV/AIDS Legal Network*, **11**, 27–8.

Mills, E.J., Nachega, J.B., Bangsberg, D.R. *et al.* (2006a). Adherence to HAART: a systematic review of developed and developing nation patient-reported barriers and facilitators. *PLoS Medicine*, **3**, e438.

Mills, E.J., Nachega, J.B., Buchan, I. *et al.* (2006b). Adherence to antiretroviral therapy in sub-Saharan Africa and North America: A meta-analysis. *JAMA*, **296**, 679–90.

Mills, E. and Siegfried, N. (2006). Cautious optimism for new HIV/AIDS prevention strategies. *Lancet*, **368**, 1236.

Mills, E., Singh, S., Wilson, K. *et al.* (2006c). The challenges of involving traditional healers in HIV/AIDS care. *International journal of STD & AIDS*, **17**, 360–3.

Montori, V.M., Devereaux, P.J., Adhikari, N.K. *et al.* (2005). Randomised trials stopped early for benefit: A systematic review. *JAMA*, **294**, 2203–9.

Mowatt, G., Grimshaw, J.M., Davis, D.A. *et al.* (2001). Getting evidence into practice: The work of the Cochrane effective practice and organization of care group (EPOC). *The Journal of continuing education in the health professions*, **21**, 55–60.

Nathan, R., Masanja, H., Mshinda, H. *et al.* (2004). Mosquito nets and the poor: Can social marketing redress inequities in access? *Tropical medicine & international health: TM & IH*, **10**, 1121–6.

Ngalande, R.C., Levy, J., Kapondo, C.P. *et al.* (2006). Acceptability of male circumcision for prevention of HIV infection in Malawi. *AIDS and Behaviour*, **10**, 377–85.

Peedicayil, A., Sadowski, L.S., Jeyaseelan, L. *et al.*: IndiaSAFE Group. Spousal physical violence against women during pregnancy. *BJOG: An International Journal of Obstetrics and Gynaecology*, **111**, 682–7.

Pottie, K., Robinson, V., Feightner, J. *et al.* (2008). Evaluation of evidence based literature and formulation of recommendations for clinical preventative guidelines for immigrant and refugees in Canada. *CMAJ* In press 2008.

Redelmeier, D.A., Guyatt, G.H., and Foldstein, R.S. (1996). On the debate over methods for estimating the clinically important difference. *Journal of Clinical Epidemiology*, **49**, 1223–4.

Sackett, D.L., Rosenberg, W.M., Gray, J.A. *et al.* (1996). Evidence based medicine: What it is and what it isn't. *BMJ*, **312**, 71–2.

Santesso, N. and Tugwell, P.S. (2003). *Knowledge translation in health and development: Research to policy strategies.* International Development Research Centre (IDRC); Canadian Coalition for Global Health Research and Institute of Population Health, University of Ottawa.

Available at: http://www.idrc.ca/uploads/user-S/10963022581KT_in_Health_and_Development.pdf Accessed 11 September 2007.

Santesso, N. and Tugwell, P. (2006). Knowledge translation in developing countries. *Journal of Continuing Education in the Health Professions*, **26**, 87–96.

Schunemann, H.J., Hill, S.R., Kakad, M. *et al.* for the WHO Rapid Advice Guideline Panel on Avian Influenza (2007). Rapid Advice Guidelines for pharmacological management of sporadic human infection with avian influenza A (H5N1) virus. *The Lancet Infectious Diseases*, **7**, 21–31.

Siddiqi, K., Newell, J., and Robinson, M. (2005). Getting evidence into practice: What works in developing countries? *International journal for quality in health care: journal of the International Society for Quality in Health Care / ISQua*, **17**, 447–54.

Siegfried, N., Muller, M., Deeks, J. *et al.* (2005). HIV and male circumcision—a systematic review with assessment of the quality of studies. *The Lancet Infectious Diseases*, **5**, 165–73.

Singh, J.A. and Mills, E.J.(2005). The abandoned trials of pre-exposure prophylaxis for HIV: What went wrong? *PLoS Medicine*, **2**, e234.

Straus, S., Haynes, R.B., Glasziou, P. *et al.* (2007). Misunderstandings, misperceptions, and mistakes. *Evidence Based Medicine*, **12**, 2–3.

Travis, P., Bennett, S., Haines, A. *et al.* (2004). Overcoming health-systems constraints to achieve the Millennium Development Goals. *Lancet*, **364**, 900–6.

Tugwell, P., Bennett, K., Sackett, D.L. *et al.* (1985). The measurement iterative loop: A framework for the critical appraisal of need, benefits and costs of health interventions. *Journal of Chronic Diseases*, **38**, 339–51.

Tugwell, P., de Savigny, D., Hawker, G. *et al.* (2006a). Applying clinical epidemiological methods to health equity: The equity effectiveness loop. *BMJ*, **332**, 358–61.

Tugwell, P., Robinson, V., Grimshaw, J. *et al.* (2006b). Systematic reviews and knowledge translation. *Bulletin of the World Health Organization*, **84**, 643–51.

Tugwell, P., Sitthi-Amorn, C., O'Connor, A. *et al.* (1995). Technology assessment. Old, new, and needs-based. *International Journal of Technology Assessment in Health Care*, **11**, 650–62.

United Nations (2001). *Millenium Development Goals*. Available at: http://www.developmentgoals.org/index.html. 1-10-2003 Accessed 31 January 2008.

Wagstaff, A. (2002). Inequality aversion, health inequalities and health achievement. *Journal of Health Economics*, **21**, 627–41.

Wawer, M.J., Reynolds, S.J., Serwadda, D. *et al.* (2005). Might male circumcision be more protective against HIV in the highly exposed? An immunological hypothesis. *Aids*, **19**, 2181–2.

Weiss, N.S. (1996). *Clinical epidemiology: The study of the outcome of illness.* Oxford University Press, Oxford.

Wells, G., Beaton, D., Shea, B. *et al.* (2001). Minimal clinically important differences: review of methods. *The Journal of Rheumatology*, **28**, 406–12.

White, K.L. (1991). *Healing the Schism: Epidemiology, medicine, and the public's health*, pp. 12–13. Springer-Verlag, New York.

Wilkins, R. and Adams, O. (1983). *Healthfulness of life.* Institute for Research on Public Policy, Montreal.

Wilkinson, D., Tholandi, M., Ramjee, G. *et al.* (2002). Nonoxynol-9 spermicide for prevention of vaginally acquired HIV and other sexually transmitted infections: Systematic review and meta-anlysis of randomised controlled trials including more than 5000 women. *The Lancet Infectious Diseases*, **2**, 613–17.

Wilkinson, R.G. (1996). *Unhealthy societies. The afflictions of inequality.* Routledge, London and New York.

World Health Organization (WHO) (2007). *Cellulose sulfate microbicide trial stopped.* Available at: http://www.who.int/mediacentre/news/statements/2007/s01/en/index.html Accessed 29 September 2007.

World Health Organization (1999). *The World Health Report 1999: Making a difference.* Geneva, ISBN 92 4 156194 7.

WHO/UNAIDS (2007). *WHO and UNAIDS announce recommendations from expert meeting on male circumcision for HIV prevention.* Available at: http://data.unaids.org/pub/PressRelease/2007/20070328_pr_mc_recommendations_en.pdf Accessed 31 January 2008.

World Health Organization (WHO) Bridging the 'Know–Do' Gap, Meeting on Knowledge Transition in global Health. Geneva.

Zwarenstein, M. and Bryant, W. (2000). Interventions to promote collaboration between nurses and doctors. *Cochrane Database of Systematic Reviews*, **2**, CD000072.

6.12

Validity and bias in epidemiological research

Sander Greenland

Introduction

Some of the major concepts of validity and bias in epidemiological research are outlined in this chapter. The contents are organized in four main sections: Validity in statistical interpretation, validity in prediction problems, validity in causal inference, and special validity problems in case–control and retrospective cohort studies. Familiarity with the basics of epidemiological study design and a number of terms of epidemiological theory, among them risk, competing risk, average risk, population at risk, and rate, is assumed. A number of textbooks provide more background and depth than can be given here; see, for example, Kelsey *et al.* (1996), Rothman and Greenland (1998), Koepsell and Weiss (2003), and Checkoway *et al.* (2004).

Despite similarities, there is considerable diversity and conflict among the classification schemes and terminologies employed in various textbooks. This diversity reflects that there is no unique way of classifying validity conditions, biases, and errors. It follows that the classification schemes employed here and elsewhere should not be regarded as anything more than convenient frameworks for organizing discussions of validity and bias in epidemiological inference. Many types of bias can be qualitatively illustrated with causal diagrams, which reveal the relationships among confounding and selection bias; for example, see Greenland *et al.* (1999), Pearl (2000), Cole and Hernán (2002), Hernán *et al.* (2004), and Glymour and Greenland (2008).

Several important study designs, including randomized trials, prevalence (cross-sectional) studies, and ecological studies, are not discussed in this chapter. Such studies require consideration of the validity conditions mentioned earlier and also require special considerations of their own. Further details of these and other designs can be found in the general textbooks cited in the preceding paragraphs. For discussions of the problems of ecological studies, see Greenland (2001, 2002, 2004a). Meta-analytic methods are discussed by Greenland and O'Rourke (2008). A number of central problems of epidemiological inference are also not covered, including choice of effect measures, problems of induction, and causal modelling. For critical discussions of effect measures by the present author, see Greenland (1987, 1999, 2002b), Greenland and Robins (1988), Greenland *et al.* (1986, 1991), Rothman and Greenland (1998, Chapter 4), and Greenland *et al.* (1999). Greenland (1998a, b) discusses problems of inductive and probabilistic inference, Greenland and Brumback (2002) review causal modelling in epidemiology, and Rothman *et al.* (2008) discuss broader issues in causal inference and philosophy.

Among the deeper problems not discussed here are the failure of conventional statistical methods to account for non-random sources of uncertainty, and the tendency of people (including scientists) to make overconfident and biased inferences in the face of uncertainty (Gilovich *et al.* 2002). Analytical approaches to these problems are discussed by Eddy *et al.* (1992) and Greenland (2005).

Inference and validity

Epidemiological inference is the process of drawing inferences from epidemiological data, such as prediction of disease patterns or identification of causes of diseases or epidemics. These inferences must often be made without the benefits of direct experimental evidence or established theory about disease aetiology. Consider the problem of predicting the risk and incubation (induction) time for acquired immunodeficiency syndrome (AIDS) among persons infected with type 1 human immunodeficiency virus (HIV-1). Unlike an experiment, in which the exposure is administered by the investigator, the date of HIV-1 infection cannot be accurately estimated in most cases; furthermore, the mechanism by which 'silent' HIV-1 infection progresses to AIDS is not known with certainty. Nevertheless, some prediction must be made from the available data if one is to prepare effectively for future health-care needs.

As another example, consider the problem of estimating how much excess risk of coronary heart disease (if any) is produced by coffee drinking. Unlike an experimental exposure, coffee drinking is self-selected; it appears that persons who drink coffee are more likely to smoke than non-users and probably tend to differ in many other behaviours as well (Greenland 1993). As a result, even if coffee use is harmless, we should not expect to observe the same pattern of heart disease in users and non-users. Thus, small effects of coffee drinking should be very difficult to disentangle from the effects of other behaviours. Nevertheless, because of the high prevalence of coffee use and the high incidence of heart disease, any effect of coffee on heart disease risk may be of considerable public health importance.

In both these examples, and in general, inferences will depend on evaluating the validity of the available studies; that is, the degree to which the studies meet basic logical criteria for absence of bias. When (as is usually the case) aspects of validity cannot be guaranteed by successful design strategies, such as blinded random assignment (which ensures that any non-comparability is random), we must evaluate the magnitude of bias that would arise from plausible violations of validity conditions.

Because biases due to misinterpretation of statistics are often neglected in textbooks yet pervade the health-sciences literature, the next subsection will describe common misinterpretations to be alert for when examining reports or analysing data. The remaining subsections will outline and illustrate major concepts of validity and bias in epidemiological research as applied in three settings: Prediction from one population to another, causal inference from cohort studies, and causal inference from case–control and retrospective cohort studies. Parallel aspects of each application will be emphasized. In particular, each problem requires the consideration of comparison bias (better known as *confounding*), follow-up bias, bias due to mismeasurement, bias due to erroneous statistical models, and bias due to erroneous statistical interpretation. (The term 'bias' is, here, used in the informal epidemiological sense, and corresponds to the formal statistical concept of inconsistency.) Case–control studies require the additional consideration of case-selection bias and control-selection bias, and are often subject to additional sources of measurement error beyond those occurring in prospective cohort studies. Similar problems arise in retrospective cohort studies.

Misinterpretations of statistics

Severe consequences can arise from failure to properly interpret statistical outputs, and failure to recognize when the output is the result of a statistical method breaking down. Unfortunately, few textbooks discuss these problems in detail, even though they can result in biases as severe as the more familiar biases discussed in the following subsections. Two problems very common in the health-sciences literature are briefly described here. Both problems as well as many others can be avoided with certain Bayesian statistical approaches. Detailed arguments for Bayesian approaches can be found in Berger and Berry (1988), Greenland (1998b, 2006), and Thomas *et al.* (2007). For an introduction to Bayesian methods that can be carried out with ordinary software, see Greenland (2006, 2007). The remainder of this subsection concerns only conventional 'frequentist' methods of significance tests, confidence intervals (CIs), *P*-values, and model fitting.

Misinterpretations of statistical significance

Many authors have noted that significance testing is fiendishly difficult to interpret correctly, so difficult that otherwise expert epidemiologists and even statisticians routinely make dramatic mistakes (Altman *et al.* 2000; Greenland 2004b). Perhaps the largest source of misreporting and misjudgment in the scientific literature, however, is the simple confusion of presence or absence of an association with presence or absence of statistical significance (Altman & Bland 1995). A common consequence of this confusion is the mistaken reporting of non-significant results as 'confirming' the null, when in reality the results are completely ambiguous. For example, a study that results in 95 per cent confidence limits for a relative risk (RR) of 0.80 and 2.0 is non-significant. Even if perfectly valid, however, it would not support the null hypothesis any more than it would support the hypothesis that the true relative risk is 1.5 (a 50 per cent increase in risk). Misinterpreting non-significant results as null is easily avoided by paying attention to the confidence limits (Altman *et al.* 2000; Rothman 1978; Thompson 1987). The limits of 0.80 and 2.0 show that the results are not 'significantly' different at the 0.05 level from any relative risk between 0.80 and 2.0. Unfortunately, mistaken claims that non-significant results support the null hypothesis of no association still pervade the field, especially in important policy and legal applications of statistics to epidemiology (Greenland 2004).

A converse misinterpretation is to say that two groups showed different results because they had different statistical significance. As an example, one article abstract (Park *et al.* 2007) reported that an inverse association with colorectal cancer was 'seen for total vitamin D intake in men (RR = 0.72, 95% CI: 0.51, 1.00; *P* for trend = 0.03) but not in women' (the estimate compares the highest quintile of vitamin D intake to the lowest). Examination of Table 3 of the paper reveals, however, that the corresponding relative risk for women was 0.89 with 95 per cent confidence limits of 0.63 and 1.27, which means that the association for women was in fact inverse, just as in men (0.89 = 11 per cent lower risk in the highest quintile than in the lowest). Although it was not significantly different at the 0.05 level from 1 (the null), it was also not significantly different from the relative risk of 0.72 seen for men; nor was it significantly different from any relative risk from 0.63 to 1.27. One way to summarize these results would have been to state that an inverse association was observed in both men and women, but that it was weaker and non-significant for women. An even better interpretation is that the study had too few subjects to detect whether men and women actually differ with respect to the relation of vitamin D to colorectal cancer. Such honest reports of study weaknesses are not common, however.

An opposite misinterpretation of the one just illustrated is to claim that two results are *not* significantly different because their confidence intervals overlap. It is true that they will not be significantly different if the interval from either group contains the point estimate from the other group (as in the preceding example, in which the men's point estimate of 0.72 falls within the women's limits of 0.63 and 1.27). Nonetheless, if the intervals overlap but neither interval contains both point estimates, one cannot determine significance without conducting a direct test of the difference in results. Finally, the two groups will be significantly different if their confidence intervals do not overlap.

Misinterpretations such as just described arise in part from the enduring use of a cut-off value such as 0.05 to declare presence or absence of significance, and the corresponding use of 95 per cent to determine the width of a confidence interval (which is just the collection of all values that are not significant at the 0.05 level). In reality, there is a continuum of degrees of significance, as measured by the *P*-value ('significance level'), and any cut-off value is both arbitrary and distortive (Rothman & Greenland 1998). Thus, some authors have encouraged a movement away from classifying associations 'significant' or 'non-significant', towards presenting instead the actual *P*-value for the null hypothesis and other values of interest (e.g. Poole 1987a,b; Goodman 1993).

Even if one presents *P*-values, however, the complexities and subtleties of determining and interpreting significance become even worse when multiple tests are involved (the 'multiple comparisons' problem). Here, adjustments for the multiplicity of tests can worsen certain problems even as it addresses others, for example, by worsening power even as it protects the validity (alpha level) of the tests. It may also shift the null hypothesis being tested to one that, if understood, might be seen as irrelevant to the scientific question at hand. For a discussion of these issues and further references, see Rothman and Greenland (1998). Many of these problems can be avoided by shifting to a multilevel (hierarchical) approach for the analysis (Greenland 2000).

Sparse-data bias

Most epidemiologic studies collect data on so many variables that any thorough stratification (tabulation) of the data on those variables will result in 'sparse data', in which many if not most cell counts may be very small. Classical epidemiological methods such as standardization break down in the face of this sparsity. Although modelling was developed to address problems of sparse data, it is not a sure fix. Conventional methods for fitting risk and rate models such as maximum likelihood (ML), weighted least squares, and generalized estimating equations (GEE) are 'large-sample' (asymptotic) techniques, meaning that they have sample-size requirements for valid performance. In the context of say logistic regression (the most common method in epidemiology), this means that among other things there are sufficient numbers of cases and non-cases observed at all levels of categorical variables in the model.

A serious problem is that when there are too few cases or non-cases in a given category a coefficient estimate based on that category may 'blow up', taking on a value that is much too large in absolute magnitude. This problem can arise in both unconditional and conditional logistic regression (Greenland *et al.* 2000). In a similar fashion, certain estimates may become inflated when there are too many variables in the model relative to the number of cases and non-cases. This hazard is especially severe when the data are divided into subgroups for separate analysis, for example, separating men and women instead of modelling effects with a variable for gender, or when 'interaction' (product) terms are used in the model. In almost all reports, the inflated estimates if 'statistically significant' are misinterpreted as representing strong effects rather than being recognized as statistical artefacts.

To spot these problems, investigators should check tables of the variables in the model against the outcome, and beware of estimates obtained when the observed numbers in each category fall below 4 or 5, or when the ratios of the number of cases and non-cases to the number of variables in the model fall below 4 or 5. Various methods for *shrinkage estimation* (including random-coefficient, hierarchical, multilevel, ridge, penalized, and Bayesian regression) can be used as an alternative to collapsing categories or deleting variables from the model to avoid sparse-data bias (Rothman & Greenland 1998; Greenland 2000b, 2007).

Validity and bias in prediction problems

Turning now to more traditional topics, the following prediction problem will be used to illustrate several basic concepts of validity. A health clinic for homosexual men is about to begin enrolling HIV-l-negative men in an unrestricted programme that will involve retesting each participant for HIV-1 antibodies at six-month intervals. We can expect that, in the course of the programme, many participants will seroconvert to positive HIV-1 status. Such participants will invariably ask difficult questions, such as: What are my chances of developing AIDS over the next five years? How many years do I have before I develop AIDS? In attempting to answer these questions, it will be convenient to refer to such participants (i.e. those who seroconvert) as the target cohort. Even though membership of this cohort is not determined in advance, it will be the target of our predictions. It will also be convenient to refer to the time from HIV-1 infection until the onset of clinical AIDS as the AIDS incubation time. We could provide reasonable answers to a participant's questions if we could accurately predict AIDS incubation times, although we would also have to estimate the time elapsed between infection and the first positive test.

There might be someone who responds to the questions posed here with the following anecdote: 'I've known several men just like the ones in this cohort, and they all developed AIDS within five years after a positive HIV-1 test'. No trained scientist would conclude from this anecdote that all or most of the target cohort will develop AIDS within five years of seroconversion. Of course, one reason is that the men in the anecdote cannot be 'just like' men in our cohort in every respect: They may have been older or younger when they were infected; they may have experienced a greater degree of stress following their infection; they may have been heavier smokers, drinkers, or drug users; and so on. In other words, we know that the anecdotal men and their post-infection life events could not have been exactly the same as the men in our target cohort with respect to all factors that affect AIDS incubation time, including measured, unmeasured, and unknown factors. Furthermore, it may be that some or all of the men referred to in the anecdote had been infected long before they were first tested, so that (unlike men in our target cohort) the time from their first positive test to AIDS onset was much shorter than the time from seroconversion to AIDS onset.

Any reasonable predictions must be based on observing the distribution of AIDS incubation times in another cohort. Suppose that we obtain data from a study of homosexual men who underwent regular HIV-1 testing, and we then assemble from these data a study cohort of men who were observed to seroconvert. Suppose also that most of these men were followed for at least five years after seroconversion. We cannot expect any member of this study to be 'just like' any member of our target cohort in every respect. Nevertheless, if we could identify no differences between the two cohorts with respect to factors that affect incubation time, we might argue that the study cohort could serve as a point of reference for predicting incubation times in the target cohort. Thus, we shall henceforth refer to the study cohort as our reference cohort.

Note that our reference and target cohorts may have originated from different populations; for example, the clinic generating the target cohort could be in New York, but the study that generated the reference cohort may have been in San Francisco. Of course, for both the target and reference cohorts, the actual times of HIV-1 infection will have to be imputed, based on the dates of the last negative and the first positive tests.

Suppose that our statistical analysis of data from the reference cohort produces estimates of 0.05, 0.25, and 0.45 for the average risk of contracting AIDS within two, five, and eight years of HIV-1 infection. What conditions would be sufficient to guarantee the validity of these figures as estimates or predictions of the proportion of the target cohort that would develop AIDS within two, five, and eight years of infection. If by 'valid' we mean that any discrepancy between our predictions and the true target proportions is unbiased or purely random (unpredictable in principle), the following conditions would be sufficient:

(C) *Comparison validity*—The distribution of incubation times in the target cohort will be approximately the same as the distribution in the reference cohort.

(F) *Follow-up validity*—Within the reference cohort, the risk of censoring (i.e. follow-up ended by an event other than AIDS) is not associated with risk of AIDS.

(M) *Measurement validity*—All measurements of variables used in the analysis closely approximate the true values of the variables. In particular, each imputed time of HIV-1 infection closely approximates the true infection time, and each reported time of AIDS onset closely approximates a clinical event defined as AIDS onset.

(Sp) *Specification validity*—The distribution of incubation times in the reference cohort can be closely approximated by the statistical model used to compute the estimates. For example, if one employs a lognormal distribution to model the distribution of incubation times in the reference cohort, this model should be approximately correct.

The first condition concerns the external validity of making predictions about the target cohort based on the reference cohort. The remaining conditions concern the internal validity of the predictions as estimates of average risk in the reference cohort. The following subsections will explore the meaning of these conditions in prediction problems.

Comparison validity

Comparison validity is probably the easiest condition to describe, although it is difficult to evaluate. Intuitively, it simply means that the distribution of incubation times in the target cohort could be almost perfectly predicted from the distribution of incubation times in the reference cohort, if the incubation times were observed without error and there was no loss to follow-up. Other ways of stating this condition are that the two cohorts are comparable or exchangeable with respect to incubation times, or that the AIDS experience of the target cohort can be predicted from the experience of the reference cohort.

Confounding

If the two cohorts are not comparable, some or all of our risk estimates for the target cohort based on the reference cohort will be biased as a result. This bias is sometimes called *confounding*. There has been much research on methods for identifying and adjusting for such bias; see the textbooks cited earlier.

To evaluate comparison validity, we must investigate whether the two cohorts differ on any factors that influence incubation time. If so, we cannot reasonably expect the incubation time distributions of the two cohorts to be comparable. A factor responsible for some or all of the confounding in an estimate is called a confounder or confounding variable, the estimate is said to be confounded by the factor, and the factor is said to confound the estimate.

To illustrate these concepts, suppose that men infected at younger ages tend to have longer incubation times and that the members of the reference cohort are on average younger than members of the target cohort. If there were no other differences to counterbalance this age difference, we should then expect that members of the reference cohort will on average have longer incubation times than members of the target cohort. Consequently, unadjusted predictions of risk for the target cohort derived from the reference cohort would be biased (confounded) by age in a downward direction. In other words, age would be a confounder for estimating risk in the target cohort, and confounding by age would result in underestimation of the proportion of men in the target cohort who will develop AIDS within five years.

Now suppose that we can compute the age at infection of men in the reference cohort, and that within one-year strata of age, for instance, the target and reference cohorts had virtually identical distributions of incubation times. The age-specific estimates of risk derived from the reference cohort would then be free of age confounding and so could be used as unconfounded estimates of age-specific risk for men in the target cohort. Also, if we wished to construct unconfounded estimates of average risk in the entire target cohort, we could do so via the technique of age standardization.

To illustrate, let P_x denote our estimate of the average risk of AIDS within five years of infection among members of the reference cohort who become infected at age x. Let W_x denote the proportion of men in the target cohort who are infected at age x. Then the estimated average risk of AIDS within five years of infection, standardized to the target cohort's age distribution, is simply the average of the age-specific reference estimates P_x weighted by the age distribution (at infection) of the target cohort; algebraically, this average is the sum of the products W_xP_x over all ages and is denoted by $\Sigma_x W_x P_x$. Considered as an estimate of the overall proportion of the target cohort that will contract AIDS within five years of HIV-1 infection, the standardized proportion $\Sigma_x W_x P_x$ will be free of age confounding.

The preceding illustration brings forth an important and often overlooked point: When one employs standardization to adjust for potential biases, the choice of standard distribution should never be considered arbitrary. In fact, the standard distribution should always be taken from the target cohort or the population about which inferences will be made. If inferences are to be made about several different groups, it may be necessary to compute several different standardized estimates.

Methods for removing bias in estimates by taking account of variables responsible for some or all of the bias are known as adjustment or covariate control methods. Standardization is perhaps the oldest and simplest example of such a method; methods based on multivariate models, which will are discussed, are more complex.

Unmeasured confounders

If all confounders were measured accurately, comparison validity could be achieved simply by adjusting for these confounders (although various technical problems might arise when attempting to do so). Nevertheless, in any non-randomized study, we would ordinarily be able to think of a number of possible confounders that had not been measured or had been measured only in a very poor fashion. In such cases, it may still be possible to predict the direction of uncontrolled confounding by examining the manner in which persons were selected into the target and reference cohorts from the population at large. If the cohorts are derived from populations with different distributions of predictors of the outcome, or the predictors themselves are associated with admission differentially across the cohorts, these predictors will become confounders in the analysis.

To illustrate this approach, suppose that HIV-1 infection via an intravenous route (e.g. through needle sharing) leads to shorter incubation times than HIV-1 infection through sexual activity. Suppose also that the reference cohort had excluded all or most intravenous drug users, whereas the target cohort was non-selective in this regard. Then incubation times in the target cohort will on average be shorter than times in the reference cohort owing to the presence of intravenously infected persons in the target cohort. Thus we should expect the results from the reference cohort to underestimate average risks of AIDS onset in the target cohort.

Random sampling and confounding

Suppose, for the moment, that our reference cohort had been formed by taking a random sample of the target cohort. Can predictions about the target made from such a random sample still be confounded? With the definition of confounding given here, the answer is yes. To see this, note for example that by chance alone men in our sample reference cohort could be younger on average than the total target; this age difference would in turn downwardly bias the unadjusted risk predictions if men had longer incubation times at younger ages.

Nevertheless, random sampling can help to ensure that the distribution of the reference cohort is not too far from the distribution of the target cohort. In essence, the probability of severe confounding can be made as small as necessary by increasing the sample size. Furthermore, if random sampling is used, any confounding left after adjustment will be accounted for by the standard errors of the estimates, provided that the correct statistical model is used to compute the estimates and standard errors. We shall examine the latter condition under the subsection on specification validity.

Follow-up validity

In any cohort study covering an extended period of risk, subjects will be followed for different lengths of time. Some subjects will be lost to follow-up before the study ends. Others will be removed from the study by an event that precludes AIDS onset, which in this setting is death before AIDS onset from fatal accidents, fatal myocardial infarctions, and so on. Because subjects come under study at different times, those who are not lost to follow-up or who die before developing AIDS will still have had different lengths of follow-up when the study ends; traditionally, a subject still under follow-up at the end of study is said to have been 'withdrawn from study' at this the time.

Suppose that we wish to estimate the average risk of AIDS onset within five years of infection. The data from a member of the reference cohort who is not observed to develop AIDS but is also not followed for the full five years from infection are said to be censored for the outcome of interest (AIDS within five years of infection). Consider, for example, a subject killed in a car crash two years after infection but before contracting AIDS: The incubation time of this subject was censored at two years of follow-up.

Follow-up validity means that over any span of follow-up time, risk of censoring is unassociated with risk of the outcome of interest. In our example, follow-up validity means that over any span of time following infection, risk of censoring (loss, withdrawal, or death before AIDS) is unassociated with risk of AIDS. All common methods for estimating risk from situations in which censoring occurs (e.g. person-years, life table, and Kaplan–Meier methods) are based on the assumption of follow-up validity. Given follow-up validity, we can expect that, at any time t after infection, the distribution of incubation times will be the same for subjects lost or withdrawn at t and for subjects whose follow-up continues beyond t.

Violations of follow-up validity can result in biased estimates of risk; such violations are referred to as follow-up bias or biased censoring. To illustrate, suppose that younger reference subjects tend to have longer incubation times (i.e. lower risks) and are lost to follow-up at a higher rate than older reference subjects. In other words, lower-risk subjects are lost at a higher rate than higher-risk subjects. Then, after enough time, the average risk of AIDS in the observed portion of the reference cohort will tend to be overestimated; that is, higher than the average risk occurring in the full reference cohort (as the latter includes both censored and uncensored subject experience).

The follow-up bias in the last illustration would not affect the age-specific estimates of risk (where age refers to age at infection). Consequently, the age bias in follow-up would not produce bias in age-standardized estimates of risk. More generally, if follow-up bias can be traced to a particular variable that is a predictor of both the outcome of interest and censoring, bias in the estimates can be removed by adjusting for that variable. Thus, some forms of follow-up bias can be dealt with in the same manner as confounding.

Measurement validity

An estimate from a study can be said to have measurement validity if it suffers from no bias due to errors in measuring the study variables. Unfortunately, there are sources of measurement error in nearly all epidemiologic studies, and nearly all sources of measurement error will contribute to bias in estimates. Thus, evaluation of measurement validity primarily focuses on identifying sources of measurement error and attempting to deduce the direction and magnitude of bias produced by these sources.

To aid in the task of identifying sources of measurement error, it can be useful to classify such errors according to their source. Errors from specific sources can then be further classified according to characteristics that are predictive of the direction of the bias they produce. One classification scheme divides errors into three major categories, according to their source:

1. *Procedural error*, arising from mistakes or defects in measurement procedures
2. *Proxy-variable error*, arising from using a 'proxy' variable as a substitute for an actual variable of interest
3. *Construct error*, arising from ambiguities in the definition of the variables

Regardless of their source, errors can be divided into two basic types, differential and non-differential, according to whether the direction or magnitude of error depends on the true values of the study variables. Two different sources of error may be classified as dependent or independent, according to whether or not the direction or magnitude of the error from one source depends on the direction or magnitude of the error from the other source. Finally, errors in continuous measurements can be factored into systematic and random components. As described in the following subsections, these classifications have important implications for bias.

Procedural error

Procedural error is the most straightforward to imagine. It includes errors in recall when variables are measured through retrospective interview (e.g. mistakes in remembering all medications taken during pregnancy). It also includes coding errors, errors in calibration of instruments, and all other errors in which the target of measurement is well defined and the attempts at measurement are direct but the method of measurement is faulty. In our example, one target of measurement is HIV-1 antibody presence in blood. All available tests for antibody presence are subject to error (false negatives and false positives), and these errors can be considered to be procedural errors of measurement.

Proxy-variable error

Proxy-variable error is distinguished from procedural error in that use of proxies necessitates imputation and hence virtually guarantees that there will be measurement error. In our example, we must impute the time of HIV-1 infection. For instance, we might take as a proxy the infection time computed as six weeks before the midpoint between the last negative test and the first positive test for HIV-1 antibodies. Even if our HIV-1 tests are perfect, this measurement incorporates error if (as is certainly the case) time of infection does not always occur six weeks before the midpoint between the last negative and first positive tests.

Construct error

Construct error is often overlooked, although it may be a major source of error. Consider our example in which the ultimate target of measurement is the time between HIV-1 infection and onset of AIDS. Before attempting to measure this time span, we must unambiguously define the events that mark the beginning and end of the span. While it may be reasonable to think of HIV-1 infection as a point event, the same cannot be said of AIDS onset. Symptoms and signs may gradually accumulate, and then it is only by convention that some point in time is declared the start of the disease. If this convention cannot be translated into reasonably precise clinical criteria for diagnosing the onset of AIDS, the construct of incubation time (the time span between infection and AIDS onset) will not be well defined let alone accurately measurable. In such situations, it may be left to various clinicians to improvise answers to the question of time of AIDS onset, and this will introduce another source of extraneous variation into the final 'measurement' of incubation time.

Differential and non-differential error

Errors in measuring a variable are said to be differential when the direction or magnitude of the errors tend to vary across the true values of other variables. Suppose, for example, that recall of drug use during pregnancy is enhanced among mothers of children with birth defects. Then, a retrospective interview about drug use during pregnancy will yield results with differential error, as false-negative error will occur more frequently among mothers whose children have no birth defects.

Another type of differential error occurs in the measurement of continuous variables when the distribution of errors varies with the true value of the variable. Suppose, for example, that women more accurately recall the date of a recent cervical-smear (Papanicolaou) test than the date of a more distant test. Then, a retrospective interview to determine length of time since a woman's last cervical smear test would tend to suffer from larger errors when measuring longer times.

Errors in measuring a variable are said to be non-differential with respect to another variable if the magnitudes of errors do not tend to vary with the true values of the other variable. Measurements are usually assumed to be non-differential if neither the subject nor the person taking the measurement knows the values of other variables. For example, if drug use during pregnancy is measured by examining pre-partum prescription records for the mother, it would ordinarily be assumed that the error will be non-differential with respect to birth defects discovered postnatally. Nevertheless, such 'blind' assessments will not guarantee non-differential error if the measurement scale is not as fine as the scale of the original variable (Flegal *et al.* 1991; Wacholder *et al.* 1991) or if there is a third uncontrolled variable that affects both the measurement and the other study variables.

Dependent and independent error

Errors in measuring two variables are said to be dependent if the direction or magnitude of the errors made in measuring one of the variables is associated with the direction or magnitude of the errors made in measuring the other variable. If there is no association of errors, the errors are said to be independent.

In our example, errors in measuring age at HIV-1 infection and AIDS incubation time are dependent. Our measure of incubation time is equal to our measure of age at AIDS onset minus our measure of age at infection; hence, overestimation of age at infection will contribute to underestimation of incubation time, and underestimation of age at infection will contribute to overestimation of incubation time. In contrast, in the same example, it is plausible that the errors in measuring age at infection and age at onset are independent.

Misclassification and bias towards the null

Measurement of a binary (dichotomous) variable is called better than random if, regardless of the true value, the probability that the measurement yields the true value is higher than the probability that it does not. In other words, the measurement is better than random if it is more likely to be correct than incorrect, no matter what the true value is. Given two binary variables, better-than-random measurements with independent non-differential errors cannot inflate or reverse the association observed between the variables. In other words, any bias produced by independent non-differential error in better-than-random measurements can only be towards the null value of the association (which is one for a relative-risk measure) and not beyond.

If either variable has more than two levels, then (contrary to assertions in most pre-1990 literature) the preceding conditions are not sufficient to guarantee that the resulting bias will only be towards the null and not beyond (Dosemeci *et al.* 1990). Despite this insufficiency, knowing that errors are independent and non-differential can increase the plausibility that any resulting bias is towards the null, although it should not increase the plausibility that the observed association is in the correct direction (Gustafson & Greenland 2006). For further discussions of measurement error and bias toward the null, see Flegal *et al.* (1991), Wacholder *et al.* (1991), Weinberg *et al.* (1994), and Rothman and Greenland (1998).

There is one important situation in which the assumption of independent non-differential measurement error and hence bias towards the null have particularly high plausibility: In a double-blind clinical trial with a dichotomous treatment and outcome, successful blinding of treatment status during outcome evaluation should lead to independence and non-differentiality of treatment and outcome measurement errors. Successful blinding thus helps to ensure (although it does not guarantee) that any bias produced by measurement error contributes to underestimation of treatment differences (conservative bias).

Systematic and random components of error

For well-defined measurement procedures on continuous variables, measurement errors can be subdivided into systematic and random components. The systematic component (sometimes called the bias of the measurement) measures the degree to which the procedure tends to underestimate or overestimate the true value on repeated application. The random component is the residual error left after subtracting the systematic component from the total error.

To illustrate, suppose that in our study HIV-1 infection time was unrelated to time of antibody testing and that the average time of HIV-1 seroconversion was eight weeks after infection. Then, even if one used a perfect HIV-1 test, a procedure that estimated infection time as six weeks before the midpoint between the last negative and first positive test would on average yield an estimated infection time that was two weeks later than the true time. Thus, the systematic component of the error of this procedure would be +2 weeks. Because AIDS incubation time is AIDS onset time minus HIV-1 infection time, use of this procedure would add −2 weeks (i.e. a two-week underestimation) to the systematic component of error in estimating incubation time.

Each of the components of an error, systematic and random, may be differential (i.e. may vary with other variable values) or non-differential, and may or may not be independent of the error components in other variables. We shall not explore the consequences of the numerous possibilities. However, one important (but semantically confusing) fact is that, for certain quantities, independent and non-differential systematic components of error will not harm measurement validity in that they will produce no bias in estimation.

To illustrate, suppose that in our example we wish to estimate the degree to which AIDS incubation time depends on age at HIV-1 infection. Suppose also that the systematic components of the measurements of incubation time and age of infection are −2 weeks and +2 weeks (as mentioned), and do not vary with true incubation time or age at measurement (i.e. the systematic components are non-differential). Then, the systematic components, being equal, will cancel out when we compute differences in incubation time and differences in age at infection. Because only these differences are used to estimate the association, the observed dependence of incubation time on age at infection will not be affected by the systematic components of error (although it may be biased by the random components of error).

Specification validity

All statistical techniques, including so-called 'distribution-free' or 'non-parametric' methods as well as basic contingency table methods, are derived by assuming the validity of a sampling model or error distribution. A common example is the binomial model, which is discussed in all the textbooks cited in the introduction. For parametric methods, the sampling model is a mathematical formula that expresses the probability of observing the various possible data patterns as a function of certain unknown constants (parameters). Although the parameters of this model may be unknown, the mathematical form of this model incorporates only known or purely random aspects of the data-generation process; unknown systematic aspects of this process (such as most follow-up and selection biases) will not be accounted for by the model.

All parametric statistical techniques also assume a structural model, which is a mathematical formula that expresses the parameters of the sampling model as a function of study variables. A common example is the logistic model (Kelsey *et al.* 1996; Rothman & Greenland 1998; Checkoway *et al.* 2004; Hosmer & Lemeshow 2000; Jewell 2004). The structural model is most often incorporated into the sampling model, and the combination is referred to as the statistical model. An estimate can be said to have specification validity if it is derived using a statistical model that is correct or nearly so.

If either the sampling model or the structural model used for analysis is incorrect, the resulting estimates may be biased. Such bias is sometimes called *specification bias*, and the use of an incorrect model is known as model misspecification or specification error. Even when misspecification does not lead to bias, it can lead to invalidity of statistical tests and confidence intervals.

The true structural relation among the study variables is almost never known in studies of human disease. Furthermore, in the absence of random sampling and randomization, the true sampling process (i.e. the exact process leading people to enter and stay in the study groups) will also be unknown. It follows that we should ordinarily expect some degree of specification error in an epidemiological analysis. Minimizing such error largely consists of contrasting the statistical model against the data and against any available information about the processes that generated the data, such as prior information on demographic patterns of incidence.

Many statistical techniques in epidemiology are based on assuming some type of logistic model. Examples include all the popular adjusted odds ratios, such as the Woolf, maximum likelihood, and Mantel–Haenszel estimates, as well as tests for odds ratio heterogeneity. Classical 'indirect' adjustment of rates and other comparisons of standardized morbidity ratios depend on similar multiplicative models for their validity (Breslow & Day 1987).

The degree of bias in traditional epidemiologic analysis methods when the model assumptions fail has not been extensively studied. A few traditional methods, such as directly standardized comparisons and the Mantel–Haenszel test, remain valid under a wide variety of structural models. In addition, risk regression has been extended to situations involving more general models than assumed in classical theory (Breslow & Day 1987; Hastie & Tibshirani 1990). Leamer (1978) and White (1993) give more details on the effects of specification error in multiple regression problems, and Maldonado and Greenland (1994) and Greenland and Maldonado (1994) examine the implications of specification error in epidemiology.

Summary of prediction example

The example in this subsection provides an illustration of the most common threats to the validity of predictions. The unadjusted estimates of AIDS risk may be confounded if the target and reference cohorts differ in composition, and may also be biased by losses to follow-up or use of an incorrect statistical model. Finally, our predictions are likely to be compromised by errors in measurements. These sources of error should be borne in mind in any attempt to predict AIDS incidence.

Validity and bias in causal inference

All the bias problems in prediction arise in studies of causation; confounding, follow-up bias, measurement errors, and specification errors must be considered. In fact, as we shall see, problems of causal inference can be viewed as a special type of prediction problem, namely prediction of what would happen (or what would have happened) to a population if certain characteristics of the population were (or had been) altered.

To illustrate the validity issues in causal inference, we shall consider the hypothesis that coffee drinking causes acute myocardial infarction. This hypothesis can be operationally interpreted in a number of ways, such as

1. *There are people for whom the consumption of coffee results in their experiencing a myocardial infarction sooner than they might have, had they avoided coffee.*

Although this hypothesis is appealingly precise, it offers little practical guidance to an epidemiological researcher. The problem lies in our inability to recognize an individual whose myocardial infarction was caused by coffee drinking. It is quite possible that myocardial infarctions precipitated by coffee use are clinically and pathologically indistinguishable from myocardial infarctions due to other causes. If so, the prospect of testing this hypothesis with purely physiological evidence is not good.

We could overcome this impasse by examining a related epidemiologic hypothesis; that is, a hypothesis that refers to the distribution of disease in populations. One of many such hypotheses is

2. *Among five-cup-a-day coffee drinkers, cessation of coffee use will lower the frequency of myocardial infarction.*

This form not only involves a population (five-cup-a-day coffee drinkers) but also asserts that a mass action (coffee cessation) will reduce the frequency of the study disease. Thus, the form of the hypothesis immediately suggests a strong test of the hypothesis: Conduct a randomized intervention trial to examine the impact of coffee cessation on myocardial infarction frequency. This solution has some profound practical limitations, not least of which would be persuading anyone to give up or take up coffee drinking to test a speculative hypothesis.

Having ruled out intervention, we might consider an observational cohort study. In this case, our epidemiological hypothesis must refer to natural conditions, rather than intervention. One such hypothesis is

3. *Among five-cup-a-day coffee drinkers, coffee use has elevated the frequency of myocardial infarction.*

There have been many conflicting cohort and case–control studies of coffee and myocardial infarction. The present discussion will be confined to the issues arising in the analysis of a single study. For a review of issues arising in the analysis of multiple studies (meta-analysis) using the coffee–myocardial infarction literature as an example, see Greenland (1994) and Greenland and O'Rourke (2008).

Consider a cohort study of coffee and first myocardial infarction. At baseline, a cohort of people with no history of myocardial infarction is assembled and classified into subcohorts according to coffee use (e.g. never-drinkers, ex-drinkers, occasional drinkers, one-cup-a-day drinkers, two-cup-a-day drinkers, etc.). Other variables are measured as well: Age, gender, smoking habits, blood pressure, and serum cholesterol. Suppose that at the end of 10 years of monitoring this cohort for myocardial infarction events, we compare the five-cup-a-day and never-drinker subcohorts, and obtain an unadjusted estimate of 1.22 for the ratio of the person-time incidence rates of first myocardial infarction among five-cup-a-day drinkers and never-drinkers (with 95% CIs of 1.00 and 1.49). In other words, it appears that the rate of first myocardial infarction among five-cup-a-day drinkers was 1.22 times higher than the rate among never-drinkers. (Hereafter, myocardial infarction means first myocardial infarction, risk means average risk, and rate means person-time incidence rate.)

The estimated rate ratio of 1.22 may not seem large. Nevertheless, if it accurately reflects the impact of coffee use on the five-cup-a-day subcohort, this estimate implies that persons drinking five cups a day at baseline suffered a 22 per cent increase in their myocardial infarction rate as a result of their coffee use. Given the high frequency of both coffee use and myocardial infarction in many populations, this could represent a substantial health impact. Therefore, we would want to perform a careful evaluation of possible bias in the estimate.

As in the AIDS example, we can proceed by examining a series of conditions sufficient for validity of the estimate as a measure of the effect of coffee:

(C) *Comparison validity (no confounding)*—If the members of the five-cup-a-day subcohort had instead never drunk coffee, their distribution of myocardial infarction events over time would have been approximately the same as the distribution among the never-drinkers.

(F) *Follow-up validity*—Within each subcohort, the risk of censoring (i.e. follow-up ended by an event other than myocardial infarction) is not associated with the risk of myocardial infarction.

(M) *Measurement validity*—All measurements of variables used in the analysis closely approximate the true values of the variables.

(Sp) *Specification validity*–The distribution of myocardial infarction events over time in the subcohorts can be closely approximated by the statistical model on which the estimates are based.

These four conditions are sometimes called *internal validity conditions* because they pertain only to estimating effects within the study cohort rather than to generalizing results to other cohorts. They are sufficient but not necessary for validity, in that certain violations of the conditions will not produce bias in the effect estimate (although most violations will produce some bias).

The meaning of these conditions for an observational cohort study of a causal hypothesis is explored in the following subsections. An important phenomenon known as *effect modification*, which is relevant to both internal validity and generalizability, will also be discussed following comparison validity.

Comparison validity

In our example, comparison validity means that the distribution of myocardial infarctions among never-drinkers accurately predicts what would have happened in the coffee-drinking groups had the members of these groups never drunk coffee. Another way of stating condition C is that the five-cup-a-day and never-drinker subcohorts would be comparable or exchangeable with respect to myocardial infarction times if no one had ever drunk coffee, or that there is no confounding (Greenland *et al.* 1999).

Despite its simplicity, comparison validity depends on the hypothesis of interest in a very precise way. In particular, the research hypothesis (hypothesis 3 in the preceding subsection) is a statement about the impact of coffee among five-cup-a-day drinkers. Thus, this subcohort is the target cohort, and never-drinkers serve as the reference cohort for making predictions about this target.

To illustrate further the correspondence between comparison validity and the hypothesis at issue, suppose for the moment that our research hypothesis was

> *4. Among never-drinkers, five-cup-a-day coffee use would elevate the frequency of myocardial infarction.*

In examining this hypothesis, the never-drinkers would be the target cohort and the coffee drinkers would be the reference cohort. Thus, the comparison validity condition would have to be replaced by a condition such as

> (C') If the never-drinkers had drunk five cups of coffee per day, their distribution of myocardial infarctions would have been approximately the same as the distribution among five-cup-a-day drinkers.

Other ways of stating condition C' are that the five-cup-a-day and never-drinker subcohorts would be comparable or exchangeable with respect to time to myocardial infarction if everyone had been five-cup-a-day drinkers, and that the myocardial infarction experience of five-cup-a-day drinkers accurately predicts what would have happened to the never-drinkers if the latter had drunk five cups a day.

Confounding

Failure to meet condition C results in a biased estimate of the effect of five-cup-a-day coffee drinking on five-cup-a-day drinkers, a condition sometimes referred to as confounding of the estimate. Similarly, failure to meet condition C' results in a biased estimate of the effect that five-cup-a-day drinking would have had on never-drinkers.

To evaluate potential confounding, we must check whether the subcohorts differed at baseline on any factors that influence time to myocardial infarction. If so, we could not reasonably expect the myocardial infarction distributions of the subcohorts to be comparable, even if the subcohorts had the same level of coffee use. In other words, we could not expect condition C (or C') to hold, and so we should expect our estimates to suffer from confounding. This is so, regardless of whether adjustment appears to change the association of coffee use and myocardial infarction (Greenland *et al.* 1999).

Some studies have found a positive association between cigarette smoking (an established risk factor for myocardial infarction) and coffee use (Greenland 1993). It also seems a *priori* sensible that a person habituated to a stimulant such as nicotine would be attracted to coffee use as well. Thus, we should expect to see a higher prevalence of smoking among coffee users in our study.

Suppose then that, in our cohort, smoking is more prevalent among five-cup-a-day subjects than never-drinkers. This elevated smoking prevalence should have led to elevated myocardial infarction rates among five-cup-a-day drinkers, even if coffee had no effect. More generally, we should expect the myocardial infarction rate among never-drinkers to underestimate the myocardial infarction rate that five-cup-a-day drinkers would have had if they had never drunk coffee. The result would be an inflated estimate of the impact of coffee on the myocardial infarction rate of five-cup-a-day drinkers. Similarly, we should expect the myocardial infarction rate among five-cup-a-day drinkers to overestimate the myocardial infarction rate that never-drinkers would have had if they had drunk five cups a day.

Adjustment for measured confounders

As in the prediction problem, we can stratify the data on potential confounders with the objective of creating strata within which confounding is minimal or absent. We can also employ standardization to remove confounding from estimates of overall effect. Again, some care in the selection of the standard is required.

To illustrate, let R_{xz} denote the estimated rate of myocardial infarction among cohort members who drank x cups of coffee per day and smoked z cigarettes per day at baseline, with R_{0z} denoting the estimated rate among never-drinkers. Let W_{xz} denote the proportion of person-time among x-cup-per-day drinkers that was contributed by z-cigarette-per-day smokers. Finally, let R_{xc} be the crude (unadjusted) rate observed among cohort members who drank x cups per day at baseline, with R_{0c} denoting the estimated crude rate among never-drinkers.

Suppose for the moment that any change in coffee-use patterns would have negligible impact on the person-time distribution of smoking in the cohort. The predicted (i.e. expected) rate among five-cup-a-day drinkers had they never drunk coffee, adjusted for confounding by smoking, is the average of the smoking-specific estimates from the never-drinker (reference) subcohort weighted by the smoking distribution of the five-cup-per-day (target) cohort. Algebraically, this average is the following sum (over z):

$$\Sigma_z W_{5z} R_{0z},$$

This sum is commonly termed the rate in the never-drinkers standardized to the distribution of smoking among five-cup-a-day drinkers. Such terminology obscures the fact that the sum is a prediction about the five-cup-a-day drinkers, not the never-drinkers.

Given the last computation, a smoking-standardized estimate of the increase in myocardial infarction rate produced by coffee drinking among five-cup-per-day drinkers is the rate ratio standardized to the five-cup-per-day smoking distribution:

$$\Sigma_z W_{5z} R_{5z} / \Sigma_z W_{5z} R_{0z}$$

This formula reveals a property common to a simple standardized rate ratio: The same weights W_{xz} must be used in the numerator and denominator sums. Some insight into this formula can be obtained by noting that the crude rate R_{5c}, among the five-cup-a-day drinkers, is equal to

$$\Sigma_z W_{5z} R_{5z}$$

so that the standardized rate ratio can be rewritten as

$$R_{5c} / \Sigma_z W_{5z} R_{0z}.$$

This version shows that the ratio is a classical observed (crude) over expected ratio, or standardized morbidity ratio (SMR). Another standardized rate ratio is

$$\Sigma_z W_{0z} R_{5z} / \Sigma_z W_{0z} R_{0z}$$

This differs from the previous standardized ratio in that the weights are taken from the never-drinkers (W_{0z}) instead of five-cup-a-day drinkers (W_{5z}). Insight into this formula can be obtained by noting that the numerator sum is simply a prediction (expectation) of what would have happened to the never-drinkers if they had been five-cup-a-day drinkers, and the denominator sum is equal to the crude rate R_{0c}, among never-drinkers. Thus, the last standardized ratio is a smoking-standardized estimate of the increase in the myocardial infarction rate that five-cup-a-day drinking would have produced among the never-drinkers.

Standardization is appealingly simple in both justification and computation. Unfortunately, if the number of cases occurring within the confounder categories tends to be small (under five or so), the technique will be subject to various technical problems including possible bias. These problems can be avoided by broadening confounder categories or by not adjusting for some of the measured confounders. Unfortunately, both these strategies are likely to result in incomplete control of confounding. To avoid having to adopt these strategies, many researchers attempt to control confounding by using a multivariate model. This remedy has problems of its own, some of which we shall address in the subsection on specification validity.

Another problem is that standardized procedures (as well as typical modelling procedures) take no account of potential exposure effects on the adjustment variables or their distribution. Thus, in the preceding example, to justify use of the fixed weights W_{xz} we had to invoke the dubious assumption that changes in coffee use would only negligibly affect the smoking distribution. We shall briefly discuss this issue in the subsection on intermediate variables.

Unmeasured confounders

Among the possible confounders not measured in our hypothetical study are diet and exercise. Suppose that 'health conscious' subjects who exercise regularly and eat low-fat diets also avoid coffee. The result will be a concentration of these lower-risk subjects among coffee non-users and a consequent overestimation of coffee's effect on risk.

Confounding by unmeasured confounders can sometimes be minimized by controlling variables along the pathways of their effect. For example, if exercise and low-fat diet lowered myocardial infarction risk only by lowering serum cholesterol and blood pressure, control of serum cholesterol and blood pressure would remove confounding by exercise and dietary fat. Unfortunately, such control may also generate bias if the controlled variables are intermediates between our study variable and our outcome variable.

If external information is available to indicate the relationship in our study between an unmeasured confounder and the study variables, we can attempt to use an indirect method to adjust for the confounder; even if external information is unreliable or unavailable, we can examine the sensitivity of our results to unmeasured confounders (Greenland & Lash 2008). Finally, we can evaluate the impact that uncertainty about unmeasured confounders should have on our final inferences about the effect (Greenland 2003; Greenland & Lash 2008).

Randomization and confounding

Suppose, for the moment, that the level of coffee use in our cohort had been assigned by randomization and that the participants diligently consumed only their assigned amount of coffee. Could our estimates of coffee effects from such a randomized trial still be confounded? By our earlier definition of confounding, the answer is yes. To see this, note for example that by chance alone the five-cup-a-day drinkers could be older on average than the never-drinkers; this difference would in turn result in an upward bias in the unadjusted estimate of the effect of five cups a day, because age is an important risk factor for myocardial infarction.

Nevertheless, randomization can help to ensure that the distributions of confounders in the different exposure groups are not too far apart. In essence, the probability of severe confounding can be made as small as necessary by increasing the size of the randomized groups. Furthermore, if randomization is used and subjects comply with their assigned treatments, any confounding left after adjustment will be accounted for by the standard errors of the estimates, provided that the correct statistical model is used to compute the effect estimates and their standard errors (Greenland 1990; Robins 1988).

Intermediate variables

In effect estimation, we must take care to distinguish intermediate variables from confounding variables. Intermediate variables represent steps in the causal pathway from the study exposure to the outcome event. The distinction is essential, for control of intermediate variables can increase the bias of estimates.

To illustrate, suppose that coffee use affects serum cholesterol levels (as suggested by the results of Curb *et al.* 1986) Then, given that serum cholesterol affects myocardial infarction risk, serum cholesterol is an intermediate variable for the study of the effects of coffee on this risk. Now suppose that we stratify our cohort data on serum cholesterol levels. Some coffee drinkers will be in elevated cholesterol categories because of coffee use and so will be have an elevated risk of myocardial infarction, yet these subjects will be compared with never-drinkers in the same stratum who are also at elevated risk due to their elevated cholesterol. Therefore, the effect of coffee on the risk of myocardial infarction via the cholesterol pathway will not be apparent within the cholesterol strata, and so cholesterol adjustment will contribute to underestimation of the effect of coffee on risk of myocardial infarction. Analogously, if coffee affected the risk of myocardial infarction by elevating blood pressure, blood pressure adjustment will contribute to underestimation of the effect of coffee. Such underestimation can be termed *overadjustment bias.*

Intermediate variables may also be confounders and thus present the investigator with a severe dilemma. Consider that most of the variation in serum cholesterol levels is not due to coffee use and that much (perhaps most) of the association between coffee use and cholesterol is not due to the effects of coffee, but rather to factors associated with both coffee and cholesterol (such as exercise and dietary fat). This means that serum cholesterol may also be viewed as a confounder for the coffee–myocardial infarction study and that estimates unadjusted for serum cholesterol will be biased unless they are also adjusted for the factors contributing to the coffee–cholesterol association.

Suppose that a variable is both an intermediate and a confounder. It will usually be impossible to determine how much of the change in the effect estimate produced by adjusting for the variable is due to introduction of overadjustment bias and how much is due to removal of confounding. Nevertheless, a qualitative assessment may be possible in some situations. For example, if we know that the effects of coffee on serum cholesterol are weak and that most of the association between coffee and serum cholesterol is due to confounding of this association by uncontrolled factors (such as exercise and diet), we can conclude that the cholesterol-adjusted estimate is the less biased of the two. Alternatively, if we have accurately measured all the factors that confound the coffee–cholesterol association, we can control these factors instead of cholesterol to obtain an estimate free of both overadjustment bias and confounding by cholesterol. Finally, if we have multiple measurements of coffee use and cholesterol over time, techniques are available that adjust for the confounding effects of cholesterol but do not introduce overadjustment (Robins & Greenland 1994; Robins *et al.* 2000).

Direct and indirect effects

Often, one may wish to estimate how much of the effect under study is indirect relative to an intermediate variable (in the sense of being transmitted through the intermediate), or how much of the effect is direct relative to the intermediate (i.e. not mediated by the intermediate). For example, we might wish to estimate how much of the effect of coffee on myocardial infarction risk is due to its effect on serum cholesterol, or how much is due to the effects of coffee on cardiovascular variables other than cholesterol.

One common approach to this problem is to adjust the coffee–myocardial infarction association for serum cholesterol level via ordinary stratification or regression methods and then use the resulting estimate as the estimate of the direct effect of coffee. This procedure is potentially biased as it may introduce new confounding by determinants of serum cholesterol, even if these determinants did not confound the total (unadjusted) association (Cole & Hermán 2002; Glymour & Greenland 2008; Robins & Greenland 1992). Nonetheless, given sufficient data, it is possible to obtain separate estimates for direct and indirect effects using special stratification or modelling techniques (Robins & Greenland 1994; Kaufman *et al.* 2005).

Effect modification (heterogeneity of effect)

Estimation of effects usually requires consideration of effect-measure modification, which is also known as effect modification, effect variation, or heterogeneity of effect. As an example, suppose that drinking five cups of coffee a day elevated the myocardial infarction rate of men in our cohort by a factor of 1.40 (i.e. a 40 per cent increase), but elevated the myocardial infarction rate of women by a factor of only 1.10 (i.e. a 10 per cent increase). This situation would be termed modification (or variation or heterogeneity) of the rate ratio by gender, and gender would be called a modifier of the coffee–myocardial infarction rate ratio.

As another example, suppose that drinking five cups of coffee a day elevated the myocardial infarction rate in men in our cohort by a factor of 400 cases per 100 000 person-years but elevated the rate in women by a factor of only 40 cases per 100 000 person-years. This situation would be termed modification of the rate difference by gender, and gender would be called a modifier of the coffee–myocardial infarction rate difference.

As a final example, suppose that drinking five cups of coffee per day elevated the myocardial infarction rate in our cohort by a factor of 1.22 in both men and women. This situation would be termed homogeneity of the rate ratios across gender.

Effect modification and homogeneity are not absolute properties of an effect, but instead are properties of the way that the effect is measured. For example, suppose that drinking five cups of coffee per day elevated the myocardial infarction rate in men from 1000 cases per 100 000 person-years to 1220 cases per 100 000 person-years, but elevated the rate in women from 400 cases per 100 000 person-years to 488 cases per 100 000 person-years. Then the gender-specific rate ratios would both be 1.22, homogeneous across gender. In contrast, the gender-specific rate differences would be 220 cases per 100 000 person-years for males and 88 cases per 100 000 person-years for females, and so are heterogeneous or 'modified' by gender. Examples such as this one show that one should not equate effect modification with biological concepts of interaction such as synergy or antagonism (Rothman & Greenland 1998).

Effect modification can be analysed by stratifying the data on the potential effect modifier under study, estimating the effect within each stratum, and comparing the estimates across strata. There are several potential problems with this approach. The number of subjects in each stratum may be too small to produce stable estimates of stratum-specific effects, particularly after adjustment for confounder effects. Estimates may fluctuate wildly from stratum to stratum owing to random error. A related problem is that statistical tests for heterogeneity in stratified data have extremely low power in many situations, and therefore are likely to miss much if not most of the heterogeneity when used with conventional significance levels (such as 0.05). Finally, the amount of bias from confounding, loss to follow-up, measurement error, and other sources may vary from stratum to stratum, in which case the observed pattern of modification will be biased.

Effect modification and generalizability

Suppose that we succeed in obtaining approximately unbiased (internally valid) estimates from our study. We can then confront the issues of generalizability (external validity) of our results. For example, we can ask whether they accurately reflect the effect of coffee on myocardial infarction rates in a new target cohort. We can view such a question as a prediction problem in which the objective is to predict the strength of the effects of coffee in the new target cohort. From this perspective, generalizability of an effect estimate involves just one additional validity issue, namely confounding of the predicted effect by effect modifiers.

Suppose that the rate increase (in cases per 100 000 person-years) produced by coffee use is 400 for males and 40 for females among five-cup-a-day drinkers in both our study cohort and the new target. If our study cohort is 70 per cent male while the new target is only 30 per cent male, the average increase among five-cup-a-day drinkers in our study cohort would be $0.7 \times 400 + 0.3 \times 40 = 292$, whereas the average increase in the new target would be only $0.3 \times 400 + 0.7 \times 40 = 148$. Thus, any valid estimate of the average increase in our study cohort will tend to overestimate greatly the average increase in the new target. In other words, modification of the effect of coffee by gender confounds the prediction of its effect in the new target. This bias can be avoided by making only gender-specific predictions of effect or by standardizing the study results to the gender distribution of the new target population.

Follow-up validity

In our example, follow-up validity means that follow-up is valid within every subcohort being compared. In other words, over any span of time during follow-up, risk of myocardial infarction within a subcohort is unassociated with censoring risk in the subcohort. Given follow-up validity, we can expect that, at any follow-up time t, the myocardial infarction rates in a subcohort will be the same for subjects lost or withdrawn at t and subjects whose follow-up continues beyond t.

In fact, we should expect follow-up to be biased by cigarette smoking: Smoking is associated with mortality from myocardial infarction and from many other causes; the association of smoking with socio-economic status might also produce an association between smoking and loss to follow-up. The result would be elevated censoring among high-risk (smoking) subjects. As a consequence, unadjusted estimates of the risks of myocardial infarction will underestimate those risks in the complete subcohorts (as the latter includes both censored and uncensored subject experience). If the degree of underestimation varies across subcohorts, bias in the relative-risk estimates will result.

In fact, the degree of underestimation should vary in this example because of the variation in the prevalence of smoking across subcohorts. Nevertheless, this variation is not necessary for smoking-related censoring to produce biased estimates of absolute effect. For example, if smoking-related censoring produced a uniform 15 per cent underestimation of the myocardial infarction rate in each subcohort, all rate differences would also be underestimated by 15 per cent.

Analogous to control of confounding, any bias produced by the association of smoking with myocardial infarction and censoring can be removed by smoking adjustment. As before, if adjustment is by standardization, the standard distribution should be chosen from the target subcohort.

Because the same correction methods can sometimes be applied, some authors classify follow-up bias as a form of confounding. Nevertheless, the two phenomena are reversed with respect to the causal ordering of the third variable responsible for the bias: Confounding arises from an association of the study exposure (coffee use) with other exposures (such as smoking) that affect outcome risk; in contrast, follow-up bias arises from an association between the risk of the study outcome (myocardial infarction) and risks of other end points (such as other-cause mortality or loss to follow-up) that are affected by exposure, and thus is classified as a form of selection bias by many authors (Kelsey *et al.* 1996; Hernán *et al.* 2004). In this regard, note that certain forms of follow-up bias cannot be removed by adjustment, and thus do not resemble confounding (Hernán *et al.* 2004; Glymour & Greenland 2008). These problems are discussed in the statistics literature under the heading dependent competing risks and resemble the selection-bias problems of case–control studies (discussed later).

Measurement validity

Unlike gender, the continuous variables of coffee use, cigarette use, blood pressure, cholesterol, and age are time-dependent covariates. With the exception of age (whose value at any time can be computed from birth date), this fact adds considerable complexity to measuring these variables and estimating their effects.

Consider that we cannot reasonably expect a single baseline measurement, no matter how accurate, to summarize adequately a subject's entire history of coffee drinking, smoking, blood pressure, or cholesterol. Even if the effect of a subject's history could be largely captured by using a single summary number (e.g. total number of cigarettes smoked), the baseline measurement may well be a poor proxy for this ideal and unknown summary. For these reasons, we should expect proxy-variable errors to be very large in our example.

Proxy-variable error in the study variables

The degree of proxy-variable error in measuring the study variables depends on the exact definitions of the variables that we wish to study. In turn, this definition should reflect the hypothesized effect that we wish to study. To illustrate, consider the following acute-effect hypothesis:

> *Drinking a cup of coffee produces an immediate rise in short-term myocardial infarction risk. In other words, coffee consumption is an acute risk factor.*

This hypothesis does not exclude the possibility that coffee use also elevates long-term risk of myocardial infarction, perhaps through some other mechanism; it simply does not address the issue of chronic effects.

One way to examine the hypothesis would be to compare the myocardial infarction rates among person-days in which one, two, three, or more cups were drunk with the rate among person-days in which no coffee was drunk (adjusting for confounding and follow-up bias). If we had only baseline data, baseline daily consumption would have to serve as the proxy for consumption on every day of follow-up. This would probably be a poor proxy for daily consumption at later follow-up times where more outcome events occur. A 'standard' analysis, which only examines the association of baseline coffee use with myocardial infarction rates, is equivalent to an analysis that uses baseline consumption as a proxy for consumption on all later days. Thus, estimates from a standard analysis would suffer large bias if considered as estimates of the acute effects of coffee.

The proxy-variable error in this example could easily be differential with respect to the outcome: Person-days accumulate more rapidly in early follow-up, where the error from using baseline consumption as the proxy is relatively low; in contrast, myocardial infarction events accumulate more rapidly in later follow-up, where the error is probably higher. This difference in accumulation illustrates an important general point: Errors in variables can be differential, even if the variables are measured before the outcome event. Such phenomena occur when errors are associated with risk factors for the outcome; in our example, the error is associated with follow-up time and hence age. In turn, such associations are likely to occur when measurements are based on proxy variables.

Suppose now that we examine the following chronic-effect hypothesis:

> *Each cup of coffee drunk eventually results in a long-term elevation of myocardial infarction risk.*

This hypothesis was suggested by reports that coffee drinking produces a rise in serum lipid levels (Curb *et al.* 1986); it does not address the issue of acute effects. One way to examine the hypothesis would be to compare the myocardial infarction rates among person-months with different cumulative doses of coffee (perhaps using a lag period in calculating dose; e.g. one might ignore the most recent month of consumption). If we had only baseline data, however, baseline daily consumption would have to be used to construct a proxy for cumulative consumption at every month of follow-up. This construction could be done in several different ways. For example, we could estimate the subjects' cumulative doses up to a particular date by multiplying their baseline daily consumption by the number of days that they had lived between age 18 and the date in question. This estimate assumes that coffee drinking began at age 18 and the baseline daily consumption is the average daily consumption since that age. We should expect considerable error in such a crude measure of cumulative consumption.

The degree of bias in estimating chronic effects could be quite different from the degree of bias in estimating acute effects. Furthermore, as discussed in the following, the errors in each proxy will make it virtually impossible to discriminate between acute and chronic effects.

Measurement error and confounding

If a variable is measured with error, estimates adjusted for the variable as measured will still be somewhat confounded by the variable. This residual confounding arises because measurement error prevents construction of strata that are internally homogeneous with respect to the true confounding variable (Greenland 1980).

To illustrate, consider baseline daily cigarette consumption. This variable can be considered a proxy for consumption on each day of follow-up or can be used to construct an estimate of cumulative consumption (analogous to the cumulative coffee variable discussed in the preceding). Suppose that we stratify the data on a cumulative smoking index constructed from the baseline smoking measurement. Within any stratum of the index, there would remain a broad range of cumulative cigarette consumption. For example, two subjects who were age 40 and smoked one pack a day at baseline would receive the same value for the smoking index and so end up in the same stratum. However, if one of them stopped smoking immediately after baseline, while the other continued to smoke a pack a day, after 10 years of follow-up the former subject would have ten less pack-years of cigarette consumption than the continuing smoker.

Suppose now that cumulative cigarette consumption is positively associated with cumulative coffee consumption. Then, even within strata of the smoking index, we should expect subjects with high coffee consumption to exhibit elevated myocardial infarction rates simply by virtue of having higher levels of cigarette consumption. As a consequence, the estimate of the effect of coffee adjusted for the smoking index would still be confounded by cumulative cigarette consumption.

In some cases, a study variable may appear to have an effect (or no effect) only because of poor measurement of an apparently unimportant confounder. This can occur, for example, when an important confounding variable is measured with a large amount of non-differential error. Such an error would ordinarily reduce the apparent association of the variable with the exposure, and would also make the variable appear to be a weak risk factor, perhaps weaker than the study exposure. This in turn would make the variable appear to be only weakly confounding, in that adjustment for the variable as measured would produce little change in the result. However, this appearance would be deceptive because adjustment for the variable as measured would eliminate little of the actual confounding by the variable.

As an example, suppose that coronary proneness of personality was measured only by the baseline yes or no question: Do you consider yourself a hard-driving person? Such a crude measure of the original construct would be unlikely to show more than a weak association with either coffee use or myocardial infarction, and adjusting for it would produce little change in our estimate of the effect of coffee. Suppose, however, that coronary-prone personalities have an elevated preference for coffee. Such a phenomenon would lead to a concentration of coronary-prone persons (and hence, a spuriously elevated myocardial infarction rate) among coffee drinkers, even after stratification on the response to the question.

One would ordinarily expect adjustment for a non-differentially misclassified confounder to produce an estimate lying somewhere between the crude (unadjusted) estimate and the estimate adjusted for the true values of the confounder (Greenland 1980). Unfortunately, if the true confounder has more than two levels, it is possible for adjustment by the misclassified confounder to be more biased than the crude estimate (Brenner 1993). It is also possible for adjustment by factors that affect misclassification to worsen bias (Greenland & Robins 1985).

Measurement error and separation of effects

Because of their impact on the effectiveness of adjustment procedures, measurement errors can severely reduce our ability to separate different effects of the study variable. Suppose in our example that we wished to estimate the relative strength of acute and chronic effects of coffee. To do so, we must take account of the fact that acute and chronic effects will be confounded. When examining acute effects, person-days with high coffee consumption will occur most frequently among persons with high cumulative coffee consumption. As a consequence, if cumulative coffee consumption is a risk factor, it will be a confounder for estimating the acute effects of coffee consumption. By similar arguments, if coffee consumption has acute effects, these will confound estimates of the chronic effects of cumulative consumption.

Unfortunately, both cumulative and daily consumption are measured with considerable error. As a result, any effect observed for one may be wholly or partially due to the other, even if the other has little or no apparent effect.

Repeated measures

One costly but effective method for reducing the degree of proxy-variable error in measuring time-dependent variables is to take repeated (serial) measurements over the follow-up period and ask subjects to report their pre-baseline history of such variables at the baseline interview. In our example, subjects could be asked about their age at first use and level of consumption at different ages for coffee and cigarettes; they could then be recontacted every year or two to assess their current consumption. Of course, not all subjects may be willing to cooperate with such active follow-up, but the penalties of some extra loss may be far outweighed by the benefit of improved measurement accuracy.

Errors in assessing incidence

An important form of measurement error in assessing incidence is misdiagnosis of the outcome event. In the AIDS example, a false-positive diagnosis of AIDS would result in underestimation of incubation time, whereas a false-negative diagnosis would result in overestimation. In the present example, false-positive errors would result in overestimation of myocardial infarction rates, whereas false-negative errors would result in underestimation. These errors will be of particular concern when the study depends on existing surveillance systems or records for detection of outcome events.

There are special cases in which the errors will induce little or no bias in estimates, provided the errors have little effect on the person-time observed. If the only form of misdiagnosis is false-negative error, the proportion of outcome events missed in this fashion is the same across cohorts, and if there is no follow-up bias, then the relative-risk estimates will not be distorted by the underdiagnosis. Suppose in our example that all recorded myocardial infarction events are true myocardial infarctions, but that in each subcohort 10 per cent of myocardial infarctions are missed. The myocardial infarction rates in each subcohort will then be underestimated by 10 per cent; nevertheless, if we consider any two of these rates, say R_0 and R_5, the observed rate ratio will be

$$\frac{0.9R_5}{0.9R_0} = \frac{R_5}{R_0}$$

which is undistorted by the underdiagnosis of myocardial infarction. Nonetheless, if coffee primarily induced 'silent' myocardial infarctions and these were the most frequently undiagnosed events, the effect of coffee would be underestimated.

Analogously, if the only form of misdiagnosis is false-positive error, the rate of false positives is the same across cohorts, and if there is no follow-up bias, then rate differences will not be distorted by the overdiagnosis. Suppose that the rate of false positives in our example is R_f in all subcohorts; then, if we consider any two true rates, say R_0 and R_5, the observed rate difference will

$$(R_5 + R_f) - (R_0 + R_f) = R_5 - R_0,$$

which is undistorted by the overdiagnosis of myocardial infarction. However, if there is non-differential underdiagnosis of myocardial infarction, as is probably the case in our example, the rate difference will be underestimated.

Specification validity

As noted earlier, the use of a statistical method based on an incorrect model (specification error) can lead to bias in estimates and improper performance of statistical tests and interval estimates. All statistical techniques, including non-parametric methods, must assume some sort of model for the process generating the data; however, in the absence of randomization or random sampling, it will rarely be possible to identify a 'correct' sampling model. In addition, structural assumptions are rarely (if ever) exactly satisfied. Thus, some specification error should be expected. As before, minimization of specification error must rely on checking the model against the data and against background information about the processes generating the data.

Recall that the unadjusted rate ratio estimates for five-cup-a-day versus never-drinkers is 1.22 in the present example, with 95 per cent confidence limits of 1.00 and 1.49, and a P value of 0.05. Suppose that these figures were obtained by conventional person-time methods (Rothman & Greenland 1998; Hastie & Tibshirani 1990). These methods are based on a binomial sampling model for the number of cases who drank five cups a day at baseline, given the combined total number of cases among five-cup-a-day and never-drinkers. In our example, the validity of this model depends on the assumption that the myocardial infarction rate remains constant within subcohorts over the follow-up period. It follows that the model (and hence the statistics given earlier) cannot be valid in our example; the subcohort members grow older over the follow-up period, and hence the myocardial infarction rates must increase with follow-up time.

The invalidity just noted can be rectified by stratifying either on follow-up time or the variable responsible for the change in rates over follow-up time (here, age). The stratification need only be fine enough to ensure that the myocardial infarction rate change within strata is negligible over follow-up. As noted earlier, however, we must also adjust for smoking and perhaps other factors responsible for confounding or follow-up bias. If we stratify finely enough to remove all the bias from these sources, the resulting estimates would be undefined or so unstable that they would tell us nothing about the association of coffee and myocardial infarction.

The standard solution to such problems is to compute adjusted estimates using regression models. These are structural models representing a set of assumptions (usually rather strong ones) about the joint effects of the study variables. Such models allow estimates and tests to be extracted from what would otherwise be hopelessly sparse data, at a cost of a greater risk of bias arising from violations of the assumptions underlying the models (Robins & Greenland 1986). For further details of cohort modelling, see Breslow and Day (1987), Hosmer and Lemeshow (2000), Kelsey *et al.* (1996), Rothman and Greenland (1998), Checkoway *et al.* (2004), and Jewell (2004).

Summary of cohort example

The example used in this subsection provides an illustration of the most common threats to the validity of effect estimates from cohort studies. The unadjusted estimates of the effect of coffee on myocardial infarction will be confounded by many variables (such as smoking), and there will be follow-up bias. As a result, the number of variables that must be controlled is too large to allow adequate control using only stratification. The true functional dependence of myocardial infarction rates on coffee and the confounder is unknown, so that estimates based on multivariate models are likely to be biased. Even if this bias is unimportant, our estimates will remain confounded because of our inability to measure the key confounders accurately. Finally, our inability to summarize coffee consumption accurately would further bias our estimates, making it impossible to separate acute and chronic effects of coffee use reliably.

Given that there are several sources of bias of unknown magnitude and different directions, it would appear that no conclusions about the effect of coffee could be drawn from a study such as the one described in the preceding, other than that coffee does not appear to have a large effect. This type of result—inconclusive, other than to rule out very large effects—is common in thorough epidemiological analyses of observational data. In particular, inconclusive results are common when the data being analysed were collected for purposes other than to address the hypothesis at issue, for such data often lack accurate measurements of key variables.

Special issues in case–control studies

The practical difficulties of cohort studies have led to extensive development of case–control study designs. The distinguishing feature of such designs is that sampling is intentionally based on the outcome of individuals. In a population-based or population-initiated case–control study, one first identifies a population at risk of the outcome of interest, which is to be studied over a specified period of time or risk period. As in a cohort study, one attempts to ascertain outcome events in the population at risk. Nevertheless, unlike a cohort study, one selects persons experiencing the outcome event (cases) and a 'control' sample of the entire population at risk for ascertainment of exposure and covariate status.

In a case-initiated case–control study, one starts by identifying a source of study cases (e.g. a hospital emergency room is a source of myocardial infarction cases). One then attempts to identify a population at risk such that the source of cases provides a random or complete sample of all cases occurring in this population. Study cases recruited from the source occur over a risk period; controls are selected in order to ascertain the distribution of exposure in the population at risk over that period. Case–control studies may also begin with an existing series of controls (Greenland 1985). Regardless of how a case–control study is initiated, evaluation of validity must ultimately refer to a population at risk that represents the target of inference for the study.

Relative-risk estimation in case–control studies

The control sample may or may not be selected in a manner that excludes cases. If persons who become cases over the risk period are ineligible for inclusion in the control group (as in traditional case–control designs), a 'rare disease' assumption may be needed to estimate relative risks from the case–control data. In contrast, if persons who become cases over the risk period are also eligible for inclusion in the control group (as in newer case–control designs), the rare disease assumption can be discarded. These points are discussed in the textbooks cited at the beginning of this chapter.

The basics of case–control estimation will be illustrated using the following example. We wish to study the effect of coffee drinking on rates of first myocardial infarction and we have selected a population for study (e.g. all residents aged 40–64 in a particular town) over a one-year risk period. At any point during the risk period, the population at risk comprises persons in this selected population who have not yet had a myocardial infarction.

Suppose that the average number of never-drinkers in the population at risk was 20 000 over the risk period, the average number of five-cup-a-day drinkers was 10 000, there were 120 first myocardial infarctions among never-drinkers, and there were 90 first myocardial infarctions among five-cup-a-day drinkers. Then, if one observed the entire population without error, the estimated rates among never-drinkers and five-cup-a-day drinkers would be:

$$\frac{120}{20000 \text{ person–years}} = \frac{90}{10000 \text{ person–years}}$$

Thus, if we observed the entire population, the estimated rate ratio would be:

$$\frac{90/10000\,\text{person–years}}{120/20000 \text{ person–years}} = \frac{90/120}{10000/20000 \text{ person–years}} = 1.50$$

This estimate depends on only two figures: The relative prevalence of five-cup-a-day versus never-drinkers among cases (90/120), and the same relative prevalence in the person-years at risk (10 000/20 000). These two relative prevalences are often called the case exposure odds and the population exposure odds.

The first relative prevalence (numerator) could be estimated by interviewing an unbiased sample of all the new myocardial infarction cases that occur over the risk period, and the second relative prevalence (denominator) could be estimated by interviewing an unbiased sample of the population at risk over the risk period. The ratio of relative prevalences from the case- and control-sample interviews would then be an unbiased estimate of the population rate ratio of 1.50. This estimate is called the *sample odds ratio*.

Three points about the preceding argument should be carefully noted. First, no rare disease assumption was made. Second, the control sample of the population at risk was accumulated over the entire risk period (rather than at the end of the risk period); such sampling is called *density sampling* (Rothman & Greenland 1998) or *risk-set sampling* (Breslow & Day 1987). Third, because of the density sampling, someone may be selected for the control sample, and yet have a myocardial infarction later in the risk period and become part of the case sample as well. Methods for carrying out density sampling can be found in the textbooks cited at the beginning of this chapter.

Validity conditions in case–control studies

The primary advantages of case–control studies are their short time frame and the large reduction in the number of subjects needed to achieve the same statistical power as a cohort study. The primary disadvantage is that more conditions must be met to ensure their validity (in addition to the four listed in the cohort study example), and hence, there are more opportunities for bias to arise.

Suppose that our case–control study data yield an unadjusted rate-ratio estimate (odds ratio) of 1.50, with 95 per cent confidence limits of 1.00 and 2.25. The following series of conditions would be sufficient for the validity of this figure as an estimate of the effect of drinking five cups of coffee a day (versus none) on the myocardial infarction rate:

(C) *Comparison validity*—If five-cup-a-day drinkers in the population at risk had instead drunk no coffee, their distribution of myocardial infarction events over time would have been approximately the same as the distribution among never-drinkers.

(F) *Follow-up validity*—Within each subpopulation defined by coffee use, censoring risk (i.e. population membership ended by an event other than myocardial infarction, such as emigration or death from another cause) is not associated with myocardial-infarction risk.

(Se) *Selection validity*—This has two components:

1. *Case-selection validity*—If one studies only a subset of the myocardial infarction cases occurring in the population over the risk period (e.g. because of failure to detect all cases), this subset provides unbiased estimates of the prevalence of different levels of coffee use among all cases occurring in the population over the risk period.
2. *Control-selection validity*—The control sample provides unbiased estimates of the prevalences of different levels of coffee use in the population at risk over the risk period.

(Sp) *Specification validity*—The distribution of myocardial infarction events over time in the subpopulations can be closely approximated by the statistical model on which the estimates are based.

(M) *Measurement validity*—All measurements of variables used in the analysis closely approximate the true values of the variables.

Issues of comparison validity, follow-up validity, specification validity, effect modification, and generalizability in case–control studies parallel those in follow-up studies, and so will not be discussed here. Case–control studies are vulnerable to certain problems of measurement error that are less severe or do not exist in prospective cohort studies. We shall discuss these problems first, and then examine selection validity and modelling. Finally, we shall briefly discuss analogous issues in retrospective cohort studies.

Retrospective ascertainment

A special class of measurement errors arises from the retrospective ascertainment of time-dependent variables; that is, attempting to measure past values of the variables. Retrospective ascertainment must be based on individual memories, existing records of past values, or some combination of the two. Therefore, such ascertainment usually suffers from faulty recall, missing or mistaken records, or lack of direct measurements in existing records.

Retrospective ascertainment may be an important component of a cohort study. For example, the cohort study of coffee and myocardial infarction discussed earlier could have been improved by asking subjects about their coffee use and smoking prior to the start of follow-up. This information would allow one to construct better cumulative indices than could be constructed from baseline consumption alone, although the resulting indices would still incorporate error due to faulty recall.

Unless records of past measurements are available for all subjects, measurements on cases and controls must be made after the time period under study as subjects are not selected for study until after that period. Thus, unlike cohort studies, most case–control studies of time-dependent variables depend on retrospective ascertainment. Considering our example, there may be much more error in determining daily coffee consumption ten years before interview than one month before interview; one might then expect case–control studies to be more accurate for studying acute effects than for studying chronic effects. Nonetheless, if acute and chronic effects are heavily confounded, the elevated inaccuracies of long-term recall will make it impossible to disentangle short-term from long-term effects. As illustrated earlier, this confounding can arise in a cohort study. Nevertheless, in a cohort study, such confounding can be minimized by taking repeated measurements. In contrast, such confounding would be unavoidable in a case–control study based on recall, even if detailed longitudinal histories were requested from the subjects.

The preceding observations should be tempered by noting that some case–control studies have access to exposure measurements of the same quality as found in cohort studies and that the exposure measurements in some cohort studies may be no better than those used in some case–control studies. For example, a cohort study in which measurements are derived by abstracting routine medical records would suffer from no less measurement error than a case–control study in which measurements are derived by abstracting the same records.

Outcome-affected measurements

One common potential problem in case–control studies is outcome-affected recall, often termed *recall bias*. This term refers to the differential measurement error that originates when the outcome event affects recall of past events. Examples arise in case–control studies of birth defects, for instance. If the trauma of having an affected child either enhances recall of prenatal exposures among case mothers or increases the frequency of false-positive reports among them, estimates of relative risk will be upwardly biased by effects of the outcome on case recall. This bias may be counterbalanced by other biases, such as recall bias among controls, making the final direction and magnitude of bias due to faulty measurements hard to predict (Drews & Greenland 1990).

One method commonly proposed for preventing bias due to outcome-affected recall is to restrict controls to a group believed to have recall similar to the cases. Unfortunately, one usually cannot tell to what degree this restricted selection corrects the bias from outcome-affected recall. Even more unfortunately, one usually cannot tell if the selection bias produced by such restriction is worse than the recall bias one is attempting to correct (Swan *et al.* 1990; Drews *et al.* 1990.

A problem similar to outcome-affected recall can occur when the outcome event affects a psychological or physiological measurement. This is of particular concern in case–control studies of nutrient levels and chronic disease. For example, if colon cancer leads to a drop in serum retinol levels, the relative risk for the effect of serum retinol will be underestimated if serum retinol is measured after the cancer develops. Errors of this type can be viewed as proxy-variable errors in which the post-outcome value is a poor proxy for the pre-outcome value of interest.

Selection validity

Selection validity is straightforward to understand but can be extraordinarily difficult to verify. A violation of the selection validity conditions is known as selection bias. Many case–control designs and field methods are devoted to avoiding such bias (Kelsey *et al.* 1996; Rothman & Greenland 1998; Koepsell & Weiss 2003; Schlesselman 1982).

In some instances, it may be possible to identify a factor or factors that affect chance of selection into the study. If in such instances we have accurate measurements of one of these factors, we can stratify on (or otherwise adjust for) the factor and thereby remove the selection bias due to the factor. Because of this possibility, some authors classify selection bias as a form of confounding. Nevertheless, there are some forms of selection bias that cannot be removed by adjustment. These points will be illustrated in the following subsections.

Case-selection validity

Case-selection bias can be minimized (although may still be large due to non-participation) if one can identify every case that occurs in the population at risk over the risk period. This requires a surveillance system for the outcome of interest, such as a population-based disease registry. In our coffee–myocardial infarction example, we would probably have to construct a myocardial infarction surveillance system from existing resources, such as emergency room admission records, ambulance service records, and paramedic records.

Even if all cases of interest can be identified, selection bias may arise from failure to obtain information on all the cases. In our example, many cases would be dead before interview was possible.

For such cases, there are only two alternatives: Attempt to obtain information from some other source, such as next of kin or co-workers, or exclude such cases from the study. The first alternative increases measurement error in the study. The second alternative will introduce bias if coffee affects risk of fatal and non-fatal myocardial infarction differently, or if coffee affects risk of myocardial infarction survivorship. To illustrate, suppose that coffee drinking reduced one's chance of reaching the hospital alive when a myocardial infarction occurred. Then, the prevalence of coffee use among myocardial infarction survivors would under-represent the prevalence among all myocardial infarction cases. Underestimation of the rate ratio would result if fatal myocardial infarction cases were excluded from the study.

It might seem possible to remove the case-selection bias in this example by redefining the study outcome as non-fatal myocardial infarction. This does not remove the bias, however; it only leads to its reclassification as a bias due to differential censoring (here classified as a form of follow-up bias). In a study of non-fatal myocardial infarction, fatal myocardial infarction is a censoring event associated with risk of non-fatal myocardial infarction; if fatal myocardial infarction is also associated with coffee use, the result will be underestimation of the rate ratio for non-fatal myocardial infarction. More generally, it is usually not possible to remove bias by placing restrictions on admissible outcomes.

Unfortunately, exclusion is the only alternative for cases that refuse to participate or cannot be located. In our example, if such cases tend to be heavier coffee users than others, underestimation of the rate ratio would result. However, suppose that, within levels of cigarette use, such cases were no different from other cases with respect to coffee use. Then, adjustment for smoking would remove the selection bias induced by refusals and failures to locate cases. (Of course, such adjustment would require accurate smoking measurement, which is a problem in itself.)

Bias that arises from failure to detect certain cases is sometimes called *detection bias*. If our surveillance system used only hospital admissions, many out-of-hospital myocardial infarction deaths would be excluded, and a detection bias of the sort described here could result.

Control-selection validity

Control-selection bias can be minimized (although may still be large due to non-participation) if one can potentially identify every member of the population at risk at every time during the risk period. In such a situation, one could select controls with one of many available probability sampling techniques, using the entire population at risk as the sampling frame. Unfortunately, such situations are exceptional.

Many studies attempt to approximate the ideal sampling situation through use of existing population lists. An example is control selection by random digit dialling; here, the list (of residential telephone numbers) is not used directly but nevertheless serves as a partial enumeration of the population at risk. This list excludes people without telephone numbers. In our example, if people without telephones drink less coffee than people with telephones, a control group selected by random digit dialling would over-represent coffee use in the population at risk. The result would be underestimation of the rate ratio.

One could redefine the population at risk in the previous example so that the telephone-related selection bias did not exist by restricting the study to persons with telephones. This would require excluding persons without telephones from the case series. The resulting relative-risk estimate would suffer no selection bias. The only important penalty from this restriction is that the resulting estimate might apply only to the population of persons with telephones, which is a problem of generalizability rather than a problem of selection validity. In a similar fashion, it is often possible to prevent confounding or selection bias by placing restrictions on the population at risk (and hence, the control group). In such instances, however, one must take care to apply the same restrictions to the case series and avoid using restrictions based on events that occur after exposure (Rothman & Greenland 1998; Poole 1999).

Even if all members of the population at risk can be identified, selection bias may arise from failure to obtain information on all people selected as controls. The implications are the reverse of those for case-selection bias. In our example, if controls who refuse to participate or cannot be located tend to be heavier coffee users than other controls, overestimation of the rate ratio would result. This should be contrasted with the underestimation that results from the same tendency among cases.

More generally, one might expect an association of selection probabilities with the study variable to be in the same direction for both cases and controls. If so, the resulting case- and control-selection biases would be in opposite directions and so, to some extent, they would cancel one another out, although not completely. To illustrate, suppose that among cases the proportions who refuse to participate are 0.05 for five-cup-a-day drinkers and 0.02 for never-drinkers, and among controls the analogous proportions are 0.20 and 0.10. These refusals will result in the odds of five-cup-a-day versus never-drinkers among cases being underestimated by a factor of $0.95/0.98 = 0.97$; this in turn results in a 3 per cent underestimation of the rate ratio. Among controls, the odds will be underestimated by a factor of $0.80/0.90 = 0.89$; this results in a $1/0.89 = 1.12$, or a 12 per cent overestimation of the rate ratio. The net selection bias in the rate ratio estimate will then be $0.97/0.89 = 1.09$, or 9 per cent overestimation.

For further discussions of control-selection validity, see the textbooks cited in the beginning of this chapter, and also Schlesselman (1982), Savitz and Pearce (1988), Swan *et al.* (1992), and Wacholder *et al.* (1992).

Matching

In cohort studies, matching refers to selection of exposure subcohorts in a manner that forces the matched factors to have similar distributions across the subcohorts. If the matched factors are accurately measured and the proportion lost to follow-up does not depend on the matched factors, cohort matching can prevent confounding by the matched factors, although there are statistical reasons to control the matched factors in the analysis (Weinberg 1985).

In case–control studies, however, matching refers to selection of subjects in a manner that forces the distribution of certain factors to be similar in cases and controls. Because the population at risk is not changed by case–control matching, such matching does not by itself prevent confounding by the matched factors. In fact, it is now widely recognized that case–control matching is a form of selection bias (Rothman & Greenland 1998; Glymour & Greenland 2008). This bias can be removed by adjusting for the matching factor; to the extent the factor has been closely matched and accurately measured, this adjustment also controls for confounding by the factor.

As an example, suppose that our population at risk is half male, that the men tend to drink less coffee than the women, and that about 75 per cent of our cases are men. Unbiased control selection should yield about 50 per cent men in the control group. However, if we matched controls to cases on gender, about 75 per cent of our controls would be men. Because men drink less coffee than women and men would be over-represented in the matched control group, the matched control group would under-represent coffee use in the population at risk. Note, however, that matching does not affect the gender-specific prevalence of coffee use among controls, and so the gender-specific and gender-adjusted estimates would be unaffected by matching. In other words, the selection bias produced by matching could be removed by adjustment for the matching factor.

The conclusion to be drawn is that matching can necessitate control of the matching factors. Thus, in order to avoid increasing the number of factors requiring control unnecessarily, one should limit matching to factors for which control would probably be necessary anyway. In particular, matching is usually best limited to known strong confounders, such as age and gender in the preceding example (Rothman & Greenland 1998; Schlesselman 1982).

More generally, the primary theoretical value of matching is that it can sometimes reduce the variance of adjusted estimators. However, there are circumstances in which matching can facilitate control selection and so is justified on practical grounds. For example, neighbourhood controls may be far easier to obtain than unmatched general population controls. In addition, although neighbourhood matching would necessitate use of a matched analysis method, the neighbourhood-matched results would incorporate some control of confounding by factors associated with the neighbourhood (such as socio-economic status and air pollution).

Special control groups

It is not unusual for investigators to select a special control group that is clearly not representative of the population at risk if they can argue that (1) the group will adequately reflect the distribution of the study factor in the population at risk or (2) that the selection bias in the control group is of the same magnitude of (and so will cancel with) the selection bias in the case group. The first rationale is common in case–control studies of mortality in which persons dying of other selected causes of death are used as controls; in such studies, selection validity can be assured only if the causes of death of controls are unrelated to the study factor. The second rationale is common in studies using hospital cases and controls; in particular, selection validity can be assured in such studies if the control conditions are unrelated to the study factor, and the study disease and the control conditions have proportional exposure-specific rates of hospital admission (Schlesselman 1982).

Selection into a special control group usually requires membership in a small and highly select subset of the population at risk. Thus, use of a special control group requires careful scrutiny for mechanisms by which the study factor may influence entry into the subset. See Schlesselman (1982) and Kelsey *et al.* (1996) for discussions of practical issues in evaluating special control groups, and Rothman and Greenland (1998) for validity principles in mortality case–control studies (so-called proportionate mortality studies).

Case–control modelling

The most popular model for case–control analysis is the logistic model. Details of logistic modelling for case–control analysis are covered in many textbooks, including Breslow and Day (1980), Schlesselman (1982), Kelsey *et al.* (1996), Rothman and Greenland (1998), Hosmer and Lemeshow (2000), and Jewell (2004).

One important aspect of case–control modelling is that matched factors require special treatment. For example, suppose that matching is done on age in five-year categories and age is associated with the study exposure. To control for the selection bias produced by matching, one must either employ conditional logistic regression with age as a stratifying factor, or else enter indicator variables for each age-matching category into an ordinary logistic regression (the latter strategy has the drawback of requiring about ten or more subjects per age stratum to produce valid estimates). Simply entering age into the model as a continuous variable may not adequately control for the matching-induced bias.

Summary of case–control example

The example in this subsection provides an illustration of the most common threats to validity in case–control studies (beyond those already discussed for cohort studies). After adjustments for possible confounding and follow-up bias (along the lines described for the cohort study), there may still be irremediable selection bias, especially if we use only select case groups (e.g. myocardial infarction survivors) or control groups (e.g. hospital controls). In addition, retrospective ascertainment will lead to greater measurement error than prospective ascertainment, and some of this additional error may be differential.

Given the even greater number of potential biases of unknown magnitude and different directions, it would appear that (as in the cohort example) no conclusions about the effect of coffee could be drawn from a study such as the one described, other than that coffee does not have a large effect. Again, this is a common result in thorough epidemiological analyses of observational data.

Special issues in retrospective cohort studies

Two major types of cohort studies can be distinguished depending on whether members of the study cohort are identified before or after the follow-up period under study. Studies in which all members are identified before their follow-up period are called *concurrent* or *prospective* cohort studies, and studies in which all members are identified after their follow-up period are called *historical* or *retrospective* cohort studies.

Similar to case–control studies, retrospective cohort studies often require special consideration of retrospective ascertainment and selection validity. In particular, retrospective cohort studies that obtain exposure or covariate histories from post-event reconstructions are vulnerable to bias from outcome-affected measurements. Suppose, for example, that a study of cancer incidence at an industrial facility had to rely on company personnel to determine the location and nature of various exposures in the plant during the relevant exposure periods. If these personnel were aware of the locations at which cases worked (as when a publicized 'cluster' of cases has occurred), biased exposure assessment could result. Such problems can also occur in a prospective cohort study if exposure or covariate histories are based on post-event reconstructions.

Retrospective cohort studies can also suffer from selection biases analogous to those found in case–control studies. Suppose, for example, that a retrospective cohort study relied on company records to identify members of the cohort of plant employees.

If retention of an employee's records (and hence identification of the employee as a cohort member) were associated with both the exposure and outcome status of the employee, the exposure–outcome association observed in the incomplete study cohort could poorly represent the exposure–outcome association in the complete cohort of plant employees.

Conclusion

Uncertainty about validity conditions is responsible for most of the inconclusiveness inherent in epidemiological studies. This inconclusiveness can be partially overcome when multiple complementary studies are conducted; that is, when new studies are conducted under conditions that effectively limit bias from one or more of the sources present in earlier studies. Ideally, after enough complementary studies have been conducted, each known or suspected source of bias might have been rendered unimportant in at least one study. If at this point all the study results appear consistent with one another (which is not the case for coffee and myocardial infarction, although the studies of smoking and lung cancer provide a good example), the epidemiological community may reach some consensus about the existence and strength of an effect.

Even in such ideal situations, however, one should bear in mind that consistency is not validity. For example, there may be some unsuspected source of bias present in all the studies, so that they are all consistently biased in the same direction. Alternatively, all the known sources of bias may be in the same direction, so that all the studies remain biased in the same direction if no one study eliminates all known sources of bias. Such problems can be addressed tentatively via sensitivity analysis or the more elaborate methods of risk analysis and bias analysis (Eddy *et al.* 1992; Greenland 2005; Greenland & Lash 2008). For these and other reasons, many authors warn that all causal inferences should be considered tentative, at least if drawn from observational epidemiological data alone (Rothman & Greenland 1998; Rothman 1988).

Acknowledgement

The author wishes to thank I. Hertz-Picciotto, P. Kass, J. Kelsey, G. Maldonado, S. Norrell, J. Schlesselman, and A. Walker for their helpful comments on earlier versions this chapter, and K. Hoggatt for her comments on the present version.

References

Altman D.G., Bland J.M. Absence of evidence is not evidence of absence. *British Medical Journal* 1995;**311**:485.

Altman D.G., Machin D., Bryant T.N. *et al.*, editors. *Statistics with confidence.* London: BMJ Books; 2000.

Berger J.O., Berry D.A. Statistical analysis and the illusion of objectivity. *American Scientist* 1988;**76**:159–65.

Brenner H. Bias due to nondifferential misclassification of a polytomous confounder. *Journal of Clinical Epidemiology* 1993;**46**:57–63.

Breslow N.E., Day N.E. Statistical methods in cancer research. I: The analysis of case control studies. Lyon: IARC; 1980.

Breslow N.E., Day NE. Statistical methods in cancer research. II: The analysis of cohort data. Lyon: IARC; 1987.

Checkoway H., Pearce N., Kreibel D. *Research methods in occupational epidemiology.* 2nd ed. New York (NY): Oxford University Press; 2004.

Cole S.R., Hermán M.A. Fallibility in estimating direct effects. *International Journal of Epidemiology* 2002;**31**:163–5.

Curb J.D., Reed D.M., Kautz J.A. *et al.* Coffee, caffeine, and serum cholesterol in Japanese men in Hawaii. *American Journal of Epidemiology* 1986;**123**:648–55.

Dosemeci M., Wacholder S., Lubin J.H. Does nondifferential misclassification of exposure always bias a true effect towards the null value? American Journal of Epidemiology 1990;132:746–8.

Drews C.D., Greenland S. The impact of differential recall on the results of case-control studies. *International Journal of Epidemiology* 1990;**19**:1107–12.

Drews C.D., Greenland S., Flanders W.D. The use of restricted controls to prevent recall bias in case-control studies of reproductive outcomes. *Annals of Epidemiology* 1993;**3**:86–92.

Eddy D.M., Hasselblad V., Schacher R. Meta-analysis by the confidence profile method. New York (NY): Academic Press; 1992.

Flegal K.M., Keyl P.M., Nieto E.J. Differential misclassification arising from nondifferential errors in exposure measurement. *American Journal of Epidemiology* 1991;**134**:1233–44.

Gilovich T., Griffin D., Kahneman D. Heuristics and biases: the psychology of intuitive judgment. New York (NY): Cambridge University Press; 2002.

Glymour M.M., Greenland S. Causal diagrams. In: Rothman K.J., Greenland S., Lash T.L., editors. *Modern Epidemiology.* 3rd ed. Philadelphia (PA): Lippincott; 2008.

Goodman S.N. P-values, hypothesis tests, and likelihood: implications for epidemiology of a neglected historical debate. *American Journal of Epidemiology* 1993;**137**:485–96.

Greenland S. The effect of misclassification in the presence of covariates. *American Journal of Epidemiology* 1980;**112**:564–9.

Greenland S. Control initiated case-control studies. *International Journal of Epidemiology* 1985;**14**:130–4.

Greenland S. Interpretation and choice of effect measures in epidemiologic analyses. *American Journal of Epidemiology* 1987;**125**:761–8.

Greenland S. Randomization, statistics, and causal inference. *Epidemiology* 1990;**1**:421–9.

Greenland S. A meta-analysis of coffee, myocardial infarction, and coronary death. *Epidemiology* 1993;**4**:366–74.

Greenland S. A critical look at some popular meta-analytic methods. *American Journal of Epidemiology* 1994;**140**:290–6.

Greenland S. Induction versus popper: substance versus semantics. *International Journal of Epidemiology* 1998a;**27**:543–8.

Greenland S. Probability logic and probabilistic induction. *Epidemiology* 1998b;**9**:322–32.

Greenland S. The relation of the probability of causation to the relative risk and the doubling dose: A methodologic error that has become a social problem. *American Journal of Public Health* 1999;**89**:1166–9.

Greenland S. Principles of multilevel modelling. *International Journal of Epidemiology* 2000a;**29**:158–67.

Greenland S. When should epidemiologic regressions use random coefficients? *Biometrics* 2000b;**56**:915–21.

Greenland S. Ecologic versus individual-level sources of confounding in ecologic estimates of contextual health effects. *International Journal of Epidemiology* 2001;**30**:1343–50.

Greenland S. A review of multilevel theory for ecologic analyses. *Statistics in Medicine* 2002a;**21**:389–95.

Greenland S. Causality theory for policy uses of epidemiologic measures. In: Murray CJL, Salomon JA, Mathers CD *et al.*, editors. *Summary measures of population health.* Cambridge (MA): Harvard University Press/WHO; 2002b. p. 291–302.

Greenland S. The impact of prior distributions for uncontrolled confounding and response bias: a case study of the relation of wire codes and magnetic fields to childhood leukemia. *Journal of the American Statistical Association* 2003;**98**:47–54.

Greenland S. Ecologic inference problems in studies based on surveillance data. In: Stroup DF, Brookmeyer R, editors. *Monitoring the health of populations: statistical principles and methods for public health surveillance.* New York (NY): Oxford University Press; 2004a. p. 315–40.

Greenland S. The need for critical appraisal of expert witnesses in epidemiology and statistics. *Wake Forest Law Review* 2004b; **39**:291–310.

Greenland S. Multiple-bias modelling for analysis of observational data (with discussion). *Journal of the Royal Statistical Society Series A* 2005;**168**:267–308.

Greenland S. Bayesian perspectives for epidemiologic research. *I: Foundations and basic methods. International Journal of Epidemiology* 2006;**35**:765–78.

Greenland S. Bayesian methods for epidemiologic research. II: Regression analysis. International Journal of Epidemiology 2007;**36**:195–202.

Greenland S., Brumback B.A. An overview of relations among causal modelling methods. *International Journal of Epidemiology* 2002;**31**:1030–7.

Greenland S., Gustafson P. Adjustment for independent nondifferential misclassification does not increase certainty that an observed association is in the correct direction. *American Journal of Epidemiology* 2006;**164**:63–68.

Greenland S., Lash T.L. Bias analysis. In: Rothman K.J., Greenland S., Lash T.L., editors. *Modern Epidemiology*. 3rd ed. Philadelphia (PA): Lippincott; 2008.

Greenland S., Maclure M., Schlesselman J.J. *et al.* Standardized coefficients: a further critique and a review of alternatives. *Epidemiology* 1991; **2**:387–92.

Greenland S., Maldonado G. The interpretation of multiplicative model parameters as standardized parameters. *Statistics in Medicine* 1994;**13**:989–99.

Greenland S., O'Rourke K. Meta-analysis. In: Rothman K.J., Greenland S., Lash T.L., editors. *Modern Epidemiology*. 3rd ed. Philadelphia (PA): Lippincott; 2008.

Greenland S., Pearl J., Robins J.M. Causal diagrams for epidemiologic research. *Epidemiology* 1999b;**10**:37–48.

Greenland S., Robins J.M. Confounding and misclassification. *American Journal of Epidemiology* 1985;**122**:495–506.

Greenland S., Robins J.M. Conceptual problems in the definition and interpretation of attributable fractions. *American Journal of Epidemiology* 1988;**128**:1185–97.

Greenland S., Robins J.M., Pearl J. Confounding and collapsibility in causal inference. *Statistical Science* 1999a;**14**:29–46.

Greenland S., Schlesselman J.J., Criqui M.H. The fallacy of employing standardized regression coefficients and correlations as measures of effect. *American Journal of Epidemiology* 1986;**123**:203–8.

Greenland S., Schwartzbaum J.A., Finkle W.D. Problems from small samples and sparse data in conditional logistic regression analysis. *American Journal of Epidemiology* 2000;**151**:531–9.

Hastie T., Tibshirani R. *Generalized additive models*. New York (NY): Chapman and Hall; 1990.

Hernán M.A., Hernandez-Diaz S., Robins J.M. A structural approach to selection bias. *Epidemiology* 2004;**15**:615–25.

Hosmer D.W., Lemeshow S. *Applied logistic regression*. 2nd ed. New York (NY): Wiley; 2000.

Jewell N. *Statistics for epidemiology*. Boca Raton (FL): Chapman and Hall/CRC; 2004.

Kaufman S., Kaufman J.S., MacLehose R.F. *et al.* Improved estimation of controlled direct effects in the presence of unmeasured confounding by intermediate variables. *Statistics in Medicine* 2005;**24**:1683–702.

Kelsey J.L., Whittemore A.S., Evans A.S. *et al. Methods in observational epidemiology*. 2nd ed. New York (NY): Oxford University Press; 1996.

Koepsell T.D., Weiss N.S. *Epidemiologic methods*. New York (NY): Oxford University Press; 2003.

Leamer E.E. *Specification searches*. New York (NY): Wiley; 1978.

Maldonado G., Greenland S. A comparison of the performance of model-based confidence intervals when the correct modell form is unknown. *Epidemiology* 1994;**5**:171–82.

Park S.Y., Murphy S.P., Wilkens L.R. *et al.* Calcium and vitamin D intake and risk of colorectal cancer: The Multiethnic Cohort Study. *American Journal of Epidemiology* 2007;**165**:784–93.

Pearl J. *Causality: models, reasoning and inference*. Cambridge: Cambridge University Press; 2000.

Poole C. Exceptions to the rule about non-differential misclassification (abstract). *American Journal of Epidemiology* 1985;**122**:508.

Poole C. Beyond the confidence interval. *American Journal of Public Health* 1987a;**77**:197–9.

Poole C. Confidence intervals exclude nothing. *American Journal of Public Health* 1987b;**77**:492–3.

Poole C. Controls who experienced hypothetical causal intermediates should not be excluded from case-control studies. *American Journal of Epidemiology* 1999;**150**:547–51.

Robins J.M. Confidence intervals for causal parameters. *Statistics in Medicine* 1988;**7**:773–85.

Robins J.M., Greenland S. The role of model selection in causal inference from nonexperimental data. *American Journal of Epidemiology* 1986;**123**:392–402.

Robins J.M., Greenland S. Identifiability and exchangeability for direct and indirect effects. *Epidemiology* 1992;**3**:143–55.

Robins J.M., Greenland S. Adjusting for differential rates of prophylaxis therapy for PCP in high- versus low-dose AZT treatment arms in an AIDS randomized trial. *Journal of the American Statistical Association* 1994;**90**:737–49.

Robins J.M., Hernán M.A., Brumback B. Marginal structural models and causal inference in epidemiology. *Epidemiology* 2000;**11**(**5**):550–60.

Rothman K.J. A show of confidence. *New England Journal of Medicine* 1978;**299**:1362–3.

Rothman K.J. *Causal inference*. Chestnut Hill (MA): Epidemiology Resources; 1988.

Rothman K.J. and Greenland S., editors. *Modern epidemiology*. 2nd ed. Philadelphia (PA): Lippincott-Raven; 1998.

Rothman K.J., Greenland S., Poole C., Lash T.L. Causation and causal inference. In Rothman KJ, Greenland S, Lash TL, eds. *Modern Epidemiology*, 3rd ed. Philadelphia: Lippincott-Williams-Wilkins, 2008, 51–70.

Savitz D.A., Pearce N. Control selection with incomplete case ascertainment, American Journal of Epidemiology 1988;127:1109–17.

Schlesselman J.J. *Case-control studies: design, conduct, analysis*. New York (NY): Oxford University Press; 1982.

Slud E., Byar D. How dependent causes of death can make risk factors appear protective. *Biometrics* 1988;**44**:265–70.

Swan S.H., Shaw G.R., Schulman J. Reporting and selection bias in case-control studies of congenital malformations. *Epidemiology* 1992;3:356–63.

Thomas D.C., Witte J.S., Greenland S. Dissecting complex mixtures: who's afraid of informative priors? Epidemiology 2007;18:186–90.

Thompson W.D. Statistical criteria in the interpretation of epidemiologic data. *American Journal of Public Health* 1987;**77**:191–4.

Wacholder S., Dosemeci M., Lubin J.H. Blind assignment of exposure does not always prevent differential misclassification. *American Journal of Epidemiology* 1991;**134**:433–7.

Wacholder S., McLaughlin J.K., Silverman D.T. *et al.* Selection of controls in case-control studies. *American Journal of Epidemiology* 1992;**135**: 1019–50.

Weinberg C.R. On pooling across strata when frequency matching has been followed in a cohort study. *Biometrics* 1985;**41**:103–16.

Weinberg C.R., Umbach D., Greenland S. When will non-differential misclassification preserve the direction of the trend? American Journal of Epidemiology 1994;140:565–71.

White H. *Estimation, inference, and specification analysis*. New York (NY): Cambridge University Press; 1993.

6.13

Causation and causal inference

Katherine J. Hoggatt and Sander Greenland

Introduction

This chapter offers an introduction to causal inference theory as relevant to public health research. Causal inference can be viewed as a prediction problem, addressing the question of what the likely outcome under one action vs. an alternative action is. Although asking these types of questions is very natural, answering them requires careful thought in both the statement of the causal hypothesis and the techniques used to attempt an answer. This chapter discusses these complexities, with further discussion in Chapter 6.12 ('Validity and bias in epidemiological research'). More thorough coverage of these issues can be found in Chapters 2, 4, and 9 of Rothman *et al.* (2008).

The chapter reviews considerations that have been invoked in discussions of causality based on epidemiologic evidence. It then describes the potential-outcome (counterfactual) framework for cause and effect, showing how measures of effect and association are distinguished in that framework. The framework illustrates problems inherent in attempts to quantify the changes in health expected under different actions or interventions. The chapter concludes with a discussion of how research findings may be translated into policy.

The study of cause and effect

Starting in childhood, people acquire a notion of cause and effect that is based on the observation of one event always or often following another. Children observe that flipping a switch consistently results in the light going on and readily assign a cause and effect interpretation to these relations. Nonetheless, such naïve equation of 'variation in tandem' with causation will too often conflate causation with mere association.

The emergence of modern science led to increasingly sophisticated observational and experimental methods to distinguish causal from non-causal association. By the twentieth century, these developments led to formal theories of causation. A formal theory of causation facilitates application of deductive reasoning to the process of causal inference. Of great importance, it allows us to define precisely the difference between causation and association and gives guidance on how to pose causal questions and test causal hypotheses; it does not, however, provide a basis for 'proving' causality, nor can it model the entire process of causal inference.

As Hume (1739) realized and discussed at length, there is no deductive way to prove causality. Thus, causal inference can only be a speculative, inductive process whose output is a theory of cause and effect. Indeed, the history of science shows that all theories, including causal ones, are necessarily provisional and that future evidence may lead to rejecting previously 'established' causal relations (Kuhn 1970). The primary distinction of causal theories is that they provide comparative predictions about the consequences of alternative interventions (e.g. dietary supplementation vs. none) rather than singular predictions of events assuming no intervention (e.g. forecasts of cold epidemics).

Those working in public health or policy must often make decisions on how to proceed in the face of equivocal evidence. The question then arises of how to weigh the evidence in favour of cause and effect to determine, say, whether smoking should be banned in bars to prevent lung cancer in bar workers, whether pregnant women should be told to take folic acid to prevent neural tube defects in their offspring, or whether postmenopausal women should be prescribed hormone replacement therapy (HRT) to prevent heart disease. In each of these cases, the final decision by health or policy professionals was made in the absence of definitive proof of causality, relying instead on the imperfect evidence gleaned from scientific studies.

Because of its central importance, causal inference is often confused with the more complex process of rational decision-making. While causal inference is a crucial input to decision-making, decision-making also depends on the costs and benefits of the outcomes. For example, it is believed that banning smoking in bars is unlikely to have strong adverse health consequences and that the economic impacts are small enough to be of debatable importance. This perceived imbalance of benefits and costs is a major basis for a proposed ban. In contrast, recommendations that doctors prescribe hormone replacement therapy (HRT) for the prevention of heart disease must acknowledge that HRT could have serious side effects on women's health. The recommendations are easily challenged if the costs are shifted according to individual preferences and values.

Such examples show that multiple effects should be considered when policy makers evaluate the evidence of cause and effect based on epidemiologic studies. Nonetheless, most attempts to formalize the process of causal inference focus on single endpoints.

This single-endpoint view must be understood thoroughly before considering multiple endpoints.

Hill's considerations

While there is no sufficient set of criteria for determining causality, many authors have attempted to list considerations that should be weighed when advancing causal arguments. Among these, the best known in epidemiology are by Sir Austin Bradford Hill (Hill 1965), which are closely related to the considerations found in the first US Surgeon General's report on smoking and health (1964). Hill's article has been widely misinterpreted as providing necessary conditions ('criteria') for causation to be inferred; see Phillips and Goodman (2004) for a discussion of this and other misinterpretations. In Hill's own words, the considerations were not meant to be a checklist or set of criteria, but rather simply 'points to consider', namely: (1) strength, (2) consistency, (3) specificity, (4) temporality, (5) biologic gradient, (6) plausibility, (7) coherence, (8) experimental evidence, and (9) analogy; we shall discuss each of these in turn.

Strength

The strength of an association may be considered important because it is harder to explain away strong effects as complete artefacts of biases such as confounding. There is no general rule for how large an association needs to be to be credible, but, for example, it has been reported that many epidemiologists would be sceptical of a identifying a new risk factor for cancer if its risk ratio were less than 3 (Taubes 1995). Nonetheless, there are many smaller associations that are generally agreed to reflect causal effects. This is in part because they have been replicated in a variety of populations using different designs and in part because of considerations other than strength. Examples include the association between smoking and heart disease and between environmental tobacco smoke and lung cancer. Similarly, there are several well-known examples of relatively strong non-causal associations. One example is the association between birth order and Down's syndrome: Maternal aging, which is strongly associated with infant birth order, has since been accepted as the actual cause of the syndrome.

Consistency

A consistent finding is an association reported across multiple populations, over time, and using different study designs. Although the presence of a consistent result is often taken as a compelling argument for causality, the argument can be specious; for example, an inverse association of beta-carotene with cancer was seen across epidemiologic studies but failed to be replicated in subsequent randomized trials. Conversely, the absence of consistency does not imply the absence of a causal effect. Acute effects may be submerged in studies that examine only chronic exposure, and some agents may operate only in highly susceptible subpopulations. For example, the effect of coffee use on myocardial infarction risk remains controversial, in part because most of the large cohort studies perceived as providing 'negative' evidence have had little power to detect acute effects (Greenland 1993).

Specificity

In Hill's formulation, specificity can refer either to a cause having a single effect or an effect having a single cause. The limitations of this criterion are apparent even in the case of smoking and lung cancer. Although the smoking and lung cancer association is stronger (on the ratio scale) than the association between smoking and, say, heart disease, there is general agreement today that smoking can increase the risk of many diseases, including heart disease and other cancers.

Specificity can strengthen a causal inference if a competing non-causal hypothesis would predict a non-specific association. For example, some have argued that screening for certain cancers is ineffective in and of itself for reducing cancer mortality, and the apparent protective effect after adjustment for lead-time reflects the fact that those people who choose to undergo regular screenings are generally more health conscious and therefore at a lower risk for cancer due to their 'healthy lifestyle'. If a specific screening instrument, say a mammogram, were shown to be associated with lower mortality from breast cancer but not lower mortality due to cancers in other sites, it could strengthen the inference that mammography is indeed useful in preventing breast-cancer deaths. Although such issues can in theory be addressed via randomized trials, the controversy surrounding trials of mammography (Freedman *et al.* 2004) shows that in practice similar considerations will arise even with randomized treatment assignment.

Temporality

Temporality means that a cause must necessarily precede its effect. This positive assertion is inarguable, but an observation that in a specific case a putative cause (X) followed the hypothesized effect (Y) is not a definitive argument against causality. Rather, it may simply reflect that in a given instance Y occurred before X. Thus temporality is a definitive criterion for non-causality only if we know that X *cannot* come before Y.

Biologic gradient

A biologic gradient is a dose-response relation between an exposure and an outcome. Though most epidemiologists think of a 'linear' or monotonic dose-response association as strengthening a causal inference, this need not be the case. There may be a sharp increase in risk for specific outcomes at low to moderate doses of a given exposure that tapers off at higher doses, or there may be no adverse effect until saturation of detoxification mechanisms is reached, resulting in increased risk only at higher doses.

Many substances show non-monotonic trends with outcomes in a manner consistent with their hypothesized biologic effects; for example, very low and very high doses of certain vitamins may increase the risk of death, a fact consistent with what we know about the biologic properties of these vitamins. In addition, an apparent dose-response gradient, even if monotonic or linear, does not prove the observed associations are genuine rather than artefacts of confounding. If a confounder is positively associated with the exposure, an apparent dose-response relation between exposure and outcome could simply reflect the dose-response relation between the confounder and outcome.

Plausibility

A plausible association is one that conforms to the current scientific understanding of the relation between a putative cause and its effect. This understanding can be informed by other epidemiologic studies, animal studies, biology, toxicology, etc. The limitation of plausibility as a criterion for assessing causality is that current scientific understanding can be incomplete or wrong. The observation that cholera occurs in outbreaks does not support the inference that it is caused by miasmas, despite miasma theory being the dominant idea in the early nineteenth century for how infectious agents were transmitted.

Coherence

Hill used the term 'coherence' to mean that the hypothesized causal relation of exposure to disease is not in conflict with the current scientific understanding of the disease process. Hill emphasized that an absence of coherent information was not a strong argument against causality. If an observed association apparently conflicts with current scientific understanding of a disease process, it may be that the understanding is mistaken rather than that the association is non-causal. For example, at the time it was made, the observation that shallow inhalers of cigarette smoke had increased rates of lung cancer relative to deep inhalers seemed to contradict the understanding of lung cancer aetiology. Subsequent research on lung cancer, however, found that the cells affected by cigarette smoke tended to be in upper respiratory tract, which was in fact consistent with the observed association for shallow inhalers.

Conversely, coherence is a very fallible argument in support of causality. The theory that the inverse association of beta-carotene with cancers observed in epidemiologic studies represented a preventive effect was quite coherent with contemporary theories of antioxdants and cancer, but this hypothesis was nonetheless refuted by subsequent randomized trials.

Experimental evidence

In modern discussions, 'experimental evidence' often refers to either human or animal experiments, which themselves are very different categories of evidence. This type of evidence may be limited or absent. For many exposures, human experimentation is impractical or unethical, and, for many disease processes, no suitable animal model exists.

Hill seemed to have a different notion of experiment in mind, however, one more akin to classical writers such as Mill (1862). Hill discussed the evidence for causality that can be obtained by examining the association between exposure and disease when the potentially harmful exposure has been reduced or removed. Although these types of before-and-after comparisons can be valuable, they are misleading if there are time-varying confounders that drive the observed associations.

Analogy

Analogy refers to drawing inferences about the association between a given exposure and disease based on what is known about other exposure-disease relations. Based on what is known about the health effects of cigarette smoking, we might expect that inhalation of other combustibles (e.g. marijuana) would have similar effects, even in the absence of studies on the subject. Analogy can be a useful scientific tool for generating new hypotheses about disease processes; however, its utility for assessing causality is limited by the understanding and imagination of the scientist.

For reasons such as those just discussed, Hill and other critical thinkers have discouraged taking his 'viewpoints' as a checklist for causality. Hill's 'criteria' may be useful in generating testable hypotheses that can bear on a discussion of causality, but none of them is sufficient to justify a causal inference, and only one, temporality, is a necessary condition for claiming that an observed association is causal.

Despite the ongoing popularity of Hill's considerations—sometimes in modified form—for making causal inferences (e.g. Giovannoni & Ebers 2007), there is no general agreement on which considerations should be used in making causal inferences, nor in how to use a given set (Weed & Gorelic 1996; Holman *et al.* 2001). Some have argued that such aids to inference amount to little more than common sense (Phillips & Goodman 2006) or may even harm the inferential process (Lanes & Poole 1984). Others have used the considerations to develop deductive hypotheses or predictions that can be directly tested (Maclure 1985; Weed 1986). Finally, researchers may use different considerations or deploy them differently based on the specifics of the inferences being made, showing that, in practice, the considerations are more like values than objective inferential tools (Poole 2001).

Formal approaches to causal inference

Implicit in the discussion of causal considerations is the idea that there is a well-defined notion of what constitutes cause and effect. Perhaps the oldest non-circular set of definitions arises from the potential-outcome or counterfactual framework. The potential-outcome model specifies what happens to individuals or populations under alternative actions or interventions and also makes explicit the problems in operationally defining causes (Greenland 2002, 2005; Hernán 2005). This model of causation is also useful in defining methodologic concepts such as confounding; this is discussed further in Chapter 6.12 ('Validity and bias in epidemiological research') and also Chapter 4 of Rothman *et al.* (2008).

Potential outcomes and counterfactual causality

Causal inference can be viewed as a prediction problem. For example, a public health researcher may wish to predict how the rates of lung cancer among bar workers would change if an indoor smoking ban was enacted. The counterfactual model allows us to formalize questions such as 'Will a smoking ban decrease the rates of lung cancer in 10 years beyond what can be expected in the absence of a ban?'

In discussions of potential outcomes, three components must be defined:

- A target of interest, either an individual or group, that will be the subject of the study of causation
- A list of possible interventions or actions (x_0, x_1, etc.) that could have been applied to the target over some time span of interest
- An outcome measure (Y) taken after implementation of the intervention or action

If x_a is the actual action taken from among possible actions x_0, $x_1, \ldots, x_n$, a potential-outcome model posits that, for an action, x_a, there is a well-defined outcome, $Y(x_a)$, that would have followed from that specific action x_a. This outcome is often termed a 'potential outcome'.

As an example, suppose the treatment of interest is sending to members of an insurance plan, on their fiftieth birthday, a mail-in home sampling kit to screen for stool blood, a possible indicator of colon cancer. Suppose $X = 1$ if the kit is supplied to a person, and $X = 0$ if not. Ordinary analyses might examine one outcome variable, such as $Y = 1$ if the person dies of colon cancer by age 60 and

$Y=0$ if the person does not die by this age. But a potential-outcome analysis considers one outcome variable for every treatment being compared: For $X=1$, we consider the outcome $Y(1)=1$ if the person dies of colon cancer by age 60 *when sent the kit* and $Y(1)=0$ if the person does not die *when sent the kit*. Similarly, for $X=0$ we consider the outcome $Y(0)=1$ if the person dies of colon cancer by age 60 *when not sent the kit* and $Y(0)=0$ if the person does not die *when not sent the kit*. Offering the kit is then beneficial for the person with respect to these outcomes if $Y(1)=0$ but $Y(0)=1$, which is to say if the person would not die of colon cancer by age 60 if sent the kit but *would so die* if the kit *was not sent*. Presumably, such a benefit would arise because the kit, if sent, would be received, used, and would lead to detection of and intervention for an otherwise fatal tumour.

The potential-outcome model is widely used in statistical discussions of causality, and it has become increasingly popular in epidemiology and other fields. Yet, it is not without controversy, largely because at most only one potential-outcome variable can be observed for each person. That observable potential outcome is the one corresponding to the treatment actually received; all the other potential outcomes are unobserved, and hence are 'missing data'. Understandably, the incompleteness of the data under the model is upsetting to practitioners, and the inevitable missingness requires reconsideration of many conventional statistical methods. Such reconsiderations have, however, led to innovative methods for previously intractable problems, such as the estimation of effects of time-varying treatment regimes.

There are also a number of aspects of the model that are often misrepresented as limitations but are not. For example, the model does *not* require that outcomes be well-defined for any possible intervention; it simply requires that the outcomes be well-defined for those interventions of interest. If, in a study of motorcycle-crash fatalities, we wish to estimate the effect of a helmet law mandating fines for non-use versus no law, we do not need to specify any other actions (such as a law mandating jail time for non-use). Also, and contrary to some misunderstandings, the potential-outcome model is not inherently deterministic: Although the model is quite often introduced and taught using deterministic language, a potential outcome could instead be the parameter of a probability distribution, for example the probability of disease.

Causes and effects

The term 'effect' is sometimes used to specify the outcome of a causal process. A researcher may describe lung cancer or heart disease as two possible effects of cigarette smoking. A quantitative definition of an effect is a numerical contrast in outcome measures corresponding to different actions or interventions, e.g. $Y(x_1)$ and $Y(x_0)$. The numerical contrast is called a *measure of effect*. In the earlier example, if x_1 is the absence of a helmet law and x_0 is the presence of a helmet law, then $Y(x_1)-Y(x_0)$ could be the fatality-rate difference for motorcycle crashes and $Y(x_1)/Y(x_0)$ could be the fatality-rate ratio.

Thus, under a potential-outcome model, an effect is a contrast in outcomes corresponding to *two* different actions in *one* single target. Effects must be defined with respect to a clearly specified alternative or reference condition. To say that smoking one pack of cigarettes a day increases the risk for lung cancer and heart disease would be incorrect without specifying the alternative: Smoking one pack a day may be harmful relative to not smoking, and this would seem the implicit reference condition, but it would likely be protective relative to smoking two packs a day. Statements about the effects of causes are likely to be ambiguous or meaningless unless both the index and reference actions are stated explicitly.

It follows that an action cannot be considered inherently causal, and it can only be deemed causal when the outcome associated with it is compared to the outcome associated with an alternative action. Consider a person with depression who is prescribed an anti-depressant medication. The weeks following initiation of treatment are thought to be periods of increased risk for suicide. If this person commits suicide in the period following treatment initiation, some would say the anti-depressant caused the suicide. Given that the person was depressed to begin with, it is possible that he would have committed suicide even if he had not been prescribed the medication, in which case the anti-depressant did not cause the suicide in reference to the alternative of no prescription. If instead of being prescribed an anti-depressant, however, the individual had been hospitalized, he may not have committed suicide, in which case the anti-depressant treatment may be considered a cause of his suicide, but only in reference to the alternative action of hospitalization.

A second important point is that because an effect is a contrast in outcomes for one target, we can observe at most one of the actions and its corresponding outcome. The other treatments, which are not observed, are *counterfactual* (contrary to fact), and as a consequence their corresponding potential outcomes are not observed (although if there is no effect they may equal the observed outcome). These alternative potential outcomes can only be estimated.

If the index and reference actions lead to identical outcomes, then the index action is said to have no effect on the target. When an action has an effect, describing it as causal or preventive depends on which outcome we are referring to. If smoking a pack a day for 20 years (versus none) causes an individual to die at age 70, then this smoking likewise prevents survival past age 70. In parallel, if not smoking prevents death at age 70 relative to smoking a pack a day for 20 years, it causes that individual to survive past age 70.

Confounding and measures of association

Our inability to observe the potential outcome of more than one action fundamentally limits our ability to make causal inferences. In any attempt to estimate a causal effect, at least one potential outcome, corresponding to a counterfactual action, must be estimated or predicted rather than measured. In practice, this is accomplished by measuring outcomes in other individuals who actually experience the reference action. In experiments and in cohort studies, these individuals are often called the control subjects.

For example, on July 1, 2000, Florida weakened its existing motorcycle helmet use law to exempt individuals over the age of 21 who had at least US$10 000 in insurance in case of an accident. To estimate the effect of weakening the helmet law in Florida, we could compare (contrast) the rates of motorcycle crash fatalities before and after the change. Instead of the fatality rate in 2001, had the law not been changed, we use the fatality rate in 1999 before the law changed. This is no longer a measure of effect, because it is not a contrast of the outcomes of two different actions in a single group. Instead, it is a *measure of association*, which is a contrast of outcomes in two or more different groups. We use this measure of association as a substitute for the corresponding measure of effect. The amount of *confounding* is the difference between the measure of association and the measure of effect that it is intended to represent.

Confounding is a serious threat to our ability to make causal inferences. Nonetheless, we can often determine factors that contribute to the difference between the measure of association and the measure of effect. In our example, these would be reasons why the motorcycle fatality rates in 1999 would differ from those in 2001, had the helmet law never changed. These factors are commonly known as *confounders*.

When confounders are measured, analytic methods can be used to minimize the amount of confounding from those factors and thus strengthen our inferences. The most basic methods are based on stratifying the observations on values of these confounders. *Standardization* then averages across outcomes in the index and reference groups using a shared (standard) weighting scheme (Rothman *et al.* 2008). Other methods make special assumptions to combine measures of association across strata. In all these approaches, the resulting summary comparison across the strata is said to be *adjusted* for the confounders used to create the stratification.

An adjusted measure of association will be a good estimate for the desired measure of effect only insofar as we have controlled for (e.g. stratified on) the important confounding factors. If there are other factors that contribute to important differences between the counterfactual (alternative) outcome and the observed outcome used as a substitute, then the measure of association will remain a biased estimate for the measure of effect. In the case of the helmet law and the motorcycle crash fatalities, one would have to ask if all the important factors contributing to changes in the rate of crash fatalities *other than the change to the helmet law* had been measured and properly controlled. To the extent we are uncertain or doubtful about our measurement and control of confounders, we would have to doubt the validity of the adjusted association as an estimate of the measure of effect (see Chapter 6.12, 'Validity and bias in epidemiological research').

Practical uses of causal inference

Academic discussions of cause and effect often focus on the 'effects' of changes that have no realistic interpretation as actions (e.g. elimination of lung cancer) or actions that are not realistic options (e.g. achieving a 'smoke-free society'). Even when discussions focus on the impact of feasible interventions, they are often based on unrealistic assumptions about their consequences, for example assuming 100 per cent compliance with a given treatment or behaviour-modification programme.

As an extreme example, some discussions centre on the expected health impact if a given disease or outcome could be removed. Such discussions are irrelevant and often misleading for policy formulation. For example, in a discussion of the 'burden of disease due to lung cancer', a rough ranking of actions and questions from irrelevant and unrealistic to most relevant would be:

- Directly eliminating lung cancer (e.g. 'How many deaths could be prevented if we could eliminate lung cancer?')
- Removing risk factors for lung cancer (e.g. 'How many deaths could be prevented if we could eliminate cigarette smoking?')
- Applying an intervention to an entire population (e.g. 'If we could implement a given smoking-cessation programme to the entire smoking population of a nation, how many deaths could be prevented?')
- Applying an intervention that will produce a small change in risk behaviours in part of a population (e.g. 'If we could implement a given smoking-cessation programme in a targeted group of motivated individuals, how many deaths could be prevented?')

We will discuss each of these actions in turn.

Removing outcomes

Discussions of the burden of disease often focus on the expected change in population health that might be expected if certain diseases or outcomes could be removed from a population, e.g. in discussions of survival if one could 'eliminate' a certain type of cause-specific mortality. For example, suppose Y represents cause of death, with $Y=y_1$ for death from myocardial infarction (MI) and $Y=y_0$ for death from other causes ('competing risks'). An individual will eventually experience one but not both of these outcomes, so at least one must be counterfactual.

Now suppose Z represents years of survival past age 50. Z is a measure of the burden of myocardial infarction among those who reach age 50. The value Z will take depends not only on the value of Y but also on how that value (y_1 or y_0) is brought about. Suppose a man with a sedentary lifestyle and poor diet died from an MI at age 54, so that we observe $Z(y_1)=4$ (the number of years lived past the age of 50). The value of $Z(y_0)$ would then be the number of years lived past age 50 *if the MI death had been prevented*. This value would depend critically on how the MI death was prevented. If the man had taken up a regime of physical activity and a healthy diet in his twenties, $Z(y_0)$ could be considerably larger than $Z(y_1)$ because the regime would lower his risk of many causes of death besides MI. If instead the MI death was prevented by medical care at the time the MI occurred, $Z(y_0)$ and $Z(y_1)$ may not differ by much because the man would remain at an increased risk for future MI, cancer, and other potentially fatal diseases.

When the outcomes are not directly manipulable, any prediction based on the hypothesized removal of the outcomes needs to consider not just the fact of the outcome removal but also the method used to remove it (Kalbfleisch & Prentice 2002; Greenland 2002, 2005; Hernan 2005). Even if we can define a realistic intervention for removal of the outcome with few side effects, there is little basis to assume that removal of a particular outcome in a given group yields a risk profile similar to that for other individuals who did not have the intervention yet do not experience the removed outcome. Unfortunately, standard statistical procedures for analysing these types of data make the assumption that the risk profiles are similar (an assumption of 'independent competing risks'). Thus, it is reasonable to expect that even if we can conceive of an intervention that will prevent a specific outcome, estimates of effect in light of this outcome removal will likely be biased if estimation is based on the experience of those who do not experience the outcome in the absence of the intervention. In sum, to estimate the effects of outcome removal, one must study successfully treated individuals.

Removing risk factors

Consider the debate on obesity and mortality. Numerous studies have reported increases in mortality associated with having a body mass index (BMI) over 30 (the cutpoint for obesity) relative to a 'normal' BMI of 20–24.9. Some authors have used these findings to ascribe a causal role for obesity in mortality and have gone on to assert that getting people to lose weight will save lives. But suppose not all individuals who go from a BMI of over 30 to a BMI of (say) 24 lose weight in the same way. Some might start exercising and eating more healthfully, in which case lower mortality may in fact result. Others might undergo gastric bypass surgery or become chronic users of amphetamines, each of which are known to confer some mortality risk.

Unfortunately, studies that examine only the association of BMI with mortality tell us nothing about the impact of different interventions to change BMI. To obtain a relevant causal inference, one must specify an intervention aimed at reducing BMI and then compare the mortality outcomes under that intervention to outcomes under a reference intervention (such as doing nothing). The resulting measure of association, as an estimate of a measure of effect, would *not* be a contrast in outcomes of persons at different levels of BMI, it would be a contrast in outcomes under *specific interventions* among persons who started with the same BMI.

The very idea of the 'health effects of BMI' suffers from confusion of the effects of interventions (e.g. a diet and exercise regime) with the downstream results of intermediate outcomes (e.g. changes in BMI). A change in BMI is not an intervention, thus one cannot unambiguously define the causal effect a change in BMI. A similar problem arises if one considers the effect on lung cancer incidence if more people were non-smokers. As with BMI, a researcher would need to specify an intervention (e.g. nicotine patches, hypnotherapy, medication, etc.) before discussing the possible result of getting smokers to quit.

When conceptualizing exposures in observational studies as interventions, as opposed to protocols in clinical trials, there are limitations to how detailed the description can be, making vagueness about the hypothetical intervention unavoidable (Robins & Greenland 2000). Nevertheless, moving away from thinking of outcomes such as BMI as potential causes—as opposed to intermediates—is necessary for making policy-relevant causal inferences from observational data.

A related problem arises in discussing the causal effects of personal characteristics. For example, considerable debate has surrounded the question of whether it is meaningful to speak about factors such as race or sex as being possible causes of effects (Holland 1986; Greenland 2005). Although it might seem natural to ask whether a disease like hypertension is caused by a person's race, studies that contrast rates of hypertension in different racial groups do not adequately address this question. To ameliorate the racial disparities in hypertension, we would first need to identify feasible interventions. For this goal, discussing race as a cause is of no help, because changing the race of individuals is not an option.

Identifying and evaluating feasible interventions

Even when an exposure is an intervention, the discussion of its effects can be complicated if there is treatment non-compliance. In practice, apart from occasional mandates, treatments are only prescribed or recommended, therefore prescription or recommendation is all that can be studied and implemented. What a subject actually chooses to do in response to the assigned treatment is a function not only of the assignment but also of other factors, many if not most of which are infeasible to modify (such as the subject's age).

If the researcher wishes to understand the effects of received treatment rather than treatment assignment, it is important to realize that received treatment is an outcome, not an intervention, and is thus subject to the problems described above for intermediate outcomes such as BMI. Special techniques are available for studying the effects of received treatment (e.g. instrumental variables, g-estimation—see Greenland 2000 and Greenland *et al.* 2008 for elementary discussions of these topics). Nonetheless, effects estimated by these techniques are those expected under ideal conditions and will likely overestimate the effects that will be seen in field implementation. The most relevant causal hypotheses for policy makers and health practitioners concern the changes in outcome to be expected under the implementation of feasible interventions, subject to all their compliance problems.

Estimating field effects of feasible interventions is difficult but doing so at least avoids the unrealism and biases that arise from pretending that subject characteristics or behaviour are under direct or perfect control of health practitioners or society. In studying these types of interventions, the effect measure of interest will be a contrast in outcomes corresponding to different levels of the intervention (e.g. whether or not to fund a given programme), rather than the 'received treatment' discussed above. Thus the question is not what would happen if people were to comply with the intervention they were assigned, but rather what would result if people were offered a given treatment at a given cost.

Studies that address causal hypotheses about feasible interventions face profound methodologic difficulties. If the intervention is not assigned at random (e.g. if individuals who participate in a given intervention are volunteers, and their outcomes are compared to those who chose not to participate), the resulting measure of association is likely to be confounded and will therefore be a poor estimate of the desired measure of effect. The measure of association can also be distorted due to refusals, loss to follow-up, and measurement error, among other things. These threats to validity are discussed in Chapter 6.12 ('Validity and bias in epidemiological research') and in epidemiologic methods texts such as Rothman *et al.* (2008).

Problems in generalizing the results from a particular study to the target population of interest are not given detailed attention in many textbooks, yet they are of great concern for policy making. The target populations for policy are always different from study populations, for at the very least the target population is defined in terms of future experience, whereas study results are always based on the past. Even if there are no time trends, however, factors such as the compliance rate and response to the intervention may depend on the characteristics of the individuals involved in a given study. The results from a study may therefore not be applicable to other populations, each of which may be composed of a different mix of individuals.

This problem of population heterogeneity is sometimes framed as an issue of 'effect modification', meaning that the measure of the intervention effect depends on characteristics of the individual or the population (Chapter 4 in Rothman *et al.* 2008). In theory, the solution is to identify factors responsible for the effect modification, stratify on these factors, estimate effect measures within the stratified groups, and predict the likely impact of an intervention in a target population by standardizing the stratified estimates based on the distribution of the factors in the target population. This approach is not wholly satisfactory, however, because it can be difficult to identify all the important sources of effect modification, and there are always severe data limitations on the number of factors can be studied in this fashion.

From research to policy and beyond

This chapter has reviewed some of the considerations necessary in making causal inferences relevant to public health. These considerations are not crucial in all or even most studies, especially if the explicit goal of the study is to report associations rather than to estimate causal effects and thus provide data for subsequent evaluations (Greenland *et al.* 2004). Nonetheless, results from epidemiologic studies are often used as inputs for policy and judicial decisions. To name just a few examples, studies on the link between smoking and lung cancer have led to labelling of cigarette packs and bans on indoor smoking; results linking air pollutants to disease and mortality have informed emissions standards; and findings on the connection between vitamin deficiencies and adverse health outcomes have led to fortification of milk, cereals, and flour.

It is thus important for public-health researchers as well as policy makers to understand the fundamentals of causal inference, especially the often neglected issues of defining meaningful and feasible interventions. It is equally important for researchers to understand that scientific research is done to inform policy making, not to set policy. Apart from outbreak investigations, no single study is capable of establishing a causal relation or fully informing either individual or policy decisions. Those decisions should be based on a careful consideration of the entire relevant scientific and policy literature and must address cost-benefit considerations as well as purely scientific issues.

References

Freedman, D.A., Petitti, D.B., and Robins, J.M. (2004). Point-counterpoint. On the efficacy of screening for breast cancer. *International Journal of Epidemiology*, **33**, 43–55.

Giovannoni, G., and Ebers, G. (2007). Multiple sclerosis: the environment and causation. *Current Opinion in Neurology*, **20**, 261–8.

Greenland, S. (1993). A meta-analysis of coffee, myocardial infarction, and coronary death. *Epidemiology*, **4**, 366–74.

Greenland, S. (2000). An introduction to instrumental variables for epidemiologists. *International Journal of Epidemiology*, **29**, 722–9. (Erratum: 2000, **29**, 1102).

Greenland, S. (2002). Causality theory for policy uses of epidemiologic measures. In *Summary measures of population health* (C.J. Murray, J.A. Salomon, C.D. Mathers *et al.*, eds.). Harvard University Press/ World Health Organization, Cambridge.

Greenland, S. (2005). Epidemiologic measures and policy formulation: Lessons from potential outcomes (with discussion). *Emerging Themes in Epidemiology*, **2**, 1–4.

Greenland, S., Gago-Domiguez, M. and Castellao, J.E. (2004). The value of risk-factor ('black-box') epidemiology (with discussion). *Epidemiology*, **15**, 519–35.

Greenland, S., Lanes, S.F., and Jara, M. (2008). Estimating efficacy from randomized trials with discontinuations: The need for intent-to-treat design and g-estimation. *Clinical Trials*, **5**, 5–13.

Hernán, M.A. (2005). Hypothetical interventions to define causal effects—afterthought or prerequisite? *American Journal of Epidemiology*, **162**, 618–20.

Hill, A.B. (1965). The environment and disease: association or causation? *Proceedings of the Royal Society of Medicine*, **58**, 295–300.

Holland, P.W. (1986). Statistics and causal inference. *Journal of the American Statistical Association*, **81**, 945–60.

Holman, C.D.J., Arnold-Reed, D.E., de Klerk, N., McComb, C., and English, D.R. (2001). A psychometric experiment in causal inference to estimate evidential weights used by epidemiologists. *Epidemiology*, **12**, 246–50.

Hume, D. (1739). *A treatise of human nature.* Oxford University Press, Oxford, 1888; 2nd edition, 1978.

Kalbfleisch, J.D., and Prentice, R.L. (2002). *The statistical analysis of failure-time data*, 2nd edition. Wiley, New York.

Kuhn, T.S. (1970). *The structure of scientific revolutions*, 2nd edition. University of Chicago Press, Chicago.

Lanes, S.F. and Poole, C. (1984). 'Truth in packaging?' The unwrapping of epidemiologic research. *Journal of Occupational Medicine*, **26**, 571–4.

Maclure, M. (1985). Popperian refutation in epidemiology. *American Journal of Epidemiology*, **121**, 343–50.

Mill, J.S.A. (1862). *System of logic, ratiocinative and inductive*, 5th edition. Parker, Son and Bowin, London. (Cited in: Clark, D.W., and MacMahon, B. (eds.) (1981). *Preventive and community medicine*, 2nd edition. Little, Brown, Boston. Chapter 2.).

Phillips, C.V. and Goodman, K.J. (2004). The missed lessons of Sir Austin Bradford Hill. *Epidemiologic Perspectives and Innovation* (online journal), **1**, 3.

Phillips, C.V. and Goodman, K.J. (2006). Causal criteria and counterfactuals; nothing more (or less) than scientific common sense. *Emerging Themes in Epidemiology* (online journal), **3**, 5.

Poole, C. (2001). Causal values. *Epidemiology*, **12**, 139–41.

Robins, J.M. and Greenland, S. (2000). Comment on 'Causal Inference Without Counterfactuals' by Dawid AP. *Journal of the American Statistical Association*, **95**, 477–82.

Rothman, K.J., Greenland, S., and Lash, T.L. (2008). *Modern epidemiology*, 3rd edition. Lippincott-Williams-Wilkins, Philadelphia.

Taubes, G. (1995). Epidemiology faces its limits. *Science*, **269**, 164–9.

United States Department of Health, Education and Welfare. (1964). *Smoking and health: report of the Advisory Committee to the Surgeon General of the Public Health Service.* Government Printing Office, Washington. PHS Publ No. 1103.

Weed, D.L. (1986). On the logic of causal inference. *American Journal of Epidemiology*, **123**, 965–79.

Weed, D.L. and Gorelic, L.S. (1996). The practice of causal inference in cancer epidemiology. *Cancer Epidemiology, Biomarkers & Prevention*, **5**, 303–11.

6.14

Systematic reviews and meta-analysis

Matthias Egger, George Davey Smith, and Jonathan Sterne

Abstract

Systematic reviews are 'studies of studies' that are done using a systematic approach to minimize bias and random error. Similar to other research, the problem to be addressed and the collection and analysis of the data should be detailed in a study protocol. This should include eligibility criteria for studies to be included, a comprehensive search strategy for such studies, and an assessment of their methodological quality. Systematic reviews may, or may not, include meta-analysis, a statistical combination of results from several studies to produce a single estimate of the effect of an intervention. Systematic reviews allow for a more objective appraisal of the evidence than traditional, narrative reviews and may contribute to resolve uncertainty and identify areas where further studies are needed. Meta-analysis, if appropriate, will enhance the precision of estimates of intervention effects, leading to reduced probability of false negative results, and potentially to a timelier introduction of effective interventions. Meta-analyses are, however, liable to numerous biases both at the level of the individual trial ('garbage in, garbage out') and the dissemination of trial results (publication bias and other reporting biases). Meta-analysis should be performed only within the framework of carefully conducted systematic reviews. The thoughtful consideration of heterogeneity between study results is an important aspect of systematic reviews and meta-analyses, and particularly important in meta-analyses of observational studies.

The volume of data that need to be considered by practitioners and researchers is constantly expanding. In many areas it has become simply impossible for the individual to read, critically evaluate and synthesize the state of current knowledge, let alone keep updating this on a regular basis. Reviews have become essential tools for anybody who wants to keep up with the new evidence that is accumulating in his or her field of interest. However, since Mulrow (Mulrow 1987) drew attention to the poor quality of narrative review articles in the 1980s, it has become clear that conventional reviews are an unreliable source of information. Since then there has been increasing focus on formal methods of systematically reviewing studies, to produce explicitly formulated, reproducible, and up-to-date summaries of the effects of healthcare interventions. This is illustrated by the sharp increase in the number of reviews that used formal methods to synthesize evidence (Fig. 6.14.1). This chapter discusses terminology and scope, provides some historical background, and examines the potentials and pitfalls of systematic reviews and meta-analysis.

Systematic review, overview, or meta-analysis?

A number of terms are used concurrently to describe the process of systematically reviewing and integrating research evidence, including 'systematic review', 'meta-analysis', 'research synthesis', 'overview', and 'pooling'. A systematic review is a review that has been prepared using a documented systematic approach to minimizing biases and random errors. A systematic review may, or may not, include a meta-analysis: A statistical analysis of the results from independent studies, which generally aims to produce a single, typical estimate of a treatment effect. The distinction between systematic review and meta-analysis is important because it is always

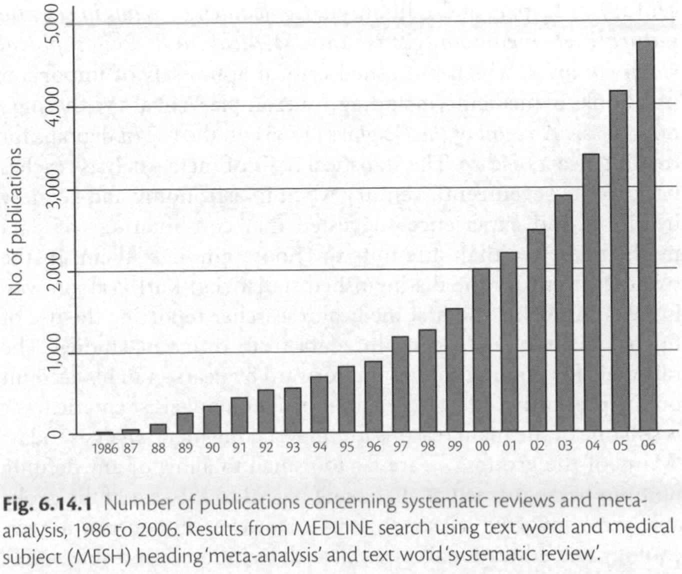

Fig. 6.14.1 Number of publications concerning systematic reviews and meta-analysis, 1986 to 2006. Results from MEDLINE search using text word and medical subject (MESH) heading 'meta-analysis' and text word 'systematic review'.

appropriate and desirable to systematically review a body of data, but it may sometimes be inappropriate, or even misleading, to statistically pool results from separate studies.

The scope of meta-analysis

A clear distinction should also be made between meta-analysis of randomized controlled trials and meta-analysis of epidemiological studies. Consider a set of trials of high methodological quality that examined the same intervention in comparable patient populations: Each trial will provide an unbiased estimate of the same underlying treatment effect. The variability that is observed between the trials can confidently be attributed to random variation and meta-analysis should provide an equally unbiased estimate of the treatment effect, with an increase in the precision of this estimate. A fundamentally different situation arises in the case of epidemiological studies, for example case-control studies, cross-sectional studies, or cohort studies. Due to the effects of confounding and bias, such observational studies may produce estimates of associations that deviate from the truth beyond what can be attributed to chance.

The fundamental difference that exists between observational studies and randomized controlled trials does not mean that the latter are immune to bias. As discussed below publication bias and other reporting biases may distort the evidence from both trials and observational studies. Bias may also be introduced if the methodological quality of clinical trials is inadequate. While systematic reviews have clear advantages over conventional reviews, it is crucial to understand the limitations of meta-analysis and the importance of exploring sources of heterogeneity and bias. Also, we believe that there continues to be a place for narrative reviews and editorials that express an informed but subjective opinion about how a particular body of evidence should be interpreted.

Historical notes

Efforts to compile summaries of research for medical practitioners who struggle with the amount of information that is relevant to medical practice are not new. Chalmers and Tröhler (Chalmers 2000) drew attention to two journals published in the eighteenth century in Leipzig and Edinburgh, *Comentarii de rebus in scientia naturali et medicina gestis* and *Medical and Philosophical Commentaries*, which published critical appraisals of important new books in medicine, including, for example, William Withering's now classic *Account of the Foxglove* (1785) on the use of digitalis for treating heart disease. The statistical basis of meta-analysis reaches back to the seventeenth century when in astronomy and geodesy intuition and experience suggested that combinations of data might be better than attempts to choose amongst them. In the twentieth century the distinguished statistician Karl Pearson was, in 1904, probably the first medical researcher reporting the use of formal techniques to combine data from different studies. The rationale for pooling studies put forward by Pearson in his account on the preventive effect of serum inoculations against enteric fever is still one of the main reasons for undertaking meta-analysis today: 'Many of the groups . . . are far too small to allow of any definite opinion being formed at all, having regard to the size of the probable error involved' (Pearson 1904). However, in contrast to psychology and educational research, such techniques were not widely used in medicine until the 1980s, when meta-analysis became increasingly popular in cardiology, oncology, and perinatal medicine. In the 1990s, the foundation of the Cochrane Collaboration (Box 6.14.1) facilitated numerous methodological developments and helped establish systematic reviews and meta-analysis as important tools in research and policy making.

Why do we need systematic reviews?

A patient with myocardial infarction in 1981

A likely scenario in the early 1980s, when discussing the discharge of a patient who had suffered an uncomplicated myocardial infarction, is as follows: A keen junior doctor asks whether the patient should receive a beta-blocker for secondary prevention of a future cardiac event. After a moment of silence the consultant states that this was a question which should be discussed in detail at the Journal Club on Thursday. The junior doctor is told to assemble and present the relevant literature. It is late in the evening when she makes her way to the library. The MEDLINE search identifies four clinical trials. When reviewing the conclusions from these trials, the doctor finds them to be rather confusing and contradictory (Table 6.14.1). Her consultant points out that the sheer amount of research published makes it impossible to keep track of and critically appraise individual studies. He recommends a good review article. Back in the library, the junior doctor finds an article which the *British Medical Journal* published in 1981. This narrative review concluded that 'Thus, despite claims that they reduce arrhythmias, cardiac work, and infarct size, we still have no clear evidence that beta-blockers improve long-term survival after infarction despite almost 20 years of clinical trials' (Mitchell 1981).

The junior doctor is relieved. She presents the findings of the review article, the Journal Club is a full success, and the patient is discharged without a beta-blocker.

Narrative reviews

Traditional narrative reviews have a number of disadvantages that systematic reviews may overcome. First, the classical review is subjective and therefore prone to bias and error. Mulrow (1987) showed that among 50 reviews published in the mid-1980s in leading general medicine journals, 49 reviews did not specify the source of the information and failed to perform a standardized assessment of the methodological quality of studies. Our junior doctor could have consulted another review of the same topic, published in the *European Heart Journal* in the same year. This review concluded that 'it seems perfectly reasonable to treat patients who have survived an infarction with timolol' (Hampton 1981). Without guidance by formal rules, reviewers will inevitably disagree about issues as basic as what types of studies it is appropriate to include and how to balance the quantitative evidence they provide. Selective inclusion of studies that support the author's view is common. It is thus hardly surprising that reviewers using traditional methods often reach opposite conclusions and miss small, but potentially important, differences (Mulrow 1987). In controversial areas the conclusions drawn from a given body of evidence may be associated more with the speciality of the reviewer than with the available data. By systematically identifying, scrutinising, tabulating, and perhaps integrating all relevant studies, systematic reviews allow a more objective appraisal, which can help to resolve uncertainties when the original research, classical reviews, and editorial comments disagree.

Box 6.14.1 The Cochrane Collaboration

Funded in 1993, the Cochrane Collaboration (www.cochrane.org) is a unique international organization whose aim is to help people make well-informed decisions by preparing, maintaining, and promoting systematic reviews in all areas of healthcare, including treatment, prevention, screening, and rehabilitation. At present, there are nearly 15 000 people participating in the collaboration, in nearly 100 countries. The main work is done in one of about 50 review groups that take on the task of preparing and maintaining reviews. These reviews generally focus on the findings from randomized trials, and most include one or several meta-analyses. There are also 12 Cochrane fields, including a Cochrane health promotion and public health field, which cut across the scope of review groups and help identify potential reviewers and topics. The coverage of Cochrane reviews is continually improving, with over 3000 reviews available at the beginning of 2008. The reviews are published in the Cochrane Database of Systematic Reviews, which is part of The Cochrane Library, an electronic publication available on Wiley Interscience (http://www.thecochranelibrary.com). Cochrane reviews are indexed in Medline. The Cochrane Library also includes a large register of controlled trials, the Cochrane Central Register of Controlled Trials, and a register of methodological studies.

The logo of the Cochrane Collaboration (Fig. 6.14.2) illustrates a systematic review of seven RCTs of a short, inexpensive course of a corticosteroid given to women about to give birth too early, comparing the intervention with placebo. A schematic representation of the forest plot is shown. The first of these RCTs was reported in 1972, the last in 1980. The diagram summarizes the evidence that would have been revealed, had the available RCTs been reviewed systematically a decade later: It indicates strongly that corticosteroids reduce the risk of babies dying from the complications of immaturity. Because no systematic review of these trials had been published until 1989, most obstetricians had not realized that the treatment was so effective, reducing the odds of the babies of these women dying from the complications of immaturity by 30–50 per cent. As a result, tens of thousands of premature babies have probably suffered and died unnecessarily, and needed more expensive treatment than was necessary. By 1991, seven more trials had been reported, and the picture had become still stronger.

A similar collaboration, the Campbell Collaboration, was set up to prepare systematic reviews of high-quality research conducted worldwide on effective methods and interventions in the fields of social welfare and social work, education and learning, and crime and delinquency (see www.campbellcollaboration.org).

Limitations of a single study

A single study often fails to detect, or exclude with certainty, a modest, albeit relevant, difference in the effects of two therapies. A trial may thus show no statistically significant treatment effect when in reality such an effect exists—it may produce a false negative result. In many trials there is a substantial probability of missing a clinically relevant difference in outcome (Freiman *et al.* 1992; Thornley & Adams 1998). The number of patients included in trials is thus often inadequate. In some cases, however, the required sample size may be difficult to achieve. A drug which reduces the risk of death from myocardial infarction by 10 per cent could delay many thousands of deaths each year in the United Kingdom alone. However, in order to detect such an effect with 90 per cent certainty over 10 000 patients in each treatment group would be needed.

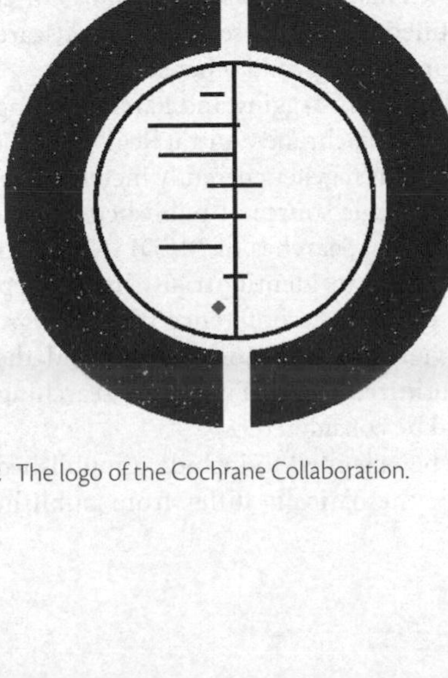

Fig. 6.14.2 The logo of the Cochrane Collaboration.

The meta-analytic approach appears to be an attractive alternative to such a large, expensive, and logistically problematic study. Data from patients in trials evaluating the same or a similar drug in a number of smaller, but comparable, studies are considered. In this way the necessary number of patients may be reached, and relatively small effects can be detected or excluded with confidence. Systematic reviews can also contribute to considerations regarding the applicability of study results. If many trials exist in different groups of patients, with similar results being seen in the various trials, then it can be concluded that the effect of the intervention under study has some generality. By putting together all available data, meta-analyses are also better placed than individual trials to answer questions regarding whether or not an overall study result varies

Table 6.14.1 Conclusions from four randomized controlled trials of beta-blockers in secondary prevention after myocardial infarction

◆ '*The mortality and hospital readmission rates were not significantly different in the two groups. This also applied to the incidence of cardiac failure, exertional dyspnoea, and frequency of ventricular ectopic beats*.' Reynolds et al. British Heart Journal (1972)
◆ '*Until the results of further trials are reported long-term beta-adrenoceptor blockade (possibly up to two years) is recommended after uncomplicated anterior myocardial infarction*.' Multicentre International Study, BMJ (1977)
◆ '*The trial was designed to detect a 50 per cent reduction in mortality and this was not shown. The non-fatal reinfarction rate was similar in both groups*.' Baber et al. British Heart Journal (1980)
◆ '*We conclude that long-term treatment with timolol in patients surviving acute myocardial infarction reduces mortality and the rate of reinfarction*.' The Norwegian Multicentre Study Group, *New England Journal of Medicine* (1981)

among subgroups—e.g. among men and women, older and younger patients, or participants with different degrees of severity of disease.

A more transparent appraisal

An important advantage of systematic reviews is that they render the review process more transparent. In traditional narrative reviews it is often not clear how the conclusions follow from the data examined. In an adequately presented systematic review it should be possible for readers to replicate the quantitative component of the argument. To facilitate this, it is valuable if the exclusion of potentially relevant studies is justified and the data included in meta-analyses are either presented in full or made available to interested readers. The increased openness required leads to the replacement of unhelpful descriptors such as 'no clear evidence, 'some evidence of a trend', 'a weak relationship', and 'a strong relationship'. Furthermore, performing a meta-analysis may lead to reviewers moving beyond the conclusions authors present in the abstract of papers, to a thorough examination of the actual data.

The epidemiology of results

The tabulation, exploration, and evaluation of results are important components of systematic reviews. As discussed in more detail below, this can be taken further to explore sources of heterogeneity and test new hypotheses that were not posed in individual studies. This has been termed the 'epidemiology of results' where the findings of an original study replace the individual as the unit of analysis (Jenicek 1989). Systematic reviews can thus lead to the identification of the most promising or the most urgent research question, and may permit a more accurate calculation of the sample sizes needed in future studies. This is illustrated by an early meta-analysis of four trials that compared different methods of monitoring the foetus during labour (Chalmers 1979). The meta-analysis led to the hypothesis that, compared with intermittent auscultation, continuous foetal heart monitoring reduced the risk of neonatal seizures. This hypothesis was subsequently confirmed in a randomized trial of almost seven times the size of the four previous studies combined (MacDonald *et al.* 1985).

What was the evidence in 1981?

What conclusions would our junior doctor have reached if she had had access to a systematic review and meta-analysis of the beta-blocker trials? A total of 13 such trials had in fact been published by the end of 1981. Using meta-analysis to combine the results of these 13 trials, the relative risk of mortality comparing patients treated with beta-blocker with those treated with placebo is estimated at 0.78 (95 per cent confidence intervals 0.69–0.88, $P<0.001$). Thus conclusive evidence of the life-saving potential of this treatment, though available, was ignored.

Steps in carrying out systematic reviews

Developing a review protocol

Systematic reviews should be viewed as observational studies of the evidence. The steps involved, summarized in Box 6.14.2, are similar to any other research undertaking: Formulation of the problem to be addressed, collection and analysis of the data, and interpretation of the results. Likewise, a detailed study protocol which clearly states the question to be addressed, the subgroups of interest, and the methods and criteria to be employed for identifying and selecting relevant studies and extracting and analysing information should be written in advance. This is important to avoid bias being introduced by decisions that are influenced by the data. For example, studies which produced unexpected or undesired results may be excluded by *post hoc* changes to the inclusion criteria. Similarly, unplanned data-driven subgroup analyses may produce spurious results. The review protocol should ideally be conceived by a group of reviewers with expertise both in the content area and the science of research synthesis.

Objectives and eligibility criteria

The formulation of detailed objectives is at the heart of any research project. This should include the definition of study participants, interventions, outcomes, and settings. As with patient inclusion and exclusion criteria in clinical studies, eligibility criteria can then be defined for the type of studies to be included. They relate to the quality of trials and to the combinability of patients, treatments, outcomes, and lengths of follow-up. Quality and design features of clinical trials can influence their results (see below). Ideally, only controlled trials with proper patient randomization which report on all initially included patients according to the intention-to-treat principle and with an objective, preferably blinded, outcome assessment would be considered for inclusion. However, the investigation of the influence of study quality may often be an important objective of a meta-analysis. Furthermore, assessing study quality can be a subjective process, especially since the information reported is often incomplete for this purpose (Schulz 1996). It is therefore generally preferable to define only basic inclusion criteria, to assess the methodological quality of component studies, and to perform a thorough sensitivity analysis, as illustrated below.

Literature search

The search strategy for the identification of the relevant studies should be clearly delineated. Identifying controlled trials has become more straightforward in recent years. Appropriate terms to index randomized trials and controlled trials were introduced in the widely used bibliographic databases MEDLINE and EMBASE by the mid-1990s. However, tens of thousands of trial reports had been included prior to the introduction of these terms. In a painstaking effort the Cochrane Collaboration checked the titles and abstracts of almost 300 000 MEDLINE and EMBASE records which were then re-tagged as clinical trials if appropriate. It was important to examine both MEDLINE and EMBASE: The majority of journals indexed in MEDLINE are published in the United States whereas EMBASE has better coverage of European journals. Also, the results of trials indexed only in EMBASE may differ from other trials (Sampson *et al.* 2003). Finally, thousands of reports of controlled trials have been identified by manual searches ('handsearching') of journals, conference proceedings, and other sources.

All trials identified in the re-tagging and handsearching projects have been included in the Cochrane Central Register of Controlled Trials (see Box 6.14.1). This register currently includes over 500 000 records and is the best single source of published trials for inclusion in systematic reviews. Searches of MEDLINE and EMBASE are, however, still required to identify trials that were published recently. Specialized databases, conference proceedings, and the bibliographies of review articles, monographs, and the located studies should be scrutinized as well. Finally, the searching by hand of key journals should be considered.

The search should be extended to include unpublished studies, as their results may systematically differ from published trials.

Box 6.14.2 Steps in conducting a systematic review

1. Formulate the review question
2. Define inclusion and exclusion criteria, considering
   - Participants
   - Interventions and comparisons
   - Outcomes
   - Study designs and methodological quality
3. Develop the search strategy to identify relevant studies, considering the following sources
   - MEDLINE, EMBASE, and other bibliographic databases
   - Cochrane Central Register of Controlled Trials
   - World Health Organization search portal of trial registers
   - Checking reference lists of relevant articles
   - Web site of Food and Drug Administration (FDA)
   - Search by hand of key journals
   - Personal communication with experts in the field
4. Select studies
   - Have eligibility checked by >1 observer
   - Develop strategy to resolve disagreements
   - Keep log of excluded studies, with reasons for exclusions
5. Assess study quality
   - Consider assessment by >1 observer
   - Use simple checklists rather than quality scales
   - Always assess concealment of treatment allocation, blinding, and handling of patient attrition
   - Consider blinding of observers to authors, institutions, and journals
6. Extract data
   - Design and pilot data extraction form
   - Consider data extraction by >1 observer
   - Consider blinding of observers to authors, institutions, and journals
7. Analyse and present results
   - Tabulate results from individual studies
   - Examine forest plot
   - Explore possible sources of heterogeneity and bias
   - Consider meta-analysis of all trials or subgroups of trials
   - Perform sensitivity analyses, examine funnel plots
   - Make list of excluded studies available to interested readers
8. Interpret results
   - Consider limitations, including publication and related biases
   - Consider strength of evidence
   - Consider applicability
   - Consider numbers-needed-to-treat to benefit/harm
   - Consider economic implications
   - Consider implications for future research

Note: Points 1–7 should be addressed in the review protocol.

A systematic review which is restricted to published evidence may produce distorted results due to publication bias (see below). The registration of trials at the time they are established (and before their results become known) would eliminate the risk of publication bias. Trial registration has gained momentum in recent years. The 1997 US Food and Drug Administration (FDA) Modernization Act mandated registration of efficacy drug trials conducted under FDA regulations. Also, the International Committee of Medical Journal Editors (ICMJE) introduced a policy, effective from July 2005, that requires prospective trial registration as a condition of publication (De Angelis *et al.* 2004). Several web-based registers have since been established, including ClinicalTrials.gov (www.clinicaltrials.gov) and the International Standard Randomized Controlled Trial Number Registry (http://isrctn.org). The World Health Organization has built an international search portal to facilitate access to the data from all major registers (www.who.int/ictrp). In addition to trial registries, colleagues, experts in the field, contacts in the pharmaceutical industry, and other informal channels can also be important sources of information on unpublished and ongoing trials. Finally, the proceedings of relevant FDA advisory panels and other FDA, which are also available at www.fda.gov, may be useful to identify unpublished studies or unpublished data, particularly on adverse effects of treatment (Jüni 2004).

Selection of studies, assessment of methodological quality, and data extraction

Decisions regarding the inclusion or exclusion of individual studies often involve some degree of subjectivity. It is therefore useful to have two observers checking eligibility of candidate studies, with disagreements being resolved by discussion or a third reviewer.

Randomized controlled trials provide the best evidence of the efficacy of medical interventions but they are not immune to bias. The assessment of study quality is therefore an important component of systematic review. Trials with inadequate allocation concealment or lack of blinding (see Box 6.14.3 for a discussion of these concepts) tend to exaggerate estimates of intervention effects, compared with adequately concealed or adequately blinded trials (Jüni *et al.* 2001). Treatment effects may also be overestimated if some participants, for example, those not adhering to study medications, were excluded from the analysis. A large number of different scales and checklists are available to assess the quality of clinical trials. However, empirical evidence and theoretical considerations suggest that although summary quality scores may in some circumstances provide a useful overall assessment, scales should not generally be used to assess the quality of trials in systematic reviews (Jüni *et al.* 1999). Rather, the relevant methodological aspects should be identified in the study protocol, and assessed individually. Again, independent assessment by more than one observer is desirable. Blinding of observers to the names of the authors and their institutions, the names of the journals, sources of funding, and acknowledgments may also be considered but this is time consuming, and potential benefits may not always justify the additional costs.

It is important that two independent observers extract the data, so errors can be avoided. The extraction of data to calculate standardized mean differences (see below) has been shown to be particularly liable to errors. A standardized record form is needed for this purpose. Data extraction forms should be carefully designed, piloted, and revised if necessary. Electronic data collection forms and web-based forms have a number of advantages, including the combination of data abstraction and data entry in one step, and the automatic detection of inconsistencies between data recorded by different observers. However, the complexities involved in programming and revising electronic forms should not be underestimated.

Box 6.14.3 A crucial distinction: allocation concealment versus blinding in clinical trials

Allocation concealment refers to procedures that secure strict implementation of the schedule of random assignments by preventing foreknowledge of forthcoming allocations by study participants or by those recruiting them to the trial. It is always feasible to conceal allocation. Failure to conceal allocation may lead to biased selection of participants into intervention groups. Examples of procedures usually considered adequate include sequentially numbered drug containers of identical appearance; central allocation (including web-based or pharmacy-controlled randomization); and sequentially numbered, opaque, sealed envelopes. Examples of procedures usually considered inadequate include using an open random allocation schedule; assignment of envelopes without appropriate safeguards (for example, unsealed or non-opaque or not sequentially numbered); and alternation or rotation.

Blinding refers to procedures that prevent study participants, caregivers, or outcome assessors from knowing which intervention was received. Blinding of participants and caregivers may not be feasible: For example, in a trial of surgery versus radiotherapy for prostate cancer. In such circumstances it may still be possible to blind the assessment of outcomes. Blinding may reduce the risk that knowledge of the intervention received, rather than the intervention itself, affects outcomes and/or outcome measurements. Examples of procedures usually considered adequate include provision of indistinguishable placebo tablets, or use of a sham surgical procedure in the control group. An example of blinded outcome assessment is assessment of medical records to ascertain cause of death by an endpoints committee unaware of intervention status.

Meta-analysis: Presenting, combining, and interpreting results

Once studies have been selected, critically appraised, and data extracted, the characteristics of included studies should be presented in tabular form. For example, a meta-analysis of parallel group randomized trials that examined the effectiveness of beta blockers versus placebo or alternative treatment in patients who had had a myocardial infarction identified 31 trials of at least 6 months' duration, which contributed 33 comparisons of beta blocker with control groups (Freemantle *et al.* 1999). In the first table of the report, the authors presented the characteristics of each trial, including the trial acronym or first author and year of publication, average length of follow up, the name of the beta blocker tested, the level of blinding, concealment of allocation and the rate of loss to follow up.

Measures of treatment effect

The results from individual studies have to be expressed in a standardized format to allow for comparison between studies. If the endpoint is binary (for example, disease versus no disease, or dead versus alive) then relative risks or odds ratios are often calculated. The odds ratio has convenient mathematical properties, which allow for ease in the combination of data and the testing of the overall effect for statistical significance, but, the odds ratio will differ from the relative risk as the outcome becomes more common. Relative risks are more intuitively comprehensible to most people. However, as the outcome becomes more common the range of the relative risk is constrained while the odds ratio is not. The odds ratio has the further advantage that the odds ratio for non-occurrence of the outcome is exactly the inverse of the odds ratio for the outcome. Different measures such as the absolute risk reduction or the number of patients needed to be treated for one person to benefit are more helpful when applying results in clinical practice (see below).

If the outcome is continuous and measurements are made on the same scale (for example, blood pressure measured in mm Hg) the mean difference between the treatment and control groups is used. If trials measured outcomes in different ways, for example, pain on a 5-point ranking scale or on a 100-mm visual analogue scale, it is necessary to standardize the measurements on a uniform scale to allow their inclusion in meta-analysis. This is done by calculating the standardized mean difference for each study, i.e. the difference in means between the two groups divided by the pooled standard deviation of the measurements (Deeks *et al.* 2001).

Meta-analysis

Careful consideration of the combinability of the studies in question is an important step in systematic reviews (Box 6.14.2): It will not always be appropriate to combine the results from the different studies to produce a single estimate of the treatment effect. If, after careful consideration, a meta-analysis is deemed appropriate, the next step consists in estimating a typical effect by combining the data. Two principles are important. First, simply pooling the data from different studies and treating them as one large study would fail to preserve the randomization, and introduce bias and confounding. For example, a 'meta-analysis' of the literature on the role of male circumcision in HIV transmission concluded that the risk of HIV infection was lower in uncircumcised men. However, the analysis was performed by simply pooling the data from 33 diverse studies. A re-analysis stratifying the data by study found that an intact foreskin was in fact associated with an increased risk of HIV infection (O'Farrell & Egger 2000). Confounding by study thus led to a change in the direction of the association (a case of 'Simpson's paradox' in epidemiological parlance). The study unit of analysis must therefore always be maintained when combining data. Of note, several randomized trials have since conclusively shown that circumcision is associated with a substantially reduced risk of HIV transmission (Busse *et al.* 2008).

Second, simply calculating an arithmetic mean would be inappropriate. The results from small studies are more subject to the play of chance and should, therefore, be given less weight. Let us assume that we have k studies, and have derived a treatment effect estimate $\hat{\theta}$ (which might be a log odds ratio, log risk ratio, or mean difference) for each study ($i = 1$ to k). The 'fixed effects' model considers the variability between these treatment effect estimates as exclusively due to random variation, so that if all the studies were infinitely large they would give identical results. To derive a summary treatment effect estimate we calculate a weighted average of the treatment effect estimates in the individual studies:

$$\hat{\theta}_F = \frac{\sum w_i \hat{\theta}_i}{\sum w_i}$$

The subscript F denotes the fixed-effects assumption. Use of a weighted average accords with our first principle because individuals are only compared with other individuals in the same study. The usual choice of weight w_i for study i, which minimizes the variability of the summary treatment effect estimate, is inverse variance weight $w_i = 1/v_i$, where v_i is the variance of the treatment effect estimate. This accords with our second principle because the larger the study, the smaller will be the variance of the treatment effect estimate from that study. The standard error of the summary effect estimate $\hat{\theta}_F$ is:

$$\mathrm{SE}(\hat{\theta}_F) = \frac{1}{\sqrt{\sum_{i-1}^{k} w_i}}$$

This can be used to derive confidence intervals, a z statistic, and hence a P value for the null hypothesis that the true treatment effect is zero. An alternative weighting scheme, which has been shown to be more robust when data are sparse, is to use Mantel–Haenszel weights to combine relative risks or odds ratios. More details on statistical methods for meta-analysis and meta-analysis software are given by Deeks *et al.* and Sterne *et al.* (2001).

Graphical display

Results from each trial are usefully displayed together with their confidence intervals in a 'forest plot', a form of presentation developed in the 1980s by Richard Peto's group in Oxford. Figure 6.14.3 represents the forest plot for the trials of beta-blockers in secondary prevention after myocardial infarction (Freemantle *et al.* 1999). Each study is represented by a black square whose centre corresponds to the treatment effect estimate, and a horizontal line representing the 95 per cent confidence intervals of the relative risk. The confidence interval of most studies cross this line. The area of the black squares is proportional to the weight of the study in the meta-analysis: Plots that use an equally sized symbol for each study unhelpfully draw attention to the widest confidence intervals and thus the smallest studies. The solid vertical line corresponds to no effect of treatment (relative risk 1.0). If the confidence interval includes 1, then the difference in the effect of experimental and control therapy is not statistically significant at conventional levels ($P > 0.05$). In Fig. 6.14.3, the confidence interval of most studies crosses this line.

The diamond at the bottom of the graph displays the result of the meta-analysis: The centre of the diamond corresponds to the summary treatment effect estimate, while its width corresponds to the 95 per cent confidence interval. The broken line also corresponds to the summary treatment effect estimate and is included to a visual assessment of the variability of the individual studies around the summary estimate.

A logarithmic scale was used for plotting the relative risk in Fig. 6.14.3. There are a number of reasons why ratio measures are best plotted on logarithmic scales. Most importantly, the value of a risk ratio and its reciprocal, for example 0.5 and 2, which represent risk ratios of the same magnitude but opposite directions, will be equidistant from 1.0. Studies with relative risks below and above 1.0 will take up equal space on the graph and thus visually appear to be equally important. Also, confidence intervals will be symmetrical around the point estimate.

Heterogeneity between study results

The thoughtful consideration of heterogeneity between study results is an important aspect of systematic reviews. As explained above, this should start when writing the review protocol, by defining potential sources of heterogeneity and planning appropriate subgroup analyses. Once the data have been assembled, simple inspection of the forest plot is informative. The results from the beta-blocker trials are fairly homogeneous, clustering between a relative risk of 0.5 and 1.0, with widely overlapping confidence intervals (Fig. 6.14.3). In contrast, trials of BCG vaccination for prevention of tuberculosis (Colditz *et al.* 1994) are clearly heterogeneous (Fig. 6.14.4). The findings of the British trial, which indicate substantial benefit of BCG vaccination are not compatible with those from the Madras or Puerto Rico trials which suggest no effect or only a modest benefit. There is no overlap in the confidence intervals of the three trials.

The fixed-effects summary estimate is based on the assumption that the true effect does not differ between studies, and statistical tests of homogeneity (also called tests of heterogeneity) assess the evidence against this. The null hypothesis is individual study results reflect a single underlying effect, so that the differences between treatment effect estimates in individual studies are a consequence of sampling variation and simply due to chance. The test statistic is:

$$Q = \sum_{i-1}^{k} w_i \sum w_i (\hat{\theta}_i - \hat{\theta}_F)^2,$$

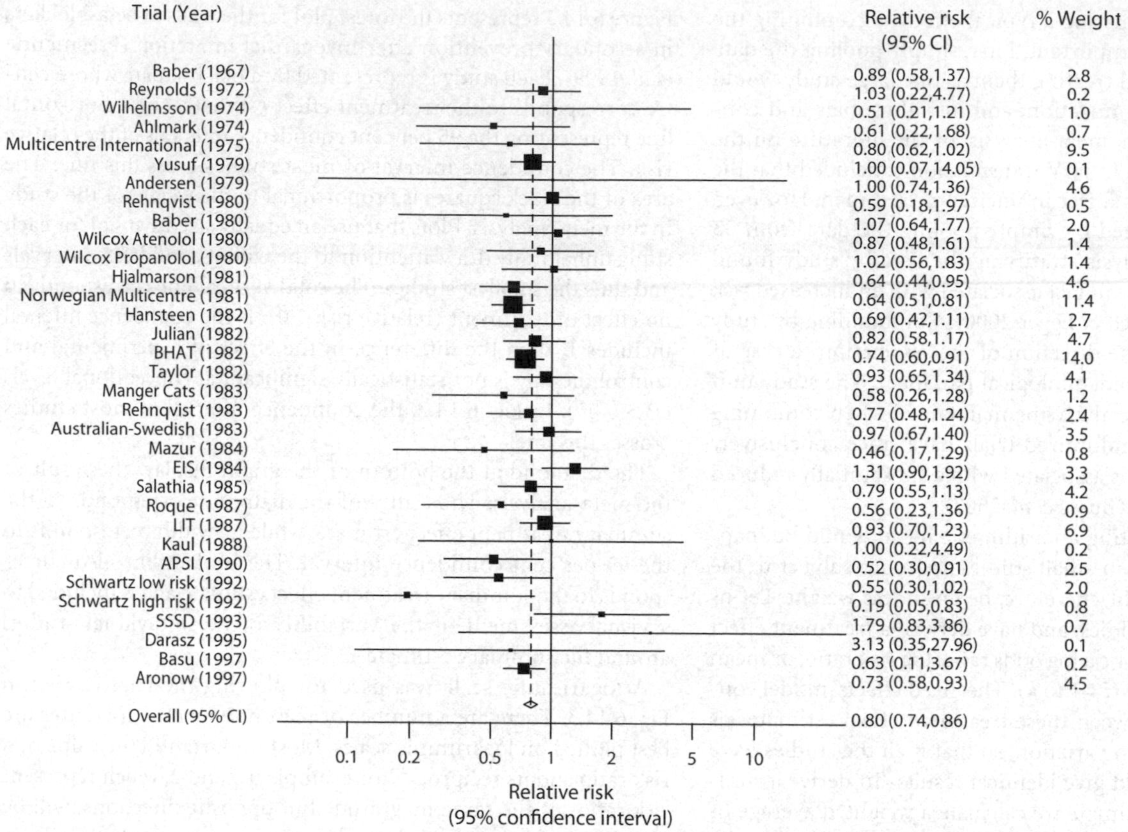

Fig. 6.14.3 'Forest plot' showing mortality results from trials of beta-blockers in secondary prevention after myocardial infarction. Trials are ordered by year of publication. The black square and horizontal line correspond to the trials' risk ratio and 95 per cent confidence intervals. The area of the black squares reflects the weight each trial contributes in the meta-analysis. The diamond represents the combined relative risk with its 95 per cent confidence interval, from fixed effects meta-analysis, indicating a 20 per cent reduction in the risk of death.

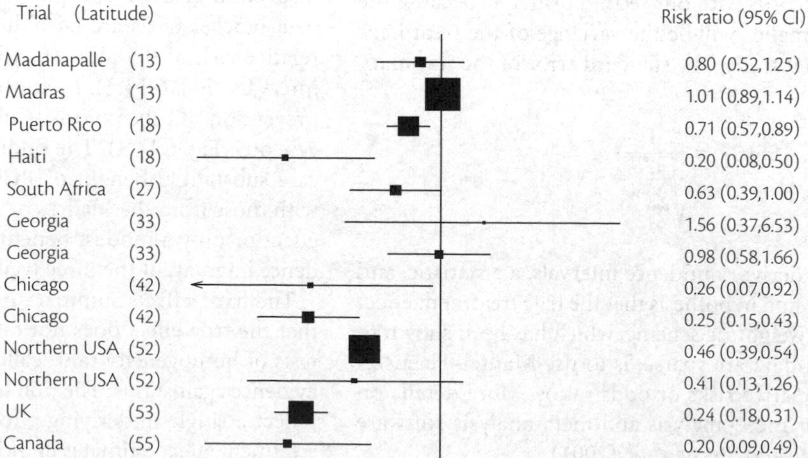

Fig. 6.14.4 Forest plot of trials of BCG vaccine to prevent tuberculosis. Trials are ordered according to the latitude of the study location, expressed as degrees from the equator. No meta-analysis is shown.

which is compared with the chi-squared distribution on (k–1) degrees of freedom. The greater the average difference between the individual study results and the summary estimate, the more evidence against the null hypothesis of a common fixed effect for all studies. The test of homogeneity gives $P=0.27$ for the beta-blocker trials but $P<0.001$ for the BCG trials. The BCG trials are an extreme example, however, and a major limitation of statistical tests of homogeneity is their lack of power—they often fail to reject the null hypothesis of homogeneous results even if substantial between-study differences exist. Reviewers should therefore not assume that a non-significant test of heterogeneity excludes important heterogeneity.

An alternative to testing for heterogeneity is to quantify it. Higgins *et al.* (2003) developed a measure of the degree of inconsistency in the studies' results, called I^2, which describes the percentage of total variation across studies that is due to heterogeneity rather than chance. It is readily calculated as $I^2 = 100$ per cent$\times(Q-\text{df})/Q$ where Q is the test statistic defined above and df the degrees of freedom. Negative values of I^2 are put equal to zero so that I^2 lies between 0 and 100 per cent. A value of 0 per cent indicates no observed heterogeneity, and larger values show increasing heterogeneity. The I^2 is 92 per cent for the BCG trials but only 12 per cent for the beta-blocker trials. Note that heterogeneity between study results should not be seen as purely a problem for systematic reviews, since it also provides an opportunity for examining why treatment effects differ in different circumstances, as discussed below.

Random-effects meta-analysis

There are a variety of statistical techniques available for meta-analysis, which can be broadly classified into 'fixed-effects' and 'random-effects' models (Deeks *et al.* 2001). Random-effects models (DerSimonian 1986) allow for between-study heterogeneity by assuming that the treatment effect varies between studies, and take this into consideration as an additional source of variation. The summary treatment effect from random-effect meta-analysis then estimates the mean about which the treatment effect in different studies is assumed to vary and thus should be interpreted differently from the results from a fixed-effects meta-analysis. In practice, random-effects estimates are derived simply by modifying the weights from the fixed-effects analysis. This leads to relatively more weight being given to smaller studies: This may be undesirable considering that small studies are more vulnerable to publication and other bias (see below). Because they assume an extra source of variability, random-effects estimates have wider confidence intervals than fixed-effects estimates.

While neither of the two models can be said to be 'correct', a substantial difference in the combined effect calculated by the fixed and random effects models will be seen only if studies are markedly heterogeneous, as in the case of the BCG trials (Table 6.14.2). Combining trials using a random-effects model indicates that BCG vaccination halves the risk of tuberculosis, whereas fixed-effects analysis indicates that the risk is only reduced by 35 per cent. This is essentially explained by the different weight given to the large Madras trial which showed no protective effect of vaccination (41 per cent of the total weight with fixed effects model, 10 per cent with random effects model, Table 6.14.2).

The use of random-effects models is often advocated if there is heterogeneity between study results. This is problematic: Rather than

Table 6.14.2 Meta-analysis of trials of BCG vaccination to prevent tuberculosis using a fixed-effects and random effects model. Note the differences in the weight allocated to individual studies

Trial	Relative risk (95% confidence interval)	Fixed effects weight (%)	Random effects weight (%)
Madanapalle	0.80 (0.52–1.25)	3.20	8.88
Madras	1.01 (0.89–1.14))	41.40	10.22
Puerto Rico	0.71 (0.57–0.89)	13.21	9.93
Haiti	0.20 (0.08–0.50)	0.73	6.00
South Africa	0.63 (0.39–1.00)	2.91	8.75
Georgia	0.98 (0.58–1.66)	0.31	3.80
Georgia	1.56 (0.37–6.53)	2.30	8.40
Chicago	0.26 (0.07–0.92)	0.40	4.40
Chicago	0.25 (0.15–0.43)	2.25	8.37
Northern United States	0.41 (0.13–1.26)	23.75	10.12
Northern United States	0.46 (0.39–0.54)	0.50	5.05
United Kingdom	0.24 (0.18–0.31)	8.20	9.71
Canada	0.20 (0.09–0.49)	0.84	6.34
Combined relative risks (95% confidence interval)		0.65 (0.60–0.70)	0.49 (0.35–0.70)

simply ignoring heterogeneity after allowing for it in a statistical model, a better approach is to scrutinize and attempt to explain it. As shown in Fig. 6.14.3, BCG vaccination appears to be effective at higher latitudes but not in warmer regions, possibly because exposure to certain environmental mycobacteria acts as a 'natural' BCG inoculation in warmer regions. In this situation it is more meaningful to quantify how the effect varies according to latitude than to calculate an overall estimate of effect which will be misleading, independent of the model used.

Cumulative meta-analysis

A useful way to show the accumulation of evidence over time is to perform a cumulative meta-analysis (Lau *et al.* 1992). Cumulative meta-analysis is defined as the repeated performance of meta-analysis whenever a new relevant trial becomes available for inclusion. This allows the retrospective identification of the point in time when a treatment effect first reached conventional levels of statistical significance.

Based on the systematic review by Freemantle *et al.* (1999), Fig. 6.14.5 shows mortality results from a cumulative meta-analysis of trials of beta-blockers in secondary prevention after myocardial infarction. A clear beneficial effect ($P<0.001$) was evident by the end of 1981. Subsequent trials in a further 15 000 patients simply confirmed this result. Similarly, Lau *et al.* (1992) showed that for the trials of intravenous streptokinase in acute myocardial infarction, a statistically significant ($P=0.01$) combined difference in total mortality was achieved by 1973. The results of the subsequent 25 studies which included the large Gruppo Italiano per lo Studio della Streptochinasi nell'Infarto Miocardico-1 (GISSI-1) (Gruppo Italiano per lo Studio della Streptochinasi nell'Infarto Miocardico (GISSI) 1986) and the Second International Study of Infarct

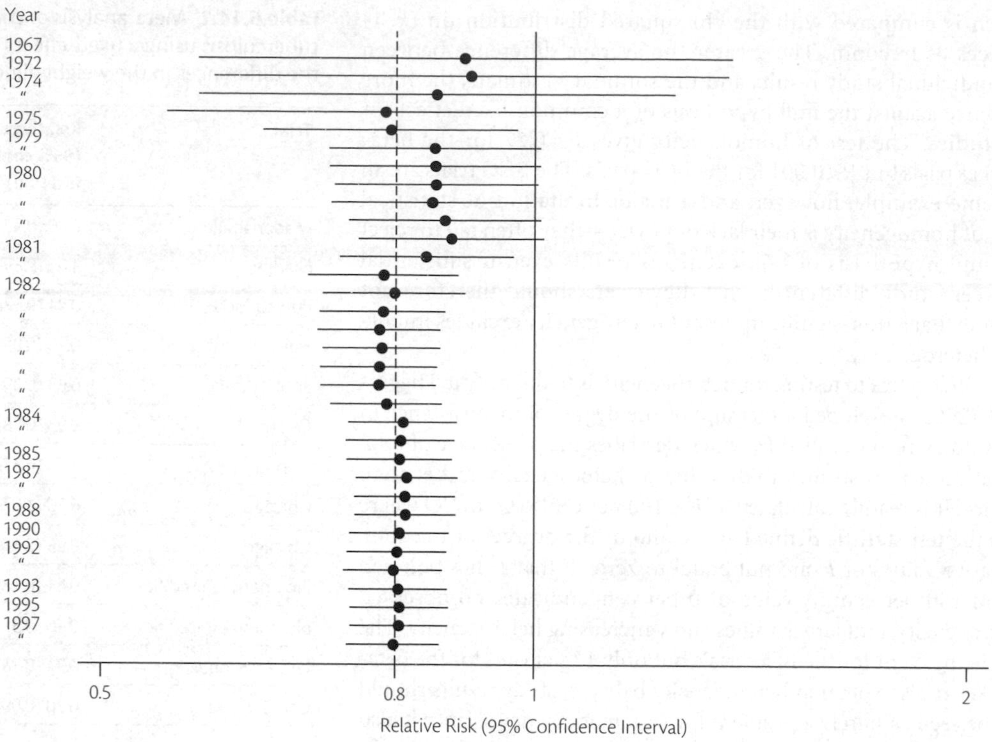

Fig. 6.14.5 Cumulative (fixed effects) meta-analysis of controlled trials of beta-blockers after myocardial infarction. A clear ($P<0.001$) reduction of mortality was evident by 1981.

Survival (ISIS-2) trials (ISIS-2 Collaborative Group 1988) and enrolled over 34 000 additional patients reduced the significance level to $P=0.001$ in 1979, $P=0.0001$ in 1986, and to $P<0.00001$ when the first mega-trial appeared, narrowing the confidence intervals around an essentially unchanged estimate of about 20 per cent reduction in the risk of death. This situation has been taken to suggest that further studies in large numbers of patients may be at best superfluous and costly if not unethical, once a statistically significant treatment effect is evident from meta-analysis of the existing smaller trials.

Another application of cumulative meta-analysis has been to correlate the accruing evidence with the recommendations made by experts in review articles and textbooks. Antman *et al.* (1992) showed for thrombolytic drugs that recommendations for routine use first appeared in 1987, 14 years after a statistically significant ($P=0.01$) beneficial effect became evident in cumulative meta-analysis. Conversely, the prophylactic use of lidocaine continued to be recommended for routine use in myocardial infarction despite the lack of evidence for any beneficial effect, and the possibility of a harmful effect being evident in the meta-analysis.

Bayesian meta-analysis

Some feel that a Bayesian approach to meta-analysis is more appropriate than the 'classical' approaches described above. Bayesian statisticians express their belief about the size of an effect by specifying some prior probability distribution before seeing the data—and then update that belief by deriving a posterior probability distribution, taking the data into account (Lilford & Braunholtz 1996). This is done by using Bayes theorem, named after the eighteenth century English clergyman Thomas Bayes. Bayesian models are available in both a fixed and random effects framework but published applications have usually been based on the random effects assumption. The confidence interval (or more correctly in Bayesian terminology: The 95 per cent credible interval which covers 95 per cent of the posterior probability distribution) will be slightly wider than that derived from using the conventional models. Bayesian approaches to meta-analysis can integrate other sources of evidence, for example, findings from observational studies or expert opinion, and are particularly useful for analysing the relationship between treatment benefit and underlying risk. The definition of prior probabilities may, however, involve subjective assessments and opinion, which runs against the principles of systematic review.

Deriving absolute measures of effect

The amount of between-study variability is usually lower for ratio than difference measures of treatment effects, so that meta-analyses are usually done using ratio measures. However, the absolute reduction in risk is a useful measure of the impact of treatment. For example, the relative risk of death associated with the use of beta-blockers after myocardial infarction is 0.80 (95 per cent confidence interval 0.74 to 0.86) (Fig. 6.14.3). The relative risk reduction, obtained by subtracting the relative risk from 1 and expressing the result as a percentage, is 20 per cent (95 per cent confidence interval 14 to 26 per cent). However, these relative measures ignore the underlying absolute risk. The risk of death among patients who have survived the acute phase of myocardial infarction varies widely.

The absolute risk reduction, or risk difference, reflects both the underlying risk without therapy and the risk reduction associated with therapy. Taking the reciprocal of the risk difference gives the number of patients who need to be treated to prevent one event, which is abbreviated to NNT or $NNT_{benefit}$ (Laupacis *et al.* 1988). The number of patients that need to be treated to harm one patient, denoted as NNH or, more appropriately, NNT_{harm} (Altman 1998) can also be calculated. It will usually be informative to calculate the

Table 6.14.3 Beta-blockade in secondary prevention after myocardial infarction. Absolute risk reductions and numbers-needed-to-treat for 1 year to prevent one death, $NNT_{benefit}$, for different levels of control group mortality

One-year mortality risk among controls (%)	Absolute risk reduction	$NNT_{benefit}$
1	0.002	500
3	0.006	167
5	0.01	100
10	0.02	50
20	0.04	25
30	0.06	17
40	0.08	13
50	0.1	10

Calculations assume a constant relative risk reduction of 20 per cent.

risk difference, NNT or NNH for a range of baseline risks reflecting the range in the component studies of the meta-analysis.

For a baseline risk of 1 per cent per year, the absolute risk difference indicates that 2 deaths are prevented per 1000 treated patients (Table 6.14.3). This corresponds to 500 patients (1 divided by 0.002) treated for 1 year to prevent one death. Conversely, if the risk is above 10 per cent, less than 50 patients have to be treated to prevent one fatal event. Many clinicians would probably decide not to treat patients at very low risk, considering the large number of patients who would have to be exposed to the adverse effects of beta-blockade to prevent one death. Appraising the NNT from a patient's estimated risk without treatment, and the relative risk reduction with treatment, is a helpful aid when making a decision in an individual patient. A nomogram to determine NNTs at the bedside is available (Chatellier *et al.* 1996) and confidence intervals can be calculated (Altman 1998). The concept has been expanded to the number of health people needed to be screened to prevent one adverse outcome (Rembold 1998).

Combining absolute effect measures in meta-analysis is often inappropriate because the combined risk difference (and the NNT calculated from it) will be applicable only to patients at levels of risk corresponding to the typical control group risk of the trials analysed. It is generally more meaningful to use relative effect measures when summarizing the evidence while considering absolute measures when applying it to a specific clinical or public health situation.

Sources of bias in systematic reviews and meta-analysis

That there are limitations to the process of systematic review and meta-analysis is illustrated by meta-analyses that reviewed the same data but reached opposite conclusions. Examples include assessments of low molecular weight (LMW) heparins in the prevention of thrombosis following surgery (Leizorovicz *et al.* 1992; Nurmohamed *et al.* 1992) or of screening mammography (Kerlikowske *et al.* 1995; Gøtzsche & Olsen 2000). In the following sections, important sources of bias are discussed in detail.

Garbage in—garbage out?

The quality of component trials is of crucial importance: If the 'raw material' is flawed, then the findings of reviews of this material may also be compromised. The biases that threaten the validity of clinical trials relate to systematic differences in the patients' characteristics at baseline (*selection bias*), unequal provision of care apart from the treatment under evaluation (*performance bias*), biased assessment of outcomes (*detection bias*), and bias due to exclusion of patients after they have been allocated to treatment groups (*attrition bias*). Empirical evidence on specific trial characteristics associated with bias in intervention effect estimates has come from collections of meta-analyses assembled in so called 'meta-epidemiologic' studies. Several such studies have found that trials with inadequate allocation concealment or lack of blinding (see Box 6.14.3) tend to exaggerate estimates of intervention effects, compared with adequately concealed or adequately blinded trials.

Different ways of dealing (or not dealing) with the methodological quality of trials sometimes explain discrepancies in the results between different systematic reviews. For example, blinding of outcome assessments was important in trials comparing LMW weight heparin with standard heparin for the prevention of postoperative deep vein thrombosis: Trials that were not double-blind showed a benefit of LMW heparin that disappeared when restricting the analysis to trials with blinded outcome assessment (Jüni *et al.* 1999). This is not entirely surprising considering that the interpretation of fibrinogen leg scanning, which is used to detect thrombosis, can be subjective. One of the two reviews of LMW heparins mentioned came to discordant conclusions because the authors chose to ignore the quality of component trials, a practice that unfortunately is still fairly common (Gerber 2007).

A recent study of a large number of meta-analyses and trials found that the bias in intervention effect resulting from inadequate allocation concealment and lack of blinding, varied according to the type of outcome assessed (Wood 2008). There was little evidence of bias in trials with all-cause mortality outcomes, or other objectively assessed outcomes. In contrast, inadequate allocation concealment and lack of blinding were associated with over-optimistic estimates of intervention effects for subjectively assessed outcomes (Wood 2008). Efforts to minimize bias thus are particularly important when objective measurement of outcomes is not feasible.

Reporting biases

The dissemination of research findings is not a dichotomous event but a continuum ranging from the sharing of draft papers among colleagues, presentations at meetings, published abstracts, to papers in journals that are indexed in the major bibliographic databases. It has long been recognized that only a proportion of research projects reach full publication in an indexed journal and thus become easily identifiable for systematic review. For example, only about half of abstracts of studies presented at conferences are later published in full (von Elm *et al.* 2003). Reporting bias is introduced when the dissemination of research findings is influenced by the nature and direction of results. When discussing these reporting biases, which are summarized in Table 6.14.4, we will denote trials with statistically significant ($P<0.05$) and non-significant results trials as trials 'positive' and 'negative' results. However, the contribution made to the totality of the evidence by trials with non-significant results is of course potentially as important as that from trials with statistically significant results.

Table 6.14.4 Definitions of different reporting biases

Type of reporting bias	Definition
Publication bias	The *publication* or *non-publication* of research findings, depending on the nature and direction of the results
Time lag bias	The *rapid* or *delayed* publication of research findings, depending on the nature and direction of the results
Multiple (duplicate) publication bias	The *multiple* or *singular* publication of research findings, depending on the nature and direction of the results
Location bias	The publication of research findings in journals with different *ease of access* or *levels of indexing* in standard databases, depending on the nature and direction of results.
Citation bias	The *citation* or *non-citation* of research findings, depending on the nature and direction of the results
Language bias	The publication of research findings *in a particular language*, depending on the nature and direction of the results
Outcome reporting bias	The *selective reporting* of some outcomes but not others, depending on the nature and direction of the results

Publication bias

In a 1979 article 'The "file drawer problem" and tolerance for null results' Rosenthal (1979) described a gloomy scenario where 'the journals are filled with the 5 per cent of the studies that show Type I errors, while the file drawers back at the lab are filled with the 95 per cent of the studies that show nonsignificant (e.g. $P > 0.05$) results'. The 'file drawer problem', more widely known as publication bias, has long been recognized in the social sciences: A review of psychology journals found that of 294 studies published in the 1950s, 97 per cent rejected the null hypothesis at the 5 per cent level ($P<0.05$) (Sterling 1959). Similar results were later found for medical and public health journals. However, the proportion of all hypotheses tested for which the null hypothesis is truly false is unknown, and surveys of published results can only provide indirect evidence of publication bias. Direct evidence is available from studies of research proposals submitted to ethics committees or institutional review boards. Seven studies of proposals submitted to institutional committees in Oxford, Sydney, Baltimore, Bern, and to national ethics committees in France and Spain found rates of publication that ranged from 31 to 67 per cent (von Elm *et al.* 2008). Five of these studies compared the probability of publication of studies that produced positive results with those that did not. Meta-analysis of the results from these five studies indicates that the probability of publication is 2.6 times greater if results are statistically significant (odds ratio 2.6, 95 per cent confidence interval 2.0–3.4) (von Elm *et al.* 2008). These studies also showed that articles may appear in print many years after approval by the ethics committee, however, there is *time lag bias* (Table 6.14.4): The positive studies are published more rapidly than negative studies.

Other reporting biases

Among published studies, the probability of identifying relevant trials for a systematic review may also be influenced by their results (Table 6.14.4). *Multiple (duplicate) publication bias*, the production of multiple publications from single studies can lead to bias in a number of ways. Most importantly, studies with significant results are more likely to lead to multiple publications and presentations, which makes it more likely that they will be located and included in a meta-analysis. The inclusion of duplicated data may therefore lead to overestimation of treatment effects, as demonstrated for trials of the efficacy of ondansetron to prevent postoperative nausea (Tramèr 1997). It is not always obvious that multiple publications come from a single study, and one set of study participants may thus be included in an analysis twice. Indeed, it may be difficult if not impossible for reviewers to determine whether two papers represent duplicate publications of one trial or two separate trials: Two articles reporting the same trial may not share a single common author (von Elm *et al.* 2004).

The perusal of the reference lists of articles is widely used to identify other publications that may be relevant. However, retrieving literature by scanning reference lists may produce a biased sample of studies, introducing *citation bias*. Several studies have shown that trials with positive results tend to be cited more often than negative trials (Gøtzsche 1987). Of note, the association is not explained by superior methodological quality of cited articles. Sampson *et al.* (2003) found that trials published in journals that are indexed in EMBASE but not in MEDLINE tended to show smaller effects of treatments compared to trials indexed in MEDLINE or MEDLINE and EMBASE. *Location bias* may thus be introduced in systematic reviews exclusively based on MEDLINE searches, although another study found little difference in effect estimates between trials indexed and not indexed in MEDLINE (Egger *et al.* 2003).

Reviews may be exclusively based on trials published in English, although language restrictions have become less common in recent years (Gerber *et al.* 2007). Investigators working in a non-English speaking country publish some of their work in local journals. It is conceivable that authors are more likely to report in an international, English-language journal if results are positive whereas negative findings are published in a local journal (*language bias*). This has been demonstrated for the German language literature. When comparing pairs of articles published by the same first author, 63 per cent of trials published in English had produced significant ($P<0.05$) results as compared to 35 per cent of trials published in German (Egger *et al.* 1997b). However, when comparing the results of trials included in meta-analyses, trials published in languages other than English tended to show somewhat more beneficial effects of the intervention (Jüni *et al.* 2002).

It has been suspected for years that not only the reporting of entire studies with 'positive' results but also the inclusion or exclusion of outcomes within study reports are subject to selection mechanisms. Such *outcome reporting bias* has received much attention recently. Among studies approved by a research ethics committee in Denmark (Chan *et al.* 2004a) or funded by the Canadian Institutes of Health Research (Chan *et al.* 2004b) statistically significant outcomes were more likely to be reported than non-significant outcomes. Similarly, a review of published trials and survey of authors showed that incompletely or unreported outcomes were more likely to be non-significant than significant

(Chan & Altman 2005). Finally, several studies have shown that the reporting of adverse events and safety outcomes in clinical trials is often inadequate and selective (Ioannidis & Lau 2001; Melander *et al.* 2003).

How important are different sources of bias?

Empirical research has shown that the importance of reporting bias and bias due to inadequate quality of trials in a particular meta-analysis is often unpredictable, and the exploration of potential sources of bias is therefore an important step in any systematic review and meta-analysis. It is nevertheless worthwhile to study and compare the overall, average size and direction of different biases by analysing many meta-analyses. A 'meta-meta-analysis' of these studies found that, on average, published trials and trials published in languages other than English will overestimate treatment effects by about 10 per cent (Egger *et al.* 2002). Larger effects are seen for concealment of allocation and blinding: Trials with inadequate or unclear concealment and trials that are not double-blind overestimate treatment effects by about 30 and 15 per cent, respectively. In general, the quality of trials thus appears to be a more important source of bias than publication bias and other reporting biases (Egger *et al.* 2002). Of note, although this has improved in recent years, many meta-analyses do not assess the quality of component studies and explore the influence of study quality (Gerber *et al.* 2007; Moher *et al.* 2007).

Investigating and dealing with bias and heterogeneity

There will often be diverging opinions on the correct method for performing a particular meta-analysis. The robustness of the findings to different assumptions, the presence of bias, and possible sources of heterogeneity should therefore always be examined.

Sensitivity analysis

A thorough sensitivity analysis of the beta-blocker after myocardial infarction meta-analysis (Freemantle *et al.* 1999) is illustrated in Fig. 6.14.6. First, the overall effect was calculated by different statistical methods, using both a fixed and a random effects model. It is evident from the figure that the overall estimate is virtually identical and that confidence intervals are only slightly wider when using the random effects model. This is explained by the relatively small amount of between trial heterogeneity present in this meta-analysis.

Methodological quality was assessed in terms of concealment of allocation of study participants to beta-blocker or control groups and blinding of patients and investigators. Figure 6.14.6 shows that the estimated treatment effect was similar in studies with concealment of treatment allocation, or studies that were described as double-blind. Publication bias is more likely to affect small studies and may therefore be examined by stratifying the analysis by study size. If publication bias is present, it is expected that of published studies, the larger ones will report the smaller effects: Smaller effects can be statistically significant in larger studies. The figure shows that this is indeed the case, with the 11 smallest trials (25 deaths or less) showing the largest effect. However, exclusion of the smaller studies has little effect on the overall estimate. Studies varied in terms of length of follow-up but this again had little effect on estimates. Finally, two trials were terminated earlier than anticipated on the grounds of the results from interim analyses. Estimates of treatment effects from trials which were stopped early because of a significant treatment difference are liable to overestimate treatment effects (Montori 2005). Bias may thus be introduced in a meta-analysis which includes such trials. Exclusion of these trials again affected the overall estimate only marginally.

The sensitivity analysis thus shows that the results from the beta-blocker meta-analysis are robust to the choice of the statistical method and to the exclusion of trials of lesser quality or of studies terminated early. It also suggests that publication bias is unlikely to have distorted its findings.

Funnel plots

Funnel plots are scatter plots in which the treatment effects estimated from individual studies on the horizontal axis are plotted against a measure of study size on the vertical axis. Such plots have long been proposed as a means of detecting publication bias (Light & Pillemer 1984). In the absence of bias, the plot should resemble a symmetrical inverted funnel, with the results of smaller studies being more widely scattered than those of the larger studies. If the plot shows an asymmetrical shape, publication bias may be present. This usually takes the form of a gap in the wide part of the funnel which indicates the absence of negative small studies. The funnel plot for the meta-analysis of the trials of beta-blockade in secondary prevention after myocardial infarction is shown in the upper panel of Fig. 6.14.7. The plot is fairly symmetrical. In contrast, the funnel plot of controlled trials of magnesium infusion in acute myocardial infarction (lower panel of Fig. 6.14.7) is clearly asymmetrical. This is an example where publication bias may explain the discrepancy between meta-analyses of smaller trials, which showed a clear treatment effect, and a very large trial (the ISIS-4 trial, ISIS-4 (Collaborative Group 1995) that showed no effect (Egger & Davey Smith 1995).

Funnel plot asymmetry does not prove the presence of bias in a meta-analysis: In interpreting funnel plots, reviewers should consider the different reasons for asymmetry listed in Table 6.14.5 (Egger *et al.* 1997a). Other types of bias can lead to asymmetry. Smaller studies are, on average, conducted and analysed with less methodological rigour than larger studies, and trials of lower quality tend to show larger effects. Heterogeneity between the treatment effects in different trials may lead to funnel plot asymmetry if the true treatment effect is larger in the smaller trials. Interventions may have been implemented less thoroughly in larger trials, thus explaining the more positive results in smaller trials. This is likely, for example, in trials of complex interventions in chronic diseases, such as rehabilitation after stroke or multifaceted interventions in diabetes mellitus. Thus the funnel plot should be seen as a generic means of examining 'small study effects' (the tendency for the smaller studies in a meta-analysis to show larger treatment effects) (Sterne *et al.* 2000). Other graphical representations, discussed in detail elsewhere, are useful to investigate bias and heterogeneity. These include Galbraith plots (Galbraith 1988) and L'Abbé plots (Song 1999).

Tests for funnel plot asymmetry

Visual inspection of funnel plots is inherently subjective. Statistical tests for funnel plot asymmetry, which examine whether the association between estimated intervention effects and a measure of study size is greater than expected by chance, can be useful to assess and quantify the evidence for asymmetry. For continuous outcomes

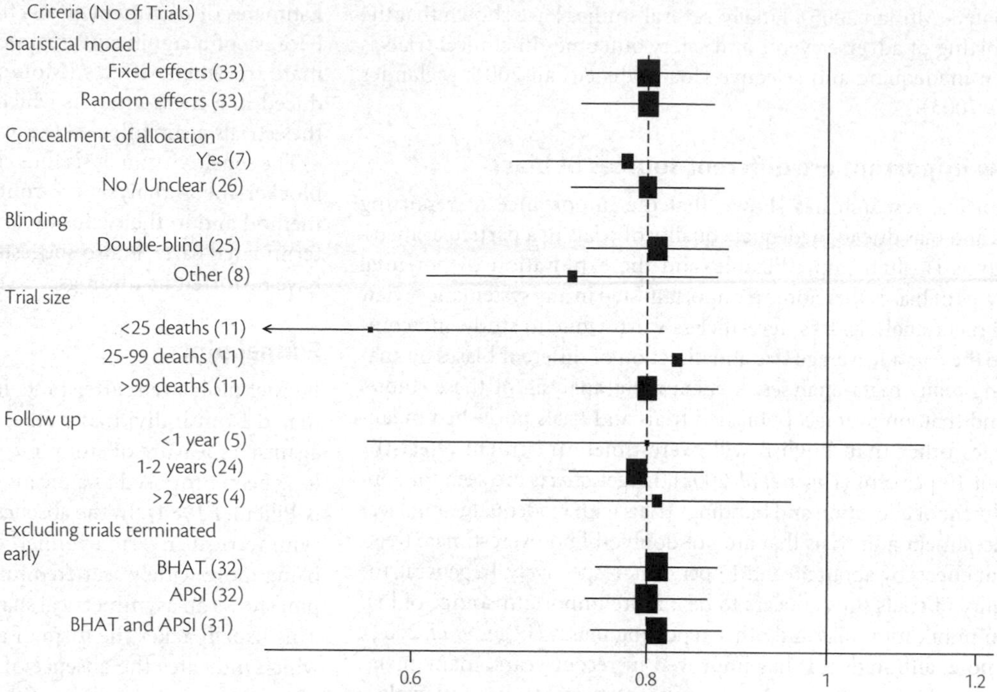

Fig. 6.14.6 Sensitivity analyses examining the robustness of the effect on total mortality of beta-blockers in secondary prevention after myocardial infarction. The dotted vertical line corresponds to the combined relative risk from the fixed effects model (0.8).

this is straightforward. We can perform a weighted linear regression of the intervention effect estimates, for example, differences in blood pressure, against their standard errors (Egger *et al.* 1997a). When outcomes are dichotomous, this approach is more problematic because the standard error of the log odds ratio is mathematically linked to the size of the odds ratio, even in the absence of small study effects (Sterne *et al.* 2000). Simulation studies have

Table 6.14.5 Possible sources of asymmetry in funnel plots

1. Selection biases
Publication bias
Delayed publication (also known as 'time-lag' or 'pipeline') bias
Location biases
Language bias
Citation bias
Multiple publication bias
Selective outcome reporting
2. Poor methodological quality leading to spuriously inflated effects in smaller studies
Poor methodological design
Inadequate analysis
Fraud
3. True heterogeneity
Size of effect differs according to study size (for example, due to differences in the intensity of interventions or differences in underlying risk between studies of different sizes)
4. Artefactual
In some circumstances, sampling variation can lead to an association between the intervention effect and its standard error.
5. Chance

shown that this may lead to false-positive test results, particularly when interventions have very large effects (Sterne *et al.* 2000; Peters *et al.* 2006). Tests that avoid the association between the log odds ratio and its standard error are therefore preferred for binary outcomes, including the modified test proposed by Harbord *et al.* (2006) or the approach proposed by Peters *et al.* (2006).

The power of tests will often be limited because many meta-analyses include few trials only (Gerber *et al.* 2007; Ioannidis & Trekalinos 2007) Therefore, even when a test does not provide evidence of funnel plot asymmetry, bias cannot be excluded with confidence. As a rule of thumb, tests for funnel plot asymmetry should be used only when there are at least 10 studies, and they should not be used if substantial heterogeneity is present between trials. Results should be interpreted in the light of visual inspection of the funnel plot. Do small studies tend to lead to more or less beneficial intervention effect estimates? Are there outliers with markedly different intervention effect estimates, or studies that are highly influential in the meta-analysis? When there is evidence of small-study effects, publication bias should be considered as one of a number of possible explanations (see Table 6.14.5). Although funnel plots, and tests for funnel plot asymmetry, may alert review authors to a problem, they do not provide a solution.

Correcting for publication bias?

The process that determines which results are published and which are not can be modelled (Iyengar & Greenhouse 1988) and such 'selection models' have been extended to estimate treatment effects corrected for the estimated publication bias. For example, Copas and Shi (2000) used such an approach to show that in epidemiological studies of passive smoking and lung cancer, allowing for the possibility of publication bias reduces the estimate of relative risk associated with passive smoking. The 'trim and fill' method is a graphical approach to identify and correct for publication bias

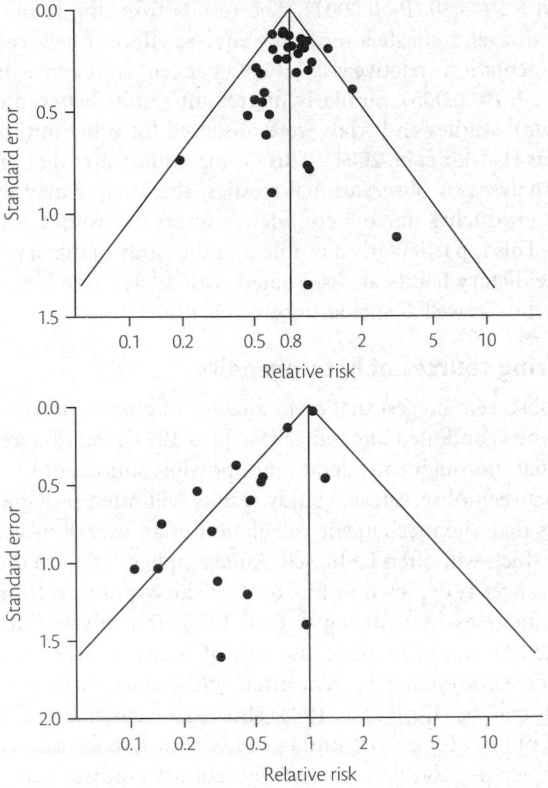

Fig. 6.14.7. Funnel plots of trials of beta-blockers in secondary prevention after myocardial infarction (upper panel) and of trials of magnesium infusion in acute myocardial infarction (lower panel). The relative risk is plotted on a logarithmic scale, to ensure that effects of the same magnitude but opposite directions will be equidistant from 1.0. Plotting against the standard error of the treatment effect emphasizes differences between the smaller studies among which publication and other biases are most likely to occur. The vertical line shows the summary estimate from the fixed effects model, diagonal lines show the expected 95 per cent confidence intervals around the summary estimate.

(Duval & Tweedie 2000). The method 'trims' (removes) the smaller studies causing funnel plot asymmetry, estimates the 'true' centre of the funnel, and then 'fills' (replaces) the omitted studies and their missing counterparts around the centre.

Whatever the method used, correcting for publication bias is problematic because the true mechanism for publication bias is unknown. Equally importantly, other reasons for small study effects other than publication bias are ignored. Therefore, 'corrected' estimates from these methods should be interpreted with great caution. Sensitivity analyses excluding smaller studies, and studies of lower methodological quality (see above and Fig. 6.14.6), will often be more helpful than either a *P* value from a test of funnel plot asymmetry, or an estimate from a statistical model that is supposedly 'corrected' for publication bias.

Spurious precision? Meta-analysis of observational studies

The randomized controlled trial is the principal research design in the evaluation of medical interventions. However aetiological hypotheses, for example, those relating common exposures to the occurrence of disease, cannot generally be tested in randomized experiments. Does breathing other people's tobacco smoke propagate the development of lung cancer, drinking coffee cause coronary heart disease, and eating a diet rich in unsaturated fat induce breast cancer? Studies of such 'menaces of daily life' (Feinstein 1988) employ observational designs, or examine the presumed biological mechanisms in the laboratory. In these situations the risks involved are generally small, but once a large proportion of the population is exposed, the potential public health implications of these associations—if they are causal—can be striking.

Analyses of observational data also have a role in medical effectiveness research. The evidence that is available from clinical trials will rarely answer all the important questions. Most trials are conducted to establish efficacy and safety of a single agent in a specific clinical situation. Due to the limited size of such trials, less common adverse effects of drugs may only be detected in case-control studies, or in analyses of databases from post-marketing surveillance schemes. Also, because follow-up is generally limited, adverse effects occurring many years later will not be identified. If years later established interventions are incriminated with adverse effects, there will be ethical, political, and legal obstacles to the conduct of a new trial. Examples for such situations include the controversy surrounding intramuscular administration of vitamin K to newborns and the risk of childhood cancer, or oral contraceptive use and breast cancer.

Meta-analysis, by promising a precise and definite answer when the magnitude of the underlying risks are small, or when the results from individual studies disagree, appears an attractive proposition both in aetiological studies and in observational effectiveness research.

Confounding, residual confounding and bias

The overall effect calculated from a group of sensibly combined and representative randomized trials will provide an essentially unbiased estimate of the treatment effect, with an increase in the precision of this estimate. A fundamentally different situation arises in the case of observational studies. Such studies yield estimates of association which may deviate from true underlying relationships beyond the play of chance. This may be due to the effects of confounding factors, the influence of biases, or both.

Those exposed to the factor under investigation may differ in a number of other aspects that are relevant to the risk of developing the disease in question. Consider, for example, smoking as a risk factor for suicide. Virtually all cohort studies have shown a positive association, with a dose response relationship being evident between the amount smoked and the probability of committing suicide. A meta-analysis of these cohorts produces very precise and statistically significant estimates of the increase in suicide risk that is associated with smoking different daily amounts of cigarettes: Relative rate for 1–14 cigarettes 1.43 (95 per cent confidence interval 1.06–1.93); for 15–24 cigarettes 1.88 (95 per cent confidence interval 1.53–2.32); 25 or more cigarettes 2.18 (95 per cent confidence interval 1.82–2.61) (Egger *et al.* 1998).

Based on established criteria, many would consider the association to be causal—if only it were more plausible. Indeed, it is improbable that smoking is causally related to suicide. Rather, it is the social and mental states predisposing to suicide that are also associated with the habit of smoking (Davey Smith *et al.* 1992). Factors that are related to both the exposure and the disease under study, confounding factors, may thus distort results. If the factor is known and has been measured, the usual approach is to control for its influence in the analysis. For example, any study assessing the influence of coffee consumption on the risk of myocardial infarction should control for smoking, since smoking is generally associated with drinking larger amounts of coffee and smoking is a cause of coronary heart disease. However, even if adjustments for confounding factors have been made in the analysis, residual confounding remains a potentially serious problem in observational research. Residual confounding arises whenever a confounding factor cannot be measured with sufficient precision—a situation that often occurs in epidemiological studies (Phillips & Davey Smith 1991). Confounding is the most important threat to the validity of results from cohort studies whereas more difficulties, in particular selection biases, arise in case-control studies.

Plausible but equally spurious findings?

Implausibility of results, like in the case of smoking and suicide, rarely protects us from reaching misleading claims. It is generally easy to produce plausible explanations for the findings from observational research. For example, observational studies have consistently shown that people eating more fruits and vegetables, which are rich in beta-carotene, and people having higher serum beta-carotene concentrations have lower rates of cardiovascular disease and cancer (Jha *et al.* 1995). Beta-carotene has antioxidant properties and could thus plausibly be expected to prevent carcinogenesis and atherogenesis by reducing oxidative damage to DNA and lipoproteins (Jha *et al.* 1995). Contrary to many other associations found in observational studies, this hypothesis could be, and was, tested in experimental studies.

A meta-analysis of the findings for cardiovascular mortality, comparing the results from six observational studies with those from four randomized trials is shown in Fig 6.14.8. For observational studies results relate to a comparison between groups with high and low beta-carotene intake or serum beta-carotene level, whereas in trials participants randomized to beta-carotene supplements were compared with participants randomized to placebo. The meta-analysis of the cohort studies shows a significantly lower risk of cardiovascular death (relative risk 0.69, 95 per cent confidence interval 0.59–0.80, $P<0.0001$). The results from the randomized trials, however, indicate a moderate adverse effect of beta-carotene supplementation (relative risk 1.12, 95 per cent confidence interval 1.04–1.22, $P=0.005$). Similarly discrepant results between epidemiological studies and trials were observed for other antioxidant vitamins (Lawlor *et al.* 2004). This example illustrates that in some meta-analyses of observational studies, the analyst may well be simply producing narrow confidence intervals around spurious results. This is particularly a problem in the study of dietary factors because dietary habits are associated with a large number of lifestyle factors as well as socioeconomic position.

Exploring sources of heterogeneity

Some observers suggest that meta-analysis of observational studies should be abandoned altogether (Shapiro 1994). We disagree, but think that thorough consideration of possible sources of heterogeneity between observational study results will often provide more insights than the mechanistic calculation of an overall measure of effect, which will often be biased. An example relating to diet and breast cancer is depicted in Fig. 6.14.9. The hypothesis from ecological analyses (Armstrong & Doll 1975) that higher intake of saturated fat could increase the risk of breast cancer generated much observational research, often with contradictory results. A meta-analysis (Boyd *et al.* 1993) showed an association for case-control but not for cohort studies (odds ratio 1.36 for case-control studies versus relative rate 0.95 for cohort studies, comparing highest with lowest category of saturated fat intake, $P=0.0002$ for difference, Fig. 6.14.9). The most likely explanation for this situation is that biases in the recall of dietary items, and in the selection of study participants, have produced a spurious association in the case-control comparisons.

Conclusions

Systematic review including, if appropriate, a formal meta-analysis is clearly superior to the narrative approach to reviewing research. Systematic reviews involve structuring the processes through which

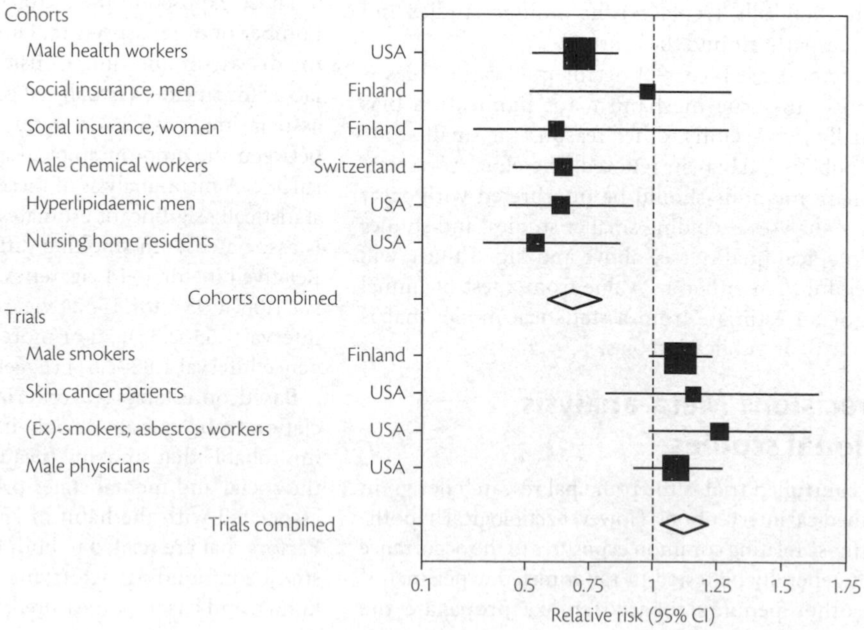

Fig. 6.14.8 Meta-analysis of the association between beta-carotene intake and cardiovascular mortality: The results from observational studies are compared to the findings of four large trials. The observational studies indicate considerable benefit whereas the findings from randomized controlled trials show an increase in the risk of death. Meta-analysis by fixed-effects model.

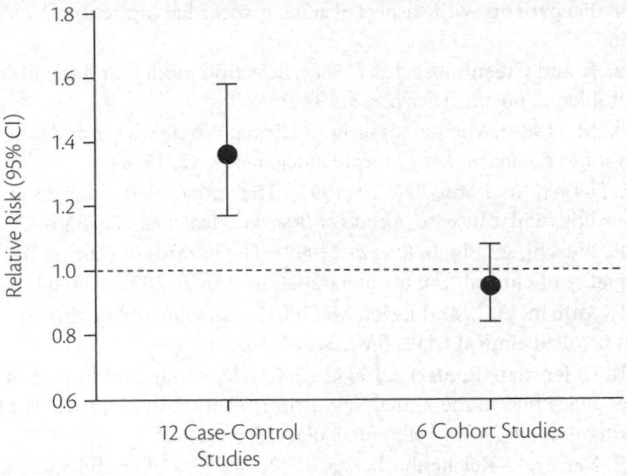

Fig. 6.14.9. An example of heterogeneity in a meta-analysis of observational studies: Saturated fat intake and cancer.

a thorough review of previous research is carried out. The issues of the completeness of the evidence identified, the quality of component studies, and the combinability of evidence are made explicit. The unprecedented effort to inject scientific principles into the process of research synthesis, which has taken place over the past decade, has improved the quality of reviews published in recent years (Gerber *et al.* 2007) although considerable room for further improvement remains (Moher *et al.* 2007). Some shortcomings of systematic review and meta-analysis are, however, a consequence of more general failings. Although various initiatives, including reporting guidelines for randomized trials (Altman 2001) and observational studies (Vandenbroucke 2007) mean that the identification and assessment of studies have become an easier task, the conduct of research and dissemination of its results continue to be an imperfect process. Finally, the suggestion that formal meta-analysis of observational studies can be misleading and that insufficient attention is often given to heterogeneity does not mean that a return to the previous practice of highly subjective narrative reviews is called for. Many of the principles of systematic reviews remain: A study protocol should be written in advance, complete literature searches should be carried out, and studies selected and data extracted in a reproducible and objective fashion. This allows for differences and similarities of the results found in different settings to be inspected, hypotheses to be formulated, and the need for future studies, including randomized controlled trials, to be defined. In summary:

- Systematic reviews allow for a more objective and reproducible appraisal of the evidence than traditional narrative reviews. The definition of eligibility criteria for trials to be included, a comprehensive search for such trials, and an assessment of their methodological quality are central components.
- Meta-analysis, if appropriate, will enhance the precision of estimates of treatment effects, leading to reduced probability of false negative results, and potentially to a more timely introduction of effective interventions. Meta-analysis is a two-stage process involving the calculation of an appropriate summary statistic for each of a set of studies followed by the combination of these statistics into a weighted average.
- Inadequate quality of studies and publication bias and other reporting biases may distort results. Concealment of treatment allocation, blinding of outcome assessment, and handling of patient attrition should be assessed and funnel plots should be examined.
- The thoughtful consideration of heterogeneity between study results is an important aspect of systematic reviews, and particularly important in systematic reviews and meta-analyses of observational studies.

References

Altman, D.G. (1998). Confidence intervals for the number needed to treat. *BMJ*, **317**, 1309–12.

Altman, D.G., Schulz, K.F., Moher, D. *et al.* (2001). The revised CONSORT statement for reporting randomized trials: Explanation and elaboration. *Annals of Internal Medicine*, **134**, 663–94.

Antman, E.M., Lau, J., Kupelnick, B. *et al.* (1992). A comparison of results of meta-analyses of randomized control trials and recommendations of clinical experts. *JAMA*, **268**, 240–8.

Armstrong, B. and Doll, R. (1975). Environmental factors and cancer incidence and mortality in different countries with special reference to dietary practices. *International Journal of Cancer*, **15**, 617–31.

Baber, N.S., Wainwright Evans, D., Howitt, G. *et al.* (1980). Multicentre post-infarction trial of propranolol in 49 hospital in the United Kingdom, Italy and Yugoslavia. *British Heart Journal*, **44**, 96–100.

Boyd, N.F., Martin, L.J., Noffel, M. *et al.* (1993). A meta-analysis of studies of dietary fat and breast cancer. *British Journal of Cancer*, **68**, 627–36.

Busse, J.W., Mills, E., Dennis, R. *et al.* (2009). Clinical epidemiology. In *Oxford Textbook of Public Health* (eds. R. Detels, R. Beaglehole, M.A. Lansang and M. Gulliford), Oxford University Press, Oxford.

Chalmers, I. (1979). Randomised controlled trials of fetal monitoring 1973–1977. In *Perinatal medicine* (eds. O. Thalhammer, K. Baumgarten, and A. Pollak), p. 260. Thieme, Stuttgart.

Chalmers, I. and Tröhler, U. (2000). Medical and philosophical commentaries, 1773–1795: A 200-year old response to the challenge of keeping abreast of the medical literature. *Annals of Internal Medicine*, **133**, 238–43.

Chan, A.W. and Altman, D.G. (2005). Identifying outcome reporting bias in randomised trials on PubMed: Review of publications and survey of authors. *BMJ*, **330**, 753.

Chan, A.W., Hrobjartsson, A., Haahr, M.T. *et al.* (2004a). Empirical evidence for selective reporting of outcomes in randomized trials: Comparison of protocols to published articles. *JAMA*, **291**, 2457–65.

Chan, A.W., Krleza-Jeric, K., Schmid, I. *et al.* (2004b). Outcome reporting bias in randomized trials funded by the Canadian Institutes of Health Research. *Canadian Medical Association Journal*, **171**, 735–40.

Chatellier, G., Zapletal, E., Lemaitre, D. *et al.* (1996). The number needed to treat: A clinically useful nomogram in its proper context. *BMJ*, **312**, 426–9.

Colditz, G.A., Brewer, T.F., Berkley, C.S. *et al.* (1994). Efficacy of BCG vaccine in the prevention of Tuberculosis. *JAMA*, **271**, 698–702.

Copas, J.B. and Shi, J.Q. (2000). Reanalysis of epidemiological evidence on lung cancer and passive smoking. *BMJ*, **320**, 417–18.

Davey Smith, G., Phillips, A.N., and Neaton, J.D. (1992). Smoking as 'independent' risk factor for suicide: illustration of an artifact from observational epidemiology. *Lancet*, **340**, 709–11.

De Angelis, C.D., Drazen, J.M., Frizelle, F.A. *et al.* (2004). Clinical trial registration: A statement from the International Committee of Medical Journal Editors. *JAMA*, **292**, 1363–4.

Deeks, J.J., Altman, D.G., and Bradburn, M.J. (2001). Statistical methods for examining heterogeneity and combining results from several studies in meta-analysis. In *Systematic reviews in health care: Meta-analysis in context* (eds. M. Egger, D.G. Smith, and D.G. Altman),. p. 285. BMJ Books, London.

DerSimonian, R. and Laird, N. (1986). Meta-analysis in clinical trials. *Controlled Clinical Trials*, **7**, 177–88.

Duval, S., and Tweedie, R. (2000). Trim and fill: A simple funnel-plot-based method of testing and adjusting for publication bias in meta-analysis. *Biometrics*, **56**, 455–63.

Egger, M. and Davey Smith, G. (1995). Misleading meta-analysis. Lessons from "an effective, safe, simple" intervention that wasn't. *BMJ*, **310**, 752–4.

Egger, M., Davey Smith, G., Schneider, M. *et al.* (1997a). Bias in meta-analysis detected by a simple, graphical test. *BMJ*, **315**, 629–34.

Egger, M., Zellweger-Zähner, T., Schneider, M. *et al.* (1997b). Language bias in randomised controlled trials published in English and German. *Lancet*, **350**, 326–9.

Egger, M., Schneider, M., and Davey Smith, G. (1998). Spurious precision? Meta-analysis of observational studies. *BMJ*, **316**, 140–5.

Egger, M., Ebrahim, S., and Smith, G.D. (2002). Where now for meta-analysis? *International Journal of Epidemiology*, **31**, 1–5.

Egger, M., Jüni, P., Bartlett, C. *et al.* (2003). How important are comprehensive literature searches and the assessment of trial quality in systematic reviews? Empirical study. *Health Technology Assessment*, **7**, 1–76.

Feinstein, A.R. (1988). Scientific standards in epidemiological studies of the menace of daily life. *Science*, **242**, 1257–63.

Freemantle, N., Cleland, J., Young, P. *et al.* (1999). Beta blockade after myocardial infarction: systematic review and meta regression analysis. *BMJ*, **318**, 1730–7.

Freiman, J.A., Chalmers, T.C., Smith, H. *et al.* (1992). The importance of beta, the type II error, and sample size in the design and interpretation of the randomized controlled trial. In *Medical uses of statistics (2)* (eds. J.C. Bailar and F. Mosteller), p. 357. NEJM Books, Boston, MA.

Galbraith, R. (1988). A note on graphical presentation of estimated odds ratios from several clinical trials. *Statistics in Medicine*, **7**, 889–94.

Gerber, S., Tallon, D., Trelle, S. *et al.* (2007). Bibliographic study showed improving methodology of meta-analyses published in leading journals 1993–2002. *Journal of Clinical Epidemiology*, **60**, 773–80.

Gøtzsche, P.C. (1987). Reference bias in reports of drug trials. *BMJ*, **295**, 654–6.

Gøtzsche, P.C. and Olsen, O. (2000). Is screening for breast cancer with mammography justifiable? [see comments]. *Lancet*, **355**, 129–34.

Gruppo Italiano per lo Studio della Streptochinasi nell'Infarto Miocardico (GISSI) (1986). Effectiveness of intravenous thrombolytic treatment in acute myocardial infarction. *Lancet*, **1**, 397–402.

Hampton, J.R. (1981). The use of beta blockers for the reduction of mortality after myocardial infarction. *European Heart Journal*, **2**, 259–68.

Harbord, R.M., Egger, M., and Sterne, J.A. (2006). A modified test for small-study effects in meta-analyses of controlled trials with binary endpoints. *Statistics in Medicine*, **25**, 3443–57.

Higgins, J.P., Thompson, S.G., Deeks, J.J. *et al.* (2003). Measuring inconsistency in meta-analyses. *BMJ*, **327**, 557–60.

Ioannidis, J.P. and Lau, J. (2001). Completeness of safety reporting in randomized trials: An evaluation of 7 medical areas. *JAMA*, **285**, 437–43.

Ioannidis, J.P. and Trikalinos, T.A. (2007). The appropriateness of asymmetry tests for publication bias in meta-analyses: A large survey. *Canadian Medical Association Journal*, **176**, 1091–6.

ISIS-2 (Second International Study of Infarct Survival) Collaborative Group (1988). Randomised trial of intravenous streptokinase, oral aspirin, both, or neither among 17 187 cases of suspected acute myocardial infarction: ISIS-2. *Lancet*, **2**, 349–60.

ISIS-4 (Fourth International Study of Infarct Survival) Collaborative Group (1995). ISIS-4: A randomised factorial trial assessing early oral captopril, oral mononitrate, and intravenous magnesium sulphate in 58 050 patients with suspected acute myocardial infarction. *Lancet*, **345**, 669–87.

Iyengar, S. and Greenhouse, J.B. (1988). Selection models and the file drawer problem. *Statistical Science*, **3**, 109–35.

Jenicek, M. (1989). Meta-analysis in medicine. Where we are and where we want to go. *Journal of Clinical Epidemiology*, **42**, 35–44.

Jha, P., Flather, M., Lonn, E. *et al.* (1995). The antioxidant vitamins and cardiovascular disease. *Annals of Internal Medicine*, **123**, 860–72.

Jüni, P., Witschi, A., Bloch, R. *et al.* (1999). The hazards of scoring the quality of clinical trial for meta-analysis. *JAMA*, **282**, 1054–60.

Jüni, P., Altman, D.G., and Egger, M. (2001). Assessing the quality of controlled clinical trials. *BMJ*, **323**, 42–6.

Jüni, P., Holenstein, F., Sterne, J. *et al.* (2002). Direction and impact of language bias in meta-analyses of controlled trials: empirical study. *International Journal of Epidemiology*, **31**, 115–23.

Jüni, P., Nartey, L., Reichenbach, S. *et al.* (2004). Risk of cardiovascular events and rofecoxib: Cumulative meta-analysis. *Lancet*, **364**, 2021–9.

Kerlikowske, K., Grady, D., Rubin, S.M. *et al.* (1995). Efficacy of screening mammography. A meta-analysis [see comments]. *JAMA*, **273**, 149–54.

Lau, J., Antman, E.M., Jimenez-Silva, J. *et al.* (1992). Cumulative meta-analysis of therapeutic trials for myocardial infarction. The *New England Journal of Medicine*, **327**, 248–54.

Laupacis, A., Sackett, D.L., and Roberts, R.S. (1988). An assessment of clinically useful measures of the consequences of treatment. *The New England Journal of Medicine*, **318**, 1728–33.

Lawlor, D.A., Davey, S.G., Kundu, D. *et al.* (2004). Those confounded vitamins: What can we learn from the differences between observational versus randomised trial evidence? *Lancet*, **363**, 1724–7.

Leizorovicz, A., Haugh, M.C., Chapuis, F.R. *et al.* (1992). Low molecular weight heparin in prevention of perioperative thrombosis. *BMJ*, **305**, 913–20.

Light, R.J. and Pillemer, D.B. (1984). *Summing up. The science of reviewing research.* Harvard University Press, Cambridge, Massachusetts, and London, England.

Lilford, R.J. and Braunholtz, D. (1996). The statistical basis of public policy: A paradigm shift is overdue. *BMJ*, **313**, 603–7.

MacDonald, D., Grant, A., Sheridan-Pereira, M. *et al.* (1985). The Dublin randomised controlled trial of intrapartum fetal heart rate monitoring. *American Journal of Obstetrics and Gynecology*, **152**, 524–39.

Melander, H., Ahlqvist-Rastad, J., Meijer, G. *et al.* (2003). Evidence b(i)ased medicine--selective reporting from studies sponsored by pharmaceutical industry: Review of studies in new drug applications. *BMJ*, **326**, 1171–3.

Mitchell, J.R.A.(1981). Timolol after myocardial infarction: an answer or a new set of questions? *BMJ*, **282**, 1565–70.

Moher, D., Tetzlaff, J., Tricco, A.C. *et al.* (2007). Epidemiology and reporting characteristics of systematic reviews. *PLoS Medicine*, **4**, e78.

Montori, V.M., Devereaux, P.J., Adhikari, N.K. *et al.* (2005). Randomized trials stopped early for benefit: a systematic review. *JAMA*, **294**, 2203–9.

Mulrow, C.D. (1987). The medical review article: State of the science. *Annals of Internal Medicine*, **106**, 485–8.

Multicentre International Study: Supplementary report (1977). Reduction in mortality after myocardial infarction with long-term beta-adrenoceptor blockade. *BMJ*, **2**, 419–21.

Nurmohamed, M.T., Rosendaal, F.R., Bueller, H.R. *et al.* (1992). Low-molecular-weight heparin versus standard heparin in general and orthopaedic surgery: A meta-analysis. *Lancet*, **340**, 152–6.

O'Farrell, N. and Egger, M. (2000). Circumcision in men and the prevalence of HIV infection: a meta-analysis revisited. *International Journal of STD & AIDS*, **11**, 137–42.

Pearson, K. (1904). Report on certain enteric fever inoculation statistics. *BMJ*, **3**, 1243–6.

Peters, J.L., Sutton, A.J., Jones, D.R. *et al.* (2006). Comparison of two methods to detect publication bias in meta-analysis. *JAMA*, **295**, 676–80.

Phillips, A.N. and Davey Smith, G. (1991). How independent are 'independent' effects? Relative risk estimation when correlated exposures are measured imprecisely. *Journal of Clinical Epidemiology*, **44**, 1223–31.

Rembold, C.M. (1998). Number needed to screen: Development of a statistic for disease screening. *BMJ*, **317**, 307–12.

Reynolds, J.L. and Whitlock, R.M.L. (1972). Effects of a beta-adrenergic receptor blocker in myocardial infarctation treated for one year from onset. *British Heart Journal*, **34**, 252–9.

Rosenthal, R. (1979). The 'file drawer problem' and tolerance for null results. *Psychological Bulletin*, **86**, 638–41.

Sampson, M., Barrowman, N.J., Moher, D. *et al.* (2003). Should meta-analysts search Embase in addition to Medline? *Journal of Clinical Epidemiology*, **56**, 943–55.

Schulz KF (1996). Randomised trials, human nature, and reporting guidelines. *Lancet*, **348**, 596–8.

Shapiro, S. (1994). Meta-analysis/Shmeta-analysis. *American Journal of Epidemiology*, **140**, 771–8.

Song, F. (1999). Exploring heterogeneity in meta-analysis: Is the L'Abbé Plot useful? *Journal of Clinical Epidemiology*, **52**, 725–30.

Sterling, T.D. (1959). Publication decisions and their possible effects on inferences drawn from tests of significance - or vice versa. *Journal of the American Statistical Association*, **54**, 30–4.

Sterne J.A.C., Gavaghan D.J., and Egger M. (2000). Publication and related bias in meta-analysis: power of statistical tests and prevalence in the literature. *Journal of Clinical Epidemiology*, **53**, 1119–29.

Sterne, J.A.C. Egger, M., and Sutton, A.J. (2001). Meta-analysis software. In *Systematic Reviews in Health Care: Meta-Analysis in Context* (eds. M. Egger, D.G. Smith, and D.G. Altman), p. 336. BMJ Books, London.

The Norwegian Multicenter Study Group (1981). Timolol-induced reduction in mortality and reinfarction in patients surviving acute myocardial infarction. *The New England Journal of Medicine*, **304**, 801–7.

Thornley, B. and Adams, C. (1998). Content and quality of 2 000 controlled trials in schizophrenia over 50 years. *BMJ*, **317**, 1181–4.

Tramèr, M.R., Reynolds, D.J.M., Moore, R.A. *et al.* (1997). Impact of covert duplicate publication on meta-analysis: a case study. *BMJ*, **315**, 635–40.

Vandenbroucke, J.P., von Elm, E., Altman, D.G. *et al.* (2004). Strengthening the Reporting of Observational Studies in Epidemiology (STROBE): explanation and elaboration. *PLoS Medicine*, **4**, e297.

von Elm, E., Costanza, M.C., Walder, B. *et al.* (2003). More insight into the fate of biomedical meeting abstracts: a systematic review. *BMC Medical Research Methodology*, **3**, 12.

von Elm, E., Poglia, G., Walder, B. *et al.* (2004). Different patterns of duplicate publication: An analysis of articles used in systematic reviews. *JAMA*, **291**, 974–80.

von Elm, E., Röllin, A., Blümle, A. *et al.* Publication and non-publication of clinical trials: Longitudinal study of applications submitted to a research ethics committee. *Swiss Medical Weekly*, 2008; **138**:197–203.

Wood, L., Egger, M., Gluud, L.L. *et al.* (2008). Empirical evidence of bias in treatment effect estimates in controlled trials with different interventions and outcomes: Meta-epidemiological study. *BMJ*, 2008; **336**:601–5.

6.15

Statistical methods

Gail Williams

Introduction

Statistics is the study of mathematically based techniques used to collect, analyse, and interpret quantitative data. In public health, this occurs in a complex of biological, clinical, epidemiological, social, ecological, and administrative systems.

Sometimes we want to describe, explore, or summarize data without extending our findings beyond the coverage of the data we have—that is, the sample. More usually, however, we want to extend, or generalize, our findings from the sample to a larger group, sometimes called the 'target' population. In this situation, we need to consider carefully two aspects of our data collection. Firstly, what was the actual source of our data, and how did we select the sample from the population? If we deliberately excluded some persons in our sampling, or made it more difficult for some than others to be included in our sample, then the sample may not represent the population equitably—we may have a *biased* sample. Secondly, we expect that if we repeat the data collection, even under identical conditions, we will get somewhat different results. This variability, called *sampling variability*, needs to be taken into account in deciding how precisely findings from our sample reflect what is happening in the population.

Owing to the ready availability of high-speed computers, development of sophisticated programming languages and statistical software, and expansion in theoretical developments, we now have access to a wider range of statistical techniques than ever before. It is important that analytical methods used are appropriate to our sampling strategy, the type of data we have collected, and the research questions we want to answer. We then usually want to generalize our results to a population. This process of drawing conclusions about populations by using samples is called *statistical inference*.

In this chapter, we discuss the basic concepts that underpin the issues raised earlier. The ideas of probability theory are heavily involved in random sampling, which takes place under the assumption of a probability model that governs the selection of the sample. As we shall see, probability models are also involved in helping us quantify the uncertainty in our sample estimates. We will also discuss a range of statistical techniques which are in common usage, outlining the underlying assumptions, and focusing on interpretation. Finally, we will reflect on the implications of analytical method for study design, in relation to study size and power.

Basic concepts

Populations, samples, and sampling

For the purpose of a discussion of statistical methods, a *population* is the complete set of entities we want to consider in our enquiry. The entities may, for example, be free-living humans, hospital patients, disease vectors, communities, or health services. A *sample* is then defined generally as a subset of a population. The sample may not be of interest in itself; it is used to provide information about the population, such as to estimate the incidence of malaria or to compare the risk of lung cancer among smokers and non-smokers. By taking a sample from the population instead of enumerating the entire population, we save resources and time. We may choose to spend some of these savings on achieving greater quality of measurement, or better follow-up of those we select, than would be the case if we attempted to use the entire population. The price paid, however, is that we can no longer make an absolute statement about the population; we have only an estimate—the sample incidence, or the excess of lung cancer in our sample of smokers.

Probability and random sampling

The solution to the concerns of obtaining an unbiased estimate and being able to quantify uncertainty entails the notion of 'fairness' in the sample selection process. A 'fair' method of sampling does not favour or discriminate against any member of the population. However, if we can quantify any 'unfairness', we can correct for this in the analysis, and so still obtain an unbiased estimate. For example, if males are twice as likely as females to be selected from a population that contains equal numbers of each, we can compile the data so that females have twice the weight. Thus, what actually matters is that we know how likely it is that individuals in a population get selected for the sample. This is formalized in terms of the *probability of selection*, for each person in a population.

In general terms, we measure probability with a single number, which has particular properties, some of which are as follows:

- Probabilities lie between 0 and 1 (or 0 and 100%).
- If the probability of the event is 0, there is no chance of the event occurring.
- If the probability of the event is 1, the event is certain to occur.
- The combined probability of a complete collection of events is 1.

A process whose outcome is unpredictable and governed by rules of probability is termed *random*. If we are drawing random lots to select one person from 100 people, we can say (before sampling) that the probability of inclusion of an individual is 1 in 100, but we can not predict exactly which individual will be included. Other classic random processes are the outcomes of coin tosses, rolls of a die, or drawing lots. We know that in the long run, provided the coin is unbiased, the chance or probability of a head is 0.5 or 50% on any one toss, but we cannot predict the outcome on any particular toss.

The word 'random' has now taken on a specialized meaning. It is being used to describe a process whose outcome (in this case, getting selected for the sample or not) is governed by the play of chance. Random does not mean 'haphazard' or 'arbitrary'.

A sample in which each person in the population has the same chance of selection is called a *simple random sample*. This can be achieved by listing all the members of the population (this list is called a *sampling frame*), applying a random process of selection, such as drawing lots or using computer-generated random numbers, and obtaining a sample of the required size. In practice, however, compiling a sampling frame can be one of the major problems to be overcome in designing a study. More generally, a sample for which we know the probability of selection (whether it is the same or not) for each person in the population is called a *probability* or *random sample*.

As we have seen, the recommended sampling techniques usually require identifying a population as the source of our sample. Thus, to obtain a sample of 7-year-old children to determine the prevalence of childhood asthma, we might begin by obtaining school class lists, but additional sources might need to be consulted. Note that it is important to keep in mind the population about which we want to draw conclusions. In the example, is it the population of 7-year-old school children or is it all 7-year-olds? In some cases, we may be only able to sample formally and statistically a restricted population (school children), but we really want to make conclusions about a wider population (all children). This wider population is sometimes referred to as the *target population*. Whether conclusions can be extrapolated to another population in a particular situation is then a matter of judgement.

If someone has no chance of being selected in the sample, and they are different with respect to the characteristics we are measuring, then we expect to have a biased sample. Similarly, if individuals vary in both their chances of selection and the characteristics of interest, we can expect to have a biased sample. We often have no way of predicting how individuals vary in terms of the characteristics being measured, but if we can control, and therefore know, the probability of selection, we control the potential for bias.

Methods of sampling which do not follow these rules are termed *non-probability samples*; here. we do not know the probability of inclusion of population units. Indeed, we often cannot define the population. These methods include convenience samples (persons waiting in outpatient departments) or haphazard samples ('persons-in-the-street').

A sample is termed a random sample because of the method of selection, not because of what it ultimately contains. We cannot determine whether a sample is random by examining it. To be certain that a sample is a probability sample, we need to know the process by which it was obtained. We may examine a randomly selected sample for observations which are deviant in some respect and we may compare some of its characteristics with those of the population, but we can never be absolutely certain that it is representative of the population.

Thus, 'random' does not equal 'representative' (although using a random method of selection, in some sense, decreases our chances of non-representativeness). In summary, the reasons for using random sampling, whether simple or complex are:

- To enable us to quantify the sampling variation using probability theory
- To ensure that we can obtain a statistically unbiased estimator of the quantity of interest

Complex sampling

Complex sampling is the term used to describe probability sampling which is not simple. A variety of methods, or their combination, may be used.

Stratified sampling is used when the population consists of a number of subpopulations or strata which vary in the quantity we are interested in. We want to sample within each one separately, in order to control the numbers we achieve from each stratum, or to take into account large variability across strata. For example, it is typical (but not universal) that urban areas have larger populations than rural areas. For sampling the population, therefore, we might first wish to stratify by rural and/or urban status, so that we can be sure of obtaining sufficient numbers in each area. If we use different sampling fractions, this means the overall sample will not be a simple random sample, because the probability of selection of units (e.g. persons) in different strata will be different, but we will still have a probability or random sample because we can, knowing the sampling fraction within strata, work out the probability of selection of any unit.

This method of sampling has another advantage, if we control the stratum sizes to closely reflect those in the population. If the quantity we are measuring varies greatly across strata, we achieve greater precision than a method which ignores this variation. In designing a stratified sampling scheme, we need to be clear about our priorities—do we want to disproportionately increase the numbers in a stratum, or do we want to control for inter-strata variability?

Cluster sampling involves selecting groups of individuals at a time, rather than individuals themselves. To obtain a random sample of persons in a city, we might first select a simple random sample of census collection districts, or suburbs, and include all persons living within the selected districts as the sample.

What would happen if we took a simple random sample from a large city? Individuals selected would be widely scattered and it would be difficult to reach them all if we have to conduct face-to-face interviews, for example; cluster sampling is much more efficient. The disadvantage is that sample may be artificially 'homogeneous'; that is, our selected persons may be more alike than if we had used a random sample.

Two-stage sampling is similar to cluster sampling except that we take a sample of the cluster instead of the whole cluster. This helps to overcome the problem of 'homogeneity' to some extent, but does create a more complex process, as we now have two sampling processes and two sampling fractions.

In some cases, the number of clusters and number from each selected cluster are carefully manipulated so that the overall probability of each population unit being selected is the same. One such method is called *sampling proportional to size*—at the first stage, units (e.g. villages) are selected with a probability proportional to their size (larger villages have larger chance of selection) and then a fixed number of individuals are selected randomly from each selected village. Another method is *proportional sampling* in which villages are selected with equal probability, and then the number of individuals selected from each selected village is proportional to the size of the village.

Cluster sampling and two-stage sampling do not require an explicit, of the whole population to be constructed. In two-stage sampling we need a list of first-stage units (e.g. census districts) and then a list only for each first-stage unit that is actually selected. This is sometimes an additional reason for the use of these staged sampling methods. If we were sampling remote undocumented populations, we would need, as part of the sampling exercise, to prepare a sampling frame. It is then efficient to carry out two-stage sampling: The first stage selects areas, villages, and/or communities, perhaps using grid references on a map. A population and/or housing census of only those areas selected would then be carried out to enable a second-stage sampling. Obviously two-stage sampling can be extended to three or more stages, for example districts, towns, households, and individuals. Finally, individuals may have very different probabilities of inclusion.

It should also be noticed that when we carry out stratified, cluster, or multistage sampling, we have the opportunity to measure entities at all levels. Thus, we may have factors that are relevant at the village level (presence of a health centre, degree of remoteness), at the household level (family income, access to piped water), or at the individual level (age, sex).

Complex sampling allows individuals to have differing probabilities of inclusion in a sample. It is imperative that we are able to calculate each person's probability of inclusion, otherwise we will not be able to make the necessary adjustments in our analysis. Thus, all information relevant to probability of inclusion must be documented in the course of the sample selection.

Complex sampling schemes require expertise and care to design, and to analyse. It is usually necessary to seek the help of a statistician in doing so. Many statistical packages now have procedures to do such analysis, and it is wise to anticipate the use of these in the construction of the data set.

We now move to considering the issue of characterizing information that we might collect on our sample. This involves some general categorizations of variable types. These will also be useful when we need to decide how we are going to present or analyse data.

Describing variables

It is useful to make a distinction between *quantitative* and *categorical* variables, because these types of variables are analysed using different techniques. This distinction is based on the kinds of *values* the variable may take. For the purpose of statistical analysis, what matters is the type of measurement of the variables; that is, whether they are measured on a numerical scale (such as age) or in categories (male or female). Sometimes a numerical variable, such as blood pressure (mm Hg), is used to derive a new variable in categories (hypertensive or not hypertensive), but it is important to realize that it is the final form of the variable that matters for analysis.

Categorical variables

A categorical variable is one whose values are expressed in mutually exclusive categories (e.g. survival status, social class, sex, religion, extent of disability). Categorical variables are further subdivided into *nominal* and *ordinal*. A nominal variable has values that are categories, with no ordering of the categories (e.g. sex, religion). The special case of a variable with two levels only (e.g. sex) is referred to as a *binary*, or *dichotomous* variable. An ordinal variable describes categories that have an underlying order (e.g. social class, extent of disability). The distinction between nominal and ordinal variables only matters when there are at least three categories because the ordering of two categories is arbitrary.

Categorical variables are usually described by *frequencies*, sometimes involving several dimensions, and usually also supplying percentages, in each value category. They may be presented in tabular form, or graphically (e.g. using bar charts or pie charts). For example, a study of child mortality examined the types of birth attendant at delivery of children in the study. This is presented in a table (Table 6.15.1), or graphically in various ways (Fig. 6.15.1)

Although the choice of graphical presentation is partly a matter of taste, bar charts tend to be used for ordinal variables (as the bars can be arranged in the appropriate order) and pie charts may be used for nominal variables (to de-emphasize order).

Quantitative variables

A quantitative variable has values expressed in numerical measurement (e.g. height, weight, blood pressure, age in years, number of previous births). These variables are further subdivided into *discrete* and *continuous* variables. A discrete variable takes only certain distinct values, usually whole numbers (e.g. number of previous births). A continuous variable take all values, usually within a certain range. (e.g. blood pressure, birthweight, serum cholesterol). These are usually measured on a scale, and it is essential to know the units of measurement.

Frequency distributions

Quantitative variables are usually described, at least initially, in a frequency distribution, which tabulates, in selected ordered, mutually exclusive and contiguous groups, the number or percentage in each group.

A study examines medical records of birthweights of children born at a major obstetric hospital in Brisbane, Australia. A sample of 500 children born at full term (39 or more weeks' gestation) in 1981 yields the corresponding birthweight, in kilograms. There are too many individual values to obtain a clear idea of birthweight for

Table 6.15.1 Community-based sample of children under 5 years of age in Bohol Province, the Philippines, 1984–86, by birth attendant at delivery

Birth attendant	Number of deliveries (n=511)	Percentage of deliveries (%)
Untrained TBA	8	1.6
Trained TBA	224	43.8
Midwife	186	36.4
Nurse	3	0.6
Physician	34	6.7
Unknown	56	11.0
Total	511	100.0

TBA = traditional birth attendant.

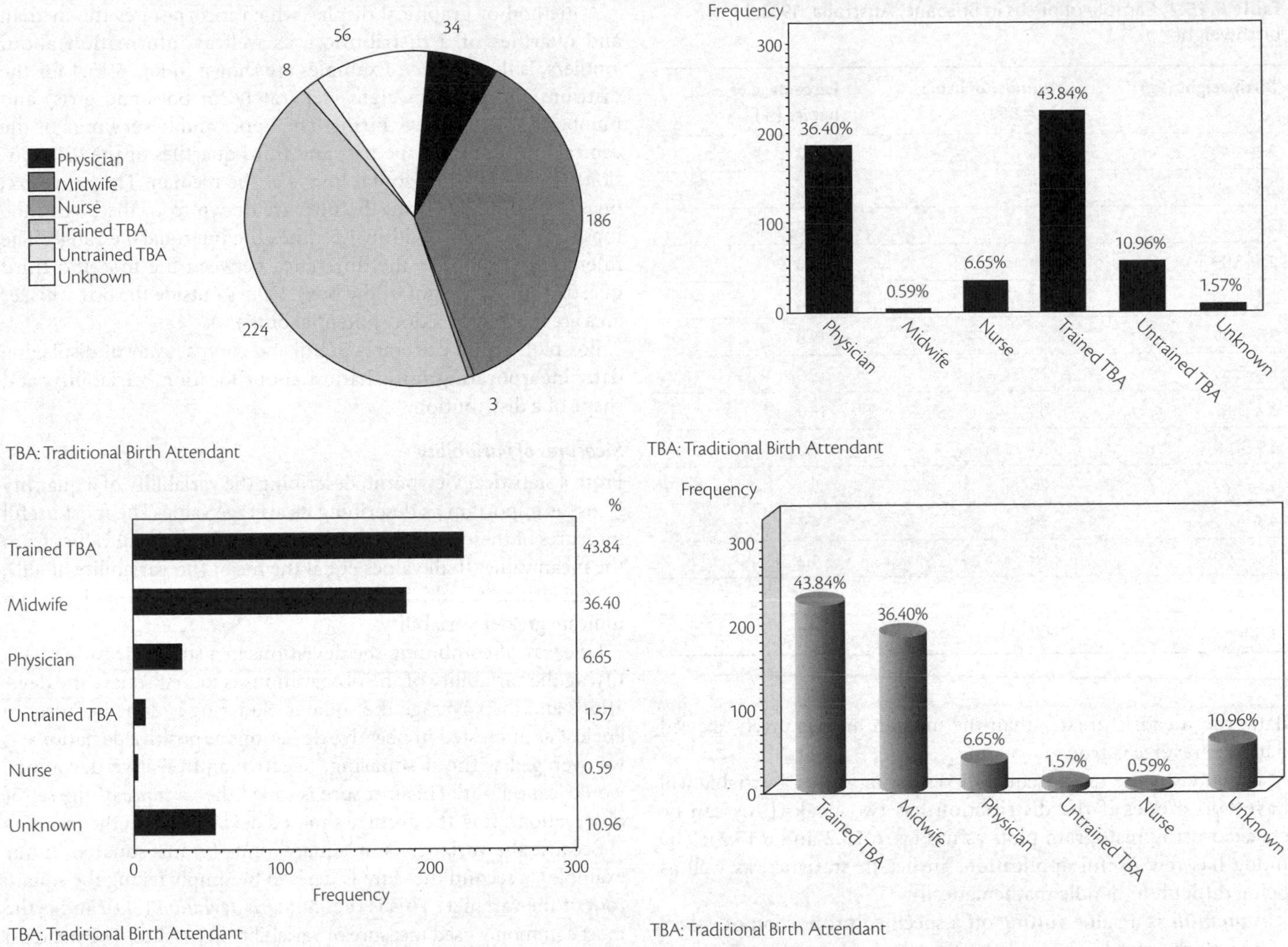

Fig. 6.15.1 Community-based sample of children under 5 years of age in Bohol Province, the Philippines, in 1984–86, by birth attendant at delivery. Alternative graphical methods of presentation.

this group from just looking at a list of 500 values. So we create a frequency distribution (Table 6.15.2), choosing suitable cut-off points for groups of birthweight.

The choice of cut-off points for groups is to some extent arbitrary. We usually want at least eight groups, and prefer them to be evenly spaced, although this is not strictly necessary. Some recommend using √N (square root of N) groups, where N is the number of data points. We may be influenced by cut-offs used for other purposes (e.g. using 2500 g as a cut-off enables us to identify 'low' birthweight babies, as commonly defined). If we want to compare our frequency distribution with that obtained in another study, we use the same cut-off points. A sample frequency distribution with very fine categories may reveal problems relating to data accuracy such as lack of sensitivity and terminal digit preference. If unexpected 'peaks' occur at regular intervals, such as when a category contains a multiple of 10, then we might become suspicious that measurements are being rounded to the nearest 10, causing those categories to be overused.

This frequency distribution is usually graphed in a histogram (Fig. 6.15.2). Constructing a frequency distribution requires a large number of values to be useful. It does, however, have the advantage that we get a picture of the shape of the distribution. This may be important when we come to choosing a method of analysis.

Not all distributions are symmetric. A variable may have a negatively skewed distribution (Fig. 6.15.3a), when the peak is pushed to the right, or a positively skewed distribution (Fig. 6.15.3b), when the peak is pushed to the left.

Measures of location

The measure most commonly used to summarize the magnitude of a quantitative variable is the *mean* (the usual arithmetic mean, or average). When some values need to be given more or less weight, a *weighted* mean may be used. When distributions are positively skewed, *geometric means* are typically used.

The *median* of a variable is the middle value of its distribution; that is, half the distribution is below, and half is above the median. The median is usually less affected than the mean by extreme values, because it takes into account only the relative ranking of observations. The mean for the distribution of 500 birthweights given in Fig. 6.15.2 is 3.49 kg, and the median is 3.47 kg; these are very similar because of the symmetry of the distribution.

When data are 'skewed', as shown in Fig. 6.15.3, the median is usually considered preferable to the mean (i.e. a better representative of the data), because the 'extreme' values may unduly influence the mean whereas the median is little affected. In positively skewed

Table 6.15.2 Sample of births in Brisbane, Australia, 1981, by birthweight

Birthweight (kg)	Number of babies (n = 500)	Percentage of babies (%)
2.3–2.49	6	1.2
2.5–2.69	10	2.0
2.7–2.89	19	3.8
2.9–3.09	63	12.6
3.1–3.29	71	14.2
3.3–3.49	94	18.8
3.5–3.69	78	15.6
3.7–3.89	65	13.0
3.9–4.09	41	8.2
4.1–4.29	26	5.2
4.3–4.49	20	4.0
4.5–4.69	6	1.2
4.7–4.89	1	0.2
Total	500	100.0

data, the mean is greater than the median; in negatively skewed data, the reverse is true.

The *mode* is the most frequently occurring value; a variable will have two modes if the distribution has two peaks (this can be checked using histogram plots as in Figs. 6.15.2 and 6.15.3). The mode has few useful applications in health statistics, as well as being difficult to handle mathematically.

A *quantile* is a value cutting off a specified proportion of values of a random variable. Common particular cases are tertiles (2 cut-off points, dividing the distribution into three equal areas of 33.3% each), quartiles (25%), quintiles (20%), deciles (10%), and percentiles (1%). Note that the median is also the 2nd quartile, the 5th decile, and the 50th percentile.

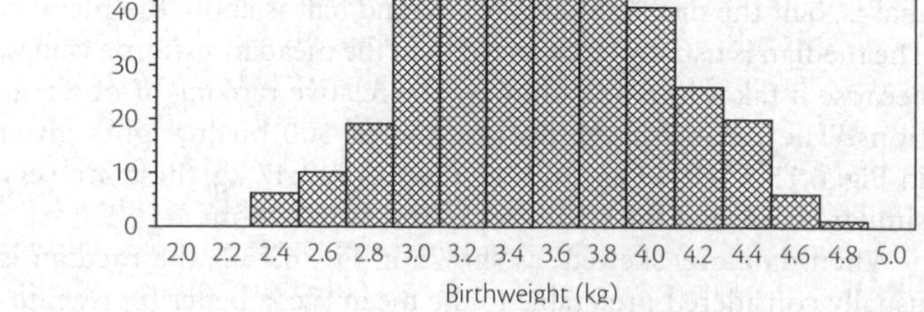

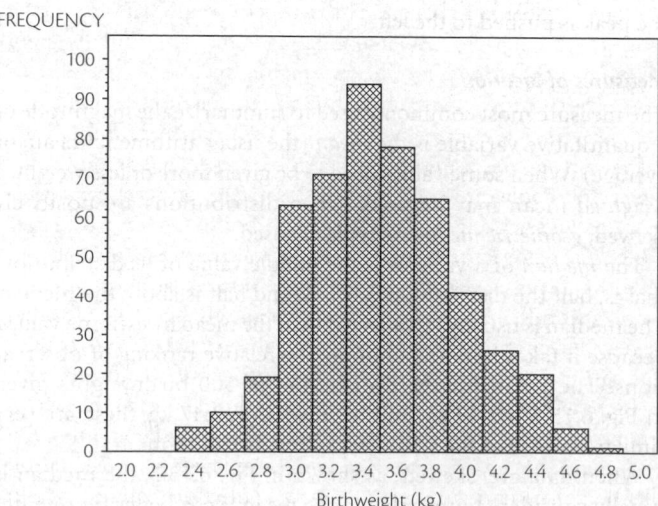

Fig. 6.15.2 Frequency distribution of birthweight; 500 babies born in Brisbane, Australia, 1981.

A method of graphical display which incorporates the median and quartiles of a distribution, as well as information about 'outliers', is the *box plot*. Examples are shown in Fig. 6.15.4 for the distributions of birthweight (separately for boys and girls) and number of previous live births. The upper and lower limits of the central box represent the first and third quartiles of the distribution. The middle horizontal line is at the median. The 'whiskers', lines extending out from the box, are drawn from the box to the most extreme point within 1.5 times the interquartile range. The interquartile range is the difference between the first and third quartiles (or the height of the box). Values outside the box whisker area are marked by a dot (potential outliers).

Box plots are an extremely useful and compact way of displaying data, incorporating information about location, variability, and shape of a distribution.

Measures of variability

From a statistical viewpoint, describing the variability of a quantity is just as important as describing its average value. The most useful measures of these examine the deviations of individual values from the mean value. If all values equal the mean (no variability at all!), all deviations would be zero; large deviations from the mean indicate greater variability.

One way of combining the deviations in a single measure quantifying the variability of the observations is to first square the deviations and then average the squares. Squaring is done because we are just as interested in negative deviations as positive deviations; if we averaged without squaring, negative and positive deviations would 'cancel out'. This measure is called the *variance* of the set of observations. It is 'the average squared deviation from the mean'.

Because the variance is in 'square' units (grams squared in our example), a second measure is derived by simply taking the square root of the variance. This is the *standard deviation* (SD), and is the most commonly used measure of variability in practice. The standard deviation for the distribution of 500 birthweights given in Fig. 6.15.2 is 0.45 kg. The standard deviation is used more commonly than the variance because it is in the same units as the original observations, whereas the variance, in square units, is more difficult to interpret. The *range* of a variable is defined as the difference between the largest and the smallest values, or loosely, as the interval defined by the smallest and largest values of the variable. For the birthweight data in Fig. 6.15.2, the range is (from the raw data) = 4.71 − 2.34 = 2.37 kg. The range is susceptible to extreme values (which are the most likely to be faulty) and depends on the number of observations; in general, the more observations, the greater the range. In practice, reporting the smallest to the largest values (2.34 to 4.71 kg) is more useful than the range itself.

The *coefficient of variation* is the ratio of the standard deviation to the mean, usually written as a percentage. It thus expresses variation in relation to location or size. For the birthweight data, the coefficient of variation is 0.45 kg/3.49 kg = 0.129 or 12.9%: The standard deviation is 12.9% of the mean birthweight.

Probability distributions

Just as a sample mean or standard deviation (if the sample is randomly drawn) reflect the population mean or standard deviation, so the observed distribution in the sample reflects the distribution of values in the population. In practice, it is found that certain distribution shapes re-occur. It turns out to be extremely useful to

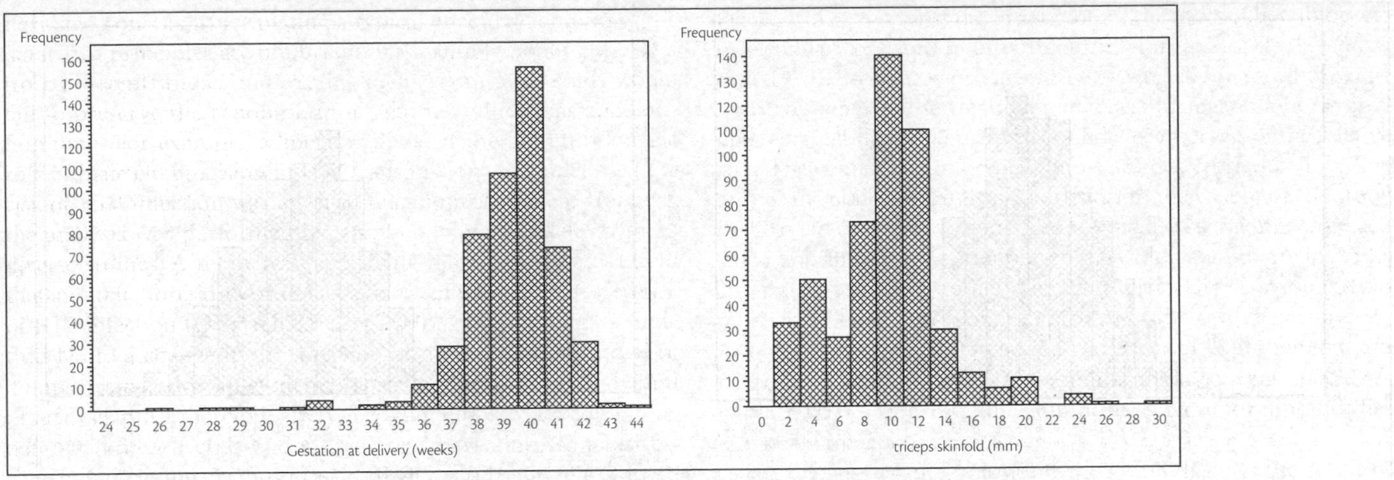

Fig. 6.15.3 Frequency distribution of (a) gestation at delivery (weeks) for 500 babies and (b) triceps skinfold thickness for 500 five-year-olds.

give a particular mathematical form to these characteristic shapes, because these forms then serve as 'models' which help us draw further conclusions from samples.

What is a probability distribution?

We saw the distribution of birthweight for a sample of 500 full-term babies born in Brisbane, Australia, followed a roughly symmetric and bell-shaped curve, and we later calculated the mean and standard deviation of that distribution of birthweight. Let us look at some other distributions, of different continuous variables, derived from some fairly large samples.

The distributions observed in Fig. 6.15.5 are of different variables, in different samples. However in each case, the shape of the distribution is somewhat similar—approximately symmetric, with a central, somewhat rounded, peak. There are some irregularities, particularly in the samples of birthweight and haemoglobin values, which are both affected by a form of rounding error, called terminal digit preference; but generally, the impression is that we have a common shape, with, of course, different means and standard deviations. We also notice that, in each case, the mean and median are similar; this is consistent with the observation of symmetry—the middle value (the median) is approximately equal to the mean.

The normal distribution

The empirical observation that distributions of continuous variables have a common shape similar to those exhibited in Fig. 6.15.5 prompted mathematicians to work on finding a mathematical or idealized representation to describe this shape.

The smooth curve so discovered the mathematical formula:

$$f(X)=\frac{1}{\sqrt{2\pi}\times(\text{SD})}\exp\left(-\frac{1}{2\times(\text{SD})^2}(X-\text{Mean})^2\right)$$

where 'exp' is the exponential (or antilog) function, and π ('pi') = 3.14159. *X* is the symbol given to the value of the variable in question (e.g. birthweight).

This formula is known as the normal distribution and is a specific case of a probability distribution; that is, a mathematical description of the behaviour of a random variable (a variable whose values

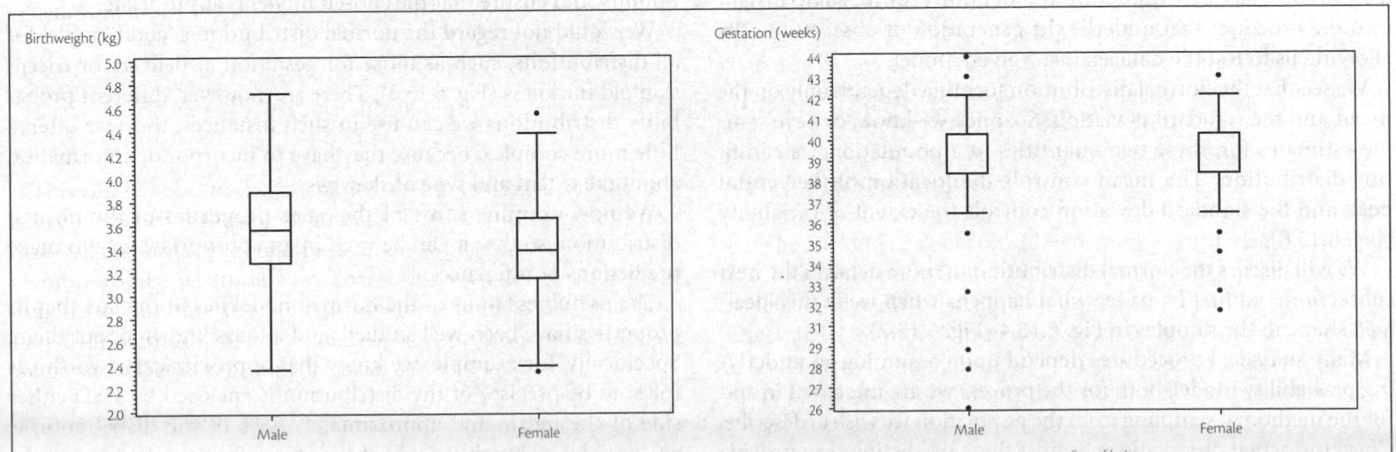

Fig. 6.15.4 Box plot of birthweights (kg) and gestation at delivery (weeks) for boys ($N=254$) and girls ($N=246$).

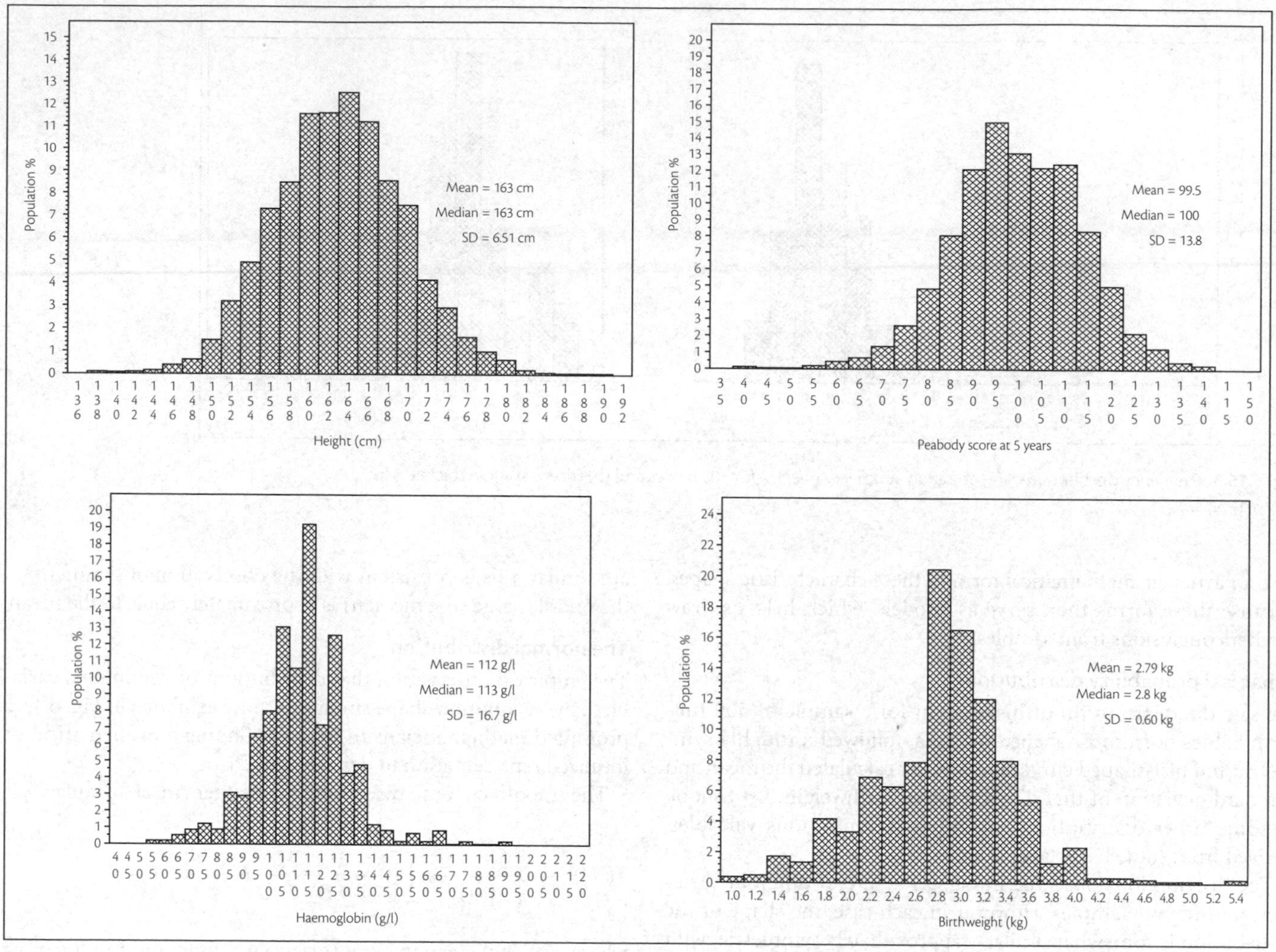

Fig. 6.15.5 Histograms for (a) heights of 8345 women, (b) language development scores of 3368 five-year-olds, (c) haemoglobin levels of 589 Filipino infants, and (d) birthweights of 813 Filipino babies.

cannot be predicted with certainty). It can be thought of as an 'idealized' description of data, and can serve as a model upon which we base our analytical approach. The purpose of having an idealized model may be to 'smooth' the data or acquire some insight into the processes that underlie the generation of observations, by allowing us to test the data against a given model.

We see that the normal distribution formula depends only on the mean and the standard deviation. So, once we know, or have sample estimates for, these two quantities in a population, we can fit this distribution. The mean controls the location of the central peak and the standard deviation controls the extent of variability (Fig. 6.15.6).

We will discuss the normal distribution in more detail in the next subsection, but first let us see what happens when we fit this idealized shape to the samples in Fig. 6.15.4 (Fig. 6.15.7).

Many statistical procedures depend upon assuming an underlying probability model, both for the process we are interested in and for the method of sampling from the population we wish to describe. Checking actual observations against these predictions can provide us with insight: If the probability model 'fits', then we may be able to use features of the model to make inferences or predictions about the population; and if the model does not 'fit', then we need to review our assumptions about the underlying process we are attempting to describe or predict. It is important that we explore options, and ensure that the chosen model is appropriate.

We would not regard the normal distribution a 'good' model for all distributions, such as those for gestation at delivery or triceps skinfold thickness (Fig. 6.15.3). There are, however, different probability distributions we can use in such instances; they are often a little more complex, because they have to incorporate information about the extent and type of skewness.

We now examine some of the basic properties of the normal distribution, so that it can be used in an appropriate way to make predictions or inferences.

The usefulness to us of the normal model lies in the fact that its properties have been well studied, and a lot is known about them. Specifically, for example, we know that approximately two-thirds (68% to be precise) of the distribution is enclosed by 1 SD either side of the mean, and approximately 95% of the distribution is enclosed by 2 SDs either side of the mean. Figure 6.15.8 shows the normal model fitted to the mean and standard deviation of the sample of birthweight.

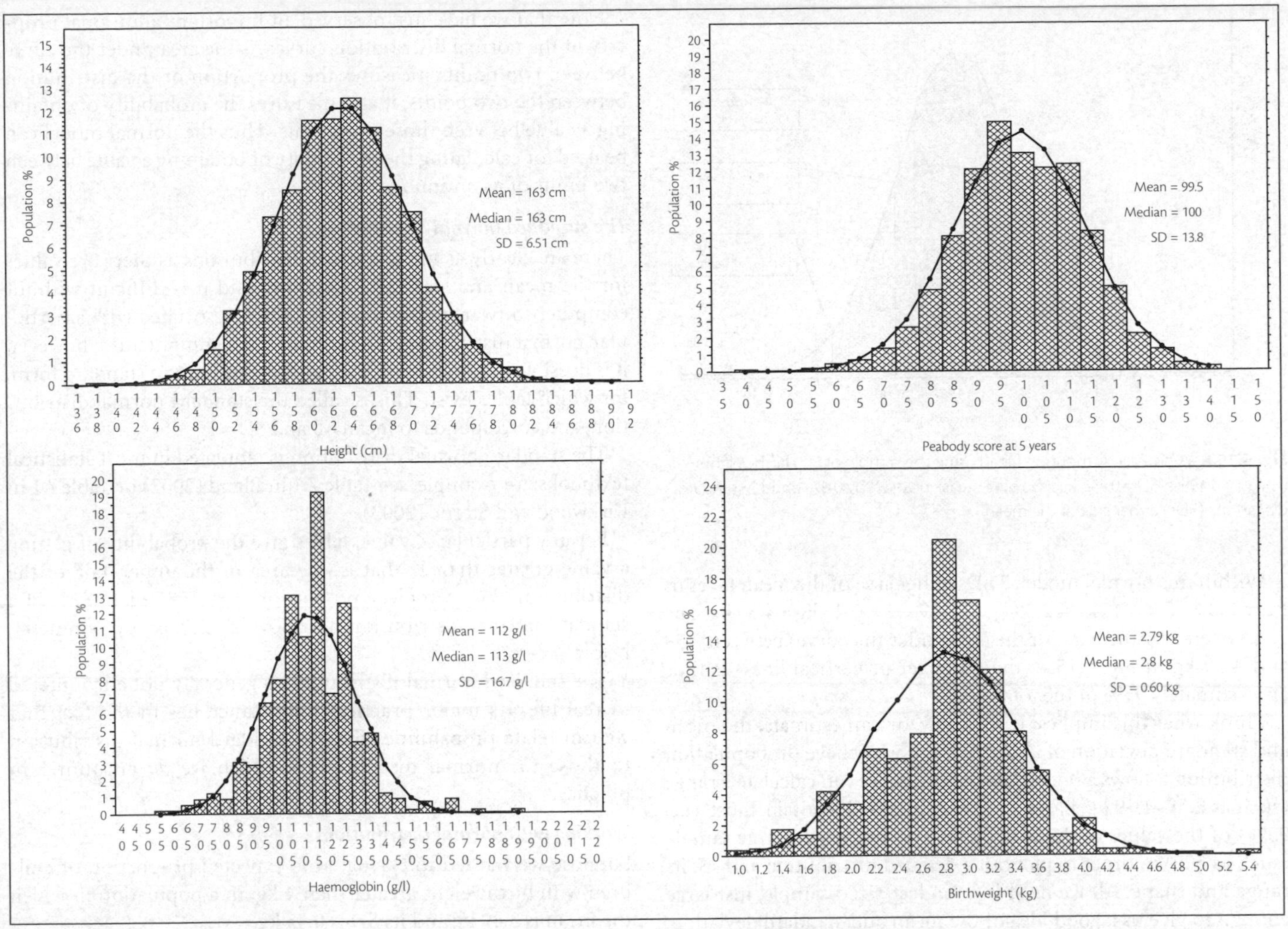

Fig. 6.15.6 Histograms and fitted normal distributions for (a) heights of 8345 women, (b) language development scores of 3368 five-year-olds, (c) haemoglobin levels of 589 Filipino infants, and (d) birthweights of 813 Filipino babies.

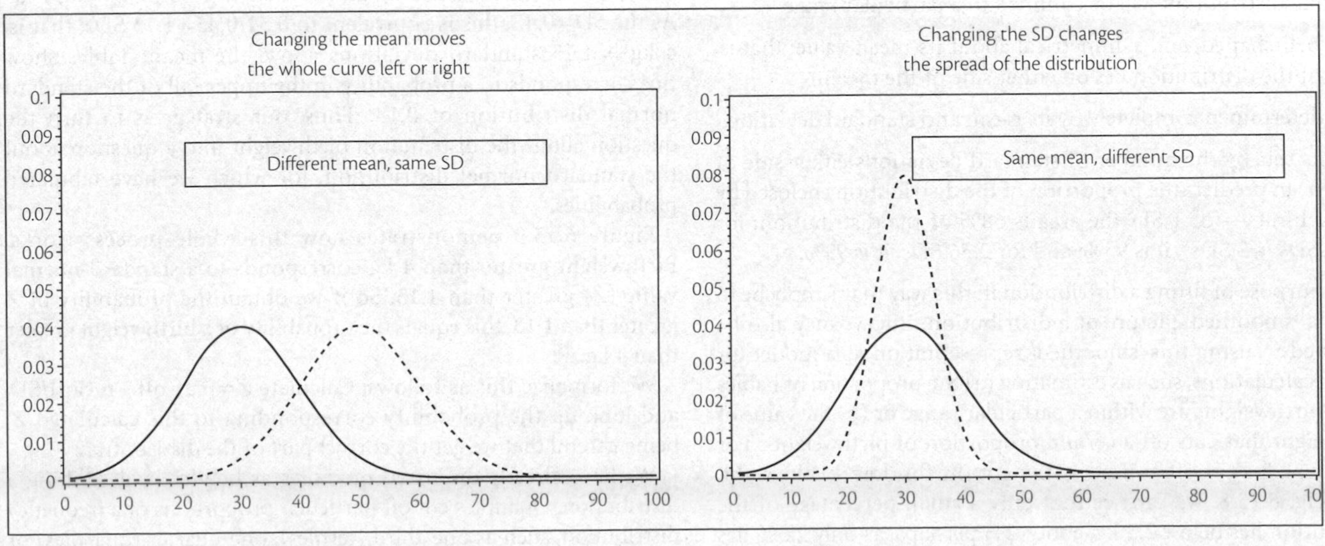

Fig. 6.15.7 The normal distribution for different mean and standard deviation (SD).

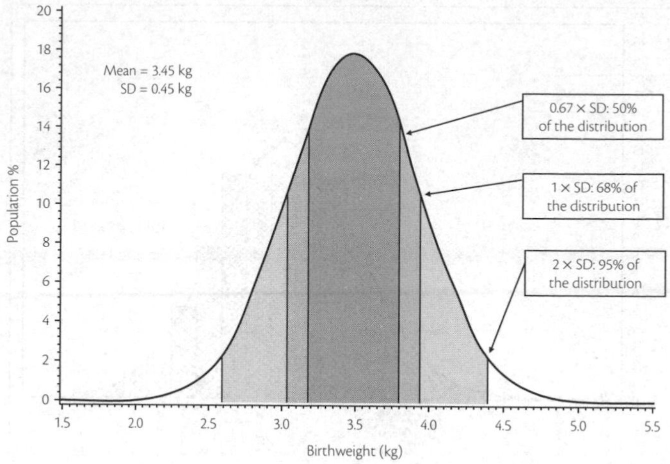

Fig. 6.15.8 A normal distribution fitted using the sample of 500 birthweights (mean=3.49 kg, SD=0.448 kg) showing areas enclosed by 0.67, 1, and 2 standard deviations (SDs) either side of the mean.

Within this normal model, 2 SDs either side of the mean takes us from 3.49 − 2 × 0.45 kg = 2.59 kg to 3.49 + 2 × 0.45 kg = 4.39 kg. The area covered by the bars (or the area under the curve) between 2.59 and 4.39 kg in Fig. 6.15.7 (the outer set of vertical lines) is thus approximately 95% of the total area.

Think what this implies: If we know, or can estimate, the mean and standard deviation of a variable, and we believe the population distribution follows a normal distribution, we can calculate a range (such as 2.59–4.39 kg, based on 2 SDs) that will contain 'most' (i.e. 95%) of the values of the variable. We do not need a large sample (such as 500) in order to plot out a detailed distribution and see its range and shape. All we need is a modest-sized sample, just large enough to give us a good idea of the mean and standard deviation, plus the assumption of a normal distribution, and we can predict the likely distribution of observations.

In summary, the descriptive properties of the normal distribution are as follows:

- It is the distribution of a continuous variable across the entire numerical scale, although in practice values from an assumed normal distribution will be confined to a particular range.
- It is bell-shaped, and symmetrical about its mean value; that is, half of the distribution lies on either side of the mean.
- It is determined completely by its mean and standard deviation.
- Limits sets by the number of standard deviations either side of the mean predicts the proportion of the distribution enclosed by these limits—for 1 SD, the area is 68% of the distribution; for 1.96 SDs (≈2 SDs), it is 95%; and for 2.56 SDs, it is 99%.

The purpose of fitting a distribution in this way may simply be to obtain a 'smoothed' picture of a distribution. But we may also be interested in using this 'smoothed' representation as a model for further calculations, such as estimating (a) the proportion of babies whose birthweights are within a particular range or (b) the value of birthweight that cuts off a certain proportion of birthweights. For example, 2.5 kg is often used as the cut-off for 'low' birthweight. From Fig. 6.15.8, we can see that only a small percentage of the distribution lies below 2.5 kg, about 2% perhaps, as only 2.5% lies below the mean—2 SD limit, just above 2.5 kg.

Note that we have just observed an important additional property of the normal distribution curve: As the area under the curve between two points measures the proportion of the distribution between the two points, it also measures the probability of obtaining a value between those two points. Thus the normal model can be used for calculating the probability of obtaining a value between two limits of a continuous variable.

The standard normal distribution

There are clearly as many normal distributions as there are values for the mean and standard deviation, and it is difficult without computer software to obtain probabilities associated with a particular normal distribution. To facilitate such computation, however, it is possible to convert any normal distribution to a standard form, for which tables exist. This is called the standard normal distribution, and corresponds to mean=0 and SD=1.

The standard normal distribution is tabulated in most statistical textbooks; for example, see Table 7.1 in Bland (2002) or Table A1 in Kirkwood and Sterne (2003).

For any particular Z value, tables give the probability of getting a value greater than Z; that is, the area in the upper 'tail' of the distribution. For example, a proportion P=0.1587 or 15.87% of a standard normal distribution lies above Z=1.0, or, by symmetry, below Z=−1.0.

The standard normal distribution is generally not encountered in real life. Its major practical importance lies in the fact that we can relate probabilities for the standard normal distribution to those for normal distributions, which we *do* encounter in practice.

Working with normal distributions

Suppose we wanted to evaluate the expected proportion of children with birthweight greater than 4 kg, in a population in which the mean is 3.49 kg and its SD is 0.45 kg.

But we do not have tables for a normal distribution when the mean is 3.49 and the SD is 0.45. We need to convert the problem to one in which the standard normal table can be applied. Remember, the standard normal table works in terms of standard deviations from the mean. So how many standard deviations is 4 kg away from the mean of 3.49 kg?

The distance between 4 kg and 3.49 kg is 4 − 3.49 kg = 0.51 kg. As the SD=0.45, this is equivalent to 0.51/0.45=1.13 SDs; that is, 4 kg is 1.13 standard deviations above the mean. Tables show this corresponds to a probability in the upper tail of the standard normal distribution of 0.13. Thus, our strategy is to turn the question about the distribution birthweight into a question about the standard normal distribution, for which we have tabulated probabilities.

Figure 6.15.9 demonstrates how this whole process works. Birthweight greater than 4 kg corresponds to a standard normal value (Z) greater than 1.13. So if we obtain the probability of Z greater than 1.13, this equals the probability of a birthweight greater than 4 kg.

We formalize this as follows: Calculate Z=[cut-off − mean]/SD, and look up the probability corresponding to this calculated Z, being careful that we get the correct part of the distribution.

We have already discussed quantiles as helpful in describing a distribution. Quantiles cut off particular proportions of a frequency distribution, such as one-third (tertiles), one-quarter (quartiles) or one-fifth (quintiles). They can be calculated from a sample frequency

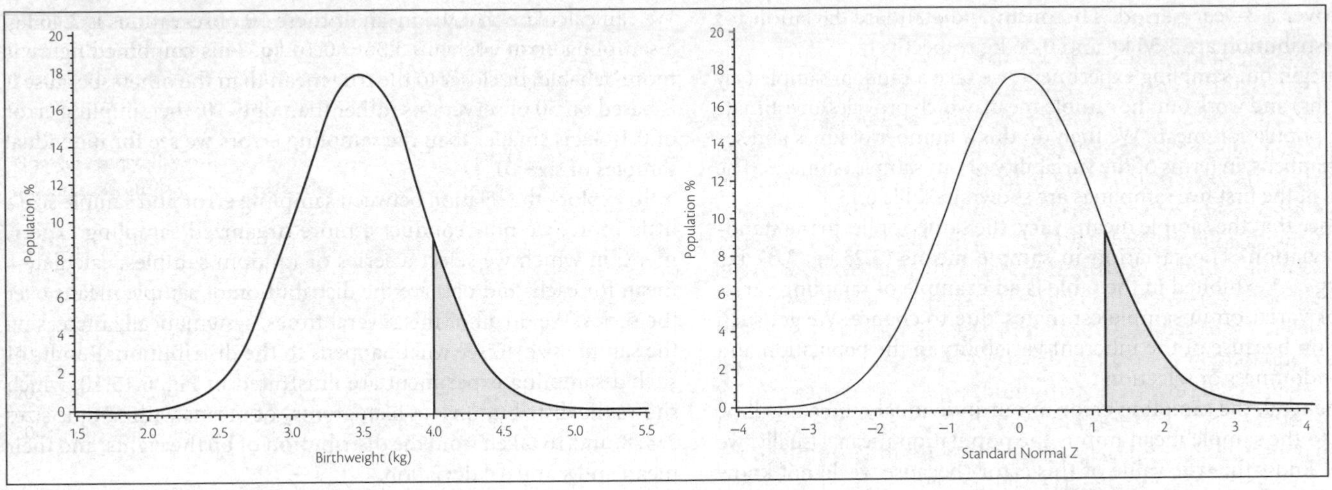

Fig. 6.15.9 Correspondence between a normal distribution fitted using the sample of 500 birthweights (mean = 3.49 kg, SD = 0.448 kg) and the standard normal distribution.

distribution by simply noting the values that correspond to the required proportions. However, now we have a new technique to achieve this, which exploits the facts that (a) we have established that birthweights have a normal distribution and (b) we can get probabilities for the normal curve.

Suppose we want to get quintiles. Looking at the probabilities-shown tables, we find that a probability of 0.20 in the upper tail corresponds to $Z = 0.84$. So we know that -0.84 and $+0.84$ correspond to the lower and upper 20% cut-offs for the distribution of Z-values: -0.84 and $+0.84$ are the lower and upper quintiles of the standard normal distribution. To see what this implies for the distribution of birthweights, we need only to remember that the Z-value gives the number of standard deviations away from the mean.

A Z-value of $+0.84$ means, for birthweight, 0.84 SDs above the mean, or $3.49 + 0.84 \times 0.45 = 3.83$ kg. Similarly $Z = -0.84$ gives us 0.84 SDs below the mean, or $3.49 - 0.84 \times 0.45 = 3.07$ kg. Thus, we would predict that 20% of babies would be lighter than 3.07 kg (the first quintile) and 20% heavier than 3.83 kg (the fourth quintile).

Summarizing the process to get a cut-off, which corresponds to a certain probability of percentage of a normal distribution, we use the following procedure:

1. For the required percentage, identify the appropriate Z-value from the standard normal table.
2. Multiply the Z-value by standard deviation.
3. Add (for values above the mean) this amount to the mean, or subtract (for values below the mean) from the mean.

It is extremely important to note that all of these examples apply only when we are reasonably sure that we have a normal distribution. If we do not have such a distribution (such as in Fig. 6.15.3), this approach will NOT give correct answers. This underlines (a) the importance of choosing the correct probability distribution, or model; and (b) the value of using probability models (in this case, to smooth the data), when they are appropriate.

An important special case when the standard normal distribution does occur in public health or clinical practice is in the assessment of nutritional status by anthropometry, in which we sometimes deal with Z-scores that are derived from standards and which measure, for example, an individual's status of height-for-age, or weight for height. In a population that matches the standards, our calculated Z-scores will be expected to have a standard normal distribution.

Sampling variability

We now examine sampling variability in a mean, using a simulated experiment, based on a known population. The purpose is to uncover rules that govern the behaviour of estimates obtained from the random sampling process. These rules have been established mathematically, and help us quantify uncertainty when we select samples, as opposed to examining an entire population. Often, we can obtain quite precise estimates, with modest-sized samples, at a considerable reduction in cost for a small loss of precision. We see how these rules contribute to the well-known practice of estimating confidence intervals and how they apply to other estimates such as prevalence. The concept of sampling variability lies at the heart of what is known as *statistical inference*.

In this process, we want to be able to say how reliable our sample estimate is. Instinctively, we feel that if the sampling method is 'fair', then we will have an 'unbiased' estimate. But also of concern is the precision of the estimate: Given it is unbiased, how close is it likely to be to the true population value (i.e. the value we would obtain if we measured everyone in the population)? Again, intuitively, we might feel this depends on the number in the sample; we would naturally expect a sample of 1000 children to provide a 'better' or more precise estimate than a sample of 100 children.

Not only can we show that larger samples provide estimates that are more likely to be 'close to' the true population value, but we can also actually quantify this, in terms of the sample size. This is extremely useful, as we shall see later, in deciding how large a sample is needed to achieve a given degree of precision.

Sampling distributions

We begin discussion of the properties of samples with an example showing what happens when we take repeated simple random samples. Let us return to an actual population of children, and their birthweight. This is now an entire series of about 7000 children born over a 3-year period. The mean and standard deviation for this distribution are 3.36 kg and 0.56 kg respectively.

To begin our sampling experiment, we take a random sample (say 10 births) and work out the sample mean, which provides an estimate of the population mean. We then do this a number of times and see what happens, in terms of the variability of our sample estimates. The results of the first five samplings are shown in Table 6.15.3.

We see that the sample means vary; the same applies to the standard deviation. The variation in sample means (3.23 kg, 3.57 kg, 3.70 kg . . .) exhibited in the table is an example of sampling variation or variation in sample estimates 'due to chance'. We get such variation because of the inherent variability in the population and the randomness of selection.

In general, the sampling error in our individual estimate will be equal to the sample mean minus the population mean. Usually, we do not know the true value of this error (because we do not know the value of population mean). In this example we do: It is the mean of the population birthweights (3.36 kg). The sampling errors are then 3.23 − 3.36 = −0.13 kg, 3.57 − 3.36 = +0.21 kg, 3.70 − 3.36 = +0.34 kg, and so on.

The question is: 'Can we conclude anything about the properties of these errors?'

Sampling error and bias

As the random sampling procedure has favoured neither high nor low birthweights (i.e. is unbiased), we expect that sampling errors will be as likely to be in one direction as another: Any particular sample mean will be as likely to be above the mean as below it. The first rule governing the behaviour of random sampling is

1. Irrespective of sample size, the sample means are expected to fluctuate evenly about the true population mean.

Sampling error and sample size

Next, let us consider the sample size. If we put our five samples together, we now effectively have a sample of 50 observations. We can calculate that the mean of these 50 observations is 3.46 kg, a sampling error of 3.46 − 3.36 = 0.10 kg. This combined figure is more 'reliable', or closer to the true mean than the others, because it is based on 50 observations rather than only 10; the sampling error of 0.10 kg is smaller than the sampling errors we see for individual samples of size 10.

To explore the relation between sampling error and sample size a little more, we now conduct a more organized sampling experiment, in which we select a series of random samples, calculate a mean for each, and observe the distribution of sample means over the series. We do all of this several times, systematically increasing the sample size, to see what happens to the distribution. Results of such a sampling experiment are illustrated in Fig. 6.15.10, which shows the distributions (as histograms) of means with sample sizes 2, 4, 8, and 16 taken from the distribution of birthweights, and their mean and standard deviation.

The distribution becomes more closely clustered around a middle value as the sample size increases. The means do not systematically increase or decrease with increasing sample size and have more variability (larger SD) when the sample size is small. The standard deviation of the means steadily decreases as sample size increases, more quickly when the sample size is small.

We have discovered a second rule governing the behaviour of random sampling:

2. The means vary less (by chance) if the sample size is large; that is, the sampling error is smaller, the larger the sample.

The practical implication of (1) and (2) is that as the sample size *N* becomes larger, our sample estimate is more likely to be closer to the population mean.

The sampling distribution of the mean

The distributions in Fig. 6.15.10 are empirical examples of sampling distributions, which describe the expected distribution of a series of samples taken from a population. In practice, of course,

Table 6.15.3 Samples of size 10 from the same population of births, mean birthweight (kg)

N	Sample 1	Sample 2	Sample 3	Sample 4	Sample 5
1	3.09	4.28	4.09	2.34	4.29
2	3.74	2.82	2.96	3.06	2.87
3	2.56	3.80	3.09	3.35	3.43
4	3.63	1.89	3.14	3.30	3.40
5	2.96	4.04	3.14	4.36	3.58
6	2.76	2.39	4.38	3.99	3.96
7	3.98	3.41	3.87	4.62	3.18
8	3.76	3.95	4.34	3.18	3.07
9	2.66	5.83	3.81	2.80	2.70
10	3.16	3.30	4.16	3.14	3.21
N	10	10	10	10	10
Mean	3.23	3.57	3.70	3.41	3.37
SD	0.51	1.10	0.56	0.71	0.48
Minimum	2.56	1.89	2.96	2.34	2.70
Maximum	3.98	5.83	4.38	4.62	4.28

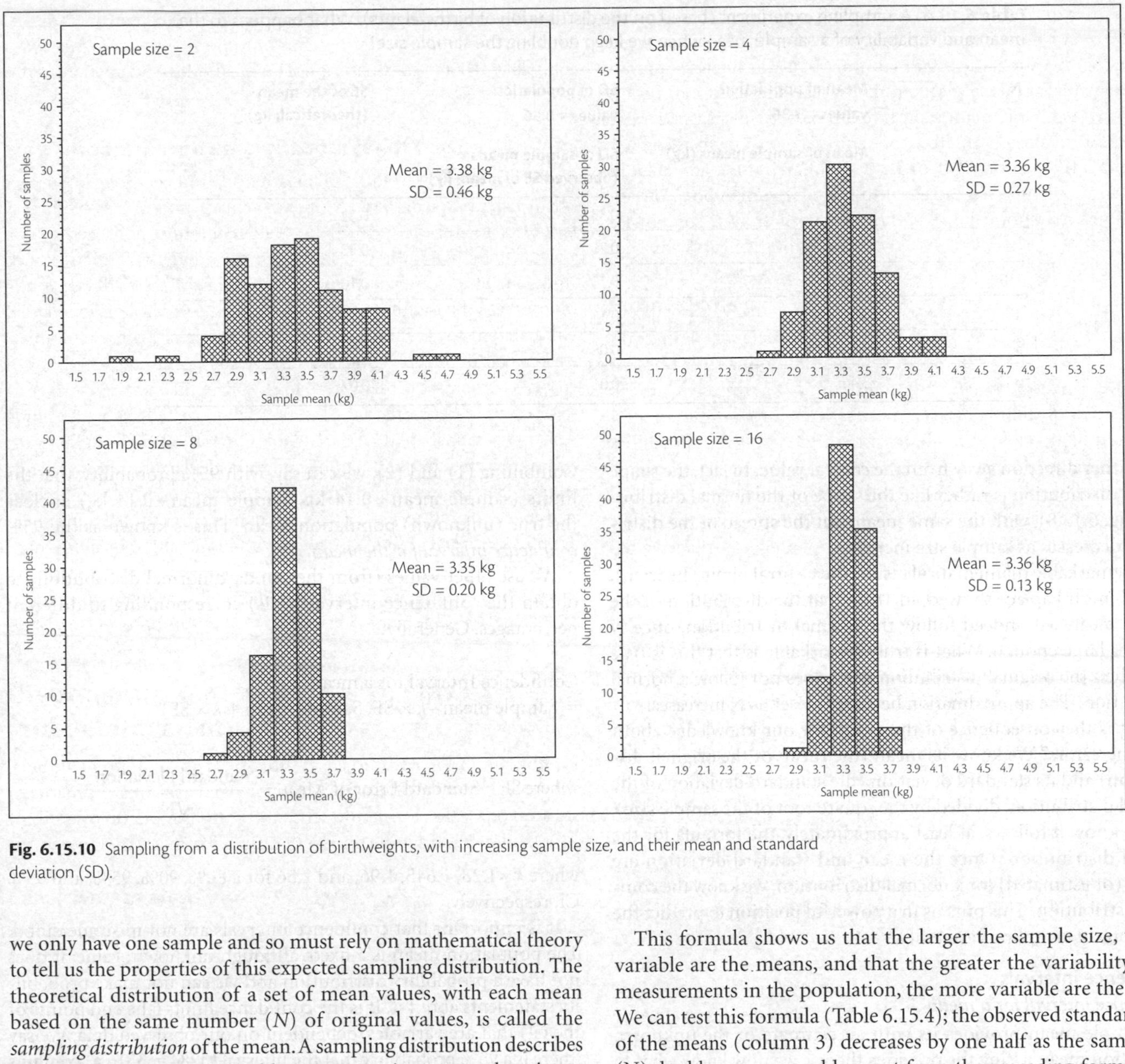

Fig. 6.15.10 Sampling from a distribution of birthweights, with increasing sample size, and their mean and standard deviation (SD).

we only have one sample and so must rely on mathematical theory to tell us the properties of this expected sampling distribution. The theoretical distribution of a set of mean values, with each mean based on the same number (N) of original values, is called the *sampling distribution* of the mean. A sampling distribution describes the chance variability we would expect to see in our sample estimate of the mean.

Both properties (1 and 2 in the preceding subsections) of the distribution of sample means have been mathematically demonstrated and further quantified. An important mathematical discovery about the expected standard deviation of the sample means revealed that the standard deviation of the means is related to the sample size (this follows also from property 1) and the standard deviation of the variable within the population. The standard deviation of a mean is more usually referred to as the *standard error of the mean* (SE), although these terms are sometimes used interchangeably.

The variability in the sample mean is defined by

$$\text{SD of the means} = \text{Standard Error of the Mean} = \frac{\text{SD of the population}}{\sqrt{N}}$$

where N is the size of the sample

This formula shows us that the larger the sample size, the less variable are the means, and that the greater the variability in the measurements in the population, the more variable are the means. We can test this formula (Table 6.15.4); the observed standard error of the means (column 3) decreases by one half as the sample size (N) doubles, as we would expect from the preceding formula and the theoretical value (column 4). This is because of the square root in the denominator of the formula.

The standard error of the mean is describing the expected variability in the behaviour of a *mean of a set of values*; on the other hand, the standard deviation of the original population describes the expected variability in the behaviour of the *original individual values*.

We now have some conclusions that help us to quantify the variability of our sample mean; summing up so far:

- We expect the sample mean to vary symmetrically around the population mean.
- We have a formula for its expected variability as expressed by a standard deviation and sample size.

Can we go any further in making predictions about the behaviour of a sample mean? Let us go back to Fig. 6.15.10. In each case, the means appear to follow a symmetric distribution, which tails

Table 6.15.4 A sampling experiment (based on the distribution of birthweights): What happens to the mean and variability of a sample mean when we keep doubling the sample size?

N	Mean of population values = 3.36 Mean of sample means (kg)	SD of population values = 0.56 SD of sample means (observed SE of mean; kg)	SE of the mean (theoretical; kg)
2	3.50	0.33	0.32
4	3.51	0.26	0.23
8	3.46	0.15	0.16
16	3.45	0.11	0.12
32	3.44	0.08	0.08
64	3.46	0.06	0.07

off in either direction away from the central value. In fact, the shape of each distribution is rather like the shape of the normal distribution (Fig. 6.15.8), with the same mean, but the spread of the distribution decreases as sample size increases.

In a remarkable mathematical result (the Central Limit Theorem), Pierre-Simon Laplace showed, in 1810, that the distribution of the sample mean will indeed follow the normal distribution, once N becomes large enough. What is truly remarkable is that this is true even when the original distribution itself does not follow a normal distribution! The approximation becomes closer as N increases.

What is the consequence of this result for our knowledge about sampling errors? We know its mean (the mean of the original distribution) and its standard deviation (the standard deviation of the original distribution, divided by the square root of the sample size), and we know it follows, at least approximately, the formula for the normal distribution. Once the mean and standard deviation are known (or estimated) for a normal distribution, we know the complete distribution. This puts us in a powerful position to predict the behaviour of sampling variability.

Confidence intervals

Confidence interval for a mean

The sample mean provides us with an estimate of the unknown population mean. Using the previous theory, we now know what to expect of its sampling variability.

Using our example of birthweights, and $N=64$, we have an expected SE of 0.07 kg. Using the assumption of a normal distribution for sample means (the Central Limit Theorem), there is a 95% chance that the error of our estimate is less than 0.14 kg (1.96×0.07). Another way of putting this is to say that there is a 95% chance that:

Sample mean − population mean < 0.14 kg, if the sample mean is greater than the population mean; and

Population mean − sample mean < 0.14 kg, if the population mean is greater than the sample mean.

Reorganizing these, with 95% probability, equivalent statements are:

1. Sample mean − 0.14 kg < population mean, if the sample mean is greater than population mean; and
2. Sample mean + 0.14 kg > population mean, if the population mean is greater than the sample mean.

Combining (1) and (2), we can say, with 95% probability, that the limits (sample mean − 0.14 kg, sample mean + 0.14 kg) enclose the true (unknown) population mean. This is known as the *95% confidence interval for the mean.*

We use other values (from the standard normal distribution) to obtain the confidence intervals (CIs) corresponding to different percentages. Generally:

Confidence Interval for a mean
$= (\text{Sample mean} - k \times \text{SE}, \text{Sample mean} + k \times \text{SE})$

$$\text{where SE} = \text{Standard Error of Mean} = \frac{\text{Standard Deviation}}{\sqrt{N}}$$

where $k=1.28$, 1.645, 1.96, and 2.56 for a 80%, 90%, 95%, and 99% CI, respectively.

It is important that confidence intervals are not misunderstood. The population mean is a fixed, although unknown, value; it does not have a probability distribution and we can not make probability statements about it. It is the confidence limits (the end points of the CI) that are variables, dependent on our observed data. We say 'there is a 95% probability that the interval (3284 g, 3516 g) contains the true mean birthweight', NOT that 'there is a 95% probability that the population mean lies within (3284 g, 3516 g)'.

In the preceding example, we used the true (usually unknown) standard deviation within the population to calculate the standard error and the confidence interval. In practice, we do not know this and therefore usually replace it with the sample standard deviation. This introduces very little error if the sample size is 50 or more. If the sample is small, we use a different multiplier for the standard error (i.e. a different k); this multiplier depends on the sample size itself, as well as the set percentage for the confidence interval, and is obtained from the t-distribution (i.e. not the standard normal distribution). This distribution is also available in textbooks. We need to specify another parameter called *degrees of freedom* (df), which depends on the sample size: For sample size N, $df=N-1$. Therefore, for $N=30$, $df=29$; for a 95% CI, we use $k=2.045$, instead of $k=1.96$.

Note that a confidence interval combines information regarding the size (location) of the parameter, the variability of values within a population, and the sample size used to estimate the parameter. It is thus a very useful quantity to summarize sample results.

Confidence interval for a proportion

If we are estimating a proportion or percentage (such as a prevalence of obesity) rather than a mean of a quantitative measure (such as birthweight), we can also obtain a confidence interval for the true proportion. The concept of a confidence interval for a mean extends to a proportion, or indeed other epidemiological measures. Let us return to the birth attendant data from the Philippines (Table 6.15.1).

We estimate that 224 of the 511 babies (43.8%) were delivered by trained traditional birth attendants. The principles underlying consideration of sampling errors for proportions are the same as for the mean. If we conducted a similar sampling experiment—taking repeated samples from a known population—we would find that the sample proportions would 'jump about', but not systematically in any direction. We would also find that this variability would be less, the larger the sample size. Indeed, the 'square root' factor still holds: The standard error of the proportions decreases according to the inverse of the square root of the sample size. The Central Limit Theorem again assures us that, provided samples are large enough, sample proportions will have, approximately, a normal distribution.

The only different feature of the process of obtaining a confidence interval for a proportion is the formula used to get the standard error of the estimate. For a proportion, we estimate its standard error by

$$\text{Standard error of a proportion (SEP)} = \sqrt{\frac{p \times (1-p)}{N}}$$

where p is the sample proportion, and N is the sample size

We use the abbreviation SEP to distinguish this from the standard error of the mean. In our example, we have $N=511$, $p=0.438$:

$$\text{Standard error of a proportion(SEP)} = \sqrt{\frac{0.438 \times (1-0.438)}{511}} = 0.022$$

The standard error of the proportion is thus 0.022, or 2.2%.

The formula for a confidence interval for a proportion is then completely analogous to that for a mean. Putting in the figures for the birth attendant data, we have for a 95% CI for the proportion of babies delivered by traditional birth attendant (TBA):

$$\begin{aligned}&\text{95\% confidence Interval for the proportion of TBA deliveries}\\&= (0.438 - 1.96 \times 0.022,\ 0.438 + 1.96 \times 0.022)\\&= (0.395,\ 0.481)\end{aligned}$$

Expressing the result in percentages, we say we have an estimate of 43.8% of deliveries by TBAs, with a 95% CI of (39.5%,48.1%). This confidence interval has the same general interpretation as earlier: It is an interval that has a 95% probability of containing the true population percentage of babies delivered by traditional birth attendants.

Basic principles and methods of comparative analysis

This subsection deals with some of the basic methods of analysis. Firstly, we consider situations in which we want to compare a set of mutually exclusive groups. This comparison may be on a number of different variable types, such as categorical or continuous health outcome, or the prevalence or mean of a risk factor. Secondly, we introduce models, aimed at examining associations of variables, or patterns of risk factors.

Group comparisons

Many research questions in public health involve comparing groups. This may be in the context of an experimental or intervention study, a designed analytical study such as a cohort study (which examines health outcomes in those with differing distributions of risk factors), a case–control study (which examines differences in distributions of risk factors in cases and controls), or a cross-sectional study. Such analyses proceed in two phases: First we describe the pattern of the data *within* each group, using methods such as those described above, and then we evaluate the comparisons *between* groups.

The comparison between groups may initially be descriptive, but then we usually want an evaluation of the 'significance' of the differences we see; that is, are the differences compatible with sampling variability alone, or are there 'real' differences between the groups, which might be due to biological or other effects[2]. We often want to go further and determine whether differences are due to 'causal' factors. The judgement of causality involves additional evidence other than statistical analysis, such as biological plausibility, magnitudes of effects, and considerations of confounding. Although statistical analysis, particularly multivariate analysis (see later), can help provide some information, the final judgement of causality is a complex one.

Some examples of research questions, how they might be framed, and the nature of the variables involved are shown in Table 6.15.5.

If a relationship is being examined, it is usually important to consider, when interpreting it, whether variables have a role (or potential role) as 'outcome', 'explanatory', or 'predictor' variables. In Table 6.15.5, birthweight, length of labour, and stage of disease are outcome variables; mother's height, number of previous births, and distance from the health centre are potentially explanatory variables ('potentially' because if it turns out there is no relationship, then one variable can hardly 'explain' the other). Notice also that a variable may take on different roles in different questions; for example, number of years of schooling is an outcome variable in question 6 and an explanatory variable in question 7. So, for the purpose of classifying variables as outcome or explanatory, what matters is the orientation of the question (which event comes first?).

The questions in Table 6.15.5 are about relationships between two variables, each of which is essentially different from the other. Sometimes, however, our question relates to whether a single variable changes over time. Suppose we are investigating the effectiveness of a dietary supplementation programme to improve the nutritional status of children. In this case, we might measure the nutritional status of each child within the sample of children before and after the supplementation programme. At first sight, this looks similar to the previous case: There are two variables, nutritional status before intervention and nutritional status after intervention. But this differs from the previous case because we are really observing one variable at two different times. We expect measurements taken on the same individual at two different times to be related. This relationship needs to be taken into account when the effect of a second variable (dietary supplementation) is being evaluated.

Table 6.15.5 Some research questions that involve relationships between two variables

Question	Variable combination
1. Does a **mother's height** influence the **birthweight** of her child?	Continuous–Continuous
2. Is there an association between **length of labour** and the **number of previous births** a woman has had?	Continuous–Discrete
3. Do people present at a later **stage of disease** if they live a greater **distance from the health centre**?	Ordinal–Continuous
4. Do different **ethnic groups** have different **calcium intake**?	Nominal–Continuous
5. Does the **number of sunburns** a person has experienced predict the **number of skin cancers** they have?	Discrete–Discrete
6. Does the **number of years of schooling** a child acquires depend on his or her **birth order** in the family?	Discrete–Ordinal
7. Does the **number of years of schooling** a girl acquires influence her **paid employment status** in later life?	Discrete–Nominal
8. Do different **socio-economic groups** present with different degrees of **disease severity**?	Ordinal–Ordinal
9. Does **diagnosis at presentation** depend on **socio-economic group**?	Nominal–Ordinal
10. Does susceptibility to **skin cancer** depend on **skin colour**?	Nominal–Nominal

The way in which these relationships are analysed depends on the types of variable combinations involved. There may be several valid methods of presentation from which to choose. Different methods of presentation and analysis are required in such cases.

Comparing proportions or percentages

When we are interested in examining the relationship between two categorical variables, the first step is usually to cross-classify them; that is, break down one variable by the values of another. This is usually displayed in a contingency table, which shows all combinations of values of the two variables. Consider an example taken from a study of skin cancer in Queensland, Australia (ref). This provided the data shown in Table 6.15.6.

Note that a contingency table should include *all* combinations of *all* categories of each variable; that is, we do not just present the numbers who have a skin cancer, for example. We are interested in examining the variability among skin types in skin cancer risk. We see that the overall incidence of skin cancer in the follow-up period is 22.7% (combining single and multiple lesions), but that incidence is higher in those who report having a skin type that sunburns, with or without tanning (21.2% and 30.6%, respectively), than in those whose skin tans without sunburning (17.3%). Differences can also be presented in a graphical form (Fig. 6.15.11).

If we repeat the skin cancer study with another sample of 1600 or so participants, we will obtain slightly different results, even if we follow exactly the same procedures. This is due to sampling variability: Within our study population, individual people with the same characteristics will have different skin cancer outcomes. How do we take this into account in our interpretation of findings?

To simplify the example, consider the comparison of the three skin type groups, combining single and multiple lesions. The first step in assessing the amount of sampling variability is to calculate what we would expect to see if people with different skin reactions instead of produced on average, the *same distribution of responses*. In other words, what would we expect to see if sampling variability was the *only* factor operating to produce variability in responses? The answer is: The same distribution of skin cancer within each skin reaction type. The results of calculating these 'expected' results are shown in Table 6.15.7.

The figures in parentheses in the table are called *expected frequencies*; that is, the numbers we would expect to see under an assumption that skin type is unrelated to skin cancer. Note that the marginal totals of observed and expected frequencies are the same. We have observed more skin cancer in the 'Always burn' group (about 27 more cases) than expected on the basis of no difference

Table 6.15.6 Numbers of people with a NMSC diagnosed on a sun-exposed site in the period 1993–2006, by skin reaction to the sun, as reported in 1992

	No NMSC	One NMSC lesion only	Multiple NMSC lesions	Total
Always burn	236 (69.4)	50 (14.7)	54 (15.9)	340
Burn, then tan	866 (78.8)	112 (10.2)	121 (11.1)	1099
Tan only	148 (82.7)	16 (8.9)	15 (8.4)	179
Total	1250 (77.3)	178 (11.0)	190 (11.7)	1618

Figures in parentheses are percentages within each skin reaction type.

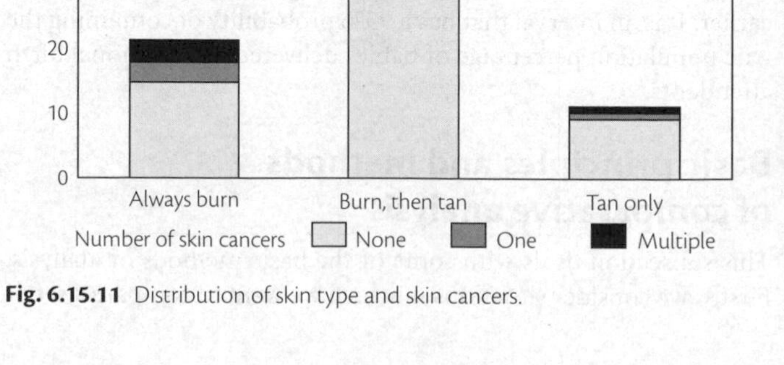

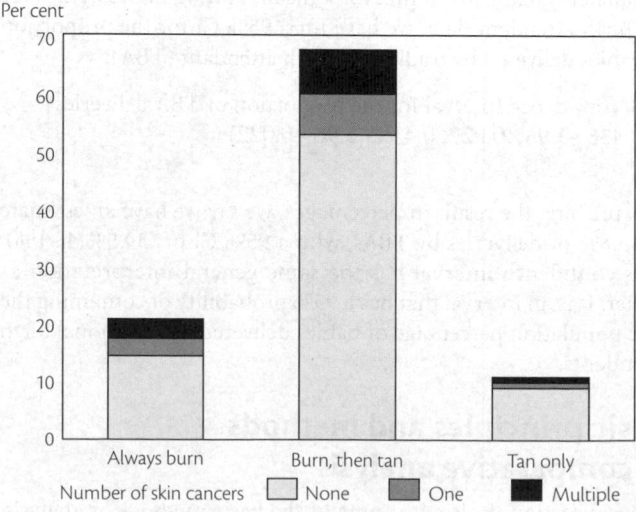

Fig. 6.15.11 Distribution of skin type and skin cancers.

Table 6.15.7 Numbers of people with a non-melanoma skin cancer NMSC diagnosed on a sun-exposed site in the period 1993–2004, by skin reaction to the sun, as reported in 1992, and numbers expected (in parentheses) if the distributions of skin reactions are the same in each group

	No NMSC lesions	One or more NMSC lesions	Total
Always burn	236 (262.7)	104 (77.3)	340
Burn, then tan	866 (849.0)	233 (250.0)	1099
Tan only	148 (138.3)	31 (40.7)	179
Total	1250	368	1618

between skin types and less in the 'Tan only' group (10 fewer cases). These differences relate either to:

(a) Sampling variability alone (i.e. no additional risk of skin cancer associated with skin type)

(b) Sampling variability *plus* an additional risk of skin cancer associated with skin type

The statement that, in the study population, skin type is unrelated to skin cancer is called the *null hypothesis*, and is the first step in any formal evaluation of the role of chance.

The Pearson chi-squared test

The statistic called the *chi-squared test statistic*, developed by Karl Pearson, enables us to summarize the differences between observed and expected frequencies, so we can make a decision as to the significance of these. Calculations are shown in Table 6.15.8.

This sum is sometimes represented by X^2. The formula for the chi-squared statistic is:

$$X^2 = \sum_{i=1}^{i=k} \frac{(O_i - E_i)^2}{E_i}$$

where k is the number of cells in the table.

The following is observed:

- The smallest value of X^2 that can occur is 0, when all individual terms have their smallest value as 0 and corresponding expected and observed frequencies are exactly equal.
- The Value of X^2 increases as differences between observed and expected frequencies increase.
- The larger the sample, the larger the value of X^2, for a given strength of association: If we double the sample size, for example, we double the calculated value of X^2.

Thus, we have a measure (X^2) that increases as the observed frequencies increasingly depart from the expected frequencies. Thus small values of X^2 are consistent with (a) above, but increases in X^2 suggest that (b) is the underlying explanation.

As shown in Table 6.15.8 the calculated value of X^2 is 16.42. But how large does X^2 need to be before we can decide in favour of (b) over (a)? Is there a cut-off point? The mathematics of this question have been solved, to the extent that for any given value of X^2 we can find the probability that this value, or one larger than it, will occur if the observed differences are due to chance alone; that is, if (a) is true. The relationship between values of X^2 and the probability of such values occurring is expressed in the *chi-squared distribution*. Tables for the chi-squared distribution are available in standard textbooks, or values can be obtained from statistical software. The probabilities depend on another parameter, the degrees of freedom (df), which depends on the number of row and column categories in the contingency table. If the table has r rows and c columns, $df = (r-1) \times (c-1)$. For Table 6.15.8, there are three rows and 2 columns: $df = (3-1) \times (2-1) = 2$.

From tabulated values or software, we find that the probability of getting $X^2 = 16.42$, or larger, is 0.0003. This probability is referred to as the *P*-value. So if (a) is the sole explanation for the observed treatment difference, the probability of seeing such a large value of X^2 is 0.0003, or 0.03% or 1 chance in 3333. This is very small, and we would feel inclined to reject (a) in favour of (b). In practice, the most common cut-off point to use in order to make this decision is $P = 0.05$ or 5%, so our inclination is supported by practice.

We then say that there is a *statistically significant difference* between skin types in risk of skin cancer ($P = 0.0003$). Alternatively, we can formally reject the null hypothesis and conclude that there is, in this case, a true difference between skin types in the risk of non-melanoma skin cancer. In order to describe the association further, we identify which cells make the most contribution to the chi-squared value. From Table 6.15.8, we see that the 'Always burn' category contributes by far the most, so we could conclude that this category is responsible for most of the statistically significant finding.

Limitations of the Pearson chi-squared test

The interpretation of the X^2 statistic with *P*-values derived from the chi-squared distribution involves an important underlying assumption—that the observed frequencies are independent. If, for example, instead of skin type we were evaluating a preventive intervention by comparing pre- and post- intervention incidence of skin cancer, the observations would not be considered to be independent, because outcomes for the same person would be expected to be related. The Pearson chi-squared test described in this subsection should not be used in such cases.

The chi-squared test is an approximate test, which depends on samples being 'large enough' to be valid. For contingency tables, 'large enough' has been found to depend on the size of the expected frequencies. The rule of thumb has emerged that if around 1 in 5 (or 20%), or more, of expected frequencies are less than 5, then the test is not a valid approximation; this rule applies to expected frequencies, not observed frequencies. This can occur in tables of any size. Thus, if one expected frequency in a 2×2 table is less than 5, the chi-square test should not be used. What should be used in these instances? Exact or permutation tests are available in many statistical packages; these are computationally intensive. However, they result in what is called an 'exact' *P*-value, which is then interpreted in the usual way.

We had decided to reject the null hypothesis based on a probability cut-off point in order to distinguish between (a) and (b). This decision might have been incorrect. It is not impossible that a value of $X^2 = 16.42$, or larger, could occur if (a) were true; it is just very unlikely (about 1 chance in 3333), and this is the basis of our decision. This type of error (rejecting the null hypothesis, concluding there is a significant difference when there is not) is a *Type 1 error*.

Table 6.15.8 Calculation of the chi-square statistic for data in Table 6.15.7

	No lesions	One or more lesions
Always burn	$\frac{(236-262.7)^2}{262.7}=2.71$	$\frac{(104-77.3)^2}{77.3}=9.22$
Burn, then tan	$\frac{(866-849.0)^2}{849.0}=0.34$	$\frac{(233-250.0)^2}{250.0}=1.16$
Tan only	$\frac{(148-138.3)^2}{138.3}=0.68$	$\frac{(31-40.7)^2}{40.7}=2.31$

$$\text{Sum of all } \frac{(\text{Observed Frequency} - \text{Expected Frequency})^2}{\text{Expected Frequency}}$$
$$= 2.71 + 9.22 + 0.34 + 1.16 + 0.68 + 2.31$$
$$= 16.42$$

Thus, statistical tests tend to be conservative; decisions are made by setting an upper limit (sometimes called the α level) on the probability that an association or difference is detected by the statistical test, when there is actually no difference or association.

The reverse error, failing to reject the null hypothesis when it is false or concluding there is no difference when there really is, is called a *Type 2 error*. This error typically arises when we have a small sample size, and our data are insufficient to detect a difference.

Table 6.15.9 summarizes the four possible outcomes from a statistical test of a hypothesis, according to whether there is a real effect (e.g. a real difference) and whether the test statistic is significant (i.e. the *P*-value is small). A Type 1 error is a false-positive finding and a Type 2 error is a false-negative finding.

Asserting that a difference, or an association, is 'significant' does not mean that the association is 'strong' or that it is causal. A statistically significant finding means that the size of the difference or association is larger than would be likely to occur by chance alone (i.e. sampling variability alone). It is essentially a statement about the data, although in formal hypothesis testing a conclusion is made about the population(s) from which the data came.

These techniques can be applied to larger contingency tables. It would still yield a single statistic, however, and further examination of the data may be needed to identify the nature of the differences.

The chi-squared test explores all variability in proportions in a contingency table. However, sometimes we want to examine a more specific type of association. In such a case, the chi-squared test may not be the best one to use. An example of such a situation occurs when we want to examine trends in proportions.

Table 6.15.9 Type 1 and Type 2 errors

		True effect (null hypothesis false)	
		Yes	**No**
Statistically significant effect (reject null hypothesis)	Yes	✓	Type 1 error (false-positive)
	No	Type 2 error (false-negative)	✓

Suppose we regarded the skin type groups (in order) in Table 6.15.7 as indicative of an increasing inflammatory reaction to sun exposure and wanted to test a hypothesis about increasing risk of skin cancer with increasing inflammatory response (rather than just variability in risk with skin type, whatever the pattern). That is, we want to regard our variable as being an ordinal variable rather than a nominal variable and we need a statistical test that specifically looks for a trend pattern. Various options are available, which usually involve assigning an increasing score to the categories of the ordinal variable. Tests for these will be discussed in the subsection for regression modelling of binary variables.

Comparing means

Suppose we want to examine whether a child's birthweight depends upon his or her mother's marital status. We know that the distribution of birthweight, a continuous variable, can be summarized by its mean and standard deviation. So we examine these same summary measures within values of the categorical variable (marital status, a nominal variable) to see how the continuous variable varies with the categorical variable. Table 6.15.10 shows the results.

Table 6.15.10 Mean, standard deviation (SD), and range of birthweight, by marital status of mother, for a group of Brisbane babies born in 1984–88

Marital status	N	Mean (kg)	SD (kg)	Minimum (kg)	Maximum (kg)
Married	363	3.57	0.42	2.33	4.85
Never married	70	3.64	0.44	2.34	5.06
Living together	53	3.38	0.42	2.27	4.18
Other	14	3.40	0.40	2.86	4.28
Total	500	3.56	0.43	2.27	5.06

Notice the principle used here: We describe the relationship between a quantitative variable and a categorical variable by first deciding how we would summarize the quantitative variable without regard to the categorical variable (e.g. using means, medians, quantiles) and then calculating these measures for each value of the categorical variable. If the frequency distribution of a continuous variable is approximately normal (as it is for birthweight), then it is described fully by its mean and standard deviation, so we would use these measures. In other cases, such as skewed distributions, we might use the median or the geometric mean as a measure of location and the inter-quartile range as a measure of variability, and present these instead of, or along with, the mean and standard deviation.

These results show that, compared to 'Married' women, women who have 'Never married' have slightly heavier babies (by 0.07 kg), whereas women 'Living together' and 'Other' have slightly lighter babies (by 0.19 kg and 0.17 kg, respectively). These differences seem comparatively small, but would be regarded as important differences (by comparison with other risk factors that decrease birthweight; e.g. smoking). Notice also that the mean for married women is very close to the overall mean, simply because they make up most (363/500=72.6%) of the sample. We can also display these results use box plots (Fig. 6.15.12).

In this example, we observe differences between means, but we need to make an assessment of the role of chance in producing these differences. We know that some variability in observed means is due to sampling error. As for the example of skin cancer and skin type, the crucial question is whether the means differ more than would be expected by chance alone.

The sampling variability of a mean is assessed by its standard error of the mean (SE) and it has earlier been used to derive a confidence interval for the true mean. We can apply these techniques to the data in Table 6.15.10, examining mother's marital status and birthweight; results are in Table 6.15.11.

In this table, we note the variability in the standard errors due to the variability in the sample size: The largest group ('Married' women) has the smallest standard error and the smallest group ('Other') has the largest standard error. Correspondingly, the confidence intervals vary greatly in their widths. This can be clearly seen graphically, as in Fig. 6.15.13.

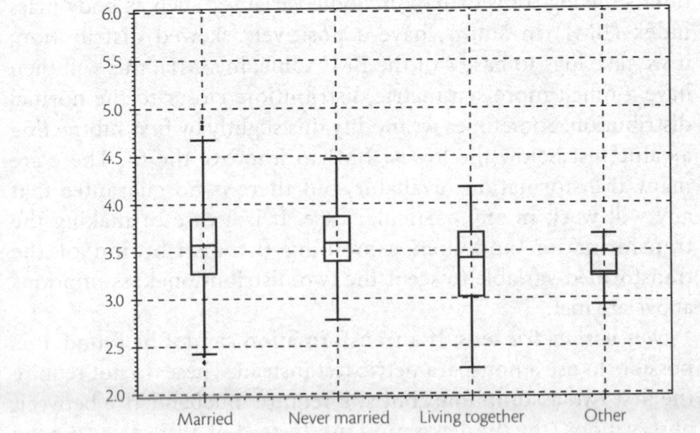

Fig. 6.15.12 Distribution of birthweights, by marital status.

Table 6.15.11 Mean birthweight (kg), standard errors (SE), and 95% confidence intervals (CI), by marital status of mother, for a sample of Brisbane babies born in 1984–88

Marital status	N	Mean (kg)	SE (kg)	95% CI
Married	363	3.57	0.022	(3.53, 3.62)
Never married	70	3.64	0.052	(3.53, 3.74)
Living together	53	3.38	0.058	(3.27, 3.50)
Other	14	3.40	0.108	(3.16, 3.63)
Total	500	3.56	0.019	(3.52, 3.59)

The cross-bars in the figure represent the means and the lines extending out represent 95% CIs. We see that for 'Married' and 'Never married' mothers the confidence intervals overlap considerably, but the 'Married' group has a very narrow confidence interval, which does not overlap the 'Living together' category. We might feel that the difference among 'Married' and the 'Never married' might be explained by sampling variability, but that the difference between 'Married' and 'Living together' categories might not. Sometimes overlap or non-overlap of confidence intervals is used in this way, but if we wish to make a formal statement about the difference between means, as we did for the skin-type groups in Table 6.15.7, then we must make a formal statistical test.

The two-sample t-test

The first step of a formal statistical test is to formulate a null hypothesis. In this case, the null hypothesis is that there is no difference between the (true) mean birthweights for the marital status groups. We observe some quite large differences in birthweights between some pairs of groups, not others. Let us first consider the difference between birthweights of children of 'Married' and 'Never married' mothers—a difference of 0.07 kg, with 'Never married' mothers having the heavier babies.

The next step involves assessing the role of chance in producing the observed difference of 0.07 kg if there is no real difference in the population means; that is, if the null hypothesis is true. As before, we need to obtain the probability of getting a difference this

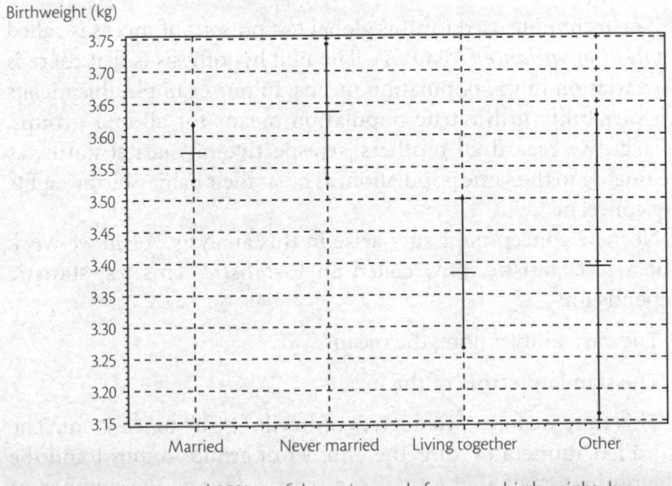

Fig. 6.15.13 Means and 95% confidence intervals for mean birthweight, by marital status.

large, if the null hypothesis is true. We evaluate this probability by calculating a t-statistic. Perhaps not surprisingly, the test statistic depends on:

- The size of the difference between the means
- The standard errors of the means

Therefore:

$$t = \frac{\text{Difference between the means}}{\sqrt{\text{Sum of}(\text{SE})^2}}$$

with degrees of freedom (df) = Sum of sample sizes − 2

This is called the *two-sample* t-*test*. The larger the difference between the two sample means, the larger the value of t; the smaller the standard errors (or the larger the sample sizes), the larger the value of t. As for the chi-squared test, once we have a calculated value and a value for the degrees of freedom, we can obtain a P-value by looking up tables or using a statistical package or programme.

For the comparison of birthweights of children whose mothers are 'Married' or 'Never married', we have:

$$t = \frac{3.57 - 3.64}{\sqrt{0.022^2 + 0.052^2}} = -1.24$$

with degrees of freedom (df) = 363 + 70 − 2 = 431

From statistical tables, we see that the P-value is >0.10 (using df = infinity [∞]). So there is quite a high probability that such a difference could occur by chance. We then attribute the observed difference to sampling variability and conclude the difference is not significant.

Analysis of variance

For the example of mother's marital status and birthweight, we could carry out more pairwise comparisons, looking at the difference between other groups. However, it is considered bad practice to 'search' for significance in this way. A more acceptable practice is to carry out a 'global' test on the set of four means, to see if there is any significant variability among the means as a set, without specifying any particular pair of means. Pairwise differences may then be examined post hoc, once overall variability has been established.

The technique used for this global test on a set of means is called *analysis of variance* (ANOVA). The null hypothesis is that there is no variation in the population means. In our example, this means no variability in the true population means for all four groups. In fact, we regard all mothers, irrespective of marital status, as belonging to the same population, as far as their babies' birthweights are concerned.

No new conceptual issues arise in this analysis. Again we work out a test statistic, now called an F-*statistic*. This test statistic depends on:

- The variability among the means
- The standard errors of the means

This time we have two degrees of freedom (df) to work out: The so-called 'numerator' df is the number of groups minus 1 and the 'denominator' df is the total sample size minus the number of groups being compared.

We would usually use a statistical package for ANOVA, which will also give us a P-value. In this case, the F-statistic is 14.01, with df = (3,497), and P = 0.0029. This is smaller than our usual cut-off point of 0.05, and we conclude that there are significant differences in birthweight among the marital status groups. These differences obviously arise from the 'Living together' and 'Other' groups.

If we had decided not to reject the null hypothesis, the matter would have ended there. When we do reject the null hypothesis, we might want to examine the pairwise differences using t-tests. Although opinions vary on this, sometimes modified versions of the t-test are used to take into account the multiple comparisons that might be involved in such examination. Multiple comparisons increase the overall risk of a type I error (i.e. finding a statistically significant result just by chance).

Assumptions of the two-sample t-test and ANOVA

The two-sample t-test and ANOVA have important underlying assumptions. These are as follows:

- If the sample size is small, the variable used to calculate the mean has a normal distribution, or if the variable does not have a normal distribution, the sample size is large enough, for the means themselves to have a normal distribution (using the Central Limit Theorem).
- The standard deviations (not the standard errors!) are approximately equal within each group.
- The samples are independent observations; that is, separate groups of individuals.

We have already established that the distribution of birthweight is quite close to a normal distribution, so the first assumption has been met. What about the second? Inspection of the 'SD' column in Table 6.15.10 assures us that this assumption has also been met—the standard deviations vary only slightly.

A statistical test, called Bartlett's test, can be used to determine whether standard deviations are significantly different. Some statistical packages automatically carry out this test when an ANOVA is requested. It is then up to the user to decide how to proceed if the standard deviations are found to be significantly different.

What do we do if the assumptions are not met? There are two main options: Transformations and non-parametric tests.

Transformations: It is sometimes possible to transform the variable to make a normal distribution, and then carry out the t-test or ANOVA on the transformed variable. A common transformation is the log transformation. Some variables, such as body mass index (BMI) in adults, have a positively skewed distribution; if we take logs to base e of the BMI value, ln(BMI), this will then have a much more symmetric distribution, closer to the normal distribution. Sometimes we modify this slightly by first subtracting a value just below the lowest BMI to improve the fit. There are many transformations available, but there is no guarantee that any will work in any particular case. It is a case of making the transformation and then examining the distribution of the transformed variable to see if the two distributional assumptions above are met.

Non-parametric tests: If a transformation cannot be found, it is possible to use a non-parametric test instead. These do not require the first two assumptions, but still require independence between observations (the third assumption). Instead of a t-test, we use the Wilcoxon–Mann–Whitney test to get a P-value for comparing two means; instead of ANOVA, we use the Kruskal–Wallis analysis of variance to obtain a *P*-value for comparing two means.

So why not use non-parametric tests all the time, and not bother about the assumptions? The reason is that if the assumptions are met and non-parametric tests are used, these tests will have less ability to detect differences between means; that is, they will result in larger *P*-values than the *t*-test or ANOVA and be less likely to reject the null hypothesis. Usually researchers want to make the maximal use of their data, and carry out the most sensitive tests possible, so they prefer to use tests based on the normal distribution if possible.

Repeated measurements of a quantitative variable

In a trial to examine the effectiveness of a dietary intervention, a subsample of 17 participants gave blood samples for researchers to determine actual vitamin A intake (μg), at baseline and 6 months later. The question is whether the use of the dietary intervention has helped increase vitamin A intake over the 6-month period.

At first sight, we might see this as a situation for a two-sample *t*-test, comparing mean at baseline and at 6 months. This is not true because the third assumption for the two-sample *t*-test—independence of the groups being compared—has not been met. The data arise from repeating measures on the same individuals, so we cannot use the two-sample *t*-test.

The data consist of vitamin A intake measured at two times: A before–after study. We can display two sets of paired measurements in a scatter plot (Fig. 6.15.14).

The scale for the first of the two measurements (i.e. time 1 or baseline) is represented on the *x*-axis and the repeated measure on the *y*-axis. We see that high values at baseline go with high values at 6 months, but our question is focused on the change between these two points—the 'intervention effect'. The diagonal line in the figure provides some information about this: We see that almost all 6 months values are higher than baseline values, although some individual differences are quite small.

As we are really interested in the change in vitamin A intake, the most appropriate summary statistic to compare paired repeated measurements of a continuous variable is the *mean change*,

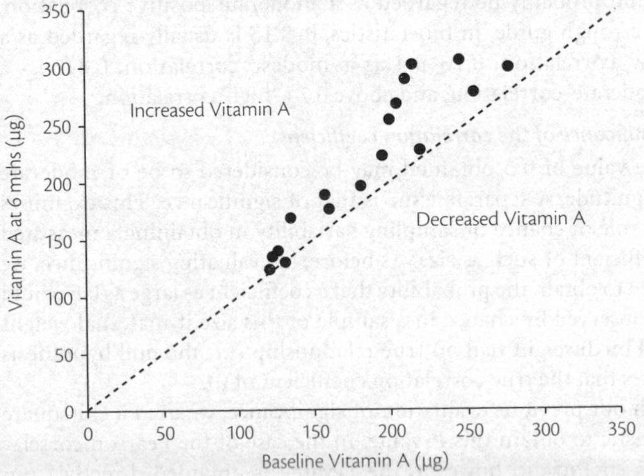

Fig. 6.15.14 Scatter plot of vitamin A levels at 6 months compared to baseline levels.

within individuals. For each of the 17 participants, we subtract baseline vitamin A levels from 6-month values. The mean and standard deviation of these individual changes are then calculated. Hence, in the situation of matched data, the exercise becomes one of summarizing one variable (i.e. change) and not two variables. In this example, the mean change in vitamin A levels was 32.1 μg, with a range of changes from −1 to +86 μg and an SD of 26.3 μg. Of course, where the distribution of the observed changes is not normal, a more valid summary would be the median.

We can go one step further and work out the standard error and a 95% CI for the mean change. The standard error of the mean change in vitamin A intake is

$$\text{SE(change)} = \frac{\text{SD(change)}}{\sqrt{N}} = \frac{26.3}{\sqrt{17}} = 6.4\,\mu\text{g}$$

with 95% Confidence Interval

$$=(\text{mean change} - 1.96 \times \text{SE(mean change)},\ \text{mean change} + 1.96 \times \text{SE(mean change)})$$
$$=(19.5, 44.6)$$

Notice that the lower limit of this 95% CI is well above zero, so we have considerable confidence that the change is positive, at least.

We can formally test the null hypothesis that the true increase is zero by calculating a *t*-statistic, as follows:

$$t = \frac{\text{Mean change}}{\text{SE(change)}}$$

This is referred to as the *paired or one-sample* t*-test*, because it assumes we have paired measures, and we want to evaluate the significance of the change (or more generally, the difference) within the paired values. The larger the mean change, the larger the value of *t*; the smaller the standard error (or the larger the sample size), the larger the value of *t*.

As for the previous *t*-test, once we have a calculated value of *t*, and its degrees of freedom (df), we can obtain a *P*-value by looking up *t*-tables or using a statistical package or programme. For the paired *t*-statistic to evaluate change within N pairs, the df is N − 1.

For the vitamin A example, we calculate that $t = 5.02$, with 16 df Tables or statistical software tells us that $P = 0.0001$. It is extremely unlikely that such a difference could occur by chance, or sampling variability, alone, with no effect attributable to the intervention. So we reject the null hypothesis and conclude that the intervention has increased dietary intake by an estimated 32.1 μg per day, with a 95% CI of (19.5 μg, 44.6 μg).

Again, this *t*-test is based on the assumption that the change in vitamin A level is normally distributed. If this assumption can not be made, a non-parametric counterpart test can be used—the Wilcoxon Signed-Rank test.

Correlation and regression

We now examine similar questions, when the variables being considered are continuous. This leads to some different measures of data presentation, and different techniques for assessing the significance and size of associations.

Scatter plots

Suppose we are interested in the relationship between birthweight and maternal weight prior to pregnancy. These are both continuous variables. The approach used for categorical variables (using a contingency table) will not do, because the values of each variable are not confined to a few categories. We could, of course, reorganize birthweight and maternal weight into several categories in each case, but this would be sacrificing a great deal of information, which seems to be a poor idea especially when we have a small sample. An efficient method of displaying such a relationship visually is to use a scatter plot in which each point represents a particular mother (weight)–child (birthweight) pair (Fig. 6.15.15).

When constructing scatter plots, it is customary to allocate the variable that is considered to 'depend on' the other (the 'outcome' variable) to the *y*-axis rather than to the *x*-axis, which then corresponds to the 'explanatory' variable. If there is no suggestion that one variable 'depends on' another, the choice of axes is arbitrary.

Figure 6.15.15 shows that heavier mothers tend to have heavier babies; that is, as maternal weight increases, birthweight tends to increase. Although such a pictorial representation of the relationship is useful, we sometimes wish to summarize the relationship more concisely, especially if we have many such relationships to discuss. This leads to the use of 'coefficients' that describe association.

Coefficients of association

Coefficients of association have been developed to provide summary indicators that measure the strength of association. These are variously applicable to categorical variables (e.g. the odds ratio) or ordinal, continuous, or discrete variables. For quantitative measures, these coefficients have a number of common properties. These include the following:

- A value of zero for the coefficient means no association.
- A negative value for the coefficient means that one variable increases as the other decreases.
- A positive value for the coefficient means that the variables increase or decrease together.
- The range of the coefficient is from −1 to +1. Attainment of −1 or +1 is said to be 'perfect association'.

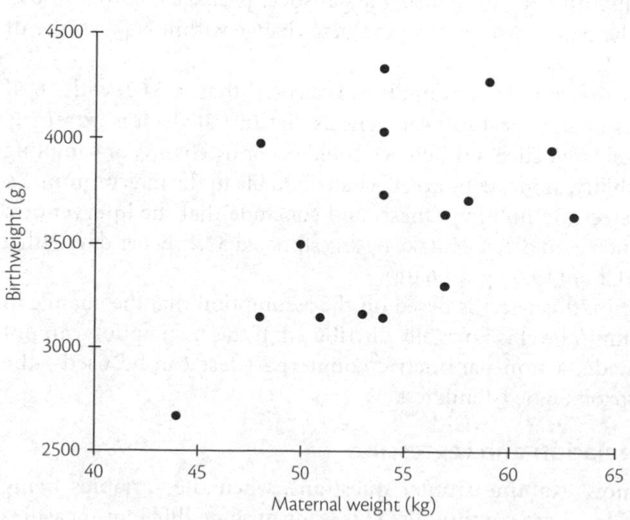

Fig. 6.15.15 Scatter plot of birthweight (g) and maternal pre-pregnancy weight (kg) for a group of 16 term Brisbane babies, born 1984–88.

For the relationship shown in Fig. 6.15.15, we would expect that any such measure of association would be a positive value, somewhat less than 1, according to the criteria mentioned here.

Pearson correlation coefficient

The most commonly used measure of association is the Pearson correlation coefficient (r). The correlation coefficient may be used to describe the linear relationship between any two continuous variables. It is estimated from a sample of N observations X_i, Y_i (where $i = 1, 2, \ldots, N$) using the formula:

$$\text{Pearson correlation coefficient } \mathrm{r} = \frac{\mathrm{Cov}(X,Y)}{\mathrm{SD}(X) \times \mathrm{SD}(Y)}$$

$$\text{where } \mathrm{Cov}(X,Y) = \frac{\sum_{i=1}^{\mathrm{N}} (X_i - \bar{X}) \times (Y_i - \bar{Y})}{\mathrm{N}}$$

$\bar{X}$ and $\mathrm{SD}(X)$ are the mean and SD of X_i

$\bar{Y}$ and $\mathrm{SD}(Y)$ are the mean and SD of Y_i

The denominator of this formula depends on the variability of X and Y separately; the numerator is the important part as it measures how X and Y vary together—if they both increase together, it will give positive results, if one increases as the other decreases, it will give negative results. The same result for r is obtained if we reverse the roles of X and Y—the correlation coefficient is symmetric.

In the example above, 'Y' is birthweight and 'X' is maternal weight, corresponding to our scatter plot in Fig. 6.15.15. The correlation coefficient is calculated by the preceding formula as +0.50. Is this a 'high' or 'strong' correlation? This will usually depend upon context; for example, researchers who expect measurements to obey tight physical laws (the relationship between temperature and pressure for a given gas, under controlled conditions) usually expect correlations to be around 0.95 before referring to them as high, whereas researchers examining correlations between social, environmental, or biological measurements which may be influenced by many variables (relationship between temperature and mortality) may feel that lower values are, all things considered, high. The value of 0.5 for the relationship between birthweight and maternal weight would probably be regarded as a 'moderate' positive correlation. As a rough guide, in biostatistics, 0–0.15 is usually regarded as a 'low' correlation, 0.16–0.4 as a 'modest' correlation, 0.41–0.7 a 'moderate' correlation, and above 0.7 a 'high' correlation.

Significance of the correlation coefficient

The value of 0.5 obtained may be considered to be of moderate magnitude. A separate issue is that of significance. This examines the role of chance or sampling variability in obtaining a measured coefficient of such as size. As before, in evaluating significance, we need to obtain the probability that a coefficient as large as 0.5 would be observed by chance in a sample of this size if maternal weight and birthweight had no true relationship (i.e. the null hypothesis states that the true correlation coefficient of 0).

In our previous evaluation of significance, we used a chi-square statistic to obtain this P-value. In the case of the Pearson correlation coefficient, however, the P-value is obtained directly from tables or a computer programme. As before, we need to supply a value for the degrees of freedom parameter. In this case, $\mathrm{df} = N - 2$, for a sample of size N, or 16 − 2 = 14. Examination of tables shows the *P*-value is just less than 0.05; the actual value is P = 0.048. As this is just less than the conventional cut-off point, the correlation coefficient could be described as 'significant' or, more completely, as 'significantly different from zero, at the 5% level'—although it would be better to state the actual *P*-value so it is clear that it is very close to 0.05.

Types of association and correlation

Figure 6.15.17 shows various types of association and how they would be described. It is important to note that the correlation coefficient measures only linear relationships; alternatively, we might say the correlation coefficient only measures that part of the relationship which is linear. A linear relationship is one in which a straight line approximates the relationship. This is so in Fig. 6.15.16, where we can imagine birthweight showing the 'average' behaviour illustrated by the dotted straight line. The line will slope upwards for positive relationships, downward for negative relationships (*r*, negative), and be horizontal if there is no linear relationship ($r = 0$). The estimation (and more about the meaning) of the line in Fig. 6.15.16 will be discussed in the next subsection.

Note that the lower right graph in Fig. 6.15.17 would give a correlation close to zero correlation for Pearson coefficient. The reason for this is that the data are non-linear, even though there does appear to be a relationship between the two variables. Thus, Pearson coefficient, in keeping with many other coefficients, only measures strength of a linear relationship. If we wanted to estimate strength of association for a non-linear relationship, we would have to specify a particular form, for example, a quadratic function.

Regression

To illustrate the regression approach to analysis, we can use the same data as that used for the discussion of correlation. Suppose we wish to 'model' the association between the two variables by fitting a straight line to the data of Figure; an obvious use for such a model is the prediction of birthweight from maternal weight.

We could simply draw 'by eye' a line that seems to fit the data (as done in Fig. 6.15.16). The disadvantage of this, apart from the element of subjectivity, is that we can not quantify the inevitable error that results from sampling variation in both our estimated line and model, and in any future value which might be predicted from it.

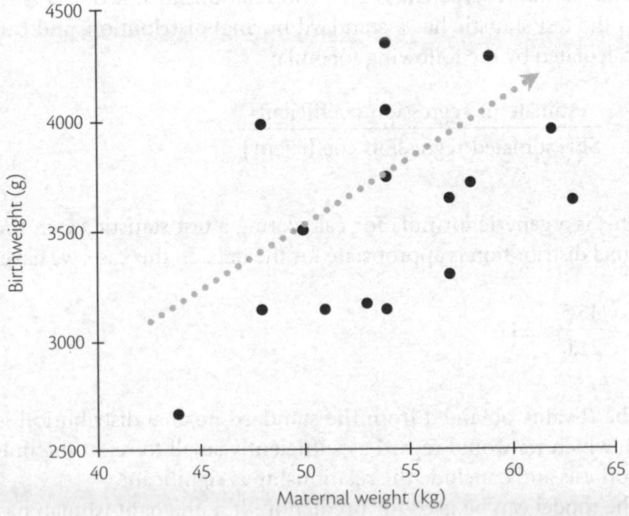

Fig. 6.15.16 Scatter plot of birthweight (g) and maternal pre-pregnant weight (kg) for a group of 16 term Brisbane babies, born 1984–1988, with line fitted 'by eye'.

Let us consider our arbitrary line fitted 'by eye' in Fig. 6.15.16. We note there will be discrepancies between the line and the dots representing the actual data. We call the vertical distance between each point and the fitted line the 'error' in the fitted line. The method used to fit the 'best' line minimizes these errors, in the sense of minimizing the sum of their squares. This is called the *method of least squares*.

In setting up a regression model for estimation, we first note that the variables now take on different roles from those adopted in a correlation analysis. One variable, usually denoted *Y*, is called the *dependent variable* (or *outcome*); this is the variable to be predicted or modelled. The other variable, usually denoted X, is sometimes called the *independent variable* (or better, the *predictor* or *explanatory variable*) and is the variable used to predict or explain *Y*.

A linear model involving one dependent and one independent variable is then expressed as:

$$Y = \alpha + \beta X + e$$

Again, *Y* has straight-line relationship with *X*. The symbols α and β represent the intercept (where the line cuts the vertical axis of the graph) and the slope of the line (the amount by which *Y* changes for a unit [e.g. 1 kg of maternal weight] change in X), respectively. β is also called the *regression coefficient*, and is a measure of how much *Y* depends on *X*; α is usually not of interest. The quantity e measures the 'error'. Given that it is very unlikely that such a simple model will describe data such as that in Fig. 6.15.15, we allow for the 'error' to have a distribution. In this case, for each value of *X*, the errors are assumed to have a normal distribution about the predicted value $\alpha + \beta X$.

The purpose of the analysis is to obtain estimates of α and β, which we will denote by *a* and *b*, using the method of least squares. When this is calculated for the birthweight data in Fig. 6.15.15, we obtain $a = 1{,}124$ and $b = 45.5$.

$$Y = 1{,}124 + 45.5\ X.$$

The fitted (least squares) regression line, in Fig. 6.15.18, shows that birthweight increases by 45.5 g for every 1 kg of mother's weight. So mothers who differ by say 10 kg in their pre-pregnancy weight would expect to have babies, on average, who differ by 455 g in birthweight.

Standard errors and confidence intervals also may be calculated for a regression coefficient. In this case, the standard error is 21 g. Using the usual formula (analogous to that for means and proportions), a 95% CI for the regression coefficient is:

Confidence Interval for a regression coefficient=
(Sample regression coefficient − 1.96 × SE, Sample regression coefficient + 1.96 × SE)

where SE = Standard Error of the regresssion coefficient

Therefore:

95% Confidence Interval
$= (45.5 - 1.96 \times 21, 45.5 + 1.96 \times 21)$
$= (4.5, 86.5)$

Although this confidence interval is quite wide, it excludes the value 0, which would correspond to no relationship between mother's weight and child's birthweight (a horizontal line on the graph).

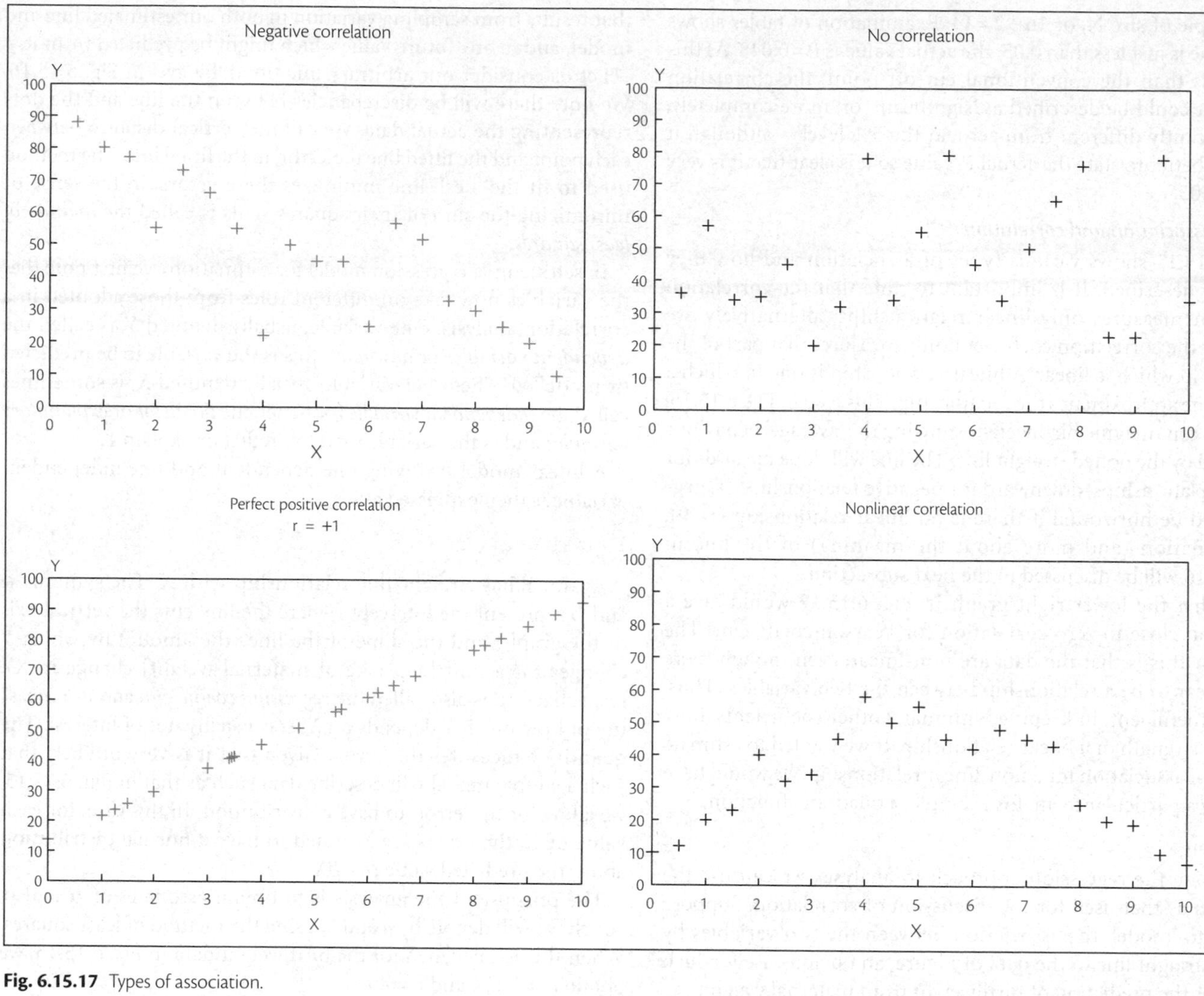

Fig. 6.15.17 Types of association.

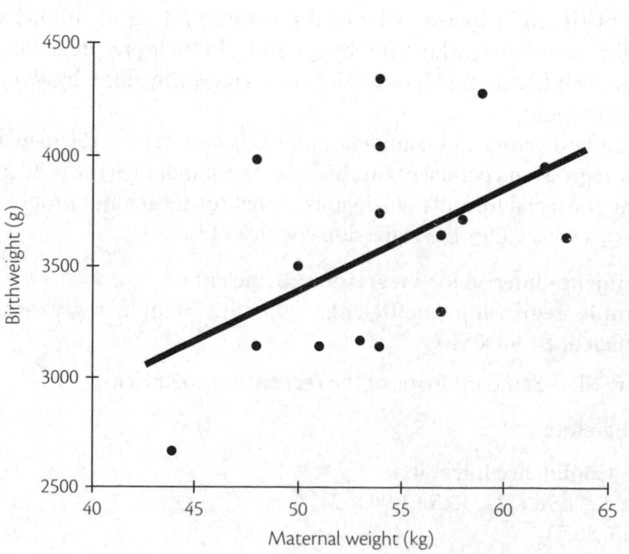

Fig. 6.15.18 Scatter plot and regression line of birthweight (g) and maternal pre-pregnancy weight (kg) fitted by least squares for a group of 16 term Brisbane babies, born 1984–88.

We can also formally test for the statistical significance of the regression coefficient. The appropriate null hypothesis is that the true regression coefficient is zero (no relationship). If this is true, then the test statistic has a standard normal distribution, and can be calculated by the following formula:

$$z = \frac{\text{estimate of regression coefficient}}{\text{SE}(\text{estimated regression coefficient})}$$

This is a generic formula for calculating a test statistic when the normal distribution is appropriate for the data. In this case, we have

$$z = \frac{45.5}{21.0} = 2.17$$

The *P*-value obtained from the standard normal distribution is 0.03, which we would regard as sufficiently small to reject the null hypothesis and conclude the relationship is significant.

The model can be used for prediction. If a pregnant woman has a pre-pregnancy weight of 50 kg, we can predict that her infant will have a birthweight of $Y = 1{,}124 + (45.5 \times 50) = 3{,}399$ g.

Assumptions of correlation and regression analyses

Correlation and regression coefficients are estimated on an assumption of a linear association. To make inferences (test hypotheses or calculate confidence intervals), however, you need to make additional assumptions. These are as follows:

- For correlation analyses, the two variables involved have joint normal distributions.
- For regression analyses, the outcome (dependent variable) has a normal distribution.
- For correlation and regression analyses, the samples are independent observations; that is, all pairs of observations are independent.

We have already established that the distribution of birthweight is quite close to a normal distribution, so the second assumption needed for regression analysis is met. What about the others? What do we do if the assumptions are not met? Again there are two main options: Transformations and non-parametric correlation coefficients.

Transformations: Transformations can be used, as described in the subsection on *t*-tests and ANOVA.

Non-parametric correlation coefficients: If a transformation cannot be found, it is possible to use a non-parametric test instead. These do not require either of the two distribution assumptions mentioned here. Instead of a Pearson correlation, we use the Kendall (τ or tau) or Spearman correlation coefficient (r_s) (ref).

The successful fitting of a straight line to the data does not establish causality. In other words, although we may be able to predict that babies whose mothers' weights differ by 1 kg will have birthweights which differ on average by 45.5 g, we cannot predict that increasing a mother's weight by 1 kg will cause an increase of 45.5 g in her child's birthweight Observing an association between an outcome and a potential risk factor is, however, the first step in examining causality; we then have to consider possible explanations, which include chance, bias, and confounding. The results of a significance test enable us to assess the role of chance, but bias and confounding are crucial to consider. Multivariate statistical modelling is one approach to examining confounding; and is dealt with later in this chapter.

Survival data

In a cohort study, if the event or disease is likely to occur in most participants, then interest centres on the actual time till the event, rather than the occurrence of the event itself. Examples include time to death following a diagnosis of breast cancer, time to remission of disease following treatment, or time to cessation of breastfeeding, in a cohort of infants. Such data are referred to as *survival data* or *failure time data*.

A person's 'survival time' is his or her time from entry in the study until the occurrence of the event. The distribution of survival times is often very skew and may be bimodal (e.g. if significant post-operative mortality is followed by increased then gradually decreasing prospects of survival).

Survival data may be *censored* if there are subjects who do not experience an event because the study ends before they experience an event, are 'lost-to-follow-up' (because of, e.g. migration or death), experience another type of event which precludes the event of interest (e.g. death from another cause), or cease to be eligible for the study (e.g. in a study of under-fives, children are no longer eligible once they reach their fifth birthday). In such instances, the person's survival time cannot be known precisely. All that is known is that it is *at least* a certain amount.

The essential feature of *survival analysis* is that it enables use of all of a person's 'at-risk' time, irrespective of whether he or she finally experiences an event. An additional feature is that it allows the incidence rate to vary for the entire period of observation.

An example of survival data occurs for child vaccination. In the early 1990s, a survey of infants was conducted in the Philippines to examine timeliness of vaccination. It was thought that vaccination coverage was high, but of concern was whether children were being vaccinated on schedule. The survey collected dates of birth and dates of vaccination (from records) for the three doses of diphtheria–pertussis–tetanus (DPT), scheduled at 6, 10, and 14 weeks. Children who had not been vaccinated by the time of the survey (perhaps because they were too young or perhaps because it was delayed) were regarded as censored for that dose. The essential data were then age at vaccination or age at the survey, if they were unvaccinated. Recorded data would be set up as shown in Table 6.15.12.

The last two columns in the table are used for the analysis. A 'flag' variable indicates whether or not a child has been vaccinated in the follow-up time, and the age at the vaccination for those who were or the age at last follow-up for those who were not vaccinated.

The approach to analysing this type of data is to divide the follow-up time into short periods, called *risk sets*, and count events that occur within the risk set, as a fraction of all persons who were present in the study for that period. The latter is particularly important: Persons will drop out of the analysis because they have experienced the event (vaccinated) or had not reached that age yet. These fractions are then manipulated in a process attributed to Kaplan and Meier (ref) to form a curve that shows the proportion of

Table 6.15.12 Format of survival data

Child ID	Birth date	DPT1?	Date DPT1	Age at DPT1 (days)	Censored?	Age to DPT1
001	01 Jan 1995	Y	22 Feb 1995	52	1	52
002	21 Jan 1995	Y	22 Mar 1995	60	1	60
003	09 Mar 1995	Y	31 May 1995	83	1	83
004	16 Apr 1995	N	—	—	0	94
005	03 Jun 1995	Y	19 Jul 1995	46	1	46

DPT1 = diphtheria–pertussis–tetanus dose 1 (usually given at 6 weeks).
Y = vaccinated.
N = unvaccinated.

persons 'surviving'—in the example, the proportion of children unvaccinated—at that time. We often use the smallest possible risk sets, which contain only one event. Sometimes, if the sample is very large, we use groups (say month of age), which gives a 'step' function. Results for fitting this curve to the Philippines vaccination data are shown in Fig. 6.15.19, with 95% CIs (ref) to show their precision.

We see that very few children in this population receive the DPT vaccinations on time (the recommended schedule is shown by the vertical lines), and by looking at the horizontal line drawn at the 'Proportion Unvaccinated' = 0.5, we see that only half of the children have received their three vaccinations at 9 weeks (instead of 6 weeks), 14 weeks (instead of 10), and 18 weeks (instead of 14). Thus, a major cause of delayed vaccination is delay in the first dose, by about a month. We could also use this analysis to estimate the ages when 'most' children are vaccinated, where 'most' ≈80%. This would occur at a horizontal line drawn at 'Proportion Unvaccinated' =0.2, which paints an even gloomier picture.

Kaplan–Meier survival curves can be formally compared using the Wilcoxon logrank test (ref). In addition, there are other approaches to analysing survival data, which we will discuss briefly the subsection on multivariate analysis.

Multivariate analysis

Normal theory regression

Having established that birthweight and maternal weight are associated, and having estimated the regression coefficient, we might be interested in further exploring the prediction of birthweight. We could perform the same analyses on a range of other variables, such as family income, tobacco, or alcohol consumption. In each case, a regression model provides us with a measure of the size of the effect (the regression coefficient, at a 95% CI) and its statistical significance (*P*-value). In this way, we might identify a collection of predictors or 'risk factors'. It is likely that these relationships will themselves be related: Consider the following example, now based on a sample of 500 births.

Regression of birthweight upon maternal pre-pregnancy weight yields:

Birthweight (g) = 2832 + 11.3 × maternal weight (kg)

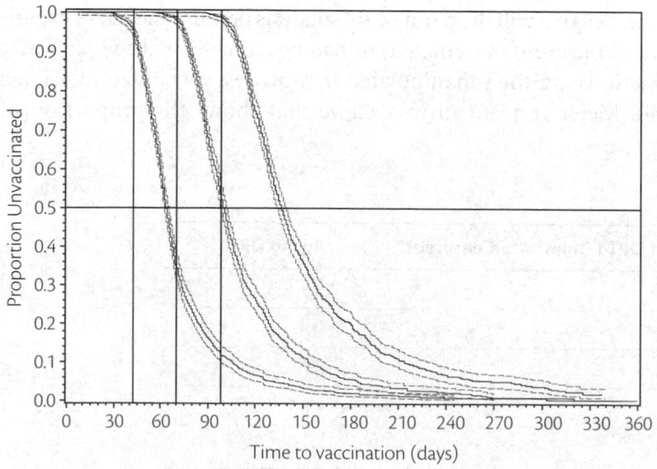

Fig. 6.15.19 Survival curves for three doses of diphtheria–pertussis–tetanus (DPT) vaccination, in relation to the expected schedule (vertical lines).

Birthweight increases by 11.3 g per kg of maternal weight, with a 95% CI of (7.9,14.8), and $P < 0.0001$, a highly significant association.

Regression of birthweight upon number of previous pregnancies yields:

Birthweight (g) = 3453 + 29.5 × number of previous pregnancies

Birthweight increases by 29.5 g per previous pregnancy, with a 95% CI of (1.7,57.4), and P=0.038, which is just below P=0.05 cut-off for significance.

But if a woman's weight increases with increasing number of pregnancies, then these two findings might be related; for example, does birthweight increase with increasing number of pregnancies because of the increasing weight of the mother, or is the effect separate?

To examine this, we set up a multivariate (or multivariable) linear model such as:

$$Y=\alpha+\beta_1 X_1+\beta_2 X_2+e$$

where β_1 and β_2 are regression coefficients indicating the dependence of Y upon variables X_1 and X_2, X_1 being maternal weight and X_2 being the number of previous pregnancies. This model is fitted in the same way as before, to obtain:

Birthweight (g) = 2830 + 11.0 × maternal weight (kg)
+ 16.9 × number of previous pregnancies

95% CIs for the maternal weight and number of previous pregnancies effects are (7.5,14.5) and (−10.3,44.0), respectively; *P*-values are <0.0001 and 0.22, respectively. We see that the maternal weight effect remains virtually the same (with a similar CI), but the effect of number of previous pregnancies has about halved, and is no longer significant.

To see why this has happened, we use our multivariate model to assess the effect of a difference in maternal weight of 1 kg on birthweight. Suppose a woman has a pre-pregnancy weight of 50 kg and one previous pregnancy, and another woman has a pre-pregnancy weight of 49 kg and no previous pregnancies. The difference in predicted birthweights associated with 1 kg of maternal weight can be evaluated using the fitted model.

For the first woman:

Predicated birthweight (g)
=2830 + 11.0 × 50 (kg) + 16.9 × 1

The second woman has no previous pregnancies; we know this has an effect on birthweight, and so she is not really comparable to the first. To make her comparable in terms of number of previous pregnancies, we use the prediction model to see what would happen if she only differed in pre-pregnancy weight; that is, we use the same number of previous pregnancies as the first woman in our prediction.

For the second woman, assuming she also had one previous pregnancy:

Predicated birthweight (g) (1 previous pregnancy)
=2830 + 11.0 × 49 (kg) + 16.9 × 1

We subtract these two equations to obtain the difference in predicted birthweight for these two women. The intercept terms cancel out in the subtraction; the terms involving maternal weight give a difference equal to the regression coefficient for maternal weight, 11.0 g. The terms involving previous pregnancy also cancel out. Thus, our regression coefficient of 11.0 g represents the effect of an addition 1 kg of maternal weight, after controlling (or adjusting) for number of previous pregnancies.

Reciprocally, the regression coefficient for number of previous pregnancies reflects the association between birthweight and number of previous pregnancies, after adjusting for the effect of maternal weight in the multivariate model. As this effect has been much decreased to the point of non-significance, we would conclude that the significant effect we saw in the first, separate analysis was due to confounding by maternal weight. A *confounding variable* is one that is associated with both the outcome variable and a predictor variable.

Thus, when a multiple regression model is fitted, we obtain estimates of the separate or 'adjusted' relationships between the outcome variable and the predictor variables. In this example, the association between birthweight and maternal weight, measured through the estimated regression coefficient, is adjusted for confounding with the other explanatory variable, number of previous pregnancies.

Essentially, no new principles emerge when this process is extended to more predictors or risk factors. We obtain a series of estimated regression coefficients, and confidence limits for the parameters, and *P*-values, each reflecting the association between the outcome and the predictor, after adjusting for all other predictors included in the analysis.

References

Bland, M. (2000). *An Introduction to Medical Statistics*. 3rd edition. Oxford University Press: Oxford.

Conover, W.J. (1999) *Practical Nonparametric Statistics*. 3rd edition. Wiley: New York.

Green, A., Williams, G.M., Neale, R. *et al.* (1999), Daily sunscreen application and betacarotene supplementation in prevention of basal-cell and squamous-cell carcinoma of the skin; a randomised controlled trial. *Lancet* 354 (9180), 72–75.

Kaplan, E.L., Meier, P. (1958) Nonparametric estimation from incomplete observations. *American Statistical Association* 53, 457–481.

Kirkwood, B.R. and Sterne, J.A.C. (2003). *Essential Medical Statistics*. 2nd edition. Blackwell Science: Massachusetts.

Miller, R.G. (1981) *Simultaneous Statistical Inference.* 2nd edition. Springer Verlag: New York.

Snedecor, G.W. and Cochran, W.G. (1989), *Statistical Methods* 8th edition, Iowa State University Press: Ames.

6.16

Mathematical models of transmission and control

Roy M. Anderson, T. Déirdre Hollingsworth, and D. James Nokes

Introduction

The aim of this chapter is to show how simple mathematical models of the transmission of infectious agents within human communities can aid the interpretation of observed epidemiological trends, guide the collection of data towards further understanding, and help in the design of programmes for the control of infection and disease. The central theme is to improve understanding of the interplay between the variables that determine the typical course of infection within an individual and the variables that control the pattern of infection and disease within communities of people. This theme hinges on an understanding of the basic similarities and differences between particular infections in terms of the number of population variables (and consequent equations) needed for a sensible characterization of the system, the typical relations between the various rate parameters (such as birth, death, recovery, and transmission rates), and the form of expression that captures the essence of the transmission process.

Model construction, whether mathematical, verbal, or diagrammatic, is in principle the conceptual reduction of a complex biological or population-based process into a more simple, idealized, and easily understandable sequence of events. Consequently, the use of mathematical modelling as a descriptive and interpretative tool is a very common exercise in scientific study. Its use, therefore, in epidemiological study should not be viewed as intrinsically difficult or beyond the comprehension of those trained in medical or biological disciplines. The reductionist approach that is inherent in model construction, which helps to define processes clearly and identify the most important components of a system, is employed in many areas of public health research and practice. The following situations, for example, are all likely to involve, at the very least, the implicit use of models to simplify and aid understanding: The assessment of the cause and severity of sporadic epidemics of *Salmonella*, hepatitis A virus food poisoning, or Legionnaires' disease; the cost-effectiveness analysis of various measures used to combat an infection within a hospital, within a community, countrywide, or globally; or the identification of the factors that control the maintenance of an endemic infection within a community.

Most epidemiological problems, by definition, are concerned with the study of populations and so involve quantitative scores of, for example, abundances and rates of spread. Thus, it is invariably necessary to convert any descriptive model of process into a more formal mathematical framework so that we work with numbers and not words. The use of a more formal structure enables us to incorporate quantitative estimates of abundances or rates, derived from experiment or field observations, into the model and to make predictions of the likely behaviour of the system under varying conditions, particularly when we are concerned with the introduction or alteration of measures to control infection or disease.

It is the step of translation from verbal or diagrammatic description into a formal mathematical framework that arouses the deepest suspicions among medical or public health workers. Quite naturally, this response is in part a consequence of the use of, what is for many, a strange symbolism to describe familiar verbal or conceptual identities. It must be remembered, however, that mathematics is the most precise language we have available for scientific study, and once a problem is formulated in mathematical terms, many techniques are available to pursue the logical consequences of the stated assumptions. The clear and unambiguous statement of assumptions is of course a particular attribute of mathematical, as opposed to verbal, description. Excessive use of symbolism or formal methods of analysis can confuse as opposed to clarify and it must be admitted that some sections of the mathematical epidemiological literature have drifted from their original moorings and sail free from the constraints of data or relevance. But to jump from this observation to the belief that mathematical models have nothing to contribute in practice to the design of public health programmes is a mistake. Sensibly used, mathematical models are no more and no less than tools for thinking about things in a precise way.

The second area of suspicion, aside from symbolism, concerns simplification. A frequent criticism of mathematical work in epidemiology is that model formulation involves too many simplifying assumptions despite known biological complexity. This is often true, and needs to be remedied, but it is in part a consequence of the infancy of the discipline and, in some cases, a result of inadequate quantitative understanding of a particular problem. There are, however, two important counter-arguments to the criticism of simplification. Firstly, and most importantly, it is often the case in biological study that a few processes dominate the generation of observed pattern despite the fact that many more can, to a lesser degree, influence the outcome. The identification of the dominant processes is an important facet of model construction and, what is termed, sensitivity analysis. The second point concerns scientific method. The process of understanding the consequences of a series of simple assumptions and building upon this by slowly adding complexity is directly analogous to the laboratory scientist's approach of carefully controlling most variables and allowing a few to vary in a planned design. Carefully building complexity on a simple framework can greatly facilitate our understanding of the major factors that influence or control a particular process or pattern.

The chapter is organized as follows. The subsection following this introduction provides a brief review of the historical development of mathematical epidemiology and outlines the types of infection that will be considered in latter subsections. The third subsection addresses the problems of model construction, design, and application. The fourth examines the major concepts in quantitative epidemiology that have been derived from mathematical study, such as threshold host densities for the persistence of an infection, the basic reproductive rate, and herd immunity. In the fifth subsection, methods are explored by which to obtain some of the basic epidemiological parameters from empirical observation. The sixth subsection turns to applied problems and considers the use of models in the design of control strategies for infection and disease, and the final subsection is reserved for concluding thoughts. Throughout, mathematical details are kept to a bare minimum and the reader interested in technical details of model construction and analysis is referred to papers in specialist journals.

Historical perspective

The application of mathematics to the study of infectious disease appears to have been initiated by Daniel Bernoulli (1760) when he used a mathematical method to evaluate the effectiveness of the techniques of variolation against smallpox. Further interest did not occur until the middle of the nineteenth century when, in 1840, William Farr effectively fitted a normal curve to smoothed quarterly data on deaths from smallpox in England and Wales over the period 1837–39 (Farr 1840). This empirical approach was further developed by John Brownlee (1906) who considered in detail the 'geometry' of epidemic curves. The origins of modern mathematical epidemiology owe much to the work of Hamer (1906), Ross (1911), Soper (1929), and Kermack and McKendrick (1927) who, in different ways, began to formulate specific theories about the transmission of infectious disease in simple but precise mathematical statements and to investigate the properties of the resulting models. Their work led to one of the cornerstones of modern mathematical epidemiology: The hypothesis that the course of an epidemic depends on the rate of contact between susceptible and infectious individuals. This led to the so-called 'mass-action' principle in which the net rate of spread of infection is assumed to be proportional to the density of susceptible people multiplied by the density of infectious individuals. In turn, this principle generated the celebrated threshold theory, according to which the introduction of a few infectious individuals into a community of susceptibles will not give rise to an epidemic outbreak unless the density or number of susceptibles is above a certain critical value (see the review by Fine 1993).

Since these early beginnings, the growth in the literature has been very rapid and reviews have been published by Bailey (1975), Becker (1979), Anderson and May (1985b, 1991), Dietz (1987), and Scott and Smith (1994). In more recent work, there has been an expansion in the range of diseases modelled and in the complexities which are included. Epidemiological models have played a key role in the design and evaluation of control programmes during the severe acute respiratory syndrome (SARS) (Lipsitch *et al.* 2003; Riley *et al.* 2003), foot and mouth disease (FMD) (Ferguson *et al.* 2001; Keeling *et al.* 2001), bovine spongiform encephalitis (BSE) and variant Creutzfeldt-Jakob disease (vCJD) (Anderson *et al.* 1996; Ferguson *et al.* 2002; Ghani *et al.* 2003) outbreaks, and in pandemic influenza planning (Longini *et al.* 2004; Ferguson *et al.* 2005; Hollingsworth *et al.* 2006). Large-scale computer-simulated spatial models of airborne transmission of infectious diseases, as reviewed by Riley (2007), are increasingly used for public health planning. Heterogeneities in transmission, whether due to biological or behavioural variability (Lloyd-Smith *et al.* 2005; Mossong *et al.* 2008), changes in transmission due to seasonality (Grassly *et al.* 2006), changing climate (Patz *et al.* 2005), the effect of heterogeneities in behaviour on the spread of sexually transmitted diseases (Garnett 1998; Eames & Keeling 2002), and changing behaviour on the outcome of outbreaks are areas of ongoing research (Ferguson 2007). The evolutionary pressures that led to the characteristics of common diseases, and which drive current pandemics, are also being investigated through a variety of approaches (Ferguson *et al.* 2003; Read & Keeling 2003; Grenfell *et al.* 2004; Fraser *et al.* 2007).

In the following subsections, we attempt to give a flavour of recent work and to distil the major conclusions that have emerged in particular areas. We have deliberately chosen to concentrate on directly transmitted viral and bacterial infections that constitute the major infectious diseases of children in developed countries and, as a consequence of the recent pandemic of AIDS, sexually transmitted infections. Our reasons are simply that the mathematical models are more highly developed in these fields in comparison with others (e.g. vector-borne infections), that theory has close contact with empirical epidemiological data in these areas, and that model structure is somewhat simpler than for other infections such as metazoan parasites.

Model construction

Definition of terms

Epidemiology

Epidemiology as a subject is concerned with the study of the 'behaviour' of an infection or disease within a population or populations of hosts (i.e. humans). Behaviour refers to observed patterns such as the incidence (the rate at which new cases arise or are reported) of infection or disease. Examples of behaviour are epidemics (a rise and subsequent fall in incidence) and endemicity (the stable maintenance of infection within the human community). The aim of the discipline is to determine the underlying processes, and understand the interactions between them, that generate observed patterns (e.g. the rate of spread of infection and the pattern of susceptibility to infection). Epidemiology is a quantitative discipline that draws on statistical techniques for parameter estimation and mathematical methods for delineating the dynamic changes that occur over time, across age classes, or through different spatial locations. The discipline also makes use of modern molecular (e.g. DNA probes and polymerase chain reaction [PCR]) and immunological (measures of the abundances of antibodies specific to an infectious agent's antigens) techniques for the detection and quantification of current and past infection or disease.

Populations

The definition and description of the host and parasite populations are of obvious importance in epidemiological studies. A population is an assemblage of organisms of the same species (or genetic type, etc.) that occupy a defined point or points in the plane created by the dimensions of space and time. The basic unit of such populations is the individual organism (i.e. parasite or human host). Populations may be divided (i.e. stratified) into a series of categories or classes, the members of which possess a unifying character or characters such as age, sex, or the stage of development. Such subdivisions may be made on spatial or temporal criteria to distinguish a local population from a larger assemblage. The boundaries in space, time, and genetic constitution between different populations are often vague, but it is important to define what constitutes the 'study population' as clearly as possible.

Natural history of infection

Mathematical models are often used to depict the rate of spread or transmission of an infectious agent through a defined human community. For their formulation, three broad classes of information are required:

1. The modes and rates of transmission of the agent
2. The typical course of events within an individual following infection
3. The demographic and social characteristics of the human community

The mode of transmission (i.e. direct, indirect, horizontal, vertical, etc.) is of obvious importance (Table 6.16.1), but if there is more than one route the relative efficiency of each in determining overall transmission must be understood. When considering microparasitic infections (e.g. viruses, bacteria, and protozoa that multiply directly within the host), it is generally not possible to measure the abundance of the pathogen within the host (i.e. the burden or intensity of infection). However, following invasion, it is important to obtain quantitative information on the typical durations of the latent and infectious periods of the infection and the incubation period of the disease it induces. As depicted in Fig. 6.16.1, the latent period is defined as the average period of time from the point of infection to the point when an individual becomes infectious to others, the infectious period denotes the average period over which an infected person is infectious to others, and the incubation period defines the average period from infection to the appearance of symptoms of disease. In practice, all these periods are variable between individuals, depending on factors such as the size of the inoculum of the infectious agent that initiates infection, the genetic background of host and parasite, past experience of infections, and the nutritional status of the host. The use of an average is an economy of thought, and where knowledge permits, models should be based on distributed latent and infectious periods. In some instances, the infectious period may be influenced by patient management practices such as the confinement of an infected person once symptoms of infection are diagnosed (e.g. measles and tuberculosis).

There are instances in the case of viral and bacterial infections when a knowledge of pathogen abundance within blood, excretions, secretions, and other tissues or organs of the host can be of importance in determining the infectivity of an infected person to susceptible contacts. A good example is provided by HIV-1. Current evidence suggests that the infectiousness of an infected person varies greatly over the long and variable incubation period of AIDS, the disease induced by the virus (Wawer *et al.* 2005), and that there is significant variability between infectiousness of different individuals due to different viral loads (Quinn *et al.* 2000) (Fig. 6.16.2). A short period of high infectiousness occurs shortly after infection, followed by a long period of variable infectiousness (perhaps many years) before it again increases as the infected patient develops symptoms of AIDS (Anderson & May 1988). In these cases, rather complex models are required to mirror the natural history

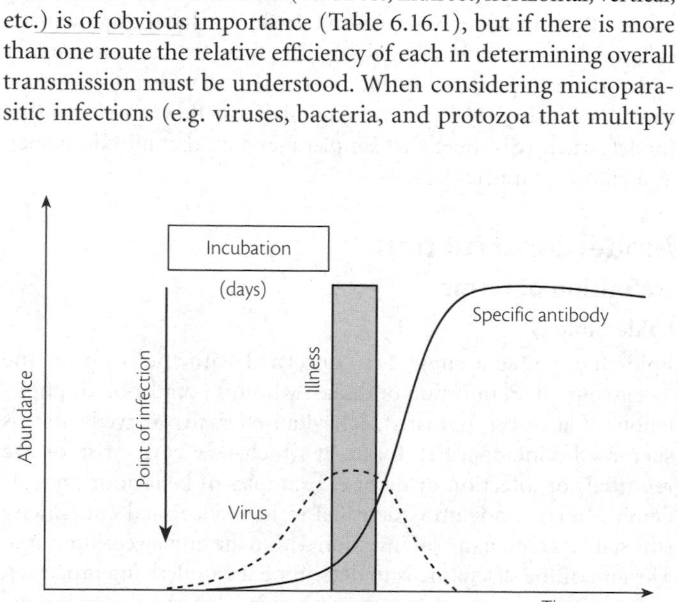

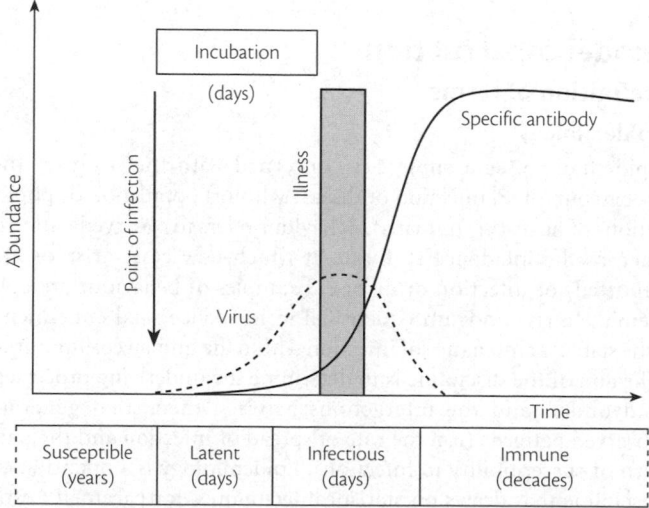

Fig. 6.16.1 Schematic representation of the typical time-course of an acute viral or bacterial infection in a host individual and the corresponding progression through infection classes (note the different time durations within each of these classes). *Source:* Nokes and Anderson (1988).

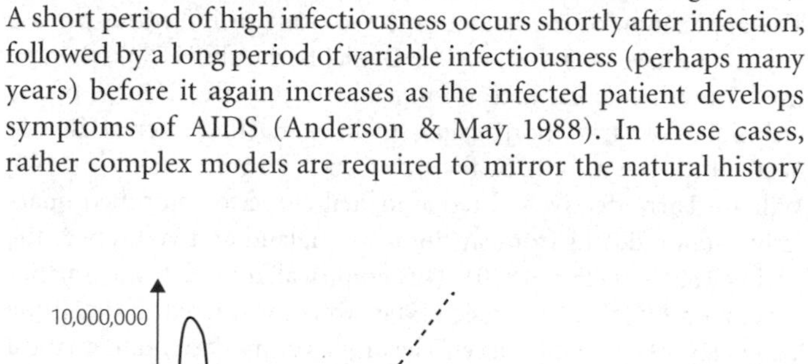

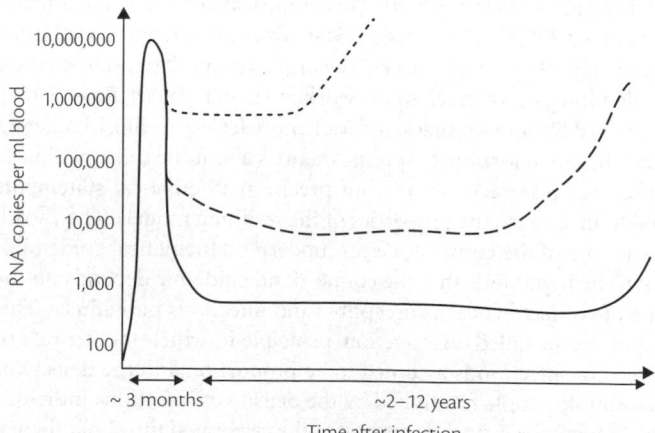

Fig. 6.16.2 Schematic of the changes in HIV-RNA concentration in the blood of an infected individual. During acute infection, viral loads and infectivity are high. During the long asymptomatic period, viral loads are at intermediate levels before rising prior to death (in the absence of treatment). High viral loads are associated with high transmission rates (Quinn *et al.* 2000) and short life expectancy (Mellors *et al.* 1996).

Table 6.16.1 Epidemiological classification of infectious diseases of public health importance in developed countries

Mode of transmission	Type of parasite	Examples (diseases or agents)
VERTICAL[a]	Micro[b]	
	Viruses	Rubella, hepatitis B, cytomegalovirus, retroviruses
	Protozoa	*Toxoplasma gondii*
HORIZONTAL		
Direct		
Close contact	Micro	
	Viruses	Measles, mumps, rubella, Epstein–Barr virus, herpes simplex-1, respiratory syncytial virus, influenza-2, varicella, common cold
	Bacteria	Diphtheria, pertussis, bacterial meningitis
	Macro[c]	
	Nematodes	*Enterobius vermicularis* (pinworm)
Environmental	Micro	
	Viruses	Hepatitis A, polio, Coxsackie
	Bacteria	Tetanus, *Shigella*, *Salmonella*, typhoid, cholera, Legionnaires' disease
	Protozoa	*Giardia intestinalis*, amoebiasis
	Macro	
	Nematodes	Pinworm
Sexual	Micro	
	Viruses	Hepatitis B, HIV, herpes simplex-2, cytomegalovirus
	Bacteria	*Neisseria gonorrhoeae*, syphilis
	Protozoa	*Trichomonas vaginalis*
Not direct		
Via other host species (zoonoses)	Micro	
	Virus	Rabies
	Protozoa	*Toxoplasma gondii*
	Macro	
	Nematodes	*Toxocara species*
	Cestodes	*Taenia solium*, *T. saginata*, *Echinococcus granulosus* (hydatid)
Vector-borne[d]	Micro	
	Viruses	Hepatitis B, HIV, Venezuelan equine encephalitis
	Bacteria	*Yersinia* species (plague)
	Protozoa	*Plasmodium* species (malaria)

[a]Inclusive of transplacental and perinatal infection.

[b]Microparasites are those that multiply directly within the host individual, usually resulting in acute infections and subsequent durable immunity to reinfection.

[c]Macroparasites are larger parasites whose reproductive stages pass out of the host. Infection intensity is thus a process of accumulation, and can be measured as worm burden.

[d]Needle transmission is included.

of infection and its implications for transmission (Fraser *et al.* 2007; Anderson 1988).

The human immune response to infection, its ability to confer protection against reinfection, and the duration of this protection have important implications for model construction. For the majority of childhood viral infections, the assumption of lifelong immunity following recovery appears to be correct. However, as one moves up a scale of parasite structural (antigenic) complexity from viruses to bacteria to protozoa, in general the duration of acquired immunity decreases. For certain infections, such as gonorrhoea, acquired immunity is absent, whereas for many protozoan infections it is of a short duration (e.g. *Plasmodium* sp.). The inability to develop effective immunity is often related to the genetic diversity of the infectious agent population (antigenic diversity) so that infection with one genetic strain fails to protect against invasions by another (e.g. *Neisseria gonorrhoea*, *Neisseria meningitidis*, and influenza viruses). The question of immunity can be complicated by a degree of cross-immunity (non-specific in character) resulting from infection by dissimilar organisms (e.g. many bacterial infections of the respiratory tract).

Demographic and behavioural characteristics of the human community are usually important in the study of transmission dynamics. For infections that confer lifelong immunity on host recovery, the rate of input by births of new susceptibles will influence the overall pattern of infection in a community. Similarly, the rate of transmission of 'close contact' infections (Table 6.16.1) will depend upon the degree of mixing between individuals and the density and age distribution of susceptibles and those infected. Heterogeneity in behaviour within a community is of particular importance in the study of sexually transmitted infections because rates of sexual-partner change vary greatly between individuals (Johnson *et al.* 1992, 1994). More generally, heterogeneity in any behaviour, whether sexual or social mixing, must be captured in model formulation.

It will be clear from the preceding comments that much quantitative detail about the natural history of infection must be understood for accurate model formulation. In many instances, such detail is not available, but model formulation can greatly facilitate our knowledge of what needs to be understood to define the transmission dynamics of a given infection. With respect to many childhood viral and bacterial infections, such as measles, rubella, mumps, pertussis, and diphtheria, a great deal is understood about the natural history, and hence, much of the work on mathematical models has focused on those infections. Their direct route of transmission, their tendency to induce lifelong immunity and, in most cases, the availability of serological or virological techniques to detect past or current infection facilitates the acquisition of quantitative data.

Units of measurement

The unit of measurement employed in epidemiological study depends on the type of infection. The most basic unit is that of the individual parasite. As already discussed, in most cases, this unit is not a practicable option for microparasitic organisms due to difficulties in detection and quantification (however, advances in molecular biology and biochemistry are generating new techniques that may be of value in the near future). As such, the most useful unit is that of the infected host, which allows the human community to be stratified on the basis of whether individuals are susceptible, infected but not yet infectious (i.e. latent or pre-patent), infectious, and recovered (i.e. immune in the case of many viral infections). Infection may be detected directly (e.g. DNA probes, virus or bacterial culture) or indirectly by the presence of antibodies specific to pathogen antigens (serological and salivary tests). Seropositivity does not necessarily discriminate between infected and recovered individuals, but for many viral and bacterial infections serological surveys of a population, perhaps stratified by age, sex, and other variables carried out longitudinally (through time via cohort monitoring) or horizontally (across age classes), provide a key measure of transmission and the broad epidemiological characteristics of the infection.

What models describe

At any point in time, a population may be classified by the density or number of susceptible, infected, and immune individuals. With the passing of time and concomitantly as individuals age, people may move from one infection class to the next. As such, with the recruitment of new susceptibles by birth and, in some cases, the loss of immunity, the population structure is a dynamic process with individuals flowing from one class to the next. Mathematical models of transmission attempt to capture the dynamic nature of these changes in the form of difference (discrete time steps) or differential (continuous time) equations (Scott and Smith, 1994 give a simple introduction). With respect to microparasitic infections for which the population is stratified or compartmentalized by infection status, the resulting models are often referred to as compartmental models. The types and numbers of compartments will depend upon the type of infectious agent and the details of its natural or life history. A number of examples are recorded in Fig. 6.16.3 in the form of flow diagrams. These diagrams form a useful intermediary step between biological comprehension and mathematical formulation.

Population rates of flow

Following the introduction of an infection into a stable population, the number or density of individuals within the various infection compartments will depend on the rates of flow between compartments such as infection and recovery rates. The size of a population in a specific compartment will depend on the magnitude of the rates that determine the entry and duration of stay. In general, the shorter the duration of stay (the higher the rate of leaving) in a particular compartment the smaller the size of the population in that category (the inverse relationship between 'standing crop' and 'rate of turnover'). If the infection attains a stable endemic equilibrium in the human community, the net input into each compartment will exactly balance the net output. The relative numbers in each compartment will be directly related to the duration of stay. Thus, for example, in the case of endemic measles in a developed country where immunity is lifelong (many decades), individuals remain in the susceptible class for an average of 4–5 years, and in the latent and infectious classes for a few days (say 7 days on average in each). As such, most people are in the immune class, followed by the susceptible class, and few individuals at any point in time are in the latent and infectious classes. Figure 6.16.4 provides a diagrammatic representation of this point.

A formal demonstration of the influence of rates of flow (or durations of stay) on the proportion of susceptibles, those infected, and immunes in a population is made possible by the translation of the flow diagram of movement between compartments (Fig. 6.16.3) into a set of coupled differential equations. Typically, these describe the rates of change with respect to time (or age or both) of the densities of infants with maternally derived immunity (due to maternal antibodies), susceptibles, infecteds not yet infectious, infectious individuals, and immunes, denoted by $M(t)$, $X(t)$, $H(t)$, $Y(t)$, and $Z(t)$, respectively, at time t (Fig. 6.16.3e). In writing down these equations, we need to define the rates of flow between compartments by a series of symbols. For example, in common notation, δ (delta) defines the loss of maternally derived immunity, that is, the average per person rate of loss of passive protection. The absolute rate of loss from or movement out of class M (Fig. 6.16.3) requires that the per capita rate (i.e. person/unit of time) be multiplied by

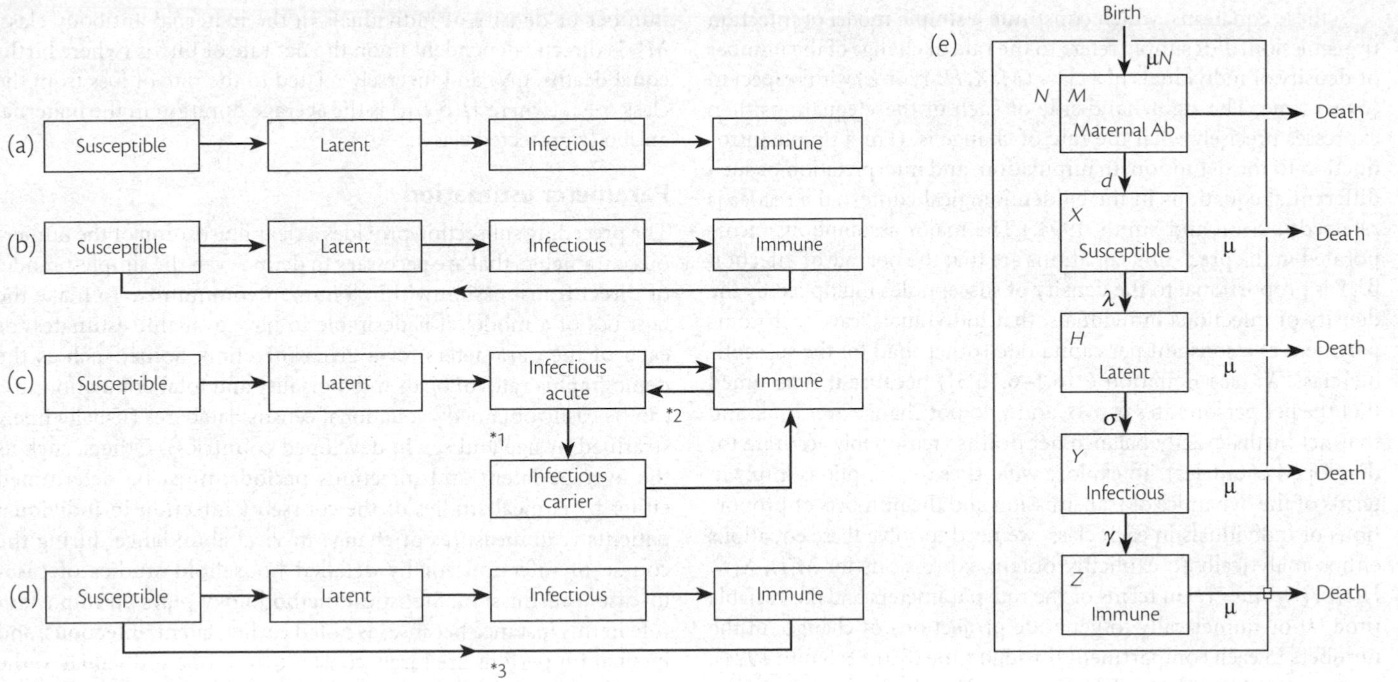

Fig. 6.16.3 Flow diagrams used to describe the movement of individuals within populations compartmentalized according to infection status to particular parasitic agents. (a) Simple model for infections inducing lasting immunity (e.g. measles, mumps, rubella, yellow fever, and poliomyelitis) or (b) in which immunity is transient and individuals subsequently return to the susceptible pool (e.g. *Neisseria gonorrhoea*, typhoid, cholera, *Trichomonas vaginalis*). (c) Many infections persist within the host for long periods of time, during which the infected individual may remain infectious (1), as is the case for carriers of hepatitis B virus, gonorrhoea, *Salmonella typhi*, and *Treponema pallidum* (syphilis), chronic tuberculosis patients, or during recrudescence of herpes viruses and malaria. The epidemiological importance of this characteristic is that it enables the perpetuation of such infections in low density communities (see discussion of the mass-action principle in the text). For other infections immunity is defence against disease but not asymptomatic reinfection (2) from which new infectious individuals arise (e.g. *Haemophilis influenzae* and *Neisseria meningitidis*). (d) Vaccination (3) has the effect of transferring individuals directly from the susceptible to the immune class. (e) More detailed description of the transmission dynamics of an acute microparasitic infection which explicitly accounts for births and deaths in the population. All neonates are born possessing maternally derived protective antibody. The net birth rate is assumed to equal the sum of the net death rates for each subpopulation (compartment), that is, births = μN, where $N = M + X + H + Y + Z$ = constant population size. The per capita rates defining movement between infection classes are described in the text.

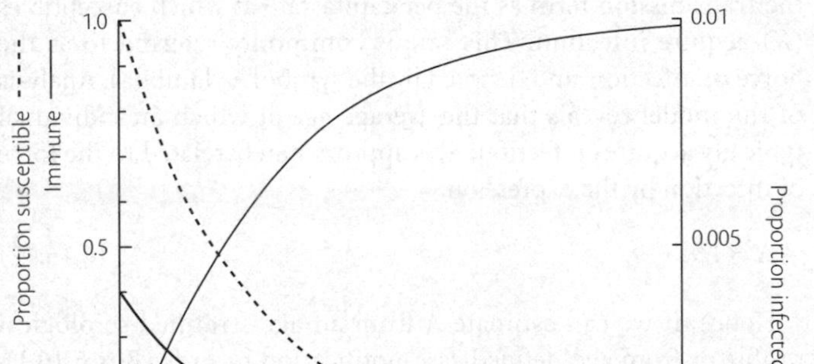

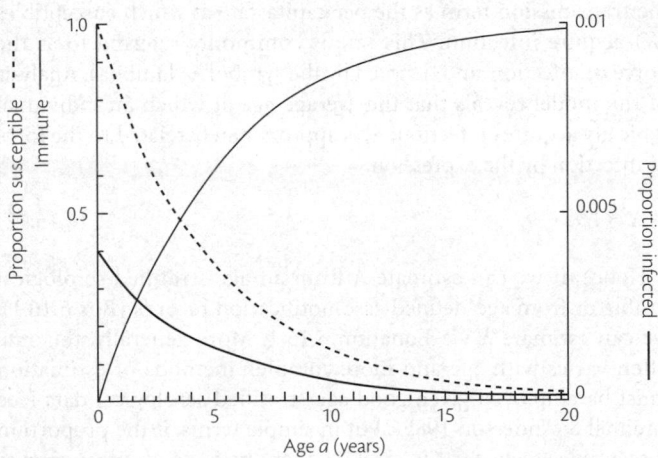

Fig. 6.16.4 The proportions of a population who are in the susceptible, infected (either latent or infectious), and immune classes for a typical childhood viral infection. In this example, which is based on measles, the force of infection, $\lambda = 0.2$ per year (corresponding to an average age at infection of 5 years) and the rate of movement from the latent class, λ, and recovery from infectiousness, λ, is 52 per year (corresponding to an average duration of stay in each of these infected classes of 1 week). Note that the proportion of the population in the infected classes is always much less than that in the susceptible or the immune classes (Fig. 6.16.1).

the size of the M subpopulation, that is, δM (expressed in persons/unit of time). If δ is the per capita rate of movement out of class M, then the average duration of maternally derived immunity is $1/\delta$. These principles apply to the other rate terms shown in Fig. 6.16.3e.

Hence, using conventional symbols, β (beta) is the transmission coefficient that defines the probability of contact and infection transfer between a susceptible and infectious person, σ (sigma) defines the per capita rate of leaving the latent class (average latent period $1/\sigma$), γ (gamma) the per capita rate of leaving the infectious class (average infectious period $1/\gamma$), and μ (mu) the natural per capita mortality rate ($1/\mu$ is average life expectancy). For developed countries, it is commonly assumed that population size is approximately constant such that net births exactly balance net deaths. Therefore, the net death rate μN (where N is the total population size $M + X + H + Y + Z$) is equated by births (hence the term μN for births in Equation 6.16.1). Additionally, it is assumed that infection does not induce an extra case mortality rate over and above natural mortality. With this notation, we can define the equations for M, X, H, Y, and Z as

$$\mathrm{d}M/\mathrm{d}t = \mu N - (\delta + \mu)M \qquad (6.16.1)$$

$$\mathrm{d}X/\mathrm{d}t = \delta M - (\beta Y + \mu)X \qquad (6.16.2)$$

$$\mathrm{d}H/\mathrm{d}t = \beta XY - (\sigma + \mu)H \qquad (6.16.3)$$

$$\mathrm{d}Y/\mathrm{d}t = \sigma H - (\gamma + \mu)Y \qquad (6.16.4)$$

$$dZ/dt = \gamma Y - \mu Z \qquad (6.16.5)$$

In these equations, which constitute a simple model of infection transmission, d/dt simply refers to the rate of change of the number or density of individuals in a class (M, X, H, Y, or Z) with respect to (over) time. The right-hand side of each of these equations then expresses precisely what the rate of change is. (For a simple introduction to the definition, manipulation, and interpretation of such differential equations in the epidemiological context, the reader is referred to Scott and Smith, 1994.) The major assumptions incorporated in the preceding equations are that the net rate of infection βXY is proportional to the density of susceptibles multiplied by the density of infectious individuals, that individuals leave each compartment at a constant per capita rate (other than for the susceptible class, X, [see Equation 6.16.1–6.16.5]) because it is assumed that the per person rates δ, μ, σ, and γ do not change over time, and that net births exactly balance net deaths (reasonably accurate for developed countries). To explore what these assumptions imply in terms of the dynamics of transmission and the numbers or proportions of individuals in each class, we need to solve these equations either analytically to explicitly obtain expressions for $M(t)$, $X(t)$, $H(t)$, $Y(t)$, and $Z(t)$ in terms of the rate parameters and the variable time (t) or numerically to generate projections of changes in the numbers in each compartment through time (Scott & Smith 1994). In the case of simple models, we can often obtain exact analytical solutions as is the case for the equation for $M(t)$ in the model defined by Equations 6.16.1–6.16.5. The solution gives us the number of infants with maternally derived protection at time t, $M(t)$:

$$M(t) = (\mu N) / (\mu + \delta) [1 - e^{-(\mu+\delta)t}] + M(0)e^{-(\mu-\delta)t} \quad (6.16.6)$$

where $M(0)$ is the number protected at time $t = 0$

More generally, the complexity of the life histories of many infections makes analytical solution difficult or impossible and numerical methods are required. Modern computers make light work of very complex models describing disease transmission (Riley 2007) and many software packages are available for the solution of sets of differential equations and now for model making. Nevertheless, in these cases, some general analytical insights can be obtained by examining the equilibrium properties of the model, which is done by setting the time derivatives (i.e. the d/dt) equal to zero, so that there are assumed to be no further changes in the number of individuals within each infection class because the flows into and out of any one category are equal. These equations can then be solved to determine the numbers at equilibrium (i.e. at stable endemicity) in each class (referred to as M^*, X^*, H^*, Y^*, and Z^*). For example, in the simple model of Equations 6.16.1–6.16.5, by simple algebraic manipulation we obtain:

$$M^* = \mu N / (\delta + \mu) \quad (6.16.7)$$
$$X^* = (\sigma + \mu)(\gamma + \mu) / \beta\sigma \quad (6.16.8)$$
$$H^* = (\gamma + \mu) Y^* / \sigma \quad (6.16.9)$$
$$Y^* = (\delta M^* - \mu X^*) / \beta X^* \quad (6.16.10)$$
$$Z^* = \gamma Y^* / \mu \quad (6.16.11)$$

where N is the constant representing the total population size.

These equilibrium solutions illustrate how the various rate parameters that determine flow between compartments influence the numbers of individuals in each compartment when the infection is at an endemic steady state. For example, based upon the assumptions in our model for an acute childhood infection (Equations 6.16.1– 6.16.5), we can suggest that at endemic equilibrium the number or density of individuals in the maternal antibody class, M^*, is directly dependent upon the net rate of births (where births equal deaths, μN) and inversely related to the rate of loss from the class $\delta + \mu$ (where $1/(\delta + \mu)$ is the average duration in the maternal antibody protected class).

Parameter estimation

The preceding subsection provides a clear illustration of the numerous parameters that are necessary to define even the simplest model of direct transmission within a human community. To make the best use of a model, it is desirable to have available estimates for each of the parameters for a given infection. Some, such as the demographic rates of birth and mortality and total population size, can be easily obtained via national census databases (usually finely stratified by age and sex in developed countries). Others, such as the average latent and infectious periods, must be determined either by clinical studies of the course of infection in individual patients (e.g. measures of change in viral abundance during the course of infection) or by detailed household studies of case-to-case transmission. Statistical methodology plays an important role in this instance because, as noted earlier, latent, infectious, and incubation periods are rarely constant from one individual to the next. Statistical estimation procedures have been developed to help derive summary statistics of these distributions (e.g. means and variances) (Bailey 1975).

Invariably, the most difficult parameter to estimate is the transmission coefficient β (see Equation 6.16.2), which is a measure of the rate of contact between members of a population plus the likelihood of infection resulting from contact. In some cases, such as certain sexually transmitted infections (e.g. gonorrhoea), direct estimates can be obtained via contact tracing methods (Hethcote & Yorke 1984). More commonly, indirect methods must be employed, often themselves based on model formulation and analysis. A simple example employs the model defined in the previous subsection by Equations 6.16.1–6.16.5. We can define the component βY of the transmission term as the per capita rate at which susceptibles (X) acquire infection. This rate is commonly referred to as the 'force of infection' and denoted by the symbol λ (lambda). Analysis of the model reveals that the average age at which an individual typically acquires infection, A, is approximately related to the force of infection by the expression:

$$A \simeq 1/\lambda \quad (6.16.12)$$

Hence, if we can estimate A from an age-stratified serological profile or from age-defined case-notification records (Box 6.16.1), we can estimate λ via Equation 6.16.1. More generally, this rate often varies with age and more complex methods of estimation must be employed given good age-stratified serological data (see Grenfell & Anderson 1985). Put in simple terms, if the proportion susceptible at age $a + 1$ is $x(a + 1)$, then the force of infection over the age interval $a \rightarrow a + 1$ (defined per unit of age) is simply:

$$\lambda = -\ln[x(a + 1) / x(a)] \quad (6.16.13)$$

With serological data finely stratified by age, under the assumption that the infection confers lifelong immunity upon recovery, Equation 6.16.13 can be used to estimate how λ changes with age in a given community. For most childhood viral and bacterial infections, λ is a function of age, changing from low values in infant

Box 6.16.1 Surveillance profiles

Two infections (i) and (ii) are at endemic equilibrium (i.e. roughly constant incidence in time) in a stationary host population (i.e. births are equal to deaths). The changes, with time or increasing age, in the proportion of the population that has experienced each infection may be estimated from longitudinal cohort or horizontal cross-sectional surveys (serological or case notifications) of individuals from birth to life expectancy *L*.

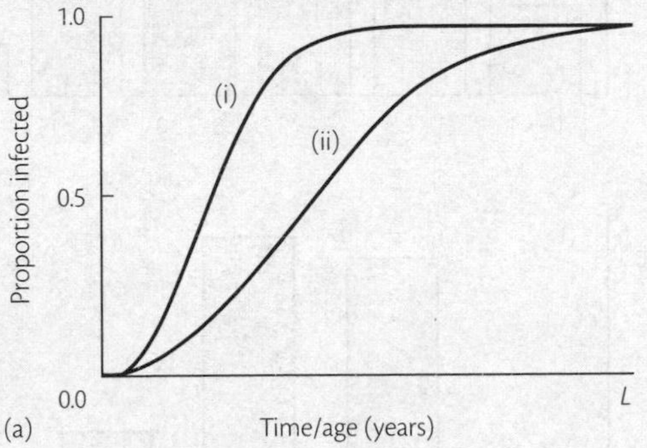

(a)

The steeper profile of (i) compared with (ii) is an indication that the basic reproductive potential R_0 of infection (i) exceeds that for infection (ii) such that:

$R_0(i) > R_0(ii)$.

Assume that each infection induces lifelong immunity; then, from the above profiles, changes with age/time in the proportion *x* susceptible to each infection are as shown in figure (b).

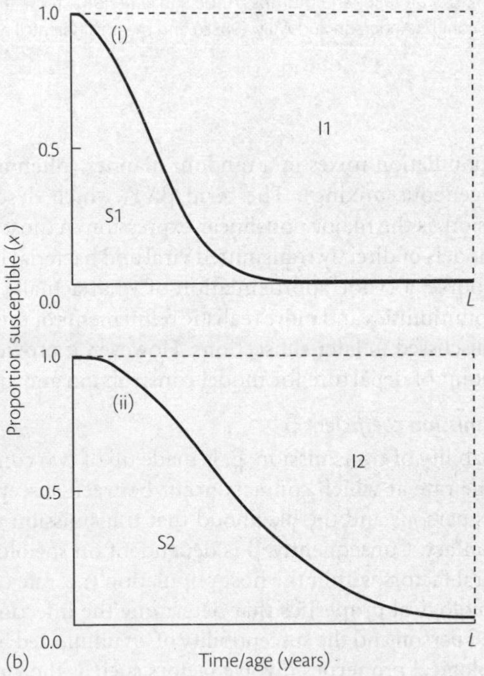

(b)

The (equilibrium) proportion of the total population susceptible to infection (i) is:

$x^*(i)$ = area S1/(area S1 area I1) and for infection (ii) it is $x^*(ii)$ area S2/(area S2 area I2).

Note that the equilibrium proportion susceptible to infection (i) (with the higher reproductive rate) is smaller than that for infection (ii) (with a lower rate of reproduction), i.e.:

$x^*(i) < x^*(ii)$.

The relationship between these two epidemiological parameters may be usefully expressed as:

$R_0(i) = 1/x^*(i)$

and

$R_0(ii) = 1/x^*(ii)$.

Summing the proportion susceptible, $x(a)$, in the above graphs for each age class from age 0 years (time 0) to *L* years, we can determine the average age at infection, *A*:

$x(a) = x(0) + x(1) + x(2) + \ldots + x(L) = A = S$

from which it can be seen that:

$A(i) < A(ii)$.

Note also that:

$R_0(i) = L/A(i) = L/S1$

and

$R_0(ii) = L/A(ii) = L/S2$.

(See also eqns (6.16.12) and (6.16.13), and Anderson and May (1983), for estimation of the force of infection from surveillance profiles.)

Summary examples

Assume infection (i) is measles and infection (ii) is rubella in the United Kingdom with average life span *L* of 75 years. If S1 = 5 and S2 = 10, then $A(i)$ = 5 years and $A(ii)$ = 10 years, and:

$x^*(i) = 5/75 = 0.066'$ $x^*(ii) = 10/75 = 0.133'$.

Therefore:

$R_0(i) = 1/0.066' = 15$

or

$R_0(i) = 75/5 = 15$

and

$R_0(ii) = 1/0.133' = 7.5$

or

$R_0(ii) = 75/10 = 7.5$.

The implications of this difference in the basic reproductive rate of infection to the proportion of the population that must be vaccinated in order to eradicate each infection can be seen in Fig. 6.16.11.

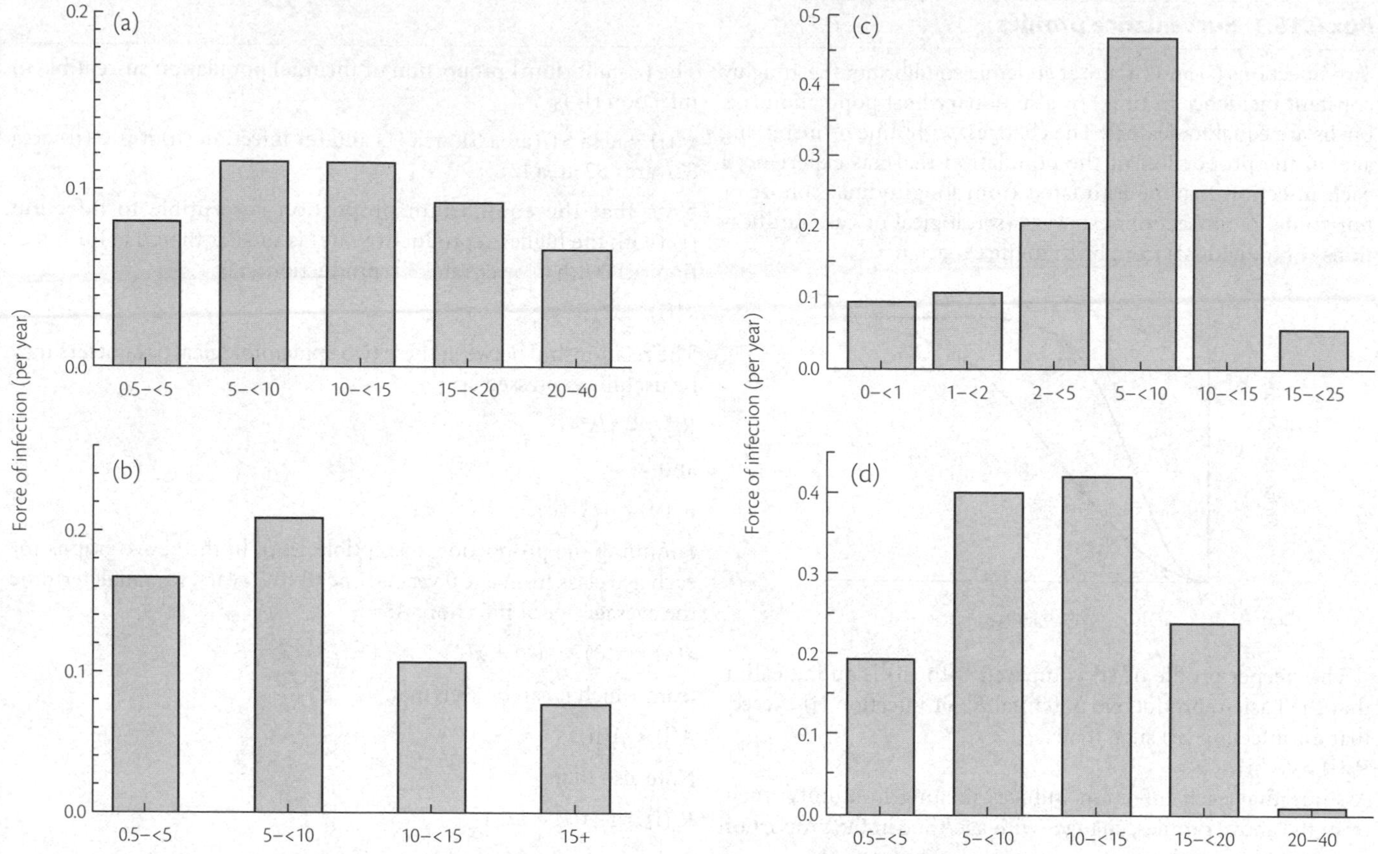

Fig. 6.16.5 Examples of the age-dependent nature of the per susceptible rate of transmission for common childhood viral and bacterial infections. Graphs (a) and (b) derive from horizontal cross-sectional serological surveys in the United Kingdom, of rubella (Nokes *et al.* 1986) and mumps (Anderson *et al.* 1987) respectively. Graphs (c) and (d) provide estimates based on case-notification data for England and Wales for whooping cough (Anderson and May 1985b) and measles (Grenfell and Anderson 1985) respectively.

classes to high in child-to-young teenage classes and back to low in adult age classes (Fig. 6.16.5). This is thought to reflect patterns of intimate contact via attendance at school and play activities.

Further complications may arise if rates of contact or transmission vary through time, perhaps due to seasonal factors such as the aggregation and dispersal of children at term and school holiday periods (Yorke *et al.* 1979; Anderson 1982; Bolker & Grenfell 1993). The problems of parameter estimation are considered in more detail in a later subsection.

Concepts in quantitative epidemiology

The incidence of infection and disease

Transmission by direct contact and the law of mass action

When close contact between infectious and susceptible individuals is necessary for transmission, the number of new cases in a population that arise in a unit of time (i.e. incidence of infection) is often assumed to be approximately given by the density (or number) of susceptibles, X, multiplied by the density (or number) of infectious persons, Y, multiplied by the probability of an effective (infectious) contact between an infectious person and a susceptible, β—that is, βXY. This relationship is commonly referred to as the 'law of mass action' by analogy with particles colliding within an ideal gas system (Box 6.16.2). The basic assumption implicit in this concept is that the population mixes in a random manner (often referred to as homogeneous mixing). The term βXY, which describes net transmission, is the major non-linear expression in most compartmental models of directly transmitted viral and bacterial infections. It is, of course, a crude approximation of what actually occurs in human communities and more realistic refinements of this assumption are discussed in later subsections. However, it provides a convenient point of departure for model construction and analysis.

The transmission coefficient β

The probability of transmission, β, is made up of two components, namely the rate at which contacts occur between susceptible and infectious persons and the likelihood that transmission will result from a contact. Consequently, β is dependent on sociological and behavioural factors within the host population (i.e. rate of mixing) and the biological properties that determine the infectiousness of an infected person and the susceptibility of an uninfected individual. These biological properties involve factors such as the virulence of the infectious agent and the genetic background as well as the nutritional status of the human host.

Incidence estimates

The incidence of infection, I, can be measured by direct observation of new, usually symptomatic, cases, such as notifications of measles or pertussis. Unfortunately, however, measures of incidence tell us

Box 6.16.2 The law of mass action and the incidence of infection

Imagine susceptible and infectious individuals behaving as ideal gas particles within a closed system with no immigration or emigration and occupying a defined space, where X is the number of particles of one gas (i.e. susceptibles), γ is the number of particles of a second gas (i.e. infectious people), and β is the collision coefficient for the formation of molecules of a new gas from one molecule each of the original gases (i.e. new cases of infection) (figure (a)).

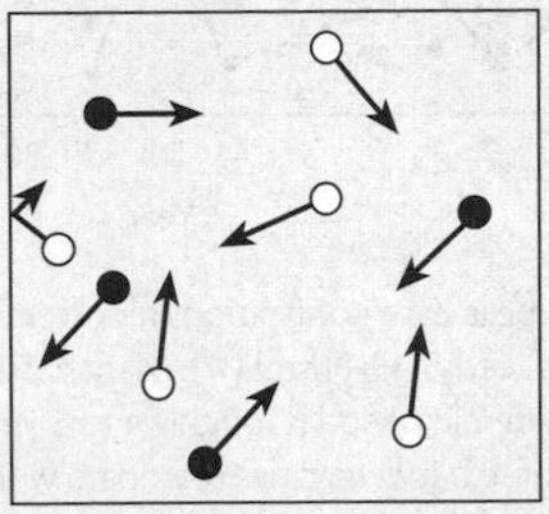

(a)

Gas particles (individuals) are mixing in a homogeneous manner such that collisions (contacts) occur at random. The law of mass action states that the net rate of production of new molecules (i.e. cases), I, is simply

$I = \beta XY$.

The coefficient β is a measure of (i) the rate at which collisions (contacts) occur and (ii) the probability that the repellent forces of the gas particles can be overcome to produce new molecules, or, in the case of infection, the likelihood that a contact between a susceptible and an infectious person results in the transmission of infection. Under these assumptions, the incidence of infection will be increased by larger numbers (or densities) of infectious and susceptible persons and/or high probabilities (β) of transmission (figure (b)).

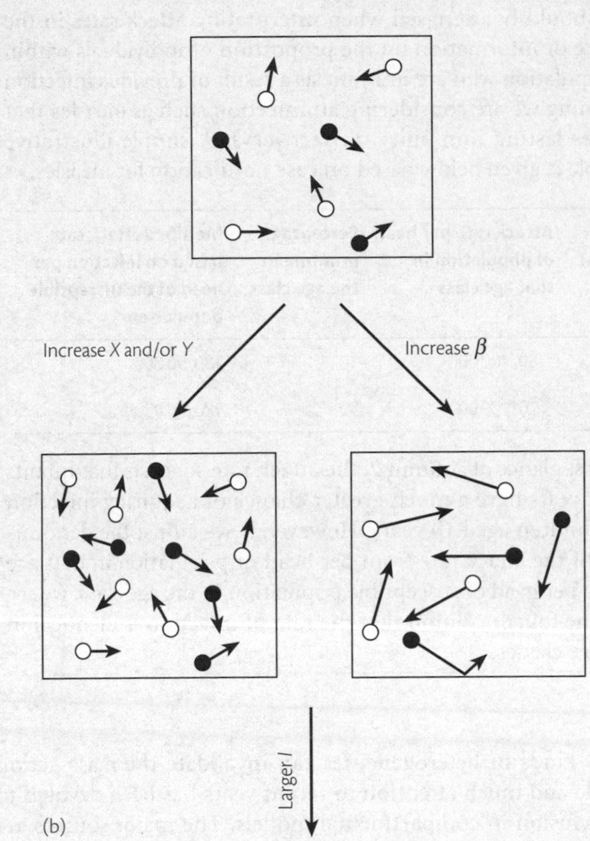

(b)

neither about the respective densities of susceptibles and infectious people, nor about the magnitude of the transmission coefficient β. It is common practice in epidemiology for I to be expressed as the number of cases per unit of population (usually 100 000 people in a defined class, such as age or sex) over a defined period of time such as 1 year (e.g. 5/100 000 per annum). Such measures are often referred to as attack rates (AR). However, they are a rather poor measure of the intensity of transmission within a population because they take no account of the proportion of the community (or age or sex class) that is susceptible to infection (Box 6.16.3). A better measure of the rate at which susceptibles acquire infection is provided by a parameter termed 'the force of infection', commonly denoted by the symbol λ. It simply defines the probability that a susceptible individual will acquire infection over a short period of time (i.e. per susceptible [equal to per capita] rate of infection) and, in the terminology of the mass-action principle, is defined as $\lambda = \beta Y$. Here, β might be thought of as the force of infection for one infectious person in a community. Estimates of this rate, λ, can be derived from age-stratified serological profiles or case notifications (Anderson & May 1991; Grenfell & Anderson 1985; Anderson & May 1983) (Fig. 6.16.5).

Validity of the mass-action principle

Despite the simplicity of the notion of homogeneous mixing implicit in the mass-action principle of transmission, the predictions of simple compartmental models based on this assumption often mirror observed epidemiological patterns surprisingly well (Anderson & May 1982). In part, this is a consequence of increased travel, movement, and mixing within many societies in developed countries. Measles epidemics, for example, are often synchronous in England and Wales, with a clear distinction in all parts of these regions between years of high incidence and years of low incidence (Fig. 6.16.6). However, the less able an infection is to spread through a particular population (lower R_0; see the following subsection) the more important are slight deviations from homogeneous mixing, resulting in a lower degree of synchrony of epidemics in a country (Fig. 6.16.7). The assumption is most appropriate for infections that are spread by close contact between individuals, such as respiratory infections transmitted by contaminated droplets and nasopharyngeal secretions. In such cases, the survival of the infectious agent in the external environment is of very short duration (i.e. minutes). As such, there is no significant reservoir of infectious stages to maintain transmission in the absence of infectious persons.

Box 6.16.3 Interpreting attack rates

Care should be exercised when interpreting attack rates in the absence of information on the proportion of individuals within the population who are immune as a result of previous infection (assuming we are considering an infection such as measles that induces lasting immunity on recovery). A simple illustrative example is given below based on case notification for measles.

Age (years)	Attack rate per head of population in that age class	Percentage immune in the age class	Modified attack rate based on infection per head of the susceptible population
2	180/100 000	10	180/90 000
10	20/100 000	90	180/90 000

At a first glance at column 2, the attack rate suggests that infants aged 2 years have a much greater chance of acquiring infection than children aged 10 years. However, if we adjust the denominator of the attack rate from per head of population in that age class to per head of susceptible population in the age class, we see from the fourth column that the rate of infection is identical in both age classes.

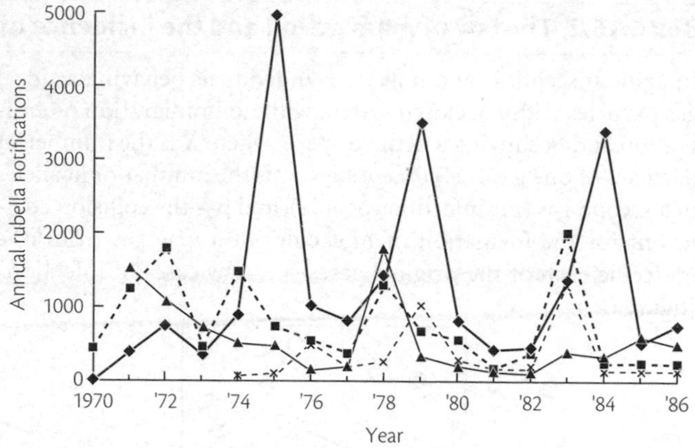

Fig. 6.16.7 Annual rubella case notifications reported by four city health authorities in England: Leeds (♦), Bristol (■), Manchester (▲), and Newcastle (×). The dominant interepidemic period is roughly 4 to 5 years with peak incidence often slightly out of phase between cities (compare with Fig. 6.16.6).
Source: Communicable Disease Surveillance Centre, London.

Many kinds of heterogeneities can invalidate the mass-action principle and much attention in recent years has been devoted to their inclusion in compartmental models. The major sources are heterogeneities arising from age-related factors, which determine contact and mixing patterns (i.e. 'who mixes with whom'), and spatial factors, such as differences in population densities in urban and rural areas of a country (Anderson & May 1991; Ferguson *et al.* 2005; Anderson & May 1984; May & Anderson 1984). Such sources of heterogeneity are very important in the design of control policies based, for example, on mass vaccination, and models have been developed to assess their impact.

Heterogeneity in behaviour is of particular importance in the study of sexually transmitted infections such as gonorrhoea and HIV. One of the major determinants of the rate of spread of such infections is the distribution of the rate of sexual-partner change within a defined community (Fig. 6.16.8). These distributions are typically highly heterogeneous in character (i.e. the variance in the rate of partner change is much greater in value than the mean rate of partner change). Most people have few different sexual partners in a lifetime (or over a defined period of time) and a few have many. The activities of individuals in the 'tail' of the distribution (the highly sexually active) are clearly important for the persistence and spread of infection because those with many partners are both more likely to acquire infection and more likely to transmit it to others.

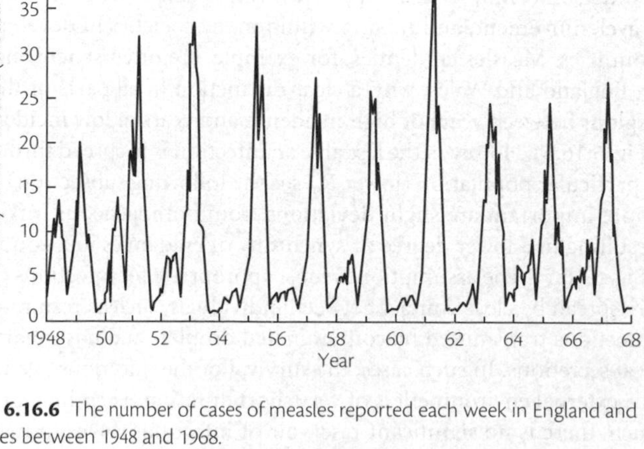

Fig. 6.16.6 The number of cases of measles reported each week in England and Wales between 1948 and 1968.
Source: Office of Population Census and Surveys, London.

Simple theory based on compartmental models of the transmission of infections such as gonorrhoea and HIV assumes that the net rate at which infection is spread in, for example, a male homosexual community, is determined by the proportion of infectious persons (Y/N, where N is the total size of the sexually active population) multiplied by the density of susceptibles, X, multiplied by a transmission coefficient, β. This coefficient is defined as the probability that a sexual contact (per partner) results in transmission, B, multiplied by the effective rate of sexual-partner change, c (which determines contacts). If the population mixed homogeneously, this effective rate would simply be the mean rate of sexual-partner change, m. When great heterogeneity in rates of partner change is present within a population, the effective rate must be defined in terms of this variability as well as the mean rate of activity. If we assume that the population is divided into classes with different rates of partner change and that partners are chosen (from any class) in proportion to their representation in the population multiplied by the rate of partner change in each group (an assumption of 'proportional mixing'; see Anderson *et al.* 1986; May & Anderson 1987; Garnett *et al.* 1992; Gupta & Anderson 1992), then the effective rate of partner change, c, is given by

$$c = m + (s^2/m) \qquad (6.16.14)$$

where m is the mean rate of partner change and s^2 is the variance in the rate

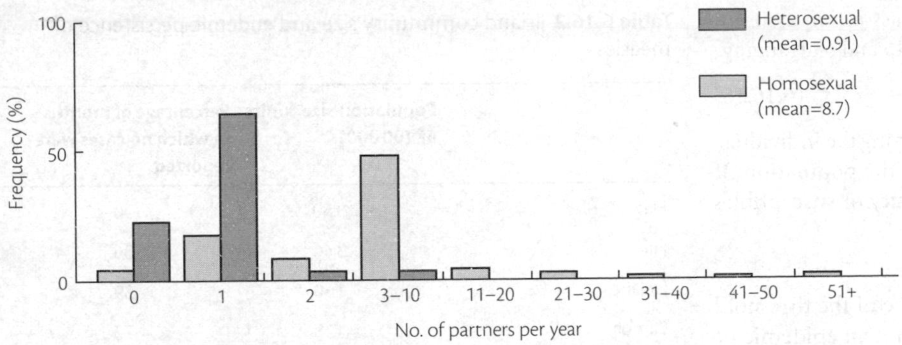

Fig. 6.16.8 Variation in the numbers of different sexual partners per year revealed from surveys of the male homosexual and the heterosexual communities in the United Kingdom, 1986 (Anderson, 1988). The skewed distribution observed in each instance (an indication that although the majority of individuals have few partners, a few have very many), and the mean rate of sexual-partner change (indicated), are both of significance to the perpetuation and rate of spread of sexually transmitted diseases in the community.

The importance of variability in contact is clear from this simple equation. For example, suppose the mean rate per year is unity but the variance is five times greater. If we assumed that homogeneous mixing occurred, our estimate of the effective rate would be 1, but if we take account of heterogeneity, the effective rate is six times as large. The influence of the small proportion of highly sexually active individuals on the overall transmission rate is very significant.

Transmission thresholds and the basic reproductive rate of infection

The basic reproductive rate of infection R_0

A key measure of the transmissibility of an infectious agent is provided by a parameter termed the basic reproductive rate (or also, in the literature, the basic reproduction number or ratio) and denoted by the symbol R_0. It measures the average number of secondary cases of infection generated by one primary case in a susceptible population. Its value is defined by the number of susceptibles present with which the primary case can come into contact, X, multiplied by the length of time the primary case is infectious to others, D, multiplied by the transmission coefficient, β (rate of effective mixing):

$$R_0 = \beta XD \qquad (6.16.15)$$

Note that R_0 is a dimensionless quantity (i.e. the units of measurement cancel out) that defines the potential to produce secondary cases (in a totally susceptible population) per generation time (i.e. the average duration of the infection).

The basic reproductive rate is of major epidemiological significance because the condition $R_0 = 1$ defines a transmission threshold below which the generation of secondary cases is insufficient to maintain the infection within the human community. For values above unity, the infection will trigger an epidemic and, with a continual input of susceptibles, will result in endemic persistence. A further quantity of interest is the effective reproductive rate, R, which defines the generation of secondary cases in a population that contains susceptibles and immunes (as opposed to just susceptible individuals). If the prevalence or incidence of infection is stable through time, R must equal unity in value, a situation in which each primary case gives rise, on average, to a single secondary infectious individual.

Factors that influence R_0

The simple expression $R_0 = \beta XD$ (appropriate for directly transmitted infections under the mass-action assumption) provides a framework for assessing how different epidemiological factors influence transmission success. Clearly, high transmission coefficients, long periods of infectiousness, and high densities of susceptibles enhance the generation of secondary cases. Note that its value depends not only on the properties that define the course of infection in an individual (i.e. the duration of infectiousness, D), but also on attributes of the host population such as the density of susceptibles, X, and the component of β that determines the rate of contact or mixing. A good example of the influence of population level characteristics is provided by the rate of transmission of the measles virus in urban centres in developed and developing countries. The more rapid rise in the proportion of children who have experienced infection, with age, in developing countries by comparison with developed regions is in part a consequence of higher population densities and poorer living conditions (McLean & Anderson 1988a).

Principles of control

The threshold condition for persistence of an infection, defined by $R_0 = 1$, captures the essence of the problem of control. To eradicate an infection, we must reduce the value of the basic reproductive rate below unity. Similarly, to reduce incidence, the value of R_0 must be reduced below the level that pertains prior to the introduction of control measures. Reductions can be achieved by reducing the infectious period D by, for example, the isolation of infectious persons (perhaps recognized by clinical symptoms of disease), reducing the number or density of susceptibles, usually by immunization, and by altering the social and behavioural factors that determine transmission such as improving living conditions to reduce overcrowding (in the case of sexually transmitted infections, education can serve to reduce rates of sexual-partner change or promote the use of condoms to lower the probability of transmission).

The threshold density of susceptibles

It is clear from the definition of R_0 given above that to maintain the value of the basic reproductive rate above unity the density of susceptibles in the population must exceed a critical value.

More precisely, this critical level X_T is (for the mass-action assumption) obtained by setting $R_0 = 1$ in Equation 6.16.15 and rearranging:

$$X_T = 1/\beta D \tag{6.16.16}$$

The aim of mass vaccination, aside from protecting the individual, is to lower the density of susceptible people in the population. If eradication is the aim of control, then the density of susceptibles must be reduced to less than X_T in value.

Critical community size

The magnitude of R_0 and, concomitantly, the size of the threshold density of susceptibles determines whether or not an epidemic of an infection will occur when introduced into a given community. In practice, however, for infections that induce lasting immunity in those who recover, the long-term endemic persistence of infection will depend on the renewal of the supply of susceptibles by new births or, to a lesser extent, by immigration. As such, the net birth rate in a community, which is itself dependent on the total population size or theoretically, as stated earlier, the incidence of cases of a sexually transmitted disease, will influence the likelihood of persistence. There is, therefore, a critical community size for the endemic persistence of a given infection. In certain island communities, immigration of susceptibles and infectious individuals may also play a role in the long-term persistence of a given infection (Anderson & May 1986, 1991; Black 1966). These factors are of growing significance as rates of population movement increase as a result of, for example, improved air transport services. Table 6.16.2 provides an example of the relationship between community size and the likelihood of the endemic persistence of the measles virus.

The concepts of a threshold density of susceptibles and a critical community size are most relevant for directly transmitted viral and bacterial infections that induce lasting (i.e. lifelong) immunity. The production of long-lived infective stages or the use of vectors (such as mosquitoes) lessens the importance of the human population density for the persistence of an infection. In the case of sexually transmitted infections, simple models suggest that there is no critical density of susceptibles for persistence because the magnitude of R_0 can be approximately given by:

$$R_0 = BcD \tag{6.16.17}$$

where c is the effective rate of sexual-partner change, D is the average duration of infectiousness, and B is the transmission probability per partner contact (Anderson *et al.* 1986).

This is simple to arrive at theoretically. If, as stated earlier, the incidence of cases of a sexually transmitted disease is defined as:

$$I = BcXY/N \tag{6.16.18}$$

then following the introduction of a single infectious person ($Y = 1$), infectious over a period D, into a totally susceptible population ($N = X$), the number of secondary cases will be represented by Equation 6.16.17. The dependence upon the number of susceptibles is lost. Biologically, this is more difficult to grasp, but it does seem reasonable that the rate of sexual-partner change should be more important to the potential for spread of a sexually transmitted disease than the number of susceptibles in the population.

Regulation of infection within human communities

The regulation (i.e. modulation or control) of the incidence or prevalence of a particular infection within a human community is largely determined by the level of herd immunity (i.e. the proportion of the population immune to infection) and the net rate of input of new susceptible individuals. A simple example serves to illustrate this point. Consider a closed population with no inflow or outflow of susceptible, infected, or immune individuals. If the densities of susceptibles, infecteds, and immunes at time t are defined by $X(t)$, $Y(t)$, and $Z(t)$, respectively, then under the mass-action assumption of transmission, the rates of change in the densities with respect to time can be captured by three coupled differential equations:

$$dX/dt = -\beta XY \tag{6.16.19}$$
$$dY/dt = \beta XY - \gamma Y \tag{6.16.20}$$
$$dZ/dt = \gamma Y \tag{6.16.21}$$

It is assumed, here, that there is no latent period of infection (individuals are infectious once infected), that the average duration of infectiousness is given by $D = 1/\gamma$, where γ is the rate of recovery from infection, that immunity is lifelong, and that no losses occur due to mortality. If we start with a totally susceptible population and introduce a few infecteds, the occurrence of an epidemic will depend upon the magnitude of the basic reproductive rate R_0 ($R_0 = \beta XD$) and, concomitantly, whether or not the density of susceptibles exceeds the critical threshold value X_T ($X_T = 1/\beta D$) (Fig 6.16.9). Assuming that R_0 is greater than unity, an epidemic will occur, but

Table 6.16.2 Island community size and endemic persistence of measles

	Population size (units of 100 000)	Percentage of months in which no cases were reported
Hawai	5.50	0
Fiji	3.46	36
Iceland	1.60	39
Samoa	1.18	72
Solomon	1.10	68
Fr. Polynesia	0.75	92
New Caledonia	0.68	68
Guam	0.63	20
Tonga	0.57	88
New Hebrides	0.52	70
Gilbert and Ellice	0.40	85
Greenland	0.28	76
Bermuda	0.41	49
Faroe	0.34	68
Cook	0.16	94
Niue	0.05	95
Nauru	0.03	95
St Helena	0.05	96
Falkland	0.02	100

Source: Anderson (1982b).

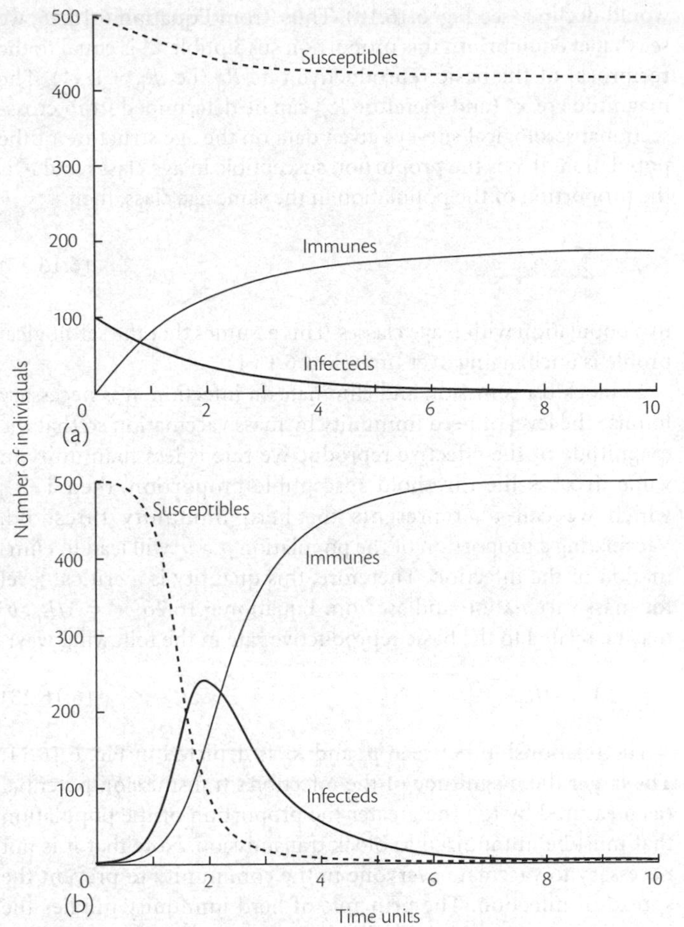

Fig. 6.16.9 Conditions for an epidemic. (a) Host density (susceptibles) below the threshold level (at time 0, $X = 500$, $Y = 100$, $Z = 0$, $\beta = 0.0001$, $\gamma = 1$, $R_0 = 0.005$, X_T 10000). (b) Host density above the threshold level (at time 0, $X = 500$, $Y = 1$, $Z = 0$, $\beta = 0.01$, $\gamma = 1$, $R_0 = 5$, $X_T = 100$).

as time progresses the density of susceptibles will decline ($X \rightarrow Y \rightarrow Z$) until the effective reproductive rate R is less than unity (i.e. susceptible numbers fall below the threshold X_T) and the infection dies out.

For the persistence of the infection, one of two things must happen. Firstly, suppose that susceptibles are continually introduced into the population at a net rate bN, where b is the per capita birth rate, and that natural mortalities occur in each class at a per capita rate μ. For simplicity, we further assume that net births exactly balance net deaths ($bN = \mu N$) to maintain the total population at a constant size. With these assumptions and provided that $R_0 \geq 1$, we find that the infection persists in the population (Fig. 6.16.10a) with an endemic equilibrium density of susceptibles again equal to X_T and equilibrium densities of infecteds, Y, and immunes, Z, given by:

$$Y^* = [\mu / (\mu + \gamma)]\,(N - X_T) \qquad (6.16.22)$$

$$Z^* = (\gamma / \mu) Y^* \qquad (6.16.23)$$

Secondly, suppose that there are no new births and no mortality but that immunity is of short duration such that individuals leave the immune class, Z, to regain the susceptible class, X, at a per capita rate α (alpha), where $1/\alpha$ is the average duration of immunity. We again find that the infection can persist (Fig. 6.16.10b) (provided that $R_0 \geq 1$) with equilibrium densities of infecteds and immunes of:

$$Y^* = [\alpha / (\alpha + \gamma)]\,(N - X_T) \qquad (6.16.24)$$

$$Z^* = (\gamma / \alpha) Y^* \qquad (6.16.25)$$

Note that the faster the loss of immunity (α is large) the higher the equilibrium density of infecteds and the lower Z^*.

These two examples show how the net input of susceptibles and the degree of herd immunity (as controlled by the duration of immunity to reinfection following recovery) influence the likelihood that an infection will persist endemically after the initial epidemic has swept through a susceptible population following the introduction of an infection. In these simple models of the transmission of direct-contact infections, the density of infecteds tends to exhibit oscillatory behaviour after the introduction of infection due to the rise and fall in the density of susceptibles taking the effective reproductive rate above and below unity in value.

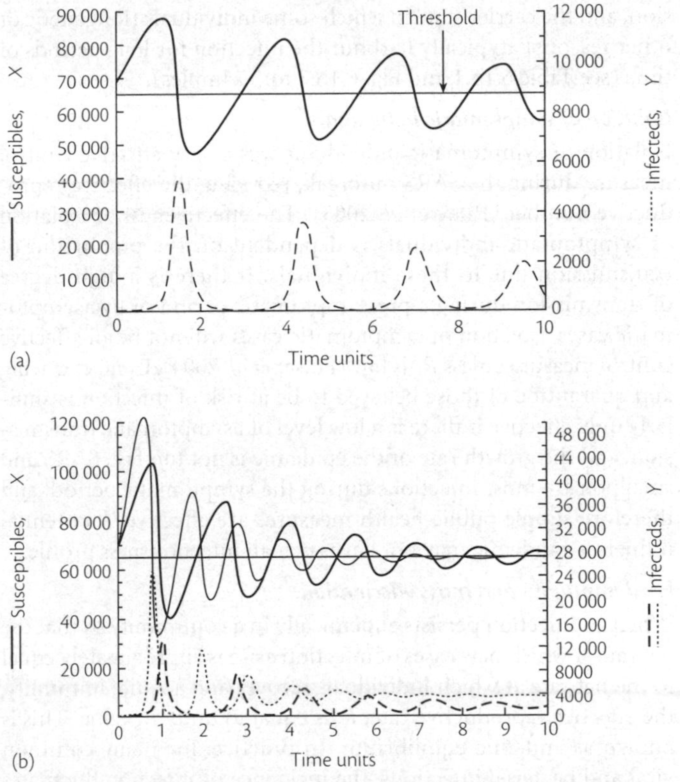

Fig. 6.16.10 Conditions for the persistence of an infection in a community. In each case solid curves represent susceptible numbers and dashed lines are infected. (a) Renewal of susceptibles by births (initial conditions: $X = 70000$, $Y = 1$, $Z = 930000$, $\beta = 0.0004$, $\gamma = 26$, $\mu = 0.02$, $\alpha = 0$, $R_0 = \beta N/(\mu + \gamma) \simeq 15$, $X = 65050$). Notice that the numbers of susceptibles oscillates above and below the threshold susceptible number, X_T (marked) and that each epidemic starts when susceptible numbers exceed the threshold, X_T, and subsequently decays as susceptibles fall below the threshold, X_T. Oscillations of X and Y (and Z, not shown) gradually damp over time towards the predicted equilibrium values X^*, Y^*, and Z^* (see text), (b) Renewal of susceptibles through waning immunity, at rate α of 0.05 (thick lines) or 0.1 (thin lines) (corresponding average durations of immunity are 20 and 10 units of time respectively) (other initial settings as for (a) above except for no mortality, i.e. $\mu = 0$). Notice that for the two different rates of loss of immunity the equilibrium susceptible numbers are the same ($X^* = X_T$) since waning immunity has no impact on R_0. However, a higher rate of loss of immunity does result in an increase in numbers of infecteds at equilibrium, Y^*.

These oscillations are seen to damp down, settling to the equilibrium values given analytically (e.g. Equations 6.16.22–6.16.25). This propensity to exhibit oscillatory behaviour is more apparent if the infection is of short duration such that infection prevalence is sensitive to the availability of susceptibles and induces long-lasting immunity as it takes some time, under these circumstances, for new births or loss of immunity replenish the supply of susceptibles such that R is again above unity in value. Maintenance of these oscillations over the longer period would require a force to be applied periodically—in reality, this might be derived from seasonal changes in mixing rates as a result of school opening and closing. In Fig. 6.16.10, it should be noted that the numbers infected, Y, are always increasing when susceptibles, X, exceed the threshold X_T (thus $R < 1$) and are always on the decrease when $X < X_T$ (when $R < 1$). Hence, infection is being driven by the availability of susceptibles.

Other factors that can promote long-term persistence include the production of infective stages that are able to survive for long periods in the external environment, sexual transmission, vertical transmission (from mother to unborn offspring), vector transmission, and the carrier state in which some individuals (for genetic or other reasons) atypically harbour the infection for long periods of time (see Table 6.16.1 and Fig. 6.16.3 for examples).

Isolation of symptomatic individuals

Isolation of symptomatic individuals was a very effective control measure during the SARS outbreak, reducing the effective reproductive number (Riley *et al.* 2003). The effectiveness of isolation of symptomatic individuals is dependent on the proportion of transmission due to these individuals. If there is a high degree of transmission during a pre-symptomatic period or by asymptomatic cases, isolation of symptomatic cases will not be an effective control measure unless R_0 is low (Fraser *et al.* 2004). Contact tracing and quarantine of those believed to be at risk of infection is similarly only effective if there is a low level of asymptomatic transmission, and the growth rate of the epidemic is not too fast. SARS and smallpox are most infectious during the symptomatic period, and therefore simple public health measures are effective. A potential influenza pandemic may not have such an infectiousness profile.

Herd immunity and mass vaccination

When an infection persists endemically in a community so that the net rate at which new cases of infection arise is approximately equal to the net rate at which individuals recover and acquire immunity, the effective reproductive rate, R, is equal to unity in value. This is known as endemic equilibrium. In practice, for many common viral and bacterial infections, the incidence of infection fluctuates both on seasonal and longer-term cycles. The effective reproductive rate therefore fluctuates below and above unity in value as the incidence and density of susceptibles change (see Figs. 6.16.6. and 6.16.10). However, the average value over a series of incidence cycles (both seasonal and longer term) will be approximately equal to unity in the absence of control intervention or changing social and demographic patterns. The effective reproductive rate is reduced below the basic reproductive rate in relation to the fraction of contacts that are with susceptible individuals $x = X/N$, that is, by the simple equation:

$$R = R_0 x \tag{6.16.26}$$

At equilibrium, when R is on average unity, the proportion susceptible represents a threshold, x^*, below which infection rates would decline (see Fig. 6.16.10). Thus, from Equation 6.16.26, we see that at equilibrium this proportion susceptible x^* is equal to the reciprocal of the basic reproductive rate R_0 (i.e. $R_0 \approx 1/x^*$). The magnitude of x^* (and therefore R_0) can be determined from cross-sectional serological surveys given data on the age structure of the population. If x_i is the proportion susceptible in age class i and p_i is the proportion of the population in the same age class, then:

$$x^* = \sum_{i=1}^{n} x_i p_i \tag{6.16.27}$$

in a population with n age classes. This assumes that the serological profile is unchanging over time (Box 6.16.1).

To block transmission and eliminate an infection, it is necessary to raise the level of herd immunity by mass vaccination so that the magnitude of the effective reproductive rate is less than unity in value. If x^* is the threshold susceptible proportion, then $1-x^*$, which we call p_c, represents the herd immunity threshold. Vaccinating a proportion of the population $p > p_c$ will lead to elimination of the infection. Therefore, this quantity is a critical level for mass vaccination and as, from Equation 6.16.26, $x^* = 1/R_0$, p_c may be related to the basic reproductive rate in the following way:

$$p_c = 1 - 1/R_0. \tag{6.16.28}$$

The relationship between p_c and R_0 is depicted in Fig. 6.16.11: The larger the magnitude of the infection's transmission potential (as measured by R_0) the greater the proportion of the population that must be immunized to block transmission. Note that it is not necessary to vaccinate everyone in the community to prevent the spread of infection. The principle of herd immunity implies the indirect protection of the individual conferred by the protection (i.e. vaccination) of the population. The mechanism underlying this concept is that of the critical density of susceptibles required to maintain the magnitude of the reproductive rate above unity in value.

Age at vaccination

In general, immunization programmes are introduced by focusing on cohorts of children so that the level of immunization coverage

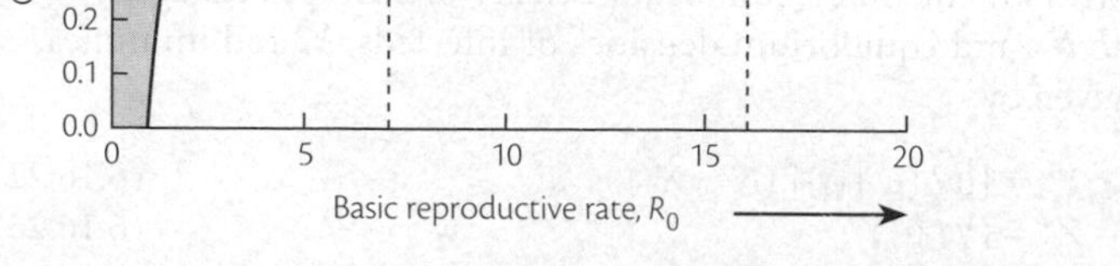

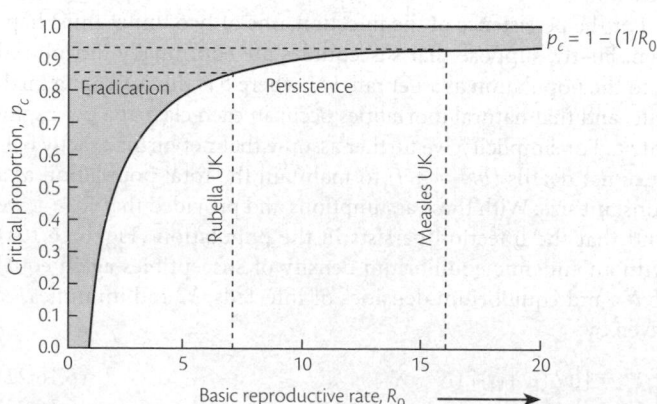

Fig. 6.16.11 Relationship between the proportion of the population vaccinated at or near birth and the likelihood of an infection persisting or, alternatively, being eliminated. Infectious agents with high basic reproductive rates in defined communities will be more difficult to control by mass vaccination as illustrated by the example of measles and rubella in the United Kingdom.
Source: Nokes and Anderson (1988).

is built up over many years of routine vaccination, that is, as children pass some age gateway. In these circumstances, p_c of Equation 6.16.28 must be interpreted as the proportion of each cohort vaccinated as soon after birth as is practically feasible, taking account of the need to immunize after the decay in maternally derived specific antibody. For most viral infections, the average duration of protection against infection provided by maternal antibodies is approximately six months. Clearly, it will take many years of cohort immunization to achieve the desired level of artificially induced herd immunity. A further complication is that it is often the case that the average age at vaccination is higher than what is epidemiologically ideal, resulting from the desire to link vaccination with a delivery opportunity (such as first attendance at school) or variation in the age of delivery resulting perhaps from inefficiency in the coordination system or motivation of the population. In this case, simple mathematical models suggest that the level of vaccination coverage required to eradicate the infection under a policy that vaccinates (with a vaccine with 100 per cent efficacy) at an average age of V years is:

$$p > [1 + (V/L)] / [1 + (A/L)] \quad (6.16.29)$$

where L is human life expectancy and A is the average age at which the infection was acquired prior to the introduction of vaccination (Anderson & May 1983). It is clear from this expression that transmission cannot be interrupted unless the average age at vaccination, V, is less than the average age at infection, A, prior to control.

Imperfect vaccines

Various forms of vaccine failure can be specified. At the time of delivery, only a proportion of individuals may respond by generating protective immunity post-immunization. This has been called vaccine 'take' (McLean & Blower 1993). In addition, a proportion of those who initially 'take' still may not be able to fend off an infection if exposed. This might be thought of as an exposure–dose-dependent phenomenon, and a vaccine exhibiting this effect might be said to provide only a 'degree' of protection. Finally, vaccine-induced immunity may wane with the passing of time such that a previously protected individual once again becomes susceptible. Therefore, a vaccine may only confer protection for a particular duration.

The impact of these three vaccine failings is to reduce the effectiveness or impact of a specified level of vaccination coverage and therefore increase the level of coverage required to achieve elimination of the infection. This new required vaccination proportion, $p\hat{}$, of an imperfect vaccine, may be related to the critical proportion that needs to be effectively vaccinated for elimination, p_c, in the form:

$$p\hat{} = p_c/\varphi \quad (6.16.30)$$

where φ is the effective vaccine efficacy,[61] defined as:

$$\varphi = \omega_1\omega_2\,[\mu / (\mu + \omega_3)] \quad (6.16.31)$$

Here, ω_1 is the 'take', ω_2 is the 'degree', $1/\omega_3$ is the 'duration' (where ω_3 is the rate of waning vaccine-induced immunity), and μ is the death rate. The effects of 'take' and 'degree' are clearly going to be in direct proportion to their magnitude. For example, if a vaccine is being used to interrupt transmission of an infection with an 0 value of 10 (for which, from Equation 6.16.28, the critical proportion to be effectively immunized, p_c, is 0.9) but only 90 per cent of those vaccinated respond (i.e. $\omega 1 = 0.9$), then the new proportion needing to be vaccinated is $0.9/0.9 = 1.0$, that is, 100 per cent coverage. The effect of a vaccine waning over time is less obvious but may be seen from Fig. 6.16.12. Here, vaccine impact f due to the waning immunity effect (for a vaccine which has perfect 'take' and 'degree') is related to the rate of loss of vaccine-induced immunity, expressed as the time taken for 10 per cent of those vaccinated to lose protection. We can see from this graph that even a slight waning of immunity may cause a very significant reduction in the impact of a vaccine; for example, if 10 per cent of those effectively vaccinated at birth lose their immunity by age 30 years, vaccine impact is reduced by 20 per cent (i.e. $\varphi = 0.8$ from Fig. 6.16.12), and in our example of an infection with $R_0 = 10$, 100 per cent vaccination in infants would not be sufficient to eliminate transmission.

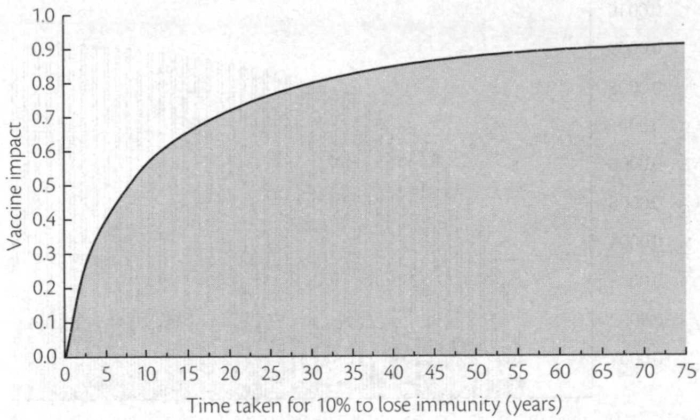

Fig. 6.16.12 The impact of an imperfect vaccine. The time taken for 10 per cent of individuals to lose their immunity after vaccination is related to the impact of a vaccine, $\phi = \mu/(\mu + \omega)$ (the vaccine is assumed to have perfect 'take' and 'degree'). Here, the proportion whose immunity has waned in τ years, p_τ is related to the rate of loss of immunity by the expression $p_\tau = \exp(-\omega\tau)$.

As a final note of caution, the components that make up the term vaccine impact, φ, have a compounding effect because they are multiplied by one another. Thus, even if each is individually of little significance, the compounded effect on impact may still be very significant.

The prevalence of infection and the basic reproductive rate

A further epidemiological feature arising from the existence of a critical density of susceptibles to maintain infection concerns the relationship between the magnitude of the basic reproductive rate and the prevalence of infection in a population in which the infectious agent persists endemically. As depicted in Fig. 6.16.13, simple models predict that the relationship is non-linear, so that a marked reduction in the endemic prevalence or incidence will only occur as the transmission potential is reduced to an extent where it approaches the threshold level $R_0 = 1$. The practical implication is that we should not expect the decline in the incidence of infection induced by mass vaccination to be directly proportional to the level of vaccination coverage. The greatest changes are predicted to occur when coverage attains high levels.

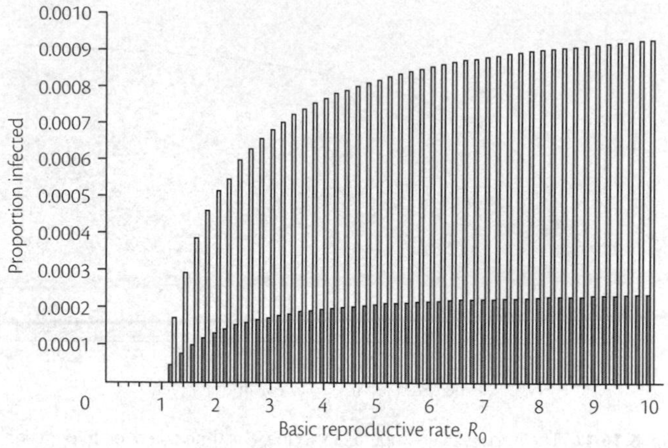

Fig. 6.16.13 Predicted changes in the equilibrium proportion of a population infected (i.e. the stable endemic prevalence of an infection) as the transmission potential of the microparasitic agent varies. For infections where there is no loss of immunity, the level of the plateau of prevalence is dependent upon the rate of input of new susceptibles (i.e. the birth rate, *b*) and the duration of infectiousness, $1/\gamma$. In the figure, $b = 1/75$ per year and $\gamma = 52$ per year (i.e. a 1-week infectious period) (closed bars) or $\gamma = 13$ per year (i.e. a 4-week period) (open bars). An important point to observe is that the greatest changes in the proportion infected occur over the first few increments of R_0 (irrespective of the magnitude of *b* or γ.)

Inter-epidemic period *T*

Many viral and bacterial infections that induce lasting immunity to reinfection and which have high transmission potentials (large R_0) tend to exhibit oscillatory fluctuations in incidence. A good example is that of measles, which in the United Kingdom prior to mass vaccination oscillated on a seasonal basis (owing to the aggregation and disaggregation of children for school term and holiday periods, respectively) and a longer-term two-year cycle with years of high incidence separated by years of low incidence (Anderson *et al.* 1984) (Fig. 6.16.6). Time-series analyses reveal that these longer-term cycles for infections such as measles, mumps, rubella, and pertussis are not due to chance fluctuations but arise as a result of the dynamic interaction between the net rates of acquisition of infection and immunity on recovery.

Simple models based on the mass-action assumption suggest that the inter-epidemic period, *T*, of the longer-term cycles is determined by the generation time of the infection, *k*, defined as the sum of the latent and infectious periods and the transmission potential of the infection inversely measured by the average age at infection, *A*, where

$$T=2\pi(Ak)^{1/2} \qquad (6.16.32)$$

This simple prediction matches well the observation for a variety of common childhood infections prior to mass vaccination (i.e. the two-year cycles of measles, the three-year cycles of mumps, the four- to five-year cycles of rubella, and the three- to four-year cycles of pertussis). Non-seasonal oscillation arises as a consequence of the exhaustion of a supply of susceptibles, as an epidemic passes through a population, plus the time lag that arises before new births replenish the pool to trigger the next epidemic. As such, the inter-epidemic period is also influenced by the birth rate of the community (which influences the average age of infection, *A*, in Equation 6.16.32). For example, in developing countries such as Kenya with high birth rates, measles tends to cycle on a one-year time scale in urban centres as opposed to the two-year cycle in the United Kingdom prior to control (McLean & Anderson 1988b).

Parameter estimation

Survey data

Survey data on the incidence or prevalence of infection (past or current) can be obtained in a variety of ways. Longitudinal (i.e. through time) data can be acquired by monitoring a cohort of people through time and recording infection as it occurs. Horizontal (i.e. one point in time) and cross-sectional (i.e. across age and sex classes) data can be acquired by a survey at one point in time or over a short interval of time, by the examination of different age classes within the population. Such surveys are of most use when based on serological examinations to determine the proportion of individuals in a given age class who have antibodies specific to the antigens of a particular infectious agent. These cross-sectional serological profiles reflect the proportion in each age class who have, at some time in the past, experienced infection. Case-notification data stratified by age and sex, and recorded over a set interval of time such as one year, can be accumulated to indicate what proportion of the cases occurs by any given age. This may then be used to infer changes in the proportion who experience infection as a function of age. Such data are clearly less reliable than serological information because they are dependent on a lack of bias in reporting efficiency by age class. Bias is to be expected if the seriousness of the disease induced by infection changes with age (e.g. rubella in women and mumps in men) or where the incidence of subclinical (i.e. undetectable) infections is age dependent.

An alternative to the use of serum for the detection of specific antibodies to infectious agents is saliva. More specifically, when looking for systemic antibodies (e.g. IgG and IgM), the fluid that collects around the gums and under the tongue (as distinct from salivary gland secretions) is rich in serum antibodies. This is known as gingivocrevicular exudate or secretion. The disadvantage of using salivary fluid for antibody detection is the low concentration of immunoglobulin it contains relative to serum. IgG in whole saliva is approximately 1000-fold less concentrated than in serum, although in crevicular fluid it may only be five-fold more dilute (Mortimer & Parry 1991). In recent years, highly sensitive assays have been developed to overcome the dilution problems and, accompanied by developments in devices for the collection of crevicular fluid samples, have now been successfully employed in the detection of antibodies to a variety of infections, including measles, rubella, and mumps (Perry *et al.* 1993; Brown *et al.* 1994), human parvovirus, hepatitis B virus (core antibodies) (Parry *et al.* 1989), and HIV (Holmstrom *et al.* 1990; Behets *et al.* 1991; van den Akker *et al.* 1992).

The advantages of using saliva over serum are numerous and associated largely with the collection procedure. For example, sampling is non-invasive and is more acceptable, which will assist in response level, the collection process is easier and can be carried out by non-technical personnel, and there is lower risk to both subject and investigator (Mortimer & Parry 1991). Surveys based on saliva collection offer great potential in the fields of epidemiology and surveillance, including the measurement of population immunity in the evaluation of the impact of vaccination programmes on infection prevalence in assessing the rate of spread of infections, such as HIV, through communities. The opportunity for longitudinal surveillance will be beneficial to studies of spatial and temporal patterns of disease spread and salivary diagnosis will become increasingly useful in outbreak investigation and control.

When conducting surveys, a number of points should be borne in mind. Firstly, sample sizes should be as large as practically possible, finely stratified by age (preferably infants to elderly people). How large will depend upon what we wish the accuracy or power (see Sokal & Rohlf 1981) of subsequent analyses to be, but 25–50 per yearly age class is a rough working estimate. Secondly, the incidence of infection may oscillate on a seasonal or longer-term basis. As such, it is good practice to carry out surveys that span epidemic and inter-epidemic years. Thirdly, systematic changes through time may occur in a given population due to social, behavioural, economic, or other changes. Examples include the observed reduction in the incidence of hepatitis A in northern European countries over the past few decades due to improved standards of hygiene and the rise in the incidence of gonorrhoea in certain developed countries during the 1960s and 1970s due to changes in sexual behaviour (e.g. increased rates of sexual-partner change). Basic reproductive rates and rates of infection may therefore change through time irrespective of the impact of control measures.

The basic reproductive rate of infection

The individual estimation of the component parameters that determine the magnitude of the basic reproductive rate, R_0, is fraught with many problems. In the case of directly transmitted viral and bacterial infections, we require a knowledge of the transmission coefficient, β, the density of susceptibles, X, and the average duration of infectiousness. In practice, it is often easier to use indirect methods to arrive at estimates of R_0 by employing serological data finely stratified by age. As discussed in relation to Equation 6.16.13, measurements of the proportion susceptible to infection at different ages, $x(a)$, provide estimates of the age-dependent forces of infection, $\lambda(a)$. These in turn can be used to obtain an estimate of the average age, A, at which an individual typically acquires infection. Mathematical models can be used to define a relationship between the magnitude of R_0 and the average age at infection. In the simplest case, the relationship is of the form

$$R_0 = Q/A \qquad (6.16.33)$$

where Q denotes the reciprocal of the net birth rate of the community

In developed countries where net births are approximately equal to net deaths, the quality Q is equal to the average life expectancy (from birth) L (Anderson & May 1985a). More generally, if maternally derived antibodies provide protection for an average of F years, R_0 is related to A by the expression

$$R_0 = Q\,/\,(A - F) \qquad (6.16.34)$$

A simple example of the use of this equation is provided by the transmission of the measles virus in the United Kingdom prior to the introduction of mass vaccination. In this case, the values of A, L, and F were 5 years, 75 years, and 0.5 years, respectively, leading to an R_0 estimate of between 16 and 17. The inverse relationship between R_0 and A makes good intuitive sense—infections with high transmission potentials will tend to have low average ages at infection and vice versa. These notions are depicted in Box 6.16.1, and Table 6.16.3 lists some estimates of R_0, A, L, and the critical

Table 6.16.3 Epidemiological parameters for a variety of childhood infections in developed countries in the absence of mass vaccination

Infection	Average age at infection A (years)	Location and date	Data type	Life expectancy L (years)	R_0[a]	p_c (%)
Measles	5.0	England & Wales, 1948–68	Case notifications	70	15.6	94
	5.5	United States, large families, 1957	Serology	70	14.0	93
	8.0	United States, small families, 1957	Serology	70	9.3	89
Whooping cough	4.5	England & Wales, 1944–78[b]	Case notifications	70	17.5	94
	4.9	United States, urban, 1908–17	Case notifications	60	13.6	93
	6.5	United States, rural, 1908–17	Case notifications	60	10.0	90
Chicken pox	8.6	United States, urban, 1913–17	Case notifications	60	7.4	86
	6.8	United States, urban, 1943	Case notifications	70	11.1	91
Mumps	7.0	United Kingdom, urban, 1977	Serology	75	11.5	91
	5.7	Netherlands, urban, 1980	Serology	75	14.4	93
	9.9	United States, urban, 1943	Case notifications	70	7.4	86
Diphtheria	10.4	United States, 1912–28	Case notifications	60	6.1	84
Rubella	10.8	England, urban, 1980–84[c]	Serology	75	7.3	86
	10.2	East Germany, 1972	Serology	70	7.2	86
Scarlet fever	8.0	United States, urban, 1908–17	Case notifications	60	8.0	88
	12.3	United States, rural, 1918–19	Case notifications	60	5.1	80

Parameter definitions given in text (data from a variety of sources).

[a] $R_0 = L/(A-F)$ where F is duration of maternally derived protection, assumed to last for 6 months in all cases. Note that no consideration of age-dependent forces of infection is given (see text).

[b] Encroaches on to vaccination era.

[c] Male serology—only females vaccinated under selective immunization policy.

level of vaccination coverage to block transmission, p_c, for a variety of common infectious agents in defined localities.

An alternative method to that outlined in the preceding is based on the prediction of simple models that the magnitude of R_0 is related to the fraction of the population susceptible to infection, x^*, when the infection has attained its endemic equilibrium. The relationship is simply

$$R_0 = 1/x^* \qquad (6.16.35)$$

and arises from the fact that at equilibrium the effective reproductive rate is equal to unity in value (see Equation 6.16.26). Note that Equations 6.16.33 and 6.16.35 imply that the average age at infection, A, is inversely related to the equilibrium fraction of susceptibles in a population, x^*, required to ensure each primary case gives rise on average to at least one secondary case (see Box 6.16.1). In general, however, the method based on estimating the average age at infection is the better one given good age-stratified serological data.

Latent and infectious periods

Two sources of data are available to estimate latent and infectious periods. The first is derived from clinical, virological, and immunological studies of the course of infection in individual patients. For some common microparasitic infections, the presence of the infectious agent in host tissues, excretions, and secretions can be directly assessed. Durations of antigenaemia in body fluids and secretions or of infective particles in specific cells will, in many instances, reflect the period over which an infected person is infectious to others (although this is, of course, not always the case as, for example, with the latent herpes viruses).

Alternatively, statistical methods can be employed in the study of transmission within small groups of individuals. The classic data on measles, collected by Hope Simpson (1952) in the Cirencester area of England during the years 1946–52, record the distribution of the observed time interval between two cases of measles in 219 families with two children under the age of 15 years. The bulk of these observations represent case-to-case transmissions within a family. However, in a small number of families, in which the observed interval is only a few days, it may be assumed that these cases are double primaries, that is, both children having been simultaneously infected from some outside source. Statistical methods, based on chain binomial models, can be used to derive estimates of the latent, infectious, and incubation periods (Bailey 1973). A rough guide to these periods for various common viral and bacterial infections is presented in Table 6.16.4. Some of these estimates are based on detailed analyses of case-to-case data whereas others are more speculative.

Sexually transmitted infections

Rather different problems in parameter estimation, to those outlined in the preceding, are presented by sexually transmitted infections. By way of illustration and given the topicality of the infection, we focus on HIV. The characteristics of most sexually transmitted diseases cause their epidemiology to differ from that of common childhood viral and bacterial infections. Firstly, the rate at which new infections are produced does not appear to be closely correlated with population density. Secondly, the carrier phenomenon in which certain individuals harbour asymptomatic infection is often important. Thirdly, many sexually transmitted diseases induce little or no acquired immunity on recovery. Fourthly, net transmission depends on the degree of heterogeneity in sexual activity prevailing in the population and the degree to which individuals in one sexual activity class (perhaps defined in terms of the rate of sexual-partner change) mix with those in the same and in different classes (i.e. 'who has sex with whom').

The basic reproductive rate, R_0, in its simplest form is determined by the transmission probability, B, multiplied by the effective rate of sexual-partner change, c, multiplied by the average duration of infectiousness, D. Heterogeneity in sexual activity is a major influence on the magnitude of transmission success. Recent national surveys of sexual attitudes and lifestyles suggest that most people have few different sexual partners and a few have many (ACSF 1992; Anderson & May 1988; Johnson *et al.* 1994). The distributions of reported numbers of sexual partners per defined period of time therefore tend to be skewed, with a long right-hand tail where a few individuals report many partners (Fig. 6.16.14). As pointed out earlier, under these circumstances the variance in partner numbers, s^2,

Table 6.16.4 Average duration of infection classes for a variety of microparasites

Infectious disease	Latent period $1/\sigma$ (days)	Infectious period $1/\gamma$ (days)	Incubation period[a] (days)
Measles	6–9	6–7	11–14
Chicken pox	8–12	10–11	13–17
Rubella	7–14	11–12	16–20
Hepatitis A	13–17	19–22	30–37
Mumps	12–18	4–8	12–26
Polio	1–3	14–20	7–12
Smallpox	8–11	2–3	10–12
Influenza	1–3	2–3	1–3
Scarlet fever	1–2	14–21	2–3
Whooping cough	6–7	21–23	7–10
Diphtheria	2–5	14–21	2–5

[a]Time to appearance of symptoms.
Source: Anderson (1982b).

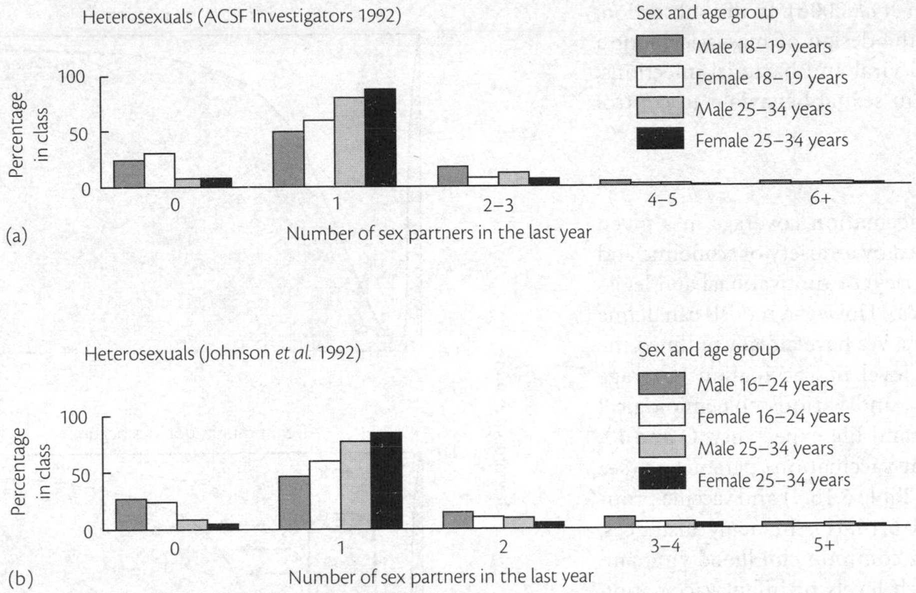

Fig. 6.16.14 Frequency distributions of the reported number of different sexual partners over the previous year in two surveys in (a) France (ACSF 1992) and (b) Britain (Johnson et al. 1992) of sexual attitudes and lifestyles, stratified by age and sex. The similarities in the results of the two surveys are striking.

is much greater in value than the mean, m, and the effective rate of sexual partner change, c, is defined as $c = m + (s^2/m)$ (as in Equation 6.16.14). It follows that those with high rates of sexual-partner change play a disproportionate role (relative to their proportional representation in a community) in the spread of infection. In the case of HIV, each component of R_0 is difficult to measure due to the sensitivity and the practical difficulties associated with the study of sexual behaviour and the long and variable incubation period of the disease, AIDS, induced by the infection. Over the long incubation period, infectiousness appears to vary widely for an individual and between individuals (Fraser *et al.* 2007).

More generally, certain of the parameters that determine the magnitude of R_0 may vary between the sexes. This is certainly the case for gonorrhoea (Hethcote & Yorke 1984), and it may be true for HIV. In these circumstances, when considering transmission via heterosexual contact, the basic reproductive rate adopts the form:

$$R_0 = (B_1 B_2 c_1 c_2 D_1 D_2) \qquad (6.16.36)$$

where the subscripts 1 and 2 denote males and females, respectively.

Further complications arise in the definition of the case reproductive number, R_0, when we take into account the pattern of mixing between different strata of the sexually active population. For example, in light of the data presented in Fig. 6.16.14 concerning heterogeneity in reported rates of sexual-partner acquisition per year in France and Britain, it seems sensible to stratify the population by the rate of sexual-partner change into low-, medium-, and high-'activity' classes. The magnitude of any epidemics of a sexually transmitted disease and the endemic level of infection in a community will depend on the degree to which the small number of people with high rates of sexual-partner change mix with the medium- and low-activity classes. If mixing is random across activity classes, the infection will be widely disseminated in the community. However, if mixing is highly assortative (i.e. like with like), the infection will tend to be restricted to the small proportion of individuals in the high-activity class (the so-called 'core' group) with a few cases in the other classes. The prevailing pattern of mixing is therefore of great importance in determining the prevalence of a sexually transmitted disease and the degree to which it is disseminated in a defined community. Recent studies of mixing patterns based on contact tracing via sexually transmitted disease clinics suggest that mixing is more assortative than random in character (Garnett & Anderson 1993). Once mixing is taken into account, it is necessary to redefine transmission success in terms of the number of secondary cases of infection in group i generated by contact with infectives in group j, R_{0ij}, where

$$R_{0ij} = p_{ij} BcD \qquad (6.16.37)$$

Here, p_{ij} is the probability that a susceptible in group i has a sexual contact with someone in group j. Again, more generally, the population is structured by other variables such as age, ethnicity, area of residence, and educational attainment. Here again, behavioural studies suggest a degree of assortative mixing with respect to the choice of sexual partner—except in contact with commercial sex workers.

Models and the design of control programmes

Mathematical models can be of help in defining the targets for a control programme, in interpreting observed epidemiological changes under the impact of control, and in discriminating between different approaches (Garnett *et al.* 1992; Gupta & Anderson 1992; Nokes & Anderson 1987, 1988, 1991, 1992, 1993) Epidemiological models have played a key role in the design and evaluation of control programmes during the SARS (Lipsitch *et al.* 2003; Riley *et al.* 2003), FMD (Ferguson *et al.* 2001; Keeling *et al.* 2001) and BSE and vCJD (Anderson *et al.* 1996; Ferguson *et al.* 2002; Ghani *et al.* 2003) outbreaks and in pandemic influenza planning (Longini *et al.* 2004;

Ferguson *et al.* 2005; Hollingsworth *et al.* 2006). In this subsection, we consider two themes, namely, the design of mass vaccination programmes to control childhood viral and bacterial infections, and education to induce changes in sexual behaviour to control sexually transmitted diseases.

Impact of mass vaccination

In practical terms, the level of vaccination coverage in a given community or country is determined by a variety of economic and logistical factors (developing countries) or motivational and legislative issues (industrialized countries). However, models can define the ideal goal of a given programme. We have already outlined the relationship between the critical level of vaccination coverage required to block transmission, p_c, and various epidemiological (R_0), demographic (net birth rate and life expectancy, Q and L), and logistical (V, the average age at vaccination) parameters (see Equations 6.16.28 and 6.16.29, and Table 6.16.3) and vaccine properties (see Equations 6.16.30 and 6.16.31). In many instances, the high transmission potentials of common childhood viral and bacterial infections imply very high levels of infant vaccination coverage if transmission is to be interrupted. If vaccine efficacy is less than 100 per cent (e.g. the current pertussis vaccines), then problems may arise in attaining these targets even if legislation enforces vaccination of all children before entry to school (as in the United States). Models emphasize the point that to obtain the best effects very high levels of coverage should be aimed at with vaccination at as young an age as is practically feasible given the complications presented by the presence of maternally derived antibodies in infants.

Aside from defining targets for vaccination coverage, models can assist in interpreting the impact of a given programme on epidemiological parameters such as the incidence of infection, the average age at infection, and the inter-epidemic period. In a later part of this subsection we consider the principles underlying an alternative approach to mass vaccine intervention, that of pulsed immunization across age cohorts, which has recently met with such success in controlling polio and measles in Central and South America.

Incidence of infection

Immunization has the direct effect of reducing the number of cases of infection as a result of the protection of the vaccinated individuals ($X \rightarrow Z$; see Fig. 6.16.3d). Because this reduces the number of infectious persons in the vaccinated population, an indirect effect is a reduction in the net rate of transmission of the virus or bacterium. This is the principle of herd immunity, where susceptibles gain protection from the vaccinated proportion of the population. Provided the infection is able to persist endemically (i.e. the level of coverage is less than that required for eradication), models suggest that the equilibrium proportion of susceptibles in the population will remain constant irrespective of the level of coverage below the critical point for eradication. This prediction is illustrated in Fig. 6.16.15. The level of coverage simply reduces the proportion of seropositive individuals who have acquired immunity via infection as opposed to via vaccination. As mentioned earlier (see Fig. 6.16.13), the manner in which the incidence declines as the level of coverage rises is non-linear in form with the most dramatic reductions occurring as the proportion vaccinated approaches the critical point for the interruption of transmission. As the level of coverage approaches the critical point, the proportion of immune persons who possess vaccine-induced immunity approaches unity.

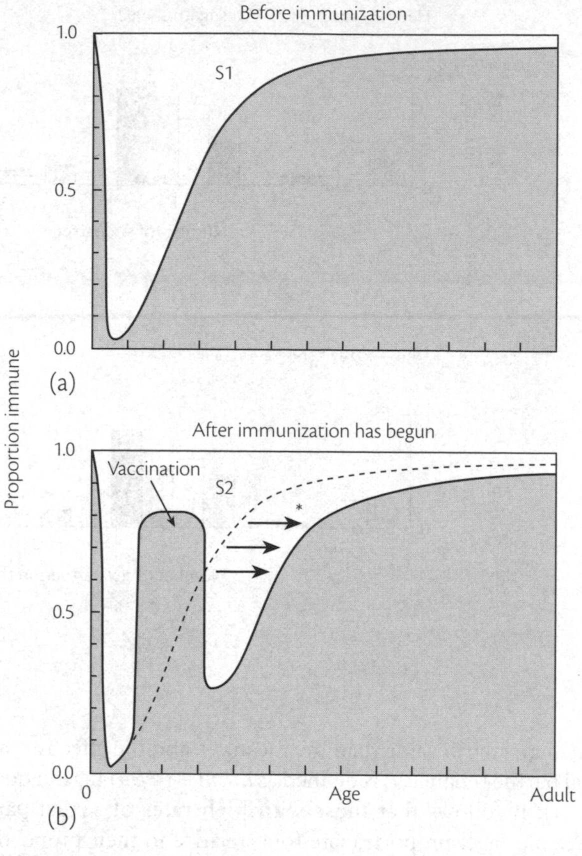

Fig. 6.16.15 Diagrammatic representation of the predicted impact of mass immunization (against a typical childhood viral or bacterial infection) on the age distribution of susceptibility in a population. Before immunization (a) there is a 'valley' of susceptibles (S1) in the young age classes. Attempts to fill in this valley by vaccination (b) reduces the rate of transmission of the infection thus lowering the probability of unvaccinated individuals being infected. As a consequence there is an upward shift in the ages of susceptibles (*) from that pertaining before vaccination (dotted line). Two points are important: (i) the number or proportion of susceptibles after immunization has begun (area S2) is roughly unchanged from that which existed before immunization (area S1) and (ii) the average age of susceptibles increases.
Source: Nokes and Anderson 1988.

The average age at infection

As a direct result of reducing the net rate of transmission, vaccination acts to increase the average age at which susceptibles acquire infection over that pertaining prior to control (i.e. by reducing the probability of coming into contact with an infectious person). Observation now bears out the expectation of an increased average age of susceptibles and of infection as a result of mass vaccination programmes. The example in Fig. 6.16.16 shows the pre-vaccination (1982) serological profile (or distribution of susceptibles by age) for rubella in Finland (Fig. 6.16.16a) and the profile (for males only) in 1986, four years after mass infant measles, mumps, and rubella (MMR) vaccine was introduced (Fig. 6.16.16b) (Ukkonen & Von Bonsdorf 1988). The similarity with Fig. 6.16.15 is striking. Also shown in Fig. 6.16.16 is the changing distribution of diagnosed

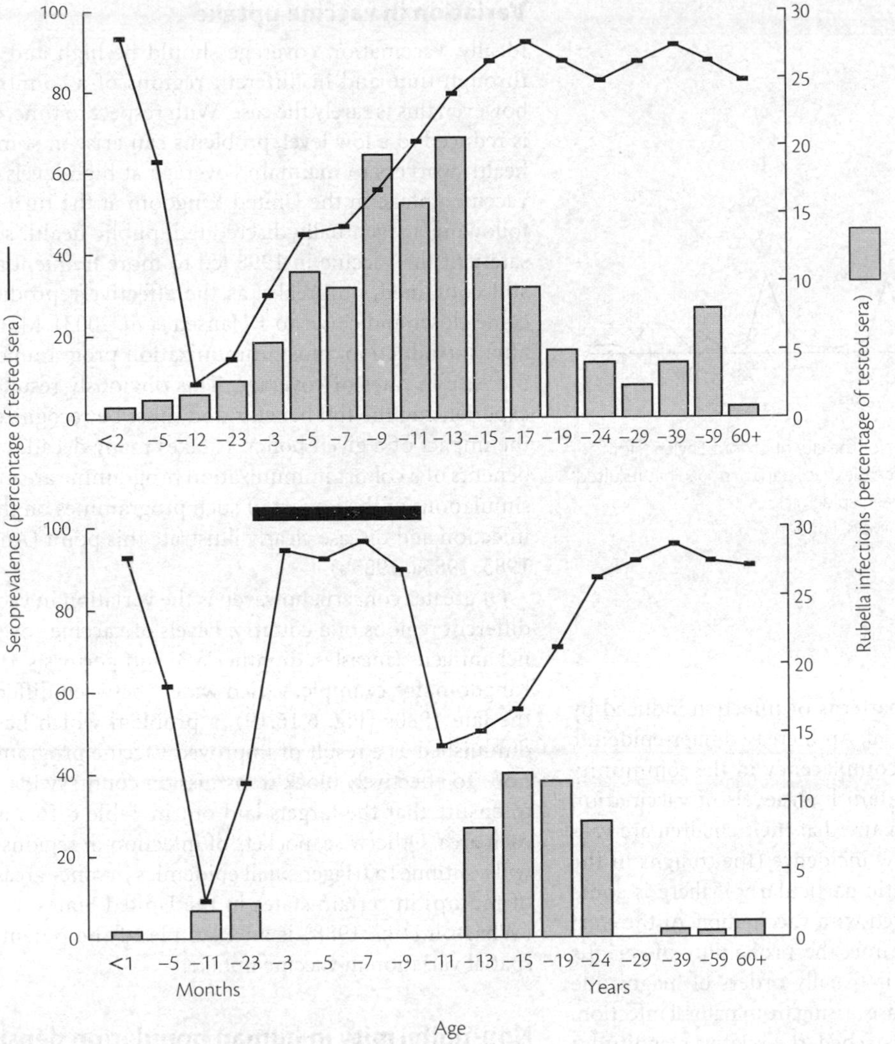

Fig. 6.16.16 The observed impact of mass immunization against rubella in Finland (Ukkonen and Von Bonsdorf 1988). (a) The prevaccination (1982) age seroprevalence of specific rubella antibodies (line) with the age distribution of diagnosed cases (bars). (b) Four years after mass infant MMR vaccination was introduced with the age range affected shown by the solid bar (data for males only) (other details as for (a)). *Source:* Nokes and Anderson 1993.

rubella cases, with a marked increase in the average age. Later, we discuss how this change in the age distribution of the incidence of infection can influence the incidence of disease arising from infection if older people differ in their vulnerability to complications and concomitant morbidity when compared with younger people.

Inter-epidemic period

Simple models also predicted that a reduction in the transmission rate in a vaccinated population will act to lengthen the inter-epidemic period over that pertaining prior to control (Anderson & May 1983). This may be shown easily using our model in Fig. 6.16.10 if a proportion of all individuals entering the population are vaccinated at the time of birth (starting from time unit 5 onwards), resulting in an increase in the time taken for susceptibles to build up to threshold numbers and, hence, an increase in the interval between epidemics (Fig. 6.16.17). This pattern has been observed in various vaccinated communities (Fig. 6.16.18).

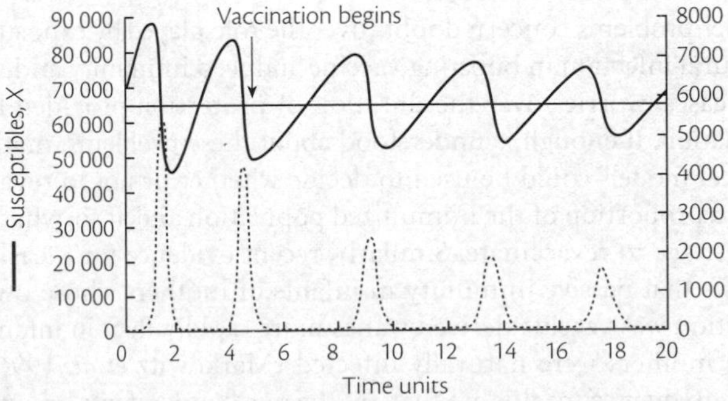

Fig. 6.16.17 Predicted impact of vaccination on the interepidemic period. Vaccination of 50 per cent of all births was introduced at time 5 into the model given in Fig. 6.16.10 (with the same initial settings).

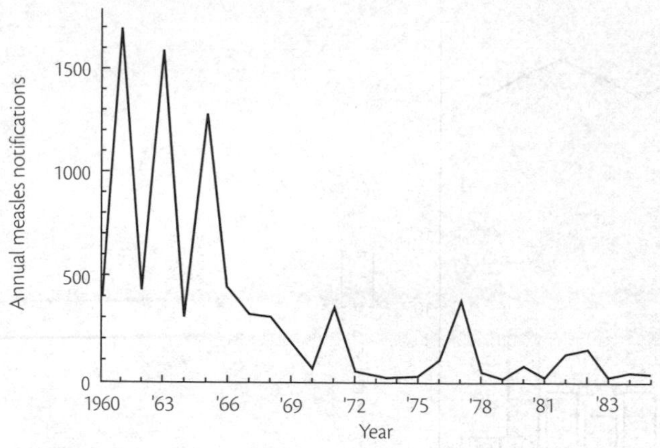

Fig. 6.16.18 Annual measles notifications for the city of Oxford, England, for the period 1960 to 1985. The introduction of measles vaccination in 1966 has resulted in a significant increase in the period between epidemics.
Source: Office of Population Census and Surveys, London.

Cautionary notes

The changes in epidemiological patterns of infection induced by vaccination are not always beneficial. An increased inter-epidemic period, for example, can induce complacency in the community with respect to the need to maintain high levels of vaccination coverage. Motivating parents to ensure that their children are vaccinated during long periods of low incidence (the troughs in the epidemic cycle) can be problematic particularly if there is some small but measurable risk associated with vaccination. At the start of a mass immunization programme, the probability of serious disease arising from vaccination is usually orders of magnitude smaller than the risk of serious disease arising from natural infection. As the point of eradication is approached, the relative magnitudes of these two probabilities must inevitably be reversed. The optimum strategy for the individual (not to be vaccinated) therefore becomes at odds with the needs of society (to maintain her immunity) (Nokes & Anderson 1991). This issue—which was central to the decline in the uptake of pertussis vaccine in the United Kingdom during the mid-to-late 1970s—can be overcome by legislation to enforce vaccination (as in the United States), but its final resolution is only achieved by global eradication of the disease agent so that routine vaccination can cease.

Other problems concern doubts over the role played by exposure to natural infection in boosting vaccine-induced immunity and, in some cases, worries over the duration of protection provided by vaccination. If enough is understood about these problems, mathematical models could be used to decide whether or not to revaccinate a proportion of the immunized population and, if so, what is the best age to revaccinate. Similarly, recent evidence for measles suggests that passive immunity in infants of mothers whose own protection was vaccine derived wanes more rapidly than in infants whose mothers were naturally infected (Markowitz *et al.* 1996). The consequences of this are that, on the one hand, infants become susceptible to infection at an earlier age than was previously the case, but on the other hand, it may allow for the lowering of the age of vaccine delivery. The merits of this latter issue could well be addressed using mathematical models.

Variation in vaccine uptake

Ideally, vaccination coverage should be high and constant both through time and in different regions of a country. In practice, however, this is rarely the case. With respect to time, once incidence is reduced to a low level, problems can arise in stimulating public health workers to maintain coverage at high levels. Falling MMR vaccine uptake in the United Kingdom at the turn of the century following a, eventually discredited, public health scare about the safety of the vaccine in 1998 led to more frequent and larger, but still contained, outbreaks, as the effective reproductive number came closer and closer to 1 (Jansen *et al.* 2003). More importantly, after introduction, most immunization programmes show a slow increase in rates of coverage. This obviously results in a delay in experiencing the full benefits and must be recognized in assessing the impact of a given policy. It takes many decades before the full benefits of a cohort immunization programme are manifest. Model simulations of the impact of such programmes on the incidence of infection and disease clearly illustrate this point (Anderson & May 1983, 1985a, 1985b).

Of greater concern, however, is the variation in vaccine uptake in different regions of a country. Levels of vaccine coverage for sentinel antigens (measles, diphtheria 3, and pertussis 3) in the United Kingdom, for example, varied widely between different regions in the late 1980s (Fig. 6.16.19), a problem which has been greatly diminished as a result of improved vaccine programme coordination. To effectively block transmission countrywide, it is necessary to ensure that the targets laid out in Table 6.16.3 are attained in each area. Otherwise, pockets of infection in regions of low uptake will continue to trigger small epidemics in other areas. The upsurge of mumps in certain states in the United States in the late 1980s (Wharton *et al.* 1988) is an example of the potential hazards of spatial variation in vaccine uptake.

Non-uniformity in human population density

Non-uniformity in the spatial distribution of humans, with some people living in dense aggregates and others living in isolated or small groups, can lead to heterogeneity in transmission rates. Models suggest that this can result in the transmission potential of an infection (R_0) being greater on average than suggested by estimation procedures, which assume spatial homogeneity (Anderson & May 1984; May & Anderson 1984). Under these circumstances, theory suggests that the optimal solution appears to involve 'targeting' vaccination coverage in relation to group size with dense groups receiving the highest levels of coverage. The optimal programme is defined as that minimizing the total, communitywide number of immunizations needed for elimination or for a defined level of control. This strategy reduces the overall proportion that must be vaccinated to block transmission, compared with that estimated on the assumption of spatial homogeneity. This conclusion has practical significance for the control of infections such as measles and pertussis in some developing countries, where rural–urban differences in population density tend to be much more marked than in developed countries (Anderson & May 1991). It is probable that in many regions of Africa and Asia, diseases such as measles cannot persist endemically in rural areas without frequent movement of people between low-density (rural) and high-density (urban) populations. Under these circumstances, transmission might be blocked in both regions by high levels of mass immunization in the urban centres alone.

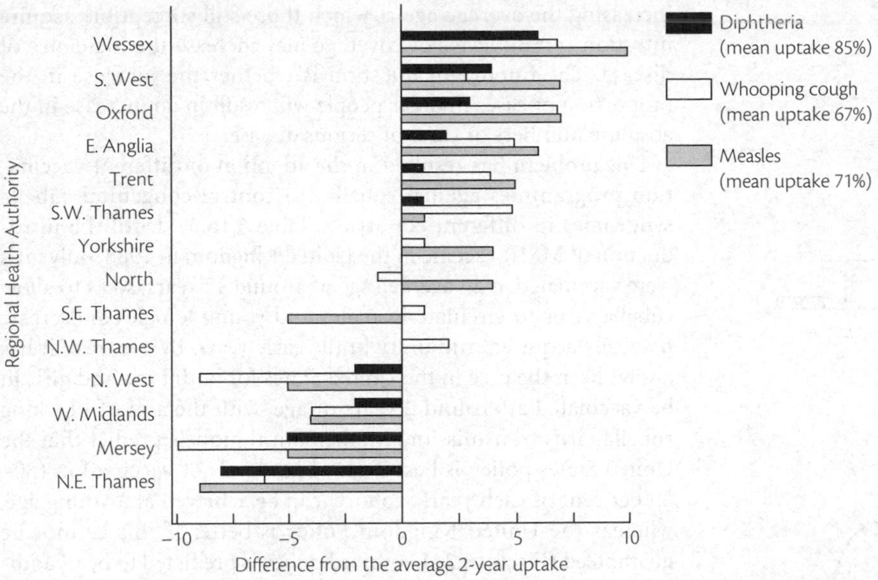

Fig. 6.16.19 Regional variation in immunization uptake for sentinel agents in England, 1986.
Source: Nokes and Anderson, 1988.

Age-dependent factors

Analyses of case-notification records and serological profiles suggest that, for many common infections (measles, rubella, and pertussis), the per capita rate of infection, $\lambda(a)$, depends on the ages of susceptible individuals, changing from a low level in the 0- to 5-year age classes, via a high level in the 5- to 15-year age classes, back to a lower level in the adult age classes (see Fig. 6.16.5). This is of interest both because it reflects behavioural attributes of human communities and because of its impact on the predicted level of vaccination required to eliminate transmission. The high levels of the force of infection in the 5–15-year-old classes are thought to arise as a consequence of frequent and intimate contacts within school environments (Anderson & May 1985b; Nokes *et al.* 1986; Anderson *et al.* 1987). Theoretical studies, which take account of age dependence in the force of infection, predict somewhat lower rates of vaccination than those arrived at under the simple mass-action assumption (Table 6.16.3). However, it should be emphasized that the values listed in Table 6.16.3 provide a good first approximation of the targets to be obtained in a vaccination programme. The reason why the observed age-related changes in the force of infection influence the predicted level of coverage relates to the tendency for mass vaccination to shift the age distribution of susceptibility (Figs. 6.16.15 and 6.16.16). Susceptibles who avoid infection and vaccination may move from an age class with a high force of infection into an older class with a lower rate.

Does mass vaccination always reduce disease incidence?

The risk of complications arising from infection is often dependent upon the age at which exposure occurs. The newborn are particularly vulnerable due to their immunological immaturity and are therefore more likely to suffer morbidity and even mortality (Fig. 6.16.20). Protection by maternally derived antibody moderates the risk during this time of great vulnerability but, in developing countries, factors such as malnutrition and high incidences of secondary 'opportunist' infections can result in high mortality rates as a result of infant and childhood viral and bacterial infection. In general, where the risk of serious disease is higher in the young than old people, mass vaccination will always act to reduce the incidence of disease.

In developed countries, case fatalities are much less common and the greatest problem is morbidity and the risk of serious disease. Of particular concern are infections for which the risk of severe complications increases with age (Fig. 6.16.21). Whether this trend is important depends on the quantitative details of such factors as how risk changes with age, the average age at which the vaccine is

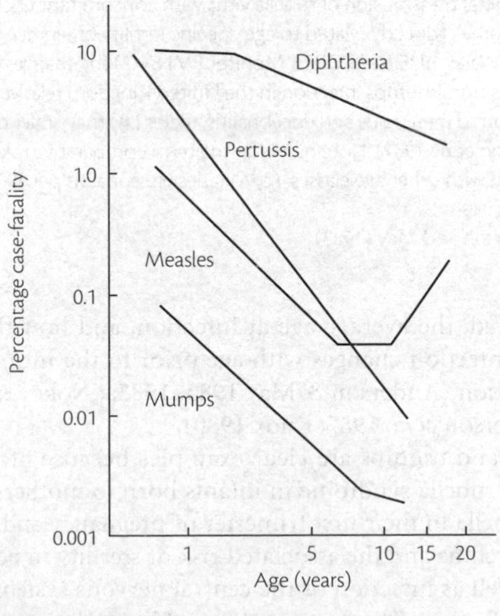

Fig. 6.16.20 Age-dependent mortality associated with infection from a variety of childhood viruses and bacteria.
Source: MIMS (1987).

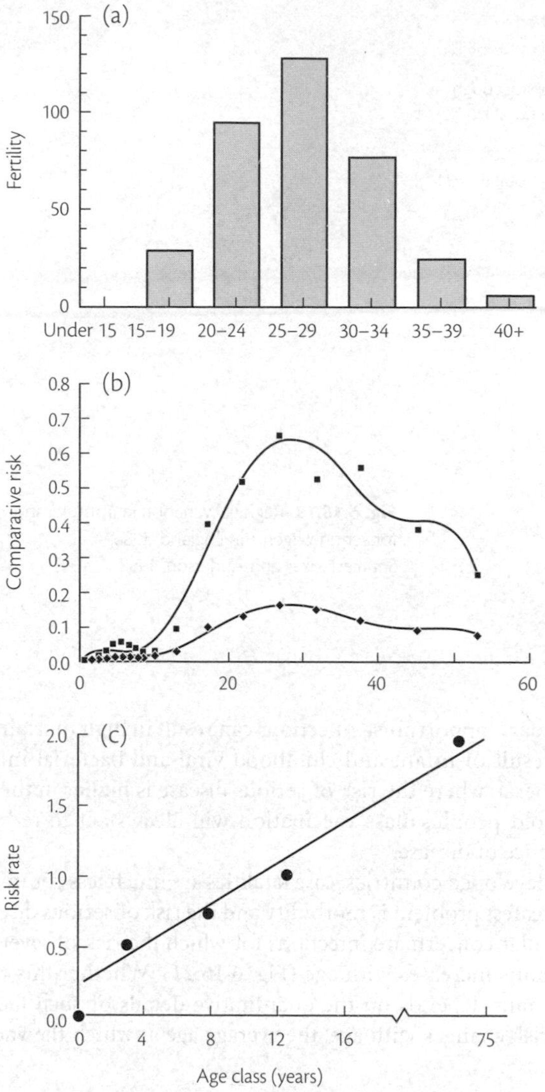

Fig. 6.16.21 Age-dependent risk of complications from infection: (a) the likelihood of fetal transmission of rubella virus with concomitant risk of congenital rubella syndrome is directly related to age-specific fertility of women (data for England and Wales 1985 from OPCS Monitor FMI 86/2) (b) changes in the risk of complications from mumps infection in the United Kingdom relative to age and sex. In addition to meningitis and encephalitis, males (■) may suffer orchitis (data from Anderson et *al.* 1987). Note here that the term comparative risk, refers to the risk compared with other age classes. (c) Measles encephalitis per 100 000 cases in the United States.
Source: Anderson and May (1983).

administered, the average age at infection, and how the rate (or force) of infection changes with age prior to the introduction of immunization (Anderson & May 1983, 1985a; Nokes & Anderson 1991; Anderson *et al.* 1987; Knox 1980).

Rubella and mumps are clear examples because of the risk of congenital rubella syndrome in infants born to mothers who contracted rubella in their first trimester of pregnancy and the occurrence of orchitis and the associated risk of sterility in postpubertal males as well as infection of the central nervous system following mumps infection. The crux of the problem relates to how mass vaccination changes the age profile of the incidence of infection. Any level of coverage will reduce the incidence of infection but by increasing the average age at which those still susceptible acquire infection certain levels of coverage may increase the incidence of disease. The important question is whether the increase in the proportion of cases in older people will result in an increase in the absolute numbers of cases of serious disease.

This problem has resulted in the adoption of different vaccination programmes against rubella (to control congenital rubella syndrome) in different countries (Table 6.16.5). Until the introduction of MMR vaccine in the United Kingdom in 1988, only girls were vaccinated at an average age of around 12 years, so as to allow rubella virus to circulate in males and young females and create naturally acquired immunity in the early years. By contrast, it has always been the case in the United States for both boys and girls to be vaccinated at around 2 years of age, with the aim of blocking rubella virus transmission. Mathematical models predict that the United States policy is best if very high levels of vaccination (80–85 per cent of each yearly cohort) can be achieved at a young age, whereas the United Kingdom policy is better if this cannot be guaranteed (Fig. 6.16.22). A mixed policy is predicted to be of additional benefit over the selective policy alone if moderate to high levels of vaccine uptake among boys and girls can be achieved at a young age (60 per cent) (Anderson & Grenfell 1986).

The process of using mathematical models to evaluate the impact of a particular mass vaccination policy in a community is detailed in Box 6.16.4, in this case for mumps. At the time of the introduction of MMR infant vaccination in the United Kingdom in November 1988, studies as these suggested that provided moderate to high levels of coverage (60–65 per cent) could be achieved the change in policy was unlikely to increase the incidence of serious disease (Anderson *et al.* 1987). Following the implementation of the MMR vaccine, coverage rose from the level of uptake for measles vaccine at the time of around 70 per cent by age 2 years

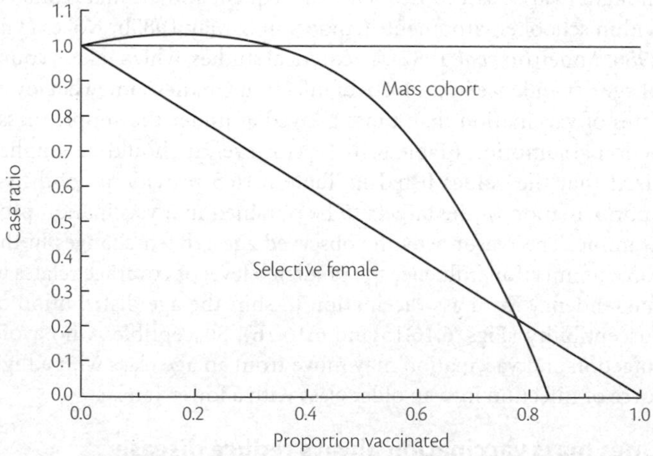

Fig. 6.16.22 Effectiveness of different rubella immunization programmes. Changes in the predicted case ratio (i.e. the average number of rubella infections in pregnant women after the introduction of immunization divided by average prevaccination number) under increasing levels of coverage for two types of policy, namely, selective immunization of girls of average age 12 years or mass vaccination of children (aged 2 years). Low to medium levels of uptake favour adoption of a selective immunization programme compared with mass vaccination which has the undesirable effect of increasing the average age at infection.

Table 6.16.5 Strategies of rubella immunization

	Selective	Mass cohort
Aim	Eliminate congenital rubella, not rubella infection	Eliminate rubella infection, and so congenital rubella
Age at vaccination	Prepubertal girls (10–15 years)	Boys and girls of 1–2 years
Philosophy	(i) Build upon levels of herd immunity attained through childhood (ii) Reduce the proportion of susceptible women of childbearing age (ii) Allow continued circulation of virus in male and young female segments of the population	(i) Reduce circulation of wild virus in community, especially children (ii) Lower the probability of susceptible women catching infection via the action of herd immunity
Overall incidence of infection	Very little impact at any level of coverage	(i) Reduction in cases in a non-linear manner as vaccine level increases (see Fig. 6.16.13) (ii) Increase in average age at infection
Other concerns	(i) Cannot eradicate congenital rubella unless 100 per cent of women 'at risk' are immune (via infection in childhhod or immunization) (ii) Herd immunity largely natural with continued re-exposure to infection and boosting of antibody response	(i) Proportion of remaining cases increases in older age classes, hence possible to increase congenital rubella at certain levels of immunization (ii) Herd immunity ultimately all vaccine induced. Less solid? No boosting of immunity by re-exposure to virus
Which policy?	Suitable for lower levels of vaccination coverage (see Fig. 6.16.22)	Suitable if high levels of uptake can be achieved (see Fig. 6.16.22)
Country (as example)	United Kingdom (prior to the introduction of the combined measles, mumps, and rubella (MMR) combined childhood vaccination)	United States

(the level of update for measles vaccine at the time) to 90 per cent within the space of two years.

Thoughts have now turned to the required strategy for elimination of these three infections and use is being made of mathematical models to explore the possible options, such as a two-dose schedule (Babad *et al.* 1995). For rubella, and specifically for the issue of when to remove the selective arm of the vaccination strategy, we now have the example from the Scandinavian countries to guide our policy. Data from Finland, for example, clearly show the need to continue schoolgirl vaccination until the cohorts with high-level immunity through infant vaccination span the entire high-fertility age groups. Note that this concurs with predictions made prior to the observations becoming available (Nokes & Anderson 1987).

The strategy of pulse vaccination

The use of the alternative strategy of pulse vaccination as a method of control of childhood vaccine-preventable diseases has gained prominence in the early 1990s largely as a result of success in the Americas against polio and measles (De Quadros *et al.* 1991). Pulse vaccination may be defined as the repeated application of vaccine across a wide age range (Agur *et al.* 1993; Nokes & Swinton 1995) and usually takes the form of vaccination days or campaigns repeated once or twice yearly in which all children under a specified age (e.g. 15 years) are offered vaccine (usually irrespective of vaccination history). Repeated vaccination days or weeks in Central and South America have seen the elimination of polio from the region since 1991 and very marked reductions in measles incidence. Although a basic understanding of the rationale underlying pulse vaccination guided its use in the Latin American context, there is good reason to seek greater quantitative insight into the underlying mechanism of action prior to advocating more widespread use in other regions with different social patterns and health infrastructure.

Remember that it is the presence of a threshold density or proportion of susceptibles in a population that enables endemic persistence of acute vaccine-preventable infections (i.e. infections requiring close contact to effect transmission and which develop lasting immunity following recovery). Vaccination of a fraction of an endemic proportion susceptible lowers the effective reproductive rate below unity and incidence declines (this may be quite a considerable reduction if a pulse is administered across a wide age range.) The lowering of the number of infectious persons in the population results in a lowering of the force of infection acting upon susceptibles. In turn, fewer infections lead to a buildup once more in susceptible numbers to the threshold level. The principle behind pulse vaccination rests upon these simple conditions. The aim of repeatedly pulsing is to maintain susceptible numbers below the threshold density or fraction and thereby maintain a continual decline in incidence (i.e. by maintaining $R \geq 1$). In practical quantitative terms, we are interested in the timing of successive pulses to achieve this objective.

Box 6.16.4 Epidemiology and control of mumps virus infection

Incidence of infection

Mumps is typical of the childhood viral infections with peak incidence in the young age classes and relatively few cases occurring in adulthood (figure (a)).

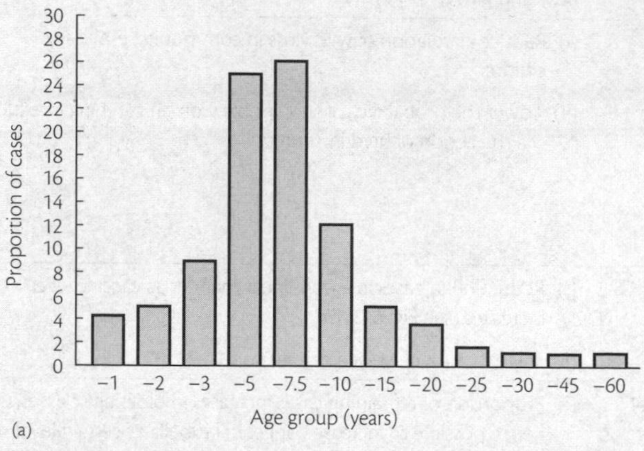

Information of this sort, obtained from age-specific case notification data or age-serological profiles, is used to derive age-dependent rates of transmission as shown in Fig. 6.16.5(b) in the main text.

Incidence of disease

Various types of complications are associated with mumps virus infection (figure (b)). In the prevaccination era mumps was the most common cause of viral meningitis in the United Kingdom, and is also a significant cause of encephalitis and, in postpubertal males, of orchitis.

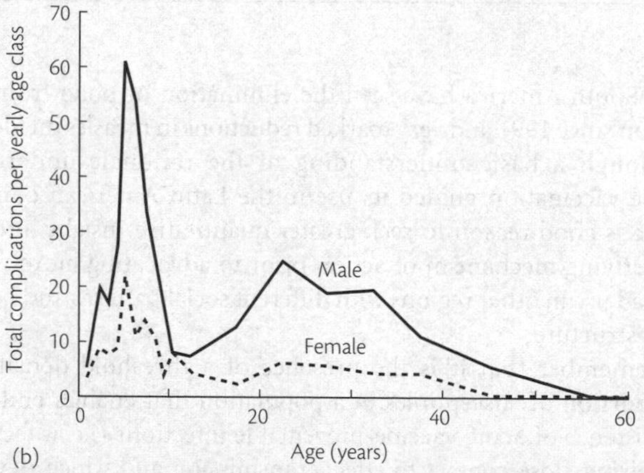

Scaling these age-complication data by the proportion of cases of infection in the corresponding age classes (shown above), it is possible to drive the relative risk of complications from infection, as shown in Fig. 6.16.21(b) in the main text. What becomes apparent from these data analyses is that, although fewest cases of infection occur in the older age classes, there remain substantial numbers of cases of complications, such that infection in older persons runs a considerably greater risk of resulting in complications when compared with infection in the young.

Mass vaccination and the incidence of infection

Figure (c) shows the predicted numbers of cases of mumps infection across a wide range of age classes, through time, before and after the introduction of a programme of mass cohort immunization (60 per cent of 2-year-olds). The force of infection is assumed to remain constant with age at 0.15 per year (corresponding to an average age at infection before immunization of 6.7 years). The epidemic peaks in the prevaccine period show the majority of cases occurring in the youngest age classes. Subsequent to the initiation of immunization two changes should be noted: (a) the obvious and expected decline in infection incidence (particularly in the young), and (b) an increase in the age at which the remaining cases occur, indicated by the wave of infections migrating, in time, into the older age classes. The implications of this shift in the age distribution of cases on the incidence of disease are addressed below.

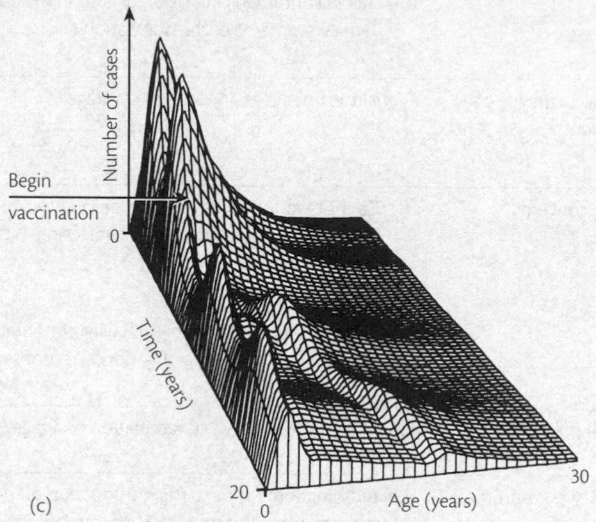

Mass vaccination and the incidence of disease

The effect of a rise in the proportion of cases in the older age classes (predicted above) on the incidence of complications is dependent upon two things: (a) the level of cohort immunization that can be attained, and (b) the age-dependent nature of the risk of complications seen in Fig. 6.16.21. Simulations that help to unravel this problem are shown in figure (d) (adapted from Anderson et *al.* 1987), recording the change in the predicted risk ratio (i.e. the average number of complications after immunization has begun divided by the average number of complications occurring before) over various levels of childhood immunization (note that the risk ratio is unity for no benefit from immunization). Obviously there is little benefit to be obtained by vaccination at less than 60 per cent, and indeed vaccination at anything less than 70 per cent is potentially hazardous when considering orchitis alone. Such a phenomenon is a direct result of the combination of increased average age at infection and of the risk of complications with age.

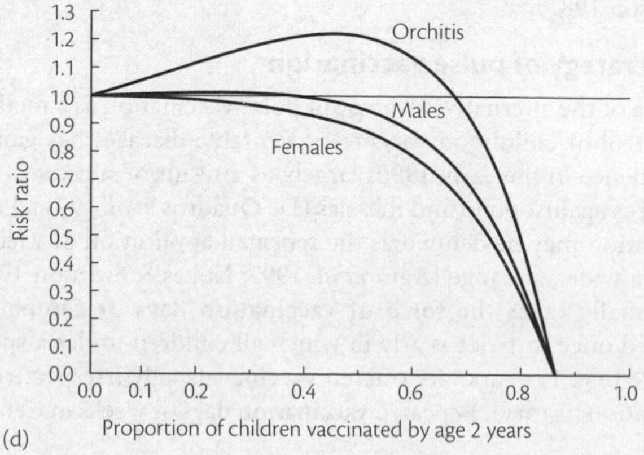

The interpulse interval depends upon three factors: What fraction of the population is susceptible at endemic equilibrium, how much of this susceptible population is immunized as a result of the campaign, and how rapidly are susceptibles replenished after a campaign. Translating these into epidemiological terms, we note that the proportion of the susceptible population vaccinated in a single pulse is $p'x^*$, where p' is the vaccination coverage and x^* is the endemic fraction susceptible (related to the basic reproductive rate in the form $x^* = 1/R_0$). In addition, if the total population is approximately constant in size, then, ignoring any further infection, the rate of replenishment of susceptibles by births is equal to the death rate, $\mu = 1/L$ (where L is life expectancy at birth). Therefore, the minimum time taken after pulsing to recover the equilibrium fraction, that is, the interpulse period T_v (Nokes & Swinton 1995), is:

$$T_v = p'x^*L \qquad (6.16.38)$$

and, as $x^* = 1/R_0 = A/L$, we obtain:

$$T_v = p'A \qquad (6.16.39)$$

This gives the common-sense result that if all susceptibles were to be immunized by a pulse of vaccine, that is, $p' = 1.0$, then the time taken to recover the threshold fraction would be equivalent to the average age at infection. The higher the average age at infection, that is, the lower the transmission potential of the infection, the higher the endemic fraction susceptible and the consequent increase in the permitted interval between pulses. An observation from this analysis is that it is possible to eliminate an infection using a pulse vaccination proportion, p', which is less than the critical level of coverage predicted to be required for a continuous immunization process. The reason for this is that by vaccinating repeatedly across an age range, some individuals will receive multiple opportunities to receive the vaccine and there is therefore a buildup of vaccine-induced immunity with increasing age.

One complication that ought to be considered is the effect of combining a routine vaccination programme with a pulse regime (Nokes & Swinton 1995). Clearly, if a fraction of susceptibles are being vaccinated at or near to birth, then the rate of replenishment of susceptibles following a pulse will be lowered. It may be shown that, provided that the vast majority of individuals acquire immunity some time during their lives, the interpulse period in the presence of a routine vaccination programme in which a proportion p are vaccinated is:

$$T = p'A/(1-p) \qquad (6.16.40)$$

In other words, the pulse interval is lengthened in direct relation to the new fraction of births that are susceptible, $(1 - p)$.

Major simplifying assumptions underlie these simple relationships for the interpulse period. It is assumed that a proportion p' of susceptibles of any age are vaccinated and that on successive occasions each individual in a population has the same likelihood of being vaccinated. Such assumptions entail that the expressions given provide simple guidelines to aid understanding. Models of greater complexity are required, which expand upon these ideas to give more practical guidelines (Nokes & Swinton 1995).

Monitoring the impact of control programmes

There is an ever-growing need to establish a coordinated surveillance programme to monitor the impact of control programmes against microparasitic infections (Nokes & Cutts 1993). The needs include the following:

1. To establish the impact of a specified control programme on a particular outcome variable, such as incidence of infection. This is of increasing importance as control programmes near their goals of elimination, where indicators of process, such as vaccination coverage, simply do not relate well enough to outcome.
2. To establish the accuracy of outcome indicators, such as notifications of infectious disease, the efficiency of which commonly fall off dramatically as incidence declines. This is crucial to the identification of outbreaks (and perhaps areas of low vaccine uptake) and to the validation of elimination targets, for example, surveillance of acute flaccid paralysis as a marker for poliomyelitis.
3. To monitor the appearance of wild-type variants, either introduced from other countries or which have gained selective advantage over persisting strains in the presence of high selective pressure of vaccination or chemotherapy.

Various modern tools are now at our disposal to assist in this process. For example, saliva antibody assays that are being used to confirm clinical diagnoses and may be useful in establishing longitudinal surveillance systems and molecular probes by which to identify the origins of strains in infection outbreaks and the arrival of variants able to circulate in the presence of high-level vaccine-associated immunity.

Mathematical models have a key role to play in this area of epidemiology. They facilitate the assessment of the impact of mass vaccination programmes through their predictive capability, where suitable outcome indicators may not be available (e.g. infections with poor differential diagnosis) or may only be measurable many years after a programme has begun (e.g. hepatitis B virus and the occurrence of hepatic disorders). In addition, models can be used to explore the potential (and the time course) for strain variants to establish themselves in highly vaccinated populations, where they would otherwise normally be out-competed by a dominant (higher R_0) strain, for which immunity through vaccination is more solid.

During an outbreak of an infectious disease, such as SARS or influenza A, real-time estimation of the impact of public health control policies is a crucial tool for informing policy. During the SARS outbreak in 2003, the effective reproductive number was estimated for Hong Kong (Riley *et al.* 2003) and Singapore (Lipsitch *et al.* 1996). These estimates showed the rapid effectiveness of public health control measures in these settings. There are several methods for estimating R during an epidemic (Ferguson *et al.* 2001; Howard & Donnelly 2000; Wallinga & Teunis 2004; Cauchemez *et al.* 2006). Many require reliable estimates of the time from one individual becoming infected to causing onward infections (Wallinga & Lipsitch 2007).

Changes in sexual behaviour and the transmission of sexually transmitted infections

The current pandemic of HIV and AIDS, and the absence of effective drugs and a vaccine to combat infection, has focused much attention in recent years on how to induce changes in sexual behaviour via education and media publicity campaigns to slow the spread of infection. The most important behaviour relevant to the rate of spread is the distribution of the rates of acquiring new sexual partners within a defined population (Fig. 6.16.8). A major characteristic of this behaviour is the heterogeneity between individuals within a given community. A central question in this problem is whether it is best to aim health educational programmes at the whole population, with the aim of reducing average rates of sexual-partner change, or whether it is best to target education at high-risk groups such as those with very high rates of sexual-partner change (in either male homosexual or heterosexual communities). This is a complicated question and its resolution depends, in part, on a detailed quantitative knowledge of the pattern of sexual behaviour within a given population. However, simple mathematical models can help to provide some clues to the resolution of this issue.

Of particular importance in understanding the dynamics of transmission of HIV is determining how sexual behaviour influences the magnitude of the basic reproductive rate, R_0. As discussed earlier, for a sexually transmitted disease such as HIV, the magnitude of R_0 is (in simple terms) defined by the probability of transmission per partner contact, B, multiplied by the effective rate of sexual-partner change, c, multiplied by the average duration of infectiousness, D, of an infected person. As noted earlier, the variance in the rate of sexual-partner acquisition is typically much larger in value than the mean, and hence, those with high rates of partner change play a disproportionate role (relative to their proportional representation within a sexually active population) in the spread of infection (Fig. 6.16.14). This simple theoretical result suggests that greater benefit is to be gained (in terms of reducing R_0) by targeting education at those with higher than average rates of sexual-partner change. In practice, the identification of such individuals is problematic in the absence of detailed survey data that relate this behaviour to other characteristics. The surveys of sexual behaviour that have been completed to date show a strong age dependency (with young adults having the highest rates of sexual-partner change) but little else of help in identifying correlates (ACSF 1992; Johnson *et al.* 1992). However, attendees at sexually transmitted disease clinics are an important target group, because sexually transmitted diseases other than HIV are more frequently present among those with high rates of partner change. Small changes in behaviour in the highly sexually active are likely to have a major impact on the prevalence of sexually transmitted diseases in a community.

Conclusion

We have glossed over much detail and ignored many complications in model formulation and analysis in this chapter. The interested reader is therefore urged to consult the source references. Our aim has been to define, as simply as possible, the central concepts underpinning the study of the transmission dynamics of infectious diseases and the major conclusions that have emerged from the development and analysis of mathematical models of transmission and control.

The recent convergence of mathematical theory and observation in epidemiology has created a powerful set of tools for the study of the population biology of infectious disease agents. At present, the potential value of these techniques is not widely appreciated by public health scientists and medical personnel. Many people have rightly criticized models that pursue the mathematics for its own sake, making only perfunctory attempts to relate the findings to epidemiological data. But, there is a converse danger which is less widely understood. The complexities of the course of infection within an individual and its spread between people are such that years of clinical experience and the most refined intuition will not always yield reliable insights into the factors that control the transmission dynamics of a given infectious agent and how these are influenced by perturbations introduced by control measures. Moreover, insensitive use of a computer will not always help in understanding these problems, because if a computer is given inappropriate instruction it will usually give inappropriate answers. What is needed, in our view, is increased collaboration between epidemiologists and mathematicians, with the models being founded on data (and with their predictions being tested against available facts) and with verbal hypotheses being founded on clear mathematical statements of the assumptions. We hope that the contents of this chapter stimulate interest towards this goal.

References

ACSF. AIDS and sexual behaviour in France. *Nature* 1992;**360**:407–9.

Agur Z., Cojocaru L., Mazor G. *et al.* Pulse mass measles vaccination across age cohorts. *Proceedings of the National Academy of Sciences (USA)* 1993;**90**:11698–702.

Anderson R.M., Crombie J.A., Grenfell B.T. The epidemiology of mumps in the UK: a preliminary study of virus transmission, herd immunity and the potential effect of immunization. *Epidemiology and Infection* 1987;**99**:65–84.

Anderson R.M., Donnelly C.A., Ferguson N.M. *et al.* Transmission dynamics and epidemiology of BSE in British cattle. *Nature* 1996;**382**:779–88.

Anderson R.M., Grenfell B.T., May R.M. Oscillatory fluctuations in the incidence of infectious disease and the impact of vaccination: time series analysis. *Journal of Hygiene (Cambridge)* 1984;**93**:587–608.

Anderson R.M., Grenfell B.T. Quantitative investigation of different vaccination policies for the control of congenital rubella syndrome (CRS) in the U.K. *Journal of Hygiene (Cambridge)* 1986;**96**:305–33.

Anderson R.M., May R.M., McLean A.R. Possible demographic consequences of AIDS in developing countries. *Nature* 1988;**332**:228–34.

Anderson R.M., May R.M. Age-related changes in the rate of disease transmission: implications for the design of vaccination programmes. *Journal of Hygiene (Cambridge)* 1985a;**94**:365–436.

Anderson R.M., May R.M. Directly transmitted infectious diseases: control by vaccination. *Science* 1982;**215**:1053–60.

Anderson R.M., May R.M. Epidemiological parameters of HIV transmission. *Nature* 1988;**333**:514–22.

Anderson R.M., May R.M. *Infectious diseases of humans: dynamics and control*. Oxford University Press; 1991.

Anderson R.M., May R.M. Spatial, temporal and genetic heterogeneity in host populations and the design of immunization programmes. *IMA Journal of Mathematics Applied in Medicine and Biology* 1984;**1**:233–66.

Anderson R.M., May R.M. The invasion, persistence and spread of infectious diseases within animal and plant communities. *Philosophical Transactions of the Royal Society of London* 1986;**314**:533–70.

Anderson R.M., May R.M. Vaccination against rubella and measles: quantitative investigations of different policies. *Journal of Hygiene (Cambridge)* 1983;**90**:259–325.

Anderson R.M., May R.M. Vaccination and herd immunity to infectious diseases. *Nature* 1985b;**318**:323–9.

Anderson R.M., Medley G.F., May R.M. *et al.* A preliminary study of the transmission dynamics of the human immunodeficiency virus (HIV), the causative agent of AIDS. *IMA Journal of Mathematics Applied in Medicine and Biology* 1986;**3**:229–63.

Anderson R.M. Directly transmitted viral and bacterial infections of man. In: Anderson R.M., editor. *Population dynamics of infectious diseases—theory and applications*. London: Chapman and Hall; 1982. p. 1–37.

Anderson R.M. Epidemiology of HIV infection: variable incubation plus infectious periods and heterogeneity in sexual activity. *Journal of the Royal Statistical Society Series A* 1988;**151**:66–93.

Babad H.R., Nokes D.J., Gay N.J. *et al.* Predicting the impact of measles vaccination in England and Wales: Model Validation and Analysis of Policy Options. *Epidemiology and Infection* 1995;**114**:319–44.

Bailey N.T.J. Estimation of parameters from epidemic models. In: Bartlett MS, Hiorns RW, editors. *Mathematical theory of the dynamics of biological populations*. London: Academic Press; 1973. p. 253.

Bailey N.T.J. *The mathematical theory of infectious diseases and its implications*. London: Griffin; 1975.

Becker N. The uses of epidemic models. *Biometrics* 1979;**35**:295–305.

Behets F.M., Eddie B., Quinn T.C. Detection of salivary HIV-1-specific IgG antibodies in high risk populations in Zaire. *Journal of Acquired Immune Deficiency Syndromes* 1991;**4**:183–7.

Bernoulli D. Essai d'une nouvelle analyse de la mortalité causée pour la verole et des avantages de L'incubation pour la prevenir [A new analysis of smallpox mortality and the benefits of incubation for its prevention]. *Memoires Mathematiques et Physiques de l'Academie Royale des Sciences (Paris)* 1760;**1**:1–45.

Black F.L. Measles endemicity in insular populations: critical community size and its evolutionary implications. *Journal of Theoretical Biology* 1966;**2**:207–11.

Bolker B.M., Grenfell B.T. Chaos and biological complexity in measles dynamics. *Philosophical Transactions of the Royal Society of London B—Biological Sciences* 1993;**251**:75–81.

Brown D.W.G., Ramsay M.E.B., Richards A.F. *et al.* Salivary diagnosis of measles: a study of notified cases in the UK, 1991–3. *British Medical Journal* 1994;**308**:1015–17.

Brownlee J. Statistical studies in immunity: the theory of an epidemic. *Proceedings of the Royal Society of Edinburgh* 1906;**26**:484–521.

Cauchemez S., Boelle P.Y., Thomas G. *et al.* Estimating in real time the efficacy of measures to control emerging communicable diseases. *American Journal of Epidemiology* 2006;**164**:591–7.

De Quadros C.A., Andrus J.K., Olive J-M. *et al.* Eradication of poliomyelitis: progress in the Americas. *Pediatric Infectious Disease Journal* 1991;**10**:222–9.

Dietz K. Mathematical models for the control of malaria. In: Wensdorfe W.H. and MacGregor J.A., editors. *Malaria*. Edinburgh: Churchill Livingstone; 1987. p. 1087.

Eames K.T., Keeling M.J. Modelling dynamic and network heterogeneities in the spread of sexually transmitted diseases. *Proceedings of the National Academy of Sciences (USA)* 2002;**99**:13330–5.

Farr W. *Progress of epidemics. Second report of the Registrar General of England and Wales*. London: Her Majesty' Stationery Office; 1840. p. 91–8.

Ferguson N. Capturing human behaviour. *Nature* 2007;**446**:733.

Ferguson N.M., Cummings D.A., Cauchemez S. *et al.* Strategies for containing an emerging influenza pandemic in Southeast Asia. *Nature* 2005;**437**:209–14.

Ferguson N.M., Cummings D.A., Fraser C. *et al.* Strategies for mitigating an influenza pandemic. *Nature* 2006;**442**:448–52.

Ferguson N.M., Donnelly C.A., Anderson R.M. Transmission intensity and impact of control policies on the foot and mouth epidemic in Great Britain. *Nature* 2001;**413**:542–8.

Ferguson N.M., Galvani A.P., Bush R.M. Ecological and immunological determinants of influenza evolution. *Nature* 2003;**422**:428–33.

Ferguson N.M., Ghani A.C., Donnelly C.A. *et al.* Estimating the human health risk from possible BSE infection of the British sheep flock. *Nature* 2002;**415**:420–4.

Fine P.E.M. Herd immunity: history, theory, practice. *Epidemiologic Reviews* 1993;**15**:265–302.

Fraser C., Hollingsworth T.D., Chapman R. *et al.* Variation in HIV-1 set-point viral load: epidemiological analysis and an evolutionary hypothesis. *Proceedings of the National Academy of Sciences (USA)* 2007;**104**:17441–6.

Fraser C., Riley S., Anderson R.M. *et al.* Factors that make an infectious disease outbreak controllable. *Proceedings of the National Academy of Sciences (USA)* 2004;**101**:6146–51.

Garnett G.P., Anderson R.M. Contact tracing and the estimation of sexual mixing patterns: the epidemiology of gonococcal infections. *Sexually Transmitted Diseases* 1993;**20**:181–91.

Garnett G.P., Swinton J., Brunham R.C. *et al.* Gonococcal infection, infertility and population growth: II. *The influence of heterogeneity in sexual behaviour. IMA Journal of Mathematics Applied in Medicine and Biology* 1992;**9**:127–44.

Garnett G.P. The influence of behavioural heterogeneity on the population level effect of potential prophylactic type 1 human immunodeficiency virus vaccines. *Journal of the Royal Statistical Society Series A Statistics in Society* 1998;**161**:209–25.

Ghani A.C., Ferguson N.M., Donnelly C.A., Anderson R.M. Factors determining the pattern of the variant Creutzfeldt-Jakob disease (vCJD) epidemic in the UK. *Proc R Soc Lond Ser B-Biol Sci.* 2003;**270**(1516):689–98.

Grassly N.C., Fraser C. Seasonal infectious disease epidemiology. *Proceedings* 2006;**273**(1600):2541–50.

Grassly N.C., Fraser C. Mathematical models of infectious disease transmission. *Nature Reviews* 2008;**6**(6):477–87.

Grenfell B.T., Anderson R.M. The estimation of age-related rates of infection from case notifications and serological data. *Journal of Hygiene* 1985;**95**:419–36.

Grenfell B.T., Pybus O.G., Gog J.R., Wood J.L.N., Daly J.M., Mumford J.A. *et al.* Unifying the epidemiological and evolutionary dynamics of pathogens. *Science* 2004;**303**(5656):327–32.

Gupta S., Anderson R.M. Sex, AIDS and mathematics. *New Scientist*; 1992 Sep **12**:34–8.

Hamer W.H. Epidemic disease in England. *Lancet* 1906;**i**:733–9.

Hethcote H.W., Yorke J.A. Gonorrhoea: transmission dynamics and control. *Lecture Notes in Biomathematics* 1984;**56**:1–105.

Hollingsworth T.D., Ferguson N.M., Anderson R.M. Will travel restrictions control the international spread of pandemic influenza? Nature and Medicine 2006;**12**:497–9.

Hollingsworth T.D., Anderson R.M., Fraser C. HIV-1 transmission, by stage of infection. *Journal of Infectious Diseases* 2008;**198**:687–93.

Holmstrom P., Syrjanen S., Laine P. *et al.* HIV antibodies in whole saliva detected by ELISA and Western blot assays. *Journal of Medical Virology* 1990;**30**:245–8.

Hope Simpson R.E. Infectiousness of communicable diseases in the household. Lancet1952;**i**:1145–55.

Howard S.C., Donnelly C.A. Estimation of a time-varying force of infection and basic reproduction number with application to an outbreak of classical swine fever. *Journal of Epidemiology and Biostatistics* 2000;**5**:161–8.

Jansen V.A.A., Stollenwerk N., Jensen H.J. *et al.* Measles outbreaks in a population with declining vaccine uptake. *Science* 2003;**301**:804–4.

Johnson A.M., Wadsworth J., Wellings K. *et al. Sexual attitudes and lifestyles*. Oxford: Blackwell Scientific; 1994.

Johnson A.M., Wadsworth J., Wellings K. *et al.* Sexual lifestyles and HIV risk. *Nature* 1992;**360**:410–12.

Keeling M.J., Woolhouse M.E., Shaw D.J. *et al.* Dynamics of the 2001 UK foot and mouth epidemic: stochastic dispersal in a heterogeneous landscape. *Science* 2001;**294**:813–7.

Kermack W.O., McKendrick A.G. A Contribution to the mathematical theory of epidemics. *Proceedings of the Royal Society of London Series A* 1927;**115**:700–21.

Knox E.G. Strategy for rubella vaccination. *International Journal of Epidemiology* 1980;**9**:13–23.

Lipsitch M., Cohen T., Cooper B. *et al.* Transmission dynamics and control of severe acute respiratory syndrome. *Science* 2003;**300**:1966–70.

Lloyd-Smith J.O., Schreiber S.J., Kopp P.E. *et al.* Super-spreading and the effect of individual variation on disease emergence. *Nature* 2005;**438**:355–9.

Longini I.M., Jr. Nizam A., Xu S. *et al. Containing pandemic influenza at the source. Science* 2005;**309**:1083–7.

Longini I.M., Jr., Halloran M.E., Nizam A. *et al.* Containing pandemic influenza with antiviral agents. *American Journal of Epidemiology* 2004;**159**:623–33.

Markowitz L.E., Albrecht P., Rhodes P. *et al.* Changing levels of measles antibody titers in women and children in the United States: Impact on response to vaccination. *Pediatrics* 1996;**97**:53–8.

May R.M., Anderson R.M. Spatial heterogeneity and the design of immunization programs. *Mathematical Biosciences* 1984;**72**:83–111.

May R.M., Anderson R.M. The transmission dynamics of HIV infection. *Nature* 1987;**326**:137–42.

McLean A.R., Anderson R.M. Measles in developing countries. *Part I. Epidemiological parameters and patterns. Epidemiology and Infection* 1988a;**100**:111–33.

McLean A.R., Anderson R.M. Measles in developing countries. *Part II. The predicted impact of mass vaccination. Epidemiology and Infection* 1988b;**100**:419–42.

McLean A.R., Blower S. Imperfect vaccines and herd immunity to HIV. *Proceedings of the Royal Society London Series B* 1993;**253**:9–13.

Mellors J., Rinaldo C., Gupta P. *et al.* Prognosis in HIV-1 infection predicted by the quantity of virus in plasma. *Science* 1996;**272**:1167–70.

Mortimer P.P., Parry J.V. Non-invasive virological diagnosis: are saliva and urine specimens adequate substitutes for blood? Reviews in Medical Virology 1991;1:73–8.

Mossong J., Hens N., Jit M. *et al.* Social contacts and mixing patterns relevant to the spread of infectious diseases. *PLoS Medicine* 2008;**5**:e74.

Nokes D.J., Anderson R.M., Anderson M.J. Rubella epidemiology in south-east England. *Journal of Hygiene (Cambridge)* 1986;**96**:291–304.

Nokes D.J., Anderson RM. Application of mathematical models to the design of immunization strategies. *Reviews in Medical Microbiology* 1993;**4**:1–7.

Nokes D.J., Anderson R.M. Mathematical models of infectious agent transmission and the impact of mass vaccination. *Reviews in Medical Microbiology* 1992;**3**:187–95.

Nokes D.J., Anderson R.M. Rubella vaccination policy: a note of caution. *Lancet* 1987;**i**:1441–2.

Nokes D.J., Anderson R.M. The use of mathematical models in the epidemiological study of infectious diseases and in the design of mass immunization programmes. *Epidemiology and Infection* 1988;**101**:1–20.

Nokes D.J., Anderson R.M. Vaccine safety versus vaccine efficacy in mass immunization programmes. *Lancet* 1991;**338**:1309–12.

Nokes D.J., Cutts F.T. Immunizations in the developing world: strategic challenges. *Transactions of the Royal Society of Tropical Medicine and Hygiene* 1993;**87**:353–4,398.

Nokes D.J., Swinton J. The control of childhood infection by pulse vaccination: an epidemiological approach. *IMA Journal of Mathematics Applied in Medicine and Biology* 1995;**12**:29–53.

Parry J.V., Perry K.R., Panday S. *et al.* Diagnosis of hepatitis A and B by testing saliva. *Journal of Medical Virology* 1989;**28**:255–60.

Patz J.A., Campbell-Lendrum D., Holloway T. *et al.* Impact of regional climate change on human health. *Nature* 2005;**438**:310–7.

Perry K.R., Brown D.W.G., Parry J.V. *et al.* Detection of measles, mumps and rubella antibodies in saliva using antibody capture radioimmunoassay. *Journal of Medical Virology* 1993;**40**:235–40.

Quinn T.C., Wawer M.J., Sewankambo N. *et al.* Viral load and heterosexual transmission of human immunodeficiency virus type 1. *Rakai Project Study Group. New England Journal of Medicine* 2000;**342**:921–9.

Read J.M., Keeling M.J. Disease evolution on networks: the role of contact structure. *Proceedings of the Royal Society of London Series B—Biological Sciences* 2003;**270**:699–708.

Riley S., Fraser C., Donnelly C.A. *et al.* Transmission dynamics of the etiological agent of SARS in Hong Kong: impact of public health interventions. *Science* 2003;**300**:1961–66.

Riley S. Large-scale spatial-transmission models of infectious disease. *Science* 2007;**316**:1298–301.

Ross R. *The prevention of malaria*. 2nd ed. London: Murray; 1911.

Scott M.E., Smith G., editors. *Parasitic and infectious diseases epidemiology and ecology*. 1st ed. London: Academic Press; 1994.

Sokal R.R., Rohlf F.J. *Biometry*. 2nd ed. San Francisco (CA): WH Freeman; 1981.

Soper M.A. Interpretation of periodicity in disease prevalence. *Journal of the Royal Statistical Society A* 1929;**92**:34–61.

Ukkonen P., Von Bonsdorf C.H. Rubella immunity and morbidity: effects of vaccination in Finland. *Scandinavian Journal of Infectious Diseases* 1988;**20**:255–9.

van den Akker R., van den Hoek J.A., van den Akker W.M. *et al.* Detection of HIV antibodies in saliva as a tool for Epidemiological studies. *AIDS* 1992;**6**:953–7.

Wallinga J., Lipsitch M. How generation intervals shape the relationship between growth rates and reproductive numbers. *Proceedings of the Royal Society of London Series B—Biological Sciences* 2007;**274**:599–604.

Wallinga J., Teunis P. Different epidemic curves for severe acute respiratory syndrome reveal similar impacts of control measures. *American Journal of Epidemiology* 2004;**160**:509–16.

Wawer M.J., Gray R.H., Sewankambo N.K. *et al.* Rates of HIV-1 transmission per coital act, by stage of HIV-1 infection, in Rakai, Uganda. *Journal of Infectious Diseases* 2005;**191**:1403–9.

Wharton M., Cochi S.L., Hutcheson R.H. *et al.* A large outbreak of mumps in the post vaccine era. *Journal of Infectious Diseases* 1988;**158**:1253–60.

Yorke J.A., Nathanson N., Pianigiani G. *et al.* Seasonality and the requirements for perpetuation and eradication of viruses in populations. *American Journal of Epidemiology* 1979;**109**:103–23.

6.17

Public health surveillance

Ruth L. Berkelman, Patrick S. Sullivan, and James W. Buehler

Abstract

Public health surveillance is the epidemiological foundation for modern public health. Surveillance data resulting from the continuous monitoring of the occurrence of a disease or condition underlie what public health actions are taken and reflect whether these actions are effective. Surveillance may also include monitoring of risk factors associated with adverse health events. A surveillance system should be designed to meet the needs of a prevention and control programme, which generally include a description of the temporal and geographical trends in the occurrence of a health event in a particular population. Most importantly, surveillance systems should identify changes in disease occurrence and in its characterization (for example, changes in antimicrobial resistance, changes in mortality). The data should be useful for substantiating patterns of both endemic and epidemic disease.

General principles that underlie the practice of surveillance are essentially the same for all countries, regardless of economic development. Defining the objectives of a surveillance system depends on what information is needed, who needs it, and how it will be used. Implementing a system will require a balance of competing interests, and a clear statement of objectives will provide a framework for subsequent decisions. Public health surveillance data are collected in many ways, depending on the nature of the health event under surveillance, potential methods for identifying the disease, the population involved, the resources available, and the goals of the programme. The widespread use of the Internet and electronic media has led to innovations in public health surveillance reaching far beyond traditional methods of disease monitoring on an individual patient basis. The performance of surveillance systems can be assessed by using a series of attributes, including sensitivity, timeliness, representativeness, positive predictive value, acceptability, flexibility, simplicity, and costs. Systems should be periodically or continually assessed as part of quality assurance. Surveillance provides a stimulus to keep prevention and control activities moving rapidly and in the right direction, guiding the response to individual cases as well as public policy. The term 'surveillance' is derived from the French word meaning 'to watch over' and, as applied to public health, means the close monitoring of the occurrence of selected health conditions in the population. Although surveillance methods were originally developed as part of efforts to control infectious diseases, basic concepts of surveillance have been applied to all areas of public health.

Definition

In 1963, Langmuir defined disease surveillance as 'the continued watchfulness over the distribution and trends of incidence through the systematic collection, consolidation, and evaluation of morbidity and mortality reports and other relevant data' together with timely and regular dissemination to those who 'need to know' (Langmuir 1963). In 1968, the twenty-first World Health Assembly described surveillance as the systematic collection and use of epidemiological information for the planning, implementation, and assessment of disease control; in short, surveillance implied 'information for action' (WHO 1968). Surveillance should begin when there exists or is likely to occur a public health problem for which programmes for prevention and control of a health event have been or may need to be initiated. A critical component of surveillance is that surveillance systems include the ongoing collection, analysis, and use of health or health-related data as part of a public health prevention or control programme.

History

The idea of collecting data, analysing them, and considering a reasonable response stems from Hippocrates. When writing on disease occurrence, Hippocrates made a distinction between the steady state, the endemic state, and the abrupt change in incidence—the epidemic. Possibly, the first public health action that can be attributed to surveillance occurred in the 1300s when public health authorities in a port near the Republic of Venice prevented passengers from coming ashore during the time of epidemic bubonic plague in Europe. The first Bill of Mortality was issued in London in 1532 as a consequence of fear of a plague epidemic. John Graunt's treatise *Natural and Political Observations on the Bills of Mortality* published in 1662 is generally recognized as one of the first documents to describe use of numerical methods for monitoring public health. In 1776, Johann Peter Frank advocated a more extensive monitoring of health in Germany that would support public health efforts related to the health of schoolchildren, prevention of injuries, maternal and child health, and public water and sewage disposal.

William Farr is recognized as the founder of the modern concept of surveillance. As Superintendent of the Statistical Department of the General Registrar's Office in Great Britain from 1839 to 1879, he collected, analysed, and interpreted vital statistics and disseminated the information in weekly, quarterly, and annual reports. He did not stop with publication of official reports, but regularly contributed papers to medical journals and even used the public press to achieve effective action (Langmuir 1976).

In the nineteenth century, Farr's efforts at health monitoring were extended by Edwin Chadwick, who investigated the relationship between environmental conditions and disease. Chadwick was followed by Louis Rene Villerme, who analysed the relation between poverty and mortality in Paris. In the United States, Lemuel Shattuck also published data that related deaths, infant and maternal mortality, and infectious diseases to living conditions. He further recommended standardized nomenclature for cause of disease and death, and the collection of health data that included sex, age, locality, and other demographic factors. The first international list of causes of death was developed in 1893 (Eylenbosch & Noah 1988).

Increasingly, elements of surveillance were applied to aid in detecting epidemics and in preventing and controlling infectious diseases. In 1899 the United Kingdom began compulsory notification of selected infectious diseases. National morbidity data collection on plague, smallpox, and yellow fever was initiated in 1878 in the United States, and by 1925 all states were reporting weekly to the United States Public Health Service on the occurrence of selected diseases.

Similar reporting activities were occurring in Europe at about the same time. In 1907 the Office International d'Hygiene Publique, predominantly composed of European member states, was created (WHO 1958). The office was to disseminate information in a monthly bulletin on the occurrence of selected diseases, most notably cholera, plague, and yellow fever. In the succeeding decades, other diseases were recommended for surveillance in step with the International Sanitary Regulations. However, many of the morbidity and mortality reporting systems were largely developed for long-term archival functions.

Since the early 1950s, the critical importance of surveillance to public health efforts has been demonstrated frequently. In 1955 acute poliomyelitis among recipients of the poliomyelitis vaccine in the United States threatened national vaccination programmes that had just begun. In collaboration with state health departments, the American Centers for Disease Control (CDC) developed an intensive national surveillance system, and at one point a daily report was being issued regarding poliomyelitis cases. The surveillance data assisted epidemiologists in demonstrating that the problem was limited to a single manufacturer of the vaccine and allowed the vaccination programme to continue with a resulting dramatic decline in cases of acute poliomyelitis in the United States in successive years (Langmuir 1963). During the worldwide malaria control programme, surveillance was used to determine areas of continued transmission and to focus spraying efforts, as well as to document those areas without malaria (Raska 1966). With the subsequent decline in malaria control efforts, surveillance data have documented the re-emergence of malaria in many areas of the world. In so doing, these data contributed to renewed interest in malaria control at the beginning of the twenty-first century.

Surveillance was also the foundation for the successful global campaign to eradicate smallpox. When the campaign began in 1967, efforts were focused on achieving a high vaccination level in countries with endemic smallpox; however, it was soon evident that a programme based on surveillance to target vaccinations in limited areas would be more efficient. Smallpox reporting sources, usually medical facilities, were contacted on a routine basis, and thus a reporting network was firmly established in most countries. In addition, other reporting sources were often established, including markets, schools, police, agricultural extension workers, and others. In 1973, as the goal of eradication neared, a systematic house-to-house search for cases was established in India and subsequently used widely in Pakistan and Bangladesh (Henderson 1976).

The potential usefulness of surveillance as a public health tool to address problems beyond infectious disease was emphasized in 1968 when the 21st World Health Assembly recommended the application of surveillance principles to a wider scope of problems, including cancer, atherosclerosis, and social problems such as drug addiction (WHO 1968). Many of the principles of surveillance traditionally applied to acute infectious diseases have also been applied to chronic diseases and conditions, although some differences in surveillance techniques have been observed. Even though chronic diseases may have long latency periods, trends in their incidence may change relatively quickly, and surveillance can play a key role in detecting these changes when effective interventions are applied (Berkelman & Buehler 1990). In addition to the increased scope of health problems under surveillance, the methods of surveillance have expanded from general disease notification systems to include survey techniques, sentinel health-provider systems, and other approaches to data collection. Beyond disease notification, an ideal surveillance system provides analyses of risk factors for disease and injury.

In 1981, shortly after the disease later named AIDS was recognized, national surveillance was begun in the United States and other countries. Even before the aetiological agent, HIV, was identified, surveillance data contributed to identifying modes of transmission, population groups at risk for infection, and, equally important, population groups not at risk for infection. These data were instrumental in directing public health resources to programmes, preventing spread of HIV, and averting widespread public hysteria (Jaffe *et al.* 1983).

The need for a strong infrastructure for surveillance systems is currently being re-emphasized not only as countries face the emergence and re-emergence of infectious diseases (Berkelman *et al.* 1994; Heymann & Rodier 1998) but also as a result of the increasing threat of biological terrorism. Epidemics such as Severe Acute Respiratory Syndrome (SARS) and avian influenza with their accompanying threats to health, trade, and security have led the World Health Assembly to adopt revised International Health Regulations in 2005; these regulations require the reporting of measures (for example, border screening, and quarantine) that countries implement in response to events that may constitute a public health emergency of potential international scope (Baker & Fidler 2006).

The dramatic growth in information technology has made possible more efficient data collection as well as more rapid and sophisticated analyses. Geographical information systems are in widespread use. The explosive development of technology has included the development of high-capacity storage devices, expansion of the capabilities of the Internet, use of local- and wide-area networks for entry of surveillance data at multiple computers simultaneously, and development of new programming tools, video and computer integration, and voice and pen input. Integration of healthcare and other systems, including data standards, is increasingly sought to allow maximal use of these advancements.

In addition, the biotechnology revolution is benefiting public health surveillance through rapid, automated, sensitive, and portable sampling and assay systems and DNA-based diagnostic tools. Such innovation is permitting earlier detection and characterization of disease or disease risk (for example, novel pathogens). New genetic technologies are also leading health communities to consider enhancing surveillance capacity for collecting and analysing information stemming from community-based assessments of genomic variation, and to assess how this information is integrated with disease reporting in assessing disease burden.

Purposes of surveillance

A surveillance system should be designed to meet the needs of a prevention and control programme (Table 6.17.1). These needs usually include a description of the temporal and geographical trends in the occurrence of a health event in a particular population. Most importantly, surveillance systems should identify changes in disease occurrence and in its characterization (for example, changes in antimicrobial resistance, changes in mortality). The data should be useful for substantiating patterns of both endemic and epidemic disease. In infectious diseases, a downward trend in total cases of tuberculosis may still be of concern if cases of multi-drug resistant tuberculosis are concurrently increasing; thus, surveillance for drug resistance is an important component of surveillance programmes for tuberculosis. Likewise, surveillance data for cases of diabetes type II must incorporate information on changes in screening asymptomatic individuals in order to accurately determine changes in the incidence of diabetes.

The role of surveillance in guiding public health programmes is illustrated by the first major national disease control activity initiated by the CDC—the Malaria Eradication Programme. Surveys in the mid-1930s had established malaria to be an endemic problem deeply rooted in the south-eastern part of the United States. An extensive chlorophenothane (DDT) spraying programme was launched after the Second World War, and surveillance was instituted in 1947. Data from this surveillance system established rapidly that endemic malaria had essentially disappeared, probably even before the DDT programme was underway (Langmuir 1963).

Table 6.17.1 Purposes of public health surveillance

To define public health priorities
To characterize disease patterns by time, place, and person
To detect epidemics
To suggest hypotheses
To identify cases for epidemiological research
To evaluate and guide prevention and control programmes, including assessment of effectiveness and/or adverse consequences.
To facilitate planning, including projection of future trends and healthcare needs

In this case, surveillance was used as the basis for dismantling a public health programme and redirecting public health resources to problems of higher priority.

The need for surveillance may continue for a disease even when prevention and control programmes are cut back, particularly for infectious diseases such as tuberculosis, dengue fever, or malaria whose incidence may change quickly. Generally, the more quickly re-emergence of a disease is detected, the more quickly and efficiently the disease can be controlled.

Surveillance data are also useful for evaluating the effectiveness of prevention and control programmes and of regulations or laws modified or initiated to address public health concerns (for example, safety of food and water, alcohol-related motor vehicle injuries). Monitoring of changes in the incidence of the disease or condition is necessary, and monitoring associated risk factors (food and water sanitation, physical activity, self-reports of drinking alcohol and driving) may also be useful in assessing interventions. The rapid decline in morbidity from many infectious diseases in certain populations has been related directly to vaccination campaigns that were conducted as a result of surveillance data on disease incidence. Measurement of the impact of an intervention on a specific disease outcome may be difficult when the aetiology of the disease is multifactorial, but the impact of an intervention on disease outcome, including its incidence and severity, remains the ultimate test of policy.

Assessment of the burden of disease, including its incidence (that is, the number of people newly affected each year) and its current and projected prevalence (that is, the number of people affected by the disease at any point in time), is essential to planning public health programmes. For example, in the 1980s, surveillance for AIDS was critical to the forecasting of the future impact of that disease in the United States. With the ageing of the population, projections of disease prevalence in the elderly are being emphasized. A current issue is the impact of major treatment programs on the long-term course of disease in the population such as HIV and tuberculosis, when adequate public health measures may not be in place to prevent continued spread or development of antimicrobial resistance.

Surveillance may be initiated to identify risk factors associated with disease and to suggest hypotheses for further investigation; cases identified through surveillance are sometimes used in case–control studies, as in the early studies of toxic shock syndrome and the AIDS epidemic (Shands *et al.* 1980). Effective preventive actions were formulated based on such research even before the aetiological agent, a toxigenic strain of *Staphylococcus aureus* was discovered.

Establishing a surveillance system

Establishing a surveillance system requires a statement of objectives, definition of the disease or condition under surveillance, and implementation of procedures for collecting, interpreting, and disseminating information. Surveillance systems can be considered as information loops, or cycles, that involve healthcare providers, public health agencies, and the public. A weakness in any part of the loop or information chain weakens the entire surveillance process. For example, if public health measures mandate that cryptosporidiosis must be reported, the surveillance system will be successful only if laboratories have the capacity to diagnose the infection (Berkelman *et al.* 1994). Likewise, if diagnoses on a hospital discharge record are coded incorrectly, surveillance data based on these records will propagate these inaccuracies.

The information cycle begins when cases occur and is completed when information about these cases is made available and is used for prevention and control. This process may involve multiple cycles, ranging from the local response to individual cases to the development of national policies based on information aggregated from many cases. Essential to the completion of the surveillance cycle is the return of information to constituents and policy makers (Langmuir 1963). In addition, in most circumstances, data that do not compromise privacy or confidentiality should be placed in the public domain to allow it to be as fully analysed and disseminated as possible.

The likelihood that effective interventions can be found, can prevent the occurrence of disease, or can alleviate the course of existing disease is an important consideration in determining whether a surveillance system will be useful. Surveillance data can also indicate the need for legislation (for example, the use of surveillance data on traumatic head injuries to influence legislation regarding mandatory use of bicycle helmets in children) or the need for more resource allocation if a problem poses an increasing health threat (for example, extensively drug-resistant tuberculosis).

Health priorities for surveillance must be continually evaluated as new infections emerge (for example, SARS), the population is exposed to new hazards (for example, new consumer products, environmental contamination), and other health conditions change. Surveillance for the disease or condition, as well as for associated risk factors and prevention services, should be considered. As the threat of terrorism increases globally, existing surveillance systems are being assessed for their usefulness and new ones are being established, including, environmental surveillance of threat agents (for example, Biowatch program in the United States (www.dhs.gov; accessed 25 July 2007).

Public health surveillance in under-resourced countries: Special considerations

General principles that underlie the practice of surveillance are essentially the same for all countries. These include the steps of system design and the principle of collecting information for action. However, the availability of data sources and resources vary widely among countries. Of interest, the revised international health regulations, which were adopted by the World Health Organization in May 2005 and came into force in June 2007, provide a powerful mandate to strengthen surveillance systems globally (Baker & Fidler 2006).

Tracking disease trends (particularly infectious diseases) has been the main reason surveillance systems have been initiated in under-resourced countries; surveillance data are also needed to establish rational public health priorities and to evaluate the impact of large-scale prevention and treatment programmes, such as those established for malaria, tuberculosis, and HIV/AIDS. Many infectious diseases and other conditions of public health import occur in settings with only rudimentary healthcare and few laboratory resources. With large-scale treatment programmes underway, the need for adequate laboratory infrastructure has become even more critical, in large part to assure that the treatment is appropriate, that the diagnosis is accurate, and that the microbes are not becoming resistant to the therapy being dispensed. Lack of definitive diagnoses may hinder surveillance and response efforts as well as result in inappropriate therapy and adverse consequences, such as increases in drug resistance.

Successful surveillance systems have been developed and maintained for targeted conditions; their success is partly dependent on features that may include sufficient resources, simplicity of reporting procedures, personal rapport with people in the network, regular feedback, and visible intervention upon reporting specific conditions. Programmes to eradicate polio make extensive use of surveillance to monitor the progress toward reaching their goals, and a major accomplishment of the polio eradication programme has been to develop a global integrated virologic surveillance network (Pallansch & Sandhu 2006). Eradication programmes must rely on targeted surveillance, which becomes more important (and expensive) as the target disease approaches eradication.

In many under-resourced countries, the process of linking surveillance to objectives highlights the need for mortality data and the absence of vital registration. The most basic health statistics are limited in many low- and middle-income countries, with death registration inadequate or non-existent. Use of the verbal autopsy, which uses a caretaker interview to determine the cause of death, may assist in following mortality patterns in places without routine death registration (Kumar *et al.* 2006). Sensitivity in establishing an accurate cause of death may be lower for some acute febrile conditions such as malaria than for conditions such as maternal causes, injuries, tuberculosis, and AIDS. In addition, different techniques in conducting verbal autopsies as well as geographic location may result in quite different sensitivities for specific conditions (Setel *et al.* 2006). An alternative and potentially simple and rapid approach to assess morbidity is to survey hospitals periodically for the number of admissions attributed to a particular condition. Again, the success of such surveys is largely dependent on the accuracy of diagnosis.

Other sources of health information may include the United Nations International Children's Emergency Fund (UNICEF), the World Health Organization (WHO), international conferences, non-governmental organizations, and population laboratories (for example, the International Centre for Diarrhoeal Disease Research, Bangladesh). Although some health problems are similar in many under-resourced settings, relying on data from other countries or districts to assess burden of disease across larger areas can often create major problems when there are large geographical and temporal differences in the incidence of the condition, such as for hepatitis C.

The design of surveillance systems must consider such issues as resources available, security, geography, population dispersion and mobility, type of health system, and literacy. Problems (more common but not unique to under-resourced countries) may include limited personnel available for public health, multiple vertical systems, lack of laboratory capacity, and infrastructure and communications constraints (for example, lack of equipment, supplies, or electrical power).

Solutions to address the lack of personnel for public health and prevention have included voluntary systems (using community health workers, traditional birth attendants, or village volunteers). More familiar solutions are public health training programmes designed to meet human resource gaps. Concerns about the cost-effectiveness of short-term training have resulted in establishing long-term programmes to build capacity within countries. Applied field epidemiology training programmes have been applauded for boosting the number of trained personnel (Cardenas *et al.* 2002).

Concurrently, the increase in availability of computers to analyse and transmit surveillance data and the decrease in the cost of such technology offer increased opportunities for surveillance. Epi Info is a freely available computer program designed to assist public health data management and analysis (Dean 1999); this tool has been used successfully in both well-resourced and under-resourced countries, and is available in 16 languages. Epi Info and other information systems should be seen as tools to be used to provide data to policy-makers and others to inform decisions that will improve health.

The gap in surveillance between well-resourced countries and under-resourced countries needs to be closed as quickly and efficiently as possible. The use of cellular phones and hand-held devices is proving useful in many areas, leveraging the international telecommunication system; few additional resources are needed to provide for collection of information and for two-way exchange of information needed for response.

Surveillance system objectives

Defining the objectives of a surveillance system depends on what information is needed, who needs it, and how it will be used. Implementing a system will require a balance of competing interests, and a clear statement of objectives will provide a framework for subsequent decisions. For example, the desire to collect detailed information about cases may compete with needs to assess the number of cases rapidly. Thus, if the primary objective is to obtain rapid case counts, less information may be collected about each case to avoid delays in reporting; alternatively, automated electronic reporting may effectively resolve reporting delay issues (for example, laboratory records). The objectives of a surveillance system will be shaped by its target population and its constituents, the nature of prevention and control programmes, and the health problem under surveillance.

Target population

A surveillance system seeks to identify health events within a specified population. This population may be defined on the basis of where people live, work, attend school, or use healthcare services. Alternatively, the population may be defined on the basis of where health events occur. For example, a surveillance system that monitors newborn health as a measure of prenatal care services would focus on deliveries to women who live within a community and not on women who live elsewhere but deliver in the community's hospitals. In contrast, surveillance of traffic injuries aimed at identifying roadway hazards could include all injuries that occur in a community, regardless of whether affected people are community residents.

In some cases, target populations for public health surveillance may be animals. For example, animal surveillance systems for West Nile virus and avian influenza have been developed, recognizing that these pathogens of concern to human health also infect animals and may serve to alert public health authorities of potential transmission to humans.

Constituents of surveillance systems

Surveillance systems are likely to have many constituents, including healthcare providers, public health professionals, researchers at academic health centres, politicians, the media, the public, and others with diverse perspectives and uses for surveillance data. Because these diverse needs cannot always be satisfied, the primary or most important constituents should be identified as the system is established.

Nature of public health programmes

The objectives of surveillance systems will be shaped by the public health programmes they serve. For example, a programme to eradicate an infectious disease requires intensive surveillance in the later stages of the campaign that emphasizes identification of all people with the disease (Hinman & Hopkins 1998). In contrast, an educational programme to influence behaviour may depend on a surveillance system that describes the practices of a sample of people in a community.

Health problems under surveillance

It is necessary to decide exactly what disease or health problem will be under surveillance, using such criteria as the magnitude of the public health problem (or potential magnitude) as well as the capacity to prevent or control the disease or condition through public health actions. Surveillance may frequently be conducted for any of several points along a spectrum, ranging from exposure to an adverse outcome. It is important to consider which manifestation(s) or stage(s) of a disease should be under surveillance. For example, manifestations of ischaemic heart disease include abnormal diagnostic tests in the absence of symptoms, angina pectoris, acute myocardial infarction, and (sudden) death. If the goal of surveillance is to assess the burden of the disease on healthcare systems, a broad definition that encompasses various manifestations may be appropriate. If the purpose is to monitor trends in the disease, a more limited and severe manifestation, such as myocardial infarction, may be the appropriate target for surveillance. Alternatively, attention may be focused on risk factors for cardiovascular disease, such as hypertension, smoking, cholesterol levels, and physical activity.

For disease with long latent periods, it may be desirable to choose surveillance events that are as early in the course of disease as feasible. The main challenge is ascertainment of events that cause lower morbidity and for which there is incomplete screening.

Newer surveillance initiatives for HIV/AIDS involve reporting of asymptomatic HIV infection (Glynn *et al.* 2007), and, in some areas, HIV incidence as determined through serologic assay (Lee & McKenna 2007). These changes move surveillance efforts closer to the leading edge of the epidemic, and increase the usefulness of surveillance data for directing prevention efforts.

Case definition

The case definition is fundamental to any surveillance system because it is the formal answer to the question of what manifestations of a disease or condition are under surveillance (CDC 1997) (see http://www.cdc.gov/epo/dphsi/casedef; accessed 25 July 2007). It is both a criterion for determining who is counted and a guide to local health departments for case investigations and follow-up. It ensures that the same measure is used across geographical areas. The case definition must be sufficiently inclusive (sensitive) to identify people who require public health attention but sufficiently exclusive (specific) to avoid unnecessary diversion of that attention. In addition, the case definition must be usable by all people on whom the system depends for case reporting.

Case definitions may also change over time as new knowledge is gained or as the purpose of the surveillance changes. One example is AIDS surveillance; surveillance changed as more knowledge was gained. The first definition of AIDS published in 1982 by CDC was highly specific as it was necessary to focus attention on aetiology of the condition, and it was undesirable to weaken epidemiologic studies by including individuals who did not definitively have the abnormal condition. Once the viral aetiology was discovered and a test available, sensitivity of the case definition was a high priority as the assessment of the extent of the condition was critical. Thus, the revision of the definitions in both 1985 and 1987 reflected the expansion of knowledge of the conditions that were associated with HIV status and accompanying immunodeficiency. As numbers of persons with AIDS swelled together with more effective treatment becoming available, the definition was further revised in 1993 to simplify reporting and to encompass those who needed treatment with antiviral therapy. In 2007, the case definition was again revised by CDC to reflect advancements in diagnostic technologies and algorithms (CDC 2008).

In another example, the focus of surveillance changed over time. During the course of the poliomyelitis eradication campaign, different definitions have been used, with a less specific definition needed when cases of poliomyelitis are common. Following successful vaccination campaigns and a large reduction in disease incidence, case definitions for poliomyelitis required more specificity, which in turn required laboratory confirmation of cases of acute flaccid paralysis, and as further progress was made in eradication, isolates were also genetically sequenced (Pallansch & Sandhu 2006).

A similar range of possible case definitions also exists for surveillance systems that focus on adverse health exposures rather than disease outcomes. For example, in a surveillance system that addresses occupational hazards, exposure to a harmful substance may be monitored by self-report of workers, by company log-books of manufacturing procedures, or by routine measurement of substances in the work environment, on workers' clothing, or in specimens collected from workers. Each of these possible case definitions would require different levels of cooperation from the company or workers, and each may be subject to unique limitations that could bias surveillance.

The flow of information

Surveillance systems may rely on multiple data sources that may be collected primarily for purposes other than public health, and this trend is growing as more resources are put into electronic healthcare data systems that are standardized. Many of the most useful surveillance systems, however, continue to depend on data acquired explicitly for surveillance purposes and rely on a sequential flow of these data through the full surveillance cycle. Each facet of this process should be carefully planned, as described below.

Reporters

People responsible for reporting cases may be all healthcare providers in a defined area, selected providers, or people at specific institutions (for example, clinics, healthcare organizations, laboratories, hospitals, schools, factories). In addition to communicating case reports, reporters may be responsible for collecting specimens needed by public health agencies for laboratory confirmation or application of molecular epidemiological techniques (for example, serogrouping meningococcal infection). Reporting is increasingly being automated from laboratories and healthcare settings; however, there still is frequently a need for an individual to be designated at a facility as responsible for assuring that data transfer is complete and accurate.

Data collection instruments

The desire to collect detailed information must be tempered by the need to limit data to items that can be reliably and consistently collected and analysed over the long term. Forms or other data collection instruments that are too detailed and too complicated will not be welcomed by those on whom the surveillance system must depend. This is independent of whether the forms are computerized, although computerization may make the process more acceptable to reporters. In addition, computerized systems that exist for other purposes (for example, patient records) may permit more detailed collection of data without additional burden to the reporter, but may overwhelm those responsible for analysis.

Standards for exchanging information are critical to the future utility of all public health surveillance and information systems. Many coding systems currently used in public health are not compatible with the needs of other organizations. In 1996, the American Congress passed the Health Insurance Portability and Accountability Act to encourage the development of standards for data related to healthcare. The passage of this legislation together with increased attention to use of electronic medical record systems for public health monitoring has increased the level of activity related to integration of clinical and public health information in the United States (Office of the National Coordinator for Health Information Technology, http://hhs.gov/healthit; accessed 21 June 2007).

Timing

Surveillance systems provide data on a regular basis, ranging from daily to annually. Whatever periodicity is used should be specified and adhered to by participants in all phases of the surveillance loop; reporting should occur even when the number of reported cases is zero. To contain an outbreak of meningococcal meningitis, the health department must receive reports of cases quickly (i.e. within 24 h) so that necessary control measures may be taken immediately. In contrast, a breast cancer registry evaluating the effectiveness of targeted screening services for breast cancer may collect and analyse data on a quarterly basis or even less frequently. With increasing computerization and Internet use, reporting at the time of case identification is becoming a reality.

Aggregation of data

Surveillance data may be in the form of individual patient (or other case) records or aggregate counts and tabulations. For example, there may be a need at the local level to maintain records on individual people to direct follow-up services. In addition, individual data permit more flexibility of analysis than aggregate data, and computerization has facilitated transfer of case-specific data at all levels.

Data transmission

The mode of data transmission will depend on both the need for timeliness and availability of resources. In many health agencies in well-resourced and under-resourced countries, reliance on postage of forms or facsimile transmission continues to exist. Since the 1990s, the Internet has increasingly been used in surveillance systems, facilitating transmission of data. In addition, computerization may facilitate and enhance regular and personal contact among public health officials, healthcare providers, and others who participate in such activities as closed (for example, Epi-X) or open electronic mail systems (see, for example, ProMED mail) (M'ikanatha *et al.* 2006).

Data management and dissemination

The following issues in data management and dissemination should be considered in planning for storage, analysis, and dissemination of surveillance information.

Updating records

Surveillance data often need to be updated. Information that was initially unattainable may become available, follow-up investigations yield supplemental information, people initially classified as meeting or not meeting a case definition may be reclassified, errors in reporting may be identified and corrected, and duplicate case reports may be recognized and culled. One approach to handling these and other changes is to maintain both provisional and final records.

Selecting measures for time and place

A case report may include dates, such as those of the onset of disease, the diagnosis, the report to local health authorities, and the report to regional or national health authorities. Analyses of surveillance data may be based on the date of any of these events. However, if there are, for example, long delays between dates of diagnosis and report, analyses of trends based on date of diagnosis will be unreliable for the most recent periods. Similarly, surveillance data may be tabulated on the basis of the site of occurrence of the health event, the site of diagnosis, or the residence of people reported.

Confidentiality/privacy

Preventing inappropriate disclosure of surveillance data is essential both to the privacy of people with reported cases of disease and to the trust of participants in the surveillance system. The protection of confidentiality begins with limiting collection of identifying information and transmission to a minimum and includes ensuring the physical security of surveillance records, the discretion of surveillance staff, and legal safeguards. Surveillance programmes may have explicit standards and guidelines to promote consistent practices which protect the security and confidentiality of surveillance data (see, for example Centers for Disease Control and Prevention and Council of State and Territorial Epidemiologists. Technical Guidance for HIV/AIDS Surveillance Programs, Volume III: Security and Confidentiality Guidelines. Atlanta, Georgia: Centers for Disease Control and Prevention; 2006. Available at http://www.cdc.gov/hiv/topics/surveillance/resources/guidelines/guidance/pdf/Security_and_Confidentiality_v3.pdf; accessed 25July 2007). To elicit public health surveillance information from the public and from healthcare providers, strong laws that assure a careful procedure for maintaining and reporting data are frequently necessary to ensure the privacy of personal information. Further, public health uses of data require definition, and should arise from a broad consensus of stakeholders in clinical medicine, public health, and the community (Fairchild *et al.* 2007). Adequate protection for electronic health information is also needed. Protection of privacy must be balanced with the needs for public health surveillance.

Physical protection of records is accomplished by rules of conduct for people involved in the design, development, operation, or maintenance of any surveillance system. For example, confidential records should be kept locked up at all times when not in use. When confidential records are in use, they must be kept out of the sight of people not authorized to work with the records. Except as needed for operational purposes, copies of confidential records should not be made. When confidential surveillance records are in the possession of others, provision should be made for their protection. Sometimes forgotten in the discussion of health information privacy is the concept that use of electronic information systems can often improve the security of data.

Provision of data containing identifiers of individuals or establishments should be held to the minimum number deemed essential to perform public health functions. Categories should be sufficiently broad to avoid inadvertent identification of an individual person or institution. Data should be as widely available as possible in accordance with the need to protect confidentiality and privacy.

Initiating and maintaining participation

Public health agencies have historically depended on the ongoing cooperation of others to identify and report cases. Whether reporting has been required by law, is voluntary, or is financially rewarded, most reporting has traditionally taken time and effort. Even with electronic reporting, many surveillance systems require contact of public health professionals with the reporting sources. Dissemination of reports that document the usefulness of surveillance data is likely to be a key to initiating and maintaining participation in the system. In addition to professional meetings and other personal contacts, electronic mail affords an excellent route of informal communication with reporters.

Reporting may be required by law. Although legal mandates may not guarantee reporting, they establish the authority under which health agencies conduct surveillance. In addition, reporting laws and regulations may identify not only those who are required to report cases but also those who may report cases without fear of liability for violation of privacy. Statutes may also protect health agencies from forced disclosure of the identity of people with particular diseases.

Organizational structure

If the surveillance loop of data collection, analysis, interpretation, and feedback is to function as a continuous process, an organizational structure is required. Such a structure depends on the resources available (for example, the number of personnel and their level of training; the technology available for communication and data management) as well as the number and type of diseases, health conditions, or risk factors under surveillance. In one example of a simple form of reporting, the organizational structure requires healthcare providers to report a single disease or health event on a regular basis to a co-ordinating public health authority. A more complex form would include a network of reporting units dealing concurrently with problems related to many diseases. In any case, the structure must allow data to be gathered from various sources and evaluated by epidemiologists in time for appropriate action to be taken. Automated systems may be in place to 'flag' the data if the number of cases in a category reaches a certain threshold; the statistical flag will alert the epidemiologist to the need for further evaluation. This is particularly true for diseases that are common (for example, influenza) or data that encompass a large number of conditions and variables (for example, emergency department diagnoses). The information must be routinely disseminated to a targeted audience, that includes those stakeholders involved in reporting and those who are responsible for prevention and control programmes. Implicit in collection of data by public health authorities may also be the expectation to investigate and control increases in disease incidence (for example, legionellosis) to prevent and control the disease under surveillance.

The structure should provide support for training of key personnel in surveillance through seminars, distance-based learning, or other venues that give field and central staff the opportunity to review procedures and to resolve operational problems. Appropriate technical support, such as provision of diagnostic reagents, laboratory space, and computers and other electronic equipment, must also be ensured. Finally, the need for periodic or preferably, ongoing evaluation of the surveillance systems should be recognized.

Delegating tasks to international, national, regional, and local health authorities should depend on information needs and resources at each level. Particular attention should be directed to the local level because primary responsibility for information collection and public health responsibilities are usually local. Central agencies are responsible for guiding, as well as co-ordinating, data collection procedures; they ensure that surveillance data are collected using standardized methodology such that the data from one geographical area can be reliably compared with data from another area and such that the data can be aggregated into regional or national summaries. Also, because many monitoring efforts for non-infectious conditions (for example, traffic injuries, water contamination) often involve governmental agencies other than public health agencies (for example, police authorities, environmental protection agencies), there needs to be effective co-ordination between health authorities and other appropriate authorities.

Surveillance systems and data collection

Public health surveillance data are collected in many ways, depending on the nature of the health event under surveillance, potential methods for identifying the disease, the population involved, the resources available, and the goals of the programme. Some surveillance systems may rely on a single source of data with alternate data sources being used periodically or in an ongoing way to evaluate or to monitor and to enhance the completeness of routine surveillance data.

In *case surveillance* systems, all cases of a health condition that have been recognized through clinical or laboratory examinations are eligible for reporting to the surveillance systems. For other surveillance purposes, it may be acceptable to collect more detailed information on a subset of all cases. In a *supplemental surveillance* system, detailed information about health behaviours or molecular characteristics of an infectious agent is obtained. For example, in the United States, the HIV/AIDS case surveillance system aims to collect basic demographic and clinical information on all persons diagnosed with HIV infection (Glynn *et al.* 2007), and supplemental surveillance systems may provide information on HIV subtype, resistance patterns, behaviours among persons living with HIV infection, clinical outcomes of HIV infection, and met and unmet resource needs. Where possible, supplemental surveillance systems should use rigorous methods to increase the representativeness of data on a subset of cases.

Notification systems

Notifiable disease reporting is the surveillance approach traditionally used by public health programmes. A system of notification is based on laws or regulations by health authorities that require reporting of selected diseases or conditions, usually infectious, to the health department to support and direct prevention and control programmes. Notification reporting may be instituted at many levels (local, national, and international). Ultimately, under a system of notification, the reporting will be most useful and most accurate for diseases if surveillance is supported and emphasized at a local level. People or institutions with responsibility for reporting to the public health authority often include doctors, other healthcare providers, coroners and medical examiners, laboratories, and hospitals. Historically, doctors and other healthcare workers such as infection control practitioners have been most important to systems of notification. Reliance on laboratory reporting and on computerized records collected primarily for other reasons is increasing.

In any country, the extent of notification activities depends on the availability and use of facilities and resources—trained staff, laboratory and other equipment, epidemiological services, and liaison with healthcare providers and other key reporters—as well as the health priority of the disease and method of diagnosis. The case must first be diagnosed and reliance on empiric diagnosis and treatment with broad-spectrum antibiotics for many infectious conditions may hinder public health surveillance. If diagnosed, reports are often initiated by healthcare providers or other reporting source; for some diseases for which more complete reporting is sought, public health professionals may contact major reporting sources and/or review laboratory or other relevant records to ensure that diagnosed cases are ascertained. These systems of reporting have been described as passive and active respectively, but the distinctions are not always clear. Data for many surveillance programmes represent a mixture of both active and passive reporting.

Reporting is incomplete for most notifiable diseases. If people are asymptomatic or have only mild symptoms, they will not usually seek healthcare, and as noted above, they may not acquire a laboratory diagnosis even if they seek medical care. In addition, patients and doctors may conceal diseases that carry a social stigma. Healthcare providers may also fail to report because they may be unaware of regulations or because they may treat the symptoms without a complete laboratory investigation. Completeness of reporting may also be significantly influenced by factors such as medical community interest and publicity; the most important factor is probably the intensity of surveillance efforts. Many incomplete data may serve their purpose, however. Epidemics, as well as general temporal and geographical trends, can be determined as long as the proportion of cases detected remains consistent over time and across geographical areas. Problems with lack of representativeness and heterogeneity of reporting characteristics as often seen in surveillance (for example, bacterial sexually transmitted infections) may limit the usefulness of incomplete data for evaluation of programmes and setting priorities (Lowndes 2004).

The potential for re-emergence of infectious diseases requires continued vigilance and capacity to respond, even though the control programme may not be a high public health priority (for example, plague). As new infectious agents are recognized, the need to expand the notifiable disease system to prevent and control these agents effectively has been recognized in many countries. Furthermore, as international travel and commerce facilitate the rapid spread of pathogens from one part of the globe to another, the need for improved international communicable disease surveillance has become apparent. The 2005 revision of the international health regulations will support these improvements. (Heymann & Rodier 1998; http://www.who.int/csr/ihr/en; accessed 27 July 2007).

Infectious conditions continue to dominate the list of notifiable diseases in most countries, although in some countries (for example, Canada) other diseases and conditions may also have to be notified to health authorities. Adverse drug reactions, occupational injuries, pesticide poisonings, and specified malignancies, among others, may be required to be reported, particularly in high-income countries (Koo & Wetterhall 1996).

Healthcare provider networks

Networks of healthcare providers have been organized for several decades, primarily to gather information on selected health events. Most have been organized by practising doctors on a voluntary basis; in many European countries, these networks have formed firm relationships with both public health authorities and academic centres. The strengths of sentinel provider systems include the commitment of the participants, the possibility of collecting longitudinal data, the flexibility of the system to address a changing set of conditions, and the ability to gain information on all patient–provider encounters, regardless of severity of illness. The most severe limitation of this type of system is that the population served by these doctors may not be representative of the general population. In addition, the illness must be fairly common to provide representative incidence data from a small sample of doctor contacts.

Example: The British Paediatric Surveillance Unit (BPSU)

The BPSU (http://bpsu.inopsu.com/publications/annual_report.html (accessed 21 March 2007) was initiated in 1986 through the collaboration of several agencies: The Institute of Child Health, the Royal College of Paediatric and Child Health, and the Health Protection Agency. The BPSU has enabled paediatricians to participate in the surveillance of emerging problems and in studies of uncommon disorders. It provides a mechanism by which new diseases can be detected quickly and monitored. The reporting system involves the mailing of a monthly card which contains the disorders currently being surveyed; the system has been limited to 12 conditions. Examples of conditions under surveillance have included HIV infection and AIDS, insulin-dependent diabetes mellitus, acute flaccid paralysis, and new variant Creutzfeldt–Jakob disease in children.

Example: Rotavirus sentinel surveillance

China has the second highest number of deaths due to rotavirus infection in the world. With a licensed vaccine in hand, China developed a sentinel surveillance system for rotavirus infection among children hospitalized in any of six hospitals. Such a surveillance system will be useful in assessing the impact of rotavirus vaccine administration as well as assessing the economic burden of rotavirus and the emergence of new strains (Fang *et al.* 2005).

Laboratory surveillance

Laboratory surveillance may be conducted as part of a notifiable diseases system, sentinel surveillance system, or other system. Diagnosis is the cornerstone for many diseases, and the use of molecular tools and drug sensitivity testing has further advanced our ability to detect epidemics amongst cases that otherwise may have been considered sporadic or unrelated. The use of molecular tools to enhance surveillance of pathogens is growing in many countries to facilitate epidemiologic linkage. PulseNet serves as a network of public health laboratories that performs DNA 'fingerprinting' on bacteria that may be foodborne. The network permits rapid comparison of these 'fingerprint' patterns through an electronic database. For example, similar pulsed field gel electrophoresis patterns of *E. coli* 0157:H7 bacteria isolated from ill people suggest that the bacteria come from a common source as with a widely distributed contaminated food product (Swaminathan *et al.* 2001; http://www.cdc.gov/PULSENET; accessed July 27, 2007).

Molecular methods are also increasingly applied in surveillance of the HIV epidemic, either as a laboratory adjunct to case reporting, or as a supplemental surveillance system. For example, surveillance systems in Canada (Jayaraman *et al.* 2006) routinely characterize newly diagnosed HIV infections with respect to the HIV subtype.

Disease registries

Registries are comprehensive longitudinal listings of people with particular conditions. They often include detailed information about diagnostic classification, treatment, and outcome. Registries were initially established primarily for epidemiological research on individual diseases or conditions to develop aetiological hypotheses and to identify cases for further research (Weddell 1973). Registries have also been used to ensure the provision of appropriate care and to evaluate changing patterns of medical care; unlike other disease information systems, they cut across the different levels of severity of illness and may provide information over time about individual people. Recently, the value of registries for monitoring disease incidence and its distribution, as well as for evaluating the effectiveness of targeted screening programmes, has been more widely recognized.

To focus on selected diseases or conditions, registries often develop a constituency that promotes participation and reporting. Most registries rely on numerous sources of data for case detection including, but not limited to, hospitals, laboratories, and death records; few registries rely primarily on doctor notification.

Example: Birth defects

Surveillance for birth defects was first initiated in response to the thalidomide tragedy; registries were established to provide reliable baseline rates for specific birth defects and to detect increases in the prevalence of birth defects as a means of rapidly identifying human teratogens. The CDC has conducted birth defects surveillance in metropolitan Atlanta since 1967 by using multiple sources of ascertainment of all serious birth defects observed in stillborn and liveborn infants or recognized by signs and symptoms apparent in the first year of life (Correa-Villasenor *et al.* 2003).

The International Clearinghouse for Birth Defects Surveillance and Research consists of 40 registries globally (Botto *et al.* 2006). The International Clearinghouse conducts a spectrum of surveillance activities that includes monitoring of selected conditions (for example, orofacial clefts) and the exchange of 'rumours', cluster information, and findings of still unpublished studies. They serve as an example of the intersection of surveillance and research with their assessment of the potential teratogenicity of first-trimester use of medications (the MADRE project).

Health information systems

Surveillance systems often depend on existing health data collection systems; these systems may be either integral to surveillance or serve as an adjunct to surveillance for specific diseases or conditions. Lack of accuracy and specificity in these existing data systems remains a concern, however, and most surveillance systems continue to need additional data collection systems to meet the needs of specific prevention and control programmes. For example, an increase in deaths attributed to 'cirrhosis', on death certificates, may be the result of an infectious agent, alcohol use, or other toxin. The occurrence of bladder cancer may or may not be related to a particular environmental exposure. These data are useful as an adjunct to surveillance systems; they are also increasingly used to provide situational awareness through syndromic surveillance.

There is frequently a lengthy interval between death and collection and analysis of death certificates, which may make such vital statistics less useful for surveillance purposes when more current data are needed. However, summary vital data can be rapidly collected. For example, weekly reporting of deaths from 121 American cities to CDC has been integral to the surveillance of influenza epidemics in that country (Choi & Thacker 1981) (Fig. 6.17.1) (http://www.cdc.gov/mmwr/preview/mmwrhtml/mm5523a2.htm, CDC 2006; accessed 25 July 2007). In addition, automated systems for coding mortality information are both expanding and improving internationally.

Medical examiner and coroner reports

For a more detailed description of circumstances surrounding deaths (including autopsy reports, toxicology studies, and police reports), medical examiner and coroner records may be useful. In the United States, these reports are most representative of deaths caused by intentional and unintentional injuries and other unnatural causes. These records have been used for surveillance of such conditions as heat-wave-related mortality, sudden unexplained death syndrome in Southeast Asian refugees, and alcohol-related injuries. Systematic necropsy examinations have also been useful in ascertaining the contribution of tuberculosis to mortality of HIV-infected individuals in West Africa. Antibody determinations performed on post-mortem medical examiner samples may be useful for estimating population prevalence of infectious diseases (for example, dengue) (Rigau-Perez *et al.* 2006).

Insurance records and workers' compensation claims

Insurance records and workers' compensation claims have been useful for surveillance of injuries and illnesses in specific geographical locales. Because regulations governing completion and submission of forms differ both among and within jurisdictions, data derived from these systems cannot easily be compared. In addition, the use of medical claims data for surveillance may be limited by the accuracy of diagnostic recording.

The severity of reported injury also varies and reporting is also influenced by regulations outlining eligibility for workers' compensation, and other legislation related to compensation and medical care, rehabilitation of those injured at work, and the degree of fear of job loss resulting from absence from work. Data from these systems generally provide an underestimate of the actual incidence or prevalence of the health condition under surveillance; the underestimate may be of a considerable degree (Fan *et al.* 2006).

Surveys of health behaviour

Behavioural data can be collected from the general population, from populations at particular risk for the health condition of interest, and from populations affected by the health condition of interest (Davy 2006). Household surveys of the general population, such as the Behavioral Risk Factor Surveillance System conducted in the United States (http://www.cdc.gov/brfss; accessed 25 July 2007) or the General Household Survey in England and Wales (Twigg 1999), have provided information at the national level on personal health practices such as alcohol use and smoking, disabilities, and doctor encounters. Inclusion of behavioural measures has been advocated by the World Health Organization for HIV and sexually transmitted infection surveillance programmes. Increasingly, demographic and health surveys are conducted to include both

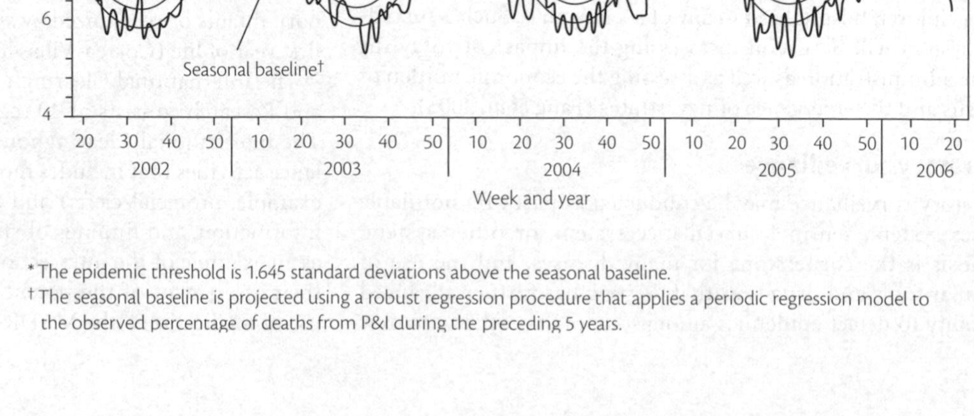

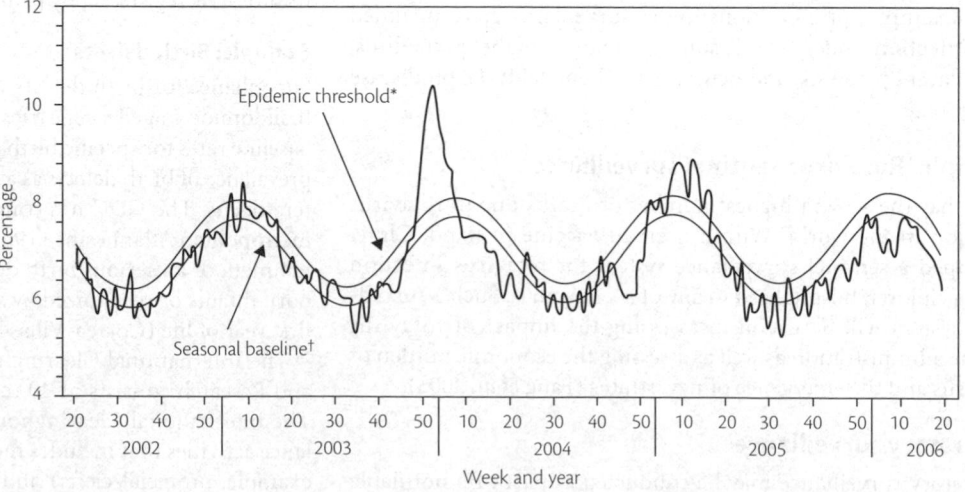

Fig. 6.17.1 Percentage of deaths attributed to pneumonia and influenza (P&I) reported by the 122 Cities Mortality Reporting System, by week and year—United States, 2002–2006.
Source: MMWR, Volume 55/No. 23, June 16, 2006.

* The epidemic threshold is 1.645 standard deviations above the seasonal baseline.
† The seasonal baseline is projected using a robust regression procedure that applies a periodic regression model to the observed percentage of deaths from P&I during the preceding 5 years.

behavioural and biologic measures, and to use sampling methods that provide representative data on a population level (Central Bureau of Statistics, Nairobi, Kenya 2003).

In high-income countries, where most residences have telephones, telephone interviews have the advantages of lower cost and ease of supervising interviewers. Interview surveys conducted by telephone and in person can obtain personal health-related information with only minor differences in the reported prevalence of various health conditions between the two techniques.

Surveys of populations at special risk may also play an important role in guiding public health response. Such systems may be relatively simple, in the form of episodic surveys of convenience samples (for example, episodic convenience samples of men who have sex with men attending gay bars in Scotland) (Williamson *et al.* 2007) or may be formalized as ongoing surveillance systems. Such surveys can provide data on levels of risk behaviours, on adoption of desired preventive behaviours, and on exposure to public health prevention messages.

Syndromic surveillance

A growing number of public health agencies have been prompted by concerns about the threat of bioterrorism to invest in 'syndromic surveillance' with an initial aim in their development to detect epidemics more quickly than traditional approaches (CDC 2004).

Syndromic surveillance involves monitoring of trends in illness syndromes or other manifestations of illness, such as healthcare seeking behaviours, that may be apparent before diagnoses are established. Because these systems emphasize timeliness of the entire surveillance process, often enabling daily or even more frequent assessments of trends in health-related events, they generally rely on electronic information systems. Such systems use automated methods to harvest electronically stored data, apply statistical tools to detect aberrant trends, and make information rapidly available to epidemiologists using Internet-based systems. Despite this emphasis on automation, these systems still require human judgment to interpret reports and determine what level of further assessment or response is warranted when statistical alerts are generated.

In using the term 'syndromic surveillance' to describe this approach, it is worth noting that surveillance of disease syndromes has long been used in public health, especially in situations where broad criteria are used to identify possible cases of high-priority diseases, where infrastructure constraints do not allow for surveillance based on confirmed diagnoses, or when surveillance is established for newly recognized conditions of unknown aetiology (http://www.cdc.gov/ncidod/eid/vol10no7/pdfs/03-1035_04-0125.pdf; accessed 25 July 2007). Another term that has come into increasing use to describe the approach is 'biosurveillance', although that term has also been used as a synonym for public health surveillance in general.

The most commonly used method of syndromic surveillance in the United States has been to monitor the presenting complaints of patients seeking emergency department care (Fig. 6.17.2) (Heffernan *et al.* 2004) Algorithms are used to scan the electronically recorded text of patients' 'chief complaints', which are classified into various syndrome categories, such as 'fever', 'respiratory disease', 'vomiting', 'diarrhoea', or 'rash'. For example, a parent may bring a child to a hospital emergency department because of concern about fever and tell the triage nurse, 'My baby feels hot'. The algorithm would scan for the text sequence 'h-o-t' to categorize the patient into a febrile illness syndrome category, while simultaneously excluding from that category the patient who states, 'I was shot'. These algorithms attempt to account for variations in professional lingo, abbreviations, slang, or misspellings. Following the onset of illness, a person may miss work or school, purchase over-the-counter medications, telephone a healthcare provider, visit a doctor's office or clinic, go to a hospital emergency department, or be admitted to a hospital. In our increasingly automated world, each of these and many other health-related events are likely to generate some form of electronic record that could theoretically be used for health surveillance. Indeed, a wide mix of data sources are being used or tested for use in syndromic surveillance (Mandl *et al.* 2004).

Attention has increasingly focused on the utility of syndromic surveillance for detecting epidemics arising from non-intentional events. To date, experience has been mixed and largely anecdotal. In some instances, outbreaks of mild or moderate disease severity have been detected using syndromic surveillance; in other instances, outbreaks detected through other means have been missed by syndromic surveillance (Buehler *et al.* 2003). For the purpose of early detection, critics of syndromic surveillance have challenged the wisdom of investments in this method, noting in particular its cost may be excessive when false alarms result in unnecessary investigations. Proponents counter that its utility extends beyond epidemic detection, including use of syndromic surveillance to monitor trends in seasonal viral illnesses such as influenza or norovirus infections, to monitor the course of epidemics regardless of

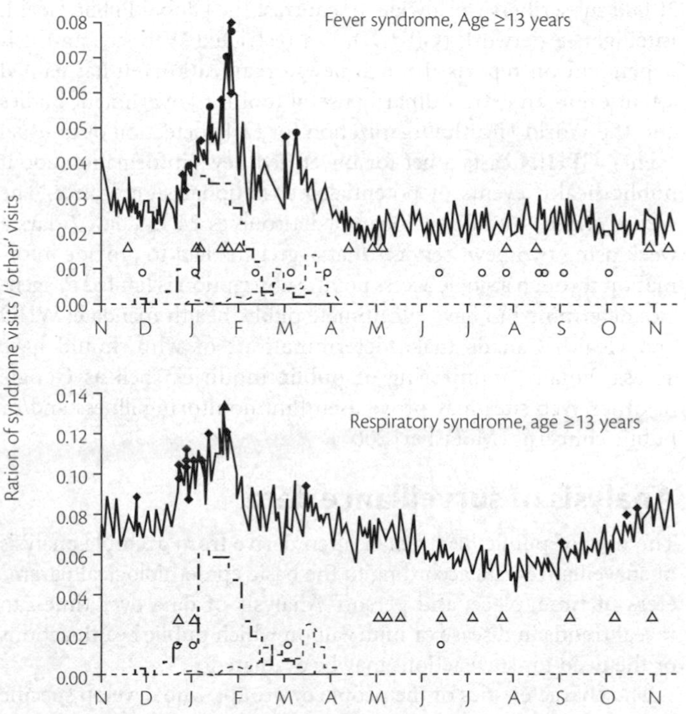

Fig. 6.17.2 Trends in emergency department visits for fever and respiratory syndromes, New York City, November 1, 2001–November 14, 2002. Plots show the daily ratio of syndrome visits to other (noninfectious disease) visits. ◆, citywide signal; Δ, spatial signal by hospital; O, spatial signal by patient's home zip code; – · –, influenza A; – – – – –, influenza B isolates (weekly number identified in New York residents by World Health Organization collaborating laboratories). *Source*: Emerging Infectious Diseases, Volume 10/No. 5, May 2004.

how they are detected, or to conduct surveillance for a spectrum of health conditions beyond infectious diseases. This broader role for syndromic surveillance has been termed 'situational awareness' monitoring.

Research, development, and evaluation of syndromic surveillance are ongoing. Virtually every dimension of syndromic surveillance is the focus of efforts to identify optimal methods, including data sources, syndrome classification criteria, statistical methods, and approaches to assessing statistical alerts. Ultimately, the current practice of syndromic surveillance may prove to be a waypoint in the evolution of potential interfaces between public health and healthcare information systems. Healthcare providers are collaborating in some areas to electronically link access to patients' medical records across multiple providers. These networks have been called 'regional health information organizations' or 'health information exchanges' (Public Health Informatics Institute 2005).

Internet-based approaches to surveillance

The widespread use of the Internet and electronic media has led to innovations in public health surveillance reaching far beyond traditional methods of disease monitoring on an individual patient basis. The first major inroad was ProMed (Program for Monitoring Emerging Diseases) initiated in 1994 such that individuals could communicate with one another on a public Web site, with a moderator assuring the professionalism of the Web site. The system is sponsored by the International Society for Infectious Diseases (Madoff & Woodall 2005). Information posted on ProMed includes alerts, reports of epidemics, and local observer reports, with over 30 000 subscribers worldwide. In contrast the Global Public Health Intelligence network (GPHIN), is a restricted Web site, and it is dependent on reports through news organizations. It has gained attention as an extraordinarily useful tool for government bodies and the World Health Organization for early detection of unusual events. GPHIN casts a net for unverified news information about public health events of potential international significance. The secure system monitors global media sources 24 h a day, 7 days a week using two news services that aggregate data to provide information through a single access point. Subscription is limited to agencies determined to have a legitimate public health mandate; WHO and Health Canada make determinations of who should have access. Finally, monitoring of public inquiries such as Google or other Web sites may prove useful in monitoring illness and/or public concerns (Motashari 2007).

Analysis of surveillance data

The uses of public health data often derive from a simple analysis of surveillance data according to the basic epidemiological parameters of time, place, and person. Analysis of data over time can reveal trends in disease or injury upon which public health actions or the need for such actions may be evaluated.

The characteristics of the people or groups who develop specific diseases or sustain specific injuries are important in understanding the disease or injury, identifying those at high risk, and targeting intervention efforts. For example, disparities in health (incidence or severity of disease) among members of different population groups highlight the need to identify cultural, economic, or social factors associated with these health problems.

When combined with appropriate population information, morbidity or mortality rates can be calculated to compare risks of disease and the magnitude of various health problems. Often rates are examined in broad age groups that are selected to reflect the different sets of conditions affecting mortality rates in each group (Doll 1974). Proper analysis of surveillance data can also assist in determining aetiology, setting priorities, determining modes of transmission, risk factors associated with disease, and opportunities for prevention or control, detecting epidemics, monitoring long-term trends, making projections of future disease occurrence, and evaluating effectiveness of interventions.

Typically, public health surveillance data are completed, summarized, and reported over specified time intervals (for example, weeks, months, or years) and may be mapped. Methods applicable to such time series data can be used to separate true temporal trends in the underlying risk from the random fluctuations, or 'noise'. The surveillance data should be plotted over the time during which they were collected. A clearer picture of this possible trend and of meaningful short-term patterns in these data are more evident if the random day-to-day variation in the number of cases is reduced. Smoothing potentially highlights meaningful patterns in collections of observed data by reducing the level of random noise (Devine & Parrish 1998). More advanced methods for analysis of surveillance data by time includes autoregressive time series techniques (Box & Jenkins 1976), generalized regression methods, and Bayesian modelling (Stroup & Thacker 1993). In addition, forecasts may be made by using regression and time series analyses, for example as for the surveillance of influenza (Fig. 6.17.2) (Serfling 1963; Choi & Thacker 1981; CDC 1999), or analyses may combine information from several surveillance series. In addition, methods (for example, Bayesian techniques) that incorporate information in addition to the data themselves, such as changes in a surveillance case definition or surveillance information from contiguous data, can be useful when applied to public health surveillance data.

The approach to the prevention and control of disease and injury is often determined by circumstances unique to 'place': The geographical distribution of the disease or of its causative exposures or risk-associated behaviour. The analysis of surveillance data by place has long used dot density maps, and geographic information systems are improving the ability to monitor disease occurrence, health inequalities, environmental exposures, and related health risks, and advance hypothesis generation about the associative causation of disease aetiologies and outcomes. For example, from the American Bureau of the Census national digital street and geographical boundary files, or Topologically Integrated Geographic Encoding and Referencing (TIGER) system, epidemiologists can translate or geocode street addresses into unique latitude and longitude locations. These locations then can be examined with computationally rigorous spatial statistical data analysis techniques using geographical information systems. Expanding computational opportunities permit dynamic space–time modelling of georeferenced data on the extent, structure, and association of diseases and suspected covariates (Anselin 1998). Statistical models of cancer incidence have been developed that incorporate potential predictors of spatial and temporal variation of cancer occurrence and that account for delay in case reporting (Pickle *et al.* 2007).

Epidemic detection and cluster analysis

Many epidemics are detected by astute healthcare providers who observe an increase in disease occurrence often before disease reports are received, assembled, and reviewed by health departments. The ongoing surveillance process between health practitioners and health departments increases the likelihood that providers will contact the health department when they suspect an outbreak or any unusual occurrence of disease.

Surveillance is most likely to detect epidemics in situations where cases, despite their aetiological link, are occurring over a wide geographic area over a relatively gradual period, or among a well-defined subgroup with links among cases (for example, epidemiological links or similar molecular patterns of isolates) that would not be apparent to individual practitioners.

A frequent concern of the analysis of surveillance data is whether an apparent cluster of health events in time is significant and unlikely to have occurred by chance alone. Although the application of cluster detection methods is growing, many of these methods require further examination and their use in surveillance remains controversial (Devine & Parrish 1998). Most of these methods involve a comparison of observed incidence with a historical baseline and may involve clustering in time (Stroup & Thacker 1993), clustering in space, or clustering in both time and space (Besag & Newell 1991). The rapidly evolving practice of syndromic surveillance has fostered renewed attention to the development of statistical methods for detecting temporal and spatial-temporal aberrations in disease trends (International Society for Disease Surveillance; www.syndromic.org; accessed 25 July 2007).

Statistical limitations of surveillance data

Surveillance data have traditionally had specific characteristics that have made application of standard statistical techniques difficult. First, reporting bias may produce data that are not representative of the population.

Second, under-reporting may be considerable, particularly in a voluntary system of notification. When another independent source of data is available (for example, hospital discharge, vital statistics), the total number of cases actually occurring can be estimated (Cormack 1963) but has had limited success in public health surveillance. In addition, specific information for each case may be incompletely reported and imputation may be needed.

Provisional data increase the timeliness and hence may increase the usefulness of public health surveillance data to epidemiologists; current provisional data should be compared with historical provisional data to avoid bias since provisional data may differ markedly from final data. To enhance the usefulness of provisional data for recent periods, epidemiologists may compare these data retrospectively with confirmed data to estimate what final data for recent periods will eventually reveal. A model can incorporate this consistent under-reporting to permit more accurate estimation of the final data from provisional data.

Role of surveillance data in evaluation of community interventions

The ease with which trends in disease occurrence can be linked to interventions depends on both the disease and the intervention. The success of an immunization campaign can usually be easily inferred from surveillance data; however, such inferences become difficult when several factors contribute to a change in disease occurrence. Analyses are also difficult because of constraints such as migration and variable acceptance of interventions in the community. In addition, combining data from several communities with similar public health programmes will strengthen the assessment of programme effectiveness.

Mathematical models can be used to elucidate the complexities of evaluating community interventions. Such models have been used most extensively for infectious diseases. Ecological spatial studies of tuberculosis incidence using socio-economic indicators have been conducted using hierarchical Bayesian models to estimate the relative risk of the occurrence of tuberculosis (Souza *et al.* 2007). Models have also been developed for predicting the decline of mortality rates due to cirrhosis using population changes in levels of consumption of alcohol (Skog 1984), for cardiovascular disease using changes in cigarette consumption in a population (Kullback & Cornfield 1976), and for blood lead levels given changes in legislation banning lead from petrol (Annest *et al.* 1983).

Linkage of surveillance data to other information sources

Given the complexity of establishing new data and information systems, there is increasing interest in the combination of existing databases for surveillance purposes. Linkage of datasets has facilitated calculation of rates, such as birthweight-specific death rates that can be calculated following linkage of birth and death certificates (McCarthy *et al.* 1980); linkage of HIV and tuberculosis records (Ahmed *et al.* 2007), and linkage of records for injury surveillance (Clark 2004). A study assessing characteristics of unmatched maternal and baby records in linked birth records and hospital discharge data suggests that studies using linked data should examine and report on the characteristics of unmatched data and recognize them as a source of potential bias. In some countries, a unique number may be assigned to an individual at birth to serve as a reference number for any contact with healthcare services.

Techniques involved in data linkage are often complex and are based on matching records by comparison of key data fields (Newcombe 1988; Newgard 2006). When record systems are linked, the probability that the record linkage is correct must be determined, with the degree of certainty of a correct linkage depending on the comparisons of the individual identifiers such as name or initials, date or year of birth, sex, and race/ethnicity, and address. These methods of probabilistic record linkage are more likely than phonetic coding systems to identify people already reported, though they often require a decision to be made on the part of the system operator as to whether the reported matches are valid. Any linked set will normally contain a small number of pairs that should not have been linked and, conversely, will have missed a few pairs that should have been linked. An advantage of probabilistic data matching is that records may frequently be linked even when parts of the identifying information are either incomplete, miscoded, or misspelled.

Dissemination of data

Communication of surveillance data is an essential step in the surveillance chain. The purpose of the communication and the audience targeted must be defined. Appropriate feedback must be given to those providing the data to demonstrate their usefulness and to stimulate further reporting. People providing the data should be credited for their contributions and acknowledged for their provision of accurate and complete data. Public health professionals, policy-makers, or others who may be responsible for taking action or setting the direction of public health programmes in response to surveillance data must receive the information that they need from the surveillance system on a timely basis and in an appropriate format for their use. In addition, these data should be available as widely as possible to all who may be interested in analysis and interpretation of these data. Web sites are increasingly used to disseminate surveillance data as with the US CDC's *Morbidity and Mortality Weekly Report* (www.cdc.gov/MMWR; accessed 25 July 2007), the WHO's *Weekly Epidemiological Record* (www.who.int/wer; accessed 25 July 2007), and the European CDC's *Eurosurveillance* (http://www.eurosurveillance.org/; accessed 25 July 2007).

Surveillance data provide information for action, and this tenet is embedded in WHO's Global Outbreak Alert and Response Network. This Network is a technical collaboration of existing institutions and networks who pool human and technical resources for the identification, confirmation, and response to outbreaks of international importance (www.who.int/csr/outbreaknetwork/en; accessed 23 July 2007).

The data must be provided on a regular basis, with the frequency of surveillance reports dependent on the nature of the surveillance system, the characteristics of the disease process (for example, surveillance reports on measles are required more frequently than reports on cancer), and the public health impact of the disease. For diseases and other health events requiring major policy decisions (for example, removal of lead paint from older homes), it may be useful to provide frequent updates to remind policy-makers of the potential for prevention. Provisional data should be accepted for dissemination, since rapid turn-around of data is usually more important than absolute accuracy and completeness; rarely have provisional data driven major public health decisions in directions different from those that would have been based on final data.

The format for dissemination varies with the target audience; a creative design will help to make the information stand apart from other documents and receive greater attention. Most policy-makers and clinicians would prefer to see the data interpreted using graphics accompanied by an abbreviated summary text. The important role that graphs and maps can play in visually decoding large quantities of data has been clearly demonstrated, with graphic displays giving the reader an understanding of large and complex datasets not conveyed easily in other ways (Tukey 1977; Tufte 1983; Dean *et al.* 1998). Many epidemiologists and other scientists, including mathematicians projecting the future course of diseases, find the more detailed raw data most useful. Comparison with previous years or previous periods (for example, experience of the last 12 months compared with experience of the previous 12 months) is often helpful.

Evaluation of surveillance systems

Traditionally, surveillance systems have been periodically evaluated to ensure that important public health problems are under surveillance and that useful information for disease prevention and control is collected. Evaluation may also be considered in a broader strategy of continuous quality assurance (Krause 2006). An evaluation of a surveillance system should include a review of its objectives, a detailed description of its operation, an assessment of its performance, and recommendations. If the evaluation is part of a broader system of quality assurance, an integrated feedback loop that continues in real-time may have more impact on the improvement of the system than a more formal assessment conducted infrequently. Surveillance systems should contribute to the prevention and control of adverse health events, and the system should be assessed as to how its use fits with the explicitly defined objectives of the surveillance system.

The performance of surveillance systems can be judged by using a series of attributes, including sensitivity, timeliness, representativeness, positive predictive value, acceptability, flexibility, simplicity, and costs (CDC 2001). The importance of individual attributes will vary among systems, and efforts to improve on a system's performance on one attribute may compete with efforts to improve its performance on another. Thus the evaluation of surveillance systems should not focus solely on the extent to which each attribute is achieved but rather on the attainment of the appropriate balance of attributes.

Sensitivity

The sensitivity of a surveillance system is most often judged by its completeness of case reporting. If all people who meet the surveillance case definition in the target population are detected by a surveillance system, then the sensitivity of the surveillance system is often reported as 100 per cent. Sensitivity of surveillance systems is often measured by comparing routinely collected case reports with data obtained by special case-finding methods (Silk & Berkelman 2005). Sensitivity may also be defined in other ways such as the percentage of outbreaks detected and the percentage of all cases of disease occurrence that are reported. In the latter instance the denominator would include all cases of a disease whether or not they are diagnosed. For example, it is estimated in many countries that fewer than 10 per cent of persons with Legionnaires' disease are diagnosed and reported.

Timeliness

Timeliness refers to the entire surveillance cycle, ranging from how quickly cases are reported to the distribution of surveillance reports. The need for timeliness is dependent on the condition (for example, the assessment of timeliness would be quite different for meningitis than for cancer). Electronic communication has the capacity to improve timeliness significantly. In addition to describing how quickly the steps of the surveillance process are completed, the timeliness of a surveillance system can also be used to describe its functionality, (for example, how quickly a system detects an important change in disease trends).

Representativeness

Representativeness is a measure of how well reported cases in a population reflect all cases that actually occurred in the population. This comparison often requires independent surveillance, which ascertains as many cases as possible in the population for a given time period. Surveillance reporting is rarely complete, and cases that are reported may differ from unreported cases in terms of demographic characteristics, site or use of healthcare services, or risk exposures (Alter *et al.* 1987). Representativeness of surveillance data is also affected by the quality of descriptive data that accompany case reports. Incomplete or incorrect data on surveillance forms limit representativeness.

Positive predictive value

People with reported cases of disease may not actually have the disease in question. This may reflect incorrect diagnoses (false positives), a lack of specificity in the case definition, or errors in the interpretation of the case definition. If all people reported as cases had the disease in question, then the positive predictive value would be 100 per cent. As with other characteristics such as sensitivity and timeliness, the concept of positive predictive value can be extended to the detection of epidemics in a surveillance system. If change in disease occurrence is used as an indicator to trigger investigations, then a high frequency of 'false alarms' would indicate a low predictive value for epidemic detection.

Acceptability

Surveillance systems depend on the co-operation of many people over a long period. If procedures are easy to follow and useful information is returned to participants, then acceptability is likely to remain high. The acceptability rate may also depend on the disease under surveillance, for example, if there is stigma attached to the disease, such as HIV or other sexually transmitted diseases, there may be underreporting.

Flexibility

The circumstances under which surveillance systems operate are subject to change, ranging from logistical constraints to information needs as well as changes in the understanding of disease (for example, AIDS). Surveillance systems should have sufficient flexibility to accommodate these changes.

Simplicity

Simplicity is desirable throughout the entire cycle in surveillance systems and is closely tied to other attributes such as acceptability, flexibility, and costs.

Costs

A description of the time requirements and costs of a surveillance system is useful. Evaluation of the costs and benefits of aggressive versus less aggressive case-finding methods in surveillance of selected notifiable diseases has yielded different conclusions that vary according to specific local circumstances (Vogt *et al.* 1986).

The evaluation of a surveillance system should conclude with an assessment of its structure and usefulness, considering its mix of attributes in relation to its objectives. Recommendations should state whether the system should be continued and what specific changes, if any, should be made.

Conclusion

Public health surveillance has historically galvanized and guided prevention and control programmes ranging from smallpox eradication and immunization campaigns for childhood diseases to programmes to prevent HIV infection and AIDS. Surveillance has also taken on increased visibility and importance in evaluating and guiding prevention and control efforts for non-infectious diseases and conditions. Surveillance provides a stimulus to keep prevention and control activities moving rapidly and in the right direction, guiding the response to individual cases as well as public policy.

Effective public health interventions depend upon a continuing and reliable source of information; resources should be allocated for the maintenance of the surveillance systems and for their regular evaluation. The data must be timely and representative of the population; they must be analysed and interpreted with feedback to the reporters and disseminated as widely as possible, including to those formulating and implementing public health policy. Resources devoted to surveillance data used to direct prevention and control activities must be balanced with resources needed to implement those activities.

Acknowledgements

The authors wish to thank Dr Donna Stroup for her contributions as an author on this chapter in the previous editions of this book.

References

Ahmed, A.B., Abubakar, I., Delpech, V. *et al.* (2007). The growing impact of HIV infection on the epidemiology of tuberculosis in England and Wales. *Thorax*, **62**, 672–676.

Alter, M.J., Mares, A., Hadler, S.C. *et al.*(1987). The effect of underreporting on the apparent incidence and epidemiology of acute viral hepatitis. *American Journal of Epidemiology*, **125**, 133–9.

Annest, J.L., Pirkle, J.L., Makuc, D. *et al.* (1983). Chronological trend in blood lead levels between 1976 and 1980. *New England Journal of Medicine*, **308**, 1373–7.

Anselin, L. (1998). Exploratory spatial data analysis in a geocomputational environment. In *Geocomputation, a primer* (eds. P. Longley, S. Brooks, R. McDonnell, and M. MacMillan M), pp. 77–94. Wiley, New York.

Baker, M.G. and Fidler, D.P. (2006). Global public health surveillance under new international health regulations. *Emerging Infectious Diseases*, **7**, 1058–65.

Berkelman, R.L. and Buehler, J.W. (1990). Public health surveillance of noninfectious chronic diseases: the potential to detect rapid change in disease burden. *International Journal of Epidemiology*, **19**, 628–35.

Berkelman, R.L., Bryan, R.T., Osterholm, M.T. *et al.* (1994). Infectious disease surveillance: a crumbling foundation. *Science*, **264**, 368–70.

Besag, J. and Newell, J. (1991). The detection of clusters in rare diseases. *Journal of the Royal Statistical Society*, **154**, 143–55.

Botto, L.D., Robert-Gnansia, E., Siffel, C. *et al.* (2006). Fostering international collaboration in birth defects research and prevention: a perspective from the International Clearinghouse for Birth Defects Surveillance and Research. *American Journal of Public Health*, **96**, 774–80.

Box, G. and Jenkins, G. (1976). *Time series analysis: forecasting and control.* Holden-Day, Oakland, CA.

Buehler, J.W., Berkelman R.L., Hartley, D.M., and Peters, C.J. (2004). Syndromic surveillance. *Emerging Infectious Diseases*, **10**, 1333–1334.

Cardenas, V.M., Roces, M.C., Wattanasri, S. *et al.* (2002). Improving global public health leadership through training in epidemiology and public health: The experience of TEPHINET. Training Programs in Epidemiology and Public Health Interventions Network. *American Journal of Public Health*, **92**, 196–7.

CDC (Centers for Disease Control) (1997). Case definitions for infectious conditions under public health surveillance. *Morbidity and Mortality Weekly Report*, **46**, 1–55.

CDC (Centers for Disease Control and Prevention) (1999). Update: Influenza activity—United States and worldwide, 1998–1999 season, and composition of the 1999–2000 influenza vaccine. *Morbidity and Mortality Weekly Report*, **48**, 374–8.

CDC (Centers for Disease Control and Prevention) (2001). Updated guidelines for evaluating public health surveillance systems. *Morbidity and Mortality Weekly Report*, **50**, 1–35.

CDC (Centers for Disease Control and Prevention) (2004). Framework for evaluating public health surveillance systems for early detection of outbreaks, Recommendations from the CDC Working Group. *Morbidity Mortality Weekly Report*, **53**(RR05),1–11. Available at: http://www.cdc.gov/mmwr/preview/mmwrhtml/rr5305a1.htm (accessed on 23 July 2007).

CDC (Centers for Disease Control and Prevention) (2006).Update: Influenza activity—United States and worldwide, 2005–06 Season, and Composition of the 2006–07 Influenza Vaccine. *Morbidity Morality Weekly Report*, **55**, 648–53.

CDC (Centers for Disease Control and Prevention) (2008) Revised Surveillance Case Definitions for HIV Infection, Incorporating the HIV Classification System and the AIDS Case Definition for Adults and Adolescents, HIV Infection Among Children Aged <18 Months, and HIV Infection and AIDS Among Children >18 Months but <13 Years, United States. *Morbidity and Mortality Weekly Report*. In press.

Central Bureau of Statistics, Nairobi, Kenya. Kenya Demographic and Health Survey 2003: Preliminary report. Available at: http://www.cbs.go.ke/downloads/pdf/Kenya_Demographic_and_Health_Survey_2003_Preliminary_Report.pdf (accessed on 23 July 2007).

Choi, K. and Thacker, S.B. (1981). An evaluation of influenza mortality surveillance, 1962–1979. I. Time series forecasts of expected pneumonia and influenza deaths. *American Journal of Epidemiology*, **113**, 215–26.

Clark, D.E. (2004). Practical introduction to record linkage for injury research. *Injury Prevention*, **10**,186–91.

Cormack, R.M. (1963). The statistics of capture–recapture. *Ocean Marine Biology Annual Review*, **6**, 455–506.

Correa-Villasenor, A., Cragan, J., Kucik, J. *et al.* (2003). The Metropolitan Atlanta Congenital Defects Program: 35 years of birth defects surveillance at the Centers for Disease Control and Prevention. *Birth Defects Research. Part A, Clinical and Molecular Teratology*, **67**, 617–24.

Davy, M. (2006). Time and generational trends in smoking among men and women in Great Britain, 1972-2004/05, *Health Statistics Quarterly*, **32**, 35–43.

Dean, A.G., Shah, S.P., and Churchill, J.E. (1998). DoEpi. Computer-assisted instruction in epidemiology and computing and a framework for creating new exercises. *American Journal of Preventive Medicine*, **14**, 367–71.

Dean, A.G. (1999). Epi info and Epi Map: Current status and plans for Epi info 2000. *Journal Public Health Management Practice*, **5**, 54–7.

Devine, O. and Parrish, R.G. (1998). Monitoring the health of a population. In Stroup DS, Teutsch SM, ed. *Statistics in public health* pp. 59–91. Oxford University Press, New York.

Doll, R. (1974). Surveillance and monitoring. *International Journal of Epidemiology*, **3**, 305–14.

Eylenbosch, W.J. and Noah, N.D. (eds.) (1988). *Surveillance in health and disease.* Oxford University Press, Oxford.

Fairchild, A.L., Gable, L., Gostin, L.O. *et al.* (2007). Public goods, private data: HIV and the history, ethics, and uses of identifiable public health information. *Public Health Reports*, **122** (Suppl 1), 7–15.

Fan, Z.Y., Bonauto, D.K., Foley, M.P. *et al.* (2006). Underreporting of work-related injury or illness to workers' compensation: individual and industry factors. *Journal of Occupational and Environmental Medicine*, **48**, 914.22.

Fang, Z.Y., Wang, B. *et al.* (2005). Sentinel hospital surveillance for rotavirus diarrhea in the People's Republic of China, August 2001-July 2003. *Journal of Infectious Diseases*, **1** (Suppl 1), S94–9.

Glynn, M.K., Lee, L.M., and McKenna, M.T. (2007). The status of national HIV case surveillance, United States 2006. *Public Health Reports,* **122** (Suppl 1), 63–71.

Heffernan, R., Mostashari, F., Das, D. *et al.* (2004). Syndromic surveillance in public health practice, New York City. *Emerging Infectious Diseases*, **10**, 858–64.

Henderson, D.A. (1976). Surveillance of smallpox. *International Journal of Epidemiology*, **5**, 19–28.

Heymann, D.L. and Rodier, G.R. (1998) Global surveillance of communicable diseases. *Emerging Infectious Diseases*, **4**, 362–5.

Hinman, A.R. and Hopkins, D.R. (1998). Lessons from previous eradication programs. In *The eradication of infectious diseases* (eds. W.R. Dowdle and D.R. Hopkins), pp. 19–32. Wiley, New York.

Jaffe, H.W., Choi, K., Thomas, P.A. *et al.* (1983). National case control study of Kaposi's sarcoma and *Pneumocystis carinii* pneumonia in homosexual men: Epidemiologic results. *Annals of Internal Medicine*, **99**, 293–8.

Jayaraman, G.C., Archibald, C.P., Kim, J. *et al.* (2006). A population-based approach to determine the prevalence of transmitted drug-resistance HIV among recent versus established HIV infections: Results from the Canadian HIV strain and drug resistance surveillance program. *Journal of Acquired Immune Deficiency Syndromes*, **42**, 86–90.

Koo, D. and Wetterhall, S.F. (1996). Historical and current status of the National Notifiable Diseases Surveillance System. *Journal of Public Health Management and Practice*, **2**, 4–10.

Krause, G. (2006). From evaluation to continuous quality assurance of surveillance systems. *Eurosurveillance* 11 Available at: www.eurosurveillance.org/em/vlln11/1111-222.asp (accessed 31 J uly 2007).

Kullback, S. and Cornfield, J. (1976). An information theoretic contingency table analysis of the Dorn study of smoking and mortality. *Computers and Biomedical Research*, **9**, 409–37.

Kumar, R., Thakur, J.S. Rao B.T. *et al.* (2006). Validity of verbal autopsy in determining causes of adult deaths. *Indian Journal of Public Health*, **50**, 90–4.

Langmuir, A.D. (1963). The surveillance of communicable diseases of national importance. *New England Journal of Medicine*, **268**, 182–92.

Langmuir, A.D. (1976). William Farr: founder of modern concepts of surveillance. *International Journal of Epidemiology*, **5**, 13–18.

Lee, L.M. and McKenna, M.T. (2007). Monitoring the incidence of HIV infection in the United States. *Public Health Reports*, **122** (Suppl 1), 72–9.

Lowndes, C.M. and Fenton, K.A. (2004). Surveillance sytems for STIs in the European Union: facing a changing epidemiology. *Sexually Transmitted Infections*, **80**, 264–71.

Madoff, L.C. and Woodall, J.P. (2005). The Internet and the global monitoring of emerging diseases: Lessons from the first 10 years of ProMED-mail. *Archives of Medical Research*, **36**, 724–30.

Mandl, K.D., Overhage, J.M., Wagner, M.M. *et al.* (2004). Implementing syndromic surveillance: a practical guide informed by the early experience. *Journal of the American Medical Informatics Association*, **11**, 141–50. Available at: http://www.pubmedcentral.nih.gov/picrender.fcgi?artid=353021&blobtype=pdf (accessed 28 July 2007)

McCarthy, B.J., Terry, J., Rochat, R.W. *et al.* (1980). The under-registration of neonatal deaths: Georgia, 1974–1977. *American Journal of Public Health*, **70**, 977–82.

M'ikanatha, N.M., Rohn, D.D., Robertson, C. *et al.* (2006). Use of the internet to enhance infectious disease surveillance and outbreak investigation. *Biosecurity Bioterrorism*, **4**, 293–300.

Motashari, F. (2007). Can internet searches provide useful data for public health surveillance? *Advances in Disease Surveillance*, **2**, 209.

Newcombe, H.B. (1988). *Handbook of record linkage.* Oxford University Press, Oxford.

Newgard, C.D. (2006). Validation of probabilistic linkage to match de-identified ambulance records to a state trauma registry. *Academic Emergency Medicine*, **13**, 69–75.

Pallansch, M.A. and Sandhu, H.S. (2006). The eradication of polio – Progress and challenges. *New England Journal of Medicine*, **355**, 2508–11.

Pickle, L.W., Hao, Y., Jemal, A. *et al.* (2007). A new method of estimating United States and state-level cancer incidence counts for the current calendar year. *CA: A Cancer Journal for Clinicians*, **57**, 30–42.

Public Health Opportunities in Health Information Exchange. Topics in Public Health Informatics (2005). Available at: http://www.phii.org/resources/doc/Opportunities_0605.pdf (accessed 31 July 2007).

Raska, K. (1966). National and international surveillance of communicable diseases. *World Health Organization Chronicle*, **20**, 315–21.

Rigau-Perez, J.G., Torres, J.V., Hayes, J.M. *et al.* (2006). Medical examiner samples:
A source for dengue surveillance. *Puerto Rico Health Sciences Journal.*, **25**, 67–9.

Serfling, R.E. (1963). Methods for current statistical analysis of excess pneumonia-influenza deaths. *Public Health Reports*, **78**, 494–506.

Setel, P.W., Rao, C., Hemed, Y. *et al.* (2006). Core verbal autopsy procedure with comparative validation results from two countries. *PLoS Medicine*, **3**, e268.

Shands, K.N., Schmid, G.P., Dan, B.B. *et al.* (1980). Toxic-shock syndrome in menstruating women: association with tampon use and *Staphylococcus aureus* and clinical features in 52 cases. *New England Journal of Medicine*, **303**, 1430–42.

Silk, B. and Berkelman, R.L. (2005). A review of strategies to enhance completeness of reporting. *Journal of Public Health Management and Practice* **11**, 191–200.

Skog, O. (1984). The risk function for liver cirrhosis from lifetime alcohol consumption. *Journal of Studies on Alcohol*, **45**, 199–208.

Souza, W.V., Carvalho, M.S., Albuquerque Mde, F. *et al.* (2007). Tuberculosis in intra-urban settings: A Bayesian approach. *Tropical Medicine & International Health*, **12**, 323–30.

Stroup, D.F. and Thacker, S.B. (1993). A Bayesian approach to the detection of aberrations in public health surveillance data. *American Journal of Epidemiology*, **4**, 435–43.

Swaminathan, B., Barrett, T.J., Hunter, S.B. *et al.* and the CDC PulseNet Task Force. (2001). PulseNet: The Molecular Subtyping Network for Foodborne Bacterial Disease Surveillance, United States. *Emerging Infectious Diseases*, **7**, 382–9.

Tufte, E.R. (1983). *The visual display of quantitative information.* Graphics Press, Cheshire, CT.

Tukey, J.W. (1977). *Exploratory data analysis.* Addison-Wesley, Reading, MA.

Twigg, L. (1999). Choosing a national survey to investigate smoking behavior: making comparisons between the General Household Survey, the British Household Panel Survey and the Health Survey for England. *Journal of Public Health Medicine*, **21**, 14–21.

Vogt, R.L., Clark, S.W., and Kappel, S. (1986). Evaluation of the state surveillance system using hospital discharge diagnoses, 1982–1983. *American Journal of Epidemiology*, **123**, 197–8.

Weddell, J.M. (1973). Registers and registries: A review. *International Journal of Epidemiology*, **2**, 221–8.

WHO (World Health Organization) (1958). *The first ten years of the World Health Organization.* WHO, Geneva.

WHO (1968). *Report of the technical discussions at the 21st World Health assembly on 'National and global surveillance of communicable diseases'.* WHO, Geneva.

Williamson, L.M., Dodds, J.P., Mercey, D.E. *et al.* (2006). Increases in HIV-related sexual risk behaviour among community samples of gay men in London and Glasgow: How do they compare? *Journal of Acquired Immune Deficiency Syndromes*, **42**, 238–41.

SECTION 7

Social science techniques

7.1

Sociology and psychology in public health

Myfanwy Morgan, Margaret Reid, and Jane Ogden

Abstract

This chapter examines the perspectives and methods of the disciplines of medical sociology and health psychology, both of which have a long history of research into public health issues. The section on sociology first traces its common history and links with medical public health. It then describes structural and social action perspectives and more recent theories that link structure and agency, and illustrates how these inform both the questions posed and explanations derived. Sociological and psychological research involves both quantitative and qualitative methods. However the chapter focuses particularly on qualitative methods, as these involve a radical departure from the assumptions and methods of quantitative research and are less familiar to epidemiologists and other clinical scientists. Particular attention is given to ethnographic and participant action research and to data collection through interviews, observation, and focus groups. Procedures for sampling and data analysis and issues of validity in qualitative research are also briefly discussed.

Sociological perspectives and methods of investigation are illustrated by research in two areas: Individuals' meanings and experiences of chronic illness, and an in-depth exploration of the role of inequalities in terms of the role of the local social environment in relation to health and health behaviours. The section on psychology focuses on social cognition models (Health Belief Model and Theory of Planned Behaviour) and the Self Regulatory Model and illustrates these models in relation to the links between obesity and diet and the development of interventions to change behaviours. Finally, some conclusions are drawn regarding the future development of medical sociology and health psychology in public health.

Introduction

Sociology and psychology share a number of common interests and areas of study in the public health field. These include issues relating to the psychosocial environment as causes of disease, help-seeking behaviours and adherence with treatment. Other shared interests include issues relating to ageing and disability, as well as effective health promotion interventions and the measurement of health status and quality of life. However, each discipline is characterized by its own perspectives and concepts, and by differences in their focus and explanations. Whereas psychology is primarily concerned with the personality, motivations, and behaviours of individuals, sociology focuses on social groups and organizations and the wider socioeconomic and political structures within which they are embedded.

This chapter describes the theoretical perspectives and methods of investigation that characterize sociological and psychological studies in the health field. Each section also has examples of the applications of these disciplines to particular areas of public health; topics relating to the sociology part are chronic illness and health and place, and those relating to psychology are health promotion and lifestyle changes.

Sociology in public health

Medical sociology as a specialized sub-field of sociology has partly developed alongside public health. Both medical sociology and public health frequently trace the origins of their common interests in the role of economic, social, political, and cultural factors in health and disease patterns to the nineteenth century struggles of physicians and public health reformers like Virchov in Germany, Chadwick in the United Kingdom, Shattuck in the United States, and Coronel in The Netherlands. The development by social scientists and public health specialists of systematic studies to examine the social distribution and causes of non-infectious conditions (such as lung cancer, bronchitis, and coronary heart disease), as well as questions relating to the organization and provision of health services, dates from the late 1940s in both Britain and the United States. This was encouraged by changing patterns of disease, increasing concerns about the social conditions and health of populations, and developments in social science survey techniques.

The period of rapid growth of medical sociology began in the 1950s in the United States and about a decade later in the United Kingdom. The founding of an international journal, *Social Science and Medicine*, which forms a marker in the development of the discipline, occurred in 1966. However, from the early 1960s the paths of sociology and medical public health specialists began to diverge, with each pursuing their separate concerns and disciplinary developments. During this period medical sociology was increasingly critical of the assumptions and limitations of the biomedical model, what were viewed as overly individualistic approaches to health promotion and the power of professions. However from the mid-1980s, sociology and public health experienced a new phase of shared interests. This largely reflected the adoption by public health of a broader social model of the causes of ill health and appropriate interventions, exemplified by the development of what is often referred to as the 'new public health'. This is an approach that sees many contemporary health problems as social (or *structural*) and environmental rather than individual, and therefore requires healthy public policies (in terms of housing, the environment, food policies, and so on) to support the promotion of health. The move towards a more social and participative model of healthcare was also encouraged by broader changes in society. These include greater importance attached to patients having a more active role in treatment choices and in assessing the outcomes of healthcare, local communities having a voice in determining local needs and priorities, and more community-based initiatives (see section on Sociology and place).

Sociologists are now likely to team up with other social scientists, for example, anthropologists and social geographers, as well as with medical public health specialists, to address public health problems. Indeed it is increasingly difficult to determine precise disciplinary boundaries, as sociology, psychology, and public health medicine each draw on concepts and explanations developed in the other disciplines, and over time these become part of the accepted wisdom in the field. For example, the sociological distinction between disease and patients' experience of illness is now commonplace and subjective health status measures are employed routinely in assessing the outcome of medical care. Similarly, effective health education is accepted to require not merely the provision of health advice but also to address people's personal beliefs and take account of the situation and context of their lives. More generally, qualitative methods are no longer confined to sociologists and anthropologists and are increasingly employed by public health doctors and other medical specialists. However, while acknowledging the considerable overlap and collaboration between the disciplines involved in studying public health issues (referred to collectively as multi-disciplinary public health specialists), this section focuses on what is distinctive about sociological investigations and describes the perspectives, methods of investigation employed, and questions addressed.

Sociological perspectives

The broad conceptual framework for sociological investigations comprises theories of the nature and workings of society. However, sociology rather than taking a single unified approach is characterized by different paradigms and theories. These influence the way of 'seeing' the social world and inform questions asked about particular aspects of health, medicine, and healthcare, as well as guiding the choice of methods of research. Sociological theories are broadly divided into structural and social action theories.

Structural theories

Structural theories share a common focus on the structure of society and its institutions, and regard society as constraining and shaping the beliefs, values, and patterns of behaviour of social groups. They also emphasize the objective nature of social phenomena and the possibility of applying quantitative methods in their study (see section on Sociological methods). However, structural theories differ in their view of the nature of society and the relationships between groups. They can be broadly divided into consensual theories that assume a consensus of values and goals, which forms the basis of social solidarity and co-operation, and conflict theories that emphasize the struggle for advantage between different groups in society.

Consensual theories, most notably that of functionalism, played an important role in the early development of sociology. An American sociologist, Talcott Parsons, undertook an analysis of society from a functionalist perspective and applied his approach to the study of societies' response to illness (Parsons 1951). Parsons identified illness as dysfunctional for the smooth running of society because he argued that sick people are not able to fulfil their normal social roles (work roles, familial roles, community activities, and so on). Parsons thus depicted illness as a social as well as a biological phenomenon. He identified the mechanisms evolved by society to manage and control the amount of illness in society as being the special status and role assigned to sick people (the 'sick role') and the complementary role for doctors. He argued that the sick person was granted certain rights (e.g. he or she would be exempt from normal duties) but also that specific expectations were made of them, including the commitment to recover from the illness. Reciprocal expectations were described for doctors. It can be argued that the ambivalent responses often displayed to conditions such as alcoholism, overdoses, and AIDS are explained by society's unwillingness to view such conditions as sickness and therefore to grant such people the privileges of the sick role. Others have noted a new category of individual who is not sick nor a patient but who occupies a 'liminal position betwixt the health and the sick' (Scott *et al.* 2005). This includes users of the cancer genetic services whose high risk of breast cancer places them in this vulnerable position.

Functionalist theory proposed a view of society in which the various parts worked together fairly harmoniously and some inequality in economic rewards was justified by the greater expertise and training required by some occupations. However, by the late 1960s conflict theories were more in keeping with the tenor of the times. Conventional Marxism emphasized the inherent conflict between different groups in society and was influential in many European countries in 1960s and 1970s, whereas other critical and conflict theories now assume much greater importance. Differences between functionalist and conflict approaches can be illustrated in relation to the professions. From a functionalist perspective professions are seen as being in the public interest through their high level of expertise, service orientation, altruistic values, and trust. In contrast, a more critical position emphasizes the ways in which the professions construct their power in terms of the type of expertise they lay claim to, and the ways in which they use their autonomy to serve self-interest, including setting up boundaries around the profession. These sociological approaches are still useful tools to understand how professions develop today, for example, in terms of challenges to medical autonomy and dominance, and the increasing professionalization of other occupational groups including the ways in which the nursing professions (nursing, midwifery) are becoming 'expert' in public health.

Whereas consensual and conflict theories were developed to explain the nature and workings of industrial society, new challenges for sociological theory have been presented by the recent period of rapid and extensive social change leading to a 'post-modern' era. This process has been likened to the industrial revolution, in that it involves the transformation of the major institutions of society and permeates all aspects of everyday life and self-identity. Movement into post-modernity is driven by a process of 'globalization', which involves changes in the economic, technological, and social spheres. 'New social movements' have emerged from these changes (Allsopp *et al.* 2002). In the field of health and illness, this is demonstrated by a rise in strong health consumer groups, who take, and expect, a more participative approach to health policy. Examples include consumer groups that have fought to have certain drugs made more widely available and to assist consumers in understanding the therapeutic function of drugs for conditions such as breast cancer.

Social action theories

Social action theories are based on a fundamentally different view of the social world from structural theories. Whereas structural theories regard the world as having an existence independent of our perception of it and the aim is therefore to establish the truth about how the social world operates, social action theories regard the social world as consisting of a series of representations. Their aim is therefore to understand subjective meanings, with social action forming a product of how individuals interpret the world and interact with others on the basis of these meanings. They also emphasize the fluidity that exists, with individuals having the ability to select, interpret, and bestow meaning upon their interactions with others. Such self-direction is however always limited by the actions and expectations of others, with the result that individuals engage in processes of 'negotiation, impression management, and meaning creation'.

Social action theories like other perspectives comprise different theoretical positions, most notably those of symbolic interactionism, phenomenology, ethnomethodology, and social constructionism. These traditions differ in their origins and underlying philosophical assumptions, and give differing accounts of the ways in which social actors make sense of the social world (for further reading on these theories, see Annandale 1998; Layder 2006). However they all emphasize subjectivity and the existence of multiple realities rather than a single 'truth' and are thus associated with the use of qualitative methods to elicit respondents to describe their own perceptions and reasons for actions (see section on Qualitative research). For example, Richards and her colleagues explored why men and women from deprived areas in Glasgow, Scotland, failed to present to the doctor with chest pain, based on in-depth interviews with 15 respondents from affluent and 15 from deprived communities (Richards *et al.* 2002). Those from deprived areas reported a greater perceived vulnerability to heart disease, reflecting greater exposure to premature morbidity and mortality in family members from heart disease, and an identification with cardiac stereotypes. Respondents also thought that the doctor might chastise them for their risk behaviours (e.g. smoking).

Another sociological tradition adopts an extreme relativist position and holds that social and human reality are socially constructed realities. This approach is exemplified by Foucault, who viewed disease entities as products of social reasoning and social practices. To call a set of symptoms 'bronchitis' or 'coronary heart disease' is therefore merely how medical science, in a given time and place with the aid of laboratory tests and theories, has come to define it. All knowledge is therefore contingent, with medical belief systems, like other belief systems, being created as a result of reasonings that are socially imbued. This approach has also informed analyses of the social construction of official mortality statistics, that can be viewed as products of not only technical and organizational shortcomings but also of the understandings that produce and inform the implementation of coding procedures.

Structure and agency

A development in sociological theory is an attempt to overcome traditional theoretical divisions, and to bring together notions of structure with a social action perspective. A key theoretical approach is Bourdieu's concepts of capital, habitus, and field (Bourdieu 1977). Bourdieu views people living in particular cultures or social classes as carrying the 'influence' of that environment into their behaviour in terms of local knowledge, type of attitude towards work and marriage, and so on. This in turn influences their anticipation of what they want and can achieve, although individuals are not aware of how their attitudes, values, and actions are shaped by these wider structural influences. Sociologists are increasingly applying these theories in the health field. For example, Angus and colleagues (2005) drew on Bourdieu's notion of habitus to explore families' experience of receiving long-term care.

Sociological methods

Sociological investigations employ a range of methods that belong to two main research traditions, those of quantitative and qualitative research. Each is derived from a set of philosophical assumptions, or epistemologies, with issues around qualitative research being the more debated and discussed. This section describes the key features of these traditions and how they contribute to the understanding of public health. It pays particular attention to qualitative methods as these involve a radical departure from the assumptions and methods of quantitative research and are less familiar to epidemiologists and other clinical scientists.

Quantitative research

Quantitative methods derive from a positivist philosophy, of which a key element is the view that social phenomena are objective and external to the individual and thus take the form of social 'facts'. Quantitative research in sociology therefore conforms to the broader principles of scientific research shared by public health and other clinical sciences. It assumes that there is an objective reality that can be measured, and that studies are reliable and valid.

There is a move in the sociology of health and illness towards greater use of qualitative methods, although there continues to be a solid contribution to public health by social scientists using quantitative techniques.

Assumptions and procedures

Quantitative and qualitative traditions are distinct along a number of dimensions (see Table 7.1.1). Studies using quantitative methods require the research question to be predefined, so that the study tests a precise hypothesis or set of research questions. It is also essential at this stage to define the variables, such as social class or 'working women', since these variables have to be translated into categories that can be incorporated into the study design and instruments and which have meaning for the study. Setting out the

Table 7.1.1 Quantitative and qualitative research

	Quantitative	Qualitative
View of the world	Social reality exists as objective, measurable phenomena, external to the individual (positivism)	Social reality is subjectively interpreted and experienced (interpretive)
Logic of enquiry	Deductive based on testing formal hypotheses to establish causal relationships	Inductive reasoning with understanding of social processes derived from data
Research design	Quantitative, with sample selection, data collection, and analyses based on scientific procedures and ensuring repeatability and generalizable results	Qualitative, based on detailed study of social processes of groups of interest to elicit interpretations and responses
Validity	Corresponds to an objective reality	Corresponds to subjective reality; other terms include trustworthiness credibility, plausibility

research questions and defining the independent variables are critical stages in the research process. To carry out a quantitative study, the researcher(s) therefore need to be aware of all the options that are available to the subject responding to the questionnaire, since lack of fit between the subject's preference and the options set out in the questionnaire decreases the validity of the study. Sociologists bring to such research a knowledge of the meanings and significance of concepts such as social class, gender, ethnicity, age, social support, and poverty, which are of value in examining and interpreting health inequalities, variations in uptake of services, or variations in the incidence of particular disease conditions between males and females, while a particular contribution of psychology has been in the development of validated measures.

Data collection

Some data may be drawn from 'secondary' sources, such as routinely collected hospital statistics, government surveys, and census data. More commonly primary data is collected, often involving a survey based on a self-completed or interview-administered questionnaire. The questionnaire is a central part of the researcher's armoury in the maintenance of reliability, since all respondents receive the same questionnaire and the same letter of introduction. As importantly, the measurement (for example, alcohol consumption, attitudes towards pain) should be precisely specified through carefully devised questions. Questions allow only a limited range of responses, while some studies also incorporate validated measures including psychometric tests (for example, measuring anxiety or depression) and other measures relating to social support, quality of life, health status, and so on. Statistical analysis of the data aims to test hypotheses, establish prevalence, and identify statistically significant differences between groups, such as identifying differences in attitudes to preventive heath care among manual and non-manual occupational groups.

Many public health issues have been addressed with the survey approach. These involve local or national studies and cross-sectional studies, or longitudinal cohort studies such as the 1946 British birth cohort (Kuh & Ben-Shlomo 2004) (For detailed description of methods of data collection in quantitative research, see Bowling 2002).

Qualitative research

Qualitative research is most often associated with interpretive or social action perspectives that emphasize the existence of multiple social realities rather than a single truth. They therefore aim to understand these differing meanings, preferences, and reasons for actions. Qualitative methods, although recently gaining greater acceptability and use in the health field, have a long tradition in sociology. They were employed in many of the early sociological studies undertaken in the 1940s in the United States, and form the general approach of anthropological research. These approaches are particularly appropriate where there is a need to develop a greater in-depth understanding of an issue or explore the beliefs and behaviours of different groups in the population (see textbooks by Silverman 2004; Green & Thorogood 2004).

Research designs

Many qualitative studies employ a single method of data collection, with semi-structured interviews being most common. These are usually undertaken at one point in time but occasionally follow-up interviews are undertaken to examine possible changes in beliefs and practices or to explore particular issues in greater depth. Three research designs that require particular comment are ethnography, action research, and the use of mixed quantitative and qualitative methods.

Ethnography

This was traditionally employed by anthropologists in studying small communities, and often involved spending many months or even years living in the community and observing the social structure and local culture. A major form of data collection was through observation, with the aim of seeing the world through the eyes of the local community and understanding how beliefs and practices are embedded in local cultures. Subsequently this method has been applied to studying modern societies. It is particularly suited to the study of small communities such as hospital wards and clinics, and in understanding the beliefs and cultures of minority groups. Ethnography is also used to study characteristics of local communities that influence health and well-being (see section on Sociology and place).

Central to ethnography is the emphasis on the researchers' immersion in the field, with observation generally forming the main method of data collection, supplemented by interviews and occasionally the analysis of written documents (minutes of meetings, medical records, time charts, etc). An example is an ethnographic study of the interpersonal, cultural, and organizational dimensions of a transitional rehabilitation scheme that explored the perspectives of the three key stakeholders: The older people, care home managers, and a variety of rehabilitation staff. Fieldwork involved participant observation, analysis of documents, and interviews with 55 people (Hart *et al.* 2005). Observational studies provide valuable data on actions and interactions tied to particular situations and circumstances, but have the drawback of being labour-intensive and therefore relatively expensive.

Participatory action research (PAR) and user involvement

Action research is often described as 'a style of research rather than a specific method'. Its distinctive element is its aim to *change* practice as well as studying it. Three key features of action research are: Its participatory character (requires participants to perceive a need for change and be willing to play an active part in the research and change process); its democracy (requires participants to be seen as equals with the researcher and to be consulted on the action process and methods of evaluation which is negotiated with participants); and its contribution to both social science knowledge and local change (the former requires that the report is presented with considerable contextual detail to aid generalization) (see Meyer 2000).

Action research may use a number of different methods to capture the process of change and to evaluate the nature of any changes that have occurred. The unpredictable nature of action research necessitates a flexible rather than a rigid research design. The action research cycle is in some ways similar to the audit cycle, in that data are systematically and successively collected in order to evaluate progress towards a series of planned changes, with different phases of the study sometimes having different goals and using different methods.

An action research approach is common in community work, but has also been employed in identifying problems in clinical practice, helping to develop potential solutions, and facilitating change within the health services. An example is the Canadian Regional Health Authorities use of action research to build a macro-level priority-setting framework within a large, complex health organization. This formed a seven-stage process, involving qualitative data collection methods of document review, participant observation, in-depth interviews, and focus groups (Patten *et al.* 2006).

Even if research is not designed as a participatory action project it is becoming increasingly common to include the participants, or the wider community from which they were selected, as recognized stakeholders in the research process. This is associated with increasing emphasis on the involvement of users or community representatives on steering groups as well as in the actual conduct of research and interpretation of findings.

Mixed methods

The increasingly complex problems facing public health often necessitates a range of methods, and frequently involves both quantitative and qualitative approaches to achieve a broader understanding and offset the weaknesses of particular methods. (For a detailed discussion of mixed methods studies, see Tachakkoni & Teddlie 2003).

Study numbers and sampling

Respondents in qualitative research may be selected through *purposive* sampling, which is the deliberate choice of respondents or setting to represent a wide range of opinion or experience. For example a study group to explore the range of views regarding personal continuity in primary care might be *purposively* selected to ensure that respondents comprise men and women, older and younger people, members of ethnic minorities, and frequent and infrequent attenders at primary care. *Theoretical* sampling is based on a previously developed hypothesis or theory. For example, if it is hypothesized that there are differences in attitudes and perceived barriers to exercise among men in non-manual and manual occupations, sampling would aim to ensure that these two groups were equally represented and broadly comparable in terms of age and the known presence of coronary risk factors if this is hypothesized to have an important influence. *'Snowball'* sampling is occasionally used when individuals under study are difficult to access using normal routes (for example studying homeless individuals) and respondents may therefore introduce other potential respondents.

In qualitative research the size of the sample is difficult to assess in advance and partly depends on the aims of the study. For example, a study may involve eliciting very detailed accounts from a relatively small number of respondents (say 15–20), or 30–50 respondents may be *purposively* selected to identify the variation in experiences, such as cancer patients experiencing different types of care or people from different ethnic groups. The term 'theoretical saturation' was initially introduced in relation to grounded theory to describe the point at which a conceptually dense theoretical account of the field of interest had been reached. However this term is now often used more loosely, with the *saturation* point being reached, and the numbers studied therefore being sufficient, when little new comes out of additional interviews.

Data collection

Methods of primary data collection in qualitative research mainly comprise interviews, focus groups, and observational work, although available records and other documentary sources may also be analysed.

Interviews

Interviews are a central tool of the qualitative researcher. They may take a number of forms but all give greater flexibility than the structured interview of quantitative research and require a more active role for the fieldworker. Most often used is the semi-structured (or semi-standardized) interview. In this the researcher starts with a list of topics and questions to be asked (often identified through earlier pilot interviews), although the order may alter and the researcher may probe for more information and follow-up a line of thinking with a respondent. At the other end of the 'structure' continuum is the non-standardized or unstructured interview, representing a 'guided conversation'. This form of interview gives greater flexibility in terms of the issues discussed. It may for example just require that the respondent 'gives an account of their help-seeking from first noticing symptoms', with prompting and probing as necessary by the researcher.

Interviews in qualitative research are usually tape-recorded and subsequently transcribed. The process is lengthy; interviews may last from 30 min to 2 or 3 h and it is generally reckoned that a 1-h interview takes 5 h to transcribe with further time to check the transcription. This contributes to the perception of qualitative research as slow and time-consuming. Analysis (see below) is also a lengthy process.

Focus groups

Focus groups form an alternative to the personal interview. They have been employed by sociologists since the 1950s, but initially became mainly known as the tool of market researchers where they were used to carry out rapid checks on public attitudes (for example, in relation to consumer goods or political attitudes). However, focus groups have now achieved a new status as a valid research tool. The method brings together a group of individuals (usually six to eight), often selected with reference to age, gender, and other criteria, to discuss a series of topics, using the group or collective interaction to produce insights (see Bloor *et al.* 2001).

Focus groups have found a niche as a research tool for investigating patient and consumer views in the development of health policy. They also have the advantage of redressing the power imbalance in fieldwork situations, and therefore often provide an appropriate format for research with children and with young adults. Focus groups are also suitable for studying topics on which people may not have pre-formed ideas or when little is known about a topic, with much therefore being gained from the discussion among group members.

A skilled facilitator may use a number of techniques to encourage participation from group members, and elicit not only the views and experiences of group members but also areas where conflict arises and disagreements expressed. To facilitate free discussion and communication during the short time of the group, the researcher must establish trust with members of the group, emphasizing the confidential nature of the study and ensuring that individuals understand the purpose of the group.

Drawbacks of focus groups include the practical difficulties of getting people together at a particular location and time and the 'self-selection' of individuals who may be willing to turn up to discuss their views and beliefs with a series of strangers. To avoid these difficulties an existing group may be used as the basis for discussion, such as a group of pensioners, mother and toddlers, or a support group who meet regularly. However it is important that 'gatekeepers' do not select individuals seen to be appropriate for the exercise and to recognize that the heterogeneity or homogeneity of groups can change the dynamics of groups and issues raised (e.g. groups of doctors and nurses, or doctors and separately nurses, professionals, and lay people, etc).

Observation

All qualitative researchers may use observation as an adjunct to other methods of data collection, for example, when visiting an interviewee in the home or the work place, the 'observant' interviewer would note the context of the interviewee's life. However, observation is a specific method, with its own logic and rules, that is undertaken in ethnographic studies following the tradition of social anthropology (see section on Ethnography).

Documentary sources

Written materials such as records of meetings or routine clinic data often form one source of data in an ethnographic or multi-method study. However written documents may also form the subject of qualitative analysis, where the emphasis is to analyse the dominant '*discourses*' or ways of constructing social phenomena. Examples include an analysis of medical and disability rights, discourses in genetics based on major journals and textbooks in the field (Shakespeare 1999), and a textual analysis of the official National Service Framework for coronary heart disease, which identified differences between managers, clinicians, and politicians and public health, in their aspirational values (e.g. efficiency, effectiveness, autonomy/choice, equity).

Data analysis

Data analyses are an ongoing feature of qualitative research, with processes of transcribing and coding suggesting concepts and relationships. The raw material for qualitative researchers can be in the form of transcriptions from (tape-recorded) interviews or focus groups, notes written by the researcher(s) from interviews and field notes in which they have recorded their fieldwork experiences, and occasionally diaries kept by the respondents themselves. Because of the importance of researchers' immersion in the field and understanding the context of interviews, those who have conducted the fieldwork ideally undertake the analysis.

Initially a set of codes or categories is identified from the data that appear of relevance for the research question. Within an extended set of codes it may be appropriate to construct subdivisions, such as dividing up the types of 'coping strategies' or different types of communication with the general practitioner, if the data provide examples of such divisions. There is no hard-and-fast rule about coding the data, some preferring quite complex systems and others starting with quite a broad basic framework. The important—and distinctive—feature of most qualitative research is that the data suggest the codes, rather than the researchers working to a prior hypothesis of what they wish to examine. The researcher will then apply this coding system to all the transcripts, either by hand, or by using one of a number of computer packages available to aid this process. These packages can be time-consuming to master but generally help the next stage of the analysis, which is to develop themes from the codes.

The themes identified in a qualitative study may be based around one or more codes; thus one theme in a study of patients with heart disease could be the different ways in which patients manage their medication taking. Much research rests at this point in the analysis and remains quite 'literal', reporting at a fairly concrete level of what the data have shown. However, many qualitative researchers will try to create some 'higher-order' theory from their research drawing on conceptual categories and frameworks drawn from their discipline.

Whereas much qualitative analysis adopts a form of thematic analysis, there are distinctive traditions and varieties of qualitative methods and analysis. Grounded theory as a form of analysis was developed and elaborated in the 1960s by Glaser and Strauss (1965). Grounded theory refers to theory which has been 'worked up' through an iterative process, involving reviewing the data to derive hypotheses that are then tested in the field, repeating the process with revised hypotheses until the theory is supported fully within the data. Although many researchers claim that they use this method, true grounded theory demands a commitment to data analysis and time in the field that is beyond the limit of many researchers.

A variant of grounded theory that is now widely used in health services research is framework analysis (Ritchie & Spencer 1994). This involves summarizing and classifying data within a thematic framework with the aim of preserving the integrity of respondents' narratives throughout the analysis and producing charts that contain summaries of data across cases by theme.

Validity

A key area of debate is the validity or truth of the interpretation of qualitative research, which has led to a number of specific techniques being recommended to assure quality, including the use of more than one coder, and the conduct of 'respondent validation' that involves checking if respondents or similar people agree with the researcher's interpretation of the data. The concept of 'triangulation' is also often advocated, with the notion that the use of multiple sources of data (interviews, observation, and routine data) to approach the same issue will support those achieved from another method in corroborating an overall interpretation. However, the way in which methodologies from different traditions actually combine together as a form of validation is still debated. There are also differing views regarding the value of the increasing availability of checklist approaches to assess quality (Dixon-Woods *et al.* 2007).

Some dislike the term 'validity' with its connotations of the existence of a single truth and prefer to suggest that the way in which the soundness of study should be assessed is by using concepts of plausibility, credibility, trustworthiness, and the nature of generalizations made from the data. Clarity of exposition of method is regarded as the key. Researchers undertaking qualitative research are also trained to be reflexive about their role, reflecting critically upon the ways in which interaction with the respondents/field situation may influence the data collected. (For issues on validity and quality in qualitative research, see Seale (1999)).

Whereas there is currently considerable emphasis on ensuring that methods of qualitative research and their detailed reporting satisfy technical process criteria, the key contribution of qualitative research lies in its contribution to conceptual development and explanation, with inferences and explanations drawn from one setting holding in other similar settings. Examples include the generalizability of Goffman's (1963) notion of 'stigma' and coping strategies to a wide range of physical and mental health problems, and evidence from a synthesis of qualitative studies of lay experiences of diabetes of the identification across studies of the strategies for achieving a balance in their lives and to attain a sense of well-being and control (Campbell *et al.* 2003). Indeed the main problem with the quality of qualitative research has been argued to lie not in the methods but in the misguided separation of method from theory, with a need for more widespread application of concepts and knowledge originating in source disciplines.

Synthesis

The need to establish a hierarchy of evidence for clinical practice and policy, and thus support evidence-based medicine and evidence-based healthcare, has led to an emphasis on methods of appraising and synthesizing the findings from research. Synthesis traditionally focused on quantitative studies, particularly randomized controlled trials. However there is now a recognized need to synthesize the findings of qualitative research and incorporate this into the evidence base.

The aim of synthesizing qualitative research has led to the development of new methods, although these are still at an early stage. One of the most widely cited approaches to qualitative synthesis is Noblitt and Hare's (1988) method of meta-ethnography. This essentially involves a re-analysis of the concepts that were the outcomes of original analyses reported in good quality published studies on similar topics. Subsequent stages of meta-ethnography involve comparing these concepts/themes across studies and examining how they are related (*reciprocal or refutational relationship*), with the aim of producing an overall interpretation or *line of argument* that integrates the findings of different studies. The process of qualitative synthesis is therefore in principle similar to that of analysing and interpreting primary data, with the main difference being that it focuses at the level of the emergent concepts rather than the primary data (see Pound *et al.* 2005).

A recent development is the synthesis of both qualitative and quantitative research on a particular topic. This may be undertaken through a narrative review, the translation of qualitative findings into a quantitative framework using the case survey method or Bayesian meta-analysis, or both sets of data are analysed and synthesized within a qualitative framework, generally based on the principles of meta-ethnography (for a detailed review of methods, see Mays *et al.* 2006). The choice of approach depends on the aim of the review, the specific questions to be addressed, and the nature and balance of the evidence available (i.e. mainly quantitative or qualitative).

Areas of sociological investigation

The sociology of health and illness covers a wide range of topics and involves the study of health and illness at three levels: The 'individual' level (e.g. perceptions of health, meanings, and responses to illness and interactions with health providers), the 'social' level (e.g. inequalities in health among social groups and the delivery of care), and the 'societal' level (e.g. social forces shaping healthcare systems and approaches to health promotion). This section provides examples of the application of sociological perspectives and methods of investigation in relation to individuals' meanings and experiences of chronic illness and the impact of the local social environment on health and health behaviours. The aim is not to provide a comprehensive review of these topics, but rather to illustrate the ways in which different perspectives and approaches focus attention on different issues and types of explanations.

Chronic illness: Meanings and identity

The social dimensions of chronic illness and disability have formed a major area of study by public health specialists, sociologists, psychologists, and others. This has included research concerned with the conceptualization and measurement of 'disability' and provision of informal care, and studies investigating individuals' personal experiences and ways of coping with chronic illness. This section provides a brief overview of one area of research informed by social action theories, namely the impact of chronic illness on the individual's self-identity. Research in this area has identified the importance of responding to individuals' social meanings. People who themselves experienced a chronic condition are often best placed to understand the realities of life and advise on needs and forms of support, which is now increasingly accepted as an important approach to care.

Biographical disruption

A key concept describing the early impact or crisis of illness is Bury's (1982) notion of 'biographical disruption'. This concept recognizes that the onset of chronic illness is a 'critical situation' that can be drastically disruptive to the structures of everyday life, and represents an assault both on the person's physical self and self-identity. Aspects of disruption were identified as first, the disruption of taken-for-granted assumptions and behaviours through the effects of disruptive symptoms on everyday life at home or work, which bring concerns about bodily states and decisions regarding seeking help to the forefront of consciousness. Second, disruption arises from the symbolic significance of chronic illness and the need for a fundamental rethinking of the person's biography and self-concept.

Responses to disruption involve the mobilization of cognitive, material, and social resources, particularly the individuals' social networks, in facing and responding to an altered situation. At a cognitive level, responses involve what has been termed *narrative reconstruction* (Williams 1984). This describes ways in which individuals attempt to give meaning and achieve a sense of order from the fragmentation produced by chronic illness, through attempting to link up and interpret their illness and answer questions of 'why me' and 'why now?' in terms of different aspects of their biography. In this way people attempt to realign present and past, and self with society. Central to this is patients' search for the causes of their illness to make sense or render intelligible the biographical disruption.

Reconstruction may draw on various sources of explanation. For example, a qualitative study examining beliefs about coronary heart disease demonstrated awareness of lifestyle risk factors, although explanations in the popular culture focused on being a 'worrier by nature' which in turn led to inappropriate behaviours, the influence of a 'divine plan' and 'luck' which also reduced the significance of lifestyle (Davison *et al.* 1992). Patients' attempts to derive meanings of illness onset from aspects of their biography and from notions of cause prevalent in the wider lay culture may explain the apparent resistance of some patients to clinical explanations of the 'cause' of their condition. It may also explain resistance to health promotion messages regarding the importance of stopping smoking, changing diet and exercise, if these clinical risk factors are not viewed by the lay population as the most important influences on health risks, or if they regard a condition such as heart disease as an acute or episodic disease rather than a life-long chronic illness (Ononeze *et al.* 2006).

Suffering and loss of self

Whereas the notion of biographical disruption and narrative reconstruction mainly focuses on the crisis of illness onset and the change from a 'normal' identity to that of a chronically ill person, 'loss of self' can be viewed as an aspect of chronic illness that is a more pervasive and continuing experience. Charmaz (1983) in her classic study of chronically ill persons observed that whereas severely disabled people largely spoke of suffering in terms of a language of loss, respondents who had improved were more likely to see their suffering as a path to knowledge and self-discovery.

Other research has examined the impacts of stigmatized medical conditions, based on Goffman's (1963) notion of stigma as a condition or attribute that is viewed as unacceptable and marks the individual as unacceptable or inferior, leading to a changed self-image or 'spoiled' identity. This research has examined cross-cultural variations in the nature and severity of stigma and the impacts and responses of stigma bearers. Examples include research on epilepsy (Scambler & Hopkins 1986), mental illness (Wright *et al.* 2007), HIV/AIDS (Parker & Aggleton 2004), tuberculosis (Mak *et al.* 2006), and leprosy (Barrett 2005). These studies describe the impacts of 'felt' stigma or the shame surrounding a stigmatized condition, and people's fears or actual experiences of 'enacted' stigma in terms of discrimination, avoidance, and exclusion. They also describe the differing ways in which individuals (and families) cope with stigma. This usually involves acceptance of societal meanings and responses of concealment, normalization, or withdrawal from interaction with outsiders who do not possess the stigmatizing condition, but may occasionally involve rejection of the negative societal meanings as demonstrated by disability activists and pressure groups for particular conditions such as HIV/AIDS and mental illness.

Adaptation and self-management

The success of the individual's adaptation to chronic conditions is demonstrated by a survey indicating that 54 per cent of people with serious disabilities reported that they experience a good or excellent quality of life (Albrecht & Devlieger 1999). Factors associated with such positive assessments were people's ability to understand their condition, take control, and introduce order and predictability. Moreover it is increasingly acknowledged that many patients with chronic disease are 'experts' in their own right as they have gained the life skills to cope with their chronic condition. This view has underpinned the introduction of lay-led chronic disease self-management programmes in the US (Lorig *et al.* 1999) and a similar model launched in the UK as *The Expert Patient Programme* (Department of Health 2001). 'Expert patient' and other chronic disease management programmes aim to build on patients' own expertise to support others in a similar situation in their own self-management. This is achieved through increasing their confidence and motivation to use their skills to organize their lives and to work in partnership with health professionals and share responsibility for treatment.

Sociology and place

Communities have long been studied by social scientists, but until the early 1990s there was little research that directly examined the impact of the local social environment on human health. Instead 'place' effects emerged only as a residual category, or what remained after investigators had controlled for other characteristics. Macintyre and her colleagues (2002) in an important position paper noted a 'resurgence of interest' in the role of place in understanding people's health status and debates regarding the relative importance of people and place characteristics that relate to broader concerns about the increasing inequalities in health observed in some Westernized societies. This change in focus was made possible by developments in statistics and multi-level modelling techniques, together with methodological developments in social geography including geographical information systems (GIS), and in the political realm by the emergence of what has been termed the 'new public health'.

The change of focus to the study of communities, social environments, and 'place' has led to a blurring of discipline boundaries, involving sociologists, anthropologists, geographers, and epidemiologists, and involves both quantitative analyses and qualitative methods which attempt to explain why certain areas may be seen as healthy or less healthy environments. Observation, perhaps not surprisingly, becomes a more dominant method when investigating the physical aspects of neighbourhoods, and data gathering may also include noting 'the amount of graffiti, litter and dog mess as well as the level of vegetation and greenery' (Ellaway *et al.* 2005). A variety of structured approaches drawn from the geographical sciences have also been used to undertake the systematic review of neighbourhood features, including use of a 'site survey checklist' (Weich *et al.* 2001).

Food choices and physical exercise

Concerns over growing obesity of western populations and the perceived poor diet of many individuals living in deprivation provided the stimulus to explore whether availability and cost of food in local retail outlets was one explanation for poor diets in low socioeconomic areas. Using a Scottish-based system of deprivation categories and Glasgow postcode sectors, the researchers mapped types of food shops in different areas within the city, and found that prices did not differ greatly by area of deprivation (Cummins & Macintyre 2002). When they did, they tended to be cheaper in poorer areas. Foods cheaper in poorer areas, however, were more likely to be high fat, high sugar foods.

A number of innovative studies from different disciplines have also investigated the ways in which the contextual aspects of local neighbourhoods may facilitate or inhibit physical exercise. Investigating walking and cycling, Pikora and her Australian colleagues undertook 31 semi-structured interviews and a Delphi study with experts to establish the relative importance of specific environmental factors and their influence on walking and (separately) cycling (Pikora *et al.* 2003). For walkers, personal safety, the attractiveness of the street, and the presence of community and commercial facilities in the neighbourhoods were found to be most important, whereas for cyclists the presence of a continuous route and traffic safety were the most significant. Krenichyn (2006) confirmed that many of the above features were also of central importance to her US study based on interviews with 41 women of different ages and ethnic groups using a New York park for exercise.

These and other studies represent an investigation of our urban landscape in a much more detailed form than previously. Moreover, despite the range of disciplines and geographical location of studies there is considerable similarity of findings in terms of the importance of the condition of the environment, the safety, the aesthetics, amenities, types of activities possible, and characteristics of the surrounding areas.

Social capital

Neighbourhoods comprise not only physical features and amenities but also social relationships. For example, exploration of urban parks not only highlighted the space for members of a community to come together, but also their contribution to the 'social capital' of the neighbourhood. Putnam defined social capital as 'the features of social organization, such as trust, norms and networks that can improve the efficiency of society by facilitating coordinated actions' (Putman 1993, 167). Despite lack of agreement over its central meaning, the core components of the social capital of an area are social support and networks, which enable trust and norms of reciprocity to be established.

Two studies linking social capital with physical exercise reflect the range of approaches used in research on 'place' and health. Linstrom *et al.* (2003) carried out a multilevel modelling exercise using data from a cross-sectional postal survey in Malmo, with 3377 people aged 20–80 years, to investigate the influence of social capital and individual factors on the level of leisure time *in*activity in Malmo neighbourhoods. The researchers found that what they took to be individual measures of social capital (country of origin, educational level, and social participation) were more important influences on activity than contextual area characteristics. A very different methodological approach was taken in an anthropological study of Italian cyclists (Whitaker 2005). Cycling remains popular in northern Italy, in particular, where it is seen as a form of transport, an accepted form of exercise (with the older men admired for their abilities and speed), and a form of social capital. An in-depth analysis of 22 older cyclists using interviews and long-term observation was undertaken to explore why older men (the study is only about men) continue cycling long after they would in many other countries. Whitaker confirms that 'the social aspects of cycling are among the most important ones discussed by the men in this study', with the social capital element evidenced by the popular group cycling, and the large membership of cycling clubs.

Research on the physical and psycho-social characteristics of communities has identified some important relationships with health status. However there is a need for greater theoretical development and conceptualisation of 'place' and 'social capital' and for their precise operationalisation. Similarly, the effects of residential environment on health and health-related behaviours appear complex and may depend on age, gender and other factors (Stafford *et al.* 2005).

Psychology in public health

Psychological research and theory has always included the study of health in its remit but until relatively recently the focus has been on mental health through the work of clinical psychologists and their interest in problems such as anxiety, depression, psychosis, and phobias. This section, however, is concerned with the role of psychological factors in understanding physical health problems and is most studied within the field of health psychology (see Ogden 2007). Health psychologists study the impact of psychology in all areas of health and illness including the role of belief and behaviours in becoming ill, the experience of being ill, contact with health professionals, coping with illness, compliance with a range of interventions, and the role of psychology in recovery from illness, quality of life, and longevity. This has many direct implications for public health including the management and prevention of chronic illness and the development of interventions to changes in health-related behaviours including diet, exercise, smoking, screening uptake, and alcohol consumption. This section first outlines some key psychological theories, and then describes some of the research methods used to develop and test these theories. The application of psychology to the healthcare setting is then illustrated in relation to diet and obesity and the development of interventions to change behaviour.

Methods of research

Psychological research draws upon many of the same research designs and methodologies as sociology and epidemiology including trials, surveys, interviews, and focus groups. Perhaps the one area that is more unique to psychology than any other is the laboratory experiment. Psychology has always used laboratory experiments as means to explore the impact of changing the independent variable on the dependent variable within a controlled setting. Laboratory studies are closely aligned to randomized controlled trials as they enable conclusions to be drawn about causality, but offer a more managed environment than trials in a clinical setting. Laboratory experiments have been used in a range of areas within health psychology such as stress, pain perception, eating behaviour, and smoking cessation. For example, stress can be induced by interventions such as an intelligence task as a means to explore its consequences; pain can be induced by placing the hand in icy water as a means to see which factors can modify pain perception and participants can be asked to eat certain foods in the laboratory to explore their impact upon weight gain or subsequent feelings of hunger and fullness. These experiments enable self-report, behavioural and physiological measures to be taken in a controlled environment so that conclusions about cause and effect can be made. Such experiments are often criticized for being artificial and not naturalistic, for using small participant numbers, and involving an unrepresentative sample. However, they do enable all variables to be manipulated, measured, or held constant in a way that surveys of clinical trials cannot.

Psychological theory

Health psychology utilizes a range of theories which are either home grown or have been drawn from other aspects of psychology including social psychology, cognitive psychology, and biological psychology. In particular, it emphasizes the role of learning through both operant and classical conditioning and the development of cognitions and emotions that impact upon subsequent behaviour. Its focus on beliefs, emotions, and behaviour therefore provides a more holistic approach to understanding physical health than the more traditional biomedical model.

This section focuses on two main theoretical perspectives: Social cognition models and the self- regulatory model.

Social cognition models

Health behaviours are defined as any behaviour that may either promote health or protect from illness and include eating, smoking, alcohol consumption, adherence to medication, screening, or exercise. Health psychology uses structured models of health beliefs as a means to predict these behaviours. These are often social cognition models as they regard cognitions as being shared by individuals within the same society. Two social cognition models, the health belief model (HBM) and the theory of planned behaviour (TPB), are described below.

The health belief model (HBM)

The HBM was developed initially by Rosenstock (1966) and further by Becker and colleagues throughout the 1970s and 1980s (Becker & Rosenstock 1987). It was derived from subjective expected utility (SEU) theory which suggested that behaviours result from a rational weighing up of the potential costs and benefits of that behaviour.

The HBM predicts that behaviour is a result of a set of core beliefs. These have been redefined over the years. The current version of the HBM suggests that behaviour is predicted by beliefs in: Susceptibility to illness (e.g. 'my chances of getting lung cancer are high'); the severity of the illness (e.g. 'lung cancer is a serious illness'); the costs involved in carrying out the behaviour (e.g. 'stopping smoking will make me irritable'); the benefits involved in carrying out the behaviour (e.g. 'stopping smoking will save me money'); cues to action, which may be internal (e.g. the symptom of breathlessness), or external (e.g. information in the form of health education leaflets); 'health motivation' (e.g. 'I am concerned that smoking might damage my health'), and perceived control (e.g. 'I am confident that I can stop smoking').

Several studies support the HBM. For example, perceived barriers are identified as the best predictors of clinic attendance for screening, and perceived barriers and perceived susceptibility are the best predictors of breast self-examination. Research also provides support for the role of cues to action in predicting health behaviours, and indicates that informational input in the form of fear-arousing warnings may change attitudes and health behaviour in such areas as dental health, safe driving, and smoking (see Abraham & Sheeran 2005).

The HBM is however not without its problems. Although the HBM provides a useful framework for research it has been criticized for the absence of the individual's social context and for neglecting the role of past behaviour. To overcome limitations of the HBM some researchers have turned to using the Theory of Planned Behaviour (Ajzen 1988) as a predictor of health behaviour, as this locates individual's behaviour within their social context.

The theory of planned behaviour (TPB)

The TPB proposes that behavioural intentions ('plans of action in pursuit of behavioural goals') are a result of the following beliefs: Attitude towards a behaviour (e.g. 'exercising is fun and will improve my health'); subjective norm (e.g. 'people who are important to me will approve if I lose weight and I want their approval'); perceived behavioural control, which is composed of a belief that the individual can carry out a particular behaviour based upon a consideration of internal control factors (e.g. skills, abilities, information) and external control factors (e.g. obstacles, opportunities), both of which relate to past behaviour.

According to the TPB, these three factors predict behavioural intentions, which are then linked to behaviour. The TPB also states that perceived behavioural control can have a direct effect on behaviour without the mediating effect of behavioural intentions. The TPB has been used to assess a variety of health-related behaviours including speeding behaviour, the uptake and maintenance of exercise, healthy eating, and smoking behaviours (see Armitage & Conner 2000).

People however, not only have beliefs about their behaviour but also beliefs about their health and illness, often known as illness cognitions or illness representations. Such beliefs may also impact upon health- related behaviours such as smoking or diet. Further, they also influence the ways in which individuals adjust to their illness and whether they take their medication, seek help from health professionals, and attend medical or surgical interventions. These beliefs are often studied within the framework of the Self Regulatory Model (SRM), which is considered next.

The self regulatory model (SRM)

Leventhal and his colleagues (Leventhal *et al.* 1997) defined illness cognitions as 'a patient's own implicit common sense beliefs about their illness'. They proposed that these cognitions provide patients with a framework or a schema for coping with and understanding their illness, and telling them what to look out for if they become ill. Using interviews with patients suffering from a variety of different illnesses, Leventhal and his colleagues identified five cognitive dimensions of these beliefs: Identity (the medical diagnosis and the symptoms experienced); the perceived cause of the illness (e.g. virus, stress, or diet); time line: (i.e. acute or chronic); consequences (e.g. pain, lack of mobility, loneliness); curability and controllability (e.g. doctors will make my illness better or my treatment will not work). Leventhal incorporated his description of illness cognitions into his self-regulatory model of illness behaviour (SRM). This model is based on approaches to problem-solving and suggests that illness and symptoms are dealt with by individuals in the same way as other problems. It is assumed that given a problem or a change in the status quo the individual will be motivated to solve the problem and re-establish his/her state of normality. In terms of health and illness, if healthiness is an individual's normal state, then any onset of illness will be interpreted as a problem and the individual will be motivated to re-establish his/her state of health. This process occurs via the three stages of interpretation, coping, and appraisal.

In terms of interpretation, the SRM suggests that an individual may be confronted with the problem of a potential illness through two channels: Symptom perception (e.g. I have a pain in my chest), or social messages (e.g. the doctor has diagnosed this pain as angina). Once the individual has received information about the possibility of illness through these channels, according to theories of problem- solving, the individual is then motivated to return to a state of 'problem-free' normality. This involves assigning meaning to the problem. According to Leventhal, the problem can be given meaning by accessing the individual's illness cognitions that enable the individual to develop and consider suitable coping strategies. A cognitive representation, however, is not the only consequence of symptom perception and social messages. The identification of the problem of illness will also result in changes in emotional state. For example, perceiving the symptom of pain and receiving the social message that this pain may be related to coronary heart disease may result in anxiety. Therefore, any coping strategies have to relate to both the illness cognitions and the emotional state of the individual.

The next stage in the self-regulatory model is the development and identification of suitable coping strategies. Coping can take many forms but two broad categories of coping have been defined that incorporate the multitude of other coping strategies: Approach coping (e.g. taking pills, going to the doctor, resting, talking to friends about emotions) and avoidance coping (e.g. denial, wishful thinking). When faced with the problem of illness, the individual will therefore develop coping strategies in an attempt to return to a state of healthy normality.

Finally, the third stage of the self-regulatory model is appraisal. This involves individuals evaluating the effectiveness of the coping strategy and determining whether to continue with this strategy or whether to opt for an alternative one.

This process is regarded as self-regulatory because the three components of the model (interpretation, coping, and appraisal) interrelate in order to maintain the status quo. Therefore, if the individual's normal state (health) is disrupted (by illness), the model proposes that the individual is motivated to return the balance back to normality. This self-regulation involves the three processes interrelating in an ongoing and dynamic fashion.

The self-regulatory model describes a transition from interpretation, through illness cognitions, emotional response, and coping to appraisal. This model has primarily been used to ask: 'How do different people make sense of different illnesses?' Research, however, has also explored the impact of illness cognitions on psychological and physical health outcomes. For example, research shows that beliefs about illness relate to adherence to medication for asthma, severe haemophilia, and hypercholesterolaemia (see Ogden 2007). Research has also reported associations between illness cognitions and recovery from stroke and MI. For example, the Heart Attack Recovery Project, in New Zealand concluded that those patients who believed that their illness had less serious consequences and would last a shorter time at baseline, were more likely to have returned to work by 6 weeks and those with beliefs that the illness could be controlled or cured at baseline were more likely to attend rehabilitation classes (Petrie *et al.* 1996). A self-regulatory approach may be useful for describing illness cognitions and for exploring the relationship between such cognitions and coping, and also for understanding and predicting other health outcomes.

Psychological investigations

Obesity and diet

The increase in both adult and child obesity has been well documented. As a means to explain this increase, researchers have focused their attention on the role of the obesogenic environment and have highlighted the importance of factors such as the food industry, food advertising, food labelling, the availability of energy dense foods, and an environment which has been increasingly designed to encourage a sedentary lifestyle through the use of cars, computers, and television. Central to this change is a shift in two key behaviours; eating behaviour and physical activity. This chapter will focus on the links between obesity and diet and will explore why people eat what they eat and how this relates to obesity onset and maintenance.

Research exploring how much and what the obese eat is problematic due to the difficulty in measuring diet without changing it. However there is evidence that the obese eat relatively more fat than the non-obese, while the very process of weight gain indicates that they are eating more than their body requires (see Ogden 2003).

Within psychological research there are three main theories of eating behaviour that can help to understand why some people eat differently and more than others, and why some may become overweight and obese. These are the cognitive approach, the developmental model, and the impact of dieting on eating behaviour.

A cognitive approach to diet

Most research using a cognitive approach has drawn upon social cognition models to predict eating behaviour. For example, attitudes have been found to predict fat intake, table salt use, eating in fast food restaurants, consuming low fat milk and healthy eating conceptualized as high levels of fibre and fruit and vegetables and low levels of fat (e.g. Povey *et al.* 2000). A cognitive approach to eating behaviour therefore emphasizes the role of cognitions and explores how these cognitions predict what we eat. From this perspective we eat food because we have positive thoughts about it. The obese may over eat because they have more positive thoughts about foods that are then translated into behaviour.

A developmental approach

In contrast, a developmental approach to eating behaviour emphasizes the importance of learning in terms of both operant and classical conditioning and focuses on the development of food preferences in childhood. Social learning describes the impact of observing other people's behaviour on one's own behaviour and is sometimes referred to as 'modelling' or 'observational learning'. In one study peer modelling was used to change children's preference for vegetables (Birch 1980). The target children were placed at lunch for four consecutive days next to other children who preferred a different vegetable to themselves (peas versus carrots). By the end of the study the children showed a shift in their vegetable preference that persisted at a follow-up assessment several weeks later. The impact of social learning has also been shown in an intervention study designed to change children's eating behaviour using video- based peer modelling (Lowe *et al.* 1998). Food preferences therefore change through watching others eat. In terms of obesity, some people may over eat or eat more unhealthily because they have watched others close to them doing so.

Parental attitudes to *food and eating behaviours are also central to the process of social learning.* For example, Olivera *et al.* (1992) reported a correlation between mothers' and children's food intakes for most nutrients in pre-school children. Contento *et al.* (1993) found a relationship between mothers' health motivation and the quality of children's diets and Brown and Ogden (2004) reported consistent correlations between parents and their children in terms of reported snack food intake and eating motivation. Obesity clearly runs in families. This may reflect the transmission of eating-related attitudes and behaviours from parent to child.

Associative learning refers to the impact of contingent factors on behaviour. Some research has examined the effect of rewarding eating behaviour as in 'if you eat your vegetables I will be pleased with you'. For example, Birch *et al.* (1980) showed that if food was given to children in association with positive adult attention the preference for the food increased. Rewarding eating behaviour seems to improve food preferences. Other research has explored the impact of using food as a reward. For these studies gaining access to the food is contingent upon another behaviour as in 'if you are well behaved you can have a biscuit'. Birch *et al.* (1980) presented children with foods either as a reward, as a snack, or in a non social situation (the control). The results showed that food acceptance increased if the foods were presented as a reward but that the more neutral conditions had no effect. This suggests that using food as a reward increases the preference for that food. The relationship between food and rewards, however, appears to be more complicated than this. In an early study Lepper *et al.* (1982) told children stories about children eating imaginary foods called 'hupe' and 'hule' in which the child in the story could only eat one if he/she had finished the other. This is analogous to saying 'if you eat your vegetables you can eat your pudding'. Although parents use this approach to encourage their children to eat vegetables the evidence indicates that this may be increasing their children's preference for pudding even further as pairing two foods results in the 'reward' food being seen as more positive than the 'access' food. In terms of obesity, people may overeat and become obese because they have learned that higher fat, unhealthier foods are more rewarding than others and / or because their parents used unhealthier foods as rewards for eating the healthier foods.

The role of dieting

The final theoretical perspective that may illuminate why some people become obese is the focus on dieting and restraint theory (see Ogden 2003). Dieting is the conscious attempt to cognitively control food intake. Many people who are already obese diet as a means to lose weight. Dieting, however, may not only be a consequence of obesity but also a cause as there is evidence that dieting is often characterized by periods of overeating which is precipitated by factors such as lowered mood and eating a high calorie food. From this perspective it has been argued that attempting to eat less paradoxically causes overeating, as the process of denial and self-control makes food more attractive and creates a situation whereby the individual becomes increasingly preoccupied with eating. There is also some evidence that overeating is reflected in weight gain, particularly in women. For example, French *et al.* (1994) reported the results from a cross-sectional and longitudinal study of 1639 men and 1913 women who were involved in a worksite intervention study for smoking cessation and weight control. The cross-sectional analysis showed that a history of dieting, current dieting, and previous involvement in a formal weight loss programme were related to a higher body weight in both men and women. Similarly, the prospective analysis showed that baseline measures of involvement in a formal weight loss programme and dieting predicted increases in body weight at follow-up. However this was for women only. In particular, women who were dieting or who had been involved in a formal weight loss programme at baseline gained nearly two pounds more than those who had not. Klesges and colleagues (1992) reported similar results in their study of 141 men and 146 women who were followed up after 1 year. This showed that both the dieting men and women were heavier than their non dieting counterparts at baseline. Higher baseline weight and higher restraint scores at baseline also predicted greater weight gain at follow-up in women. If dieters perceive themselves to be overweight, but are not necessarily obese, and if dieting causes overeating and subsequent weight gain then dieting could predictably play a causal role in the development of obesity. It is possible that dieting also results in the relative over consumption of high fat foods as these are the foods that dieters try to avoid.

Obesity is therefore on the increase in both adults and children and research suggests a clear role for changes in behaviour, particularly diet. Psychological theories focusing on cognitions, learning, and the role of dieting suggest that overeating may be a result of their beliefs about food, how and what they have seen others eat, how food was presented to them in their childhood, and their subsequent attempts to diet and reduce their food intake.

Developing interventions to change health-related behaviour

Health psychology theory provides a framework for understanding behaviour and beliefs and exploring how these factors may relate to illnesses. These theories have drawn on social cognition models, implementations intentions and the self regulatory model to inform interventions aiming to change behaviours and beliefs.

Using social cognition models (SCMs)

SCMs have been developed to describe and predict health behaviours such as smoking, screening, eating, and exercise. Over recent years there has been a call towards using these models to inform and develop interventions to change behaviours. This has been based upon two observations. First, it was observed that many interventions designed to change behaviour were only minimally effective. For example, reviews of early interventions to change sexual behaviour concluded that these interventions had only small effects (e.g. Oakley *et al.* 1995) and dietary interventions for weight loss may result in weight loss in the short term but the majority show a return to baseline by follow-up (e.g. NHS Centre for Reviews and Dissemination 1997). Second, it was observed that many interventions were not based upon any theoretical framework nor were they drawing upon research that had identified which factors were correlated with the particular behaviour. Some researchers have therefore outlined how theory can be translated into interventions. In particular, Sutton (2002) describes a series of steps that can be followed to develop an intervention: (1) Identify target behaviour and target population; (2) identify the most salient beliefs about the target behaviour in the target population using open-ended questions; (3) conduct a study involving closed questions to determine which beliefs are the best predictors of behavioural intention. Choose the best belief as the target belief; (4) analyse the data to determine the beliefs which best discriminate between intenders and non-intenders. These are further target beliefs; (5) develop an intervention to change these target beliefs.

Over recent years an increasing number of behavioural interventions have drawn upon a theory of behaviour change to change behaviours such as condom use, sun cream use, and cervical cancer screening. For example, Quine *et al.* (2001) followed the steps outlined above to identify salient beliefs about safety helmet wearing for children. They then developed an intervention based upon persuasion to change these salient beliefs. The results showed that after the intervention the participants showed more positive beliefs about safety helmet wearing than the control group and were more likely to wear a helmet at 5 months follow-up.

Using implementation intentions

SCMs emphasize the relationship between the intention to behave in a certain way and actual behaviour. Research indicates, however, that intentions do not always translate into behaviour. Gollwitzer's (1993) notion of implementation intentions have been employed to strengthen this association. Gollwitzer regards carrying out an intention as involving the development of specific plans as to what an individual will do given a specific set of environmental factors.

Implementation intentions therefore describe the 'what' and the 'when' of a particular behaviour. For example, the intention 'I intend to stop smoking' will be more likely to be translated into 'I have stopped smoking' if the individual makes the implementation intention 'I intend to stop smoking tomorrow at 12.00 when I have finished my last packet'. Some experimental research has shown that encouraging individuals to make implementation intentions can actually increase the correlation between intentions and behaviour for behaviours such as reducing dietary fat. Gollwitzer and Sheeran (2006) carried out a meta-analysis of 94 independent tests of the impact of implementation intentions on a range of behavioural goals including eating a low fat diet, using public transport, exercise, and a range of personal goals. The results from this analysis indicated that implementation intentions had a medium to large effect on goal attainment. By tapping into variables such as implementation intentions it is argued that the models may become better predictors of actual behaviour.

Using the SRM

Research indicates that patients' beliefs about their illness may relate to a range of health outcomes in terms of adherence to medication, attendance at rehabilitation, return to work, and adjustment. Interventions have therefore been developed to change beliefs and promote more positive outcomes. For example, Petrie *et al.* (2002) aimed to change illness cognitions and examined the subsequent impact upon a range of patient outcomes. The intervention consisted of three sessions of about 40 min with a psychologist and was designed to address and change patients' beliefs about their myocardial infarction (MI). Throughout the intervention the information and discussion were targeted to the specific beliefs and concerns of the patient. The results showed that patients who had received the intervention reported more positive views about their MI at follow-up in terms of beliefs about consequences, time line, control/cure, and symptom distress. They were also better prepared to leave hospital, returned to work at a faster rate, and reported a lower rate of angina symptoms. The intervention therefore appeared to change cognitions and improve patients' functional outcome after MI.

Conclusion: Future directions

Both sociology and psychology are now well established as part of multi-disciplinary public health and are increasingly forging new partnerships with anthropology, social policy, and geography in studying public health issues. The particular focus of research reflects what are seen as current major public health issues, with the particular contributions of sociology and psychology being through their perspectives and concepts that guide both the formulation of research questions and the explanations and models derived. A key and continuing area of sociological investigation remains the worldwide concern with socioeconomic and gender inequalities in health, often manifest through inequities of access to healthcare, together with increasing emphasis on the health and rights to healthcare of ethnic minorities and refugee groups and issues of the provision of care for older people. This is leading to new sociological analyses of the concepts and meanings of 'ethnicity' and of 'old age', which emphasize the fluid and heterogeneous nature of these epidemiological categories. Another increasing policy focus is the importance of health promotion and health education based on behaviour change techniques to achieve risk reduction through life style change and for chronic disease management in terms of improving adherence to medication and increasing attendance for treatment and rehabilitation. Whereas much research in health psychology has emphasized theory development and the testing a range of psychological models, there is currently a drive to become more involved in interventions based on an understanding of cognitions and motivations, with health psychology thus becoming a central part of public health work. Moreover the focus of health psychology on individual behaviour is increasingly complemented by sociological research that contributes to an understanding of social structures, in terms of how inequalities are manifest and perpetuated and the significance of the local environment and its social capital for health risks and health-related behaviours.

Qualitative methods of anthropology and sociology are now increasingly employed by health psychology, and acknowledged within the public health field as mainstream methods that are valuable in providing in-depth insights into processes, beliefs, and everyday understandings of people's lives. This emphasis on qualitative methods alongside quantitative techniques is likely to continue, with possibly a greater integration of different methodological approaches. In particular there is an increasing emphasis on the evaluation of different forms of healthcare delivery that requires both traditional methods of outcomes evaluation together with an understanding of processes of implementation and patients' experiences. This is leading to a greater emphasis on both multi-methods of evaluation and new theoretically driven approaches to evaluation. Other methods are new methods of synthesizing quantitative and qualitative research are likely to become more formalized and seen as an increasingly important activity.

References

Abraham, C. and Sheeran, P. (2005) The health belief model. In *Predicting health behaviour* (eds. M. Conner and P. Norman), 2nd edition, pp. 28–80. Open University Press, Buckingham.

Ajzen, I. (1988). *Attitudes, personality and behavior*. Dorsey Press, Chicago, IL.

Albrecht, G.L. and Devlieger, P.J. (1999). The disability paradox: High quality of life against all odds. *Social Science & Medicine*, **50** (6), 757–9.

Allsopp, J., Baggott, R., and Jones, K. (2002). Health consumer groups and the national policy process. In). *Consuming health* (eds. S Henderson and A Petersen) Routledge, London.

Angus, J., Kontos, P., Dyck, I. *et al.* (2005). The experience of home; habitus and the experience of receiving long-term home care. *Sociology of Health & Illness*, **27** (2), 161–87.

Annandale, E. (1998)*The sociology of health and medicine: a critical introduction*. Polity Press, Cambridge.

Armitage, C.J. and Conner, M. (2000). Social cognition models and health behaviour: Astructured review. *Psychology and Health*, **15**, 173–89.

Banta, H.D. (2003). Considerations in defining evidence for public health (The European Advisory Committee on Health Research, World Health Organisation Regional Office for Europe). *International Journal of Technology Assessment in Health Care*, **19** (23), 559–72.

Barbour, R.S. and Barbour, M. (2003). Evaluating and synthesizing qualitative research: The need to develop a distinctive approach. *Journal of Evaluation in Clinical Practice*, **9** (2), 179–86.

Barrett, R. (2005). Self-mortification and the stigma of leprosy in Northern India. *Medical Anthropology Quarterly*, **19** (2), 216–30.

Becker, M.H. and Rosenstock, I.M. (1987). Comparing social learning theory and the health belief model. In *Advances in health education and promotion*(ed. W.B. Ward), pp. 245–9. JAI Press, Greenwich, CT.

Birch, L.L. (1980). Effects of peer models' food choices and eating behaviors on preschoolers' food preferences. *Child Development*, **51**, 489–96.

Bloor, M., Frankland, J., Thomas, M. *et al.* (2001). *Focus groups in social research*. Sage Publications, London.

Bourdieu, P. (1977). *The outline of a theory of practice*. Cambridge University Press, Cambridge.

Bowling, A. (2002). *Research methods in health: Investigating health and health services*, 2nd edition. Open University Press, Buckingham.

Brown, R. and Ogden, J. (2004). Children's eating attitudes and behaviour: A study of the modelling and control theories of parental influence. *Health Education and Research*, **19** (3), 261–71.

Bury, M. (1982). Chronic illness as biographical disruption. *Sociology of Health and Illness*, **4** (2), 167–82.

Campbell, R., Pound, P., Pope, C. *et al.* (2003). Evaluating meta-ethnography: A synthesis of qualitative research on lay experiences of diabetes and diabetes care. *Social Science and Medicine*, **56**, 671–84.

Charmaz, K. (1983). Loss of self: A fundamental form of suffering in the chronically ill. *Sociology of Health & Illness*, **5** (2), 168–95.

Contento, I.R., Basch, C., Shea, S. *et al.* (1993). Relationship of mothers' food choice criteria to food intake of pre-school children: Identification of family subgroups, *Health Education Quarterly*, **20**, 243–59.

Corrigan, P.W., Kerr, A., and Knudsen, A. (2005). The stigma of mental illness: Explanatory models and methods for change. *Applied and Preventive Psychology*, **11** (3), 179–90.

Cummins, S. and Macintyre, S. (2002). A systematic study of an urban foodscape: The price and availability of food in Greater Glasgow. *Urban Studies*, **39**, 2115–30.

Davison, C., Frankel, S., and Dabey Smith, G. (1992). The limits of lifestyle: Reassessing 'fatalism' in the popular culture of illness prevention. *Social Science and Medicine*, **34** (6), 675–85.

Department of Health (2001). *The Expert Patient: A new approach to chronic disease management in the 21st century*. Stationery Office, London.

Dixon-Woods, M., Alex, S., Shaw, R. *et al.* (2007) Appraising qualitative research for inclusion in systematic reviews: a quantitative and qualitative comparison of three methods. *Journal of Health Services Research and Policy*, **12** (1), 42–7.

Ellaway, A., Macintyre, S., and Bonnefoy, X. (2005). Graffiti, greenery and obesity in adults; secondary analysis of European cross sectional survey. *British Medical Journal*, **331**, 611–12.

Foucault, M. (1976). *The birth of the clinic: An archaeology of medical perception*. Tavistock, London.

French, S.A., Jeffery, R.W., Forster, J.L. *et al.* (1994). Predictors of weight change over two years among a population of working adults: The healthy worker project. *International Journal of Obesity*, **18**, 145–54.

Gebbie, K.M. and Hwang, I. (2000). Preparing currently employed public health nurses for changes in the health system. *American Journal of Public Health*, **90** (5), 716–21.

Glaser, B. and Strauss, A. (1967). *The discovery of grounded theory*. Aldine, Chicago.

Goffman, E. (1963). *Stigma: Notes on the management of a spoiled identity*. Prentice-Hall, Englewood Cliffs, NJ.

Gollwitzer, P.M. (1993). Goal achievement: The role of intentions. In *European Review of Social Psychology* (eds. W. Stroebe and M. Hewstone), **4**, 141–85.

Gollwitzer, P.M. and Sheeran, P. (2006). Implementation intentions and goal achievement: A meta-analysis of effects and processes. *Advances in Experimental Social Psychology*, **38**, 69–119.

Green, J. and Thorogood, N. (2004). *Qualitative methods for health*. Sage Publications, London.

Hart, E., Lymbery, M., and Gladman, J.R.F. (2005). Away from home: an ethnographic study of a transitional rehabilitation scheme for older people in the UK. *Social Science and Medicine*, **60**, 1241–50.

Klesges, R.C., Isbell, T.R., and Klesges, L.M. (1992). Relationship between dietary restraint, energy intake, physical activity, and body weight: A prospective analysis. *Journal of Abnormal Psychology*, **101**, 668–74.

Krenichyn, K. (2006). 'The only place to go and be in the city'; women talk about exercise, being outdoors and the meaning of a large urban park. *Health and Place*, **12** (4), 631–43.

Kuh, D. and Ben-Shlomo, Y. (2004). *A life course approach to chronic disease epidemiology: Tracing the origins of ill health from early to adult life*, 2nd edition. Oxford University Press, Oxford.

Layder, D. (2006). *Understanding social theory*, 2nd edition. Sage, London.

Lepper, M., Sagotsky, G., Dafoe, J.L. *et al.* (1982). Consequences of superfluous social constraints: effects on young children's social inferences and subsequent intrinsic interest. *Journal of Personality and Social Psychology*, **42**, 51–65.

Leventhal, H., Benyamini, Y., Brownlee, S. *et al.* (1997). Illness representations: Theoretical foundations. In *Perceptions of health and illness: Current research and applications* (eds. K.J. Petrie and J.A. Weinman), pp. 19–45. Harwood Academic Publishers, Amsterdam, The Netherlands.

Linstrom, M., Moghaddassi, M., and Merlo, J. (2003). Social capital and leisure time physical activity; a population based multilevel analysis. *Journal of Epidemiology and Community Health*, **57** (1), 23–8.

Lorig, K.R., Sobel, D.S., Stewart, A.L. *et al.* (1999). Evidence suggesting that a chronic disease self-management programme can improve health status while reducing hospitalization. *Medical Care*, **37**, 5–14.

Lowe, C.F., Dowey, A., and Horne, P. (1998). Changing what children eat. In *The Nation's diet: The social science of food choice* (ed. A. Murcott), pp. 57–80. Addison Wesley Longman Ltd, Harlow.

Macintyre, S., Ellaway, A., and Cummins, S. (2002). Place effects on health; how can we conceptualise, operationalise and measure them? *Social Science and Medicine*, **5**, 125–39.

Mak, W.W.S., Mo, P.K.H., Cheung, R.Y.M. *et al.* (2006). Comparative stigma of HIV/AIDS, SARS, and tuberculosis in Hong Kong. *Social Science & Medicine*, **63** (7), 1912–22.

Mattingley, C. and Garro, L.C. (eds.) (2000) *Narrative and the cultural construction of illness and healing*. University of California Press, California.

Mays, N., Pope, C., and Popay, J. (2006). Systematically reviewing qualitative and quantitative evidence to inform management and policy-making in the health field. *Journal of Health Services Research and Policy*, **10** (Suppl 1), S16–20.

Mead, G.H. (1967). *Mind, self and society*. Chicago University Press, Chicago.

Meyer, J. (2000). *Using qualitative methods in health-related action research*. Chapter 7 in Qualitative research in health care (eds. C. Pope and N. Mays), 2nd edition. BMJ Books, London.

NHS Centre for Reviews and Dissemination (1997). *Systematic Review of Interventions in the Treatment and Prevention of Obesity*. University of York, York.

Noblitt, G.W. and Hare, R.D. (1988). *Meta-ethnography: synthesising qualitative studies*. Qualitative Research Methods, Vol. 11. Sage Publications, New York.

Oakley, A., Fullerton, D., Holland, J. *et al.* (1995). Sexual health education interventions for young people: a methodological review. *British Medical Journal*, **310**, 158–62.

Ogden, J. (2003). *The psychology of eating: From healthy to disordered behaviour*. Blackwell, US / UK.

Ogden, J. (2007). *Health Psychology: A textbook*, 4th edition. McGraw Hill/ Open University Press, Buckingham.

Olivera, S.A., Ellison, R.C., Moore, L.L. *et al.* (1992), Parent-child relationships in nutrient intake: The Framingham Children's Study. *American Journal of Clinical Nutrition*, **56**, 593–8.

Ononeze, V., Murphy, A.W., Byrne, M. *et al.* (2006). Patients and health professionals' perspectives on the sociocultural influences on secondary cardiac behaviour: A qualitative study of the implications in policy and practice. *Family Practice*, **23** (5), 587–96.

Parker, R. and Aggleton, P. (2004). HIV and AIDS related stigma and discrimination: A conceptual framework and implications for action. *Social Science and Medicine*, **59** (3), 457–71.

Parsons, T. (1951). *The social system*. Free Press, New York.

Partridge, C.J. and Johnston, M. (1989). Perceived control and recovery from physical disability. *British Journal of Clinical Psychology*, **28**, 53–60.

Patten, S., Mitton, C., and Donaldson, C. (2006). Using participatory action research to build a priority setting process in a Canadian Regional Health Authority. *Social Science and Medicine*, **63**, 1121–34.

Petrie, K.J., Cameron, L.D., Ellis, C.J. *et al.* (2002). Changing illness perceptions after myocardial infraction: An early intervention randomized controlled trial. *Psychosomatic Medicine*, **64**, 580–6.

Petrie, K.J., Weinman, J.A., Sharpe, N. *et al.* (1996). Role of patient's view of their illness in predicting return to work and functioning after myocardial infarction: Longitudinal study. *British Medical Journal*, **312**, 1191–4.

Pikora, T., Giles-Corti, B., Bull, F. *et al.* (2003). Developing a framework for assessment of the environmental determinants of walking and cycling. *Social Science and Medicine*, **56**, 1693–1703.

Popay, J., Rogers, A., and Williams, G. (1998). Rationale and standards for the systematic review of qualitative literature in health services research. *Qualitative Health Research*, **8** (3), 341–51.

Pound, P., Britten, N., Morgan, M. *et al.* (2005). Resisting medicines: A synthesis of qualitative studies of medicine taking. *Social Science and Medicine*, **61** (1), 133–55.

Povey, R., Conner, M., Sparks, P. *et al.* (2000). The theory of planned behaviour and healthy eating: Examining additive and moderating effects of social influence variables. *Psychology and Health*, **14**, 991–1006.

Putman, R.D. (1993). *Making democracy work*. Princeton University Press, Princeton, New Jersey.

Quine, L., Rutter, D.R., and Arnold, L. (2001). Persuading school-age cyclist to use safety helmets: Effectiveness of an intervention based on the theory of planned behaviour. *British Journal of Health Psychology*, **6**, 327–45.

Reidpath, D.D., Burns, C., Garrard, J. *et al.* (2002). An ecological study of the relationship between social and environmental determinants of obesity. *Health and Place*, **8**, 141–5.

Richards, H., Reid, M.E., and Watt, G.C.M. (2002). Socioeconomic variation in responses to chest pain; qualitative study. *British Medical Journal*, **324**, 308–11.

Ritchie, J. and Spencer, L. (1994). Qualitative data analysis for applied policy research. In *Analyzing qualitative data* (eds. A Bryman and R.G. Burgess), pp. 173–94. Routledge, London.

Rosenstock, I.M. (1966). Why people use health services. *Millbank Memorial Fund Quarterly*, **44**, 94–124.

Rutter, D.R. and Quine, L. (2002). *Changing health behaviour: Intervention and research with social cognition models*. Open University Press, Buckingham.

Scambler, G.S. and Hopkins, A. (1986). Being epileptic: Coming to terms with stigma. *Sociology of Health and Illness*, **8**, 26–43.

Scott, S., Prior, L., Wood, F. *et al.* (2005). Repositioning the patient: The implications of being 'at risk'. *Social Science and Medicine*, **60** (8), 1869–79.

Seale, C. (1999). *The quality of qualitative research*. Sage Publications, London.

Shakespeare, T. (1999). "Losing the plot?": Medical and activist discourses of contemporary genetics and disability. *Sociology of Health and Illness*, **21**, 669–88.

Silverman, D. (2004). *Qualitative research: Theory, method and practice*. 2nd edition. Sage Publications, London.

Strauss, A. and Corbin, J. (1990). *Basics of qualitative research: Grounded theory procedures and techniques*. Sage, Newbury Park, CA.

Stafford, M., Cummins, S., Macintyre, S. *et al.* (2005). Gender differences in the association between health and neighbourhood environment. *Social Science and Medicine*, **60**, 1681–92.

Sutton, S. (2002). Using social cognition models to develop health behaviour interventions: Problems and assumptions. In *Changing health behaviour: Intervention and research with social cognition models* (eds. D. Rutter and L. Quine), pp. 193–208. Open University Press, Buckingham.

Tachakkoni, A. and Teddlie, C.B. (eds.) (2003). *Handbook of mixed methods*. Sage Publications, London.

Weich, S., Burton, E., Blanchard, M. *et al.* (2001). Measuring the built environment: Validity of a site survey instrument for use in urban settings. *Health and Place*, **7** (4), 238–92.

Whitaker, E.D. (2005). The bicycle makes the eyes smile; exercise, ageing and psychophysical well-being in older Italian cyclists. *Medical Anthropology*, **24**, 1–43.

Williams, G. (1984). The genesis of chronic illness: Narrative reconstruction. *Sociology of Health and Illness*, **6**, 175–200.

Wright, E.R., Wright, D.E., Perry, B.L. *et al.* (2007). Stigma and the sexual isolation of people with serious mental illness. *Social Problems*, **54** (1), 78–98.

7.2

Demography and public health

Emily Grundy

Abstract

The health and healthcare needs of a population cannot be measured or met without knowledge of its size and characteristics. Demography is concerned with this essential 'numbering of the people' and with understanding population dynamics—how populations change in response to the interplay between fertility, mortality, and migration. This understanding is a pre-requisite for making the forecasts about future population size and structure which should underpin healthcare planning. Analysis of both the present and the future necessitates a review of the past. The number of very old people in a population, for example, depends on the number of births eight or nine decades earlier and risks of death at successive ages throughout the intervening period. The *proportion* of very old people depends partly on this numerator but more importantly on the denominator (the size of the population as a whole)—itself a function of reproductive behaviour, mortality, and net migration from yesterday back through time. The number of births in a population depends not just on current patterns of family building, but also on the number of women 'at risk' of reproduction—itself a function of past trends in fertility and mortality. Similarly, the number of deaths (and their distribution by cause) is strongly influenced by age structure.

Formal or pure demography is largely concerned with answering questions about how populations change and how these changes can be measured. The broader field of population studies embraces the questions of why these changes occur, and with what consequences.

This chapter presents information on demographic methods and data sources, in the context of their application to health and population issues, together with information on demographic trends and their implications and the major theories about demographic change in order to elucidate the complex inter-relationship between population change and human health.

Global issues

Figure 7.2.1 shows that the world's population has been growing at an unprecedented rate and was estimated to comprise some 6.12 billion persons in 2000 (UN 2007). While it took an estimated 123 years (from 1804 to 1927) for the world to increase its population from 1 to 2 billion, the increase from 5 to 6 billion was achieved in a tenth of the time (1987–1999). The United Nation's medium

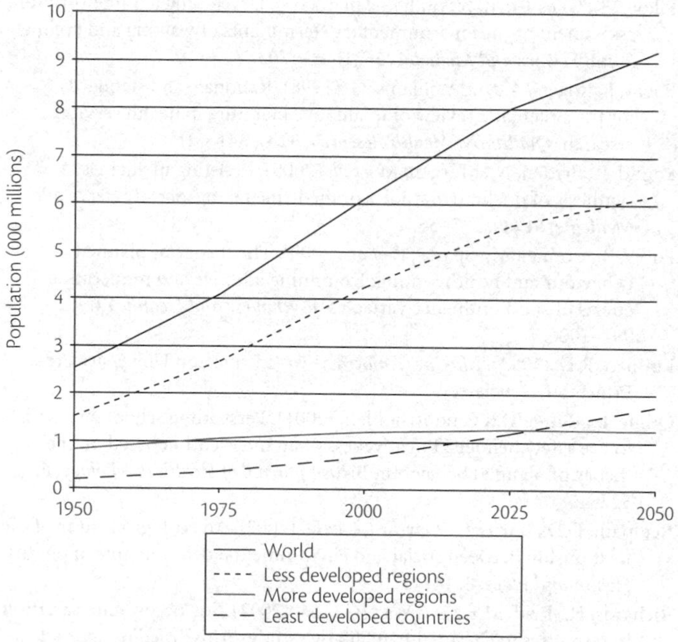

Fig 7.2.1 Population and projected population of the world and more, less, and least developed regions, 1950–2050.
Data source: UN 2007.

projection suggests a further increase of some three billion by 2050 (UN 2007). Looking further into the future, there now seems a good chance that the twenty-first century will be the one in which global population growth will cease (Lutz *et al.* 2001).

This prospect of global population stability masks huge differences between regions and between richer and poorer countries. Most recent growth in population has been in the less developed world; and, barring an abrupt change in trends, future growth will be concentrated in the poorest countries. Between 1950 and 2000, 76 per cent of world population growth occurred in countries currently designated by the United Nations as less developed (excluding the least developed, see Box 7.2.1 for definitions); 13 per cent in least developed countries and 11 per cent in more developed regions. Between 2000 and 2050 medium-term projections suggest that population growth in more developed regions will account for only 2 per cent of the total with 64 per cent occurring

Box 7.2.1 Country and regional classifications by level of development

The United Nations classifies countries into 'more' and 'less' developed and also identifies a group of 50 'least developed' countries. The more developed category includes all of Europe, North America, Australia, New Zealand, and Japan. The least developed countries are mostly in sub-Saharan Africa but also include Afghanistan, Bangladesh, Cambodia, and Myanmar. The classification has some anomalies in that some wealthy Asian and near-Eastern countries are counted as less developed (e.g. Republic of Korea, Singapore, Cyprus, Israel), whereas some poorer former Eastern bloc countries are treated as more developed (e.g. Albania, Belarus, Bulgaria).

The World Bank employs a classification based on gross national income per capita which divides countries into high-, middle-, and low-income groups, with a subdivision of the middle into upper and lower. Some of the countries (principally from Eastern Europe) classified by the UN as developed fall into middle-income categories, while some of the UN less developed group are classified by the World Bank as middle income (principally Latin American) or high income (some Southeast Asian).

Membership of the Organisation for Economic Co-operation and Development (OECD) is also sometimes used as an indicator of developed country status; members include Russia and Mexico, both of which are classified by the World Bank as middle- rather than high-income countries.

The Human Development Index compiled by the United Nations Development Programme takes into account factors other than income, such as school enrolment, literacy, and levels of mortality.

Regional groupings employed by different international agencies also vary slightly.

Further details of all these classifications are available on the relevant organizations' Web sites.

in less developed countries and 35 per cent in the least developed countries. These projections imply that by 2050 the share of the world's population living in currently more developed regions will account for only 14 per cent of total world population—compared with 32 per cent a century earlier, while the representation of those in the poorest countries will have increased from 8 per cent of the total in 1950 to 19 per cent in 2050.

While some regions grapple to deal with the needs of rapidly growing populations, such as large increases in requirements for child health services and schools, others face challenges arising from population ageing and, in some cases, population decline. By 2025 approaching a quarter of the populations of a number of European countries will be aged 65 or more (UN 2007) and if current very low rates of fertility persist, in some countries, such as Japan and Italy, a third or more of the population will be aged 65 and over by 2050 (UN 2007, constant fertility assumption).

These hugely differing rates of growth are a consequence of differences in vital rates, and associated large variations in age structures, which are illustrated for regions and selected countries within them in Table 7.2.1. In Europe as a whole, and some Southeast Asian countries, such as Japan, the Republic of Korea, and Singapore,

Table 7.2.1 Indicators of fertility, mortality, and age structure: World regions and selected countries, 2005

Region/ country		Proportion (%) of population aged:		Total fertility rate	Life expectancy at birth (years)
		<15	65 and over		
Africa		41	3	4.8	51
	Sub-Saharan	43	3	5.3	49
	Northern	32	5	2.6	72
Asia		28	6	2.4	68
	India	32	5	2.9	67
	China	21	8	1.7	72
	Japan	14	19	1.4	81
	Indonesia	29	5	2.4	70
	South Korea	19	9	1.3	77
Australia		20	13	1.8	80
Europe		16	16	1.4	75
	Italy	14	19	1.3	80
	Poland	16	13	1.2	75
	Germany	14	19	1.4	79
	Sweden	17	17	1.7	80
	Ukraine	15	16	1.4	68
	United Kingdom	18	16	1.7	78
Latin America & Caribbean		29	6	2.4	72
	Brazil	26	6	1.9	72
	Chile	25	8	2.0	77
	Guatemala	42	4	3.9	69
North America		20	13	2.0	78
	United States	21	12	2.1	78
World		28	7	2.6	65

Data from US Census Bureau, Population Division, International Programs Center, International Data Base http://www.census.gov/ipc/www/idbnew.html.

women on average have only 1.4 children or fewer, (a more detailed explanation of the derivation of the total fertility rate is given in Box 7.2.2) and people aged 65 and over outnumber children under 16. In sub-Saharan Africa, women on average have more than five children each, 40 per cent or more of the population is aged 15 or under and only 3 per cent aged 65 or more.

Levels of mortality, and associated differences in age and cause distribution of death, also vary markedly. In some high-income countries average life expectancy at birth is close to 80, in some sub-Saharan countries it is below 45. Figure 7.2.2 shows the distribution of deaths by age for four countries which range from the very poor (Malawi) to the very rich (Japan). In Malawi, 50 per cent of all

Box 7.2.2 Fertility measure

Definitions

Fertility: The childbearing performance of individuals, couples, or populations

Fecundity: The physiological capability of producing a live birth

Parity: The number of children previously born alive (or sometimes number of previous confinements) to a woman or couple. Nulliparous women are those who have borne no children.

Measures

Crude birth rate (CBR): The ratio of births in a year (other specified period) to the average population in the same year/period (mid-year population), expressed per 1000

$$\text{CBR} = \frac{\text{number of births}}{\text{mid-year population}} \times 1000$$

General fertility rate (GFR): Births to women aged 15–44/49 in a year/period per 1000 women aged 15–44/49 in the same period.

$$\text{GFR} = \frac{\text{number of births to women aged } 15-44/49}{\text{mid-year population of women aged } 15-44/49} \times 1000$$

Age-specific fertility rate (ASFR): Number of births to women aged x (or x to $x + n$) per 1000 women aged x (or x to $x + n$). 'n' refers to the length of an age interval. ASFRs are frequently calculated for five year age groups from 15–19 to 40–44 or 45–49

$$\text{ASFR} = \frac{\text{births to women aged } x}{\text{mid-year population of women aged } x} \times 1000$$

Total (period) fertility rate (TFR/TPFR): The sum of the age-specific fertility rates for all reproductive age groups for a particular period (usually a year), conventionally expressed per woman. The TFR indicates how many children a woman would have if throughout her reproductive life, she had children at the age specific rates prevalent in the specified year or period

$$\text{TRF} = \sum_{x=15}^{45-49} fx$$

where 'fx' is the age-specific fertility rate at age x. If rates for age groups, rather than single years, are used then the sum of the age-specific rates must be multiplied by the number of single ages included in the group (usually five).

$$\text{TRF} = 5\,x \sum_{x=15-19}^{45-49} fx$$

Parity progression ratio: The probability of a women of parity x progressing to parity $x + 1$

deaths in a year are deaths of infants and children aged under 5; in Japan the equivalent proportion is 0.5 per cent. Conversely 60 per cent of all deaths in Japan and 45 per cent of all deaths in Chile, now a middle-income country, are deaths of people aged 75 and over; equivalent proportions for Egypt and Malawi are 25 per cent and less than 5 per cent respectively. These variations have enormous implications for health and healthcare priorities in, and beyond, the populations concerned. Divergence in population growth between regions of the world is also fuelling mass migration, which itself has implications for global population health.

Closely related to variations in the distribution of deaths by age (and differences in levels of mortality) are differences in the cause structure of death. As shown in Fig. 7.2.3, communicable diseases, maternal and perinatal conditions, and nutritional deficiencies account for 72 per cent of all deaths in sub-Saharan Africa but only 6 per cent in Europe. Conversely, non communicable diseases are responsible for 21 per cent of deaths in Sub Saharan Africa, 51 per cent in Southeast Asia, but 86 per cent in Europe. While in parts of the world communicable diseases and reproductive and child health present the most pressing public health problems; in others concerns about the prevalence of age-related degenerative diseases predominate.

The watershed that separates populations with high fertility, relatively high mortality, young age structures, and rapid growth, from those with low vital rates, older age structures, and slow or no growth, is conceptualized as the demographic transition. Identifying, and explaining, this and associated profound changes in health has been a central pre-occupation of modern demography. Before turning to the causes, progress, and consequences of these transformations, the basic methods and materials of demographic analysis must be considered and the issue of population dynamics—how populations change—addressed.

Demographic data and methods of analysis

In the seventeenth century John Graunt, a London merchant, used data from the London Bills of Mortality to devise an early life table. This pioneering work led to him being dubbed the 'father of modern demography'. However, Graunt was handicapped by the fact that although he had information on *numbers* of deaths, he lacked data on the population at risk and could not compute death *rates*. Essentially all demographic analysis requires data both on the population 'stock' and on 'flows' in and out—births, deaths, and migration. The traditional sources of information on the former are population censuses and, for the latter, vital registration systems.

Population censuses

Head counts of the population have an ancient history but the first 'modern' censuses were undertaken in Scandinavia in the eighteenth century. In England and Wales, the first census was undertaken in 1801, although a question on age was not included until 1841. Censuses spread throughout Europe during the nineteenth century and most of the rest of the world in the twentieth. As well as basic questions about age, sex, marital status, and place of residence, data on other characteristics such as employment, education, and housing are often collected. The United Nations recommends that censuses be conducted at least decennially in years ending in 0 or 1.

Censuses have many strengths and are often the only source of data for small areas or population sub-groups. Although primarily

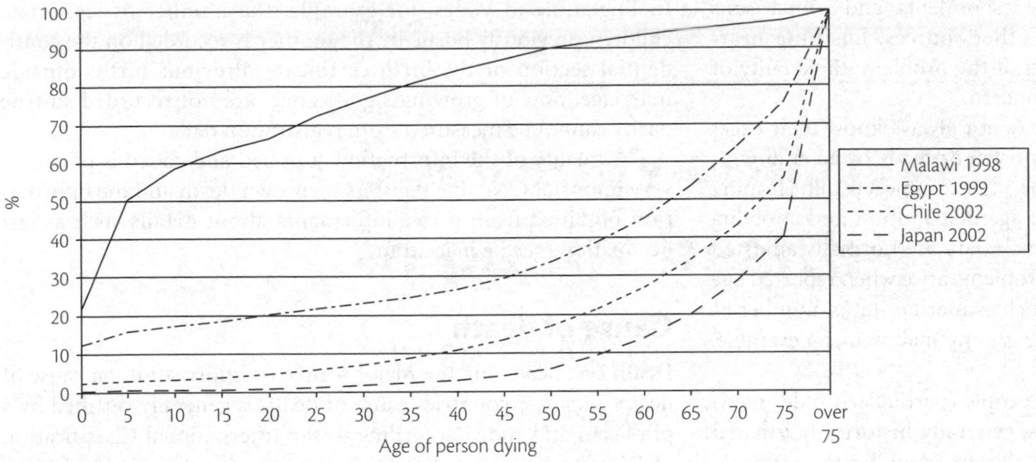

Fig. 7.2.2 Distribution of deaths by age, Malawi 1998, Egypt 1999, Chile 2002, Japan 2002.
Data source: UN 2004.

a tool for collecting data on population 'stock', censuses have also been used to find out about vital events. Many countries use censuses to provide data on recent internal migration (through questions on place of residence one or more years earlier) and immigration (through questions on country of birth and/or date of entry for those born elsewhere). Indirect estimation techniques developed by Brass and others mean that questions on number of children borne and number who have died, on widowhood and orphanhood, can be used to assess mortality levels and trends (UN 1983; Preston *et al.* 2001).

Against the strengths of censuses must be set the huge costs of collecting and processing census data and the problems involved in ensuring it is of reasonable quality. Approaches to reducing cost (and improving quality) include use of sample censuses, either for the census as a whole, as in China, or for more detailed questions,

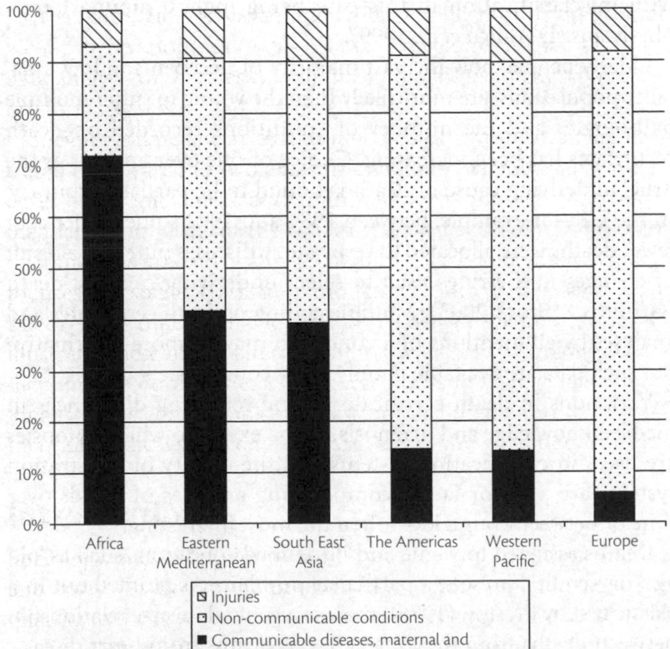

Fig.7.2.3 Distribution (%) of deaths by cause group and world region, 2004.
Data Source: WHO 2004.

as in the United States. The twenty-first century is likely to see more countries adopting alternatives as the information required by governments becomes more complex and the difficulties of collecting it in a timely fashion on a mass scale escalate. Census taking requires not only a reasonable administrative infrastructure, but also the co-operation of the population to be enumerated. Some countries, including Germany and the Netherlands, have given up taking censuses because the latter is lacking and now rely on large scale surveys or 'virtual censuses' based on population registration data.

When censuses are taken, difficulties arising from errors and omissions are common, even in countries with a long history of census taking. Some of the groups that policy makers and health professionals may be most keen to know about are among those least likely to be included. Young, geographically mobile adults; recent (especially unauthorized) immigrants; members of minority ethnic groups; infants and the very old are the groups most likely to be under-enumerated. In the 1991 UK census an estimated 1.2 million people were missed, including 10 per cent of males in their 20s and 8 per cent of those aged 85 or more. In 2001 over a fifth of the Inner London population was missed, although a system of imputation was used to adjust for this in published results.

Groups such as seasonal migrants, military personnel, people temporarily away from home, and those with more than one residence also present particular problems. Not only are they more likely to be missed, but a decision has to be made about whether they should be assigned to their place of usual or legal residence (assuming it can be determined), or counted as belonging to the place of enumeration. The former system is termed *de jure*, the latter *de facto*. The issue of assigning people to some place of usual residence is important as often resources are distributed on the basis of population size and characteristics. Moreover, it is essential to try and ensure that demographic events recorded in one system (vital registration) are attributed to the population actually 'at risk' of experiencing them. In richer countries, for example, most deaths occur in hospitals which may draw patients from a wide area. If no attempt is made to assign these decedents to the locality where they lived prior to hospital admission, areas including large hospitals will appear to have very high mortality rates while in others recorded mortality will be artificially low.

Assessment of under-enumeration is usually achieved through census validation surveys (surveys of a sample of census addresses in which intensive efforts are made to contact non-respondents and check information supplied by respondents) and comparisons with population estimates from other sources. Ensuring near-complete enumeration is only part of the problem; the quality of the data collected is also a major concern.

In many populations, people may not always know their exact age and some approximation is reported or made by an enumerator. 'Heaping' on ages ending in 0 or 5 is a common result. Heaping can be detected by looking at the age distribution and applying various tests of consistency and such data are normally adjusted before publication. More serious problems arise when reported age is based on other characteristics, such as marital status, number of children or grandparent status, as clearly any analysis of, for example, age at first marriage, will be biased.

Overstatement of age by elderly people (particularly older men) is common. There are some areas, generally historically isolated regions of small islands, with unusually large numbers of extremely aged people, but in general investigations into reported 'super-longevity' in particular populations have shown that age mis-statement, rather than yoghurt-eating, lie behind them (Garson 1991). Age mis-statement is not confined to poorer countries. In the United States, large discrepancies have been found between the number of very elderly people in the census and the number estimated from other sources, such as Medicare records.

Other characteristics may be 'mis-stated' because individuals' perceptions of their status do not match official classification systems. Thus in England and Wales, it is clear from linked census data that quite high proportions of divorced men revert to describing themselves as single (never-married). How people describe their ethnicity has also been found to vary over time and often does not fit with official classifications (Rosenberg *et al.* 1999).

Differential age misreporting between census and other sources, such as death certificates, presents a further difficulty. Numerator–denominator discrepancies may introduce serious bias into the analysis of mortality at advanced ages, or by characteristics such as occupationally defined social class, marital status, or ethnicity (Fox & Goldblatt 1982; Rosenberg *et al.* 1999).

Vital registration

Data on demographic events, as well as on population characteristics, are needed. In richer countries these are drawn from vital registration. Compulsory registration of births and deaths was established in most European countries during the nineteenth century. In England and Wales, for example, civil registration was introduced in 1837. Subsequent improvements to the system included those following the 1874 *Births and Deaths Registration Act*, which made parents legally responsible for registering births and required attending physicians to supply information on cause of death. Other revisions have since been made, for example, the inclusion of first mother's and later father's age on the confidential section of birth certificates. Most high-income countries have well-established registration systems with complete, or very near complete, coverage. In poorer parts of the world, however, many people have no need for certificates of birth or marriage. Consequently, vital registration systems are frequently seriously incomplete or non-existent, although there are some exceptions, and some countries, including India and China, have sample registration systems for selected areas. Even in well-established systems, the fact that registration is undertaken primarily for administrative reasons may mean that demographically relevant details are not recorded. In England and Wales, for example, the number of legitimate children previously borne by the mother is recorded on the confidential section of the birth certificate. Previous births outside marriage, now of growing significance, are not recorded so true parity cannot be measured from registration data.

The quality of the information supplied and coded is of course very important. No one registers their own death and the information obtained from proxy informants about details such as last occupation may be inaccurate.

Cause of death

Death certificates are the major source of information on cause of death. In richer countries cause of death is generally certified by a physician and coded according to the International Classification of Diseases. There is substantial scope for error and inconsistency at the various stages involved in assigning cause of death. The International Classification of Diseases (ICD), which originated from work undertaken by the nineteenth century British medical statistician, William Farr, is now on its tenth revision; each revision has been associated with changes particularly affecting certain causes of death. The introduction of ICD-10 in 2001 represented the largest change in ICD coding for some 50 years.

'Fashions' and national preferences also seem to influence assignment of cause of death, as illustrated in a number of classic papers in which case studies of deaths were distributed to physicians in different countries. Place of death may also be important. In Britain an apparent rise in respiratory disease mortality among elderly people in the 1950s and 1960s was found to largely reflect the increased proportion of deaths occurring in hospital. The hospital doctors who filled out the death certificates were more likely than family doctors to ascribe the deaths of elderly people to bronchopneumonia. A more recent Italian study also showed differences in classification, and misclassification, by different types of physician with misclassification in this case being highest among family physicians (D'Amico *et al.* 1999).

Elderly people, now the vast majority of decedents in low mortality populations, are more likely than the young to suffer multiple pathologies and the number of conditions recorded on death certificates has been increasing. Choice of one over another as the 'true' underlying cause of death is bound to be partially arbitrary. In the UK, for example, between 1984 and 1992 some 25 per cent fewer deaths were allocated to respiratory diseases purely as a result of changes in the rules used to select underlying cause of death (Griffiths & Brock 2003). Multiple coding of death certificates and analyses by all mentions of a condition may be more informative but such data are available in only a few countries.

Variations in death certificate coding reflecting differences in medical knowledge and diagnosis, in the extent to which autopsies are used, in classification systems and the quality of registration systems are a major factor complicating analyses of trends over time or between countries—often the most interesting.

Deaths assigned to vague and ill-defined conditions such as 'old age' or 'senility' present a particular problem. As pointed out in a classic text by Preston (1976), there is a general inverse relationship between deaths from these 'causes' and deaths from heart disease, suggesting that part of the twentieth century epidemic in heart disease mortality in richer countries may reflect improvements in death certification. Figure 7.2.4 shows the proportion of all deaths in England and Wales assigned to circulatory diseases and to ill-defined causes in age groups over 65 from 1911–15 to 2001–05. Early in the twentieth century large proportions of deaths among the very old were assigned to ill-defined categories and declines in this proportion were associated with increases in the proportion attributed to circulatory diseases. The proportion of ill assigned deaths in the oldest group aged 80 and over was, however, slightly higher in 2001–05 than in the preceding period, reflecting increased assignment to 'old age' as a cause. Reasons for this are unclear, although the cessation in 1993 of further enquiry into vague causes of death may have been a small contributory factor. Use of this 'cause of death' may have subsequently reversed again in response to the public enquiry into the case of Harold Shipman, a British family doctor whose serial murder of elderly patients was not detected for many years—an illustration of the importance of surveillance of deaths for reasons other than epidemiological or demographic investigation (Griffiths & Brock 2003).

In countries which lack adequate certification and registration systems, data on deaths by cause are seriously limited. Attempts have been made to develop protocols for collecting information from lay informants which can be used to assign cause of death (Wang *et al.* 2007). However, although this approach has been useful in a number of small-scale investigations, its widespread application would be extremely costly.

Other data sources

Many countries have a range of government surveys which provide more detailed information on, for example, health-related behaviour, family building strategies, or reasons for migration than it would be possible to collect in a census. In poorer countries, where other data sources are scarcer, surveys often present the best source of data on basic demographic parameters. Data quality is potentially better in a survey than a census, as it is more likely that well-trained interviewers can be used. The World Fertility Survey (WFS), an international population research programme launched in 1972 to determine fertility levels throughout the world, and its successor, the Demographic and Health Survey Programme (DHS), have been particularly valuable in providing data for a range of countries, including many lacking adequate vital registration systems. Other approaches to data capture include multi-round surveys, in which respondents are asked about events since last contact, and dual-record systems which involve two independent data collection systems (one often a multi-round survey), the results of which are then combined. This method allows some estimation of missed events to be made, but is expensive. These approaches are described in more detail in most demographic textbooks (Preston *et al.* 2001; Rowland 2003; Siegel & Swanson 2004).

The raw materials of demography relate to individuals' most personal experiences—sexual activity, family formation, birth control, reproduction, marital breakdown, illness, and death. All of these occur in a social framework which attaches value to some of these behaviours and stigmatizes others. Not surprisingly, respondents in censuses and surveys may be reluctant to disclose non-marital pregnancies, illegal abortions, illegal migration, or deaths of relatives from AIDS. Concealment has also been the policy of some national governments which have treated demographic data as official secrets.

As well as allowing for these personal and political factors, the enormous potential complications arising from people's uncertainties about age or other 'basic' characteristics; uncertain recollections of prior events, and the vast scope for administrative errors of various kinds have to be considered. In this context the demographer's traditional obsession with data quality becomes understandable. Real current questions turn on such issues. In the United States, for example, death rates for African-Americans are higher than those for whites until the age of 75 or so when they appear to 'cross-over'. This has been interpreted as an effect of selective survival. As the health challenges faced by African-Americans are greater on average than those faced by whites, it is argued that only the most robust African-Americans survive to old

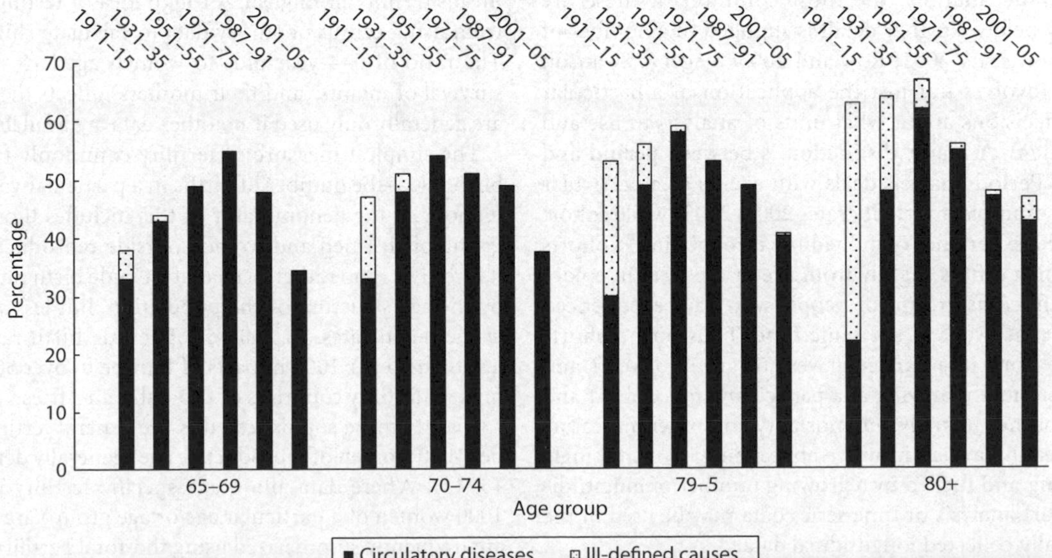

Fig. 7.2.4 Percentage of all deaths due to circulatory diseases and ill-defined causes, age groups 65–69 to 80+, England and Wales, 1911–1915 to 2001–2005.
Data Source: OPCS/ONS Mortality Statistics, various years.

age and so their mortality thereafter is lower than that of whites. However, detailed investigation has shown that this 'cross-over' is at least partly an artefactual result of differences between ethnic groups in the extent of age misreporting in censuses and on death certificates (Preston *et al.* 1996).

Differences in perceptions and reporting of health status are also problematic. The 1991 UK censuses for example, included a question which asked whether a person had 'any long-term illness, health problem or handicap which limits his/her daily activities or the work he/she can do'. The same question was repeated in 2001, except that the term 'disability' was substituted for handicap. In 2001 the proportions reporting limiting long-term illness were considerably higher than in 1991; it is unclear to what extent this reflects the slight change in the question, the inclusion of an additional question about self-rated health in 2001 which may have prompted people to think more about health status, or a real change in prevalence. Similar problems have bedevilled attempts to make international comparisons of health status as, even if questions are harmonized, it is clear that the ways people respond to them are not (Robine & Jagger 2003).

The statistics produced in series like the *United Nations Demographic Yearbooks* have their origins in what is or has been *done* by millions of people, mediated by what is *said* about these events and experiences, further filtered by how this is *recorded*, processed, and analysed. Some assessment of data quality is given in the *United Nations Demographic Yearbooks*, but sometimes users may pay insufficient attention to this. Apart from this series, and a range of other UN publications, a number of other organizations produce international reference works and databases. These include the World Health Organization (WHO), the World Bank, the Organization for Economic Co-operation and Development (OECD), Eurostat, and The United States Census Bureau for International Research. In most cases the data available in these series are available on line and free of charge.

The analysis of demographic data

A standard array of techniques and measures forms the basis of much demographic analysis, the most common of these are described briefly below. Further detail is supplied in a number of textbooks (Preston *et al.* 2001; Rowland 2003; Siegel & Swanson 2004). Analysis involves not just the application of a particular technique, but decisions about what units of analysis to use and how to group them. A major distinction is between **period** and **cohort** analysis. Period analysis deals with events of a particular time period (for example, mortality rates 2000–2005) while cohort analyses follow the experience of individuals through time. Cohorts in this sense (which differs slightly from use of the term in epidemiology) are defined as groups of people who have experienced the same significant event at the same time. Thus birth cohorts comprise people born in a particular year or group of years and marriage cohorts those marrying at a particular time. Cohort and life-course approaches to analysing mortality and other indicators of population health have an intuitive appeal and are increasingly used, both fuelling and fuelled by a growing number of longitudinal studies. Cohort analysis of time series data may be used in the absence of specially collected longitudinal data.

Cohort and period are two of the dimensions which 'place' persons in time; the third is age. Duration effects (such as duration of marriage or length of exposure to a particular pathogen) may also be important. Models in which age, period, and cohort effects are considered separately have been used in mortality analyses, but less so in analyses of reproductive behaviour (Hobcraft *et al.* 1982). Cohort effects may be substantial and, unless allowed for, may mask relationships between age and various risks. Differences in the smoking behaviour of cohorts, for example, have a major effect on the relationships between age and smoking-related disease observed at different periods.

Other decisions about whether to use individuals, families, households, or geographic areas as units of analysis are often constrained by data availability. Until relatively recently most census data were only available as aggregate tabulations. The growing availability of microdata—individual level information—has greatly extended the scope of demographic analysis. Other innovations include the development of sample record linkage systems, such as the ONS Longitudinal Study in England and Wales (Fox & Goldblatt 1982). In these data sets individuals' census records are linked with their vital registration records so numerator denominator biases in, for example, the analysis of mortality are avoided. The recently established Scottish Longitudinal Study additionally includes linked information on hospital admissions. In Nordic countries the whole population has been assigned personal identification numbers facilitating linkage of information from a range of registers. Linkage to use of health and care services is also available in some countries, such as Finland.

These advances have greatly extended the material available for analyses of variations in demographic behaviour, and their consequences. They have also raised complex security and confidentiality issues fuelling debate over appropriate restrictions on access to data.

The measurement of fertility

Fertility means the childbearing performance of a woman, couple, or population. Generally only live births are included. The term fecundity, by contrast, is used to refer to the physiological capability of producing a live-born child. Confusingly in the Franco-phone world, the meaning of these terms is reversed so fécundité in French means fertility in English. A rough idea of fertility may be gained from using census or survey data to calculate child woman ratios: The ratio of 0–4-year-olds to women aged 15–49. However the survival of infants (and their mothers) affects these ratios, so they are generally only used if no other data are available.

The simplest measure of fertility commonly used is the crude birth rate—the number of births in a particular year per 1000 population. As the denominator of this includes those not 'at risk' of giving birth (men and women outside reproductive age groups), it is really a ratio rather than a rate. Crude birth rates are influenced by the age structure of the population, but less seriously so than crude death rates. In 2000–2005, crude birth rates ranged from less than 10 per 1000 in parts of Europe to over 50 per 1000 in the highest-fertility countries of sub-Saharan Africa.

Slightly more sophisticated is the general fertility ratio—births per 1000 women of reproductive age (generally defined as 15–49 or 15–44). Where data allow, age-specific fertility rates (births per 1000 women of a particular age or age group) are preferred. These are frequently summarized using the Total Fertility Rate. Where, as is usually the case, period data are used to calculate this, it indicates how many children women in a hypothetical cohort would have if they experienced current age-specific fertility rates throughout their reproductive life. This measure is sometimes explicitly denoted TPFR (total period fertility rate). In low-mortality populations a TFR of 2.1 is taken to indicate *replacement level* fertility as, under this regime, a cohort of women would be succeeded by a cohort of daughters of the same size (after some allowance for mortality and the fact that 105–106 boys are born for every 100 girls). Fertility levels in much of the developed world have been below this level for some 30 years. In 2005, TFRs were lowest in Eastern and Southern Europe and the richer countries of Southeast Asia, being 1.3 or lower in the Ukraine, Belarus, Bulgaria, Greece, Poland, Korea, Slovakia and Slovenia, the Czech Republic, and Italy, and between 1.3 and 1.5 in a large number of other countries including Germany, Italy, Russia, Japan, Spain, and Singapore. TFRs are highest in sub-Saharan Africa; in 2005 Niger, Mali, Liberia, and Uganda were among those with TFRs close to, or above, 7.

One difficulty with the TFR is that it is affected by changes in the 'tempo' rather than the 'quantum' of childbearing. If women start delaying their fertility but 'catch up' later, there will be a divergence between cohort and period measures, as the latter will be based partly on the behaviour of earlier cohorts whose timing of births was different. Similarly, if women have children earlier TFRs will rise, even if eventual family sizes remain unchanged. For this reason, many statistical offices use cohort, rather than period, measures of fertility as the basis for projections. Although apparently a technical matter, considerable controversy surrounds this issue, particularly in France where it has inspired front-page articles in *Le Monde* and acrimonious resignations of demographers. This reflects a longstanding French pro-nationalist tradition and concern about low fertility. In this context it is vital to know whether recent trends in fertility, as measured by TFRs, are partly an artefactual result of changes in the timing of births or whether they really indicate a change in final family size.

More sophisticated measures of fertility include parity progression ratios. These indicate the probability of proceeding from one birth to another (for example, what proportion of mothers with two children progress to having a third). Parity progression ratios are normally calculated for cohorts who have completed, or nearly completed, their childbearing but it is also possible to use data on births by birth order to derive period progression ratios (Bongaarts & Feeny 1998).

Marriage patterns may have a major influence on fertility and in the past demographers often preferred to calculate age-specific **marital** fertility rates (and TFRs and other measures) on the grounds that the unmarried population is not 'at risk' (or at reduced risk) of childbearing. Changes in marital fertility indicative of deliberate attempts to limit family size are regarded as one of the defining features of the fertility 'transition' (see below) and so distinguishing these from changes due to variations in the 'at risk' (married population) has been particularly emphasized. However, rises in non-marital childbearing mean that restricting analyses to marital fertility is generally no longer appropriate.

Reproduction rates

In the long term, populations grow if mothers replace themselves with one or more (surviving) daughters and decline if they fail to achieve this. Theoretically, it would also be possible to measure the replacement of fathers by sons, but in practice the difficulties involved in obtaining paternity data make this infeasible. Reproduction rates thus relate only to female fertility, i.e. births of daughters. The gross reproduction rate (GRR) is derived in the same way as the TFR except that age-specific birth rates based only on births of daughters are used in the calculation. The net reproduction rate (NRR) makes an allowance for mortality; specifically the chance that a daughter will survive to the age her mother was when she was born. The NRR cannot be calculated unless both age-specific fertility and mortality data are available (although it can be approximated using the GRR and appropriate life table survival data). Changes in either fertility or mortality (or both) will mean a divergence between period measures (based on the experience of a hypothetical cohort) and the experiences of real cohorts.

Summary information on measures of fertility and reproduction are summarized in Boxes 7.2.2 and 7.2.3.

The measurement of mortality

As for fertility, the simplest measure of mortality is the crude mortality rate, deaths per 1000 population. This is strongly influenced by age structure. Although life expectancy at birth in the more developed regions of the world in 2000–2005 was some 12 years longer than in less developed regions (76 and 64 years, respectively), crude death rates—deaths per 1000 population of all ages—were in fact higher in the more developed regions (10.2 compared with 8.4 in less developed regions) (United Nations (UN) 2007). Age- (and sex-) specific rates, or measures based on them, are therefore much to be preferred if data are available to calculate them. Both direct and indirect standardization are sometimes used to make comparisons between populations with different age and sex structures.

Standardized mortality ratios (SMRs) are calculated using indirect standardization. This involves selecting a set of 'standard' age-specific mortality rates, for example those for a national population, and applying these to the numbers of people in the relevant

Box 7.2.3 Reproduction ratios

Measures

Gross reproduction rate (GRR): The sum of the age-specific female fertility rates (births of daughters), for all reproductive age groups for a particular period (usually a year) conventionally expressed per woman. The GRR indicates how many daughters a woman would have if, throughout her reproductive life, she had children at the age-specific rates prevalent in the specified year of period. The GRR can be calculated either by summing female age specific fertility rates, (relating to births of daughters rather than all births) or using the formula

$$GRR = TFR \times \text{Proportion of female births}$$

The proportion of female births can be taken as 0.488 (100/205) in the absence of more detailed information.

Net reproduction rate (NRR): The average number of daughters that would be borne, according to specified rates of mortality and of bearing daughters, by a woman subject through life to these rates. The NRR employs the same fertility data as the GRR, but also takes into account the effects of mortality. An NRR of 1 indicates that a population's fertility and mortality levels would result in exact replacement of mothers by daughters.

age groups in the sub-population of interest—for example, the population of a particular region. This yields an 'expected' number of deaths—the number of deaths there would be in the sub-population if age-specific death rates were the same as those in the standard population. The ratio of observed to expected deaths, conventionally multiplied by 100, gives the SMR. Thus an SMR of 124 indicates that mortality in the sub population is 24 per cent higher than in the standard population, allowing for age differences. SMRs are useful summary measures of differences in mortality, but give no indication of the *level* of mortality.

Age-specific death rates are calculated using the numbers of deaths at age x (or between ages x and $x + n$) in a particular year as the numerator and the mid-year population of the same age as the denominator. The rate is conventionally expressed per 1000 or per 100 000 population. The mid-year population is used as a measure of the average population at risk on the assumption that deaths are evenly distributed throughout the year. For some age groups, notably infants, this assumption is invalid. In low-mortality populations deaths in the first three days of life may account for half or more of all deaths in the first year of life. Moreover, information on the size of population aged less than 1 normally comes from birth data (since in 9 out of 10 years relevant census data will not be available). For these reasons live births in a particular year are conventionally used as the denominator of the infant mortality rate while deaths to infants aged less than 1 constitute the numerator. Some infants dying in a given year will have been born in the previous year and some born in the year in question will die the following year. This can cause distortions if there are large annual fluctuations in numbers of births (or infant deaths) and often 3-year averages are preferred. Deaths at very old ages are also not evenly distributed throughout the year and an adjustment is normally made to allow for this.

Infant mortality rates (IMRs) were very high in some parts of historical Europe (300 or even 400 deaths per 1000 live births in regions of Russia and Germany at the end of the nineteenth century) (van de Walle 1986). In England and Wales, where declines in infant mortality came late in relation to declines in other age groups, the infant mortality rate at the start of the twentieth century stood at some 140 infant deaths per 1000 live births. Infant mortality in high-income countries is now extremely low—fewer than five infant deaths per 1000 live births in many European countries and in Singapore. There have also been huge falls in infant mortality in many poorer countries; in 2005 China and India had IMRs of 23 and 56, respectively (WHO 2007). Rates remain high in some of the very poorest countries: Over 150 deaths per 1000 live births in parts of sub-Saharan Africa.

Variations on this scale have substantial demographic impacts. Infant mortality has also attracted particular interest because of links with fertility behaviour and as an indicator of public health conditions. Particularly in this latter context, perinatal, early and late neo-natal, and post neo-natal mortality rates are often distinguished where data allow (see Box 7.2.4).

Box 7.2.4 Mortality measures

Measures

Crude death rate: The ratio of deaths in a year (other specified period) to average population in the same year/period (mid-year population), expressed per 1000

$$\text{CDR} = \frac{\text{number of deaths}}{\text{mid-year population}} \times 1000$$

Age specific mortality rate (ASMR): number of deaths to persons aged x (or x to $x + n$) per 1000 persons aged x (or to $x + n$)

$$\text{ASMR} = \frac{\text{deaths to persons aged } x}{\text{mid-year population of persons aged } x} \times 1000$$

Standardized mortality ratio (SMR): the ratio (× 100) of observed to expected deaths in a study population. Expected deaths are calculated by applying a set of standard age-specific mortality rates to the age distribution of the study population. Standardized ratios are only useful for comparisons. They have no intrinsic meaning.

$$\text{SMR} = 100 \times \frac{\Sigma r_i}{\Sigma n_i\, p_i} = \frac{\text{observed}}{\text{expected}}$$

Infant mortality rate (IMR):

$$\frac{\text{number of deaths to infants ages} < 1 \text{ year in year}}{\text{number of live births in year } x} \times 1000$$

sometimes decomposed into *neonatal mortality rates* (deaths of live born infants during the first 4 weeks) and *post-neonatal* mortality (from 4 to 52 weeks)

The *perinatal mortality rate* measures late foetal deaths (stillbirths) and early neonatal deaths relative to live births.

$$\text{Perinatal mortality rate} = \frac{\text{stillbirths} + \text{deaths under 1 week}}{\text{stillbirths} + \text{live births}} \times 1000$$

Stillbirths used to refer to deaths of foetuses of 28 or more weeks' gestation, however an earlier threshold of 24 weeks is now more generally used.

Life tables

Life table analysis is a core demographic technique and life tables provide one of the most powerful tools for analysing mortality and other non-renewable processes.

Life tables show the probability of dying (and surviving) between specified ages. They also allow the calculation of various other indicators, including expectation of life. If complete data on the mortality of a birth cohort are available, then a cohort life table may be constructed. However, the use of cohort life tables is obviously only possible retrospectively. More commonly period life tables, based on mortality rates at a particular time, are calculated. These life tables show death (and survival) probabilities for a hypothetical cohort with an arbitrary radix (number of babies at the beginning) usually set to 10 000, 100 000, or some other multiple of 100.

Specific notation, summarized in Box 7.2.5, is used in life table analysis. The basis of the table is a set of probabilities of dying—${}_nq_x$—which are calculated from age-specific death rates. x here refers

Box 7.2.5 Life table measures and notation

x	=	age attained last birthday
l_x	=	number of survivors at age x, so l_{65} is the number of persons alive at age 65 in the hypothetical life table population
l_0	=	the radix of the life table (hypothetical number of babies), usually 100 000
$_nq_x$	=	probability of dying between age x and $x+n$, so $_4q_1$ is the probability of dying between age 1 and 5 for a person aged 1
$_np_x$	=	probability of surviving between ages x and $x+n$, so $_{20}p_{65}$ is the probability of surviving from age 65 to age 85 for a person aged 65
$_nd_x$	=	number of deaths between age x and $x+n$
$_nL_x$	=	number of person years lived between x and $x+n$
Tx	=	total number of person years lived after age x
e^0_{0x}	=	expectation of life at age x, so e^0_0 is expectation of life at birth

to age at the start of an interval whose length is specified by n. Thus $_5q_{50}$ refers to the probability of someone alive at 50 dying between age 50 and age 55. The complement of $_nq_x$—the probability of surviving is denoted $_np_x$. The (hypothetical) number of survivors at each age is given by l_x; thus l_0 equals the radix (of 100 000) and l_{75} the number of survivors at age 75. The number of person years lived in an interval ($_nL_x$) and the total number of person years lived after a particular age (T_x) are often not shown in published tables but are steps on the way to the calculation of e_x—life expectancy at age x.

This measure provides an indicator of mortality which is very largely independent of the age structure of the population. This makes it more useful than either a standardized mortality ratio (which gives no indication of level) or a crude death rate (which is strongly influenced by age structure). Life expectancy either at birth (e_0) or further life expectancy at a particular age, say 65 (e_{65}), is calculated by dividing total person-years lived after age 0 or 65 (T_0 or T_{65}) and dividing it by the number of survivors aged 0 (l_0) or 65 (l_{65}).

Values of life expectancy at birth are sometimes (mis)interpreted as indicators of usual age at death in a particular population. In very low mortality populations where most deaths occur within a relatively small range of ages (see the example of Japan in Fig. 7.2.1), there will be a close correspondence between median and modal ages of death and life expectancy at birth (which is a mean value). However in populations such as Malawi where so many deaths occur in infancy, there will be a wide divergence. There is sometimes confusion too about the interpretation of values of further life expectancy at a particular age. This is derived from information about the probabilities of death and survival at *subsequent* ages, and so is not influenced by deaths at earlier ages and it is erroneous to think that, for example, the further life expectancy of someone aged 65 will equal life expectancy at birth minus 65. The divergence will be greatest in populations with high mortality rates at young ages. In 2000–2002, for life example, female life expectancy at birth in the United States was 80.4 years but the further life expectancy of women aged 65 was 19.2 years. The equivalent figures in 1900–1901 were 49 and 12 years.

Model life tables

Patterns of age-specific death rates show similarities whatever the level of mortality. Death rates tend to be higher in infancy than later childhood and rise with age from around the age of puberty, although in the oldest age groups rates of increase tend to flatten out. Because of the tendency for death rates at one age to be associated with death rates at other ages in a given population, it is possible to derive hypothetical schedules, called **model life tables**, describing variations in mortality by age and sex, normally in terms of a limited number of parameters which allow for particular features of the mortality pattern of the population considered. Model life tables are derived from empirical data from countries where these are available. They are extremely useful aids for the estimation of mortality by age in populations with defective data. They are also used (in conjunction with fertility data) to show the outcomes of particular fertility and mortality regimes on, for example, population age structure. All demography texts give further details of their derivation and application.

Other applications of life table analysis

Life tables are widely used to analyse probabilities associated with events other than death, such as risks of divorce or contraceptive use failure rates and discontinuation rates and in estimates of disability-free or healthy life expectancy. Many chronic conditions associated with ageing, such as musculoskeletal and sensory impairments, may have serious implications for health status but are not directly life-threatening. Life table methods are used to decompose total life expectancy into 'healthy' and 'unhealthy' or 'disabled' components. This can be done using cross-sectional data on morbidity prevalence in conjunction with mortality data, although this has some limitations. More sophisticated (and data demanding) multi-state approaches which allow transitions both to and from disabled states have also been pursued (Manton *et al.* 2006). Despite these technical advances, there is still controversy about *trends* in indicators of the health status of populations, including disability. To a large extent this debate arises from measurement problems and the difficulties involved in making comparisons between health indicators derived in different ways, a further reminder of the importance of data quality and measurement.

Multiple decrement life tables allow 'decrements' from more than one event—for example different causes of death. Cause elimination life tables are also used to identify the 'pure' severity of a particular cause of death. Multi-state models allow analysis of a range of transitions, particularly those where re-entries into a particular state, such as being married or living in a certain region, are possible. These more sophisticated applications of course require more detailed data.

The measurement of migration

In many countries, migration is the predominant influence on the spatial distribution of the population. In Asia and Latin America recent rural to urban migration has resulted in the phenomenal growth of cities, often lacking the infrastructure to meet the needs of the expanding population for basic services such as sanitation and power. In 2005 half (49 per cent) of the world's population lived in urban areas compared with 29 per cent in 1950 (UN 2006a).

Measuring migration represents particular difficulties. The classical definition of internal migration is a permanent or semi-permanent move across an administrative boundary. Use of this definition means that the extent of migration recorded depends partly on the size of administrative areas. In a country divided into many small areas a move over 5 km will count as migration, while in countries divided into fewer larger ones a move over 50 km may not. This means that international comparison of internal migration rates is potentially misleading. Even the distinction between international (between country) and internal (within country) migration may be problematic if boundaries are contested or changing. The temporal dimension to migration presents further difficulties; what constitutes permanent or semi-permanent migration and how should groups such as seasonal migrants be treated?

The reason for defining migration as a move over a boundary is largely pragmatic. Often only moves of this kind are recorded; moreover this is the information required by local administrations. For research purposes, analyses of *all* moves (preferably with an indication of distance moved) may often be preferred. Some countries have registration systems in which changes of address are recorded (with varying completeness and immediacy). More commonly censuses are used to find out about migration. Questions on usual address 1 or 5 years ago allow the proportion of **movers** in the population to be measured (except for those aged less than one or five). These data also allow gross flows—inflows *and* outflows—between pairs of areas to be measured. **Moves**, as opposed to **movers**, are not directly measured as someone moving several times in the reference period cannot be distinguished from someone moving only once. Those leaving an address and later returning to it cannot be identified either. This means that the length of the reference period used is important; the proportion of movers in the 5 years preceding a census will **not** equal five times the proportion moving in 1 year before the same census.

In the absence of direct census data, estimates of migration can be made indirectly using the 'balancing equation' referred to below. Differences in the size of a population at two points in time not accounted for by natural increase or depletion must be due to migration (or data errors). If vital registration data are available, then both births and deaths can be taken into account. If they are lacking, then the survival of groups enumerated in the first of a pair of censuses must be estimated from a life table and the number of expected survivors compared with the number enumerated in the second census (obviously ageing must be allowed for, so the number of 20–29-year-olds in the first census will be compared with 30–39-year-olds 10 years later). These methods only allow estimation of **net** migration (balance between in-migration and out-migration). Their major weakness lies in the fact that the residual population balance assumed to be due to migration may in fact reflect differences in the quality of the two censuses considered or errors in the estimates of survival used.

Survey data are also used to measure migration and potentially provide illuminating information on the reasons for, and consequences of, migration. However, as migration over long distances is a relatively rare event, even large samples may yield relatively few migrants. A similar problem besets samples of international travellers, such as the UK International Passenger Survey, designed to estimate flows of international migrants through port or border surveys. Tourists and business travellers comprise the vast bulk of people entering or leaving so surveys are an inefficient way of identifying immigrants and emigrants. Unfortunately, other data are often lacking as legal and administrative record systems are frequently concerned with citizenship and right of abode rather than international migration *per se* (and virtually never with emigration).

International migration is also difficult to deal with because it is affected by policies and events outside the country and is often a sensitive political issue. Patterns may vary hugely, witness recent mass movements of refugees and other groups of international migrants. Within the larger countries of Europe, Switzerland has the highest proportion of 'foreign' residents—24 per cent in 2006—and 60 per cent of Swiss population growth in the past 20 years has been due to net immigration. In an interesting reversal of historic patterns, in 2005 Ireland and Spain were the European countries with the highest levels of net immigration, both with rates at over 10 per 1000 population (OECD 2006). In many other Western European countries, particularly Germany and the UK, rates of immigration increased during the 1980s and 1990s and, as in Switzerland, have contributed to population growth (Coleman & Rowthorn 2004).

Population dynamics

Any population comprises those who have made an entry and not yet exited. When whole populations of defined geographic areas are considered, the only means of entry are birth or immigration and the only means of exit death or emigration.

The most basic method of demographic analysis is the decomposition of overall population change ($P_t - P_0$) into its components (B, D, I, E):

$$P_t - P_0 = B - D + I - E$$

where P_t = population at an end of period; P_0 = population at the beginning of a period; and B, D, I, E represent respectively births, deaths, immigrations, and emigrations during the same period (I–E is referred to as net migration). Population subgroups may be similarly defined in terms of entries and exits. Entry to the population aged 75–84 is through ageing (passage from 74 to 75); exit is through further ageing (84 to 85) or death. This simple accounting equation is an important one, both methodologically and as a formal reminder of the need to consider *past* as well as current events.

Of the three demographic determinants of population size, structure and growth, fertility is nearly always of much greater importance than either mortality or migration. Every birth represents not just an addition to the current generation of children, but also potentially an exponentially increasing augmentation in the size of future generations. Death carries no such promise of future return. The third determinant—migration—is generally not of significant magnitude to have a major impact on national populations, although there are exceptions and at the sub-national level migration may have a large effect.

For social and biological reasons fertility, mortality, and migration have interactive effects. Decreases in mortality among those with reproductive potential, for example, influence not just the size of the age group affected at the time, but also the size of succeeding generations.

Declines in male mortality, particularly in populations where large age differences between spouses are common and remarriage of widows is rare, will similarly tend to increase fertility by effectively increasing the proportion of women of reproductive age who are still married. Conversely, reductions in fertility clearly reduce the risk of maternal mortality and may have further positive effects on the survival of mothers, infants, or both. Age at motherhood also influences rates of population growth. The average age of mothers at the birth of their daughters is termed the mean length of a generation and is generally around 29 years. A shorter interval will mean more rapid generational succession (and faster population growth); a longer one will have the opposite effect.

Migration has an effect on both the other demographic parameters because migrants differ from the general population. International migrants are generally young and in good health and often may move from relatively high fertility populations to low fertility populations. As a result immigrants may serve to (temporarily) 'rejuvenate' the host population and, at least initially, have higher fertility and lower mortality. In England and Wales, for example, 22 per cent of births in 2006 were born to mothers themselves born outside the UK. Despite the disadvantages they often face, mortality of immigrant groups is generally lower than that of host populations because of the differential selection of immigrants. The degree of selection tends to vary according to difficulties and distance to be overcome in making an international move. For all these reasons the demographic characteristics of population sub-groups largely comprising immigrants and their immediate descendants may vary substantially from those of the population as a whole. In the United Kingdom in 2001–2002, for example, 38 per cent of the population of Bangladeshi origin was aged under 16 compared with 20 per cent of the population as a whole, reflecting both the relatively high fertility of Bangladeshi born women in the UK and the fact that most migration from Bangladesh has been in the period since 1975.

Population projections

Population projections represent one of the most widely used outputs of demographic analysis. Strictly speaking a projection simply represents the outcome of applying various assumptions about future fertility, mortality, and migration and so differs from a **forecast**, which implies prediction. However, projections are often treated as forecasts and the degree of uncertainty inherent in them is not always sufficiently recognized, although the production of probabilistic forecasts makes this more explicit (Lutz *et al.* 1998). The most common method of projection is the component method, based on the balancing equation ($P_t = P_0 + B - D + I - E$). Assumptions are made about the three components of change—births, deaths and migration—and applied to age and sex groups within the initial population to give a projection of future size and structure. To a large extent assumptions are based on recent trends together with other information on, for example, survey data on fertility intentions or (sometimes) models of change in particular causes of death. Forecasting fertility is generally regarded as the most problematic area of projection; projections of the future population size of the United Kingdom varied widely during the 1955–1974 period when birth rates first rose and then fell. Recently greater attention has been paid to the errors that have been made in forecasting mortality in developed countries. This has little effect on age groups in which survival is high, but can have quite substantial impacts on forecasts of the number of elderly people. At the sub-national level migration is an important, and sometimes quite volatile, element which is hard to predict, especially by those in central statistical offices lacking local knowledge.

Population growth

Changes in the size of a population produced by the surplus (or deficit) of births over deaths are termed natural increase (or decrease). A common indicator of growth is the crude rate of natural increase–the difference between the crude birth rate (annual births per 1000 population) and the crude death rate (annual deaths per 1000 population). If net migration is zero, this will be the same as the growth rate of the population—the overall annual change in the population divided by the population size—(conventionally expressed as a percentage). In several European countries, including Germany, Greece, Poland, Portugal, and the Russian Federation, deaths now outnumber births. In others births still outnumber deaths even though fertility rates have been below the level required for *long-term* replacement for 30 years or more. This apparent paradox largely reflects the fact that the number of births is a function of the number of potential mothers, as well as of their fertility patterns. If the former is increasing, so too may the numbers of births, even if women have fewer children each.

The young age structures of many populations in the developing world mean that these populations have a huge built-in potential for growth. Population *momentum* is the measure which gives the ratio of the ultimate size a given population would achieve to current population size if fertility were to immediately fall to replacement level. Even allowing for the devastating effect of HIV/AIDs-related mortality, the population of sub-Saharan Africa is expected to increase from 0.7 billion to 1.7 billion between 2005 and 2050 (UN 2007), a consequence of both population momentum and high levels of fertility. In some low fertility countries there are now concerns about 'negative momentum'—the prospect of decline in population even if fertility rates increase somewhat—because of successively smaller cohorts of women in childbearing age groups.

Intrinsic rate of natural increase: Stable population theory

Early in the twentieth century Lotka (1907) demonstrated mathematically that a population closed to migration and subject to unchanging age-specific fertility and mortality rates for a long period would eventually have a fixed age structure (in which the proportion in each age group remained unchanged) and would grow at a constant rate. This type of population is called a *stable* population. The fixed age structure of a stable population is independent of the initial age structure—two very different populations subject to the same unchanging rates for a long period would eventually assume the same structure. A particular variant of a stable population is a *stationary* population—one in which birth and death rates are constant and in balance and so population growth is zero. The *Lx* column of the life table is an example of a stationary population. The number of births is fixed (the radix) and the age distribution is also fixed. In non-stationary stable populations the age structure is also fixed but the size of every age group is growing at the same constant rate as the overall population and the number of births. This is called the *intrinsic rate of natural increase* and is a function of the Net Reproduction Rate and the mean length of a generation (approximated by the mean age of childbearing). Non-stationary stable populations can be calculated by adjusting the *Lx* values of a particular life table to allow for the intrinsic rate of growth. These are often published in conjunction with model life tables to show the effects of particular (unchanging) fertility and mortality regimes.

Although stable and stationary populations are theoretical constructs, real populations at various times have met the model requirements closely enough to allow stable population theory to be used to develop methods for indirectly estimating fertility and mortality in populations lacking adequate directly derived data. Stable population models are also widely used for insurance, pension, and personnel planning. One of the important results of the work of Lotka and his successors was to show theoretically that fertility is the predominant influence on age structure. This has also been demonstrated empirically.

Age structure

Population pyramids graphically illustrate the current structure of populations and in so doing, also provide insights into both the future and the past of the population. High fertility populations have a pyramid shape, with each successive cohort being larger than its predecessor. The population pyramid for Bangladesh (Fig. 7.2.5A) shows a typical pattern for a population with a history of high fertility but a recent downturn. Each successive cohort is larger than the preceding one, with the exception of the youngest. 'Old' populations, such as that of England and Wales (Fig. 7.2.5B), show a gradual tapering at the top. This shape is the result of sustained downward trends in fertility which reduce the proportion of children in more recently born cohorts in the population and so lead to a corresponding increase in the proportion of older people (survivors of larger cohorts). Bulges in population pyramids due to high numbers of births have 'echo' effects when members of large cohorts themselves have children. Thus the baby boom experienced in many populations in the post-World War II period (precise timing varies between countries) had an echo effect in the 1980s.

Historically, and apparently paradoxically, improvements in mortality in those European populations which now have high proportions of old people in fact served to *offset* the trend toward population ageing, as they chiefly benefited the young—and led to increases in the proportions surviving to have children themselves. However, although fertility has the greatest **potential** impact on age structure and population growth, in some circumstances mortality (or migration) may become a more important influence. Many populations in richer countries now have fertility at or below replacement level, life expectancies at birth close to 80 and near universal survival to the end of the (female) reproductive span. In these conditions, further improvements in mortality have the greatest impact at old ages and further population ageing occurs from the apex, rather than, or in addition to, the base of the population pyramid. Mortality changes are now the main motor of the further ageing of a number of populations with already old age structures. Table 7.2.2 shows life table survivorship based on period mortality data from England and Wales in the early 1970s and 2000s. The mortality rates of the latter period imply survival to age 85 for 40 per cent of women. Moreover, changes in survivorship between the two periods were greater at older ages than at younger, and mortality at young ages is now so low that there is little scope for demographically important further change.

Population age structures and associated rates of growth or decline, changes in age structures such as population ageing, and the speed and stage of age structural change all have important economic and health implications which have attracted considerable debate and controversy.

Many economists have pointed out that population growth has often provided a spur to human ingenuity and economic growth. Less positively, the countries which now have the youngest age structures and most rapid rates of population growth are already suffering from land degradation and in many cases constrained agricultural potential (Alexandratos 2005). Large and growing child populations also hamper efforts at improving human capital through education or improved health (Ahlburg 1994).

Reduced fertility initially produces a 'demographic dividend' or 'window' when the ratio of children to adults falls and those in prime productive ages, the survivors of larger birth cohorts, account for a higher proportion of the population. It has been argued that this dividend of lower child dependency and higher representation of adults in the prime working age groups played an important part in the rapid economic development of the 'East Asian Tigers', like the Republic of Korea and also China (Bloom *et al.* 2000). The next phase, involving high and increasing representation of older people may also bring some economic benefit in the form of

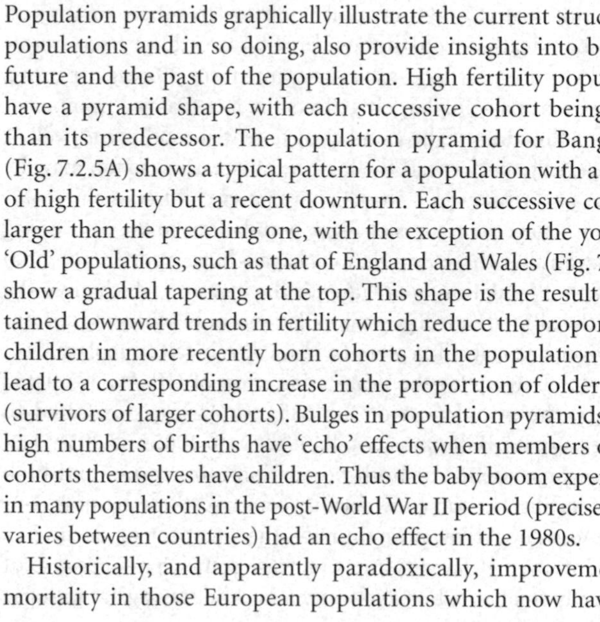

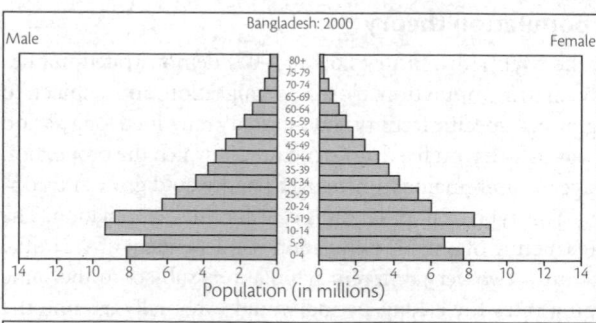

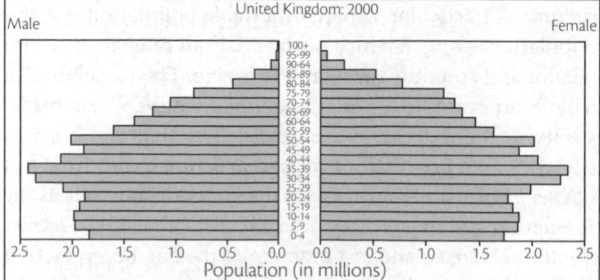

Fig. 7.2.5 Distribution of the population of (A) Bangladesh and (B) the UK by age and sex, 2000.
Source: US Census Bureau, International Data Base.

Table 7.2.2 Life table estimates of survivorship, England and Wales, 1970–72 and 2002–4

% Surviving at Age:	Males		Females	
	1970–72	2002–4	1970–72	2002–4
5	97.7	99.3	98.2	99.4
25	96.4	98.6	97.6	99.1
45	95.8	96.2	95.4	97.7
65	70.4	84.0	82.4	89.7
85	11.4	29.7	27.2	45.0

Data Source: OPCS/ONS Mortality Statistics, DHI No.24 (1992) and DHI No 37 (2007).

increased savings (by the large number of older people) and so greater capital available for investment (Mason & Lee 2006). However, population ageing is more often perceived as a challenge with potentially negative implications for both the economy and for population health (OECD 1999).

The major concerns arising from increases in the proportions of older people relate to effects on productivity and needs for support systems of various kinds, including pensions, healthcare, and long-term care. In OECD countries, healthcare expenditure is typically three to five times as high for those aged 65 and over as for those aged under 65, although there is considerable international variation in the proportion of GDP devoted to healthcare spending for older people which bears little obvious relationship to the proportion of older people in the population concerned.

In populations which have more recently moved to low fertility and low mortality regimes, the pace of demographic change has been much faster than occurred historically in Europe. The proportion of the Japanese population aged 65 or over doubled, from 7 per cent to over 14 per cent, between 1970 and 1995. In France a similar increase took 130 years to achieve. More recently, ageing populations have thus had a much shorter period in which to adapt to new public health priorities. The origins of these age structure changes lie in the demographic transition.

The demographic transition

Towards the end of the nineteenth century (earlier in France) birth and death rates started falling in a number of European countries. This is illustrated for England and Wales in Fig. 7.2.6, which shows long-term trends in fertility (TFR). Between 1871–1875 and 1911–1915 the TFR dropped from 4.8 to 2.8; by the early 1930s it was below replacement level, a development which was viewed with alarm and led to the first Royal Commission on Population. Although modern methods of contraception were lacking, it was clear that this huge drop in fertility was the result of the deliberate limitation of family size. Half of couples married in the 1870s had six or more children compared with 12 per cent of couples married in 1911–1915 (Coleman & Salt 1992). Expectation of life at birth, meanwhile, increased by some 15 years between the end of the nineteenth century and the early 1930s.

Scholars attempting to understand these profound changes sought to relate changes in demographic regimes to changes in the economic and social environment and so originated the theory of the demographic transition. The 'classical' view propounded by Notestein (1945) and others was that in 'traditional' societies fertility and mortality are both high and roughly in balance. Change is driven by economic advance which results in lower mortality. Fertility initially remains high, resulting in a rapid period of population growth. After this lag, however, fertility also falls in response to falling mortality and the erosion of 'traditional' pro-natalist values.

This classical view has since been considerably modified. The work of Coale and his collaborators in an ambitious project to track the transition in historical Europe suggested that no economic 'threshold' for fertility decline could be identified and that the pattern of decline seemed to follow regional groupings, suggesting a cultural rather than a socio-economic dimension (Coale & Watkins 1986). Falls in infant mortality, assumed to be a particularly important stimulus to fertility decline, sometimes followed rather than preceded changes in fertility. Indeed, Woods *et al.* (1989), on the basis of data from England and Wales, argued that declines in fertility led to reductions in infant mortality, rather than *vice versa*.

In short, the role of mortality decline as a trigger and the dominance of economic change have both been questioned (Cleland & Wilson 1987). Caldwell (1982) additionally argued that in non-European countries, it was not so much socio-economic modernization but 'Westernization' involving increased emphasis on the nuclear family and a change in inter-generational wealth flows (resulting in the costs of children coming to outweigh their potential benefits) that was the important trigger of fertility transition.

The huge amount of research on the historical demographic transition in Europe may seem of limited relevance to contemporary problems. However, much of the fuel for this research and debate came from post-War fears about population growth.

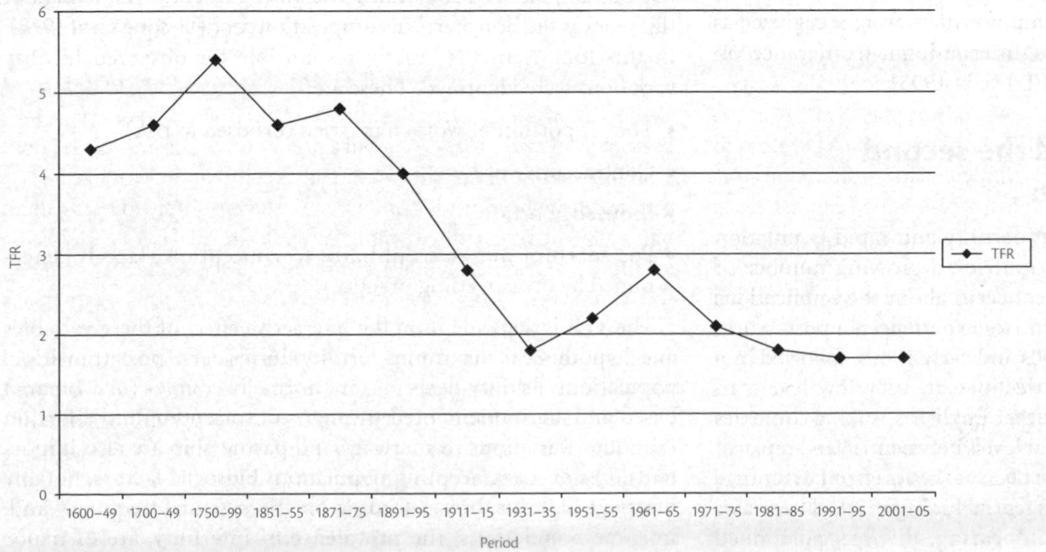

Fig. 7.2.6 Long-term trends in fertility (total fertility rate) England/England & Wales.
Data Sources: Wrigley and Schofield 1981; ONS Birth Statistics Series FM1, various years.

By 1950 significant mortality declines had been achieved or initiated throughout the world. In China, for example, expectation of life at birth increased from 43 in 1960 to over 70 by 2000. Even in sub-Saharan Africa where mortality remains unacceptably high, a gain (sadly since reversed) of nearly 10 years—from 43 to 52—was achieved between 1950 and 1990 (World Bank 1993; UN 2007). In this context it seemed imperative to discover the causes of fertility decline and use this knowledge to accelerate fertility 'adjustment' to falling mortality. Was 'development the best contraceptive' as concluded at the stormy 1974 World Population Conference, could change be achieved through intensive family planning programmes, as the Taiwanese experience seemed to suggest, or was some combination of these and other factors the key to fertility transition? Studies of societies in which the fertility transition had occurred seemed to offer the best prospect of an answer to these questions. While simple answers to complex questions are rarely forthcoming, Coale (1973) identified three factors which he considered a prerequisite for fertility decline in contemporary populations. These were: That potential parents must think it acceptable to balance the advantages and disadvantages of another child; that some advantage must be gained from reduced fertility, and that effective techniques of fertility control must be available.

It is now clear that substantial fertility declines have occurred in a number of countries with only a limited amount of development, such as Sri Lanka, Thailand, China, and more recently Bangladesh. In 1981, for example, Sri Lanka, with a per *capita* GNP of US$500, had a TFR of 2.5 (which by 2005 had fallen to 2) (World Bank 1993; UN 2007). There does nevertheless seem to be some relationship between development and fertility decline, although cultural and policy-related factors may modify this (Bryant 2007). Common factors identified in poor rural populations where fertility has fallen significantly since 1950 are well-established education systems, improvements in healthcare, some form of extra familial welfare, well-organized local government and an organized family planning programme. Potential benefits of investing more resources in fewer children, as a consequence of increasing opportunities in urban or industrial livelihoods also seem to have been important (Bryant 2007; McNicoll 2006). The education of women has been identified as a particularly important influence on both falling fertility and improved infant survival (Cleland 1990; Hobcraft 1993), and female education and empowerment were recognized as key policy objectives at the 1994 International Conference on Population and Development (ICPD) (UN 1995).

Lowest low fertility and the second demographic transition

In contrast to this scenario of high fertility and rapid population growth in some of the poorest countries, a growing number of high-income countries now have concerns about the implications of low fertility. Many of these countries experienced a post-World War II 'baby boom' during the 1950s and early 1960s, followed by a 1970s 'baby bust' when fertility declined to very low levels. In Scandinavia, France, the UK, and other English-speaking countries fertility rates have since fluctuated at levels between 1.6 and replacement level. These populations have been at the forefront of a range of family-related behavioural changes, including marked increases in cohabitation, non-marital childbearing, divorce, postponed childbearing, and increased levels of childlessness, described by some as a 'Second Demographic Transition' (van da Kaa 1987; Lesthaeghe & Niedert 2006). Such behaviours, which have become more usual among Northern European cohorts born from around the 1950s onwards, are much less prominent in Southern Europe and Southeast Asia where fertility is still very largely marital. However, it is these latter countries which now have 'lowest low' fertility—rates below 1.5—in part because marriage rates have fallen precipitously (Billari & Kohler 2004). Japan, for example, has been transformed from a society with near universal marriage in the early and mid-twentieth century to one in which a fifth of the population will remain unmarried at age 45 (Retherford *et al.* 2001). In this case the erosion of arranged marriages after World War II has played a part; changing gender roles may also be important. For a young Japanese woman with a good job of her own, the prospect of marriage to the traditional 'salaryman' who returns home late at night and contributes little to domestic or family life, may not be an attractive proposition.

The proximate determinants of fertility

One of the contributions of research into the fertility transition has been improved understanding of biosocial influences on reproduction. A huge range of social, economic, cultural, and psychological factors may influence decisions about family building strategies and family size. However, literacy rates and measures of *per capita* GNP do not beget or bear children and none of these variables can have the slightest effect unless translated into patterns of behaviour or physiological characteristics that influence the risks of conception or delivery.

Conversely, other patterns of behaviour with potentially important influences on fertility may be adopted with little or no thought to these consequences. In short social, economic, and other factors which influence fertility can only do so through the proximate determinants—the biological and behavioural factors which have a direct influence. Davis and Blake (1956), in a classic paper, distinguished a series of 'intermediate fertility variables'; factors influencing the chance of exposure to risk of pregnancy (marriage and coital frequency); factors influencing risk of pregnancy (such as contraception); and factors influencing pregnancy outcome (spontaneous and induced abortion). The most influential refinement of this work is the Bongaarts decomposition model (Bongaarts 1978). In this four elements chiefly responsible for observed fertility variations were identified. These are:

- The proportion of women married (exposed to risk)
- Contraceptive use
- Induced abortion
- Post-partum non-susceptibility to conception (largely determined by breastfeeding practice)

The TFR is dependent on the interactive effect of these variables and hypothetical maximum fertility. In modern 'post-transition' populations, fertility decisions are normally couple- (or woman-) based and are implemented through contraception and abortion (although variations in marriage and partnership are also important). In non-contracepting populations biosocial factors, notably marriage patterns, breast-feeding practices, sexual frequency and, in some populations, the prevalence of infertility, are of major importance.

Entry into marriage, or more generally any sexual union, marks entry to what has been termed the social reproductive span which nearly always comes later, often much later, than menarche and is terminated by the end of marriage. Fecundity—the potential for bearing children—decreases after the third decade, more sharply after the age of 35. In most non-contracepting populations, the average age at last birth is around 40, several years earlier than average age at menopause. Social factors, as well as biological ones, are important influences. Sexual activity may cease before menopause as a result of widowhood or separation. In some African populations continued childbearing after becoming a grandmother is disapproved of, leading to 'terminal abstinence'.

For those within the effective reproductive span—biologically capable of childbearing and in a sexual union—overall fertility is largely a function of length of intervals between births, itself largely determined by breastfeeding patterns. Among non-breastfeeding women, average duration of post-partum amenorrhea is only 1.5 to 2 months, compared with 18 months or more in rural Bangladesh where breastfeeding is protracted. In some populations, sexual activity is proscribed for breastfeeding mothers and so the period of post-partum infecundability extends beyond the period of amenorrhea.

Longer birth intervals and increased breastfeeding also have positive effects on infant and child health. Overall child mortality (deaths before the age of 5) might be reduced by as much as 30 per cent in some countries if closely spaced births were delayed (World Bank 1993; Cleland *et al.* 2006).

The epidemiological transition

Transitions from relatively high to low mortality regimes have in all populations been associated with transformations in the age, cause, and sex structure of death. Omran (1971) coined the phrase 'epidemiological transition' to describe this process. Changes in the response of societies to health and disease processes also need consideration. The term 'health transition' has been proposed as one which embraces both these phenomena.

Substantial falls in death rates from infectious and parasitic diseases; bronchitis, influenza and pneumonia; diarrhoeal diseases, and maternal mortality are all the hallmarks of the epidemiological transition. In England and Wales over half the gain in life expectancy at birth between 1871 and 1911 was due to reduced infectious disease mortality. Some 20 per cent of the total gain was due to falls in death rates from respiratory tuberculosis (Casselli 1991). The decline in these causes of death from which the young benefited more than the old meant that deaths at older ages accounted for a larger share of all deaths; the epidemiological transition in all countries which have experienced it has also been associated with larger falls in mortality among women than among men. Changes in the intra-household allocation of resources, declines in causes of death specifically or primarily affecting women (such as maternal mortality and respiratory tuberculosis), gender differences in health-related behaviour and in exposure to occupational hazards, and the possibly greater susceptibility of men to stresses associated with socio-economic changes, may all be underlying factors.

Figure 7.2.7 shows sex ratios in mortality rates by age for England and Wales in 1901 and 2004. It can be seen that the extent of female advantage was considerably greater in 2004 and most marked in young adulthood and late middle age. Although the former peak is more pronounced, the latter (and continuing differential in old age) is much more important demographically, as death rates are much higher at these older ages.

The relative contribution of various eighteenth and nineteenth century developments in promoting the historical epidemiological transition in the West remains a matter of debate. Improved nutrition, better housing and living conditions, public sanitation schemes, and specific public health initiatives, such as vaccinations all have their particular adherents (Coleman & Salt 1992). In the early twentieth century (and to some extent earlier), improved personal hygiene practices and better infant care were also very important. A common thread linking most of these factors is their relationship to overall social and economic development and improvements in standards of living. During the twentieth century, however, developments in medical technology and vector control offered the potential for 'exogenous' mortality decline less dependent on a particular country's level of income and development. One consequence was that the relationship between *per capita* income and life expectancy has shifted to the right (Preston 1975; 2007). In 1900, for example, life expectancy in the United States was about 49 and income *per capita* was about US$4800 (1991 prices). In 1990, that income *per capita* was associated with a life expectancy of about 71 years (World Bank 1993).

Many poor countries have been able to achieve remarkable falls in mortality, especially child mortality, through behavioural change, improved education of women, and introduction of relatively cheap treatments and interventions, such as immunizations and antibiotics (Caldwell 1986; Cutler *et al.* 2006). Between 1975–1980 and 2000–2005 life expectancy at birth increased from 47 to 62 in Bangladesh and from 53 to 69 in Indonesia (UN 2007) and there are now a number of low- or middle-income countries with life expectancies at birth as high as in the United States.

The process of the epidemiological transition (or at least the initial phases) is now complete or under way in much of the world and non-communicable causes of death predominate in all regions except sub-Saharan Africa (see Fig. 7.2.3). However, some recent changes have been less benign and new challenges or reversals have emerged, notably the HIV/AIDs epidemic and the health consequences of the collapse of the former Soviet Union (Olshansky *et al.* 1999; McKee 2001). Partly because of these challenges, there are signs that after a period in which risks of mortality in different parts of the world showed a tendency to converge (i.e. poorer countries caught up with richer ones), more recently there has been a trend towards divergence. Another factor in this may be that recent successes in richer countries in, for example, lowering mortality from heart disease, have to a considerable extent been achieved through treatments which are harder to 'transfer' to poor countries because of infrastructure and cost limitations (Vallin & Mesle 2004; Ford *et al.* 2007).

Recent demographic trends and public health

Population size, growth, and age structure are all outcomes of variations in demographic behaviours and all have implications for population health and well-being. In much of Europe and the richer Southeast Asian populations, population ageing will almost certainly be the predominant demographic issue of the early twenty-first century. Ageing at the individual level is a heterogeneous

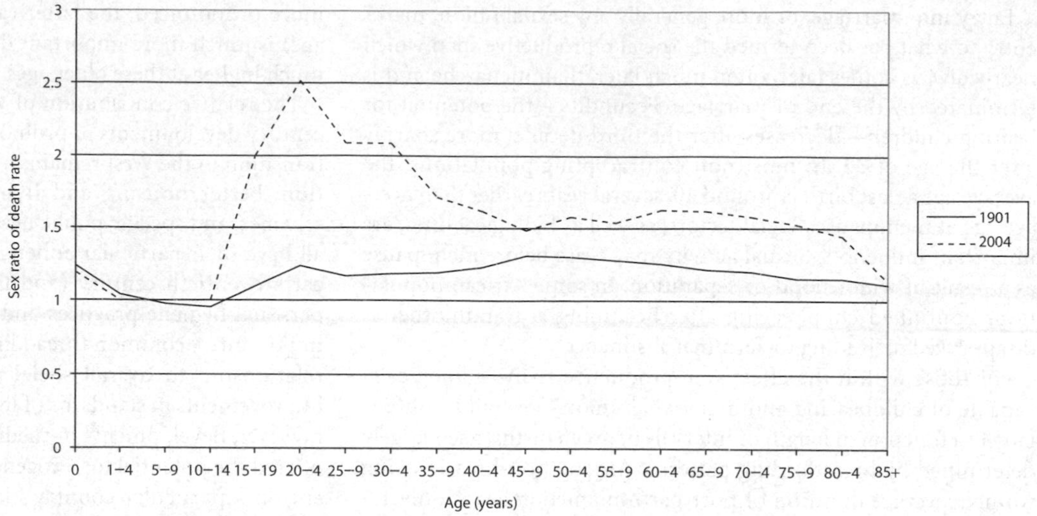

Fig. 7.2.7 Sex ratios of death rate (M/F) by age, England and Wales, 1901 and 2004.
Data Source: WHO Department of Management and Health Information.

experience not inevitably involving serious disability; however the strong association between age and risks of health impairment and disability imply growing needs for support services, even if levels of disability fall.

Changes in marriage and family patterns also have public health implications. In North America and North West Europe (and also Latin America and the Caribbean) high rates of divorce and non-marital childbearing mean that increasing proportions of children are spending at least part of their childhood in lone parent families. Although causal pathways are difficult to elucidate because of various selection effects, there is evidence indicating poorer health among lone mothers and their children, and among unmarried (especially divorced) people more generally, so these trends have some negative implications.

Continuing improvement in both child and adult mortality is projected for the poorer world, although this rests on optimistic assumptions about the course of the HIV/AIDs epidemic. In the poorest countries the interaction of rapid population growth, environmental degradation and conflict pose continuing, and possibly growing, health problems and the 'unfinished agenda' in terms of health includes providing access to contraception for women who wish to space or limit their children (Cleland 2006). In other low- and middle-income countries, patterns of tobacco use are likely to have a substantial effect on health trends in coming decades (West 2006).

Issues such as international migration, economic and cultural 'globalization', and climate change all have substantial health implications for the rest of the twenty-first century; all interact with demographic patterns and processes. Measuring these trends and assessing their effect on health and demand for healthcare requires an understanding of population dynamics and population-based measures, and suitable demographic data. Demography is thus an important component of public health.

References

Ahlburg, D.A. (1994). Population growth and poverty. In *Population and development: Old debates, new conclusions* (ed. R Cassen). Transaction Publishers, Oxford.

Alexandratos, N. (2005). Countries with rapid population growth and resource constraints: issues of food, agriculture and development. *Population and Development Review*, **31**, 237–58.

Billari, F. and Kohler, H.P. (2004). Patterns of low and lowest-low fertility in Europe. *Population Studies*, **58**, 161–76.

Bloom, E., Canning, D., and Malaney, P. (2000). Demographic change and economic growth in Asia. *Population and Development Review*, **26** (Supp) 257–90.

Bongaarts, J. (1978). A framework for analysing the proximate determinants of fertility. *Population and Development Review*, **4**, 105–32.

Bongaarts, J. and Feeny, G. (1998). On the quantum and tempo of fertility. *Population and Development Review*, **24**, 271–91.

Bryant, J. (2007). Theories of fertility decline and the evidence from development indicators. *Population and Development Review*, **33**, 101–27.

Caldwell, J. (1982). *Theory of fertility decline*. Academic Press, New York.

Casselli, G. (1991). Health transition and cause specific mortality. In *The Decline of Mortality in Europe* (eds. R. Schofield, D. Reher and A. Bideau), pp. 68–96. Clarendon Press, Oxford.

Cleland, J. (1990). Maternal education and child survival: further evidence and explanations. In *What Do We Know About Health Transition? The cultural, social and behavioural determinants of health* (eds. J. Caldwell *et al.*). pp. 400–19. Health Transition Centre, Australian National University, Canberra.

Cleland, J., Bernstein, S., Ezeh, A. *et al.* (2006). Family planning: the unfinished agenda. *Lancet*, **368**, 1810–27.

Cleland, J. and Wilson, C. (1987). Demand theories of the fertility transition. *Population Studies*, **41**, 5–30.

Coale, A. (1973). The demographic transition. In *International Population Conference 1973*. International Union for the Scientific Study of Population, Liège.

Coale, A. and Watkins, S.C. (eds.) (1986). *The decline of fertility in Europe*. Princeton University Press, Princeton, NJ.

Coleman, D. and Rowthorn, R. (2004). The economic effects of immigration into the United Kingdom. *Population and Development Review*, **30**, 579–624.

Coleman, D. and Salt, J. (1992). *The British Population: patterns, trends and processes*. Oxford University Press, Oxford.

D'Amico, M., Agozzino, E., Biagino, A. *et al.* (1999). Ill-defined and multiple causes on death certificates—a study of misclassification in mortality statistics. *European Journal of Epidemiology*, **15**, 141–8.

Davis, K. and Blake, J. (1956). Social structure and fertility: An analytic framework. *Economic Development and Cultural Change*, **4**, 211–35.

Ford, E.S., Ajani, U.A., Croft, J.B. *et al.* (2007). Explaining the decrease in U.S. deaths from coronary heart disease, 1980–2000. *New England Journal of Medicine*, **356**, 2388–98.

Fox, A.J. and Goldblatt, P.O. (1982). *Longitudinal Study: Socio-demographic mortality differentials*. HMSO, London.

Garson, L.K. (1991). The centenarian question: old age mortality in the Soviet Union 1897–1970. *Population Studies*, **45**, 265–78.

Griffiths, C. and Brock, A. (2003). Twentieth century mortality trends in England and Wales. *Health Statistics Quarterly*, **18**, 5–16.

Grundy, E.M.D. (1996). Ageing in Europe. In. *Europe's Population in the 1990s* (ed. D. Coleman). Oxford University Press, Oxford.

Hobcraft, J. (1993). Women's education, child welfare and child survival: A review of the evidence. *Health Transition Review*, **3**, 159–73.

Hobcraft, J., Menken, J., and Preston, S. (1982). Age, period and cohort effects in demography: a review. *Population Index*, **48**, 4–43.

Lesthaeghe, R.J. and Neidert, L. (2006). The second demographic transition in the United States: Exception or textbook example. *Population and Development Review*, **32**, 669–98.

Lotka, A. (1907). Relation between birth and death rates. *Science*, **26**, 21–2.

Lutz, W., Vaupel, J.W., and Ahlburg, D.A. (eds.) (1998). Frontiers of population forecasting. *Population and Development Review* (Suppl), **24**. pp. 1–198.

Lutz, W., Sanderson, W., and Sherbov, S. (2001). The end of world population growth. *Nature*, **412**, 543–6.

Manton, K.G., Gu, X., and Lamb, V.L. (2006). Long-term trends in life expectancy and active life expectancy in the United States. *Population and Development Review*, **32**, 81–105.

Mason, A. and Lee, R. (2006). Reform and support systems for the elderly in developing countries: capturing the second demographic dividend. *Genus*, **LXII**, 11–36.

McKee, M. (2001). The health consequences of the collapse of the Soviet Union. In *Poverty, inequality and health: an international perspective* (eds. D Leon and G. Walt), pp. 17–36, Oxford University Press, Oxford.

McNicoll, G. (2006). Policy lessons of the East Asian Demographic Transition. *Population and Development Review*, **32**, 1–25.

Notestein, F.W. (1945). Population: the long view. In. *Food for the World* (ed. T.W. Schulz), pp. 36–57. University of Chicago Press, Chicago.

Organisation for Economic Co-operation and Development (OECD) (1999). *Maintaining prosperity in an ageing society*. OECD, Paris.

OECD (2006). *International migration outlook, 2006 edition*. OECD, Luxembourg.

Office for National Statistics (2002). Results of the ICD-10 bridge coding study, England and Wales 1999. *Health Statistics Quarterly*, **14**, 75–83.

Omran, A.R. (1971). The epidemiologic transition: A theory of the epidemiology of population change. *Millbank Memorial Fund Quarterly*, **49**, 509–38.

Olshansky, S.J., Carnes, B., Rogers, R.G. *et al.* (1997). Infectious diseases—new and ancient threats to World health. *Population Bulletin* 52, Population Reference Bureau, Washington D.C.

Preston, S.H. (1975). The changing relation between mortality and level of economic development. *Population Studies*, **29**, 231–48.

Preston, S.H. (1976). *Mortality patterns in national populations*. Academic Press, New York.

Preston, S.H. (2007). Response: On 'The changing relation between mortality and level of economic development'. *International Journal of Epidemiology*, (advance access doi:10.1093).

Preston, S.H., Elo, I.T., Rosenwaike, I. *et al.* (1996). African-American mortality at older ages: Results of a matching study. *Demography*, **33**, 193–209.

Preston, S.H., Heuveline, P., and Guillot, M. (2001). *Demography: Measuring and modelling population processes*. Blackwell Publishers, Oxford.

Retherford, R.D., Ogawa, N., and Matsukura, R. (2001). Late marriage and less marriage in Japan. *Population and Development Review*, **27**, 65–102.

Robine, J.M., Jagger, C., and Euro-REVES Group (2003). Creating a coherent set of indicators to monitor health across Europe: The Euro-REVES 2 project. *European Journal of Public Health*, **13**(3 Suppl), 6–14.

Rogers, A., Rogers, R.G., and Belanger, A. (1990). Longer life but worse health? Measurement and dynamics. *The Gerontologist*, **30**, 640–9.

Rosenberg, H.N., Maurer, J.D., Sorlie, P.D. *et al.* (1999). Quality of death rates by race and Hispanic origin: A summary of current research 1999. *Vital Health Statistics*, **2**, 1–13.

Rowland, D.T. (2003). *Demographic methods and concepts*. Oxford University Press, Oxford.

Siegel, J.S. and Swanson, D.A. (eds.)(2004). *The methods and materials of demography*, Second edition. Academic Press, San Diego.

United Nations (UN) (1983). *Indirect techniques for demographic estimation, Manual X*. United Nations, New York.

UN (1999). *World Population Prospects, the 1998 revision*. UN, New York

UN (2002). *World population prospects: The 2000 Revision, Volume III, Analytical Report*. United Nations, New York.

UN (2006a). *World Urbanization Prospects: The 2005 Revision*. United Nations, New York.

UN (2007). *World Population Prospects: The 2006 Revision*. United Nations, New York.

US Agency for International Development (2002). Birth spacing: Research Update. USAID Bureau for Global Health, Office of Population and Reproductive Health. USAID, Washington D.C.

Vallin, J. and Mesle, F. (2004). Convergences and divergences in mortality: A new approach to health transition. *Demographic Research*: Special collection 2, 12–43, http://www.demographic-research.org/special/2/2.

van da Kaa, D.J. (1987). Europe's second demographic transition. *Population Bulletin*, **42**. Population Reference Bureau Inc., Washington, D.C.

van de Walle, F. (1986). Infant mortality and the European demographic transition. In *The decline of fertility in Europe* (eds A.J. Coale and S.C. Watkins), pp. 201–33. Princeton University Press, Princeton, N.J.

Wang, L., Yang, G., Jiemin, M. *et al.* (2007). Evaluation of the quality of cause of death statistics in rural China using verbal autopsies. *Journal of Epidemiology and Community Health*, **61**,519–26.

West, R. (2006). Tobacco control: present and future. *British Medical Bulletin*, **77–78**, 123–36.

Wolf, D.A., Hunt, K., and Knickman, J. (2005). Perspectives on the recent decline in disability at older ages. *Millbank Quarterly*, **83**, 365–95.

World Health Organisation (WHO) (1999). *The world health report 1999*. WHO, Geneva.

WHO (2007). World health statistics 2007. http://www.who.int/whosis/database/core

Woods, R.I., Watterson, P.A., and Woodward, J.H. (1989). The causes of rapid infant mortality decline in England and Wales, 1861–1921 (Part II). *Population Studies*, **43**, 113–32.

World Bank (The International Bank for Reconstruction and Development) (1993). *World Development Report 1993: Investing in health, world development indicators*. Oxford University Press, Oxford.

World Bank (2006). World development indicators 2006. http://devdata.worldbank.org/wdi2006

Wrigley, E.A. and Schofield, R.S. (1981). *The Population History of England 1541–1871: A reconstruction*. Edward Arnold, London.

Zeng Yi., Tu Ping, Gu Baochang *et al.* (1993). Causes and implications of the recent increase in the reported sex ratio at birth in China. *Population and Development Review*, **19**, 283–302.

7.3

Health promotion, health education, and the public's health

Marcia Hills and Simon Carroll

Abstract

Health promotion is a complex, ambiguous concept and set of practices. While many have linked it, primarily, to a revolution in health education, its roots go much deeper into the history of public health. It had its beginnings in the throes of the backlash against bureaucratic and professional dominance exemplified by the new social movements of the 1970s and 1980s. At its heart, health promotion is centred on the values and principles of *equity*, *participation*, and *empowerment*. These concepts are embedded in health promotion's founding document, the *Ottawa Charter for Health Promotion*. However, exactly how these values are articulated is often ambiguous. In this chapter, the authors contend that health promoters must intensify their reflection on these core values and principles; particularly in the light of the tendency to slip back into a comfortable paternalism, which reinforces existing power imbalances. We are specifically concerned with the precise interpretation of *health equity* in health promotion. In order to pursue a deeper level of reflection on the meaning of *equity*, it is argued that health promotion must engage more deeply with recent developments in political philosophy and political economy. Furthermore, health promotion must be much more active in supporting the global efforts to address equity in health and development represented by work on the United Nation's Millennium Development Goals and with the World Health Organization's Commission on the Social Determinants of Health.

Health promotion, health equity, and action on the determinants of health: An introduction

Previous attempts (Green & Raeburn 1988; Tones & Tilford 1994; Tones 2004) to situate health promotion within the broad field of public health have often used 'health education' as the starting point. This is an entirely sensible approach and we will discuss it in this chapter; however, it does tend to under-emphasize the *radical* departure health promotion aims to make from traditional public health approaches in general. Without falling into the trap of claiming health promotion means everything all at once, and therefore leave its lofty rhetoric in the realm of the aspirational yet ineffectual, we aim to place health promotion as a more central character in the ongoing saga of an increasingly globally aware public health. As one of the acknowledged founders and most determined innovators of the modern health promotion movement has unceasingly argued, health promotion, at its most persistent and radical, heralds a 'new public health', not merely a more fine-tuned and effective tool-box for a less paternalistic health education (Kickbusch 1998, 2007).

We will begin with a clear definition of health promotion, followed by an analysis of the elements of that definition. By unpacking the dense and sometimes opaque wording that define the elements of health promotion as a concept, we intend to open up some of its central, yet often hidden, connections to much broader themes in contemporary social and political movements and ideas.

Next, we will clearly situate health education and its internal critique as an important part of the history of health promotion, yet at the same time, provide more context concerning the specific historical/national trajectories that made the genesis of the modern health promotion movement a mixture of different influences, with health education being only one among others.

We will consider how health promotion manages its ambiguous relationship with the history and ideological background of public health. How does health promotion see itself in relation to the past, present, and future of public health? How one answers this question largely determines how one answers the question: What is health promotion?

We suggest that there exists a new opportunity for health promotion to reconnect with the *avant-garde* in public health. This opportunity will be examined along two broad dimensions: The question of how to achieve health equity; and, the question of health in a global political-economic context. Within this matrix, particular attention will be paid to the recent work on the social determinants of health, spearheaded by the World Health Organization's (WHO) Commission on the Social Determinants of Health, led by Sir Michael Marmot. In addition, some recent attempts to more seriously engage public health with political and moral philosophy will be considered. In both these cases, it will be argued that health promotion has a particular perspective to offer and something to learn from engaging more deeply in these debates.

In relation to the latter issues, there is an under-analysed political economy of health promotion; however, here we can only suggest some lines of inquiry and point to some that have already started.

In general, this chapter on health promotion is resolutely *critical* in the positive sense of the word. Previous surveys of the concept and practice of health promotion that provide excellent guidance to the field are available and are referenced. However, at this crucial juncture, we consider that practitioners and researchers in public health can benefit from a reflexive inquiry into the rich ambiguities and tensions that are embedded in the discourse and practice of health promotion. This is particularly the case if, as we argue, the development of health promotion *is* the development of a 'new public health'.

'Health promotion': A definition and conceptual critique

In this chapter, we will follow the *The Ottawa Charter for Health Promotion* (WHO 1986) definition of health promotion as 'the process of enabling people to increase control over, and to improve their health'. However, we will also draw upon the expanded definition in the updated *Health Promotion Glossary*, where the 'how' and 'why' *ideology* is linked to the 'what' of the *determinants of health* (WHO 1998). We believe this is crucial, because if health promotion is about anything, it is about *action* taken across the broad spectrum of health determinants, particularly directed towards the social, environmental and economic conditions that support health (WHO 1984). We reproduce here the *Glossary* definition, in full:

> *Health promotion represents a comprehensive social and political process, it not only embraces actions directed at strengthening the skills and capabilities of individuals, but also action directed towards changing social, environmental and economic conditions so as to alleviate their impact on public and individual health. Health promotion is the process of enabling people to increase control over* the determinants of health *and thereby improve their health (pp. 1–2).* [our emphasis]

The *Glossary* also emphasizes that 'participation is essential to sustain health promotion action'. It then goes on to identify the three *Ottawa Charter* strategies for health promotion: '*Advocacy* for health to create the essential conditions for health indicated above; *enabling* all people to achieve their full health potential; and *mediating* between the different interests in society in the pursuit of health'.

These strategies are supported by five priority action areas as outlined in the *Ottawa Charter*:

1. Build healthy public policy
2. Create supportive environments for health
3. Strengthen community action for health
4. Develop personal skills, and
5. Re-orient health services

As one can see from the concise definition of the *Ottawa Charter* to the expanded and revised definition of the *Glossary* we already have started the 'unpacking'. Below is a more nuanced analysis of some of the key elements in this definition: The 'process' of health promotion; 'enabling' and 'empowering'; and for what, the outcome, 'improved health'. This will be followed by an analysis of the *Ottawa Charter strategies* and its *priority action areas* (which have often been called 'action strategies').

As soon as we begin, we find ourselves in murky waters; nevertheless, we are not without some guidance. Ironically, although health promotion is, as Tones (2004) noted, an 'essentially contested concept', there has been a remarkable degree of effort, rewarded with consensus, concerning its ostensive definition. Few, if any, health promoters dispute the *Ottawa Charter*'s now canonical phrasing; and in fact, recently, an attempt to introduce a new 'Charter' for health promotion in Bangkok, Thailand (WHO 2005), caused enough commotion to force the drafters to include a reverential paean to the Ottawa document in its preamble.

The real ambiguity that surrounds the concept of health promotion is embedded in the elision of the concrete meaning of the elements that make up its agreed upon definition.

Health promotion as a process

The emphasis on *process* is important, if only because it warns against reducing health promotion to a technical function of public health. It connotes the wider meaning of the concept by signalling that the radical departure and critique of traditional public health lies in its advocacy for changing the *way* we do public health, just as much as *what* we change and *why* we change.

Health promotion, whether it be generated from an internal critique of health education or whether it is born from other sources of discontent with the way public health was being practised, is fundamentally concerned with change and, specifically, with the failure of traditional, paternalistic, and professionally dominated public health processes to bring about positive changes in health, particularly for those groups that suffer disproportionately negative health outcomes and the myriad disadvantages that are consequent. What is substituted is a call for health promoters to create a dynamic, participatory engagement with individuals and communities, to help or 'enable' them to take control over the determinants of their own health.

The first ambiguity we meet when trying to analyse this 'process' turns on whether one interprets the health promotion process as: A revamped tool box of health education techniques and social marketing devices, with a rhetorically efficient participatory gloss; or, as a values-based process of communicative interaction that has as its central premise the ethical foundation of respect for human dignity and autonomy. These are certainly polar extremes and there is no doubt that there is room for both aspects in a broad, ecumenical attitude to a diverse field of practical action. Yet, because, health promotion is a process often dominated by professionals, in a context where its supposed beneficiaries are invariably those in a position of relative powerlessness, the tendency for professionals to retreat to an insulated cocoon of technical expertise is strong. The essence of the health promotion process is a focused shift of power from professionals to the community and to individuals within their communities who historically have had less power. To do this, it is crucial that the 'process' we focus on is the one that involves negotiating values, principles, ethics, and power, not the less complicated one of transferring a packet of new skills and technical tools to a community that is presumed to lack capacity. In order to achieve this shift in power, health promoters need to begin by examining their own values and assumptions that inform their actions.

Beliefs and assumptions underlying health promotion

Health promotion practice, just like any other human activity, is influenced by the beliefs and assumptions we hold. While it is beyond the scope of this chapter to delve too deeply into this topic, we would be remiss not to at least outline how certain beliefs and assumptions influence our ability to act in health promoting ways in given situations.

Beliefs are learned through life experiences; they are what we hold as 'true'. They are convictions and they influence the way we think, feel and act. Health promotion practice relies on a set of underlying assumptions that guide those who work in the field of health promotion. Hartrick *et al.* (1994) contend health promotion is a 'way of being' that requires certain convictions in order to act in health promoting ways. These include:

1. All people have strengths and are capable of determining their own needs, finding their own answers, and solving their own problems.
2. Every person and family lives within a social-historical context that helps shape their identity and social relationships.
3. Diversity is positively valued.
4. People without power have as much capacity as the powerful to assess their own needs (people are their own experts).
5. Relationships between people and groups need to be organized to provide an equal balance of power (this includes professional/client relationships).
6. The power of defining health problems and needs belongs to those experiencing the problem.
7. The people disadvantaged by the way that society is currently structured must play the primary role in developing the strategies by which they gain increased control over valued resources.
8. Empowerment is not something that occurs purely from within (only I can empower myself), nor is it something that can be done to others (we need to empower the group). Rather, empowerment describes our intentional efforts to create more equitable relationships where there is greater equality in resources, status, and authority.
9. Shared power relations do not deny health professionals their specialized expertise and skills. Rather, professional expertise and skills are used in new ways that result in greater power equity in interpersonal and social relations.

So, for example, if we consider the first assumption in the list, believing that people are able to find their own answers and solve their own problems leads one to act in empowering ways because of the belief that people have this capacity to figure things out. On the other hand, if one believes that people need to be told what to do, or that they are not able to figure out issues on their own, it is more difficult to create conditions that are enabling. For some, it might even feel irresponsible to put people in these circumstances or to allow them to have control over these types of decisions.

Enabling and empowerment

At the time of the *Ottawa Charter*, the word 'enabling' was favoured, although later this tended to be replaced with the more direct and comprehensive concept of 'empowerment'. Essentially, this meant that a prerequisite for the new approach was that people, meaning individuals and communities, were to directly participate in the planning and implementation of health promotion activities. The assumption was based on the notion that only by genuinely participating in the health promotion process would people be 'enabled' or 'empowered' to take control of what determined their health. However, the concept of 'enabling' also referred to the more general process of changing the social, economic, and environmental conditions that made it difficult for people to become empowered. There is a deep ambiguity here: It is not clear whether more macro-scale action, at a policy level, also requires active participation of local communities. There is some room for an interpretation that tends to retain a traditional paternalism when it comes to healthy public policy, leaving the 'participatory' aspect of health promotion to the realm of 'community action'. As will be argued throughout this chapter, health promotion is constantly at risk of sliding back into this paternalistic approach, leaving the more 'complex' and high-level 'technical' decisions to the experts. Yet, if there is a direct link between human dignity, autonomy, and equity, then *all* aspects of health promotion must integrate the fundamental perspective (or even stronger, paradigm) of participation. In fact, it is argued that the rhetoric of 'empowerment' often masks a continuing bureaucratic and professional dominance of the process of improving public health (Baum 2007).

A key aspect of this ambiguity can be seen when we consider the link to health inequity. Without a genuinely participatory, empowering process, we find that it is those worst off who are left further behind as they suffer, not only a failure to affect those conditions most important to their health, but also a direct assault on their human dignity (Sennett 2003). Those who tend to manage any gains from processes that lack true participation are usually segments of the population that already have access to positions of status and have the resources and capacities to take advantage of the type of interventions on offer. The distinction here is between a situation where already disadvantaged people are assumed to be too ignorant or incapable of participating and thus have solutions imposed on them, and a situation where people of a privileged status delegate, as equals, to professional experts. This is not to say that a participatory process is not better for everyone, regardless of class position or status; rather, it is to emphasize that non-participatory processes have a disproportionate adverse effect on disadvantaged groups.

On the positive side, an empowering health promotion process leaves the ownership and control of a health promotion activity or programme in the hands of the community itself. This is particularly important in communities that have suffered historical social injustices and have thus been actively 'disempowered' (an ugly term, but an accurate one). Allowing people to participate in a genuine way in determining not only *what* they want but *how* they want to get it is demonstrably the most effective strategy for change. It is also the *only* strategy for sustaining progress in improving health and shifting control back to the community and away from a negative dependence on bureaucratic and professional power. In this model, professionals are not demons; they are just transformed from arrogant experts into supportive servants of the will of the community.

There is in these simple terms ('enable' or 'empower') the entire, complex, and ambiguous story of health promotion. All the themes that will be touched upon in this chapter can be traced back to just what is at stake in the ostensive goal of 'empowering' people to take control over what determines their health.

What is the 'health' in health promotion?

Understanding how we conceptualize health is a key reflective step in health promotion. How we think about health largely determines the types of action we take in order to promote health. We see below how different historical conceptions of health still shape the contemporary health landscape and continue to sustain ambiguities in how people approach health promotion itself. In the twentieth century, due to the relative success of the sanitation approach to public health and the emergent hegemony of the germ theory of disease, an implicit biomedical definition of health as *the absence of disease* dominated, and along with it, a narrow, individual treatment focus, centred on the healthcare system, was the preferred solution. The WHO had, in 1946, introduced the *positive* definition of health as 'a state of complete physical, mental, and social well-being and not merely the absence of disease or infirmity'. (WHO 1946). Nevertheless, this definition had little concrete impact on actual health systems, leaving the absence of disease approach to health as the default option when governments turned their attention to the public's health.

The introduction of the Lalonde report, an official document produced by the Canadian Department of Health and Welfare (Lalonde 1974), marked a significant change in thinking about health. Although the Lalonde report is recognized internationally as being the first government document to suggest that health promotion could be a key strategy for improving health, its other, more significant contribution, was to redefine how we view health. Lalonde's report argued that the healthcare system plays only a small part in determining health. The report suggested that health was determined by the interplay between human biology, healthcare organization, environment, and lifestyle. This view of health became known as the 'lifestyle or behavioural approach to health', partly because the 'environmental' dimension was either ignored or treated narrowly.

With the publication of the discussion paper on concepts and principles of health promotion (WHO 1984) and the endorsement of the *Ottawa Charter for Health Promotion* (1986), a third view of health arose: The socioecological approach. This approach defined health as 'a resource for everyday life, not the objective of living'. 'Health is a positive concept emphasizing social and personal resources as well as physical capacities' (1986, p.1). In order to reach this state of physical, mental, and social well-being, people must be able to identify and realize their aspirations, to satisfy their needs and to change, or cope, with their environment. This inextricable link between people and their environment provides the conceptual basis for this socioecological perspective on health and it forms the conceptual base for health promotion practice.

At first glance, these different views of health may appear to be developmental or historical. However, Labonté and others (Labonté 1993; Rootman & Raeburn 1994; Raeburn & Rootman 2007) argue that, in fact, all three views of health (along with many other definitions) continue to be endorsed by different people in the field of health promotion and, furthermore, that the view of health one holds influences one's health promotion practice. Figure 7.3.1 illustrates this connection between how we think about health, our view of health, and our actions (health promotion practice). For example, if we hold a view that health is the absence of disease,

From concept to action: Different approaches to health			
	Medical approach	Behavioural approach	Socio-ecological approach
Health concept	Biomedical; absence of disease or disability	Individualized; physical-functional ability; physical well-being	Positive state; connectedness; ability to do things that are important or have meaning; psychological well-being
Health determinant	Disease categories, physiological risk factors (e.g. hypertension)	Behavioural risk factors (e.g. unsafe sex)	Psychological risk factors (e.g. isolation), and socio-environmental risk conditions (e.g. poverty)
Principle strategy	Surgery, drugs, therapy, illness care, medically managed behavioural change	Advocacy for healthy lifestyle choices	Personal empowerment, small group development, community organization, coalition advocacy, political action
Programme development	Professionally managed	Negotiated with individuals, communities and professionals	Managed by community in critical dialogue with supporting professionals and agencies

Fig. 7.3.1

we are likely to talk about disease processes and risk factors and to manage the problem professionally by prescribing a treatment. If we hold a socioecological view of health, we are more likely to focus on the conditions in which the person is living, the factors that are influencing their ability to meet their needs, and to use enabling strategies to assist the person to have more control over their health.

The *Ottawa Charter* strategies

The three strategies mentioned in the *Ottawa Charter* are: *To advocate, to enable,* and *to mediate.* We have already reflected upon the second strategy as it is part of the definition of health promotion. However, a few words need to be said about the other two strategies.

The concept of *advocacy* receives very little elaboration in the *Ottawa Charter*. In the *Health Promotion Glossary*, it is stated that advocacy 'can take many forms including the use of the mass media and multi-media, direct political lobbying, and community mobilization through, for example, coalitions of interest around defined issues. Health professionals have a major responsibility to act as advocates for health at all levels in society' (WHO 1998: 6). This raises one of the many thorny issues that come up when professionals are caught between highly mobilized and often highly critical communities and a state bureaucracy that is extremely reticent about providing funding that sanctions and supports the capacity for critical attention to its policies and programmes. Even at the level of independent professional organizations, the participation and funding provided by government bodies creates a tension around the organization taking strong critical perspectives. Another aspect of this strategy, as defined in the glossary and glossed over, is the potential contradiction between activities such as 'political lobbying' and 'community mobilization'. Often, the same organization or individual will be less effective as a political lobbyist to the extent they are perceived to be directly associated with community mobilization efforts that the powerful are either indifferent to, or actively disfavour.

Mediation is an even more delicate strategy for health professionals. Its original *Glossary* definition in relation to health promotion was: 'A process through which the different interests (personal, social, economic) of individuals and communities and different sectors (public and private) are reconciled in ways that promote and protect health' (WHO 1986b). In the expanded definition of 1998, more explicit emphasis is given to the potential conflicts that often arise between the competing interests mentioned in the original definition. However, the goal of mediation as 'reconciliation' is left unchanged. While there is nothing inherently wrong with the idea of reconciliation, professionals should be extremely self-critical and reflexive when operating with this strategy. Two dangers are apparent with the strategy. First, in striving for 'reconciliation', one may simply paper over a conflict for the purposes of short-term peace, while leaving the principle reasons behind the conflict intact, thereby creating the potential for longer term embitterment and strategic action by all parties, which ultimately undermines the appearance of agreement. Second, a very real threat to equity can arise when professionals reconcile a conflict between the powerful and the powerless and end up re-enforcing the powerful at the expense of the powerless. This tendency is very strong given the fact that professionals have little to gain personally from any radical re-structuring of power relations. Despite these important caveats, mediation has become even more critical for the success of health promotion in the future, especially in relation to the new global, multi-layered context of health governance that the *Bangkok Charter* (WHO 2005) has set out to address and which will be discussed later.

The *Ottawa Charter* action areas

The priority action areas of the *Ottawa Charter* were identified as those areas that were seen at the time of the charter (and still to this day) as critical arenas for health promotion's strategic activities. We will not try and survey the myriad accomplishments of health promotion activity; rather, consistent with our general approach, we will offer a few critical comments on each action area:

Building healthy public policy

There are three elements of healthy public policy emphasized in the *Ottawa Charter*.

1. If it is true, as the Lalonde Report (1974) argued, that the determinants of health lay mainly outside healthcare itself, then it is equally true that policy action must come from policy sectors other than health. The health sector would still play an important role in public policy action to support health, but no longer exclusively.
2. Healthy public policy requires the coordinated use of all policy levers available, including 'legislation, fiscal measures, taxation, and organizational change' (WHO 1986a).
3. Healthy public policy requires the identification and removal of obstacles to the adoption of healthy public policies in non-health sectors.

Without going into a long list of efforts and results in this area, one can sum up the progress made by characterizing it as substantial and encouraging in regard to changes in the rhetoric and discourse around health, in both the developed industrial nations and in many of the global institutions responsible for improving health and development worldwide. Conversely, one can equally characterize progress as ephemeral and demoralizing when it comes to the concrete goal of 'coordinated action that leads to health, income and social policies that foster greater equity' (WHO 1986a). For a variety of reasons discussed in the section below on the political economy of health promotion, given the stark and increasingly urgent crisis of widening inequities in health both between and within societies, the collective policy response of the most powerful countries on earth has been miserly and despicable. To call it 'inadequate' is a gross understatement and an unconscionable euphemism.

When *action* finally starts to catch up with some of the lofty rhetoric behind the calls for 'health in all policies' (Ståhl *et al.* 2006), health promotion can begin to find some satisfaction in the area of building healthy public policy.

Creating supportive environments

This area forms the basis for what is called the *socioecological* approach to health. Here it is asserted that both the natural and built environments are inextricably linked with people's health. It is crucial to understand that the conceptualization of supportive environments given here is consistent with the expanded, positive understanding of health as a 'resource for everyday life'. It is not merely about threats to physical health, but involves creating conditions that allow people to have 'living and working conditions that are safe, stimulating, satisfying, and enjoyable'. This entails the complex relationships between rapidly changing technologies, working conditions, resource use, urbanization, and health (amongst many other relevant factors).

In considering progress in this area, both past endeavours and future prospects, one must take into account the lofty ambition (and some would say naiveté) of this programme of action. As a project of knowledge development, its referral to the 'complex interrelatedness' of contemporary societies is but a cipher for the entire corpus of theoretical and empirical dispute and debate within the social sciences over how to characterize what are now acknowledged to be multiple, interrelated, global, national, regional, and local processes of socioeconomic and cultural change (Held *et al.* 1999).

Of course, in the real world, we are not able to coordinate all the best knowledge sources available and neatly calculate what is best for health. In the real world, we are left with tools like 'Health Impact Assessment' (HIA) (Kemm 2006). As could be derived from the preceding paragraph, the action area of creating supportive environments can be seen as a great boon to academic productivity, both theoretical and empirical; yet, before the final judgements of the academy can be handed down (a moment that never quite seems to arrive), actions must be taken and decisions must be made. Communities and developers, politicians, and bureaucrats must decide whether to build this or that highway, license this or that mining operation, enact this or that employment regulation. We are thus forced, by the necessity to decide and act, into an inevitable reduction of complexity. The question is not whether this is a good or bad thing; it is *how*, by what *process*, is complexity reduced? Whither participation and empowerment in a field dominated by professional expertise and the cloistered secrecy of executive and administrative decision-making in both the public and private sectors?

We argue *against* the implication that instruments like HIA inevitably vitiate participatory processes (Kemm 2006). The natural tendency is always to define ahead of time, objectively, what elements of the built or natural environment are most important for enhancing people's health. From a utilitarian perspective, locally defined needs and wishes may even legitimately be ignored in the name of some greater good for a larger population. However, health promotion should always err primarily on the side of the fundamental value of the autonomy and the dignity of people and their communities. In this mode, participation is foundational, even in what are *prime facie* obvious areas for the guidance of refined professional expertise. In inquiring into the best way to protect and enhance the built and natural environment for health, the first step is to find out what people actually identify as the things that would make life 'safe, stimulating, satisfying, and enjoyable'. From the professional perspective this route has one incontestable drawback: People' are inevitably confused, ignorant, inconsistent, contradictory, and even just 'wrong'. 'People' will disagree with each other; will get annoyed or, even worse, angry; will disrespect experts, politicians, lawyers, and any number of people who 'actually know' about the issue. What is feared here is what is fondly called deliberative politics; in other words, the foundation of democratic civil society.

We are, as is universally acknowledged in the health promotion community, a long way from creating supportive environments for health, especially for those who are suffering gross inequities in social conditions and in their consequent health outcomes. What is less often acknowledged is that part of the reason this is so difficult is that we consistently exclude the very people we are meant to be helping from determining the goals, objectives, strategies, and tactics that are necessary to move from here to there. Once again, we are led to believe that the ends can justify the means; we can have non-participatory processes as long as we intend to make changes to enhance the lives of the less fortunate. That we end up in a place we did not intend, is inextricably linked to the fact that, at crucial junctures, when inevitable changes of directions and compromises are made (local development processes are a prime example), the people who have an inherent interest in speaking up for the powerless (the powerless themselves) are nowhere to be seen, or they are heard only as a distant voice of protest muffled by the closed doors of the back rooms.

Strengthening community action

This action area is at the very heart of health promotion; in fact, it can be argued that it is in this one action area where the basic principles of health promotion lie. As has been implied earlier, you can imagine participation, equity, and empowerment to be contingent add-ons to the other action areas; with strengthening community action the essential unity of all the values of health promotion are embedded as necessary features of its realization. In fact, what we see in this area is the place where the true spirit of health promotion is anchored in community development as a process. In fact, in the *Ottawa Charter* itself, there is a strange ellipsis where the term community development is introduced in the section on strengthening community action. It is as if one missed something: There is no linking phraseology relating community development to strengthening community action. This, we surmise, is no error: Strengthening community action quite simply *is* community development.

Consider a recent definition of community development as agreed upon at the International Association for Community Development at a meeting in Budapest in 2004:

> *Community development is a way of strengthening civil society by prioritising the actions of communities, and their perspectives in the development of social, economic and environmental policy. It seeks the empowerment of local communities, taken to mean both geographical communities, communities of interest or identity and communities organizing around specific themes or policy initiatives. It strengthens the capacity of people as active citizens through their community groups, organizations and networks; and the capacity of institutions and agencies (public, private and non-governmental) to work in dialogue with citizens to shape and determine change in their communities. It plays a crucial role in supporting active democratic life by promoting the autonomous voice of disadvantaged and vulnerable communities. It has a set of core values/social principles covering human rights, social inclusion, equality and respect for diversity; and a specific skills and knowledge base.* (Craig 2005: 3)

For a more sustained treatment of the need to recognize the central place processes of community development and empowerment should play in health promotion, Raeburn and Rootman's *People-Centred Health Promotion* is an essential reference (Raeburn & Rootman 1998). Raeburn and Rootman draw heavily, in their chapter on community development, on Meridith Minkler's important piece, 'Improving health through community organization' (1990).

In this seminal piece, Minkler outlines the five principles she sees as foundational to community organization or development:

- Empowerment
- Community competence
- Participation
- Issue selection
- Creating 'critical consciousness'

As is now obvious, we have run into some of these principles already. The key to these principles is that the community itself has collective control over the process of identifying issues and planning how to address them. In addition, the important notion of 'critical consciousness' is raised. This refers to the need for critical dialogue in the Freirian sense (1972); this is particularly important when working with historically oppressed or disadvantaged communities.

Developing personal skills

The new wave of health promotion has often downgraded attention to this critical aspect of its mandate. The *Ottawa Charter* tells us that health promotion 'supports personal and social development through providing information, education for health, and enhancing life skills'. However, since the *Ottawa Charter*, health promoters, with some exceptions, have tended to either ignore or aim strong criticism at the developing personal skills area. This has come about for three reasons. First, as part of the critique of health education, it was argued that individually focused education approaches were generally ineffective in bringing about health promoting behavioural change; it was felt that a switch to an emphasis on the *social* factors that influence health was necessary to overcome the limitations of traditional counselling and other interventions circumscribed by the discipline of psychology. Second, the emphasis on developing personal skills was associated with the 'victim-blaming' element that many health promoters saw as the consequence of an interpretation of the Lalonde report and other government documents (particularly, the approach taken in the UK under the Thatcher governments) in the context of the neo-liberal rolling back of the state's commitment to a strong social safety net. Finally, although developing personal skills is a central mechanism for empowering individuals to take control over their own health, many worried that, in this narrow approach, the *collective* strengthening of communities was adversely effected by too much emphasis on individual empowerment.

All of these concerns are legitimate, though in each of them there is a high risk that we will miss important opportunities by mistaking what are contingent tendencies for essential features.

As has recently been argued, the ignorance of, or even hostility to work in this area may seriously damage health promotion's potential impact (Godin 2007). First, while many health education and behaviour change approaches are limited in their effectiveness, there are some demonstrably effective interventions that should not be ignored (Kok *et al.* 1997). Furthermore, we can learn and are learning about why some approaches in this area have not been effective. Second, the fact that this area of health promotion can be enlisted as part of a more general 'victim-blaming' culture of health promotion, does not mean it must be enlisted; in fact, to the extent that genuinely empowering health education is taken seriously, the resulting improvements in self-esteem should work against victim blaming. Third, individual and community empowerment should not be a zero sum trade-off. It is only when an exclusive focus on individuals is emphasized that we will have the phenomenon of rescuing survivors from a sinking ship.

In summary, while we must be vigilant against the temptation and limitations of an individually focused, skills development approach, we must also re-engage with the most advanced and progressive elements in this area of work. If we fail to do this, we will jeopardize a key aspect of health promotion.

Reorienting health services

While we have made some important gains in the previous four areas, reorienting health services has proved more difficult. In general, throughout the world, health services remain medically dominated, cure and treatment focused, and individualistic. The *Ottawa Charter* states 'the role of the health sector must move increasingly in a health promotion direction, beyond its responsibility for providing clinical and curative services'. However, 'across the world, there appears to have been a stubborn resistance to systematic change in healthcare services and only limited examples of effective and sustainable health services reorientation' (Wise & Nutbeam 2007). Health services need to embrace an expanded mandate which is sensitive and respects cultural needs. This mandate should support the needs of individuals and communities for a healthier life, and open channels between the health sector and broader social, political, and physical environmental components.

Health services are broad and far-reaching, with the most complex service for health promotion being the acute care hospital setting. There has been some advancement in this area with the creation of the healthy hospital settings movement and there has been some research that provides evidence that it is possible to practice from a health promotion perspective even within this particularly medically dominated environment, for nurses at least (Hills 1998). However, we want to focus our attention in this chapter on the area where health promotion should flourish but has not as yet—primary healthcare. Many who work in health promotion would argue that, in fact, the *Alma Ata Declaration* (WHO 1978) was the precursor for the *Ottawa Charter*. These two documents share the same values, principles, and basic tenets; the *Alma Ata Declaration* addresses health systems more particularly while the *Ottawa Charter* has a broader mandate. But it is their relationship that provides the key to re-orienting health services. That is, primary healthcare is a place for health promotion to focus its energy in terms of re-orienting health services. In fact, the more that health promotion disassociates itself from primary healthcare, the more we give the impression that it is in the domain of medicine, not health. 'The more health promotion becomes distinct from the world of curative care, the more the latter is allowed to continue to be seen as the real work of medicine . . .' (MacDonald 1992).

We want to be clear that when we are talking about primary healthcare, we are not talking about primary care. These terms are often confused or used interchangeably. Primary healthcare refers to the philosophy and principles articulated in the *Alma Ata Declaration* (WHO 1978). It calls for universal access to health services (universality) and the removal of barriers to access such as, geographic, social, economic, or cultural (accessibility); it demands community participation in planning, operation, and evaluation of health services (participation); it requires integration across health and other sectors such as housing, education, and employment; it recognizes the power of multi-disciplinary teams working as equal partners for the health of the community; it focuses on a range of services, determined by the community, that include health promotion, primary prevention, rehabilitative, and curative (essentiality); and, it demands a commitment to equity concerning issues of power and resources (equity and access). Therefore, primary healthcare resists the conceptual and operational separation of treatment and prevention which fits the engineering model of healthcare, with prestige and often scarce resources going to clinical medicine to the neglect of prevention, promotion, and rehabilitation (MacDonald 1992).

People who work in health promotion and understand the philosophy and principles of health promotion must be involved in the development and implementation of primary healthcare. Many people working in health promotion are of the opinion that health promotion and healthcare are distinct and separate entities. They are critical of health promoters who talk about healthcare or health service delivery at the same time that they are talking about health promotion. We have a different opinion: It is necessary, not only to talk but to act as health promoters to facilitate primary healthcare reform.

Besides the *Ottawa Charter* outlining our responsibility to take up this challenge, there are two other reasons why it must be people who work in health promotion who participate in the reorientation of health systems to primary healthcare.

First, the health system is controlled by the powerful. There is a hegemony that supports a predominant treatment/cure paradigm. Power resides in these structures and with the health professionals who work in those systems. So, as advocates for equity and social justice, health promoters have a responsibility to take up this challenge. If we continue to work only in the community where we are comfortable, we will avoid confronting one of the greatest challenges of our times: Creating a health system that is based on the principles of health promotion. We are not neutral in this process. As Paulo Freire (1972) said, 'washing one's hands of the conflict between the powerful and the powerless, means to side with the powerful, not to be neutral'. Kickbusch (1989) confirms this concern. She states, 'herein lies the great historical opportunity and challenge. Maybe health promotion can break the deadlock of the health policy debate that is basically about medical care and provider dominance. It must break this deadlock by redefining the issue of health expenditure. Only in this way could health promotion be attractive to politicians as a social and ecological investment in the future' (p. 14). As she suggests, we are well beyond the burden of proof needed to claim that health promotion is successful—we have demonstrated this through our change in attitudes towards smoking, drinking, and nutrition—even if these are mainly concerns of the middle class and of high-income countries. 'Accountability and the burden of proof should now lie with the medical system to show in detail the payoff that has been received from swallowing 99 per cent of the health budget' (Kickbusch 1989, p.14).

The second reason that health promoters must take up this challenge can be summarized in one question: If health promoters do not advocate for primary healthcare based on the principles of the *Alma Ata Declaration* and the *Ottawa Charter*, what model of primary healthcare will dominate our countries?

Health promotion: History and influences

Health education

Health education plays a profound role in the history of health promotion. While it is true that health promotion is an 'essentially contested concept' claimed by a variety of different interests and actors (Green & Raeburn 1988), many of its most prolific commentators, particularly in the area of health promotion research and knowledge development, have been from the field of health education (Green & Kreuter 2005).

These writers have often been concerned with the failure of traditional health education approaches to help motivate individuals to act on health information. Following Tones, we adopt his definition of health education as: 'Any intentional activity which is designed to achieve health or illness-related learning, that is, some permanent change in an individual's capability or disposition' (Tones 2004: 7). This refers to what knowledge, attitudes, or skills can be acquired by individuals through a variety of health education processes. In relation to health promotion, key health educators have radically restructured the traditional approaches to influencing health behaviour. Most of this work has revolved around challenging what are now seen to be simplistic and mechanical models of health belief and health decision-making. At the centre of this change has been an adoption of the concept of empowerment and an advocacy for using participatory learning processes that break down the power imbalances between health professionals and lay members of society. Crucially, the relationship between devolving control, developing self-esteem, and bridging the gap between knowledge, attitude, and behaviour is highlighted.

In relation to the overall theme of health equity, the move away from traditional health education models has been critical. Without the concept of empowerment, and the development of capacities and self-esteem, the traditional 'health action model' of raising awareness and changing attitudes to health behaviours tended to exacerbate health inequalities, as the 'prepared' middle classes quickly adopted and even fetishized the new healthy practices of more exercise, less smoking, and a healthy diet. The efforts to help population groups that had both the worst health outcomes and the most intransigent health-related social conditions have not been nearly as successful.

A detailed account of these changes can be found in Tones (2004). One very important aspect of his account is how health promoters can learn, as professionals, to overcome the social gap in both power and understanding between them and the groups and individuals they aim to enable and empower. As Tones notes, the 'holy trinity' of counselling (respect, empathy and genuineness) is pertinent here. Often the more socioecological accounts of the health promotion process gloss over this crucial interactive aspect of health promotion. Whether it is with individuals or with groups, health promoters cannot act effectively without using highly developed skills of empathic understanding and facilitation. Particularly with group interactions, where often highly charged community issues are discussed, the professionals striving for neutrality and objectivity, will find themselves unable to cope with the anger and resentment felt by people who perceive a history of grave social injustice behind their 'health' problems. It is important that these basic counselling skills are imparted to health promoters-in-training before they go out into communities and work with them on issues relevant to their health.

This shift in health education from an information-giving, pamphlet distribution approach to an empowerment liberatory approach has brought renewed interest in Freire's emancipatory education paradigm (1972). Health promoters in several countries, most notably those in Brazil, have reclaimed and embraced his basic premises and have employed his dialogical problem-posing teaching strategies that help make health education more consistent with the principles and values of health promotion and the 'new' public health. Freire's (1972) model of empowerment education describes a three-stage methodology consisting of listening, participatory dialogue, and action. The consistency with health promotion is evident. Freire proposes that the main strategy of empowerment education, critical dialogue, requires us to engage in a process of problem posing rather than a process of problem solving. Problem posing is different from problem solving because it does not seek immediate solutions to problems. Rather, generative themes arising from the listening phase are 'codified' and posed as problematics to raise group consciousness about specific issues. Wallerstein and Hammes (1991) contend that this process recognizes the complexity and the time needed to create effective solutions to societal issues. 'An effective code shows a problematic situation that is many sided, familiar to participants and open-ended without solutions' (Wallerstein & Bernstein 1988, p. 383). Freire describes these as 'generative' themes because they generate energy and motivate people to act. Freire contends that, through a process of dialogue that reflects on the generative themes raised through listening, people become 'masters of their thinking by discussing the thinking and views of the world explicitly or implicitly manifest in their own suggestions and those of their comrades' (p. 95). As Wallerstein and Bernstein explain: 'The goal of group dialogue is critical thinking by posing problems in such a way as to have participants uncover root causes of their place in society—the socioeconomic, political, cultural, and historical contexts of personal lives' (p. 382).

Freire cautions that 'the liberating educator has to be very aware that transformation is not just a question of methods and techniques' (p. 35). If that were the case, we could simply substitute one set of methods for another. 'The question is in a different relationship to knowledge and to society' (Freire, p. 35).

Public health

Many health promotion researchers preface their scholarly remarks on the birth and development of health promotion with a discussion of the sometimes tortured relationship of the field to its older, more developed discipline, public health (Kickbusch 1986; Terris 1992). How this history is understood is perhaps the most telling aspect of how health promotion and its progress are viewed as a contemporary phenomenon. The argument developed below is that there has been a tendency within health promotion to tell a story of public health as a 'fall from grace'—a fall from its original reforming, perhaps even zealous, focus on the social and environmental causes of ill health, to a more restrictive, preventive biomedical era, and finally, to a broader scale but narrower scope in the 'lifestyles' approach focused on individual risk factors and behavioural change (Kickbusch 1986). Health promotion steps into the story to herald the era of a 'new public health', as a sort of re-emergence of the spirit of the nineteenth century socioenvironmental model, with a modern gloss on the more subtle socioeconomic determinants of health. The purpose of this critical analysis is to challenge this tendency to nostalgia, and to explicate some of its continuing consequences for health promotion's rather schizophrenic relationship to public health. The 'golden age' of public health was influenced by a particular philosophical and political outlook that still finds its expression today in its most modern and rigorous proponents.

As has already been alluded to, the history of health promotion conventionally begins with the publication of the *Lalonde Report*, entitled 'A new perspective on the health of Canadians' (Lalonde 1974). The report was notable because it was the first high level national government document anywhere in the world to advocate for health promotion as a basic strategy for improving population health. It was influential internationally and it set the stage for future debate with its concept of the *health field* as the articulation of the argument that the medically dominated healthcare system was only one and perhaps the least significant determinant of health, alongside biology, the physical and social environment, and individual lifestyles. The *Lalonde Report* relied explicitly for its argumentation on such critiques of the healthcare system found in 'social medicine' as those comprehensively outlined by McKeown (1976), but which had their roots in the classic public health tradition of William Petty, Johann Frank, Rudolf Virchow and William Farr (White 1991). The Report contains not only the notable (and much commented on) tension between an emphasis on individual lifestyles and the subsequently neglected socioenvironmental factors, but also an equal tension, given its own chapter heading, of 'Science versus Health Promotion'. Here it is made very clear that the 'science base' of the health field concept is epidemiology and, in this context, health promotion is seen as that type of action that must be taken even though the pertinent scientific questions have yet to be definitively answered. In some ways, this attitude allowed some initial breathing space for health promotion to prosper; however, by setting up this dichotomy, it ensured that, eventually, when 'science' made its accounting, health promotion would have its day of reckoning with epidemiology.

Meanwhile, many in the health promotion community, especially in Europe and Canada, were starting to develop an independent conceptual basis for their work, based on a rigorous reflection on the type of actions necessary to most effectively promote the health of individuals and communities. Much of this work evolved out of a complex internal critique of the failure of traditional health education approaches and a more sophisticated understanding of behavioural change (Kickbusch 1986; Tones 1993). Yet, in some countries, such as Canada, the absence of a strong health education tradition contributed strongly to a more socioecological approach to promoting health (with some of its most influential leaders being sociologists and nurses, rather than psychologists and health educators) (Green 2001). Furthermore, for a variety of complex reasons (including, again, individual leadership), much of the discourse of contemporary social movements (new leftist, feminist, gay/lesbian, environmentalist) found its way onto the official agenda of major institutions such as the World Health Organization (WHO) and Health and Welfare Canada (Labonte 1994). As has been recognized by one of the leaders in health promotion internationally, Canada provided a hybrid and fertile mixture of traditional welfare state values and innovative community activism that seemed to provide the perfect ground for a push for the new socioenvironmental approach to health promotion (Kickbusch 1994). Out of this productive interaction between European 'health promotion tourists' (Kickbusch 1986, 1994) and many able Canadian activist/public health practitioners, grew the idea and finally the accomplishment of the *Ottawa Charter for Health Promotion* (1986).

In order to fully understand the impact that the *Charter* had and continues to have, it is important to see that there was a crucial transformation from the epidemiological and bureaucratic dominance of the Lalonde Report to the emerging 'more pluralistic (and messier) social-science paradigm of human and social relations' embedded in the *Ottawa Charter* (Labonte 1994, p. 86). This shift is key to understanding the constant tension between a 'scientific' approach to health promotion and the 'values' underlying the *Charter* that is renewed each occasion that health promoters are asked to more rigorously account for their activities. It raises the uncomfortable question for those who, correctly, see the importance of reconnecting health promotion to the new public health, of just how 'new' the new public health is willing to be, when it comes to its underlying philosophical commitments.

This same tension underlies some of the confusion within the health promotion research community about how to relate to the more recent (Evans & Stoddard 1990) emphasis on 'population health' (Labonte 1997; Poland *et al.* 1998; Raphael & Bryant 2002). On the one hand, there is a justified admiration for the advocates of population health for their influential arguments about socioeconomic determinants of health, even so far as to single out progressive population health researchers such as John Frank (Raphael & Bryant 2002). On the other hand, there is the well-articulated angst about the lack of health promotion principles within the population health perspective. The critiques of the population health perspective for its lack of emphasis on values, its weak or non-existent orientation to action, and its somewhat imperious attitude to what is to count as proper 'knowledge', are all cogent and well-aimed. The question is: Why should this be a surprise? It is not enough to point out and lament the baleful influence of a replacement ideology for health promotion. Where did it come from, and why is it so influential? Furthermore, is this newly emergent approach (Evans & Stoddard 1990) really so new? How far is it simply a modern, sophisticated renaissance of that very same 'golden era' of public health that health promoters so often return to as their intellectual and moral heritage?

Although health promoters themselves (especially Canadians, who were the ones facing this challenge directly) reacted strongly and were able to defend the rationale for keeping a health promotion focus, the more incisive critiques were often too 'reactionary' and came off rhetorically as overly defensive. A more accommodating response came from within Health Canada itself with Hamilton and Bhatti (1996) introducing the concept of *population health promotion*. This was clearly an attempt to marry these two potentially adversarial positions and to cement the term health promotion as an integral component of population health that could not be ignored.

Why is it that health promotion often seems 'behind the game' in the science debate? Partly, this is due to the fact that, as Labonte says and a recent *Companion to Social Theory* attests (Turner 2000) the social science world is 'messy'. However, it may also be partially true that, for too long, health promotion has neglected its need to develop an independent 'science base' having unconsciously bought into that original Lalonde dichotomy. This is becoming increasingly clearer as many of the leading proponents in the field are pushing for more intensive theoretical development, a pressure that has become especially acute as the need for demonstrating effectiveness has increased (McQueen 2001; McQueen & Jones 2007; McQueen & Kickbusch 2007). To understand why health promotion has such a complex and ambiguous relationship to public health, it is necessary to dig more deeply into the foundations of modern public health and to unpack its driving philosophy and world-view.

Politics and philosophy in public health and epidemiology

It is crucial to understand that the roots of the modern public health epidemiologists' focus on individual risk factors and randomized controlled trials (RCTs) is not in contradiction with or a deviation from the Edwin Chadwicks, the John Simons, and the John Snows of the classical public health. Rather, the full flowering of a utilitarian calculus, an uncompromising economism, and an obdurate scepticism of anything but positivistic scientific knowledge, can be seen as the late fruit of more than three centuries of development in public health and epidemiology.

There is a dilemma and *prime facie* paradox that health promotion faces when confronting its genealogy in the history of public health. In terms of lives saved and healthy years lived, the early public health interventions to combat the spread of deadly and debilitating communicable diseases cannot be underestimated. However, it is no accident that once the environmental risk factors of the major communicable diseases were effectively neutralized, a shift in focus took place to providing preventive, immunization measures. As Kerr White (1991) so convincingly puts it, the history of public health and epidemiology can be read as successive and iterative 'redefinings of the unacceptable'. Public health has always been concerned with an economistic and utilitarian approach to the health of the population; when things start to 'cost too much', the unacceptable becomes miraculously 'visible'. To understand this history, one has to ignore the facile disciplinary chasm between public health and economics, a chasm that has only recently and tentatively been bridged (Evans *et al.* 1994). The fact is that, while economics became progressively theoretical and mathematical, public health continued the original classical liberal tradition of reformist, practical utilitarianism, most powerfully apparent in the Benthamite tradition's attempt to rationalize government and public services. There is a great irony that the humanitarian idealism (an idealism at the core of health promotion's values base) of the British 'public health doctors', such as Haygarth, Heysham, Thackrah, Baker, and Millar, was never the driving force behind concentrated public health action (Fraser 1973).

As we will discuss in the section on health promotion and social justice, public health shares with economics a default, often merely implicit, utilitarian ethics. This shared history is seldom acknowledged, but it is a history that health promotion must confront explicitly. Fortunately, and ironically, recent developments in public health have brought into question the utilitarian approach, finding it inadequate, particularly in relation to the question of health inequity (Anand *et al.* 2004). The argument fleshed out below is that health promotion must forcefully engage in helping public health move in the direction advocated for by Amartya Sen and others (Anand *et al.* 2004).

Social movements

In this section, we briefly review one of the constitutive ambiguities at the heart of health promotion—many public health practitioners in the 1970s and early 1980s were increasingly cognizant of the lack of participatory involvement of the 'public' in public health programming.

A strong feature of the so-called 'new social movements' in the post-1968 period was a trenchant critique of bureaucratic structures and an increasingly administered society alongside the traditional leftist critique of capitalism. Some public health institutions, particularly urban public health units, decided to transform local public health practice by integrating a participatory model of programming that was heavily influenced by this anti-bureaucratic critique (Labonté 1994). However, as Dupéré *et al.* (2007) argue, despite its ambitions, health promotion is still not accurately described as a 'social movement', but rather a 'professional movement that had successfully advanced a discourse about health and the production of health'. Yet, despite this acknowledged status, health promoters have recognized that much of their effectiveness depends on very high levels of social engagement. The more recent emphasis on health in the context of globalization (Labonté 2007) makes the necessity for health promotion to engage with larger social movements, particularly on the global development agenda, even more apparent.

Nevertheless, we find health promotion once again suspended between its constitutive desire to become one with the 'community' and its real position as a mediating professional fraction, often acting on behalf of formal public institutions. In the future, health promotion will have to sacrifice some of its cherished professional neutrality to choose sides, especially in its responsibility to advocate for health. While this new form of activist engagement must be balanced with the legitimacy attained from professional status, the balance must shift quite radically, given the growing threats to health represented by the inequity of contemporary societies in a globalized world.

Health promotion, health inequities, and social justice

We have, throughout this chapter, alluded to the commitment health promotion has to the principle of health equity. This is a fundamental and central value for health promoters and is often the touchstone for deciding why, where, and how to enact health promoting practice and policy. Yet, despite this nearly constant refrain, there is still confusion within health promotion about the theoretical and conceptual basis for its concern with health equity. While most, if not all health promoters, would see health equity as a basic goal of health promotion, seldom is the specific normative dimension that underlies this commitment fleshed out. The basic understanding is that health inequities are undesirable and should be eliminated because they are a set of systematic inequalities in health outcomes that are based on *unjust* inequalities of access to resources that provide for health. Here is how the *Health Promotion Glossary* describes what equity in health entails: '. . . That all people have an equal opportunity to develop and maintain their health, through fair and just access to resources for health'.

However, the definition above begs many key questions, such as: What is 'fair' and 'just' access? and, what are 'resources for health'?

While health promoters have often reflected deeply on health inequity, much of the appeal has been to an intuitive basis for supporting the elimination of inequity. We argue that this stance is no longer good enough. Health promotion must fully engage with recent work in political philosophy, particularly in the arguments surrounding the concept of social justice that have been developing since the publication of John Rawls' *A Theory of Justice* (1971). Since Rawls' groundbreaking work, an ongoing debate has taken place concerning what is the proper approach to justice for whole societies (Kymlicka 1990; Aveneri & de-Shalit 1992). More recently this debate has been expanded to consider how we are to think of justice in the global context (Nussbaum 2006). Health promoters should pay close attention to what is at stake in these debates for two reasons:

First, without an awareness of these important arguments, health promotion is liable to accept a default utilitarianism that it inherits from public health, which in turn the latter shares with orthodox economics. It is argued here that this unacknowledged utilitarianism is in direct contradiction to two profound moral intuitions that form the core of health promotion values: That it is wrong to increase overall health at the expense of the least well off; and, that human dignity and personal autonomy are overriding values.

Second, important developments in these debates are directly relevant to concerns with acting on the social determinants of health. Recent arguments have been refined concerning why and how we should address the issue of health inequity, both within and between societies (Anand *et al.* 2004; Nussbaum 2000). As health promoters, charged with the responsibility to advocate, enable, and mediate for equity in health, we should be armed with the very best arguments supporting our position.

We argue here that the most promising theoretical developments in political philosophy that have implications for health promotion are in the evolving 'capabilities' approach to social justice and equity (Nussbaum 2000, 2006; Nussbaum & Sen 1993). This approach most nearly matches the health promotion approach to health as a 'resource for everyday living'; according to this doctrine, the 'social bases for health' would count as a primary good, or capability that should, by right, be provided to all citizens (and by extension, all human beings) at a minimum standard (Nussbaum 2006). Sometimes it is just assumed that arguments for equity in health are unassailable and intuitively obvious. This is wrongheaded on two counts. First, without some substance behind what is meant by equity and what kinds of resources are to be distributed equitably, the demand for equity in health can be dismissed as either empty (meaning nothing in particular) or naïvely utopian (meaning equalizing health outcomes). Second, differing conceptions of what is just will lead to different outcomes in terms of actions to promote health. For example, unless we are very clear, 'equal opportunity' can be understood in an absolute minimalist sense and can allow powerful institutions to continue to support vast inequities in resources for everyday living. As we will see below, how we conceive of social justice has a profound impact on the types of actions we can imagine as solutions to the gross inequities in health we find across the world. Specifically, it has become apparent that the goals of health promotion are intimately related to the goals of a socially just global development agenda. Below we consider two major global efforts underway to address these issues. The first is a broader agenda of global development, led by the United Nations (UN); the second is a WHO-led Commission on the Social Determinants of Health. After reviewing these two efforts, a short reflection is offered on the political-economic context within which these efforts and other health promoting actions take place.

Millennium development goals

We have already presented an argument for the link between health and development. The creation of the Millennium Declaration and the Millennium Development Goals (MDGs) adopted by all

UN Member States in 2000, have become a universal framework for development and a vehicle by which low- and middle-income countries and their development partners can work together 'in pursuit of a shared future for all'.

In a synthesis volume, *Investing in development: A practical plan to achieve the Millennium Development Goals* (Sachs 2005), an independent advisory committee, headed by Professor Jeffrey Sachs, presented its final recommendations to the Secretary-General. This work was completed by 10 thematic Task Forces, each of which also presented its own detailed recommendations. The Task Forces comprised a total of more than 250 experts from around the world including: Researchers and scientists; policymakers; representatives of NGOs, UN agencies, the World Bank, IMF and the private sector. The secretariat plays an important advisory role in assisting low- and middle-income countries to prepare actual strategies for reaching the MDGs.

In the interim report (United Nations 2007) which marks the half way point to the target date, progress on the eight MDGs is described. As the report states, 'the results are, predictably, uneven' (p.4). The report suggests that there are some encouraging results that suggest that progress is being made 'even in those regions where the challenges are greatest'. Progress on each of the goals is described and available on the Web site (http://www.un.org/millenniumgoals/pdf/mdg2007.pdf).

Like most similar reports, the preventative health inequities reported are overwhelming and their impact is devastating. Even more discouraging is a call within the report for high-income countries to scale up their response if we are to have any hope of meeting these goals. Some feel that sub-Saharan Africa will not meet one of the MDGs (Lewis 2005).

The Commission on the social determinants of health: From evidence to action?

The Commission on Social Determinants of Health (CSDH) was established in March 2005 by the late Dr. Lee Jong-Wook, the former Director-General of the WHO, and has the endorsement of the current Director-General, Dr. Margaret Chan. The Commission's vision is 'a world in which all people have the freedom to lead lives they have a reason to value' (CSDH 2007, p. 7). The Commission describes this vision as a matter of social justice, equity, and empowerment. With a focus on action, the Commission is building a global movement for change. It is currently reviewing the global evidence base on health inequity with the intent to take action on the social determinants of health from—'structural conditions of society to the more immediate influences, at all levels from global to local, across government and inclusive of all stakeholders from civil society and the private sector' (p.8). The question that the Commission is ultimately seeking to answer is 'What would social action to tackle these inequities look like?'. Recommendations for action will be made in the Final Report in 2008.

In the interim report (CSDH 2007), the Commission sets out its goals, its plans, and some preliminary reports of evidence produced by the nine thematic knowledge networks that were created to complete this work. These Knowledge Networks include experts from each of the following areas: Globalization, Health Systems, Urban Settings, Employment Conditions, Early Child Development, Social Exclusion, Women and Gender Equity, Measurement and Evidence, and Priority Public Health Conditions. Each of the networks is reviewing evidence of what is known, what works, and why it works. These reports are available on the WHO Web site (http://www.who.int/social_determinants/knowledge_networks/final_reports/en/index.html). The descriptions and statistics contained in these reports are discouraging, to say the least. On a positive note, a critical aspect to the work that is being done by these Networks is the concerted effort to identify potential actions that can be taken to eliminate the staggering level of inequities that are reported. A detailed analysis of this work is included in the final report that is now available (http://www.who.int/social_determinants/final_report/en).

The political economy of health promotion

Much good work has been done on the 'political economy of health' (the analysis of how different politico-economic social structures affect health outcomes), yet an enormous amount is still required (Navarro 2002; Navarro & Shi 2001; Langille 2003; Raphael 2003). Furthermore, there have been some excellent analyses of the 'political economy of healthcare' (the analysis of the effect of different political and economic arrangements on the quality and differential access to health services). In this section, we outline a different question. We ask: What is it about our contemporary political and economic structures that vitiates against the implementation of health promotion strategies and actions as they are conceived in the *Ottawa Charter*?

To begin to answer this question, we need to consider the three fundamental dimensions to health promotion: Empowering communities and individuals, building health public policy, and creating supportive environments.

As has already been argued, empowerment is a key dimension of health promotion. By its very nature, empowerment aims to rebalance existing power arrangements by enabling those currently without power to gain access to the resources necessary to live fulfilled and happy lives. In order to do this with any success, health promoters must do two things: They must have a clear-headed view of existing power structures and relations; and, they must recognize, as professionals, how they themselves fit into those power relations and how they help, often unconsciously, to reproduce them.

Health promotion, to be successful, must rely on concerted action by governments around the world, both within their own territories and in cooperation to address needs that require global action, such as on climate change. However, while these wishes are often articulated (WHO 2005), seldom are we offered an analysis of the structure and dynamics of the contemporary state system in a global context. A more reflective perspective is important here, as theorists of the state argue that certain issues and certain groups, using specific strategies, are more or less likely to be successful changing the nature of hegemonic projects and reversing the direction of state policies (Jessop 2002). Health promotion must become more strategic in how it operates vis-à-vis the state; it must recognize in an explicit way the limitations and opportunities available and must integrate theoretical perspectives and practical actions in regard to one of its key areas: Building health public policy.

Finally, creating a supportive environment is even more wrapped up in the dynamics of global capitalism than all the other areas combined. The fundamental prerequisites for health as outlined in the *Ottawa Charter* are: Peace, shelter, education, food, income, a stable eco-system, sustainable resources, social justice, and equity. These are the elements that, when in adequate supply, make up many of the properties of a supportive environment for health.

Yet, each of these elements is in large part determined by the particular structure and dynamics of our global socioeconomic system.

This entails the necessity for developing an awareness of the fundamental political and economic drivers behind the dynamics of contemporary societies in both the developed and developing worlds. If, as is argued in the section on social justice above, equity in health relies on the fundamental fairness of social, political, and economic institutions, then ignoring these basic realities is no longer an option for a serious approach to health promotion.

These important insights should no longer be gained in an *ad hoc* way, as the peripheral pursuits of a few mavericks in the field, but should be seen as part of what should constitute core knowledge for competent health promoters.

Conclusion

We have chosen, quite explicitly, not to give a technical survey of the health promotion field. There are many excellent sources available that provide the reader with such information (Green & Kreuter 2005; Tones & Green 2004). Recently, two global perspectives on health promotion have been published: One covering substantive areas (Scriven & Garmen 2005); and, one covering technical research problems concerning health promotion effectiveness (McQueen & Jones 2007).

Instead, we have attempted to offer the reader a chance to reflect on a set of core conceptual issues that underlie the health promotion problematic. Below are the five key messages we want to impart about health promotion:

- Health promotion is a complex, often ambiguous concept and set of practices. Yet, in the *Ottawa Charter* health promotion finds its core values and principles; therefore, a careful examination of this core document is still the best way to comprehend the essence of health promotion.
- Health promotion has an intimate connection to health education, with many of its most important and prolific thinkers having a health education background. The revolution in health education practice is directly connected to the birth of health promotion. However, health promotion is more than just this connection and has its roots in the deep history of public health and has been invigorated by contemporary social movements.
- Health promotion is fundamentally about ethics, values and social justice. Only secondarily, is it about technical strategies for behaviour change. The foundational principles of health promotion are *equity*, *participation*, and *empowerment*.
- Health promotion is a professionally dominated movement. This requires health promotion professionals to be critical and reflexive in their practice; they must acknowledge power imbalances that favour professional dominance and work to restore power to individuals and communities.
- Health promotion must take its duty to enable people to control the determinants of their health seriously. To do this it must engage more directly with contemporary arguments in political philosophy and it must be aware of the dynamics of the global political economy and its effect on the potential for health promotion.

Some of these issues are well known, such as the problem of professional dominance; while others, such as the political economy of health promotion, or the engagement with political philosophy are areas that are either not addressed at all, or at least require much deeper reflection.

We have argued that, at its heart, health promotion is about a radical shift in values for public health. It is not that public health was never concerned with equality or alleviating the misery of the poor; arguably, the so-called 'golden age' was driven by exactly these moral questions. However, these intuitive commitments were not sufficiently followed through when it came to not just *what* outcomes to change but *how* to change them. Too much of public health, for too long, was driven by a benevolent paternalism that, particularly when it came to dealing with chronic diseases and with vulnerable populations, ended up being counter-productive. Indeed, not only was this paternalism ineffective in many areas, it was unethical. It assumed the authority of experts and professionals, not only to determine technical solutions, but to determine needs. We have learned that, if we are to take the concepts of equity and empowerment seriously and follow them through, they have profound implications for how we do public health interventions. We have learned that by addressing needs without first establishing a participatory framework that enables individuals and communities to determine those needs for themselves, we fatally undermine one of the most crucial capacities for health: Human dignity and self-respect. In relation to people living in communities that have suffered historical social injustices, this kind of paternalism further undermines dignity, and thus self-respect. As Richard Sennett says, people subjected to this disempowering process, experience 'that peculiar lack of respect which consists of not being seen, not being accounted as full human beings' (Sennett 2003).

We hope to have demonstrated that there are many barriers to realizing this change in power relations; yet, at the same time, there are very important opportunities, such as with the MDGs and the Commission on the Social Determinants of Health, where there is an increasing clamour for action to redress health inequities through empowering processes. It is notable that even the World Bank, often the subject of brutal criticism for exacerbating inequalities (Stiglitz 2003), has recently made significant moves toward recognizing the importance of reducing inequity in human development and has integrated an empowerment approach (World Bank 2006). It remains to be seen whether these gains can be translated into major policy changes and followed through with implementation; nevertheless, it is at this level where health promoters and all public health practitioners and researchers must have a strong advocacy position.

We hope that it is apparent that, in our interpretation, health promotion is much more than a set of technical public health interventions aimed at revamping traditional health education for the twenty-first century. We cannot let go of the core competencies built up by health education and other contributing fields, but we cannot be limited in our vision either. Health promotion has to face up to the fact that, while it may only be a junior partner in the global struggle to develop a more just and equitable world, when it comes to a key human capability and resource, *health*, it must take a lead role in making the argument for equity, develop and present the evidence for what *action* is necessary to achieve equity in health, and finally, to hold the powerful accountable where they fail to live up to the demands of justice for health. Embedded in health promotion is an ethical imperative to act ethically and justly. In this case, unlike most, there is no choice.

References

Anand, S., Peter, F., and Sen, A. (eds.)(2004). *Public health, ethics, and equity.* Oxford University Press, Oxford.

Aveneri, S. and de-Shalit, A. (eds.) (1992). *Communitarianism and individualism.* Oxford University Press, Oxford.

Baum, F. (2007). Cracking the nut of health equity: Top down and bottom up pressure for action on the social determinants of health. *Promotion & Education*, **14**, 90–95.

Berman, M. (1982). *All that is solid melts into air.* Penguin Books, New York.

Craig, G. (2005). Community capacity-building: Definitions, scope, measurements and critiques. OECD Paper, Prague, Czech Republic, 8 December 2005.

Commission on the Social Determinants of Health (2007). *Achieving health equity: From root causes to fair outcomes.* WHO, Geneva.

Dupéré, S., Ridde, V., Carroll, S. *et al.* (2007).

Conclusion: The rhizome and the tree. In *Health Promotion in Canada* (eds. M. O'Neill, A. Pederson, S. Dupéré and I. Rootman), pp. 371–88. Canadian Scholar's Press, Toronto.

Evans, R., Barer, M., and Marmor, T. (eds.)(1994). *Why are some people healthy and others not?* Aldine de Gruyter, New York.

Evans, R. and Stoddart, G. (1990). Producing health, consuming health care. *Social Science & Medicine*, **31**, 1347–63.

Fraser, D. (1973). *The evolution of the British welfare state.* Macmillan Press Ltd, London.

Freire, P. (1972). *Pedagogy of the oppressed.* Penguin, Harmondsworth.

Godin, G. (2007). Has the individual vanished from Canadian health promotion?. In *Health Promotion in Canada* (eds. M O'Neill, A. Pederson, S. Dupéré, and I. Rootman), pp. 367–70, Canadian Scholar's Press, Toronto.

Green, L. and Raeburn, J. (1988). Health promotion. What is it? What will it become? *Health Promotion International*, **3**, 151–9.

Green, L. and Kreuter, M. (2005). *Health promotion planning: An educational and ecological approach.* McGraw-Hill Higher Education, Toronto.

Hamilton, N. and Bhatti, T. (1996). *Population health promotion: An integrated model of population health and health promotion.* Health Promotion Development Division, Public Health Agency of Canada, Ottawa. Available at: http://www.phac-aspc.gc.ca/ph-sp/phdd/php/php.htm Accessed 7 February 2008.

Hartrick, G., Lindsey, A., and Hills, M. (1994). Family nursing assessment: meeting the challenge of health promotion. *Journal of Advanced Nursing*, **20**, 85–91.

Held, D., McGrew, A., Goldblatt, D. *et al.* (1999) *Global transformations.* Polity Press, Oxford.

Hills, M. (1998). Student experiences of nursing health promotion practice in hospital settings. *Nursing Inquiry*, **5**, 164–73.

Hills, M., Mullett, J., and Carroll, S. (2007). Community-based participatory research: Transforming multi-disciplinary practice in primary health care. *Revista Panamericana de Salud Publica/ Pan American Journal of Public Health*, **21**, 125–35.

Jessop, R. (2002) *The Future of the Capitalist State.* Polity Press, Cambridge.

Kickbusch, I. (1986). Health promotion: A global perspective. *Canadian Journal of Public Health*, **77**, 321–6.

Kickbusch, I. (1989). Back to the future: Moving public health into the 90's. Proceedings from National Symposium on Health Promotion, 1–5. BC Ministry of Health.

Kickbusch, I. (1994). Introduction: Tell me a story. In *Health promotion in Canada: Provincial, national & international perspectives* (eds. A.Pederson, M. O'Neill, and I. Rootman), pp. 8–17. WB Saunders Canada, Toronto.

Kickbusch, I. (2007). Health promotion: Not a tree but a rhizome. In *Health Promotion in Canada,* (eds. M. O'Neill, A. Pederson, S. Dupéré, and I. Rootman), pp. 363–6. Canadian Scholar's Press, Toronto.

Kemm, J. (2006). Health impact assessment and Health in All Policies. In *Health in all policies: Prospects and potentials* (eds. T. Ståhl, M. Wismar, E. Ollila, E. Lahtinen, and K. Leppo) Ministry of Social Affairs and Health, Helsinki, Finland.

Kok, G., Van Den Borne, B., and Dolan Mullen, P. (1997). Effectiveness of health education and health promotion: Meta-analyses of effect studies and determinants
of effectiveness. *Patient Education and Counseling*, **30**, 19–27.

Kymlicka, W. (1990). *Contemporary political philosophy: An introduction.* Oxford University Press, Oxford.

Labonté, R. (1993). Community development and partnerships. *Canadian Journal of Public Health*, **84**, 237–40.

Labonté, R. (1994). Death of program, birth of metaphor: The development of health promotion in Canada. In *Health promotion in Canada: Provincial, national & international perspectives* (eds. A. Pederson, M. O'Neill, and I. Rootman), pp. 72–90. WB Saunders Canada, Toronto.

Labonte, R. (1997). The population health/health promotion debate in Canada: The politics of explanation, economics and action. *Critical Public Health.* **7** (1 and 2), 7–27.

Labonté, R. (2007). Promoting health in a globalized world: The biggest challenge of all? In *Health Promotion in Canada* (eds. M. O'Neill, A. Pederson, S. Dupéré, and I. Rootman), pp. 207–22. Canadian Scholar's Press, Toronto.

Lalonde, M.(1974). *A New Perspective on the Health of Canadians.* Health and Welfare Canada, Ottawa.

Langille, D. (2003). The political determinants of health. In *Social determinants of health: Canadian perspectives* (ed. D. Raphael), pp. 283–96. Canadian Scholar's Press, Toronto.

Lewis, S. (2005). *Race against time.* Anansi Press, Toronto.

MacDonald, J. (1992). *Primary health care: Medicine in its place.* Earthscan Publications Ltd., London, UK.

McKeown, T. (1976). *The role of medicine: Dream, mirage or nemesis.* Nuffield Provincial Hospitals Trust, London.

McQueen, D. (2001). Strengthening the evidence base for health promotion. *Health Promotion International*, **16**, 261–8.

McQueen, D. and Jones, C. (eds.) (2007). *Global perspectives on health promotion effectiveness.* Springer Publications, New York, NY.

McQueen, D., Kickbusch, I., Potvin, L. *et al.* (2007). *Health and modernity: The role of theory in health promotion.* Springer Publications, New York, NY.

Minkler, M. (1990). Improving health through community organization. In *Health behavior and health education* (eds. K. Glanz, F. Lewis, and B. Rimer), Jossey-Bass, San Francisco, CA.

Navarro, V. (ed.)(2002). *The political economy of social inequalities: Consequences for health and quality of life.* Baywood Press, Amityville.

Navarro, V. and Shi, L. (2001). The political context of social inequalities and health. *Social Science & Medicine*, **52**, 481–91.

Nussbaum, M. (2000). *Women and human development.* Cambridge University Press, Cambridge.

Nussbaum, M. (2006). *Frontiers of justice: Disability, nationality, dpecies membership.* Harvard University Press, Cambridge, MA.

Nussbaum, M. and Sen, A. (eds.)(1993). *The quality of life.* Clarendon Press, Oxford.

Poland, B., Coburn, D., Robertson, A. *et al.* (1998). Wealth, equity, and health care: A critique of a population health perspective on the determinants of health. *Social Science & Medicine*, **46**, 785–98.

Raeburn, J. and Rootman, I. (2007). A new appraisal of the concept of health. In *Health promotion in Canada* (eds. M. O'Neill, A. Pederson, S. Dupéré, and I. Rootman), pp. 19–32. Canadian Scholar's Press, Toronto.

Raphael, D. (ed.)(2003). *Social determinants of health: Canadian perspectives.* Canadian Scholar's Press, Toronto.

Raphael, D. and Bryant, T. (2002). Putting the population into population health. *Canadian Journal of Public Health*, **91**, 9–12.

Rawls, J. (1971). *A theory of justice.* Harvard University Press, Cambridge, MA. Rootman, I. and Raeburn, J. (1994). The concept of health. In *Health promotion in Canada: Provincial, national & international perspectives* (eds. A. Pederson, M. O'Neill, and I. Rootman), pp. 72–90. WB Saunders Canada, Toronto.

Sachs, J. (2005). *Investing in development: A Practical plan to achieve the Millennium Development Goals: Report to the Secretary General.* United Nations, New York.

Sennett, R. (2003). *Respect: The formation of character in an age of inequality.* Penguin, London.

Shor, I. and Freire, P. (1987). *A pedagogy for liberation: Dialogues on transforming education.* Bergin & Garvey Publishers, South Hadley, MA.

Ståhl, T., Wismar, M., Ollila, E. (eds.)(2006). *Health in all policies: Prospects and potentials.* Ministry of Social Affairs and Health, Helsinki, Finland.

Stiglitz, J. (2003). *Globalization and its discontents.* WW Norton & Company, New York.

Terris, M. (1992). Concepts of health promotion: Dualities in public health theory. *Journal of Public Health Policy,* **13**, 267–76.

Tones, K. (1993). Changing theory and practice: Trends in methods, strategies and settings in health education. *Health Education,* **52**, 125–39.

Tones, K. (2004). Health promotion, health education, and the public health. In *The Oxford Textbook of Public Health* (eds. R. Detel, J. Mcewen, R. Beaglehole, and H. Tanaka). Oxford University Press, Oxford.

Tones, K. and Green, L. (2004). *Health promotion: Planning and strategies.* Sage, London.

Tones, K. and Tilford, S. (1994). *Health promotion: Effectiveness, efficiency and equity.* Chapman and Hall, London.

Turner, B. (ed.)(2000). *The Blackwell companion to social theory.* Blackwell Publishers, Malden, MA.

United Nations (2007). *The Millenium Development Goals Report.* United Nations, New York.

Wallerstein, N. and Bernstein, E. (1988). Empowerment education: Freire's ideas adapted to health education. *Health Education Quarterly,* **15**, 379–84.

Wallerstein, N. and Hammes, M. (1991). Problem posing: A teaching strategy for improving the decision-making process, *Health Education,* **22**, 250–3.

White KL (1991). *Healing the schism: epidemiology, medicine, and the public's health.* Springer-Verlag Inc., New York.

Wise, M. and Nutbeam, D. (2007). Enabling health systems transformation: What progress has been made in re-orienting health services? *Promotion & Education* (Suppl 2), 23–7.

World Health Organization (1946). *Constitution.* WHO, Geneva.

World Health Organization (1978). *Declaraction of Alma-Ata.* Paper presented at the International Conference on Primary Health Care, Alma-Ata, USSR.

World Health Organization (1984). *Health Promotion: A discussion document on the concept and principles.* WHO, European Regional Office for Europe.

World Health Organization (1986). *Ottawa Charter for Health Promotion.* WHO, Ottawa.

World Health Organization (1998). *Health Promotion Glossary.*WHO, Geneva

World Health Organization (2005). *The Bangkok Charter for Health Promotion in a* Globalized World. WHO, Geneva.

World Bank (2006). *World bank development report 2006: Equity and development.*

World Bank, Washington, D.C.

7.4

Cost-effectiveness analysis: Concepts and applications

Dean T. Jamison

Introduction

Cost-effectiveness analyses (or CEAs) in health describe interventions in terms of their cost per unit of health gain that they provide. Deaths averted provides a measure of health gain but CEAs typically use measures that take account of both years and quality of life gained. Cost and effects are typically measured from the perspective of society as a whole but other perspectives are possible. Broadly speaking CEAs are used in two distinct ways: One use provides an input into a (usually public sector) decision maker about whether to alter intervention mix or change intervention coverage levels. The second is to inform broader generalizations about health policy. This chapter provides an overview of the methods currently in use to undertake CEAs and provides an extended example—based on the Disease Control Priorities Project—that illustrates both uses.

Many of the world's poorest countries spend under US$10 per person per year on health services. High-income countries spend thousands of dollars per year. Yet across this entire expenditure range questions arise about value gained for money spent on health. Most poor countries suffer huge burdens from some mix of childhood infection, malaria, maternal deaths, tuberculosis, and HIV/AIDS. Highly effective interventions exist to address most (but not all) of these conditions. If a few additional dollars per year were available, misspending those dollars on interventions offering relatively little health gain for the money would entail lost opportunities to postpone many deaths and prevent much serious disability. High- income countries, too, face choices: Could an improved mix of interventions reduce overall costs (or at least their rate of growth) while maintaining existing levels of health? Which of the effective but usually costly new interventions emerging from the R&D pipeline should public or private insurance plans cover? Rationing of healthcare is part of our future and, in many cases, our present (Maynard & Bloom 1998).

Concern, then, with value for money (or cost-effectiveness) spans income levels. Neither is the issue one principally for the private sector, for non-governmental organizations or for the public sector. Each has a potential interest. Analysts have responded to this interest over a period of several decades and produced a substantial literature on both methods and results. The purpose of this chapter is to introduce the reader to this literature. It is often said that 'Prevention is more cost-effective than cure' or 'Tertiary facilities are not cost-effective in low-income countries'. One application of CEA involves generation of the cost-effectiveness generalizations that would support or undermine such propositions. In the second major application of CEA, analysts assess options for dealing with a particular problem—options involving scale of intervention or choice of technique. Discussion in this chapter covers both these applications.

The chapter begins with a brief discussion of background and terminology, then describes methods of cost-effectiveness analysis (hereafter CEA). The chapter then illustrates use of the methods with an application that provides a sense of results.

Background

Cost-effectiveness analysis in health comprises one part of a very much larger literature on project appraisal, i.e. on assessment of the economic desirability of alternative 'projects' from a social perspective. Another important part of this literature deals with the questions of when public sector finance is most appropriate. CEAs provide relevant information to either public or private sector decision makers by indicating the cost to them of alternatives for buying better health, information that is relevant independent of the source of finance. That said, the chapter's perspective is particularly relevant to situations where public finance is justified on grounds of avoiding insurance market failures and is explicitly designed to crowd out private spending on interventions the public sector finances for all (as in all high-income countries except the US). Table 7.4.1 lists three approaches to the economic appraisal of projects or interventions and indicates their realm of applicability.

Cost-minimization analysis examines the costs of alternative approaches to achieving a quite specific objective, e.g. the cost per infant death averted or per new HIV infection averted. The purpose is to identify the least cost way of achieving the objective and to see how both cost and choice of technique vary as the magnitude of the objective varies. (For example if one had very modest goals with respect to prevention of HIV infection the least cost approach might very well be blood screening in hospitals; more substantial goals would entail addition of more costly programmes—e.g. STD treatment, condom use—to achieve the goal at minimum total cost. Note that in this example, as will often be the case, the *average* cost per HIV infection averted will rise as the target number of infections averted rises.) Cost-minimization analysis has the virtues

Table 7.4.1 Choice of economic appraisal techniques

Economic appraisal technique	Applicability for assessing			
	Options to achieve a specific objective	**Options throughout the health sector**	**Options inside and outside the health sector**	**Intrinsic value**
1. Cost-minimization analysis	Yes	No	No	No
2. Cost-effectiveness analysis (sometimes called cost-utility analysis)	Yes	Yes	No	No
3. Cost-benefit analysis	Yes	Yes	Yes	Yes

of specificity and of ease of communication concerning results. The disadvantage becomes apparent if there is need to compare the attractiveness of efforts to reduce infant mortality rate with those to avert HIV infections: Costs can be compared but outcomes remain incommensurable.

Cost-benefit analysis, in contrast, allows comparison of projects (or interventions or investments) across the entire economy. It does so by placing monetary values on outcomes as well as inputs. Kilowatt-hours of electricity can be compared to kilograms of rice by multiplying each by its price to obtain a total value. The simple word 'price' conceals vast complexities, however, particularly when used to measure social benefits. There is an extensive literature on the theoretical methods as well as applications in different contexts of monetary valuation of benefits. Benefits and costs occur over time—with benefits usually following costs—and alternative figures of merit (e.g. present value of net benefits or the internal rate-of-return) generate orderings of outcomes by desirability. Squire (1989) and Layard and Glaister (1994) provide excellent overviews of the methods of cost-benefit analysis and the related literature. Viscusi and Aldy (2003) review the now-extensive literature on valuation of changes in annual mortality probabilities (or on the 'value of a statistical life'). Lomborg (2007) has coordinated cost-benefit analyses for a broad range of sectors, including health (Jamison 2007) in order to create a 'Copenhagen Consensus' of where the greatest benefits would accrue to social investment.

Practical difficulties associated with monetary valuation of benefits often lead analysts to utilize the much simpler methods of cost-minimization (with the concomitant limits on applicability of the results). In addition to practical difficulties there is the more fundamental problem, in assessing health intervention options, of placing dollar value on human life (or other health outcomes). Sometimes this can be noncontroversial as when Levin *et al.* (1993) use labour productivity increases associated with reducing anaemia to derive benefit measures to weigh against the costs of anaemia control. Their findings—of high dollar benefits relative to dollar costs—can either be compared with findings for interventions in other sectors or, more important, to assess intrinsic value: If benefits exceed costs the intervention is worth doing (ignoring deadweight loss from taxation and possible public sector fiscal constraints). If one can overcome practical and other problems with cost-benefit analysis its results have the virtue of standing alone in the sense of indicating intervention desirability independently of comparison to alternatives.

In the health sector, *cost-effectiveness analysis* lies between cost-minimization analysis and cost-benefit analysis (Table 7.4.1). CEA rests on a non-financial metric that will allow comparisons across the health sector. The concepts most typically used are those of the quality-adjusted life-year (QALY) or the disability-adjusted life year (DALY), which can be measured in many ways, but which then—by assigning, for example, a DALY value both to an HIV infection averted and to an infant death averted—allows costs per DALY to be compared for interventions addressing a broad range of problems. Even focussing analysis to within the health sector cannot be completely done by CEA, however. Some interventions that may be undertaken principally for health reasons, such as reducing ambient air pollution, have other outcomes, in this case reduced pollution-related corrosion and the amenity value of clean air. These outcomes elude the DALY metric but must explicitly be listed as inputs to the decision-making process.

This chapter focuses on CEA. That said, work on cost minimization will often in practice prove essential to CEA. Likewise empirical observations of what societies appear prepared to pay for a DALY, or more frequently to avert a death (which can be converted to DALYs), have increasingly been undertaken. These estimates of the value of a statistical life allow CEAs to be immediately translated into cost-benefit analyses. From experience it can be suggested that an explicit valuation of human life for cost-benefit analysis usually generates reactions that distract from a discussion of improving efficiency of resource allocation in the health sector. The interested reader, however, can turn to Viscusy and Aldy (2003) for a valuable review of the monetary valuation of health outcomes.

Part of the value of undertaking CEA lies in the ability to formulate generalizations—or to indicate their inapplicability. Doing so requires care and consistency concerning the definitions that underlie the generalizations, and this chapter attempts to be quite explicit. Table 7.4.2 provides a number of important definitions and distinctions that will be used later in the chapter. Perhaps the central point to note in Table 7.4.2 is the distinction between 'interventions' *per se* and the 'instruments of policy' that can encourage (or discourage) intervention or intended behaviour change. Although most CEAs concern intervention, some concern instruments of policy. More is needed concerning the latter which, after all, is what government can implement.

CEAs in the literature vary substantially in their underlying methodologies and assumptions and, in consequence, comparisons are frequently difficult. Yet without comparability of substantial numbers of interventions, the relative attractiveness of individual interventions remains uncertain and generalizations are difficult or impossible. To define best practice in methods and to provide a template for comparative studies, the US Public Health Service convened a major review panel in 1993. Gold *et al.* (1996) report its conclusions. Discussion in this chapter for the most part follows the Public Health Service guidelines. Garber (1999) and Newmann (2005) provide more extensive discussions of the theory, methods,

Table 7.4.2 Interventions and instruments of policy[1]

1. *Intervention categories*

The term 'intervention' is used to denote actions taken by or for individuals to reduce the risk, duration, or severity of an adverse health condition. Interventions are the proximal cause of deliberate changes in risks, duration, or severity. Instruments of policy (see below) encourage, discourage, or undertake interventions. Stopping smoking, for example, is an intervention that an individual can take to reduce risk from a range of diseases; taxing tobacco products is a potential instrument of government policy to encourage this intervention. Interventions are divided into those that are 'population-based' and those that are 'personal'.[2]

1.1 *Personal interventions* are directed to individuals and can be provided at home, at clinics (community, private, work-based, or school-based), at district hospitals, or at referral hospitals.

a) Primary prevention aims to reduce the level of one or more identified risk factors in order to reduce the probability of the initial occurrence of a disease (e.g. medication for established hypertension to prevent stroke or MI).

b) Cure of a condition aims to remove its cause and restore function to the *status quo ante*.

c) Acute management consists of time-limited interventions that decrease the severity of acute events or the level of established risk factors to minimize their long-term effect (e.g. thrombolytics for acute MI or angioplasty to reduce stenosis in coronary arteries).

d) Secondary prevention (or chronic care) consists of ongoing interventions aimed at decreasing the severity and frequency of recurrent events of chronic or episodic diseases (e.g. SSRIs for severe unipolar depression).

e) Rehabilitation aims to restore (or partially restore) physical, psychological, or social function resulting from a previous condition.

f) Palliation aims to reduce pain and suffering from a condition for which no means of cure or rehabilitation is currently available (this may range from the use of aspirin from headaches to the use of opiates to control terminal cancer pain).

1.2 *Population- based primary prevention* is directed toward entire populations or population subgroups. These interventions fall into three broad categories:

a) Personal behaviour change;

b) control of environmental hazards; or

c) population-oriented medical interventions (e.g. immunization, mass chemoprophylaxis, and screening and referral).

2. *Instruments of policy*

These are the activities that can (potentially) be undertaken by governments or other entities that wish to encourage or discourage interventions, or, importantly, to expand the menu of potential intervention. We distinguish five major instruments of policy:

2.1 Use of *information, education, and communication* (IEC) seeks to improve the knowledge of individuals (and service providers) about the consequences of their choices.

2.2 Use of *taxes and subsidies* on commodities, services, and pollutants seeks to effect appropriate behavioural responses.

2.3 Use of *regulation and legislation* seeks to limit availability of certain commodities, to curtail certain practices, and to define the rules governing finance and provision of health services.

2.4 Use of *direct expenditures* seeks to provide (or finance provision of) selected interventions (e.g. immunizations), to provide infrastructure (e.g. medical schools) that facilitates provision of a range of interventions or to provide infrastructure that influences behaviour (e.g. speed bumps).

2.5 Undertaking *research and development* (or encouraging them through subsidies) is an instrument central to the goal of expanding the range of interventions available and reducing their cost.

[1] This table was prepared with Thomas Gaziano and Sonbol Shahid-Salles.

[2] The International Epidemiology Association's *Dictionary of Epidemiology* (Last 1988) provides a helpful discussion of different types of preventive intervention but, interestingly, has no entries for 'cure' or 'rehabilitation'. Their term 'tertiary prevention', which is not used here, seems to encompass both 'rehabilitation' and 'palliation', as we define those terms.

and uses of CEA than is appropriate for this chapter, and the interested reader is referred to those reviews.

Assessing the cost-effectiveness of intervention

This section contains a discussion of general issues associated with choosing interventions, that is, with criteria for cost-effective choice. The nature of the instruments open to government to promote cost-effective intervention was delineated in Table 7.4.2. The purpose is not to provide an account of the (many) methodological issues associated with economic assessment of intervention options; rather it is simply to describe the basic concepts being applied, raise a few particular issues, and refer the reader to the relevant literature. In addition to the comprehensive work for the Public Health Service that was just mentioned, valuable additional background may be found in Drummond *et al.* (2005).

Cost-effectiveness analysis broadly and narrowly construed

A starting point for cost-effectiveness analysis broadly construed is to observe that health systems have two objectives: (1) To improve the level and distribution of health outcomes in the population, and (2) to protect individuals from financial risks that are often very substantial and that are frequent causes of poverty (WHO 1999, 2000). Financial risk results from illness-related loss of income as well as expenditures on care; the loss can be ameliorated by preventing illness or its progression and by using appropriate financial architecture for the system.

We can also consider two classes of resources to be available: Financial resources and health system capacity. To implement an intervention in a population, the system uses some of each resource. Just as some interventions have higher dollar costs than others, some interventions are more demanding of system capacity than others. In countries with limited health system capacity, it is clearly important to select interventions that require relatively little of such capacity. Human resource capacity constitutes a particularly important aspect of system capacity. Figure 7.4.1 illustrates this broadly construed vision of CE and, in its shaded region, the more narrow (standard) approach for which quantitative estimates are available. Jamison (2006) discusses further.

Although in the very short run little trade-off may exist between dollars and human resources or system capacity more generally, investing in *the development of such capacity can help make more of that resource available in the future*. An important mechanism for strengthening capacity, inherent in highly outcome-oriented programmes, may simply be to use it successfully—learning by doing.

In practice, however, literature on economic evaluation of health projects typically reports the cost per unit of achieving some measure of health outcome—QALYs or DALYs or deaths averted—and at times addresses how that cost varies with the level of intervention and other factors. This corresponds to the shaded box in Fig. 7.4.1. Pritchard (2004) and Newman (2005) provide valuable introductions to this literature. Cost-effectiveness calculations provide important insights into the economic attractiveness of an intervention, but other considerations—such as consequences for financial protection and demands on health system capacity—need to be borne in mind.

As previously indicated it is useful to consider two distinct uses for CEA. One is to inform broad policy generalizations and the other is to help assess the relative attractiveness of changes in the scale of implementation of an intervention or in the technique for addressing a specific problem. In either case the analyst must specify a base case and define the intervention as a change from that base. For policy generalizations it will typically be useful to include consideration of large changes; for addressing specific problems more modest increments will be typical. The natural base case for dealing with specific problems will usually be the status quo, and what is to be considered as 'given' for the purpose of analysis will usually be substantial (although dependent on time frame). Establishing a base case for policy generalizations is less obvious. Guidelines developed at WHO (Murray *et al.* 2000) suggest using the '. . . null set of related interventions'. Substantial practical difficulties are likely to be associated with ascertaining the consequences of no intervention, and the utility to a policy maker of trying to imagine a starting point so different from her own may be limited. In most cases a more natural approach will be to identify base cases close to current reality for policy makers in a number of paradigmatic circumstances. Incremental cost-effectiveness assessments from those bases will then provide more naturally interpretable information. In this context it will often prove important to explicitly consider the effects of doing less than is being done in the base case, thereby generating negative costs and negative effects. Such 'negative intervention' may prove highly cost-effective.[1]

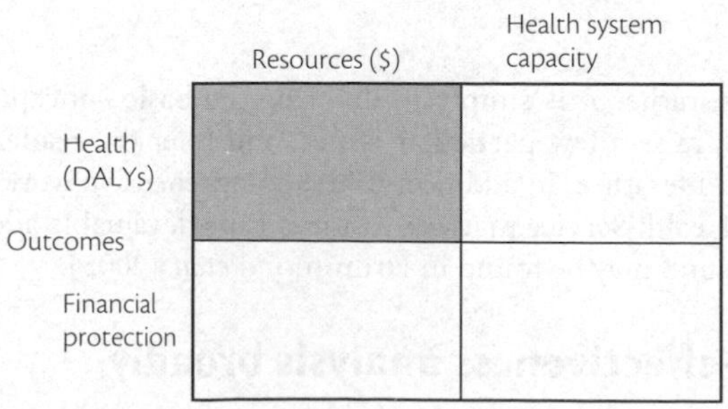

Note: The shaded box represents the domain of traditional cost-effectiveness analysis.

Fig. 7.4.1 Intervention costs and effects—a more general view.

Outcome measurement: Disability-adjusted life-years (DALYs)

A critical choice in applications of economic analysis to resource allocation is that of whether to value outcomes because of their economic benefits or because of some more proximal effectiveness measure (Table 7.4.1). To provide a clearer sense of the context for CEA it is worth a brief additional discussion of approaches to monetary valuation of health outcomes. When there are good markets for products or labour, benefits can be assessed in monetary terms by using market prices to value benefits as well as to value costs. Even when willingness-to-pay valuation cannot be assessed directly because of lack of market prices, as is often true in the health sector, questions in surveys are increasingly being used to elicit information about hypothetical willingness-to-pay (or contingent valuation). Pervasive problems of consumer ignorance of effectiveness of intervention and a widespread tendency for individuals systematically to underestimate risks (Weinstein 1989) suggest that willingness-to-pay assessments will need to be used with caution when applied to health. An alternative approach—sometimes called the human capital approach—is to view health investments as instrumental to improving economic productivity; estimates of the effect of a health intervention on productivity thus provide a lower bound to total benefits. One example comes from assessing the effect on the productivity of rubber plantation workers of correcting iron deficiencies (Levin *et al.* 1993); other examples come from assessment of the effect on economic productivity of malaria control efforts. It is worth noting that both willingness-to-pay and human capital approaches inevitably imply different values to be attached to the life of different individuals of the same age in the same country—and even greater variation across countries. Phelps and Mushlin (1991) and Garber (1999) further discuss the close relation between cost-effectiveness and cost-benefit analyses.

More typically, however, outcomes will be assessed in deaths or disability averted, rather than dollars, and the task is to come up with some measure for making such an assessment that allows comparisons across the health sector (i.e. that allows CEA), even if intersectoral comparisons (cost-benefit analyses) remain infeasible or subject to excessive ethical debate. There is now a valuable literature on how effectiveness measures to aggregate the disability-, morbidity-, and premature mortality-averting effects of interventions across the health sector might be constructed and applied. The most widely used measures are the (closely related) DALY and QALY, for disability or quality-adjusted life year. The DALY, in addition to providing the effectiveness measures for cost-effectiveness analyses, can be used with epidemiological information to assess the burden of disease in a population, as has been done for the major regions of the world (Murray *et al.* 1994; most recently updated in Lopez *et al.* 2006). Table 7.4.3 sets forth the characteristics of the main approaches to disability weighting that serve as the core of effectiveness measurement. Stouthard *et al.* (1997) provide a clear exposition of methods for disability weighting with an informative application for the Netherlands. From a practical perspective, the use of ratings based on expert judgement is probably the best that can now be done if the purpose of the analysis is to compare interventions across the sector. It is also worth noting that the construction of DALYs or QALYs requires value judgements, although they are less subject to controversy than is explicit valuation of human life. (Even measures involving mortality only, e.g. numbers of deaths averted, while they appear to be value-free, if used to measure intervention effectiveness or disease burden, rest on strong value judgements. Minimally a mortality-based measure rests on the implicit value assumption that disability is not a concern. Chapman *et al.* 2004 argue that usually, in practice, inclusion of disability weights affects relatively few cost-effectiveness analyses.)

A workable measure for effectiveness for most CEAs will be DALYs gained. The DALY gain associated with averting a death at a given age is, simply, the life expectancy at that age, with life-years gained in the future discounted back to the present (typically at a discount rate of 3 per cent per annum). Life expectancy at a given age is calculated relative to a standard low-mortality population, e.g. Japan. Unhealthy life-years are given lower weights than healthy ones, depending on degree of disability (assessed by one of the rating procedures listed in Table 7.4.3) so that the effectiveness of interventions to address morbidity or disability can be measured in terms that permit comparison with interventions that avert mortality. The QALY and DALY measures now used are particular forms of the more general concept introduced by Zeckhauser and Shepard (1976).[2] Garber and Phelps (1997) provide the basic theoretical underpinnings for cost-effectiveness analyses in health that adjust life-years for quality, and, in particular, they point to conditions allowing a dollar value to be assigned to a QALY so that, if desired, a CEA can be directly reinterpreted as a cost-benefit analysis.

Timing of outcomes can be dealt with through discounting. Johannesson (1992) provides a general discussion of discounting healthy life-years, and Cropper *et al.* (1992) report empirical assessments of time preference for saving lives. Most analysts value years of healthy life at all ages equally; this assumption can be readily relaxed, however, to give greater weight to different age. The initial variant of the QALY did provide greater relative weight to middle-aged people, but the DALY can (but need not) weight

Table 7.4.3 Alternative approaches to measuring outcomes

Approach to measurement	Cost of implementation	Possible bias	Example or application
Mortality			
Deaths averted	Very low	Highly biased against conditions involving disability; equally weights death in very old age and in middle age	Assessment of priorities in child survival (Walsh and Warren 1979)
Years of potential life lost	Very low	Highly biased against conditions involving disability	Regularly used by Centers for Disease Control and Prevention to assess burden of disease in the United States (MMWR 1992)
Disability or quality-of-life adjusted life-years (DALYs or QALYs)[1]			
Expert ratings assessment	Low	Unrepresentative experts	Ghana Health Assessment Project Team (1981)
Survey-based	Medium	NA	European quality-of-life assessments (EuroQol Group 1990)
Risk trade-offs	High	Questionable relevance of artificial gambles	Various quality-of-life assessments
Quantity-of-life trade-offs: Individual length versus quality of life	Medium/high	Probably low for patient-level decision-making	Various quality-of-life assessments
Quantity-of-life trade-offs: Across individuals	Medium	Probably low bias for social decision making	Vaccine development study (Institute of Medicine 1986); Nord (1991)

NA: Not applicable

Note: This table does not review approaches to measuring the economic benefits of changes in health status. Such measures—based, for example, on willingness to pay for reductions in the probability of adverse outcomes or on assessment of health-related determinants of labour productivity (human capital)—allow conclusions to be drawn about the inherent attractiveness of particular health interventions relative to their cost, not simply by comparison with other interventions. Tolley *et al.* (1994) and Pauly (1995) provide valuable overviews of this literature, which is briefly discussed in the text.

[1] Each of the methods for quality of life measurement—ratings, risk trade-offs, quantity-of-life trade-offs, and calibrations—can be undertaken by different groups, possibly with different results. The groups can be of 'experts', respondents to a survey or, in a clinical setting, potential patients. For the ratings method, this table comments on both expert and survey approaches: a similar breakdown could be provided for each method.

Sources: See references in final column of table.

different age groups differently. DALYs have been used for disease burden assessment and cost-effectiveness analysis in a number of recent World Bank and WHO documents (World Bank 1993; WHO 1996; WHO 2000; Murray and Lopez 1996). Lopez *et al.* (2006) report results using DALYs without age weights. Sensitivity analyses were undertaken in the initially published disease burden assessment using DALYs (Murray *et al.* 1994) and concluded that results were insensitive to age weights and discount rates over a broad range.[3]

DALYs can in principle also be weighted to reflect how equitably they are distributed in ways that are standard in project evaluation outside the health sector (Squire 1989).

Costs

Costs of inputs are generally assessed at market prices. This simple observation masks much complexity, however, both conceptually and in practice. The few paragraphs that follow highlight several important issues, but the interested reader is referred to Gold *et al.* (1996) for a more thorough treatment.

Tradeable and nontradeable inputs

For some inputs into healthcare, costs may be lower in low- and middle-income countries (for example, for semi-skilled labour). These costs are typically for inputs that cannot be traded internationally, and their existence undermines attempts to estimate costs that are not simply country-specific. Squire (1989) provides a general discussion of approaches to dealing with tradeables in project analysis through use of 'shadow prices'. His recommendations are more relevant to country-specific assessments than to cross-national comparisons.

The working conclusion of this chapter is that for tradeables (e.g. non-patented drugs, most equipment, and high-level manpower) considerations of cost variability between high- and low-income countries are of minimal significance (relative to other uncertainties).[4] For facilities and lower level manpower real costs do vary across countries, leading some analysts to conclude that costs are most usefully expressed as fractions of local per capita income—a method that assumes essentially no health sector inputs to be internationally tradeable. Barnum and Greenberg's (1993) CEA for cancer interventions is an example of an attempt to divide costs into those for traded goods and those for nontradeables. Their assessments do suggest that local costs will often be important and that those who attempt to assess the cost-effectiveness of intervention in a comparative context should pay close attention to this issue unless there is a free market for foreign exchange and the costs of nontradeables are similar to those of the comparator country. It is a matter of judgement about the extent to which costing of nontradeables undermines efforts to form generalizations across countries. One conclusion is that such generalizations are both useful and possible, but that they are best done within groups of countries with broadly similar income levels.

Patient and home provider time

Another important issue in cost analysis concerns assessment of the amount and value of time required of patients or caretakers. More attention to time costs is important both for improving cost analyses and because behavioural response to the availability of an intervention may be sensitive to time requirements. The importance of mothers' time, in particular, for compliance with child survival interventions has been stressed by Leslie (1989). Yabroff *et al.* (2007) point to the potentially substantial magnitude of patient time costs in a study from the US The Public Health Service provides recommendations for subsequent work that would help redress this omission. A related issue concerns treatment of costs that will ensue from intervention success; Levin *et al.* (1993), for example, point out that substantial food costs can result from micronutrient supplementation or parasite control: Appetites improve. The existence of such costs suggests the importance, in these cases, of broadening the definition of the intervention. Meltzer (1997) provides a theoretically complete discussion of these issues.

Costs to well-being and risks to health

Some interventions impose costs in well-being, e.g. use of condoms of reduced alcohol or cigarette consumption. Others entail direct adverse health consequences through side effects of their inherent riskiness. While little effort has been made to include these costs in CEAs for low- and middle-income countries, their existence points to issues for interventions to change behaviour.

Joint costs

A final issue concerning cost analysis is that of joint costs, that is, the situation where several interventions are essentially made available with a (partially) common set of inputs. Some authors handle this in part by defining interventions in terms of natural packages; for example, Jamison *et al.* (1993) consider the preventive intervention for polio to be diphtheria–pertussis–tetanus vaccine plus polio immunization, and assess the cost-effectiveness of that package, because polio immunization would (almost always) be given with the other vaccines. Debas *et al.* (2006) also deal with joint costs in surgical interventions by packaging, in this case by considering the 'intervention' to be the operation of the surgical ward of a district hospital for a year. Future directions for CEA will likely include much attention to large packages or 'platforms', like the surgical ward both to deal with joint costs and because of greater policy relevancy.

Other issues

CEAs for comparisons across interventions use the common metric of dollar cost per DALY gained, with the understanding that incremental costs and cost-effectiveness will likely vary across locales (even after controlling for intervention quality) because of differences in individuals, in epidemiological conditions, in delivery system characteristics, in the initial degree of penetration of the intervention into the population, and in the range of available alternatives.[5] Table 7.4.4 lists many important factors that lead to variation in incremental cost-effectiveness, and, to the extent that interventions are first applied where their cost-effectiveness is highest, these factors collectively will lead to rising costs per QALY with increased application of an intervention. Figure 7.4.2 illustrates this for control of dengue; up to a point, improved case management is most cost-effective, but beyond that point, if a higher level of control for dengue is to be sought, chemical and then environmental strategies of vector control must be introduced.

Intervention specificity and targeting

This phenomenon of rising costs per DALY comes up implicitly in many analyses; the cause of the phenomenon is, frequently, the lack of intervention specificity and, also frequently, the needs for costly targeting, case-finding, or compliance monitoring.

Table 7.4.4 Factors influencing variation in cost-effectiveness

Influencing factor	**Important examples**
Epidemiological environment	
Prevalence of condition	Screening and referral programmes for leprosy; for cervical and breast cancer.
Incidence of condition	BCG immunization for tuberculosis; preventive measures for many injuries.
Case-fatality rate	Measles immunization; oral rehydration therapy for diarrhoea.
Transmission dynamics of infectious conditions	Treatment of sexually transmitted diseases in core versus non-core groups; vector control for malaria, dengue.
Existence of competing risks or synergisms	Measles vaccination results in amplification of cost-effectiveness by strengthening individuals in a general way. Among the very young or elderly, competing risks reduce the cost-effectiveness of some targeted interventions.
Individual characteristics	
Age	Cancer treatment: More cost-effective for younger patients
Tendency to compliance	Tuberculosis chemotherapy; antihypertensive medication
Tendency to self-refer	Sexually transmitted diseases control
Levels of risk factors	High levels of hypertension and hyperlipidemin enhance intervention cost-effectiveness
Individual variation in values	Attitude toward disability relative to risk of death; can lead to individual differences in intervention effectiveness.
System characteristics	
Local costs of non-traded inputs to healthcare system	Real costs of care-intensive interventions (such as hospitalization to ensure compliance with tuberculosis chemotherapy) are low where wages are low, because most health-care personnel are relatively immobile internationally.
Generalized systemic competence	Case management of dengue haemorrhagic fever: High cost and low effectiveness in unsophisticated systems. Cost per DALY at the margin of some interventions in a system with high level of professionalism and capacity may be much lower than in less well developed systems.
Discount rate	Hepatitis B immunization: Where discount rates are high, interventions with pay-offs well into the future become relatively less attractive, and age of the patient becomes a less significant determinant of cost-effectiveness.

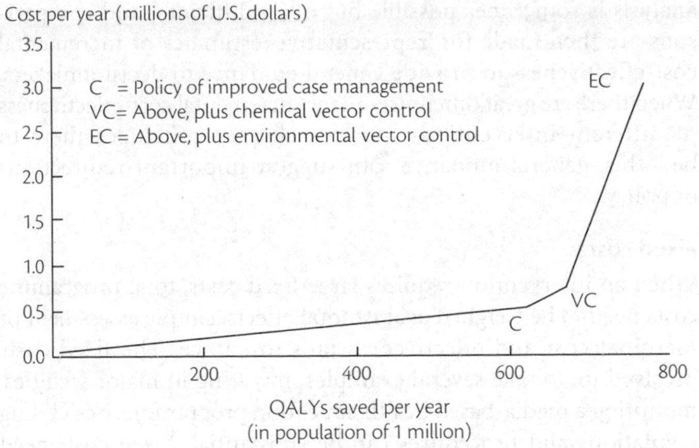

Fig. 7.4.2 Increasing cost per QALY associated with more complete control of dengue.

Intervention specificity refers to what fraction of intervention recipients would benefit assuming that the intervention is applied exactly to the individuals to whom it should be applied. Specificity will be influenced by such factors as the 'prevalence of the condition', 'incidence of condition', and 'levels of risk factors' (Table 7.4.4). Take BCG vaccination for TB as an example; many countries specify that it be applied to all newborns, but it is a benefit, *ex post*, only to that tiny fraction of children who would have died in childhood from miliary tuberculosis (TB) without it. Tuberculosis chemotherapy for sputum positives, by contrast, although costly, will virtually never be applied when unneeded; it is highly specific. Initially targeting BCG or other interventions to populations at highest risk, although inevitably at some cost, will maximize cost-effectiveness while simultaneously advancing equity objectives. Although the incremental cost per DALY gained by expanding coverage may be rising, sufficient resource availability may justify expansion.

To continue the TB example, patients who seek care, and who are then compliant with the treatment regimen, cost less than those for whom active case-finding is required or who require careful monitoring for compliance. All these factors lead to another reason for rising costs per incremental DALY gained. To take another example, oral rehydration therapy (ORT) in the hospital or clinic setting is highly cost-effective; it will only be used for severe cases of diarrhoea, and it is likely to be applied effectively by qualified medical personnel. When ORT is taken to the community, however, cost-effectiveness declines substantially, both because of a decrease in intervention specificity (mild cases will be treated unnecessarily) and because home treatment will be applied less effectively than hospital treatment in severe cases.

These points are relatively obvious, but there is often an optimistic bias toward assessing cost-effectiveness under assumptions of favourable targeting and compliance costs and of favourable intervention specificity. One might expect, as previously noted, rising marginal costs and decreasing marginal effectiveness as interventions are extended through populations; these combine to dilute cost-effectiveness. Thus favourable case cost-effectiveness estimates can be real, but their margin of applicability may be limited. In principle, it is desirable to acquire some sense of the responsiveness of intervention cost-effectiveness to a range of parameters, particularly the extent of application of the intervention. In practice, sensitivity analysis is sometimes possible but often difficult—and comparisons are then made for 'representative' estimates of incremental cost-effectiveness to provide general guidance to decisionmakers. When there are great differences in the incremental cost-effectiveness of different interventions—as this chapter concludes there to be—this 'general guidance' can suggest important redirections of policy.

Fixed costs

When an intervention requires large fixed costs, total programme costs need to be weighed against total effects; simple assessment of marginal cost and effectiveness fails to suffice. The fixed costs involved in, to take several examples, investing in major facilities, mounting a media-based health education programme, or devising regulations and procedures can be substantial. Fixed costs need not be financial; managerial or political attention to a problem may have an important fixed cost element. When fixed cost may be important, understanding the total burden of disease is necessary for estimating potential total intervention effects. By the same token, cost-effectiveness analyses will need to include consideration of large increments in intervention. (See, for examples, Barnum *et al.* (1980) for analysis of simultaneous scaling up of multiple child survival interventions or Watts and Kumaranayake (1999) for a brief discussion of scaling up AIDS control interventions in Africa.)

Disease burden assessment needs can be combined with CEA in an explicit way to help evaluate where there might be large pay-offs to R&D investments or to focused political or managerial attention on reallocation of interventions. This requires an analysis, essentially, of whether a major disease burden persists mainly because of: (1) A lack of knowledge about the disease and its determinants, (2) a lack of tools, or (3) failure to use the existing tools efficiently. Of course, more than one factor is likely in each case. Where possible, this analysis can be quantitative. Figure 7.4.3 illustrates an analytical approach recently applied (WHO 1996). Using data on the efficacy of the available cost-effective interventions, and consulting the judgement of field experts on the proportion of the population receiving effective interventions, it is possible to estimate:

- What portion of the potential burden of each disease or condition is now being averted
- What could be averted now with better use of existing cost-effective interventions
- What could be averted now, but only with interventions that are not cost-effective
- What cannot be averted with existing interventions but would require new ones

The analysis is intended to identify where the greatest needs lie, and thereby guide assessment of priorities for different major fixed commitments such as R&D or political attention. The unit of currency employed for this analysis is, once again, the DALY. While such analyses are not intended to suggest that some spurious

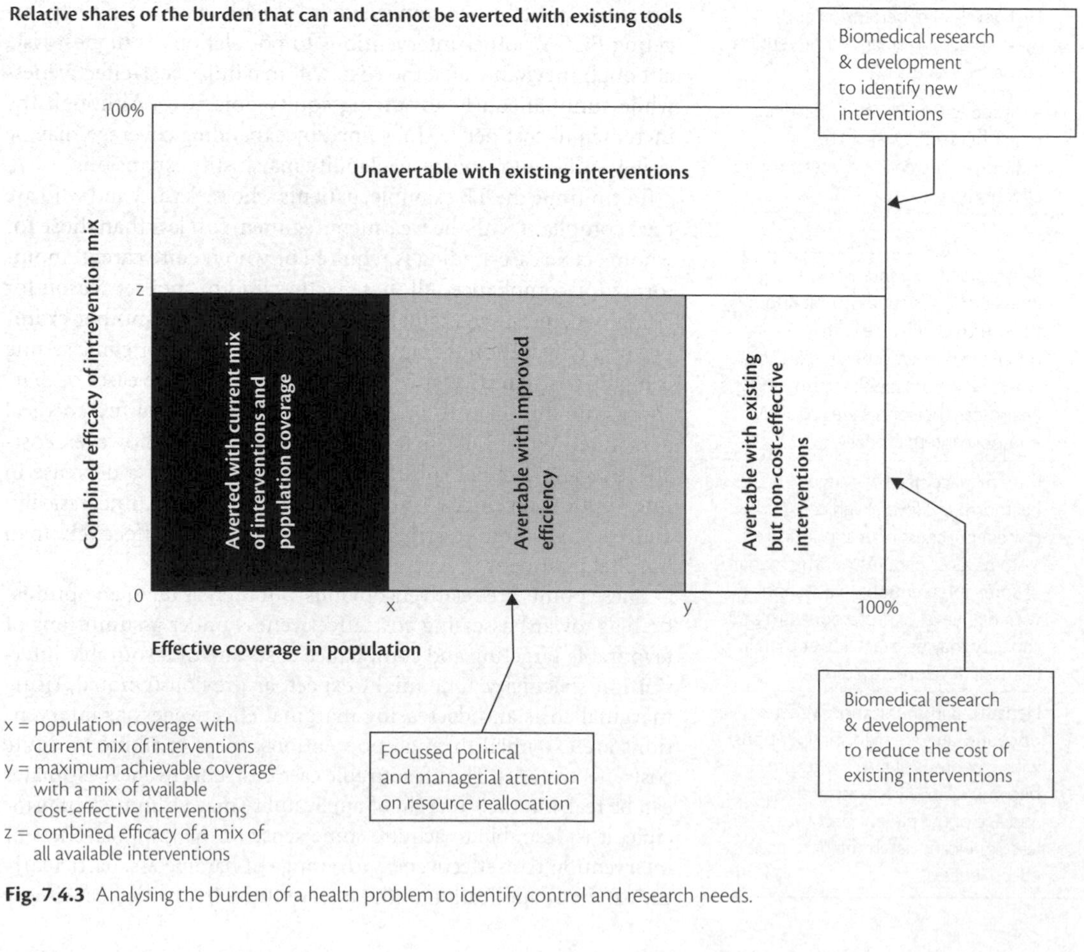

Fig. 7.4.3 Analysing the burden of a health problem to identify control and research needs.

precision can be achieved in the analysis of need, they do indicate a sense of the *relative* distribution of the effort required.

The area of the rectangle in Fig. 7.4.3 represents the total estimated disease burden in DALYs (or deaths or YLLs) from a given condition, such as diarrhoeal disease, under the counterfactual assumption that current explicit control interventions were not being applied. The horizontal axis represents the extent to which effective treatment is reaching the population—that is, how far into the population a mix of interventions is penetrating. The vertical axis represents the combined effectiveness of this mix. The subdivisions within that square represent different portions of the burden: (1) That which is being averted now by the existing mix of cost-effective interventions among the people that the intervention is reaching; (2) that which could be averted if the existing interventions were used more efficiently; (3) that which could be averted with existing tools, but not cost-effectively; and (4) that which is not avertable with existing interventions. Calculations of the relative share occupied by each subdivision can help to spell out the priorities. For example, where it is calculated that a large portion of the total burden of a certain disease cannot be averted with the existing cost-effective tools, then there is a strong case for R&D to develop new ones (if the disease burden is sufficiently large). Where it is calculated that a large fraction of the burden could be averted if existing tools were used more efficiently, *and the absolute disease burden is large*, there is a strong case for political and managerial attention to achieve fuller employment of available cost-effective interventions.

Non-health outcomes of health interventions

An additional problem in applications concerns interventions that have outcomes outside the health sector. Table 7.4.5 lists a number of important examples. CEA applied to health outcomes only will, obviously, understate the overall value of these interventions. While cost-benefit analysis would solve this problem, applicability may be difficult for reasons previously discussed. Under these circumstances a clear listing of costs, probable health effects, and non-health effects will at least inform the analysis.

Perhaps the clearest examples are control of smoking, promotion of breastfeeding, and environmental improvements. Limitation of smoking markedly reduces risk for lung cancer, ischaemic heart disease, and chronic obstructive pulmonary disease; outside the health sector it reduces (at least to some extent) property damage from fire and frees productive resources for alternative use. Breastfeeding, likewise, has multiple health effects; it enhances child immunity, reduces exposure to infection, provides balanced nutrition and, by suppressing ovulation, postpones the next pregnancy (Anderson 1990). The cost of breastfeeding, includes however, as do many health-promoting interventions, substantial amounts of mothers' time—which is not easily valued in terms, say, of wages forgone (Leslie 1992). Finally, whereas environmental interventions have beneficial health consequences, their main objectives may lie outside the health sector; World Bank (1992) provides a comprehensive discussion.[6]

Thus when interventions for health have a range of non-health outcomes, assessment of the attractiveness of these interventions

Table 7.4.5 Selected interventions with multiple outcomes

Intervention	Outcomes		
	Main health outcome	**Secondary health outcome**	**Non-health outcomes**
Provision of water supplies and sanitation	Control of diarrhoeal diseases	Control of skin, respiratory, and helminthic infections	Saving of household time; welfare improvements
Provision of soap	Control of diarrhoeal diseases	Control of skin, respiratory, and helminthic infections	Amenity
Reducing ambient air pollution	Reduced lung and vascular disease		Amenity
Reduction of vehicle speed limits	Reduced severity and incidence of crash-related injuries		Reduction in property damage from vehicle crashes; energy conservation; time costs
Control of smoking	Reduced incidence of lung cancer, heart disease, and chronic obstructive pulmonary disease	Reduced incidence of minor cancers; reduction in burn injuries	Welfare loss for current addicts, welfare gain for nonsmokers; freeing of land and labour for uses other than tobacco production
Vector control	Reduced incidence of vector-borne diseases		Improved welfare when vectors, such as mosquitoes, are nuisances
Female education	Reduced child mortality rates	Improved child growth; improved adult health	Higher levels of female productivity and earnings; improved congruence between actual and desired fertility levels
Breastfeeding	Improved child growth through improved nutrient availability and protection against diarrhoea	Protection of child against infectious disease; postponement of next pregnancy; possible long-term cognitive benefits to child	Savings in costs of infant formula and bottles; time costs for mother
Family planning services	Reduced child mortality	Reduced maternal morbidity and mortality	Economic and welfare gains from improved control of level and timing of fertility

should, ideally, quantitatively aggregate intervention effects along multiple dimensions. Likewise for clinical interventions there will frequently be joint costs (associated, for one example, with the availability of diagnostic facilities in a district hospital); again, in country-specific application, these matters can be assessed more quantitatively than they can be in a general overview.

The purpose of this section has been to introduce concepts without attempting to provide a detailed discussion of methods. In the next section an extended example of application of CEA is provided both to convey broad substantive lessons and to indicate how CEA has now become a working tool of the health policy analyst. A number of valuable handbooks on methods do exist and, as indicated earlier, this chapter is in the spirit of the US Public Health Services recommendations. Box 7.4.1 encapsulates that perspective.

An application: The disease control priorities project

This section summarizes the findings of a range of condition-specific analyses, principally relevant to low- and middle-income countries, that were undertaken initially for the World Bank's 'Health Sector Priorities Review' (Jamison *et al.* 1993) and then updated and substantially extended in the 'Disease Control Priorities Project' (DCPP) (Jamison *et al.* 2006; Laxminarayan *et al.* 2006).[7] Earlier in this chapter it was noted that dividing interventions into two broad categories—population-based primary prevention and personal—was conducive to discussing policy tradeoffs and this section is so divided. (Table 7.4.2 defined what is included in each of these categories.) The first subsection deals with population-based interventions, and the following subsection deals with personal ones. Unless otherwise specified, the assessments are of incremental cost-effectiveness from an implicitly defined typical starting point and they are designed to reach generalizable conclusions as well as to inform decision-making in a specific context. The DCPP reached a number of substantive conclusions and those are discussed to give a sense of the input CEA can make to informing policy.

Population-based primary prevention

Population-based interventions for primary were organized into three separate strategies in the DCPP—those designed to change personal behaviour, to control environmental hazards, and to deliver preventive medical services into the population (e.g. to immunize, to provide mass chemoprophylaxis to a population). In reviewing health policies, or intervention alternatives, it will often be useful to do so within each of these three broad strategies because of commonalities of logistics, policy instruments, and approaches within each. (This is true despite the frequently great diversity of conditions to be addressed within any one intervention strategy.)

Before turning to the summary of findings, the issue of joint costs (and multiple outcomes) of interventions is discussed in light of conclusions from the DCPP. The analysis upon which the DCPP was based was structured by diseases (or adverse health conditions more generally), and the issues addressed in the individual analyses thus concern the nature, cost, and effectiveness of the interventions available for dealing with each condition or its risk factors. In many cases, of course, any given intervention will address multiple conditions and, indeed, may well have important effects outside the health sector altogether.

Looking across findings of the individual chapters in the DCPP, it is clear that multiple effect and joint cost problems do complicate the task of assessing cost-effectiveness in many important instances; that said, it is more generally true that these problems are relatively minor or can be dealt with by reasonable approximations and simplifications in the analysis.

A few general conclusions on each public health approach emerged from the DCPP:

Personal behaviour change

Some personal behaviour changes that are favourable for health outcomes tend to occur naturally as incomes rise; these include, at least for many cultures, improved hygienic behaviours, increased energy intake and quality in the diet, and decreased crowding. Improvements in these behaviours are typically important for the pre-epidemiological transition diseases and can often be affected by educational interventions even though the main force driving improvements—income increases—is beyond the domain of health policy.

Other behaviours are likely either to be less dependent on income levels (for example, breastfeeding behaviour, sexual practices) or to be adversely influenced by income increases, at least for a period of time (for example, dietary excess, sedentary lifestyles, smoking, alcohol consumption). Most of these are risk behaviours for post-transition conditions. Although the natural course of development may well improve these behaviours, the Review found scope for affordable government policy to influence them. Regulatory policies and, particularly, taxation policies for tobacco, alcohol, and fatty meats show great promise for inducing behavioural change and, currently, are very much underused. Education of elites and the public are complementary instruments, not least because they generate the political will and popular support for regulation and taxation. The extremely high cost-effectiveness of smoking control makes it, perhaps, the top priority for governmental action.

Environmental hazards control

Rising incomes help with improving water supply and sanitation and that is likely to be important in prevention of a broad range of infectious and parasitic diseases. Specific investments in water supply and sanitation are unlikely, however, because of high costs to be justified in terms of health benefits alone. Vector control, however, is at least marginally cost-effective for a number of conditions (malaria, onchocerciasis, dengue) in some environments. Use of insecticide-impregnated bed nets appears particularly attractive for control of malaria-carrying mosquitoes. Industrialization introduces new hazards into the environment (lead, mercury, and the like) that can produce severe lifetime disability if not effectively controlled. Cleaner fuels and improvements in ventilation of indoor fireplaces and cookstoves can substantially reduce risks for chronic obstructive pulmonary disease (COPD); and occupational and transport safety measures are important in many specific instances. In principle, protective measures can be delivered through environmental intervention; and water fluoridation for prevention of caries is one example. Another problem is that of lead toxicity resulting from excess use of lead-based paints and combustion of gasoline with high lead content.

Box 7.4.1 US Public health service recommendations on CEA

In 1993, the US Public Health Service convened a 'Panel on Cost-Effectiveness in Health and Medicine'. The Public Health Service asked the Panel to assess the current state-of-the-art of cost-effectiveness analysis (CEA) in health and to provide recommendations for the conduct of future studies. Gold *et al.* (1996) bring together the Panel's conclusions, and their Appendix A provides a summary of recommendations. The following extracts provide the highlights of that summary.

Purpose of CEA

- CEA evaluates a given health intervention through the use of a 'cost-effectiveness ratio'. In this ratio, all health effects of the intervention (relative to a stated alternative) are captured in the denominator, and changes in resource use (relative to the alternative) are captured in the numerator and valued in monetary terms.
- CEA is an aid to decision making, not a complete procedure for making resource allocation decisions in health and medicine, because it cannot incorporate all the values relevant to such decisions.

Costs

- The major categories of resource use that should be reflected in the numerator of a C/E ratio include costs of health-care services; costs of patient time expended for the intervention; costs associated with caregiving (paid or unpaid); other costs associated with illness such as childcare or travel expenses; and costs associated with non-health impacts of the intervention (e.g. on the education system or the environment).
- Time spent seeking care or undergoing an intervention is a resource and a component of the intervention. It should be valued in monetary terms and incorporated in the numerator of a cost-effectiveness ratio. For individuals in the labour force, wages are generally an acceptable measure of time costs.
- In aggregating resource costs across time, CEAs should be conducted in constant dollars that remove general price inflation.
- 'Transfer payments' (e.g. cash transfers from tax payers to welfare recipients) associated with a health intervention redistribute resources from one individual to another. While administrative costs associated with such transfers are included in the numerator of a C/E ratio, the transfers themselves are not, since, by definition, their impact on the transferer, and the recipient cancel out.

Outcome measurement

- Incorporation of morbidity and mortality consequences into a single measure should be accomplished using QALYs. In general, since lives saved or extended by an intervention will not be in perfect health, a saved life year will count as less than one full QALY.
- In general, community preferences for health states are the appropriate ones for use. If distinct subgroup preferences are identified that will markedly affect a C/E ratio, the study should provide this information and conduct sensitivity analyses that reflect this difference.
- The health-related quality of life of those whose lives have been saved or extended by a health intervention may be influenced by characteristics such as age, gender, or race. This may affect the analysis in ways that are ethically problematic. In these instances, sensitivity analyses should be conducted to indicate explicitly how the results are affected by these characteristics.

Discounting

- Costs and health outcomes should be discounted to present value with the shadow-price-of-capital (SPC) approach to evaluating public investments. This rate (often termed the *social rate of time preference)* can be approximated by the real rate of return on long-term government bonds, and a real, riskless discount rate of 3 per cent is now appropriate. Because of the large number of previous CEAs that have adhered to a discount rate of 5 per cent, analysts should perform sensitivity analyses using 5 per cent. The discount rate should be subject to review, and possible revision, over time in light of significant changes in the underlying economic data.
- Costs and health outcomes should be discounted at the same rate.

Uncertainty

- At a minimum, univariate (one-way) sensitivity analyses should be conducted in order to determine where uncertainty or lack of agreement about some key parameter's value could have substantial impact on the CEA's conclusions.
- Where possible, where parameter uncertainty is a major concern, a reasonable confidence interval should be estimated based on either statistical methods or simulation.

Early research—reviewed in Pollitt (1990)—indicates that lead toxicity may be far more important than previously thought as a determinant of slow development and impaired mental functioning.

Immunization, mass chemoprophylaxis, and screening

Interventions that can be characterized under the headings immunization, mass chemoprophylaxis, and screening all share certain common characteristics: (1) They involve the direct administration or application of a specific technical intervention to individuals on a one-by-one basis; (2) they are directed to certain target populations; and (3) the coverage of the target population is important to produce the desired effect. Technically, each of these intervention strategies is highly efficacious when correctly applied to a compliant subject, but their actual effectiveness in low- and middle-income countries is strongly conditioned by the local administrative, managerial, and logistical capabilities, as well as by traditional cultural constraints.

Most immunization interventions are highly cost-effective; and many of them address highly prevalent conditions. Measles and tetanus vaccination appear particularly cost-effective and worthy of relatively greater attention within immunization programmes. Far more could be efficiently spent on immunization than is now being spent; and, even though costs of delivery tend to rise as more marginal populations are reached, extending immunization programmes to virtually universal coverage is likely to prove both cost-effective and a practical way of significantly improving the health of the poor.

One particularly promising application of mass chemoprophylaxis lies in the administration of anthelmintic medication and micronutrient supplements to school-age children. Here cost-effectiveness appears quite high for conditions that, although of extremely high prevalence, have only recently been seen to be of substantial importance for intellectual and physical development. A programme of chemoprophylaxis for school-age children could, like the Expanded Programme on Immunization (EPI) for younger children, be expected to serve as the starting point for an ultimately much expanded capacity to deal with the health needs of this age group.

Perhaps the most significant cancers for which treatment may be cost-effective (breast, cervical) are ones for which early screening and referral are important; so, as noncommunicable diseases become increasingly significant, this strategy will become increasingly relevant. The emerging strategies for treatment of acute respiratory infections in children all rely heavily on community-based programmes for early detection and quick referral; with increased experience, improvements in capacity for cost-effective screening and referral programmes can be expected to develop.

Personal interventions

Facilities to provide personal intervention vary continuously in size, in the degree of complexity (and range) of the conditions that they address, in the sophistication of their facilities and equipment, and in the training and skill of their staff. For conducting comparable CEAs it is useful, nonetheless, to use generally accepted terminology in categorizing facilities into three groups—clinic-level, district hospitals, and referral hospitals—while recognizing that categorization involves much simplification and that the appropriate classification structure will vary substantially from country to country. Table 7.4.6 indicates (in a very general way), for each of these three levels of facility, examples of the kinds of interventions they might address and what capacity such a facility might have for primary modes of diagnostic and therapeutic intervention.

One lesson that emerged from the DCPP is that currently CEA is severely constrained by the paucity of data relating to the effect and cost of clinical interventions in low- and middle-income environments. In the absence of such analyses, it is perhaps natural for low- and middle-income countries to import, to the extent that resources permit, the methods of case management used or being developed in high-income countries. The key phrase here is, of course, 'to the extent that resources permit'. Available resources permit importation of high-cost interventions for only a tiny proportion of a population of a low- or middle-income country. In order to extend access to services for the rapidly emerging epidemic of acquired immunodeficiency syndrome (AIDS) as well as for the impending epidemic of noncommunicable diseases, radically lower cost methods of case management will need to be developed from the rich range of technologies and procedures that now exist, or that are coming into being.

Several additional observations can be made:

- Curative care for tuberculosis and sexually transmitted diseases appears extremely cost-effective; further, such care is not now being provided to anything like the extent it should be, given the high burden of morbidity and mortality resulting from these conditions. Surgical treatment of cataract is also highly cost-effective.
- The extremely diverse range of clinical interventions of moderate cost-effectiveness (medical management of angina or diabetes are examples as is surgical management of cervical cancer) suggests that country-specific analyses of these conditions are required and that facilities capable of competently handling diverse conditions will need to be developed.
- The cost is sufficiently high for some clinical interventions to imply that even if they are effective (as is the case with coronary artery bypass grafting to deal with angina), their marginal cost-effectiveness (in this case relative to medical management) is so poor that their use should be actively discouraged until other, more cost-effective interventions can be delivered to their appropriate potential.
- Control of pain from terminal cancer could benefit perhaps 1.5 million individuals annually at acceptable costs; current legislation and standard practices greatly limit what is done in relation to what potentially could be done.
- Rehabilitation (in particular from leprosy, poliomyelitis, and injury) shows promise of being extremely cost-effective; but very little attention has been accorded rehabilitation, and little is known about how best to provide services on a population basis or what might be expected in terms of effectiveness and cost.
- Expanding access of populations to surgical services at the district hospital level appears highly cost-effective.

Again, as with the discussion of population-based primary prevention, one theme that emerges from this review of personal intervention cost-effectiveness is that of complexity and diversity. Many interventions are clearly not cost-effective, and public policy should make every effort to discourage their use. But the available evidence does suggest that a broad range of interventions, addressing a similarly broad range of conditions, *will* prove cost-effective. Many of these interventions are not now being used to anything like the extent that they should be. Likewise, much of what is currently undertaken by the clinical system is misdirected (toward interventions of low cost-effectiveness) or simply inefficiently used. Redirection of substantial resources from interventions of low cost-effectiveness toward those with very high cost-effectiveness is clearly possible; a central task of health policy must be to design implementation strategies and government policy instruments that can promote these potential efficiency gains. At the same time, however, given our at best modest understanding of how to promote efficiency, there will often be a strong case for additional resources (appropriately directed).

Lessons from the disease control priorities project

Five very broad conclusions can be drawn from the DCPP—one methodological and the other four substantive. The methodological conclusion is that it is feasible, on a broad scale, to assess systematically intervention cost-effectiveness in the health sector in a way that can provide broad policy guidance. The effort required is substantial, but results that allow broad intrasectoral assessment of intervention priorities can be obtained.

One substantive conclusion is that the available evidence points to great variation, across interventions, in marginal cost-effectiveness.

Table 7.4.6 Personal intervention: Level of facility and mode of intervention

		Intervention mode			
			Therapeutic		
Level of clinical facility	**Typical conditions addressed**	**Diagnostic**	**Medical**	**Surgical**	**Physical or psychological therapy**
Clinic (private, community, and school- and work-based)	Minor trauma; simple injections; support of population-based interventions; uncomplicated childbirth; family planning	Clinical	Short list of essential drugs (about 20)	Sutures	Important potential role for supervising physical therapy
District hospital	Complicated childbirth; fractures and burns; complicated infections; cataract; hernia; appendicitis; diabetes, hypertension, and similarly complex condition	Clinical; basic laboratory; basic radiologic facilities	Long list of essential drugs (about 200)	Capacity of dealing with abdominal surgery, many fractures, caesarean sections, some rehabilitative surgery	Design and management of more complex regimens of physical and psychological therapy
Referral hospital	More complicated medical and surgical conditions	More advanced laboratory and radiologic facilities	As above, but also specialized drugs, chemotherapy, and radiotherapy	As above but also capacity for more complicated surgery of head and chest	Support capacity for district hospitals

Laxminarayan *et al.* (2006) summarized this evidence by grouping interventions into ranges of marginal cost per DALY for different interventions in South Asia and sub-Saharan Africa. The challenge ahead is that of designing and implementing instruments of government policy that will greatly expand use of cost-effective while decreasing use of interventions that provide very little value for money.

Garber and Phelps (1997) calculate that under a reasonable range of assumptions it will make economic sense to pay for QALYs up to a cost of about twice the level of per capita income; this leads to a second substantive conclusion, which is that, in many countries, quite a broad array of specific additional intervention is likely to prove attractive by any reasonable economic standard. (Such intervention could either be financed by reallocation from non-cost-effective interventions within the health sector, or from new resources to the sector.)

The third substantive conclusion concerns the extent to which population-based preventive as opposed to personal strategies tend to be more cost-effective. Although there are some patterns (in particular, smoking control and primary prevention by way of immunization accounts for many highly cost-effective interventions), the general conclusion is that there is no especially strong reason to believe that population-based prevention or public health interventions to have superior cost-effectiveness.

The fourth substantive conclusion from the DCPP is that few cost-effective interventions in low- and middle-income countries require more specialized facilities than those available at district hospitals. Thus, even though one cannot argue in general in favour of prevention over cure or public health over clinical intervention, one *can*, at least tentatively, conclude that district hospitals and lower level facilities potentially offer almost all attractive interventions. A strong caveat here is that relatively few advanced surgical interventions were assessed. Many of the more cost-effective ones can be done in a district hospital but some may require referral facilities.

Conclusion

Multiple methods—cost-minimization analysis, cost-effectiveness analysis and cost-benefit analysis—can provide decision makers with insights into resource allocation in health. Methods for undertaking these analyses are now mature (although, of course, controversy continues on specific points). Extensive efforts over many years have yielded a large harvest of results. Among the methods in use CEA appears most relevant for many purposes, but little additional effort may be required to recast results in terms of cost-minimization or cost-benefit analyses. In short CEA and its relatives are tested, working tools for the analyst.

That said, much remains to be done that goes beyond specific individual applications, important as those remain. Parallel analyses of a broad array of interventions provide information more than in proportion to the number of interventions. Much of what has caught political attention in CEA has resulted from these larger efforts, although only few exist. Further investment in large comparative studies—taking a number of paradigmatic environments as the base case—will both generate valuable insights directly and serve as solid starting points for more tailored, country-specific efforts.

Notes

1. An example of negative intervention may be useful. Many countries now place individuals with severe mental illness in specialized mental hospitals that provide very long-term (and hence

expensive) care. An increasingly advocated alternative would be short-term inpatient care in general hospitals combined with long-term medical management on an outpatient basis. Scaling back or closing mental hospitals would gain dollars at the cost of DALYs. From the perspective of a national decisionmaker assessing the cost-effectiveness of closing down existing facilities is likely to prove more salient than would an exercise that hypothesizes no intervention as the base case and concludes that the health system should have avoided building mental hospitals in the first place. The widespread existence of mental hospitals for long-term care makes generic analysis of the desirability of closing them down valuable (perhaps for several paradigmatic environments).

2. Most procedures for measuring QALYs result in an interval scale of measurement with a scale unique up to an affine transformation. That is if q_1 is a utility function resulting from the measurement process then q_2 will equally well represent that measurement process if $q_2 = a + b\, q_1$, $b > 0$. Incremental cost-effectiveness analysis utilizing interval scales will preserve cost-effectiveness ratios under permissible transformations of the utility function. Any attempt at assessing cost-effectiveness in a more absolute way, e.g. not with respect to a stated starting point, will require a scale of measurement that is stronger in the sense that it will need to be unique up to a similarity transformation ($q_2 = b\, q_1$, $b > 0$) if cost-effectiveness ratios are to be preserved. Such a scale is called a ratio scale, which has a natural zero that interval scales lack. Use of QALYs or DALYs to measure burden of disease requires a ratio scale of measurement. The existing literature on utility measurement in health lacks an axiomatic formulation of the conditions under which such a scale will exist and, until such a formulation is undertaken, the theoretical foundation for disease burden measurement will remain shaky. See Krantz *et al.* (1971) for a thorough discussion of measurement theory, including a discussion of conditions under which two differently established interval scales on a set of outcomes can be used to generate an underlying ratio scale. These are conditions that indicate when, in the health context, utility measures generated by time trade-off method and the standard gamble method on the same set of outcomes would suffice to justify a ratio scale.

3. Existing disease burden studies (and cost-effectiveness analyses) discount life years lost from the life expectancy at the age of death to the present. For reasonable discount rates, this implies that the QALY or DALY loss associated with a death just after birth lies within 20–30 per cent of the loss associated with a death at age 20. This ratio differs substantially from the factor of 2 to 4 the limited number of empirical assessments have obtained (e.g. Institute of Medicine 1986). At the same time, deaths before birth are treated as having no loss—at patent variation with human reaction and social willingness to pay to avert late fetal death. This issue is also quantitatively important in that there are about 3.3 million stillbirths annually (over 1 million of which are in the 12 h before the expected time of birth). A conceptual approach to dealing with these two problems, and a related complete recalculation of the global burden of disease, appears in Jamison *et al.* (2006).

4. Garber (1999) discusses the question of what cost to assign pharmaceuticals (or devices) that are covered by patent. Patents confer temporary monopolies on the patent holders that allow prices to be set at levels often far above the marginal cost of production and packaging. This provides incentives for new product development. If a CEA uses the market price of a patented drug as its measure of cost then, clearly, it cannot properly be considered an incremental CEA. Garber (1999) argues that if the CEA is undertaken from a consumer perspective the practical approach will nonetheless be to use market prices (or whatever price can be negotiated by an influential purchaser) for costs. Pharmaceutical companies often adopt 'tiered' pricing regimes that result in lower prices in low-income countries. This will be profit-maximizing from the company's perspective and will result in patented drug prices in developing countries being much closer to the marginal cost of production—thereby attenuating the problem Garber raises. For this reason CEA's from a low-income country perspective should not treat patented drugs as tradeables.

5. Practical work in CEA often devotes substantial effort to defining and structuring the set of alternatives (Garber 1999, pp. 13–17). One result will often be to demonstrate that one or more alternatives are in some sense dominated by other alternatives under consideration. What techniques should be chosen early (i.e. under very tight budget constraints) and which ones added later can be assessed. Finally only in the context of considering closely related options can the attractiveness of a more costly but better technique be assessed. An example concerned an analysis of the attractiveness of coronary artery bypass grafts (CABG) in Brazil, which concluded that CABG for disease in the left main coronary artery was a 'good buy' because the cost per QALY was only about 25 per cent of Brazil's GDP per capita. This, however, was the cost per QALY of CABG relative to doing nothing. Medical management and (now) angioplasty are less costly but nonetheless somewhat effective alternatives to CABG. The right way to think about CABG is in terms of how much more it would cost than one of these alternatives and how many more QALYs it would buy. It is likely that considered as incremental to alternatives the cost per QALY for CABG would be far higher than the original estimate. The cost-effectiveness of any one intervention, then, can be highly sensitive to the range of alternatives being considered.

6. The extent to which environmental interventions are justified on health grounds varies. While some discussions of air quality, for example, place importance on the amenity value of clean air other emphasize health consequences. A particularly important example of the need to consider non-health outcomes, in the context of very poor environments, concerns improving water supplies (from collection of surface water, say, to wells serving a community). Unclean and inadequate water supplies undoubtedly contribute substantially to risks of diarrhoeal and other disease—diseases killing millions of people every year. Increased quantities of cleaner water will have important health benefits. Improving water supplies is, however, very costly and, in most circumstances, would appear non cost-effective relative to public health or clinical interventions to reduce child mortality. That is they would appear non cost-effective if there were no other benefits. Other benefits include time savings (usually for women) in fetching water and the amenity value (beyond the sanitary value) of the cleaner bodies, clothing, and dwellings that improved water supplies facilitate. A cost-benefit analysis, if it were feasible,

would place a monetary value on all benefits that would allow combining them. If CBA cannot be done in an acceptable way, can CEA help to inform decisions? This is probably best done through sensitivity analysis. If all the non-health benefits can be given monetary values, one can calculate the dollar value per QALY that would be required for a satisfactory rate of return to the investment in water supplies. A high value would suggest that the water supply intervention was unattractive. Alternatively one can calculate the cost of the intervention that would make the cost per QALY of improved water competitive with alternatives for reducing child mortality. If the calculated cost is much less than the actual cost this would suggest that primary justification for the water supply investment should be for its other benefits, not its health benefits, even if the other benefits cannot be valued in monetary terms.

7. In many ways the DCPP is very much in the spirit of several previous assessments (e.g. Walsh & Warren 1979), which provided an assessment of priorities for control of communicable childhood diseases in developing countries. Other recent works in this comparative spirit, but emphasizing effectiveness, include Amler and Dull (1987) and the US Department of Health and Human Services (1991), which reviewed a broad range of preventive intervention policies for the United States, and, more for clinical preventive services, the US Preventive Services Task Force (1989) review of the effectiveness of 169 interventions. The state of Oregon in the United States rank ordered over 700 interventions, using cost-effectiveness and other criteria, for the purpose of rationing limited public resources to provide healthcare for the poor; Strosberg and others (1992) discuss many facets of the Oregon plan. Jha *et al.* (1998) assessed the relative cost-effectiveness of 40 potentially important interventions in the West African context. The Harvard 'life saving' project assessed cost per life saved of several hundred preventive options (Tengs 1996). Udvarhelyi *et al.* (1992) provide a comprehensive review of medical cost-effectiveness and cost-benefit studies from the perspective of their methodological adequacy. All these approaches to the analytic evaluation of health practices fall within the general area of CEA. Once somewhat comparable cost-effectiveness assessments are available for a range of interventions then analyses focusing on only a limited set of interventions can be put into the context provided by existing studies. For example, careful analysis for the sub-Saharan Africa context of malaria control (Goodman *et al.* 1999) and HIV-1 transmission interruption (Kumarayake & Watts 2000) both benefit from and contribute to an increasing understanding of intervention cost-effectiveness in Africa.

References

Amler, R.W. and Dull, H.B. (eds.) (1987). *Closing the gap: The burden of unnecessary illness.* Oxford University Press, New York.

Anderson, M.A. (1990). Nature and magnitude of the problem of suboptimal breastfeeding practices. Paper presented at the International Policymakers Conference on Breastfeeding, Florence, Italy, 30 July–1 August 1990.

Barnum, H. (1987). Evaluating healthy days of life gained from health projects. *Social Science and Medicine*, **24**, 833–41.

Barnum, H. and Greenberg, E.R. (1993). Cancers. In *Disease control priorities in developing countries* (eds. D.T. Jamison, W.H. Mosley, A.R. Measham and J.R. Bobadilla), pp. 529–60. Oxford University Press for the World Bank, Oxford.

Bloom, D.E., Canning, D., and Jamison, D.T. (2004). Health, wealth and welfare. *Finance and Development*, **41**, 10–15.

Briscoe, J. and de Ferranti, D. (1988). *Water for rural communities.* Washington, D.C.

Chapman, R.H. Berger, M., Weinstein, M.C. *et al.* (2004). When does Quality-Adjusting Life Years matter in cost-effectiveness analysis? *Health Economics*, **12**, 429–36.

Cropper, M.L., Aydede, S.K., and Portney, P.R. (1992). Rates of time preference for saving lives. *American Economic Review*, **82**, 469–72.

Debas, H.T., Gosselin, R., McCord, C. *et al.* (2006). Surgery. In *Disease control priorities in developing countries* (eds. D.T. Jamison, J. Breman, A. Measham, G. Alleyne, M. Claeson, D.B. Evans *et al.*), 2nd edition, pp. 1245–60. Oxford University Press, Oxford and New York.

Drummond, M.F., Sculpher, M.J., Torrance, G.W. *et al.*(2005). *Methods for the economic evaluation of health care programs.* 3rdedition. Oxford University Press, Oxford.

EuroQol Group (1990). EuroQol—A new facility for the measurement of health-related quality of life. *Health Policy*, **16**, 199–208.

Feachem, R.G., Kjellstrom, A.T., Murray, C.J.L. *et al.* (1992). *The health of adults in the developing world.* Oxford University Press, New York.

Garber, A.M. (1999). Advances in cost-effectiveness analysis of health interventions. In *Handbook of health economics* (eds. J.P. Newhouse and A.J. Culyer). North Holland, Amsterdam.

Garber, A.M. and Fuchs, V.R. (1991). The expanding role of technology assessment in health policy. *Stanford Law and Policy Review*, **3**, 203–9.

Garber, A.M. and Phelps, C.E. (1997). Economic foundations of cost-effectiveness analysis. *Journal of Health Economics*, **16**, 1–31.

Garber, A.M.,Weinstein, M.C., Torrance, G.W. *et al.* (1996). Theoretical foundations of cost-effectiveness analysis. In *Cost-Effectiveness in Health and Medicine* (eds. M.R. Gold, J.E. Siegel, L.B. Russell, and M.C. Weinstein), pp. 25–53. Oxford University Press, New York.

Ghana Health Assessment Project Team (1981). Quantitative method of assessing the health impact of different diseases in less developed countries. *International Journal of Epidemiology*, **10**, 73–80.

Gold, M.R., Siegel, J.E., Russell, L.B. *et al.* (eds.)(1996). *Cost-effectiveness in health and medicine.* Oxford University Press, New York.

Goodman, C.A., Coleman, P.G., and Mills, A.J. (1999). Cost-effectiveness of malaria control in sub-Saharan Africa. *Lancet*, **354**, 378–85.

Institute of Medicine (1986). *New vaccine development: Establishing priorities.* Vols. 1 and 2. National Academy Press, Washington, D.C.

Jamison, D.T. (2006). Investing in health. In *Disease Control Priorities in Developing Countries* (eds. D.T. Jamison, J. Breman, A. Measham, G. Alleyne, M. Claeson, D.B. Evans *et al.*), 2nd edition, pp. 3–34. Oxford University Press, Oxford and New York.

Jamison, D.T. (2007). Disease control. In *Solutions for the world's biggest problems: Costs and benefits* (ed. B. Lomborg), pp. 295–344. Cambridge University Press, Cambridge.

Jamison, D.T., Shahid-Salles, S., Jamison, J.S. *et al.* (2006). Incorporating deaths near the time of birth into estimates of the global burden of disease. In *Global burden of disease and risk factors* (A.D. Lopez, C.D. Mathers, M. Ezzati, D.T. Jamison, and C.J.L. Murray), pp. 427–62. Oxford University Press, New York.

Jamison, D.T., Mosley, M.H., Measham, A.R. *et al.* (eds.)(1993). *Disease control priorities in developing countries.* Oxford University Press for the World Bank, Oxford.

Jha, P., Bangura, O., and Ransom, K. (1998). The cost-effectiveness of forty health interventions in Guinea. *Health Policy and Planning*, **13**, 249–62.

Krantz, D.H., Luce, R.D., Suppes, P. *et al.* (1971). *Foundations of measurement, volume I, additive and polynomial representations.* Academic Press Inc., New York.

Kumaranayake, L. and Watts, C. (2000). Economic costs of HIV/AIDS prevention activities in sub-Saharan Africa. *AIDS*, **14**, S1–S14.

Last, J.M. (ed.)(1988). *A dictionary of epidemiology*. 2nd edition. Oxford University Press for the International Epidemiological Association, New York.

Laxminarayan, R., Mills, A.J., Breman, J.G. *et al.* (2006). Advancement of global health: Key messages from the Disease Control Priorities Project. *Lancet*, **367**, 1193–1208.

Layard, R. and Glaister, S. (1994). Introduction. In *Cost-Benefit Analysis* (eds. R. Layard and S. Glaister), pp. 1–56. Cambridge University Press, Cambridge, UK.

Leslie, J. (1989). Women's time: A factor in the use of child survival technologies? *Health Policy and Planning*, **4**, 1–16.

Levin, H.M., Pollitt, E., Galloway, R. *et al.* (1993). Micronutrient deficiency disorders. In *Disease control priorities in developing countries* (eds. D.T. Jamison, W.H. Mosley, A.R. Measham, and J.L. Bobadilla), pp. 421–54. Oxford University Press for the World Bank, Oxford.

Lindert, P.H. (2004). *Growing public: Social spending and economic growth since the eighteenth century.* Vol. 1. Cambridge University Press, Cambridge, U.K.

Lomborg, B. (ed.)(2007). *Solutions for the world's biggest problems: Cost and benefits*. Cambridge University Press, Cambridge, U.K.

Lopez, A.D., Mathers, C.D., Ezzati, M. *et al.* (eds.) (2006). *Global burden of disease and risk factors*. Oxford University Press, New York.

Luce, B.R., Manning, W.G., Siegel, J.E., and Lipscomb, J. (1996). Estimating costs in cost-effectiveness analysis. In. *Cost-effectiveness in health and medicine* (eds. M.R. Gold, L.B. Russell, J.E. Siegel, and M.C. Weinstein), pp. 176–213. Oxford University Press, New York.

Maynard, A. and Bloor, K. (1998). *Our certain fate: Rationing in health care.* Office of Health Economics, London.

Meltzer, D. (1997). Accounting for future medical costs in medical cost-effectiveness analysis. *Journal of Health Economics*, **16**, 33–64.

MMWR (Morbidity and Mortality Weekly Report)(1992). Years of potential life lost before ages 65 and 85—United States, 1989-1990. *MMWR(Morbidity and Mortality Weekly Report)*, **41**, 313–15.

Murray, C.J., Evans, D., Acharya, A. *et al.* (2000). Development of WHO guidelines on generalized cost-effectiveness analysis. *Health Economics*, **9**, 235–51.

Murray, C.J., Jamison, D.T., and Lopez, A.D. (1994). The global burden of disease in 1990: Summary results, sensitivity analysis and future directions. *Bulletin of the World Health Organization*, **72**, 495–509.

Newmann, P.J. (2005). *Using cost –effectiveness analysis to improve health care*. Oxford University Press, Oxford.

Nord, E. (1991). The relevance of QALYs in prioritizing between different patients. Paper presented at the 12th Nordic HESG meeting, Copenhagen, August.

Patel, M.S. (1989). Eliminating social distance between North and South: Cost-effective goals for the 1990s. Staff Working Paper 5. UNICEF, New York.

Phelps, C.E. and Mushlin, A.I. (1991). On the (near) equivalence of cost-effectiveness and cost-benefit analysis. *International Journal of Technology Assessment in Health Care*, **7**,12–21.

Pritchard, C. (2004). Developments in economic evaluation in health care: A review of NEED. Office of Health Economics, OHE Briefing No. 40, London.

Russell, L.B., Siegel, J.E., Daniels, N.E. *et al.* (1996). Cost-effectiveness analysis as a guide to resource allocation in health: Roles and limitations. In *Cost-effectiveness in health and medicine* (eds. M.R. Gold, J.E. Siegel, L.B. Russell, and M.C. Weinstein), pp. 3–24. Oxford University Press, New York.

Shepard, D.S. and Halstead, S.B. (1993). Dengue (with notes on Yellow Fever and Japanese Encephalitis). In *Disease control priorities in developing countries* (eds. D.T. Jamison, W.H. Mosley, A.R. Measham, and J.L. Bobadilla), pp. 303–20. Oxford University Press for the World Bank, Oxford.

Squire, L. (1989). Project evaluation in theory and practice. In *Handbook of Development Economics* (eds. H.B. Chenery and T.N. Srinivasan), Vol. 2. North Holland, Amsterdam.

Strosberg, M.A., Weiner, J.M., and Baker, R. *et al.* (eds.)(1992). *Rationing America's medical care: The Oregon plan and beyond*. The Brookings Institution. Washington, D.C.

Stouthard, M.E., Essink-Bot, M.L., Bonsel, G.J. *et al.* (1997). *Disability weights for diseases in The Netherlands.* Erasmus University, Department of Public Health, Rotterdam.

Tengs, T.O. (1996). Enormous variation in the cost-effectiveness of prevention: Implications for public policy. *Public Health*, **2**, 13–17.

Udvarhelyi, I.S., Colvitz, G.A., Rai, A. *et al.* (1992). Cost-effectiveness and cost-benefit analyses in the medical literature. *Annals of Internal Medicine*, **116**, 238-44.

USDHHS (U.S. Department of Health and Human Services) (1991). *Healthy people 2000: National health promotion and disease prevention objectives*. U.S. Government Printing Office, Washington, D.C.

U.S. Preventive Services Task Force (R. S. Lawrence, Chairman) (1989). *Guide to clinical preventive services*. Williams and Wilkins, Baltimore.

Viscusi, W.K. and Aldy, J.E. (2003). The value of a statistical life: A critical review of market estimates from around the world. *Journal of Risk and Uncertainty*, **27**, 5–76.

Walsh, J.A. and Warren, K.S. (1979). Selective primary health care—an interim strategy for disease control in developing countries. *New England Journal of Medicine*, **301**, 967–74.

Watts, C. and Kumaranayake, L. (1999). Thinking big: Scaling up HIV-1 interventions in sub-Saharan Africa. *The Lancet*, **354**,1492.

Weinstein, M.C. (1995). From cost-effectiveness ratios to resource allocation: Where to draw the line? In *Valuing health care: Costs, benefits, and effectiveness of pharmaceuticals and other medical technologies* (eds. F.A. Sloan), pp. 77–97. Cambridge University Press, Cambridge, U.K.

Weinstein, N.D. (1989). Optimistic biases about personal risks. *Science*, **246**, 1232–3.

World Bank (1992). *World development report 1992: Development and the environment*. World Bank, Washington, D.C.

World Bank (1993). *World Development Report 1993. Investing in Health*. World Bank, Washington, D.C.

World Health Organization (1996). *Investing in health research and development*. Report of the Ad Hoc Committee on Health Research Relating to Future Intervention Options. Document TDR/Gen/96.1. Geneva.

World Health Organization (1999). *World health report 1999: Making a difference*. WHO, Geneva.

World Health Organization (2000). *World health report 2000: Health systems: Improving performance*. WHO, Geneva.

Yabroff, K.R., Davis, W.W., Lamont, E.B. *et al.* (2007). Patient time costs associated with cancer care. *Journal of the National Cancer Institute*, **4**, 643–56.

Zeckhauser, R. and Shepard, D. (1976). Where now for saving lives? *Law and Contemporary Problems*, **40**, 5–45.

7.5

Governance and management of public health programmes

Diana Bontá and Meredith Cagle

Abstract

Societies must have a system and capacity in place to carry out essential public health functions. This system comprises public health's infrastructure and is directed by governance and management of public health services. Together, governance and management work to achieve the core public health functions. Governance and management are also challenged to address social injustice issues and must work to eliminate the root cause of health inequities. Worldwide, public health systems exist with varying degrees of governance structure. Whether the system is robust and well developed or fragmented and limited, good governance can help societies and the public health organizations within them effectively fulfil their mission and provide services that are responsive to community needs. Conversely, poor governance can lead to corruption, resulting in losses of public funds and challenges to service delivery, access, and quality of healthcare. Public health management serves as the intersection between the governance structure and the actual work activities conducted within the system. Various theories have been developed to describe the work and skills of managers. Public health management is challenged to apply the unique characteristics of general managerial concepts within the nonprofit arena. Bridging the gaps in governance and management of public health systems is a challenge facing health systems worldwide. Regardless of government and management strategies, ultimately public health leaders must strive to ensure that the practical aspects needed in public health practice are not overlooked.

This chapter describes the application of governance and management of public health programmes at local, state, national, and international levels and provides both theoretical models and practical examples of their application. Its primary focus is on governance and management of public health programmes within the United States.

Introduction

Collectively, governance and management operate to achieve the core public health functions. In 1988, the Institute of Medicine's report, The Future of Public Health, identified the core public health functions as assessment, policy development, and assurance (IOM 1988). Although well conceived, many members of the public had a difficult time understanding what these core functions meant (Turnock 1996). In 1994, the Public Health Functions Steering Committee, including representatives from US Public Health Services agencies, the American Public Health Association, the Public Health Foundation, and other major public health organizations, developed the framework for the Essential Services (Public Health Functions Steering Committee 1994). The Essential Services provide a working definition of public health and a guiding framework for the responsibilities of local public health systems. They are:

1. Monitor health status to identify community health problems.
2. Diagnose and investigate health problems and health hazards in the community.
3. Inform, educate, and empower people about health issues.
4. Mobilize community partnerships to identify and solve health problems.
5. Develop policies and plans that support individual and community health efforts.
6. Enforce laws and regulations that protect health and ensure safety.
7. (a) Link people to needed personal health services; and (b) Assure the provision of healthcare when otherwise unavailable.
8. Assure a competent public health and personal healthcare workforce.
9. Evaluate effectiveness, accessibility, and quality of personal and population-based health services.
10. Research for new insights and innovative solutions to health problems (Public Health Functions Steering Committee 1994).

Detels in Chapter 1.1 *(The scope and concerns of public health)* outlines other public health concerns in addition to the above: Prevent disease and injuries; reduce health disparities and assure access for all to healthcare; promote and protect a healthy environment; plan and prepare for natural and man-made disasters; reduce interpersonal violence and aggressive war; and increase environmental stewardship (Detels 2009). Public health at its best is social justice.

Societies must have a system and capacity in place to carry out essential public health functions. This system comprises public health's infrastructure and is directed by governance and management of public health services. Governance and management of public health programmes are far reaching issues that apply to local health jurisdictions as well as international agencies such as the World Health Organization. For example, the decisions made by government, non-government agencies (NGOs), health officials, and others may impact the economy; have an effect on the spread and sequelae of disease; influence trade and travel; provide the identification of new microbes and/or mutations of existing agents; create new laboratory diagnostics and technology; alter treatment; or affect future legislation.

Health and well-being are requirements for human development. Social injustice occurs when policies or actions adversely affect the societal conditions in which people can be healthy. Often, this occurs when those who control access to opportunities and resources block the underprivileged and the powerless from gaining fair and equitable access to opportunities and resources (Levy 2006). Outcomes of social injustice include a range of adverse health consequences demonstrated by disparities in health status and health services access among or between populations. Factors related to social injustice, such as poverty, illiteracy, and lack of health insurance, contribute to higher rates of disease, disability, and death (Levy 2006).

The public health system must be challenged to address the root cause of health inequities and to reduce social injustice through appropriate public health policies, programmes, and services at all government levels (Plough 2006). Using theoretical knowledge about the role of social injustice in increasing health risks and poor health outcomes to develop and implement broad and sustainable changes in public health policy and practice is critical to affecting significant reductions in health disparities (Plough 2006).

The US National Association of City and County Health Officials (NAACHO) defines health inequities as 'systemic, avoidable, unfair, and unjust differences in health status and mortality rates, as well as in the distribution of disease and illness across population groups' (Hofrichter 2006). In *Tackling Health Inequities Through Public Health Practice* (2006), NAACHO utilized seven basic assumptions in developing the handbook for action. These assumptions are shared here because they are also suited to setting the stage for the consideration of the governance of public health systems and the managerial challenges of providing health for all within that system:

- Health is an end in itself, an asset or resource required by everyone, and critical to human development and well-functioning communities.
- Equity in health status benefits everyone.
- Health is a social concept, not only a medical one, and therefore would be usefully defined broadly, for example, demonstrating its connection to quality of life and well-being.
- Population health outcomes are primarily the result of social and political forces, not lifestyles or behaviour.
- Health is a collective public good, actively produced by institutions and social policies.
- An accumulation of negative social conditions and lack of fundamental resources contribute to health inequities, and include economic and social insecurity, racial and gender inequality, lack of participation and influence in society, unfavourable conditions during childhood, absence of quality and affordable housing, unhealthy conditions in the workplace and lack of control over the work process, toxic environments, and inequitable distribution of public goods.
- Addressing health inequities effectively will require an emphasis on root causes and social injustice, the latter having to do with inequality and hierarchical divisions within the population (Hofrichter 2006).

Defining governance

Governance is the structure and process by which a governing body makes decisions, determines strategic direction, and defines roles within the organization or society. It concerns the role all stakeholders play in the decision-making process.

The United Nations Development Programme (UNDP) (2004) defines governance as:

> *the system of values, policies and institutions by which a society manages its economic, political and social affairs through interactions within and among the state, civil society and private sector. It is the way a society organizes itself to make and implement decisions—achieving mutual understanding, agreement and action. It comprises the mechanisms and processes for citizens and groups to articulate their interests, mediate their differences and exercise their legal rights and obligations. It is the rules, institutions and practices that set limits and provide incentives for individuals, organizations and firms. Governance, including its social, political and economic dimensions, operates at every level of human enterprise, be it the household, village, municipality, nation, region or globe.*

Definitions of governance are broader than its application to public health systems. However, the indicators of good governance can be justly applied to public health. In a policy paper entitled 'Governance for sustainable human development' the UNDP (1997) outlined eight major characteristics of good governance:

- Participation
- Rule of law
- Transparency
- Responsiveness
- Consensus oriented
- Equity and inclusiveness
- Effectiveness and efficiency
- Accountability

The section below defines those characteristics and seeks to demonstrate how those indicators apply to public health.

Participation

Good governance necessitates representation of the people, both men and women, either directly through informed and organized participation, or through legitimate intermediate institutions of representation.

At a national or federal level, an example of participation in public health governance would be the opportunity to vote for a legislative representative who values the impact made by effective public health practices and will serve as a voice for the public in policy and law making related to public health issues. At a more regional or local level, participation in the governance of public health could be seen at the public comment period of a board of health meeting. Another example would be a community forum in which a structured format is used to provide attendees with accurate information about the topic and allow individuals an opportunity to provide feedback. It is important that a system based on 'good governance' is mindful to include representation for the disenfranchised and vulnerable, as even if the process for participation is democratic and open, there is no guarantee that these population needs will be considered.

Another means by which society participates in governance is through advocacy. Public health advocacy is the application of information and resources to effect systemic changes that reduce death or disability in groups of people (Christoffel 2000). When individuals and communities are educated and empowered to participate in the governing process through the provision of information and tools, their involvement is able to effectively influence the public health system to make significant changes. The development of new legislation, regulations, and policies, as well as the rescinding of ineffective or discriminatory laws are examples of system changes propelled by the work of advocacy groups. Americans for Nonsmokers' Rights (ANR) is an example of a national organization dedicated to advocating for nonsmokers' rights through an action-oriented programme of policy and legislation (http://www.no-smoke.org). Since 1976, ANR has been advocating for clean indoor air ordinances to protect nonsmokers in thousands of communities and states, and providing assistance to countries and communities around the world to do the same. ANR's strategy to inform, educate, provide technical assistance, and develop and disseminate 'best practice' guidelines has influenced significant changes in the tobacco use arena.

Rule of law

Fair and legal frameworks that are enforced impartially are required for good governance. Protection of human rights, especially those of minorities, is a basic and fundamental right within this framework.

From the World Health Organization's International Health Regulations (2005) to health code regulations and local ordinances, rules exist to provide a framework for addressing public health issues. Public health focuses on the population as a whole and is concerned with encouraging and supporting a healthy community. Nevertheless, it is critical that personal rights be considered and respected. While public health jurisdictions and governance systems vary from region to region, public health authorities, as a whole, have the responsibility and the authority to enact rules and regulations to influence individual behaviour (tobacco use restriction laws, for example). Public health leaders are required to understand, implement, and enforce health and safety statues and regulations. Vaccination laws, communicable disease reporting, and investigation are examples of instances where the rights and privacy of an individual are balanced with protecting the public's health.

With the threat of newly emerging infectious diseases such as pandemic influenza and severe acute respiratory syndrome (SARS), or an act of bioterrorism causing a disease epidemic, the potential need for voluntary or compulsory quarantine is significant. Although the legal basis to implement and enforce quarantine may exist, the planning and implementation of quarantine presents a number of challenges for the governing system (Blendon *et al.* 2006). While quarantine may be used as a public health tool to prevent or limit the spread of highly infectious diseases that can lead to death or serious illness, public health officials must consider the logistics and costs of quarantine. For example, where will the quarantine period be spent? Will quarantined individuals be able to communicate with family and friends? How will their health status be monitored and how will basic needs be met? Additionally, the direct costs of quarantine such as stipends to financially compensate quarantined individuals, resources, personnel time, and economic productivity, and indirect costs like social stigma, curtailment of civil liberties (restriction on freedom of movement), and declining personal and community mental health must be balanced with the benefits of a quarantine (MMWR 2003; Blendon *et al.* 2006).

The existence of a governance structure, which includes policies and procedures, that account for these legal and ethical issues that undoubtedly arise at all levels within the public health system, will assist in ensuring that the rules are applied and enforced to every extent possible and for the achievement of the greater good—the public's health. Regardless of the strength and attributes of the governance structure, the application of policies and procedures is in the hands of individuals and, thus, is subject to individual interpretation and action. Nevertheless, the stronger the system, the greater the likelihood that the 'rule of law' may be achieved.

Transparency

Transparency means that decisions and their enforcement are completed in a way that adheres to rules and regulations. The public's right for freely available and accessible information on matters and decisions that affect them is a fundamental element of transparency.

Transparency relates to the way an organization does business both internally and externally. Organizations that operate 'transparently' establish trust with the communities they serve. An example of how transparency can be applied to the public health governance system is the design and implementation of a restaurant inspection programme. In California, a local city health department undertook a process to develop a restaurant inspection reporting system. The development of the process included meeting with the local business association, restaurant association, consumers, and city officials. The process of developing and implementing a food facility inspection programme was conducted in an open and publicly transparent manner through the provision of educational, technical, legal, and scientific information about the inspection process. It also included discussions about the benefits and challenges of implementing a restaurant grading system versus an inspection summary report system. The outcome of the process included the implementation of enhanced food facility inspecting criteria and a summary report, which outlines specific violations related to food handling, temperature control, and employee and establishment hygiene and cleanliness. The programme also ensures a system of checks and balances for proper inspection and facility follow-up and code enforcement, as well as timely corrections to violations. Additionally, to avoid potential corruption—kick-backs to inspectors to give restaurants a more favourable report, for example—environmental health inspectors' assignments are routinely rotated to avoid the development of relationships that could lead to biased or influenced inspections. Ultimately, the development of the food facilities inspection programme and its implementation were conducted in a transparent manner that allowed all stakeholders a voice and insight in the process and its findings.

In contrast, an individual's right to privacy must always be balanced with transparency. For example, in an epidemiological investigation of a sexually transmitted disease outbreak, one must consider when the potential harm to the public's health outweighs the individual's right to privacy. And, even if it is determined that the greater good may potentially come at the individual's expense, it is not prudent for public health officials to issue health alerts and media interviews with specific details of personal information. A consideration for what is 'sufficient information' should be made. In such cases, transparency may be somewhat limited, yet it still exists.

Responsiveness

Governance of programmes and services including preparedness and response to emerging threats, disease outbreaks, environmental health hazards, and natural and man-made disasters including bioterrorist attack require that public health officials act and serve the community and its stakeholders within a reasonable timeframe. This is known as responsiveness in governance, and makes provision for integrating community needs and input in order to address issues and concerns of members of the community. Additionally, public health responsiveness to such matters allows for representation of a broad range of stakeholders. This includes, but is not limited to, public health employees, the public at large, government agencies, non-profit organizations, hospitals and clinics, healthcare providers, laboratories, police, fire and other safety agencies, businesses, legislators, and many more. Public health services are not implemented effectively without a mechanism for responding to stakeholders' concerns. In addition to public health programmes and services that measure health indicators and/or oversee regulatory functions in a community (e.g. vital records, prenatal care, immunization, water quality, safe housing, and hazardous material), public health programmes are usually designed in response to local needs and specific populations and in accordance to state and federal standards and mandates, as well as health code regulations.

The scope and responsibilities of the public health system are continually changing to reflect and address epidemiological and demographic transitions in a community, as well as emerging and potential threats to the public health system. One example of this is the Bioterrorism Preparedness Cooperative Agreement of the US Centers for Disease Control and Prevention (CDC), which provides funding to state and local health departments, and US Territories to increase public health capacity and improve its infrastructure through specific critical tasks, which address broad-based public health programmes. This includes planning, epidemiology and surveillance, laboratory capacity, health alert network, risk communication, and training and education. To be responsive in the face of potential biological attacks and/or infectious disease outbreaks, public health governing bodies need to ensure that the public health infrastructure is adequate. The laboratory, surveillance, and epidemiologic capacity of the public health system are critical and drive public health response in emergencies and non-emergency situations alike. Additionally, the ability to disseminate risk communications and health information in a timely fashion should be considered. Communication methods such as telephone, facsimile, and email are basic tools to ensure responsiveness. In addition to technological enhancements, public health systems need to consider their ability to provide services to communities with limited access to public health services due to travel distance and ease, business hours, and cultural and linguistic barriers. The Internet, radio and television, and print media may also serve as an effective means of outreach and dissemination of information, especially when developed and implemented for specific needs of the population.

Consensus oriented

The organizational culture and practice of public health lends itself to be consensus oriented in its governance of programmes and services. This is especially true of programmes that are based on national consensus of health, human and social standards of specific outcome measures and health indicators (e.g. the United States' Healthy People 2010, which embodies national health objectives designed to identify the most significant preventable threats to health and to establish national goals to reduce these threats).

When approaching a broad range of public health issues, strategic planning or stakeholder hearings are undertaken to further identify target areas for a community to achieve. For example, a local health department in the United States convened community hearings to determine funding priorities for social service programmes. This was accomplished through a series of meetings where interested parties were provided the opportunity to provide recommendations on current and future areas of need. This included soliciting community input and feedback and conducting a needs assessment to identify gaps in services and populations in most need of those services. As a neutral body to oversee this process, the Board of Health and Human Services reviewed the findings of the community hearings and determined funding priorities and services. Proposals were then solicited, which allowed social and human service agencies the opportunity to submit proposals for grant funding based on the identified priorities. Proposals were evaluated based on a number of criteria including the proposed community to be served, organizational ability to fulfil programmatic and grant mandates, feasibility of programme evaluation, and other standards. The Board of Health and Human Services' funding recommendations were then reviewed and approved by the City Council. Interested parties were able to again comment on the recommendations. The governing process for determining social service funding was designed to achieve a broad consensus on what was in the best interest of the community overall.

Needs assessment processes are important strategies for public health officials to use in identifying and building consensus. Whether used to gather information on a specific issue (e.g. social service programmes), or on a community as a whole, the process can provide significant information about a community's priorities. Due to legislative mandates, funding streams and other government or funding organization applied restrictions, public health practitioners often enter a community prepared to deal with a specific pre-determined health issue. While the epidemiologic data may indicate that the issue is a significant one, the community may not recognize it as a priority. It is important then, to consider whether or not the community support exists to make the public health programme a success.

Equity and inclusiveness

Like other elements of governance, effective public health programmes ensure equity and inclusiveness of the scope, reach, and delivery of services. Although many believe public health services exist to provide services only to indigent populations, the fact is that public health is integrated into the fabric of the entire community, impacting individuals of all sociodemographic backgrounds. Thus, the most effective programmes are inclusive of all members of society by providing opportunities for all groups, especially the most vulnerable, to improve their health and well-being.

Public health jurisdictions must continue to analyse the demographic changes in their community so that programmatic functions evolve with these transitions. This includes monitoring indicators such as race/ethnicity, age and gender distribution, cultural and linguistic variations, patterns of disease, vital statistics, and population density.

Another element of equity and inclusiveness is dissemination of information, as well as appropriately delivered services. Public health jurisdictions are required to provide information in alternative formats for specific need populations, such as visual and/or hearing impaired or in foreign languages. Also, it is important to remember that not all households have access to the Internet, or may not subscribe to cable television where critical information may be posted or aired. Therefore, the use a broad range of mediums and greater outreach methods must be utilized to ensure that all members of the community have access to public health information, especially critical information that provides precautionary measures to avoid illness and/or injury. When considering the possible consequences of overlooking this vital element of governance, equity, and inclusiveness is a measure of the outreach and impact a public health jurisdiction has in a community.

Effectiveness and efficiency

The utilization and leveraging of human, financial and other resources to ensure that core public health functions, programmatic, regulatory, and community needs are standard operating procedures in most public health organizations. The effectiveness and efficiency of delivering these basic elements will vary based on the overall quality of governance of each jurisdiction.

With increasing pressure to do more with less, public health departments operate and provide more far-reaching and higher quality services with reduced resources and limited operational capacities. Nonetheless, organizations must do the best possible job at protecting the public's health on these limited resources. Public health departments at all government levels should consider the outcomes of providing services by establishing partnerships with private businesses, community organizations, or other public agencies (Reich 2000). Partnerships often result in greater participation, better utilization of resources, and increased efficiency in service delivery.

One method by which public health organizations can measure the effectiveness and efficiency of programmatic and regulatory functions is evaluation. This may be as basic as formative evaluation or enumerating the number of clients served to more detailed assessments of programmatic interventions and improvements in the public's health. Programme evaluation is an essential organizational practice in public health, but does not always measure effectiveness and efficiency. Evaluation must be practised consistently and integrated into programmatic efforts. Evaluating programmes on an ongoing basis may enhance decision making, lead to additional funding opportunities and expand and improve services to the community.

Accountability

The characteristics of good governance are not mutually exclusive. They are integrated together and continuously evolve with changing demographics, programmes and services, community needs, allocation of resources, and advanced practices in public health standards. In essence, public health organizations are accountable to meeting these changing demands and maintain a level of proficiency in order to protect the public's health.

One method of public health accountability is driven by an effort to improve the performance of public health organizations. In the United States, this effort is led by the CDC, which is leading a coalition of national public health organizations to develop, promote, and achieve national public health performance standards. These recognized performance standards were developed to improve the quality of public health practice and the performance of public health systems. The National Public Health Performance Standards are an effort to ensure accountability through organized monitoring and assessment of public health programmes and services. The standards are designed to increase capacity and foster infrastructure building. The standards also promote participation in the development and implementation of programmatic enhancements to meet new challenges, changing needs, public health workforce leadership development, broad and more frequent dissemination of information of public health issues, and incorporating strategic directions for future efforts (DHHS 2006).

The public health system must develop a governance structure that is responsive to the needs and demands of the community it serves. Community members need to be considered not just for their service needs but also for their role as active participants in decision-making. The public health system needs to have the capacity to respond to complex social and economic issues as well as evolving public health threats and challenges.

Overall, good governance in public health enables an organization to effectively fulfil its mission. Within the public health system, each organization must develop its own definition of good governance to meet its vision, mission, needs and values. When essential public health functions are met, governance of public health jurisdictions leads to a trusted and valued organization within a community. An effective organization's governing body is connected to its workforce, community members, stakeholders, and other community leaders. When properly integrated into the infrastructure of an organization, public health programmes are able to focus on their strategic direction and adapt more easily to both internal and external dynamics.

Corruption in governance

Transparency International has defined corruption as 'the abuse of entrusted power for private gain' (Transparency International 2007). Corruption in the health sector results in significant losses of public funds and undermines service delivery, access, and quality of healthcare. Examples of corruption in the public health sector include: Staff absenteeism; poor management; informal payments or tips for health services and bribery of medical professionals; and corrupt practices including misuse of public funds, fraudulent billing of insurance companies or government, irregularities in supply procurement, petty theft and selling of positions and promotions (Lewis 2006; Savedoff & Hussman 2006).

Savedoff and Hussman (2006) identified several characteristics that make health systems vulnerable to corruption. First, an imbalance of information, between health professionals and their patients, and between health supply companies (pharmaceutical and medical device) and public officials provide opportunities for abuse.

Uncertainty in health markets also makes it difficult to manage resources. Perhaps most significantly, the complexity of health systems, especially the large number of stakeholders involved, can both provide opportunities for corruption and create challenges in detection and prevention.

All health systems are vulnerable to corruption. However, the forms of abuse and corruption will vary depending on the structure of the public health system. In the United States, for example, where the financing of health services is separate from the provision of services, corruption is largely focused on abuses that alter the flow of payments and reimbursements (Savedoff & Hussman 2006). Within the US public health system, Medicaid and Medicare exist as entitlement programmes for the poor and elderly. The reimbursement system of the programmes is highly automated, where the filing of claims and issuing of payments are made with no human component. This lack of accountability has led to abuse and fraudulent billing.

In developing or transition countries where the public health system is integrated, where the government is responsible for establishing and providing the healthcare directly, corruption occurs due to a variety of factors but is largely focused on informal, or illegal, payments for services (Savedoff & Hussman 2006). Poor infrastructure such as the inability to secure and control pharmaceuticals and other supplies provides opportunities for theft, or transportation and access issues resulting in high levels of absenteeism, as well as a lack of training among staff. Kickbacks in the purchase of medical supplies and equipment also lead to corruption and abuse within the public health system (Lewis 2006).

Simply, corruption results when governance is poor (Lewis 2006). Systems that operate without sufficient accountability, transparency, participation, and enforcement of rule of law are more likely to experience significant corruption.

Public health systems and infrastructure

Since its inception, the World Health Organization (WHO) has been the coordinating body for international disease detection and response efforts. WHO's efforts have been largely aimed at limiting the international spread of public health epidemics and emergencies before they affect travel and trade, yet until recent revisions, control was focused at national borders and was based on passive notification and control measures. Prior to 2005, the International Health Regulations (1969) were limited to the notification and response to cases of cholera, plague and yellow fever. In 2005, WHO members approved revisions of the International Health Regulations, which increased the stringency of national disease reporting requirements, as well as allowed WHO to bypass state parties to collect information about outbreaks (WHO 2005). State parties must now notify the WHO of all events that may constitute a public health emergency of international concern.

Worldwide, public health systems exist with varying degrees of governance structure. Public health systems may be sophisticated and well planned out, fragmented, or limited. A country's capacity to provide and implement an ongoing and robust public health system is dependent on several factors including a country's government structure, resources and gross national and domestic product, infrastructure, health indicator status, and sociodemographics, to name a few.

In most regions, the Ministry of Health or Department of Health plays the role of providing information, improving health awareness and education, ensuring the accessibility of health services, and monitoring the quality of health services. The ministry is also involved in disease control and illness prevention, and coordinating the utilization of resources. These objectives are accomplished through the formulation and enforcement of health laws, regulations, and policies. Additionally, the ministry of health may conduct overall health planning for regional health programmes. Typically, within the Ministry or Department, there is a specific branch dedicated to overseeing the public health of the region. As an example, Box 7.5.1 describes the governance structure of the US public health system.

Effect of politics on public health governance

As high-level public health positions are often government appointed, the effect of a change in political office may affect both the long-term and short-term objectives of the public health system. For instance, in the United States, each state's governor frequently appoints state health department directors. When the governor changes, the health department director may or may not continue in the position depending on the political alliance of the involved parties. Additionally, even if the state health department director is from the same political party as the incoming governor, there is no guarantee that the director will remain in place or that the public health objectives will stay the course. Thus, the ability to achieve public health objectives established by the health department director under the direction of a governor is potentially limited to the length of political office.

At a local level, politics play a role when there is conflict between the governing body (e.g. the City Council), advisory groups (e.g. Board of Health or issue specific planning councils), local health department management, or other players (e.g. Mayor or City Manager). Similar to the state level example, the challenge to the public health system may be a result of changes in political positions (e.g. new City Council members). An important role of the local health department is to educate political officials about the public health system and issues. Nonetheless, the individual viewpoint of the elected officials or the desire to respond favourably to what they believe is their constituencies' beliefs will influence, either positively or negatively, their commitment to the public health department's objectives.

Management of public health programmes

What is management?

Management is the intersection between governance and the actual work activities performed by employees. A public health manager has the responsibility for coordinating their workforce and resources to achieve a given programme's goals and objectives. These goals and objectives may be legislated by regulatory programmes (e.g. enforcement of environmental health laws), grant-funded programmes monitored by county, state, or federal agencies, established by a governing body (e.g. board of health), or determined by the health department director with their management team. Public health managers must work to set the course for successful implementation and achievement of the identified goals and

Box 7.5.1 Governance structure of the United States public health system

Though variations across local, regional, state, and national levels exist, the overall organization and structure of the US public health system is assembled to promote health and well-being among a population and address threats and other health concerns that may impact a community. The system consists of an array of congruent and independently operated governmental and nongovernmental entities that include:

- Over 3000 county and city health departments and local boards of health
- 59 state and territorial health departments
- Tribal health departments
- More than 160 000 public and private laboratories
- Parts of multiple federal departments and agencies
- Hospitals and other healthcare providers
- Volunteer organizations (Lister 2005)

The public health delivery system begins with a limited federal role, with national, state, and local levels of authority. Federal government exercises authority primarily through policy development, funding decisions, and regulatory enforcement. Federal health agencies are able to formulate and implement a national health policy agenda and to allocate health resources across broad public priorities.

The Department of Health and Human Services (DHHS), the US government's principal agency for public health activities, plays a national role in protecting the health of all Americans and providing essential human services, especially for those who are least able to help themselves. The DHHS includes more than 300 programmes and operated an annual budget of US$698 billion in fiscal year 2007. The DHHS works closely with state and local public health jurisdictions, and many DHHS-funded services are provided at the local level by state or county agencies, or through private sector grantees (DHHS 2007).

Working with states and other partners, the US CDC provides a system of health surveillance to monitor and prevent disease outbreaks (including bioterrorism preparedness), implement disease prevention strategies, and maintain national health statistics. Other programmes include immunization services, workplace safety, and environmental disease prevention. CDC takes the lead to protect against international disease transmission, with personnel stationed in more than 25 foreign countries (CDC 2007).

In the United States, public health activities are based in law. The federal government influences public health practice through its power to tax and spend and its responsibility for regulating interstate commerce (Grad 2005). Using its authority to regulate commerce, the federal government is able to pass laws and regulations and set policies and standards to protect the environment, ensure food and drug safety, and promote occupational health and safety (IOM 1988; Grad 2005; Lister 2005). Its power to tax and spend for the general welfare provides the federal government an opportunity to influence certain behaviours (e.g. raising taxes on cigarettes discourages smoking) and to provide service-oriented programmes, such as financing of personal health services through Medicaid and Medicare programmes (Lister 2005; IOM 1988). Through the financing of various public health initiatives, the federal government can also set conditions on the expenditure of federal funds. In this way, the federal government is able to exercise considerable influence on public health practice.

States are the principal governmental entity responsible for protecting the public's health within the United States (IOM 1988). State governments participate in public health regulatory activities and carry out substantial responsibilities in public health programme administration and resource allocation (Lister 2005). States have governmental authority to carry out most of their responsibilities through their 'police power'—the 'power to provide for the health, safety, and welfare of the people' (Grad 2005). The state's police power generally involves the delegation of authority, to local health agencies. Delegation of public health authority can be classified into three categories: (1) A centralized approach in which states have extensive legal and operational control over local authorities; (2) a decentralized approach in which local governments are delegated significant control; and (3) a hybrid approach in which some public health responsibilities are provided directly by the state, while others are assumed by the localities (Lister 2005).

A 1997 CDC survey of local and state health departments reported that all 50 states, the District of Columbia, and eight territories have state health agencies (SHAs), which are responsible for the administration of public health services within their jurisdictions. The organization of SHAs typically follows one of two models: A freestanding, independent agency responsible directly to the governor or the board of health, or as a component of a superagency. Nearly two-thirds (62 per cent or 31 states) report that the SHA is an independent government agency, and in 19 (38 per cent) states and the District of Columbia, it is a state government superagency. Of the seven territories for which information is available, SHAs are independent agencies in six territories and a component of a superagency in one territory (CDC 1997).

Local health departments (LHDs) are the 'frontline' of the public health system (IOM 1988). Local government agencies usually have the primary responsibilities of implementing public health activities to the community it serves. This decentralization of public health service delivery, bringing services and public officials closer to people, helps ensure a higher level of responsiveness and customization leading to increased satisfaction. One benefit to this structure is the ability to develop locally designed programmes to meet specific needs of the local jurisdiction's constituency. The ability to accomplish this is usually governed by the ease of transparency and collaborative efforts among a greater number of stakeholders at this level, which translate into more neatly defined services for specific populations.

A 2005 Profile of Local Health Departments Survey by NAACHO characterized LHD governance by state, using three categories: All LHDs are units of the SHA; all LHDs are units of local government; and some LHDs are units of the SHD and some are units of local government (mixed). Seventy-nine per cent of LHDs are units of local government; 21 per cent of LHDs are units of the state health agency (Leep 2006).

objectives and ensure staff understands what must be accomplished to ensure deliverables are met on a timely basis. Managers are responsible for aligning employees behind the jurisdiction's vision and mission, programme's strategic direction, creating a positive work environment, and establishing conditions to encourage employee success and reduce risk of failure.

Management theory

Henri Fayol, a French management theorist, proposed the primary functions by which management operates. These management functions include:

1. *Planning*: Deciding what has to happen in the future and creating action plans
2. *Organizing and staffing*: Optimizing the use of resources to enable the successful implementation and achievement of plans
3. *Leading/motivating*: Getting others to play an effective role in achieving plans; motivating people to perform tasks to accomplish objectives
4. *Controlling*: Continually assessing and checking progress against established plans and objectives and modifying based on feedback (Bateman & Zeithaml 1993)

This classical view of management provides a practical definition of what managers do. However, it is not necessarily a complete picture. In 1966, Henry Mintzberg began his research to describe more accurately what managers do. His work led to the description of the basic content of managerial work in terms of 10 roles. Within these 10 roles, all managerial activities were found to involve one or more of three basic behaviours—interpersonal contact, information processing, and decision-making (Mintzberg 1971; Mintzberg 1975).

Interpersonal roles are those elements of a manager's behaviour that focus on and foster interpersonal relationships. These roles originate directly from the formal authority and status associated with the management position. Responsibilities involving interpersonal roles are imperative to the smooth operation of an organization. Using the status of the position, the manager interacts both internally and externally of the organization, building relationships, creating networks, and influencing others.

The first interpersonal role, the *figurehead*, is associated directly with the legal authority of the management position. As the head of an organizational unit, from health department director to clinic manager to programme manager, managers complete some tasks of a ceremonial nature. The director presents pins to employees achieving significant years of service with the health department to recognize their commitment. The clinic manager provides a facility tour for individuals from a local school of public health. The programme manager attends an open house at a community agency. While these responsibilities could be delegated to a subordinate, the completion of these tasks positions the manager to be successful in their other roles.

As a *leader*, managers are responsible for providing motivation and leadership to staff. In many cases, managers are directly responsible for the recruitment, hiring, and training of staff. More importantly, a good manager provides development opportunities for the workforce. In day-to-day operations, the staff members look to their manager to provide them overall direction, approval, and feedback.

Managers have a *liaison* role that includes establishing networks and relationships with external partners. These are valuable relationships, and an unspoken norm in business in general, which leads to reciprocity of information and positive considerations for the organization. The liaison role is devoted to creating information systems outside of the organization or unit. These external relationships create reciprocity of human resource time, deliverables, and information. This role may include serving on a board of directors for a community agency, participating as a member of an advisory board, or simply having coffee with another manager.

Informational roles are devoted to the processing of information. Mintzberg described the manager as the 'nerve centre of the organizational unit'. As a manager, the individual has an opportunity to acquire information through their myriad roles, such as liaison.

An effective manager is constantly seeking useful information from the environment through established contacts both within and outside the organization. In the *monitor or nerve centre* role, the manager obtains information, typically in verbal form.

Once the information is gathered, the manager becomes the *disseminator*. The manager is able to direct the information as s/he determines to be most appropriate. Typically, the knowledge is passed to individuals who would not otherwise have access to the information. The manager may have garnered information from outside sources that will benefit the organization. S/he also shares information within the unit to staff that may not otherwise interact. For example, in a public health agency, the epidemiology manager may be aware of food-borne illness reports, talk to the environmental health manager, and learn that the restaurant inspection programme has found multiple violations at a food establishment mentioned in several epidemiological investigations.

As *spokesperson*, the manager provides some of the information outside of the unit or organization. His/her role includes informing influential people. In public health, this may be seen when the health department director is interviewed by a local news outlet for information on influenza vaccinations or provides information on the health status of the community to a legislator.

The ***decisional*** roles are based on the manager's formal authority to commit to new courses of action and the information gathered as the organizational nerve centre. Four functions describe the decisional roles of a manager.

Managers are constantly seeking to improve the unit or organization and must frequently adapt to changing conditions. As *entrepreneur*, the manager initiates new projects. The manager may: Delegate responsibility for the new project; delegate work but retain final approval; or actively supervise the new project.

Even the best manager cannot anticipate the consequences of all decisions. Thus, the manager becomes the *disturbance handler*, responsible for responding to the unanticipated changes.

As *resource allocator* the manager determines how resources—time, money, opportunities—will be divided. The resource allocator is responsible both for structuring the use of their own time, and for determining the work of employees. In this role, the manager must consider the availability of resources, the impact of the decisions, and the acceptability of the choices to those who influence organization. For example, the manager must consider the assignment of projects to motivate employees as well as getting the project done. Or when budgets are reduced, where do the cuts come from and how do those changes affect the remaining people, programmes, and services?

Managers, especially those in executive level positions, spend a great deal of time in negotiations. As *negotiator*, public health managers may find themselves negotiating the scope of work and budget with a funding source; determining an employee's salary; or working with another manager to decide who should provide what service and to whom.

Mintzberg's identification of the managerial roles assists in providing a framework to describe the work of all managers, including those in public health.

Management skills

To manage an organization, skills in accounting, financial management, human resources, strategic and programme planning, operations research, economics, communication, and monitoring outcome measures are essential. Development, analysis, interpretation, and evaluation of government policies require analytic skills and social skills, as well as a deep understanding of politics.

Managers have also been described based on the kinds of skills exhibited in carrying out their job effectively (Katz 1955). In this context, skill is defined as 'an ability which can be developed, not necessarily inborn, and which is manifested in performance, not merely in potential'. Katz suggests that effective management is dependent on the following three basic developable skills:

- *Technical*: Technical skill involves specialized knowledge, analytical ability, and the ability to use tools and methods to accomplish specific managerial tasks. A public health laboratory manager, for example, must not only be able to manage people, but will need to have the technical mastery and skill to perform specific laboratory diagnostic procedures, use complex and expensive instrumentation, and analyse and interpret test results.
- *Interpersonal/human*: Interpersonal skills are among the most critical skills. Without this fundamental human characteristic, a manager's ability to lead, motivate, and communicate with other people may be limited and jeopardize the effectiveness and efficiency of staff performance. Despite a manager's level of technical proficiency, an effective manager must be able to communicate both within the work unit to employees, equals, and superiors, and outside the work unit with clients, public, and community partners.
- *Conceptual*: Conceptual skill is the ability to see the organization as a whole, to understand the full range of organizational objectives and activities, and to make decisions while accounting for the effect on various components both within and outside the organization. In a retrospective commentary, Katz recognizes that conceptual skill may be more an innate ability than previously considered. Nonetheless, training opportunities such as job rotation and interdepartmental activities may enhance an individual's conceptual skills (Katz 1974).

Overall, managers should be active participants in the department or organizations for which they are responsible. They should be intimately involved in key decisions and activities and have a deep understanding of delegated tasks.

Management in the nonprofit organization

Not-for-profit organizations have some unique characteristics that challenge the application of general managerial concepts. In an article by Newman and Wallender (1976), the authors identify these characteristics.

1. *Service is intangible and hard to measure. Difficulty is often compounded by the existence of multiple service objectives.*

One often hears that when public health is properly functioning, it is not visible. While some public health functions and services provided are easily measurable (e.g. the number of vaccinations per year, intake numbers of clients seen by clinic), most public health services are not quantifiable. Ongoing evaluation of programmes, services, and interventions over time plays an important role in making inferences of public health benefit to the community from services such as food facility inspection, reduction of teen birth rates, decrease in infant death rates, and increase in prenatal care within the first trimester. By the same token, enumerating progress may not equate to lower disease rates or better outcomes. In fact, with new and patient-friendly diagnostic methods, rates of certain infectious diseases may rise, indicating more disease in a community. If the surveillance system is collecting a large amount of disease data, is the public health system doing a better job at encouraging and facilitating data reporting? Or are the disease prevention programmes failing to do their job? Public health managers must be aware of this extraordinary challenge of evaluating programme effectiveness and justifying the work of public health to individuals who are not as aware of this challenge.

An increase in disease cases may not translate into an increase in risky health behaviours among a jurisdiction's residents, but may be an indicator of positive outreach and better surveillance methods. Nevertheless to counter the increase of reported cases of a given disease in the community (e.g. acute and/or chronic hepatitis B, HIV/AIDS, or other sexually transmitted diseases), public health must also be prepared to respond through education, risk communication, and healthcare referrals for treatment.

2. *Customer influence may be weak. Often the enterprise has a local monopoly and payments by customers may be a secondary source of funds.*

An example of weak customer influence is that health department clients may pay only a portion of the cost of treatment (e.g. a clinic co-pay) or no direct fees at all (health education programme). Therefore, health department officials need to consider the source of their funding, such as government agencies, taxpayers, foundations, and ensure that their needs are satisfied.

Consider the implementation of an HIV prevention social marketing campaign in a California city as another example of weak customer influence (http://www.hivstopswithme.org). Although research demonstrated the effectiveness of 'sex-positive' messages, the target population or 'customers' had little influence on the decision-making process of whether or not to implement the campaign. Rather, the city government (which had ultimate influence over the health department director decision) was more greatly influenced by its experiences with the general public that would not be supportive of the campaign. Ultimately, the campaign messages needed to be modified to meet the influence of all customers versus the target audience. In the for-profit arena, marketers are interested in the influence their messages will have on the targeted consumers, not how the people they are not trying to influence will feel about their message.

3. *Strong employee commitment to professions or to a cause may undermine their allegiance to the enterprise.*

'That's not what I was hired to do' is unfortunately heard often among the public health workforce. Among specially trained or professional positions, there are ideas about what the specific responsibilities of a job include and when asked to perform in areas considered outside of their scope, employees may reject the opportunity. It is important for managers to convey how the role they play will influence the greater 'good' of the organization or how it provides a job enrichment opportunity. Government positions further lend themselves to this challenge. When certain positions are paid extra for specific skills, such as the ability to speak another language or specialized education, then others with those skills but without the 'credentialing' may challenge management.

4. *Resource contributors may intrude into internal management—notably fund contributors and government.*

As much of public health services and programmes are supported either partially or fully by the government, therefore the public and government officials have an opportunity to provide input, guidance, and restrictions on how it is spent. The challenge is that those giving the input or determining the restriction are not necessarily public health experts and their input may go against the overall public health mission and strategic plan developed by management.

Much of public health work is also grant (public or private) funded. Therefore, there may be competing ideas on how the work should be completed. The type of evaluation required may impact the implementation of the programme or service. Funders may specify the type of credentialing or skills required by staff. This type of influence on public health work is simply a reality and a challenge to be met by the public health manager.

5. *Restraints on the use of rewards and punishments result from items 1, 3, and 4 above.*

Public health organizations must rely heavily on personal commitment of employees to shared goals. If you cannot easily measure service, it is difficult to recognize, reward or punish an individual. Thus, how do you reward an employee in a government or non-profit organization? Often financial incentives such as bonuses or pay increases are used in other businesses (you make the company money, you get more money). But in public health, service is hard to measure—you cannot use taxpayer or grant money to award a bonus, and civil service or non-profit regulations limit pay increases, so how do you motivate an employee? The desire of professionals (doctors, nurses, therapists) to self-motivate may come in the form of completing a certain number of hours toward continuing education or getting experience and then moving on to another agency.

6. *Charismatic leaders and/or the 'mystique' of the enterprise may be important means of resolving conflict concerning objectives and overcoming restraints.*

A dynamic and forceful individual may be influential enough that values are accepted by others who make decisions. A strong conviction about the importance of a particular service mission and the unusual capacity of the enterprise to provide that service may play a role in addressing the restraints of rewards and punishments or encouraging employees to focus on the mission of the organization versus their individual position. Working at a non-profit or regional health department that is recognized as a leader in the community, state, or nation is also a motivating factor for employees.

Management in public health

As management is about achieving objectives, the public health manager's overall job is to guide the establishment of programmes, services, and infrastructure that allow the workforce to accomplish core public health functions. Indeed, the governing body (if it exists and is properly functioning) will also have specific goals and objectives that steer the course of management's work, but the overarching goal of any public health programme should be the achievement of the essential public health functions.

The public health manager—whether managing an agency, department, division, unit, or programme—must fulfil certain responsibilities. Overall, managers must ensure that local departments achieve federal and state public health goals. Additionally, the public health manager needs to have a clear mission and vision, and a strategic plan for the administration of the agency or programme.

In doing so, managers need to work within the legal framework established for public health issues. Therefore, they must have a thorough understanding of the guidelines of health codes, laws and regulations, and enforcement options. Managers must make decisions about implementation of regulations where options exist (e.g. use of quarantine for certain communicable diseases, issuing public health alerts). Additionally, public health managers must be knowledgeable about the boundaries of their jurisdiction.

The public health manager also functions under the governing structure. At the directorate level, the manager likely works under the direction of a Board of Health, a City Council or, in a non-profit organization, a Board of Directors. In local governance, it is the public health director's or manager's responsibility to educate members of the board of health, non-public health government officials, community members, and other stakeholders about the organization or programme mission, specific health issues, and emerging threats. The local health department typically provides technical support to the governing body. The manager must stay focused on public health and not be swayed into conducting 'non-public health' activities.

While typically only the highest level public health manager reports directly to the governing body, it is common for managers at all levels to work with the input and/or accountability to some 'external' body such as an advisory board, a community planning body, or a citizens' board. These collaborations may help improve the transparency, participation, and accountability of the public health programme. Managed well, these collaborations provide an opportunity to gather information about the community or the population to be served by the public health programme. Nevertheless, the public health manager must be cognizant of the competing priorities and conflicts of interest that may exist.

Public health infrastructure is composed of many agencies and disciplines; these players must work together to respond to the public health needs of a community. This assembly of partners may include government agencies, non-government agencies, medical practitioners, human service organizations, community non-profits, the media, the community, and funders. Collaborations may exist because of some type of regulations (e.g. grant requirement), or develop more organically out of the need to respond to a public health issue. Collaborations may exist to ensure systems are present to link people to needed health services and assure the provision of healthcare. Whatever the reason for their initial formation, collaborations need to be actively managed and should improve the organization's effectiveness. New collaborations will develop in response to evolving public health issues.

Management challenges to enhance public health systems

Bridging the gaps in governance and management of public health systems is a challenge facing health authorities worldwide. When illness, injury, and death can be prevented, it is the role of the public health workforce to bridge the gaps in an unfinished agenda that continues to present new and growing concerns. Public health is a global public good. Discoveries in one part of the world benefit all of humankind. Likewise, basic prevention and control measures of disease and disability can also be factors that sustain societies from outbreaks and subsequent human and economic loss.

Technology and infrastructure

Today's public health workforce is tasked with added responsibilities to keep up with the growing pace of technological advances, changing communication methods, enhanced training, increasing need for interagency collaboration, more stringent federal government demands on local agencies, and shrinking funding sources and resources. Both government and non-governmental funding sources are insufficient to support the demands on managers to provide sufficient and effective public health services.

The invention of the Internet, new and user-friendly computer applications, and other technological developments in the areas of health alert networks, web-based technology, and paperless medical records systems are value-added tools for the public health workforce. The pressure to understand and apply technological advances into government agencies whose infrastructure is not designed to keep pace presents a significant challenge. However, public health agencies are experts at leveraging financial, human and other resources to sustain their essential functions and build capacity along the way. One example of this in the United States is the utilization of public health emergency management grants (DHHS 2006). These grants have bridged several gaps in public health capacity and infrastructure building. Although intended to address bioterrorism and public health outbreaks, many public health agencies have utilized these grants to increase technological capacity including paperless medical records and health information exchange. Other benefits of these grants include greater partnerships and collaboration among regional local public health departments, hospitals, academia, non-profit organizations, private businesses, and other first responders (e.g. fire and police).

Managers will face increasing issues of handling aging public health facilities and infrastructure. The challenge of creating new facilities that will have to accommodate changing needs for many years is significant. What does a new facility need to look like? What laboratory services will be included? What public health programmes or services will be offered, needed, or available? Managers will need to develop plans for the future of public health when that future is uncertain. To meet this challenge, public health systems may consider looking toward a business model like that of Kaiser Permanente. In order to streamline the development and building of hospitals, Kaiser created a template with approved building plans that are used as a starting point for all new hospital facilities. The benefits of this model include a faster, more efficient permitting process. Kaiser is also being a 'good neighbour' and responsible business through the use of sustainable and renewable resources and plans for mitigating the environmental impact (Kaiser 2007).

Changing spectrum of disease and health emergencies

Public health response to the anthrax attacks in the United States in the fall of 2001 increased the visibility of public health nationally. And as a first responder discipline, public health has risen to the challenge by training staff on incident command systems and other emergency response applications. Health jurisdictions have enhanced laboratory diagnostics and the ability to transfer data or results through new platforms of technology. Additionally, the development of response plans to wide-scale biological events that require mass prophylaxis and that have been successfully exercised enhanced collaborative efforts with partnering agencies that would be involved in the response and recovery of such incidents.

Public health officials will have to work to preserve the prevention focus of public health in a time where the spectrum of what falls under the 'public health' umbrella is widening. Chronic disease prevention, for example, has become a notable source of funding and programmes with increases in diabetes prevention programme. While this expansion is important, especially in light of the ageing population of the United States, the public health community must ensure that this increasing focus on chronic disease prevention does not negatively impact efforts toward communicable disease control.

The changing spectrum of public health priorities also applies to transitional economies, which face both a rise in the burden of non-communicable diseases and the unfinished agenda of communicable disease and high maternal/infant mortality.

The health workforce

At a time of increasing demands and expectations of the public health community, the public health workforce within the United States is declining (Perlino 2006) and there is concern about their skills and competencies (HRSA 2005). Severe shortages in the number of epidemiologists, nurses, laboratory personnel, and environmental health specialists have been found (Perlino 2006). Budget constraints have been identified as the most significant barrier to adequate staffing of governmental public health agencies. Other challenges of recruitment include a lack of qualified candidates, non-competitive salaries, and lengthy processing times for new hires (HRSA 2005). Training in core public health concepts as well as training on specific public health issues of bioterrorism and disaster preparedness has been identified as unmet needs among the public health workforce (HRSA 2005).

At the centre of any effective public health programme is its staff. Public health emergency management grants have provided health jurisdictions with the opportunity to increase the level and frequency of training of its workforce. This includes training of the essential functions of public health, core competencies by discipline, and other elements that can appropriately and effectively be linked back to preparedness and response. Without an appropriately trained, dedicated workforce, public health programmes cannot operate effectively.

Like most managers, public health managers must deal with workforce development issues such as hiring, training and developing, dealing with problem employees, managing conflict, mentoring, rewarding and motivating employees, handling problem employees, and operating within union and civil service rules. Public health managers also must manage people of various skills and educational levels—from volunteers and lay workers to professionals and medical personnel. Individuals working in public health may have limited, if any, public health training. Therefore, managers must provide training opportunities that provide a general orientation to public health. They must also provide on-the-job technical training for specific tasks.

Management is required to possess a high level of skill, and pass on instruction to subordinates in order for them to apply practical approaches to day-to-day services. Effective managers must foster an attitude that education is a lifelong process. It does not end with a degree and is not renewed with continuing education units. Some of the best training comes from job experience and managers should consider the appropriateness and feasibility of providing training opportunities to staff by challenging them with new responsibilities and projects.

Healthcare reform and financing

Management is also tasked with keeping up with the latest legislation that may impact the future of their programmes. Public health funding at the state and federal levels is based on tax revenues. Funding for local health departments, however, may come from a variety of sources, including revenues from local government; revenues from state government (state direct); federal funds passed through to local health agencies by state agencies (federal pass-through funds); direct funding from federal agencies (e.g. CDC, Health Resources and Services Administration, Substance Abuse and Mental Health Services Administration); reimbursement from Medicare, Medicaid, and other insurers; regulatory and patient personal fees; and other sources (e.g. funding from private foundations) (NAACHO 2007). Therefore the public health manager must be aware of the timing and sources of funding. Federal, state, and local government, and private foundation grant cycles vary, as well as the terms of the grant. Specific regulations regarding the use of funds also vary from source to source, and even programme to programme. Managers are challenged not just to demonstrate the appropriate use of funds, but also to balance resources. They must consider where the funding comes from and the competing influence and needs of the sources, as well as how the resources are distributed and shared.

Proposals for healthcare reform will influence public health services and could potentially reduce or eliminate the need for the provision of core public health services. In California, for example, Governor Schwarzenegger unveiled a healthcare proposal that 'promotes a healthier California through prevention and wellness and universality of coverage' (http://gov.ca.gov/pdf/press/Governors_HC_Proposal.pdf). Key programme elements include the promotion and prevention, wellness and health coverage for all Californians, and improving affordability and cost containment. If the Governor's healthcare reform efforts are successful, the need for categorical programmes such as immunizations, HIV care, and the Women, Infant and Children Program could be significantly affected, as individuals currently receiving services under these programmes would have access to more comprehensive health coverage.

Conclusion

Public health governance and management systems throughout the world are striving to apply theoretical knowledge about good governance, the impact of social injustice on increased health risks and poor health outcomes, and management theories to develop and implement far-reaching and sustainable changes in public health policy and practice to affect significant reductions in health disparities and improve the health of the public overall. While the challenges for developing and maintaining strong public health systems can be overwhelming, great progress is made by various organizations in different parts of the world every day.

- Good governance can help societies and the public health organizations within them effectively fulfil their mission and provide services that are responsive to community needs.
- Systems that operate with poor governance, especially without sufficient accountability, transparency, participation, and enforcement of rule of law, are more likely to experience significant corruption.
- Bridging the gaps in governance and management of public health systems is a challenge facing health authorities worldwide. When illness, injury, and death can be prevented, it is the role of the public health workforce to bridge the gaps in an unfinished agenda that continues to present new and growing concerns.
- Public health managers need to be aware of and understand the societal influences and changes that impact the public health industry. Healthcare reform, bioterrorism preparedness, legislative changes, the influence of media, emerging diseases, and other public health and societal issues require that the public health manager continuously understand these changes so that they are able to respond with appropriate and effective programmes and services.

References

Americans for Nonsmokers' Rights (2007). Americans for nonsmokers' rights: About us. http://www.no-smoke.org Accessed 20 July 2007.

Bateman, T.S. and Zeithaml, C.P. (1993). Managers and Organizations. In *Management: Function and strategy*, pp. 5–29. Irwin, Illinois.

Blendon, R.J., DesRoches, C.M., Cetron, M.S. *et al.* (2006). Attitudes toward the use of quarantine in a public health emergency in four countries. *Health Affairs—Web Exclusive*. **25**, W15–W25.

Carrin, G. and James, C. (2004). Reaching universal coverage via social health insurance: Key design features in the transition period. Health Financing Policy Issue Paper. World Health Organization, Geneva.

Centers for Disease Control and Prevention (2003). Use of quarantine to prevent transmission of severe acute respiratory syndrome—Taiwan, 2003. *Morbidity and Mortality Weekly Report*. **52**, 680–3.

Centers for Disease Control and Prevention (2007). Trends in tuberculosis incidence—United States, 2006. *Morbidity and Mortality Weekly Report*. **56**, 245–50.

Crane, D.P. and Jones, Jr. W.A. (1982). *The public manager's guide*. Bureau of National Affairs, Washington, DC.

Department of Health and Human Services, Centers for Disease Control and Prevention (2006). Public health emergency preparedness cooperative agreement AA154. Available at: www.bt.cdc.gov/planning/coopagreement/pdf/fy06announcement.pdf. Accessed on May 26, 2007.

Detels, R. (2009). The scope and concerns of public health. In *Oxford Textbook of Public Health* (eds. R. Detels *et al.*), Oxford University Press, Oxford.

Grad, F.P. (2005). Constitutional and legal sources of public health powers. In *Public health law manual*, pp. 10–26. American Public Health Association, Washington DC.

HIV stops with me (2007). HIV stops with me social marketing campaign. http://www.hivstopswithme.org/default.aspx?t=EN&l=longbeach. Accessed on 14 June 14 2007.

Hofrichter, R. (ed.)(2006). Chapter 1—Introduction. In *Tackling health inequities through public health practice: A handbook for action*, pp. 11–31. National Association of County and City Health Officials, Washington D.C.

Human Resources Services Administration (2005). *Public health workforce study*. U.S. Department of Health and Human Services.

Innovations in Governance and Public Administration (2206). *Replicating what works*. Department of Economic and Social Affairs, United Nations. New York.

Institute of Medicine (1988). *The future of public health*. National Academy Press, Washington D.C.

Johnson, J.A. and Breckon, D.J. (2007) Evolution of management and administrative leadership theories. In *Managing health education and promotion programs: Leadership skills for the 21st century*, pp. 11–25. Jones and Bartlett, Massachusetts.

Kaiser Permanente (2007). *Building health care for the 21st century*. Kaiser Permanente Southern California Region, Strategic Planning and Consulting.

Katz, R.L. (1974). Skills of an effective administrator. *Harvard Business Review*, **52**, 90–102.

Kaul, I., Grunberg, I., and Stern, M.A. (eds.) (1999). *Global public goods*. Oxford University Press, New York.

Leep, C.J. (2006). *2005 National profile of local health departments*, pp. 1–73. National Association of County and City Health Officials. Washington D.C.

Levy, B.S. and Side, V.W. (eds.)(2006). Nature of social injustice and impact on public health. In *Social injustice and public health*. pp. 5–21, Oxford University Press, New York.

Lewis, M. (2006). Governance and corruption in public health care systems. Working paper number 78. Center for Global Development.

Lister, S.A. (2005). *An overview of the U.S. public health system in the context of emergency preparedness*. CRS Report for Congress. March 17, 2005.

Mintzberg, H. (1971). Managerial work: Analysis from observation. *Management Science*, **18**, B97–B110.

Mintzberg, H. (1975). The manager's job: Folklore and fact. *Harvard Business Review*, **53**, 49–61.

Newman, W.H. and Wallender, H.W. (1978). Managing not-for-profit enterprises. *Academy of Management Review*, **3**, 24–31.

Perlino, C.M. (2006). *The public health workforce shortage: Left unchecked, will we be protected*? American Public Health Association, Washington D.C.

Plough, A. (2006). Promoting social justice through public health policies, programs, and services. In *Social injustice and public health* (eds. B.L. Levy and V.W. Sidel), pp.418–31, Oxford University Press, New York.

Public Health Functions Steering Committee (1994). Public health in America, 1994.

Public Health Workforce Study (2005). Bureau of Health Professions, Health Resources and Services Administration. January 2005.

Reich, M.R. (2000). Public-private partnerships for public health. *Nature Medicine*, **6**, 617–20.

Savedoff, W. and Hussman, K. (2006). Why are health systems prone to corruption? In Transparency International's *Global corruption report*. pp. 3–16, Pluto Press, London.

Sparrow, M. (2006). Corruption in health care systems: The US experience. In Transparency International's *Global corruption report*, pp. 16–24, Pluto Press, London.

Transparency International (2007). Transparency International. http://www.transparency.org/about_us Accessed on 22 June 2007.

Turnock, B.J. (1996). What is public health? In *Public health: What it is and how it works*. Aspen Publishers, Maryland.

United Nations Development Programme (1997). Governance for sustainable human development: A UNDP policy document. Available at: http://mirror.undp.org/magnet/policy Accessed on 26 May 2007.

World Health Organization (2004). *Regional overview of social health insurance in South-East Asia*. WHO, New Delhi.

World Health Organization (2005). *International health regulations*. WHO, Geneva.

7.6

Public health sciences and policy in high-income countries

Tim Tenbensel and Peter Davis

Abstract

The very nature of public health research, as it has evolved since the early 1900s, has increasingly required active intervention in public policy processes in order for the research insights generated by public health to have practical application. However, as in many other areas of public policy, policies regarding public health are typically only marginally influenced by research. This gap between research and policy can be perplexing and frustrating to public health researchers. The academic enterprise of policy studies, which draws from the social science disciplines of politics, sociology, and economics, can shed a great deal of light regarding why the gap exists and what might be done about it.

The chapter begins with an introduction into the broad topic of the role of public health research in policy ('Introduction: Getting from research to policy'). The main theme advanced in this chapter is that research is best considered as one of a myriad of factors including values, interests, and institutions that influence policy. The bulk of this chapter ('Power' and 'Processes') provides an overview of the key insights and conceptual frameworks that have been generated by policy studies. This material boils down to answers to two basic questions—who has *power* over public policy and why? ('Power'); and (ii) what is the nature of public policy *processes?* ('Processes'). The picture that develops from this overview is that public health in high income countries has been very successful at defining policy problems, but meets very significant obstacles on the road to translating the definition of problems into concrete policy action.

The final quarter of this chapter ('Research to policy informed by policy studies') returns the focus to the role of research in public policy, drawing on the material outlined in 'Power' and 'Processes' regarding power and process. Research is important for its capacity to contribute to policy *arguments.* However, while research may be an increasingly necessary component of policy arguments, it is rarely sufficient. The key to maximizing the impact of research in policy is to develop arguments that successfully integrate research-based knowledge with an understanding of values and practical political exigencies. Few public health researchers have the capacity to develop all of these components. Therefore it is imperative that relationships and alliances are built with other participants in policy processes such as government agencies and interest groups that are capable of supplementing public health research expertise.

Introduction: Getting from research to policy

Public health, research, and policy

Despite the long involvement of public health researchers and practitioners in social action and despite their reliance on at least a rudimentary level of knowledge about social and political context, the active participation of the social and policy sciences in public health work is of fairly recent origin (Mechanic 1995). The core public health sciences have been of a more technical kind, principally epidemiology and biostatistics, together with related clinical and laboratory disciplines. Such a narrow disciplinary base, however, came to be seen as unsustainable for two reasons. First, it was realized that the traditional interventions of disease prevention need to be adequately contextualized if they are to be delivered effectively (Schmid *et al.* 1995). The effectiveness, as opposed to the efficacy, of such interventions is not something that can just be left to simple improvisation in the field. Second, with the growing salience of the chronic and non-communicable diseases in the high income countries, issues of health promotion are now much more important, and these have brought with them an irreducibly and strongly behavioural dimension to the public health sciences (O'Neill & Pederson 1992). The decade of the 1990s brought with it the realization that traditional public health and health promotion needed further supplementation. Accordingly, a new 'population health' paradigm has emerged which incorporates concerns with health outcomes of whole populations, inequalities of outcomes within populations, and the determinants of these patterns (Glouberman & Millar 2003).

With each additional layer to the enterprise of public health there has been a greater imperative for the public health community to engage in public policy. Health promotion required advocates to compete for health sector resources, often at the same time that many countries were attempting to control health system costs. The population health framework requires an even greater understanding of public policy as many of the determinants of population health and health inequalities, as well as the possible solutions are shaped by policy dynamics. This population health imperative to engage with policy goes well beyond the bounds of health policy into the domains of economic, education, housing, transport, and income support policy as part of 'healthy public policy'.

The worlds of research and policy

Public health researchers know that their research has significant policy implications, and are therefore keen to see the fruits of research translated and incorporated into public policy decisions. Such hopes and expectations are not unique to public health. However, those who have studied the interconnection between research and policy have consistently found that research findings produced within academia are seldom utilized in policy (Landry 2003). According to Jonathan Lomas, '(t)he general picture is one of poorly connected worlds lacking knowledge of (and respect for) the other' (2007). Currently, the push to strengthen the role of research in policy is captured by the catchphrase 'evidence-based policy' (EBP) (Davies *et al.* 2000).

Why is there such a seeming disconnection between the worlds of research and policy? Such a question has routinely occupied the minds of those who have studied and participated in public policy processes for the past 60 years, and some of the most insightful commentary has come from those who have done both (Ellwood 2003). Essentially, policymakers and researchers operate in environments shaped by fundamentally different priorities, motivations, definitions of success, and time-frames.

Most high income countries are parliamentary democracies and the world of policy in democratic societies is characterized by conflicting values and conflicting interests. Policy is fundamentally shaped by politics and most, if not all, policy decisions are potentially subject to opposition and criticism. Governments, and those public officials who hold key positions in them, require knowledge that can be used to support and justify potentially contentious policy decisions.

The world of research remains fundamentally shaped by the traditional concept of the role of the scientist as a 'dispassionate creator of knowledge'. Under this view science is value-free, its findings are of universal application, and scientists are expected to retain a position of objectivity, keeping their personal prejudices at a distance from their work and avoiding public controversy. To an important extent these prescriptions for personal behaviour serve to insulate scientific work from extraneous dispute, thus focusing argument and controversy on matters of common scientific discourse to which agreed methodologies and data can be brought to bear. This is the conventional view of the laboratory sciences.

Beyond this, however, these prescriptions for the scientific role are quite understandable given the very real uncertainty there is about the interpretation of scientific findings once they come to be applied in the public arena. In the paradigmatic scientific research setting, findings are generated under carefully controlled—frequently experimental laboratory—conditions. These conditions are not replicated in the real world where they are applied. Nevertheless, it is in these 'real world' circumstances that the carefully nurtured aura of value neutrality is breached because at this point scientific application touches upon the frequently competing interests of different groups in the community (Greenberg 1992). Such an environment is not generally conducive to producing 'usable knowledge' (Lindbom & Cohen 1979) for policy. The incentives for researchers do not necessarily help. The sorts of research valued by government agencies typically do not coincide with the types of research rewarded by scholarly journals.

However, there is a rather different divide between research and policy that comes into play whenever researchers openly advocate particular policy directions. Over the past 20–30 years, many public health researchers, particularly in the areas of tobacco, alcohol, and latterly obesity, have been highly visible advocates for particular policy initiatives that are seen as appropriate responses to the problems they help to define and diagnose. These advocates often become frustrated with what they see as the slow progress of public health issues through policy, and the fact that policy changes tend to be piecemeal and incremental rather than large-scale.

As an example, public health research has highlighted the environmental factors that shape rates of obesity—a constellation of increased prevalence of energy-dense foods, which itself is attributable to marketing; and changes in the environment for physical activity. Largely on the basis of this research, a number of measures, including restrictions on advertising, taxation of energy-dense foods, and new regimes of labelling foods have been proposed (Lang & Rayner 2007). Although a few jurisdictions have made policy moves in these directions, public health advocates have been generally disappointed. According to Swinburn *et al.* (2005), 'no country has yet developed and implemented a coherent programme of action to prevent further weight gain in the population and to manage its current obesity burden'. Existing government responses tend to emphasize measures aimed at entreating individuals to change lifestyle and dietary habits, and are less focused on changing the environmental conditions that have been identified (Wang & Brownell 2005).

From the perspective of those more central to policy decision-making, public health voices are simply one element of the cacophony of demands for policy change from an enormous variety of sources. Politicians and public officials are typically cautious, knowing that many solutions proposed by public health advocates are likely to provoke fierce opposition from business, big and small, whose economic well-being will be affected. They know that many citizens will object to what they see as unwarranted government interference in private decisions. They know from experience that untried policy ideas can have unintended consequences.

Towards an understanding of public policy

How can researchers better understand the world of policy? A useful starting point has been suggested by John Lavis, a Canadian policy scholar at the forefront of efforts to bridge the worlds of research and policy (Lavis 2006). The three basic components of policy are *ideas, interests,* and *institutional arrangements.* Research and other forms of evidence ('is' statements) are regarded as a sub-category of *ideas,* alongside values ('ought' statements). In portraying the place of research in policy process in this way, Lavis is emphasizing that there is much more that shapes policy besides research.

As public policy is ultimately rooted in a democratic framework, values cannot and should not be quarantined from policy processes. This places some inherent limits to the ideal of evidence-based policy. The issue of fluoridation illustrates this. The adjustment of fluoride levels in central water supplies has been shown to be a safe and effective public health measure for preventing tooth decay for over 50 years. And yet, once the technical health issues have become secondary to wider political considerations of safety and individual rights, adoption of this measure has often been subject to value debate (Winstanley 2005). If public opinion and public values 'trump' scientific expertise, that may be entirely legitimate in a democracy.

In response, many champions of more rational policy processes have argued that scientific research should be the deciding factor in policy once a society determines which value objectives are most important (Alexander 1986). So, for example, if it can be established that improved oral health for the population is more important to the public than personal choice, then fluoridation is an optimal policy. However, such a neat demarcation between spheres of science and values is highly unrealistic (Lindblom 1959). Debates about values occur simultaneously with debates about evidence. It is rarely the case that societies collectively agree about what should be done *before* determining the best way to achieve it. Value debates evolve over time and frequently do not get resolved as such, even though some value positions strengthen over time and others weaken.

In any case, public health at its core is a value-laden enterprise as well as a scientific enterprise. Improving the health of the population is clearly a value that can stand in relation to, and in competition with, other important societal values in particular policy contexts. Over the past century, the public health community has been active in articulating and promoting the values of population health, and more recently, the reduction of health disparities. To the extent that policymakers have come to regard these as valued objectives, this is in large part due to the value-based arguments developed by the public health community.

Nevertheless, there are many instances in which public health research evidence has little effect on policy even when public opinion broadly supports policy measures advocated by the public health community. In these cases, such as efforts to raise the minimum legal age for alcohol consumption, it is the involvement of affected interests more than public values that present the major obstacle to policy change. Indeed, the bulk of policy studies literature suggests that understanding the interplay of interests is the most useful place to start in understanding policy dynamics.

It is easy to conclude that policy that is driven more by interests than by research is inherently problematic. However, some influential understandings of democracy give interest groups a central place as the building blocks of democratic policymaking. Because interests are opposed by other interests, policy in a democratic society emerges from the processes of interplay and conflict. Debates are cross-cutting, no particular group has a pervasive influence across all issues all the time. This perspective is known as 'pluralism'. Whether or not this is an entirely plausible account of how policy is made (and most policy scholars would doubt this), organized interests have a legitimate place in policy processes because they enable people to protect their livelihood when it is threatened. Can particular interests be regarded as illegitimate policy actors? Public health advocates have successfully cast the tobacco industry as a 'pariah'. But it has taken decades to achieve this and, in any case other industries whose interests are threatened by public health are not as unambiguously problematic as tobacco. While the power of particular interests may be problematic (and we will explore issues of power below) it is difficult, in a democratic context, to argue that such interests should not have some presence in policy processes, particularly when and where livelihoods are affected.

Understanding public policy: Power and processes

There is no single technique of studying policy, given the enormous variety of dynamics and processes characterizing the development of policy across different policy arenas and different jurisdictions. Instead, the academic study of policy is an eclectic activity which incorporates insights and concepts across the range of social sciences, most notably political science, sociology, and economics. Reducing to basics, the two most significant concepts in the study of policy are *power* and *processes*. The study of power provides the toolkit for unpacking the 'interests' and 'institutions' components of Lavis's model of policy.

Not all interests and values affect policy equally. Understanding power is fundamental to understanding how public policy develops and changes, and to increasing the likelihood of desired policy changes. For many in the public health community, as for many other researchers, there is almost something distasteful, even underhand, about acknowledging the role that power and political position might play in achieving what appear to be self-evidently laudable and highly noble public objectives (such as saving lives and preventing illness and disease). In contrast, a policy studies approach views power as inevitable and unavoidable. Support must be mobilized, resources transferred, regulations instituted, programmes established, and administrative interventions sustained and carried through to successful completion (Williams-Crowe & Aultman 1994). At every point, issues of power, position, and politics are crucial.

Analysis of power, however, needs to be supplemented with an understanding of process. Policy should not be viewed as the result of the brute translation of power into action. In specific circumstances, powerful actors and interests may 'play their hand' badly, while those with seemingly limited power achieve unexpected successes. Many policy developments are highly contingent and unpredictable. For those policies that do follow a more straightforward and predictable trajectory, it is still important to understand how policy processes unfold.

Finally, before embarking on a tour through the key concepts of policy studies, it is important to distinguish between two types of policy analysis. (Buse *et al.* 2005) Analysis *of* policy is primarily an academic enterprise, in which the student of policy sits 'outside' looking in. It is essentially a retrospective exercise, and attempt to understand what has happened (Buse *et al.* 2005). Analysis *for* policy implies engagement and involvement in policy from a 'partisan' standpoint. It is 'usually carried out to inform the formulation of a policy or anticipate how a policy might fare if introduced (e.g. how other actors might respond to the proposed changes)' (Buse *et al.* 2005). Analysis *of* policy is important inasmuch as it provides an essential platform for analysis *for* policy. The following two sections cover the most important concepts that form the basis of analysis *of* policy. Section 'Research to policy informed by policy studies' shows how this material can be used to underpin analysis *for* policy.

Power

Having said that understanding power is fundamental to understanding policy, those who study policy are not of one mind as to *how* to understand power. There is a plethora of approaches to power that can be found in political science and sociology more generally. While this means that it is difficult to arrive at a definitive diagnosis of power in any particular situation, this diversity of approaches and concepts serves to strengthen the quality of studies of policy, and provides a diverse toolkit of concepts, all of which can provide a useful basis for analysis *for* policy.

Focus on 'policy actors'

An obvious and important place to start in exploring power relationships is to identify the various organizations, groups and individuals—the policy actors—that participate in policy processes. The most important categories of policy actors are politicians, government agencies, and their officials and interest groups.

Politicians and political parties are the visible tip of the policy process iceberg. In many cases, their influence is relatively minor in comparison to other types of policy actors. Under democratic systems of governance, it is expected that democratically elected representatives form the basis of governments and that these governments are constitutionally entitled to formulate and implement public policy. Exactly what role politicians play in policy is largely determined by the design of governmental institutions (see Section 'Institutions' below). In most political systems apart from the USA, only a minority of elected politicians play an influential role in policy, and often that role is circumscribed by the role that they occupy. The partisan composition of government is also an essential consideration, as major political parties often differ in the degree to which they prioritize particular public health concerns.

Government agencies and public officials are crucial figures in policy processes. While, symbolically speaking, the legislature is important for imparting public support to policy proposals, and while the executive plays a central role as the embodiment of political leadership, appointed officials largely drive the detail of policy formulation. In principle they are answerable to elected politicians in the executive arm of government, but there is a limit to the extent to which generalist politicians can effectively maintain scrutiny over specialist advisers and bureaucrats supposedly at their command. Historically, many important policy measures, such as the emergence of social welfare systems in Sweden and Britain, were principally developed and sponsored by public officials with minimal input from politicians (Heclo 1974).

Government agencies have characteristic interests that correspond to their role in the structure of government. As such, health agencies frequently find themselves pitted against revenue departments on public health issues, especially where sizeable proportions of government revenue are sourced from taxes and excises on tobacco, alcohol, and gambling (Seelig & Seelig 1998).

Interest groups can be defined as groups that organize in order to influence public policy, but are not political parties. They are active in shaping policy by providing independent (i.e. non-governmental) sources of policy ideas and directions, as critics of existing policy, as sounding boards for the feasibility of policy proposals, and often they play a crucial role in policy implementation. A crude but useful distinction can be made between two broad types of interest groups. 'Sectional' interest groups are those that have well-defined economic interests and include organizations representing particular industry or business sectors, employer organizations, employee, and professional organizations. 'Advocacy' interest groups are advocates of value-based causes. Advocacy interest groups are usually defined in terms of the specific cause they promote or in terms of their identity, be it geographic, ethnic, gender, or based on a particular health condition. Public health has spawned a great many advocacy groups which have close ties to public health researchers.

A policy actor focus allows one to map the positions of various actors on particular issues. Most proposed changes to policy are likely to have beneficial effects for some groups and categories of the population, and have adverse effects for others. Itemizing the policy actors whose interests and values may be affected is a useful starting point for analysis of policy.

In doing so, it is necessary to take into account important differentials in power between policy actors. The distribution of costs and benefits of changes to policy is a crucial consideration (Wilson 1973). In situations in which the benefits of policy changes are distributed diffusely across many, but where the costs are borne by a few, the few can be expected to lobby strongly against such changes, particularly if they have the resources to do so. Generally, sectional groups are relatively well-resourced, as they are able to draw on financial contributions from member firms, employees, or professionals. Advocacy groups on the other hand, tend to be much smaller in scale, less well-resourced, and more dependent on member commitment.

Many key public health issues including tobacco, alcohol, and obesity fit this profile. Tobacco control is an instance where a professional consensus on the case for intervention is not in question and where a relatively sophisticated and policy-relevant conceptualization of the issue has been developed. Yet, formidable obstacles to progress in this area remain because of the powerful constituency against regulatory and policy change that is nurtured by the tobacco companies. Controls on advertising, price increases, and the creation of smoke-free environments, have all been opposed by the industry. Similarly, the alcohol and food industries have been very active in other areas of public health concerned with diet and alcohol consumption. The public health task is made very much more difficult in these circumstances since a single, powerful opponent can work at a number of levels of the policy process to block public health initiatives.

In contrast, public health lacks a powerful, united, and consistent political constituency. This is partly because some of the greatest achievements of public health are nearly invisible; death, disease, and injury averted are hard to relate to and quantify (Remington 1990). Furthermore, there are no major, cohesive, and articulate constituencies that recognize and openly acknowledge the benefit they derive from public health initiatives (apart from those they employ), and there are many groups whose interests may be affronted by energetic public health action. Therefore, on political grounds alone, policy initiatives in public health are difficult to mount and sustain.

A structural focus

A policy actor framework focusing predominantly on policy actors can go some way towards understanding the policy dynamics of these public health issues, but it also has limitations. Although some groups may exert more power than others, a background assumption is that the exertion of power itself is generally visible to the tutored observer. An alternative way of understanding power involves identifying underlying structures of power that are not readily visible. While multiple interest groups may be present and apparent, the real work of politics and strategic choice comes down to a few key players with the power to influence the final outcome.

Structural power can also be thought of as involving broader societal forces which may or may not take the form of particular organizations. The dynamics between these deeper structural forces ultimately shape public policy. Surface dynamics between government agencies and interest groups should be viewed as the product of these deeper structural forces. In health policy literature, three types of structural interest are characteristically identified—business, medicine, and the state.

The first structural force that is significant is that of the state itself. The term state is in many ways synonymous with government but it is used to denote a constellation of agencies and institutions that is more enduring than particular elected governments. In most high income countries, states play a key role in the funding, provision and/or regulation of the health sector (Blank & Burau 2004). From their central position in health sectors, states have particular interests in fostering healthy populations so as to help maximize economic productivity, and in exerting some control over the cost of health systems.

Social theorists have long regarded business as structurally powerful because it performs key functions in the economy as a whole. Governments still stand or fall in large part on their capacity to foster conditions for economic growth. Economic growth, in turn, is primarily driven by business decisions to invest, produce, and employ (Lindblom 1977). Governments must always consider the downstream economic and political consequences of following policies that adversely affect some or all sectors of business. Since the 1970s, increasing globalization has added a new and arguably even stronger element to the power of business. Changes in the international economy, best indicated by the increasing power of international financial markets, have placed significant constraints on the capacity of states to respond to some domestic needs. Particularly in health systems which are tax-funded, the power of global markets restricts government capacity to expand spending on health.

In contrast, the medical profession is a structural interest that increases expansionary pressures in health systems and is capable of resisting efforts to control costs. Government policies in health must be crucially sensitive to the interests of medical professionals (Salter 2004). As with business, such resistance might not require the presence of powerful interest groups representing the profession; it may simply be the result of the pervading logic of the way in which the health system is organized. For example, where governments have attempted to ground health policy more squarely within a population health framework, the structural weight of the medical profession is a significant barrier to the shift of resources away from curative medicine towards population health (Marmor *et al.* 1994).

Many analysts of health policy take structural forces as their starting point. An early, influential outline of this view was advanced by Robert Alford (1975) who characterized health policy as a field of contending interests made up of the *dominant interests* of the medical profession, the *challenging interests* of the funders of health care—the state and/or private insurers; and the *repressed interests* of the broader community. More recently, sociologist Donald Light (1995) has suggested that health policy is fundamentally shaped by the interplay of 'countervailing powers' between the state and medicine. Ultimately, the power of business, medicine, and the state varies according to context. Each may, in particular circumstances, be internally divided, while in other circumstances structural power might not be particularly relevant.

A discourse focus

Under both the pluralist and structuralist approaches, power is regarded as a thing which different actors and interests possess more or less of (Hindess 1996). This would suggest that all we need to do is to find a way of measuring how much power particular groups have. More recent developments in social and political theory suggest that power is better understood as something that is fluid, qualitative, and relational' rather than 'quantitative'. Power operates through a variety of channels, and often power can operate in ways that would not be recognized if we only focused on actors and interests.

A key idea to have emerged over the past two decades is that power operates through discourse—i.e. the language people use to describe the world. The very act of naming things in particular ways reflects the operation of power. For example, referring to the recipients of healthcare services as clients rather than patients indicates a shift from one way of thinking and talking to another. In many respects this emphasis on language is not that new. Structural approaches usually emphasized how ideology was a key way in which dominant groups achieve and maintain power. But in the newer discourse understanding of power, there does not need to be a particular group or category 'pulling the strings' so to speak. While some groups may consciously use language to further their interests and objectives, discourse also takes on a life of its own. According to this approach, one particularly powerful discourse since the 1980s has been labelled as neo-liberal. Neo-liberalism is a language of choice in which people actively construct their lives and identities through conscious choices. This is one explanation for why there has been much interest in developing market mechanisms in health policy. In this sense, broader shifts in discourse have significant implications for policy.

Using a discourse approach to power, public health has been cast in a rather different light to policy actor and structural approaches in which it is generally regarded as lacking substantial influence over policy. According to Peterson and Lupton (1996), the new public health is closely aligned to a discourse of 'risk' that has become very powerful in recent decades. Peterson and Lupton also claim that the new public health discourse also fits very well with neo-liberal discourse. Whether or not we are witnessing the ascendancy of public health in an era of neo-liberalism, however, is somewhat debatable. While some health promotion models appropriate the language of choice, the framework of population health with its emphasis on population-based approaches is frequently at odds with a discourse in which choice is paramount. Others have identified the discourse of 'privacy' as a significant counterweight to public health policy agendas (Annas 1999). This discourse focus suggests that the most important long-term policy battles for public health advocates are battles over language.

Integrating actors and structure

The most fruitful approaches to the analysis of power and public policy combine insights from the policy actor and structural approaches, and take discourse into account. One very useful concept is that of the policy network (Marsh & Rhodes 1992). Members of networks are in regular interaction on their common issues of interest, although the regularity and coherence may vary greatly. In some areas, where interests are well defined and of long standing, the policy networks that have formed are highly integrated and stable. In some instances such networks are so small, stable, and predictable that they have been termed 'iron triangles', referring to their longevity and intractability.

The concept of a tight policy community is relevant to the discussion of power and its distribution; this particular form of policy network derives from a structural interest configuration of power. Policy actors that are not included in the policy core will only have a peripheral influence on policy. Clearly, power and influence are concentrated in this set of circumstances, and policy debates are promoted in a highly stylized and predictable fashion. Nothing much will change until, and unless, there is some significant shift in the balance of power (for instance, a change of government, or an international event, or a new ally to the coalition).

An alternative set of interacting relationships to that based on the structural interest model is the issue network, an association based on a wide range of loosely connected groups. This follows a more pluralistic concept of power distribution. Issue networks are perhaps more common in the health arena, since the health sector exhibits such a wide range of issues around which local and small special interest groups can coalesce.

Policy networks as defined here—ranging from the cohesive and predictable sets of actors to broader and looser associations—provide the framework of allegiances, interest, and ideology that help to define the parameters within which policy is formulated. Debates, public and private, take place among the principal actors, and these debates in turn help to shape the progress of policy (Read 1992).

The analysis by Read (1992) of the politics of tobacco policy in Britain in the 1980s remains one of the best examples of this type of approach. Read depicted an inner policy core consisting of sectional interest groups representing the tobacco and advertising industries alongside key government agencies, notably Treasury and the Department of Trade and Industry. Opponents such as the British Medical Association, the advocacy group Action on Smoking and Health (ASH) and the Department of Health had more peripheral roles.

Another approach that developed during the 1990s, known as the advocacy coalition framework (Sabatier & Jenkins-Smith 1999) gives an even more elegant way of depicting the dynamics of issues such as tobacco control that have been evident in many high income countries since the 1970s (Sato 1999). This approach proposes a model of policy dynamics consisting of competing coalitions, each of which coalesce around particular core values. Usually one coalition is identified as dominant, although this may change over time. Thus, in the 1980s tobacco policy could be characterized by a dominant coalition based on protection of tobacco interests which was aligned against a public health coalition. More recently, the advocacy coalition framework has been used to depict the conflict between these coalitions at a transnational level (Farquharson 2003; Princen 2007). In a similar vein, Hajer (1995) has drawn on the concept of discourse to describe policy dynamics as 'discourse coalitions'.

Institutions

An analysis of power can tend to emphasize the raw ingredients of group relations and positional influence. Power can be seen as a force that emanates from the brute facts of material resources and privileged social position. Thus the emphasis in the previous section is on advocacy groups, lobbyists, and governmental agencies as actors in a dynamic field of power relations. Such an approach emphasizes the role of actors with distinct interests and capabilities. Yet, the interaction of these agencies, and to some extent their source of power, is shaped by institutions. In other words, the patterns of interaction between agencies are shaped, though not ultimately determined, by relatively established rules and processes that are socially sanctioned and often legally enshrined (Immergut 1992).

In the case of the policy process there is a clear organizational context through which policy issues are channelled. In the case of the advanced Western democracies this means understanding the respective roles of the different arms of government—executive and legislature—and of the bureaucracy. For example, a very important distinction has to be drawn between the differing policy capacities of the executive and the legislature, respectively. The executive arm of government is in a position to formulate and carry out policy, but it cannot on its own necessarily secure political legitimacy, full financial support (where this is taxpayer-funded), or legal sanction (for instance, a change in the law). These are functions of the legislature. Crucially, it is important for the purposes of political symbolism that key policy changes are publicly debated and passed through the legislature.

In presidential systems the separation of powers between the executive and the legislature means that a legislative majority cannot be taken for granted, and hence there is more room for negotiation and bargaining. A further distinction needs also to be drawn between federal and unitary systems of government. The capacity for making consistent and coherent policy is much more difficult in federal systems because of the distinct sets of responsibilities and jurisdictions at national and state levels. This means that there is a frequent requirement for negotiation and considerable opportunity for jurisdictional disputes. If we add to its presidential and federal nature the lack of party discipline in the American system, then consistent, coherent, and long-term policy development would seem to be difficult indeed (Steinmo & Watts 1995).

Federal and unitary systems have different strengths and weaknesses. Leichter (1991) compared these fundamental differences in political structures for the United States and Great Britain across a number of major health promotion issues (smoking, alcohol, road safety, and HIV/AIDS). While the unitary nature of the British political system encouraged clarity and decisiveness in policymaking, it did not necessarily lead either to greater creativity or to the 'right' result (as judged from a conventional public health perspective). Indeed, the multiple nature of the American political system meant that, while federal initiatives on health promotion might be blocked at the centre, experimentation with a diversity of interventions could take place at the level of the individual state. While clarity, coherence, and decisiveness might not have been apparent in the American context, creativity, inventiveness, diversity, and local ownership were.

One important characteristic of institutional structures in which formal decision-making power is diffused is that there are multiple venues for policy action. This enables policy actors to engage in 'venue shopping', i.e. looking for the part of the institutional structure that is most likely to achieve results. In the US, the legal system has been an attractive venue for public health advocates and one which ultimately produced a sizeable shift in the balance of power on tobacco. Political systems with more concentrated formal power enhance decisive policymaking when political conditions are favourable for public health advocates, but have fewer venues for policy decisions when conditions are unfavourable. With this in mind, public health advocacy coalitions in European countries are increasingly looking to the European Union as a venue for policy change (Princen 2007).

In many respects the key element of the institutional framework for the purposes of policy-making is the bureaucracy, and the structure of the bureaucracy itself becomes a key factor in the policy process. In the case of the health bureaucracy, officials usually retain a host of formal committees and informal advisory groups in order to nurture links with key constituencies in the sector and to maintain competency and intelligence in a range of policy and technical areas. Beyond this there are important distinctions to be made within the health bureaucracy—functionally between public health and healthcare, for example, and operationally between policy advice and service delivery. Apart from the health ministry there are other sections of the bureaucracy that are important to health policy-making. For example, the finance ministry will typically set the fiscal parameters for health funding, the transport ministry will be important for certain public health campaigns, education, and environmental health for others, and the police and judiciary for still others. Any attempt to negotiate the policy process requires a full understanding of these organizational intricacies. Indeed, most public health initiatives require intersectoral allegiances and partnerships of this kind for their success.

A key institutional consideration in the role of public health concerns the way in which the health system in general, and public health in particular, is funded. In high income countries in which health is predominantly tax-funded, such as most English-speaking and Scandinavian countries, public health tends to have a higher institutional profile, and sits alongside healthcare services. In countries in which social insurance funds are the primary source of health funding, public health is further separated from other health services.

Finally, however health is funded, the overall design of the public sector can have a significant impact on public health capacity. For instance, the decision to devolve Ontario's public health functions to a local government level restricted the province's capacity to deal with the SARS crisis in 2003 (Deber *et al.* 2007). Conversely, the creation of a stand-alone public health advisory body in New Zealand in the 1990s had the unintended effect of isolating the public health function from the rest of the health bureaucracy, and ultimately weakening the voice of public health in policy (Hutt & Howden-Chapman 1998).

Processes

A rough map of policy processes

The most common 'map' of policy processes is that of the 'policy cycle'. The policy cycle orders the parts of the policy process into a sequence that begins with problem definition, moves through agenda-setting, policy formulation, decision-making, implementation, and evaluation. This should not be regarded as an accurate depiction of what actually happens, as few policies follow the whole of this trajectory. It is better used as a device to break complex policy processes down into bite-sized areas of inquiry.

Problem definition

Policy problems are 'socially constructed' (Spector & Kitsuse 1987). That is to say, they do not arrive fully formed on governmental agendas. Instead, policy problem definitions are subject to numerous social processes. Child abuse, for example, was not defined as a public policy issue in high income countries prior to the early 1960s (Nelson 1984). This does not mean that the phenomenon now defined as child abuse did not take place prior to the 1960s. Barbara Nelson's book shows how medical professionals were instrumental in naming and framing something that had been hitherto considered as the concern of private individuals and families rather than as a public concern.

The starting point for definitions of new policy problems is the naming of an undesirable situation or phenomenon. It certainly helps if those who propose problem definitions are able to demonstrate that a situation is getting worse, and this usually requires that the phenomenon can be measured in order to demonstrate deterioration.

Central to all definitions of public problems is an assertion that some greater harm is being, or will be, suffered unless policy action is taken. It is important that this harm must be considered as harm to the public body in some way, not merely as harm to individuals. This requires problems to be expressed in terms of social and economic aggregates or health outcomes. Thus, when obesity is framed as a public policy issue, public health advocates emphasize broader projected social and economic effects such as increased health expenditure and lost worker productivity (Wang & Brownell 2005).

The third essential element of policy problem definition is the attribution of causes. If harm is being suffered, but the causes of that harm are unknown, then it is unlikely to gain policy traction until the causes are better understood. The likelihood of identifying and crafting appropriate policy interventions is higher if causal factors are amenable to intervention. The attribution of causes is an area in which public health science makes a prominent contribution. Public health research into the causes of obesity has generated extensive information on the contribution of energy-dense foods and sedentary lifestyles. Further back in the causal change, the increasing prevalence of energy-dense foods and sedentary lifestyles is attributed to a range of environmental factors (Wang & Brownell 2005).

Finally, advocates of particular problem definitions must also develop arguments as to why the problem requires *governmental* action and intervention. While it may be accepted that obesity is a societal problem, it does not necessarily follow that it is the role of government to develop solutions. So what makes a problem a concern of government? One powerful way of answering this question stems from the discipline of economics. Most policy issues are concerned, at some level, with the distribution of scarce resources. Generally, economists regard markets as the most *efficient* mechanism for the distribution of goods and services provided certain conditions are met. Market failure occurs if the required conditions are not met. For economists, this provides the most compelling justification for government interventions in areas that otherwise would be considered as private. For example, many goods and services have 'negative externalities'—additional costs that are borne by society generally rather than the consumer or purchaser. This argument has been applied to justify government intervention to tackle obesity (Rashad 2005). A less restrictive way of justifying government action is based on the idea that public policy is essentially a democratic enterprise. In other words, a sufficient case for government involvement is that a significant proportion of the public think that government should act. Nevertheless, there are no clear guidelines as to what constitutes 'sufficient' public support.

Most policy problem definitions are likely to be challenged, particularly if there are groups who see adverse effects for the interests and/or values they represent. Problem definitions are contested on any or all of the grounds outlined above. Opponents may question that there is a problem or take issue with how it is measured. They can question the accuracy of the predicted effects. Most importantly they are likely to contest the causes and the case for government intervention. Stone (2002) developed a framework to show that some 'causal stories' have greater traction. When causes are regarded as accidental or unintentional, the imperative for policy action is weaker because such causal factors are beyond the control of governments. If however, causes are framed as intentional it strengthens the argument that policy should address the actions of those deemed responsible.

Over the past 50 years, public health advocates have been very successful at reframing phenomena such as road deaths, work injuries, and tobacco-related cancers as intentional where once they had been considered accidental. This has continued in attempts to classify the causes of rising rates of obesity as intentional—the direct result of food industry practices—in order to strengthen the case for policy responses. Food and advertising industry representatives, on the other hand, emphasize the complexity of causes—thus portraying the causes of obesity as inadvertent or accidental.

The science behind specific problem definitions is routinely challenged, often with competing research. Alternatively, opponents may attempt to render the science and research irrelevant by challenging the value basis of the problem definition. For example, activists in the USA have attempted to reframe the obesity issue as one of diversity and acceptance of 'the right to be fat', drawing on previous successes of anti-discrimination movements (Saguy & Riley 2005).

The resolution of many key public health issues turns on the particular value framework within which they are viewed by the public. Whether it be the fencing of private swimming pools, gun control, or restrictions on smoking and drinking, a primary aspect of the public definition of these issues is whether they are seen as matters of health and safety or controversies impinging on the expression of individual rights (Burris 1997). For advocacy groups, lobbyists, and governmental agencies involved in these controversies, positioning of the issue in relation to these two value complexes becomes crucial and much energy is devoted to presenting the issue in the appropriate light (Chapman & Lupton 1994). Again, certain groups are greatly advantaged because of their material resources (which enables them to run public relations campaigns), their access to the media, or relevant cultural assets (such as positive public image, high social status), and these can become crucial in issue definition and agenda setting.

Agenda-setting

Of course, there are a plethora of definitions of public policy problems, advanced by various policy actors, circulating at particular time. However the attention of policymakers and the wider public is inevitably limited. Some issues may never make the policy agenda, while others rise and fall in importance over time. The term 'policy agenda' is a useful metaphor; however, the term can be applied to quite distinct areas. Students of policy typically distinguish between those issues that are widely discussed in the public domain (the public or systemic agenda) and those that receive the attention of key public officials and political decision-makers (the formal agenda) (Birkland 2001).

The public agenda is mostly driven, or at least substantially mediated, by the media. The formal agenda responds to different stimuli such as new research and the dynamics within policy communities. While the two agendas operate according to rather different logics, they are not completely separate. Obesity has only reached the public agenda relatively recently. US and Australian studies indicate that media coverage of obesity increased sharply during 2002 (Schlesinger 2005; Nathan *et al.* 2005). Many issues reach the formal agenda via the public agenda due to the incentives of electoral competition. If governments and legislators are seen as unresponsive to public demands for policy action, this creates opportunities for other politicians to make the running.

While the dynamics of the public agenda can be a catalyst for policy change, students of policy tend to be more interested in the dynamics of the formal agenda. Power dynamics operate at the level of agenda-setting. The history of tobacco control, for example, is largely a history of a battle in which tobacco interests have fought hard to keep successive tobacco control measures off governmental agendas (Givel 2006).

There are other reasons why issues do not make the agenda that may be more about values and less about interests. For instance, US and Canadian environmental and public health advocates were reluctant to press for action on the presence of dioxin in breast milk for fear that publicizing this problem would have wider repercussions of lowering rates of breastfeeding across the wider population (Harrison 2001).

The inevitable limits to 'the policy agenda space' means that within the domain of public health, not all issues receive attention at any one time. Frequently, public health policy priorities are contingent and subject to highly ad hoc processes. These may include unexpected developments (e.g. AIDS, SARS) or public agenda dynamics which throw up 'diseases of the month'. Competition between public health issues often means that key players in government agencies filter demands for attention, and that access to these individuals is a crucial determinant of agenda status.

Formulation

Agenda status means that policymakers are paying attention to a particular problem—but it does not necessarily mean that policy action will be taken. Even if solutions are devised, it does not follow that they will be satisfactory to those who first defined the problem. In formulation, the focus is on devising possible solutions to policy problems. The generation of solutions might be seen to follow straightforwardly from the definition of the problem. Thus, if there is an outbreak of a contagious disease, the appropriate response may be to develop or adapt a vaccine. This may well be an appropriate technical solution, but devising policy solutions requires attention to a far broader range of factors. In the case of new problems, or existing problems about which there is new knowledge, the definitional process and the development of feasible policy options are particularly crucial.

The advent of HIV/AIDS presented a novel problem that could not be ignored and for which there were no clear policy precedents. Problem definition proceeded to policy development at a reasonably low political threshold, only requiring high-level political support once a series of relatively unprecedented policy options were proposed. Many public health problems, however, are long-standing and do not offer any clear-cut technical solutions. Still more intractable are issues of health inequalities and social determinants of health (Marmot & Wilkinson 1999). Wilkinson (2007) has recently lamented that in the UK, after almost a decade of government initiatives, policy has not had an impact on these problems. These are problems in search of the right policy prescription. The mobilization of political resources has been evident, but the principal requirement of a feasible policy option has not (Exworthy *et al.* 2003).

Finally, there are those public health problems about which a clear problem definition and policy options have emerged, but that await the correct political climate (window of opportunity). For example, according to Berridge (1999) passive smoking was a 'scientific fact waiting to emerge'. The public acceptability of passive smoking was shaped by a complex number of factors, only one of which was the scientific evidence. It was consistent with a growing individualistic and environmental ethos, giving medical and scientific legitimacy to a position that had originated from a moral, and then a personal rights, issue.

The development of policy proposals is often a highly contingent and unpredictable process, typically reliant on the capacity of policy 'entrepreneurs' to craft and broker novel combinations. One of the most useful ideas for understanding the feasibility of policy is that of the policy 'primaeval soup' in which different policy ideas and proposals develop, mutate and combine together (Kingdon 2003). The advocacy coalition framework discussed earlier also views policy formulation as the product of dynamic interaction between policy actors. For Sabatier and Jenkins-Smith (1993), 'policy learning' takes place when participants in competing coalitions broker particular policy initiatives that do not threaten the core values of each coalition but nevertheless move the policy process forward. Sato's (1999) analysis of tobacco policy in Japan shows how these ideas can be applied in a public health context.

Decision-making

Decision-making lies at the heart of the policy process since it alone can precipitate a formal change in policy settings. However, it should be noted that a decision not to alter an existing policy may be just as important as a decision to institute changes formally (Bachrach & Baratz 1963). Thus, the decision not to prosecute a tobacco company that is transgressing existing legislation, for example, has nearly as much effective force as a decision to change the legislation.

Policy decision-making is generally a highly complex process. For the purposes of analysing policy, it is useful to identify broad 'ideal types' of decision-making in order to provide a template against which actual decision-making processes can be compared. For the past 50 years, two particular templates have had the most currency. The first of these is the rationalist model of decision-making. The rationalist model is driven by the production and consideration of evidence. Under this model, the evaluation of alternative policy options needs to be synoptic and all-embracing, if it is properly to co-ordinate all aspects of the issue under consideration. In this sense rational decision-making takes into account longer-term strategic objectives (Alexander 1986). A proposed advantage of rationalist policy processes is that it can provide a basis for major shifts in policy direction if such shifts are supported by available evidence.

A classic example of rationalist policymaking is when government agencies are engaged in deciding which new pharmaceutical products are to be purchased in publicly funded health systems. In a number of high income countries (e.g. Australia and New Zealand) such decisions are made on the basis of cost-benefit, or cost-utility analysis (Davis 2004). In principle, public health services could also be prioritized in this way, provided there is sufficient robust information regarding the costs and benefits of the range of interventions.

Under the rationalist model, the input of technical experts and analysts, either employed or contracted by government agencies is highly valued. Therefore it is not surprising that this model appeals to researchers. By contrast, the input of other types of policy actors is typically regarded as problematic for policymaking. Nevertheless, in most contexts the concept of rational decision-making is probably best considered a normative one; that is, a desirable objective, rather than providing an accurate description of actual decision-making processes. Decision-makers are limited by the availability of information on the one hand, and the competing demands, interests, and values of various policy actors, be they government agencies, sectional interest groups, or advocacy interest groups, on the other.

At the other end of the spectrum are decisions that are made on the basis of negotiation, bargaining, and compromise between the various stakeholders. It has been argued that this style of decision-making—the stakeholder model—is both a better description of the policy process as it is, and a reasonable guide as to how policy should be conducted. Most decisions in the health sector are largely determined by interactions between stakeholders. As a consequence, policy change is typically incremental rather than large-scale. There are two reasons why stakeholder decision-making processes are likely to be the norm. First, there is the inertia of existing arrangements and power relations, such that it is more likely both to achieve agreement and to secure a shift in resources at the margin, and in smaller scale, than in a major and thoroughgoing fashion. Second, decision-makers are often conscious that decisions that are made without the buy-in of interests who are most affected are likely to run into obstacles when they are implemented (see Section 'Implementation' below).

For some prominent scholars of policy, such a model of decision-making is entirely appropriate and desirable. Lindblom (1959), for example, argued that 'mutual partisan adjustment' among contending interests was preferable to the rational synoptic model because rationalism would require a concentration and centralization of policy authority in government that is not consistent with democratic ideals. Decisions made through mutual partisan adjustment, according to Lindblom, were both more practical and robust than those which excluded relevant stakeholders. In response, advocates of a more rationalist approach argue that the problem with such a style of decision-making is that it does little to maintain or ensure the overall coherence of policy.

Realistically a pure rationalist approach is likely to occur only in circumstances where decision-makers are provided with a relatively simple (and therefore rare) set of policy circumstances, where there is broad agreement regarding the nature of a problem and where relevant evidence is readily available and can be used to decide which policy option is optimal. As an ideal, this model remains attractive to those involved in public health policy-making, at least as an organizational tool for policy appraisal. Nevertheless, the most effective policy approach is likely to be 'mixed scanning', involving a mix of rational planning and incremental adjustment (Etzioni 1967). Indeed, it is usually possible to find some elements of rationalism intermingled with stakeholder bargaining and negotiation and incrementalism in any particular policy decision. For example, in the 2000s many high income countries have legislated to ban smoking in bars, clubs, and restaurants. This is a significant policy change that is primarily based on epidemiological evidence regarding second-hand smoke (SHS). Yet it is not the optimal strategy for reducing SHS morbidity and mortality. An optimal strategy would also ban smoking in domestic premises. Such a policy at this point in time, however, would place a large burden on a range of stakeholders (e.g. police, local government), as well as stirring opposition from civil libertarian groups. Clearly, decision-makers, as well as public health advocates have chosen the achievable over the optimal.

The debate between advocates of the rationalist and stakeholder models can give the misleading impression that any occurrence of large-scale policy change is an indication of a rationalist decision-making process. Kingdon's approach (2003) outlined earlier suggests another possibility—that large-scale policy change can take place, but that this may have little to do with whether or not it has been decided upon through a synoptic, rational process. Rather, policy change occurs when 'windows of opportunity' open that can be taken advantage of by policy *entrepreneurs* who lie in wait for them. Some windows are predictable, such as the election of new governments known to be sympathetic to particular problem definitions and policy proposals. Others, however, are highly unpredictable, and may be opened when particular events focus public and political attention on problems that had previously had little profile.

Nor do the stakeholder and rationalist models exhaust the range of 'ideal types' of decision-making processes. Indeed, both have been subject to challenge on the grounds that they privilege insider policy expertise and limit the capacity of citizens to shape policy decisions. Since the 1970s and 1980s another model has been advanced which posits that citizens should have a more direct role in policy decisions rather than having their values and interests mediated by politicians, government agencies, and interest groups. Associated mechanisms include petitions, referenda, citizens' juries, and forums. While these arguments have had some practical impact, rationalist and stakeholder processes remain the dominant models of policymaking.

Implementation

In most cases effective decision-making does entail some change to existing policy settings. This is usually the desired outcome in much public health policy since typically the promotion of public health objectives involves some modification to a status quo that is dominated by economic and individualistic values (Burris 1997). This being so, the key to policy success is the implementation process. Traditionally, this part of the policy cycle was viewed as relatively unproblematic, being seen as principally an administrative function. However, a series of studies revealed that the objectives of many programmes—agreed and sanctioned in formal policy—were not being achieved in practice. From this insight sprang the study of implementation and a closer assessment of policy design and policy instruments (Pressman & Wildavsky 1984).

The nature of the problems that policy is addressing are usually complex, multifaceted, and sometimes quite intractable. The greatest likelihood of implementation success is in circumstances where the policy has relatively simple technical features, represents a relatively marginal change to the status quo, is implemented by a single agency, has a clear single objective, and is of short duration. It also helps if the policy does not upset powerful interest groups and has relatively low visibility with the public (Walt 1994).

As with decision-making, therefore, there is a tension between rationalist and stakeholder imperatives. Policies can be fundamentally reformulated at the implementation stage because implementation frequently depends on the co-operation of particular groups. For example, the successful implementation of HIV screening for newborns is crucially dependent on the co-operation of doctors and/or midwives. If these frontline staff regard the requirement as an additional imposition which takes away from what they perceive to be their core responsibilities, they are likely to give this task low priority. For reasons such as this, it is important that key stakeholders have some buy-in to the policy change. This may be easier in some situations than others. Sometimes, policy change is decided upon precisely to change the behaviour of providers and stakeholders and in such cases the priorities of decision-makers and implementers are likely to be in direct conflict.

Such conflicts are more likely if certain kinds of policy instruments are utilized. Thus, 'command and control' policy instruments such as regulation and legislation are more likely to provoke implementation resistance than 'softer' mechanisms that draw on voluntary, family, and community endeavours. Many public health matters naturally lend themselves to the deployment of regulatory policy instruments and/or the direct provision of services. Typically, a public health initiative requires change to existing patterns of behaviour or activities. Frequently this involves some regulatory or administrative intervention and usually this can only be delivered and enforced by an officially sanctioned agency of the state. A striking departure from this tradition was the almost universal reliance on non-statutory mechanisms in the response to HIV/AIDS across high income countries (Kirp & Bayer 1992). Indeed, non-governmental organizations are playing an increasingly important role as partners in public health initiatives (Walt 1994).

Evaluation

While the study of implementation focuses on what happens after a policy decision is made, evaluation refers to formal attempts to determine whether the policy succeeded or failed in meeting desired objectives. Yet this final stage of the policy cycle is often never attempted, particularly in the case of large-scale policy changes. However, evaluation is generally more common for smaller, 'programme' initiatives such as vaccination or screening initiatives. Evaluation is considered to be an essential element of evidence-based policy, as information generated through the implementation of programmes should inform decisions to continue, amend, or discontinue particular initiatives. This logic seems straightforward but examples of termination of policies based on evaluation evidence are rare in policy. This is because initiatives are rarely 'owned' by a single policy actor. In policy environments in which there are multiple stakeholders it is unlikely that there are a clear set of policy objectives agreed by all stakeholders. Therefore, evaluation, as with decision-making and implementation is also shaped by the interplay between rationalist (top-down) and stakeholder (bottom-up) imperatives.

Research to policy informed by policy studies

From the excursion into the insights and conceptual models of policy studies in Sections 'Power' and 'Processes', there are two major implications for public health. First, public health has been clearly influential in the definition of policy problems. Indeed, other communities of researchers are likely to be envious of public health's hit rate. Second, and in contrast, public health advocates generally face much greater hurdles in translating problem definitions informed by their research into policy, particularly where benefits are diffuse and the costs are concentrated. With this in mind we can return more specifically to the role of research in policy in order to suggest some ways of thinking that can be helpful to those who wish to engage in analysis *for* policy and see research have a greater impact on policy.

Three perspectives on research to policy

There is a wealth of useful material that has explored the relationship between scientific and social scientific research and public policy. The following discussion takes as its foundation the three prevailing conceptions of the role of research in policy outlined by Carol Weiss (1991). The first conception of 'research as data' carries with it the expectation that research data 'speaks for itself' in that it has policy implications that should be recognized and acted upon by policymakers. For example, such an idea of the appropriate role of research would imply policymakers are obliged to respond when presented with data that the rate of overweight and obese children shows a continual rise.

For Weiss, those who expect that research data should generate policy action are likely to be perennially disappointed. Values and interests typically take precedence over data as 'research findings were useful primarily when they helped policy actors to do what they already wanted to do' (Weiss 1991). Data does makes a difference to policy in situations in which there is broad social consensus on the nature of the problem, and on values and goals, and/or where two or three clear alternatives are compared in order to test which policy option is optimal. In other words, research as data is influential when the policy environment conforms to expectations of a rationalist policy process. As outlined above, such circumstances are rare.

The second view of the relationship between research and policy is the 'research as ideas' model, which Weiss also refers to as research for 'enlightenment'. Rather than expecting policy to be adjusted by the accretion of new data, the key way in which academic research influences policy is through the gradual acceptance and adoption of 'big ideas', which amount to new high-level definitions of policy problems or the reframing of prevailing definitions. Examples of such big ideas over the past 20–30 years include 'global warming' and the 'unsustainability of health sector growth'. As Weiss notes, policy research as ideas is characterized by the 'stripping away' of 'most of the paraphernalia of research' such as methodology or analytical techniques (Weiss 1991). What remains is a relatively simple and clear message that is digestible to policy actors.

The 'research as ideas' model is most likely to apply in the early stages of policy discussion, or when existing policy is in disarray or when there is a high degree of uncertainty (Weiss 1991). She also notes that research as ideas is particularly suited to decentralized institutional settings where 'a relatively simple idea can travel further and faster than detailed data'. As the enlightenment model suggests that research as ideas has a substantial impact on problem definition and, possibly, agenda-setting, public health can claim many successes in transferring big ideas such as population health, population-based approaches, and the reduction of health disparities into the health policy arena. However, the take-up of influential ideas by policymakers does not necessarily mean that they survive intact. As a recent study into the impact of research into health inequalities has shown, the journey of these ideas into policy may also be fractured or partial (Smith 2007).

A third characterization is that of 'research as arguments' and this starts from the basis that research is inextricably bound up in broader political dynamics. In this model, research is consciously married to advocacy and researchers forge ties with other policy actors in the process of engaging in political policy battles. Because of this, research is valuable for its capacity to contribute to compelling arguments. By all means, researchers and their allies can stand on the objectivity of scientific research knowing that this is a powerful rhetorical tool. To do otherwise, Weiss notes, would amount to 'unilateral disarmament'. But they must also expect that their opponents will also enlist allies from the research community.

The notion of research as argument is also consistent with the policy networks and advocacy coalition frameworks discussed above. Clearly, this model applies when political conflict is high, but it also can be important to justify when decisions have been made. Research as argument is also important where there are policy actors who are crucial to implementation but may be ambivalent about the decision (Weiss 1991).

Politicization of research is also more likely when the research community itself is divided, either within a particular discipline, or along disciplinary lines (Buse *et al.* 2005). The fault lines of substantive policy debates often coincide with epistemological and methodological debates among researchers. In this model, researchers need to hone their rhetorical and argumentative skills, or develop alliances with those who are adept at translating research into persuasive policy arguments.

Research in the context of knowledge for policy

Weiss's framework provides a starting point for thinking about the question of how the impact of research on policy can be maximized. Even though not all policy issues are highly contested, thinking of research in the context of policy argument is a very useful habit. In using the word 'argument', we are not assuming that all policy contexts are adversarial, as might be suggested by the politicized model, although we know they often are. The key point is that any policy issue has the potential to become politicized. The term 'argument' is also used in its broader, philosophical sense, denoting a coherent set of propositions. Policy arguments are basic building blocks of policy processes. Research is best considered as one (and by no means the only) activity that contributes to the construction of policy argument. What, then, makes a good policy argument?

In a recent influential work titled *Making Social Science Matter,* the Danish scholar Bent Flyvbjerg (2001) resurrected Aristotle's three 'intellectual virtues'—*episteme, techne, and phronesis. Episteme* denotes objectively verifiable knowledge produced according to the prescriptions of scientific method. *Techne* denotes 'practical-technical' know-how and skills. This type of knowledge, according to Flyvbjerg, is 'concrete, variable, and context-dependent'. It is knowledge gained from experience and practice. In policy terms, this type of knowledge has been described as the knowledge of 'street-level officials', or those on whom successful policy implementation depends. *Techne* knowledge also includes awareness of pragmatic, political exigencies. The third type of knowledge, *phronesis* is 'a sense of the ethically practical'. Phronetic knowledge addresses value questions such as: Where are we going?; is this desirable?; and what should be done?. In policy terms, this translates as an understanding of public values, although one that is not derived from abstract philosophical principles but on 'consideration, judgement, and choice' in specific contexts.

What does this mean for public health researchers? Effective policy argument integrates all three types of knowledge because all three types of knowledge are typically in play in policy debate (Tenbensel 2006). A useful analogy is that of a card game involving tricks and trumps such as Bridge, Whist, or Euchre. In such games, players that only concentrate on playing their preferred suit are unlikely to be very successful. Skilled cardplay involves the flexible utilization of all the available suits. We will return to this analogy in the conclusion, after we have considered the role that research plays in the production of each type of knowledge.

Of the three types of knowledge, *epistemic* knowledge is the one primarily founded upon a basis of research. As such, the production of *epistemic* knowledge is the strong suit of public health. However, epistemic knowledge is generally founded in disciplinary bodies of knowledge, and there remains the question of how knowledge produced through different disciplinary frameworks adds up (Tenbensel 2004). Frequently, different bodies of epistemic research support are used to support quite different policy arguments For example, clinical research trial evidence is sometimes counterposed against evidence from observational studies (say, in dealing with the question of whether exposure to environmental contaminants is a cause of cancer).

Of particular importance is the relationship between public health domains of epidemiology and more 'generic' disciplines, particularly economics. For example, research evidence may suggest that population-based vaccination campaigns are an effective means for dealing with an outbreak of a contagious disease. However, economists will ask how cost-effective this is compared to other possible interventions. They might also ask whether the amount of money required for vaccination campaigns could produce greater benefits elsewhere in the health sector (or even beyond). One key implication is that public health research with an interdisciplinary base is more likely to be robust in policy environments characterized by conflicts over evidence, because it increases the likelihood of being able to respond to contending arguments based on other types of *epistemic* evidence.

Where *epistemic* knowledge supports differing policy implications, the difference is often simply founded on divergent values. As indicated earlier, most public health research addresses *phronetic* questions, although this dimension of the research is not always explicitly articulated—after all, there are limited incentives to outline the value foundations of one's work in scientific publications. The value-based elements of public health have expanded as the enterprise of public health has developed. Normative arguments about the importance of population health as a policy goal, the benefits of population-based approaches, and the reduction of health inequalities have each made some impact on policymakers in high income countries.

Explicit articulation of the value bases *(phronesis)* of public health and population health can often help to sharpen policy argument. Consequently, public health advocates sometimes engage in research in gauging public support for proposed measures such as regulating workplace exposure to second-hand smoke, or controlling exposure to sugary drinks in schools. While such research can often be useful, particularly when governments are actively sponsoring such changes, it is rarely decisive when governments are ambivalent, because most public opinion research generated by any policy advocate is inevitably regarded with scepticism. As the advocacy coalition framework suggests, public health advocates need allies in government agencies that share key public health values. Without this, appealing to the court of public opinion is rarely effective.

Typically, the weakest suit for public health is *techne;* however, questions that address *techne* issues are central to public policy deliberations. Such questions include: What are the practical implications of suggestions for policy reform?; which organizations will have to change what they do?; how are they likely to react?; who will these changes adversely affect and how will they react?; will this matter politically?; how feasible is the course of action proposed?

Some of these questions, particularly those regarding the practical feasibility and effectiveness of particular initiatives can be answered through public health research. This has been a particularly important strand of health promotion research. However, many public health researchers still see this type of research as only weakly developed. Rychetnik and Wise (2004) note that while there is extensive research on the magnitude and aetiology of public health problems, research on the effectiveness of actual policy initiatives is scant. The obesity example illustrates this. The prevailing public health research paradigm of 'problem-oriented' research attempts to definitively nail down the aetiology of the obesity epidemic, and the relationship between causal factors. Such a primarily *epistemic* research agenda, by itself, is insufficient and may act as a significant obstacle to the development of potential policy approaches (Robinson & Sirard 2005). Essentially, these authors are calling for a greater emphasis on researching *techne* questions. Among policy evaluation researchers, a strong argument has been developed that whether or not particular programmes work is highly dependent on context (Boaz & Pawson 2005), echoing Flybjerg and Aristotle's emphasis on the contextual basis of *techne* knowledge.

Public health researchers clearly are not in the best position to answer other *techne* questions such as political feasibility, and some aspects of implementation, as it is not where their expertise lies. But if they are to construct convincing policy arguments, these questions still need to be answered. If not, then this amounts to a weakness that can be easily exploited by policy adversaries. Given that it is likely to be government agencies that do have to think through the practical *techne* implications of policy proposals such as fat taxes and regulating advertising to children (in the event of public health advocates successfully getting such measures on the policy agenda), public health advocates need to be aware of the political exigencies faced by such bodies. This highlights the need to develop stronger linkages between researchers and policymakers to facilitate better mutual understanding.

The development of institutionalized linkages between researchers and government has been emphasized by those who have argued that the divide between the 'two communities' of research and policy is at the heart of the problem of lack of research influence (Lavis 2006; Lomas 2007). Other policy scholars have argued that this distinction is overemphasized (Buse *et al.* 2005), particularly given the wide range of policy cases that involve competing policy communities or advocacy coalitions where contending coalitions each have their own constellation of researchers *and* government agencies and interest groups. However, this criticism only serves to underline the importance of strong linkages between researchers and those involved more directly in policy processes.

Developing constructive, integrated policy arguments is not a guarantee of success. Rather, in the context of power relations and institutional structures, the development of such arguments improves the chances of success and is something that is within the control of public health advocates. Furthermore, the capacity to generate coherent and persuasive policy argument to shape discourse is itself one important source of power in policy.

Conclusion

The main message of this chapter has been to emphasize that the role of research-based knowledge must be understood in the context of a much wider range of factors that shape policy. The card game metaphor provides a neat way of pulling together the various concepts and ideas outlined in this chapter.

Research evidence may give public health advocates some strong cards in the game, but these cards on their own will never be sufficient to shape the outcome of policy. To expect powerful research-based knowledge regarding the rates of obesity and smoking to translate directly into policy is akin to expecting that holding the ace and king of spades is sufficient to win a hand of cards. While these may be potentially powerful cards, whether they are effective or not depends on many things, including a mix of factors both within and beyond the control of the player.

The player has some control over the hand of cards they hold and how it is played. Having a good hand of cards is analogous to having an integrated set of arguments. Arguments correspond to 'ideas' in the Lavis scheme. The challenge of policy is to develop *ideas* that integrate knowledge about what is *(episteme)*, what works *(techne)*, and what should be done *(phronesis)*. But good arguments alone do not guarantee policy success. Arguments are marshalled in the broader policy context, which is beyond the control of researchers, in which the structure of opportunities and constraints are moulded by *interests* and *institutions.* Institutions are the rules of the game, and interests define the positions of opponents and allies.

With an understanding of these basic elements, the next step is to grasp the dynamic features of the policy game. An understanding of power equates to the ability to infer what cards other players have, what their strengths are (the basis of their power), and whether or not it is possible to prevent their powerful cards from having an impact. An understanding of process enables a player to focus on the whole game from problem definition to implementation and evaluation. Ultimately, the two things that matter most are the development of a hand that incorporates different types of knowledge and the nurturing of alliances with players that have complementary strengths. When and where public health research is integrated into the broader policy context along these lines, the chances of successfully shaping policy can only be enhanced.

References

Alexander, E. (1986). *Approaches to planning: Introducing current planning theories, concepts and issues.* Gordon & Breach, New York.

Alford, R.R. (1975). *Health care politics: Ideological and interest group barriers to reform.* The University of Chicago Press, Chicago and London.

Annas, G.J. (1999). *Is privacy the enemy of public health? Health Affairs,* **18**, 197–8.

Berridge, V. (1999). Passive smoking and its pre-history in Britain: Policy speaks to science? *Social Science and Medicine,* **49**, 1183–96.

Birkland, T.A. (2001). *An introduction to the policy process : Theories, concepts, and models of public policy making.* M.E. Sharpe, Armonk, N.Y.

Blank, R.H. and Burau, V. (2004). *Comparative Health Policy.* Palgrave, Basingstoke.

Boaz, A. and Pawson, R. (2005). The perilous road from evidence to policy: Five journeys compared. *Journal of Social Policy,* **34**, 175–94.

Burris, S. (1997). The invisibility of public health: population-level measures in a politics of market individualism. *American Journal of Public Health,* **87**, 1607–10.

Buse, K., Mays, N., and Walt, G. (2005). *Making health policy.* Open University Press, Maidenhead.

Chapman, C. and Lupton, D. (1994). *The fight for public health. Principles and practice of media advocacy.* BMJ Publishing, London.

Davies, H., Nutley, S., and Smith, P. (eds.) (2000). *What works?: Evidence-based policy and practice in public services.* The Policy Press, Bristol.

Davis, P. (2004). "Tough but fair"? The active management of the New Zealand drug benefits scheme by an independent Crown agency. *Australian Health Review,* **28**, 171–81.

Deber, R., Millan, K., Shapiro, H. *et al.* (2007). A cautionary tale of downloading public health in Ontario: What does it say about the need for national standards for more than doctors and hospitals? *Healthcare Policy,* **2**, 60–75.

Dror, Y. (1968). *Public policymaking reexamined.* Chandler Pub. Co., San Francisco; Science Research Associates distributors. Chicago.

Ellwood, D.T. (2003). From research to social policy and back again: Translating scholarship into practice through the starry eyes of a Sometimes scarred veteran. *Social Policy Journal of New Zealand,* **20**, 6–28.

Etzioni, A. (1967). Mixed-scanning: A 'third' approach to decision-making. *Public Administration Review,* **27**, 385–92.

Exworthy, M., Blane, D., and Marmot, M.(2003). Tackling health inequalities in the united kingdom: The progress and pitfalls of policy. *Health Services Research,* **38**, 1905–21.

Farquharson, K. (2003). Influencing policy transnational: Pro- and anti-tobacco global advocacy networks. *Australian Journal of Public Administration,* **62**, 80–92.

Flyvbjerg, B. (2001). *Making Social Science Matter.* Cambridge University Press, Cambridge.

Givel, M. (2006). Punctuated equilibrium in Limbo: The tobacco lobby and U.S. state policymaking from 1990 to 2003. *Policy Studies Journal,* **34**, 405–18.

Glouberman, S. and Millar, J. (2003). Evolution of the determinants of health, health policy, and health information systems in Canada. *American Journal of Public Health,* **93**, 388–92.

Greenberg, M. (1992). Impediments to basing government health policies on science in the United States. *Social Science and Medicine,* **35**, 531–40.

Hajer, M.A. (1995). *The politics of environmental discourse: Ecological modernization and the policy process.* Clarendon Press, Oxford.

Harrison, K. (2001). Too close to home: Dioxin contamination of breast milk and the political agenda *Policy Sciences,* **34**, 35–62.

Heclo, H. (1974). *Social policy in Britain and Sweden.* Yale University Press, New Haven CT.

Hindess, B. (1996). *Discourses of power.* Blackwell, London.

Hutt, M. and Howden-Chapman, P. (1998). *Old wine in new bottles: The Public Health Commission and the making of New Zealand alcohol policy*. Institute of Policy Studies, Wellington.

Immergut, E.M. (1992). *Health politics: Interests and institutions in Western Europe*. Cambridge University Press, Cambridge.

Kingdon, J.W. (2003). *Agendas, alternatives, and public policies*. HarperCollins College Publishers, New York.

Kirp, D.L. and Bayer, R. (eds.)(1992). *AIDS in the industrialized democracies. passions, politics, and policies*. Rutgers University Press, New Brunswick, NJ.

Landry, R., Lamari, M., and Amara, N. (2003). The extent and determinants of the utilization of university research in government agencies. *Public Administration Review*, **63**, 192–205.

Lang, T. and Rayner, G. (2007). Overcoming policy cacophony on obesity: An ecological public health framework for policymakers. *Obesity Reviews*, **8**, 165–81.

Lavis, J.N. (2006). Research, public policymaking, and knowledge-translation processes: Canadian efforts to build bridges. *Journal of Continuing Education in the Health Professions*, **26**, 37–45.

Leichter, H.M. (1991). *Free to be foolish. Politics and health promotion in the United States and Great Britain*. Princeton University Press, Princeton.

Light, D. (1995). Countervailing powers: A framework for professions in transition. In *Health professions and the state in Europe* (eds. T. Johnson, G. Larkin, and M. Saks), pp. 7–24. Routledge, London.

Lindblom, C. (1959). The science of muddling through. *Public Administration Review*, **19**, 79–88.

Lindblom, C. (1977). *Politics and markets*. Basic Books, New York.

Lindblom, C.E. and Cohen, D.K. (1979). *Usable knowledge: Social science and social problem solving*. Yale University Press, New Haven CT.

Lomas, J. (2007). The in-between world of knowledge brokering. *British Medical Journal*, **334**, 129–32.

Marmor, T., Barer, M.L., and Evans, R.G. (1994). The determinants of a population's health: What can be done to improve a democratic nation's health status? In *Why are some people healthy and others not: The determinants of health of populations* (eds. R.G. Evans, M.L. Barer, and T. Marmor).Aldine De Gruyter, New York.

Marmot, M. and Wilkinson, R.G. (eds.)(1999). *Social determinants of health*. Oxford University Press, Oxford.

Marsh, D. and Rhodes, R.A.W. (1992). *Policy networks in British government*. Oxford University Press, Oxford.

Mechanic, D. (1995). Emerging trends in the application of the social sciences to health and medicine. *Social Science and Medicine*, **40**, 1491–6.

Nathan, S.A., Develin, E., Grove, N. *et al*. (2005). An Australian childhood obesity summit: the role of data and evidence in 'public' policy making. *Australia and New Zealand Health Policy*, **2**, 1–10.

Nelson, B. (1984). *Making an issue of child abuse*. University of Chicago Press, Chicago.

O'Neill, M. and Pederson, A.P. (1992). Building a methods bridge between public policy analysis and health public policy. *Canadian Journal of Public Health*, **83** (Suppl 1), S25–30.

Petersen, A. and Lupton, D. (1996). *The new public health: Health and self in the age of risk*. Allen & Unwin, St Leonards, NSW.

Pressman, J.L. and Wildavsky, A.B. (1984). *Implementation: How great expectations in Washington are dashed in Oakland*. University of California Press, Berkeley, CA.

Rashad, I. (2005). Whose fault is it we're getting fat? Obesity in the United States. *Public Policy Research*, **12**, 30–6.

Read, M. (1992). Policy networks and issue networks: The politics of smoking, In *Policy networks in British government* (eds. D. Marsh and R.A.W. Rhodes RAW), pp. 124–48. Oxford University Press, Oxford.

Remington, R.D. (1990). From preventive policy to preventive practice. *Preventive Medicine*, **19**, 105–13.

Robinson, T.N. and Sirard, J.R. (2005). Preventing childhood obesity: A solution-oriented research paradigm. *American Journal of Preventive Medicine*, **28**, 194–201.

Rychetnik, L. and Wise, M. (2004). Advocating evidence-based health promotion: Reflections and a way forward. *Health Promotion International*, **19**, 247–57.

Sabatier, P.A. and Jenkins-Smith, H.C. (eds.)(1993). *Policy learning and change: An advocacy coalition approach*. Westview Press, Boulder.

Saguy, A.C. and Riley, K.W. (2005). Weighing both sides: Morality, mortality, and framing contests over obesity. *Journal of Health Politics Policy and Law*, **30**, 869–923.

Salter, B. (2004). *The new politics of medicine*. Palgrave Macmillan, Basingstoke.

Sato, H. (1999). The advocacy coalition framework and the policy process analysis: The case of smoking control in Japan. *Policy Studies Journal*, **27**, 28–44.

Schlesinger, M. (2005). Weighting for Godot. *Journal of Health Politics, Policy and Law*, **30**, 785–801.

Schmid, T.J., Pratt, M., and Howze, E. (1995). Policy as intervention: Environmental and policy approaches to the prevention of cardiovascular disease. *American Journal of Public Health*, **85**, 1207–11.

Princen, S. (2007). Advocacy coalitions and the internationalization of public health policies. *Journal of Public Policy*, **27**, 13–33.

Seelig, M.Y. and Seelig, J.H. (1998). 'Place your bets!' on gambling, government and society. *Canadian Public Policy*, **24**, 91–106.

Smith, K.E. (2007). Health inequalities in Scotland and England: The contrasting journeys of ideas from research into policy. *Social Science and Medicine*, **64**, 1438–49.

Spector, M. and Kitsuse, J. (1987). *Constructing social problems*. Aldine de Gruyter, New York.

Steinmo, S. and Watts, J. (1995). It's the institutions, stupid! Why comprehensive national health insurance always fails in America. *Journal of Health Politics, Policy and Law*, **20**, 329–71.

Stone, D.A. (1997). *Policy paradox : The art of political decision making*. W.W. Norton, New York.

Swinburn, B., Gill, T., and Kumanyika, S. (2005). Obesity prevention: A proposed framework for translating evidence into action. *Obesity Reviews*, **6**, 23–33.

Tenbensel, T. (2004). Does more evidence lead to better policy? The implications of explicit priority-setting in New Zealand's health policy for evidence-based policy. *Policy Studies*, **25**, 189–207.

Tenbensel, T. (2006). Policy knowledge for policy work. In *The work of policy: An international survey* (ed. Colebatch HK), pp. 199–215. Lexington Books, Lanham; University Press, New York.

Walt, G. (1994). *Health policy. An introduction to process and power*. Zed Books, London.

Wang, S.S. and Brownell, K.D. (2005). Public policy and obesity: The need to marry science with advocacy. *Psychiatric Clinics of North America*, **28**, 235–52.

Weiss, C.H. (1991). Policy research: Data, ideas or arguments. In *Social sciences and modern states: National experiences and theoretical crossroads* (ed. P. Wagner), pp. 307–32. Cambridge University Press, New York.

Wilkinson, R. (2007). The challenge of prevention: A response to Starfield's "Commentary: pathways of influence on equity in health". *Social Science and Medicine*, **64**, 1367–70.

Williams-Crowe, S.M. and Aultman, T.V. (1994). State health agencies and the legislative policy process. *Public Health Reports*, **109**, 361–7.

Wilson, J.Q. (1973). *Political organizations*. Sage, Beverly Hills, CA.

Winstanley, A. (2005). The not-so-hidden politics of fluoridation. *Policy and Politics*, **33**, 367–85.

7.7

Public health sciences and policy in low- and middle-income countries

Lindiwe Makubalo, Mary Ann Lansang[1], and J. Peter Figueroa

Abstract

Public health sciences contributed significantly to improving the health of individuals and communities in the twentieth century through evidence-informed policy. Now, more recently emerging public health challenges such as HIV and AIDS, SARS, human influenza, the increase in non-communicable diseases, and the globalization of public health are placing new and increased demands on technical requirements, and on the disciplines required to help craft appropriate policies to address new and evolving public health demands. This chapter argues the need to advance from a more traditional paradigm of public health to a more inclusive approach that incorporates a range of disciplines from outside of the traditional public health domain. This inclusive approach should be more responsive to the changing nature of public health needs in the twenty-first century. Examples are provided of how sciences outside of the public health tradition contributed to improved policy development and resolution of health problems. Challenges related to the public health sciences are identified. These include: Increasing health demands requiring strong collaboration among already stretched disciplines that do not traditionally interact; the need for national-level training for health policy development in low- and middle-income countries; advocacy and capacity building for policy and health systems research; and the development of new collaborative arrangements at global and regional levels. A model of how public health sciences might contribute more effectively to policy development is proposed.

Introduction

The public health sciences provide the scientific foundation for improving the health of the public and for understanding the determinants of health. More specifically, public health sciences focus on: (1) the epidemiology, control and prevention of diseases and their consequences; (2) health promotion, prevention and rehabilitation; and (3) the structure and function of health systems that guide health policy and programmes.

In low- and middle-income countries, public health sciences play an important role in informing and influencing health policy and, ultimately, in disease control and achieving better health outcomes. Unfortunately there has not been much discussion on how public health sciences in these countries could better contribute to addressing the changing needs and growing challenges in public health. There has not even been much of an appraisal of the disciplines that would be needed to strengthen the dynamic and expansive demands placed on public health in the twenty-first century.

Meanwhile there is a major concern that many low- and middle-income countries are already lagging behind in the race towards achieving public health targets, if the Millennium Development Goals (MDGs) are used as a benchmark of the progress in achieving public health objectives (WHO 2005). The countries that are lagging are those countries that have the greatest constraints with regard to finances, infrastructural arrangements, and human resources. The extent to which realignment of expertise and resources to strengthen the public health response to new health challenges remains to be determined, but most would argue that assembling together and re-organizing the diverse disciplines that contribute to meeting the objectives of health into a much expanded 'public health' approach, would greatly benefit health outcomes. Inclusion of other disciplines that have not traditionally enjoyed a central place in policy development and public health can potentially contribute significantly to successful outcomes in the field of public health.

Low- and middle-income countries are confronted with serious health and development challenges to which there are no easy answers. In particular, low-income countries, which account for only 2 per cent of global health spending or an estimated US$30 per capita per annum on average (World Bank 2005; Lopez *et al.* 2006),

[1] M. A. Lansang, chapter co-author, currently works at The Global Fund to Fight AIDS, Tuberculosis and Malaria. The views expressed in this chapter are those of the named authors and do not necessarily reflect the decisions or stated policy of The Global Fund.

experience severe underlying poverty and under-development. Chapter 1.1 (by Roger Detels) has addressed the broader contextual factors that underlie poverty and under-development and that have a major impact on health policy and health delivery. These factors are varied but relate to climatic change and natural disasters, failing national economies brought on by armed conflict, poor security, political instability, weak governance, imprudent spending, and weak stewardship. In addition, global trade policies, unfair conditions of trade, and conditional ties of lending impact negatively on the ability of many countries to sustain reasonable levels of health.

As a consequence low- and middle-income countries are faced with low life expectancy levels and an overwhelming disease burden, estimated at 56 per cent of the global total. In most instances, the millennium health indicators show high levels of child and infant deaths in these countries. Most of these deaths, an estimated 41 per cent of the world's child deaths, occur in sub-Saharan Africa and 43 per cent in South Asia. Furthermore, the decline in deaths in these regions has slowed from an estimated 2.5 per cent per year between 1960 and 1990 to only 1.1 per cent per year in the 1990–2001 period. However there is a growing concern that some of these declines in infant death rates may slow down or even be offset because many low-income countries in particular have not been able to prevent malnutrition or achieve the health system coverage required to prevent malaria and vaccine-preventable diseases such as pneumonia, and in some instances because of the contribution that mother-to-child transmission of HIV to childhood diseases associated with HIV and AIDS (WHO 2005).

There are an estimated 2.7 million deaths due to malaria each year. HIV/AIDS, TB, malaria, and childhood diseases continue to be responsible for high infant and child mortality rates and weigh heavily on these fragile health systems, where high bed occupancy rates and high costs of medicines (particularly medications for chronic diseases such as anti-retroviral drugs) are a major burden. HIV and AIDS, affecting 38.6 million cases worldwide, have the highest burden in low- and middle-income countries. Countries with the highest burden such as Botswana report an infection prevalence of approximately 38 per cent among women attending antenatal clinics. TB infection rates are highest in Asia and sub-Saharan Africa, with 74 million new cases per year, or approximately 84 per cent of the global TB burden (UNAIDS 2006).

Control of vaccine-preventable diseases is a concern because millions of children in these countries continue to die or suffer ill health despite established and affordable interventions like vaccines and prevention tools. There are available evidence-based interventions that can potentially prevent two-thirds of child deaths worldwide, but the global coverage for most of these interventions is less than 50 per cent (Jones *et al.* 2003). Progress in the control of diseases has been marred by weak health systems that are neither able to cope with demand nor provide efficient delivery systems especially to urban slums, informal settlements, or remote and difficult-to-reach rural communities. These health systems barriers include weak policy environments and governance, political instability, and deficiencies in human resources, financing, drug and supply systems, and health information systems (Travis *et al.* 2004).

Epidemic-prone diseases such as cholera remain a threat in many low- and middle-income countries, where once again preparedness is often inadequate and health systems are unable to maintain early warning systems and response mechanisms that match the speed with which such epidemics as cholera multiply and spread. Moreover with increasing globalization, global health emergency response agreements are mounting pressure on countries, regardless of their levels of socioeconomic development, to respond to the most recent developments on the public health agenda, in particular preparedness against severe acute respiratory syndrome (SARS), avian influenza, and other potential pandemics. Since bioterrorist activities could be launched from anywhere in the globe, countries are also challenged to put in place policies and mechanisms against less traditional health domains such as bioterrorism. For many low-income countries the probabilities of achieving adequate levels of preparedness and response systems may be remote in the face of more basic socioeconomic and health needs, and yet more compelling in the face of the higher epidemic potential in these countries.

As if these challenges are not formidable enough, most low- and middle-countries are experiencing changing epidemiological profiles, resulting in a triple burden of communicable and infectious diseases, non-communicable diseases, and trauma and conditions resulting from injuries. The growing burden of non-communicable diseases such as hypertension, diabetes, coronary artery disease, stroke, and cancers, particularly in middle-income countries, places another set of demands on health services in terms of treatment and chronic care. Effective public health interventions are needed to prevent further escalations in non-communicable diseases and chronic health conditions. Mathers and Loncar (2006) estimate a rise in global deaths from non-communicable diseases from 59 per cent in 2002 to 69 per cent in 2030, with cerebrovascular disease and ischaemic heart disease being among the top three causes of death in low- and middle-income countries by 2030. The management of chronic diseases needs alternative health delivery and care models. Existing models that are more traditional and geared to providing preventive interventions, care, and treatment of communicable diseases can barely cope without the pressure of adjusting to the provision of services for prevention and care of chronic conditions. The rising disease trends and challenges, associated with weak health systems contexts, demand new approaches and paradigms for health policy processes and systems.

Public policy environments in low- and middle-income countries

Equitable, effective, and well-functioning health systems are critical for driving health services and enabling countries to achieve their health goals. The response to the overwhelming picture of disease and ill health in low- and middle-income countries is hampered by factors in the public policy environment and inadequacies of the health system. The World Health Report (2000), which focused on the role of health systems, raised much global interest and debate on the factors contributing to weak performance of health systems and concluded that effective health development cannot take place outside of well-functioning health systems, effective stewardship, and overall social and economic development.

Low- and middle-income countries differ in their level of socioeconomic development and political contexts. It is widely accepted that there is a correlation between poor income of individuals and low socioeconomic development levels and health. However, Cuba is an example of a society where income redistribution and a clear focus on policy objectives increased life expectancy and improved health indicators in only 15 years (Waitzkin 2000). Many countries have adopted egalitarian health policies where free services are provided to all or provided for vulnerable groups in particular, younger children and infants, women, and the disabled. However the pressure on the budgets of low- and middle-income countries has led to ongoing debates on the most appropriate pro-poor policies and health strategies, with some opting for social health insurance schemes. In practice, however, even those countries that aspire towards more egalitarian policies are constrained by sociopolitical and contextual factors. The policies are not always pro-poor as the countries may be under-resourced and health services under-funded. Many countries with small economies and a large informal sector have a limited ability to tax, resulting in high out-of-pocket payments for health by the citizens who can afford to pay whilst others simply do without formal healthcare.

Unfortunately, equitable redistribution of available resources is often difficult to achieve. There is often a focus on improved access to healthcare services. Whilst physical access is important, having access to services does not in itself produce health as inequalities may be rooted in other levels such as gender, race, or ethnic group.

Initiatives such as the Commission on the Social Determinants of Health continue to underscore the importance of health equity and the 'causes of the causes' of ill health (Commission on Social Determinants of Health 2007). It is well accepted that health improvements in many high-income countries correlated with socioeconomic development and ultimately the latter was more contributory to health improvements seen in the twentieth century than drugs, vaccines, and other technological advances. In the context of low- and middle-income countries, it has been shown that availability of safe water, sanitation, adult literacy, in particular education of mothers of infants, contribute very significantly to improved health.

Aside from the profound influence of social determinants of health, health reforms in many low- and middle-income countries in the 1980s and 1990s had a strong influence in shaping health policy and systems in these countries. The range of reforms in state management, referred to as the new public management (NPM), involved changes in organizational structure (e.g. moves towards managerial autonomy or corporatization of public entities) and introduction of market processes (e.g. through privatization or market-simulating reforms within the public sector). Government's role was redefined from that of direct service to one of stewardship, oversight, and regulation (Khaleghian & Das Gupta 2004).

Whereas in highly centralized management structures, the policy arena is generally top-down, with limited interactions and information from other stakeholders, the policy arena tends to have a wider range of stakeholders in decentralized or more progressive systems where academic and research institutions, non-governmental and people's organizations, professional associations of healthcare providers, and the media have achieved some regular channels for engagement. For effective, knowledge-based policymaking and implementation, the engagement of more stakeholders is desirable. However, despite health reforms, most low- and middle-income countries still do not have effective management structures and technical resources in place to systematically organize and analyse inputs from different stakeholders and use them for effective policymaking and planning. The multiplicity of players and their complex interactions, in the face of weak health systems in many low- and middle-income countries, can thus pose severe constraints on policy making in these countries.

The health sector is human resource-intensive and yet, in low- and middle-income countries, the sector is highly beset with human resource challenges that include: Worker shortages, skill-mix imbalances, maldistribution of skills between densely populated urban settings and rural areas, difficult work environments, and weak knowledge base (Chen *et al.* 2004). The highly contentious issue of human resource migration, usually from the southern hemisphere to the northern hemisphere countries or from low-income countries to middle-income countries, is often highest on the agenda in recent international discussions on human resources for health. The Global Human Resources for Health initiative (http://www.who.int/hrh/en; accessed 20 August 2007) and the Joint Learning Initiative (Chen *et al.* 2004) observed that mobilization and strengthening of human resources for health have been neglected, reaching health crisis proportions particularly in some of the less resourced countries of the world. These initiatives have argued for concerted global action to reverse the human resource crisis in many countries. This should go hand in hand with national policies and supportive environments for workforce development.

Low- and middle-income countries also have to contend with two major forces that have a profound influence on the financing of the health sector: Overseas development assistance and the private sector. For these countries, public sector expenditures for health constitute only 26–51 per cent of total health expenditures (Jamison 2006). Particularly, in the case of low-income countries where the average per capita expenditure for health is only US$19 per year (Hecht 2006), funds from overseas development assistance can constitute a significant resource for health expenditures. Paradoxically, the countries that are most in need of health financing assistance tend to be the same ones where development assistance is less effective because of weak health systems and inadequate policy contexts to implement programmes, environments, and institutions (Jamison 2006). Multiple development agencies with competing and uncoordinated programmes and interests as well as varying reporting and performance requirements tend to overwhelm the health systems and absorptive capacity of recipient countries. They may also distort the countries' health priorities in favour of programmes supported by development agencies, other funding agencies, and international health institutions (Travis 2004).

Moreover, a bewildering array of strategies and performance assessment schedules proposed by multilateral and bilateral agencies and other funding agencies pose a challenging menu for policy reform and programmes in low- and middle-income countries. The evolving menu has ranged from health sector reform that focused on financing and decentralization, global initiatives that offered packages of interventions, or specific disease-control programmes, to more recent movements that have supported health systems strengthening, integrated health service delivery, poverty reduction support credits, and sector-wide approaches (Hecht 2006).

The private sector can also be a major player in low- and middle-income countries, particularly in relation to the national policy on pharmaceuticals or the national tobacco policy. The stakeholders in these arenas include the pharmaceutical or tobacco companies, commodity distributors, healthcare practitioners, and consumers. In relation to drugs and vaccines, there are many contentious and unresolved issues such as issues of pricing and access, inclusion of drugs in national formularies, regulation and quality assurance, intellectual property rights, counterfeit drugs, parallel importation, taxation, and financing. It is a timely development for low- and middle-income countries that the Intergovernmental Working Group on Public Health Innovation and Intellectual Property (WHO 2007) has been established and will now attempt to broker the process to resolve some of these issues and promote the use of flexibilities in trade-related aspects of public health. In general, however, low- and middle-income countries have weak national drug policies and regulatory frameworks that are unable to provide effective governance over competing public and market interests.

Finally, the policy making process itself presents major challenges. These challenges are more severe in low- and middle-income contexts. In all critical steps of the policy and practice pathway described by Bowen and Zwi (2005), from the availability, timeliness, appreciation, and understanding of evidence to its dissemination and utilization (Fig. 7.7.1), deficiencies are observed in these settings. More specifically, although the public health sciences play a potentially important role in providing the best evidence for decision making, only a small and tenuous cadre of public health scientists in these countries are generally able and available to collect, analyse, and synthesize relevant evidence, and translate them to policy recommendations. Many of the individual, organizational, and system level conditions for policy to be implemented are weak or absent, particularly in low-income settings. These include weak leadership, distrust, vested interests, patronage, political expediencies and pressure, corruption, poor information management systems, and weak partnerships. Where there may be exceptional leaders and champions of evidence-informed policy making, the rapid turnover of these policy makers and officials retards organizational learning and growth.

In general, different skills and levels of expertise are required to support policy development at various levels of the health system. At the 'macro' level is national policy development, which is often seen as the most complex as it is more closely linked to sociopolitical and economic processes of government. At a 'meso' level, exemplified by district and sub-district level policy processes, policymaking is often more closely linked to programme development. The interplay between national and local policy making can be particularly challenging in decentralized health systems where the needs, demands, and resources at the local level may not necessarily reflect national policies and strategies. At the 'micro' level, public health sciences also have a role in developing policies for clinical and public health practice, in particular in providing the evidence-base for appropriate clinical and public health interventions and facilitating consensus building and implementation among health practitioners. Overall, the health policy environment is dependent on the governance structures and mechanisms of the country. Many low- and middle-income countries are marked by political upheavals, civil wars and violence, lack of accountability and transparency, corruption, and lack of a free and/or responsible media, all of which weaken the ability to effectively formulate and implement policy and programmes that will improve the health of the public. For many of these countries, the fundamental challenge is to address the troubled political context in which health policy development takes place. The countries that are not beset with such political upheavals face the challenge of transforming and evolving from colonialist cultures to systems that embrace more internationally accepted democratic policies.

It is interesting to note though that even in the midst of such huge development challenges, there are important examples of countries, particularly middle-income countries, that have been extremely progressive and proactive in introducing legislation and social practices on the basis of available evidence, even ahead of some of the more economically developed countries—for example, banning tobacco advertising, introducing restrictions on tobacco usage in public places, and creating a tobacco-free environment.

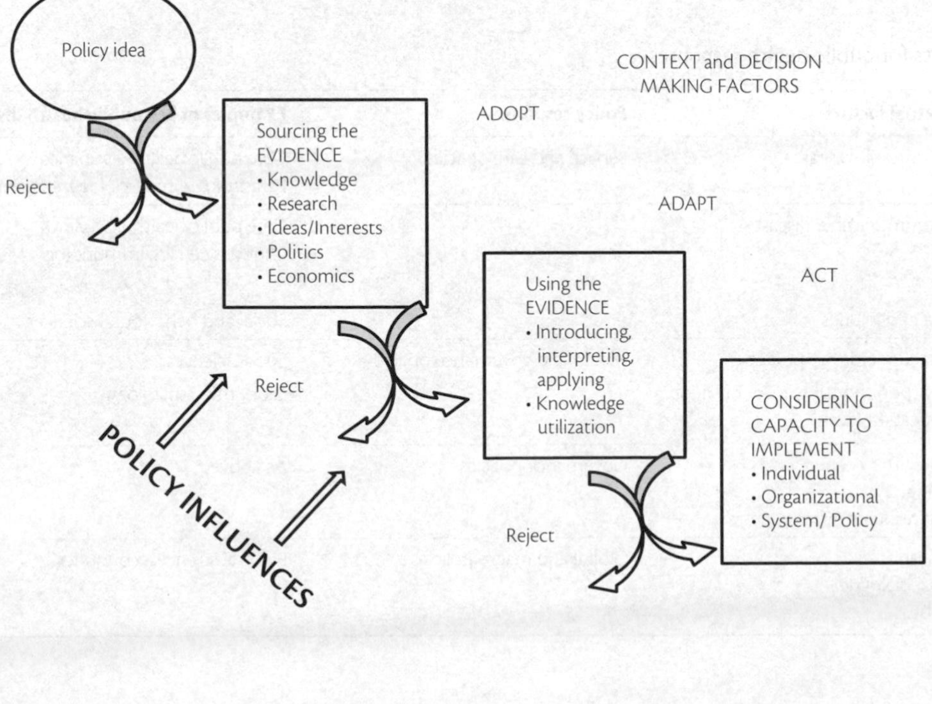

Fig. 7.7.1 The evidence-informed policy and practice pathway
Source: Bowen and Zwi (2005).

The changing landscape of public health sciences

If the field of public health is to be the driving force towards finding effective solutions to the complex challenges that low- and middle-income countries face, then there is a compelling need to expand and broaden the traditional scope of the public health sciences beyond the so-called 'core' disciplines to include a wider spectrum of disciplines and skills. In addition to epidemiology and biostatistics, public health sciences cover many other disciplines in the health sciences including biomedical and clinical research, as well as biology, physics, chemistry, economics, anthropology, psychology, sociology, demography, and the humanities.

Table 7.7.1 shows the changing context of public health responses. Historically public health focused more on disease agents and mechanisms of action in disease transmission. Last (2005) provides an interesting account of the contribution of non-public-health professionals to public health. For instance, Theophrastus Bombastus von Hohenheim, a chemist, contributed to our understanding of how dust could result in the acquisition of lung diseases; Edward Jenner, an English family doctor, published an inquiry into the causes and effect of the viriolae vaccine in 1798; and Ignaz Semmelweiss used statistical analysis and germ theory to describe puerperal sepsis in obstetric wards. Ronald Ross, who trained in surgery and parasitology in 1897, described the all-important role of the *Anopheles* mosquitoes in the transmission of malaria parasites to humans (Chernin 1988), eventually leading to vector control as an important strategy for malaria control. Thus in the early days the scope of public health sciences, though not recognized as a discipline, was wide and encompassed individuals from disparate disciplines. In later years, as the field of public health became more clearly defined, there was a recognition that it covered core disciplines such as epidemiology, biostatistics, parasitology, clinical and laboratory sciences. The basic biological sciences that have contributed to public health have since expanded to include ecology, immunochemistry, molecular biology, genomics, proteomics, and bioinformatics.

There are examples of institutions that grew from a limited public health science scope into larger centres with a range of disciplines involved in responding to the changing needs of public health. The Caribbean Epidemiology Center (CAREC), for instance, grew from a response to poliomyelitis and typhoid fever outbreaks in Trinidad and Tobago in 1971. In collaboration with other Caribbean islands, and the Pan American Health Organization (PAHO), the Center has grown, housing a number of public health disciplines to better respond to new health challenges.

The Unites States of America's Centers for Disease Control (CDC) celebrated its 60th year of existence in 2006, having evolved from a small centre for malaria control agency in 1946. The CDC has expanded from a cadre of entomologists and engineers in the 1940s to inclusion of epidemiologists, veterinarians, microbiologists, and medical officers in the 1970s, to the latest addition of economists, behavioural and social scientists, molecular biologists, statisticians, urban planners, informatics specialists, and other scientists, altogether representing approximately 25 scientific disciplines. This process of inclusion is still in progress as the CDC plans for its public work force in the coming decade (Lee & Popovic 2006).

In spite of the rapid advances in science and technology, applications of the basic sciences to public health have not at all been straightforward. Major knowledge gaps stand in the way of progress towards disease control or, even more difficult, eradication. For example, the increasing burden of illness from HIV/AIDS-related diseases demonstrates that even when interventions to prevent infections are known, successes in controlling infections are still relatively moderate because behaviour modification is so difficult to achieve. In the case of HIV and AIDS, behavioural interventions such as safe sex, condom use, and maintaining mutually faithful partners have been widely publicized for many years, yet translation from knowledge to practice has been slow and, from the increasing incidence trends, difficult to achieve. Similarly, with respect to tobacco consumption behavioural change has been slow and most successes have been catapulted by stringent measures such as implementation of tobacco legislation. Public health disciplines that focus on

Table 7.7.1 Changing policy contexts for public health responses

Health contexts	Contextual factors	Policy response	Examples of key public health disciplines
Disease burden	Communicable diseases	Service and care policies	Core public health disciplines Parasitology, immunology, epidemiology
	Non-communicable diseases Trauma and injuries		Core public health disciplines Clinical sciences, immunology + Social and behavioural sciences
National health contexts	National underdevelopment Poverty (poor housing, poor nutrition, low education levels)	Macro and governance policies	Social sciences: Economics, sociology
	Weak health systems Financing Human resource infrastructure	Governance policies	As above
Regional and global health context	Globalization Regional dialogue New diseases	Global and macro policies	Political science, economics

developing and refining skills on the knowledge-to-behavioural-change gap need to be strengthened.

An unfinished public health agenda relates to increasing the knowledge and understanding of the social determinants of health. Examples of factors for which we need more information are: The types of societies people live in, their organization and culture, traditional beliefs, and age-old customs and behaviours of individuals when faced with an ecosystem of competing risks. These factors, which can also determine the uptake of health technologies, have a major impact on effective delivery of health and on policy processes.

There are also health systems issues that have to be addressed, such as organizational behaviours, availability of resources, health financing options, and improving access to care and scale up of interventions. These have progressed to questions on how to finance these programmes on a large scale, how to access financing from development agencies and other finance institutions, and even how to free up other local resources in order to take successes to scale.

These much broader issues have challenged many national and local governments in low- and middle-income countries to approach health policy development in the context of health sector reform. Box 7.7.1 illustrates the expanded set of disciplines and skills in focus areas that are needed to help attain the objectives of health sector reform in the Philippines. Clearly, public health scientists from different disciplines will need to collaborate closely to achieve synergies in policy formulation, programme planning and implementation, and evaluation.

Challenges for the public health sciences

Multidisciplinary approach

The disciplinary scope of the public health sciences has broadened through the years, spurred by a better understanding of the determinants of health and the imperative to work collaboratively to combat new and increasingly complex global health threats. A multidisciplinary base is all the more important in developing and effectively communicating the evidence base for policy making within the unique socioeconomic and political contexts of low- and middle-income countries (Beaglehole 2004).

Rather than parallel contributions from the public health sciences, however, the ability to cross-disciplinary boundaries and collaborate in providing a comprehensive but comprehensible evidence base for policy makers is an important challenge for public health practitioners.

Box 7.7.1 Potential contributions of public health sciences to health sector reform in the Philippines

Components and objectives of 'FOURmula One for Health'*	Examples of public health disciplines	Examples of focus areas for study
Health financing To secure more, better, and sustained investments in health to provide equity and improve health outcomes, especially for the poor.	◆ Health economics ◆ Management sciences	◆ Social protection mechanisms ◆ Cost-effectiveness analyses of interventions ◆ National health accounts ◆ Poverty and equity analysis ◆ Budget and investment planning
Health regulation To assure access to quality and affordable health products, devices, facilities and services, especially those commonly used by the poor	◆ Biomedical and laboratory sciences	◆ Health technology assessment ◆ Benchmarking ◆ Practice guideline development
Service delivery To improve the accessibility and availability of basic and essential health care for all, particularly the poor.	◆ Epidemiology and biostatistics ◆ Demography ◆ Biomedical, clinical, and laboratory sciences ◆ Sociobehavioral sciences—sociology, anthropology, psychology ◆ Management sciences ◆ Communications	◆ National health and demographic surveys ◆ Health information systems ◆ Health services research ◆ Health needs assessment ◆ Consumer satisfaction surveys ◆ Behaviour change communication ◆ Monitoring and evaluation
Governance To improve local health systems performance and coordination, enhance effective private–public partnerships, and improve national capacities to manage the health sector.	◆ Political science ◆ Law ◆ Management sciences ◆ Public health informatics ◆ Communications	◆ Political mapping ◆ Policy analysis ◆ Knowledge management ◆ Public–private partnerships ◆ Capacity development

* 'FOURmula One for Health' is the Philippine Department of Health's implementation framework for health sector reforms.
Source (for Column 1): Department of Health, Philippines, http://www2.doh.gov.ph/f1primer/F1-Page.htm (accessed 14 July 2007).

For example, the discovery of SARS and the containment of the outbreak required the close collaboration of hundreds of scientists from across the globe and spanned the disciplines of epidemiology, the clinical sciences, molecular virology, pharmacology, vaccinology, biochemistry, bioethics, health economics, social sciences, and so on. In the global fight against HIV and AIDS there is an understanding that finding a therapeutic solution lies in a good understanding of the human immunodeficiency virus. It is well accepted however that global containment of HIV lies squarely on prevention of new infections. To achieve this objective, which has such a huge behavioural modification element, will require strong collaboration and synergy of different disciplines.

Wider collaborative links

In addition to good disciplinary collaboration, developing equal partnerships with government agencies, non-governmental organizations, and community groups is critical to the success of public health programmes. Collaboration and dialogue with funding agencies are also important so that resources are appropriately allocated and managed.

Partnership development is easier said than done. Many apparent partnerships have been nominal or, worse, neo-colonial, with the agenda of the dominant party taking the lead, and leaving the indigenous public health scientists and practitioners ill-prepared to take over and sustain the programme after the external funding ceases. The continuing challenge is for all potential partners to jointly create a constructive environment of mutual trust and respect, and accept joint responsibility for decision-making and action. These partnerships will need to extend beyond the professionals and public health experts to communities.

Effective partnership development is exemplified by the work such as at the international level of the People's Health Movement in Bangladesh. This movement was founded in 2000 with people from 90 countries. Characterized as a movement, which grew from the grass roots upwards, and representing numerous sectors and types of expertise such as education, health, and agriculture, it has been particularly strong in social mobilization at the grass root level. It has partnered with health authorities, grassroots organizations, and other national and international networks to strengthen and re-define Primary Healthcare and other important public health initiatives. This organization spearheaded the drawing up of a People's Charter for Health, contributed to policy change in countries, and participated in discussions at the international level. An evaluation of the people's movement suggests that one of its major strengths has been to translate community needs and thus enable the participation of the marginalized in many countries, particularly in Asia, to influence health programmes (http://www.phmovement.org/about/phmevaluation). An example at the national level is the Philippine Coalition against Tuberculosis (PhilCAT, www.philcat.org), which demonstrates how government, academic, non-governmental and private organizations and institutions have banded together to influence TB policy and control in the country. Established in 1994 with 12 founding members consisting of representatives from the Department of Health, professional societies, and the pharmaceutical industry, it has grown to a coalition of 67 member organizations. The varied skill-mix of its membership (control programme staff, local governments, epidemiologists, chest specialists, infectologists, microbiologists, social scientists, health economists, educators, and NGOs) has been instrumental in enabling active participation towards the formulation of the Comprehensive and Unified Policy for TB Control in the Philippines and in producing other policy documents and recommendations related to TB control, particularly in the area of public–private mix models for directly observed treatment, short course (DOTS) (Mantala 2003).

Information and methodological challenges

For low- and middle-income countries, the lack of complete, reliable, timely, and valid data and information on local and national disease burdens and risk factors continues to be a real challenge. National health infrastructure systems in most developing countries remain poor, inadequate, and unable to produce information for planning and policy development. These systems span areas such as disease surveillance systems, vital registration systems, and confidential enquires. Strengthening infrastructure and training to ensure functional vital registration systems and the availability of routine health statistics is critical. Disciplines that are traditionally more quantitative should become more involved in predicting disease trends and strengthening the health information systems. These scientists should work more closely with health personnel to help translate statistics from being mere statistical reports as produced by most central statistical offices in low-income countries to becoming health information and, better still, knowledge that can be applied to health problems.

In this regard, in many low- and middle-income countries there is a gap between initiatives that aim at collecting information and those that translate this information into useable knowledge.

Whilst there are examples of countries that have made some progress in strengthening health information systems, there are more that still face major challenges. In recent years, however, there have been encouraging developments that have addressed this gap, such as burden of diseases estimates (Lopez 2006), or worked to strengthening country capacity for national demographic health surveys, establish demographic surveillance sites in member countries of the INDEPTH Network (http://www.indepth-network.net), and more recently, the improvement of health information systems through the global Health Metrics Network (http://www.who.int/healthmetrics/en/). However, there continue to be controversies on health statistics that are generated at both global and national levels, requiring more investments into country health information systems and more methodological work on the generation and use of health statistics (Boerma 2007; Murray 2007) as well as closer collaboration of international organizations with national information authorities and experts in the compilation and estimation of country-specific statistics.

Greater numbers of longitudinal studies and randomized controlled trials are now conducted in low- and middle-income countries, but more attention should be given to the training of indigenous scientists on methodological and ethical issues in the conduct of such studies (Lansang 2004). In addition attention needs to be given to the development of national guidelines for Good Clinical Practice (GCP), ethics, and others to assist local researchers in planning and conducting scientifically valid and ethical studies. Moreover oversight mechanisms such as the South African National Clinical Trials Register, a compulsory and open register provides an important resource to potential research participants, investigators, and policy makers on ongoing clinical trials in the country (Makubalo 2006).

Systematic reviews and meta-analyses have provided better estimates of the robustness of the effectiveness of health interventions

(Volmink 2004), but there are still far too few systematic reviews on public health interventions applicable to low- and middle-income countries and taking equity issues into consideration. The integration of qualitative techniques with quantitative methods is critical in building and communicating the evidence and developing consensus for policy development. Even in high-income countries this is a challenge and there is a need for greater development and application of these skills to strengthen public health.

The limitations that exist in the knowledge and information domain are not only the limited numbers of professionals in each area. In many low- and middle-income countries access to literature can be difficult. Access to the Internet can greatly improve the situation in this regard but increasingly the library and information sciences and funders will need to become more involved in the public health arena, in particular to promote open access publishing of journals to enable health professionals of different backgrounds to have access to published literature. Examples of global and regional initiatives to improve access through Web-based technology are provided in the chapter on 'Web-based public health information dissemination and evaluation' (Siegel *et al.* 2008).

The need for health policy and systems research (HPSR)

The methodological challenges above underscore the need to refine and improve the existing knowledge bases but research is also needed to develop new methodological paradigms for generating new knowledge for policy and for translating knowledge into policy.

In 1996, the WHO *Ad Hoc* Committee on Health Research identified health policy and systems research as a priority (WHO 1996). This eventually led to the establishment of the global Alliance on Health Policy and Systems Research (http://www.who.int/alliance-hpsr/en), currently a programme under the auspices of WHO. However, support for health policy and systems research remains inadequate. With only a few global initiatives in these areas, Travis *et al.* (2004) cite several reasons for the lack of support at both national and global levels, namely:

- Health systems issues, such as planning or accountability, do not always draw the same level of public attention as concrete or emotive issues such as child mortality or immunization campaigns.
- There are differing views on the types of questions amenable to scientific enquiry.
- Health-systems research answers require long periods of study and may be uncertain.
- Generalization to other countries and settings can be difficult;
- Funding sources generally support disease-specific interventions.
- Systemic evaluations of health systems reforms can be difficult to design and defend.
- Limited research capacity and career structure in low- and middle-income countries.
- The right questions are not being asked and policy makers are not adequately engaged into the process.

In the context of global efforts towards attainment of the Millennium Development Goals, the Mexico Summit in 2004 and the World Health Assembly in 2005 made a renewed call for supporting health policy and systems research as a mechanism to achieve these objectives. Some of the priority areas for action cited by the Alliance on Health Policy and Systems Research include: Defining and standardizing the HPSR field; developing HPSR capacity; increasing funding; and promoting evidence-informed policy making (Alliance HPSR 2007). In addition, Mills (2006) proposed some priority areas for research: Circumstances under which health systems reforms are likely to improve efficiency and equity of service delivery; impact of reforms on health outcomes; characteristics of delivery strategies that are likely to achieve and maintain high coverage for specific intervention in various epidemiological, health system and cultural contexts; types of governance and institutional arrangements that will support the achievement of health improvements for the poor; and costs of capacity strengthening in health policy and systems research.

Whilst global and international initiatives have identified important research priorities, priority setting at regional and in particular at national level poses the greatest and most important challenge. Priority setting using the Essential National Health Research strategy was advocated and supported by the Council on Health research for Development (COHRED) in the 1990s (Working Group on Priority Setting, COHRED 1997). For many of the low- and middle-income countries supported by COHRED, health systems research issues were invariably listed as priorities. The priority setting exercises also underscored the difficulty of balancing national priorities against global and international priorities, underscoring the need for a stronger voice for advocating for country priorities, including health policy and systems research, as part of global agenda setting.

The need for training

The need to promote a public health domain territory with more porous boundaries allowing for incorporating disciplines which were not part of the public health tradition requires long-term planning, particularly in training and education institutions. Apart from the contribution that the migration of healthcare personnel has made to the scarceness of public health professionals, the current general workforce crisis is particularly acute in relation to the issue of public health training and education. Training institutions should seriously consider increasing the discourse and exposure regarding the concepts, principles, and challenges in public health to a broad range of disciplines within and beyond the 'health' field. This could serve as a point of contact and as a mechanism to draw interest in the application of the public health sciences to actual health problems.

Research would need to be done on the required competencies of the public health workforce, the training resources required, formal recognition of new disciplines, career structures, and so on. Not only is there a need to develop programmes that would accommodate less traditional disciplines into the public health arena, there is a need to revisit training of existing public health professionals in relation to the changing needs of public health. Sadana *et al.* (2007) argue that public health training has existed for such a long time, yet there is little systematic evidence that current approaches adequately prepare public health professionals to improve health through effective and equity-oriented health programmes.

Building indigenous capacity for HPSR in low- and middle-income countries is also important in bringing about a sustainable system of evidence-informed decision-making in low- and middle-income countries. A postal/web survey of 176 institutions in low- and middle-income countries that produced HPSR capacity showed inadequate training, experience, and critical mass of researchers to effectively engage in policy development (Block & Mills 2003). The range of HPSR-related disciplines present within the institutions varied, having 9 on the average, predominantly in public health, economics, statistics, epidemiology, medicine, and sociology. Less than one-third had researchers with training in demography, anthropology, and communications (Block & Mills 2003).

The uptake of HPSR by policy makers is an even greater challenge. This has been attributed mainly to the lack of a strong evidence-based culture within policy and programme development in low- and middle-income countries (Hennink & Stephenson 2005). In a systematic review of 24 studies in 10 countries on this issue, the following were identified as barriers to the use of evidence (Innvaer *et al.* 2002):

- Absence of personal contact between researchers and policy-makers
- Lack of timeliness/relevance of research
- Mutual distrust, including perceived political naivety of scientists and scientific naivety of policy-makers
- Power and budget struggles
- Poor quality of research
- Political instability or high turnover of policymaking staff

The need to apply new tools and technological advances

A growth in the information technology (IT) industry has resulted in major developments in IT enabling some of these technologies to become central to the concept of e-health. Telemedicine and the use of mobile technologies such as mobile telephones have enormous potential in public health. In Asia and Africa, Singapore and South Africa, respectively, have taken the lead in developing infrastructure and the application of these tools to public health (Prakash 2000; Telemedicine Task Force 2007).

There are examples of the use of telemedicine to provide primary care services such as tele-radiology or tele-pathology in remote facilities that do not have physicians and specialists to consult on site. Similarly mobile cellular phones are used to send short message services (SMS) which alert patients to take their medicines or remind them about their next visit (Atun 2006; bridges.org 2005). Smart card technology has been seen to offset the age-old problem of patient files being misplaced in health facilities and ensuring that patient records are thus easily accessible at any point of care. Whilst these technologies are available a more integrated approach among the public health disciplines is required to better align and enable the public sector to maximize the technologies for decision-making and public health advantage. The arena of information technologies is one that is considered outside the sphere of health but could make significant contributions. Whilst this tremendous potential exists, there is clearly a need for the experts in this field to work closely with policy makers and public health practitioners in low- and middle-income countries to identify the needs and enable more relevant and feasible applications of these tools to the advancement of public health.

Contributions of public health sciences to policy: Some examples

Although many political, methodological, and resource challenges confront public health scientists, examples of how public health sciences have directly contributed to evidence-informed policy are on the rise. The selected cases here illustrate the multidisciplinary nature of information for policy, the importance of partnerships and collaboration, and the need for strategies for knowledge translation.

The Onchocerciasis Control Programme (OCP)

This programme was established in West Africa by the World Health Organization in 1974 (WHO 2006). Confronted with a huge challenge of a disease which causes blindness, severe illness, and death. Stretched over 11 countries, 30 million people and 1 200 000 sq. km and largely covering communities in the poorest and most difficult-to-reach geographical locations, OCP drew together expertise from various disciplines including epidemiology, parisitology, entomology, statistics, vector biology, and public health to map out the problem. In particular, a discipline that has become increasingly important, mathematicians working closely with epidemiologists and entomologists, played an important role in the success of the programme. The Onchosim model was developed to quantify the duration and costs of vector control as well as simulate the dynamics and interactions of transmission cycles. These were critical contributions to intervention activities such as the aerial larviciding used to control transmission. The disease burden was reduced drastically through a concerted effort of vector control and management.

Having achieved its objectives and targets, the programme was handed over to countries under the auspices of the African Programme for Onchocerciasis Control (APOC) where a strong community involvement component involving social and behavioural science methods have managed to bring about community-directed treatment using ivermectin as a safe and efficient treatment and prevention delivery mechanism within existing health systems. A major success of the programme was its ability to build in and therefore result in significant socioeconomic development (WHO 2002; Winnen *et al.* 2002).

Access to generic medicines

The public health epidemics and pandemics that are experienced by low- and middle-income countries call for a widespread use of generic medicines for treatment. Even with the price of some medicines such as antiretroviral drugs falling in price, the cost is still out of reach for many of these countries. The issue of access has become particularly heightened by the potentially high demand for antiretroviral drugs and the Trade Related Intellectual Property Rights (TRIPs) agreements. Pharmaceutical companies have maintained that branded pharmaceuticals would need to be purchased from them (at higher costs) even though generic medicines have been available at much more accessible and affordable prices.

The changing nature of issues that confront public health in recent years is exemplified by the increasing contribution of specialists in public health law. This has evolved way beyond being an administrative support for drafting contracts and agreements of service. Countries facing a huge burden of disease on one hand and very limited health budgets on the other are working in synergy with colleagues in complementary disciplines to deal with contentious issues of patent rights, intellectual property, and innovation. An important global landmark in this area occurred in a legal case where the Pharmaceutical Manufacturers Association (PMA) representing 39 pharmaceutical companies filed a lawsuit against the government of South Africa. This challenge aimed against legislation to enable parallel importation of the generic equivalent but less costly medicines than those with brand names. Various interest groups representing disciplines such as pharmacists, researchers, economists, clinicians, and so on worked consistently to ensure that the legislation to increase access to medicines would be achieved (Berger 2004).

The local and international pressure over a 3-year period resulted in the PMA withdrawing the case. This was seen as a major victory for the South African government and partners. Beyond that the outcome had far-reaching implications for access of medicines in low- and middle-income countries. The role of the legal profession in health has found increasing importance during times when interests such as patient protection have a more profound role on public heath than was the case in the past (Kasper 2005). The Doha agreement of the World Trade Organization was subsequently a turning point for middle-income countries with manufacturing capability. The work of the WHO Intergovernmental Working Group on Intellectual Property Rights, Innovation and Public Health (IGWG) will also have a significant role in shaping public health for the future.

Mexican health reform, 2003–2006

The health sector reform experience in Mexico is an outstanding example of policy and action based on evidence generated from various disciplines related to the public health sciences. Reform in the Mexican health system was motivated by increasing pressures on the national health system from the double burden of communicable and non-communicable diseases as a result of a 'protracted and unequal epidemiological transition' (Frenk 2006). Work in the 1990s by health specialists and economists, led by the National Institute of Public Health (INSP) and the Mexican Health Foundation (FUNSALUD) in collaboration with the Harvard University and the World Bank, showed a heavy reliance on out-of-pocket spending for health in the country, leading to catastrophe and impoverishment for many Mexican families. Their analyses were based on seven rounds of the National Household Income and Expenditure Survey (NHIES) from 1992 onwards, undertaken every 2 years by the National Institute for Statistics, Geography and Informatics. This large body of information fed into the World Health Organization's work on health system performance, with focus on fairness of financing, and into the development of *Seguro Popular* (Popular Health Insurance) in 2001. The reform of the General Health Law in 2003, which took effect in January 2004, established the System for Social Protection in Health (SSPH), including the expansion of *Seguro Popular*. SSPH aimed to increase financial protection by offering publicly provided health insurance to some 50 million Mexicans, mostly the poor, in a span of 7 years. In monitoring and evaluating the ongoing health reform, econometricians analysed time trends from NHIES and performed regression analysis using data from National Survey of Health and Nutrition and the NHIES. The initial analyses indicate reductions in poverty coinciding with the institution of SSPH and integrated social programmes such as *Oportunidades*, increased use of health services by insured people, and a negative association between out-of-pocket catastrophic health spending and coverage of *Seguro Popular* (Gakidou *et al.* 2006; Knaul *et al.* 2006). This unfolding success story would not have been possible without the rich collaboration of public health specialists, policy analysts, economists, other social scientists, epidemiologists, and statisticians.

Tobacco control in South Africa

Tobacco consumption is increasing at an alarming rate in most low- and middle-income countries. Health education messages in most countries have not been effective particularly against the lure of tobacco advertising; tobacco use has increased among the youth where single stick sales have made cigarettes more easily accessible. South Africa is an example of a country that has been able to contain the tobacco problem. An anti-tobacco lobby comprising government public health experts from various disciplines including behavioural scientists, epidemiologists, legal practitioners, health promotion practitioners along with counterparts from non-governmental organizations mounted pressure on the tobacco industry. This resulted in the enactment of the Tobacco Control Act in South Africa and the banning of tobacco advertising. Between 1993 and 1999 average cigarette consumption fell by 20 per cent. The average number of packs consumed by smokers slid from 223 to 176. The smoking rate has been reduced in all groups particularly among the 16–24-year-old group. In its review of the South African experience, the University of Cape Town concluded that a strong Ministry of Health backed by numerous anti-smoking groups from various disciplines is necessary to overcome the opposition by industry and related groups (van Walbeek 2000). Globally, it is expected that the framework convention on tobacco control will provide the motivation for harnessing the combined strength of all public health disciplines in preventing further public health challenges resulting from tobacco consumption.

Research to policy: The Tropical Medicine Research Unit (TMRU) in Jamaica

The TMRU was established in Kingston, Jamaica, in 1956 by the Medical Research Council, UK, to understand 'the basic metabolic changes which occur in childhood malnutrition', which was the leading cause of death among young children in the Caribbean at that time. In 1970, the TMRU was handed over to the University of the West Indies (UWI). Thirty per cent of all paediatric admissions to the University Hospital of the West Indies, Jamaica, were malnourished and 20 per cent of the severely malnourished children admitted to the TMRU died. Within two decades, deaths among such admissions to TMRU were rare due to the research conducted there. In 1972, TMRU staff and paediatric colleagues from UWI and the Children's Hospital in Kingston drafted a manual for the treatment of malnutrition in hospitals, which was field-tested in four rural hospitals in Jamaica. This manual played an important role in improving the treatment of malnutrition in Jamaica, throughout the Caribbean and internationally. In 1973, the Fifth Caribbean Health Ministers Conference called for the development of a plan to address 'the large preventable waste of life caused by gastroenteritis and malnutrition in children under two years of age'. A Technical Group Meeting was held in 1974 to formulate a 'Strategy and Plan of Action to Combat Gastroenteritis and Malnutrition in Children under Two Years of Age'. This historic and far-sighted document helped to galvanize Caribbean governments to develop comprehensive programmes to address the leading cause of death and morbidity among young children. The research at TMRU provided the evidence that children need not die from severe malnutrition and contributed to the considerable technical and political will that formulated and implemented this far-reaching public health campaign throughout the Caribbean. In addition, the research done by TMRU over the years provided substantial input for three major WHO technical publications on the management of malnutrition as well as a sustained campaign led by WHO to reduce malnutrition in low- and middle-income countries, including in times of war and famine (Figueroa 2007).

Responding to the challenges

The complex scenario of public health challenges calls for a broad-based multifaceted response. At the global and regional levels, there is an increasing need for dialogue to take place between low- and middle-income countries on the one hand and high-income countries on the other on policy issues such as governance, health financing, human resources, and intellectual property. These efforts can be facilitated through international bodies such as the World Health Organization (WHO).

Many high-level global initiatives aimed at addressing different key domains have emerged. Amongst them is the WHO Commission for the social determinants of health whose work continued until 2008 (http:/www.who.int/social determinants). This commission seeks to gain a better understanding of those factors that need to be addressed in order to improve health even though they may not be directly a health sector responsibility. Another significant initiative was the Commission on Macroeconomics and Health (Sachs JD/WHO 2001) whose role was to place health at the centre of the international development agenda. Several global health funding mechanisms such as the Gates Foundation and the Global Fund have placed special focus on malaria, HIV, and TB, which are seen as the primary disease challenges in low- and middle-countries today. Cross-cutting domains have also been addressed through global initiatives, for example, the Global Health Financing Initiative (http://www3.brookings.edu/global/about_global_health.pdf), which is engaged in active dialogue on issues such as user fees, community-based insurance and national insurance; and the Joint Learning Initiative (http://www.globalhealthtrust.org/JLI.htm), which created a multi stakeholder forum to landscape the problem of health human resources and recommend strategies. Health policy initiatives such as the Alliance for Health Policy and Systems Research have recognized that there are many gaps in our understanding of the factors that enable health systems to function optimally and effectively. The Alliance aims to promote and undertake relevant research and strengthen multi-disciplinary research capacity to develop appropriate solutions to address health policy and systems weaknesses.

Emerging public health challenges such as avian influenza, SARS, and even bioterrorist threats are demanding new health legislation, regulations, new structures and operational mechanisms, regional reference laboratories or centres of excellence, and advanced rapid response reporting mechanisms, all of which require effective and efficient regional collaboration and coordinated regional responses.

In low- and middle-income countries, there has been an increase in regional groupings such as The African Union Health Conference or the Association of Southeast Asian Nations (ASEAN), which are active in formulating regional policies based on national and regional positions. These are important in lobbying at the global level, for example, at the World Health Assembly and in major global funding bodies. Regional forums have also been involved in peer-review mechanisms and target setting, for example, for the health-related Millennium Development Goals. All these policy-related functions and activities require a broad range of policy development skills and competencies.

At the national level, in-country inter-sectoral responses have become increasingly more important. Programmes that deal with health determinants such as sanitation and safe water supply and timely responses to natural disasters have to collaborate with other ministries and departments such as those responsible for environmental affairs, social welfare and social development, housing, treasury, and finance. Public health officials must be able to advocate effectively for health concerns and mainstream health agendas, using language that is understandable to various sectors.

A large number of country initiatives and programmes have been developed to address single domains or a multiplicity of policy domains in health. For example, Levine *et al.* (2004) showcased 17 cases of successful public health in action in the book *Millions Saved: Proven Successes in Global Health*, proving that 'national governments can get the job done—a finding that contrasts with the view that governments in poor countries are inefficient at best and corrupt at worst. The public sector was integral to the successful delivery of services in most of the cases'. Their analysis of 7 key elements of success in these 17 scaled-up programmes suggests that the public health sciences were important in 6 of the 7 factors for success, i.e. effective communication with the political leadership; technological innovation within an effective delivery system at a sustainable price; technical consensus about the appropriate biomedical or public health approach; good management on the ground; and effective use of information.

Conclusion

Low- and middle-income countries have an important role to play in global health. Mapping the successes and challenges in public health, it is evident that some gains have been made in health in the last 50 years. These gains are however constantly threatened by new global health emergencies and the re-emergence of diseases that have once been thought to be on the verge of control or eradication. These create tremendous demands on national health systems to promote, formulate, and implement appropriate and evidence-based policies.

The public health sciences have an important role to play in this complex scenario. The frameworks, technical expertise, skills, and new knowledge required to be applied to these complex situations need to emerge from the public health sciences. There is a compelling need to take a wider perspective on the range of disciplines that could contribute to health impact and health gains, develop better methodological approaches, promote closer collaboration among stakeholders, build and strengthen health policy and systems research, and increase the quality and quantity of training in the public health sciences in low- and middle-income countries.

References

Alliance for Health Policy and Systems Research (2007). *What is health policy and systems research and why does it matter?* (Policy brief). Available at: http://www.who.int/alliance-hpsr/resources/AllBriefNote1_5.pdf accessed on 29 September 2007.

Arrow, K.J., Panosian, C.B., Gelband, H. (eds.)(2004). *Saving lives, buying time: Economics of malaria drugs in an age of resistance (executive summary)*. National Academy of Sciences. (Document TDR/Gen/96.1).

Atun, R.A. and Sittampalam, S.R. (2006). A review of the characteristics and benefits of SMS in delivering healthcare. Moving the debate forward. The Vodafone Policy Paper Series Number 4, 18–28.

Beaglehole, R., Bonita, R., Horton, R. *et al.* (2004). Public health in the new era: Improving health through collective action. *Lancet*, **363**, 2084–6.

Berger, J.M. (2004). Using the law to increase access to treatment for HIV/AIDS: lessons from South Africa. *International Conference on Aids, 15: abstract no, MoPEe4044.*

Boerma, J.T. and Stansfield, S.K. (2007). Health statistics: Are we making the right investments? *Lancet*, **369**, 779–86.

Bowen, S. and Zwi, A.B. (2005). Pathways to "evidence-informed" policy and practice: a framework for action. *PLoS Medicine*, **2,** e166. Available at: www.plosmed.org DOI:10.1371/journal.pmed.0020166 accessed 14 July 2007).

Bridges.org 2005). Executive summary—Testing the use of SMS reminders in the treatment of tuberculosis. Available at http://www.bridges.org/publications/11/exec_summary accessed 20 August 2007.

Commission on Social Determinants of Health (2007). *Achieving health equity: From root causes to fair outcomes (Interim statement).* World Health Organization, Geneva, Switzerland. Available at: http://www.who.int/social_determinants/en accessed on 29 September 2007.

Daniels, N., Kennedy, B., Kawachi, I. (2000). Justice is good for our health. *Boston Review,* **25**(1), 4–19.

Datta, S. (1993). Applications of O.R. in health in developing countries: A review. *Social Science & Medicine,* **37**(12) Dec, 1441–50.

European Observatory on Health Care Systems (1999). *Health care systems in transition: United Kingdom.* European Observatory on Health Care Systems, Copenhagen.

Figueroa, J.P. (2007). The impact of the tropical metabolism research unit on governments. In *The tropical metabolism research unit, The University of the West Indies, Jamaica, 1956–2006: The house that John built* (eds. T. Forrester, S. Walker, and D. Picou). Ian Randle Publishers, Kingston, Jamaica.

Frenk, J. (2006). Bridging the divide: Global lessons from evidence-based health policy in Mexico. *Lancet,* **368**, 954–61.

Gakidou, E., Lozano, R., Gonzales-Pier, E. *et al.* (2006). Assessing the effect of the 2001–06 Mexican health reform: an interim report card. *Lancet,* 368, 1920–35.

Gonzalez Block, M.A. and Mills, A. (2003). Assessing capacity for health policy and health systems research in low and middle income countries. *Health Research Policy and Systems,* **1**, 1. Available at: http://www.health-policy-systems.com/content/1/1/1 Last accessed 20 August 2007.

Hamilton, P. and Diggory, P. (1979). The Caribbean Epidemiology Centre (CAREC). *Bulletin of the Pan American Health Organization,***13**, 187–94.

Hecht, R. and Shah, R. (2006). Recent trends and innovations in development assistance for health. In *Disease control priorities in developing countries* (eds. D.T. Jamison, J.G. Breman, A.R. Measham *et al.*), pp. 243–57. Oxford University Press, New York.

Hennink, M. and Stephenson, R. (2005). Using research to inform health policy: Barriers and strategies in developing countries. *J Health Commun,* **10**, 163–180. doi: 10.1080/10810730590915128.

Innvaer, S., Vist, G., Trommald, M. *et al.* (2002). Health policy-makers' perceptions of their use of evidence: A systematic review. *Journal of Health Services Research &* Policy, **7**, 239–44.

Jamison, D.T. (2006). Investing in health. In *Disease control priorities in developing countries*(eds. D.T. Jamison, J.G. Breman, A.R. Measham *et al.*),pp. 3–34. Oxford University Press, New York.

Jones, G., Steketee, R.W., Black, R.E. *et al.* and Bellagio Child Survival Study Group (2003). How many child deaths can we prevent this year? *Lancet,* **362**, 65–71.

Kaster, T. (2005). Developing countries must stand firm on people over patents. *South Bulletin.* Vol. 11, 30 April 2001. Available at: http://www.southcentre.org

Khaleghian, P. and Das Gupta, M. (2004). *Public management and the essential public health functions.* World Bank Policy Research Working Paper Series 3220. Available at: http://www-wds.worldbank.org/external/default/WDSContentServer/IW3P/IB/2004/04/21/000009486_20040421095725/Rendered/PDF/wps3220Publicmgt.pdf accessed on 29 September 2007.

Knaul, F.M., Arreola-Ornelas, H., Mendez-Carniado, O. *et al.* (2006). Evidence is good for your health system: Policy reform to remedy catastrophic and impoverishing health spending in Mexico. *Lancet,* **368**, 1828–41.

Lansang, M.A. and Dennis, R.(2004). Building capacity in health research in the developing world. *Bulletin of the World Health Organization,* **82**, 764–70.

Last, J. (2005). A brief history of advances toward health. In Gunn, S.W.A., Mansourian, P.B., Davies, A.M., Piel, A., Sayers B.McA., eds. *Understanding the Global Dimensions of Health.* Springer Science + Business Media. pp. 3–14.

Lee, L.M. and Popovic, T. (2006). Preface: 60 years of public health science at CDC. *Morbidity and Mortality Weekly Report,* **55** (SUP02), 1.

Levine, R. (2004). What Works Working Group *Millions saved: proven successes in global health.* Center for Global Development, Washington, D.C.

Lopez, A.D., Mathers, C.D., Ezzati, M. *et al.* (2006). *Global burden of disease and risk factors.* Oxford University Press, New York.

Makubalo, L.E. (2006). Registering clinical trials in South Africa: A Web based clinical trial register. Department of Heath Report. South Africa.

Mantala, M.J. (2003). Public–private mix DOTS in the Philippines. *Tuberculosis (Edinb.),* **83**, 173–6.

Mills, A., Rasheed, F., and Tollman, S. (2006). Strengthening health systems. In *Disease control priorities in developing countries* (eds. D.T. Jamison, J.G. Breman, A.R. Measham *et al.*), pp. 84–102. Oxford University Press, New York.

Moore, D., Castillo, E., Richardson, C. *et al.* (2003). *Determinants of health status and the influence of primary health care services in Latin America,* 1990-98. *The International journal of health planning and management,* **18**, 279–92.

Moynihan, R. (2004). *Using health research in policy and practice: Case studies from nine countries.* Milbank Memorial Fund, New York.

Murray, C.J.L. (2007). Towards good practice for health statistics: Lessons from the Millenium Development Goal health indicators. *Lancet,* **369**, 862–73.

Prakash, B. (2000). Information and communication technology in developing countries of Asia. Asian Development Bank, Manila, Philippines.

Sachs, J.D. (2001) WHO: Macroeconomics and health: Investing in health for economic development: Report of the Commission of Macroeconomics and Health.

Sadana, R., Mushtaque, A., Chowdhury, R. *et al.* (2007). Strengthening public health education and training to improve global health. *Bulletin of the World Health Organization,* **85**, 163.

Shann, F. and Steinhoff, M.C. (1999). Vaccines for children in rich and poor countries in *Lancet,* **354** (Suppl II), 7–11.

Siegel, E.R., Wood, F.B., Scott, J.C. *et al.* (2009). Web-based public health information dissemination and evaluation. In *Oxford Textbook of Public Health* (eds. R. Detels, R. Beaglehole, M.A. Lansang, M. Gulliford). Oxford University Press, Oxford.

Stearns, B.P. (2007). Combating disease and promoting health: A report on Forum 10—Cairo, 29 October–2 November 2006. Global Forum for Health Research, Geneva.

Travis, P., Bennett, S., Haines, A. *et al.* (2004). Overcoming health-systems constraints to achieve the Millennium Development Goals. *Lancet,* **364**, 900–6.

Turmen, T., and Clift, C. (2006). Public health, innovation, and intellectual property rights. *Bulletin of the World Health Organization*, 84, 338.

UNAIDS (2006). *Report on the global AIDS epidemic.* Geneva, Switzerland.

United Nations (2007). *Millennium Development Goals Report 2007.* United Nations, New York.

Volmink, J., Siegfried, N., Robertson, K., Gulmezoglu A.M. (2004). Research synthesis and dissemination as a bridge to knowledge management: The Cochrane Collaboration. *Bulletin of the World Health Organization*, **82**, 778–83.

Walbeek, C. (2000). *The economics of tobacco control in South Africa project The Framework Convention on Tobacco Control.* Afrec Center for Applied Field Fiscal Research, South Africa pp. 1–5.

Winner, M., Plaisier, A.P., Alley, E.S. *et al.* (2002). Can ivermectin mass treatment eliminate onchocerciasis? *Bulletin of the World Health Organization*, 80, 384–91.

Working Group on Priority Setting, Council on Health Research for Development (2000). Priority setting for health research: Lessons from developing countries. *Health Policy and Planning*, **15**, 130–6.

World Health Organization (1996). Ad Hoc committee on health research relating to future intervention options. *Investing in health research and development.* (Document TDR/Gen/96.1). WHO, Geneva, Switzerland.

World Health Organization (1999). *The World Health Report 1999: Making a Difference.* Geneva, Switzerland.

World Health Organization (2002). *Success in Africa: The onchocerciasis control programme in West Africa, 1974 – 2002.* Geneva, Switzerland.

World Health Organization (2005). *Health and the Millennium Development Goals.* Geneva, Switzerland.

World Health Organization (2007). *The World Health Report 2007: A safer future—Global public health security in the 21st century.* WHO, Geneva, Switzerland.

World Health Organization (2007). *World Health Statistics 2007.* Geneva, Switzerland.

SECTION 8

Environmental and occupational health sciences

8.1

Environmental health issues in public health

Chien-Jen Chen

Abstract

Human beings live in complex environments. The importance of environmental factors in human health has long been investigated. Both genetic and environmental factors are involved in the development of human diseases, but the relative importance of environmental factors in comparison with genetic factors varies as a continuous spectrum for various diseases. Environmental causes of disease include physical, chemical, biological, behavioural, and social components. Human behavioural responses to environments are also important in determining the occurrence of various diseases. Three disease models have been proposed to describe the interaction between host and agents in environments. The epidemiologic triangle model emphasizes the importance of a unique agent for a specific disease, the ecological wheel model points to host–environment interactions and the multifactorial aetiology of environmental diseases, while the evolutionary spiral model highlights the progression of multistage pathogenesis with differing multifactorial aetiology at various stages of the disease natural history. Environmental health hazards are assessed through ecological studies, cross-sectional surveys, case-control studies, cohort studies, and intervention studies. Consistent findings in both observational and interventional studies at aggregate and individual levels may provide strong evidence of causation between the disease and environmental agents. These study designs are illustrated by the elucidation and confirmation of the pleiotropic health effects of arsenic in drinking water and the multifactorial aetiology of hepatitis B-related hepatocellular carcinoma. Molecular and genomic biomarkers are used to explore the gene–environment interaction in the development of environmental diseases. They include the biomarkers of internal dose and biologically effective dose of exposure to environmental agents; the molecular, cellular, histological, and preclinical biomarkers of health effect; and genetic and acquired susceptibility to environmental diseases. Environmental health intervention may not only promote public health but also yield long-term social benefits other than health. Global partnerships need to be strengthened to achieve interrelated goals of health, environmental sustainability, and development.

Environment and health: Historical perspective

Human beings live in complex environments. The importance of environmental factors in human health has long been investigated. Hippocrates in his classical writing *On Airs, Waters and Places* emphasized the relevance of the environment to human health (Hippocrates 1950). He pointed out the influence of seasons and weather, location of residence and nature of water on human health and occurrence of epidemics. The seasonality of infectious diseases and the geographical clustering of endemic diseases have long been documented since ancient time worldwide. Several theories had been hypothesized to explain the unique distribution of various diseases in time and place. The contagion theory proposed both direct and indirect contact with sick people or animals might transmit diseases. Both isolation and quarantine had been suggested to prevent the spread of diseases based on the contagion theory. Although they might have reduced the risk of spread of infectious diseases by ships, the strategies evolved from contagion theory had never stopped the outbreak of many infectious diseases.

The miasma theory proposed that dirty living environments, unclean drinking water, and poor ventilation due to overcrowding might cause the occurrence of various diseases (Hamlin 1998). This led to environmental sanitary reforms aimed at removing miasma by contributing to a cleaner environment in Europe. The hygienic movement emphasized the importance of implementing a safe drinking water supply and sewage disposal system. The *Public Health Act* enacted in Britain in 1848 was considered the first example of governmental involvement in public health affairs. However, a large-scale outbreak of cholera still occurred in London despite its well-constructed sewage disposal system and much improved environmental sanitation in the 1850s. Through a carefully designed survey John Snow published his famous epidemiological study on cholera in 1855 (Snow 1936) while the germ theory was still in its infancy. He identified the consumption of contaminated drinking water as the cause of the cholera outbreak. The removal of the handle which pumped contaminated water 'magically' prevented the spread of the disease. The relocation of sources of drinking water successfully controlled cholera outbreak. This was a pioneering epidemiological study in the identification of environmental factors in the disease outbreak.

In the late nineteenth century, the development of germ theory led to the discovery of many specific infectious agents for human diseases. It also led to the development of several drugs for treatment of diseases, and the improvement in sanitation and disinfection to control outbreaks of diseases. Koch's postulates (Koch 1891), which emphasize a one-to-one relationship between cause and disease, were well accepted as criteria for the identification of causal agents of infectious diseases. Effective control of several infectious diseases through identification of specific agents, discovery of chemical and biological drugs, invention of preventive and therapeutic vaccines had improved life quality and longevity of human beings. The discovery of animal reservoirs and vectors of infectious agents led to the control of vector through environmental sanitation and disinfection. More and more biological and mechanical vectors have been identified for various viral, bacterial, and parasitic diseases since then. Control of vectors in the environment using pesticides became an important task for the prevention of infectious diseases. For example, malaria was eradicated in Taiwan through the detection and treatment of infected cases and use of the insecticide DDT. However, the widely used pesticides polluted the environments and became hazardous to wild animals and humans.

Life expectancy in most countries increased significantly after the 1950s, when conventional infectious diseases have been controlled through the widespread use of various vaccines and antibiotics. The major diseases that threaten human life have gradually shifted from infectious to chronic degenerative disease. Environmental factors with exposures through lifestyle habits, dietary intakes, and environmental pollution play important roles in the development of the chronic diseases including cancers, cardiovascular diseases, and neurological disorders. There are multiple risk factors in the complex pathogenesis of chronic diseases. For examples, risk factors for ischaemic heart diseases included hypertension, diabetes, hyperlipidemia, cigarette smoking, obesity, lack of exercise, and environmental pollutants including arsenic. Some environmental pollutants may cause several chronic diseases in multiple organ systems. For example, arsenic in drinking water has been documented to induce cancers of the skin, bladder, kidney, and lung, blackfoot disease, ischaemic heart disease, stroke, hypertension, diabetes, mental retardation, neurological disorder, and cataract. The classical Koch's postulates for judging the cause of disease are less applicable for the identification of complicated aetiology of chronic diseases. Hill's criteria including the strength, dose–response relationship, temporality, specificity, and biological plausibility of the association between risk factor and disease have been widely adopted for the identification of causes of various diseases (Hill 1953).

Endemic diseases are often characterized by their unique geographical clustering. This clustering may be associated with biological or chemical agents prevailing in local environments. Some parasitic diseases such as schistosomiasis have long been documented to be endemic in areas where the ecological system maintains the life cycle of the parasites. The interruption of the life cycle through the identification and treatment of affected patients, eradication of vectors, and improvement of environmental sanitation may decrease the prevalence of these endemic parasitic diseases. Some endemic diseases such as, goitre and blackfoot disease are caused by the excessive or deficient intake of certain chemicals in the environment. High concentration of fluoride and arsenic in well water has been identified as the cause of fluorosis and blackfoot disease, respectively. The supply of surface water with low concentration of these chemicals had decreased the occurrence of the diseases. As low intake of iodine was the cause of endemic goitre, salt iodization has been implemented to prevent it.

The workplace environment has long been documented to induce occupational diseases. Ramazzini published his seminal treatise on disease of workers (Raffle *et al.* 1987). Scrotum cancer had long been considered a disease of chimney sweeps. The poor working environment in the nineteenth century brought reform attempts in Europe, but specific regulations to protect workers against occupational diseases were mostly implemented in the twentieth century. Occupational hazards may spread from the workplace to its adjacent environments. For example the explosion of chemical plants in Bhopal, India, and nuclear power plant in Chernobyl, Ukraine, resulted in environmental disasters. In addition to the immediate casualties, both events also increased the risk of a number of chronic diseases in residents living near the plants where catastrophic accidents occurred. The health hazards induced by long-term exposure to industrial wastes are usually more insidious than those resulting from acute environmental disasters. Environmental pollution by industrial waste has been well documented to cause Itai-itai disease and Minamata disease in Japan. The chronic poisoning by heavy metals in industrial waste has become an important issue in environmental health. Soil and water contamination by widely used agricultural chemicals have brought significant threats to human health, wild animal life, and ecological sustainability. Air pollution has increased the risk of pulmonary diseases including asthma and chronic bronchitis.

The strikingly increased emission of carbon dioxide in recent decades has resulted in the global warming and climate changes. Meteorological disasters including snowstorms, hurricanes, floods, sand storms, and forest fires have had serious consequences for public health. Other environmental disasters including earthquakes, tsunami, and landslides are also detrimental to human health. In addition to the heavy immediate casualties, these natural environmental disasters threaten the function and efficiency of food, water and electricity supply systems, ambulance and healthcare systems, sewage and waste disposal, and the control of infectious diseases. Protecting public health through proper environmental management is becoming a lasting challenge.

Causes of environmental diseases: Natural and human components

Both genetic and environmental factors are involved in the development of human diseases, but the relative importance of environmental factors in comparison with genetic factors varies as a continuous spectrum for various diseases. Environmental factors seem to play a small role in the development of genetic diseases compared with infectious diseases or accidents. However, exposure to environmental factors may trigger the clinical manifestation of genetic diseases such as phenylketonuria and glucose-6-phosphate dehydrogenase deficiency. Environmental influences on human health are through exposures to physical, chemical, and biological risk factors, and through related changes in human behavioural responses to those factors. The World Health Organization has released a country-by-country analysis of the impact of environmental factors on health (Pruss-Ustun & Corvalan 2006). These data show huge inequalities but also demonstrate that in every country, people's health could be improved by reducing environmental risks including pollution, hazards in the work environment, UV radiation, noise, agricultural risks, climate and ecosystem change. It is estimated that 13 million deaths worldwide could be prevented every year by making environments healthier. Reducing environmental risks could save as many as four million lives a year in children alone, mostly in developing countries. In some countries, more than one-third of the disease burden could be prevented through environmental improvements. In 23 countries worldwide, more than 10 per cent of deaths were due to two environmental risk factors: Unsafe water, including poor sanitation and hygiene; and indoor air pollution due to solid fuel used for cooking. Around the world, children under 5 years were the main victims and made up 74 per cent of deaths due to diarrhoea and lower respiratory infections. Proper environmental management is the key to prevent the quarter of all illnesses, which are directly caused by environmental factors.

Human beings live in environments with many causes of diseases as shown in Table 8.1.1. Environmental causes of disease include physical, chemical, biological, behavioural, and social components. The physical component includes non-ionizing and ionizing radiation, noise, vibration, pressure, humidity, and temperature. Ionizing radiation includes α and β particles, γ rays, and X rays. Ionizing radiation may induce spontaneous abortion, congenital malformation, cancers, and hematopoietic disorders through its effects on genetic damages and chromosomal aberrations. Non-ionizing radiation includes ultraviolet rays, visible light, infrared rays, microwave and electromagnetic fields. Ultraviolet rays may induce skin cancer and cataract; while electromagnetic field may induce some cancers. The chemical components include heavy metals, organic solvents, agricultural chemicals, polycyclic hydrocarbons, and chlorinated organic compounds. Their health effects may be classified as acute toxigenicity, subacute toxigenicity, chronic toxigenicity, carcinogenicity, mutagenicity, and teratogenicity. Some chemicals have environmental toxicity, while some may persist in the environment and result in bioaccumulation. Biological components include viruses, bacteria, fungi, parasites, allergens, arthropods, as well as plant and animal toxicants. A number of infectious diseases of various organ systems are caused by biological agents. In addition to the acute and subacute symptoms and signs, these infectious agents also induce chronic diseases such as cancers of the nasopharynx, stomach, liver, bladder, cervix, uterus, and lymphoid and soft tissue, pulmonary diseases, cardiovascular diseases, as well as neurological disorders.

Human behaviours in response to physical, chemical, and biological factors in environments are also important in the determination of a number of diseases as shown in Table 8.1.2. Built environments, occupational settings, agricultural methods and irrigation schemes, water supply system, sewage and waste disposals, healthcare system, anthropogenic climate changes and ecosystem degradation, as well as individual behaviours of hand-washing, occupational safety, and safe sex all play very important roles in the development of environmental health hazards. For example, using cleaner fuel such as gas or electricity, using better cooking devices, improving the ventilation, or modifying people's behaviour (such as keeping children away from smoke) could have a major impact on respiratory infections and diseases among women and children. As estimated by the World Health Organization, reducing levels of air pollution (measured by PM10) as set out in the Air Quality Guidelines would save an estimated 865 000 lives per year. The household interventions could dramatically reduce the death rate. Interventions at the community or national level would involve promoting household water treatment and safe storage, and introducing energy policies, which favour development and health.

Several disease models have been proposed to describe the interaction between an individual (host) and a disease cause (agent) in the environment (Table 8.1.3). The traditional epidemiological triangle emphasizes the equal importance of host, agent, and environment, which are located in three angles of the epidemiological mode as shown in Table 8.1.3. Host factors may include biological characteristics such as age, gender, ethnicity, genetic composition, anthropometric characteristics, and nutritional and immune status; sociodemographic characteristics such as marital status, educational level, occupation, profession, and socioeconomic status; behavioural characteristics such as dietary habits, lifestyles, personality, and social activity. The agent factor may include the physical,

Table 8.1.1 Natural components of causes for environmental diseases

Component	Category
Physical	Ionizing radiation (α-particles, β-particles, γ-rays, χ-rays)
	Non-ionizing radiation (ultraviolet rays, visible light, infrared rays, microwave, electromagnetic field)
	Noise
	Vibration
	Pressure
	Humidity and temperature
	Earthquakes and landslides
	Typhoons and hurricanes
	Snow-storms and sand storms
Chemical	Heavy metals
	Organic solvents
	Agricultural chemicals
	Polycyclic hydrocarbons
	Chlorinated organic compounds
Biological	Viruses
	Bacteria
	Fungi
	Parasites
	Allergens
	Arthropods
	Animal and plant toxins

Table 8.1.2 Human components of causes for environmental diseases

Component	Category
Behavioural	Substance abuse (alcohol, tobacco, betel, drugs)
	Dietary intake (malnutrition, over-nutrition)
	Personal hygiene
	Occupational protection practice
	Stressful life events
	Sports and exercise
	Personal communication and networking
Social	Housing and home safety
	Water supply system
	Sewage and waste disposal
	Transportation system
	Agricultural and irrigational methods
	Working environment
	Industrial hygiene and safety
	Anthropogenic pollution and climate changes
	Ecosystem degradation
	Schooling system
	Healthcare system
	Social welfare and criminal prevention

Table 8.1.3 Disease models describing host–environment interaction

Model	Illustration	Components	Characteristics
Epidemiological triangle	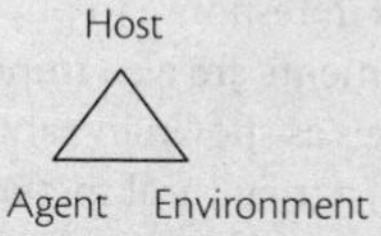	Host	Biological: Age, gender, race, genetic composition, nutritional status, immune status, anthropometric characteristic Sociodemographic: Marital status, education, occupation, profession, socioeconomic status Behavioural: Dietary habits, lifestyles, personality, social activities
		Agent	Physical Chemical Biological Social
		Environment	Family School Working place Recreation place
Ecological wheel	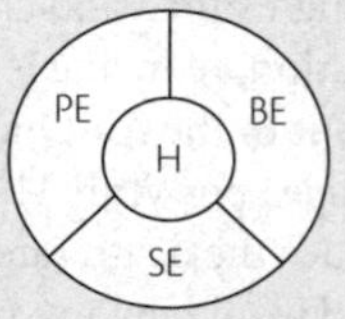	Host	Genes Behaviours
		Physicochemical environment	Energy and chemical substances Living and working infrastructure Public facilities
		Biological environment	Infectious agents Animal reservoir Vectors Infected carriers
		Social environment	Culture Customs Social networks
Evolutionary spiral	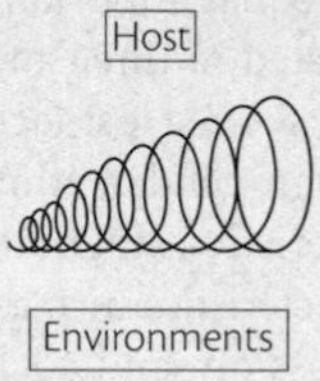	Chronology/stage	Initiation → Promotion → Progression
		Health effects/lesions	Molecules → Cells → Tissues → Organs → Systemic illness
		Host	Genes Behaviours
		Environments	Physicochemical environment Biological environment Social environment

chemical, biological, and social characteristics of causal agent of disease. Environmental factors may include living and working environments including family, school, workplace, and recreation place. The epidemiological triangle model is widely used to develop various strategies to prevent the occurrence of diseases. Host factors may be strengthened through the improvement in nutritional status, optimal rest and exercise, personal hygiene, active and passive immunization, chemopreventive treatment, and so forth. Agent factors may be controlled through disinfection and sterilization, antibiotic use, prevention of drug resistance. Environmental factors may be improved through clean housing and work places, safe water and food supply, hygienic sewage and waste disposal, and others.

The epidemiological triangle model emphasizes the specific causal agent of a specific disease. This model is most appropriate for infectious diseases because the infectious agent is the necessary cause of a given infectious disease. The one-to-one relationship between agent and disease is obvious under this circumstance. However, the triangle model is not appropriate for chronic degenerative diseases. Most chronic diseases have multiple causes. A single agent is neither necessary nor sufficient to induce the disease. The ecological wheel model was proposed to describe the host–environment interaction for the development of diseases as shown in Table 8.1.3. The wheel model includes an axle (host factors) surrounded by a tyre (environmental factors). No unique single agent is specified for a disease in this model. Environmental factors are further classified into those from the physicochemical environment including energy and chemical substances, living and working infrastructure, public facilities; biological environmental factors including infectious agents, animal reservoir, vectors and infected carriers; social environmental factors including culture, customs, and social networks. Genetic factors are located in the core of the host with the rest of host factors including lifestyle, personality, dietary intake, and immunity. This disease model emphasizes the importance of ecological balance in the maintenance of the health status of a host. The relative importance of host and various environments varies by diseases. For example, genetic factors are most important for the highly inheritable diseases; the biological environment for various infectious diseases; and the social environment for accidents. This model also describes the interrelationship among host and various environments.

The ecological wheel does not take the time dimension of disease development into consideration. The development of both acute and chronic diseases follows a specific temporal sequence. This usually starts from contact of causal agent with target cells, through the structural and functional changes as well as proliferation of causal agent and transformed cells, the development of lesions in affected tissues or organs, the onset of clinical symptoms and signs, to the development of systemic illness. There are various agents and environment factors involved at different stages of the pathogenesis. For example, the multistage process of carcinogenesis may be classified into initiation, promotion, progression, invasion, and metastasis. An evolutional spiral model has been proposed to describe host–environment interactions over the entire period of disease development as shown in Table 8.1.3 (Chen 1999). At the initial stage, both cause and molecular or cellular change are simple and small, and causal relationship tends to be one-to-one. Along with the disease progression, both causes and affected lesions are getting more and more complicated at different stages, which involve complex host–environment interactions.

The evolutional spiral model is most appropriate for the description of multistage pathogenesis with a multifactorial aetiology. As shown in Fig. 8.1.1, the development of hepatocellular carcinoma is a multistage process with the involvement of multiple risk factors. A healthy individual may be infected by infectious agents such as hepatitis B and C virus in early life and become a carrier without any symptom and sign. The carrier may start to develop chronic hepatitis, liver cirrhosis, and even hepatocellular carcinoma in the adulthood. During the disease development period, there exist host and environmental factors to influence the disease progression at various stages. Chemical carcinogens including aflatoxins, benzo(a)pyrene, and 4-aminobipheyl as well as micronutrients such as carotenoids and selenium are involved in hepatocarcinogenesis. Host factors including humoral and cellular immunity, xenobiotic metabolism, hormones, susceptibility genes, and even practice of immunization and early screening are also involved to modify the pathogenic process. This example illustrates how physicochemical, biological, and social environments are important in the entire period of the hepatocarcinogenesis.

Ecological studies: Identification of environmental health hazards at aggregate level

Geographical clustering of endemic diseases in a small area is a most important characteristic of environmental health hazards. An extremely high prevalence of an endemic disease in a confined area always leads to the exploration of unique environmental risk factors. Ecological studies are often used to compare the morbidity or mortality of environmental disease between endemic and non-endemic areas. In ecological studies, aggregate attributes such as the morbidity of residents in exposed and unexposed areas, rather than individual attributes such as the health status of exposed and unexposed subjects, are analysed and compared. Ecological studies tend to compare health indices in areas with and without the environmental exposure, or to examine quantitatively the correlation between health indices and environmental exposure in many areas. Some environmental characteristics or comorbidity rates may be used as surrogate variables of the causal agents to elucidate the relationship between the disease risk and the causal agent. The interpretation of ecological studies may be limited by the potential existence of ecological fallacy, when the agent–disease correlation observed at the aggregate level may not consistently be found at the individual level. However, ecological studies are frequently used to explore causal agents of environmental diseases.

Blackfoot disease is an endemic peripheral vascular disorder confined to a limited area on the southwest coast of Taiwan. Clinically the disease starts with numbness or coldness of one or more extremities and intermittent claudication, which progresses to black discoloration, ulcer, and gangrene. In the end stages of the disease, spontaneous amputation of the distal parts of the affected extremities is common. The disease was hyperendemic in four neighboring townships in southwestern Taiwan. As the water from shallow wells (6–8 m in depth) in this area has high salinity, residents in some villages had started to use water from artesian wells (100–200 m deep) since 1920s. The use of artesian well water was found to be associated with the occurrence of the blackfoot disease, and water samples from artesian wells of the endemic area was found to have high arsenic concentration ranged from 0.35 to 1.14 mg/l. Based on the analysis of mortality data, residents in the endemic area of blackfoot disease had a significantly elevated mortality from cancers of the bladder, kidney, skin, lung, and liver as shown in Table 8.1.4. Compared with the general population in Taiwan, the standardized mortality ratios for cancer of the bladder, kidney, skin, and lung were greater than three-fold among residents in the endemic area (Chen *et al.* 1985).

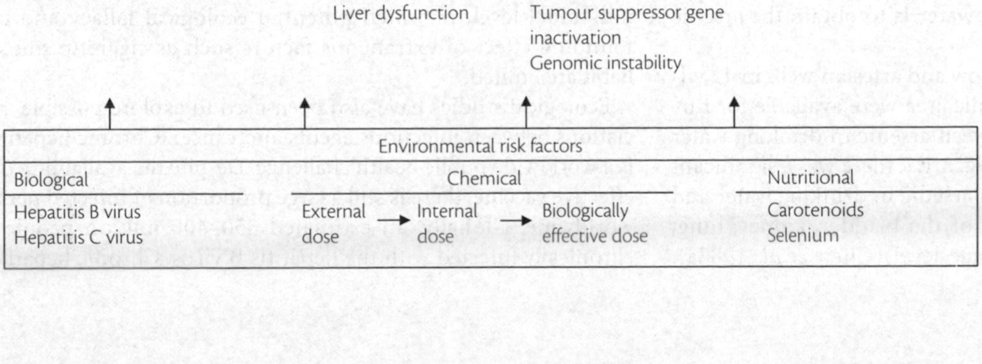

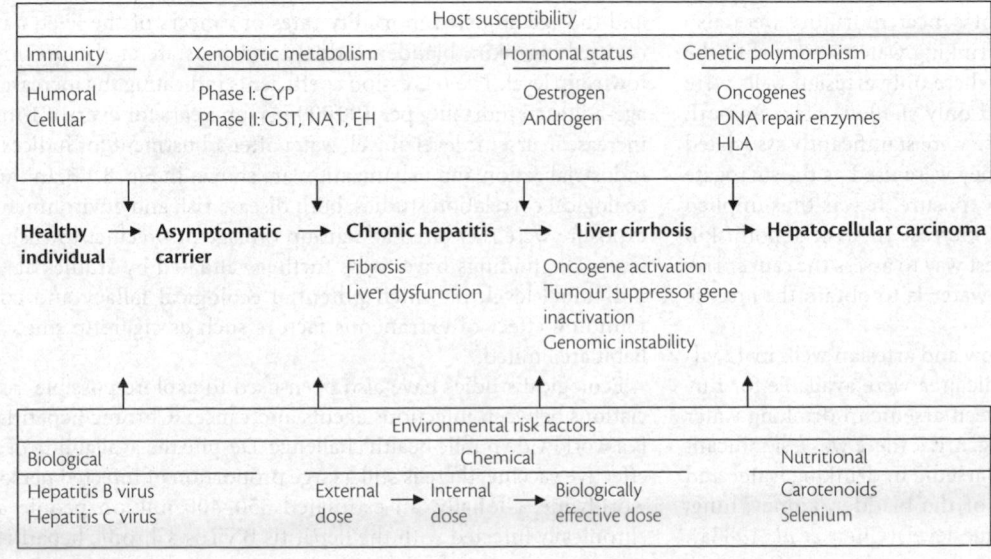

Fig. 8.1.1 Multistage hepatocarcinogenesis with a multifactorial aetiology.

Table 8.1.4 Age-standardized mortality ratios for skin and internal cancers in the endemic area of blackfoot disease by different geographical levels[1]

Cancer	Gender	Blackfoot disease endemic area	Township by blackfoot disease endemicity[2]				Village by blackfoot disease endemicity[3]			Village by types of wells as major drinking water source[4]		
			Very high	High	Medium	Low	High	Medium	Low	Artesian only	Both	Shallow only
Skin	Male	5.3	8.4	8.3	5.3	1.3	11.2	6.5	2.2	10.9	6.5	2.2
	Female	6.5	6.8	15.7	3.6	1.9						
Bladder	Male	11.0	13.8	15.6	10.7	6.1	40.3	17.2	3.8	26.3	11.2	4.5
	Female	20.1	38.0	34.6	16.1	5.6						
Kidney	Male	7.7	14.0	12.4	8.2	4.8	14.9	7.7	3.2	9.2	7.5	3.3
	Female	11.2	14.7	22.5	8.5	3.2						
Lung	Male	3.2	3.8	5.3	2.6	1.7	6.2	3.1	1.8	4.6	2.8	1.8
	Female	4.1	6.3	6.8	3.3	1.9						
Liver	Male	1.7	1.6	1.9	1.7	1.6	3.0	1.5	1.3	2.0	1.8	1.4
	Female	2.3	1.8	2.3	2.5	2.4						

[1] Mortality rates of general population in Taiwan were used as the standard rates to calculate standardized mortality ratio (Taiwan = 1.0)

[2] Four townships including Peimen, Husehchia, Putai, and Ichu with blackfoot disease prevalence of 5.67, 3.87, 2.02, and 0.64 per 1000, respectively. Age-standardized mortality ratios were calculated for males and females, respectively.

[3] A total of 84 villages were classified into three groups by blackfoot disease prevalence: 0, 0.1–5.0, and >5.0 per 1000, respectively. Age–gender–standardized mortality ratios were calculated.

[4] A total of 84 villages were classified into three groups by type of wells used as major drinking water source: Artesian wells only, both artesian and shallow wells, and shallow wells only. Age–gender–standardized mortality ratios were calculated.

Source: Chen *et al.* (1985).

As the four townships in this endemic area had different prevalence of blackfoot disease, cancer mortality was further compared among townships. It was found that the higher the blackfoot disease prevalence of a township, the greater the age-standardized mortality ratios for cancers of the skin, bladder, lung, and liver of the township. As 84 villages in these four townships also had different prevalence of blackfoot disease and used different type of well water, more refined analyses of cancer mortality at village level were carried out. A significant dose–response relationship between the prevalence of blackfoot disease and the age–sex–standardized mortality ratios for cancers of the skin, bladder, kidney, lung, and liver was observed at the village level as shown in Table 8.1.4. Furthermore, biological gradients of cancer mortality were also found by the type of wells used as drinking water source with the highest cancer mortality in villages where only artesian wells were used and the lowest in villages used only shallow wells. As both blackfoot disease and artesian well use were significantly associated with the arsenic in drinking water, they were used as the surrogate environmental variable for arsenic exposure. It was thus implied that arsenic in drinking water might increase the risk of both skin and internal cancers. However, the best way to assess the cancer risk associated with arsenic in drinking water is to obtain the arsenic levels in drinking water from wells.

The arsenic levels in water of shallow and artesian wells in 42 villages of the blackfoot disease endemic area were available for further analysis of the association between arsenic in drinking water and cancer mortality. As shown in Fig. 8.1.2, there was a significant dose–response relationship between arsenic in drinking water and age-adjusted mortality for cancers of the bladder, kidney, lung, skin, liver, and prostate at the village level (Chen *et al.* 1988a). A significant dose–response relationship was also observed between arsenic in drinking water and age-adjusted mortality for cardiovascular diseases and peripheral vascular diseases at the village level (Wu *et al.* 1989). In another ecological correlation study on age-adjusted cancer mortality of 314 precincts and townships in Taiwan (Chen & Wang 1990), the arsenic level in water of 83656 wells was tested to derive the average arsenic level in well water in each precinct or township. Both cancer deaths and mid-year population in all study precincts and townships were obtained from the national death certification and household registration system. Based on the weighted multiple regression analysis, there were significant correlations between the average arsenic level in well water and the age-adjusted mortality rates of cancers of the liver, nasal cavity, lung, skin, bladder, kidney, and prostate at the precinct/township level. The regression coefficients indicating the increase in age-adjusted mortality per 100000 person-years for every 0.1 mg/l increase in arsenic level of well water after adjustment for indices of industrialization and urbanization are shown in Fig. 8.1.3. In these ecological correlation studies, both disease risk and environmental exposure were measured at a group (village or precinct/township) level. The findings have to be further validated by studies at the individual level, in which potential ecological fallacy and confounding effect of extraneous factors such as cigarette smoking habit are limited.

Ecological studies have also been used to explore possible associations between infectious agents and cancer. Chronic hepatitis B is a worldwide public health challenge. Despite the availability of an effective vaccine, there is still a large proportion of infected persons worldwide. Globally, an estimated 350–400 million people are chronically infected with the hepatitis B virus. Chronic hepatitis B

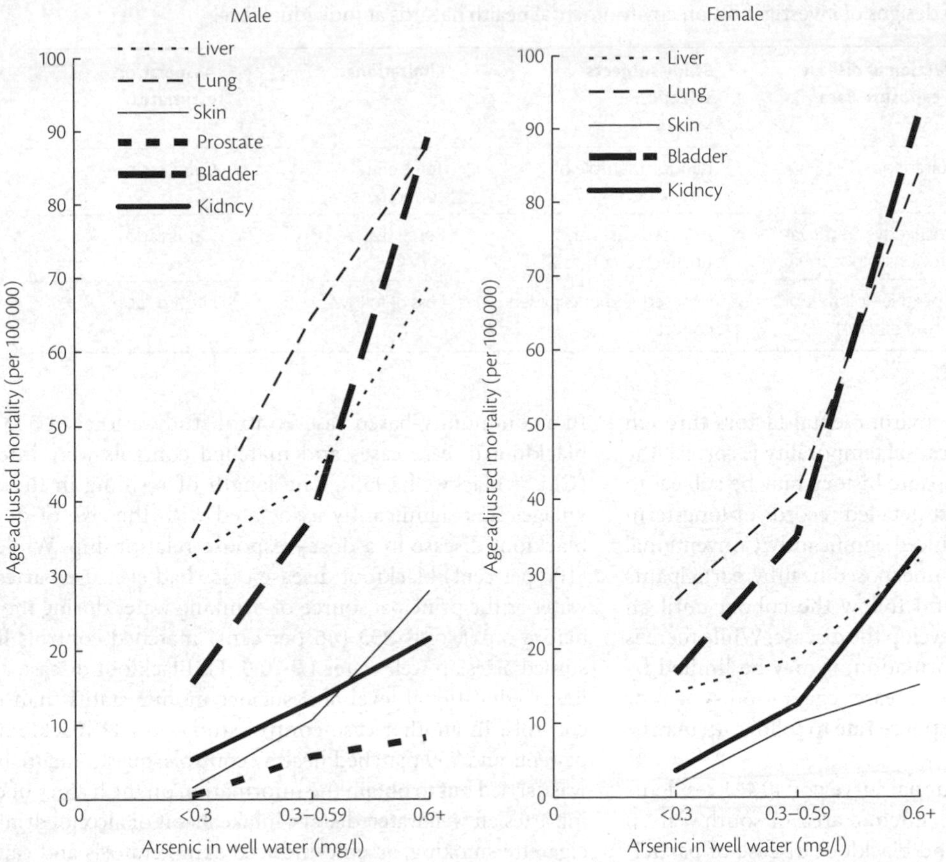

Fig. 8.1.2 Age-adjusted mortality from skin and internal cancers in 42 blackfoot disease-endemic villages by arsenic level in well water.
Source: Chen *et al.* (1988a).

is particularly prevalent in the Asia-Pacific and sub-Saharan Africa regions, where infection is predominantly acquired either during the perinatal period or in the early childhood years. The countries with high incidence of liver cancer are also clustered in the Asia-Pacific and sub-Saharan Africa regions. The significant ecological correlation between the mortality from liver cancer and the prevalence of chronic hepatitis B was also observed among townships in Taiwan. These ecological study findings suggest the importance of chronic hepatitis B in the development of liver cancer, specifically hepatocellular carcinoma. The seroprevalence of antibodies against *Helicobacter pylori* was found to be associated with the mortality from gastric cancer in Taiwan, suggesting *Helicobacter pylori* infection may be a causal agent of gastric cancer. However, the ecological correlation observed at the aggregate level needs further validation by studies at the individual level.

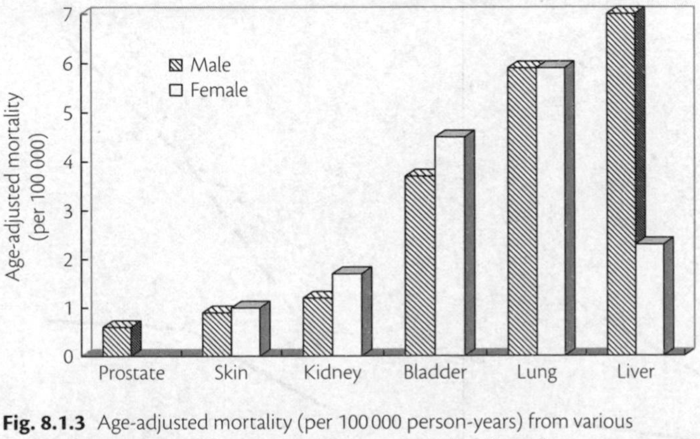

Fig. 8.1.3 Age-adjusted mortality (per 100 000 person-years) from various cancers for every 0.1 mg/l increase in average arsenic level in well water among residents in 170 townships of southwestern Taiwan.
Source: Chen and Wang (1990).

Cross-sectional surveys and longitudinal studies: Assessment of environmental health hazards at individual level

Several different study designs have been used to assess the environmental health hazards at the individual level as shown in Table 8.1.5. Based on the time of the collection of disease risk and environmental exposure data, these may be classified into cross-sectional and longitudinal studies. Cross-sectional studies collect the data of disease and exposure at the same time. The most common type of cross-sectional studies is the environmental health survey, in which participants are enrolled from exposed and unexposed areas to collect the information on health status, exposure to environmental factors, and potential confounding factors. Morbidity estimates from cross-sectional surveys represent disease prevalence rather than incidence. As the disease and exposure data are collected simultaneously, the causal temporality of disease and exposure needs further evaluation. If the environmental exposure is quite consistent over a long period of time before the onset of the disease, the assessment of temporality may be considered correct. Longitudinal studies may be further classified into case-control and cohort studies according to the enrolment of study participants. Conventional case-control studies recruit incident cases and matched controls from healthcare institution or community, and

Table 8.1.5 Major study designs of investigation on environmental health hazards at individual level

Temporality between disease and exposure	Collection of disease and exposure data	Study subjects selection	Limitations	Association estimates
Cross-sectional	Simultaneous	Random sample of population	Temporal correctness	Odds ratio
Longitudinal/cross-sectional	Retrospective (retrieval of previous exposure)	Affected cases and unaffected controls	Recall bias	Odds ratio
Longitudinal	Prospective (follow-up of future disease)	Exposed and unexposed cohorts	Loss of follow-up	Hazard ratio

collect the history of exposure to environmental factors through questionnaire interview. While the causal temporality is correct, the information on environmental exposure history may be subject to recall and other biases. If there exist detailed records of long-term exposure history, the bias may be reduced significantly. Conventional cohort studies recruit exposed and unexposed healthy participants from community or workplace, and follow the cohort until an adequate number of participants develop the disease. While there is no recall bias of the exposure information, it may be limited by losses of follow-up. If there exist the disease registration system or regular health examinations, the response rate to follow-up may be increased.

In a community-based cross-sectional survey of 40 421 residents in 37 villages of blackfoot disease endemic area in southwestern Taiwan, the status of skin cancer and blackfoot disease of participants and arsenic in well water were examined during the survey (Tseng 1977). As shown in Fig. 8.1.4, there was a significant dose–response relationship of skin cancer and blackfoot disease with arsenic in drinking water in most age and sex groups. There was a significant co-existence of both skin cancer and blackfoot disease. In a community-based case-control study, a total of 353 pairs of blackfoot disease cases and matched controls were interviewed (Chi & Blackwell 1968). The length of residing in the endemic villages was significantly associated with the risk of developing blackfoot disease in a dose–response relationship. While all 353 (100 per cent) blackfoot disease cases had ever used artesian well water as the principal source of drinking water during the 15 years before onset, only 233 (66 per cent) matched controls had consumed artesian well water ($P<0.001$). Blackfoot disease cases had lower educational level and socioeconomic status than matched controls. In another case-control study on 241 blackfoot disease patients and 759 matched healthy controls, questionnaire interview was carried out to obtain the information on the history of consuming artesian well water, dietary intake, habit of alcohol drinking and cigarette smoking, arsenic-induced skin keratosis and cancer, and blackfoot disease in first degree relatives (Chen *et al.* 1988b). There was a significant dose–response relationship between the risk of developing blackfoot disease and the duration of consumption of artesian well water. In addition, arsenic-induced skin lesions, family history of blackfoot disease, and undernourishment were also

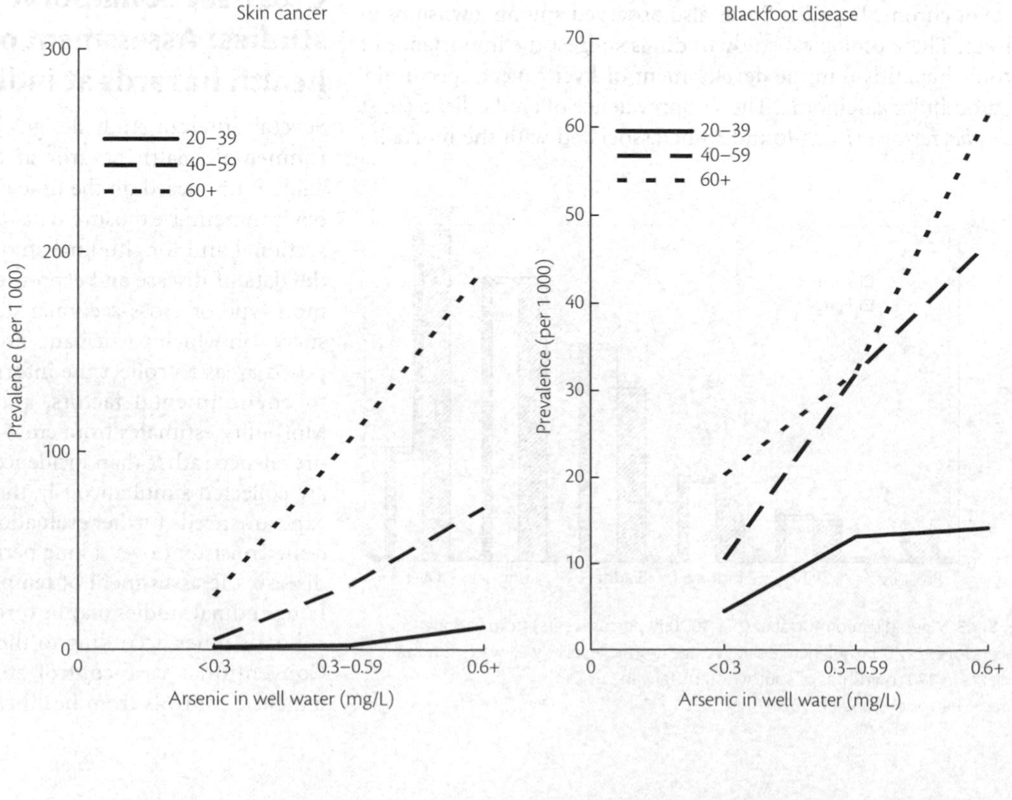

Fig. 8.1.4 Dose–response relationship between arsenic in well water and prevalence of skin cancer and blackfoot disease.
Source: Tseng (1977).

associated with the development of blackfoot disease independent of the duration of consuming artesian well water.

In a cohort study on cause-specific mortality of 789 blackfoot disease patients followed for 15 years (Chen *et al.* 1988b), age–sex–standardized mortality ratios were derived for blackfoot disease patients using the mortality rates of the general population in Taiwan and the blackfoot disease endemic area as the standard rates, respectively. As shown in Table 8.1.6, patients of blackfoot disease had significantly increased mortality from cardiovascular disease and cancers of the bladder, skin, lung, and liver compared to two reference populations. In another case-control study on cancers of bladder, lung, and liver in the endemic area of blackfoot disease (Chen *et al.* 1986), the duration of consuming artesian well water was significantly associated with three cancers in a dose–response relationship after adjustment for age and sex as shown in Fig. 8.1.5.

A community-based health survey study was carried out in three blackfoot disease-hyperendemic villages to examine the associations between arsenic in drinking water and various chronic diseases. A total of 1571 residents aged over 30 years were interviewed by public health nurses, and 1071 of them participated in the health examination. Residents in these villages started using artesian wells as the principal drinking source in the early 1910s, and shifted to public water supply system using surface water from distant reservoir in the early 1970s. The arsenic level in water of artesian wells of the blackfoot disease hyperendemic villages were surveyed in the early 1960s. As residents in a given village shared few wells together, the median arsenic level in water of shared wells was used as the level of arsenic in drinking water for residents of the village. As a participant might migrate from one village to another, a detailed life history of residence and consumption of artesian well water was obtained through a structured questionnaire interview. The cumulative arsenic exposure was derived by the formula $\Sigma(C_i \times D_i)$;

Table 8.1.6 Age-standardized mortality ratios for cancers and vascular diseases in blackfoot disease patients compared with two populations

Disease	Standardized mortality ratio in blackfoot disease patients	
	Taiwan population as reference[1]	Endemic area population as reference[2]
Skin cancer	28.5**	4.5*
Bladder cancer	38.8***	2.6**
Kidney cancer	19.5	1.6
Lung cancer	10.5***	2.8**
Liver cancer	4.7***	2.5**
Prostate cancer	17.3	2.7
Peripheral vascular disease	12.4***	3.5***
Cardiovascular disease	2.1***	1.6**
Cerebrovasular disease	1.2	1.1

1 Mortality rates of general population in Taiwan were used as the standard rates (Taiwan = 1.0)

2 Mortality rates of population in blackfoot disease-endemic area were used as the standard rates (endemic area = 1.0)

Source: Chen et al. (1988b)

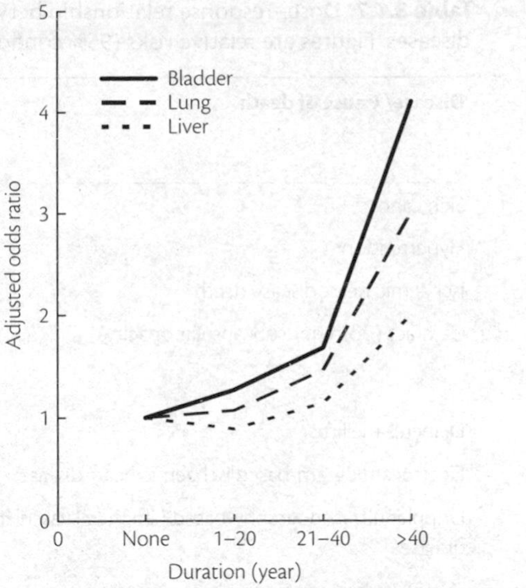

Fig. 8.1.5 Dose–response relationship between mortality from cancers of the bladder, Lung, and liver and duration of consuming artesian well water.
Source: Chen *et al.*(1986).

where C_i was the median arsenic level in water of shared wells of a village in which the participant inhabited, and D_i was the duration of drinking artesian well water in the village during the consecutive period *i*. The average arsenic exposure level in drinking water of a participant was derived by $\Sigma(C_i \times D_i)/\Sigma(D_i)$. Residents in hyperendemic villages of blackfoot disease had a significantly higher age-specific prevalence of diabetes mellitus (Lai *et al.* 1994) and hypertension (Chen *et al.* 1995) than residents in the non-endemic area. Furthermore, there was a significant dose–response relationship between the cumulative arsenic exposure and prevalence of diabetes mellitus (Lai *et al.* 1994), hypertension (Chen *et al.* 1995), Doppler ultrasonography-based peripheral vascular disease (Tseng *et al.* 1996), duplex ultrasonography-based carotid atherosclerosis (Wang *et al.* 2002), electrocardiogram-based ischaemic heart disease (Tseng *et al.* 2003), and cataract (See *et al.* 2007) as shown in Table 8.1.7. Follow-up studies also found a significant biological gradient of incidence of skin cancer (Hsueh *et al.* 1997) and lethal ischemic heart disease (Chen *et al.* 1996a) with the increasing cumulative arsenic exposure as also shown in Table 8.1.7.

In another survey of well-water arsenic and health status in northeastern Taiwan, a total of 8102 residents in four townships participated in the study. Residents in these townships had their own tube wells in their backyards. The arsenic levels in well water of these households were tested in the early 1990s. The public water supply system using surface water was implemented in this northeastern endemic area in the early 1990s, and its coverage was as high as 95 per cent in 2000. Cerebrovascular disease, especially cerebral infarction, was identified from home-visit personal interview and ascertained through the review of hospital medical records as shown in Table 8.1.7 (Chiou *et al.* 1997). In several cohort studies of participants enrolled from the endemic areas of arseniasis in southwestern and eastern Taiwan, the occurrence of cancers were identified and ascertained through the computerized data linkage with national cancer registry and death certification profiles. A dose–response relationship was observed between long-term arsenic exposure from drinking well water and incidence of

Table 8.1.7 Dose–response relationship between cumulative arsenic exposure and risk of various diseases. Figures are relative risks (95% confidence intervals).

Disease/ Cause of death	Cumulative arsenic exposure			
	Low	Medium	Medium high	High
Skin cancer[1]	1.0 (reference)	2.8 (0.3–31.9)	2.6 (0.3–22.9)	7.6 (1.0–60.3)
Hypertension[2]	1.0 (reference)	0.9 (0.2–3.3)	2.4 (0.8–6.9)	3.6 (1.4–9.6)
Ischaemic heart disease death[3]	1.0 (reference)	2.5 (0.5–11.4)	4.0 (1.0–15.6)	6.5 (1.9–22.2)
Cataract (posterior subcapsular opacity)[4]	1.0 (reference)	2.2 (0.4–12.1)	4.8 (1.0–22.2)	5.7 (1.2–26.3)
	Low	Medium	High	
Diabetes mellitus[5]	1.0 (reference)	6.6 (0.9–51.0)	10.1 (1.3–77.9)	
Electrocardiogram-based ischaemic heart disease[6]	1.0 (reference)	1.6 (0.5–5.3)	3.6 (1.1–11.7)	
Doppler ultrasonography-based peripheral vascular disease[7]	1.0 (reference)	2.8 (0.9–9.1)	4.3 (1.3–14.5)	
Dupplex ultrasonography-based carotid atherosclerosis[7]	1.0 (reference)	1.8 (0.8–3.8)	3.1 (1.3–7.4)	
Cerebral infarction[8]	1.0 (reference)	2.7 (1.2–5.8)	3.4 (1.4–8.1)	

[1] Follow-up study in southwestern Taiwan, arsenic level stratified as 0, 0.1–10.6, 10.7–17.7, >17.7 mg/l-years
[2] Survey in southwestern Taiwan, arsenic level stratified as 0, 0.1–6.3, 6.4–10.8, 10.9–14.7 mg/l-years (two groups >14.7 mg/l-years are not shown here)
[3] Follow-up study in southwestern Taiwan, arsenic level stratified as 0, 0.1–9.9, 10.0–19.9, >19.9 mg/l-years
[4] Survey in southwestern Taiwan, arsenic level stratified as 0, 0.1–12.0, 12.1–20.0, >20.0 mg/l-years
[5] Survey in southwestern Taiwan, arsenic level stratified as 0, 0.1–15.0, >15.0 mg/l-years
[6] Survey in southwestern Taiwan, arsenic level stratified as 0, 0.1–14.9, >14.9 mg/l-years
[7] Survey in southwestern Taiwan, arsenic level stratified as 0, 0.1–19.9, >19.9 mg/l-years
[8] Survey in northwestern Taiwan, arsenic level stratified as <0.1, 0.1–4.9, >4.9 mg/l-years

Sources: Skin cancer (Hsueh *et al.* 1997), hypertension (Chen *et al.* 1995), ischaemic heart disease death (Chen *et al.* 1996a), cataract (See *et al.* 2007), diabetes mellitus (Lai *et al.* 1994), electrocardiogram-based ischaemic heart disease (Tseng *et al.* 2003), Doppler ultrasonography-based peripheral vascular disease (Tseng *et al.* 1996), duplex ultrasonography-based carotid atherosclerosis (Wang *et al.* 2002), and cerebral infarction (Chiou *et al.* 1997)

urothelial carcinoma (Chiou *et al.* 2001) and lung cancer (Chen *et al.* 2004) (Fig. 8.1.6). It is important to be aware of temporal variations in concentration of causal agent in various environmental media, individual variation in frequency and quantity of contact with the contaminated environmental media, and variation in detection limit of various exposure assessment methods. It is essential to ensure accuracy in the assessment of exposure to environmental factors in all cross-sectional surveys, case-control studies, and cohort studies in order to identify and characterize the environmental health hazards efficiently and effectively.

Several case-control studies have assessed the association between risk of hepatocellular carcinoma chronic and seropositivity of hepatitis B surface antigen (HBsAg) (Chen *et al.* 1997; You *et al.* 2004). The association between hepatocellular carcinoma and HBsAg serostatus was statistically significant in all cross-sectional case-control studies. As the serostatus of HBsAg was determined at the same time of the diagnosis of hepatocellular carcinoma, it might not reflect the serostatus long before the onset of the disease. However, most HBsAg-seropositive participants become chronic carriers in early childhood, the causal temporality between HBsAg seropositivity and hepatocellular carcinoma is likely to be correct. Another case-control study further evaluated the importance of hepatitis Be antigen (HBeAg) in the development of hepatocellular carcinoma (Chen *et al.* 1991). The relative risk of hepatocellular carcinoma was 58-fold for those who were seropositive for both HBsAg and HBeAg, 17-fold for seropositives for HBsAg only compared with the seronegative on both markers as reference. As both HBsAg and HBeAg disappear gradually with increasing age, their seroprevalence estimated at the onset of hepatocellular carcinoma is much lower than those in childhood or young adulthood. An insurance-based cohort study on 3454 chronic HBsAg carriers and 19 253 non-carriers in northern Taiwan had confirmed the high risk of hepatocellular carcinoma for chronic HBsAg carriers compared with the non-carriers showing a relative risk greater than 100-fold (Beasley *et al.* 1981). Another community-based cohort study on 2361 carriers and 9532 non-carriers of HBsAg in seven townships in Taiwan confirmed the importance of HBeAg serostatus in the development of hepatocellular carcinoma in addition to HBsAg serostatus (Yang *et al.* 2002). These observational studies suggest the most effective and efficient way to reduce the risk of hepatocellular carcinoma in Taiwan is to prevent the infection of hepatitis B virus through vaccination and anti-viral treatment.

Intervention studies: Validation of environmental health hazards through prevention and intervention

It is unethical to implement experimental studies on human beings to validate environmental health hazards identified from observational

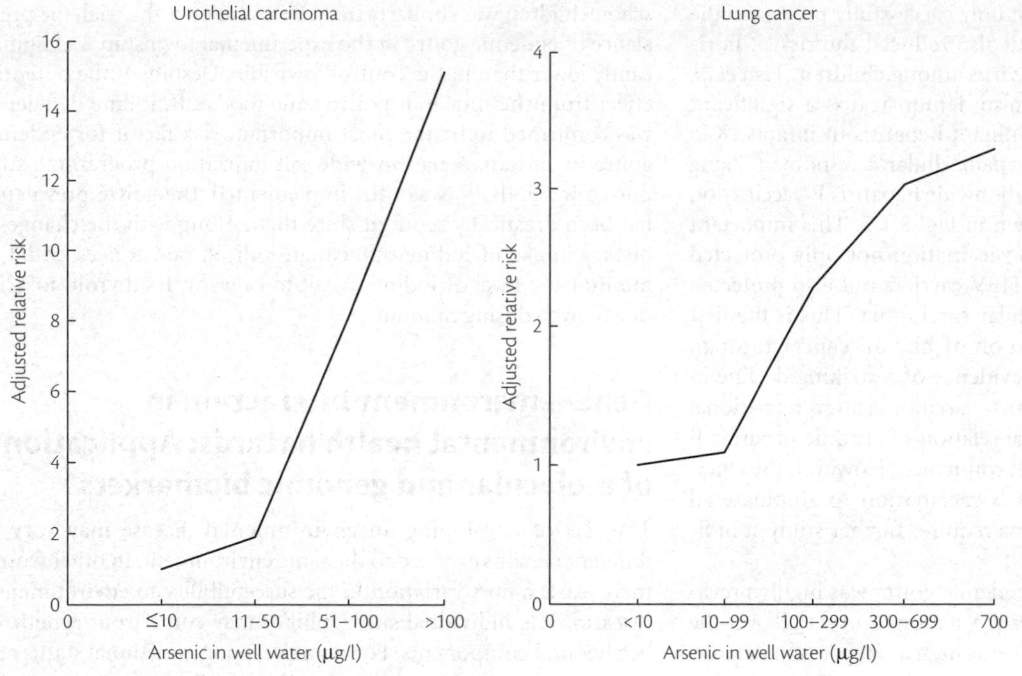

Fig. 8.1.6 Dose–response relationship between the arsenic level in well water and multivariate-adjusted relative risk of urothelial carcinoma and lung cancer incidence.
Source: Urothelial carcinoma (Chiou *et al.* 2001) and lung cancer (Chen *et al.* 2004).

studies mentioned above. However, interventions that remove environmental hazards may be evaluated for possible effects on disease risk. Intervention studies may be classified as individual or cluster trials depending on whether individual subjects or clusters such as households, schools, or communities are allocated to the intervention. Intervention studies may also be classified as controlled and uncontrolled trials depending on the inclusion of a comparable control group or not. In controlled trials, the effect of intervention on environmental health hazards is evaluated by the comparison of disease occurrence between experimental and control groups. In uncontrolled trials, the effect of intervention is assessed by the comparison of disease occurrence of the experimental group before and after the intervention.

The implementation of a public water supply system, which used uncontaminated surface water from distant reservoir, in the blackfoot disease endemic area of southwestern Taiwan was started in the early 1960s and completed in the 1970s. The arsenic-induced health hazards identified from observational studies could thus be validated through the comparison of the secular changes in morbidity and mortality of arsenic-induced diseases in the endemic and non-endemic areas. In a series of studies, cause-specific standardized mortality ratios of residents in the blackfoot disease endemic from 1971 to 2003 were calculated using the general population in Taiwan as the standard population. Cumulative sum techniques were used to detect the occurrence of changes in the standardized mortality ratios. A significant decline in mortality from ischaemic heart disease (Chang *et al.* 2004), renal disease (Chiu & Yang 2005), peripheral vascular disease (Yang 2006), and cancers of the lung (Chiu *et al.* 2004a), kidney (Yang *et al.* 2004), and bladder (Yang *et al.* 2005) was observed for both males and females in the southwestern endemic area of blackfoot disease. A significant decline in mortality from liver cancer (Chiu *et al.* 2004b) and diabetes mellitus (Chiu *et al.* 2006) was observed for females but not males. Based on the reversibility criterion, it was concluded that associations between arsenic exposure and various health hazards was likely to be causal. Although the findings are quite consistent with observational studies mentioned above, there are several issues that need further clarification: (1) Classification of underlying causes of death may vary by area and time. It is necessary to examine whether the variation in the classification of underlying causes in death certificates are comparable in different areas over the study period. (2) Competing causes of death may be quite different between the endemic area and Taiwan as a whole. Arsenic has a pleiotropic health effect to induce various cancers, circulatory diseases, diabetes mellitus, hypertension, renal disease, and so forth. A person may die with several arsenic-induced diseases. It is thus difficult to select an underlying cause of death for an arsenic-exposed person. (3) Mortality of a disease is a function of the incidence and fatality of the disease. High mortality may imply an increased incidence and/or an elevated fatality. It is better to analyse incidence rather than mortality to clarify the causal association between agent and disease. (4) Risk factors other than arsenic may be important confounding factors, such as habits of cigarette smoking and alcohol drinking, chronic infection of hepatitis viruses, and obesity status. They are not taken into consideration in the mortality analysis. It is more convincing to compare the secular changes in the incidence of arsenic-induced diseases after the implementation of public water supply system. Furthermore, age–cohort–period analysis may also help in the identification of susceptible ages at exposure to arsenic and the assessment of reversibility effect of intervention.

A nationwide vaccination programme aimed to eradicate hepatitis B virus was launched on July 1, 1984, in Taiwan (Chien *et al.* 2006). It was the first universal hepatitis B vaccination programme for newborns in the world. During the first two years (July 1984 to June 1986) of the programme, only newborns born to high-risk (HBsAg-positive) mothers were vaccinated. All newborns have been vaccinated since July 1986. The programme was further extended to the preschool children who did not receive vaccination at the neonatal stage since 1987. There has been a dramatic decrease in the HBsAg carrier rate and hepatitis B virus infection rate among children and adolescents born after 1984 as shown in Fig. 8.1.7, demonstrating the programme not only successfully prevented the perinatal transmission of HBV but also reduced the risk of horizontal transmission of hepatitis B virus among children (Hsu *et al.* 1999). Recent studies in Taiwan also demonstrated a significant decline in the mortality from fulminant hepatitis in infants (Kao *et al.* 2001) and the incidence of hepatocellular carcinoma (Chang *et al.* 1997) in children since the nationwide hepatitis B vaccination programme was launched as shown in Fig. 8.1.7. This important finding demonstrated hepatitis B vaccination not only protected children from becoming chronic HBV carriers but also protected them from developing hepatocellular carcinoma. This is the first study to demonstrate the prevention of human cancer through vaccination. Through the strong evidence of a striking decline in childhood incidence of hepatocellular carcinoma after the national vaccination programme, the causal relation of chronic hepatitis B to hepatocellular carcinoma is well confirmed. However, the elucidation of the failure of hepatitis B vaccination to eliminate all childhood hepatocellular carcinoma requires further study at individual rather than national level.

Before the Second World War, endemic goitre was highly prevalent in mountainous areas in Taiwan. A national survey all over the Taiwan Island showed the prevalence as high as 70 per cent in some aboriginal townships in mountainous areas. The prevalence of goitre in pigs was found to be significantly higher in the goitre-endemic area than non-endemic area. It was debated whether dietary deficiency in iodine or goitrogenic foodstuff intake was the major cause of endemic goitre. The use of iodine tablet was found to be effective to lower the prevalence of endemic goitre in schoolchildren, it was considered costly and inconvenient. In order to identify an effective and efficient prevention strategy at the community level, a controlled community intervention trial on iodized salt was carried out in two townships in northern Taiwan (Chen *et al.* 1976). All the dietary salt used in experimental and control townships was strictly provided by the research team. Before the implementation of the community trial, the endemic goitre prevalence among schoolchildren was similarly high. One year after the trial, the prevalence of endemic goitre in the experimental township was significantly lower than in the control township. Despite of the potential effect from the intake of goitrogenic foodstuff, iodine deficiency was confirmed to be the most important risk factor for endemic goitre in Taiwan. A nation-wide salt iodization programme supported by UNICEF was thus implemented, the goitre prevalence has been drastically reduced since then. Along with the change in dietary intake of iodine other than iodized salt, it is essential to monitor the level of iodine in salt to prevent the thyroid toxicity due to over-dosing of iodine.

Gene–environment interaction in environmental health hazards: Application of molecular and genomic biomarkers

The risk of developing an environmental disease may vary in different persons exposed to the same environment. In other words, there exists a host variation in the susceptibility to environmental diseases. The individual susceptibility may come from genetic or behavioural components. For example, poor nutritional status and arsenic methylation capability may modify the risk associated with arsenic-induced health hazards including cancers and cardiovascular diseases. Multiple risk factors including cigarette smoking habit, aflatoxin exposure, antioxidant deficiency, and serum androgen level are all important risk factors to the hepatitis B-induced hepatocellular carcinoma. Some environmental cofactors are difficult to detect and quantify unless biomarkers are used. In order to elucidate the preclinical lesions of environmental diseases for their early detection and prompt intervention; changes in structures and functions of macromolecules, cells, tissues, and organ systems in response to exposures to environmental risk factors are studied intensively in recent decades. Along with the advances in genomic biotechnology, the polymorphisms and mutations of genes of host

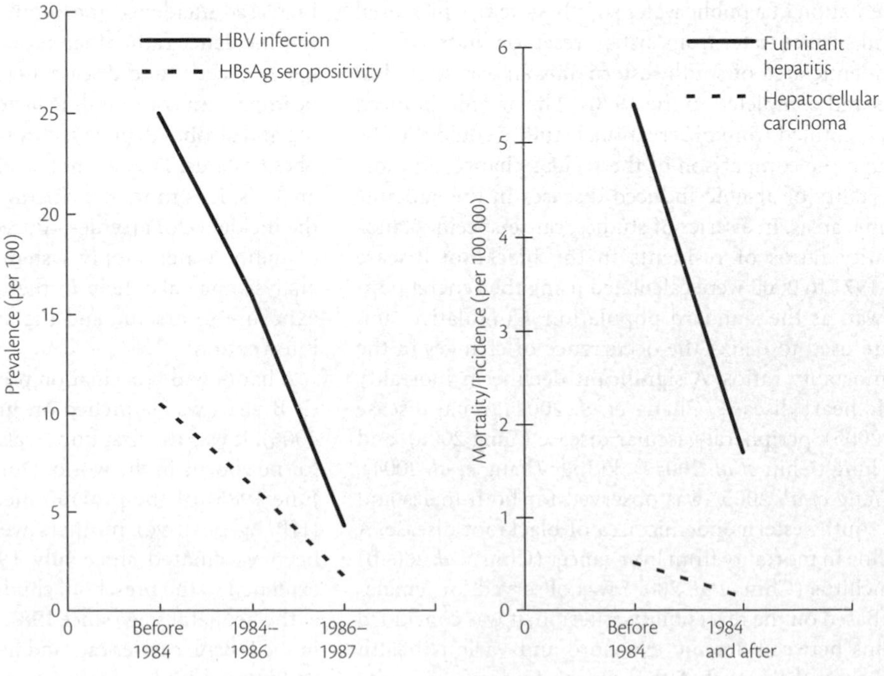

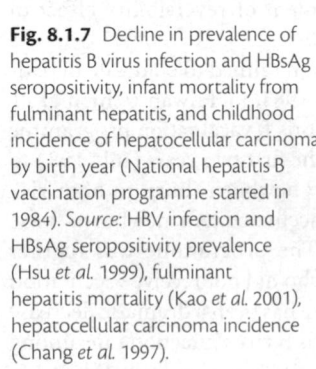

Fig. 8.1.7 Decline in prevalence of hepatitis B virus infection and HBsAg seropositivity, infant mortality from fulminant hepatitis, and childhood incidence of hepatocellular carcinoma by birth year (National hepatitis B vaccination programme started in 1984). *Source*: HBV infection and HBsAg seropositivity prevalence (Hsu *et al.* 1999), fulminant hepatitis mortality (Kao *et al.* 2001), hepatocellular carcinoma incidence (Chang *et al.* 1997).

and biological agents are explored extensively to examine the gene–gene and gene–environment interactions.

Various biomarkers of exposure, effect, and susceptibility of human diseases have been identified and applied in studies on environmental health hazards. These include the molecular dosimetry of internal dose and biologically effective dose of exposure to environmental risk factors; the characterization of early biological effects, altered structures and functions of target organs, and preclinical lesions; as well as the identification of genetic and acquired susceptibility to diseases. As the development of chronic arsenic poisoning is a multistage pathogenesis, a series of biomarkers of arsenic-induced health hazards have been developed and studied as shown in Table 8.1.8 (Chen *et al.* 2005). There are several biomarkers of short-term internal dose for ingested arsenic including levels of arsenic in blood, urine, hair, and finger or toe nails. Arsenic in urine, hair, and nails are better biomarkers for short-term exposure than arsenic in blood. The cumulative arsenic exposure to arsenic from drinking water was found to be significantly associated with urinary levels of monomethylarsonic acid and dimethylarsinic acid; but not with arsenite, arsenate, and organic arsenic. Skin hyperpigmentation and palmoplantar hyperkeratosis are characteristic dermatological lesions induced by long-term exposure to arsenic. They are excellent biomarkers for long-term exposure to ingested arsenic. The proportion of monomethylarsonic acid in total urinary arsenic level is an important marker for the biologically effective dose of ingested arsenic. The biomarkers of molecular changes induced by ingested arsenic include plasma levels of reactive oxidants and inflammatory molecules such as chemokine C-C motif ligand 2/monocyte chemotactic protein-1 (CCL2/MCP1). The arsenic-induced cellular changes include sister chromatid exchanges, micronuclei and chromosomal aberrations in peripheral lymphocytes and urothelial cells; as well as chromosomal loss and gain detected by comparative genomic hybridization and loss of heterozygosity in urothelial cells. Biomarkers of subclinical changes include carotid atherosclerosis, QT prolongation and increased dispersion detected by electrocardiogram, retarded peripheral neural conduction, and retarded neurobehavioural function. The biomarkers of susceptibility to arsenic-induced health hazards include low serum level of carotenes and genetic polymorphisms of enzymes involved in xenobiotic metabolism, arsenic methylation, oxidative stress, and DNA repair.

In the multistage hepatocarcinogensis of chronic hepatitis B, there are many other risk factors that modify the risk of developing hepatocellular carcinoma (Chen & Chen 2002). Biomarkers associated with hepatitis B-induced hepatocellular carcinoma are shown in Table 8.1.9. HBV infection markers include HBsAg, HBeAg, antibodies against hepatitis B core antigen (anti-HBc), antibodies against HBsAg (anti-HBs), antibodies against e antigen (anti-HBe), as well as serum HBV DNA level. Different HBV infection markers have different associations with the development of hepatocellular carcinoma. In addition to the seropositivity of HBsAg and HBeAg, serum HBV DNA level is associated with an increased risk of liver cirrhosis and hepatocellular carcinoma in a dose-response relationship (Iloeje *et al.* 2006; Chen *et al.* 2006). Different genetic characteristics of hepatitis B virus are also associated with different risk of liver cirrhosis and hepatocellular carcinoma. The genotype C, basal core promoter A1762T/G1764A mutant, and pre-S mutant of hepatitis B virus are significantly associated with an increased risk of liver diseases; while the precore stop codon G1896A mutant is associated with a decreased risk. Both quantitative and qualitative characteristics of hepatitis B virus are important in the development of hepatocellular carcinoma. Such gene–gene interactions between human host and various infectious agents need further elucidation.

Dietary exposure to aflatoxins and habits of cigarette smoking, alcohol drinking, and betel quid chewing have been found to

Table 8.1.8 Biomarkers of exposure, effect, and susceptibility of arsenic-induced health hazards

Category	Group	Biomarkers
Exposure	Internal dose	
	Short-term	Arsenic in urine, hair, and nail
	Long-term	Relative proportion of Monomethylarsonic acid and
	Biologically effective dose	dimethylarsinic acid in urine
		Skin hyperpigmentation and hyperkeratosis
		Monomethylarsonic acid in urine
Effect	Molecular changes	Reactive oxidants in blood Inflammatory molecules in blood
	Cellular changes	Sister chromatid exchanges, micronuclei, chromosomal aberrations in target cells Chromosomal loss/gain and loss of heterozygosity in target cells
	Subclinical changes	QT abnormality in electrocardiogram Carotid atherosclerosis Retarded peripheral neural conduction Retarded neurobehavioural function
Susceptibility	Genetic susceptibility	Xenobiotic metabolism enzymes DNA repair enzymes Oxidative stress-related enzymes
	Acquired susceptibility	Serum carotene level

Table 8.1.9 Biomarkers associated with hepatitis B-induced hepatocellular carcinoma

Category	Group	Biomarkers
Exposure	Hepatitis B virus	HBsAg/HBeAg seropositivity HBV DNA (viral load) HBV genotype HBV mutants
	Aflatoxins	Urinary levels of metabolites and guanine adducts Serum level of albumin adducts
	Tobacco smoke	DNA adducts of 4-aminobiphenyl and polyaromatic hydrocarbons
Effect	Asymptomatic carriers	HBsAg-seropositivity and normal ALT
	Chronic hepatitis	Elevate ALT, liver fibrosis
	Liver cirrhosis	Liver fibrosis, cirrhosis, failure
Susceptibility	Immunity	Anti-HBs-seropositivity
	Hormonal status	Serum levels of androgen and oestrogen/progesterone
	Genetic polymorphisms	HLA Xenobiotic metabolism enzymes DNA repair enzymes Hormone metabolism enzymes and receptors
	Nutritional intake	Serum levels of carotenoids and selenium

increase the risk of hepatitis B-related hepatocellular carcinoma. Due to the difficulties in measuring dietary exposure to trace amount of aflatoxins and environmental exposures to tobacco smoke, several biomarkers are used for the molecular dosimetry of aflatoxin and tobacco smoke exposures. These include metabolites in urine as biomarkers for internal dose, and macromocule adducts as biomarkers for biologically effective dose. The hepatic DNA adducts of 4-amino-biphenyls and polyaromatic hydrocarbons are used to measure the biologically effective dose of exposures to tobacco smoke, while DNA and albumin adducts of aflatoxin B_1 were used as biomarkers of biologically effective dose. There is a dose–response relationship between exposure to these hepatotoxins and risk of hepatocellular carcinoma. There exist significant synergistic effects on hepatocellular carcinoma between chronic hepatitis B and environmental hepatotoxins. The hepatocarcinogenesis progresses from asymptomatic carrier status, chronic hepatitis, liver cirrhosis to hepatocellular carcinoma. Several biomarkers may be used for the detection of various precancerous lesions.

The effect of environmental hepatotoxins on the hepatitis B-induced hepatocellular carcinoma is modified by genetic polymorphisms of enzymes related to xenobiotic metabolism. Genetic polymorphisms of cytochrome P450 (CYP) enzymes 1A1 and 2E1, glutathione S-transferase (GST) M1 and T1, *N*-acetyltransferase 2 were found to modify the associations with hepatocellular carcinoma for chemical carcinogen exposure and low micronutrient intake among those with chronic HBV infection. As shown in Fig. 8.1.8, a significant dose–response relationship between risk of hepatocellular carcinoma and serum level of aflatoxin B_1 albumin adducts is observed in chronic hepatitis B virus carriers with null genotype of glutathione S-transferase (GST) M1 or T1, but no dose–response relationship is observed for carriers with wild genotypes (Chen *et al.* 1996b). Elevated serum testosterone level is associated with an increase the risk of HCC. This association is modified by genetic polymorphisms of androgen receptor (Yu *et al.* 2000). The highest risk of hepatitis B-related hepatocellular carcinoma was observed among those who have elevated serum level of testosterone and high-risk genotype of androgen receptor. Furthermore, the combination of putative high-risk genotypes of androgen receptor, CYP17, and steroid 5α-reductase is associated with highly elevated risk of hepatocellular carcinoma suggesting a significant effect of gene–gene interaction in human host (Yu *et al.* 2001). Low serum levels of micronutrients including carotenes and selenium are associated with an increased risk of hepatitis B-related hepatocellular carcinoma. The interactive effects on human health between biological and chemical agents in the environment are complicated and deserve further scrutiny.

Most environmental health hazards are influenced by the interaction between host gene and environment factor exposure. Figure 8.1.9 shows four hypothetical examples of gene–environment

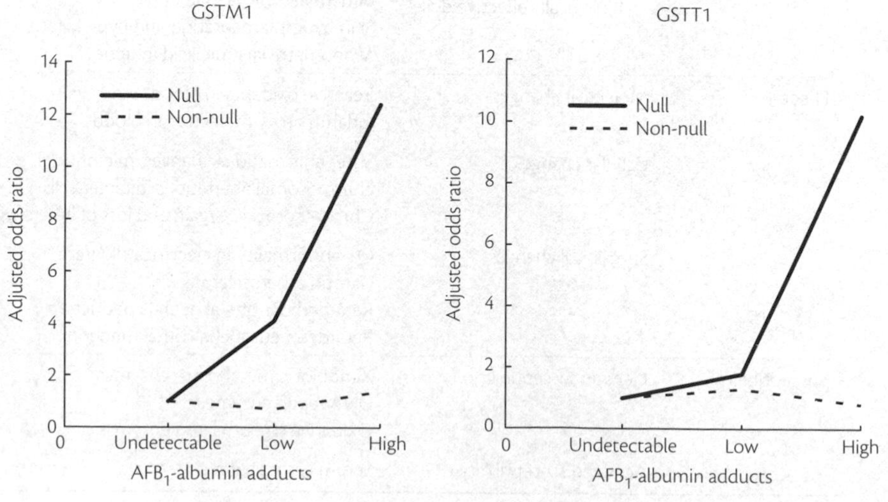

Fig. 8.1.8 Modifying effect of genotypes of glutathione S-transferase (GST) M1 and T1 on the dose–response relationship between serum level of aflatoxin B_1(AFB_1)–albumin adducts and risk of hepatocellular carcinoma.
Source: Chen *et al.* (1996b).

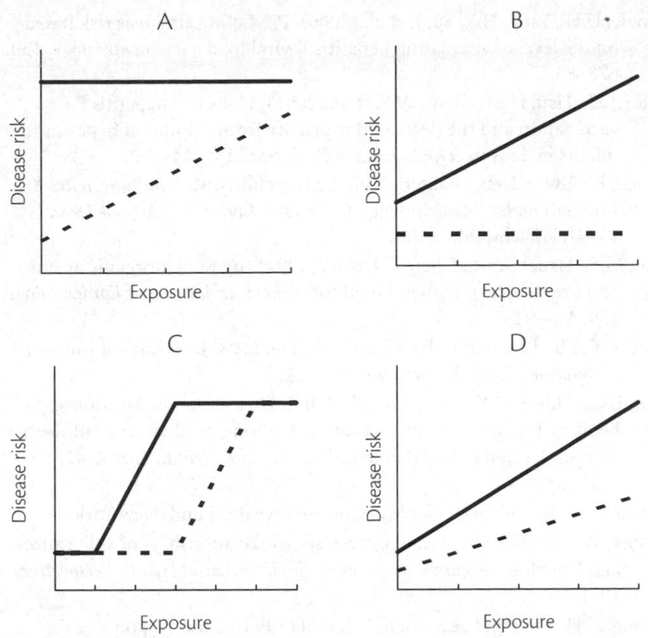

Fig. 8.1.9 Environmental disease risk by exposure dose and susceptible genotype (____ high risk, ... low risk). Panel A, relative risk decreases with exposure dose; Panel B, relative risk increases with exposure dose; Panel C, relative risk is highest at medium exposure dose; Panel D, relative risk remains constant throughout the exposure dose range.

interaction in the development of environmental diseases. In panel A, persons with the high-risk genotype have consistently high risk of disease and those with low-risk genotype have a dose–response relationship between disease risk and environmental exposure. The relative disease risk for the high-risk genotype compared with the low-risk genotype decreases with the increase in environmental exposure. In panel B, persons with low-risk genotype have consistently low risk of disease and those with the high-risk genotype have an increasing disease risk with the increase in environmental exposure; showing an increasing relative risk with the increase in environmental exposure. In panel C, the dose–response relationship was observed for both high-risk and low-risk genotypes with a shift of the dose–response curve from the left for high-risk genotype to the right for low-risk genotype; showing the highest relative risk at medium exposure and a decreasing relative risk toward low and high exposures. In panel D, there is a constant relative risk over the entire spectrum of environmental exposure. Comprehensive and intensive study on interaction between environmental agents and host genomics may provide accurate information for individualized prevention of environmental health hazards.

Promotion of public health through environmental health intervention

All human beings inhabit the unique 'global village', environmental pollution or infectious disease outbreaks in one country may result in environmental disaster and health hazards in both adjacent and remote countries. Public health can be promoted through environment health intervention including the prevention of air, water, and soil pollution with chemicals or biological agents; the reduction in exposures to ultraviolet, ionizing radiation, noise and electromagnetic fields; improvement of built environments including housing, land use patterns, and roads; minimization of carbon dioxide emission, global warming, severe climate change, and ecosystem deterioration; optimization of agricultural methods and irrigation schemes; and promotion of occupational safety and security, and so forth. Many environmental health interventions are more cost-effective compared with other kinds of health-sector efforts. These interventions often yield long-term benefits in addition to immediate health improvement. Reduction in burden of environmental diseases may help the eradication of extreme poverty and hunger, the achievement in universal primary education, the promotion of gender equality and women empowerment, the reduction in child mortality, the improvement in maternal health, the maintenance of environmental sustainability, and the control of epidemics including AIDS/HIV, malaria, tuberculosis, and other infectious diseases. Global partnerships need to be strengthened to achieve interrelated goals of health, environmental sustainability, and development.

References

Beasley, R.P., Hwang, L.Y., Lin, C.C. *et al.* (1981). Hepatocellular carcinoma and hepatitis B virus: A prospective study of 22,707 men in Taiwan. *Lancet*, **2**, 1129–33.

Chang, C.C., Ho, S.C., Tsai, S.S. *et al.* (2004). Ischemic heart disease mortality reduction in an arseniasis-endemic area in southwestern Taiwan after a switch in the tap-water supply system. *Journal of Toxicology and Environmental Health. Part A*, **67**, 1353–61.

Chang, M.H., Chen, C.J., Lai, M.S. *et al.* and Taiwan Childhood Hepatoma Study Group (1997). Nationwide hepatitis B vaccination and the incidence of hepatocellular carcinoma in children in Taiwan. *The New England Journal of Medicine*, **336**,1855–9.

Chen, C.J. (1999). *Epidemiology: Principles and methods.* Lian-Chin, Taipei.

Chen, C.J., Chuang, Y.C., Lin, T.M. *et al.* (1985). Malignant neoplasms among residents of a blackfoot disease-endemic area in Taiwan: High-arsenic artesian well water and cancers. *Cancer Research*, **45**, 5895–9.

Chen, C.J., Chuang, Y.C., You, S.L. *et al.* (1986). A retrospective study on malignant neoplasms of bladder, lung and liver in blackfoot disease endemic area in Taiwan. *British Journal of Cancer*, **53**, 399–405.

Chen, C.J., Kuo, T.L., and Wu, M.M. (1988a). Arsenic and cancers (letter). *Lancet*, **1**, 414–15.

Chen, C.J., Wu, M.M., Lee, S.S. *et al.* (1988b). Atherogenicity and carcinogenicity of high-arsenic artesian well water: Multiple risk factors and related malignant neoplasms of blackfoot disease. *Arteriosclerosis, Thrombosis, and Vascular Biology*, **8**, 452–60.

Chen, C.J., Liang, K.Y., Chang, A.S. *et al.* (1991). Effects of hepatitis B virus, alcohol drinking, cigarette smoking and familial tendency on hepatocellular carcinoma. *Hepatology*, **13**, 398–406.

Chen, C.J., Hsueh, Y.M., Lai, M.S. *et al.* (1995). Increased prevalence of hypertension and long-term arsenic exposure. *Hypertension*, **25**, 53–60.

Chen, C.J., Chiou, H.Y., and Chiang, M.H. (1996a). Dose-response relationship between ischemic heart disease mortality and long-term arsenic exposure. *Arteriosclerosis, Thrombosis, and Vascular Biology*, **16**, 504–10.

Chen, C.J., Yu, M.W., Liaw, Y.F. *et al.* (1996b). Chronic hepatitis B carriers with null genotypes of glutathione S-transferase M1 and T1 polymorphisms who are exposed to aflatoxins are at increased risk of hepatocellular carcinoma. *American Journal of Human Genetics*, **59**, 128–34.

Chen, C.J., Yu, M.W., and Liaw, Y.F. (1997). Epidemiology and multifactorial etiology of hepatocellular carcinoma. *Journal of Gastroenterology and Hepatology*, **12**, S294–S308.

Chen, C.J., Hsu, L.I., Shih, W.L. *et al.* (2005). Biomarkers of exposure, effect and susceptibility of arsenic-induced health hazards in Taiwan. *Toxicology and Applied Pharmacology*, **206**, 198–206.

Chen, C.J., Yang, H.I., Su, J. *et al.* (2006). Risk of hepatocellular carcinoma across a biological gradient of serum hepatitis B virus DNA level. *Journal of the American Medical Association*, **295**, 65–73.

Chen, C.J. and Chen, D.S. (2002). Interaction of hepatitis B virus, chemical carcinogen and genetic susceptibility: Multistage hepatocarcinogenesis with multifactorial etiology (Editorial). *Hepatology*, **36**, 1046–9.

Chen, C.J. and Wang, C.J. (1990). Ecological correlation between arsenic level in well water and age-adjusted mortality from malignant neoplasms. *Cancer Research*, **50**, 5470–4.

Chen, C.L., Hsu, L.I., Chiou, H.Y. *et al.* (2004). Ingested arsenic, cigarette smoking and lung cancer risk: A follow-up study in arseniasis-endemic areas in Taiwan. *Journal of the American Medical Association*, **292**, 2984–90.

Chen, K.P., Lee, T.Y., Hsu, P.Y. *et al.* (1976). Studies on the effect of salt iodization on endemic goiter, Taiwan. I. Mass survey on goiter of school children. *Journal of the Formosan Medical Association*, **75**, 471–82.

Chi, I.C. and Blackwell, R.Q. (1968). A controlled retrospective study of blackfoot disease, an endemic peripheral gangrene disease in Taiwan. *American Journal of Epidemiology*, **88**, 7–24.

Chien, Y.C., Jan, C.F., Kuo, H.S. *et al.* (2006). Nationwide hepatitis B vaccination program in Taiwan: Effectiveness in 20 years after it was launched. *Epidemiologic Reviews*, **28**, 126–35.

Chiou, H.Y., Huang, W.I., Su, C.L. *et al.* (1997). Dose-response relationship between prevalence of cerebrovascular disease and ingested inorganic arsenic. *Stroke*, **28**, 1717–23.

Chiou, H.Y., Chiou, S.T., Hsu, Y.H. *et al.* (2001). Incidence of transitional cell carcinoma and arsenic in drinking water: A follow-up study of 8,102 residents in an arseniasis-endemic area in northeastern Taiwan. *American Journal of Epidemiology*, **153**, 411–18.

Chiu, H.F. and Yang, C.Y. (2005). Decreasing trend in renal disease mortality after cessation from arsenic exposure in a previous arseniasis-endemic area in southwestern Taiwan. *Journal of Toxicology and Environmental Health. Part A*, **68**, 319–27.

Chiu, H.F., Ho, S.C., and Yang, C.Y. (2004a). Lung cancer mortality reduction after installation of tap-water supply system in an arsenic-endemic area in Southwestern Taiwan. *Lung Cancer*, **46**, 265–70.

Chiu, H.F., Ho, S.C., Wang, L.Y. *et al.* (2004b). Does arsenic exposure increase the risk for liver cancer? *Journal of Toxicology and Environmental Health. Part A*, **67**, 1491–1500.

Chiu, H.F., Chang, C.C., Tsai, S.S. et al. (2006). Does arsenic exposure increase the risk for diabetes mellitus? *Journal of Occupational and Environmental Medicine*, **48**, 63–67.

Hamlin, C. (1998). *Public health and social justice in the age of Chadwick: Britain, 1800–1854*. Cambridge University Press.

Hill, A.B. (1953). Observation and experiment. *The New England Journal of Medicine*, **248**, 995–1001.

Hippocrates (1950). *Airs, waters, places*. In *The medical works of Hippocrates* (trans. J. Chadwick, W.N. Mann), pp. 90–111. C. C. Thomas, Springfield, Illinois.

Hsu, H.M., Lu, C.F., Lee, S.C. *et al.* (1999). Seroepidemiologic survey for hepatitis B virus infection in Taiwan: The effect of hepatitis B mass immunization. *The Journal of Infectious Diseases*, **179**, 367–70.

Hsueh, Y.M., Chiou, H.Y., Huang, Y.L. *et al.* (1997). Serum beta-carotene level, arsenic methylation capability and incidence of arsenic-induced skin cancer. *Cancer Epidemiology, Biomarkers & Prevention*, **6**, 589–96.

Iloeje, U.H., Yang, H.I., Su, J. *et al.* (2006). Predicting cirrhosis risk based on the level of circulating hepatitis B viral load. *Gastroenterology*, **130**, 678–86.

Kao, J.H., Hsu, H.M., Shau, W.Y. *et al.* (2001). Universal hepatitis B vaccination and the decreased mortality from fulminant hepatitis in infants in Taiwan. *The Journal of Pediatrics*, **139**, 349–52.

Koch, R. (1891). Ueber bakteriologische Forschung. *Verhandlungen des X. Internationalen Medicinischen Congresses Berlin, 4-9 August 1890, 35–47*. Hirschwald, Berlin.

Lai, M.S., Hsueh, Y.M., Chen, C.J. *et al.* (1994) Ingested inorganic arsenic and prevalence of diabetes mellitus. *American Journal of Epidemiology*, **139**, 484–92.

Raffle, P.A.B., Lee, W.R., McCallum, R.I. *et al.* (1987). *Hunter's diseases of occupations*. Little Brown, Boston, MA.

See, L.C., Chiou, H.Y., Lee, J.S. *et al.* (2007). Dose-response relationship between ingested arsenic and cataract among residents in southwestern Taiwan. *Journal of Environmental Science and Health. Part A*, **42**, 1843–51.

Snow, J. (1936). *Snow on Cholera*. Commonwealth Fund, New York.

Tseng, W.P. (1977). Effects and dose-response relationships of skin cancer and blackfoot disease with arsenic. *Environmental Health Perspectives*, **19**, 109–19.

Tseng, C.H., Chong, C.K., Chen, C.J. *et al.*(1996). Dose-response relationship between peripheral vascular disease and ingested inorganic arsenic among residents in blackfoot disease endemic villages in Taiwan. *Atherosclerosis*, **120**, 125–33.

Tseng, C.H., Chong, C.K., Tseng, C.P. *et al.* (2003). Long-term arsenic exposure and ischemic heart disease in arseniasis-hyperendemic villages in Taiwan. *Toxicology Letters*, **137**, 15–21.

Wang, C.H., Jeng, J.S., Yip, P.K. *et al.* (2002). Biological gradient between long-term arsenic exposure and carotid atherosclerosis. *Circulation*, **105**, 1804–9.

Pruss-Ustun, A. and Corvalan, C. (2006). Preventing disease through healthy environments: Towards an estimate of the environmental burden of disease. World Health Organization, Geneva.

Wu, M.M., Kuo, T.L., Hwang, Y.H. *et al.* (1989). Dose-response relation between arsenic concentration in well water and mortality from cancers and vascular diseases. *American Journal of Epidemiology*, **130**, 1123–32.

Yang, C.Y. (2006) Does arsenic exposure increase the risk of development of peripheral vascular diseases in humans? *Journal of Toxicology and Environmental Health. Part A*, **69**, 1797–804.

Yang, C.Y., Chiu, H.F., Wu, T.N. *et al.* (2004). *Archives of Environmental Health*, **59**, 484–8.

Yang, C.Y., Chiu, H.F., Chang, C.C. et al. (2005). *Environmental Research*, **98**, 127–32.

Yang, H.I., Lu, S.N., You, S.L. *et al.* (2002). Hepatitis B e antigens and the risk of hepatocellular carcinoma. *The New England Journal of Medicine*, **347**, 168–74.

You, S.L., Yang, H.I., and Chen, C.J. (2004). Seropositivity of hepatitis B antigen and hepatocellular carcinoma. *Annals of Medicine*, **36**, 215–24.

Yu, M.W., Cheng, S.W., Lin, M.W. *et al.* (2000). Androgen-receptor CAG repeat, plasma testosterone levels, and risk of hepatitis B-related hepatocellular carcinoma. *Journal of the National Cancer Institute*, **92**, 2023–8.

Yu, M.W., Yang, Y.C., Yang, S.Y. *et al.* (2001). Hormonal markers and hepatitis B virus-related hepatocellular carcinoma risk: a nested case-control study among men. *Journal of the National Cancer Institute*, **93**, 1644–51.

8.2

Radiation and public health

Leeka Kheifets, Myles Cockburn, and Manjit Dosanjh

Abstract

This chapter reviews sources, health effects, and policies for limiting human exposure to ionizing and non-ionizing radiation. Technological developments involving exposure to electromagnetic fields bring social and economic benefits to large sections of society but the health consequences of these developments can be difficult to predict and manage. Biological effects and our knowledge of the health effects of these forms of energy varies: For ionizing radiation, ultraviolet radiation, and power frequency fields numerous state-of-the art epidemiologic and toxicologic investigations, covering a variety of endpoints, have been undertaken. While numerous studies of static and radiofrequency fields have been completed, much of the key research is yet to be done; and for intermediate frequencies, only scant information is available.

Of numerous health effects that have been studied in relation to various aspects of radiation, cancer has received the most attention and appears to be an outcome with the strongest link to exposures at most frequencies. The International Agency for Research on Cancer (IARC) classified ionizing radiation as a 'known' or Group 1 carcinogen; ultraviolet radiation was classified as 'probable human carcinogen', or a Group 2A carcinogen; while extremely low frequency magnetic fields have been classified as a 'possible human carcinogen', or a Group 2B: Static fields as well as extremely low frequency electric fields have been assigned Group 3 (not classifiable as to carcinogenicity to humans). Intermediate frequencies, radio frequency fields, and infrared radiation have not yet been evaluated as to their carcinogenic potential.

Insufficient knowledge and inconsistency in the existing data presents difficulties in the development of public health policies. Additional issues include balancing benefits of technologies to the society overall with potential risks to individuals. As it is not possible to eliminate exposure to ionizing radiation, these exposures are kept to a practical minimum. Most recommend avoiding solar UV exposure in order to facilitate the prevention of skin cancers. However, because recent literature suggests beneficial effects of solar UV exposure it is critical to develop and adopt a well-balanced set of recommendations regarding this exposure. For ELF magnetic fields, given exposure prevalence, considerable scientific uncertainty and limited public health impact, only very low-cost precautionary measures are justified. For RF, while health risks have not been identified, potential risk could affect a large number of people because of the ubiquitous nature of the exposure. Thus given important gaps in knowledge and availability of no to low cost measures for mobile phones precautionary measures can and should be adopted. Higher risks are more acceptable in medical applications, which employ a variety of frequency and bring direct benefit to individuals.

Introduction

The electromagnetic spectrum encompasses frequencies that range from above approximately 10^{20} hertz (Hz) for ionizing radiation at the high end of the spectrum to static fields and power frequencies of 50–60 Hz at the low end. Between the two ends of the spectrum, in order of decreasing frequency, are ultraviolet radiation, visible light, infrared radiation, microwaves, and radio waves (Fig. 8.2.1). This chapter reviews sources and health effects of human exposure to radiation within the electromagnetic spectrum, and reviews policies for limiting human exposure where appropriate.

The focus of research and our knowledge of the health effects of these forms of energy has been driven, at least partly, by the prevalence of exposure to the general public, although valuable additional information has been derived from occupational studies of high exposure. Our understanding varies: For ionizing radiation, ultraviolet radiation, and extremely low frequency fields (ELF) numerous state-of-the art epidemiologic and toxicologic investigations, encompassing a variety of endpoints, have been undertaken; although numerous studies of static and radiofrequency fields (RF) have been completed, much of the key research is yet to be done; for infrared radiation and intermediate frequencies only scant information is available.

Technological developments involving exposure to electromagnetic fields bring social and economic benefits to large sections of society but the health consequences of these developments can be difficult to predict and manage. As countries increase their capacity to generate and distribute electricity, and take advantage of the many new technologies—such as telecommunications—to improve lifestyle and work efficiency exposures to electric and magnetic fields from 0 to 300 GHz (non-ionizing radiation) has been increasing rapidly. In this chapter, our main emphasis is on exposures common in the everyday life rather than occupational exposures. When relevant we also consider separately exposures from medical applications, as these exposures are commonly higher, but carry a different risk/benefit ratio for the exposed individuals.

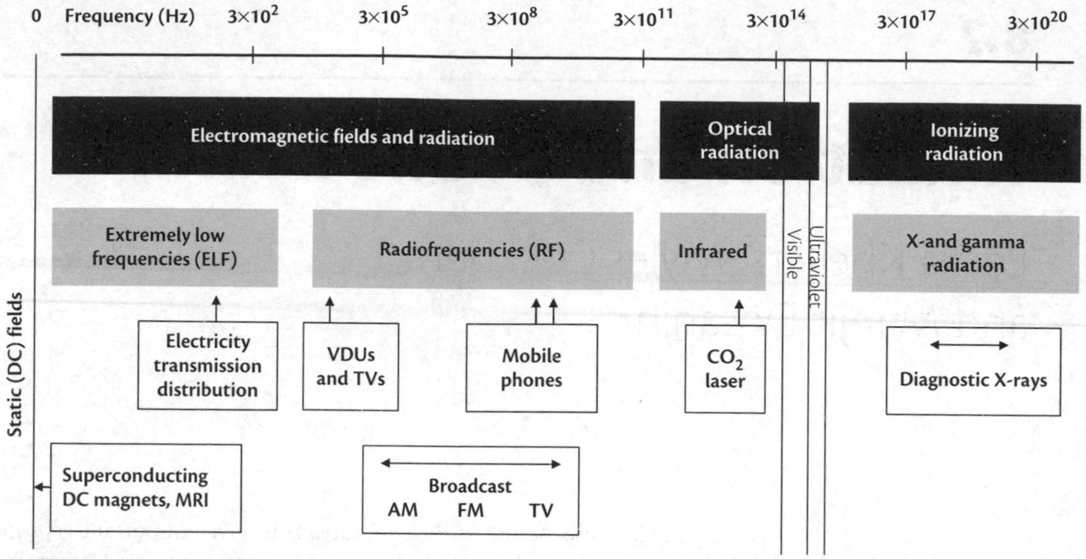

Fig. 8.2.1 Major sources and electromagnetic spectrum.

Static fields

Sources and environmental levels

For a steady current in a circuit corresponding to the zero-frequency (static fields), the charge density at any point of the circuit is constant, and therefore the electric fields are constant in time. Since magnetic fields are created by moving electric charges, magnetic fields are also constant for static fields. The unit of measurement for magnetic fields is tesla (T). Another commonly used unit in engineering sciences is gauss (G); one T is equivalent to 10000 G. Environmental exposure levels are described in microtesla (μT), or 10^{-6} T.

There is a natural static magnetic field that originates from the electric current flowing in the upper layer of the Earth's core, as well as solar activity and atmospheric processes. There are significant local differences in the strength of this field: The vertical component of the field reaches a maximum of about 70 μT at the magnetic poles, and approaches zero at the magnetic equator; conversely the horizontal component is close to zero at the poles and is a maximum of just over 30 μT at the magnetic equator.

In addition to the earth's magnetic field are man-made magnetic fields of significantly higher strength. Major sources of exposure to the general public are transportation and Magnetic Resonance Imaging (MRI). High occupational exposures to static fields are encountered in several industrial processes including aluminium and chlorine production, gas welding, and in research.

In general, electrified railway systems produce some of the largest static field levels encountered by the general public. Magnetic flux densities of up to 1 mT have been reported inside Italian high-speed trains (Grandolfo & Veccia 1996). Static fields up to several tens of microtelsa have been reported inside trams operating on direct current (EC 1996). Modern magnetic levitation (maglev) systems use very high fields (around 1 T) directly on the rails; inside the trains fields vary between 50 μTand 10 mT depending on the cabin design.

MRI systems have proliferated in recent years and there are currently many thousands world wide. The static magnetic fields are in the range of 0.2–3 T for systems for routine clinical use. MRI also utilizes much smaller time-varying gradient magnetic fields and radio frequency radiation. Medical applications with the potential of using fields up to 10 T and higher are being developed (Simon & Szumowski 1992; Polk & Postow 1996; Gowland 2005).

Sources of exposure that are either relatively uncommon or small include steel construction materials, high voltage DC transmission lines, headphones and telephone speakers, and steel-belted radial tires. Use of magnetic plasters, blankets, and mattresses for therapeutic properties have surface magnetic flux densities of about 50 mT, but decay quickly within a few millimetres and are not used widely (EC 1996).

Health effects

Cancer

The few epidemiological studies published to date leave a number of unresolved issues concerning the possibility of increased cancer risk from exposure to static magnetic fields. These studies have been carried out almost exclusively on workers exposed to static magnetic fields generated by equipment using large DC currents. Assessment of exposure has been poor, and the number of participants in the studies has been very small. Most of the studies were conducted in aluminium or other smelter plants. The limitations of these studies to provide useful information is supported by the lack of clear evidence for increased risk due to other, more established, carcinogenic factors present in some of these work environments: Aluminium reduction creates coal tar, pitch volatiles, fluoride fumes, sulphur oxides, and carbon dioxide. Although some welders are exposed to relatively high static fields in some processes, they are also exposed to fumes, ELF and RF magnetic fields. A small but significantly elevated risk of brain tumours (Kheifets *et al.* 1995) but not for leukaemia (Kheifets *et al.* 1997) for welders (RR:1.25; 95 per cent-CI = 1.06 – 1.47) was reported in a meta-analyses of occupational EMF exposure. However, most of the studies on welders do not provide enough information to determine the type of welding used, limiting the usefulness of these data in a review of potential health effects of static magnetic field exposure. Other work environments, for example MRI technicians, with a potential for high fields have not been adequately evaluated. In short: There is insufficient information for proper risk assessment of the impacts of static magnetic fields on cancer. Evidence from animal carcinogenesis studies is inconclusive, in the few studies that have been carried out.

Other outcomes

Even less information is available on other outcomes such as reproductive health. One study examined fertility and pregnancy outcomes in female MRI operators, where the potential for exposure to relatively large static fields of up to ~1 T may have existed. The risk of miscarriage for pregnancies during MRI work was slightly increased compared to work in other jobs and was considerably higher than the risk of homemakers (Evans *et al.* 1993), but the study is methodologically weak. Several indicators of reproductive health were studied in aluminium and metal workers with inconsistent results in studies with numerous methodological limitations. No adverse effects have been demonstrated in animal studies, but there are few good studies, especially with exposures in excess of 1 T.

Policy and prevention

Exposure to equipment generating large static electric fields is uncommon. Exposures to large static magnetic fields (up to several tens of mT) occur as a result of the industrial use of DC electric currents, for example in welding and electrolytic processes, and less commonly in high energy physics laboratories and experimental fusion reactors. Few countries have developed exposure guidance.

However exposure may be becoming more common. With the advent of superconductor technology in the latter part of the twentieth century, it has been possible to develop large electromagnets capable of generating fields in excess of 1 T. Patient exposure to fields of 1–2 T during clinical MRI diagnostic procedures is now routine and will increase in the future, as technology develops. Most MRI use involves relatively short scans of less than 1 h, and there are usually clear benefits to the individual being scanned, hence the approach to guidance on exposure is different to that adopted for occupational and public exposure, because of the different risk/benefit ratio to the individual concerned.

ICNIRP (1994) recommended a time-weighted average exposure to magnetic fields of 200 mT during the working day for occupational exposures, with a ceiling value of 2 T. For extremities a ceiling value of 5 T is considered acceptable. For the general public, a 'continuous exposure limit' of 40 mT is given. This is in effect a ceiling value, although 'occasional access to special facilities where magnetic flux densities exceed 40 mT can be allowed under controlled conditions, provided that the appropriate occupational exposure limit is not exceeded'.

Extremely low-frequency (ELF)

Sources and environmental levels

Extremely low frequency electro-magnetic fields (ELF EMF) are associated with all aspects of the production, transmission, and use of electricity. The fields are imperceptible to humans and are ubiquitously present in modern societies. ELF EMF are composed of two separate components, electric fields and magnetic fields. Electric fields are created by electric charges and are measured in volts/metre (V/m). Typical residential exposure levels are under 10 V/m. In the immediate vicinity of electric appliances, exposure levels can reach as high as several hundreds of V/m, whereas exposure levels immediately under high-tension power lines can reach several kilovolts per meter (kV/m) i.e. several thousand V/m.

Average magnetic field exposures in the workplace have been found to be higher in electrical occupations which include power and telephone line workers, electricians, and electrical engineers, among others, than in other occupations such as office workers. Exposures range from 0.4 to 0.6 μT for electricians and electrical engineers to approximately 1.0 μT for power line workers, and above 3 μT for welders, railway engine drivers, and textile workers. By contrast, typical residential exposure levels are around 0.1 μT. In the immediate vicinity of electric appliances that are in use, magnetic fields could be as high as several hundreds of μT but are usually only of short duration.

Health effects

Since the late 1970s, numerous epidemiologic studies of varying quality have investigated possible health risks from residential and occupational exposure to both electric and magnetic fields.

Cancer

An association between higher-than-average magnetic field exposure levels and leukaemia risk is reported in most of the approximately 20 epidemiologic studies investigating childhood leukaemia and ELF EMF fields. A robust biologic hypothesis to explain this association is lacking. In 2000, two independently conducted pooled analyses of previously published studies showed a statistically significant, approximately two-fold increase in childhood leukaemia risk for average residential exposure levels above 0.3 or 0.4 μT, compared to the lowest exposure category of ≤ 0.1 μT (Ahlbom *et al.* 2000; Greenland *et al.* 2000). Risk increases this small are notoriously hard to evaluate in epidemiology because it is usually difficult to achieve enough precision to distinguish a small risk from no risk. Such small effect estimates, compared to larger ones, are also more likely to result from inadvertent error, or bias, that can occur in epidemiologic studies (Greenland & Kheifets 2006). Selection bias, which can arise in the process used to select or enrol study participants might explain some of the observed association (Mezei & Kheifets 2005). Given: (1) The small associations observed in studies of magnetic fields and childhood leukaemia; (2) a limited understanding of causal risk factors for childhood leukaemia; (3) methodological difficulties in an assessment of a non-memorable and highly variable exposure; and (4) the potential for selection bias, a conclusive interpretation of these findings remains a challenge. The lack of a robust biophysical mechanism that would explain how environmental magnetic fields could cause cancer and a lack of support from laboratory investigations also argue that the findings might be a result of study design and measurement issues rather than being truly causal. However, the remarkable consistency of epidemiologic studies is difficult to dismiss, disregard, or explain away.

Results for other cancers, such as adult leukaemia (occupational exposures only) and adult and childhood brain cancer, are less consistent than those for childhood leukaemia. For breast cancer a biologic mechanism has been proposed, but has not been confirmed in recent epidemiologic studies which strongly argue against an association (WHO EHC 2007).

Other health outcomes

A number of additional health outcomes, particularly motor neuron diseases, reproductive outcomes, and cardiovascular disease, have also been investigated in epidemiologic studies.

Motor neuron diseases and reproductive outcomes have not been sufficiently investigated and studies that have been conducted are characterized by methodological difficulties. Although several studies have observed an increased risk of amyotrophic lateral sclerosis in electrical occupations which might be associated with electric shocks, magnetic fields, or both, the results are inconsistent and lack supportive laboratory evidence.

Epidemiologic investigation of cardiovascular diseases has been motivated by biologically based hypotheses which stemmed from two independent lines of evidence: (1) Magnetic fields were reported to reduce the normal heart rate variability in human experiments, and (2) Several prospective cohort studies have suggested that reductions in some components of heart rate variability are associated with increased risk for heart disease, overall mortality rate in survivors of myocardial infarction, and sudden cardiovascular death. Thus it was hypothesized that occupational exposure to magnetic fields increases the risk for cardiac arrhythmia-related conditions and acute myocardial infarction, but not chronic cardiovascular disease. Although an initial study appeared to support this hypothesis, recent larger and more rigorous studies have found no effects and have failed to confirm earlier findings, which suggest that ELF magnetic fields do not play a role in the development of cardiovascular diseases (Kheifets *et al.* 2007).

Policy and prevention

During the past decade, a number of national and international expert panels, including ones assembled by the US National Institute of Environmental Health Sciences (NIEHS) and the International Agency for Research on Cancer (IARC) and the World Health Organization (WHO) have reviewed the evidence on the potential relationship between exposure to ELF EMF and various adverse health outcomes (National Institute of Environmental Health Sciences 1999; International Agency for Research on Cancer 2002; World Health Organization 2007). Evaluations by these expert panels generally agree that short-term, adverse effects do not occur at exposures to magnetic fields below 100 μT. Current guidelines are based on avoiding the risks to health that result from the interaction of the induced fields and currents with electrically excitable nerve tissue, particularly that of the central nervous system. For general public exposure, the reference levels for power frequency electric and magnetic fields are of the order of 5 kV/m and 100 μT, respectively. These values are well above levels encountered in most environments,

Based on these intensive reviews, both the NIEHS, IARC, and WHO classified ELF magnetic (but not electric) fields as a 'possible human carcinogen', or a Group 2B carcinogen. This classification was based both on epidemiologic evidence showing a consistent association between exposure to ELF magnetic fields and childhood leukaemia even though laboratory studies in animals and cells, do not support an association between exposure to ELF magnetic fields and cancer. The NIEHS assessment (but not the IARC or WHO assessments) concluded that there was also sufficient epidemiologic evidence for an association between adult chronic lymphocytic leukaemia and occupational exposure to ELF magnetic fields to warrant a classification as a 'possible human carcinogen'.

Several risk characterization attempts have indicated that the public health impact of residential magnetic fields on childhood leukaemia is likely to be limited (Kheifets *et al.* 2006). Positing sensitivity and bias models for methodologic problems in the epidemiologic studies and accounting for uncertainties regarding field levels that may have effects, suggest that, in light of the available data, both no public health impact and a large impact remain possibilities (Greenland & Kheifets 2006).

The combination of widespread exposures, established biological effects from acute, high-level exposures, and the possibility of leukaemia in children from low-level, chronic exposures have made it necessary but difficult to develop consistent public health policies. In view of these uncertainties, it might be advisable to adopt general no- and low-cost measures to reduce exposure (WHO 2007).

Intermediate frequency

Intermediate frequency (IF) exposures occur in the range 300 Hz to 10 MHz, partially encompassing frequencies also assigned to very low frequency (VLF; 0.3–30 kHz); and high (3–30 MHz) ranges.

Because few biological studies of exposures to intermediate frequencies have been conducted, exposure guidelines have largely been extrapolated from the encompassing ELF (at the low end) and RF (at the high end) limits.

Sources and environmental levels

IF exposures are common from occupational appliances such as induction heaters (used in the heating of metals prior to manipulation) and plasma heaters. Smaller exposures occur from induction heating elements in residential cooking appliances. Television, radio, and other communications transmitters can emit IF, but they are discussed in the section on RF, which constitutes the much more common wavelengths of exposure from such sources. Indirect exposures from medical equipment (e.g. MRI machines and magnetic bone stimulators where pulses may drop to IF levels) may occur rarely. Direct exposures to IF may also occur from surgical equipment used for tissue cutting and cauterizing.

Common exposures to IF occur in proximity to devices that read magnetic cards or buttons for identification purposes (Polichetti & Vecchia 1998), and similarly, from anti-theft devices that read magnetic identification tags. Very small exposures are obtained from television screens (and CRT computer monitors).

Health effects

Since exposure level and proximity to the source (i.e. the method by which IF is conducted to the relevant tissue), together determine the IF levels in tissue knowledge, of both is important in determining the biological effects of IF exposure levels in humans.

Biological effects in humans can be either thermal when frequency is sufficient to induce a heating response or non-thermal, (i.e. cell membrane excitation or electroporation), when frequency does not induce a heating response.

Findings for the impact of IF on cancer in humans are inconsistent. A number of epidemiologic studies of IF (and other wavelengths) exposure from televisions and CRT monitors on reproductive effects, have not found an impact.

Policy and prevention

Because of the limited data currently there are no specific recommendations for limiting exposure to IF, other than those extrapolated from EMF at extremes of the IF range (ELF and RF).

Radiofrequency radiation

Sources and environmental levels

With rapid advances in EMF technologies and communications, people are increasingly exposed to frequencies in the radiofrequency (RF) range. RF fields are produced by radio and TV broadcasts, mobile phone base stations, and other communication infrastructure. The most prevalent and rapidly growing exposure is to handheld mobile telephones. This technology typically uses frequencies from 450 to 2500 MHz, although new technology may broaden this band. Other sources of exposure to the general population are radio and television transmitters which operate at between 200 kHz and 900 MHz. Radio and TV signals are broadcast to a large area from comparatively few sites (Neubauer *et al.* 2006). Compared to radio and TV transmitters, mobile phone base stations cover a smaller area, and produce much lower emissions, but are vastly more common in many countries. Residential exposures also come from wireless monitors used in children's cribs, cordless phones, and Wi-Fi (wireless Internet connections) commonly used at home and in schools. Occupational exposures include RF PVC welding machines, plasma etchers, and military and civil radar systems. All operate at different frequencies.

Handheld mobile phones available since the late 1980s became widely used by the general population only in the late 1990s. Currently there are more than 2.5 billion mobile phone users worldwide, with a penetration in some countries reaching 80 per cent. Exposure from mobile phones is concentrated to the part of the head closest to the handset and the antenna. The exposure declines rapidly with distance; exposures from mobile phone base stations are several orders of magnitude lower than from the phones. Because of this, most research has focused on mobile phones. For RF sources other than the mobile phones typical power densities outdoors would be 0.01–1 mW/m^2, but could be orders of magnitude higher (i.e. 100 mW/m^2 and above). For the whole body exposure, mobile phone base stations can be the largest individual source of RF, but other sources such as radio or TV transmitters can result in comparable or greater exposures depending on where the measurements are taken. Indoor levels are often lower than outdoor exposures by orders of magnitude; for example, in Europe, a median indoor power density of 0.005 $mW\ m^{-2}$ has been reported. Note that the exposure from base stations differs from that of mobile phones; base stations expose the whole body, but the exposure duration is considerably longer. Perhaps more importantly, base station exposure has been a subject of much concern to the public because it is not under the control of the public and its presence is not perceived to be of direct individual benefit.

Population exposure to RF fields has been less completely characterized than exposures to ELF fields. This is due to: (1) Technical challenges (lack of adequate measuring equipment); (2) the rapid evolution of the technology (frequency, coding schemes); and (3) to new patterns of use (duration of calls, text messaging). However, the main reason ELF sources are better understood than RF sources is that they have been studied more.

Health effects

Since RF radiation induces heating in body tissues and imposes a heat load on the whole body, prevention of excessive heating serves as a basis for most international guidelines for human exposure. Studies of the interaction of RF with tissue in the range used for mobile phones have led to the proposal of many different non-thermal mechanisms for RF interaction. Generally, it is thought that non-thermal interactions are unlikely to be biologically significant at the RF levels below guidance values, but much of the ongoing research is directed towards non-thermal mechanisms.

Cancer

Epidemiological studies of health effects related to RF exposure from mobile phones have primarily focused on cancer, especially brain tumours. Because the technology is relatively new, the number of studies, particularly for long-term exposure with sufficient latency is limited. Currently it is only possible to evaluate short-term effects of mobile phone exposure; the majority of studies have found no effects on either brain or parotid gland tumour risk (Feychting *et al.* 2004). Exposure assessment remains problematic: Substantial random error has been shown for even short-term recall of mobile phone use; and information bias appears to affect at least the reporting of the side of the head where the phone is commonly used. Also, some studies may be compromised by a non-representative control group, caused by an increased participation of mobile phone users. Results for acoustic neuroma are more suggestive albeit inconsistent (Takebayashi 2006; AGNIR 2003).

There are no studies of cancer risk related to mobile phone base stations, but a few studies have assessed cancer risk in relation to radio and TV transmitters (Ahlbom *et al.* 2004). Often driven by a previously identified cancer cluster, these analyses are based simply on distance from the source and often include an extremely small number of cases. It is therefore not surprising that such studies have been uninformative. More rigorous investigations might be feasible with a development of new instruments capable of capturing personal RF exposure (Neubauer *et al.* 2006).

Although occupational studies have been performed over a longer time period we are only beginning to measure and learn about RF exposures in various occupations, and the exposure may not always be relevant for an assessment of effects of mobile phone frequencies. Although some increased risks have been found in certain studies, there is no consistent evidence of risk increases for any cancer sites. The studies have several methodological weaknesses: None of the studies have made measurements of the actual RF exposure for the subjects included; exposure classification has often been based on the job title alone; and no or only limited control of confounding has been made (Ahlbom *et al.* 2004).

All of the studies have reported null results for carcinogenicity in normal animals at exposure levels compatible with mobile phones, while controversy still exists about the carcinogenic effects of RF radiation in a transgenic mouse model (Goldstein *et al.* 2002a, 2002b).

Other outcomes

It is well established in animal studies that hyperthermia during pregnancy can cause embryonic death, abortion, growth retardation, and developmental defects; in particular development of the central nervous system is especially susceptible. Serious health effects in humans are associated only with greatly elevated body temperatures (>40°C) and such temperature rises are well above the maximum allowable for public RF exposure.

Numerous studies have evaluated developmental effects of RF fields on mammals, birds, and other non-mammalian species

(AGNIR 2003; Heynick & Merritt 2003). These studies have shown that RF fields are teratogenic at exposure levels that are high enough to cause significant increases in temperature. There is no consistent evidence of effects at non-thermal exposure levels, although a few studies have evaluated possible effects on postnatal development using sensitive endpoints, such as behavioural effects.

Several studies of occupational RF exposure, primarily to physiotherapists, have reported an increased risk of congenital malformations but no specific type of malformation has been consistently reported and there is a potential for recall bias in these studies. When a pregnant woman is using hands-free equipment, small exposure to the foetus from a mobile phone kept in a pocket, handbag, or belt by the hip is possible. The only epidemiologic study of cell phones use in pregnancy and early childhood found that Exposure to cell phones prenatally—and, to a lesser degree, postnatally - was associated with behavioural difficulties such as emotional and hyperactivity problems around the age of school entry. The observed associations may be non causal and due to unmeasured confounding; however, if they are real they would have major public health implications (Divan *et al.* 2008).

Possible health effects based in part on anecdotal reports of numerous symptoms such as headaches and sleep disturbance from continuous whole body RF exposure from base stations is an area of major public concern. Because of numerous methodologic shortcomings, data regarding effects of such RF exposure on symptoms are inadequate for assessment at present.

Policy and prevention

Guidance on exposure for the general public is intended to restrict local tissue temperature rises to acceptable levels and currently is set to 0.08 Wkg^{-1}, for the whole body, and 2 Wkg^{-1}, for the head. Most reviews conclude that the scientific evidence available to date does not give cause for concern. However this area of research has important gaps. Mobile telephones have only been in widespread use for a relatively short time and therefore, the possibility remains that long-term RF exposures from mobile telephony can have adverse health effects. More importantly, many of the health outcomes are yet to be studied and research on potential detrimental effects on children is particularly sparse. Continued research on low levels of RF is needed.

The need for Public Health policy coupled with the paucity of data, particularly for children regarding the long-term health effects of mobile phone use, suggests that low-cost precautionary measures are appropriate. Mobile phone use is increasingly common among school children, and teenagers may be among the heaviest mobile phone users today with some exposures close to guideline limits (Kheifets *et al.* 2005). Exposure can be reduced by restricting the length of calls, or by using 'hands-free' devices to keep mobile phones away from the head and body.

Infrared radiation

Sources and environmental levels

Infrared radiation (IR) occurs at wavelengths between 780 nm and 1 mm. The IR spectrum is conventionally broken down into three separate categories: IR 'A' (780nm –1.4 μm); IR 'B' (1.4–3 μm); and IR 'C' (3 μm–1mm), which are arbitrary categories based loosely on the biological potential of each range in humans (see below).

Primary sources of IR are man-made: Heating devices, lights (LEDs), some designs of sauna, industrial sources (also related to heat production, particularly in glass-making and steel/iron industries), and from communication devices using IR wavelengths to transfer data. There have been relatively few studies of the health effects of IR, other than those showing that the wavelengths involved are unlikely to impact humans (other than ocular damage in specific applications, and with heat-related illness in special cases, discussed below).

Health effects

IR has the ability to penetrate human skin, although only IR-A penetrates further than about 1 mm. Most studies suggest that the main effect of exposure to IR in humans is the generation of heat, with little evidence of any adverse effects on DNA or other biological processes.

Harmful effects

The main detrimental effect of IR is on the eye (with potential for damage to the lens, cornea, and retina). There is considerable evidence of IR-induced cataract, in industries with extremely high exposures (glass workers (Lydahk & Philipson 1984), iron and steel workers (Lydahk & Philipson 1984)). Most non-industrial exposures to IR appear insufficient to cause cataract or other eye damage. Some IR heaters do not have an accompanying light source, and so do not 'warn' the user that exposure is occurring, but there is no evidence that they cause ocular damage (McItyre *et al.* 1993).

Workers exposed to high levels of IR also have to contend with hyperthermic effects (rise in body temperature), which are similar to those in any industry involving physical activity in warm environments. Subsequently, the exposure limits in those occupations instead rely on ensuring that body temperatures are managed.

It is thought that either the amount of exposure in the home (from heating lamps and other non-industrial sources) is insufficient to produce heat-related damage on the skin, or removing oneself from the exposure source (an 'aversion' response) causes one to avoid exposure that would otherwise cause a burn. There is some evidence of a 'delay' in skin burning effect when the original exposure was insufficient to burn the skin, but the circumstances under which this might occur are unclear.

IR is not considered relevant in the initiation of skin cancer although it might contribute to development of skin cancer by reducing DNA repair ability (Dewhirst *et al.* 2003). Evidence of this is scant. It has been hypothesized that IR might accelerate UV-induced skin carcinogenesis (Edwards *et al.* 1999).

Beneficial effects

Exposure to IR appears to improve microcirculation, mostly via warmth, but perhaps also via some other mechanism of improving blood flow unrelated to temperature (Yu *et al.* 2006). One study has demonstrated that exposure to IR improves lactation (Ogita *et al.* 1990). For centuries there has been a general belief that IR exposure (in heat chambers or sauna) improves general health, although there have been no randomized or longitudinal studies showing this to be the case.

Policy and prevention

There are various international standards for limiting exposure to IR that are provided separately for IR-A, B, and sometimes C

(The International commission on Non-Ionizing Radiation Protection 2006). These limits based on combinations of wavelength and time of exposure, are most appropriate for industrial applications where exposures are extreme and measurable. Avoiding the heat-generating effects of IR tends to be accomplished by innate human response prior to the occurrence of thermal injury to the skin when humans react to avoid exposure. This is not true for exposures causing cataract, so specific recommendations exist for wearing protective eye coverings and limiting exposure to IR, again largely in occupational settings with extreme exposures, but also assuming that any exposure of the eye to IR is potentially harmful.

There are currently no recommendations for limiting or avoiding exposures to IR in saunas and other recreational exposures, other than to limit exposure to avoid heat-related illness which is the main outcome of over-exposure to IR from these sources. There has been little research conducted on the health effects of IR exposure in sauna use (Meffert & Piazena 2002). One recommendation that the use of saunas be limited following UV exposures (van der Leun & de Gruijl 2002) has been suggested based on the possibility that the effects of UV exposure are accelerated with IR exposure.

Ultraviolet radiation

Sources and environmental levels

Ultraviolet radiation (UV) is non-ionizing and invisible to the eye. The most common source of human exposure to UV is from the sun, but man-made sources are becoming more common.

Solar UV is conventionally categorized into UVA (400–320 nm), UVB (320–280 nm), and UVC (280–250 nm), based on energy potential for damage in human skin. Wavelengths within the UV spectrum penetrate human skin to varying degrees; UVA penetrates deep into the dermis and has a long-term cumulative effect, while UVB affects only the upper levels of skin (epidermis).

UVC is absorbed by the atmosphere and does not reach the earth's surface. Most UVB is also absorbed by the atmosphere: The amount that arrives at the earth's surface is determined by the time of year, time of day, location on the earth's surface, and atmospheric conditions. UVB reaching the earth's surface has a marked peak in summer and in the middle of the day. By contrast, the diurnal and seasonal peaks of UVA reaching the earth's surface are less pronounced (McKenzie *et al.* 2003). Neither UVA nor UVB are completely absorbed or blocked by cloud cover.

As well as direct exposure to UV from the sun, environmental exposure also occurs indirectly, from reflection off any solid, light coloured surface such as concrete or snow. Reflected UV from light-coloured surfaces tends to have increased intensity compared to direct UV. UV penetrates into water but a small amount of UV is also reflected from the surface of water.

UVB breaks ozone, O_3, into oxygen, O_2, and a single reactive O molecule. It is probable that in certain geographical locations there are marked increases in UVB exposure over time due to the depletion of ozone in the atmosphere (thought to result from increasing concentrations of chlorofluorocarbons and other ozone-destroying chemicals).

Exposure to UV comes from a variety of man-made sources in occupational, medical, cosmetic, and other settings. Occupational exposures include: Exposure to mercury vapour lamps; arc-welding; commercial bacteriocidal UV lamps; and, in printing from finishing inks. Recent studies have shown that exposure to UV-transilluminators, which use UV to aid in the visualization of products from gel electrophoresis procedures, can result in substantial UV exposures for laboratory personnel (Akbar-Khanzadeh & Jahangir-Blouchian 2005). Man-made sources of UV are used in phototherapy for skin (e.g. psoriasis) and immune disorders. Dental polymerizing equipment also uses UV to bond materials together. Sometimes medical personnel as well as patients are exposed.

Cosmeticians use sunlamps and sun beds and thereby provide exposure to UV and the public at large is exposed to UV in daily life by fluorescent lamps.

Health effects

Exposure to UV has both harmful and beneficial effects. Recent research attempts to balance the relative importance of UV exposure in both preventing and causing skin diseases, immunological diseases, and cancers (Krause *et al.* 2006).

Harmful effects

Animal and human studies have demonstrated measurable effects of UV at the cellular level. Both UVA and UVB have been shown to modify DNA at all levels of the epidermis and dermis. Low doses of UVA induce p53 expression in basal keratinocytes, whereas higher doses affect all layers of the epidermis (Burren *et al.* 1998).

Cancer: Skin cancer (non-melanoma skin cancer (NMSC) and melanoma)

The impact of solar radiation on the skin is well documented. Differing wavelengths of UV, from 250 to 400 nm, can have as much as a 4-fold difference in their potential to produce sun burn or DNA damage in the skin.

While there are various studies implicating only UVB in the development of melanoma and NMSC (De Fabo *et al.* 2004), *in vivo* and *in vitro* studies suggest the full UV spectrum may be involved. DNA damage that initiates melanoma or affects modulation of cell division and cell death that promotes melanoma development and invasiveness may occur (Wang *et al.* 2001). UVB directly damages DNA by forming photoproducts (cyclobutane pyrimidine dimmers), photosensitizes cells, and probably affects cell function including transcription, DNA replication, and cell cycle progression (Garinis *et al.* 2005). UVA initiates single strand DNA breaks (Wang *et al.* 2001) and causes mutation (Ramos *et al.* 2004). UVB is directly absorbed by the DNA and causes two adjacent pyrimidine bases to chemically bond. Both cyclobutane–pyrimidine dimers (CPDs; ~75 per cent of damage products), such as thymine dimers, and 6–4 pyrimidine photoproducts (the remaining 25 per cent) impair the ability of DNA polymerase to replicate the DNA. UVA is less efficient in inducing DNA damage because UVA wavelengths are not absorbed; instead the action of UVA likely occurs by secondary photoreactions of existing DNA photoproducts or via indirect photosensitizing reactions.

A multitude of ecological epidemiologic studies have noted that melanoma rates tend to vary with latitude and altitude, as one might expect if solar UV radiation were involved (Rigel *et al.* 1999; Boniol *et al.* 2005). Moreover, migration studies have noted that a higher potential UV exposure in childhood appears to further increase risk (Mack & Floderus 1991; Whiteman *et al.* 2001), although recent analytic studies indicate exposures over the entire life span are probably equally important (Solomon *et al.* 2004; Fears *et al.* 2002).

Most epidemiologic studies have shown increased risk of melanoma with greater time spent outdoors (Walter *et al.* 1999), with increased self-reported sun exposure behaviour (Bastuji & Diepgen 2002) and with an increase in outdoor recreational activity (Osterlind *et al.* 1988). While sunburn (an indicator of excessive UVB exposure) has been shown in many retrospective studies to increase melanoma risk (Elwood & Jopson 1997), not all studies have identified sun burn as a risk factor (Pfahlberg *et al.* 2001). Moreover, outdoor workers constantly exposed to sunlight have a lower, not higher, risk of melanoma (Goodman *et al.* 1995). This may be explained by an 'intermittent exposure hypothesis', where long-term consistent exposure to solar radiation results in skin reaction (tanning) that protects against melanoma by increasing pigmentation and reducing dose to the dermis, whereas short intermittent (and presumably excessive) exposures result in damage without the chance of protection (Armstrong 1988).

Use of tanning beds or sunlamps appears to increase risks of melanoma and some NMSCs (squamous cell skin cancers) particularly if exposure occurs in young adulthood or earlier, but not other (basal cell) skin cancers (International Agency for Research on Cancer Working Group on artificial ultraviolet and skin 2007).

Non-cancer outcomes

Short-term exposure to UV (particularly in the range 210–320 nm) can result in photokeratitis and conjunctivitis in the eyes, and there is some evidence of an increase in cataract occurrence with exposure to UV (particularly UVA). UV exposure may increase risk of dermatomyositis, an inflammatory myopathy characterized by rash and muscle weakness. UV exposure (particularly to UVB) appears to activate human papilloma virus and a number of other viruses, most likely via immune suppression.

Beneficial effects

UV exposure enhances Vitamin D synthesis and has both local and systemic immunosuppressive effects in humans. These mechanisms are thought to explain much of the apparent association between UV exposure and protection from multiple sclerosis, type 1 diabetes, and rheumatoid arthritis, all of which appear to benefit from Vitamin D supplementation. Whether or not UV exposure is required in order to enjoy that benefit remains to be demonstrated.

Protective effects of UV exposure have been shown for some cancers (Krause *et al.* 2006) (colon, prostate, breast, ovary, non-Hodgkin's lymphoma, and for survival after the diagnosis of melanoma), and while this could also be related to a Vitamin D pathway, the mechanism remains unknown.

Policy and prevention

Limiting exposure to solar UV

Most cancer control agencies worldwide have made recommendations on how best to avoid solar UV exposure in order to facilitate the primary prevention of skin cancers. These include avoiding outdoor activity between the hours of 10 am and 4 pm (although the specificity of this time frame varies in effectiveness depending on location on the earth's surface and time of year). Most recommendations include seeking shade, wearing long-sleeved shirts, long pants and wide-brimmed hats, and the adoption of sun-resistant fabrics, as many common fabrics do not block out all UV.

Excessive exposure to UVA is characterized by long-term outdoor activity, whereas excessive UVB exposure can be obtained by short-term exposure around mid-day and in summer. Few current recommendations for limited solar UV exposure take into account this difference, and it is unclear how best to frame such a public health message to achieve that aim.

The use of sunscreen, which either reflects or blocks UVA and UVB, is also widely advocated, along with recommendations on its appropriate application and reapplication (after exercise, swimming, and long periods in the sun), and the correct Sun Protection Factor (SPF) to use. SPF is an index of the sunscreen's ability to protect against erythema (reddening of the skin), and most recommendations involve using a sunscreen with an SPF of 15 or greater (resulting in protection for 15 times the duration that unprotected skin provides). Most recommendations advocate the use of sunglasses that block a broad spectrum of UV.

Limiting exposure to sun beds and tanning lamps

The International Agency for Research on Cancer (IARC) has recently recommended avoiding sun bed and tanning lamp use, and suggested that policymakers consider limiting sun bed and tanning lamp access for young adults and children (International Agency for Research on Cancer Working Group on artificial ultraviolet and skin 2007).

Limiting occupational exposures

The International Commission on Non-Ionising Radiation Protection (ICNIRP) recommends values for limiting exposure to UV in occupational settings, and a number of recent studies have evaluated how well those recommendations have been implemented. Most occupational exposures appear to be well controlled (and in the case of treatment-related occupational exposures for medical care, for the patient as well), with the exception of laboratory exposures in the increasingly common use of UV-transilluminators.

Achieving well-balanced recommendations

Because recent literature suggests beneficial effects of UV exposure (particularly solar UV exposure), it is critical to develop and adopt a well-balanced set of recommendations regarding exposure limitations. While the evidence that solar UV exposure causes non-melanoma skin cancers appears to justify avoiding UV exposure, doing so could result in compromising Vitamin D status and impacting some immunosuppressive diseases, and perhaps some cancers. Demonstrating the need for balance is the paradoxical finding that while UV exposure appears to increase melanoma risk, it also appears to diminish the risk of recurrence of melanoma.

An additional need for well-balanced recommendations regarding the avoidance of solar UV exposure revolves around the competing risk to many chronic diseases of reduced physical activity: How do we communicate a balanced message of avoiding excessive solar UV exposure (reducing time spent outdoors) while maintaining outdoor physical activity? These issues require deeper understanding of the mechanisms, both harmful and beneficial, of UV exposure, and a well-weighted consideration of their relative importance.

Ionizing radiation

Ionizing radiation consists of electromagnetic radiation—e.g. X-ray, gamma-ray—or of subatomic particles such as protons, neutrons, alpha-particles, pions, electrons, and muons. For radiation to be ionizing, the particles must have high enough energy to eject electrons from atoms, thus creating ions. The ionizing radiation exposure is measured as quantity of absorbed dose and its International System unit is J/kg, commonly referred to as the gray (Gy).

The amount of energy per-unit-length transferred by charged particles passing through a living cell or tissue is called the linear energy transfer (LET) of the radiation. For example gamma and X-rays and electrons and muons (which are the most abundant elementary charged particles reaching sea-level) are considered to be sparsely ionizing—or low-LET—because only a few ionization events are generated along their track when they traverse the cell. On the other hand neutrons and accelerated heavy charged particles from machines like a cyclotron are termed high-LET radiations because they transfer a large amount of energy along their short track as they traverse the cell producing a high density of ionizations. Measurement units commonly used are defined and listed in Table 8.2.1.

In biology, the different ionization capability of the radiation and the different response of the various organs become relevant in addition to the absorbed dose. The equivalent and the effective dose—which take into account the ionization power of a given type of radiation and also the susceptibility of various organs and tissues to radiation damage—are measured in sievert (Sv). For low-LET radiation (X-rays and gamma-rays) the effective dose is equal to the absorbed dose.

Sources and environmental levels

Background radiation dose to human beings worldwide is about 2.4 mSv/year (UNSCEAR 2000) with different sources contributing the fractional amounts as summarized in Fig. 8.2.2. Globally about 80 per cent of the annual dose has a natural origin, namely from cosmic rays and terrestrial sources. Radon which constitutes more than 40 per cent of total background dose, is inhaled and therefore is listed as source of internal exposure.

There are important variations to the background dose depending on altitude and the nature of rock and soils. There exist on earth areas where radiation doses exceed 20 mSv (Kerala, India) and can go up to 130 mSv (Ramsar, Iran) therefore, the population there is living in areas of truly high radiation background.

Table 8.2.1 Quantities and doses units of ionizing radiation

Quantity dose	Unit	Definition
Absorbed dose	Gray (Gy)	Energy deposited in tissue (1 J/kg)
	rad	1 rad = 100 erg/g = 0.01 Gy
Equivalent dose	Sievert (Sv)	Absorbed dose weighted for the ion density (potency) of the radiation
	rem	1 rem = 0.01 Sv
Effective dose	Sievert (Sv)	Equivalent dose weighted for the sensitivity of the exposed organ(s)
Collective effective dose	Person-Sv	Effective dose applied to a population
Committed effective dose	Sievert (Sv)	Cumulative effective dose to be received from a given intake of radio-activity
Radioactivity	Becquerel (Bq)	One disintegration per second
	Curie (Ci)	37 billion disintegrations per second

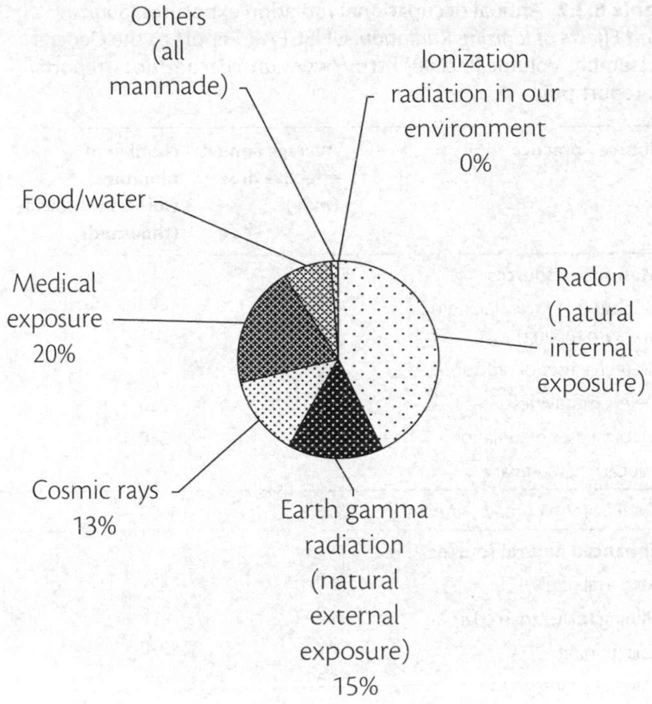

Fig. 8.2.2 Percentage contribution from different sources to the total effective dose of ionizing radiation exposure to the world population
Source: www.who.int/ ionizing_radiation

Cosmic radiation

The Earth and all living organisms are continually bombarded by radiation from outer space. Cosmic radiation consists mostly of protons and alpha particles with smaller contributions from heavier nuclei. These primary cosmic rays interact with the atmosphere and create secondary particulate radiations: Protons, neutrons, pions, etc. Unstable particles and their decay products reach the surface of the Earth. Human exposure is largely from muons, neutrons, and electrons. Exposures vary depending on altitude (since the amount of atmosphere affects the interaction of the primary cosmic rays), latitude, and solar cycle (which affects the flux of primary particles).

The dose rate from cosmic radiation on aeroplanes flying at conventional cruising altitude of 10 000–12 000 m is approximately one hundred times higher than that at ground level. Airline workers, flying for 600–800 h per year, receive a 2 to 5 mSv per year. This dose on average is higher than that of most of the other workers (see Table 8.2.2 on occupational radiation exposures, UNSCEAR 2000), including nuclear power plant workers (WHO, Radiation and Environmental Health, Cosmic Radiation 2005).

External terrestrial sources

Most material on Earth contains radioactive nuclei but most non-radon-related radiation is received as gamma-rays mainly emitted from potassium isotopes and isotopes present in the uranium and thorium decay chains.

Table 8.2.2 Annual occupational radiation exposures (*Sources and Effects of Ionizing Radiation*. UNSCEAR Report to the General Assembly, Volume II, 2000) http://www.unscear.org/docs/reports/gareport.pdf

Source / practice	Average annual effective dose (mSv)	Number of monitored workers worldwide (thousands)
Man-made sources		
Nuclear fuel cycle (including	1.8	800
uranium mining)	0.5	700
Industrial uses of radiation	0.2	420
Defence activities	0.3	2320
Medical uses of radiation	0.1	360
Education/veterinary		
Total from man-made sources	0.6	4600
Enhanced natural sources		
Air travel (crew)	3.0	250
Mining (other than coal)	2.7	760
Coal mining	0.7	3910
Mineral processing	1.0	300
Above ground workplaces (radon)	4.8	1250
Total from natural sources	1.8	6500

Radon

Radon is a natural radioactive gas produced by the decay of radium, which in turn is produced in the ^{238}U decay chain. Found in air, it is often the largest contributor to an individual's background radiation. The concentration of radon in a home depends on the quantity of radon-producing uranium in the underlying soil and surrounding rocks and building materials. Radon gas enters houses through cracks and accumulates in the basement while its level is the lowest in the upper floors of buildings. It should be noted that radon is an indoor and closed space problem only and that increased ventilation reduces the risk from radon.

Man-made radiation sources

The main man-made contribution to environmental exposure has come from the testing of nuclear weapons in the atmosphere mainly between 1945 and 1980. It has been estimated that the world average annual effective dose reached a peak of 0.15 mSv in 1963 and since then it has decreased to about 0.005 mSv in 2000 (UNSCEAR 2000).

Since 1950, it is also necessary to add radiation of industrial origin to environmental levels mainly coming from nuclear power stations producing electricity, which results in exposure of about 0.01–0.02 mSv/year and from coal burning and extraction with additional exposure of 0.01 mSv/year.

It should be noted that the exposure to the personnel working in such environments has been approximately halved since the 1970s because of the improved care and safety regulations. (UNSCEAR 1988, 1993, 1996, 2000).

Exposure from medical procedures

In the past 100 years, diagnostic radiology, nuclear medicine, and radiation therapy have evolved techniques that form essential tools for all branches and specialities of medicine. The inherent properties of ionizing radiation provide many benefits but also may cause potential harm.

Medical interventions and examinations are now the largest contributor to man-made exposure and accounting globally for about 20 per cent of the total dose in the general population, this fraction being much higher for developed countries. The ranges of the absorbed or effective doses in medical procedures are given in Table 8.2.3 (NRC 2006).

Diagnostic radiology

Modern diagnostic radiology assures earlier, more precise diagnosis, and to monitor the progression of a large number of diseases. Screening procedures (such as mammography) are beneficial for specific populations who are at a higher risk from certain diseases. In addition, a number of interventional radiologically driven procedures (such as angioplasty) introduced in the last 10–20 years, contribute significantly to the effectiveness of treatment of serious and life threatening diseases of the cardiovascular, central nervous systems, and other organs. Diagnostic radiology using normal X-rays, computed tomography (CT), positron emission tomography (PET) have significantly improved the staging and accuracy of diagnosis. Such improvements can be critically important in effecting cures but result in high exposure and therefore should be used with care.

Nuclear medicine uses radioactive isotopes specifically developed to be taken up predominantly by one organ, or type of cell in the body in the diagnosis and treatment of a range of diseases. Following their uptake into the body for diagnostic purposes they are followed either by external measurements, resulting in images of their distribution, or by activity measurements in blood, urine, or other substrate. The information obtained is of functional character and is not readily obtainable or is less precisely obtained by other methods. Nuclear medicine provides diagnostic information in cardiology, endocrinology, urology, in detecting and staging cancer as well as other diseases. Most of the currently used methods are chosen because they show high sensitivity and specificity (ICRP 93 2004).

Radiation therapy (RT) for cancer treatment

Appropriate use of radiotherapy cures many lives every year and in the case of palliative treatment substantially reduces suffering. There are also some non-malignant diseases whose treatment by radiation is also a method of choice.

RT is a widely used and cost-effective treatment for cancer which generally conserves tissue function. With increasing cancer incidence in an aging population, the role of radiotherapy will further increase over the next decades. The main aim of radiation therapy is to deliver a maximally effective dose of radiation to a designated tumour site while reducing coincident exposure of surrounding healthy tissues as much as possible.

It should be noted that radiotherapy may be accompanied by adverse side effects of the treatment. Some of these effects are unavoidable and often resolve spontaneously after treatment. Side effects may occur and result from the proximity of sensitive normal tissues to the treatment field. Most of the side effects of conventional radiotherapy are predictable and expected and one of the aims of modern IMRT (intensity modulated radiation therapy) is to reduce the side effects to a minimum by sparing normal tissues (Hall 2006).

Table 8.2.3 Estimated range of absorbed/effective doses from Diagnostic Radiation Exposures (National Research Council 2006. *Health Risks from exposure to low levels of ionizing radiation, BEIR VII Phase 2*)

Procedure range of:	Conventional simple X-rays	Conventional complex X-ray	Computed tomography (CT)	Angiography	Interventional procedures	Internal emitters
Type of examination	◆ Chest films ◆ X-rays of bones and skull ◆ X-ray of abdomen	◆ GI series ◆ Barium enema ◆ Intravenous urogram	◆ Head injuries ◆ Whole-body examinations	◆ Coronary ◆ Aortic ◆ Peripheral ◆ Carotid ◆ Abdominal	◆ Angioplasties with stent placement ◆ Percutaneous dilatations ◆ Closures ◆ Biopsy procedures	◆ Radioisotope studies
Absorbed doses	0.02–10 mGy	3–10 mGy	5–15 mGy	10–200 mGy	10–300 mGy	3–14 mSv (Effective dose)

Radiation effects on cells and tissues

Mechanisms

The energy deposited within a cell by ionizing radiation damages the cell and this may result in its death or in the creation of cell changes (mutations, deletions, chromosomal aberrations), which can affect the normal functioning of the cells and tissue.

In deterministic effects, the probability of causing harm is a function of the dose which is minimal at small doses, but for doses above a certain level the probability increases steeply resulting in total cell death. Furthermore, above the threshold, the severity of the harm will increase with dose. Thresholds for these effects are often at doses ranging from a fraction of a Gy to a few Gy per year but the exact dose at which these cell effects occur depends on both the cell development, and the cell and tissue type.

For stochastic effects there is no threshold and they are all-or-none rather than incremental and may result when an irradiated cell is modified rather than killed. Modified somatic cells may subsequently, sometimes after a prolonged delay, develop into a cancer. There are repair mechanisms to overcome this but the probability of a cancer, resulting from radiation, increases with increasing dose and is often assumed to have no threshold, although the absence of such a threshold is the subject of a lively debate. When the damage occurs in a cell whose function is to transmit genetic information to later generations, this type of stochastic effect is called hereditary.

DNA damage and repair

The inactivation of biological cells by ionizing radiation is mainly due to DNA damage.

For sparsely ionizing radiation these ionization events are distributed over the irradiated cells and produce biochemical damage such as DNA single and double strand breaks as well as base damage and protein lesions.

Damage to DNA in the nucleus is the main initiating event by which radiation causes long-term harm to the cells and tissues. Double stranded breaks are most likely to result in lethal damage. Damage to other cellular components may result in malfunction of the cellular processes.

Late normal tissue effects, including in particular the risk of cancer, are of importance and specific areas of research related to the biological radio-toxicity of critical organs (especially the central nervous system), individual radio sensitivities to radiation carcinogenesis, and the analysis of effects in mixed radiation fields still require more research (NRC 2006; ICRP 2007).

Numerous genes including those for DNA damage repair and cell cycle regulation are involved in cellular response to overcome DNA damage. If the genes coding for a repair protein or for cell cycle arrest are mutated or damaged, there may be insufficient repair or complete lack of repair if the cell cycle is not delayed. One gene that plays a critical role is TP53 tumour suppressor gene, which normally controls both cell cycle arrest and apoptosis (programmed cell death). It acts as a guardian for the cell and if the damage cannot be repaired it triggers cell death: Hence changes in TP53 are critical (Lane 1992).

Cell lethality occurs when the primary lesion cannot be repaired and yields either premature cell aging and differentiation or results in apoptosis. For sparsely ionizing radiation, apoptosis can occur when the DNA lesions are produced in a localized cluster as, for example, in the vicinity of an internalized gamma-producing isotope.

External beams of heavy charged particles produce localized clusters due to the large number of ionizations per unit length along their path; the density of ionizations depends on the velocity and on the charge of the particle. Generally with decreasing velocity the interaction time with the target electrons increases and this yields a greater energy deposition toward the end of each particle trajectory. Like the sparsely ionizing radiation, high LET radiation produces single and double strand breaks; it has, however, a higher probability of producing multiple strand breaks at distances of a limited number of base pairs and therefore the result is a more intense biological effect (ICRP 92).

At the present time, direct evidence of a radiation-associated initiating event due to damage to DNA leading to development of human tumours is limited. The basic assumption is that ionizing radiation interacts with DNA and if this damage is not repaired or if it is incorrectly repaired this may act as an initiating event in tumourigenesis. Mutation in some genes often results in changes in their expression and this may lead to alterations in the biochemical balance of the cell. This, in turn, can compromise the normal functioning of the cell itself as well as bring about changes in proliferation and differentiation, and hence increase the risk of cancer.

Health effects of ionizing radiation

Radiation has always been a natural part of our environment. Natural and artificial sources are identical in their nature and their effect. It is challenging to distinguish between cancers occurring from radiation exposure (both man-made and naturally occurring) and from other causes (NRC 2006; UNSCEAR 2000; ICRP 92).

For example, in Britain elevated childhood leukaemia rates have been reported near some nuclear reactors. Similarly other small studies have also found an increased incidence of childhood leukaemia near some nuclear power stations in Germany and France. However, the results of multi-site studies do not support the hypothesis of an increased risk of leukaemia related to nuclear discharge. The reasons for these increases, or clusters, are unclear and are a cause of controversy and debate (Laurier *et al.* 2002; Zahm & Devesa 1995). These studies highlight the fact that effects from low exposure are still under discussion.

Despite these uncertainties with the effects of low radiation doses, much is understood and known about health effects of radiation since radiation damage has been studied extensively.

The atomic bomb survivors of Hiroshima and Nagasaki continue to be the major source of information on radiation-induced cancer incidence and non-cancer mortality. Genetic aspects of biological risk of chronic multifactorial diseases (e.g. coronary heart disease and diabetes mellitus) due to radiation exposure have also been reported. Epidemiological data from specific radiation accidents are becoming available and are contributing to our understanding of the significance of the mode and rate of the radiation received. These data are important since most occupational radiation exposures are at considerably lower doses where large uncertainty regarding health effects remains (UNSCEAR 1982, 1988, 1993, 1996).

The accident at the Chernobyl nuclear power plant in 1986 was the most serious in history of the nuclear power industry causing a huge release of radioactivity. The highest radiation was received by the emergency workers and about one thousand people were exposed to doses ranging from 2 to 20 Gy. This was fatal for some of these workers. In fact, among them, 28 people died in 1986 due to acute radiation sickness and 19 more have died in the period 1987–2004, although it should be said that one cannot confirm that these latter deaths were due to a direct consequence of exposure to radiation (UNSCEAR 2000; Chernobyl's Legacy 2006).

The lens of the eye is very sensitive to ionizing radiation and may result in opacity (cataracts) at effective doses from 2 Sv. From the Chernobyl data there is evidence for doses as low as 250 mSv causing opacity. Evidence from other data such as astronauts and patients with CT-scans of the head lends support to such low-dose effect.

Progress has also been made in the estimation of genetic effects of radiation, especially since advances in human molecular biology have been incorporated into genetic risk estimation and it is possible to project risks for all classes of genetic diseases. Advances in cell and molecular biology have also contributed new information and newly identified mechanisms through which cells respond to radiation-induced damage as well as the close association between DNA damage and response and cancer development.

Cancer in humans

Radiation-associated cancer in humans has generally been studied in populations/groups that have been exposed to doses higher than the normal background. The majority of such data has come from the atomic bomb survivors as well as medical irradiated patients and those who have been occupationally exposed.

A limited amount of data is also available on the effects of exposure to natural radiation sources.

- For the inhabitants of the areas with high background levels there is no documented evidence to indicate particular health risks. It should be noted that detailed studies capable of detecting a small effect have not been carried out in these populations. In addition, suggestions that exposure to high levels of natural background radiation can induce radio adaptive response resulting in radio resistance (Mortazavi *et al.* 2001) can complicate interpretation of such studies should they be undertaken.
- As already stated, airline crew members receive on average a higher radiation dose than most other workers. An extensive study of cabin crew in Europe (Zeeb *et al.* 2002) showed no measurable increase in mortality that could be attributed to cosmic radiation. It should be noted that there exists also conflicting data from other more limited studies which found some increased risk in breast cancer. In general air travellers will be exposed to lower amounts of cosmic radiation due to the limited flying time and therefore have lower risk of harmful effects from cosmic irradiation than airline workers.
- The major risk of radon inhalation is lung cancer. This has been demonstrated by a number of studies conducted on uranium miners. Recent studies estimate that 6–15 per cent of lung cancers are caused by radon and this is the second most important factor in causing lung cancer, following cigarette smoking. Furthermore lung cancer incidence seems to increase linearly with increasing dose of radon (Darby *et al.* 2005; WHO, Radon Fact Sheet No. 291 2005).

Although the cancer risk estimates have not changed much since 1990 (NRC 1990), the confidence in estimates has increased due to increased epidemiological and biological data.

Available data indicates that an exposure of more than 200 mSv in adults and 100 mSv in children/infants results in excesses of cancer. However, uncertainty remains for doses lower than 100 mSv. Existing epidemiological data on the effects of the X-ray irradiation *in-utero* remain inconclusive.

It is known that ionizing radiation can cause cancer in almost any organ although some sites are more sensitive than others, notably blood (leukaemia), thyroid, and breast. Better understanding has also been reached in terms of differences due to gender and age. Although the difference in absolute risks between men and women is not large, women have somewhat greater sensitivity for solid tumours. Children, on the other hand, have both higher absolute and relative risk. In fact they are considered to be more sensitive to radiation-induced cancer than are adults by almost a factor of 10 (ICRP, Pub 60). This depends on the anatomic site of the cancer and the age at exposure. The risk of breast cancer was highest for Japanese women exposed during puberty, although the risk also increased in women who were younger than 10 years old (an age at which girls have little or no breast tissue) at the time of the explosion. Children are found to be particularly sensitive to thyroid cancer and this has been demonstrated by the Chernobyl studies (UNSCEAR 2000; Chernobyl's Legacy 2006).

Effective doses to the population evacuated from the Chernobyl area in 1986 were estimated to be about 33 mSv on average (Chernobyl's Legacy 2006). It is now known that the main health impact of the Chernobyl accident has been an increase in childhood thyroid cancer resulting from the high intake of radioactive iodine found in contaminated milk. By 2002, about 4000 thyroid cancers in children have been diagnosed and most of these are due to the accident. In contrast, there has been no clearly demonstrated increase of leukaemia and solid cancer tumours in the population around Chernobyl (2000 UNSCEAR Chernobyl's Legacy 2006). However, this conclusion by IAEA and WHO is being challenged by many activists.

One of the most recent and extensive studies of occupational workers (15 country study) was published by Cardis *et al.* (2005) and it suggests that the radiation workers in the nuclear industry face a small increase in the probability of developing cancer.

Ionizing radiation and risk of hereditary effects in humans

There is still no direct evidence that radiation exposure in humans results in an inheritable disease to their off-spring. Studies in experimental animals demonstrate that this occurs and therefore this risk continues to be included in radiation effects (NRC 2006).

Risks and benefits of the use of ionizing radiation in medicine

The magnitude of risk from radiation is dose-related, with higher amounts of radiation being associated with higher risks. The undisputed health benefits of diagnostic X-ray and nuclear medicine may be accompanied by a generally modest risk of harmful effects. This fact has to be taken into account while using ionizing radiation sources in diagnosis.

The risk mentioned above is particularly important for children. In fact they are still growing rapidly and therefore more sensitive to radiation-induced cancer than adults; in addition they have a longer perspective life span and hence the possibility of side-effects arising from such diagnostic procedures is likely to be higher (Brenner *et al.* 2001, Rosen 2001). Therefore, care should be taken to minimize the number of unnecessary X-rays, including dental X-rays, and in optimizing the CT exposure settings when this procedure is indicated.

Experience shows that appropriate selection of conditions, under which ionizing radiation is used in medicine, results in health benefits substantially outweighing the harmful side effects. Indeed, in the recent past, it was felt that there was an over use of dental X-rays in children. A raised awareness with the health professionals of this occurrence has resulted in more careful and timely examinations. Improved digital imaging which results in lower X-ray exposure is being developed and is beginning to be used.

In radiation therapy, large amounts of radiation are required and therefore the risk of radiation-related adverse effects is measurably higher. This is particularly relevant for deeply seated tumours, tumours closely located to critical organs, and in paediatric tumours.

One newly emerging method is the use of charged ions (protons and light ions), with their unique physical and radiobiological properties, which allows highly conformal treatment of various kinds of tumours, while delivering minimal doses to large volumes of surrounding healthy tissues. This means that they can cause severe damage to the DNA in cancer cells while sparing both traversed and deeper healthy tissue. This characteristic also enables them to be used for a more accurate irradiation of the tumour (Amaldi & Kraft 2006).

Topics related to ionizing radiations of public concern

Recent terrorist events have raised concern about the possibility of a terrorist attack involving radioactive materials, possibly through the use of a 'dirty bomb'. The idea behind a dirty bomb is to spread radioactive material into some populated area. Dirty bombs (technically known as Radiological Dispersion Bombs) are devices that use conventional explosives to spread radioactive material (WHO Fact sheet on Radiological Dispersion Device 2003). The primary danger from a dirty bomb would be the blast itself. It is difficult to assess how much of an effect on health might come from the radiation when the source type and activity are unknown. At the levels of most probable sources, not enough radiation would be present in a dirty bomb to cause significant illness. Dirty bombs are designed to spread fear and panic. It is widely believed that most of the harmful effect would come from these conventional explosives rather than from ionizing radiation and furthermore the contamination would occur in a limited area.

To be used in nuclear power plants, the naturally occurring uranium needs to be enriched in the isotope ^{235}U. Depleted uranium is what remains after the removal of the enriched fraction. Compared to the natural uranium it emits less gamma radiation and its contribution to the increase in radiation exposure over natural background is considered negligible (WHO Fact sheet N°257 2003). Contamination from the use of depleted uranium munitions has been studied after the conflict in Kosovo (Depleted Uranium in Kosovo Post-Conflict Environmental Assessment 2001; United Nations Environment Programme) and the conclusions are that the harmful effects are mainly caused by the chemical toxicity rather than by radiation.

Policy and prevention

Recommendations by international commission on radiation protection (ICRP) (2007)

In March 2007, ICRP approved a new set of recommendations for protection against ionizing radiation after carrying out an extended world-wide consultation and these replace the previous recommendations of 1990 (Pub 60). The new recommendations include recent biological and physical information and trends in the setting of radiation standards. However, the overall estimate of the risk of harmful effects after exposure to radiation remains basically the same.

The three key principles of radiological protection remain (i) the justification of activities that could cause or affect radiation exposures, (ii) the optimization of protection in order to keep doses as low as reasonably achievable, and (iii) the use of dose limits. The recommendations state:

(a) No practice involving exposures to radiation should be adopted unless it produces sufficient benefit—to the exposed individuals or to society—to offset the radiation detriment it causes.

(b) In relation to any particular source within a practice, the magnitude of individual doses, the number of people exposed, and the likelihood of incurring exposures where these are not certain to be received should all be kept as low as reasonably achievable, economic and social factors being taken into account.

(c) The exposure of individuals resulting from the combination of all the relevant practices should be subject to dose limits, or to some control of risk in the case of potential exposures. Hence ensuring that no individual is exposed to radiation risks that are judged to be unacceptable from these practices in any normal circumstances. (Individual dose and risk limits.)

Table 8.2.4 Recommended dose limits (from ICRP 2007)

Type of limit	Occupational	Public
Effective dose	20 mSv per year, averaged over defined periods of 5 years	1 mSv in a year
Annual equivalent dose in		
Lens of the eye	150 mSv	15 mSv
Skin	500 mSv	50 mSv
Hands and feet	500 mSv	-

The restrictions on effective dose are sufficient to ensure the avoidance of deterministic effects in all body tissues and organs as shown in Table 8.2.4.

The basis for the control of the occupational exposure of women who are not pregnant is the same as that for men. However, once pregnancy has been declared, the foetus should be protected and the equivalent dose limit to the surface of the woman's abdomen (lower trunk) is 2 mSv for the remainder of the pregnancy.

There has been considerable effort to raise awareness and thereby reduce the rate of lung cancer caused by radon, including the launching of the International Radon Project by WHO (WHO, International Radon Project 2005).

Recommendations for medical exposure

Medical exposures are intended to provide a direct benefit to the exposed individual. If the practice is justified and the protection optimized, the dose in the patient will be as low as is compatible with the medical purposes. Therefore dose limits are generally not applied to medical exposures.

However, there is considerable opportunity for dose reductions in diagnostic radiology using the techniques of optimization of protection and this is important since the second largest exposure to individuals is from medical exposures and this is increasing particularly in the developed countries. Therefore, consideration should be given to the use of dose limits, and investigation levels, selected by the appropriate professional or regulatory agency, for application in common diagnostic procedures. The limits need to be applied with flexibility to allow higher doses when clinically desired.

Conclusions

The nature, frequency, and severity of adverse effects on human health caused by exposure to ionizing and non-ionizing radiation varies depending on the intensity and other exposure parameters and is highly frequency dependent. Potential effects range from rapidly fatal injuries to birth and hereditary defects, cancer, and other chronic diseases. Many effects occur only at high levels and are controlled or reduced by applicable exposure standards. In this chapter, our main emphasis is on exposures common in the everyday life and on long-term effects, which are typically of most concern to the public.

The International Agency for Research on Cancer (IARC) classified ionizing radiation as a 'known' or Group 1 carcinogen; ultraviolet radiation was classified as 'probable human carcinogen', or a Group 2A carcinogen; while extremely low frequency magnetic fields have been classified as a 'possible human carcinogen', or a Group 2B: Static fields as well as extremely low frequency electric fields have been assigned Group 3 (not classifiable as to carcinogenicity to humans). Intermediate frequencies, radiofrequency fields, and infrared radiation have not yet been classified as to their carcinogenic potential.

As it is not possible to eliminate exposure to ionizing radiation, these exposures are kept to a practical minimum. Most recommend avoiding solar UV exposure in order to facilitate the prevention of skin cancers. Because recent literature suggests beneficial effects of solar UV exposure it is critical to develop and adopt a well-balanced set of recommendations regarding this exposure. For ELF magnetic fields given exposure prevalence, considerable scientific uncertainty, and limited public health impact very low-cost precautionary measures are justified. For RF, while health risks have not been identified, potential risk could affect a large number of people because of the ubiquitous nature of the exposure. Thus, given the important gaps in knowledge and availability of no- to low-cost measures, such as use of hands-free device to reduce exposures from mobile phones, such measures can and should be adopted.

Rigorous studies capable of addressing knowledge gaps are urgently needed, particularly for emerging technologies such as mobile phones, MRI exposures, and modern magnetic levitation (maglev) systems.

Acknowledgements

We are grateful to Lawrence Goldstein, Hans-Georg Menzel, Giulio Magrin for helpful comments and to May Gadallah for help in manuscript preparation.

Reference

AGNIR (2003). Health effects from radiofrequency electromagnetic fields. *Report of an independent Advisory Group on Non-ionising Radiation*, 14. NRPB, Chilton, UK.

Ahlbom, A., Day, N., Feychting, M. *et al.* (2000). A pooled analysis of magnetic fields and childhood leukaemia. *British Journal of Cancer*, **83**, 692–8.

Ahlbom, A., Green, A., Kheifets, L. *et al.* (2004). Epidemiology of health effects of radiofrequency exposure. *Environmental Health Perspectives*, **112**(17), Dec.,1741–54.

Akbar-Khanzadeh, F. and Jahangir-Blourchian, M. (2005). Ultraviolet radiation exposure from UV-transilluminators. *Journal of Occupational & Environmental Hygiene*, **2** (10), 493–6.

Amaldi, U. and Kraft, G. (2006). Particle accelerators take up the fight against cancer. CERN Courier, Dec 2006.

Anane, R., Dulou, P.E., Taxile, M. *et al.* (2003). Effects of GSM-900 microwaves on DMBA-induced mammary gland tumors in female Sprague-Dawley rats. *Radiation Research*, 160(4), Oct., 492–7.

Armstrong, B. (1988). Epidemiology of malignant melanoma: intermittent or total accumulated exposure to the sun? *Journal of Dermatologic Surgery & Oncology*, **14** (8), 835–49.

Bastuji-Garin, S. and Diepgen, T. (2002). Cutaneous malignant melanoma, sun exposure, and sunscreen use: epidemiological evidence. *British Journal of Dermatology*, **146** (Suppl. 61), Apr., 24–30.

Boniol, M., De Vries, E., Cobergh, J. *et al.* (2005). Seasonal variation in the occurrence of cutaneous melanoma in Europe: influence of latitude. An analysis using the EUROCARE group of registries. *European Journal of Cancer*, **41**(1), 126–32.

Brenner, D.J., Elliston, C.D., Hall, E.J. *et al.* (2001). 'Estimated risks of radiation-induced fatal cancer from pediatric CT', *American Journal of Roentgenology*, **176**, 289–96.

Burren, R., Scaletta, C., Frenk, E. *et al.* (1998). Sunlight and carcinogenesis: Expression of p53 and pyrimidine dimers in human skin following UVA I, UVA I + II and solar simulating radiations. *International Journal of Cancer*, **76**(2), 201–6.

Cardis, E., Vrijheid, M., Blettner, M. *et al.* (2005). Risk of cancer after low doses of ionising radiation—retrospective cohort study in 15 countries. *British Medical Journal*,[online], 331:77, doi:10.1136/bmj.38499.599861.E0
Available from: http://www.bmj.com/cgi/content/abstract/331/7508/77

Chernobyl's Legacy (2006). Health, Environmental and Socio-economic Impacts. *Chernobyl Forum*, a UN-organized body made up of representatives from the IAEA, WHO, UNDP, UNEP, World Bank, FAO, UNEP, UN-OCHA, UNSCEAR, Belarus, Russian Federation, Ukraine.

Darby, S., Hill, D., Auvinen, A., Barros-Dios J.M. *et al.* (2005). Radon in homes and risk of lung cancer: Collaborative analysis of individual data from 13 European case-control studies. *BMJ*, **330**, 223–30.

De Fabo, E., Noonan, F., Fears, T. *et al.* (2004). Ultraviolet B but not ultraviolet A radiation initiates melanoma. *Cancer Research*, **64**(18), 6372–6.

Dewhirst, M., Viglianti, B., Lora-Michiels, M. *et al.* (2003). Basic principles of thermal dosimetry and thermal thresholds for tissue damage from hyperthermia. *International Journal of Hyperthermia*, **19**(3), 267–94.

Divan H., Kheifets L., Obel C., Olsen J. (2008) 'Prenatal and postnatal exposure to mobile phone use and behavioral problems in children at the age of seven', *Epidemiology*, 19(4), 523–529.

Edwards, C., Gaskell, S., Hill, S. *et al.* (1999). Effects on human epidermis of chronic suberythemal exposure to pure infrared radiation. *Archives of Dermatology*, **135**(5), 608–9.

Elwood, J. and Jopson, J. (1997). Melanoma and sun exposure: An overview of published studies. *International Journal of Cancer*, - **73** (2), 198–203.

Environmental Health Criteria (2006). *Static fields*. World Health Organization, Monograph, vol. 232, Geneva.

European Commission (EC) (1996). *Non-ionizing radiation; sources exposure and health effects*. B-1049 Brussels.

Evans, J., Savitz, D., Kanal, E. *et al.* (1993). Infertility and pregnancy outcome among magnetic resonance imaging workers. *Journal of Occupational Medicine*, **35** (12), 1191–5.

Fears, T., Bird, C., Guerry, D. *et al.* (2002). Average midrange ultraviolet radiation flux and time outdoors predict melanoma risk. *Cancer Research*, **62** (14), 3992–6.

Feychting, M., Ahlbom, A., and Kheifets, L. (2004). EMF and Health. Invited Contribution to *Annual Review of Public Health*, **26**, 165–89.

Garinis, G., Mitchell, J., Moorhouse, M. *et al.* (2005). Transcriptome analysis reveals cyclobutane pyrimidine dimers as a major source of UV-induced DNA breaks. *European Molecular Biology Organization Journal (EMBO)*, **24**, 3952–62.

Goldstein, L., Kheifets, L., van Deventer, E. *et al.* (2002a). Comments of the paper "Long-term exposure of Eμ-Pim 1 transgenic mice to 898.4 MHz microwaves does not increase lymphoma incidence. *Radiation Research*, **158**, 357–64.

Goldstein, L., Kheifets, L., van Deventer, E. *et al.* (2002b). Further Comments of the paper "Long-Term exposure of Eμ-Pim1 transgenic mice to 898.4 MHz microwaves does not increase lymphoma incidence. Comments on Letter to the editor, *Radiation Research*, **159** (6), 835.

Goodman, K., Bible, M., London, S. *et al.* (1995). Proportional melanoma incidence and occupation among white males in Los Angeles County (California, United States). *Cancer Causes & Control*, - **6**, (5), 451–9.

Gowland, P.A. (2005). Present and future Magnetic Resonance sources of exposure to static fields. Progress in Biophysics and Molecular Biology. *Progress in Biophysics and Molecular Biology*, **87**(2–3), 175–83.

Grandolfo, M. and Vecchia, P. (1996). Static electric and magnetic fields: Sources, physical interactions, and bioeffects. In *Non-Ionizing Radiation, Proceedings of the 3rd International Non-Ionizing Radiation Workshop*(ed. R. Mathes, Baden, Austria).

Greenland, S., Sheppard, A.R., Kaune, W.T. *et al.* (2000). A pooled analysis of magnetic fields, wire codes, and childhood leukaemia. *Epidemiology*, **11**, 624–34.

Greenland, S. and Kheifets, L. (2006). Leukemia attributable to residential magnetic fields: Results from analyses allowing for study biases. *Risk Analysis*, **26**, 471–81.

Hall, E. (2006). 'Intensity-modulated radiation therapy, protons, and the risk of second cancers', *International Journal of Radiation Oncology Biology Physics*, **65** (1), 1–7.

Heynick, L.N. and Merritt, J.H. (2003). Radiofrequency fields and teratogenesis. *Bioelectromagnetics*, Suppl 6, S174–86.

ICNIRP (1994). Guidelines on limits of exposure to static magnetic fields. *Health Physics*, **66**, 100–6.

International Agency for Research on Cancer Working Group on artificial ultraviolet light and skin (2006). The association of use of sun beds with cutaneous malignant melanoma and other skin cancers: A systematic review. *International Journal of Cancer*, **120** (5), 1116–22.

International Association of Cancer Registries (IARC) (2002). Non-ionizing radiation, Part 1: Static and extremely low-frequency (ELF) electric and magnetic fields. *Monographs of the Evaluation of Carcinogenic Risks to Humans*, vol. 80. Lyon, France.

International Commission on Radiological Protection (ICRP) (1990). *Recommendations of the ICRP*. ICRP Publication 60:1990. Pergamon, Elsevier Science, Oxford, UK.

International Commission on Radiological Protection (ICRP) (2003). *Relative biological effectiveness (RBE), quality factor (QF), and radiation weighting factor (WR)*. A report of the International Commission on Radiological Protection. ICRP Publication 92: Ann ICRP vol.33, pp.1–117.

International Commission on Radiological Protection (ICRP) (2004). *"Managing patient dose in digital radiology"*, Publication 93, Annals of ICRP, Elsevier Science.

International Commission on Radiological Protection (ICRP) (2007). *Recommendations. Annals of the ICRP)* **37** (6), Elsevier Science.

Kheifets, L., Afifi, A., Buffler, P. *et al.* (1995). Occupational electric and magnetic field exposure and brain cancer: a meta-analysis. *Journal of Occupational And Environmental Medicine*,**37** (12), 1327–41.

Kheifets, L., Afifi, A., Buffler, P. *et al.* (1997). Occupational electric and magnetic field exposure and leukemia. A meta-analysis. *Journal of Occupational And Environmental Medicine*, **39** (11), 1074–91.

Kheifets, L., Afifi, A., and Shimkhada, R. (2006). Public health impact of extremely low frequency electromagnetic fields. *Environmental Health Perspectives*, **114**, 1532–7.

Kheifets, L., Ahlbom, A., Feychting, M. *et al.* (2007). Extremely low-frequency magnetic fields and heart disease: Review and commentary. *Scandinavian Journal of Work Environment and Health*. **33** (1), Feb.,5–12.

Kheifets, L., Repacholi, M., Saunders, R. *et al.* (2005). Sensitivity of children to EMF. *Pediatrics*, **116** (2), August, e303–13.

Kheifets, L., Sahl, J., Shimkhada, R. *et al.* (2005). Developing policy in the face of scientific uncertainty: Interpreting 0.3 μT or 0.4 μT cut points from EMF epidemiologic studies. *Risk Analysis*, **25**, 927–35.

Krause, R., Matulla-Nolte, B., Esser, M. *et al.* (2006). UV radiation and cancer prevention: What is the evidence?. *Anticancer Research*, **26** (4A), 2723–7.

Lane, D.P. (1992). p53, guardian of the genome. *Nature* **358**, 15–16.

Laurier, D., Grosche, B., and Hall, P. (2002). Risk of childhood leukaemia in the vicinity of nuclear installations findings and recent controversies. *Acta Oncologica*, **41**, 14–24.

Lydahl, E. and Philipson, B. (1984). Infrared radiation and cataract II. Epidemiologic investigation of glass workers. *Acta Ophthalmologica*, **62**, (6), 976–92.

Lydahl, E. and Philipson, B. (1984). Infrared radiation and cataract. I. Epidemiologic investigation of iron- and steel-workers. *Acta Ophthalmologica*, **62**, (6), 961–75.

Mack, T. and Floderus, B. (1991). Malignant melanoma risk by nativity, place of residence at diagnosis, and age at migration. *Cancer Causes & Control*, **2**, (6), 401–11.

McIntyre, D., Charman, W., and Murray, I. (1993). Visual safety of quartz linear lamps. *Annals of Occupational Hygiene*, **37**, (2), 191–200.

McKenzie, R., Björn, L., Bais, A. *et al.* (2003). Changes in biologically active ultraviolet radiation reaching the Earth's surface. *Photochemical & Photobiological Sciences*, **2** (1), 5–15.

Meffert, H. and Piazena, H. (2002). Effects of artificial infrared raditaion on human beings. *Acta Dermalogica*, **28**, 187–92.

Mezei, G. and Kheifets, L. (2005). Selection bias and its implications for case-control studies: a case study of magnetic field exposure and childhood leukaemia. *International Journal of Epidemiology*, **35**, 397–406.

Mortazavi, S., Ghiassi, N., and Beitollahi, M. (2001). Very High Background Radiation Areas (VHBRAs) of Ramsar: Do we need any regulations to protect the inhabitants? *Proceedings of the 34th midyear meeting, Radiation Safety and ALARA Considerations for the 21st Century*, California, USA, 177-182. Available from:http://www.angelfire.com/mo/radioadaptive/ramsar.html.

National Institute of Environmental Health Sciences (NIEHS) (1999). *NIEHS Report on Health Effects from Exposure to Power-Line Frequency Electric and Magnetic Fields*. National Institute of Environmental Health Sciences, National Institutes of Health: Research Triangle Park, NC, NIH Publication, no. 99-4493.

National Research Council (NRC) (2006). *Health risks from exposure to low levels of ionizing radiation, BEIR VII Phase 2*. National Academies Press, Washington, DC.

National Research Council (NRC) (1990). *Health effects of exposure to low levels of ionizing radiation: BEIR V*. National Academies Press, Washington, DC.

Neubauer, G., Feychting, M., Hamnerius, Y. *et al.* (2006). Feasibility of future epidemiological studies on possible health effects of mobile phone base stations. *Bioelectromagnetics*, **28** (3), 224–30.

Ogita, S., Imanaka, M., Matsuo, S. *et al.* (1990). Effects of far-infrared radiation on lactation. *Annals of Physiological Anthropology*, **9** (2), 83–91.

Osterlind, A., Tucker, M., Stone, B. *et al.* (1988). The Danish case-control study of cutaneous malignant melanoma. II. Importance of UV-light exposure. *International Journal of Cancer*, **42**, (3), 319–24.

Pfahlberg, A., Kolmel K-F., and Gefeller, O. (2001). Timing of excessive ultraviolet radiation and melanoma: epidemiology does not support the existence of a critical period of high susceptibility to solar ultraviolet radiation- induced melanoma. *British Journal of Dermatology*, **144** (3), 471–5.

Polichetti, A. and Vecchia, P. (1998). Exposure of the general public to low-and medium-frequency electromagnetic fields. In: *Proceedings of the 3rd COST 244bis workshop on the intermediate frequency range* (eds. L. Miro and R. de Seze). April 25–26 1998, Paris.Polk, C. and Postow, E. (1996). *Biological effects of electromagnetic fields*. CRC Press, Florida.

Ramos, J., Villa, J., Ruiz, A. *et al.* (2004). UV dose determines key characteristics of nonmelanoma skin cancer. *Cancer Epidemiology, Biomarkers & Prevention*, **13** (12), 2006–11.

Repacholi, M.H., Basten, A., Gebski, V. *et al.* (1997). Lymphomas in E mu-Pim1 transgenic mice exposed to pulsed 900 MHZ electromagnetic fields. *Radiation Research*, **147** (5), May, 631–40.

Rigel, D., Rigel, E., and Rigel, A. (1999). Effects of altitude and latitude on ambient UVB radiation. *Journal of the American Academy of Dermatology*, **40** (1), 114–6.

Rosen, N.S. (2001). Taking care of children. *American Journal of Roentgenology*, **177**, 715–17.

Simon, J.and Szumowski, J. (1992). Proton (fat/water) chemical shift imaging in medical magnetic resonance imaging. Current status. *Investigative Radiology*, **27** (10), 865–74.

Solomon, C.C., White, E., Kristal, A.R. *et al.* (2004). Melanoma and lifetime UV radiation. *Cancer Causes & Control*, **15** (9), 893–902.

Takebayashi, T., Akiba, S., Kikuchi, Y. *et al.* (2006). Mobile phone use and acoustic neuroma risk in Japan. *Occupational and Environmental Medicine*, **63** (12), 802–7.

The International Commission on Non-Ionizing Radiation Protection (2006). ICNIRP statement on far infrared radiation exposure. *Health Physics*, **91** (6), 630–45.

United Nations Scientific Committee on the Effects of Atomic Radiation (UNSCEAR) (1982). *Ionizing Radiation: Sources and Biological Effects*. The 1982 Report to the General Assembly with Annexes. United Nations, New York.

United Nations Scientific Committee on the Effects of Atomic Radiation (UNSCEAR) (1988). *Sources, Effects, and Risks of Ionizing Radiation*. The 1988 Report to the General Assembly with Annexes. United Nations, New York.

United Nations Scientific Committee on the Effects of Atomic Radiation (UNSCEAR) (1993). *Sources and Effects of Ionizing Radiation*. Report to the General Assembly, with Scientific Annexes. United Nations, New York.

United Nations Scientific Committee on the Effects of Atomic Radiation (UNSCEAR) (1996). *Sources and Effects of Ionizing Radiation*. Report to the General Assembly with Scientific Annex. United Nations, New York.

United Nations Scientific Committee on the Effects of Atomic Radiation (UNSCEAR) (2000). *Sources and Effects of Ionizing Radiation*. UNSCEAR Report to the General Assembly, Volume II: Effects. United Nations, New York.

United Nations Scientific Committee on the Effects of Atomic Radiation (UNSCEAR) (2001). *Hereditary Effects of Radiation*. The 2002 Report to the General Assembly with Scientific Annex. United Nations, New York.

Van der Leun, J. and de Gruijl, F. (2002). Climate change and skin cancer. *Photochemical & Photobiological Sciences*, **1** (5), 324–6.

Walter, S., King, W., and Marrett, L. (1999). Association of cutaneous malignant melanoma with intermittent exposure to ultraviolet radiation: results of a case-control study in Ontario, Canada. *International Journal of Epidemiology*, **28** (3), 418–27.

Wang, S.Q., Setlow, R., Berwick, M. *et al.* (2001). Ultraviolet A and melanoma: A review. *Journal of the American Academy of Dermatology*, **44** (5), 837–46.

Whiteman, D., Whiteman, C., and Green, A. (2001). Childhood sun exposure as a risk factor for melanoma: A systematic review of epidemiologic studies. *Cancer Causes & Control*, **12**(1), 69–82.

World Health Organization (2007). *Extremely low frequency (ELF) fields. Environmental Health Criteria, 238. 2007* [online] Geneva, World Health Organization. 430 p. Available at: <http://www.who.int/peh-emf/publications/elf_ehc/en/index.html>.

World Health Organization (2005). *Radiation and Environmental Health, Information sheet Cosmic Radiation and Air travel, Nov 2005* [online]. Geneva World Health Organization. Available at:<http://www.who.int/ionizing_radiation/env/cosmic/WHO_Info_Sheet_Cosmic_Radiation.pdf>

World Health Organization (2003). *The International Radon Project (IRP)*. Geneva, World Health OrganizationAvailable at: <www.who.int/ionizing_radiation/env/radon/en/>

World Health Organization (2003), *Depleted uranium Fact sheet N° 257* [online]. January 2003,Geneva, World Health Organization. Available at: <http://www.who.int/mediacentre/factsheets/fs257/en/>.

World Health Organization (2005). *Radon and cancer Fact sheet N° 291* [online], June 2005. Geneva, World Health Organization. Available at: < http://www.who.int/mediacentre/factsheets/fs291/en/index.html>World Health Organization (2006), *Health effects of the Chernobyl accident: an overview.*

Fact sheet N° 303[online], April 2006, Geneva, World Health Organization. Available at: < http://www.who.int/mediacentre/factsheets/fs303/en/>

World Health Organization (2003). *Radiological Dispersion Device (Dirty Bomb)*[online]. Geneva, World Health Organization. Available at: < http://www.who.int/ionizing_radiation/en/WHORAD_InfoSheet_Dirty_Bombs21Feb.pdf >

Yu, S.Y., Chiu, J.H., Yang, S.D. *et al.* (2006). Biological effect of far-infrared therapy on increasing skin microcirculation in rats. *Photodermatology, Photoimmunology & Photomedicine*, **22**, (2), 78–86.

Zahm, S.H. and Devesa, S.S. (1995). Childhood cancer: Overview of incidence trends and environmental carcinogens. *Environmental Health Perspectives*, **103**, 177–84.

Zeeb, H., Blettner, M., Langner, I. *et al.* (2002).'Mortality from Cancer and Other Causes among Airline Cabin Attendants in Germany, 1960–1997'. *American Journal of Epidemiololgy*, **156**, 556–65.

8.3

Control of microbial threats: Population surveillance, vaccine studies, and the microbiological laboratory

Frank Sorvillo and Shira Shafir

Scope and burden of infectious diseases

Globally, the burden of infectious diseases remains staggering, exacting an enormous toll in terms of morbidity, mortality, and disability, as well as resulting in significant economic costs and impeding development. Although data are imperfect, annually an estimated 12–13 million deaths, many of them preventable, are caused by infectious agents. Worldwide, five of the top eight causes of years of life lost are infectious diseases and the impact as measured in disability-adjusted life years (DALYs) is substantial (Table 8.3.1) (Lopez & Mathers 2006; World Health Organization 2004). The toll of infectious agents on children is particularly high. In 2001, an estimated 10.6 million children died, 99 per cent of whom lived in low- and middle-income countries (Black *et al.* 2003). Over 50 per cent of these deaths were attributable to acute respiratory infections, diarrhoea, measles, malaria, and HIV/AIDS (Lopez *et al.* 2006). The ancillary tragic effects of infectious agents including infertility, adverse birth outcomes, and disfigurement are considerable. Although exact figures are difficult to determine, it has been estimated that the global economic burden for tuberculosis alone is a massive US$12 billion annually and for malaria an estimated US$14 billion on the African continent alone (World Health Organization 2005). Even in developed countries, where public health measures have led to substantial reductions in the impact of infectious diseases, the toll from food-borne, sexually transmitted, nosocomial, blood-borne, and emerging infections remains high.

Table 8.3.1 Estimated annual mortality and disability-adjusted life years (DALYs) for leading infectious diseases

Disease	Estimated number of deaths (millions)	DALYs (thousands)
Respiratory diseases	> 2	94 037
Tuberculosis	1.6–2.6	36 040
Malaria	1–3	42 280
Diarrhoeal diseases	1.5–2.5	62 451
HIV/AIDS	2.5–3.5	88 429

2001 data for the DALYs. (WHO 2002.)

Types of microbial threats

Important microbial threats include traditional infectious diseases, emerging and re-emerging agents, microbial resistance, the intentional use of infectious agents (bioterrorism), and pathogens linked to chronic conditions. Nosocomial, food-borne, waterborne, zoonotic, and arthropod-borne infections are among the traditional, emerging, and bioterrorism threats.

Traditional infectious diseases

Traditional infectious diseases such as measles, diarrhoeal diseases, and acute respiratory infections continue to be important and preventable causes of significant human suffering, particularly in the developing world. Despite the availability of an effective vaccine, deaths from measles still total over 500 000 globally each year (Centers for Disease Control and Prevention 2005). Respiratory infections are responsible for widespread morbidity and disability, and annually cause an estimated 2 million deaths, principally among children (Mulholland 2003). Diarrhoeal illnesses take 3 million lives, exacerbate malnutrition, and impede child development (Keusch *et al.* 2007). Infectious diseases continue to cause significant mortality in developed countries as well (Redelings *et al.* 2005).

Emerging infectious diseases

Emerging and re-emerging agents are newly recognized infections or traditional pathogens that have become resurgent. In the past three decades more than 30 new infectious diseases have been identified. The most prominent of these is HIV/AIDS, which has caused 40 million deaths and infected an estimated 200 million worldwide in just 25 years since it was first recognized. Severe acute respiratory syndrome (SARS), caused by a previously unrecognized coronavirus, was first identified in late 2002 and by spring 2003 a serious multi-country epidemic was unfolding (Mazzulli *et al.* 2004). Eventually, over 30 countries on 5 continents were affected, with over 8000 cases and nearly 800 deaths being reported. Moreover, long-recognized diseases such as malaria and tuberculosis have re-emerged with force. Approximately 40 per cent of the world's population has been exposed to malaria and over 100 countries have been impacted, with 1–3 million deaths (mostly children less than 5 years old in Africa) and an estimated 500 million acute episodes annually (Breman *et al.* 2004; Nahlen *et al.* 2005).

Microbial resistance

Antimicrobial resistance is a serious and growing threat in both developed and developing countries. Resistance of infectious agents can lead to increases in mortality, duration of illness, disease transmission, and treatment costs (Okeke *et al.* 2005). Key resistant organisms exist across the various pathogen types and include *Staphylococcus aureus*, *Salmonella enterica* serotype Typhi, *Vibrio cholerae*, *Shigella* sp., *Streptococcus pneumoniae*, *Neisseria gonorrhoeae*, influenza A (including avian influenza), and multi-drug-resistant *Mycobacterium tuberculosis* and *Plasmodium falciparum*.

Infectious causes of chronic diseases

Infectious agents have been increasingly implicated as causes of important chronic conditions including cancer (e.g. hepatitis C virus [HCV], human papilloma virus [HPV]), peptic ulcer (*Helicobacter pylori*), arthritis (*Borrelia burgdorferi*), and heart disease (e.g. *Trypanosoma cruzi*, *Chlamydia pneumoniae*) (Smolinski *et al.* 2003; O'Connor *et al.* 2006) (Table 8.3.2). Infection is second, only to tobacco, as a cause of cancer (Parsonnet 1999). The availability of hepatitis B immunization and recent licensure of an HPV vaccine demonstrates the potential for the control of selected chronic diseases through immunization. It is likely that the recognized role of infectious agents as causes of chronic diseases will expand.

Table 8.3.2 Selected chronic diseases linked to infectious agents

Disease	Agent
Cervical cancer	HPV
Hepatocellular carcinoma	HBV, HCV
Chronic liver disease	HBV, HCV
Kaposi's sarcoma	Human herpes virus 8
Leukaemia	HTLV 1
Burkitt" lymphoma	Epstein–Barr virus
Bladder cancer	*Schistosoma haematobium*
Peptic ulcer and gastritis	*Helicobacter pylori*
Heart disease	*Trypanosoma cruzi, Chlamydia pneumoniae*
Dementia	Prions
Arthritis	*Borrelia burgdorferi*
Guillain–Barré syndrome	*Campylobacter jejuni*
Whipple's disease	*Tropheryma whippelii*

Intentional use

The potential for bioterrorism, or the intentional use of microbes to cause harm, has gained significant attention and considerable national funding. Bioweapons have a long history of use, and the anthrax mail attacks in late 2001 in the United States demonstrated the resultant anxiety and financial burden of a bioterrorist event even in the face of just 22 confirmed cases (Jernigan *et al.* 2002). The Centers for Disease Control and Prevention (CDC) has published a list of potential bioterrorism agents; a variety of other microbes can conceivably be used in such attacks as well (Centers for Disease Control and Prevention 2000).

Control of microbial threats

A wide array of approaches are available to respond to microbial threats. These include methods such as sanitation, water treatment, personal hygiene, reduction or treatment of reservoir hosts, vector control, environmental interventions, hospital infection-control efforts, and improved nutrition. This chapter focuses on population surveillance, vaccine studies, and the role of the microbiological laboratory in responding to infectious disease problems. Other methods of control and response are presented in detail in Chapter 12.6 (Kim-Farley 2008).

Population surveillance

Surveillance is the collection and analysis of data on the occurrence of disease (or related factors such as behaviours and vector populations) and is the most important and fundamental of activities necessary for control of microbial threats (Buehler 1998; Thacker & Birkhead 2002). An effective surveillance system identifies where disease is occurring, who is being affected, and provides direction on the prioritization of resources for control efforts. Successful targeting of interventions and pursuit of reasonable strategies for control are not possible without a clear understanding of the occurrence, extent, and types of infectious diseases that impact on a community (Table 8.3.3). Surveillance also provides information that enables an evaluation of the effectiveness of ongoing interventions. Ultimately, public health action, either immediate (e.g. removal of a contaminated food product or providing prophylaxis) or long term (e.g. immunization programmes), is taken on the basis of surveillance information. Given this, surveillance is considered

Table 8.3.3 Selected goals of surveillance systems

Assess disease burden.
Determine populations at risk.
Target control efforts.
Evaluate effectiveness of control programmes.
Identify emerging infections.
Detect outbreaks and epidemics.
Monitor microbial resistance.
Recognize acts of bioterrorism early.
Measure and monitor risk factors.
Evaluate vector, reservoir, and intermediate host populations.

the foundation of control measures and among the most essential of public health functions. There has been increasing recognition of the need for evidence-based, data-driven public health decision making; good surveillance systems can provide such data.

Components of surveillance systems

Effective surveillance systems have several key components (Teutsch *et al.* 2000). These include clearly defined objectives, sound case definitions, defined data source(s), established data collection mechanism(s), an efficient data collection instrument (typically a questionnaire), field testing of methods (including piloting of questionnaires), implementation of data quality standards, development of a relevant analysis plan, and identification of a dissemination mechanism for results (Centers for Disease Control and Prevention 1997, 2001). A high level of completeness and timeliness are other important characteristics of sound population surveillance systems. The success of a surveillance system is dependent on its sensitivity to detect disease occurrence, the acceptability of participants such as physicians and hospitals, flexibility of the system to address new questions, and whether the data collected is representative of disease occurrence in the target population.

A commitment to comprehensive and timely surveillance requires dedicated resources including adequate funding and training of epidemiologists and other public health staff. Successful microbial disease surveillance systems must also have a strong laboratory component. The role of the microbiology laboratory is discussed in detail later in this chapter.

Active and passive surveillance approaches

Generally, surveillance systems can be classified as passive or active in nature. In passive surveillance methods, health authorities depend on the reporting of infectious diseases by practitioners and/or laboratories. Often, there is a list of notifiable diseases that are required by law to be reported. Passive surveillance is notorious for significant under-reporting and considerable lag times (Kimball *et al.* 1980; Ewart *et al.* 1995; Standaert *et al.* 1995).

Active surveillance is far more time- and labour-intensive. In active surveillance approaches, public health staff search for cases of communicable diseases by routinely contacting health-care providers, clinics, laboratories, and hospitals, or by regularly visiting health-care facilities to review medical logs and records for the occurrence of selected diseases. Increasingly, electronic transfer of data, where available, is facilitating such active surveillance methods. Other approaches include establishing sentinel reporting sites in the community and conducting surveys. Active surveillance methods are typically more complete and timely but may often require considerable resources. A number of newer, innovative approaches to surveillance have been pursued because of concerns over the possible intentional use of infectious agents and are discussed under novel surveillance methods.

Sources of surveillance data

There are many different types of data sources for population surveillance, each with advantages and disadvantages (Table 8.3.4). The principal sources are discussed in the following.

Traditional morbidity reporting

Health-care providers: Historically, the most common source of communicable disease surveillance information has been through the passive reporting of cases by health-care providers.

Table 8.3.4 Types of data sources for population surveillance systems

Passive reporting from health-care providers
Active contact of providers
Electronic transfer of data from health-care providers
Laboratory reporting (passive)
Electronic transfer of data from laboratories
Syndromic surveillance
Population and subgroup surveys
Sentinel systems
Mortality records
Pharmacy records
Absenteeism records (school and business)
Media reports
Internet reports
Enhanced surveillance at mass gatherings

Many countries require the reporting of selected infectious diseases (Thacker & Birkhead 2002). For example, laws and statutes make mandatory the reporting of 50–130 notifiable diseases to state health departments in the United States. Although such passive systems are adequate for selected (usually severe) diseases, they suffer from significant completeness and timeliness issues. For example, studies of measles in Los Angeles County and shigellosis in Washington, DC found that only about 30 per cent of the cases were reported (Kimball *et al.* 1980; Ewart *et al.* 1995). Standaert and colleagues (1995) reported a median lag time of 24 days in the reporting of invasive disease caused by *Neisseria meningitidis* and *Haemophilus influenzae*, two infections for which effective prophylaxis of contacts is available. Active surveillance conducted by public health staff can improve the performance of morbidity surveillance. More recently, health authorities have explored the transfer of data from central computerized systems of clinicians and acute-care sites (Travers *et al.* 2003).

Laboratories: Laboratory reporting is another useful adjunct for case identification, and the electronic transfer of data from laboratories offers the potential for improving sensitivity and reducing lag times. Moreover, laboratories provide important surveillance for the emergence of microbial resistance as well as genetic characterization of agents that can assist in the determination of the source of infection. A genetic match between organisms isolated from patients and a suspect source provides strong implicating evidence. Laboratory information may also be useful in predicting outbreak or pandemic potential, as in characterization of influenza isolates. However, laboratory data may suffer from a lack of clinical and demographic information, and the expanding use of large regional laboratories can complicate case allocation to the appropriate geographic jurisdictions. PulseNet is a system designed to detect food-borne disease case clusters by pulsed-field gel electrophoresis (PFGE). This can facilitate early identification of common-source outbreaks and assist epidemiologists in their investigation by enabling separation of outbreak-associated cases from sporadically occurring, non-outbreak related cases. The utility of PulseNet was recently demonstrated in detecting an outbreak of *Escherichia coli* O157:H7 that was linked to fresh spinach across several states in the United States (Centers for Disease Control and Prevention 2006).

Absenteeism: School and business absenteeism data can provide useful surveillance information for conditions such as influenza, which cause widespread community illness (Lenaway & Ambler 1995; Takahashi *et al.* 2001). Use of such data has been employed for influenza surveillance activities in a wide variety of jurisdictions. Given that reporting is typically voluntary, individual schools or businesses may not comply for every reporting period, and consequently, establishment of meaningful baselines is difficult. Nevertheless, as a crude measure, and one that can be combined with other data sources, such information can be valuable.

Hospital discharge data: Use of hospital discharge data, although typically not timely, can provide beneficial information on the burden of infectious diseases and are useful in evaluating the completeness of other surveillance data sources (Huff *et al.* 1996). Given that it reflects disease severe enough to warrant hospitalization, such data can be an important community indicator but will lack sensitivity as a surveillance tool for less virulent infections.

Mortality data: Mortality data is a population-based data source that is vital for measuring the burden of disease and targeting control efforts against the most severe conditions as well as for evaluating the impact of interventions. In many countries, mortality data are routinely collected and readily accessible in electronic format for analysis purposes. Although historically death certificate data have been used primarily to measure the burden of chronic diseases, increasingly, health jurisdictions are utilizing data on cause of death for assessing infectious disease problems (Redelings *et al.* 2005; McCoy *et al.* 2004). Typically, long lag times prevent the use of mortality data for immediate response purposes; however, the implementation of electronic, web-based systems for death registration offer the promise of timely availability of mortality data that can be directed to health authorities on a near real-time basis. Routinely collected mortality data are generally not available in developing countries. Consequently, data on leading causes of death must rely on other methods, such as surveys.

Birth registries: Information from birth registries can also be useful both directly and indirectly for measuring infectious disease occurrence. Most registries contain data on the occurrence of foetal death, congenital anomalies, including congenital syphilis, and low birth weight. Increasing evidence indicates an important role of infectious agents in inducing premature birth and low birth weight. Such data may therefore augment standard surveillance activities.

Syndromic surveillance: Syndromic surveillance is an approach that collects data on the occurrence of syndromes, such as pneumonia or rash-like illnesses, before a definitive diagnosis is made (Buehler *et al.* 2003; Buehler 2004). Such a method, which often uses emergency department data (Travers *et al.* 2003), theoretically can result in earlier detection of outbreaks of disease and promote more rapid public health response. Concern over the potential for bioterrorism has heightened the interest in syndromic surveillance among public health officials. However, such systems may have problems with specificity (false-positive cases and outbreaks), and debate over the utility of syndrome-based systems persists.

Sentinel systems: Sentinel systems typically employ a series of volunteer providers or health-care facilities who agree to report selected conditions. This approach has been used for influenza surveillance purposes where providers report cases of influenza-like illness and/or provide specimens for confirmatory testing and characterization of strains. Given that influenza is not reportable in most jurisdictions, such alternative approaches are necessary for surveillance purposes. Because sentinel systems are voluntary, participation can often be erratic, and therefore, the establishment of baselines and the analysis of data can be problematical. Sentinel surveillance of animals is also routinely used to detect possible activity of important infectious agents. Assessing the seroconversion of sentinel chickens to viral infections such as St. Louis encephalitis and West Nile viruses can detect local activity before human cases occur (Buckley *et al.* 2007). In Peru, cysticercosis control activities have used sentinel pigs as a means of detecting environmental contamination with the eggs of *Taenia solium* (Gonzalez *et al.* 1994). Pathogen surveillance of both wild and domestic animals can also be important in early identification of potential emerging infections (Kuehn 2006).

Environmental testing: The surveillance of water sources through testing for evidence of faecal contamination has been a routine and standard method to evaluate waterborne disease risk. More recently, testing of selected foods, such as ready-to-eat meats and soft cheeses, for Listeria monocytogenes has been used to identify risk foods and reduce contamination and transmission of food-borne diseases (Peng & Shelef 2002).

Surveys: The use of surveys, including population-based and subgroup approaches, can provide valuable data on the occurrence of disease or risk behaviours. Examples of such surveys include the following:

The Behavioural Risk Factor Surveillance System (BRFSS), initiated in 1984, is an annual, ongoing telephone health-survey system, tracking health conditions and risk behaviours in the United States (Li *et al.* 2004). Conducted by the 50 state health departments as well as those in the District of Columbia, Puerto Rico, Guam, and the US Virgin Islands, BRFSS provides data on the self-reported prevalence of a variety of behaviours and diseases. Federal, state, and local health officials and researchers use this information to track health risks, identify emerging problems, and direct intervention programmes.

The National Health and Nutrition Examination Survey (NHANES) is a population-based survey that is conduced every 10 years by the National Center for Health Statistics to survey the dietary habits and health of US residents (Alter *et al.* 1999). Mobile examination centres collect data on height and weight as well as other information. The National Health Interview and California Health Interview surveys are other interview-based efforts that are conducted on a regular basis in the United States.

Similarly, environmental surveys to assess the population of selected vectors and reservoir animals, as well as determine types of infection and prevalence rates, can provide valuable information for targeting control efforts and assessing potential future threats (Kuehn 2006).

Geographic information systems (GISs): Mapping the geographic occurrence of disease is a vital surveillance tool, and GISs are the powerful, modern-day equivalent of John Snow's classic 'spot map' of cholera cases in London. The GIS is a computer-based system that can present the geographic distribution of diseases coupled with other key information including topography, climate, vegetation, water sources, housing, vectors, or any spatial variable for which data are available. Such 'layering' of information can be invaluable in identifying risk factors and sources of infection as well as for targeting and assessing intervention efforts (McKee *et al.* 2000). The GIS is more than just a visualization tool: Sophisticated statistical analyses, including assessment of space–time clustering, and diffusion models can also be applied using GIS technology.

Novel surveillance approaches

A number of novel approaches to active surveillance, propelled by concerns over bioterrorism, have been implemented in an effort to improve the completeness and timeliness of infectious disease surveillance (Pavlin *et al.* 2003; Desenclos 2006). Among these include the following:

Electronic Surveillance System for the Early Notification of Community-Based Epidemics (ESSENCE I): In 1999, the Walter Reed Army Institute of Research created ESSENCE I to detect and track infectious disease outbreaks among approximately 9 million military active-duty personnel, their dependents, and retirees (Pavlin *et al.* 2004). Using electronic data from all military treatment facilities, selected International Classification of Diseases (ICD-9) codes indicating infectious diseases are grouped into similar diagnostic categories (Lober *et al.* 1993).

ESSENCE II: An expanded version of ESSENCE I that integrates data from a variety of diverse sources including military ambulatory visits and prescription medications, and merges them with civilian emergency department chief-complaint records, school-absenteeism data, over-the-counter and prescription medications sales, civilian ambulatory visits, veterinary health records, and health department requests for influenza testing (Lomabardo *et al.* 2004).

Real-time Outbreak and Disease Surveillance (RODS): RODS is a computer-based public health surveillance system for early detection of infectious disease outbreaks. It uses clinical (chief complaint) and demographic data collected at patient registration at selected emergency departments and acute-care facilities (Estacio 2006). Data are transferred electronically in real time. The RODS system automatically classifies the registration chief complaint into one of seven syndrome categories.

Public health liaisons: Assigning public health workers to emergency departments and acute-care clinics with the sole purpose of collecting data on infectious diseases or syndromes provides staff who are dedicated to surveillance and therefore does not rely on possibly overburdened clinicians. This approach, sometimes termed 'drop-in surveillance', may be particularly useful during special high profile and/or large-scale events such as the Olympic Games or political conventions. As with other methods, establishing baseline levels and thresholds for detecting outbreaks can be problematic.

Web-based field collection: Historically, field collection of data including clinical, demographic, exposure, and geographic information has relied on paper data-collection methods. Such systems are cumbersome, inefficient and, because of the need to transcribe into computer systems, can be fraught with error. The feasibility of using PDAs and laptop computers with wireless Internet connections for field collection of data has been demonstrated (*Lober et al.* 1993). Such an approach can improve the timeliness and accuracy of information and allow more rapid response, particularly to emergency situations.

BioWatch: BioWatch is an environmental surveillance effort employed in the United States that uses a network of air samplers maintained by the Environmental Protection Agency to detect possible dispersal of an airborne bioterrorism agent (Estacio 2006). These devices are placed in densely populated areas of undisclosed cities. Filters from the samplers are removed at least once each day and transported to a designated laboratory that is part of the Laboratory Response Network, where the samples are analysed using PCR technology. A positive result from these tests would trigger an immediate evaluation to rule out a possible false-positive finding. If the initial test result is confirmed, agent-specific response activities, including antibiotic prophylaxis or administration of vaccines, would be initiated.

Global surveillance programmes

Infectious diseases are not constrained by political or other artificial boundaries. The SARS epidemic is a recent example of the ready movement of people and infection. In just a few months, a major outbreak in southern China became an epidemic halfway around the globe in Toronto. This event underscores the importance of establishing robust global surveillance efforts (Table 8.3.5).

Global Public Health Intelligence Network (GPHIN): Among the most innovative of surveillance approaches is the GPHIN implemented by the Public Health Agency of Canada. GPHIN is a secure, Internet-based 'early warning' system that monitors global media reports including news wires and Web sites gathering preliminary reports of potential public health significance in seven languages on a real-time, continuous basis. The information is initially evaluated by an automated process and then analysed by the Public Health Agency of Canada GPHIN officials. Identified reports that may have serious public health consequences are immediately forwarded to users, which include the global public health community.

Early Warning and Response System (EWRS): EWRS, an Internet-based system, was established in 1998 by the European Union to ensure rapid communication between public health authorities

Table 8.3.5 Selected global surveillance systems

Global Public Health Intelligence Network (GPHIN)
Early Warning and Response System (EWRS)
Global Emerging Infections System (GEIS)
Global Influenza Surveillance Network
Program for Monitoring Emerging Diseases (ProMed)
Global Outbreak Alert and Response Network (GOARN)
Pacific Public Health Surveillance Network (PACNET)

of EU Member States for the control of communicable disease-related events (Guglielmetti *et al.* 2006). Between 1998 and December 2005, a total of 583 messages regarding 396 events were circulated through the EWRS.

Global Emerging Infections System (GEIS): The US Department of Defense's GEIS is a programme that uses data from the international medical and research units of the Department of Defense. Established in 1997, its principal mission is to identify infectious diseases that may be a threat to US military forces.

Global Influenza Surveillance Network: Coordinated by the World Health Organization, this network serves as a global alert mechanism for the emergence of influenza viruses with pandemic potential. One hundred and sixteen institutions from 87 countries are recognized by the WHO as National Influenza Centers (NICs) (World Health Organization 2007). Annually, the NICs collect more than 175 000 patient samples and submit approximately 2000 viruses to the WHO Collaborating Centers in Australia, United Kingdom, United States, and Japan for antigenic and genetic analyses. Such work is essential to the early recognition of antigenic changes that are important for effective vaccine development and recognition of possible pandemic emergence. Also established is the Global Avian Influenza Network for Surveillance, which targets surveillance for influenza strains in migratory birds (Kuehn 2006).

Program for Monitoring Emerging Diseases (ProMED): The International Society for Infectious Diseases established ProMED in 1994 as a means to take advantage of the Internet for rapidly identifying new diseases, outbreaks, and epidemics (Madoff 2004). ProMED-Mail is a free service that serves as a central site for news, updates, and discussions of outbreaks of emerging and re-emerging diseases that affect human, animal, and plant health. Information is gleaned through staff review of official and unofficial Internet sites as well as emails from subscribers. A panel of expert 'moderators' reviews and interprets the reports and provides commentary. ProMED, which currently has over 32 000 members from more than 150 different countries, posted the first public description of the SARS epidemic.

Global Outbreak Alert and Response Network (GOARN): GOARN is a WHO-sponsored collaboration of existing institutions and networks that pools resources for the rapid identification, confirmation, and response to outbreaks of international importance (World Health Organization 2007). It links technical and operational capabilities from scientific institutions of WHO Member States, medical and surveillance initiatives, regional technical networks, networks of laboratories, United Nations organizations (e.g. UNICEF, UNHCR), the Red Cross (International Committee of the Red Cross, International Federation of Red Cross and Red Crescent Societies, and national societies), and international humanitarian non-governmental organizations (e.g. Médecins sans Frontières, International Rescue Committee, Merlin and Epicentre).

Analysis of surveillance data

Routine, ongoing analysis of surveillance data is critical to infectious disease control efforts. An important component of effective analysis is establishing reasonable case definitions. Frequently, both confirmed cases (through laboratory data) and presumptive cases (typically based on clinical manifestations) are defined. Among the most vital, and often overlooked, aspects of analysis is the necessity for quality control in the collection, recording, and management of data. The most sophisticated analyses may be meaningless without accurate and reliable information. This requires a carefully constructed data-collection instrument, a well-designed data-entry system to reduce errors that may include cross-field edit checks and/or double data entry, and a data-management scheme (e.g. detection of duplicates) to further ensure a high degree of data quality.

Most analyses of surveillance data are generally descriptive and straightforward (Buehler 1998). Tallying disease frequencies and calculation of rates, with descriptive analysis of the standard epidemiologic variables of person, place, and time, is often sufficient. Ongoing evaluation of the occurrence of disease that rises above baseline, or expected, levels is important in detecting possible outbreaks. Such analyses may range from simple techniques including visual assessment to more sophisticated approaches such as time-series analysis (Grijalva *et al.* 2007).

In some cases, more detailed information and special approaches such as case–control or cohort studies, may be needed beyond what are routinely performed. These may include attempts to assess and control for confounding factors when comparing groups. Such efforts may require the use of matched and/or multivariate analyses. Other sophisticated analyses include multilevel modelling that can simultaneously take into consideration both individual and group-level factors (Diez-Roux & Aiello 2005).

Surveillance analysis can be conducted by manual tabulation or, more commonly, through simple computer-aided programmes. Hand tallying increases the potential for error and must be done carefully. EpiInfo™, a free software programme produced by CDC, is used in many countries and jurisdictions for entering and analysing surveillance data and EpiMap, a companion product, can be used for mapping such data.

In the analysis and interpretation of surveillance data, it is essential for public health authorities to be aware of the caveats and limitations of such information. Reported or detected occurrence of infectious diseases in a community will usually be a minimal estimate of actually occurring disease (Fig. 8.3.1). Not all persons infected will manifest clinically apparent illness. Among those that

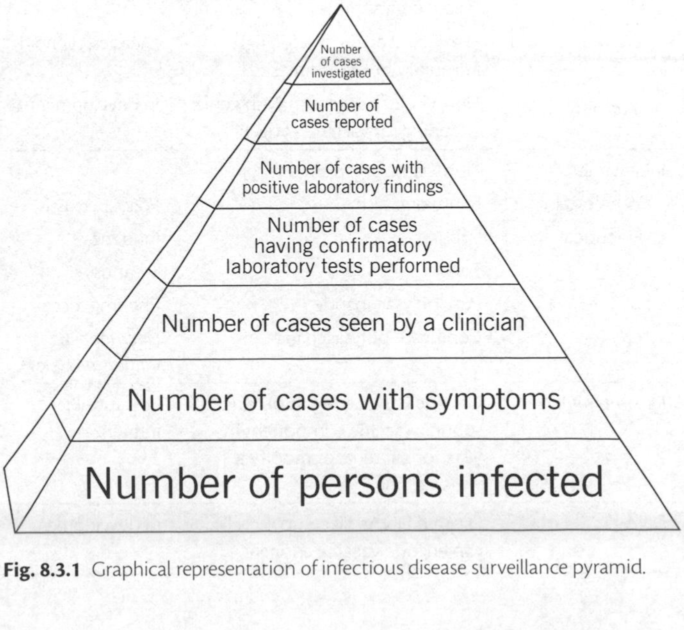

Fig. 8.3.1 Graphical representation of infectious disease surveillance pyramid.

do develop symptoms, not all will seek medical attention. Moreover, for those that are seen by a clinician, typically only a limited number of patients will have laboratory tests performed to identify the infectious agent. In addition, the sensitivity and specificity of laboratory tests must be considered in the evaluation of the reported data (Sorvillo & Nahlen 1990). Therefore, significant misclassification of disease is inevitable. Misclassification of key demographic and exposure variables must also be expected.

A final problem, not widely recognized, is the inherent uncertainty and error in population estimates and the potential errors that can result when calculating rates of disease (Rollin *et al.* 2007). Although the availability and accuracy of population information in under-resourced countries is particularly problematical, this is an issue that must be considered even in jurisdictions that have routine collection of census data.

Problems/needs

To be effective, surveillance systems require political and economic support. Funding, training, ensuring case and patient confidentiality, improved Web-based systems, and use of emerging information technology will be continuing challenges. Resources for population surveillance are particularly needed for developing countries. Ultimately, given the imperfections of individual surveillance methods, the best approaches are those that integrate data from multiple sources.

Vaccine studies for control of microbial threats

A wide array of vaccines are currently available or in development (Table 8.3.6). It is not a hyperbole to suggest that vaccines have been responsible for reducing the burden of human disease and suffering more than any other medical intervention. Moreover, the cost-effectiveness of immunization is striking (Masingnani *et al.* 2003): It has been estimated that for every US$1 spent on the measles-mumps-rubella (MMR) vaccine US$21 is saved in direct medical costs, and the diphtheria–tetanus–pertussis (DTP) vaccine results in a US$24 return for US$1 expenditure (Ehreth 2003).

Table 8.3.6 General types of vaccines and their characteristics with examples.

Vaccine type	Characteristics	Vaccine examples
Live	Viable organism	
Live attenuated	Weakened agent producing immunity but not disease	Measles, typhoid
Vector	Non-virulent organism with genes encoding for vaccine antigens	In development
Inactivated	Non-viable organism or product	
Whole-cell	Entire organism	Polio, pertussis
Fractional	Subunit	Influenza
	Toxoid	Tetanus
	Pure polysaccharide	Pneumococcus
	Conjugate polysaccharide	*Haemophilus influenzae* type B
Recombinant	Genetic engineering to produce subunit vaccine component in yeast or bacteria, or modify a live virus vaccine	Hepatitis B, influenza
DNA	Plasmid DNAs taken up by cells can encode vaccine antigens	In development

Table 8.3.7 Estimated global mortality from selected infectious diseases for which effective vaccines are available.

Disease	Estimated annual deaths
Measles	500 000
Rotavirus infection	600 000
Hepatitis B infection	2 000 000
Tetanus	511 000
Pneumococcal infection	814 000
Meningococcal infection	171 000[a]
Pertussis	300 000
Haemophilus influenzae type B infection	114 000
Rubella	100 000[b]

[a] Number of bacterial meningitis deaths. (Jodar *et al.* 2002.)
[b] Cases of congenital rubella syndrome.

Yet, vaccine-preventable infections continue to cause widespread global disease and considerable mortality (Table 8.3.7). Despite some notable successes, traditional infectious agents for which effective vaccines exist still exact a heavy toll in developing nations and cause periodic outbreaks of disease in industrialized countries as well. Moreover, for many important infectious diseases, including long-standing established microbial threats, emerging infections, and agents likely to be used in a bioterrorism event, vaccines do not exist or are less than optimal.

Vaccine studies across a wide array of issues are critical for expanding the historic successes of immunization efforts in controlling infectious diseases. These studies will need to address areas such as vaccine development, including the use of new technologies, alternative methods of production and administration, evaluation of efficacy and effectiveness in various population groups and settings, efforts to improve our understanding of the immune response to infectious agents, vaccines for reservoir animals, methods to reduce vaccine-related adverse events, approaches to education and acceptance of vaccines, and overcoming social, economic, and political barriers.

Diseases with effective vaccines

Many important traditional infectious agents are readily preventable through immunization. Safe and effective vaccines exist for polio, measles, mumps, rubella, tetanus, diphtheria, hepatitis A and B, and pneumococcal, meningococcal, and rotavirus infections, as well as other agents. Yet measles kills approximately 500 000 annually and causes severe disability, including blindness, deafness, brain and lung damage, and stunted growth and development, among children who survive the disease. Worldwide, an estimated 350 million people are chronic carriers of HBV, many of whom will develop hepatocellular carcinoma and end-stage cirrhosis. Approximately 2 million deaths attributable to HBV occur each year (Kao & Chen 2002). *Streptococcus pneumoniae* accounts for roughly 814 000 deaths among children less than 5 years of age in developing countries annually (Scott 2007). Globally, about 100 000 infants are born with congenital rubella syndrome each year (Robertson *et al.* 2003).

Pertussis affects roughly 50 million annually with approximately 300 000 deaths, mostly among infants, and increased incidence among adults and adolescents has been reported over the past decade (Caro *et al.* 2005). Although dated, an estimate of the worldwide tetanus burden for 1990 suggested a total of 679 000 cases and 511 000 deaths, 427 000 of which occurred among neonates (Galazka *et al.* 2004). Rotavirus is responsible for 29–45 per cent of the hospitalizations for diarrhoea in children less than 5 years of age and causes over 600 000 deaths annually (Parashar *et al.* 2006). *Haemophilus influenza* type B accounts for an estimated 350 000–500 000 deaths among children each year (World Health Organization 2001). Although considerable progress has been made towards polio eradication, this disease remains active in several countries, and mumps, varicella, and meningococcal infection also continue to exact a considerable toll.

Selected diseases without vaccines or with suboptimal vaccines

Effective vaccines have not been developed, or are less than optimal, for a number of the most important infectious causes of global morbidity and mortality including malaria, tuberculosis, HIV/AIDS, respiratory syncytial virus, and hepatitis C virus (HCV) infections. Moreover, vaccines are unavailable or suboptimal for most of the recently emergent infections and potential bioterrorism agents and few have effective treatment options.

The global impact of malaria is staggering and historic control approaches have been complicated by resistance of both the *Plasmodium* parasite (to chemotherapy) and anopheline vectors (to pesticides). Although aggressive efforts have been made to develop an effective malaria vaccine, using a variety of approaches to attack the different stages of the parasite, success has been elusive (Graves & Gelband 2006). Most vaccine efficacy studies have demonstrated little or no protection from infection, and in those studies where reduction in disease has been observed, such effects have been modest.

It is estimated that over 2 per cent of the world's population is infected with HCV, representing 123 million people (Global Burden of Disease Working Group 2004) , approximately 10 per cent of whom will go on to develop cirrhosis or hepatocellular carcinoma. Unfortunately, therapy is less than optimal and a vaccine is lacking for this viral infection. Moreover, there are significant challenges to vaccine development. The fact that HCV can produce chronic infection despite an active immune response, and the capacity for RNA viruses such as HCV to mutate resulting in significant antigenic heterogeneity, are major obstacles that must be overcome (Lechmann & Liang 2000).

Respiratory syncytial virus (RSV) is the leading cause of bronchitis and bronchiolitis in infants and has increasingly been recognized as an important cause of severe lower respiratory tract infection in the elderly as well. Worldwide, an estimated 463 000 children die of RSV infection each year (Openshaw *et al.* 2005). Early trials of several candidate RSV vaccines failed to attain the desired safety and protection against natural infection. Some vaccine types either failed to elicit immunogenicity or resulted in exaggerated disease on natural exposure to the virus. Recent formulations of candidate RSV vaccines have focused on subunit vaccines, preparations employing adjuvants, live attenuated vaccines, genetically engineered live attenuated vaccines, and polypeptide vaccines (Pollack & Karoon 2004).

Tuberculosis (TB) infects approximately one-third of the world's population and is a leading cause of premature death. Although the BCG vaccine is currently used for tuberculosis in some countries, effectiveness is suboptimal. Moreover, treatment of tuberculosis is long and expensive, and drug-resistant strains (including multidrug resistance) of *M. tuberculosis* are increasing. In addition, the HIV pandemic has exacerbated transmission and complicated control efforts. TB is now the leading cause of death among persons with HIV infection, accounting for 25 per cent of the AIDS deaths worldwide (Corbett *et al.* 2003). Several promising efforts to develop a new TB vaccine include live attenuated vaccines, subunit formulations, and vector-based approaches (Girard *et al.* 2005).

In just 25 years since its emergence, HIV/AIDS has become one of the most devastating and intractable pandemics in human history. It is the leading cause of death among adults in the countries of sub-Saharan Africa, and a leading cause of death globally. Combination therapy can prolong survival but is not a cure and remains costly and unavailable to many in high-prevalence areas of the developing world. The persistence of HIV infection, despite a robust but ineffective natural immune response, reflects the inherent challenges of vaccine development. Recent phase III trials of monomeric HIV-1 envelope gp120 vaccine failed to demonstrate efficacy and underscored the inability of neutralizing antibodies to suppress infection (Garber *et al.* 2004). Similarly, the failure of cytotoxic T cells to control HIV infection indicates that approaches to stimulate protective cell-mediated immunity will be challenging as well. Moreover, the genetic diversity of HIV as well as its capacity for change present significant additional hurdles to the development of a successful AIDS vaccine.

Effective vaccines for potential bioterrorism threats are also needed (Cieslak *et al.* 2000). Current anthrax vaccines include *Bacillus anthracis* live spore preparations (the former Soviet Union) and cell-free filtrate-derived products (the United States and the United Kingdom). Given the sizable occurrence (2.4–3.9 per cent) of local adverse reactions and the need for repeated boosters with some vaccine preparations (six-dose primary series for the US vaccine), considerable effort has been devoted to the development of new anthrax vaccines including recombinant, mutant-strain, purified protective antigen (PA), and DNA plasmid preparations.

Although an effective formalin-inactivated plague vaccine was formerly available in the United States, it is no longer being produced. Moreover, local reactions were common and immunity short-lived, necessitating booster doses. In addition, evidence suggests that this vaccine may not provide protection against aerosol exposure, which is the most likely route of dissemination as a bioweapon. Current efforts are focused on evaluating recombinant subunit vaccines as well as live attenuated preparations of the agent, *Yersinia pestis*.

Tularemia, caused by *Francisella tularensis*, can also be disseminated via the airborne route. Although a live attenuated vaccine commonly referred to as the 'live vaccine strain' is available, the preparation is suboptimal. Concerns regarding genetic instability of the vaccine and reversion to virulence or loss of immunogenicity coupled with the required scarification method of administration have accelerated attempts to produce improved vaccines.

Although smallpox was eradicated in 1977, stocks of the virus may exist outside of the WHO-authorized repositories, and there exists the potential use of smallpox in a bioterrorist attack. Vaccinia, the historic smallpox vaccine, was effective enough to result in eradication. However, only relatively small amounts of vaccine currently exist and this supply is gradually losing potency. Moreover, the former method of vaccine production through harvesting from calf lymph is no longer an acceptable process. Early results from a phase-1 trial of cell-culture-derived vaccinia vaccine have demonstrated immunogenicity in both vaccinia-naive and non-naive groups (Greenberg *et al.* 2005).

Many important emerging infections also lack effective vaccines. The potential spread of influenza A H5N1 with its demonstrated capacity to cause severe and fatal human infection, the observed rapid resistance to available antiviral therapy, and concerns regarding its possible adaptation to a strain that can be readily transmitted from person to person, underscore the need to pursue vaccine studies for the control of potentially pandemic influenza strains (Poland 2006). Although effective inactivated and live attenuated vaccines exist, the frequent antigenic changes of the influenza A virus, the challenge in identifying potential epidemic and pandemic strains, and the considerable lag time required for vaccine production present significant impediments to control (Stephenson *et al.* 2006).

Vaccines and therapies are also lacking for many other emerging infectious agents that can cause serious and fatal infection including SARS, Nipah virus, the filoviruses, and *Baylisascaris procyonis* (Whalen 1996).

Vaccine studies for the control of microbial threats

Vaccine studies are needed across a host of scientific, logistical, operational, and epidemiologic arenas. Some of these are discussed next:

Heat-stable vaccine preparations

Currently, the need to refrigerate most vaccines and maintain a cold chain complicates immunization efforts, especially in developing countries. The availability of heat-stable vaccine preparations would reduce the complexity and cost of vaccination and significantly promote the control of vaccine-preventable diseases (Grand Challenges in Global Health 2007). Studies to develop such vaccines, including encapsulating in heat-resistant bacterial spores and promoting temperature stabilization through the use of polymers, are in progress. Continued efforts to design and evaluate heat-stable vaccine preparations are needed.

Evaluation of needle-free mechanisms of delivery

Most vaccines require administration through needle and syringe. Such a method of delivery can result in transmission of blood-borne pathogens including HIV, HBV, and HCV through re-use of inadequately sterilized needles or accidental needle-stick injuries. Moreover, needle and syringe administration is costly and requires considerable logistical support. Needle-free methods of vaccine delivery including mucosal (oral, nasal, or aerosol) or transcutaneous approaches would provide considerable advantages. These benefits would include cost savings, ease of administration, improved logistics, reduced risk of transmission of blood-borne agents, improved access, increased patient compliance, and expanded vaccine coverage.

Multivalent vaccines

Many vaccine preparations are monovalent, which necessitates repeated administration of separate vaccines to ensure protection. The use of multivalent vaccine preparations, that is, combining multiple antigens into a single dose, can improve efficiency of delivery, promote increased coverage rates, and reduce the cost of immunization (Grand Challenges in Global Health 2007). Further study of the feasibility and effectiveness of such an approach is needed.

Single-dose vaccines

Many vaccines require repeated boosters to provide continuing immunity. If equivalent or greater protection could be elicited with a single dose of vaccine, it would have considerable financial and programmatic benefits, and would reduce the operational and logistical challenges encountered with vaccines requiring multiple doses (Grand Challenges in Global Health 2007). Ideally, single-dose vaccines should be effective in neonates. Improving knowledge of the immune response and development of effective adjuvants may be necessary to realize success towards this goal.

Adjuvants

Ideally, vaccination should induce a strong immune response and provide long-term protection. Vaccine adjuvants are substances that can enhance the immune system response, reduce the amount of antigen or the number of immunizations required, and improve efficacy in immunocompromised persons (including newborns, the elderly, persons with HIV and other immune deficits) and otherwise low responders. Adjuvants can also provide an antigen delivery system for mucosal administration. Few adjuvants (alum, virosomes, liposomes) are currently licensed for use, and their effect on boosting immunity is generally modest. Other, more immunologically potent compounds, such as Freund's (complete adjuvant) and LPS, have been abandoned because of adverse local and systemic reactions (Aguilar & Rodriguez 2007). Additional work to understand the mechanisms of action of adjuvants and efforts to develop better compounds that can safely and effectively boost the immune system are warranted.

Studies to improve understanding of the immune response to infectious agents

Generating the most effective immune response to neutralize infectious agents is critical to ensuring optimal control of vaccine-preventable diseases. Determining conserved epitopes that result in high-affinity antibody and robust T-cell responses is the key to such efforts. Basic science studies of immunity and immune mechanisms are crucial. Although our knowledge of immunology has progressed considerably, additional understanding of markers of immunity and the mechanisms to induce a protective immune response are needed. Such information can help to guide development of vaccines as well as advanced diagnostic and prognostic tests.

Vaccine production and delivery in plants

One of the most promising new methods for production and delivery of vaccine antigens is via transgenic edible plants (Tacket 2005; Jiang *et al.* 2007). Plant geneticists can introduce genes coding for specific microbial proteins that are expressed in plant tissues including the edible parts. Production of vaccine components in plants offers a number of advantages in manufacturing, packaging, transporting, storage, and product stability. It would also avoid the potential for exposure to contaminant pathogens that may be found in human or animal cell-derived vaccines. Moreover, vaccine can be delivered orally, when the product is consumed, offering the benefits of needle-free administration. Studies have demonstrated that such oral administration can elicit an immune response, and the potential for developing a strong mucosal immunity, which represents the portal of entry for many pathogens, is appealing.

Reverse vaccinology

Vaccine studies are needed to expand on recent genome-based laboratory innovations. In traditional vaccine development, a pathogen is cultivated, antigenic components are isolated, tested for immunogenicity, and then vaccine is produced through culturing the agent in large quantities or by using recombinant technology. More recently, the ability to sequence the entire genome of microbes has allowed a reverse approach to vaccine development (Scarselli *et al.* 2005). Starting from the whole genome, computer-generated (in silico) predictions of the entire set of potential vaccine antigens can be made. These antigens are then cloned and screened for immunogenicity. Such an approach is faster and more thorough than conventional methods and can be used to develop vaccines for agents that are not cultivable. More studies of this promising reverse-vaccinology approach are warranted.

DNA vaccines

These are plasmid DNAs that can be taken up by cells of an inoculated host. These plasmids encode antigens that can be expressed in cells and induce an immune response (Herrmann 2006). DNA vaccines have distinct advantages including ease of production with relatively simple molecular biologic techniques, stability and temperature resistance, induction of cytotoxic T-cell response, no risk of infection, and effectiveness in the presence of maternal antibodies. Moreover, these vaccines can be administered in a variety of ways including via the mucosal route. Additional studies of this promising vaccine approach are warranted, including methods designed to improve the magnitude of the immune response.

Efficacy and effectiveness studies in developing countries

Expanded study to assess the efficacy and effectiveness of vaccines in developing countries is needed. Malnutrition and undernutrition in such countries may result in reduced immune response, and therefore, results observed in wealthier countries may not be applicable (Clemens & Jodar 2005). Other factors, including logistical and programmatic issues, may also mean that vaccines will not perform as well in resource-limited countries.

Vaccines targeting resistant microbes

Given the increasing resistance of pathogenic agents to antimicrobial therapy and the challenges of continuing to develop new drugs, the use of vaccines that specifically target resistant organisms offers an important method for addressing this critical problem (Heath & Breathnach 2002). Additional efforts to develop such vaccines and to assess their impact on reducing the burden of disease caused by resistant agents are warranted. Studies targeting *Streptococcus pneumoniae*, *Staphylococcus aureas*, and *Pseudomonas aeruginosa* would be of particular value.

Animal models for live attenuated vaccines

Live attenuated vaccines typically result in a more robust immune reaction and greater protection. However, given the potential risks in the testing of such vaccines, including reversion to virulence and possible significant adverse reactions, studies are needed to develop reliable animal model systems to evaluate live attenuated vaccine preparations (Grand Challenges in Global Health 2007).

Animal vaccines

Many important microbial threats are zoonoses (e.g. salmonellosis, rabies). The control of infectious agents in animals that serve as sources of human infection can promote control efforts for zoonotic diseases. Enhanced efforts are needed in the study of vaccines for reservoir animals. Such initiatives can aid in the development of complementary human vaccines as well.

Assessment of vaccination coverage levels

Critical to the success of any immunization programme is determining vaccination coverage levels to assess populations at risk. Although such studies are often very basic in nature, they are essential for appropriately targeting immunization efforts and controlling vaccine-preventable diseases. Assessment of community levels of vaccination must be routinely conducted and may include not only history of immunization but also laboratory testing to measure immunity. More sophisticated statistical and survey techniques such as those used by the US National Immunization Survey can provide more accurate estimates of vaccine coverage levels (Simpson *et al.* 2001), but such methods may not be economically or logistically feasible for widespread implementation.

Transmission-blocking vaccines

These vaccines represent a novel disease control approach that immunizes a host, not for development of immunity and protection of the host but to interfere with the pathogen's development in the vector, which blocks subsequent transmission. Such an approach is being pursued for malaria by targeting the sexual stage (gametocytes) of Plasmodium, which is necessary for the development of sporozoites (the infectious stage for humans) in the vector mosquito. Uptake of anti-gametocyte antibodies can impede sexual development in the mosquito and reduce malaria transmission. Transmission-blocking vaccines may be useful for other infectious disease threats as well and can be put into practice in combination with other control strategies.

Analysis considerations

A number of important epidemiologic issues should be considered when approaching analysis of vaccine studies. Halloran (1998) has drawn attention to the value of assessing the impact of immunization programmes through direct, indirect, total, and overall effects. Direct effect reflects the impact of the vaccination in generating individual immunity and protecting the person immunized. Indirect effect is the protection afforded to non-immunized persons by boosting herd immunity. This reduces the level of exposure and transmission, thereby 'indirectly' providing protection. Total effect is a combination of both direct and indirect effects. Overall effect refers to the effect on the population as a whole.

In vaccine efficacy and effectiveness studies, the use of confirmatory laboratory tests or 'validation samples' can improve estimation, especially for diseases such as influenza, where laboratory testing of all presumptive cases may not be practical (Halloran & Longini 2001). However, given that confirmatory laboratory samples may not be randomly obtained, Bayesian techniques can be useful in estimating vaccine efficacy in such circumstances (Scharfstein *et al.* 2006). Bayesian approaches may also be of value in estimating vaccine efficacy in small trials of a highly efficacious vaccine where few, if any, immunized subjects develop disease (Chu & Halloran 2004).

The considerable future promise of vaccines for the control of microbial threats will require expansion of current studies and initiation of new efforts. In addition, continuing work to overcome economic and political barriers will be necessary to realize this promise.

Role of the microbiological laboratory

The microbiological laboratory plays a key role in both passive and active surveillance as well as in outbreak detection. Early recognition of microbial threats is essential for ensuring effective containment, reduction of casualties, and drug or vaccine development (Kaufmann *et al.* 1997). Control of microbial threats requires development of enhanced laboratory capabilities to ensure rapid detection of agents. Of particular importance are the rapid microbiological techniques, such as immunoassay, microscopy, and molecular testing (Canton 2005). Microbiological tests can be divided into two categories: Those that directly identify the infectious agent and those that indirectly identify the infectious agent. Indirect methods are preferable when either they are more expeditious or when a pathogen cannot be cultivated in laboratory media.

Direct techniques

Culture

Culture is the most commonly used technique for the identification of microbial threats in laboratories, clinics, and health-care facilities worldwide, particularly in developing countries. Over the past few decades, due to the discovery of additional media components, the ability to control certain environmental conditions, and the use of growth-promoting factors, culture techniques have improved substantially, thereby increasing the sensitivity of these techniques (Mukamolova *et al.* 1998). Although claims have been made that the skills and resources necessary to correctly carry out culture techniques, as well as staining and microscopy, are present at nearly every laboratory in the world (Henchal *et al.* 2001), this may only apply for reference laboratories or government-run facilities. In rural areas where many infectious diseases are present, the laboratories are rudimentary and may not have appropriate incubators and facilities to make sterile culture media (Liu *et al.* 2003). Additionally, even if a laboratory and the appropriate equipment are available, lack of training and experience may hinder accurate diagnosis. Even in those laboratories worldwide with the necessary equipment and skill, time is a key factor because culture techniques require growth of the organism. Hence, results typically cannot be obtained in less than 18 hours and may take as long as six weeks for some slow-growing organisms such as mycobacteria.

Viral isolation

Viral isolation is typically the first step in the identification of an emerging or re-emerging viral infection, and was a critical step in the recent outbreaks of haemorrhagic fevers in Europe (Pugliese *et al.* 2007).

Direct microscopy

For a number of parasitic diseases (malaria, babesiosis), identification by direct microscopy remains the most rapid as well as the most sensitive and specific method (Dumler *et al.* 2007). Diagnosis can be obtained within minutes; however, accuracy requires highly trained and skilled microscopists. Microscopic techniques can also be used when coupled with staining as a preliminary step in the identification of bacterial agents.

Molecular techniques

Although isolation and subculture for bacterial identification have long been the mainstay of the microbiological laboratory and virus isolation and subsequent antigenic serotyping is the accepted gold standard for diagnosis of viral infection, such techniques can take a minimum of 36 hours before they yield useful data (Krafft & Kulesh 2001). Furthermore, for many infectious agents, cultivation in the laboratory is not possible, or takes many weeks. Molecular techniques, particularly those that have been developed during the last two decades, have been shown to be essential for identifying emerging pathogens, and for characterizing their virulence determinants and antibiotic-resistance genes. Because they typically do not require culture of the organism, they can be implemented quickly, allowing a more rapid laboratory response.

Polymerase chain reaction (PCR) is a widely accepted molecular technique that uses nucleic acid amplification to increase minute amounts of DNA into detectable quantities. RT-PCR, which involves reverse transcription of the genetic material, must be used if the target genetic material is RNA. PCR and RT-PCR offer increased sensitivity and the ability to confirm the presence of an infectious agent in any sample, as long as primers are available for the specific infectious agent. The specificity of PCR is determined by the choice of primers, and in order to choose and synthesize suitable primers, the sequence of target DNA must be known, which is currently one of the greatest limitations of PCR. However, PCR can be a powerful tool for initial screening of a large number of suspected infectious agents when regions of highly conserved nucleotide sequences are used in the development of primers (Examples of the Laboratory Response Network in Action 2007).

Indirect methods

Immunodiagnostic techniques

Immunodiagnostic methods, including immunofluorescence, enzyme-linked immunosorbent assay (ELISA), and Western blotting, are regularly used to confirm the clinical diagnosis by characterizing the immune response of the infected host to the agent. However, they lack the sensitivity of molecular and culture techniques to detect microbial threats. Furthermore, because many infectious agents are immunologically cross-reactive, immunodiagnostic techniques may also be limited by poor specificity (Mukamolova *et al.* 1998). Additionally, immunodiagnostic techniques are often serologic assays that rely on detection of antibodies in a patient's serum. Because it can take 2–4 weeks for an individual to mount such an immune response, immunodiagnostic techniques can also be constrained by time. However, these methods are powerful in that they allow for screening of several different infections simultaneously and can be useful in conducting seroprevalence studies.

The Laboratory Response Network (LRN)

The LRN is a network of more than 150 state, federal, military, food, and environmental testing laboratories in the United States that was established by the CDC and is a cooperative effort between the Association of Public Health Laboratories and the Federal Bureau of Investigation. Although originally established under a presidential directive to combat biological and chemical terrorism, the LRN maintains an integrated network of state and local public health, federal, military, and international laboratories that can respond to a wide variety of public health emergencies. The network functions by helping to increase the number of trained laboratory technicians in state and local public health facilities, distributing standardized test methods and reagents to local laboratories, promoting the acquisition of advanced technologies, and supporting facility improvements. Examples of recent efforts of the LRN include the testing of over 125 000 samples following the anthrax attacks of 2001 and the developing of an H5N1 assay and reagent kit as well as PCR primers for SARS (Examples of the Laboratory Response Network in Action).

Role of the laboratory in developing countries

Laboratories in developing countries are often underequipped, understaffed, and unable to meet the demand for accurate and timely information. Late detection on the part of the microbiological laboratory can translate into a delayed response by health officials and a missed opportunity for early control of an outbreak. Although culture techniques are most often used in developing countries, technological advances such as ELISA and molecular techniques have potential for use in developing countries because they typically increase the speed at which a diagnosis is made, and in the case of techniques such as ELISA and rapid diagnostic tests, they allow diagnosis to be made away from major medical centres. However, for such advances to be useful, changes in the curricula of laboratory technicians are necessary in order to make well-informed use of the new technology (Ebrahim, 1992).

In an effort to address the lack of capacity and expertise against emerging threats in developing countries, the WHO's Department of Communicable Diseases, Surveillance, and Response opened an office in Lyon, France in order to strengthen diagnostic and surveillance capabilities in these countries. The office administers a two-year training programme for senior laboratory staff focused on enhancing the capacity of national public health laboratories, supporting field epidemiology training programmes, and improving the capacity to detect and respond to disease outbreaks. It is estimated that the programme has trained over 150 specialists from 45 countries since its creation in 2001. During the course of the programme, participants receive training in essential diagnostic practices and techniques with the expectation that upon completion they will be able to utilize these skills to rapidly identify epidemic and endemic infectious diseases as well as train laboratory technicians in their home countries (Hamburg *et al.* 2003). The programme partners with the leading infectious disease laboratories in the world including, among others, the CDC, Institute Pasteur (France), and the London School of Tropical Medicine and Hygiene.

Given that the limited resources and infrastructure preclude the availability of comprehensive microbiological services in every region of a country, the use of sentinel hospitals in selected areas should be considered (Archibald & Reller 2001). Such sentinel sites should have wide-ranging laboratory capabilities, including the ability to assess microbial resistance, and employ strict quality-control standards. These sites are usually government affiliated with close ties to the Ministry of Health, characteristics that can promote collaborations with agencies including the WHO and the US Agency for International Development.

Rapid tests for infectious agents that are easy to use and have high sensitivity and specificity can mitigate the absence of diagnostic laboratory capacity. However, few such 'point-of-care' tests are currently available. This lack of availability of rapid and affordable diagnostic tests undercuts the successful treatment and control of microbial threats in developing countries.

Ultimately, the successful control of microbial threats requires accurate and timely diagnosis. This can only be achieved if clinical and public health laboratories are adequately staffed with qualified professionals who are specially trained public health microbiologists and who are supervised by competent laboratory directors (Peterson *et al.* 2001).

The global impact of infectious diseases continues to be staggering in terms of the cost of morbidity, mortality, economic losses, and impeded development. Control of microbial threats requires a complex, multifaceted, and interdisciplinary approach. Population surveillance, vaccine studies, and the microbiological laboratory are three cornerstones of control and critical to the mitigation of infectious diseases.

References

Aguilar J.C., Rodriguez E.G. Vaccine adjuvant revisited. *Vaccine* 2007;**25**:3753–62.

Alter M.J., Kruszon-Moran D., Nainon O.V. *et al.* The prevalence of hepatitis C virus infection in the United States, 1988 through 1994. *New England Journal of Medicine* 1999;**341**:556–62.

Archibald L.K., Reller L.B. Clinical microbiology in developing countries. *Emerging Infectious Diseases* 2001;**7**:302–5.

Black R.E., Morris S.S., Bryce J. Where and why are 10 million children dying every year? Lancet 2003;361:2226–34.

Breman J.G., Alilio M.S., Mills A. Conquering the intolerable burden of malaria: what's new, what's needed: a summary. *American Journal of Tropical Medicine and Hygiene* 2004;**71** Suppl **2**:1–15.

Buckley A., Dawson A., Gould E.A. Detection of seroconversion to West Nile virus, Usutu virus and Sindbis virus in UK sentinel chickens. *Virology Journal* 2007;**3**:71.

Buehler J.W., Berkelman R.L., Hartley D.M. *et al.* Syndromic surveillance and bioterrorism-related epidemics. *Emerging Infectious Diseases* 2003;**9**:1197–204.

Buehler J.W. Review of the 2003 National Syndromic Surveillance Conference—lessons learned and questions to be answered. Morbidity and Mortality Weekly Report 2004:53 Suppl:18–22.

Buehler J.W. Surveillance. In: Rothman K., Greenland S., editors. *Modern epidemiology*. Philadelphia (PA): Lippincott-Raven; 1998.

Canton R. Role of the microbiology laboratory in infectious diseases surveillance, alert and response. *Clinical Microbiology and Infection* 2005;**11** Suppl **1**:3–8.

Caro J.J., Getsios D., Payne K. *et al.* Economic burden of pertussis and impact of immunization. *Pediatric Infectious Disease Journal* 2005;**24**:S48–54.

Centers for Disease Control and Prevention. Biological and chemical terrorism: strategic plan for preparedness and response. *Morbidity and Mortality Weekly Report* 2000;**49**:1–14.

Centers for Disease Control and Prevention. Case definitions for infectious conditions under public health surveillance. *Morbidity and Mortality Weekly Report* 1997;RR-**10**:46.

Centers for Disease Control and Prevention. Ongoing multi-state outbreak of Escherichia coli serotype O157:H7 infections associated with consumption of fresh spinach—United States, September 2006. *Morbidity and Mortality Weekly Report* 2006;**55**:1045–6.

Centers for Disease Control and Prevention. Progress in reducing measles mortality. *Morbidity and Mortality Weekly Report* 2005;**54**:200–3.

Centers for Disease Control and Prevention. Updated guidelines for evaluating public health surveillance systems: recommendations from the Guidelines Working Group. *Morbidity and Mortality Weekly Report* 2001;RR**13**:1–35.

Chu H., Halloran M.E. Bayesian estimation of vaccine efficacy. *Clinical Trials* 2004;**1**:306–14.

Cieslak T.J., Christopher G.W., Kortepeter M.G. *et al.* Immunization against potential biological warfare agents. *Clinical Infectious Diseases* 2000;**30**:843–50.

Clemens J., Jodar L. Introducing new vaccines into developing countries: obstacles, opportunities and complexities. *Nature Medicine* 2005;**11**:S12–15.

Corbett E.L., Watt C.J., Walker N. *et al.* The growing burden of tuberculosis. *Global trends and interactions with the HIV epidemic. Archives of Internal Medicine* 2003;**163**:1009–21.

Department of Vaccines and Biologicals, World Health Organization. *Estimating the local burden of* Haemophilus influenza *type B (HIB) disease preventable by vaccination. A rapid assessment tool.* [Online]. Available from: http://whqlibdoc.who.int/hq/2001/WHO_V&B_01.27.pdf

Desenclos J.C. Are there "new" and "old" ways to track infectious diseases hazards and outbreaks? Eurosurveillance 2006;**11**:206–7.

Diez-Roux A.V., Aiello A.E. Multilevel analysis of infectious diseases. *Journal of Infectious Diseases* 2005;**191**:S25–33.

Dumler J.S., Madigan J.E., Pusterla N. *et al.* Ehrlichioses in humans: epidemiology, clinical presentation, diagnosis and treatment. *Clinical Infectious Diseases* 2007;**45**:S45–51.

Ebrahim G.J. Laboratory services in developing countries. *Journal of Tropical Pediatrics* 1992;**38**:50–1.

Ehreth J. The global value of vaccination. *Vaccine* 2003;**21**:596–600.

Estacio P.L. Surge capacity for health care systems: early detection, methodologies and process. *Academic Emergency Medicine* 2006;**13**(**11**):1135–7.

Ewart D., Westman S., Frederick P.D. *et al.* Measles reporting completeness during a community-wide epidemic in inner-city Los Angeles. *Public Health Reports* 1995;**110**:161–5.

Galazka A., Birmingham M., Kurian M. *et al.* Tetanus. In: Murray C.J.L., Lopez A.D., Mathers C.D., editors. *Global epidemiology of infectious diseases*. Geneva: World Health Organization; 2004.

Garber D.A., Silvestri G., Feinberg M.B. Prospects for an AIDS vaccine: three big questions, no easy answers. *Lancet Infectious Diseases* 2004;**4**:397–413.

Girard M.P., Fruth U., Kieny M.P. A review of vaccine research and development: tuberculosis. *Vaccine* 2005;**23**:5725–31.

Global Burden of Disease Working Group 2004

Gonzalez A.E., Gilman R., Garcia H.H. *et al.* Use of sentinel pigs to monitor environmental Taenia solium contamination. *The Cysticercosis Working Group in Peru. American Journal of Tropical Medicine and Hygiene* 1994;**51**:847–50.

Grand Challenges in Global Health. [Online]. 2007. Available from: http://www.gcgh.org/channels/gcgh

Graves P., Gelband H. Vaccines for preventing malaria (blood stages). *[Online]. Cochrane Database Systematic Reviews* 2006 Oct 18;(**4**): CD006199.

Greenberg R.N., Kennedy J.S., Clanton D.J. *et al.* Safety and immunogenicity of new cell-cultured smallpox vaccine compared with calf-lymph derived vaccine: a blind, single-centre, randomized controlled trial. *Lancet* 2005;**365**:398–409.

Grijalva C.G., Nuorti K.J.P., Arbogast P.G. *et al.* Decline in pneumonia admissions after routine childhood immunization with pneumococcal conjugate vaccine in the USA: a time series analysis. *Lancet* 2007;**369**:1179–86.

Guglielmetti P., Coulombier D., Thinus G. *et al.* The Early Warning and Response System for communicable diseases in the EU: an overview from 1999 to 2005. *Eurosurveillance* 2006;**11**:215–20.

Halloran M.E., Longini I.M. Using validation sets for outcomes and exposure to infection in vaccine field studies. *American Journal of Epidemiology* 2001;**154**:391–8.

Halloran M.E. Infectious disease epidemiology. In: Rothman K., Greenland S., editors. Modern epidemiology. Philadelphia (PA): Lippincott-Raven; 1998.

Hamburg M., Lederberg J., Smolinski M. Addressing the threats: conclusions and recommendations. *Microbial threats to health: emergence, detection and response*. Joseph Henry Press; 2003.

Heath P.T., Breathnach A.S. Treatment of infections due to resistant organisms. *British Medical Bulletin* 2002;**61**:231–45.

Henchal E.A., Teska J.D., Ludwig G.V. *et al.* Current laboratory methods for biological threat agent identification. *Clinics in Laboratory Medicine* 2001;**21**:661–78.

Herrmann J.E. DNA vaccines against enteric infections. *Vaccine* 2006;**24**:3705–8.

Huff L., Bogdan G., Burke K. *et al.* Using hospital discharge data for disease surveillance. *Public Health Reports* 1996;**111**:78–81.

Jernigan D.B., Raghunathan P.L., Bell B.P. *et al.* Investigation of bioterrorism-related anthrax, United States 2001: epidemiologic findings. *Emerging Infectious Diseases* 2002;**10**:1019–28.

Jiang X.L., He Z.M., Peng Z.Q. *et al.* Cholera toxin B protein in transgenic tomato fruit induces systemic immune response in mice. *Transgenic Research* 2007;**16**:169–75.

Jodar L., Feavers I.M., Salisbury D. *et al.* Development of vaccines against meningococcal disease. *Lancet* 2002;**359**:1499–508.

Kao J.H., Chen D.S. Global control of hepatitis B virus infection. *Lancet Infectious Diseases* 2002;**2**:395–403.

Kaufmann A.F., Meltzer M.I., Schmid G.P. The economic impact of a bioterrorist attack: are prevention and postattack intervention programs justifiable? Emerging Infectious Diseases 1997;**3**:83–94.

Keusch G.T., Fontaine O., Bhargava A. *et al.* Diarrheal diseases. *Disease Control Priorities Project*. [Online]. 2007. Available from: http://www.dcp2.org/pubs/DCP/19/

Kimball A.M., Thacker S.B., Levy M.E. Shigella surveillance in a large metropolitan area: assessment of a passive reporting system. *American Journal of Public Health* 1980;**70**:164–6.

Kim-Farley R.J. Global strategies for control of communicable diseases. In: Detels R., McEwen J., Beaglehole R. *et al.*, editors. *Oxford textbook of public health*. 5th ed. New York (NY): Oxford University Press; 2008.

Krafft A.E., Kulesh D.A. Applying molecular biological techniques to detecting biological agents. *Clinical Laboratory Medicine* 2001;**21**:631–60.

Kuehn B.M. Animal-human disease targeted to stop pandemics before they start. *Journal of the American Medical Association* 2006;**295**:1987–9.

Lechmann M., Liang T.J. Vaccine development for hepatitis C. *Seminars in Liver Disease* 2000;**20**:211–26.

Lenaway D.D., Ambler A. Evaluation of a school-based influenza surveillance system. *Public Health Reports* 1995;**110**:333–7.

Li Y.C., Norton E.C., Dow W.H. Influenza and pneumococcal vaccination demand responses to changes in infectious disease mortality. *Health Services Research* 2004;**39**:905–25.

Liu H., Detels R., Yin Y. *et al.* Do STD clinics correctly diagnose STDs? An assessment of STD management in Hefei, China. *International Journal of STD and AIDS* 2003;**14**:665–71.

Lober W.B., Bliss D., Dockrey M.R. *et al.* Communicable disease case entry using PDAs and public wireless networks. AMIA Annual Symposium Proceedings 2003;916.

Lomabardo J.S., Burkom H., Pavlin J. ESSENCE II and the framework for evaluating syndromic surveillance systems. *Morbidity and Mortality Weekly Report* 2004;**53** Suppl:159–65.

Lopez A.D., Mathers C.D., Jamison D.T. *et al.* Global and regional burden of disease and risk factors, 2001. *Lancet* 2006;**367**:1747–57.

Lopez A.D., Mathers C.D. Measuring the global burden of disease and epidemiological transitions: 2002–2030. *Annals of Tropical Medicine and Parasitology* 2006;**100**:481–99.

Madoff L.C. ProMED-mail and early warning system for emerging disease. *Clinical Infectious Disease* 2004;**39**:227–32.

Masingnani V., Lattanzi M., Rappuoli R. The value of vaccines. *Vaccine* 2003;**21**:S110–3.

Mazzulli T., Kain K., Butany J. Severe acute respiratory syndrome. *Archives of Pathology and Laboratory Medicine* 2004;**128**:1346–50.

McCoy L., Sorvillo F., Simon P. Varicella-related mortality in California, 1988–2000. *Pediatric Infectious Disease Journal* 2004;**23**:498–503.

McKee K.T., Jr., Shields T.M., Jenkins P.R. *et al.* Application of a geographic information system to the tracking and control of an outbreak of shigellosis. *Clinical Infectious Diseases* 2000;**31**:728–33.

Mukamolova G.V., Kaprelyants A.S., Young D.I. *et al.* A bacterial cytokine. *Proceedings of the National Academy of Sciences USA* 1998;**95**: 8916–21.

Mulholland K. Global burden of acute respiratory infections in children: implications for intervention. *Pediatric Pulmonology* 2003;**36**: 469–74.

Nahlen B.L., Korenromp E.L., Miller J.M. *et al.* Malaria risk: estimating clinical episodes of malaria. *Nature* 2005;**437**:E3.

O'Connor S.M., Taylor C.E., Hughes J.M. Emerging infectious determinants of chronic diseases. *Emerging Infectious Diseases* 2006;**12**:1051–7.

Okeke I.N., Laxminarayan R., Bhutta Z.A. *et al.* Antimicrobial resistance in developing countries. *Part 1: recent trends and current status. Lancet Infectious Diseases* 2005;**5**:481–93.

Openshaw P.J., Tregoning J., Harker J. RSV 2005: global impact, changing concepts, and new challenges. *Viral Immunology* 2005;**18**:749–51.

Parashar U.D., Gibson C.J., Bresee J.S. *et al.* Rotavirus and severe childhood diarrhea. *Emerging Infectious Diseases* 2006;**12**:304–6.

Parsonnet J., editor. Introduction. In: *Microbes and malignancy: infection as a cause of human cancers*. New York (NY): Oxford University Press; 1999.

Pavlin J.A., Mostashari F., Kortepeter M.G. *et al.* Innovative surveillance methods for rapid detection of disease outbreaks and bioterrorism: results of an interagency workshop on health indicator surveillance. *American Journal of Public Health* 2003;**93**:1230–5.

Pavlin J.A., Murdock P., Elbert E. *et al.* Conducting population behavioral health surveillance by using automated diagnostic and pharmacy data systems. *Morbidity and Mortality Weekly Report* 2004;**53** Suppl:166–72.

Peng H., Shelef L.A. Automated simultaneous detection of low levels of listeriae and salmonellae in foods. *International Journal of Food Microbiology* 2002;**63**:225–33.

Peterson L.R., Hamilton J.D., Baron E.J. *et al.* Role of clinical microbiology laboratories in the management and control of infectious diseases and the delivery of health care. *Clinical Infectious Diseases* 2001;**32**(**4**):605–11.

Poland G.A. Vaccines against avian influenza—a race against time. *New England Journal of Medicine* 2006;**354**:1411–3.

Pollack F.P., Karoon R.A. The future of respiratory syncytial virus vaccine development. *Pediatric Infectious Disease Journal* 2004;**23**:S65–73.

Pugliese A., Beltramo1 T., Torre D. Emerging and re-emerging viral infections in Europe. *Cell Biochemistry and Function* 2007;**25**:1–13.

Redelings M., Sorvillo F., Simon P. A population-based analysis of pneumococcal disease mortality in California, 1989–1998. *Public Health Reports* 2005;**120**:157–64.

Robertson S., Featherstone D.A., Gacic-Dobo M. *et al.* Rubella and congenital rubella syndrome: global update. *Pan American Journal of Public Health* 2003;**14**:306–15.

Rollin L., McCoy L., Redelings M. *et al.* Impact of different population estimates on burden of disease analyses. *Public Health Reports* 2007. In press.

Scarselli M., Giuliani M.M., Abdu-Bobie J. *et al.* The impact of genomics on vaccine design. *Trends in Biotechnology* 2005;**23**:84–91.

Scharfstein D.O., Halloran M.E., Chu H. On estimation of vaccine efficacy using validation samples with selection bias. *Biostatistics* 2006;**7**: 615–29.

Scott J.A. The preventable burden of pneumococcal disease in the developing world. *Vaccine* 2007;**25**:2398–405.

Simpson D.M., Ezzati-Rice T.M., Zell E.R. Forty years and four surveys: how does our measuring measure up? American Journal of Preventive Medicine 2001;20:6–14.

Smolinski N.S., Hamburg M.A., Lederberg J., editors. *Microbial threats to health emergence, detection and response*. Washington (DC): Institute of Medicine; 2003.

Sorvillo F.J., Nahlen B. Lyme disease. *New England Journal of Medicine* 1990;**322**:474–5.

Standaert S.M., Lefkowitz L.B., Jr., Horan K.M. *et al.* The reporting of communicable diseases: a controlled study of Neisseria meningitidis and Haemophilus influenzae infections. *Clinical Infectious Diseases* 1995;**20**:30–6.

Stephenson I., Gust I., Pervikov Y. *et al.* Development of vaccines against influenza H5. *Lancet* 2006;**6**:450–60.

Tacket C.O. Plant-derived vaccines against diarrheal diseases. *Vaccine* 2005;**23**:1866–9.

Takahashi H., Fujii H., Shidno N. *et al.* Evaluation of the Japanese school health system for influenza. *Japanese Journal of Infectious Diseases* 2001;**54**:27–30.

Teutsch, Steven M., Churchill R.E., editors. *Principles and practice of public health surveillance*. Oxford University Press; 2000.

Thacker S.B., Birkhead S.G. Surveillance. In: Gregg M.B., editor. *Field epidemiology*. New York (NY): Oxford University Press; 2002.

Travers D.A., Waller A., Hass S.W. *et al.* Emergency department data for bioterrorism surveillance electronic data availability, timeliness, sources and standards. AMIA Annual Symposium Proceedings 2003;664.

Whalen R.G. DNA vaccines for emerging infectious diseases: what if? Emerging Infectious Diseases 1996;2:168–75.

World Health Organization. Annex table 3: Burden of disease in DALYs by cause, sex and mortality stratum in WHO regions, estimates for 2002. *World health report* 2004: *reducing risks, promoting healthy life*. [Online]. Available from: http://www.who.int/whr/2004/annex/topic/en/annex_3_en.pdf

World Health Organization. Global Influenza Surveillance Network. 2007. [Online]. Available from: http://www.who.int/csr/disease/influenza/surveillance/en/

World Health Organization. Global Outbreak Alert and Response Network. 2007. [Online]. Available from: http://www.who.int/csr/outbreaknetwork/en/

World Health Organization. The burden of tuberculosis: economic burden. [Online]. Available from: http://www.who.int/trade/distance_learning/gpgh/gpgh3/en/index7.html

World Health Organization. *World malaria report* 2005. [Online]. Available from: http://rbm.who.int/wmr2005/html/1-1.htm.1_1_1

8.4

The science of human exposures to contaminants in the environment

Paul J. Lioy

Abstract

The basic principles of the emerging field of exposure science are outlined and discussed, and the methods used to define human contact with chemical, biological, or physical agents found in the environment are described. The chapter provides several definitions and describes approaches to conducting research on exposure and its ultimate assessment for various applications in environmental health. The discussion of exposure science touches on the strategies for measuring exposure for single or multiple routes of entry into the body. The chapter also highlights the methods needed to collect samples from various points of entry into the body, and the types of methods needed for collecting samples either indirectly (microenvironmental) or directly (biological markers) to quantify exposure. A discussion on the ways human behaviour and human activities can increase or decrease contact with various agents, including pesticides, and how this information improves the assessment of exposure is included. Further, the process continuum that leads from the source of an agent to the exposure and eventual health effects is discussed. The exposures can be derived from single or multiroute contacts with an environmental contaminant associated with one or more media (air, soil, etc.) or route of entry into the body (inhalation, ingestion). Finally, there is a brief discussion of the opportunities for modelling exposure and dose, a brief description of the use of various approaches to analyse data, and a few illustrations of the uncertainties that must be addressed within an analysis.

Introduction

The presence of chemical, biological, and physical agents in the environments in which people live, work, and play may cause illness. Therefore, it is essential to develop and employ reliable methods that define the intensity and duration of contact with such agents and assess the likelihood of a role in disease aetiology. In a recent editorial, Barr (2006, p. 473) has provided a definition of human exposure science: 'the study of human contact with chemical, physical, or biological agents occurring in their environments that advances knowledge of the mechanisms and dynamics of events either causing or preventing adverse human health outcome'. The field of exposure science is associated with epidemiology, risk assessment, and disease intervention and prevention (National Research Council 1991a; Graham *et al.* 1992; Sexton *et al.* 1992; Ott 1995a; Lioy 1999), and the scientists and engineers who conduct these studies now are called exposure scientists, previously called analysts (National Research Council 1985, 1991b, c) or exposurologists (Ott 1995a). The kinds of exposures examined by exposure science are illustrated in Fig. 8.4.1. The traditional terms—industrial hygienists and radiation health physicists—refer specifically to those individuals who conducted exposure assessments in the various workplaces and who provided much of the fundamental technical bases for the first sets of field studies. Thus, exposure science expands upon these concepts by including the entire human environment (Wakefield 2000).

Exposure measurement techniques may be indirect or direct (National Research Council 1991c). Indirect techniques include sampling locations (microenvironments), where contact may occur with a contaminant, and/or the administration of survey instruments, such as time or activity questionnaires. Direct techniques include personal monitors worn by individuals and samples of blood, urine, and other bodily fluids, which permit measurements of exposure and dose for specific individuals (Barr *et al.* 2005). The number of people examined and analyses conducted during such experiments can be daunting. Thus, the field has been developing exposure models and, now, source-to-dose models to provide estimates for large populations, and to understand basic principles (McCurdy 2000; Furtaw 2001; Price & Chaisson 2005; Georgopoulos & Lioy 2006).

The measurement of the concentration of physical, chemical, radioactive, and/or biological agents in air, water, food, and so on, and the estimation of human behaviours and their use in estimating energy expenditure using instruments such as time or activity pattern diaries (McCurdy 2000; McCurdy *et al.* 2000) have helped improve the development of models that can predict not only exposure but also dose. Currently, it is feasible to trace an agent from the source through pathways into exposed people. Figure 8.4.2 illustrates the 'flow' of a contaminant through the points of contact, to

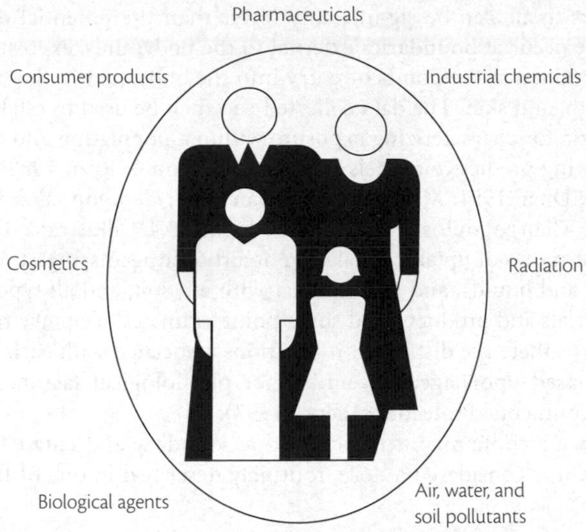

Fig. 8.4.1 Types of exposures that may be experienced by the general population.

the exposure, and to the dose that can appear inside the body. The domain-related scientific and professional disciplines—environmental science, exposure science, toxicology, and epidemiology—are also illustrated in Fig. 8.4.2.

This chapter describes the principles of exposure science starting with concepts and theory. The types of exposure measurements and estimates needed for the applications to environmental health will also be illustrated using, in varying detail, information about lead, benzene, trihalomethanes, pesticides, airborne particulate matter, infectious agents, and alternate fuels. Finally, some observations will be made concerning the future of exposure science in public health practice.

Basic principles

Over the past twenty years, the theoretical and conceptual bases for exposure assessment, and now science, have evolved from simple mathematical expressions that consider exposure and dose, to complex mechanistic descriptions of exposure and dose equations and concepts that can describe multiple routes of contact with a toxic agent. The aim, as described in Fig. 8.4.2, is to establish a relationship between the release of an agent that can cause, or is suspected of causing, human health effects and a dose that may cause an adverse health outcome (Lioy 1990; Lioy & Pellizzari 1995).

Some pollutants, such as ozone, are not emitted into the environment but are formed from their chemical precursors. In such cases, it is necessary to establish a relationship between the release of precursors of the toxicant, the conditions under which the toxicant is formed, and the health effect. Study of the effects of

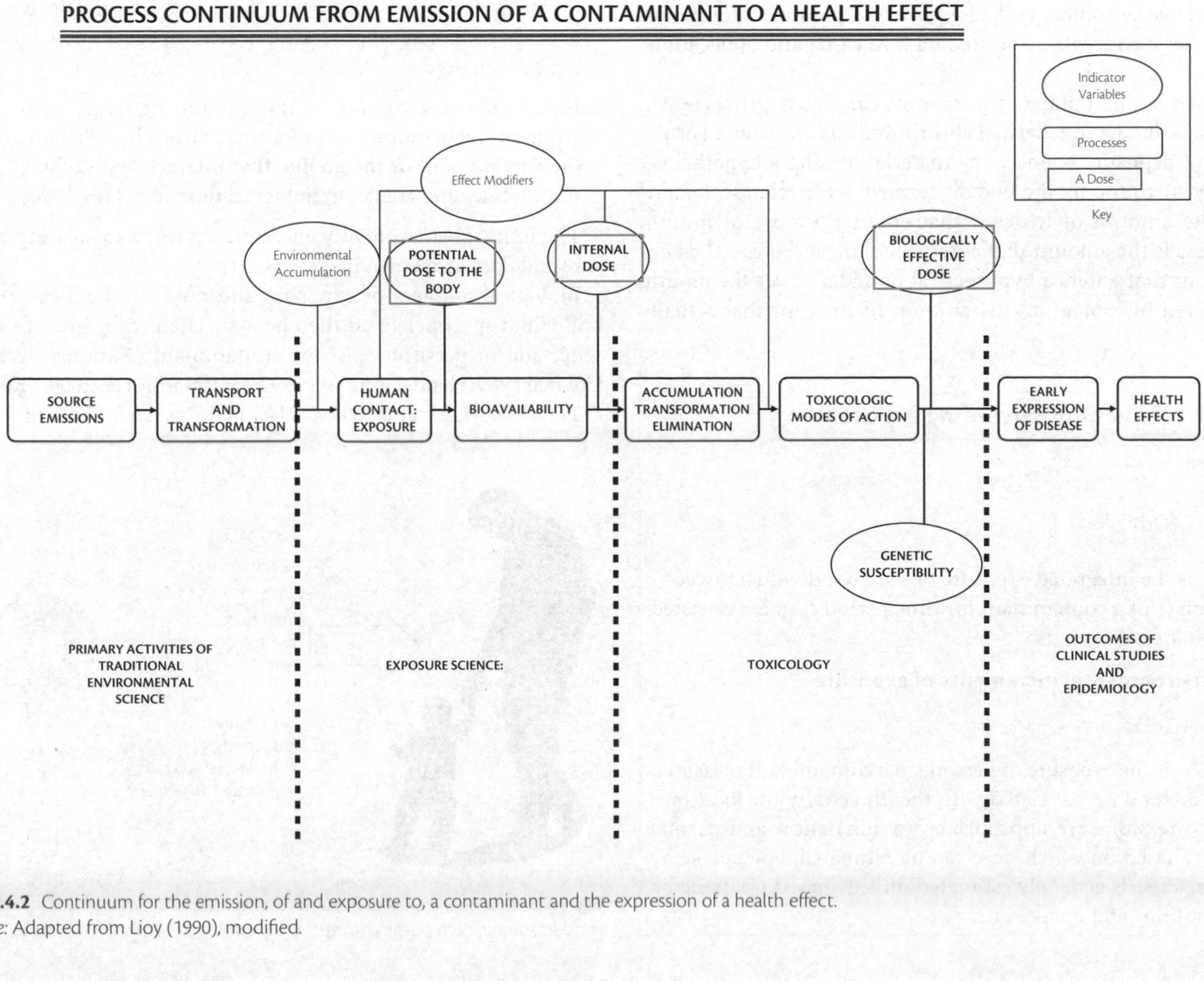

Fig. 8.4.2 Continuum for the emission, of and exposure to, a contaminant and the expression of a health effect.
Source: Adapted from Lioy (1990), modified.

exposure on ecological receptors can have important implications for human health. Ecological effects can have indirect effects on human health, and can also serve as sentinels of human exposure. Ecological effects can also have significant environmental justice implications, because the lives of some tribal and disadvantaged human populations are more closely linked to ecological health than that of the general population. An example of the linkage between human and ecosystem exposures was published by Jorgenson (2001). She examined environmental deposition through to epidemiological information on aldrin and diedrin in the United States.

Exposure to a contaminant is defined as the 'contact at a boundary between a human and the environment at a specific concentration over an interval of time' (National Research Council 1991c). Based on this definition, the types of integral or summation equations needed to estimate or describe exposure were identified, and are presented in Box 8.4.1. The integral equation is an exact expression of an individual's exposure, over the course of time, and the summation provides an approximate representation of exposure. The integral equation requires knowledge of the instantaneous concentration of the toxicant, which is generally available only from modelling studies, whereas the summation requires knowledge of time-averaged concentrations, which are often available from the application of direct and indirect measurement techniques. Generalized versions of these equations can be used to estimate exposures in modelling studies and can be found in Georgopoulos and Lioy (1994), Ott (1995a), and Zartarian *et al.* (1997b). Recently, Zartarian *et al.* (2005) have completed the first glossary on exposure science-related terminology. These provide a point of information on many basic concepts associated with research and applications in the field.

In principle, the uptake of a toxicant can occur primarily via three routes: Inhalation, dermal absorption, and ingestion. For the purpose of exposure science, any material passing a hypothetical boundary surrounding the body is termed *potential dose*. *Inhaled dose* is the amount of toxicant that enters the nose or mouth, *dermal dose* is the amount that enters the skin, and *ingested dose* is the amount that enters a hypothetical boundary over the mouth. As suggested by 'potential', the amount of toxicant that actually enters tissue can be significantly lower than the potential dose. These occur at boundaries external to the body; thus, exposure is determined at the points of entry into the body, that is, the nose, mouth, and skin. The data collected can then be used to establish criteria for characterizing exposure within a population and constructing predictive models (Ott 1982; Sexton & Ryan 1988; Ott 1990; Duan 1991; McKone 1991; Ryan 1991; Georgopoulos *et al.* 1997; Georgopoulos & Lioy 2006). Figure 8.4.3 illustrates three major routes of uptake: Inhalation of airborne agents, ingestion of food and liquids, and skin contact with air, soil, and all types of materials and products, and some point estimates of uptake rates. Clearly, there are distribution functions associated with each that are based upon age, sex, and other physiological factors (US Environmental Protection Agency 1997).

Once a contaminant has crossed a boundary and entered the body, it is considered a dose, routinely described in one of three ways:

1. *Potential dose* is the amount of material that enters a hypothetical external boundary around a receptor on a surface, which can potentially cause an effect on the surface or can be transferred to another organ or tissue. The entire mass (100 per cent) is assumed to cause a biological response.
2. *Internal dose* is the amount of material that actually enters one or more tissues; *target tissue dose* is the amount of toxicant that actually reaches sensitive tissue in which the toxic response occurs or is estimated to be available for absorption by an organ or tissue, or absorption on a surface, and is available to undergo biological processes, which can cause altered physiological function.
3. *Biologically effective dose* is the amount of target tissue dose required for manifestation of a toxic effect. It is the amount of the contaminant or metabolite that interacts with cellular macromolecules and alters physiological function (Lioy 1990).

The units most frequently encountered when calculating exposure and dose are shown in Table 8.4.1.

Biological markers of exposure and dose can be measured in body fluid specimens and then be associated with time of occurrence and/or persistence of the contaminant (National Research Council 1989; Henderson *et al.* 1992; Hoffmann *et al.* 2000a; Korrick *et al.* 2000; Maier *et al.* 2004; National Research Council 2006).

Box 8.4.1 Equations governing exposure

Exposure

$$E_j = \int_{t_1}^{t_2} C_j(t)\mathrm{d}t$$

where E_j is the integrated exposure of the *i*th individual to a concentration C of a contaminant for time period t_1 to t_2 associated with a biological response.

Microenvironmental increments of exposure

$$\Delta E_{ji} = C_{ji}(\Delta t)\Delta t_i$$

where $\Delta E_{j,i}$ is the exposure of person *i* to a contaminant measured over an interval Δt associated with the *j*th activity (or location). These expressions are appropriate for inhalation and dermal exposure, based on which dose can be estimated. For uptake by ingestion, dose is generally estimated directly based upon media concentrations and uptake rate.

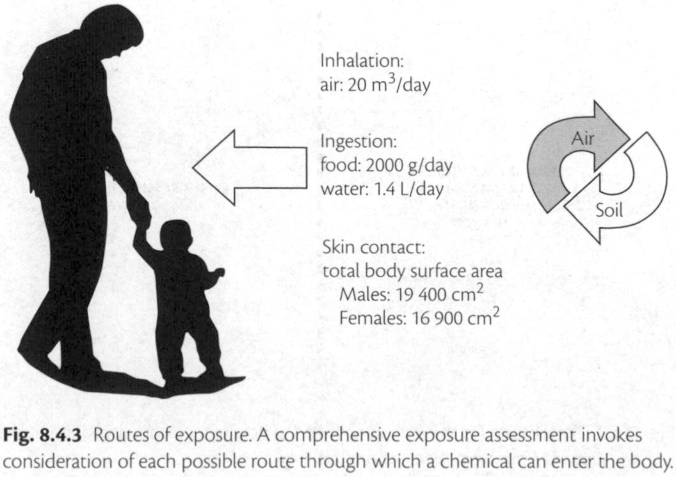

Fig. 8.4.3 Routes of exposure. A comprehensive exposure assessment invokes consideration of each possible route through which a chemical can enter the body.

Table 8.4.1 Examples of units used to express exposure and dose

Variable	Typical units	
Concentration in media	mg/kg	(food)
	mg/l	(water)
	μg/m³ and fibres/m³	(air)
	mg/100 cm²	(contaminated surface)
	mg/g or per cent	(fraction by weight in consumer products)
Time increments	min, h, day, year, 70 years (lifetime)	
Rate of intake	l/day	
	l/h	
	mg/kg body weight ingested per day (or per meal)	
	mg inhaled per hour	
	minutes	
Quantity available for absorption (potential dose)	mg inhaled, total	
	mg inhaled per kg body weight	
	mg ingested, total	
	mg ingested per kg body weight	
	mg on skin, total	
	mg/cm² skin area	
	mg injected or implanted/kg body weight	
Concentration in body tissues	μg/ml blood fibres/ml lung tissue	
Body burden	μg in bone (example)	
Organ dose	mg to liver (example)	

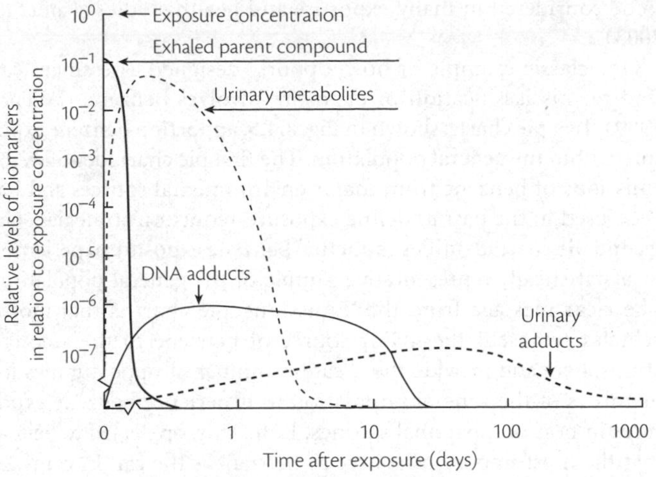

Fig. 8.4.4 Hypothetical relationships between different biological markers of exposure and time after a single exposure.
Source: Henderson *et al.* 1992.

Henderson *et al.* (1992) published the first conceptual framework for describing the persistence of different types of markers in the body. Recent advances and discussions on genomics and proteomics have suggested the need to consider other biomarkers of exposure to enhance current approaches (Burse *et al.* 2000; Poirier *et al.* 2000; Seifert *et al.* 2000a, b; Freeman *et al.* 2005; Weis *et al.* 2005).

The general time course of elimination of each type of marker is illustrated in Fig. 8.4.4. The results indicate that exhaled parent compounds yield the highest levels of biomarker concentrations relative to exposure concentration. Adducts spend the longest time in the body. The term *markers of exposure* is currently used to describe most of the above biomarkers, but in actuality the level of a contaminant or transformed product present in the body is defined as a dose (National Research Council 1989, 1992). In recent years, the measurement of exposure from biological samples has increased, and is providing ranges of values for members of the general population (Centers for Disease Control and Prevention 2005).

Methodologies

Accurate measurement or estimation of baseline information about the plausibility of human contact with the contaminant of concern assists in establishing the data-quality objectives for studying any particular problem. In the selection of the appropriate measurement 'tools', the analyst also needs to take into account factors such as the sensitivity and specificity of a technique for each medium or route studied, and the ease of sample handling and collection. In some situations, simple techniques such as survey instruments (e.g. time and location or activity questionnaire) are extremely valuable in acquiring semi-quantitative data for the characterization of exposure (Carpenter & Huston-Stein 1980; Lebowitz *et al.* 1989; National Research Council 1991c; Freeman *et al.* 1991, 1997; Zartarian *et al.* 1997a, 1998; Cohen-Hubal *et al.* 2000; McCurdy 2000). In other cases, more complex techniques such as microenvironmental or personal monitors are used to establish the primary route by which human contact occurs with a contaminant (Seifert & Abraham 1983; Akland *et al.* 1985; Spengler *et al.* 1985; National Research Council 1991a; Clayton *et al.* 1993; Lioy 1993; Valerio *et al.* 1997; Gurunathan *et al.* 1998; Edwards & Lioy 1999; Pellizzari *et al.* 1999; Hoffmann *et al.* 2000; Freeman *et al.* 2001a, 2001b, 2004; Rodes *et al.* 2001; Royster *et al.* 2002; Khoury & Diamond 2003; Gustafson *et al.* 2005; Heinrich *et al.* 2005; Hore *et al.* 2005). It is important to note, however, that all types of techniques do not have to be employed in a single study. Those selected would depend upon the data-quality objectives and the hypotheses being tested for a particular study.

The issue of contact with contaminants found in multiple media (e.g. soil/air) has increased awareness and the desire to obtain measurements on multiple routes of exposure, and to ensure that exposure–response relationships are constructed for media or routes of the greatest concern (Georgopoulos *et al.* 1997; Georgopoulos & Lioy 2006). The data gathered will also improve a manager's ability to prioritize strategies for intervention and the eventual reduction of exposure. The linkage of exposure science with environmental health problems leads to a tacit point: It is not scientifically sound to prejudge which is the most important medium or route of concern for a particular contaminant (Lioy 1990, 2006; National Research Council 1991c). Avoiding this pitfall will make it possible to obtain a broader view of a problem and improve the selection of measurement and analytical techniques. In the past, many studies have focused on a limited number of routes, and frequently have led to poorly identified exposures, and eventually the selection of inappropriate remedial solutions. In particular, the chemistry and physical chemistry of the indoor environment needs to be considered in many exposure and health studies (Fan *et al.* 2003).

One classic example of how a poorly designed assessment can lead to misclassification of exposure involves benzene (Wallace 1989). Two pie charts, shown in Fig. 8.4.5, apportion benzene exposure within the general population. The first pie chart identifies the emissions of benzene from major environmental sources and has been used in the past to define exposure-reduction strategies. The second pie chart identifies the actual benzene exposure experienced by a statistically representative sample of the general population. The clear message from the 'Emissions' pie chart is that motor vehicles represent the major source of benzene to the ambient atmosphere and provide the greatest number of opportunities for members of the general population to experience benzene exposures in non-occupational settings. From this, one is led to believe that the most important source of benzene is the car. In contrast, measurements made within personal monitoring studies have shown that the predominant source contributing to benzene exposure (>50 per cent) is cigarette smoke, with only 20 per cent of the exposures caused by automobile emissions 'Exposures' pie chart, Fig. 8.4.5. Thus, potentially high exposures to benzene would be misclassified or ignored in current strategies to reduce benzene that are based primarily upon emissions data. Regulators or health officials would benefit from data collected on individual or population activities to help identify the 'true' major source of exposure.

Another illustration of the manner in which improved exposure assessment data provided better information on how commuters come in contact with a contaminant concerns the fuel additive methyl tertiary butyl ether (MTBE). This compound is an oxygenate designed to reduce carbon monoxide emission and is representative of other chemicals found in new or reformulated fuels. In this instance, many initial studies on oxygenated fuel were conducted to estimate the environmental levels of MTBE or other hydrocarbons caused by car tail-pipe emissions. However, experiences of the general public and petrol-pump workers with petrol oxygenated by MTBE at 15 per cent by volume, have suggested that the highest exposures to the driver or passengers in a car, or to garage workers, were derived from evaporative emissions released by the engine compartment or petrol tank into the interior of the car, or in microenvironments adjacent to petrol service pumps. This is in contrast to the typical tail-pipe emissions scenario used in exposure assessments for motor vehicle fuels. Experiments conducted using cars that followed a typical commuter route and then had the petrol tank filled at some point during the trip are illustrated in Fig. 8.4.6 (Lioy *et al.* 1994). The results showed that the highest exposures to MTBE occurred during a tank refill. The approach used in the study demonstrated the importance of both personal and microenvironmental analyses in providing insight on what can lead to high exposures of evaporative emissions. Other examples exist for dermal and ingestion exposure; however, the main point is not to demonstrate all misclassifications of exposure that can or have occurred, but to recognize that when a study is designed, it must evaluate the possibility that a variety of sources and routes can affect exposure. This will improve the detection of, and source apportionment of, emissions, and determine how each contributes to the intensity of human contact with the contaminants of concern.

A recent example of difficulties in establishing the magnitude and extent of exposures comes from the 2001 attack on the World Trade Center (WTC). The aftermath of the attack provided some important insights into the potential application of exposure science in the future (Lioy *et al.* 2002; Oktay *et al.* 2003; Offenberg *et al.* 2004; Yiin *et al.* 2004; Geyh *et al.* 2005; Lioy 2006; Lioy & Georgopoulos 2006). It opened up the issue of acute exposure and health effects (Prezant *et al.* 2002; Herbert *et al.* 2006), which was first manifested by the acute-response WTC cough, and the subsequent variety of longer-term effects experienced by workers who had not worn or only periodically worn respirators. The research by Lioy and Georgopoulos (2006) also showed that the event had four categories of outdoor exposures and indoor exposures. Each would affect the intensity of exposure–response relationship. From the standpoint of applications, it demonstrated a need to develop flexible strategies and methods for measuring the severity of acute exposures more precisely, especially to 'non-' traditional air pollutants or 'supercoarse' particles (>10 cm in diameter), and the need to develop sensors for highly toxic pollutants that can assist in establishing the levels of concern after an event. The benchmark for some could be the Acute Exposure Guideline levels (AEGLs) (National Research Council 2001–2004). However, this still leaves a vacuum for a 'supercoarse' particle guideline.

Approaches used in exposure analysis

Determination of human contact or the potential contact with a contaminant is not an integral part of traditional environmental quality measurements. Usually, there are criteria available for making environmental quality measurements, which establish a statistically representative sampling scheme for determining the areal extent of

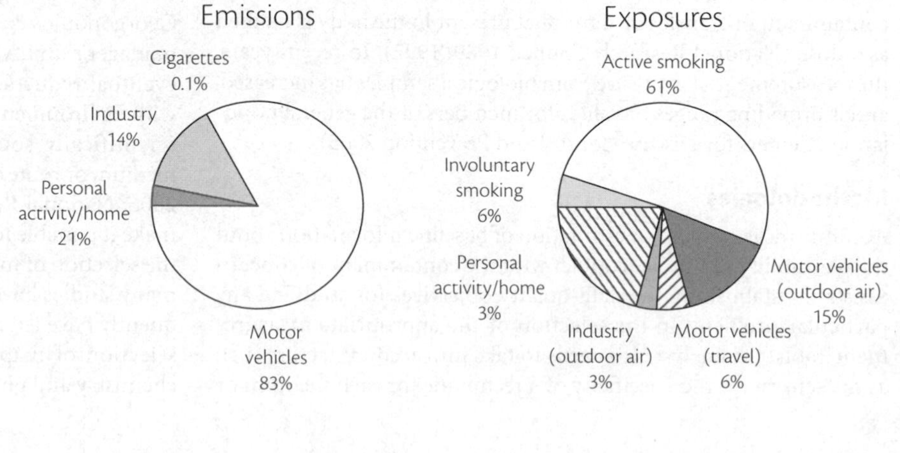

Fig. 8.4.5 Benzene emissions versus exposures. 'Personal activity/home' refers to benzene from materials such as paints, adhesives, and marking pens. For individuals who do not actively smoke, the 'active smoking' contribution to exposure is zero, and the other exposure categories increase proportionally.
Source: Wallace (1989).

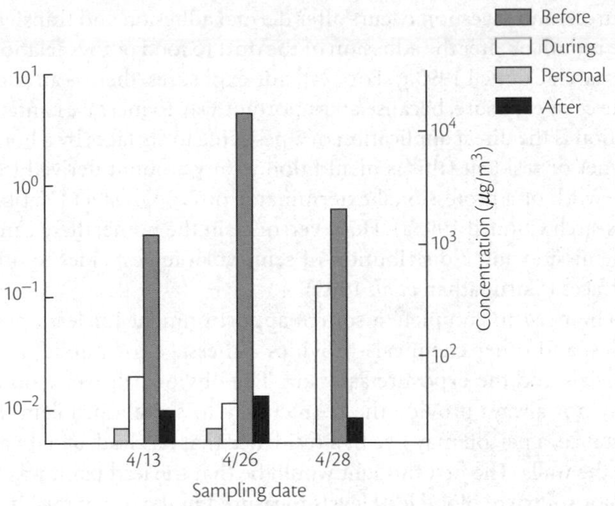

Fig. 8.4.6 MTBE microenvironmental and personal exposure samples during commuter refuelling

contamination, and establishing long-term concentration trends within an environmental medium (Ott 1977; Lioy 1990; Anderson-Sprecher *et al.* 1994; Ott *et al.* 2007). Unfortunately, these measurements do not provide data that can be used to assess exposure directly. Historically, an assessment of exposure was based primarily on the concentration of a contaminant found in an environmental medium at a single sampling site for a prescribed sampling period. However, little or no information was provided on the duration of contact or the probability of contact with the contaminant by people spending time in the location where the measurements were being made. More representative historical examples of exposure measurements would be the breathing zone samples collected in occupational settings; however, the concentrations were much higher.

In many cases, environmental quality measurements continue to provide the only data available for calculating exposure–response relationships within various public health-related studies; for example, air pollution (National Research Council 2004). These data have been used in applications within epidemiology or risk assessment, and have yielded results with a high degree of uncertainty. Also, environmental quality data are rarely collected using strategies that ensure the duration of the measurements is coupled with the relevant biological response time to the presence of a contaminant in the body. As stated previously, the latter point is critical for exposure analysis. All too often, environmental quality measurement programmes are based upon a regulatory requirement for determining compliance to a regulation, and/or the limits of detection and collection capacity of a sampler. Some advances have been made, most notably in water pollution, in which there are more concerns for the levels of substances found in actual drinking water samples. These are used to establish the level of risk to a pollutant or series of pollutants.

The major paradigm shift in framework for exposure analyses, which started in about 1990, has led to the expanded use of personal monitoring and/or microenvironmental monitoring for the development of exposure databases. Both types of monitors are more intrusive than the devices used for monitoring environmental quality as the sample is taken: (a) at or from the individual; (b) in an area occupied by the individual; or (c) from objects used, worn, or eaten by an individual. The samples also require the acquisition of time-resolved data on where and how individuals spend their time (Lebowitz *et al.* 1989; National Research Council 1991c; Freeman *et al.* 1997; Zartarian *et al.* 1997).

A hierarchy of exposure measurements is presented in Table 8.4.2, and emphasizes that personal monitoring provides the best data for completing an exposure assessment (National Research Council 1991c). The table should be reviewed with some caution, however, as in some studies even weak metrics of exposure may be adequate for examining the exposure–health effects relationships. The weak metrics are clearly useful in situations where an isolated source significantly affects a specific community, or a major event or episode has caused health effects. In addition, some techniques currently used for personal exposure could alter a person's usual activity patterns. For instance, personal samplers for particles are usually bulky and cannot be worn comfortably during periods of outdoor and indoor exercise (Lioy 1993). Therefore, based upon needs of a study, it can be safely stated that the exposure analyst has a virtual toolbox of techniques to ensure that measurements can be used successfully to answer a public health question (Lioy 1992, 1999; Sexton *et al.* 1995a).

Another component critical to an exposure analysis is the identification of the study population. In contrast to studies on environmental quality, for which minimal information is required on the population of concern, examination of exposure requires the selection of either a probability-based sample of the general population with possibilities for oversampling of specific subgroups, or a specific subgroup of the population that exhibits characteristics of susceptibility, or is potentially at the high end of exposure to a contaminant. The latter is a major challenge because it is difficult a priori to select the high-end exposure groups, greater than the 90th percentile (US Environmental Protection Agency 1992a). Work completed by Williams *et al.* (2000a,b) attempted to deal with these

Table 8.4.2 Hierarchy of exposure measurements, estimates, and surrogates

	Type of metric	Approximation of human exposure
1.	Quantified personal and biomarker monitoring	Accurate
2.	Quantified area measurements in the vicinity of a person's activities	Accurate to precise
3.	Quantified modelling estimates of contact with contaminates	Precise
4.	Quantified area of ambient measurements in the vicinity of population of concern	Moderate
5.	Surrogates of exposure source use, frequency of contact	Fair
6.	Distance of a source from a residence (other locations) and duration of residence	Fair
7.	Residence or employment in a geographic area in a reasonable proximity to source	Poor activity
8.	Residence or employment in a defined geographical area containing a major source	Poor

Source: Adapted from NRC (1991c).

issues by sampling personal exposures for a group of elderly individuals who lived in an assisted living centre.

Typical sampling plans based on the general population or populations at risk are illustrated in Table 8.4.3. The selection of a susceptible subgroup is more difficult as detailed information is required on the physical or physiological characteristics of interest before selections can be made for entry into a study. Some of the major questions that need to be addressed for properly selected susceptible or sensitive individuals are shown in Table 8.4.4.

Media and routes of exposure

The preceding discussion generally described the environmental media and routes of entry to the body needed to characterize exposure. Each has been examined over the years to provide information on the magnitude and extent of environmental problems. For exposure assessment, there is a special need to know how each medium or route is associated with the degree to which individuals or members of a population come into contact with a contaminant. Many types of sources can impact each medium, and some of the more common issues are shown in Table 8.4.5. Clearly, inorganic or organic emissions can come from industrial processes, commercial activities, personal use and activities, disposal activities, and nature.

It is evident that the environmental media that can lead to contact with a contaminant include air, water, soil, and food as people routinely come into contact with these daily. However, it may be surprising that a contaminant originally released in one medium may, directly or indirectly, utilize multiple routes of entry to the body. An exception is the inadvertent or purposeful injection of a biological or chemical contaminant. This important point is illustrated in Table 8.4.6 for the contaminants lead and pesticides.

Lead can be emitted by sources that have direct impact on the air, water, soil, and food; it may then be transported to and deposited in another medium, and thereby be made available to indirectly cause exposures via multiple routes of entry to the body. From the standpoint of public health, the situation is complicated because there is no easy formula available to determine the route of entry, or to apportion the sources contributing to lead burden. In the case of house dust, lead can be derived from indoor and outdoor sources, and ingestion occurs after dermal adhesion and transfer to the mouth or after the adhesion of the dust to food or toys (National Research Council 1993a). For pesticide exposures, there is an added source of exposure, because an important way to increase contamination is the direct application of a pesticide to surfaces by a homeowner or resident (this is in addition to any amount derived from the work of a professional exterminator or crop duster) (National Research Council 1993a). However, once in the home, there can be re-emission and redistribution of semi-volatile pesticides to other surfaces (Gurunathan *et al.* 1998).

The need to complete a source apportionment for lead, pesticides, and other chemicals provides a message for public health officials and the exposure assessor: The obvious answer (source) may not always provide the correct way to solve a problem. For instance, a person may live in a residence that has lead-based paint on the walls. The first thought would be that the lead paint was the major source of blood lead levels measured in the occupants. If the painted surface is isolated or intact, however, the source that could cause an increase in blood lead may be street dust and/or soil in the neighbourhood. Therefore, source apportionment plays a crucial part in linking the point of emission through the route of exposure to an internal or biologically effective dose (previously illustrated in Fig. 8.4.2).

An example of how exposure and risk derived from multiple routes of entry can be underestimated is associated with regulations or public health warnings for potable water supplies. In the 1970s, potential exposures and health risks were based solely on the quantity of the contaminant ingested by drinking the water (US Environmental Protection Agency 1980), and the assumed consumption of 2L of water per day, which is unusual for most members of the general population. Public health warnings on the use of contaminated water supplies, for example, wells with water containing contaminants leached from hazardous waste sites, stated that individuals using a particular water supply 'should not drink the water'. If scientists and regulators had seriously considered all the opportunities for contact with potable water prior to estimating the risk, they would have included two other routes of exposure: Dermal and inhalation (Brown *et al.* 1984). Only after studies by Andelman (1985), which focused on the shower as a route for

Table 8.4.3 Summary of sampling strategies for exposure measurements

Sampling design	Condition for most useful application
Haphazard sampling	Only valid when target population and exposure is homogeneous in space and time; hence not generally recommended
Purposive sampling	Target population well defined and homogeneous, so sample-selection bias is not a problem; or specific microenvironmental or personal samples selected for unique value and interest, rather than for making inferences to wider population
Probability sampling	
Simple random sampling	Homogeneous population
Stratified random sampling	Homogeneous population with strata (subregions); might consider strata as domains of study
Systematic sampling	Frequently most useful: trends over time and space must be quantified; can easily be adapted to total exposure
Multistage sampling	Target population large and homogeneous; simple random sampling used to select contiguous groups of population units
Cluster sampling	Economical when population units cluster (e.g. schools of fish); ideally, cluster means are similar in value, but concentrations within clusters should vary widely. Anticipate high-end exposures
Double sampling	Must be strong linear relation between variable of interest and less expensive or more easily measured variable

Table 8.4.4 Defining high-exposure populations

Data collection methods
Choice of method
◆ Purposive exposure study
◆ Applied, or response, epidemiology
◆ Targeted case-control or cohorts
◆ Registries
◆ Reference population surveys
◆ Complete enumeration
Sampling design
◆ Representative
◆ Convenient
Detecting small populations or rare events
Defining subgroups of the population
Cultural characteristics
◆ Cultural identity
◆ Heterogeneity within categories
◆ Sensitive information
◆ Cultural habits or rituals
◆ Choice of appropriate indicator
Susceptibility characterizations
◆ Race
◆ Gender
◆ Age
◆ Disease state
◆ Population on family genetics
◆ Occupations (participation or avoidance)
Population
◆ Mobility
◆ Estimation of local population size
◆ Intermarriage
◆ Assimilation
◆ Daily living activities
◆ Proximity to a source or source region
◆ Observation of any effects

Table 8.4.5 Typical sources of contaminants that can be present in various media

Air (outdoor)	
Smelters	Atmosphere reactions
Power plants	Space heating
Petrochemical	Car
Plants	Trucks
Chemical	Transportation
Manufacturing	Water treatment
Paper and pulp	Plants
Cement plants	Autobody repair
Municipal incinerators	Mining operations
Degreasing operations	
Air (indoor)	
Passive smoking	Deodorizers
Household products	Rugs
Indoor combustion	Ventilation system
Disinfectants	Water contaminants
Paint	Paint removers
Water	
Landfills	Domestic waste
Hazardous waste sites	Agriculture
Chemical plants	Agriculture run-off
Pesticides production	Underground storage
Food process industry	Urban street run-off
Sewage treatment	Water system
Septic tank	Sealants
Soil	
Hazardous wastes	Yard clean-up and maintenance
Underground storage tanks	Buried underground
Domestic waste	Storage
Industrial dumping	
Food	
Garden soil	Insufficient food preparation
Agricultural soil	Pesticide residuals
Insufficient food cleaning	Unapproved packaging
Injection	
Contaminated needles and objects	Contaminated products
Contaminated fluids	Spills and transportation

inhalation exposure, and by Jo *et al.* (1990) and Weisel *et al.* (1993b), which demonstrated that significant human exposures to volatile organics occurred via inhalation and dermal route during showering or bathing, did the public health practice and environmental regulations embrace the concept of total exposure. The results have led to the concept that individuals should 'just not use contaminated water'. According to Jo *et al.* (1990), at least half of an individual's internal dose derived from chloroform found in a public water supply could be just from one 10-min shower per day. Obviously, more and varied uses of the water would lead to higher or lower daily internal doses. This work has been extended by Xu and Weisel (2005) to haloketones in showers.

The importance of both the dermal and inhalation routes is demonstrated in Fig. 8.4.7, for the concentration of chloroform found in exhaled breath after using a swimming pool. Integration of the

Table 8.4.6 Pathways of exposure

Contaminant	Medium or pathway	Source
Lead	Outdoor air	Industrial Automobile
	Indoor air	Infiltration of outdoor air
	Outdoor soil	Air deposition Flaking paint Hazardous waste
	Outdoor dust	Air deposition Flaking paint Soil resuspension
	House dust	Tracked dust Paint flaking Air filtration
	Food utensils/ food preparation	Dust deposition Dust contact Pottery/glasses
	Clothing	Surface contact Laundering of clothes
	Water	Water pipes Water supply
	Food	Grown in contaminated soil Preparation
Pesticides	Outdoor air	Spraying of crops or yards
	Indoor air	Spraying of plants Outdoor air filtration
	Outdoor soil	Air deposition Direct spraying of plants/vegetation
	Outdoor dust	Air deposition Resuspension of soil
	House dust	Indoor spraying Tracked outdoor dust/soil Outdoor air filtration
	Food	Surface deposition Fruit/vegetable contamination
	Food preparation	Surface dust (outdoor/house)
	Water	Run-off from soil Water supply

area under the curve indicates that both routes made similar contributions to an internal dose, even though there is a much slower rate of chloroform accumulation by the dermal route (Georgopoulos *et al.* 1997; Kim & Weisel 1998). The concept of single and multiple route exposures has led to the introduction of new measurement tools for long-term exposure characteristics: Aggregate exposure and cumulative exposure. These can be defined as:

- Aggregate exposure: The extent of contact or exposure of a defined population to a given chemical by all relevant routes and all relevant sources.
- Cumulative exposure: The extent of contact or exposure of a defined population to multiple chemicals with common toxic effects found in at least one media and one or more sources (US Environmental Protection Agency 2001b, 2003).

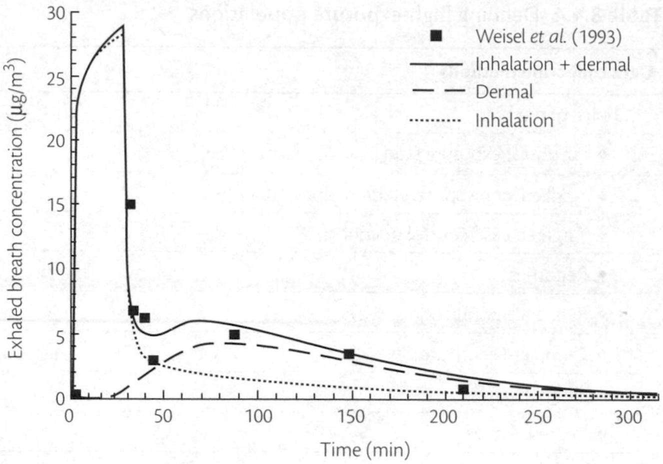

Fig. 8.4.7 Exhaled breath concentration of chloroform following inhalation and dermal absorption in a swimming pool (air concentration 100 μg/m^3, water concentration 150 μg/l).

Techniques

The measurement process used to establish the presence of a contaminant in one or more of the media or routes mentioned in the preceding subsection can become complex and require the application of a variety of techniques. Two primary categories exist for exposure measurements: Direct and indirect techniques (Fig. 8.4.8) (National Research Council 1991c). These categories correspond to the types of methods being used to collect data or estimate exposure in field studies and modelling simulations, respectively. The main differences between these two types of techniques are associated with the proximity of the measurement or estimate of exposure to the individual, and the qualitative or quantitative nature of the information. At present, there is no uniformity in the quality and quantity of techniques available for any category of indirect or direct measurements. In fact, there are major instrumentation needs for each environmental medium and route of exposure. This is not to say that there is a lack of sampling and analytical equipment to measure chemical, physical, and biological agents in various environmental media. However, many have been designed to provide environmental quality measurements rather than human exposure measurements. This is an important point and is substantiated by the fact that many of the currently available techniques are too bulky to be used in applications requiring either microenvironmental and/or personal measurements (Lioy 1993). However, microsensor development should begin to improve this situation in the future (Weis *et al.* 2005).

In many cases, personal monitors still require optimization for a number of parameters. A list of general technical criteria that must be met to develop these monitors is shown in Table 8.4.7 (National Research Council 1991c). It is apparent that the techniques must be compact, and each must have low detection limits and sufficient time resolution in order to obtain human exposures for the chemical (s) under consideration. These three features are difficult to achieve simultaneously in a single device. For example, as an instrument is miniaturized, the substrate available for sample collection or the detection volume available for instrumental analyses (e.g. a photocell) is reduced. Consequently, the detection limits will rise and/or the time necessary to collect an adequate sample will increase,

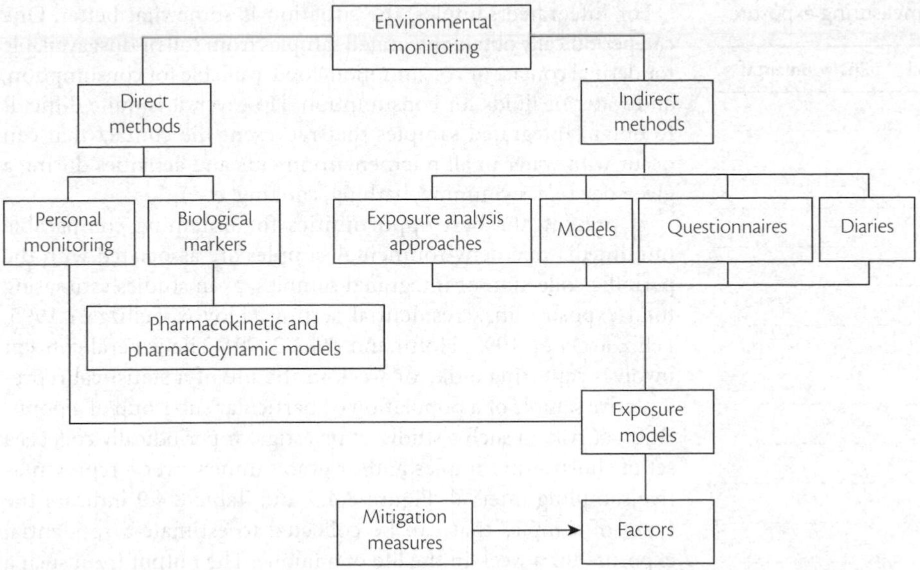

Fig. 8.4.8 Possible approaches for analysis of air contaminant exposures.
Source: NRC (1991c).

which can preclude their use in specific applications; for example, low-level short-term exposure or acute exposures. Such incompatibilities can only be eliminated by conducting basic research prior to the development of a sampling programme that will employ a device in any particular application. Sometimes, there may be 'off-the-shelf' devices available for use in an application or study, but the possibilities have been limited for most media and routes of exposure. During the mid-1970s, because of the increased concern about health problems associated with indoor air pollution, technology developed rapidly and microenvironmental and personal

Table 8.4.7 Methods criteria

Factor	Ideal condition
Sensitivity	Detects analytes at levels below those causing adverse health effect; sensitivity 0.1× level of interest; range 0.1–10× level of interest; precision and accuracy ±5%; easy and accurate calibration
Selectivity	No response to similar compounds that might be present simultaneously with the analyte of interest, or can differentiate multiple compounds in single device
Rapidity	Short sampling and analysis times compared with biological response time or with significant changes in contaminant concentration; response time 90% in less than 30s; RS232 or equivalent output
Operation	Few complex components to change in the field, quick releases, low noise
Comprehensiveness	Sensitive to all contaminants that could result in a similar adverse health effect
Portability	Sampling and analysis device is rugged and can be worn without modifying the normal behaviour of individual; lower power consumption; battery operated; stabilization time less than 15 min; temperature range −20 to 40°C; humidity range zero to 100%
Cost	Cost of sampling and analysis is not prohibitive; inexpensive; readily available components; few consumables; low maintenance

air measurements were available for the detection of traditional contaminants (e.g. volatile organics, fine particles, and carbon monoxide). Others are being developed for agents such as microbiological aerosols. Some of the personal monitors are based on passive sampling techniques whereas other sampling systems use an active pump (Seifert & Abraham 1983; Ryan *et al.* 1986; Samet *et al.* 1987, 1988; Jantunen *et al.* 1998; Hoffmann *et al.* 2000b; Weisel *et al.* 2005).

Before the concept of total exposure became a starting point for the design of field studies and risk assessments, the following measurement issue received little attention: How comparable are the data collected by various techniques used across more than one medium or route of entry into the body? Unfortunately, there is no complete answer because of the many different types of physical, chemical, and biological agents that exist and the nature of the emissions, transport, accumulation, and transformation processes that can affect the occurrence of biologically significant exposures. A summary of the types of techniques employed for collecting microenvironmental and personal samples is shown in Table 8.4.8. To illustrate the problem of obtaining comparable measurements, Table 8.4.8 can be used to examine the situation as it currently exists for microenvironmental monitors. For microenvironmental studies of air pollution, there exist both continuous and integrating monitors; the devices have high resolution and low detection limits for specific compounds, for example, metals and volatile organics. The data can easily be used to estimate the direct inhalation exposure. However, for other media, there are very few comparable techniques available for completing events with even quasi-continuous monitors. In fact, there are no continuous monitors currently available for these sampling media that operate without the constant use of a technician as a personal shadow. For example, a subject could take a surface soil sample at every location that he or she came into contact with soil during the day (Hawley 1985). Alternately, the person would be required to have a trained technician directly shadow his or her movements during the sampling in order to collect the appropriate surface soil samples, or provide dermal contact samples similar to those experienced by the subject. In either case, the approach is very cumbersome and can lead to many errors.

Table 8.4.8 General availability of monitors for measuring exposure

Type/route	Personal	Micro-environmental	Environmental
Inhalation/gases			
C	+	+	+
I	+	+	+
Pesticides			
C	–	+	+
I	+	+	+
Ingestion			
Food			
C	–	–	–
I	+	+	+
Water			
C	–	–	–
I	–	+	+
Soil and dust			
C	–	–	–
I	–	+	+
Dermal			
Water			
C	–	–	–
I	–	+	+
Soil and dust			
C	–	–	–
I	–	+	+

C, continuous monitor; I, integrated monitor; –, not available; +, available.

For integrated samples, the situation is somewhat better. One can periodically obtain integrated samples from soil or dust available for dermal contact or consumption, food available for consumption, and water or fluids for consumption. However, it is quite difficult to obtain integrated samples that represent the contact that can occur with water in all microenvironments and activities during a given day (e.g. swimming, bathing, cooking, etc.)

At present, the best opportunities for obtaining comparable multimedia microenvironmental samples are associated with the periodic collection of integrated samples, as in studies estimating total exposure in a residential setting (Lioy & Pellizzari 1995; Pellizzari *et al.* 1995; Hoffmann *et al.* 2000). The general concept involves capturing a day or week in the life of a statistical representative sample of a population or particular subgroup of a population at risk. In such a study, an investigator periodically collects a set of short-term samples and/or grab samples over a representative sampling interval. Figure 8.4.9 and Table 8.4.9 indicate the types of samples that can be collected to estimate a residential exposure for a week in the life of a family. The output from such a measurement study will be a series of microenvironmental samples that are analysed for the chemicals of concern. The data are then used as inputs to exposure scenarios of specific environmental contaminants in residential settings. They can also be used to construct total exposure estimates using variants to the summation equations given in Box 8.4.1.

One major component of this type of study is the application of questionnaires, which must include a time/activity log that is completed by the members of the household during the time of field sampling. The data are essential for reducing uncertainties that are inherent in the application of generic exposure scenarios to site- or person-specific assessments.

Activity logs have become customized to address the exposures that can occur for specific chemicals (Freeman *et al.* 1991; McCurdy *et al.* 2000; US Environmental Protection Agency 2001a), in addition

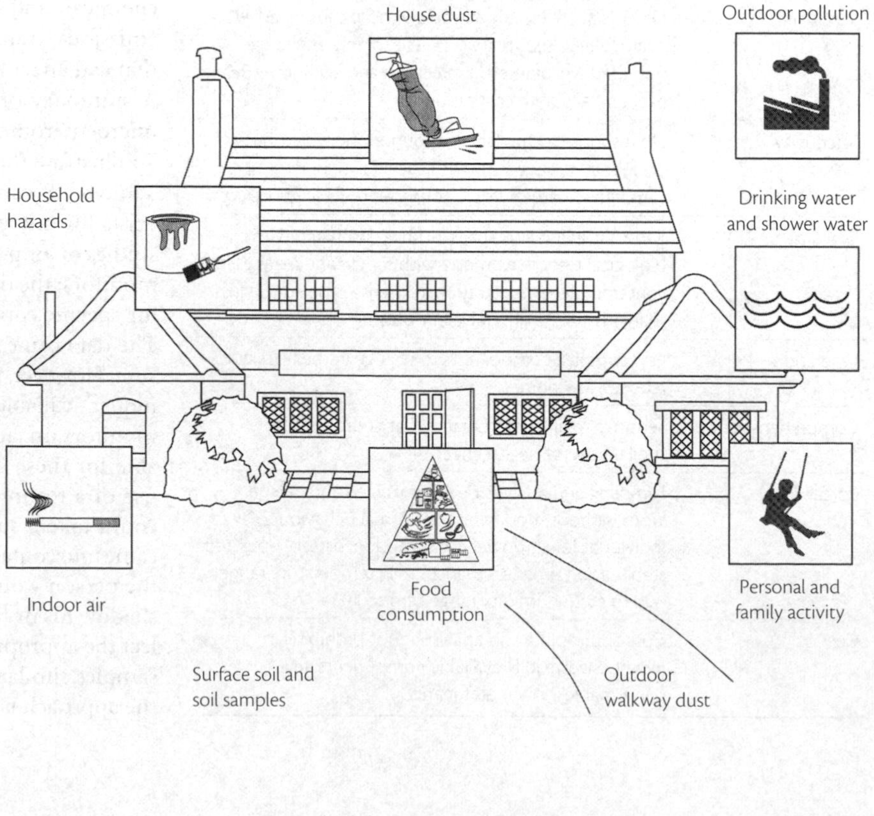

Fig. 8.4.9 Types of integrated microenvironmental sentinel for home exposure to metals, pesticides, and/or volatile organics.

Table 8.4.9 Sampling strategy

Types of samples	Location	Duration
Indoor air	Two high-use rooms	1–7 days
Outdoor air	Breathing zone in yard	1–7 days
Soil	Yard surface	Composited grab
	0–2-cm gridded yard sweep	
	Subsurface	
	0–100-cm gridded dig	
Dust	Flat interior surface	Integrated wipe
	Rugs on interior floor	Integrated vacuum
	Flat exterior walkways	Integrated sweeps
Water	Drinking water	Daily tap water (1 litre)
	Shower water	10–30 min
	Bath water	Daily bath water
Food	Kitchen-prepared and -consumed meals	1–7-day duplicate diet
Activity patterns	Residential actions or events	Daily diary

to logs that address generic issues on contact with environment contaminants (e.g. frequency of personal product use and contact with volatile components, frequency and duration of outdoor activities). For instance, in a study of residential exposure, typical questions for a week-long study of chromium exposure would include the following:

1. Were any of the following used in the house today: (a) vacuum, (b) carpet sweeper, (c) broom, (d) dust cloths/mops, (e) wet mops, (f) other house cleaning, (g) laundry?
2. Did you notice any green, yellow, red, or orange deposits or stains on the walls or floors of your home?
3. If you noticed these deposits, were you or members of your family in the room or rooms with these deposits for more than 10 minutes at a time?

Results obtained by these types of methods can be validated by video records, technician observations (Reed *et al.* 1999; Tulve *et al.* 2002; Shalat *et al.* 2003), and fluorescent tracer studies (Fenske *et al.* 1991). During the chromium study, validation was obtained via observations made by a trained technician (Freeman *et al.* 1991). However, there are a number of issues that must be considered when using children in exposure studies, some of which are discussed by Sexton (2005).

Although not shown in Fig. 8.4.9, a residential microenvironmental study can easily be expanded to include personal monitoring and biological monitoring. Some of the more common are used to measure organic and inorganic chemicals in blood and urine. These samples will provide personal integrated or time series data for the duration of the sampling period (e.g. a day or a week). Biological monitoring data provide baseline information on the residents and can be used to determine if they have been 'truly' in contact with a contaminant. If a residential experiment is to be repeated one or more times, biological marker data can be valuable in pharmacokinetic model simulations for some contaminants. Follow-up biological monitoring samples can also allow the analyst to establish any incremental changes in dose.

Biological monitoring is currently used to measure selected heavy metals in blood and urine, volatile organics in blood, and pesticides in blood and urine in studies at hazardous waste sites, other research studies, and within the National Health and Nutrition Examination Survey (NHANES), and was previously used in the National Human Exposure Assessment Survey (Pellizzari *et al.* 1995; Pirkle *et al.* 1995). Further, the Centers for Disease Control and Prevention (CDC) extensively tested for a variety of agents during the NHANES (Centers for Disease Control and Prevention 2005). There are also some techniques available for the measurement of metabolites and DNA adducts (National Research Council 1989, 1991c; Ashley *et al.* 1992), some of which are associated with polycyclic aromatic hydrocarbons. The future of biological marker measurements was recently summarized by Schmidt (2006). A first-order analysis of the data would be to determine the change in contaminant level for a bodily fluid that could be associated with a change in the type of intensity of exposure that occurred at the residence. A second-order analysis would involve the application of pharmacokinetic models (Caudill *et al.* 1992; Hoffmann *et al.* 2000; Kieszak *et al.* 2002).

In 1993, the National Academy of Sciences (NAS) published a report (National Research Council 1993a) arguing that children are a highly susceptible population for exposure to pesticides. This remains a continuing concern (Needham & Sexton 2000; Quackenboss *et al.* 2000; Schneider & Freeman 2001; Barr *et al.* 2005; Hore *et al.* 2005) because both in terms of surface-to-volume ratio and physiological function, children are different from adults, and children may be more susceptible to exposure to environmental contaminants. Their way of interacting with the world is different from adults, and they spend more time on the floor and take baths rather than showers. Further, infants and toddlers are more likely to mouth objects and exhibit hand-to-mouth behaviours, and have substantially greater food and fluid consumption when expressed as grams or litres per kilogram of body weight than adults (US Environmental Protection Agency 1997; Freeman *et al.* 1997; National Research Council 1993b; Tsang & Klepeis 1996). Because of their close contact with floors and carpets, the concept of a well-mixed air environment may not be appropriate for the air they breathe. The air inhaled close to a carpet may have very different concentrations of chemicals than the air inhaled 4 or 5 feet (120–150cm) from the floor, where the inlets of air samplers are typically placed. The prolonged hot baths of toddlers and school children in combination with the greater surface-to-volume ratio produces potentially greater exposure to volatile organic compounds in water than an adult receives in his or her 5- to 10-min shower. The mouthing behaviours of children become a constant means of incidentally ingesting contaminants on their hands or the objects that they put in their mouths.

In response to the issues raised by the National Academy of Sciences report (National Research Council 1993a), the methods used in exposure assessment had to be changed in new directions as interest in children's exposure to environmental contaminants evolved. Previously, when children were the target population of interest (primarily lead-exposure studies), information about the children was obtained from parents or caregivers. This allowed acquisition of global knowledge about exposure activities such as identifying the microenvironment in which the child spent time or macroactivities such as whether or not the child took a bath or played in a sandbox. The amount of time spent in a microenvironment, submerged in a bath, or in contact with sand could not effectively be obtained from parents as the parents are often not present with the child, much less timing the events. The temporal information obtained from parents is at best 'guesstimates'. The introduction of tools for obtaining a characterization of aggregate exposure has helped to design studies that look at all aspects of the exposure characterization, pesticides being a prime example (US Environmental Protection Agency 2001b).

Collecting information from children also has problems as often the target population is so young that self-reports cannot be obtained. Even children as old as 10 or 12 years have difficulty with concepts of time, and reportage using real-time diaries has not been entirely successful (Cohen-Hubal *et al.* 2000; Tulve *et al.* 2002). Younger children not only have limited concepts of time but also may not have the ability to read and complete diaries, or verbally express themselves in response to an interviewer (Cohen-Hubal *et al.* 2000).

Additional problems with understanding children's exposure to environmental contaminants have emerged as the source of exposure has shifted from outdoor and/or indoor air pollutants to waterborne and dust- or soil-borne contaminants, and the routes of exposure have shifted from inhalation to dermal contact, and dietary and non-dietary ingestion. To understand these sources and routes of exposure, information is needed about not only microenvironments but also microactivities, such as contact with dust and soil or mouthing objects and fingers (Cohen-Hubal *et al.* 2000). Additional sources of exposure in the child's environment may be the toys the child plays with and mouths (Gurunathan *et al.* 1998). The dynamic character of semi-volatile chemicals such as pesticides means that surfaces and objects not directly sprayed may become reservoirs and future sources of exposure. Understanding the potential exposure from these surfaces and objects requires collection of information about microactivities, which has seldom been done.

Although parental reportage of time and activity information about their children continues to be used, parental responses are now being supplemented, if not supplanted, by observational methods (Zartarian *et al.* 1997, 1998; Reed *et al.* 1999). Videotaped observations can be used to verify parental responses, quantify use of microenvironments, and collect frequency and duration data about microactivities. Reed *et al.* (1999) found that even a simple event such as hand washing was not accurately reported by either parents or day-care teachers. The adult reports were perhaps influenced by expectations rather than reality. Mouthing behaviours of children that contribute to children's exposure to dust- and soil-borne contaminants can only be accurately quantified by an observational technique. The independently conducted observational studies by Zartarian *et al.* (1998) and Freeman *et al.* (2001b) found very similar frequencies of activities among toddlers in a Californian farm community and in urban and suburban New Jersey. The children in these studies made hundreds of hand contacts with surfaces and objects in their environment every hour, maximizing the opportunity of contact with contaminants. Part of the evolution in exposure assessment prompted by the NAS report is to think of exposure to a contaminant or family of contaminants from all potential media; that is, to aggregate the individual's exposure to air, food, soil, dust, water, and other contaminated media. For the child, the 'other media' may be a major pathway, but for which there are presently few data and for which activities may have a large influence on exposure. This example of children just illustrates the needs of one subgroup of the general population. In the future, investigators will need to fill in major blanks for culture-, gender-, and age-specific behaviours that can influence individual or subpopulation exposure.

Data analysis and models

Once microenvironmental and/or personal exposure data have been acquired in a field study or estimated by a model, there are a number of analyses that can be used to place the data in a form that is helpful for examining a public health issue. The levels of analysis are dependent upon the types and amount of data available from a particular study or a series of companion or comparative studies (US Environmental Protection Agency 1989a; Burke *et al.* 2001). A parallel issue is the form of the data necessary for the application of interest; for example, epidemiology or risk assessment. For instance, the data can be reported as exposure using the units of concentration and time (μg/m^3 per h) or as a time-weighted average (μg/m^3 per day). Then, depending upon the amount of data available, a distribution of exposure can be constructed and particular statistical quantities calculated from that data. Information derived from a distribution of exposures is shown in Fig. 8.4.10 (US Environmental Protection Agency 1992a), and includes the mean exposure (=50th percentile), the high-end exposure (>90th percentile), the form of the exposure distribution curve, and the worst possible case estimate (bounding estimate) of exposure.

If the database includes information that can be examined across pathways or routes of exposure, the result will be estimates of total exposure across each medium or each route of entry into the body. The data collected representing a day or week of a family, and Table 8.4.9 and Fig. 8.4.9, can be used to determine the microenvironmental increments to total exposure. Theoretically, an integrated exposure can be derived from microenvironmental exposures by the summation formula given in Box 8.4.1.

Risk assessment applications require at least one further level of analysis: A dose calculated from the exposure level. The result can then be used in a risk characterization analysis, and as stated

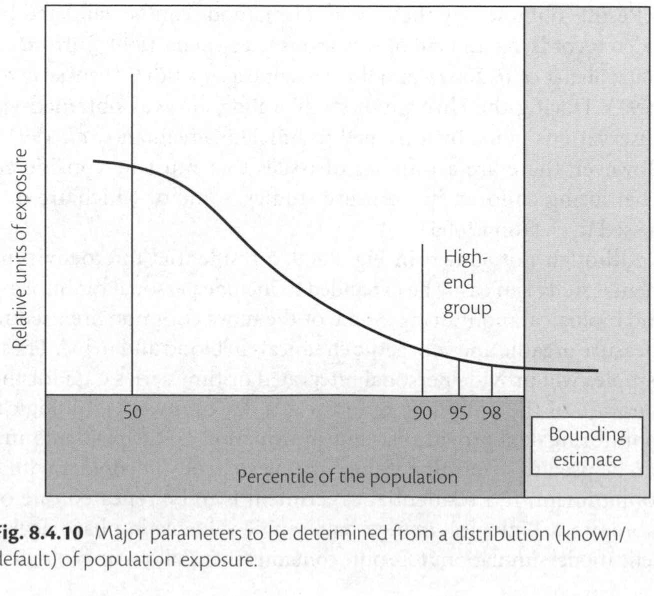

Fig. 8.4.10 Major parameters to be determined from a distribution (known/default) of population exposure.

earlier, these calculations can be one of three forms: Potential, internal, or biologically effective dose. The general forms of the equations needed to calculate dose from exposure data are shown in Box 8.4.2. Based upon the ancillary information and parameters needed to complete such calculations (e.g. absorption rate), the value most frequently calculated is the potential dose. In rare instances, the biologically effective dose can be calculated, but there are large uncertainties in the values used for factors to complete such calculations (e.g. repair rate) (Lioy 1990).

A second reason for calculating a dose from the exposure data is to place units of measurement in a form that is consistent for comparisons between each route of entry. A typical form for dose is micrograms of contaminant per kilogram of body weight per unit of time. The format makes it easier to compare intensity of the contact with the amount that has been deposited within the body for different routes of entry. These data can also be used to determine which of the exposures encountered were at levels that may cause a biological effect.

As shown in Box 8.4.2, unless the investigator has acquired biological marker data, the determination of a dose requires information on a series of variables or factors that may only be measurable in detailed exposure assessment studies (American Industrial Health Council 1994; US Environmental Protection Agency 1997). An update on such factors was published by the US Environmental Protection Agency in 2002 on a CD-ROM and it continues to be updated periodically. Examples of factors needed to complete dose calculations include breathing rate, skin absorption rate, ingestion rate, internal absorption rate, elimination rate, and repair rates. Obviously, it is easier to acquire data on breathing or ingestion rate than on cellular repair mechanisms. In fact, there are no methods currently available that can quantify cellular repair.

Box 8.4.2 Generalized equations governing exposure and dose

Integrated exposure

$$E = \int_{t_1}^{t_2} C(t)\,\mathrm{d}t$$

where E is exposure, $C(t)$ is time-variant concentration, and t_1, t_2 are time periods of exposure associated with a specific biological response.

Potential dose

$$D_{\mathrm{p}} = \int_{t_2}^{t_1} C(t) f(t)\,\mathrm{d}t$$

where D_{P} is the potential dose and $f(t)$ is the contact rate.

Internal dose

$$D_{\mathrm{i}} = \int_{t_1}^{t_2} C(t) f(t) g_{\mathrm{ab}}\,\mathrm{d}t$$

where D_{i} is the internal dose and g_{ab} is the absorption function (e.g. skin, lung membrane, gut).

Target tissue dose

$$D_{\mathrm{T}} = \int_{t_1}^{t_2} C(t) f(t) g_{\mathrm{pk}}\,\mathrm{d}t$$

where D_{T} is the target tissue dose and g_{pk} is the pharmacokinetic model (accounts for absorption, distribution, and elimination processes).

Biologically effective dose

$$D_{\mathrm{BE}} = \int_{t_1}^{t_2} f(x) g(ab) p(\mathrm{as,rd,me,el}) C(t)\,\mathrm{d}t$$

where $p(\mathrm{as,rd,me,el})$ is a function based on nature of assimilation, repair, elimination, and/or metabolism.

A type of data that is not usually available for dose calculations, but could be obtained, is the bioavailability of a contaminant in the matrix that contains it (e.g. soil) (Ruby *et al.* 1993; Wainman *et al.* 1994; Hamel *et al.* 1998; Ellickson *et al.* 2002). This value depends upon the amount of a contaminant that can be extracted from the matrix (e.g. soil) by bodily fluids found within the digestive system or the lung.

As it is not possible to routinely acquire data in a field study on accumulation or elimination rates, or absorption factors, dose calculations employ what have been conventionally described as generic exposure factors (single values or a distribution of values).

Based upon the type of dose calculation, the number of exposure factors selected can be minimal or extensive. These are driven by the data quality objectives, the amount of data available, the anticipated variability of the activities affecting the dose, and the types of individual or population characteristics considered to be of importance. Once these types of information have accumulated and the purpose and objectives of the analyses have been established, the analyst can complete either a point estimate of a dose or a distributional estimate of a dose.

Point estimates of exposure require the application of an equation similar to those found in Box 8.4.2 for each route of exposure and each microenvironment that can lead to an individual having contact with chemicals. For example, selection of ingestion exposure, inhalation exposure, and dermal exposure scenarios can provide an estimate of the potential or, with additional data, an internal dose of a contaminant by completing a calculation similar to that illustrated in Box 8.4.3 (US Environmental Protection Agency 1989a). Results can then be summed for all microenvironments and media to obtain point estimates of exposure for a hypothetical or representative member of the local population. One can also develop a distribution of dose point estimates based upon exposure measurements (e.g. personal monitoring) and/or estimates of exposure using exposure factors characteristic of the population of concern.

There has been a distinct move away from relying exclusively on point estimates of exposure and dose. This is done primarily to reduce the uncertainties that surround identifying a 'most exposed individual' (US Environmental Protection Agency 1992a), which was frequently used to describe the person exposed to everything over a lifetime. In fact, exposure scientists are now being encouraged to employ distributional analyses by the frequency distributions of all or selected factors needed to estimate particular exposures or doses. This has led to the use of Monte Carlo techniques for combining the selected distributions of parameters or variables (Marnicio *et al.* 1991; Johnson & Capel 1992b; Hattis & Burmaster 1994; Ott 1995b). On the surface, this appears to be a step forward in the development of exposure or dose databases especially for risk assessment applications. However, there are some

Box 8.4.3 Point estimate of potential dose

◆ Ingestion of chemicals in water or beverages:

$$\text{potential dose}=\frac{CW \times IR \times EF \times ED}{BW \times AT}\ \text{mg/kg/day}$$

where CW is the chemical concentration in water, IR is the ingestion rate (L/day), EF is the exposure frequency (days/year), ED is the exposure duration (years), BW is the body weight (kg), and AT is the averaging time (period over which exposure is averaged) (days).

◆ Chemicals in soil:

$$\text{potential dose}=\frac{CS \times IR \times CF \times FI \times EF \times ED}{BW \times AT}\ \text{mg/kg/day}$$

where CS is the chemical concentration in soil (mg/kg), IR is the ingestion rate (mg soil/day), CF is the conversion factor (10^6 kg/mg), FI is the fraction ingested from contaminated source (unitless), EF is the exposure frequency (days/years), ED is the exposure duration (years), BW is the body weight (kg), and AT is the averaging time (period over which exposure is averaged) (days).

◆ Inhalation of airborne (vapour-phase) chemicals:

$$\text{potential dose}=\frac{CA \times IR \times ET \times EF \times ED}{BW \times AT}\ \text{mg/kg/day}$$

where CA is the contaminant concentration in air (μg/m^3), IR is the inhalation rate (m^3/h), ET is the exposure time (h/day), EF is the exposure frequency (days/year), ED is the exposure duration (years), BW is the body/weight (kg), and AT is the averaging time (period over which exposure is averaged) (days).

◆ Dermal contact with chemicals in soil:

$$\text{potential dose}=\frac{CS \times CF \times SA \times AF \times ABS \times EF \times ED}{BW \times AT}\ \text{mg/kg/day}$$

where CS is the chemical concentration in soil (mg/kg), CF is the conversion factor (10^6 kg/mg), SA is the skin area (cm^2), AF is the soil-to-skin adherence factor (mg/cm^2), ABS is the absorption factor (unitless), EF is the exposure frequency (days/years), ED is the exposure duration (years), BW is the body weight (kg), AT is the averaging time (period over which exposure is averaged) (days).

'landmines' buried in the analysis of distributions that employ the random selection of points to establish a distribution of exposure. Figure 8.4.11 illustrates the general concept of combining distributions of independent variables to establish an overall distribution of one dependent variable; in our case, exposure or dose.

At first glance, this seems to be a relatively simple task, because Monte Carlo techniques, available in many computer programmes, combine the points along each known or approximated variable distribution and produce a final distribution that represents the exposure or dose. There are inherent statistical limitations to Monte Carlo analyses that must be examined prior to selecting the distributions used in applications of a particular set of exposure data, and these have been outlined by many researchers (Marnicio *et al.* 1991; Johnson & Capel 1992b; Hattis & Burmaster 1994; Ott 1995a). Beyond the statistical constraints, there are other informational issues that must be evaluated to ensure that the estimates are plausible and realistic; included is the evaluation of the usefulness of the values that combine across distributions to simulate either the high-end exposures or low-end exposures. An example of a distribution of an exposure factor—fish ingestion—is shown in Fig. 8.4.12. It is clear that there is a tendency towards biomodality (American Industrial Health Council 1994). The shape of the curve indicates different consumption patterns for subgroups of a population. Thus, proper utilization of the data requires knowledge of consumption activities within a potentially affected population.

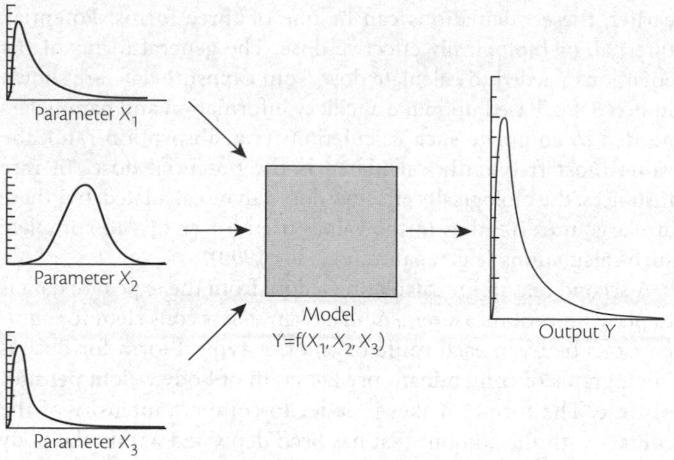

Fig. 8.4.11 Representation of Monte Carlo analysis used to construct a dependent variable distribution Y.

Evaluations of distributional data must also ascertain whether or not all projected exposures or doses can occur and whether they can occur for the situation or activity under investigation. At a minimum, sensitivity analyses should be conducted on the tails of the variable distributions used to estimate the exposure or dose. For example, an acute toxin (such as cyanide or ozone) at sufficient concentration to induce a biological response (death or asthma attack, respectively) over a short period of time would not logically be coupled with a contact period equivalent to a week or more. An 82-year-old grandparent or unathletic person would not be spending too much time engaging in activities with a high ventilation rate of 1.5m^3/h when the outdoor ozone concentration exceeds 150ppb. Finally, a child would not be spending 24h a day over a 12-year period sitting on the grounds of a hazardous waste site. These examples may seem somewhat absurd, but if the appropriate constraints are not placed on a distributional analysis of exposure, these types of results, or worse, will be propagated through a computer programme and reported as part of the estimated distribution of exposure or dose.

Although distributional analyses are more likely to be conducted for risk assessments, they are of value in epidemiological studies. A specific case is the comparison of biological marker data for a contaminant or metabolite with a dose estimated from external exposure measurements. In intervention studies, distributional data are of immense value for comparing a point measurement of exposure or dose (individual or affected subgroups) with the values observed and/or estimated for a much larger population (Lioy 1992).

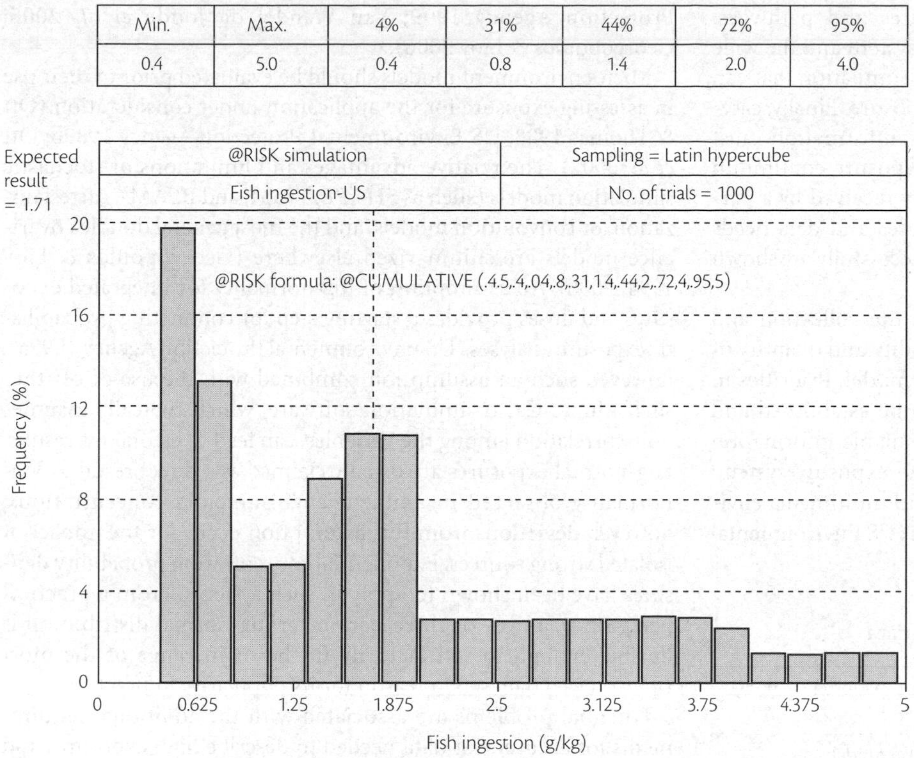

Fig. 8.4.12 Distribution of fish ingestion.
Source: AIHC (1994).

Exposure modelling

Predictions of an exposure or potential dose have been based on emissions, environmental transport, and fate modelling (Thibodeaux 1979; Javandel *et al.* 1984; Cohen 1989), and population time or location and activity pattern modelling combined with microenvironmental quality modelling (Duan 1991; Pardi 1992; Patrick 1994; US Environmental Protection Agency 1999; Roy *et al.* 2003). This is called prognostic assessment. Prediction of exposure can also be carried out based on modelling of biomarker data (Georgopoulos & Lioy 1994, 2006), which is called diagnostic assessment. Whenever possible, both microenvironmental and biomarker data should be used, because these data are from independent sources, and should therefore result in the reduction of overall uncertainty (Roy & Georgopoulos 1998). An excellent set of references on many new modelling tools are summarized in the article by Georgopoulos and Lioy (2006).

As noted in the subsection on basic principles, the overarching aim is to relate environmental releases to adverse health effect. Although it is possible to relate exposure with toxic effects, more direct relationships can be increasingly obtained by using potential dose, internal dose, and target tissue dose, respectively. Calculation of target tissue dose requires the application of a pharmacokinetic model (sometimes referred to as toxicokinetic model) that describes the uptake, distribution, metabolism, and elimination of the toxicant. Pharmacokinetic models used in exposure assessments are generally compartmental models, which are empirically based, or physiologically based pharmacokinetic (PBPK) models that have a mechanistic basis and represent the major tissues of the body as separate compartments linked by anatomically correct blood flow (Georgopoulos & Lioy 2006).

The fraction of an internal dose that reaches the target tissue can be highly dependent upon the route of uptake, and PBPK models are a natural choice for estimating the target tissue dose for each route of uptake. For example, the fraction of an ingested internal dose that reaches the liver will generally be much greater than that of an internal dermal dose. A further advantage of a PBPK formulation is that it is amenable to interspecies scale-up, which is an important attribute because ethical and practical reasons generally preclude the intentional dosing of humans with toxic substance. Thus, a PBPK model for humans can be developed on the basis of a PBPK model in laboratory animals (Ramsey & Andersen 1984). Moreover, PBPK models can be adapted to reflect the inherent variability in human populations. Model parameters are generally formulated as functions of body weight, and in principle, this can be extended to other covariates such as age, height, and sex. Physiologically-based models that relate exposure to internal and target tissue dose have been successfully applied to predict doses for a variety of toxicants. Both traditional 'lumped' parameter (ordinary differential equation) formulations as well as 'refined' distributed parameter (particle and ordinary differential equation) schemes have been used for the inverse problem of dose to exposure medium to reconstruction (Georgopoulos & Lioy 1994; Georgopoulos *et al.* 1994). This approach utilizes time profiles of biomarker concentrations found in excreted fluids following exposure to reconstruct the single and/or multimedia or multiroute exposures experienced by an individual (e.g. simultaneous inhalation and dermal absorption of a volatile organic present in air and water).

A detailed exposure assessment may also require resource-intensive data collection studies or model-based simulations to characterize one or more of the following: Source attributes, toxicant properties, geographical domain of influence attributes, population composition and/or stratification, population time and/or location patterns and activity patterns, macroenvironmental media properties and concentrations, microenvironmental media properties and concentrations, and the exposure routes and pathways. Consequently, the complexity of the exposure system and the wide range of information requirements necessitate simulation that can describe the exposure to dose or the dose to exposure. Finally, case-specific requirements of available mechanistic information must be available to link each component of the exposure continuum (Fig. 8.4.2) and then estimate doses potentially received by a particular population. The overall types of analyses and data needs required to complete an exposure simulation successfully are shown in Table 8.4.10 (Patrick 1994).

A general modelling framework can guide the collection and analysis of new data; on the other hand, the quality and quantity of available data limits the sophistication of any model. Priorities in data collection and model development must be established and the options must be explored for analysing available information and for modelling various components of the exposure system; that is, components of both single-medium and multimedia environmental and environmental exposure models (US Environmental Protection Agency 1999; Van Wendel de Joode *et al.* 2005; Georgopoulos & Lioy 2006).

Table 8.4.10 Exposure modelling: concepts and data

Analytical solution	Method for solving differential equations in a model using classical tools of algebra and calculus
Boundary conditions	Input values used to initialize the model
Calibration	The process of using a set of observed data to adjust the structure and/or internal coefficients of a model such that the output values are accurate with respect to a known value
Causation	The independent change in the value of one variable causes a predictable change in the value of dependent variables
Deterministic model	A model in which the variations in the variables do not include a random component—there is one output for each set of inputs
Equilibrium	A system that is not exchanging energy or matter with its surrounding and is in equilibrium with the surroundings
Model	A theoretical construct attempting to relate an identified system to the data and information available to simulate the system
Numerical solution	Method for solving differential equations using numerical approximation techniques
Sensitivity analysis	The investigation of changes in dependent variable values resulting from changes in values in independent variables and in the posited relationships among variables
Stability	The ability of a numerical integration method to iterate to a solution
Steady state	The case where input to a system is balanced by output; A model in which no variables change for the time period under consideration
Stochastic model	A model in which the variation in one or more variables includes a random component
Verification	Testing of a model following initial calibration to evaluate mode

Adapted from Patrick (1994).

Microenvironment models should be evaluated prior to their use in assessing exposure for the application under consideration (Ott & Thomas 1988; US Environmental Protection Agency 1989b; Ott *et al.* 2007). The relative advantages and limitations of stochastic simulation models (such as SHAPE, TRIM, and BEAM), cartesianization, or convolution models, and the most general double covariance models are summarized elsewhere (Georgopoulos & Lioy 1994, 2006). An assumption of log-normality for integrated exposures and doses provides a starting step for conducting probabilistic exposure analyses (US Environmental Protection Agency 1992a); however, such an assumption combined with the use of off-the-shelf Monte Carlo simulation software, which typically assumes non-correlation among the variables, can lead to erroneous results. Log-normal exposures are usually claimed as a direct result of log-normality observed in ambient environmental concentrations; however, deviations from this assumption occur for the impact of isolated strong sources. Exponential concentration probability densities have been shown to apply in such systems. From a practical perspective, a two- or three-parameter log-normal distribution is flexible enough to satisfactorily fit the main range of the most right-skewed data sets, a reason for its popularity in practice.

Potential problems are associated with the additional requirements for accuracy of data needed to describe high exposures and doses. It is exactly in this range for which assumptions on independence (typical in Monte Carlo simulations) are less valid. One solution in any analysis is to use asymptotic distributions of extremes, such as Gumbel's double-exponential distribution, for the high ends ('distribution tails') of concentration and exposure time.

Practical application of exposure science has been mainly driven by generic or 'typical' assumptions (e.g. a person eating large quantities of waste throughout his or her life). However, as data evolve, management requirements for information obtained from large-scale, comprehensive exposure assessment programmes such as the National Human Exposure Assessment Survey (NHEXAS) will be overwhelming in comparison with today's standards for routine exposure data management (Sexton *et al.* 1995b). Consequently, state-of-the-art information management tools must be evaluated and used to organize, utilize, and interpret exposure-related data efficiently. These include geographical information systems, interactive scientific visualization systems, distributed relational database management systems, and object-oriented environments for data and model integration.

Exposure probabilities for individuals and populations

Exposure distributions (probability density functions and cumulative distribution functions of exposure) for an individual express the probability that an individual will experience a given level of exposure over a specified duration (such as a day, year, or lifetime). The exposure distribution for a population expresses the probability that a fraction of the population will experience a given level of exposure. Exposure distributions can vary significantly among individuals in a population, resulting in multimodal distributions for a population. For example, the distribution of exposure in a population can be biomodal when a fraction of the population is occupationally exposed at levels much greater than environmental levels experienced by the other fraction of the population. Consequently, population strata need to be characterized to achieve the data quality objectives. Exposure distributions that should be developed include individuals expected to experience the highest long-term exposures, individuals expected to experience the highest short-term exposures, and special or susceptible segments of the population.

As mentioned in the previous subsection, log-normal distributions of exposures are commonly employed, and they also have been suggested as a 'default' when case-specific information is not available (Johnson & Capel 1992b). The log-normal distribution possesses many advantageous properties, such as positivity (the probability of a negative exposure is zero), left-skewedness (implying that the average exposure is less than the median exposure), and mathematical properties that are well known because the log-normal distribution is closely related to the normal distribution. However, its adoption in a particular study should be with caution because log-normality of a random variable implies that the randomness in the underlying processes is multiplicative. Other alternatives, such as asymptomatic distributions for extreme values (e.g. bi-exponential), could potentially provide more appropriate information for risk analyses.

Attributes related to the potential target population and sensitive subpopulations should include: (a) plausible contact patterns with the contaminants for different routes of exposure; (b) spatial population distribution stratification by age, sex, and so on; and (c) identification of subgroups of people sharing potentially similar exposure patterns. As stated earlier, identification of time–activity patterns for potentially exposed populations, such as school children versus adults, men versus women, office workers versus outdoor workers, and so on, and of spatial distributions of target population groups are essential for exposure characterization.

Uncertainty analysis

Exposure assessments are inherently uncertain, because of limitations in the precision with which nature can be observed and the randomness inherent in nature. Uncertainty and the closely related concept of variability are means of quantifying the lack of knowledge regarding a quantity of interest, which in exposure assessment can be any variable affecting the estimation of exposure. Uncertainty generally refers to a lack of knowledge of a quantity due to limitations in available quantification techniques, whereas variability is a means of representing the lack of knowledge of a quantity due to unavailability of a measurement on the specific instance of the quantity. For example, an exposure assessment involving contaminated soil will be uncertain, because of a lack of knowledge regarding the relevant concentration of contaminant in soil resulting from (a) imprecision in contaminant concentrations measured in soil samples and (b) variability in measured concentrations in several randomly selected representative samples. The variability in soil concentrations results in uncertainty in exposure because it is not possible a priori to predict the exact concentrations in soil that actually cause the exposure. Although it is useful to conceptualize these two sources of uncertainty in exposure, ultimately however it does not matter whether the lack of knowledge is due to uncertainty or variability, because they are both represented using probability distribution functions and their effect on the exposure is estimated by propagating the uncertainty through a exposure model in an identical manner. However, it is important to acknowledge explicitly that exposure assessments are inherently uncertain, and therefore, exposure estimates should be probabilistic wherever possible. One of the main benefits of conceptualizing uncertainty as arising due to imprecision and variability is the reduction of uncertainty by identifying and filling data gaps. The identification of data gaps usually involves a sensitivity analysis to determine the contribution of individual variables to the overall uncertainty in the exposure assessment. Reduction of uncertainty due to imprecision can only be effected by improving instrumentation, whereas it may be possible to reduce the uncertainty in exposure assessments due to variability in underlying factors by stratifying the population from which the samples are drawn (see Table 8.4.3). Knowledge of the population probability distribution functions can be used to judge the appropriateness of stratification of the population into smaller groups. For example, bimodal distributions are an indication that there are at least two subpopulations that are more homogeneous. This type of information is important in identifying subgroups by age, sex, race, and so on, and locating susceptible subgroups exposed to a contaminant.

Frequency distributions can be affected by a small sample size. In some cases, only a few data points are available for quantities such as the mean, variance, and distribution. However, a confidence interval can only be calculated when the mean and variance of the distribution are known with certainty (e.g. based on large numbers of samples or data). A small sample size will increase the uncertainty in the mean and the variance. Calculation of tolerance intervals is one method for identifying sources of uncertainty (Mandel 1969).

Uncertainty about the underlying distribution of a variable can limit the application of standard statistical tests. Most tolerance and confidence intervals assume a normal distribution for all measurements. In cases where measurement error dominates the observed variance, this assumption may be reasonable; however, when there is significant interindividual variability, a skewed distribution can result. In this case, tolerance and confidence intervals based on an assumption of normality will not provide valid information error. Thus, it is important to view statistical tests as only one component in determining the accuracy of the exposure data.

Conclusion

The field of exposure science and its application to public health practices provides information and an understanding of the variety of ways an individual or population comes into contact with a contaminant. The approach must be framed within a conceptual framework that involves multiple disciplines and interdisciplinary studies. Calculations of exposure and dose are data intensive, and often require situation-specific or site-specific data to characterize exposure accurately. Finally, the scientific approaches employed to establish measurement and modelling procedures must consider information on biological mechanisms or health outcomes.

Acknowledgements

The author thanks Dr Natalie Freeman from the University of Florida, and Dr Amit Roy and Bristol Myer Squibb for their original contributions and assistance. The author also thanks the many scientists who have conducted exposure science research over the years to help improve our current understanding of human exposure and human exposure science.

References

Akland G.G., Hartwell T.D., Johnson R.R. *et al.* Measuring human exposure to carbon monoxide in Washington, DC, and Denver, Colorado, during the winter of 1982–1983. *Environmental Science and Technology* 1985;**19**(10):911–18.

American Industrial Health Council. *Exposure factors handbook*. Washington (DC): American Industrial Health Council; 1994.

Andelman J.B. Inhalation exposure in the home to volatile organic contaminants of drinking water. *Science of the Total Environment* 1985;**47**:443–60.

Anderson-Sprecher R., Flatman G.T., Borgman L. Environmental sampling: a brief review. *Journal of Exposure Analysis and Environmental Epidemiology* 1994;**4**(**2**):115–31.

Ashley D.L., Bonin M.A., Cardinali F.L. *et al.* Determining volatile organic compounds in human blood from a large sample population by using purge and trap gas chromatography/mass spectrometry. *Analytical Chemistry* 1992;**64**(**9**):1021–9.

Barr D.B. Expanding the role of exposure science in environmental health. *Journal of Exposure Science and Environmental Epidemiology* 2006;**16**:473.

Barr D.B., Wang R.Y., Needham L.L. Biological monitoring of exposure to environmental chemicals throughout life stages: requirements and issues for the National Children's Study. *Environmental Health Perspectives* 2005;**113**:1083–91.

Brown H.S., Bishop D.R., Rowan C.A. The role of skin absorption as a route of exposure for volatile organic compounds (VOCs) in drinking water. *American Journal of Public Health* 1984;**74**(**5**):479–84.

Burke J.M., Zufall M.J., Ozkaynak H. A population exposure model for particulate matter: case study results for PM(2.5) in Philadelphia, PA. *Journal of Exposure Analysis and Environmental Epidemiology* 2001;**11**(**6**):470–89.

Burse V.W., Najam A.R., Williams C.C. *et al.* Utilization of umbilical cords to assess in utero exposure to persistent pesticides and polychlorinated biphenyls. *Journal of Exposure Analysis and Environmental Epidemiology* 2000;**10**(**6** Pt **2**):776–88.

Carpenter G.J., Huston-Stein A. Activity, structure and se-typed behavior in preschool children. *Child Development* 1980;**51**:862–72.

Caudill S.P., Pirkle J.L., Michalek J.E. Effects of Measurement error on estimating biological half-life. *Journal of Exposure Analysis and Environmental Epidemiology* 1992;**2**(**4**):463–76.

Centers for Disease Control and Prevention. *Third national report on human exposure to environmental chemicals*. Atlanta (GA): National Center for Environmental Health; 2005.

Clayton C.A., Perritt R.L., Pellizzari E.D. *et al.* Particle total exposure assessment methodology (PTEAM) study: distribution of aerosol and element concentrations in personal, indoor and outdoor air samples in a Southern California community. *Journal of Exposure Analysis and Environmental Epidemiology* 1993;**3**:227–50.

Cohen Y. Multimedia and intermedia transport modeling concepts in environmental monitoring. In: Allen D, Kaplan IR, Cohen Y, editors. *Intermediate pollutant transport modeling and field measurements*. New York (NY): Plenum; 1989.

Cohen-Hubal E.A., Sheldon L., Burke J. *et al.* Children's exposure assessment: a review of factors influencing children's exposure, and the data available to characterize and assess that exposure. *Environmental Health Perspectives* 2000;**108**:475–86.

Duan N. Stochastic microenvironmental models for air pollution exposure. *Journal Exposure Analysis and Environmental Epidemiology* 1991; **1**:235–57.

Edwards R., Lioy P. The EL sampler: a press sampler for the quantitative estimation of dermal exposure to pesticides in house dust. *Journal of Exposure Analysis and Environmental Epidemiology* 1999;**9**:521–9.

Ellickson K.M., Schopfer C.J., Lioy P.J. The bioaccessibility of low level radionuclides from two Savannah river site soils. *Health Physics* 2002;**83**(**4**):476–84.

Fan Z., Lioy P.J., Weschler C. *et al.* Ozone initiated reactions with volatile organic compounds under simulated indoor conditions. *Environmental Science and Technology* 2003;**37**:1811–21.

Fenske R.A., Curry P.B., Wandelmaier F. *et al.* Development of dermal and respiratory sampling procedures for human exposure to pesticides in indoor environments. *Journal of Exposure Analysis and Environmental Epidemiology* 1991;**1**:11–30.

Freeman N., Waldman J., Lioy P.J. Design and evaluation of a location and activity log used for assessing personal exposure to air pollutants. *Journal of Exposure Analysis and Environmental Epidemiology* 1991;**1**(**3**):327–38.

Freeman N., Ettinger A., Berry M. *et al.* Hygiene-and food-related behaviors associated with blood lead levels of young children from lead-contaminated homes Journal of Exposure Analysis and Environmental Epidemiology 1997;**7**:103–18.

Freeman N., Sheldon L., Jimenez M. *et al.* Contribution of children's activities to lead contamination of food. *Journal of Exposure Analysis and Environmental Epidemiology* 2001a;**11**:407–13.

Freeman N., Jimenez M., Reed K. *et al.* Quantitative analysis of children's microactivity patterns: the Minnesota children's pesticide exposure study. *Journal of Exposure Analysis and Environmental Epidemiology* 2001b;**11**:501–9.

Freeman N., Shalat S., Black K. *et al.* Seasonal pesticide use in a rural community on the U.S.-Mexico border. *Journal of Exposure Analysis and Environmental Epidemiology* 2004;**14**:473–8.

Freeman N., Hore P., Black K. *et al.* Contributions of children's activities to pesticide hand loadings following residential pesticide application. *Journal of Exposure Analysis and Environmental Epidemiology* 2005;**15**(**1**):81–8.

Furtaw E.J., Jr. An overview of human exposure modeling activities at the USEPA's National Exposure Research Laboratory. *Journal of Toxicology and Industrial Health* 2001;**17** (5–10):302–14.

Georgopoulos P., Lioy P. Conceptual and theoretical aspects of human exposure and dose assessment. *Journal of Exposure Analysis and Environmental Epidemiology* 1994;**4**(**3**):253–85.

Georgopoulos P.G., Lioy P.J. From a theoretical framework of human exposure and dose assessment to computational system implementation: the Modeling ENvironment for TOtal Risk Studies (MENTOR). *Journal of Toxicology and Environmental Health B Critical Reviews* 2006;**9**(**6**):457–83.

Georgopoulos P., Roy A., Gallo M.A. Reconstruction of using physiologically based pharmacokinetic models. *Journal of Exposure Analysis and Environmental Epidemiology* 1994;**4**:1–20.

Georgopoulos P.G., Walia A., Roy A. *et al.* Integrated exposure and dose modeling and analysis system.1. Formulation and testing of microenvironmental and pharmacokinetic components. *Environmental Science and Technology* 1997;**31** (1):17–27.

Geyh A.S., Chillrud S., Williams D.L. *et al.* Assessing truck driver exposure at the World Trade Center disaster site: personal and area monitoring for particulate matter and volatile organic compounds during October 2001 and April 2002. *Journal of Occupational and Environmental Hygiene* 2005;**2**(**3**):179–93.

Graham J., Walker K., Berry M. *et al.* Role of exposure databases in risk assessment. *Archives of Environmental Health* 1992;**47**:408–21.

Gurunathan S., Robson M., Freeman N. *et al.* Accumulation of chlorpyrifos on residential surfaces and toys accessible to children. *Environmental Health Perspectives* 1998;**106**(**1**):9–16.

Gustafson P., Barregard L., Lindahl R. *et al.* Formaldehyde levels in Sweden: personal exposure, indoor, and outdoor concentrations. *Journal of Exposure Analysis and Environmental Epidemiology* 2005;**15**(**3**):252–60.

Hamel S., Buckley B., Lioy P.J. *et al.* Bioaccessibility of met als in soils for different liquid for soil ratios in synthetic gastric fluids. *Environmental Science and Technology* 1998;**32**:358–62.

Hattis D., Burmaster D. Some thoughts on choosing distributions for practical risk analyses. *Risk Analysis* 1994;**14**:713–30.

Hawley J. Assessment of health risk from exposure to contaminated soils. *Risk Analysis* 1985;**5**:282–302.

Heinrich J., Holscher B., Seiwert M. *et al.* Nicotine and cotinine in adults' urine: the German Environmental Survey 1998. *Journal of Exposure Analysis and Environmental Epidemiology* 2005;**15** (**1**):74–80.

Henderson R., Bechtold W., Maples K. Biological markers as measure of exposure. *Journal of Exposure Analysis and Environmental Epidemiology* 1992;**2** Suppl 2:1–14.

Herbert R., Moline J., Skloot G. *et al.* The World Trade Center disaster and the health of workers: five-year assessment of a unique medical screening program. *Environmental Health Perspectives* 2006;**114**(12):1853–8.

Hoffmann K., Krause C., Seifert B. *et al.* The German Environmental Survey 1990/92 (GerES II): sources of personal exposure to volatile organic compounds. *Journal of Exposure Analysis and Environmental Epidemiology* 2000a; **10**(**2**):115–25.

Hoffmann K., Becker K., Friedrich C. *et al.* The German Environmental Survey 1990/1992 (GerES II): cadmium in blood, urine and hair of adults and children. *Journal of Exposure Analysis and Environmental Epidemiology* 2000b;**10**(**2**):126–35.

Hore P., Robson M., Freeman N. *et al.* Chlorpyrifos accumulation patterns for child-accessible surfaces and objects and urinary metabolite excretion by children for 2 weeks after crack-and-crevice application. *Environmental Health Perspectives* 2005;**113**(**2**):211–9.

Jantunen M., Hanninen O., Katsouyianni K. *et al.* Air pollution exposure in European cities: the EXPOLIS study. *Journal of Exposure Analysis and Environmental Epidemiology* 1998;**8**:495–518.

Javandel I., Doughty C., Tsang C. *Groundwater transport: handbook of mathematical models*. Washington (DC): American Geophysical Union; 1984. Water Sources Monograph 10.

Jo W.K., Weisel C.P., Lioy P.J. Routes of chloroform exposure and body burden from showering with chlorinated tap water. *Risk Analysis* 1990;**10**(**4**):575–70.

Johnson T., Capel J. A Monte Carlo approach to simulating residential occupancy periods and its applications to the general US population. Research Triangle Park (NC): US Environmental Protection Agency; 1992b. EPA/450/3-92/011.

Jorgenson J.L. (2001) 'Aldrin and dieldrin: a review of research on their production, environmental deposition and fate, bioaccumulation, toxicology, and epidemiology in the United States.' *Environmental Health Perspectives*, 109 Suppl 1, 113–39.

Khoury G.A., Diamond G.L. Risks to children from exposure to lead in air during remedial or removal activities at Superfund sites: a case study of the RSR lead smelter Superfund site. *Journal of Exposure Analysis and Environmental Epidemiology* 2003;**13**(**1**):51–65.

Kieszak S.M., Naeher L.P., Rubin C.S. *et al.* Investigation of the relation between self-reported food consumption and household chemical exposures with urinary levels of selected non-persistent pesticides. *Journal of Exposure Analysis and Environmental Epidemiology* 2002;**12**:(6):404–8.

Kim H., Weisel C.P. Dermal absorption of dichloro- and trichloroacetic acids from chlorinated water. *Journal of Exposure Analysis and Environmental Epidemiology* 1998;**8**:555–75.

Korrick S.A., Altshul L.M., Tolbert P.E. *et al.* Measurement of PCBs, DDE, and hexachlorobenzene in cord blood from infants born in towns adjacent to a PCB-contaminated waste site. *Journal of Exposure Analysis and Environmental Epidemiology* 2000;**10**(**6** Pt **2**):743–54.

Lebowitz M., Quackenboss J., Kollander M. *et al.* Standard question naira for estimation of indoor concentrations. *Journal of Air Pollution Control Association* 1989;**2**(**39**):1411–9.

Lioy P.J. The analysis of total human exposure for exposure assessment: a multi-discipline science for examining human contact with containments. *Environmental Science and Technology* 1990;**24**:938–45.

Lioy P.J. Exposure analysis and the biological response to a contaminant: a melding necessary for environmental health sciences. *Journal of Exposure Analysis and Environmental Epidemiology* 1992;**2** Suppl **1**:19–24.

Lioy P.J. Measurement of personal exposure to air pollution: status and needs, measurement challengers in atmospheric chemistry. Washington (DC): 1993.

Lioy P.J. The 1998 ISEA Wesolowski Award lecture. *Exposure analysis: reflections on its growth and aspirations for its future. International Society of Exposure Analysis. Journal of Exposure Analysis and Environmental Epidemiology* 1999;**9**(**4**):273–81.

Lioy P.J. Employing dynamical and chemical processes for contaminant mixtures outdoors to the indoor environment: the implications for total human exposure analysis and prevention. *Journal of Exposure Science and Environmental Epidemiology* 2006;**16**(**3**):207–24.

Lioy P.J., Pellizzari E. Conceptual framework for designing a national survey of human exposure. *Journal of Exposure Analysis and Environmental Epidemiology* 1995;**5**:425–44.

Lioy P.J., Georgopoulos P. The anatomy of the exposures that occurred around the World Trade Center site: 9/11 and beyond. *Annals of the New York Academy of Sciences* 2006;**1076**:54–79.

Lioy P.J., Weisel C.P., Jo W-K *et al.* Microenvironmental and personal measurements of methyl-tertiary butyl ether (MTBE) associated with automobile use activities. *Journal of Exposure Analysis and Environmental Epidemiology* 1994;**4**(**4**):427–41.

Lioy P.J., Weisel C.P., Millette J.R. *et al.* Characterization of the dust/smoke aerosol that settled east of the World Trade Center (WTC) in lower Manhattan after the collapse of the WTC 11 September 2001. *Environmental Health Perspectives* 2002;**110**(**7**):703–14.

Lioy P.J., Pellizzari E., Prezant D. (2006) 'The World Trade Center aftermath and its effects on health: understanding and learning through human-exposure science'. *Environmental Science and Technology*, **40**, (22), 6876–85.

Maier A., Savage R.E., Jr, Haber L.T. Assessing biomarker use in risk assessment—a survey of practitioners. *Journal of Toxicology and Environmental Health A* 2004;**67**(**8–10**):687–95.

Mandel J. *The statistical analysis of experimental data*. North Chelmsford (MA): Courier Dover Publications; 1969.

Marnicio R., Hakkinen P., Lutkenhoff S. *et al.* Risk analysis software and databases: review of Riskware'90 Conference and Exhibition. *Risk Analysis* 1991;**11**:545–60.

McCurdy T. Conceptual basis for multi-route intake dose modeling using an energy expenditure approach. *Journal of Exposure Analysis and Environmental Epidemiology* 2000;**10**(**1**):86–97.

McCurdy T., Glen G., Smith L. *et al.* The national exposure research laboratory's consolidated human activity database. *Journal of Exposure Analysis and Environmental Epidemiology* 2000;**10**(**6** Pt **1**):566–78.

McKone T.E. Human exposure to chemicals from multiple media and through multiple pathways: research overview and comments. *Risk Analysis* 1991;**11**:5–10.

National Research Council. *Epidemiology and air pollution*. Washington (DC): National Academies Press; 1985.

National Research Council. *Biologic markers in pulmonary toxicology*. Washington (DC): National Academies Press; 1989.

National Research Council. *Environmental epidemiology*. Vol 1: Public health and hazardous wastes. Washington (DC): National Academies Press; 1991a.

National Research Council. *Frontiers in assessing human exposures to environmental toxicants*. Washington (DC): National Academies Press; 1991b.

National Research Council. *Human exposure assessment for airborne pollutants: advances and opportunities*. Washington (DC): National Academies Press; 1991c.

National Research Council. *Biologic markers of immunotoxicology*. Washington (DC): National Academies Press; 1992.

National Research Council. *Pesticides in the diets of infants and children*. Washington (DC): National Academies Press; 1993a.

National Research Council. *Measuring lead exposure in infants, children, and other sensitive populations*. Washington (DC): National Academies Press; 1993b.

National Research Council. *Acute exposure guideline levels for selected airborne chemicals*. Washington (DC): National Academies Press; 2001–2004.

National Research Council. *Air quality management in the United States*. Washington (DC): National Academies Press; 2004. p. 1–401.

National Research Council. *Human biomonitoring for environmental chemicals*. Washington (DC): National Academies Press; 2006. p. 1–215.

Needham L.L., Sexton K. Assessing children's exposure to hazardous environmental chemicals: an overview of selected research challenges and complexities. *Journal of Exposure Analysis and Environmental Epidemiology* 2000;**10**(**6** Pt **2**):611–29.

Offenberg J.H., Eisenreich S.J., Gigliotti C.L. *et al.* Persistent organic pollutants in dusts that settled indoors in lower Manhattan after September 11, 2001. *Journal of Exposure Analysis and Environmental Epidemiology* 2004;**14**(**2**):164–72.

Oktay S.D., Brabander D.J., Smith J.P. *et al.* WTC geochemical fingerprint recorded in New York Harbor sediments. *EOS Transactions American Geophysical Union* 2003;**84**:21–5.

Ott W.R. Development of criteria for citing air monitoring stations. *APCA Journal* 1977;**27**(**6**):543–7.

Ott W.R. Concepts of human exposure to air pollution. *Environment International* 1982;**7**:179–96.

Ott W.R. Total human exposure: basic concepts, EPA field studies and future research needs. *Journal of the Air and Waste Management Association* 1990;**40**(**7**):966–75.

Ott W.R. Human exposure assessment: the birth of a new science. *Journal of Ex.posure Analysis and Environmental Epidemiology* 1995a;**5**:449–72.

Ott W.R. *Environmental statistics and data analysis*. Boca Raton (FL): CRC Press; 1995b. p. 1–313.

Ott W.R., Thomas J., Mage D. *et al.* Validation of the Simulation of Human Activity and Pollutant Exposure (SHAPE) model using paired days from the Denver, CO, Carbon Monoxide field study. *Atmospheric Environment* 1988;**22**(10):2102–3.

Ott W.R., Steinemann A.C., Wallace L.A. *Exposure analysis*. Boca Raton (FL): CRC Press; 2007. p. 1–533.

Pardi R. IMES: A system for identifying and evaluation computer models for exposure assessment Risk Analysis 1992;11:319–21.

Patrick D. *Toxic air pollution handbook*. New York (NY): Van Nostrand Reinhold; 1994.

Pellizzari E., Lioy P., Quackenboss J. *et al.* Population-based exposure measurements in EPA region 5: a phase I field study in support of the National Human Exposure Assessment Survey. *Journal of Exposure Analysis and Environmental Epidemiology* 1995;**5**(**3**):327–58.

Pellizzari E.D., Clayton C.A., Rodes C.E. *et al.* Particulate matter and manganese exposures in Toronto, Canada. *Atmospheric Environment* 1999;**33**:721–34.

Pirkle J.L., Needham L.L., Sexton K. Improving exposure assessment by monitoring human tissues for toxic chemicals. *Journal of Exposure Analysis and Environmental Epidemiology* 1995;**5**(**3**):405–24.

Poirier M., Santella R., Weston A. Carcinogen macromolecular adducts and their measurement. *Carcinogenesis* 2000;**21**:353–59.

Prezant D.J., Weiden M., Banauch G.I. *et al.* Cough and bronchial responsiveness in firefighters at the World Trade Center site. *New England Journal of Medicine* 2002;**347**(**11**):806–15.

Price P.S., Chaisson C.F. A conceptual framework for modeling aggregate and cumulative exposures to chemicals. *Journal of Exposure Analysis and Environmental Epidemiology* 2005;**15**:(6):473–81.

Quackenboss J., Pellizzari E., Shubat P. *et al.* Design strategy for assessing multi-pathway exposure for children: the Minnesota children's pesticide exposure study (MNCPES). *Journal of Exposure Analysis and Environmental Epidemiology* 2000;**10**:145–58.

Ramsey J., Andersen M. A physiologically based description of the inhalation pharmacokinetics of styrene in rats and humans. *Toxicology and Applied Pharmacology* 1984;**73**:159–75.

Reed K., Jimenez M., Freeman N. *et al.* Quantification of children's hand and mouthing activities through a videotaping methodology. *Journal of Exposure Analysis and Environmental Epidemiology* 1999;**9**:513–20.

Rodes C., Newsome J., Vanderpool R. *et al.* Experimental methodologies and preliminary transfer factor data for estimation of dermal exposures to particles. *Journal of Exposure Analysis and Environmental Epidemiology* 2001;**11**:123–39.

Roy A., Georgopoulos P.G. Reconstructing week-long exposures to volatile organic compounds using physiologically based pharmacokinetic models. *Journal of Exposure Analysis and Environmental Epidemiology* 1998;**8**(**3**):407–22.

Roy A., Georgopoulos P.G., Ouyang M. *et al.* Environmental, dietary, demographic, and activity variables associated with biomarkers of exposure for benzene and lead. *Journal of Exposure Analysis and Environmental Epidemiology* 2003;**13**(**6**):417–26.

Royster M.O., Hilborn E.D., Barr D. *et al.* A pilot study of global positioning system/geographical information system measurement of residential proximity to agricultural fields and urinary organophosphate metabolite concentrations in toddlers. *Journal of Exposure Analysis and Environmental Epidemiology* 2002;**12**(**6**):433–40.

Ruby M., Davis A., Link T. *et al.* Development of an in vitro screening test to evaluate the "in vitro" bioaccessibility of ingested mine-wasted lead. *Environmental Science and Technology* 1993;**27**:2870–7.

Ryan P. An overview of human exposure modeling. *Journal of Exposure Analysis and Environmental Epidemiology* 1991;**1**:453–74.

Ryan P., Spengler J., Letz R. Estimating personal exposures to NO_2. *Environment International* 1986;**12**:395–400.

Samet J.M., Marbury M.C., Spengler J.D. Health effects and sources of indoor air pollution. *Part I. American Review of Respiratory Disease* 1987;**136**(**6**):1486–508.

Samet J.M., Marbury M.C., Spengler J.D. Health effects and sources of indoor air pollution. *Part II. American Review of Respiratory Disease* 1988;**137**(**1**):221–42.

Schmidt C.W. Signs of the times: biomarkers in perspective. *Environmental Health Perspectives* 2006;**114**(12):A701–5.

Schneider D., Freeman N. Childhood environmental health risks: a state-of-the-art conference. *Archives of Environmental Health* 2001;**56**(**2**):103–10.

Seifert B., Abraham H. Use of passive samplers for the determination of gaseous organic substances in indoor air at low concentration levels. *International Journal of Environmental Analytical Chemistry* 1983;**13**:234–54.

Seifert B., Becker K., Helm D. *et al.* The German Environmental Survey 1990/1992 (GerES II): reference concentrations of selected environmental pollutants in blood, urine, hair, house dust, drinking water and indoor air. *Journal of Exposure Analysis and Environmental Epidemiology* 2000a;**10**:(6 Pt 1):552–65.

Seifert B., Becker K., Hoffmann K. *et al.* The German Environmental Survey 1990/1992 (GerES II): a representative population study. *Journal of Exposure Analysis and Environmental Epidemiology* 2000b;**10**(**2**):103–14.

Sexton K., Ryan P.B. Human exposure to air pollution: Methods, measurements and models. In Watson A, Bates RR, Kennedy D (Editors) *Air Pollution, the Automobile, and Public Health*. National Academy Press, Washington DC, 1988; pp. 203–238.

Sexton K., Selevan S., Wagener D. *et al.* Estimating human exposures to environmental pollutants: availability and utility of existing databases. *Archives of Environmental Health* 1992;**47**:398–407.

Sexton K., Callahan M., Bryan E. Estimating exposure and dose to characterize health risks: the role of human tissue monitoring in exposure assessment. *Environmental Health Perspectives* 1995a;**103**(supplement 3):13–29.

Sexton K., Kleffman D.E., Callahan M.A. An introduction to the National Human Exposure Assessment Survey (NHEXAS) and related phase I field studies. *Journal of Exposure Analysis and Environmental Epidemiology* 1995b;**5**(**3**):229–32.

Sexton K., Greaves I., Church T. *et al.* A school-based strategy to assess children's environmental exposures and related health effects in economically disadvantaged urban neighborhoods. *Journal of Exposure Analysis and Environmental Epidemiology* 2000;**10**(**6** Pt **2**):682–94.

Sexton K. Comparison of recruitment, retention, and compliance results for three children's exposure monitoring studies. *Journal of Exposure Analysis and Environmental Epidemiology* 2005;**15**(**4**):350–6.

Shalat S.L., Donnelly K.C., Freeman N.C. *et al.* Nondietary ingestion of pesticides by children in an agricultural community on the US/Mexico border: preliminary results. *Journal of Exposure Analysis and Environmental Epidemiology* 2003;**13**(**1**):42–50.

Spengler J.D., Treitman R., Mage D. *et al.* Personal exposures to respirable particulates and implications for air pollution epidemiology. *Environmental Science and Technology* 1985;**19**:700–7.

Thibodeaux L. Chemodynamics: environmental movement of chemicals in air, water, and soil. New York (NY): Wiley; 1979.

Tsang A.M., Klepeis N.E. Descriptive statistics tables from a detailed analysis of the National Human Activity Pattern Survey (NHAPS) data. Las Vegas (NV): US Environmental Protection Agency; 1996. EPA/600/R-96/148.

Tulve N., Suggs J., McCurdy T. *et al.* Frequency of mouthing behavior in young children. *Journal of Exposure Analysis and Environmental Epidemiology* 2002;**12**:259–64.

US Environmental Protection Agency. Federal Register 79318–79.1980.

US Environmental Protection Agency. *Exposure factors handbook.* Washington (DC): US Environmental Protection Agency; 1989a. NTIS PB90-106774.

US Environmental Protection Agency. Benzene exposure assessment model (BEAM): interim report. Las Vegas (NV): Environmental Measurements and Surveillance Laboratory; 1989b.

US Environmental Protection Agency. *Guidelines for exposure assessment.* 1992a. Federal Register 57(104):22888–22938.

US Environmental Protection Agency. *Exposure factors handbook.* Washington (DC): US Environmental Protection Agency; 1997.

US Environmental Protection Agency. Total Risk Integrated Methodology (TRIM) expo. Research Triangle Park (NC): US Environmental Protection Agency; 1999. Technical Support Document EPA-453/D-99-001.

US Environmental Protection Agency. Consolidated human activities database. [Online]. 2001a. Available from: http//www.epa.gov/chadnet1/index.html

US Environmental Protection Agency. *Principles for performing aggregate exposure and risk assessments.* Washington (DC): US Environmental Protection Agency; 2001b. p. 1–79. Item 6043.

US Environmental Protection Agency. *Framework for cumulative exposure assessment.* Washington (DC): US Environmental Protection Agency; 2003. EPA630/P-02/001F.

Valerio F., Pela M., Lazarotto A. *et al.* Preliminary evaluation, using passive tubes, of carbon monoxide concentrations in outdoor and indoor air and street shops in Greece. *Atmospheric Environment* 1997;**32**:2871–76.

Van Wendel de Joode B., van Hemmen J.J., Meijster T. *et al.* Reliability of a semi-quantitative method for dermal exposure assessment (DREAM). *Journal of Exposure Analysis and Environmental Epidemiology* 2005;**15**(**1**):111–20.

Wainman T., Hazen R.E., Lioy P.J. The extractability of Cr(VI) from contaminated soil in synthetic sweat. *Journal of Exposure Analysis and Environmental Epidemiology* 1994;**4**(**2**):171–81.

Wakefield J. Human exposure assessment: finding out what's getting in. *Environmental Health Perspectives* 2000;**108**(**1**):A24–6.

Wallace L.A. Major sources of benzene exposure. *Environmental Health Perspectives* 1989;**82**:165–9.

Weis B.K., Balshaw D., Barr J.R. *et al.* Personalized exposure assessment: promising approaches for human environmental health research. *Environmental Health Perspectives* 2005;**113**(**7**):840–8.

Weisel C., Jo W., Lioy P. Utilization of breath analysis for exposure and dose estimates of chloroform. *Journal of Exposure Analysis and Environmental Epidemiology* 1993b;**2** Suppl 1:55–69.

Weisel C.P., Zhang J., Turpin B.J. *et al.* Relationship of Indoor, Outdoor and Personal Air (RIOPA) study: study design, methods and quality assurance/control results. *Journal of Exposure Analysis and Environmental Epidemiology* 2005;**15**:123–37.

Williams R., Suggs J., Creason J. *et al.* The 1998 Baltimore Particulate Matter Epidemiology-Exposure Study: part 2. *Personal exposure assessment associated with an elderly study population. Journal of Exposure Analysis and Environmental Epidemiology* 2000a;**10**(**6** Pt **1**):533–43.

Williams R., Suggs J., Zweidinger R. *et al.* The 1998 Baltimore Particulate Matter Epidemiology-Exposure Study: part 1. *Comparison of ambient, residential outdoor, indoor and apartment particulate matter monitoring. Journal of Exposure Analysis and Environmental Epidemiology* 2000b;**10**(**6** Pt **1**):518–32.

Xu X., Weisel C.P. Human respiratory uptake of chloroform and haloketones during showering. *Journal of Exposure Analysis and Environmental Epidemiology* 2005;**15**(**1**):6–16.

Yiin L.M., Millette V.A., Ilacqua V. *et al.* Comparisons of the dust/smoke particulate that settled inside the surrounding buildings and outside on the streets of southern New York City after the collapse of the World Trade Center, 11 September 2001. *Journal of the Air and Waste Management Association* 2004;**54**:515–28.

Zartarian V.G., Ott W.R., Duan N. A quantitative definition of exposure and related concepts. *Journal of Exposure Analysis and Environmental Epidemiology* 1997a;**7**:411–38.

Zartarian V., Ferguson A., Ong C. *et al.* Quantifying videotaped activity patterns video translation software and training methodologies. *Journal of Exposure Analysis and Environmental Epidemiology* 1997b;**7**:535–42.

Zartarian V., Ferguson A., Leckie J. Quantified dermal activity data from a 4-child pilot field study. *Journal of Exposure Analysis and Environmental Epidemiology* 1997c;**7**:543–52.

Zartarian V., Ferguson A., Leckie J. Quantified mouthing activity data from a four-child pilot field study. *Journal of Exposure Analysis and Environmental Epidemiology* 1998;**8**:543–53.

Zartarian V., Bahadori T., McKone T. Adoption of an official ISEA glossary. *Journal of Exposure Analysis and Environmental Epidemiology* 2005;**15**(**1**):1–5.

8.5

Occupational health

David Koh and Dean Baker

Abstract

Workers constitute a large and important group, accounting for up to half of the world's population. Occupational health, which involves the 'promotion and maintenance of the highest degree of physical, mental, and social well-being of workers in all occupations' is thus an important component of public health practice.

Work-related injuries and illnesses are estimated to kill 2.2 million people worldwide each year. Globally, there are about 270 million occupational accidents and 170 million victims of work-related illnesses annually. Many cases are unrecognized or not reported. The overall economic losses from work-related injuries and illnesses account for approximately 4 per cent of the world's GNP.

At the workplace, workers may suffer from occupational diseases which may affect almost all organ systems, and are caused by exposure to specific hazards at the workplace; work-related diseases with 'multifactorial' aetiology, where factors in the work environment may play a role, together with other risk factors in the development or aggravation of such diseases, and/or general diseases affecting the working population.

Disease prevention and health promotion in the workforce begin with assessment of the risk of work, and recognition of vulnerable populations including, for example, workers in developing nations, migrant workers, child labour, women workers, or impaired workers. Managing the risks of work may be via primary prevention including elimination of the hazard or substitution with a safer alternative, engineering controls, redesign of the work station or process, administrative controls, education of workers, improved and safer work practices, use of personal protective equipment, good personal hygiene practices, and pre-employment or preplacement examinations; secondary prevention including periodic health monitoring, detection of evidence of excessive exposure, biological tests of excessive exposure or early effect, and removal of the worker from further exposure; and/or tertiary prevention including planning for emergency response, rehabilitation and return to work, workers compensation. Health promotion at the workplace—which includes promoting healthy lifestyles and community action for health, and creation of conditions that make it possible to live a healthy life—is also important.

Increasingly, occupational health practice has evolved to encompass environmental health issues. Hence the term occupational and environmental health might more accurately describe this important aspect of public health.

Introduction

Workers constitute a large and important population. The World Health Organization (WHO) estimated in 2007 that the global labour force was half of the world's population (about 3300 million) (WHO 2007a). The officially registered working population includes 60–70 per cent of the world's adult males and 30–60 per cent of adult females. Most people between the ages of 22 and 65 spend approximately 40 per cent of their waking hours at work (Leigh *et al.* 1997).

Occupational health, as defined by a joint committee of the WHO and the International Labour Organization, involves the 'promotion and maintenance of the highest degree of physical, mental and social well-being of workers in all occupations' (Forsmann 1983). This definition emphasizes the term health rather than disease, and further implies a multidisciplinary responsibility as well as a mechanism for the provision of health services for the working population. As practised today, the cornerstones of occupational health practice are health protection and health promotion of those who work. In many countries, such activities extend beyond the worker to include his or her family members.

History and development

The Italian physician Bernardino Ramazzini (1633–1714) is often described as the 'Father of Occupational Medicine'. His publication *De Morbis Artificum Diatriba*, which appeared in 1700, was the seminal text in occupational medicine. Ramazzini stated that according to Hippocratic teaching, 'When you come to a patient's house, you should ask him what sort of pain he has, what caused them, how many days he has been ill, whether the bowels are working, and what sort of food he eats'. Following this citation, Ramazzini wrote: 'I may venture to add one more question: *What occupation does he follow?*' Ramazzini described many occupational illnesses that are still seen today, and furthermore, described the principles for their control.

The industrial revolution and occupational health

The major event that profoundly influenced the development of occupational health was the industrial revolution in the eighteenth century. Dramatic social changes during this period occurred in the western world. These transformations related to newly introduced industrial processes and the setting up of factories, which in turn set in motion a variety of social changes. Previously, most work was done by craftsmen in rural cottage industries. The industrial revolution resulted in work being carried out in factories in urban centres.

Effects were seen both within the community, as well as in the individual worker. Family life was disrupted, with men leaving their families and moving to work in new industrial areas. In industrial areas, health and social problems emerged—such as poor housing and sanitation, alcoholism, prostitution, and poverty. Inside factories, individuals were exposed to long hours of work and uncontrolled occupational hazards; and faced the risk of accidents at work. Child labour and apprenticeship of young children were commonplace, and there was an absence of labour legislation.

As problems of industrialization grew, people of influence and political power campaigned to improve working conditions. Occupational health legislation appeared towards the end of the eighteenth century, and progressively developed to protect the health and rights of workers.

Today, the same phenomena seen during the industrial revolution are being replicated in some developing nations. Even in industrialized nations, the similar problems are still encountered by migrant workers and other deprived sectors of their society.

Occupational health legislation

The first environmental cancer was described by Percival Pott over 200 years ago. This cancer—scrotal skin cancer—occurred in chimney sweeps, and was caused by exposure to polycyclic aromatic hydrocarbon compounds in soot. An early piece of English legislation was the *Act for Better Regulations of Chimney Sweeps and their Apprentices, 1788.* This act stipulated a minimum age of 8 years for chimney sweeps; provided for inspections and hearing of complaints, required that the master not 'misuse or evil treat' the apprentice, and stated that the master 'shall at least once in every week, cause the said apprentice to be thoroughly washed and cleansed from soot and dirt'.

The *Health and Morals of Apprentices Act, 1802* applied to apprentices in the cotton and woollen industry. It limited work to 12 h a day, specified factory walls to be washed and rooms to be ventilated, and allowed voluntary factory inspections by visitors. The *Factory Act, 1819* set 9 years as a minimum age for the worker and limited work hours. Other work environments were covered by other legislation, such as the *Mines Act, 1842*, which prohibited females from working in mines, and allowed for government inspection.

Many countries today have comprehensive occupational health legislation. For example, in the United States, the *Occupational Safety and Health Act* was passed by Congress in 1970. Its goal was 'to assure as far as possible every working man and woman in the nation safe and healthful working conditions'. The *Health and Safety at Work Act*, enacted in 1974 in the United Kingdom, provides a broad legislative framework for the protection of workers through specific regulations. The European Union (EU) adopted a policy in 1989 on the 'Fundamental Social Rights of Workers', emphasizing the need for safety and health protection in the workplace, improvements in living and working conditions, and provision of social protection for workers.

Another recent development of occupational health legislation aims to ensure that employers do not discriminate against applicants and employees with disabilities. One example of this type of legislation is the *Disability Discrimination Act, 1995* in the United Kingdom. Employers should also make reasonable accommodations for a known impairment; unless it would cause undue hardship, such as incurring significant difficulty or expense.

Occupational diseases, injury, and work-related ill health

In most nations, there is no completely reliable source of information on the extent of work-related injuries and diseases. Even so, the International Labour Office (ILO) estimates that work-related injuries and illnesses kill 2.2 million people worldwide each year. Globally, there are about 270 million occupational accidents and 170 million victims of work-related illnesses annually (ILO 2005). An estimated 160 million new cases of work-related diseases occur each year worldwide.

At the workplace, three categories of diseases may be noted in workers. These are:

(1) Occupational diseases: These are caused by exposure to specific hazards at the workplace. However, in some situations these occupational diseases may also occur among the general community as a consequence of contamination of the environment from the workplace, e.g. lead, pesticides. Occupational diseases are cause-specific—e.g. asbestos causes asbestosis.

(2) Work-related diseases: Work-related diseases are 'multifactorial' in origin, where factors in the work environment may play a role, together with other risk factors in the development or aggravation of such diseases. These diseases have a complex aetiology.

(3) General diseases affecting the working population: These are medical conditions prevalent in the community such as malaria, hereditary haemolytic anaemia, or diabetes mellitus, without a causal relationship with work. The unhealthy worker may not be able to be as productive as his healthy counterpart. Furthermore, work may have a deleterious or aggravating effect on the medical condition.

Table 8.5.1 shows the differences between occupational and work-related diseases.

Table 8.5.1 Differences between occupational and work-related diseases

Work-related diseases	Occupational diseases
Occurs largely in the community	Occurs mainly among working population
'Multifactorial' in origin	Cause specific
Exposure to workplace may be a factor	Exposure to workplace is essential
May be notifiable and compensable	Notifiable and compensable

Major types of occupational disease and injury

Occupational illness can affect virtually every organ system. Occupational diseases of the lung and skin are common since these organs have substantial surface areas in direct contact with toxic substances. Noise-induced hearing loss and musculoskeletal disorders are among the most common disorders arising from physical factors in the workplace. Occupational cancer is a major concern because of the high mortality associated with many forms of cancer. Increasing attention has been paid in recent years to diseases affecting the neurological, reproductive, and immunological systems.

Occupational lung diseases

The lung is an easily accessible target organ for airborne toxic substances. Major categories of occupational lung disease include the 'dust diseases' of the lung or pneumoconioses, lung cancer, occupational asthma, industrial bronchitis and other effects of irritants, and infections. Silicosis is the most common pneumoconiosis worldwide. Exposure to silica occurs in a wide variety of work situations such as sandblasting, mining, milling, pottery work, foundry work and work using abrasives. In the United States, over 1 million workers are at risk for developing silicosis each year; more than 200 workers die from silicosis and hundreds more become disabled (NIOSH 2006). The International Agency for Research on Cancer (IARC) has classified crystalline silica as a known human carcinogen (IARC 1997).

Asbestos is another important cause of pneumoconiosis and other lung diseases. Asbestos has been responsible for over 200 000 deaths in the United States and will cause millions more deaths worldwide (Collegium Ramazzini 2004). All forms of asbestos cause asbestosis, a progressive fibrosis of the lungs. All forms of asbestos can also cause lung cancer and malignant mesothelioma. Peto and colleagues (1999) estimate there will be more than 500 000 asbestos-related malignant mesothelioma cancer deaths in Western Europe over the next 35 years. Given the long latency, the future burden of mortality resulting from asbestos will be substantial even if all future exposure were to be eliminated completely.

Bronchial asthma affects about 5–16 per cent of the population in developed countries (Masoli 2004). Population-based estimates in the United States suggest that 15–23 per cent of new-onset asthma cases in adults are work related (NIOSH 2004). In some jurisdictions, occupational asthma has become the most prevalent occupational lung disease, exceeding silicosis and asbestosis. Even so, prevalence studies of occupational asthma usually underestimate the number of affected workers because these workers tend to quit jobs where they suffer such symptoms, although their asthma symptoms and signs may continue even after leaving work.

Many gases, fumes, and aerosols are directly toxic to the respiratory tract by causing acute inflammation. Examples include soluble irritants, e.g. hydrogen chloride, ammonia, sulphur dioxide, which produce effects in the eyes, nasopharynx, and large airways. Less soluble irritants, e.g. nitrogen dioxide, ozone, and phosgene, produce few upper respiratory symptoms, but in high exposure can cause a toxic pneumonitis. Long-term exposure can lead to lung fibrosis.

Occupational cancer

Based on a review of IARC classification, there are 28 definite, 27 probable, and 110 possible human occupational carcinogens. They include chemical substances (e.g. benzene and asbestos), physical hazards (e.g. ionizing radiation), and biological hazards (e.g. viruses). It is estimated that approximately 16 million workers in the EU are exposed to carcinogens at work. The most common cancers due to these workplace exposures are cancers of the lung, bladder, skin, pleura (mesothelioma), liver, haematopoietic tissue, bone, and soft connective tissue.

Occupational cancer accounts for about 4–20 per cent of all cancers in developed countries. The large variability in the estimates arises from differences in data sets used and the assumptions applied. The most commonly accepted estimate is 4 per cent with a plausible range, based on the best quality studies, being 2–8 per cent. However, if one considers only the adult population in which exposure to occupational carcinogens almost exclusively occurs, the proportion of cancer attributed to occupation would increase to about 20 per cent among those exposed (Pearce *et al.* 1998).

Occupational skin disorders

Skin disorders are among the most commonly reported occupational diseases. Approximately one worker per thousand is affected (LaDou 2007). The most common occupational skin disorder is irritant contact dermatitis. Although skin disorders are relatively easily diagnosed, occupational skin diseases are believed to be underreported, so that the actual rate is many times higher than officially reported (NIOSH 2007). Occupational skin disorders are unevenly distributed among industries. A worker in agriculture, forestry, fishing, or manufacturing has three times the risk of developing a work-related skin disease as a worker in other industries.

Occupational infectious diseases

Much attention about infectious diseases has focused on healthcare settings, although infections can be transmitted in other work places, such as research laboratories and animal processing facilities. Within healthcare settings, awareness has grown about the risk of infection by hepatitis, the human immunodeficiency virus (HIV), and tuberculosis (*Mycobacterium tuberculosis*). Needlestick injuries accounted for about 40 per cent of hepatitis B and hepatitis C infections and 4.4 per cent of HIV infections in healthcare workers (Nelson *et al.* 2005). An increased risk of HIV infection has been shown to exist in settings in which workers may be exposed to blood or body fluids (NIOSH 1996).

Transmission of *M. tuberculosis* is a recognized risk in healthcare facilities. After years of declining incidence rates, multidrug-resistant (MDR) tuberculosis re-emerged as a major occupational health problem during the 1990s in major cities in the United States which serve populations with high rates of MDR tuberculosis (CDC 1999).

Emerging infectious diseases also pose a risk to healthcare workers. One example is severe acute respiratory syndrome (SARS), which is caused by a coronavirus. In the 2003 worldwide outbreak of SARS, 20 per cent of patients were healthcare workers (Koh *et al.* 2003). Currently there is concern about risk of infection among healthcare workers caring for patients with avian influenza (Schultsz *et al.* 2005; WHO 2007b).

Infectious diseases can be especially prevalent in developing countries, resulting in higher risks for workers in these countries. Some of the infections result directly from the work, while others are indirectly related to work. Examples include vector-borne diseases like malaria; water- and food-borne diseases resulting from poor sanitation and inadequate potable water; and zoonoses among agricultural workers.

Occupational reproductive disorders

The overall contribution of occupational exposures to reproductive disorders is not known because there has been little research in this area until recently. More than 84 000 chemical compounds are in the workplace, and about 2000 are added every year. Only about 4000 have been evaluated for reproductive toxicity, and among these, few have been sufficiently evaluated for human reproductive effects. Most of the studies were conducted on animals (Lawson *et al.* 2003). Very few studies have been done on physical and biological agents that may affect fertility and pregnancy outcomes.

It is well documented that lead (Pb) and the pesticide dibromochloropropane cause testicular injury with resultant reduction in sperm count. Also, Pb can cross the placenta in a pregnant woman worker to cause neurological impairment in the foetus. Other substances associated with documented adverse reproductive outcomes include methyl mercury, solvents such as carbon disulphide, carbon monoxide, oestrogens, anaesthetic gases, antineoplastic drugs, ethylene oxide, ethylene glycol ethers, polychlorinated biphenyls, and physical agents such as ionizing radiation (Windham 2007).

Occupational exposures can cause a wide range of reproductive disorders in both males and females. Effects of exposures in males include altered sperm number, shape or function; altered sperm transfer; and altered hormones or sexual performance. Exposures in females may cause menstrual disorders, infertility, chromosomal aberrations, breast milk alteration, early onset of menopause, and suppressed libido.

Reproductive disorders also include adverse effects on the offspring of the exposed worker. Potential foetal effects from maternal exposures include preterm delivery, foetal loss, prenatal death, low birth weight, altered sex ratio of livebirths, congenital malformations, childhood malignancies, infant or childhood illness, and developmental disabilities.

Occupational noise-induced hearing loss

High levels of occupational noise are a persistent problem in all regions of the world. In Germany, 12–15 per cent of the workforce are exposed to hazardous noise levels (Concha-Barrientos 2004). In the EU, noise-induced hearing loss is one of the most commonly reported occupational disease—20 per cent of the workers report they were exposed to high levels of noise for at least half of their working hours. The prevalence of noise exposure is especially high in the manufacturing and construction industries—40 per cent of workers in these sectors are exposed. In the United States, about 30 million workers are exposed to hazardous noise levels at work (NIOSH 2004).

Industries such as manufacturing, mining, construction, transportation, agriculture, and the military are at the highest risk for noise-induced hearing loss. In developed countries, increasing awareness has led to greater implementation of protective measures, whereas in developing countries, industrialization may herald an increase in average noise levels (Concha-Barrientos 2004).

Occupational traumatic injuries

These injuries include such events as amputations, fractures, severe lacerations, eye losses, acute poisonings, and burns. ILO estimates that 2 million people die every year from work-related accidents and illnesses. For every fatal accident, there are another 500–2000 injuries, depending on the occupation (ILO 2002). In Great Britain, the rate of nonfatal major injuries reported in 2005–2006 was 100.3 per 100 000 workers. European Statistics at Work reported about 4.7 million accidents at work in the EU which resulted in three or more days away from work in 2001, and about 4900 fatal accidents at work (European Communities 2004).

Work-related diseases

Work-related diseases are diseases in which workplace factors may be associated in their occurrence, but need not be the only risk factor in each case. Common work-related diseases include: Hypertension, ischaemic heart disease, psychosomatic illnesses, musculoskeletal disorders, and non-specific respiratory disease. In these diseases, work may be associated with their causation or may aggravate a pre-existing condition.

Work-related diseases are more common than pure 'occupational diseases'. While prevention of occupational diseases is possible by the elimination of the workplace hazard, work-related diseases cannot be entirely prevented by only addressing occupational hazards.

Work-related musculoskeletal disorders

Work-related musculoskeletal disorders include both acute and chronic injury to the musculoskeletal system, other than acute trauma. These conditions are one of the leading problems affecting workers. In the United States, musculoskeletal disorders account for 34 per cent of all nonfatal occupational injuries and illnesses involving days away from work (NIOSH 2004). More than half of the working population develops low-back injury at some time in their working career. Musculoskeletal injuries are the principal cause of disability of people in their working years.

According to the Labour Force Survey in Great Britain, musculoskeletal disorders accounted for about 75 per cent of self-reported work-related illness in 2005–2006. The commonest musculoskeletal complaint was back pain. Among the 7000 cases assessed per year for industrial injuries disablement benefits, vibration white finger and carpal tunnel syndrome were among the largest categories (HSE 2006).

In the EU, 53 per cent of workers reporting work-related illness had musculoskeletal disorders. About 17–46 per cent of workers report exposure to the risk factors for musculoskeletal diseases. The 1999 Labour Force Survey reported that about 4 million European workers suffered from a work-related musculoskeletal problem (European Communities 2004).

Stress-related ill health

Job stress has been defined as the 'harmful physical and emotional responses that occur when the requirements of the job do not match the capabilities, resources or needs of the worker' (NIOSH 1999). In terms of the magnitude of the problem, NIOSH (1999) reports that:

- 25 per cent of employees view their jobs as the number one stressor in their lives.
- 75 per cent of employees believe that today's worker has more 'on-the-job' stress than a generation ago.
- Problems at work are more strongly associated with health complaints; than any other life stressor—more than even financial or family problems.

- Workers who take time off work because of stress, anxiety, or a related disorder will be off the job for about 20 days.

Individual and situational factors, such as balance between work and family life, social support, individual outlook, and personality, can affect the likelihood of developing stress. However, working conditions often play a significant, and sometimes major role in the causation of stress.

Workplace stress-related hazards (WHO 2003) consist of factors in both work content as well as context. Work content encompasses job content (e.g. meaningless, unpleasant tasks), workload (under as well as overload) and working under time pressure, work schedules (e.g. long, unsociable, inflexible working schedules), degree of participation in decision making, and lack of control of work. Work context includes concerns about career development, status and salary, the individual's role in the organization, issues relating to interpersonal relationships, the organizational culture/climate, and conflict or lack of support in the home–work interface.

Averse health outcomes of job stress are wide ranging, from increased risk of cardiovascular disease, musculoskeletal disorders, psychological disorders (e.g. emotional distress, depression, insomnia), impaired immune function, gastrointestinal disorders (e.g. ulcers), cancer, and even suicide. The organization may face a decrease in work commitment, an increase in absenteeism, lowered productivity, and increasing complaints and poor public image.

General diseases affecting the working population

There are general diseases prevalent in every community. These include infections such as HIV-AIDS, tuberculosis, and malaria, or non-communicable diseases and lifestyle-related diseases such as diabetes mellitus, cardiovascular disease, cancer, and malnutrition. Such diseases may not be caused by work exposures, but can affect work productivity. Workplace factors may also influence the medical condition.

Estimates of cost and economic loss

Total economic losses due to occupational injuries and illnesses are large. The ILO estimated that overall economic losses from work-related injuries and illnesses in 1997 were approximately 4 per cent of the world's gross national product (GNP). According to recent estimates, the cost of work-related health loss and associated productivity loss may amount to several percent of total GNP of a country. For example, the Health and Safety Executive (HSE) has estimated the cost of occupational illness and injury to the British economy to between £13.1 billion to £22.2 billion in 2001–02 (HSE 2004).

In the United States, the direct cost of workplace injuries and illnesses was estimated to be US$45.8 billion, and the indirect costs ranging from US$137.4 to US$229 billion. The National Safety Council estimated that the cost of work injuries in 2002 was US$1060 per worker, with a national total of US$146.6 billion. In addition, employer costs for providing workers' compensation rose from US$52.8 to US$72.9 billion between 1998 and 2002 (NIOSH 2005).

Under-recognition of occupational ill health

Although recording of workplace injuries is reasonably accurate in most developed countries, surveillance systems generally result in substantial under-estimates of actual cases of occupational illness. One explanation for under-recognition of occupational disease is the inherent difficulty in diagnosing occupational diseases and in establishing cause-and-effect relationships. The link between occupation and disease may sometimes be unclear, because most occupational diseases are not distinct clinically and pathologically from diseases associated with non-occupational aetiologies. For example, skin cancer caused by polycyclic aromatic hydrocarbons is similar in appearance to that caused by sunlight. Similarly, solvent-induced encephalopathy may easily be attributed to old age. Only in rare instances, such as the associations between asbestos and mesothelioma (Selikoff *et al.* 1964) and between vinyl chloride monomer and angiosarcoma of the liver (Creech & Johnson 1974), is the causal association between occupational exposure and disease readily established on clinical grounds alone.

Another cause of the under-recognition of occupational disease is that the majority of chemicals in commerce have never been evaluated with regard to their potential toxicity. Only 7 per cent of the approximately 80 000 chemicals commonly used in industry have been screened for toxicity, and less than half of these have been studied thoroughly (LaDou 2007). Such toxicity testing often concentrate primarily on high-dose, acute effects, and on the long-term risk of cancer. Toxicity testing of reproductive, neurological, and other adverse effects remains quite limited.

The long latency which typically elapses between occupational exposure and onset of illness is a third factor which may obscure the occupational aetiology of chronic disease. For example, few occupational cancers appear within 10 or even 20 years of first exposure. Similarly, chronic neurotoxic effects of solvents may become evident only after decades of exposure. In such instances, it is unlikely that the worker will be diagnosed as having a disease of occupational origin.

Lack of awareness among health practitioners about the hazards found at work is a fourth cause of underestimation of occupational disease, reflecting the fact that most physicians are not adequately trained to suspect work as a cause of disease (Institute of Medicine 1988; Goldman *et al.* 1999). Very little time is devoted in most medical schools to teaching physicians to take a proper occupational history, to recognize symptoms of common industrial toxins, or to recall known associations between occupational exposures and disease.

Compounding this lack of medical awareness is the limited ability of many workers to provide an accurate report of their exposures. Workers may have had multiple toxic exposures in a variety of jobs over a working lifetime. In most countries, there are no requirements to inform workers of the hazard of the materials with which they work. Even in the United States, employers' reporting requirements remain limited under the Hazard Communication Standard and state right-to-know laws. In many instances, a patient may not know about all his or her past occupational exposures.

Finally, given the potential financial liability associated with the finding that a disease is of occupational origin, employers may be resistant to recognizing the work-relatedness of a disorder, especially in cases where personal habits or non-occupational pursuits are possible contributory factors. Since employers are often in the best position to recognize causal associations between workplace exposures and disease, this conflict of interest represents an obstacle to obtaining accurate estimates of the burden of occupational illness.

Globalization and workers' health

Globalization is defined as an 'increase in the total world economic activity as a consequence of the liberalization of trade and the elimination of the hindrances to the transfer of capital, goods, and services across the national border' (Rantanen 2000).

Rapid technological innovation and the proliferation of multinational organizations are driving the formation of a global economy that has a substantial impact on workers' safety and health. Technological change is creating fundamental transformations in the ways corporations organize production, trade goods, invest capital, and develop new products. Technology allows virtually instantaneous communication among widely dispersed operations. Advanced manufacturing technologies have changed patterns of productivity and employment. Improved air and sea transportation has greatly accelerated the flow of peoples and goods. These developments have created greater interdependence among firms and nations. At the same time, the rapid rate of innovation means that competitive advantages are fleeting and companies must function with ever increasing efficiency to survive in the global economy.

The strategy is for corporations to be agile and rapidly responsive to market demands (Menzies 1998). This strategy has led to concepts such as computer-integrated manufacturing, just-in-time manufacturing, and lean production. Quality circles, total quality management, and other 'cultural training' programmes train workers to identify with the competitive goals of management. New technologies have been implemented to increase productivity and make flexible work schedules possible. However, these technologies can also mean loss of control for workers, increased work speed, and more repetitious work—each of which has been associated with increased job stress (Schnall *et al.* 2000). Employment is both more flexible and less secure as corporations use technology to ensure that individual workers are dispensable and that they conform to the competitive needs of the corporation. Consequently, there has been a dramatic growth in contracted work and non-standard forms of employment, such as part-time and home-based work.

Shift work and irregular work hours have increased significantly among those who are employed. About 20 per cent of workers in the EU countries engage in shift work, and about the same number are involved in some night work (European Communities 2004). The ILO found that one in five (or 614.2 million) workers worldwide put in more than 48 h of work a week, often earning only a bare minimum (ILO 2007b).

The contingent workforce (which includes self-employed, temporary, and part-time workers) typically have less training about hazards, less access to occupational health services, and less access to other social services (e.g. medical and unemployment insurance or programmes). It is difficult under these circumstances for traditional forms of labour protection, such as government regulations and representation by unions, to function efficiently.

The global economy has also led to shifts in the distribution of occupational hazards among regions of the world. In the industrially developed nations, the principal shift has been from a manufacturing-based economy to an economy that is based on the provision of services and transfer of information. Consequently, exposure to classical hazards such as silica, asbestos, and heavy chemicals are becoming less important in these nations, while exposure to new synthetic materials and solvents, as well as the ergonomic exposures associated with repetitive work before computer terminals, have become more important (Mustard 1997). In developing nations, major hazards have resulted from the export of dangerous industries, materials, and occupations from the industrially developed nations. In some instances, this export can lead to devastating disasters such as the explosion in the chemical plant at Bhopal, India, that killed several thousand people. Another example is the international boom in the microelectronics industry, which now employs hundreds of thousands of workers worldwide, occasionally under poorly controlled and exploitative conditions. Multinational corporations account for 70 per cent of world trade. They play a dominant role in global manufacturing and trade and carry a large responsibility for economic development (LaDou 2007).

The global economy has led to the negotiation of trade agreements, such as the North American Free Trade Agreement, which define conditions of work in the context of trade facilitation and barriers. In some cases, agreements have led to standards that raise the level of protection to workers in countries where previously such protections were minimal; however, in many cases, agreements have encouraged de-unionization and movement away from work protections in order to 'harmonize' protections at a low, but common level among trading partners (Armstrong 1998). A major challenge for nations and international organizations is to implement policies that balance the demands of the global market economy with appropriate protections for workers' health and well-being.

Globalization affects nations selectively. Countries such as China, Argentina, Brazil, India, and the Philippines have seen economic growth and reduction in poverty rates in the past 20 years through globalization. On the other hand, 2 billion people in countries such as Pakistan and much of Africa are becoming more isolated from the world community and are seeing stagnant economies and increasing poverty (LaDou 2007).

Special populations of workers

Recognition has increased that workplace hazards impact disproportionately on some worker populations—such as those in developing nations, as well as child labourers, women workers, and impaired workers (IPEC 1999). These populations are especially impacted because of the interaction between their work roles and broader roles in society, as well as by their particular exposures in the workplace.

Workers in developing nations

More than 80 per cent of workers in the global workforce are from the developing world (Rosenstock 2005). Workers' health should be viewed in the context of national development. Occupational health policy makers in many nations must consider a balance between adverse impacts on workers' health and the economic advantages of rapid development by allowing foreign investigators access to low-cost labour and conditions of weak labour protections.

The relationship between workers' health and development is complex for many reasons (Jeyaratnam 1998). For example, workers in many developing countries may be affected by poor nutrition or endemic diseases, such as malaria, in which work may aggravate the condition, or which make the worker more susceptible to the effects of workplace exposures. Workers in these countries also generally have lower educational backgrounds and are often inadequately trained to handle the new technologies and potential hazards. There may be high turnover with little management investment in worker training.

Working conditions in tropical developing countries may present special hazards because of climate and building ventilation issues in production facilities. Much of the production equipment is imported from developed countries so that replacement parts and service may be unavailable. The machinery may be used or considered obsolete for use in the developed countries, while new and safer equipment may be unavailable or too expensive.

The social organization of work in developing countries also affects workers' health. In addition to the large number of workplaces with a small number of workers, large proportions of the workforce work in the 'informal' sector. This sector consists of small, often home-based businesses that have no government registration and oversight. For example, recent estimates of the proportion of informal non-agricultural employment were about 58 per cent for Latin America and 75 per cent in sub-Saharan Africa. The informal economy accounts for 90 per cent of women working in non-agricultural sectors in India and Indonesia, and 95 per cent in Benin, Chad, and Mali (Rosenstock 2005).

Finally, countries of the developing world may have access to advanced technologies from the developed world without having developed legal or administrative infrastructure to control their adverse impacts on the work force (Jeyaratnam 1998). Even if developing countries adopt standards and legislation from more developed nations, there often is a shortage of trained personnel to recognize and manage workplace hazards.

Child labour

Children are an important population of workers worldwide. The ILO estimated that in 2004 there were 218 million children who were engaged in economic activity, with at least 126 million of them in hazardous work (ILO 2006a). Sub-Saharan Africa has the highest proportion of children engaged in economic activities, at about 26 per cent. Child labour also exists in many industrialized countries. Child labour has become an important issue because the children are often exploited in the workplace and denied basic human rights, such as access to education. Additionally, many children work in dangerous jobs and they may be more susceptible to workplace hazards (Warshaw 1998).

Poverty is the primary reason why children work. Poor households need the money, and children commonly contribute around 20–25 per cent of family income. Furthermore, if the family has a tradition of engaging in a hazardous occupation, it is likely that the children will continue in the trade.

Many children work in hazardous occupations and are at greater risk of suffering ill effects than adult workers. These children may have greater exposure to hazards than adult workers in the same occupation because children tend to be given the most menial jobs, which may involve higher exposures to toxic substances. Children are more susceptible to the same hazards faced by adult workers because they differ from adults in their anatomical, physiological, and psychological characteristics. Children using hand tools designed for adults run a higher risk of fatigue and injury. Personal protective equipment may also not fit and provide adequate protection. Furthermore, children may not be as aware as adults of workplace dangers, or as knowledgeable of precautions to be taken at work. Children are also more vulnerable to psychological and physical abuse than are adults, and suffer deeper psychological damage when they are denigrated or oppressed.

A resurgence of child labour is occurring in developed nations as well. Each year in New York State, for example, more than 1000 children receive workers' compensation awards for injuries incurred on the job; over 40 per cent of these awards each year are for permanent disability (Belville *et al.* 1993).

The issue of child labour has received increasing attention (Warshaw 1998; IPEC 1999). This is reflected in the number of organizations involved in the cause of children and child workers. For example, the International Programme on the Elimination of Child labour (IPEC) was launched in 1992 and, as of 1999, developed into a 90 country alliance. The aim of IPEC is the elimination of child labour, giving priority to its worst forms. The 'worst forms' comprise all forms of slavery or practices similar to slavery; the use, procurement or offering of a child for prostitution or production of pornography; the use, procurement, or offering of a child for illicit activities; and work which is inherently likely to harm the health, safety, or morals of children (IPEC 1999). Withdrawing children from the worst forms of child labour requires improved legislation and enforcement, improved methodologies for identifying the children, rehabilitation of the children, provision of viable alternatives to the children, and raising awareness at all societal levels.

The effort of IPEC in the elimination of child labour is beginning to pay off. The last 4 years have seen an 11 per cent reduction in the number of child labourers. Hearteningly, the greatest drop has been in the number of children involved in hazardous work. The number of children in the 5–14 age group involved in hazardous work has fallen by 33 per cent. The number of children at work in Latin America and the Caribbean has declined the most, by two-thirds in the last 4 years. However, the rate of child labour is still disparately high in sub-Saharan Africa (ILO 2006a).

Women workers

About 42 per cent of the global workforce is female (Messing 2006). Women are a special worker population because of the significant interplay between their roles in society, socioeconomic condition, and occupation. Women's roles in virtually all societies are defined in relation to their reproductive functions and responsibilities as family caregivers. Paid employment of women has increased in most countries, but this employment has increased the conflict between paid work and women's traditional family responsibilities. In many societies, early marriage, repeated child bearing, low education, and poverty all disproportionately impact on women workers (Loewenson 1999). The dual roles of women as workers and unpaid caregivers is especially challenging for sole-support mothers, who comprise 20–30 per cent of households worldwide.

Employment of women in most societies is characterized by occupational segregation, under-employment—doing seasonal and part-time work below their level of education, and barriers to advancement. Occupational segregation means that women tend to be clustered into a small number of occupations while being under-represented in most others (Stellman 1999). For example, professional women tend to be in teaching, nursing, and other healthcare specialities. In manufacturing, women tend to have jobs in assembly and small machine operations. Women in developing countries tend to be employed in sectors such as agriculture, textiles and clothing, food processing, and social services (Loewenson 1999). Compared with men, women work for smaller industries or organizations, have less opportunity for work control, and face the psychological demands of people-oriented or machine-paced work

(Paltiel 1998). Women are more likely to work in the informal sector, in specific types of informal work such as domestic work, street vending, and sex work, with their accompanying low social status and lack of legislative protection. While some countries have enacted laws prohibiting gender discrimination, many countries still have formal restrictions on women's employment.

Gender differences are observed in the rates of occupational injuries and illnesses, but these differences are primarily because of differences in the conditions of work or exposures, rather than due to genetic differences (Stellman 1999). As mentioned, women tend to work in different occupations than men, with a different distribution of hazards. Even when employed in the same industry, women generally do different jobs or different tasks from men so their exposures may be different. Even when doing the same task, women may have different levels of exposure because of variation in the effectiveness of engineering controls and personal protective equipment—which are generally designed for men.

Impaired workers

Around 470 million people with disabilities are in the working age group. Many people can make constructive contributions in the workplace although they have some type of physical impairment. In the United Kingdom, the *Disability Discrimination Act, 1995* prohibits employers from discriminating against applicants and employees with disabilities. Employers also should make reasonable accommodations for a known impairment.

A number of countries (e.g. China, Cambodia, and Tanzania) have established legislation for people with disabilities, prohibiting discrimination and covering various aspects of the rights of disabled people, including employment. Some countries (e.g. France, Germany, and Japan) go one step further and impose quotas on some enterprises to employ a certain percentage of disabled persons. Other countries, e.g. India and Japan, use employment promotion measures to ensure workplace accessibility and provide employment services in the form of job placement agencies. Singapore provides tax reductions as a financial incentive to compensate employers for any financial burden resulting from the employment of disabled persons (ILO 2007a). In 2006, the UN adopted a Convention on the Rights of Persons with Disabilities (ILO 2006b).

Reasonable accommodations are changes made to the work environment, job responsibilities or conditions of work that provide opportunities for workers with special needs to perform essential job functions. Reasonable accommodation can cover the special needs of persons with impairments or those workers with chronic or recurrent disease, including persons with AIDS. Accommodation may include technical assistance devices; customization, including personal protective equipment and clothing; and changes to processes, location, or timing for essential job functions. Surveys conducted by DuPont showed that employees with disabilities perform equally or better compared to employees with no disabilities. Additional adjustments in the workplace were required by only 4 per cent of disabled persons of employable age (ILO 2007a).

Migrant workers

There are an estimated 150–190 million migrants in the world—2 per cent of the world's population—including migrant workers, refugees, asylum seekers, and permanent immigrants. The number has increased dramatically with globalization. The vast majority of migration is from developing to developed countries. Three-quarters of all migrants lived in 28 countries in 2005, with one in five migrants living in the United States. Many migrants move to seek work. According to the UN, 'migrant workers' are persons who are to be engaged, are engaged, or have been engaged in remunerated activities in a State of which they are not nationals (UN 1990). Some migrant workers stay permanently in their new countries, while many return to their original homes after working for a period of time.

Migrant workers are a particularly vulnerable population for many of the same reasons that were described for workers in developing countries, e.g. they may be affected by poor nutrition and endemic diseases, they often have lower educational backgrounds, and they are inadequately trained for the potential work hazards. Migrant workers face additional obstacles because they may not speak the language of the host country; they often are not familiar with the health and safety practices and regulations, nor their rights in the host country; they may have temporary housing and limited access to medical care and other social services; they may be impacted by racism and xenophobia in their workplaces and communities; and they may not have full legal status, which makes them vulnerable to exploitation (Holmes 2006; McKay *et al.* 2006).

The UN and other international agencies have established programmes to monitor the status of migrants, including migrant workers. In July 2003, the UN 'Convention on the Protection of the Rights of All Migrant Workers and Their Families' entered into force. The Committee on Migrant Workers (CMW), which is linked with the UN, monitors implementation of the convention. Interestingly essentially all of the countries that ratified or signed the convention are countries of origins of migrants. The migrant-receiving nations of Europe and the United States have not ratified the convention, although there is growing awareness in Europe of the importance of addressing the rights of migrants. A key concept in the convention is that migrant workers are entitled to enjoy their human rights regardless of their legal status. In particular, the convention seeks to put an end to the illegal or clandestine recruitment and trafficking of migrant workers and to discourage the employment of migrant workers in undocumented situations, in which they are most vulnerable to exploitation (OHCHR, from: www.unhchr.ch/html/menu2/6/cmw/features.htm).

Assessing the risk of work

Health protection begins with an assessment of risk. Risk assessment is a structured and systematic procedure that is dependent upon the correct identification of hazards and an appropriate estimation of the risks arising from them (HSE 1995). The purpose for risk assessment is to ensure that a valid decision can be made for measures necessary to control exposure to substances hazardous to health arising in the workplace. Risk assessments are legal requirements in many countries. It can be either a qualitative or quantitative process.

Expertise, effort, and detail required for risk assessment depends on the nature and degree of risk, and the complexity of the work process. Adequate controls are determined based on several factors, such as the toxicity of substance, numbers exposed, acceptability of risk, legal requirements, costs, and availability of control measures.

Hazard and risk

There is a distinction between the terms 'hazard' and 'risk'.

A *hazard* is a substance, agent, or physical situation with a potential for harm in terms of injury or ill health, damage to property, damage to the environment, or a combination of these. Hazards can be

Table 8.5.2 Types of hazards at the workplace and their health effects

Type of hazard	Examples	Health effect
Physical	Noise Local vibration	Noise-induced hearing loss Traumatic vasospastic disease
Chemical	Various chemicals, e.g. solvents, heavy metals	Intoxications, fibroses, cancers, allergies, nervous system damage
Biological	Bacteria, fungi, viruses	Infections, allergies
Ergonomic	Repetitive work, work–rest schedules	Musculoskeletal injuries mental stress, lowered productivity and work quality
Psychosocial	Organizational stress, conflicts	Work dissatisfaction, burnout, depression

physical, chemical, biological, ergonomic, or psychosocial in nature (Table 8.5.2). *Hazard identification* is the process of recognizing that a hazard exists and defining its characteristics.

Risk relates to the likelihood of the harm or undesired event occurring, and the consequences of its occurrence. It is the probability that the substance or agent will cause adverse effects under the conditions of use and/or exposure, and the possible extent of harm. It is thus a function of both exposure to the hazard and the likelihood of harm from the hazard. *Extent of risk* covers the population that might be affected by the risk, the numbers exposed, and the consequences.

Risk assessment is the process of estimating the magnitude of risk, and deciding if the risk is tolerable or acceptable. A tolerable risk may not always be acceptable. It merely refers to a willingness to live with a risk to secure certain benefits, and in the confidence that the risk is being properly controlled (Sadhra & Rampal 1999). The levels of tolerability of risk are different for different countries, and in different working populations and the general public.

Risk assessment process

The process of risk assessment and management should take into account both routine and non-routine activities and conditions, including foreseeable emergency situations. Hazards that are intrinsic to these situations or generated by such activities should be identified.

Exposed persons should be identified, including non-employees and those who are susceptible and therefore at higher risk because of illness or other medical conditions. Existing control measures, if any, should be evaluated.

The health risks from the hazards should be determined and assessed, and a decision made if the risk is acceptable or tolerable. Unacceptable risks should be eliminated or reduced with new or improved control measures, and their effectiveness monitored. Such a process should be a team effort, involving the workers themselves as well as personnel with the relevant expertise. If needed, further corrective actions should be implemented. At the same time, workers should be informed of the hazards, risks, and appropriate measures that can be taken to protect themselves.

The steps for risk assessment for chemical, biological, ergonomic, and psychosocial hazards may differ, as illustrated by the following examples. The assessments for chemical or physical exposures are generally more objective and precise than the assessment for psychic stressors. As an example, an initial assessment for a chemical exposure might include the following steps:

1. List substances in the area to be assessed.
2. Determine which are actually used.
3. Evaluate workers concerns.
4. Assess the tasks of workers, their exposure, and methods of handling.
5. Obtain suppliers' data sheets.
6. Evaluate data sheets.
7. Inspect places where the substances are handled.
8. Evaluate method of control.
9. Perform environmental monitoring for the chemical if needed.
10. Decide on acceptability or tolerability of risk, and if further control measures are needed.

The assessment of psychosocial factors at work is more complex. It may include the evaluation of organizational dysfunction, work conditions, as well as a study of indicators such as sickness absence, staff turnover, and measurement of stress-related illness among employees. The identification of work stressors should review design of tasks, management style, interpersonal relationships, work roles, career concerns, and environmental conditions. Questionnaires to staff can be carried out using validated instruments—e.g. the Finnish Occupational Stress Questionnaire.

Environmental monitoring

Environmental or ambient monitoring in the workplace is undertaken to measure external exposure to harmful agents. The monitoring is to ensure that exposure is kept within 'permissible levels' so as to prevent the occurrence of disease.

Permissible levels or occupational exposure limits (OELs)

Permissible levels, or OELs, are standards that are available for many of the common hazards found in workplaces. Standards are available for the commonly encountered physical as well as chemical hazards. Standards can also be found for some substances of biological origin, including cellulose, some wood, cotton and grain dusts, proteolytic enzymes, and vegetable oil mists.

Permissible levels are based on the following considerations: (i) the physical and chemical properties of substance, including the nature and amount of impurities; (ii) toxicological studies; and (iii) available human data. The concept of permissible levels assumes that for each substance there is a level of exposure at or below which the exposed worker does not suffer any health impairment.

Permissible levels have their limitations. As such every effort must be made to keep exposure levels as low as reasonably practicable and the permissible level is a level above which exposure should not occur. This level could also be mandated by legislation. However, such levels may be based on incomplete information. Previously unsuspected health risks have arisen from substances assumed to be comparatively safe, for example, glycol ethers in the electronic industry and the risk of spontaneous abortions. The use of exposure standards for working conditions depends on good professional judgement, and hence should be used and interpreted only by trained persons.

Different countries have different exposure limits. The process of standard setting, nomenclature, and applicability would necessarily differ. For example, different approaches were taken in setting standards in the USSR and the United States in the 1970s (Levy 1999). The USSR standards, which were lower than those set in the United States at that time, were maximum allowable concentrations based on an absence of development of any disease or deviation from normal. In contrast, the US approach allowed for minor physiological adaptive changes. In addition, the principle in the USSR was that standards should be based entirely on health and not on technological and economic feasibility. In the United States, economic and technological feasibility were important considerations in the development of the standards.

Another consideration would be to take into account the situation for which the standards were set. For example, standards that are set for an 8-h working day would not be applicable for a 12-h working day. Furthermore, exposure to several hazards simultaneously may occur. In such situations, there may be interactions, with possible synergistic or additive effects. This would then require more stringent control of each individual hazard.

The method of environmental monitoring is also important. The choice of the correct collecting devices, sampling strategy, and analysis of the collected samples in accredited laboratories with proper quality control are important considerations that have to be addressed.

The type of persons exposed should also be considered. These include variations in age, gender, pre-existing disease, genetic make-up, and social habits (e.g. smoking) influence individual susceptibility. Some permissible limits, such as the threshold limit values (TLVs) of the American Conference of Governmental Industrial Hygienists (ACGIH), are derived to protect the majority of, but not all exposed persons. Susceptible individuals may still suffer health effects even at levels below the recommended TLV.

In spite of these limitations, sensible use of environmental standards can often result in practical control of many common workplace hazards so that the majority of workers are protected. Supplementary measures, such as biological monitoring, will ensure a safety net to identify workers with excessive body burdens or who have early health impairments.

The proprietary TLV developed by the ACGIH is one of the best known and widely used of the OELs. The TLVs are updated and published annually. They are derived from information from industrial experience, as well as studies in both animal and human populations. The TLVs of some chemicals, with their accompanying notations, are listed in Table 8.5.3.

Exposure limits for combined exposures

The toxicity of substances of variable composition, for example, welding fumes, is dependent on factors such as the welding process and electrodes used, and the particular alloy that is welded. The TLV given, which is based on total particulate concentration, would be adequate only if no toxic elements are present in the welding rod, metal or its coating, and the welding conditions are not conducive to the formation of toxic gases.

Threshold limit values for chemical mixtures can be computed if components in the mixture have either similar toxic effects or independent toxic effects, using the appropriate correction formulae. Exposures to a combination of factors, such as physical and chemical agents, may result in interaction of these agents, and place added stress on the exposed person. For example, among exposed workers, interactions between physical and psychosocial risk factors can

Table 8.5.3 Threshold limit values of selected agents (ACGIH 2007)

Substance	TWA[a]	STEL/C[b]	TLV basis—critical effects
Acetylene	-	-	Asphyxiation
Acetylene tetrabromide	1 ppm	-	Irritation, liver
Acrylamide	0.03 mg/m³	-	CNS, dermatitis
Asbestos (all forms)	0.1 f/cc	-	Asbestosis, cancer
n-butyl acrylate	2 ppm	-	Irritation, reproductive
Chlorine	0.5 ppm	1 ppm	Irritation
Chloroacetone	-	1 ppm	Irritation
Lead chromate			
as Pb	0.05 mg/m³	-	Cancer, CVS, reproductive
as Cr	0.012 mg/m³	-	
Mercury			
Alkyl compounds	0.01 mg/m³	0.03 mg/m³	CNS
Aryl compounds	0.1 mg/m³	-	CNS, neuropathy, vision, kidney
Inorganic forms, including metallic Hg	0.025 mg/m³	-	CNS, kidney, neuropathy, vision, reproductive, GI
Welding fumes	5 mg/m³	-	Metal fume fever, irritation
Wood dust			
All species except Western red cedar	1 mg/m³	-	Cancer, irritation, mucostasis, dermatitis
Western red cedar	5 mg/m³	10 mg/m³	Irritation, dermatitis, asthma

[a] TWA—time-weighted average

[b] STEL/C—short-term exposure limit ceiling

increase the risk of developing work-related musculoskeletal disorders (Devereux *et al.* 1999).

Managing the risk of work

Prevention of occupational disease can take place at various levels, such as at the national level, or at the level of the workplace itself. The aim is to reduce the occurrence of occupational disease by eliminating the cause or by controlling exposure to safe levels in order to prevent damage to the health of workers. Customarily several levels of prevention are recognized.

Primary prevention aims to reduce the occurrence of disease by eliminating the cause of disease or reducing exposure to safe levels that prevent it from causing damage, for example, banning the use of asbestos or reduction of noise at its source to levels that do not cause noise-induced deafness. Primary prevention with regard to chemicals requires either (i) elimination of toxic materials and their replacement by less hazardous substitutes or (ii) use of tight processes and controls, such as complete enclosure or ventilation at the source of aerosol generation.

Secondary prevention aims to detect situations of early effects of disease before they manifest as clinical symptoms and signs in order to take corrective action, for example, regular monitoring of blood lead (BPb) levels among exposed workers or regular audiograms among noise-exposed workers. Successful secondary prevention depends on the ability to identify work-related illness efficiently and effectively through screening workers at high risk for occupational disease.

Tertiary prevention aims to minimize the consequences in persons who already have disease. This activity is largely a curative and rehabilitative procedure and depends on proper and appropriate treatment. Tertiary prevention depends on the development and wide application of appropriate diagnostic techniques for identification of persons with already established occupational illness.

Prevention on all three levels requires information on the potential effects of specific occupational exposures, as well as data on the industries, occupations, and geographical areas in which hazardous substances are used. The hierarchy of strategies for preventing occupational diseases is as follows:

- A. Primary prevention
  - Elimination of the hazard
  - Substitution with a safer alternative
  - Engineering controls
  - Redesign of the work station or process
  - Administrative controls
  - Education of workers
  - Improved and safer work practice
  - Use of personal protective equipment
  - Personal hygiene
  - Pre-employment or Pre-placement examinations
- B. Secondary prevention
  - Periodic health monitoring
  - Detection of evidence of excessive exposure
    - Biological tests of excessive exposure
    - Biological tests of early effect
- C. Tertiary prevention
  - Planning for emergency response
  - Rehabilitation and return to work
  - Workers compensation

Primary prevention

The most important prevention strategy is the primary prevention of exposure to toxic chemical, physical, biological, or psychosocial hazards. Reductions in exposure can be accomplished by using the techniques listed below, in descending order of preference.

Control of new hazards

Animal toxicity studies of chemicals to be used in industry are a reasonable predictor of potential health hazards to humans. On the basis of such studies, legislation in manufacturing nations would control the usage of such chemicals in industrial processes. One limitation is that such controls apply only to the new chemicals that are to be introduced into the market. For instance, it is estimated that only 10 per cent of pesticides in current usage have undergone such toxicological evaluation (Koh *et al.* 2001).

Control of known hazards

Several countries have legislation to ban the use of substances known to be harmful to human health. The UN has compiled a consolidated list of products whose consumption and sale have been banned, withdrawn, severely restricted, or not approved by governments. This publication constitutes a tool that helps governments keep up-to-date with regulatory decisions taken by other governments and assists them in considering the scope for eventual regulatory action. The United Nations Environment Program (UNEP) in 1989 has evolved a procedural mechanism of Prior Informed Consent (PIC) to inform government of banned agents such that these governments could take appropriate action for their control. By such means, the UN system attempts to prevent importing countries from unknowingly using substances banned in countries for health reasons.

At the national level, there may be rules that regulate the import, storage, sale, and transport of legislated substances through a licensing system, for example, for pesticides. Some substances may be subjected to import controls.

Control of hazards at the workplace

Total elimination of the hazard

This method eliminates the health risk completely, and has been used for substances that are carcinogenic (e.g. asbestos, benzene), or those that can cause serious health effects (e.g. cadmium). In the United Kingdom, the HSE had regulated in the mid-1980s that solder should be substituted with solder low in, or without, cadmium (Mason *et al.* 1999).

Substitution of the hazard

Substitution of the hazard with a less toxic alternative is another feasible option. In the case of processes which use solvents, such as degreasing operations, a less toxic solvent such as 1,1,1 trichloroethane can be used, instead of the more toxic trichloroethylene or tetrachloroethane.

Another method could be the substitution of the hazard to a form that reduces risk of exposure for example changing the particle size or other physical characteristic of a toxic chemical so that it is less easily inhaled or absorbed.

Selection of a less hazardous process or equipment also represents a meaningful control strategy. For example, substitution of a continuous process for an intermittent process almost always results in a decrease of exposure. Where an entire process does not need to be changed to reduce hazards, equipment substitution may achieve the desired reduction in exposure. An example is use of a degreaser with a low-speed hoist in lieu of dipping parts by hand.

Engineering controls

Automation, enclosure, or segregation of a work process, the use of dampeners or mufflers to reduce vibration or noise, reducing the open surface area for the evaporation of volatile toxic agents have been some of the successful engineering control measures used.

Ventilation is one of the most effective and widely used control measures. Control of hazards by ventilation is usually further subdivided into two categories: Local exhaust ventilation and general exhaust ventilation. The approach for implementing ventilation controls is: (1) Conduct an engineering study to evaluate sources of exposure, (2) develop an engineering design, (3) install a system based on the design, and (4) evaluate the completed system to ensure that the air contaminant has been effectively controlled.

Isolation is defined as the interposing of a barrier between a hazard and workers who might be injured or made ill by the hazard. Isolation may refer to storage of materials, such as flammable liquids, enclosure or removal of equipment to another area (such as noisy generators), or isolation of processes or of the workers themselves (e.g. by enclosing a sawmill worker in a sound-proof ventilated booth to protect him from noise and wood dust). The petroleum industry, for example, uses automated remote processing in plants based on centralized computer control of process equipment. Workers are thus largely isolated from hazards except in maintenance operations and during process upsets.

Suppressing the substance by processes such as 'wetting' of dusty operations is another example of an engineering control. Alteration of work practices can help to reduce exposure to hazards. An example is vacuuming cotton lint off spinning machines rather than blowing it off with compressed air, a practice which creates airborne dust particles.

Redesign of the work station or process

Workstation redesign to reduce unnecessary and repetitive bending, or to prevent excessive stretching to the limit of the range of movement of the workers, can minimize ergonomic hazards. Among computer operators, use of adjustable equipment, positioning of the workstation to reduce glare, and appropriate work rest pauses can prevent the development of eyestrain and musculoskeletal complaints.

Administrative controls

Administrative controls may be a viable alternative or an additional measure to reduce worker exposure to occupational hazards. This could take the form of job enlargement or job rotation, restriction of hours of work at a hazardous operation, or temporary job reassignment.

With administrative controls, the level of exposure to the hazard is not diminished; instead, the duration of exposure is reduced and exposure is spread more widely among the work-force. For example, if the air standard for inorganic lead is 50 mg/m^3 based on an 8-h day, a worker could permissibly be exposed to 100 mg/m^3 for 4 h and then rotated to a job without lead exposure as an administrative control. A common use in industry of administrative controls is to reduce overall noise exposure through rotation. Given the typical demands of production and the potential for misuse, administrative methods of controls are not an optimal mode of control.

Education of workers

Training of workers to recognize work hazards, how to work safely, and what to do in the event of an emergency or when occupational diseases occur, is another important aspect of prevention. For example, metalworkers are often exposed to skin contact with coolants and soluble oils. Different workers performing the same job can have variable skin contact with coolants, ranging from almost negligible exposure to almost total constant skin contact with the coolants (Wassenius *et al.* 1998). This variation can be explained by differences in hazard awareness, attitude, and practice of safe working techniques in different workers.

- The 'right to know' concept refers to the mandatory sharing of information regarding workplace exposure to toxic substances between employers and workers, regulatory agencies, and in some cases communities near a workplace. The fundamental assumption in the right-to-know concept is that this transfer of information will prompt activity that will improve worker health. In fact, there have been several instances of workers themselves playing a direct role in the discovery of occupational health problems. Two examples are the discovery of lung cancer in workers exposed to bis(chloromethyl) ether (Figueroa *et al.* 1973) and sterility in workers exposed to dibromochloropropane (Whorton 1977).
- The right of workers to know about potential hazards necessarily implies a corresponding duty on employers to provide that information. Employers' duties can be considered in three ways. First, the duty to generate or retain information means that an employer would be required to perform environmental or medical monitoring and to retain the records pertaining to that monitoring for a specified period of time. This duty is specified under some of the Occupational Safety and Health Administration (OSHA) comprehensive standards, such as those for asbestos and lead. Second, the duty to disclose information on request means that an employer must provide copies of exposure or biological monitoring data to a worker or worker representative if that information is requested. For example, the OSHA Access to Employee Exposure and Medical Records Standard attempts to ensure that exposure, medical, and biological monitoring records are preserved and workers have access to them. Third, the duty to inform refers to an employer's or manufacturer's obligation to disclose information about potential toxic substances in the workplace. Under the OSHA Hazard Communication Standard, employers have a duty to inform workers of the identity of the substances with which they work through labelling the product containers and disclosing the source of supply through the use of Material Safety Data Sheets (MSDSs). The standard also requires that workers must be trained in methods to detect the presence of hazardous chemicals, the hazards of the chemicals, and protective measures.

Use of personal protective devices

The use of personal protective equipment is often widely practised. It has its merits, a major one being its relative inexpense, and is especially useful for situations of short-term or occasional exposure to occupational hazards. Respirators, gloves, protective clothing, ear plugs, and muffs are all common forms of personal protective equipment in use throughout industry. They can play an important role, provided that carefully designed personal protective equipment programmes are in place and the equipment itself is frequently and regularly checked.

Protective devices have to be properly selected to be effective against specific hazards, e.g. the choice of an appropriate glove for use with a particular solvent. Workers have to be trained to use the equipment correctly and to ensure that it is working effectively, such as respirator fit testing in the use of respirators. Worker compliance in the use of these devices has to be high, or its protective effects may be less than desired. Compliance can be an issue, because of discomfort, especially for workers in hot and humid climates. Finally, protective devices have to be properly maintained and replaced when necessary.

It is important to recognize that programmes of personal protection never constitute as efficient a means of protection as engineering or process controls. Personal protective equipment is intended to reduce exposures to toxic substances which have already been dispersed in the workplace as the result of inadequate control at source. Unfortunately, programmes for personal protective equipment, such as respirator programmes, often are ill defined, given inadequate attention, and used in lieu of engineering controls, with poor maintenance of the necessary equipment.

Personal hygiene

Programmes for encouraging personal hygiene constitute another approach to reducing exposure. In some instances, management may require showers and a change to clean clothes at the end of the working day. Several US OSHA standards, such as the occupational lead standard, require management to provide such facilities. A subtle but potentially important route of exposure is ingestion of toxic agents by eating, smoking, or applying cosmetics in the work place. To prevent such exposure, separate eating facilities outside production areas should be provided. Workers should be encouraged to wash their hands before eating or smoking.

Pre-employment or pre-placement examinations

Pre-placement or pre-employment medical examinations are undertaken to achieve proper job placement according to the mental and physical capabilities of the worker, and to prevent damage to susceptible workers. Such tests are also undertaken for other objectives—e.g. to protect other workers and the general public, for insurance purposes, and to obtain baseline information on fitness. Pre-placement examinations should not be used as a means to discriminate workers and deny employment.

Education of workers should be given during these assessments. Those who work have a right to know the potential hazards and risks in their work and workplaces. They should be educated on these matters and be given information on how to safeguard their health. Immunization against diseases that may possibly be contracted on the job, and for which an effective vaccine is available, should also be given. An example is the immunization of health-care personnel exposed to the hepatitis B virus.

There are genetic disorders which can be identified and may make a worker more vulnerable to certain workplace exposures—e.g. people with red cell glucose-6-phosphate dehydrogenase deficiency are at risk for haemolytic anaemia and more susceptible to haemolytic agents. Persons with serum total α1-antitrypsin deficiency may be susceptible to respiratory irritants (Koh & Jeyaratnam 1998).

Similarly, evidence of other behaviours (e.g. smoking, alcohol consumption) and diseases (e.g. chronic bronchitis, liver, kidney disease), may increase the susceptibility of workers exposed to certain toxicants. Biological monitoring of the worker ideally begins at the pre-employment examination stage, as can be continued periodically (see below).

Secondary prevention

Secondary prevention aims to detect situations of early effects of disease before they manifest as clinical symptoms and signs. Upon early detection, corrective action can be taken, such as removal of the worker from further exposure. In most instances, early effects of disease can be reversed if corrective action is promptly taken.

Biological monitoring

Biological monitoring and environmental monitoring complement each other in the assessment of health risk in the exposed worker. It is a useful tool in the prevention and management of ill health among workers (Morgan 1997). One major feature of biological, as compared to environmental, monitoring is that for a particular individual, it takes into account exposure from all routes of absorption. For example, for workplace exposure to organic solvents, skin absorption may be a significant route of entry of the solvent into the body, and ambient environmental air monitoring might be less useful as an indicator of exposure than biological monitoring.

Furthermore, environmental monitoring at the workplace would not account for non-occupational or extra-occupational exposures. A person working in a noisy environment could be additionally exposed to noise in a second job, hobby, or non-occupational activity, e.g. reserve military service.

While some consider any procedure (e.g. periodic X-rays, blood tests, symptom enquiry, etc.) used to monitor exposed workers as biological monitoring, others make a distinction between biological monitoring and effects monitoring.

Biological monitoring

Biological monitoring refers to the measurement and assessment of workplace agents, their metabolites or effects either in tissues, secreta, excreta, expired air, or any combinations of these for the purpose of evaluating exposure and health risk (Meister 2007). The specific chemical, or its breakdown product, can be measured, to detect the total body burden of the substance. The method of measurement of these substances must be validated and there should be a means to interpret the results obtained in terms of the extent of exposure, and risk to health.

Biological effect monitoring

This refers to the measurement and assessment of early biological effects, of which the relationship to health impairment has not yet been established, in exposed workers to evaluate exposure and/or other health risk compared to an appropriate reference.

Some examples of include detection of alterations in enzyme levels (e.g. cholinesterase for workers exposed to organophosphorus or carbamate pesticides), or other biochemical changes such as delta aminolaevulinic acid in urine of workers exposed to inorganic lead, or beta 2 microglobulin in the urine of cadmium exposed workers.

In the early stages, these changes need not necessarily cause any direct pathological damage to the individual, but rather, reflect situations of excessive exposure. These changes are often reversible on removal of the worker from further exposure.

Health effects monitoring (health surveillance)

Health effects monitoring is 'the periodic physiological or clinical examination of exposed workers with the objective of protecting and preventing occupationally related diseases' (Aw 1995). These examinations detect early clinical effects in exposed workers. Examples include audiometry for noise exposed workers, clinical examination for skin lesions in workers exposed to polycyclic aromatic hydrocarbon compounds in tar, pitch, and bitumen, and chest X-rays for workers exposed to pneumoconiosis producing dusts. Figure 8.5.1 illustrates and summarizes the terminology and levels of prevention that are used in occupational health practice.

Biological exposure limit value

The measurement value obtained by biological monitoring is evaluated as a health risk by comparing it with the corresponding biological exposure limit value. A set of values have been developed by the ACGIH, which include results of biological monitoring as well as biological effects monitoring. The Biological Exposure Index (BEI) is described as in general representing the 'levels of determinants which are most likely to be observed in specimens collected from a healthy worker who has been exposed to chemicals in the same extent as a worker with inhalation exposure to the TLV'.

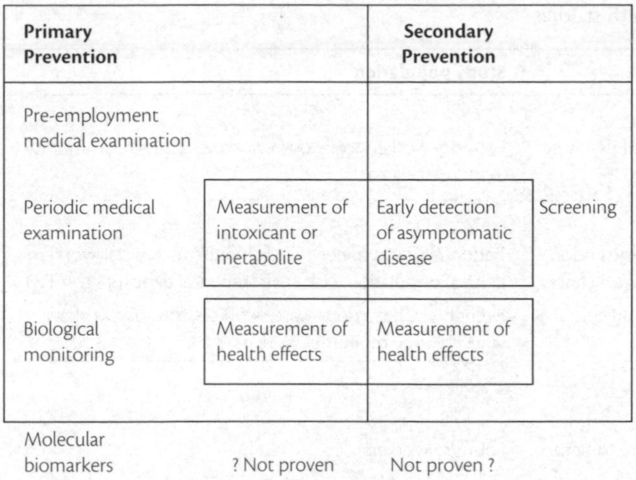

Primary Prevention
Secondary Prevention
Pre-employment medical examination
Periodic medical examination
Measurement of intoxicant or metabolite
Early detection of asymptomatic disease
Screening
Biological monitoring
Measurement of health effects
Measurement of health effects
Molecular biomarkers
? Not proven
Not proven ?

Fig. 8.5.1 Summary of terminology and levels of prevention in occupational disease.

Exceptions would be made for chemicals for which TLVs are based on non-systemic effects, for example, irritation; and for chemicals with significant routes of entry via additional routes of entry (usually percutaneous absorption).

The ACGIH cautions that 'BEIs do not indicate a sharp distinction between hazardous and non-hazardous exposures. Due to biological variability, it is possible for an individual's measurements to exceed the BEI without incurring an increased health risk'. It further states that BEIs are not intended for use as a measure of adverse effect or diagnosis of occupational disease. However, if measurements of the individual or group of workers persistently exceed the BEIs, the cause of the excessive values should be investigated, and measures should be taken to reduce the exposure. Biological exposure indices (as used by ACGIH) for some toxicants are shown in Table 8.5.4.

Technological advances in molecular biology over the last few decades have offered more sophisticated techniques that can be used to study the role of specific exogenous agents and host factors in causing ill-health. These advances have resulted in the development of newer molecular biomarkers of exposure, response, and

Table 8.5.4 Biological exposure indices (BEIs) of some chemical toxicants (ACGIH 2007)

Intoxicant	BEI	Source	Sampling time
Carbon monoxide			
Carboxyhaemoglobin	3.5% of haemoglobin	Blood	End of shift
Carbon monodixe	20 ppm	Exhaled air	End of shift
Cadmium and inorganic compounds	5 μg/g creatinine	Urine	Not critical
	5 μg/L	Blood	Not critical
n-hexane			
2,5 hexanedione	5 μg/g creatinine	Urine	End of shift
Lead	30 μg/100 ml	Blood	Not critical
Mercury (inorganic)	35 μg/g creatinine	Urine	Pre-shift
	15 μg/l	Blood	End of shift/week
Phenol	250 mg/g creatinine	Urine	End of shift

genetic susceptibility. These include measurements for structural gene damage, gene variation, and gene products in cells and body fluids, e.g. oncogenes and tumour suppressor genes, DNA adducts, gene products, and genetic polymorphisms and metabolic phenotypes in environmentally exposed populations (Koh *et al.* 1999).

An understanding of biochemistry and genetics at the molecular level, specific knowledge on metabolism and mechanisms of action, and epidemiology is important. This is necessary in order to address the major question of validation and relevance of these molecular biomarkers. For example, the availability of genetic tests to identify susceptible workers raises issues of ethics, individual privacy, right to work, and the relevance of such tests. Several studies have presented data on the association of environmental measurements and various biomarkers for internal and biologically effective dose, genetic polymorphisms, and early response markers (Table 8.5.5). Given the limitations of individual molecular biomarkers in assessing health risk, and the multifactorial nature of environmental disease, it is likely that a combined approach which examines several of these biomarkers simultaneously will increase our understanding of the complex issue of disease mechanisms and further refine the process of risk assessment.

Periodic medical examinations

Periodic medical examinations may be required for some occupational groups in order to achieve primary, or failing that, secondary prevention of disease. In many countries, certain categories of employees must undergo statutory periodic medical examinations. These examinations are usually for workers exposed to known hazards such as noise, radiation, asbestos, silica, heavy metals, and specific toxic chemicals.

For some countries, only properly qualified health personnel, with additional postgraduate training in occupational health, are empowered to perform the examinations, and issue fitness to work certificates. The results of the examinations have to be kept for a specified period of time, and copies sent to the relevant government body.

The objective of statutory medical examinations is to prevent special groups of 'at risk' workers from developing serious occupational diseases. Regular health examinations, which are specific for the type of hazard the worker is exposed to, are conducted. Workers found to have signs of overexposure to any hazard; or with early signs of disease can be removed from further exposure. They can be given alternative work until they are fit to return to their former jobs. Furthermore, if signs of overexposure are detected, further control measures can be taken to reduce the exposure at source, and prevent other workers from being similarly affected.

Sometimes, special groups of workers are required to undergo periodic medical examinations for other reasons, such as to certify ongoing fitness to work in order to protect the health of the public, e.g. professional drivers and food handlers.

Post illness or injury evaluation

An evaluation of the health status of the employee returning to work after a prolonged absence from work due to illness or injury is important. This is to ensure that the worker has sufficiently recovered from the illness or injury, and is fit to return to work. Two issues to consider would be:

- Can the worker perform his/her duty without adverse health and safety risks to himself/herself or fellow workers?
- Should he/she return to full-time unrestricted duty, or should some modified, restricted or alternative duty be given?

Table 8.5.5 Examples of molecular biomarkers measured in occupational health studies

Molecular biomarkers	Application	Study population
Exposure marker		
PAH–DNA adduct	Workplace and community exposures and exposure to cigarette smoke, and risk of lung cancer	Foundry workers, coke oven workers, general community in industrial areas
Early effect markers		
p53 tumour suppressor gene or its protein product	Specific fingerprint mutation in certain gene codon and risk of liver, breast, lung, and oesophageal cancer	Radon-exposed miners, vinyl chloride monomer workers, general population with environmental exposure to AFB1
H-*ras* and K-*ras* gene or its protein product	Increased risk of various cancers, e.g. lung, liver, and bladder	Firefighters, hazardous waste workers, foundry workers, vinyl chloride monomer workers
Host susceptibility markers		
CYP1A1 polymorphism	Increased risk of lung cancer with exposure to Benzo pyrene	Foundry workers
NAT2 polymorphism	Increased risk of bladder cancer	Workers exposed to arylamine and hydrazine

Notification of occupational diseases

Most countries require the statutory notification of occupational diseases to the government. Notification should be done on the suspicion of occupational disease. The notified case is subsequently investigated and confirmed by the relevant government specialists. Either the employer or health practitioner who sees the worker can notify. In many countries, a list of notifiable occupational diseases is available.

Notification serves as an additional means of control of occupational diseases, undertaken by occupational health and safety professionals in the public sector. It initiates a chain of events, which often includes investigation and confirmation of the index case, and active case finding of other affected persons. Recommendations for specific preventive measures at the workplace are then prescribed. The authorities would follow up by ensuring that the recommendations have been implemented. If necessary, further evaluation of the effectiveness of the preventive measures can be made.

Figure 8.5.2 summarizes the continuum of various means of prevention in occupational health practice.

Tertiary prevention

Tertiary prevention activities are largely curative and rehabilitative procedures. Workers should be removed from further exposure, and the appropriate medical treatment given if indicated. Examples of appropriate treatment include the rendering of first aid promptly after an injury, chelation for severe cases heavy metal overexposure, and hyperbaric treatment for cases of compressed air illness.

Planning for emergency response

Occupational health personnel can also assist in planning for disasters in the workplace and community. In addition to consideration of first aid and acute healthcare, other aspects, such as the fire and emergency response services are essential in dealing with disasters at the workplace and that may spill over to affect the community. Planning and practice drills should be done jointly with the relevant local community agencies.

Rehabilitation

Rehabilitation of workers is another important aspect of occupational healthcare. Management, fellow workers, occupational health professionals, and the injured worker have to work together to ensure that suitable alternative duties are provided, and that any work restrictions or physical limitations are understood. There should be clear short- and long-term goals in rehabilitation, and alternative duties should be meaningful and contribute to production (ACOM and ACRM 1987). Sometimes, the use of external rehabilitation resources may be needed.

Workmen's compensation

In many countries, workers who are injured at work, or fall ill from hazardous work exposures are eligible for compensation. Employers who carry out economic activities through labour and machines create an environment that may be likely to cause ill health in the employees. Thus employers should be liable for payment of compensation to workers if they are injured or fall sick because of the work. Legislation concerning employment injury benefits is often called a *Workmen's Compensation Act*. Employers may be required to insure against their liability under the act.

Workers' compensation is a legal system designed to provide income support, medical payments, and rehabilitation payments to workers injured on the job, as well as to provide benefits to survivors of fatally injured workers. Essentially, all industrialized countries and many others have workers' compensation programmes. In some countries, certain categories of workers, e.g. domestic helpers, may be excluded. Other countries may have social insurance to give protection to employment injury victims. The principle of social insurance is that of sharing of risks and pooling financial resources. A social insurance scheme establishes a public channel through a government department or government supervised body, which oversees procedures of screening, determination of award and payment of benefits.

Benefits are payable for temporary incapacity or permanent incapacity, and survivors' benefits for those killed at work. Guidelines for assessment of disability are available in most countries.

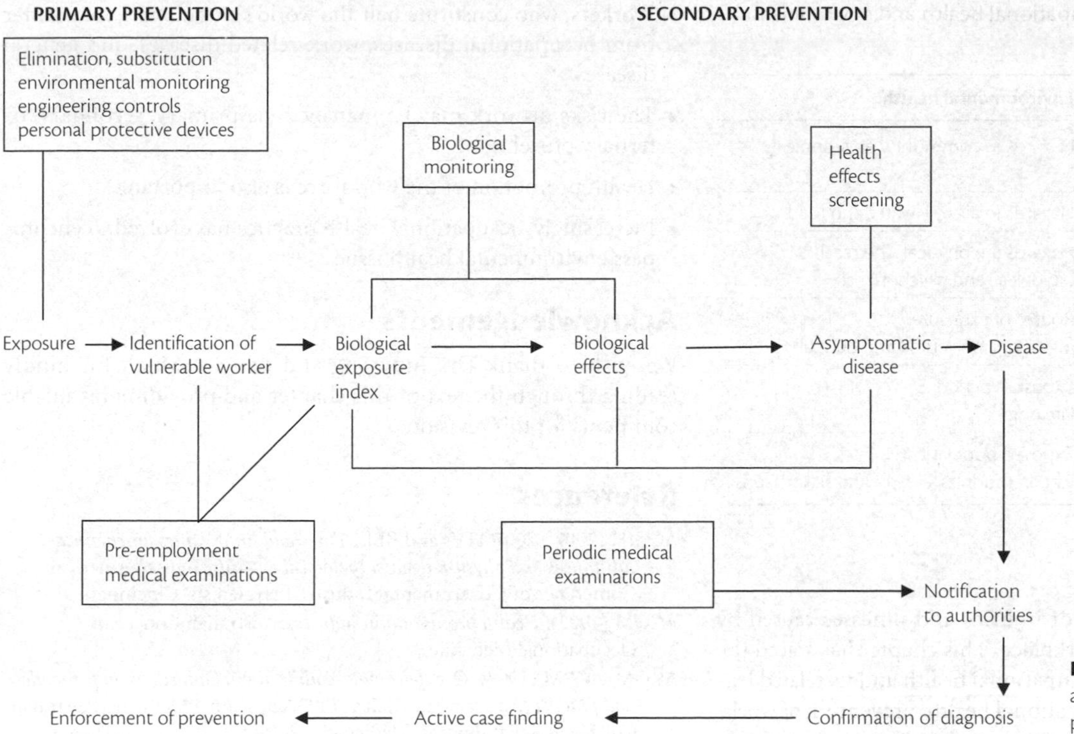

Fig. 8.5.2 Continuum of preventive actions in occupational health practice.

The final assessments for disability are made when the workers' medical condition has stabilized, and not likely to improve or deteriorate further. Besides Workmen's Compensation and social insurance schemes, injured workers can sue their employer through common law and claim benefits. This can be a long process, and the worker has to prove negligence on the part of the employer. In general, workers who have claimed benefits from Workmen's Compensation are not allowed further recourse through this action.

Health promotion at the workplace

Occupational health practitioners have long recognized health promotion to be an integral part of a comprehensive occupational healthcare system (ACOM 1983). However, the definition of what really constitutes 'health promotion' is sometimes unclear, as definitions of health promotion differ consequent to the continual evolution of the basic concept of health.

The WHO defines health promotion in its broadest sense as 'the process of enabling people to increase control over, and to improve their health'. Health promotion is seen as a continuum ranging from the treatment of disease, to the prevention of disease including protection against specific risks, to the promotion of optimal health (WHO 1988).

This definition appears somewhat vague but it does highlight the essence of health promotion. It involves the population as a whole, in the context of their everyday life, rather than focusing on people at risk for specific diseases. Health promotion is the social action dimension of health development, other dimensions being biomedical and technological interventions embodied in public health practice (WHO 1991).

It is a process of activating communities, policy-makers, professionals, and the public for health supportive policies, systems, and ways of living. It is manifested by promoting healthy lifestyles and community action for health, and by creating conditions that make it possible to live a healthy life.

From occupational health to environmental health

The recent growth in interest in environmental health has created a dilemma as to its identity as a speciality in the field of health. The public interest in environmental health was not matched by a well-developed speciality in the health field which could respond to its needs and concerns.

Increasingly, occupational health practice today has evolved to encompass environmental health issues as well. This is because of several reasons. First, many sources of pollution originate from the workplace. Second, in many other instances, the distinction between the work environment, the home environment, and the general environment may not be clearly defined—e.g. in agriculture and small-scale industries, often a clear demarcation does not exist between the workplace and home.

Furthermore, there are several areas of common ground between occupational and environmental health (Jeyaratnam 1994). A comparison of the factors in the work environment influencing the health of the working population (occupational health) and that of the general environment affecting the health of the community (environmental health), is shown in Table 8.5.6. It is evident that there exist several areas of similarity between the work environment and the general environment affecting health.

Occupational health practitioners have the necessary skills in clinical medicine, toxicology, hygiene, epidemiology, and preventive health to position themselves for the management of environmental health concerns.

Table 8.5.6 Comparison of occupational health and environmental health

Occupational health	Environmental health
Hazards in workplace environment	Hazards in community environment
Hazards largely in air	Hazards in air, soil, water, and food
Hazards are physical, chemical, biological, and psychosocial	Hazards are physical, chemical, biological, and psychosocial
Routes of exposure: Inhalation and dermal	Routes of exposure: Ingestion, inhalation, and dermal
Exposure period: 8 h/day for working life	Exposure period: Lifelong
Exposed population: Adults, usually healthy	Exposed population: Children, adults, elderly, and sick persons

Conclusion

Workers suffer a broad range of injuries and illnesses caused by hazards encountered in the workplace. This chapter has traced the history and development of occupational health and its related legislation. In the practice of occupational health, prevention of work-related and occupational disease is a key objective. The priority in prevention of occupational diseases should be to effect primary prevention. When this fails, secondary prevention activities are undertaken to contain damage. However, health protection is not the only occupational health concern. Health promotion in the working population is another important activity. The workplace is an ideal setting for health promotion activities, and appropriate lifestyle interventions can prevent many of the common causes of morbidity in society.

Despite the existence protective legislation in many countries, the burden of injury and illness on workers remains significant. It is essential for medical practitioners and public health programmes to recognize, prevent, and manage work-related injuries and illnesses. There is need for international co-ordination of occupational health protection for workers, given the increasing globalization of the world economy. Several approaches have been proposed to address this issue. For example, there should be harmonization of health, safety, and environmental standards in a way that does not unfairly impose a competitive disadvantage on the newly industrialized nations. Governments and multinational corporations should share the most advanced technologies and resources. Rather than allowing companies to manufacture products banned for use in their own country, governments in developed nations should provide financial incentives for their industries to develop and export safer products and technologies. At a minimum, international systems should be established to ensure complete notification of potential hazards, including labelling the contents of raw materials and products.

Finally, the practice of occupational health today has extended beyond the domain of the workplace, into the general environment. Hence, the term 'occupational and environmental health' might more accurately describe this important aspect of public health.

Key points

- 2.2 million work-related deaths, 270 million occupational accidents, and 170 million work-related illnesses occur annually.
- Workers, who constitute half the world's population, may suffer from occupational diseases, work-related diseases, and general diseases.
- The risks of work may be managed via primary, secondary, or tertiary prevention.
- Health promotion of the workforce is also important.
- Increasingly, occupational health practice has evolved to encompass environmental health issues.

Acknowledgements

We wish to thank Drs Judy Sng and Lee See Muah for kindly reading through the text of this chapter and providing invaluable comments for this revision.

References

ACGIH (2007). 2007 TLVs and BEIs. *Threshold limit values for chemical substances and physical agents. Biological exposure indices*. American Conference of Governmental Industrial Hygienists. Cincinnati.

ACOM (1983). *Health promotion in industry*. Australian College of Occupational Medicine.

ACOM, ACRM (1987). *Occupational rehabilitation. Guidelines on principles and practice*. Australasian College of Occupational Medicine, Australian College of Rehabilitation Medicine.

Armstrong, P. (1998). Transformation in markets and labour. In *Encyclopaedia of occupational health and safety* (ed. J. Stellman), 4th edition, pp. 24.1–24.21. International Labour Office, Geneva.

Aw, T.C. (1995). Biological monitoring. In *Occupational hygiene* (eds. J.M. Harrington and K. Gardiner), 2nd edition, pp. 276–86. Blackwell Science Ltd., Oxford.

Belville, R., Pollack, S.H, Godbold, J.H. *et al.* (1993). Occupational injuries among working adolescents in New York State. *Journal of the American Medical Association*, **269**, 2754–9.

CDC (1999). Progress toward the elimination of tuberculosis—United States, 1998. *Morbidity and Mortality Weekly Report*, **48**, 732–6.

Collegium Ramazzini (2004). *Call for an international ban on asbestos: Statement update*. Eleventh Collegium Ramazzini Statement.

Concha-Barrientos, M., Campbell-Lendrum, D., and Steenland, K. (2004). *Occupational Noise: Assessing the burden of disease from work-related hearing impairment at national and local levels*. (WHO Environmental Burden of Disease Series, No. 9). World Health Organisation, Geneva.

Creech, J.L. Jr. and Johnson, M.N. (1974). Angiosarcoma of liver in the manufacture of polyvinyl chloride. *Journal of Occupational Medicine*, **16**, 150–1.

Devereux, J.J., Buckle, P.W., and Vlachonikolis, I.G. (1999). Interactions between physical and psychosocial risk factors at work increase the risk of back disorders: an epidemiological approach. *Occupational and Environmental Medicine*, **56**, 343–53.

European Communities (2004). *Work and health in the EU: A statistical portrait*. European Communities, Luxembourg.

Figueroa, W.G., Raszkowski, R., and Weiss, W. (1973). Lung cancer of chloromethyl methyl ether workers. *New England Journal of Medicine*, **228**, 1096–7.

Forsmann, S. (1983). Occupational health. In *Encyclopaedia of occupational health and safety* (ed. L. Parmeggiani) Vol. 2., 3rd edition, pp. 1491–3.

Goldman, R.H., Rosenwasser, S., Armstrong, E. (1999). Incorporating an environmental/ occupational medicine theme into the medical school curriculum. *Journal of Occupational and Environmental Medicine*, **41**, 47–52.

Holmes, S.M. (2006). An ethnographic study of the social context of migrant health in the United States. *PLoS Medicine*, **3**(10), e448. DOI:10.1371/journal.pmed.0030448.

HSE (1995). *Generic terms and concepts in the assessment and regulation of industrial risks. Health and Safety Executive.* HMSO. London.

HSE (2004). *Interim update of the "Costs to Britain of Workplace Accidents and Work-related Ill Health". Economic advisers unit. Health and Safety Executive.* HMSO. London.

HSE (2006). *Health and safety statistics 2005/06. Health and Safety Executive.* London.

IARC (1997). *Working group on the evaluation of carcinogenic risks to humans: Silica, some silicates, and coal dust and para-aramid fibrils.* International Agency for Research on Cancer, Lyon, France.

ILO (2002). *Press release: Work related fatalities reach 2 million annually. ILO Reference no. ILO/02/23.* International Labour Organisation, Geneva.

ILO (2005). *World day for safety and health at work 2005: A Background Paper.* International Labour Office, Geneva.

ILO (2006a). *The end of child labour: Within reach. Global report under the follow-up to the ILO Declaration on fundamental principles and rights at work.* International Labour Organisation, Geneva.

ILO (2006b). *Press release: ILO welcomes new UN Convention on rights of people with disabilities. ILO Reference no. ILO/06/58.* International Labour Organisation, Geneva.

ILO (2007a). *Equality at work: Tackling the challenges. Global report under the follow-up to the ILO Declaration on fundamental principles and rights at work.* International Labour Organisation, Geneva.

ILO (2007b). *Working time around the world. Press release on 7th June 2007. ILO reference no. ILO/07/29.* International Labour Organisation, Geneva.

Institute of Medicine (1988). *Role of the primary care physician in occupational and environmental medicine.* National Academy Press, Washington, DC.

IPEC (1999). *IPEC action against child labour – achievements, lessons learned and indications for the future (1998-1999).* International Labour Office, Geneva.

Jeyaratnam, J. (1994). Editorial: Occupational and environmental health. *Journal of Occupational Medicine (S'pore)*, **6**, 1–2.

Jeyaratnam, J. (1998). Occupational health trends in development. In *Encyclopaedia of occupational health and safety* (ed. J. Stellman), 4th edition, pp. 20.1–20.28. International Labour Office, Geneva.

Koh, D. and Jeyaratnam, J. (1998). Biomarkers, screening and ethics. *Occupational Medicine*, **48**, 27–30.

Koh, D., Seow, A., and Ong, C.N.(1999). New techniques in molecular epidemiology and their relevance to occupational medicine. *Occupational and Environmental Medicine*, **56**, 725–9.

Koh, D., Chia, K.S., and Jeyaratnam, J. (eds.) (2001). *Textbook of occupational medicine practice*. 2nd edition. World Scientific, Singapore.

Koh, D., Lim, M.K., and Chia, S.E. (2003). SARS: Health care work can be hazardous to health. *Occupational Medicine (London)*, **53**(4), 241–3.

LaDou, J. (2007). The practice of occupational medicine. In *Current occupational and environmental medicine* (ed. J. LaDou), 4th edition, pp. 1–6. McGraw-Hill.

Lawson, C.C., Schnorr, T.M., Daston, G.P. *et al.* (2003). An occupational reproductive research agenda for the third millennium. *Environmental Health Perspectives*, **111**(4), 584–92.

Leigh, J.P., Markowitz, S.B., Fahs, M. *et al.* (1997). Occupational injury and illness in the United States. *Archives of Internal Medicine*, **157**, 1557–68.

Levy, L.S. (1999). Standard setting in occupational health. In *Occupational health risk assessment and management* (eds. S. Sadhra and K.G. Rampal), pp. 118–28. Blackwell Science Ltd. Oxford.

Loewenson, R.H. (1999). Women's occupational health in globalization and development. *American Journal of Industrial Medicine*, **36**, 34–42.

Masoli, M., Fabian, D., Holt, S. *et al.* (2004). Global burden of asthma. Global initiative for asthma (GINA).

Mason, H.J., Williams, N., Armitage, S. *et al.* (1999). Follow up of workers previously exposed to silver solder containing cadmium. *Occupational and Environmental Medicine*, **56**, 553–8.

McKay, S., Craw, M., and Chopra, D. (2006). *Migrant workers in England and Wales: an assessment of migrant worker health and safety risks.* Health & Safety Executive (HSE Books), Suffolk, England. (www.hsebooks.co.uk)

Meister, R.K. and Zheng, Y. (2007). Biologic Monitoring. In *Current occupational and environmental medicine* (ed. J. LaDou), 4th edition, pp. 629–40. McGraw-Hill.

Menzies, H. (1998) Globalizing technologies and the decimation / transformation of work. In *Encyclopaedia of occupational health and safety*(ed. J. Stellman), 4th edition, pp. 24.1–24.21. International Labour Office, Geneva.

Messing, K. (2006). *Gender equality, work and health: A review of the evidence.* World Health Organisation, Geneva.

Morgan, M.S. (1997). The biological exposure indices: A key component in protecting workers from toxic chemicals. *Environmental Health Perspectives*, **105**(Suppl 1), 105–15.

Mustard, F. (1997). The economy and social equity in a period of major technoeconomic change. *Scandinavian Journal of Work, Environment and Health*, **23**(Supp 4), 10–15.

Nelson, DI., Concha-Barrientos, M., Driscoll-T. *et al.* (2005). The global burden of selected occupational diseases and injury risks: Methodology and summary. *American Journal of Industrial Medicine*, **48**(6), 400–18.

NIOSH (1996). *National occupational research agenda update. (DHHS (NIOSH) Publication No. 96-115).* National Institute for Occupational Safety and Health, Cincinnati.

NIOSH (1999). *Stress at work. DHSS (NIOSH) Publication No. 99-101.* National Institute for Occupational Safety and Health, Cincinnati.

NIOSH (2004). *Worker health chartbook 2004. (NIOSH Publication No. 2004-146).* National Institute for Occupational Safety and Health, Cincinnati.

NIOSH (2005). *A Compendium of NIOSH economic research: 2002-2003. (NIOSH Publication No. 2005-112).* National Institute for Occupational Safety and Health, Cincinnati.

NIOSH (2006). *Silicosis - Working with cement roofing tiles: A silica hazard. (NIOSH Publication No. 2006-110).* National Institute for Occupational Safety and Health, Cincinnati.

NIOSH (2007). *NORA (National Occupational Research Agenda): Disease and injury. NORA priority reseach areas.* National Institute for Occupational Safety and Health, Cincinnati. Available at: http://www.cdc.gov/niosh/docs/96-115/diseas.html

Paltiel, F. (1998). Shifting paradigms and policies. In *Encyclopaedia of occupational health and safety* (ed. J. Stellman), 4th edition, pp. 24.1–24.21. International Labour Office, Geneva.

Pearce, N., Boffetta, P., and Kogevinas, M. (1998). Cancer – introduction. In *Encyclopaedia of occupational health and safety* (ed. J. Stellman), 4th edition, pp. 2.1–2.18. International Labour Office, Geneva.

Peto, J., Decarli, A., La Vecchia, C. *et al.*(1999). The European mesothelioma epidemic. *British Journal of Cancer*, **79**, 666–72.

Rantanen, J. (2000). *Impact of Globalisation on Occupational Health. Keynote Address. 26th International Congress on Occupational Health. 27 Aug-1 Sep 2000.* Singapore. Book of Keynote Addresses, pp. 3–16.

Rosenstock, L., Cullen, M.R., and Fingerhut, M. (2005). Advancing worker health and safety in the developing world. *Journal of Occupational and Environmental Medicine*, **47**, 132–6.

Sadhra, S. and Rampal, K.S. (eds.) (1999). *Occupational health. Risk assessment and management.* Blackwell Science Ltd., Oxford.

Schnall, P.L., Belkic, K., Landsbergis, P. *et al.* (eds.) (2000). The workplace and cardiovascular disease. *Occupational Medicine: State of the Art Reviews*, **15**, 1–334.

Schultsz, C., Vo C.D., Nguyen, V.V.C. *et al.* (2005). Avian influenza H5N1 and healthcare workers [letter]. *Emerging Infectious Diseases*. Available from http://www.cdc.gov/ncidod/EID/vol11no07/05-0070.htm

Selikoff, I.J., Churg, J., Hammond, E.C. (1964). Asbestos exposure and neoplasia. *Journal of the American Medical Association*, **188**, 22.

Stellman, J. (1999). Women workers: The social construction of a special population. *Occupational Medicine: State of the Art Review*, **14**, 559–80.

United Nations (1990). *Convention on the protection of the rights of all migrant workers and members of their families.* Ratified 1 July 2003. (www.ohchr.org/english/law/cmw.htm)

Warshaw, L. (1998). Precarious employment and child labour. In *Encyclopaedia of occupational health and safety* (ed. J. Stellman), 4th edition, pp. 24.1–24.21. International Labour Office, Geneva.

Wassenius, O., Jarvholm, B., Engstrom, T. *et al.* (1998). Variability in the skin exposure of machine operators exposed to cutting fluids. *Scandinavian journal of work, environment & health*, **24**, 125–9.

WHO (1988). *Health promotion for working populations.* Technical Report Series 765. Geneva.

WHO (1991). *Action for public health. Health promotion in developing countries.* WHO/HED/91.1.

WHO (2003). *Work organization and stress. Protecting workers health series No.3.* World Health Organization, Geneva.

WHO (2005). *Number of work-related accidents and illnesses continues to increase.* Joint news release by World Health Organisation and International Labour Organisation, Geneva.

WHO (2007a). *Workers' health: Draft global action plan. Sixtieth world health assembly, provisional agenda item 12.13.* World Health Organization, Geneva.

WHO (2007b). *Avian influenza, including influenza A (H5N1), in humans: WHO interim infection control guideline for health care facilities.* World Health Organisation, Geneva.

Whorton, D., Krauss, R.M., Marshall, S. *et al.* (1977). Infertility in male pesticide workers. *Lancet*, **2** (8051), 1259–61.

Windham, G.C. and Osorio A.M. (2007). Female reproductive toxicology, male reproductive toxicology. In *Current occupational and environmental medicine*, (ed. J. LaDou), 4th edition, pp. 384–412. McGraw-Hill.

8.6

Ergonomics and public health

Laura Punnett

Abstract

Ergonomics is the application of scientific knowledge about human physical and psychological capacities and limitations to the design of products, systems, and environments for comfort, safety, and ease of use. Ergonomic principles can—and should—be applied to the workplace, transportation vehicles and throughways, consumer products, and complex systems ranging from healthcare delivery to nuclear power plants to international aviation. Tools and other items for use at work and at home should be designed to fit the full range of the population in body size, strength, and aerobic capacity. Task and system design should further take account of human requirements in sensory perception (vision, hearing, and touch), cognition and memory, and psychosocial environment. All human characteristics display variability from person to person that is only partly explained by gender, age, ethnicity, and training or experience.

Occupational ergonomics receives special attention in many countries because of the risk of musculoskeletal disorders, such as back pain and tendonitis, associated with job demands such as heavy lifting, repetitive motions, and vibration exposure. Work stations, equipment (operating controls and display devices), and tools can accommodate the human body so that they are easy to use without error, fatigue, or injury. Jobs that permit variations in motion patterns and work routines, offer sufficient rest and recovery, encourage learning and using new skills, and facilitate rather than impede positive interactions among co-workers will promote both physical and mental health. The physical environment should be optimized in terms of temperature, lighting, and background noise to achieve workplace safety, optimized physiological endurance, and mental concentration. Work schedules other than a standard 40-h, 5-day work week are increasingly common in the global 24/7 economy. The health consequences include sleep disruption, digestive disorders, loss of mental concentration and risk of injury, and elevated risk of obesity and heart disease. Flexibility in selecting one's own work schedule mitigates some of these hazards, but overtime work is often not voluntary and economic competition pressures many professionals to maintain electronic communication with the workplace even during supposed leisure time. In fact, productivity suffers when individuals do not have sufficient recovery time; more broadly, the application of ergonomics principles to the workplace often—but not always—improves efficiency and reduces costs, both directly and as a result of improved employee health. Developing countries tend to have fewer resources for occupational health and safety in general, including for risk analysis, standard-setting, and enforcement. However, ergonomics measures are not always expensive and can promote both worker protection and enhanced productivity and sustainability of the national enterprise.

Overview

Definition

Ergonomics is an applied, multi-disciplinary scientific field concerned with the design of jobs, products, systems, and environments to be compatible with human needs, abilities, and limitations. A work process, device, or complex system that is badly designed, or not designed at all, may lead to injury, illness, discomfort, fatigue, frustration, and/or boredom for the user. According to the International Ergonomics Association (2000), ergonomics (or human factors) is 'concerned with the understanding of interactions among humans and other elements of a system, and [is] the profession that applies theory, principles, data and methods to design in order to optimize human well-being and overall system performance'. The ergonomist's design goals may simultaneously encompass multiple characteristics of a tool or process, such that it should be easy and satisfying to use; not fatiguing or injurious; promoting user learning rather than error; and promoting work quality and productivity. Thus the contributing research fields range from kinesiology to psychology to engineering to epidemiology.

Brief history

The earliest tools were made by their own users and thus were likely designed to fit the user's characteristics as closely as possible within the constraints of the technology of that time. In contrast, modern equipment is typically manufactured in large batches rather than for a designated individual and all too often is designed on a one-size-(does not)-fit-all template. Some of the health consequences of excessive physical load and highly repetitive motions were recognized nearly three centuries ago, in the work of Dr. Bernardino Ramazzini (1713). In modern times, the professional field was defined in 1949 with the establishment of the Ergonomics Society in the United Kingdom (Murrell 1965). Ergonomics research had begun as early as 1915 in this country with the establishment of the Industrial Fatigue Research Board. Fatigue was to be prevented through proper allocation of rest breaks and suitable working hours, and thus improved efficiency of production would be achieved. During the First World War, the productivity of the British ammunition factories was shown to increase in parallel with a reduction of weekly working hours (Vernon 1921). The practice of measuring the range of body sizes in a population originated even earlier, in the field of physical anthropology; early uses of such data included military forces' determination of the appropriate size of equipment, from boots to aeroplane cockpits.

Thus the first modern applications of ergonomics were in the defence industry, both in the United Kingdom and in the United States. One important impetus to further development was the nature of the problems encountered during the Second World War with technological change, such as the introduction of new weapons. Some new systems were found to perform poorly because of a mismatch between humans and technology. Previously attempts had been made to fit humans to new technology by means of training and information, but neither one could be used to their full capacity with this approach. When knowledge of human capabilities was employed in system design, efficiency and accuracy were vastly improved.

From productivity and safety in military systems, the focus of research and applications in ergonomics has broadened considerably over the years. After the Second World War, the concepts of ergonomics were applied to manufacturing and physically strenuous jobs in other sectors, such as mining and forestry. High aerobic demands and heavy manual handling characterized these jobs, and problems with general fatigue, accidents, and low back pain were widespread.

In modern manufacturing, many such tasks have been mechanized; work reorganization and the use of new technology have reduced aerobic demands in traditionally 'heavy work'. However, these changes have also resulted in increased prevalence of static body positions and repetitive movements, with an accompanying pattern of musculoskeletal problems affecting the neck, shoulder, arm, and hand. Similar problems are encountered in the office environment, especially among people performing data entry work (Punnett & Bergqvist 1997). Meanwhile, a substantial minority of the global working population still performs physically strenuous jobs, even in developed countries, especially in mining, agriculture, transportation, and construction, and so-called service jobs in health care, food preparation, and cleaning. In the developing world, of course, lower levels of capitalization mean an even higher physical workload. While the first four 'heavy' sectors are typically male-dominated and recognized as hazardous, service jobs such as in healthcare or hospitality tend to employ more women and are often perceived as clean and safe, even when they require high physical capacity in a psychologically adverse work climate.

Since the 1970s, issues such as human–computer interaction and health consequences of poor ergonomics, especially in the occupational setting, have grown in importance. Much more attention is given now than previously to work organization issues ('macroergonomics') and prevention of technological system failure, as well as techniques for implementing ergonomic improvements through worker participatory processes.

In the present day the advantages of good ergonomics can be seen in occupational settings, in public life, and in homes. Reduction of heavy lifting and handling of objects through lifting devices, the introduction of ergonomically designed office furniture and computer keyboards and pointing devices, and the improved design of transportation systems are examples that bear witness to these advances. Much remains to be done, however, to ensure safe, healthy, and productive workplaces, homes, and public spaces.

The 'human–machine' system

The central paradigm in ergonomics is the interaction of the person with the work environment, or the 'human–machine–environment system' (Fig. 8.6.1). In this system, the 'machine' presents information to the person, often via one or more displays; the information is perceived by the operator's sensory apparatus (e.g. vision or hearing); the operator uses his or her cognitive capacity and memory to decide on a suitable response, which is transferred to the 'machine' as a motor activity, such as pushing buttons or handling objects. The machine's response involves additional information to the operator, and so on (Kroemer and Grandjean 1997, Chapter 3).

Of course, people at work interact not only with devices but also with the physical and social environment, including with other people. Thus the system may also respond through speech, signs (sign interpretation), or touch; alternatively there may be other responses or input from society via road traffic signs, books, or other means. The operator's response can then be any form of motor activity, like talking, writing, steering a car, or typing on a keyboard, or mental activity.

A key feature of the human–machine concept is that humans perform their actions as part of a system that is in dynamic equilibrium. The aim of the system is to perform efficiently and without mishap, which requires an optimization of the interface between the person and the 'machine' (now a metaphor for any other component of the system). Thus feedback or information must be presented in a way that can be perceived easily and without mistakes, and physical controls must be designed to comply with the person's strength, body dimensions, and natural range of motion. The environment should be conducive to task performance, with attention to temperature, background noise, and psychosocial conditions. Efficiency also implies an optimal allocation of tasks between humans and 'machines', so that each component of the system performs the task for which he/she/it is best suited (Oborne *et al.* 1993; Mital *et al.* 1994). For example, humans are usually superior to machines in recognition of subtle patterns, decision-making requiring experience, and creativity, while machines are often superior in activities that require high force, both precision and endurance, or high consistency in repeating an action.

This system has traditionally been presented as a closed loop, where deviations from the desired 'state' of the system are corrected. Humans or operators were seen as elements of the system whose task is to respond to the feedback from the 'machine'. The quality of the response depends, of course, on their individual physiological, anatomical, sensory, and cognitive capacity. In a complex system with high demands on safety, like a nuclear power plant or chemical process industry, it is crucial that the operator does not deviate from the desired response to an anticipated situation. Nevertheless, in modern ergonomics it is acknowledged that the individual has a more central role. This 'person-centred' philosophy sees the operator as the one who initiates action, controls, and dominates the system. The human being contributes an ability to anticipate and predict what may happen within the system (Oborne *et al.* 1993), as well as his or her own concepts of the purpose of the system, which may build upon and improve the original design goals (Karasek & Theorell 1990). Training of the power plant or

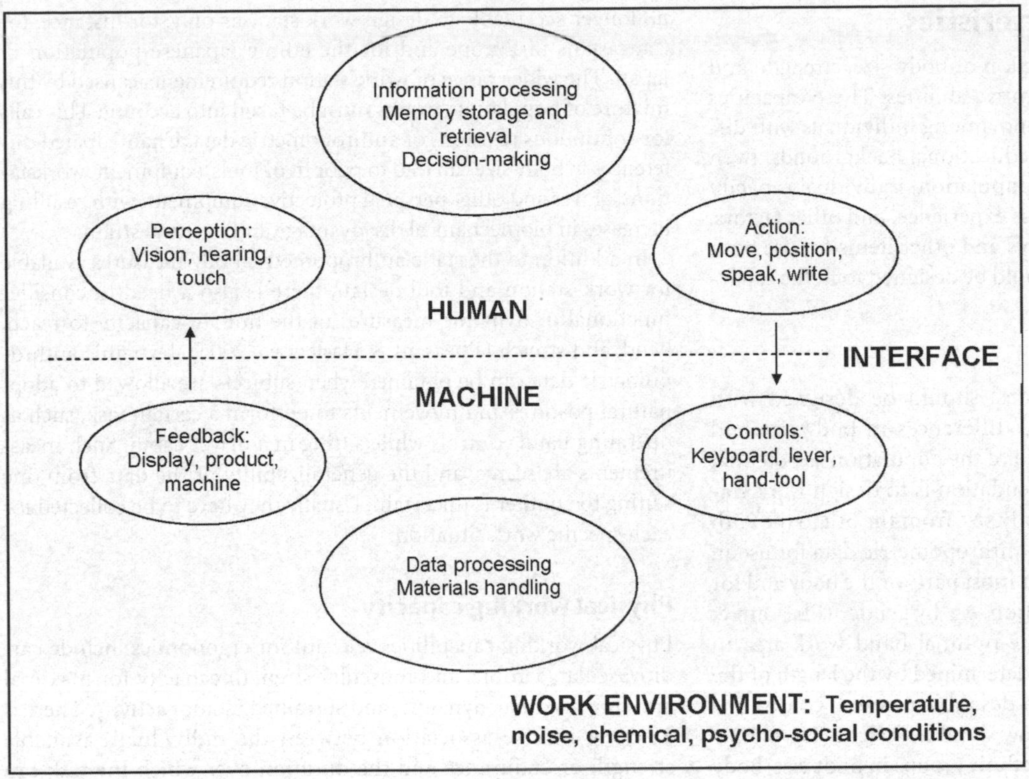

Fig. 8.6.1 The human–machine–environment system.

chemical process operator need not only teach automatic responses to a variety of 'standard' situations but instead may seek to enhance critical thinking and problem-solving skills, while design of the process displays and controls should take account of the operators' knowledge, expectations, and needed information.

Ergonomics as an applied, interdisciplinary field

One important characteristic of ergonomics is that it is both a scientific area of research and a practical area of application. Another is that ergonomics is multi-disciplinary and requires knowledge in at least three main areas: Anatomy and physiology; psychology; and technology. Although it is impossible to have extensive knowledge in all these fields, the ergonomist must be able to integrate knowledge from areas other than that of his or her own basic training. In large ergonomic problem-solving projects, a teamwork approach, with representatives of several disciplines with a common ergonomics perspective, is often most successful.

There are some differences in professional focus in different parts of the world. The psychological aspects of ergonomics, especially cognitive and sensory perception issues, often referred to as 'human factors', dominated research in the United States for many years, and many US practitioners have a background in engineering rather than in health sciences. Manufacturing systems and consumer issues have received much attention in research from the United Kingdom and Japan. Work physiology has dominated research in the rest of Europe, especially in the Nordic countries, while Francophone ergonomists put more emphasis on the worker's integrated, subjective experience. These varying emphases reflect differences in scientific traditions, industrial structures, and types of legislation related to occupational injuries and illness.

In research, some basic questions have to be tackled separately by psychologists, physiologists, and engineers. However, most ergonomic research is applied to field settings, whether for occupational or consumer problems, and therefore requires a truly multi-disciplinary approach. Dialogue among the disciplines is essential to establish common frames of reference. Joint training in ergonomics, where students with varying backgrounds can meet, develop a common outlook, and learn to appreciate the contributions of each other, is key to strengthening multi-disciplinary research and problem-solving skills.

The future of ergonomics

In a short period of time, ergonomics has grown to become an important area of scientific research and practical applications. This is especially true for working life, but special ergonomic applications for consumers, for people with physical or mental disabilities and older people, for leisure and sports, and for developing countries are also emerging. Thus ergonomics, through its effects on health, safety, and well-being, has a large impact on public health.

The International Ergonomics Association, which was formed by a number of national societies, has issued minimum requirements for training and practical experience in ergonomics, to be fulfilled by those researchers, consultants, and others who wish to be approved as 'European Ergonomists'. Similar requirements have been developed for the United Kingdom, the United States, and Australia. Professional qualifications like these are likely to raise the quality of ergonomics work still further, although still there are geographical and professional differences regarding the areas of expertise considered most important.

Relevant human characteristics

Human capacity for work is a function of body size, strength, and fitness, and sensory as well as cognitive abilities. These capacities vary by age, between the genders, and among individuals with different hereditary, nutritional, and educational backgrounds. Even within a specific subgroup of the population, individual capacity varies with health, training, previous experience, and other factors. Therefore work tasks, as well as tools and other items for use both in occupational and private life, should be designed to fit the capacities of a wide range of people.

Anthropometry

Work stations, tools, and machines, should be designed with enough adjustability to individual differences in body size and shape in order to include virtually all of the population as potential users. The most common recommendation is to design work stations and tools to fit the range in body size from the 5th to the 95th percentile of the adult population. Anthropometric data for use in work-station design are available for most parts of the body and for some specific subsets of the population, e.g. by gender (Pheasant & Haslegrave 2005). For example, the optimal hand work area in front of a person is rather small, as determined by the length of the arm segments in combination with desirable postural constraints such as keeping the upper arms below shoulder height (Fig. 8.6.2).

There are large variations among ethnic groups in body size, body proportions, and limb length as a proportion of body height. With the increased mobility of population groups around the world, it is no longer acceptable to design work stations only, for instance, for Caucasians in Europe and for the ethnic Japanese population in Japan. The wider range of work-station requirements caused by this mixture of population groups must be taken into account. This calls for continuous revisions of anthropometric data. Unanticipated differences in body size can lead to poor fit of tools, equipment, workstations, gloves and other personal protective equipment, with resulting increases in biomechanical disadvantage and postural strain.

In addition to the static anthropometric body measures available for work-station and tool design, there is also a need to consider functional or dynamic measures of the human capacity to reach, bend, and stretch (Pheasant & Haslegrave 2005). Dynamic anthropometric data can be obtained when subjects are allowed to adopt natural postures and movements to perform a certain task, such as operating hand controls while sitting in a driver cabin. Such measurements are scarce, and the generalizability of the data from one setting to another is uncertain. Usually they have to be collected for each specific work situation.

Physical working capacity

Physical working capabilities relevant for ergonomics include cardiovascular, aerobic, and muscular strength capacity for maximal and sub-maximal, dynamic, and sustained (static) activity. There is a strong inverse association between the individual's available strength or endurance and the duration over which the task can be sustained without fatigue. Human physical capacity is seldom taxed up to 100 per cent, except for all-out life-saving operations.

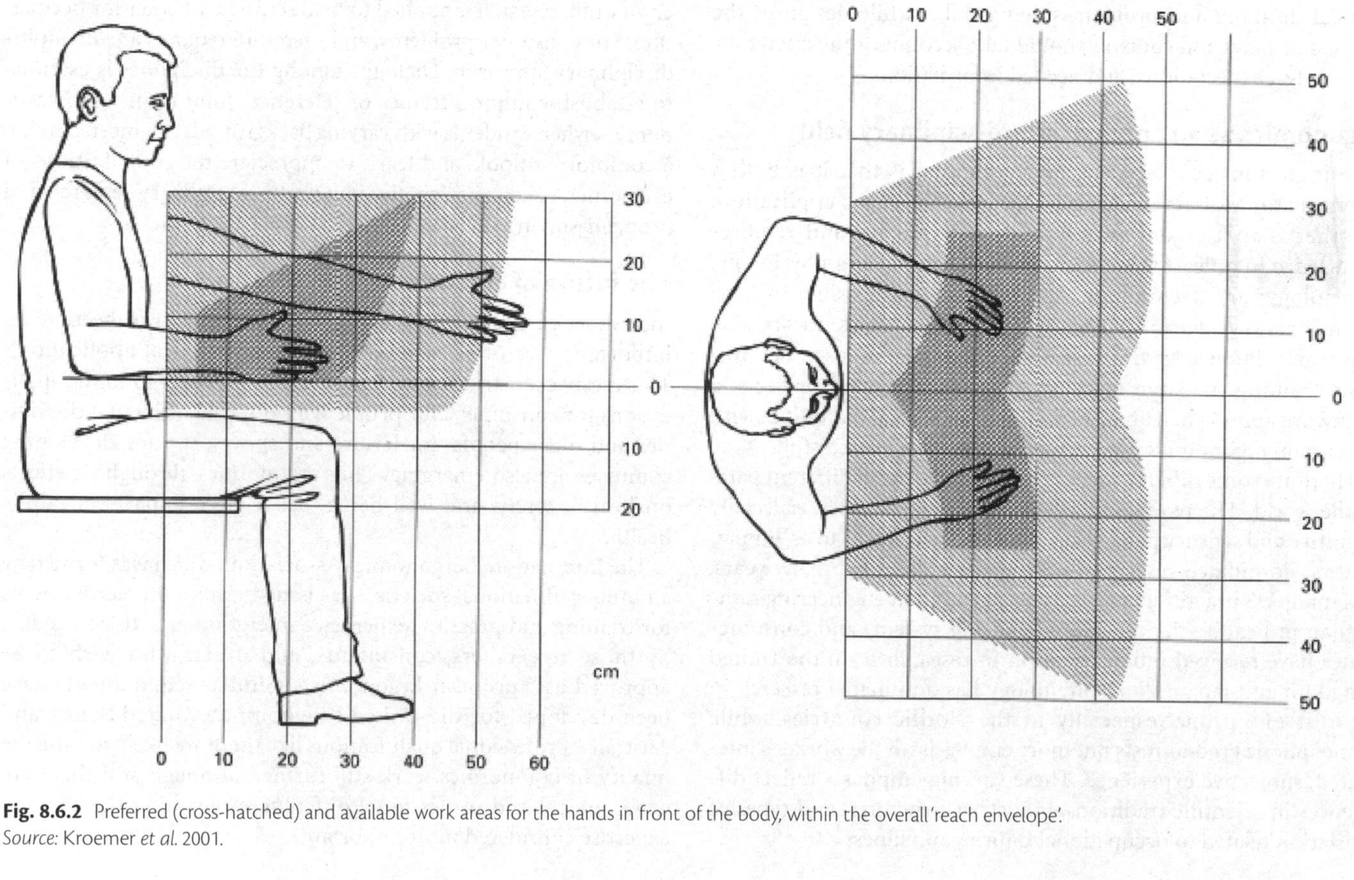

Fig. 8.6.2 Preferred (cross-hatched) and available work areas for the hands in front of the body, within the overall 'reach envelope'.
Source: Kroemer *et al.* 2001.

More commonly, we use from a few per cent of capacity up to as much as 50 per cent in physically demanding jobs.

Most physical capacities demonstrate a peak at around age 20–30 years and a gradual decline by about 30 per cent at least to the age of 60 (Åstrand *et al.* 2003). Women usually have on average a 30 per cent lower maximal aerobic power (expressed in litres of oxygen uptake per minute) than men, and about 30–50 per cent lower maximal muscle strength. However, at a given level of relative sub-maximal exertion, there is no gender difference. The ratio in static strength ranges from 35 to 85 per cent, depending on the tasks and muscles involved (Chaffin *et al.* 2006, Chapter 6); it is smaller when men and women have similar industrial experience or athletic training (Messing & Stevenson 1996). There are large inter-individual differences in capacity, related to factors such as heredity, physical training, and health status. In all, gender, age, weight, and height together explain only about one-third of the variability in human strength.

Overall, the occupationally active population demonstrates higher capacities then the general population, since the latter includes those too ill or otherwise impaired to work. There are also differences between occupational groups, with higher values often found in those who perform physically demanding tasks (Åstrand *et al.* 2003). This difference appears to be caused mainly by selection, since physically demanding jobs do not usually contain work tasks strenuous enough to introduce a training effect (Torgén *et al.* 1999). Moreover, differences between occupations are most obvious in young age groups. In some (but not all) studies, muscle strength shows a larger decrease with age in blue collar than white collar workers, which may be attributable to a combination of musculoskeletal trauma and 'wear and tear' among those performing physically heavy work (Era *et al.* 1992).

Physically fit workers exhibit higher productivity and less fatigue in strenuous jobs than less fit workers (Åstrand 1967b). However, among women performing electronics assembly work, there was no evidence that low muscle strength predicted upper extremity musculoskeletal disorders (MSDs) (Jonsson *et al.* 1988). Other studies have been similarly inconclusive as to whether or not muscle strength is protective against back or other musculoskeletal disorders, and some have even shown higher muscle force capacity to be a risk factor, rather than protective (Barnekow-Bergkvist *et al.* 1998; Keyserling *et al.* 1980; Kujala *et al.* 1996; Leino *et al.* 1987; Malchaire *et al.* 2001; Mikkelsson *et al.* 2006). Stronger muscles are capable of generating higher internal forces, but they do not necessarily produce greater mechanical resistance in vulnerable soft tissues such as nerves and spinal discs. Therefore, pre-employment strength testing cannot be recommended on a scientific basis as a way to select workers unlikely to develop musculoskeletal disorders. Among people in jobs with substantial exposure to ergonomic stressors, individual factors like muscle strength or flexibility appear to be of less importance for the risk of developing MSDs (Hagberg *et al.* 1995).

Neuromuscular function in precision tasks and the effect of motor control and skill training are areas of rapidly developing research, and it may develop in the future that these capacities are also relevant to the risk of musculoskeletal disorders.

Sensory perception

Vision, hearing, and touch are all-important factors in our perception of the environment and thus our ability to respond appropriately to cues from machines, displays, warning signs, and information received from other sources, including people. Taste and smell are less important for ergonomics but may be life-saving in toxic environments.

The critical aspect of vision for most perceptual needs is the ability to focus the eye, through contraction of the ocular muscles (accommodation), in order to see objects of varying sizes at distances ranging from very near to very far away. Visual acuity is also affected by the level of illumination, the contrast between the object and its background, and the time available for viewing (Kroemer & Grandjean 1997).

With the evolution of electronic devices offering more and more complex displays, the design of visual information presentation is no longer as simple as ensuring adequate size and contrast. Concurrently, advances in neuroscience have permitted new questions to be addressed in the growing field of 'visual cognition', such as how we recognize and remember faces or three-dimensional moving objects and how visual images compete successfully for our attention.

At the same time, the sensory input from vision should not be overemphasized, in that sound or touch stimuli might sometimes fill the same purpose. Ergonomics for handicapped individuals has many examples of successful switches from vision to hearing (e.g. traffic signals) and from vision to touch (e.g. Braille).

Both the perception of sensations (e.g. light or sound) and the interpretation of that sensory information vary among people because of physiological differences but also their training, attitudes, and experiences. With advancing age, the sensitivity of the eye to light and of the ear to sound are reduced; therefore, the elderly require clearer signals in order to perceive important information easily and accurately.

Cognitive capacity

According to the human–machine system model, information is perceived through the sensory organs and then processed in the brain, leading to a decision on what action to take. The capacity to process information and make decisions (cognitive capacity) requires short-term (working) memory for processing and long-term memory for storage of relevant experience and knowledge (Wickens *et al.* 2004, Chapter 6). Cognitive capacity is a function of education and experience as well as physiological integrity of the central nervous system.

Aging is associated with a continuous, gradual decline in cognitive functions such as speed of information processing, working memory, long-term memory, and time-sharing (the ability to coordinate two simultaneous activities) (Salthouse 1996). However, it is usually not until the age of around 65 years that noticeable change occurs. On the other hand, vocabulary and linguistic ability increase across the life span. With increasing age the variation around mean values of cognitive capacities appears to increase, probably because of the training effects of different life styles, jobs, and levels of continuing mental exercise. Neurophysiological and psychological research indicate that it is the brain's 'hardware' (number of brain cells) that decline with age, rather than the 'software' (quality of processing). Correlations between cognitive functioning (memory, speed, and verbal ability) and physiological markers such as sensory functioning (i.e. visual and auditory acuity), grip strength, reaction time, and balance with advancing age suggest that the latter may reflect the physiological integrity of the aging nervous system ('biological age'), although this is still being debated. Even though the memory deteriorates slowly, experience and life management skills ('crystallized intelligence') can compensate for reduced capacity, especially in complex decision-making (Rabbitt 2005).

Relevant work environment characteristics

Work station and equipment design

Work stations, equipment, tools, and other objects should be designed in a way that facilitates their use, permits variations in work routines, does not give fatigue, and leads to high efficiency. Common effects of poor work-station design are twisted and bent neck and trunk postures and elevated arms, leading to fatigue, musculoskeletal and other disorders (see below). In the office this applies to the dimensions of the computer and furniture, in industry to machines and tools as well as to supports, and in a kitchen to the layout and the usability of cleaning equipment.

The correct height of a work surface depends on the nature of the task performed (Kroemer and Grandjean 1997, Chapter 3). For precision work, the hands must be held relatively close to the eyes or visuomotor coordination. However, since working with elevated arms is tiring, arm support must be provided. For light manual work with less visual precision, such as on an assembly line, the working area should be close to elbow height (standing or sitting). When lifting or other heavy work is performed, the working height should be even lower (Fig. 8.6.4). Frequent changes between sitting, standing, and walking reduce fatigue; many modern workplaces have work surfaces where the height can be adjusted for both standing and sitting. A minimum requirement is that the height can be adjusted to fit both a tall man and a small woman.

Standing work

The advantage of a standing posture is that the combined mobility of the trunk and arms permits a much larger reach and work area than is possible in the sitting position. Another advantage is that much larger forces can be exerted, especially if the work area is relatively low so that the arms can be held straight and the trunk weight can be used. Conversely, standing work is tiring for the legs, especially for older people and for those with peripheral circulatory problems in the legs. Static standing for at least half the work day is also a risk factor for spontaneous abortion and premature labour among pregnant workers (Gold & Tomich 1994). When work is performed standing and walking it can be made less fatiguing if shoes are changed a few times a day and if the floor is not hard—concrete floors are extremely tiring.

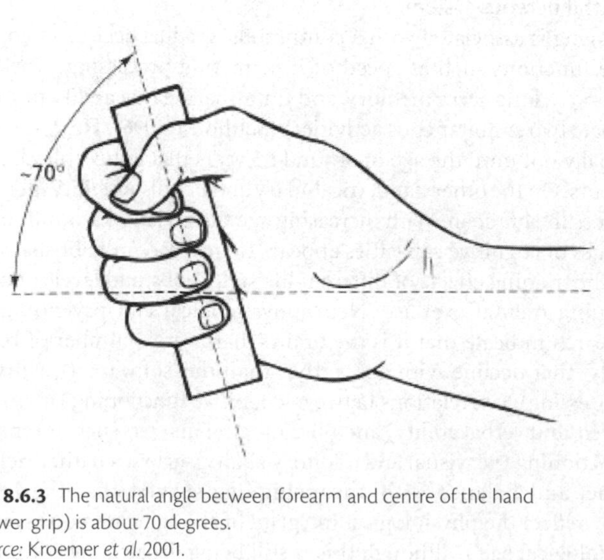

Fig. 8.6.3 The natural angle between forearm and centre of the hand (power grip) is about 70 degrees.
Source: Kroemer *et al.* 2001.

Seated work

Sitting is preferred by most people for prolonged tasks because it is less tiring for the legs. On the other hand, in many jobs sitting implies confined and static postures with elevated shoulders and arms, and frequent or sustained twisting and bending of the neck. The optimal horizontal work area in front of a seated person is even smaller than for standing work. In general, commonly occurring work tasks should not be performed beyond forearm reach, to avoid postural strain and because much less force can be exerted. For example, every tool, handle, or equipment lever should be usable with the hand at a neutral angle relative to the forearm (Fig. 8.6.3). The basic posture in sitting (Hansson 1987; Kroemer & Grandjean 1997) requires that:

- The shoulders are relaxed, the upper arms are nearly vertical alongside the torso, and the forearms are flexed about 100° at the elbows (i.e. angled slightly below horizontal).
- The forearm and hand form a straight line, or alternatively the hand can be slightly extended (angled upward) but should not be bent sideways toward the little finger.

The head posture in seated work is frequently static, especially when fine manual tasks or visually intensive work, such as computer operation, are performed. The line of vision should be horizontal or somewhat below horizontal, and the seated workplace must also provide sufficient leg space, because sitting with the trunk twisted to accommodate the legs requires static muscle exertion and is very tiring. For the seated worker, no equipment is more important than a well-padded, fully adjustable chair. However, no seated posture—even with good furniture—can be maintained for prolonged periods.

Repetitive work and rest time

Lack of recovery time after performance of repetitive work or sustained loading is believed to be an important factor in the aetiology of work-related musculoskeletal disorders, especially of the arm, wrist, and hand. Highly routinized, short-cycle tasks are associated with physiological fatigue and delayed cardiovascular recovery after work (Frankenhaeuser & Johansson 1976). Prolonged repetitive tasks should be avoided by providing frequent breaks and alternative tasks that do not tax the same tissues. Repetitive tasks should not be machine-paced; the individual should be allowed to set his or her own pace and to vary it over the course of the day, as fatigue sets in. Tasks that require precision, force exertion, *and* speed in combination with repetitiveness especially imply particularly high risk (Kilbom 1994).

Piece-work, or performance-based pay, is a wage system explicitly designed to increase worker productivity. Just the effort to work faster, even without an actual increase in speed, may lead to higher tension in the involved muscles. Elevated levels of adrenaline and noradrenaline excretion result, indicating sympathetic nervous system activity and probably relevant to experiences of fatigue and psychological stress that follow. In a large cohort of garment workers, long-term work disability due to cardiovascular and to

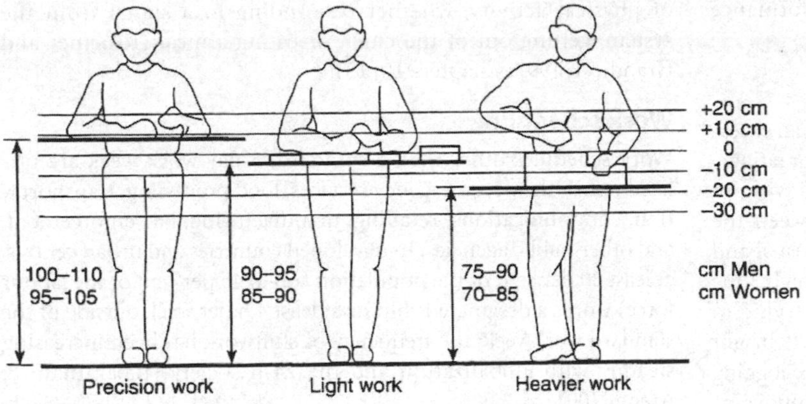

Fig. 8.6.4 Recommended height for benches for standing work. The reference line (=0) is the height of the elbows above the floor, which averages 1050 mm for men and 98 mm for women in Western populations.
Source: Kroemer and Grandjean 1997.

musculoskeletal disease both increased in relation to years in piece-rate versus hourly wage employment (Brisson 1989).

Manual handling

Manual handling of loads—lifting, lowering, holding, carrying, pushing, and pulling—is an important risk factor for low back and other musculoskeletal disorders, in particular. The US National Institute of Occupational Safety and Health has developed a Lifting Equation for estimating the acceptability of a two-handed lift based on the weight of the object, its horizontal distance from the body, the degree of asymmetry, the height of the object, the vertical distance that it is moved, and the frequency of lifting (Waters *et al.* 1993). Although this equation does not apply to all lifting situations, its dissemination has increased awareness about the interactions among these factors in manual handling and how to prioritize them for intervention. A similar assessment procedure is incorporated into the U.K. Manual Handling Operations Regulations issued by the Health and Safety Executive (HSE 2007). Apart from minimizing object weight and distance from the body, manual handling tasks should be designed to eliminate trunk bending and twisting, remove obstructions, provide good coupling of the load and the worker, and eliminate uneven or slippery surfaces.

Case study on manual handling in nursing (Ljungberg *et al.* 1989)

The importance of work-station design, technical lifting aides, and work organization was studied among nursing aides in two hospital geriatric wards. The traditional ward had cramped work spaces, narrow corridors, and small lavatories with room for only one nursing aide to help the patient. Mobile hoists were available but the space was so cramped that they were seldom used. In the modern ward, both corridors and rooms were spacious and about 50 per cent of the beds had motorized overhead hoists for lifting patients. Moreover, the modern ward had a new work organization incorporating 'group-care', in which a senior nurse and two aides shared the responsibility for 12 patients, whereas work at the traditional ward was more like an 'assembly line'.

Patient handling workload was compared between the two wards. The vertical force in each lifting and carrying manoeuvre, as well as the time for each lift, was measured using wooden shoes instrumented with strain gauges. The work performed in lifting was considerably less in the modern ward, whether expressed as total weight lifted per hour, the duration of each lift, or the proportion of lifts with uneven distribution of weight between right and left leg (Table 8.6.1).

It was not possible to distinguish whether the differences in work organization, use and availability of technical aids, or work-station layout most accounted for these large differences; most likely it was a combination of all three. The important point is that physical stresses due to manual handling can be substantially reduced.

Physical environment

Extremes of temperature and humidity, poor lighting, vibrations, noise, low frequency sound, and slippery or unstable ground conditions can all severely influence working capacity, endurance, and mental concentration. This is partly because these factors require additional physiological resources in addition to the work task. For instance, heat reduces blood circulation available for working muscles, cold reduces motor precision, and vibrations and slippery ground require extra muscle exertion to stabilize the body. Lighting, in addition to its impact on vision, also plays an important role in synchronizing the biological clock, for example diurnal rhythms of hormones like cortisol and melatonin, which in turn affect states of alertness and mood (van Bommel 2006).

Background noise, even at low frequency and at levels too low to cause hearing loss, has a number of other adverse consequences. Noise interferes with mental concentration, information processing and communication, and performance of complex tasks, and accuracy of perception. Health effects include elevated catecholamine secretion, psychological symptoms, hypertension and ischaemic heart disease (Babisch 2006; Stansfeld & Matheson 2003). In children, such as in community studies of chronic aircraft noise exposure, noise delays physical growth and impairs reading

Table 8.6.1 Workload of nursing aides in lifting and carrying patients: A comparison between two geriatric hospital wards in Sweden

	Traditional ward	Modern ward
Number of lifts/h	30	14
Number of lifts/h with asymmetric uplift	14.8	7.5
Cumulated vertical force per hour (N)	2880	1660
Average duration of each lift (s)	10.5	4.8
Time spent in lifting (% of working day)	8.6	1.9

comprehension, long-term memory, and academic performance (Kawada 2004; Stansfeld & Matheson 2003).

Information perception and processing

Work with poorly presented sensory information requires an excessively high level of attention, leading to errors, stress, and/or fatigue. In order to enable humans to respond to sensory stimuli without missing information or overreacting, the contrast between the relevant information and the 'noise' caused by irrelevant visual and hearing stimuli, that is the 'signal to noise ratio', must be high. One common example of inadequate signal to noise ratio is trying to read text on computer screens with too little contrast or with bright lights surrounding the screen. In leisure time activities like jogging and cycling, music from earphones can camouflage important safety information from traffic.

Unfortunately, large-scale accidents bring to public attention the need to present information, both in workplaces and public places, in a way that is easily understandable and compatible with human comprehension (see case studies below). Warning signs must use symbols and icons familiar to people: The colour red signifies something forbidden while green means acceptable or safe to proceed; and the symbol for radioactivity is well known to most. Deficiencies in such conceptual compatibility are especially noteworthy in many computer programmes. Movement compatibility implies that there is a concordance between the movement of a control or a lever, and the ensuing movement of a machine or tool; for instance, you turn the wheel to the right when you want to make a right turn (Kroemer and Grandjean 1997, Chapter 9). Spatial compatibility reflects human expectations with regard to the relative positioning of displays and controls and the understanding of 'high' versus 'low' measurements; high values are expected to be at the top of, or at the right-handed side of, a display, whereas low values are expected to be represented at the bottom or the left end.

Good quality visual display is important to avoid both fatigue and error. Sources of direct or indirect glare should be screened from the viewer. Work at a visual display terminal, especially for prolonged periods, requires that the screen be of high quality with good contrast, no flicker, and adjustable in height (see *Seated work* above.)

Information on any display or sign (whether auditory or visual) should be coded in a way that accentuates the crucial information, while redundant information is suppressed. Recommendations for the design of warning signs and labels have been given by Lehto (1992). The schematic representation of the very complex London subway is a good example of a simplified, schematic, yet easily understandable system. Information should be organized in such a way that it is easy to compare and relate to previous training and work experience, and so that it can be stored in the long-term memory and retrieved in a suitable form for use later.

The quality of information processing can be further improved by undivided attention to the task and high motivation. Thus care should be taken when presenting information so that attention is not divided between simultaneous or conflicting demands. Another task design issue that impacts information intake and response is that of prolonged vigilance, which arises when a job requires monitoring of continuous processes for long periods of time during which there is little or no physical activity. The decline in physiological alertness or arousal progresses until the introduction of physical activity, whether responding to a signal from the system, getting out of the chair, or eating a meal (Kroemer and Grandjean 1997, Chapters 10, 13).

Work scheduling

Work schedules other than a standard, 5-day work week are utilized in healthcare, emergency services, food processing, transportation, communications, retailing, manufacturing, law enforcement, and other public agencies. In developed countries and urban centres, at least 20 per cent of the population (up to 45 per cent of the labour force) works a designated shift or at least 4 h per week outside of the standard workweek; the frequency of shiftwork has been increasing steadily with globalization and the 24-h society (Rajaratnam & Arendt 2001).

There is a wide range of potential social and health consequences, including fatigue, increased risk of occupational or transportation injury, reduced mental well-being, and quality and quantity of family and leisure time (work–family imbalance). Sleep disorders are the most obvious and consistently reported health problem. Many shift workers also experience gastrointestinal and digestive disorders. Shift workers, compared to day workers, are at greater risk of coronary heart disease and associated risk factors, including poor diet, adverse serum lipid and lipoprotein cholesterol profiles, and tendency to male central obesity (Steenland 2000). Cognitive and neuropsychological functioning has been shown to decrease with duration of shiftwork (Rouch *et al.* 2005). Flexibility in selecting one's own work schedule mitigates the adverse health effects of irregular schedules (Costa *et al.* 2004). Among female hospital workers with child-care responsibilities, those dissatisfied with their work schedules experienced worse mental health than their colleagues (Estryn-Behar *et al.* 1990).

A related issue is the total number of hours worked per week. The International Labour Organization estimated that 22 per cent of the global workforce (in over 50 countries), or 614.2 million workers, are working 'excessively' long hours—i.e. more than 48 h a week (Lee *et al.* 2007). Some of this is due to white collar professionals whose work boundaries have become porous because of ubiquitous telecommunication media, while at the other end of the socioeconomic spectrum many low-wage workers hold two jobs, sometimes both with irregular schedules and/or in the informal sector, simply in an attempt to make ends meet. In the countries studied by the ILO, men tended to work longer average hours for wages than women, who continued to carry primary responsibility for 'unpaid' household work and care for family members. Again, the variety of health effects of overtime work include stress and fatigue, disrupted sleep, more smoking, and higher risk of injury and cardiovascular disease (Johnson & Lipscomb 2006). Family life, work productivity, and equality between the sexes may also suffer (Lee *et al.* 2007).

Organizational design and management

Work organization—that is, the leadership style (democratic or authoritarian), the hierarchical structure of the organization (flat or high pyramid), the influence of employees on decisions about the work process, the distribution of work tasks among employees, the industrial relations within the organization, the wage/salary negotiating system, the level of technology, and skill utilization—all influence the immediate physical workload and psychosocial environment of individual employees (Sauter *et al.* 2002). These features of the work environment may also be referred to as organizational design and management or as 'macroergonomics' (Hendrick & Kleiner 2001).

'Psychological job demands' refer to features such as work pace, time pressure in processing or responding to information, conflicting demands, mental overload, and the emotional impact of responsibility for another's well-being. 'Job control', or decision latitude, reflects the individual's decision-making opportunities and discretion over skill use, i.e. the ability to control one's own work process (timing, sequence, etc.), to coordinate with others and to decide which skills to utilize to accomplish the job. The two most widely used paradigms for the psychosocial conditions of work are the Demand–Control–Support model (Karasek & Theorell 1990), in which high job demands in combination with low decision latitude result in residual job strain and positive interpersonal relations may have a buffering effect, and the more recent Effort–Reward Imbalance model, in which high efforts combined with low extrinsic and intrinsic rewards produce psychological strain (Siegrist 1996). Studies based on either of these models have shown that psychosocial job strain is a powerful predictor of cardiovascular morbidity and of mental health problems (Schnall 2000; Stansfeld & Candy 2006); it may also play a role in musculoskeletal disorders and acute occupational injury (Bongers *et al* 2006; d'Errico *et al.* 2007). The relationship of work organization factors with psychosocial strain has also been demonstrated by intervention studies showing that interventions which increase worker participation in decision-making can resolve strain linked to high levels of demands over which the worker had no control (Karasek & Theorell 1990).

In addition to the health effects mediated by psychological stress, organizational features of work have other implications for occupational health and safety. Examples include the work scheduling issues discussed above; failure to adjust for overtime hours in determining compliance with permissible chemical exposure levels; piece-work as a disincentive for workers to take rest breaks or utilize safety measures that require extra time (Lilley *et al.* 2002); night work and unprotected exposure to the risk of assault; and job rotation as a disincentive for continuous use of personal protective equipment (Bell & MacDonald 2003).

Organizations that promote employee initiatives, support development of skills and experience, and let employees exercise choice regarding quality and quantity of work adapt more easily to structural changes in society and appear to maintain a higher level of innovation. The underlying philosophy is that humans not only need bread and clothing for satisfaction and full development; when the above additional demands are met people can contribute more to the aims of the organization.

The full consequences of work organized along these lines are not yet fully realized—some disadvantages may follow, for example, for persons with little initiative. Moreover, stress levels may increase above acceptable levels when individuals feel pressured to be as creative and productive as possible. There is no doubt, however, that work organization has a profound influence on employee productivity, well-being, and health (MacDonald *et al.* 2008).

Cost-effectiveness of ergonomic measures in the workplace

Well-designed ergonomic systems often improve efficiency and productivity in industry, both directly and as a result of improved employee health (Oxenburgh *et al.* 2004). In the workplace, productivity, safety, and health may not always be parallel outcomes (Frick 1997). However, there are many situations in which these goals go hand in hand, at least over the longer term.

To evaluate cost-effectiveness, the costs of ergonomic improvements like re-engineering of work stations and tools, introduction of new production methods and work reorganization can be compared with the past or expected costs of leaving the work system unchanged. Potentially hidden costs that should be balanced against the expenses of improvements include sick-leave rate, compensation claims, staff turnover, and productivity (quantity and quality).

Case study on cost-effectiveness from the hospitality sector (Oxenburgh 2004)

Hotel house keepers work for low wages under substantial time pressure to clean hotel rooms; the work involves heavy lifting, pushing and pulling and many awkward postures (Milburn & Barrett 1999; Lee & Krause 2002). A four-star hotel had seen a significant increase in workers' compensation costs due to back and arm musculoskeletal disorders among room attendants. These were almost entirely female, many from Southeast Asia, and about one-third were contract staff from an outside agency rather than full-time employees. These short-term employment arrangements led to difficulties with training and quality maintenance, which were worsened by high turnover among the full-time staff.

An ergonomics specialist was brought in who facilitated worker participation in the change process. Committees of house keepers plus the hotel's occupational health manager evaluated risk factors and determined better work methods, which were incorporated into a revised training procedure. Other improvements implemented by the hotel included better trolleys (linen carts) and vacuum cleaner heads; regular maintenance; and collection of used linen from the trolleys by an extra employee. Contract labour was replaced in part by part-time employees (5-h shifts). The injury rate, severity, and absenteeism were all markedly reduced, producing a measurable increase in productive hours worked; in addition, labour turnover dropped from 60 per cent to 40 per cent per year. The costs of improvements were paid back in only 6 weeks.

Ergonomics and public health

Musculoskeletal disorders (MSDs)

MSDs are widespread in many countries, with substantial costs and impact on quality of life. In the United States, Canada, and Finland, more people are disabled from working as a result of musculoskeletal disorders than from any other group of diseases (Badley *et al.* 1994; Pope *et al.* 1991; Rempel & Punnett 2006; Riihimäki 1995).

Accurate data on the incidence and prevalence of musculoskeletal disorders are difficult to obtain, and the true magnitude is likely underestimated. In addition, regional differences have been noted in the relative frequency of different diagnoses and affected body regions. These may be related to variations in clinical practice, the circumstances under which the disorders were first noted, or the occupational health legislation and compensation systems in each jurisdiction. Criteria for diagnosis and for evaluating work-relatedness and completeness of reporting vary among countries, making statistical comparisons difficult. However, where record-keeping systems have been developed, MSDs are often the single largest group of recorded and/or compensated work-related diseases, representing a third or more of all registered occupational diseases in the United States, the Nordic countries, and Japan (Bernard 1997; Pope *et al.* 1991; Vaaranen *et al.* 1994). From 15 to 49 per cent of all MSDs in the Nordic countries in 1991 were attributable to working conditions, and their cost represented approximately 1 per cent of gross national product (Hansen 1993).

Some industries and occupations have MSD rates up to three or four times higher than the overall frequency. High-risk sectors include nursing facilities; air transportation; mining; food processing; leather tanning; and heavy and light manufacturing of vehicles, furniture, appliances, electrical equipment, electronic products, textiles, apparel, and shoes (Bernard 1997). Upper extremity musculoskeletal disorders are highly prevalent in manual-intensive occupations such as clerical work, postal sorting, cleaning, industrial inspection, and packaging (Rempel & Punnett 2006). Back and lower limb disorders occur disproportionately among truck drivers, warehouse workers, aeroplane baggage handlers, construction trades, nurses, nursing aides and other patient-care workers, and operators of cranes and other large vehicles (Pope *et al.* 1991).

The work-relatedness of musculoskeletal disorders has been discussed extensively (Armstrong *et al.* 1993; Hagberg *et al.* 1995; Bernard 1997; Buckle & Devereaux 1999; International Commission for Occupational Health, Musculoskeletal Committee 1996; National Research Council 2001; Sluiter *et al.* 2000). Experimental science and epidemiology converge regarding the increased risk of work-related musculoskeletal disorders that results from heavy lifting; repetitive hand motion; static work, such as to maintain the body in a fixed posture; vibration; and any of these in combination with each other or with an undesirable thermal environment. The question is unresolved whether or not psychosocial strain has an independent contribution, separate from the physical stressors with which it is often correlated.

Most MSD research has been carried out in more developed countries, where large-scale data bases and research infrastructure support data collection and comparison across the range of economic sectors. It might be supposed that occupation-specific risks are actually higher in the developing world, where general working conditions are poorer and physical workload is higher due to lower levels of mechanization and capital investment in ergonomic improvements. However, the limited evidence permitting cross-national comparisons does not show a clear trend by level of economic development (Punnett *et al.* 2005). It is possible—but not confirmed—that under-reporting is also more pronounced in less developed countries and thus obscures any general effect of labour- versus capital-intensive production.

Work-related disorders of the upper extremity are in some countries referred to as 'repetition strain injury' or 'cumulative trauma disorders'. These terms are intended to convey that the cause is repetitive work or the accumulation of micro-trauma over a period of time, but they are clinically imprecise and even misleading, since musculoskeletal disorders can also occur as a result of high-intensity exposure for relatively brief periods. It is generally acknowledged that the aetiology of these disorders in the population is multifactorial and may involve risk factors both on and off the job. A more useful term is 'work-related musculoskeletal disorders', which reflects the idea that the work environment contributes substantially to causation in the population, although with varying importance among individuals (WHO 1985). Work-related disorders are thus distinguished from specific 'occupational' disorders where a single factor is both necessary and sufficient to cause the disease (e.g. mesothelioma from asbestos exposure).

Work-related musculoskeletal disorders comprise a wide range of inflammatory and degenerative diseases, including some less well-described states of pain and functional impairment. Common clinical disease entities are tendinitis and related conditions, myalgia, nerve entrapment syndromes, low back pain, sciatica, and arthrosis. Body regions most commonly involved are the low back, neck, shoulder, forearm, and hand, although recently the lower extremity has received more attention.

Inflammations of tendons and surrounding tissues (tendinitis, peritendinitis, tenosynovitis), especially in the forearm and wrist, elbow, and shoulder, have a high prevalence and incidence in occupations with prolonged periods of repetitive and static work loads (Kurppa *et al.* 1991). Tendon strain accumulates as a function of work pace (the frequency and duration of mechanical loading), the level of muscular effort, and recovery time between exertions (Goldstein *et al.* 1987). Tendon disorders may have an acute or insidious onset, depending on the intensity of the loading. Recovery is usually complete, but some workers develop chronic disorders.

Myalgia, or pain and functional impairment of muscles, occurs especially in the shoulder and neck region in occupations with large static demands, when performing precision work with the hands or work with the arms elevated (Winkel & Westgaard 1992). The forearm muscles may also be affected in hand-intensive tasks (Ranney *et al.* 1995).

Nerve entrapment syndromes cause pain or other symptoms and loss of sensibility and strength. The most common of these is carpal tunnel syndrome (Hagberg *et al.* 1992; Viikari-Juntura & Silverstein 1999). It occurs in work tasks that require prolonged, repetitive, and forceful gripping or wrist bending, especially if combined with exposure to local vibration. With continued exposure, functional impairment may become permanent.

Degenerative joint disease, or osteoarthrosis (OA), commonly occurs in the spine, especially in the neck and low back regions, as well as in the hand, hip, and knee joints. This disorder is common in the general population at older ages. However, several factors at work, especially heavy physical work, manual handling of objects, prolonged stooping and bending, and possibly exposure to whole-body vibration (especially while seated) increase the risk of spinal degeneration and accelerate the disease process (Felson 1999; Rossignol 2004; Vingård 1991). Kneeling, squatting, and knee bending; striking with the knee; stair climbing; heavy lifting and other 'heavy physical work' are risk factors for OA of the knee and hip (Jensen & Eenberg 1996). The course of these disorders is chronic, and usually exposure to risk factors at work has lasted for many years before symptoms occur.

Acute traumatic injuries in the workplace

Both acute injuries and chronic disorders have essentially the same aetiologic agents, namely, physical energy transmitted to the human body in doses harmful to tissues. Despite the traditional focus on individual behaviour as the cause, it is increasingly recognized that workplace factors, such as poor machine and tool design and lack of adequate maintenance and house-keeping, contribute to many injuries at work. For example, instructions and warning signs are often not designed in accordance with ergonomic principles regarding visual perception and information processing, and they may not be provided in all of the languages spoken within the workforce. Physical work load is relevant in several ways: Fatigue may lead to reduced attention and motor coordination; musculoskeletal trauma may itself manifest as an acute incident (e.g. low back strain) or may lead to an acute episode (e.g. inability to handle a heavy load may result in loss of balance and a slip or fall). The contributions of the physical and psychosocial environment include noise, which interferes with concentration and communication, and piece-rate wages, which encourage bypassing of safety procedures and equipment (Sundström-Frisk 1984; Moll van Charante & Mulder 1990; Melamed *et al.* 1999). Injury prevention therefore requires attention to all aspects of ergonomics: Technical redesign, information processing demands, physical work environment, and reorganization of work procedures. For these reasons, many now reject the term 'accident' altogether, because it implies an unforeseeable or random occurrence, in favour of 'acute injury' or 'incident', concepts more compatible with the public health approach of identifying preventable risk factors.

A high incidence of occupational injuries in industry was the original impetus for occupational health and safety legislation in many countries. Despite the past century of professional attention to occupational injuries, and dramatic declines in most developed countries, this preventable source of mortality continues to produce over 300 000 deaths per year worldwide (WHO 2002, pp. 74–5). Table 8.6.2 summarizes the 2006 official statistics on reported occupational injuries and illnesses in the United States (Bureau of Labor Statistics 2008). The four largest categories of workplace fatality involved falls, being struck by objects, highway accidents, and homicides. (Motor vehicle accidents are counted as work-related in the United States if vehicle operation is necessary in the job.) In contrast, overexertion was by far the most common type of non-fatal incident, followed by falls and being struck by objects. (The fact that MSDs may result either from overexertion or from acute trauma explains why they are labelled as 'illnesses' in some national surveillance systems and as 'injuries' in others.) Among the non-fatal acute incidents, falls to a lower level were relatively infrequent but had the highest median number of days away from work (14 days per case), compared to only 4–5 days per case for struck by or against an object.

Table 8.6.2 Proportion of reported occupational injuries and illnesses by type of event or exposure: United States, 2006 (US Bureau of Labor Statistics)

	Fatalities (n=5 840)	**Non-fatal incidents with lost or restricted work days (n=1 183 500)**
Transportation	42%	5%
Contact with object or equipment (struck by or against)	17%	28%
Fall	14%	20%
Assault	13%	2%
Exposure to harmful substance or environment	9%	5%
Fires and explosions	3%	1%*
Overexertion or bodily reaction	0%	39%

* Fire or explosion plus all other types of event

Cardiovascular disease and other chronic conditions

The impact of psychosocial 'job strain' on physiologic stress response, mental strain, coronary heart disease, hypertension, and other heart disease risk factors is well-established (Karasek & Theorell 1990; Belkic *et al.* 2004) (see 'Organizational design and management'). While estimates of the proportion of cardiovascular disease (CVD) due to job strain vary greatly among studies, as much as 23 per cent (over 150 000 deaths per year in the US) might potentially be preventable if the level of job strain in all jobs was reduced just to the national average for all occupations. The economic costs (e.g. absenteeism, lost productivity) are difficult to estimate but could be as high as several hundred billion dollars per year in the US alone (Karasek & Theorell 1990).

Shiftwork is another established risk factor for CVD; possible mechanisms include poor sleep quality, disruption of circadian rhythm, unhealthy eating patterns, and altered metabolism (Steenland 2000). The CVD risk is even greater when other occupational exposures, such as noise or airborne contaminants, are present simultaneously.

Mental health problems, such as anxiety and depression, and job dissatisfaction have also been associated with occupational features such as low decision latitude or rewards (especially relative to job demands); emotional labour (having to regulate or manage emotions in job-specific ways, as in most care-taking work) (Brotheridge & Lee 2003); fear of assault, discrimination or harassment; work-family imbalance; and job insecurity (Janzen *et al.* 2007a, b; Parker & Griffin 2002; Tsutsumi *et al.* 2001; Wadsworth *et al.* 2007).

For the pregnant worker, physically demanding tasks such as heavy lifting interfere with uteroplacental blood flow and may precipitate uterine contractility later in pregnancy. Such work has been associated with preterm birth (before 37 weeks gestation) and hypertension or preeclampsia (Mozurkewich *et al.* 2000). Prolonged standing and shiftwork also increase the risk of preterm birth; psychosocial strain is also physiologically relevant (Omer & Everly 1988), although the epidemiology is not conclusive (Hedegaard *et al.* 1996).

Ergonomic applications in transportation systems

Traffic accidents are one of the leading causes of death and disability today. In the United States, traffic injury is second only to cancer in the total financial cost to the community of major disabilities and deaths. Even in some developing countries where infectious disease is still a significant cause of death, traffic injury accounts for a percentage of all deaths similar to that in some highly motorized countries (WHO 2002, p. 72).

Traffic incidents are often blamed on 'human error'. The car driver 'disregarded' the warning sign, the truck driver stepped on the brakes 'too late', the signal box attendant 'forgot' the coming train, and so on. What if the warning sign was obscured because of the car design and the position of the sign, the truck driver was just entering a tunnel with sudden (relative) darkness, and the signal box attendant was tired because of having to work double shifts? Transportation systems can be designed in a way that takes human limitations into consideration, instead of relying on unrealistic instructions, rules, and regulations that are not compatible with human capacities.

Traffic incidents have a complex causality, and ergonomics can play an important role for prevention through the design of vehicles and traffic signs, and the engineering of roads and railways. Because of the high speed of movement in traffic, the design of transportation systems has special requirements. Speed places excessive demands on reaction time, short-term memory and vision of both drivers and pedestrians, although these demands can be moderated by the design of the road system (Dewar & Olson 2007).

Reaction time can be reduced by encouraging familiarity, because drivers reset faster to a familiar situation, and by reducing the number of alternatives. For example, unusual intersection layouts and a large number of exits from a roundabout require longer response times.

Short-term memory is crucial for driver performance because most of the driving task relies on information that is never stored in long-term memory. Therefore, warning signs should require an immediate response, drivers should be frequently reminded of control information which varies along the road (for example speed limits), and the driver should be allowed to respond to one stimulus before the next is imposed.

Of all information required by a vehicle driver, 90 per cent is supplied by vision. As the amount of visual information is nearly without limit, the driver must continuously select the most important cues to help in his or her driving. As the data processing demands increase, the driver tends to be overloaded and to miss some information or to shed part of it. This situation also takes place immediately after a situation of overload. Thus the departure side of an intersection may be relatively more accident prone than the approach side, which also implies that pedestrian crossings and bus stops should not be placed after intersections. Only 1–1.5 fixations of vision per second are realistic in driving. Road traffic signs must therefore be separated in time and space and must only be used for the most necessary information. They must be within the field of vision of the driver which, when moving at a certain speed, implies a narrower field both horizontally and vertically than for a stationary observer. Delineation, that is, markings of road alignment immediately ahead, is especially important at the approach to curves and crests, and for elderly drivers whose visual capacity is often reduced.

The design of the driver cabin directly influences traffic safety by the degree of visibility that it affords to the driver. Cabin design should provide a comfortable seated posture in which the driver can reach all of the hand and foot controls and is protected from vibration (Pheasant & Haslegrave 2005). Traffic safety is also influenced by circumstances as varied as fatigue, training of drivers and pedestrians, legislation, traffic density, weather conditions, and ill health and medications of the driver (Dewar & Olson 2007; Kroemer & Grandjean 1997).

Consumer product design

The design of products, implements, and entire systems for use by the general population increasingly involves ergonomics. Some important applications that influence the health or safety of the consumer include the design of furniture and kitchen utensils, floor coverings, hand-held tools and containers. As in the workplace, injuries often happen as a consequence of several factors simultaneously—consider slipping and falling due to a combination of slippery floors and carrying a bulky, wobbly object that obscures one's vision. In the kitchen, problems may occur due to unsuitable working heights, poor lighting, and ambiguous labelling of stove controls. Examples of poor ergonomic design of consumer products include: Carrying purchases in plastic bags whose handles cut into your fingers; trying to open containers that require excessive pinch force; and sorting paper money of different denominations but the same size and colour. In all of these situations, better design would reduce discomfort and fatigue, make the task less time-consuming, and reduce the risk of mistakes.

As with industrial tools, devices for the home should be designed to fit the anthropometry, strength, and endurance of the entire population. Information and warning signs must similarly be understandable to populations with large variations in sensory and cognitive capacity, cultural background, and level of schooling. All areas of design must be considered: A product or an implement must be shaped and marked in a way that explains its function; safety devices must be designed without demands on previous training and experience; and size, weight, and grips must fit a wide variety of human body sizes. Design for the public therefore requires even more sophisticated considerations than design for the workplace, where the user population is better defined in terms of physical and psychological capacities and where additional training can be given to selected groups.

This area is becoming increasingly important, partly as a consequence of product liability legislation enacted in many Western countries. The manufacturer of any product can be made economically responsible for a user's injury if it can be demonstrated that deficient design of the product was responsible or that the user could not have been expected to know of the risk. There are also market considerations; since a consumer device is purchased by the end user, that user (unlike most workers) has the opportunity to choose for him or herself among available designs, and comfort and ease of use are usually important criteria for the purchaser.

Although usually not described in ergonomic terms, many implements and tools used in sports and leisure time have been developed with an ergonomics approach, emphasizing high levels of achievement and absence of accidents and injuries. Some examples are hand-grip fit in golf clubs and tennis rackets to improve force output and reduce the risk of epicondylitis, and the development of sport shoes to reduce impact forces and periostial and tendon inflammation.

Design for the elderly and people with physical or mental disability

In recent years there have been advances in design for rehabilitation and for people with physical or mental disabilities, with primary emphasis on compensating for reduced physical capacity such as muscle strength and precision, hearing, vision, and mobility (Kroemer 2005). In the future, more emphasis should also be put on compensating for longer reaction times and reduced cognitive capacity. Computer use, for example, is often out of reach both for people with disabilities and for the elderly because of demands on vision and rapid information processing, and the increasing use of unfamiliar symbols. In a recent survey of commercially available products intended for elderly people, it was found that many of them were inappropriate or inadequate to perform the task for which they were intended (Gardner *et al.* 1993). Some did not perform the intended job; others introduced hazards that could have led to serious accidents but which could have been avoided easily by simple consumer trials and redesign.

In the same way that a disabled individual may have a decrement in only one of many functional capacities, an elderly person may have most functions well preserved. There is therefore no need to distinguish between ergonomics for people with physical or mental disabilities and the elderly. In fact, it would make more economic sense if all products were designed for use by the full range of the population, including those with limited abilities as well as the more able-bodied (Haigh 1993).

One group of ergonomists and designers in Sweden, Ergonomi-Design Gruppen, have successfully designed a range of products for people with disabilities and the elderly (Benktzon 1993). Modification of products such as knives, walking sticks, and cutlery have made people with reduced strength and mobility of the hand or arm more self-sufficient in their everyday life. The design process is stepwise, starting with thorough documentation of the functional ability of groups with different types of disabilities, preparing a range of test tools, prototype testing, and finally manufacturing. The same approach has been used in the redesign of products for crafts workers and others with repeated and prolonged use of tools and implements. Small design details can be of vital importance for safety, comfort, and usability. Pliers, screwdrivers, and butcher's knives with improved grip surface and grip diameter, and a coffee pot with its centre of gravity closer to the hand, are other commercial products developed by the group. These all reduce the load on the forearm and hand, improving comfort and decreasing fatigue, and therefore have been widely adopted. Solutions originally created for the elderly or for people with physical or mental disabilities have frequently been found acceptable to a broader range of users (Benktzon 1993).

Public health implications of complex technological environments—two case studies

Most people have heard about disasters in high-tech environments such as the nuclear power plants in Japan, Chernobyl (Russia), and Three Mile Island (US). Such disasters can be ascribed to the combined effects of design defects, conflicts between safety and productivity goals, poor operating and maintenance procedures, and inadequate training (Reason 1990). Ergonomics is central in the causality of many of these accidents because of poor system design, which was not compatible with human capacity and its limitations. The operators or workers involved are often victims, but the reason these disasters are widely publicized and analysed is that the public—the third party—is exposed to risks without the ability to protect itself. The following two case studies illustrate that serious 'accidents' can and will happen when technical systems have not been designed and implemented with consideration to human limitations.

Urban tram collision

In a tram accident in Sweden, 13 people died and 29 were taken to hospital when a tram raced downhill along the track with the brakes disconnected. All those killed or injured were waiting at the next stop, or were pedestrians or car passengers happening to pass downhill. The tram had been taken out of service because of a breakdown in the overhead power supply. As the electric power had been cut, the normal electrodynamic brakes did not function and mechanical brakes had automatically taken over. The traffic supervisor in charge of the removal of the tram decided to use the down-slope to move the tram further down to where the power was intact. However, the mechanical brakes first had to be released, which could be done by a simple handgrip from the outside of each carriage. The intention was to use the mechanical brakes again further down. However, for the mechanical brakes to be functional again they had to be refilled with pressurized air, which could only be done when under electrical power. As a consequence, once they had been released the tram driver could not stop the tram from racing down the track.

This incident appears to be a typical example of so-called 'human error'. However, the subsequent investigation revealed several errors in the design of the system (Haverikommission 1992). The drivers and supervisors knew that the mechanical brakes must not be released unless the tram was secured by other means, but they did not know why; nor did they know how the brakes were constructed or what the consequences might be of disconnecting the mechanical brakes. Moreover, they had been given no formal training in emergency procedures of this nature. The mechanical brakes had been designed with an external release mechanism that was easily accessible but without any warning signs. This case is an unfortunate example of the combined effects of deficiencies in technical design and training and emergency procedures that could have been avoided by the application of ergonomic principles.

Unnecessary patient death in a hospital emergency room

A 74-year-old woman died in the emergency department (ED) of an American hospital where she had arrived by ambulance after fainting at home. The ED physician suspected that she might have fainted due to an undiagnosed heart arrhythmia, so she was connected to a bedside heart monitor and kept overnight for observation. The woman was checked by her nurse at 3:30 AM and found to be fine. At the time of the next routine check, two hours later, the patient's heart and breathing had stopped and emergency resuscitation procedures were unsuccessful. Her death was eventually determined (Fairbanks *et al.* 2008) to result primarily from a hidden feature of the heart monitor, so that an important alarm could be unintentionally disabled without making the ED staff aware of this.

The initial assumption of the hospital staff was that the arrhythmia alarm on the heart monitor had failed. However, analysis of the stored data showed that this was not correct; the monitor had recorded the arrhythmia but the arrhythmia alarm was in the 'off' position, although the nurse had turned off only the heart-rate alarm. The investigation showed that the monitor had a faulty design, in that deactivation of the two alarms (heart-rate and arrhythmia) was coupled, but there was no feedback to the users to alert them that disabling one would automatically disable the other. The bedside monitor had a label in very small font saying, 'ALL ARRH ALARMS OFF', but the message did not stand out in the display and was easily missed.

There is no medical rationale for designing the device in this way, and none of the ED staff was aware of it. The manufacturer stated that the ED nurse manager had been informed at the time of installation (almost a decade ago), but there was no written documentation of it, including in the operator's manual, and there had been substantial staff turnover since the purchase.

At the time of the incident the central monitoring unit at the nurses' station indicated that the arrhythmia alarm had been turned off, but this was also a small text message on a busy screen. The design of the monitor apparently did not conform to standard human factors guidelines for ensuring legibility through large enough font size or for denoting critical information, such as using a special colour (e.g. red), a flashing display, or an accompanying auditory signal (Kroemer & Grandjean 1997, Chapter 9; Wickens *et al.* 2004, Chapter 8).

Other human factors and work organization issues in the ED permitted the deactivation and the arrhythmia itself to go unnoticed, losing the opportunity to intervene early enough to save the patient's life. The central nursing station had numerous monitors for 20 ED patient rooms, and many of these had alarms–resulting in competing visual and auditory displays and information overload. Such a situation is not unique to the healthcare environment; similar problems have been previously described in industrial settings (Wickens *et al.* 2004, Chapter 8). The monitor displays were positioned very high on the wall and not in the normal viewing area. Again, most ergonomics textbooks offer recommendations for equipment selection and workstation layout to facilitate perception and appropriate prioritization of the most critical information. These address issues such as placement of monitors (close enough to read, with the most important ones at eye height), provision of redundant signals for information that should not go overlooked), and consistency among displays so that experience with one model does not lead to misinterpretation of another.

Obviously the design of the monitor, as well as the nurse's understanding of how it functioned, were both faulty. Insufficient training had been provided to the users about how the critical alarm switch functioned. However, the patient's death was initially attributed to human error on the part of the nurse. The eventual hospital response included re-positioning of the display, reconfiguration of the monitor so that the heart alarm cannot be turned off, staff training, and a formal apology to the patient's family. This case emphasizes the need for unambiguous designs of medical devices with consistent markings and design and positioning of displays that facilitate prioritizing information appropriately. The application of ergonomic principles in the design of this monitor, as well as for other devices and systems used throughout the healthcare system, is necessary for the avoidance of similar 'accidents'.

Ergonomics in developing countries

In developing countries, especially with high rates of unemployment, occupational safety and health is commonly disregarded by employers (Nuwayhid 2004). In some countries the regulations themselves are inadequate; in others there are strong regulations that are not enforced because labour inspectors are scarce and have limited resources. Medical surveillance of occupational conditions is often lacking as well. As in developed countries, knowledge and resources for occupational health are especially scarce in small and middle-sized companies. Ergonomics needs therefore to be promoted not only as a means to improve safety but also to forward social progress; should emphasize practical, low-cost problem-solving (ILO 1996); and must stem from local initiatives to be effective. Ergonomics may also sometimes help to fulfil other management goals, such as high productivity, but the right of workers to have safe working conditions must be respected for its own sake (United Nations 1976) regardless of the economic implications.

Because of the great need for improvements and the scarcity of ergonomists in developing countries, the International Labour Organization has developed a training programme targeting entrepreneurs and workers of small and medium-sized enterprises, 'Work Improvement in Small Enterprises (WISE)' (Thurman *et al.* 1988). The programme focuses on the simultaneous improvement of working conditions and productivity and encourages low-cost, voluntary measures using locally available materials and skills. Eight themes were selected: Materials storage and handling; workstation design; machine safety; control of hazardous substances; lighting; welfare facilities and services (drinking water, rest areas, etc.); work premises (housekeeping and physical environment); and work organization. The training methods emphasize joint worker–manager participation in action learning and sharing of experience. Technical support offers advice on priority-setting and hands-on guidance to implement practical improvements. In order to sustain the interest of managers and workers, it is important for them to see possible productivity gains and to learn to use their own ideas and skills (Kogi 2006).

Implementing change

Legislation, standards, and guidelines

National legislation concerning ergonomic factors varies widely between different countries. Traditionally, legislation in occupational health focuses on quantitative data, such as the concentrations of chemical substances, or minimum physical dimensions of barriers and guardrails as safety measures. The application of strict quantitative risk assessment in ergonomics has proved controversial for several reasons especially related to the multiplicity of physical risk factors, lack of standardized assessment protocols for each of them and uncertainties in quantifying the interactions among them for different health outcomes (Fallentin *et al.* 2001; Kilbom 1999; Viikari-Juntura 1997). At the same time, regulations are desirable because voluntary actions by forward-thinking employers only cover a small proportion of the workforce in any single country, and because those measures generally lag behind technological changes rather than anticipating future health effects.

As an alternative approach, some countries have adopted performance standards based on functional requirements and desired outcomes, for example, that a certain work process must not produce injuries and must comply with safe handling. Such an approach could more feasibly address work organization as well, rather than focusing only on micro-ergonomic issues (Kilbom 1999).

Intense effort is under way in the European Community to develop directives relevant for ergonomics (Buckle & Devereaux 1999); some have already been presented for machine work (89/392/EEC), manual handling (90/269/EC), working time (93/104/EC), use of visual display terminals (Dul & de Flaming 1994), and vibration (2002/44/EC). In the United States, a national ergonomics programme standard for prevention of musculoskeletal disorders was proposed in 1999 but did not stand.

International occupational standards are also continually being developed and refined; these are generally not legally binding. The International Organization for Standardization (ISO) issues standards complementary to the European Community directives and has addressed many topics covered in this chapter, such as illumination, noise, whole-body and hand-arm vibration, the thermal environment, the needs of persons with disabilities, and child safety (http://www.iso.ch). Other examples of voluntary guidelines are the Threshold Limit Values® issued by the American Conference of Government Industrial Hygienists on hand activity level and manual lifting (ACGIH 2007).

Large manufacturing or scientific organizations often develop codes of practice or guidelines for the specific area of their activity. These can be made more precise, relating to the conditions at hand at a certain organization, and are therefore useful for the practitioner (for example, Mital & Kilbom 1992; Winkel & Westgaard 1992; Kilbom 1994).

In the public sector, intensification of product liability legislation in many countries has given better tools for consumers in pursuing safety.

Training

Effective ergonomics programmes in the workplace emphasize engineering controls, especially the ergonomic design of workstations, equipment, tools, and work re-organization, along with a participatory process that engages the workers' knowledge and empowers them to identify and remedy hazards (Hagberg *et al.* 1995). Thus both professional expertise and worker education are required.

The labour inspectorate is, in most countries, the organization responsible for the follow-up of ergonomics legislation. Since inspectors are usually poorly trained in ergonomics, this surveillance is often ineffective. In countries with a well-developed occupational health service (e.g. the Nordic countries), physiotherapists and safety engineers are usually well trained in ergonomics and perform valuable work. In the US, plant nurses has traditionally provided such services in large companies.

Sometimes the occupational health service is unable to sufficiently the development of new work situations—the effort is reactive rather than proactive. For improved ergonomic conditions, both at workplaces and for the public, those responsible for developing technical systems need more training in ergonomics. Production engineers, designers, architects, and systems engineers (in computing), and personnel managers are seldom exposed to ergonomics in their technical education. Since few universities provide postgraduate degrees in ergonomics there is so far an unfulfilled need for training, which is even more pronounced in developing countries.

Education of workers to recognize hazards and participate in work redesign processes is essential, although there is little consensus on the specific goals or methods for worker education in occupational health and safety. To be effective, worker education should involve two-way dialogue, value experiential knowledge, recognize the organizational nature of many hazards, and assist workers to develop strategies for corrective action (Wallerstein & Weinger 1992).

Participatory approaches

In recent years it has been proved repeatedly that improvements of ergonomic conditions are most efficiently achieved when all those using a particular system are also involved in its improvement (Haines *et al.* 2002; Hignett *et al.* 2005). For example, 'expert' advice from a short-term consultant frequently results in failure if not supported by the experience of those manufacturing or using the product. The knowledge of the consumer or the worker is often unspoken but can be used for product and system improvement in practical trials. The group of people involved in a workplace ergonomics programme should include not only the product designer and manufacturing engineer but also the workers, the occupational health staff, those who sell and promote the product, and its users. Technical expertise and guidance should be offered in an ongoing manner, since it is not easy for the worker or consumer to predict new hazards that may arise from a change in design.

Conclusion

The design of tools, equipment, and complex systems to be compatible with human needs, abilities and expectations is increasingly important in the modern world. Failure to apply these principles impacts negatively on people in their workplaces, in transit, and at home. The necessary knowledge basis exists, to a large extent, although the extent to which it is utilized varies widely among countries and types of applications. Legal requirements appear to be necessary to achieve protection from occupational injury and illness, while market incentives may motivate improved design of many consumer devices.

Acknowledgement

This chapter was originally written for the Third Edition by Åsa Kilbom. Dr Punnett's revisions were undertaken with her consent but without her review of specific changes.

References

ACGIH (2007). *TLVs7 and BEIs7: Documentation of the Threshold Limit Values and Biologiocal Exposure Indices.* American Conference of Governmental Industrial Hygienists, Cincinnati, OH, USA.

Armstrong, T.J., Buckle, P., Fine, L.J. *et al.*(1993). A conceptual model for work-related neck and upper-limb musculoskeletal disorders. *Scandinavian Journal of Work Environment and Health*, **19**, 73–84.

Åstrand, I. (1967b). Degree of strain during building work as related to individual aerobic work capacity. *Ergonomics*, **10**, 293–303.

Åstrand, P.O., Rodahl, K., Dahl, H.A., and Stromme, S.B. (2003). *Textbook of work physiology: Physiological bases of exercise* (ed. P.O. Åstrand) 4th edition. Human Kinetics Publishers, Champaign, IL.

Babisch, W. (2006). Transportation noise and cardiovascular risk: Updated review and synthesis of epidemiological studies indicate that the evidence has increased. *Noise Health*, **8**, 1–29.

Badley, E.M., Rasooly, I., and Webster, G.K. (1994). Relative importance of musculoskeletal disorders as a cause of chronic health problems, disability, and health care utilization: Findings from the 1990 Ontario Health Survey. *The Journal of Rheumatology*, **21**, 505–14.

Barnekow-Bergkvist, M., Hedberg, G.E., Janlert, U. *et al.* (1998). Determinants of self-reported neck-shoulder and low back symptoms in a general population. *Spine*, **23**, 235–43.

Belkic, K. L., Landsbergis, P.A., Schnall, P.L. *et al.* (2004). Is job strain a major source of cardiovascular disease risk? *Scandinavian Journal of Work Environment and Health*, **30**, 85–128.

Bell, J.L. and MacDonald, L.A. (2003). Hand lacerations and job design characteristics in line-paced assembly. *Journal of Occupational and Environmental Medicine*, **45**, 848–56.

Benktzon, M. (1993). Designing for our future selves: The Swedish experience. *Applied Ergonomics*, **24**, 19–27.

Bernard, B.P. (ed.) (1997). *Musculoskeletal disorders and workplace factors: A critical review of epidemiologic evidence for work-related musculoskeletal disorders of the neck, upper extremity, and low back*, Department of Health and Human Services, National Institute for Occupational Safety and Health, Cincinnati, OH.

Bongers, P.M., Ijmker, S., van den Heuvel, S.*et al.* (2006). Epidemiology of work related neck and upper limb problems: Psychosocial and personal risk factors (part I) and effective interventions from a bio behavioural perspective (part II). *Journal of Occupational Rehabilitation*, **16**, 279–302.

Brisson, C., Vinet, A., Vezina, M.*et al.* (1989). Effect of duration of employment in piecework on severe disability among female garment workers. *Scandinavian Journal of Work Environment and Health*, **15**, 329–34.

Brotheridge, C.M. and Lee, R.T. (2003). Development and validation of the Emotional Labour Scale. *Journal of Occupational and Organizational Psychology*, **76**, 365–79.

Buckle, P.W. and Devereaux, J. (1999). *Work-related neck and upper limb musculoskeletal disorders*, European Agency for Safety and Health at Work, Luxembourg.

Bureau of Labor Statistics, U.S. Department of Labor, Survey of Occupational Injuries and Illnesses. Accessed on June 10, 2008, at: http://www.bls.gov/iif/oshwc/cfoi/cfch0005.pdf (fatalities) and http://www.bls.gov/iif/oshwc/osh/case/osch0036.pdf (non-fatal incidents).

Chaffin, D.B., Andersson, G.B.J., and Martin, B.J. (2006). *Occupational biomechanics*, 4th edition. John Wiley & Sons, New York.

Costa, G., Akerstedt, T., Nachreiner, F. *et al.* (2004). Flexible working hours, health, and well-being in Europe: some considerations from a SALTSA project. *Chronobiology International*, **21**, 831–44.

d'Errico, A., Punnett, L., Cifuentes, M.*et al.* and Phase.in Healthcare Team. (2007). Hospital injury rates in relation to socioeconomic status and working conditions. *Occupational and Environmental Medicine*, **64**, 325–33.

Dewar, R.E. and Olson, P.L. (2007) *Human factors in traffic safety*, 2nd edition. Lawyers and Judges Publishing, Tucson AZ.

Dul, J. and de Flaming, P (1994). A review of ISO and CEN standards on ergonomics. In *Proceedings of the 12th Triennial Congress of the International Ergonomics Association*, pp. 131–33. Human Factors Association of Canada, Toronto, Canada.

Era, P., Lyyra, A.L., Viitasalo, J.T. *et al.* (1992). Determinants of isometric muscle strength in men of different ages. *European Journal of Applied Physiology*, **64**, 84–91.

Estryn-Behar, M., Kaminski, M., Peigne, E. *et al.* (1990). Stress at work and mental health status among female hospital workers. *British Journal of Industrial Medicine*, **47**, 20–8.

Fairbanks, R.J., Caplan, S.H., Hildebrand, J.M. (2008) Heart monitor user interface characteristics and an unnoticed patient death in the emergency department. Proceedings of the HEPS (Healthcare Systems, Ergonomics, and Patient Safety) Conference.

Fallentin, N., Viikari-Juntura, E., Waersted, M. *et al.* (2001). Evaluation of physical workload standards and guidelines from a Nordic perspective. *Scandinavian Journal of Work Environment and Health*, **27** (Suppl 2), 1–52.

Felson, D.T. (1999) Occupation-related physical factors and osteoarthritis. In *Rheumatic diseases and the environment* (eds. L.D. Kaufman and J. Varga), pp. 189–95. Oxford University Press, New York.

Frankenhaeuser, M. and Johansson, G. (1976). Task demand as reflected in catecholamine excretion and heart rate. *Journal of Human Stress*, **3**, 15–23.

Frick, K. (1997). Can managers see any profit in health and safety? *New Solutions: A Journal of Environmental and Occupational Health Policy*, **7**, 32–40.

Gardner, L., Powell, L., and Page, M. (1993). An appraisal of a selection of products currently available to older consumers. *Applied Ergonomics*, **24**, 35–9.

Goldstein, S.A., Armstrong, T.J., Chaffin, D.B. *et al.* (1987). Analysis of cumulative strain in tendons and tendon sheaths. *Journal of Biomechanics*, **20**, 1–6.

Hagberg, M., Morgenstern, H., and Kelsh, M. (1992). Impact of occupations and job tasks on the prevalence of carpal tunnel syndrome: A review. *Scandinavian Journal of Work Environment and Health*, **18**, 337–45.

Hagberg, M., Hendrick, H., Silverstein, B. *et al.* (1995). *Work related musculoskeletal disorders (WMSDs): A reference book for prevention.* Taylor & Francis, London.

Haigh, R. (1993). The ageing process: a challenge for design. *Applied Ergonomics*, **24**, 9–14.

Haines, H., Wilson, J.R., Vink, P. *et al.* (2002). Validating a framework for participatory ergonomics (the PEF). *Ergonomics*, **45**, 309–27.

Hansen, S.M. (1993). *Arbeidsmiljo og samfundsokonomi.* Nordisk Ministerråd, Nord 1993:22.

Hansson, J.-E. (1987). Funktionell anatomi, antropometri och biomekanik. In *Människan i arbete.* (eds. N. Lundgren, G. Luthman, and K. Elgstrand) pp. 92-118. Almqvist & Wiksell, Stockholm.

Haverikommissionen (1992). *Spårvägnsolycka* 1992-03-12. Swedish Board of Accident Investigation Report no J 1992:1, Stockholm.

Hedegaard, M., Henriksen, T.B., Secher, N.J. *et al.* (1996). Do stressful life events affect duration of gestation and risk of preterm delivery? *Epidemiology*, **7**, 339–45.

Hignett, S., Wilson, J.R., and Morris, W. (2005). Finding ergonomic solutions—participatory approaches. *Occupational Medicine (London)*, **55**, 200–7.

Health and Safety Executive (2007). *Manual handling assessment chart (MAC) Tool.* Accessed at: http://www.hse.gov.uk/msd/mac/index.htm.

International Ergonomics Association Council (2000). *What is Ergonomics.* On-line at: http://www.iea.cc/browse.php?contID=what_is_ergonomics (accessed June 20, 2007).

ILO (1996). *Ergonomic checkpoints: Practical and easy-to-implement solutions for improving safety, health and working conditions.* International Labour Organization, Geneva.

Hendrick, H.W. and Kleiner, B.M. (2001). *Macroergonomics - An introduction to work system design.* Human Factors and Ergonomics Society, Santa Monica, CA.

Janzen, B.L., Muhajarine, N., and Kelly, I.W. (2007). Work-family conflict, and psychological distress in men and women among Canadian police officers. *Psychological Reports*, **100**, 556–62.

Janzen, B.L., Muhajarine, N., Zhu, T. *et al.* (2007). Effort-reward imbalance, overcommitment, and psychological distress in Canadian police officers. *Psychological Reports*, **100**, 525–30.

Jensen, L.K. and Eenberg, W. (1996). Occupation as a risk factor for knee disorders. *Scandinavian Journal of Work Environment and Health*, **22**, 165–75.

Johnson, J.V. and Lipscomb, J. (2006). Long working hours, occupational health and the changing nature of work organization. *American Journal of Industrial Medicine*, **49**, 921–9.

Jonsson, R.G., Persson, I., and Kilbom, Å. (1988). Disorders of the cervicobrachial region among female workers in the electronics industry. A two-year follow up. *International JournaI of lndustrial Ergonomics*, **3**, 1–12.

Karasek, R.A. and Theorell, T. (1990). *Healthy work. Stress, productivity and the reconstruction of working life.* Basic Books, New York.

Kawada, T. (2004). The effect of noise on the health of children. *Journal of Nippon Medical School*, **71**, 5–10.

Keyserling, W.M., Herrin, G.D., and Chaffin, D.B. (1980). Isometric strength testing as a means of controlling medical incidents on strenuous jobs. *Journal of Occupational Medicine*, **22**, 332–6.

Kilbom, Å. (1994). Repetitive work of the upper extremity: Part 1 - Guidelines for the practitioner. Part II - The scientific basis (knowledge base) for the guide. *International Journal of lndustrial Ergonomics*, **14**, 51–86.

Kilbom, Å. (1999). Possibilities for regulatory actions in the prevention of musculoskeletal disorders. *Scandinavian Journal of Work Environment and Health*, 25(Suppl 4) 5–12.

Kogi, K. (2006). Participatory methods effective for ergonomic workplace improvement. *Applied Ergonomics*, **37**, 547–54.

Kroemer, K.H.E. and Grandjean, E. (1997). *Fitting the task to the human: A textbook of occupational ergonomics (Fifth edition).* Taylor & Francis, Bristol, PA, and London.

Kroemer, K.H.E. (2005). *'Extra-ordinary' ergonomics: How to accommodate small and big persons, the disabled and elderly, expectant mothers, and children.* CRC Press.

Kujala, U.M., Taimela, S., Viljanen, T. *et al.* (1996). Physical loading and performance as predictors of back pain in healthy adults: A 5-year prospective study. *European Journal of Applied Physiology*, **73**, 452–8.

Kurppa, K., Viikari-Juntura, E., Kuosma, E. *et al.* (1991). Incidence of tenosynovitis or peritendinitis and epicondylitis in a meat-processing factory. *Scandinavian Journal of Work Environment and Health*, **17**, 32–7.

Lee, P.T. and Krause, N. (2002) The impact of a worker health study on working conditions. *Journal of Public Health Policy*, **23**, 268–85.

Lee, S., McCann, D., and Messenger, J.C. (2007). *Working time around the world: Trends in working hours, laws, and policies in a global comparative perspective*. Routledge, London and International Labour Organization, Geneva.

Lehto, M. (1992). Designing warning signs and warning labels. Part I: Guidelines for the practitioner. Part II: The scientific basis for the guide. *International Journal of Industrial Ergonomics*, **10**, 78–95.

Leino, P., Aro, S., and Hasan, J. (1987). Trunk muscle function and low back disorders: A ten-year follow-up study. *Journal of Chronic Diseases*, **40**, 289–96.

Lilley, R., Feyer, A.-M., Kirk, P. *et al.* (2002). A survey of forest workers in New Zealand: Do hours of work, rest, and recovery play a role in accidents and injury? *Journal of Safety Research*, **33**, 53–71.

Ljungberg, A.-S., Kilbom, Å., and Hägg, G. (1989). Occupational lifting by nursing aides and warehouse workers. *Ergonomics*, **32**, 59–78.

Lundberg, A. (1992). *Dialysmålet—ett öppet såt i svensk rättskipning.* Private Report.

MacDonald, L.A., Härenstam, A., Warren, N.D. *et al.* (2008). Incorporating work organization into occupational health research – An invitation for dialogue. *Occupational and Environmental Medicine*, 65,1–3.

Malchaire, J. B., Cock, N., and Vergracht, S. (2001). Review of the factors associated with musculoskeletal problems in epidemiological studies. *International Archives of Occupational and Environmental Health*, **74**, 79–90.

Melamed, S., Yekutieli, D., Froom, P. *et al.* (1999). Adverse work and environmental conditions predict occupational injuries. *American Journal of Epidemiology*, **150**, 18–26.

Messing, K. and Stevenson, J. (1996). Women in Procrustean beds: Strength testing and the workplace. *Gender, Work and Organization*, **3**, 156–67.

Mikkelsson, L.O., Nupponen, H., Kaprio, J. *et al.* (2006). Adolescent flexibility, endurance strength, and physical activity as predictors of adult tension neck, low back pain, and knee injury: A 25 year follow up study. *British Journal of Sports Medicine*, **40**, 107–13.

Milburn, P.D. and Barrett, R.S. (1999). Lumbosacral loads in bedmaking. *Applied Ergonomics*, **30**, 263–73.

Mital, A. and Kilbom, Å. (1992). Design, selection and use of hand tools to alleviate trauma of the upper extremities. *International Journal of lndustrial Ergonomics*, **10**, 1–21.

Mital, A., Motorwala, A., Kulkarni, M. *et al.* (1994). Allocation of functions to humans and machines in a manufacturing environment. Part I - Guidelines for the practitioner. *International Journal of lndustrial Ergonomics*, **14**, 3–29.

Moll van Charante, A.W. and Mulder, P.G.H. (1990). Perceptual acuity and the risk of industrial accidents. *American Journal of Epidemiology*, **131**, 652–63.

Mozurkewich, E.L., Luke, B., Avni, M. *et al.* (2000). Working conditions and adverse pregnancy outcome: A meta-analysis. *Obstetrics & Gynecology*, **95**, 623–35.

Murrell, K.F.H. (1965). *Ergonomics - Man in his working environment.* Chapman & Hall, London.

National Research Council, & Institute of Medicine. (2001). *Musculoskeletal disorders and the workplace: Low back and upper extremities.* Panel on Musculoskeletal Disorders and the Workplace. Commission on Behavioral and Social Sciences and Education. National Academy Press, Washington, D.C.

Nuwayhid, I.A. (2004). Occupational health research in developing countries: A partner for social justice. *American Journal of Public Health*, **94**, 1916–21.

Oborne, D.J., Branton, R., Leal, F. *et al.*(1993). *Person-centred ergonomics. A Brantonian view of human factors.* Taylor & Francis, London.

Omer, H. and Everly, G.S. (1988). Psychological factors in preterm labor: Critical review and theoretical synthesis. *American Journal of Psychiatry*, **145**, 1507–13.

Oxenburgh, M., Marlow, P.S.P., and Oxenburgh, A. (2004). *Increasing productivity and profit through health and safety*, 2nd edition. CRC Press, London & Boca Raton, FL, USA.

Park, D.C., Lautenschlager, G., Hedden, T. *et al.* (2002) Models of visuospatial and verbal memory across the adult life span. *Psychology and Aging*, **17**, 299–320.

Parker, S.K. and Griffin, M.A. (2002). What is so bad about a little name-calling? Negative consequences of gender harassment for overperformance demands and distress. *Journal of Occupational Health Psychology*, **7**, 195–210.

Pheasant, S. and Haslegrave, C.M. (2005). *Bodyspace: Anthropometry, ergonomics,and the design of work*, 3rd edition. CRC Press, London & Boca Raton, FL. USA.

Pope, M.H., Andersson, G.B.J., Frymoyer, J.W.*et al.* (eds.) (1991). *Occupational low back pain: Assessment, treatment and prevention*, Mosby-Year Book, Inc., St. Louis, MO.

Punnett, L. and Bergqvist, U. (1997). *Visual display unit work and upper extremity musculoskeletal disorders. A review of epidemiological findings.* National Institute of Working Life, Solna, Sweden.

Punnett, L., Prüss-Üstün, A., Nelson, D.I. *et al.* (2005). Estimating the global burden of low back pain attributable to combined occupational exposures. *American Journal of Industrial Medicine*, **48**, 459–69.

Rabbitt, P.M. (2005). Cognitive gerontology: cognitive change in old age. Introduction. *Quarterly Journal of Experimental Psychology A*, **58**, 1–4.

Rajaratnam, S.M.W. and Arendt, J. (2001). Health in a 24-h society. *Lancet*, **358**, 999–1005.

Ramazzini, B. (1713). *Diseases of workers.* Reprinted (1993) by OH&S Press, Thunder Bay, Canada.

Ranney, D., Wells, R., and Moore, A. (1995). Upper limb musculoskeletal disorders in highly repetitive industries: Precise anatomical physical findings. *Ergonomics*, **38**, 1408–23.

Reason, J. (1990). *Human error.* Cambridge University Press, Cambridge.

Rempel, D.M. and Punnett, L. (2006). Epidemiology of wrist and hand disorders. In *Musculoskeletal disorders in the workplace: Principles and practice* (eds. M. Nordin, G.B.J. Andersson, and M.H. Pope), 2nd edition, pp. 421–30. Mosby-Year Book, Inc., Philadelphia, PA.

Riihimäki, H. (1995). Back and limb disorders. *Epidemiology of work related diseases*, (ed. C. McDonald), pp. 207–38. BMJ Publishing Group, London.

Rodgers, S.H. (1987). Recovery time needs for repetitive work. *Seminars in Occupational Medicine*, **2**, 19–24.

Rossignol, M. (2004). Primary osteoarthritis and occupation in the Quebec national health and social survey. *Occupational and Environmental Medicine*, **61**, 729–35.

Rouch, I., Wild, P., Ansiau, D. *et al.* (2005). Shiftwork experience, age and cognitive performance. *Ergonomics*, **48**, 1282–93.

Salthouse, T.A. (1996). The processing-speed theory of adult age differences in cognition. *Psychological Review*, **103**, 403–28.

Sauter, S.L., Brightwell, W., Colligan, M.J. and NORA Organization of Work Team. (2002). *The changing organization of work and the safety and health of working people. Knowledge gaps and research directions.* National Institute for Occupational Safety and Health (NIOSH), U.S. Department of Health and Human Services, Cincinnati, OH.

Schnall, P., Belkic, K., Landsbergis, P.*et al.* (eds.)(2000). The workplace and cardiovascular disease. *Occupational medicine: State of the art reviews*, Hanley & Belfus, Philadelphia.

Scientific Committee for Musculoskeletal Disorders of the International Commission on Occupational Health (1996). Musculoskeletal disorders: Work-related risk factors and prevention. *International Journal of Occupational and Environmental Health*, **2**, 239–46.

Siegrist, J. (1996). Adverse health effects of high-effort/low-reward conditions. *Journal of Occupational Health Psychology*, **1**, 27–41.

Sluiter, J.K., Rest, K.M., and Frings-Dresen, M.H.W. (2000). *Criteria document for evaluation of the work-relatedness of upper extremity musculoskeletal disorders*. SALTSA Joint Programme for Working Life Research in Europe and Academic Medical Center, University of Amsterdam, Amsterdam.

Stansfeld, S. A. and Matheson, M. P. (2003). Noise pollution: non-auditory effects on health. *British Medical Bulletin*, **68**, 243–57.

Stansfeld, S. and Candy, B. (2006). Psychosocial work environment and mental health--a meta-analytic review. *Scandinavian Journal of Work Environment and Health*, **32**, 443–62.

Steenland K. (2000). Shift work, long hours, and cardiovascular disease: A review. *Occupational Medicine: State of the Art Reviews*, **15**, 7–17.

Sundström-Frisk, C. (1984). Behavioural control through piece-rate wages. *Journal of Occupational Accidents*, **6**, 49–59.

Thurman, J.E., Louzine, A.E., and Kogi K. (1988) *Higher productivity and a better place to work. Action manual & Trainers' manual*. International Labour Organization, Geneva (http://www.ilo.org/public/english/protection/condtrav/workcond/wise/wise.htm).

Torgén, M., Punnett, L., Alfredsson, L. *et al.* (1999). Physical capacity in relation to present and past physical load at work: a study of 484 men and women aged 41 to 58 years. *American Journal of Industrial Medicine*, **36**, 388–400.

Tsutsumi, A., Kayaba, K., Theorell, T. *et al.* (2001). Association between job stress and depression among Japanese employees threatened by job loss in a comparison between two complementary job-stress models. *Scandinavian Journal of Work Environment and Health*, **27**, 146–53.

United Nations (1976). International Covenant on Economic, Social and Cultural Rights (Article 7). Office of the High Commissioner for Human Rights, United Nations, Geneva. (Accessed at http://www.unhchr.ch/html/menu3/b/a_cescr.htm on October 5, 2007.)

Vaaranen, V., Vasama, M., Toikkanen, J. *et al.* (1994). *Ammattitauditi 1993 (Occupational diseases in Finland l993)*. Institute of Occupational Health, Helsinki.

Van Bommel, W.J.M. (2006). Non-visual biological effect of lighting and the practical meaning for lighting for work. *Applied Ergonomics*, **37**, 461–6.

Vernon, H.M. (1921). *Industrial fatigue and efficiency*. Routledge, London.

Viikari-Juntura, E. (1997). The scientific basis for making guidelines and standards to prevent work-related musculoskeletal disorders. *Ergonomics*, **40**, 1097–1117.

Viikari-Juntura, E. and Silverstein, B.A. (1999). Role of physical load factors in carpal tunnel syndrome. *Scandinavian Journal of Work Environment and Health*, **25**, 163–85.

Vingård, E., Hogstedt, C., Alfredsson, L. *et al.* (1991). Coxarthrosis and physical work load. *Scandinavian Journal of Work Environment and Health*, **17**, 14–19.

Wadsworth, E., Dhillon, K., Shaw, C. *et al.* (2007). Racial discrimination, ethnicity and work stress. *Occupational Medicine (London)*, **57**, 18–24.

Wallerstein, N. and Weinger, M. (1992). Health and safety education for worker empowerment. *American Journal of Public Health*, **22**, 619–35.

Waters, T.W., Putz-Anderson, V., Garg, A. *et al.* (1993). Revised NIOSH equation for the design and evaluation of manual lifting tasks. *Ergonomics*, **36**, 749–76.

Wickens, C.D., Lee, J.D., Liu, Y., and Becker, S.E.G. (2004). *An Introduction to Human Factors Engineering (2nd ed.)*. Pearson Prentice Hall, Saddle River NJ, USA.

Winkel, J. and Westgaard, R. (1992). Occupational and individual risk factors for shoulder-neck complaints: Part I - Guidelines for the practitioner. Part II - The scientific basis (literature review) for the guide. *International Journal of Industrial Ergonomics*, **10**, 79–104.

WHO (1985). *Identification and control of work related diseases*. World Health Organisation, Technical Report Series no 714, Geneva.

WHO (2002). *The World Health Report 2002: Reducing risks, promoting healthy life*. World Health Organisation, Geneva.

8.7

Toxicology and risk assessment in the analysis and management of environmental risk

Bernard D. Goldstein

Abstract

Risk-based decision making increasingly has global dimensions, extending from the international management of chemical risks to the sustainable development of our planet. Environmental risk assessment is firmly based on toxicological sciences with input from other public health disciplines. Increasing understanding of how the human genotype and phenotype affects absorption, distribution, metabolism, and excretion of external agents, including foods, is providing insight into answers to the oldest human question about disease: 'Why me?' The risk paradigm components of hazard assessment, dose–response analysis, exposure assessment, and risk characterization, and the toxicological concepts on which they are based, have proven durable in approaching increasingly complex environmental hazards. Newer approaches to managing risk, such as the precautionary principle, and newer challenges ranging from nanotechnology to the health impacts of global climate change, are necessitating more systematic thinking on how best to protect human health and the environment.

Introduction

The goal of this chapter is to synthesize toxicology and risk assessment as a basis for comprehension of human health risks posed by chemical and physical agents in the environment. Disciplines other than toxicology, such as epidemiology and exposure assessment, also are of signal importance to understanding risk, and for many specific chemical and physical agents will provide the major basis for the information underlying risk assessment and risk management.

Environmental risk analysis is a broad field, encompassing risks to ecosystems and materials as well as to human health. Only human health risks will be considered in this chapter. However, the unity of human and environment health is unambiguous. Risk to ecosystems can often serve as a warning about human health risk. As just one example, the concern about the impact of acid deposition on trees and lakes preceded by about two decades the recognition that relatively low atmospheric concentrations of the same fine particulates responsible for acid deposition are a human health risk.

Toxicology has two important roles in environmental risk management: Ascertainment of cause and effect relationships linking chemical and physical agents to adverse effects in humans or the general environment, and the development of techniques capable of preventing these problems. Toxicologists usually approach questions of disease causation by starting with the chemical or physical agent and studying its effects in laboratory animals or in test tube systems. One of the more exciting aspects of modern toxicology is the development of tools, primarily through molecular biology, capable of probing the extent to which a given disease in an individual is caused by a chemical or other environmental factor. This reversal of approach, in which we start with disease and move toward determining the cause, is enabled by the increasing ability of epidemiology to link subtle biological markers indicative of early effects to biological markers indicative of exposure.

Toxicology is also an important discipline in the primary and secondary prevention of human health effects. Understanding the mechanisms by which chemical agents cause biological effects can result in toxicological tests useful to prevent the development of harmful chemicals, or the early detection of potential adverse effects.

General concepts of toxicology relevant to risk assessment

Toxicology is the science of poisons. Knowledge about poisons extends back to the beginning of history as humans became aware of the toxicity of natural food components. The bible contains injunctions concerning poisons, including how to avoid them. Greek and Roman history gives evidence of the use of poisons as an instrument of statecraft, an approach that was extended in the middle ages with such notable practitioners as the Borgias. Toxicologists tend to view Paracelcus, a sixteenth-century alchemist and a bit of a charlatan, as their ancestor, crediting him with the first law of toxicology, that the dose makes the poison. There are two other major maxims that underlie modern toxicology: That chemicals have specific biological effects, a maxim that has been credited to Ambrose Pare (Goldstein & Gallo 2001); and that humans are members of the animal kingdom.

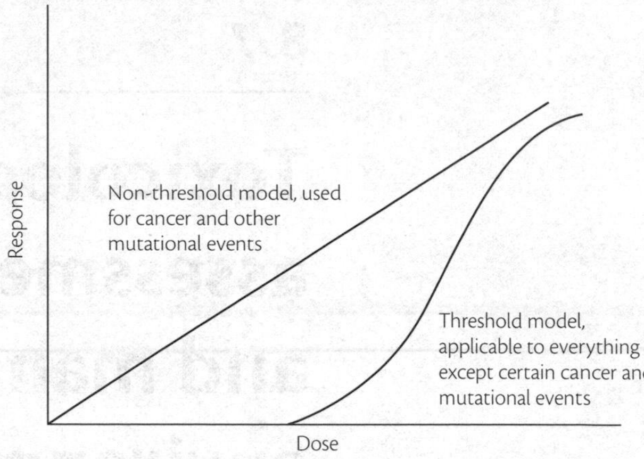

Fig. 8.7.1 Dose–response curve.

The 'laws' of toxicology

The following section discusses 'laws' and general concepts of toxicology pertinent to understanding how a chemical or physical agent acts in a biological system (Table 8.7.1). The focus will be on the biological response, rather than on the intrinsic properties of the agent.

The dose makes the poison

Central to toxicology is the exploration the relation between dose and response. As a generalization, there are two types of dose–response curves (see Fig. 8.7.1). One is an S-shaped curve that is characterized by having at lowest doses no observed effect and, as the dose increases, the gradual development of an increasing response. This is followed by a linear phase of increase in response in relation to dose and, eventually, a dose level at which no further increase in response is observed. Of particular pertinence to environmental toxicology is that this curve presumes that there is a threshold level below which no harm whatsoever is to be expected. There is an ample scientific base for the existence of thresholds for specific effects. For example, if one drop of undiluted sulphuric acid is splashed on the skin it is capable of producing a severe burn. Yet one drop of pure sulphuric acid in a bathtub of water is sufficiently dilute to be without effect. Thresholds for an adverse effect will differ among individuals based upon a variety of circumstances, some of which are genetically determined and others may represent stages of life or specific circumstances. In the example of sulphuric acid on the skin, there are genetically determined differences in susceptibility related to the protective presence of skin hair; babies will be more susceptible than adults; and skin that is already damaged will be at particular risk. This S-shaped dose–response curve is assumed to fit all toxic effects except those that are produced by direct reaction with genetic material.

The second general type of dose–response curve covers those endpoints caused by persistent changes in the genes. This occurs in cancer, in which a somatic mutation occurring in a single cell results in a clone of cancer cell progeny, or in inherited mutations of the genetic components of cells involved in reproduction. It is believed that a single change in DNA can alter the genetic code in such a way to lead to a mutated cell. It therefore follows that any single molecule of a carcinogenic chemical, or packet of physical energy such as ionizing radiation, that can alter DNA is theoretically capable of causing a persistent mutation. The presumption that every single molecule or ionizing ray has the possibility of changing a normal cell to a cancerous cell implies that there is no absolutely safe dose. The resultant dose–response curve starts at a single molecule, i.e. it has no threshold below which the risk is zero. As a further simplification, the shape of the curve can be linearly related to dose in that the risk of two molecules of a DNA-altering chemical causing a mutation is conceivably twice that of one molecule, and so on until a dose level results in dead cells.

Table 8.7.1 The three 'laws' of toxicology

◆	The dose makes the poison
◆	Chemicals have specific effects
◆	Humans are animals

Specificity of effects

That chemical and physical agents have specific effects is in essence no different than recognizing that possession of a gun does not make one a murder suspect if the victim has been stabbed to death. The law of specificity is well understood by the general public in terms of drugs: Aspirin will help with your headache but is useless for constipation, while laxatives have the opposite effect. However, various surveys suggest that the selectivity of effects of environmental chemicals is not well understood by the lay public; many believing that a chemical that can cause cancer in a particular organ can cause cancer and other diseases anywhere in the body.

The specificity of effects is due both to chemistry and to biology. Understanding the relationship between chemical structure and biological effect has been central to both pharmacology and toxicology. Structure activity relationships (SAR) are often used as a means to design a chemical with a specific effect that might be useful as a therapeutic agent. SAR is also used to predict whether a new chemical being readied for manufacture might be of potential harm. While SAR is a useful tool which is being improved through modern computational approaches, its predictive value remains too limited to be used without recourse to additional testing of a potentially toxic agent. For example, only one simple methyl group separates toluene from benzene, with only the latter causing bone marrow damage and leukaemia; ethanol from methanol, the latter causing metabolic acidosis and renal failure; and hexane from either n-heptane or n-pentane, with only n-hexane being responsible for peripheral nerve damage. These examples of specificity reflect both the formation of toxic metabolites, such as active species derived from the metabolism of benzene, and the interaction of a chemical or its metabolite within specific biological niches, such as the diketone metabolite of n-hexane within neuronal axons.

Specificity of effects is also conferred by cellular processes that lead certain cells to be more of a target to environmental agents. For example, red blood cells have an iron-containing protein known as haemoglobin that is responsible for the delivery of oxygen. Toxicity through alteration of efficient oxygen delivery occurs through certain specific mechanisms. One is through the oxidation of the reduced ferrous form to the ferric form of iron, known as methaemoglobin, which can no longer carry oxygen. This occurs with a limited number of agents or their metabolites that once within the red blood cell are capable of oxidizing intracellular iron. Another specific mechanism of interference with oxygen delivery by haemoglobin is exemplified by carbon monoxide. This otherwise relatively inert gas has a physical chemistry that sufficiently resembles oxygen so that it is able to tightly combine with the oxygen combining site of haemoglobin, thereby displacing oxygen. There are many other examples in which in essence a normal body process is disrupted by an exogenous chemical through a specific chemical alteration, such as oxidation or covalent addition, or by fitting into a niche designed through evolution to accommodate a necessary internal chemical which it superficially resembles.

Humans are animals

The conceptual foundation for extrapolating from animals to humans is a central facet of modern toxicology. The basic principles of cell function are common to all of biology. All cells must obtain energy, build structure, and release waste. Cell function in complex organisms such as humans is highly specialized, but there is still a great deal of similarity in cellular and organ function among mammals facilitating extrapolation of effects from one species to another. In general, the specificity of toxic effects is relatively similar across mammals, e.g. a kidney poison in one species is likely to be a kidney poison in another, although there are certainly exceptions. However, dose–response considerations often vary substantially, reflecting differences in adsorption, distribution, metabolism, excretion, function, and target organ susceptibility among species. Understanding the factors responsible for inter-species differences greatly facilitates extrapolation from animals to humans. Once elucidated, the role of different absorption rates, metabolism, or other factors can be taken into account, often through a mathematical approximation that has come to be called physiologically based pharmacokinetics (or toxicokinetics). One of the greatest threats to the public health value of toxicological sciences comes from animal rights activists who intentionally ignore the major positive impact of animal toxicology on the well-being and lifespan of animals, including pet dogs and cats.

Pathways of exogenous chemicals within the body

The four major processes governing the impact of an exogenous chemical within the human body are absorption, distribution, metabolism, and excretion. All can vary greatly among different individuals, and within the same individual depending upon stage of life and circumstances. These variations are among the major reasons for differences among humans in susceptibility to risks due to exposure to chemical and physical agents. The increased understanding of how the human genotype and phenotype affects absorption, distribution, metabolism, and excretion of external agents, including foods, is providing insight into answers to the oldest human question about disease: 'Why is this happening to me?' (Omenn 2000).

Absorption

Absorption of a chemical into the body occurs through ingestion, inhalation, and across the skin. Depending upon the specific chemical, the route of exposure can have major implications on the extent of absorption and the resultant toxicity. For example, almost 100 per cent of inhaled lead-containing fine particles are absorbed into the body as compared to a much smaller percent of ingested lead. Internal factors also can affect absorption, particularly from the gastrointestinal tract. In the case of lead absorption, iron and calcium deficiencies, which are common in children in inner city areas where lead is prevalent, both produce an increase in absorption of ingested lead. The matrix of the exposure agent also may have an effect. For example, the rate at which benzene in gasoline is absorbed through the skin will likely be increased by oxygenated components of the gasoline mixture; and the absorption of dioxins from contaminated soil can vary enormously (Umbreit *et al.* 1986). Often, a single route of absorption is dominant. But, in many instances, more than one route is important. For example, exposure to chlorinated disinfection products in drinking water systems, or gasoline contamination of well water through a leaky underground storage tank, is usually thought of solely in terms of the ingestion of water. However, during showering there is likely to be both inhalation and transdermal absorption, and if groundwater is contaminated there can be offgassing from soil into the home. Epidemiological studies of the potential adverse consequences of water contamination need to take all of these exposure routes into account (Arbuckle *et al.* 2002).

Distribution

Once inside the body, distribution of the chemical occurs through different pathways. In part, this depends upon the route of absorption. Most compounds absorbed in the gastrointestinal tract go directly to the liver and may go no further, while inhaled agents first go to the lung or other parts of the respiratory tract. Distribution also depends upon the chemical and physical properties of the agents. Small particles tend to be distributed deep within the respiratory tract while larger particles get filtered out in the nose or upper respiratory tract. Chemicals that are poorly soluble in water, e.g. oils, usually distribute within fatty tissues. Only certain types of compounds are able to penetrate from the blood to the brain. Distribution will often depend upon organ-specific factors, such as a specific pump located in the thyroid gland that facilitates uptake of iodine and which makes the thyroid particularly vulnerable to the adverse impact of radioactive iodine.

Metabolism

Metabolism in the narrowest sense of the term refers to alteration of chemicals by the body. The major metabolic function of the body is to alter food into energy or structural materials. Metabolism of xenobiotics is often protective, converting unwanted absorbed materials into chemical forms that are readily excretable. Thus, a fat soluble agent can often be converted into water-soluble agents capable of being excreted in the urine. However, for certain classes of chemicals, metabolism is central to toxicity through conversion of relatively inactive compounds into harmful agents. Various carcinogens, including polycyclic organic hydrocarbon components of soot and the leukemogen benzene, require metabolic activation.

All organs appear to have metabolic capability, often related both to organ function and to susceptibility to toxic agents. Understanding the specifics of the enzyme and enzyme families responsible for metabolism within cell types is important to the question of why chemicals have specific effects in specific organs.

Genomics and proteomics applied to metabolism is often known as 'metabolomics'. In the case of benzene, about 50 per cent of the body burden is exhaled unmetabolized and about 50 per cent is metabolized into potentially toxic metabolites. Slowing down benzene metabolism leads to an increase in the relative amount that is exhaled rather than metabolized, and thus a decrease in bone marrow toxicity An apparent genetically-determined increase in benzene metabolism to toxic metabolites, or a decrease in the detoxification of these metabolites, increases hematological risk in humans—with both polymorphisms together appearing to be at least additive and perhaps multiplicative in increasing risk (Rothman *et al.* 1997; Kim *et al.* 2007).

Excretion

Excretion from the body can occur through a variety of different routes, primarily the gastrointestinal tract for unabsorbed compounds and for compounds dissolved in bile; and the urine for water soluble agents of appropriate molecular weight and charge. Significant loss of volatile compounds can occur through the respiratory tract. Other routes of excretion include sweat and lactation, the latter unfortunately putting the infant at risk.

Risk assessment

Risk assessment has evolved from two separate streams of toxicological reasoning: Originally for toxic agents implicitly or explicitly assumed to have a threshold; and then for carcinogens. The safety assessment of chemicals developed from simplified approaches such as studies on laboratory animals in which the dose capable of killing 50 per cent of the animals (the LD50) was determined. This observed dose was used as a basis for extrapolating to permissible levels in humans, often using three separate ten-fold 'safety factors'. These protective factors were based on the concern that humans could be more sensitive as a species than were the laboratory animals; that there was a greater variability in sensitivity among humans than among genetically inbred laboratory animals all raised in a similar environment; and that there would be adverse non-lethal effects that should be avoided. More recently, a presumptive ten-fold safety factor has been added specifically to protect children in recognition of their greater risk to certain chemicals (National Research Council 1993).

The inherent assumption in the 'safety factor' approach is that there is a threshold dose level below which there are no adverse effects. As discussed above, increased understanding of the mechanisms of carcinogenesis has led to the recognition that a single mutation could be the basis for the entire cancer process. As each molecule of a carcinogen at least theoretically could cause this mutation, a threshold could not be assumed, and, as a simplification, there is no level of exposure that is without risk, however tiny.

Almost all DNA damage is repaired by efficient cellular processes. Some unrepaired mutations are lethal to the cell—as dead cells do not reproduce they cannot be the basis for cancer or for inherited abnormalities. The majority of mutations are silent in that they have no discernible effects. Accordingly, the risk of any one molecule actually causing cancer is infinitesimally small—literally trillions of molecules of carcinogens are inhaled with every cigarette, yet only a minority of cigarette smokers develop cancer. Yet, the assumption that the risk is not zero has a major impact on communicating to the public about cancer risk due to chemical and physical carcinogens.

There are circumstances in which cancer causation does depend upon exceeding a threshold level of a chemical (e.g. the mechanism by which saccharin causes bladder cancer in laboratory animals appears to proceed through the precipitation of saccharin in the bladder which requires a dose sufficient to exceed the physicochemical processes determining saccharin solubility). However, the prudent management of cancer risk usually assumes that the carcinogen is 'guilty until proven innocent' of having no risk-free level. In essence, the burden of proof is on industry to scientifically demonstrate that their cancer-causing chemical does have a threshold.

In the late 1970s, the US Environmental Protection Agency (EPA) developed a Carcinogen Assessment Group that developed many of the basic approaches to cancer risk assessment now in use. Three concurrent and related events led to the adoption of formal approaches to risk assessment by EPA and other federal agencies. Some of these agencies, such as the FDA, had their own risk assessment processes, with FDA's exploration of the safety of food additives under the leadership of Dr Arnold Lehman being particularly of note (Stirling & Junod 2002). The three events were:

(1) In 1980, a US Supreme Court decision narrowly overturned OSHA's attempt to develop a more stringent benzene standard following OSHA's recognition that benzene was a carcinogen. The court's decision called for a risk assessment as a means to determine the extent of harm on which the agency should base its decision.

(2) The original appointee of President Reagan to head the EPA resigned in disgrace in 1983, in part because of the perception that she had distorted scientific findings in order to favour her political positions.

(3) The NAS released its report, known as the Red Book, that laid out a formal process for the assessing of risks (NRC 1983).

The definitions of the four major components of risk assessment are shown in Table 8.7.2.

Table 8.7.2 Components of risk assessment

(1) Hazard identification: The determination of whether a specific chemical or physical agent is causally linked to a specific endpoint of concern; i.e. specificity, or the second law of toxicology.
(2) Dose–response evaluation: The determination of the relation between the magnitude of exposure and the probability of occurrence of the specific endpoint of concern; i.e. the dose makes the poison, or the second law of toxicology.
(3) Exposure evaluation: The determination of who and how many people will be exposed; through which routes; and the magnitude, duration, and timing of the exposure.
(4) Risk characterization: The description of the nature and often the magnitude of the human risk, including attendant uncertainty.

Hazard identification

Hazard is an intrinsic property of a substance or situation. Risk depends on both hazard and exposure; e.g. rattlesnakes are intrinsically hazardous to humans, garter snakes are not—but if one is living in an area with no rattlesnakes there is no exposure and therefore no risk. Hazard for a specific endpoint can be related to exposure of the target organ; e.g. asbestos is a hazard for lung cancer as inhaled fibres get into the lung, but asbestos is not thought to be a hazard for liver cancer as asbestos fibres are unlikely to penetrate the GI tract to the liver.

A weight of evidence approach is often used by regulatory and quasi-scientific bodies to identify a hazard. In essence, a panel of scientists is asked to judge whether sufficient evidence exists to identify an agent or condition as having a risk of a specific effect in humans, or in some other target such as an ecosystem. The US approach to permitting the marketing of a new chemical is to have an internal EPA scientific group review the chemical structure and other data submitted by industry. Similarly, FDA relies heavily on an advisory committee process to review evidence of efficacy and toxicity before approving a new pharmaceutical agent or medical device.

Formal weight-of-evidence approaches have been particularly useful in evaluating potential human carcinogens. One well-known process for hazard identification for of a carcinogen is that of the International Agency for Research on Cancer (IARC) of the World Health Organization. IARC convenes expert panels that during a week-long meeting evaluate the evidence for carcinogenicity of specific chemical compounds or defined mixtures (e.g. diesel fuel, wood dust). The effort is focused on the weight of the evidence for carcinogenicity based upon carefully framed criteria considering animal toxicology, epidemiology, mechanistic information, and exposure data—but not on the potency of the compound as a cancer causing agent. IARC has recently increased the weight it places on understanding toxicological mechanisms in assigning its score (Cogliano 2004). This information is used internationally to decide governmental regulatory approaches at the workplace or general environment. In the United States, the IARC ranking has no official status but carries much weight with US regulators as does a similar process used by the National Toxicology Program for its semi-annual Report on Carcinogens (National Toxicology Program 2007).

Note that relatively few chemicals are capable of causing cancer in humans. Of the perhaps 70 000–1 00 000 chemicals in commerce, well less than one hundred are known human carcinogens. To a large extent this represents the success of environmental health science in providing tools that guide chemical manufacturers away from new chemicals that are potentially carcinogenic. Early application in the chemical development process of simple test batteries evaluating the potential for mutagenesis or other predictors of cancer causation provides a responsible chemical industry with the means to avoid producing carcinogens or other potentially harmful products—and the means to avoid the regulatory and toxic tort consequences of harming the public. The value of this primary preventive approach depends upon the availability of effective toxicological test batteries. Such tests are based upon a basic understanding of the chemical and biological processes underlying toxic effects. Unfortunately, the investment in using standardized test batteries for high production volume chemicals, and the major increase in such investments due to the new EU REACH legislation (see below) has not been accompanied by recognition of the need to develop better and more effective tests to protect the public. Newer advances in molecular toxicology provide many opportunities to improve these test batteries (NAS 2007).

A key issue facing risk management is how to proceed in the presence of hazard data with no evidence of toxicity. Rapid advances in analytical chemistry coupled with the fragmentation of authority, at least in the United States, among different environmental agencies, has made this issue particularly challenging. The CDC National Center for Environmental Health Division of Laboratory Sciences is perhaps the world's leading analytical laboratory capable of detecting ever smaller amounts of an increasing number of chemicals in blood and other biological fluids. This analytical capacity for blood and urine samples has been coupled to the National Health and Nutrition Examination (NHANES) survey which also provides medical and sociodemographic information (Centers for Disease Control and Prevention 2005). This work provides an opportunity for surveillance for environmental exposures that is of major public health significance. Environmental organizations have emphasized the importance of body burden to risk management (e.g. see Environmental Working Group 2007). However, the health impact, if any, of our body burden for most of these chemicals remains unknown. The disclaimer language of the CDC report puts it very well:

> *The measurement of an environmental chemical in a person's blood or urine does not by itself mean that the chemical causes disease. Advances in analytical methods allow us to measure low levels of environmental chemicals in people, but separate studies of varying exposure levels and health effects are needed to determine which blood or urine levels result in disease* (Centers for Disease Control and Prevention 2005).

Unfortunately, there appears to be little coordination with the National Institute of Environmental Health Sciences or with the US Environmental Protection Agency to obtain these needed studies, reflecting the fragmentation of the US federal approach to environmental risk.

Dose–response evaluation

The key issues in dose–response evaluation involve how to extrapolate from the high doses at which an effect is observed in an animal or epidemiological study, to the usually much lower levels of risk which are of public or policy concern. Crucial to extrapolation are assumptions about the shape of the dose–response curve, i.e. threshold, linear non-threshold, sublinear, or supralinear. It must be emphasized that the levels of risk desired by our society, for example in the range of one in ten thousand to one in one million lifetime, are usually too low to be scientifically verifiable. This is particularly true as the endpoints of concern cannot be solely attributed to the environmental hazard under consideration. The following example is given in part to justify my contention that environmental risk assessment primarily is aimed at approaching problems of broad societal concern at risk levels too low to be scientifically verifiable. It also provides an opportunity to give an example of a risk assessment.

Based upon extrapolation from both epidemiologic and animal studies, the potency of benzene is estimated by the USEPA to result in a range of 2.2–7.8 in one million increase in the lifetime risk of leukaemia of an individual who is exposed for a lifetime to 1 μg/m^3 benzene in air (USEPA 2007). A reasonable average benzene outdoor level for the US population is approximately 3 μg/m^3, which would predict a risk of 6.6–23.4 in one million lifetime caused by this benzene exposure. Regulatory approaches that decrease that outdoor background level by two-thirds to 1.0 μg/m^3 benzene nationwide would be estimated to decrease the risk of benzene-induced leukaemia by two-thirds. This would mean that nationwide there would be 4.4–15.6 less cases of leukaemia lifetime for every one million Americans, or approximately 10 in one million lifetime. Assuming a 70-year lifetime, and 350 million Americans, one can estimate that there would be 50 fewer cases of leukaemia a year nationwide as a result of a two-thirds decrease in outdoor benzene levels. This is a very small percent of the 24 800 new cases of leukaemia in 2007 estimated by the American Cancer Society. While preventing that number of leukaemia cases is socially desirable, there are no current epidemiological or animal toxicology methods that could scientifically validate these assumptions. Note the further complication that our unregulated and highly variable indoor exposure to benzene, as well as to many other volatile organic compounds, far exceeds outdoor exposure for most of the US population. In fact, the major reason for a decrease in personal benzene exposure in the US has been the decline in cigarette smoking for smokers, and its restriction from public places for non-smokers.

The challenge posed by extrapolation from animals to humans is increasingly being met by advances in understanding of the dynamics of absorption, distribution, metabolism, and excretion of external chemicals in humans, including the use of 'metabolomics'. The ability to use metabolomics and toxicokinetics to increase understanding of the relevance of animal data to human dose–response evaluation enhances the value of animal toxicology for dose–response evaluation.

Exposure evaluation

Exposure evaluation is central to the management of environmental risks. Understanding the pathways of exposure allows interdiction of the exposure pathway—prevention of human exposure to a harmful chemical is synonymous with prevention of human risk. New advances in the field of exposure science are beginning to have major impact in our understanding and preventing risk. These advances are particularly crucial to understanding aggregate and cumulative risk (USEPA 2003; International Life Sciences Institute 1999). Aggregate risk takes into account the different pathways of exposure for the same chemical (see 'Distribution', above). Cumulative risk describes the multiple effects of different agents through different routes, in essence an assessment of the impact of the soup of external synthetic and natural chemicals in which we all live. Cumulative risk assessment is particularly pertinent to environmental justice considerations.

The central importance of exposure assessment in understanding risk is exemplified by investigations of potential adverse health consequences due to inhalation of pollutants resulting from the World Trade Center terrorist event. Careful evaluation of disease endpoints in relation to exposure pathways is central to unravelling the highly political and litigious issue of whether responders or the general public have an increased incidence of disease from inhaling the dust generated by the explosion or the clean up. New protocols and tools to assess exposure resulting from man-made or natural disasters are being developed (Lioy *et al.* 2006).

Risk characterization

Many challenges are presented through the seemingly straightforward process of characterizing the risk estimated through the hazard identification, dose–response evaluation, and exposure evaluation steps. First, those doing the characterization are given an opportunity to put their 'spin' on the findings, e.g. the public is likely to respond differently to the characterization that something is '99 per cent free of risk' than to the numerically equivalent characterization that there is a 'one percent likelihood of a serious consequence including death'. (For a detailed discussion of risk communication, see Chapter 8.8 of this volume, by Baruch Fischhoff.) There is also the challenge of characterizing who is at risk—reporting the risk in terms of the entire exposed general public can trivialize the risk to a highly sensitive subpopulation, such as asthmatics. Further, risk can be displaced from one country to another, as was recently observed when the dumping of hazardous waste, illegally sent from Europe to the Ivory Coast, reported to have caused 9000 acute illnesses and 6 deaths in Abidjan (Greenpeace 2006). Compounding the issue is that the Ivory Coast, not having its own expertise, had to use its scanty funds to hire a European company to retrieve, ship, and process the toxic waste (United Nations Environmental Program 2006).

There is also a long-standing debate on the extent to which numerical uncertainty, rather than a simple qualitative statement of the major sources of uncertainty, should be a routine part of risk characterization. Those in favour of routinely providing numerical boundaries that quantify the extent of uncertainty point out that the many estimates and default assumptions in a risk assessment provide wide ranges of uncertainty that should be presented to the risk manager and the general public. Those in favour of a more restricted use of quantitative uncertainty analysis, including this author, point out that most risk assessments are scoping activities aimed at considering alternatives or developing priorities. Further, major societal decisions are made on numerical estimates for which no uncertainty factors are given (e.g. the gross domestic product, unemployment estimates). There is no disagreement that the qualitative issues underlying uncertainty in a risk analysis should always be transparent to the risk manager and to the affected stakeholders.

The future of risk assessment

Risk assessment as a formal process to evaluate environmental agents has been evolving, particularly during the last few decades where more sophisticated approaches to cancer risk assessment and to cumulative and aggregate risk have developed. Using molecular toxicology to replace standard default assumptions is particularly promising (NAS 2007). Just as in other natural sciences, newer advances in data handling and informatics provide the opportunity to assess larger and more complex databases. Advances in epidemiologic methodology using biological indicators of exposure and effect based upon ecogenetics and other molecular biological techniques should be particularly fruitful (Omenn 2000). Conceptually, our genetic make-up is what loads the gun—but it is the environment that pulls the trigger. Identification of subpopulations sensitive to environmental factors will challenge regulatory and legal interpretation of the many environmental health laws that are aimed at protecting susceptible populations. Global harmonization of risk assessment has been under way for decades and will particularly be needed to avoid the use of environmental health principles as a façade for trade barriers. Attempts are under way to apply to toxicology the formal evidence-based approaches now coming into use in medicine. It will be a challenge to use such processes for risk assessments that depend heavily on extrapolation to levels of risk below those that are readily observable, i.e. the evidence will be indirect. Reviews of recent directions in risk assessment can be found in a series of articles commemorating the twentieth anniversary of the NAS Red Book (Johnson & Reisa 2003) and in Goldstein (2005).

The regulatory approach to protecting worker health from toxic chemicals is often based upon both a measurable workplace standard and a subtle measure of effect. Thus for benzene, there is a 1 ppm time-weighted average workplace air standard as well as a requirement for routine blood counts. The latter informs the former both in terms of whether unmeasured exposures may be occurring, and whether a reconsideration of the allowable external standard is needed. In contrast, environmental standards are almost always measures of external pollutant emissions or ambient levels. Such standards are surrogates for the desired goal of avoiding adverse consequences to human health and the environment. Achieving a level of scientific knowledge that would permit the direct evaluation of subtle biological precursors of adverse effects would be a desired route to develop emission standards that are truly protective. Much work in this area is in progress under the rubric of environmental health indicators.

Human history of protecting against the consequences of environmental agents in essence is the history of catching up on the adverse effects of otherwise beneficial new technology—starting with the human use of fire. One of the more challenging new technologies with potential for beneficial and adverse consequences is that of nanotechnology. Decreasing the size of particles can result in unexpected new physicochemical properties, in part due to a very high surface-to-volume ratio (Helland *et al.* 2007). The debate is unresolved about whether current toxicological testing schemes and regulatory processes are adequate to protect against the potential harm of nanotechnology products.

The precautionary principle and/or/versus risk assessment

The precautionary principle has been advanced as a new approach to environmental risk that, at least to some of its advocates, is a replacement or at least a supplement for risk assessment. Impetus to utilize the precautionary principle was given by the 1992 Rio Declaration on the Environment and Development which provided the definition shown in Box 8.7.1 (United Nations Environmental Programme 1992).

There are many variants of this definition and an extensive literature devoted to developing a more rigorous definition of the precautionary principle. To some, the precautionary principle is merely a means to build more public health protection into quantitative risk analysis, with additional prudent defaults and safety factors to protect at risk populations, and a further focus on uncertainty. To others, the precautionary principle is a new way of addressing environmental risk which is more democratic than risk assessment, better allows for dealing with complexity and uncertainty, and more likely to provide timely and preventive interventions (Martuzzi 2007; Tickner & Ketelson 2001). Some of the important approaches advocated by the precautionary principle, such as transparency and involvement of stakeholders, has also been advocated by many under the rubric of risk assessment and management. For example, the Presidential/Congressional Commission on Risk Assessment and Risk Management (1997), mandated under the 1990 US Clean Air Act amendments, developed a framework for environmental health risk management that has six steps: Formulation of the problem within the context of public or ecosystem health; analysis of the risks; determination of options for risk management; action on the decision; and evaluation of the outcome—all to be performed collaboratively and transparently with stakeholders. Of note is that the precautionary principle puts the burden of proof on corporations to prove the safety of their products rather than on governments or concerned citizens to prove harm. The European Union's advocacy of this principle includes incorporation of a statement in support of the precautionary principle in its founding documents, although without any definition being advanced.

Box 8.7.1 Definition of the precautionary principle in the Rio Declaration on the environment and development

In order to protect the environment, the precautionary approach shall be widely applied by States according to their capabilities. Where there are threats of serious or irreversible damage, lack of full scientific certainty shall not be used as a reason for postponing cost-effective measures to prevent environmental degradation.

Source: United Nations Environmental Programme (1992)

Two examples that provide practical insight into the often confusing debate about the precautionary principle and/or/versus risk assessment are those of the 1990 US Clean Air Act amendments concerning hazardous air pollutants (HAPs), and the new EU legislation that is in the process of redoing how the EU, and the rest of the world, tests the safety of chemicals, known as Registration, Evaluation, Authorisation and Restriction of Chemical Substances (REACH).

The 1990 amendments to the US Clean Air Act provided a complete overhaul of the regulation of hazardous air pollutants (HAPs; in essence all air pollutants other than those for which outdoor air pollutant standards are set, such as ozone and particulates). Previously, the burden of proof was on the government to show that a specific HAP was harmful. Frustration with the torturous process that had regulated relatively few air pollutants led to Congress providing a list of 185 air pollutants that were to be regulated unless an industry was able to prove safety to the satisfaction of EPA, also after a torturous regulatory process—a switch in the burden of proof consistent with the precautionary principle.

Further, the 1990 Clean Air Act amendments replaced risk assessment as the guiding principle for regulatory control of emissions by the requirement for a maximum available control technology for all sources—irrespective of the extent of risk imposed. Although clearly consistent with the precautionary principle, the principle was not mentioned in the debates.

REACH was developed after a long and often rancorous debate, with its proponents focusing on the precautionary principle as a rationale for the new legislation. REACH imposes significant burdens on industry to develop data, assess risk, and provide information about virtually all chemicals in use, including constituents of product mixtures. No distinction is made between newly developed chemicals or those long available in commerce—a contrast with the US Toxic Substances Control Act whose weakness in this regard has led to the inadequate testing of compounds such as methyl tert-butyl ether (MTBE) before their inappropriate release into the environment (Goldstein & Erdal 2000). REACH is heavily dependent upon developing a toxicological data base on virtually every compound and constituent to which exposure might occur. The cost is estimated at about 3–6 billion US dollars over the first 11 years for obtaining the data and registering the compounds. Risk assessment, based on both toxicity and exposure, is used extensively throughout the process, including setting priorities for data needs and making decisions on regulatory approaches. Unfortunately, there is no provision for obtaining the research needed to improve the underlying science on which effective toxicological testing is based.

These two examples suggest that the precautionary principle is both a significant aspect of US regulation, and that even a risk management approach derived so directly from the precautionary principle can be firmly based on risk assessment. Hammitt *et al.* (2005) reviewed EU and US regulations and concluded that despite the great attention given to the precautionary principle in the EU, there is no significant difference in the extent of precaution in US and EU regulations.

In addition to definitional issues, there are other major concerns about the precautionary principle. These are summarized in Table 8.7.3. First, what does the precautionary principle add to standard public health concepts? The precautionary principle is very welcome as an enthusiastic restatement of these concepts which provides an impetus and rallying point for actions that protect public health and the environment, even if nothing new is added to our understanding of the forces responsible for public health action and inaction. Perhaps of greater potential consequence is the treatment of science by some of the major advocates of the precautionary principle, a treatment which at times borders on deconstructionism (Martuzzi 2007; Goldstein 2007). It is true, but also trite and usually trivial, that scientists have values which inform their activities.

Table 8.7.3 Questions about the precautionary principle

◆ What does it add to standard public health concepts?
◆ Is it true that complex scientific questions are unsolvable and, if so, is the precautionary principle needed to act in the face of scientific uncertainty?
◆ In view of its frequent use to justify trade barriers, is it still possible to advocate the precautionary principle as an antidote to biased decision-making?

Even in the face of uncertain science, there is no evidence that the precautionary principle is needed to decrease risk. One example often used of scientific uncertainty for which the precautionary principle is said to be pertinent is that of the health and environmental risks of endocrine disruptors, a particularly challenging problem in view of the need to consider the interactive effects of multiple chemicals with a wide range of additive, synergistic, and antagonistic interactions (Kortenkamp 2007). Yet the United States banned the production of PCBs in 1976 despite the opposition, then and now, of industry on the grounds of uncertain science. The continual decline in body burdens of PCBs and dioxins have been accomplished based on regulatory decisions that were made without recourse to the precautionary principle. Advancing the science needed for decision-making must remain a major goal for environmental public health, including actions taken under the precautionary principle (Foster *et al.* 2000; Goldstein & Carruth 2003; Grandjean *et al.* 2004).

Unfortunately, the precautionary principle has been tainted through misuse by the European Union to justify agricultural trade barriers. The examples go well beyond the US, Canada, and other countries winning well-publicized World Trade Organization judgements against the EU on hormone-treated beef or genetically modified foods—judgements that specifically took the EU to task for using the precautionary principle to replace or ignore public health science. Perhaps most egregious is the EU's use of the precautionary principle to increase the stringency of their aflatoxin standards to well below those of any other nation or international organization (Goldstein 2007). Aflatoxin is produced by a fungus that grows on agricultural produce, particularly when wet. To the benefit of EU agricultural interests, US$700 million/year worth of agricultural produce has been excluded from sub-Saharan Africa, the world's poorest nations,. The FAO/WHO Codex Alimentarius Commission's Joint Expert Committee on Food Additives found no significant health benefit for the more stringent EU aflatoxin standard which, based upon risk analysis, would decrease the amount of cancer in 500 million Europeans by one case every other year. The recent failure of the Doha round of trade talks, a particular loss to sustainable development of less developed countries, has been in part ascribed to the failure of the rest of the world to be willing to trust the EU not to use the precautionary principle to manufacture reasons to avoid free trade in agricultural products. Clearly, the precautionary principle is not a protection against the misuse of science.

The primary missing ingredient in the approach to ever more complex environmental challenges, including such broader issues as global warming, is a systems-based approach incorporating the best science focusing on the most important questions. Unfortunately, the fragmented national and international approaches to environmental issues are producing piecemeal efforts that are falling further behind in protecting public health and the environment. Perhaps the need to respond to the challenges of global climate change will lead to a more systematic international effort.

Conclusions

Understanding the web of environmental cause and effect relations is an increasing challenge in a shrinking globe. Advances in toxicology, filtered through an appropriate appreciation of the optimal approaches to analyse and present risks to an involved public, are crucial to protecting public health and the environment.

References

Arbuckle, T.E., Hrudey, S.E., Krasner, S.W. *et al.* (2002). Assessing exposure in epidemiologic studies to disinfection by-products in drinking water: Report of an international workshop. *Environmental Health Perspectives*, **110** (Suppl 1) 53–60.

Centers for Disease Control and Prevention (2005). *Third national report on human exposure to environmental chemicals*. Atlanta, GA.

Cogliano, V.J. (2004). Current criteria to establish human carcinogens. *Seminars in Cancer Biology*, **14**, 407–12.

Environmental Working Group (2007). *Body burden*. http://www.ewg.org/featured/15. Accessed Dec 9, 2007.

Foster, K.R., Vecchia, P., and Repacholi, M.H. (2000). Science and the precautionary principle. *Science*, **288**, 979–81.

Goldstein, B.D. (2003). Risk characterization and the red book. *Journal of Human and Ecological Risk Assessment* (August 2003 special issue to commemorate the 20th anniversary of the NRC Red Book). **9**, 1283–9.

Goldstein, B.D. (2005). Advances in risk assessment and communication. *Annual Review of Public Health*, **26**, 141–63.

Goldstein, B.D. (2007). Problems in applying the precautionary principle to public health. *Occupational and Environmental Medicine*, **64**, 571–4.

Goldstein, B.D. and Carruth, R.S. (2003). Implications of the precautionary principle to environmental regulation in the United States: Examples from the control of hazardous air pollutants in the 1990 Clean Air Act Amendments. *Law & Contemporary Problems*. **66**, 247–61.

Goldstein, B.D. and Carruth, R.S. (2003). Implications of the precautionary principle: Is it a threat to science? *European Journal of Oncology*, **2**, 193–202.

Goldstein, B.D. and Erdal, S. (2000). MTBE as a gasoline oxygenate: Lessons for environmental public policy. *Annual Review of Energy and the Environment*, **25**, 765–802.

Goldstein, B.D. and Gallo, M.A. (2001) Paré's law: The second law of toxicology. *Toxicological Sciences*, **60**, 194–5.

Grandjean, P., Bailar, J.C., Gee, D. *et al.*(2004) Implications of the Precautionary Principle in research and policy-making. *American Journal of Industrial Medicine*, **45**, 382–5.

Greenpeace (2006). *Toxic waste in Abidjan*. http://www.greenpeace.org/international/news/ivory-coast-toxic-dumping/toxic-waste-in-abidjan-green

Hammitt, J.K., Wiener, J.B. Swedlow, B. *et al.* (2005). Precautionary regulation in Europe and the United States: a quantitative comparison, *Risk Analysis*, 25, 1215–28.

Helland, A., Wick, P., Koehler, A. *et al.* (2007) Reviewing the environmental and human health knowledge base of carbon nanotubes. Environmental Health Perspectives, 115, 1125–31.

International Life Science Institute (1999). *A framework for cumulative risk assessment; Workshop report*. ILSI Risk Science Institute, Washington, DC.

Johnson, B.L.and Reisa, J.J. (2003). Essays in commemoration of the 20th anniversary of the National Research Council's risk assessment in the federal government: Managing the process. *Human Ecological Risk Assessment*, **9**, 1093–9.

Kim, S., Lan, Q., Waidyanatha, S. *et al.* (2007) Genetic polymorphisms and benzene metabolism in humans exposed to a wide range of air concentrations. *Pharmacogenetics and Genomics*, **17**, 789–801.

Kortenkamp, A. (2007). Ten years of mixing cocktails: A review of combination effects of endocrine-disrupting chemicals. *Environmental Health Perspectives*, **115**(Suppl 1), 98–105.

Lioy, P., Pellizzari, E., and Prezant, D. (2006). The World Trade Center aftermath and its effects on health: Understanding and learning through human exposure science. *EnvIronmental Science and Technology*, **40**, 6876–85.

Martuzzi, M. (2007). The precautionary principle: In action for public health. *Occupational and Environmental Medicine*, **64**, 569–70.

National Research Council (1983) *Risk assessment in the federal government: Managing the process*. National Academy Press, Washington, DC.

National Research Council (1993) *Pesticides in the diets of infants and children*. National Academy Press, Washington, DC.

National Research Council (2007). *Toxicity testing in the 21st century*. National Academy Press. Washington, DC.

National Toxicology Program (2007). *Report on carcinogens*. http://ntp.niehs.nih.gov/index.cfm?objectid=72016262-BDB7-CEBA-FA60E922B18C2540 Accessed Dec 1, 2007.

Omenn, G.S. (2000). Public health genetics: an emerging interdisciplinary field for the post-genomic era. *Annual Review of Public Health*, **21**, 1–13.

Presidential/Congressional Commission on Risk Assessment and Risk Management (1997). *Framework on Environmental Health and Risk Management*. Final Report. Vol. 1

Rothman, N., Smith, M.T., Hayes, R.B. *et al.* (1997) Benzene poisoning, a risk factor for hematological malignancy, is associated with the NQO1 609C -->T mutation and rapid fractional excretion of chlorzoxazone. *Cancer Research*, **57**, 2839–42.

Stirling, D. and Junod, S. (2002). Profiles in toxicology: Arnold J. Lehman. *Toxicological Sciences*, **70**, 159–60.

Tickner, J. and Ketelson, L. (2001). Democracy and the precautionary principle. *Science and Environmental Health Network*, **6**, 1–6. http://www.sehn.org/Volume_6-3.html. Accessed Nov 14, 2007

Umbreit, T.H., Hesse, E.J., and Gallo, M.A. (1986). Bioavailability of dioxin in soil from a 2,4,5-T manufacturing site. *Science*, **232**, 497–9.

United Nations Environmental Programme (1992) *Rio Declaration on environment and development*, Principle 15. http://www.unep.org/Documents.Multilingual/Default.asp?DocumentID=78&ArticleID=1163; Accessed, December 22, 2007

United Nations Environmental Programme Press Release (2006). *Liability for Cote d'Ivoire hazardous waste clean-up*. http://www.unep.org/Documents.Multilingual/Default.asp?DocumentID=485&ArticleID=5430&l=en Accessed December 22, 2007

University of Pittsburgh European Union Center of Excellence and Graduate School of Public Health (2007). *REACH, A New EU Approach to Chemical Safety: Lessons for the US*. Conference Chair, BD Goldstein. http://www.ucis.pitt.edu/euce/events/policyconf/07/PDFs/ReachReport.pdf Accessed December 22, 2007

US Environmental Protection Agency *Integrated Risk Information System: Benzene CASRN 71-43-2* http://www.epa.gov/iris/subst/0276.htm#carc; Accessed November 28, 2007

US Environmental Protection Agency (2003). *Framework for Cumulative Risk Assessment*. EPA/630/P-02/001F. Risk Assess. Forum, Washington, DC http://www.epa.gov/fedrgstr/EPA-PEST/1999/November/Day-10/6043.pdf

Woodruff,T.J., Axelrad, D.A., Kyle, A.D. *et al.* (2003). *America's children and the environment. Measures of contaminants, body burdens and illnesses*. US Environmental Protection Agency, EPA 240-R-03-001

8.8

Risk perception and communication

Baruch Fischhoff

Abstract

Public health depends on laypeople's ability to understand the health-related choices that they and their societies face. The study of *risk perception* examines that ability. The study of *risk communication* examines the processes that determine how communication with lay people enhances or degrades their decision-making ability. Although focused on decisions involving risk, that research necessarily considers potential benefits as well, including the benefits of reducing risks (e.g. through medical treatment, lifestyle changes, or improved air quality). Communication is seen as a two-way process. Without listening to people, it is impossible to understand what they know and value, hence impossible to provide them with relevant information in a comprehensible form. The basic science of *behavioural decision research* describes the general processes that find specific expression in risk-related decisions. It provides the conceptual framework, methodology, and theory for this chapter.

Risk perception and communication research is conceptually straightforward. First, characterize the decisions that people face, in sufficiently precise terms to identify the information that is most critical to them. Second, describe people's existing beliefs and values, in sufficiently precise terms to understand their roles in risk-related choices. Third, develop and empirically evaluate communications designed to bridge the critical gaps between what people know and what they need to know, in order to have the best chance of making choices that achieve what they value. These steps are interdependent. For example, descriptive research can reveal unexpected goals, obstacles, and capabilities, forcing revision of the decision analysis; communication failures can force additional research regarding decision-making processes.

Executing a communication research programme requires four kinds of expertise: (a) *subject matter specialists*; (b) *risk and decision analysts*, for characterizing choices and identifying critical information; (c) *behavioural scientists*, for characterizing existing beliefs and values, then designing and empirically evaluating communications; and (d) *communication practitioners*, for executing sustainable programmes. Individuals with each kind of expertise should have final authority in their domain.

Behavioural decision research provides extensive guidance on two topics central to this endeavour. One is identifying potential threats to risk-related decision making, along with an understanding of the underlying behavioural processes that communications must address. The second is the measurement procedures needed to ensure that people have been properly understood, when creating and evaluating communications. Without proper measurement, it is impossible to assess and address people's information needs. A particular risk is underestimating laypeople's decision-making competence, thereby denying them the opportunity for active participation in health decisions. That risk is aggravated when communications are disseminated without proper evaluation, after which their audience is held responsible for failing to understand content that was neither clear nor relevant. One should no more release untested communications than untested pharmaceuticals. The chapter seeks to reduce those risks, while helping experts to help laypeople to choose wisely.

Introduction

Many health risks arise from deliberate decisions by individuals trying to make choices that balance health and other concerns. Some choices are made as individuals. They include whether to wear bicycle helmets and seat belts, whether to read and follow safety warnings, whether to buy and use condoms, and how to select and cook food. Other choices are made as citizens. They include whether to protest the siting of hazardous waste incinerators and halfway houses, whether to support fluoridation and "green" candidates, and whether to allow sex education.

Sometimes, single choices have large effects (e.g. buying a safe car, taking a dangerous job, getting pregnant). Sometimes, small effects accumulate over multiple choices (e.g. exercising, avoiding transfats, wearing seatbelts, using escort services). Sometimes, health-related choices focus on health; sometimes, not (e.g. purchasing homes that require long commutes, choosing friends who exercise regularly, joining religious groups opposed to vaccination).

Making health-related decisions wisely requires understanding the associated risks and benefits. This chapter reviews the research base for characterizing and improving that understanding. Following convention, these are called *risk perception* and *risk communication*, respectively. However, the basic principles also apply to perception and communication regarding the potential benefits of health-related decisions (e.g. lifestyle changes that reduce risks).

Psychologists sometimes reserve 'perception' for direct physiological responses to stimuli, using 'judgement' for the translation of that response into observable estimates. A currently active research topic is identifying the conditions under which judgement surrenders entirely to perception (Lowenstein *et al.* 2001). Perceptions could prevail either when passions run high or when judgement fails to yield satisfactory choices. This chapter emphasizes judgement, hoping to expand the envelope of deliberative processes in personal and public health decisions.

Inaccurate judgements about risks can hurt people. So can inaccurate beliefs about those judgements. If people's understanding is overestimated, then they may face impossibly hard choices (e.g. among unfamiliar medical alternatives, without adequate information). If people's understanding is underestimated, then they may be needlessly denied the right to choose. As a result, the chapter assumes (a) that descriptive statements about people's beliefs must be disciplined by empirical evidence and (b) that evaluative statements about the adequacy of people's understanding must be founded on rigorous analysis of what they need to know, in order to make good choices. To these ends, the chapter emphasizes methodological safeguards against misguided assessments.

The next section, 'Quantitative Assessment', treats judgements about how big risks are. The following section, 'Qualitative Assessment', treats beliefs about the processes that create and control risks, on the basis of which people produce and evaluate quantitative estimates. Both sections address both measurement issues and barriers to understanding. The section on 'Creating Communications' provides a structured approach for developing communications about health-related decisions, focused on individuals' greatest information needs. The 'Conclusion' section considers the strategic importance of risk communication in risk management. Access to research on complementary social and emotional processes might begin with Krimsky and Golding (1992), Peters and McCaul (2005), and Slovic (2001).

Quantitative assessment

Estimating risk magnitude

A common complaint among experts is that 'the public doesn't realize how small (or large) Risk X is'. There is empirical evidence demonstrating examples of such biases (Slovic 2001). However, that evidence has typically been collected in settings designed to reveal biases, in order to help researchers study the processes that create them. As a result, the prevalence and magnitude of bias in published studies need not reflect their prevalence and magnitude in life. Generalizing from research decisions to real-world ones requires matching the conditions in each. Looking at one widely cited study in some detail shows how that matching might proceed, while introducing some general principles and results.

Participants

Lichtenstein *et al.* (1978) asked people to estimate the annual number of deaths in the US from 30 causes (e.g. botulism, tornadoes, motor vehicle accidents). These 'people' were members of the League of Women Voters and their spouses, making them older than the proverbial college sophomores often studied by psychologists. Age might affect *what* people think, as a result of education and experience. It is less likely to affect *how* they think. Many cognitive processes seem to be widely shared, once people pass middle adolescence, unless they suffer some impairment (Fischhoff 2008; Reyna & Farley 2006).

One widely shared class of cognitive processes is relying on judgemental *heuristics*, or rules of thumb, when asked to infer unknown quantities (Gilovich *et al.* 2003; Kahenman *et al.* 1982). One well-known heuristic is *availability*, whereby people assess an event's probability by how easily instances come to mind. Although more available events are often more likely, media coverage (among other things) can make events disproportionately available, inducing biased judgements. How people generate instances, using their memory and imagination, should reflect general cognitive processes. However, the contents of those memories and images should vary with individuals' experiences. So should their trust in information sources—and attempts to adjust for bias.

Lichtenstein *et al.* (1978) elicited judgements with two *response modes*. One asked people to pick the more frequent of two paired causes of death and, then, to estimate the ratio of their frequencies. The second asked people for the number of deaths. It began by giving the answer for one cause (either electrocution or motor vehicle accidents). That *anchor* was designed to provide a feeling for annual death rates—after pretests found that people often knew little about these statistics. Figure 8.8.1 shows results with the second method.

Results

(a) Relative risk judgements were consistent, across the two response modes. Risks given higher frequency estimates were typically judged more likely, when paired with risks given lower frequency estimates. The ratios of the direct estimates were similar to the directly estimated ratios. Thus, these people seemed to have an internal 'scale' of relative risk, which they expressed consistently even with these unfamiliar tasks.

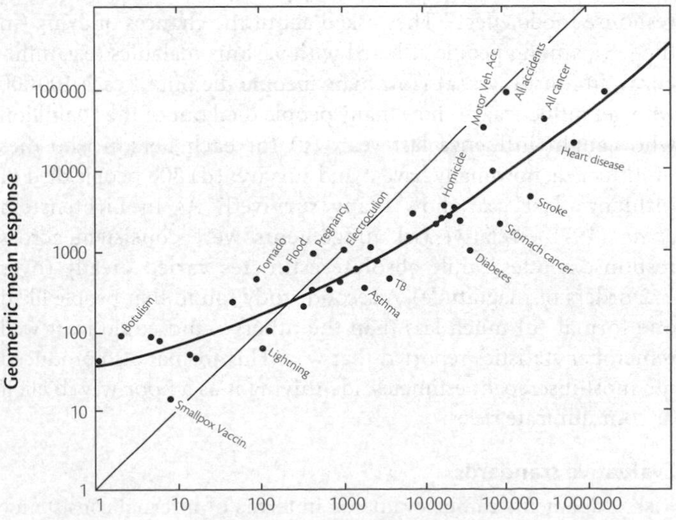

Fig. 8.8.1 Best quadratic fit line to geometric mean judgements of the annual toll from 40 causes of death in the United States, compared to best available statistical estimates.
Source: Lichtenstein *et al.* (1978).

(b) Absolute risk judgements were affected by the anchor. People told that 50 000 people die annually from auto accidents gave estimates two to five times higher than did people told that 1000 die annually from electrocution. Thus, people seemed to have less feeling for absolute frequency, rendering them sensitive to implicit cues in how questions are posed (Poulton 1989; Schwarz 1999).

(c) Absolute risk judgements were less dispersed than the corresponding statistical estimates. While the latter varied over six orders of magnitude, individuals' estimates typically ranged over 3–4. That compression could reflect anchoring, if judgements were drawn toward the value that was given for perspective. Overall, people overestimated small frequencies and underestimated large ones. That pattern might change with different anchors. For example, a lower anchor (e.g. botulism deaths) would, likely, reduce (or even eliminate) overestimation of small frequencies, while increasing underestimation of large ones.

(d) Relative and absolute risk judgements seemed to reflect availability bias. For any statistical frequency, some causes of death consistently received higher estimates (e.g. homicide, tornadoes, flood). These causes were disproportionately reported in the news media and as personal experiences. When told of availability bias, participants could not improve their judgements, consistent with the finding that tracking frequency is an automatic process (e.g. Koriat 1993).

Lichtenstein *et al.* (1978) found some response patterns that were procedure invariant (e.g. relative risk judgements) and some that were not (e.g. absolute estimates). A century of psychophysics research (Poulton 1989) has identified procedural factors that can affect quantitative judgements. Determining their effects in specific settings requires dedicated studies. The practical importance of any bias depends on the decision. Shifting fatality estimates by a factor of 2 might tip some decisions, but not others.

Fischhoff and MacGregor (1983) provide another example of response mode effects. They asked about the chances of dying (in the US), among people afflicted with various maladies (e.g. influenza), in four ways: (a) How many people die out of each 100 000 who get influenza; (b) how many people died out of the 80 million who caught influenza last year; (c) for each person who dies of influenza, how many have it and survive; (d) 800 people died of influenza last year, how many survived? As in Lichtenstein *et al.* (1978), relative risk judgements were consistent across response modes, while absolute estimates varied greatly (over 1–2 orders of magnitude). A second study found that people liked one format (c) much less than the others—and could least well remember statistics reported that way. This format also produced the most discrepant estimates, identifying it as a poor way to elicit or communicate risks.

Evaluative standards

Risk judgements can be evaluated in terms of internal consistency (e.g. whether estimates increase with increasing exposure) or accuracy. Without sound risk estimates (see Chapter 8.7, Toxicology and risk assessment in the analysis and management of environmental risk), one cannot evaluate accuracy. For example, after the 9/11 attacks, some critics claimed that some Americans had increased their risk level by flying, rather than driving. These claims were based on historical risk statistics. However, at that time, no one knew how safe aviation was (the fleet was grounded), while traffic deaths are disproportionately high among the young, elderly, and drinkers—not the drivers who were shifting transportation modes. Even if the historical statistics were valid, decisions involving risks can reflect other factors as well. Any additional risk of driving might have been justified for someone who was financially strapped by the declining economy or wary of flight delays (with added security hassles). Without understanding all elements of a choice, one cannot judge its reasonableness.

Probability judgements

The sensitivity of quantitative judgements to procedural details might suggest avoiding them, in favour of verbal quantifiers (e.g. likely, rare). Unfortunately, such terms have their own problems, namely, being interpreted differently across people and situations, unless usage norms have evolved (Budescu & Wallsten 1995; Schwarz 1999).

Table 8.8.1 shows verbal and quantitative judgements of seven risks, provided by a fairly homogeneous group (US undergraduates). The quantitative response mode explicitly offered probabilities as low as 0.01 per cent—using a linear scale for 1 –100 per cent and expanding 0–1 per cent with log scales from 1:100 to 1:10 000. The qualitative response mode used typical labels (1 = very unlikely; 2 = unlikely; 3 = somewhat unlikely; 4 = somewhat likely; 5 = likely; 6 = very likely). Comparing the two response modes revealed a nonlinear relationship: The median probabilities corresponding to the qualitative responses were 0.01 per cent for 'very unlikely', 0.5 per cent for 'unlikely', 5 per cent for 'somewhat unlikely', 25 per cent for 'somewhat likely', 60 per cent for 'likely', and 96 per cent for 'very likely'.

Some researchers hesitate to elicit probabilities, lest they exceed laypeople's cognitive capabilities. That hesitation is strengthened by (research and anecdotal) evidence of lay innumeracy. However, even imperfect measures can have value, if their strengths and weaknesses are understood. The research literature on probability

Table 8.8.1 Comparison of numerical verbal and statistical risk estimates ('Please estimate your personal risk to the following events in the next 3 years'.)

Risk	Quantitative (Probability) Response (Median %)	Verbal response Median	Verbal response Mean	Statistical risk Estimate (probability in %)
Electrocution	0.1	1.0	1.67	0.015
Cancer	0.3	2.0	2.09	0.06
Flu	55.0	5.0	4.72	86.2
Car Injury	10.0	3.0	3.38	4.7
Herpes	0.1	1.0	1.73	4.1
AIDS virus/sexual	0.02	1.0	1.41	0.2

Source: Linville *et al.* (1993).

elicitation is enormous (O'Hagan *et al.* 2006). Results relevant to public health researchers and practitioners include:

(a) Numeric probability judgements can be as reliable and acceptable to users as verbal ones. Woloshin *et al.* (1998) found this, comparing linear and log-linear probability scales with verbal ones, for judgements of medical events.

(b) People often prefer to provide verbal judgements and to receive quantitative ones. Quantitative responses require more effort and entail greater accountability (Erev & Cohen 1990).

(c) Probability judgements often have good construct validity, correlating sensibly with other variables. For example, Fischhoff *et al.* (2000) found higher probabilities of pregnancy among US teens reporting more sexual activity and high probabilities of being arrested among teens reporting more violent lives.

(d) Misinformation and mistaken inferences can bias probability judgements. For example, availability can contribute to unwarranted optimism. Our own carefulness (e.g. in avoiding traffic accidents or bad investments) is more 'available' to us than is that of others.

(e) Probability judgements can be deliberately biased, when people respond strategically. For example, Christensen-Szalanski and Bushyhead (1993) found physicians overestimating the probability of pneumonia, perhaps fearing that the healthcare system would ignore unlikely cases. Probability of precipitation forecasts may show an 'umbrella bias', overstating chances, to keep people from being caught unprotected (Lichtenstein *et al.* 1982).

(f) Transient emotions can affect judgements. For example, anger increases optimism, fear the opposite (Lerner & Keltner 2001), with effects large enough to tip close decisions.

(g) Judgements for the probability of being correct are moderately correlated with actual knowledge. For example, Fischhoff *et al.* (1977) elicited probabilities for successfully choosing the larger of two causes of death (from Lichtenstein *et al.* 1978). Correct choices received higher probabilities. Overall, people were *overconfident* (e.g. with 75 per cent correct choices, when 90 per cent confident). Overconfidence is typical with hard tasks, underconfidence with easy ones.

(h) Probability judgements can vary by response mode. Differences have been found with odds and probabilities, probabilities and relative frequencies, and judgements of individual or grouped items (Griffin *et al.* 2003).

(i) Some numerical values are treated specially. For example, people seldom use fractional values (motivating the log-linear scale); when uncertain what to say, people sometimes offer 50, meaning 50–50 and not a numeric probability (Bruine de Bruin *et al.* 2000).

(j) Probability judgement processes mature by middle adolescence. For example, teens show no greater optimism bias than adults, despite the common belief in adolescent invulnerability (Quadrel *et al.* 1993). Fischhoff *et al.* (2000) found that teens, unlike adults, greatly exaggerate the probability of premature death.

(k) There are stable individual differences in the ability to use probabilities. They correlate with performance on other tasks, as well as life outcomes that might reflect decision-making competence (Bruine de Bruin *et al.* 2007).

(l) The use of probabilities can sometimes be taught. Lichtenstein and Fischhoff (1980) found improvement after a single round of intense feedback.

A test of any measure is its predictive validity. Even though risk decisions often involve choices among options with non-risk consequences, Brewer *et al.* (2007) found that risk judgements alone sometimes have predictive value. In the contexts of smoking (Viscusi 1992) and breast cancer (Black *et al.* 1995), researchers argue that advertising has worked too well, leading to exaggerated fears, a claim supported by unduly high probability judgements (even after deleting apparently non-numeric 50s).

Defining risk

Studies like Lichtenstein *et al.* (1978) measure risk perceptions, if 'risk' means 'chance of death'. However, even among experts, 'risk' has multiple meanings (Fischhoff *et al.* 1984; National Research Council 1996). For those who focus on fatalities, 'risk' might be measured in probability of death, expected life years lost, total deaths, or deaths per person exposed (or per hour of exposure). Each definition entails an ethical position. For example, *life-years lost* places extra weight on deaths of young people, whereas *probability of death* disregards age. Focusing on lost life expectancy increases concern for deaths by injury (e.g. drowning, driving, workplace hazards), relative to deaths from the cumulative effects of chronic illnesses. Adding morbidity and psychological trauma would heighten concern for alcohol and illegal drugs, which can ruin lives without ending them.

Unless such definitional issues are recognized, people can unwittingly speak past one another, when addressing 'risks'. Clarifying definitional issues has been central to risk research. Before reviewing some results, it is worth noting that 'risk' is sometimes used as a discrete variable, treating activities as risky or not. That shorthand says little, without knowing the threshold of concern. Calls for 'safe' products can be unfairly ridiculed, by treating them as demanding zero-risk. Critics of cost-benefit analysis have offered various *precautionary principles*, for avoiding risks too uncertain to countenance. However, they have limited use until one specifies the threshold of concern and procedures for assessing compliance (DeKay *et al.* 2002).

Catastrophic potential

One early risk perception study asked experts and laypeople to estimate the US 'risk of death' from 30 activities and technologies (Slovic *et al.* 1979). These judgements correlated more strongly with statistical estimates of average-year fatalities for experts than for laypeople. However, when asked to estimate average-year fatalities, laypeople responded like experts. Inspection suggested that laypeople interpreted 'risk of death' to include catastrophic potential, reflecting the expected deaths in non-average years. If so, then experts and laypeople agreed about routine deaths (which have relatively good scientific estimates) and disagreed about possible anomalies (for which the science is much weaker). Such potentially reasonable disagreement would be obscured by the casual assumption that any disagreement between experts and laypeople reflects lay ignorance (National Research Council 1989).

The moral principle underlying this definitional disagreement could mean valuing deaths more when lost at once than when lost individually. Slovic *et al.* (1984) found, however, that catastrophic potential worries people because it suggests technologies that might spin out of control. An aversion to deep uncertainty should be less controversial.

Dimensions of risk

Beginning with Starr (1969), many features, like uncertainty and catastrophic potential, have been suggested as affecting definitions of risk. In order to reduce the set to manageable size, Fischhoff *et al.* (1978) had members of a liberal civic organization rate 30 hazards on nine such features. Factor analysis on mean ratings identified two *dimensions*, accounting for 78 per cent of the variance. Similar patterns emerged with students, members of a conservative civic organization, members of a liberal women's organization, and risk experts. Figure 8.8.2 plots factor scores within the common factor space for these four groups.

Hazards high on the vertical factor (e.g. food colouring, pesticides) were rated as new, unknown, and involuntary, with delayed effects. Hazards high on the horizontal factor (e.g. nuclear power, commercial aviation) were rated as fatal to many people, if things go wrong. The factors were labelled *unknown* and *dread*, respectively. They might be seen as capturing the cognitive and emotional bases of people's concern, respectively.

Many studies, using this 'psychometric paradigm' have found roughly similar dimensions, despite differing elicitation mode, scaling techniques, items, and participants (Slovic 2001). When a third dimension emerges, it appears to reflect the scope of the threat, labelled *catastrophic potential.* Hazards' position in the space correlates with attitudes toward them, such as the desired stringency of regulation. Analyses of mean responses are best suited to predicting aggregate (societal) responses. Individual differences have also been studied (e.g. Vlek & Stallen 1981).

Risk comparisons

The multidimensionality of risk means that hazards similar on some dimensions may still evoke (and deserve) quite different responses. This fact is neglected in appeals to accept a risk because one has accepted another risk with some similarities (Fischhoff *et al.* 1984). Such risk comparisons sometimes present many hazards, in quantities posing equal statistical risks (e.g. both a tablespoonful of peanut butter and 50 years living by a nuclear power plant create a one-in-a-million risk of premature death). Box 8.8.1 shows such potential flaws in risk comparisons.

One way to improve the legitimacy of risk comparisons is to involve users in setting them. Following this strategy, the US Environmental Protection Agency (1993) promoted some 50 regional, state, and national risk-ranking exercises, in which citizens deliberated priorities on dimensions of their choosing, supported by technical staff providing relevant analyses. Participants' freedom to choose dimensions made individual exercises more relevant, while reducing comparability across exercises. Florig *et al.* (2001) developed a method for standardizing such comparisons, based on the risk dimensions research (Table 8.8.2). The UK government has endorsed a variant (HM Treasury 2005).

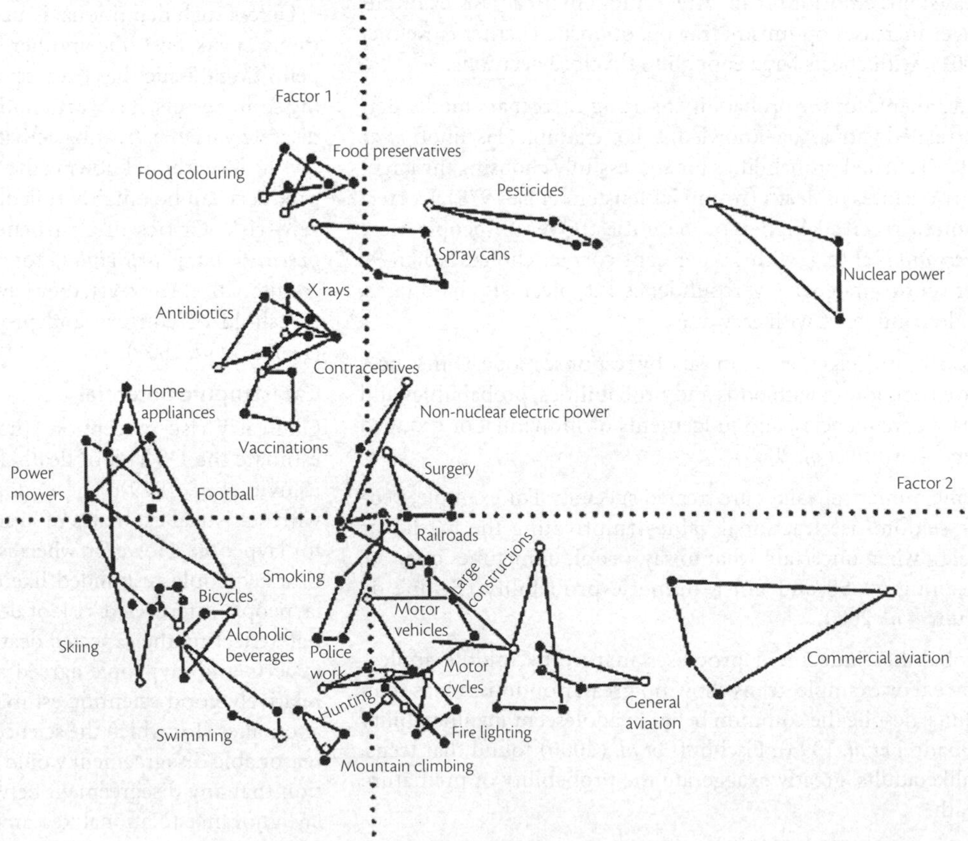

Fig. 8.8.2 Location of 30 hazards within the two-factor space obtained from League of Women Voters, student, active Club, and expert groups. Respondents evaluated each activity or technology on each of nine features. Ratings were subjected to principal components factor analysis, with a varimax rotation. Connected lines join or enclose the loci of four group points for each hazard. Open circles represent data from the expert group. Unattached points represent groups that fall within the triangle created by the other three groups. *Source*: Slovic *et al.* (1985).

Box 8.8.1 Risk comparisons

One . . . legitimate purpose [for risk comparisons] is giving recipients an intuitive feeling for just how large a risk is by comparing it with another, otherwise similar, risk that recipients understand. For example, roughly one American in a million dies from lightning in an average year (NOAA 1995). 'As likely as being hit by lightning' would be a relevant and useful comparison for someone who has an accurate intuitive feeling for the probability of being hit by lightning, faces roughly that 'average' risk, and considers the comparison risk to be like death by lightning in all important respects. It is not hard to imagine each of these conditions failing, rendering the comparisons irrelevant or harmful:

(a) Lightning deaths are so vivid and newsworthy that they might be overestimated relative to other, equally probable events. But 'being struck by lightning' is an iconic very-low-probability risk, meaning that it might be underestimated. Where either occurs, the comparison will mislead.

(b) Individual Americans face different risks from lightning. For example, they are, on the average, much higher for golfers than for nursing-home residents. A blanket statement would mislead readers who did not think about this variability and what their risk is relative to that of the average American.

(c) Death by lightning has distinctive properties. It is sometimes immediate, sometimes preceded by painful suffering. It can leave victims and their survivors unprepared. It offers some possibility of risk reduction, which people may understand to some degree. It poses an acute threat at some very limited times but typically no threat at all. Each of those properties may lead people to judge them differently—and undermine the relevance of comparisons with risks having different properties.

(d) It is often assumed that the risks being used for comparison are widely considered acceptable at their present levels. The risks may be accepted in the trivial sense that people are, in fact, living with them. But that does not make them acceptable in the sense that people believe that they are as low as they should or could be . . .

The second conceivable use of risk comparisons is to facilitate making consistent decisions regarding different risks. Other things being equal, one would want similar risks from different sources to be treated the same. However, many things might need to be held equal, including the various properties of risks . . . that might make people want to treat them differently despite similarity in one dimension . . .

The same risk may be acceptable in one setting but not another if the associated benefits are different (for example, being struck by lightning while golfing or working on a road crew). Even when making voluntary decisions, people do not accept risks in isolation but in the context of the associated benefits. As a result, acceptable risk is a misnomer except as shorthand for a voluntarily assumed risk accompanied by acceptable benefits.

Source: National Research Council (2006).

Table 8.8.2 A standard multi-dimensional representation of risks

Number of people affected	Degree of environmental impact	Knowledge	Dread
Annual expected number of fatalities:	Area affected by ecosystem stress or change	Degree to which impacts are delayed	Catastrophic potential
0–**450**–600 (10% chance of zero)	**50** km^2	**1–10** years	**1000** times expected annual fatalities
Annual expected number of person-years lost	Magnitude of environmental impact	Quality of scientific understanding	Outcome equity
0–**9000**–18 000 (10% chance of zero)	**modest** (15% chance of large)	**medium**	**medium** (ratio = 6)

Source: Adapted from stimuli used in research reported by Willis *et al.* (2005).

Qualitative assessment

Event definitions

Once defined, 'risk' can be estimated. That requires specifying the conditions for its observation. For example, when estimating the 'risk' of pregnancy, conditions include the frequency and timing of intercourse, contraceptives used, and partners' physical state. Unless laypeople are given similar detail, when asked to judge risks, they cannot convey their beliefs. Unfortunately, many survey questions leave respondents guessing at their meaning. Consider, for example, 'How likely do you think it is that a person will get the AIDS virus from sharing plates, forks, or glasses with someone who had AIDS?' US college students answered this question (taken from a prominent national survey), then were asked what they had inferred about the kind and amount of sharing. They generally agreed about the kind, with 82 per cent choosing 'sharing during a meal' from a set of options. However, they disagreed about the frequency (a single occasion, 39 per cent; several occasions, 20 per cent; routinely, 28 per cent; uncertain, 12 per cent) (Fischhoff 1996). Thus, they were, effectively, answering different questions, whose meaning could only be guessed by those hearing their responses.

Laypeople are, similarly, left guessing when experts communicate risks ambiguously (Fischhoff 1994). For example, McIntyre and West (1992) found that teens knew that 'safe sex' was important, but disagreed about what it entailed. Downs *et al.* (2004b) found that teens interpret 'it can only take once' as meaning that they will get pregnant after having sex once. If they do not, some infer that they are infertile, encouraging unsafe sex. Murphy *et al.* (1980) found people divided over whether '70 per cent chance of rain' referred to (a) the area receiving rain, (b) the time it would rain, (c) the chance of some rain anywhere, or (d) the chance of some rain at the weather station (the correct answer). Fischhoff (2005a) describes procedures for improving and evaluating event definitions, so that experts and laypeople understand one another well enough to be talking about the same thing.

Supplying details

The details that people infer, when given ambiguous risk questions or messages, reveal their intuitive theories. For example, when teens thought aloud while judging the probabilities of ambiguous events based on survey questions (e.g. having an accident after drinking and driving, getting AIDS through sex), they typically noticed many unstated details, usually focusing on ones that would affect scientific risk estimates (Fischhoff 1994). For example, they wondered about the 'dose' of most risks (e.g. the amount of drinking and driving), which was not stated in any of the questions. An exception was not thinking about the amount of sex when judging the risks of pregnancy and HIV transmission. Teens seemed to believe that an individual is either vulnerable or not (consistent with Downs *et al.* 2004b and other results reported there). Sometimes they considered variables that were not clearly related to risk, such as how well partners know one another. In an interactive DVD that reduced adolescent sexual risks, Downs *et al.* (2004a) addressed how partners could fail to self-diagnose STIs.

Cumulative risk—A case in point

There is no full substitute for directly studying the beliefs that people bring to and take away from risk messages. However, the research literature provides a basis for anticipating those beliefs. For example, the optimism bias is so widespread with events where some personal control seems feasible that one can assume that people see themselves as facing less risk when told (or asked) about others' risk. Similarly, teens' insensitivity to the amount of sex, when judging STI risks, reflects a well-known insensitivity to how risks accumulate over repeated exposure. Thus, people cannot be expected to infer the accident risk from repeatedly driving without a seat belt (Slovic *et al.* 1978) or the pregnancy risk from having sex with generally effective contraceptives (Shaklee & Fischhoff 1990). One corollary of this insensitivity is not realizing the cumulative impact of small differences in single-exposure risks (e.g. slightly better ontraceptives, wearing a seat belt). People similarly underestimate exponential growth (e.g. Frederick 2005). Some people have difficulty with the mental arithmetic; others see no risk–exposure relationship.

For example, Linville *et al.* (1993) had college students judge the probability of transmission from an HIV-positive man to a woman from 1, 10, or 100 cases of protected sex. For one case, the median estimate was 0.10, much higher than then-current public health estimates—despite using a log-linear response mode that facilitated making very low probability judgements. The median estimate for 100 contacts was 0.25, a more accurate estimate, but one that reveals typical under-accumulation. Studies that asked about just one or just 100 exposures would reveal very different pictures of lay beliefs. Conversely, risk messages could convey very different pictures if they reported risks of just one or just 100 exposures. A complete picture requires providing and asking about both exposures.

Mental models of risk processes

The role of mental models

As mentioned, when people lack explicit information about the magnitude of risks (and benefits), they must infer it. Judgemental heuristics, like availability, provide one class of inferential rules, deriving quantitative estimates from experience. Other inferences are derived from people's *mental models* of the processes creating and controlling risks. Those intuitive theories serve other functions, beyond providing estimates useful for (relatively) well-formulated decisions. They allow people to follow issues in the news media, participate in discussions, feel competent to make decisions, and generate choice options.

The term 'mental model' is often applied to intuitive theories that are well enough elaborated to generate predictions or explanations in diverse circumstances. Mental models have a long history in psychology, studied for topics as diverse as how people understand physical processes, international tensions, complex equipment, energy conservation, interpersonal relations, and drug effects (Ericsson & Simon 1993).

If mental models contain 'bugs', they can produce erroneous conclusions, even for otherwise well-informed individuals. For example, not realizing how quickly the risks of pregnancy and STIs accumulate with additional sex acts could undermine other knowledge. Bostrom *et al.* (1992) found that many people know that radon is a colourless, odourless, radioactive gas. Unfortunately, people also associate radioactivity with permanent contamination. However, this (widely publicized) property of high-level waste is not shared by radon, whose relevant by-products have short half-lives. Not realizing this, homeowners might not bother to test, believing that they could do nothing if they found a problem and not knowing that the rapid decay means rapid energy release.

Different methods have evolved for eliciting mental models of different processes. With health risks, the initial measurement challenge is determining the factors that people consider relevant. Morgan *et al.* (2001) offer a strategy that has been used for varied risks. It begins by creating a formal model, summarizing scientific knowledge of the processes affecting risk levels. It should be sufficiently precise in specifying its variables and relationships so that quantitative predictions could be computed, were its data needs met (Fischhoff *et al.* 2006). A common formalism is the influence diagram (Howard 1989). Figure 8.8.3 shows part of an influence diagram for radon. An arrow means that the value of the variable at its head depends on the value of the variable at its tail. Thus, the lungs' particle clearance rate depends on individuals' smoking history. Other examples include STIs (Fischhoff *et al.* 1998), breast implants (Byram *et al.* 2001), sexual assault (Fischhoff 1992), Lyme disease, falls, sexual assault, breast cancer, vaccination, infectious disease, and nuclear energy sources in space (Downs *et al.* 2008; Fischhoff 2005b; Morgan *et al.* 2001).

The research continues with open-ended individual interviews, structured around the model. Interviews begin very generally, asking what respondents know about the topic, then requesting elaboration on each issue they raise. The tone is non-judgemental, seeking to understand respondents' perspectives, not evaluate them. Interviews proceed to ask about exposure, effect, and mitigation issues—topics so basic that mentioning them would correct an oversight, rather than introduce foreign concepts. Once these general topics have been exhausted, more specific issues are raised (e.g. 'How does the amount of sex [or number of partners] affect HIV risk?'; 'What does 'safe sex' mean?'). Another technique is having people think aloud while sorting diverse photographs by their relevance, hoping to evoke neglected topics, without inducing improvised ones. For example, seeing a supermarket produce counter led some respondents to say that radon in the air or soil might contaminate plants (Bostrom *et al.* 1992).

Once transcribed, interviews are coded into the expert model of the risk, adding elements raised by respondents. Those additions might be errors or reflections of lay expertise (e.g. about their own behaviour, unstudied side effects, or how equipment really works). Once mapped, lay beliefs can be analysed in terms of their accuracy, relevance, specificity, and focus. Coding for accuracy can reveal beliefs that are correct and relevant, clearly wrong, too vague to evaluate, correct but peripheral (suggesting misplaced attention), and broadly relevant (e.g. radon is a gas). Bostrom *et al.* (1992) interviewed individuals drawn from civic groups. Most knew that radon is a gas (88 per cent), which concentrates indoors (92 per cent), is detectable with a test kit (96 per cent), comes from underground (83 per cent), and can cause cancer (63 per cent). However, many also believed erroneously that radon affects plants (58 per cent), contaminates blood (38 per cent), and causes breast cancer (29 per cent). Few (8 per cent) mentioned that radon decays.

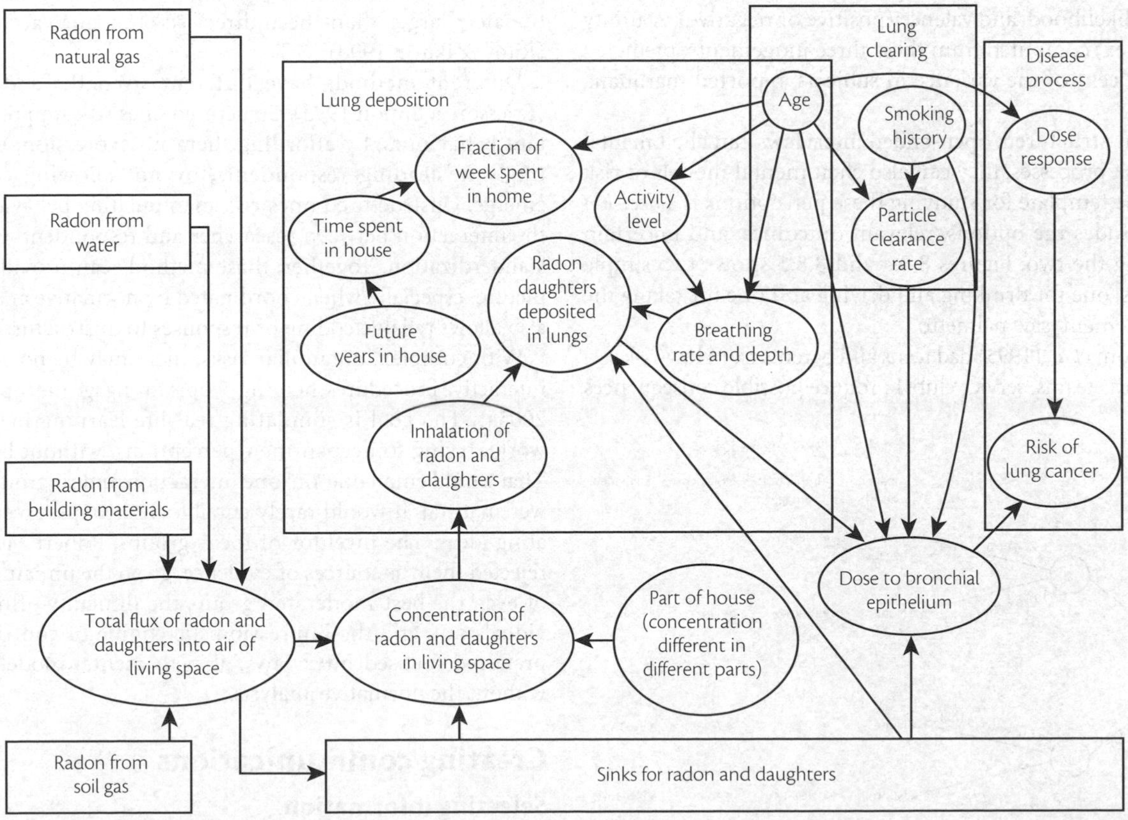

Fig. 8.8.3 Expert influence diagram for health effects of radon (in a home with a crawl space). This diagram was used as a standard and as an organizing device to characterize the content of lay mental models. *Source:* Morgan *et al.* (1992).

The robustness of these interview results was examined (and generally confirmed) in larger samples, using structured questionnaires that reflected the content and wording of the interview.

From risk beliefs to risk decisions

As mentioned, reasonable decisions should reflect all the outcomes possibly arising from the possible choices. That context is also needed to assess the adequacy of risk perceptions. Some decisions require precision, others just a rough idea. For example, von Winterfeldt and Edwards (1986) showed that decisions with continuous options (e.g. invest US$X) are often insensitive to imprecision in individual input variables (i.e. probabilities, values)—although multiple, correlated errors have cumulative effects. Dawes *et al.* (1989) showed that choices with discrete outcomes (e.g. graduate candidates) are often insensitive to how predictors are weighted, when using simple linear (weighted sum) models. As a result, any model that considers the probability and magnitude of consequences should have some success in predicting behaviour, if applied by researchers familiar with the topics on people's minds. On the other hand, because many such models will do reasonably well, it is difficult to distinguish among them or to gain insight into underlying processes.

Feather (1992) provides a general account of such *expectancy-value* (probability-consequence) models, in which decisions are predicted by multiplying ratings of the likelihood and of the (un)desirability of seemingly relevant consequences. The health-belief model and theory of reasoned action fall into this general category. For example, Bauman (1980) had seventh graders rate 54 possible consequences of using marijuana, in terms of their importance, likelihood, and valence (positive or negative). A 'utility structure index', computed from these three judgements, predicted about 20 per cent of the variance in subjects' reported marijuana usage.

Just as semi-structured, open-ended interviews can elicit mental models of risk processes, they can also elicit mental models of risk decisions. The template for studying these perceptions is a *decision tree*, that includes the options, relevant outcomes, and uncertain events linking the two. Figures 8.8.4 and 8.8.5 shows two simple decision trees, one for drinking and driving and one for taking the dietary supplement, saw palmetto.

Beyth-Marom *et al.* (1993) had teens and parents from low-risk settings (e.g. sports teams, service clubs) produce possible consequences

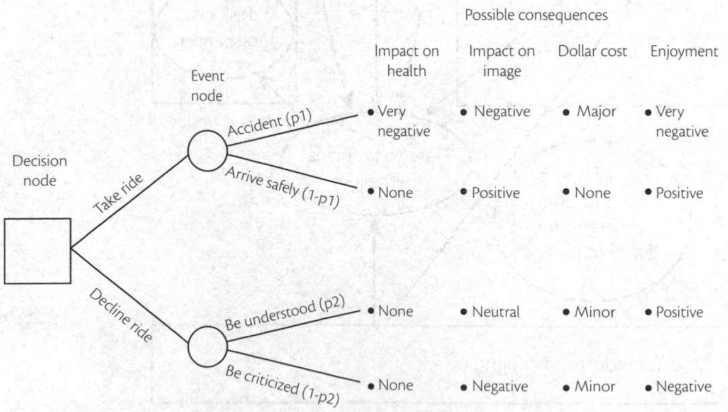

Fig. 8.8.4 A simple decision tree for whether to ride with friends who have been drinking
Source: Fischhoff & Quadrel 1991.

of accepting or rejecting a risky option (e.g. drinking and driving, smoking marijuana). Although accepting and rejecting are formally complementary, they can stimulate different thoughts (Schwarz 1999). Here, accepting the risky options evoked more consequences (suggesting that action was more evocative), a higher ratio of bad to good consequences (suggesting that its risks were more available), and fewer references to social consequences. Making some choices repeatedly evoked different consequences than did doing them once (e.g. more social reactions for repeatedly 'accepting an offer to smoke marijuana at a party'). Teens and parents responded similarly, except that parents mentioned more long-term consequences (e.g. ruining career prospects). These different conceptualizations would be hidden with structured surveys, eliciting ratings of fixed, predetermined consequences.

Fischhoff (1996) reports a study imposing even less structure, with teens describing three difficult personal decisions, in their own terms. These descriptions were coded in terms of their content (what choices trouble teens) and structure (how they were formulated). None of the 105 teens mentioned a choice about drinking-and-driving, while many described drinking decisions. Few decisions had option structures as complicated as Fig. 8.8.4. Rather, most had but one option (e.g. whether to attend a party with drinking). Judging by Beyth-Marom *et al.*'s (1993) results, teens looking at that one option saw a different decision than teens focusing on another possible option (e.g. not attending the party, going somewhere else) or multiple ones. Experimental research has found that the opportunity costs (foregone benefits) of neglected options are less visible than their direct consequences (Thaler 1991). For example, the direct risks of vaccinating children can loom disproportionately larger than the indirect risks of not vaccinating them (Ritov & Baron 1990).

Different methods have different strengths and weaknesses (Ericsson & Simon 1993). Structured ones risk suppressing important behaviours, by affording them no expression, while unwittingly misleading respondents, by not allowing confusion to emerge. Unstructured ones risk manipulating behaviour, through the interaction between researcher and respondent, while lacking standardization. Together, these methods can provide a rounded picture, especially when coordinated by normative analysis (which also allows reliable coding of responses to unstructured methods).

With complex, unfamiliar risks, there may be no substitute for interactive procedures, helping people to engage the topic (Fischhoff 2005a). The goal is simulating real-life learning in a beneficent world, trying to deepen their perceptions, without biasing them. That would entail one-on-one interaction, unless group experience were natural. It would rarely entail focus groups, except for generating ideas. The inventor of focus groups, Robert Merton (1987) rejected them as sources of evidence, given the unnatural discourse of even the best-moderated group, the difficulty of hearing individuals out, and the impressionistic coding of contributions. He preferred focused interviews, akin to mental models interviews without the normative analysis.

Creating communications

Selecting information

Communication design should begin by selecting its content. The gold standard is a normative analysis, identifying the information most relevant to the specific choices facing recipients. In practice,

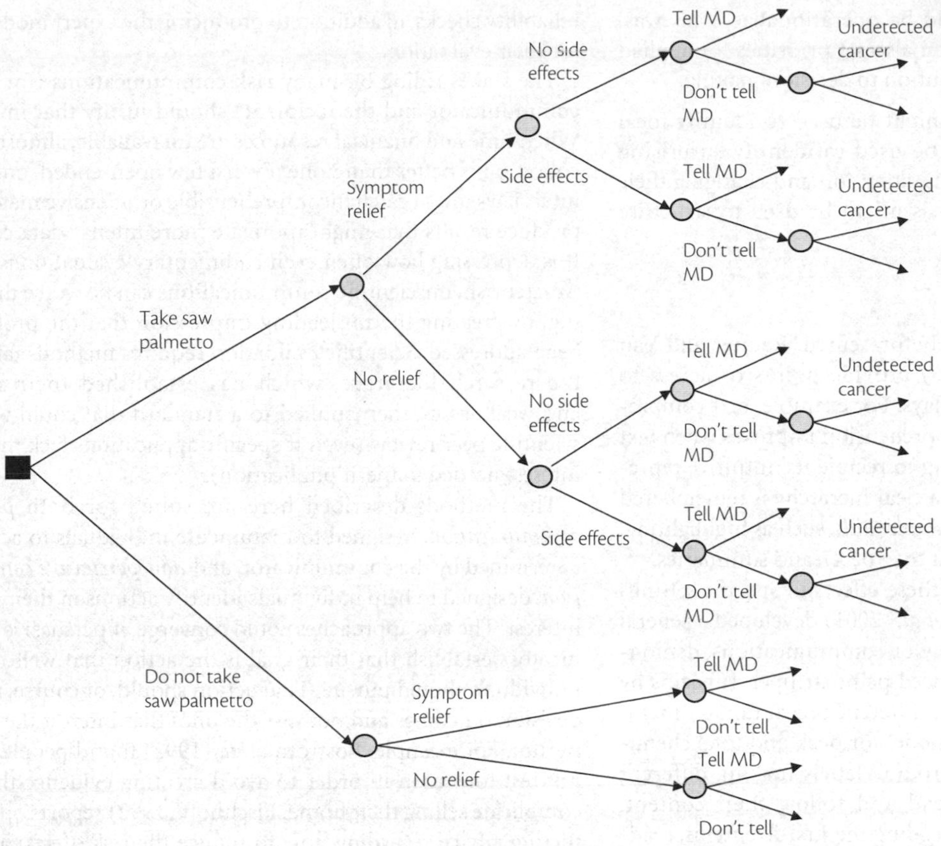

Fig. 8.8.5 A simple decision tree for whether to take saw palmetto for benign prostatic hyperplasia. *Source:* Eggers & Fischhoff 2004.

the process is disturbingly ad hoc, with self-appointed experts intuiting 'what people ought to know'. Not only can poorly chosen information waste recipients' time; it can also erode their faith in experts (and the institutions employing them). It has opportunity costs, taking the place of needed content. It allows recipients to be judged unfairly, if they seem unable to learn, when they are actually denied a meaningful chance or are uninterested in information that seems irrelevant to them, even if experts deem it important. The Institute of Medicine's landmark report, *Confronting AIDS* (1986), despaired over a survey finding that only 41 per cent of the public knew that a virus caused AIDS. Yet, one might ask what practical value that information has (and what 'a virus' meant for those who answered correctly). Florig and Fischhoff (2007) find that an official list of emergency provisions is outside many individuals' budget. Their analysis also shows that even those who can afford the stockpile might see it as not worth the cost, given the minuscule probability of proving effective.

Here are three approaches to determining what to say:

- *Complete mental models, by bridging the gaps between expert and lay mental models.* That could mean adding missing concepts, correcting mistakes, strengthening correct beliefs, and de-emphasizing peripheral ones. Following the method given above: (a) Define the universe of relevant expert knowledge; (b) elicit current beliefs; and (c) assess the centrality of imperfect beliefs.
- *Ensure appropriate confidence in beliefs.* The most dangerous beliefs are those held with too great or too little confidence. The appropriateness of confidence can be assessed by comparing judged probabilities of being correct with actual ones. Then focus communication on cases where overconfidence could cause poor choices or under-confidence could prevent sound ones. Routinely communicating how well facts are known might improve the appropriateness of recipients' confidence. For example, a meta-analysis (Fortney 1988) concluded, with great confidence, that oral contraceptives may increase a non-smoking woman's life expectancy by up to 4 days and decrease it by up to 80 days. Moreover, the existing research base was so large that no conceivable study could materially change those bounds. That might be enough for some choices. Probability of precipitation forecasts (Murphy *et al.* 1980) show the value of providing information about definitiveness.
- *Provide information in the order of its expected impact on decisions.* Value-of-information analysis determines a fact's expected contribution to decision outcomes. It can create a 'supply curve', prioritizing facts by their value. For example, Merz *et al.* (1993) examined the potential risks of carotid endarterectomy. Scraping out the artery to the head can reduce stroke risk, but also cause many problems. The research created a population of hypothetical patients, varying in their physical condition and health preferences, all of whom would want the procedure, were there no side effects. The analysis found that only three possible side effects (death, stroke, facial paralysis) were likely and severe enough that considering them should change many decisions. Although nothing should be hidden, communications should get these few facts across. Arguably, the materiality standard in

medical informed consent could be operationalized this way. Value-of-information analysis can also set priorities for applied research, by clarifying its contribution to decision making.

Value-of-information analysis might be used to identify focal facts. Calibration analysis might be used to identify surprising facts, capable of grabbing recipients' attention and changing their behaviour. A mental model analysis might be used to structure explanatory materials.

Formatting information

Once selected, information must be presented. Reimer and Van Nevel (1999) and Wogalter (2006) provide points of access to research regarding alternative displays. For example, text comprehension research finds that (a) comprehension improves when text has a clear structure, corresponding to recipients' intuitive representation; (b) information leading a clear hierarchy is remembered best; and (c) readers benefit from *adjunct aids*, such as highlighting, advanced organizers (showing what to expect), and summaries.

As elsewhere, the magnitude of these effects in specific settings must be studied empirically. Riley *et al.* (2001) developed a general method for evaluating the adequacy of communications, demonstrated with methylene chloride-based paint stripper. It begins by estimating the risks to users taking different precautionary measures (using an inhalation-uptake model for peak and total chemical exposure). It then evaluates product labels making different assumptions about how users read and follow their content. Possible reading patterns include reading the first five items, reading instructions only, reading highlighted material only, and reading every word. Their prevalence can be assumed or observed in actual use. How well people follow what they read can be estimated from mental models interviews or observation studies. The study found widely varying risk for the same product, depending on their labels. Some provided critical, useful precautionary information for all readers, while some provided it for just some readers (e.g. those looking for warnings), and others hardly provided it at all.

Evaluating communications

However sound their theoretical foundations, communications must be empirically evaluated (National Research Council 1989; Slovic 2001). One should no more release an untested health communication than an untested drug. Indeed, communications could be seen as part of drugs, shaping how they are chosen, used, and monitored. Arguably, that evidence should be part of regulatory filings for approval and part of post-licensing surveillance, especially for drugs available over-the-counter or used off-label. A minimum standard is that recipients understand the content when initially read. More ambitious tests include remembering it later, demonstrating active mastery by making inferences in novel situations, and reaching personally optimal choices.

Evaluating what people learn from communications faces the same challenges as measuring their current risk perceptions. One wants to avoid restricting the expression of non-expert beliefs, suppressing inconsistent beliefs, and changing beliefs through cues embedded in how questions and answers are phrased. Table 8.8.3 summarizes approaches to reader-based evaluation. Open-ended interviews are the best way to reduce these threats. However, performing them to scientific standards is labour intensive. It entails conducting, transcribing, and coding interviews, with suitable reliability checks, in addition to producing the expert model needed for their evaluation.

The stakes riding on many risk communications (for both the communicator and the recipient) should justify that investment. When time and financial resources are unavailable, almost any data collection is better than none. Even a few open-ended, one-on-one interviews might catch incomprehensible or offensive material, and produce results that might motivate more intense data collection. It is depressing how often even rudimentary evaluation is missing. Amateurish, unscientific communications can be worse than nothing, by creating the misleading impression that the problem has been addressed. Scientific evaluation requires methods taken from the research literature, which has established their strengths and weaknesses, then applied to a standard that could withstand scientific peer review (even if specific applications lack the general interest needed to merit publication).

The methods described here are suited for both *persuasive communication*, designed to manipulate individuals to act in ways determined by the communicator, and *non-persuasive communication*, designed to help individuals identify actions in their own best interest. The two approaches could converge, if persuasive communicators establish that their goal is the action that well-informed individuals should pursue. That action should, of course, reflect all decision outcomes and not just the ones that interest the communicator. For example, Bostrom *et al.* (1992) found people who did not test for radon in order to avoid creating evidence that could complicate selling their home. Fischhoff (1992) reports on the conflicting advice regarding how to reduce the risk of sexual assault, apparently reflecting advisors' different views on women's goals and the division of responsibility among women and society, as well as on the effectiveness of possible actions. Slovic and Fischhoff (1983) describe how reasonable individuals may 'defeat' safety measures by gaining more benefit from a product (e.g. driving faster with a car that handles better)—even if that does not satisfy the safety engineers.

Managing communication processes

In order to communicate effectively organizations require four kinds of expertise:

a. *Subject matter specialists*, who can identify the processes creating and controlling risks (and benefits).

b. *Risk and decision analysts*, who can estimate the risks (and benefits) most pertinent to decision makers (based on subject matter specialists' knowledge).

c. *Behavioural scientists*, who can assess decision makers' beliefs and goals, guide the formulation of communications, and evaluate their success.

d. *Communication practitioners*, who can manage communication products and channels, getting messages to audiences and feedback from them.

These experts' work must be coordinated, so that they play appropriate roles. For example, behavioural scientists should not revise text (for improved comprehensibility), without having subject matter specialists check that the content has not been changed; subject matter specialists should not slant the facts according to their pet theories of how the public needs to be alarmed or calmed.

Table 8.8.3 Data collection options for reader-based evaluations of risk communications

	Strengths	Weaknesses
Concurrent		
Think-aloud protocol	Protocols identify specific problems with text content and organization; can produce surprises	Costly, time-consuming; difficult to analyse; samples usually small
Retrospective		
Open-ended	Least reactive—avoids structuring answers for respondents	Coding scheme necessary—data potentially difficult to analyse
Interview	Identifies how reader structures knowledge, is less reactive than most methods	Costly, time-consuming; samples usually small
Short questions, recall	Measures what 'sticks' in readers' minds; can measure how readers assign importance	May not elicit information used in actual decision-making; responses driven by context; difficult to analyse
Problem solving (scenarios)	Elicits decision-making information and strategies	Frames problems for respondents—may be reactive
Closed-ended	Data structured, hence easier and cheaper to collect and analyse; large samples more feasible	Potentially reactive—may misrepresent respondents' knowledge and attitudes
Knowledge tests (true–false, multiple-choice)	Can verify specific misconceptions and beliefs; data readily comparable	Costly; difficult to design valid questions and response scales

Source: Bostrom *et al.* (1994).

Without qualified experts, these roles will be filled by amateurs, imperiling the communicating organization and its public.

Conclusion

Effective risk communication is essential to managing risks in socially acceptable ways. Without it, individuals are denied the best chances of making sound choices, before, during, and after problems arise. As a result, they may suffer avoidable injuries, along with the insult of feeling that the authorities have let them down, by failing to create and disseminate the information that they need, in a timely, comprehensible way. One should no more expose individuals to an untested risk communication than to an untested drug.

Effective risk communication focuses on the decisions that people face. Without that focus, one cannot know what information they need. Sound risk management requires not only communicating that information, but also creating it, both through risk analyses, summarizing existing research (Chapter 8.7, Toxicology and risk assessment in the analysis and management of environmental risk), and new research creating the basis for risk analyses (most other chapters in the textbook).

As a result, risk communication is not just an afterthought, letting the public know what the experts and authorities have decided. Rather, it is central to risk management, providing a disciplined way of communicating decision makers' needs to policy makers. It begins the process by analysing risks from decision makers' perspectives, giving formal representation to the situations they face and the help they need. That analysis also helps to ensure that individuals are judged fairly, when evaluating their risk perceptions and decisions.

This chapter has focused on measurement. In part, that is because the research relevant to each risk domain entails details specific to those decisions. Separate chapters could cover the details for diabetes, drugs, driving, etc. In part, that is because good measurement is essential to good science. Moreover, the methods are sufficiently general and well understood that they could be applied in any domain. Given a well-characterized decision or risk, it is relatively straightforward, if technically demanding, to assess lay (or expert) perceptions.

Given good measurement of risk and benefit perceptions, risk-related choices can often be roughly predicted with a simple linear model (Dawes *et al.* 1989). More precise prediction requires more detailed understanding of the processes shaping these beliefs, as well as an understanding of the emotional, social, economic, and other processes impinging on specific decisions. Prediction may not be that important, if the public health goal is helping people to make the best choices, given their circumstances—or to empower them to change those circumstances.

Meeting the risk perception and communication challenge requires coordinating the activities of four kinds of experts: Subject matter specialists, risk and decision analysts, behavioural scientists, and communication practitioners. Without them, risk communication will be mismanaged. With them, organizations will have access to the reservoirs of knowledge in their respective disciplines. For example, behavioural scientists trained in decision making will also know something about cognitive, health, and social psychology, as well as whom to call for more.

Although innovative research continues in these constituent fields, the initial challenge for risk communication is taking advantage of what is known already. There is no good reason for the measurement of risk perceptions and the evaluation of risk communications to use less than the readily available methods described here. There is no good reason to ignore well-established results, such as the multidimensional character of 'risk', the problems with verbal quantifiers, and the need to help people to understand how risks mount up through repeated exposure. Ad hoc communications might reflect sound intuition, but they deserve less trust than scientifically developed ones.

By definition, better risk communication should help its recipients to make better choices. It need not make the communicators' lives easier—recipients may discover bonafide disagreements with the communicators and their institutions. What it should do is avoid conflicts due to misunderstanding, increasing the light-to-heat ratio in risk management, leading to fewer but better conflicts (Fischhoff 1995).

Summary

- Risk communication is central to public health. Without it, individuals are denied the opportunity to make the best possible choices for themselves, their families, and their society.
- Scientifically sound risk communication requires (a) explicit analysis of the decisions facing people; (b) empirical assessment of individuals' relevant beliefs, values, and decision-making processes; and (c) development and empirical evaluation of communications focused on the facts critical to individuals' choices.
- Risk research should reflect the century of research into basic processes of judgement and decision making, both to ensure the robustness of its results and to take advantage of its knowledge for identifying and overcoming potential barriers to risk-related decisions.
- Unless measured appropriately, lay risk perceptions may be judged unfairly, leading professionals to be unduly critical of laypeople's decision-making capabilities.
- Only by understanding the decisions that individuals face can health research produce the information that people need.

Acknowledgement

The preparation of this chapter was supported by US National Science Foundation Grant SES 0433152. The views expressed are the author's.

References

Bauman, K.E. (1980). *Predicting adolescent drug use: Utility structure and marijuana*. Praeger, New York.

Beyth-Marom, R., Austin, L., Fischhoff, B. *et al.* (1993). Perceived consequences of risky behaviors. *Developmental Psychology*, **29**, 549–63.

Black, W.C., Nease, R.F., and Tosteson, A.N.A. (1995). Perceptions of breast cancer risk and screening effectiveness in women younger than 50 years of age. *Journal of the National Cancer Institute*, **8**, 720–31.

Bostrom, A., Atman, C.J., Fischhoff, B. *et al.* (1994). Evaluating risk communications: Completing and correcting mental models of hazardous processes. Part 2. *Risk Analysis*, **14**, 789–98.

Bostrom, A., Fischhoff, B., and Morgan, M.G. (1992). Characterizing mental models of hazardous processes: A methodology and an application to radon. *Journal of Social Issues*, **48**(4), 85–100.

Brewer, N.T., Chapman, G.B., Gibbons, F.X. *et al.* (2007). Meta-analysis of the relationship between risk perception and health behavior: The example of vaccination. *Health Psychology*, **26**, 136–45.

Bruine de Bruin, W., Fischhoff, B., Halpern-Felsher, B. *et al.* (2000). Expressing epistemic uncertainty: It's a fifty-fifty chance. *Organizational Behavior and Human Decision Processes*, **81**, 115–31.

Bruine de Bruin, W., Parker, A., and Fischhoff, B. (2007). Individual differences in adult decision-making competence (A-DMC). *Journal of Personality and Social Psychology*. **92**, 938–56.

Budescu, D.F. and Wallsten, T.S. (1995). Processing linguistic probabilities: General principles and empirical evidence. In *Decision making from the perspective of cognitive psychology* (eds. J.R. Busemeyer, R. Hastie, and D.L. Medin), pp. 275–316. Academic Press, New York.

Byram, S., Fischhoff, B., Embrey, M. *et al.*(2001). Mental models of women with breast implants regarding local complications. *Behavioral Medicine*, **27**, 4–14.

Christensen-Szalanski, J. and Bushyhead, J. (1993). Physicians' misunderstanding of medical findings. *Medical Decision Making*, **3**, 169–75.

Dawes, R.M., Faust, D., and Meehl, P. (1989). Clinical versus actuarial judgment. *Science*, **243**, 1668–74.

DeKay, M.L., Small, M.J., Fischbeck, P.S. *et al.* (2002). Risk-based decision analysis in support of precautionary policies. *Journal of Risk Research*, **5**, 391–417.

Downs, J.S., Murray, P.J., Bruine de Bruin, W. *et al.* (2004a). An interactive video program to reduce adolescent females' STD risk: A randomized controlled trial. *Social Science and Medicine*, **59**, 1561–72.

Downs, J.S., Bruine de Bruin, W., Murray, P.J. *et al.* (2004b). When "it only takes once" fails: Perceived infertility predicts condom use and STI acquisition. *Journal of Pediatric and Adolescent Gynecology*, **17**, 224.

Eggers, S.L. and Fischhoff, B. (2004). Setting policies for consumer communications: A behavioral decision research approach. *Journal of Public Policy and Marketing*, **23**, 14–27.

Erev, I. and Cohen, B.L. (1990). Verbal versus numerical probabilities: Efficiency, biases and the preference paradox. *Organizational Behavior and Human Decision Processes*, **45**, 1–18.

Ericsson, K.A. and Simon, H.A. (1993). *Verbal reports as data*. MIT Press, Cambridge. MA.

Feather, N. (1982). *Expectancy, incentive and action*. Erlbaum, Hillsdale, NJ.

Fischhoff, B. (2005a). Cognitive processes in stated preference methods. In *Handbook of Environmental Economics* (eds. K-G Mäler and J. Vincent), pp. 937–68. Elsevier, Amsterdam.

Fischhoff, B. (2005b). Decision research strategies. *Health Psychology*, **21**, S9–S16.

Fischhoff, B. (1996). The real world: What good is it? *Organizational Behavior and Human Decision Processes*, **65**, 232–48.

Fischhoff, B. (1995). Risk perception and communication unplugged: Twenty years of process. *Risk Analysis*, **15**, 137–45.

Fischhoff, B. (1994). What forecasts (seem to) mean. *International Journal of Forecasting*, **10**, 387–403.

Fischhoff, B. (1992). Giving advice: Decision theory perspectives on sexual assault. *American Psychologist*, **47**, 577–88.

Fischhoff, B., Bruine de Bruin, W., Guvenc, U. *et al.* (2006). Analyzing disaster risks and plans: An avian flu example. *Journal of Risk and Uncertainty*. **33**, 133–51.

Fischhoff, B., Downs, J., and Bruine de Bruin, W. (1998). Adolescent vulnerability: A framework for behavioral interventions. *Applied and Preventive Psychology*, **7**, 77–94.

Fischhoff, B., Parker, A., Bruine de Bruin, W. *et al.* (2000). Teen expectations for significant life events. *Public Opinion Quarterly*, **64**, 189–205.

Fischhoff, B. and MacGregor, D. (1983). Judged lethality: How much people seem to know depends upon how they are asked. *Risk Analysis*, **3**, 229–36.

Fischhoff, B. and Quadrel, M.J. (1991). Adolescent alcohol decisions. *Alcohol Health & Research World*, **15**, 43–51.

Fischhoff, B., Slovic, P., and Lichtenstein, S. (1977). Knowing with certainty: The appropriateness of extreme confidence. *Journal of Experimental Psychology: Human Perception and Performance*, **3**, 552–64.

Fischhoff, B., Slovic, P., Lichtenstein, S. *et al.* (1978). How safe is safe enough? A psychometric study of attitudes towards technological risks and benefits. *Policy Sciences*, **8**, 127–52.

Fischhoff, B., Watson, S., and Hope, C. (1984). Defining risk. *Policy Sciences*, **17**, 123–39.

Florig, K. and Fischhoff, B. (2007). Individuals' decisions affecting radiation exposure after a nuclear event. *Health Physics*, **92**, 475–83.

Florig, H.K., Morgan, M.G., Morgan, K.M. *et al.* (2001). A deliberative method for ranking risks. *Risk Analysis*, **21**, 913–22.

Fortney, J. (1988). Contraception: A life long perspective. In *Dying for love*. National Council for International Health, Washington, DC.

Frederick, S. (2005). Cognitive reflection and decision making. *Journal of Economic Perspectives*, **19**(4), 25–42.

Gilovich, T., Griffin, D., and Kahneman, D. (eds.) (2003). *Judgment under uncertainty II: Extensions and applications.* Cambridge University Press, New York.

Griffin, D., Gonzalez, R., and Varey, C. (2003). The heuristics and biases approach to judgment under uncertainty. *Blackwell handbook of social psychology*. Blackwell, Boston.

HM Treasury. (2005). *Managing risks to the public.* Author, London.

Howard, R.A. (1989). Knowledge maps. *Mananagement Science*, **35**, 903–22.

Institute of Medicine (1986). *Confronting AIDS*. National Academy Press, Washington, DC.

Kahneman, D., Slovic, P., and Tversky, A. (eds.) (1982). *Judgment under uncertainty: Heuristics and biases*. Cambridge University Press, New York.

Krimsky, S. and Golding, D. (1992). *Theories of risk*. Praeger, New York.

Koriat, A. (1993). How do we know that we know? *Psychological Review*, **100**, 609–39.

Lerner, J.S. and Keltner, D. (2001). Fear, anger, and risk. *Journal of Personality and Social Psychology*, **81**, 146–59.

Lichtenstein, S. and Fischhoff, B. (1980). Training for calibration. *Organizational Behavior and Human Performance*, **26**, 149–71.

Lichtenstein, S., Fischhoff, B., and Phillips, L.D. (1982). Calibration of probabilities. In *Judgment under uncertainty: Heuristics and biases* (eds. D. Kahneman, P. Slovic, and A. Tversky), pp. 306–39. Cambridge University Press, New York.

Lichtenstein, S., Slovic, P., Fischhoff, B. *et al.* (1978). Judged frequency of lethal events. *Journal of Experimental Psychology: Human Learning and Memory*, **4**, 551–78.

Linville, P.W., Fischer, G.W., and Fischhoff. B. (1993). AIDS risk perceptions and decision biases. In *The social psychology of HIV infection* (eds. J.B. Pryor and G.D. Reeder), pp. 5–38. Erlbaum, Hillsdale, NJ.

Loewenstein, G., Weber, E., Hsee, C. *et al.* (2001). Risk as feelings. *Psychological Bulletin*. **127**, 267–86.

McIntyre, S. and West, P. (1992). What does the phrase "safer sex" mean to you? Understanding among Glaswegian 18 year olds in 1990. *AIDS*, **7**, 121–6.

Merton, R.F. (1987). The focussed interview and focus groups. *Public Opinion Quarterly*, **51**, 550–66.

Merz, J., Fischhoff, B., Mazur, D.J. *et al.* (1993). Decision-analytic approach to developing standards of disclosure for medical informed consent. *Journal of Toxics and Liability*, **15**, 191–215.

Morgan, M.G., Fischhoff, B., Bostrom, A. *et al.* (1992). Communicating risk to the public. *Environmental Science and Technology*, **26**, 2048–56.

Morgan, M.G., Fischhoff, B., Bostrom, A. *et al.* (2001). *Risk communication: The mental models approach.* Cambridge University Press, New York.

Murphy, A.H., Lichtenstein, S., Fischhoff, B. *et al.* (1980). Misinterpretations of precipitation probability forecasts. *Bulletin of the American Meteorological Society*, **61**, 695–701.

National Research Council (2006). *Scientific review of the proposed risk assessment bulletin from the Office of Management and Budget.* National Academy Press, Washington, DC.

National Research Council (1996). *Understanding risk: Informing decisions in a democratic society*. National Academy Press, Washington, DC.

National Research Council (1989) *Improving risk communication*. National Academy Press, Washington, D.C.

O' Hagan, A., Buck, C.E. Daneshkhah, A. *et al.* (2006). *Uncertain judgements: eliciting expert probabilities*. Wiley, Chichester.

Peters, E. and McCaul, K.D. (eds.) (2005). Basic and applied decision making in cancer. *Health Psychology*, **24**(4), S3.

Poulton, E.C. (1989). *Bias in quantifying judgment*. Lawrence Erlbaum, Hillsdale, NJ.

Quadrel, M.J., Fischhoff, B., and Davis, W. (1993). Adolescent (in)vulnerability. *American Psychologist*, **48**, 102–16.

Reimer, B., and Van Nevel, J.P. (eds). Cancer risk communication. *Journal of the National Cancer Institute Monographs*, **19**, 1–185.

Reyna, V. and Farley, F. (2006). Risk and rationality in adolescent decision making: Implications for theory, practice, and public policy. *Psychology in the Public Interest*, **7**(1), 1–44.

Riley, D.M., Fischhoff, B., Small, M. *et al.* (2001). Evaluating the effectiveness of risk-reduction strategies for consumer chemical products. *Risk Analysis*, **21**, 357–69.

Ritov, I. and Baron, J. (1990). Satus quo and omission bias. Reluctance to vaccinate. *Journal of Behavioral Decision Making*, **3**, 263–77.

Schwarz, N. (1999). Self reports. *American Psychologist*, **54**, 93–105.

Shaklee, H. and Fischhoff, B. (1990). The psychology of contraceptive surprises: Judging the cumulative risk of contraceptive failure. *Journal of Applied Psychology*, **20**, 385–403.

Slovic, P. (2001). *Perception of risk*. Earthspan, London.

Slovic, P. and Fischhoff, B. (1983). Targeting risk. *Risk Analysis*, **2**, 231–8.

Slovic, P., Fischhoff, B., and Lichtenstein, S. (1985). Characterizing perceived risk. In *Perilous progress: Managing the hazards of technology* (eds. R.W. Kates, C. Hohenemser, and J. Kasperson), pp. 91–125. Westview, Boulder, CO.

Slovic, P., Fischhoff, B., and Lichtenstein, S. (1979). Rating the risks. *Environment*, **21**(4), 14–20, 36–9.

Slovic, P., Fischhoff, B., and Lichtenstein, S. (1978). Accident probabilities and seat-belt usage: A psychological perspective. *Accident Analysis and Prevention*, **10**, 281–5.

Slovic, P., Lichtenstein, S., and Fischhoff, B. (1984). Modeling the societal impact of fatal accidents. *Management Science*, **30**, 464–74.

Starr, C. (1969). Societal benefit versus technological risk. *Science*, **165**, 1232–8.

Thaler, R. (1991). *Quasi-rational economics*. Russell Sage Foundation, New York.

USEPA (1993). *A guidebook to comparing risks and setting environmental priorities*. Author, Washington, DC.

Viscusi, K. (1992). *Smoking: Making the risky decision*. Oxford University Press, New York.

Vlek, C. and Stallen, P.J. (1981). Judging risks and benefits in the small and in the large. *Organizational Behavior and Human Performance*, **28**, 235–71.

von Winterfeldt, D. and Edwards, W. (1986). *Decision analysis and behavioral research*. Cambridge University Press, New York.

Willis, H.H., DeKay, M.L., Fischhoff, B. *et al.* (2005). Aggregate and disaggregate analyses of ecological risk perceptions. *Risk Analysis*, **25**, 405–28.

Wogalter, M. (2006). *The handbook of warnings*. Lawrence Erlbaum Associates, Hillsdale, NJ.

Woloshin, S., Schwartz, L.M., Byram, S. *et al.* (1998). Scales for assessing perceptions of event probability: A validation study. *Medical Decision Making*, **14**, 490–503.

SECTION 9

Major health problems

9.1

Gene–environment interactions and public health

Paolo Vineis and Rodolfo Saracci

Searching for disease genes

Twentieth-century developments

The establishment of the role of genes in the hereditary causation of disease followed almost immediately the independent rediscovery in 1900, after 35 years of oblivion, of Mendel's laws by three botanists, de Vries, Correns, and Tschermak (1950). In 1902, Archibald Garrod published in *The Lancet* a paper titled 'The incidence of alkaptonuria, a study of chemical individuality', in which he noted both the all-or-none character of the disease and its familial and discontinuous inter-generational distribution. Each day, affected subjects excreted several grams of homogentisic acid, a metabolite of tyrosine which imparts a black colour to deposited urine, while normal subjects did not excrete any. Garrod consulted William Bateson, one of the first British geneticists who propounded the general relevance of Mendel's laws across the living world (he also coined the word 'genetics'). He pointed out that the observed data could be readily explained in terms of a Mendelian inheritance pattern. Alkaptonuria became the first recognized example of a recessive condition in humans (Harris 1959). Garrod subsequently produced a considerable body of research on inherited biochemical disorders, culminating in the publication of the book *Inborn Errors of Metabolism*, in which the concept of genetically determined biochemical variations in humans was developed. The nature of these variations brings into focus the complementary and necessary role of the environment in disease causation: Alkaptonuria requires the presence of tyrosine and phenylalanine in the diet and, at least in theory, could be relieved by a selectively restricted diet. Porphyrias, conditions also investigated by Garrod, are now known to depend on the deficiency of any of the seven enzymes in the biosynthetic pathway of the haeme, the oxygen-carrying moiety of haemoglobin: Crises are precipitated by external factors like the absorption of barbiturates or sulphonamides that accelerate the synthesis of the haeme above the catalytic capacity of the defective enzyme, resulting in the accumulation of noxious precursor metabolites.

Garrod had opened a new field of research which by the middle of the past century had thrown light on a substantial number of inherited diseases, identified phenotypically by characteristic biochemical disorders and genetically by Mendelian patterns of familial segregation and transmission. Among these of particular importance were early pharmacogenetic observations (Harris 1959). Abnormal sensitivity to the muscle relaxant succinylcholine, used in anaesthesia, resulted in prolonged apnoea due to inadequate inactivation of the drug by a defective cholinesterase enzyme: The defect appeared inherited as an autosomal recessive trait. Plasmatic level of the antituberculosis drug isoniazid showed a wide inter-individual variation for a fixed administered dose: Subjects could be divided into fast and slow acetylators (inactivators) of the drug, with slow acetylator behaving as an autosomal recessive trait. Primaquine, an antimalarial drug, caused haemolytic crises in subjects defective in glucose-6-phospahate dehydrogenase (G-6-PD), an enzyme central to the aerobic metabolism of red cells: In this case, the defective trait appeared X-linked with incomplete dominance.

In the first years of the twentieth century also, the blood groups of the ABO system were recognized as individually different and inheritable traits. By the mid-1920s, the pattern of inheritance had become clear, involving only one locus with three alleles (A, B, and O), the first demonstrable case of multiallelic inheritance in humans. These firmly identified heritable traits, either normal like the blood groups or pathological like a host of biochemical disorders, are almost always monogenic, with a direct and constant, or marginally variable, correspondence between phenotype and genotype (in a given environment). The same applies to the vast number of (uncommon) clinical syndromes, from Tay–Sachs disease to Marfan's syndrome to neurofibromatosis, inventoried in McKusick's reference book *Mendelian Inheritance in Man* (McKusick 1998). The persistence in a population of rare alleles with pathological effects could be understood in terms of history of mutation of normal alleles balanced by selective pressure keeping the abnormal alleles at low equilibrium level (say a frequency of <1 per cent). It was much less clear, however, whether selection could play any role in the persistence of frequent polymorphic alleles, like those of the ABO blood groups, with no obvious pathological effects. Association studies were carried out to search for subtler effects, in the form of increased risk of (or 'susceptibility to') common diseases.

These consistently showed, for instance, an association of blood groups O with gastric, duodenal, and stomal ulcer, findings that can today be related to differential affinity of *Helicobacter pylori* for the gastric mucosa mediated by blood group antigens (Borén *et al.* 1993). A paper by Lower *et al.* (reprinted in 2007) marked in 1979 a clear step forward in the investigation of susceptibility to a common disease, bladder cancer, when exposure to an environmental pathogen occurs. Lower *et al.* argued, on the basis of a detailed consideration of the activation and inactivation (detoxification) metabolism of aromatic amines, that slow N-acetylators of aromatic amines, a phenotype with a Mendelian segregation, should have—other things been equal—a higher risk of bladder cancer than fast acetylators when exposed to aromatic amines in the environment. They tested the hypothesis in a case–control study in urban Denmark and rural Sweden finding an odds ratio of 1.7 for the association of the slow acetylator phenotype with bladder cancer in urban Denmark and an odds ratio of 1.1 in rural Sweden. They attributed the difference to the different levels of exposure to aromatic amines from occupational and environmental sources in the two study locations. As noted in a commentary (Vineis 2007), this explanation is questionable since studies have generally failed to show an association between air pollution and bladder cancer and occupational exposure to aromatic amines is uncommon. However, the argument underlying the explanation is of interest as it stresses the role of environmental exposures to detect an increase susceptibility to disease development.

The contemporary scene

Advances in molecular genetic technologies in the last quarter of the twentieth century have remarkably improved the ability to locate genes in chromosomes and allowed for the first time to clone and sequence genes in DNA samples. This has led to the completed sequence of the human genome in 2003 and has opened new avenues for the study of common diseases, such as ischaemic heart disease, diabetes, and cancers, whose complex determination results from the interplay of heritable polygenic and environmental factors. Genetic epidemiology linkage studies of these diseases, in which the co-segregation within families of the disease with genetic markers of known segregation pattern and chromosomal location is analysed, are being largely superseded by association studies. These may investigate the association of disease with an allele presumed, from existing biological knowledge, to functionally affect the disease (candidate gene) or, often, with some allele in 'linkage disequilibrium' with it (i.e. tightly associated with it because it is located at a closely proximate site, no recombination occurring between the loci of the two alleles). With this approach and the availability of a dense chromosomal map of marker alleles, like the single-nucleotide polymorphisms (SNPs), the exploration of all regions of the genome has become feasible. The efficiency of the search is being further facilitated by the fact that SNPs in linkage disequilibrium with each other tend to be passed together in a block (haplotype) from parents to offspring. The International HapMap Project has completed a map of haplotypes making possible to choose for testing only selected single SNPs ('tagging' SNPs) within each haplotype, as these imply the presence of all other SNPs in the block as well of any functionally disease-related mutation. Concurrently the testing technology has undergone a vertiginous advancement: High-throughput platforms allowing the simultaneous determination of half a million SNPs are available and this, combined with the tagging SNP approach, has paved the way to 'genome-wide association' (GWA) studies. In these the search of disease-related alleles is not any more focused on candidate genes but covers bit by bit the whole genome.

A successful story concerning the use of high-throughput genetic technologies to screen for new associations is represented by the region 8q24. Family-based linkage studies, association studies, and studies of tumours had already highlighted human chromosome 8q as a genomic region of interest for a prostate cancer susceptibility loci. Recently, a locus at 8q24, characterized by both a SNP and a microsatellite marker, has been shown to be associated with prostate cancer risk in Icelandic, Swedish, and US samples (Witte 2007). These data suggest that the locus on chromosome 8q24 harbours a genetic variant associated with prostate cancer and that the microsatellite marker is a stronger risk factor for aggressive prostate cancers defined by poorly differentiated tumour morphology. Evidence has now been provided that colon cancer might also be associated with the same region. Using a multistage genetic association approach comprising 7480 affected individuals and 7779 controls, researchers have identified markers in chromosomal region 8q24 associated with colorectal cancer (Zanke *et al.* 2007). This example is interesting for several reasons, including (a) 'reverse genetics', i.e. the possibility that aetiologic pathways for cancers that elude epidemiological research can be discovered starting from the observation of genetic susceptibility; and (b) 'pleiotropy', the ability of certain gene variants to increase or modulate the risk for different diseases.

Recently the results of a large genome-wide association study have been published (The Wellcome Trust Case Control Consortium 2007), involving 2000 cases of each of seven common diseases and 3000 shared controls. Case–control comparisons identified 24 independent association signals at a high level of statistical significance ($P < 5 \times 10^{-7}$): One in bipolar disorder, one in coronary heart disease, nine in Crohn's disease, three in rheumatoid arthritis, seven in type 1 diabetes, and three in type 2 diabetes. On the basis of prior findings and of the limited replication already performed the authors interpret almost all of the signals as reflecting genuine susceptibility effects. Also in this study some loci identified by the signals are implicated in more than one disease, i.e. show pleiotropy.

Given the strong momentum that this high-tech research has gained more GWA studies will come forward in the near future. In addition important new sources of variability have been discovered all along the human genome, notably the copy-number variants (CNV), involved in gene expression, ready to be explored in relation to disease. A recent comment stated: 'The avalanche of recent data provided by genome-wide association studies represents a quantum leap in information about the inherited component of certain diseases' (Hunter & Kraft 2007). No doubt the environmental components can be submerged and lost sight of within the avalanche.

Genes or environment?

Genes and heredity

Genes have to do with heredity, but what is the relationship between the two? A confusion, still largely present in the literature and regularly echoed in the lay press, concerning heredity vs. genetic causation is emblematically represented by the debate that took place around IQ after the publication of The Bell Curve by Herrnstein and Murray (1994). As it was pointed out by Block (1995), the basic confusion in this book and in many other similar papers was between heritability and genetic determination. Heritability has to do with similarity of observable traits between parents and the offspring, while a characteristic is 'genetically determined' if it is coded in and caused by the genes within a 'normal' environment. Two extreme examples are the following: (a) the number of fingers in humans is totally genetically determined and the rare deviations from five fingers are caused by defects of development, e.g. from thalidomide; they are congenital but not heritable; (b) wearing skirts among European populations has a very strong heritability, as it occurs only in women (with the exception of the odd Scotsmen). Hence, it is related to having an XX rather than a XY chromosomal pair but it is not genetically determined (Block 1995). Such misconceptions are clearly relevant to the discussion about the heritability vs. genetic determination of diseases. For example, studies of twins which often do not rule out similar environmental exposures for the pair, cannot be used to automatically infer that cancer or schizophrenia are due to pathologic genetic variants in DNA. In fact the environment itself is inherited, for example in the case of the propensity to wear skirts. The same argument applies to claims that IQ has 60 per cent heritability, academic performance 50 per cent or occupational status 40 per cent: These figures do not mean that such characteristics are inherited through genes (DNA), i.e. there is genetic determination, but only that there is a substantial association between the characteristic in the index subject and the same characteristic in the parents.

Genes and disease

The role of genes in causing human disease is often misunderstood. In 1972, a key paper by Lewontin drew attention on the mistakes of partitioning nature and nurture (Lewontin 1972). Genetic determinism, namely the contention that the causal determination of a disease is due to a gene and nothing else, is a fundamental misconception.

There are several objections to it, in particular:

(1) The sequence of information in genes is 'per se' insufficient to dictate how gene products give origin to a new organism; much depends on a cascade of interacting events, pre-mRNA alternative splicing, a large number of different types of RNA, gene–gene interactions and the pre-natal environment, i.e. biological phenomena that encompass but expand much beyond the gene sequence.

(2) Genetic pathways completely specify an abnormal function of the organism only on rare occasions, namely for 'monogenic' diseases like sickle-cell anaemia or Huntington's chorea. In these cases the cell does not have compensatory mechanisms to overcome the metabolic alteration and influences from environmental variations within the range experienced by the human species are negligible. These are the only situations in which the simplified paradigm 'one gene-one disease' is valid. In all other cases diseases are due to the interplay of gene variations with environmental variations, the latter being often dominant. The phenomenon of availability of multiple metabolic pathways, controlled by different genes, that allow the cell and the organism to adequately overcome damages caused by the environment, represents an early conquest of human evolution. As the geneticist Bailey stated, the implication of gene *robustness* is the inability of many genes (or signals, or regulatory interactions) to have any significant effect over the phenotype unless a number of other genes are simultaneously altered (Fox Keller 2000). This is a complementary phenomenon to the already mentioned *pleiotropy* by which most genes have multiple functions.

A simple correspondence between genotype and phenotype subsumed when exploring the role of genes in disease may in fact almost completely break down. For example, some African populations—such as the Ethiopians, show multiple gene copies (multiduplication) of genes such as CYP2D6. This phenomenon has been attributed to diet-related selection during the evolutionary history of these populations (famine and the need to adapt their detoxifying metabolic capacities to toxicants in the only food available). However, often they tend to have a slow rather than a rapid metabolizer phenotype, as would be expected. To reconcile the genotype–phenotype gap, and to determine if environmental factors are responsible for the observed differences, the genotype and phenotype of CYP2D6 among Ethiopians living in Sweden were assessed and compared to data from Ethiopians living in Ethiopia and Swedish Caucasians (Aklillu *et al.* 2002). A comparison of the debrisoquine metabolizing ability among individuals of the same CYP2D6 genotype revealed that Swedes exhibited the highest rate of debrisoquine metabolism, followed by Ethiopians in Sweden and Ethiopians in Ethiopia. It has been speculated that inhibitory dietary factors may explain the differences seen between the different groups and that these components in the past might have contributed to dietary stress-mediated selection of duplicated and multiduplicated active CYP2D6 genes, as frequently seen in Ethiopians. These results indicate a significant influence of environmental factors in shaping the difference in the relation between CYP2D6 genotype and phenotype (metabolic capacity) between Caucasians and Black Africans.

Notwithstanding these considerations genetic determinism is still at least implicit in a large number of investigations, when certain traits or diseases are straightaway attributed to genes or even to a single gene.

A clear example is the so called 'fragile X syndrome', a condition in which 1 out of 1000 males develops a serious mental retardation (Abbeduto *et al.* 2007; Penagarikano *et al.* 2007). When their X chromosome is observed under the microscope, it appears as lacking a fragment, a characteristic named 'fragile site'. These observations led to the conclusion that chromosome X carries a gene implicated in the development of the central nervous system. Several research groups started work to isolate the gene also in the hope that new prenatal screening strategies could be developed to avoid the birth of children with the syndrome. The gene was identified in 1991 and it received the name of FMR-1 (fragile X mental retardation-1). In the meantime, the syndrome was assigned a spectrum that went much beyond reality to include anti-social and criminal behaviours: The denomination 'crime gene' ensued. However, after the isolation of the gene it became evident that things were much more complex. Expressivity of the gene turned out to be variable: Children with the same defect (repetition of three letters in the DNA sequence, CGG) may have very serious neurological defects, while others may be absolutely normal. These children are sometimes hyperkinetic, or have difficulties in concentrating, but—contrary to some claims—there is no firm evidence of criminal behaviour. Currently the disorder is interpreted as mainly caused by the expansion of the trinucleotide sequence CGG located in the 5′ UTR of the FMR1 gene on the X chromosome. The abnormal expansion of this triplet leads to hypermethylation and consequent silencing of the FMR1 gene, and the absence of the encoded protein (FMRP) is the basis for the phenotype. FMRP appears to play an important role in synaptic plasticity by regulating the synthesis of proteins encoded by certain mRNAs localized in the dendrite. Around the one specific and clearly genetically based condition (lack of FMRP) there are a number of minor forms and other phenotypes that have little resemblance to the genetically based disorder.

Genes and environment

There is a large consensus among scientists that only a minor fraction of diseases, of the order of about 5 per cent is monogenic while the vast majority of cases are due to the interplay or 'interaction' of genetic and environmental factors, the latter being often dominant.

Models of gene–environment interactions

Some useful models describing gene–environment interactions as they manifest at the level of disease occurrence have been proposed by Ottman (Fig. 9.1.1) (Ottman 1996): These models portray five different and general biological situations, rather than entering in the details of disease-specific pathogenetic mechanisms. A similar approach has been used by Yang and Khoury (1997) who present a typology of six models describing in terms of relative measures of association in epidemiological studies (relative risks) different ways in which genes and the environment can interact.

In Ottman's Model A the effect of the genotype is to produce or increase expression of an environmental 'risk factor' that can also be produced non-genetically. For example, in phenylketonuria (PKU) subjects homozygous for the autosomal recessive allele are deficient in the enzyme necessary to convert dietary phenylalanine into tyrosine. If left untreated, i.e. without dietary restriction, these subjects develop high levels of blood phenylalanine (regarded as the internal environment 'risk factor') which causes mental retardation. High blood levels of phenylalanine and mental retardation may, however, even occur in subjects without the deficient genotype, e.g. children who had intrauterine exposure to high blood levels because the mother is affected by the enzyme deficiency. In the pathway from gene to disease the high blood level of phenylalanine is an intermediate variable which can however also be induced by *a separate and independent mechanism*. Model A therefore typifies an absence of interaction.

In Model B, the genotype exacerbates the effect of the environmental factor, but there is no effect of genotype in unexposed persons. For example, xeroderma pigmentosum (XP) is an autosomal recessive disorder in which exposure to UV light causes a large number of skin cancers because of a defect of DNA repair enzymes. However, the risk of skin cancer is increased with UV exposure also in people without XP.

In Model C, the environmental factor exacerbates the effect of genotype but there is no effect of the environmental factor in persons with the low-risk genotype. For example, an autosomal dominant disorder, porphyria variegata, is characterized by skin problems of variable severity. Exposure to barbiturates, which is innocuous in persons without the condition, precipitates an acute crisis that may involve even paralysis and death.

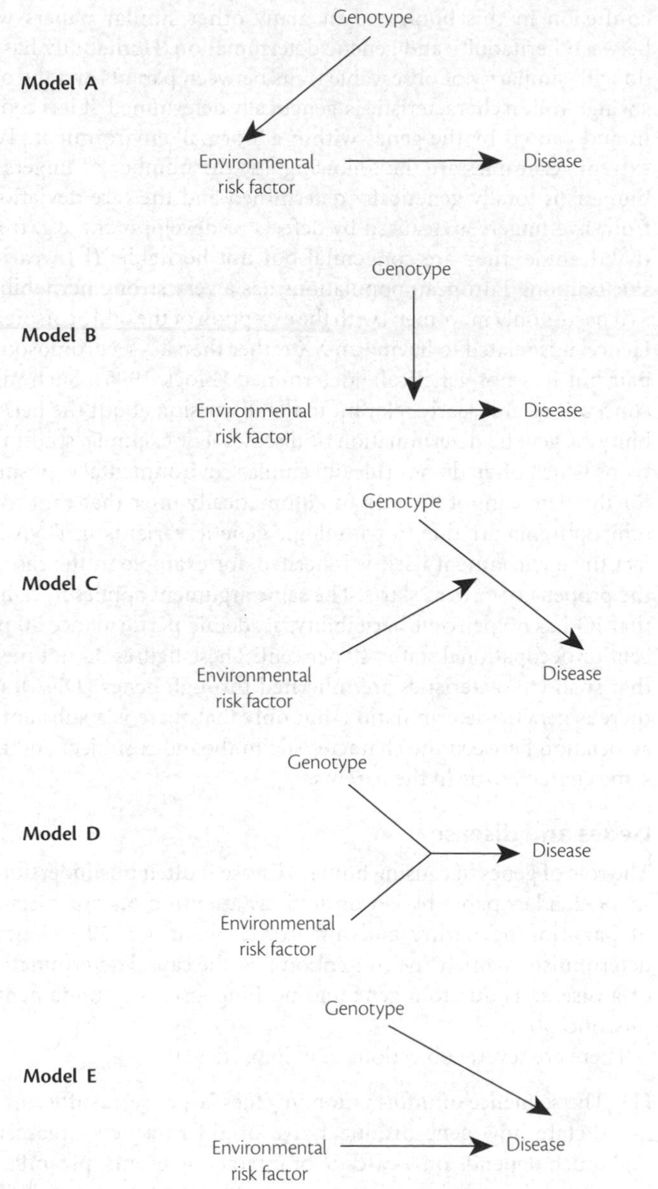

Fig. 9.1.1 Five general models of gene–environment interaction (from Ottman).

In Model D, both genotype and the environmental factor are required to increase risk. As already mentioned, G-6-PD deficiency is an X-linked recessive disorder with incomplete penetrance: Individuals are asymptomatic unless, for example, they eat fava beans, in which case they develop severe haemolytic anaemia. Fava beans, however, do not produce any symptoms without the deficiency.

Finally, in Model E, both the genotype and the environmental factor have a separate effect in disease risk, but when they occur together the risk is higher or lower than when they occur alone. For example, COPD risk is increased in smokers without alpha-1-antitrypsin deficiency and in non-smokers with the deficiency, but risk is increased to a greater extent in smokers with the deficiency. It is likely that many cases of gene–environment interactions relevant to common diseases belong to this category.

A population story: Native Americans and the metabolic syndrome

Investigating gene–environment interactions may play a role not only in elucidating disease development and individual susceptibility, but also in understanding why certain populations or subgroups show high risks of disease. A classical example, worth some detailed consideration, is represented by 'Native Americans' and other genetically well-defined population.

Native American (NA) populations have rates of chronic diseases such as those encompassed by the 'metabolic syndrome' that are higher than in other populations with similar lifestyles. It had been suggested that this is due to a genetic predisposition coupled with rapid environmental changes as their lifestyle became more Westernized (Wendorf 1989). More recently, it has been hypothesized that Native Americans have a relatively large number of gene variants that modify environmental factors to cause chronic disease (Nagi *et al.* 1998). Accordingly, the Native American population could be considered to be a 'natural laboratory' for the thesis that chronic diseases are caused by gene–environment interactions. The metabolic syndrome is a good example of a complex of chronic conditions. Its prevalence has been increasing and is higher in Native Americans than in other populations living a similar lifestyle (Ford *et al.* 2002; Resnick 2002).

In 1999, the World Health Organization defined metabolic syndrome as the presence of diabetes or impaired glucose tolerance or insulin resistance, plus two of the following: Obesity, dyslipidaemia, hypertension, or microalbuminuria (Isomaa 2003). Having one of these traits increases the risk of having another, and there is a consequential high risk of cardiovascular disease and increased incidence of type 2 diabetes mellitus (T2DM) (Greenlund *et al.* 1999).

The metabolic syndrome is a complex condition and many genes could contribute to its development (Reilly & Rader 2003). Genes that have been reported to be involved are those controlling both energy metabolism and storage and inflammatory pathways. Genes that improve the efficiency of energy storage, especially as fat, are often referred to as 'thrifty genes'. These would have been selected when our ancestors were hunter–gatherers and lived in times of alternating feast and famine (Zimmet & Thomas 2003). It has also been suggested that physical inactivity may alter gene expression in some way that leads to derangement of metabolism and metabolic syndrome (Booth *et al.* 2002). There are various genes that have shown differences in expression due to exercise, including genes that encode for intermediates in insulin signalling and energy metabolism and enzymes that are involved in lipid metabolism. These genes could also be candidate genes for causing metabolic syndrome (Bray 2000).

It has been hypothesized that when modern humans began to spread across the globe 100 000 years ago these genetic divergences occurred due to the selection pressures of the different geographical areas and social groups in which they were living. Genes/mutations that made it more likely for an individual in a group to reach reproductive age and be successful in finding a mate became more common in that group (Olson 2002). Concerning Native Americans, there is some debate surrounding the settlement of the Americas. It is likely that the initial settlers migrated from Asia probably through Siberia and then moved south. It is also possible that some settlers also came from Europe (Olson 2002). When the ancestors of the Native Americans migrated south, they did so in a particularly harsh environment, so it is possible that those genes giving an efficient energy metabolism would have been selected for in this population (Wendorf 1989).

Over the past 50 years, Native American populations have become increasingly Westernized. The main changes that have come with the Western lifestyle are those in physical activity and diet. For example, a community initiative in Mohawk Native Americans has shown that over the last 50 years they had become less physically active and that the availability of foods high in fat and calories has increased (Hood *et al.* 1997).

A study of diabetes prevalence and behavioural risk factors in Native Americans showed that their prevalence of diabetes was 2.5 times higher than in whites. The prevalence of obesity was also higher. However the prevalence of risk factors such as a sedentary lifestyle and smoking were similar in Native Americans and Caucasian populations (Muneta *et al.* 1993). This suggests that Native Americans might have a higher frequency of gene variants that interact with the environment causing them to have the high prevalence of metabolic syndrome. Or, alleles that are beneficial with a traditional lifestyle (and so would have been selected in these populations) may be disadvantageous in the context of a Western lifestyle.

In light of these hypotheses the exploration has developed of genetic causes of cardiovascular disease, obesity or type 2 diabetes in Native Americans populations. At the time of writing there are already more than 25 published papers investigating a spectrum of genes. Four papers (Aguilar *et al.* 1999; Kataoka *et al.* 1996; Thompson *et al.* 1997; Vozarova *et al.* 2003) found variation between Native Americans and Caucasians in the frequency of an allele associated with metabolic syndrome. In each case the frequency of the allele positively associated with metabolic syndrome was higher in the Native American population. Additionally, Knowler *et al.* (1988) found an allele with a negative association with type 2 diabetes that was associated with the presence of Caucasian admixture.

Methodological issues

The investigation of the effects, separate and joint, of genes and environment confronts a number of methodological issues (Thomas 2004).

Errors of measurement

First, measurement of genes (genotyping) and of environmental agents are usually prone to different degrees of error. Genotyping is in general more accurate than the majority of methods used to measure environmental exposures. This implies a lower degree of classification error that in turn means an easier identification of associations with disease. Table 9.1.1 (Armstrong *et al.* 1994) shows the attenuation that a true association, expressed as true odds ratio, undergoes as a consequence of errors of measurement, expressed as imperfect (i.e. less than 1 per cent or less than 100 per cent) sensitivity and specificity; the error is assumed to be non-differential, applying equally to cases and controls. The observable odds ratio for an environmental exposure is likely to be markedly attenuated, as in the first line of the table, as a sensitivity of 60 per cent and a specificity of 90 per cent are realistic, and perhaps even optimistic for measurements of environmental exposures. The attenuation for the genetic exposure, i.e. for genotyping, is more likely to be as in the last lines of the table (for example, the common genotyping method Taqman has 96 per cent sensitivity and 98 per cent specificity): The observable odds ratios are materially higher than those in the first line and much closer to the true ones, making a true association, namely the point estimate of the odds ratio, more likely to show-up for the genetic than for the environmental variable. Whether the estimate is statistically significant at a chosen probability level depends also on the prevalence of the exposure (whose effect on the attenuation of the true odds ratio is shown in Table 9.1.1): The power of the study to detect an odds ratio as significantly deviating from unity is higher for exposures with frequencies of 40–50 per cent (as for the slow acetylator phenotype of NAT2 or the GSTM1 null variant of GSTM) than for rare exposures, of the order of 1–10 per cent, as is often the case for environmental exposures in the general population. Again this favours the detectability of associations of disease with genetic traits more than with environmental exposures and has obvious consequences for the size of studies. When both genetic traits and environmental exposure are investigated within the same study, as typically occurs when one of the aims is to explore gene–environment interactions, the size of the study which has a good power for detecting gene–disease associations may be vastly underpowered for detecting associations of environmental exposures with disease, and the study may become 'de facto' worthless for this purpose and, related to this, for an adequate exploration of the interaction.

Testing of multiple hypotheses

While accurate genotyping measurements make easier the detection of gene–disease associations it also contributes to enhancing the chance of false positive results if, as is more and more the case, associations between each of the hundred or thousands of genetic variants and disease phenotype are tested. If a thousand association tests are performed and the conventional level of statistical significance of, say, $P = 0.01$, is used one expects merely by chance to find 10 associations with $P < 0.01$ when none is real. The problem becomes dramatic with the genome-wide association studies in which hundred of thousands or even millions of SNP-to-disease association tests are performed. As pointed out in recent papers (Wacholder *et al.* 2004; Thomas & Clayton 2004), the issue is not one of finding an appropriate level of statistical significance for the multiple testing of a single global null hypothesis (as in the classical theory of multiple testing) but for multiple hypotheses, one for each SNP-to-disease association. In the light of reasonable assumptions on the 'a priori' probability of an association being real and of the power of the study, values of P of the order of 10^{-7} have been worked out as significance threshold to separate real from false associations (however associations with less extreme P values may still be worth considering for replication studies, particularly when supported by information on biological mechanism).

Interactions

Further problems arise when the joint effects of genes and environment are considered, namely 'gene–environment interactions'. This label—GEI—has become current for any study involving genotyping as well as some measures of environmental factors. The term interaction lends itself to confusion as it has several meanings: Biological, statistical, and public health (Saracci 1980).

In a biological sense, it indicates how two or more agents—genetic and/or environmental—cooperate in a biological mechanism to produce an effect. Specific mechanistic models of interactions translating into observable patterns of disease occurrence have been developed for communicable diseases but much less commonly for non-communicable diseases: The multistage carcinogenesis model is one example.

In a statistical sense the presence of an interaction indicates that the observed data actually deviate in respect to a model of joint effect assumed to adequately summarize the data. The interaction is designated as 'qualitative' or 'non-removable' if the deviation consists of the reversal of the effect of an agent, for example, the hypotensive effect of a drug being changed into an hypertensive effect in the presence of a genetic variant controlling a metabolizing enzyme. If the deviation consists instead of an amplification or reduction of the effect expected under the model, the interaction is designated as 'quantitative' and can be removed by an appropriate change of the scale of measurement on which the effect is expressed, for instance changing the scale from arithmetic to logarithmic. The additive and the multiplicative models are the two summarizing models most employed in epidemiology. Unfortunately, it has been

Table 9.1.1 Effect of non-differential misclassification of a dichotomous exposure on the observable odds ratio (ORobs) (from Armstrong *et al.* 1994)

			OR true = 1.5	OR true = 2	OR true = 4
Exposure sensitivity	**Exposure specificity**	**Prev.**	**OR obs.**	**OR obs.**	**OR obs.**
0.6	0.9	0.1	1.17	1.34	1.93
0.6	0.9	0.5	1.24	1.42	1.86
0.6	0.99	0.1	1.40	1.79	3.20
0.6	0.99	0.5	1.30	1.54	2.12
0.9	0.9	0.1	1.24	1.48	2.41
0.9	0.9	0.5	1.38	1.73	2.85
0.9	0.99	0.1	1.45	1.89	3.61
0.9	0.99	0.5	1.43	1.82	3.11

Note: 'Prev.' is the exposure prevalence among non-diseased subjects.

shown that each of them may arise from a variety of underlying mechanistic models so that, contrary to hopes, the observation of joint responses to several agents, e.g. a gene and an environmental exposure, throws scarce light on the biological pathways involved. Even the different models outlined by Ottman and by Khoury *et al.* previously mentioned, which are more specific than the additive and multiplicative models may prove difficult to distinguish by means of epidemiological data.

In the additive model, the incidence rate resulting from the joint exposure to several agents equals the sum of the basic population rate (no agent present) plus the excess rate associated with each of the agents: The incidence rate is the fundamental expression of the disease occurrence in a population, hence anything larger or smaller than this baseline sum can be regarded as an interaction, notably in a public health sense.

In the multiplicative model, the relative risk due to the two exposures is simply the product of the relative risk for the separate exposures. In a case–control study, the same relationship holds for the odds ratios. This multiplicative relation is the basis of the logistic regression, commonly used in the analysis of epidemiological data from studies with multiple exposure variables. In the context of a GEI study, it presents an additional interesting feature: If the distributions in the source population of the genotypes and of the environmental factors are independent, errors in environmental exposure measurement have as the only effect the driving of the data toward a multiplicative relation (probably this being the reason why in practice the data very often conform to a multiplicative model) (Clayton & McKeigue 2001). Under the same assumption of independent distributions of genotypes and environmental exposures in the source population it becomes possible to explore the GEI only among cases ('case-only' study design). If in this type of study no association is found (namely an odds ratio of 1) between genotype and environmental exposure among the cases of a disease, the inference can be made that the joint effect of the two agents is multiplicative: Hence, the 'case-only' design can be used to screen for genes and environmental factors acting (at least) multiplicatively, a point not always clearly understood. In fact both from a biological and a public health viewpoint this multiplicative, i.e. more than merely additive, joint effect may be in itself of interest.

Focusing on the joint effect of a gene and an environmental agent could also help in detecting weak overall effects. If the gene variant acts only in the presence of an environmental exposure, i.e. exhibits a supramultiplicative interaction, the possibility of detecting its effects depends on having correctly measured the environmental variable as well. Suppose the gene variant has an odds ratio of 4 for the association with a disease among subjects who also are exposed (in an independent way) to an environmental agent, and an odds ratio of 1 among those not so exposed. If there is no information on the environmental exposure, which is in fact present in 50 per cent of the subjects, the odds ratio for the main effect of the gene variant will show up as 2.5; if however the environmental exposure is present in only 10 per cent of the subjects (a more realistic situation for many environmental agents) the odds ratio for the main effect will be reduced to 1.3, a weak effect hardly detectable. Knowledge of environmental variables may thus enhance the power of detecting the effects of genetic variables (and vice versa). This advantage, however, needs to be looked at with caution: Unless existing biological knowledge allows one to pinpoint the subgroups where one should expect to observe the highest risks a mere blind search will contribute to inflate the problem of multiple hypotheses testing previously discussed (Clayton & McKeigue 2001).

The importance of measuring environmental exposures

Many investigations labelled as studies on 'gene–environment interactions' are under way in different parts of the world, and the subject also currently appears as one of the leading items in grant calls from NIH or EU. Most of these studies employ similar methods and technological supports for genotyping while the assessment of exposure to environmental agents is extremely variable, being for example state of the art for dietary intake in the EPIC investigation, but not in other studies, nor for other exposures. Unless the size of these studies is calculated to achieve an adequate power of detection for associations of disease with the variables most affected by classification errors, i.e. the environmental ones (diet, pollutants, etc.) it can be safely predicted that such studies will come up with a number of genetic associations but very few credible environmental associations with disease. In addition as the majority of genetic polymorphisms are believed to act through biological interaction with environmental agents, it may also become difficult to make sense of genetic observations if the environmental component is substantially misclassified.

Accurate and precise measurements of environmental exposures meet objective problems as they are targeted on free-living populations with great variability of exposures and changes in time. These measurements often involve recall of complex information—such as diet—or extrapolation from few points in space and time—such as for air pollution data. For rare exposures (that may be relevant for the involved subjects) these difficulties are even greater. The solution lies in empowering exposure assessment, by investing—much more than many investigators have done until now—in robust and validated exposure measurement procedures. This implies that epidemiologists collaborate not only with geneticists and molecular biologists, but also with environmental scientists. Large efforts have already been made in the field of nutrition, but not yet in other areas of environmental exposures. Novel research-based measurement methods should be developed, for example those derived from metabolomics or the identification of specific DNA adducts, to detect signatures left within body fluids by metabolic processes and/or external exposures e.g. air pollutants. Also in the actual measurement process repeated measurements of the same environmental variables, as well as combined measurements of different variables, will reduce misclassification.

Mendelian randomization

Not only exposures to environmental agents are imperfectly measured but the relation of environmental exposures to disease is prone to confounding. Mendelian randomization (MR) is a way to exploit genetic testing in epidemiology to overcome some of the limitations of observational epidemiology. MR has been suggested (Davey Smith & Ebrahim 2003) as a way to overcome confounding by exploiting the random allocation of alleles from parents to the offspring. Because of chromosome separation at meiosis and of recombination, at long-term equilibrium—i.e. after many generations—alleles at different loci on the same or on different chromosomes become (under some reasonable assumptions about the mating pattern in the population) all independently and randomly distributed in the population. Hence one should not expect that alleles, in general, are associated with any particular exposure and as a consequence an association between a gene variant and a disease should not be subject to the confounding by environmental, behavioural or socioeconomic factors that plague observational epidemiological studies. Also 'reverse causation' (the disease inducing the exposure rather than the exposure inducing the disease) would be excluded by MR.

An interesting example of MR concerns dairy products, lactase and prostate cancer. It has been suggested that the intake of milk could increase the risk of prostate cancer. In an international ecological study in 42 countries, Ganmaa *et al.* (2002) found a strong correlation between milk intake and the incidence of prostate cancer ($r = 0.71$). Analytical studies are overall positive, with odds ratios in the order of 1.6–5.1 in both case–control and cohort studies (Chan *et al.* 1998). The mechanism which is hypothesized is the inhibitory effect of calcium on the conversion of 25 (OH) vitamin D to 1,25 (OH)2 vitamin D. The latter has an antiproliferation effect in human prostate cells (Skowronski *et al.* 1993). Also, a protective effect of ultraviolet radiation on prostate cancer has been suggested and is consistent with this proposed mechanism (Hanchette & Schwartz 1992). However, milk intake is subject to considerable measurement error and the association with prostate cancer could be due to confounders such as dietary habits or exposures/behaviours associated with social class.

If it can be shown that a genetic variant (e.g. related to lactase persistence) that affects milk intake is associated with prostate cancer, this will be indirect but unconfounded evidence on the role of milk in prostate carcinogenesis. The autosomal lactase gene (LTC) presents a two allele T and C polymorphism and lends itself to this exercise as it controls the lactose metabolizing lactase enzyme and its persistence or non-persistence in adults. In a study on the geographic distribution of allele frequencies for the lactase gene (Sacerdote *et al.* 2007) it was hypothesized: (a) a north-to-south gradient for the T allele frequency for LTC in Italy, based on previous observations of such a gradient in Europe; (b) a lower intake of milk (but not yoghurt or cheese, in which lactose is hydrolysed) among carriers of the CC genotype for LTC. Overall, the LTC gene T allele frequency was around 21 per cent in Northern Italy and 9 per cent in Southern Italy, i.e. much lower than in Northern Europe (80 per cent in the UK). Food intake was associated with gene variants. A statistically significant association was evident for ice-cream and LTC variants ($P = 0.004$), less so for milk intake. The next step will be to examine the association between lactase and prostate cancer. If an association between the T allele and cancer will be found, then the 'MR triangle' will have been completed, i.e. it will be reasonable to infer that the involvement of milk in prostate cancer aetiology is real and not confounded, or biased because of inaccurate measurement. The concept of 'MR triangle' refers to the fact that the strategy implies looking at the association between: (a) exposure and disease (usually the first to be investigated and found), (b) exposure or its metabolites and gene variants and (c) gene variants and disease.

Like for any method there are, however, limitations with this approach, whose real relevance will become clearer as the method becomes applied in different circumstances. The Achilles heel of MR is probably the fact that many genes are pleiotropic, i.e. have multiple effects: Hence an association gene variant-disease may occur not via the path involving the exposure of interest but via one of the other gene-dependent paths. Confounding thrown out by the door using MR would reenter by the window through pleiotropy. The opposite case of no association found between the gene variant and the disease would also be open to several possibilities: (a) the relationship between exposure and disease was in fact confounded or biased; (b) the phenotype is only partially related to the tested allele, and other haplotypes/gene variants are also involved; (c) penetrance/expression of the gene depends on circumstances, including for example diet (as the example of CYP2D6 in Ethiopians suggests); (d) the power of the study could be too limited to show an association.

Public health applications and perspectives

A number of potential public health applications flowing from the investigation of gene–environment interactions may be imagined, the common element of which is by definition the identification of subjects carrying different gene variants through genetic testing within families already known to be at high risk of disease or genetic screening in the general population The former is well established within clinical genetics (though the new developments may pose new specific problems) while the latter opens perspectives worth discussion.

Preventing disease in high-risk subjects: Rose's framework for prevention

A theoretical and practical discussion took place several years ago about the selection of high-risk subjects groups for the implementation of preventive measures. Particularly important in this discussion was Geoffrey Rose's setting out the main advantages and disadvantages of such a 'high-risk group' preventive strategy. The strategy presents two main advantages:

- It produces interventions that are appropriate to the particular individuals identified and consequently has the potential advantage of enhanced subject motivation in complying with the intervention requirements (e.g. changing diet, taking a drug, etc.)
- It offers in principle a more cost-effective use of limited resources and a more favourable ratio of benefits to risks.

However the 'high-risk' strategy has some serious disadvantages and limitations. First, as in all screening, it may meet problems with compliance, with a tendency for the response to be greatest amongst those who are often least at risk of the disease (this, however, is unlikely to apply for genetic screening). A second disadvantage is that this strategy is palliative and temporary. It does not seek 'to alter the underlying causes of the disease but rather to identify individuals who are particularly susceptible to those causes' (Rose 1985). There is another, third, related and more crucial reason why the predictive basis of the 'high-risk' strategy of prevention could be weak, as well illustrated, for example, by the case of breast cancer in relation to parity and other reproductive factors. Women at the highest risk for these factors generate a relatively small proportion of the cases, too few to justify pre-screening for the identification of high-risk women to whom to offer mammography. The lesson from this and numerous other examples is that *a large number of people at a small risk may give rise to more cases of disease than the small number who are at a high risk.* To the extent that this situation is common—as it appears to be—it limits the utility of the 'high-risk' approach to prevention, and is certainly relevant to the issue of screening for 'low-penetrant' gene variants. How far it is relevant needs some closer consideration, through specific examples, as Rose's concepts were formulated when the field of gene–environment interactions and susceptibility due to low-penetrance genes was in its infancy, at least for major chronic diseases.

Screening for genetic susceptibility: Number needed to screen and treat

To assess the role of a gene–environment interaction and screening in a population knowledge of the penetrance of the genetic trait (variant allele) and of its frequency is needed. Penetrance is expressed by the absolute risk of disease among individuals carrying the gene variant. So, high penetrance means high individual risk, which tends to be a feature of rarer gene variants or mutations. A useful measure for assessing the utility of an intervention is to estimate the number needed to treat (NNT) to prevent an event, which is equal to the inverse of the absolute risk reduction (Vineis *et al.* 2001). If screening is applied before intervening, NNT and frequency may be combined to compute the number needed to screen (NNS) to prevent one case of, say, cancer. The NNS in high-risk families for a high-penetrant gene (BRCA1) of breast cancer has been calculated (the expression 'genetic testing' rather than 'genetic screening' would be more appropriate in this situation). The cumulative (lifetime) risk of breast cancer was found as high as 80 per cent in some studies and in some populations among mutation carriers (in high-risk families) and the frequency of mutations in high-risk families is about 50 per cent. Based on results from randomized trials it can be assumed that tamoxifen or raloxifene halve this risk. In this situation it can be calculated that one needs to treat 2.5 (i.e. $1/[0.8 \times 0.5]$) mutation carriers and test 5 (i.e. $1/[0.8 \times 0.5 \times 0.5]$) family members to prevent one cancer. If instead the general population would be screened the NNS would change greatly. In the general population, however, the cumulative risk in carriers of mutations that do not all confer the same very high risk, turns out to be lower than 80 per cent and in the order of 40 per cent: This implies, with tamoxifene or raloxifene halving it, an absolute risk reduction of 20 per cent and a number needed to treat of five mutation carriers. However, since only 0.2 per cent of the general population are mutation carriers, the NNS is 2500 to prevent one cancer. One might discuss whether this substantial NNS (which even with a highly specific test may involve a number of false-positives) would make BRCA1 a realistic target for screening in the general population. However, with dwindling cost and ease of high throughput genotyping technology this calculus may change in future, at least among certain populations known to be at higher risk of carrying mutations.

Calculations along similar lines have been considered for low-penetrance genes (Vineis *et al.* 2001). For example, in the occupational context workers exposed to polycyclic aromatic hydrocarbons (PAHs) might hypothetically be screened for the null variant of the GSTM1 gene, which through a deficit of detoxification of the PAHs may entail an increased risk, of the order of 30 per cent, of lung cancer. Through screening subjects found to have the null genotype can be excluded from jobs that expose them to PAHs (maybe not hiring them at all). From a prevention viewpoint there is, however, a basic though subtle difference of this scenario in respect to the just mentioned case of BRCA1. In the latter the aim is to identify women who test positive and are at (much) higher risk of breast cancer than other women in order to offer them intensive treatment (e.g. continuous surveillance plus mastectomy when it becomes necessary); no demonstrable benefit would follow instead by the same treatment (unless universal prophylactic mastectomy would be adopted) for women testing negative. In contrast, in the workplace scenario the treatment would be radical—no exposure at all to PAHs—for those testing positive, while workers testing negative, who could also obviously benefit from the same measure (or in any case from a reduction in exposure) would not receive the treatment and be left at risk. In this situation a comparison of different preventive strategies simply in terms of NNT and NNS is not adequate and needs to be expanded taking into account costs, direct and indirect, tangible and intangible.

For example in a simulation study, Bartell and colleagues showed that genetic screening for chronic beryllium disease with HLA-DPB1*0201 may give health benefits that outweighed financial costs only if avoidance of one case of the disease is valued at US$1 million or higher in a US context (Bartell *et al.* 2000). Yet, their estimate of the predictive value of the screening might have been unrealistically high and might not have correctly weighed the harmful effects of false-positive results.

Screening for genetic susceptibility to environmental exposure to arsenic

Arsenic is an exposure that is important both for industrial workers and for the general population in wide areas of the world. The identification of high-risk groups could in principle be extremely useful to overcome the practical difficulties and the costs of primary prevention in affected populations.

Chronic exposure to arsenic is known to cause non-melanocytic skin and internal tumours in humans. Exposure to arsenic commonly occurs in occupational and environmental settings. Although occupational exposure to arsenic occurs in a variety of industrial settings the predominant source of arsenic exposure for more than 100 million people worldwide, including nearly 70 million in Bangladesh and the adjoining part of India, has been from contaminated drinking water (Rahman *et al.* 2001). Given the magnitude of the problem, which the WHO labelled as the largest mass poisoning in human history, the issue of risk reduction of arsenic-induced health problems has become an important research and policy topic. Since millions of people already accrued chronic exposure, and their risk of cancer has increased several fold, measures of secondary and even tertiary prevention also become pertinent in addition to primary prevention. The ability to isolate 'high-risk' groups would contribute enormously to the development of an effective preventive strategy. For this reason the knowledge of mechanisms of arsenic carcinogenesis can help. Several studies have examined the role of oxidative stress and DNA repair genes on the susceptibility to arsenic carcinogenicity as expressed by premalignant skin lesions. In these studies, carriers of certain polymorphisms in oxidative stress genes of myeloperoxidase (MPO) and catalase (CAT) as well as in the DNA repair gene xeroderma pigmentosum complementation group D (XPD) have been shown to have a 3 to 11-fold higher risk of premalignant skin lesions than the non-carriers (Ahsan *et al.* 2003).

Arsenic has a dose-dependent effect on skin and internal tumours. The risk of cancer among arsenic exposed population is ~1 per cent but the risk for premalignant skin lesions is much higher, up to more than 10 per cent, depending on the dose and duration of exposure.

Let us make an extreme assumption, i.e. the relative risk for premalignant lesions is 11, the highest estimate in literature, and that the cumulative risk of such lesions is 10 per cent in subjects with wildtype (normal) polymorphisms. Also assume two kinds of interventions: (a) one that leads to a 50 per cent decrease in the risk of skin lesions, and (b) one leading to a 100 per cent decrease. (These assumptions, useful for the sake of the example, are probably too extreme and unrealistic, since a relative risk of 11 is more compatible with a high-penetrant gene than with a low-penetrant gene.) As the calculations in Table 9.1.2 show: (a) if an intervention is implemented (improving the quality of water) that reduces the risk of premalignant lesions by 50 per cent, 20 subjects with wildtype genotype need to be 'treated' (NNT) to prevent one lesion, given that the cumulative risk of lesions is 10 per cent for the wildtype; (b) if the intervention is 100 per cent effective, then the NNT is 10, i.e. for every 10 treated persons (wildtype) one case is prevented. If screening for a gene variant that multiplies the risk of skin lesions by 11 (entailing a cumulative risk close to 100 per cent) is applied and a preventive intervention 50 per cent effective, the NNT is 2 for subjects testing positive, i.e. for every two persons screened and found positive one is 'saved'. However, in order to identify the subjects with the variant gene one needs to actually screen the population: With a prevalence of 20 per cent of the variant, the NNS is 10 for an intervention with 50 per cent efficacy and 5 with an intervention of 100 per cent. In the absence of screening, the NNT in the total population is the weighted mean of the NNT among subjects testing negative and subjects testing positive: 16.4 for 50 per cent efficacy and 8.2 for 100 per cent efficacy of the preventive effort. Hence even with (unrealistically) extreme assumptions the screening strategy would entail, with a 50 per cent effective intervention, screening 10 people and treating 2 to prevent one premalignant lesion to be contrasted with treating 16.4 without the screening: These comparative figures (and the same applies for those for a 100 per cent effective intervention) offer no support for the screening strategy unless the costs of screening and targeted

Table 9.1.2 Calculation of the number needed to screen for a hypothetical highly penetrant gene among subjects exposed to arsenic. Two assumptions are made, that the preventive intervention has 50% (a) or 100% (b) efficacy (from Vineis *et al.*).

	Gene			
	Wildtype		**Variant**	
	(a)	**(b)**	**(a)**	**(b)**
Relative risk for gene	1.0	1.0	11	11
Cumulative risk of premalignant lesions (%)	10	10	100	100
Risk reduction (%)	50	100	50	100
Cumulative risk after intervention (%)	5	0	50	0
Absolute risk reduction (%)	5	10	50	100
NNT	20	10	2	1
Carrier frequency (%)	80	80	20	20
NNS	25	12.5	10	5
NNT in the absence of screening	16.4	8.2		

intervention on the subjects testing positive would be orders of magnitude inferior to the intervention for everybody, i.e. general improvement of the water quality entailing a substantial reduction of exposure to arsenic.

In this particular example if a high-risk strategy would be considered as an option, rather than genetic screening (because of uncertainties in NNT and NNS), identification of the at-risk population through screening for arsenic exposure of the population by testing drinking water and biological samples (urine, hair or nail) for arsenic would be more practical. Since the distribution of arsenic exposure is somewhat less individual-specific (unlike genetic polymorphisms), instead of genetically tailored individual-level interventions household-level interventions (provision of safe wells) may turn out to be more promising. For many arsenic affected areas where 50–90 per cent of the population are exposed (e.g. in Bangladesh, West Bengal, India, inner Mongolia, and certain provinces of China) several community-level interventions (e.g. community wells, supply water, and, in addition, food fortification with antioxidants or other anti-arsenic nutrients) are warranted. Needless to say, provision of good-quality water, a primary good, entails also a number of other benefits for the population.

Screening for subjects claimed to be genetically susceptible: The NicoTest

A recent example illustrates how weakly supported findings might translate into shaky 'predictive medicine' under the pressure of commercial interests. In 2004, a private firm from Oxford (G-Nostics) put on the market a kit for the identification of the carriers of a genetic variant of the gene DRD2, involved in the syndrome of nicotine addiction. The carriers of the variant would be more susceptible to developing addiction, but also to responding to a treatment with nicotine patches, and then should be treated as really 'sick' people. There were some observations from studies of the DRD2 gene that genetic variants related to relatively decreased dopaminergic tone in the mesocorticolimbic system are associated with increased risk for relapse to smoking following a cessation attempt. The offer of the test was, however, mainly based on the results of a randomized experiment, the most persuasive type of clinical investigation. Overall 1532 heavy smokers had been randomly allocated to two arms, the first receiving the nicotine patch, and the second other types of anti-smoking treatments. Subsequently (after 8–10 years), 755 (49.3 per cent) of these subjects agreed to donate a blood sample for genetic determinations. At this point, the researchers noted that those who quit smoking with the use of a patch were predominantly subjects with the genetic variant of DRD2, who came to be regarded as the best target for this kind of dissuasion intervention. The difference between carriers of the variant and 'normal' subjects was strong (a proportion of quitting two–three times higher) and statistically significant. However, the effectiveness of the dissuasion intervention, i.e. quitting smoking, was evaluated at short time (between 1 and 12 weeks) (Johnstone *et al.* 2004), while it is well known that relapses occur in a substantial proportion within the first 6–12 months. Also, in two other randomized trials, carried out in two culturally very diverse populations (African Americans and Japanese) (McBride *et al.* 2002; Hamajima *et al.* 2004), knowledge of genotype did not influence the success rate of smoking cessation.

It is worth noting the potential problems and the slippery slope that could be created on the basis of premature introduction into practice, based on wholly inadequate evidence, of a test like the NicoTest (incidentally, the DRD2 genotype seems of relevance also to the propensity to develop obesity) (Morton *et al.* 2006). It is not far-fetched to imagine that there might be a category of people who, being told that they have a greater genetic resistance to the effectiveness of the nicotine patch and other anti-smoking devices, will end up with thinking they have no hope of quitting; other people might instead wrongly come to think that, based on their genetic make-up, they are generally protected from the effects of smoking and for the same reason may not give up. A worrying scenario would develop if this type of testing based on flimsy evidence would extend to other characteristics, for example the propensity to develop obesity or antisocial behaviours. An approach that is typical of clinical medicine (pharmacogenetics) would be automatically extended to behaviours like smoking, thus suggesting that these complex behaviours simply belong to the category of 'disease'. Addictions and behaviours that are hazardous to health, and even antisocial, arise from an interaction between the environment and individual susceptibility, including the genetic form. The two aspects cannot be simplistically disentangled, and to dissociate them may lead to a dangerous slippery slope including: A stigma towards minorities (for carriers of the susceptibility genes); increasing conflicts around the eligibility for insurance of carriers of such genes; a widespread climate of irresponsibility, since the fault for diseases and behaviours is attributed to genes; and the diffusion of a model of causality more and more influenced by hard natural sciences rather than social and political determinants of the most significant events in people's lives.

Ethical issues (Vineis *et al.* 2005)

Screening for low-penetrant genes also raises a number of important ethical and social issues which need to be considered in any decision about implementation. The following analysis of arguments for and against such screening is centred on workers but similar considerations apply to environmentally exposed populations.

Arguments in favour of the availability of genetics testing in the workplace

The use of genetic screening in employment is hardly objectionable when it aims at directly protecting a wider 'public interest', i.e. public safety. An example might be screening those who are to be responsible for flying planes or working in air traffic control for mutations conferring a low risk of fatal cardiac arrhythmia on the rationale that whilst unlikely, the occurrence of such failure would have serious implications for public safety.

Apart from such cases there are some ethical arguments which have been put forward in favour of the use, or at least the availability, of genetic screening of workers. Perhaps the strongest of these draws its strength from a long-standing belief that employers and indeed legislators, have a duty, where this is possible, to protect employees, particularly those who are vulnerable, from avoidable risks in the workplace. Duties of this kind have been stressed in employment legislation in the United Kingdom and many other countries for well over a century; e.g., in the Factory Act 1851 (outlawing child labour under the age of 8) and the Mines Act 1842 (outlawing women, girls, and boys under 10 working in mines).

If employers have a duty of care for their employees it follows that when a test or screen is known to be effective, employers have an obligation to use it to improve the safety of workers and potential workers. This may also imply that where such tests or screens do exist, but are not used, the employers may be vulnerable to legal challenge. Indeed such a case has recently occurred in the United States where the Dow Chemical Company was sued by the widow of a deceased employee for failing to include the employee in a cytogenetic testing programme which might have detected his development of leukaemia from exposure in the workplace to benzene at an early stage (Brandt-Rauf & Brandt-Rauf 2004).

A second set of ethical arguments in favour of the availability of screening or testing arises from the broad duty of respect for freedom of choice, i.e. autonomy. It could be argued that making an informative test available, either commercially or in the workplace, would enable workers to make informed choices about the kinds of jobs they take—about whether or where to work. In at least one legal jurisdiction this right has been established legally. In the case of *International Union UAW v Johnson Controls Inc.*, it was decided that the choice of whether or not to work in a hazardous environment—while pregnant in this case—was reserved for workers to make themselves and was not for their potential employers to decide (Desmond & Gardner-Hopkins 2001). Freedom of choice arguments claim that to deny workers access to informative tests is unacceptably paternalistic. On the other side, the concern has been raised that creating a situation in which workers are free to use tests but employers are not would lead to 'adverse selection' (Human Genetics Commission 2002), i.e. employees who know about their risks (while employers, and insurers, do not) may use this asymmetry to their advantage. This may be particularly relevant in contexts, such as the United States, where healthcare insurance is related to employment. As a consequence, 'genetic transparency' has been advocated, where both parties should have access to such information (Diver & Cohen 2001).

A third argument for the use of genetic screening in the workplace might be that this has the potential to bring about important economic advantages through increased safety and reduced healthcare costs. Again, this might be of particular relevance to companies operating in a country such as the United States where health insurance is tied to employment. But, taking economic advantage in the broader sense, such an argument might also be made in the context of countries with publicly funded healthcare (Vineis *et al.* 2005, p. 139).

Arguments against the use of genetic testing in the workplace

Despite the arguments put forward for the availability and use of genetic screening in the workplace under certain conditions, there are a number of important arguments against it which provide grounds for concern and extreme caution should such screening be contemplated for implementation.

The first and strongest argument against the use of genetic testing in employment is that it carries the potential to lead to increased discrimination. There is indeed, good evidence that this is already happening. Recently, for example, the US Equal Employment Opportunity Commission filed suit against the Burlington Northern Santa Fe Railroad Co. for defying the 'Americans with Disability' Act (case settled in 2002 for US$2.2 million) on the grounds that the company required employees to submit blood samples to test them for genes predisposing to the carpal tunnel syndrome. It was also argued, successfully, that the company failed to obtain adequate informed consent and in some cases threatened employees with dismissal for failing to comply (Vineis *et al.* 2005, p. 139). This is one amongst many examples of such discrimination (p. 146).

Discrimination might also arise out of the *selective* use of genetic screening. For example, if there is a shortage of people willing to work in a particularly dangerous process, testing may be withheld for economic reasons in order to maintain a needed workforce.

In general, arguments about discrimination arise out of concern that genetic screening in employment may lead to a situation in which a person's genetic make-up determines work opportunities (Davis 2004): Individuals who test 'positive' may as a result become less employable, less insurable, and vulnerable in a number of different and important respects. Such concerns do not arise solely out of the nature of genetics or of genetic information but also out of the social and political realities of the world in which people live and work. Arguments about freedom of choice, for example, may sound attractive in the abstract, but policies based on freedom of choice divorced from an awareness of the broader social context have the potential to favour the wealthy, the highly educated, and the 'genetically normal'. Not everyone, for example, has the choice about where to work: Lack of skills, lack of mobility, living in an area of high unemployment, may make it impossible for those who are rejected from local employment to find a job elsewhere.

Second, in addition to its potential to lead to increased discrimination, the use of genetic screening in the workplace may lead to an increased likelihood of invasion of privacy and confidentiality of workers, for example in the writing of references or the provision of information for the purposes of insurance. Moreover, the standards of security and confidentiality in relation to the use of genetic information and samples may be less rigorously monitored in the context of employment than in, for example, medical research. Indeed, examples already exist of samples being tested for outcomes other than that for which they were taken. For example, in the case of *Norman-Bloodsaw v Lawrence Berkeley Laboratory employees* provided blood and urine samples for cholesterol testing but in fact some of these samples were subsequently tested for syphilis, pregnancy and sickle-cell trait (Michie *et al.* 2003).

A third set of arguments against the use of genetic screening for low-penetrant genes in the workplace arises out of concerns that the information provided by such tests is likely to be extremely difficult to interpret and/or to communicate. To begin with there is the question about the extent to which such testing is likely to produce information of any real value for use in the workplace. In addition the question arises of how risk information, particularly in the case of low-penetrant genes associated with a mild increase in disease risk, is to be communicated to employers and to employees in a way that is understandable or usable. Finally there is a good deal of evidence that even in the case of single gene disorders where the mode of inheritance and risk are, by comparison, clear, those tested have a tendency to misunderstand the implications of test results, especially when these are negative.

The fourth and final set of arguments against the use of genetic screening in the workplace is that it may easily become a diversion from the responsibility of employers and legislators to ensure that the working environment is safe for all of those who work there. Instead of using resources to identify workers who may be genetically at lesser risk, the focus should be on finding ways to make the workplace safe for all. Of course, quite similar arguments apply to environmentally exposed populations, with the added proviso that these include subjects often particularly vulnerable, like children, very old people, or pregnant women.

Conclusion

At present, knowledge of gene–environment interactions and of genetic susceptibility to disease in presence of environmental exposures does not support the view that screening for genetic variants—especially of low-penetrance genes—in order to identify subjects and subgroups at higher risk in the general population may be a practical and useful (or ethically recommendable) prevention strategy. Research in this area, however, is undergoing an extremely fast evolution and a reassessment of the evidence at short intervals is necessary.

Acknowledgements

This work was made possible by a grant to ECNIS (Environmental Cancer Risk, Nutrition and Individual Susceptibility), a network of excellence operating within the European Union 6th Framework Program, Priority 5: 'Food Quality and Safety' (Contract No 513943). We wish to acknowledge Sarah Teague, Michael Parker, and Habibul Ahsan for thoughtful contributions.

References

Abbeduto L., Brady N., Kover S.T. (2007) Language development and fragile X syndrome: profiles, syndrome-specificity, and within-syndrome differences. *Mental Retardation and Development Disabilities Research Review*, **13**, 36–46.

Aguilar C.A., Talavera G., Ordovas J.M. *et al.* (1999). The apolipoprotien E4 allele in not associated with an abnormal lipid profile in a Native American population following its traditional lifestyle. *Atherosclerosis*, **142**, 409–14.

Ahsan H., Chen Y., Wang C. *et al.* (2003) DNA repair gene XPD and susceptibility to arsenic-induced hyperkeratosis. *Toxicology Letters*, **143**, 123–31.

Aklillu E., Herrlin K., Gustafsson L.L. *et al.* (2002) Evidence for environmental influence on CYP2D6-catalysed debrisoquine hydroxylation as demonstrated by phenotyping and genotyping of Ethiopians living in Ethiopia or in Sweden. *Pharmacogenetics*, **12**, 375–83.

Armstrong B.K., White E., and Saracci R. (1994) *Principles of exposure measurement in epidemiology*. 2nd edition. Oxford University Press, Oxford.

Bartell S.M., Ponce R.A., Takaro T.K. *et al.* (2000) Risk estimation and value-of-information analysis for three proposed genetic screening programs for chronic beryllium disease prevention. *Risk Analysis*, **20**, 87–99.

Block N. (1995) How heritability misleads about race. *Cognition*, **56**, 99–128.

Booth F.W., Chakravarthy M.V., and Spanenberg E.E. (2002) Exercise and gene expression: physiological regulation of the human genome through physical activity. *Journal of Physiology*, **543**, 399–411.

Borén T., Falk P., Roth K.A. *et al.* (1993). Attachment of *Helicobacter pylori* to human gastric epithelium mediated by blood group antigens. *Science*, **262**, 1892–5.

Brandt-Rauf P.W. and Brandt-Rauf S.I. (2004) Genetic testing in the workplace: ethical, legal and social implications. *Annual Review of Public Health*, **25**, 139–53.

Bray M.S. (2000) Genomics, genes, and environmental interaction: the role of exercise. *Journal of Applied Physiology*, **88**, 788–92.

Chan J.M., Giovannucci E., Andersson S.O. *et al.* (1998) Dairy products, calcium, phosphorous, vitamin D, and risk of prostate cancer (Sweden). *Cancer Causes & Control*, **9**, 559–66.

Clayton D. and McKeigue P.M. (2001) Epidemiological methods for studying genes and environmental factors in complex diseases. *Lancet*, **358**, 1356–60.

Davey Smith G. and Ebrahim S. (2003) 'Mendelian randomization': can genetic epidemiology contribute to understanding environmental determinants of disease? *International Journal of Epidemiology*, **32**, 1–22.

Davis D.S. (2004) Genetic research and communal narratives. *Hastings Center Report*, **34**, 40–9.

Desmond J. and Gardner-Hopkins J.D. (2001) Unemployable genes: genetic discrimination in the workplace. *Auckland University Law Review*, **9**, 435–68.

Diver C.S. and Cohen J.M. (2001) Genephobia: what is wrong with genetic discrimination? *University PA Law Review*, **149**, 1439–82.

Ford E.S., Giles W.H., and Dietz W.H. (2002) Prevalence of the metabolic syndrome among US adults: findings from the Third National Health and Nutrition Examination Survey. *JAMA*, **287**, 356–9.

Fox Keller E. (2000) *The century of the gene*. Harvard University Press, Cambridge, MA.

Ganmaa D., Li X.M., Wang J. *et al.* (2002) Incidence of testicular and prostate cancers in relation to world dietary practices. *International Journal of Cancer*, **98**, 262–7.

Greenlund K.J., Valdez R., Casper M.L. *et al.* (1999) Prevalence and correlates of the insulin resistance syndrome among Native Americans. The Inter-Tribal Heart Project. *Diabetes Care*, **22**, 441–7.

Hamajima N., Atsuta Y., Goto Y. *et al.* (2004) A pilot study on genotype announcement to induce smoking cessation by Japanese smokers. *Asian Pacific Journal for Cancer Prevention*, **5**, 409–13.

Hanchette C.L. and Schwartz G.G. (1992) Geographic patterns of prostate cancer mortality. Evidence for a protective effect of ultraviolet radiation. *Cancer*, **70**, 2861–9.

Harris H. (1959) *Human biochemical genetics*. Cambridge University Press, Cambridge.

Herrnstein R.J. and Murray C. (1994) *The Bell Curve: Reshaping of American Life by Differences in Intelligence*. Simon and Schuster, New York.

Hood V.L., Kelly B., Martinez C. *et al.* (1997) A Native American community initiative to prevent diabetes. *Ethnicity & Health*, **2**, 277–85.

Human Genetics Commission. (2002) Inside Information: balancing interests in the use of personal genetic data. (Accessed on 1 July 2008 on: www.hgc.gov.uk)

Hunter D.J. and Kraft P. (2007) Drinking from the fire hose – statistical issues in genomewide association studies. *New England Journal of Medicine*, **357**, 436–9.

Isomaa B. (2003) A major health hazard: the metabolic syndrome. *Life Sciences*, **73**, 2395–411.

Johnstone E.C., Yudkin P.L., Hey K. *et al.* (2004) Genetic variation in dopaminergic pathways and short-term effectiveness of the nicotine patch. *Pharmacogenetics*, **14**, 83–90.

Kataoka S., Robbins D.C., Cowan L.D. *et al.* (1996) Apolipoprotein E polymorphism in American Indians and its relation to plasma lipoproteins and diabetes. The Strong Heart Study. *Arteriosclerosis, Thrombosis & Vascular Biology*, **16**, 918–25.

Knowler W.C., Williams R.C., Pettitt D.J. *et al.* (1988) Gm3;5,13,14 and type 2 diabetes mellitus: an association in American Indians with genetic admixture. *American Journal of Human Genetics*, **43**, 520–6.

Lewontin R. (1972) The analysis of variance and the analysis of causes. *American Journal of Human Genetics*, **26**, 400–11.

Lower G.M., Jr, Nilsson T., Nelson C.E. *et al.* (2007). N-acetyltransferase phenotype and risk in urinary bladder cancer: approaches in molecular epidemiology. Preliminary results in Sweden and Denmark. *International Journal of Epidemiology*, **36**, 11–17.

McBride C.M., Bepler G., Lipkus I.M. *et al.* (2002) Incorporating genetic susceptibility feedback into a smoking cessation program for African-American smokers with low income. *Cancer Epidemiology Biomarkers & Prevention*, **11**, 521–8.

McKusick V.A. (1998) *Mendelian inheritance in man*, 12th edn. Johns Hopkins University Press, Baltimore.

Michie S., Smith J.A., Senior V. *et al.* (2003) Understanding why negative genetic test results sometimes fail to reassure. *American Journal of Medical Genetics*, **119**, 340–7.

Morton L.M., Wang S.S., Bergen A.W. *et al.* (2006) DRD2 genetic variation in relation to smoking and obesity in the Prostate, Lung, Colorectal, and Ovarian Cancer Screening Trial. *Pharmacogenetics and Genomics*, **16**, 901–10.

Muneta B., Newman J., Wetterall S. *et al.* (1993) Diabetes and associated risk factors among Native Americans. *Diabetes Care*, **16**, 1619–20.

Nagi D.K., Foy C.A., Mohamed-Ali V. *et al.* (1998) Angiotensin-1-converting enzyme (ACE) gene polymorphism, plasma ACE levels, and their association with the metabolic syndrome and electrocardiographic coronary artery disease in Pima Indians. *Metabolism*, **47**, 622–6.

Olson S. (2002) *Mapping human history: unravelling the mystery of Adam and Eve*. Bloomsbury Publishing, London.

Ottman R. (1996) Gene-environment interaction: definitions and study designs. *Preventive Medicine*, **25**, 764–70.

Penagarikano O., Mulle J.G., Warren S.T. (2007) The pathophysiology of fragile X syndrome. *Annual Review of Genomics and Human Genetics*. May 3, **8**, 109–29.

Rahman M.M., Chowdhury U.K., Mukherjee S.C. (2001) Chronic arsenic toxicity in Bangladesh and West Bengal, India--a review and commentary. *Journal of Toxicology and Clinical Toxicology*, **39**, 683–700.

Reilly M.P. and Rader D.J. (2003) The metabolic syndrome: more than the sum of its parts? *Circulation*, **108**, 1546–51.

Resnick H. (2002) Metabolic Syndrome in American Indians. *Diabetes Care*, **25**, 1246–7.

Rose G. (1985) Sick individuals and sick populations. *International Journal of Epidemiology*, **14**, 32–8.

Sacerdote C., Guarrera S., Smith G.D. *et al.* (2007) Lactase persistence and bitter taste response: instrumental variables and Mendelian randomization in epidemiologic studies of dietary factors and cancer risk. *American Journal of Epidemiology*, **166**, 576–81.

Saracci R. (1980) Interaction and synergism. *American Journal of Epidemiology*, **112**, 465–6.

Skowronski R.J., Peehl D.M., and Feldman D. (1993) Vitamin D and prostate cancer: 1,25 dihydroxyvitamin D3 receptors and actions in human prostate cancer cell lines. *Endocrinology*, **132**, 1952–60.

The Wellcome Trust Case Control Consortium. (2007). Genome-wide association study of 14,000 cases of seven common diseases and 3,000 shared controls. *Nature*, **447**, 661–84.

Thomas D.C. (2004) *Statistical Methods in Genetic Epidemiology*. Oxford University Press, New York.

Thomas D.C. and Clayton D. (2004) Betting odds and genetic associations. *JNCI*, **96**, 421–3.

Thompson D.B., Ravussin E., Bennet P.H. *et al.* (1997). Structure and sequence variation at the human leptin receptor gene in lean and obese Pima Indians. *Human Molecular Genetics*, **6**, 675–9.

Tschermak E. (1950). Concerning artificial crossing in 'Pisum Sativum'. *Genetics*, **35**, 42–7 (translation of the original 1900 publication in German).

Vineis P. (2007). Commentary: First steps in molecular epidemiology: Lower *et al.* 1979. *International Journal of Epidemiology*, **36**, 20–22.

Vineis P., Ahsan H., Parker M. (2005) Genetic screening and occupational and environmental exposures. *Occupational and Environmental Medicine*, **62**, 657–62.

Vineis P., Schulte P., and McMichael A.J. (2001) Misconceptions about the use of genetic tests in populations. *Lancet*, **357**, 709–12.

Vozarova B., Fernandez-Real J.M., Knowler W.C. *et al.* (2003). The interleukin-6 (-174) G/C promoter polymorphism is associated with type-2 diabetes mellitus in Native Americans and Caucasians. *Human Genetics*, **112**, 409–413.

Wacholder S., Chanock S., Garcia-Closas M. *et al.* (2004) Assessing the probability that a positive report is false: an approach for molecular epidemiology studies. *JNCI*, **96**, 434–42.

Wendorf M. (1989) Diabetes, the ice free corridor, and the Paleoindian settlement of North America. *American Journal of Physical Anthropology*, **79**, 503–20.

Witte J.S. (2007) Multiple prostate cancer risk variants on 8q24. *Nature Genetics*, **39**, 579–80.

Yang Q. and Khoury M.J. (1997) Evolving methods in genetic epidemiology. III. Gene-environment interaction in epidemiologic research. *Epidemiological Review*, **19**, 33–43.

Zanke B.W., Greenwood C.M., Rangrej J. *et al.* (2007). Genome-wide association scan identifies a colorectal cancer susceptibility locus on chromosome 8q24. *Nature Genetics*, **39**, 989–94.

Zimmet P. and Thomas C.R. (2003) Genotype, obesity and cardiovascular disease—has technical advancement outstripped evolution? *Journal of Internal Medicine*, **254**, 114–25.

9.2

Cardiovascular and cerebrovascular diseases

Russell V. Luepker and Kamakshi Lakshminarayan

Abstract

Cardiovascular diseases, conditions of the heart and blood vessels, are leading causes of morbidity and mortality throughout the world. Largely diseases of lifestyle and affluence, they account for a majority of deaths in some industrialized countries. They are a coming epidemic in the developing world as communities and individuals attain richer and less healthy lifestyles. The leading cardiovascular diseases are coronary heart disease, hypertension, stroke, and heart failure. They are frequently interconnected with the underlying pathology atherosclerosis, a condition damaging medium and large arteries. There are also other important diseases which, while less common, present considerable health burden including rheumatic heart disease, peripheral artery disease, cardiomyopathy, and congenital heart disease.

Unlike many lifestyle related conditions, the causes or risk factors for the leading cardiovascular diseases are well known. They are diet resulting in hyperlipidemia, elevated blood pressure leading to hypertension, diabetes mellitus, physical inactivity, and cigarette smoking. There are also other identified characteristics but this group of risk factors underlies the epidemic. As well studied conditions, much is known about the pathophysiology of risk factors and cardiovascular disease. In addition, knowledge from clinical trials dictates treatment of risk for primary and secondary prevention. Few chronic diseases had such an extensive scientific basis for the prevention and treatment. Prevention starts at the community level where unhealthy diets, smoking and physical inactivity can be confronted and reduced. Clinical presentations of individual risk factors such as hypertension, hyperlipidemia and diabetes mellitus can be treated with lifestyle modification and/or medication. The implementation of prevention programmes at the community and clinic level results in population-wide changes and disease reduction. The potential for continuing improvement in the industrialized world and blunting the epidemic in the developing world is substantial.

Introduction

Cardiovascular and cerebrovascular diseases are the leading causes of death and disability in most industrialized countries and they are increasingly prevalent in the developing world. The principal cardiovascular diseases are related to atherosclerosis: Coronary heart disease, athero-thrombotic stroke, and peripheral vascular disease. Hypertension, haemorrhagic stroke, heart failure, rheumatic heart disease, cardiomyopathy, and congenital heart disease are also common. The patterns on distributions of these diseases vary in different regions; however, coronary heart disease, stroke and heart failure are frequently pre-eminent, leading to widespread population morbidity and mortality.

The rise of the cardiovascular diseases is attributed to a number of factors. The gradual reduction and elimination of infectious disease leading to increased longevity. Cardiovascular diseases are usually chronic conditions mainly affecting older populations. Additionally, atherosclerotic-related diseases are associated with affluent lifestyles. The widespread availability of rich foods leads directly to elevated blood lipids. Surplus food and reduction in habitual physical activity results in obesity, also encouraging hyperlipidaemia, hypertension and diabetes. In countries where affluence is growing, these diseases are found first among the wealthy. However, cardiovascular disease gradually affects all segments of the population as affluent living conditions prevail.

These shifts have led to changing patterns of cardiovascular diseases worldwide. In many industrialized countries, the rates of cardiovascular disease are falling, in others still rising. In most developing countries, the rates are rising associated with greater affluence and reduced infectious diseases.

The rise in cardiovascular and cerebrovascular diseases was a phenomenon of the twentieth century in the industrialized world. It threatens to be the leading cause of death and disability worldwide in the twenty-first century. Public health can and does play a leading role in the prevention of these diseases. Since risk factors for these diseases are identifiable and readily modified in healthy individuals at the population level, the sources of this epidemic can be confronted. The elimination of these diseases is possible and is a major public health challenge for the coming period.

Burden of cardiovascular diseases mortality

Cardiovascular disease is the leading cause of death in many countries and rising in many others. Figure 9.2.1 depicts mortality for cardiovascular disease including stroke, cancer, and all causes in 2002 for men and women combined in selected countries. Cardiovascular diseases account for around 50 per cent of the deaths in many countries (WHO 2007). For example, in the United States,

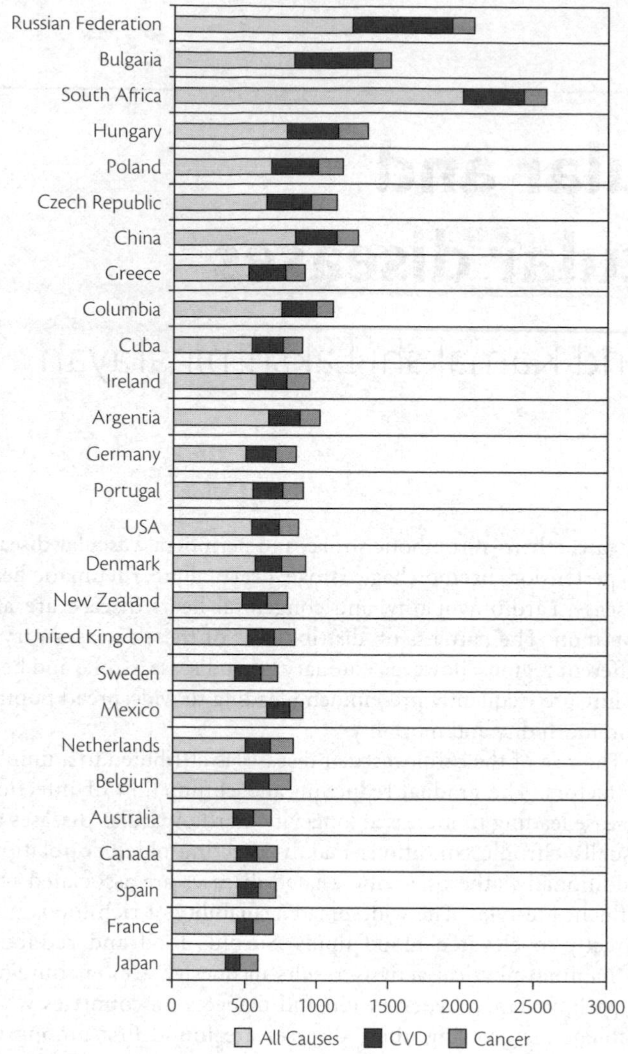

Fig. 9.2.1 Mortality for CVD, cancer, and all causes by selected country, age standardized to WHO population (age 35–74) (Year 2002).

as in many Western European countries, coronary heart disease accounts for approximately half of the cardiovascular deaths, while stroke and other causes provide the remainder. In Sweden, coronary heart disease and stroke are about equal. In Japan, stroke is more common. In Egypt, infectious cardiac diseases are important causes, however, atherosclerotic diseases are increasing (WHO 2007; AHA 2007). These differences in distributions of cardiovascular disease mortality are associated with different circumstances in those countries and differing methods of classifying death. They also reflect age and sex distributions of the populations, as most cardiovascular diseases are strongly associated with increasing age.

Although rarely appreciated by clinicians, the majority of cardiovascular disease mortality occurs outside of hospitals as 'sudden' death (McGovern *et al.* 1996; Tunstall-Pedoe *et al.* 1996). It may occur at home, in a public place, at work and during ambulance transport. Even those who reach the hospital alive have high rates of mortality which may approach 100 per cent in some categories (e.g. myocardial rupture).

Morbidity

While death is a common outcome of cardiovascular disease, non-fatal disease is also prevalent. As shown in Table 9.2.1, the total population with prevalent cardiovascular disease is estimated to be over 71 million in the United States in 2003 (NHLBI 2006). Hypertension is most common, but there are over 13 million people with coronary heart disease and 5 million with congestive heart failure. Stroke is estimated to include 5.5 million current victims in the population.

The magnitude of this problem is also shown in Fig. 9.2.2, which describes trends in non-fatal and fatal coronary heart disease hospital admissions over time in Southeastern New England in the United States. The rates reflect the age and sex differences in coronary heart disease (Derby *et al.* 2000). More people are surviving previously fatal attacks.

These common diseases now have many high-technology procedures designed to ameliorate the conditions and reduce symptoms. Many can prolong life. These medical procedures and treatments include cardiac surgery, angioplasty, angiography, pacemakers, implanted defibrillators, sophisticated diagnostic testing, and pharmaceuticals. Between the cost of this care and the lost productivity resulting from morbidity and mortality, cardiovascular disease represents an enormous economic burden, as shown in Fig. 9.2.3, for the United States in 2006 (AHA 2007). The total is over US$430 billion.

Disease trends

The epidemic of cardiovascular disease is largely a phenomenon of the twentieth century, and trends within this century are apparent. The Monitoring Trends and Determinants in Cardiovascular Disease (MONICA) study demonstrated that coronary heart disease rose or fell in different nations during the 1980s and 1990s (Tunstall-Pedoe *et al.* 1999). In selected countries, different patterns continue to be observed for coronary heart disease from 1970 to 2005 (Fig. 9.2.4) (NHLBI 2006). A downward trend was noted in the United States with coronary heart disease rates peaking in the mid-1960s and falling substantially since that time (Table 9.2.2) (NHLBI 2006). Stroke peaked earlier, declined slowly and then began a precipitous age-adjusted decline in the 1970s. Non-cardiovascular disease

Table 9.2.1 Prevalence of common cardiovascular and lung diseases, US, 2004

Disease	Number
Cardiovascular diseases[a]	79 400 000
Hypertension[b]	72 000 000
Coronary heart disease	15 800 000
Heart failure	5 200 000
Stroke	5 700 000
Congenital heart disease[c]	1 000 000

[a] Includes hypertension, CHD, heart failure, and stroke.

[b] Systolic blood pressure ≥140 mm Hg, diastolic blood pressure ≥90 mm Hg, on antihypertensive medication, or told twice of having hypertension.

[c] Range from 650 000 to 1 300 000 (Am Hrt J 2004;147:425–439).

Sources: National Health and Nutrition Examination Survey (NHANES) of NCHS and National Health Interview Survey of NCHS, except as noted.

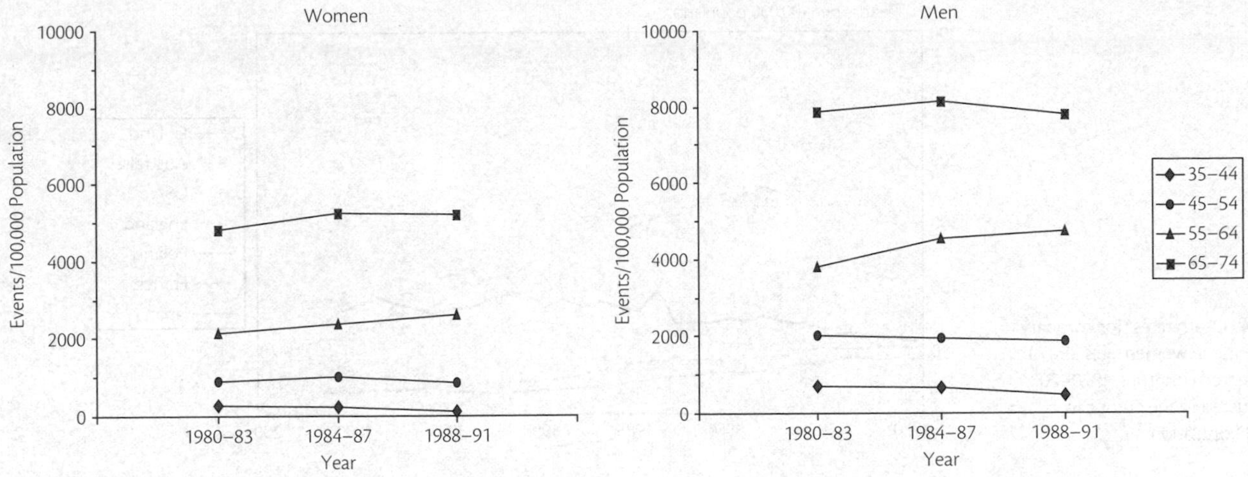

Fig. 9.2.2 Total discharges and deaths with ICD-9 code 410-414 in men and women, by age, Southeastern New England, 1980–91.

declined somewhat, but accounted for only a small fraction of the improvements in age-adjusted population mortality. With age-adjusted mortality falling, driven by a decline in cardiovascular disease, the result has been increased longevity in many populations. However, absolute mortality (not adjusted for age) has not fallen as much, as the disease is pushed into older age groups (Luepker 1994).

Disease definitions and classification

Cardiovascular disease

The leading cause of cardiovascular disease is atherosclerosis, a pathology affecting the walls of large and medium arteries. This disease process begins with injury and deposits of cholesterol in the arterial wall associated with inflammation and cellular infiltration. The arterial channel narrows with these deposits sometimes becoming 'hardened' with calcification. The result is an obstruction of blood flow and inadequate perfusion with diminished oxygen supply. Acute obstruction may occur with clots forming on the diseased vessel walls. In organs such as the heart or brain, which are dependent on a constant blood supply and oxygen, an acute obstruction can lead to irreversible damage to the tissue dependent on that supply. Temporary interruption or diminished flow will result in other symptoms. In the heart, loss of blood supply leads to myocardial infarction with death of heart muscle. In blood vessels of the extremities, atherosclerotic disease can limit blood flow resulting in symptoms of pain on exertion. In extreme cases, loss of blood supply can lead to gangrene and loss of a limb.

Other cardiovascular diseases have their own pathology which is described in later sections.

Stroke

Stroke is a heterogeneous entity and can be broadly divided into ischaemic strokes caused by blockage or occlusion of blood vessels and haemorrhagic stroke caused by a rupture of blood vessels. Ischaemic strokes are further subdivided based on mechanism of causation into those due to (i) atherosclerotic stenosis or occlusion of large cervico-cerebral vessels, (ii) cardio-embolism, (iii) small vessel disease, i.e. lacunes caused by the lipohyalinosis of and micro-atheromata from small penetrating arteries and (iv) less common, miscellaneous group of mechanisms including non-atherosclerotic vasculopathies, central nervous system infections such as *Cryptococcus*, certain hypercoagulable states, and disorders

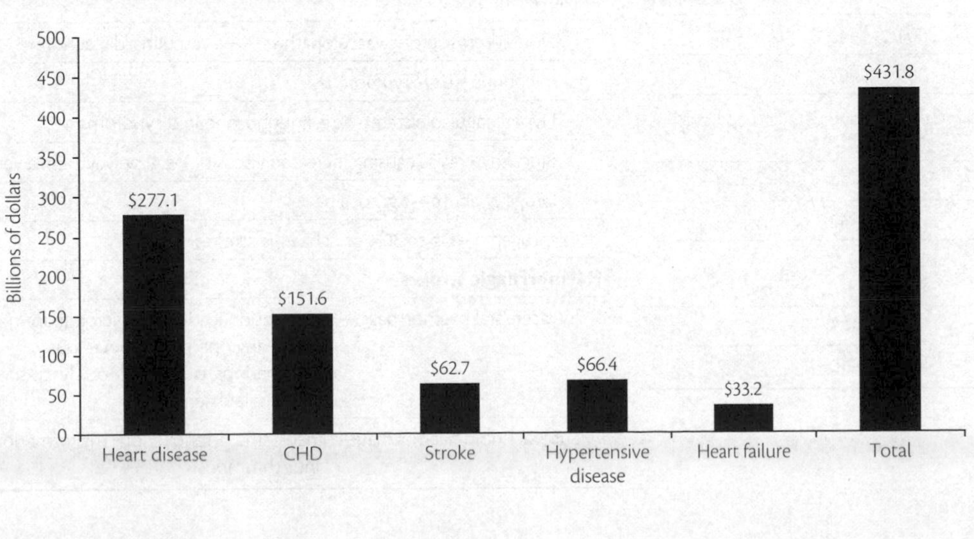

Fig. 9.2.3 Estimated direct and indirect costs of cardiovascular disease (CVD) and stroke in the United States, 1998.

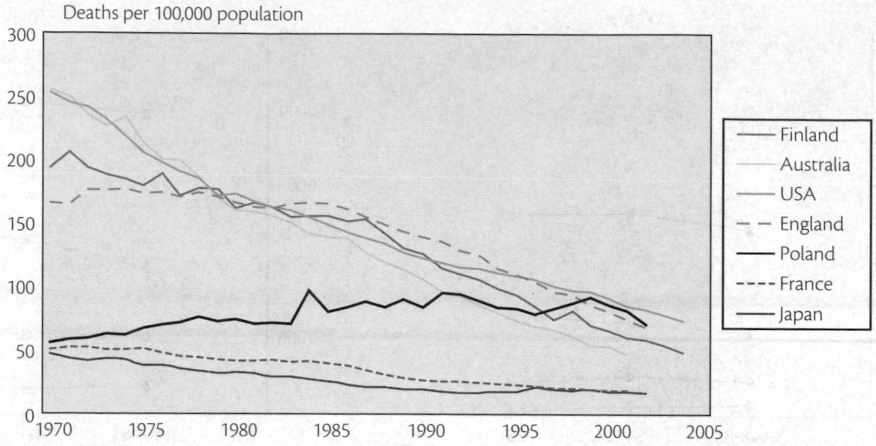

Fig. 9.2.4 Death rates* for coronary heart disease in women ages 35–74 years, selected countries, 1970–2004
*Age-adjusted to the European Standard Population.

of the cellular components of blood including sickle cell disease and polycythemia vera. Up to a third of all ischaemic strokes do not have an identified mechanism despite extensive evaluation. Haemorrhagic strokes can be subdivided based on location of haemorrhage into (i) subarachnoid haemorrhages commonly caused by the rupture of berry aneurysms into the subarachnoid space and (ii) intra-parenchymal haemorrhages caused by bleeding into the substance of the brain from a variety of reasons (Table 9.2.3).

Coronary heart disease

A vast body of research enhances the understanding of the aetiology, prevention, and treatment of coronary heart disease (AHA 2007). Important observations are summarized below:

1. Population-based studies show wide differences between countries and groups within those countries (Fig. 9.2.1).
2. Between and within populations, lipids, blood pressure, cigarette smoking, diabetes, and other characteristics are highly predictive of coronary heart disease events in individuals (Keys 1980). These risk factors are first evidenced in youth and track into adulthood. That is, high-risk youth are likely to become high-risk adults (Luepker *et al.* 1999).
3. Studies of large-scale migrations from one culture to another demonstrate that an increase in risk factors and coronary heart disease is observed when individuals migrate from a low- to high-risk culture and assume the lifestyle of that new culture (Kagan *et al.* 1974).
4. Population patterns in coronary heart disease are changing rapidly (Fig. 9.2.5).
5. Changes in coronary heart disease patterns are associated with a reduction in risk characteristics leading to decreased incidence

Table 9.2.2 Death rates[a] for cardiovascular and non-cardiovascular diseases, US, 1963, 1984, and 2004

Cause of death	1963	Rate[a] 1984	2004	Percent Change 1963–2004	Percent Change 1983–2004
All causes	1346	982	801	−40	−18
Cardiovascular diseases	805	488	289	−64	−41
Coronary heart disease	478	268	150	−69	−44
Stroke	174	83[b]	50	−71	−40
Other	153	137	88	−42	−36
Noncardiovascular diseases	541	495	512	−5	4
COPD and asthma	16	34[c]	42	153	24
Other	524	462	471	−10	2

[a] Age-adjusted; rate per 100 000 populations.
[b] Comparability ratio (1.0502) applied.
[c] Comparability ratio (1.0411) applied.
Source: Vital Statistics of the United States, NCHS.

Table 9.2.3 Stroke subtypes and pathophysiological causes

Ischemic strokes
Large vessel atherosclerosis or stenosis of cranio-cerebral vessels
Cardio-embolism
Small vessel disease (Lacunar strokes)
Miscellaneous
Non-atherosclerotic vasculopathies—e.g. vasculitis, dissection
Infectious—e.g. *Cryptococcus*
Hypercoagulable states—e.g. antiphospholipid syndrome
Blood dyscrasias causing increased viscosity—e.g. polycythemia vera
Drugs of abuse—e.g. cocaine
Cryptogenic—Up to 30% of ischaemic strokes
Haemorrhagic strokes
Intracerebral haemorrhage—hypertension leading to microaneurysms, amyloid angiopathy, arteriovenous malformations, trauma, blood dyscrasias (e.g. acute leukaemia)
Subarachnoid haemorrhage—aneurysms, arteriovenous malformations, sinus thrombosis

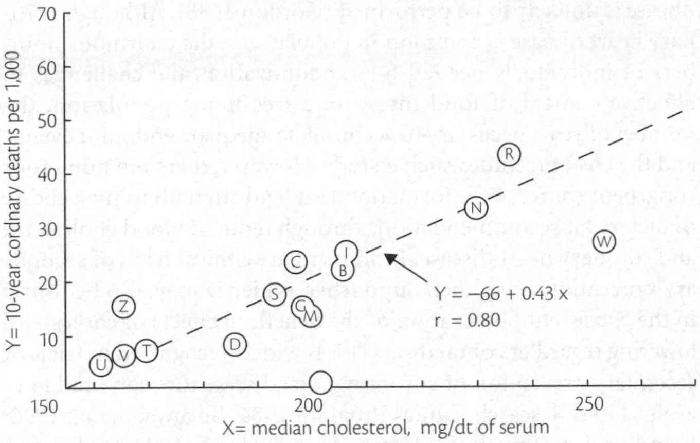

Fig. 9.2.5 Coronary death and cholesterol.
E=East Finland, R=American railroad, N=Zutphen, W=West Finland, I=Italian railroad, B=Belgrade, C=Crevalcore, S=Slavonia, G=Corfu, M=Montegiorgio, D=Dalmatia, K=Crete, Z=Zrenjanin, T=Tanushimaru, V=Velika Krsna, U=Ushibuka
Coronary heart disease age-standardized 10-year death rates of the cohorts versus the median serum cholesterol levels (mg per dl) of the cohorts. All men judged free of coronary heart disease at entry.
Source: Keys, A. Seven Countries 1980.

and to improved medical care, leading to increased survival after an initial clinical event.

6. Clinical trials demonstrate conclusively that a reduction in coronary heart disease mortality and morbidity results from the lowering of traditional risk factors (cholesterol, blood pressure, cigarette smoking) by either behavioural and/or pharmaco-logical methods. This occurs in both primary and secondary trials.

The rationale for disease prevention is found in many observations. Environmental factors encourage population-wide changes in behaviour resulting in mass elevations of risk. As populations live longer, this chronic disease is manifest following prolonged and sustained exposure to risk factors. Widespread genetic susceptibility also plays an important role in the setting of an unfavourable environment. Prevention of coronary heart disease is well founded based on these scientific observations. It begins with primary prevention or prevention of risk factor elevation in the first place (Luepker 1999). It includes identification and reduction of risk in high-risk individuals without manifest disease signs or symptoms. Finally, it rests on the identification of those who continue to be at high-risk after a coronary heart disease diagnosis. Well-established population and medical strategies are tested to implement prevention and the epidemic could be controlled with widespread and effective implementation of current knowledge.

Risk factors for atherosclerosis and coronary heart disease

There are numerous known risk factors playing a role in the development of atherosclerosis. Risk factors are characteristics discovered initially in prospective epidemiological studies. The aetiological role of risk factors is supported by laboratory experimental data and confirmed in clinical trials reducing risk in humans. Risk factors predict disease and frequently play a causal role in the pathological process. These include diet, lipids, obesity, physical inactivity, diabetes, hypertension, tobacco smoking, and others.

Diet

There is substantial evidence to support a causal association of habitual dietary intake with coronary heart disease. Much of that evidence is found in studies comparing populations. However, there is also evidence within populations to suggest the role of individual dietary intake in coronary heart disease morbidity and mortality. Human feeding experiments add evidence as do animal studies. A number of components of habitual diet have been considered. These include fats, dietary cholesterol, carbohydrates, fibre, alcohol, protein, and caloric excess. Information regarding diet and coronary heart disease is summarized here:

1. Habitual food intake varies greatly between populations. These differences are related to population prevalence of coronary heart disease (Keys 1980).
2. While more difficult to study, individual eating patterns are also associated with coronary heart disease (Keys 1980).
3. When all components of diet are considered, the type and amount of fat intake is the most important component in preventing coronary heart disease.
4. The association of dietary fat with coronary heart disease is predominantly through the effects of saturated fats and cholesterol on blood lipids.
5. Eating patterns are changing in many cultures, leading to improving coronary heart disease rates in some and worsening in others.
6. Clinical trials of secondary prevention find diet change useful in lowering coronary heart disease.
7. Laboratory animal studies of non-human primates are congruent with human diet–disease relationships.

Fat

The evidence is strong for the effect of diet between populations. The best known is the Seven Countries Study. This research compared habitual food intake in samples from among seven national populations (Keys 1980). This study demonstrated great variability in habitual food intake and a clear association of fatty acids and dietary cholesterol with blood cholesterol levels. Those blood cholesterol levels were a strong predictor of coronary heart disease in initially healthy populations followed more than 25 years (Blackburn & Jacobs 1984).

So central is the association of diet with blood cholesterol level, that many investigators suggest a cholesterol-raising diet is essential for mass expression of coronary heart disease (Blackburn & Jacobs 1984). These conclusions rest on data showing a diet with increased animal fats, specifically saturated fat and cholesterol, is found in populations where disease rates are high. Conversely, populations where these dietary components are low show a decreased incidence of coronary heart disease. Changes in diet seem to precede rising or falling coronary heart disease rates. Such is the case in the United States where diet is changing associated with falling blood cholesterol and coronary heart disease (CDC 2006) (Table 9.2.4). Additional evidence comes from observations in other international studies, where countries such as Japan have elevated levels of blood pressure and cigarette smoking, important coronary heart disease risk factors,

Table 9.2.4 Nutrient intake in the United States (1971–2002)

	1971–1975	1976–1980	1988–1994	1999–2002
Saturated fat (g/day)	31	31	27	25
Total fat (g/day)	87	87	80	78

but fail to manifest high rates of coronary heart disease. The Japanese have lower population levels of blood cholesterol (Keys 1980).

Observations on migrating populations show the same conclusions. The Japanese living in Japan have low cholesterol levels and low rates of coronary heart disease. As they move to Hawaii and the United States, they progressively assume the lifestyle of those Westernized cultures and experience elevations in blood cholesterol, obesity and coronary heart disease rates similar to the local population (Kagan *et al.* 1974). Again, the assumption of a high-fat Western diet is associated with increased coronary heart disease.

While the associations between diet and coronary heart disease are very strong in between population comparisons, the data are more conflicting in studies within populations. Here, studies of food intake or eating patterns of individuals modestly predict subsequent disease, if at all. There are several well-recognized reasons for this apparent paradox.

Supportive evidence comes from metabolic ward feeding studies. Here, individuals fed controlled diets of known composition for prolonged periods, show a clear relationship between type and quantity of fat intake and blood cholesterol levels. This relationship is best described by the Keys' formula which relates the intake of saturated fats, polyunsaturated fats, and dietary cholesterol to blood cholesterol levels (Keys *et al.* 1974). The Keys formula is calculated using the formula: $1.35\ (2S - P) + 1.5Z$ where S is the percentage of dietary calories from saturated fatty acids, P is the percentage of dietary calories from polyunsaturated fatty acids, and Z is the square root of dietary cholesterol in mg/1000 kcal.

More recent studies have provided increased detail including information on monounsaturated fats, and specific fatty acids including *trans*-fatty acids (Ascherio *et al.* 1994; Ginsberg *et al.* 1998). Trans-fatty acids, often the result of the chemical saturation process to harden fats, have a significant cholesterol raising effect.

Given clear and consistent associations in between population studies and feeding experiments involving fat, why has such an association not emerged in free-living populations? There are several reasons postulated. Among these is the difficulty of measurement of habitual food intake in individuals. While this measure is relatively simple in societies which have little variation in foods, it is particularly difficult in societies where unlimited foods are available and composition is highly variable on a daily basis. Individual data collection, such as 24-h recalls, fail to characterize usual intake adequately. Food frequency approaches which characterize longer periods of time are susceptible to recall bias and difficulty in determining 'average intake'.

There are also individual factors in the response to dietary intake. Even when food intake is carefully controlled, the digestion and absorption process may vary between individuals and genetic factors may play a role. Thus, two individuals eating the same diet may have a different cholesterol response.

It is generally acknowledged that a large-scale trial of reducing dietary fat intake for the primary prevention of coronary heart disease is unlikely to be performed (Gordon 1988). Although coronary heart disease is common in populations, the enormous numbers of individuals needed for randomization, the challenges to effective control of food intake in a free-living population, the number of years necessary to accumulate adequate endpoint events, and the cost, precludes such a study. However, there are numerous congruent sources of information that lend strength to the validity of dietary fat recommendations through reduced blood cholesterol and coronary heart disease. Prominent are clinical trials of secondary prevention using diet. Supportive evidence may also be found in the consistent observation of the beneficial effects of cholesterol lowering regardless of method. This is widely recognized in trials of secondary prevention of coronary heart disease through lipid lowering (Lipid Research Clinics Program 1984; Buchwald *et al.* 1990; Scandinavian Simvastatin Survival Study Group 1994; Sacks *et al.* 1996; LIPID Study Group 1998), but also studies of primary prevention with lipid-lowering medications (Shepherd *et al.* 1995; Downs *et al.* 1998).

The recognition that usual food intake is a behaviour strongly related to culture and food availability has resulted in community-based public health strategies to improve dietary intake. The North Karelia and Stanford Three Town Studies were among the first to use public and health professional education about dietary fat to reduce blood cholesterol (Farquhar *et al.* 1977; Puska *et al.* 1995). In both studies, an improved eating pattern with reduced animal fats (saturated fats and cholesterol) resulted in reduced average blood cholesterols in these small communities. Larger studies in medium-sized cities in Europe and the United States showed similar results. Strong favourable secular trends in control communities resulted in modest differences in blood cholesterol levels (GCP Research Group 1988; Farquhar *et al.* 1990; Luepker *et al.* 1994; Carleton *et al.* 1995).

Protein

Comparisons between populations in countries show an ecological correlation between dietary proteins, particularly animal protein and mortality from coronary heart disease. However, there is little evidence that this association is causal. Metabolic ward experiments of men under isocholoric condition, with fat intake held constant while protein intake varied between 5 and 20 per cent of daily calories, found no change in blood cholesterol levels (University of Minnesota, unpublished data).

These observations and others suggest that associations observed between populations are the result of animal fat associated with animal protein, rather than the effect of the protein itself. Specifically, consumption of fat from animals and high-fat milk products result in elevated blood cholesterol, rather than their high protein content. In coronary heart disease, it is generally agreed that dietary protein is not a factor in coronary heart disease.

Carbohydrates

A positive association is found between population intake of refined sugars and coronary heart disease. This relationship is confounded by many other dietary components and, importantly, the association of high levels of refined sugars with the usual diet of Westernized industrial countries. In the absence of a plausible biological connection between refined sugars and atherosclerosis, the association may actually be that of the high animal fat intake also found in those societies. However, refined sugars have other deleterious effects such as dental disease.

Complex carbohydrates are negatively associated with coronary heart disease. Higher intake is found with low coronary heart disease mortality. These are also confounded by fat intake and other dietary factors. There is a plausible biological mechanism by which complex carbohydrates may affect coronary heart disease. Foods having high levels of carbohydrates, such as fruits and vegetables, also contain fibre including pectins in fruit, bran fibre, and guar gum. These play a role in the absorption of fat and cholesterol in the intestines. Observational studies and clinical trials have demonstrated that increased fibre intake is associated with lower cholesterol levels (Jenkins *et al.* 1993). It is important to note that increased fibre intake is best attained by consumption of healthy fruits and vegetables, rather than dietary supplements.

Alcohol

There is a continuing debate regarding the effects of alcohol consumption on cardiovascular disease including coronary heart disease. Alcohol has several associations with coronary heart disease including: (1) the association of alcohol consumption with increased blood pressure and the risk of stroke (Criqui 1987); (2) the association of alcohol consumption with increased high-density lipoprotein cholesterol and levels of triglycerides (Gordon *et al.* 1981); (3) the effect of alcohol on haemostatic factors including fibrinogen, platelet aggregation and fibrinolysis (Meade *et al.* 1987); (4) Large doses of alcohol lead to addiction and other severe diseases. These include cardiovascular diseases such as congestive cardiomyopathy, cardiac arrhythmias, and sudden death (Regan 1990).

Given these findings, why is there controversy about alcohol intake? It principally stems from epidemiological research which shows moderate intake of alcohol is associated with lower risk of coronary heart disease when compared to non-drinkers. Numerous studies support this observation after adjusting for other risk factors and confounders, which stimulates this debate. One controversy focuses on the type of alcoholic beverage containing this benefit. Some have suggested wine is the essential form, while others find that other alcoholic beverages such as beer and spirits are equally implicated (Colditz 1990). It is still not certain whether it is the ethanol or some other component in the beverage. Studies of alcohol consumption are also fraught with difficulties. In many, report of consumption is inaccurate with long-term consumption as difficult to ascertain as for other foods. There is also a suggestion that people who are ill eliminate their alcohol consumption as the result of their illness, confusing cause and effect. Finally, there are social factors associated with the intake of certain beverages, particularly the use of wine among the more affluent.

In summary, while there are observational studies associating alcohol intake with lower coronary heart disease rates and plausible biological mechanisms are available, there are also concerns regarding the recommendation of alcoholic beverages as a preventive strategy for coronary heart disease. These rest in the potential for addiction, vehicular accidents, and negative effects on a number of organ systems, including the cardiovascular system.

Vitamins, minerals, and food supplements

Coronary heart disease has many advocates of oral supplements for treatment and prevention. Vitamins, minerals, and other food supplements are promoted as a simple easy way to avoid disease. There are numerous manufacturers who are willing to fulfil this 'need'. However, most of these substances are untested in a rigorous and controlled manner. Among those considered are vitamins C and E, β-carotene, copper, iron, selenium, fish oil, and fibre.

Observational studies show benefit and/or harm for some supplements (Ascherio & Hunter 1994; Kritchevsky *et al.* 1995; Stampfer & Rimm 1995; Ascherio *et al.* 1999). Very few have been submitted to clinical trials. When this has occurred, either in healthy subjects or those with coronary heart disease, the results have been mixed and usually negative (Omenn *et al.* 1996; Hennekens *et al.* 1996; Collins *et al.* 2002; Lee *et al.* 2005). The need for more trials is recognized.

Homocysteine has been evaluated as a risk factor for coronary heart disease. It is a product of methionine metabolism and observational studies consistently show elevated blood homocysteine in association with coronary heart disease (Boushey *et al.* 1995). The exact mechanism for this association is uncertain. Supplementation with vitamins B6, B12, and folate appears to lower homocysteine levels (Osganian *et al.* 1999). Recently in the United States and other nations, folate supplementation was added to many grain products to prevent birth defects. This should result in lower population levels of homocysteine (Boushey *et al.* 1995; Osganian *et al.* 1999). Unfortunately, several large clinical trials of vitamin supplementation in patients with known cardiovascular disease and stroke failed to show treatment advantages (Toole *et al.* 2004; Lonn *et al.* 2006; Bonaa, *et al.* 2006).

Blood lipids

The preponderance of population, clinical, and experimental data indicate that blood lipids play a causal role in atherosclerosis and resulting coronary heart disease. Mass elevations in blood lipids appear to be a necessary factor for mass coronary heart disease. The research underlying these statements is summarized below.

1. Mean levels and distributions of blood lipids which vary widely between populations (Keys 1980) demonstrate a strong graded relationship between levels of total serum or plasma cholesterol and coronary heart disease. The low-density lipoprotein fraction of cholesterol is most atherogenic.
2. High-density lipoprotein cholesterol is inversely related to coronary heart disease. Higher levels are associated with less disease. High-density lipoprotein cholesterol is strongest as a predictor of coronary heart disease in populations where total cholesterol and disease risk is high (NIH 2002).
3. Although the mechanisms are poorly understood, there is a growing consensus that serum triglycerides, as measured in the fasting state, are associated with coronary heart disease (NIH 2002).
4. Blood cholesterol levels among youth after puberty parallel those of the adult population (Luepker 1999).
5. Blood cholesterol levels continue to be predictive among adults over the age of 65 years, although the relative risk is reduced (Abbott *et al.* 1997).
6. Blood cholesterol can be lowered among adults with moderate changes in diet and loss of weight.
7. Clinical trials with lipid-lowering agents among those with moderate to severe blood cholesterol elevations demonstrate reduced coronary heart disease associated with lower cholesterol levels. This occurs both in individuals with coronary heart disease and those without evidence of clinical disease. It is particularly true

of the newer statin drugs, but also with other methods (Scandinavian Simvastatin Survival Study 1994; Shepherd *et al.* 1995; Multiple Risk Factor Intervention Trial Research Group 1996; Sacks *et al.* 1996; Downs *et al.* 1998; LIPID Study Group 1998).

8. A progressive fall in blood cholesterol in the United States is associated with changes in the habitual diet during the last 25 years (Carroll *et al.* 2005; Arnett *et al.* 2005).

Population studies of blood lipids consistently show a positive association of mean blood cholesterol with coronary heart disease. As shown in Fig. 9.2.5, comparisons between different national groups show a significant association between blood cholesterol levels in health and coronary heart disease events among middle-aged men (Keys 1980). Similarly, data from the Multiple Risk Factor Intervention Trial, where over 356 000 healthy middle-aged men were followed over time, blood cholesterol predicted coronary heart disease outcomes in a progressive and continuous way as shown in Fig. 9.2.6 (Neaton *et al.* 1992). This continued gradation of blood cholesterol levels and disease suggest that lower blood cholesterol is better but there is no discrete point at which relative risk is sharply higher.

Lipids are insoluble in a water medium, namely blood. They are carried as lipoprotein particles in combination with proteins. Total cholesterol is the most widely used blood measure. It represents that chemical entity regardless of the carrier protein. Total cholesterol is commonly divided into three major components based on the density of the particles: Low-density lipoprotein cholesterol, high-density lipoprotein cholesterol, and very low-density lipoprotein cholesterol. Each of these fractions is associated with specific protein carrier molecules. Low-density lipoprotein is the largest component of total cholesterol and is the atherogenic fraction. High-density lipoprotein comprises a smaller fraction and is inversely related to coronary heart disease, with higher levels of high-density lipoprotein associated with less disease. The very low-density lipoprotein contains modest amounts of cholesterol, but is the main carrier for triglycerides. Triglycerides are the major method by which fat is transported and stored in the body.

There is considerable research on subfractions of these lipoproteins and the protein carriers which transport them. While important in research, these subfractions—including lipoprotein A, apolipoprotein E, B-lipoprotein, high-density lipoprotein 2, and high-density lipoprotein 3—and many others are not established measures for clinical use nor are they relevant for public health strategies at this time.

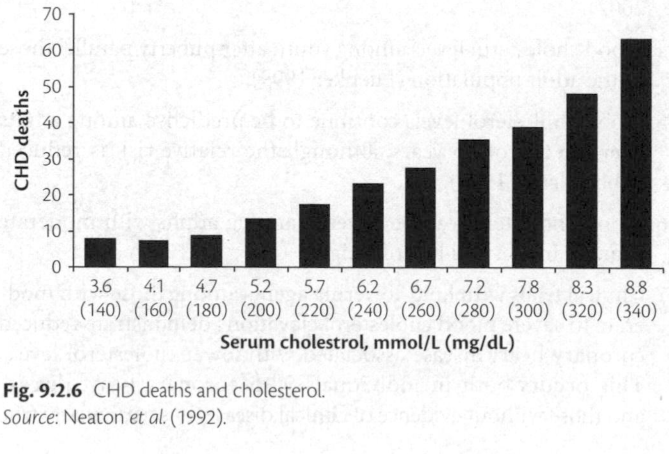

Fig. 9.2.6 CHD deaths and cholesterol.
Source: Neaton *et al.* (1992).

There are numerous trials designed to lower blood cholesterol or its subfractions. Dietary trials are noted above. The majority of trials have been in high-risk individuals by virtue of elevated blood cholesterol or known coronary heart disease. The trials take many years and are costly; however, the results are consistent and clear. The Coronary Drug Project enrolled men between 30 and 64 years old who had a previous myocardial infarction. The nicotinic acid treatment group showed significant lower mortality compared to those on placebo at 15 years after the study began (Canner *et al.* 1986). Many early trials occurred before the more powerful cholesterol lowering drugs—the statins. With the use of statins, much larger effects of cholesterol reduction are observed with accompanying greater reductions in coronary heart disease events. In primary prevention, the West of Scotland Coronary Prevention Study is of particular interest (Shepherd *et al.* 1995). Randomizing 6595 men with moderately elevated cholesterol to placebo or pravastin, investigators observed significant reductions in serum total cholesterol and low-density lipoprotein cholesterol concentrations. Significantly fewer major coronary events were observed with lower total mortality in the treatment group compared to the controls. Similarly, the Airforce/Texas Coronary Atherosclerosis Prevention Study studied healthy subjects with modest increases in blood cholesterol. With lovastatin, significant reductions in cholesterol, coronary events and all causes of mortality were observed (Downs *et al.* 1998).

A number of large secondary prevention trials using statin therapy to lower cholesterol have also been completed, including the Scandinavian Simvastatin Survival Study (Scandinavian Simvastatin Survival Study 1994). It demonstrated a significant reduction in all causes of mortality, coronary heart disease mortality, coronary events and revascularization procedures in patients with known coronary heart disease. The Cholesterol and Recurrent Events trial and the Long-Term Intervention with Fibrostatin in Ischaemic Disease trial also demonstrated lipid reductions associated with fewer major coronary events (Sacks *et al.* 1996; LIPID Study Group 1998). The MRC/BHF Heart Protection Study resulted in a 25 per cent reduction in cardiovascular events with simvastatin in 20 536 high-risk adults (Collins *et al.* 2002).

There have also been two important secondary prevention trials with gemfibrozil, a fibric acid derivative. A Finnish trial among men with known coronary heart disease resulted in a significant reduction of coronary events associated with increased high-density lipoprotein cholesterol and decreased triglycerides. Total cholesterol results were variable (Frick *et al.* 1987). A more recent treatment study of men with average total and low-density lipoprotein cholesterol but low high-density lipoprotein cholesterol with gemfibrozil also produced positive results. High-density lipoprotein cholesterol increased in the treatment group compared to placebo. Coronary events were reduced. Serum triglycerides also fell significantly, raising questions about the relative importance of the two lipid effects (Rubins *et al.* 1999).

There is consistent evidence from clinical trials of the benefits of lower total cholesterol and low-density lipoprotein cholesterol. There is also a suggestion that raising high-density lipoprotein cholesterol and lowering triglycerides add to these beneficial effects.

While recognizing that population-wide reductions in blood cholesterol would have the greatest benefits, there are also clinical indicators of elevated blood cholesterol requiring aggressive and pharmacological management. This includes both high-risk individuals who are disease free and those who have known coronary heart disease. The Adult Treatment Panel (ATP III) of the United States National Cholesterol Education Program has suggested levels appropriate for further diagnosis and treatment (NIH 2002). These are seen in Table 9.2.5. This report also adds 'coronary heart disease risk equivalents'. In addition to prevalent coronary heart disease, peripheral artery disease, carotid artery disease, abdominal aortic aneurysm, and diabetes are considered as factors requiring more aggressive treatment. The report also includes other risk factors for coronary heart disease (e.g. smoking) in a combined risk score which directs prevention strategies. The European Society of Cardiology made similar recommendations for prevention (Wood *et al.* 1998).

Blood pressure

Considerable epidemiological, clinical, and experimental data find high blood pressure or hypertension to be a major risk factor for coronary heart disease. Hypertension is also strongly predictive of other diseases including stroke, renal failure, and congestive heart failure. It is also widely recognized that treatment of hypertension to lower blood pressure reduces cardiovascular disease. The problem is common, and large portions of the population have hypertension and/or are currently under treatment. The important observations about hypertension are as follows:

1. Population studies find a modest relationship between hypertension and coronary heart disease mortality between countries (Keys 1980) but within populations, coronary heart disease is strongly related to both systolic and diastolic blood pressures.
2. Levels of blood pressure among youth track into adulthood.
3. For those with fixed hypertension, clinical trials demonstrate that treatment to reduce blood pressure reduces stroke, coronary heart disease, congestive heart failure, cardiovascular disease, and total mortality.
4. Treatment for hypertension is widely available; however, many individuals are neither diagnosed nor effectively treated (Chobanian *et al.* 2003).

Elevated blood pressure plays an important role in a number of diseases. The effect of sustained mechanical forces associated with elevations in blood pressure leads to target organ damage in the heart, brain, kidneys, and other organs. The origins of high blood pressure are not well understood, however, associations with obesity, physical inactivity, salt intake, and alcohol intake suggest behavioural factors play an important role. Genetic factors are also apparent, but the considerable prevalence of hypertension suggests that any hereditary characteristics are very common in most populations.

In international studies, systolic blood pressure predicts coronary heart disease outcomes between populations in a modest but linear fashion (Keys 1980). Many populations worldwide have highly prevalent hypertension including the Japanese, Chinese, Africans, and others (over 50 per cent in some adult groups).

Within populations, blood pressure is predictive of cardiovascular disease outcomes including coronary heart disease (Chobanian *et al.* 2003). Early studies focused on diastolic blood pressure, but more recently systolic blood pressure, which appears to be more reliably measured, has assumed increasing importance for diagnosis and treatment (Fig. 9.2.7).

While hypertension is common, its prevalence has not changed significantly in recent years. However, in the past 20 years, detection, treatment and control of high blood pressure has progressively improved. As shown in Table 9.2.6, awareness, treatment and control of blood pressure have substantially increased. In the 1990s, however, there was an apparent levelling of effect in the United States with many still unaware and ineffectively treated (Chobanian *et al.* 2003; Luepker 2006).

Lifestyle modifications including weight, exercise, and diet offer the potential for preventing hypertension. They have also been found to be effective at lowering moderate hypertension with little risk and minimal cost. Even though lifestyle factors alone may not control high blood pressure, they can reduce the amount of antihypertensive drugs deemed necessary (Neaton *et al.* 1993). Excess body weight is associated with elevation in blood pressure. Weight reduction can reduce blood pressure in obese individuals with hypertension (Neaton *et al.* 1993). Therefore, it is widely recommended that weight reduction is an important part of hypertension control. Physical inactivity also plays a role in hypertension with unfit individuals having up to 50 per cent increased risk of developing high blood pressure. Moderate physical activity aids in controlling weight and may actually lower blood pressure (NIH 1996). Dietary factors may also play a role in precipitating or reducing hypertension. Alcohol use raises blood pressure. The National High Blood Pressure Education Program recommends no more than 30 ml of ethanol as beer, wine, or whisky per day for men and 15 ml per day for women (Chobanian *et al.* 2003).

Salting of food as a method of preservation is well established over many centuries. However, modern food preservation methods do not require salt and it is mainly an acquired taste. Unfortunately, the human kidney was developed in the setting of low sodium and high potassium diets. Hence, the body is well designed to retain, but not excrete sodium, which it effectively does. The need for sodium is quite small and many times the amount required is consumed in processed food (Blackburn & Prineas 1983).

Salt intake is particularly relevant to hypertension. Population surveys demonstrate strong associations between population blood pressure and salt intake (INTERSALT Cooperative Research Group 1988). Migration studies where salt intake is greatly increased among people who migrate from low to high salt cultures is associated with increasing prevalence of hypertension (Joseph *et al.* 1983).

Table 9.2.5 ATP III classification of total cholesterol, LDL cholesterol, and triglycerides

Total cholesterol (mg/dL)		LDL cholesterol (mg/dL)		Triglycerides (mg/dL)	
		<100	Optimal	<150	Normal
<200	Desirable	100–129	Near optimal/ above optimal	150–199	Borderline high
200–239	Borderline high	130–159	Borderline high	200–499	High
≥240	High	160–189	High	≥500	Very high
		≥190	Very high		

Source: National Cholesterol Education Program. Third Report of the National Cholesterol Education Program Expert Panel on: Detection, Evaluation, and Treatment of High Blood Cholesterol in Adults (Adult Treatment Panel III). NIH Pub. 02-5215. Bethesda, MD: National Heart, Lung, and Blood Institute, 2002.

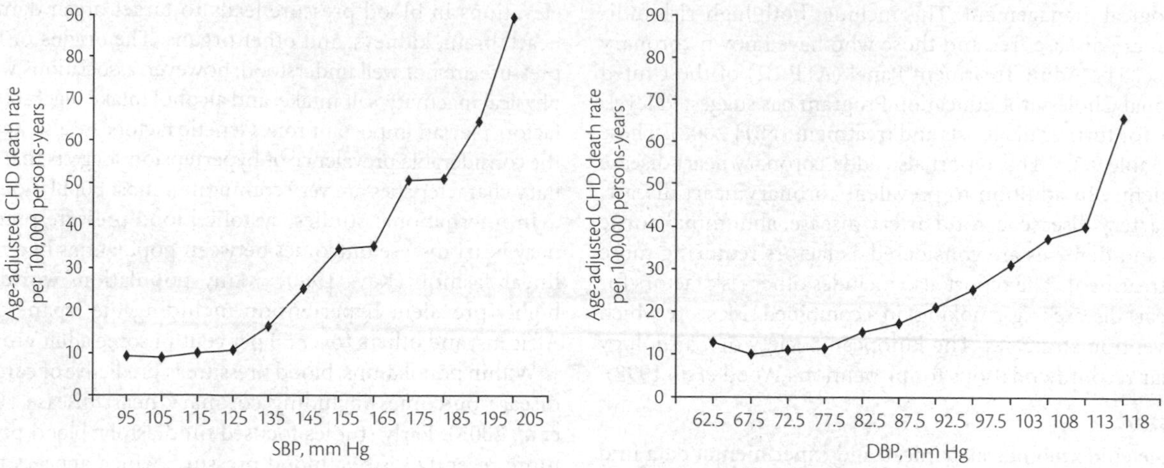

Fig. 9.2.7 CHD and blood pressure.
Source: Neaton *et al.* (1992).

Clinical studies have found that restriction in salt results in lower blood pressure. Marked sodium depletion, as practised in an earlier era, can even reduce blood pressure among severe hypertensives, and sodium restriction enables high blood pressure to be controlled with lower doses of antihypertensive drugs. In some patients, salt restriction may control mild-to-moderate hypertension without resorting to drugs.

Despite widespread information about the role of salt, considerable debate remains. The US National Dietary Goals recommend no more than 6 g of sodium chloride daily (Chobanian *et al.* 2003). This remains significantly more than humans need, but well below the average intake. As the use of processed foods increases, salt may play an undiminished or even increasing role in hypertension.

The decision to initiate pharmacological treatment of high blood pressure depends on a variety of factors, including the absolute level of blood pressure, the presence of cardiovascular disease, target organ damage and the presence of other coronary heart disease risk factors. The benefits of pharmacological treatment have been demonstrated for coronary heart disease, stroke, heart failure, renal disease, and all causes of mortality (Furberg 2002). There was debate over the generalizability of hypertension trials to older adults and other groups; it is generally believed that all populations will benefit from blood pressure lowering. There are many medications currently available for hypertension treatment, however, diuretics are recommended for initiating treatment as they have the longest clinical trial experience and a proven record of reducing morbidity and mortality in clinical trials (Chobanian *et al.* 2003; Furberg 2002). Other agents may be added if blood pressure is not adequately controlled (Chobanian *et al.* 2003).

There is some debate regarding what constitutes a normal blood pressure and, hence, what requires pharmacological treatment. Most agree that 120/80 represents a normal blood pressure in an adult. The recommendations for blood pressure classification and treatment among adults over the age of 18 years of the United States National High Blood Pressure Education Program are shown in Table 9.2.7 (Chobanian *et al.* 2003). The European recommendations are somewhat different, but in a similar range (Wood *et al.* 1998).

Cigarette smoking

Tobacco use is a worldwide problem associated with many diseases. While best known for causing lung cancer, cigarette use has a larger

Table 9.2.6 Trends in awareness, treatment, and control of high blood pressure in adults with hypertension aged 18–74 years*

	National Health and Nutrition Examination Surveys, weighted %			
	1976–1980	1988–1991	1991–1994	1999–2000
Awareness	51	73	68	70
Treatment	31	55	54	59
Control†	10	29	27	34

* Data from the National Heart, Lung, and Blood Institute and data for National Health and Nutrition Examination Surveys.
† Systolic blood pressure of less than 140 mm Hg and diastolic blood pressure of less than 90 mm Hg.
Source: Chobanian *et al.* (2003).

Table 9.2.7 Classification and management of blood pressure for adults aged 18 years or older

BP classification	Systolic BP, mm Hg*		Diastolic BP, mm Hg*
Normal	<120	and	<80
Prehypertension	120–139	or	80–89
Stage 1 hypertension	140–159	or	90–99
Stage 2 hypertension	≥160	or	≥100

* Treatment determined by highest BP category.
Source: Chobanian *et al.* (2003).

effect on mortality and morbidity from coronary heart disease. Some of the salient observations on tobacco use are as follows:

1. Cigarette smoking addicts 20–80 per cent of adult men worldwide, with a somewhat lower proportion of adult women addicted.
2. Comparisons between populations often find no association between coronary heart disease and the prevalence of cigarette smoking. However, the individual association of cigarette smoking to coronary heart disease is strong.
3. Cigarette smoking is falling in some countries but rising in many, and is a growing epidemic in developing nations.
4. Cigarette smoking begins in youth and gradually increases until it becomes nicotine addiction.
5. The main mechanisms by which cigarette smoking affects coronary heart disease are as a chronic promoter of atherosclerotic lesions and as an acute risk factor increasing sympathetic stimulation and enhancing clotting.
6. While randomized population trials of cigarette use have not been performed, cigarette smoking cessation is associated with reduced coronary heart disease mortality.
7. There is growing evidence that environmental tobacco smoke or second-hand smoke has a deleterious effect on exposed non-smokers.

Tobacco use through cigarette smoking is one of the major causes of disease and disability in the world. In the United States, there are approximately 47 million adult smokers, and it is estimated that 430 000 deaths annually are associated with cigarette smoking (USDHHS 1998*a*). These victims are replaced by the teenagers who begin the smoking habit. In the United States, the direct medical costs of smoking are estimated to be over US$60 billion/year, with similar indirect costs.

Cigarette smoking is linked to the major cardiovascular diseases including myocardial infarction, sudden death, stroke and peripheral vascular disease (USDHHS 1997). These associations are found across age, gender and ethnic groups (USDHHS 1997; Neaton & Wentworth 1992). The relationship of coronary heart disease mortality to smoking status is shown in Fig. 9.2.8. One of the most important findings is the association of cigarette smoking with

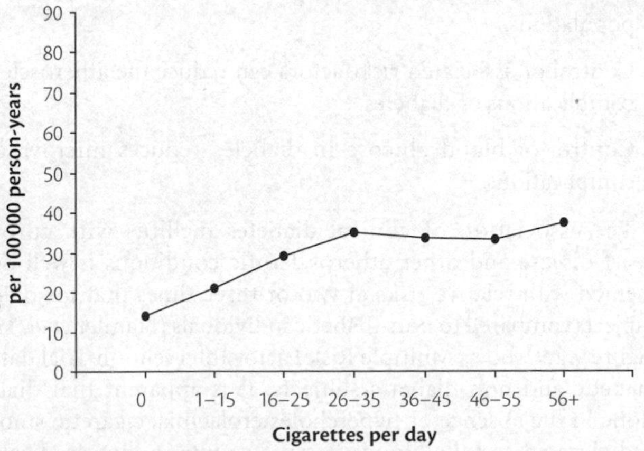

Fig. 9.2.8 Cigarette smoking and CHD
Source: Neaton *et al.* (1992).

sudden unexpected death among younger individuals. Similarly, acute myocardial infarction in younger individuals (less than 50 years of age) is very strongly associated with tobacco use. The interaction of cigarette smoking with other risk factors such as cholesterol, diet, obesity, hypertension, lipids, diabetes, and ECG abnormalities is also well demonstrated (Multiple Risk Factor Intervention Trial Research Group 1996). Among the strongest pieces of evidence is the observation that continued cigarette smoking after myocardial infarction is predictive of recurrent events and death (Hermanson *et al.* 1988), and those who quit smoking dramatically reduce their chance of a second event or death (Hermanson *et al.* 1988; USDHHS 1990).

The mechanisms by which tobacco and the constituents of tobacco smoke affect cardiovascular disease are still debated. Both acute and chronic mechanisms probably contribute. Firstly, there is evidence that smoking plays a direct role in the atherosclerotic process. This is shown by the Pathological Determinants of Atherosclerosis in Youth Study of 1443 autopsies of men and women aged 15–34 years who died of trauma (McGill *et al.* 1997). Fatty abdominal and aortic streaks and raised lesions were associated with cigarette use in this otherwise healthy population. This may be the result of injury to the arterial endothelium from smoking (McGill *et al.* 1997). More acutely, the immediate pharmacological effects of nicotine and carbon monoxide are well known. Platelet adhesion, acute coronary constriction and tachycardia are commonly cited (Meade *et al.* 1987). Finally, there is the rapid improvement in patients observed after smoking cessation.

In recent years, the focus has shifted to environmental tobacco smoke which affects non-smokers in public and private settings. A number of recent studies suggest consistent and increased relative risk of cardiovascular disease among those exposed to environmental tobacco smoke (Table 9.2.8). While it is difficult to measure exposure to environmental tobacco smoke, the consistency of these studies is suggestive and reinforces the effort to control cigarette smoking in public settings (Steenland *et al.* 1996).

Programmes to control tobacco use have focused on prevention and cessation. Smoking prevention programmes in the schools have received considerable attention and met some success (Perry

Table 9.2.8 Cohort studies of environmental tobacco smoke and CHD

Source	Year	Location	Cases/population	Adjusted RR (CI)
Garland	1985	United States	19/695	2.7 (0.7–10.5)
Svendsen	1987	United States	88/1245	2.2 (0.72–6.92)
Helsing	1988	United States	1358/19 035	M 1.31 (1.05–1.64) F 1.24 (1.10–1.40)
Hole	1989	United Kingdom	53/7987	2.01 (1.2–3.4)
Layard	1995	United States	1389/2916	M 0.97 (0.73–1.28) F 0.99 (0.84–1.16)
Tunstall-Pedoe	1995	United Kingdom	70/2,278	2.7 (1.3–5.6)
Steenland	1996	United States	3819/309 599	M 1.22 (1.07–1.40) F 1.10 (0.96–1.27)
Kawachi	1997	United States	152/32 046	F 1.91 (1.11–3.28)

et al. 1992). Cessation interventions among adults have emphasized behavioural and pharmacological strategies (Fiore *et al.* 1996). These have included nicotine replacement therapy, medications, social support, and skills training/problem solving. In addition, widespread restriction of smoking reduces the societal support for the behaviour.

In summary, cigarette smoking is an addictive behaviour leading to many health-impairing effects including coronary heart disease. Elimination of cigarette smoking would significantly improve the health of any population.

Overweight and obesity

Excess body weight as fat is increasingly recognized for its importance in the development of cardiovascular diseases. On a population level, overweight and obesity have become common among all adults in industrialized countries and the affluent in developing countries. Several important observations include the following:

1. Overweight and obesity are associated with increased mortality.
2. Obesity is associated with elevated blood pressure, hyperlipidaemia, diabetes mellitus, and insulin resistance. Reduction in body fat diminishes the level of each of these risk factors.
3. Increasing body weight is a worldwide problem and is the result of excess food in the setting of reduced physical activity.

Obesity is commonly described as excess body fat; however, the exact proportion of fat rendering one overweight or obese is debated. Body mass index, which is weight in kilograms divided by height in meters squared, is a commonly used standard. Expert panels suggest a body mass index above 25 is classified as overweight and above 30 as obese (Eckel & Krauss 1998; USDHHS 1998*b*). More recently, visceral adiposity has been proposed as a better marker for obesity as a predictor of cardiac risk (Freedman 1995). Visceral adiposity is simply measured by the waist to hip ratio, using the circumference of these two sites. Other more complex methods to determine body fat are available but require sophisticated instruments.

Overweight and obesity are an increasing problem in much of the world. In recent years, overweight and obesity measured in national surveys have substantially increased in the United States (Ogden *et al.* 2006). Men are more likely to be overweight (body mass index greater than 25 kg/m^2) but women are more likely to be obese (body mass index greater than 30 kg/m^2). Ethnic minorities, such as African Americans, and Mexican Americans living in the United States, have similar, if not greater, adiposity (Ogden *et al.* 2006).

The association of obesity with mortality is well established. For the severe or morbidly obese, lifespan is significantly reduced (Sjostrom 1992). For the less severely obese, the debate is that of obesity as an independent risk factor for cardiovascular disease or as one which operates through other known risk factors (Harris *et al.* 1997; Solomon & Manson 1997). The question is a scientific one rather than one of public health.

Obesity and overweight affects lipoprotein metabolism through higher low-density lipoprotein cholesterol, increased triglycerides and lower levels of high-density lipoprotein cholesterol. Weight reduction accomplished through diet is associated with significant improvement in lipids (Dattilo & Kris-Etherton 1992). The association of weight and blood pressure is also well established. In the Nurses Health Study, one unit in body mass index was associated with a 12 per cent increase in the risk of hypertension (Huang *et al.* 1998). Other observational studies consistently show this relationship (Dyer & Elliott 1989). Weight loss is well demonstrated to reduce blood pressure. This includes even modest reductions in weight (Trials of Hypertension Prevention Collaborative Research Group 1997). In addition, recent research suggests that a diet lower in fat and higher in fruits and vegetables also results in lower blood pressure among the mildly hypertensive (Krauss *et al.* 1998). In each of these studies, weight reduction via diet allows the reduction of antihypertensive medications.

Insulin resistance is the underlying condition associated with adult-onset or type II diabetes. Obesity is a crucial factor in the development of insulin insensitivity and increased interabdominal fat is implicated (Krauss *et al.* 1998). The current epidemic of diabetes is associated with the increase in obesity. Weight loss can be critical to the control of adult-onset diabetes. Both insulin resistance and hyperglycaemia are significantly reduced when patients lose weight (Paisey *et al.* 1998). This may result in the ability to reduce diabetic therapy.

Clinicians are well aware of the difficulty of obtaining significant and sustained weight loss among patients, consequently obesity prevention is a better strategy. By reducing the increased adiposity that occurs with age, many of the sequelae and difficulty of losing weight as an adult would be avoided (National Task Force on Prevention and Treatment of Obesity 1994). For those who are obese, both control of calorie intake and increase in calorie expenditure through physical activity is essential.

Diabetes, hyperglycaemia, and hyperinsulinaemia

The insulin era, allowing patients to live longer, revealed a strong association between diabetes and cardiovascular diseases, particularly those caused by atherosclerosis. Large vessel disease associated with diabetes results in myocardial infarction, stroke, and peripheral vascular disease. Microvascular disease is associated with retinopathy, renal disease and cardiomyopathy. In addition to strong associations with known cardiovascular risk factors, diabetes is an independent predictor of disease (Stamler *et al.* 1993). Salient observations regarding diabetes are as follows:

1. Diabetes and hyperglycaemia are strongly related to atherosclerosis, obesity, and abnormal lipid patterns.
2. Diabetes is increasing along with obesity in susceptible populations.
3. Control of associated risk factors can reduce the atherosclerotic complications of diabetes.
4. Control of blood glucose in diabetes reduces microvascular complications.

The association of clinical diabetes mellitus with coronary heart disease and other atherosclerotic conditions is well documented with relative risks at two or three times that for diabetic subjects compared to non-diabetic individuals (Stamler *et al.* 1993). Figure 9.2.9, shows Multiple Risk Factor Intervention Trial data for diabetic and non-diabetic subjects. It is apparent that diabetes alone in the absence of hypercholesterolaemia, cigarette smoking and elevated systolic blood pressure results in increased relative risk of cardiovascular disease mortality. The effect of diabetes is magnified when associated with these other risk characteristics.

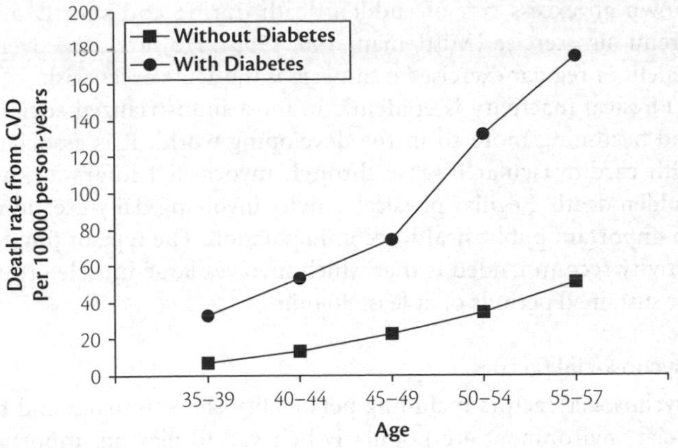

Fig. 9.2.9 CVD mortality and diabetes.
Source: Stamler *et al.* (1993).

It was believed that diabetes combined with the use of a high-fat, low-carbohydrate, and low-fibre diet increased vascular complications. It is now clear that the deleterious effects of the disease itself on the endothelium and coagulation abnormality play an important direct role (Sowers *et al.* 1994). It was also observed that diabetes is strongly associated with classical risk factors. People with diabetes have elevated levels of triglycerides and low-density lipoprotein cholesterol with decreased levels of high-density lipoprotein cholesterol. There is also a high prevalence of obesity and hypertension among people with diabetes (Lehto *et al.* 1997).

Cross-cultural comparisons present a more complicated picture. They indicate that factors other than the glucose insulin disorder itself result in atherosclerosis. Evidence is presented in the apparently low rates of atherosclerosis in diabetic Eastern Jews, Chinese, and south-west American Indians. The Pima Indians are a classical example of a population exposed to calorie abundance, excessive obesity, and diabetes, but little cardiovascular disease.

In healthy people, glucose intolerance alone is weak and inconsistently associated with cardiovascular disease risk. However, increased insulin levels were found to predict coronary heart disease in Australia, France, and Finland, and it is postulated to be the cause of excess coronary heart disease among South Asian immigrants to the United Kingdom (Hughes 1990).

The treatment of diabetes is based on control of blood glucose and treatment of associated risk factors. Lifestyle strategies, weight loss, and physical activity can be effective at reducing blood glucose and controlling the associated risk factors. This is particularly true in type II diabetes. For type I diabetes, insulin for glucose control and control of associated risk factors can reduce some diabetic complications.

Pharmacological control of type II diabetes has produced mixed results. The original University Group Diabetes Program reported an increased rate of myocardial infarction with the use of first-generation sulphonylureas in the setting of effective blood glucose control (UGDP 1975). Later trials with newer oral agents did not observe this complication (UKPDS 1995). The Diabetes Control and Complication Trial studied glucose control in insulin dependent diabetes. Microvascular complications were significantly reduced (DCCT Research Group 1993). Large vessel disease was also reduced, but the differences were not significant. More recently, a meta-analysis of clinical trials of a popular oral hypoglycemic, rosiglitazone, revealed a significant increase in myocardial infarction and an increase in death from cardiovascular causes (Nissen & Wolski 2007).

The control of blood lipids in diabetes has been shown to be particularly effective in the setting of increased LDL cholesterol. This is true for primary prevention (Downs *et al.* 1998) and secondary prevention in type 2 diabetes (Pyorala *et al.* 1997; Goldberg *et al.* 1998).

The relationship between diabetes, atherosclerosis and coronary heart disease is well established in people with clinical diabetes living in affluent industrialized cultures. Data from other cultures suggest that other factors are at work. The use of lifestyle strategies, control of other risk factors and pharmacological measures in diabetes is the standard of care and may reduce cardiovascular complications of this disease.

Physical inactivity

Physical inactivity has assumed increasing importance as a risk factor for cardiovascular disease. As society has become more mechanized, sedentary lifestyle is the norm. Operating through other risk factors such as obesity, hypertension, hyperlipidaemia and diabetes, physical inactivity is associated with cardiovascular disease. However, it may be independently associated as well. Several important observations regarding physical inactivity include the following:

1. Physical inactivity is associated with acute myocardial infarction and sudden death both for the initial event and recurrent events. Regular activity is associated with reduced events.
2. Physical activity at work is declining.
3. Physical activity in leisure time, while increasing, is still not widespread.
4. Physical inactivity begins with declining exercise among youth as they reach teenage years.
5. Physical inactivity is associated with known risk factors including hyperlipidaemia, hypertension, diabetes mellitus, and obesity.

Two of the primary activities of human beings are obtaining and consuming food. Historically, this took considerable physical energy in hunting or farming activities, only a few very affluent were spared from activity. The past two centuries have witnessed a dramatic transition as farming has become more efficient. Mechanized transportation has eliminated the use of physical activity to move from place to place and in the workplace machines do most or all heavy labour. The result has been a rising tide of physical inactivity.

Much of the information on physical inactivity comes from observational studies. A meta-analysis of observational studies selected for quality, measurement and follow-up showed a significant and graded relationship between physical inactivity and the risk of first coronary heart disease event. They calculated a relative risk of 1.9 compared with sedentary individuals (Powell *et al.* 1987). The Multiple Risk Factor Intervention Trial of over 12 000 men demonstrated similar relationships with those with regular leisure time physical activity having lower risk of coronary heart disease and death (Leon *et al.* 1987) (Table 9.2.9). While there are many observational studies, there is general agreement that a primary prevention trial of physical activity is unlikely to be feasible and public health recommendations must come from available data.

Table 9.2.9 Mortality and leisure-time physical activity—men

	Tertile of LTPAs		
End points	**1 (lowest)**	**2**	**3 (highest)**
	Age-adjusted risk ratios		
CHD death	1.00	0.63‡(0.43–0.86)	0.64‡(0.47–0.88)
Sudden death	1.00	0.63‡(0.42–0.93)	0.65‡(0.44–0.96)
All-cause deaths	1.00	0.71‡(0.57–0.88)	0.83‡(0.67–1.01)

Source: Leon *et al.* (1987).

There are more data for secondary prevention. Observational studies find that individuals who continue with regular physical activity after myocardial infarction have lower relative risk than those who are sedentary (NIH 1996). These studies are confounded by disease severity associated both with physical inactivity and mortality. Those who are most ill are less likely to exercise and more likely to have increased recurrent events and mortality. For this reason, a number of randomized clinical trials of cardiac rehabilitation after myocardial infarction have been performed. These demonstrate lower mortality associated with exercise, but most studies have been small and underpowered. A meta-analysis by Oldridge *et al.* of 10 randomized trials found significant improvement associated with cardiac rehabilitation programmes lasting at least 6 weeks (Oldridge *et al.* 1988).

Physical activity is believed to function through a number of biological and physiological mechanisms. It operates through other cardiovascular risk factors including lipoproteins, carbohydrate metabolism, clotting factors, and obesity. It may result in lower blood pressure and aid in smoking cessation. In addition to its effects on other risk characteristics, physical activity is thought to increase epicardial artery diameter, increase coronary blood flow, and decrease myocardial work and oxygen demand. The heart may work more efficiently and be better able to function under stressful circumstances.

There is considerable debate over public health recommendations for physical activity. Some of the issues include the amount, type, and duration of physical activity needed to obtain beneficial cardiovascular effects. There is also the independent issue of fitness. Finally, the association of vigorous physical activity with sudden death has increased concerns regarding advice. Considering these factors, several recommendations have emerged in recent years (NIH 1996). These suggest that moderate physical activity such as brisk walking for 30 min on most days of the week is adequate to produce significant benefit in a sedentary society. More vigorous physical activity can be recommended; however, only moderate cardiovascular gains accrue from this addition (NIH 1996). The activity should be of sufficient vigour to increase the heart rate and breathing rate. Regular physical activity will lead to increased fitness; however, much of the association with fitness may be genetically determined rather than the result only of training (Blair *et al.* 1989). Nonetheless, observational studies do show that physical fitness is associated with lower rates of cardiovascular disease (Blair *et al.* 1989).

Finally, safety considerations are crucial in advising physical activity for individuals or public health recommendations. Research has shown an excess risk of sudden death during and shortly after strenuous exercise (Mittleman *et al.* 1993). However, the overall benefit of regular exercise far outweighs the acute excess risk.

Physical inactivity is epidemic in most industrialized societies and becoming more so in the developing world. It is associated with cardiovascular disease through myocardial infarction and sudden death. Regular physical activity involving daily exertion is an important public health recommendation. The type of physical activity recommended is that which involves large muscle groups for sustained periods of at least 30 min.

Psychosocial factors

Psychosocial factors including personality characteristics and the social environment are popularly believed to play an important role in cardiovascular disease. There are also many professionals who believe that these factors influence the major diseases of modern life. Despite this widespread belief, it has been difficult to demonstrate causal connections to coronary heart disease or other diseases. This may be due to difficulties in measurement, confounders, or less than convincing biological mechanisms. Nonetheless, emotional states of anger, aggression, fear, anxiety, and depression are associated with physiological changes which may affect cardiovascular disease. Certain personality types may precipitate or aggravate these factors. There are three major areas that have received attention and will be briefly discussed here. They are type A behaviour, hostility and social support.

Type A behaviour

Type A behaviour is characterized by aggressiveness, competitive drive, preoccupation with deadlines, and time urgency. Historically, it is measured by a structured interview (Friedman & Rosenman 1959). There are also other methods including self-reported inventories and questionnaires. Data in the 1980s found type A behaviour to be associated with coronary heart disease in the Western Collaborative Group Study and the Framingham Study (Rosenman *et al.* 1975; Haynes *et al.* 1980). In the Western Collaborative Group Study, a prospective cohort of 3000 men was assessed by the structured interview. The relative risk of fatal and non-fatal coronary heart disease was approximately 2 for type A men. The Framingham Study used a self-administered questionnaire to evaluate type A behaviour. Relative risk for coronary heart disease was similar to that found in the Western Collaborative Group Study (Haynes *et al.* 1980).

Following these initial observations, a number of other studies attempted to replicate these results. A summary of 14 angiography studies found an equal balance of positive and null associations (Dimsdale *et al.* 1981). Several larger prospective studies done in the 1980s failed to confirm earlier findings using either self-administered instruments or the structured interview (Case *et al.* 1985; Shekelle *et al.* 1985a,b). A reanalysis of the original Western Collaborative Group data also questioned the original results (Ragland & Brand 1988). In an intervention study to look at behaviour patterns and recurrent coronary heart disease, performed by the originators of the type A behaviour interview, coronary heart disease outcomes were reduced, but this study has not been replicated (Friedman *et al.* 1984).

Current evidence for type A behaviour is mixed and while there continues to be widespread belief about its importance, there is inadequate evidence to make public health or clinical recommendations regarding its detection and treatment.

Hostility

Initial enthusiasm about type A behaviour findings led to an attempt to find critical elements accounting for the observed coronary heart disease differences. Studies in selected groups found an association between hostility and coronary heart disease (Barefoot *et al.* 1983). Many studies used parts of the type A behaviour construct. Others used the Minnesota Multi-Phasic Personality Index and its 'Cook Medley Hostility Subscore'. Six prospective studies using the Cook Medley instrument have been published with three positive and three negative findings (Shekelle *et al.* 1983; McCranie *et al.* 1986; Hecker *et al.* 1988; Hearn *et al.* 1988; Leon *et al.* 1988; Barefoot *et al.* 1989).

Recent research suggests that anger or hostility is an acute rather than a chronic risk factor and associated with plaque rupture (Muller *et al.* 1997). This research may provide further insights into this characteristic.

Social support

A number of observational studies find social support or a supportive environment associated with lower coronary heart disease risk. Scandinavian studies found a strong relationship between social support and mortality in men (Orth-Gomer & Johnson 1987). Disentangling the role of social support from prevalent illness, economic factors and personality types is difficult but it is apparent from observational studies that those who report substantial support network, including a supportive spouse, have better coronary heart disease outcomes.

An intervention study of 2481 post MI patients (ENRICHD) evaluated cognitive behaviour therapy to improve social support (Berkman *et al.* 2003). Measures of psychosocial outcomes were significantly improved but there were no differences in recurrent myocardial infarction or mortality.

Acute coronary heart disease risk factors

Most of the risk factors discussed are associated with the underlying disease process, atherosclerosis. If atherosclerosis is prevented, then coronary heart disease, as a clinical event, is rare. However, since many individuals have atherosclerosis by middle-age or older years, there has been an increasing search for factors which lead to the transition from chronic atherosclerotic disease to acute ischaemia, myocardial infarction, and sudden death. These are indicators of sub-clinical arterial disease burden and acute risk factors or triggers.

There were two initial observations leading to these insights. The first related to the pathophysiology of the atherosclerotic plaque. While large and obstructing plaques are clearly related to disease, it was also found that small non-obstructive lesions can rupture, form a nidus for clot, and ultimately obstruct the coronary artery. This phenomenon was more likely to result in death than traditional obstructive lesions causing chronic ischaemia and angina pectoris (Fuster *et al.* 1992). The second observation was that of a morning peak in acute myocardial infarction, sudden death, and stroke. This suggested there were identifiable circumstances associated with disease manifestation (Muller *et al.* 1987). Further work in this field suggested that sympathetic stimulation with activation of clotting as a potential underlying mechanism. A number of factors were implicated. They included heavy exertion, sexual activity, anger, and other factors (Mittleman *et al.* 1993). Some of the characteristics are modified with aspirin use or β-blockers (Willich *et al.* 1993).

In summary, it is likely that more will be learned about these risk factors and treatment found to prevent events in individuals with established atherosclerotic disease. This should not be confused with true primary prevention where the atherosclerotic process is prevented.

Stroke risk factors

Risk factors for stroke can be broadly classified into non-modifiable risk factors such as age, gender, race and ethnicity, and genetic factors, and, modifiable risk factors such as hypertension, hyperlipidemia, smoking, diabetes, and others discussed below. There are several salient observations about stroke including:

1. Stroke rates vary between ethnic groups and countries as do stroke subtypes.
2. Hypertension is the strongest modifiable risk factor for stroke.
3. Drug treatment of hypertension can significantly reduce stroke incidence and recurrence.

Age

Stroke is a disease of older adults and advanced age is associated with increased stroke incidence, prevalence, and mortality. The United States Framingham study (Wolf *et al.* 1991) showed that the risk of stroke increased with age and that this increased risk persisted after adjustment for risk factors associated with increased age including blood pressure, diabetes, smoking, heart disease and atrial fibrillation. The adjusted relative risk for every decade increase in age after 55 years was 1.66 in men and 1.93 in women. This association with increased age has been shown in other geographic/ethnic cohorts. A population-based study from Taiwan estimated an annual incidence of 2.6/100 000 in those in the 36–44 years age group and 1417/100 000 in those aged 75 and older (Hu *et al.* 1992). Data from a stroke registry in Malmö, Sweden similarly showed incident stroke rates of 10/100 000 in those younger than 45 years of age to rates greater than 1700/100 000 in the very elderly (85 years and older) (Jerntrop *et al.* 1992). The association of increased stroke incidence with age is most marked for ischaemic stroke and intra-parenchymal haemorrhages and less so for strokes due to sub-arachnoid haemorrhages (Jerntrop *et al.* 1992). The rise in stroke incidence with age contributes to increased age-associated stroke prevalence and stroke mortality. For example, the stroke prevalence in the NHANES study increased from 0.5 per cent to those in the 20–39-year age category to 12-15 per cent among those in the 80+ age groups. Similarly, stroke mortality increased from 0.5 per 100 000 in those 15–24 years of age to 360/100 000 in those 65 years and older according to United States census data. This association of stroke risk with age has public health implications as the population ages.

Sex

Stroke incidence is higher in men with an overall male/female ratio ranging from 1.15 to 1.3 depending on the population studied (Sacco *et al.* 2001) There appears to be an age effect with the male/female difference shrinking or even reversing in older age groups (Brown *et al.* 1996). Stroke prevalence and mortality are also modestly higher in men than in women though stroke survival per se appears to be higher in men (Brown *et al.* 1996).

Geography and ethnicity

Stroke mortality shows a wide geographic variation with the highest rates reported in Eastern European countries (Fig. 9.2.10)

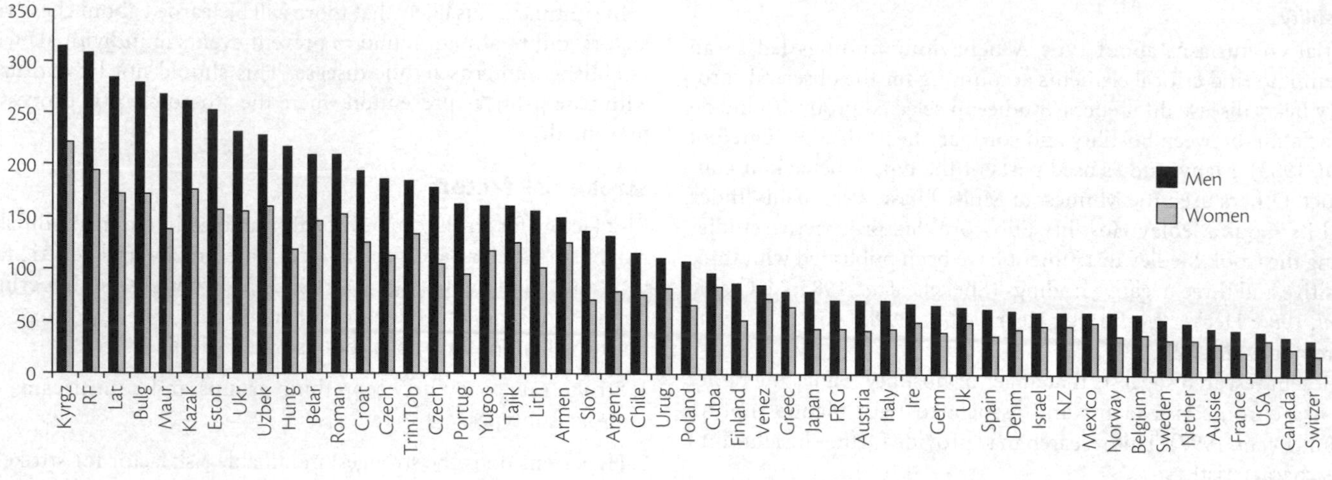

Fig. 9.2.10 Age-standardized stroke mortality per 100 000 men and women in the 1990s.
Source: Sarti *et al.* (2000).

(Sarti *et al.* 2000). The high mortality is a reflection of both higher incidences as well as higher case fatality rates (WHO 2003). There are ethnic differences in stroke mortality even within the same geographical area. For example, there is an excess of stroke mortality among African-Americans compared to Whites in the United States, even after adjustment for county of residence (Howard *et al.* 2001). Stroke mortality has continued to decline in many western countries over the last few decades though a few eastern European countries have shown a rising mortality trend (WHO 2003).

The distribution of stroke subtypes shows geographic and ethnic differences as well. For example, in the United States, pooled data from various population-based studies estimate that ischaemic strokes comprise 87 per cent of all strokes and haemorrhagic strokes comprise the remaining 13 per cent (AHA 2007). Studies from Japan (Sankai *et al.* 1991) and China (Zhang *et al.* 2003) have shown an estimated higher proportion of haemorrhagic strokes in those populations, in the range of 30–48 per cent. An epidemiological study from Malmö, Sweden examined the relative proportion of different subtypes in sub-populations defined by country of birth. This study found that while 12 per cent of all strokes were haemorrhages in those born in Sweden, up to 34 per cent were haemorrhages in immigrants to Malmö who were born in China (Khan *et al.* 2004). These variations in geographic and ethnic groups may be due to different risk profiles including genetic, dietary, or other environmental factors.

Genetic factors

Various genetic epidemiological studies have shown familial aggregation of stroke, though, many traditional stroke risk factors such as diabetes, hypertension, hyperlipidemia and cardiac disease also aggregate in families. Brass *et al.* (1992) analysed male twin pairs and found a fivefold increase in stroke prevalence in monozygotic twins compared to dizygotic twins. The Danish Twin study on the other hand reported a more modest effect in the range of 2.1 for relative risk of stroke death in mono vs. dizygotic twins (Bak *et al.* 2002). A recent systematic review focusing on ischaemic stroke also suggests a modest effect with monozygotic twins being 1.6 times more likely to be concordant for stroke than dizygotic twins (Flossmann *et al.* 2004). Many of the twin studies did not subtype stroke and this may have diluted the effect. There are well-documented monogenic disorders associated with stroke such as the Notch-3 mutation on chromosome 19 leading to cerebral autosomal dominant arteriopathy with subcortical infarcts and leukoencephalopathy, the Icelandic form of amyloid angiopathy due to a Cystatin C point mutation on chromosome 20 associated with hereditary intra-cerebral haemorrhage. However, the overall contribution of monogenic disorders to the burden of stroke appears to be small (Sacco *et al.* 2001). The exact contribution of genetic factors to stroke risk as well as the interaction of genetic and environmental factors is still under investigation.

Hypertension

Hypertension is the most important modifiable stroke risk factor. The age-adjusted relative risk for stroke was increased at least 3-fold in hypertension with a blood pressure ≥ 160/95 and 1.5-fold with blood pressure between 140/90 and 160/95 (Wolf *et al.* 1998). The stroke risk is proportional to the level of hypertension. The Framingham study estimated the relative risk of stroke associated with every 10 mmHg increase in systolic blood pressure was 1.9 for men and 1.7 for women, even after adjustment for other risk factors (Wolf *et al.* 1991). Hypertension increases the risk in both ischaemic and haemorrhagic strokes. Both systolic and diastolic blood pressure levels are related to increased stroke risk. In people with diastolic hypertension (diastolic BP ≥ 95 mmHg) increase in levels of systolic blood pressure is associated with increased stroke risk. However, the converse is not true. In patients with systolic hypertension (systolic BP ≥ 160 mmHg) stroke risk does not increase with increasing levels of diastolic blood pressure (Wolf *et al.* 1998). Control of hypertension has been shown to reduce the risk of stroke in multiple clinical trials using a wide variety of anti-hypertensive agents. A review of eighteen long-term clinical trials examining beta-blockers and diuretics found that low-dose diuretics, high-dose diuretics and beta-blockers were all effective in reducing stroke risk when compared to placebo. The relative risk of stroke for various anti-hypertensive agents versus placebo ranged from 0.49 to 0.71 (Psaty *et al.* 1997). Other studies have shown angiotensin converting enzyme inhibitors, angiotensin receptor blockers and calcium channel blockers to be effective in reducing stroke risk in people with hypertension. The treatment of isolated systolic hypertension in the elderly has been shown to reduce overall stroke risk as well as the risk of ischaemic and haemorrhagic strokes separately (Perry *et al.* 2000; Staessen *et al.* 1997). The INDANA meta-analysis showed that blood pressure lowering drug interventions reduced the risk of stroke recurrence in stroke survivors consistently across multiple studies, (relative risk of stroke in those treated with anti-hypertensive therapy versus placebo controls = 0.72).

Diabetes

Diabetes mellitus is an independent risk factor for ischaemic stroke. The Honolulu Heart Program found a twofold increase in the relative risk of thrombo-embolic stroke in those with diabetes mellitus compared to those without even after adjustment for other risk factors (Abbott *et al.* 1987). There was no association between diabetes and haemorrhagic stroke. Similarly, the Framingham study showed diabetes to be an independent risk factor for stroke with a relative risk ranging from 1.4 to 1.7 (Wolf *et al.* 1991). Tight glycemic control in both type 1 and type 2 diabetes has been shown to delay the onset of microvascular complications such as diabetic retinopathy, nephropathy and neuropathy (UKPDS 1998; DCCT 1993). The effect of such glycemic control on stroke prevention has not been reported though recent results from the Diabetes Control and Complications Trial indicate significant reduction in a combined end-point of non-fatal myocardial infarction, stroke, or cardiovascular death with intensive diabetes therapy in patients with Type I diabetes (risk reduction 57 per cent; Nathan *et al.* 2005). The United Kingdom Prospective Diabetes Study showed that tight blood pressure control reduced stroke risk by 44 per cent in patients with type 2 diabetes (UKPDS 1998). Other studies have shown the beneficial effect of angiotensin converting enzyme inhibitors and angiotensin receptor blockers in reducing cardiovascular mortality and stroke rates in patients with diabetes (HOPE 2000; Dahlof *et al.* 2002).

Blood lipids

The relationship between lipid levels and stroke risk is complex and the nature of the relationship varies by stroke subtype. There is epidemiological evidence for increased haemorrhagic stroke risk with very low cholesterol levels. The Honolulu Heart Study showed that there was an inverse relationship between serum cholesterol levels and the risk of intra-cranial haemorrhage after adjustment for other risk factors (Kagan *et al.* 1980). Similar results were reported in a 10-year study of a rural population from Japan (Tanaka *et al.* 1982) and in the Multiple Risk Factor Intervention Trial (Iso *et al.* 1989). The MRFIT trial showed an interaction between high diastolic blood pressure and low serum cholesterol. The relation between total cholesterol and ischaemic stroke has been equivocal. There was a modest association between elevated serum cholesterol and thrombo-embolic stroke in the Honolulu Heart Program with a relative risk of 1.4 between the highest and lowest cholesterol quartiles (Benfante *et al.* 1994). The Framingham study did not find a significant relationship between ischaemic stroke and total cholesterol or its sub-fractions (Wolf *et al.* 1991). Other studies have shown associations between cholesterol subfractions and ischaemic stroke. The Northern Manhattan Stroke Study and the Oxfordshire Community Study both found a protective effect of high HDL-cholesterol levels on ischaemic stroke risk (Sacco *et al.* 2001; Qizilbash *et al.* 1991). Extra-cranial carotid atherosclerosis, an important risk factor for ischaemic stroke has been shown to be associated with elevated LDL-cholesterol levels and inversely related to HDL-cholesterol levels (Salonen *et al.* 1988). The recently published Stroke Prevention by Aggressive Reduction in Cholesterol Levels trial showed that treatment with a 3-hydroxy-3-methylglutaryl coenzyme A reductase inhibitor (atorvastatin) reduced the risk of recurrent strokes despite a small increase in the incidence of haemorrhagic stroke (Amarenco *et al.* 2006).

Cardiovascular disease

Cardiovascular disease is an independent risk factor for stroke with a relative risk estimated at 1.7 after adjustment for other risk factors (Wolf *et al.* 1991). Cardiovascular disease is primarily associated with ischaemic stroke. Specific entities associated with stroke include atrial fibrillation, coronary artery disease, acute myocardial infarction, congestive heart failure, dilated cardiomyopathy, significant right-to-left intra-cardiac shunts, left ventricular hypertrophy, and valvular heart disease. Atrial fibrillation, an independent risk factor for stroke, is estimated to increase the ischaemic stroke risk 5-fold. Rheumatic heart disease with mitral and tricuspid valvular involvement is the most common pre-disposing factor for atrial fibrillation in developing countries where rheumatic fever is common (Vora 2006). In contrast, atrial fibrillation is a disease related to atherosclerosis in western countries. For example, in the United States where rheumatic heart disease is uncommon, the incidence of atrial fibrillation in the United States ranges from less than 1 per 1000 patient years in those under 40–19.2 per 1000 patient years in those over 65. The aging of the population and the improved survival after myocardial infarction has led to projections of an increased atrial fibrillation burden in developed countries over the next few decades (Go *et al.* 2001). The risk of thromboembolism in atrial fibrillation patients with rheumatic valvular heart disease is in the order of 17–18 per cent per year (Vora 2006). In non-rheumatic atrial fibrillation, stroke risk varies from <2 per cent per year in otherwise healthy individuals in the 50–59 age range to over 10 per cent in the elderly in the presence of other co-morbidities such as hypertension and diabetes mellitus. Warfarin anti-coagulation has been shown to reduce stroke risk by 60–65 per cent in unselected patients with non-valvular atrial fibrillation and such anti-coagulation is recommended in eligible patients with risk factors for thromboembolism (Hart *et al.* 2003). This therapy, however, remains under-utilized (Lakshminarayan *et al.* 2006).

Cigarette smoking

Tobacco smoking is a worldwide problem, and cigarettes are associated with a substantial increase in stroke risk. The effect of tobacco smoking on stroke risk varies by stroke sub-type. Comparing current smokers to never smokers in the Nurses Health Study, Kawachi *et al.* estimate an adjusted relative risk of 4.85 for sub-arachnoid haemorrhage, 2.53 for ischaemic stroke and 1.24 for cerebral haemorrhage (Kawachi *et al.* 1993). A meta-analysis examining cigarette smoking and stroke risk also estimates a higher relative risk for sub-arachnoid haemorrhage compared (2.9), compared to ischaemic stroke (1.9) and intra-cerebral haemorrhage (0.7). The stroke risk due to tobacco smoking declines after smoking cessation and approaches that of non-smokers 2–4 years post-cessation.

Alcohol

Like tobacco smoking, the association between alcohol consumption and stroke risk appears to vary by stroke subtype. The Honolulu Heart Program study showed that both light and heavy alcohol use were associated with a significant increase in haemorrhagic stroke risk after adjustment for other risk factors (relative risk 2–3 compared to non-drinkers). The association was stronger for sub-arachnoid haemorrhages. In contrast, moderate alcohol consumption (up to two drinks per day) was associated with a decreased ischaemic stroke risk (odds ratio 0.51) in the NOMASS study (Sacco *et al.* 1999). The NOMASS study also found an increased risk of ischaemic stroke associated with heavy alcohol use (odds ratio 2.96) and the data suggested a J-shaped relation between alcohol consumption and ischaemic stroke risk.

Physical activity

Physical activity has been shown to reduce stroke risk in both men and women. The Framingham study showed that medium and high levels of physical activity were protective against stroke when compared to low levels of activity, but did not show a similar protective effect in women (Kiely *et al.* 1994). The Nurses Health Study however showed that physical activity was associated with a significant reduction in the risk of total stroke as well as ischaemic stroke and that the reduction was dose-related, i.e. the effect was more substantial at higher levels of activity (Hu *et al.* 2000).

Heart failure

Heart failure is a clinical constellation of signs and symptoms resulting from circulatory and neural responses to cardiac dysfunction. It is increasing in prevalence in many areas of the world. Manifest by inadequate pumping ability by the heart, heart failure can have multiple underlying aetiologies including ischaemic heart disease, hypertension, non-ischaemic cardiomyopathy, infection, diabetes mellitus, and others (Cowie *et al.* 1999). Several observations about the population patterns of include:

1. Population prevalence of heart failure is directly related to the prevalence and types of underlying cardiovascular conditions. Coronary heart disease is a leading cause in developed countries.
2. Population rates of heart failure vary widely because of the differing definitions and classification systems used to describe cases.
3. Population levels of heart failure are rising as more individuals survive acute myocardial infarction and chronic hypertension.
4. Heart failure is predominantly a disease of older adults and the mortality is similar to serious cancers.
5. Treatment of heart failure has improved as randomized clinical trials have demonstrated the utility of new drugs.

Research into heart failure is hampered by variability in case definition. Symptoms, signs, radiological studies, tests of ventricular performance, and tests of exercise capacity have all been utilized. All methods have limitations and are particularly poor in the classification of mild heart failure. The diagnosis may be commonly confused with obesity-related dyspnoea, poor physical condition, myocardial ischaemia, pulmonary disease, or other conditions.

There are several studies of heart failure incidence. The Framingham Study and the Gothenberg Study are examples of the cohort approach (Eriksson *et al.* 1989; Ho *et al.* 1993a). These were able to identify incident cases prospectively and characterize them at the time of diagnosis. Studies in Finland, Holland, and Rochester, Minnesota, are examples of a population approach (Mosterd *et al.* 1999; Remes *et al.* 1992; Senni *et al.* 1998). These studies find significant differences in incidence, which ranges from 100 to 500 per 100 000 population per year, and that incidence increases sharply with age.

There are more data available on heart failure prevalence. Rates also vary widely due to differences in methodology and case definition. Observed prevalence in industrialized societies ranges from 300 to 2000 individuals per 100 000 population (unadjusted for age) and 3000 to 13 000 per 100 000 population for those over the age of 65 years (Cowie *et al.* 1997). Of particular interest are the data from the American National Health Interview Survey which show a self-report prevalence ranging from 0.1 per cent for adults aged 18–39 to 5.5 per cent for those 75 years and above (Ni 2003). Self-report may underestimate true prevalence. Heart failure prevalence appears to be rising, largely attributed to increased survival from acute myocardial infarction (Graves & Gillum 1996).

Mortality from heart failure is substantial with the Framingham Study reporting 5-year survival of 25 per cent for men and 38 per cent for women in an early analysis (Ho *et al.* 1993*b*). Among individuals with heart failure (age greater than 55 years), 61 per cent of women and 28 per cent of men were still alive 15 years later. However, the validity of heart failure diagnosis on death certificates has been questioned (Cowie *et al.* 1997). Because heart failure is a constellation of signs, symptoms and physiological changes, it is often not considered among the underlying causes of death. For example, in the United Kingdom, heart failure is never used as an underlying cause of death (Cowie *et al.* 1997). In the United States, heart failure is categorized as a cause of death and rose from 10 000 in 1968 to 58 000 deaths in 2004 (NHLBI 2006).

Previously, hypertension was the most common underlying cause of heart failure, but there has been a shift to coronary heart disease as a more common aetiology. Hypertensive cardiovascular disease with left ventricular hypertrophy results in a 15-fold greater risk of developing heart failure (Kannel *et al.* 1994). Coronary heart disease, particularly when manifested as myocardial infarction, also leads to increased heart failure with damaged and dysfunctional myocardial muscle. In the Framingham Study, approximately 20 per cent of those who survived myocardial infarction developed heart failure within 5–6 years (Kannel 1987). Diabetes mellitus with heart failure also increased in prevalence (Ho *et al.* 1993a; Levy *et al.* 1996; Davis *et al.* 1997). While these are the major causes of heart failure in industrialized societies, in many nations other diseases play an important role including rheumatic heart disease, cardiomyopathy and pulmonary heart disease.

As most heart failure is a late consequence of an underlying cardiovascular disease, primary treatment should consist of prevention of that underlying disease whether it is hypertension, coronary heart disease, rheumatic heart disease, or other conditions. If these conditions are adequately controlled, heart failure is uncommon. However, there are currently many individuals with these diseases who have heart failure as the primary cause of their limitation and disability. Treatment with diuretics and digitalis are widely used, however, these are aided by modern drugs (Cohn 1996). In recent clinical trials, heart failure treated with vasodilators, beta blockers and angiotensin-converting enzyme inhibitors has reduced mortality and increased function, leading to optimism for long-term therapy for heart failure (Johnson *et al.* 1993; Cohn 1996).

Rheumatic fever and heart disease

For centuries, rheumatic fever with resulting rheumatic heart disease was the leading cause of cardiovascular morbidity and mortality worldwide. It continues as an important problem in areas where poverty, overcrowding, malnutrition, and lack of medical care are found (Hanna *et al.* 2005; Kurahara *et al.* 2006; WHO 2004). Although much less common than previously, it is still a problem even in industrialized countries where outbreaks can occur.

During the 1960s, the incidence of acute rheumatic fever ranged from 23 to 55 per 100 000 urban children aged 2–14 years in the United States. Currently, it is less than 2 per 100 000 with a prevalence of rheumatic heart disease of less than 1 per 1000 school-aged children (Dajani 1991). In other parts of the industrialized world, such as Scandinavia, similar low rates are found (WHO 1988). However, in some areas of South America, the prevalence of acute rheumatic fever is significantly higher, ranging from 1 to 10 per cent of school-aged children (PAHO 1970). Similar high rates are seen in areas of Asia and Africa (WHO 2004). Reported prevalence of rheumatic heart disease in school children in these areas ranges from 1 to 78/1000 (WHO 2004). The mechanisms by which this infection produces the clinical syndrome of acute rheumatic fever and subsequent rheumatic heart disease is well studied (WHO 2004). A group A streptococcal infection of the throat (tonsillopharyngitis) can be followed, in approximately 3 weeks, by an episode of acute rheumatic fever. In outbreak situations, rheumatic fever occurs in up to 3 per cent of those with a throat infection; however, it is usually much lower (Siegel *et al.* 1961). The rheumatic fever attack results in an inflammatory reaction which involves the heart, joints and/or the central nervous system. Of those with acute rheumatic fever, at least 50 per cent develop some manifestation of carditis, and this proportion rises when more sophisticated diagnostic methods are used (Dajani 1991). The diagnosis of acute rheumatic fever is made principally from the clinical findings using the revised Jones Criteria. These include combinations of the major manifestations of carditis, polyarthritis, chorea, erythema marginatum, and/or subcutaneous nodules. Other manifestations include arthralgias and fever. Laboratory findings of acute phase reactants including elevated erythrocyte sedimentation rate and C-reactive proteins are common. A positive throat culture for streptococcal antigen and/or increased streptococcal antibody titre aid in making the diagnosis. These criteria may not be sufficiently sensitive in industrialized countries where clinical patterns have changed significantly so that arthritis may be the only presentation. In addition, a significant portion of individuals do not have a symptomatic preceding infection (Wannamaker 1973).

Rapid antigen tests for the diagnosis of group A streptococcal throat infections are highly specific, but less sensitive. While a positive test suggests the need for treatment, a negative test indicates the need for a throat culture (Dajani *et al.* 1995). Antibody tests can confirm a recent group A streptococcal infection.

Primary prevention of acute rheumatic fever is the recommended approach. Throat cultures should be performed on all patients with tonsillopharyngitis and those with a positive culture for group A streptococcal infections treated (Dajani *et al.* 1995). Antibiotic treatment can effectively prevent acute rheumatic fever even when given up to 9 days from the onset of the infection (Denny *et al.* 1950). The recommended treatment schedule by the American Heart Association is found at http://www.americanheart.org. Antibiotic treatment can be either oral or by injection.

In individuals with a history of acute rheumatic fever, the likelihood of secondary attacks with additional damage is common, estimated to be approximately 50 per cent of those with streptococcal infections. For this reason, prophylaxis with an antibiotic is recommended (Dajani *et al.* 1995).

If group A streptococcal infections are appropriately detected and treated, rheumatic heart disease can be effectively prevented. In those where it is not prevented, lifelong valvular heart disease results in diminishing function and premature mortality.

Congenital heart disease

Malformations of the heart and cardiovascular system present at birth are among the more common of congenital defects. They are the result of genetic and/or environmental factors. These malformations frequently have significant haemodynamic consequences and may result in severe illness and/or death (Friedman 1997).

Congenital heart disease includes a wide variety of malformations of the cardiovascular system including the septal, heart valve, and great vessels defects. The true incidence of moderate-to-severe congenital heart disease is difficult to determine but approximates 6 per 1000 live births in the United States (Friedman 1997; Hoffman & Kaplan 2002). This is probably an underestimate, as much congenital heart disease is not discovered until adulthood, is mild, or is fatal prior to birth (Hoffman & Kaplan 2002). In addition, the 0.6 per cent incidence does not include mitral valve prolapse or non-obstructive bicuspid aortic valves, both of which are common. Males are more likely to have congenital heart disease than females, but the pattern differs by defect type (Samanck 1994).

Genetic transmission plays an important role in congenital heart disease. Family studies find that the offspring of parents with congenital heart disease have an increased malformation incidence ranging from 1.4 to 16.1 per cent (Ferencz 1986). Identical twins are both affected 25–30 per cent of the time. However, despite the known genetic clustering and the identification of disorders associated with single genes, it is estimated that only 10 per cent of congenital heart disease has an identifiable genetic origin (Noonan 1978).

Maternal infections are an important etiology of congenital heart disease. Rubella is commonly implicated when it occurs in the first 2 months of pregnancy with congenital malformations in about 80 per cent of live births. Subclinical maternal Coxsackie and other virus infections are also implicated in congenital heart disease.

There are many exposures associated with increased incidence of congenital heart disease. Acute hypoxia, residence at high altitudes, high carboxyhaemoglobin levels and cigarette smoking are among potential causes. X-ray exposure is associated with Down syndrome and other congenital defects. Metabolic defects including diabetes and phenylketonuria are associated with increases in congenital defects.

Diet- and drug-associated exposures are also implicated. They include the well-known examples of thalidomide and folic acid antagonists. Dextroamphetamines, anticonvulsants, lithium chloride, alcohol and progesterone/oestrogen are suspected as teratogens acting in the first trimester of pregnancy. Certain pesticides and herbicides are implicated (Zierler 1985).

The overall incidence of congenital heart disease appears to have remained stable although the distribution of defect types may be changing. There are unexplained increases in ventricular septal defect and patent ductus arteriosis. Rubella-related disease is declining, perhaps the result of widespread vaccination for that disease.

The most effective strategy for congenital heart disease is prevention including genetic counselling for families with congenital heart disease, rubella immunization, and avoidance of exposure to known teratogens. Of particular importance are avoidance of alcohol abuse and cigarette smoking.

For many that were born with congenital heart disease, modern medical and surgical techniques can provide palliation, if not a cure. For the most severe cases, heart and heart–lung transplants are assuming increasing importance.

Cardiomyopathy and myocarditis

Cardiomyopathy and myocarditis are a diverse set of diseases that have, as a central feature, pathological involvement of the heart muscle. Heart failure is the frequent outcome of this condition. Cardiomyopathies account for a substantial portion of cardiovascular disease related deaths in developing countries. However, they are becoming more common in industrialized nations with increasing rates of ischaemic cardiomyopathy associated with coronary heart disease.

There are numerous known causes of myopathy as detailed in a recent report by the WHO (Richardson *et al.* 1996). The WHO advocates that the term 'cardiomyopathy' be reserved for myocardial dysfunction of unknown aetiology; however, it is commonly applied even when the aetiology is known (Richardson *et al.* 1996).

The natural history of cardiomyopathy varies according to the type. Many cases begin with an acute phase where inflammation of the myocardium is common (myocarditis). The widespread use of endomyocardial biopsy has been of some assistance in identifying and classifying myocarditis (Fowles 1985). In many cases, the initial myocarditis is probably undetected because it is mild. There are clinical courses ranging from minimal heart failure to a brief rapid course leading to death. Investigators at the Mayo Clinic in Olmsted County, Minnesota, found an incidence of idiopathic dilated cardiomyopathy of 6 per 100 000 person years (Shabeter 1983). Overall prevalence in the United States was 35.3 per 100 000 population (Gillum 1986).

The prevalence of cardiomyopathy appears to be increasing in the United States. However, it is uncertain whether this is an actual increase or improved diagnostic methods and greater clinical sensitivity. For many cases, a specific cause is not known.

Cardiomyopathy is grouped into three major types: (a) dilated, characterized by dilatation of the ventricles and contractual dysfunction with heart failure; (b) hypertrophic, with left ventricular hypertrophy and well-preserved cardiac function; (c) restrictive, with impaired diastolic filling frequently due to scarring of the myocardium of the ventricle. The dilated cardiomyopathy pattern is most commonly observed, although there is considerable overlap between types (Keren & Popp 1992).

Alcohol abuse is an important environmental cause of cardiomyopathy in the United States accounting for approximately 8 per cent of all cases (Okada & Wakafuji 1985). This may operate through a direct toxic effect, thiamine deficiency, or additives such as cobalt in alcoholic beverages. Abstinence may halt or reverse this disease (Okada & Wakafuji 1985). Viral infections are a very commonly observed cause of cardiomyopathy. Coxsackie virus, echo virus, influenza, and polio are frequently implicated (Levine 1979). These diseases begin as acute myocarditis and then progress to a chronic condition which results in dilated cardiomyopathy.

Hypertrophic cardiomyopathy is detected by the use of echocardiographic techniques. This condition uncommonly causes difficulty for patients and is usually well managed with medication (Wigle 1988). Chagas' disease is caused by the protozoan *Trypanosoma cruzi*. Beginning as a myocarditis, its clinical manifestations are manifest many years later. The disease is most prevalent in Central and South America with over 20 million thought to be infected with the parasite (Morris *et al.* 1990; Hagar & Rahimtoola 1995). This disease may also be found in non-endemic areas through migration, contaminated blood products and tourism (Hagar & Rahimtoola 1995). Treatment is available for the acute parasitic infections; however, the cardiomyopathy cannot be directly treated.

Schistosomiasis is a parasitic infection epidemic in the Nile and Yangtze basins. It may involve a majority of the population in certain endemic areas. Chronic pulmonary embolization of the parasite leads to pulmonary hypertension, right ventricular hypertrophy and right ventricular heart failure. Direct involvement of the myocardium is rare. New medications can be of assistance in controlling the infection and prevention is the principal strategy employed.

Prevention programmes for cardiovascular disease and stroke

Research in the prevention of cardiovascular diseases and stroke at the individual level resulted in more advanced programmes at the individual and community level than any other chronic disease. Core to this understanding is the risk factor model and the identification of disease predictors using epidemiological techniques. The finding of modifiable risk factors such as hypertension and demonstration of modification by interventions forms the basis for causality, treatment, and public policy recommendations. The demonstration of environmental and behavioural factors in the genesis of increased disease risk also points to specific strategies. For the high-risk individual patient, smoking cessation, blood pressure control, and cholesterol reduction form the basis of medical therapy to prevent disease events. For the high-risk community, facilitation of smoke-free buildings, healthy diets, regular physical activity are among the prevention strategies (Farquhar *et al.* 1990; Luepker *et al.* 1994; Carleton *et al.* 1995; Puska *et al.* 1995). The dramatic reduction in cardiovascular disease and stroke observed in some industrialized countries is directly linked to community wide and individual patient changes.

Summary

Cardiovascular disease and stroke is a leading cause of morbidity and mortality worldwide. While rates are declining in some industrialized nations, they are rising in the developing world resulting in a continued epidemic. Much is known about the prevention of cardiovascular disease and stroke. The major risk factors are known and effective interventions at the community and individual levels available. If these preventive strategies were widely applied, the epidemic could be controlled. There is an important role for public health in the prevention of cardiovascular disease and stroke.

References

Abbott R.D., Donahue R.P., MacMahon S.W. *et al.* (1987). Diabetes and the risk of stroke. The Honolulu Heart Program. *Journal of the American Medical Association*, **257**, 949.

Abbott R.D., Sharp D.S., Burchfiel C.M. *et al.* (1997). Cross-sectional and longitudinal changes in total and high-density-lipoprotein cholesterol levels over a 20-year period in elderly men: the Honolulu Heart Program. *Annals of Epidemiology*, **7**, 417–24.

Amarenco P., Bogousslavsky J., Callahan A. *et al.* (2006). High-dose Atorvastatin after stroke or transient ischemic attack. *New England Journal of Medicine*, **355**, 549.

American Heart Association (2007). *Heart Disease and Stroke Statistics - 2007 Update*. Dallas, Texas.

Arnett D.K., Jacobs Jr., D.R., Luepker R.V. *et al.* (2005). Twenty-year trends in serum cholesterol, hypercholesterolemia, and cholesterol medication use: the Minnesota Heart Survey, 1980-1982 to 2000-2002. *Circulation*, **112**, 3884–91.

Ascherio A. and Hunter D.J. (1994). Iron and myocardial infarction. *Epidemiology*, **5**, 135–7.

Ascherio A., Hennekens C.H., Buring J.E. *et al.* (1994). Trans-fatty acids intake and risk of myocardial infarction. *Circulation*, **89**, 94–101.

Ascherio A., Rimm E.B., Hernan M.A. *et al.* (1999). Relation of consumption of vitamin E, vitamin C, and carotenoids to risk for stroke among men in the United States. *Annals of Internal Medicine*, **130**, 963–70.

Bak S., Gaist D., Sindrup S.H. *et al.* (2002). Genetic liability in stroke: a long-term follow-up study of Danish twins. *Stroke*, **33**, 769.

Barefoot J.C., Dahlstrom W.G., and Williams R.B. (1983). Hostility, coronary heart disease incidence and total mortality: a 25-year follow-up study of 255 physicians. *Psychosomatic Medicine*, **45**, 59–63.

Barefoot J.C., Dodge K.A., Peterson B.L. *et al.* (1989). The Cook-Medley hostility scale: item content and ability to predict survival. *Psychosomatic Medicine*, **51**, 46–57.

Benfante R., Yano K., Hwang L.J. *et al.* (1994). Elevated serum cholesterol is a risk factor for both coronary heart disease and thromboembolic stroke in Hawaiian Japanese men. Implications of shared risk. *Stroke*, **25**, 814.

Berkman L.F., Blumenthal J., Burg M. *et al.* (2003) Effects of treating depression and low perceived social support on clinical events after myocardial infarction: the Enhancing Recovery in Coronary Heart Disease Patients (ENRICHD) Randomized Trial. *Journal of the American Medical Association*, **289**, 3106–16.

Blackburn H. and Jacobs D. (1984). Sources of the diet–heart controversy: confusion over population versus individual correlations. *Circulation*, **70**, 775–80.

Blackburn H. and Prineas R.J. (1983). Diet and hypertension: anthropology, epidemiology, and public health implications. *Progress in Biochemical Pharmacology*, **19**, 31–79.

Blair S.N., Kohl H.W., Paffenbarger Jr R.S. *et al.* (1989). Physical fitness and all-cause mortality: a prospective study of healthy men and women. *Journal of the American Medical Association*, **262**, 2395–401.

Bonaa K.H., Njolstad I., Ueland P.M. *et al.* (2006). Homocysteine lowering and cardiovascular events after acute myocardial infarction. *New England Journal of Medicine*, **354**, 1578–88.

Boushey C.J., Beresford S.A., Omenn G.S. *et al.* (1995). A quantitative assessment of plasma homocysteine as a risk factor for vascular disease. Probable benefits of increasing folic acid intakes. *Journal of the American Medical Association*, **274**, 1049–57.

Brass L.M., Isaacsohn J.L., Merikangas K.R. *et al.* (1992). A study of twins and stroke. *Stroke*, **23**, 221.

Brown R.D., Whisnant J.P., Sicks J.D. *et al.* (1996). Stroke incidence, prevalence, and survival: secular trends in Rochester, Minnesota, through 1989. *Stroke*, **27**, 373.

Buchwald H., Matts J.P., Fitch L.L. *et al.* for the Program on the Surgical Control of the Hyperlipidemias (POSCH) Group (1992). Changes in sequential coronary arteriograms and subsequent coronary events. *Journal of the American Medical Association*, **268**, 1429–33.

Buchwald H., Varco R.L., Matts J.P. *et al.* (1990). Effective lipid modification by partial ileal bypass reduced long-term coronary heart disease mortality and morbidity: five year post-trial follow-up report from POSCH. *New England Journal of Medicine*, **323**, 946–55.

Canner P.L., Berge K.G., Wenger N.K. *et al.* (1986). Fifteen year mortality in Coronary Drug Project patients: long-term benefit with niacin. *Journal of the American College of Cardiology*, **8**, 1245–55.

Carleton R.A., Lasater T.M., Assaf A.R. *et al.* and the Pawtucket Heart Health Program Writing Group (1995). The Pawtucket Heart Health Program: community changes in cardiovascular risk factors and projected disease risk. *American Journal of Public Health*, **85**, 777–85.

Carroll M.D., Lacher D.A., Sorlie P.D. *et al.* (2005). Trends in serum lipids and lipoproteins of adults, 1960–2002. *Journal of the American Medical Association*, **294**, 1773–81.

Case R.B., Heller S.S., Case N.B. *et al.* (1985). Type A behavior and survival after acute myocardial infarction. *New England Journal of Medicine*, **312**, 737–41.

Centers for Disease Control and Prevention, National Center for Health Statistics. National Health and Nutrition Examination Survey (NHANES): NHANES I, II, III, 1999–2000 and 2001–2002.

Chobanian A.V., Bakris G.L., Black H.R. *et al.* (2003). Seventh report of the Joint National Committee on Prevention, Detection, Evaluation, and Treatment of High Blood Pressure. *Journal of the American Medical Association*, **289**, 2560–2571.

Cohn J.N. (1996). The management of chronic heart failure. *New England Journal of Medicine*, **335**, 490–8.

Colditz G.A. (1990). A prospective assessment of moderate alcohol intake and major chronic diseases. *Annals of Epidemiology*, **1**, 167–77.

Cowie M.R., Mosterd A., Wood D.A. *et al.* (1997). The epidemiology of heart failure. *European Heart Journal*, **18**, 208–25.

Cowie M.R., Wood D.A., Coats A.J. *et al.* (1999). Incidence and aetiology of heart failure; a population-based study. *European Heart Journal*, **20**, 421–8.

Criqui M.H. (1987). The roles of alcohol in the epidemiology of cardiovascular diseases. *Acta Medica Scandinavica*, **717** (Suppl), 73–85.

Dahlof B., Devereux R.B., Kjeldsen S.E. *et al.* (2002). Cardiovascular morbidity and mortality in the Losartan Intervention For Endpoint reduction in hypertension study (LIFE): a randomised trial against atenolol.see comment. *Lancet*, **359**, 995.

Dajani A., Taubert K., Ferrieri P. *et al.* (1995). Treatment of acute streptococcal pharyngitis and prevention of rheumatic fever: a statement for health professionals. Committee on Rheumatic Fever, Endocarditis, and Kawasaki Disease of the Council on Cardiovascular Disease in the Young, The American Heart Association. *Pediatrics*, **96**, 758–64.

Dajani A.S. (1991). Current status of nonsupportive complications of group A streptococci. *Pediatric Infectious Disease Journal*, **105**, S25–7.

Dattilo A.M. and Kris-Etherton P.M. (1992). Effects of weight reduction on blood lipids and lipoproteins: a meta-analysis. *American Journal of Clinical Nutrition*, **56**, 320–8.

Davis R.C., Hobbs F.D.R., McLeod S. *et al.* (1997). Heart failure prevalence in patients in 'high-risk' groups. *European Heart Journal*, **18**, 597.

DCCT (Diabetes Control and Complications Trial) Research Group (1993). The effect of intensive treatment of diabetes on the development and progression of long-term complications in insulin-dependent diabetes mellitus. *New England Journal of Medicine*, **329**, 977–86.

Denny F.W., Wannamaker L.W., Brink W.R. *et al.* (1950). Prevention of rheumatic fever: treatment of the preceding streptococcic infection. *Journal of the American Medical Association*, **143**, 151–3.

Derby C.A., Lapane K.L., Feldman H.A. *et al.* (2000). Sex-specific trends in validated coronary heart disease rates in Southeastern New England, 1980–1991. *American Journal of Epidemiology*, **151**, 417–29.

Dimsdale J.E., Gilbert J., Hutter A.M. *et al.* (1981). Predicting cardiac morbidity based on risk factors and coronary angiographic findings. *American Journal of Cardiology*, **47**, 73–6.

Downs J.R., Clearfield M., Weis S. *et al.* (1998). Primary prevention of acute coronary events with lovastatin in men and women with average cholesterol levels: results of AFCAPS/TexCAPS. Air Force/Texas Coronary Atherosclerosis Prevention Study. *Journal of the American Medical Association*, **279**, 1615–22.

Dyer A.R. and Elliott P. (1989). The INTERSALT Study: relations of body mass index to blood pressure. *Journal of Human Hypertension*, **3**, 299–308.

Eckel R.H. and Krauss R.M. (1998). American Heart Association call to action: obesity as a major risk factor for coronary heart disease. *Circulation*, **97**, 2099–100.

Eriksson H., Svardsudd K., Larsson B. *et al.* (1989). Risk factors for heart failure in the general population: the study of men born in 1913. *European Heart Journal*, **10**, 647–56.

Farquhar J.W., Fortmann S.P., Flora J.A. *et al.* (1990). Effects of community-wide education on cardiovascular disease risk factors: the Stanford Five-City Project. *Journal of the American Medical Association*, **264**, 359–65.

Farquhar J.W. Maccoby N. Wood P.D. *et al.* (1977). Community education for cardiovascular health. *Lancet*, **1**, 1192–5.

Ferencz C. (1986). Offspring of fathers with cardiovascular malformations. *American Heart Journal*, **111**, 1212–13.

Fiore M.C., Bailey W.C., Cohen S.J. *et al.* (1996). *Smoking cessation*. Clinical practice guideline No. 18. United States Department of Health and Human Services, Public Health Service, Agency for Health Care Policy and Research. AHCPR Publication No. 96–0692.

Flegal K.M. (1996). Trends in body weight and overweight in the US population. *Nutrition Reviews*, **54**, S97–S100

Flossmann E., Schulz U.G., and Rothwell P.M. (2004). Systematic review of methods and results of studies of the genetic epidemiology of ischemic stroke. *Stroke*, **35**, 212.

Fowles R.E. (1985). Progress of research in cardiomyopathy and myocarditis in the USA. International Symposium on Cardiomyopathy and Myocarditis. *Heart Vessels*, **1**, 5–7.

Freedman D.S. (1995). Relation of body fat distribution to ischemic heart disease. The National Health and Nutrition Examination Survey I (NHANES I) Epidemiologic Follow-up Study. *American Journal of Epidemiology*, **142**, 53–63.

Frick M.H., Elo O., Haapa K. *et al.* (1987). Helsinki Heart Study: primary-prevention trial with gemfibrozil in middle-aged men with dyslipidemia. *New England Journal of Medicine*, **317**, 1237–45.

Friedman M. and Rosenman R.H. (1959). Association of specific overt behavior pattern with blood and cardiovascular findings: blood cholesterol level, blood clotting time, incidence of arcus senilis, and clinical coronary artery disease. *Journal of the American Medical Association*, **169**, 1286–96.

Friedman M., Thorensen C.E., Gill J.J. *et al.* (1984). Alteration of type A behavior and reduction in cardiac recurrences in post-myocardial infarction patients. *American Heart Journal*, **108**, 237–48.

Friedman W.F. (1997). Congenital heart disease in infancy and childhood. In *Heart disease: a textbook of cardiovascular medicine* (ed. E. Braunwald), (5th ed), pp. 877–962. Saunders, Philadelphia.

Furberg C.D., Wright J.T., Davis B.R. *et al.* (2002). Major outcomes in high-risk hypertensive patients randomized to angiotensin-converting enzyme inhibitor or calcium channel blocker vs diuretic - The Antihypertensive and Lipid-Lowering Treatment to Prevent Heart Attack Trial (ALLHAT). *Journal of the American Medical Association*, **288**, 2981–2997

Fuster V., Badimon L., Badimon J. *et al.* (1992). Mechanisms of disease: the pathogenesis of coronary artery disease and the acute coronary syndromes. *New England Journal of Medicine*, **326**, 310–18.

GCP Research Group (1988). GCP German Cardiovascular Prevention study. *Design, methods, results*. Program Report. Scientific Institute of the German Medical Association (WIAD), Bonn, Germany.

Gillum R.F. (1986). Idiopathic cardiomyopathy in the United States, 1970–1982. *American Heart Journal*, **111**, 752–5.

Ginsberg H.N., Kris-Etherton P., Dennis B. *et al.* (1998). Effects of reducing dietary saturated fatty acids on plasma lipids and lipoproteins in healthy subjects: the DELTA Study, protocol 1. *Arteriosclerosis, Thrombosis and Vascular Biology*, **18**, 441–9.

Go A.S., Hylek E.M., Phillips K.A. *et al.* (2001). Prevalence of diagnosed atrial fibrillation in adults: national implications for rhythm management and stroke prevention: the Anticoagulation and Risk Factors in Atrial Fibrillation (ATRIA) Study. *Journal of the American Medical Association*, **285**, 2370.

Goldberg R.B., Mellies M.J., Sacks F.M. *et al.* (1998) Cardiovascular events and their reduction with pravastatin in diabetic and glucose-intolerant myocardial infarction survivors with average cholesterol levels: subgroup analyses in the cholesterol and recurrent events (CARE) trial. The Care Investigators. *Circulation*, **98**, 2513–9.

Gordon T. (1988). The diet–heart idea. *American Journal of Epidemiology*, **127**, 220–5.

Gordon T., Ernst N., Fisher M. *et al.* (1981). Alcohol and high-density lipoprotein cholesterol. *Circulation*, **64**, (Supplement III), 63–7.

Graves E.J. and Gillum B.S. (1996). 1994 Summary: National hospital discharge survey: advance data. *National Center for Health Statistics*, **278**, 1–12.

Hagar J.M. and Rahimtoola S.H. (1995). Chagas' heart disease. *Current Problems in Cardiology*, **20**, 825–924.

Hanna J.N., Heazlewood R.J. (2005). The epidemiology of acute rheumatic fever in Indigenous people in north Queensland. *Australia and New Zealand Journal of Public Health*, **29**, 313–7.

Harris T.B., Launer L.J., Madans J. *et al.* (1997). Cohort study of effect of being overweight and change in weight on risk of coronary heart disease in old age. *British Medical Journal*, **314**, 1791–4.

Hart R.G., Halperin J.L., Pearce L.A. *et al.* (2003). Lessons from the Stroke Prevention in Atrial Fibrillation trials. *Annals of Internal Medicine*,**138**, 831–8.

Haynes S.G., Feinleib M., and Kannel W.B. (1980). The relationship of psychosocial factors to coronary heart disease in the Framingham Study. III. Eight-year incidence of coronary heart disease. *American Journal of Epidemiology*, **111**, 37–58.

Hearn M.D., Murray D.M., and Luepker R.V. (1988). Hostility, coronary heart disease, and total mortality. A 33-year follow-up study of university students. *Journal of Behavioral Medicine*, **12**, 105–21.

Heart Outcomes Prevention Evaluation Study Investigators (2000). Effects of ramipril on cardiovascular and microvascular outcomes in people with diabetes mellitus: results of the HOPE study and MICRO-HOPE substudy. *Lancet*, **355**, 253–9.

Hecker M.H.L., Chesney M.A., Black G.W. *et al.* (1988). Coronary prone behaviors in the Western Collaborative Group Study. *Psychosomatic Medicine*, **50**, 153–64.

Hennekens C.H., Buring J.E., Manson J.E. *et al.* (1996). Lack of effect on long-term supplementation with beta carotene on the incidence of malignant neoplasms and cardiovascular disease. *New England Journal of Medicine*, **334**, 1145–9.

Hermanson B., Omenn G.S., Kronmal R.A. *et al.* (1988). Beneficial six-year outcome of smoking cessation in older men and women with coronary artery disease: results from the CASS registry. *New England Journal of Medicine*, **319**, 1365–9.

Ho K.K., Pinsky J.L., Kannel W.B. *et al.* (1993a). The epidemiology of heart failure: the Framingham Study. *Journal of the American College of Cardiology*, **22**, 6A–13A.

Ho K.K., Anderson K.M., Kannel W.B. *et al.* (1993b). Survival after the onset of congestivec heart failure in Framingham Heart Study subjects. *Circulation*, **88**, 107–15.

Hoffman J.I. and Kaplan S. (2002). The incidence of congenital heart disease. *Journal of the American College of Cardiology*, **39**, 1890–900.

Howard G., Howard V.J. for the Reasons for Geographic And Racial Differences in Stroke Investigators (2001). Ethnic disparities in stroke: the scope of the problem. *Ethnicity & Disease*, **11**, 761.

Hu F.B., Stampfer M.J., Colditz G.A. *et al.* (2000). Physical activity and risk of stroke in women. *Journal of the American Medical Association*, **283**, 2961.

Hu H.H., Sheng W.Y., Chu F.L. *et al.* (1992). Incidence of stroke in Taiwan. *Stroke*, **23**, 1237.

Huang Z., Willett W.C., Manson J.E. *et al.* (1998). Body weight, weight change, and risk for hypertension in women. *Annals of Internal Medicine*, **128**, 81–8. 1150.

Hughes L.O. (1990). Insulin, Indian origin and ischemic heart disease (editorial). *International Journal of Cardiology*, **26**, 1–4.

INTERSALT Cooperative Research Group (1988). INTERSALT: an international study of electrolyte excretion and blood pressure: results for 24 h urinary sodium and potassium excretion. *British Medical Journal*, **297**, 319–28.

Iso H., Jacobs D.R., Jr., Wentworth D. *et al.* (1989). Serum cholesterol levels and six-year mortality from stroke in 350,977 men screened for the multiple risk factor intervention trial. *New England Journal of Medicine*, **320**, 904.

Jenkins D.J.A., Wolever T.M.S., Rao A.V. *et al.* (1993). Effect on blood lipids of very high intakes of fiber in diets low in saturated fat and cholesterol. *New England Journal of Medicine*, **329**, 21–6.

Johnson G., Carson P., Francis G.S. *et al.* (1993). Influence of prerandomization (baseline) variables on mortality and on the reduction of mortality by enalapril: Veterans Affairs Cooperative Study on Vasodilator Therapy of Heart Failure (V-HeFT II). *Circulation*, **87**, VI32–VI39.

Joseph J.G., Prior I.A.M., Salmond C.E. *et al.* (1983). Elevation of systolic and diastolic blood pressure associated with migration: the Tokelau Island Migrant Study. *Journal of Chronic Disorders*, **36**, 507–16.

Kagan A., Popper J.S., and Rhoads G.G. (1980). Factors related to stroke incidence in Hawaii Japanese men. The Honolulu Heart Study. *Stroke*, **11**, 14.

Kagan A., Harris B.R., Winkelstein W. *et al.* (1974). Epidemiologic studies of coronary heart disease and stroke in Japanese men living in Japan, Hawaii and California: demographic, physical, dietary and biochemical characteristics. *Journal of Chronic Disorders*, **27**, 345–64.

Kannel W.B. (1987). Epidemiology and prevention of cardiac failure: Framingham Study insights. *European Heart Journal*, **8**, 23–6.

Kannel W.B., Ho K., and Thom T. (1994). Changing epidemiological features of cardiac failure. *British Heart Journal*, **72**, S3–9.

Kawachi I., Colditz G.A., Stampfer M.J. *et al.* (1993). Smoking cessation and decreased risk of stroke in women. *Journal of the American Medical Association*, **269**, 232.

Keren A. and Popp R.L. (1992). Assignment of patients into the classification of cardiomyopathies. *Circulation*, **86**, 1622–33.

Keys A. (ed.) (1980). *Seven countries: a multivariate analysis of death and coronary heart disease*. Harvard University Press, Cambridge, MA.

Keys A., Grande F., and Anderson J.T. (1974). Bias and misrepresentation revisited—'perspective' on saturated fat. *American Journal of Clinical Nutrition*, **27**, 188–212.

Khan F.A., Zia E., Janzon L. *et al.* (2004). Incidence of stroke and stroke subtypes in Malmo, Sweden, 1990–2000: marked differences between groups defined by birth country. *Stroke*, **35**, 2054.

Kiely D.K., Wolf P.A., Cupples L.A. *et al.* (1994). Physical activity and stroke risk: the Framingham Study. *American Journal of Epidemiology*, **140**, 608.

Krauss R.M., Wonston M., Fletcher R.N. *et al.* (1998). Obesity: impact of cardiovascular disease. *Circulation*, **98**, 1472–6.

Kritchevsky S.B., Shimakawa T., Tell G.S. *et al.* (1995). Dietary antioxidants and carotid artery wall thickness: the ARIC Study. *Circulation*, **92**, 2142–50.

Kurahara D.K., Grandinetti A., Galario J. *et al.* (2006). Ethnic Differences for Developing Rheumatic Fever in a Low-Income Group Living in Hawaii. *Ethnicity and Disease*, **16**, 357–361.

Lakshminarayan K., Solid C.A., Collins A.J. *et al.* (2006). Atrial fibrillation and stroke in the general medicare population: a 10-year perspective (1992 to 2002). *Stroke*, **37**, 1969.

Lee I.M., Cook N.R., Gaziano J.M. *et al.* (2005). Vitamin E in the primary prevention of cardiovascular disease and cancer: the Women's Health Study: a randomized controlled trial. *Journal of the American Medical Association*, **294**, 56–65.

Lehto S., Ronnemaa T., Haffner S.M. *et al.* (1997). Dyslipidemia and hyperglycemia predict coronary heart disease events in middle-aged patients with NIDDM. *Diabetes*, **48**, 1354–9.

Leon A.S., Connett J., Jacobs Jr. D.R. *et al.* (1987). Leisure time physical activity levels and risk of coronary heart disease and death: the Multiple Risk Factor Intervention Trial. *Journal of the American Medical Association*, **258**, 2388–95.

Leon G.R., Finn S.E., Murray D. *et al.* (1988). Inability to predict cardiovascular disease from hostility scores of MMPI items related to type A behavior. *Journal of Consulting and Clinical Psychology*, **56**, 597–600.

Levine H.D. (1979). Virus myocarditis: a critique of the literature from clinical, electrocardiographic and pathologic standpoints. *American Journal of Medical Sciences*, **277**, 132–43.

Levy D., Larson M.G., Vasan R.S. *et al.* (1996). The progression from hypertension to congestive heart failure. *Journal of the American Medical Association*, **275**, 1557–62.

Long-term Intervention with Pravastatin in Ischaemic Disease (LIPID) Study Group (1998). Prevention of cardiovascular events and death with pravastatin in patients with coronary heart disease and a broad range of initial cholesterol levels. *New England Journal of Medicine*, **339**, 1349–57.

Lonn E., Yusuf S., Arnold M.J. *et al.* (2006). Homocysteine lowering with folic acid and B vitamins in vascular disease. *New England Journal of Medicine*, **354**, 1567–77.

Luepker R.V. (1994). Epidemiology of atherosclerotic diseases in population groups. In *Primer in preventive cardiology* (ed. T.A. Pearson, M.H. Criqui, R.V. Luepker, A. Oberman, and M. Winston), pp. 1–10. American Heart Association, Dallas, TX.

Luepker R.V. (ed.) (1999). Proceedings from primordial prevention of cardiovascular disease risk factors: an international symposium honoring the career and research of Henry Blackburn, MD. *Preventive Medicine*, **29**.

Luepker R.V., Arnett D.K., Jacobs Jr, D.R. *et al.* (2006). Trends in blood pressure, hypertension control, and stroke mortality: The Minnesota Heart Survey. *American Journal of Medicine*, **119**, 42–49.

Luepker R.V., Jacobs D.R., Prineas R.J. *et al.* (1999). Secular trends of blood pressure and body size in a multi-ethnic adolescent population: 1986 to 1996. *Journal of Pediatrics*, **134**, 668–74.

Luepker R.V., Murray D.M., Jacobs Jr. D.R. *et al.* (1994). Community education for cardiovascular disease prevention: risk factor changes in the Minnesota Heart Health Program. *American Journal of Public Health*, **84**, 1383–93.

McCranie E.W., Watkins L.O., Brandsma J.M. *et al.* (1986). Hostility, coronary heart disease incidence, and total mortality: lack of an association in a 25-year follow-up study of 478 physicians. *Journal of Behavioral Medicine*, **9**, 119–25.

McGill H.C., McMahan C.A., Malcom G.T. *et al.* for the PDAY Research Group (1997). Effects of serum lipoproteins and smoking on atherosclerosis in young men and women. *Arteriosclerosis and Thrombosis Vascular Biology*, **17**, 95–106.

McGovern P.G., Pankow J.S., Shahar E. *et al.* for the Minnesota Heart Survey Investigators (1996). Recent trends in acute coronary heart disease mortality, morbidity, medical care and risk factors. *New England Journal of Medicine*, **334**, 884–90.

Meade T.W., Imeson J., and Stirling Y. (1987). Effects of changes in smoking and other characteristics on clotting factors and the risk of ischaemic heart disease. *Lancet*, **2**, 986–8.

Mittleman M.A., Maclure M., Tofler G.H. *et al.* for the Determinants of Myocardial Infarction Onset Study Investigators (1993). Triggering of acute myocardial infarction by heavy physical exertion: protection against triggering of regular exertion. *New England Journal of Medicine*, **329**, 1677–83.

Morris S.A., Tanowitz H.B., Wittner M. *et al.* (1990). Pathophysiological insights into the cardiomyopathy of Chagas' disease. *Circulation*, **82**, 1900–9.

Mosterd A., Hoes A.W., de Bruyne M.C. *et al.* (1999). Prevalence of heart failure and left ventricular dysfunction in the general population; The Rotterdam Study. *Eur Heart J*, **20**, 447–55.

Muller J.E., Kaufmann P.G., Luepker R.V. *et al.* (1997). Mechanisms precipitating acute cardiac events: Review and recommendations of an NHLBI workshop. *Circulation*, **96**, 3233–9.

Muller J.E., Ludmer P.L., Willich S.N. *et al.* (1987). Circadian variation in the frequency of sudden cardiac death. *Circulation*, **75**, 131–8.

Multiple Risk Factor Intervention Trial Research Group (1996). Mortality after 16 years for participants randomized to the Multiple Risk Factor Intervention Trial. *Circulation*, **94**, 946–51.

Nathan D.M., Cleary P.A., Backlund J.Y. *et al.* for the Diabetes Control and Complications

Trial/Epidemiology of Diabetes Interventions and Complications (DCCT/EDIC) Study Research Group (2005). Intensive diabetes treatment and cardiovascular disease in patients with type 1 diabetes. *New England Journal of Medicine*, **353**, 2643–53.

National Task Force on Prevention and Treatment of Obesity (1994). Towards prevention of obesity: research directions. *Obesity Research*, **2**, 571–84.

Neaton J.D. and Wentworth D. for the Multiple Risk Factor Intervention Trial Research Group (1992). Serum cholesterol, blood pressure, cigarette smoking, and death from coronary heart disease: Overall findings and differences by age for 316099 white men. *Archives of Internal Medicine*, **152**, 56–64.

Neaton J.D., Grimm Jr R.H., Prineas R.J. *et al.* (1993). Treatment of mild hypertension study: final results. *Journal of the American Medical Association*, **270**, 713–24.

NHLBI (National Heart, Lung, and Blood Institute) (2006). Morbidity and Mortality: 2006 Chart book on cardiovascular, lung, and blood diseases. Bethesda, MD: National Institutes of Health.

NIH (2003). Prevalence of self-reported heart failure among US adults: results from the 1999 National Health Interview Survey. *American Heart Journal*, **146**, 121–8.

NIH (2002). *Third Report of the* National Cholesterol Education Program *Expert Panel on Detection, Evaluation, and Treatment of High Blood Cholesterol in Adults (Adult Treatment Panel III)*. US Department of Health and Human Services.
NIH Publication No. 02–5215. National Institutes of Health, Washington, DC.

NIH Consensus Conference (1996). Physical activity and cardiovascular health. *Journal of the American Medical Association*, **276**, 241–6.

Nissen S.E. and Wolski K. (2007). Effect of rosiglitazone on the risk of myocardial infarction and death from cardiovascular causes. *New England Journal of Medicine*, **356**, 2457–71.

Noonan J. (1978). Twins, conjoined twins and cardiac defects. *American Journal of Diseased Children*, **132**, 17–18.

Ogden C.L., Carroll M.D., Curtin L.R. *et al.* (2006). Prevalence of overweight and obesity in the United States, 1999-2004. *Journal of the American Medical Association*, **295**, 1549–55.

Okada R. and Wakafuji S. (1985). Myocarditis in autopsy. International Symposium on Cardiomyopathy and Myocarditis. *Heart Vessels*, **1**, 23–9.

Oldridge N.B., Guyatt G.H., Fischer M.E. *et al.* (1988). Cardiac rehabilitation after myocardial infarction. Combined experience of randomized clinical trials. *Journal of the American Medical Association*, **260**, 945–50.

Omenn G.S., Goodman G.E., Thornquist M.D. *et al.* (1996). Effects of a combination of beta carotene and vitamin A on lung cancer and cardiovascular disease. *New England Journal of Medicine*, **334**, 1150–5.

Orth-Gomer K. and Johnson J.V. (1987). Social network interaction and mortality: a six year follow-up study of a random sample of the Swedish population. *Journal of Chronic Disorders*, **40**, 949–57.

Osganian S.K., Stampfer M.J., Spiegelman D. *et al.* (1999). Distribution of and factors associated with serum homocysteine levels in children: Child and Adolescent Trial for Cardiovascular Health. *Journal of the American Medical Association*, **281**, 1189–96.

PAHO (Pan American Health Organization) (1970). *Fourth Meeting of the Working Group on Prevention of Rheumatic Fever*, Quito, Ecuador.

Paisey R.B., Harvey P., Rice S. *et al.* (1998). An intensive weight loss programme in established type 2 diabetes and controls: effects on weight and atherosclerosis risk factors at 1 year. *Diabetic Medicine*, **15**, 73–9.

Perry H.M., Jr., Davis B.R., Price T.R. *et al.* (2000). Effect of treating isolated systolic hypertension on the risk of developing various types and subtypes of stroke: the Systolic Hypertension in the Elderly Program (SHEP). *Journal of the American Medical Association*, **284**, 465.

Perry C.L., Kelder S.H., Murray D.M. *et al.* (1992). Community-wide smoking prevention: long-term outcomes of the Minnesota Heart Health Program and the Class of 1989 Study. *American Journal of Public Health*, **82**, 1210–16.

Powell K.E., Thompson P.D., Caspersen C.J. *et al.* (1987). Physical activity and the incidence of coronary heart disease. *Annual Review of Public Health*, **8**, 253–87.

Psaty B.M., Smith N.L., Siscovick D.S. *et al.* (1997). Health outcomes associated with antihypertensive therapies used as first-line agents. A systematic review and meta-analysis. *Journal of the American Medical Association*, **277**, 739–45.

Puska P., Tuomilehto J., Nissinen A. *et al.* (ed.) (1995). *The North Karelia Project: 20 year results and experiences*. Helsinki University Printing House.

Pyorala K., Pedersen T.R., Kjekshus J. *et al.* (1997). Cholesterol lowering with simvastatin improves prognosis of diabetic patients with coronary heart disease. A subgroup analysis of the Scandinavian Simvastatin Survival Study (4S). *Diabetes Care*, **20**, 614–20.

Qizilbash N., Jones L., Warlow C. *et al.* (1991). Fibrinogen and lipid concentrations as risk factors for transient ischaemic attacks and minor ischaemic strokes. *British Medical Journal*, **303**, 605.

Ragland D.R. and Brand R.J. (1988). Coronary heart disease mortality in the Western Collaborative Group Study. Follow-up experience of 22 years. *American Journal of Epidemiology*, **127**, 462–75.

Regan T.J. (1990). Alcohol and the cardiovascular system. *Journal of the American Medical Association*, **264**, 377–81.

Remes J., Reunanen A., Aromaa A., and Pyorala K. (1992). Incidence of heart failure in Eastern Finland: a population-based surveillance study. *European Heart Journal*, **13**, 588–93.

Richardson P., McKenna W., Bristow M. *et al.* (1996). Report of the 1995 World Health Organization/International Society and Federation of Cardiology Task Force on the Definition and Classification of cardiomyopathies. *Circulation*, **93**, 841–2.

Rosenman R.H., Brand R.J., Jenkins C.D. *et al.* (1975). Coronary heart disease in the Western Collaborative Group Study: final follow-up experience of 8.5 years. *Journal of the American Medical Association*, **233**, 872–7.

Rubins H.B., Robins S.J., Collins D. *et al.* (1999). Gemfibrozil for the secondary prevention of coronary heart disease in men with low levels of high-density lipoprotein cholesterol. Veterans Affairs High-Density Lipoprotein Cholesterol Intervention Trial Study Group. *New England Journal of Medicine*, **341**, 410–18.

Sacco R.L., Benson R.T., Kargman D.E. *et al.* (2001). High-density lipoprotein cholesterol and ischemic stroke in the elderly: the Northern Manhattan Stroke Study. *Journal of the American Medical Association*, **285**, 2729.

Sacco R.L. and Boden-Albala B. (2001). Stroke Risk Factors. In M. Fisher (ed). *Stroke Therapy*. Boston Butterworth-Heinemann, 1–23.

Sacco R.L., Elkind M., Boden-Albala B. *et al.* (1999). The protective effect of moderate alcohol consumption on ischemic stroke. *Journal of the American Medical Association*, **281**, 53.

Sacks F.M., Pfeffer M.A., Moye L.A. *et al.* (1996). The effect of pravastatin on coronary events after myocardial infarction in patients with average cholesterol levels. Cholesterol and Recurrent Events Trial Investigators. *New England Journal of Medicine*, **335**, 1001–9.

Salonen R., Seppanen K., Rauramaa R. *et al.* (1988). Prevalence of carotid atherosclerosis and serum cholesterol levels in eastern Finland. *Arteriosclerosis* **8**, 788–92.

Samanck M. (1994). Boy:girl ratio in children born with different forms of cardiac malformation: a population-based study. *Pediatric Cardiology*, **15**, 53–7.

Sankai T., Miyagaki T., Iso H. *et al.* (1991). A population-based study of the proportion by type of stroke determined by computed tomography scan. *Nippon Koshu Eisei Zasshi - Japanese Journal of Public Health*, **38**, 901.

Sarti C., Rastenyte D., Cepaitis Z. *et al.* (2000). International trends in mortality from stroke, 1968 to 1994. *Stroke*, **31**, 1588–1601.

Scandinavian Simvastatin Survival Study (1994). Randomized trial of cholesterol lowering in 4444 patients with coronary heart disease: the Scandinavian Simvastatin Survival Study (4S). *Lancet*, **344**, 1383–9.

Senni M., Tribouilloy C.M., Rodeheffer R.J. *et al.* (1998). Congestive heart failure in the community: a study of all incident cases in Olmsted County, Minnesota, in 1991. *Circulation*, **98**, 2282–9.

Shabeter R. (1983). Cardiomyopathy: How far have we come in 25 years? How far yet to go? *Journal of the American College of Cardiology*, **1**, 252–63.

Shekelle R.B., Hulley S.B., Neaton J.D. *et al.* (1985*a*). The MRFIT behavior pattern study. I. Type A behavior and incidence of coronary heart disease. *American Journal of Epidemiology*, **122**, 559–70.

Shekelle R.B., Gale M., and Norusis M. (1985*b*). Type A score (Jenkins Activity Survey) and risk of recurrent coronary heart disease in the Aspirin Myocardial Infarction Study. *American Journal of Cardiology*, **56**, 221–5.

Shekelle R.B., Gale M., Ostfeld A.M. *et al.* (1983). Hostility, risk of coronary heart disease, and mortality. *Psychosomatic Medicine*, **45**, 109–14.

Shepherd J., Cobbe S.M., Ford I. *et al.* for the West of Scotland Coronary Prevention Study Group (1995). Prevention of coronary heart disease with pravastatin in me with hypercholesterolemia. *New England Journal of Medicine*, **333**, 1301–7.

Siegel A.C., Johnson E.E., and Stollerman G.H. (1961). Controlled studies of streptococcal pharyngitis in a pediatric population: 1. factors related to the attack rate of rheumatic fever. *New England Journal of Medicine*, **265**, 559–66.

Sjostrom L.V. (1992). Mortality of severely obese subjects. *American Journal of Clinical Nutrition*, **55**, 516S–23S.

Solomon C.G. and Manson J.E. (1997). Obesity and mortality: a review of the epidemiologic data. *American Journal of Clinical Nutrition*, **66**, 1044S–50S.

Sowers J.R., Sowers P.S. and Peuler J.D. (1994). Role of insulin resistance and hyperinsulinemia in development of hypertension and atherosclerosis. *Journal of Laboratory and Clinical Medicine*, **123**, 647–52.

Staessen J.A., Birkenhager W.H. and Fagard R. (1997). Implications of the Systolic Hypertension in Europe (Syst-Eur) Trial for clinical practice. *Nephrology Dialysis Transplantation*, **12**, 2220.

Stamler J., Vaccaro O., Neaton J.D. *et al.* (1993). Diabetes, other risk factors, and 12-year cardiovascular mortality for men screened in the Multiple Risk Factor Intervention Trial. *Diabetes Care*, **16**, 434–44.

Stampfer M.J. and Rimm E.B. (1995). Epidemiologic evidence for vitamin E in prevention of cardiovascular disease. *American Journal of Clinical Nutrition*, **62**, 1365S–9S.

Steenland K., Thun M., Lally C. *et al.* (1996). Environmental tobacco smoke and coronary heart disease in the American Cancer Society CPS-II cohort. *Circulation*, **94**, 622–8.

Tanaka H., Ueda Y., and Hayashi M. (1982). Risk factors for cerebral hemorrhage and cerebral infarction in a Japanese rural community. *Stroke*, **13**, 62.

Toole J.F., Malinow M.R., Chambless L.E. *et al.* (2004). Lowering homocysteine in patients with ischemic stroke to prevent recurrent stroke, myocardial infarction, and death: the Vitamin Intervention for Stroke Prevention (VISP) randomized controlled trial. *Journal of the American Medical Association*, **291**, 565–75.

Trials of Hypertension Prevention Collaborative Research Group (1997). Effects of weight loss and sodium reduction intervention on blood pressure and hypertension incidence in overweight people with high normal blood pressure: the Trials of Hypertension Prevention, phase II. *Archives of Internal Medicine*, **157**, 657–67.

Tunstall-Pedoe H., Kuulasmaa K., Mahonen M. *et al.* (1999). Contribution of trends in survival and coronary-event rates to changes in coronary heart disease mortality: 10-year results from 37 WHO MONICA project populations: monitoring trends and determinants in cardiovascular disease. *Lancet*, **353**, 1547–57.

Tunstall-Pedoe H., Morrison C., Woodward M. *et al.* (1996). Sex differences in myocardial infarction and coronary deaths in the Scottish MONICA population of Glasgow 1985 to 1991: presentation, diagnosis, treatment, and 28-day case fatality of 3991 events in men and 1551 events in women. *Circulation*, **93**, 1981–92.

UGDP (University Group Diabetes Program) (1975). A study of the effects of hypoglycemic agents on vascular complications in patients with adult onset diabetes. V. Evaluation of phenoformin therapy. *Diabetes*, **24**, 65–184.

UKPDS (United Kingdom Prospective Diabetes Study) Group (1995). UKPDS 13: relative efficacy of randomly allocated diet, sulphonylurea, insulin, or metformin in patients with newly diagnosed non-insulin dependent diabetes followed for three years. *British Medical Journal*, **310**, 83–8.

UK Prospective Diabetes Study Group (1998). Tight blood pressure control and risk of macrovascular and microvascular complications in type 2 diabetes: UKPDS 38. *British Medical Journal*, **317**, 703.

USDHHS (United States Department of Health and Human Services) (1990). *The health benefits of smoking cessation: a report of the Surgeon General*. DHHS Publication No. CDC-90-8416. USDHHS, Centers for Disease Control, Center for Chronic Disease Prevention and Health Promotion, Office on Smoking and Health, Washington, DC.

USDHHS (United States Department of Health and Human Services) (1997). *Changes in cigarette-related disease risks and their implication for prevention and control*. NIH Publication No. 97–4213. Monograph 8. USDHHS, Public Health Services, National Institutes of Health, National Cancer Institute, Washington, DC.

USDHHS (United States Department of Health and Human Services) (1998*a*). *Targeting tobacco use: the nation's leading cause of death: at-a-glance*. Centers for Disease Control and Prevention, Washington, DC.

USDHHS (United States Department of Health and Human Services) (1998*b*). *Clinical guidelines on the identification, evaluation, and treatment of overweight and obesity in adults: the evidence report*. USDHHS, Public Health Service, National Institutes of Health, National Heart, Lung, and Blood Institute, Washington, DC.

USDHHS (United States Department of Health and Human Services). National Heart, Lung, and Blood Institute. National High Blood Pressure Education Program (2003). Available at: http://www.nhlbi.nih.gov/about/nhbpep/index.htm. Accessed March 5, 2003.

Vora A. (2006). Management of atrial fibrillation in rheumatic valvular heart disease. *Current Opinion in Cardiology*, **21**, 47.

Wannamaker L.W. (1973). The chain that links the heart to the throat. *Circulation*, **48**, 9–18.

WHO (World Health Organization) (1988). *Cardiomyopathies*.Technical Report Series No. 764. Report of a WHO Expert Committee. WHO, Geneva.

WHO (World Health Organization) (2004). *Rheumatic fever and rheumatic heart disease*. Technical Report Series No. 923. WHO, Geneva.

WHO (World Health Organization) (2003). *MONICA Monograph Multimedia Sourcebook*. Tunstall-Pedoe H (ed). Geneva, Switzerland.

WHO/Europe, European mortality database (MDB), June 2007.

Wigle E.D. (1988). Hypertrophic cardiomyopathy 1988. *Modern Concepts in Cardiovascular Disease*, **57**, 1–6.

Willich S.N., Maclure M., Mittleman M. *et al.* (1993). Sudden cardiac death. Support for a role of triggering in causation. *Circulation*, **87**, 1442–50.

Wolf P.A. and D'Agostino R.B. (1998). Epidemiology of stroke. In Barnett H.J.M., Mohr J.P., Stein B.M., Yatso F.M. (eds). *Stroke - pathophysiology, diagnosis and management*. New York: Churchill-Livingstone, 3–28.

Wolf P.A., D'Agostino R.B., Belanger A.J. *et al.* (1991). Probability of stroke: a risk profile from the Framingham Study. *Stroke*, **22**, 312.

Wood D., De Backer G., Faergeman O. *et al.* (1998). Prevention of coronary heart disease in clinical practice. *European Heart Journal*, **19**, 1434–1503.

Zhang L.F., Yang J., Hong Z. *et al.* for the Collaborative Group of China Multicenter Study of Cardiovascular E (2003). Proportion of different subtypes of stroke in China. *Stroke*, **34**, 2091.

Zierler S. (1985). Maternal drugs and congenital heart disease. *Obstetrics and Gynecology*, **65**, 155–65.

9.3

Neoplasms

Paolo Boffetta and Carlo La Vecchia

Abstract

Neoplasms are a group of diverse diseases with complex distributions in human populations and with different aetiological factors. Current knowledge of the causes of human neoplasms and the development of control strategies have led to the elaboration of lists of recommendations for their prevention. A comprehensive strategy for cancer control might lead to the avoidance of a sizeable proportion of human cancers, and the greatest benefit can be achieved via tobacco control.

Nevertheless, neoplasms will continue to be a major source of human disease and death. Considerable efforts are made in the public and private domains to develop effective therapeutic approaches. Even if major discoveries in the clinical management of cancer patients will be accomplished in the near future, the changes will mainly affect the affluent part of the world population. Prevention of the known causes of cancer remains the most promising approach in reducing the consequences of cancer, in particular in countries with limited resources. Control of tobacco smoking and of smokeless tobacco products, reduced overweight and obesity, moderation in alcohol intake, increased physical activity, avoidance of exposure to solar radiation and control of known occupational carcinogens are the main approaches we currently have to reduce the burden of human neoplasms.

Introduction

Neoplasms include a family of diseases, several hundreds of which can be distinguished in humans by localization, morphology, clinical behaviour, and response to therapy. Whether considered from a biological, clinical or public health viewpoint, it is the invasive nature of many of these diseases which is of dominant importance.

Benign neoplasms represent localized growths of tissue with predominantly normal characteristics: In many cases they cause minor symptoms and are amenable to surgical therapy. Benign tumours, however, can become clinically very important when they occur in organs in which compression is possible and surgery cannot be easily performed (e.g. the brain), and when they produce hormones or other substances with a systemic effect (e.g. epinephrine produced by benign pheochromocytoma). Relatively little is known about the distribution and causes of most benign neoplasms and, with the exception of benign brain neoplasms, they will not be further discussed in this chapter.

Malignant neoplasms are characterized by progressive growth of tissue with structural and functional alterations with respect to the normal tissue. In some cases, the alterations can be so important that it becomes difficult to identify the tissue of origin. A peculiarity of most malignant tumours is the ability to migrate and colonize other organs (metastatization) via blood and lymph vessel penetration. The presence and extension of metastases are often the critical factors to determine the success of therapy and the survival of cancer patients.

The pace of growth of malignant neoplasms varies widely, and asymptomatic neoplasms are often found at autopsy of individuals deceased from other causes. The long process of carcinogenesis justifies the efforts to develop and apply screening approaches for early detection of selected subclinical neoplasms in healthy individuals.

At the molecular level, the process of malignant transformation is characterized by alterations in several genes that are responsible for the control of the replication cycle of the cell and other regulatory functions. Many cancer-related genes have been identified, and the distribution of their alterations varies among different neoplasms. However, neoplasms which are morphologically and clinically identical often include different genetic alterations, showing that the malignant transformation may result from the accumulation of genetic damage through different pathways.

Most malignant neoplasms in adults arise from epithelial tissues and are defined as carcinomas. In practice, however, the terms 'malignant neoplasm', 'malignant tumour' and 'cancer' are used interchangeably. Neoplasms are classified according to the International Classification of Diseases—Oncology (WHO 1990) into topographical categories (according to the organ where the neoplasm arises) and morphological categories (according to the characteristics of the cells). More and more often, neoplasms are characterized at the clinical level according to phenotypic aspects (e.g. presence of receptors, expression of genes) and genetic alterations (e.g. mutation in a given gene).

The identification of the determinants of cancer relies on two complementary approaches, the epidemiological and the experimental. The epidemiological approach has produced both general and specific evidence for the role of different types of agents in

Table 9.3.1 Ratio of the 20th and 80th percentile in the ranking of country-specific estimated age-standardized incidence rates of selected cancers (Globocan 2002)

Cancer	Men	Women
Oral cavity	3.5	2.7
Nasopharynx	5.5	5.1
Oesophagus	4.4	7.3
Stomach	3.9	3.1
Colon-rectum	6.1	6.0
Liver	5.1	4.2
Pancreas	5.5	4.2
Lung	9.3	6.4
Melanoma	8.5	9.0
Breast	–	2.8
Cervix	–	3.5
Corpus uteri	–	4.8
Ovary	–	2.3
Prostate	5.8	–
Bladder	4.2	3.4
Kidney	6.6	4.8
Nervous system	6.0	4.4
Non-Hodgkin's lymphoma	2.1	1.8
Leukaemia	2.8	2.4

cancer causation. The evidence of a more general nature derives from the observations of considerable variation of the incidence rates of most cancers in different populations, defined according to geographical area. Table 9.3.1 reports the ratio of the 80th to the 20th percentile of the ranking of country-specific incidence rates of selected cancers, as estimated in the Globocan 2002 project (Ferlay *et al.* 2004). For all gender-specific rates but one, the ratio is above 2, and for several neoplasms it is close to 10. This comparison is based on stable figures, but masks ever larger variations among very-high-risk and very-low-risk areas, which for many neoplasms may reach 100- or even 1000-fold differences. Variations are also shown within countries or according to other characteristics such as ethnic group, religion, social class. For instance, when contrasted with other religious groups, the Mormons of Utah and the Seventh-Day Adventists of California exhibit low rates for cancers of the respiratory, gastrointestinal, and genital systems. This marked variation in rates according to different axes of exploration is unlikely to be explained chiefly by concomitant genetic variations, and points to the role of lifestyle determinants.

Finally, changes in incidence rates in time, particularly when they take place over a few decades, are incompatible with a genetic explanation, as changes in the genes of a population pool require longer intervals. Recorded incidence rates are affected by diagnostic changes and mortality rates are, in addition, affected by changes in treatment effectiveness; however, marked trends like the one for lung cancer (Fig. 9.3.1) are most likely to reflect real changes in cancer rates, pointing to the importance of non-genetic factors.

Genetic determinants of cancer have also been demonstrated. Several inherited conditions carry a very high risk of one or several cancers. High-penetrance genes are identified through family-based and other linkage studies. These conditions, however, are rare and explain only a small proportion of human cancers. Genetic factors, however, are likely to play an important role in interacting with non-genetic factors to determine individual cancer risk.

The understanding of the molecular and cellular mechanisms of carcinogenesis has greatly advanced in recent years. According to a widely accepted model, cells have to acquire six characteristics to become fully malignant (Hanahan *et al.* 2000). These include the ability to produce growth signals (several known oncogenes mimic growth signalling), the lack of sensitivity to antigrowth signals [the Retinoblastoma (RB) protein and its homologues play a key role in the ability of the cell to decide whether to proliferate, to be quiescent, or to enter into a postmitotic state, based on external signalling], resistance towards programmed cell death or apoptosis (in many cases via inactivation of the p53 protein), immortalization (normal cells have a limited replication potential, that is related to the length of the telomeres: In malignant cells overexpression of telomerases circumvents it), stimulation of blood vessel production (by changing the balance of angiogenesis inducers and countervailing inhibitors) and ability to invade and metastasize. The acquisition of these neoplastic characteristics typically occurs by alterations of relevant genes, but an inability to maintain genomic integrity (so-called genomic instability, which includes reduced ability to repair DNA damage) is an additional feature of malignant cells, as accumulation of random mutations in genes involved in all the functions mentioned above would be a too rare event for the development of cancer during the normal lifespan. A final point to consider is the heterogeneity of neoplastic genetic alterations: The acquisition of the different biological capabilities of the neoplastic cell can appear at different times, and the particular sequence in which capabilities are acquired can vary widely, even among the same type of tumours.

The identification of carcinogens via the laboratory relies on three types of tests: (i) long-term (often lifetime) carcinogenicity tests in experimental animals, most commonly rodents (mice, rats, hamsters), (ii) short-term tests assessing the effect of chemical agents on a variety of endpoints belonging to three general classes: DNA damage, mutagenicity and chromosome damage, and (iii) mechanistic test, aimed at identifying the intermediate steps in the compound-specific carcinogenic process.

These tests are valuable to the extent that such effects may reflect underlying events in the carcinogenic process. Indeed, consistent positivity in tests measuring DNA damage, mutagenicity and chromosomal damage is usually regarded as indicating potential carcinogenicity of the tested agent. Results of laboratory tests constitute useful supporting evidence when adequate epidemiological data for the carcinogenicity of an environmental agent exist (for example, vinyl chloride), but they become all the more essential when the epidemiological evidence is non-existent or inadequate in quality or in quantity. In the latter case, although no universally accepted criteria exist to automatically translate data from long-term animal tests or short-term tests in terms of cancer risk in humans, an evaluation of the risk can be made on a judgmental basis using all available scientific evidence. This policy has been applied by the International Agency for Research on Cancer (IARC) in a systematic programme of evaluation of the carcinogenic risk of chemicals to man. Within this programme of IARC Monographs, agents are classified in group 1

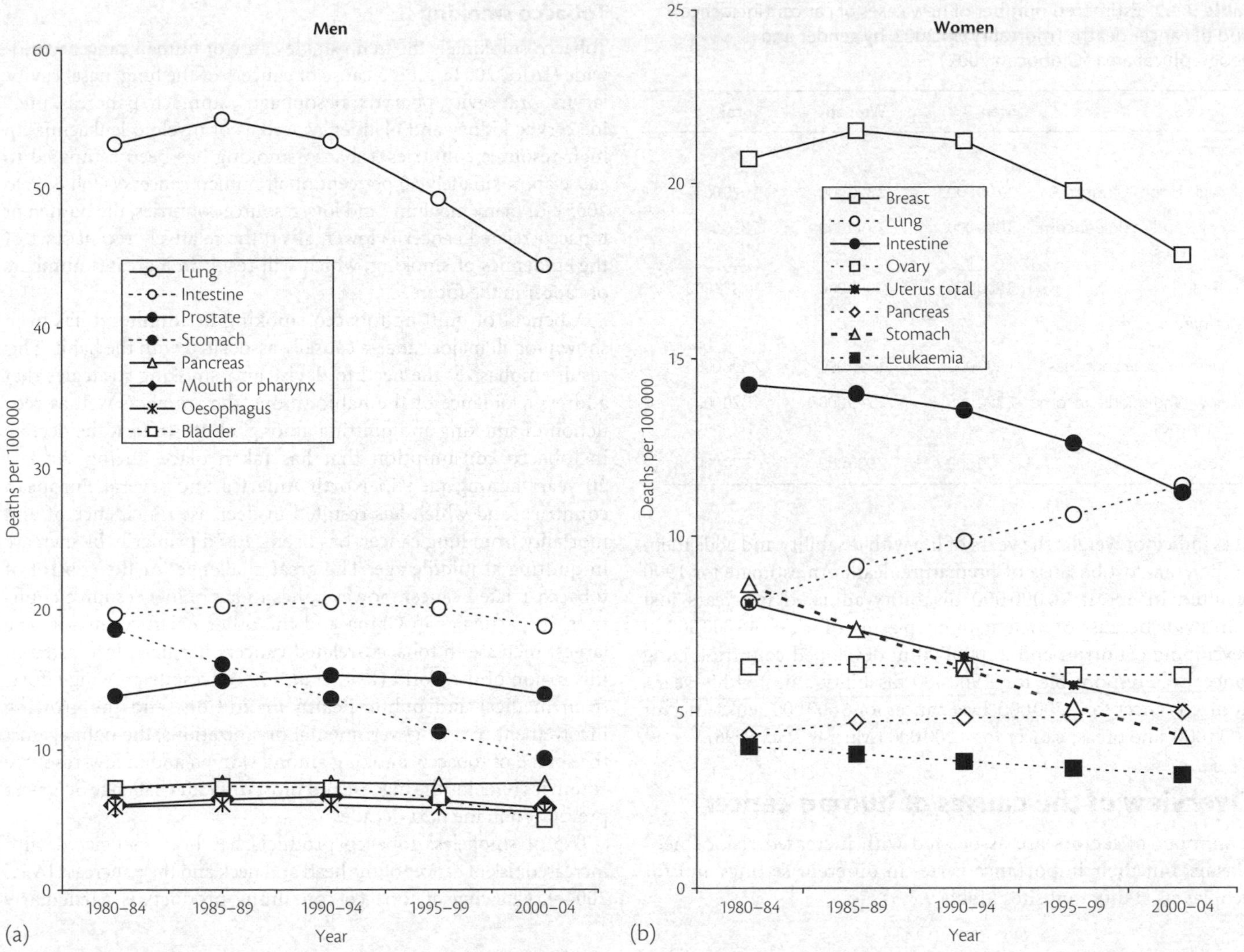

Fig. 9.3.1 Trends in mortality from major cancers in the European Union, 1980–2002. *Source:* Levi et al. (2004a).

(established human carcinogen), 2A (probable human carcinogens), 2B (possible human carcinogens) and 3 (not classifiable as to carcinogenicity to humans) (http://monographs.iarc.fr/index.php). Agents are commonly classified in group 1 when the evidence of their carcinogenicity in humans, derived from epidemiological studies, is considered sufficient, and are classified in group 2A when the evidence in humans is limited and the agent is an experimental carcinogen. Agents in group 2B include mainly experimental carcinogens for which the human evidence is inadequate or non-existent. Between 1972 and 2006, 96 volumes presenting evaluations (and re-evaluations) for 932 chemical, physical and biological agents and groups of agents, as well as exposure circumstances such as occupations, have been published. A total of 101 agents have been classified in group 1, 69 in group 2A, and 245 in group 2B. The complete list of agents, with their evaluations can be found on the Monographs web site.

The global burden of neoplasms

The number of new cases of cancer which occurred worldwide in 2002 has been estimated at about 10 860 000 (Table 9.3.2) (Ferlay *et al.* 2004). Of these, 5 800 000 occurred in men and 5 060 000 in women. About 5 020 000 cases occurred in high-resource countries (North America, Japan, Europe including Russia, Australia, and New Zealand) and 5 830 000 in low- and medium-resource countries. Among men, lung, stomach, colorectal, prostate, and liver cancers are the most common malignant neoplasms (Fig. 9.3.2), while breast, colorectal, cervical, lung, and ovarian cancers are the most common neoplasms among women (Fig. 9.3.3).

The number of deaths from cancer was estimated at about 6 720 000 in 2002 (Table 9.3.2) (Ferlay *et al.* 2004). No global estimates of survival from cancer are available: Data from selected cancer registries suggest wide disparities between high- and low-resource countries for neoplasms with effective but expensive treatment, such as leukaemia, while the gap is narrow for neoplasms without an effective therapy, such as lung cancer (Berrino *et al.* 1999; Kosary *et al.* 1995; Sankaranarayanan *et al.* 1998) (Fig. 9.3.4). The overall 5-year survival of cases diagnosed during 1985–1989 in European Union countries was 41 per cent (Berrino *et al.* 1999).

One complementary approach in assessing the global burden of neoplasms is to estimate the loss in disability-adjusted life-years.

Table 9.3.2 Estimated number of new cases of cancer (incidence) and of cancer deaths (mortality) in 2002, by gender and geographical area (Globocan 2002)

	Men	Women	Total
Incidence			
High-income countries	2 700 000	2 320 000	5 020 000
Low- and middle-income countries	3 090 000	2 740 000	5 830 000
Total	5 800 000	5 060 000	10 860 000
Mortality			
High-income countries	1 500 000	1 190 000	2 690 000
Low- and middle-income countries	2 280 000	1 740 000	4 020 000
Total	3 790 000	2 930 000	6 720 000

This indicator weighs the years of life with disability and adds them to the years lost because of premature death. An estimate for 1990 resulted in about 70 000 000 disability-adjusted life-years lost worldwide because of malignant neoplasms, of which 48 000 000 in developing countries and 22 000 000 in developed countries. Lung cancer was responsible for 8 900 000 disability-adjusted life-years, stomach cancer for 7 700 000, liver cancer for 6 600 000, leukaemia for 4 600 000, and breast cancer for 4 200 000 (Murray *et al.* 1996).

Overview of the causes of human cancer

A number of factors are associated with increased risk of neoplasms, but their importance varies in different settings and for neoplasms at different sites (Table 9.3.3).

Tobacco smoking

Tobacco smoking is the main single cause of human cancer worldwide (IARC 2004a). It is a cause of cancers of the lung, nasal cavity, larynx, oral cavity, pharynx, oesophagus, stomach, pancreas, uterine cervix, kidney and bladder, as well as of myeloid leukaemia. In high-resource countries, tobacco smoking has been estimated to cause approximately 30 per cent of all human cancers (Doll & Peto 2005). In many medium- and low-resource countries, the burden of tobacco-related cancer is lower, given the relatively recent start of the epidemics of smoking, which will result in a greater numbers of cancer in the future.

A benefit of quitting tobacco smoking in adulthood has been shown for all major cancers causally associated with the habit. This result emphasizes the need to devise anti-smoking strategies that address avoidance of the habit among the young as well as reduction of smoking and quitting among adults. In fact, the decline in tobacco consumption that has taken place during the last 20 years among men in North America and several European countries, and which has resulted in decreased incidence of and mortality from lung cancer, has been caused primarily by increase in quitting at middle age. The great challenge for the control of tobacco-related cancer, however, lies today in low-resource countries, in particular in China and the other Asian countries: The largest increase in tobacco-related cancers has been forecasted in this region of the world (Peto *et al.* 1999). Despite growing efforts from medical and public health institutions and the growing involvement of non-governmental organizations, the fight against the spread of tobacco smoking among women and in low-resource countries remains the biggest and most difficult challenge of cancer prevention in the next decades.

Use of smokeless tobacco products has been associated with increased risk of cancer of the head and neck and the pancreas (IARC 2004c). Chewing of tobacco-containing products is particularly

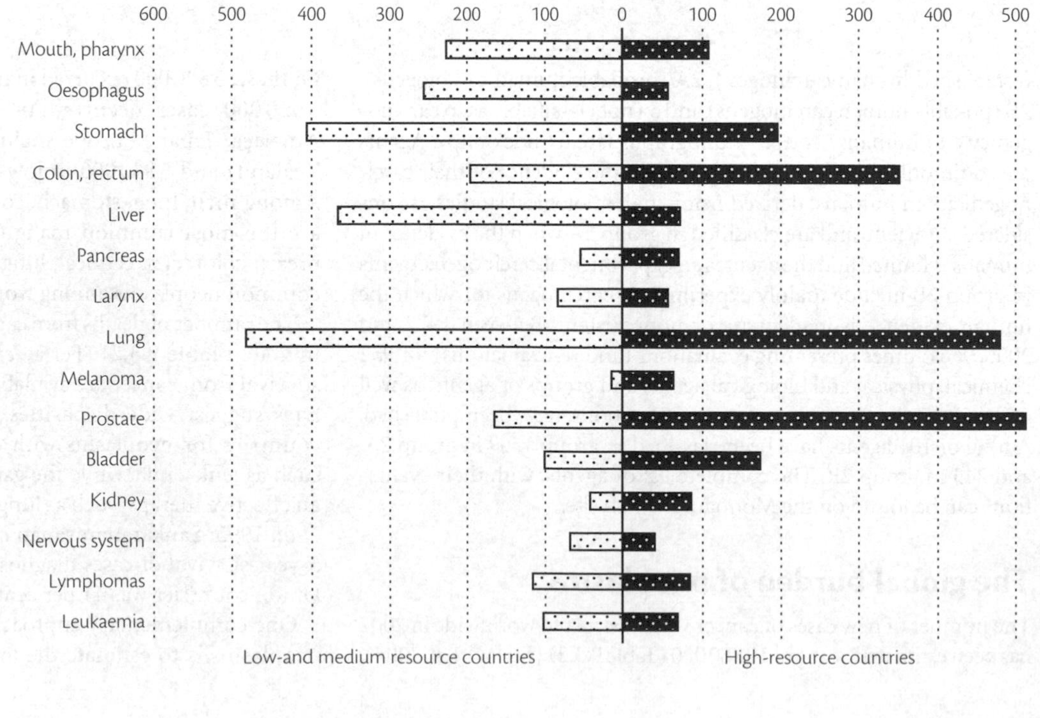

Fig. 9.3.2 Estimated number of new cancer cases (x1000), 2002. Men.

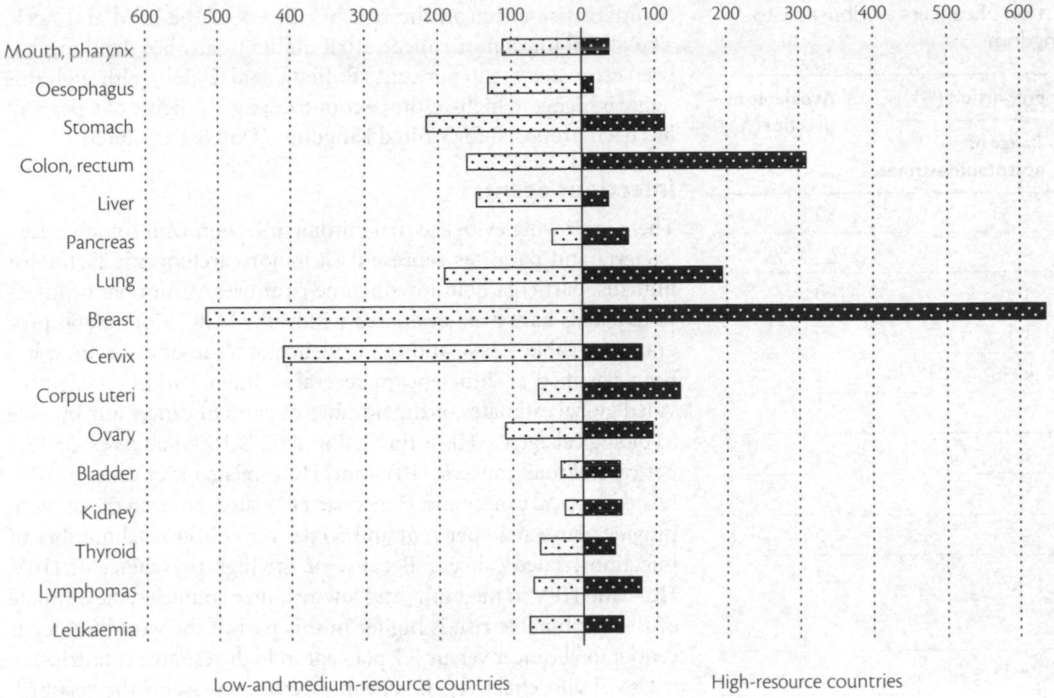

Fig. 9.3.3 Estimated number of new cancer cases (x1000), 2002. Women.

prevalent in Southern Asia, where it represents a major cause of oral and pharyngeal cancer.

Dietary factors

Despite considerable research efforts in recent years, the exact role of dietary factors in causing human cancer remains largely obscure. For no dietary factor other than alcohol and aflatoxin (a carcinogen produced by some fungi in certain tropical areas) there is sufficient evidence of an increased or decreased risk of cancer. In particular, a role of intake of fat or other nutrients in determining breast and colorectal cancer risk has not been confirmed by recent studies (Marques-Vidal *et al.* 2006; Michels *et al.* 2007). There is limited evidence for a protective role of vegetable and fruit intake for cancers of the mouth and pharynx, oesophagus, stomach, colorectum, larynx, lung, ovary (vegetables only), bladder (fruit only), and bladder (IARC 2003), and there is evidence suggestive lack of cancer-preventive activity for preformed vitamin A (IARC 1998b) and for β-carotene when used at high doses (IARC 1998a). Systematic reviews have concluded that nutritional factors may be responsible for about one fourth of human cancers in high-resource countries, although,

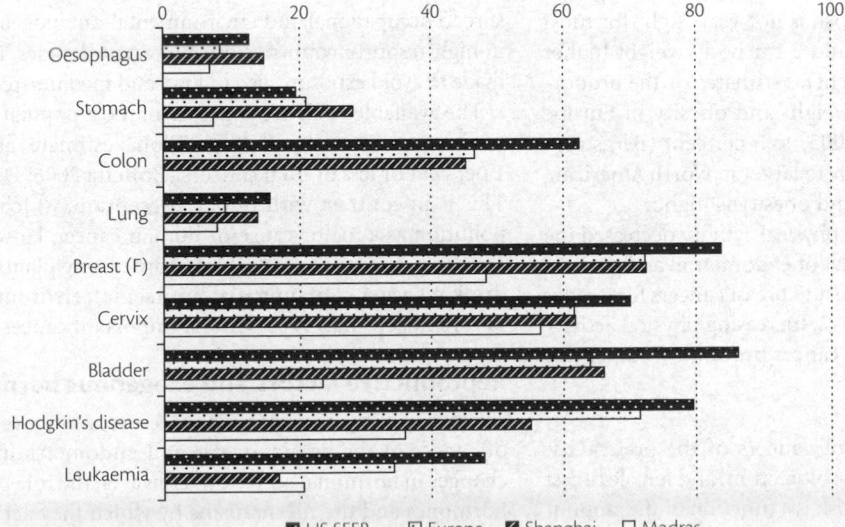

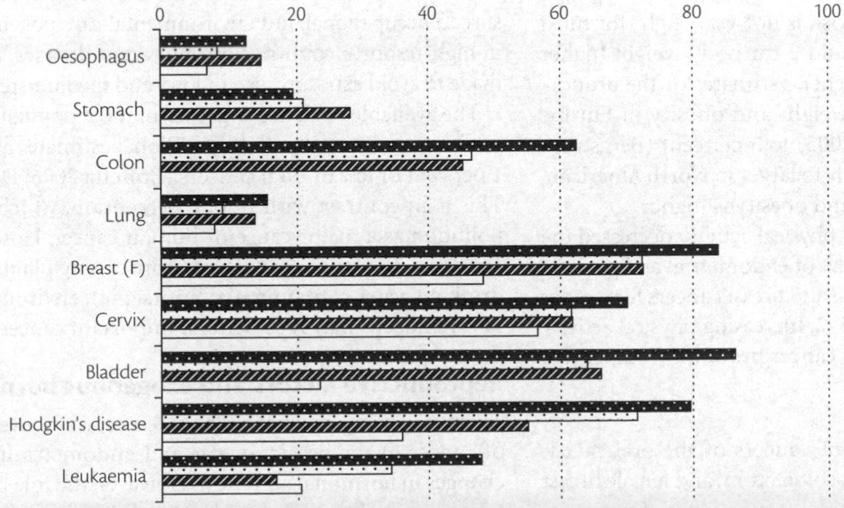

Fig. 9.3.4 Five-year relative survival from cancer in selected populations.

Table 9.3.3 Estimate of the proportion of cancers attributable to major risk factors in the United Kingdom

Risk factor	Attributable proportion (%)		Avoidable in practice (%)
	Best estimate	Range of acceptable estimates	
Tobacco smoking	30	27–33	30
Alcohol drinking	6	4–8	6*
Ionizing radiation	5	4–6	<1
Ultraviolet light	1	1	<1
Infections	5	4–15	1
Medical drugs	<1	0–1	<1
Occupation	2	1–5	<1
Pollution	2	1–5	<1
Diet and obesity	25	15–35	2
Reproduction and other hormonal factors	15	10–20	<1
Physical inactivity	<1	0–1	<1

* Total avoidance of alcohol would increase overall mortality as the increase in cardiovascular mortality would exceed the reduction in cancer mortality.
Source: Doll & Peto (2005).

because of the limitations of the current understanding of the precise role of diet in human cancer, the proportion of cancers known to be avoidable in practicable ways is much smaller (Doll & Peto 2005). The only justified dietary recommendation for cancer prevention is to reduce total caloric intake, which would contribute to a decrease in obesity, an established risk factor for human cancer.

Obesity and physical exercise

There is sufficient evidence for a cancer preventive effect of avoidance of weight gain, based on a decreased risk of cancers of the colon, gall-bladder, post-menopausal breast, endometrium, kidney, and oesophagus (adenocarcinoma) (IARC 2002b). It is likely that obesity exerts a carcinogenic effect in conjunction with other factors such as insulin resistance, low physical activity and menopausal status. The magnitude of the excess risk is not very high (for most cancers the RR ranges between 1.5 and 2 for body weight higher than 35 per cent above the ideal weight). Estimates of the proportion of cancers attributable to overweight and obesity in Europe range from 2 per cent (Doll & Peto 2005) to 5 per cent (Bergstrom *et al.* 2001). However, this figure is likely to larger in North American, where the prevalence of overweight and obesity is higher.

Increased workplace or recreational physical activity decreased the risk of colon and breast cancers and that of endometrial and prostate cancers (IARC 2002b). The RR of colon and breast cancers for regular versus no activity is in the order of 1.5–2. Increasing physical activity should be part of any comprehensive cancer prevention strategy.

Alcohol drinking

Alcohol drinking increases the risk of cancers of the oral cavity, pharynx, larynx, oesophagus and liver, colorectum, and female breast (Baan *et al.* 2007). For all cancer sites, risk is a function of the amount of alcohol consumed. Alcohol drinking and tobacco smoking show an interactive effect on the risk of cancers of the head and neck. The global burden of cancer attributable to alcohol drinking has been estimated at 3.6 per cent (Boffetta *et al.* 2006b), although this figure is higher in high-resource countries; e.g. the figure of 6 per cent has been proposed for United Kingdom (Doll & Peto 2005).

Infectious agents

There is growing evidence that chronic infection with some viruses, bacteria and parasites represents a major carcinogenic factor for humans, particularly in low-income countries. A number of infectious agents have been evaluated within the IARC Monograph programme (Table 9.3.4), and the evidence of a causal association has been classified as sufficient for several of them. Parkin (2006) provided global estimates of the number of cases of cancer attributable to biological agents. His estimate for 2002 is 1 900 000 cases, or 17.8 per cent of total cancers. HBV- and HCV-related liver cancer, HPV-related cervical cancer and Helicobacter-related stomach cancer each provide between 20 per cent and 30 per cent of the total number of infection-related cancers. Because of the high prevalence of HBV, HCV and HPV in medium- and low-resource countries, the estimate of the attributable risk is higher in this part of the world (26.3 per cent of total cancer versus 7.7 per cent in high-resource countries).

Use of safe, effective, and cheap vaccines represents the best preventive strategy for cancers caused by viruses, and HBV and HPV infection can be effectively prevented today. Chronic infection with *Helicobacter pylori* can be prevented by eradication treatment and sanitation measures, and changes in dietary practices (e.g. avoidance of raw fish) can prevent infection by carcinogenic parasites.

Occupation and pollution

Approximately 40 occupational agents, groups of agents and mixtures have been classified as carcinogenic by IARC (Table 9.3.5). While some (e.g. *bis*-chloro methylethers) represent today a historic curiosity, exposure is still widespread for carcinogens such as asbestos, arsenic, and silica. Estimates of the global burden of cancer attributable to occupation in high-resource countries result in figures in the order of 2–3 per cent (Doll & Peto 2005; Steenland *et al.* 2003). However, these cancers concentrate in some sectors of the population (mainly male blue-collar workers), among whom they may represent a sizable proportion of total cancers. Furthermore, unlike lifestyle factors, exposure is involuntary. In fact, reduction of exposure to occupational and environmental carcinogens has taken place in high-resource countries during recent decades. Efforts should be made to avoid exposure also in low- and medium-resource countries.

The available evidence suggests, in most populations, a small role of air, water and soil pollutants. Global estimates are in the order of 1 per cent or less of total cancers (Boffetta 2006; Doll & Peto 2005). This is in contrast with public perception, which often identifies pollution as a major cause of human cancer. However, in selected areas (e.g. residence near asbestos processing plants or in areas with drinking water contaminated by arsenic), environmental exposure to carcinogens may represent an important cancer hazard.

Reproductive factors and exogenous hormones

There is a strong association between reproductive history and risk of cancer of the breast, ovary, and endometrium, which reflects changes in hormonal secretion. However, the role played by specific hormones and the mechanisms by which they act are still unclear. The reproductive factors with the strongest effect on breast cancer

Table 9.3.4 Assessment of associations between infections and human cancer, from IARC 1994a (Monographs Vol. 59), 1994b (Vol. 61), 1996 (Vol. 67), 1997b (Vol. 70), and in press (Vol. 90)

	Evidence[a]	Target organs[b]	IARC Monographs Vol.
Viruses			
Hepatitis B virus	S	Liver	59
Hepatitis C virus	S	Liver	59
Hepatitis D virus	I	Liver	59
Human papilloma virus type 16	S	Cervix, vulva, vagina, penis, anus, oral cavity, oropharynx	90
Human papillomavirus types 18, 31, 33, 35, 39, 45, 51, 52, 56, 58, 59, 66	S	Cervix	90
Human papilloma virus types 6, 11	L	(Larynx, vulva, penis, anus)	90
Human papilloma virus, genus-beta types	L	(Skin)	90
Human immunodeficiency virus 1	S	Kaposi's sarcoma, non-Hodgkin's lymphoma	67
Human immunodeficiency virus 2	I		67
Human T-cell lymphotrophic virus I	S	Adult T-cell leukaemia/ lymphoma	67
Human T-cell lymphotrophic virus II	I		67
Epstein–Barr virus	S	Burkitt's lymphoma, Hodgkin's disease, nasopharynx	70
Human herpes virus 8	L	(Kaposi's sarcoma)	70
Bacterium			
Helicobacter pylori	S	Stomach	61
Parasites			
Schistosoma haematobium	S	Bladder	61
Schistosoma japonicum	L	(Liver, stomach)	61
Schistosoma mansoni	I		61
Opistorchis viverrini	S	Liver	61
Opistorchis felineus	I		61
Clonorchis sinensis	L	Liver	61

[a] I, inadequate; L, limited; S, sufficient.
[b] Established target organs without brackets; suspected target organs in brackets.

risk are parity and age at first full-term pregnancy. Nulliparity or low parity is also related to increased risk of endometrial and ovarian cancer. In contrast, high parity is associated to an increased risk of cervical cancer. Oestrogenic stimulation is probably a major cause of breast cancer, as shown by the strong reduction in breast cancer risk among women enrolled in randomized trials of tamoxifen, and antioestrogenic drug. Exogenous oestrogens and progestins given in combination as hormone replacement therapy (HRT) in menopause and in steroid contraceptives increase the risk of breast and ovarian cancer (IARC 2005b). The risk is present, but considerably smaller, for use of oestrogen-only HRT. In contrast, unopposed oestrogens are strongly related to endometrial cancer. OC exert a consistent and long-term protection against ovarian and endometrial cancer, but current used of OC is associated to an increased risk of cervical and liver cancer (IARC 2005b). No detailed estimates are available of the contribution of reproductive factors to the global burden of cancer, and given the uncertainties in the definition of the relevant circumstances of exposure, proposed figures for high-resource countries range from 3 per cent (Harvard Center for Cancer Prevention 1996) to 15 per cent (Doll *et al.* 2005). An effect of sex hormones on testicular and prostate cancer is plausible, but the epidemiological evidence is currently inadequate to draw any conclusion.

Perinatal and growth factors

Excess energy intake early in life is probably associated with an increased risk breast and colon cancer. The role of attained height, growth factors and other factors such as insulin resistance in this association is unclear. In addition, high birth weight has been associated with an increased risk of breast and prostate cancer. The implications of these findings for preventive strategies will be clarified by a more complete understanding of the underlying carcinogenic mechanisms.

Ionizing and non-ionizing radiation

Ionizing radiation causes several neoplasms, including in particular acute lymphocytic leukaemia, acute and chronic myeloid leukaemia and cancers of the breast, lung, bone, brain and thyroid (IARC 2000). Theoretical considerations and extrapolations from high doses lead to the conclusion that is a threshold below which no excess cancer risk is present is unlikely, although the quantification

Table 9.3.5 Occupational agents, classified by the IARC Monographs programme as carcinogenic to humans (www.monographs.iarc.fr)

Agents, mixture, circumstance	Main industry, use
Agents, groups of agents	
4-Aminobiphenyl	Pigment
Arsenic and arsenic compounds	Glass, metal, pesticide
Asbestos	Insulation, filter, textile
Benzene	Chemical, solvent
Benzidine	Pigment
Benzo[a]pyrene	Combustion processes
Beryllium and beryllium compounds	Aerospace
Bis(chloromethyl)ether and chloromethyl methyl ether	Chemical intermediate
1,3 Butadiene	Chemical
Cadmium and cadmium compounds	Dye/pigment
Chromium[VI] compounds	Metal plating, dye/pigment
Ethylene oxide	Sterilant
Formaldehyde	Chemical
Gallium arsenide	Microelectronics
2-Naphthylamine	Pigment
Nickel compounds	Metallurgy, alloy, catalyst
Radon-222 and its decay products	Mining
Silica, crystalline	Stone cutting, mining, glass, paper
Talc containing asbestiform fibres	Paper, paints
2,3,7,8 Tetrachlorodibenzo-para-dioxin	Chemical
Vinyl chloride	Plastics
X- and γ-radiation	Medical
Mixtures	
Coal-tar pitches	Construction, electrode
Coal-tars	Fuel
Mineral oils, untreated and mildly treated	Metal
Shale oils	Shale oil production
Soot	Pigment
Wood dust	Wood
Exposure circumstances	
Aluminium production	
Auramine, manufacture of	
Boot and shoe manufacture and repair	
Chimney sweeping	
Coal gasification	
Coal-tar distillation	
Coke production	
Furniture and cabinet making	
Haematite mining (underground) with exposure to radon	
Iron and steel founding	
Isopropyl alcohol manufacture (strong-acid process)	
Magenta, manufacture of	
Painter (occupational exposure as a)	
Paving and roofing with coal-tar pitch	
Rubber industry	
Strong-inorganic-acid mists containing sulphuric acid (occupational exposure to)	

of the excess risk at low doses, at which most people are commonly exposed, is difficult. For most individuals, the main exposure is natural radiation, including indoor radon, although artificial sources (e.g. radiotherapy) might be important in particular cases. The estimates of the contribution of ionizing radiation to human cancer in high-resource countries are in the order of 3 per cent (Harvard Center for Cancer Prevention 1996) to 5 per cent (Doll & Peto 2005).

Solar (ultraviolet, UV) radiation is carcinogenic to the skin. Over 90 per cent of skin neoplasms are attributable to sunlight; because of the low fatality of non-melanocytic skin cancer, solar radiation is responsible for only about 1 per cent of total cancer deaths (Doll & Peto 2005). Avoidance of sun exposure, in particular during childhood, is an important cancer preventive behaviour. The evidence of a carcinogenic effect of other types of non-ionizing radiation, in particular electric and magnetic fields, is inconclusive.

However, high rates of cancer motility have been observed in regions with low UV radiation, and among African-Americans. This has been related to anti-cancers effects of vitamin D, which is produced by the skin through solar UV-B radiation exposure. Vitamin D, and in particularly its most active forms 1,25 $(OH)_2D$, has been inversely related to the risk of colorectal, breast and prostate cancers (Giovannucci 2005b; Tuohimaa *et al.* 2007). There are also suggestion that sunlight exposure, and hence vitamin D, may favourably influence cancer prognosis and survival (Lim *et al.* 2006).

Medical procedures and drugs

The drugs that may cause or prevent cancer fall into several groups. Many cancer chemotherapy drugs are active on the DNA, which might also result in damage to normal cells. The main neoplasm associated with chemotherapy treatment is leukaemia, although the risk of solid tumours might also be increased. A second group of carcinogenic drugs includes immunosuppressive agents, notably used in transplanted patients. NHL is the main neoplasm caused by these drugs. The carcinogenic effects of HRT and OC are discussed above. Phenacetin-containing analgesics increase the risk of cancer of the renal pelvis.

No precise estimates are available for the global contribution of drug use to human cancer. It is unlikely, however, that they represent more than 1 per cent in high-resource countries (Doll & Peto 2005). Furthermore, the benefits of therapies are usually much greater than the potential cancer risk.

Use of ionizing radiation for diagnostic purposes is likely to carry a small risk of cancer, which has been demonstrated only for childhood leukaemia following intrauterine exposure. Radiotherapy increases the risk of cancer in the irradiated organs. There is no evidence of an increased cancer risk following other medical procedures, including mammography and surgical implants.

Genetic factors

A number of inherited mutations of a high-penetrance cancer gene increase dramatically the risk of some neoplasms (see sections on specific neoplasms). However, these are rare conditions in most populations and the number of cases attributable to them is rather small.

Familial aggregation has been shown for most types of cancers, in non-carriers of known high-penetrance genes. This is notably the case for cancers of the breast, colon, prostate and lung. The RR is in the order of 2–4, and is higher for cases diagnosed at young age. Although some of the aggregation can be explained by shared risk factors among family members, it is plausible that a true genetic component exists for most human cancers. This takes the forms of an increased susceptibility to endogenous and exogenous carcinogens. The knowledge of low-penetrance genes responsible for such susceptibility is still very limited, although research has currently focused on genes encoding for metabolic enzymes, DNA repair, cell cycle control and hormone receptors. Current estimates of the global contribution of genetic factors to human cancer are in the range of 5–10 per cent, of which less than 1 per cent is attributable to high-penetrance genes.

Principles of cancer prevention

Primary prevention

Many determinants of malignant neoplasms, including UV radiation, ionizing radiation, tobacco smoking, alcohol drinking, a number of viruses and parasites, and a number of chemicals, industrial processes and occupational exposures, are sufficiently well established to constitute logical priorities for preventive action. Two more reasons add weight to this priority: Some of the agents are responsible for sizeable proportions of the cancers occurring today, and for many agents it is in principle feasible to reduce or even to completely eliminate exposure. If this is taken as the objective of preventive action, some practical points are helpful in guiding such action.

First, although epidemiological data in most cases do not allow a direct estimate of the risk of cancer at low doses, it is reasonable (at least from a preventive point of view) to assume that the dose (exposure)–risk relationships for agents acting through damage to DNA is linear with no threshold (Peto *et al.* 1991). Second, the carcinogenic effect is not equally dependent on the dose rate (dose per unit of time) and on duration of exposure. For example, in regular smokers, the incidence rate of lung cancer depends more strongly on duration of exposure, increasing with the fourth power of it, than on dose rate, increasing only with the first or second power of it (Peto 1977).

Furthermore, as illustrated above, the carcinogenic process may be represented as a succession of stages, taking place in the time span from first exposure to a carcinogenic agent to the appearance of clinical cancer. In its simplest form, as first brought out in mouse skin carcinogenesis experiments, the multistage process reduces to two stages: An irreversible 'initiation' stage inducing malignant cells, and a 'promotion' stage which propagates these cells into a malignant growth. A third stage of 'progression', characterized by an increased rate of growth and metastases, as well as an increase in chromosomal changes in the cell, has also been observed. Formal statistical multistage models of carcinogenesis have provided a useful framework to interpret on a common basis of (postulated) mechanism both experimental and epidemiological observations. As the stages are assumed to occur in a specific sequence, some may be described as 'early' and some as 'late'. Epidemiological observations indicate that, for example, smoking has both an early stage effect, as indicated by the existence of a minimum interval of several years before an increase in risk of lung cancer becomes manifest, and a late stage effect, as indicated by the decrease in risk (with respect to continuous smokers) soon after stopping smoking.

The attribution of causality to specific agents (as done when, for instance, smoking is said to be the cause of some 30 per cent of all cancers) is complicated by their interactive effects. This is particularly relevant when considering the relative effectiveness of removing (or reducing) exposure to one of two (or more) jointly-acting agents. Whenever a positive interaction (synergism) occurs between two (or more) hazardous exposures, there is an enlarged possibility of preventive action; the effect of the joint exposure can be attacked in two (or more) ways, each requiring the removal or reduction of one of the exposures; moreover, the larger the size of the interaction relative to the total effect, the more these ways of attack tend to become equal in effectiveness.

Finally, reducing exposure to carcinogens can be implemented in two major ways: By elimination of the carcinogen or its substitution with a non-carcinogen, or by impeding by various means the contact between the carcinogen and people. Reduction of exposure depends in each case on technical and economical considerations.

Cancer prevention strategies have evolved from a predominant environmental and lifestyle approach to a model that matches individual-oriented actions with public health interventions. Advances in identifying, developing and testing agents with the potential either to prevent cancer initiation, or to inhibit or reverse the progression of initiated lesions support this approach. Encouraging laboratory and epidemiologic studies, along with studies of secondary endpoints in prevention trials, have provided a scientific rationale for the hypothesis. Promising results have been reported for various types of cancer, in particular among high-risk individuals (Greenwald 2005).

Secondary prevention

Given the limitations still constraining the primary prevention of many cancers, early detection needs to be considered as a secondary and alternative option, based on the reasonable expectation that the earlier the diagnosis and the stage at which a malignancy is discovered, the better the prognosis. This implies that an effective treatment for the disease exists and that the less advanced the cancer at the pre-clinical stage, the better the scope for treatment, and the better the prognosis. This latter aspect cannot be taken for granted.

Before a screening programme can be adopted on a large scale, a number of other requirements need to be fulfilled. First of all, a screening test (that is, a relatively simple and rapid test aimed at the presumptive identification of pre-clinical disease) must be available that is capable of correctly identifying cases and non-cases. In other words, both sensitivity and specificity should be high, approaching 100 per cent. While high sensitivity is obviously important, given that the very purpose of screening is to pick up, if possible, all cases of a cancer in its detectable pre-clinical phase, it is specificity that plays a dominant role in the practical utilization of the test within a defined population. As the prevalence of a pre-clinical cancer to be screened in well-defined populations is often in the range of 1 to 10 per 1000, if a test is used with a specificity of 95 per cent, then 5 per cent of results will be false-positives. In other words, for every case which will turn out at the diagnostic work-up to be a true cancer (assuming 100 per cent sensitivity), there will be 5–50 cases falsely identified as such and ultimately found not to be cancers. This situation is likely to prove unacceptable due to too high psychological and economical costs. One solution is an increase in specificity, for example by developing better tests or combinations of tests, or by changing the criterion of positivity of a given test to make it more stringent (this necessarily decreases sensitivity). In addition, one might select populations with relatively high prevalence of the cancer ('high-risk' groups), so as to increase the number of the true positives. Whatever the group on which the programme operates, additional requirements are that the test is safe, easily and rapidly applicable, and acceptable in a broad sense to the population to be examined. It has also to be cheap, but what is or is not cheap is better evaluated within a cost-effectiveness analysis of different ways of preventing a cancer case or death, an issue not further discussed here.

If these requirements are met, still nothing is known about the possible net benefit in outcome deriving from the screening programme (in fact, screening test plus diagnostic work-up plus treatment, as applied in a given population). To evaluate benefit, several measures of outcome can be assessed. An early one, useful but not sufficient, is the distribution by stage of the detected cancer cases which, if the programme is ultimately to be beneficial, should be shifted to earlier, less invasive stages of the disease in comparison with the distribution of the cases discovered through ordinary medical care. A second measure of outcome is the survival of cases detected at screening compared with the survival of cases detected through ordinary medical care. This is a superficially attractive but usually equivocal criterion, to the extent that a screening may only advance the time of diagnosis (and therefore the apparent survival time), without postponing the time of death ('lead-time bias'). A final outcome (and the main test of the programme) is the site-specific cancer mortality in the screened population compared with the mortality in the unscreened population.

Correct, unbiased comparison of this outcome, and thus unbiased measure of the effect of the screening programme, should in principle be made within the framework of a randomized controlled trial, in which two groups of subjects are randomly allocated to the screening programme and to no screening (that is, receiving only the existing medical care system) or to two alternative screening programmes, for instance, entailing different tests or different intervals between periodical examinations. Unfortunately, largely due to pressures to adopt a large scale screening programmes hoped to be effective, a situation has often arisen where withholding screening to a group has been regarded as unethical or socially unacceptable, thus preventing the conduct of a proper experiment. Very few randomized trials evaluating the effectiveness of screening programmes are available. Comparisons made through non-randomized experiments or through observational studies.

In addition to lead-time bias, three types of bias are peculiar to the assessment of screening programmes. Because of self-selection, persons who elect to receive early detection may be different from those who do not: For instance, they may belong to better educated classes, be generally healthier and health conscious, and this could produce a longer survival independent of any effect of early detection. In addition, cancers with longer pre-clinical phases, which may mean less biological aggressiveness and better prognosis, are, in any case, more likely to be intercepted by a programme of periodical screening than cancers with a short pre-clinical phase, and a rapid, aggressive clinical course (length bias). Finally, because of criteria of positivity adopted to maximize yield of early cases, a number of lesions which in fact would never become malignant growths are included as 'cases', thus falsely improve the survival statistics (over-diagnosis bias).

Distribution, causes, and prevention of selected neoplasms

This section includes a review of the descriptive epidemiology of the most important malignant neoplasms. It also includes an overview of the current state of knowledge about the risk factors and the strategies for primary and secondary prevention. We chose a global approach, which excludes important local aspects of the descriptive epidemiology, the aetiology and the prevention of neoplasms. All incidence and mortality rates are standardized to the world population. We report estimates for 2002 since more recent data are available only for selected regions and countries.

Cancer of the stomach

Stomach cancer was the fourth most frequent cancer worldwide in 2002, accounting for approximately 930 000 new cases or 8.5 per cent of the global cancer burden (Ferlay *et al.* 2004). High incidence areas, with rates above 25/100 000 in men and 15/100 000 in women, are found in Central and Eastern Europe, Portugal, Eastern Asia and parts of South America. The highest observed rates are found in Japan, with an incidence rate in 1990 of 78/100 000 in men and 33/100 000 in women. Low-incidence areas include Eastern and Northern Africa, North America and South and Southeast Asia (IARC 2002a). The rates are approximately twice as high among men as among women and are also 2–3 times higher among groups of low socioeconomic status.

Migrants tend to maintain the high risk of their home country; their offspring tend to acquire a risk closer to their host country. The most striking feature of the epidemiology of stomach cancer is the dramatic decline in its incidence and mortality which has been observed in most countries over the past century. The decline is apparent for both sexes, and has occurred earlier in countries which currently have a low risk. This continuous dramatic decline, as well as the results from migrant studies, suggests a strong environmental influence on the disease.

The reasons for the generalized decline in gastric cancer rates are complex and not completely understood. Almost certainly, these include a more varied and affluent diet and better food conservation, including refrigeration, as well as the control of *Helicobacter pylori* infection. Whether improved diagnosis and treatment has also played some role on the favourable trends in gastric cancer, particularly over most recent calendar periods, however, remains open to question.

Several intervention trials have also been conducted involving nutrient supplements and stomach cancer. In one of these trials, which was conducted in a Chinese population known to be micronutrient deficient, a combination supplement of β-carotene, vitamin E and selenium did result in a small reduction in the risk of stomach cancer (Blot 1997), but recent findings on the issue on other, better nourished populations, are largely negative (Plummer *et al.* 2007).

Regarding beverages, no evidence has been found that black tea, coffee or alcohol influence the risk of stomach cancer. Throughout the world there is a strong and consistent correlation between consumption of salt and salted foods and stomach cancer incidence. A large number of studies that have examined this relationship have generally found an increased risk of approximately twofold for frequent consumption of salt and salted foods. The relationship is biologically plausible given that salt may lead to damage of the protective mucosal layer of the stomach.

An increased risk of gastric cancer is associated with *H. pylori*. The biological plausibility of a causal association is also supported by a strong association between *H. pylori* and precancerous lesions, including chronic and atrophic gastritis and dysplasia. Given that the prevalence of infection is very high, especially in developing counties and among older cohorts, *H. pylori* can explain over 50 per cent of all new cases of gastric cancer that occur, or over 5 per cent of all cancer cases globally (Parkin 2006). There are, however, still some uncertainties regarding this association. The extent to which different strains of *H. pylori*, for example those containing the *cagA* gene, have different carcinogenic potential is unclear (Kato *et al.* 2007).

Another important cause of stomach cancer is tobacco smoking. Smokers have a 50–60 per cent increased risk of stomach cancer, as compared to non-smokers. This relationship would indicate that smoking is responsible for approximately 10 per cent of all cases (IARC 2004a).

Primary prevention of stomach cancer by dietary means is feasible by encouraging high-risk populations to decrease consumption of cured meats and salt preserved foods. Prevention may also be feasible through eradication of *H. pylori* infection, particularly in childhood and adolescence, by avoiding mother to child transmission. Screening and early detection of stomach cancer have been developed in Japan with use of X-ray photofluorography to identify possible early lesions, followed by gastroscopy.

Colon cancer

Cancer of the intestine is the most frequent human neoplasm in non-smokers of both sexes combined and its rates are high in particular in developed countries. Most cancers of the intestine occur in the large intestines, while cancer of the small intestine is rare. Of colorectal cancers, approximately two-thirds originate from the colon and one third from the rectum and the rectosigmoid junction. Most cancers of the intestine are of adenocarcinoma type, that is, originate from the glandular cells. Other histological types include carcinoids, sarcomas and lymphomas.

When taken together, cancers of the colon and rectum accounted in 2002 for an estimated 1 020 000 new cases and 530 000 deaths worldwide (Ferlay *et al.* 2004). They represent the fourth most frequent malignant disease in terms of incidence and the third for mortality.

The highest rates of colon cancer (around or above 30/100 000 in men and 25/100 000 in women) are recorded in Oceania, the United States (in particular among Blacks) and Western Europe. Rates in developing countries are lower (5–15/100 000) (IARC 2002a). In most populations, rates are higher in men than in women, with a ratio in the order of 1.5; however, given the predominance of women at older ages, the number of cases is similar in the two genders. A small increase in the incidence of colon cancer has been observed during the last decades in most populations, but mortality has been declining in North America and Western Europe over the last two decades (Fernandez *et al.* 2005).

The predominant histological type of malignant neoplasms of the colon is adenocarcinoma. This neoplasm is usually preceded by a polyp, or adenoma, less frequently by a small area of flat mucosa exhibiting various grades of dysplasia. The malignant potential of an adenoma is increased by a surface diameter greater than 1 cm, by villous (rather than tubular) organization and by severe cellular dysplasia. Carriers of one adenoma larger than 1 cm have a 2–4 times increased risk of developing colon cancer; this risk is further doubled in carriers of multiple adenomas. On a geographical basis, the prevalence of adenomas detected during colonoscopy closely parallels the incidence of colon cancer.

Migrant studies suggest that dietary factors are responsible for a substantial proportion of colorectal cancer; however, recent evidence from perspective studies provides only limited evidence in favour of a role of specific foods and nutrients (Marques-Vidal *et al.* 2006). The strongest evidence concerns an increased risk for high intake of meat and of smoked, salted or processed foods. A protective role of high intake of fruits and vegetables has been reported, but is still open to discussion Vitamin D, and in particular its most active form, 25(OH) D has been inversed related to colorectal cancer risk (Giovannucci 2005).

Several studies have associated tobacco smoking with an increased risk of colonic adenoma. For colon cancer, a modest increased risk following prolonged heavy smoking has been shown in some of the largest prospective studies (IARC 2004a).

Increased use of aspirin and other anti-inflammatory drugs is likely to have reduced the incidence of colorectal cancer (Bosetti *et al.* 2006). Hormone therapy in menopause and other female hormones, including OC, have been inversely related to colon cancer risks, and hence may also play some protective role. In addition life-style factors, such as physical activity, and avoidance of overweight and obesity reduce the risk of the disease.

Patients with ulcerative colitis and Crohn's disease are at increased risk of colon cancer. The overall RR has been estimated in the range of 5–20, and it is higher for young age at diagnosis, severity of the disease, and presence of dysplasia. The contribution of shared genetic and environmental factors in the genesis of the two inflammatory conditions and of colon cancer is not known. Diabetes and cholecystectomy have been associated with a moderate (1.5–2-fold) increased risk of (right-sided) colon cancer, possibly due to continuous secretion of bile. Patients with one cancer of the colon have a double risk to develop a second primary tumour in the colon or rectum, and the relative (though not the absolute) risk is greater for early age at first diagnosis. In women, an association has been shown also with cancers of the endometrium, ovary and breast, possibly due to shared hormonal or dietary factors.

There are several rare hereditary conditions that are characterized by a very high incidence of colon cancer. Familial adenomatous polyposis, due to inherited or de-novo mutation in the adenomatous polyposis colon gene on chromosome 5, is characterized by a very high number of colonic adenomas and a cumulative incidence of colon or rectal cancer close to 100 per cent by age 55. Other, rarer, diseases characterized by colonic polyposis, among other features, are Gardner's syndrome, Turcot syndrome and juvenile polyposis. All these hereditary conditions, although very serious for the affected patients, account for no more than 1 per cent of colon cancers in the general population.

Two syndromes characterized by hereditary non-polyposis colon cancer, that is, with increased familial risk of colon cancer in the absence of adenomas, have been described. Lynch syndrome I is characterized by increased risk of cancer of the proximal (right) colon, and is due to inherited mutation in one of two genes involved in DNA repair. Patients of Lynch syndrome II have also an increased risk of extra-colonic neoplasms, mainly of the endometrium and the breast. As a whole, hereditary non-polyposis colon cancer may account for a sizeable proportion of cases of colon cancer in Western populations. In addition to these hereditary conditions, first-degree relatives of colon cancer patients have a 2–3-fold increased risk of developing a cancer of the colon or the rectum.

Cancer of the rectum

The distribution of cancer of the rectum, including the recto-sigmoid junction and the anus, parallels the distribution of colon cancer: The highest rates are recorded in Oceania, North America and central Europe and are in the order of 20/100 000 in men and 10/100 000 in women (IARC 2002a). In most populations, incidence rates have been stable in recent decades. The male-to-female ratio is close to 2.

Most biological and epidemiological features of rectal cancer resemble those described for colon cancer, including the pre-neoplastic role of adenomas and non-polypoid dysplastic mucosa, the presence of familial syndromes, the increased risk among patients with chronic inflammatory bowel diseases, and the likely protective role of dietary factors and physical activity. In addition, several studies have provided evidence, although not fully consistent, of an association between elevated intake of alcohol, and increased risk of colorectal adenoma and adenocarcinoma (Baan *et al.* 2007).

Surveillance via flexible colonoscopy, involving removal of adenomas, is a secondary preventive measure for colorectal cancer. An additional approach consists in the detection of faecal occult blood. The method suffers from low specificity and, to a lesser extent, low sensitivity, in particular in the ability to detect adenomas. However, trials have shown a reduced mortality from colorectal cancer after annual test, although this is achieved at a high cost due to an elevated number of false positive cases. Current recommendations for individuals aged 50 and over include either annual faecal occult blood testing or once colonoscopy (Boyle *et al.* 2003).

Cancer of the liver and biliary tract

The epidemiology of liver cancer is made complex by the large number of secondary tumours, which are difficult to separate from primary liver cancers without histological verification. The most common histological type of liver malignant neoplasm is hepatocellular carcinoma (HCC). Other forms include: (i) childhood hepatoblastoma, and (ii) adult cholangiocarcinoma (originating from the intrahepatic biliary ducts) and (iii) angiosarcoma (from the intrahepatic blood vessels). Cancers of the extrahepatic biliary ducts are of the adenocarcinoma type. Most HCC originate from cirrhotic tissue.

The incidence of liver cancer is high in all low-resource regions of the world, with the exception of Northern Africa and Western Asia. The highest rates (above 40/100 000 in men and above 10/100 000 in women) are recorded in Thailand, Japan and certain parts of China. In most high-resource countries, age-standardized rates are below 5/100 000 in men and 2.5/100 000 in women. Intermediate rates (5–10/100 000 in men) are observed in areas of Southern and Central Europe (IARC 2002a). Rates are 2–3-folds higher in men than women, and the difference is stronger in high-incidence than in low-incidence areas. The estimated worldwide number of new cases of liver cancer in 2002 is 630 000, of which more than 80 per cent are from developing countries (55 per cent from China alone) (Ferlay *et al.* 2004). Given the poor survival from this disease, the estimated number of deaths is similar to that of new cases (600 000): Liver cancer is the second most frequent cause of neoplastic death in low-resource countries.

Incidence and mortality from primary liver cancer have been rising among middle age men in the United States (El Serag 2004), but not consistently in Europe (Bosetti *et al.* 2008), over the last few decades.

Incidence rates of biliary tract cancer are high (above 3/100 000 in men and above 5/100 000 in women) in Central Europe, South America, Japan, and Western Asia. In the United States, rates are higher among people of American-Indian, Hispanic, and Japanese origin than in other groups. Most of the geographical variation is accounted for by cancer of the gall-bladder, which represents the majority of biliary tract cancers. Rates of gall-bladder cancer in women are generally higher than in men, while other biliary tract cancers are slightly more frequent in men.

Hepatocellular carcinoma

Chronic infections with hepatitis B virus (HBV) and hepatitis C virus (HCV) are the main causes of HCC (Fig. 9.3.5). The risk increases with early age at infection (in high-risk countries, most HBV infections occur perinatally or in early childhood), and the presence of cirrhosis is a pathogenic step. HBV is the main agent in China, Southeast Asia and Africa, while HCV is the predominant virus in Japan and Southern Europe. The most frequent routes of HCV transmission are parenteral HCC and sexual, while perinatal infection is rare. The estimated risk of developing HCC among infected subjects, relative to uninfected, ranged between 10 and 50 in different studies. On a global scale, the fraction of liver cancer cases attributable to HBV is 54 per cent, the one attributable to HCV is 31 per cent (Parkin 2006).

Ecological studies have shown that the incidence of HCC correlates not only with HBV and HCV infection, but also with contamination of foodstuff with aflatoxins, a group of mycotoxins produced by the fungi *Aspergillus flavus* and *Aspergillus parasiticus*, which cause liver cancer in many species of experimental animals. Contamination originates mainly from improper storage of cereals, peanuts and other vegetables and is prevalent in particular in Africa, Southeast Asia and China (London *et al.* 2006).

Alcohol intake increases the risk of HCC. The most likely mechanism is through development of cirrhosis, although alternative mechanisms such as alteration in activation and detoxification of carcinogens may also play a role. Alcoholic cirrhosis is probably the most important risk factors for HCC in populations with low prevalence of HBV and HCV infection and low exposure to aflatoxins, such as North America and Northern Europe (La Vecchia 2007). The association between tobacco smoking and HCC is now established, with a RR of the order of 1.5 to 2 for tobacco smoking on liver carcinogenesis (IARC 2004a).

Use of oral contraceptives (OC) greatly increases the risk of liver adenomas, and is associated with the risk of HCC, although the absolute risk is likely to be small (IARC 2005b). Case reports have associated use of anabolic steroids with development of liver cancer, but the evidence is not conclusive at present. An increase in iron storage in the body is a likely cause of HCC: The evidence comes from studies of patients with hemochromatosis or other disorders of iron metabolism. The effect of iron overload seems to be

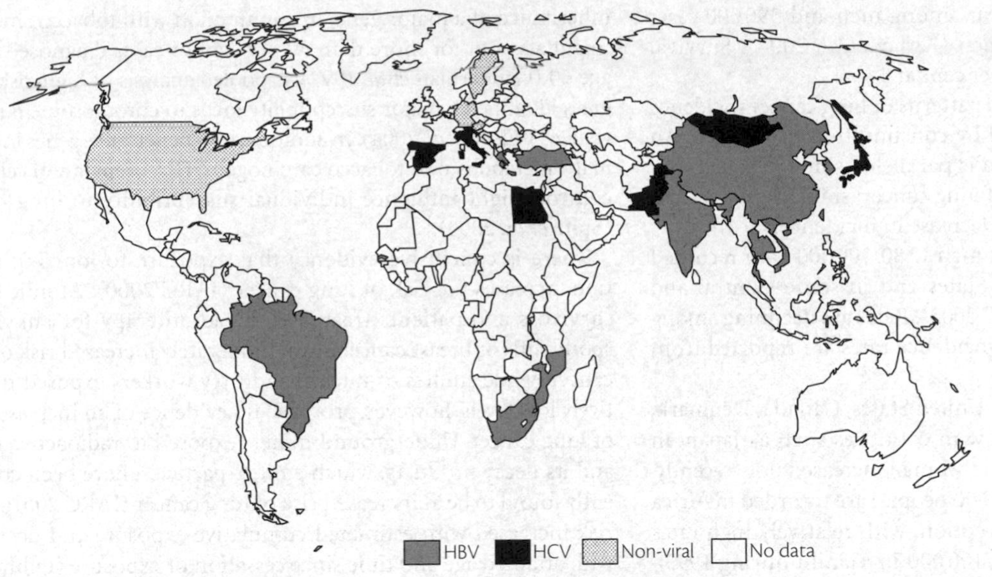

Fig. 9.3.5 Predominant causes of hepatocellular carcinoma (hepatitis B virus, hepatitis C virus, and seronegative for both) by country.*

independent from development of cirrhosis and may interact with HBV infection.

Diabetes is also related to an excess risk of HCC and the increased prevalence of overweight and obesity, and consequently of diabetes, is several populations may have had some role in recent unfavourable trends in North America and other areas of the world.

Other types of primary liver cancer

Infestation with the liver flukes, *Opistorchis viverrini* and *Clonorchis sinensis*, is the main known cause of cholangiocarcinoma, that is rare in most populations but relatively frequent in infested areas in Southeast Asia. Infection occurs via consumption of improperly cooked fish. Exposure to thorotrast, a contrast medium containing radioactive thorium used for angiography in Europe and Japan during 1930–1955, resulted in an increase of cholangiocarcinoma and of liver angiosarcoma. Workers exposed to vinyl chloride, a monomer used in the chemical industry for production of the plastic polymer, polyvinyl chloride, experience an increased risk of angiosarcoma. The identification of clusters of cases of liver angiosarcoma in these workers has led to a drastic reduction in occupational exposure to vinyl chloride.

Cancer of extrahepatic biliary ducts

The main known risk factor for cancer of the gall-bladder is the presence of gallstones. The RR is in the order of 3, and it is higher in patients with large (>3 cm in diameter) rather than small (<1 cm) stones. In Western populations, most gallstones are formed by cholesterol, and their formation is associated with hypersecretion and saturation of cholesterol in the bile. The possible causes of cholesterol saturation (obesity, multiple pregnancies and other hormonal factors) are also associated with increased risk of gall-bladder cancer. An additional role of gall-bladder hypomotility in stone formation is likely. In Asia, the main types of gallstone are formed by bilirubin salts and have as risk factor bacterial infection of the biliary system: Their association with gall-bladder cancer, however, is not clear (Hsing *et al.* 2006).

Fewer data are available on risk factors for cancer of extrahepatic biliary ducts. Infestation with the liver flukes causing intrahepatic cholangiocarcinoma, and history of ulcerative colitis are established risk factors but explain only a small proportion of these cancers. Tobacco smoking and diabetes have been suggested as additional causes. The incidence of gall-bladder cancer has increase in Europe during the last two decades (Jepsen *et al.* 2007).

Prevention

The strong role in liver carcinogenesis of infection with HBV, a virus for which effective and cheap vaccines are available, indicates that a large proportion of liver cancers are preventable. In high-prevalence areas, HBV vaccination has to be introduced in the perinatal period. In the last decades, many countries from Asia, Southern Europe and, to a lesser extent, Africa have expanded the national childhood vaccination programme to include HBV. A similar primary preventive approach is not available for HCV. Control of transmissions is however feasible and medical treatment of carriers with interferon might represent an alternative approach (which is also available for HBV carriers).

Control of aflatoxin contamination of foodstuffs represents another important preventive measure. While this is easily achieved in high-income countries, its implementation is limited by economic and logistic factors in many high-prevalence regions. Control of alcohol drinking and tobacco smoking represents additional primary preventive measures.

Cholecystectomy is an obvious mean to prevent gall-bladder cancer. The removal of the gall-bladder in asymptomatic patients, however, is not justified, with the possible exception of high-risk circumstances such as large stones and calcified gall-bladder. The increased rate of cholecystectomy in many high-resource countries is probably responsible for the temporal decreasing trend of gall-bladder cancer (Randi *et al.* 2006).

Lung cancer

Lung cancer was a rare disease until the beginning of the twentieth century. Since then, its occurrence has increased rapidly and this neoplasm has become the most frequent malignant neoplasm among men in most countries, and represents the most important cause of cancer death worldwide. It accounts for an estimated 960 000 new cases and 850 000 deaths each year among men and 390 000 cases and 330 000 deaths among women (Ferlay *et al.* 2004). Survival from lung cancer is poor (5–10 per cent at 5 years).

The geographical and temporal patterns of lung cancer incidence are to a large extent determined by consumption of tobacco. An increase in tobacco consumption is paralleled some decades later by an increase in the incidence of lung cancer; similarly, a decrease in consumption is followed by a decrease in incidence.

The highest incidence rates in men (>80/100 000) are recorded among Blacks from the United States and in some Central and Eastern European countries (IARC 2003). Rates are declining among men in and Europe. The lowest incidence rates are reported from Africa and Southern Asia.

Rates in women are high in the United States, Canada, Denmark, and the United Kingdom, and low in countries such as Japan, in which the prevalence of smoking in women increased only recently. The lowest rates (<3 cases per 100 000 people) are recorded in Africa and India. China is a notable exception, with relatively high rates recorded among women (e.g. 37/100 000 in Tianjin during 1993–1997; (IARC 2003), despite a low prevalence of smoking.

The main histological types of lung cancer are squamous cell carcinoma, small cell carcinoma, adenocarcinoma and large cell carcinoma. Over the last decades, the proportion of squamous cell carcinomas, which used to be the predominant type, has decreased and an increase of adenocarcinomas has taken place in both genders.

A carcinogenic effect of tobacco smoke on the lung has been demonstrated in the 1950s and has been recognized by public health and regulatory authorities since the mid 1960s (IARC 2004a). The risk of lung cancer among smokers relative to the risk among never-smokers is in the order of 30-fold or more. This overall risk reflects the contribution of the different aspects of tobacco smoking: Average consumption, duration of smoking, time since quitting, age at start, type of tobacco product and inhalation pattern, with duration being the dominant factor. As compared to continuous smokers, the excess risk decreases in ex-smokers after quitting, but a small excess risk is likely to persist in long-term quitters throughout life. In the United Kingdom, the cumulative risk of lung cancer of a continuous smoker is 16 per cent and it is reduced to 10, 6, 3, and 2 per cent among those who stopped at age 60, 50, 40, and 30, respectively (Peto *et al.* 2000). Smokers of black (air-cured) tobacco cigarettes are at higher risk of lung cancer than smokers of blond (flue-cured) tobacco cigarettes. A causal association with lung cancer has been shown also for consumption of cigars, cigarillos, pipe, bidis, water pipe, and other smoking tobacco products.

An association has been shown in many studies between exposure to involuntary smoking and lung cancer risk in non-smokers. The magnitude of the excess risk among non-smokers exposed to involuntary smoking is in the order 20 per cent (IARC 2004a).

There is limited evidence that a diet rich in vegetables and fruits exerts a protective effect against lung cancer (IARC 2003). In particular, a protective effect has been suggested for intake of cruciferous vegetables, possibly because of their high content in isothiocyanates (IARC 2004b). Despite the many studies of intake of other foods, such as cereals, pulses, meat, eggs, milk, and dairy products, the evidence is inadequate to allow a judgement regarding the evidence of a carcinogenic or a protective effect.

A positive familial history of lung cancer has been found to be a risk factor in several studies. Segregation analyses suggest that inheritance of a major gene, in conjunction with tobacco smoking, might account for more than 50 per cent of cases diagnosed below age 60 (Gauderman *et al.* 1997). A pooled analysis of high-risk pedigrees identified a major susceptibility locus to chromosome 6q23–25 (Bailey-Wilson *et al.* 2004). In addition, low-penetrance genes involved in the metabolism of tobacco carcinogens, DNA repair and cell cycle control might influence individual susceptibility to lung cancer (Spitz *et al.* 2006).

There is conclusive evidence that exposure to ionizing radiation increases the risk of lung cancer (IARC 2000). Atomic bomb survivors and patients treated with radiotherapy for ankylosing spondylitis or breast cancer are at moderately increased risk of lung cancer, while studies of nuclear industry workers exposed to relatively low levels, however, provided no evidence of an increased risk of lung cancer. Underground miners exposed to radioactive radon and its decay products, which emit α-particles, have been consistently found to be at increased risk of lung cancer (IARC 2001a). The risk increased with estimated cumulative exposure and decreased with attained age and time since cessation of exposure (Lubin *et al.* 1994).

The risk of lung cancer is increased among workers employed in several industries and occupations. For several of these high-risk workplaces, the agent (or agents) responsible for the increased risk have been identified. Of these, asbestos and combustion fumes are the most important. Occupational agents are responsible for an estimated 5–10 per cent of lung cancers in industrialized countries.

Patients with pulmonary tuberculosis are at increased risk of lung cancer; it is not clear whether the excess risk is due to the chronic inflammatory status of the lung parenchyma or to the specific action of the Mycobacterium. Chronic exposure to high levels of fibres and dusts might result in lung fibrosis (e.g. silicosis and asbestosis), a condition which entails an increase in the risk of lung cancer. Chronic bronchitis and emphysema have also been associated with lung cancer risk.

There is abundant evidence that lung cancer rates are higher in cities than in rural settings (Speizer *et al.* 1994). Although this pattern might result from confounding by other factors, notably tobacco smoking and occupational exposures, the combined evidence from analytical studies suggests that urban air pollution might be a risk factor for lung cancer, although the excess relative risk is unlikely to be larger than 20 per cent in most urban areas.

Indoor air pollution is thought to be responsible for the elevated risk of lung cancer experienced by non-smoking women living in several regions of China and other Asian countries. The evidence is strongest for coal burning in poorly ventilated houses, but also burning of wood and other solid fuels, as well as fumes from high-temperature cooking using unrefined vegetable oils such as rapeseed oil (IARC 2006). In other parts of the world, indoor exposure to radon decay particles may entail a sizeable increase of risk.

Control of tobacco smoking remains the key strategy for the prevention of lung cancer. Reduction in exposure to occupational and environmental carcinogens (in particular indoor pollution and radon), as well as increase in consumption of fruits and vegetables are additional preventive opportunities. No screening approaches are effective to reduce lung cancer mortality (Bach *et al.* 2007).

Cancer of the skin

There are four main types of skin cancer: SqCC, arising from the epidermal cells, basal cell carcinoma, from basal cells forming sebaceous glands, melanoma, arising from melanocytes, and Kaposi's sarcoma, arising from endothelial cells. SqCC and basal cell carcinoma share pathological, clinical and aetiological features, and are often combined under the definition of non-melanocytic skin cancer.

Non-melanocytic skin cancer

Given the simplified diagnostic and therapeutic procedures (often treated in outpatient clinics and physicians' offices) of most non-melanocytic skin cancers, reporting of cases to registries is frequently incomplete, and many cancer registries do not attempt to provide incidence figures. The very good prognosis (a more than 95 per cent survival rate in most populations) makes mortality figures useless to estimate incidence. Population-based data incidence derive therefore from ad-hoc surveys. A survey conducted in the United States in the late 1970s estimated an age-adjusted incidence rate of SqCC of 68/100 000 in White men and 24/100 000 in white women; corresponding figures for basal cell carcinoma were 258 and 155/100 000. Rates in Blacks were about 100 times lower than in Whites, and SqCC predominates. The comparison with a similar survey conducted in the early 1970s revealed a 4–5 per cent increase in incidence of basal cell carcinoma per year, which can be attributed, at least in part, to improved diagnostic and surveillance procedures. SqCC rates increased little during the same period. Rates in Whites approximate those of all other malignant neoplasms combined. Even higher rates have been recorded in Ireland and among Whites living in countries with high solar exposure, such as Australia and South Africa, while black populations have consistently low rates.

Between 75 per cent and 90 per cent of both SqCC and basal cell carcinomas in Whites are localized on the face, head and neck. In Blacks, the lower extremities are the most frequent location of SqCC.

Solar radiation is the main known risk factor for non-melanocytic skin cancer. For squamous cell carcinoma, the cumulative dose of ultraviolet radiation, disregarding dose rate, appears to be the predominant risk factor, while for basal cell carcinoma sun exposure and sunburning during childhood are the main determinants of subsequent risk. The effect of solar radiation has been shown following occupational, recreational and involuntary exposure. A strong excess of skin cancer has also been shown in psoriasis patients treated with psoralen in combination with ultraviolet radiation A. Solar keratosis is a precursor lesion of SqCC of the skin (not of basal cell carcinoma): It occurs in those areas of the skin exposed to solar radiation. The cumulative progression rate of keratosis to carcinoma (usually through a phase of carcinoma *in situ*, or Bowen's disease) is in the order of 5 per cent. Skin pigmentation is a modifying factor of the carcinogenic effect of ultraviolet radiation, with people with light pigmentation having the greatest risk (Karagas *et al.* 2006).

An excess risk of basal carcinoma, but not SqCC, has been shown following exposure to ionizing radiation (studies of medical personnel, uranium miners, radiotherapy patients and atomic bomb survivors): The shape of the dose–response appears to be linear without threshold (Levi *et al.* 2006). Exposure to arsenic and its inorganic compounds has been linked to an excess of skin cancer in people exposed occupationally, from drinking water or from drugs used in the past. Mixtures of polycyclic aromatic hydrocarbons (coal tar, tar pitch, soot, creosote, lubricating and cutting oils) are also carcinogenic to the skin: An excess of non-melanocytic cancer has been shown in classical occupational epidemiological studies among workers such as chimney sweeps, machine operators and roofers.

Skin cancer occurs in Asian countries as a consequence of burn scars produced by traditional heating devices kept in close contact to the skin: Kangri in Kashmir, India, kairo in some areas of Japan and kang in northern China. It is possible that polycyclic aromatic hydrocarbons released by the burning material interact with heat in causing the cancer.

Immunodeficiency increases the risk of SqCC of the skin, as it has been shown in patients treated with immunosuppressive drugs following renal transplant or other conditions. Xeroderma pigmentosum and the nevoid basal cell carcinoma syndrome are rare hereditary conditions characterized by a very high incidence of skin cancer. In the former syndrome, the mechanism is a reduced capacity to repair damage to DNA. The action of immunodeficiency and genetic predisposition may be via an enhancement of the carcinogenic effect of ultraviolet and ionizing radiation, since the neoplasms occur on parts of the body exposed to the sun.

Avoidance of sun exposure, in particular during the middle of the day, is the primary preventive measure to reduce the incidence of skin cancer. There is no adequate evidence of a protective effect of sunscreens, possibly because use of sunscreens is associated with increased exposure to the sun. The possible benefit in reducing skin cancer risk, however, should be balanced against possible favourable effects of ultraviolet radiation in promoting vitamin D metabolism. Control of occupational skin carcinogens has taken place in many industries, although high exposure circumstances may still take place in developing countries. Avoidance of drinking water with a high arsenic level should be a priority in contaminated areas. Secondary prevention can be achieved by regular skin examination, in particular for high-risk individuals: However, there is a lack of controlled trials on skin cancer screening.

Malignant melanoma

Malignant melanomas occur most frequently on the trunk in men and on the lower limbs in women. While pathologists distinguish several histological types of melanoma, these are likely to represent different stages of the same condition. A special type of melanoma, however, is the rare lentigo malignant melanoma, which occurs on the head and neck, in areas with sun damage.

An estimated 160 000 new cases of malignant melanoma occurred worldwide in 2002 (Ferlay *et al.* 2004). The incidence is highest (in the order of 25/100 000) in Australia, it ranges between 5 and 10/100 000 in other parts of Oceania, in North America and in Northern and Western Europe, and is below 5/1 000 000 in the other regions of the world. In general, the incidence is low in dark-skinned populations (IARC 2002a). In many White populations, there has been an increase in incidence until the 1990s, with a recent levelling off: This pattern was not observed in non-White populations.

There is strong evidence of a carcinogenic role of ultraviolet radiation in determining malignant melanoma. Intermittent exposure to the sun seems to play a more important role than total cumulative exposure.

Exposure to fluorescent lamp is not associated to the risk of melanoma, but artificial sources of Ultraviolet Radiation (UBV) have been related to excess risk.

Light colour of hair and eyes and skin complexion are risk factors for melanoma. Colour of hair seems to be the main predictor of risk, with RR in the range of 1.5–2 for blond hair and 2–4 for red hair as compared to dark or brown hair. Freckling is likely to be an additional risk factor. Skin response to sun exposure and propensity to burn (or poor ability to tan) have also been associated to melanoma risk, with a RR in the range 1.5–4. However, pale complexion and propensity to burn are strongly correlated, and the available data are inadequate to completely separate these two factors.

Presence of a high number of nevi is the strongest risk factor for melanoma. Assessment of the number and type of nevi is not straightforward, and misclassification is likely to affect studies on nevi and melanoma. The RR is in the order of 10 for the category at highest number of nevi. Their number depends on sun exposure, in particular intermittent exposure and sunburns: Exposure in childhood is more important than exposure in adulthood. In subjects with familial melanoma, large atypical nevi, referred to as dysplastic nevi, might be found. Individuals with dysplastic nevi and familial melanoma have a very high risk of melanoma. In subjects without familial melanoma, presence of dyspastic nevi seems to be a risk factor independent from number of total nevi (Gruber *et al.* 2006).

The number of atypical nevi and the risk of melanoma are increased among immunosuppressed patients. There is no clear evidence of a role of any other risk factor, including dietary factors and exogenous hormones, in the aetiology of melanoma. There is a 2 to 5 increased risk of melanoma in subjects with an affected relative, which is independent from exposure to solar radiation. Several putative high-risk genes have been proposed to explain the increased familial risk.

Reducing of solar and other sources of UBV exposure, especially in childhood, is the major primary preventive measure that can be recommended. Early diagnosis, in particular of thin lesions, is associated with better survival: Screening via medical examination is justified in high-risk individuals, defined according to familial history, type of skin and reaction to solar radiation.

Cancer of the breast

Over 80 per cent of the neoplasms of the breast originate from the ductal epithelium, while a minority originates from the lobular epithelium. However, the proportion of ductal carcinomas has been increasing over recent calendar periods. Five-year survival from breast cancer has slowly increased in high-resource countries, where it now achieves 85 per cent, following improvements in screening practices and treatments. Survival in low-resource countries remains poor, in the order of 50–60 per cent.

Breast cancer is the most common cancer among women worldwide: The estimated number of new cases in 2002 was 640 000 in developed countries and 510 000 in developing countries (Ferlay *et al.* 2004). It is also the most important cause of cancer deaths among women, causing an estimated 410 000 deaths worldwide. The incidence of breast cancer is low (less than 20/100 000) in most countries from sub-Saharan Africa, in China and in other countries of East Asia, except Japan. The highest rates (70–90/100 000) are recorded in North America, Australia, and Northern and Western Europe, in Brazil and Argentina (IARC 2002a). The incidence of breast cancer has grown rapidly during the last decades in many low-resource countries and slowly in medicinal high-resource countries. Mortality rates have remained fairly stable between 1960 and 1990 in most of Europe and the Americas, with however appreciable declines since the early 1990s. The incidence increases linearly with age up to menopause, after which a further increase is less marked (high-resource countries) or almost absent (low-resource countries) (Fig. 9.3.6). Women from high social class have consistently higher rates than women from low social class, the difference being in the order of 30–50 per cent.

The cumulative number of ovarian cycles is a determinant of breast cancer risk, and there is an increased risk for early age at menarche and late age at menopause. Artificial menopause exerts a similar or somewhat stronger protective effect than natural menopause (Colditz *et al.* 2006).

Pregnancy increases in the short term the risk of breast cancer, probably because of increase in the level of free oestrogens during the first trimester. Overall, there is a protective role of early age at first pregnancy and a small residual protective effect of other pregnancies. An additional protective effect of lactation has been shown in several populations. In a collaborative reanalysis of 47 studies, breast cancer risk decreased by 4.3 per cent for each year of lactation (Collaborative Group on Hormonal Factors in Breast Cancer 2002). Epidemiological studies indicate a lack of association between spontaneous or induced abortions and breast cancer.

Current and recent users of OC have a modest increase (i.e. about 25 per cent) in risk of breast cancer as compared to never users. Furthermore, 10 or more years after stopping use of OC the risk levels off to approach that of never users (IARC 2008). This is of particular importance, since most women who use OC are young and have low baseline incidence of breast cancer. Therefore, their increased risk during and shortly after OC use is little relevant (La Vecchia *et al.* 2001). With further reference to exogenous hormones, the evidence derived both from observational epidemiological studies (cohort and case–control) and randomized clinical trials indicates that the risk of breast cancer (mainly ductal cancer) is elevated among women using (combined) Hormonal Replacement Therapy (HRT) (IARC 2005c). Several epidemiological investigations consistently reported higher risks among current users of HRT, increasing from 1.1 to 1.6 according to their duration of use. The risk of breast cancer is reduced after cessation of use, and levels off after 5 or more years since quitting HRT. The Women's Health Initiative, a randomized controlled trial conducted on postmenopausal women, provided comprehensive information on the risk of breast cancer in users of conjugated oestrogen alone or in combination with progestin. In the oestrogen-alone trial, after about 7 years of follow-up, there was no significant difference in

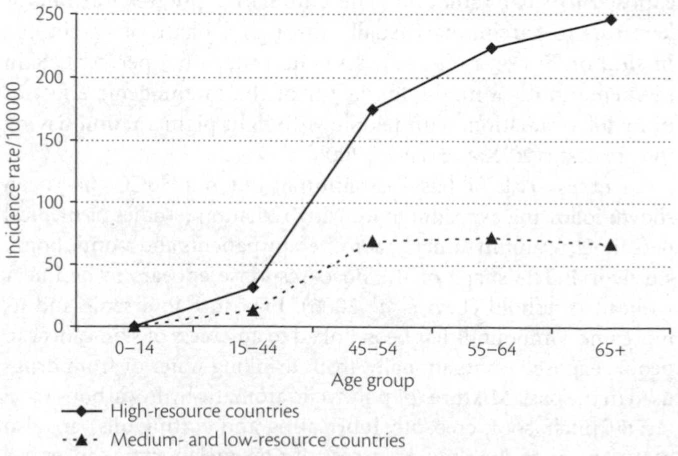

Fig. 9.3.6 Age-specific incidence rates of breast cancer by region of the world, 2002.

breast cancer incidence comparing conjugated oestrogen users to the placebo group (Stefanick *et al.* 2006). On the other hand, a higher incidence of invasive breast cancer was observed in the oestrogen plus progestin group as compared to women receiving placebo (Chlebowski *et al.* 2003).

The combined evidence from reproductive factors points towards an important role of endogenous hormones in breast carcinogenesis. A direct assessment of the role of oestrogen and testosterone is also available from recent prospective studies collecting data of biological samples. Oestradiol concentrations in the blood have been directly associated with breast cancer risk in post-menopausal women, whereas data are fewer and results are less consistent in pre-menopausal women. The association might be stronger with oestrogen and progesterone receptor positive tumours. Comparable findings have been reported for measures of testosterone and other androgens, but the data are inconsistent for all endogenous hormones across major cohort studies.

Women suffering from the two most common benign breast diseases, fibrocystic disease and fibroadenoma carry a 2–3-fold increased risk of breast cancer.

A history of breast cancer in first degree relatives is associated with a 2–3-fold increased risk of the disease. Most of the role of familial history is likely to result from low-penetrance genes associated with hormonal metabolism and regulation, DNA damage and repair. There is some evidence of an increased risk of breast cancer associated with polymorphisms of genes involved in the biosynthesis of oestradiol, particularly the CYP19 gene. Several other low-penetrance genes have been analysed, but studies have generally reported null or inconsistent findings. In addition, breast cancer risk is greatly increased in carriers of mutations of several high-penetrance genes, in particular BRCA1, BRCA2, ATM, CHECK2 and p53. Although the cumulative lifetime risk in carriers of these genes is over 50 per cent, they are rare in most populations and explain only a small fraction (2–5%) of total cases. There are exceptions, however, such as Ashkenazi Jews, among whom high-risk BRCA1 or BRCA2 mutations are responsible for an estimated 12 per cent of breast cancers.

Although a role of nutrition in breast cancer risk has been suggested by international comparisons, the combined evidence from epidemiological studies is inconclusive for most aspects of diet, including intake of fruit and vegetables, total fat, saturated fat and fibres (Michels *et al.* 2007). Similarly, results on micronutrients have been elusive, although there is some evidence of a protective role played by folate and phytooestrogens, particularly isoflavones and dietary lignans. Furthermore, vitamin D, and in particular serum 25(OH) D levels, have been inversely related to breast cancer risk (Giovannucci 2005). Hormonal levels and nutritional factors during the intrauterine period and childhood are also likely to be important in breast carcinogenesis (Lagiou *et al.* 2006). In fact, energy intake during childhood is one of the determinant of adult height, which in turn has been directly associated with breast cancer risk in most epidemiological studies.

Besides height, other anthropometric factors are involved in the aetiology of breast cancer (Lagiou *et al.* 2006). An increased risk with increasing weight during adult life has been consistently reported among women older than 60, but not among younger women. Body mass index is associated to breast cancer, the relation being inverse in pre-menopausal and direct in post-menopausal women (IARC 2002b). Several studies reported a modifying effect of HRT use on the relation between body weight and weight gain and breast cancer in post-menopausal women. The increase in risk of breast cancer observed for a high body weight and/or weight gain was stronger or limited to non-users of HRT.

Many lifestyle factors have been investigated as possible causes of breast cancer. Alcohol drinking is an established aetiological factor. Consumption of three or more alcoholic drinks per day carries an increased risk in the order of 30–50 per cent, with each daily drink accounting for an about 10 per cent higher risk. It is likely that both overweight and heavy alcohol drinking act on breast cancer through mechanisms involving hormonal level or metabolism. Tobacco smoking does not carry an increased risk of breast cancer. A high level of physical activity, on the other hand, is likely to moderately decrease the risk. Studies of occupational factors and of exposure to organochlorine pesticides have failed to provide evidence of an aetiological role.

Less than 1 per cent of all cases of breast cancer occur in men. The incidence provides limited evidence of geographical and interracial variations, with no clear correlation with incidence in women. Conditions involving high oestrogen level, such as gonadal dysfunction, alcohol abuse and obesity, are risk factors for breast cancer in men. BRCA2 mutations are more frequent than BRCA1 in male familial breast cancers.

Control of weight gain and of overweight and obesity or post-menopausal women would have favourable implications in breast cancer risk.

Tamoxifen, an anti-oestrogen drug used in chemotherapy, has shown a chemopreventive action against breast cancer, although its use is recommended in women with a previous breast cancer only. Aspirin and other nonsteroidal anti-inflammatory drugs might also have a chemopreventive effect on breast cancer risk, although results from epidemiological studies are heterogeneous (Bosetti *et al.* 2006).

The most suitable approach for breast cancer control is secondary prevention through mammography. The effectiveness of screening by mammography in women older than 50 years has been demonstrated, and programmes have been established in various countries (Boyle *et al.* 2003). The effectiveness in women younger than 50 is not yet demonstrated, though there is some evidence for a reduction in risk of dying from breast cancer in women aged 40–49 years that undergo annual mammography. Other screening techniques, including breast self examination, have not been proven to reduce breast cancer mortality.

Cancer of the female genital organs

The female genital organs comprise the ovaries and their annexes, the uterus, the vagina and the external genitals. The uterus is composed of two parts, the cervix and the corpus, which have very distinct physiological and pathological features. Cancers of the cervix and corpus of the uterus are different histologically, clinically, and aetiologically. However, the distinction between cervix and corpus is often neglected in records used for epidemiological purposes, such as death certificates. Today in Europe and North America, most cancers of the uterus without further specification are likely to be cancer of the corpus. This, however, may not have been the case in the past and in other countries, and this fact complicates temporal and geographical comparisons.

Cancer of the uterine cervix

Cervical cancer is a major public health problem in many low- and medium-resource countries. Incidence rates are high

(20–40/100 000) in sub-Saharan African and Latin American countries, as well as in India and Southern Asia. In China, the Middle East, northern Africa and high-resource countries, rates are in the order of 5–15/100 000 (IARC 2002a). This results in a number of cases each year in excess of 370 000, 78 per cent of which occur in developing countries, where cervical cancer represents the second most common female neoplasm after breast cancer. The number of estimated cancer deaths in low- and medium-resource countries (230 000 in 2002) exceeds that from breast cancer (Ferlay *et al.* 2004). Incidence and mortality rates have decreased steadily in high-resource countries, but an upturn in incidence has been observed among young women. Few data on temporal trends are available from low-resource countries, but incidence has likely decreased during recent decades. In high-risk countries, rates increase up to age 60, while in low-resource countries there is little increase above age 50. In most countries, cervical cancer hits preferentially women of lower education and social class.

Most cervical cancers originate from the area of squamous metaplasia called transformation zone, which is adjacent to the junction between the columnar epithelium of endometrial origin and the cheratinizing epithelium of vaginal origin. Most invasive cancers are SqCC or mixed adeno-squamous tumours. Invasive carcinoma is preceded by inflammatory and condylomatous atypia, mild dysplasia (also called cervical intraepithelial neoplasia of grade 1, or CIN 1), moderate dysplasia (CIN 2), severe dysplasia, and carcinoma *in situ* (CIN 3) (Schiffman *et al.* 2006).

Chronic infection with HPV is a necessary cause of cervical cancer. Using sensitive molecular techniques, virtually all tumours are positive for the virus, while the prevalence in non-diseased women represents 5–40 per cent in the different populations (Clifford *et al.* 2005). Different types of HPV exist, and those associated with cervical cancer are mainly types 16, 18, 31, and 45. In particular, HPV 16 is a main carcinogen in many populations, while the distribution of other types varies by geographical region (Fig. 9.3.7). Differences in prevalence of HPV infection explain much of the descriptive epidemiology of cervical cancer (geographical patterns, high risk in low social class, etc.). The host response to HPV infection is important in determining its possible carcinogenic effect; immunosuppression, as present in transplanted patients and Human Immunodeficiency Virus (HIV) infected individuals, increases the risk of dysplasia, carcinoma *in situ* and invasive neoplasms.

Sexual characteristics of women (early age at first intercourse and high number of sexual partners) and of their male partners (high number of sexual partners, presence of genital diseases and contact with prostitutes) are risk factors for cervical cancer in many populations. They reflect an increased likelihood of HPV infection, in particular at young age.

Studies of infection with other agents, in particular Chlamydia and Herpes Simplex 2, have failed to provide consistent evidence of an effect independent from HPV. An increased risk, of the order of twofold, has been detected among long-term current or recent users of OC, which is not completely explained by sexual behaviour or HPV infection. However, there is no residual association 5–10 years after stopping OC use. Consequently, the public health implications of OC use on cervical cancer risk are limited in time. Condom and diaphragm, on the other hand, exert a protective effect, possibly via prevention of HPV infection.

Tobacco smoking has also an independent effect, with a RR of 1.5–1.6 for current smokers, also once HPV infection was taken into account (IARC 2004a). A possible protective effect of a diet rich in fruits and vegetables has been suggested in a few studies, but the role of diet on cervical cancer risk is probably modest and largely undefined.

Cytological examination of exfoliated cervical cells (the Papanicolaou smear test) is effective in identifying precursor lesions, resulting in a decrease in incidence of and mortality from invasive cancer. Cytological smears are not applicable, however, in countries with limited availability of cytologists and pathologists, including in many countries with high prevalence of HPV infection and high incidence of invasive cancer. Alternative approaches for secondary prevention have therefore been proposed, including visual inspection of the cervix with possible enhancement of precursor lesions

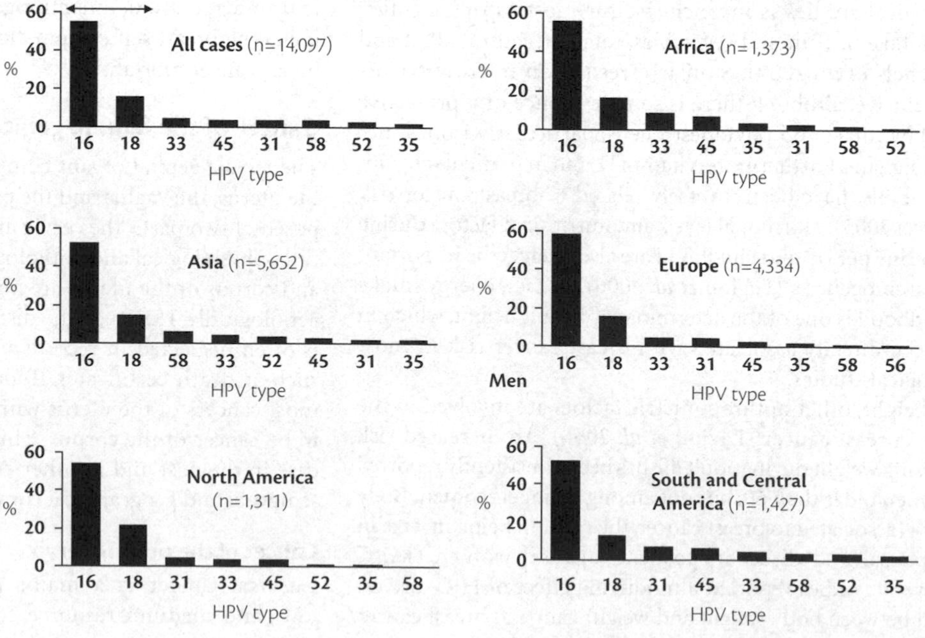

Fig. 9.3.7 Most common HPV types in 14 097 cases of invasive cervical cancer by region.
Source: Clifford et al. 2005.

by acetic acid, but their efficacy on cervical cancer prevention remains unproven. Use of HPV testing as a screening method, either as a first choice for general application or as the triage method of inconclusive cytological diagnoses, is also under investigation. The primary method for prevention of cervical cancer for future generations, however, is likely to become HPV vaccination. One vaccine against HPV 16, 18, 6, and 11 is now available, and another against HPV 16 and 18 is in the late stage of testing (The Future II Study Group 2007). The final impact of the effect of such vaccination is complicated by the geographical variations in the distribution of HPV types (Clifford *et al.* 2005).

Cancer of the uterine corpus

Cancer of the endometrium is the most frequent malignant neoplasm of the uterine corpus, while sarcomas, originating from the muscular tissue, are relatively rare. The descriptive epidemiology of cancer of the uterine corpus is complicated by the large proportion of hysterectomized women in high-resource countries. The number of new cases occurring in 2002 worldwide was estimated in the order of 200 000, of which two thirds occurred in high-resource countries (Ferlay *et al.* 2004). The number of deaths is in the order of 50 000. Incidence rates are relatively high (10–15/100 000) in Europe and North America, while they are below 5/100 000 in most African countries, in the Caribbean, and in China. It is a cancer of postmenopausal women. In the United States, the incidence is higher in Whites as compared to Blacks, while the opposite applies to mortality (IARC 2002a).

Nulliparity, infertility and late age at menopause are associated with a 2–3-fold increased risk of endometrial cancer. The evidence regarding other reproductive factors, including age at menarche, is less consistent. Medical conditions resulting in high endogenous oestrogen levels (including oestrogen-secreting tumours and polycystic ovarian syndrome) have been consistently associated to an increased endometrial cancer risk. Studies of blood oestrogen levels, however, are too sparse to be conclusive (Cook *et al.* 2006).

An increased risk of endometrial cancer was reported in the 1970s, followed by a decline up to the 1990s. This trend in incidence parallels the patterns of postmenopausal unopposed oestrogen use. Combined contraceptives, on the other hands, reduce the risk of endometrial cancer by about 50 per cent (La Vecchia *et al.* 2001). Use of oestrogen replacement therapy is associated with a 2-fold increase in risk of endometrial cancer. The strength of the association depends on the dose and the duration of use. Addition of progestin to oestrogen replacement therapy may protect from the increased risk of endometrial cancer, but it may also reduce the beneficial effects of oestrogens on cardiovascular disease and osteoporosis (IARC 2005c). An increased risk of endometrial cancer has also been shown among breast cancer patients treated with tamoxifen at a relatively high dosage (30 to 40 mg) or for a long period of time (5 or more years), though results are not consistent for low dosages and short period of tamoxifen use.

An increased risk of endometrial cancer has been consistently reported among obese as compared to lean women (IARC 2002b) depending on the measure used to evaluate overweight, endometrial cancer risk increases 2–10-fold. An increased risk in the order of 50 per cent to 100 per cent has also been reported among women with diabetes and hypertension, which does not seem to be fully explained by increased weight in these patients. A decreased risk of endometrial cancer has been reported among smokers in many populations, particularly among post-menopausal women: This result has been attributed to an anti-oestrogenic activity of smoking. The results of studies of diet and endometrial cancer have been inconsistent. Several other potential risk factors have been addressed, including alcohol and coffee drinking, and history of gall-bladder disease, without conclusive evidence of an association.

Current knowledge suggests that an impact on primary prevention of endometrial cancer can be made by avoidance of overweight minimizing the use of unopposed oestrogens.

Ovarian cancer

Most malignant neoplasms of the ovary originate from the coelomic epithelium; less frequent tumours originate from the germ cells (dysgerminomas and teratomas) and the follicular cells (granulosa cell tumours). The estimated number of new cases worldwide in 2002 was in the order of 200 000, that of deaths 125 000 (Ferlay *et al.* 2004). High incidence rates (in the order of 10–12/100 000) are found in Western and Northern Europe and in North America; the lowest rates (below 3/100 000) are from China and Central Africa (IARC 2002a). In high-risk countries the rates have remained stable in recent decades.

Late age at menarche is a risk factor, but its effect on ovarian cancer risk is modest. Lifelong number of menstrual cycles has also been associated with ovarian cancer risk, suggesting that ovulation may be implicated in the process of ovarian carcinogenesis. Several studies showed a direct relation between risk of ovarian cancer and early menarche and late age at menopause (Hankinson *et al.* 2006).

Nulliparity and low parity are related to ovarian cancer. Most studies showed a decline in risk associated with number of full-term pregnancies beyond the first one, thus suggesting that additional risk reduction is conferred by events accompanying each pregnancy.

The protection afforded by combined OC is also established, and is most important from a public health perspective, feature of epithelial ovarian cancer. The overall estimated protection is approximately 40 per cent in ever OC users and increases with duration of use. The favourable effect of OC against ovarian cancer risk persists for at least 15–20 years after OC use has ceased, and it is not confined to any particular type of OC formulation (La Vecchia *et al.* 2001). The issue of fertility drugs and ovarian cancer has also attracted lively interest, but the findings of various studies remain inconsistent. Hormone therapy in menopause has also been related to increased ovarian cancer risk (Anderson *et al.* 2003).

Potential links between ovarian cancer and diet were originally suggested on the basis of international differences or correlation studies. The role of diet on ovarian cancer incidence and mortality rates and trends remains, however, unquantified.

There have long been clinical observations suggesting familial aggregations of ovarian cancer. Besides the clustering of ovarian cancer, an excess of breast cancer and a more general excess of several cancers (including colon and endometrium) have been described. These patterns are consistent with an autosomal dominant gene with variable penetration. The estimated RR from case–control studies that included data on family history range between 3 and 5. Two tumour-suppressor genes have been identified, BRCA1 on chromosome 17q and BRCA2 on chromosome 13q, whose autosomal dominant transmitted mutations confer a high risk of breast and ovarian cancer. BRCA1 may account for 5 per cent of ovarian cancers below age 50, and 2 per cent between age 50 and 70. The prevention of ovarian cancer is currently hampered by the limited knowledge of its causes and the lack of availability of early diagnostic techniques.

Cancer of the male genital organs

Prostate cancer

Cancer of the prostate is the most common malignant neoplasm in men from North America, where the incidence is as high as 100/100 000. In other high-resource countries, the incidence is in the order of 20–40/100 000, and in most low- and medium-resource countries it is below 30/100 000, and it can be as low as 5/100 000 in Southern and Eastern Asia (IARC 2002a). The estimated number of new cases occurring worldwide in 2002 is estimated to be about 680 000 (Ferlay *et al.* 2004). Mortality rates show less variability among regions, suggesting that the number of non-fatal cases diagnosed in different countries varies depending on screening and other diagnostic procedures. The estimated number of deaths is 220 000, 60 per cent of which occur in high-resource countries. The incidence of prostate cancer increased slowly during the last decades in most populations; in the United States and Canada, and subsequently in Europe and other high-resource regions of the world a very rapid increase has been observed since the mid-1980s. The disease is more common in African Americans than in European Americans. In most countries, it is more common among affluent groups of the population.

The descriptive epidemiology of prostate cancer is highly dependent on the adoption of Prostate Specific Antigen (PSA) testing. Prostate cancer incidence has shown substantial changes following the introduction of PSA testing, with major increases due to the detection of large number of prevalent cases, followed by substantial declines. The changes in trends have been much smaller for mortality, but both in the United States and in Western Europe, peak rates were observed in the early 1990s, with a levelling off thereafter (Levi *et al.* 2004b).

The recent trends in prostate cancer mortality in Europe are consistent with a favourable impact of improved diagnosis, and well as of advancements in therapy, on prostate cancer mortality in Western Europe and North America.

Carriers of BRCA1 and BRCA2 mutations have a 4–5-fold increased risk of prostate cancer. More in general, history of prostate cancer in first-degree relatives carries a 2–3-fold increased risk of developing the same neoplasm. Similar associations, of smaller magnitude, are also suggested for family history of breast and colon cancers (Negri *et al.* 2005). Recently, genetic variants entailing an increased risk of prostate cancer have been identified within the 8q24 region (Amundadottir *et al.* 2006; Gudmundsson *et al.* 2007a; Haiman *et al.* 2007; Yeager *et al.* 2007) and possibly the 17q12 region (Gudmundsson *et al.* 2007b).

It has been shown in several populations that the risk of the disease increases with number of sexual partners and number of encounters with prostitutes, and with previous history of syphilis and gonorrhoea. Serological studies of HPV 16 and HPV 18 have shown an increased risk among positive subjects. It is not clear at present, however, whether syphilis and HPV are causal factors or markers of infection with other sexually transmitted agents.

A possible protective role of high intake of vegetables has been suggested in several studies; high intake of meat, diary products, total fat, and saturated fat might represent a risk factor. The evidence concerning other dietary factors, including fruit intake and intake of specific micronutrients, is inconclusive at present, including that of lycopene, a retinoid present in particular in tomatoes which has been found to be associated with a reduced risk in a few (but not other) studies, and calcium which has been associated with elevated risk, possibly on account of its influence on vitamin D balance (Giovannucci 2005). An increased risk of the disease has been repeatedly reported among subjects with a high weight or body mass (Platz *et al.* 2006).

The wide geographical variability of prostate cancer strongly suggests that environmental factors likely related to diet and other lifestyle factors, such as physical activity, are important determinants of the disease. Primary prevention, however, is hampered by the fragmentary knowledge of its precise causes. Secondary prevention has been proposed, based on digital rectal examination and measurement of PSA. There is no evidence from controlled trials that either procedure decreases the mortality from prostate cancer (Boyle *et al.* 2003). Despite this lack of evidence, these procedures, in particular the PSA testing, have gained popularity in many countries, and are the cause of the steep increase in number of diagnosed cased since the mid-1980s in North America and other high-resource countries. It is unclear whether the decrease in mortality reported since the mid-1990s in the United States and in Western Europe can be partly attributed to a beneficial effect of unplanned use of PSA testing, but it is likely due mainly to improved treatment of the disease.

Testicular cancer

Some 95 per cent of malignant neoplasms of the testis arise from the germinal tissue. About half of the germinal neoplasms are seminomas, while the remaining comprise teratomas and a variety of rare lesions. Testicular cancer is common in young age, and its incidence decreases after age 30 (Fig. 9.3.8). Teratomas and other non-seminomatous neoplasms predominate before age 15, after which most tumours are seminomas. Incidence rates are high (3/100 000 or more) in Latin America and Western Europe and are low (1/100 000 or less) in most of Africa and in Eastern and Southern Asia (IARC 2002a). In the United States, rates are higher in European Americans than in African Americans. The global number of new cases in 2002 has been estimated at 50 000, that of deaths at 9000 (Ferlay *et al.* 2004). The incidence has increased in most countries during the last decades, with evidence of a birth cohort effect. In many countries, the risk if higher in the more affluent groups of the population.

Cryptorchism is the best known cause of testicular cancer (Sarma *et al.* 2006). The RR is in the order of 2 to 5; this risk factor might

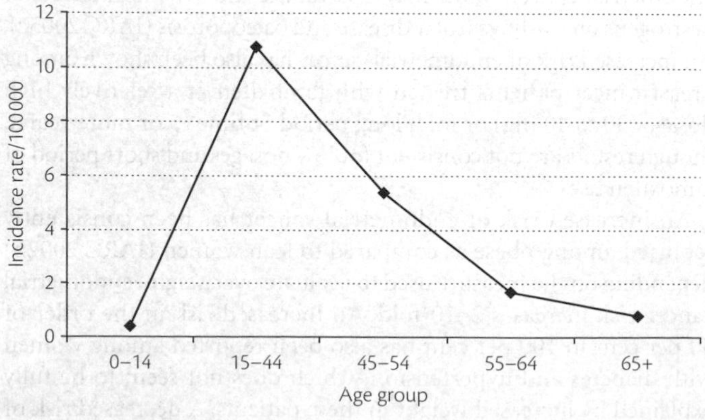

Fig. 9.3.8 Age-specific incidence rates of testicular cancer, United States 2002.

be responsible for up to 10 per cent of all cases of testicular cancer. The risk is lower when orchiopexy is performed before age 10 than at older ages (Pettersson *et al.* 2007). This suggests that micro-environmental factors might be responsible for the development of cancer in the undescended testis. Several rare diseases in gonadal differentiation, including Klinefelter's syndrome, increase the risk of non-germinal tumours of the testis. Exposure to elevated oestrogen levels during pregnancy, from either endogenous or exogenous origin, might be a risk factor for testicular cancer, although the evidence of an association is not fully consistent among studies. Familial aggregation has also been shown for different types of testicular cancer.

The limited knowledge about the causes of testicular cancer makes it difficult to devise effective preventive strategies, with the exception of early surgical treatment of cryptorchism.

Testicular cancer, particularly seminomas and teratomas in young men, is one of the most curable neoplasms if adequate treatment is adopted. Substantial differences in mortality from this neoplasm were found between Western and Eastern European countries, probably due to different availability of the expensive drugs required to treat testicular cancer (Levi *et al.* 2003). Likewise mortality from testicular cancer substantially declined in North America, but less so in Central and South America (Bertuccio *et al.* 2007). Widespread adoption of efficacious therapy worldwide is therefore a priority to avoid unnecessary deaths from testicular cancer in young men.

Childhood cancer

Acute lymphoblasts leukaemia and acute myeloid leukaemia account for the large majority of childhood leukaemias, and hence for over 50 per cent of all childhood cancers in most population.

Several chromosomal rearrangements are present in childhood leukaemia, and Down syndrome and ataxia-telangeciasia appreciably increase the risk of both types of leukaemia. In utero diagnostic radiation was associated to the risk of both types of childhood leukaemia, but the doses have substantially decreased over the last few decades, and consequently the public health implications are now minor. Childhood leukaemia is directly related to higher socioeconomic status, and both types of leukaemias have been related to a rare and late response to infection, though the pathogenic agent has and not been established. The role of other risk factors, including non-ionizing radiation, maternal smoking, paternal occupation, exposure to benzene or pesticides remains unclear (Ross *et al.* 2006).

Central nervous system cancers of various histologic types account for about one in six childhood cancers. They have been associated to nitrosamines, polyoma viruses, and pesticides, but the evidence is not conclusive and there is no established cause. Except for astrocitoma survival is relatively lower than for most other childhood cancers.

Hodgkin lymphoma (HL) in children has also been related to higher socioeconomics status, and shows a genetic predisposition. Its prognosis has substantially improved over the last few decades, and now survival is over 90 per cent in high-resource countries.

Most non-Hodgkin lymphoma (NHL) in children are high-grade tumours, including lymphoblastic lymphoma, Burkitt lymphoma and anaplastic lymphoma. Burkitt lymphoma accounts from most cases diagnosed in Africa, and is related to EBV infection. Apart from genetic factors (ataxia-telangectasia, Wiscott Aldrich syndrome), no other risk factor is known.

Table 9.3.6 European code against cancer

Many aspects of general health can be improved, and many cancer deaths prevented, if we adopt healthier lifestyles:

1. Do not smoke; if you smoke, stop doing so. If you fail to stop, do not smoke in the presence of non-smokers.
2. Avoid obesity.
3. Undertake some brisk, physical activity every day.
4. Increase your daily intake and variety of vegetables and fruits: eat at least five servings daily. Limit your intake of foods containing fats from animal sources.
5. If you drink alcohol, whether beer, wine, or spirits, moderate your consumption to two drinks per day if you are a man or one drink per day if you are a woman.
6. Care must be taken to avoid excessive sun exposure. It is specifically important to protect children and adolescents. For individuals who have a tendency to burn in the sun active protective+ measures must be taken throughout life.
7. Apply strictly regulations aimed at preventing any exposure to known cancer-causing substances. Follow all health and safety instructions on substances which may cause cancer. Follow advice of National Radiation Protection Offices.

There are public health programmes that could prevent cancers developing or increase the probability that a cancer may be cured:

8. Women from 25 years of age should participate in cervical screening. This should be within programmes with quality control procedures in compliance with *European Guidelines for Quality Assurance in Cervical Screening.*
9. Women from 50 years of age should participate in breast screening. This should be within programmes with quality control procedures in compliance with *European Guidelines for Quality Assurance in Mammography Screening.*
10. Men and women from 50 years of age should participate in colorectal screening. This should be within programmes with built-in quality assurance procedures.
11. Participate in vaccination programmes against hepatitis B virus infection.

Other types of childhood cancer include soft tissue sarcoma, neuroblastoma, renal cell cancers (Wilms tumour), bone tumours (osteosarcoma, Ewing sarcoma) germ cell cancers, hepatoblastoma and RB. The latter is related to the RB gene.

The advancements in treatment of childhood cancer were later and inadequate in Eastern Europe in South America, and in most all middle and low resource countries. At ages 15–19 years, a different proportional composition of various neoplasms is observed, with a rise of testicular cancer in boys, germ cell ovarian neoplasms in girls and, mostly, bone cancer in both genders combined. Nonetheless, mortality from all neoplasms, as well as from leukaemias, declined by over 50 per cent since the late 1960s in North America at in Western Europe, while in Eastern Europe and in other low and middle resource areas of the world some decline in cancer mortality was observed only during the last two decades, again reflecting the delayed and inadequate adoption of efficacious treatment for various cancers. This is reflected also within each neoplasm, including the ones most amenable to treatment, such as HL or leukaemia, and calls for urgent widespread adoption of modern and integrated treatment for childhood and adolescent cancers worldwide.

Conclusion

Neoplasms are a group of diverse diseases with complex distributions in human populations and with different aetiological factors. Current knowledge of the causes of human neoplasms and the development of control strategies have led to the elaboration of lists of recommendations for their prevention (Table 9.3.6). A comprehensive strategy for cancer control might lead to the avoidance of a sizeable proportion of human cancers, and the greatest benefit can be achieved via tobacco control. However, such a strategy would imply major cultural, societal, and economic changes. More modest objectives for cancer prevention should focus on the neoplasms and the exposures that are prevalent in any given population. For example, vaccination of children against HBV is likely to be the most cost-effective cancer prevention action in many countries of Africa and Asia.

Neoplasms will continue to be a major source of human disease and death. Considerable efforts are made in the public and private domains to develop effective therapeutic approaches. Even if major discoveries in the clinical management of cancer patients will be accomplished in the near future, the changes will mainly affect the affluent part of the world population. Prevention of the known causes of cancer remains the most promising approach in reducing the consequences of cancer, in particular in countries with limited resources. Control of tobacco smoking and of smokeless tobacco products, reduced overweight and obesity, moderation in alcohol intake, increased physical activity, avoidance of exposure to solar radiation, and control of known occupational carcinogens are the main approaches we currently have to reduce the burden of human neoplasms.

References

Amundadottir L.T., Sulem P., Gudmundsson J. *et al.* (2006). A common variant associated with prostate cancer in European and African populations. *Nat Genet*, **38**, 652–658.

Anderson G.L., Judd H.L., Kaunitz A.M. *et al.* (2003). Effects of estrogen plus progestin on gynecologic cancers and associated diagnostic procedures: the Women's Health Initiative randomized trial. *JAMA*, **290**, 1739–1748.

Baan R., Straif K., Grosse Y. *et al.* (2007). Carcinogenicity of alcoholic beverages. *Lancet Oncol*, **8**, 292–293.

Bach P.B., Jett J.R., Pastorino U., Tockman M.S., Swensen S.J., Begg C.B. (2007). Computed tomography screening and lung cancer outcomes. *JAMA*, **297**, 953–961.

Bailey-Wilson J.E., Amos C.I., Pinney S.M. *et al.* (2004). A major lung cancer susceptibility locus maps to chromosome 6q23-25. *Am J Hum Genet*, **75**, 460–474.

Bergstrom A., Pisani P., Tenet V., Wolk A., Adami H.O. (2001). Overweight as an avoidable cause of cancer in Europe. *Int J Cancer*, **91**, 421–430.

Berrino F., Capocaccia R., Esteve J. *et al.* (1999). Survival of Cancer Patients in Europe: the EUROCARE-2 Study. *IARC Sci. Publ.* No. 151. IARC, Lyon.11

Bertuccio P., Malvezzi M., Chatenoud L. *et al.* (2007). Testicular cancer mortality in the Americas, 1980-2003. *Cancer*, **109**, 776–779.

Blot W.J. (1997). Vitamin/mineral supplementation and cancer risk: international chemoprevention trials. *Proc Soc Exp Biol Med*, **216**, 291–296.

Boffetta P. (2006). Human cancer from environmental pollutants: the epidemiological evidence. *Mutat Res*, **608**, 157–162.

Boffetta P., Hashibe M. (2006a). Alcohol and cancer. *Lancet Oncol*, **7**, 149–156.

Boffetta P., Stayner L. (2006b). Pleural and Peritoneal Neoplasms. In Schottenfeld D., Fraumeni J.F., eds. Cancer Epidemiology and Prevention. Oxford University Press, New York. pp.659–673.

Bosetti C., Gallus S., La Vecchia C. (2006). Aspirin and cancer risk: an updated quantitative review to 2005. *Cancer Causes Control*, **17**, 871–888.

Bosetti C., Levi F., Boffetta P., Lucchini F., Negri E., La Vecchia C. (2008). Trend in mortality from hepatocellular carcinoma in Europe, 1980-2004. *Hepatol*, **48**, 137–145.

Boyle P., Autier P., Bartelink H. *et al.* (2003). European Code Against Cancer and scientific justification: third version (2003). *Ann Oncol*, **14**, 973–1005.

Chlebowski R.T., Hendrix S.L., Langer R.D. *et al.* (2003). Influence of estrogen plus progestin on breast cancer and mammography in healthy postmenopausal women: the Women's Health Initiative Randomized Trial. *JAMA*, **289**, 3243–3253.

Clifford G.M., Gallus S., Herrero R. *et al.* (2005). Worldwide distribution of human papillomavirus types in cytologically normal women in the International Agency for Research on Cancer HPV prevalence surveys: a pooled analysis. *Lancet*, **366**, 991–998.

Colditz G.A., Baer H.J., Tamimi R.M. (2006). Breast Cancer. In Schottenfeld D, Fraumeni JF, eds. Cancer Epidemiology and Prevention. Oxford University Press, New York. pp.995–1012.

Collaborative Group on Hormonal Factors in Breast Cancer (2002). Breast cancer and breastfeeding: collaborative reanalysis of individual data from 47 epidemiological studies in 30 countries, including 50302 women with breast cancer and 96973 women without the disease. *Lancet*, **360**, 187–195.

Cook L.S., Weis N.S., Doherty J.A., Chen C. (2006). Endometrial Cancer. In Schottenfeld D, Fraumeni JF, eds. Cancer Epidemiology and Prevention. Oxford University Press, New York. pp.1027–1043.

Doll R., Peto R. (2005). Epidemiology of cancer. In Warell D.A., Cox T.M., Firth J.D., eds. Oxford Textbook of Medicine. Volume 3. 4th Edition. Oxford University Press, New York. pp.193–218.

El Serag H.B. (2004). Hepatocellular carcinoma: recent trends in the United States. *Gastroenterology*, **127**, S27–S34.

Ferlay J., Bray F., Pisani P., Parkin M. (2004). Cancer Incidence, Mortality and Prevalence Worldwide. Globocan 2002. IARC CancerBase N°5, version 2.0. IARC Press, Lyon.

Fernandez E., La Vecchia C., Gonzalez J.R., Lucchini F., Negri E., Levi F. (2005). Converging patterns of colorectal cancer mortality in Europe. *Eur J Cancer*, **41**, 430–437.

Gauderman W.J., Morrison J.L., Carpenter C.L., Thomas D.C. (1997). Analysis of gene-smoking interaction in lung cancer. *Genet Epidemiol*, **14**, 199–214.

Giovannucci E. (2005). The epidemiology of vitamin D and cancer incidence and mortality: a review (United States). *Cancer Causes Control*, **16**, 83–95.

Greenwald P. (2005). Lifestyle and medical approaches to cancer prevention. *Recent Results Cancer Res*, **166**, 1–15.

Gruber S.B., Armstrong B.K. (2006). Cutaneous and ocular melanoma. In Schottenfeld D, Fraumeni JF, eds. Cancer Epidemiology and Prevention. Oxford University Press, New York. pp.1196–1229.

Gudmundsson J., Sulem P., Manolescu A. *et al.* (2007a). Genome-wide association study identifies a second prostate cancer susceptibility variant at 8q24. *Nat Genet*, **39**, 631–637.

Gudmundsson J., Sulem P., Steinthorsdottir V. *et al.* (2007b). Two variants on chromosome 17 confer prostate cancer risk, and the one in TCF2 protects against type 2 diabetes. *Nat Genet*, **39**, 977–983

Haiman C.A., Patterson N., Freedman M.L. *et al.* (2007). Multiple regions within 8q24 independently affect risk for prostate cancer. *Nat Genet*, **39**, 638–644.

Hanahan D., Weinberg R.A. (2000). The hallmarks of cancer. *Cell*, **100**, 57–70.

Hankinson S.E., Danforth K.N. (2006). Ovarian. In Schottenfeld D., Fraumeni J.F., eds. Cancer Epidemiology and Prevention. Oxford University Press, New York. pp.1013–1026.

Harvard Center for Cancer Prevention (1996). Harvard report on cancer prevention, Volume 1: Causes of human cancer. *Cancer Causes Control*, **7**, S3–S58.

Hsing A.W., Rashid A., Devesa S.S., Fraumeni J.F. (2006). Biliary tract cancer. In Schottenfeld D., Fraumeni J.F., eds. Cancer Epidemiology and Prevention. Oxford University Press, New York. pp.787–800.

IARC (1998a). IARC Handbooks of Cancer Prevention. Volume 3. Vitamin A. IARC Press, Lyon. pp.1–261.

IARC (1998b). IARC Handbooks of Cancer Prevention. Volume 2. Carotenoids. IARC Press, Lyon. pp.1–326.

IARC (2000). X-radiation and y-radiation. In IARC Monographs on the Evaluation of Carcinogenic Risks to Humans. Volume 75. Ionizing radiation, Part 1: X- and Gamma (y)-Radiation, and Neutrons. IARC, Lyon. pp.121–362.

IARC (2001a). IARC Monographs on the Evaluation of Carcinogenic Risks to Humans. Volume 78. Ionizing radiation, Part 2: Some internally deposited radionuclides. IARC Press, Lyon. pp.1–563.

IARC (2002a). Parkin DM, Whelan SL, Ferlay J, Teppo L, Thomas DB, eds. Scientific Publication No. 155. Volume 8. Cancer Incidence in Five Continents. IARC, Lyon. pp.1–781.

IARC (2002b). IARC Handbooks of Cancer Prevention. Volume 6. Weight Control and Physical Activity. IARC Press, Lyon. pp.1–315.

IARC (2003). IARC Handbooks of Cancer Prevention. Volume 8. Fruit and Vegetables. IARC Press, Lyon. pp.1–376.

IARC (2004a). Tobacco smoke. In IARC Monographs on the Evaluation of the Carcinogenic Risks to Humans. Volume 83. Tobacco Smoke and Involuntary Smoking. IARC, Lyon. pp.51–1187.

IARC (2004b). IARC Handbooks of Cancer Prevention. Volume 9. Cruciferous Vegetables, Isothiocyanates and Indoles. IARC Press, Lyon. pp.1–262.

IARC (2004c). IARC Monographs on the Evaluation of Carcinogenic Risks to Humans. Volume 89. Smokeless Tobacco Products. IARC, Lyon. pp.**708**–708.

IARC (2005b). Combined Estrogen-Progestogen Contraceptives. In IARC Monographs on the Evaluation of Carcinogenic Risks to Humans. Volume 91. Combined Estrogen-progestogen Contraceptives and Combined Estrogen-progestogen Menopausal Therapy. IARC, Lyon. pp.1–22. In press.

IARC (2005c). Combined Estrogen-Progestogen Menopausal Therapy. In IARC Monographs on the Evaluation of Carcinogenic Risks to Humans. Volume 91. Combined Estrogen-progestogen Contraceptives and Combined Estrogen-progestogen Menopausal Therapy. IARC, Lyon. pp.1–11. In press.

IARC (2006). IARC Monographs on the Evaluation of Carcinogenic Risks to Humans. Volume 95. Household Combustion of Solid Fuels and High-temperature Frying. IARC, Lyon. pp.977–978.

Jepsen P., Vilstrup H., Tarone R.E., Friis S., Sorensen H.T. (2007). Incidence rates of intra- and extrahepatic cholangiocarcinomas in Denmark from 1978 through 2002. *J Natl Cancer Inst*, **99**, 895–897.

Karagas M.R., Weinstock M.A., Nelson H.H. (2006). Keratinocyte carcinomas (basal and squamous cell carcinomas of the skin). In Schottenfeld D, Fraumeni JF, eds. Cancer Epidemiology and Prevention. Oxford University Press, New York. pp.1230–1250.

Kato I., Canzian F., Plummer M. *et al.* (2007). Polymorphisms in genes related to bacterial lipopolysaccharide/peptidoglycan signaling and gastric precancerous lesions in a population at high risk for gastric cancer. *Dig Dis Sci*, **52**, 254–261.

Kosary C.L., Ries L.A.G., Miller B.A., Hankey B.F., Harras A., Edwards B.K. (1995). SEER Cancer Statistics Review, 1973-1992: Tables and Graphs. NIH Publication No. 96-2789. National Cancer Institute, Bethesda.

La Vecchia C. (2007). Alcohol and liver cancer. *Eur J Cancer Prev*, **16**, 495–497

La Vecchia C., Altieri A., Franceschi S., Tavani A. (2001). Oral contraceptives and cancer: an update. *Drug Saf*, **24**, 741–754.

Lagiou P., Adami H.O., Trichopoulos D. (2006). Early life diet and the risk for adult breast cancer. *Nutr Cancer*, **56**, 158–161.

Levi F., Lucchini F., Boyle P., Negri E., and La Vecchia C. (2003). Testicular cancer mortality in Eastern Europe. *Int J Cancer*, **105**, 574–574.

Levi F., Lucchini F., Negri E., La Vecchia C. (2004a) Trends in mortality from major cancers in the European Union, including acceding countries. *Cancer*, **101**, 2843–2850.

Levi F., Lucchini F., Negri E., Boyle P., La Vecchia C. (2004b). Leveling of prostate cancer mortality in Western Europe. *Prostate*, **60**, 46–52.

Levi F., Randimbison L., Maspoli M., Te V.C., La Vecchia C. (2006). High incidence of second basal cell skin cancers. *Int J Cancer*, **119**, 1505–1507.

Lim H.S., Roychoudhuri R., Peto J., Schwartz G., Baade P., Moller H. (2006). Cancer survival is dependent on season of diagnosis and sunlight exposure. *Int J Cancer*, **119**, 1530–1536.

London W.T., McGlynn K.A. (2006). Liver Cancer. In Schottenfeld D., Fraumeni J.F., eds. Cancer Epidemiology and Prevention. Oxford University Press, New York. pp.763–786.

Lubin J.H., Liang Z., Hrubec Z. *et al.* (1994). Radon exposure in residences and lung cancer among women: combined analysis of three studies. *Cancer Causes Control*, **5**, 114–128.

Marques-Vidal P., Ravasco P., Ermelinda C.M. (2006). Foodstuffs and colorectal cancer risk: a review. *Clin Nutr*, **25**, 14–36.

Michels K.B., Mohllajee A.P., Roset-Bahmanyar E., Beehler G.P., Moysich K.B. (2007). Diet and breast cancer: a review of the prospective observational studies. *Cancer*, **109**, 2712–2749.

Murray C.J., Lopez A.D. (1996). Evidence-based health policy--lessons from the Global Burden of Disease Study. *Science*, **274**, 740–743.

Negri E., Pelucchi C., Talamini R. *et al.* (2005). Family history of cancer and the risk of prostate cancer and benign prostatic hyperplasia. *Int J Cancer*, **114**, 648–652.

Parkin D.M. (2006). The global health burden of infection-associated cancers in the year 2002. *Int J Cancer*, **118**, 3030–3044.

Pettersson A., Richiardi L., Nordenskjold A., Kaijser M., and Akre O. (2007). Age at surgery for undescended testis and risk of testicular cancer. *N Engl J Med*, **356**, 1835–1841.

Peto R. (1977). Epidemiology, multistage models and short-term mutagenicity tests. In Origins of human cancer. In Hiatt H.H., Watson J.D., Winsten J.A., eds. Cold Spring Harbor Laboratory, *Cold Spring Harbor*, pp.1403–1428.

Peto J., Decarli A., La Vecchia C., Levi F., Negri E. (1999). The European mesothelioma epidemic. *Br J Cancer*, **79**, 666–672.

Peto R., Darby S., Deo H., Silcocks P., Whitley E., Doll R. (2000). Smoking, smoking cessation, and lung cancer in the UK since 1950: combination of national statistics with two case-control studies. *BMJ*, **321**, 323–329.

Peto R., Gray R., Brantom P., and Grasso P. (1991). Effects on 4080 rats of chronic ingestion of N-nitrosodiethylamine or N-nitrosodimethylamine: a detailed dose-response study. *Cancer Res*, **51**, 6415–6451.

Platz E.A., Giovannucci E. (2006). Prostate Cancer. In Schottenfeld D., Fraumeni J.F., eds. Cancer Epidemiology and Prevention. Oxford University Press, New York. pp.1128–1150.

Plummer M., Vivas J., Lopez G. *et al.* (2007). Chemoprevention of precancerous gastric lesions with antioxidant vitamin supplementation: a randomized trial in a high-risk population. *J Natl Cancer Inst*, **99**, 137–146.

Randi G., Franceschi S., La Vecchia C. (2006). Gallbladder cancer worldwide: geographical distribution and risk factors. *Int J Cancer*, **118**, 1591–1602.

Ross J.A., Spector L.G. (2006). Cancers in Children. In Schottenfeld D., Fraumeni J.F., eds. Cancer Epidemiology and Prevention. Oxford University Press, New York. pp.1251–1268.

Sankaranarayanan R., Black R.J., Swaminathan R., Parkin D.M. (1998). An overview of cancer survival in developing countries. In: Sankaranarayanan R., Black R.J., and Parkin D.M., eds. Cancer Survival in Developing Countries. IARC Sci Publ No. 145, Lyon. pp.135–173.

Sarma A.V., McLaughlin J.C., Schottenfeld D. (2006). Testicular Cancer. In Schottenfeld D., Fraumeni J.F., eds. Cancer Epidemiology and Prevention. Oxford University Press, New York. pp.1151–1165.

Schiffman M.H., Hildesheim A. (2006). Cervical Cancer. In Schottenfeld D., Fraumeni J.F., eds. Cancer Epidemiology and Prevention. Oxford University Press, New York. pp.1044–1067.

Speizer F.E., Samet J.M. (1994). Air pollution and lung cancer. In Epidemiology of lung cancer. Volume 74. Lung Biology in Health Disease. Marcel Dekker, New York. pp.131–150.

Spitz M.R., Wu X., Wilkinson A., Wei Q. (2006). Cancer of the Lung. In Schottenfeld D, Fraumeni JF, eds. Cancer Epidemiology and Prevention. Oxford University Press, New York. pp.638–658.

Steenland K., Burnett C., Lalich N., Ward E., Hurrell J. (2003). Dying for work: The magnitude of US mortality from selected causes of death associated with occupation. *Am J Ind Med*, **43**, 461–482.

Stefanick M.L., Anderson G.L., Margolis K.L. *et al.* (2006). Effects of conjugated equine estrogens on breast cancer and mammography screening in postmenopausal women with hysterectomy. *JAMA*, **295**, 1647–1657.

The Future II Study Group (2007). Quadrivalent vaccine against human papillomavirus to prevent high-grade cervical lesions. *N Engl J Med*, **356**, 1915–1927.

Tuohimaa P., Pukkala E., Scelo G. *et al.* (2007). Does solar exposure, as indicated by the non-melanoma skin cancers, protect from solid cancers: Vitamin D as a possible explanation. *Eur J Cancer*, **11**, 1701–1712.

WHO (1990). International Classification of Diseases for Oncology (ICD-O). World Health Organization, Edition 2, Geneva.

Yeager M., Orr N., Hayes R.B. *et al.* (2007). Genome-wide association study of prostate cancer identifies a second risk locus at 8q24. *Nat Genet*, **39**, 645–649.

9.4

Chronic obstructive pulmonary disease and asthma

Jeroen Douwes, Marike Boezen, and Neil Pearce

Abstract

In this chapter, we will describe definitions of chronic obstructive pulmonary disease (COPD) and asthma, possible mechanisms, time trends, and population patterns of prevalence, and evidence regarding the causes of both diseases. COPD and asthma are highly prevalent non-malignant respiratory conditions that have increased dramatically in the past few decades, both in Western and non-Western societies. They have a profound impact on the quality of life for patients and their families, and COPD is also a major cause of death.

The major causal risk factor for COPD is tobacco smoke, although a substantial proportion of COPD is also caused by occupational exposures and indoor environmental exposures, particularly in middle- and low-income countries. Although cigarette smoking is the major risk factor for COPD, usually only a relatively small proportion of smokers develop COPD, a pattern which may be explained by genetic susceptibility factors. Similar to asthma, COPD prevalence differs greatly between countries and these differences are not explained by cigarette smoking alone. Nonetheless, smoking cessation is the most effective way to halt global increases in the prevalence of COPD. Improved indoor ventilation measures to reduce indoor pollutants in houses of most middle- and low-income countries are also effective ways to reduce morbidity and mortality, particularly in the developing world.

A large number of potential risk factors for asthma have been identified including genetic factors, allergen exposure, demographic parameters, diet, obesity, indoor and outdoor pollution, passive and active tobacco smoking, occupational exposures, viral infections, and the use of paracetamol (acetaminophen). However, none of these risk factors on their own appear to explain the substantial global increases in asthma prevalence observed over the last few decades. They also cannot explain the significant differences in asthma prevalence between countries. Interestingly, recent studies have shown that the increase in asthma prevalence appears to have levelled off in many high-income countries, with some even showing a decrease. The reasons for this are unclear. Understanding why these changes in prevalence are occurring, and ascertaining which elements of the 'package' of twentieth-century economic development and lifestyle changes are responsible, is essential in order to develop effective intervention programmes to halt the current global asthma epidemic.

Introduction

The most common non-malignant respiratory conditions characterized by airway dysfunction are often collectively referred to as obstructive airway diseases and comprise several clinical disease entities including chronic obstructive pulmonary disease (COPD) and asthma. Both conditions are highly prevalent and have increased dramatically in the past few decades, both in Western and non-Western societies (Douwes & Pearce 2002; Mannino & Buist 2007). They have a profound impact on the quality of life for patients and their families. In addition, COPD accounts for several million premature deaths per year worldwide (Lopez *et al.* 2006a).

COPD is usually defined as airflow obstruction due to inflammation of the peripheral airways and lung parenchyma, in which the airflow limitation is not fully reversible and progresses over time. Asthma is a heterogeneous chronic inflammatory disorder of the airways involving airflow limitation, which is variable and reversible. Thus, the critical difference between the definitions of the two conditions is whether airflow obstruction is reversible. However, it is now well recognized that airway obstruction in some asthmatics is only partially reversible. Also, acute and chronic reversibility of airway obstruction has been described in COPD patients. COPD and asthma are therefore partially overlapping conditions that share some clinical features. They also share some common risk factors including various environmental and occupational exposures. Based on these similarities, it has been suggested that COPD and asthma should not be considered as separate diseases rather as different expressions of the same disease entity. This theory, proposed in 1961 and known as the *Dutch hypothesis*, has since been heavily debated with compelling arguments both in favour (Kraft 2006) and against (Barnes 2006).

In this chapter, we will describe both conditions in parallel. We first consider definitions, possible mechanisms, time trends, and population patterns of prevalence. Then, we consider the evidence regarding risk factors for exacerbations as well as the initial development of both diseases.

Definitions

COPD

Traditionally, COPD has been defined as 'irreversible airflow obstruction due to chronic bronchitis and emphysema, which progresses over time' (Petty 2006). Emphysema was already described in the seventeenth and eighteenth century (Petty 2006), and one of the first reports of chronic bronchitis as a serious and disabling disorder appeared in 1814 (Badham 1814). It was only a few years later that Laënnec (1821) made the observation that chronic bronchitis and emphysema often occurred in the same subject at the same time (Petty 2002, 2006). However, it was not until about 150 years later that Burrows *et al.* (1966) suggested labelling the spectrum of chronic bronchitis and emphysema as 'chronic obstructive lung disease', or COPD as it is currently most often referred to. A few years before that, the CIBA Guest Symposium (1959) and the American Thoracic Society symposium (Committee on Diagnostic Standards for Nontuberculous Respiratory Diseases 1962) proposed the first definitions of chronic bronchitis and emphysema, respectively. Our current definitions are still largely based on these initial definitions; that is chronic bronchitis is defined clinically as 'the presence of chronic productive cough for at least three consecutive months in two consecutive years'; emphysema, on the other hand, is defined in pathological terms as 'an increase in the size of the distal airspaces and destruction of their walls without obvious fibrosis' (American Thoracic Society Committee on Diagnostic Standards 1962).

The most recent definitions of COPD as reported in the American Thoracic Society (ATS), European Respiratory Society (ERS), and the Global Initiative for Chronic Obstructive Lung Disease (GOLD) guidelines emphasize the inflammatory response to noxious particles and gases as the predominant pathological feature of the disease, and have parted from the definition of COPD as being a syndrome of chronic bronchitis and emphysema. The widely accepted GOLD definition states that COPD is:

> *A preventable and treatable disease with some significant extra pulmonary effects that may contribute to the severity in individual patients. Its pulmonary component is characterized by airflow limitation that is not fully reversible. The airflow limitation is usually progressive and associated with an abnormal inflammatory response of the lung to noxious particles or gases* (Rabe *et al.* 2007)

Although no longer specifically included in the definition, it is still recognized that chronic bronchitis and emphysema are important causes of the chronic airflow limitation characteristic of COPD. The three main components (inflammation, airflow limitation that is not fully reversible, and a gradual loss of lung function over time) represent the major pathophysiological events leading to the symptoms typically expressed by those with COPD: Chronic and progressive cough, sputum production, and dyspnoea (difficult or laboured breathing). Cough and sputum production may precede the development of airflow limitation by many years, but fixed airflow obstruction may also develop without these symptoms (Petty 2006).

Clinical COPD

Spirometry is an essential tool in the clinical diagnosis of COPD and there are well-accepted standardized guidelines (Miller *et al.* 2005). In COPD, the maximum volume of air that can be forcibly expired (forced vital capacity [FVC]) is generally not affected, or only marginally affected; the volume of air exhaled in the first second of expiration (forced expiratory volume in one second [FEV_1]), on the other hand, is significantly reduced and is a clear marker of airway obstruction. COPD is therefore defined based on the post-bronchodilator FEV_1/FVC ratio. A cut-off point of 0.7 (i.e. 70 per cent) is widely used (Rabe *et al.* 2007), but this has not been clinically validated. Also, it is well recognized that using a fixed FEV_1/FVC ratio to define COPD independent of age has the potential for significant misclassification, with underdiagnosis in younger adults and overdiagnosis in the elderly (Medbo & Melbye 2007). Bronchodilator treatment prior to spirometry is important because it establishes whether obstruction is irreversible and distinguishes it from asthma in which obstruction is mostly reversible.

The degree of severity of COPD (defined as a FEV_1/FVC < 70 per cent) is usually based on the patient's FEV_1. The 2006 GOLD criteria classify COPD severity into four stages (Rabe *et al.* 2007):

Stage I, mild: $FEV_1 \geq 80$ per cent predicted.

Stage II, moderate: 50 per cent $\leq FEV_1 \geq 80$ per cent predicted.

Stage III, severe: 30 per cent $\leq FEV_1 \geq 50$ per cent predicted.

Stage IV, very severe: $FEV_1 < 30$ per cent predicted *or* $FEV_1 < 50$ per cent predicted *plus* chronic respiratory failure (i.e. arterial pressure of oxygen [PaO_2] less than 8 kPa [60 mm Hg] with or without arterial pressure of CO_2 [$PaCO_2$] greater than 6.7 kPa [50 mm Hg] while breathing air at sea level).

Previous GOLD guidelines also listed a 'Stage 0, at risk' level, which included those with respiratory symptoms such as chronic cough and sputum production but normal lung function. This is no longer included in the 2006 guidelines as there is insufficient evidence that the individuals who meet these criteria necessarily progress on to Stage I.

Despite the well-accepted guidelines for diagnosis, and the availability of inexpensive and convenient hand-held spirometers, COPD remains a significantly underdiagnosed disease particularly in younger people and women (Halbert *et al.* 2006). This is largely because those with mild COPD often have no symptoms, or they have symptoms that are not perceived by patients and healthcare providers as abnormal, therefore not warranting a spirometric assessment. Similarly, subjects may be less likely to be diagnosed with COPD if there is no history of smoking, one of the best-known risk factors for COPD.

Defining COPD in epidemiological surveys

In population-based surveys, COPD is often defined on the basis of (1) self-report of a doctor diagnosis of COPD, bronchitis, or emphysema; (2) self-report of respiratory symptoms; and (3) spirometry with or without prior bronchodilator treatment. It has repeatedly been shown that self-reports of a clinical diagnosis significantly underestimate the true disease prevalence (Chapman *et al.* 2006). In a recent meta-analysis using population-based prevalence estimates during the period 1990–2004, it was shown that spirometric criteria resulted in an almost twofold higher prevalence estimate compared with patient-reported COPD; i.e., 9.2 per cent versus 4.9 per cent, respectively (Halbert *et al.* 2006). This is probably largely due to the general underdiagnosis of COPD by most general practitioners.

Spirometric assessment to define COPD is therefore superior to a clinical assessment without spirometry, or a self-report of doctor-diagnosed COPD. However, the use of bronchodilators significantly complicates large population-based spirometry surveys and many studies therefore do not collect post-bronchodilator measurements. The implications of failing to check for reversibility of airflow obstruction (using pre- and post-bronchodilator spirometry) may, however, result in an overestimation of the prevalence. For example, in a study in a random population sample of 2235 Norwegian adults aged 26–82 years, the prevalence of COPD based on post-bronchodilator measurements was 7 per cent compared to 9.6 per cent for pre-bronchodilator measurements (Johannessen *et al.* 2005). Thus, post-bronchodilator spirometry to determine the diagnosis of COPD in population-based studies is strongly recommended.

Asthma

The word 'asthma' comes from a Greek word meaning 'panting' (Keeney 1964), but reference to asthma can also be found in ancient Egyptian, Hebrew, and Indian medical writings (Unger & Harris 1974; Ellul-Micallef 1976). Asthma has puzzled and confused physicians and patients from the time of Hippocrates to the present day. There were clear observations of patients experiencing attacks of asthma in the second century and evidence of disordered anatomy in the lung as far back as the seventeenth century (Willis 1678).

The definition of asthma initially proposed at the Ciba Foundation conference in 1959 (CIBA Foundation Guest Symposium 1959) and endorsed by the American Thoracic Society in 1962 (American Thoracic Society Committee on Diagnostic Standards 1962) is that 'asthma is a disease characterized by wide variation over short periods of time in resistance to flow in the airways of the lung'. Although these features receive lesser prominence in some current definitions, as the importance of airways inflammation is appropriately recognized, they still form the basis of the recent Global Initiative for Asthma (GINA) description of asthma, as follows:

> *A chronic inflammatory disorder of the airways in which many cells and cellular elements play a role. The chronic inflammation is associated with airway hyperresponsiveness that leads to recurrent episodes of wheezing, breathlessness, chest tightness, and coughing, particularly at night or in the early morning. These episodes are usually associated with widespread, but variable, airflow obstruction within the lung that is often reversible either spontaneously or with treatment.* (Global Initiative for Asthma 2006)

These three components—chronic airways inflammation, reversible airflow obstruction, and enhanced bronchial reactivity—form the basis of current definitions of asthma. They also represent the major pathophysiological events leading to the symptoms of wheezing, breathlessness, chest tightness, cough, and sputum by which physicians clinically diagnose this disorder.

Clinical asthma

There is no single test or pathognomic feature that defines the presence or absence of asthma. Furthermore, the variability of the condition means that evidence of it may or may not be present on the day, or at the time, that someone is assessed. Thus, a diagnosis of asthma is made on the basis of the clinical history, combined with physical examination and respiratory function tests over a period of time. Several studies have found the prevalence of physician-diagnosed asthma to be substantially lower than the prevalence of asthma symptoms in the community (e.g. Asher *et al.* 1998). This is not surprising because a clinical diagnosis of asthma can only be made if a person presents him or herself to a doctor. This requires an initial self assessment of the symptoms (in terms of severity and frequency), as well as access to a doctor once a self-assessment has been made. Several medical consultations may then be required. Thus, diagnosed asthma is dependent not only on morbidity but also on patient perception of their symptoms, physician practice, and the availability of healthcare.

There are a number of tests that may facilitate the diagnosis and monitoring of asthma. Measurements of lung function are the most frequently used and provide important information on airflow limitation including variability, reversibility, and severity. Airflow limitation is most often measured using spirometry or a peak flow (PEF) meter. Spirometry is the preferred method. Pre- and post-bronchodilator treatment is important because it will establish whether obstruction is irreversible and will distinguish it from COPD in which obstruction is mostly reversible. Reversibility of $FEV_1 \geq 12$ per cent and ≥ 200 mL from the pre-bronchodilator value is generally accepted as a valid indication of asthma (Global Initiative for Asthma 2006). However, due to the highly variable nature of the condition, repeated lung function tests are required. PEF meters are inexpensive and easy to use, but they are less precise and may underestimate the degree of airflow limitation (Aggarwal *et al.* 2006).

In subjects with asthma symptoms but normal lung function, bronchial hyperresponsiveness (BHR) testing is often used as a diagnostic aid. BHR constitutes airway narrowing to non-specific stimuli, such as exercise, cold air, and chemical irritants, and can be measured as airway responsiveness to histamine, methacholine, adenosine-5'-monophosphate (AMP), hypertonic saline or exercise challenge (de Meer *et al.* 2004a). However, although BHR is related to asthma, it may occur independently of asthma, and vice versa (Pearce *et al.* 2000a), which makes this test of limited use for individual asthma diagnostics.

More recently, an increasing number of tests are available to measure non-invasive markers of airway inflammation including sputum induction tests (Simpson *et al.* 2006), exhaled NO tests (Taylor *et al.* 2006), and measurements of inflammatory markers in exhaled breath condensate (Kharitonov & Barnes 2006). Although these may be useful in establishing asthma phenotypes (Simpson et al. 2006; Douwes et al. 2002a) and determining optimal treatment (Smith *et al.* 2005), they have as yet to be demonstrated to aid in asthma diagnosis. Also, with the exception of the exhaled NO test, all other tests require rigorous validation before they can be applied in clinical practice.

The degree of severity is commonly classified using GINA criteria (Global Initiative for Asthma 2006), which subdivide asthma into four categories:

Intermittent: Symptoms less than once a week, brief exacerbations, nocturnal symptoms not more than twice a month, FEV_1 or PEF ≥ 80 per cent predicted, FEV_1 or PEF variability < 20 per cent.

Mild persistent: Symptoms more than once a week but less than once a day, exacerbations may affect activity and sleep, nocturnal symptoms more than twice a month, FEV_1 or PEF ≥ 80 per cent predicted, FEV_1 or PEF variability < 20–30 per cent.

Moderate persistent: Symptoms daily, exacerbations may affect activity and sleep, nocturnal symptoms more than once a week, daily use of inhaled short-acting $\beta 2$-agonist, FEV_1 or PEF = 60–80 per cent predicted, FEV_1 or PEF variability > 30 per cent.

Severe persistent: Symptoms daily, frequent exacerbations, frequent nocturnal asthma symptoms, limitation of physical activities, FEV_1 or PEF ≤ 60 per cent predicted, FEV_1 or PEF variability > 30 per cent.

Defining asthma in epidemiological surveys

Defining and diagnosing asthma in population-based epidemiological surveys of asthma prevalence or incidence poses even greater difficulties than defining asthma in individual patients. Thus, comparisons of diagnosed asthma between populations are fraught with difficulty as the differences in diagnostic practice may be as great in magnitude as the real differences in asthma morbidity.

Thus, asthma prevalence surveys usually focus on self-reported (or parental reported) 'asthma symptoms' rather than diagnosed asthma. Standardized questionnaires on asthma symptoms have therefore become the cornerstone of large studies of the incidence or prevalence of asthma (Burney *et al.* 1994; Asher *et al.* 1995). This approach allows a large number of participants to be surveyed without great cost, in a short time period. Wheezing, chest tightness, breathlessness, and coughing are all symptoms clinically associated with asthma, but epidemiological studies have shown that wheezing is the most important symptom for the identification of asthma, and the majority of questionnaires used to assess asthma prevalence are based on this symptom (Pearce *et al.* 1998).

An alternative approach to symptom questionnaires has been to use more 'objective' measures such as bronchial responsiveness testing, either alone or in combination with questionnaires. In particular, it has been suggested that asthma should be defined in epidemiological studies as symptomatic BHR (Toelle *et al.* 1992). However, some have criticized the use of BHR as a more valid assessment of asthma (Pearce *et al.* 2000a).

Mechanisms, prevalence, and risk factors of COPD

Mechanisms of COPD

Patients with COPD have an impaired ability to exhale air from their lungs. COPD includes emphysema, chronic bronchitis, or a combination of both conditions. Emphysema is characterized by loss of elasticity of the lung tissue and destruction of structures supporting the alveoli. As a result, the small airways collapse during exhaling, which leads to obstruction and trapping of air in the lungs. Chronic bronchitis involves an inflammation of the airways in the lungs resulting in thick mucus, which plugs up the airways and makes it difficult to efficiently inhale air into the lungs.

COPD is a major cause of death throughout the world and is accompanied by a large personal, societal, and economic burden. Patients experience poor physical functioning and live with distressing symptoms that require frequent hospital admission as the disease progresses. They are frequently unable to work and may become socially isolated and depressed. In the Confronting COPD survey, 80 per cent of the patients had two or more symptoms on most or all days, such as breathlessness (45 per cent), cough (46 per cent), and sputum production (40 per cent) (Rennard *et al.* 2002). Just over two thirds of the patients were breathless when walking up a flight of stairs, and one third were breathless getting washed or dressed. In addition, 39 per cent of the patients woke due to their symptoms at least a few nights each week.

As well as living with the daily symptoms of stable disease, patients live with the fear of exacerbations, which are common for all levels of lung disease. Exacerbations are associated with significant mortality, lead to frequent hospitalization, and are a major determinant of COPD costs.

Smoking is the major risk factor for its development, and therefore COPD is largely (but not exclusively) attributable to this environmental factor, with the exception of the genetic predominance of the alpa-1-antitrypsine (AAT) deficiency gene, in which carriers need no further environmental smoke exposure to develop a phenotypic expression of COPD. AAT deficiency accounts for only a minimal number of COPD cases worldwide (<1 per cent); thus, the majority of the COPD cases are due to smoking. However, genetics may also play a role in the development of COPD. In particular, although cigarette smoking is clearly the major risk factor for development of COPD, only a small proportion of smokers develop COPD. These 'susceptible smokers' show premature onset of lung function decline and, to a lesser extent, more rapid rates of decline later in life (Tager *et al.* 1988) In non-smokers, FEV_1 declines at a mean rate of approximately 30 mL/year during adult life, whereas in smokers this is increased to 30–45 mL/year. Within a subset of susceptible cigarette smokers, the rate of decline is 80–100 mL/year, and only 10–20 per cent of Caucasian chronic heavy cigarette smokers develop symptomatic COPD.

The deleterious effect of smoking is due to the fact that cigarette smoke contains a large amount of free radicals, which disturbs the reduction–oxidation balance in the lungs, leading to elevated oxidative stress (Kirkham & Rahman 2006). Such an oxidant overdose can injure lung tissue directly by oxidation of cellular components, or indirectly by promoting neutrophilic inflammation and tissue degradation, subsequently affecting lung function (Kirkham & Rahman 2006; MacNee 2005).

Prevalence of COPD

Up to 2001, only about 30 prevalence surveys of COPD had been reported. This is in sharp contrast with asthma, which has been much more extensively studied with hundreds of reported prevalence studies (Chapman *et al.* 2006). The establishment of the Burden of Obstructive Lung Disease (BOLD) initiative (described later in this subsection), and other recent international initiatives to assess the global burden of COPD, will allow more valid comparisons of the prevalence of COPD over time and across nations in the near future. In the following, we summarize the most important studies currently available.

European epidemiological studies of COPD show prevalence estimates of 4–11 per cent (Vestbo 2004). These differences in prevalence estimates are presumed to be attributable to differences in risk exposures or population characteristics, but methods and definitions used to measure COPD may also play a role. Definitions of COPD used in these studies vary from doctor's diagnosis of COPD to more rigid definitions based on pathology and/or pulmonary lung function testing. Definitions based on spirometry are the least influenced by local diagnostic practice, but are nevertheless subject to variation based on the lung function parameters selected (Vestbo 2004).

Halbert *et al.* (2006) assessed the reasons for conflicting prevalence estimates described in the literature. They selected studies that had (1) estimated population-based COPD prevalences and (2) clearly described the methods used to obtain these estimates. In total, 32 studies presenting prevalence data for COPD were identified and reviewed, representing 17 countries and 8 World Health Organization (WHO) regions. Prevalence estimates were based on spirometry (11 studies), respiratory symptoms (14 studies), patient-reported disease (10 studies), or expert opinion.

The reported prevalence of COPD ranged from 0.23 to 18.3 per cent, with the lowest prevalences (0.2–2.5 per cent) being those based on expert opinion. Sixteen studies had measured rates that could confidently be extrapolated to an entire region or country; all of these 16 studies were conducted in Europe or North America, and in most the prevalence was between 4 and 10 per cent. A recent analysis of the data of the Vlagtwedde and Vlaardingen population-based cohort of Dutch Caucasians (van Diemen *et al.* 2005) reported that based on spirometry 13.4 per cent of all subjects had COPD as defined by GOLD stage II or higher, corresponding to $FEV_1/FVC < 70$ per cent and $FEV_1 < 80$ per cent predicted (see the section title 'Definitions').

Although the most accurate prevalence data are from Western countries, estimates suggest that about half of the approximately 2.7 million deaths in 2000 were in the Western Pacific Region, with the majority occurring in China. About 400 000 deaths occur each year from COPD in industrialized countries (Lopez *et al.* 2006b). Lopez *et al.* recently noted that the increase in global COPD deaths between 1990 and 2000 (0.5 million) is partially real, and may partially be due to better diagnostic methods and more extensive data availability in 2000. The regional COPD prevalence in adults in 2000 was estimated to vary from 0.5 per cent in parts of Africa to 3–4 per cent in North America (Soriano *et al.* 2000).

Halbert *et al.* (2006) recently quantified the global prevalence of COPD by performing a systematic review and random effects meta-analysis. They searched for studies published during 1990–2004, and identified 101 prevalence estimates from 28 countries. The pooled prevalence of COPD was 7.6 per cent, the prevalence of chronic bronchitis alone was 6.4 per cent, and the prevalence of emphysema alone was 1.8 per cent. The pooled prevalence of COPD based on spirometry was 8.9 per cent, with the most commonly used spirometric definitions being those of the Global Initiative for Chronic Obstructive Lung Disease.

The BOLD initiative developed standardized methods for estimating COPD prevalence and is currently one of only a few studies with truly comparable international prevalence estimates (Buist *et al.* 2007). The study included 9425 participants from 12 centres in 12 countries including China, Turkey, Austria, South Africa, Iceland, Germany, Poland, Norway, Canada, the United States, the Philippines, and Australia. Using identical methods, the study showed considerable variation in COPD prevalences, with GOLD stage II or higher COPD (post-bronchodilator $FEV_1/FVC < 70$ per cent) in women ranging from 5.1 per cent in Guangzhou, China, to 16.7 per cent in Cape Town, South Africa. In men, it ranged from 8.5 per cent in Reykjavik, Iceland, to 22.2 per cent in Cape Town, South Africa. Using a similar study design, the Latin American Project for the Investigation of Obstructive Lung Diseases (PLATINO) studied the prevalence of COPD among 5315 study participants in five Latin American centres (Mexico, Venezuela, Brazil, Chile, and Uruguay) (Menezes *et al.* 2005). Crude prevalence rates of COPD ranged from 7.8 per cent in Mexico City, Mexico, to 19.7 per cent in Montevideo, Uruguay. Interestingly, age and smoking did not fully explain the international variation in disease prevalence, suggesting an important role of additional risk factors.

Although COPD is considered to be mainly present in the elderly, it is not a disease of the elderly alone. In the Confronting COPD study, the presence of COPD based on doctor's diagnosis and presence of symptoms in younger age groups has also been described (Rennard *et al.* 2002); a phenomenon that was confirmed in the European Community Respiratory Health Survey (ECRHS) which verified COPD diagnosis with spirometric testing in random population samples of younger age (<45 years) (Vestbo 2004).

Future prevalence and burden of COPD

Although it is recognized that the burden of COPD is high, an accurate estimate of COPD prevalence data is hampered by both underdiagnosis and misdiagnosis. Mortality data are also likely to underestimate the impact of COPD because many COPD patients do not have this recorded on their death certificate due to inconsistent use of International Classification of Disease (ICD) codes (Vestbo 2004). However, despite this under-reporting, it is clear that COPD is one of the most common causes of death.

Assessing the future prevalence and burden of COPD requires taking changing population distributions and smoking habits into account. For example, Feenstra *et al.* (2001) used a dynamic multistage life table model to compute projections for the Netherlands. Changes in the size and composition of the population were predicted to increase COPD prevalence from 21/1000 in 1994 to 33/1000 in 2015 for men, and from 10/1000 to 23/1000 for women. Changes in smoking behaviour would reduce the projected prevalence to 29/1000 for men, but would increase it to 25/1000 for women. The model estimated the unavoidable increase in the burden of COPD, an increase that is greater for women than for men (142 per cent and 43 per cent increase in prevalence, respectively) (Watson *et al.* 2003). This greater increase in prevalence of COPD in women compared to men might also be associated with more severe COPD in women.

Vestbo *et al.* examined survival after admission due to COPD in 267 men and 220 women who had participated in the Copenhagen City Health Study and who were hospitalized with a discharge diagnosis of COPD. The crude five-year survival rate after a COPD admission was higher in women (52 per cent) than in men (37 per cent). However, estimations of the overall mortality due to COPD in the next decade showed that COPD mortality of women was expected to exceed that of men. A similar trend was observed in the United States. Thus, with the expected global increase in female mortality from COPD, it is predicted that COPD mortality rates for females will soon equal or exceed those for males (Watson *et al.* 2003; Crockett et al. 1994; Mannino *et al.* 1997; Vestbo *et al.* 1998; Vestbo 2002).

Irrespective of the expected greater increase in prevalence of COPD in women compared to in men, women are less likely to receive a COPD diagnosis than men when presenting to a physician (Watson *et al.* 2003). This gender bias results in a further underdiagnoses of COPD in women, as shown by Chapman *et al.* (2001). They found that spirometry not only reduced the risk of underdiagnosis but also limited the effects of gender bias.

Risk factors for COPD

In the past few decades, the environmental risk factors for COPD—that is, smoking, air pollution, occupational exposure, childhood respiratory illness, diet, and exposure to respiratory allergens—have been studied in detail. Also, the presence of respiratory symptoms, increased numbers of eosinophils, and increased airway responsiveness were all found to be significant predictors of reduced level of FEV_1 (Wang *et al.* 2004).

Cigarette smoking

The WHO has estimated that 73 per cent of all COPD mortality in high-income countries is caused by smoking; the estimate for low- and middle-income countries was 40 per cent (Lopez *et al.* 2006a). Tobacco smoke, therefore, is the most important cause of COPD. In fact, there is a well-established association between current and cumulative smoking and COPD, and several cohort studies have shown that adult smokers experience a faster FEV_1 decline than non-smokers. This excess decline in lung function may return to normal levels of ageing-related decline after smoking cessation (Camilli *et al.* 1987).

Women and children are considered to be particularly sensitive to the effects of inhaled tobacco smoke (Xu *et al.* 1994). A recent study also demonstrated a significant (10.7 per cent) reduction in FEV_1 due to environmental tobacco smoke among children with smoking parents compared to children of non-smoking parents. This latter finding emphasizes the importance of environmental tobacco smoke in childhood (Tager *et al.* 1983).

What has been the most striking about the epidemiology of COPD is the change in prevalence in women over the past decade (Lopez & Murray 1998). As a result of changes in smoking habits in recent decades, the prevalence of COPD in women in the United Kingdom reached the same level as that of men in the previous decade (Lopez *et al.* 2006b). A similar pattern is seen in the United States with respect to female mortality and this is expected to be reflected in other European countries in the near future (Halbert *et al.* 2003). Nonetheless, as noted in the preceding subsection, women with COPD are less likely to be diagnosed and treated (Miravitlles *et al.* 2005). General practitioners, in particular, consider the diagnosis of COPD less frequently in women than in men although presenting with the same risk factors and clinical symptoms (Miravitlles *et al.* 2006).

The pattern, until recently, of greater COPD prevalence among males than females is likely to be explained by the traditionally higher rates of smoking among men (Watson *et al.* 2003). This is supported by an increase in the prevalence of COPD in the past ten years among females, which is attributed to the fact that the rates of smoking among women have significantly increased in more recent times (Kemm 2001). Moreover, females now take up smoking at younger ages, thereby increasing their risk of developing smoking-related disease.

Few data are available on the incidence of COPD according to smoking habits. Analysis of the Copenhagen City Heart Study confirmed a higher incidence of COPD among smokers than non-smokers with 27 per cent of the participants who continued to smoke over a 25-year period developing COPD as defined by GOLD stage II–IV COPD, compared with 5.7 per cent of the non-smokers (Lokke *et al.* 2006). The longitudinal Vlagtwedde and Vlaardingen cohort study with a follow-up of 25 years also showed that persistent cigarette smokers (OR = 1.99; 95% CI = 1.68,2.35), recidivist smokers (OR = 1.96; 95% CI = 1.34,2.86), variable pipe or cigar smokers (OR = 2.11; 95% CI = 1.52,2.91), and subjects who stopped smoking (OR = 1.39; 95% CI = 1.08,1.80) had an increased risk of developing COPD compared to never-smokers. The risks of developing COPD in sustained ex-smokers (OR = 0.98; 95% CI = 0.79,1.22), starters (OR = 1.62; 95% CI = 0.87,2.99), brief smokers (OR = 1.22; 95% CI = 0.76,1.94), and persistent pipe or cigar smokers (OR = 1.41; 95% CI = 0.98,2.04) were not significantly different from the risk in the never-smokers. Therefore, it was concluded that, taking longitudinal smoking habits into account, subjects who had quit smoking between two successive surveys still had an increased risk of developing COPD compared with never-smokers, whereas sustained ex-smokers were no longer at risk of developing COPD.

Other environmental risk factors

In addition to smoking, the rate of decline in lung function is also determined by several other environmental factors. For example, occupational exposure to dusts, gases, and fumes has been shown to be associated with the rate of decline in FEV_1 and the development of COPD. In fact, a 2003 report by an ad hoc committee of the American Thoracic Society reviewing occupational studies on COPD estimated that 15–20 per cent of the COPD cases were caused by occupational factors (Balmes 2005). More recent studies suggest that these estimates could even be higher. For example, analyses of data collected in the Third National Health and Nutrition Examination Survey (NHANES III) suggest that approximately 20 per cent of the COPD cases in the United States are attributable to work-related exposures (Hnizdo *et al.* 2002). The proportion was even higher (approximately 30 per cent) among never-smokers. Combined exposures to smoking and occupational factors have been shown to have greater than additive effects (Trupin *et al.* 2003). Some examples of occupational risk factors for COPD are coal dust, silica dust, oil mists, welding fumes, and organic dusts including cotton, grain, and wood (Balmes 2005).

Indoor air pollutants are another important risk factor for COPD, particularly in low-income countries where biomass fuels (wood and crop residues) and coal fuels are often used for heating and cooking without appropriate ventilation (Liu *et al.* 2007). WHO estimates suggest that indoor smoke from biomass fuels may cause 35 per cent of all COPD cases in low- and middle-income countries (Lopez *et al.* 2006a). COPD is also related to outdoor pollution levels, but the attributable risk is expected to be relatively small (Tashkin *et al.* 1994).

Genetic risk factors

Genetic risk factors have been studied in detail only recently. COPD is a disease that is predominantly expressed at later ages and genetic factors are also more difficult to study, because the parents of individuals with COPD have often already died and the children of subjects with COPD are likely to be too young to have significant fixed airway obstruction (van Diemen & Boezen 2007). In the past decade, genetic studies on COPD have therefore usually included small numbers of subjects and applied various definitions of disease, hampering a valid comparison between studies. Also, small sample sizes increase the likelihood of spurious results, because genotyping in small sample sizes can lead to positive results in a predefined number of studies (e.g. 5 per cent, if = 0.05 is accepted). Thus, it is not surprising that many positive results from genetic studies of COPD have not been replicated (Boezen & Postma 2007). In addition, there may be a bias towards lack of publication of negative findings.

Lack of replication might also be due to the apparent difficulties of extrapolating results from one population to another. For example, associations found in Asians may be missed in Caucasian populations as a result of lower prevalences of the polymorphisms under study in Caucasians (Boezen & Postma 2007).

More recently, several large population-based cohort studies have been conducted in which excess decline in lung function leading to development of COPD was studied prospectively. These studies have the advantage of being able to assess different mechanisms that can lead to poor lung function. For example, subjects may have experienced an unusually high rate of decline in lung function, or alternatively they may not have attained the normal maximal level of lung function, or the age of onset of decline may have been unusually early. Genetic factors may affect any one, or a combination, of these different patterns of lung function loss. Therefore, it is of crucial importance to study the genetic contribution to lung function loss in a longitudinal population-based study design, covering the time span during which these different patterns and their underlying causes evolve (van Diemen & Boezen 2007).

To date, most studies on the genetics of COPD have focused on genes that are involved in the processing of various tobacco smoke products, affect the degree of oxidative stress, or are involved in the protease–anti-protease balance. In particular, variations in the enzymes that detoxify cigarette smoke products, and are thus protective against oxidative stress, might explain why only a small proportion of smokers develop COPD. For example, a polymorphism in exon 5 of the glutathione S1-transferase (GST) P1 that affects its catalytic activity was significantly more common in men with irreversible airway obstruction than in those without (Hayes *et al.* 2005). More recently, an association between COPD and a short tandem repeat polymorphism in the haeme oxygenase-1 gene promoter has been described, which results in an up-regulation of haeme oxygenase-1 upon exposure to reactive oxygen species in cigarette smoke (Takahashi *et al.* 2004). As haeme oxygenase is more expressed in lung tissue of individuals with COPD, a genetic variation in this gene may also contribute to its development. Moreover, mutations in enzymes that generate protective antioxidants have also been associated with the development of COPD.

Detoxifying enzymes such as microsomal epoxide hydrolase (mEH) and cytochrome P 4501A1 (CYP1A1) are important protective factors against oxidative stress and may also play a role in COPD. There are about 50 known CYP genes, and the CYP3 and CYP1 genes are expressed in lung tissue and have an important role in the detoxification of inhaled substances such as cigarette smoke. CYP3A5 and CYP3A4 may be of particular interest; CYP3A5 is the predominant CYP3A form in human airways and CYP3A4 is expressed in about 20 per cent of the individuals, with considerable variation of pulmonary expression occurring in both CYPs between individuals (Anttila *et al.* 1997; Yamada *et al.* 2000). Slow detoxification of epoxide derivatives of cigarette smoke components may contribute as well. In addition, enzymes affecting the degree of oxidative stress due to exogenous (cigarettes) or endogenous reactive oxygen species, as well as mutations in enzymes that generate protective antioxidants, may be associated with the development of COPD (Barnes 1999; Sandford *et al.* 2002; Boezen & Postma 2004). Finally, genes involved in the protease–anti-protease balance are likely to play a role in COPD development.

Mechanisms, prevalence, and risk factors of asthma

Allergy, atopy, and asthma

Asthma is almost universally regarded as an atopic disease involving allergen exposure, IgE-mediated sensitization with a Th_2 lymphocyte response, and subsequent IL 5-mediated eosinophilic airways inflammation, resulting in enhanced bronchial reactivity and reversible airflow obstruction (asthma) (Douwes *et al.* 2002a). As a consequence, asthma is often described as an allergic disease and grouped together with other 'allergic diseases' such as rhinitis and eczema. This assumption is increasingly being challenged (Pearce *et al.* 1999; Ronchetti *et al.* 2007; Weinmayr *et al.* 2007), and there is growing interest in other (non-allergic and non-eosinophilic) inflammatory mechanisms that may be involved in producing the final common pathway of enhanced bronchial reactivity and reversible airflow obstruction that characterizes asthma (Simpson *et al.* 2006, 2007; Douwes *et al.* 2002a; Berry *et al.* 2007).

Respiratory allergy

Allergy can be defined as 'adverse acute or chronic hypersensitivity reactions resulting from immunologic sensitization with production of immunoglobulin (Ig) E against a specific agent or allergen'. Thus, the term *allergy* refers to symptomatic conditions (allergic asthma, rhinitis, etc.) whereas the term *sensitization* refers to an individual's immune status assessed by *in vivo* or *in vitro* diagnostic tests. Symptoms can be induced by inhalation of allergens, even at very low concentrations. Individuals who are not sensitized to these allergens will usually not show symptoms even with very high exposure. Symptoms in sensitized subjects are caused by inflammatory reactions initiated by allergen-specific IgE antibodies present in the airways. Only a proportion of sensitized subjects show symptoms and are thus also allergic. It can take weeks to years between first encounter with an allergen and the development of an allergy.

Allergic asthma is caused by IgE-mediated inflammatory mechanisms in which a large number of cells play a role including mast cells, eosinophils, T lymphocytes, dendritic cells, and macrophages. Briefly, the sensitization process involves the adaptive (or acquired) immune system wherein allergens interact with dendritic cells in the airway mucosa, which migrate to the regional lymph nodes where the allergens are presented to B and T cells. This results (through T helper-2 [Th_2] responses) in the production of allergen-specific IgE. Once allergic, a subject can develop symptoms minutes after being exposed. This is known as the early-phase allergic reaction and symptoms develop as a result of mast cell degranulation and release of inflammatory mediators through allergen IgE–antibody complexes on the surface of mast cells, causing contraction of bronchial smooth muscle and oedema in the airways. Clinically, this results in a decreased lung function and symptoms of wheeze, shortness of breath, chest tightness, and coughing.

During the late phase of the allergic reaction (4–8 h after exposure), eosinophil-related inflammatory reactions are particularly important. A critical step in this late-phase reaction is the activation of Th_2 cells, which release several pro-inflammatory cytokines including IL-5 resulting in the influx and activation of eosinophils. This reaction is characterized by the development of a non-specific bronchial hyperresponsiveness (BHR) that can continue for several days. Repeated exposures can result in more permanent BHR.

Atopy

'Atopy' (allergic sensitization) is a common term for IgE-mediated sensitization and/or allergic reaction. In population studies, this term is used to indicate the predisposition of individuals to produce increased levels of specific or total IgE after exposure to common allergens such as house-dust mite, pet and various food allergens. It is usually assessed by using skin prick tests or specific serum IgE against common allergens, and it can therefore be defined either in terms of skin prick text positivity or elevated serum IgE levels (Pearce *et al.* 1999). Depending on the definition, about 20–40 per cent of the people in affluent countries are atopic.

In population studies, atopy is often associated with an increased risk of asthma (Pearce *et al.* 1999), but the association is stronger in Westernized countries than in developing countries (Weinmayr *et al.* 2007).

Aeroallergens

Many macromolecules (particularly proteins) of non-human origin, including those of animals (e.g. arthropod proteins, animal dander, proteins in excreta), plants (e.g. pollens, latex dust), and microorganisms (e.g. spores of fungi such as *Alternaria, Aspergillus*, and *Penicillium*), can act as allergens by inducing a specific IgE response and provoke allergic reactions in sensitized subjects.

Dust mites produce the predominant inhalant allergens in many parts of the world. The most common mite species that produce allergens are *Dermatophagoides pteronyssisus* and *D. farinae*. The major allergens produced by *D. pteronyssisus* (called Der p 1 and Der p 2) are proteases present in high amounts in faecal pellets. *D. farinae* produces as its major allergen Der f 1. Elevated levels of these allergens have been detected in house dust, mattress dust, and bedding in damp homes (Van Strien *et al.* 1994).

Other important inhalant allergens include proteins associated with cats and dogs, cockroaches, grass and tree pollens, and fungi such as *Alternaria*. Allergens in the occupational environment can range from cow urinary proteins in farming situations to fungal enzymes in the biotechnology and bakery industry. Low molecular weight chemicals such as diisocyanates (e.g. tolueen diisocyanate, TDI) can also cause occupational allergic asthma, but the specific immunological mechanisms have not yet been resolved.

Is asthma an allergic disease?

Ten years ago, it was widely believed that asthma was an atopic disease caused by allergen exposure. The fundamental aetiological mechanism was that allergen exposure, particularly in infancy, produced atopic sensitization and continued exposure resulted in asthma through the development of eosinophilic airways inflammation, bronchial hyperresponsiveness, and reversible airflow obstruction. In recent years, it has become increasingly evident that this picture is, at best, too simplistic (Ronchetti *et al.* 2007; Weinmayr *et al.* 2007). A systematic review of population-based studies (Pearce *et al.* 1999) has shown that the proportion of asthma cases that are attributable to atopy (defined as skin prick test positivity) is usually less than one half (Table 9.4.1). Standardized comparisons across populations or time periods also show only weak and inconsistent associations between the prevalence of asthma and the prevalence of atopy. For instance, a comparison of asthma and atopy among 9–11-year-olds in Albania and the United Kingdom (Priftanji *et al.* 2001) showed large differences in the prevalence of current wheeze (4.4 per cent and 9.7 per cent, respectively) and exercise-induced bronchial reactivity (0.8 per cent and 5.4 per cent) but not in skin prick test positivity (15 per cent and 17.8 per cent), suggesting that large variations in asthma prevalence can occur without differences in the frequency of atopy. This was confirmed by the International Study on Allergies and Asthma in Children (ISAAC; see subsection on the same), which showed that the association between atopy and asthma symptoms differed strongly among populations, but increased with economic development (Weinmayr *et al.* 2007). In this study, the fraction of current wheeze attributable to atopy ranged from 0 per cent in Ankara (Turkey) to 93.8 per cent in Guangzhou (China) (Figs. 9.4.1a and 9.4.1b); the overall proportion of asthma cases that were attributable to atopy was only 40.7 per cent in affluent countries and 20.3 per cent in non-affluent countries. Moreover, the ECRHS (see subsection on the same) showed that asthma attributable to atopy in adults ranged from 4 to 61 per cent between individual study centres with an overall estimate of only 30 per cent for all centres combined (Sunyer *et al.* 2004).

Also, Martinez (1998) questions whether the association of atopy with asthma is causal, on the basis that the development of sensitization after 8 years is not associated with an increased asthma risk, whereas if the association of sensitization and asthma was causal, one would not expect the age at which sensitization occurs to be of major importance.

Recent studies using sputum induction and/or bronchoalveolar lavage (BAL) techniques to measure and characterize airways inflammation in asthmatics have also demonstrated that less than 50 per cent of the asthma cases are attributable to eosinophilic airways inflammation, the hallmark of allergic asthma (Simpson *et al.* 2006; Douwes *et al.* 2002a). Thus, evidence from studies of eosinophilia and asthma is consistent with that from studies of atopy and asthma: In both instances, at most about one half of the asthma cases appear to be due to 'allergic' mechanisms. This further adds to the evidence that allergic mechanisms may not be the only, or the most important, underlying mechanism for asthma.

Non-allergic mechanisms

As noted earlier, a substantial proportion of all asthma cases have an underlying pathology that is clearly different from that observed in 'classic' allergic asthma (Simpson *et al.* 2006; Douwes *et al.* 2002a). Patients may have severe and persistent asthma in the absence of eosinophilic inflammation, and may experience an exacerbation of asthma without an increase in eosinophilic inflammation (Turner *et al.* 1995). Repeated assessments of airways inflammation over time have shown that the non-eosinophilic asthma phenotype is reproducible both in the short (4 weeks) and

Table 9.4.1 Summary of nine population-based studies in children and seven population-based studies in adults: proportions of asthmatics and non-asthmatics who are atopic, and per cent of asthma cases attributable to atopy

Age-group	Non-asthmatics atopic (per cent)	Asthmatics atopic (per cent)	Pooled relative risk	Cases attributable to atopy (per cent)
Children	29	58	3.4	38
Adults	24	54	3.7	37

Source: Adapted from Pearce *et al.* How much asthma is really attributable to atopy? *Thorax* 1999;**54**:268–72.

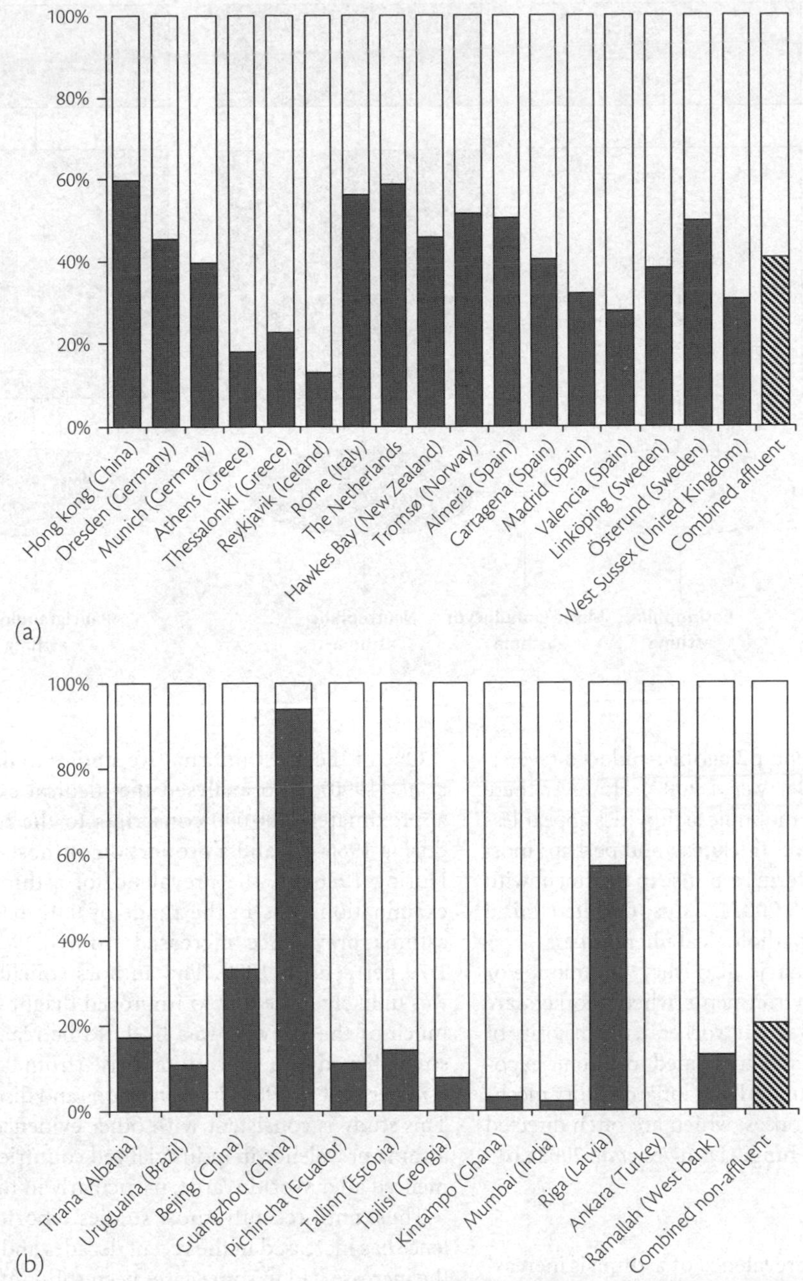

Fig. 9.4.1 The ISAAC Phase II-estimated fractions (per cent) of current wheeze attributable to atopy for all affluent countries (A) and non-affluent countries (B). (Adapted from Weinmayr *et al.* Atopic sensitization and the international variation of asthma symptom prevalence in children. *American Journal of Respiratory and Critical Care Medicine* 2007;**176**:565–74.).

long-term (1–5 years) (Simpson *et al.* 2006). However, the underlying mechanisms of non-eosinophilic and non-allergic asthma are not fully elucidated. One recent study in 93 non-smoking adult asthmatics found sputum airway eosinophilia in 41 per cent of all asthma cases, 20 per cent had elevated levels of neutrophils, 8 per cent had a mixed inflammatory profile with both cell types being elevated, and the remainder (31 per cent) had no signs of airway inflammation with both eosinophil and neutrophil levels within the normal range (Simpson *et al.* 2006). This suggests that asthma can be categorized into four inflammatory subtypes based on sputum eosinophil and neutrophil proportions: Eosinophilic asthma, neutrophilic asthma, mixed granulocytic asthma, and paucigranulocytic asthma (Simpson *et al.* 2006).

The common pathophysiological features of neutrophilic asthma involve an IL 8-mediated neutrophil influx and the subsequent neutrophil activation is a potent stimulus to increased airway hyperresponsiveness (Simpson *et al.* 2007). Although the stimuli that trigger this response are diverse (endotoxin, ozone, particulates, virus infection), the common features are consistent with activation of innate immune mechanisms (involving Toll-like receptors and CD14) rather than IgE-mediated activation of acquired immunity (Fig. 9.4.2).

There is also the potential for combined activation of both innate and allergen-specific inflammatory mechanisms in asthma. This may be the case in mixed granulocytic asthma (Fig. 9.4.2), and may explain the ability of ozone and NO_2 to potentiate allergen-induced asthmatic responses (Jenkins *et al.* 1999). The pathophysiological mechanisms involved in paucigranulocytic asthma are not clear.

Clinically, the eosinophilic and non-eosinophilic phenotypes are very similar with only marginal differences in lung function, airway

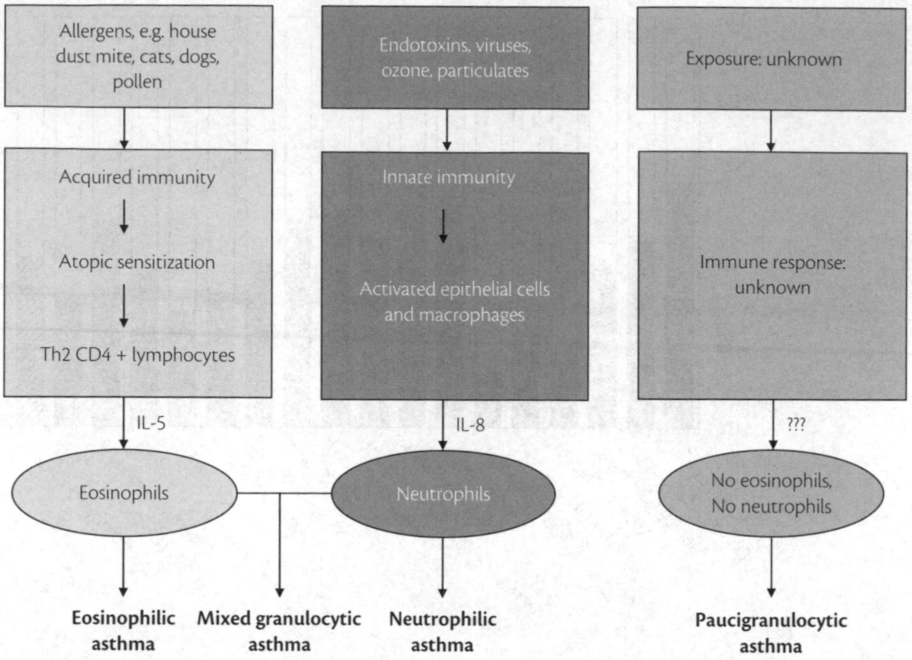

Fig. 9.4.2 The inflammatory pathways of various asthma phenotypes.

hyperreactivity, corticosteroid use, and β2 agonist-induced reversibility in FEV_1 (Simpson *et al.* 2006; Berry *et al.* 2007). However, there are also distinct differences: Non-eosinophilic asthmatics appear less atopic, have normal subepithelial-layer thickness, and perhaps most importantly, they have a poor short-term response to treatment with inhaled corticosteroids (Berry *et al.* 2007). Thus, despite clinical similarities, they represent distinct pathological phenotypes.

Non-allergic occupational asthma is also very common. For instance, in many occupational environments where workers are exposed to organic dust (e.g. farmers, grain workers), the majority of asthma cases are non-IgE-mediated, and are related to chronic exposure to environmental irritants. The underlying inflammatory mechanisms involve innate immune responses, which are often directed against constituents of bacteria and fungi (Douwes *et al.* 2002a,b).

Asthma time trends

It has long been suspected that the prevalence of asthma is increasing not only in industrialized countries but also in developing countries (Pearce *et al.* 2000c). However, this has been a particularly difficult issue to resolve because of the lack of systematic standardized studies measuring changes in asthma prevalence over time, and some reviewers have argued that the increases in reported prevalence are largely due to increased awareness, labelling, and diagnosis of asthma symptoms (Magnus & Jaakkola 1997). Nevertheless, most studies, which have determined the prevalence of asthma symptoms using the same methodology in the same community at different times, have reported that asthma prevalence has increased in the recent decades and that the magnitude of the increase has in some cases been substantial (Table 9.4.2). Although methodological differences in these studies make it difficult to compare the magnitude of the differences in asthma prevalence between countries, the trend of increasing prevalence among populations in countries of widely differing lifestyles and ethnic groups is generally consistent.

One of the most informative studies to date is that of Haahtela *et al.* (1990), who analysed the medical examination reports of approximately 900 000 conscripts to the Finnish defence forces during 1966–89, and a proportion of those examined in 1926–61. During 1926–61, the prevalence of asthma recorded at call-up examinations was in the range of 0.02–0.08 per cent. However, asthma prevalence increased from 0.29 per cent in 1966 to 1.79 per cent in 1989. The authors concluded that the increase was unlikely to be due to improved diagnostic methods, and that much of the increase was likely to be real. This conclusion was strengthened by a concomitant rise (from 0.12 per cent in 1966 to 0.75 per cent in 1989) in exemptions and discharges due to asthma. This study is consistent with other evidence that the increases in asthma prevalence in industrialized countries appear to have commenced after World War II, particularly in the 1960s and 1970s.

Thus, until recently, most studies reported that asthma prevalence has increased in the recent decades and that the magnitude of the increase had in some cases been substantial (Table 9.4.2).

However, several recent studies have reported either no increase or even a decrease in asthma prevalence over the last ten years. For instance, Bollag *et al.* (2005) examined time trends in consultations for asthma in primary care in Switzerland and found that overall consultation rates for asthma increased from 1989 to 1994, then stabilized, and have declined since 2000. The observation that asthma incidence might be falling is in agreement with several other studies that showed similar time trends for asthma and hay fever (Pearce & Douwes 2005). The best indication of what is currently happening globally is provided by the Phase III of the ISAAC study, the results of which are discussed in the following subsection.

International prevalence comparisons

The causes of the international time trends in the prevalence of asthma are unclear, and are currently a major focus for asthma epidemiology worldwide. An important component of this research process involves standardized international prevalence comparisons

Table 9.4.2 Changes in asthma prevalence in children and young adults

Country	Period	Asthma prevalence		Reference
		1st study	2nd study	
Australia	1964–1990	19.1%	46.0%	Robertson *et al.*
	1982–1992	10.4%	28.6%	Robertson *et al.*
	1992–2002	28.6%	23.7%	
	1987–1992	5.6%	9.3%	Campbell *et al.*
	1992–1995	9.3%	11.4%	Adams *et al.*
Canada	1980–1983	3.8%	6.5%	Infante-Rivard *et al.*
	1980–1990[c]	140/10 000	256/10 000[a]	Manfreda *et al.*
		125/10 000	254/10 000[b]	
England	1956–1975	1.8%	6.3%	Morrison Smith
	1966–1990	18.3%	21.8%	Whincup *et al.*
	1973–1986	2.4%	3.6%	Burney *et al.*
	1978–1991	11.1%	12.8%	Anderson *et al.*
England and Wales	1970–1981	11.6%	20.5%[a]	Fleming and Crombie
		8.8%	15.9%[b]	
Finland	1961–1986	0.1%	1.8%	Haahtela *et al.*
France	1968–1982	3.3%	5.4%	Perdrizet *et al.*
Germany	1991–1996	3.7%	4.1%	von Mutius *et al.*
Israel	1986–1990	7.9%	9.6%	Auerbach *et al.*
Italy	1983–1993/5	2.9%	4.4%	Ciprandi *et al.*
Japan	1982–1992	3.3%	4.6%	Nishima
Netherlands	1989–1993	13.4%	13.3%	Mommers *et al.*
	1993–1997	13.3%	11.9%	
	1997–2001	11.9%	9.1%	
New Zealand	1969–1982	7.1%	13.5%	Mitchell
	1975–1989	26.2%	34.0%	Shaw *et al.*
Papua New Guinea	1973–1984	0.0%	0.6%	Dowse *et al.*
Scotland	1964–1989	10.4%	19.8%	Ninan and Russell
	1989–1994	19.8%	25.4%	Omran and Russell
Spain	1994–2003	9.3%	9.3%	Garcia-Marcos *et al.*
Sweden	1971–1981	1.9%	2.8%	Aberg
	1979–1991	2.5%	5.7%	Aberg *et al.*
Tahiti	1979–1984	11.5%	14.3%	Liard *et al.*
Taiwan	1974–1985	1.3%	5.1%	Hsieh and Shen
United Kingdom	1991–1998	33.9%	27.5%	Anderson *et al.*
United States	1964–1983[d]	183/100 000	284/100 000	Yunginger *et al.*
	1971–1976	4.8%	7.6%	Gergen *et al.*
	1981–1988	3.1%	4.3%	Weitzman *et al.*
	1983–1992	9.2%	15.9%	Farber *et al.*
Wales	1973–1988	4.0%	9.0%	Burr *et al.*

[a]Men, [b]women, [c]prevalence rates per 10 000 subjects, [d]incidence rates per 100 000 subjects.

(Pearce *et al.* 1998). The key problem is to gain information on large numbers of people in random samples collected in a comparable manner across social groups, regions, and countries. Thus, comparisons of asthma prevalence are increasingly being based on a simple comparison of symptom prevalence in a questionnaire survey of a large number of people, followed by more intensive testing of factors related to asthma (e.g. BHR) and risk factors for asthma (skin prick test positivity, serum IgE, and environmental exposures) in a subsample, and a repeat of the prevalence survey over time. This approach has been used in the international survey of asthma prevalence in adults (Burney *et al.* 1994) and in the ISAAC study (Asher *et al.* 1995; Pearce *et al.* 1993; Ellwood *et al.* 2005).

The European Community Respiratory Health Survey (ECRHS)

In each centre of the ECRHS, a representative sample of 3000 adults, aged 20–44 years, completed a Phase-I screening questionnaire seeking information on asthma symptoms and medication use (Burney *et al.* 1994). Individuals answering 'yes' to waking with an attack of shortness of breath, an attack of asthma, or current asthma medications were defined as 'asthmatic'. A random subsample of 600 subjects and an additional sample of up to 150 'asthmatic' individuals were then studied in more detail in Phase II, with measurements of skin prick tests to common allergens, serum total and specific IgE, bronchial responsiveness to inhaled methacholine, as well as an additional questionnaire on asthma symptoms and medical history, occupation and social status, smoking, the home environment, and the use of medications and medical services. The Phase-I results (Burney *et al.* 1996) included data from 48 centres, predominantly in Western Europe, with only 9 centres from 6 countries (Algeria, Iceland, India, New Zealand, Australia, and the United States) being from outside Europe. Phase II was conducted in 37 centres in 16 countries (Burney *et al.* 1996).

The International Study of Asthma and Allergies in Childhood (ISAAC)

The ISAAC study (Asher *et al.* 1995; Ellwood *et al.* 2005) had a similar study design to that of the ECRHS study, with a simple Phase-I survey and a more in-depth Phase-II survey. However, in order to obtain the maximum possible participation across the world, Phase I (which was conducted in 155 centres in 56 countries) was separated from Phase II (which was conducted in a smaller number of centres), and the Phase-I questionnaire modules were designed to be simple and inexpensive to administer. In addition, a video presentation of clinical signs and symptoms of asthma was developed (Shaw *et al.* 1995) in order to minimize translation problems. The populations of interest were schoolchildren aged 6–7 years and 13–14 years within specified geographical areas. The Phase-I findings, involving more than 700 000 children, showed striking international differences in asthma symptom prevalence (Asher *et al.* 1998; Beasley *et al.* 1998). Figure 9.4.3 shows the international patterns of 12-month period prevalence of wheezing in 13–14 year olds (based on the question 'Have you had wheezing or whistling in the chest in the last 12 months?')

ISAAC Phase II was conducted in 30 centres in 22 countries and involved parental questionnaires (n = 54 439), skin prick tests (n = 31 759), and serum IgE measurements (n = 8951). House dust samples to measure indoor allergens were also collected (Weinmayr *et al.* 2007).

Phase III involved a repeat of the Phase-I survey after an interval of 5–10 years in 106 centres in 56 countries among children aged 13–14 years (n = 304 679) and in 66 centres in 37 countries among children aged 6–7 years (n = 193 404) (Asher *et al.* 2006; Pearce *et al.* 2007). It was found that international differences in asthma symptom prevalence have reduced, particularly among 13–14-year-olds, with decreases in prevalence in English-speaking countries and Western Europe and increases in prevalence in regions where prevalence was previously low (Fig. 9.4.4). Although there was little change in the overall prevalence of current wheeze, the percentage of children reported to have had asthma increased significantly, possibly reflecting greater awareness of this condition and/or changes in diagnostic practice. The asthma symptom prevalence increases in Africa, Latin America, and parts of Asia indicate that the global burden of asthma is continuing to rise, but the global prevalence differences are lessening.

What do the ECRHS and ISAAC studies show?

The ISAAC and ECRHS studies provide, for the first time, a picture of global patterns of asthma prevalence, and identify the key phenomena which future research must address and attempt to explain:

1. Both studies show a particularly high prevalence of reported asthma symptoms in English-speaking countries (Fig. 9.4.3); that is, the British Isles, New Zealand, Australia, the United States, and Canada (Asher *et al.* 1998; Burney *et al.* 1996). This is unlikely to be entirely due to translation problems, because the same pattern was observed in the ISAAC video questionnaire (Asher *et al.* 1998).
2. The ISAAC study showed that centres in Latin America also had particularly high symptom prevalence (Fig. 9.4.3). This finding is of particular interest in that the Spanish-speaking centres of Latin America showed higher prevalences than Spain itself, in contrast with the general tendency for more affluent countries to have higher prevalence rates.
3. Among the non-English-speaking European countries, both studies show high asthma prevalence in Western Europe, with lower prevalences in Eastern and Southern Europe. For example, in the ISAAC study, there is a clear northwest–southeast gradient within Europe, with the highest prevalence in the world being in the United Kingdom, and some of the lowest prevalences in Albania and Greece (Asher *et al.* 1998). The West–East gradient was particularly strong; in particular, there was a significantly lower prevalence in the former East Germany than in the former West Germany.
4. Africa and Asia generally showed relatively low asthma prevalence (Fig. 9.4.3). In particular, prevalence was low in developing countries such as China and Indonesia, whereas more affluent Asian countries such as Singapore and Japan showed relatively high asthma prevalence rates. Perhaps the most striking contrast is between Hong Kong and Guangzhou, which are close geographically and involve the same language and predominant ethnic group: Hong Kong (the more affluent city) had a 12-month period prevalence of wheeze of 10.1 per cent compared with 2 per cent in Guangzhou (the less affluent city).
5. In contrast to the asthma findings, the highest prevalences of rhinitis were reported from centres scattered throughout most regions of the world, including Western Europe, Africa, North America, and Southeast Asia; the highest prevalences of eczema were generally in centres of high latitude, including

Scandinavia and New Zealand, although there were some notable exceptions including some centres in South America and Africa (Ethiopia). Thus, although the prevalences of these conditions were correlated, the association was not particularly strong and there were numerous centres that had high prevalence for asthma but not for rhinitis and/or eczema, and vice versa, suggesting that the major risk factors are different for these related disorders, or that they involve different latency periods and time trends.

6. The ISAAC Phase II showed that the link between atopic sensitization and asthma symptoms differed strongly between populations

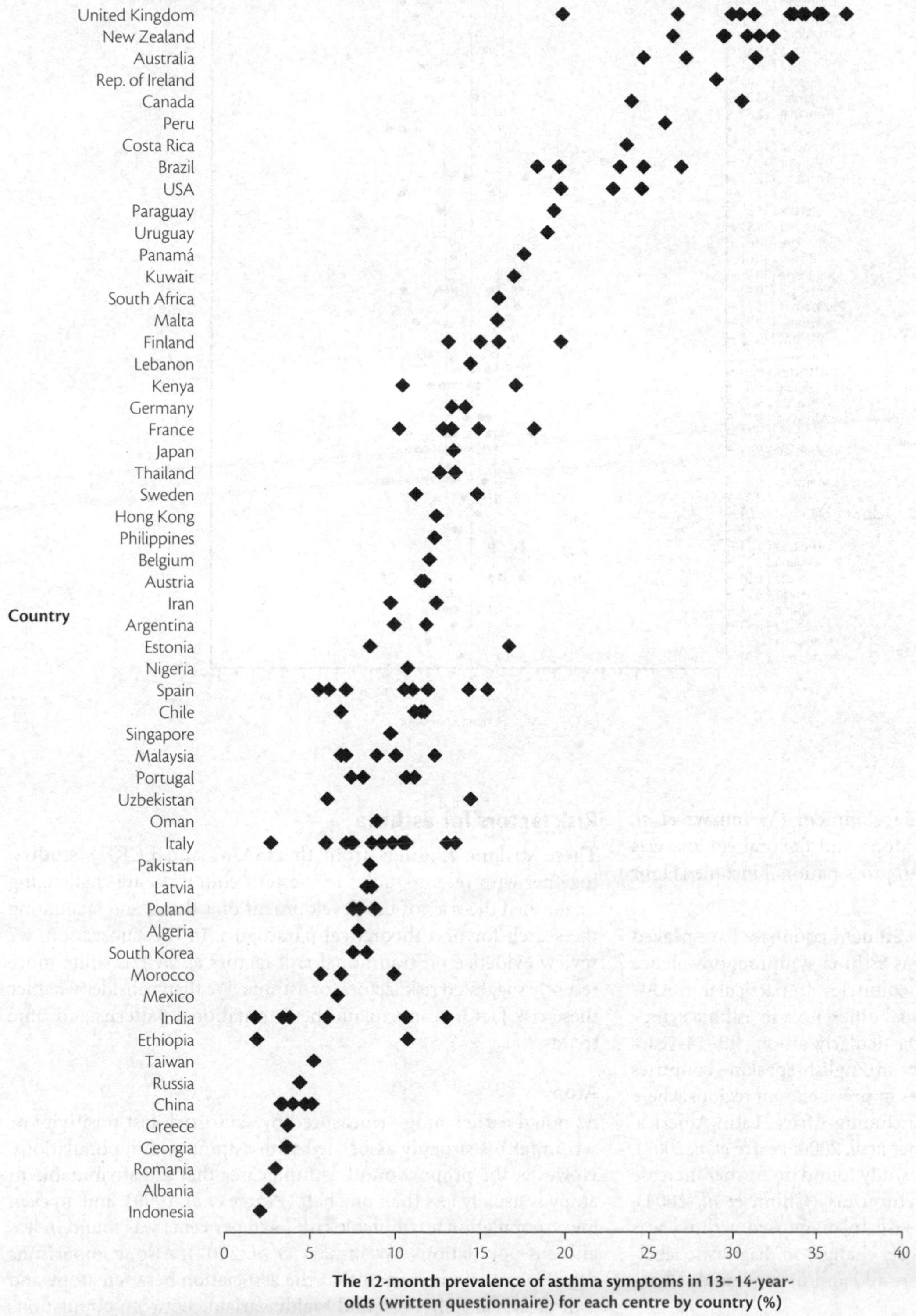

Fig. 9.4.3 Wheeze in the previous 12 months among 13–14-year-olds for each centre by country (per cent), ordered according to the mean prevalence for all centres in the country (from ISAAC 1998a).

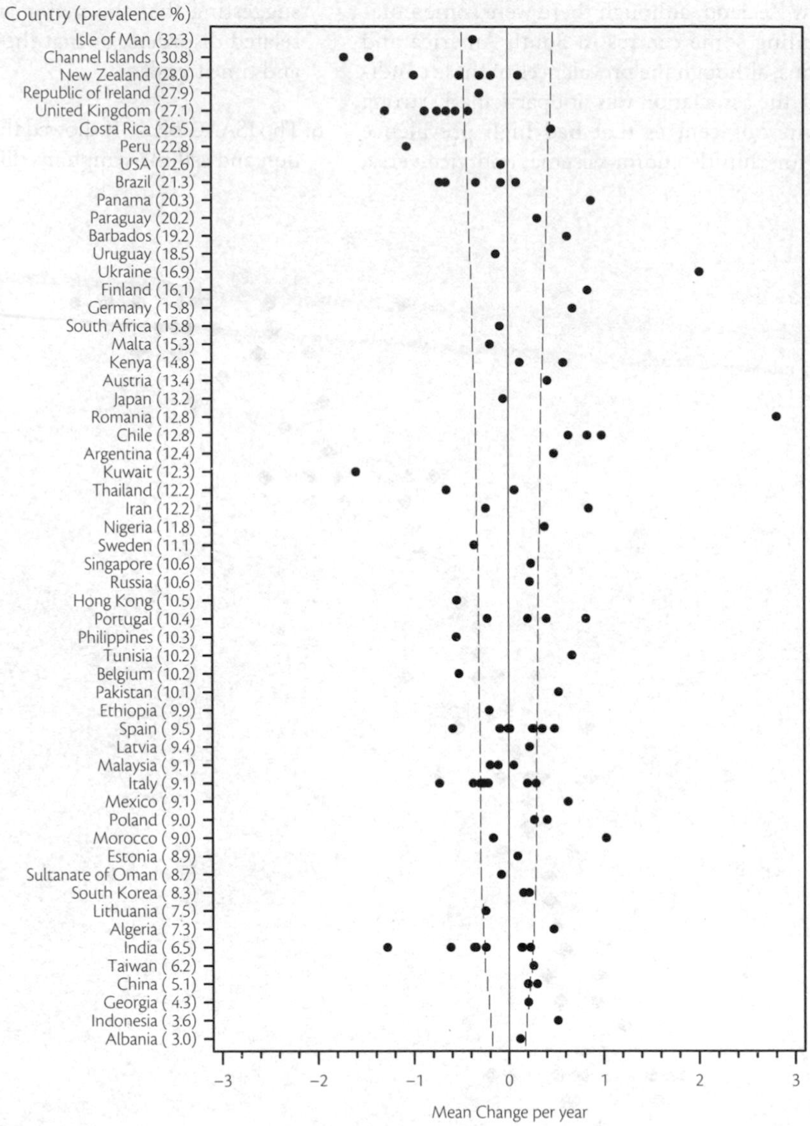

Fig. 9.4.4 Ranking plot showing the change per year in the 12-month prevalence (per cent) of current wheeze among 13–14-year-olds for each centre by country, with countries ordered by their average prevalence (for all centres combined) across Phase I and Phase III. The plot also shows the confidence interval about zero change (dashed lines) for a given level of prevalence (i.e. the average prevalence across Phase I and Phase III) given a sample size of 3000 and no cluster sampling effect. (From Pearce *et al.* Worldwide trends in the prevalence of asthma symptoms: Phase III of the International Study of Asthma and Allergies in Childhood (ISAAC). *Thorax* 2007;**62**:758-66.)

and increased with economic development (Weinmayr *et al.* 2007); the association between atopy and flexural eczema was also weak and positively linked to gross national income (Flohr *et al.* 2007).

7. The asthma prevalences in many affluent countries have peaked or even begun to decline, whereas asthma symptom prevalence continues to rise in less affluent countries. In particular, ISAAC Phase III showed that international differences in asthma symptom prevalence have reduced, particularly among 13–14-year-olds, with decreases in prevalence in English-speaking countries and Western Europe and increases in prevalence in regions where prevalence was previously low including Africa, Latin America, and parts of Asia (Fig. 9.4.4) (Asher *et al.* 2006; Pearce *et al.* 2007). Similarly, Phase II of the ECRHS study found no further increase in current or severe asthma symptoms (Chinn *et al.* 2004). Nonetheless, a significant increase in diagnosed asthma was observed, which most likely reflects changes in diagnostic labelling and/or medical treatment for mild and/or moderate asthma (Weiland & Pearce 2004).

Risk factors for asthma

These striking findings from the ISAAC and ECRHS studies, together with recent studies in Western countries, are challenging established theories of the development of asthma, and facilitating the search for new theoretical paradigms. In this subsection, we review evidence on traditional risk factors as well as some more recently suggested risk factors for asthma. We then consider whether these risk factors can explain the international patterns and time trends.

Atopy

As noted earlier, atopy (measured by skin prick test positivity or serum IgE) is strongly associated with asthma within populations. However, the proportion of asthma cases that are attributable to atopy is usually less than one half (Pearce *et al.* 1999), and an even lower population attributable risk (~20 per cent) was found in less affluent populations (Weinmayr *et al.* 2007). Also, comparisons across populations suggest that the association between atopy and asthma is relatively weak and highly variable between populations

(Weinmayr *et al.* 2007; Sunyer *et al.* 2004). Furthermore, although atopy may be a risk factor for asthma, it is not a classic environmental 'exposure' (e.g. indoor allergen exposure, smoking, air pollution), which could by itself explain increases in asthma prevalence; rather, it represents a biological response to various exposures (e.g. allergen exposure), which is modified by susceptibility factors (genetic and/or environmental).

Genetic factors

Asthma is multifactorial in origin and influenced by multiple genes and environmental factors. Thus, it is not inherited in the simple Mendelian fashion that is characteristic of single-gene disorders. A particular genetic factor may affect one or more aspects of the complex aetiological processes potentially involved in asthma including atopic sensitization, bronchial hyperresponsiveness (BHR), airway inflammation, innate immunity, and so on. Whether this genetic potential is expressed will depend upon various factors, including whether sufficient exposure to environmental factors occurs. Investigating possible genes for the individual aetiological factors is also fraught with difficulties, because control of these factors (e.g. IgE production and BHR) are also multifactorial (Zamel *et al.* 1996). Also, as noted earlier, asthma is an extremely heterogeneous disease including a variety of phenotypical and clinical manifestations, which are likely to be associated with different (combinations of) genes. Another potential source of phenotypic variability is that asthma development, exacerbations, and progression may involve different environmental triggers and genetic factors.

Currently, a number of genome-wide linkage studies have identified several chromosomal regions associated with asthma susceptibility; the regions with the strongest evidence include chromosome 2q, 5q, 6q, 11q, 12q, and 13q (Bierbaum & Heinzmann 2007). A large number of candidate genes have been described, with only some confirmed in subsequent independent studies; these include IL4, IL13, CD14, and ADRB2 on chromosome 5; HLA-DRB1, HLA-DBQ1, and TNF on chromosome 6; FCER1B on chromosome 11; IL4RA on chromosome 16; and ADAM33 on chromosome 20 (Bierbaum & Heinzmann 2007). However, some of these potentially interesting findings need further replication in other populations.

Demographic factors

There are a variety of demographic factors that are associated with asthma including age (Anderson *et al.* 1992), gender (Anderson *et al.* 1992), and ethnicity (Pattemore *et al.* 2004). Age is the demographic factor that is most strongly related to asthma symptom prevalence, with symptoms usually declining at or before the onset of puberty (Kimbell-Dunn *et al.* 1999).

Asthma incidence and prevalence are consistently lower among females than males before age 12 years, whereas during adolescence and adulthood there is evidence of higher incidence and prevalence among females (Kimbell-Dunn *et al.* 1999). One possible explanation is that the average age of onset in childhood and adolescence may be later for females. Levels of cord blood IgE are lower at birth in girls than in boys (Weeke 1992), indicating a lower risk of the subsequent development of asthma. Some authors have noted that boys have smaller airways relative to lung size than girls, and that this may explain the greater frequency and severity of lower respiratory tract illness in boys, even though infection rates are similar for both sexes (Martinez *et al.* 1988). Alternatively, it is possible that boys have more exposure to factors that increase asthma incidence or duration. On the other hand, the relatively higher prevalence (or smaller reduction in prevalence) among females than males after puberty could be due to hormonal influences on allergic predisposition, airway size, inflammation, and smooth muscle vascular functions (Redline & Gold 1994). Premenstrual asthma may be especially relevant to the hormonal involvement of asthma as it may not only cause asthma exacerbations but may thereby also affect the frequency and duration of asthma symptoms, resulting in an increase in the prevalence of 'current asthma'.

Studies in the 1960s and 1970s suggested that asthma is more common in children in the higher social classes. There has been less evidence of social class differences as the diagnosis of asthma has become more widespread (Littlejohns & Macdonald 1993), even though diagnostic labelling of wheezing in adults differs by social class (Littlejohns *et al.* 1989). However, severe asthma appears to be more common in children in the lower social classes (Stewart *et al.* 2001) and in some disadvantaged ethnic groups (Pattemore *et al.* 2004), and low socioeconomic status is associated with hospital admissions for asthma (Watson *et al.* 1996) and with reduced lung function in adults. This could represent either a greater prevalence of asthma in disadvantaged groups, increased severity due to environmental factors (e.g. environmental tobacco smoke, nutrition, occupational exposures) (Eagan *et al.* 2002; Ellison-Loschmann *et al.* 2007), or inadequate disease management and poor access to healthcare (Ellison-Loschmann & Pearce 2006).

Obesity

The specific mechanisms linking body weight and asthma are unclear, but several have been proposed including (1) common aetiologies, (2) co-morbidities, (3) mechanical factors, and (4) adipokines (i.e. cytokines secreted by adipose tissue) (Shore 2007). Similar to asthma, the prevalence of overweight and obesity have increased dramatically in the past few decades in many regions of the world (Burney 2002). Studies have shown associations between body weight and asthma in both adults (Braback *et al.* 2005) and children (von Mutius *et al.* 2001). Prospective studies of children suggest that obesity precedes asthma, signalling a causal link (Gilliland *et al.* 2003; Gold *et al.* 2003), as do studies showing associations between asthma and both weight gain and weight loss in adults (Hakala *et al.* 2000). Nonetheless, some studies have failed to show an association (Brenner *et al.* 2001) whereas others showed an association only in one gender (Mannino *et al.* 2006). Several reported an association only with respiratory symptoms (e.g. wheeze), but not BHR (Bustos *et al.* 2005), although this may merely indicate that obesity increases asthma risk through mechanisms other than BHR. Obesity may also increase severity in subjects with pre-existing asthma (Akerman *et al.* 2004).

Diet

Many studies have investigated the effects of breastfeeding on allergies and asthma with some studies showing protective effects, some showing no effect, and others suggesting that breastfeeding is a risk factor (Friedman & Zeiger 2005). A recent long-term longitudinal study found that exclusive breastfeeding was associated with a slightly reduced risk of asthma and atopy at age 7 years, but an increased risk at age 14 and 44 (Matheson *et al.* 2007). An infant cohort study in New Zealand showed that breastfeeding did not protect against atopy and asthma and may even increase the risk at age 9–26 years (Sears *et al.* 2002). A recent cluster randomized trial reported similar findings for allergies and asthma at age 6.5 years (Kramer *et al.* 2007).

Other nutritional factors may also play a role in the aetiology of asthma. In particular, it has been speculated that the increase in asthma prevalence may be due to a change in dietary patterns in the past few decades; that is, as cultures become more 'Westernized', they have shifted from a tradition of growing and consuming local foods to consuming more processed foods with an overall increase in the intake of refined sugars, fats, and additives, and a reduction in the intake of fresh fruits, vegetables, and fish. Several observational studies have shown protective effects of fruit and vegetables, whole grain products, and fish (Devereux 2007), and these findings are consistent with an ecologic analysis of the ISAAC Phase-I survey (Ellwood *et al.* 2001). Fruit, vegetables, and whole-grain products are rich in antioxidants and may reduce airway inflammation by protecting the airways against both endogenous and exogenous oxidants (Devereux 2007). Fish oils are rich in n-3 polyunsaturated fatty acids, which may also protect against airway inflammation and subsequent symptoms of asthma (Devereux 2007). However, recent dietary supplement studies focusing on antioxidants and n-3 fatty acids have not showed convincing evidence of a protective effect on allergies and asthma (Reisman *et al.* 2006; Almqvist *et al.* 2007).

Outdoor air pollution

The role of outdoor air pollutants (particulate matter, ozone, nitrogen dioxide, and sulphur dioxide) in asthma and other diseases has been extensively studied and debated. An association between measures of distance to major roads or traffic density and asthma symptoms has been demonstrated in a number of European countries (World Health Organization 2005). Also, a large number of studies have reported associations between direct measurements of air pollution levels and exacerbation of pre-existing asthma, both in children and adults (World Health Organization 2005; Boezen *et al.* 1999). Some studies, including a recent birth cohort study (Brauer *et al.* 2007), have also suggested that air pollution may cause *new onset* of asthma and allergic disease. In particular, several large prospective studies have suggested a role of ozone (McDonnell *et al.* 1999, 2002), although significant associations with some asthma outcomes were also shown for PM2.5, soot, and NO_2 (Brauer *et al.* 2007). Nonetheless, although it is clear that air pollution can provoke exacerbations in pre-existing asthma and a negative association between outdoor air pollution and asthma prevalence at the population level has been shown (Asher *et al.* 1998), the weight of evidence does not currently support a *major* role of outdoor air pollution as a cause of the initial development of asthma.

Tobacco

Similarly, the evidence for a role of tobacco smoke in asthma is strongest for increases in severity in children who already have asthma, whereas the evidence for the initial occurrence of asthma (incidence) is less conclusive. In particular, several recent reviews and meta-analyses differ in their conclusions about the role of second-hand tobacco smoke (SHS). The US Environmental Protection Agency (EPA) and the Californian EPA concluded that SHS was causally associated with the development of asthma in children (US Environmental Protection Agency 1992; Office of Environmental Health Hazard Assessment 1997). The 2006 Surgeon General's report on 'health effects from involuntary exposure to tobacco smoke' (US Department of Human Health and Human Services 2006) concluded that the evidence was suggestive but not sufficient to infer a causal relationship. This analysis was based on a previous meta-analysis conducted by Strachan and Cook (Strachan & Cook 1998) and did not include the most recent epidemiological studies. However, the most recent meta-analysis including studies published between 1970 and 2005 concluded that household SHS exposure was positively and consistently associated with the incidence of new-onset asthma (Vork *et al.* 2007) not only in younger but also older children.

The evidence on active smoking as a risk factor is also conflicting, with some studies reporting only exacerbations (Siroux *et al.* 2000) whereas others have also documented a dose-related risk of new-onset asthma in adolescents and adults (Eagan *et al.* 2002).

Overall, it therefore appears that environmental tobacco smoke is a cause of asthma exacerbations, and that it may also be involved in the development of asthma itself.

Indoor air pollution

Little is currently known about the contribution of indoor air pollutants (other than environmental tobacco smoke) to the incidence and prevalence of asthma. The range of potential pollutants is large, the determinants of ambient levels involve a complex interaction of lifestyle and building factors, and precise measurement of airborne concentrations is difficult. Nitrogen dioxide from burning fossil fuels has by far received the most attention, and sulphur dioxide from burning sulphur-containing coal or gas, mosquito coil smoke, and formaldehyde from wood preparation have also been considered. Particulates from open or closed wood and coal-burning fires have received less attention in developed countries, but have been studied in developing countries, where very high indoor levels have been encountered.

Damp indoor environments and indoor fungal exposure may also play a role, as demonstrated in a large number of studies conducted across many geographical regions (Douwes & Pearce 2003). However, although it has been concluded that the evidence for a causal association between dampness and respiratory morbidity is strong, it is not clear whether indoor dampness *causes* or 'only' *exacerbates* pre-existing respiratory conditions such as asthma (Douwes & Pearce 2003).

Occupational exposures

Occupational asthma (OA) is the most common occupational respiratory disease in developed countries. For example, asthma accounted for 28 per cent of the cases reported to the United Kingdom Surveillance of Work-Related and Occupational Respiratory Diseases (SWORD) project (Meredith *et al.* 1991). Estimates of the total proportion of adult asthma thought to be occupational in origin range from 2 to 15 per cent in the United States, 15 per cent in Japan (Chan-Yeung & Malo 1994), 5 per cent in Spain (Kogevinas *et al.* 1996), 2 to 3 per cent in New Zealand (Fishwick *et al.* 1997), and 2 to 6 per cent in the United Kingdom (Meredith & Nordman 1966). More than 250 agents have been identified as causes of OA (see http://www.remcomp.com/asmanet/asmapro/asmawork.htm and http://www.state.nj.us/health/eoh/survweb/wra/agents.shtml). Some of the most common occupational asthmagens include flour and grain dusts, wood dusts, latex allergens, and isocyanates.

Respiratory viral infections

Viral infections are common causes of exacerbations of asthma (Johnston *et al.* 1995). In fact, respiratory viral infections are detected in the majority of asthma exacerbations (80–85 per cent in children and 75–80 per cent in adults); of these, about 60 per cent are rhinoviruses (Johnston 2007). There is also a strong association between viral infections and hospital admission for asthma among both children and adults.

Viral infections may also be involved in the development of asthma, but the evidence is less clear. Several long-term longitudinal studies have shown that respiratory syncytial virus (RSV) infections increase the risk of subsequent recurrent wheezing and asthma in early childhood (Stein *et al.* 1999; Sigurs *et al.* 2005). However, this risk may progressively decrease with increasing age (Stein *et al.* 1999). Other viruses have also been associated with asthma development including human rhinovirus (HRV), which may in fact be a more important risk factor than RSV (Lemanske *et al.* 2005). The mechanisms of viral-induced asthma are poorly understood, but it has been speculated that impaired innate immune responses may play a crucial role (Johnston 2007).

Paracetamol

It has been reported that prenatal paracetamol (or acetaminophen) use during pregnancy is a risk factor for asthma, wheezing, and total IgE in the offspring at 6–7 years of age (Shaheen *et al.* 2002, 2005). Similarly, several cross-sectional and longitudinal studies have reported that paracetamol use is associated in a dose-dependent manner with an increase in asthma in children and also new-onset asthma in adults (Shaheen *et al.* 2000; Barr *et al.* 2004). Furthermore, national per-capita consumption of acetaminophen was ecologically associated with the prevalence of wheeze, diagnosed asthma, and bronchial hyperresponsiveness in Western Europe (Newson *et al.* 2000). Some of these associations may have been due to confounding (e.g. confounding by indication), but this is unlikely to fully explain the positive associations in birth cohort studies (Shaheen *et al.* 2002; Shaheen *et al.* 2005), and longitudinal studies among adults that focused on new-onset asthma (Barr *et al.* 2004). The underlying mechanisms are unclear, but it has been suggested that paracetamol decreases glutathione levels in the lungs, which may predispose to oxidative injury, bronchospasm, and an increased Th_2 response (Shaheen *et al.* 2002). Interestingly, the use of paracetamol has increased considerably (replacing aspirin) since the 1970s and 1980s (Varner *et al.* 1998), suggesting that the increased used of paracetamol may account for some of the increasing prevalence of childhood asthma.

Allergens

Indoor allergens, particularly house-dust mite allergens, are perhaps the group of possible asthma risk factors that have received the greatest attention. It is well established that, in sensitized asthmatics, allergen exposure can trigger asthma attacks and that prolonged exposure can lead to the prolongation and exacerbation of symptoms. However, most studies among children show only weak associations between allergen exposure and current asthma, even when the analyses are restricted to atopic patients and allergen avoidance has been accounted for (Pearce *et al.* 2000b). Also, secondary intervention trials have had mixed results (Gotzsche *et al.* 1998).

In fact, although there is good evidence for asthma exacerbations, the evidence for new-onset asthma is much weaker (Pearce *et al.* 2000b). The key study linking allergen exposure in infancy to the subsequent development of asthma is that of Sporik *et al.* (1990), who followed 67 children with a family history of atopy. They found an association between dust mite allergen levels and mite sensitization, and an association between exposure to more than 10 μg/g in the first year of life and a history of wheezing, although this association was not statistically significant (OR = 2.3, p = 0.17). There were marginally non-significant associations with 'active wheezing and BHR' (p = 0.08) and with 'receiving medication' (p = 0.10).

More recent longitudinal birth cohort studies found little or no association between early dust mite allergen exposure and asthma later in childhood (Burr *et al.* 1993; Corver *et al.* 2006; Tepas *et al.* 2006). For example, Burr *et al.* (1993) conducted a longitudinal study among 453 infants in South Wales with a family history of allergic diseases. Doctor-diagnosed asthma and wheezing at age 7 was neither associated with mite allergen exposure as determined in the first 12 months nor with dust mite levels measured at 7 years of age (odds ratios were not given). Similarly, in the German Multicentre Allergy Study, levels of mite and cat allergens in early life remained strongly related to specific sensitization at age 3–7 years, but no dose–response relationship between allergen exposure and any measure of asthma or wheeze at 7 years of age was found (Lau *et al.* 2000, 2002) Dust mite allergens are therefore unlikely to play a major role in the initial development of asthma.

There are several other indoor and outdoor allergens that have been suggested to be associated with the development of asthma, including cat, dog, cockroach, and *Alternaria* allergens. However, the evidence for a causal relationship is even weaker than for house-dust mite allergens (Pearce *et al.* 2000b). In fact, several studies even reported a protective effect on the development of asthma of pet keeping early in life.

Can the traditional risk factors explain the international patterns and time trends?

There is little evidence that the traditional risk factors can account for the global prevalence increases or the international prevalence patterns that have been observed. The increases in asthma prevalence cannot be due to genetic factors because they are occurring too rapidly, and the rapidity of the increases indicates that genetic factors alone are unlikely to account for a substantial proportion of asthma cases (Douwes & Pearce 2002), although genetic susceptibility to changing environmental exposures may play an important role.

The global patterns of asthma prevalence are also inconsistent with the hypothesis that air pollution is a major risk factor for the development of asthma (Asher *et al.* 1998, 2006; Beasley *et al.* 1998). Regions such as China and Eastern Europe, which have some of the highest levels of traditional air pollution such as particulate matter and SO_2, generally have lower asthma prevalence than the countries of Western Europe and North America, Australia, and New Zealand, which have lower levels of pollution. It also appears very unlikely that the international prevalence patterns can be explained by differences in smoking (Mitchell *et al.* 2001), or in occupational exposures.

Allergen exposure is the risk factor that has perhaps received the most attention as a possible cause of the global increases in prevalence of asthma and allergies. In particular, it has been suggested

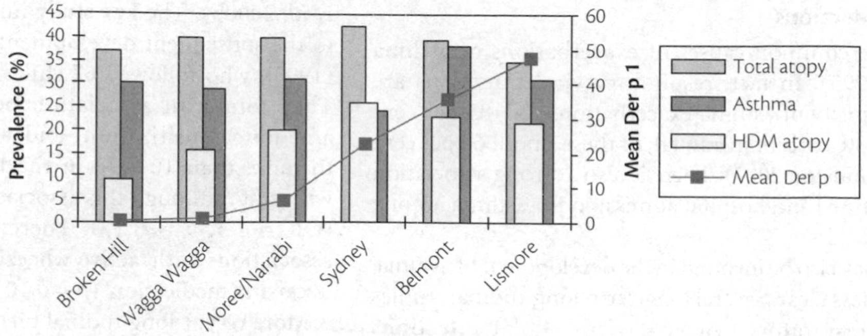

Fig. 9.4.5 Mean Der p 1 levels and prevalence (per cent) of house-dust mite (HDM) atopy, total atopy, and asthma in six areas of Australia.

that increases in indoor allergen exposures, through changes in lifestyle such as wall-to-wall carpeting, cold water washing, greater time spent indoors watching television, and so on, could account for the global increases in asthma prevalence (Sporik *et al.* 1990). However, the only study of English homes at two time points (1979 and 1989) did not demonstrate any change in house-dust mite allergen levels (Butland *et al.* 1997), but marked increases have been observed in Australian studies (Peat *et al.* 1996).

The ISAAC (Asher *et al.* 1998) and ECRHS (Burney *et al.* 1996) studies have consistently found uniformly high levels of asthma prevalence in centres in English-speaking countries, even though there is a wide variation in house-dust mite levels across these countries (Martinez 1997). In geographical areas in which dust mite exposure is very low or absent, including desert regions and mountainous regions, the prevalence of asthma is as high or even higher than that in other areas where house dust mite exposure is high (Martinez 1997).

Other available evidence on the association between allergen exposure and the subsequent risk of asthma at the population level is also less than persuasive. For example, Leung *et al.* (1997) reported that asthma prevalence was high in Hong Kong (6.6 per cent for asthma ever) and low in San Bu, China (1.6 per cent), but exposures to house-dust mite allergen were similar in Hong Kong and San Bu. Similarly, Fig. 9.4.5 shows data from six Australian surveys in centres with widely differing levels of mite allergen exposure; the overall prevalences of sensitization and asthma were both unrelated to the levels of house-dust mite allergen (Der p 1) exposure in the six centres. The dominant allergen varied between regions, but there was little overall difference in the prevalence of sensitization or of asthma despite the major differences in mite allergen levels. Similarly, Von Mutius *et al.* (1994) found that asthma was significantly higher in Munich, West Germany (5.9 per cent) than in Leipzig, East Germany (3.9 per cent), and this paralleled the pattern of skin prick test positivity (19.2 and 7.3 per cent); however, house-dust mite allergen levels were similar in the East and the West (Hirsch *et al.* 1998).

The other asthma risk factors (e.g. diet, obesity, and/or paracetamol) may significantly contribute to the observed time trends and international patterns of asthma prevalence, but the current evidence for this is scant.

Towards a new paradigm

Thus, for many of the traditional risk factors, there is evidence that they may exacerbate pre-existing asthma, but the evidence that they may be involved in the initial development of asthma is limited. Also, there is little evidence that these factors account for the global prevalence increases.

Recent research has, therefore, shifted attention from allergens that may cause sensitization and/or provoke asthma attacks to factors that may 'programme' the initial susceptibility to asthma, through allergic or non-allergic mechanisms. This also, in part, involves a shift of attention from risk factors for asthma to protective factors, and the possible role of the loss of protective factors in the global increases in asthma prevalence (Pearce *et al.* 2000c).

The 'hygiene hypothesis' has been prompted by evidence that overcrowding and unhygienic conditions were associated with a lower prevalence of atopy, eczema, hay fever, and asthma (Strachan 1989). Having a large number of siblings (especially older siblings) and attendance at day-care centres were determined to be particularly protective (Ball *et al.* 2000). An increase in infections has been proposed as an explanation for these findings (Martinez 1994), and several studies have in fact shown a direct association between infections (e.g. hepatitis A, measles) or immunization with BCG and a lower prevalence of atopy and allergies (Shaheen *et al.* 1996; Matricardi *et al.* 1997). However, the results for airborne viruses (measles, mumps, rubella, and chickenpox) and BCG vaccination are inconsistent (Alm *et al.* 1998; Matricardi *et al.* 2000).

Exposure to specific microbial agents with strong pro-inflammatory properties such as bacterial endotoxin have also been suggested to be protective (Douwes *et al.* 2004). A study of 61 infants showed that allergen-sensitized infants had significantly lower house dust endotoxin levels than non-sensitized infants and levels correlated with IFN-γ producing T helper 1 cells (Th_1) but not with IL-4, IL-5, or IL-13 producing cell proportions (Th_2) (Gereda *et al.* 2000). Studies in both rural and non-rural environments reported a significant inverse association between indoor endotoxin levels and atopic sensitization (Gehring *et al.* 2001), hay fever, and atopic asthma (Braun-Fahrlander *et al.* 2002). In contrast, a birth cohort study conducted by the same researchers found that early endotoxin exposure was associated with an *increased* risk of atopy at the age of 2 years (Bolte *et al.* 2003) However, two similar birth cohort studies found a protective effect on atopy in 2-year-olds (Bottcher *et al.* 2003) and asthma symptoms in 4-year-olds (Douwes *et al.* 2006). Thus, despite some inconsistencies in the available evidence, which may be related to the hypothesized bimodal effect of endotoxin on the Th_1/Th_2 balance (Eisenbarth *et al.* 2002), it appears that endotoxin exposures may protect against atopy and allergic asthma.

Although most of the evidence points towards LPS, other pathogen-associated molecular patterns (PAMPs) may be equally (or more) important. There is evidence that exposure to peptidoglycans, CpG containing DNA, and certain viruses may also reduce the risk of atopic disease (Douwes *et al.* 2005). The evidence for these PAMPs is, however, scarce.

In addition to specific agents with potential protective effects, subpopulations have been identified with low atopy and asthma rates compared to the general populations. For instance, it has been documented that children with an anthroposophic lifestyle in Sweden (Alm *et al.* 1999) and children raised on farms with livestock in Europe, Canada, and Australia have less atopy and asthma (Braun-Fahrlander *et al.* 2002). Similar effects have also been shown in adult farmers (Douwes *et al.* 2007). Contact with animals was shown to be particularly protective. It is currently not clear which specific factors associated with animal contact confer protection, but specific microbial exposures have been hypothesized to be involved either through ingestion (lactobacilli) or inhalation (endotoxin). Ingestion of lactobacilli through consumption of unpasteurized milk may be important because they have the ability to colonise the human gut (Johansson *et al.* 1993), and may subsequently modify the immune development in a non-atopic Th_1 direction (Björkstén *et al.* 1999). However, various other microbes of the gut flora may play a role as well (Bottcher *et al.* 2000; Björkstén *et al.* 2001).

Furthermore, several studies in Europe have shown that the presence of pets in the home early in life was inversely associated with atopy (Hesselmar *et al.* 1999). Another study showed that having had a cat before the age of 18 protected against atopy to outdoor allergens, airway hyperreactivity, current wheeze, and current asthma (de Meer *et al.* 2004b). These results should, however, be interpreted with caution, because avoidance behaviour (removal of pets in the families with sensitized and/or symptomatic children) may have contributed to this inverse association. However, in a recent longitudinal study in which subjects with childhood asthma at enrolment were excluded from the analyses, the protective effects actually increased (de Meer *et al.* 2004b), whereas a decrease would be expected if selective avoidance was a major issue. At present, it is not clear which specific exposures and immunological mechanisms underlie the observed protective effects of pet ownership, but increased microbial exposure may play a role.

In other parts of the world (Guinea-Bissau and Nepal), it has been shown that pigs and cattle in the home are associated with less atopy (Shirakawa *et al.* 1997; Melsom *et al.* 2001). This is in line with observations that animal contact among farmers' children may confer protection, and as hypothesized for the farmers' children, increased endotoxin exposures may play a role (Douwes *et al.* 2002b).

Although the specific immune mechanisms are not clear, it is believed that microbial exposure may affect T lymphocytes, which have an important function in controlling immune responses including help for B-cell production of antibodies (IgE, IgG, IgA, IgM). T helper 2 (Th_2) cells stimulate B cells to produce IgE upon allergen stimulation whereas T helper 1 cells (Th_1) inhibit this process. The initial interpretation was that growing up in a more hygienic environment with less microbial exposure may enhance atopic (Th_2) immune responses, whereas microbial pressure would drive the response of the immune system—which is known to be skewed in an atopic Th_2 direction during foetal and perinatal life—into a Th_1 direction and away from its tendency to develop atopic immune responses (Martinez & Holt 1999). More recently, an alternative interpretation has been offered, which involves a reduction in activity of T regulatory cells resulting in a reduced immune suppression and subsequently an up-regulation of both Th_1 and Th_2 immunity. However, at this stage, the immunological mechanisms underlying the observed epidemiological associations (see the following subsection) remain largely unclear (Romagnani 2004).

Can the 'hygiene hypothesis' explain the international patterns and time trends?

With the large proportion of asthma that is not attributable to atopy or allergy, it is questionable whether the 'hygiene hypothesis' on its own can explain the large increases observed over the last decades or the global prevalence patterns, particularly because there is some evidence that non-atopic asthma may have increased more than atopic asthma (Thomsen *et al.* 2004). Also, although housing conditions are unlikely to have become more hygienic in US inner-city populations, asthma prevalence has increased significantly in those populations, particularly among African Americans living in poverty (Crater *et al.* 2001). Finally, the hygiene hypothesis is unlikely to explain why asthma prevalence is now apparently falling, as exposures to factors that have previously been identified as being 'protective' (family size, endotoxin exposure, infectious diseases, pets, etc.) are likely to have decreased in more recent times rather than increased. Also, there is no indication that exposures to suspected risk factors such as environmental tobacco smoke, house-dust mites, and air pollution have significantly decreased. These findings, thus, further emphasize the potential limitations of the current hygiene hypothesis. Nevertheless, whatever mechanism is involved, it is becoming increasingly clear that the 'package' of changes associated with Westernization may be contributing to the global increases in asthma susceptibility and prevalence.

Conclusion

What do these epidemiological findings tell us about the major causes of asthma and COPD?

The prevalence of COPD is still increasing particularly among women, and future projections indicate that the global burden of COPD will increase even further. The major causal risk factor is tobacco smoke, but a substantial proportion of COPD is also caused by occupational and indoor exposures, particularly in middle- and low-income countries. Only a minority of the persistent smokers develop COPD; that is, those who are likely to be genetically susceptible for cigarette smoking. Similar to asthma, large international differences are observed in COPD prevalence even when identical assessment methods are used, and these are not explained by age or cigarette smoking alone. Further understanding is required why some smokers develop COPD, and others do not, and what causes the striking differences in the global prevalence of COPD. However, we do know how to prevent COPD in the majority of cases; that is, smoking cessation is the most effective way to prevent the development of COPD and reduce disease progression.

In contrast, there are major gaps in our current understanding of asthma aetiology. Although atopic sensitization is strongly associated with asthma, it appears to account for less than one half of all cases, and there is little evidence that the traditional environmental asthma risk factors account for international prevalence increases. Recent decades have seen decreasing family size, increased hygiene, shift in dietary patterns, as well as increasing use of medical interventions such as immunization, antibiotics, and use of paracetamol. It seems that as a result of this 'package' of changes in the intrauterine and infant environment, we are seeing an increased susceptibility to the development of asthma and/or allergy. However, more recently, the increase in asthma prevalence appears to have levelled off in many high-income countries, with some even showing a decrease. The reasons for this are unclear. Understanding why these changes are occurring, and ascertaining which elements of the 'package' of twentieth-century economic development and lifestyle changes are responsible, is essential in order to develop effective intervention programmes to halt the current global asthma epidemic.

Key points

- COPD and asthma have increased dramatically in the past few decades, both in Western and non-Western societies.
- Smoking cessation and improved indoor ventilation measures to reduce indoor pollutants in houses of most middle- and low-income countries are the most effective ways to halt global increases in the prevalence of COPD.
- Asthma is a very heterogeneous disease with less than half of the asthma cases attributable to allergic mechanisms.
- Asthma prevalence differs greatly between countries with the highest prevalences in English-speaking countries and considerably lower prevalences in most low-income countries.
- The increases in asthma prevalence observed in the past few decades appear to have levelled off in many high-income countries in the last decade, with some even showing a decrease.
- Although risk factors for asthma exacerbations have been well identified, the main factors causing new-onset asthma are still only poorly understood, thus hampering the development of an effective prevention programme.

Acknowledgements

The Centre for Public Health Research is supported by a Programme Grant from the Health Research Council of New Zealand, and Jeroen Douwes is supported by a Sir Charles Hercus Research Fellowship from the Health Research Council (HRC) of New Zealand.

Author contributions

Jeroen Douwes has contributed to all sections of this chapter. Marike Boezen has primarily contributed to the COPD subsection, and Neil Pearce primarily to the asthma subsection.

References

Aberg N., Hesselmar B., Alberg B. *et al.* Increase in asthma, allergic rhinitis and eczema in Swedish schoolchildren between 1979 and 1991. *Clinical and Experimental Allergy* 1995;**25**:815–9.

Aberg N. Asthma and allergic rhinitis in Swedish conscripts. *Clinical and Experimental Allergy* 1989;**19**:59–63.

Adams R., Ruffin R., Wakefield M. *et al.* Asthma prevalence, morbidity and management practices in South Australia, 1992–1995. *Australian and New Zealand Journal of Medicine* 1997;**27**:672–9.

Aggarwal A.N., Gupta D., Jindal S.K. The relationship between FEV_1 and peak expiratory flow in patients with airways obstruction is poor. *Chest* 2006;**130**:1454–61.

Akerman M.J., Calacanis C.M., Madsen M.K. Relationship between asthma severity and obesity. *Journal of Asthma* 2004;**41**:521–6.

Alm J.S., Lilja G., Pershagen G. *et al.* BCG vaccination does not seem to prevent atopy in children with atopic heredity. *Allergy* 1998;**53**:537.

Alm J.S., Swartz J., Lilja G. *et al.* Atopy in children of families with an anthroposophic lifestyle. *Lancet* 1999;**353**:1485–8.

Almqvist C., Garden F., Xuan W. *et al.* Omega-3 and omega-6 fatty acid exposure from early life does not affect atopy and asthma at age 5 years. *Journal of Allergy and Clinical Immunology* 2007;**119**:1438–44.

American Thoracic Society Committee on Diagnostic Standards. Definitions and classification of chronic bronchitis, asthma and pulmonary emphysema. *American Review of Respiratory Disease* 1962;**85**:762–8.

Anderson H.R., Butland B.K., Strachan D.P. Trends in prevalence and severity of childhood asthma. *British Medical Journal* 1994;**308**:1600–4.

Anderson H.R., Pottier A.C., Strachan D.P. Asthma from birth to age 23—incidence and relation to prior and concurrent atopic disease. *Thorax* 1992;**47**:537–42.

Anderson H.R., Ruggles R., Strachan D.P. *et al.* Trends in prevalence of symptoms of asthma, hay fever, and eczema in 12–14 year olds in the British Isles, 1995–2002: questionnaire survey. *British Medical Journal* 2004;**328**:1052–3.

Anttila S., Hukkanen J., Hakkola J. *et al.* Expression and localization of CYP3A4 and CYP3A5 in human lung. *American Journal of Respiratory Cell and Molecular Biology* 1997;**16**:242–9.

Asher M.I., Anderson H.R., Stewart A. *et al.* Worldwide variations in the prevalence of asthma symptoms: International Study of Asthma and Allergies in Childhood (ISAAC). *European Respiratory Journal* 1998;**12**:315–35.

Asher M.I., Keil U., Anderson H.R. *et al.* International Study of Asthma and Allergies in Childhood (ISAAC): rationale and methods. *European Respiratory Journal* 1995;**8**:483–91.

Asher M.I., Montefort S., Bjorksten B. *et al.* Worldwide time trends in the prevalence of symptoms of asthma, allergic rhinoconjunctivitis, and eczema in childhood: ISAAC phases one and three repeat multicountry cross-sectional surveys. *Lancet* 2006;**368**:733–43.

Auerbach I., Springer C., Godfrey S. Total population survey of the frequency and severity of asthma in 17 year old boys in an urban area in Israel. *Thorax* 1993;**48**:139–41.

Badham C. An essay on bronchitis: with a supplement containing remarks on simple pulmonary abscess. 2nd ed. London: J Callow; 1814.

Ball T.N., Castro-Rodriguez J.A., Griffith K.A. Siblings, day care attendance and the risk of asthma and wheezing during childhood. *New England Journal of Medicine* 2000;**343**:538–43.

Balmes J.R. Occupational contribution to the burden of chronic obstructive pulmonary disease. *Journal of Occupational and Environmental Medicine* 2005;**47**:154–60.

Barnes P.J. Against the Dutch hypothesis: asthma and chronic obstructive pulmonary disease are distinct diseases. *American Journal of Respiratory and Critical Care Medicine* 2006;**174**:240–3.; discussion 243–4.

Barnes P.J. Genetics and pulmonary medicine. *9: Molecular genetics of chronic obstructive pulmonary disease. Thorax* 1999;**54**:245–52.

Barr R.G., Wentowski C.C., Curhan G.C. *et al.* Prospective study of acetaminophen use and newly diagnosed asthma among women. *American Journal of Respiratory and Critical Care Medicine* 2004;**169**:836–41.

Beasley R., Keil U., Von Mutius E. *et al.* Worldwide variation in prevalence of symptoms of asthma, allergic rhinoconjunctivitis and atopic eczema: ISAAC. *Lancet* 1998;**351**:1225–32.

Berry M., Morgan A., Shaw D.E. *et al.* Pathological features and inhaled corticosteroid response of eosinophilic and non-eosinophilic asthma. *Thorax* 2007;**62**:1043–9.

Bierbaum S., Heinzmann A. The genetics of bronchial asthma in children. *Respiratory Medicine* 2007;**101**:1369–75.

Björkstén B., Naaber P., Sepp E. *et al.* The intestinal microflora in allergic Estonian and Swedish 2-year-old children. *Clinical and Experimental Allergy* 1999;**29**:342–6.

Björkstén B., Sepp E., Julge K. *et al.* Allergy development and the intestinal micro flora during the first year of life. *Journal of Allergy and Clinical Immunology* 2001;**108**:516–20.

Boezen H.M., Postma D.S. Genetics of COPD. In: Dekhuijzen PNR, editor. *Chronic obstructive pulmonary disease*. Alphen aan de Rhijn, the Netherlands: Van Zuijden Communications; 2004.

Boezen H.M., Postma D.S. Tumour necrosis factor and lymphotoxin A polymorphisms: a relationship with COPD and its progression? *European Respiratory Journal* 2007;**29**:8–10.

Boezen H.M., van der Zee S.C., Postma D.S. *et al.* Effects of ambient air pollution on upper and lower respiratory symptoms and peak expiratory flow in children. *Lancet* 1999;**353**:874–8.

Bollag U., Capkun G., Caesar J. *et al.* Trends in primary care consultations for asthma in Switzerland, 1989–2002. *International Journal of Epidemiology* 2005;**34**:1012–8.

Bolte G., Bischof W., Borte M. *et al.* Early endotoxin exposure and atopy development in infants: results of a birth cohort study. *Clinical and Experimental Allergy* 2003;**33**:770–6.

Bottcher M.F., Bjorksten B., Gustafson S. *et al.* Endotoxin levels in Estonian and Swedish house dust and atopy in infancy. *Clinical and Experimental Allergy* 2003;**33**:295–300.

Bottcher M.F., Nordin E.K., Sandin A. *et al.* Microflora-associated characteristics in faeces from allergic and non-allergic infants. *Clinical and Experimental Allergy* 2000;**30**:1590–6.

Braback L., Hjern A., Rasmussen F. Body mass index, asthma and allergic rhinoconjunctivitis in Swedish conscripts-a national cohort study over three decades. *Respiratory Medicine* 2005;**99**:1010–4.

Brauer M., Hoek G., Smit H.A. *et al.* Air pollution and development of asthma, allergy and infections in a birth cohort. *European Respiratory Journal* 2007;**29**:879–88.

Braun-Fahrlander C., Riedler J., Herz U. *et al.* Environmental exposure to endotoxin and its relation to asthma in school-age children. *New England Journal of Medicine* 2002;**347**:869–77.

Brenner J.S., Kelly C.S., Wenger A.D. *et al.* Asthma and obesity in adolescents: is there an association? *Journal of Asthma* 2001; **38**:509–15.

Buist A.S., McBurnie M.A., Vollmer W.M. *et al.* International variation in the prevalence of COPD (the BOLD Study): a population-based prevalence study. *Lancet* 2007;**370**:741–50.

Burney P., Chinn S., Luczynska C. *et al.* Variations in the prevalence of respiratory symptoms, self-reported asthma attacks, and use of asthma medication in the European Community Respiratory Health Survey (ECRHS). *European Respiratory Journal* 1996;**9**:687–95.

Burney P., Chinn S., Rona R.J. Has the prevalence of asthma increased in children? Evidence from a national study of health and growth, 1973–86. *British Medical Journal* 1990;**300**:1306–10.

Burney P. The changing prevalence of asthma? *Thorax* 2002;**57** Suppl **2**: II36–II39.

Burney P.G.J., Luczynska C., Chinn S. *et al.* The European Community Respiratory Health Survey. *European Respiratory Journal* 1994; **7**:954–60.

Burr M.L., Butland B.K., King S. *et al.* Changes in asthma prevalence: two surveys 15 years apart. *Archives of Disease in Childhood* 1989;**64**: 1452–6.

Burr M.L., Limb E.S., Maguire M.J. *et al.* Infant-feeding, wheezing, and allergy—a prospective-study. *Archives of Disease in Childhood* 1993;**68**:724–8.

Burrows B., Fletcher C.M., Heard B.E. *et al.* The emphysematous and bronchial types of chronic airways obstruction. *A clinicopathological study of patients in London and Chicago. Lancet* 1966;**1**:830–5.

Bustos P., Amigo H., Oyarzun M. *et al.* Is there a causal relation between obesity and asthma? Evidence from Chile. *International Journal of Obesity (London)* 2005;**29**:804–9.

Butland B.K., Strachan D.P., Anderson H.R. The home environment and asthma symptoms in childhood: two population based case-control studies 13 years apart. *Thorax* 1997;**52**:618–24.

Camilli A.E., Burrows B., Knudson R.J. *et al.* Longitudinal changes in forced expiratory volume in one second in adults. Effects of smoking and smoking cessation. *American Review of Respiratory Disease* 1987;**135**:794–9.

Campbell D., Ruffin R., Mcevoy R. *et al.* South Australian asthma prevalence survey [abstract]. *Australian and New Zealand Journal of Medicine* 1992;**22**:A658.

Chan-Yeung M., Malo J.L. Epidemiology of occupational asthma. In: Busse W, Holgate ST, editors. *Asthma and rhinitis*. Oxford: Blackwell Scientific; 1994. p. 44–57.

Chapman K.R., Mannino D.M., Soriano J.B. *et al.* Epidemiology and costs of chronic obstructive pulmonary disease. *European Respiratory Journal* 2006;**27**:188–207.

Chapman K.R., Tashkin D.P., Pye D.J. Gender bias in the diagnosis of COPD. *Chest* 2001;**119**:1691–5.

Chinn S., Jarvis D., Burney P. *et al.* Increase in diagnosed asthma but not in symptoms in the European Community Respiratory Health Survey. *Thorax* 2004;**59**:646–51.

CIBA Foundation Guest Symposium. Terminology definitions, classification of chronic pulmonary emphysema and related conditions. *Thorax* 1959;**14**:286–99.

Ciprandi G., Vizzaccaro A., Cirillo I. *et al.* Increase of asthma and allergic rhinitis prevalence in young Italian men. *International Archives of Allergy and Immunology* 1996;**111**:278–83.

Committee on Diagnostic Standards for Nontuberculous Respiratory Diseases. Definitions and classification of chronic bronchitis, asthma and pulmonary emphysema. *American Review of Respiratory Disease* 1962;**85**:762–9.

Corver K., Kerkhof M., Brussee J.E. *et al.* House dust mite allergen reduction and allergy at 4 yr: follow up of the PIAMA-study. *Pediatric Allergy and Immunology* 2006;**17**:329–36.

Crater D.D., Heise S., Perzanowski M. Asthma hospitalization trends in Charleston, South Carolina, 1956 to 1997: twenty-fold increase among black children during a 30-year period. *Paediatrics* 2001;**108**:E97.

Crockett A.J., Cranston J.M., Moss J.R. *et al.* Trends in chronic obstructive pulmonary disease mortality in Australia. *Medical Journal of Australia* 1994;**161**:600–3.

de Meer G., Marks G.B., Postma D.S. Direct or indirect stimuli for bronchial challenge testing: what is the relevance for asthma epidemiology? *Clinial and Experimental Allergy* 2004a;**34**:9–16.

de Meer G., Toelle B.G., Ng K. *et al.* Presence and timing of cat ownership by age 18 and the effect on atopy and asthma at age 28. *Journal of Allergy and Clinical Immunology* 2004b;**113**:433–8.

Devereux G. Early life events in asthma—diet. *Pediatric Pulmonology* 2007;**42**:663–73.

Douwes J., Gibson P., Pekkanen J. *et al.* Non-eosinophilic asthma: importance and possible mechanisms. *Thorax* 2002a;**57**:643–8.

Douwes J., Le Gros G., Gibson P. *et al.* Can bacterial endotoxin exposure reverse atopy and atopic disease? *Journal of Allergy and Clinical Immunology* 2004;**114**:1051–4.

Douwes J., LeGros G., Gibson P. *et al.* On the hygiene hypothesis: regulation down, up, or sideways? [reply] *Journal of Allergy and Clinical Immunology* 2005;**115**:1326–1326.

Douwes J., Pearce N., Heederik D. Does environmental endotoxin exposure prevent asthma? [comment] *Thorax* 2002b;**57**:86–90.

Douwes J., Pearce N. Asthma and the Westernization 'package'. *International Journal of Epidemiology* 2002;**31**:1098–102.

Douwes J., Pearce N. Is indoor mold exposure a risk factor for asthma? [comment] *American Journal of Epidemiology* 2003;**158**:203–6.

Douwes J., Travier N., Huang K. *et al.* Lifelong farm exposure may strongly reduce the risk of asthma in adults. *Allergy* 2007;**62**:1158–65.

Douwes J., van Strien R., Doekes G. *et al.* Does early indoor microbial exposure reduce the risk of asthma? The Prevention and Incidence of Asthma and Mite Allergy birth cohort study. *Journal of Allergy and Clinical Immunology* 2006;**117**:1067–73.

Dowse G.K., Turner K.J., Stewart G.A. *et al.* The association between Dermatophagoides mites and the increasing prevalence of asthma in village communities within the Papua New Guinea highlands. *Journal of Allergy and Clinical Immunology* 1985;**75**:75–83.

Eagan T.M., Bakke P.S., Eide G.E. *et al.* Incidence of asthma and respiratory symptoms by sex, age and smoking in a community study. *European Respiratory Journal* 2002;**19**:599–605.

Eisenbarth S.C., Piggott D.A., Huleatt J.W. *et al.* Lipopolysaccharide-enhanced, toll-like receptor 4-dependent T helper cell type 2 responses to inhaled antigen. *Journal of Experimental Medicine* 2002;**196**:1645–51.

Ellison-Loschmann L., Pearce N. Improving access to health care among New Zealand's Maori population. *American Journal of Public Health* 2006;**96**:612–7.

Ellison-Loschmann L., Sunyer J., Plana E. *et al.* Socioeconomic status, asthma and chronic bronchitis in a large community-based study. *European Respiratory Journal* 2007;**29**:897–905.

Ellul-Micallef R. Asthma: a look at the past. *British Journal of Diseases of the Chest* 1976;**70**:112–6.

Ellwood P., Asher M.I., Beasley R. *et al.* The International Study of Asthma and Allergies in Childhood (ISAAC): phase three rationale and methods. *International Journal of Tuberculosis and Lung Disease* 2005;**9**:10–6.

Ellwood P., Asher M.I., Bjorksten B. *et al.* Diet and asthma, allergic rhinoconjunctivitis and atopic eczema symptom prevalence: an ecological analysis of the International Study of Asthma and Allergies in Childhood (ISAAC) data. ISAAC phase one study group. *European Respiratory Journal* 2001;**17**:436–43.

Farber H.J., Wattigney W., Berenson G. Trends in asthma prevalence: the Bogalusa Heart Study. *Annals of Allergy, Asthma and Immunology* 1997;**78**:265–9.

Feenstra T.L., van Genugten M.L., Hoogenveen R.T. *et al.* The impact of aging and smoking on the future burden of chronic obstructive pulmonary disease: a model analysis in the Netherlands. *American Journal of Respiratory and Critical Care Medicine* 2001;**164**:590–6.

Fishwick D., Pearce N., D'Souza W. *et al.* Occupational asthma in New Zealanders: a population based study [comment]. *Occupational and Environmental Medicine* 1997;**54**:301–6.

Fleming D.M., Crombie D.L. Prevalence of asthma and hay fever in England and Wales. *British Medical Journal (Clinical Research Edition)* 1987;**294**:279–83.

Flohr C., Weiland S.K., Weinmayr G. *et al.* The role of atopic sensitization in flexural eczema: findings from the International Study of Asthma and Allergies in Childhood phase two. *Journal of Allergy and Clinical Immunology* 2008;**121**:141–7.

Friedman N.J., Zeiger R.S. The role of breast-feeding in the development of allergies and asthma. *Journal of Allergy and Clinical Immunology* 2005;**115**:238–48.

Garcia-Marcos L., Quiros A.B., Hernandez G.G. *et al.* Stabilization of asthma prevalence among adolescents and increase among schoolchildren (ISAAC Phases I and III) in Spain. *Allergy* 2004;**59**:1301–7.

Gehring U., Bolte G., Borte M. *et al.* Exposure to endotoxin decreases the risk of atopic eczema in infancy: a cohort study. *Journal of Allergy and Clinical Immunology* 2001;**108**:847–54.

Gereda J.E., Leung D.Y., Thatayakitom A. Relation between house-dust endotoxin exposure, type 1 T-cell development, and allergen sensitisation in infants at high risk of asthma. *Lancet* 2000; **355**:1680–3.

Gergen P.J., Mullally D.I., Evans R., III. National survey of prevalence of asthma among children in the United States, 1976 to 1980. *Pediatrics* 1988;**81**:1–7.

Gilliland F.D., Berhane K., Islam T. *et al.* Obesity and the risk of newly diagnosed asthma in school-age children. *American Journal of Epidemiology* 2003;**158**:406–15.

Global Initiative for Asthma. Global strategy for asthma management and prevention. [Online]. 2006. Available from: *http://www.ginasthma.org*

Gold D.R., Damokosh A.I., Dockery D.W. *et al.* Body-mass index as a predictor of incident asthma in a prospective cohort of children. *Pediatric Pulmonology* 2003;**36**:514–21.

Gotzsche P.C., Hammarquist C., Burr M. House dust mite control measures in the management of asthma: meta-analysis. *British Medical Journal* 1998;**317**:1105–10.

Haahtela T., Lindholm H., Bjorksten F. *et al.* Prevalence of asthma in Finnish young men. *British Medical Journal* 1990;**301**:266–8.

Hakala K., Stenius-Aarniala B., Sovijarvi A. Effects of weight loss on peak flow variability, airways obstruction, and lung volumes in obese patients with asthma. *Chest* 2000;**118**:1315–21.

Halbert R.J., Isonaka S., George D. *et al.* Interpreting COPD prevalence estimates: what is the true burden of disease? *Chest* 2003;**123**:1684–92.

Halbert R.J., Natoli J.L., Gano A. *et al.* Global burden of COPD: systematic review and meta-analysis. *European Respiratory Journal* 2006;**28**:523–32.

Hayes J.D., Flanagan J.U., Jowsey I.R. Glutathione transferases. *Annual Review of Pharmacology and Toxicology* 2005;**45**:51–88.

Hesselmar N., Aberg N., Aberg B. *et al.* Does early exposure to cat or dog protect against allergy development? Clinical and Experimental Allergy 1999;29:611–7.

Hirsch T., Range U., Walther K.U. *et al.* Prevalence and determinants of house dust mite allergen in East German homes. *Clinical and Experimental Allergy* 1998;**28**:956–64.

Hnizdo E., Sullivan P.A., Bang K.M. *et al.* Association between chronic obstructive pulmonary disease and employment by industry and occupation in the US population: a study of data from the Third National Health and Nutrition Examination Survey. *American Journal of Epidemiology* 2002;**156**:738–46.

Hsieh K.H., Shen J.J. Prevalence of childhood asthma in Taipei, Taiwan and other Asian Pacific countries. *Journal of Asthma* 1991;**25**:73–82.

Infante-Rivard C., Esnaola Sukia S., Roberge D. *et al.* The changing frequency of childhood asthma. *Journal of Asthma* 1987;**24**:283–8.

Jenkins H.S., Devalia J.L., Mister R.L. *et al.* The effect of exposure to ozone and nitrogen dioxide on the airway response of atopic asthmatics to inhaled allergen: dose- and time-dependent effects. *American Journal of Respiratory and Critical Care Medicine* 1999;**160**:33–9.

Johannessen A., Omenaas E.R., Bakke P.S. *et al.* Implications of reversibility testing on prevalence and risk factors for chronic obstructive pulmonary disease: a community study. *Thorax* 2005;**60**:842–7.

Johansson M.L., Molin G., Jeppsson B. Administration of different Lactobacillus strains in fermented oatmeal soup: in vivo colonization of human intestinal mucosa and effect on the indigenous flora. *Applied Environmental Microbiology* 1993;**59**:15–20.

Johnston S.L., Pattemore P.K., Sanderson G. *et al.* Community study of role of viral-infections in exacerbations of asthma in 9–11 year-old children. *British Medical Journal* 1995;**310**:1225–9.

Johnston S.L. Innate immunity in the pathogenesis of virus-induced asthma exacerbations. *Proceedings of the American Thoracic Society* 2007; **4**:267–70.

Keeney E.L. The history of asthma from Hippocrates to Meltzer. *Journal of Allergy and Clinical Immunology* 1964;**35**:215–26.

Kemm J.R. A birth cohort analysis of smoking by adults in Great Britain 1974–1998. *Journal of Public Health Medicine* 2001;**23**:306–11.

Kharitonov S.A., Barnes P.J. Exhaled biomarkers. *Chest* 2006;**130**:1541–6.

Kimbell-Dunn M., Pearce N., Beasley R. Asthma. In: Hatch M, editor. *Women and health*. San Diego(CA): Academic Press; 1999. p. 724–39.

Kirkham P., Rahman I. Oxidative stress in asthma and COPD: antioxidants as a therapeutic strategy. *Pharmacology and Therapeutics* 2006; **111**:476–94.

Kogevinas M., Anto J.M., Soriano J.B. *et al.* The risk of asthma attributable to occupational exposures—a population-based study in Spain. *American Journal of Respiratory and Critical Care Medicine* 1996;**154**:137–43.

Kraft M. Asthma and chronic obstructive pulmonary disease exhibit common origins in any country! *American Journal of Respiratory and Critical Care Medicine* 2006;**174**:238–40.; discussion 243–4.

Kramer M.S., Matush L., Vanilovich I. *et al.* Effect of prolonged and exclusive breast feeding on risk of allergy and asthma: cluster randomised trial. *British Medical Journal* 2007;**335**:815.

Laënnec R. *A treatise on the disease of the chest* [translated from the French by J Forbes]. London: T and G Underwood; 1821.

Lau S., Illi S., Sommerfeld C. *et al.* Early exposure to house-dust mite and cat allergens and development of childhood asthma: a cohort study. Multicentre Allergy Study Group. *Lancet* 2000; **356**:1392–7.

Lau S., Nickel R., Niggemann B. *et al.* The development of childhood asthma: lessons from the German Multicentre Allergy Study (MAS). *Paediatric Respiratory Reviews* 2002;**3**:265–72.

Lemanske R.F., Jr., Jackson D.J., Gangnon R.E. *et al.* Rhinovirus illnesses during infancy predict subsequent childhood wheezing. *Journal of Allergy and Clinical Immunology* 2005;**116**:571–7.

Leung R., Ho P., Lam C.W.K. *et al.* Sensitization to inhaled allergens as a risk factor for asthma and allergic diseases in Chinese population. *Journal of Allergy and Clinical Immunology* 1997;**99**:594–9.

Liard R., Chansin R., Neukirch F. *et al.* Prevalence of asthma among teenagers attending school in Tahiti. *Journal of Epidemiology and Community Health* 1988;**42**:149–51.

Littlejohns P., Ebrahim S., Anderson R. Prevalence and diagnosis of chronic respiratory symptoms in adults. *British Medical Journal* 1989; **298**:1556–60.

Littlejohns P., Macdonald L.D. The relationship between severe asthma and social-class. *Respiratory Medicine* 1993;**87**:139–43.

Liu S., Zhou Y., Wang X. *et al.* Biomass fuels are the probable risk factor for chronic obstructive pulmonary disease in rural South China. *Thorax* 2007;**62**:889–97.

Lokke A., Lange P., Scharling H. *et al.* Developing COPD: a 25 year follow up study of the general population. *Thorax* 2006;**61**:935–9.

Lopez A., Mathers C., Ezzati M. *et al.* *Global burden of disease and risk factors.* Washington (DC): The World Bank; 2006a.

Lopez A.D., Murray C.C. The global burden of disease, 1990–2020. *Nature Medicine* 1998;**4**:1241–3.

Lopez A.D., Shibuya K., Rao C. *et al.* Chronic obstructive pulmonary disease: current burden and future projections. *European Respiratory Journal* 2006b;**27**:397–412.

MacNee W. Pulmonary and systemic oxidant/antioxidant imbalance in chronic obstructive pulmonary disease. *Proceedings of the American Thoracic Society* 2005;**2**:50–60.

Magnus P., Jaakkola J.J.K. Secular trend in the occurrence of asthma among children and young adults: critical appraisal of repeated cross sectional surveys. *British Medical Journal* 1997;**314**:1795–99.

Manfreda J., Becker A.B., Wang P.Z. *et al.* Trends in physician-diagnosed asthma prevalence in Manitoba between 1980 and 1990. *Chest* 1993;**103**:151–7.

Mannino D.M., Brown C., Giovino G.A. Obstructive lung disease deaths in the United States from 1979 through 1993. An analysis using multiple-cause mortality data. *American Journal of Respiratory and Critical Care Medicine* 1997;**156**:814–8.

Mannino D.M., Buist A.S. Global burden of COPD: risk factors, prevalence, and future trends. *Lancet* 2007;**370**:765–73.

Mannino D.M., Mott J., Ferdinands J.M. *et al.* Boys with high body masses have an increased risk of developing asthma: findings from the National Longitudinal Survey of Youth (NLSY). *International Journal of Obesity (London)* 2006;**30**:6–13.

Martinez F.D., Holt P.G. Role of microbial burden in aetiology of allergy and asthma. *Lancet* 1999;**354**:12–5.

Martinez F.D., Morgan W.J., Wright A.L. *et al.* Diminished lung-function as a predisposing factor for wheezing respiratory illness in infants. *New England Journal of Medicine* 1988;**319**:1112–7.

Martinez F.D. Complexities of the genetics of asthma. *American Journal of Respiratory and Critical Care Medicine* 1997;**156**:S117–22.

Martinez F.D. Gene by environment interactions in the development of asthma. *Clinical and Experimental Allergy* 1998;**28**:21–5.

Martinez F.D. Role of viral infections in the inception of asthma and allergies during childhood: could they be protective? *Thorax* 1994;**49**:1189–91.

Matheson M.C., Erbas B., Balasuriya A. *et al.* Breast-feeding and atopic disease: a cohort study from childhood to middle age. *Journal of Allergy and Clinical Immunology* 2007;**120**:1051–7.

Matricardi P.M., Rosmini F., Ferrigno L. Cross-sectional retrospective study of prevalence of atopy among Italian military students with antiboides against hepatitis A virus. *British Medical Journal* 1997;**314**:999–1003.

Matricardi P.M., Rosmini F., Riondino S. *et al.* Exposure to food borne and orofecal microbes versus airborne viruses in relation to atopy and allergic asthma. *British Medical Journal* 2000;**320**:412–7.

McConnell R., Berhane K., Gilliland F. *et al.* Asthma in exercising children exposed to ozone: a cohort study. *Lancet* 2002;**359**:386–91.

McDonnell W.F., Abbey D.E., Nishino N. *et al.* Long-term ambient ozone concentration and the incidence of asthma in non smoking adults: the AHSMOG Study. *Environmental Research* 1999;**80**:110–21.

Medbo A., Melbye H. Lung function testing in the elderly—can we still use $FEV_1/FVC < 70\%$ as a criterion of COPD? *Respiratory Medicine* 2007;**101**:1097–105.

Melsom T., Brinch L., Hessen J.O. Asthma and indoor environment in Nepal. *Thorax* 2001;**56**:477–81.

Menezes A.M., Perez-Padilla R., Jardim J.R. *et al.* Chronic obstructive pulmonary disease in five Latin American cities (the PLATINO study): a prevalence study. *Lancet* 2005;**366**:1875–81.

Meredith S., Nordman H. Occupational asthma: measures of frequency from four countries. *Thorax* 1966;**51**:435–40.

Meredith S.K., Taylor V.M., McDonald J.C. Occupational respiratory disease in the United Kingdom 1989—a Report to the British Thoracic Society and the Society of Occupational Medicine by the Sword Project Group. *British Journal of Industrial Medicine* 1991;**48**:292–8.

Miller M.R., Hankinson J., Brusasco V. *et al.* Standardisation of spirometry. *European Respiratory Journal* 2005;**26**:319–38.

Miravitlles M., de la Roza C., Naberan K. *et al.* Attitudes toward the diagnosis of chronic obstructive pulmonary disease in primary care. *Archives of Bronconeumology* 2006;**42**:3–8.

Miravitlles M., Ferrer M., Pont A. *et al.* Characteristics of a population of COPD patients identified from a population-based study. *Focus on previous diagnosis and never smokers. Respiratory Medicine* 2005;**99**:985–95.

Mitchell E.A., Stewart A.W., ISAAC Phase One Study Group. The ecological relationship of tobacco smoking to the prevalence of symptoms of asthma and other atopic diseases in children: The International Study of Asthma and Allergies in Childhood (ISAAC). *European Journal of Epidemiology* 2001;**17**:667–73.

Mitchell E.A. Increasing prevalence of asthma in children. *New Zealand Medical Journal* 1983;**96**:463–4.

Mommers M., Guekjens-Sijstermans C., Swaen G.M.H. *et al.* Trends in the prevalence of respiratory symptoms and treatment in Dutch children over a 12 year period: results of the fourth consecutive survey. *Thorax* 2005;**60**:97–9.

Morrison Smith J. The prevalence of asthma and wheezing in children. *British Journal of Diseases of the Chest* 1976;**70**:73–7.

Newson R.B., Shaheen S.O., Chinn S. *et al.* Paracetamol sales and atopic disease in children and adults: an ecological analysis. *European Respiratory Journal* 2000;**16**:817–23.

Ninan T.K., Russell G. Respiratory symptoms and atopy in Aberdeen school children: evidence from two surveys 25 years apart. *British Medical Journal* 1992;**304**:873–5.

Nishima S. A study on the prevalence of bronchial asthma in school children in western districts of Japan—comparison between the studies in 1982 and in 1992 with the same methods and same districts, the Study Group of the Prevalence of Bronchial Asthma and the West Japan Study Group of Bronchial Asthma. *Arerugi* 1993; **42**:192–204.

Office of Environmental Health Hazard Assessment. *Health effects of exposure to environmental tobacco smoke*. California Environmental Protection Agency; 1997.

Omran M., Russell G. Continuing increase in respiratory symptoms and atopy in Aberdeen schoolchildren. *British Medical Journal* 1996; **312**:34.

Pattemore P.K., Ellison-Loschmann L., Asher M.I. *et al.* Asthma prevalence in European, Maori, and Pacific children in New Zealand: ISAAC study. *Pediatric Pulmonology* 2004;**37**:433–42.

Pearce N., Ait-Khaled N., Beasley R. *et al.* Worldwide trends in the prevalence of asthma symptoms: phase III of the International Study of Asthma and Allergies in Childhood (ISAAC). *Thorax* 2007;**62**:758–66.

Pearce N., Beasley R., Burgess C. *et al. Asthma epidemiology: principles and methods.* New York (NY): Oxford University Press; 1998.

Pearce N., Beasley R., Pekkanen J. Role of bronchial responsiveness testing in asthma prevalence surveys. *Thorax* 2000a;**55**:352–4.

Pearce N., Douwes J., Beasley R. Is allergen exposure the major primary cause of asthma? *Thorax* 2000b;**55**:424–31.

Pearce N., Douwes J., Beasley R. The rise and rise of asthma: a new paradigm for the new millennium? *Journal of Epidemiology and Biostatistics* 2000c;**5**:5–16.

Pearce N., Douwes J. Asthma time trends—mission accomplished? International Journal of Epidemiology 2005:34:1018–9.

Pearce N., Pekkanen J., Beasley R. How much asthma is really attributable to atopy? *Thorax* 1999;**54**:268–72.

Pearce N., Weiland S., Keil U. *et al.* Self-reported prevalence of asthma symptoms in children in Australia, England, Germany and New Zealand: an international comparison using the ISAAC protocol. *European Respiratory Journal* 1993;**6**:1455–61.

Peat J.K., Tovey E., Toelle B.G. *et al.* House dust mite allergens—a major risk factor for childhood asthma in Australia. *American Journal of Respiratory and Critical Care Medicine* 1996;**153**:141–6.

Perdrizet S., Neukirch F., Cooreman J. *et al.* Prevalence of asthma in adolescents in various parts of France and its relationship to respiratory allergic manifestations. *Chest* 1987;**91**:104S-6S.

Petty T. The history of COPD. *International Journal of COPD* 2006;**1**:3–14.

Petty T.L. COPD in perspective. *Chest* 2002;**121**:116S-20S.

Priftanji A., Strachan D., Burr M. *et al.* Asthma and allergy in Albania and the UK. *Lancet* 2001;**358**:1426–7.

Rabe K.F., Hurd S., Anzueto A. *et al.* Global strategy for the diagnosis, management, and prevention of chronic obstructive pulmonary disease: GOLD executive summary. *American Journal of Respiratory and Critical Care Medicine* 2007;**176**:532–55.

Redline S., Gold D. Challenges in interpreting gender differences in asthma. *American Journal of Respiratory and Critical Care Medicine* 1994;**150**:1219–21.

Reisman J., Schachter H.M., Dales R.E. *et al.* Treating asthma with omega-3 fatty acids: where is the evidence? A systematic review. *BMC Complementary and Alternative Medicine* 2006;**6**:26.

Rennard S., Decramer M., Calverley P.M. *et al.* Impact of COPD in North America and Europe in 2000: subjects' perspective of Confronting COPD International Survey. *European Respiratory Journal* 2002; **20**:799–805.

Robertson C.F., Heycock E., Bishop J. *et al.* Prevalence of asthma in Melbourne schoolchildren: changes over 26 years. *British Medical Journal* 1991;**302**:1116–8.

Robertson C.F., Roberts M.F., Kappers J.H. Asthma prevalence in Melbourne schoolchildren: have we reached the peak? *Medical Journal of Australia* 2004;**180**:273–6.

Romagnani S. The increased prevalence of allergy and the hygiene hypothesis: missing immune deviation, reduced immune suppression, or both? *Immunology* 2004;**112**:352–63.

Ronchetti R., Rennerova Z., Barreto M. *et al.* The prevalence of atopy in asthmatic children correlates strictly with the prevalence of atopy among non-asthmatic children. *International Archives of Allergy and Immunology* 2007;**142**:79–85.

Sandford A.J., Joos L., Pare P.D. Genetic risk factors for chronic obstructive pulmonary disease. *Current Opinion in Pulmonary Medicine* 2002; **8**:87–94.

Sears M.R., Greene J.M., Willan A.R. *et al.* Long-term relation between breastfeeding and development of atopy and asthma in children and young adults: a longitudinal study. *Lancet* 2002;**360**:901–7.

Shaheen S.O., Aaby P., Hall A.J. Cell-mediated immunity after measles in Guinea-Bissau: historical cohort srudy. *British Medical Journal* 1996;**313**:969–74.

Shaheen S.O., Newson R.B., Henderson A.J. *et al.* Prenatal paracetamol exposure and risk of asthma and elevated immunoglobulin E in childhood. *Clinical and Experimental Allergy* 2005;**35**:18–25.

Shaheen S.O., Newson R.B., Sherriff A. *et al.* Paracetamol use in pregnancy and wheezing in early childhood. *Thorax* 2002;**57**:958–63.

Shaheen S.O., Sterne J.A., Songhurst C.E. *et al.* Frequent paracetamol use and asthma in adults. *Thorax* 2000;**55**:266–70.

Shaw R., Woodman K., Ayson M. *et al.* Measuring the prevalence of bronchial hyper-responsiveness in children. *International Journal of Epidemiology* 1995;**24**:597–602.

Shaw R.A., Crane J., O'Donnell T.V. *et al.* Increasing asthma prevalence in a rural New Zealand adolescent population: 1975–89. *Archives of Disease in Childhood* 1990;**65**:1319–23.

Shirakawa T., Enomoto T., Shimazu S. *et al.* The inverse association between tuberculin responses and atopic disorder. *Science* 1997;**275**:77–9.

Shore S.A. Obesity and asthma: lessons from animal models. *Journal of Applied Physiology* 2007;**102**:516–28.

Sigurs N., Gustafsson P.M., Bjarnason R. *et al.* Severe respiratory syncytial virus bronchiolitis in infancy and asthma and allergy at age 13. *American Journal of Respiratory and Critical Care Medicine* 2005;**171**:137–41.

Simpson J.L., Grissell T.V., Douwes J. *et al.* Innate immune activation in neutrophilic asthma and bronchiectasis. *Thorax* 2007;**62**:211–8.

Simpson J.L., Scott R., Boyle M.J. *et al.* Inflammatory subtypes in asthma: assessment and identification using induced sputum. *Respirology* 2006;**11**:54–61.

Siroux V., Pin I., Oryszczyn M.P. *et al.* Relationships of active smoking to asthma and asthma severity in the EGEA study. *Epidemiological study on the genetics and environment of asthma. European Respiratory Journal* 2000;**15**:470–7.

Smith A.D., Cowan J.O., Brassett K.P. *et al.* Use of exhaled nitric oxide measurements to guide treatment in chronic asthma. *New England Journal of Medicine* 2005;**352**:2163–73.

Soriano J.B., Maier W.C., Egger P. *et al.* Recent trends in physician diagnosed COPD in women and men in the UK. *Thorax* 2000;**55**:789–94.

Sporik R., Holgate S.T., Plattsmills T.A.E. *et al.* Exposure to house-dust mite allergen (Der-P-I) and the development of asthma in childhood—a prospective-study. *New England Journal of Medicine* 1990;**323**:502–7.

Stein R.T., Sherrill D., Morgan W.J. *et al.* Respiratory syncytial virus in early life and risk of wheeze and allergy by age 13 years. *Lancet* 1999;**354**:541–5.

Stewart A.W., Mitchell E.A., Pearce N. *et al.* The relationship of per capita gross national product to the prevalence of symptoms of asthma and other atopic diseases in children (ISAAC) [comment]. *International Journal of Epidemiology* 2001;**30**:173–9.

Strachan D.P., Cook D.G. Parental smoking and childhood asthma: longitudinal and case-control studies. *Thorax* 1998;**53**:204–12.

Strachan D.P. Hay fever, hygiene, and household size. *British Medical Journal* 1989;**299**:1259–60.

Sunyer J., Jarvis D., Pekkanen J. *et al.* Geographic variations in the effect of atopy on asthma in the European Community Respiratory Health Study. *Journal of Allergy and Clinical Immunology* 2004;**114**:1033–9.

Tager I.B., Segal M.R., Speizer F.E. *et al.* The natural history of forced expiratory volumes. Effect of cigarette smoking and respiratory symptoms. *American Review of Respiratory Disease* 1988;**138**:837–49.

Tager I.B., Weiss S.T., Munoz A. *et al.* Longitudinal study of the effects of maternal smoking on pulmonary function in children. *New England Journal of Medicine* 1983;**309**:699–703.

Takahashi T., Morita K., Akagi R. *et al.* Heme oxygenase-1: a novel therapeutic target in oxidative tissue injuries. *Current Medicinal Chemistry* 2004;**11**:1545–61.

Tashkin D.P., Detels R., Simmons M. *et al.* The UCLA population studies of chronic obstructive respiratory disease: XI. *Impact of air pollution and smoking on annual change in forced expiratory volume in one second. American Journal of Respiratory and Critical Care Medicine* 1994;**149**:1209–17.

Taylor D.R., Pijnenburg M.W., Smith A.D. *et al.* Exhaled nitric oxide measurements: clinical application and interpretation. *Thorax* 2006;**61**:817–27.

Tepas E.C., Litonjua A.A., Celedon J.C. *et al.* Sensitization to aeroallergens and airway hyperresponsiveness at 7 years of age. *Chest* 2006;**129**:1500–8.

Thomsen S.F., Ulrik C.S., Larsen K. *et al.* Change in prevalence of asthma in Danish children and adolescents. *Annals of Allergy, Asthma and Immunology* 2004;**92**:506–11.

Toelle B.G., Peat J.K., Salome C.M. *et al.* Toward a definition of asthma for epidemiology. *American Review of Respiratory Disease* 1992;**146**:633–7.

Trupin L., Earnest G., San Pedro M. *et al.* The occupational burden of chronic obstructive pulmonary disease. *European Respiratory Journal* 2003;**22**:462–9.

Turner M.O., Hussack P., Sears M.R. *et al.* Exacerbations of asthma without sputum eosinophilia. *Thorax* 1995;**50**:1057–61.

Unger L., Harris M.C. Stepping stones in allergy. *Annals of Allergy* 1974;**32**:214–30.

US Department of Human Health and Human Services. The health consequences of involuntary exposure to tobacco smoke: a report of the Surgeon General. Atlanta (GA): US Department of Human Health and Human Services, Centers for Disease Control and Prevention, Coordinating Centre for Health Promotion, Office on Smoking and Health; 2006.

US Environmental Protection Agency. *Respiratory health effects of passive smoking: lung cancer and other disorders*. Washington (DC): Office of Research and Development, US Environmental Protection Agency; 1992.

van Diemen C.C., Boezen H.M. Genetic epidemiology of reduced lung function. In: Postma D.S., Weiss S.T., editors. *Genetics of asthma and chronic obstructive pulmonary disease*. New York (NY): Informa Healthcare USA; 2007. p. 218.

van Diemen C.C., Postma D.S., Vonk J.M. *et al.* A disintegrin and metalloprotease 33 polymorphisms and lung function decline in the general population. *American Journal of Respiratory and Critical Care Medicine* 2005;**172**:329–33.

Van Strien R.T., Verhoeff A.P., Brunekreef B. *et al.* Mite antigen in house dust: relationship with different housing characteristics in The Netherlands. *Clinical and Experimental Allergy* 1994;**24**:843–53.

Varner A.E., Busse W.W., Lemanske R.F. Jr. Hypothesis: decreased use of pediatric aspirin has contributed to the increasing prevalence of childhood asthma. *Annals of Allergy, Asthma and Immunology* 1998;**81**:347–51.

Vestbo J., Prescott E., Lange P. *et al.* Vital prognosis after hospitalization for COPD: a study of a random population sample. *Respiratory Medicine* 1998;**92**:772–6.

Vestbo J. COPD in the ECRHS. *Thorax* 2004;**59**:89–90.

Vestbo J. Epidemiology. In: Voelkel NF, MacNee W, editors. *Chronic obstructive lung disease*. Hamilton, Canada: BC Decker Inc; 2002. p. 41–55.

Von Mutius E., Martinez F.D., Fritzsch C. Skin test reactivity and number of siblings. *British Medical Journal* 1994;**308**:692–5.

von Mutius E., Schwartz J., Neas L.M. *et al.* Relation of body mass index to asthma and atopy in children: the National Health and Nutrition Examination Study III. *Thorax* 2001;**56**:835–8.

von Mutius E., Weiland S.K., Fritzsch C. *et al.* Increasing prevalence of hay fever and atopy among children in Leipzig, East Germany. *Lancet* 1998;**351**:862–6.

Vork K.L., Broadwin R.L., Blaisdell R.J. Developing asthma in childhood from exposure to secondhand tobacco smoke: insights from a meta-regression. *Environmental Health Perspectives* 2007; **115**:1394–400.

Wang X., Mensinga T.T., Schouten J.P. *et al.* Determinants of maximally attained level of pulmonary function. *American Journal of Respiratory and Critical Care Medicine* 2004;**169**:941–9.

Watson J.P., Cowen P., Lewis R.A. The relationship between asthma admission rates, routes of admission, and socioeconomic deprivation. *European Respiratory Journal* 1996;**9**:2087–93.

Watson L., Boezen H.M., Postma D.S. Differences between males and females in the natural history of asthma and COPD. *European Respiratory Monthly* 2003;**25**:50–73.

Weeke E. Epidemiology of allergic diseases in children. *Rhinology* 1992;**30** Suppl **13**:5–12.

Weiland S.K., Pearce N. Asthma prevalence in adults: good news? *Thorax* 2004;**59**:637–8.

Weinmayr G., Weiland S.K., Bjorksten B. *et al.* Atopic sensitization and the international variation of asthma symptom prevalence in children. *American Journal of Respiratory and Critical Care Medicine* 2007;**176**:565–74.

Weitzman M., Gortmaker S.L., Sobol A.M. *et al.* Recent trends in the prevalence and severity of childhood asthma. *Journal of the American Medical Association* 1992;**268**:2673–7.

Whincup P.H., Cook D.G., Strachan D.P. *et al.* Time trends in respiratory symptoms in childhood over a 24 year period. *Archives of Disease in Childhood* 1993;**68**:729–34.

Willis T. Pharmaceutice rationalis [the operations of medicine in humane bodies]. London: Dring, Harper, and Leigh; 1678.

World Health Organization. *Air quality guidelines, global update 2005*. Particulate matter, ozone, nitrogen dioxide and sulphur dioxide. Copenhagen: WHO Regional office for Europe; 2005.

Xu X., Weiss S.T., Rijcken B. *et al.* Smoking, changes in smoking habits, and rate of decline in FEV_1: new insight into gender differences. *European Respiratory Journal* 1994;7:1056–61.

Yamada N., Yamaya M., Okinaga S. *et al.* Microsatellite polymorphism in the heme oxygenase-1 gene promoter is associated with susceptibility to emphysema. *American Journal of Human Genetics* 2000;**66**:187–95.

Yunginger J.W., Reed C.E., O'Connell E.J. *et al.* A community-based study of the epidemiology of asthma. *Incidence rates, 1964–1983. American Review of Respiratory Disease* 1992;**146**:888–94.

Zamel N., McClean P.A., Sandell P.R. *et al.* Asthma on Tristan de Cunha: looking for the genetic link. *American Journal of Respiratory and Critical Care Medicine* 1996;**153**:1902–6.

9.5

Obesity

Philip James

Abstract

Obesity is of increasing public health importance. Recent increases in life expectancy in high-income countries may be threatened by the rapid rise in the prevalence of obesity and associated health problems, including diabetes mellitus. Obesity has also emerged as an increasing concern in many middle-income countries. This chapter begins by analysing definitions of obesity, including older standard values of weight-for-height, more recent classifications based on body mass index (BMI) for adults and children, as well as classifications of abdominal obesity based on waist circumference. The association of anthropometric indices with ethnic origins is discussed and the rationale for population-specific criteria for abdominal obesity is outlined. Application of these criteria in population surveys from 191 countries around the year 2000 suggest that there were about 1.1 billion overweight and obese adults in the world of whom 320 million were obese with BMI of 30 kg/m^2 or more. More than half of overweight people are in middle- or low-income countries. About 10 per cent of boys and 9 per cent of girls aged 5–17 years are overweight, based on recently developed international standard criteria. Obesity is associated with a range of morbidity including well-known associations with diabetes and coronary heart disease and less appreciated impacts on respiratory function, sleep, and back and joint pains that contribute to diminished physical activity. Obesity is estimated to be one of the three risk factors that contribute most to the global burden of disability-adjusted life years lost (DALYs). Preventive interventions must target adults as well as children because it is in adult life that the greatest increases in obesity and its complications occur. Overweight and obesity result from small errors in energy balance, which lead to weight increments and the persistence of weight gain. In high-income countries, physical activity and energy expenditure have declined due to decrease in physical activity in work, commuting, and domestic activities while leisure-time physical activities have remained stable. Overall energy intakes have been declining. Interventions to reduce overweight and obesity must be made at individual, community, and societal levels. These may include changes in the physical environment that promote safe physical activity; economic measures using incentives or taxes to promote change; policy interventions to encourage, for example, breast feeding within healthcare settings; and sociocultural interventions including strategies for health promotion.

Introduction

The prevalence of obesity and overweight has been increasing rapidly in high-income countries, especially over the last decade. This increase is of great public health concern because projections suggest that as substantial further increases in obesity occur, the morbidity associated with obesity and its complications will threaten gains in life expectancy made as a result of the earlier decline in cardiovascular diseases. Overweight and obesity are also increasing rapidly in middle-income countries and in some low-income country populations. There is therefore a need to intervene on the growing epidemic of obesity with some urgency.

This chapter analyses the problem of obesity from the public health perspective. The chapter begins by considering definitions of overweight and obesity for adults and children. Definitions of abdominal obesity that are relevant in different populations are also described. The second section of the chapter presents estimates and projections for the prevalence of overweight and obesity, as well as estimates for the burden of disease and healthcare costs associated with obesity. The final section of the chapter outlines principles of energy balance in the context of trends in physical activity and energy intakes. This information may be used to inform potential interventions at the individual, community, and societal levels.

Definitions of obesity

The classification of obesity was originally based on analyses of death rates for those taking out life insurance policies with the US Metropolitan Life Insurance Company before the World War II. At that time, weights and heights were taken in light indoor clothing and wearing shoes with an additional subjective assessment by the doctor of whether the man or woman had a small, medium, or large frame size. It was then considered that somebody had a substantial increased risk if they were 20 per cent overweight but it was often unclear whether the normal weight should be the mid or upper level of the weight range for the man or woman of a particular frame size. These data were then recalculated by the UK Department of Health/MRC group in the early 1970s to provide BMI data after adjustments were made for the clothes and shoes (James 1976). To these data were later added those collected for the Build Study and the Royal College of Physicians (London) in their

1983 report highlighted for the first time the substantial public health significance of the prevailing rates of overweight and obesity based on taking a BMI of 30 as indicative of obesity. The value of 30 was 20 per cent above the now accepted upper normal BMI limit of 25, no specification now being made for using frame size in subcategorizing the risk. The upper normal limit of BMI 25 was taken from analyses of US (Royal College of Physicians 1983; Garrow 1981) mortality statistics but the separate analysis of male and female smokers then proved important in displaying the same U-shaped curves as those observed in non-smokers but with rates at a consistently higher level. Thus, the mortality risk of a smoker with a BMI of 22 was roughly equivalent to that of a non-smoker who had a BMI of 30. Then the World Health Organization (WHO) in 1995 accepted the BMI as the appropriate method for crudely assessing degrees of underweight and overweight but took a lower limit of 18.5 for distinguishing normal from underweight. This followed a series of earlier international analyses of adults' capacity to engage in heavy agricultural work which set the limit at 18.5, whereas the propensity to infections only became apparent in the available South American, African, and Asian studies when the BMI was below 17. This BMI value therefore became the next cut-off point signifying undernutrition (James *et al.* 1988) (Table 9.5.1) (National Institutes of Health 1998).

It was not until the WHO Expert Consultation on obesity in 1997 that the implications of overweight and obesity were accepted by WHO as a global problem (World Health Organization 2000). At that time, there was considerable discussion about the appropriateness of the choice of BMI cut-offs because in the United States it was accepted by physicians that there were so many heavy adults that perhaps one should only consider an individual overweight in national terms if their BMI was 28 or more. The Japanese, however, were pressing for a lower BMI cut-off and by the year 2000 the WPRO branch of WHO had accepted an upper cut-off of 23 for Asians (WHO/IASO/IOTF 2000); above this value, the risks of diabetes and hypertension in particular were unacceptably high. This was generally accepted following the WHO Singapore meeting in 2002 (WHO Expert Consultation 2004) but has not been applied on a regional basis, although numerous national bodies in Asia take the lower BMI criteria for granted and use Table 9.5.1 as the approach to clinical and public health decision making.

More recently, mortality data from the United States involving nationally representative data from the NHANES series of surveys have produced controversial findings using new modelling techniques to assess whether modest degrees of overweight are inducing increased mortality rates (Flegal *et al.* 2007). The BMIs associated with the lowest death rates were about 25–28, and the risk of death associated with high BMIs seemed to be falling on a secular basis. These findings are intriguing but need to be taken with some caution because it was shown many years ago that identifying the mortality effects of overweight (BMIs 25–29.9) required many years of follow-up with very substantial numbers of subjects (James 1976) and in practice the apparent secular decline in death rates also involved progressively shorter periods of follow-up in Flegal's study (Flegal *et al.* 2007). The recent analyses take account of the first of two forms of statistical bias: (a) the reverse causation phenomenon whereby some of those with lower weights are already ill, and (b) the subjects' progressive increase in weight during the period of observation (Greenberg 2006). Once these corrections are made in other surveys, then more modest degrees of overweight are on a cohort basis associated with a clear increase in mortality. Thus, the British Whitehall study with over 18 000 men, but followed for up to 35 years, showed that all-cause and ischaemic heart disease mortality rates (but not stroke death rates) were increased in the overweight

Table 9.5.1 The NIH and Asian adaptations of the WHO criteria for classification of overweight and obesity with their associated risks

		Disease risk*			
		Europids (NIH)		**Asians**	
Classification	**BMI kg/m²**	**Waist circumference**		**Waist circumference**	
		≤102 cm (M) ≤88 cm (W)	≥102 cm (M) >88 cm (W)	<90 cm (M) <80 cm (W)	≥90 cm (M) ≥80 cm (W)
Underweight	<18.5		—	Low (but increased risk of other clinical problems)	Average
Asian normal	18.5–22.9		—	Average	Increased
Asian overweight	23–24.9			Increased	Moderate
Asian obesity grade I	25–29.9			Moderate	Severe
Asian grade II	≥30			Severe	Very severe
Europid normal	18.5–24.9				
Europid overweight	25–29.9	Increased	High		
Europid obese class 1	≥30	High	Very high		
Europid obese class 2	30–34.9	Very high	Very high		
Europid obese class 3	≥35	Extremely high	Extremely high		

* Disease risk specified by NIH as relating to type 2 diabetes, hypertension, and cardiovascular disease. M = Men W = Women.

group (Batty *et al.* 2006). Another recent integrated analysis of 33 cohorts involving nearly a third of a million adults, followed for an average of 7 years from the Asia-Pacific region and including Australasia and Pacific Islanders, showed that the risk of fatal and non-fatal cardiovascular disease, particularly ischaemic stroke and ischaemic heart disease increased progressively from a BMI of 20, whereas the impact on haemorrhagic stroke was not evident until BMIs were in the region of 30 (Asia Pacific Cohort Studies Collaboration 2004). As in many of these studies, the first 3 years of follow-up in all the cohorts had to be discarded because those who were already ill had lower BMIs and early deaths so without this adjustment the curves were J-shaped. Similarly when over half a million US subjects who had never smoked were followed for up to 10 years by the American Cancer Society there was a remarkably rapid increase in death rates related to earlier BMIs (albeit self reported) of ≥25 (Adams *et al.* 2006). This relationship was more evident when the follow-up periods were long; the avoidance of the marked confounding effects of smoking again proved important.

Given that the focus on specifying the disadvantages of excess weight gain was originally dependent on information from those who took out life insurance policies, it is not surprising that the mortality criteria dominated earlier thinking on classifying appropriate weights for height. Later, it will be shown that a somewhat different perspective emerges when account is taken of the physical impact of weight gain or that of diseases that either only develop or are amplified in their effects when weight gain occurs.

From a public health perspective the development of the original criteria for assessing the risk from excess weight neglected the fact that the classification of excess weight used a classic clinical categorical approach when in practice there are progressive increases in the risk as the BMI increases. Thus, the precise choice of cut-off point is arbitrary: The health hazards are progressive and not substantially changed at any particular cut-off point. Furthermore, there are age-dependent changes in the relationship of BMI to total mortality (see below) and the classic co-morbidities intrinsically linked to an excess BMI, e.g. diabetes, hypertension, gall stones, and coronary heart disease are linearly related to BMI from a BMI nadir of about 19 or 20 in prospective studies of professional groups of men and women. Thus, the choice of an upper normal value of 24.9 for individuals is very generous and this value is quite different from the optimum population mean BMI which, as in the latest WHO report, should be between 21 and 23. Non-smoking individuals are likely to have an optimum life expectancy and disability-free life if their BMIs remain at about 20 throughout life.

Other criteria for classifying excess weight gain: Abdominal obesity

It has been recognized for many decades that the distribution of body fat was a useful clinical guide to the likelihood of risk and the waist–hip ratio was frequently advocated as a valuable tool. More recently the INTERHEART international case–control study of coronary heart disease has shown that the waist–hip ratio (W/HR) was a far more sensitive measure of risk with several analyses then being cited to indicate that fat deposition on the hips was protective so that the risk associated with a high waist circumference was reduced by the extent to which fat was also laid down peripherally (Yusuf *et al.* 2005). The superiority of the WHR compared with other indices of risk in part relates to the fact that different populations have very different skeletal and muscle masses so the ratio not only allows for the differential effect of central and peripheral fat distribution but also standardizes the risk for populations of very different sizes. From a simple clinical point of view and a practical public health approach, waist circumference alone is simpler to measure, does not require complex calculations, and overcomes the need to measure the hip circumference which in some societies is a culturally problematic measure to make except with female physicians taking considerable care.

The original choice of waist circumference (WC) was made so that the different values for men and women's waist cut-off points corresponded with the BMI cut-offs for overweight and obesity i.e. 25 and 30. These are the values which WHO then adopted (Table 9.5.1) for classifying—at least in Caucasians—excess abdominal fat. With the Asian focus on specifying lower normal BMI ranges, however, new WC values were proposed for Asians based on statistical calculations of the sensitivity and specificity of detecting hypertension or diabetes at different WC levels. More recently, the International Diabetes Federation in proposing new criteria for specifying the metabolic syndrome—which signifies a collection of risk factors including dyslipidaemia, hypertension, diabetes, and abdominal obesity—adapted the different values proposed for different ethnic groups despite their being derived very differently (Table 9.5.2). Thus, the women's WC limit for normality in Japan is based on the WC needed to find >100 cm^2 area of intra-abdominal fat on CT scanning, this value being taken as the marker of the absolute risk of men and women having a high risk

Table 9.5.2 Different waist circumference cut-off points selected by the International Diabetes Federation as part of their assessment of the metabolic syndrome

Country/ethnic group	Waist circumference (cm)	
Europids* In the United States, the ATP III values (102 cm male; 88 cm female) are likely to continue to be used for clinical purposes.	Male Female	≥94 ≥80
South Asians Based on a Chinese, Malay, and Asian-Indian population	Male Female	≥90 ≥80
Chinese	Male Female	≥90 ≥80
Japanese**	Male Female	≥85 ≥90
Ethnic South and Central Americans	Use South Asian recommendations until more specific data are available.	
Sub-Saharan Africans	Use European data until more specific data are available.	
Eastern Mediterranean and Middle East (Arab) populations	Use European data until more specific data are available.	

ATP—Adult Treatment Panel

* In future epidemiological studies of populations of Europid origin, prevalence should be given using both European and North American cut-points to allow better comparisons.

** Originally different values were proposed for Japanese people but new data support the use of the values shown above.

Source: International Diabetes Federation. A new worldwide definition of the Metabolic syndrome, 2005, 11. Available from: http://www.idf.org.

of a coronary artery diseases (James 2005). This contrasts with the general approach where the relative risk of a complication of a high WC determines the values chosen.

The criteria for specifying the metabolic syndrome differs markedly between different national and global groups but it is now generally accepted that different WC values are needed for different ethnic groups because of their increased absolute risk of diabetes and hypertension at the same WC. There is now increasing evidence that not only is there a strong genetic influence on fat distribution but in addition environmental factors including smoking and alcohol consumption amplify the propensity to abdominal obesity with early nutritional and other handicaps, demonstrated for example by low birth weights, being a marked promoter of subsequent abdominal obesity when even modest weight is gained in adult life. Thus, Indian, Chinese, and Hispanic populations with a marked history of early childhood malnutrition are particularly liable to display abdominal obesity even when their BMIs are within the normal WHO BMI range of <25. Thus, the unusual susceptibility of the major populations of the world to greater disability on adult weight gain than Caucasians living in Northern Europe or North America may require a much broader public health perspective involving the whole life cycle (see later).

Children's criteria for overweight and obesity

There were no acceptable criteria for overweight and obesity in children except those generated by WHO for the first time in 1995 when the same statistical criteria as those developed for underweight or childhood malnutrition were invoked. This essentially depended on arbitrarily classifying a child as underweight for their age, underheight for age, or underweight for height by defining any individual falling within the mean ±2 SDs as 'normal' and those outside these limits as 'abnormal'. Thus, the >2 SD for weight for height was taken as indicative of overweight and the reference data were based on a composite US data set which had become the WHO reference growth curves. They reflected the findings from a series of meticulous surveys of US children deemed to be healthy and growing adequately after World War II. No specific health criteria were therefore used in specifying the normal range. Furthermore, at that time WHO was wholly occupied with establishing national surveillance systems for monitoring only the under-5-year-olds so that they could assess progress in tackling the national and global prevalence of protein–energy malnutrition (PEM). PEM was originally specified as those having a low weight for age, but then more sophisticated approaches emerged in the 1970s to assess the prevalence of wasting i.e. low weight for heights and stunting—low heights for age. Thus, at that time, there were no coherent analyses of overweight in the under-5-year-olds and almost no data on older children. This reflected the paediatric view at that time that overweight and obesity in children was not a public health issue and any obese child needed clinical evaluation to see if they had an associated genetic disease.

Developing an international classification of overweight and obesity in children

The International Obesity Task Force (IOTF) group which had collected data on adult prevalences of overweight and obesity from the developing as well as the developed world for the WHO consultation on obesity then recognized the need to develop a new classification system for overweight and obesity in children (Cole *et al.* 2000) because it had become clear that the obesity issue in children had been neglected. After a detailed analysis of the options (Dietz & Bellizzi 1999), the BMI index was again chosen as useful because it had already been applied to children (Must *et al.* 1991), and Cole's method (Cole & Green 1992) for developing smooth percentile BMI curves on a sex-specific basis throughout childhood made simpler analyses possible. Many countries, e.g. Japan, and some in Europe, North America, and the Middle East, were also beginning to use either a 90th, 95th, or 97th BMI percentile as the basis for distinguishing obese children from normal; only Australia used the 85th percentile as a cut-off point (Guillaume 1999). The IOTF concluded that one could develop an approach which linked the childhood and adult definitions by taking, at age 18 years, those percentiles which corresponded to BMIs of 25 and 30 and using these same percentiles throughout the childhood age range for specifying overweight and obesity in childhood in girls and boys separately. Table 9.5.3 sets out the cut-off points to be used for this classification. This assumes that individual boys and girls will tend to retain the same percentile as they grow (see below).

The IOTF chose data from six countries, i.e. the original NHANES I data from the United States, UK data, and surveys from the Netherlands, Hong Kong, Singapore, and Brazil. This choice could have been improved by the inclusion of data on well-fed children of Indian and African origin, but suitable data were not available. The composite percentile cut-off points chosen from the six data sets are now being used routinely in many parts of the world. These IOTF overweight cut-off points correspond approximately to the 90th and 95th centiles for British and Dutch males, respectively, but the obesity cut-off points are above the 97th centile for almost all the assessed national surveys. It is not surprising, therefore, that by selecting the much higher percentile value for obesity there is likely to be much greater variability at these extreme values.

There have been concerns about the use of BMI in a standardized form as an index of body fatness in children from different societies because of the different ages for the onset of puberty (Dietz & Bellizzi 1999). Reilly *et al.* (2000), however, using UK data and body impedance measures of total fat, assessed the sensitivity and specificity of the IOTF BMI cut-off points for overweight and obesity. They showed that there was excellent specificity and sensitivity for the overweight cut-off points, but lower sensitivity for the higher obesity cut-off point (Table 9.5.4).

Tracking of body fat and BMI into adult life

The usefulness of the age- and sex-specific BMI cut-off points in the IOTF reference values and the adult BMI 25 and 30 cut-off points would be amplified if children in practice do grow along the same percentiles for both body fat and BMI through childhood into adult life. This issue was not straight forward because Rolland-Cachera *et al.* (1987) produced a detailed study of 164 subjects monitored from the age of one month to adult life. Only 41–42 per cent of pre-school children remained into adult life in their original category of being lean, medium, or fat if these categories were defined based on the 25th and 75th centiles of BMI. Rolland-Cachera *et al.* therefore focused on the issue of 'fat-rebound' in

Table 9.5.3 The IOTF cut-off points by age and sex for children from 2 to 18 years designed to pass through BMIs of 25 and 30 when aged 18 years

Age years	Child's BMI percentile corresponding to BMI 25 when adult		Child's BMI percentile corresponding to BMI 30 when adult	
	Boys	Girls	Boys	Girls
2	18.41	18.02	20.09	19.81
2.5	18.13	17.66	19.60	19.55
3	17.89	17.56	19.57	19.36
3.5	17.69	17.40	19.39	19.23
4	17.55	17.28	19.29	19.15
4.5	17.47	17.19	19.26	19.12
5	17.42	17.15	19.30	19.17
5.5	17.45	17.20	19.47	19.34
6	17.55	17.34	19.78	19.65
6.5	17.71	17.53	20.23	20.08
7	17.92	17.75	20.63	20.51
7.5	18.16	18.03	21.09	21.01
8	18.44	18.39	21.60	21.57
8.5	18.76	18.69	22.17	22.18
9	19.10	19.07	22.77	22.81
9.5	19.46	19.45	23.19	23.36
10	19.84	19.86	24	24.11
10.5	20.20	20.29	24.57	24.77
11	20.55	20.74	25.10	25.42
11.5	20.89	21.20	25.58	26.05
12	21.22	21.68	26.02	26.67
12.5	21.56	22.14	26.43	27.24
13	21.91	22.58	26.84	27.76
13.5	22.27	22.98	27.25	28.20
14	22.62	23.34	27.63	28.87
14.5	22.96	23.66	27.98	28.87
15	23.29	23.94	28.10	29.11
15.5	23.60	24.17	28.60	29.29
16	23.90	24.34	28.68	29.43
16.5	24.19	24.54	29.14	29.56
17	24.46	24.70	29.41	29.69
17.5	24.73	24.85	29.70	29.84
18	25	25	30	30

Source: Cole *et al.* (2000).

pre-pubertal school children. Guo and Chumlea (1999), however, had shown from US longitudinal studies that the probability of children with high BMIs still being overweight and obese at the age of 35 rose markedly throughout childhood. Thus, the probability of being overweight when aged 35 was 0.3 in 5-year-old children

Table 9.5.4 Sensitivity and specificity of overweight and obesity based on the IOTF BMI cut-off points for boys and girls and based on impedance estimates of body fat

	Sensitivity (%, n)	Specificity (%, n)
Boys		
Overweight	90 (90/100)*	92 (1756/1910)
Obesity	46 (46/100)**	99 (1901/1910)
Girls		
Overweight	97 (94/97)	84 (1543/1841)
Obesity	72 (72/97)	99 (1813/1841)

Significant differences in sensitivity between the sexes *$P < 0.05$ **$P < 0.01$
Source: Reilly *et al.* (2000).

with a BMI on the 95th percentile, about 0.35 at 10 years, 0.5 at 15 years, and about 0.7 at the age of 18. Systematic reviews of the evidence, e.g. by Power *et al.* (1997) and Parsons *et al.* (1999), have not found much evidence for the value of selective monitoring in the pre-pubertal phase for predicting the emergence of obesity if this is based on detailed analyses of weight rebound. Power's analyses showed that the older the children studied, the greater was the risk of their continuing to be obese in adult life. Once children were over 5 years of age, being obese incurred a great risk of this persisting, with the majority remaining obese into adult life (Table 9.5.5). Barlow and Dietz (1998) have also emphasized the value of concentrating on children over at least the age of 3. IOTF therefore chose to concentrate on children aged 5 and over and a consensus seems to have emerged that, for the present, one should focus on children of school age for predicting the risk of obesity persisting into adult life.

New definitions of 'normal' weight gain in children

WHO has recently undertaken a new approach to defining the normal growth of children (WHO Child Growth Standards 2007) which traditionally has been seen by many paediatricians to be very different in different countries and ethnic groups. The original WHO criteria, based on US data, were used as a reference because it had become evident that when the environmental conditions improved in many societies, the growth of children increasingly conforms with that set out in the WHO reference tables. WHO then established a major multinational study involving children in California, Norway, India, Oman, Ghana, and Brazil. Normal babies delivered at full term by healthy, non-smoking mothers who agreed to breastfeed their babies exclusively for at least 4 months were monitored carefully, with specific advice being given relating to immunization and other rearing practices. Further cohorts of preschool children from similar environments were also chosen so that, over a period of 6.5 years, it was possible to obtain data on 8400 children's growth patterns. It was surprising to find that whatever the ethnic background, the children's growth was almost identical and the variability in growth was far less than in the data bases normally used for producing growth charts. This implies that if one takes the latest WHO ±2 SD values, then the new estimates of underweight and overweight prevalences will be greater. This particularly applies to the prevalence of overweight children because

Table 9.5.5 The likelihood of children continuing to be overweight as adults ranked by age of first measurement

Study number	Age of monitoring		% still obese as adults	
	As children	As 'adults'	Males	Females
3	<1	20–30	36	-
5	1–5	19–26	27	-
7	7	14	90	87
7	7	16	63	62
11	7	33	43	63
6	7	35	40	20
9	1–14	10–23	42	66
8	2–14	10–24	43	-
4	9–10	31–35	57	64
11	11	33	54	64
2	9–13	42–53	63	-
1	10–13	29–34	74	72
6	13	35	40	30
4	13–14	31–35	77	70
10	13–17	27–31	58	-
11	16	33	64	78

Source: Data rearranged from Power *et al.* (1997) with study numbers as in their analysis. The proportion of obese adults who had been originally overweight as a child was usually 3–10 fold lower than the corresponding probability of overweight children maintaining their excess weight into adulthood.

in both children and adults there is an increasingly skewed distribution of weights as the average weight for age rises.

This new set of growth curves from WHO establishes for the first time a standard rather than a reference set of growth curves since it is being taken to imply that all children from any ethnic group, provided they have the advantages of exclusive breastfeeding and appropriate environmental conditions with suitable immunization and dietary patterns, will grow at almost identical rates. This is a proposition which is not accepted by many paediatricians or policy-makers in lower-income countries.

Later in 2007, WHO issued a further proposal on the appropriate growth of children from 5 to 20 years of age. This new set of criteria is surprisingly still based on US data, despite detailed examination of other growth curves from many international sources. However, the care with which the early US growth rates were monitored and the fact that the growth charts chosen link well with the charts for breastfed children <5 years is WHO's justification for now providing, for the first time, standard or reference growth charts for children throughout the world. As yet, only a few countries have begun to adapt their policies to incorporate the new concepts for the under-5-year-olds. What is already clear, however, is that with such small SDs for the variability in the growth of well-nourished non-infected children, the new WHO practice of taking the 85th and 95th percentiles corresponding very approximately to 1 SD and 2 SDs as cut-offs for 'at risk' and 'overweight' children will mean that far more children will be now designated as overweight. In fact, the cut-off points chosen are very close to those percentiles chosen for the IOTF analyses at the age of 18–20 years, but there are differences in the actual BMI values between the different estimates at younger ages. The WHO charts are presented in Fig. 9.5.1.

The prevalence of adult overweight and obesity

The original assessment of the global prevalence of overweight and obesity for WHO in 1996 was based on crude analyses which showed that obesity had become a global problem. The Millennium analyses by IOTF and WHO, based on a sifting of data and some interpolation of data from 191 countries revealed that there were about 1.1 billion overweight and obese adults in the world, of whom about 320 million were obese with a BMI of 30 or more (James *et al.* 2004). Different regions varied markedly in their prevalence. Surprisingly the developing world is making an even greater contribution than the developed world: If the whole of the developing world comprises all countries other than Japan, and those in Europe, North America, and Australasia, then 54 per cent of the world's 1105 million overweight (i.e. BMI 25–29.9) and 46 per cent of the world's 312 million obese are in the lower-income countries. The problem in these countries is therefore beginning to match the problem of cardiovascular diseases where the developing countries have a far greater burden than that of the affluent world.

The nutrition transition

There is now a recognized major increase in obesity rates associated with the economic development of a country and particularly the urbanization of populations in the developing world (Popkin 2006). The development of overweight and obesity varies markedly. Early Brazilian studies showed that, in poorer communities, middle-aged women are the first to become overweight and then as the economy develops women become progressively heavier with men then also beginning to catch up. In poor societies, the more affluent have a higher prevalence of obesity with the average BMI of the population increasing progressively as national incomes rise to about a GDP of US$5000 then peaks in women at US$15 000 and in men at US$17 000 (Ezzati *et al.* 2005). Figure 9.5.3 shows that the average BMI rises with progressive urbanization and this also leads to a fall in the proportion of household income spent on food. Then, as societies develop, there is a progressive reversal of the socioeconomic gradient so that the more affluent women become slimmer and then both men and women in wealthy environments have lower obesity rates than the poor. Ethnic differences within countries are well documented but this often links to their socioeconomic status rather than to any relationship with ethnicity.

As the increase in the average weight of the population rises, the proportion of obese individuals goes up markedly because of the marked skewing of the BMI distributions as illustrated originally by Rose using data from the INTERSALT studies (Rose 1991). Figure 9.5.4 shows these data and also highlights the fact that the most genetically sensitive members of the community are those found in the upper distributions for their society.

Table 9.5.6 provides an illustration of the age-related adult changes in the prevalences in some of the regions of the world. It is noteworthy that the main increase occurs in the 20–40-year-old group.

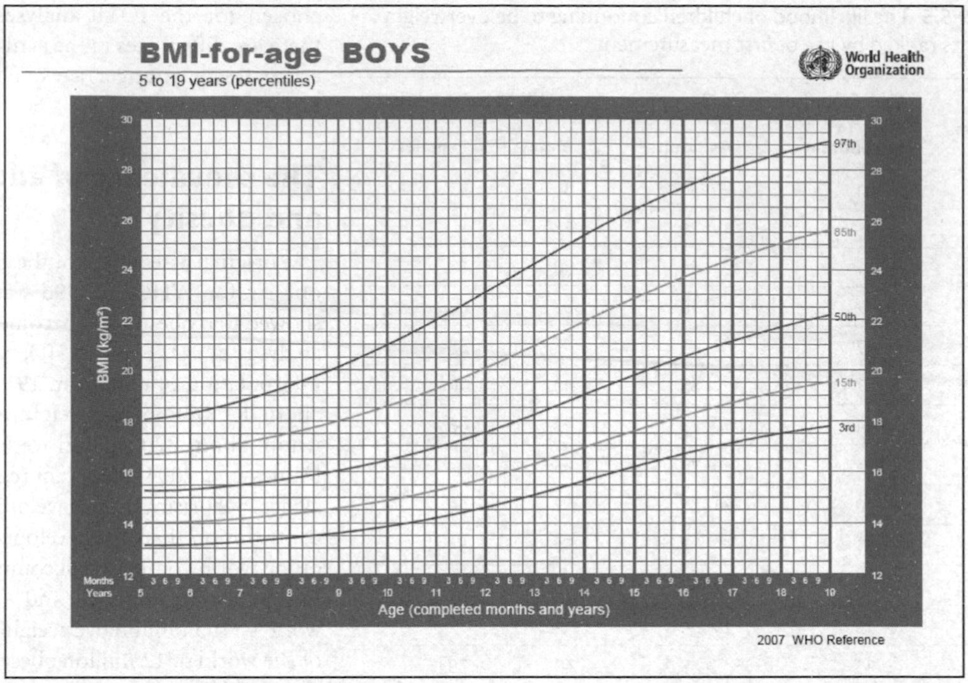

(a)

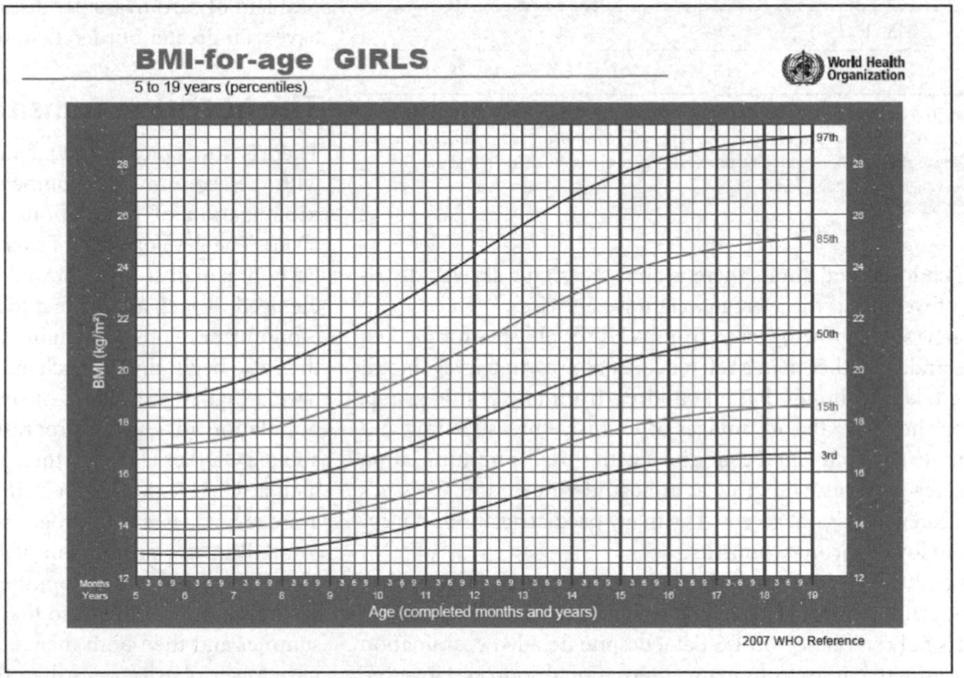

(b)

Fig. 9.5.1 New WHO children's growth charts.

Childhood prevalences on obesity

The preliminary analyses show that about 10 per cent of boys and 9 per cent of girls aged 5–17 years in the world are overweight, i.e. a total of 118 million overweight and obese children based on the IOTF criteria. The latest available regional prevalences for overweight and obesity using the IOTF international set of definitions (Wang & Lobstein 2006) are given in Table 9.5.7.

The health hazards associated with excess weight

Data relating to all the major risk factors were collected by different groups for WHO, the data then being collated according to standard protocols to take account of the different population age structures. These data were collated on a subregional basis by extrapolating to obtain estimates based on analogous countries and measured age

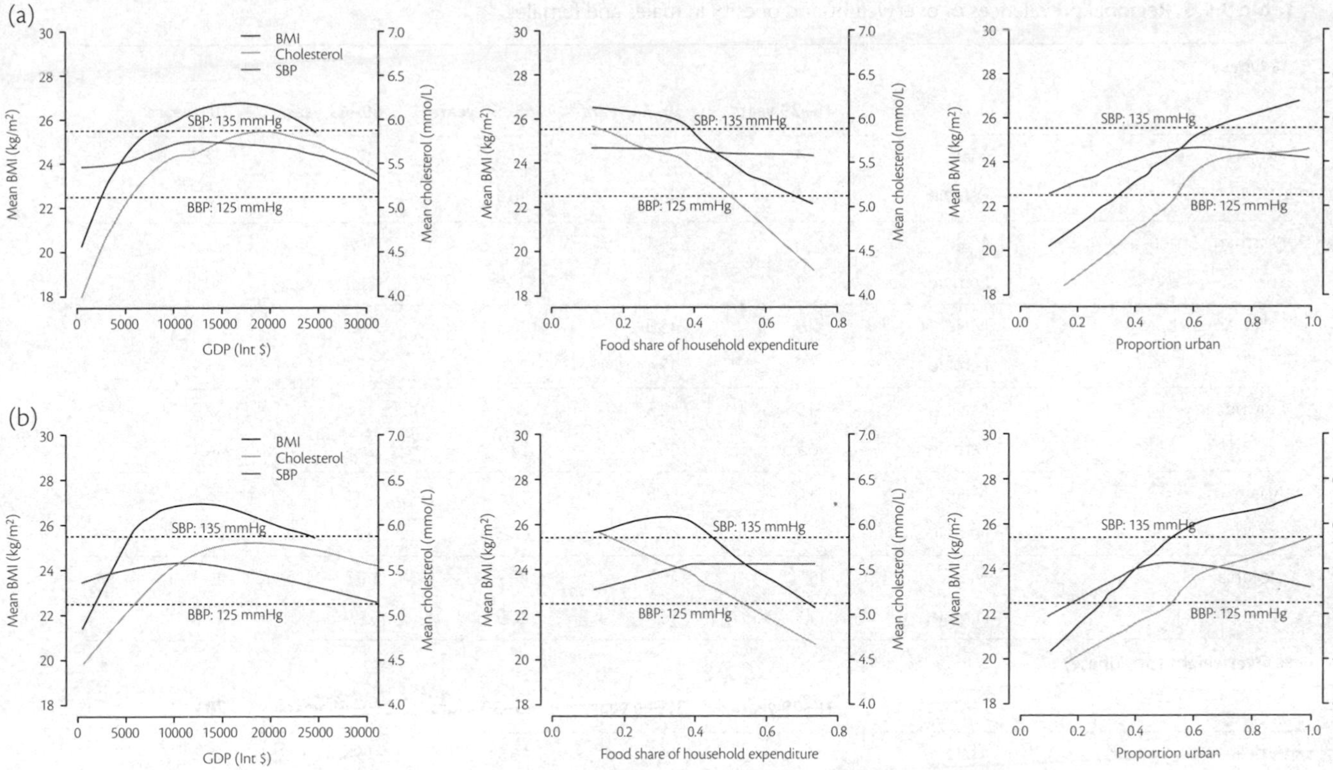

Fig. 9.5.2 (a) Males; (b) Females.
The relationship of mean population BMI, systolic blood pressure (SBP), and total cholesterol with average national income, food share of household expenditure, and proportion of population in urban areas. National income was measured as gross domestic product (GDP). Taken from Ezzati *et al.* (2005).

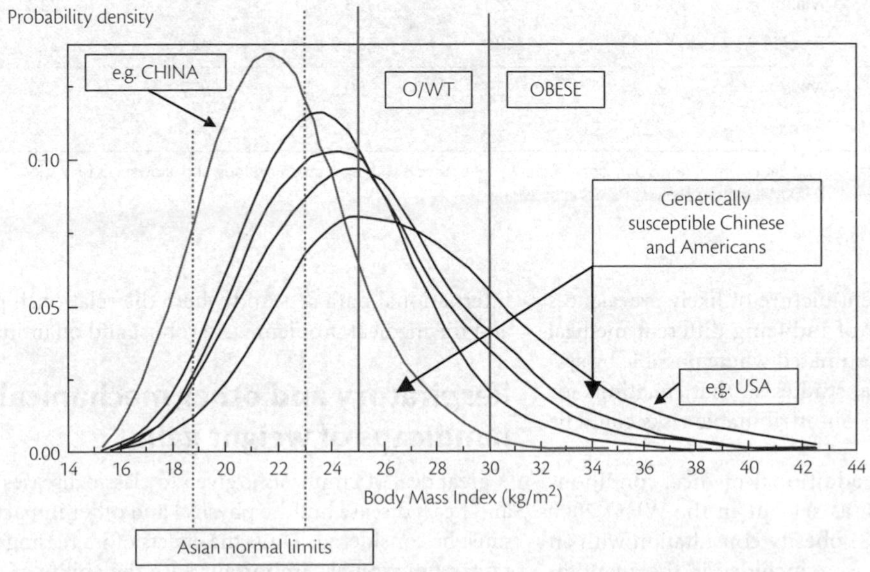

Fig. 9.5.3 The skewed distribution of BMI with increases in the average population BMI. Cross-sectional data taken from the INTERSALT study (Rose 1991) to illustrate the progressive marked increase in obesity rates for modest increases in mean BMI. Those in the upper BMI range for each population distribution represent the genetically susceptible individuals to weight gain. The usual Caucasian cut-offs for overweight and obesity are shown together with the Asian upper limit of 'normal' BMI.

Table 9.5.6 Regional prevalences of overweight and obesity in males and females

% Obese

		18–29 years	30–44 years	45–59 years	60–69 years	70+ years
Africa	Male	4.4	5.4	6.6	7.7	2.7
	Female	6.3	13.8	16.4	16	10.1
Northern America	Male	26.6	29.1	34.3	30.4	29.9
	Female	27.7	31.1	37.9	30.7	30.5
Latin America	Male	7.9	13.6	16.3	14.9	8.3
	Female	8.9	17.4	23.2	23.7	15.9
Europe	Male	4.9	12.5	20	16.6	7.8
	Female	6.8	16.3	27	26.7	14.1
Asia	Male	1.6	4.8	6	6.4	3.1
	Female	2.2	6	8.3	9.5	6.7
Oceania	Male	15	16.2	20.7	20.8	16.3
	Female	11.3	16.2	26.9	28.9	22.5

% Overweight (pre-obese)

		18–29 years	30–44 years	45–59 years	60–69 years	70+
Africa	Male	9.3	14.1	16.9	16.8	12.3
	Female	16.1	21.1	23.3	17.9	12.2
Northern America	Male	26.6	29.1	34.3	30.4	29.9
	Female	27.7	31.1	37.9	30.7	30.5
Latin America	Male	24.4	34.9	34.1	36.4	30.7
	Female	21.4	30.4	35.1	29	32.4
Europe	Male	27.2	42.4	47.7	47	45.8
	Female	17.2	28.7	36.4	38.8	38.1
Asia	Male	14.2	23.1	26	25.6	20.3
	Female	9.7	18.8	21.9	22.4	27
Oceania	Male	42.2	45.3	50.5	51.7	52.2
	Female	22.3	24.5	33.1	36.8	36.9

Unpublished updates of IOTF estimates using data from national or regional representative surveys with age standardization and allowances for national population differences as in the original WHO Millennium analyses (James *et al.* 2004).

and sex differences so that a coherent picture of likely prevalences could be obtained. Then the risks of inducing different medical problems with excess weight were estimated where possible by systematic analyses of epidemiological studies so that equations for deriving the proportion of population-attributable risks could be obtained.

Table 9.5.8 compares the list of additional medical conditions associated with excess weight gain as set out in the WHO 2000 (National Institutes of Health 1998) obesity consultation with an indication of those diseases which were included in the quantitative analyses for the WHO Millennium assessment of the risk factors contributing to the global burden of disease. The differences relate to the fact that quantitative estimates of the risks at different BMI levels could only be applied to conditions where there were international data sets and where the relationships between BMI and the medical problem were robust and quantifiable.

Respiratory and other mechanical handicaps of weight gain

A great deal of emphasis is given to classic diseases such as diabetes and heart disease but the physical and other impacts of weight gain must be considered. Thus, the effects of increasing weight on respiratory function are important with the ability of overweight children and adults to engage in strenuous physical activity becoming more limited the greater their weight increase. Thus, very obese adults, when asked to walk slowly, are already using up to 60 per cent of their maximum exercise capacity, and this can only be sustained

Table 9.5.7 Prevalence of overweight and obesity in school-age children based on latest available data, and estimated for 2006 and 2010 based on population-weighted annualized increases in prevalence and the use of IOTF criteria for overweight and obesity

WHO region (dates of most recent surveys)	Most recent surveys		Projected 2006		Projected 2010	
	Overweight (inc obesity) %	Obesity %	Overweight (inc obesity) %	Obesity %	Overweight (inc obesity) %	Obesity %
Africa (1987–2003)	1.6	0.2	4.1	1.3	7.9	2.2
Americas (1988–2000)	29.7	11	44.4	15.4	50.8	17.4
Eastern Mediterranean (1992–2001)	22.1	4.2	37.9	8.9	44.3	10.9
Europe (1992–2003)	19.6	4.6	29.5	7.6	35.9	9.6
Southeast Asia (1997–2002)	10.9	1.9	18.1	4	24.4	6
West Pacific (1993–2000)	16.4	3.7	27.4	7.1	33.9	9.1

Source: Wang & Lobstein (2006).

for a while. It is therefore not surprising that obese adults are often found to be doing less than normal-weight individuals because their physical exertions are very energy consuming. For those with any degree of respiratory impairment, weight gain is also a marked handicap. Thus, asthmatic patients and those with chronic obstructive respiratory disease can show a marked improvement in exercise tolerance and comfort if they lose weight. One further feature of weight gain is the far greater tendency to develop sleep apnoea, which is associated with a large neck and a tendency to obstruct breathing. This leads to their stopping breathing for increasing lengths of time, particularly at night. This seemingly innocuous problem is actually a major medical handicap associated with drug-resistant hypertension because of the persistent induction of the sympathetic nervous system by the repeated anoxia. When severe, it is not only associated with a higher mortality but can be the cause of traffic accidents as abdominally obese adults with thick necks fall asleep as they drive their vehicles.

Back and joint pains are another major problem leading to greater time off work for overweight and obese patients. The mechanical force on joints and the strain on the muscular skeletal system is marked leading to time off work and reactive depression among many overweight and obese subjects.

Table 9.5.8 The relative risk* of health problems associated with obesity

Greatly increased (relative risk much greater than 3)	Moderately increased (relative risk 2–3)	Slightly increased (relative risk 1–2)
NIDDM†	CHD†	Cancers: Breast† in postmenopausal women; endometrial†; colon†
Gallbladder disease	Hypertension†	Reproductive hormone abnormalities
Dyslipidaemia	Osteoarthritis (knees)†	Polycystic ovary syndrome
Insulin resistance	Hyperuricaemia and gout	Impaired fertility
Breathlessness		Low back pain due to obesity
Sleep apnoea		Increased risk of anaesthesia complications Fetal defects associated with maternal obesity

* All relative risk values are approximate;

† quantitative data in relation to different degrees of excess weight were available for these conditions which allowed them to be used in the assessment of the Millennium analyses of the global burden of disease. WHO Technical Report Series 894 (2000).

The medical and other costs of excess weight

There have been many estimates of the economic costs of obesity conducted by academic and government groups based on the direct costs of medical treatment of obesity and on the proportion of the other diseases, e.g. diabetes and hypertension which can theoretically be attributed to excess weight. A simpler scheme is shown in Fig. 9.5.5 where the observed medical costs of individuals was monitored on an annual basis as part of an assessment of the different annual medical costs at different extreme levels of obesity in the United States (Arterburn *et al.* 2005). It is clear that the least medical costs are incurred by individuals with BMIs within the normal range and that there is then a modest but steady increase in the costs at greater BMIs. If, however, the prevalences of these different groups is considered then the greatest absolute costs are incurred in the modest overweight group because this represents such a large proportion of the population.

The principal risk factors which affect both premature mortality and disability considered together as DALYs can then be assessed from data on mortality and national statistics for the prevalence of different medical conditions. Figure 9.5.6 provides the latest update on the dominance of different risk factors produced by the conjoint World Bank/WHO/CDC group in 2006 for the more affluent countries of the world (Lopez *et al.* 2006). By 2006, excess weight (calculated from the optimum of BMI 21) had climbed to the third most important factor and even if one includes all the poor countries

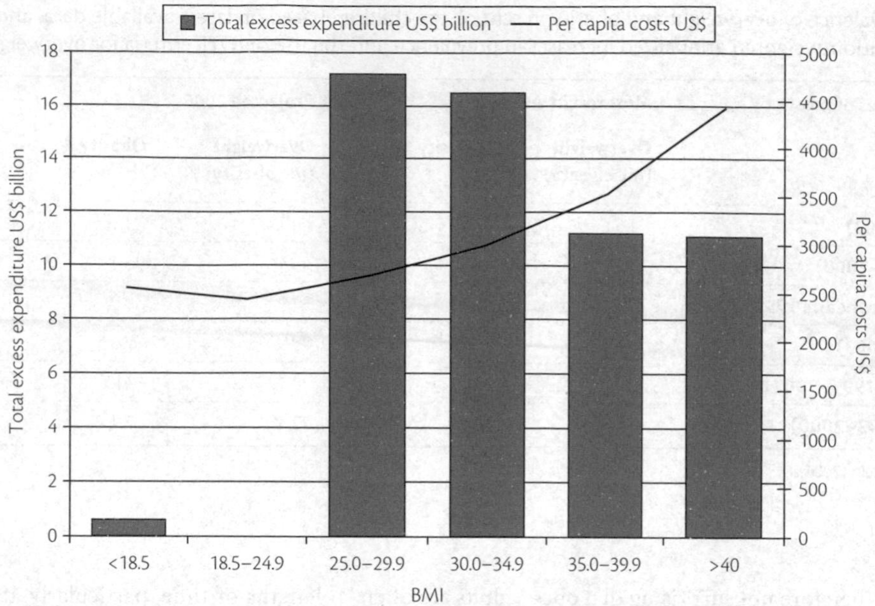

Fig. 9.5.4 The relationship between the annual costs per head of medical care in US adults and the estimated extra costs for the whole of each population group outside the normal weight range.
The curvilinear line reflects the increase in medical costs from about US$2500 per head per annum when at normal weight up to US$4500 for those with morbid obesity. The histograms then represent the impact of the different prevalences of the population within each BMI category on the total national cost in billions of US dollars for the BMI category within the population. Recalculated from data in Arterburn *et al.* (2005).

in analyses excess weight gain still comes out within the top 10 global risk factors. Further reappraisals are now being considered for the year 2010.

The estimations of the DALYs attributable to excess weight gain as conducted by WHO are sometimes considered unusual in that, as with blood pressure, total blood cholesterol, or any other risk factor, the challenge was to identify the optimum value to which the average population should ideally strive. For systolic blood pressure, the optimum value was estimated to be 115 mmHg, and for total blood cholesterol, 3.8 mmol/l. These values are very different from what one finds in clinical management guidelines, but illustrate the difference between pragmatic clinical judgements about what is possible on the basis of current management systems and what can be considered ideal from a public health perspective. So, the choice of BMI 21 as the optimum median population BMI was made in an analogous way.

Ethnic differences in susceptibility to chronic diseases on weight gain

Recently, Asian investigators have returned to this issue and considered with very large data sets whether the Asian community is really more susceptible to disease at different rates than Europids. This stems from the concern about the high prevalence of diabetes and hypertension at very modest increases in BMI. Figures 9.5.7a and b show that both type 2 diabetes and hypertension are markedly amplified by weight gain (Huxley *et al.* 2007). Similar relationships have been found in analyses of the Mexican national surveys which also showed that Mexicans as well as Asians are far more susceptible to increases in abdominal obesity at even normal BMIs than US non-Hispanic whites (Sanchez-Castillo *et al.* 2005).

While this ethnic difference is seen by most investigators as indicative of genetic factors, Barker and his colleagues suggested a

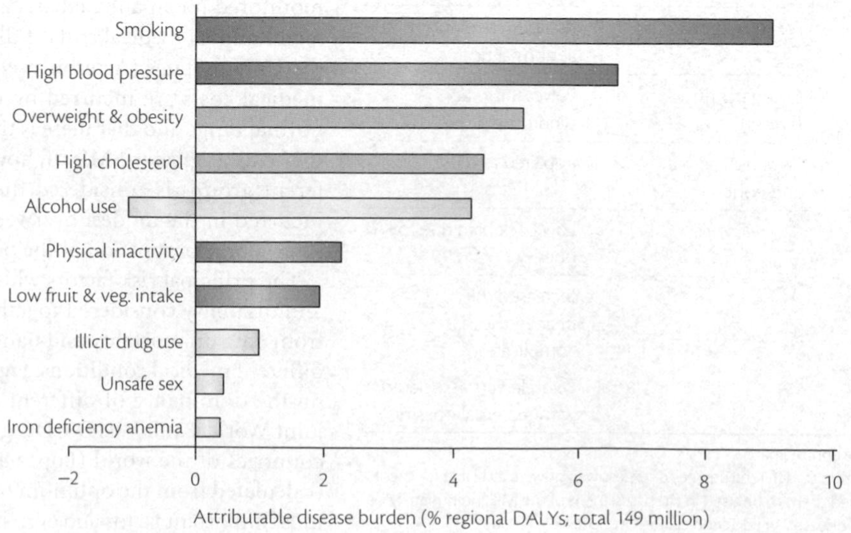

Fig. 9.5.5 The 2006 estimates of the relative importance of different risk factors contributing to the burden of diseases in high-income countries
Source: Lopez *et al.* (2006).

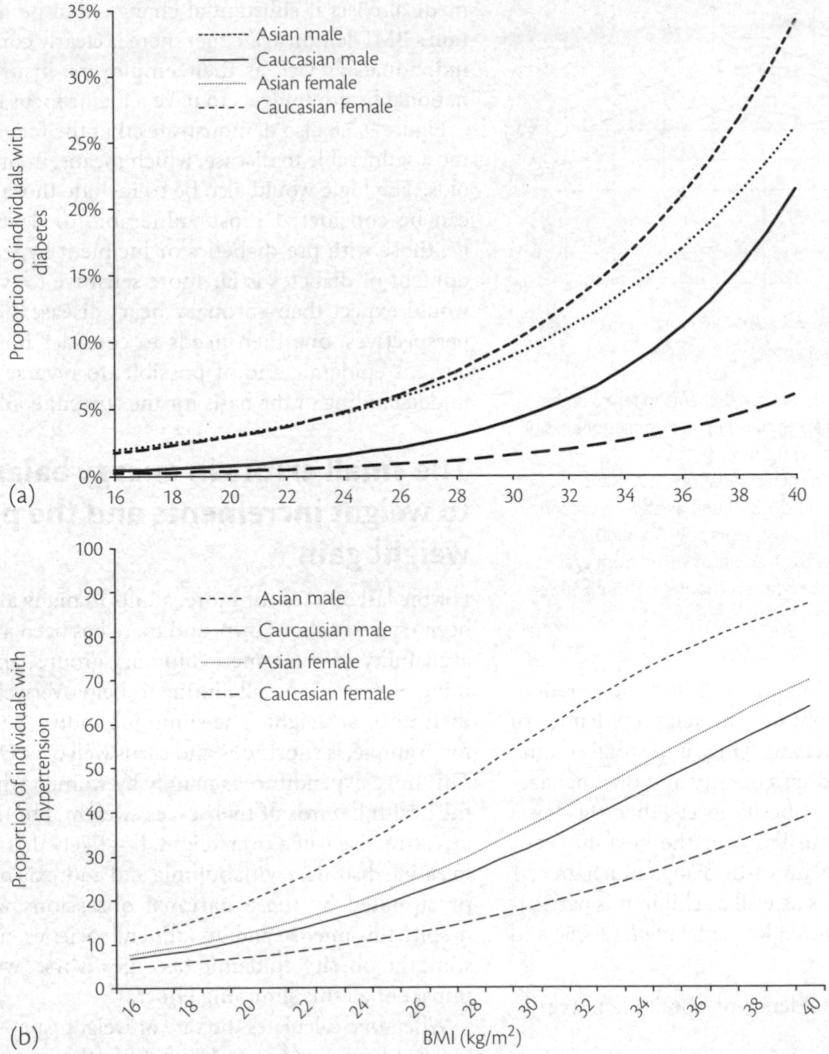

Fig. 9.5.6 The increased risk of (a) diabetes and (b) hypertension in Asian compared with Caucasian men and women in relation to their BMI. 7a) Diabetes 7b) Hypertension *Source:* Huxley *et al.* (2007).

foetal nutrition hypothesis where environmental factors both in utero and early foetal life are of exceptional importance in amplifying the risk of abdominal obesity and the development of diabetes and hypertension and cardiovascular disease (Barker 2004). Thus, systematic analyses of the relationship between birth weight and the prevalence of adult hypertension have shown a clear inverse relationship between the two in the majority of more than 80 studies from all over the world, and this is very evident in children from both developed and developing countries (Law *et al.* 2001). New evidence suggests that even mental illness in adult life is perhaps amplified by events early in the life cycle through modulation of the stress and other responses to the programming of hypothalamic and other responses (Eero Kajantie *et al.* 2007). Although both diabetes and hypertension are amplified in adult life by increases in BMI the gradient of effect rather than the absolute differences may not be very different in differing societies. Therefore the amplification in the absolute but not relative risk in adult life of particular levels of BMI may well prove to be based on differences in foetal programming which in turn may be markedly affected by the mother's nutrition before and during pregnancy and subsequent changes in infantile and later childhood growth.

Projections of the obesity epidemic and its consequent morbidity and costs

Recently, the UK government in an unusual programme 'Foresight' has considered not only the basis of the epidemic but its likely evolution. They calculated costs on the basis of current trends, using national BMI data sets of high quality based on weights and heights measured by trained observers yearly over a 10-year period with 10 000–20 000 children and adults each year in England. These data provide the opportunity to project by non-linear regression analysis the changes in the distribution of BMI by age and sex in the years to come (Fig. 9.5.8) (McPherson *et al.* 2007). As in most countries, the progressive shift in the distribution of BMI seems to be unremitting; so, given the wealth of data and the proposed continued effects of the factors stimulating obesity, the future magnitude of the epidemic and its consequences and costs can be predicted with some confidence. The analyses also allow modelling to assess the potential value of different interventions, e.g. a selective approach to preventing obesity in different age groups.

Although the prevention of obesity on children is publicly and therefore politically appealing, it is not likely to bring rapid changes

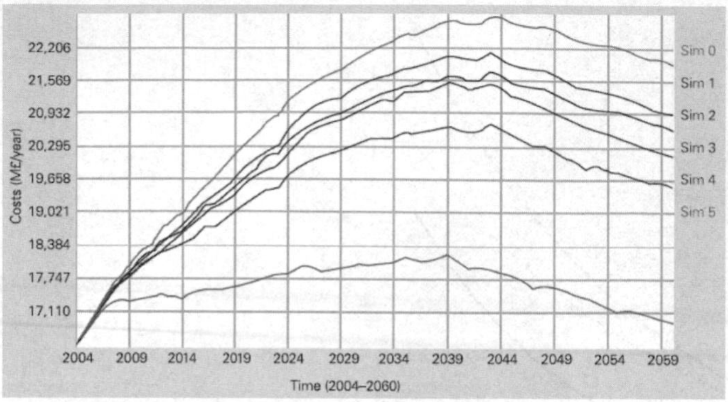

Fig. 9.5.7 The UK Foresight's modelling of the relative benefits in terms of the different effects of age related interventions for minimizing the impact of obesity related disease on the National Health costs in England.
Simulation 0 (top line): No interventions; and then simulations 1, 2, 3, and 4 reflect interventions where there were 1, 2, 4, and 8 BMI unit average reductions, respectively, achieved in the population aged 15–50 years only. Scenario 5 shows the comparison with scenario 4 but with all adults involved from ages 15 to 100 years. This highlights the importance of interventions in those >50 years.
Source: McPherson *et al.* (2007).

in the public health of the population and will do little to reduce the escalating health costs of the obesity-inducing epidemics of diabetes and hypertension now underway. Thus, if the total emphasis is put on the prevention of children's obesity and one manages to stop any further deterioration in obesity levels, then this has a negligible impact on the disease burden over the next 40 years, whereas intervention from 18 years onwards brings much greater benefits, Therefore, a focus on adults as well as children is particularly useful for several reasons, as noted by Seidel *et al.* (2005) and Gill (2002):

(a) The sharpest increase in the incidence of obesity is in (early) adulthood.

(b) Adults usually continue to gain weight during adulthood.

(c) Adult weight gain is almost always fat gain, except in athletes in training.

(d) The relative risks for many diseases associated with obesity decrease with age, but the absolute and population-attributable risks for disease increase with age.

(e) Interventions in children and adolescents need to be maintained for many more years or decades in order to have a considerable effect on the number of new cases of type 2 diabetes mellitus, heart disease, or cancer, compared with interventions in older individuals.

(f) Adults who are parents act as role models and have other responsibilities for the diet and physical activity behaviours of children.

These concepts have been reinforced by the UK's Foresight modelling (McPherson *et al.* 2007). Figure 9.5.8 shows that inducing such effective changes at the community level, so that the average BMI of the population is reduced by a whole 4 BMI units, produces a major and dramatic effect, but this has never been seen except perhaps in Cuba during their financial crisis when food deprivation was widespread throughout the country. Nevertheless, the remarkable differences in the medical burden and therefore medical costs if substantial changes can be made in the population's BMI demonstrate that there is clearly considerable benefit for individuals as well as their employers, insurance companies, or national health budgets to have a major focus on adults.

Figure 9.5.8 also demonstrates that the focus should be on those most vulnerable to disease, which means, in practice, the >50 years olds. The logic would also be to include those below 50 years who can be considered most vulnerable to developing the disease, i.e. those with pre-diabetics or incipient hypertension. The development of diabetes is far more sensitive to weight change as one would expect than coronary heart disease. Given these different perspectives, one then needs to consider how to counteract the current epidemic and, if possible, to reverse it. This requires an understanding of the basis for the current epidemic.

The small errors in energy balance leading to weight increments and the persistence of weight gain

For the last 30 years or more, adults in many affluent societies have been trying to slim down, and there has been a huge increase in the availability of magazines, voluntary groups, and commercial slimming organizations, all aiming to help overweight adults return to their normal weight. The slimming industry in the United States, for example, is enormous and earns well over US$100 billion yearly. This huge expenditure is mainly by women who consider not only the health hazards of their excess weight, but the fact that they feel less attractive when overweight. It is likely that the marked increase in eating disorders with bulimia and anorexia nervosa has also been precipitated by these national obsessions with slimming. Yet, despite this intense and, in affluent societies, nation-wide effort to slim, the obesity epidemic becomes worse, with little sign of the impact of all this slimming effort.

When one calculates the rate of weight gain—which may amount to 0.5–1 kg per year in early adult life, this amounts to a yearly accumulation of about 3500–7000 kcal. This in turn means that, on average, the discrepancy between energy intake and energy expenditure is only in the range of 10–20 kcal/day—this now being called the 'energy gap'. The energy gap amounts to a discrepancy in energy balance of only about 0.4–0.8 per cent of normal food intake per day. This concept of only small changes in energy storage being responsible often leads to the idea that simple small measures—cutting down food a bit and going for a short walk daily—will stop this weight gain.

These small discrepancies actually show how remarkable the normal regulation of energy balance is. Thus, our expenditure in all activity may vary daily by 200–300 kcal, depending on how much walking or leisure time activity we undertake but the variation in food intake is much more marked and can vary easily by 1000 kcal/day. Hence, the discrepancies in energy balance with fat accumulation represent the residual effect of extremely complex neuro-hormonal regulatory mechanisms operating on a short-, medium-, and long-term basis to preserve energy balance. However, the mechanisms which avoid weight loss are multiple and much more robust than those that limit weight gain.

Physical inactivity

The obvious thermodynamic principles of energy balance require that one recognizes the influence of both dietary change and the reduction in physical activity. The collapse in the demand for physical exertion came with cheaper cars for personal transport and multiple mechanical and electrical aids to remove the physical demands in the home and at work. Then with the advent of computers and television it is now clear that in many affluent societies one can earn an excellent wage and have enjoyable leisure without any physical exertion at all.

The evidence for current trends in physical activity varies, but most affluent countries have noted relatively stable rates or slight declines in leisure time physical activity over recent decades (Brownson *et al.* 2005) and in general the rates of sedentariness, defined as an absence of leisure time physical activity (LTPA), have remained rather stable. Of more importance to total energy expenditure has been the decline in the other domains of physical activity. Thus, the number of people involved in heavy occupational physical activity has declined dramatically, with more than a 50 per cent reduction in 'heavy work' in Norwegian adults since the mid-1980s, this change being associated with increases in sedentary work (Anderssen *et al.* 2007). Other countries have noted marked increases in car usage and other motorized transport, at the expense of more active commuting through walking or cycling trips (Fox & Hillsdon 2007). One study even reported a 6 per cent increase in the risk of obesity for every hour spent commuting by car each day (Frank *et al.* 2004). Limited data are available on domestic settings, but with increases in technologically sophisticated labour-saving devices, and reduced time spent in preparing meals and carrying out household tasks (predominantly through increases in dual adult working households), it seems that energy expenditure on domestic tasks and yard/garden work is likely to have reduced as well (Brownson *et al.* 2005).

For some European countries, the increase in obesity was delayed by up to a decade, notably in the Netherlands and Scandinavian countries (IOTF slides 2007). This might have been due to high rates of active commuting, especially cycling, as nutritional differences are not apparent compared with several other Western European countries (UK Parliament Select Committee on Health Third Report 2007). A few countries have demonstrated increasing trends in LTPA. For example, Finland and Canada have shown increasing LTPA trends over 25 years, and Singapore over about 10 years (Barengo *et al.* 2006; Craig *et al.* 2004). These comparisons are reliable within-country, even if they are not comparable between countries, due to the different physical activity measures used (Craig *et al.* 2003). Yet, despite these increases in LTPA, all of these countries have observed increases in obesity rates that were similar to demographically matched countries which did not have increases in LTPA (Cutler *et al.* 2003; Borodulin *et al.* 2007; Belanger-Ducharme & Tremblay 2005). Thus, in Finnish adults, the rates of increase in obesity were marginally but not substantially faster among the inactive and in Norway (leisure time defined) active and inactive adults gained weight at roughly similar rates from 1990. Therefore, in spite of LTPA increases, the increasing obesity rates develop either because of the impact of increases in energy intake, or because of substantial reductions in energy expenditure for tasks during the normal non-leisure times of day.

Evidence for the transformation of our diets is easier to document but the mistake made by doctors, scientists, and policy makers is to assume that we can measure the diet with sufficient accuracy to discern an energy imbalance of 10–20 kcal/day, i.e. <1 per cent of normal daily intake and expenditure. Whatever the interplay of changes in intake and energy expenditure under the usual environmental conditions before 1980, children and adults on average were able to maintain their energy balance unless they became ill and anorexic. At that time, it also seems clear that there was sufficient demand for physical work both in the home and in the usual range of occupations for people's appetite regulatory centres to be repeatedly operating to ensure that sufficient food was eaten to satisfy energy needs.

It now seems clear that, with the removal of the need for physical activity to earn one's living, the prevailing pressure on most people's brain regulatory systems has been to attempt to limit intake. It seems reasonable to accept that we have already moved away from the fabled large meals of our ancestors. Indeed, within our lifetime in relatively sophisticated environments, the meals and portions served in restaurants—at least in Europe—have become smaller, because that is what consumers seem to want. Thus, data from national food surveys in the United Kingdom showed a progressive fall in consumption even when allowances were made for the greater amount of food now eaten outside the home. Similarly, there are many people now who do not bother with breakfast, and this may well be a behavioural adaptation to a brain system which is trying to stop us eating so much. However, there have been remarkable changes in the normal food systems with an ever-increasing tendency to eat outside the home and to buy rather than make at home the range of meals which busy women and men still wish to consume. This means that populations have become far more dependent on manufactured processed foods and on decisions based on information about the nature of the purchased food.

The biological as well as societal maintenance of obesity

Unfortunately, in addition to these social issues there is now very good evidence that, as weight gain occurs, particularly in older adults, there is a 'resetting' of the regulatory system, so that weight loss is resisted. As weight gain occurs, this extra weight includes 25 per cent lean tissues which once laid down require additional daily energy for their maintenance. Thus, people's weight should plateau as soon as their increased weight compensates for the small discrepancy in intake. Unfortunately, this is not as effective as we would wish because weight gain usually continues and slowly the neuroregulatory systems progressively adjust as though they prefer to maintain the excess weight. The adaptation is progressive so that in due course the additional 10 kg extra weight then demands a permanent extra daily intake of 200–300 kcal/day. This adaptive mechanisms does not occur after the acutely overfeeding of young adults because they spontaneous return after the overfeeding stops to their previous body weights but this is not seen when older adults are acutely overfed (Roberts *et al.* 1994; Roberts & Rosenberg 2006).

Putting overweight and obese individuals on a slimming diet then immediately leads to the switching on of acute hormonal, hypothalamic regulated responses involving both the thyroidal axis and the autonomic nervous system which simulate the response to semi-starvation within 2–4 days even though the obese may have 0.25–1 million extra kcal stored. The brain mechanism which increases the drive to eat is also activated immediately.

A reflection of this persistent adaptive change in the brain of obese people is that most slimming overweight individuals readily regain the weight which they have taken so much trouble to lose. Those who are successful in maintaining their weight loss find that

Table 9.5.9 The contributors to the development of obesity as set out by WHO and categorized by the level of evidence for each contributor

Evidence	Decreases risk	No relationship	Increases risk
Convincing	Regular physical activity High-dietary NSP (fibre) intake		High intake of energy-dense nutrient-poor foods Sedentary lifestyles
Probable	Home and school environments that support healthy food choices for children** Promoting linear growth Breastfeeding		Heavy marketing of energy-dense foods** and fast-food outlets Adverse social and economic conditions (in developed countries, especially for women) Sugar-sweetened soft drinks and fruit juices
Possible	Low-glycaemic index foods	Protein content of the diet	Large portion sizes High proportion of food prepared outside the home (Western countries) 'Rigid restraint/periodic disinhibition' eating patterns
Insufficient	Increasing eating frequency		Alcohol

** Associated evidence and expert opinion

Source: Table taken from Diet, Nutrition and the Prevention of Chronic Diseases, WHO 2003, TRS 916.

they have to obsessively monitor their food intake and purchasing habits and deliberately engage in 2000–3000 kcal per week exercise to avoid gaining weight (Wing 2004)! The individuals describe a continuous battle to maintain their normal weight, so on this basis it is far more likely that the biological adaptation observed experimentally contributes to and amplifies the continuing environmental pressures which in susceptible individuals promote weight regain. These adaptive problems therefore seem to explain why the obesity epidemic continues to increase despite the desire of so many adults to lose their excess weight. This indicates a need for prevention to become a very high priority.

An evaluation of all the principal factors contributing to the obesity epidemic was set out by WHO in an Expert Technical report (World Health Organization 2003) (Table 9.5.9), which became a politically sensitive document because it highlighted again the inappropriateness of the prevailing high sugar intakes which in the earlier WHO 797 report in 1990 had led to a sustained campaign by sugar organizations to pressure governments—particularly the United States—to negate its implications. Now, sugar intakes are being linked by WHO not only to the prevalence of dental caries but also to the development of obesity.

Preventive strategies: The options

The analyses already presented on the impact of changes in population BMIs at different ages have emphasized the importance of tackling not just obesity but also overweight. The strategies may initially be considered on the basis of rectifying the major societal forces which currently promote the epidemic. The multiplicity of factors promoting the epidemic is dramatically revealed in the UK Foresight exercise. The specific factors with seemingly the greatest impact were highlighted, and it then became clear that in terms of both physical activity and the intake of energy there are very powerful forces that the individual does not control. This analysis led to the United Kingdom's designation of obesity as a 'passive' normal response of humans to the prevailing inappropriate environment. This then means that those who successfully remain lean throughout life are either genetically fortunate or they have the advantage in educative, social or financial terms to withstand the environmental forces and often create for themselves what is in effect a healthy 'microenvironment'.

The UK Foresight assessment of the key processes which contribute to the development of the epidemic cannot be used to simply specify that abolishing or reversing these forces will lead to useful prevention strategies. Thus, the introduction of the car, mechanical aids, the computerization of so many processes, and the advent of Internet-related communications have all contributed substantially to reducing the need of each of us to engage in physical activity by perhaps 750–1000 kcal or more on a daily basis. Nevertheless, nobody would consider reversing these developments as a coherent public health strategy for combating obesity. Hence, the issue is how best to combine current understanding of: (a) the most effective initiatives on the basis of either coherent trials or on the basis of a suitable model backed by an understanding of the underlying processes; (b) the most cost-efficient initiatives; (c) the most feasible initiatives on the basis of the features of the country's societal organization, cultural perceptions, and political system; and (d) whether there are other policy initiatives in the areas affecting food and physical activity which need to be integrated or, if conflicting, resolved.

Age-related issues: Childhood prevention

It was evident from Fig. 9.5.8 that successful measures in middle aged and older adults are likely to have an impact on public health rapidly: Selectively focusing primarily on the prevention of childhood overweight and obesity had very little impact on the burden of ill health nationally for decades. The current focus on childhood overweight/obesity has been justified, however, on several grounds:

(a) Public health measures are seen to be immediately relevant, given the fact that neither the public nor most policy makers blame the individual child for their predicament, and only a few try to assign blame to their parents. Therefore, this childhood focus has a politically useful place in persuading the public and politicians to do something other than advocating treatment.

(b) It is readily recognized that in older children excess weight gain confers on the affected group a far higher medical burden in their life time and a much greater probability of an early death than if one simply is concerned about the middle aged and older person. So a successful strategy can have a substantial impact for the individual concerned.

(c) The focus on children also chimes with the routine mantra that the key to the problem of obesity is 'education' so clearly there is merit in educating the child so that they 'do not behave' like their parents.

(d) If one is to focus on a group in society then school aged children are a useful choice because one is guaranteed to be able to reach them in most societies through a school mediated initiative.

Childhood prevention initiatives

These have been reviewed by Lobstein (2008) and by Brown *et al.* (2007). Table 9.5.10 summarizes the different types of programme which have shown some success as judged by short-term studies. This approach has been helped by the fact that the impact on weight gain of changes in children's environment can be documented relatively easily given their normal rates of growth. Studies lasting only a year or two are therefore valuable but whether the benefits can then be considered to last remains uncertain.

Table 9.5.10 Interventions for the prevention of overweight and obesity in school children*

Weight outcomes
1. The evidence of effectiveness of multi-component school-based interventions is equivocal.
2. School-based physical activity interventions (physical activity promotion and reduced television viewing) may help children maintain a healthy weight.
3. There is limited evidence from one UK-based study to suggest interventions to reduce consumption of carbonated drinks containing sugar.
Diet and physical activity outcomes
4. There is a body of evidence to suggest that school-based multi-component interventions addressing various aspects of diet and/or activity in the school, including the school environment (a 'whole-school approach'), are effective in improving physical activity and dietary behaviour, at least while the intervention is in place.
5. There is a body of evidence to suggest that short-term and long-term school-based interventions to improve children's dietary intake may be effective, at least while the intervention is in place. This includes interventions aiming to increase fruit and vegetable intake, improve school lunches, and/or promote water consumption.
6. UK-based evidence suggests that school children with the lowest fruit and vegetable intake at baseline may benefit the most from school-based dietary interventions.
7 There is a body of evidence from multi-component interventions to suggest that short-term and long-term school-based, physical activity-focused interventions may be effective, at least while the intervention is in place.

* *Source:* Brown *et al.* (2007).

Approaches to prevention: Is there a logic to the chosen initiatives?

A simpler overview than the United Kingdom's Foresight collation of different options is presented in Fig. 9.5.9, where the IOTF prevention group (Kumanyika *et al.* 2002) highlighted the different environmental systems which affect the environmental impact on both the diet and physical activity. Then, Swinburn (Egger & Swinburn 1997) developed the ANGELO framework for working out how to consider the different aspects of implementation at the different levels of influence on physical activity and diet. This depended on defining the options both at the micro and macro levels in terms of four overall areas of action:

(a) *Physical* changes, e.g. in the design of the environment for physical activity involving play areas, safe pedestrian and cycling friendly streets, or in terms of diet which is affected by food availability in shops within easy reach of poor families

(b) *Economic*, which might involve incentives or taxes or other economic measures at either a local or national level

(c) *Political*, e.g. specifying the requirement for baby-friendly hospitals to promote breastfeeding

(d) *Sociocultural*, e.g. involving changes to the health promotion and other national or local programmes and the involvement of major cultural figures to change perceptions of what is reasonable

This ANGELO approach was then taken further by WHO Euro (Robertson *et al.* 2004) to ensure that this approach to nutritional issues was integrated with other policy areas. On the energy expenditure side of energy balance there is a clear concordance of the need to promote physical activity with the new demand for societal mechanisms to limit climate change where national transport systems, e.g. trains and the use of buses is given much higher priority than car use. This then automatically requires more routine walking by the general public. In terms of food, Table 9.5.11 illustrates how the different levels of action can be classified and then how to consider the role of a ministry of government in taking responsibility for these actions.

This approach now allows a logical analysis of the options but still does not necessarily provide a clear approach to the choice of preventive measures. Some appear on the basis of collated evidence from previous initiatives to be good options whereas others are much more of an unknown entity. Given this uncertainty one can then develop a scheme of integrated public health actions judged on the basis of the likely impact and then the risk involved in implementing the various initiatives (Hawe & Shiell 1996). This approach, as illustrated in Table 9.5.12, was then used by Gill *et al.* (2006) to establish a set of obesity prevention priorities for New South Wales, Australia.

Identifying the evidence for effective prevention strategies by systematic review, if based on the demand to demonstrate conclusively the coherence of evidence from community or group interventions over a 12-month period at least, is sparse as set out in a recent review (Hawkes *et al.* in press) for the World Cancer Research Fund. Table 9.5.13 shows the current perceptions based on physiological studies, observational studies and mechanistic evidence, and Table 9.5.10 provided the outcome of one (in school children) of the five reviews of interventions. This illustrates how limited the data are when the criteria are based on having several properly controlled and preferably randomized groups in the community. It is also important to recognize that randomized controlled trials assess

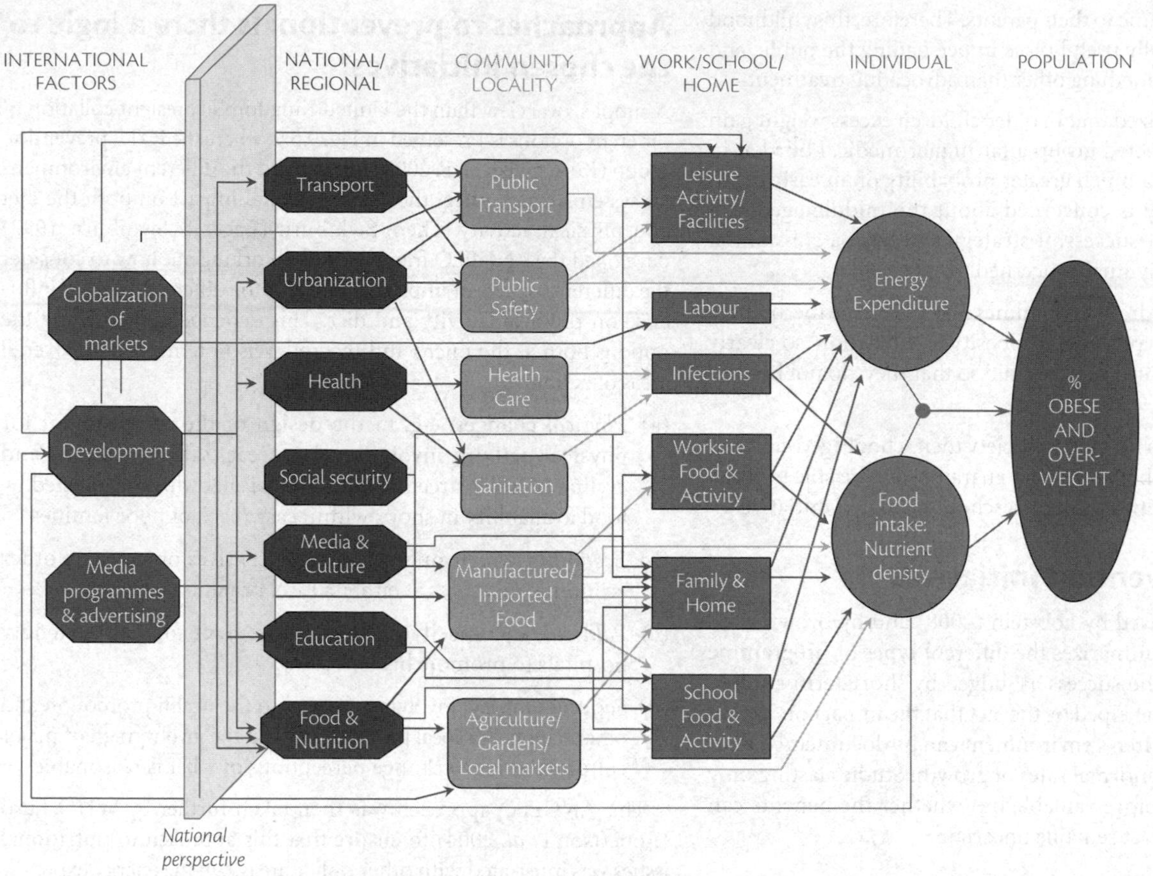

Fig. 9.5.8 Societal policies and processes influencing the population prevalence of obesity.
Source: Modified from Kumanyika *et al.* (2002).

the efficacy of interventions but do not necessarily inform policy makers about their effectiveness when implemented on a wider public health basis. Even when this is undertaken, however, one still has to work out the cost effectiveness because initiatives, particularly at the grass roots level, can be very costly once one has taken into account all the checks and arrangements and training that are involved.

The State of Victoria, Australia, building on the NSW initiatives, undertook meticulous analyses of the costs having established a set of principles for determining effectiveness (Haby *et al.* 2006). Figure 9.5.10 shows the relative potential effectiveness of ten possible initiatives affecting school children in relation to the degree of uncertainty, and then Table 9.5.14 sets out the relative cost-effectiveness of these community-related initiatives in ranked order of cost-effectiveness (ACE Obesity 2006). The reason why TV advertising tops the list is because the options are calculated on the basis of the cost to the consumer or government and not to industry. Thus, restricting TV advertising has the benefit of modifying the input to practically all children because almost all watch TV—often for several hours a day. So, changes in the regulation, when implemented, will have an immediate potential impact on practically every child in most countries. Restricting access to the TV has also been shown to limit the development of obesity because it limits very sedentary behaviour during viewing time and the loss of the usual intense marketing of inappropriate foods may also play a role. This marketing has been shown to induce confusion about nutrition, alter attitudes favouring the advertised goods, change purchasing practices in favour of the foods marketed and distort the children's diets (Hastings *et al.* 2003); the additional bonus of a government-directed ban on marketing is that the initiation of these measures simply requires a government regulation which then has to be followed. There is then no cost in terms of educating schools, parents, and children. This illustrates the fact that government intervention using conventional mechanisms for adjusting societal rules or habits usually automatically involve few direct costs. Thus, the more that can be undertaken by governmental processes which require industry or businesses or governmental workers to change their practices affecting food and activity, the lower the potential cost compared with individually related initiatives, e.g. involving health education or personal trainers or other focused and individually based advice to individual consumers.

Upstream measures for obesity prevention: The price, availability, and marketing of foods

In developing a food business, it is well recognized that, apart from producing a product that is attractive, there are three key features which determine their increasing turnover:

(a) The price of their product

(b) Its pervasive availability for consumers

(c) Intense marketing

Table 9.5.11 An illustration of the STEFANI (STrategies for Effective Food And Nutrition Initiatives) model developed by WHO (Euro) for action by (a) the Ministry of Health and (b) other ministries on diet

	Dietary quality; physical activity	Food safety	Environment
(A) Ministry of Health—direct responsibilities			
Physical	Appropriately accessible health centres Promoting access to appropriate self-monitoring, e.g. weight, BP	Catering in hospitals; monitoring facilities	Fluoridation systems for water Facilities for iodizing salt
Economic	Primary health payments for specific targets in management	Penalties for providing unsafe food	Subsidize iodine for iodination purposes
Policy	Baby-friendly hospitals Dietary guidelines establishing fortification policies Establish policies on health claims, e.g. functional foods	Health impact of multi-sectoral food safety policies	Establish specific guidelines for toxicants and contaminants in soil, water, and primary food products HIA of agrochemical use
Sociocultural	Health education	Promote concept of limited clinical antibiotic use	Promote new concept of health impact of new traffic policy
(B) Other ministries—specified on a national basis			
Physical	Ensuring playgrounds in schools, suitable cycling and road systems; urban planning; sports facilities. Designated urban areas for local food production	Provision of appropriate local abattoirs. Proper public toilet and sanitary facilities. Proper catering facilities based on stringent hygiene requirements	Urban planning: Green spaces, cycle paths, parks, playgrounds, lead free Establish facilities for farmers' markets
Economic	Re-evaluate taxation and subsidy policies	Establish appropriate penalties for inappropriate hygiene	Reform CAP. Finance new public transport systems. Promote urban agriculture, new outlets for high-quality, affordable foods in deprived areas
Policy	HIA of CAP Food labelling with appropriate, understandable health-related information	Establish criteria for ensuring pathogen- and contaminant-free access to the food chain. Establish systematic HACCP for food chain, systematic surveillance, and mechanisms for emergency response	Reform CAP Develop soil improvement, clean water, agricultural recycling, planting, fertilizer, pesticide, water use policies
Sociocultural	Promote physical activity in the workplace. Create breastfeeding time and space in the workplace with NGO help	Establish new criteria for excluding antibiotics as growth promoters and specifying veterinary use Educational initiatives for safety of fast-food outlets, and modifying nutrient composition, and limiting and ensuring appropriate food waste disposal	Change attitudes to cycle path use, pedestrian areas. Educational initiatives for caterers, communal use of school recreational facilities

Source: Taken from the WHO Euro report Robertson *et al.* (2004) and inspired by the ANGELO model Egger and Swinburn (1997).

Table 9.5.12. A planning approach to developing a portfolio of public health options: weighing up potential gains and risks

Increasing returns/health gains ↑		
Very high gain—low uncertainty *Not found*	High gain—moderate uncertainty *1. Very promising*	High gain—high uncertainty *3. Promising*
Moderate gains—low uncertainty *Not found*	Moderate gain—moderate uncertainty *2. Promising*	Moderate gains—high uncertainty *4. Some promise*
Low gain—low uncertainty *Treatment options*	Low gain—moderate uncertainty *Inappropriate*	Low gain—high uncertainty *Inappropriate*
	Increasing uncertainty or risk →	

Source: Hawe & Sheill (1996) by Gill *et al.* (2007).

Table 9.5.13 Components of diet and physical activity deemed to be important determinants of overweight and obesity based only on observational and mechanistic evidence

Evidence	Decreases risk of overweight and obesity	Increases risk of overweight and obesity
Convincing	Increased* total physical activity	
Probable	Breastfeeding (in terms of preventing obesity in child from 5 years of age); diets rich in low energy-dense foods (wholegrain cereals and cereal products; foods rich in non-starch polysaccharides and dietary fibre)	Frequent large portions of energy-dense foods; sugary drinks

*Increased over time, rather than simply 'high'.
Source: Brown et al. (2007).

These three factors—price, availability, and marketing—have also been repeatedly shown to be important in the public health initiatives for the effective limiting of smoking and alcohol consumption. The same clearly now applies to the issue of obesity because even children respond to cheaper options by purchasing more; e.g. of fruit in a school setting (French *et al.* 2001). It is also clear that the cost of foods in a Western environment is inversely related to the nutritional quality of the product; the greater the energy density of the food, i.e. in terms of kcal/g, the cheaper it is (Drewnowski & Specter 2004; Maillot *et al.* 2007).

The cost of foods in Western environments has been changing steadily over the last four to five decades as a result of government policies which were set out after World War II. The aim was to promote the production and consumption of ever cheaper meat, milk, butter, fats, and oils, as there was widespread disruption of food supplies during World War II, which rapidly became national

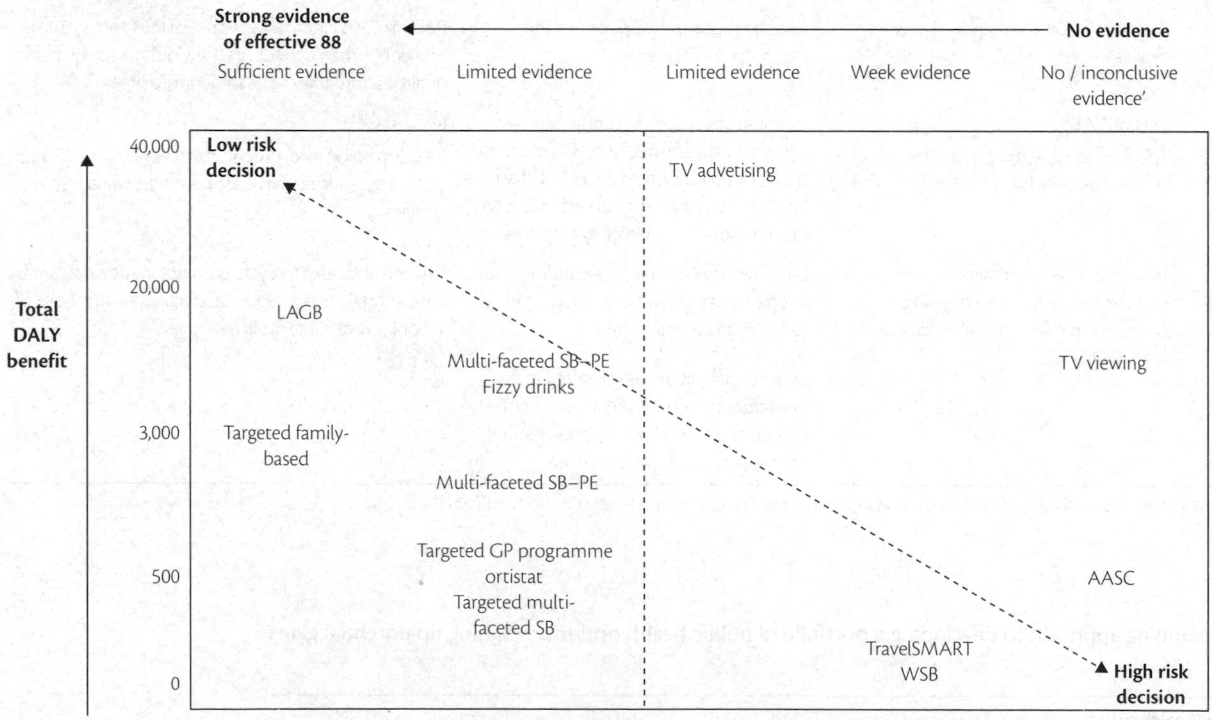

Fig. 9.5.9 The evaluation of different initiatives to prevent childhood obesity
The area to the left of the vertical dotted line signifies stronger evidence i.e. sufficient evidence or limited evidence that is unlikely to be due to chance. To the right of the line there is limited evidence of effectiveness but theoretical reasons why the intervention should work (Haby *et al.* 2006).
AASC—Active After School Communities programme
GP—General practitioner
LAGB—Laparoscopic adjustable gastric banding
PE—Active physical education
SB—School-based
WSB—Walking school bus

Table 9.5.14 Differences in estimated cost-effectiveness from different initiatives in the prevention of obesity in children in the state of Victoria, Australia

Intervention	Cost in AU$ for each DALY saved
Restrict TV advertising	4
Soft drink education intervention at school	3000
School education to reduce TV viewing	3000
School programme targeting overweight and obese children	3000
Family-based programme for the obese child	4000
Add physical education	7000
Gastric banding for severely obese adolescents	10 000
School multiple interventions, but no physical education	14 000
Medical treatment with drugs, e.g. orlistat	14 000
Doctors targeting the overweight children	32 000
After-school community programmes	90 000
Cycling (Travel SMART Schools)	260 000
Walking buses to school	770 000

Victoria State analyses announced by the Minister of Health, Australia, September 2006.
Source: ACE Obesity (2006).

security issues. This led to a pervasive system of agriculture support involving direct grants, subsidies, free research and advisory services, guaranteed prices for food purchased by marketing boards for several decades, and continuing EU and US export subsidies (Elinder 2005; Shoonover & Muller 2006). It is not surprising therefore that there has been a remarkable transformation of food costs which have made fruits and vegetables more expensive in relative terms and fats, meat, sugars, and oils much cheaper. The poorer sections of the community in responding to their biological desire to satisfy their intrinsic energy needs purchase the cheapest products which are therefore richer in fat and sugars. This practice then tends to lead to 'passive over-consumption' because of the relatively poor satiety effects of fats and sugars—the latter particularly when provided in soft drinks between meals. The purchasing patterns of the poorer sections of society are much more price-sensitive; they are spending a much higher proportion of household income on food and normally attempt to minimize these costs to allow more flexibility for purchasing other household needs.

These economic constraints require an integrated approach before satisfactory dietary changes can be supported. Putting a higher price on fat- and sugar-rich foods will be a regressive measure, i.e. poorer households will pay more as with taxes on tobacco and alcohol. An integrated economic package needs to be developed, so that the poorer section of society obtains more financial support by other means. Then the alteration of relative food prices still induces changes, particularly in the poorer sections of the community. If the appropriate foods are then also made more readily available, the poorer sections of the community will respond. Thus, in Finland, the vegetables provided with main meals at canteens and restaurants are included in the general price of the main meal. Thus, the poorer sectors of the community particularly benefited, and the combined public health measures in Finland led to a trebling in the average vegetable intake of the population over a 15-year period. In parallel with these changes, there was a marked reduction in the prevalence of hypertension and a progressive fall in cardiovascular diseases. Such practical measures at a community level will probably need reinforcing by changes in policies affecting the whole food chain from food labelling with appropriate instantly understandable symbols such as the traffic light labelling scheme proposed by the UK Food Standards Agency through to more complex arrangements affecting agricultural policies. These more upstream measures are only now being considered, but post-World War II policies relating to agriculture and other food policies, e.g. for school food, appear to have had marked and deleterious effects on public health over the last half century.

References

ACE Obesity (2006) Assessing the cost effectiveness of obesity interventions in children and adolescents. Summary of results. Published by the Victorian Government Department of Human Services Melbourne, Victoria 2006. www.health.vic.gov.au

Adams, K.F., Schatzkin, A., Harris, T.B., *et al.* (2006) Overweight, obesity, and mortality in a large prospective cohort of persons 50 to 71 years old. *New England Journal of Medicine*, **355**, 763–78.

Anderssen, S.A., Engeland, A., Sogaard, A.J., *et al.* (2007) Changes in physical activity behaviour and the development of body mass index during the last 30 years in Norway. *Scandinavian Journal of Public Health*, 1–9.

Arterburn, D.E., Maciejewski, M.L., Tsevat, J. (2005) Impact of morbid obesity on medical expenditures in adults. *International Journal of Obesity*, **29**, 334–9.

Asia Pacific Cohort Studies Collaboration (2004) Body mass index and cardiovascular disease in the Asia-Pacific Region: an overview of 33 cohorts involving 310 000 participants. *International Journal of Epidemiology*, **33**, 751–8.

Barengo, N.C., Nissinen, A., Pekkarinen, H., *et al.* (2006) Twenty-five-year trends in lifestyle and socioeconomic characteristics in Eastern Finland. *Scandinavian Journal of Public Health*, **34**, 437–44.

Barker, D.J. (2004) The developmental origins of well-being. *Phil Trans R Soc Lond B*, **359**, 1359–66.

Barlow, S.E., Dietz, W.H. (1998) Obesity evaluation and treatment: Expert committee recommendations. *Pediatrics*, **102**, 1–11.

Batty, G.D., Shipley, M.J., Jarrett, R.J., *et al.* (2006) Obesity and overweight in relation to disease-specific mortality in men with and without existing coronary heart disease in London: the original Whitehall study. *Heart*, **92**, 886–92.

Belanger-Ducharme, F., Tremblay, A. (2005) Prevalence of obesity in Canada. *Obesity Reviews*, **6**, 183–6.

Borodulin, K., Makinen, T., Fogelholm, M., *et al.* (2007) Trends and socioeconomic differences in overweight among physically active and inactive Finns in 1978–2002. Preventive Medicine, **45**, 157–62.

Brown, T., Kelly, S., Summerbell, C. (2007) Prevention of obesity: a review of interventions. *Obesity Reviews*, **8** (suppl), 127–30.

Brownson, R.C., Boehmer, T.K., Luke, D.A. (2005) Declining rates of physical activity in the United States: what are the contributors? *Annual Review of Public Health*, **26**, 421–43.

Cole, T.J., Green, P.J. (1992) Smoothing reference centile curves: the LMS method and penalized likelihood. *Statistics in Medicine*, **11**, 1305–19.

Cole, T.J., Bellizzi, M.C., Flegal, K.M., *et al.* (2000) Establishing a standard definition for child overweight and obesity worldwide: international survey. *British Medical Journal*, **320**, 1240–3.

Craig, C.L, Marshall, A.L., Sjostrom, M., *et al.* (2003) International Physical Activity Questionnaire: 12-country reliability and validity. *Medicine & Science in Sports & Exercise*, **35**, 1381–95.

Craig, C.L., Russell, S.J., Cameron, C., *et al.* (2004) Twenty–Year Trends in Physical Activity among Canadian Adults. *Canadian Journal of Public Health*, **95**, 59–63.

Cutler, D., Glaeser, E., Shapiro, J. (2003) Why have Americans become more obese?, *Journal of Economic Perspectives*, **17**, 93–118.

Dietz, W.H., Bellizzi, M.C. (1999) Assessment of childhood and adolescent obesity. *American Journal Clinical Nutrition*, **70**(suppl), 117–175S.

Drewnowski, A., Specter, S.E. (2004) Poverty and obesity: the role of energy density and energy costs. *American Journal of Clinical Nutrition*, **79**, 6–16.

Eero Kajantie, F., Feldt, K., Räikkönen, K., *et al.* (2007) Body size at birth predicts hypothalamic-pituitary-adrenal axis response to psychosocial stress at age 60 to 70 years. *Journal of Clinical Endocrinology and Metabolism.*, **92**, 4094–100. Epub 2007 Sep 11.

Egger, G., Swinburn, B. (1997) An "ecological" approach to the obesity pandemic. *British Medical Journal*, **315**, 477–80.

Elinder, L.S. (2005) Obesity, hunger and agriculture: the damaging role of subsidies. *British Medical Journal*, **331**, 1333–6.

Ezzati M., Hoorn S.V., Lawes C.M.M., *et al.* (2005) Rethinking the "diseases of affluence" paradigm: Economic development and global patterns of nutritional risks obesity and other cardiovascular risk factors 2005 in relation to economic development. *PLoS Medicine*, **2**, 0404–0412.

Flegal, K.M., Graubard, B.I., Williamson, D.F., *et al.* (2007) Cause-specific excess deaths associated with underweight, overweight, and obesity. *JAMA*, **298**, 2028–37.

Fox, K.R., Hillsdon, M. (2007) Physical activity and obesity. *Obesity Review*, **8**(S1), 115–21.

Frank, L.D., Andresen, M.A., Schmid, T.L. (2004) Obesity relationships with community design, physical activity, and time spent in cars. *American Journal of Preventive Medicine*, **27**, 87–96.

French, S.A., Story, M., Jeffery, R.W. (2001) Environmental influences on eating and physical activity. *Annual Review of Public Health*, **22**, 309–35.

Garrow, J.S. (1981) *Treat Obesity Seriously. A Clinical Manual.* Churchill Livingstone, New York.

Gill, T. (2002) The importance of preventing weight gain in adulthood. *Asia Pacific*, **11**(suppl), S632–6.

Gill, T., King, L., Webb, K. (2006) Best options for promoting healthy weight and preventing weight gain in NSW. NSW Dept of Health at www.health.nsw.gov.au

Greenberg, J.A. (2006) Correcting biases in estimates of mortality attributable to obesity 1. *Obesity*, **14**, 2071–9.

Guillaume, M. (1999) Defining obesity in childhood: current practice. *American Journal of Clinical Nutrition*, **70**(suppl), 126–30S.

Guo, S.S., Chumlea, W.C. (1999) Tracking of body mass index in children in relation to overweight in adulthood. *American Journal of Clinical Nutrition*, **70**, 145–148S.

Haby, M.M., Vos, T., Carter, R., *et al.* (2006) A new approach to assessing the health benefit from obesity interventions in children and adolescents: the assessing cost-effectiveness in obesity project. *International Journal of Obesity*, **30**, 1463–75.

Hastings, G., Stead, M., McDermott, L., *et al.* Review of research on the effects of food promotion to children. Final report prepared for the Food Standards Agency, 2003. http://www.food.gov.uk/multimedia/pdfs/foodpromotiontochildren1.pd

Hawe, P., Shiell, A. (1996) Preserving innovation under increasing accountability pressures. The health promotion investment portfolio approach. *Health Promotion Journal of Australia*, 5, 4–9.

Hawkes, C., Asfaw, A., Bauman, A., *et al.* Evidence on the determinants of dietary patterns, nutrition and physical activity, and the interventions to maintain or to modify them: A systematic review. WCRF (in press).

Huxley, R., James, W.P.T., Barzi, F., *et al.* on behalf of the Obesity in Asia Collaboration Ethnic comparisons of the cross-sectional relationships between measures of body size with diabetes and hypertension (2007) In James W.P.T. and Chen C.M. Obesity in China. *Obesity Reviews* (in press).

IOTF slides: Trends in obesity (Europe) http://www.iotf.org/database/TrendsinObesityPrevalence.htm [accessed July 2007].

James, W.P.T, Ferro-Luzzi, A., Waterlow, J.C. (1988) Definition of chronic energy deficiency in adults. Report of a Working Party of the International Dietary Energy Consultative Group. *European Journal of Clinical Nutrition*, **42**, 969–81.

James, W.P.T. (1976) (Compiler) *Research on Obesity*. A Report of the DHSS/MRC Group. H.M.S.O, London.

James, W.P.T. (1976) *Research on Obesity*. A Report of the DHSS/MRC Group. Compiled by James WPT, HMSO, London.

James, W.P.T. (2005) Assessing obesity: are ethnic differences in body mass index and waist classification criteria justified? *Obesity Reviews.*, **6**, 179–81.

James, W.P.T., Jackson-Leach, R., Ni Mhurchu, C., *et al.* (2004) Overweight and obesity (high body mass index). In: Ezzati M., Lopez A.D., Rodgers A., Murray C.J.L. (eds.) *Comparative Quantification of Health Risks. Global and Regional Burden of Disease Attributable to Selected Major Risk Factors*, Chapter 8, Volume 1. World Health Organization, Geneva.

Kumanyika, S., Jeffery, R.W., Morabia, A., *et al.* (2002) Public Health Approaches to the Prevention of Obesity (PHAPO) Working Group of the International Obesity Task Force (IOTF). Obesity prevention: the case for action. *International Journal of Obesity*, 26, 425–36.

Law, C.M., Egger, P., Dada, O., *et al.* (2001) Body size at birth and blood pressure among children in developing countries. *International Journal of Epidemiology.*, **30**, 52–7.

Lobstein T. (2008) The prevention of obesity in childhood and adolescence. In: Bray G.A., Bouchard C. (eds.) *Handbook of Obesity: Clinical Applications*. 3rd Edition. Informa Healthcare, New York, p. 131–156.

Lopez, A.D., Mathers, C.D., Ezzati, M., *et al.* (eds.) (2006) *Global Burden of Disease and Risk Factors*. New York: Oxford University Press.

Maillot, M., Darmon, N., Vieux, F., *et al.* (2007) Low energy density and high nutritional quality are each associated with higher diet costs in French adults. *American Journal of Clinical Nutrition*, 2007, **86**, 690–6.

McPherson, K., Marsh, T., Brown, M. (2007) Foresight. Tackling Obesities: Future choices – modelling future trends in obesity and the impact on health. www.foresight.gov.uk

Must, A., Dallal, G.E., Dietz, W.H. (1991) Reference data for obesity: 85th and 95th percentiles of body mass index (wt/ht2) and triceps skinfold thickness. *American Journal of Clinical Nutrition*, **53**, 839–46.

National Institutes of Health 1998: Clinical Guidelines on the Identification, Evaluation and Treatment of Overweight and Obesity in Adults: the Evidence Report. US Department of Health & Human Services, National Institutes of Health, National Heart, Lung and Blood Institute, USA.

Parsons, T.J., Power, C., Logan, S., *et al.* (1999) Childhood predictors of adult obesity: a systematic review. *International Journal of Obesity*, **23** (Suppl), S1–107.

Popkin, B.M. (2006) Global nutrition dynamics: the world is shifting rapidly toward a diet linked with noncommunicable diseases. *American Journal of Clinical Nutrition*, **84**, 289–98.

Power, C., Lake, J.K., Cole, T.J. (1997) Measurement and long-term health risks of child and adolescent fatness. *International Journal of Obesity*, **21**, 507–26.

Reilly, J.J., Dorosty, A.R., Emmett, P.M. and the ALSPAC Study Team (2000) Identification of the obese child: adequacy of the body mass index for clinical practice and epidemiology. *International Journal of Obesity*, **24**, 1623–7.

Roberts, S.B., Rosenberg, I. (2006) Nutrition and aging: changes in the regulation of energy metabolism with aging. *Physiological Review*, **86**, 651–67.

Roberts, S.B., Fuss, P., Heyman, M.B., *et al.* (1994) Control of food intake in older men. *JAMA*, **272**, 1601–6. Erratum in: *JAMA*, **273**, 702.

Robertson, A., Tirado, C., Lobstein, T., *et al.* Food and Health in Europe: a new basis of action. WHO 2004, European Series No 96.

Rolland-Cachera, M.F., Deheeger, M., Guilloud-Bataille, M., *et al.* (1987) Tracking the development of adiposity from one month of age to adulthood. *Annals of Human Biology*, **14**, 219–29.

Rose, G. (1991) Population distributions of risk and disease. *Nutrition Metabolism and Cardiovascular Diseases*, **1**, 37–40.

Royal College of Physicians (1983) Obesity – A Report of the Royal college of Physicians. *Journal of the Royal College of Physicians of London*, **17**.

Sanchez-Castillo, C.P., Velasquez-Monroy O., Lara-Esqueda A., *et al.* (2005) Diabetes and hypertension increases in a society with abdominal obesity: results of the Mexican National Health Survey 2000. *Public Health Nutrition.*, **8**, 53–60.

Seidell, J.C., Nooyens, A.J., Visscher, T.L.S. (2005) Cost-effective measures to prevent obesity: epidemiological basis and appropriate target groups. *Proceedings of the Nutrition Society*, **64**, 1–5.

Shoonover, H., Muller, M. (2006) Food without thought. How US food policy contributes to obesity. Institute for Agriculture and Trade Policy. Minneapolis, USA

UK Food Standards Agency. Signposting labelling scheme. http://www.food.gov.uk/foodlabelling/signposting

UK Parliament Select Committee on Health Third Report 2006–2007. http://www.publications.parliament.uk/pa/cm200304/cmselect/cmhealth/23/2306.htm. Accessed June 2007:. n 307, Sections 305–309

Wang, Y., Lobstein, T. (2006) Worldwide trends in childhood overweight and obesity. *International Journal of Pediatric Obesity*, **1**, 11–25.

WHO Child Growth Standards. WHO, Geneva, 2007.

WHO Expert Consultation (2004) Appropriate body-mass index for Asian populations and its implications for policy and intervention strategies. *Lancet*, **363**, 157–63.

WHO/IASO/IOTF (2000) The Asia-Pacific perspective: redefining obesity and its treatment. February 2000. Health Communications, Australia PTY Ltd. Full document available from: http://www.idi.org.au/obesity_report.htm

Wing, R.R. (2004) Behavioural approaches to the treatment of obesity. In *Handbook of Obesity. Clinical Applications*. (ed Bray, G.A. and Bouchard, C. 2nd Edition), Marcel Dekker, New York. pp. 147–67.

World Health Organization (WHO) (1995) *Physical Status: The Use and Interpretation of Anthropometry*. Tech. Rep. Series 854.

World Health Organization. (2000) *Obesity: Preventing and Managing the Global Epidemic*. WHO Technical Report Series No. 894. WHO, Geneva.

World Health Organization. *Diet, Nutrition and the Prevention of Chronic Diseases*. Report of a Joint WHO/FAO Expert Consultation. WHO Technical Report Series No. 916. World Health Organization, Geneva, 2003.

Yusuf, S., Hawken, S., Ôunpuu, S., *et al.* on behalf of the INTERHEART Study Investigators (2005) Obesity and the risk of myocardial infarction in 27 000 participants from 52 countries: a case-control study. *Lancet*, **366**, 1640–49.

9.6

The epidemiology and prevention of diabetes mellitus

Nigel Unwin and Paul Zimmet

Abstract

Diabetes mellitus is a heterogeneous disease characterized by raised blood glucose. The current classification recognizes two main types: Type 1, due to destruction of the insulin-producing cells of the pancreas and typically requiring exogenous insulin for survival; and type 2, representing 85–95 per cent of all diabetes, and due to a combination of resistance to the action of insulin and diminished insulin production. Currently, around 250 million people worldwide have diabetes, 6 per cent of the adult population, and this figure will increase markedly over the coming years as populations age and become increasingly overweight and sedentary, the major risk factors for type 2 diabetes. Contrary to popular perception over 70 per cent of people with diabetes live in low- or middle-income countries, and most new cases of diabetes over the coming decades will be in such countries. Diabetes reduces life expectancy by around 15 years in type 1 diabetes and 10 years in type 2 and in many populations is the major cause of lower limb amputation, visual loss and renal failure. It is a major source of expenditure in health systems the world over and also impacts upon economic productivity. It was recently estimated that in 2007 diabetes cost India 2.1 per cent of its gross domestic product. Prevention, or at least delayed onset, of type 2 diabetes through behavioural or pharmacological measures has been convincingly demonstrated in several trials. At best these trials were able to achieve a 60 per cent reduction in incidence. The prevention of type 1 diabetes remains the subject of research. Nonetheless, a substantial reduction in the incidence of complications in people with diabetes is possible, including reductions in cardiovascular disease events, visual loss, lower limb amputation and renal failure. However, achieving these reductions requires well organized and resourced health care, and good education and support to people with diabetes in managing their condition. Diabetes is one of the major public health challenges of the twenty-first century, a fact recognized in 2006 by a United Nations resolution.

Definition, classification, and diagnosis

Diabetes is a metabolic disease characterized by hyperglycaemia (raised blood glucose) resulting from defects in insulin secretion, insulin action, or both (American Diabetes Association 2004). Insulin, produced by the beta cells of the pancreatic islets of Langerhans, is the main hormone regulating blood glucose levels, and is released in response to rising blood glucose following eating or drinking. Insulin has wide-ranging metabolic effects, which include the stimulation of glucose uptake into skeletal muscle and liver, and key roles in lipid and protein metabolism.

Prior to the late 1970s, there was little consistency in the classification of, or diagnostic criteria for, diabetes. In the mid-1930s, Himsworth (1936) had proposed that there were at least two clinical types of diabetes, insulin-sensitive and insulin-insensitive, the former being due to insulin deficiency. Confirmation of his clinical observations came with Bornstein's development of a bioassay for insulin (Bornstein & Lawrence 1951). The Nobel Prize-winning discovery of a radioimmunoassay for insulin a decade later saw the confirmation of Bornstein's observations (Berson & Yalow 1963). The widespread acceptance of the terms *juvenile-onset* and *maturity-onset* diabetes at this time was affirmation of the concept that there were at least two major forms of the disease.

However, since 1979 and 1980, the American Diabetes Association (ADA) and the World Health Organization (WHO), respectively, have produced a series of recommendations on both classification and diagnosis. These recommendations have changed over time to reflect the latest scientific evidence. There are small but important differences between the WHO and ADA recommendations. Most parts of the world tend to follow the recommendations of WHO, but those of the ADA are also followed in many places outside the United States. In the description that follows, we therefore focus on the recommendations of WHO (World Health Organization 1999, 2006) but in appropriate places describe how those of the ADA differ.

The classification of diabetes is based on current understandings of its underlying aetiology. There are two main types of diabetes. Type 1 diabetes results from destruction of the insulin-producing cells (beta cells) in the pancreas. This is usually, but not always, associated with detectable auto-antibodies to components of the beta cell. Type 2 diabetes, which accounts for 85–95 per cent of all diabetes, results from a combination of resistance to the action of insulin, particularly at skeletal muscle, liver, and fat tissue, and insufficient insulin production by the pancreas. There are several other rarer types of diabetes with specific aetiologies, such as maturity onset diabetes of the young, associated with specific single gene defects, and diabetes associated with toxicity to certain drugs. Gestational diabetes refers to diabetes that is diagnosed for the first time during pregnancy.

A classification of diabetes is shown in Fig. 9.6.1 (World Health Organization 2006). It is worth remembering that, as is the case for many conditions, our current understandings of the aetiologies of diabetes remain incomplete, and the classification described here may well change in the future. For example, distinction between type 1 and type 2 diabetes is not always clear cut. The term 'double diabetes' has recently been used to describe the situation in some children and adolescents in which insulin resistance, associated with obesity, is accompanied by auto-antibodies to the beta-cell (Pozzilli & Buzzetti 2007), although rather than 'double diabetes', it is also hypothesized type 1 and type 2 diabetes are the same disorder of insulin resistance, set against different genetic backgrounds (Wilkin 2001), with one background leading to autoimmune destruction of the beta cells of the pancreas and what is currently called type 1 diabetes.

In adults, diabetes which clinically appears to be type 2 diabetes may be accompanied by auto-antibodies to the beta cells and follow a relatively rapid course to insulin dependency. This type of diabetes has received various names, including latent autoimmune diabetes of adults (LADA) (Tuomi *et al.* 1993) and type 1.5 (Palmer & Hirsch 2003). If all this seems a bit confusing, it makes the point that a classification of diabetes based on aetiology is work in progress, while at the present time the categories of type 1 and type 2 remain useful and widely used.

For clinical practice, it is often useful to stage people with diabetes according to their requirements for insulin as follows:

- Insulin required for survival (virtually all of these will have type 1 diabetes)
- Insulin required for adequate metabolic control but not survival (most of these will have type 2 diabetes, but some will have type 1 diabetes in which there remain some functioning beta cells)
- Insulin not required, and treatment adequate without drugs or drugs other than insulin (the vast majority will have type 2 diabetes, but some may have type 1 diabetes before the beta cell destruction has advanced very far)

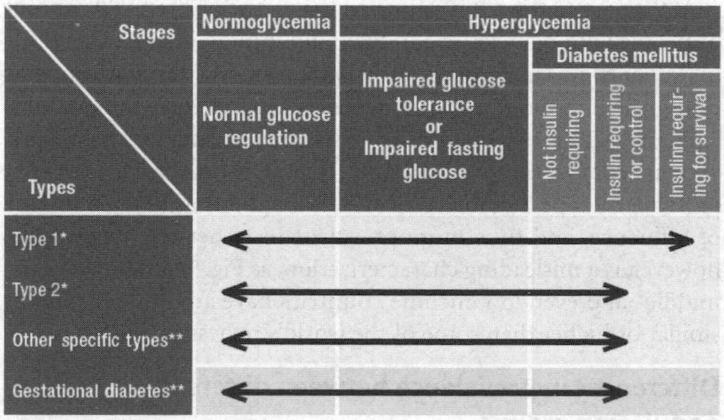

Fig. 9.6.1 The relationship between aetiological types of diabetes and clinical stages of hyperglycaemia.

* Even after presenting in an acute crisis, such as ketoacidosis, these patients can briefly return to normoglycaemia without requiring specific therapy

** In rare instances, patients in these categories (e.g. Vacor toxicity, type 1 diabetes presenting in pregnancy) may require insulin for survivial.

Source: World Health Organization (2006).

The relationships between the current aetiological classification and clinical stages of diabetes are shown in Fig. 9.6.1. The clinical staging includes a category called 'intermediate hyperglycaemia', in which blood glucose is considered above normal but below the diagnostic thresholds for diabetes. This category should not be considered as a clinical entity but rather as a risk category, identifying as it does, people at high risk of developing type 2 diabetes and cardiovascular disease, and providing a potential target for preventive interventions.

Diagnosis

The diagnosis of diabetes is based on blood glucose levels. Diagnostic thresholds, following current WHO recommendations (World Health Organization, 1996, 2006 are shown in Table 9.6.1. The 'gold standard' diagnostic test or reference method is the oral glucose tolerance test (OGTT). In brief, an OGTT involves the measurement of fasting glucose, followed by a drink containing a fixed quantity of glucose, and the measurement of blood glucose 2 hours after that drink. Undertaking an OGTT is time consuming and relatively expensive (compared to fasting glucose alone). Largely for these pragmatic reasons, the ADA recommends using fasting glucose alone as the main diagnostic test. Unfortunately, however, around one-third of individuals who have diabetes will have an abnormal result after an OGTT but fasting glucose below the diabetes threshold (Decode Study Group 1999). In other words, using fasting glucose alone misses about one-third of individuals with diabetes. Similarly, with fasting glucose, it is impossible to identify those who fall into the category of intermediate hyperglycaemia based on the post glucose challenge result (impaired glucose tolerance (IGT)), and as is discussed later much of the evidence on preventing type 2 diabetes is in individuals with IGT.

Table 9.6.1 WHO criteria for the diagnosis of diabetes and intermediate hyperglycaemia

Diabetes	
Fasting plasma glucose 2-hour plasma glucose*	≥7 mmol/l (126 mg/dl) or ≥11.1 mmol/l (200 mg/dl)
Impaired glucose tolerance (IGT)	
Fasting plasma glucose 2-hour plasma glucose*	<7 mmol/l (126 mg/dl) and ≥7.8 and <11.1 mmol/l (140 mg/dl and 200 mg/dl)
Impaired fasting glucose (IFG)	
Fasting plasma glucose 2-hour plasma glucose*	6.1–6.9 mmol/l (110–125 mg/dl) and (if measured) <7.8 mmol/l (140 mg/dl)

* Venous plasma glucose 2 hours after ingestion of 75 g oral glucose load (OGTT). If 2-hour plasma glucose is not measured, status is uncertain as diabetes or IGT cannot be excluded.

NB: The WHO criteria for gestational diabetes are diabetes (as defined above) or IGT.

Source: World Health Organization (2006).

There is also good evidence that the risk of cardiovascular disease associated with raised blood glucose is more strongly related to blood glucose after a glucose load than to fasting glucose (Decode Study Group 2001). It is for all these reasons that WHO continues to recommend using an OGTT as the main diagnostic test.

The thresholds for diabetes (Table 9.6.1) are based largely on epidemiological evidence that demonstrates an association between the diagnostic blood glucose levels and the presence of the typical small blood vessel complications of diabetes (e.g. diabetic retinopathy) (World Health Organization 2006). Because there is error in the measurement of blood glucose, and natural biological variation in its levels, the diagnosis of diabetes in someone without symptoms (such as polyuria and polydipsia) should only be made on the basis of two tests on separate occasions. In the presence of symptoms, the diagnosis of diabetes may be based on a casual (non-fasting, non OGTT) blood glucose level. It is worth noting that while the diagnostic cut points for diabetes are of necessity precisely defined (i.e. to the nearest tenth of a mmol per litre of glucose) different studies suggest somewhat different cut points often differing by at least one mmol per litre (Tapp *et al.* 2006).

The rationale for the cut points defining intermediate hyperglycaemia is less clear than that for those defining diabetes. Both fasting and 2 hours post challenge glucose are continuously related to the future risk of diabetes and cardiovascular disease—there is no evidence for thresholds and there is a strong argument for using the actual glucose value as part of a risk score for future diabetes or cardiovascular disease (Unwin *et al.* 2002; World Health Organization 2006). However, at present, this is not the case. The cut point for IGT is based on analyses published in the early 1980s on data from the Pima Indians on the risk of incident diabetes (Bennett *et al.* 1982). Impaired fasting glucose (IFG) was introduced in 1997 by the ADA (The Expert Committee on the Diagnosis and Classification of Diabetes Mellitus 1997), followed by WHO in 1999 (World Health Organization 1999). The cut point for IFG proposed in 1997, and still used by WHO, was based on physiological data of the level above which first phase insulin secretion is lost in response to intravenous glucose (The Expert Committee on the Diagnosis and Classification of Diabetes Mellitus 1997). However, in 2003, ADA recommended a lowering of the cut point for IFG, based partly on wishing to make the prevalence of IFG more similar to IGT and partly to improve the sensitivity of IFG as a predictor of future diabetes (American Diabetes Association 2004). WHO reviewed the classification of intermediate hyperglycaemia in 2006 and decided that the evidence was not strong enough to follow the ADA and lower the IFG cut point (World Health Organization 2006).

Incidence, prevalence, and trends

Both the WHO and the International Diabetes Federation (IDF) produce global estimates of the number of people with diabetes and how their numbers are expected to increase in the future (Wild *et al.* 2004; International Diabetes Federation 2006). These estimates are based on extrapolation from studies in which blood glucose was tested and thus include people with diagnosed and undiagnosed diabetes. This is important because in many populations more than half the people with diabetes (Harris 1993), sometimes as many as 80 or 90 per cent (Aspray *et al.* 2000), have not been diagnosed. The age specific prevalences of diabetes from these epidemiological studies are applied to United Nations population figures and projections in order to give national, regional, and global estimates. The methodologies used by WHO and IDF are essentially the same, although relatively minor differences do exist in the criteria used to select the prevalence studies that are the basis of the estimates, and this leads to small differences in the estimated number of people with diabetes.

The most recent estimates are those of IDF, who estimate that in 2007 there were 246 million people globally with diabetes, 3.7 per cent of total global population, and that 5.9 per cent of the global adult population (age range 20–79 years) has diabetes. Figure 9.6.2 shows the prevalence of diabetes in adults across the world. The prevalence of diabetes rises steeply with age (see Fig. 9.6.3). Most people with diabetes, between 85 and 95 per cent depending on the population, have type 2 diabetes. Some studies have described differences in prevalence between men and women. For example, a pooled analysis of 13 European cohorts reported a higher prevalence in men than women in the age range 40–59, but higher in women above the age of 70 (The Decode Study Group 2003). However, such sex differences are not consistent across populations. For example, in Fig. 9.6.3, based on over 40 studies worldwide (Wild *et al.* 2004), the prevalence is similar in men and women across the age groups up to the age of 70. Above 70 the prevalence is marginally (1–2 per cent) higher in women.

IDF estimates that by 2025 the number of people with diabetes will have increased to 380 million. This estimate is based on demographic trends (increasing population size, and an increasing elderly population), and increasing urbanization. The projected increase does not specifically include trends in risk factor levels, such as obesity for type 2 diabetes, nor does it include the fact that people with diabetes may survive longer, at least in developed parts of the world, than in the past. Trends in risk factors will be partly accounted for by including trends in urbanization, but it is clear that obesity is increasing within urban centres the world over (Popkin 2002; Popkin & Gordon-Larsen 2004). Thus, the current global projections for the number of people with diabetes are likely to be conservative. Globally, most of the increase in the number of people with diabetes will occur in middle-aged adults in developing countries, illustrated in Fig. 9.6.4 using data available from the WHO.

At the present time, it is estimated that between 70 and 80 per cent of people with diabetes live in low- and middle-income (developing) countries. This proportion will increase as a result of population growth in developing countries, ageing of their populations, and increasing exposure to risk factors for type 2 diabetes associated with mechanization and urbanization (Unwin 2007). Diabetes, particularly type 2 diabetes, is often thought of as being a disease of affluence, and thus more prevalent in richer countries. This, however, is a misleading characterization, as Fig. 9.6.2 shows. Many middle- and even low-income countries have a prevalence that is similar or higher than some of the world's richest nations.

Differences in prevalence between different population groups

There are large differences in the prevalence of type 2 diabetes between different population groups. For example, in developing countries, the prevalence tends to be several fold higher in urban compared to rural areas (Wild *et al.* 2004). In most developed countries the prevalence is inversely related to socioeconomic position, with the highest prevalence in those of lowest socioeconomic

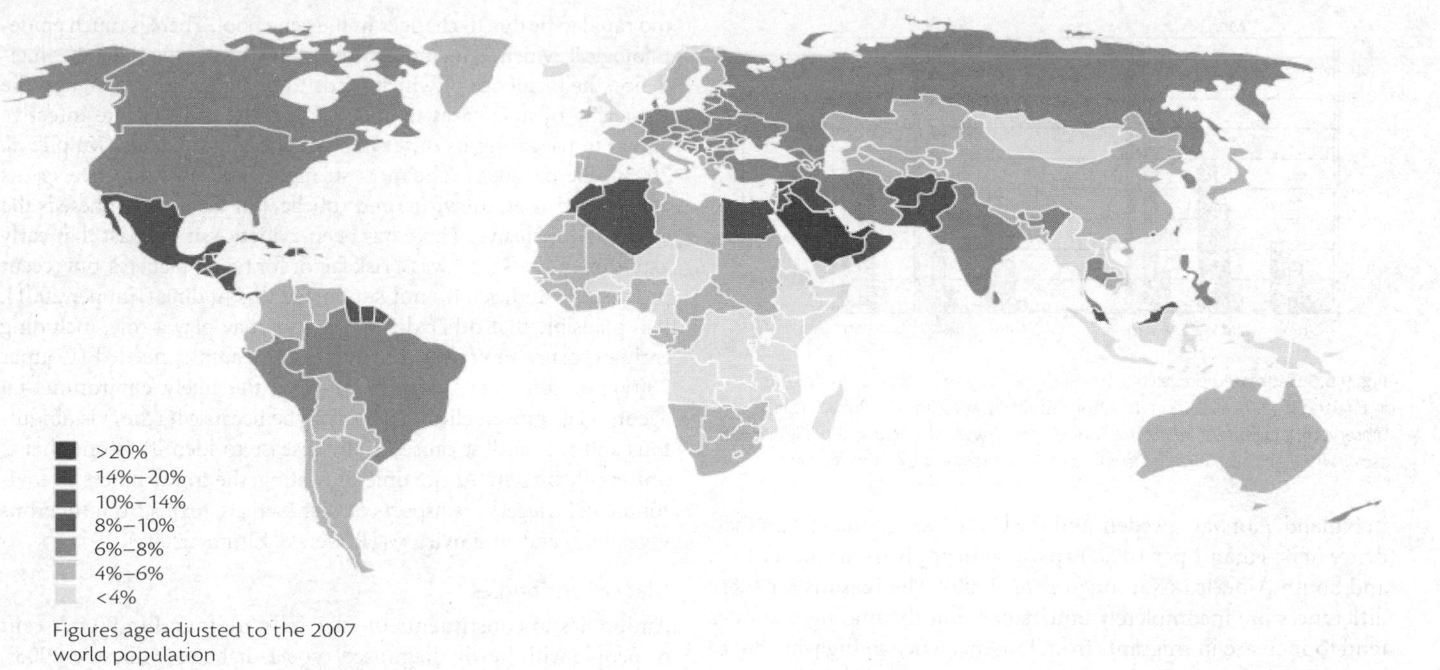

Fig. 9.6.2 The global prevalence (%) of diabetes in adults (20 in 79 years) in 2007. *Source: Diabetes Atlas*, third edition © International Diabetes Federation (2007).

position (Larranaga *et al.* 2005; Whitford *et al.* 2003; Evans *et al.* 2000; Connolly *et al.* 2000; Kumari *et al.* 2004). In some developing countries, there is evidence that diabetes prevalence is positively related to socioeconomic status, with the more affluent sections of society having the higher prevalence (Xu *et al.* 2006; Abu Sayeed *et al.* 1997; Herman *et al.* 1995). It is expected that with further economic development the socioeconomic patterning of type 2 diabetes will be similar in all countries, with the poorest groups having the highest prevalence. There is evidence from several middle-income countries that obesity, the strongest risk factor for type 2 diabetes, is now becoming more common in the less well off (Popkin 2004).

Finally, there are marked differences in diabetes prevalence between some ethnic groups living within the same regions and countries. For example, in England, most studies have found that the prevalence in people of South Asian and African Caribbean origin is 2–4-fold higher than in people of European origin living in the same area (Oldroyd *et al.* 2005) (see Fig. 9.6.5). In North America, African and Hispanic Americans (Kenny *et al.* 1995) have higher levels of type 2 diabetes than white Americans, with some of the highest rates of all in the indigenous peoples of North America (Gohdes 1995).

Incidence of type 1 diabetes

Unlike type 2 diabetes, in which the incidence is highest in adults and rises with age, the incidence of type 1 diabetes is highest in children, and in most populations peaks between the ages of 5–14 years (International Diabetes Federation 2006; Karvonen *et al.* 2000). Internationally there are huge differences, up to 300-fold, in the incidence of type 1 diabetes. For example, an incidence of greater than 20 per 100 000 per year (in those aged 14 years or less) is found

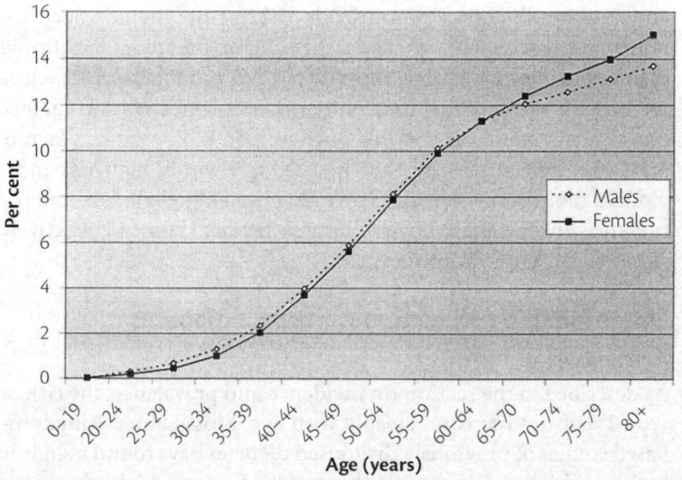

Fig. 9.6.3 The global prevalence of diabetes by age and sex in the year 2000. *Source*: Wild et al. (2004).

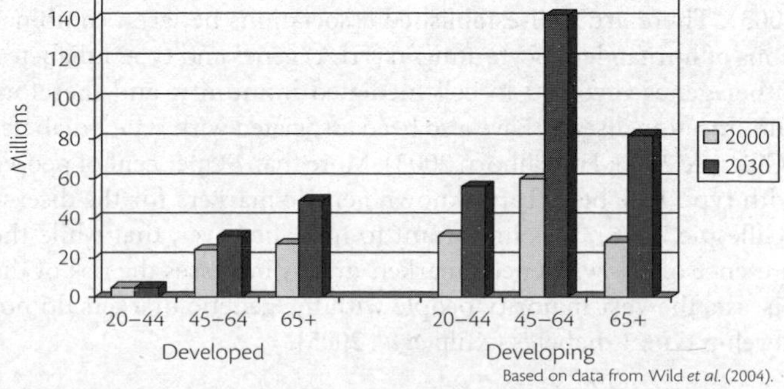

Fig. 9.6.4 Estimated number of adults by broad age group with diabetes in developed and developing countries.

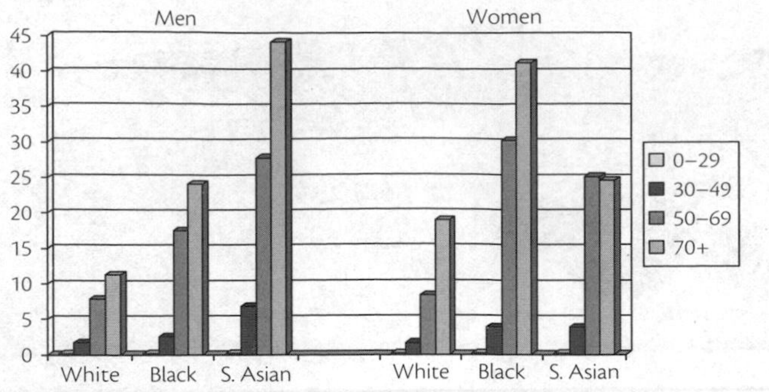

Fig. 9.6.5 Estimated prevalence (%) of diabetes by age, sex and ethnic group in England in 2007. Based on data from Yorkshire and Humber Public Health Observatory Diabetes Prevalence Model (http://www.yhpho.org.uk/PBS_diabetes.aspx), with special thanks to David Merrick for providing age-specific data.

in Finland, Norway, Sweden, and the United Kingdom, and an incidence of less than 1 per 100,000 per year in populations from China and South America (Karvonen *et al.* 2000). The reasons for these differences are incompletely understood, but the finding that rates tend to increase in migrants from low-incidence to high-incidence areas (Knip *et al.* 2005) suggests that environmental factors account for at least some of the difference. There is also evidence from several parts of the world, including the United Kingdom, that the incidence of type 1 diabetes is increasing (Onkamo *et al.* 1999), particularly in younger children, again suggesting the influence of environmental factors.

Risk factors

There are strong genetic and environmental (in its broadest sense) influences on the risk of both type 1 and type 2 diabetes, and it is the interaction between the two that results in the onset of the disease. The specific environmental influences on the risk of type 2 diabetes are relatively well understood (essentially certain behaviours and their physiological consequences), whereas those for type 1 diabetes remain frustratingly elusive.

Risk factors for type 1 diabetes

Familial and genetic

The lifetime risk of type 1 diabetes is roughly 6 per cent if a first degree relative has the condition, such as a sibling, compared to roughly 0.4 per cent (depending on the population) if a first degree relative is not affected. If a monozygotic twin has type 1 diabetes, the lifetime risk in the other twin is around 50 per cent (Hirschhorn 2003). There are well-established associations between combinations of human leukocyte antigen (HLA) genes and type 1 diabetes. Other genes involved in cell-mediated immunity, and therefore autoimmune disease, have also been associated with type 1 diabetes (Gillespie 2006; Hirschhorn 2003). More than 90 per cent of people with type 1 diabetes carry known genetic markers for the disease (Gillespie 2006). It is important to note, however, that while the presence of known genetic markers greatly increases the risk of the disease, the vast majority people with the genetic markers do not develop type 1 diabetes (Knip *et al.* 2005).

Environmental factors

The importance of environmental factors is indicated by the changing incidence of type 1 diabetes (described above) at a rate that is far too rapid to be due to changes in the gene pool. There is much epidemiological evidence, including the seasonality of type 1 diabetes incidence, the incidence of which tends to be higher in winter, and the clustering of new cases in space and time, to implicate infective agents in triggering its onset in susceptible individuals (Knip *et al.* 2005; Gillespie 2006). The most strongly implicated infective agents are enteroviruses, rotavirus, and rubella, but for none of these is the evidence conclusive. There has been evidence in the past that early exposure to cow's milk was a risk factor for type 1 diabetes, but recent prospective studies have not supported this finding (Couper 2001). It is plausible that other dietary factors may play a role, including early exposure to cereals, but further research is needed (Couper 2001). In summary, identification of the likely environmental agent(s) has proved elusive. This may be because it (they) is ubiquitous and the hardest cause of any disease to identify is one that is universally present. At the time of writing, the frontrunners as environmental triggers are aspects of diet (cereals, toxins from tuberous vegetables) and enteroviruses (Rewers & Zimmet 2004).

Islet cell antibodies

Antibodies to constituents of islet cells are found in 90 per cent of people with newly diagnosed type 1 diabetes (Gillespie 2006). They include islet-cell antibodies (ICA), anti-GAD (glutamic acid decarboxylase), anti-insulin, and so called IA2 (anti-tyrosine-phosphatase-like protein **IA2**). In those without diabetes, the presence of two or more antibodies carries a high risk of progression to overt diabetes, whereas the presence of a single antibody appears to carry little additional risk (Kukko *et al.* 2005).

Identifying individuals at high risk of type 1 diabetes

A combination of family history, genotyping, and measurement of islet cell antibodies can identify a group of individuals in whom around half will develop type 1 diabetes over five years (Diabetes Prevention Trial—Type 1 Diabetes Study Group 2002). This, however, is a costly and labour intensive exercise and currently only worthwhile as a means of identifying high risk individuals for trials of preventive measures, and none of the measures for prevention so far tested have been found to work.

Risk factors for type 2 diabetes

It is useful to divide risk factors for type 2 diabetes into unmodifiable and modifiable. Unmodifiable risk factors include age, sex, family history, genetic markers, history of previous gestational diabetes, and ethnicity. The most important modifiable risk factors are obesity and physical inactivity; others include certain dietary constituents, smoking, and low birth weight. Biological risk factors are also important as they can be used to identify high-risk individuals. Biological risk factors include raised blood glucose and the presence of several cardiovascular risk factors (known collectively as 'the metabolic syndrome').

Unmodifiable risk factors for type 2 diabetes

Age and sex

As described in the section on incidence and prevalence, the risk of type 2 diabetes increases steeply with age. Most United Kingdom-based studies of previously diagnosed diabetes have found a slightly higher prevalence in men, whereas studies in which glucose is measured either find no sex difference or a slightly higher prevalence in women.

Familial and genetic

The strong familial clustering of type 2 diabetes, suggestive of important genetic influences, has been known for many years (Zimmet 1992). For example, the presence of type 2 diabetes in a parent or sibling tends to double the risk type 2 diabetes. Until recently, however, identifying genetic markers for type 2 diabetes has proved difficult, and the markers identified could account for only a few percent of the genetic risk (Permutt *et al.* 2005; Almind *et al.* 2001). The use of genome-wide approaches is likely to change this picture rapidly. Recently, for example, a genome-wide approach identified four genetic loci that accounted for 70 per cent of the genetic risk of type 2 diabetes in the populations studied (Sladek *et al.* 2007).

Previous gestational diabetes

Women with gestational diabetes tend to be older, more overweight, have a family history of diabetes, and be from an ethnic group with high prevalence of diabetes (Buchanan & Xiang 2005). Following delivery, glucose levels return to normal in around 90 per cent of women, but over the next 10 years, as many as 70 per cent go on to develop diabetes (Buchanan & Xiang 2005; Kim *et al.* 2002).

Ethnicity

As described previously, there are marked differences in the prevalence of type 2 diabetes by ethnic group. It is far from clear what underlies these differences, how much is related to differences in environment (including behaviours), and how much to differences in genetic susceptibility (Oldroyd *et al.* 2005).

Modifiable risk factors for type 2 diabetes

Obesity, physical inactivity, and aspects of diet

The relationship between overweight and obesity and the risk of type 2 diabetes is continuous, very strong, and is apparent below conventional cut points for overweight (Vazquez *et al.* 2007; Hartemink *et al.* 2006). There is a large body of evidence suggesting that it is the distribution of body fat that is particularly important in determining the risk of type 2 diabetes (and indeed cardiovascular disease), with the greatest risk associated with abdominal obesity (Despres 2001).

There is good evidence that physical activity lowers the risk of type 2 diabetes independently of obesity level. Regular moderate or vigorous activity has been associated with a 30–50 per cent reduction in the risk (Jeon *et al.* 2007) of developing type 2 diabetes. Physical activity is hard to measure accurately, particularly if assessed by questionnaire, as it is in most studies, and it is possible that its protective effect is even greater.

There is also evidence that the composition of the diet, over and above its calorific value, influences the risk of type 2 diabetes. Increased risk has been associated with diets low in fibre and high in saturated fat (Parillo & Riccardi 2004), and conversely intervention studies support the hypothesis that high-fibre–low-saturated-fat diets can help to prevent diabetes (Lindstrom *et al.* 2006b). High-glycaemic index foods have also been associated with an increased risk of type 2 diabetes (Hodge *et al.* 2004). There is evidence that moderate alcohol intake (Wannamethee *et al.* 2003; Parillo & Riccardi 2004) and coffee consumption (Salazar-Martinez *et al.* 2004; Smith *et al.* 2006) both reduce the risk of type 2 diabetes.

Smoking

Several studies have found that smoking increases the risk of type 2 diabetes by 50 per cent or more (Rimm *et al.* 1995; Sargeant *et al.* 2001; Carlsson *et al.* 2004; Foy *et al.* 2005).

Birth weight and intrauterine environment

Several studies have found an inverse association between birth weight and the risk of type 2 diabetes in adulthood (Phillips *et al.* 2006). It has been hypothesized that lower birth weight represents poorer foetal nutrition and that this has a programming effect on aspects of physiology and metabolism. However, there is also evidence for an alternative hypothesis, which is that low birth weight is associated with an increased genetic susceptibility to insulin resistance and type 2 diabetes (Frayling & Hattersley 2001; Hattersley & Tooke 1999). While debate continues on the nature of the relationship, it seems clear that birth weight, and other markers of early life experience, are substantially less important than adult behavioural risk factors (Parker *et al.* 2003; Boyko 2000).

Biological risk factors

There is a continuous positive relationship between blood glucose level (both fasting and post glucose challenge) and the risk of developing type 2 diabetes—the higher the level, the greater the risk (Unwin *et al.* 2002). As described above, WHO currently defines two non-diabetic risk categories based on glucose level (see Table 9.6.1): IFG and IGT. The potential benefits of identifying and intervening in people with IGT and IFG are discussed in the section on prevention.

There is a strong tendency for several metabolic and cardiovascular risk factors to cluster within the same individuals. This clustering is strongly associated with abdominal obesity and insulin resistance (Unwin 2006), and has been labelled 'the metabolic syndrome' (Alberti *et al.* 2005). Core features of the metabolic syndrome include abdominal obesity; raised blood glucose, blood pressure, and triglycerides; and low HDL cholesterol. The presence of the metabolic syndrome in those without diabetes strongly predicts its development (Laaksonen *et al.* 2002).

Risk scores

Several research groups have derived 'risk scores' based on some of the risk factors described above in order to help predict who is at high risk of developing type 2 diabetes (Glumer *et al.* 2004; Lindstrom & Tuomilehto 2003; Griffin *et al.* 2000).

Health consequences

Mortality and life expectancy

People with diabetes have a substantially higher mortality than people without diabetes, and this is found across all age groups. The relative risk of death is 4–6-fold higher at ages 20–29 years, falls with age but is still 40–80 per cent higher at ages 70–79 years (Roglic *et al.* 2005). Most, but not all, studies have found that the relative risk of death is higher in women (i.e. compared to women without diabetes) than in men (i.e. compared to men without diabetes). It should be noted that the number of good longitudinal studies able to properly compare mortality rates in people with and without diabetes are relatively small and largely limited to wealthier countries. The relative mortality in poorer countries, where diabetes prevalence is increasing rapidly (Wild *et al.* 2004) but where health care coverage is often wholly inadequate, may be even greater.

The higher mortality rates in people with diabetes across all age groups lead to substantial reductions in life expectancy. For example, in a North of England population, it was estimated that type 2 diabetes at age 40 results in 8 years lost life expectancy in both men and women, and a loss of 4 years at age 60 (Roper *et al.* 2001).

Recent data on loss of life expectancy in people with type 1 diabetes are hard to find. Widely quoted figures are from a critical review published in 1984 (Panzram 1984) which found that loss of life expectancy was at least 15 years, whatever the age of diagnosis, with some evidence that it may be over 25 years in those diagnosed under the age of 15. However, at least in developed countries, the picture may have improved since then, with some evidence that the difference in mortality between people with type 1 diabetes and those without diabetes, while still substantial, has decreased (Nishimura *et al.* 2001).

The proportion of deaths attributable to diabetes is not known with accuracy because diabetes is frequently not recorded on death certificates. Estimates of the number of deaths due to diabetes have been made using the relative risk of death in people with diabetes compared to those without, the known prevalence of diabetes and the underlying population mortality. These suggest that in most parts of the world diabetes is responsible for 5–10 per cent of all deaths in adults (Roglic *et al.* 2005). In the United Kingdom, it is estimated that diabetes accounted for 7.7 per cent of all adult deaths in 2007.

Cardiovascular disease

People with diabetes are at greatly increased risk of diseases of the large arteries, including the coronary and cerebral arteries and those supplying the lower limbs. The risk of cardiovascular disease in people with diabetes is 2–4-fold higher than in people without diabetes (Folsom *et al.* 1997, 1999; Stamler *et al.* 1993), and this fact accounts for much of the increased mortality associated with diabetes (Roglic *et al.* 2005). In most populations, well over 50 per cent of deaths in people with diabetes are from cardiovascular disease. For example, in people with diabetes in Teesside, England, 59 per cent of deaths in men and 74 per cent in women were due to cardiovascular disease (Roper *et al.* 2002).

Diabetic eye disease

In developed countries, diabetes is the leading cause of blindness in people aged over 25 years (Klein & Klein 1995). Twenty years after diagnosis, virtually 100 per cent of people with type 1 diabetes have diabetic retinopathy (Klein 1997; Roy *et al.* 2004), and when blood pressure and blood glucose control are poor, it is estimated that 75 per cent will develop proliferative retinopathy, the most severe form, during their lifetime. In type 2 diabetes, between 40 and 60 per cent are expected to develop retinopathy during their lifetime, with around 10 per cent developing proliferative retinopathy (Klein 1997; Eye Diseases Prevalence Research Group *et al.* 2004).

Diabetes also increases the risk of cataracts and open-angle glaucoma (Klein & Klein 1995).

Diabetic renal disease

Diabetes is the single leading cause of renal failure in developed countries, responsible for 40–50 per cent of all new patients requiring dialysis in North America, and 15–33 per cent in Europe and Australia (Atkins 2005). In cross-sectional surveys in Europe, around 1 in 10 people with type 1 diabetes, and 1 in 7 with type 2 diabetes, have evidence of overt nephropathy (International Diabetes Federation 2006). Approximately 30 per cent of people with diabetes with overt nephropathy will progress to end-stage renal failure (Atkins 2005). Large increases in the number of new cases of end-stage renal failure associated with diabetes have been documented in developed countries such as Australia. These increases largely reflect the increasing prevalence of type 2 diabetes. Figure 9.6.6 shows the year-on-year increase over the past 20 years in the number of people with diabetes and end-stage renal disease in Australia, with virtually all the increase being associated with type 2 diabetes, and not type 1.

Neuropathy and diabetic foot problems

The nerve damage associated with diabetes can affect both peripheral and autonomic nerves and thus affect digestion, urination, heart and blood pressure responses, erectile function, and peripheral sensation and musculature (Little *et al.* 2007). Diabetic foot problems are a result of peripheral neuropathy, often, but not always, compounded by peripheral vascular disease (Edmonds *et al.* 1996). In cross-sectional studies, peripheral neuropathy is found in 1 in 5 to more than a third of people with diabetes (International Diabetes Federation 2006). During their life time, roughly 15 per cent of people with diabetes develop a foot ulcer and of these 5–15 per cent go on to amputation (Edmonds *et al.* 1996). In developed countries, diabetes is the single-most important cause of non-traumatic lower limb amputation, accounting for 40–60 per cent of all

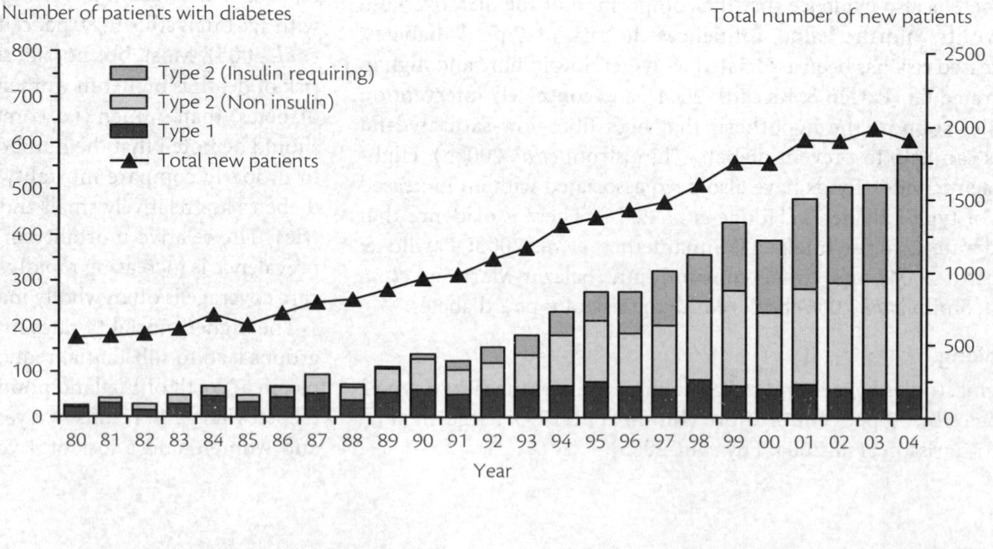

Fig. 9.6.6 Incidence of diabetes-related end-stage renal failure: Australia 1980–2004.
Source: Atkins (2005).

amputations (Global Lower Extremity Amputation Study Group 2000), and people with diabetes have a 15-fold-risk of amputation compared to people without diabetes (Edmonds *et al.* 1996).

Erectile dysfunction

Diabetes increases the risk of erectile dysfunction in men. A recent study (Bacon *et al.* 2002) found that type 1 diabetes increased the risk threefold, and type 2 diabetes increased the risk by a third. The same study found that the prevalence of erectile dysfunction in men with diabetes was around 50 per cent.

Depression

Depression is more common in people with diabetes than in people without. A recent study reported diagnosed depression in 18 per cent of people with type 2 diabetes compared to 11 per cent in age and sex matched controls (Nichols & Brown 2003). Depression in people with diabetes is associated with more complications and poorer self care (Lin *et al.* 2004).

Economic impact of diabetes

Although there is a lack of robust studies into the economic impact of diabetes, it is clear that the cost of diabetes to individuals and their carers, to health services, and to national economies is substantial. On average, a person with diabetes uses more health care resources than a person without diabetes—around 1.5–3 times more, depending on age (International Diabetes Federation 2006). This fact, along with knowledge of the prevalence of diabetes and the overall health care budget, has been used to derive estimates of the average health care expenditure per person with diabetes and the overall cost to the health care system (Williams 2005; International Diabetes Federation 2006). For example, it has been estimated that, in 2007, the cost of diabetes to the health care system was between 4.4 and 8.8 billion international dollars (ID) in the United Kingdom; 6.1–10.9 billion in India; 14.8–26.9 billion in China; and 119.3–213.8 billion in the United States (International Diabetes Federation 2006). The costs of diabetes care increase dramatically with the presence of complications, being 2–3-fold higher with the presence of either micro- or macro-vascular complications, and 5–6-fold higher with the presence of both micro- and macro-vascular complications than in people with diabetes without complications (Williams 2005).

Diabetes, as with any other chronic illness, may limit employment and impact upon the income of people with it and the people caring for them. A study in the United Kingdom found that, in people with type 2 diabetes aged less than 65 years, 7 per cent lost income because of diabetes. They lost on average £13 800 per year (at 1998 values) and their carers lost £11 000 per year (Holmes *et al.* 2003). A recent study, from the Economist Intelligence Unit, estimated the total economic impact of diabetes, both in terms of costs to the health care system and in terms of lost productivity. The findings suggested that, in 2007, the United Kingdom lost 0.4 per cent of its total gross domestic product to diabetes, the United States 1.2 per cent, and India 2.1 per cent (Economist Intelligence Unit 2007).

Prevention of diabetes and its complications

Prevention of type 1 diabetes

Just as our knowledge of the environmental triggers for type 1 diabetes remains elusive, so does our knowledge of how to prevent it in humans. Interventions that have been evaluated in individuals at high risk of diabetes have included nicotinamide therapy and low-dose insulin, but neither was effective. Other options currently being evaluated include the use of immunosuppressant therapy in individuals at high risk (Gillespie 2006). In those with type 1 diabetes, pancreatic transplantation is of proven benefit, but comes with the drawbacks common to all organ transplantation. At the time of writing, beta cell regeneration is a major area of investigation that holds promise (Gillespie 2006).

Prevention of type 2 diabetes

There is excellent evidence that type 2 diabetes can be prevented, or at least its onset delayed, in individuals at high risk of type 2 diabetes. Interventions aimed at modifying behaviours and pharmacological interventions have both been shown to be effective, and at best to reduce the incidence of type 2 diabetes by 50–60 per cent. The findings of some of the major trials are summarized in Table 9.6.2. Overall, interventions promoting behavioural change were as effective as pharmacological interventions, a conclusion supported by a recent meta-analysis (Gillies *et al.* 2007). Aspects of behavioural change that were promoted included weight loss (in those overweight and obese), increased physical activity, and a low total and saturated fat and high-fibre diet. Follow-up from the Finnish Diabetes Prevention Study suggests, not surprisingly, that the more of the behavioural goals that were achieved, the lower the long-term risk of type 2 diabetes (Lindstrom *et al.* 2006a).

Targeting individuals at high risk of diabetes, based on impaired glucose tolerance or impaired fasting glucose, is unlikely to have a large (e.g. 50 per cent or greater) impact on the overall population incidence of type 2 diabetes. This is because roughly 40–60 per cent of new cases of type 2 diabetes arise in people who had normal glucose tolerance 3–5 years earlier (Unwin *et al.* 2002). Other approaches to identifying and targeting individuals at high risk may improve this, but there seems little doubt that it is only through population-based measures aimed at reducing overweight and obesity and increasing physical activity that a large impact on the incidence of type 2 diabetes will be achieved. The potential impact of population-wide measures was illustrated in an analysis from EPIC-Norfolk, a UK cohort of 24 155 subjects. It assessed the association between the achievement of five 'diabetes healthy behaviour prevention goals' (BMI < 25 kg/m2), fat intake < 30 per cent of energy intake, saturated fat intake < 10 per cent of energy intake, fibre intake ≥ 15 g/1000 kcal, physical activity > 4 hours/week) and the risk of developing diabetes at follow-up (mean 4.6 years). Diabetes incidence was inversely related to the number of goals achieved. None of the participants who met all five of the goals developed diabetes, whereas diabetes incidence was highest in those who did not meet any goals. If the entire population were able to meet one more goal, the total incidence of diabetes would be predicted to fall by 20 per cent (Simmons *et al.* 2006).

As reviewed elsewhere in this Textbook, achieving population-wide changes to reduce the incidence of diabetes and related chronic non-communicable diseases presents major challenges. Despite increasing awareness in many parts of the world amongst both policy makers and the general public of the importance of obesity as a risk factor for diabetes and other adverse health outcomes, there is not yet a single population-wide example where the trend towards increasing levels of obesity has been reversed. This includes high-income countries in which there is a multi-billion-dollar 'diet industry' (Arterburn 2006) ostensibly aiming to help people achieve and

Table 9.6.2 Summary of some of the major prevention trials in people at high risk of type 2 diabetes

Study/authors	Date	Setting	Population	Intervention	Trial groups	Relative risk reduction
Da Qing IGT and Diabetes Study (Pan *et al.* 1997)	1997	China	N=577 Chinese men and women aged over 25 years with IGT	Lifestyle	- Control group - Diet only - Exercise only - Diet and exercise	31% (diet) 46% (exercise) 42% (diet and exercise)
Finnish Diabetes Prevention Study (DPS) (Tuomilehto *et al.* 2001)	2001	Finland	N=552 overweight Finnish men and women aged 40–65 years with IGT	Lifestyle	- Control group - Lifestyle	58% (lifestyle)
Diabetes Prevention Program (DPP) (Knowler *et al.* 2002)	2002	United States	N=3234 overweight American men and women including 45% of African, Hispanic, Asian or Native American descent aged over 25 years with IGT	Lifestyle/ pharmaceutical	- Control group - Metformin (850 mg twice daily) - Lifestyle	31% (metformin) 58% (lifestyle)
STOP-NIDDM Trial (Chiasson *et al.* 2002)	2002	Multi-centre	N=1368 overweight Europid men and women aged 40-70 years with IGT	Pharmaceutical	- Control group - Acarbose (100 mg three times daily)	25%
Troglitazone in Prevention of Diabetes (TRIPOD) (Buchanan *et al.* 2001)	2002	United States	N=266 Hispanic-American women aged ≥18 years with previous gestational diabetes in last 4 years	Pharmaceutical	- Control group - Troglitazone (400 mg daily)	56%
XENical in the Prevention of Diabetes in Obese Subjects (XENDOS) study (Torgerson *et al.* 2004)	2004	Sweden	N=3305 obese Swedish men and women aged 40–60 years with normal glucose tolerance (79%) or IGT (21%)	Pharmaceutical	- Control group (placebo and lifestyle) - Lifestyle and orlistat (120 mg three times daily)	45% (lifestyle and orlistat) in those with IGT
The Indian Diabetes Prevention Program (IDPP-1) (Ramachandran *et al.* 2006)	2006	India	N=531 Asian Indian men and women aged 35–55 years with IGT	Lifestyle/ pharmaceutical	- Control - Lifestyle - Metformin - Metformin and lifestyle	29% (lifestyle) 26% (metformin) 28% (metformin and lifestyle)
Dream trail investigators (DREAM Trial Investigators *et al.* 2006)	2006	Multi-centre	N=5269 men and women, >30 years, with IFG/IGT	Pharmaceutical	Control group Rosiglitazone 8 mg	60% reduction in diabetes incidence or death

(Thanks to Dr R. Simmonds who compiled this table.)

maintain weight loss. This highlights the considerable challenges in achieving population-wide changes in diet and physical activity, and thus reductions in obesity, and it is clear that it will require much more than raising awareness and providing information. This was put succinctly in the 1997 WHO report on obesity (World Health Organization 1997), when it stated that, 'what has been demonstrated . . . is that approaches that are firmly based on the principle of personal education and behaviour change are unlikely to succeed in an environment in which there are plentiful inducements to engage in opposing behaviours'. It went on to suggest that, 'It would therefore seem appropriate to devote resources to programmes which focus on reducing the exposure of the population to obesity promoting agents by addressing the environmental factors such as transportation, urban design, advertising and food pricing'.

The need to change the 'obesogenic environment' (Egger & Swinburn 1997) if the obesity epidemic is to be reversed is now widely accepted. It is the basis for the World Health Organization's Global Strategy on Diet, Physical Activity and Health, which was mandated by the World Health Assembly in 2002 and then accepted in 2004 (World Health Organization 2004). There are some examples to draw on where policy measures have led to, or at least been associated with, improvements in diet and physical activity (Willett *et al.* 2006) although not with declines in obesity. They include community based, multi-faceted approaches, such as undertaken in Finland (Puska *et al.* 1985) and Singapore (Cutter *et al.* 2001), both associated with declines in at least some aspects of CVD risk. Despite such examples, there remains in general a lack of hard evidence on what approaches are effective in achieving population-wide changes in diet and physical activity. In acknowledgement of

- **Advocacy**
  - Supporting national associations and non-governmental organizations
  - Promoting the economic case for prevention
- **Community support**
  - Providing education in schools regarding nutrition and physical activity
  - Promotion opportunities for physical activity through urban design (e.g. to encourage cycling and walking)
- **Fiscal and legislative measures**
  - Examining food pricing, labelling, and advertising
  - Enforcing environmental and infrastructure regulation, e.g. urban planning and transportation policy to enhance physical activity
- **Engagement of private sector**
  - Promoting health in the workplace
  - Ensuring healthy food policies in food industry
- **Media communication**
  - Improving level of knowledge and motivation of the population (press, TV, and radio)

Fig. 9.6.7 Recommendations from the International Diabetes Federation for population-wide measures for the prevention of type 2 diabetes.

this, one of the guiding principles of the WHO strategy on Diet, Physical Activity and Health is to seek stronger evidence for what types of policy change are effective in promoting healthier diets and increased levels of physical activity. The strategy aims to use this evidence to advocate for change, supporting countries to develop frameworks for action that are appropriate to their own circumstances. General guidance on a package of measures aimed at producing population-wide changes has been produced by both WHO (World Health Organization 2005) and the IDF (Fig. 9.6. 7) (Alberti *et al.* 2007).

Prevention of diabetes-related complications

There is excellent evidence that the increased morbidity and mortality in people with diabetes, compared to those without, can be significantly reduced (Venkat Narayan *et al.* 2006). This evidence includes approaches to reducing the incidence of complications and to limiting their progression and impact once they exist. A summary of the main interventions and estimates of their effectiveness for preventing diabetes related complications is provided in Table 9.6.3 (Venkat Narayan *et al.* 2006). Control of blood glucose, blood pressure, blood lipids, and the avoidance of smoking are core; with specific measures to reduce the incidence of sight-threatening retinopathy, morbidity and loss of the lower limbs, and progression to end stage renal disease.

A detailed discussion of how to achieve reductions in morbidity and mortality in people with diabetes and the contents of good diabetes care is beyond the scope of this chapter. There are many sources of guidance on this, including the National Service Framework on Diabetes for England (Roberts 2007), the Global Guideline for Type 2 diabetes from the International Diabetes Federation (International Diabetes Federation: Clinical Guidelines Taskforce 2005), and a forthcoming report from the WHO (World Health Organization, forthcoming). However, it is worth making the following points here. People with diabetes play the central role in managing their condition (as with most chronic conditions), and thus core to effective diabetes care is empowering people with diabetes with the knowledge and support they need to do this. Effective health care for diabetes, in common with many other chronic conditions (Epping-Jordan *et al.* 2004), requires a well-functioning health care system, with good communication between many

Table 9.6.3 Examples of treatment strategies and relative reductions in morbidity and mortality in people with diabetes

Strategy	Estimated benefit
Glycaemic control in people with HbA1c greater than 9 per cent	Reduction of 30 per cent in microvascular disease per 1 per cent drop in HbA1c
Glycaemic control in people with HbA1c greater than 8 per cent	Reduction of 30 per cent in microvascular disease per 1 per cent drop in HbA1c
Blood pressure control in people whose pressure is higher than 160/95 mmHg	Reduction of 35 per cent in macrovascular and microvascular disease per 10 mmHg drop in blood pressure
Cholesterol control in people with total cholesterol > 5.2 mmol l^{-1}	Reduction of 25–55 per cent in coronary heart diseases events; 43 per cent fall in death rate
Annual screening for microalbuminuria	Reduction of 50 per cent in nephropathy using ACE inhibitors for identified cases
Annual eye examinations	Reduction of 60 to 70 per cent in serious vision loss
Foot care in people with high risk of ulcers	Reduction of 50 to 60 per cent in serious foot disease
Aspirin use	Reduction of 28 per cent in myocardial infarctions, reduction of 18 per cent in cardiovascular disease
ACE inhibitor use in all people with diabetes	Reduction of 42 per cent in nephropathy; 22 per cent reduction in cardiovascular disease

Source: Based on Venkat Narayan *et al.* (2006).

different specialities and levels of care. Finally, it is an accurate generalization to state that diabetes is care is currently suboptimal the world over (Venkat Narayan *et al.* 2006), in both rich and poor countries. In rich countries, suboptimal care includes inadequate coverage of basic preventive measures, such as regular eye and foot examinations, as well as room for much better control of glucose, blood pressure, and lipids. In poor countries, inadequate care includes no care at all for a large proportion of people with diabetes, including, in many parts of the world, lack of, or intermittent access to, insulin leading to the death of those who require it for survival (Yudkin 2000). It is not hyperbole to state that diabetes presents one of the major public health challenges of the twenty-first century, one that has reached the attention of the United Nations in its call for coordinated global action (Unite for Diabetes 2006).

References

Abu Sayeed, M., ALI, L., Hussain, *et al.* (1997) Effect of socioeconomic risk factors on the difference in prevalence of diabetes between rural and urban populations in Bangladesh. *Diabetes Care*, **20**, 551–5.

Alberti, K.G.M.M., Zimmet, P., and Shaw, J. (2005) The metabolic syndrome: a new worldwide definition. *Lancet*, **366**, 1059–62.

Alberti, K.G.M.M., Zimmet, P., and Shaw, J. (2007) International Diabetes Federation: a consensus on Type 2 diabetes prevention. *Diabetic Medicine*, **24**, 451–63.

Almind, K., Doria, A., and CR., K. (2001) Putting the genes for type II diabetes on the map. *Nature Medicine*, **7**, 277–9.

American Diabetes Association (2004) Diagnosis and classification of diabetes mellitus. *Diabetes Care*, **27**, 5S–10S.

Arterburn, D. (2006) The BBC diet trials. *British Medical Journal*, **332**, 1284–5.

Aspray, T.J., Mugusi, F., Rashid, S., *et al.* & Essential Non-communicable Disease Health Intervention (2000) Rural and urban differences in diabetes prevalence in Tanzania: the role of obesity, physical inactivity and urban living. *Transactions of the Royal Society of Tropical Medicine & Hygiene*, **94**, 637–44.

Atkins, R.C. (2005) The epidemiology of chronic kidney disease. *Kidney International*, **67**, S14–8.

Bacon, C.G., Hu, F. B., Giovannucci, E., *et al.* (2002) Association of type and duration of diabetes with erectile dysfunction in a large cohort of men. *Diabetes Care*, **25**, 1458–63.

Bennett, P., Knowler, W., Pettitt, D., *et al.* (1982) Longitudinal studies of the development of diabetes in the Pima Indians. In *Advances in Diabetes Epidemiology* (ed. E. ESCHWEGE), Amsterdam, Netherlands, Elsevier Biomedical Press.

Berson, S.A. and Yalow, R.S. (1963) Antigens in insulin determinants of specificity of porcine insulin in man. *Science*, **139**, 844–5.

Bornstein, J. and Lawrence, R. D. (1951) Plasma insulin in human diabetes mellitus. *British Medical Journal*, **2**, 1541–4.

Boyko, E.J. (2000) Proportion of type 2 diabetes cases resulting from impaired fetal growth. *Diabetes Care*, **23**, 1260–4.

Buchanan, T., Xiang, A., Peters, R., *et al.*(2001) Protection from type 2 diabetes persists in the TRIPOD cohort eight months after stopping troglitazone. *Diabetes*, **50**, A81.

Buchanan, T.A. & Xiang, A.H. (2005) Gestational diabetes mellitus. *Journal of Clinical Investigation*, **115**, 485–91.

Carlsson, S., Midthjell, K., Grill, V., *et al.* (2004) Smoking is associated with an increased risk of type 2 diabetes but a decreased risk of autoimmune diabetes in adults: an 11-year follow-up of incidence of diabetes in the Nord-Trondelag study. *Diabetologia*, **47**, 1953–6.

Chiasson, J., Josse, R., Gomis, R., *et al.* (2002) Acarbose can prevent the progression of impaired glucose tolerance to type 2 diabetes mellitus: results of a randomised clinical trial, The STOP-NIDDM Trial. *Lancet*, **359**, 2072–7.

Connolly, V., Unwin, N., Sherriff, P., *et al.* (2000) Diabetes prevalence and socioeconomic status: a population based study showing increased prevalence of type 2 diabetes mellitus in deprived areas. *Journal of Epidemiology & Community Health*, **54**, 173–7.

Couper, J.J. (2001) Environmental triggers of type 1 diabetes. *Journal of Paediatrics & Child Health*, **37**, 218–220.

Cutter, J., Tan, B.Y. & Chew, S.K. (2001) Levels of cardiovascular disease risk factors in Singapore following a national intervention programme.[see comment]. *Bulletin of the World Health Organization*, **79**, 908–15.

Decode Study Group (1999) Is fasting glucose sufficient to define diabetes? Epidemiological data from 20 European studies. The DECODE-study group. European Diabetes Epidemiology Group. Diabetes Epidemiology: Collaborative analysis of Diagnostic Criteria in Europe. *Diabetologia*, **42**, 647–654.

Decode Study Group (2001) Glucose tolerance and cardiovascular mortality: comparison of fasting and 2-hour diagnostic criteria. *Archives of Internal Medicine*, **161**, 397–405.

Despres, J.P. (2001) Health consequences of visceral obesity. *Annals of Medicine*, **33**, 534–541.

Diabetes Prevention Trial—type 1 Diabetes Study Group (2002) Effects of insulin in relatives of patients with type 1 diabetes mellitus. *New England Journal of Medicine*, **346**, 1685–91.

Dream Trial Investigators, Gerstein, H.C., Yusuf, S., *et al.* (2006) Effect of rosiglitazone on the frequency of diabetes in patients with impaired glucose tolerance or impaired fasting glucose: a randomised controlled trial. *Lancet*, **368**, 1096–105.

Economist Intelligence Unit (2007) The silent epidemic: an economic study of diabetes in developed and developing countries. London, Economist Intelligence Unit.

Edmonds, M., Boulton, A., Buckenham, T., *et al.* (1996) Report of the diabetic foot and amputation group. **13**, S27–S42.

Egger, G. & Swinburn, B. (1997) An "ecological" approach to the obesity pandemic. *British Medical Journal*, **315**, 477–480.

Epping-Jordan, J.E., Pruitt, S.D., Bengoa, R., *et al.* (2004) Improving the quality of health care for chronic conditions. *Quality & Safety in Health Care*, **13**, 299–305.

Evans, J.M., Newton, R.W., Ruta, D.A., *et al.* (2000) Socio-economic status, obesity and prevalence of Type 1 and Type 2 diabetes mellitus. *Diabetic Medicine*, **17**, 478–80.

Eye Diseases Prevalence Research Group, Kempen, J.H., O'Colmain, B.J., Leske, M.C., *et al.* (2004) The prevalence of diabetic retinopathy among adults in the United States. *Archives of Ophthalmology*, **122**, 552–63.

Folsom, A.R., Rasmussen, M.L., Chambless, L.E., *et al.* (1999) Prospective associations of fasting insulin, body fat distribution, and diabetes with risk of ischemic stroke. The Atherosclerosis Risk in Communities (ARIC) Study Investigators. *Diabetes Care*, **22**, 1077–83.

Folsom, A.R., Szklo, M., Stevens, J., *et al.* (1997) A prospective study of coronary heart disease in relation to fasting insulin, glucose, and diabetes. The Atherosclerosis Risk in Communities (ARIC) Study. *Diabetes Care*, **20**, 935–42.

Foy, C.G., Bell, R.A., Farmer, D.F., *et al.* (2005) Smoking and incidence of diabetes among U.S. adults: findings from the Insulin Resistance Atherosclerosis Study. *Diabetes Care*, **28**, 2501–7.

Frayling, T.M. & Hattersley, A.T. (2001) The role of genetic susceptibility in the association of low birth weight with type 2 diabetes. *British Medical Bulletin*, **60**, 89–101.

Gillespie, K.M. (2006) Type 1 diabetes: pathogenesis and prevention. *CMAJ*, **175**, 165–70.

Gillies, C.L., Abrams, K.R., Lambert, P.C., *et al.* (2007) Pharmacological and lifestyle interventions to prevent or delay type 2 diabetes in people with impaired glucose tolerance: systematic review and meta-analysis. *BMJ*, 334, 299.

Global Lower Extremity Amputation Study Group (2000) Epidemiology of lower extremity amputation in centres in Europe, North America and East Asia. The Global Lower Extremity Amputation Study Group. *British Journal of Surgery*, **87**, 328–37.

Glumer, C., Carstensen, B., Sandbaek, A., *et al.* (2004) A Danish diabetes risk score for targeted screening: the Inter99 study. *Diabetes Care*, **27**, 727–33.

Gohdes, D. (1995) Diabetes in North American Indians and Alaska Natives. IN NATIONAL DIABETES DATA GROUP (Ed.) *Diabetes in America.* Second ed. Washington, National Institutes of Health.

Griffin, S. J., Little, P. S., Hales, C. N., *et al.* (2000) Diabetes risk score: towards earlier detection of type 2 diabetes in general practice. *Diabetes/Metabolism Research Reviews*, **16**, 164–71.

Harris, M. (1993) Undiagnosed NIDDM: Clinical and public health issues. *Diabetes Care*, **16**, 642–652.

Hartemink, N., Boshuizen, H.C., Nagelkerke, N.J.D., *et al.* (2006) Combining risk estimates from observational studies with different exposure cutpoints: a meta-analysis on body mass index and diabetes type 2. *American Journal of Epidemiology*, **163**, 1042–52.

Hattersley, A.T. & Tooke, J.E. (1999) The fetal insulin hypothesis: an alternative explanation of the association of low birthweight with diabetes and vascular disease. *Lancet*, **353**, 1789–92.

Herman, W.H., Ali, M.A., Aubert, R.E., *et al.* (1995) Diabetes mellitus in Egypt: risk factors and prevalence. *Diabetic Medicine*, **12**, 1126–31.

Himsworth, H.P. (1936) Diabetes mellitus: its differentiation into insulin-sensitive and insulin-insensitive types. *Lancet*, **i**, 127–130.

Hirschhorn, J. N. (2003) Genetic epidemiology of type 1 diabetes. *Pediatric Diabetes*, **4**, 87–100.

Hodge, A.M., English, D.R., O'dea, K., *et al.* (2004) Glycemic index and dietary fiber and the risk of type 2 diabetes. *Diabetes Care*, **27**, 2701–6.

Holmes, J., Gear, E., Bottomley, J., *et al.* (2003) Do people with type 2 diabetes and their carers lose income? (T2ARDIS-4). *Health Policy*, **64**, 291–296.

International Diabetes Federation (2006) Diabetes Atlas: third edition. Brussels, International Diabetes Federation.

International Diabetes Federation: Clinical Guidelines Taskforce (2005) Global Guideline for Type 2 Diabetes. Brussels, International Diabetes Federation.

Jeon, C.Y., Lokken, R.P., Hu, F.B., *et al.* (2007) Physical activity of moderate intensity and risk of type 2 diabetes: a systematic review. *Diabetes Care*, **30**, 744–52.

Karvonen, M., Viik-Kajander, M., Moltchanova, E., *et al.* (2000) Incidence of childhood type 1 diabetes worldwide. *Diabetes Care*, **23**, 1516–1526.

Kenny, S., Aubert, R. & Geiss, L. (1995) Prevalence and Incidence of Non-Insulin-Dependent Diabetes. In National Diabetes Data Group (Ed.) *Diabetes in America.* Second ed. Washington, National Institutes of Health.

Kim, C., Newton, K.M. & Knopp, R.H. (2002) Gestational diabetes and the incidence of type 2 diabetes: a systematic review. *Diabetes Care*, **25**, 1862–8.

Klein, R. (1997) The epidemiology of diabetic retinopathy. In *Textbook of Diabetes* (eds. Pickup, J. and Williams, G.). London, Blackwell Scientific Publications.

Klein, R. & Klein, B. E. (1995) Vision disorders in diabetes. In *Diabetes in America* (ed. National Diabetes Data Group). Second ed. Bethesda, USA, National Institutes of Health.

Knip, M., Veijola, R., Virtanen, S. M., *et al.* (2005) Environmental triggers and determinants of type 1 diabetes. *Diabetes*, **54**, S125–36.

Knowler, W.C., Barrett-Connor, E., Fowler, S.E., *et al.* & Diabetes Prevention Program Research Group (2002) Reduction in the incidence of type 2 diabetes with lifestyle intervention or metformin. *New England Journal of Medicine*, **346**, 393–403.

Kukko, M., Kimpimaki, T., Korhonen, S., *et al.* (2005) Dynamics of diabetes-associated autoantibodies in young children with human leukocyte antigen-conferred risk of type 1 diabetes recruited from the general population. *Journal of Clinical Endocrinology & Metabolism*, **90**, 2712–7.

Kumari, M., Head, J. & Marmot, M. (2004) Prospective study of social and other risk factors for incidence of type 2 diabetes in the Whitehall II study. *Archives of Internal Medicine*, **164**, 1873–80.

Laaksonen, D.E., Lakka, H.-M., Niskanen, L.K., *et al.* (2002) Metabolic syndrome and development of diabetes mellitus: application and validation of recently suggested definitions of the metabolic syndrome in a prospective cohort study. *American Journal of Epidemiology*, **156**, 1070–7.

Larranaga, I., Arteagoitia, J.M., Rodriguez, J.L., *et al.* & The Sentinel Practice Network Of The Basque Country (2005) Socio-economic inequalities in the prevalence of Type 2 diabetes, cardiovascular risk factors and chronic diabetic complications in the Basque Country, Spain. *Diabetic Medicine*, **22**, 1047–53.

Lin, E.H.B., Katon, W., Von Korff, M., *et al.* (2004) Relationship of depression and diabetes self-care, medication adherence, and preventive care. *Diabetes Care*, **27**, 2154–60.

Lindstrom, J., Ilanne-Parikka, P., Peltonen, M., *et al.* (2006a) Sustained reduction in the incidence of type 2 diabetes by lifestyle intervention: follow-up of the Finnish Diabetes Prevention Study. *The Lancet*, **368**, 1673–9.

Lindstrom, J., Peltonen, M., Eriksson, J.G., *et al.* (2006b) High-fibre, low-fat diet predicts long-term weight loss and decreased type 2 diabetes risk: the Finnish Diabetes Prevention Study. *Diabetologia*, **49**, 912–20.

Lindstrom, J. & Tuomilehto, J. (2003) The diabetes risk score: a practical tool to predict type 2 diabetes risk. *Diabetes Care*, **26**, 725–31.

Little, A.A., Edwards, J.L., & Feldman, E.L. (2007) Diabetic neuropathies. *Practical Neurology*, **7**, 82–92.

Nichols, G.A. & Brown, J.B. (2003) Unadjusted and adjusted prevalence of diagnosed depression in type 2 diabetes. *Diabetes Care*, **26**, 744–9.

Nishimura, R., Laporte, R.E., Dorman, J.S., *et al.* (2001) Mortality trends in type 1 diabetes. The Allegheny County (Pennsylvania) Registry 1965-1999. *Diabetes Care*, **24**, 823–7.

Oldroyd, J., Banerjee, M., Heald, A., *et al.* (2005) Diabetes and ethnic minorities. *Postgraduate Medical Journal*, **81**, 486–90.

Onkamo, P., Vaananen, S., Karvonen, M., *et al.* (1999) Worldwide increase in incidence of Type I diabetes—the analysis of the data on published incidence trends [erratum appears in Diabetologia 2000 May;43(5):685]. *Diabetologia*, **42**, 1395–403.

Palmer, J. P. & Hirsch, I.B. (2003) What's in a Name: Latent autoimmune diabetes of adults, type 1.5, adult-onset, and type 1 diabetes. *Diabetes Care*, **26**, 536–8.

Pan, X., Li, G., Hu, Y.H., *et al.* (1997) Effects of Diet and Exercise in Preventing NIDDM in People With Impaired Glucose Tolerance. The Da Qing IGT and Diabetes Study. *Diabetes Care*, **20**, 537–44.

Panzram, G. (1984) Epidemiologic data on excess mortality and life expectancy in insulin-dependent diabetes mellitus--critical review. *Experimental & Clinical Endocrinology*, **83**, 93–100.

Parillo, M. & Riccardi, G. (2004) Diet composition and the risk of type 2 diabetes: epidemiological and clinical evidence. *British Journal of Nutrition*, **92**, 7–19.

Parker, L., Lamont, D.W., Unwin, N., *et al.* (2003) A lifecourse study of risk for hyperinsulinaemia, dyslipidaemia and obesity (the central metabolic syndrome) at age 49-51 years.[erratum appea rs in *Diabetic Medicine*. 2003 Sep;20(9):781]. *Diabetic Medicine*, **20**, 406–15.

Permutt, M.A., Wasson, J., & Cox, N. (2005) Genetic epidemiology of diabetes *J. Clin. Invest*, **115**, 1431–1439.

Phillips, D.I.W., Jones, A., & Goulden, P.A. (2006) Birth weight, stress, and the metabolic syndrome in adult life. *Annals of the New York Academy of Sciences*, **1083**, 28–36.

Popkin, B.M. (2002) The shift in stages of the nutrition transition in the developing world differs from past experiences! *Public Health Nutrition*, **5**, 205–14.

Popkin, B.M. (2004) The nutrition transition: an overview of world patterns of change. *Nutrition Reviews*, **62**, S140–S143.

Popkin, B.M. & Gordon-Larsen, P. (2004) The nutrition transition: worldwide obesity dynamics and their determinants. *International Journal of Obesity & Related Metabolic Disorders*, **28**, s2–9.

Pozzilli, P. & Buzzetti, R. (2007) A new expression of diabetes: double diabetes. *Trends in Endocrinology & Metabolism*, **18**, 52–7.

Puska, P., Nissinen, A., Tuomilehto, J., *et al.* (1985) The community-based strategy to prevent coronary heart disease: conclusions from the ten years of the North Karelia project. *Annual Review of Public Health*, **6**, 147–93.

Ramachandran, A., Snehalatha, C., Mary, S., *et al.* (2006) The Indian Diabetes Prevention Programme shows that lifestyle modification and metformin prevent type 2 diabetes in Asian Indian subjects with impaired glucose tolerance (IDPP-1). *Diabetologia*, **49**, 289–97.

Rewers, M. & Zimmet, P. (2004) The rising tide of childhood type 1 diabetes—what is the elusive environmental trigger?[comment]. *Lancet*, **364**, 1645–7.

Rimm, E.B., Chan, J., Stampfer, M.J., *et al.* (1995) Prospective study of cigarette smoking, alcohol use, and the risk of diabetes in men. *BMJ*, **310**, 555–9.

Roberts, S. (2007) *Working together for better diabetes care:clinical case for change.* London, Department of Health.

Roglic, G., Unwin, N., Bennett, P.H., *et al.* (2005) The burden of mortality attributable to diabetes: realistic estimates for the year 2000. *Diabetes Care*, **28**, 2130–5.

Roper, N.A., Bilous, R.W., Kelly, W.F., *et al.* (2001) Excess mortality in a population with diabetes and the impact of material deprivation: longitudinal, population based study. *British Medical Journal*, **322**, 1389–1393.

Roper, N.A., Bilous, R.W., Kelly, W.F., *et al.* (2002) Cause-specific mortality in a population with diabetes: South Tees Diabetes Mortality Study. *Diabetes Care.*, **25**, 43–48.

Roy, M.S., Klein, R., O'Colmain, B.J., *et al.* (2004) The prevalence of diabetic retinopathy among adult type 1 diabetic persons in the United States. *Archives of Ophthalmology*, **122**, 546–51.

Salazar-Martinez, E., Willett, W.C., Ascherio, A., *et al.* (2004) Coffee consumption and risk for type 2 diabetes mellitus. *Annals of Internal Medicine*, **140**, 1–8.

Sargeant, L.A., Khaw, K.T., Bingham, S., *et al.* (2001) Cigarette smoking and glycaemia: the EPIC-Norfolk Study. *International Journal of Epidemiology*, **30**, 547–54.

Simmons, R., Harding, A.H., Jakes, R., *et al.* (2006) How much might achievement of diabetes prevention behaviour goals reduce the incidence of diabetes if implemented at the population level? *Diabetologia*, **49**, 905–11.

Sladek, R., Rocheleau, G., Rung, J., *et al.* (2007) A genome-wide association study identifies novel risk loci for type 2 diabetes. *Nature*, **445**, 881–5.

Smith, B., Wingard, D.L., Smith, T.C., *et al.* (2006) Does coffee consumption reduce the risk of type 2 diabetes in individuals with impaired glucose? *Diabetes Care*, **29**, 2385–90.

Stamler, J., Vaccaro, O., Neaton, J.D., *et al.* (1993) Diabetes, other risk factors, and 12-yr cardiovascular mortality for men screened in the Multiple Risk Factor Intervention Trial. *Diabetes Care*, **16**, 434–44.

Tapp, R.J., Zimmet, P.Z., Harper, C.A., *et al.* (2006) Diagnostic thresholds for diabetes: The association of retinopathy and albuminuria with glycaemia. *Diabetes Research and Clinical Practice*, **73**, 315–21.

The Decode Study Group (2003) Age- and Sex-Specific Prevalences of Diabetes and Impaired Glucose Regulation in 13 European Cohorts. *Diabetes Care*, **26**, 61–9.

The Expert Committee on the Diagnosis and Classification of Diabetes Mellitus (1997) Report of the Expert Committee on the Diagnosis and Classification of Diabetes Mellitus. *Diabetes Care*, **20**, 1183–97.

Torgerson, J.S., Hauptman, J., Boldrin, M.N., *et al.* (2004) XENical in the Prevention of Diabetes in Obese Subjects (XENDOS) Study: A randomized study of orlistat as an adjunct to lifestyle changes for the prevention of type 2 diabetes in obese patients. *Diabetes Care*, **27**, 155–61.

Tuomi, T., Groop, L. C., Zimmet, P.Z., *et al.* (1993) Antibodies to glutamic acid decarboxylase reveal latent autoimmune diabetes mellitus in adults with a non-insulin-dependent onset of disease. *Diabetes*, **42**, 359–62.

Tuomilehto, J., Lindstrom, J., Eriksson, J. G., *et al.* & Finnish Diabetes Prevention Study Group (2001) Prevention of type 2 diabetes mellitus by changes in lifestyle among subjects with impaired glucose tolerance. *New England Journal of Medicine*, **344**, 1343–50.

Unite for Diabetes (2006) Resolution adopted by the General Assembly: 61/225. World Diabetes Day.

Unwin, N. (2006) The metabolic syndrome. *Journal of the Royal Society of Medicine*, **99**, 457–62.

Unwin, N. (2007) Diabetes and the good, the bad and the ugly of globalization. *International Diabetes Monitor*, **19**, 5–10.

Unwin, N., Shaw, J., Zimmet, P., *et al.* (2002) Impaired glucose tolerance and impaired fasting glycaemia: the current status on definition and intervention. **19**, 708–23.

Vazquez, G., Duval, S., Jacobs, D.R., JR., *et al.* (2007) Comparison of Body Mass Index, Waist Circumference, and Waist/Hip Ratio in Predicting Incident Diabetes: A Meta-Analysis. *Epidemiol Rev*, **29**, 115–28.

Venkat narayan, K.M., Zhang, P., Kanaya, A.M., *et al.* (2006) Diabetes: The Pandemic and Potential Solutions. In *Disease control priorities in developing countries* (eds. Jamison, D.T., Breman, J.G., Measham, A.R., *et al.*), Second ed. Washington/New York, World Bank/Oxford University Press.

Wannamethee, S.G., Camargo, C.A., JR., Manson, J.E., *et al.* (2003) Alcohol drinking patterns and risk of type 2 diabetes mellitus among younger women. *Archives of Internal Medicine*, **163**, 1329–36.

Whitford, D.L., Griffin, S.J. & Prevost, A.T. (2003) Influences on the variation in prevalence of type 2 diabetes between general practices: practice, patient or socioeconomic factors? *British Journal of General Practice*, **53**, 9–14.

Wild, S., Roglic, G., Green, A., *et al.* (2004) Global prevalence of diabetes: estimates for the year 2000 and projections for 2030. *Diabetes Care*, **27**, 1047–53.

Wilkin, T.J. (2001) The accelerator hypothesis: weight gain as the missing link between Type I and Type II diabetes.[see comment]. *Diabetologia*, **44**, 914–22.

Willett, W.C., Koplan, J.P., Nugent, R., *et al.* (2006) Prevention of Chronic Disease by Means of Diet and Lifestyle Changes. In Jamison, D.T., Breman, J.G., Measham, A.R., *et al.* (Eds.) *Disease control priorities in developing countries.* Second ed. Washington/New York, World Bank/ Oxford University Press.

Williams, R. (2005) Medical and economic case for prevention of type 2 diabetes and cardiovascular disease. *Eur Heart J Suppl*, **7**, D14–17.

World Health Organization (1997) Obesity: preventing and managing the global epidemic - Report of a WHO consultation on obesity. Geneva, World Health Organization,.

World Health Organization (1999) Definition, diagnosis, and classification of diabetes mellitus and its complications. Report of a WHO consultation. Part 1: Diagnosis and classification of diabetes mellitus. Geneva.

World Health Organization (2004) Global Strategy on Diet, Physical Activity and Health. Geneva, World Health Organization.

World Health Organization (2005) Preventing chronic diseases: a vital investment: WHO global report. Geneva, World Health Organization.

World Health Organization (2006) Definition and diagnosis of diabetes mellitus and intermediate hyperglycemia: report of a WHO/IDF consultation. Geneva, World Health Organization.

World Health Organization (Forthcoming) Prevention of diabetes mellitus and its complications. Geneva, World Health Organization.

Xu, F., Yin, X.M., Zhang, M., *et al.* (2006) Family average income and diagnosed Type 2 diabetes in urban and rural residents in regional mainland China. *Diabetic Medicine*, **23**, 1239–46.

Yudkin, J. S. (2000) Insulin for the world's poorest countries. *Lancet*, **355**, 919–21.

Zimmet, P. Z. (1992) Kelly West Lecture 1991. Challenges in diabetes epidemiology—from West to the rest. *Diabetes Care*, **15**, 232–52.

9.7

Public mental health

Benedetto Saraceno,
Melvyn Freeman, and Michelle Funk

Abstract

Mental health is an integral part of health. Consequently, public mental health is critical to achieving better health in populations. The prevalence of mental disorder is substantial with around 450 million people worldwide suffering from neuropsychiatric conditions. Suicide is among the leading causes of death in 15–45-year-olds. Moreover, mental disorder makes a considerable independent contribution to the burden of disease worldwide—accounting for 13 per cent of the global burden of disease. By 2030, it is estimated that unipolar depression will be the second-highest cause of disability-adjusted life years (DALYs) lost. Globally, the majority of people who need mental health care do not receive it. This 'service gap' is far highest in middle- and low-income countries. There are, however, cost-effective treatments available, and it has been estimated that the benefits of a basic specified package of treatment could lead to a reduction of 2000–3000 DALYs lost per million population. Inadequate and inappropriate mental health systems and services are a major cause of poor mental health outcomes. Decentralization of services and integration of mental health into general health care are critical to improve mental health status in populations. In middle- and low-income countries, additional trained personnel and facilities are required, especially in general health care. Though there are multiple determinants of mental disorder, social and economic factors are fundamental. Poverty, gender discrimination and violence/war are amongst the most important of these. Understanding social determinants is important for planning services; to initiate prevention and promotion; for advocacy and for the information of sectors outside of health that need to assist in improving mental health—such as social development, labour, education, and housing. Finding appropriate and adequate promotive and preventive interventions in mental health is increasing but remains an important area of growth. Given the inextricable connections between mental and physical health, and the importance of mental disorder as a health problem in its own right, this chapter shows that public mental health is central to improved global health.

Introduction

More than 60 years after health was defined in the preamble of the Constitution of the World Health Organization (WHO) as 'a state of complete physical, *mental*, and social well-being, and not merely the absence of disease or infirmity' (WHO 1946), there is still considerable consensus regarding the merit of this definition. Notwithstanding, most countries have not effectively translated this broad conceptualization into health policies and practice. Of particular relevance for this chapter, the 'mental' in the definition has been neglected in public health. This, we maintain, has impeded the realization of better health (both mental and physical) in populations. Nevertheless, public mental health is a rapidly growing discipline and we envisage that it will make a far more substantial contribution to the health status of populations in the future.

There are many reasons for past and current neglect of mental health in health (Saraceno *et al.* 2007). Critical contributory factors include historical deficiencies in information about prevalence, impact, and effective interventions for prevention and treatment and the stigma and discrimination associated with 'abnormalities of the mind'. However, increasing evidence from the study of the epidemiology and burden of mental disorder; mounting knowledge of the relationships between mental and physical health; better understanding of and information on the determinants of mental ill health; increased evidence with regard to prevention and promotion; comprehensive evidence of effective (including cost-effective) interventions for mental disorder and a growing consensus regarding more humane and more efficient ways of organizing mental health systems and services are all contributing to the growing realization that public mental health is vital to improving the health of populations. Though certainly considerably more effort is still needed to 'unblock' various obstacles to the full recognition of mental health as a key public health issue (such as stigma of mental disorder and political commitment to service development in mental health), the reality that mental health interventions are central to health is gaining momentum.

What is mental health, mental disorder, and public mental health?

Developing a consensus around a definition for mental health has proved far more elusive than that attained for health. According to WHO, from a cross-cultural perspective mental health is nearly impossible to define (WHO 2001). Different groups of people value and aspire to different states of well-being and hence mental health is necessarily a matter of ideology. For example, a person who independently achieves great wealth through striving to be better than anyone else and who overcomes all competitors in achieving personal goals may be regarded in one culture as the epitome of success and possibly reflecting superior mental health status. However, in a milieu where collective action and the success of the whole community is valued above individual attainment, the same aspirations and behaviour may be perceived as emotionally astray or even disturbed. Nonetheless, mental health usually includes notions such as subjective well-being, perceived self-efficacy, autonomy, competence, intergenerational dependence, and self-actualizing of one's intellectual and emotional potential (WHO 2001). It has recently been suggested that mental or psychological well-being is part of '... an individual's capacity to lead a fulfilling life and that this includes the ability to study, work or pursue leisure interests, and to make day-to-day personal or household decisions about educational, employment, housing and other choices' (WHO 2006b).

Over a number of years, attempts to define and categorize mental and behavioural *disorders* has also proved difficult. However, classification and diagnostic systems such as the International Classification of Mental Disorders (ICD-10) (WHO 1992) and the Diagnostic and Statistical Manual for Mental Disorders DSM -IV-TR (American Psychiatric Association 2000) now allow for a far more scientific categorization of mental disorder and the separation of abnormal or pathological conditions from 'normal' functioning. Mental and behavioural disorders are generally regarded as 'clinically significant conditions characterized by alterations in thinking, mood (emotions) or behaviour associated with personal distress and/or impaired functioning' (WHO 2001). Notwithstanding there is still considerable debate with regard to the impacts of the 'medicalization' of disorder brought about through these instruments, whether diagnostic categories are valid cross-culturally and the importance of the meanings that cultures attribute to symptoms.

Kovel comments that classification and diagnostic instruments such as DSM and ICD encourage the objectification of people. They 'promulgate a structure in which one is simply to observe from the outside ... and it fosters the discourse of the medical disease in which what is wrong with the person is the disorder that he/she *has*' (Kovel 1988). Thinking about a person in this way is not only 'superficial and instrumental' but encourages the practitioner to forget firstly that the patient has agency and secondly that there are social roots of mental disorder.

While applying diagnostic systems of symptom clusters can be extremely helpful, particularly as this informs treatment, categories may not always have good cultural 'fit' and the treatment required may also be culture specific (see the section 'Brief historical overview of mental health services'). The term 'culture bound syndrome' has been used to describe disturbed behaviour, highly specific to certain cultural systems, which does not conform to Western nosological entities. Given this complexity, diagnosis, especially within cultures that are foreign to individuals, can be fraught with difficulties. Public mental health is concerned with reducing the incidence, prevalence, and impacts of mental disorders and improving the mental health status of populations. In the section 'Mental health as a public health priority', we show that mental and behavioural disorders are indeed a major public health concern. Equally though, optimizing mental health (positive mental health) is an important goal for achieving healthy populations. Furthermore, given the inseparable interrelationship between mental and physical health, public mental health also aims to optimize physical health through mental and behavioural interventions (see the section 'Treatment efficacy'). The tools of public mental health are no different from other areas of public health; epidemiology, health promotion and prevention, health systems and services development, health economics, and monitoring and evaluation—all play important roles.

Mental health as a public health priority

Different criteria have been used at different times and by different experts in order to decide what health problem is, or should be, regarded as a public health priority. We will show that there is compelling evidence using various criteria and perspectives for prioritizing mental health. These include epidemiological data on mental health, co-morbidity with physical health, treatment efficacy, gaps in current treatment, impacts on individuals and their families, and the ideology of health.

Prevalence of mental disorder

WHO estimates that about 450 million people worldwide suffer from neuropsychiatric conditions (WHO 2001). Mental and behavioural disorders are found in all countries, in women and men at all stages of life, amongst the rich and poor, and amongst rural and urban people.

Surveys to determine the prevalence of mental disorder have been carried out since the end of the World War II; however, the use of a range of different diagnostic instruments and methods have made it difficult to make cross-national comparisons or even assess longitudinal changes within countries. Moreover, different studies have measured 'point prevalence' (people who have a condition at a point in time), 'period prevalence' (presence of disorder in a particular time period such as one year), or 'lifetime prevalence' (having suffered from a disorder at some point in their lives) and, unless it is made very clear in the study what is being measured, and this has not always been the case, comparisons are difficult. Analysis by WHO in 2000 indicated a 10 per cent point prevalence of neuropsychiatric conditions in adults (WHO 2001) and that around 25 per cent of individuals will develop one or more mental or behavioural disorders in their lifetime.

Most studies have found the overall prevalence of mental disorder to be almost the same for men and women. However, almost all studies show a higher prevalence of depression amongst women than men with a ratio of between 1.5:1 and 2:1 as well as higher rates of most anxiety and eating disorders. On the other hand, men have higher rates of attention deficit hyperactivity disorder, autism, and substance abuse disorders (Hyman *et al.* 2006).

In the 1990s, the World Health Organization Composite International Diagnostic Interview (WHO CIDI) was used to determine both prevalence of mental disorder in countries and to assess cross-country differences. While prevalence varied widely, in most countries, more than one third of respondents were found to have had a mental disorder in their lifetime. In 1998, WHO established the World Mental Health (WMH) Survey Consortium to refine the CIDI and conduct mental health surveys around the world. The instrument was modified to measure not only prevalence but also severity, impairment and treatment (WHO 2004). Twenty-eight countries, including both high- and lower-income countries in each region of the world participated in the survey. More than 200 000 interviews were conducted. Results of the first 14 countries that had completed the survey were reported in 2004 (WHO World Mental Health Survey

Table 9.7.1 Twelve-month prevalence of WMH CIDI disorders and proportion with mild severity

Country[1]	Percentage prevalence of any mental disorder (95% CI)	Of mild severity[2] (95% CI)
China (Beijing)	9.1 (6–12.1)	5.3 (3.2–7.3)
China (Shanghai)	4.3 (2.7–5.9)	1.8 (0.6–3)
Belgium	12 (9.6–14.3)	6.4 (5–7.7)
Colombia	17.8 (16.1–19.5)	5.9 (5.1–6.8)
France	18.4 (15.3–21.5)	9.7 (7.3–12.1)
Germany	9.1 (7.3–10.8)	4.5 (3.2–5.9)
Italy	8.2 (6.7–9.7)	4.5 (3.2–5.9)
Japan	8.8 (6.4 –11.2)	3.2 (1.7–4.7)
Lebanon	16.9 (13.6–20.2)	6.1 (3.6–8.7)
Mexico	12.2 (10.5–13.8)	4.9 (4–5.8)
Netherlands	14.9 (12.2–17.6)	8.8 (6.1–11.5)
Nigeria	4.7 (3.6–11.2)	3.8 (2.8–4.8)
Spain	9.2 (7.8–10.6)	5.3 (9.4–6.7)
Ukraine	20.5 (17.7–23.2)	8.2 (6.4–10.1)
United States	26.4 (24.7–28)	9.2 (8.1–10.3)

Source: Adapted from World Mental Health Survey Consortium (2004).

[1] Though all sites measured mental disorder in adults there are substantial cross-national differences in age structure between countries with more younger people assessed in developing countries.

[2] Severity was assessed in terms of ability to carry out normal daily activities and rated as severe, moderate, or mild in terms of the Sheehan Disability Scale or the Global Assessment of Functioning.

Consortium 2004). This included three countries in the Americas, seven in Europe, one in the Middle East, one in Africa, and two in Asia. Six countries were classified by the World Bank as less developed and the others developed.

As seen in Table 9.7.1, the overall prevalence varied from 4.3 per cent in Shanghai, China, to 26.4 per cent in the United States with a 9.1–16.9 per cent inter-quartile range (WHO 2004). The most common disorders found were anxiety and depression (with a high level of co-morbidity). In all but one country, anxiety disorder had the highest prevalence (2.4–18.2 per cent) followed by depression (0.8–9.6). Importantly the proportion of disorders classified as mild is substantial—from 33.1 per cent in Colombia to 80.9 per cent in Nigeria. However in cases of serious mental disorder most respondents reported at least 30 days in the past year where they were totally unable to carry out their usual activities.

It has been recognized by the designers of the WMHS that some of the variation found may be attributable to extraneous factors. For example, perceived stigma is likely to have played an important part in the lower prevalence rate observed in those countries were mental health stigma is highest (Kessler *et al.* 2006).

Determining the prevalence of serious mental disorder, such as schizophrenia, usually requires more specialized and specific studies than the one above and a number have been conducted. A systematic review by Saha and colleagues (Saha *et al.* 2005) identified 188 studies conducted between 1965 and 2002. Table 9.7.2 shows the mean estimates found.

Table 9.7.2 Mean (95% confidence interval) estimates of the population prevalence (%) of schizophrenia[1]

Point prevalence	0.46 (0.19–1)
12-month prevalence	0.33 (.13–.82)
Lifetime prevalence	0.4 (.16–1.2)
Lifetime morbid risk	0.72 (.31–2.7)

Source: Adapted from Saha et al. (2005)

[1] A systematic review of 188 studies conducted in 46 countries was conducted. All studies that reported primary data on the prevalence of schizophrenia between 1965 and 2002 were included.

No significant differences were found between males and females and between urban, rural, and mixed sites. In terms of economic status, the prevalence estimates from lower-income countries were significantly lower than both 'emerging' and high-income sites.

Not many prevalence studies have been conducted on psychotic disorders other than schizophrenia, though the lifetime prevalence of bipolar disorder, like schizophrenia is often assumed to be about 1 per cent (Perälä *et al.* 2007). A recent comprehensive study of psychotic and bipolar I disorders in Finland found a lifetime prevalence of psychotic disorders of 3.06 per cent. Lifetime prevalence of schizophrenia was 0.87 per cent, schizoaffective disorder 0.32 per cent, schizophreniform disorder 0.07 per cent, delusional disorder 0.18 per cent, bipolar I disorder 0.24 per cent, major depressive disorder with psychotic features 0.35 per cent, substance-induced psychotic disorder 0.42 per cent, and 0.21 per cent for psychotic disorders due to a medical condition (Perälä *et al.* 2007).

Mortality

Causes of mortality are sometimes used to determine priority levels of different disorders. While mental disorders in themselves have relatively low mortality rates, mental disorders, particularly depression and substance abuse, are associated with more than 90 per cent of all cases of suicide (Bertolote *et al.* 2004) and the incidence of suicide is substantial. WHO has reported that in 2000 around 1 million people died from suicide. The 'global' mortality rate was 16 per 1000—or a death through suicide every 40 seconds. Global suicidal rates for 2006 are shown in Fig. 9.7.1. Nearly 20 times this number attempt suicide. Moreover official suicide rates are usually substantially underestimated. In an Indian study using surveillance with validated verbal autopsy, the observed rates exceeded official national estimates tenfold (Aaron *et al.* 2004).

According to WHO, suicide is among the three leading causes of death among 15–45-year-olds (men and women). The numbers of suicides has increased by 60 per cent over a 45-year period. In 2002, it was estimated that self-inflicted injuries were the fourteenth highest cause of all deaths. Projections to 2030 suggest that this will rise to twelfth place in the causes of death (Mathers & Loncar 2006).

Raised non-suicide-related mortality has also been found in, for example, people living with schizophrenia, bipolar disorder, and dementia (Heila *et al.* 2005; Ösby *et al.* 2001; Dewey & Saz 2001). A major investigation by the Disability Rights Commission (England and Wales) found that people with learning disabilities and mental health problems do not live as long as other citizens. Individuals with serious mental health problems were more likely to get strokes and coronary heart disease before 55 years of age and to survive for

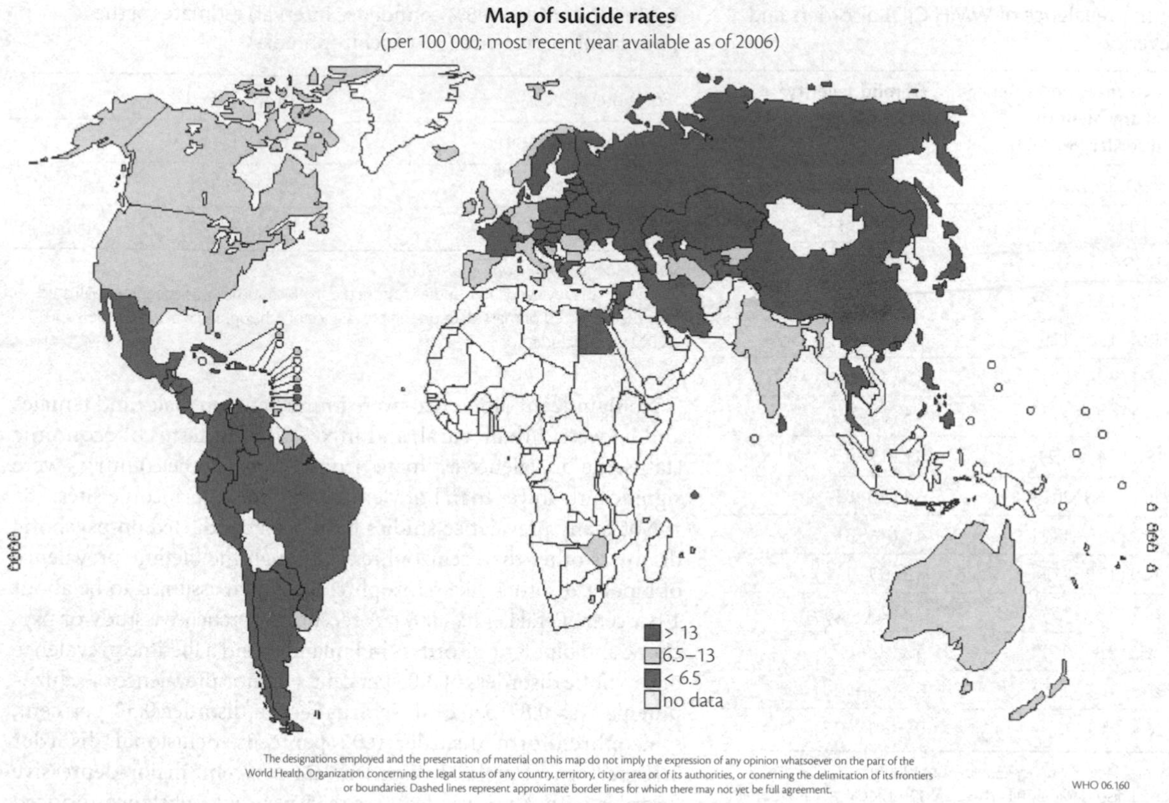
Map of suicide rates
(per 100 000; most recent year available as of 2006)
> 13
6.5–13
< 6.5
no data
The designations employed and the presentation of material on this map do not imply the expression of any opinion whatsoever on the part of the World Health Organization concerning the legal status of any country, territory, city or area or of its authorities, or conerning the delimitation of its frontiers or boundaries. Dashed lines represent approximate border lines for which there may not yet be full agreement.
WHO 06.160

Fig. 9.7.1 Map of suicide rates.
Source: WHO webpage on Suicide Prevention: http://www.who.int/mental_health/prevention/suicide/suicideprevent/en/index.html

less than 5 years thereafter (Disability Rights Commission 2006). Reasons for this include the fact that people with serious mental disorder often live in social deprivation (see the subsection 'Social determinants of mental (ill) health'), but also that the health services discriminate against people with mental health problems. They are less likely to receive medical checks and to be provided with evidence-based treatment.

Burden of disease

While morbidity and mortality are important measures for making health decisions, they fail to take into account important variables necessary for health planning. In response, a joint initiative of the WHO, the World Bank and Harvard University designed and conducted the Global Burden of Disease study. The GBD approach uses a summary measure—DALY—to quantify the burden of disease. DALYs combine the years of life lost due to premature mortality (YLL) in the population and the years lost to due to disability (YLD) for incident cases of the health condition.

The prominence of mental and neurological disorders from the GBD study relative to other disorders was a major revelation to many people and countries. When the DALY figures were first published in 1993, most countries found a major mismatch between the burden of mental health (10.5 per cent of all DALYs lost) and the prominence and attention given it. This was because traditionally only incidence/prevalence and mortality were measured in most international and national statistics. While these indices were well suited to acute diseases that either resulted in death or full recovery, mental and behavioural disorders, which more often cause disability, did not feature prominently. With the loss of 'healthy life' being elevated, mental and neurological disorders were catapulted into the limelight. Moreover projections showed that the burden due to mental disorders was likely to substantially increase relative to other health conditions. In 2002, mental and substance use disorders accounted for 13 per cent of the GBD (WHO 2004). When taking only the disability component of the burden of disease into account, mental and neurological conditions accounted for 30.8 per cent of all years lived with disability.

In 2006, Mathers and Loncar published an update of earlier DALY figures and projections on the burden of disease (Mathers & Loncar 2006). Estimates are now available up to 2030. Importantly for public mental health, as predicted, the relative burden of mental disorder is rising and is set to rise even further. By far the highest mental health cause of DALYs lost is unipolar depressive disorder and this disorder alone is likely to be the second-highest cause of all DALYs lost by 2030—second only to HIV/AIDS. In high-income countries, depression will become the single-highest cause of DALYs lost.

In Table 9.7.4, the three leading causes of DALYs lost, projected to 2030, by income group, are presented. Crucially unipolar depressive disorder is amongst the top three causes of DALYs lost in high-, middle-, and low-income countries.

Interrelationship between physical and mental health

Over the past 20 years, a fundamental and inseparable interconnection between mental and physical health has been established (WHO 2001) While thoughts, feelings, and behaviour have a major impact on physical health, physical health strongly influences mental health and well-being. There are two key pathways through which the physical and mental interact—firstly through physiological systems such

Table 9.7.3 Changes in ranking for leading causes of DALYs lost, 2002 and 2030—World

Disease or injury	2002 rank	2030 rank	Change in rank
Perinatal conditions	1	5	−4
Lower respiratory infections	2	8	−6
HIV/AIDS	3	1	+2
Unipolar depressive disorder	4	2	+2
Diarrhoeal diseases	5	12	−7
Ischaemic heart disease	6	3	+3
Cerebrovascular disease	7	6	+1
Road traffic accidents	8	4	+4
Malaria	9	15	−6
Tuberculosis	10	25	−15
COPD	11	7	+4
Congenital abnormalities	12	20	−8
Hearing loss, adult onset	13	9	+4
Cataracts	14	10	+4
Violence	15	13	+2
Self-inflicted violence	17	14	+3

Source: Adapted from Mathers *et al.* (2006).

Table 9.7.4 Leading causes of DALYs lost by income group—2030

Income group	Rank	Disease or injury	Per cent total DALYs lost
World	1	HIV/AIDS	12.1
	2	Unipolar depressive disorder	5.7
	3	Ischaemic heart disease	4.7
High-income countries	1	Unipolar depressive disorder	9.8
	2	Ischaemic heart disease	5.9
	3	Alzheimer and other dementias	5.8
Middle-income countries	1	HIV/AIDS	9.8
	2	Unipolar depressive disorder	6.7
	3	Cerebrovascular disease	6.0
Low-income countries	1	HIV/AIDS	14.6
	2	Perinatal conditions	5.8
	3	Unipolar depressive disorder	4.7

Source: Adapted from Mathers *et al.* (2006).

as neuroendocrine and immune functioning, and secondly through health behaviour (WHO 2001). However, these pathways are not independent in that behaviour may affect physiology, while physiological functioning may in turn affect health behaviour.

There are numerous examples of how mental health status may impact on physical health and vice versa. At least one-third of all somatic symptoms remain medically unexplained. Common symptoms include pain, fatigue, and dizziness, while defined syndromes include irritable bowel syndrome, fibromyalgia, chronic fatigue syndrome, chronic pelvic pain, and tempero-mandibular joint dysfunction (Prince *et al.* 2007). Somatization is present in around 15 per cent of patients seen in primary care and is independently associated with poor-health-related quality of life and increased healthcare utilization (Barsky *et al.* 2005).

A review by Prince *et al.* has shown strong evidence from population-based research for moderate to strong prospective associations between depression and anxiety and coronary heart disease outcomes including angina and non-fatal and fatal myocardial infarctions. They also showed strong evidence that depression is an independent risk factor for stroke. Depression is increased after myocardial infarction, mostly in the first month after the event. There is also strong evidence for co-morbidity between mental disorder and diabetes. The prevalence of diabetes among people with schizophrenia has consistently been found to be in the order of 15 per cent compared to a typical community prevalence of 2–3 per cent (Holt *et al.* 2005).

The interrelationships between physical and mental health are highly complex. Here, we illustrate five important mechanisms of this relationship through the example of mental health and HIV/AIDS.

Mental health status increases the risk of infection

In the United States, people with severe mental illness are nearly 20 times more likely to be infected with HIV than the general population (McKinnon & Rosner 2000). Reasons for this include a lack of appreciation of risk, impaired social interactions, low levels of assertiveness, low use of condoms, injecting drug use, multiple partners, sexual activity within closed environments such as institutions, and homelessness. Though this relationship has not been documented in low- and middle-income countries, and though the ratio would inevitably be lower, the reasons for high-risk sexual behaviour and the chances of transmission within psychiatric institutions pertain at least as much to people in low- and middle-income countries as they do to those in high-income countries. High risk of infection is also not limited to severe mental disorder. In South Africa, depression in youth has been significantly correlated with risky sexual behaviour (Moghraby *et al.* 2005).

HIV infection directly affects the central nervous system functioning

The HIV virus has numerous direct impacts, including on the central nervous system. HIV dementia and minor cognitive disorder are common in people living with HIV/AIDS who are not taking anti-retroviral treatment with between 30 per cent and 50 per cent of HIV-seropositive individuals experiencing cognitive-motor problems (Grant *et al.* 1999). HIV invades the brain early in the infection process and in a certain proportion of people psychotic symptoms manifest—especially in late-stage AIDS. Manic episodes are above the population norm in people with HIV (around 5 per cent), especially at more advanced stages of the disease (Catalan *et al.* 2000). It is clear that a disease that attacks the immune system of the body also has direct 'mental' manifestations.

Psychological impacts

Studies of the mental health status of people infected with HIV have consistently found higher prevalence of mental health problems than is found in community or clinic samples. From the research thus far it has not been possible to reliably separate out people who may have had a pre-existing mental disorder from those that may have developed mental disorder following a positive HIV diagnosis. Moreover the extent to which mood and anxiety disorder may be caused directly by the viral infection itself is not clear. However, we know from qualitative research that receiving a diagnosis of HIV and living with the disease can be highly psychologically distressing.

High levels of major depression, mild depressive disorder, and dysthymia have all been found in seropositive individuals. Bing and his co-researchers found a 36 per cent one-year prevalence of depression among a large national sample of HIV-positive men and women in the United States (Bing *et al.* 2001). This is substantially higher than found in the general population. Ciesla and colleagues conducted a meta-analysis of studies comparing HIV-positive and HIV-negative samples and found that major depressive disorder occurred nearly twice as often among people living with HIV (Ciesla & Roberts 2001). In a review of studies of mental health problems of HIV infected people in developing countries, Collins *et al.* also found a significantly higher prevalence of depressive symptoms among HIV-positive people compared with controls (Collins *et al.* 2006).

Feelings of anxiety and distress are a normal and arguably even a healthy response to a diagnosis of HIV. However anxiety may reach clinical levels and impair overall functioning and people's capacity for adequate self care. The prevalence of anxiety disorders in studies in the United States range from negligible to around 40 per cent. Anxiety can be provoked by the unpredictability of the virus and by certain 'milestones' such as initial diagnosis, first opportunistic infection, declining CD4 count or the onset or progression of an AIDS defining illness.

Influencing the course of the disease

To maintain good health a person living with HIV/AIDS (PLHA) must engage in a number of 'health promoting' behaviours and maintain a 'positive' attitude towards themselves and towards the virus. For example, a PLHA must engage in protected sex to avoid reinfection, they should eat nutritious food, refrain from excessive use of alcohol, not smoke cigarettes, immediately seek treatment for opportunistic infections when needed, and, if they are on antiretroviral treatment (ART), they must adhere to their medication regimen.

A review by Uldall *et al.* (2004) found a number of studies that showed that poor mental health was a barrier to ART adherence. This association was particularly significant in women. At least eight studies have showed that adherence to antiretroviral medication is adversely affected by mood disturbance. In addition, research indicates associations between poor adherence and generalized anxiety disorder, panic disorder, post-traumatic stress disorder (PTSD), recent trauma, and social phobia.

Side effects of medication

Another way that the physical and the mental interact is when medication is given to treat a physical problem and there are mental side effects. (Of course, the opposite is often also true whereby medication given to treat a mental condition has physical side effects such as tardive dyskinesia.) In a minority of patients receiving anti-retroviral therapy, mania and psychosis can occur due to the medication they receive such as AZT, 3TC, efavirenz, abacavir, and nevirapine. Patients who have had multiple episodes of depression are at particular risk of having negative reactions to efavirenz.

Treatment efficacy

Having effective (including cost-effective) treatments available is another crucial component of whether a health condition should be prioritized. Most mental disorders can be effectively treated and at a cost that justifies intervention. Whiteford suggests that the burden of illness on the individual and society combined with treatment efficacy could be used as the basis of decisions to allocate resources (Whiteford 2000). Interventions that demonstrate the greatest health gain for the lowest cost would be the most highly prized. Mental health interventions fall into this category.

A recent analysis by the WHO of the comparative effectiveness and costs of pharmacological and psychosocial interventions for reducing the burden of mental disorders found the following (WHO 2006a):

Pharmacological interventions

Both conventional neuroleptic and newer 'atypical' antipsychotic drugs are effective in treating psychosis. Both types of medication have similar efficacy though the former are less expensive. It is therefore recommended that in countries with limited resources (and until such time as newer drugs come off their patents) conventional neuroleptic drugs should be provided.

Both older tricyclic anti-depressants (TCAs) and selective serotonin reuptake inhibitors (SSRIs) are effective in treating depression. Costs and effectiveness of medication vary in different contexts, and therefore the drug treatment of choice should be driven by patient or clinical preferences and local costs.

Psychosocial interventions

Psychosocial treatment, alongside pharmacological treatment for severe disorders such as schizophrenia and bipolar affective disorder, is expected to result in substantial health gains. A combined strategy is more cost-effective than pharmacotherapy on its own.

Psychotherapy is expected to be as cost-effective as most medication for people with depression or anxiety disorders.

Case management

It is expected that long-term maintenance treatment of depression with pharmacological and psychosocial interventions is a more cost-effective strategy than episodic treatments as it prevents a proportion of recurrent depressive episodes.

The mental health service gap

Another reason to prioritize a condition is if the gap between the existence of a condition and the numbers of people being treated for it (especially if effective treatments are available), or programmes to prevent it, is high. Kohn and colleagues reviewed community-based psychiatric epidemiology studies and calculated the median rates of untreated cases of various mental disorders (Kohn *et al.* 2004). The median treatment gaps are found in Table 9.7.5.

These figures are major underestimates of the gaps globally as most of the data available are from high-income countries that have far greater availability of services. For example, in the only condition where a figure was available for Africa, there was a 67 per cent treatment gap for major depression compared with a 45.4 per cent gap for Europe. In the World Mental Health Survey, 35.5–50.3 per cent of serious cases of mental disorder in high-income countries and 76.3–85.4 per cent in middle- and low-income countries received no treatment in the 12 months before the interview (WHO World Mental Health Survey Consortium 2004).

Table 9.7.5 Treatment gaps for mental disorder—world

Mental disorder	Median treatment gap[1]
Schizophrenia and other non-affective psychotic disorders	32.2%
Depression	56.3%
Dysthymia	56%
Bipolar disorder	50.2%
Panic disorder	55.9%
Generalized anxiety disorder	57.5%
Obsessive compulsive disorder	57.3%
Alcohol abuse and dependence	78.1%

Source: Adapted from Kohn *et al.* (2004)

[1] Treatment gap represents the absolute difference between the true prevalence of a disorder and the treated proportion of individuals over 15 affected by the disorder.

Clearly, the majority of people needing mental health interventions are not receiving it. Some of the reasons for the gap include a lack of identification of mental health problems by health workers; sufferers themselves not seeking treatment due to stigma, fear, or lack of knowledge that they have a treatable condition; lack of or unavailability of resources; seeking assistance elsewhere due to cultural beliefs; affordability; and poor health systems that do not allow or encourage treatment in the community. For many people, the only time they might receive treatment is if they become so disruptive in their families or communities that they are given involuntary treatment.

Personal and family impacts

The GBD study estimated that, in 2000, mental and neurological disorders accounted for 30.8 per cent of all years lived with disability—with depression accounting for 12 per cent of all disability (WHO 2004). This though does not capture the economic and psychological stress to individuals and their families resulting from this disability.

'Days out of role' is a very important measure of the macroeconomic impacts of mental disorder (WHO 2006a); however, for individuals and families, this very often means a direct and personal loss of income (especially where there are no or poor unemployment benefits). Moreover, a family member, often a woman spouse or parent, has to take time off from income-generating activities to care for the person with mental disorder. Income into the family is hence further eroded. Furthermore, due to the person's mental disorder there are additional health care and usually transport costs (to get to a treatment centre) that need to be paid for (Patel & Kleinman 2003). As mental disorder is often chronic, these costs may be ongoing. In addition, in many countries, insurance payouts for mental disorder are limited (even discriminatory relative to other health problems). Thus, health care may become even less accessible and less available with time—and so the condition deteriorates and the need for care increases. The result of this cycle is often a 'drift' into poverty, with little chance for a person to move back to their pre-mental disorder life situation.

Being ill with any condition can be psychologically debilitating. This is exacerbated if one is forced out of work by one's condition and one has to become dependent on others. But when this condition is also quite frightening to oneself and one sometimes feels out of control, when the condition is shrouded in stigma, where blame is often put on the ill person themselves and where appropriate treatment is not readily available (WHO 2001), the condition can become psychologically devastating to the individual concerned.

For families too, having a person develop and live with mental disorder, can be frightening, extremely disruptive, and a major economic burden. Especially where information and support are not available, family members may be inclined to just want to get rid of the person or to restrain or seclude them. Families too often become the object of discrimination. It has been found that carers who provide someone with substantial support are twice as likely to have mental health problems as those they are caring for (Singleton *et al.* 2007).

In many countries, access to and knowledge of treatment is so poor that it is only when the ill person becomes so disruptive in their family and community and they can no longer be dealt with, that help is sought. At this point, the patient is often unwilling or unable to cooperate and so involuntary care and treatment is required. Poor service accessibility hence results in higher proportions of people receiving care without their consent than would otherwise be the case.

Ideology of health

There is no health without mental health. This seemingly simple assertion, which flows directly from the WHO definition of health, contains a number of important inter-related meanings and has major practical implications for health and health services. Firstly, any reference to health or ill-health or any health condition invariably includes a mental health component. Hence, where a person has developed or contracted a 'physical' disease (communicable or non-communicable), or has even been physically injured, there is usually also a mental aspect that needs consideration. This is important—whether mental health may have been a risk factor of the presenting problem (for example, depression underlying risky sex behaviour resulting in HIV/AIDS or an alcohol problem resulting in a car accident), or is a secondary outcome. Mental health should thus be integral to *all* health assessments and treatment. Secondly, the assertion implies that a state of optimal health also implies a state of optimal mental health. Initiatives directed at attaining good population health should thus include considerations of mental health. Thirdly, if a state of health includes both physical and mental health, then clearly there can be no 'health' if mental disorder is present. Attending to mental health problems should therefore have parity with regard to treatment and prevention of physical conditions. Finally, following from the above points, health policy, health systems, and health service development should always include a mental health component. Hence, there should not only be no health without mental health, but no health *service* that does not provide mental health. Brundtland, a previous Director-General of the WHO, commented that 'talking about health without mental health is a little like tuning an instrument and leaving a few discordant notes' (WHO 2001).

The highly complex nature of human beings involves interacting biological, social, and *mental* components, and to accurately understand and improve human health, all three elements, and the interactions between them, need focus (WHO 2001). Critically, human beings are not mechanical automatons that 'break down' from time to time, but are dynamic and active beings that substantially shape their own state of health and illness. For example, a person's eating habits, the amount of exercise they do, whether they avoid dangerous situations such as drinking and driving or having unsafe sex, and whether they take the medication that is prescribed and in the manner instructed, and whether they seek health care at an early stage of an illness are all fundamental to healthy human states and rely irrevocable on human agency—though decisions are often not taken at a conscious level and are often made without adequate information. People may also be limited in what they can do by their socioeconomic conditions.

Clearly then, mental factors, including personal volition and individual behaviour, are as important to states of health as are biological and social factors. Importantly though, mental states do not have an independent existence from the biological and the social and are in themselves shaped in interaction with these elements. Similarly, the mental states shape the biological and the social components. Hence, while it is useful to theoretically separate out the 'contributors' to health, this is an analytic exercise rather than an empirical one. The interacting process between the components begins at birth and stops only at death. Yet, despite this 'empowering' people to make 'healthy' decisions is seldom seen as an important health intervention (Peterson & Swartz 2002).

In addition to the impacts on health through behaviour, as previously seen, physical and mental states of well-being mutually affect each other (see the section 'Interrelationship between physical and mental health').

Mental disorders, like other health problems, also have physical, psychological, and social components. Hence, in treating and preventing mental disorder, all three components must also be considered. The mental aspect of health probably captures that which is 'most human' in health and without which much of human health care may be likened to veterinary medicine. Considering human health without mental health then is fundamentally flawed, and health policy, systems, and services that neglect the 'mental' side will inevitably be less effectual in improving the health status of populations than those that include mental health.

Cost effectiveness of treatment for mental disorders

The economic costs associated with mental disorder are considerable. Conservative estimates across the 15 countries of the European Union found mental health costs to be at least 3–4 per cent of gross national product. The majority of costs occur outside the health sector, being due to lost employment, absenteeism, poor performance, and premature retirement (McDaid 2005). These costs account for between 60 per cent and 80 per cent of the total economic impact. Millions of working days are lost because of mental health. In France, in 2000, nearly 32 million working days were lost due to depression alone. Though estimates are not available from lower-income countries it is likely that the costs of mental disorders as a proportion of the overall economy are also high (WHO 2001).

Given the high estimates of the burden of mental disorders and cost-effective treatments available (see the subsection 'Treatment efficacy'), Hyman *et al.* calculated the burden that could be averted by efficacious treatment for schizophrenia, bipolar disorder, depression, and panic disorder. A model was developed that included giving no treatment at all, current treatment, and scaled-up treatment. The model derived the number of additional healthy years gained (equivalent with DALYs averted) each year compared with the outcome of no treatment at all (Hyman *et al.* 2006). In Table 9.7.6, the estimated costs and effects of a package consisting of a basic mental health services for the four conditions is outlined. The authors estimate that the benefit of this package would be an annual reduction of 2000–3000 DALYs per million population at a cost of US$3 million to US$9 million (that is US$3–4 per capita in sub-Saharan Africa and South Asia, and US$7–9 per capita in Latin America and the Caribbean). This means that for every US$1 million invested in such a mental health package, 350–700 healthy years of life would be gained over no intervention.

However, even if healthy life years could be gained, how affordable would such mental health interventions be? When set against the gross domestic product per capita, the WHO have found that:

- The interventions recommended in the package for depression and anxiety can be considered very cost-effective. Each healthy year gained costs less than one year of average per capita income.
- Older anti-psychotic and mood-stabilizing drugs as part of community-based interventions can be considered moderately cost-effective for severe mental disorders. Each healthy year gained costs less than three times average income.
- Atypical anti-psychotic drugs at current international prices, especially if delivered in hospital based settings, are not cost-effective in the context of most low- and middle-income countries as each healthy year gained costs significantly more than three times average annual income.

While mental health interventions do not compare favourably in terms of the above affordability criteria with health actions such as vaccinations or tuberculosis control, the WHO estimates that there is just as much economic justification for mental health care as there is for anti-retroviral therapy for AIDS, glycaemic control of diabetes, and cholesterol control with statins (WHO 2006b).

Mental health systems and services

Two critical reasons for poor mental health status of populations is that people do not receive care when they need it (care is not available or accessible) and when treatment is provided it is not given effectively or efficiently. These problems can primarily be attributed to inadequate and inappropriate health systems and services for the delivery of mental health, though personal and social reasons (such as stigma) also inhibit good care.

Brief historical overview of mental health services

Different cultures have viewed mental illness from vastly different perspectives, and hence there has not been one history of mental health care but many highly diverse examples. Still today, the provision of mental health services is often based on misunderstandings about the causes, consequences, and treatment of people with mental disorders. According to Tyrer *et al.*, some of the earliest reports of 'madness' date back to the Anglo-Saxon period where it was generally thought that people exhibiting symptoms of mental disorder were possessed by the devil (Tyrer & Steinberg 1998). Accordingly, the treatment, when available, centred around the practice of exorcism. Those that were not afforded this 'luxury of leniency' were either left to wander aimlessly in a neglected state or were punished by being chained up, beaten, or ultimately burned at stake. In medieval times, in the United Kingdom, there was a shift towards acknowledging that the mad were in fact ill and were treated together with other people who were ill.

Table 9.7.6 Estimated costs and effects of a package consisting of basic mental health services, by region

	Sub-Saharan Africa	Latin America, Caribbean	Middle East, North Africa	Europe, Central Asia	South Asia	East Asia, Asia-Pacific
Total effect (DALYs averted per year per 1 million population)						
Schizophrenia: older antipsychotic drug plus psychosocial treatment	254	373	364	353	300	392
Bipolar; older mood-stabilizing drug plus psychosocial treatment	312	365	322	413	346	422
Depression: proactive care with newer antidepressant drug (SSRI; generic)	1174	1953	1806	1789	1937	1747
Panic disorder: newer antidepressant drug (SSRI; generic)	245	307	287	307	284	330
Total effect of interventions	1985	2998	2779	2862	2867	2891
Total cost (US$ million per year per 1 million population)						
Schizophrenia: older antipsychotic drug plus psychosocial treatment	0.47	1.81	1.61	1.32	0.52	0.75
Bipolar; older mood-stabilizing drug plus psychosocial treatment	0.48	1.80	1.23	1.39	0.62	0.95
Depression: proactive care with newer antidepressant drug (SSRI; generic)	1.80	4.80	3.99	3.56	2.81	2.59
Panic disorder: newer antidepressant drug (SSRI; generic)	0.15	0.27	0.21	0.23	0.16	0.20
Total effect of interventions	2.9	8.7	7	6.5	4.1	4.5
Cost-effectiveness (DALYs averted per US$1 million expenditure)						
Schizophrenia: older antipsychotic drug plus psychosocial treatment	544	206	226	267	574	
Bipolar; older mood-stabilizing drug plus psychosocial treatment	647	203	262	298	560	
Depression: proactive care with newer antidepressant drug (SSRI; generic)	652	407	452	502	690	
Panic disorder: newer antidepressant drug (SSRI; generic)	1588	1155	1339	1350	1765	

Source: Adapted from Hyman *et al.* (2006).

In traditional Chinese medicine, mental disorders were considered, in the same way as physical disorders, to be due to imbalances in the internal organs. The treatment of mental illness was aimed at restoring physiological function and balance (Chang *et al.* 2002). Specialized treatment for the mentally ill was introduced to China by foreign missionaries in the late 1800s, with the establishment of the first asylums. According to Chang *et al.* in the 1950s, the health of the people of China became symbolically intertwined with the health of the new regimen with psychiatric treatment linked with achieving the goals of the 'collective good' and assisting the patient to fulfill his or her prescribed role in society. Unique models have since developed taking into account the cultural, social, political and resource factors in the country. For example the 'Shanghai model' involves inter alia community mental health networks that provide follow-up and rehabilitation in the community. Rehabilitation is implemented through guardianship networks consisting of trained volunteers who supervise individual patients, maintain treatment schedules and provide family support (Chang *et al.* 2002).

Meanings given to behaviour and the resultant intervention is also well illustrated through examination of 'bizarre' behavioural symptoms in isiZulu-speaking communities in South Africa. The syndromes of '*amafufunyana*' and '*ukuthwasa*' are relatively common, and the 'symptoms' of both overlap with ICD 10 and DSM IVTR schizophrenia and other psychotic disorders (Niehaus *et al.* 2004). However, these conditions are understood very differently from allopathic interpretations of mental disorder, and indeed from each other. *Ukuthwasa* is understood as a form of ancestor possession that signifies a calling to become a healer. By removing herself (it is usually a women) to live with a healer/teacher and become a healer herself, the *Thwasa* sufferer is able to overcome the symptoms. On the other hand, *amafufunyana* is caused by spirit possession. Rituals to appease the ancestors usually need to be performed to rid the person of the cause of the usually uncontrollable behaviour exhibited.

The first documented moves to treat people with mental illness in segregated facilities in the United Kingdom was at the turn of the fifteenth century, when the first hospital for the treatment of people with mental illness was set up—Bethlem Hospital. In Europe, during the eighteenth and nineteenth centuries, people with mental illness were moved to large asylums that were built for this purpose. This trend was later exported to Africa, the Americas, and Asia (WHO 2001). The initial aims of these asylums were therapeutic but soon turned into impersonal institutions (Tyrer & Steinberg 1998). At the peak of institutional care in the mid-twentieth century, hundreds of thousands of people were kept in institutions. In the United Kingdom and the United States alone, there were 1 55 000 and 5 59 000 people in asylums, respectively (Hafner & an der Heiden 1989).

In the mid-twentieth century, there was a major ideological and organizational shift away from large institutions towards more community-based care and treatment. Many reasons have been given for this change including the introduction of neuroleptics in the mid-1950s; fiscal considerations (institutional care was seen as expensive); sociological criticisms and an increase in human rights advocacy and the anti-psychiatry movement (Tyrer & Steinberg 1998; Prior 1991; Drew & Funk 2006). It is likely that all of these factors played some role. In any event, in countries that had very high asylum bed to population ratios, significant decreases of bed numbers occurred.

Probably the most radical example of the move away from large mental asylums occurred in Italy. In 1978, 'Psichiatrica Democratica' under the leadership of Franco Basaglia came to fruition through Law 180. The law stated that no patient could be admitted to existing psychiatric asylums and demanded that all chronic patients be gradually discharged from hospital. All existing psychiatric hospitals were to be unlocked and the civil liberties of patients returned to them. Provision was made for 15 beds (maximum) in general hospitals. Importantly, the pressures that brought the changes came predominantly from community groups. The fact that this reform was a social movement towards integrating and accepting the mentally ill into the community distinguishes this experience from any other deinstitutionalization and remains a central ingredient of the Italian success (Scheper-Hughes & Lovell 1986).

All the above examples illustrate how the social and political environment and the cultural meanings ascribed to mental disorder have shaped and continue to shape the treatment and care approach.

Current mental health services

Formal mental health services in many parts of the world, especially in poorer countries, are characterized by poor accessibility, inadequate resources, and far from optimal organization of services. Most people with mental disorders do not have medical care for their conditions (Funk *et al.* 2005). Many people rely on traditional remedies and traditional healers for their mental health care.

Availability of mental health professionals is a major inhibitor to treatment. Table 9.7.7 shows the median number of psychiatrists, psychiatric nurses, and psychologists working in mental health per 1 00 000 population per region (WHO 2005).

People with mental disorders often access health care in large isolated mental health institutions. A disproportionate proportion of most country's mental health budget is spent in these institutions (WHO 2001). However, in Table 9.7.8, it can be seen that despite significant discharge of patients from psychiatric hospitals in higher-income countries and a concomitant development of community mental health services, there are still far more beds per capita in high-income than in lower-income countries. Hence, though the vast majority of mental health resources in low- and middle-income countries are indeed spent on psychiatric hospitals, these facilities still have far fewer beds per 10 000 population than is available in higher-income countries. Though for low- and middle-income countries, moving resources out of psychiatric hospitals is a necessity as additional resources for much needed mental health care in the community is often not available, reduction of bed numbers is from an already very low base.

Table 9.7.7 Median number of mental health professionals per 1 00 000 population in WHO regions

Region	Psychiatrists	Psychiatric nurses	Psychologists
Africa	0.04	0.2	0.05
Americas	2	2.6	2.8
Eastern Mediterranean	0.95	1.25	0.6
Europe	9.8	24.8	3.1
Southeast Asia	0.2	0.1	0.03
Western Pacific	0.32	0.5	0.03
World	1.2	2	0.6

Source: WHO Mental Health Atlas 2005 (WHO 2005).

Accessibility of services

There are a number of reasons why access to services may be limited. Here we consider only two issues: Geographical and financial access.

Geographical accessibility

Primary care is usually the first access point for people needing health care. Many countries have put considerable effort into providing health care as near to people's homes or places of work as possible through initiatives such as community or village health worker programmes and the expansion of health posts and clinics to underserved areas. Health posts or clinics have extended their hours to make it easier for working people to access and to treat people when they fall ill outside of normal working hours. However, many (if not most) of these primary care initiatives have not included mental health.

Table 9.7.8 Hospital beds for mental disorder for WHO regions

Region	Median hospital beds for mental disorder per 10 000 population	Per cent of beds in mental hospitals
Africa	0.34	73%
Americas	2.6	80.6%
Eastern Mediterranean	1.07	83%
Europe	8	63.5%
Southeast Asia	0.33	82.7%
Western Pacific	1.06	60.1%
World	1.69	68.6%

Source: WHO Mental Health Atlas 2005 (WHO 2005).

The principle of 'no health without mental health' has not been applied. Some of the reasons put forward regarding why mental health has not been included are that health workers are not trained or supported to do mental health interventions, staff do not have time for mental health and reluctance and fear amongst health workers to see people with mental health problems due to the 'otherness' of mental health. Similarly, most general hospitals do not admit and treat people with mental health problems. Staff at general hospitals are often reluctant to admit people with mental health problems into the general wards as patients with mental disorder are perceived as being disruptive (and sometimes are) and no dedicated psychiatric wards have been set up.

Poor accessibility at primary care and general hospital levels forces people to either not receive care at all or to try and access care at a centralized psychiatric hospital. However, because of the work pressures that people at the psychiatric institutions are under and because the hospital is usually designated as a 'specialist' level, even if the patient does manage to get to the hospital, they are often turned away as the hospital has many more severe cases that have to be dealt with. The outcome of the limited primary care service is that the less severe problems become more severe. When this occurs, the patient may finally receive care at the psychiatric hospital (but by this time often as an involuntary patient). Then, because of the distance of the hospital from the community, family and other community members may not be able to visit the patient, and the patient may lose contact with them. Moreover, if hospitalization has become necessary because the person became disruptive, the family and community often do not want the individual back when they do recover. In many countries, there are no community facilities for the person to be (down) referred to; hence, the progression that started when the person could not access primary or general hospital care continues with the individual becoming a chronic patient in the institution. The alienation of this experience then psychologically 'institutionalizes' them, and discharge becomes even more difficult. Early and accessible care may have prevented this progression with minimal harm to the person concerned and would have been considerably less expensive to the state!

Financial accessibility

Different countries have different policies on the financing of health care and mental health care in particular. Where mental health services are not free, this has critical consequences for accessibility. It will be shown (see the section 'Understanding the determinants of mental health') that many people who need mental health services are poor, and even if they did not start that way, many drift into poverty. In addition, because many mental health conditions are chronic, health expenses tend to be relatively high. For an individual, ongoing medication and occasional hospitalization may be required.

Moreover, especially where mental health care is not obtainable at a local level (but also then), there may be a number of additional costs for the individual and their family. For example, transport to the facility to get medication and review may be prohibitive. Furthermore, because of their condition, the patient may need to be accompanied to the place they receive care. The accompanying person would then also endure transport costs, they may also have to take leave from their employment to accompany the patient, both the patient and the person accompanying them may need to buy food and so forth. As a result of these expenses, the person may be denied access to mental health care. As in the geographical accessibility scenario, the consequences of not accessing treatment due to no finances is often 'false economy', as the person may land up in expensive and long-term care.

Pyramid of services—an optimal mix for mental health

WHO have put forward a 'pyramid of services' (Fig. 9.7.2) that provides an optimal mix of services required by people with mental disorders (Funk *et al.* 2004). This model is based on the premise that no single service can meet all mental health needs. In fact, without

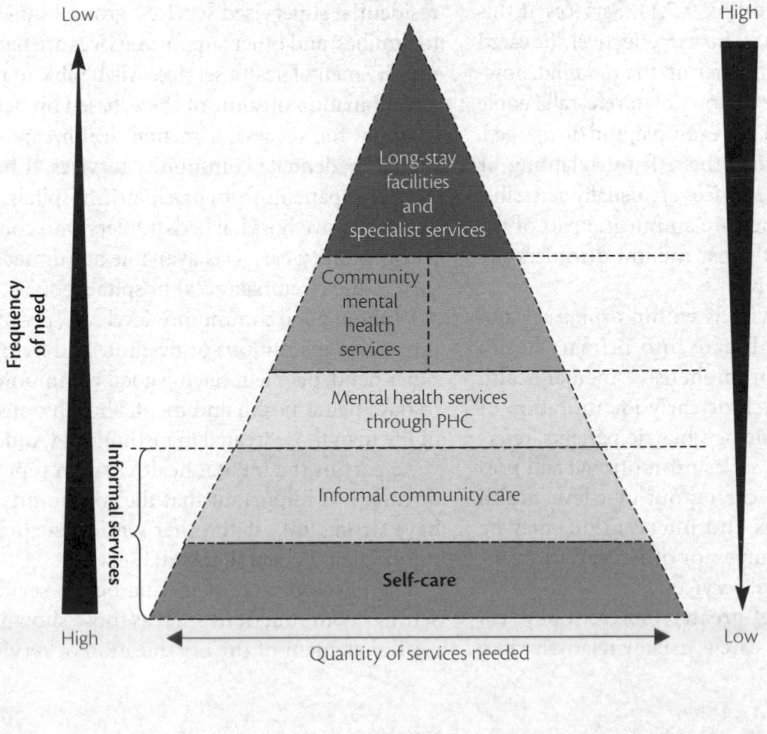

Fig. 9.7.2 Optimal mix of services.
Source: Funk et al. (2004).

Box 9.7.1 Examples of providers of informal community mental health services (WHO 2003)

- Traditional healers
- Village of community workers
- Family members
- Self-help and other user groups
- Advocacy services
- Lay volunteers providing parental and youth education on mental health issues and screening for mental disorders (including suicidal tendencies) in clinics and schools
- Religious leaders proving health information on trauma reactions in complex emergencies
- Day care services provided by relatives, neighbours, or retired members of local communities
- Humanitarian aid workers in complex emergencies

any one of these service levels, and referrals up and down the pyramid, the 'system' breaks down, and the other parts are unable to function effectively and efficiently.

At the bottom of the pyramid, and where most care is provided, is *self-care*. Most people can manage their own mental health problems themselves or with help from family or friends. However to facilitate the autonomy and ability of people to care for themselves, the health service or non-governmental organizations need to provide information to people. This should be available and accessible to all people through, for example radio shows or pamphlets that are distributed in languages and literacy levels that people understand.

Informal community mental health services are services provided in the community but that are not part of the formal health and welfare system. Examples of this are traditional healers, professionals in other sectors such as teachers, police, village health workers, services provided by non-governmental organizations, user and family associations, lay-persons, and so forth (see Box 9.7.1). Services at this level are important in preventing people who can effectively be cared for at this level from making demands further up the pyramid, however it is also an extremely important level for 'down referral'. People who may have been treated in a hospital, for example, and discharged, often need informal support to prevent them from relapsing or needing care at a higher level. Informal services are usually accessible and acceptable to the community as they are an integral part of the community. It can be seen then that most mental disorders are dealt with outside of the medical system.

The first 'formal' mental health service is within *primary health care*. The integration of mental health care into primary health services is a critical component of comprehensive mental health care. Essential services at this level include early identification of mental disorders, management of stable psychiatric patients, referral to other levels where required, as well as promotional and prevention activities. Depending on who carries out first-level health care in a particular country, activities and interventions may be carried out by general practitioners, nurses, or other staff that provide assessment, treatment, and referral services.

Mental health services at this level greatly increases physical accessibility as first-level general health care is usually relatively close to where people live. In addition, the person can be treated as a whole person who may have co-morbid physical and mental health problems. We have previously emphasized the importance of interacting physical and mental health problems. Seeking and receiving treatments part of a general health care is also often less stigmatizing for an individual, especially where having a mental disorder is regarded as shameful. Services are therefore more acceptable to users than having to be treated in a psychiatric facility. From a clinical perspective, it has been found that most common mental disorders can be treated at primary care level. In situations where there are few trained mental health practitioners, an integrated approach substantially increases the chances of being treated for mental disorders.

Integration of mental health into primary health care requires careful training and supervision of staff. Staff needs to be equipped with knowledge and skills that enable them to provide mental health care through training provided as part of initial health worker training as well as ongoing in-service training (WHO 2003). Additionally, they have to be adequately supervised and supported. Health workers often feel ill-equipped and reluctant to undertake mental health in addition to other health care and so ongoing assistance is essential. Critically too, where psychotropic medication is needed, this must be available at this level. This means that these drugs need to become an integral part of the supply, storage, and distribution chain and provision must be made for the prescription of necessary drugs at this level.

Where there is no integrated first-level care, addition pressures are put on the higher levels of care. People are inappropriately referred to levels of care that should be dealing with more complex problems and where there is no early identification of problems, treatment or prevention, and promotion, more people become seriously ill and need to be treated at the higher levels.

The next level of the pyramid has two complementary components, the first is *formal community mental health services* and the second is *mental health services in general hospitals*.

In addition to the informal services that are commonly provided in communities for people with mental disorder, additional formal community services such as day centres, rehabilitation services, hospital diversion programmes, mobile crisis teams, therapeutic and residential supervised services, group homes, home help, assistance to families, and other support services are needed. While not all community mental health services will be able to provide all these services, a combination of some of these, based on needs and requirements, is essential for successful mental health care. Where there are no or highly inadequate community services, it becomes very difficult to discharge patients from psychiatric hospitals, thus 'clogging up' scarce and expensive hospital beds. Others who could avoid hospitalization if community care was available are unnecessarily (though necessary in the circumstances) hospitalized.

Without good community-level care, people often land up either in inhumane institutions or destitute and living on the streets. On the other hand, people receiving good community care have been shown to have better health and mental health outcomes and better quality of life than those treated in institutions (Anderson *et al.* 1993).

As part of the mental health system represented by the pyramid of care, it is important that the community mental health services have strong links with other services such as the primary care and informal and general hospital services.

The development of mental health services in general hospital settings with functions such as those shown in Box 9.7.2 is another critical element of the organization of services. Given the nature of

Box 9.7.2 Mental health services offered in general hospitals (WHO 2003)

- Acute inpatient care
- Crisis stabilization care
- Partial (day/night) hospital programmes
- Consultation/liaison services for general medical patients
- Intensive/planned outpatient programme
- Respite care
- Expert consultation/support/training for primary care services
- Multidisciplinary psychiatric teams linked with other local and provincial sectors (schools, employers, correctional services, welfare) and non-governmental organizations in intersectoral prevention and promotion initiatives
- Specialized units/wards for persons with specific mental disorders and for related rehabilitation programmes

mental disorders, for a number of people some hospitalization at some time (or times) during acute phases of their condition will be necessary. As with integrated primary mental health care, mental health care in general hospitals is more accessible and acceptable than in dedicated psychiatric hospitals. In any country, especially low- and middle-income countries, there are likely to be only a few dedicated psychiatric hospitals and these are usually situated in urban areas—albeit often somewhere out of town. These hospitals are very often not geographically or financially accessible to patients or families wishing to visit them (see the subsection 'Accessibility of services'). There is also often high stigma associated with these facilities which are often the butt of highly discriminatory jokes or references. While clearly the issues of stigma needs to be directly dealt with, until such time as stigma around mental disorder and particularly psychiatric hospitals does change, most people prefer to get treatment in a general hospital. Any co-morbid conditions can also more easily be treated, and special investigations can be conducted.

At the peak of the pyramid, providing services at the highest cost to the least number of people are *long-stay facilities and specialist services.*

A small minority of people with mental disorders require more specialist care than can be provided at general hospital level. Especially in low- and middle-income countries, where there are very few mental health professionals, and certainly not enough highly skilled people to be available in every general hospital, it is necessary to refer people with therapy-resistant or complex presentations to specialized mental health centres—or hospitals where mental health specialists are available. Moreover, a small group of people require ongoing nursing care in a residential facility due to their mental disorder. This, however, is a far cry from 'old style' mental institutions.

Psychiatric institutions have a history of serious human rights violations, poor clinical outcomes, and inadequate rehabilitation programmes. They are also costly and consume a disproportionate proportion of mental health expenditure. The WHO have thus recommended replacing these institutions with a network of services in the community and, for the majority, care in general hospitals where hospitalization is warranted.

Understanding the determinants of mental health

Mental disorders are caused by a combination of biological, psychological and social factors (WHO 2001) and the interactions between them (see the subsection 'Interrelationship between physical and mental health'). Neuroscientists and geneticists have made significant progress regarding biological determinants of mental disorder while psychological research and insight have added substantially to our understanding of mental disorder and human behaviour. For example biochemical and morphological abnormalities of the brain associated with various disorders such as schizophrenia, autism, mood and anxiety disorders are currently being identified through postmortem analysis and noninvasive neuroimaging. Moreover, research identifying risk-conferring genes for mental disorder is underway and it seems that initial results are promising (Hyman *et al.* 2006). Furthermore, improved understanding of the structure and functioning of the brain has led to major advances in psychotropic medications. From a psychological perspective, comprehensive explanations of human dysfunction and behaviour have been translated into effective therapies that improve mental health status.

While all health is determined by biological, psychological, and social factors, in various respects, the aetiology of mental disorder is even more complex than for many physical disorders. The balance between the three domains is often weighted differently for mental health than physical heath with a stronger influence of psychological and social factors. Moreover, cultural differences (including different belief systems regarding the causes of disease and how they can be cured), language, and power relations between provider and patient are also often different when a disorder manifests 'mentally' rather than physically. Stigma is another major public health concern that most disorders do not carry to the same extent as mental disorders do. All these impact on the course and outcome of mental disorders. In the following section, we look primarily at the social determinants of mental (ill) health, as these are of the most specific concern to public mental health.

Social determinants of mental (ill) health

Research in mental health has tended to focus more on the psychological or the biological determinants of mental ill-health than the social determinants. This has led to an imbalanced focus on the use of biomedical interventions and/or a focus on treating the individual to the neglect of altering aspects of the wider social environment. Part of the reason for this imbalance in focus relates to the real difficulties in altering the social environment (especially the macro social environment) since, quite often, these are not within the control of public health practitioners. However, redressing this imbalance can make a highly significant contribution to public health or public mental health and in improving social development.

In this section, we examine four critical ways through which an understanding of the social determinants of mental health can improve public mental health.

1. Careful and scientific documentation of social and economic determinants informs mental health service planning.

Planners of mental health services need to know the extent of mental disorders within a country and whether there are differences between groups of people, but they also need to know what the reasons for these differences are. In addition, they need to be aware of particular 'vulnerable' groups so that they can put in appropriate prevention programmes where possible, identify problems at an early stage and/or allocate resources where they are most needed.

For example, poor and deprived people have a high incidence of mental and behavioural disorders (WHO 2001). Whether this is due to the impacts of poverty on the poor or to a 'drift' of the mentally ill into poverty is often debated, but in all likelihood both are true and in fact they are inextricable.

Patel and Kleinman reviewed 11 studies that examined the relationship between poverty and common mental disorders (Patel & Kleinman 2003). They found that the mean prevalence rates of depression and anxiety disorders varied between 20 per cent and 30 per cent with almost all studies showing a significant relationship between prevalence and various indicators of poverty. The association between poverty and common mental disorders was found to occur in all societies regardless of their levels of development, however they found no 'absolute level' that could be correlated with mental disorder.

Severe mental disorders such as schizophrenia are also highest in people living in lowest socioeconomic circumstances. Saraceno and Barbui showed that people with the lowest SES have eight times higher relative risk for schizophrenia than those in the highest SES groups (Saraceno & Barbui 1997).

Poverty cannot be said to 'cause' mental disorder as most people living in poverty do not have a mental disorder, however it does increase the risk of developing a mental disorder. Poverty and common mental disorders interact with one another in setting up a vicious cycle of poverty and mental illness (Saraceno & Barbui 1997). People are simply more likely to develop mental disorders in conditions of poverty. Moreover the ability of the person to confront or overcome their poverty condition, including getting treatment, is exacerbated if the person has a mental disorder, thus a 'vicious' cycle of poverty/mental health is created.

Access to treatment and rehabilitation is profoundly affected by poverty. People who can afford treatment, whose family members are able to support them financially and emotionally, who can go to rehabilitation therapy, have access to housing, job opportunities, and so forth have a considerable recovery advantage. Where a person has minimal financial means they often put an additional financial and emotional burden on the family. The need to plan services directed at people in poverty is evident.

Another example of how an understanding of social determinants can assist intervention planning is in conflict and post-conflict situations. Wars have significant mental health impacts on both soldier and civilian populations. Baingana *et al.* report that conflicts cause widespread insecurity due to forced displacement, sudden destitution, the break-up of families and communities, collapsed social structures and breakdown in the rule of law and may last even after the conflicts have ended (Baingana *et al.* 2005). People in war situations may also have experienced or witnessed killings, injuries, or amputations and gender-based violence. In addition, displaced peoples, whether internally or as refugees in other countries often have difficulties adjusting to losses incurred and the new circumstances they find themselves in. Symptoms of mental dysfunction associated with conflicts include sleeplessness, fear, nervousness, anger, aggression, depression, flashbacks, alcohol and substance abuse, suicide, and domestic and sexual violence (Baingana *et al.* 2005). Increased rates of PTSD and depression have consistently been found (Murthy & Lakshminarayana 2006). Most recently, Hoge *et al.* (2004) found that soldiers returning from combat in Afghanistan were more likely to have self-reported alcohol abuse problems than pre-deployment troops, while soldiers serving in Iraq had significantly higher rates of depression, anxiety, and PTSD than either troops that had not been deployed or were deployed in Afghanistan (Hoge *et al.* 2004). Differences between the troops in Iraq and Afghanistan were attributed to the higher direct combat exposure in Iraq.

Studies examining impacts on non-combatants has increased significantly in the past two decades. Table 9.7.9 summarizes studies that have addressed this issue.

Research has clearly demonstrated that war is a major social determinant of poor mental health. Although there is little that public health experts can do to prevent or stop wars, an important public mental health contribution that can be made is to assist the planning of services for people who require help as a result of the impacts of war.

2. Programmes for prevention of mental disorder and promotion of mental health can be organized around the information and knowledge about social determinants of mental health.

The mental health impacts of major social determinants of mental ill health can, to some extent at least, be mitigated through understanding these causes in a nuanced way and adapting interventions based on evidence from public health research. In their review of mental health and poverty, Patel and Kleinman (2003) showed that mental health was related to income insecurity including fear of losing employment, drop in income, and fear of land loss. High levels of hopelessness mediated by shame, stigma, and the humiliation of poverty were also found to decrease people's psychological ability to cope. Some evidence was also found that social change through changing lifestyles, shifts from rural to urban areas, and lack of social support linked to change played an important role in the development of common mental disorders. The factor that they found had the most consistent relationship with poor mental health was low education. This level of information can be used to prevent mental health problems developing.

Taking the need for social support as an example of risk for the development of common mental disorder, it is highly feasible for public mental health practitioners to identify poor and vulnerable individuals and assist them in accessing support. In situations of rapid urbanization, for instance, many people lose contact with their support systems and often also their cultural roots and practices. Simply organizing get-togethers of people with similar backgrounds and providing transport can be highly cost effective from a mental health perspective but may also enable people who, because of their poor mental health status were unable to become economically productive, to more easily engage in work activities.

Helping people to acquire economic security has been shown to improve psychological well-being. The non-governmental organization BRAC in Bangladesh has developed programmes for poverty alleviation targeting credit facilities, gender equity, basic health care, nutrition, education, and human rights. By, amongst other things, alleviating the stress of being indebted to informal moneylenders, the mental health of many women has been improved (Chowdhury & Bhuiya 2001).

Providing literacy to women is another example where it has been shown that mental health can be promoted through social interventions. Cohen has demonstrated that providing women with information about and ideas from wider worlds, and by empowering them through literacy, it was possible to increase their sense of pride, self-worth, and purpose, and they were more able to exercise greater control of their lives (Cohen 2002).

Table 9.7.9 Impacts of non-combatants of war†

Country/territories/areas	Population surveyed	Results
Afghanistan*	Adult household members aged 15 and above. 62% had experienced at least four trauma events in previous 10 years	Depression—67.7% Anxiety—72.2% PTSD—42%
Afghanistan*	Adults 15 and over. Nearly half had experienced traumatic events	Depression—38.5% Anxiety—51.8% PTSD—20.4%
Cambodia*	Adults in displaced persons camp	Depression—55% PTSD—15%
Cambodia*	Young people traumatized at ages 8–12 followed up 3 years later	Depression—41% PTSD—48%
Iraq*	Kurdish families in camps	PTSD in children—87% in caregivers—60%
Israel*	Subjects exposed to war-related trauma	At least one PTSD symptom—76.7% Acute stress disorder—9.4%
Kenya**	Internally displaced people	PTSD—80.2%
Kosovo*	Adults 15 and over	PTSD—17.1%
Lebanon*	Adults 18–65 in communities exposed to war	Major depression—16.3–41.9%
Rwanda*	Community-based sample	PTSD—24.8%
Sri Lanka*	Civilian population	Somatization—41% PTSD—27% Anxiety disorder—26% Major depression—25%
Uganda	Civilian population	Depression—52% Anxiety—60% PTSD—39.9%
West Bank and Gaza Strip*	10–19-year-old children	97.5% had varying levels of PTSD
West Nile region**	Refugees	PTSD—male 31.6% —female 40.1%

* Extracted from Murthy and Lakshminarayana (2006).
** Extracted from Njenga *et al.* (2006).
† Neither the methods utilized nor the ages of respondents are standardized across these studies. This figure is thus not intended to give cross-country comparisons, but rather illustrates prevalence found in different studies.

3. Associations and impacts on mental health can be utilized by politicians, economists, and activists to *advocate* for social change.

The evidence for social determinants having negative mental health impacts alone is unlikely to bring about large social changes. However, when considered together with other reasons for change, the evidence for mental health impacts can add significant weight to arguments for change and can be constructively utilized in advocacy for change. A good example to illustrate this is in the field of women's mental health.

Women have around a 1:1.5 or 1: 2 times higher levels of depression than men. While some variation is no-doubt attributable to biological factors, for example, in the case of post-natal depression, the social role that women play in most societies is critical. Freeman comments that the traditional role of women as primarily the bearers and rearers of children, inferior and obedient to men (socially and sexually), whose productive labour has been within the household and without power in social and political decisions, leaves many women feeling disempowered, dehumanized, and without dignity. Without an internal sense of worth, power, and value, many women withdraw into a depressed existence (Freeman 2007). He remarks further that even where there have been changes in labour market roles for women, rather than meaning equality with men it has usually resulted in women having to do 'double work shift'—that is, work both at home and in formal employment. Often without recognition, and even censure from the male partner for not carrying out domestic duties adequately, this often results in severe psychological and physical stress. Given traditional gender roles, working-women may also experience guilt about neglecting their children—leading to further stress and internal conflict. Added to this are high levels of domestic violence. The impacts of abuse, especially in the longer term, are often more sorely experienced on a psychological than a physical level. Undoubtedly, gender discrimination and violence towards women have serious negative impacts on women's mental health.

Analysis of gender discrimination and its consequences reveals numerous economic, social, and health reasons for change. However, the additional fact and evidence for increased prevalence of mental health problems as a result of gender discrimination provides more convincing evidence and reasons which politicians and activists could use in efforts to attain gender equity.

4. Information on social determinants provides the necessary information and impetus for authorities outside of health, that have an indirect responsibility with respect to health, to act accordingly.

Public mental health practitioners do not often have the means to bring about changes to improve mental health; however, they have the information necessary to inform authorities outside of health to make appropriate interventions. For example, because of the high correlation between mental disorder and poverty, special social programmes are usually needed. For example, people may require supported or subsidized housing or to be placed in special skills and job creation programmes or to be supported within the mainstream work environment. Public mental health practitioners have a major responsibility to communicate and persuade officials in departments outside of health to take direct responsibility for providing the necessary social support. Similar to public health practitioners who need to engage authorities involved in water and sanitation supplies to prevent physical diseases, public mental health practitioners too have an important role to play in conveying messages around social actions to be taken to improve people's mental health.

Substance abuse is both a classified disorder in itself and, according to increasing evidence, certain substances such as cannabis may be a direct cause of psychosis (Fergusson *et al.* 2002). Factors that lead individuals to abuse substances include interacting social, psychological, and biological phenomena. Controlling the use of substances and thereby preventing mental disorder thus requires complex intersectoral collaborations involving both supply and demand characteristics. Clearly, while health must care and treat abusers—which also forms part of secondary and tertiary prevention—and must lead in prevention programmes such as media campaigns, the social determinants are linked to issues such as poverty and gangsterism that must be addressed primarily outside of the health system.

Prevention and promotion in mental health

A key part of any public health programme is to prevent disease/disorder wherever possible and to promote good health. This is also true of public mental health. The WHO suggests that it is useful to conceptualize three categories of primary prevention in mental health—i.e. *universal prevention* (targeting the general public or a whole population); *selective prevention* (targeting individuals or subgroups of the population whose risk of developing a mental disorder is significantly higher than that of the rest of the population); and *indicated* prevention (targeting persons at high risk who are identified as having minimal but detectable signs or symptoms foreshadowing mental disorder or biological markers indicating predisposition for mental disorder). In addition, there should be secondary prevention (interventions to reduce the prevalence, i.e. all specific treatment-related strategies) and tertiary prevention (interventions that reduce disability and includes all forms of rehabilitation as well as prevention of relapses of the illness).

Mental health promotion usually refers to positive mental health, rather than mental ill health, whereas prevention refers to reducing the incidence, prevalence and recurrence of mental disorder. However, there is no clear line between avoiding disease and improving health and well-being. An activity aimed at promoting mental health in a population may also decrease the incidence of disorder or prevent relapse in certain people. As there are numerous determinants of health relating to the actions of individuals as well as social and environmental factors, the objectives of mental health promotion and prevention are to foster the individual, social and environmental qualities that enhance mental health and make sure that factors that may lead to mental health problems are avoided (Herrman 2001; WHO 2004).

Research evidence regarding the impacts and outcomes of promotion and prevention in mental health is somewhat limited but has grown significantly since the early 1980s. While the importance of theory, anecdotes, and personal reports in designing and assessing prevention and promotion programmes cannot be discounted, governments and donors usually need more rigorous evidence to warrant major expenditure and it is important to research, monitor and evaluate preventive interventions. The WHO has collated a number of studies that document successful mental health promotion and disorder prevention strategies (WHO 2002). Some examples of good practice are shown in Box 9.7.3. Up to now, most of the research on prevention and promotion has been conducted in high-income countries, and it is unclear to what extent many of these interventions can be transported into different cultural and economic settings. Some research though is now being conducted in less well-resourced countries. While 'prevention is better than cure' in all situations, in countries with the highest rates of mental disorder and also the least resources for treatment, the need for prevention is even more profound.

Given the close relationships between mental and physical health that have been emphasized in this chapter, not surprisingly prevention programmes can also be combined. For example, the CHAMP (Collaborative HIV/AIDS Adolescent Mental Health Project), adapted in South Africa as the AmaQhawe programme, is a developmentally-timed programme targeting pre-adolescent children and their caregivers that strengthens personal influences (such as assertive and refusal skills) and interpersonal family influences such as caregiver–child communication, caregiver warmth, and active monitoring of children, with the primary aim of reducing risky behaviour in adolescents. Through improved personal well-being and better relationships, including better communication between parents and children around sensitive issues such as sex, transmission of HIV can be reduced (Petersen & Govender 2007).

In 2007, the National Institute for Health and Clinical Excellence in the United Kingdom collated all systematic reviews, syntheses, meta-analyses, and review papers that dealt with non-pharmacological interventions aimed at promoting positive mental health and preventing disorder in adults (Taylor *et al.* 2007). Some of their key findings were:

- Following counselling within primary care, people with broad psychological and psychosocial problems showed modest improvements in psychological symptoms in the short term compared with the usual GP care—though recipients of counselling were highly satisfied with the intervention.

Box 9.7.3 Examples of mental health promotion and prevention programmes where scientific evidence of benefit had been found—adapted and selected from the WHO (WHO 2002, 2004)

For mothers during pregnancy and perinatal period

- Home visits during pregnancy and early infancy addressing factors such as maternal smoking, poor social support, parenting skills, and early child–parent interactions has shown positive health, social, and economic outcomes.
- Prenatal and postnatal visits by nurses and community workers to mothers reduced child abuse, led to better vocational adjustment, and better educational achievement in the children.
- Early monitoring of growth development by mothers, along with proper maternal advice by educators and nurses, resulted in better cognitive competence and lower behaviour problems.
- Early stimulation programmes by mothers prevented slow developmental growth in preterm infants and improved growth.
- Breastfeeding, which improves bonding and attachment, has significant benefits to child development.
- Nutrient supplements can prevent neurological impairment (e.g. salt iodization).

For children, adolescents, and schools

- Home visiting programmes for high-risk mothers can prevent child physical abuse and neglect and self-defence for school-aged children can prevent child sexual abuse.
- Self-esteem and life skills can be improved through pro-social behaviour, school based curricula, and improvement of school climate. Training teachers to improve detection of problems and facilitate appropriate intervention provides additional advantages.
- Restructuring the school environment can improve emotional and behavioural functioning of pupils.
- Aggressive behaviour and violence can be reduced through parent training, focused interventions in elementary schools, and comprehensive mental health promotion in primary and middle schools.
- Anxiety disorders can be prevented through individual- and family-based interventions with 'at risk' groups.
- Depression and hopelessness amongst adolescents can be reduced through a resilience-building school-based programme.
- Suicide can be prevented through comprehensive school-based prevention programmes. This includes changing school policy, providing teacher education, parent education, stress management, and providing life skills and a crisis team.

Adults and elderly

- Stress management programmes at work have been found to be effective in preventing adverse mental health outcomes.
- Assistance to individuals who have lost their jobs have been shown to have positive effects on rates of re-employment, quality, and pay of jobs obtained, and to reduce depression and distress.
- Awareness of mental disorder in communities can promote early help seeking behaviour and identification and treatment of severe mental disorder.
- Reducing access to the means to commit suicide is the clearest way for preventing suicide.
- Suicide can be prevented through prescription of psychotropic medicines.
- Head and other injuries can be prevented through legislation around helmets and seat belts.
- Marital and parenting counselling to couples and 'would-be' parents can prevent marital stress and child abuse and promote better parenting.
- Caregivers of people with mental disorder who were taught better coping skills showed reduced incidence of depression and somatic complaints.
- Widowed people who were supported and helped with locating community resources developed relationships quicker and showed fewer depressive symptoms.

- Workplace interventions involving either early referral to occupational health services or group-based information and role play sessions can be effective in reducing sickness absence.
- Stress-reducing interventions in the workplace, focused either on the individual or the organization, can help reduce work-related stress.
- Cognitive behavioural interventions are more effective in improving people's skills for coping than relaxation techniques.
- Family interventions where there is a member with a psychiatric disorder can have a modest positive effect on variables related to the relatives' burden of care.

- Cognitive-behavioural parenting programmes are effective in improving measures related to parental psychological health.
- Mass media campaigns, particularly those that include community activities, can have beneficial effects on attitudes towards, and knowledge of, mental health issues. They can also impact on an individual's behavioural intentions and support enhancing behaviours to improve their own well-being.
- Participation in physical activity is positively associated with mood, emotion, and psychological well-being.

Despite important developments in mental health promotion and the prevention of disorder, this is still a significant growth area for public mental health—both in terms of research that informs focused prevention and promotion programmes and interventions based on existing knowledge.

Stigma: A major public health challenge

One of the principal obstacles to mental health taking its 'rightful' place in health, is the stigma attached to it. Given that a primary goal of public health is to identify and ameliorate the causes of ill health in a population, addressing stigma is undoubtedly a critical public mental health concern. Stigma prevents people from acknowledging any mental health problem and hence seeking care and treatment; providers are reluctant to treat people with mental disorder; people with mental disorder are alienated from and discriminated against by their families and communities and many people experience rampant harassment (Berzins *et al.* 2003). Stigma from communities is an important reason for institutionalization of people with mental disorder. As a result of all these factors, the mental health status of populations is compromised.

The extent of stigma is well illustrated in the following two studies. In the United Kingdom, it was found that community respondents perceived people with schizophrenia as unpredictable (77.3 per cent) and dangerous (71.3 per cent). People with range of mental disorder were perceived as difficult to talk to (Crisp *et al.* 2000). In Nigeria, 96.5 per cent of community respondents believed that people with mental illness are dangerous. Most respondents would not tolerate even basic social contacts with a mentally person with 82.7 per cent saying they would be afraid to have a conversation with a mentally ill person and only 16.9 per cent would even consider marrying a person with mental illness (Gureje *et al.* 2005).

Public mental health has not found adequate solutions to the issue of stigma. Changing media responses, promoting the idea that mental illness is an illness like any other, and community campaigns educating populations about mental disorder have made some headway, but finding innovative ways to redress stigma of mental disorder remains a major challenge for public mental health.

Conclusion: Will greater emphasis on public mental health make a difference to global health?

It is not only conceptually incorrect to consider health without mental health, but there are major practical ramifications in neglecting the 'mental' side of health. Some of the reasons are highlighted in Box 9.7.4, and discussed below:

- There is a high prevalence of mental disorder which takes a significant toll on individuals, families, and the economy. Mental disorder has been shown to have a very significant burden socially and economically. Unipolar depression is currently ranked as carrying the fourth highest burden of all diseases and by 2030 will become the second-highest cause of all DALYs lost. It is only through concerted public health interventions that a problem of this magnitude can be addressed—especially given major human resource constraints in mental health.
- Human behaviour or agency is fundamental to health. Health promoting behaviours are dependent, to some extent at least, on healthy mental states. Moreover, the human behaviour change that is necessary to improve health of populations falls squarely in the realm of public mental health. The development of this area is critical for the health of populations.
- There are inextricable links between physical and mental health. Without adequate consideration to improving mental health, physical health is undermined, and vice versa. This applies as much to public health as to clinical health.
- Prevention of mental ill-health and prevention of mental disorder is possible. This public health approach is necessary to meaningfully improve mental health status of populations. In addition, prevention of physical diseases can benefit from promoting mental health and preventing mental disorder.
- Accessible, affordable, and acceptable mental health care requires mental health systems, and services that take account of culture, available resources, and an optimal mix of levels of care. Public mental health is needed to facilitate this.
- From health economics, we know that there are cost-effective interventions for mental health and that these are indeed affordable. This information needs to be incorporated into health care delivery.

Recognition of the role that public mental health can play in improving the health of populations is increasing. However, to fully contribute to improving health of populations, what is already known needs to be much more vigorously promoted, advocated, and implemented, and progress with regard to the many gaps still existing in public mental health research and practice needs to be advanced with some urgency.

Box 9.7.4 Five key points in public mental health

- Mental disorder has a high prevalence and burden.
- Mental disorders develop through interaction of biological, psychological, and social factors. The social factors are the least studied and understood but are critically important to improving mental health.
- Mental and physical health are inextricably linked. Health as a whole will benefit from improved mental health, and particularly public mental health interventions.
- Mental health promotion and prevention of disorder show promise, but are areas for further growth and development.
- Mental health systems development and economics have the potential to positively and substantially change the lives of people with mental disorder. However, this will require greater use of advocacy and fundamental shifts in people's attitudes (including at a political and health planning level).

References

Aaron R., Joseph A., Abraham S. *et al.* (2004). Suicides in young people in rural southern India. *Lancet,* **363**, 1117–18.

American Psychiatric Association (2000). *Diagnostic and Statistical Manual for Mental Disorders. Fourth edition. Text revision (DSM-IV-TR).* American Psychiatric Association, Washington DC.

Anderson J., Dayson D., Wills W. *et al.* (1993). The TAPS project 13: clinical and social outcomes of long-stay psychiatric patients after one year in the community. *British Journal of Psychiatry,* **162** (suppl), 45–56.

Baingana F., Bannon I., and Thomas R. (2005). *Mental Health and Conflicts: Conceptual Framework and Approaches.* World Bank, Washington.

Barsky A.J., Orav E.J., and Bates D.W. (2005). Somatization increases medical utilization and costs independent of psychiatric and medical comorbidity. *Archives of General Psychiatry,* **62**, 903–10.

Bertolote J.M., Fleischmann A., De Leo D. *et al.* (2004). Psychiatric diagnoses and suicide: revisiting the evidence. *Crisis,* **25**, 147–55.

Berzins K.M., Petch A., and Atkinson J.M. (2003). Prevalence and experience of harassment of people with mental health problems living in the community. *British Journal of Psychiatry,* **183**, 526–33.

Bing E.G., Burnam M.A., Longshore D. *et al.* (2001). Psychiatric disorders and drug use among human immunodeficiency virus-infected adults in the United States. *Archives of General Psychiatry,* **58**, 721–8.

Catalan J., Meadows J., and Douzens A. (2000). The changing pattern of mental health problems in HIV infection: the view from London. *AIDS Care,* **12**, 333–43.

Chang D., Yifeng X., Kleinman A. *et al.* (2002). Rehabilitation of Schizophrenia Patients in China: The Shanghai Model. In Cohen A., Kleinman A. and Saraceno B. *World Mental Health Casebook,* pp. 27–50. Kluwer Academic, New York.

Chowdhury A. and Bhuiya A. (2001). Do poverty alleviation programs reduce inequities in health? The Bangladesh experience. In Leon D., Walt G. eds. *Poverty, Inequality and Health.* Oxford University Press, Oxford.

Ciesla J.A. and Roberts J.E. (2001). Meta analysis of the relationship between HIV infection and risk for depressive disorders. *American Journal of Psychiatry,* **158,** 725–30.

Cohen A. (2002). 'Our Lives were Covered in Darkness': The Work of the National Literacy Mission in Northern India. In Cohen A., Kleinman A. and Saraceno B. *World Mental Health Casebook.* Kluwer Academic, New York.

Collins P., Holman A., Freeman M. *et al.* (2006). What is the relevance of mental health to HIV/AIDS care and treatment programs in developing countries? a review of the literature. *AIDS,* **20**, 1571–82.

Crisp A.H., Gelder M.G., Rix S. *et al.* (2000). Stigmatisation of people with mental illnesses. *British Journal of Psychiatry,* **177**, 4–7.

Dewey M.E. and Saz P. (2001). Dementia, cognitive impairment and mortality in persons aged 65 and over living in the community: a systematic review of the literature. *International Journal of Geriatric Psychiatry,* **16**, 751–61.

Disability Rights Commission (2006). *Equal Treatment: Closing the Gap – A formal investigation into physical health inequalities experienced by people with learning disabilities and/or mental health problems.* Disability Rights Commission, Stratford upon Avon.

Drew N. and Funk M. (2006). Commentary on The Israeli Model of the 'District Psychiatrist' A Fifty-Year Perspective. *Israel Journal of Psychiatry Related Sciences,* **43**, 189–94.

Fergusson D.M., Poulton R., Smith P.F. *et al.* (2002). Cannabis and Psychosis. *British Medical Journal,* **332**, 172–5.

Freeman M. (2007). Mental health and social change. In Visser M. *Contextualising Community Psychology in South Africa.* Van Schaik Publishers, Pretoria.

Funk M., Drew N., Saraceno B. *et al.* (2005). A framework for mental health policy, legislation and service development: addressing needs and improving services. *Harvard Health Policy Review,* **6**, 57–69.

Funk M., Saraceno B., Drew N. *et al.* (2004). Mental health policy and plans: promoting an optimal mix of services in developing countries. *International Journal of Mental Health,* **33**, 4–16.

Grant I., Marcotte T.D., and Heaton R.K. (1999). Neurocognitive complications of HIV Disease. *Psychological Science,* **10**, 191–5.

Gureje O., Lasebikan V.O., Ephraim-Oluwanuga O. *et al.* (2005). Community study of knowledge of and attitude to mental illness in Nigeria. *British Journal of Psychiatry,* **186**, 436–41.

Hafner H. and an der Heiden W. (1989). The evaluation of mental health care systems. *British Journal of Psychiatry,* **155**, 12–17.

Heilä H., Haukka J., Suvisaari J. *et al.* (2005). Mortality among patients with schizophrenia and reduced psychiatric hospital care. *Psychological Medicine,* **35**, 725–32.

Herrman H. (2001). The need for mental health promotion. *Australian and New Zealand Journal of Psychiatry,* **35**, 709–15.

Hoge C., Catro C., Messer S.C. *et al.* (2004). Combat duty in Iraq and Afghanistan: mental health problems, and barriers to care. *New England. Journal of Medicine,* **351**, 13–22.

Holt R.I., Bushe C., and Citrome L. (2005). Diabetes and schizophrenia 2005: closer to understanding the link? *Journal of Psychopharmacology,* **19** (6 Suppl), 56–65.

Hyman S., Chisholm D., Kessler R. *et al.* (2006). Mental Disorders. In 2nd ed. *Disease Control Priorities Related to Mental, Neurological, Developmental and Substance Abuse Disorders.* WHO, Geneva.

Kessler R.C., Haro J.M., Heeringa S.G. *et al.* (2006). The World Health Organization World Mental Health Survey Initiative. Editorial. *Epidemiologia e Psichiatria Sociale,* **15**, 161–6.

Kohn R., Saxena S., Levav I. *et al.* (2004). The treatment gap in mental health care. *Bulletin of the World Health Organization,* **82**, 858–66.

Kovel J. (1988). A critique of DSM-111 Research in Law. *Deviance and Social Control,* **9**, 127–46.

Mathers C.D. and Loncar D. (2006). Projections of Global Mortality and Burden of Disease from 2002 to 2030. *PLos Medicine,* **3**, 2011–30.

McDaid D. (2005). *Policy Brief. Mental Health 1. Key issues in the development of policy and practice across Europe.* WHO on behalf of the European Observatory on Health Systems and Policies, Brussels.

McKinnon K. and Rosner J. (2000). Severe mental illness and HIV/AIDS. In Cournos F and Forstein M (Eds) *What Mental Health Practitioners Need to Know About HIV and AIDS.* Jossey-Bass, San Francisco.

Moghraby O., Ferri C., and Prince M. (2005). Risk behaviour in school-based adolescents. Presented at the *Second Annual International Mental Health Conference at the Institute of Psychiatry: Mental Health and the Millennium Development Goals,* August 31st–September 2nd 2005.

Murthy R.S. and Lakshminarayana R. (2006). Mental health consequences of war: a brief review of research findings. *World Psychiatry,* **5**, 25–30.

Niehaus D., Oosthuisen P., Lochner C. *et al.* (2004). A Culture-Bound Syndrome 'Amafufunyana' and a Culture Specific Event 'Ukuthwasa': Differentiated by a Family History of Schizophrenia and other Psychiatric Disorders. *Psychopathology,* **37**, 59–63.

Njenga F., Nguithi A., and Kang'Ethe R. (2006). War and mental disorders in Africa. *World Psychiatry,* **5**, 38–9.

Ösby U., Brandt L., Correia N. *et al.* (2001). Excess Mortality in Bipolar and Unipolar Disorder in Sweden. *Archives of General Psychiatry,* **58**, 844–50.

Patel V. and Kleinman A. (2003). Poverty and common mental disorders in developing countries. *Bulletin of the World Health Organization*: 609–15.

Perälä J., Suvisaari J., Saarni S. *et al.* (2007). Lifetime prevalence of psychotic and bipolar I disorders in a general population. *Archives of General Psychiatry,* **64**, 19–28.

Petersen I. and Govender K. (2007). Health and health promotion. In Visser M. *Contextualising Community Psychology in South Africa.* Van Schaik, Pretoria.

Peterson I. and Swartz L. (2002). Primary health care in the era of HIV/AIDS. Some implications for health systems reform. *Social Science and Medicine,* **55**, 1005–13.

Prince M., Patel V., Rahman A. *et al.* No health without mental health – a slogan with substance. *Lancet* (in press).

Prior L. (1991). Community verses hospital care: the crisis in psychiatric provision. *Social Science and Medicine,* **32**, 483–9.

Saha S., Chant D., Welham J. *et al.* (2005). A Systematic Review of the Prevalence of Schizophrenia. *PloS Medicine,* **2**, 413–33.

Saraceno B. and Barbui C. (1997). Poverty and mental illness. *Canadian Journal of Psychiatry,* **42**, 285–90.

Saraceno B., van Ommeren M., Batniji R. *et al.* Barriers to improving mental health services in low and middle income countries. *Lancet* (in press).

Scheper-Hughes N. and Lovell A.M. (1986). Breaking the circuit of social control: lessons in public psychiatry from Italy and Franco Basaglia. *Social Science and Medicine,* **23**, 159–78.

Singleton N., Maung N.A., Cowie A. *et al.* (2007). Mental Health or Carers. Quoted in Taylor L, Taske N, Swann C and Waller S. *Public Health interventions to promote positive mental health and prevent mental health disorders among adults.* National Institute for Health and Clinical Excellence, London.

Taylor L., Taske N., Swann C. *et al.* (2007). *Public health interventions to promote positive mental health and prevent mental health disorders among adults. Evidence briefing.* National Institute for Health and Clinical Excellence, London.

Tyrer P. and Steinberg D. (1998). *Models for Mental Disorder: Conceptual Models in Psychiatry, 3rd Edition.* John Wiley & Sons Canada, Ltd.

Uldall K., Palmer N., Whetten K. *et al.* (2004). Adherence in people living with HIV/AIDS, mental illness and chemical dependency – a review of the literature. *AIDS Care,* **16** (Suppl. 1), 71–96.

Whiteford H. (2000). Unmet need: a challenge for governments. In Andrews G and Henderson S (Eds) *Unmet need in psychiatry.* Cambridge University Press, Cambridge.

WHO (1946). *Constitution of the World Health Organization,* adopted by the International Health Conference, New York, 19 June to 22 July, and signed on 22 July 1946. WHO, Geneva.

WHO (1992) *The ICD Classification of Mental and Behavioural Disorders.* WHO, Geneva.

WHO (2001). *World Health Report 2001. Mental Health: New Understanding, New Hope.* WHO, Geneva.

WHO (2002). *Prevention and Promotion in Mental Health.* WHO, Geneva.

WHO (2003). *Organization of Services for Mental Health.* WHO, Geneva.

WHO (2004). *World Health Report 2004. Changing History.* WHO, Geneva.

WHO (2005). *Mental health Atlas 2005.* WHO, Geneva.

WHO (2006a) *Dollars, DALYs and Decisions: Economic Aspects of the Mental Health System.* WHO, Geneva.

WHO (2006b). *Economic Aspects of the Mental Health System: Key Messages to Health Planners and Policy Makers.* WHO, Geneva.

WHO World Mental Health Survey Consortium (2004). Prevalence, severity and unmet need for treatment of mental disorders in the World Health Organization World Mental Health Surveys. *Journal of the American Medical Association,* **291**(21), 2581–90.

9.8

Dental public health

Zoe Marshman and Peter G. Robinson

Abstract

Dental public health is concerned with preventing oral disease, promoting oral health and improving the quality of life through the organized efforts of society. Oral health is an important public health problem as dental diseases including dental caries, periodontal disease, oral neoplasms, and dento-facial trauma are common, have significant impact on individuals and wider society, and are largely preventable. Individual risk factors for oral disease are largely equivalent to the risk factors for other common diseases namely diet, tobacco, and alcohol use, accidents, ineffective oral hygiene and limited exposure to fluoride. In common with many other diseases, many of these risks are patterned by social and economic factors. Oral health promotion involves a common risk factor approach which may be based on the principles of the Ottawa Charter. Examples include reducing the consumption of sugars through regulation of advertising and labelling of foods, training dental care professionals to give alcohol and tobacco advice, preventing accidents damaging the mouth through promotion of impact-absorbing surfaces for play areas, and the provision of mouthguards for use during contact sports. Good oral hygiene and optimal exposure to fluoride is promoted through provision of low cost fluoride toothpastes and other sources of fluoride including community fluoridation schemes of water, salt, and milk. Dental services are involved in the prevention and treatment of dental disease with the additional aim of improving the quality of life of affected individuals. Opportunities for clinical prevention include sealing the biting surfaces of teeth and the application of fluoride varnishes. Dental services are increasingly expanding the use of dental care professionals other than dentists to improve access to services. Non-specialist personnel can be trained to provide atraumatic restorative techniques, a method of restoring decayed teeth that does not rely on expensive equipment or electricity. To ensure their effectiveness and efficiency, dental services should provide high-quality, evidence-based patient management.

Dental public health: A definition

Dental public health is the science and art of preventing oral disease, promoting oral health, and improving the quality of life through the organized efforts of society. Major areas of dental public health activity include the following:

- Measures of oral health
- Determinants of oral health status
- Prevention and control of oral disease
- Promotion of oral health
- Policy and service development and prioritization
- Evaluation of the effectiveness of oral health services and treatment modalities
- Evidenced-based commissioning

In some countries, the specialty also involves provision of services to special population subgroups.

These activities may be divided into three broad groups: Oral health needs and demands assessment; oral health promotion; and the planning, commissioning, and evaluation of dental services. All have relevance in both developing and developed countries, although the emphasis will vary according to social conditions, the burden of disease, organization of health services, geographical factors, and the economy.

Oral health needs and demands assessment

This includes improving knowledge of the distribution and determinants of oral disease, identifying those determinants that are amenable to change, and understanding the impacts of oral diseases and conditions.

Oral health promotion

Dental public health focuses on improving oral health by identifying opportunities at community and national levels for evidence-based programmes aimed at improving diet and nutrition, hygiene, tobacco use, and ensuring optimal exposure to fluorides.

Planning, management, and evaluation of dental health services

This area involves using knowledge about disease levels and needs for care to plan and design dental services and to evaluate them to ensure they meet the needs of communities within the constraints of healthcare and political systems.

This chapter describes these three main areas of dental public health activity in relation to the epidemiology, aetiology, and management of the four oral conditions of the greatest public health importance: Dental caries; periodontal diseases; oral cancer; and oro-facial trauma. Approaches to oral health promotion will be outlined within a common risk factor approach. First, we discuss the relevance of oral health for public health.

The importance of oral health

Oral health is often a low priority for individuals, policy makers, and public health specialists. In fact, oral health poses important public health problems because oral diseases have significant impacts on individuals and the community, they are widespread, and the two most common diseases: Tooth decay (dental caries) and gum (periodontal) diseases are almost entirely preventable. The impacts of oral disease range from mortality to effects on general health and quality of life. Oral diseases are associated with a considerable burden to both individuals and the community in terms of lost economic productivity.

Impacts of oral disease

Mortality from oral cancer is related to the site in the mouth and the timing of the diagnosis, but 5-year survival is still less than 50 per cent. In addition to mortality, oral disease affects other aspects of general health. Limited dietary choice and calorific and micronutrient intake are direct consequences of conditions such as xerostomia, poorly fitting dentures, loss of teeth in early childhood caries, and oral developmental disorders.

Oral diseases also directly affect our quality of life and a considerable effort has been made to assess the extent to which oral disorders compromise aspects of daily living (Locker 2004). Dental pain is very common. In the United Kingdom, 40 per cent of dentate adults and 26 per cent of 12-year-olds reported oral pain in the past 12 months (Nuttall & Steele 2001; Nuttall & Harker 2004). Even the appearance of the mouth is hugely important. It affects our self-esteem, our willingness to interact with others, and influences the judgements other people make about us, and good dental appearance is regarded as a requirement for some prestigious occupations.

The economic costs of dental disease are difficult to calculate. As well as the direct costs of disease and treatment there are indirect costs which might include reduced employment or promotion expectations and opportunities, limitation of academic achievement, and the total societal burden through loss of economic productivity. The direct costs are between 0.2 per cent and 1 per cent of the gross national product in developed countries (van Amerongen *et al.* 1993). The United Kingdom is at the lower end of this range, yet the National Health Service in England and Wales (population 54 million) budget for dentistry is in excess of £2 billion (US$3.9 billion). This sum is all the more surprising when it is considered that only about 50 per cent of the population are registered with an NHS dentist. The cost of treatment provided outside the NHS is not known, but may be an additional £1 billion. Annually, over 20 million work days and 51 million school hours are lost in the United States alone due to oral disease and its treatment (Department of Health and Human Services 2000). These data equate to one and a half hours for each employee annually. Low-income families are more likely to lose time from work and school because of dental disease, and so these impacts of oral disease compound the inequalities that already exist in health, income, and educational attainment.

Frequency of oral disease

Despite decreasing prevalence of dental caries over the last three decades, 40 per cent of 5-year-olds in the United Kingdom have evidence of clinically significant tooth decay (Pitts & Harker 2004). Periodontal diseases are even more common. More than 80 per cent of adults have inflamed gums (gingivitis), and most have evidence of destruction of the attachment between tooth and bone (periodontitis).

Oral cancer is the eighth most common cancer worldwide, and its incidence is increasing particularly in some Western European countries. The highest reported incidence rates are in India and Sri Lanka where the mouth is the most common site comprising up to 40 per cent of all cancers.

Prevention

Finally, the two most common oral diseases are almost entirely preventable. Clinically significant dental caries occurs only in the presence of excess dietary sugar. The incidence of disease is low when the intake of free sugar is less than 15–20 kg/year, which equates to 6–10 per cent of energy intake (Moynihan & Petersen 2004). This dietary control of tooth decay can be supplemented by the use of fluorides, which reduce the disease whether presented in drinking water or in toothpastes. Likewise, the presence of dental plaque is necessary for destructive periodontal disease. Targets for oral cleanliness have been calculated which appear to be compatible with freedom from periodontal disease throughout life (Burt *et al.* 1985). Slightly higher levels of plaque might be compatible with acceptably low levels of periodontal disease.

Therefore, in terms of prevalence, impact on individuals and society and the possibility of effective interventions, oral health has considerable public health significance.

Dental caries

Dental caries is the demineralization of tooth substance by acid metabolites of oral bacteria. In the very early stages the lesion appears as a chalky white spot on the tooth. If the lesion progresses, the surface of the tooth breaks down leading to cavitation. If the caries reaches the underlying dentine, it can spread more readily through the porous and less mineralized tissue towards the pulp. Infection of the pulp may allow the passage of bacteria along the root canals to the alveolar bone.

The direct consequences of this process are destruction of the tooth, pain, and a possible dental abscess. Dentine is sensitive to physical, thermal, and osmotic stimuli. When it is exposed by cavitation there may be transient pain associated with hot or cold drinks or sweet foods. Later, as the pulp becomes inflamed, the discomfort may be spontaneous, exquisitely painful, and of longer duration. In a dental abscess pressure to the tooth is transmitted to the infected alveolus and the unfortunate person avoids biting or knocking the tooth.

Four factors are necessary for the development of caries: Dietary sugars, a susceptible tooth surface, the microflora of dental plaque, and adequate time.

The evidence implicating sugars in the aetiology of dental caries is convincing. Rugg-Gunn's (1993) encyclopaedic review classifies this evidence methodologically into human observational studies, human interventional studies, animal experiments, enamel slab experiments, plaque pH studies, and incubation experiments. Dietary sugars are essential if the caries is to be of clinical relevance. Dental plaque, a substance that forms on the tooth surface, which is composed mainly of bacteria, particularly *Streptococcus mutans*, metabolize sugars and so produce acids. With each exposure to sugar the plaque pH falls sharply and rises slowly back to normal levels over the following hour. It follows that caries incidence is related to the frequency of intake of sugars.

At high pH, there is remineralization of the tooth, especially in the presence of fluoride. Saliva plays a crucial protective role against caries by simple dilution, by buffering plaque acid and by acting as a source of minerals and chemical and immunological plaque inhibitory factors. For these reasons dental caries is more frequent in the sites less accessible to the saliva: In the pits and fissures of posterior teeth and between these teeth and also in people with restricted salivary flow.

Epidemiology

Caries of the permanent dentition is traditionally measured with the DMF index that records the number of decayed missing and filled teeth. A more precise index records the number of surfaces affected (DMFS). A similar index is used to record the status of the deciduous dentition (DMF). As the index aggregates both disease and treatment experience it is sensitive to the treatment decisions of dentists and so less valid with increasing age. Since each of the categories is equally weighted it is insensitive to both the severity of the disease and outcomes of treatment.

Nonetheless, the DMFT has been used for 60 years and will continue to be so for some years to come. This does not mean that DMF scores of yesteryear are directly comparable with those of today as the criteria for judging a tooth as carious have changed. Previously caries was diagnosed using a sharp dental probe to determine whether there was cavitation of the tooth. If no cavity was judged to be present, the tooth was classed as 'caries free'. More recently, the international convention has become to diagnose caries from much earlier stages, before frank cavitation when caries has visibly progressed into dentine. Sharp probes are no longer used, to prevent damage to the tooth surface. If no caries is visible, the tooth is now judged as having 'no obvious caries'. The changes in the detection thresholds reflect changes of the philosophies of the management of dental caries from an emphasis on early intervention to a more preventive approach.

Although dental caries can be found in the teeth of archaeological remains, dental caries as it is known today did not emerge until sugar became widely available. Disease levels rose during the seventeenth century and reached epidemic proportions in the nineteenth and twentieth centuries in some populations with near universal experience in some generations in many countries. Since systematic data have been collected the typical pattern has been one of high levels of caries in developed countries associated with exposure to sugars. In the mid-1970s, levels in many developed countries began to fall dramatically, for example in the United Kingdom mean DMFT of 12-year-olds decreased from 4.8 to 0.8 between 1973 and 2003 (Pitts & Harker 2004).

This fall in caries prevalence in developed countries appears to have slowed in the early to mid-1980s in the deciduous dentition. The mean dmft of 5-year-olds in England and Wales fell from 4 to 1.8 between 1973 and 1983, but now appears stable at around 1.6 (Pitts & Harker 2004). Nevertheless, children and young adults (that is, under the age of 40 years) have better oral health than preceding generations. As these cohorts age there will be commensurate improvements in adult oral health.

Data on caries levels aggregated at the national level provide useful information, but can mask important trends. The fall in caries prevalence has polarized inequalities in oral health. In times of high disease prevalence, the disease was almost universal and inequalities were manifest merely as differences in the number of teeth affected in an individual. With lower disease prevalence, a minority of people carry the burden of most of the disease. Data from the United States highlight the difference in proportion of people with at least one untreated, decayed tooth between those above and before the poverty level (Fig. 9.8.1) (Department of Health and Human Services 2000). It is often suggested that 80 per cent of the dental caries in the United Kingdom is concentrated in 20 per cent of the population, particularly those from poor socioeconomic areas. While this statement may be an oversimplification of a more complex picture it serves to illustrate that, as for most important diseases, dental caries and its consequences are increasingly diseases of the poor (Watt 2007).

Although data are scarce, there are concerns of increasing levels of caries in children in some countries undergoing economic growth and nutrition transition while caries levels remain low in countries where a poor economy restricts consumption of sugars. Surveys in Africa show that caries levels in 12-year-olds are still relatively low although aggregated national data may mask local variations, particularly, high caries levels in urban areas. Of particular concern is the fact that 90 per cent of the caries in that continent remains untreated.

Treatment of dental caries

Until the nineteenth century, the only useful treatment for dental caries was extraction of the affected tooth. Since then there has been a transition to restorative care in which the infected parts of the tooth are removed and replaced with an inert obdurating filling. During the latter half of the twentieth century, technology has moved forward, dentists have been keen to make use of innovations, and some patients have been willing to pay for them. The result is that in developed countries operative treatment for adults is increasingly complex and technology intensive. Badly decayed teeth can now be restored with a range of adhesive tooth coloured materials that are either formed in the mouth or prepared in laboratories and then fitted. Originally, missing teeth could only be replaced with removable dentures. Now they can be replaced with bridges that adhere to the remaining teeth or with prostheses supported by osseo-integrated implants that project out through the gingivae.

These treatments provided by dentists might reduce the social impact of dental caries on affected people, but play a very minor role in preventing the disease. Dental services explained 3 per cent of the reduction in caries levels in industrialized countries during the

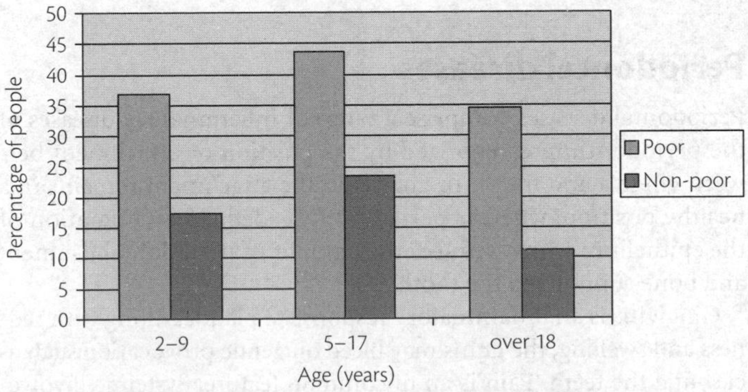

Fig. 9.8.1 Percentage of people above and below the poverty level, with at least one untreated, decayed tooth.
Source: Department of Health and Human Services (2000), United States. Poor is defined as an annual income below the US poverty level.

1970s compared to the 65 per cent contribution made by broader socioeconomic factors and the availability of fluoride toothpastes (Nadanovsky & Sheiham 1994).

In developing countries, the necessary infrastructure is often not available for complex treatment of carious teeth. In some areas the atraumatic restorative technique (ART) is the only sustainable method because the decay is removed only with hand instruments. The cavities are then filled with glass ionomer cements that are hand mixed with water. Upon insertion, the filling adheres to the tooth, gradually leaking fluoride to prevent secondary disease around the cavity. All the instruments can be carried in a small case, and treatment can be provided painlessly, at low cost, without either local anaesthesia, electricity, or expensive dental equipment. Non-dentists can be trained in the technique in a matter of weeks using manuals available from the World Health Organization. The technique is most suitable for exactly the types of cavities found in many developing countries with low caries levels (Yip *et al.* 2001).

Implications of changes in caries prevalence

The low prevalence of disease experienced in the developed world over the last 15 years has profound implications for the management of dental caries. When the incidence of the disease is low proportionately more caries affects the accessible occlusal surfaces of the teeth. Fissure sealants can be applied to these surfaces to prevent caries and are still cost-effective at low caries levels (Armfield & Spencer 2007). Only simple restorations are needed to treat existing disease at these sites. The disease also progresses more slowly, so allowing deferred operative treatment whilst attempting to prevent the spread of the lesion. Many lesions are detected at an earlier stage so that new dental materials can be used in minimally invasive techniques.

The lower levels of disease mean that the costs of some dental services might be reduced. Increasing the intervals between dental examinations is safe and effective for children and adults with low disease incidence (National Institute for Health and Clinical Excellence 2004). Since most of the restorations required by children are relatively simple, the number and costs of dentists can be reduced by using less highly-trained dental care professionals (DCPs). The reduced burden of disease may allow general dental practitioners to become more involved in health promotion, to place a greater emphasis on prevention and place a greater emphasis on quality. Conversely, there are still many people more than approximately 40 years of age who have suffered the ravages of dental caries and its treatment. These people will continue to need and demand increasingly complex treatment for decades to come.

Periodontal diseases

Periodontal diseases comprise a range of inflammatory diseases of the periodontium categorized by the position of attachment between gingiva and tooth. In gingivitis, the attachment remains in a healthy position, whereas periodontitis is defined by migration of the epithelium which reduces the amount of periodontal ligament and bone supporting the tooth.

Gingivitis is an inflammatory response to plaque. Along with redness and swelling, the gums may bleed on gentle provocation such as cleaning the teeth. Pain is an uncommon feature. Systemic involvement including hormonal changes, skin diseases, and medication use may modify these diseases or cause other gingival changes. The disease is exceedingly common.

In periodontitis, the loss of periodontal attachment is manifest by deepening of the pockets between the gingivae and teeth and by recession of the gingivae. In severe cases, the supporting structures are so depleted that the teeth become loose. The disease is rarely painful unless an acute infection complicates a periodontal pocket ('a lateral periodontal abscess') or if the exposed root surfaces are temperature sensitive.

Mild periodontal pocketing is common. For example, it is seen in half or more of UK and US adults (Department of Health and Human Services 2000; Morris *et al.* 2001). Severe periodontitis is much less frequent. Lost attachment or pockets of 6 mm or more (thought to be sufficient to threaten tooth survival) are seen in less than 8 per cent of US and UK adults (Department of Health and Human Services 2000; Morris *et al.* 2001). The disease is more frequent and severe in countries where tooth cleaning practices are less sophisticated.

One other periodontal disease has public health importance. Acute necrotizing ulcerative gingivitis (ANUG, Vincent's infection or 'trenchmouth') causes necrosis, ulceration, soreness and bleeding of the gingivae. The ulcerated papillae may have a grey slough and there may be a characteristic foetor. Lymphadenopathy and mild fever are variable findings. In many developed countries ANUG is a disease of young adults. There are no good incidence data, but anecdotally, it has become less frequent among some developed populations in recent years. A variant of the disease is associated with HIV infection. ANUG is also seen in African children where it can progress in the absence of treatment. In severe cases necrosis may extend over adjacent and contiguous tissues to cause gross destruction of oral and facial tissues (known as cancrum oris or noma).

Pathogenesis

The pathogenesis of periodontitis involves the interaction of plaque pathogens with the host's immune system. Dental plaques are consistently implicated in the aetiology of periodontal diseases. Considerable research is devoted to determining which, if any, specific pathogens are responsible for periodontal destruction (the 'specific plaque hypothesis'). Dental plaque is ubiquitous, but destructive disease occurs only in a minority of people. Plaque is therefore not sufficient cause for periodontitis and technology-intensive research may divert attention from the important determinants of periodontal disease susceptibility.

It is now clear that tobacco exerts an independent deleterious effect. In addition, periodontal treatment is less effective in smokers (Reibel 2003). Stress is also a risk factor in periodontal disease. Greater occupational stress is associated with progression of periodontitis and ANUG has been noted among soldiers on difficult postings, students during exam terms, and people with other negative life events.

Periodontitis often takes decades to become clinically detectable. Accordingly, it is more common and severe with advanced years because age confounds disease duration. Periodontitis is not a consequence of age; it is associated with poor oral hygiene irrespective of age and does not progress in adults with good oral hygiene.

In the last few years periodontal diseases have been linked to a number of other health problems including cardiovascular diseases, stroke, pre-term birth, and low birth weight. A number of authors have gone so far as to suggest that periodontal diseases are independent risk factors for these diseases with many reports focusing on the biological plausibility of these associations. Epidemiological evidence supporting links between periodontal and other diseases suffers from a huge range of possible variables, the potential for misclassification and other sources of bias. Whilst efforts have been made to control for socioeconomic and lifestyle factors, residual confounding resulting from a failure to account fully for these variables seems inevitable. Specific cardiovascular risk factors such as tobacco use, obesity, and lower serum HDL-cholesterol are more common among people with high dental disease experience (Sanders *et al.* 2005). Some of these factors such as tobacco smoking are independent risk factors for both cardiovascular and periodontal diseases, whereas others may be linked less directly.

This area of research is exciting periodontal researchers. Systematic reviews of these possible links have been conducted, yet for the meantime, methodological complexity prevents firm conclusions being drawn (Beck & Offenbacher 2005; Xiong *et al.* 2006).

Treatment

For the majority of people the progression of periodontal destruction is compatible with the retention of a natural dentition into old age. Targets for oral cleanliness have been calculated that appear to be compatible with freedom from periodontal disease throughout life or with acceptably low levels of periodontal disease (Burt *et al.* 1985).

A significant minority of people (perhaps 5–15 per cent) may lose teeth as a result of periodontal diseases and considerable effort is spent by dentists and dental hygienists attempting to prevent and treat them. Both the prevention and treatment of periodontal diseases focus on the mechanical removal of plaque. Dental professionals attempt to bring this about by instructing patients in the use of toothbrushes and dental floss. Adjunctive services provided by dental services include the removal of calcified plaque (calculus) as it may harbour micro-organisms and provide a mechanical barrier to inhibit effective self-care and planning the surfaces of the roots to remove the superficial layers which might be contaminated with bacterial toxins. In some cases the architecture of the periodontium may be surgically adjusted to excise diseased tissue and allow the entry of toothbrush bristles and dental floss into inaccessible areas. In recent times, a technique known as guided tissue regeneration (GTR) has used membranes of synthetic material to prevent epithelial cells proliferating down the root surface after periodontal surgery.

Systematic reviews are beginning to provide an evidence base for periodontal therapy although there may be considerable Hawthorne effects reflecting differences between the effectiveness of treatment provided routinely in primary care and its efficacy in clinical trials conducted in university departments. There are also few long-term studies showing effects on tooth retention.

Interventions aimed at improving oral hygiene produce only short-term changes that are not sustained (Watt & Marinho 2005). Powered toothbrushes with a rotation oscillation action assist self-care although their long-term benefits on periodontal health have yet to be evaluated (Robinson *et al.* 2005). The most common professional procedure to prevent and treat periodontal diseases, the removal of calculus by scaling and polishing, has not been evaluated using contemporary standards of research. Nor is there compelling evidence of benefits from professional mechanical plaque removal alone over simple oral hygiene instruction to prevent periodontal diseases (Needleman *et al.* 2005a). Another common treatment, subgingival debridement, remains untested in randomized controlled trials, but showed modest short-term reductions in pocket depths in other controlled studies (Van der Weijden & Timmerman 2002) and a systematic review of GTR indicated that the mean level of attachment gained is less than 1 mm with eight sites needing to be treated to regain 2 mm in one site (Needleman *et al.* 2005b).

Oral neoplasms

Benign neoplasms in the oral cavity include papillomas, polyps, and various types of granuloma. This section will deal principally with malignant neoplasms, of which approximately 90 per cent are squamous cell carcinomas. They may occur on the lip, tongue, gingivae, oral floor, or elsewhere in the mouth. The site is often related to the aetiological factors. Lesions may present as swellings, ulcers, or red or white patches and many are painless until they become large. Significantly, survival is related to the stage of the disease at presentation. Five-year survival is less than 50 per cent.

Malignant change is often seen in a number of lesions which precede the development of the tumour. These premalignant lesions present as leukoplakias and erythroplakias of unknown origin. Malignant change is also seen, albeit infrequently, in oral lichen planus and hyperplastic candidiasis.

Overall incidence worldwide for males has been estimated at an age standardized rate of 6.42 per 100 000 population with dramatic variation between and within countries (World Health Organization 2001) (Table 9.8.1). Men are more susceptible than women in almost all populations, independent of the effects of tobacco use.

Variations in the incidence of oral malignancy are largely explained by varying exposure to three major risk factors. Cancer of the lower lip is strongly associated with exposure to sunlight especially in people with fair skin. Tobacco use, whether chewed or smoked, predisposes to intra-oral cancer. The high incidence of oral cancer among southern Asians is largely accounted for by the addition of tobacco to betel quid or 'paan'. There are dose–response relationships for the duration of use and type of tobacco inhaled. Alcohol is also an independent aetiological factor and has a synergistic relationship with tobacco use.

In the past, oral cancer was predominantly a disease of older people (over 60 years). However, there is now evidence of an increased incidence in those less than 45 years with a suggestion that oral cancer in this younger age-group may be a distinct and more aggressive disease entity (Conway 2006).

Because early intervention determines survival in oral cancer, and many cases are preceded by premalignant lesions, there is a strong argument for case finding as a method of disease control.

Table 9.8.1 Oral cancer in males—age standardized rate per 100 000 population

	Rate per 100 000
Worldwide	6.42
India	12.6
Thailand	4.6
China	0.7

Source: World Health Organization (2001).

However, active screening does not appear to be justified in part because of the low incidence of the disease (Downer *et al.* 2006). Opportunistic screening, when patients may already visit the dentist for a dental check up, may be viable.

Dento-facial trauma

Trauma to the teeth is common and frequently causes fracture of the tooth or supporting bone or bodily movement of the tooth including complete avulsion. In many cases the long-term survival of the tooth is threatened. As the anterior and most visible teeth are most often involved the result is disfiguring. Worldwide the prevalence of dento-facial trauma is approximately 10–15 per cent. Risk factors include contact sports, bicycle/skateboard accidents, falls, violence and poor environments such as overcrowding. Clinical features of protruding upper front teeth and inadequate lip coverage also put individuals at risk. The peak age for trauma is early adolescence with boys experiencing more injuries than girls.

Trauma to deciduous teeth is managed by monitoring in case any consequent infection threatens the permanent tooth developing beneath it. In permanent teeth, adhesive fillings can be used to protect sensitive fractured teeth and calcium hydroxide dressings may be placed to allow continued root development in immature teeth. For permanent teeth that have been knocked out, timely first-aid is crucial. They should be replaced in the socket as soon as possible or else placed in a suitable container of milk or normal saline. Dental care should be sought immediately as the long term survival rates of avulsed teeth are greatest if the tooth is replanted within 30 minutes. The tooth should be held in place by non-rigid splint to adjacent teeth for 7–10 days. Systemic antibiotic and anti-tetanus treatments are required. The need for almost immediate care means that skilled emergency dental services should be available wherever possible. Unfortunately dento-facial trauma is not limited to office hours.

The cost of treating dento-facial trauma has been estimated at US$3.2–3.5 million per million subjects (Andreasen 1997) and in the United Kingdom the average total cost of treating one patient with a dental traumatic injury has been estimated at £856 (US$1665) (Wong & Kolokotsa 2004).

Oral health promotion

Because oral diseases are brought about by people's behaviours, dentistry has traditionally adopted health education as the central thrust of prevention. Toothbrushing and sugar reduction messages have been repeated *ad nauseam* in both chairside and public education campaigns. But dental educators became disillusioned with the recognition that health education cannot readily change these behaviours which are largely determined by our social and cultural environment. Indeed, health education carries its own dangers of disempowerment and victim-blaming and may increase inequalities in oral health (Watt 2007).

Closer examination of the causes of oral disorders reveal the potential value of community-based approaches to maintain oral health by acting on the wider determinants of health. Oral disease is brought about by the consumption of sugars, ineffective oral cleaning, tobacco and alcohol use, limited exposure to fluoride, and stress. The determinants of oral health are largely equivalent to the determinants of health in general, and there are many opportunities for wider social and environmental action to play an invaluable role in promoting oral health. There is an increasing recognition that a 'common-risk factor' approach is fundamental to the integrated approach to oral health promotion (Sheiham & Watt 2000). The key principle behind this approach is that controlling a number of risk factors through multidisciplinary action can have a major impact on a large number of chronic diseases. This approach then reduces duplication, saves resources, and improves effectiveness.

An additional consideration is that preventive strategies that focus on individuals does not appear to be suitable for dental caries and periodontal diseases since there are, as yet, no effective ways of identifying which individuals are at high risk of developing the diseases (Rose 1992; Watt 2007). Whilst individuals at high risk for dental disease cannot be identified with adequate sensitivity and specificity, it is possible to identify at risk populations. In these situations, it can be cost-effective to target preventive interventions at people in specific socioeconomic groups, attending particular schools or living in an area with high disease incidence (Burt 1998). However, a strategy of targeted interventions should take place within a common risk factor approach that addresses general health conditions for the whole population. Such an approach will reduce social inequalities and will provide a multiplicity of benefits, especially as risk factors for oral and general health tend to be clustered in the same groups (Sanders *et al.* 2005). It also avoids the limitations inherent in attempting to identify and treat differently those individuals at high risk for disease. Finally, a recognition of the social context in which personal choices are made avoids the social iatrogenesis of describing oral heath in individual terms (Dickson 1995). Dentistry has been quick to adopt approaches which would now be recognized as health promoting. For example, fluoride levels in water supplies were adjusted to prevent dental caries as early as 1945 (Dean *et al.* 1950).

Health promotion, the process of enabling people to take control over and to improve their health', has five broad actions as outlined in the Ottawa Charter: Creating supportive environments, building healthy public policy, strengthening community action, developing personal skills and reorienting health services (World Health Organization 1984, 1986). Within this approach Sheiham (1995) suggested six policy areas relevant to oral health that are used in this review (Box 9.8.1).

With the growing emphasis on evidence-based healthcare oral health promotion must increasingly demonstrate its effectiveness. Repeated systematic reviews have aimed to identify oral health promotion practices which yield demonstrable health gains or modified knowledge or behaviours (Sprod *et al.* 1996; Kay & Locker 1997). These reviews reveal a paucity of evidence with few reports of well-designed studies in which the intended outcome was health gain. The most robust studies tended to focus on programmes in which the intended outcome was improved knowledge or modification of the behaviours of individuals. Even these studies, which might be termed 'health education' usually involved a relatively short follow-up. The main finding from meta-analysis was the effectiveness of fluoride to prevent caries (Kay & Locker 1997). A less rigorous approach adopted by Sprod and colleagues (1996) allowed exploration of other avenues of activity and research, but still concluded there was little evaluative literature on broader approaches to health promotion.

Other chapters in this text will consider the evaluation of health promotion in some detail, but it needs to be stressed that key features of broader approaches to health promotion may render them

Box 9.8.1 Policy areas relevant to oral health promotion (Sheiham 1995)

1. Use of fluoride
   - Including water, milk, salt, tablets/drops, toothpaste, mouthrinses, and varnishes/gels
2. Food and health policies to reduce sugars consumption
   - National policies recommending proportion of energy intake from sugars and frequency of intake
   - Regulation of advertising and labelling of foods
3. Community approaches to improve body hygiene including oral cleaning
   - Emphasis on toothbrushing with fluoride toothpaste
4. Smoking cessation
   - Advice and support from dental team members
5. Policies on reducing accidents
   - Use of impact-absorbing materials
   - Mouthguards for contact sports
6. Ensuring access to appropriate preventive care
   - Ensuring clinical effectiveness
   - Equity of access
   - Appropriate skill mix

unsuitable for evaluation by randomized controlled trials. Health promotion inevitably takes place in 'real world' settings rather than the strictly controlled environment of randomized controlled trials, many other factors and considerable time often intervene between the intervention and a health outcome and the need for strictly specified outcomes in trials mitigates against the ethos of a common risk factor approach. These factors have led the World Health Organization (1998) to conclude that: 'The use of RCTs to evaluate health promotion initiatives is, in most cases, inappropriate, misleading and unnecessarily expensive'. Even the keenest advocates of RCTs acknowledge that they are unsuitable for evaluating legislative and policy changes (Rosen *et al.* 2006). Other approaches to evaluating health promotion involve other research designs and the use of underlying theory to guide the design of evaluations and the selection of intermediate indicators as proxies of health outcomes (Tones & Tilford 2001).

The use of fluoride

The presence of fluoride at the interface between plaque and dental enamel inhibits the development of caries. To be most effective fluoride should be present both before the teeth start to develop and then continuously throughout life. These findings suggest its effect is derived from a combination of modes of action. Three modes currently receive the most attention: The effect of fluoride on plaque metabolism; the effect of its incorporation during tooth development and its effect on the dynamics of demineralization and remineralization after tooth development.

Water fluoridation

Beneficial effects of fluoride on dental health were discovered as a consequence of investigations of endemic developmental defects of the teeth in Colorado. McKay implicated the water supplies in the aetiology of the staining and pits and discovered that the teeth with defects were less susceptible to dental caries than those without (McKay 1933). The staining was shown to be due to fluoride which existed in some of McKay's samples at levels as high as 14 parts per million (ppm). This staining (now known as dental fluorosis) is hypomaturation or hypomineralization of the teeth caused by chronic ingestion of fluoride during tooth development. It has a variety of presentations from small white flecks on the tooth to larger yellow/brown defects.

Dean and colleagues went on to demonstrate an inverse relationship between dental caries and the fluoride concentration of drinking water (and the associated fluorosis) in two cross-sectional ecological studies (now called the '21 cities studies'). The first intervention trial of fluoridation started in Grand Rapids in 1945 (Dean *et al.* 1950). Since then, similar studies have taken place in many countries including the United Kingdom, the Netherlands and Australia. Worldwide around 400 million people now receive water from a fluoridated water supply and water fluoridation has been designated one of the ten most important public health measures currently available (Centers for Disease Control and Prevention 1999). Dean originally suggested that the optimal concentration for water fluoridation was 1 ppm (1 mg/l), the recommended optimal range of fluoride is now 0.6–1 ppm F.

A systematic review of the effectiveness and safety of water fluoridation included the results of 88 studies (83 of which were cross-sectional) from 30 different countries. Study areas above 5 ppm F were excluded (McDonagh *et al.* 2000). Overall, the included studies were judged to be of low to moderate quality, mainly because of the lack of appropriate adjustment for the effect of confounding factors. Bearing in mind the concerns about the quality of the included studies, water fluoridation was associated with a median increase of 14.6 per cent in the proportion of children without caries experience and a median reduction in dmft/DMFT of 2.25 teeth. For one extra child to be 'caries-free', six children would need to be exposed to water fluoridated at 1 ppm F. Water fluoridation was also found to have an effect over and above that of other sources of fluoride, particularly toothpaste.

A direct dose–response relationship was found between water fluoridation and dental fluorosis. At 1 ppm F, the prevalence of fluorosis was estimated to be 48 per cent and for fluorosis of aesthetic concern 12.5 per cent. The number of additional people who would have to be exposed to water fluoridation at this level for one additional person to develop fluorosis of any level was six. Other possible negative effects considered included bone fracture, cancer, Down syndrome, senile dementia, and goitre. No clear evidence of these potential effects was found, but interpretation of the results of these studies was difficult due to the quality of the primary data.

The cost-effectiveness of water fluoridation depends on the baseline level of caries and the capital costs of the necessary equipment. In areas where water is supplied to large numbers of people via a single source, fluoridation is more cost-effective than in areas supplied by many smaller water sources. In the United Kingdom, water fluoridation is recommended for those areas where the mean DMFT of 5-year-olds is greater than 2 and where water schemes cover approximately 200 000 residents (Sanderson 1998).

Further high-quality research into the safety, efficacy, cost-effectiveness (McDonagh *et al.* 2000), and impact of fluoridation on quality of life has been recommended (Medical Research Council 2002).

The introduction of water fluoridation schemes has been opposed by active antifluoridationist lobbies. Such groups tend to be small, but very enthusiastic and vociferous, with an impact which is often disproportionate to their size or the support they garner. The main arguments against water fluoridation include the safety concerns investigated in the York Review together with ethical objections concerning infringement of individual liberties.

Those against fluoridation argue that it is unethical to fluoridate water supplies as this infringes on the individual's freedom of choice and removes the rights of adults to refuse medical treatment. The claim of fluoridation being an attempt at 'mass medication' is made frequently. The ethical objections to water fluoridation have been discussed by applying the four principles that encompass most of the moral aspects of healthcare, that is; respect for autonomy, beneficence, non-maleficence and justice (Jones & Lennon 1997) (Table 9.8.2).

Opponents claim water fluoridation represents a loss of autonomy, but those proposing fluoridation suggest that in society, some reduction of individual freedom is accepted for the overall good of the community. Anti-fluoridationists argue the only members of society to potentially benefit from water fluoridation are dentate individuals particularly children. Those in favour of fluoridation acknowledge that edentulous people will not benefit, but fluoridation will 'do no harm' to any members of society. On the principle of justice, some claim that imposing water fluoridation is not fair on those against it. Proponents counter this argument by suggesting that the reduction in inequalities in dental health that fluoridation potentially provides is a just way of helping those least able to help themselves.

The debate about fluoridation is an interesting one. Anti-fluoridationists tend to come from relatively healthy middle-class groups. Because children in these groups have the lowest caries experience they have the least to benefit from the intervention. Unfortunately, their effect is to maintain social inequalities in health. Anti-fluoridationist arguments are often alarmist and sometimes unorthodox from the viewpoint of scientists. Unfortunately, public debates between pro- and anti-fluoridationists often end in pro-fluoridationists attempting to refute, in detailed scientific terms, an extensive list of claims. With the current mistrust of science it can be difficult to make such a position attractive in the face of very emotional arguments. Some proponents of fluoridation avoid open debate with anti-fluoridationists for this reason.

Table 9.8.2 Summary of ethical arguments about water fluoridation

	For	Against
Autonomy	Some reduction of individual freedom accepted for overall good of the community	Loss of autonomy
Beneficence	Those most in need gain benefit	Only dentate individuals benefit
Non-maleficence	Fluoridation 'does no harm'	Fluoridation causes adverse health effects
Justice	Fluoridation reduces inequalities	Fluoridation is not fair

Source: Jones & Lennon (1997).

Other vehicles for administering fluoride

Fluoride milk

Fluoride has been added to milk as an alternative to water since the 1950s in many countries worldwide. These schemes vary in the age at which children start drinking the milk, the number of years over which it is consumed, the number of days a year the milk is consumed, and the concentration of fluoride added (Marino *et al.* 2006). A systematic review to determine the effectiveness of fluoridated milk for preventing caries on a community basis found insufficient studies of good quality to make a definitive conclusion, but stated fluoridated milk may be beneficial for the permanent dentition (Yeung *et al.* 2005).

Fluoride salt

Salt fluoridation was first used in Switzerland in the 1950s. In certain cantons and in some Latin American countries, all salt for human consumption is fluoridated. Other European countries including France only sell fluoridated salt for domestic use. The typical concentration is 250 ppm F. Several cross-sectional studies report fluoride salt to be effective at reducing caries (Jones *et al.* 2005).

Fluoride tablets/drops

Fluoride tablets/drops use also began in the 1950s. They have been used as dietary supplements with different countries having different dosing regimens (based on child's age, weight, caries-risk, fluoride in the water). Their effectiveness has not been confirmed by any well-designed trials or systematic reviews and the available studies fail to account for confounding factors. There is some evidence that when sucked to maximize the topical dose a preventive effect is observed in deciduous teeth.

Others problem with fluoride supplementation include compliance of individuals and their families and risk of fluorosis. Many of the people most susceptible to caries find the dosing schedules difficult to maintain and taken as a daily bolus fluoride supplements increase the risk of fluorosis (Ismail & Bandekar 1999). These concerns have led to a reduction in the use of tablets/drops as a public health measure.

Topical fluorides

Topically applied fluoride includes delivery systems where fluoride is applied to tooth surfaces at high concentrations for a local protective effect. A series of systematic reviews of trials have investigated the effectiveness of various topical fluorides expressing the effectiveness in terms of the preventive fraction (the difference in caries increments between the intervention and control groups expressed as a percentage of the increment in the control group) (Table 9.8.3).

Fluoride toothpaste

Toothpaste is the most widespread source of fluoride and the decline in caries experience in children in some countries has been attributed to its regular use. The fluoride compounds and concentrations found in toothpastes vary between brands and between countries. The usual concentration is 1000–1500 ppm F with higher (over 2000 ppm F) and lower (less than 600 ppm F) formulations available. They present a good vehicle for the frequent low dose application of fluoride and their effectiveness of fluoride toothpaste in reducing caries in children has been confirmed with a PF of 24 per cent (Marinho *et al.* 2003a). The risk of fluorosis from toothpaste can be minimized by using a smear of paste and supervising children under 6 years of age.

The use of fluoride toothpaste has a distinct disadvantage over water fluoridation as a broad preventive strategy. It relies on people brushing their teeth. In developed countries, poor oral hygiene and high caries incidence are *associated* (although not necessarily causally) and so the people who have most to benefit from the use of fluoride toothpastes are less likely to use them frequently. In developing countries there may not be a tradition of tooth cleaning with toothpastes and western proprietary brands are likely to be expensive. However, cheap locally made pastes can be profoundly effective (Yee *et al.* 2003).

Fluoride mouthrinses

Fluoride mouthrinses have been used extensively for the past 30 years. School-based programmes were common in certain countries although individual home use now predominates. Mouthrinsing is not recommended for children under 6 years of age, due to the risk of fluoride ingestion. The two main concentrations available are 0.05 per cent (230 ppm F) sodium fluoride used daily and 0.2 per cent (900 ppm F) sodium fluoride weekly. The effectiveness of mouthrinses in children has also been confirmed with a PF of 26 per cent (Marinho *et al.* 2003b).

Fluoride varnishes/gels

Topically applied fluoride varnishes and gels have been used widely for over two decades both as part of community-based programmes and on an individual basis. Fluoride varnishes are professionally applied with the two most commonly used varnishes containing 22 600 ppm F or 7000 ppm F. A systematic review of trials has confirmed the effectiveness of topical varnishes although the included studies were of poor quality. The PF in permanent teeth was 46 per cent (Marinho *et al.* 2002a).

Fluoride gels can be professionally or self-applied under supervision. The most commonly used gel is a professionally applied 12 300 ppm F acidulated phosphate fluoride (APF). Due to the risk of excessive ingestion this gel is not recommended for young children. The effectiveness of professionally-applied and self-applied gels have been reviewed with a prevented fraction of 28 per cent (Marinho *et al.* 2002b).

Diet

Dietary sugars are a necessary cause of clinically significant decay. However, evidence that health education can reduce their intake and so reduce the incidence of caries is lacking (Kay & Locker 1997). Many studies of health education interventions have used self-reported sugar consumption as the primary outcome with the obvious danger of ascertainment bias. Studies that have measured clinical outcomes have combined health education approaches with the use of fluorides and thus the independent effect of the health education cannot be assessed.

Some of the data that implicate sugars in the aetiology of caries suggest that restriction of dietary sugar is preventive. For example, per capita sugar supplies and caries experience data correlate significantly in simple national ecological comparisons. A children's home in Australia had a dietary regimen with almost no sugar and the children had very low caries levels until they were allowed to make their own food choices at the age of 12. Likewise, caries levels fell in parallel with the availability of sugar during World War II (Rugg-Gunn 1993).

Table 9.8.3 Relative effectiveness of sources of topical fluoride

Source	ppm F	Prevented fraction (%)
Toothpaste	500–1500	24
Mouthrinse	230–900	26
Varnish	7000–22 000	46 (permanent) 33 (deciduous)
Gel	12 300	28

Source: Marinho *et al.* (2002a, 2002b, 2003a, 2003b).

Whether these findings can be translated into effective public health strategies remains uncertain. A health-directed food policy seems logical. A common risk factor approach might impact on dental diseases as well as obesity, diabetes and cardiovascular diseases. Possible strategies fall within the framework of education, substitution, regulation, pricing, or provision (Sanderson 1984). However, few countries have such policies in place, and the resources of health advocates are very limited in comparison to those of the affluent and powerful lobby of the commercial food industry. Despite these difficulties, it is by operating at this level that public health might have its greatest impact.

In addition to approaches aimed at individuals, education can take the form of authoritative dietary guidelines to inform national policies, community initiatives, and caterers. The World Health Organization recommends countries to formulate their own specific goals to reduce the amount of free sugars, recommending a maximum of no more than 10 per cent of energy intake. In addition, the frequency of consumption of foods containing free sugars should be limited to a maximum of four times per day (Moynihan & Petersen 2004).

Dietary sugars can be substituted with artificial sweeteners to reduce caries increments. Sales of sugar-free carbonated drinks in Europe and North America demonstrate the compatibility of this tactic with commercial interests. However, substitution of dietary sugars has only limited potential in oral health promotion. The manufacture of many food stuffs relies on the bulk and other specific properties of sugars. In addition, some sweeteners have side effects and resistance to the extended use of artificial sweeteners persists.

Regulation of advertising and labelling of foods in tandem with the effective use substitution is illustrated by a partnership between dentists and the confectionery industry in Switzerland. The *Zahnfreundlich* (toothfriendly) logo is used to label non-acidogenic confectionery (Rugg-Gunn 1997). The label is well recognized by children, is commonly seen on confectionery, and is thought to have been effective in reducing levels of decay (Marthaler 1990). Fiscal policies might be used to discourage manufacture and sale of sugar-containing products. All of the above approaches and direct consumer pressure can be brought to bear on caterers and retail outlets to provide food in a way that makes the healthy choices the easier choices. There are numerous other examples of approaches which may reduce sugars consumption and an exhaustive list is presented by Sheiham (1995).

Oral cleaning

Plaque is a necessary cause of periodontal diseases and so it seems logical that tooth cleaning should be the cornerstone of their management and prevention. Interventions aimed at improving oral hygiene can be successful and achieve a commensurate reduction in gingival inflammation (Kay & Locker 1997; Watt & Marinho 2005). Interestingly, interventions carried out in dental surgeries have been more effective than school-based interventions. However, most studies have had short follow-up periods and the effectiveness of even the best interventions diminishes with time. Therefore, few data show that attempts to improve oral hygiene to prevent destructive disease are effective. Nonetheless, there remains a consensus that the best public health approach to improve periodontal health remains with improved oral hygiene.

The relationship between plaque removal and tooth decay is much more contentious. In a carefully designed trial, professional oral cleaning did not demonstrate any additional preventive effect above a standard preventive programme of fissure sealants and locally applied topical fluoride received by the control groups (Arrow 1997). Sutcliffe's (1996) traditional review considered the effect of research methods on the observed relationship between oral cleaning and dental caries and concluded that there was 'no unequivocal evidence that good oral cleanliness reduces caries experience'. This area of research is fraught with difficulty. As well as the difficulties of measuring dental disease, studies are susceptible to selection bias, leakage of intervention, and the likely confounding effects between self-reported behaviours, diet and oral hygiene. Studies where professional cleaning has been effective have used pastes containing fluoride.

What is known is that brushing with a *fluoride* toothpaste is effective in preventing caries. Therefore, brushing as it is currently practised in most developed countries combats both caries and periodontal diseases, and is to be encouraged.

The systematic reviews cited earlier demonstrated that it is difficult to achieve sustainable changes in oral hygiene behaviour. A study of teenagers found good oral hygiene to be associated with not smoking, exercise, healthy eating, managing in school, and having confidence in one's family (Schou 1998). These types of findings invite the common risk factor approach in which oral cleanliness is promoted as both a health related and health directed behaviour where cleaning ones teeth makes one feel and look nice and is part of a part positive and healthy lifestyle. Toothbrushing is a habit learnt as a young child and is therefore difficult to change later in life. This behaviour is often an established routine before the child has seen a dentist, and interventions via healthcare workers and social agencies working with young children and their mothers may be useful.

Smoking cessation

The role of smoking in the aetiology of oral cancers and periodontal diseases has already been discussed. Johnson has listed 20 oral conditions either directly or indirectly associated with tobacco smoking (Johnson 1997). In addition to the well-known benefits to cardiovascular and respiratory health, cessation of smoking almost eliminates the increased risk of oral cancer within 5–10 years.

Many of the oral conditions such as stained teeth, receding gums, and altered taste are readily perceptible to the individual and may encourage or reinforce the desire to stop smoking. The dental team are also often aware of the personal and social circumstances (e.g. pregnancy or a new job) that prompt people to give up. Therefore, smoking cessation is another area where it is particularly appropriate for dentistry to become integrated into a common risk factor approach. As clinicians, the dental team can be effective in supporting smoking cessation by providing advice (Carr & Ebbert 2006).

Prevention of accidents

Several strategies can be used to reduce trauma to teeth. Playground surfaces can be made of impact-absorbing materials which cushion against trauma. The use of mouthguards is compulsory for some sports in some countries. Mouthguards not only prevent dental injuries, but also prevent laceration of the facial soft tissues against the teeth, reduce the risk of mandibular fracture and may protect the cranial cavity. Mouthguards are usually made of a copolymer of polyvinyl acetate and polyethylene. The most basic type may be obtained prefabricated in a range of sizes. A more sophisticated type may be adapted to fit the mouth, typically by softening it in hot water first. Custom-made devices constructed on models made from impressions of the teeth are the most comfortable and can be made to support the lower teeth and mandible during trauma.

As immediate first-aid for dental trauma, particularly avulsed teeth, is so important for the long-term survival of the traumatized teeth, informing athletes and their teachers and trainers of the need for immediate action can reduce the impact of the trauma.

Unfortunately, orthodontic treatment of protruding front teeth is complex and prolonged, but can be justified in children of 8 or 9 years to reduce the risk of trauma (Welbury 1996).

Ensuring access to appropriate preventive care

There has been disillusionment with the biomedical model of healthcare. By focusing on the diseases of individuals, it was criticized for emphasizing the hierarchy of professionals over lay people and treatments rather than prevention. All of these things have taken place with substantial economic and social costs and yet medical care was said to make a relatively small contribution to health (McKeown 1976; Illich 1976).

Within this view, the biomedical approach distracts attention from the wider social, political, and economic determinants of health. The Primary Health Care Approach (PHCA) recognized that these determinants are more important than medical interventions (World Health Organization 1978).

Whilst dental services are rarely designed to deliver benefits at the public health level, they are just as susceptible to the criticisms of the medical model of healthcare. Dental treatment has made a relatively small contribution to aspects of oral health. For example, orthodontic treatment is often advocated on the basis of social and psychological benefit; however, a recent 20-year follow-up study of orthodontic treatment was unable to find evidence to support such a benefit (Kenealy *et al.* 2007). Data from the 1970s show that dental services explain 3 per cent of the variation in oral health of 12-year-olds in developed countries, compared to the 65 per cent contribution made by broader socioeconomic factors (Nadanovsky & Sheiham 1994, 1995). Furthermore, the interventions used in dentistry may also be clinically inappropriate. Dentistry has adopted a surgical approach to treatment with a cycle of placing and replacing fillings. It has long been recognized that the quality of many fillings is not high and that even the decisions to place fillings are idiosyncratic (Elderton & Nuttall 1983). Since fillings are often replaced several times over a lifetime, the remaining tooth is increasingly damaged with each new filling.

Clinical dental services also neglect the determinants of disease. With its emphasis on personal behaviour and even with the search for specific periodontal pathogens, clinical dentistry and some dental research diverts attention from the factors that determine oral health and disease.

Dental services are also costly. National Health Service dentistry costs £2 billion per year for the 54 million people living in England and Wales. Compared to the potential costs of treatment the resources available are few and are likely to reduce in future. Curative services serve those who can afford them. In addition to creating dependence on professionals, the services become focused on those with least health problems.

The problems of medical and dental care exist in parallel; therefore, the same kinds of changes are applicable to both. There are too few resources, the resources that are available are still poorly allocated, services still congregate around the wealthy people, ordinary people have little control over own health, and health professionals still do not trust people to make good decisions about their health. All of these points apply to dentistry. In every country of the world, there are people who cannot attend and or cannot afford dental treatment in its current guise. Even in countries with well-developed socialized systems of dental care, there are major inequalities in oral health (Watt & Sheiham 1999).

Views about the relative role of health services remain polarized. From one perspective, too narrow a focus on 'health service issues' contributes to the failure of public health to improve population health (Holland 2002; Beaglehole & Bonita 2004). The 'post-new public health' view argues that preventive and curative measures prolong life expectancy and maintain and improve the quality of life. Bunker (2001) estimated the increases in life expectancy attributable to clinical care by calculating increases resulting from declines in disease-specific death rates and from specific treatments. His conclusions may have been optimistic in both generalizing from results achieved in research trials to routine practice with patients with complex problems and in underestimating the continuing role of social and other environmental factors in health (Frankel 2001; Tudor Hart 2001).

At a population level, it remains exceedingly difficult to distinguish the effects of medical care from those of other health determinants. In addition, clinical services offer advantages other than those of life expectancy (or tooth survival). As we gain greater knowledge of the effects of specific clinical and public health interventions, we can regard the direct opposition of the two approaches as a false dichotomy (Frankel 2001). The key decisions are to select which interventions can improve the health of the population.

Unfortunately, as this review has shown, when compared to medicine, the benefits and costs of clinical dentistry at either an individual or population level are relatively unknown. Some check is required to counter the assumption that the principle way to improve the oral health of a population is via the provision of more dental treatment. Dental services remain overdue for an evaluation and reorientation. A more holistic practice of dentistry will also ensure that services are more equitable and appropriate.

Public health specialists can contribute to increasing the effectiveness of services and facilitating equity of access to services when needed. For example, clinical dentistry can have a role in reducing the psycho-social impacts of oral disease (Awad *et al.* 2000; Robinson *et al.* 2005). For this reason, it is essential that we generate a greater understanding within dentistry of the nature of oral health. The movement to identify more relevant measures of oral health to assess treatment need and the outcomes of care should be encouraged. The evidence-based approach, the use of clinical governance, and managed care should provide both the impetus and the means to ensure that only effective and efficient interventions are used.

Dental surgeries are a natural health-related setting for health promotion. Practice-based oral health promotion activities provide an opportunity to increase knowledge and promote self-esteem and empowerment. Their role could be expanded by adopting a common risk factor approach. However, practice-based health promotion is only useful for those who attend the services and may exclude those people with the greatest need who do not. In addition, there needs to be a change in emphasis in health education from the prescriptive approaches that ignore the needs of people they serve and so blame the victims. Patients should not feel they are being chastised or told to do things. A more effective approach would be a patient-centred model which respects patients' autonomy and seeks their active participation in defining their needs (Croucher 1989).

Specific changes that could be made to ensure access to dental services can still be categorized in the framework used by Penchansky and Thomas (1981). Services must be available, accessible, affordable, acceptable, and accommodating. This framework is broadly compatible with the characteristics of dental services as seen within Andersen's (1995) behavioural model of access.

Clearly people cannot use services that do not exist, so increasing their availability has a direct effect on service use. One way of making dental services more available at limited cost is to delegate care to other DCPs. In developed countries the majority of treatment required falls within the remit of DCPs. It is therefore not cost-effective to employ highly trained and highly paid dentists to undertake this less demanding and repetitive work. A number of countries including Australia, New Zealand, Canada, and the United Kingdom employ dental care professionals with a limited repertoire of treatment options (variously called school dental nurses, dental auxiliaries, and dental therapists) who provide high quality care at lower cost. Similar data exist for dental hygienists. DCPs work under the supervision of a dentist. By reducing the level of supervision required and expanding there role, the availability of care can be increased whilst limiting costs. Dental hygienists can work independently without reducing either the quality of treatment or patients' satisfaction with it. Likewise, hygienists can be trained to conduct clinical examinations in dental surveys with no compromise to the quality of the data (Kwan *et al.* 1996).

Clearly the expanded use of DCPs threatens the monopoly on the provision of dental treatment held by dentists and the profession has been a frequent barrier to their wider use. For example, executives of the American Dental Association have recently advocated a free market dental system with subsidized treatment for disadvantaged families rather than a needs-based system using DCPs in areas with an undersupply of care (Bramson & Guay 2005).

One particular aspect of dentistry in many countries that could be revised is the system of payment of fees to dentists for each item of service provided. Fee-per-item service payments encourage dentists to work quickly and have been associated (in the past at least) with over-treatment. This system of payment tends to encourage the curative technical approach to treatment, unless there is a specific fee for prevention. On the other hand, services based on capitation per patient enrolled reduce restorative treatment, increase preventive care with no evidence of 'supervised neglect' (Johansson *et al.* 2007).

The acceptability of dental services was highlighted in a qualitative study of people who did not go to the dentist (Gregory *et al.* 2007). As well as being influenced by the perceived accessibility of care, participants were swayed by their trust in dentistry and their perceptions of oral health as a commodity. For these people at least, greater marketing may have been counter-productive in encouraging use of dental services.

Middle- and low-income countries

Whilst the prevalence of dental caries in many developing countries is still low, other diseases such as oral cancer and dental fluorosis are more common than in most developed countries. Non-industrialized countries also suffer from a shortage of resources including workforce, appropriate technology and universally available power supplies. For example, the dentist: Population ratio in many countries in Africa is less than 1 to 100 000 population compared to 1 to 1100 population in many Scandinavian countries. Over the last two decades, the additional burden of meeting the costs of the infection control implications of the HIV epidemic have exacerbated any deficiencies in resources.

The traditional curative approach to dental health is limited in any setting but these limitations are more extreme when they are exported to the developing world. The surgical approach to dentistry used in industrialized countries is technology intensive and requires an infrastructure of continuous power and water supply. It involves expensive equipment that is difficult to use and maintain. Dentists, therefore, need to treat patients who can help them recoup their costs. These pressures limit the availability of services and contribute to the inequalities in their provision. Hobdell (1993) described this situation as 'trying to implement a type of oral healthcare developed mainly in the last century in another part of the world using equipment and materials developed for use in an entirely different socioeconomic and political setting'. Large parts of the western model of dental care may be inappropriate in developing countries, including an over-emphasis of clinical surveys in healthcare planning. Services based on normative assessment limit community participation in healthcare and ignore the sociodental implications of oral disease. They may also over complicate healthcare. In one notorious example, survey data were used to calculate the periodontal treatment needs of children in Kenya (Manji & Sheiham 1986). Using the World Health Organization model the treatment proposed would have used the entire dental workforce of Kenya for up to 21 years, allowing for no other care. Services could concentrate on the relatively few conditions that comprise the bulk of oral health problems: Toothache (not *tooth decay*), trauma, oral infections, and neoplasms (Hobdell 1993).

The primary healthcare approach is still relevant to oral healthcare in all countries but it is particularly applicable to the developing world. It has five principles: An equitable distribution of services; community involvement in health; a focus on prevention; the use of appropriate technology and a multi-sectoral approach. *The Berlin Declaration on Oral Health and Oral Health Services in Deprived Communities* provides comprehensive guidelines for planning, implementing and evaluating oral health projects within this framework (Mautsch & Sheiham 1995). It was conceived by the Oral Health Alliance: An international network which provides support and information to colleagues working in this field. Specific examples of activities within this framework are presented below.

Equitable distribution

Tudor Hart's (1971) 'Inverse care law' between the availability of services and the need for them also occurs in dentistry. It is particularly extreme in countries where there are wide disparities between rich and poor. In Africa 80 per cent of the trained professional personnel live and work in affluent neighbourhoods in cities although the same proportion of the population lives in rural areas (Thorpe 1993). The scope for other dental care professionals in developing countries may be greater since advocates of their use may not have to compete with the well established political lobbies of dentists which exist in industrialized nations. DCPs can be used to provide simple, but essential treatments to extend the availability of services and reduce inequalities in access.

Models exist for identifying the types of personnel needed for oral healthcare in deprived communities along with training and evaluation methods (Samarawikrama 1995). Such models consider the frequency of problems, the difficulties encountered in undertaking the different roles and the identification of the difficulties themselves.

Community development

Community involvement means that people are allowed to take control of their own health and is necessary if programmes are to thrive. It is perhaps the most difficult aspect of the PHCA since it requires that health professionals must relinquish their traditional hierarchical role. In addition, individuals and communities often regard health as beyond their control and may not regard oral health as a priority. There are isolated examples of wide involvement in oral health. In Glasgow, Scotland, community-based Oral Health Action Teams—partnerships of parents, teachers, nursery nurses, health visitors and dentists—have reduced levels of caries in young children in deprived areas of the city (Blair 2004).

Focus on prevention

Prevention is universally accepted as an essential component of healthcare. However, if prevention is to avoid the existing system in which people are passive recipients of information and preventive therapies, it must adopt the principles of health promotion.

Appropriate technology

'Appropriate technology' is sometimes taken to mean 'cheap' and 'second rate'. It is neither of these things, but is an approach which recognizes the needs and resources of the local community. For example, the ART referred to earlier combines these requirements with new knowledge of the process of dental caries and developments in dental materials science (Frencken *et al.* 1966).

Multisectoral approach

We have seen how an effective health strategy might involve a number of departments of both national and local governments, water providers, the educational system, community members, and healthcare workers. All of the approaches to health promotion outlined in the second part of this essay must be integrated. However, integration should mean more than using the resources of other sectors to promote oral health. Such an approach often means that dentists simply get teachers to provide dental health education which carries the risk of not truly involving the other sectors (Mautsch & Sheiham 1995).

Conclusions and future developments in dental public health

Our understanding of the importance of oral health and its significance as a public health concern continues to grow. There is a greater knowledge than ever before of the nature of the oral diseases that threaten health (dental caries, periodontal diseases, oral cancer, and dento-facial trauma), the epidemiology of those diseases, and the factors that determine them. Moreover, we are starting to accumulate a body of evidence on the effectiveness of health promotion and treatment strategies. Those strategies include the use of fluoride; food and health policies to reduce sugar consumption; and community approaches to improve body hygiene including oral cleaning, smoking cessation, policies on reducing accidents, and ensuring access to appropriate preventive care. Many of these strategies could work in common with approaches to the promotion of general health.

Many oral health strategies discussed in this review do not involve clinical dental services. Dentistry lags behind medicine in recognizing the relative impotence of clinical dentistry to bring about oral health for populations and a greater awareness of its potential harm. The evidence of effectiveness should be used to identify beneficial interventions and should help re-orientate dentistry from its traditional curative approach that focuses on the responsibility of clinicians and their individual patients. In so doing we may be able to move toward a more shared responsibility in which all participate.

It is important that all these strands of information are combined. Perhaps most important of all, we need a more universal understanding of what is meant by 'oral health' and its relationship with oral disease. The ways we measure health and the outcomes of interventions will determine not only which interventions we choose but whether we choose to intervene at all.

Future developments in dental public health can be considered in four areas: Trends in oral health, the deprofessionalization of dentistry, technological developments, and relationships between oral and general healthcare delivery.

Two trends in oral health have been observed. Some countries, particularly developing countries, may be experiencing increases in dental caries. Any increases are related to the adoption of western dietary patterns high in sugars. Even if these trends are currently limited to more affluent city dwellers, they represent worrying concerns for the future. The increase in treatment needs created by these trends is likely to place an unaffordably high burden on developing economies. To some extent, this burden will be moderated by the low levels of perceived need in communities unused to receiving dental treatment. However, if disability and handicap brought about by oral disease is to be minimized, then appropriate methods of treating it will be required. Numerous examples now exist of dental care professionals being used to provide a limited range of treatments in both the developed and developing world. DCPs can be trained quicker to provide care to similar standards to dentists, but at greatly reduced costs. Food and health policies could also be used in countries with rising caries levels to control imports, the production and sale of cariogenic foods and drinks while encouraging the use of traditional foods.

In many developed countries, the decreased caries incidence witnessed over the last two decades appears to have stabilized in young children. The trend may have stabilized but its effects will continue to change dentistry for decades to come. When coupled with demographic changes, changed attitudes towards oral health and the preservation of teeth seen in developing countries over the last 50 years, this trend produces an interesting pattern. On the one hand, there is a growing and ageing group of younger people whose treatment needs will remain lower in terms of volume and complexity than preceding generations. On the other hand, there is a large group of older people who will live for longer and retain many heavily restored teeth. These people will require more care, some of it more complex, than the generations that preceded them. It is difficult to predict whether there will be a net change in the need for dental care or in which direction such a change would be. One likely change will be a greater emphasis on specialization within dentistry. The majority of the young people's needs will comprise simple one surface fillings that could be placed by DCPs. However, this change could be offset by the more complex demands of older people seeking dental implants and treatment for root caries and tooth wear that may remain in the domain of specialists.

A dominant political direction over recent years has been the deprofessionalization of dentistry. This trend is manifest in several different forms. In many developed countries, patients are demanding 'rights' as consumers of care. These demands are complemented by the application of marketing theory to dentistry, which places consumer satisfaction as an essential criterion in business success. Thus, patients have been directly and indirectly implicated in moves to regulate the way in which dentists market themselves and have ensured that patient satisfaction is an active concern of dentists. Similar principles are cornerstones of new public health. Health promotion takes public involvement in oral health well beyond clinical dentistry. Even within clinical care, satisfaction is an integral part of the process of care rather than just an outcome. Other agencies, such as governments and insurance companies, are increasingly involved in healthcare. Externally applied measures to minimize the costs of care and increase the accountability of healthcare organizations whilst assuring the quality of care all serve to reduce professional power within dentistry.

This trend of deprofessionalization is likely to continue and may help to make oral care more relevant to the needs of the people it serves. Professions resist any tendency to undermine their power. This reaction could present an opportunity for dental public health to facilitate and manage the deprofessionalization of dentistry.

A number of technological developments may also influence oral health and care. The ART shows considerable potential for providing simple, inexpensive, and effective treatment for the type of minimal caries seen in developing countries. Because the technique requires minimal training and equipment, it will allow services to be provided in relatively small and isolated communities. If the technique is used by partially skilled staff it may also contribute to the deprofessionalization of dentistry in these countries; it will certainly reduce the cost.

In developed countries, osseo-integrated implants are increasingly used to support dental prostheses. By providing a stable and retentive base for both single and multiple tooth prostheses, implants show great potential for reducing the handicap brought about by oral disease (Awad *et al.* 2000). One disadvantage is that, for the time being at least, implant treatment demands considerable specialist expertise, and is costly. Implants may therefore become a treatment limited to those who can afford them and thus contribute to inequalities in oral health.

Oral healthcare is becoming increasingly integrated with the delivery of other services. In policy terms greater integration can be seen as part of a multidisciplinary approach (World Health Organization 1978). There are many examples of integration at the level of clinical service provision. Dental surgeries may be linked with other clinical services in health centres. In some cases, dentists invite other types of healthcare workers into their practices to provide services. At a broader level of health promotion, integration is particularly compatible with a common risk factor approach to disease. Health educators and health promoters recognize the value of involving other healthcare workers, teachers, and other community workers, either as original deliverers or reinforcers of their messages. Oral health also becomes a consideration of local and national governments with debates about fluoridation of water supplies and whether agricultural and fiscal policy are used to promote oral health. It is the role of specialists in dental public health to act as advocates at all these levels.

References

Andersen, R.M. (1995) Revisiting the behavioral model and access to medical care: Does it matter? *Journal of Health and Social Behavior*, **36**, 1–10.

Andreasen, J.O. and Andreasen, F.M. (1997) *Textbook and Color Atlas of Traumatic Injuries to the Teeth.* Munksgaard, Copenhagen.

Armfield, J.M. and Spencer, A.J. (2007) Community effectiveness of fissure sealants and the effect of fluoridated water consumption. *Community Dental Health*, **24**, 4–11.

Arrow, P. (1997) Control of occlusal caries in the first permanent molars by oral hygiene. *Community Dentistry and Oral Epidemiology*, **25**, 278–83.

Awad, M.A., Locker, D., Korner-Bitensky, N., *et al.* (2000) Measuring the effect of intraoral implant rehabilitation on health related quality of life in a randomised controlled clinical trial. *Journal of Dental Research*, **79**, 1659–63.

Beck, J.D., Offenbacher, S. (2005) Systemic effects of periodontitis: epidemiology of periodontal disease and cardiovascular disease. *Journal of Periodontology*, **76** (Suppl.), 2089–100.

Beaglehole, R., Bonita, R. (2004) *Public Health at the Crossroads*. Cambridge University Press, Cambridge.

Blair, Y., Macpherson, L.M., McCall, D.R., *et al.* (2004) Glasgow nursery-based caries experience, before and after a community development-based oral health programme's implementation. *Community Dental Health*, **21**, 291–8.

Bramson, J.B., Guay, A.H. (2005) Comments on the proposed pediatric oral health therapist. *Journal of Public Health Dentistry*, **65**, 123–27.

Bunker, J.P. (2001) The role of medical care in contributing to health improvements within societies. *International Journal of Epidemiology*, **30**, 1260–1263.

Burt, B.A. (1998) Prevention policies in the light of the changed distribution of dental caries. *Acta Odontologica Scandinavia*, **56**, 179–86.

Burt, B.A., Ismail, A.I., and Eklund, S.A. (1985) Periodontal disease, tooth loss, and oral hygiene among older Americans. *Community Dentistry and Oral Epidemiology*, **13**, 93–6.

Carr, A.B., Ebbert, J.O. Interventions for tobacco cessation in the dental setting. *Cochrane Database of Systematic Reviews* 2006, Issue 1. Art. No.: CD005084. DOI: 10.1002/14651858.CD005084.pub2.

Centers for Disease Control and Prevention. (1999) Ten Great Public Health Achievements - United States, 1900-1999. *MMWR CDC Surveillance Summaries*, **48**, 241–243.

Conway, D.I., Stockton, D.L., Warnakulasuriya, K.A., *et al.* (2006) Incidence of oral and oropharyngeal cancer in United Kingdom (1990-1999) - recent trends and regional variation. *Oral Oncology*, **42**, *586–92.*

Croucher, R. (1989) *The Performance Gap*. Health Education Authority, London.

Dean, H.T., Arnold, F.A. Jr., Jay, P., *et al.* (1950) Studies on mass control of dental caries through fluoridation of the public water supply. *Public Health Reports*, **65**, 1403–8.

Department of Health and Human Services (2000) *Oral Health in America: A report of the Surgeon General.* Washington: Department of Health and Human Services.

Dickson, M. (1995) Oral Health Promotion In *Promoting oral health in deprived communities* (ed. Mautsch, W. and Sheiham, A.), pp. 175–86. Deusche Stiftungfur Internationale Entwicklung, Berlin.

Downer, M.C., Moles, D.R., Palmer, S., *et al.* (2006) A systematic review of measures of the effectiveness of screening for oral cançer and precancer. *Oral Oncology*, **42**, 551–60

Elderton, R.J. and Nuttall, N.M. (1983) Variation among dentists in planning treatment. *British Dental Journal*, **154**, 201–6.

Frankel, S. (2001) Commentary: Medical care and the wider influences upon population health: a false dichotomy. *International Journal of Epidemiology*, **30**, 1267–8.

Frencken, J.E., Pilot, T., Songpaisan, Y., *et al.* (1996) Atraumatic restorative treatment (ART): rationale, technique, and development. *Journal of Public Health Dentistry*, **56**, 135–40.

Gregg, T.A. and Boyd, T.H (1998) Treatment of avulsed permanent teeth in children. *International Journal of Paediatric Dentistry*, **8**, 75–81.

Gregory, J., Gibson, B., Robinson, P.G. (2007) The relevance of oral health for attenders and non-attenders: a qualitative study. *British Dental Journal*, 202, E 18.

Hobdell, M.H. (1993) Essential elements of a primary oral health care model. In *Promotion of Oral Health in the African Region. Proceedings of Workshop held in Nairobi, Kenya, 2–6 August 1993* (ed. Akpabio, S.P.), pp. 99–108. Commonwealth Dental Association, London.

Holliser, M.C. and Weintraub, J.A. (1993) The association of oral status with systemic health, quality of life, and economic productivity. *Journal of Dental Education*, **57**, 901–12.

Holland, W.W. (2002) A dubious future for public health? *Journal of the Royal Society of Medicine*, **95**, 182–8.

Illich I. (1976) *Limits to Medicine*. Penguin, London.

Ismail, A.I. and Bandekar, R.R. (1999) Fluoride supplements and fluorosis: a meta-analysis. *Community Dentistry and Oral Epidemiology*, **27**, 48–56.

Johansson, V. Axtelius, B., Soderfeldt, B., *et al.* (2007) Financial systems' impact on dental care: a review of fee-for-service and capitation systems. *Community Dental Health*, **24**, 12–20.

Johnson, N.W. (1997) Oral cancer: practical prevention. *FDI World*, **6**, 6–13.

Jones, S., Burt, B. A., Petersen, P. E., *et al.* (2005) The effective use of fluorides in public health. *Bulletin of World Health Organization*, **83**, 670–6.

Jones, S. and Lennon, M. A. (Eds.) (1997) Fluoridation. Community Oral Health. Bath, Wright.

Kay, E.J. and Locker, D. (1997) *Effectiveness of oral health promotion: a review*. Health Education Authority, London.

Kenealy, P.M., Kingdon, A., Richmond, S., *et al.* (2007) The Cardiff dental study: A 20-year critical evaluation of the psychological health gain from orthodontic treatment. *British Psychological Society*, **12**, 17–49.

Kwan, S.Y., Prendergast, M.J., and Williams, S.A. (1996) The diagnostic reliability of clinical dental auxiliaries in caries prevalence surveys – a pilot study. *Community Dental Health*, **13**, 145–49.

Locker, D. (2004) Oral health and quality of life. *Oral Health & Preventive Dentistry*, **2** (Suppl.), 247–53.

Manji, F. and Sheiham, A. (1986) CPITN findings and the manpower implications of periodontal treatment needs for Kenyan children. *Community Dental Health*, **3**, 143–51.

Marino, R., Villa A., and Weitz, A. (2006) Dental Caries Prevention using Milk as the vehicle for Fluorides: The Chilean Experiences. Melbourne, Australia: School of Dental Science, The University of Melbourne.

Marinho, V.C.C., Higgins, J.P.T., Logan, S., *et al.* (2002a) Fluoride varnishes for preventing dental caries in children and adolescents. *Cochrane Database of Systematic Reviews.* Issue 1. Art. No.: CD002279. DOI: 10.1002/14651858.CD002279.

Marinho, V.C.C., Higgins, J.P.T., Logan, S., *et al.* (2002b) Fluoride gels for preventing dental caries in children and adolescents. *Cochrane Database of Systematic Reviews.* Issue 1. Art. No.: CD002280. DOI: 10.1002/14651858.CD002280

Marinho, V.C.C., Higgins, J.P.T., Logan, S., *et al.* (2003a) Fluoride toothpastes for preventing dental caries in children and adolescents. *Cochrane Database of Systematic Reviews.* Issue 1. Art. No.: CD002278. DOI: 10.1002/14651858.CD002278.

Marinho, V.C.C., Higgins, J.P.T., Logan, S., *et al.* (2003b) Fluoride mouthrinses for preventing dental caries in children and adolescents. *Cochrane Database of Systematic Reviews.* Issue 3. Art.No.: CD002284. DOI: 10.1002/14651858.CD002284.

Marthaler, T.M. (1990) Changes in the prevalence of dental caries: How much can be attributed to changes in diet. *Caries Research*, **24**, 212–23.

Mautsch, W. and Sheiham, A. (1995) *Promoting Oral Health in Deprived Communities.* Zahnmedizinische Entwicklungshilfe e.V., Berlin.

McDonagh, M., Whiting, P., Bradley, M., *et al.* (2000) *A Systematic Review of Public Water Fluoridation.* York: Publications Office, NHS Centre for Reviews and Dissemination, University of York.

McKay, F.S. (1933) Mottled enamel: The prevention of its further production through a change of water supply at Oakley, Idaho. *Journal of the American Dental Association*, **20**, 1137–49.

McKeown, T. (1976) *The Role of Medicine: Dream, Mirage or Nemesis?* The Nuffield Provincial Hospitals Trust, London.

Medical Research Council. (2002) *Water Fluoridation and Health.* Medical Research Council, London.

Moynihan, P. and Petersen, P.E. (2004) Diet, nutrition and the prevention of dental diseases. *Public Health Nutrition*, **7**, 201–26.

Morris, A.J., Steele, J., and White, D.A. (2001) The oral cleanliness and periodontal health of UK adults in 1998. *British Dental Journal*, **191**, 186–92.

Nadanovsky, P. and Sheiham, A. (1994) The relative contribution of dental services to the changes and geographical variations in caries status of 5- and 12-year-old children in England and Wales in the 1980s. *Community Dental Health*, **11**, 215–23.

Nadanovsky, P. and Sheiham, A. (1995) Relative contribution of dental services to the changes in caries levels of 12-year-old children in 18 industrialized countries in the 1970s and early 1980s. *Community Dentistry and Oral Epidemiology*, **23**, 331–9.

National Institute for Health and Clinical Excellence (2004) *Dental recall-recall interval between routine dental examinations.* National Institute for Health and Clinical Excellence, London.

Needleman, I., Suvan, J., Moles, D.R., *et al.* (2005a) A systematic review of professional mechanical plaque removal for prevention of periodontal diseases. *Journal of Clinical Periodontology*, **32** (Supplement), 229–82.

Needleman, I., Tucker, R., Giedry-Leeper, E., *et al.* (2005b) Guided tissue regeneration for periodontal intrabony defects - a Cochrane Systematic Review. *Periodontology 2000*, **37**, 106–123. doi:10.1111/j.1600-0757.2004.37101.x

Nuttall, N., Steele, J.G., Pine, C.M., *et al.* (2001) The impact of oral health on people in the UK in 1998. *British Dental Journal*, **190,** 121–126.

Nuttall, N. and Harker, R. (2004) *Impact of oral health- Children's Dental Health in the United Kingdom 2003. http://www.statistics.gov.uk/downloads/cdh5_Impact_of_oral_health.pdf* Accessed 19th March 2007.

Penchansky, R. and Thomas, J.W. (1981) The concept of access. Definition and relationship to consumer satisfaction. *Medical Care*, **19**, 127–40.

Pitts. N. and Harker, R. (2004) *Obvious decay experience. Children's Dental Health in the United Kingdom 2003. http://www.statistics.gov.uk/children/dentalhealth/downloads/cdh_dentinal_decay.pdf.* Accessed 19th March 2007.

Reibel, J. (2003) Tobacco and oral diseases. Update on the evidence, with recommendations. *Medical Principles and Practice*, **12** (Suppl. 1), 22–32

Robinson, P.G., Deacon, S.A., Deery, C., *et al.* Manual versus powered toothbrushing for oral health. *The Cochrane Database of Systematic Reviews* 2005, Issue 2. Art. No.: CD002281.pub2. DOI: 10.1002/14651858.CD002281.pub2.

Robinson, P.G., Pankhurst, C.L., Garrett, E.J. (2005) Randomized-controlled trial: effect of a reservoir biteguard on quality of life in xerostomia. *Journal of Oral Pathology and Medicine*, **34**, 193–7.

Rose, G. (1992) *The Strategy of Preventive Medicine.* Oxford University Press, Oxford.

Rosen, L., Manor, D., Engelhard, D., *et al.* (2006) In defense of the randomized controlled trial for health promotion research. *American Journal of Public Health*, **96**, 1181–6.

Rugg-Gunn, A. (1997) Nutrition, dietary guidelines and food policy in oral health. In *Community Oral Health* (ed. Pine, C.), pp. 206–20. Wright, Oxford.

Rugg-Gunn, A.J. (1993) *Nutrition and Dental Health.* Oxford University Press, Oxford.

Samarawikrama, D.Y.D. (1995) Appropriate technology, personnel and training. In *Promoting Oral Health in Deprived communities* (ed. Mautsch, W. and Sheiham, A.), pp. 347–61. Deusche Stiftungfur Internationale Entwicklung, Berlin.

Sanders, A.E., Spencer, A.J., and Stewart, J.F. (2005) Clustering of risk behaviours for oral and general health. *Community Dental Health*, **22,** 133–40.

Sanderson, M.E. (1984) Strategies for implementing NACNE recommendations. *Lancet*, **10**, 1352–6.

Sanderson, D. (1998) *Water fluoridation - an economics perspective.* York: York Health Economics Consortium. University of York.

Schou, L. (1998) Behavioural aspects of dental plaque control measures: an oral health promotion perspective. In *European workshop on mechanical plaque control* (eds Lang, N.P., Attstrom, R., and Loe, H.), pp. 287–99. Quintessence, Chicago.

Sheiham, A. (1995) Development of oral health promotion strategies In *Turning Strategy into Action* (ed. Kay, E.), pp. 9–46. Eden Bianchi Press, Manchester.

Sheiham, A. and Watt, R.G. (2000) The common risk factor approach: a rational basis for promoting oral health. *Community Dentistry and Oral Epidemiology*, **28,** 399–406.

Smith, S.E., Warnakulasuriya, K.A., Feyerabend, C., *et al.* (1998) A smoking cessation programme conducted through dental practices in the UK. *British Dental Journal*, **185**, 299–303.

Sprod, A., Anderson, R., and Treasure, E.T. (1996) *Effective Oral Health Promotion: Literature Review.* Health Promotion Wales, Cardiff.

Sutcliffe, P. (1996) Oral cleanliness and dental caries In *Prevention of oral disease* (ed. Murray, J.J.), pp. 68–77. Oxford University Press, Oxford.

Thorpe, S.J. (1993) Oral health status and trends in Africa – A WHO overview. In *Promotion of oral health in the African region. Proceedings of workshop held Nairobi, Kenya, 2–6 August 1993* (ed. Akpabio, S.P.), pp. 72–6. Commonwealth Dental Association, London.

Tones, K. and Tilford, S. (2001) *Health Promotion. Effectiveness, Efficiency and Equity.* Nelson Thornes Ltd, Cheltenham.

Tudor Hart, J. (1971) The inverse care law. *Lancet*, **1**, 405–12.

Tudor Hart, J. (2001) Commentary: Can health outputs of routine practice approach those of clinical trials? *International Journal of Epidemiology*, **30,** 1263–7.

van Amerongen B.M., Schutte G.J.B. and Alpherts W.C.J. (1993) *International dental key figures: A dynamic and relational data base analyzing oral health care.* Key Figure, Amsterdam.

Van der Weijden, G.A. and Timmerman, M.F. (2002) A systematic review on the clinical efficacy of subgingival debridement in the treatment of chronic periodontitis. *Journal of Clinical Periodontology*, **29** (Suppl. 3), 55–71.

Watt, R. and Marinho, V.C. (2005) Does oral health promotion improve oral hygiene and gingival health? *Periodontology 2000*, **37**, 35–47.

Watt, R. and Sheiham, A. (1999) Inequalities in Oral Health: A review of the evidence and recommendations for action. *British Dental Journal*, **187**, 6–12.

Watt, R. (2007) From victim blaming to upstream action: tackling the social determinants of oral health inequalities. *Community Dentistry and Oral Epidemiology*, **35**, 1–11.

Welbury, R.R. (1996) The prevention of dental trauma. In *The prevention of oral disease* (ed. Murray, J.J.), pp. 147–52. Oxford University Press, Oxford.

WHO/UNICEF (1978) *Primary Health Care, Alma-Ata 1978*. World Health Organization, Geneva.

Wong, F.S. and Kolokotsa, K. (2004) The cost of treating children and adolescents with injuries to their permanent incisors at a dental hospital in the United Kingdom. *Dental Traumatology*, **20**, 327–33.

World Health Organization (1984) *Health Promotion: A Discussion Document on the Concepts and Principles*. World Health Organisation Regional Office for Europe, Copenhagen.

World Health Organization (1986) *Ottawa Charter for Health Promotion*. World Health Organisation, Geneva.

World Health Organization (1998) *Health Promotion Evaluation: Recommendations to policy makers*. World Health Organisation, Geneva.

World Health Organization (2001) *Global Oral Health Data Bank*. Geneva: World Health Organization.

World Health Organization (1980) *Risk factors and comprehensive control of chronic diseases. Report ICP/CVD 020(2)*. Geneva: World Health Organization.

Xiong, X., Buekens, P., Fraser, W.D., *et al.* (2006) Periodontal disease and adverse pregnancy outcomes: a systematic review. *British Journal of Obstetrics and Gynaecology*, **113**, 135–43.

Yee, R., McDonald, N., and Walker, D. (2003) An advocacy project to fluoridate toothpastes in Nepal. *International Dental Journal*, **53**, 220–30.

Yeung, C.A., Hitchings, J.L., Macfarlane, T.V., *et al.* (2005) Fluoridated milk for preventing dental caries. *Cochrane Database of Systematic Reviews*. Issue 3. Art. No.: CD003876. DOI: 10.1002/14651858.CD003876.pub2.

Yip HK, Smales RJ, Ngo HC, Tay FR, Chu FC. (2001) Selection of restorative materials for the atraumatic restorative treatment (ART) approach: a review. *Special Care Dentistry*, **21**, 216–21.

9.9

Musculoskeletal diseases

Jennifer L. Kelsey and Marian T. Hannan

Abstract

Musculoskeletal conditions are a major cause of impairment, disability, health care utilization, and loss of economic productivity throughout the world. Among adults, *osteoarthritis* is one of the leading causes of disability worldwide. Risk factors include increasing age and the female sex, as well as obesity, malalignment and repetitive loading of joints, and previous congenital and developmental conditions and injuries involving joints. Reduction of exposure to these factors, when possible, should retard the development and progression of osteoarthritis. *Rheumatoid arthritis*, although less common, often results in significant disability. It is considered to be of autoimmune aetiology, with a strong genetic component. The incidence and severity are associated with a specific amino acid sequence on several human leukocyte antigen (HLA) DRB1 alleles. New drugs are helping to alleviate symptoms and inhibit structural damage.

Osteoporosis, a common condition in older people, predisposes to fractures. Among the risk factors are increasing age, the female sex, thinness, low oestrogen concentrations, frailty and poor health, and to a lesser extent, low calcium and vitamin D intake, and lack of physical activity. Prevention of falls in older people can reduce the frequency of osteoporosis-associated fractures. *Low back and neck pain* affect the majority of the people throughout the world at some time during their lives. Heavy manual labour and exposure to whole-body vibration are major risk factors, and reduction in these activities should reduce the frequency of low back and neck pain. *Foot disorders* represent a variety of structural, biomechanical, skin, and sensory conditions as well as manifestations of systemic diseases such as arthritis, diabetes mellitus, and peripheral vascular disease. Wearing appropriate shoes and weight reduction are possible preventive measures for some common structural foot problems.

Disorders of adolescents and children include conditions associated with the adolescent growth spurt such as scoliosis and slipped epiphysis, injuries such as childhood fractures, and conditions of infants such as developmental dislocation of the hip.

Musculoskeletal conditions are common in all age groups, but their greatest impact is on the elderly. The number of elderly persons is rapidly increasing worldwide, especially in developing countries. Thus, the burden of musculoskeletal conditions will become substantially greater over the next several decades. Application of known methods of prevention at all levels and development of new preventive methods are urgently needed.

Magnitude of the problem

Musculoskeletal diseases are common, affect both sexes and all age groups, and are responsible for a substantial amount of impairment, disability, and economic burden throughout the world. These disorders range from minor aches and pains to chronic disabling conditions. Although they are occasionally fatal, their main effects are on the quality of life and economic productivity.

The World Health Organization (WHO) uses disability-adjusted life years (DALYs), which are the sum of the years of life lost from premature mortality and the years of life lived with disability, as an indicator of the burden of disease. Table 9.9.1 shows that throughout the world musculoskeletal diseases account for a large number of DALYs, including almost 9 000 000 in developed regions and about 21 000 000 in developing regions in 2001 (Brooks 2006). These estimates do not include fractures and other injuries, which are classified separately by the WHO under trauma.

High-income countries

In high-income countries, musculoskeletal conditions affect almost all people at some time during their lives. In the United States, musculoskeletal conditions are the most frequently reported impairment, defined as a chronic or permanent defect representing a decrease or loss of ability to perform various functions. Each year,

Table 9.9.1 Estimated number of disability-adjusted life years (DALYs) in the developing and developed regions of the world, 2001

Region	Number of DALYs[a]
Developing regions	21 076 000
Developed regions	8 723 000
Total	29 798 000

[a] DALYs are the sum of the years of life lost from premature mortality and the years of life lived with disability.

Source: Modified from Brooks P.M. The burden of musculoskeletal disease—a global perspective. *Clinical Rheumatology* 2006;**25**:778–81.

about 14 per cent of the population of all ages reports a musculoskeletal impairment (Praemer *et al.* 1999). The prevalence of musculoskeletal impairments increases with age. Among those aged 85 years and older, the annual prevalence is 20 per cent, with impairments of the back or spine and lower extremity or hip accounting for slightly more than half of the musculoskeletal impairments. Among impairments, musculoskeletal disorders are the leading cause of days of restricted activity and days in bed.

A survey in the United Kingdom found that 17 per cent of adults report a long-standing musculoskeletal disorder (Bowling 1996). The most important areas of life affected by long-standing disorders of the musculoskeletal system are ability to move around, stand, walk, and go shopping (24 per cent), and to participate in social and leisure-time activities (24 per cent). The ability to work is also a major issue (17 per cent), particularly for those of working age.

Acute injuries of the musculoskeletal system, including fractures, dislocations, sprains, and strains, are also common. According to the US Health Interview Survey (Praemer *et al.* 1999), 14.5 musculoskeletal injuries occur per 100 people per year of sufficient severity to warrant medical care or at least one half day of restricted activity.

Musculoskeletal conditions generate substantial health care utilization. About 11 per cent of all hospitalizations in short-stay hospitals in the United States are attributed to musculoskeletal conditions (Praemer *et al.* 1999). Fractures, arthritis, intervertebral disc disorders, and other back problems are responsible for the greatest number of hospitalizations. The population aged 65 years and older accounts for 44 per cent of the hospitalizations for musculoskeletal conditions. Among visits to physicians in office-based practice, musculoskeletal conditions rank first, accounting for 17 per cent of all office visits. Fifteen per cent of the visits to hospital outpatient departments and 26 per cent of the visits to emergency departments are attributable to musculoskeletal conditions.

In addition, a significant and increasing number of people throughout the industrialized world are using complementary and alternative medicine. In a national sample of adults in the United States, 48 per cent of those with back pain, 27 per cent of those with arthritis, 57 per cent of those with neck problems, and 24 per cent of those with sprains and strains had used complementary and alternative medicine for their condition in the past year (Eisenberg *et al.* 1998).

The monetary cost of these diseases to society is substantial, especially because of the decreased productivity of those affected. Felts and Yelin (1989) reported that costs of musculoskeletal diseases accounted for 1 per cent of the gross national product in the United States. Badley (1995) noted that musculoskeletal diseases account for 32 per cent of all chronic disability costs in Canada.

Middle- and low-income countries

The impact of musculoskeletal diseases on the work and personal lives of people in middle- and low-income countries is also enormous, but only limited data are currently available on this impact. As in industrialized countries, pain, disability, and loss of employment are major problems. In Bangladesh, for instance, 26 per cent of those surveyed had musculoskeletal pain at the time of the survey, most commonly in the low back, knees, hips, and shoulders (Haq *et al.* 2005). The two most common musculoskeletal disorders were osteoarthritis of the knees and non-specific low back pain. In an urban area of Indonesia, the prevalence of pain in the joints, back, or neck was 31 per cent, and in a rural area, 24 per cent. Among those with pain, 78 per cent in the urban area and 75 per cent in the rural area had to discontinue work because of the pain; these high percentages reflect the preponderance of jobs requiring manual labour in both urban and rural areas (Darmawan *et al.* 1992). Work-related problems, many of which can be prevented with proper ergonomic techniques, are particularly common in developing countries (Ahasan *et al.* 1999). In a survey in Thailand, about 50 per cent of the female workers in five industries (garment, fertilizer, pharmaceutical, textile, and cigarettes) reported low back symptoms, most of which could be attributed to the work environment (Chavalitsakulchai & Shahnavaz 1993).

In addition, because common musculoskeletal conditions such as osteoarthritis and osteoporosis are most prevalent at older ages and because the numbers of elderly in developing countries are rapidly increasing, the burden of musculoskeletal conditions in these areas will become even greater. For instance, in the early 1990s it was estimated that about half of the estimated 1 660 000 hip fractures worldwide occurred in Europe and North America, but by 2050 it is predicted that three quarters of the 6 260 000 hip fractures will occur in other parts of the world, with almost two thirds occurring in Asia and Latin America (Cooper *et al.* 1992). In younger age groups, the increasing frequency of accidents related to motor vehicles in low- and middle-income countries is resulting in a steep increase in the number of severe injuries, many of which involve the musculoskeletal system (Beveridge & Howard 2004). Thus, the burden of musculoskeletal conditions will continue to rise substantially over the next few decades in these countries.

Some common problems in epidemiologic studies of musculoskeletal conditions

Conducting epidemiologic studies of musculoskeletal conditions even in high-income countries presents several difficulties not experienced to the same extent in studies of other important chronic diseases such as cancer and coronary heart disease. First, because many musculoskeletal conditions are not fatal, have a gradual onset, and often do not even come to medical attention, ascertainment of representative cases for epidemiologic study may be difficult. Consequently, many studies of musculoskeletal diseases are based on the experiences of particular clinics or hospitals. However, cases representative of those occurring in the general population are needed in order to provide an accurate description of disease occurrence, aetiology, and progression in the community.

Even if all cases coming to medical attention within a defined geographic area are included in a study, unless the disease under study almost invariably comes to medical attention, the factors that bring persons with a given condition to medical attention often cannot be separated from factors that may be related to disease aetiology. For instance, it may be difficult to know whether psychological characteristics of persons seeking care for low back pain are involved in the aetiology of low back pain or if they are related to the care-seeking behaviour among those with low back pain. A person may also report low back pain only in order to obtain worker's compensation. A person may say that he or she has low back pain, but the researcher or practitioner cannot know with certainty when no radiographic or other signs are apparent. Even if objective evidence of an abnormality is present, interpretation may be difficult. For instance, as the majority of the asymptomatic people in the general population show evidence of bulging or protruding intervertebral discs on magnetic resonance imaging, even such imaging may be of limited value without clinical evidence of pathology.

Sometimes, a condition for which medical care is virtually always sought, and for which case ascertainment is therefore relatively easy, is used as a surrogate for a disease for which medical care is not necessarily sought. For instance, hip fracture, which is almost always seen in a hospital, is used as a surrogate for osteoporosis. Hip fracture, however, usually depends not only on whether a person has poor bone quality, but also on whether the person falls and how he or she falls. Thus, the risk factors for osteoporosis and hip fracture will overlap, but they also differ in some respects.

The diagnostic criteria used for a disease may differ from one study to another, making it difficult to compare results. To address this problem for major arthritic disorders, expert committees were established to develop and then periodically revise diagnostic criteria for several diseases. The comparability of cases from one study to another increases when the diagnostic criteria are uniformly applied; however, this is not always the case, and as the criteria change over time, it may not be possible to examine corresponding changes in disease frequency.

Diseases that constitute one end of a continuous distribution, such as osteoporosis and scoliosis, present other problems. To define cases of these conditions, relatively arbitrary cut-off points aimed at classifying individuals as 'diseased' and 'normal' are employed, which has made comparisons of prevalence among countries more meaningful. Nevertheless, some investigators may choose different cut-off points, precluding comparison. In addition, people with values just above or just below the cut-off point are actually quite similar to each other, yet one group is considered diseased and the other is not.

Labels for diseases once considered a single entity may become irrelevant when subcategories of the disease are more clearly delineated. For instance, what was once called 'juvenile rheumatoid arthritis' is now known to comprise several subtypes, each with its own aetiology. Much information may be lost when several distinct entities are considered as one disease, as exemplified by studies of low back pain that do not consider the contribution of many different disease processes, such as sprains and strains, intervertebral disc herniations, osteoarthritis, and osteoporosis.

Another concern relates to study design. Cross-sectional studies are often undertaken, such as of the relation between neuromuscular abnormalities and scoliosis. Results from such studies, however, are difficult to interpret because it is not known whether the neuromuscular abnormalities lead to curvature of the spine, whether curvature of the spine leads to neuromuscular defects, or whether some other factor leads to both. Cross-sectional studies of psychological symptoms and low back pain and of obesity and osteoarthritis present similar difficulties in interpretation. In such situations, longitudinal studies, despite their great expense, are needed.

Problems in conducting epidemiologic studies of musculoskeletal diseases are considerably magnified in low-income countries. Because of money and staff shortages, many studies are based in hospitals or clinics. However, in many developing countries, most people do not seek care from a physician or in a hospital unless the disease is quite severe; instead, care may be obtained from community-based nurses. In a survey in the Philippines it was found that most people who sought treatment for rheumatic complaints were seen by someone other than a physician. Only 23 per cent had seen a general practitioner, and 2 per cent saw a rheumatologist. Care from a physician is frequently not available, accessible, or affordable (Dans *et al.* 1997). Some countries have no rheumatologists at all. Patriarchal societies may limit access to medical care for women, and relatively few women survive to old age. Consequently, both comparisons of disease frequency in men and women within such countries and comparisons with other countries may be difficult to interpret (Hameed *et al.* 1995; Farooqi & Gibson 1998). In addition, even when affected individuals are seen by qualified medical personnel, the diagnostic criteria vary considerably (Ferraz 1995).

If community surveys are undertaken in low-income countries, many difficulties are likely to be encountered. Poor training of personnel, inadequate facilities, limited ability to reach populations for study, a low level of public support, political instability, and bureaucratic rigidity are often encumbrances to epidemiologic studies (Ferraz 1995). The diagnostic tests used in such surveys must be simple and inexpensive. If the study is being conducted in a tropical region, reagents and tests used in other geographic areas may not work because of the heat. In addition, pain, complaints, and manifestations of disability may vary cross-culturally, and measures of disability often require modification. Risk factors may also be quite different in low-income countries.

Finally, great variation in disease frequency and risk factor prevalence occurs among and within developing countries. In north Pakistan, for instance, osteoarthritis of the knee is an especially common complaint; fibromyalgia, low back pain, and soft-tissue rheumatism are the next most common, mainly among the urban poor (Farooqi & Gibson 1998). Thus, not only should one avoid generalizing from one country to another, but frequently one cannot generalize from one part of the same country to another part.

Selected musculoskeletal disorders of adults

Osteoarthritis

Osteoarthritis, also known as degenerative joint disease, is a gradual deterioration of the joint cartilage with proliferation and remodelling of subchondral bone. Any of the joint tissues may be involved, including synovium, joint capsule, periarticular muscles, sensory nerve endings, and ligaments. The usual symptoms are pain and stiffness, followed by loss of function. The typical radiographic appearance of the joint includes osteophyte formation, joint space narrowing, and subchondral sclerosis. Single joints may be affected, with the hands, knees, feet, hips, and spine most commonly involved. Generalized osteoarthritis is defined as having three or more affected joint groups.

Several pathologic features of osteoarthritis, including the proliferative bone changes, may represent attempted repair responses in an injured joint. Osteophytes, for example, may result from a reactive response of cartilage and bone to abnormal mechanical loading, conferring protection to a damaged joint by reducing instability (Arden & Nevitt 2006).

Estimates of osteoarthritis prevalence have generally used an individual's report of pain or decreased articular movement in the joint and/or radiographs of the joint. According to the United States Health Interview Survey, an estimated 22 per cent of adults have osteoarthritis (Centers for Disease Control and Prevention 2006). The proportions affected in Caucasian populations in various high-income countries are quite similar, but hip osteoarthritis may be less common in Africa and Asia than in the Western countries. Knee osteoarthritis shows less geographical variation than hip and hand osteoarthritis, possibly reflecting the importance of injury as a cause of knee disease. Most studies of osteoarthritis have been conducted in developed countries. Worldwide symptom-based prevalence is estimated at 10 per cent among men and 18 per cent among women aged 60 years and older (Woolf & Pfleger 2003). The prevalence of symptomatic osteoarthritis in Turkey is 15 per cent among adults aged 50 years and older (Kacar *et al.* 2005).

Osteoarthritis is the leading cause of disability in the United States (Centers for Disease Control and Prevention 2001). As the populations of low-income countries age, osteoarthritis will become an increasing burden in these populations as well. The WHO has predicted that osteoarthritis will become the fourth leading cause of disability worldwide by the year 2020 (Woolf & Pfleger 2003).

Many individuals with radiographic evidence of osteoarthritis are asymptomatic. In the United States, European, and Asian populations, roughly 50 per cent of the adults with radiographic evidence of knee osteoarthritis report knee pain; discrepancy between radiographic evidence of osteoarthritis and pain has been noted for the hands and hips as well (World Health Organization 2003).

Risk factors

Prevalence increases steeply with age in all populations, especially after 50 years. On autopsy, almost everyone 65 years or older has at least one joint with features of osteoarthritis. Individual joints show the same age-related rise in osteoarthritis prevalence, with the hip showing a later rise than the knee. Women are at least twice as likely to be affected as men, especially for hand and knee osteoarthritis, and particularly after age 50 years.

Overweight persons are at increased risk for osteoarthritis of several sites, most notably the knees and hands. In the United States, obese persons have double the prevalence of osteoarthritis at most sites compared with persons of normal weight, especially at the knee (Centers for Disease Control and Prevention 2006); the higher prevalence exists whether osteoarthritis is defined by symptom or radiograph. Longitudinal studies show that increased weight precedes the occurrence of hand or knee osteoarthritis and is not merely a consequence of it. Furthermore, overweight persons with knee osteoarthritis are at higher risk of experiencing progressive disease than persons who are not overweight. Weight loss reduces the risk of symptomatic knee disease (Centers for Disease Control and Prevention 2006).

Repetitive loading of joints, particularly in certain occupations and sports, is a strong risk factor for osteoarthritis. It has long been noted that miners often develop osteoarthritis of the elbows and knees, cotton pickers of particular joints in the fingers, farmers of the hips, and dockworkers of the fingers, elbows, and knees. Specific on-the-job activities that predispose to knee and hip osteoarthritis are knee bending, squatting, kneeling, stair climbing, heavy lifting, and carrying heavy loads (Cooper *et al.* 1994). In high- and low-income countries, hip osteoarthritis is more frequent among farmers than among persons in non-farming occupations. These risks are cumulative, and evidence indicates increasing risk with greater number of years spent in such occupations.

Studies of recreational and competitive athletes suggest that frequent exercise, including jogging or moderate low-impact running, is not a detectable risk factor for hip and knee osteoarthritis in those with normal joints. However, these activities may increase the risk in those with previous joint injuries or developmentally defective joints. Prolonged decreased joint use and decreased loading generate changes that make cartilage more vulnerable to injury.

Congenital and developmental disorders and injuries involving joints, particularly if not treated early, greatly increase the likelihood of developing osteoarthritis in the affected joint. Prior inflammatory joint disease is also a risk factor. Greater grip strength appears to increase the risk for osteoarthritis of the hands, whereas muscle weakness may be a risk factor for other sites such as the knees and hips. Nutritional factors, high bone mineral density, and low concentrations of serum oestradiol have been linked to osteoarthritis in some studies, but the evidence is not conclusive (Arden & Nevitt 2006).

Genetic susceptibility is considered to be important (Arden & Nevitt 2006); multiple genes are likely to be involved in the aetiology of osteoarthritis. Polymorphisms of the type II collagen gene (Col2A1) are of particular interest because type II collagen is a major constituent of the articular cartilage. The vitamin D and oestrogen receptor genes may contribute as well. Genes encoding other structural proteins of the cartilage matrix and bone as well as cartilage growth factors are under study.

Prevention

Preventive measures include weight loss, reduction of repetitive biomechanical stress on the joints, and prevention and early treatment of congenital, developmental, and adult diseases involving the joints. Techniques for avoiding sports-related joint trauma include providing appropriate protection and padding for contact sports and modifying game rules to minimize contact that is associated with joint trauma. Developing and maintaining adequate muscle strength is an important mechanism to minimize joint stress.

To decrease pain and stiffness and reduce functional limitations, several steps may be taken, depending on the severity of the disease (Bartlett *et al.* 2006). Self-management, which incorporates self-care and self-treatment, is one of the first-line non-pharmacologic treatment options for management of osteoarthritis. Self-care and self-treatment may include education, exercise, healthy eating, and over-the-counter remedies, as well as pain coping skills. Studies in the United States, United Kingdom, and China show that arthritis self-management programmes improve health behaviours and health status. Weight reduction has been shown to protect against both the development and progression of osteoarthritis. Therapy can involve the use of analgesics, nutriceuticals, and/or non-steroidal anti-inflammatory drugs to control symptoms of pain, combined with physical and occupational therapy to maintain joint range of motion, muscle strength, and an individual's ability to perform everyday activities. Other steps may include steroid injections into joints or minor surgery. Finally, joint replacement surgery of the hips and knees has been highly successful for those with severe osteoarthritis.

Rheumatoid arthritis

Rheumatoid arthritis is a chronic inflammatory joint disorder characterized by proliferative synovitis leading to destruction of the articular cartilage and bony erosions. Symptoms typically include pain and stiffness of multiple joints (particularly the small joints of the hands and feet), soft-tissue swelling, increased temperature of affected joints, decreased range of motion, weakness, and fatigue. Systemic manifestations of rheumatoid arthritis include vascular, renal, and eye complications. The diagnostic classification system generally used is the 1987 American College of Rheumatology revised criteria (Bartlett *et al.* 2006).

Rheumatoid arthritis is usually not a fatal disorder. The clinical course is variable, but as the disease progresses, most people with rheumatoid arthritis develop functional limitations, physical disabilities, and sometimes early mortality.

The prevalence of rheumatoid arthritis in the United States and Western Europe ranges from 0.5 to 1 per cent. There is evidence of a decline in rheumatoid arthritis incidence over the last few decades in US and European populations (Bartlett *et al.* 2006). The prevalence is similar among African-Americans and Caucasian Americans, but greater prevalence of rheumatoid arthritis has been reported among several Native American tribes. Lower prevalence has been reported among some Asian populations, and Asians may also have milder disease compared to Caucasians (Lau *et al.* 1996).

Risk factors

Overall, the incidence among females is about twice that of males, although this gender gap decreases with age. Over the age of 60 years, women are affected about 1.5 times more often than men (Rasch *et al.* 2003).

Rheumatoid arthritis is considered to be of autoimmune aetiology, and genetic factors are important. Genetic studies have focused primarily on autoimmune aspects of the disease, especially the role of the human leukocyte antigen (HLA) alleles. HLA-DR4 was the first allele to be associated with rheumatoid arthritis, and it is now known that the incidence and severity of rheumatoid arthritis are associated with a specific amino acid sequence on several HLA-DRB1 alleles called the *rheumatoid arthritis shared epitope* (Bartlett *et al.* 2006).

Although the potential contribution of genetic susceptibility is widely recognized, questions remain regarding the triggering events that lead to rheumatoid arthritis and its patterns of expression. Infectious agents have been proposed but none have been definitively linked with rheumatoid arthritis. Oral contraceptives may retard the progression from mild to severe disease. Previous blood transfusion, obesity, and cigarette smoking may be associated with increased risks (Bartlett *et al.* 2006).

Prevention

No viable primary or secondary prevention measures are available for rheumatoid arthritis. Treatment includes the use of analgesics and/or non-steroidal anti-inflammatory drugs to control pain and stiffness, physical therapy to maintain and improve joint range of motion, and occupational therapy to maximize the individual's ability to perform daily activities. Disease-modifying drugs, including gold, penicillamine, and sulfasalazine, are believed to inhibit cytokines. These drugs produce a slow response and a high level of toxicity, and thus typically have not been taken for long periods of time. Methotrexate has somewhat better properties, but is still not used for lengthy periods. Nevertheless, use of these drugs early in the disease course and aggressive escalation of therapy based on objective evidence of continued disease activity have greatly improved the course of the disease (Emery 2006).

In addition, the discovery that the pro-inflammatory cytokine tumour necrosis factor α (TNF-α) plays a major role in pathogenesis has led to the use of TNF-α antagonists in the treatment of rheumatoid arthritis. These agents have been shown to be highly effective in reducing symptoms and signs and in inhibiting structural damage in patients who have not responded to disease-modifying anti-rheumatic drugs, including methotrexate. Cases of severe and disabling rheumatoid arthritis require careful and integrated health care delivery, as many of these drugs have significant toxicity and the potential for serious side effects. In addition, patients with severe disease may require more support services, assistive devices, and possibly surgical interventions at relatively young ages.

Osteoporosis and associated fractures

Osteoporosis is a skeletal disorder characterized by compromised bone strength, predisposing to an increased risk of fracture. Fractures of the hip, vertebrae, and distal radius are particularly common. The WHO has defined osteoporosis as bone mineral density more than 2.5 standard deviations below the mean value of peak bone mass in young adults of the same sex. Using the WHO definition, the estimated prevalence of osteoporosis in the femoral neck among women aged 50 years and older was found to be 18 per cent in the United States (Looker *et al.* 1997), from 8 to 22 per cent in various Latin American countries (Morales-Torres & Gutiérrez-UrenÞa 2004), 44 per cent in Saudi Arabia (Sadat-Ali *et al.* 2004), and 29 per cent for low-income Indian women (Shatrugna *et al.* 2005). As discussed later in this subsection, different lifestyle characteristics in these various regions are believed to contribute to the variations in prevalence.

In addition to low bone mass, other aspects of bone quality that affect fracture risk include structural properties such as the size and shape of bone, microarchitectural properties such as trabecular thickness and connectivity, cortical thickness and porosity, material properties such as mineralization, collagen composition, and damage accumulation (Seeman & Delmas 2006).

Osteoporosis-associated hip fractures in older people are particularly common and disabling. Globally, hip fracture incidence rates vary considerably and are highest among whites in northern Europe and North America, slightly lower among Asians living in economically developed areas such as Hong Kong and the United States, still lower among Hispanics and Blacks in the United States and in South America, and the lowest in less developed areas of Asia such as China as well as in Africa. In general, the ratio of female to male incidence rates is greater in the areas with the highest incidence rates. Table 9.9.2 shows age-adjusted incidence rates for females and males in selected countries among people of age 50 years and

Table 9.9.2 Age-adjusted incidence rates per 100 000 of hip fracture among females and males aged 50 years and older in selected localities

Locality	Females	Males
Beijing, China	96	107
Porto Alegre, Brazil	202–327.2	104.7–169.6
Budapest, Hungary	316	251
Hong Kong	428.3	269.6
Reykjavik, Iceland	696.6	348.7

Age adjusted to the 1990 non-Hispanic white US population.
Source: Modified from Schwartz A.V., Kelsey J.L., Maggi S., *et al.* International variation in the incidence of hip fractures: cross-national project on osteoporosis for the World Health Organization Program for Research on Aging. *Osteoporosis International* 1999;**9**:242–53.

older (Schwartz *et al.* 1999). Hip fracture incidence rates in Beijing, China, are among the lowest in the world. However, in China and other developing countries (World Health Organization 2003), age-adjusted hip fracture incidence rates appear to be rising. With the increasing numbers of elderly in these countries, the numbers of hip fractures will be dramatically increasing.

Risk factors

In most areas, osteoporosis is much more common among females than males. In both sexes, prevalence increases markedly with age, but the increase in prevalence occurs about 10 years earlier for females than males. Table 9.9.3 shows prevalence by age among females in the United States (Melton 1995). A particularly rapid decrease in bone mass occurs in females in the years immediately following menopause, suggesting that loss of oestrogen is an important aetiological factor in women.

Bone mass in later adulthood, when fracture risk is the greatest, depends on bone mass in young adulthood, when bone mass is at its peak, and the rate of loss of bone mass after the peak is reached. Heredity is an important determinant of bone mass in childhood, adolescence, and early adulthood, but the role of genetics in loss of bone mass at older age is less certain; multiple genes are probably involved, each with a small effect. Although results of studies are not entirely consistent, it appears that modifiable risk factors such as weight, calcium intake, and physical activity also affect premenopausal bone mass, but to a lesser extent than heredity. Premenopausal oophorectomy results in loss of bone mass if menopausal hormone therapy is not used.

In postmenopausal women, the evidence is strong that the risk for low bone mass or hip fracture is increased by prolonged immobility, prolonged corticosteroid use, a history of a previous fracture, a history of falls, maternal history of an osteoporotic fracture, very low concentrations of endogenous oestradiol, poor self-rated health, poor vision, use of psychotropic drugs, and cigarette smoking. Probable risk factors include tallness, a recent increase in the frequency of falls, high alcohol consumption, and high caffeine consumption. Strong protective factors include obesity and menopausal hormone therapy, and to a lesser extent, calcium supplements, adequate dietary calcium consumption, adequate vitamin D intake, adequate vitamin D metabolism, physical activity, and use of thiazide diuretics.

Risk factors appear to be similar in low- and middle-income countries, but special circumstances make certain risk factors of particular importance in some areas. In Middle Eastern countries such as Saudi Arabia and Turkey, inadequate levels of vitamin D are found in most postmenopausal women, probably because of their clothing and a reclusive lifestyle. In other regions, such as low-income areas of India, poor nutrition and failure to maintain adequate body weight may increase the risk for osteoporosis and fractures (Shatrugna *et al.* 2005; Morales-Torres 2007). On the other hand, lack of physical activity may not be an important risk factor in areas where levels of physical activity are high.

Most fractures of sites other than the spine depend on whether a person falls and how the person falls. Among the risk factors for falls in older adults are problems with balance and gait, limited muscle strength, deficiencies in vision, arthritis, depressive symptoms, orthostasis, cognitive impairment, and the use of multiple prescription medications. As the number of these risk factors increases, so does the risk of falling (Tinetti 2003). How a person falls also affects the likelihood that a fracture will occur and which skeletal site is fractured. Falling sideways or straight down and landing on the hip or leg, for instance, greatly increase the risk of a hip fracture. Breaking the fall with a hand decreases the risk of hip fracture, but increases the risk of lower forearm fracture (Nevitt & Cummings 1993). Frail women are more likely to fracture their hip whereas healthier active women are more likely to fracture their lower forearm. Falls from heights or on hard surfaces increase the risk for fracture.

Table 9.9.3 Percentage of Rochester, Minnesota, women with bone mineral measurements in the spine, hip, or mid-radius more than 2.5 standard deviations below the mean for young normal women

Age group (years)	Percentage
50–59	14.8
60–69	21.6
70–79	38.5
≥80	70
Total[a]	30.3

[a] Age adjusted to the 1990 US white women population aged 50 years or older.
Source: Modified from Melton LJ. III. How many women have osteoporosis now? *Journal of Bone and Mineral Research* 1995;**10**:175–7.

Prevention

Primary prevention includes trying to achieve high bone mass at younger ages by having a diet adequate in calcium and vitamin D and engaging in sufficient physical activity. Once loss of bone mass has begun, calcium supplementation can provide a small amount of protection, especially in those with low dietary calcium intake (Jackson *et al.* 2006). Moderate physical activity, such as brisk walking, is often recommended for older people to reduce loss of bone mass, but at most this probably has a modest beneficial effect.

Because only a small amount of protection is provided by increased dietary calcium consumption, calcium supplementation, and physical activity, much attention has been focused on the use of pharmaceutical agents to retard loss of bone mass and to reduce the risk of fractures in older adults. Menopausal hormone therapy, once used effectively for this purpose, is no longer recommended because of its association with an increased risk for other major diseases such as breast cancer, coronary heart disease, and pulmonary embolism. Other agents commonly used for retarding loss of bone mass and possibly reducing the risk for fractures are bisphosphonates, the selective oestrogen receptor modulator raloxifene, and for severe osteoporosis, parathyroid hormone.

Although bisphosphonates, including alendronate, ibandronate, and risedronate, have been shown to reduce loss of bone mass in the hip and spine, randomized trials among women have shown that bisphosphonates protect against fracture only in those who already have very low bone mass (Cummings *et al.* 1998). A recent extension of an earlier randomized trial (Black *et al.* 2006) suggests that little additional benefit on bone mineral density and fracture risk is gained from using alendronate for an additional five years after the first five years of treatment in most women. In addition, compliance is a problem because alendronate has to be taken in a rather strict manner to achieve maximal absorption and avoid unpleasant upper gastrointestinal effects.

The selective oestrogen receptor modulator raloxifene has been shown to reduce loss of bone mass in the hip and spine and to protect against vertebral fractures in women regardless of their baseline bone mass, but not against non-vertebral fractures, including hip fracture (Ettinger *et al.* 1999). Teriparatide, a recombinant human parathyroid hormone that acts through increasing bone formation, may be useful in reducing risk for vertebral and non-vertebral fractures in those with severe osteoporosis, but its use is approved for a maximum of only two years because its long-term effects are not known. Thus, available evidence suggests that none of these agents is useful in the primary prevention of osteoporosis, although each has utility as a therapeutic agent.

In low- and middle-income countries, the cost of these pharmaceutical agents precludes their widespread use for treatment. Rather, inexpensive primary prevention measures such as supplemental calcium and vitamin D, attainment of adequate body weight, exercise, avoidance of smoking and alcohol abuse, and fall prevention programmes could be useful preventive measures, but extensive education of high-risk populations is needed (Morales-Torres 2007).

Regarding secondary prevention, in high-income countries screening women in the perimenopausal and postmenopausal years for high fracture risk by measuring their bone mass, usually with dual-energy X-ray absorptiometry, has achieved some popularity in recent years. However, many questions have been raised about the usefulness of such screening, such as who should be screened, whether multiple measurements over time are needed, what other information on risk should be obtained along with the measure of bone mass, and what therapy should be used in those with various degrees of low bone mass. Ultrasonography, usually of the heel bone, provides information about bone architecture and elasticity as well as bone mineral density, and has been found to predict fracture (Hans *et al.* 1996). As ultrasound is less expensive and radiation-free compared to other methods of measuring bone mass, it is possible that it will be used more widely for screening in the future. At present, however, there is no consensus that any screening method should be used for healthy women in the general population.

Finally, reducing the frequency and impact of falls among those with osteoporosis is another potential means of reducing the incidence of fracture. Table 9.9.4 shows strategies demonstrated in randomized trials to be effective in reducing the occurrence of falls among elderly persons living in the community (Tinetti 2003). Preventive measures may differ somewhat from one country to another. For instance, in countries such as Iran (Abolhassani *et al.* 2006) where older people and particularly women spend little time outdoors, preventive efforts should focus on indoor rather than outdoor risk factors for falls.

Table 9.9.4 Strategies found in randomized trials to be effective in decreasing the number of falls among the elderly living in the community

Strategy	Estimated risk reduction (per cent)
Health care based	
Balance and gait training and strengthening exercise	14–27
Reduction in home hazards after hospitalization	19
Discontinuation of psychotropic medication	39
Multifactorial risk assessment with targeted management	25–39
Community-based	
Specific balance or strength exercise programmes	25–49

Source: Modified from Tinetti M.E. Preventing falls in elderly persons. *New England Journal of Medicine* 2003;**348**:42–9.

Low back pain

About 75–85 per cent of adults in Western countries have low back pain during their lifetime. In the United States, around 15–20 per cent of adults experience low back pain during the course of a year, about 1 per cent are chronically disabled because of low back pain, and another 1 per cent are temporarily disabled. About 5 per cent of workers lose one or more workdays because of low back pain and 2 per cent have compensable back injuries each year. Back pain is the most frequently reported reason for a physician visit in the United States (Andersson 1998).

Most low back problems resolve within 2–4 weeks, and almost 90 per cent resolve within 12 weeks (Andersson 1998). Recurrences are common, however, and low back pain often becomes a chronic problem with intermittent, usually mild exacerbations. In a study of English patients seen by general practitioners for low back pain, after one year only 25 per cent had no disability even though most were no longer seeking care for their problem from their practitioner (Croft *et al.* 1998). In a small proportion of cases, the pain becomes constant and severe.

The prevalence of low back pain is also high in low-income areas of the world. In a community-based study in rural China, the percentage having low back pain during the course of a year was 65 per cent (Barrero *et al.* 2006); it was 61 per cent for tannery workers in India (Öry *et al.* 1997), 56 per cent in a steel industry in South Africa (Van Vuuren *et al.* 2005), and 36 per cent in an urban population in Turkey (Gilgil *et al.* 2005).

As noted earlier, the category low back pain consists of a variety of entities with somewhat different aetiologies. However, almost all studies have considered low back pain as a whole, so the general category is considered here unless otherwise mentioned.

Risk factors

The best predictor of low back pain is a history of low back pain. First episodes of low back pain most frequently occur among persons in the age range 20–39 years, but the proportion of the population reporting low back pain (either old or new) is relatively uniform across the working years. If only cases seeking medical care or compensation are considered, low back pain is seen more frequently among males than females in Western countries, but in surveys in the general population, males and females are affected with approximately equal frequency (Biering-Sorenson 1982). Persons in lower social classes are more likely to report low back pain than those in higher classes, probably because of their tendency to have jobs requiring heavy physical labour.

In Western countries, people who do heavy manual labour are at increased risk for low back pain. Lifting objects of 25 lb or more appears to be particularly detrimental. Specific activities that probably further increase the risk are frequent lifting of heavy objects while bending and twisting the body, holding heavy objects away from the body while lifting, and failing to bend the knees while lifting (Andersson 1981; Kelsey *et al.* 1984). Driving motor vehicles either on or off the job and exposure to whole-body vibration increase the risk for low back pain (Pope *et al.* 1998). A recent review (Lis *et al.* 2007) indicates that sitting by itself does not increase the risk for low back pain, but sitting in combination with other exposures such as whole-body vibration and awkward posture increases the risk. Cigarette smoking has been found in many studies to be associated with an increased risk. Psychological attributes such as low social support in the workplace and low job satisfaction may increase risk (Hoogendoorn & van Poppel 2000).

Many risk factors in middle- and low-income countries are similar to those in high-income countries. In rural China, having been a farmer, reporting moderate or heavy physical stress, and being exposed to vibration were associated with low back pain (Barrero *et al.* 2006). In urban Turkey, cigarette smoking was related to the occurrence of low back pain (Gilgil *et al.* 2005). Among steel workers in a factory in South Africa, carrying heavy loads, bulky manual handling, twisting and bending, kneeling and squatting, prolonged sitting, and working on slippery and uneven surfaces conferred increased risks (Van Vuuren *et al.* 2005). Heavy manual lifting was also a risk factor among tannery workers in India (Öry *et al.* 1997). Within low-income countries, back pain is particularly prevalent in various types of workshops, factories, and storage facilities, which have been referred to as 'enclosed workshops' (Volinn 1997). As indicated earlier, in a survey in Thailand about 50 per cent of the female workers in the garment, fertilizer, pharmaceutical, textile, and cigarette industries reported low back symptoms (Chavalitsakulchai & Shahnavaz 1993). Worldwide, at least 37 per cent of low back pain has been attributed to occupational factors; Table 9.9.5 presents the relative risks upon which this estimate is based (Punnett *et al.* 2005).

In Western countries, predictors of disability from low back pain include previous episodes of law back pain, long duration of pain, a history of past disability and hospitalizations, an onset of pain attributable to trauma, lack of recognition and respect at work, low supervisory support, unemployment, other disabilities, self-reported poor health, low educational level, heavy physical demands on the job, dissatisfaction with the job, whether insurance payments are being received, the perception of fault, and whether a lawyer has been retained (Deyo & Diehl 1988; Cats-Baril & Frymoyer 1991; Wickstrom & Pentti 1998). Little information is available on predictors of disability in low-income countries, but in the South-African steel factory mentioned previously, heavy manual handling, kneeling and squatting, and working on slippery and uneven surfaces were associated with disability from low back pain (Van Vuuren *et al.* 2005).

Table 9.9.5 Relative risk for low back pain by selected occupational category

Occupational category	Relative risk
Managers and professionals	1 (referent)
Clerical and sales workers	1.38
Production workers	2.39
Service workers	2.67
Farmers	5.17

Source: Modified from Punnett L., Prüss-Üstün A., Nelson D.I., *et al.* Estimating the global burden of low back pain attributable to combined occupational exposures. *American Journal of Industrial Medicine* 2005;**48**:459-69

Prevention

Various approaches have been used for the primary prevention of low back pain in the workplace, and these measures are applicable to high-, middle-, and low-income countries. Low back X-rays and medical examinations have not proved useful as predictors of who will develop back pain on the job. However, careful selection of workers for jobs involving heavy manual work by strength testing may be helpful (Keyserling *et al.* 1980). It has been found that training workers to bend their knees while lifting does not reduce the likelihood of low back injuries, in part because of poor compliance. A better approach may be to redesign jobs to minimize bending and twisting motions while lifting and to reduce the amount of weight that must be lifted (Snook 1988). Redesigning jobs in these ways may also allow injured workers to return to work sooner. Other ways of reducing the frequency of back pain may include smoking cessation, improved physical fitness, moving around from time to time in situations requiring prolonged exposure to one position, vibration dampening, and use of motor vehicles with good lumbar support and positioning.

To reduce the likelihood of acute back pain progressing to chronic back pain, it is important for those affected to continue their normal activity to the extent that they are able (Malmivaara *et al.* 1995). Upon return to work, however, the worker should avoid activities that may exacerbate the problem, such as heavy lifting or staying in one position for long periods of time.

Neck pain

Neck pain has been less well studied than low back pain, and as with low back pain, a variety of conditions can result in neck pain. In high-income countries, about 60–70 per cent of the adults report having experienced neck pain at some time during their lives (Côté *et al.* 1998). Most neck pain is mild, but as with low back pain, episodes may be recurrent, and about 5 per cent of the cases result in disability. Little information is available from middle- and low-income countries.

Risk factors

Some studies report that males and females are affected with approximately equal frequency, whereas others show a female excess. Chronic neck pain and disability from neck pain occur more often in females than males. Neck pain occurs most frequently in young adulthood, and some evidence suggests that its prevalence decreases with age (Côté *et al.* 1998; Leclerc *et al.* 1999).

Only a few studies have been undertaken to identify other risk factors for neck pain, and many of the risk factors appear to be similar to those for low back pain. Prolonged exposure to awkward postures may be associated with mild neck pain. For instance, in Hong Kong, frequent use of video display units with a fixed keyboard height requiring a bent neck was found to result in neck pain (Yu & Wong 1996). Other risk factors for either general neck pain or herniated cervical disc found in one or more studies (Kelsey *et al.* 1984; Magnusson *et al.* 1996; Krause *et al.* 1997) include heavy lifting, cigarette smoking, driving motor vehicles, exposure to whole-body vibration, and psychological distress, psychosomatic problems, and headaches (Leclerc *et al.* 1999). One study (Krause *et al.* 1997) found that particularly detrimental were vehicles in which seat adjustment was difficult.

Prevention

Little research has been undertaken on predictors of disability from neck pain and on primary prevention. However, it would appear that reduction in the amount of heavy lifting, cigarette smoking, awkward positions (especially at video display units), prolonged driving in motor vehicles, and exposure to other sources of whole-body vibration should reduce the incidence.

Foot disorders

Foot disorders represent a number of structural or biomechanical conditions, skin conditions, manifestations of systemic disease, and sensory conditions. Structural problems include bunions, flat feet, hammer toes, overlapping toes, and high arches. Systemic diseases often seen with foot symptoms include arthritis, diabetes mellitus, and peripheral vascular disease. Foot complications of diabetes may be caused by ischaemia, neuropathy, and susceptibility to infection. Foot ulcers are common in persons with peripheral vascular disease, vascular insufficiency, or trauma. Peripheral vascular disease is associated with colour changes and oedema, and may cause inadequate blood flow with symptoms of pain or numbness (Karpman 1995).

In the United States, foot and toe symptoms are among the top twenty reasons for physician office visits among persons aged 65–74 years (US Department of Health and Human Services 1997). Karpman (1995) has reported that up to 80 per cent of elderly patients are afflicted with a bunion, hammer toe deformity, callus, or other structural deformity. A population-based study (Clarke 1969) of adults 18–90 years of age in the United Kingdom found that 60 per cent of those surveyed reported a painful foot problem, yet a podiatric examination found 85 per cent to have some foot condition. The most frequent foot disorders were bunions, arthritis, claw toes, hammer toes, overlapping toes, and aching, swollen feet that might have arisen from a general condition such as peripheral vascular disease. In this study, women reported foot pain (71 per cent) more often than men (53 per cent). Of those reporting foot disorders, about half reported foot pain and approximately 10 per cent reported that their foot condition limited at least one of their daily activities. Another US population-based study (Dunn *et al.* 2004) noted that the most prevalent foot conditions were toe deformities, bunions, and toe infection or maceration. A study of geriatric patients in Hong Kong found that half had foot deformities (Hung *et al.* 1985).

In an Australian study of older adults (Menz & Lord 2001), foot problems were associated with slower walking speed and poor balance. A British study (Clarke 1969) found that 40 per cent of adults aged 65 years and older reported difficulty walking, and 16 per cent stated that their difficulty in walking was due to trouble with their feet. Studies in other localities (Benvenuti *et al.* 1995; Leveille *et al.* 1998) also report that older people with foot problems have difficulty walking, standing, and with everyday activities. A study in Beijing (Cummings *et al.* 1997) found that 38 per cent of women aged 80 years and older and 18 per cent of women aged 70–79 years were affected by deformities resulting from previous foot binding and that these deformities caused substantial disability in standing and balance. There are few, if any, other studies of the prevalence of or disability from foot disorders in low- or middle-income countries.

Risk factors

Women are more likely to have foot pain than men, but it is not known whether this is because of a higher prevalence of primary foot deformities or underlying disease. An Italian study (Benvenuti *et al.* 1995) reported that 56 per cent of women over 65 years of age had foot pain compared to 24 per cent of older men. The Third National Health and Nutrition Examination Survey in the United States (US Department of Health and Human Services 1996) reported that 60 per cent of women over age 65 years had bunions compared to 40 per cent of men. Additionally, older women are more likely to have arthritis than men, and the foot is the fourth most commonly affected site in those with osteoarthritis.

Structural foot deformities are thought often to be caused by long-term use of ill-fitting shoes. Shoes with an improper fit worn over years, or other stress to the feet, can result in various deformities including bunions, hammer toes, and claw toes, in turn leading to muscle maladaption and progression of the deformity (Karpman 1995).

The only other risk factor consistently linked with painful foot disorders is obesity. Obesity has a major effect on soft-tissue structures such as tendon and cartilage.

Little is known of how the foot might affect physical functioning of the lower extremity in adults. Extrapolating from clinical studies of patients with diabetes, it is thought that even slight deformities of the feet can lead to impaired balance, changes in gait, and pain. Foot disorders may often be overlooked as an important cause of falls, poor balance, and walking problems.

Prevention

Primary prevention measures include appropriate footwear that protects and supports the foot without confining the toes, as well as weight loss in those who are obese to reduce biomechanical stress on the foot. These aspects become even more important in those whose health is compromised by diabetes, arthritis, vascular disease, or other chronic systemic disease.

Once people have foot pain, interventions should be directed to both the location of the pain and underlying muscle, tendons, or ligaments. These interventions vary by foot disorder and may include heel lifts, gel inserts, injection with pain-relieving medications, orthotic devices, and avoidance of activity that irritates the tenderness. Other tertiary prevention measures are aimed at reduction of pain, inflammation, and maladaptive response and include use of foot inserts, stretching and strengthening exercises, non-steroidal anti-inflammatory drugs, short-term cast immobilization, joint injection, reduction of weight bearing, and other measures to reduce symptoms. Finally, adaptive shoes as well as surgical options may be considered for long-term foot disorders. Prompt diagnosis and early treatment may lessen the possible long-term maladaption and structural disability seen with many foot disorders.

Selected musculoskeletal disorders of adolescents and children

Adolescent idiopathic scoliosis

The Scoliosis Research Society defines scoliosis as a lateral spinal curve of greater than 10 degrees as measured by the Cobb angle on a radiograph taken with the person standing. The curvature is usually associated with rotation of the vertebrae. In Western countries, about 2–3 per cent of the adolescents develop curves of 10 degrees of more before growth ceases, and 2 per 1000 children develop curves of 30 degrees or more (Miller 1999). Prevalence estimates of 1 per cent in Nigeria (Jenyo & Asekun-Olarinmoye 2005) and 3 per cent in Mostar, Bosnia, and Herzegovina (Ostojic *et al.* 2006) have been reported. Those with large curvature usually develop spinal osteoarthritis in their adult years. Lung and heart complications may also occur. Additional progression of curves sometimes takes place in adults with scoliosis.

Risk factors

The ages at which adolescent idiopathic scoliosis is most frequently diagnosed are 11–14 years in girls and 14–16 years in boys, the difference in ages reflecting the earlier onset of the adolescent growth spurt in females. The ratio of females to males among the more severe cases seen at surgery is around 4–5 to 1, but curves of less than 15 degrees are seen with about equal frequency in females and males. Reports from surgical case series indicate that curves occur most frequently at the thoracic level, but school screening programmes that identify mild as well as severe cases have found curves to be most common at the thoracolumbar level.

The risk of scoliosis in first-degree relatives of cases is about three to four times that in children from the general population, but the mode of inheritance is unclear. A prospective study in Finland (Nissinen *et al.* 1993) identified several factors that may predict the development of scoliosis, including the female sex, trunk asymmetry as indicated by large rip humps on the forward-bend test (see Prevention for a description), the degree of thoracic kyphosis, the degree of lumbar lordosis in boys, and probably standing height, sitting height, recent increase in sitting height, and early age at gain in sitting height. Once girls reach menarche, their risk is considerably reduced.

Specific mechanisms hypothesized to be involved in the development of scoliosis, but for which the evidence is not conclusive, include connective tissue abnormalities, particularly of collagen, proteoglycan, and elastic fibres; a growth or functional defect within skeletal muscle; neuromuscular abnormalities including of proprioception, postural equilibrium, oculovestibular function, and vibratory sensation; central nervous system asymmetries; hormonal characteristics involving growth hormone and melatonin; and biomechanical imbalances and abnormalities in vertebral bodies, muscles of the ribs and trunk, ligaments, and intervertebral discs (Miller 1999).

Once a curve has developed, several risk factors for progression have been identified, including double curves as opposed to single curves, thoracic curves, larger curves, the female sex, skeletal immaturity, the absence of a sacral tilt, leg length inequality, early chronological age, and low bone mass (Hung *et al.* 2005).

Prevention

No means of primary prevention are known. Therefore, secondary prevention by screening in schools has become widespread and is in fact required by law in many localities in the United States. The assumption of the screening programme is that if cases of scoliosis are detected early, they can be treated conservatively and surgery can be avoided.

The forward-bend test has been used for screening for many years in high-income countries. It is simple and affordable in developing countries such as Nigeria (Jenyo & Asekun-Olarinmoye 2005) as well as in high-income countries. In the forward-bend test, the child's back is examined while the child bends forward from the waist. In scoliosis, the rotation of vertebrae that is often associated with the lateral curvature results in prominent ribs on the concave side of the curve. Accordingly, in this test, evidence of a 'rib hump' is considered positive for scoliosis. Recently, the scoliometer, an inclinometer used to measure axial trunk rotation during forward bending, has been introduced as a screening test and to monitor curve progression, but only limited evaluation has been undertaken to date.

School screening programmes identify relatively large numbers of children with possible curvature in their spine. Positive tests are followed by X-ray examination for a more definitive diagnosis. Curves of 5–19 degrees are generally monitored by subsequent X-rays every few months. If a curve progresses to 20–25 degrees or more, treatment is usually started to prevent further progression. Methods of treatment include exercises, braces, external or internal muscle stimulators, and especially for curves of greater than 40 degrees, surgery.

Despite the widespread acceptance of screening for scoliosis, its effectiveness has been questioned (US Preventive Services Task Force 1993; Goldberg *et al.* 1995). Many children screened as positive are not followed up for definitive diagnosis. Many false positives occur even with the forward-bend test, resulting in an excess of X-ray examinations and considerable expense and anxiety. A report from a screening programme in Ireland (Goldberg *et al.* 1995) indicates that the positive predictive value of the forward-bend test is only 8 per cent; that is, of every 100 forward-bend tests classified as positive, only 8 develop clinically significant scoliosis. It is uncertain whether school screening programmes have actually caused a reduction in the number of cases of severe curvature that require surgery. Disagreement exists about the optimal ages for screening and about whether males should be screened at all. Criteria for referral for diagnosis and treatment need to be better specified, and improved training and evaluation of the nurses who do the screening is needed. In view of all these uncertainties, the US Preventive Services Task Force (US Preventive Services Task Force 1993) did not recommend either for or against routine screening for scoliosis in adolescents, and routine screening is not recommended by the United Kingdom National Screening Committee.

Slipped capital femoral epiphysis

In slipped capital femoral epiphysis, the head of the femur is displaced backward and downward off the diaphysis. The actual separation takes place through the layer of hypertrophied cartilage next to the zone of calcified cartilage of the epiphyseal plate. The usual symptoms are pain, stiffness, limp, and a limited range of motion of the hip joint. Slipped epiphysis usually occurs during the adolescent growth spurt, and does not occur once the epiphysis is fused to the shaft of the femur. In northern urbanized areas, about 1 in 1000 males and 1 in 1800 females are diagnosed with a slipped epiphysis over the age range at risk (Jerre *et al.* 1996).

Risk factors

Most cases occur between the ages of 10–17 years in males and 8–15 years in females. The median age at diagnosis is 13 for males and 11–12 for females, the earlier age in females corresponding to their earlier onset of puberty. Males are affected more frequently than females, although the male to female ratio appears to have decreased over time and varies from one geographic area to another. In males, the left hip is affected about twice as frequently as the right, whereas in females the left and right hips are affected with approximately equal frequency. In both sexes, about 20–25 per cent of the cases are bilateral.

Slipped epiphysis appears to be particularly common among the Maori of New Zealand (Stott & Bidwell 2003). Worldwide, Polynesian and Black children have higher incidence rates than White children, whereas residents of Asia (including the Indian subcontinent), the Near East, and north Africa have lower rates (Loder 1996). The incidence in Japan is reported to have increased considerably in the past 25 years, a trend in all likelihood attributable to the increased prevalence of childhood and adolescent obesity (Noguchi *et al.* 2002).

About half of those with slipped epiphysis have weights at or above the 95th percentile for their age (Loder 1996). Children with slipped epiphysis tend to have undergone slower skeletal maturation than average for their age (Sorenson 1968). They tend to be tall for their age at the time of diagnosis, but at maturity their heights are almost normal for their chronological age (Hansson *et al.* 1987). Familial aggregation of cases has been noted by several investigators.

Most of the established risk factors for slipped epiphysis are related either to a weakening of the epiphyseal plate or to an increase in the shearing stress on the plate. The epiphyseal plate is weaker during periods of rapid growth, such as during the adolescent growth spurt. The growth spurt in males is of greater magnitude and of longer duration than that in females, and the male growth spurt is more likely to have periods of acceleration and deceleration

A deficit of sex hormones relative to the growth hormone brings about a widening of the epiphyseal plate and a reduction in the shearing force needed to displace the epiphysis. Oestrogens protect against slipped epiphysis, whereas androgens are protective only in large doses after prolonged exposure. Slowly maturing children are exposed for a longer period to high levels of growth hormone relative to sex hormones than are children who mature faster. Tall children also have a longer exposure to growth hormone relative to sex hormones (Morscher 1968).

During adolescence the epiphyseal plate changes from a horizontal to an oblique plane, so that it becomes more vulnerable to stress from superincumbent weight. Children who are overweight put more stress on their plate than lighter children.

Prevention

Reducing the prevalence of adolescent obesity would have a large impact on the number of cases of slipped epiphysis. No screening tests are available, but slipped epiphysis should be considered in adolescents who have a limp and hip or knee pain or restriction of motion in the hip. The contralateral hip in children with slipped epiphysis in one hip needs to be carefully monitored, especially if the first slipped epiphysis occurred at an early age (Loder 1996). Early diagnosis is important, as slight displacement treated early by pinning the hip has a favourable prognosis, whereas cases that are diagnosed late and that have severe displacement usually have early onset of osteoarthritis of the hip and permanent disability.

Childhood fractures

In the United States, about 1 in 36 persons of age 18 years or younger fractures a bone each year (Praemer *et al.* 1999). In South Wales, about 64 per cent of boys and 39 per cent of girls can expect to fracture a bone by 15 years of age (Lyons *et al.* 1999). Except when rare complications occur, most fractures heal quickly in children, and the younger the age, the more rapid the healing.

Risk factors

Among children, incidence rates of fracture peak at about age 14 years in boys and age 11 years in girls (Cooper *et al.* 2004). Throughout childhood, incidence rates are higher in males than females. In one study (Brudvik & Hove 2003), the ratio of male to female fracture cases rose from 1.1 among children less than age 6 years to 2.1 in those of ages 13–15 years. Most forms of trauma associated with fractures are more common in boys than girls.

Fractures of the radius and ulna are the most frequent of the childhood fractures. Other common sites are the carpals, hands, feet, humerus, and clavicle (Cooper *et al.* 2004; Brudvik & Hove 2003). Children who have one fracture are at increased risk of having an additional fracture.

In a series of childhood fracture cases in Wales, sports and leisure-time activities accounted for 36 per cent of fractures, assaults for 3.5 per cent, and road traffic accidents for 1.4 per cent (Lyons *et al.* 1999). In a study in Norway (Brudvik & Hove 2003), fractures in children under 6 years of age most commonly occurred indoors at home (32 per cent), outdoors near the home (23 per cent), and outdoors in kindergarten (17 per cent). Among school children, fractures were most common outdoors near the home (23 per cent), outdoors at school (20 per cent), and indoors at school (10 per cent), mainly in school gymnastics. The activities associated with fractures included soccer, bicycling, handball, volleyball, basketball, and rollerblading or skateboarding. Over time, rollerblading and skateboarding, along with snowboarding, have been accounting for increasing proportions of fractures, and a high proportion of the injuries associated with these sports are fractures (Brudvik & Hove 2003).

Little information is available from low- and middle-income countries, but injuries from falls and road traffic incidents are the leading causes of disease burden among children of ages 5–14 years in these countries (Beveridge & Howard 2004). In a study that included children from Ethiopia, Peru, Vietnam, and India (Howe *et al.* 2006), fractures in very young children were found to be associated with chronic mental disease in the caregiver, the father not living in the household, and a long-term health problem in the child.

Prevention

Preventing accidents and reducing the impact on bones when accidents do occur are key to decreasing the number of fractures in children, including decreasing the number of sports and recreational injuries; falls; bicycle, motorcycle, and automobile accidents; child-battering injuries; and other childhood traumas. Many fractures resulting from falls on hard surfaces could be reduced by the use of impact-absorbing surfaces in playgrounds. Many distal forearm fractures, the most common fracture site in children, could be prevented by the use of wrist guards while engaging in such activities as soccer, rollerblading, skateboarding, and snowboarding, although some evidence indicates that the number of fractures in the forearm just above the brace might be increased (Lyons *et al.* 1999; Brudvik & Hove 2003).

Developmental dysplasia of the hip

Developmental dysplasia of the hip includes a spectrum of abnormalities in which the femoral head and the acetabulum are either in improper alignment or grow abnormally. Long-term complications include osteoarthritis, difficulty walking, and chronic pain.

The diagnosis is made shortly after birth in about 80 per cent of cases, whereas about 20 per cent of cases are diagnosed later, especially when the child starts to walk. From 60 to 80 per cent of hips identified as abnormal or suspicious for developmental dysplasia by physical examination and over 90 per cent of those identified with mild dysplasia by ultrasound in the newborn period resolve spontaneously and require no intervention (US Preventive Services Task Force 2006).

Considerable variation occurs in the frequency of developmental dysplasia of the hip from one geographic area to another and from one racial or ethnic group to another. Using data collected before screening at birth became widespread, in most North American and western European countries as well as in Australia, New Zealand, and Israel, prevalence rates of around 1 per 1000 to 10 per 1000 births were found. In the Navajo, Apache, and Cree-Ojibwa of North America, and the Lapps, as well as in Hungary, northern Italy, Brittany, and the Faroe Islands, rates from 10 per 1000 to 100 per 1000 births were reported. On the other hand, developmental dysplasia of the hip was rare among blacks in South Africa, the West Indies, and Uganda, and among Chinese living in Hong Kong (reviewed in Kelsey (Kelsey 1982)). It must be kept in mind that the nature of the neonatal examination of the infant, the experience of the examiner, the timing of the examination, and the criteria for developmental dysplasia of the hip could all affect these figures.

Risk factors

Risk factors for developmental dysplasia of the hip have been reviewed (Storer & Skaggs 2006). Females are affected about four to six times more frequently than males. In the United States, whites are affected more often than blacks. First-born children are at higher risk than later-born children; in pregnancies after the first, the ligaments and other tissues in and around the maternal uterus have already been stretched during previous pregnancies, allowing more foetal movement. In unilateral cases, the left hip is affected more frequently than the right, probably because the left hip is positioned against the maternal spine more often than is the right hip.

Familial aggregation occurs, and both hereditary and environmental factors are believed to contribute to the familial excess. Infants with developmental dysplasia of the hip are considerably more likely to have been born by breech delivery than other infants. *In utero* postural deformities and oligohydramnios are also associated with an increased risk.

Prevention

No means of primary prevention are known, but screening of newborns either by serial physical examination using the Ortolani or Barlow procedures or by ultrasonography is now widely used. In the Ortolani test, the hip is placed in flexion and gently adducted and then abducted. The Ortolani test is considered positive if a palpable jerk and an audible click are heard as the head of the femur returns to the acetabulum. Some physicians consider just an audible click to be a positive test. The Barlow test involves exerting gentle downward pressure over the lesser trochanter with the hip in flexion and adduction; an unstable hip will shift from the acetabulum and a sensation similar to the Ortolani sign is produced. When the leg is allowed to abduct, the hip is reduced. Because many hips noted to be unstable at birth soon become stable spontaneously, these tests are often repeated at around three weeks. Infants who are positive by either the Ortolani or Barlow test are generally treated with braces, splints, or harness for 2–4 months. Routine checks of the hips of these infants should be performed until they are walking well. If diagnosis is delayed until after the neonatal period, surgery is usually required and the prognosis is poorer.

Although screening for developmental dysplasia of the hip by the Ortolani or Barlow tests is routine in many localities, the US Preventive Services Task Force (US Preventive Services Task Force 2006) concluded that the evidence for the effectiveness of these tests is insufficient to recommend their use for routine screening. First, the Task Force could find no direct evidence that screening leads to a reduced need for surgery or improved functional outcomes. Second, because the majority of hips that are abnormal at birth resolve spontaneously within 2–8 weeks, intervention is not needed for most of those screened as positive. Third, the accuracy of the screening tests is difficult to assess because of variable definitions of a positive test and the lack of a practical confirmatory gold standard for a positive result. Fourth, the effectiveness of both surgical and non-surgical interventions is uncertain because of the high rate of spontaneous resolution and various deficiencies in the studies examining the effectiveness of surgery. Fifth, the potential harm from screening has not been well evaluated, such as the possibility that the procedures themselves could dislocate a hip, the radiation exposure from follow-up radiography, parental psychosocial stress, and false-positive tests that result in unnecessary and possibly harmful follow-up and treatment, including the risks associated with surgery. The training and experience of physicians performing the tests and interventions vary considerably.

Ultrasound, in which a defined image of the bony and cartilaginous hip can be examined, has become widely available for screening for developmental dysplasia of the hip. Ultrasound may be of value in following up infants who have shown hip instability on clinical examination (Elbourne *et al.* 2002), but its use for routine screening and even its use in high-risk infants are controversial. Some of the problems are that ultrasound is expensive, cases developing after the neonatal period will not be detected if ultrasound is done only in newborns, and the vast majority of hips classified as positive on ultrasound develop normally. It is unclear how an infant with a normal clinical examination but with abnormal ultrasonogram should be treated. In addition, better training is needed to improve the scans and their interpretation.

Conclusion

The global impact of musculoskeletal diseases, though now substantial, will become much greater over the next several decades. Musculoskeletal diseases are common at all ages, but their greatest impact is on the elderly. The number of people aged 65 years or older in the world is expected to more than double between 2007 and 2035, for a total of about 1.16 billion people of age 65 years and older in 2035 (US Census Bureau 2007). Thus, musculoskeletal diseases will account for an increasing portion of health care costs. In addition to the development and application of better methods of primary prevention, much more needs to be done to limit the pain and disability among the large number of those already affected and to help people learn how best to cope with these frequently lifelong disabilities. Musculoskeletal disorders are often not given high priority in developing countries, despite the large amount of disability they cause and their high monetary cost to the community.

Several measures could be undertaken on the basis of current knowledge. For instance, total joint replacements of the hip and knee are highly successful and cost-effective operations for disabled people in high-income countries, but are not widely used in low-income countries because of cost and limited resources (Brooks 2006). Ergonomic improvements and better training in the workplace could now be instituted in many regions. In addition, more information on the most important musculoskeletal problems and risk factors in specific geographic areas is needed if limited funds are to be used wisely. Thus, we are at a time when more epidemiologic and clinical research is needed and when current knowledge could be much more widely applied to reduce the frequency and burden of musculoskeletal diseases throughout the world.

References

Abolhassani F., Moayyeri A., Naghavi M. *et al.* Incidence and characteristics of falls leading to hip fracture in Iranian population. *Bone* 2006;**39**:408–13.

Ahasan M.R., Mohiuddin G., Vayrynen S. *et al.* Work-related problems in metal handling tasks in Bangladesh: obstacles to the development of safety and health measures. *Ergonomics* 1999;**42**:385–96.

Andersson G.B.J. Epidemiologic aspects of low-back pain in industry. *Spine* 1981;**6**:53–60.

Andersson G.B.J. Epidemiology of low-back pain. *Acta Orthopaedica Scandinavica Supplement* 1998;**281**:28–31.

Arden N., Nevitt M.C. Osteoarthritis: epidemiology. *Best Practice and Research Clinical Rheumatology* 2006;**20**:3–25.

Badley E.M. The economic burden of musculoskeletal disorders in Canada is similar to that for cancer, and may be higher [Editorial]. *Journal of Rheumatology* 1995;**22**:204–6.

Barrero L.H., Hsu Y.H., Terwedow H. *et al.* Prevalence and physical determinants of low back pain in a rural Chinese population. *Spine* 2006;**31**:2728–34.

Bartlett S.J., Bingham C.O., Maricic M.J. III *et al. Clinical care in the rheumatic diseases*. 3rd ed. Atlanta (GA): Association of Rheumatology Health Professionals; 2006.

Benvenuti F., Ferrucci L., Guralnik J.M. *et al.* Foot pain and disability in older persons: an epidemiologic survey. *Journal of the American Geriatrics Society* 1995;**43**:479–84.

Beveridge M., Howard A. The burden of orthopaedic disease in developing countries. *Journal of Bone and Joint Surgery* 2004;**86**A:1819–22.

Biering-Sorenson F. Low back trouble in a general population of 30-, 40-, 50-, and 60-year-old men and women. *Study design, representativeness, and basic results. Danish Medical Bulletin* 1982;**29**:289–99.

Black D.M., Schwartz A.V., Ensrud K.E. *et al.* Effects of continuing or stopping alendronate after 5 years of treatment. The Fracture Intervention Trial Long-term Extension (FLEX): a randomized trial. *Journal of the American Medical Association* 2006;**296**:2927–38.

Bowling A. The effects of illness on quality of life: findings from a survey of households in Great Britain. *Journal of Epidemiology and Community Health* 1996;**50**:149–55.

Brooks P.M. The burden of musculoskeletal disease—a global perspective. *Clinical Rheumatology* 2006;**25**:778–81.

Brudvik C., Hove L.M. Childhood fractures in Bergen, Norway: identifying high-risk groups and activities. *Journal of Paediatric Orthopaedics* 2003;**23**:629–34.

Cats-Baril W.L., Frymoyer J.W. Identifying patients at risk of becoming disabled because of low-back pain. The Vermont Rehabilitation Engineering Center predictive model. *Spine* 1991;**16**:605–7.

Centers for Disease Control and Prevention. Prevalence of disabilities and associated health conditions among adults—United States, 1999. *Morbidity and Mortality Weekly Report* 2001;**50**:120–5.

Centers for Disease Control and Prevention. Prevalence of doctor-diagnosed arthritis and arthritis-attributable activity limitation–United States, 2003–2005. *Journal of the American Medical Association* 2006;**296**:2671–2.

Chavalitsakulchai P., Shahnavaz H. Musculoskeletal disorders of female workers and ergonomics problems in five different industries of a developing country. *Journal of Human Ergology (Tokyo)* 1993;**22**:29–43.

Clarke M. Trouble with feet. In: Titmuss RM, editor. *Occasional papers on social administration*. London: Bell G and Sons; 1969. vol 29. p.1–182.

Cooper C., Campion G., Melton L.J. III. Hip fractures in the elderly: a worldwide projection. *Osteoporosis International* 1992;**2**:285–9.

Cooper C., Dennison E.M., Leufkens H.G. *et al.* Epidemiology of childhood fractures in Britain: a study using the general practice research database. *Journal of Bone and Mineral Research* 2004;**19**:1976–81.

Cooper C., McAlindon T., Coggon D. *et al.* Occupational activity and osteoarthritis of the knee. *Annals of the Rheumatic Diseases* 1994;**53**:90–3.

Côté P., Cassidy J.D., Carroll L. The Saskatchewan Health and Back Pain Survey. The prevalence of neck pain and related disability in Saskatchewan adults. *Spine* 1998;**23**:1689–98.

Croft P.R., Macfarlane G.J., Papageorogiou A.C. *et al.* Outcome of low back pain in general practice: a prospective study. *British Medical Journal* 1998;**316**:1356–9.

Cummings S.R., Black D.M., Thompson D.E. *et al.* Effect of alendronate on risk of fracture in women with low bone density but without vertebral fractures: results from the Fracture Intervention Trial. *Journal of the American Medical Association* 1998;**280**:2077–82.

Cummings S.R., Ling X., Stone K. Consequences of foot binding among older women in Beijing, China. *American Journal of Public Health* 1997;**87**:1677–9.

Dans L.F., Tankeh-Torres S., Amante C.M. *et al.* The prevalence of rheumatic diseases in a Filipino urban population: a WHO-ILAR COPCORD Study. *Journal of Rheumatology* 1997;**24**:1814–9.

Darmawan J., Valkenburg H.A., Muirden K.D. *et al.* Epidemiology of rheumatic diseases in rural and urban populations in Indonesia: a World Health Organisation-International League Against Rheumatism COPCORD study, stage 1, phase 2. *Annals of the Rheumatic Diseases* 1992;**51**:525–8.

Deyo R.A., Diehl A.K. Psychosocial predictors of disability in patients with low back pain. *Journal of Rheumatology* 1988;**15**:1557–64.

Dunn J.E., Link C.L., Felson D.T. *et al.* Prevalence of foot and ankle conditions in a multiethnic community sample of older adults. *American Journal of Epidemiology* 2004;491–8.

Eisenberg D.M., Davis R.B., Ettner S.L. *et al.* Trends in alternative medicine use in the United States, 1990–1997. Journal of the American Medical Association 1998;**280**1569–75.

Elbourne D., Dezateux C., Arthur R. *et al.* Ultrasonography in the diagnosis and management of developmental hip dysplasia (UK Hip Trial): clinical and economic results of a multicentre randomised controlled trial. *Lancet* 2002;**360**:2009–17.

Emery P. Treatment of rheumatoid arthritis. *British Medical Journal* 2006;**332**:152–5.

Ettinger B., Black D.M., Mitlak B.H. *et al.* Reduction of vertebral fracture risk in postmenopausal women with osteoporosis treated with raloxifene. Results from a 3-year randomized clinical trial. *Journal of the American Medical Association* 1999;**282**:637–45.

Farooqi A., Gibson T. Prevalence of major rheumatic disorders in the adult population of north Pakistan. *British Journal of Rheumatology* 1998;**37**:491–5.

Felts W., Yelin E. The economic impact of the rheumatic diseases in the United States. *Journal of Rheumatology* 1989;**16**:867–84.

Ferraz M.B. Tropical rheumatology. Epidemiology and community studies: Latin America. *Baillieres Clinical Rheumatology* 1995;**9**:1–9.

Gilgil E., Kaçar C., Bütün B. *et al.* Prevalence of low back pain in a developing urban setting. *Spine* 2005;**30**:1093–8.

Goldberg C.J., Dowling F.E., Fogarty E.E. *et al.* School scoliosis screening and the United States Preventive Services Task Force. *Spine* 1995;**20**: 1368–74.

Hameed K., Gibson T., Kadir M. *et al.* The prevalence of rheumatoid arthritis in affluent and poor urban communities of Pakistan. *British Journal of Rheumatology* 1995;**34**:252–6.

Hans D., Dargent-Molina P., Schott A.M. *et al.* Ultrasonographic heel measurements to predict hip fracture in elderly women: the EPIDOS prospective study. *Lancet* 1996;**348**:511–4.

Hansson L.I., Hagglund G., Ordeberg G. Slipped capital femoral epiphysis in southern Sweden, 1910–1982. *Acta Orthopaedia Scandinavica* 1987;**226**:1–67.

Haq S.A., Darmawan J., Islam M.N. *et al.* Prevalence of rheumatic diseases and associated outcomes in rural and urban communities in Bangladesh: a COPCORD study. *Journal of Rheumatology* 2005;**32**: 348–53.

Hoogendoorn W.E., van Poppel M.N., Bongers P.M. *et al.* Systematic review of psychosocial factors at work and private life as risk factors for back pain. *Spine* 2000;**25**:2114–25.

Howe L.D., Huttly S.R.A., Abramsky T. Risk factors for injuries in young children in four developing countries: the Young Lives Study. *Tropical Medicine and International Health* 2006;**11**:1557–66.

Hung L.K., Ho Y.F., Leung P.C. Survey of foot deformities among 166 geriatric inpatients. *Foot and Ankle* 1985;**5**:156–64.

Hung V.W.Y., Qin L., Cheung C.S.K. *et al.* Osteopenia: a new prognostic factor of curve progression in adolescent idiopathic scoliosis. *Journal of Bone and Joint Surgery* 2005;**87**A:2709–16.

Jackson R.D., LaCroix A.Z., Gass M. *et al.* Calcium plus vitamin D supplementation and the risk of fractures. *New England Journal of Medicine* 2006;**354**:669–83.

Jenyo M.S., Asekun-Olarinmoye E.O. Prevalence of scoliosis in secondary school children in Osogbo, Osun State, Nigeria. *African Journal of Medicine and Medical Sciences* 2005;**34**:361–4.

Jerre R., Karlsson J., Henrikson B. The incidence of physiolysis of the hip. A population-based study of 175 patients. *Acta Orthopaedica Scandinavica* 1996;**67**:53–6.

Kacar C., Gilgil E., Urhan S. *et al.* The prevalence of symptomatic knee and distal interphalangeal joint osteoarthritis in the urban population of Antalya, Turkey. *Rheumatology International* 2005;**25**:201–4.

Karpman R.R. Foot problems in the geriatric patient. *Clinical Orthopedics* 1995;**316**:59–62.

Kelsey J.L., Githens P.B., Walter S.D. *et al.* An epidemiologic study of acute prolapsed cervical intervertebral disc. *Journal of Bone and Joint Surgery* 1984;**66**A:907–14.

Kelsey J.L., Githens P.B., White A.A. III *et al.* An epidemiological study of lifting and twisting on the job and risk for acute prolapsed lumbar intervertebral disc. *Journal of Orthopaedic Research* 1984;**2**:61–6.

Kelsey J.L. *Epidemiology of musculoskeletal disorders*. New York (NY): Oxford University Press; 1982.

Keyserling W.M., Herrin G.D., Chaffin D.B. Establishing an industrial strength testing program. *American Industrial Hygiene Association Journal* 1980;**41**:730–6.

Krause N., Ragland D.R., Greiner B.A. *et al.* Physical workload and ergonomic factors associated with prevalence of back and neck pain in urban transit operators. *Spine* 1997;**22**:2117–26.

Lau E.M.C., Symmons D.P.M., Croft P. The epidemiology of hip osteoarthritis and rheumatoid arthritis in the Orient. *Clinical Orthopaedics and Related Research* 1996;**323**:81–90.

Leclerc A., Niedhammer I., Landre M.F. *et al.* One-year predictive factors for various aspects of neck disorders. *Spine* 1999;**24**:1455–62.

Leveille S.G., Guralnik J.M., Ferrucci L. *et al.* Foot pain and disability in older women. *American Journal of Epidemiology* 1998;**148**:657–65.

Lis A.M., Black K.M., Korn H. *et al.* Association between sitting and occupational LBP. *European Spine Journal* 2007;**16**:283–98.

Loder R.T. The demographics of slipped capital femoral epiphysis. An international multicenter study. *Clinical Orthopaedics and Related Research* 1996;**322**:8–27.

Looker A.C., Orwoll E.D., Johnston C.C. Jr. *et al.* Prevalence of low femoral bone density in older U. S. adults from HNANES III. *Journal of Bone and Mineral Research* 1997;**12**:1761–8.

Lyons R.A., Delahunty A.M., Kraus D. *et al.* Children's fractures: a population based study. *Injury Prevention* 1999;**5**:129–32.

Magnusson M.L., Pope M.H., Wilder D.G. *et al.* Are occupational drivers at an increased risk for developing musculoskeletal disorders? *Spine* 1996;**21**:710–7.

Malmivaara A., Häkkinen U., Aro T. *et al.* The treatment of acute low back pain—bed rest, exercises, or ordinary activity? *New England Journal of Medicine* 1995;**332**:351–5.

Melton L.J. III. How many women have osteoporosis now? *Journal of Bone and Mineral Research* 1995;10:175–7.

Menz H.B., Lord S.R. The contribution of foot problems to mobility impairment and falls in community-dwelling older people. *Journal of the American Geriatrics Society* 2001;**49**:1651–6.

Miller N.H. Cause and natural history of adolescent idiopathic scoliosis. *Orthopedic Clinics of North America* 1999;**30**:343–52.

Morales-Torres J., Gutiérrez-UrenÞa S. The burden of osteoporosis in Latin America. *Osteoporosis International* 2004;**15**:625–32.

Morales-Torres J. Strategies for the prevention and control of osteoporosis in developing countries. *Clinical Rheumatology* 2007;**26**:139–43.

Morscher E. Strength and morphology of growth cartilage under hormonal influence of puberty. *Reconstructive Surgery and Traumatology* 1968;**10**:3–104.

Nevitt M.C., Cummings S.R. Type of fall and risk of hip and wrist fractures: the Study of Osteoporotic Fractures. *Journal of the American Geriatrics Society* 1993;**41**:1226–34.

Nissinen M., Heliövaara M., Seitsamo J. *et al.* Trunk asymmetry, posture, growth, and risk of scoliosis. A three-year follow-up of Finnish prepubertal school children. *Spine* 1993;**18**:8–13.

Noguchi Y., Sakamaki T., the Multi-center Study Committee of the Japanese Pediatric Orthopaedic Association. Epidemiology and demographics of slipped capital femoral epiphysis in Japan: a multicenter study by the Japanese Paediatric Orthopaedic Association. *Journal of Orthopaedic Sciences* 2002;**7**:610–7.

Öry F.G., Rahman F.U., Katagade V. *et al.* Respiratory disorders, skin complaints, and low-back trouble among tannery workers in Kanpur, India. *American Industrial Hygiene Association Journal* 1997;**58**:740–6.

Ostojic Z., Kristo T., Ostojic L. *et al.* Prevalence of scoliosis in school-children from Mostar, Bosnia and Herzegovina. *Collegium Antropologicum* 2006;**30**:59–64.

Pope M.H., Magnusson M., Wilder D.G. Low back pain and whole body vibration. *Clinical Orthopaedics and Related Research* 1998;**354**:241–8.

Praemer A., Furner S., Rice D.P. *Musculoskeletal conditions in the United States*. Rosemont (IL): American Academy of Orthopaedic Surgeons; 1999.

Punnett L., Prüss-Üstün A., Nelson D.I. *et al.* Estimating the global burden of low back pain attributable to combined occupational exposures. *American Journal of Industrial Medicine* 2005;**48**:459–69.

Rasch E.K., Hirsch R., Paulose-Ram R. *et al.* Prevalence of rheumatoid arthritis in persons 60 years of age and older in the United States: effect of different methods of case classification. *Arthritis and Rheumatism* 2003;**48**:917–26.

Sadat-Ali M., Al-Habdan I.M., Al-Mulhim F.A. *et al.* Bone mineral density among postmenopausal Saudi women. *Saudi Medical Journal* 2004;**25**:1623–5.

Schwartz A.V., Kelsey J.L., Maggi S. *et al.* International variation in the incidence of hip fractures: cross-national project on osteoporosis for the World Health Organization Program for Research on Aging. *Osteoporosis International* 1999;**9**:242–53.

Seeman E., Delmas P.D. Bone quality—the material and structural basis of bone strength and fragility. *New England Journal of Medicine* 2006;**354**:2250–61.

Shatrugna V., Kulkarni B., Kumar P.A. *et al.* Bone status of Indian women from a low-income group and its relationship to the nutritional status. *Osteoporosis International* 2005;**16**:1827–35.

Snook S.H. Approaches to the control of back pain in industry: job design, job placement, and education/testing. Spine: State of the Art Reviews. *Occupational Back Pain* 1988;**2**:45–59.

Sorenson K.H. Slipped upper femoral epiphysis. *Acta Orthopaedica Scandinavica* 1968;**39**:499–517.

Storer S.K., Skaggs D.A. Developmental dysplasia of the hip. *American Family Physician* 2006;**74**:1310–6.

Stott S., Bidwell T. Epidemiology of slipped capital femoral epiphysis in a population with a high proportion of New Zealand Maori and Pacific children. New Zealand Medical Journal 2003;**116**:U647.

Tinetti M.E. Preventing falls in elderly persons. *New England Journal of Medicine* 2003;**348**:42–9.

US Census Bureau. International database [Online]. 2007.

US Department of Health and Human Services, National Center for Health Statistics. *National Ambulatory Medical Care Survey, 1995 summary*. Hyattsville (MD): Centers for Disease Control and Prevention; 1997.

US Department of Health and Human Services, National Center for Health Statistics. *Third National Health and Nutrition Examination Survey, 1988–94* [NHANES III Examination Data File, CD-ROM]. Public Use Data File Documentation Number 76200. Hyattsville (MD): Centers for Disease Control and Prevention; 1996.

US Preventive Services Task Force. Screening for adolescent idiopathic scoliosis: review article. *Journal of the American Medical Association* 1993;**269**:2667–72.

US Preventive Services Task Force. Screening for adolescent idiopathic scoliosis: policy statement. *Journal of the American Medical Association* 1993;**269**:2664–6.

US Preventive Services Task Force. Screening for developmental dysplasia of the hip: recommendation statement. *Pediatrics* 2006;**117**: 898–902.

Van Vuuren B.J., Becker P.J., van Heerden H.J. *et al.* Lower back problems and occupational risk factors in a South African steel industry. *American Journal of Industrial Medicine* 2005;**47**:451–7.

Volinn E. The epidemiology of low back pain in the rest of the world: a review of surveys in low-and middle-income countries. *Spine* 1997;**22**:1747–54.

Wickstrom G.J., Pentti J. Occupational factors affecting sick leave attributed to low-back pain. *Scandinavian Journal of Work, Environment and Health* 1998;**24**:145–52.

Woolf A.D., Pfleger B. Burden of major musculoskeletal conditions. *Bulletin of the World Health Organization* 2003;**81**:646–56.

World Health Organization. *Prevention and management of osteoporosis*. WHO technical report series 921. Geneva: World Health Organization; 2003.

World Health Organization. *The burden of musculoskeletal conditions at the start of the new millennium*. WHO technical report series 919. Geneva: World Health Organization; 2003.

Yu I.T.S., Wong T.W. Musculoskeletal problems among VDU workers in a Hong Kong bank. *Occupational Medicine* 1996;**46**:275–80.

9.10

Neurologic diseases, epidemiology, and public health

Walter A. Kukull and James Bowen

Abstract

This chapter presents information for selected neurological conditions by referring to current or classic research papers. Conditions such as headache have substantial public health impact because of the age groups affected, the prevalence, and the associated lost economic productivity. Multiple sclerosis (MS), a relatively common neurologic disease, can affect individuals in young adulthood, decrease their productivity and ultimately make them dependent on others. Traumatic brain injury occurring in youth or young adulthood can cause years of extra medical care in addition to lost productivity among those who survive the immediate event. Epilepsy may have onset throughout the life course, it may result from trauma or may be caused by specific genes, among other causes. While there are intractable forms of epilepsy, great strides have been made in seizure control enabling patients to lead relatively full and normal lives. Neurodegenerative diseases, such as Parkinson's disease (PD) and Alzheimer's disease (AD), rob productivity, functional ability, and independence from older individuals; they also force huge increases in health care costs. Without question neurologic diseases have substantial public health impacts.

Introduction

Included in this chapter are brief descriptions of some selected neurological disorders along with a discussion of their general epidemiology. Several themes cut across all of the sections. Case diagnosis is critical to epidemiologic study of neurological diseases and disorders. Diagnosis is, however, difficult for many neurological diseases because specific histologic evidence or antemortem biologic markers may not exist and clinical diagnosis must be relied upon. Variation in clinical criteria can lead to misclassification of disease. As a case series includes more misclassification of disease diagnoses, the ability to recognize risk factors becomes reduced. Standardization of clinical criteria is one method to reduce the amount of misclassification; in practice, standardization across unrelated sites is difficult to achieve, however.

Case ascertainment and selection for inclusion are more substantial problems for the validity of most epidemiologic studies. If an incidence study must rely on death certificates in order to count new cases, and the course of disease is long, the characteristics of cases identified in that way are likely to be skewed and will reflect factors associated with survival. The method of identifying and including cases in a case–control study is important because if identification is associated with exposure history, selection bias could result and the findings could then be spurious. Can all cases identified from a particular study base be enrolled in the study at hand? Usually not; many persons decline to participate in studies. Frailty, age, ethnicity, gender, education, and a host of other factors influence participation. If any of those participation factors are systematically related to exposure status, an uncontrolled bias may result, also. Case identification methods are critical to cohort studies (and intervention trials) as well. Failure to start with a cohort that is free of the disease of interest will potentially bias results. Lack of, or differential sensitivity or specificity in screening or diagnosing disease during cohort follow-up will lead to miss-estimated incidence and to distorted risk factor relationships. The choice of controls in a case–control study also determines the size of the measure of effect. Selection of appropriate controls is even more difficult than selection of cases. Controls should be selected from the same study base that gave rise to the cases. In fact, if persons we would have available to select controls from were to contract the disease under study we would expect that they would be included as cases in our study. Briefly, that is how case and control definition may be used to define the underlying study base, as well.

Obtaining valid estimates of exposures for analytic risk factor studies is of great importance. For most neurological diseases, exposure determination is complicated by insidious and indeterminate onset of disease, obscuring the temporal relationship between exposure and disease. Long past exposure histories are difficult to construct and validate, especially in diseases that affect memory. Self report histories and those obtained from proxies are often the basis for risk factor inference, but may be flawed by distorted recollection or recall bias. Actual records, for example of medication history or occupational exposures, are seldom available. Biological markers of exposure (except for genotype) are difficult to obtain; and some may be affected by disease. Peripheral markers, if available may not correspond to exposure levels in neuronal tissue. Biopsy may not be feasible or possible and autopsy, while often the gold standard for diagnosis, may reflect cumulative disease processes, leaving the picture additionally confusing.

As one leaves major research institutions or attempts to begin epidemiologic research studies in less developed countries, the problems grow in magnitude. Differences in available facilities and local practices are likely the easiest to overcome. Addressing political concerns and suspicions to gain cooperation necessary to begin a study may take additional time and preparation. Case detection, acquisition and exposure measurement still remain critical but the difficulty in obtaining acceptable levels of each is increased by an order of magnitude.

In following sections, we discuss the current descriptive and analytic research for a number of neurological disorders. We also provide a brief appraisal of the public health burden for these conditions.

Headache

Clinical overview

The pathogenesis of most headaches is poorly understood. Therefore, the nosology of headaches is based on the cause of headaches in those types that the cause is known, and the clinical picture in those in which the cause is unknown. The International Headache Society (IHS) classification, second edition, is currently the most commonly used system of classifying headaches (Table 9.10.1) (..2004a) It is important to realize that this system is used to classify individual headaches. Patients may suffer from more than one type of headache with each headache type fulfilling one of the IHS classifications. In fact, most headache patients have more than one type of headache. The IHS classification contains a large number of conditions in which the headaches are symptomatic of neurologic or systemic diseases. Headaches associated with these conditions are comparatively rare. Idiopathic conditions are far more common and include migraine (with or without aura), tension-type headaches and cluster headaches. Because these idiopathic headaches are the overwhelming majority, they have the greatest impact on epidemiologic studies.

Table 9.10.1 International Headache Society, abbreviated classification of headache

1. Migraine
1.1 Migraine without aura
1.2 Migraine with aura
2. Tension-type headache
3. Cluster headache and chronic paroxysmal hemicrania
4. Miscellaneous headaches unassociated with structural lesion
5. Headache associated with head trauma
6. Headache associated with vascular disorders
7. Headache associated with nonvascular intracranial disorder
8. Headache associated with substances or their withdrawal
9. Headache associated with noncephalic infection
10. Headache associated with metabolic disorder
11. Headache or facial pain associated with disorder of cranium, neck, eyes, ears, nose, sinuses, teeth, mouth, or other facial or cranial structures
12. Cranial neuralgias, nerve trunk pain, and deafferentation pain
13. Headache not classifiable

Migraine without aura was previously named common migraine. It is an episodic headache that, as its name suggests, has no aura. The headache may be unilateral or bilateral. Some have throbbing pain while others have constant non-throbbing pain. Nausea, vomiting, or diarrhoea may occur. The pain often builds over a few hours. The typical length of the headache is 4–72 h.

Migraine with aura was previously named classic migraine. The identifying feature of this type of headache is the aura. This consists of an alteration of neurologic function that usually precedes the headache. The aura most commonly consists of changes in vision with a central area of visual loss surrounded by a rim of shimmering light (the scintillating scotoma). Non-visual auras may also occur including paresthesias, numbness, weakness, aphasia, or vertigo. Auras usually precede the headache by about 20 min, though the timing may vary. The headache resembles that seen in migraine without aura. It is most commonly, though not always, unilateral. It is most often throbbing and often associated with nausea and vomiting. It typically lasts a few hours. It is episodic and may have premonitory symptoms preceding the headache and aura.

Tension-type headaches, the most common type of headache, are usually bilateral and have a sensation of pressure or a tight band around the head. They are less likely to have premonitory symptoms and less likely to have nausea or vomiting. They do not have auras. They usually last longer than migraine headaches and typically last an entire day or even several days. They build up more slowly than migraine headaches. Episodic and chronic subtypes are recognized.

Cluster headaches are named after the tendency to occur in clusters lasting weeks to months. However, other types of headaches may also occur in clusters and the diagnosis is made based on the characteristics of the headache rather than the clustering. The headache develops abruptly. During a cluster, it usually occurs between one and eight times a day, often at the same time of day. The pain is more short-lived than that of other idiopathic headaches and generally subsides within 3 h. The pain is often more severe than that seen with migraine and patients are often agitated during the attack.

As previously noted, patients often suffer from more than one type of headache. In a single patient, less severe headaches tend to be tension-type while more severe headaches are migraine. There is also a tendency for patient's headaches to change over time with the headache pattern being classic migraine in youth but more closely matching that of tension-type headaches with time. These headaches may increase in frequency with age and become chronic daily headaches. Some term these headaches as 'transitioned migraines'. This term is not included in the International Headache Classification and many of these cases are actually due to medication overuse.

Prevalence

Recent studies have assessed the prevalence of headache and migraine in many countries. Most recent studies have used the IHS criteria to determine probable diagnosis. Characteristics of the samples selected and analytic designs have differed, sometimes substantially, raising questions of comparability.

The 1-year prevalence of all types of headache varies widely between different studies, from 20 to 90 per cent (Stovner *et al.* 2007). Migraine varied from 3 to 24.6 per cent, tension-type headache from 9.8 to 72.3 per cent, and chronic headache from 0.5 to 7.3 per cent. Much of this variability can be attributed to differences in methodology including survey methods, case definition, and the study population involved. Several large population-based studies have been completed. A survey of 5000 adults in the United Kingdom (Boardman *et al.* 2006) found that 71 per cent had suffered a headache in the past 3 months, with 76 per cent having headaches over a 1-year period. In a Spanish study, a mail-in survey followed by clinical evaluations found that 77 per cent had headaches, with 4.7 per cent having headaches 15 or more days per month (Castillo *et al.* 1999). The head-HUNT study began with all people 20 years of age or older, who resided in a single county in Norway. Of 51 383 respondents, the 1-year prevalence of all headaches was 38 per cent and of migraine was 12 per cent (Hagen *et al.* 2000).

Several studies have evaluated the prevalence of migraine. This reflects the availability of survey instruments that have been validated to identify migraine in study populations. The 1-year period prevalence of migraine is approximately 12 per cent (Rasmussen 1995). The American Migraine Prevalence and Prevention study assessed 162 576 individuals by mail survey (Lipton *et al.* 2007). It found a 1-year prevalence rate of migraine in men of 5.6 per cent and in women of 17.1 per cent. Prevalence peaked at 30–39 years of age, and was higher in whites and in those with lower incomes. Only 68 per cent of women and 57 per cent of men reported their migraines to a physician. Of those that did, approximately 40 per cent did not receive a correct diagnosis of migraine (Lipton *et al.* 1998). These estimates compare favourably with other studies that included both treated and untreated, self-reported headache. Gobel *et al.* (1994) selected a representative sample of 5000 persons from among 30 000 households in Germany. Using IHS criteria, approximately 71 per cent of the subjects reported any history of headache. The lifetime prevalence of migraine was 27.5 per cent. This survey did not rely on access to medical care and so may estimate the underlying lifetime prevalence of both treated and untreated migraine. Merikangas *et al.* (1994) studied the prevalence of headache in persons aged 29–30 in Zurich, Switzerland, again using the IHS criteria. Migraine with aura had a 1-year prevalence of 3.3 per cent and migraine without aura showed a 1-year prevalence of 21.3 per cent. Franceschi *et al.* (1997) studied an elderly population (mean age 73 years) in Italy to determine whether increasing age would affect reported prevalence. Although 18 per cent of subjects admitted to 'troublesome' headaches in the past, only 6 per cent were currently bothered by headache and 1 per cent met HIS criteria for current migraine. These results leave the impression that headache problems in young adulthood, may not persist into old age. However, in order to adequately evaluate change in the frequency of headache events with age would require a cohort study design instead of a cross-sectional one. O'Brien *et al.* (1994) drew a stratified sample in Canada, selecting 2922 subjects for a telephone interview based on IHS criteria. The prevalence of migraine was 7.8 per cent in male and 24.9 per cent in females; only about 46 per cent of those with migraine were reported to have ever contacted a physician for their problem. Within women, the peak prevalence was seen in the 40–44-year age group. A recent meta-analysis included 24 population-based studies of migraine (Stewart *et al.* 1995). Most of the variation in prevalence estimates, among the studies included, was accounted for by age and gender differences along with case definition. Stewart concluded that after accounting for age gender and case definition, migraine prevalence estimates were stable across the studies included in the meta-analysis. Thus, despite variations in design and case ascertainment methods, there appears to be a gender difference and age-related differences that appear with some consistency in a number of countries. Many people apparently do not mention their headaches to physicians, and physicians often do not correctly identify headache subtypes.

Osuntokun *et al.* (1992) applied a screening questionnaire to more than 18 000 persons in Nigeria. The questionnaire was not strictly the IHS criteria but reportedly showed high sensitivity and specificity when compared to the gold standard neurologist examination for headache. Much lower lifetime prevalence of migraine (5.3%) was reported in this study than in those primarily comprised of Caucasians. No gender difference was noted, also in contrast to the studies reported above. Stewart *et al.* (1996a) compared migraine prevalence in Caucasians, African Americans, and Asian Americans living in the United States. The study involved about 12 000 persons aged 18–65 selected from Baltimore County, Maryland, selected by random digit dialling, and interviewed by telephone. Observed prevalence of migraine in Caucasians was 20.4 per cent for women and 8.6 per cent for men; among African Americans: 6.2 per cent in women and 7.2 per cent in men; and among Asian-Americans: 9.2 per cent in women and 4.2 per cent in men. Despite obvious geographic, and sociodemographic differences as well as methodologic differences between the two studies (Stewart *et al.* 1996a; Osuntokun *et al.* 1992), there appears to be a suggestion that susceptibility to migraine may be affected by ethnicity.

There are far fewer studies on tension-type headaches. Up to 89 per cent of people suffer tension-type headaches at some point in their lives, but for most, this is infrequent. About 25 per cent have tension-type headaches weekly while only 2–3 per cent of the population has chronic tension-type headaches (Lyngberg *et al.* 2005a). The 1-year prevalence appears to be increasing, though the factors leading to this increase are not entirely clear. About half of people with tension-type headaches improve within a decade (Lyngberg *et al.* 2005b).

Cluster headaches are the least common of the idiopathic headache disorders. In Germany, the 1-year prevalence of cluster headache was 0.119 per cent (Katsarava *et al.* 2007). However, an Italian survey found a higher rate of cluster headache of 0.279 per cent overall, 0.227 per cent in women and 0.338 per cent in men (Torelli *et al.* 2005). In San Marino, a point prevalence rate of 0.056 per cent was found in 1999. A previous survey in 1985 found a rate of 0.069 per cent indicating the rates remained approximately stable over the time interval (Tonon *et al.* 2002).

Familial and genetic risks

The influence of genetic constitution on the occurrence of migraine has been investigated principally by studies of familial aggregation and by twin studies. While these classic methods provide general clues concerning whether a genetic component to the disease may exist, their lens is generally not of sufficient resolution to identify specific genes or linked markers. Progress in molecular genetics is providing remarkable discoveries for many diseases. Preliminary reports of rare mutations in the mitochondrial genome and associations with polymorphic forms of serotonergic and dopaminergic genes and migraine are as yet unsubstantiated, but may be more carefully evaluated and tested in the future.

Two recent twin studies based in the Danish Twin Registry (Gervil *et al.* 1999; Ulrich *et al.* 1999) compared concordance rates of migraine without aura and migraine with aura, respectively. Twin pairs with one member affected by a specific type of migraine were selected from the registry. Both monozygotic (MZ) and dizygotic (DZ) twins (same sex) were selected for study and the occurrence of migraine was determined by interview and/or examination. The overall lifetime prevalence of migraine with aura for MZ and DZ twins was 7 per cent, similar to population surveys. The concordance in MZ twins was 34 per cent compared to 12 per cent for DZ twins. For migraine without aura the pairwise concordance for MZ twins was 28 per cent, compared with 18 per cent for DZ. This indicates a potential genetic contribution to migraine. But, because there is substantially less than 100 per cent concordance among MZ twins the modifying influence of environmental factors may also be important in migraine aetiology. Ziegler *et al.* (1998) studied MZ and DZ, female twin pairs, raised together ($n = 154$) and apart ($n = 43$). This classical twin study design showed that concordance was higher for MZ than DZ twins whether raised together or raised apart. Zeigler *et al.* concluded that about 50 per cent of the variance was explained by genetic factors and the remaining half was due to 'nonshared environmental factors', and measurement error. This conclusion was confirmed in a recent update to this study (Russell *et al.* 2007).

Stewart *et al.* (2006) examined familial aggregation in first degree relatives of migraine probands and first-degree relatives of unaffected control subjects. The relative risk (RR) of migraine in first degree relatives of migraineurs was 1.88 (95 per cent confidence interval [CI] 1.30–2.72] compared to relatives of a control group. The relative risk was higher in relatives of those whose headaches began before 16 years of age (RR = 2.50; 95% CI 1.65–3.79) than those whose headaches began later (RR = 1.44; 95% CI 0.93–2.23). The risk in relatives of those with severe headaches had a relative risk of 2.38 (95% CI 1.56–3.62) while relatives of those with less severe pain had a relative risk of 1.52 (0.99–2.34).

Recently, individual genetic alleles have been linked to various types of headache. Though each of these account for only a small proportion of headaches, they serve as important models for understanding the pathogenesis of these disorders. A study by Nyholt *et al.* (..1998) was based on three large multigenerational families. It shows linkage between headaches and a locus on the X-chromosome (Xq) (Nyholt *et al.* 1998). Some polymorphisms of the angiotensin-converting enzyme (ACE) and matrix metalloproteinase (MMP) genes may increase the risk of headache, while other polymorphisms decrease the risk (Kara *et al.* 2007). Polymorphisms of the 5,10-methylenetetrahydrofolate reductase gene have been reported to increase the risk of headaches, migraine with aura, migraine without aura, and tension-type headache (Kara *et al.* 2003). Alleles of the dopamine b-hydroxylase gene have also been linked to migraine (Lea *et al.* 2000). It is expected that rapid progress will be made in understanding the genetic underpinnings of this group of diseases and that this will influence future treatment strategies.

Risk factors for headaches

Stress or psychological factors are often cited as contributing to tension-type headaches. However, the frequency of these factors is similar in patients with migraine and tension-type headaches. With chronicity, psychological changes increase in frequency, suggesting that psychological issues are secondary to chronic headaches rather than causative.

Breslau and Davis (1993) and Breslau *et al.* (1994) conducted a longitudinal study in 1007 young adults to observe the association between migraine and major depression. She reported a significant threefold increased risk of major depression among those with a history of migraine and also a threefold increased risk for migraine among those with prior depression. This finding raised the possibility that the two disorders may have mechanisms in common. Pine *et al.* (1996) reported a similar longitudinal study that followed 776 persons aged 9–18 (in 1983) for up to 9 years. They reported that in subjects with no history of 'chronic impairing headache', those with major depression at baseline had a tenfold risk of developing such headaches during follow-up. Breslau *et al.* (2000) conducted another study to clarify the association between severe headache or migraine and depression. In this longitudinal study, persons with severe headache experienced approximately a threefold increased risk of first onset depression but those with major depression at baseline experienced no significantly increased risk of severe headache. However, the previously reported 'bi-directional' association between migraine and depression was replicated. The issues of migraine and depression have recently been reviewed (Frediani & Villani 2007).

In a case–control study, Scher found that chronic daily headaches were more common in women, whites, and those with less education. An improvement in headache frequency after 1 year was more common in those with higher education, non-whites, and those who were married (Scher *et al.* 2003). Migraine is higher in those with lower education and socioeconomic levels, though it is not known whether this is a cause or an effect of the headaches (Hagen *et al.* 2002a). However, in adolescents with a family history of migraine, the prevalence of migraine is the same in low- vs. high-income groups (OR 0.97, 95% CI 0.81–1.15) suggesting that genetic factors overwhelm environmental risk factors in those genetically susceptible. In contrast, those without a family history of migraine have a lower prevalence of headaches within those from the higher-income group (OR –0.49, 95% CI 0.38–0.63) suggesting a socioeconomic contribution in those who are not genetically predisposed to the disease (Bigal *et al.* 2007). One of the strongest risk factors for headaches is prior headaches (RR = 4.15), but difficulty sleeping (did not reach significance) and caffeine intake (NS) are also factors (Boardman *et al.* 2006). Pain in other areas of the body are associated with headache (RR = 1.43, 95% CI 1–2)

Stroke and migraine

Data from the Physicians Health Study (Buring *et al.* 1995) and from the National Health and Nutrition Examination Survey (Merikangas *et al.* 1997) support a significantly increased risk of stroke in persons with a history of migraine. Because of the relatively high prevalence of migraine among young women the occurrence of stroke in that population is of some concern. In a World Health Organization case–control study sample, Chang *et al.* (1999) reported an approximately threefold increased odds ratio for history of migraine in young women with ischaemic stroke as compared to controls. Tietjen (2000) cautions that the relationship between migraine and stroke may be complicated by the contribution of additional risk factors, such as cigarette smoking and oral contraceptives, and possibly by genetic factors as well. In the Stroke Prevention in Young Women study, a case–control investigation of migraine and stroke was undertaken (MacClellan *et al.* 2007). Women who had migraine with visual aura had a relative risk of having an ischaemic stroke of 1.5 (95% CI 1.1–2), but there was no increased risk in those with migraine without aura. The odds ratio for those with more than 12 headaches per year was 1.7 (95% CI, 1.1–2.8) and 1.3 (95% CI, 0.8–1.9) in those requiring bedrest or absence from work. In the Women's Health Study, those having a history of migraine with aura had a hazard ratio of 1.53 (95% CI 1.02–2.31) for all strokes and 1.71 (95% CI 1.11–2.66) for ischaemic strokes (Kurth *et al.* 2005). There was no increase in risk for those having migraine without aura. Additional study may be needed to adequately describe the true relationship between migraine and stroke.

Costs and public health impact

The estimated 23 million persons with migraines in the United States may miss 150 million workdays each year with an associated cost of up to US$17 billion (Cady 1999; Hu *et al.* 1999). Many more persons suffer with decreased effectiveness at work than actually miss work days; this results in additional hidden loss of productivity due to migraine (Schwartz *et al.* 1997). Estimates of costs are challenging because of differences in the methodology used to determine prevalence and indirect costs of lost wages, decreased productivity while at work with a headache, and related factors. Insufficient data exists to calculate results for tension-type headache in Europe, but an estimate of migraine costs has been performed. This found a range of direct costs over 1 year from €12 in the United Kingdom, to 68 in the Netherlands, using 2004 prices. Indirect costs ranged from €80 in Sweden to €850 in Germany. Indirect costs included lost wages and decreased productivity on days worked with headache. Only migraine was evaluated. Workers lost on average 2.5 workday/patient/year due to HA and had a reduced work efficiency of 65 per cent during 4.1 additional days (Berg & Stovner 2005). New treatments are relatively effective but only a minority of persons consult physicians for their problem or receive the effective medications (Lipton 1998). Early recognition and treatment of migraine may significantly limit societal and personal costs (Cady 1999).

Health-related quality of life is lower in those with migraine, and this is related to the frequency of attacks (Wang *et al.* 2001). There are many challenges in making cost determinations due to limits on available epidemiological data (Leonardi *et al.* 2005). However, the best estimate suggests that migraine accounts for 1.4 per cent of all years of healthy life lost worldwide. It is the nineteenth leading cause of years of healthy life lost in men and twelfth in women. This major public health issue deserves continued attention.

Traumatic brain injury

Clinical overview

Traumatic brain injury (TBI) is commonly divided into categories by mechanism of action: Penetrating or closed head injuries. These also may be characterized as resulting from direct contact injuries or from concussive 'acceleration deceleration' types of injuries (Werner & Engelhard 2007). Among penetrating injuries, greater tissue damage is caused by high velocity penetrating objects than by lower velocity ones. Both penetrating and closed injuries may perturb or impair cerebral blood flow (CBF) leading to ischaemia and altered cerebral metabolism. Impaired CBF resulting from cerebral vasospasm predicts poorer outcome and may occur in approximately 30 per cent of TBI cases (Werner & Engelhard 2007). Brain contusions may lead to both blood vessel and cell membrane injury resulting in vasogenic or cytotoxic edema. Hydrocephalus may develop due to blockage of the routes of normal cerebrospinal fluid flow. Finally, closed head injuries may lead to diffuse axonal injury. Diffuse axonal injury results in balls of axonal material occurring at axon transection sites or sites of altered axonal flow. Therefore, much of the neurological damage due to TBI does not occur at the time of impact but grows with impaired cerebral perfusion and other factors in the hours and days after the injury itself. Treatment or prevention of the insults that are the physiological result of the injury may ultimately decrease morbidity and mortality.

The symptoms of focal head injuries have been thought to be determined by the site of injury. However, Power *et al.* (2007) have shown that among children aged 6–14 the severity of the injury is a better predictor of neurobehavioural outcome than is location.

For mild head injuries, including skull fracture, concussion, and unspecified intracranial or head injury (Bazarian *et al.* 2005), the severity of the injury is usually measured by the degree of post-traumatic amnesia. Amnesia lasting less than 5 min is classified as very mild, less than 1 h is mild, 1–24 h is moderate, 1–7 days is severe, more than 7 days is very severe and more than 4 weeks is extremely severe. Mild and severe head injuries are usually classified by the Glasgow Coma Scale: Scores of 13–15 are minor, 9–12 are moderate, 5–8 are severe, and 4 or less are very severe; and by length of coma (Sherer *et al.* 2007).

Incidence and prevalence

The CDC estimates that 1.57 million persons (95% CI = 1.37–1.77 million) suffered a TBI in 2003 in the United States (538.2 per 100 000 population), approximately 51 000 of those resulted in death (TBI mortality 17.5 per 100 000 population) based on all reported emergency department visits, hospitalizations and deaths. The numbers of TBIs reported during each of the previous 5 years were not statistically significantly different. TBI incidence among children aged 0–4 was the highest of all age groups at 1188.5 per 100 000, while hospitalization and death rates were highest among those aged 65 and older. Falls accounted for 32 per cent of TBIs, motor vehicle traffic for 19 per cent, struck by/against events 18 per cent and assaults 10 per cent. Men experienced about 1.5 times greater rate of TBI than women (Rutland-Brown *et al.* 2006). Cassidy *et al.* (2004) compiled a review of more than 160 published studies to estimate the occurrence of mild TBI. They found that approximately 70–90 per cent of all treated TBIs are likely to be mild and which results in an expected rate for treated mild TBI of 100–300 per 100 000 population. Because most mild TBIs are not hospitalized however, Cassidy *et al.* further estimate that overall population rate for mild TBI might approach 600 per 100 000 population. This may have implications for the occurrence of post traumatic epilepsy also, as a related neurological public health problem.

Incidence of TBI in Europe was the subject of a recent review (Tagliaferri *et al.* 2006); the authors compared 23 European studies and noted that the incidence varied from about 546 per 100 000 to about 91 per 100 000. Reasons for the reported wide variation in incidence were thought to depend at least in part on case definition, inclusion criteria and methodological differences between the studies. Generally speaking, most of the incidence rates ranged between 150/100 000 and 300/100 000 with a mean value of 243/100 000. The mean incidence changed only modestly if the two most extreme observed rates were excluded from the calculation, to 235/100 000 (Tagliaferri *et al.* 2006). Based on that conservative estimate of hospitalized TBI incidence and a European population of 330 million, then 775 500 new TBI cases would occur each year. If for these cases injury-related morbidity remained active for 10 years then about 7.8 million prevalent TBI cases would be expected in Europe (Tagliaferri *et al.* 2006).

Reports from investigators associated with the CDC have focused on the incidence of TBI hospitalizations (only), based on a 15-State surveillance system (..2006). During 2002, the age-adjusted annual TBI hospitalization incidence rate (also adjusted for false-positives) was 79 per 100 000 population. Age-specific rates varied substantially from 264.4 per 100 000 among those aged 75 years or older to 103.3 among those aged 15–24, the next highest incidence age group. Unintentional falls accounted for 203.9 per 100 000 of the TBI hospitalizations among person aged 75 of more. Motor Vehicle Traffic incidents were also a prominent cause of TBI hospitalization among those aged 75+, but the rate for 15–24-year olds was approximately double that of any other age group. TBI hospitalization associated with assault was nearly six times higher for males than females across all age groups 15–64. Sadly, females aged 0–4 years showed approximately twice the TBI hospitalization rate due to assault as any other female age group. The proportion of in-hospital deaths (13%) and the proportion needing continuing health-care assistance after discharge (68%) were greatest among those aged 75 years or greater (..2006).

Risk factors

Falls

Falls are either the first or second most common cause of TBI, depending in part of the age group chosen for comparison. The incidence of TBI resulting from falls increases dramatically with advanced age. An analysis of hospitalizations resulting from nonfatal TBI showed that while the all ages incidence of these events was approximately 21 per 100 000 population (in California, 1996–99), age-specific rates ranged from about 13.6 per 100 000 in persons aged less that 65 years, to 41.8 in those aged 65–74, to 104 in those aged 75–84 and then more than doubled to 223 per 100 000 among those aged 85 years or older (..2003). Among the elderly, who suffer TBI as a result of falls co-morbidity with several other conditions is relatively common (Coronado *et al.* 2005). Use of four or more medications may significantly increase of TBI from falling.

Falls are an important cause of TBI among very young also. The 15-State CDC surveillance system allowed calculation of TBI hospitalization rates due to unintentional falls for children aged 0–11 months compared to those aged 12–23 months. Fall-related TBI hospitalizations were 71.5 per 100 000 person-years in the younger group as compared to 36.5 per 100 000 person-years in the older group. Skull fracture with or without intracranial injury predominated in those aged less than 1 year while nonspecific concussion injuries were most common in the older group (Eisele *et al.* 2006). Careful examination of the consistency of reported mechanisms of the injury with the resulting pathology is often necessary to discriminate whether the TBI may have been due to an unintentional falls or inflicted trauma. Among toddlers and older young children. falls from stairs, furniture and playground equipment become more common; however, these are more often associated with hospitalization than with mortality. Among older children, motor vehicle accidents contribute substantially more to TBI than falls do (Keenan & Bratton 2006).

Vehicle accidents

A report constructed by the CDC based on TBI which led to an emergency department visit, hospitalization or death in 2003, showed that overall motor vehicle accidents (19%) were second only to falls (32%) as a cause of TBI based on a total overall estimate of TBI of between 1.37 million and 1.77 million events (Rutland-Brown *et al.* 2006). Injuries resulting from motor vehicle accidents whether occurring to occupants or as pedestrian or cyclist vs. motor vehicle, result in many of the more severe TBIs. Mandatory seatbelt and child seat laws could have an effect on reducing occupant injuries, while bicycle and motorcycle helmet use may reduce the occurrence of TBI in those constituent categories (Rezendes 2006). In the United States, between 1975 and 2004, states which have repealed motorcycle helmet laws have shown a 12 per cent increase in motorcycle fatalities while those that have instituted such laws have experienced an 11 per cent reduction in motorcycle fatalities (Houston & Richardson 2007). Elderly individuals generally appear to be at higher risk of poor outcome or more severe TBI resulting from motor vehicle traffic (Thompson *et al.* 2006).

Violence

Assaults are estimated to have accounted for approximately 10 per cent of the TBIs occurring in the United States in 2003 or roughly 160 000 TBIs (Rutland-Brown *et al.* 2006). As much as 20 per cent of TBI may be the result of violence, roughly half of these are due to firearms. The age group at highest risk is 15–24 years. While males appear to be more likely to sustain an injury due to violence, women may be more likely to die as a result. Generally, community violence indicates an increased opportunity that TBI will be involved. Durkin *et al.* (1996) describes the incidence of paediatric severe nonfatal assault in North Manhattan (NYC) as approximately 60 per 100 000 (about 30 per 100 000 due to firearms). Among adolescents, firearms were the most common method of serious assault and carried more than a tenfold increased fatality risk. A similar study of general trauma was conducted in Los Angeles County (Demetriades *et al.* 1998). In that study, homicides accounted for 45 per cent of traumatic deaths compared to 32 per cent resulting from traffic accidents. The incidence of firearm-related injury or death was 42 per 100 000. The homicide rate varied dramatically by age and ethnic group. Overall it was about 14 per 100 000, but rose to 73 per 100 000 in African-American males and further to 164.2 per 100 000 among 15–34-year-old African American males. While this study speaks to trauma and homicide generally, Lam and MacKersie (1999) states that among children admitted to hospitals 75 per cent are admitted because of trauma and as many as 70 per cent of paediatric trauma deaths are due to head injury. Also, firearms may be involved in a substantial proportion of TBI, hence, the relevance of these statistics.

Abuse and domestic violence are important causes of TBI among women and among children (Monahan & O'Leary 1999). Monahan estimates that about 35 per cent of the 2–3 million women battered each year by their domestic partner sustain TBI as a result. The sequellae of these injuries may be difficult to document because they may include behavioural and cognitive deficits as well as the acute physical problems. Abusive head trauma may also be an under-recognized problem among very young children. Keenan *et al.* (2003) found that physical abuse may be the most frequent cause of TBI in children aged less than 2 years with an estimated incidence rate of approximately 17 per 100 000 person-years; infants had a higher incidence that older children and boys were at somewhat greater risk than girls. Children born to younger mothers or who were part of multiple births also showed greater risk (Keenan *et al.* 2003). So-called 'shaken baby syndrome' and other forms of physical abuse may result in TBI as well as in spinal cord injury.

Sports injuries account for a relatively small proportion of serious TBI. Between 2001 and 2005, approximately 208 000 emergency department visits each year in the United States were the result of sports and recreational activities (..2007b). The majority of these injuries occurred among children aged 10–14 years, closely followed by those aged 15–19 years. Hospital admission resulted in approximately 10 per cent of these incidents. Among the more frequent causes were riding horses, bicycles or motorized bikes, and all terrain vehicles along with ice skating and sledding (..2007b). However, many mild head injuries may go unreported, and it is unclear what the long-term risk of such injuries may be.

A comprehensive review of mild TBI was accomplished by Holm *et al.* (2005) for the World Health Organization Task Force on Mild TBI. Mild TBI resulting from most sports injuries resolve relatively spontaneously with 'no objective evidence' of cognitive deficits remaining longer that several months. However, Holm *et al.* (2005) caution that better designed and more objective studies are needed to adequately characterize the outcomes.

War and sociopolitically directed violence

By the end of 2007, over a million US and UK men and women have served in the wars in Iraq and Afghanistan, resulting in thousands of deaths and tens of thousands of severe injuries. The local populations of those countries have suffered perhaps several orders of magnitude greater numbers of casualties. Similarly, around the world, there are almost daily, similar situations involving sociopolitical violence which may also affect large numbers. Injuries related to explosive blasts may account for many or most of these (Warden 2006) and lasting results of these types of injuries could have important individual and public health consequences for many years to come. Not only do blasts account for much of the observable and immediate injuries, but they may also lead to more mild or unreported TBI that can be coupled with post-traumatic stress disorder (PTSD) (Okie 2005). In addition, manifestation of sequellae may be dependent upon the age at which the injury occurred, with younger people tending to develop psychotic symptoms, middle aged developing anxiety and depression and older individuals developing cognitive deficits (Keltner & Cooke 2007). It is not clear whether the younger and middle-aged persons who may have experienced TBI or blast-related TBI will ultimately be at higher risk for dementia and developing cognitive impairment as they enter ages 60–80, for example, but it would be consistent with head trauma as a risk factor for dementia (Mehta *et al.* 1999). Of course, there is also the potential for developing epilepsy as a result of TBI possibly due to blast, though it may be more commonly due to other mechanisms.

Implications for public health

Both mild and severe TBI impact the public health. Severe TBI may frequently result in death or long-term disability. The potential years of productive life lost, due to TBI varies with its cause, and causes are differentially age-related. Personal costs experienced by victims of TBI have no monetary cost estimate; lost opportunities for education and employment, changed or foregone personal relationships, psychological distress may all result from TBI (Colantonio *et al.* 1998). Further, the risk of seizures following TBI is increased up to seventeen-fold in patients with severe injuries (Annegers *et al.* 1998). While injuries related to motor vehicles and falls are the most common, those who are most severely affected, have the poorest outcomes and require the most continuing care, tend to be the very young and the elderly. Sports injuries despite their public visibility, especially when severe, and because of their occurrence in active and otherwise healthy individuals, tend to be mild, resolving and carry few sequellae. Sociopolitically related TBIs could be source of unexpected public health burden in the future with the potential long-term development of PTSD, psychiatric symptoms, cognitive deficits and degenerative dementias or other neurological disorders. While the actual short-term case fatality rate for TBI may be high, that in itself does not describe the major cost.

Epilepsy

Clinical overview

The International League Against Epilepsy (ILAE) classification system for epilepsy, proposed in 1985 and revised in 1989 (Table 9.10.2), is currently the most commonly used classification for epileptic syndromes (..1989). Syndromes may be classified according to the characteristics of the individual seizures. They are divided into location-related seizures (formerly named partial or local seizures) that begin in a localized part of the brain, and generalized epilepsies that begin diffusely in the brain. The areas of brain initially involved determine the symptoms of location-related seizures. Location-related seizures may (simple partial) or may not (complex partial seizures) be associated with altered consciousness. They may secondarily generalize after a focal onset.

Generalized seizures are those that begin in widespread areas of the brain. The most common type of generalized seizure is noted for muscle stiffening followed by jerking (tonic–clonic). Generalized seizures were formerly called *grand mal* seizures. Absence seizures (formerly *petit mal*) consist of brief episodes of staring and lack of responsiveness. Myoclonic seizures involve brief jerks of muscles rather than repetitive clonic movements. Tonic seizures involve a generalized muscle stiffening. Atonic seizures involve sudden loss of muscle tone.

9.10.2 The international league against epilepsy classification of epileptic seizures

I. Partial (focal, local) seizures
A. Simple partial seizures
B. Complex partial seizure (with impairment of consciousness)
C. With impairment of consciousness at onset
D. Partial seizures evolving to secondarily generalized seizures
II. Generalized seizures
A. Absence seizures
B. Myoclonic seizures
C. Clonic seizures
D. Tonic seizures
E. Tonic–clonic seizures
F. Atonic seizures
III. Unclassified epileptic seizures

Recently, a diagnostic scheme has been proposed that emphasizes different ways (or axes) of classifying seizure and epileptic syndromes. Axis 1 describes the ictal semiology, axis 2 the seizure type, axis 3 the syndromic diagnosis, axis 4 the aetiology, and axis 5 the degree of impairment (Engel 2001). The terminology in this scheme has changed to focal seizures and generalized seizures.

Incidence and prevalence

Aspects of epilepsy epidemiology have been reviewed by a number of contemporary authors (e.g. Jallon & Latour 2005). Epidemiological studies of epilepsy are challenged by the difficulty in making a correct diagnosis and the sophisticated technology required for proper diagnosis and classification. For example, Uldall *et al.* studied all cases of paediatric epilepsy admitted to a tertiary centre in Denmark (Uldall *et al.* 2006). Of 223 children admitted, 87 (39%) did not have epilepsy on sophisticated EEG monitoring. Of the 184 cases in which there was no doubt expressed about the diagnosis of epilepsy on admission, 30 per cent were found to not have epilepsy. There is also difficulty with standardizing case ascertainment. For example, a recent study found a mean prevalence of 8.2/1000 for active epilepsy defined as those having a seizure within the past 5 years or on antiepileptic drugs (Svendsen *et al.* 2007). This rate fell to 5.3/1000 if the definition was changed to having a seizure within the past 5 years regardless of medication status. Nevertheless, the incidence of epilepsy has been estimated to be 46/100 000/year (range 32–71) (Hirtz *et al.* 2007). This rises to 57/100 000/year in children (range 41–65 per 100 000). The prevalence is estimated to be 7.1/1000 (range 4–8.9). Below, we present several studies that focus on the incidence and prevalence of epilepsy.

Hauser *et al.* (1996) reported the age-adjusted incidence of epilepsy as 44 per 100 000 person-years, based on data from the Rochester Epidemiology Project spanning approximately a 50-year period up to 1980. Reassessment in that same population in 1980–84 yielded a consistent though slightly higher estimate of epilepsy incidence (Zarrelli *et al.* 1999). Importantly, Hauser noted that the incidence and prevalence of epilepsy and unprovoked seizures decreased with calendar time among children and increased among the elderly. The prevalence of active epilepsy among those aged 75 or older was reported as 1.5 per cent (as of January 1980). About 1 per cent of persons under age 20 experienced epilepsy (Hauser 1995), and their prognosis was generally favourable with most achieving control within 2 years. Kramer *et al.* (1998) reported the distribution of different seizure types, among 440 children with two or more unprovoked seizures, attending the paediatric neurology clinic in Tel Aviv. Partial seizures accounted for 52 per cent and primary generalized seizures 33 per cent. This is in general agreement with a prospective German study where an annual incidence of 60.3/100 000 was seen in children aged 1 month to 15 years (Freitag *et al.* 2001). Focal (partial) seizures accounted for 58 per cent of these.

Olafsson and Hauser (1999) conducted a survey in rural Iceland, determining the prevalence of recurrent unprovoked seizures. Records of primary care physicians and neurologists were used for case identification. The crude age adjusted prevalence was 4.8 per 1000 population. The British national child development study followed all 17 733 children who were born during a single week in 1958 in England, Scotland, and Wales (Kurtz *et al.* 1998). A screening survey asking about symptoms consistent with seizures was supplemented by medical records. The cumulative incidence by age 23 was 8.4/1000 (95% CI 6.8–10). The prevalence of 'active' epilepsy, defined as having a seizure within the past 2 years or currently taking anticonvulsant medications, at age 23 was 6.3/1000 (95% CI 4.9–7.7). Christensen *et al.* studied cases through the Danish Civil Registration System (Christensen *et al.* 2007). This system identifies patients who were inpatients or outpatients in Danish hospitals, but not those in private practitioner's offices. The diagnosis was determined by the International Classification of Disease (ICD-10) coding, which depended on the diagnosis of the admitting physician. In recent years, this study found an incidence of epilepsy of 83.3/100 000/year.

Another method of case ascertainment was used by Nicoletti *et al.* (1998, 1999) to study epilepsy and other neurologic conditions in Bolivia. For this study a 'door-to-door survey' was conducted; 10 000 persons were screened, approximately 1000 were referred to neurologists and of those 112 were determined to have active epilepsy, leading to a prevalence estimate of 11.1 per 1000. In contrast to studies reported above (Hauser *et al.* 1996), the highest prevalence occurred in the 15–24-year age group (20.4 per 1000). Regardless of the shift in peak occurrence the prevalence appears dramatically higher than in other studies. A telephone survey of random households was conducted in a minority community of New York City (Kelvin *et al.* 2007). The age-adjusted prevalence of active epilepsy was 5/1000. Differences in racial groups were noted with rates of 5.2 in Blacks, 5.9 in Whites and 6.3 in Hispanics. These rates contrast with those found in other regions. In Southern Italy a survey of physician's records found a point prevalence rate of 3.13 (95% CI 2.2–4.2) (Gallitto *et al.* 2005). These researchers speculated that the low rate may, in part, be due to a cultural prejudice regarding epilepsy. Differences in study methodology, survey methods, case definition, the availability of sophisticated medical technology in a community, and cultural differences make epilepsy studies particularly challenging.

Mortality

Persons with epilepsy may experience two to three times the risk of death as their unaffected counterparts, Sperling *et al.* (1999) examined the relationship between recurrent seizure and risk of death; they compared persons whose seizures had been eliminated by surgery to those with recurrent seizures. The standardized mortality ratio (SMR) for persons with recurrent seizure was approximately fourfold higher than expected. A longitudinal study conducted in the Netherlands (Shackleton *et al.* 1999) enrolled newly diagnosed epilepsy patients (n=1355) who were followed a mean of 28 years. Overall they observed a threefold excess in all cause mortality, and a sevenfold increase among those under age 20. Loiseau *et al.* (1999) studied short-term mortality after first afebrile, provoked, or unprovoked seizure (n=804). After 1 year of follow-up, no deaths had occurred among patients with idiopathic seizures. Increased SMRs were observed for those with provoked seizures or seizures related to other CNS disorders. Some of the risk of death in epilepsy reflects underlying diseases like brain neoplasms and cerebrovascular disease. However, there is also an increased mortality compared to the non-epileptic population due to accidents (often drowning and burns) and suicide (Lhatoo & Sander 2005).

Sudden unexplained death in persons with epilepsy (SUDEP) (Annegers & Coan 1999) is a substantial risk in younger aged persons as compared to people without epilepsy. Much of the excess risk may be associated with seizure severity with greater severity leading to greater risk of death (Annegers & Coan 1999). Careful definition of SUDEP is necessary as is attention to methodologic detail; early findings may have been the result of selection bias and similar problems,. The incidence of SUDEP varies between 0.9 and 1.5/1000 person-years for people with epilepsy (Tomson *et al.* 2005) In a population-based study in Rochester, Minnesota, all persons diagnosed with epilepsy between 1935 and 1994 were followed to determine cause of death. SUDEP rates were compared to the rate of sudden unexplained death in the general population for ages 20–40. Although the SUDEP death rate exceeded the expected by 23.7 times, it was still a rare cause of death accounting for only 1.7 per cent of the deaths in the epilepsy cohort. Nilsson *et al.* (1999) investigated SUDEP in Sweden focusing on risk factors. They found that patients with 50 seizures per year were about 10 times more likely to succumb to SUDEP than patients with 2 or fewer seizures. Risk of SUDEP was also substantially increased with the number of concomitant antiepileptic drugs, and among those who had frequent medication changes. Compared to the general population the cohort of epilepsy patients experienced an all-cause mortality approximately 3.6 times greater than the general population with the majority of the excess mortality due to malignant neoplasms; diseases of the circulatory, respiratory, and digestive systems; injury; and poisoning (Nilsson *et al.* 1997). Though seizure severity has been linked to SUDEP, other factors are also associated with it including prone positioning, respiratory factors, and cardiac factors (Nashef *et al.* 2007). Genetic risks including mutations in ion channel genes have been postulated as risk factors, but to date clear links with SUDEP have not been made (Nashef *et al.* 2007). Tomson *et al.* provides a current review (Tomson *et al.* 2005).

Infectious causes of epilepsy

In developing countries, infections are a much more important cause of epilepsy than in the United States and Europe (Senanayake & Roman 1993), and the overall prevalence of epilepsy may approach 57 per 1000 population. Parasitic, bacterial, and viral infections contribute substantially to the prevalence, but hereditary factors, perinatal damage, head trauma, and toxic exposures also play important aetiologic roles. From a public health view, the excess risk attributable to many of these exposures is potentially preventable (Senanayake & Roman 1993).

An example of an important infectious risk factor is *Taenia solium* cysticercosis (from pork tapeworm) which can lead to neurocysticercosis. Palacio *et al.* (1998) examined a series of 643 epilepsy patients in Columbia, of those 376 had serologic tests for cysticercosis. The prevalence of antibody was 17.5 per cent among late onset epilepsy patients. Among patients with no CT-scan evidence of neurocysticercosis only 2.7 per cent had antibody. However, a similar study conducted in Honduras (Sanchez *et al.* 1999) raises questions as to the validity of the serology antibody tests in predicting neurocysticercosis. Sanchez *et al.* conclude CT-scan findings of neurocycticercosis are necessary for diagnosis. Even though *T. solium* is a frequent exposure in the population as indicated by serology, neurocystericosis is not always the result. A different view is presented by Bern *et al.* (1999). They combined data from 12 population-based community studies in Peru and showed a seroprevalence of 6–24 per cent. The high seroprevalence was presented as evidence for the prevalence of neurocysticercosis. Bern *et al.* estimated a burden of 23 000 to 39 000 symptomatic neurocysticercosis cases in Peru. Extrapolating from these data, Bern *et al.* concluded that cysticercosis is a formidable cause of neurologic disease in Latin America. Whether seropositivity is synonymous with neurocysticercosis appears controversial. The common occurrence of the *T. solium* cyst may account for an important fraction of epilepsy in Latin American countries. Though serological testing may not firmly establish the role of *T. solium* in epilepsy, it is believed to be an important cause of epilepsy, particularly in developing countries.

Genetics

Rapid progress is being made in determining the genetic contributions to epileptic disorders. Several authors have recently reviewed this field (Crino 2007). A number of types of epilepsy have now been explained as genetic disorders. However, these are rare forms of epilepsy and the genetic contribution to the majority of cases remains unexplained. There is some degree of consensus, however, that idiopathic generalized epilepsies are likely to have a genetic aetiology (Steinlein 1999). First-degree relatives of people with epilepsy have a two- to fourfold increase in epilepsy risk (Annegers *et al.* 1982). However, the absence of clear genetic contributions to many forms of epilepsy, and the presence of differing phenotypes resulting from a given genotype emphasizes the importance of environmental factors in epilepsy. Most of the study of genetics in epilepsy has been directed towards primary generalized epilepsies. This reflects the belief that primary generalized epilepsy is often due to some 'brainwide' disorder that would be more likely due to a genetic disorder. Localized seizures more often reflect focal brain disease that is less likely to be due to a genetic mutation. However, it should be kept in mind that in some cases genes may have focal influences on the brain (Dobyns *et al.* 1999). A number of epilepsies have now been shown to be due to channelopathies, mutations in ion channels (Avanzini *et al.* 2007). It is expected that additional genes will soon be identified that cause epilepsy, or that influence environmental epileptic factors.

Costs and public health burden

The costs of epilepsy are often categorized as direct and indirect (Begley *et al.* 2000). The direct costs refer to those specifically involved with epilepsy treatment; the indirect costs include lost work days and unrealized earnings. Begley *et al.* (2000) estimates that 181 000 new cases of epilepsy in the United States in 1995 will result in a lifetime cost of US$11.1 billion. The 2.3 million prevalent cases, in 1995, resulted in an annual cost of US$12.5 billion. Indirect costs may account for 85 per cent of the total, and the largest share of direct costs is attributable to patients with intractable epilepsy (Begley *et al.* 2000). Annegers *et al.* cautions that cost figures may derive from different methodologies between United States and Europe, which may influence the degree of comparability (Annegers *et al.* 1999). With regard to the quality of life reported by persons with epilepsy, Leidy *et al.* (1999) report that seizure frequency is inversely associated with health-related quality of life. Seizure-free individuals report a quality of life similar to the general population; however more seizures lead to a poorer quality of life, regardless of additional comorbidity, and irrespective of gender. Effective seizure control appears to be important in reducing costs as well as increasing patient quality of life.

Dementia

Clinical overview

Dementia presents with a progressive loss of a person's usual and customary cognitive function from any of several domains. This often begins with memory problems in AD but could also begin with language deficits or disinhibition in frontotemporal lobar degeneration, or with deficits in executive function in vascular cognitive impairment, or with sleep disorders or hallucinations in Lewy body disease, additional symptoms may initially predominate where other dementias may be the underlying cause. Regardless of the beginning domain, initial cognitive impairment associated with dementia tends to progress and affect other cognitive domains with time. Behavioural changes may be prominent, including agitation, wandering, personality change or depression, as well as sleep disturbances and psychiatric symptoms. In late stages of dementia, patients frequently become completely dependent on others. Various definitions of dementia have been used in past research studies, but the Diagnostic and Statistical Manual, Edition IV (DSM-IV) is one of the most commonly used now (APA & AMA Task Force on DSM-IV 1994). The DSM-IV criteria for dementia require memory impairment and one or more additional cognitive disturbance, because of the memory predominance, it is often criticized as being too specific for AD, despite the other domains involved. These other domains involve aphasia (language disturbance), apraxia (impaired ability to carry out motor activities despite intact motor function), agnosia (failure to recognize or identify objects despite intact sensory function) and disturbances in executive functioning (i.e. planning, organizing, sequencing, abstracting). The cognitive deficits must be severe enough to cause significant impairment in social or occupational functioning and represent a significant decline from a previously attained level of functioning. The DSM criteria were originally constructed to provide for mutually exclusive diagnostic subgroups, but that schema is becoming more problematic as the research community now understands that more than one underlying dementia causes may coexist and the location of the specific pathologies in the brain may determine the clinical picture expressed. Furthermore, the clinical diagnosis of AD was originally conceptualized within the DSM criteria as a diagnosis of exclusion, however that view now, is becoming rapidly obsolete.

Dementia represents the severe decline from a usual or customary degree of cognitive function enjoyed in a person's adult life; it may have many causes including neurodegenerative, vascular, infectious, and traumatic, to name a few. Among the neurodegenerative dementias that predominate with aging are AD, Lewy body disease (dementia with Lewy bodies [DLB] or PD dementia), and frontotemporal lobar degeneration (FTLD) dementias. Cerebrovascular disease may co-exist with and contribute to any of these or may be a primary cause on its own as vascular dementia, still considered to be the second most frequent cause of dementia. Prion disease, and associated spongiform encephalopathies (e.g. Creutzfeldt–Jakob disease [CJD] and variant CJD) are potentially transmissible from ingestion of animal tissue or from contact or transplantation of human tissue. HIV infection and other infections causing encephalitis may affect wider age groups and specific populations or exposure groups. Though AD, vascular dementia, Lewy body disease, and FTLD are likely to be the most common and well known, there are many other disorders and insults which can result in dementia including drug-induced conditions, alcoholism, Huntington's disease, amyotrophic lateral sclerosis, subdural hematoma, brain tumours, hydrocephalus, B_{12} deficiency, multiple medical conditions, hypothyroidism, and neurosyphilis.

Current criteria for the clinical diagnosis of dementia and AD, specifically, are applied relatively consistently by research studies and have been active for some time (American Psychiatric Association and American Psychiatric Association Task Force on DSM-IV). Neuropathological criteria for the diagnosis of AD are currently accepted as those of the NIA-Reagan consensus working group (..1997a). However, possibly because of the increasing understanding that underlying causes or pathologies may co-exist and initial cognitive changes may be noted earlier in the course of disease, the primary AD criteria may soon be considered for revision (Morris 2006). Accurate identification of preclinical or asymptomatic disease is thought to provide the best opportunity to intervene with disease modifying therapies—if such effective therapies can be developed.

Mild cognitive impairment

Determination of when a particular disease is clinically evident and diagnosable is of great interest to epidemiologists as well as to those involved with clinical medicine. Certainly the principles of early detection and potential early treatment lead us to expect a better prognosis, in most conditions, if there are effective treatments. The usually gradual and insidious nature of symptom onset for AD and some other dementias, and the current practical absence of adequate asymptomatic disease pathology detection (by biologic test or neuroimaging) has forced investigators to attempt to characterize the earliest clinical features of cognitive impairment, in order to approach an earlier diagnostic threshold. For epidemiologists searching for risk factor associations this earlier threshold is somewhat of a double edged sword. If diagnosis cannot be made with certainty at the earlier point: (a) diagnostic misclassification may distort risk factor associations, (b) earlier detection may allow better determination of the critical exposure period, prior to pathological onset, when the putative risk factor could have had an initiating or promoting effect. Thus, mild cognitive impairment is often characterized as a segment of the overall, underlying disease development trajectory by some, or as a diagnostic entity representing the transitional phase from cognitively normal to demented by others.

Efforts to observe and characterize the spectrum of observable cognitive decline from mild to severe cases of dementia have been with us at least since more intense studies of the dementias developed in the late 1970s and 1980s. Those efforts began to focus on and more carefully describe the early clinical presentation of dementia in the late 1980s and 1990s, for example, Bowen *et al.* (1997). While mild impairment was well recognized, it carried many names and definitions: Age associated memory impairment, age associated cognitive decline, cognitive impairment no dementia, benign senescent forgetfulness, questionable dementia. The concept of Mild Cognitive Impairment (MCI) emerged from careful consideration of much of this prior information but also included additional intellectual structure and definition (Petersen *et al.* 1999). The original criteria for MCI included: (1) memory complaint, preferably qualified by an informant; (2) memory

Table 9.10.3 Causes of dementia

Idiopathic	Systemic disease
Alzheimer's disease	Cardiac
Frontotemporal lobar degeneration (tauopathies and non-tau ubiquitin positive)	Pulmonary
Lewy body disease	Renal
Amyotrophic lateral sclerosis	Renal failure
Focal CNS pathology	Dialysis dementia
Vascular dementia	Hepatic
Binswanger's disease	Hepatic failure
Multiple sclerosis	Hepatocerebral degeneration
Mass lesions	Wilson's disease
Tumours, multiple sites	Endocrine
Tumours, single site	Hyper/hypo thyroid
Gliomatosis cerebri	Hyper/hypo parathyroid
Abscess	Hyper/hypo adrenalism
Subdural malformation	SIADH
Hydrocephalus	Rheumatologic
Infections	Vasculitis (including SLE)
AIDS (HIV)	Giant cell arteritis
Chronic meningitis	Sarcoid
Encephalitis	Amyloid
Progressive multifocal leukoencephalopathy	Neoplastic
Subacute sclerosing panencephalitis	Metastasis
Syphilis	Carcinomatous meningitis
Lyme disease	Paraneoplastic (limbic encephalitis)
Prion disease (kuru, Creutzfeldt–Jacob, vCJD)	Associated movement disorder
Toxins	Huntington's disease
Drugs	Parkinsonian diseases
Alcohol	Parkinson's disease
Heavy metals	Progressive supranuclear palsy
Industrial toxins	Postencephalitic dementia
Domoic acid	Post-traumatic (dementia pugilistica)
Inherited disease	Diffuse Lewy body disease
Huntington's disease	Multiple-system atrophy
Gerstmann–Straussler syndrome	Myoclonus
Porphyria	Creutzfeldt–Jakob disease
Propionic aciduria	Alzheimer's
Adult onset lysosomal storage diseases	Metabolic derangement
Hexosaminidase	Other movement disorder
Arylsulfatase (MLD)	Hereditary ataxias
Kuf disease	Hereditary spastic paraplegia
Adrenoleukodystrophy	Kuru
Others	Wilson's disease
Myotonic muscular dystrophy	Seizures
Down's syndrome	Kuf disease
Hereditary ataxias	Deficiency
Hereditary spastic paraplegias	B_{12} deficiency
Cerebrotendinous Xanthomatosis	Thiamine
	Niacin (Pellagra)

impairment for age and education; (3) preserved general cognitive function; (4) intact activities of daily living; (5) not demented (Petersen *et al.* 1999). These criteria were later revised to include both memory and non-memory affected groups allowing for 'amnestic' with single and multiple cognitive domains affected and 'non-amnestic' with single or multiple cognitive domains affected (Petersen 2007). The Petersen schema allowed for MCI to represent a variety of aetiologies in addition to AD. On the non-amnestic side, it could easily include vascular cognitive impairment) as well as cognitive impairment due to frontotemporal lobar degeneration or Lewy body disease. However, the amnestic side of MCI is regarded by many to represent primarily early AD (Morris 2006). Persons diagnosed with MCI also are known to recover and not go on to develop dementia. For example, in the Cardiovascular Health Study approximately 18 per cent of those initially diagnosed with amnestic MCI recovered (Lopez *et al.* 2007).

Since the concept was solidified by Petersen *et al.* (1999), literally thousands of research papers have been generated on the topic and with the effort a good deal of controversy has ensued, as well. In part because some of the controversy was becoming counterproductive to understanding, Winblad *et al.* (2004) hosted an international working group to arrive at a consensus understanding of MCI for the international research community. The resulting comprehensive recommendations allowed for self and informant report of deficits, as well as for more objective testing to be considered. The consensus recommendation also encouraged that the potential underlying cause of the impairment might be specified, if clinical judgment would allow. Age and educational status are also important in the determination of whether current performance represents cognitive decline, but to most carefully evaluate whether decline has taken place there should also be consideration of the intra-individual change. Despite comparison of individual performance with group test norms, for example, one should also evaluate whether the individual's performance represents a change in his/her usual and customary functioning, in order to determine whether cognitive decline has taken place.

Dementia and Alzheimer's disease

Prevalence and incidence

Almost two decades ago, Evans reported prevalence estimates for dementia and AD based on a community study in East Boston (Evans *et al.* 1989). The results of this study seemed controversial because of their magnitude but they placed an heuristic upper bound on estimated prevalence of dementia in United States' communities. Prevalence rose from 3 per cent among those 65–74 years of age to 47 per cent in those over age 85. Over 80 per cent of the observed dementia was classified as AD. Evans later applied the observed rates to census data projecting that 10.3 million persons would have AD in the year 2050. Meta-analyses of prevalence studies worldwide (Fratiglioni *et al.* 1999); and individual prevalence studies seemed to show consistency within geographical regions except for some variation due to methodological differences. Generally, the prevalence proportion was reported to rise from about 0.3–1 per cent in 60–64-year-olds to 43–68 per cent in persons aged 95 or older, or often reported as a summary figure of 6 per cent to 10 per cent among persons aged 65 or older in North America (Hendrie 1998). Based on estimates like these, Brookmeyer *et al.* estimated that if disease onset could be delayed 2 years the future disease burden would be reduced by 2 million cases (Brookmeyer *et al.* 1998).

More recently, Ferri *et al.* (2005) conducted a systematic review of published studies to estimate dementia prevalence in 14 world regions, as designated by the World Health Organization. They assembled a panel of 12 experts to arrive at individual estimates for each region based on the accumulated published studies resulting from the literature search. A 'Delphi' technique was implemented and agreement between experts within region was estimated. The mean prevalence estimates for each of the 14 world regions were then used to project numbers of cases in the future, also taking into account population and mortality changes, but maintaining the agreed upon prevalence estimates, and arriving at an estimated incidence rate through the use of standard software. Given the derived incidence rates, Ferri *et al.* estimated approximately 4.6 million new cases of dementia would occur each year in the world and this would cause the number of prevalent dementia cases to double about every 20 years. However, the increase is not expected to be constant across regions. Developed regions similar to Europe and North America are expected to increase their number of prevalent cases about 100 per cent by 2040, while Latin America and Africa are expected to increase 235–393 per cent, and India, China, and the South Asia/Western Pacific regions' numbers are expected to increase 314–336 per cent. As a result, the China, South Asia, and Western Pacific regions are projected by 2040 to have three times more prevalent cases of dementia than Western Europe will have and Latin America will have as many persons living with dementia as North America will have (Ferri *et al.* 2005). These projection are for all dementias rather than being limited to a particular subtype such as AD. However, there is increasing evidence that treatable factors associated with cardiovascular disease, such as hypertension or cholesterol level or those related to diabetes may play a role not only in vascular dementia, but also in the aetiology or progression of AD (Kukull 2006). Though there remains some controversy as to the nature of these putative associations, such an association, if causal, could allow existing treatments to potentially reduce the incidence of dementia or delay its onset for some number of years as suggested by Brookmeyer *et al.* (1998) and therefore could reduce the global dementia health care burden substantially. The health care burden of dementia is represented primarily by the prevalence proportion, which is a function of disease incidence and subsequent duration of survival.

In contrast to prevalence, incidence provides a means to estimate the risk of disease and the identification of risk factors (not directly possible with prevalence data alone). Jorm and Jolley (1998) gathered data from 23 studies and produced a meta-analysis of dementia incidence. Incidence was estimated for Europe, the United States, and East Asia; dementia, AD, and vascular dementia rates were computed. Incidence rates for the United States and Europe were quite similar: 'moderate' dementia incidence rose from 3.6 per 1000 person-years (65–69 ages) to 37.7 per 1000 person-years (85–89 ages) in Europe and from 2.4 to 27.5 per 1000 person years for the same age groups in the United States. 'Mild' AD incidence was also computed ranging from 2.5 per 1000 person years (65–69 ages) to 46.1 per 1000 person-years, for Europe, compared with 6.1– 74.5 for the United States, and, 0.7– 39.7 for East Asia.

The unique character of the Rochester Epidemiology Project at Mayo Clinic has allowed for the estimation of AD and dementia incidence over an extended period. While this project did not constitute an 'active' cohort study per se, the nature of the health care system and its nearly exclusive use by the surrounding population allowed for the observation and estimation of incident cases of disease through the review of medical records. These data provide some of the few estimates of secular trends for dementia incidence in the United States. Rocca *et al.* (1998) re-analysed dementia and AD incidence data for 1975 through 1984, from the Rochester Epidemiology Project at Mayo Clinic. The results showed dementia incidence overall as 2.2 per 1000 person-years in 65–69-year-olds rising to 40.8 per 1000 person-years in those aged 90 or more. Similarly for AD, rates rose from 1.2 to 33.9 per 1000 person-years. Because of the remarkable consistency of these incidence rates with more recent active cohort studies in Europe and North America one might also have some degree of confidence in Rocca's observation that annual age-specific incidence rates have appeared to stay quite stable with time stable during the 1975–1984 time interval. After disaggregating the data for the oldest old Rocca also reported that rates appeared to continue to rise with age after age 84; they also noted that rates were similar for men and women. As data continue to accumulate with time, it will be interesting to note if the effects of, for example, anti-hypertensive and lipid-lowering agents may be seen to alter the incidence, or perhaps whether potential gains there might be offset by increases in population obesity or diabetes.

Still one of the better estimates of dementia incidence for Europe comes from the combined analysis of four large, ongoing European cohort studies of dementia and AD as reported by Launer *et al.* (1999). Cohorts enrolled in Denmark, France, the Netherlands, and the United Kingdom summed to more than 16 000 members age 65 or older at enrolment. After a mean follow-up of 2.2 years (comprising approximately 28 600 person-years), the overall incidence of dementia was 14.6 per 1000 person-years, about two-thirds of these cases were due to AD. Incidence of dementia was 2.5 per 1000 person-years at age 65–69 an rose to 85.6 per 1000 person-years in those age 90 and older. Similarly AD rose from 1.2 per 1000 person-years to 63.5 per 1000 person-years across the same age groups. Launer's report was one of the first to include combined data from large cohort studies in Europe. Over the last 5 years more cohort studies begun to report incidence figures which are consistent, generally, with the estimates above. Among the more recent well-designed cohort studies that have reported comparable incidence rates within various population groups are Kukull *et al.* 2002, Lopez *et al.* 2007, Newman *et al.* 2005, Tyas *et al.* 2006, Brayne 2006, and Ganguli *et al.* 2000. The long-standing Framingham Study, the population-based approaches of the Mayo Clinic, studies of specific religious groups and orders, and other population-based cohorts are also of tremendous importance, in addition to those mentioned earlier.

While the tendency has been to attempt to count primary cause or pathologically 'pure' cases of dementia subtypes those single aetiology cases may be less frequent than previously suspected. In studies conducted in communities, dementia aetiologies (e.g. AD, vascular, Lewy body, tauopathy) appear to comingle frequently in community dwelling cases (Schneider *et al.* 2007). This comingling is consistent with the view that features of AD, Lewy body disease and frontotemporal lobar degeneration may exist as a multiple amyloidoses resulting from aggregation of amyloid-beta (neuritic plaques), tau (neurofibrillary tangles), alpha-synuclein (Lewy bodies) and other proteins (Morimoto 2006; Trojanowski & Mattson 2003; Trojanowski & Lee 2002; Lippa *et al.* 2007).

Because identification of late stage dementia and AD holds little hope for curative or restorative treatment applications or for identification of consistent risk factors, interest has begun to focus on early identification of disease through mild cognitive impairment or simply early identification of the aetiologic cause of decline prior to the criteria-based diagnosis of dementia, as discussed in detail above. Early forms of pre-AD or dementia are difficult to distinguish from relatively benign, cognitive decline associated with aging. Distinguishing between normal persons, those with mild cognitive impairment and those asymptomatic persons with incipient, occult dementia-related pathology, now possible to some degree with newly developed neuroimaging techniques, may provide important clues about pathological onset of disease as well as inform the study of risk factors and critical periods of exposure prior to disease onset (Rowe *et al.* 2007).

Risk (and protective) factors for AD

Until the mid-1990s, most analytic observational epidemiologic studies of AD were based on a case–control design. In this design, cases of disease were identified and their exposure histories were compared to those of persons without the disease. The design itself is well accepted as a method of study. However, in the study of AD (and other dementias), problems with case ascertainment, case selection, and misclassification of disease and exposure may have caused at least some results to be biased or spurious. Now, as cohort studies of AD and dementia are beginning to emerge, findings which were viewed as consistent in case–control studies are being questioned or refuted. One example of incompatible conclusions concerns the observation of a potential protective effect for AD associated with cigarette smoking. A meta-analysis of smoking–AD studies showed a consistent decreased risk associated with smoking (Lee 1994). The majority of these studies were of the case–control design. When case–control studies rely on cross-sectional samples to obtain cases, they are most likely to encounter those cases with the longest survival after diagnosis (Rothman & Greenland 1998). Also, when decreased post diagnosis survival among cases is associated with the exposure of interest (e.g. smoking) a potential spurious excess of exposure among controls may be observed. Cohort studies, where this selection bias is eliminated (essentially) now report either 'no association' or a potential *increased* risk of AD associated with smoking. A recent and comprehensive meta-analysis of prospective studies investigating smoking as a risk factor for dementia and AD involving more than 26 000 persons followed for 2–30 years showed a significantly increased risk of AD in smokers as compared to non-smokers, relative risk = 1.79 (95% CI 1.43–2.23) (Anstey *et al.* 2007).

Head trauma has also been shown to be a relatively consistent risk factor for AD, primarily based on case–control studies. Here, selective recall or recall bias may be more important than the effect of survival, even though risk of death and/or continued cognitive impairment immediately resulting from the injury is substantial (..1998). Several longitudinal studies now show negligible risk of AD associated with head injury (Nee & Lippa 1999) though others still find some potentially increased risk sometimes modified by other factors (e.g. Schofield *et al.* 1997). Many studies of head trauma focus on injuries severe enough to cause loss of consciousness. There is little rigorous analytic investigation of mild traumatic brain injury as a potential risk factor. TBI due to blast injuries, suffered in war, provide an important cohort in which to study the future incidence of dementia and AD.

Higher educational level has been proposed as influencing decreased risk of AD, but the relationship between education and AD may be quite complex (e.g. Koepsell *et al.* 2007). Educational level influences subject's likelihood of participation in epidemiologic studies, and may do so differentially between cases and controls. Educational level influences the diagnostic process, at least in the early stages of disease, because of the individual's ability to respond correctly in testing situations. Education may influence health care usage and may result in greater income or higher occupational level. The idea that higher education confers greater 'cognitive reserve' to be accessed when disease strikes is tantalizing, though biologically unsubstantiated. Koepsell *et al.* in a clinico-pathologic study found that there was 'no evidence of larger education-related differences in cognitive function when AD neuropathology was more advanced', and concluded further that 'higher Mini-Mental State Examination scores among more educated persons with mild or no AD may reflect better test-taking skills or cognitive reserve, but these advantages may ultimately be overwhelmed by

AD neuropathology' (Koepsell *et al.* 2007). Quality of early life environment, as measured by number of siblings, area of residence was associated with developing AD in late life, but educational level was not significantly associated with risk of AD (Moceri *et al.* 2000).

Anti-inflammatory medications have been studied for their potential protective effect on AD. Even though the quality of the studies has varied with respect to determination of exposure, the results appear to have been quite consistent in showing significant associations, which if causal could be interpreted as protective (e.g. Hayden *et al.* 2007). Because of this evidence and the potential biological plausibility related to the role of inflammation in the aetiology of AD, a randomized placebo controlled prevention trial was launched, known as the AD anti-inflammatory prevention trial (ADAPT), enrolment began in 2001. The trial planned to enrolled 2625 subjects, aged 70 years or older, who had a family history of dementia and randomized them to placebo, celecoxib, or naproxsyn sodium treatment arms. The plan was to follow the enrollees for approximately 7 years; however, the trial was stopped in December 2004 because of concerns that adverse cardiovascular events which were related to use of similar anti-inflammatory drugs might also apply to the trial treatments. A preliminary analysis based on the small amount of accumulated data available following trial closure showed no significant effect of either celecoxib or naproxsyn as compared to placebo for the prevention of AD.

Oestrogen replacement therapy as a protective factor has shown a remarkably similar checkered research results history as anti-inflammatory medications, with the bulk of epidemiologic evidence favouring protection and a fair amount of biological plausibility also marshalled in its support (e.g. Henderson *et al.* 2000). Despite this large accumulation of epidemiologic and laboratory evidence supporting the potential protective effect of oestrogen against the onset of AD, the Women's Health Initiative Memory Study (a randomized controlled trial of oestrogen and oestrogen plus progestin v. placebo) showed a statistically significant increased risk of dementia among those given the active treatments (Shumaker *et al.* 2004). In the case of oestrogen as a potential treatment for AD, results also have shown no indication that oestrogen replacement therapy is an effective treatment for AD (Henderson *et al.* 2000).

Few environmental risk or protective factors for AD have been consistently described. There is much current interest in the potential for factors related to cardiovascular disease and metabolic syndrome (including diabetes) having an influence on AD and other dementias even though the exact mechanisms of interaction may not yet have been shown beyond reasonable doubt, nor have they in most cases yet reached the bar for clear and convincing evidence (Whitmer *et al.* 2007). The rationale for this approach appears to be that it is sound medical practice to treat hypertension, high cholesterol, diabetes and obesity, and if more complete and effective treatment can be accomplished it may also, secondarily, serve to reduce the occurrence of dementia.

Elevated homocysteine levels, also associated with cardiovascular disease, have been reported to increase risk of AD (Haan *et al.* 2007). Whether hyperhomocysteinemia may be related to mutations in the methylenetetrahydrofolate reductase gene or to dietary intake or to other factors is unclear. However, homocysteine levels can reportedly be modified with vitamin B_{12} and folate intake, so there may be a potentially safe, intervention to evaluate in that regard, though it seems unlikely a formal prevention trial would be mounted unless the strength and specificity of the effect might be better described along with the potential attributable fraction.

AD is likely to be heterogeneous both diagnostically and aetiologically. What results in the AD phenotype may be the sum or product of aging, environmental factors, genetic constitution, and sociodemographic experiences. Aside from the observable effect of aging dramatically increasing the risk of dementia and AD, success in finding environmental risk factors has been limited and potentially related to design and selection factors. At this point disease modifying therapies and drug targets are being developed primarily from basic science research.

Genetics and AD

Great progress was made in the genetics of AD during the late 1980s and 1990s. Since then, despite lots of activity, it has been in the doldrums regarding consistent and important results. Most of the strict genetic 'causes' of disease have been limited to so-called 'familial' AD. Familial AD behaves similar to an autosomal dominant genetic pattern and tends to affect predominantly, persons less than age 60. Familial AD, so defined appears to account for less than 5 per cent of all AD, but important clues may be learned from study of Familial disease which will apply to the more common forms of primarily late onset AD (often called sporadic—but it too may have undiscovered genetic causes). Several reviews of AD genetics describing this period of growth in greater detail include St George-Hyslop (2000).

The largest proportion of familial AD is attributed to mutations in the Presenilin 1 gene (chromosome 14) and the next largest known contribution is due to mutations in a homologous gene on chromosome 1, Presenilin 2. Very small proportion of cases is due to specific mutations in the amyloid precursor protein gene (chromosome 21). It is abnormal cleavage of the amyloid precursor protein, which results in the formation of amyloid beta (1–42) protein. Amyloid beta protein aggregates in the brain forming the characteristic plaques of AD. Important work has been published concerning identification of enzymes (for example, BACE and PS1, itself), which cleave the precursor protein abnormally forming the amyloid beta 1–42 protein (Zhao *et al.* 2007; Multhaup 2006). This work may ultimately help to identify sites for drug intervention, not only for Familial but also for non-familial AD (Octave *et al.* 2000). Perhaps one quarter to one half of familial AD is still of unknown genetic cause (Shastry & Giblin 1999).

The strongest and most consistent genetic risk factor for non-familial AD today is apolipoprotein E (APOE) genotype. The association was first described from Dr Allen Roses' laboratory (Roses 1994). APOE naturally occurs as three different alleles (epsilon 2, epsilon 3 and epsilon 4) which pair to form one of six genotypes for each individual. Genotypes containing the epsilon 4 allele are associated with increased risk of AD; homozygous epsilon 4 greatly increases risk (e.g. >eightfold). Since the initial description of increased risk associated with the epsilon 4 allele, many investigators have observed the association. Discussion of APOE genotype is now included in most risk factor studies of AD, either as a focus or as a potential confounder/effect modifier of an association. Despite the huge volume of studies including APOE genotype relatively little is known concerning how the e2, e3, and e4 alleles actually work to influence the risk of AD.

Since the discovery of the association between APOE and AD a huge number of other candidate genes, single nucleotide polymorphisms and other mutations have been examined by a variety of methods. An up-to-date meta-analysis of the studies related to most of these published associations is available through AlzGene (Bertram *et al.* 2007) (http://www.alzgene.org). It is safe to say that none of the other candidates have shown the strength or consistency of APOE.

Vascular dementia

Vascular dementia is difficult to describe clinically and neuropathologically. This may be due in part to the rather common coexistence of vascular features with AD in the elderly. The more sophisticated the search for stroke and cerebrovascular disease becomes, for example, by identifying white matter hyperintensities (WMH) through magnetic resonance imaging (MRI), the more likely such evidence will be found (Au *et al.* 2006). The clinical identification of stroke is surpassed and augmented by CT, which, in turn, has been surpassed by MRI; other specialized neuroimaging techniques may continue this progression. Hopefully, as the resolution provided by the progression from clinical to detailed imaging evidence increases, the false positive identification of stroke and cerebrovascular disease should decrease. Several different criteria have been developed to diagnose vascular dementia (American Psychiatric Association and American Psychiatric Association Task Force on DSM-IV 1994; Roman *et al.* 1993). Much of the pioneering work in the definition and recognition of vascular dementia can be attributed to Hachinski and colleagues, and the Hachinski Ischemic Score continues to be used in many research settings to indicate the extent of cerebrovascular involvement in cognitive decline (Rockwood *et al.* 2000).

Despite clinical diagnostic criteria for vascular dementia (Roman *et al.* 1993), this syndrome remains an area of controversy and uncertainty. Pathologically, vascular dementia also represents somewhat of an enigma, reportedly because of the lack of clear definitional thresholds for white matter damage, infarcts, and lesion location especially in strategic areas of the brain—vascular dementia, in effect, lacks a pathological gold standard against which to compare the clinical diagnosis or clinical criteria and measure their effectiveness (Murray *et al.* 2007). In part because of this problem application of the clinical diagnostic criteria has been shown to be difficult and potentially unreliable in practice, even when applied by well-experienced research investigators (Chui *et al.* 2000). Some of the reliability and validity problems experienced by investigators in classifying a case as 'vascular' or AD may stem from the mutual exclusion of the two conditions, imposed by the various criteria, when the conditions frequently co-exist.

Lewy body disease and frontotemporal lobar degeneration

Two additional types of dementia, Lewy body disease (McKeith 2006) and frontotemporal dementia (Cairns *et al.* 2007a) have been separated from AD based on their clinical presentations and pathology. Lewy body disease or DLB may be more common than originally thought, potentially diagnosable in up to 30 per cent of dementia cases (Tsuang *et al.* 2006). Lewy body disease often presents with fluctuating cognitive performance, visual hallucinations, REM sleep behaviour disorder and/or Parkinsonism. Memory impairment may not be as prominent in the early stages of the disease as deficits in attention, frontal sub-cortical skills and visuospatial ability.

Frontotemporal lobar degeneration includes specific disease subtypes and may be the most frequently occurring dementia in persons under age 65 (Mackenzie & Rademakers 2007). Frontotemporal dementia (FTD) represents a behavioural subtype where changes may include loss of personal awareness, loss of social graces, disinhibition, overactivity, restlessness, impulsivity, distractibility, hyperorality, withdrawal from social contact, apathy or inertia, and stereotyped or perseverative behaviours. The memory loss is variable and often appears to be due to lack of concern or effort. Frontal lobe impairments are notable including abstraction, planning, and self-regulation of behaviour. FTLD may also be associated with Parkinsonism or motor neuron disease. Pathologically, approximately 40 per cent of FTLDs are related to mutations in the microtubule associated protein tau gene (MAPT) on chromosome 17 and are therefore 'tauopathies', these include Pick's disease, corticobasal degeneration and progressive supranuclear palsy (Rademakers & Hutton 2007; Tolnay & Frank 2007). About 50 per cent of FTLDs are not tauopathies but are reactive to ubiquitin (FTLD-U) rather than mutations in MAPT (Mackenzie & Rademakers 2007). Recently, it was discovered that mutations in the progranulin gene, also on chromosome 17, were an important cause of FTLD-U disorders (Cruts *et al.* 2006; Gass *et al.* 2006) including primary progressive aphasia (Mesulam *et al.* 2007). The pathological protein involved in these disorders as well as in motor neuron disease is TDP-43 (Kwong *et al.* 2007; Cairns *et al.* 2007b). Especially in the FTLDs, location of the pathology appears to determine the clinical dementia syndrome expressed. This question of pathology and location is certainly an important focus for future elucidation. The progranulin and TDP-43 discoveries were arguably the most exciting and important findings for dementia and FTLD in recent times.

Peripheral neuropathy

Clinical overview

Though the term 'peripheral neuropathy' may refer to any disease of the peripheral nerves, it generally is used to describe a group of systemic diseases that affect the peripheral nerves rather than focal diseases affecting an isolated nerve. Most of these diseases affect longer nerves first with symptoms developing first in the feet and progressing up the legs. There are a few peripheral neuropathies that affect the shorter proximal nerves first. By the time the symptoms have reached the knees, the hands become symptomatic followed by the anterior trunk and crown of the head. The symptoms that develop depend on the type of nerve fibre involved. Involvement of motor fibres leads to weakness, muscle wasting, and hyporeflexia. If longstanding, motor neuropathies may lead to high arches (pes cavus) or hammer toes. Sensory nerve involvement leads to loss of sensation, distorted sensation (dysesthesias), or spontaneous unpleasant sensations (paresthesias). Autonomic neuropathies most commonly lead to postural hypotension but may also include sexual dysfunction, bowel dysfunction, bladder dysfunction, disorders of gastroparesis. The size of the affected nerve fibre can often be suggested by the history with disease of large fibre causing reflex loss, vibration loss, and joint position loss. Small fibre disease often leads to autonomic dysfunction, dysesthesias, loss of pain sensation, and loss of temperature sensation.

Electrodiagnostic testing is often performed to diagnose and further classify peripheral neuropathies. Nerve conduction velocities can be used to classify peripheral neuropathies into those that are demyelinating and those that are axonal. Demyelinating neuropathies lead to disproportionate slowing of nerve conduction speeds and increases in latency of responses. Axonal diseases cause disproportional loss of amplitude with relative preservation of conduction speed. Nerve conduction studies measure only the fast-conducting large diameter fibres. Electromyography (EMG) measures the electrical activity of muscle fibres. It is useful in diagnosing a number of muscle and myoneural junction diseases. The use of EMG in the diagnosis of peripheral neuropathy is primarily in recognizing the loss of innervation of muscle fibres by large myelinated neurons. Loss of innervation leads to increased insertional activity, positive waves, fibrillation potentials, polyphasic motor unit potentials, and decreased recruitment patterns. Occasionally, electrodiagnostic studies are supplemented with nerve or muscle biopsy.

Generally, polyneuropathies are the result of lesions involving many peripheral nerves and result in autonomic neuropathies, sensory loss or weakness. Mononeuropathies, as the name implies, involve a single nerve injury or entrapment. Carpal tunnel syndrome and Bell's palsy are common examples of mononeuropathies. Peripheral nerve disorders are, also, often classified as either hereditary or acquired. Charcot–Marie–Tooth syndrome is perhaps the most well-known hereditary form. Acquired nerve disorders are commonly associated with trauma or compression, diabetes, alcoholism and other nutritional and metabolic problems. They may also be related to infectious causes such as, Guillian–Barré syndrome, leprosy, Lyme disease or, HIV-infection; or, they may be caused by toxic exposures to metals (e.g. lead, mercury) or industrial chemicals or even by therapeutic drugs (e.g. anti-neoplastic agents) (Rowland & Merritt 1995).

Little is known about the epidemiology of peripheral neuropathies, though they appear to be common. Few studies have been conducted on the prevalence of these diseases, but what scant data exists finds prevalence to range from 2.4 to 8 per cent (Martyn & Hughes 1997). Prevalence increases considerably with age. Mold reported that 54 per cent of those aged 85 and older seen in practices of family practitioners had evidence of peripheral neuropathy on physician examination (Mold *et al.* 2004).

Carpal tunnel syndrome

First characterized in 1880 by James J. Putnam, carpal tunnel syndrome is probably the most common neuropathy. Carpal tunnel release surgery is also one of the most common hand surgeries performed in the United States (Rayan 1999). Franklin *et al.* reported that 'occupational' carpal tunnel syndrome (CTS) resulting from repetitive, higher impact actions may differ from CTS occurring in a non-occupational setting (Franklin *et al.* 1991). Specifically, occupational CTS appeared to occur nearly equally among men and women and at a substantially lower mean age than had been reported for non-occupational CTS (37 vs. 51 years). Based on workman's compensation records in 1984–88, an incidence of 1.74 per 1000 full-time equivalent jobs was observed (Franklin *et al.* 1991). Abbas *et al.* (1998) conducted a meta-analysis of work-related CTS. They showed that force and repetitive motion were important predictors of CTS after adjusting for study population and country of origin.

A general population estimate of CTS incidence was reported by Nordstrom *et al.* (1998). Medical records of all cases occurring in 2 years, in a defined population were reviewed and classified as definite or probable CTS. In contrast to the occupational CTS incidence observed by Franklin, as well as other previous incidence estimates Nordstrom *et al.* reported a CTS incidence of 3.46 per 1000 person-years. The apparent increase in incidence may reflect a true change in incidence or may be partially due to popular knowledge of the condition and diagnostic suspicion. Prevalence of symptoms in relation to true disease prevalence is also an important consideration (Atroshi *et al.* 1999). Reported CTS symptoms of tingling, pain, and numbness have a prevalence of about 14 per cent, whereas CTS was clinically and electrophysiologically confirmed in less than 3 per cent. Atroshi concludes that symptoms of CTS are common but only about 1 in 5 of the persons complaining of symptom is likely to actually have confirmed CTS (Atroshi *et al.* 1999).

Non-occupational factors related to the occurrence and treatment of CTS were studied by Solomon *et al.* (1999) and Stallings *et al.* (1997). Solomon found that CTS patients with inflammatory arthritis were about 3 times more likely to undergo carpal tunnel release surgery; patients with diabetes and hypothyroidism were also significantly more likely to receive surgery. Using data from a United Kingdom twin study, Hakim *et al.* reported that heredity was the single strongest predictor of CTS (Hakim *et al.* 2002). The overall prevalence was 14.2 per cent among the 4488 women. Using monozygotic and dizygotic twins, the heritability was estimated to be 0.46 (95% CI 0.34–0.58) indicating that half of the risk of CTS is due to genetic factors. Age is also related to the development of CTS. Bland found that there was a bimodal age distribution with peaks at 50–54 and 75–84 years of age (Bland & Rudolfer 2003). Obesity has been reported as a risk factor for the occurrence of CTS (Bland 2005) This association was addressed in a case–control study by Stallings *et al.* (1997). Results indicated that obesity, as determined by body mass index, was significantly more common among cases than among control subjects.

Diabetes mellitus

Diabetes is a common, yet complex cause of both mono- and polyneuropathies. Diabetes may affect up to 7 per cent of the US population, and peripheral neuropathy may affect 26–47 per cent of these (Barrett *et al.* 2007). More effective glucose control could reduce the risk to some extent (Boulton 1998a). Patients with diabetes have a higher hospital admission rate, length of stay and mortality than non-diabetics (Currie *et al.* 1998) indicating the potential human and economic cost of the disease. The cost of diabetic peripheral neuropathy, particularly in those with pain, can be substantial (Barrett *et al.* 2007).

Dyck *et al.* (1999) developed a composite score for assessing the degree of diabetic polyneuropathy, then conducted a longitudinal study of 264 diabetics to determine how hyperglycaemia related to diabetic polyneuropathy. Microvessel disease, chronic hyperglycaemia and type of diabetes were the most important predictors of polyneuropathy. Orchard *et al.* (1996) has also shown that among patients with insulin dependent diabetic, autonomic neuropathy is strongly influenced by chronic hyperglycaemia and is associated with increased mortality. A study of diabetic peripheral neuropathy in 16 European countries identified several additional risk factors: Elevated diastolic blood pressure, ketoacidosis, elevated fasting triglyceride level, and microabuminuria (Tesfaye *et al.* 1996). It is now recognized that a substantial number of patients with peripheral neuropathy of unknown cause have prediabetes with impaired fasting glucose or glucose tolerance tests (Smith & Singleton 2006). Improved diabetes control may minimize the impact of diabetic peripheral neuropathy.

Nutritional neuropathies

A number of nutritional deficiencies can lead to peripheral neuropathies. The most common is vitamin B_{12} deficiency. An epidemic of peripheral neuropathy was reported in Cuba during 1992–1993 (Roman 1994). That epidemic was said to affect over 50 000 Cubans and achieved a cumulative incidence rate of 461 per 100 000. An optic form and a peripheral form of the disease were observed. Extensive search for toxic exposures and a variety of other risk factors eventually lead to nutritional deficiency as the principal explanation for the outbreak (Roman 1994). Intervention and treatment with multivitamins, in particular B-vitamins, acted to stop the outbreak.

Peripheral neuropathy due to infection

Infection with HIV is emerging as an increasing source of a number of neurological conditions including peripheral neuropathies. There are many different types of peripheral neuropathy associated with HIV infections including diffuse peripheral neuropathy, Guillain–Barré syndrome, mononeuropathies, neuropathies due to secondary infections and neuropathies due to medications (Brew 2003). The prevalence of peripheral neuropathy reached 44 per cent in one African HIV study (Parry *et al.* 1997). Distal symmetrical polyneuropathy affects about 30 per cent of people with HIV who have CD4 counts less than 200 per μl (Tagliati *et al.* 1999). The cause of this peripheral neuropathy is uncertain, but one potential cause may be the AIDS therapy itself. Specifically, nucleosides may act, in about 15–40 per cent of patients to promote neuropathy (Brew 2003). The severity of the neuropathy may then cause patients to discontinue the needed therapy.

Guillain–Barré syndrome is due to an autoimmune attack on the peripheral nerve myelin. Previously considered an idiopathic disease, it is now recognized that a significant proportion of cases are associated with prior infections. The best documented of these infections is *Campylobacter jejuni* (Yuki 2007). Other infectious organisms have also been implicated. There appears to be molecular mimicry between gangliocides found in the organism and gangliocides found in myelin (Yuki 2007).

Though the prevalence of leprosy is declining, it remains one of the most important causes of peripheral neuropathy in the developing world (Ooi & Srinivasan 2004). Fortunately, early treatment can prevent many of the disabling and disfiguring effects of the disease. However, as the disease becomes less common, healthcare providers become increasingly unfamiliar with its early manifestations.

Parkinsonism

The Parkinson's research community is experiencing considerable controversy related to the conceptual description of idiopathic PD. Whether, as in the past the definition should be confined to the clinical motor phenotype and the pathological description of loss of dopaminergic neurons in the substantia nigra along with the occurrence there of alpha-synuclein deposits in the form of Lewy bodies or neurites, or, whether because of the widespread occurrence of these misfolded proteins throughout the body, PD should be viewed and studied more systemically (Langston 2006). The argument for expanding the view of PD continues that limiting the clinical and pathologic view of the disease itself limits the potential for research progress (Langston 2006).

Clinical overview

There are four cardinal features of Parkinsonism: Tremor, rigidity, bradykinesia, and postural gait changes. Though there are no established criteria, the diagnosis of Parkinsonism usually requires two or more of these symptoms In severe cases, patients may be unable to move (freezing) when they encounter minor obstacles such as doorways or cracks. While movement disorder specialists make the diagnosis of Parkinsonism with some degree of confidence, PD usually requires histopathologic confirmation. In an attempt to increase the accuracy and validity of clinical diagnosis, improvements in clinical diagnostic criteria have been proposed (Jankovic *et al.* 2000).

Parkinsonism includes several major subclasses: Idiopathic Parkinsonism (PD), symptomatic Parkinsonism (e.g. drug-induced, toxin-induced, and other specific causes), 'Parkinson's-plus' syndromes (e.g. multiple system atrophy; MSA), progressive supranuclear palsy), and hereditary degenerative diseases (e.g. Hallervorden–Spatz disease, Huntington disease). PD or idiopathic Parkinsonism comprises approximately 80 per cent of Parkinsonism.

Multiple System Atrophy is sometimes misdiagnosed as PD; it is a relatively rare and very debilitating condition usually involving progressive autonomic failure plus poor responsiveness to levodopa or cerebellar ataxia. The is some evidence that MSA is a synucleinopathy (Armstrong *et al.* 2006). There role of environmental toxins such as pesticides, in the pathogenesis of MSA has also been discussed but little evidence for such an association has been established to date.

Incidence and prevalence of PD

Parkinson's disease prevalence has been reported with dramatic inconsistency. Case ascertainment, age structure of the population and study design may account for some part of the variability. Certainly door-to-door screening may find more disease that relying on medical records or death certificates. Decisions regarding the inclusion of institutionalized subjects in a screening effort may also impact obtained prevalence.

Consider that PD prevalence typically has been reported in the range of about 50 per 100 000 to 200 per 100 000 population, with a maximum of about 350 per 100 000. Morgante conducted a study in Sicily and found 63 PD cases among 24 496 persons in the population base which results in a prevalence proportion of 257.2 per 100 000 (or 0.257%) (Morgante *et al.* 1992). The Rotterdam Study (de Rijk *et al.* 1995) reported identifying a total of 97 PD cases from among 6969 enrolled subjects *age 55 or older* for a crude prevalence of 1.39 per cent or 1392 per 100 000. Recently, combined results of five European studies were published (de Rijk *et al.* 1997). The combined studies included 14 636 persons *age 65 or older*; after age adjusting to the European 1991 standard population the prevalence of PD was reported as 1.6 per 100 population (presumably age 65 or older), this translates to about 1600 per 100 000. In addition, the age-specific prevalence of PD was reported to increase from 0.6 per cent in 65–69-year-olds to 3.5 per cent in 85–89-year-olds (or 600 per 100 000 to 3500 per 100 000) (de Rijk *et al.* 1997). The example above is instructive. Not only must the reader attend to differences in case ascertainment when evaluating reported prevalence estimates, but also attention should be directed to the base from which the prevalence proportion is calculated.

Incidence rates for PD and Parkinsonism carry many of the same caveats as raised (above) for prevalence. In addition, confusion is added by choosing to report incidence in terms of person-years, or per population per year, or perhaps as projected cumulative lifetime incidence. With some effort, or with some assumptions, conversions can be made, but such may not be obvious to the reader. Bower *et al.* (1999) studied the incidence of Parkinsonism and PD in Rochester, Minnesota, during 1976–1990. The overall figures for PD showed an incidence rate of 10.8 per 100 000 person-years (i.e. based on the entire age distribution population). The age-specific incidence for the 50–59 age group was 17.4 per 100 000 person-years, rising to 52.5 for 60–69 ages and peaking at 93.1 for 70–79 age group and 79.1 for 80–99-year-olds. Parkinsonism showed an overall incidence rate of 25.6 per 100 000 person years and rose from 26.5 at ages 50–59 to 304.8 per 100 000 person-years in those aged 80–99 (Bower *et al.* 1999).

Age-specific incidence rates provide critical information not available from summary rates. The strong influence of age on the disease process is evident from the Rochester, Minnesota, data: The incidence among those aged 0–29 is practically nil; while the incidence triples from 50–59 to 60–69, then nearly doubles again in the 70–79 age group (Bower *et al.* 1999). How aging contributes to the degenerative process of PD or how aging increases susceptibility to genetic and environmental risk factors is important to describe the epidemiology of Parkinsonism and PD.

Risk factors

Clear and consistent evidence of specific, strong, environmental risk factors has been evasive. However, the possibility of environmental causes was increased by the observation that 1-methyl-4-phenyl-1,2,3,6-tetrahydropyridine (MPTP), a 'designer' street drug, was observed to cause acute PD shortly after ingestion (Langston *et al.* 1983). Because the structure of MPTP and its metabolism products are somewhat similar to some pesticides and herbicides there was and is great interest in exploring the potential for those types of exposures as risk factors or causes of PD. Observations focusing on family history and familial cases, along with the rapid increase in information available on the human genome, has led to new interest in describing the genetics of PD.

Rural living, well-water consumption, and pesticide/herbicide exposure are reported relatively frequently as potential risk factors for PD, although, neither critical time periods nor duration for these exposures necessary to influence onset, nor specific mechanisms have been identified. For example, a case–control study conducted by Gorell *et al.* (1998) found about a fourfold increase in risk of PD for exposure to herbicides and insecticides and nearly a three time the risk of PD for those who had a farming occupation (but no increase for rural or farm residence, nor well-water use). Firestone *et al.* reported consistently elevated, though not statistically significant risks due to pesticide exposure raising some doubts as to the role of pesticides in PD (Firestone *et al.* 2005). Petrovitch *et al.* also have shown, in the Honolulu Asia Aging Study that the risk of PD increased significantly for long-term plantation workers as compared to those who worked on plantations 10 years or less, to approach a dose–response relationship (Petrovitch *et al.* 2002). Marder *et al.* (1998) found an association between farming, rural living and well-water in multi-ethnic case–control study, but that association held only for African Americans and not for Hispanics. Kuopio *et al.* (1999) conducted a population-based case–control study in Finland and found no association between farming, drinking water, pesticide/herbicide use, and PD.

An association between exposure to metals and PD has been described by Gorell *et al.* (1999a,b). An association was noted with manganese exposure and with copper, also with combinations of lead and iron or copper. While this association is interesting, it raises the question of whether the manganese association represented manganism rather than PD.

Smoking has been rather consistently associated with decreased risk of PD in reported reviews and in individual studies (Ritz *et al.* 2007). Reasons for the plausibility of such an association revolve around the potential action of nicotine on neurons. Although this is one of the more consistent findings, it is not completely without alternative explanations. Most epidemiologic studies of PD use 'prevalent' or existing cases in their studies. The low incidence of PD effectively precludes concentrating on only newly diagnosed cases in all but the largest of studies (or in very large cohort studies). When attempting to identify a cross-sectional sample of cases for enrolment into a case–control study, it can be shown that those patients who have had the disease the longest are the most likely to be included. The most severe, short duration or rapidly declining cases tend to be missed. If PD cases who had a history of smoking were much more likely to die than non-smoking PD cases; and at the same time if the smoking–non-smoking mortality differential was somewhat less among the controls, then, the cross-sectional sampling of cases and controls could give the spurious impression of an excess of smoking among controls. The excess numbers of smokers among controls might then be misinterpreted as a causal, protective effect. At this point, however, the PD research community appears to be relatively confident in the potential protective effect of smoking (Ritz *et al.* 2007). Because DLB represents similar molecular pathology (i.e. alpha-synuclein, Lewy bodies) which develops primarily in a different brain location, it would be interesting to test whether the apparent protective effect of smoking seen in PD could also be observed in DLB and similar Lewy body diseases.

Dietary-related factors have been shown in some studies to affect risk of PD, with more fish and vegetables appearing to protect (Gao *et al.* 2007). Coffee and caffeine intake appears to lower risk of PD even after adjusting for smoking (Ross *et al.* 2000). Dietary folate and vitamin B_{12} intake were reported as potentially protective for PD in the Rotterdam study (de Lau *et al.* 2006). The relation to dietary folate and B_{12} is somewhat consistent to similar reports concerning high homocystiene as a risk factor for AD. Also, consistent with work in AD, body mass index has been reported by researchers in Finland to increase the risk of PD (Hu *et al.* 2006). Coincidently, the occurrence of gout and hyperuricemia has been reported to protect against PD through an hypothesized link to the antioxidant properties of uric acid (de Lau *et al.* 2005; Alonso *et al.* 2007). It is not clear whether the pathway might be different for persons who are overproducers of uric acid due to one type of genetic defect, as compared to those who simply indulge in large quantities of high urate generating foods, or those whose serum uric acid levels are raised because of the use of diuretics.

Interest in pesticide exposure as a potential cause, led to a biotransformation gene approach for evaluating the occurrence of susceptible persons. Specifically, some persons may be more, or less, able to metabolize environmental toxins because of polymorphic genes involved in metabolism. One of the family of cytochrome P-450 biotransformation genes, CYP2D6 is involved in metabolism of debrisoquine (structurally similar to pesticides); some polymorphic forms are 'poor' metabolizers and others are normal or rapid metabolizers of debrisoquine. Initial studies appeared to show that poor metabolizers were at increased risk of PD but later studies and meta analyses fail to support this conclusion (Scordo *et al.* 2006; Maraganore *et al.* 2000).

A similar approach has been taken to identify susceptibles focusing on polymorphic forms of glutathione transferases (GST) which are involved in the metabolism of pesticides and other xenobiotics

Table 9.10.4 Genes associated with PD aetiology

Gene	a.k.a.	Chromosome	Occurrence
SNCA (α-Synuclein)	PARK1 or PARK4	4q21	Lewy body component Sporadic PD
PARK2 (Parkin)	PARK2	6q25–q27	Recessive; juvenile/ early onset
UCHL1	PARK5	4p14	Sporadic PD
PINK1	PARK6	1p35–p36	Recessive; rare, slowly progressive
DJ1	PARK7	1p36	Recessive; rare; early onset
LRRK2	PARK8	12p12	Sporadic PD; LBs or NFTs

(Menegon *et al.* 1998). Continued effort to identify gene environment interaction in this way may eventually prove fruitful, but success is rather limited to date.

As recently as two decades ago, it was commonly taught that PD had little genetic basis. With the explosion of genetic knowledge and technology and an understanding of some of the proteins potentially involved in pathogenesis, the picture has changed dramatically. Table 9.10.4 shows genes most commonly agreed to be involved with PD aetiology (Farrer 2006). The number of genes associated with PD will almost certainly have increased by the time this current chapter is published. Genome-wide association studies are also beginning to be mounted by investigators to further elucidate the potential genetic relationships that influence the occurrence of PD and Parkinsonism (Evangelou *et al.* 2007).

Public health impact

PD is progressive and debilitating. While initial treatments with levodopa and similar medications effectively quell most motor symptoms, their effectiveness begins to subside in about 50 per cent of patients after 3–5 years. With increasing motor problem comes increased health care cost and decreased quality of life (de Boer *et al.* 1999). For many patients, dementia also ensues as PD progresses (Marder *et al.* 1999), leading to the need for long-term care in many instances. The overlap between PD dementia and DLB is of great interest because of the potential underlying synuclein pathology and there for the potential genetic relationships as well (Rocca *et al.* 2007).

Multiple sclerosis

Clinical overview

Although multiple sclerosis (MS) is not as common as most of the neurological diseases previously discussed, it is an important cause of disability in young adults in developed countries, and is thus worthy of at least brief discussion here. The impact of this disease on society is disproportionately large because it strikes people 20–50 years of age. The impact of MS on wage earning is notable with only 21 per cent of MS patients having no work limitations and only 29 per cent remaining in the work force (Minden *et al.* 2004). In addition to the stresses the disease places on home life and employment, MS patients have substantial increases in medical costs compared to the general population (Minden *et al.* 2004). Because of lost earnings and increased healthcare costs, MS is the third leading cause of significant disability in the 20–50-year age range (LaRocca *et al.* 1984).

Clinically, MS is characterized by demyelination of central nervous system white matter tracts including motor, sensory, cerebellar, visual, brainstem, autonomic, and spinal cord pathways (Noseworthy *et al.* 2000). The symptoms may be episodic, with exacerbations and remissions, with symptoms remaining stable between exacerbations (relapsing/remitting disease) (Lublin & Reingold 1996). Alternatively, symptoms may slowly progress in the absence of exacerbations (primary progressive disease). Relapsing/remitting cases may change to include slow deterioration of the baseline in between attacks (secondary progressive disease). When the disease results in death, the immediate cause is usually infectious, secondary to urinary tract involvement or pneumonia.

At present, corticosteroids are used to shorten the length of acute relapses. Interferon beta 1a, interferon beta 1b, glateramer acetate, mitoxantrone, and natalizumab have all been shown to slow the progression of the disease. In addition to disease-modifying therapy, symptomatic treatments are often required. A multitude of new immunosuppressive and immunomodulating treatments are being tested, giving hope for more effective treatments in the future.

Definition

The criteria developed by Schumacher *et al.* (1966) and revised by Poser and Kurtzke (1991) were previously used for diagnosis. These have recently been replaced by the McDonald criteria (McDonald *et al.* 2001; Polman *et al.* 2005). These new criteria for MS retain the previous requirements for two or more episodes of neurologic deficit at different times and different locations within the nervous system. For those MS attacks used to fulfil the criteria, symptoms must be typical of those seen with MS and objective findings on examination or paraclinical tests must be present. The new criteria allow diagnosis by clinical presentation alone, but also allow MRI findings to be used to demonstrate dissemination in time or locations within the nervous system. The revised McDonald criteria have allowed the disease to be diagnosed at an earlier stage than previous criteria.

Case ascertainment

Because of the necessity for neurological expertise and special studies to make reliable diagnoses, reported worldwide prevalences may not be completely comparable, especially where differences in the availability and quality of health care exist. This is especially true in light of the highly variable clinical presentation of the disease, and the variable course. The requirement for repeated attacks before a diagnosis is made and the often vague nature of the initial clinical symptoms leads to difficulties in determining exact incidence figures in a timely manner.

Prevalence

Disease prevalence is easier to determine than incidence, particularly considering the difficulty in determining the time of onset of the disease. With the new McDonald criteria, MRI availability and increasing awareness of the disease, the time from symptom onset until diagnosis is rapidly shortening in regions with ready access to sophisticated neurological care (Marrie *et al.* 2005). The reported prevalence of MS varies widely with latitude, from one per 100 000 or less near the equator, to over 150 per 100 000 in some high latitude areas. In the Southern Hemisphere less data are available, but studies in Australia and New Zealand support a similar gradient in prevalence (Skegg *et al.* 1987). Persons who migrate in childhood from high risk to lower risk areas seem to lower their risk of MS, while migrants over age 15 retain the risk associated with their areas of origin (Alter *et al.* 1966a,b). However, the prevalence and incidence of MS in relation to latitude appears to be changing rapidly over the past few years. In the United States, nurses born in the North before 1946 had a threefold greater risk of developing MS than their Southern counterparts. In those born after 1946, there was no difference in risk between those born in the North or the South (Hernan *et al.* 1999). In a study of US veterans, the relative risk of developing MS in white men born in the North compared to those born in the South was 2.47 among World War II and Korean veterans compared to 1.97 in Vietman era veterans (Wallin *et al.* 2004) Among white women veterans, the rates fell from 3.46 to 1.52 during the same time period. The study of veterans minimizes regional and socioeconomic differences in access to healthcare. It appears that this change is due primarily to an increase in MS in the South rather than to a decrease in the North.

The prevalence of MS also appears to be changing in Europe. The North–South gradient is now less pronounced and areas that previously had low incidence rates are now increasing (Pugliatti *et al.* 2006). This is particularly notable for areas around the Mediterranean and the far North. Previously, the Middle East was considered a region of low risk for developing MS. Like low-prevalence regions in North America and Europe, this risk also appears to be changing. The prevalence of MS in Kuwait increased from 6.68/100 000 in 1993 to 14.77/100 000 in 2000 (Alshubaili *et al.* 2005). Most of this increase was due to an increase in native Kuwaitis where the prevalence was 31.15/100 000. In Asia, the prevalence of MS remains low, but this rate appears to be increasing in some regions including China (Cheng *et al.* 2007). The leveling of MS rates with latitude may reflect an improvement in case ascertainment, but it likely also reflects a true increase in MS in areas in which it was previously rare.

Risk factors

Gender

Multiple sclerois is more common in females. Approximately 75 per cent of people with MS are female. However, the increased incidence among females has not always been a feature of the disease. In the first half of the twentieth century, males predominated (Kurtzke 2005). Some of the male preponderance may be related to a tendency to misdiagnose females as hysterical during that period of time. However, most believe that there was truly a male preponderance. The gender rates of MS gradually changed to a female preponderance during the middle of the century. In a longitudinal population-based cohort of 27 074 people with MS, the proportion of cases that are female has been slowly increasing over the past 50 years (Orton *et al.* 2006). The disease is less active during pregnancy and more active during the three months immediately postpartum (Confavreux *et al.* 1998). In a case–control study of 242 MS cases nested within a large British primary care database, the incidence of MS was lower in those taking oral contraceptives during the past 3 years (OR 0.6, 95% CI 0.4–1) (Alonso *et al.* 2005). The changes in MS activity with hormones and pregnancy may be due to alterations in immune system function, but the temporal changes in gender ratios remain unexplained.

Ethnic background

In general, MS occurs with greater frequency in whites, particularly those of northern European ancestry. Other ethnic groups have a lower incidence and prevalence of MS. However, the ethnic contributions to MS risk appear to be changing also. In a study of Canadian First Nations people, the prevalence of MS has increased from 56.3/100 000 in 1994 to 99.9/100 000 in 2002 (Svenson *et al.* 2007). The prevalence of MS in blacks has increased dramatically. The relative risk of MS in black compared with white males increasing from 0.44 in World War II/Korean conflict veterans to 0.67 in Vietnam era veterans (Wallin *et al.* 2004). The relative risk among black females compared to white males increased from 1.28 to 2.86 during the same time period, essentially catching up to the risk of white females.

Genetic susceptibility

There are several types of evidence for genetic influences on susceptibility. Asian, African, and aboriginal groups seem to have lower prevalence than Caucasians, regardless of latitude of residence. In Caucasians, it has been shown that some alleles of the HLA complex are associated with MS susceptibility, particularly the HLA-DRB1.1501 locus (Haines *et al.* 1996). In addition, other groups of genes that influence the immune response or myelin structure have been investigated (Sadovnick *et al.* 1991). A study by the International MS Genetics Consortium looked at 500 000 single nucleotide polymorphisms in 12 360 subjects (Hafler *et al.* 2007). In addition to the known HLA genes, only two additional alleles, IL2RA and IL7RA, were found to be risk factors for MS. Both of these genes are involved in T cell immunity, but each accounts for only 0.2 per cent of the variance in the risk of MS.

The hereditability of MS may also be instructive. There is an extremely high rate of concordance in monozygotic twins, supporting a genetic contribution to the disease. In the Danish twin study, there was concordance for MS in 24 per cent of monozygotic twins and 3 per cent of dizygotic twins (Hansen *et al.* 2005). The standardized incidence ratio for monozygotic twins compared to nontwins was 1.23 (Hansen *et al.* 2005). This contrasts with the standardized incidence ratio of 0.78 for dizygotic twins. However, areas with a lower prevalence of MS appear to have lower concordance rates for MS in monozygotic twins (..1992). In addition to the risk in twins, there is an increased risk of MS in other first degree relatives of people with MS. In a Danish study, the relative risk of MS in first degree relatives of people with MS was 7.1 (95% CI 5.8–8.8) (Nielsen *et al.* 2005). The lifetime risk was calculated to be 2.8 per cent for male and 2.9 per cent for female first degree relatives. Some have found that the risk of MS is higher in children of MS fathers than MS mothers (OR 1.99, 95% CI 1.05–3.77) (Kantarci *et al.* 2006).

This increased rate of transmission to offspring by a subgroup in which the disease is less common (men) suggests a genetic contribution in which genes are concentrated in men with the disease. However, others have reported that the risk of MS in children whose parents have MS is similar regardless of whether the affected parent was the father or mother (Herrera *et al.* 2007). A Canadian study found that the age-adjusted risk of MS in siblings was 3.11 per cent (95% CI 2.39–3.83) (Ebers *et al.* 2004). In half siblings, the risk was 1.89 per cent (95% CI 1.36–2.41). This risk was greater for maternal half siblings (2.35%, 95% CI 1.57–3.13) than paternal half siblings (1.31%, 95% CI 0.65–1.96). These genetic studies indicate that there is an important genetic contribution to the disease, but that environmental factors also play a major role.

Environmental factors

In the presence of inherent susceptibility, some external factors seem to be associated with MS. People with MS have a later age of exposure to common childhood exanthematous diseases, and lower birth orders though not all studies have supported this finding (Bager *et al.* 2006). There have been reports of clusters of disease, thought to have been related to environmental exposures, but on investigation these supposed clusters have generally not been beyond expected variability.

The strong relationship between MS and latitude has led some to postulate that areas with less sun exposure, and thus lower levels of vitamin D, may be responsible for the disease. A North American study of monozygotic twins who were discordant for MS found that childhood activities involving sun exposure decreased the risk of MS. Nine sun-related activities were investigated (Islam *et al.* 2007). The odds ratio of developing MS ranged from 0.25 to 0.57, indicating that sun-related activities in childhood decreased the risk of developing MS in later life. Each unit increase in a sun exposure index decreased the relative risk of MS by 25 per cent. In a study of US military recruits, blood samples were obtained at entry into the military (Munger *et al.* 2006). A case–control study was then performed to evaluate premorbid vitamin D levels in those who subsequently developed MS. The odds ratio for a 50 nmol/l increase in 25-hydroxyvitamin D was 0.59 (95% CI 0.36–0.97). Thus far, it has been impossible to determine whether vitamin D deficiency causes or worsens MS, or whether MS patients develop vitamin D deficiency by avoidance of the sun. This issue is further complicated by the fact that many MS patients avoid overheating because it worsens their symptoms. Also, since the disease may be present for many years before it is diagnosed the occurrence of vitamin D deficiency prior to diagnosis cannot be taken as proof that the deficiency preceded the disease.

The relationship between MS prevalence, latitude, migration, and socioeconomic factors has led some to suggest that MS is related to the degree and timing of exposure to various infectious organisms (Fleming & Cook 2006). This hygiene hypothesis states that exposure to one or more infectious agents later in life (due to high levels of hygiene) leads to changes in the immune system that eventually lead to MS. A number of infectious agents have been postulated to cause MS. Epstein–Barr virus (EBV) is associated with MS (Ascherio & Munger 2007). MS is extremely rare in people who have never had EBV. Furthermore, those exposed to EBV later in childhood have a two- to threefold increase in risk relative to those who acquire EBV in early childhood. Antibody titres to EBV are increased in MS, often years before recognition of the disease, but this may reflect a general upregulation of the immune system. Chlamydia pneumoniae has also been suspected as a cause of MS. A case–control study within the Nurses Health Study found an odds ratio of 1.7 (95% CI 1.1–2.7) in those who were seropositive for antibodies to the organism (Munger *et al.* 2003). Human herpes virus-6 (HHV6) has also been associated with MS. Human endogenous retroviruses have also been implicated in the disease (Sotgiu *et al.* 2006). Despite these associations, to date the relationship between specific viruses and MS remains uncertain.

Trauma does not appear to explain the onset of disease (Goldacre *et al.* 2006) or exacerbations of the disease (Sibley *et al.* 1991). Smoking prior to disease onset increases the risk of MS (OR 1.22–1.51) (Hawkes 2007). However, children exposed to cigarette smoke have a higher risk of developing MS (Mikaeloff *et al.* 2007). The environmental factors that contribute to MS remain uncertain.

Overview

The risk of MS appears to be due to environmental factors acting on genetically predisposed people. Eventually, these factors lead to an immune attack on the central nervous system, resulting is symptoms. The genetic factors appear to be polygenetic. The environmental factors remain uncertain. Immunomodulating treatments have played an important role in slowing the disease, but their benefits are only partial. Much remains to be clarified about the mechanisms of the disease process, and it is hoped that a better knowledge of these mechanisms will lead to improved treatments.

Epilogue

Presenting current and useful research information on a number of neurologic conditions is a difficult task. This chapter has attempted to address that challenge, for some selected neurologic conditions . We have attempted to cite important current or classic research papers, but many potentially important references included in earlier drafts became merely stubble for Occam's razor, as wielded by the editor. Conditions such as headache and TBI have substantial public health impact because of the age groups affected, their prevalence and the lost productivity (or economic loss) related to them. Multiple sclerosis, a relatively common neurologic disease, can affect individuals in young adulthood, decrease their productivity and ultimately make them dependent on others. Traumatic brain injury occurring in youth or young adulthood can cause years of extra medical care in addition to lost productivity among those who survive the immediate event. Epilepsy may have onset throughout the life course, it may result from trauma or may be caused by specific genes, among other causes. While there are intractable forms of epilepsy, great strides have been made in seizure control enabling patients to lead relatively full and normal lives. Neurodegenerative diseases, such as PD and AD, rob productivity, functional ability and independence from older individuals; they also force huge increases in health care costs. Without question neurologic diseases have substantial public health effects.

Determining the incidence and prevalence for most of the diseases and conditions in this chapter is quite an inexact science. The conditions are often difficult to define and detect in the population and for the most part they are not regarded as 'reportable' conditions. Therefore we gain insight as to disease occurrence primarily from limited but (hopefully) well-designed and conducted studies. As mentioned in the introduction to this chapter, the epidemiologic study of neurologic conditions is a complicated matter. Problems with diagnostic inaccuracy and insidious disease onset influence our ability to observe risk factor associations; factors related to survival may be mistaken for risk/protective factors.

The recent work of the Human Genome Project and the HapMap Project has greatly influenced technology and has now made possible genome-wide studies that could not have been imagined a decade ago. The contribution to disease incidence of genes, that in and of themselves cause disease may be smaller than that of genes which act together with other genes in complex ways, or act to metabolize or potentiate environmental exposures. The interaction between genes and environment will be increasingly well studied in the future. Description of gene products and functions may lead to specific drug therapies never before possible. The genetic information presented in this chapter, while relatively current, may become obsolete quickly. The fields of genetics and molecular biology are moving rapidly. It is a challenge also for epidemiologists to apply the knowledge gained by the genetic researchers to the design and analysis of epidemiologic studies. The diagnosis of neurologic conditions may ultimately be made more accurately and earlier by incorporating as yet undiscovered genetic information. Science and the public health will benefit beyond even our current grand expectations.

Epidemiology must take advantage of these molecular advances. Many scholars have written on pros and cons of reductionism in science. Much of epidemiology lies in its public health context, and the same is likely to be true for genetic influences on neurologic diseases. Arrays of genes may identify susceptible individuals however those individuals may avoid disease unless met with specific environmental or behavioural exposures. The tasks of public health and epidemiology will still involve prevention, the non-random occurrence of disease and its environmental context—in addition to heredity. The tools to address those tasks will continue to be refined.

References

(..1989) Proposal for revised classification of epilepsies and epileptic syndromes. Commission on Classification and Terminology of the International League Against Epilepsy. *Epilepsia*, **30**, 389–99.

(..1992) Multiple sclerosis in 54 twinships: concordance rate is independent of zygosity. French Research Group on Multiple Sclerosis. *Ann Neurol*, **32**, 724–7.

(..1997a) Consensus recommendations for the postmortem diagnosis of Alzheimer's disease. The National Institute on Aging, and Reagan Institute Working Group on Diagnostic Criteria for the Neuropathological Assessment of Alzheimer's Disease. *Neurobiol Aging*, **18**, S1–2.

(..1998) Rehabilitation of persons with traumatic brain injury. NIH Consensus Statement 1998 Oct 26–28, **16**, 1–41.

(..2003) Nonfatal fall-related traumatic brain injury among older adults—California, 1996–1999. *MMWR Morb Mortal Wkly Rep*, **52**, 276–8.

(..2004a) The International Classification of Headache Disorders: 2nd edition. *Cephalalgia*, **24** Suppl 1, 9–160.

(..2006) Incidence rates of hospitalization related to traumatic brain injury—12 states, 2002. *MMWR Morb Mortal Wkly Rep*, **55**, 201–4.

(..2007a) Introduction. Guidelines for the management of severe traumatic brain injury. *J Neurotrauma*, **24** Suppl 1, S1–2.

(..2007b) Nonfatal traumatic brain injuries from sports and recreation activities—United States, 2001–2005. *MMWR Morb Mortal Wkly Rep*, **56**, 733–7.

Abbas, M.A., Afifi, A.A., Zhang, Z.W., *et al.* (1998) Meta-analysis of published studies of work-related carpal tunnel syndrome. *Int J Occup Environ Health*, **4**, 160–7.

Aisen, P.S., Schafer, K.A., Grundman, M., *et al.* (2003) Effects of rofecoxib or naproxen vs placebo on Alzheimer disease progression: a randomized controlled trial. *JAMA*, **289**, 2819–26.

Alonso, A., Jick, SS., OLEK, M. J., *et al.* (2005) Recent use of oral contraceptives and the risk of multiple sclerosis. *Arch Neurol*, **62**, 1362–5.

Alonso, A., Rodriguez, L.A., Logroscino, G., *et al.* (2007) Gout and risk of Parkinson disease: a prospective study. *Neurology*, **69**, 1696–700.

Alshubaili, A.F., Alramzy, K., Ayyad, Y. M., *et al.* (2005) Epidemiology of multiple sclerosis in Kuwait: new trends in incidence and prevalence. *Eur Neurol*, **53**, 125–31.

Alter, M., Leibowitz, U. and Halpern, L. (1966a) Multiple sclerosis in European & Afro-Asian populations of Israel. *A clinical appraisal. Acta Neurol Scand*, **42**, Suppl 19:47–54.

Alter, M., Leibowitz, U. and Speer, J. (1966b) Risk of multiple sclerosis related to age at immigration to Israel. *Arch Neurol*, **15**, 234–7.

American Psychiatric Association & American Psychiatric Association (APA & AMA) Task Force on DSM-IV (1994) Diagnostic and statistical manual of mental disorders: DSM-IV, Washington, American Psychiatric Association.

Annegers, J.F., Beghi, E. & Begley, C.E. (1999) Cost of epilepsy: contrast of methodologies in United States and European studies. *Epilepsia*, **40**, 14–8.

Annegers, J.F. and Coan, S.P. (1999) SUDEP: overview of definitions and review of incidence data. *Seizure*, **8**, 347–52.

Annegers, J.F., Hauser, W.A., Anderson, V. E., *et al.* (1982) The risks of seizure disorders among relatives of patients with childhood onset epilepsy. *Neurology*, **32**, 174–9.

Annegers, J.F., Hauser, W.A., Coan, S. P., *et al.* (1998) A population-based study of seizures after traumatic brain injuries. *N Engl J Med*, **338**, 20–4.

Anstey, K.J., Von sanden, C., Salim, A., *et al.* (2007) Smoking as a risk factor for dementia and cognitive decline: a meta-analysis of prospective studies. *Am J Epidemiol*, **166**, 367–78.

Armstrong, R.A., Cairns, N.J. and Lantos, P.L. (2006) Multiple system atrophy (MSA): topographic distribution of the alpha-synuclein-associated pathological changes. *Parkinsonism Relat Disord*, **12**, 356–62.

Ascherio, A. and Munger, K. L. (2007) Environmental risk factors for multiple sclerosis. Part I: the role of infection. *Ann Neurol*, **61**, 288–99.

Atroshi, I., Gummesson, C., Johnsson, R., Ornstein, E., Ranstam, J. & Rosen, I. (1999) Prevalence of carpal tunnel syndrome in a general population [see comments]. *JAMA*, **282**, 153–8.

AU, R., Massaro, J.M., Wolf, P.A., *et al.* (2006) Association of white matter hyperintensity volume with decreased cognitive functioning: the Framingham Heart Study. *Arch Neurol*, **63**, 246–50.

Avanzini, G., Franceschetti, S. and Mantegazza, M. (2007) Epileptogenic channelopathies: experimental models of human pathologies. *Epilepsia*, **48** Suppl 2, 51–64.

Bager, P., Nielsen, N.M., Bihrmann, K., *et al.* (2006) Sibship characteristics and risk of multiple sclerosis: a nationwide cohort study in Denmark. *Am J Epidemiol*, **163**, 1112–7.

Barrett, A.M., Lucero, M.A., LE, T., *et al.* (2007) Epidemiology, public health burden, and treatment of diabetic peripheral neuropathic pain: a review. *Pain Med*, **8** Suppl 2, S50–62.

Bazarian, J.J., Mcclung, J., Shah, M.N., *et al.* (2005) Mild traumatic brain injury in the United States, 1998–2000. *Brain Inj*, **19**, 85–91.

Begley, C.E., Famulari, M., Annegers, J.F., *et al.* (2000) The cost of epilepsy in the United States: an estimate from population-based clinical and survey data. *Epilepsia*, **41**, 342–51.

Berg, J. and Stovner, L.J. (2005) Cost of migraine and other headaches in Europe. *Eur J Neurol*, **12** Suppl 1, 59–62.

Bern, C., Garcia, H.H., Evans, C., *et al.* (1999) Magnitude of the disease burden from neurocysticercosis in a developing country. *Clin Infect Dis*, **29**, 1203–9.

Bertram, L., Mcqueen, M.B., Mullin, K., *et al.* (2007) Systematic meta-analyses of Alzheimer disease genetic association studies: the AlzGene database. *Nat Genet*, **39**, 17–23.

Bigal, M., Rapoport, A., Aurora, S., *et al.* (2007) Satisfaction with current migraine therapy: experience from 3 centers in US and Sweden. *Headache*, **47**, 475–9.

Bland, J.D. (2005) The relationship of obesity, age, and carpal tunnel syndrome: more complex than was thought? *Muscle Nerve*, **32**, 527–32.

Bland, J.D. and Rudolfer, S.M. (2003) Clinical surveillance of carpal tunnel syndrome in two areas of the United Kingdom, 1991–2001. *J Neurol Neurosurg Psychiatry*, **74**, 1674–9.

Boardman, H.F., Thomas, E., Millson, D.S., *et al.* (2006) The natural history of headache: predictors of onset and recovery. *Cephalalgia*, **26**, 1080–8.

Boeve, B.F., Silber, M.H., Parisi, J.E., *et al.* (2003) Synucleinopathy pathology and REM sleep behavior disorder plus dementia or Parkinsonism. *Neurology*, **61**, 40–5.

Boulton, A. J. (1998a) Guidelines for diagnosis and outpatient management of diabetic peripheral neuropathy.European Association for the Study of Diabetes, Neurodiab. *Diabetes Metab*, **24** Suppl 3, 55–65.

Bowen, J., Teri, L., Kukull, W., *et al.* (1997) Progression to dementia in patients with isolated memory loss. *Lancet*, **349**, 763–5.

Bower, J.H., Maraganore, D.M., Mcdonnell, S.K., *et al.* (1999) Incidence and distribution of Parkinsonism in Olmsted County, Minnesota, 1976–1990. *Neurology*, **52**, 1214–20.

Braak, H., Del tredici, K., Rub, U., *et al.* (2003) Staging of brain pathology related to sporadic Parkinson's disease. *Neurobiol Aging*, **24**, 197–211.

Brayne, C. (2006) Incidence of dementia in England and Wales: the MRC Cognitive Function and Ageing Study. *Alzheimer Dis Assoc Disord*, **20**, S47–51.

Breitner, J.C., Martin, B.K. and Meinert, C.L. (2006) The suspension of treatments in ADAPT: concerns beyond the cardiovascular safety of celecoxib or naproxen. PLoS Clin Trials, 1, e41.

Breslau, N. and Davis, G. C. (1993) Migraine, physical health and psychiatric disorder: a prospective epidemiologic study in young adults. *J Psychiatr Res*, **27**, 211–21.

Breslau, N., Davis, G.C., Schultz, L.R., *et al.* (1994) Joint 1994 Wolff Award Presentation. Migraine and major depression: a longitudinal study. *Headache*, **34**, 387–93.

Breslau, N., Schultz, L.R., Stewart, W. F., *et al.* (2000) Headache and major depression: is the association specific to migraine? *Neurology*, **54**, 308–13.

Brew, B.J. (2003) The peripheral nerve complications of human immunodeficiency virus (HIV) infection. *Muscle Nerve*, **28**, 542–52.

Brookmeyer, R., Gray, S. and Kawas, C. (1998) Projections of Alzheimer's disease in the United States and the public health impact of delaying disease onset. *Am J Public Health*, **88**, 1337–42.

Bruns, J., JR. and Hauser, W.A. (2003) The epidemiology of traumatic brain injury: a review. *Epilepsia*, **44** Suppl 10, 2–10.

Buring, J.E., Hebert, P., Romero, J., *et al.* (1995) Migraine and subsequent risk of stroke in the Physicians' Health Study. *Arch Neurol*, **52**, 129–34.

Cady, R.K. (1999) Diagnosis and treatment of migraine. Clin Cornerstone, **1**, 21–32.

Cairns, N.J., Bigio, E.H., Mackenzie, I.R., *et al.* (2007a) Neuropathologic diagnostic and nosologic criteria for frontotemporal lobar degeneration: consensus of the Consortium for Frontotemporal Lobar Degeneration. *Acta Neuropathol*, **114**, 5–22.

Cairns, N.J., Neumann, M., Bigio, E.H., *et al.* (2007b) TDP-43 in familial and sporadic frontotemporal lobar degeneration with ubiquitin inclusions. *Am J Pathol*, **171**, 227–40.

Cassidy, J.D., Carroll, L.J., Peloso, P.M.,*et al.* (2004) Incidence, risk factors and prevention of mild traumatic brain injury: results of the WHO Collaborating Centre Task Force on Mild Traumatic Brain Injury. *J Rehabil Med*, 28–60.

Castillo, J., Munoz, P., Guitera, V., *et al.* (1999) Epidemiology of chronic daily headache in the general population. *Headache*, **39**, 190–6.

Chang, C.L., Donaghy, M. and Poulter, N. (1999) Migraine and stroke in young women: case–control study. The World Health Organisation Collaborative Study of Cardiovascular Disease and Steroid Hormone Contraception [see comments]. *BMJ*, **318**, 13–8.

Cheng, Q., Miao, L., Zhang, J., *et al.* (2007) A population-based survey of multiple sclerosis in Shanghai, China. *Neurology*, **68**, 1495–500.

Christensen, J., Vestergaard, M., Pedersen, M.G., *et al.* (2007) Incidence and prevalence of epilepsy in Denmark. *Epilepsy Res*, **76**, 60–5.

Chui, H.C., Mack, W., Jackson, J.E., *et al.* (2000) Clinical criteria for the diagnosis of vascular dementia: a multicenter study of comparability and interrater reliability [see comments]. *Arch Neurol*, **57**, 191–6.

Colantonio, A., Dawson, D.R. and Mclellan, B.A. (1998) Head injury in young adults: long-term outcome. *Arch Phys Med Rehabil*, **79**, 550–8.

Confavreux, C., Hutchinson, M., Hours, M.M., *et al.* (1998) Rate of pregnancy-related relapse in multiple sclerosis. Pregnancy in Multiple Sclerosis Group. *N Engl J Med*, **339**, 285–91.

Coronado, V.G., Thomas, K.E., Sattin, R.W., *et al.* (2005) The CDC traumatic brain injury surveillance system: characteristics of persons aged 65 years and older hospitalized with a TBI. *J Head Trauma Rehabil*, **20**, 215–28.

Crino, P.B. (2007) Gene expression, genetics, and genomics in epilepsy: some answers, more questions. *Epilepsia*, **48** Suppl 2, 42–50.

Cruts, M., Gijselinck, I., Van der zee, J., *et al.* (2006) Null mutations in progranulin cause ubiquitin-positive frontotemporal dementia linked to chromosome 17q21. *Nature*, **442**, 920–4.

Currie, C.J., Morgan, C.L. and Peters, J.R. (1998) The epidemiology and cost of inpatient care for peripheral vascular disease, infection, neuropathy, and ulceration in diabetes. *Diabetes Care*, **21**, 42–8.

Dahlof, C. and Linde, M. (2001) One-year prevalence of migraine in Sweden: a population-based study in adults. *Cephalalgia*, **21**, 664–71.

De boer, A.G., Sprangers, M.A., Speelman, H.D. and De haes, H.C. (1999) Predictors of health care use in patients with Parkinson's disease: a longitudinal study. *Mov Disord*, **14**, 772–9.

De lau, L.M., Koudstaal, P.J., Witteman, J.C., *et al.* (2006) Dietary folate, vitamin B_{12}, and vitamin B6 and the risk of Parkinson disease. *Neurology*, **67**, 315–8.

De rijk, M.C., Breteler, M.M., Graveland, G.A., *et al.* (1995) Prevalence of Parkinson's disease in the elderly: the Rotterdam Study. *Neurology*, **45**, 2143–6.

De rijk, M.C., Tzourio, C., Breteler, M.M., *et al.* (1997) Prevalence of Parkinsonism and Parkinson's disease in Europe: the EUROPARKINSON Collaborative Study. European Community Concerted Action on the Epidemiology of Parkinson's disease. *J Neurol Neurosurg Psychiatry*, **62**, 10–5.

Demetriades, D., Murray, J., Sinz, B., *et al.* (1998) Epidemiology of major trauma and trauma deaths in Los Angeles County. *J Am Coll Surg*, **187**, 373–83.

Dobyns, W.B., Truwit, C.L., Ross, M.E., *et al.* (1999) Differences in the gyral pattern distinguish chromosome 17-linked and X-linked lissencephaly. *Neurology*, **53**, 270–7.

Durkin, M.S., Kuhn, L., Davidson, L.L., *et al.* (1996) Epidemiology and prevention of severe assault and gun injuries to children in an urban community. *J Trauma*, **41**, 667–73.

Dyck, P.J., Davies, J.L., Wilson, D.M., *et al.* (1999) Risk factors for severity of diabetic polyneuropathy: intensive longitudinal assessment of the Rochester Diabetic Neuropathy Study cohort. *Diabetes Care*, **22**, 1479–86.

Ebers, G.C., Sadovnick, A.D., Dyment, D.A., *et al.* (2004) Parent-of-origin effect in multiple sclerosis: observations in half-siblings. *Lancet*, **363**, 1773–4.

Eisele, J.A., Kegler, S.R., Trent, R.B., *et al.* (2006) Nonfatal traumatic brain injury-related hospitalization in very young children-15 states, 1999. *J Head Trauma Rehabil*, **21**, 537–43.

Elias, M.F., Sullivan, L.M., D'agostino, R.B., *et al.* (2005) Homocysteine and cognitive performance in the Framingham offspring study: age is important. *Am J Epidemiol*, **162**, 644–53.

Engel, J., JR. (2001) A proposed diagnostic scheme for people with epileptic seizures and with epilepsy: report of the ILAE Task Force on Classification and Terminology. *Epilepsia*, **42**, 796–803.

Evangelou, E., Maraganore, D.M. and Ioannidis, J.P. (2007) Meta-analysis in genome-wide association datasets: strategies and application in Parkinson disease. PLoS ONE, 2, e196.

Evans, D.A., Funkenstein, H.H., Albert, M.S., *et al.* (1989) Prevalence of Alzheimer's disease in a community population of older persons. Higher than previously reported [see comments]. *JAMA*, **262**, 2551–6.

Farrer, M.J. (2006) Genetics of Parkinson disease: paradigm shifts and future prospects. *Nat Rev Genet*, **7**, 306–18.

Ferri, C.P., Prince, M., Brayne, C., *et al.* (2005) Global prevalence of dementia: a Delphi consensus study. *Lancet*, **366**, 2112–7.

Firestone, J.A., Smith-Weller, T., Franklin, G., *et al.* (2005) Pesticides and risk of Parkinson disease: a population-based case–control study. *Arch Neurol*, **62**, 91–5.

Fleming, J.O. and Cook, T.D. (2006) Multiple sclerosis and the hygiene hypothesis. *Neurology*, **67**, 2085–6.

Franceschi, M., Colombo, B., Rossi, P., *et al.* (1997) Headache in a population-based elderly cohort. An ancillary study to the Italian Longitudinal Study of Aging (ILSA). *Headache*, **37**, 79–82.

Franklin, G.M., Haug, J., Heyer, N., *et al.* (1991) Occupational carpal tunnel syndrome in Washington State, 1984–1988. *Am J Public Health*, **81**, 741–6.

Fratiglioni, L., De Ronchi, D. and Aguero-Torres, H. (1999) Worldwide prevalence and incidence of dementia. *Drugs Aging*, **15**, 365–75.

Frediani, F. and Villani, V. (2007) Migraine and depression. *Neurol Sci*, **28** Suppl 2, S161–5.

Freitag, C.M., May, T.W., Pfafflin, M., *et al.* (2001) Incidence of epilepsies and epileptic syndromes in children and adolescents: a population-based prospective study in Germany. *Epilepsia*, **42**, 979–85.

Gallitto, G., Serra, S., La Spina, P., *et al.* (2005) Prevalence and characteristics of epilepsy in the Aeolian islands. *Epilepsia*, **46**, 1828–35.

Ganguli, M., Dodge, H.H., Chen, P., *et al.* (2000) Ten-year incidence of dementia in a rural elderly US community population: the Movies Project [In Process Citation]. *Neurology*, **54**, 1109–16.

Gao, X., Chen, H., Fung, T.T., *et al.* (2007) Prospective study of dietary pattern and risk of Parkinson disease. *Am J Clin Nutr*, **86**, 1486–94.

Gass, J., Cannon, A., Mackenzie, I.R., *et al.* (2006) Mutations in progranulin are a major cause of ubiquitin-positive frontotemporal lobar degeneration. *Hum Mol Genet*, **15**, 2988–3001.

Gervil, M., Ulrich, V., Kyvik, K.O., *et al.* (1999) Migraine without aura: a population-based twin study. *Ann Neurol*, **46**, 606–11.

Gobel, H., Petersen-Braun, M. and Soyka, D. (1994) The epidemiology of headache in Germany: a nationwide survey of a representative sample on the basis of the headache classification of the International Headache Society [see comments]. *Cephalalgia*, 14, 97–106.

Goldacre, M.J., Abisgold, J.D., Yeates, D.G., *et al.* (2006) Risk of multiple sclerosis after head injury: record linkage study. *J Neurol Neurosurg Psychiatry*, **77**, 351–3.

Gordon Smith, A. and Robinson Singleton, J. (2006) Idiopathic neuropathy, prediabetes and the metabolic syndrome. *J Neurol Sci*, **242**, 9–14.

Gorell, J.M., JOHNSON, C. C., RYBICKI, B. A., *et al.* (1999a) Occupational exposure to manganese, copper, lead, iron, mercury and zinc and the risk of Parkinson's disease. *Neurotoxicology*, **20**, 239–47.

Gorell, J.M., Johnson, C.C., Rybicki, B.A., *et al.* (1998) The risk of Parkinson's disease with exposure to pesticides, farming, well water, and rural living. *Neurology*, **50**, 1346–50.

Gorell, J.M., Rybicki, B.A., Cole Johnson, C., *et al.* (1999b) Occupational metal exposures and the risk of Parkinson's disease. *Neuroepidemiology*, **18**, 303–8.

Haan, M.N., Miller, J.W., Aiello, A.E., *et al.* (2007) Homocysteine, B vitamins, and the incidence of dementia and cognitive impairment: results from the Sacramento Area Latino Study on Aging. *Am J Clin Nutr*, **85**, 511–7.

Hafler, D.A., Compston, A., Sawcer, S. *et al.* (2007) Risk alleles for multiple sclerosis identified by a genomewide study. *N Engl J Med*, **357**, 851–62.

Hagen, K., Vatten, L., Stovner, L. J., *et al.* (2002a) Low socio-economic status is associated with increased risk of frequent headache: a prospective study of 22718 adults in Norway. *Cephalalgia*, **22**, 672–9.

Hagen, K., Zwart, J.A., Vatten, L., *et al.* (2000) Prevalence of migraine and non-migrainous headache—head-HUNT, a large population-based study. *Cephalalgia*, **20**, 900–6.

Haines, J.L., Ter-Minassian, M., Bazyk, A., *et al.* (1996) A complete genomic screen for multiple sclerosis underscores a role for the major histocompatability complex. The Multiple Sclerosis Genetics Group. *Nat Genet*, **13**, 469–71.

Hakim, A. J., Cherkas, L., El Zayat, S., *et al.* (2002) The genetic contribution to carpal tunnel syndrome in women: a twin study. *Arthritis Rheum*, **47**, 275–9.

Hansen, T., Skytthe, A., Stenager, E., *et al.* (2005) Concordance for multiple sclerosis in Danish twins: an update of a nationwide study. *Mult Scler*, **11**, 504–10.

Hauser, W.A. (1995) Epidemiology of epilepsy in children. *Neurosurg Clin N Am*, **6**, 419–29.

Hauser, W.A., Annegers, J.F. and Rocca, W.A. (1996) Descriptive epidemiology of epilepsy: contributions of population-based studies from Rochester, Minnesota. *Mayo Clin Proc*, **71**, 576–86.

Hawkes, C.H. (2007) Smoking is a risk factor for multiple sclerosis: a metanalysis. *Mult Scler*, **13**, 610–5.

Hayden, K.M., Zandi, P.P., Khachaturian, A.S., *et al.* (2007) Does NSAID use modify cognitive trajectories in the elderly? The Cache County study. *Neurology*, **69**, 275–82.

Henderson, V.W., Paganini-Hill, A., Miller, B. L., *et al.* (2000) Estrogen for Alzheimer's disease in women: randomized, double-blind, placebo-controlled trial. *Neurology*, **54**, 295–301.

Hendrie, H.C. (1998) Epidemiology of dementia and Alzheimer's disease. *Am J Geriatr Psychiatry*, **6**, S3–18.

Hernan, M.A., Olek, M.J. and Ascherio, A. (1999) Geographic variation of MS incidence in two prospective studies of US women. *Neurology*, **53**, 1711–8.

Herrera, B.M., Ramagopalan, S.V., Orton, S., *et al.* (2007) Parental transmission of MS in a population-based Canadian cohort. *Neurology*, **69**, 1208–12.

Hirtz, D., Thurman, D.J., Gwinn-Hardy, K., *et al.* (2007) How common are the 'common' neurologic disorders? *Neurology*, **68**, 326–37.

Holm, L., Cassidy, J.D., Carroll, L.J. and Borg, J. (2005) Summary of the WHO Collaborating Centre for Neurotrauma Task Force on Mild Traumatic Brain Injury. *J Rehabil Med*, **37**, 137–41.

Houston, D.J. and Richardson, L.E., JR. (2007) Motorcycle safety and the repeal of universal helmet laws. *Am J Public Health*, **97**, 2063–9.

Hu, G., Jousilahti, P., Nissinen, A., *et al.* (2006) Body mass index and the risk of Parkinson disease. *Neurology*, **67**, 1955–9.

Hu, X.H., Markson, L.E., Lipton, R.B., *et al.* (1999) Burden of migraine in the United States: disability and economic costs. *Arch Intern Med*, **159**, 813–8.

Islam, T., Gauderman, W.J., Cozen, W. *et al.* (2007) Childhood sun exposure influences risk of multiple sclerosis in monozygotic twins. *Neurology*, **69**, 381–8.

Jallon, P. and Latour, P. (2005) Epidemiology of idiopathic generalized epilepsies. *Epilepsia*, **46** Suppl 9, 10–4.

Jankovic, J., Rajput, A.H., Mcdermott, M.P., *et al.* (2000) The evolution of diagnosis in early Parkinson disease. Parkinson Study Group. *Arch Neurol*, **57**, 369–72.

Jorm, A.F. and Jolley, D. (1998) The incidence of dementia: a meta-analysis. *Neurology*, **51**, 728–33.

Kantarci, O.H., Barcellos, L.F., Atkinson, E.J., *et al.* (2006) Men transmit MS more often to their children vs women: the Carter effect. *Neurology*, **67**, 305–10.

Kara, I., Ozkok, E., Aydin, M., *et al.* (2007) Combined effects of ACE and MMP-3 polymorphisms on migraine development. *Cephalalgia*, **27**, 235–43.

Kara, I., Sazci, A., Ergul, E., *et al.* (2003) Association of the C677T and A1298C polymorphisms in the 5,10 methylenetetrahydrofolate reductase gene in patients with migraine risk. *Brain Res Mol Brain Res*, **111**, 84–90.

Katsarava, Z., Obermann, M., Yoon, M.S., *et al.* (2007) Prevalence of cluster headache in a population-based sample in Germany. *Cephalalgia*, **27**, 1014–9.

Keenan, H.T. and Bratton, S.L. (2006) Epidemiology and outcomes of pediatric traumatic brain injury. *Dev Neurosci*, **28**, 256–63.

Keenan, H.T., Runyan, D.K., Marshall, S.W., *et al.* (2003) A Population-Based Study of Inflicted Traumatic Brain Injury in Young Children. *JAMA*, **290**, 621–626.

Kegler, S.R., Coronado, V.G., Annest, J.L., *et al.* (2003) Estimating nonfatal traumatic brain injury hospitalizations using an urban/rural index. *J Head Trauma Rehabil*, **18**, 469–78.

Keltner, N.L. and Cooke, B.B. (2007) Biological perspectives: traumatic brain injury-war related. *Perspect Psychiatr Care*, **43**, 223–6.

Kelvin, E.A., Hesdorffer, D.C., Bagiella, E., *et al.* (2007) Prevalence of self-reported epilepsy in a multiracial and multiethnic community in New York City. *Epilepsy Res*, **77**, 141–50.

Koepsell, T.D., Kurland, B.F., Harel, O., *et al.* (2008) Education, cognitive function, and severity of neuropathology in Alzheimer disease. *Neurology*,**70**,1725–7.

Kramer, U., Nevo, Y., Neufeld, M.Y., *et al.* (1998) Epidemiology of epilepsy in childhood: a cohort of 440 consecutive patients. *Pediatr Neurol*, **18**, 46–50.

Kukull, W.A. (2006) The growing global burden of dementia. *Lancet Neurol*, **5**, 199–200.

Kukull, W.A., Higdon, R., Bowen, J.D., *et al.* (2002) Dementia and Alzheimer disease incidence: a prospective cohort study. *Arch Neurol*, **59**, 1737–46.

Kuopio, A.M., Marttila, R.J., Helenius, H., *et al.* (1999) Environmental risk factors in Parkinson's disease. *Mov Disord*, **14**, 928–39.

Kurth, T., Slomke, M.A., Kase, C.S., *et al.* (2005) Migraine, headache, and the risk of stroke in women: a prospective study. *Neurology*, **64**, 1020–6.

Kurtz, Z., Tookey, P. and Ross, E. (1998) Epilepsy in young people: 23 year follow up of the British national child development study. *Bmj*, **316**, 339–42.

Kurtzke, J.F. (2005) Epidemiology and etiology of multiple sclerosis. *Phys Med Rehabil Clin N Am*, **16**, 327–49.

Kurtzke, J.F. and Heltberg, A. (2001) Multiple sclerosis in the Faroe Islands: an epitome. *J Clin Epidemiol*, **54**, 1–22.

Kwong, L.K., Neumann, M., Sampathu, D.M., *et al.* (2007) TDP-43 proteinopathy: the neuropathology underlying major forms of sporadic and familial frontotemporal lobar degeneration and motor neuron disease. *Acta Neuropathol*, **114**, 63–70.

Lam, W.H. and Mackersie, A. (1999) Paediatric head injury: incidence, aetiology and management. *Paediatr Anaesth*, **9**, 377–85.

Langston, J.W. (2006) The Parkinson's complex: Parkinsonism is just the tip of the iceberg. *Ann Neurol*, **59**, 591–6.

Langston, J.W., Ballard, P., Tetrud, J.W., *et al.* (1983) Chronic Parkinsonism in humans due to a product of meperidine-analog synthesis. *Science*, **219**, 979–80.

Larocca, N.G., Scheinberg, L.C., Slater, R.J., *et al.* (1984) Field testing of a minimal record of disability in multiple sclerosis: the United States and Canada. *Acta Neurol Scand* Suppl, **101**, 126–38.

Launer, L.J., Andersen, K., Dewey, M.E., Letenneur, L., Ott, A., Amaducci, L.A. *et al.* (1999) Rates and risk factors for dementia and Alzheimer's disease: results from EURODEM pooled analyses. EURODEM Incidence Research Group and Work Groups. European Studies of Dementia. *Neurology*, **52**, 78–84.

Lea, R.A., Dohy, A., Jordan, K., *et al.* (2000) Evidence for allelic association of the dopamine beta-hydroxylase gene (DBH) with susceptibility to typical migraine. *Neurogenetics*, **3**, 35–40.

Lee, P.N. (1994) Smoking and Alzheimer's disease: a review of the epidemiological evidence. *Neuroepidemiology*, **13**, 131–44.

Leidy, N.K., Elixhauser, A., Vickrey, B., *et al.* (1999) Seizure frequency and the health-related quality of life of adults with epilepsy. *Neurology*, **53**, 162–6.

Leonardi, M., Steiner, T.J., Scher, A.T., *et al.* (2005) The global burden of migraine: measuring disability in headache disorders with WHO's Classification of Functioning, Disability and Health (ICF). *J Headache Pain*, **6**, 429–40.

Lhatoo, S.D. and Sander, J.W. (2005) Cause-specific mortality in epilepsy. *Epilepsia*, **46** Suppl 11, 36–9.

LIPPA, C. F., DUDA, J. E., GROSSMAN, M., *et al.* (2007) DLB and PDD boundary issues: diagnosis, treatment, molecular pathology, and biomarkers. *Neurology*, **68**, 812–9.

Lipton, R.B. (1998) Comorbidity in migraine—causes and effects. *Cephalalgia*, **18** Suppl 22, 8–11; discussion 11–4.

Lipton, R.B., B1, M.E., Diamond, M., *et al.* (2007) Migraine prevalence, disease burden, and the need for preventive therapy. *Neurology*, **68**, 343–9.

Lipton, R.B., Stewart, W.F. and Simon, D. (1998) Medical consultation for migraine: results from the American Migraine Study. *Headache*, **38**, 87–96.

Loiseau, J., Picot, M.C. and Loiseau, P. (1999) Short-term mortality after a first epileptic seizure: a population-based study. *Epilepsia*, **40**, 1388–92.

Lopez, O.L., Kuller, L.H., Becker, J.T., *et al.* (2007) Incidence of dementia in mild cognitive impairment in the cardiovascular health study cognition study. *Arch Neurol*, **64**, 416–20.

Lublin, F.D. and Reingold, S.C. (1996) Defining the clinical course of multiple sclerosis: results of an international survey. National Multiple Sclerosis Society (USA) Advisory Committee on Clinical Trials of New Agents in Multiple Sclerosis. *Neurology*, **46**, 907–11.

Lyngberg, A.C., Rasmussen, B.K., Jorgensen, T., *et al.* (2005a) Has the prevalence of migraine and tension-type headache changed over a 12-year period? A Danish population survey. *Eur J Epidemiol*, **20**, 243–9.

Lyngberg, A.C., Rasmussen, B. K., Jorgensen, T., *et al.* (2005b) Prognosis of migraine and tension-type headache: a population-based follow-up study. *Neurology*, **65**, 580–5.

Macclellan, L.R., Giles, W., Cole, J., *et al.* (2007) Probable migraine with visual aura and risk of ischemic stroke: the stroke prevention in young women study. *Stroke*, **38**, 2438–45.

Mackenzie, I.R. and Rademakers, R. (2007) The molecular genetics and neuropathology of frontotemporal lobar degeneration: recent developments. *Neurogenetics*, **8**, 237–48.

Maraganore, D.M., Farrer, M.J., Hardy, J.A., *et al.* (2000) Case–control study of debrisoquine 4-hydroxylase, N-acetyltransferase 2, and apolipoprotein E gene polymorphisms in Parkinson's disease. *Mov Disord*, **15**, 714–9.

Marder, K., Logroscino, G., Alfaro, B., *et al.* (1998) Environmental risk factors for Parkinson's disease in an urban multiethnic community. *Neurology*, **50**, 279–81.

Marder, K., Tang, M.X., Alfaro, B., *et al.* (1999) Risk of Alzheimer's disease in relatives of Parkinson's disease patients with and without dementia. *Neurology*, **52**, 719–24.

Marrie, R.A., Cutter, G., Tyry, T., *et al.* (2005) Changes in the ascertainment of multiple sclerosis. *Neurology*, **65**, 1066–70.

Martyn, C.N. and Hughes, R.A. (1997) Epidemiology of peripheral neuropathy. *J Neurol Neurosurg Psychiatry*, **62**, 310–8.

McDonald, W.I., Compston, A., Edan, G., *et al.* (2001) Recommended diagnostic criteria for multiple sclerosis: guidelines from the International Panel on the diagnosis of multiple sclerosis. *Ann Neurol*, **50**, 121–7.

Mckeith, I.G. (2006) Consensus guidelines for the clinical and pathologic diagnosis of dementia with Lewy bodies (DLB): report of the Consortium on DLB International Workshop. *J Alzheimers Dis*, **9**, 417–23.

Mehta, K.M., Ott, A., Kalmijn, S., *et al.* (1999) Head trauma and risk of dementia and Alzheimer's disease: The Rotterdam Study. *Neurology*, **53**, 1959–62.

Menegon, A., Board, P.G., Blackburn, A.C., *et al.* (1998) Parkinson's disease, pesticides, and glutathione transferase polymorphisms [see comments]. *Lancet*, **352**, 1344–6.

Merikangas, K.R., Fenton, B.T., Cheng, S.H., *et al.* (1997) Association between migraine and stroke in a large-scale epidemiological study of the United States. *Arch Neurol*, **54**, 362–8.

Merikangas, K.R., Whitaker, A.E., Isler, H., *et al.* (1994) The Zurich Study: XXIII. Epidemiology of headache syndromes in the Zurich cohort study of young adults. *Eur Arch Psychiatry Clin Neurosci*, **244**, 145–52.

Mesulam, M., Johnson, N., Krefft, T.A., *et al.* (2007) Progranulin mutations in primary progressive aphasia: the PPA1 and PPA3 families. *Arch Neurol*, **64**, 43–7.

Mikaeloff, Y., Caridade, G., Tardieu, M., *et al.* (2007) Parental smoking at home and the risk of childhood-onset multiple sclerosis in children. *Brain*, **130**, 2589–95.

Minden, K., Niewerth, M., Listing, J., *et al.* (2004) Burden and cost of illness in patients with juvenile idiopathic arthritis. *Ann Rheum Dis*, **63**, 836–42.

Moceri, V.M., Kukull, W.A., Emanuel, I., *et al.* (2000) Early-life risk factors and the development of Alzheimer's disease. *Neurology*, **54**, 415–20.

Mold, J.W., Vesely, S.K., Keyl, B.A., *et al.* (2004) The prevalence, predictors, and consequences of peripheral sensory neuropathy in older patients. *J Am Board Fam Pract*, **17**, 309–18.

Monahan, K. and O'Leary, K.D. (1999) Head injury and battered women: an initial inquiry. *Health Soc Work*, **24**, 269–78.

Morgante, L., Rocca, W.A., Di Rosa, A.E., *et al.* (1992) Prevalence of Parkinson's disease and other types of Parkinsonism: a door-to-door survey in three Sicilian municipalities. The Sicilian Neuro-Epidemiologic Study (SNES) Group. *Neurology*, **42**, 1901–7.

Morimoto, R.I. (2006) Stress, aging, and neurodegenerative disease. *N Engl J Med*, **355**, 2254–5.

Morris, J.C. (2006) Mild cognitive impairment is early-stage Alzheimer disease: time to revise diagnostic criteria. *Arch Neurol*, **63**, 15–6.

Multhaup, G. (2006) Amyloid precursor protein and BACE function as oligomers. *Neurodegener Dis*, **3**, 270–4.

Munger, K.L., Levin, L.I., Hollis, B.W., *et al.* (2006) Serum 25-hydroxyvitamin D levels and risk of multiple sclerosis. *JAMA*, **296**, 2832–8.

Munger, K.L., Peeling, R.W., Hernan, M.A., *et al.* (2003) Infection with Chlamydia pneumoniae and risk of multiple sclerosis. *Epidemiology*, **14**, 141–7.

Murray, M.E., Knopman, D.S. and Dickson, D.W. (2007) Vascular dementia: clinical, neuroradiologic and neuropathologic aspects. *Panminerva Med*, **49**, 197–207.

Nashef, L., Hindocha, N. and Makoff, A. (2007) Risk factors in sudden death in epilepsy (SUDEP): the quest for mechanisms. *Epilepsia*, **48**, 859–71.

Nee, L.E. & Lippa, C.F. (1999) Alzheimer's disease in 22 twin pairs—13-year follow-up: hormonal, infectious and traumatic factors. *Dement Geriatr Cogn Disord*, **10**, 148–51.

Newman, A.B., Fitzpatrick, A.L., Lopez, O., *et al.* (2005) Dementia and Alzheimer's disease incidence in relationship to cardiovascular disease in the Cardiovascular Health Study cohort. *J Am Geriatr Soc*, **53**, 1101–7.

Nicoletti, A., Reggio, A., Bartoloni, A., *et al.* (1998) A neuroepidemiological survey in rural Bolivia: background and methods. *Neuroepidemiology*, **17**, 273–80.

Nicoletti, A., Reggio, A., Bartoloni, A., *et al.* (1999) Prevalence of epilepsy in rural Bolivia: a door-to-door survey. *Neurology*, **53**, 2064–9.

Nielsen, N.M., Westergaard, T., Rostgaard, K., *et al.* (2005) Familial risk of multiple sclerosis: a nationwide cohort study. *Am J Epidemiol*, **162**, 774–8.

Nilsson, L., Farahmand, B.Y., Persson, P.G., *et al.* (1999) Risk factors for sudden unexpected death in epilepsy: a case–control study. *Lancet*, **353**, 888–93.

Nilsson, L., Tomson, T., Farahmand, B. Y., *et al.* (1997) Cause-specific mortality in epilepsy: a cohort study of more than 9,000 patients once hospitalized for epilepsy [see comments]. *Epilepsia*, **38**, 1062–8.

Nordstrom, D.L., Destefano, F., Vierkant, R.A., *et al.* (1998) Incidence of diagnosed carpal tunnel syndrome in a general population. *Epidemiology*, **9**, 342–5.

Noseworthy, J.H., Lucchinetti, C., Rodriguez, M., *et al.* G. (2000) Multiple sclerosis. *N Engl J Med*, **343**, 938–52.

Nourhashemi, F., Gillette-Guyonnet, S., Andrieu, S., *et al.* (2000) Alzheimer disease: protective factors. *Am J Clin Nutr*, **71**, 643S–649S.

Nyholt, D.R., Dawkins, J.L., Brimage, P. J., *et al.* (1998) Evidence for an X-linked genetic component in familial typical migraine. *Hum Mol Genet*, **7**, 459–63.

O'Brien, B., Goeree, R. and Streiner, D. (1994) Prevalence of migraine headache in Canada: a population-based survey. *Int J Epidemiol*, **23**, 1020–6.

Octave, J.N., Essalmani, R., Tasiaux, B., *et al.* (2000) The role of presenilin-1 in the gamma-secretase cleavage of the amyloid precursor protein of Alzheimer's disease. *J Biol Chem*, **275**, 1525–8.

Okie, S. (2005) Traumatic brain injury in the war zone. *N Engl J Med*, **352**, 2043–7.

Olafsson, E. and Hauser, W.A. (1999) Prevalence of epilepsy in rural Iceland: a population-based study. *Epilepsia*, **40**, 1529–34.

Ooi, W.W. and Srinivasan, J. (2004) Leprosy and the peripheral nervous system: basic and clinical aspects. *Muscle Nerve*, **30**, 393–409.

Orchard, T.J., Ce, L.L., Maser, R.E., *et al.* (1996) Why does diabetic autonomic neuropathy predict IDDM mortality? An analysis from the Pittsburgh Epidemiology of Diabetes Complications Study. *Diabetes Res Clin Pract*, **34** Suppl, S165–71.

Orton, S.M., Herrera, B.M., Yee, I.M., *et al.* (2006) Sex ratio of multiple sclerosis in Canada: a longitudinal study. *Lancet Neurol*, **5**, 932–6.

Osuntokun, B.O., Adeuja, A.O., Nottidge, V.A., *et al.* (1992) Prevalence of headache and migrainous headache in Nigerian Africans: a community-based study. *East Afr Med J*, **69**, 196–9.

Palacio, L.G., Jimenez, I., Garcia, H.H., *et al.* (1998) Neurocysticercosis in persons with epilepsy in Medellin, Colombia. The Neuroepidemiological Research Group of Antioquia. *Epilepsia*, **39**, 1334–9.

Parry, O., Mielke, J., Latif, A.S., *et al.* (1997) Peripheral neuropathy in individuals with HIV infection in Zimbabwe. *Acta Neurol Scand*, **96**, 218–22.

Petersen, R.C. (2007) Mild cognitive impairment: current research and clinical implications. *Semin Neurol*, **27**, 22–31.

Petersen, R.C., Smith, G.E., Waring, S.C., *et al.* (1999) Mild cognitive impairment: clinical characterization and outcome [published erratum appears in Arch Neurol 1999 Jun;56(6):760]. *Arch Neurol*, **56**, 303–8.

Petrovitch, H., Ross, G.W., Abbott, R.D., *et al.* (2002) Plantation work and risk of Parkinson disease in a population-based longitudinal study. *Arch Neurol*, **59**, 1787–92.

Pine, D.S., Cohen, P. and Brook, J. (1996) The association between major depression and headache: results of a longitudinal epidemiologic study in youth. *J Child Adolesc Psychopharmacol*, **6**, 153–64.

Polman, C.H., Reingold, S.C., Edan, G., *et al.* (2005) Diagnostic criteria for multiple sclerosis: 2005 revisions to the 'McDonald Criteria'. *Ann Neurol*, **58**, 840–6.

Poser, S. and Kurtzke, J.F. (1991) Epidemiology of MS. *Neurology*, **41**, 157–8.

Power, T., Catroppa, C., Coleman, L., *et al.* (2007) Do lesion site and severity predict deficits in attentional control after preschool traumatic brain injury (TBI)? *Brain Inj*, **21**, 279–92.

Pugliatti, M., Rosati, G., Carton, H., *et al.* (2006) The epidemiology of multiple sclerosis in Europe. *Eur J Neurol*, **13**, 700–22.

Rademakers, R. and Hutton, M. (2007) The genetics of frontotemporal lobar degeneration. *Curr Neurol Neurosci Rep*, **7**, 434–42.

Rasmussen, B.K. (1995) Epidemiology of headache. *Cephalalgia*, **15**, 45–68.

Rayan, G.M. (1999) Carpal tunnel syndrome between two centuries. *J Okla State Med Assoc*, **92**, 493–503.

Rezendes, J.L. (2006) Bicycle helmets: overcoming barriers to use and increasing effectiveness. *J Pediatr Nurs*, **21**, 35–44.

Ritz, B., Ascherio, A., Checkoway, H., *et al.* (2007) Pooled analysis of tobacco use and risk of Parkinson disease. *Arch Neurol*, **64**, 990–7.

Rocca, W.A., Bower, J.H., Ahlskog, J.E., *et al.* (2007) Risk of cognitive impairment or dementia in relatives of patients with Parkinson disease. *Arch Neurol*, **64**, 1458–64.

Rocca, W.A., Cha, R.H., Waring, S.C., *et al.* (1998) Incidence of dementia and Alzheimer's disease: a reanalysis of data from Rochester, Minnesota, 1975–1984. *Am J Epidemiol*, **148**, 51–62.

Rockwood, K., Wentzel, C., Hachinski, V., *et al.* (2000) Prevalence and outcomes of vascular cognitive impairment. Vascular Cognitive Impairment Investigators of the Canadian Study of Health and Aging. *Neurology*, **54**, 447–51.

Roman, G.C. (1994) An epidemic in Cuba of optic neuropathy, sensorineural deafness, peripheral sensory neuropathy and dorsolateral myeloneuropathy. *J Neurol Sci*, **127**, 11–28.

Roman, G.C., Tatemichi, T.K., Erkinjuntti, T., *et al.* (1993) Vascular dementia: diagnostic criteria for research studies. Report of the NINDS-AIREN International Workshop [see comments]. *Neurology*, **43**, 250–60.

Roses, A.D. (1994) Apolipoprotein E is a relevant susceptibility gene that affects the rate of expression of Alzheimer's disease. *Neurobiol Aging*, **15**, S165–7.

Ross, G.W., Abbott, R.D., Petrovitch, H., *et al.* (2000) Association of coffee and caffeine intake with the risk of Parkinson disease. *JAMA*, **283**, 2674–9.

Rothman, K.J. and Greenland, S. (1998) Modern epidemiology, Philadelphia, Pa., Lippincott-Raven.

Rowe, C.C., Ng, S., Ackermann, U., *et al.* (2007) Imaging beta-amyloid burden in aging and dementia. *Neurology*, **68**, 1718–25.

Rowland, L.P. and Merritt, H.H. (1995) *Merritt's textbook of neurology*, Baltimore, Williams & Wilkins.

Russell, M.B., Levi, N. and Kaprio, J. (2007) Genetics of tension-type headache: A population based twin study. *Am J Med Genet B Neuropsychiatr Genet*, **144**, 982–6.

Rutland-Brown, W., Langlois, J.A., Thomas, K.E., *et al.* (2006) Incidence of traumatic brain injury in the United States, 2003. *J Head Trauma Rehabil*, **21**, 544–8.

Sadovnick, A.D., Bulman, D. and Ebers, G. C. (1991) Parent-child concordance in multiple sclerosis. *Ann Neurol*, **29**, 252–5.

Sanchez, A.L., Lindback, J., Schantz, P.M., *et al.* (1999) A population-based, case–control study of *Taenia solium* taeniasis and cysticercosis. *Ann Trop Med Parasitol*, **93**, 247–58.

Scher, A.I., Stewart, W.F., Ricci, J.A., *et al.* (2003) Factors associated with the onset and remission of chronic daily headache in a population-based study. *Pain*, **106**, 81–9.

Schneider, J.A., Arvanitakis, Z., Bang, W., *et al.* (2007) Mixed brain pathologies account for most dementia cases in community-dwelling older persons. *Neurology*, **69**, 2197–204.

Schofield, P.W., Tang, M., Marder, K., *et al.* (1997) Alzheimer's disease after remote head injury: an incidence study. *J Neurol Neurosurg Psychiatry*, **62**, 119–24.

Schumacher, G.A. (1966) Multiple sclerosis. *Arch Neurol*, **14**, 571–3.

Schwartz, B.S., Stewart, W.F. and Lipton, R.B. (1997) Lost workdays and decreased work effectiveness associated with headache in the workplace. *J Occup Environ Med*, **39**, 320–7.

Scordo, M.G., Dahl, M.L., Spina, E., *et al.* (2006) No association between CYP2D6 polymorphism and Alzheimer's disease in an Italian population. *Pharmacol Res*, **53**, 162–5.

Senanayake, N. and Roman, G.C. (1993) Epidemiology of epilepsy in developing countries. *Bull World Health Organ*, **71**, 247–58.

Shackleton, D.P., Westendorp, R.G., Trenite, D.G., *et al.* (1999) Mortality in patients with epilepsy: 40 years of follow up in a Dutch cohort study [see comments]. *J Neurol Neurosurg Psychiatry*, **66**, 636–40.

Shastry, B.S. and Giblin, F.J. (1999) Genes and susceptible loci of Alzheimer's disease. *Brain Res Bull*, **48**, 121–7.

Sherer, M., Struchen, M.A., Yablon, S.A., *et al.* (2008) Comparison of indices of TBI severity: Glasgow coma scale, length of coma, post-traumatic amnesia. *J Neurol Neurosurg Psychiatry*,**79**, 678–85.

Shumaker, S.A., Legault, C., Kuller, L., *et al.* (2004) Conjugated equine estrogens and incidence of probable dementia and mild cognitive impairment in postmenopausal women: Women's Health Initiative Memory Study. *JAMA*, **291**, 2947–58.

Sibley, W.A., Bamford, C.R., Clark, K., *et al.* (1991) A prospective study of physical trauma and multiple sclerosis. *J Neurol Neurosurg Psychiatry*, **54**, 584–9.

Skegg, D.C., Corwin, P.A., Craven, R.S., *et al.* (1987) Occurrence of multiple sclerosis in the north and south of New Zealand. *J Neurol Neurosurg Psychiatry*, **50**, 134–9.

Solomon, D.H., Katz, J.N., Bohn, R., *et al.* (1999) Nonoccupational risk factors for carpal tunnel syndrome. *J Gen Intern Med*, **14**, 310–4.

Sotgiu, S., Arru, G., Soderstrom, M., *et al.* (2006) Multiple sclerosis-associated retrovirus and optic neuritis. *Mult Scler*, **12**, 357–9.

Sperling, M.R., Feldman, H., Kinman, J., *et al.* (1999) Seizure control and mortality in epilepsy. *Ann Neurol*, **46**, 45–50.

St George-Hyslop, P.H. (2000) Molecular genetics of Alzheimer's disease. *Biol Psychiatry*, **47**, 183–99.

Stallings, S.P., Kasdan, M.L., Soergel, T.M., *et al.* (1997) A case–control study of obesity as a risk factor for carpal tunnel syndrome in a population of 600 patients presenting for independent medical examination. *J Hand Surg [Am]*, **22**, 211–5.

Steinlein, O. K. (1999) Gene defects in idiopathic epilepsy. *Rev Neurol (Paris)*, **155**, 450–3.

Stewart, W.F., Bigal, M.E., Kolodner, K., *et al.* (2006) Familial risk of migraine: variation by proband age at onset and headache severity. *Neurology*, **66**, 344–8.

Stewart, W.F., Lipton, R.B. and Liberman, J. (1996a) Variation in migraine prevalence by race. *Neurology*, **47**, 52–9.

STewart, W.F., Simon, D., Shechter, A., *et al.* (1995) Population variation in migraine prevalence: a meta-analysis. *J Clin Epidemiol*, **48**, 269–80.

Stovner, L., Hagen, K., Jensen, R., *et al.* (2007) The global burden of headache: a documentation of headache prevalence and disability worldwide. *Cephalalgia*, **27**, 193–210.

Svendsen, T., Lossius, M. and Nakken, K.O. (2007) Age-specific prevalence of epilepsy in Oppland County, Norway. *Acta Neurol Scand*, **116**, 307–11.

Svenson, L.W., Warren, S., Warren, K.G., *et al.* (2007) Prevalence of multiple sclerosis in First Nations people of Alberta. *Can J Neurol Sci*, **34**, 175–80.

Tagliaferri, F., Compagnone, C., Korsic, M., *et al.* (2006) A systematic review of brain injury epidemiology in Europe. *Acta Neurochir (Wien)*, **148**, 255–68; discussion 268.

Tagliati, M., Grinnell, J., Godbold, J., *et al.* (1999) Peripheral nerve function in HIV infection: clinical, electrophysiologic, and laboratory findings. *Arch Neurol*, **56**, 84–9.

Tesfaye, S., Stevens, L.K., Stephenson, J.M., *et al.* (1996) Prevalence of diabetic peripheral neuropathy and its relation to glycaemic control and potential risk factors: the EURODIAB IDDM Complications Study. *Diabetologia*, **39**, 1377–84.

Thompson, H.J., Mccormick, W.C. and Kagan, S.H. (2006) Traumatic brain injury in older adults: epidemiology, outcomes, and future implications. *J Am Geriatr Soc*, **54**, 1590–5.

Tietjen, G.E. (2000) The relationship of migraine and stroke. *Neuroepidemiology*, **19**, 13–9.

Tolnay, M. and Frank, S. (2007) Pathology and genetics of frontotemporal lobar degeneration: an update. *Clin Neuropathol*, **26**, 143–56.

Tomson, T., Walczak, T., Sillanpaa, M., *et al.* (2005) Sudden unexpected death in epilepsy: a review of incidence and risk factors. *Epilepsia*, **46** Suppl 11, 54–61.

Tonon, C., Guttmann, S., Volpini, M., *et al.* (2002) Prevalence and incidence of cluster headache in the Republic of San Marino. *Neurology*, **58**, 1407–9.

Torelli, P., Beghi, E. and Manzoni, G.C. (2005) Cluster headache prevalence in the Italian general population. *Neurology*, **64**, 469–74.

Trojanowski, J.Q. and Lee, V.M. (2002) Parkinson's disease and related synucleinopathies are a new class of nervous system amyloidoses. *Neurotoxicology*, **23**, 457–60.

Trojanowski, J.Q. and Mattson, M. P. (2003) Overview of protein aggregation in single, double, and triple neurodegenerative brain amyloidoses. *Neuromolecular Med*, **4**, 1–6.

Tsuang, D., Simpson, K., Larson, E.B., *et al.* (2006) Predicting lewy body pathology in a community-based sample with clinical diagnosis of Alzheimer's disease. *J Geriatr Psychiatry Neurol*, **19**, 195–201.

Tyas, S.L., Tate, R.B., Wooldrage, K., *et al.* (2006) Estimating the incidence of dementia: the impact of adjusting for subject attrition using health care utilization data. *Ann Epidemiol*, **16**, 477–84.

Uldall, P., Alving, J., Hansen, L.K., *et al.* (2006) The misdiagnosis of epilepsy in children admitted to a tertiary epilepsy centre with paroxysmal events. *Arch Dis Child*, **91**, 219–21.

Ulrich, V., Gervil, M., Kyvik, K.O., *et al.* (1999) Evidence of a genetic factor in migraine with aura: a population-based Danish twin study. *Ann Neurol*, **45**, 242–6.

Wallin, M.T., Page, W.F. and Kurtzke, J. F. (2004) Multiple sclerosis in US veterans of the Vietnam era and later military service: race, sex, and geography. *Ann Neurol*, **55**, 65–71.

Wang, S.J., Fuh, J.L., Lu, S.R., *et al.* (2001) Quality of life differs among headache diagnoses: analysis of SF-36 survey in 901 headache patients. *Pain*, **89**, 285–92.

Warden, D. (2006) Military TBI during the Iraq and Afghanistan wars. *J Head Trauma Rehabil*, **21**, 398–402.

Werner, C. and Engelhard, K. (2007) Pathophysiology of traumatic brain injury. *Br J Anaesth*, **99**, 4–9.

Whitmer, R.A., Gunderson, E.P., Quesenberry, C.P., JR., *et al.* (2007) Body mass index in midlife and risk of Alzheimer disease and vascular dementia. *Curr Alzheimer Res*, **4**, 103–9.

Winblad, B., Palmer, K., Kivipelto, M., *et al.* (2004) Mild cognitive impairment—beyond controversies, towards a consensus: report of the International Working Group on Mild Cognitive Impairment. *J Intern Med*, **256**, 240–6.

Yuki, N. (2007) Ganglioside mimicry and peripheral nerve disease. *Muscle Nerve*, **35**, 691–711.

Zarrelli, M.M., Beghi, E., Rocca, W.A., *et al.* (1999) Incidence of epileptic syndromes in Rochester, Minnesota: 1980–1984. *Epilepsia*, **40**, 1708–14.

Zhao, J., Fu, Y., Yasvoina, M., Shao, P., *et al.* (2007) Beta-site amyloid precursor protein cleaving enzyme 1 levels become elevated in neurons around amyloid plaques: implications for Alzheimer's disease pathogenesis. *J Neurosci*, **27**, 3639–49.

Ziegler, D.K., Hur, Y.M., Bouchard, T.J., JR., *et al.* (1998) Migraine in twins raised together and apart. *Headache*, **38**, 417–22.

9.11

The transmissible spongiform encephalopathies

Richard S.G. Knight and Hester J.T. Ward

Abstract

Prion diseases are a group of animal and human diseases having disparate causes, distributions, and clinical pictures, but are unified by a common neurodegenerative pathology, the common central role of the prion protein, and a shared potential for transmissibility (even in those instances where the primary cause is apparently spontaneous or genetic). This potential transmissibility from animal to man (e.g. variant Creutzfeldt–Jakob disease [vCJD] resulting from bovine spongiform encephalopathy [BSE] dietary contamination) or from human to human (via various means, most recently by blood transfusion) gives these illnesses their specific public health importance.

Introduction

Prion diseases, also known as transmissible spongiform encephalopathies, are a group of animal and human illnesses united by broadly similar pathological features and transmissible potential (Table 9.11.1a). The most common human prion disease is Creutzfeldt–Jakob disease (CJD); this has been divided into four forms on the basis of differing clinicopathological features and cause (Table 9.11.1b). The transmissibility of prion diseases raises important public health concerns, in relation to both animal-to-human and human-to-human disease. To date, the principal occurrences of transmission have been therapy with cadaver-derived human growth hormone (hGH), surgical use of human dura mater grafts, and BSE contamination of human diet. More recently, there has been increasing concern about secondary transmission of vCJD via blood and blood products.

One form of prion disease, kuru, is exclusively an acquired human illness based on person-to-person transmission, albeit by unusual means, namely ritual mourning cannibalism. Kuru is confined to the Fore group in Papua New Guinea and, following the cessation of cannibilistic feasts, a very significant decline in the number of cases, from being the commonest cause of adult female death in the affected area to being a rarity, has been observed (Cervenakova *et al.* 1998).

The nature of prion diseases

Prion diseases are invariably progressive, ultimately fatal neurological illnesses. The underlying pathological changes in the brain are essentially neurodegenerative, involving neuronal loss, astrocytic hyperplasia, spongiform change, and deposition of an abnormal form of prion protein (the most characteristic feature of these diseases) (DeArmond *et al.* 2004). Prion protein (PrP) is a normal cellular protein encoded, in humans, by *PRNP*, the prion protein gene on chromosome 20. The precise function of the normal prion protein (PrP^{C}) is uncertain. In prion diseases, PrP^{C} undergoes a post-translational conformational change to an abnormal, disease-related, structure designated PrP^{Sc} (Prusiner 2004a). The pathogenesis of prion diseases is uncertain; the precise relationship between the protein conversion or its tissue deposition and the neuronal damage has not been established. In animals or humans affected by prion diseases, the clinical manifestations are purely neurological; there are no typical systemic responses to infection (such as fever), no detectable antibody responses, and no non-neurological symptoms (even when PrP^{Sc} is found in non-neurological tissues).

When PrP^{Sc} is obtained from prion disease tissue, it has varying molecular features. After treatment with proteases, the protease-resistant fragment has different sizes, and has been termed Type I or Type II on this basis. PrP has two glycosylation sites and thus exists in non-, mono-, and diglycosylated forms. It is now routine practice to classify prion diseases partly according to the PrP^{Sc} type and the ratio of glycoforms found, the most commonly used protein classification being Type I, Type IIA, and Type IIB (Parchi *et al.* 1996; Head *et al.* 2004). The exact significance of this protein classification is unclear and it is not entirely straightforward: Different protein types can be found in one brain (Head *et al.* 2004). However, the classification has utility; for example, Type IIB in humans is unique to vCJD. *PRNP*, and the equivalent gene in animals, is important for two reasons: Firstly, pathogenic mutations are apparently responsible for genetic forms of prion disease (Kovacs *et al.* 2002); secondly, polymorphisms in the gene have important potential effects on susceptibility to developing disease, the incubation period, and the resulting clinicopathological phenotype (Parchi *et al.* 1999).

At codon 129 of *PRNP*, an individual may code either for methionine (M) or valine (V); therefore, each person can be *PRNP*-129 MM, *PRNP*-129 MV, or *PRNP*-129 VV. The distribution of these different genotypes in normal populations shows some geographic variation (Nurmi *et al.* 2003). The significance of this is particularly illustrated by the fact that all examined cases of vCJD to date have been of the MM genotype (Clarke & Ghani 2005). In acquired

Table 9.11.1a Prion diseases: the transmissible spongiform encephalopathies

	Disease	Comments
Animal diseases	Scrapie	Natural disease of sheep and goats
	Bovine spongiform encephalopathy (BSE)	Primarily affected cattle Secondary transmission to feline species and exotic ungulates
	Feline spongiform encephalopathy (FSE)	Prion disease caused by BSE transmission to feline species
	Chronic wasting disease (CWD)	Natural disease of cervid species in North America
	Transmissible mink encephalopathy (TME)	Disease of farmed mink
	Atypical scrapie	Recently identified atypical form of scrapie in sheep
	H-type and L-type BSE	Recently described atypical forms of bovine prion disease
Human diseases	Creutzfeldt–Jakob disease (CJD)	The commonest human prion disease. Subclassified into four types (see Table 9.11.1b)
	Gerstmann-Sträussler-Scheinker syndrome (GSSS)	A genetic prion disease
	Fatal familial insomnia (FFI)	A very rare genetic prion disease
	Sporadic fatal insomnia (SFI)	Extremely rare form of prion disease with similar phenotype to FFI, but of sporadic, non-genetic occurrence
	Kuru	A disease confined to a region of Papua New Guinea, spread via cannibalistic mourning rites

prion diseases, the codon 129 genotype may affect the incubation period, as has been seen in hGH-related CJD and kuru: Individuals with either MV or VV genotypes may develop vCJD with a longer incubation period than those with the MM genotype (Cervenakova *et al.* 1998; Clarke & Ghani 2005; Huillard d'Aignaux *et al.* 2002a; Brandel *et al.* 2003). In Japan, but not in other countries, another *PRNP* polymorphism (at codon 219) has been shown to have effects on susceptibility and clinicopathological phenotyope (Shibuya *et al.* 1998).

Despite their neurodegenerative pathology, prion diseases are transmissible and this gives rise to a number of important public health concerns. In general, transmissibility is associated with PrP^{Sc} and the prevailing view is that PrP^{Sc} is either the infectious agent or its major component (Prusiner 2004b). However, the exact nature of the agent is unknown. This has important implications for research and public health protection with only two methods of detecting infectivity in tissues: Laboratory animal transmission experiments and the identification of PrP^{Sc} in the tissue. The first is

Table 9.11.1b The different types of CJD

Type	Comments
Sporadic (sCJD)	Commonest form (but with an annual mortality rate of only 1–2/million). Worldwide distribution; cause unknown. Principally affects the middle-aged and the elderly
Genetic (gCJD)	Resulting from mutations in the *PRNP* gene. Autosomal dominant inheritance
Variant (vCJD)	Due to BSE infection. Most cases in the United Kingdom. Relatively young age group affected compared to sCJD
Iatrogenic (iCJD)	Due to secondary transmission of human prion disease via medical and surgical procedures. Recently, blood transfusions implicated in vCJD transmission (see Table 9.11.2)

direct (giving definitive evidence of transmissibility) but slow and expensive, the incubation period being generally of several months in rodents, for example (Bruce 2003). There are also associated difficulties due to potential differences in susceptibility between humans and, for example, rodents. The second is simpler, quicker, and cheaper from the laboratory standpoint, but indirect (using PrP^{Sc} as a marker of infectivity). Both require appropriate tissue samples, which, in the case of human brain, are not straightforward to obtain in life and may be difficult to obtain after death, because of issues surrounding post-mortems and consent.

Surveillance of CJD

The UK National CJD Surveillance Unit (NCJDSU), Edinburgh, was established by the Department of Health in 1990 following the Southwood Committee Report (www.cjd.ed.ac.uk). The principal aim of the NCJDSU was to identify any changes in CJD in the United Kingdom, in the wake of the BSE epidemic in cattle, that could indicate transmission of BSE to man. Past records of CJD existed from a previous UK MRC-funded study that had run over a 5-year period (1980–84) and had also collected retrospective data from 1970 to 1979 (Will *et al.* 1986; Cousens *et al.* 1990). At the start of the 1990 surveillance period, cases were identified retrospectively for the period 1985–90. In 1996, the NCJDSU reported the emergence of a previously unrecognized form of CJD—vCJD (Will *et al.* 1996). The NCJDSU continues with UK CJD surveillance, identifying all cases of human prion disease, along with associated research particularly to examine risk factors for all UK cases of sCJD and vCJD, to investigate the geographic distribution of CJD, to identify mechanisms of transmission of BSE to humans, to establish short- and long-term trends, to evaluate potential risks of onward transmission, to identify novel forms of human prion diseases, and to evaluate case definitions and diagnostic tests. The UK National Prion Clinic in London has primary responsibility for the identification of UK genetic prion disease. The UK Institute of Child Health in London has primary responsibility for the identification of UK hGH-related CJD.

Many other countries have established CJD surveillance systems and there is active international collaboration that has achieved standardization of methodology, agreed case definitions, and also undertaken many research projects (www.eurocjd.ed.ac.uk)

(Pocchiari *et al.* 2004; Ladogana *et al.* 2005). The World Health Organization (WHO) has published guidelines for the diagnosis of prion diseases (World Health Organization 1998, 2002). This international approach allows the accumulation of data on significant numbers of cases in a rare disease and also provides good country comparative data; the initial identification of vCJD was undoubtedly helped by the ability to ascertain that, in 1996, similar cases had not been identified in countries other than the United Kingdom, the country principally affected by BSE.

In most of the European Union countries, cases of prion disease are subject to mandatory reporting rules, but UK surveillance is based on a relatively informal system. One problem of mandatory reporting of prion disease is the case definition for such reporting. There is no simple, non-invasive diagnostic test in life and premortem diagnosis therefore heavily depends on clinical judgement. The internationally agreed, WHO-adopted, clinical diagnostic criteria may not identify clinically atypical cases and also require experience in their application; it is difficult for individual clinicians to obtain this, given the rarity of these diseases. The reporting of definite cases will, of course, identify only those cases with either cerebral biopsy (not a common procedure) or those with autopsy. In the United Kingdom, surveillance is run by local clinicians being asked to refer 'any case suspected of being prion disease' to the NCJDSU. The NCJDSU neurologists then assess the referral, visit the case, interview the family, and review the investigations. In the UK system, about half of the referred living suspect cases are finally classified as prion disease. Pathologists are asked to refer any cases identified by biopsy or at autopsy. Referrals to the NJCDSU also come from death certificates recorded with ICD-10 codes A810 and FO21.

The clinical diagnosis of prion disease is a relatively complex matter, involving a number of neurological differential diagnoses. A number of investigations are required; one cerebrospinal fluid (CSF) test (for 14-3-3 protein) has become an important part of assessment and case classification, especially with respect to sporadic CJD (sCJD) (Green *et al.* 2006). There is a national CSF protein laboratory service located within the NCJDSU. The possibility of obtaining advice or a clinical opinion from neurologists experienced with prion disease, and the provision of CSF laboratory and neuropathological services, encourages referral of cases, including atypical ones. Overlapping, multiple methods of case ascertainment (clinical referral, laboratory test provision, pathology referral, and death certificate review) serve to ensure that surveillance is as complete as possible. The opportunity for expert, experienced advice, laboratory tests, and neuropathological studies has aided notification of suspect cases in other countries.

Sporadic CJD

Background

Sporadic CJD has a worldwide distribution with an annual mortality rate of around 1–2 per million population per year (Fig. 9.11.1) (Will *et al.* 2004). It is predominantly a disease of mid-to-late life, and with its neurodegenerative pathology, it would be placed alongside other diseases such as Alzheimer's disease, Parkinson's disease, and motor neuron disease, except for its transmissibility (Fig. 9.11.2). The typical clinical profile is of a rapidly progressing encephalopathy: The median duration in most countries is around 4 months (Pocchiari *et al.* 2004; Will *et al.* 2004). Dementia, cerebellar ataxia, and myoclonus are the most characteristic clinical features. The typical pathological findings, including spongiform change and PrP^{Sc} deposition, are confined to the central nervous system. There is, however, some clinicopathological variation, which includes the following: Presentation with a progressive isolated deficit (such as cerebellar ataxia or visual disturbance), atypically young onset, atypically long duration, and different PrP^{Sc} deposition patterns in the brain, including the presence of amyloid plaques in the brain (DeArmond *et al.* 2004; Ladogana *et al.* 2005; Boesenberger *et al.* 2005; Cooper *et al.* 2005; Cooper *et al.* 2006).

Cause

The cause is unknown. The two most favoured theories are spontaneous protein conversion and somatic *PRNP* mutation (Prusiner 2004a). The fact that sCJD is transmissible in the laboratory and can indeed be transmitted from person to person under special circumstances (such as neurosurgery) raises the question as to whether it is, in general, a naturally transmitted disease. There are three ways of exploring this possibility: Investigation of individual cases and their contacts (although this may produce essentially anecdotal evidence), statistical analysis of case clustering, and case–control studies. Despite its rarity, the epidemiology of sCJD has been studied in some detail and case–control studies have been undertaken, involving significant numbers of cases, because of both sustained surveillance over time within individual countries and international collaboration, with data pooling (Harries-Jones *et al.* 1988; Wientjens *et al.* 1996; Van Duijn *et al.* 1998; Collins

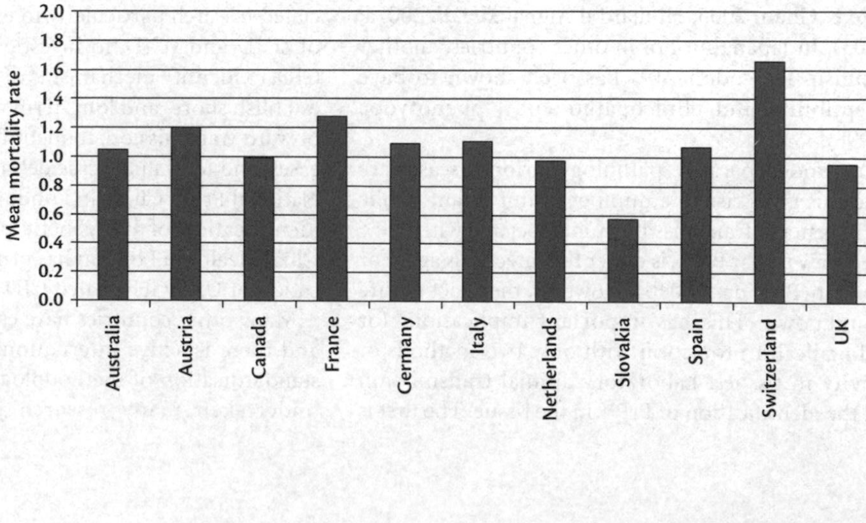

Fig. 9.11.1 Mean annual mortality rates for sCJD in several countries (1993–2006).

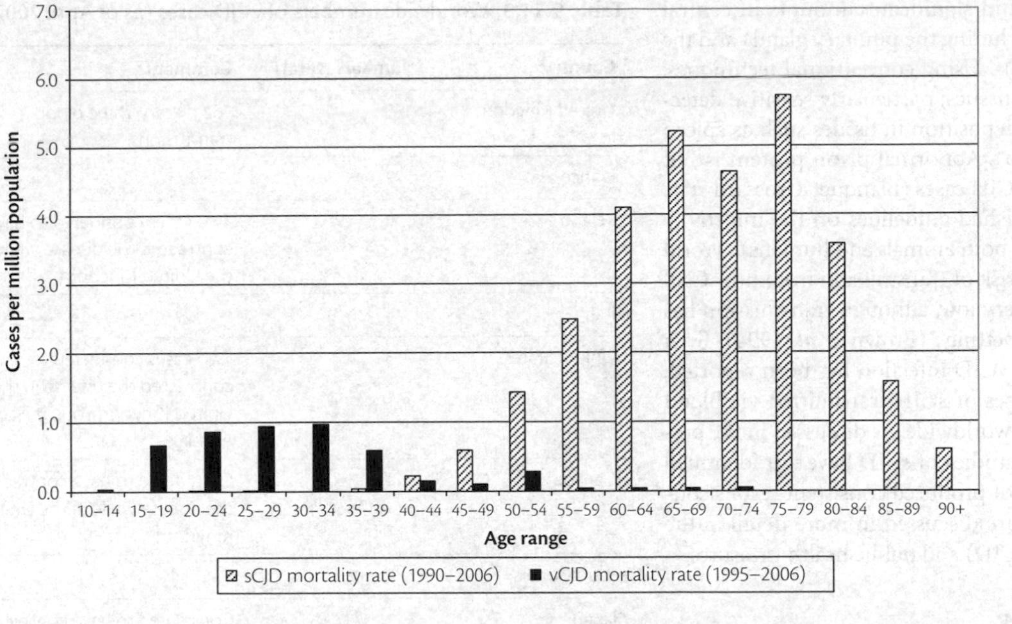

Fig. 9.11.2 Age-specific mortality rates for sCJD cases and variant Creutzfeldt–Jakob disease (vCJD) cases, by 5-year age group (the UK).

et al. 1999; Wilson *et al.* 2000; Zerr *et al.* 2000; Ward *et al.* 2002). Two large case–control studies in Australia and Europe (Collins *et al.* 1999; Ward *et al.* 2002) have shown an increased risk of sCJD associated with any surgery, which in the Australian study increased with increased number of operations. The Australian study found increased risk associated with a range of surgical procedures (carpal tunnel, eye, heart, haemorrhoid, gall bladder, hernia, hysterectomy, varicose vein), and the European study found a small increased risk associated with gynaecological surgery (and a reduced risk associated with tonsillectomy and appendicectomy). 'Other surgery' not categorized a priori into anatomical groups, such as stitches to the skin, was also shown to be associated with increased risk of sCJD in both studies.

Other smaller studies have reported varying findings related to medical risk and sCJD, but have lacked power and/or been subject to bias (Bobowick *et al.* 1973; Kondo & Kuroiwa 1982; Davanipour *et al.* 1985). Examination of clusters, or areas of high incidence of sCJD, has been carried out in various countries; some in fact proved to be due to genetic mutations rather than sCJD infection (in Slovakia, Chile, and among Libyan Jews in Israel) (Kahana *et al.* 1974; Brown *et al.* 1992; Lee *et al.* 1999). However, investigation of smaller clusters has been difficult to interpret (in Australia, England, France, Japan, and the United States) (Matthews 1975; Farmer *et al.* 1978; Will & Matthews 1982; Arakawa *et al.* 1991; Collins *et al.* 2002; Huillard d'Aignaux *et al.* 2002b). One statistical analysis of clustering of sCJD in the United Kingdom reported that cases lived closer together than might be expected by chance and the evidence for this increased the further in the past it was examined. These findings suggest that some sCJD cases may result from exposure to a common external factor years before clinical onset; however, identifying these common factors years after the event is very difficult (Linsell *et al.* 2004).

Although the prion hypothesis allows for the spontaneous conversion of PrP^{C} to PrP^{Sc}, exposure to an environmental agent, perhaps many years before disease onset, has not been ruled out. As described in the preceding subsection, case–control studies and examination of clusters have not produced convincing evidence of a route or exposure by which public health measures can be implemented to reduce the incidence of sCJD. Of course, it is possible that sCJD is a heterogeneous disease in terms of its cause.

Health risks

Although no definitive evidence that sCJD is a primarily acquired disease exists, it can certainly be secondarily transmitted. Over the years, there have been many instances of transmission, either of sCJD or presumed sCJD, through medical practice: Neurosurgical instruments, depth EEG electrodes, human dura mater grafts, corneal transplantation, and use of human-derived pituitary hormones (Brown *et al.* 2000; 2006) (Table 9.11.2).

Table 9.11.2 Summary of iatrogenic human prion disease

Procedure	Numbers reported[a]	Comments
Human growth hormone treatment	194	
Human dura mater grafts	196	Japan: 123 France: 13 Spain: 10 UK: 7
Neurosurgical instruments	4	
Depth EEG electrodes	2	
Corneal transplants	2	
Human gonadotrophin treatment	4	
Blood transfusion infection of vCJD	4	Three resulted in vCJD; one case of infection but no neurological disease at time of death.

[a] As of April 2007.
vCJD: variant Creutzfeldt–Jakob disease.

In sCJD, infectivity is present in significant amounts in central nervous system (CNS) tissue (including the pituitary gland) and the posterior eye (Peden *et al.* 2004) . Using conventional techniques, PrP^{Sc} is not found in peripheral tissues; particularly sensitive detection methods may reveal PrP^{Sc} deposition in tissues such as spleen and muscle (Glatzel *et al.* 2003a). Abnormal prion protein is not detectable in the dental pulp of sCJD cases (Blanquet-Grossard *et al.* 2000). The WHO recently published guidelines on the infectivity distribution of prion diseases (of both animals and humans) (World Health Organization 2006). The risk of transmission from non-CNS non-ocular tissues is generally very low, although transmission has been reported in experimental settings (Brown *et al.* 1994). Even though transfusion-transmitted vCJD infection has been reported, there have been no reported cases of sCJD transmitted via blood components or plasma products worldwide. As discussed in the preceding subsection, case–control studies of sCJD have not identified blood as a risk factor and have not produced consistent results concerning surgery. These matters are discussed in more detail in the subsections on iatrogenic CJD (iCJD) and public health measures.

Genetic prion diseases

Background

Human genetic prion diseases have been classified into three groups, originally according to clinicopathological characteristics: Genetic CJD, fatal familial insomnia, and Gerstmann–Staussler–Scheinker syndrome. The identification of pathogenic *PRNP* mutations allows for a more rational classification (Kovacs *et al.* 2005). The mode of inheritance is autosomal dominant. Penetrance is reportedly high, but may vary with mutation; in *PRNP* point mutation E200K, penetrance is complete (Spudich *et al.* 1995). A family history is not present in all cases (12–88 per cent); therefore, genetic prion disease cannot be absolutely excluded without *PRNP* sequencing (which can be performed straightforwardly on a blood sample) (Kovacs *et al.* 2005).

Cause

The current belief is that the mutations are directly disease causing. The idea that they represent particular susceptibility factors cannot be absolutely excluded.

Health risks

It is a curious and striking fact that an autosomally inherited gene mutation disease can potentially be transmitted to others who do not have the underlying mutation. Genetic prion disease therefore poses a public health risk one would not expect from its basic genetic cause. It is likely that the tissue distribution of infectivity is similar to that of sCJD (World Health Organization 2006). It is not known whether there is a significant risk of infection from an individual with a *PRNP* mutation in the pre-symptomatic period, but it is wise to assume that such is possibly the case. As is mentioned earlier, not all cases of genetic CJD have a recognized family history. It is assumed that iCJD results from initial sCJD cases; statistically this is probable, but it is possible that some arise from unsuspected genetic cases.

Primary variant CJD

Background

The recognition of BSE in the United Kingdom in 1986 gave rise to concerns that it could be transmitted to humans through diet, and in 1996, a new form of human prion disease (vCJD) was reported in the United Kingdom (Will *et al.* 1996). There were alarming predictions of thousands or even millions of cases of vCJD but, to date, the epidemic has, fortunately, been much more limited (Clarke & Ghani 2005; Cousens *et al.* 1997).

The earliest recognized case had symptom onset in 1994, and by April 2007, 202 people had been diagnosed with vCJD worldwide, predominantly in the United Kingdom (Table 9.11.3). The basic epidemiology of vCJD is given in Table 9.11.4 (the age distribution among UK cases is also shown in Fig. 9.11.2). It is important to note that, by international agreement, cases of vCJD are attributed to the country where they are normally resident at the time of diagnosis. Especially given the potentially very long incubation period

Table 9.11.3 Worldwide numbers of vCJD cases (as of April 2007)

Country*	Numbers (total)	Comments
United Kingdom	165	162 dietary, three blood transfusions
France	22	
Ireland	4	Two cases considered to have contracted the disease while in the United Kingdom
Italy	1	
United States	3	Two cases considered to have contracted the disease in the United Kingdom, one in Saudi Arabia
Canada	1	Considered to have contracted the disease while in the United Kingdom
Saudi Arabia	1	
Japan	1	Considered to have contracted the disease while in the United Kingdom
The Netherlands	2	
Portugal	1	
Spain	1	

* Cases attributed to country according to normal country of residence at time of illness onset; this may not be the country of exposure to infection (see 'Comments' column).

Table 9.11.4 Basic epidemiology of vCJD in the United Kingdom

Age at onset	Mean: 28 years Median: 26 Range: 12–74
Age at death	Mean: 30 years Median: 28 Range: 14–74
Duration (based on deaths)	Median: 14 months Range: 6–40
Male:Female	92:73
PRNP codon 129*	100 per cent (145 tested)

* All tested cases in other countries have also been *PRNP* codon-129.

of this illness, this is not necessarily the same as the country where they contracted the infection. For example, 3 cases of vCJD have been attributed to the United States, but none of these were thought to have been infected in that country. Judgments as to the likely country of infection have to be based on the residential history of the individual and the estimated risk of BSE infection in that country during the relevant period. After the United Kingdom, France has reported the greatest number of cases, but modelling predicts a limited size to the epidemic, and with a lower total than for the United Kingdom (Alperovitch & Will 2002).

Clinicopathological features and diagnosis

Variant CJD typically presents as an essentially psychiatric disturbance, involving depression, anxiety, social withdrawal, and sometimes, more unusual symptoms such as hallucinations or delusions. The presenting clinical features in the first hundred UK cases have been described in detail by Spencer *et al.* (2002). Symptoms such as chorea, dystonia, and painful sensory disturbances are not uncommon, and with progression, other clearly neurological features appear, including cerebellar ataxia and dementia (Will *et al.* 2004).

The clinical and neuropathological picture is significantly different from that seen in sCJD (DeArmond *et al.* 2004). One particular difference of clinical and public health importance between vCJD and other forms of CJD is that, in vCJD, lymphoreticular tissue (tonsil, appendix, other gut-associated lymphoid tissue, lymph nodes, and spleen) show significant levels of PrP^{Sc} deposition and infectivity even during the incubation period (Hilton *et al.* 1998, 2004; Ironside *et al.* 2000). Infectivity in the CNS in vCJD is thought to arise later in the incubation period and reaches much higher infectivity levels than that seen in the lymphoreticular tissues.

Definite diagnosis requires brain tissue and is usually at autopsy, but in some situations, brain biopsy is performed. Clinical diagnosis depends on the exclusion of other possible diagnoses, the presence of characteristic brain MRI findings, and in some cases, tonsil biopsy (Hill *et al.* 1999; Collie *et al.* 2003). Primary vCJD cases, that is, those considered to be due to BSE contamination of foodstuffs, are considered in this subsection. Secondary infection from primary vCJD cases has been so far identified only through blood transfusion (as of August 2008, four reported instances) and is discussed in a separate subsection.

Cause

The causal linkage of vCJD to BSE has three broad bases: vCJD and BSE have the same causative agent, the agent passed from cattle to man, and the passage was via diet (Knight 1999). There are laboratory studies showing that the BSE and vCJD agents have identical biological and molecular properties (although it has to be borne in mind that the agent itself has not been fully characterized) (Bruce *et al.* 1997; Hill *et al.* 1997). All of the epidemiological evidence suggests that the agent passed from cattle to man. BSE-infected material clearly entered human food in significant amounts. There is some support for the dietary cause from a UK case–control study, and possible routes of infection other than diet are not supported by the accumulated epidemiological data (including case–control study) (Ward *et al.* 2006). This causal explanation does not have absolute proof, but it is beyond reasonable doubt.

The main dietary vehicle remains uncertain, but the main exposure was probably via bovine mechanically recovered meat (MRM) and head meat added to pre-prepared foodstuffs, such as burgers, meat pies, and sausages. It is notable that, in the United Kingdom, MRM was prepared from vertebral columns until the end of 1995. There is evidence that such vertebral columns could have contained significant residual spinal cord and also dorsal root ganglia (both materials containing significantly high infectivity) (Will 1998).

An excess of vCJD cases in the north of the United Kingdom, compared with the south, was first described in 2001 (Cousens *et al.* 2001). The excess appears to have declined over time but still remains, with those living in the north of the United Kingdom in 1991 being about one and a half times more likely to have developed vCJD than those residing in the south (rate ratio = 1.46; 95 per cent CIs: 1.07,2.01). The difference remains when the analysis is adjusted for socio-economic status, urban and rural mix, and population density. Although regional variations in diet might explain these observed differences, results of dietary analyses were inconsistent.

Health risks

The relevant health risks can be considered in two parts: The risk of contracting vCJD from BSE infection in diet and the risk of secondary human-to-human transmission, which is discussed in detail in the subsection on secondary vCJD.

Countries have been classified according to BSE risk status by the WHO, according to their particular incidence of BSE in cattle and their potential exposure from imports originating in BSE-affected countries (www.who.int).

From before the first human cases of BSE were recognized in the United Kingdom (in 1986) to approximately mid 1996, the UK population was exposed to BSE in food containing beef and beef products, and therefore was potentially at risk of vCJD (Anderson *et al.* 1996). Although the United Kingdom has had by far the greatest number of cases of BSE in cattle, other countries have been affected as well, with the Republic of Ireland having the next greatest number of cases, France coming third, and Portugal fourth. To some extent, this has been reflected in the number of cases of vCJD to date; however, the risk to a particular country must reflect imports of bovine material from high-risk countries (particularly the United Kingdom) as well as imports of BSE-affected cattle and intrinsic occurrence of BSE. With all diseases, the number of cases identified must depend on the methods of identification. Testing for BSE in cattle was introduced at different times, and in different ways, in different countries. The numbers of reported cases of BSE in cattle depend in part on whether surveillance is passive or active and the population tested; that is, clinically suspect cases, ill animals, animals discovered dead, or healthy animals slaughtered for human consumption. The European Union introduced new testing rules in January 2001, including the need for post-mortem testing of all apparently healthy cattle over 30 months of age at slaughter for human consumption. The figures for BSE in different countries can be obtained through the World Organization for Animal Health (OIE; www.oie.int). The true figures for BSE in many countries in the past remain subject to doubt; it is clear that numbers rose significantly in a number of EU countries after the introduction of the more comprehensive testing policy in 2001. For example, in Germany, only 6 cases of BSE were reported, all in imports, between 1989 and 2000; in 2000, 7 cases were reported, followed by 125 in 2001. In Italy, only 2 cases were reported between 1989 and 2000 (both in imports); in 2001, 48 cases were reported.

Many public health measures have been implemented to prevent transmission of BSE to humans from the 1980s onwards. These can be separated into those that were put in place in order to prevent onward transmission of BSE in cattle and those that were designed to break the chain of transmission from cattle to humans.

Prevention of onward transmission of BSE in cattle

In the United Kingdom, the ban on the use of ruminant protein in feed to ruminants was introduced in 1988, which was extended to pigs and poultry in 1990. In 1994, additional measures were introduced in the United Kingdom to prevent ruminants being fed any form of mammalian protein (with specific exceptions), and in 1996, it became illegal in the United Kingdom to feed any farmed livestock, including fishes and horses, with mammalian meat and bone meal.

Harmonized EU control measures were introduced in 2001, which included the ban on feeding of processed animal proteins to animals which are kept, fattened, or bred for food production. These control measures together with domestic controls have proved successful in significantly reducing the number of BSE cases across EU member states.

Prevention of dietary transmission to humans

Since 1988, under the UK Compulsory Slaughter and Compensation Scheme, all UK cattle suspected of suffering from BSE are slaughtered and sent for diagnosis. All BSE suspects are then destroyed by incineration. In addition, all adult animals presented for slaughter are inspected by veterinary surgeons to make sure that no suspected cases are slaughtered for human consumption.

Controls have existed since 1989 in the United Kingdom that ban certain tissues (specified risk material [SRM]) from cattle, sheep, and goats from entering the human food chain. Since 1989, the European Commission, in close cooperation with its member states, has taken a series of measures to manage the risk of BSE in the European Union. In 2000, harmonized SRM controls were introduced across all EU member states, and in 2001, EU-wide regulations laying down the rules for the prevention, control, and eradication of certain forms of transmissible spongiform encephalopathy (TSE) were introduced. These controls are enforced by domestic legislation.

In 1997 in the United Kingdom, bone-in-beef and beef bones were excluded from the human food chain to protect the public from BSE infectivity, which the UK Spongiform Encephalopathy Advisory Committee (SEAC) had evidence to link to cattle bones. The continuing decline in the BSE epidemic allowed the ban on retail sales to be lifted towards the end of 1999, although it was retained for manufacturing uses of both bone-in-beef and beef bones.

In the United Kingdom in 2005, a system of BSE testing was introduced for slaughtered cattle aged over 30 months (OTM) intended for human consumption. This system replaced the OTM rule that had been in place in the United Kingdom since 1996, which prohibited the sale of beef for human consumption from OTM cattle.

At the height of the BSE epidemic, there was considerable public concern about BSE and the safety of British meat. The UK Government set up an independent committee (SEAC) of leading experts to ensure that it received the best possible scientific advice surrounding TSEs. The UK Food Standards Agency was also established to protect public health and consumers interests in relation to food. In January 1998, the UK 'BSE Inquiry' was set up to 'establish and review the history of the emergence and identification of BSE and new variant CJD in the United Kingdom, and of the action taken in response to it up to 20 March 1996; to reach conclusions on the adequacy of that response, taking into account the state of knowledge at the time' (www.bseinquiry.gov.uk). Different countries introduced human dietary protection measures at different times. For example, animal CNS material was reportedly still being used in the preparation of certain sausages in Germany in 2000 (Lucker *et al.* 2000). The present EU testing policy identifies infected animals and thereby prevents their entering human food.

The European Commission produced the TSE Roadmap in 2005 (http://ec.europa.eu/food/food/biosafety/bse/roadmap_en.pdf), which provided an outline of possible future changes to EU measures on BSE in the short, medium, and long term. Since 1995, the Commission has generated 70 primary and implementing acts setting out stringent measures to protect animal and human health at the community level. With indications of a favourable trend in the BSE epidemic, the goal for the coming years is to ensure relaxation of measures while assuring that a high level of food safety is maintained. Relaxation of measures is risk-based and aims to reflect advances in technology and evolving scientific knowledge.

Iatrogenic CJD

Background and cause

Evidence from animal studies and from humans shows that efficiency of transmission of prion diseases depends on the type of prion disease (the agent strain), the species barrier, the route of transmission, the dose of infectivity (relating to the tissue involved and the amount of that tissue), and the susceptibility of the 'host'. The concept of agent strain is a complex and controversial matter. For acquired diseases such as BSE, kuru, and vCJD, it is obviously necessary to consider the nature of the infectious agent; for diseases such as sCJD and gCJD, which are considered not to be acquired, the concept is less clear, although some sort of agent is required for their secondary transmission. Although the currently accepted theory is that the agent is based on PrP^{Sc} itself, the agent has not been finally characterized in any form of prion disease. Different strains of agent do exist, as indicated by persistent, reproducible, different biological behaviours, such as incubation period, neuropathological profile, and biochemical properties of the abnormal prion protein (Bruce 2003; Hill *et al.* 1997; Somerville *et al.* 1997; Safar *et al.* 1998). For example, scrapie infection from one source has a specific incubation period and neuropathological lesion profile distinguishable from those of scrapie from another source (Bruce 2003).

Taking BSE as the cause for vCJD, the BSE agent clearly behaves differently in humans, than the agent from sCJD. The basis of this strain variation is not yet understood. The concept of species barrier in prion disease is also incompletely understood. However, it is a commonly observed experimental feature. The ease of transmission from one species to another varies with species; the incubation period may be initially long, with shortening on serial passage in the new species (Bruce 2003). The route of transmission is very important, and there is no doubt that the most successful means overall is the inoculation of brain tissue directly into recipient brain. However, different diseases and/or agents behave differently and the BSE or vCJD agent appears to be relatively readily transmitted via blood through the intravenous route (Hunter *et al.* 2002). Further, different tissue distributions of infectivity are associated with different agents and/or diseases; for example, much greater lymphoreticular involvement exists in vCJD than in other human prion diseases. The world summary of iCJD is given in Table 9.11.2.

Two groups account for the majority of the instances: Human dura mater grafts and cadaver-derived human growth hormone treatments. Abnormal prion protein has been detected in the pituitary gland in both sCJD and vCJD (Peden *et al.* 2004). Case-to-case transmission involving brain to brain has happened rarely: Four instances of transmission related to common surgical instruments used in brain surgery and two cases related to normal usage of depth EEG electrodes. There are just two cases linked to corneal transplantation (Brown *et al.* 2006). There is no known risk of transmission of any form of prion disease by normal contact.

As noted, blood components and blood products have not yet been implicated in the secondary transmission of sCJD or gCJD. Recently, blood components have been shown to be a risk for BSE and vCJD. Animal experiments using sheep with BSE have demonstrated that whole blood transfusion is a relatively efficient means of transmission, including blood from preclinical infected animals (Hunter *et al.* 2002). The much greater involvement of lymphoreticular tissue in vCJD compared with other human prion diseases, especially with its preclinical occurrence, raises greater concerns of vCJD transmission via a wide variety of surgical procedures. The specific issue of secondary vCJD is discussed in the following.

Secondary vCJD

Background

The concern that vCJD might be a greater secondary transmission risk than other prion diseases has been justified by the occurrence of blood-transfusion-associated transmissions (Peden *et al.* 2004; Llewelyn *et al.* 2004; Wroe *et al.* 2006; Health Protection Agency 2007). To date, there has been no transmission of vCJD identified through invasive medical procedures, including dentistry, or through receipt of plasma products. The risk of vCJD secondary transmission depends on four factors: Frequency of infected individuals in the general population, presence of significant infectivity in the relevant tissue, route or mode of potential transmission, and susceptibility of the exposed individual. These four factors are considered in detail as follows.

Population prevalence of variant CJD infection

Such cases have, so far, been very limited in number and, in the United Kingdom, are currently declining in number. Naturally, these data need cautious interpretation: There are likely to be later cases in *PRNP*-129 non-MM individuals and there may be other genetic factors that affect incubation period. In addition, increasing numbers of other countries have reported vCJD cases (Table 9.11.3). At present, the chief concern regarding secondary transmission relates to individuals who are preclinically or subclinically infected. Preclinical infection undoubtedly occurs: There are two reported instances of lymphoreticular involvement prior to disease onset in the appendix (up to 2 years before onset), although one appendix specimen was negative 9 years before onset (Hilton *et al.* 1998). It is assumed that all cases of vCJD resulting from BSE dietary contamination have a potentially long period of clinically silent lymphoreticular and blood infectivity. Recently, the idea that truly subclinical vCJD infection of humans may occur has been considered, with such individuals being a clinically silent source of infection throughout their lifespan. Animal experiments have supported this notion (Bishop *et al.* 2006). Modelling of the present vCJD UK epidemic data also suggests that subclinical infection occurs (Clarke & Ghani 2005).

In addition to the three cases of clinical vCJD transmitted through blood transfusion to date, there has also been one case of vCJD transfusion-transmitted infection without clinical or neuropathological disease reported in the United Kingdom (Peden *et al.* 2004). A patient died from a non-neurological disorder five years after receiving a blood transfusion from a donor who subsequently developed vCJD. Abnormal prion protein was found in the spleen and in a cervical lymph node, but not in the brain or tonsil. The patient was a *PRNP*-129 heterozygote (MV). It is not possible to state whether this represents a truly subclinical infection or someone simply in the preclinical phase, but it proves that vCJD infection is not confined to the *PRNP*-129 methionine homozygous (MM) genotype.

Various methods of determining the prevalence of vCJD infection in the UK population have been carried out or are underway. These include the following:

Retrospective Tonsil and Appendix Study: A study examining routine surgical appendix and tonsil paraffin-embedded blocks from 1995–99 in two centres in the United Kingdom which estimated the total population prevalence of vCJD infection to be 3808 (or 237 per million) in those aged 10–30 years, with wide 95 per cent confidence intervals of 785–11 128 (or 49–692 per million) (Hilton *et al.* 2004). However, this study had recognized limitations (relative small size, only two regions in the United Kingdom, and use of fixed specimens); therefore, the UK National Anonymous Tonsil Archive was established.

UK National Anonymous Tonsil Archive: The aim of this is to establish an unlinked, anonymous archive of routine surgical tonsil specimens, from 100 000 individuals, using what would have otherwise been discarded. A further 3000 tonsil pairs are included from the National Prion Unit, London. Patients are informed of the study preoperatively and given the opportunity to opt out of the study on the routine operation consent form. The UK Health Protection Agency coordinates the study. However, the majority of the tonsillectomies are performed in those under 25 years of age and many of these individuals should have been protected by dietary measures implemented in the 1990s. Therefore, a study that will give more information regarding prevalence in the older population is being established: The UK Post-Mortem Archive.

UK Post-Mortem Archive: This is in the process of being considered in the United Kingdom. It is envisaged that relatives of people referred to the coroner (or equivalent regional official) will be asked to give consent to allow a specimen to be taken from the spleen, in the first instance, and the brain to test for abnormal prion protein. The study would be coordinated by the UK Health Protection Agency and aims to collect over 100 000 specimens, with the majority in the over-65-years age group.

Switzerland has established a cross-sectional, linked anonymous prevalence study in an attempt to determine the population prevalence of vCJD (Glatzel *et al.* 2003b). Tissues used are those obtained from tonsillectomies and autopsies.

Tissue infectivity distribution

In vCJD, the greatest levels of infectivity are found in CNS tissues, but lymphoreticular tissues contain significant levels. Other tissues contain either generally lower levels still or undetectable amounts. The most comprehensive summary of tissue infectivities has been produced by the WHO (2006).

Route of exposure

In general, the evidence, from both animal experiments and human occurrences of secondary transmission, indicates that the direct introduction of infection into the brain is the most efficient transmission route, with the shortest incubation periods. However, other routes are also clearly effective, as indicated by iatrogenic cases resulting from eye surgery and intramuscular injection of human growth hormone. In addition, the intravenous route is a relatively efficient means of infection, as shown in transfusion experiments with BSE-infected sheep and the occurrence of cases of human vCJD following blood transfusion.

Susceptibility of the exposed individual

The only definitively identified susceptibility factor is that of the *PRNP*-129 genotype, as discussed earlier. However, there may be other genetic susceptibility factors.

It is notable that the age of onset of vCJD in the United Kingdom has not changed over the epidemic period. This could suggest that susceptibility to dietary infection is age-related; there is no definitive proof of an age-related susceptibility, and if it exists, its basis is not known (Clarke & Ghani 2005). However, there are known age-related changes in gut-associated lymphoid tissue and these could be relevant. Further, there is no evidence presently to indicate that other modes of infection (e.g. blood transfusion transmission of vCJD) are affected by age at exposure.

An additional important factor in determining the scale of the public health threat from secondary transmission of CJD is to ascertain whether a self-sustaining secondary epidemic is likely. Two studies have modelled data in order to estimate whether blood transfusions could result in a self-sustaining epidemic of vCJD. The first showed that although self-sustaining epidemics were possible (basic reproductive number $R_0 > 1$), they were unlikely when only biologically plausible scenarios, in which the mean incubation period for transfusion-acquired vCJD cases was shorter or similar to that for primary (foodborne), were considered. In addition, public health interventions (leucodepletion and the ban on previously transfused donors; for details, see the next subsection) were likely to be effective (Clarke & Ghani 2005). The second model predicted that vCJD could not become endemic by transfusion alone (Dietz *et al.* 2007). Modelling of the risk of surgical transmission of vCJD demonstrated that self-sustaining epidemics were possible. Key factors determining the scale of such epidemics were the number of times a single instrument was re-used, together with the infectivity of contaminated instruments and the effectiveness of cleaning those instruments (Garske *et al.* 2006).

Public health measures to reduce secondary transmission of CJD

Invasive medical procedures, including surgery and dentistry

In 1998, the UK TSE Working Group of the Advisory Committee in Dangerous Pathogens and the Spongiform Encephalopathy Advisory Committee revised the guidance on the decontamination of instruments and handling of patients known to have CJD, or to be suspect cases of CJD or to be 'at risk' of CJD (www.advisorybodies.doh.gov.uk/acdp/tseguidance/Index.htm). The guidance covers potential exposure in the wider health-care setting, focusing on surgical transmission but including guidance to laboratory staff and mortuary attendants. It is updated online as new advice becomes available.

In addition, prompted by concerns of the theoretical risk of surgical transmission of vCJD in the United Kingdom, the National Decontamination Programme was launched in 1999 to support the NHS (in England) in improving and maintaining standards related to the re-processing of surgical instruments. The key areas of work included development of a national decontamination training scheme, provision of technical advice and guidance, and establishment of a standard output specification (www.dh.gov.uk/en/Policyandguidance/Organisationpolicy/Estatesandfacilitiesmanagement/EngineeringEnvironmentAndTechnology/DH_4118225). In 2005, ESAC-Pr (Engineering and Science Advisory Committee, for the decontamination of surgical instruments including prion removal) was formed, which aims to take forward the practical application of relevant research in the area of decontamination in relation to prion removal and deactivation (www.dh.gov.uk/en/Publicationsandstatistics/Publications/PublicationsPolicyAndGuidance/DH_072443). In the United Kingdom in 2006, the National Institute for Health and Clinical Excellence (NICE) published guidance to further reduce risk of transmission of CJD via surgery, in particular surgery involving high-risk tissues (neurosurgery and posterior ophthalmic procedures) and through neuroendoscopy.

A wholesale move to single-use instruments has not been advocated by NICE or ESAC-Pr. Apart from taking into account their cost, the question of instrument quality is paramount. In England, postoperative haemorrhage following the introduction of single-use instruments for tonsillectomy in 2001 resulted in the reversal of this recommendation shortly afterward. However, in Scotland, where significant complications were not seen, single-use instruments have been recommended for tonsillectomy since 2001, and for dental root canal treatment since 2005. Other countries in the European Union, as well as worldwide, have performed their own risk assessments and implemented various measures accordingly.

Blood, organs, and tissues

As knowledge and potential evidence of the transmission of CJD through blood and plasma product transfusion and organ and tissue transplantation has increased, various public health measures have been implemented in the United Kingdom in an attempt to reduce this likelihood (Table 9.11.5). Countries outside the United Kingdom, including the United States, Canada, New Zealand, Australia, Hong Kong, and several European countries including Germany, Switzerland, Austria, and the Republic of Ireland, have taken the precautionary step of excluding blood donors who have spent more than a defined period in the United Kingdom between 1980 and 1996.

Blood screening tests

There are currently a number of potential tests in development. Most of these are based on the detection of PrP^{Sc} in blood, as a marker of infectivity. Such tests could have a variety of uses: Diagnostic testing of symptomatic cases, individual presymptomatic diagnosis, population studies to determine the number of

Table 9.11.5 Public health measures implemented in the UK in order to reduce the likelihood of transmission of CJD through blood and plasma product transfusion and organ and tissue transplantation

◆ Withdrawal and recall of any blood components, plasma derivatives, cells, or tissues obtained from any individual who later develops vCJD (December 1997).
◆ Importation of plasma from countries other than the UK for fractionation to manufacture plasma derivatives (fully implemented in October 1999).
◆ Leucodepletion of all blood components (fully implemented in Autumn 1999).
◆ Importation of clinical fresh frozen plasma for patients born after January 1996 (fully implemented in June 2004). Extended to all patients under the age of 16 (July 2005).
◆ Exclusion of whole blood donors who state that they have received a blood component transfusion in the UK since 1st January 1980 (April 2004). Extended to whole blood and apheresis donors who may have received a blood component transfusion in the UK since 1st January 1980 (August 2004) and to any donors who have been treated with UK plasma-derived, intravenous immunoglobulin or have undergone plasma exchange. Extended to those who may have received a blood component transfusion anywhere in the world since 1 January 1980 (November 2005).
◆ Exclusion of live bone donors who have been transfused since 1 January 1980 (July 2005).
◆ Exclusion of blood donors whose blood has been transfused to recipients who later developed vCJD, where blood transfusion cannot be excluded as a source of the vCJD infection and where no infected donor has been identified (July 2005).
◆ Promotion of appropriate use of blood and tissues products and alternatives throughout the National Health Service.

infected individuals, and screening of blood donations for infection. Presently, it is the last of these that is the main driver behind test development. Although the introduction of a screening test for blood has obvious public health advantages (in line with those that have come from screening for HIV, hepatitis C, etc.), there are a number of potential problems, even leaving aside the technical difficulties of detecting a small amount of PrP^{Sc} in the complex matrix of blood that contains normal PrP^{C}. Firstly, the sensitivity of the current potential tests will be defined according to their detection target (as indicated, mostly PrP^{Sc}); this is an indirect measure of infectivity. Secondly, specificity will be difficult to determine; if a positive result is obtained in a normal, healthy individual, it is difficult to know how its significance can be easily and quickly determined. Finally, if the number of infected individuals in the population is relatively small, even a test with high sensitivity and specificity would generate a large number of false-positive results; the management of such individuals would need careful consideration.

CJD Incidents Panel

Many countries throughout the world have assessed the risk to their citizens in relation to the iatrogenic transmission of CJD, especially in view of vCJD. Based on the perceived risk, different actions have been implemented in different countries in an attempt to reduce the risk of onward transmission of CJD.

In 2000, the UK Chief Medical Officers established an expert committee—the CJD Incidents Panel. Its secretariat is provided by the Health Protection Agency on behalf of the Department of Health (http://www.hpa.org.uk/webw/HPAweb&Page&HPAwebAutoListName/Page/1204031511121?p=1204031511121). Incidents involve the potential transmission of CJD between patients through invasive medical procedures, including surgery, blood donations, and organ and tissue donations. Incidents occur when patients diagnosed with (or suspected of having) CJD, or patients identified as 'at risk' of CJD, have undergone invasive medical procedures that may have put other patients at risk.

Patients diagnosed with CJD, or those suspected of having CJD, are referred by the local clinician caring for the patient to the local Consultant in Communicable Disease Control (CCDC) using a standardized format (http://www.cjd.ed.ac.uk/guidance.htm). The CCDC gathers a full invasive medical history with the collaboration of the patient's general practitioner and refers the patient to the CJD Incidents Panel.

Action is decided upon with regards to instruments in surgical incidents and potential 'contacts' who may have been put at risk. This depends on the type of tissue involved (high, medium, or low risk), the type of operation (if surgical), when the incident occurred in relation to the incubation period, and whether 'contacts', who have been put at risk, are traceable via medical records. The CJD Incidents Panel considers individual incidents when there has been no similar incident previously for which a precedent for action has been set. Surgical instruments are quarantined and returned to medical use, destroyed, or given for research purposes.

Designation of groups 'at risk' of CJD

In the United Kingdom, the CJD Incidents Panel advises contacting patients who have been put at additional risk (to that through diet of the background population resident in the United Kingdom between 1980 and 1996) of CJD, of at least 1 per cent through exposure in an incident. Patients are told that they should take certain public health measures to prevent CJD from being spread to other patients. The risk assessment models used to derive this threshold were highly precautionary and based on a number of scientific assumptions and uncertainty. The 1 per cent threshold is seen as a public health tool and not to be used to advise individuals their exact risk of developing CJD.

Table 9.11.6 is a summary of the groups of individuals who are designated 'at risk' of CJD in the United Kingdom, at time of print. In comparison with those who have been informed that they are 'at risk' of CJD through surgery, those 'at risk' of CJD through blood and plasma product incidents are the largest group to date. Plasma product recipients, mainly haemophiliacs treated with Factor VIII,

Table 9.11.6 Groups considered 'at risk' of CJD in the United Kingdom

Surgery related:
◆ Those undergoing high- or medium-risk procedures following a case of CJD.
Transfusion related (variant only):
◆ 'Implicated' red blood cell recipients
◆ 'Implicated' plasma product recipients
◆ Red blood cell donors to cases of vCJD
◆ Other blood component recipients from donors to vCJD cases
At risk of familial forms:
◆ Two or more blood relatives affected by CJD or prion disease, or known genetic mutation in relatives or known genetic mutation in themselves.
Recipients of hormone derived from human pituitary:
◆ Growth hormone and gonadotrophin
Recipients of dura mater grafts:
◆ Those who underwent neurosurgery or operation for tumour or cyst of spine before August 1992

are by far the largest individual group 'at risk' so far. In addition, groups such as those at risk of genetic forms of CJD and recipients of human pituitary-derived growth hormones, have also been designated 'at risk' of CJD. Table 9.11.7 outlines the advice given to those designated 'at risk' of CJD in the United Kingdom.

At present, there are no routine screening tests, for example, on blood, or prophylactic treatments available for those 'at risk' of CJD. If they are developed in the coming years, they will be offered to those at risk if appropriate.

Guidance of the TSE Working Group of the Advisory Committee in Dangerous Pathogens and the Spongiform Encephalopathy Advisory Committee advises as to what precautions should be taken when caring for those 'at risk' of CJD in the health-care setting (www.advisorybodies.doh.gov.uk/acdp/tseguidance/Index.htm).

It is imperative that those designated 'at risk' are followed up for public health and research purposes. In the United Kingdom, the Health Protection Agency is coordinating two different research proposals: The first to look at the psychological and social effects of being put in an 'at risk' of CJD group and the second following up those 'at risk' of CJD over time. Ethical approval has been granted and studies have commenced.

Conclusion

Prion diseases have led to a number of public health concerns and actions, despite their general rarity. Fortunately, the number of cases of vCJD due to dietary BSE contamination is likely to be limited, but concerns remain about possible secondary transmission via blood and surgical instruments. The magnitude of this risk depends on the prevalence of preclinical or subclinical BSE or vCJD infection in the United Kingdom and other populations. A number of important public health protective measures are in place. The cause of sCJD remains uncertain. Iatrogenic transmission of sCJD is uncommon, with most cases relating to the use of cadaver-derived human growth hormone and human dura mater grafts, both of which are now avoided. The difficulties of accidental transmission of prion diseases are increased by their long incubation period (when acquired), the uncertain nature of the prion agent, the lack of direct methods of detecting the agent or infectivity, and the unusual resistance of the infection to the usual sterilization methods employed in health services.

Table 9.11.7 Advice for those designated 'at risk' of CJD in the United Kingdom

◆ Not to donate blood, organs, or tissues
◆ To tell the doctor, dentist, or nurse in charge of their care whenever they are going to have surgery or invasive medical procedures that they are in an 'at-risk' group for CJD
◆ To tell their family in case they require emergency surgery

Summary

- All prion diseases are potentially transmissible, even if the original cause is not an infection.
- The prion agent is not fully characterized; there are no simple direct methods of detecting the agent and its infectivity.
- Infectivity is resistant to many standard methods of inactivation.
- There are no simple, non-invasive, absolute diagnostic tests for human prion diseases, but experienced clinicians can achieve relatively secure clinical diagnosis in the majority of the cases.
- Many public health measures are in place in many countries; these should limit the risk of transmission from animal to man and man to man.

References

Alperovitch A., Will R.G. Predicting the size of the vCJD epidemic in France. *Comptes Rendus Biologies* 2002;**325**:33–6.

Anderson R.M., Donnelly C.A., Ferguson N.M. *et al.* Transmission dynamics and epidemiology of BSE in British cattle. *Nature* 1996;**382**:779–88.

Arakawa K., Nagara H., Itoyama Y. *et al.* Clustering of 3 cases of Creutzfeldt-Jakob disease near Fukuoka City, Japan. *Acta Neurologica Scandinavia* 1991;**84**(5):445–7.

Bishop M.T., Hart P., Aitchison L. *et al.* Predicting susceptibility and incubation time of human to human transmission of vCJD. *Lancet Neurology* 2006;**5**:393–8.

Blanquet-Grossard F., Sazdovitch V., Jean A. *et al.* Prion protein is not detectable in dental pulp from patients with Creutzfeldt-Jakob disease. *Journal of Dental Research* 2000;**79**(2):700.

Bobowick A.R., Brody J.A., Matthews M.R. *et al.* Creutzfeldt-Jakob disease: a case-control study. *American Journal of Epidemiology* 1973; **98**:381–94.

Boesenberger C., Schulz-Schaeffer W., Meissner B. *et al.* Clinical course in young patients with sporadic Creutzfeldt-Jakob disease. *Annals of Neurology* 2005;**58**:533–43.

Brandel J-P, Preece M., Brown P. *et al.* Distribution of codon 129 genotype in human growth hormone-treated CJD patients in France and the UK. *Lancet* 2003;**362**:128–30.

Brown P., Brandel J-P, Preece M. *et al.* Iatrogenic Creutzfeldt-Jakob disease: the waning of an era. *Neurology* 2006;**67**:389–93.

Brown P., Galvez S., Goldfarb L.G. *et al.* Familial Creutzfeldt-Jakob disease in Chile is associated with the codon 200 mutation of the PRNP amyloid precursor gene on chromosome 20. *Journal of the Neurological Sciences* 1992;**112**:65–7.

Brown P., Gibbs C.J., Jr., Rodgers-Johnson P. *et al.* Human spongiform encephalopathy: the National Institutes of Health series of 300 cases of experimentally transmitted disease. *Annals of Neurology* 1994;**35**:513–29.

Brown P., Preece M., Brandel J.P. *et al.* Iatrogenic Creutzfeldt-Jakob disease at the millennium. *Neurology* 2000;**55**:1075–81.

Bruce M.E., Will R.G., Ironside J.W. *et al.* Transmissions to mice indicate that 'new variant' CJD is caused by the BSE agent. *Nature* 1997;**389**:498–501.

Bruce M.E. TSE strain variation. *British Medical Bulletin* 2003;**66**:99–108.

Cervenakova L., Goldfarb L.G., Garruto R. *et al.* Phenotype-genotype studies in kuru: implications for new variant Creutzfeldt-Jakob disease (nvCJD). *Proceedings of the National Academy of Sciences USA* 1998;**95**:13239–41.

Clarke P., Ghani A.C. Projections of the future course of the primary vCJD epidemic in the UK: inclusion of subclinical infection and the possibility of wider genetic susceptibility. *Journal of the Royal Society Interface* 2005;**2**:19–31.

Collie D.A., Summers D.M., Sellar R.J. *et al.* Diagnosing variant Creutzfeldt-Jakob disease with the pulvinar sign: MR imaging findings in 86 neuropathologically confirmed cases. *American Journal of Neuroradiology* 2003;**24**:1560–9.

Collins S., Boyd A., Fletcher A. *et al.* Creutzfeldt-Jakob disease cluster in an Australian rural city. *Annals of Neurology* 2002;**52**(1):115–8.

Collins S., Law M.G., Fletcher A. *et al.* Surgical treatment and risk of sporadic Creutzfeldt-Jakob disease: a case-control study. *Lancet* 1999;**353**:693–7.

Cooper S.A., Murray K.L., Heath C.A. *et al.* Isolated visual symptoms at onset in sporadic Creutzfeldt-Jakob disease: the clinical phenotype of the 'Heidenhain variant'. *British Journal of Ophthalmology* 2005;**89**:1341–2.

Cooper S.A., Murray K.L., Heath C.A. *et al.* Sporadic Creutzfeldt-Jakob disease with cerebellar ataxia at onset in the United Kingdom. *JNNP* 2006;**77**:1273–5.

Cousens S., Smith P.G., Ward H. *et al.* Geographical distribution of variant Creutzfeldt-Jakob disease in Great Britain, 1994–2000. *Lancet* 2001;**357**:1002–7.

Cousens S.N., Harries-Jones R., Knight R. *et al.* Geographical distribution of cases of Creutzfeldt-Jakob disease in England and Wales, 1970–84. *Journal of Neurology, Neurosurgery, and Psychiatry* 1990;**53**:459–65.

Cousens S.N., Vynnycky E., Zeidler M. *et al.* Predicting the CJD epidemic in humans. *Nature* 1997;**385**:197–8.

Davanipour Z., Alter M., Sobel E. *et al.* A case-control study of Creutzfeldt-Jakob disease: dietary risk factors. *American Journal of Epidemiology* 1985;**122**:443–51.

DeArmond S.J., Ironside J.W., Bouzamondo-Bernstein E. *et al.* Neuropathology of prion diseases. In: Prusiner SB, editor. *Prion biology and diseases*. New York (NY): Cold Spring Harbour Laboratory Press; 2004. p. 777–856.

Dietz K., Raddatz G., Wallis J. *et al.* Blood transfusion and spread of variant Creutzfeldt-Jakob disease. *Emerging Infectious Diseases* 2007;**13**(1):89–96.

Farmer P.M., Kane W.C., Hollenberg-Sher J. Incidence of Creutzfeldt-Jakob disease in Brooklyn and Staten Island. *New England Journal of Medicine* 1978;**298**:283–4.

Garske T., Ward H.J.T., Clarke P. *et al.* Factors determining the potential for onward transmission of variant Creutzfeldt-Jakob disease via surgical instruments. *Journal of the Royal Society Interface* 2006;**3**:757–66.

Glatzel M., Abela E., Maissen M. *et al.* Extra neural pathologic prion protein in sporadic Creutzfeldt-Jakob disease. *New England Journal of Medicine* 2003a;**349**:1812–20.

Glatzel M., Ott P.M., Linder T. *et al.* Human prion diseases: epidemiology and integrated risk assessment. *Lancet Neurology* 2003b;**2**:757–63.

Green A., Sanchez-Juan P., Ladogana A. *et al.* CSF analysis in patients with sporadic CJD and other transmissible spongiform encephalopathies. *European Journal of Neurology* 2006;**14**:121–4.

Harries-Jones R., Knight R., Will R.G. *et al.* Creutzfeldt-Jakob disease in England and Wales, 1980–1984: a case-control study of potential risk factors. *Journal of Neurology, Neurosurgery, and Psychiatry* 1988;**51**:1113–9.

Head M.W., Bunn T.J.R., Bishop M.T. *et al.* Prion protein heterogeneity in sporadic but not variant Creutzfeldt-Jakob disease: UK cases, 1991–2002. *Annals of Neurology* 2004;**55**:851–9.

Health Protection Agency. Fourth case of transfusion-associated variant-CJD. Health Protection Report 2007;1(3).

Hill A.F., Butterworth R.J., Joiner S. *et al.* Investigation of variant Creutzfeldt-Jakob disease and other human prion diseases with tonsil biopsy samples. *Lancet* 1999;**353**:183–4.

Hill A.F., Desbruslais M., Joiner S. *et al.* The same prion strain causes vCJD and BSE. *Nature* 1997;**389**:448–50.

Hilton D.A., Fathers E., Edwards P. *et al.* Prion immunoreactivity in appendix before clinical onset of variant Creutzfeldt-Jakob disease. *Lancet* 1998;**352**(9129):703–4.

Hilton D.A., Ghani A.C., Conyers L. *et al.* Prevalence of lymphoreticular prion protein accumulation in UK tissue samples. *Journal of Pathology* 2004;**203**:733–9.

Huillard d'Aignaux J., Cousens S.N., Delasnerie-Laupretre N. *et al.* Analysis of the geographical distribution of sporadic Creutzfeldt-Jakob disease in France between 1992 and 1998. *International Journal of Epidemiology* 2002b;**31**:490–5.

Huillard d'Aignaux J., Cousens S.N., Maccario J. *et al.* The incubation period of kuru. *Epidemiology* 2002a;**13**:402–8.

Hunter N., Foster J., Chong A. *et al.* Transmission of prion diseases by blood transfusion. *Journal of General Virology* 2002;**83**:2897–905.

Ironside J.W., Hilton D.A., Ghani A. *et al.* Retrospective study of prion-protein accumulation in tonsil and appendix tissues. *Lancet* 2000;**355**:1693–4.

Kahana E., Alter M., Braham J. *et al.* Creutzfeldt-Jakob disease: focus among Libyan Jews in Israel. *Science* 1974;**183**:90–1.

Knight R. The relationship between new variant Creutzfeldt-Jakob disease and bovine spongiform encephalopathy. *Vox Sanguinis* 1999;**76**:203–8.

Kondo K., Kuroiwa Y. A case-control study of Creutzfeldt-Jakob disease: association with physical injuries. *Annals of Neurology* 1982;**11**:377–81.

Kovacs G.G., Puopolo M., Ladogana A. *et al.* Genetic prion disease: the EUROCJD experience. *Human Genetics* 2005;**118**:166–74.

Kovacs G.G., Trabattoni G., Hainfellner J.A. *et al.* Mutations of the prion protein gene: phenotypic spectrum. *Journal of Neurology* 2002; **249**:567–1582.

Ladogana A., Puopolo M., Croes E.A. *et al.* Mortality from Creutzfeldt-Jakob disease and related disorders in Europe, Australia, and Canada. *Neurology* 2005;**64**:1586–91.

Lee H-S, Sambuughin N., Cervenakova L. *et al.* Ancestral origins and worldwide distribution of the PRNP 200K mutation causing familial Creutzfeldt-Jakob disease. *American Journal of Human Genetics* 1999;**64**:1063–70.

Linsell L., Cousens S.N., Smith P.G. *et al.* A case-control study of sporadic Creutzfeldt-Jakob disease in the United Kingdom: analysis of clustering. *Neurology* 2004;**63**:2077–83.

Llewelyn C.A., Hewitt P.A., Knight R.S.G. *et al.* Possible transmission of variant Creutzfeldt-Jakob disease by blood transfusion. *Lancet* 2004;**363**:417–21.

Lucker E.H., Eigenbrodt E., Wenisch S. *et al.* Identification of central nervous system tissue in retain meat products. *Journal of Food Protection* 2000;**63**:258–63.

Matthews W.B. Epidemiology of Creutzfeldt-Jakob disease in England and Wales. *Journal of Neurology, Neurosurgery, and Psychiatry* 1975;**38**:210–13.

Nurmi M.H., Bishop M., Strain L. *et al.* The normal population distribution of PRNP codon 129 polymorphism. *Acta Neurologica Scandinavica* 2003;**108**:374–8.

Parchi P., Castellani R., Capellari S. *et al.* Molecular basis of phenotypic variability in sporadic Creutzfeldt-Jakob disease. *Annals of Neurology* 1996;**39**:767–78.

Parchi P., Giese A., Capellari S. *et al.* Classification of sporadic Creutzfeldt-Jakob disease based on molecular and phenotypic analysis of 300 subjects. *Annals of Neurology* 1999;**46**:224–33.

Peden A.H., Head M.W., Ritchie D.L. *et al.* Preclinical vCJD after blood transfusion in a PRNP codon 129 heterozygous patient. *Lancet* 2004;**364**:527–9.

Pocchiari M., Puopolo M., Croes E.A. *et al.* Predictors of survival in sporadic Creutzfeldt-Jakob disease and other human transmissible spongiform encephalopathies. *Brain* 2004;**127**:2348–59.

Prusiner S.B., editor. An introduction to prion biology and diseases. *Prion biology and diseases*. New York (NY): Cold Spring Harbour Laboratory Press; 2004a. pp. 1–87.

Prusiner S.B. Development of the prion concept. In: Prusiner SB, editor. *Prion biology and diseases*. New York (NY): Cold Spring Harbour Laboratory Press; 2004b. pp. 89–141

Safar J., Wille H., Itri V. *et al.* Eight prion strains have PrP^{Sc} molecules with different conformations. *Nature Medicine* 1998;**4**:1157–65.

Shibuya S., Higuchi J., Shin R-W *et al.* Protective prion protein polymorphisms against sporadic Creutzfeldt-Jakob disease. *Lancet* 1998;**351**:419.

Somerville R.A., Chong A., Mulqueen O.U. *et al.* Biochemical typing of scrapie strains. *Nature* 1997;**386**:564.

Spencer M.D., Knight R.S.G., Will R.G. First hundred cases of variant Creutzfeldt-Jakob disease: retrospective case note review of early psychiatric and neurological features. *British Medical Journal* 2002;**324**:1479–82.

Spudich S., Mastrianni J.A., Wrensch M. *et al.* Complete penetrance of Creutzfeldt-Jakob disease in Libyan Jews carrying the E200K mutation in the prion protein gene. *Molecular Medicine* 1995;**1**:607–13.

Van Duijn C.M., Delasnerie-Laupretre N., Masullo C. *et al.* Case-control study of risk factors of Creutzfeldt-Jakob disease in Europe during 1993–95. *Lancet* 1998;**351**:1081–85.

Ward H.J.T., Everington D., Cousens S.N. *et al.* Risk factors for variant Creutzfeldt-Jakob disease: a case-control study. *Annals of Neurology* 2006;**59**:111–20.

Ward H.J.T., Everington D., Croes E.A. *et al.* Sporadic Creutzfeldt-Jakob disease and surgery: a case-control study using community controls. *Neurology* 2002;**59**:543–8.

Wientjens D.P.W.M., Davanipour Z., Hofman A. *et al.* Risk factors for Creutzfeldt-Jakob disease: a reanalysis of case-control studies. *Neurology* 1996;**46**:1287–91.

Will R.G., Alpers M.P., Dormont D. *et al.* Infectious and sporadic prion diseases. In: Prusiner SB, editor. *Prion biology and diseases*. New York (NY): Cold Spring Harbor Laboratory Press; 2004. p. 629–671

Will R.G., Ironside J.W., Zeidler M. *et al.* A new variant of Creutzfeldt-Jakob disease in the UK. *Lancet* 1996;**347**:921–5.

Will R.G., Matthews W.B., Smith P.G. *et al.* A retrospective study of Creutzfeldt-Jakob disease in England and Wales 1970–1979 II: epidemiology. *Journal of Neurology, Neurosurgery, and Psychiatry* 1986;**49**:749–55.

Will R.G., Matthews W.B. Evidence for case-to-case transmission of Creutzfeldt-Jakob disease. *Journal of Neurology, Neurosurgery, and Psychiatry* 1982;**45**:235–8.

Will R.G. New variant Creutzfeldt-Jakob disease. *The Darlington Postgraduate Journal* 1998;**17**(1):35–42.

Wilson K., Code C., Ricketts M.N. Risk of acquiring Creutzfeldt-Jakob disease from blood transfusions: systematic review of case-control studies. *British Medical Journal* 2000;**321**:17–9.

World Health Organization. Guidelines on tissue infectivity distribution in transmissible spongiform encephalopathies. Geneva: World Health Organization; 2006. pp. 1–61.

World Health Organization. Manual for strengthening diagnosis and surveillance of Creutzfeldt-Jakob disease. Geneva: World Health Organization; 1998. pp. 1–75.

World Health Organization. The revision of the surveillance case definition for variant Creutzfeldt-Jakob disease (vCJD). Geneva: World Health Organization; 2002. pp. 1–30.

Wroe S.J., Pal S., Siddique D. *et al.* Clinical presentation and pre-mortem diagnosis of variant Creutzfeldt-Jakob disease associated with blood transfusion: a case report. *Lancet* 2006;**368**:2061–7.

Zerr I., Brandel J.P., Masullo C. *et al.* European surveillance on Creutzfeldt-Jakob disease: a case-control study for medical risk factors. *Journal of Clinical Epidemiology* 2000;**53**:747–54.

9.12

Sexually transmitted infections

Mary L. Kamb and John M. Douglas, Jr.

Sexually transmitted infections (STI) are among the world's most common diseases. More than 20 organisms and at least as many syndromes are recognized as being transmissible through vaginal, anal, or oral sex, including human immunodeficiency virus infection (HIV), discussed separately in Chapter 9.13 (Table 9.13.1). Globally, annual incidence of bacterial STI is exceeded only by diarrhoeal diseases, malaria, and lower respiratory infections (World Health Organization 2007). In the United States, two bacterial STI, chlamydia and gonorrhoea, are the first and second most commonly reported of all notifiable diseases (CDC 2006). Even so, the burden of bacterial STI is small when compared to that of viral STI such as human papillomavirus (HPV) and herpes simplex virus-2 (HSV-2), the former leading to persistent long-term infection in many and the latter resulting in lifelong infection in all those infected.

Given the high burden of STI, it is not surprising to find that regardless of a nation's resources, STI symptoms rank among the top five disease categories for which adults seek health-care services (Dallabetta *et al.* 2007). It is less well-recognized that STI are associated with substantial public health costs because of their profound effects on reproductive health outcomes, causation of a variety of malignancies, and the role they play in enhancing HIV transmission (Over & Piot 1996; World Health Organization 2007). In developing nations, STI are among the most important causes of years of healthy productive life lost overall (Over & Piot 1993, 1996), and for women of reproductive age, STI-associated disability adjusted life years lost is exceeded only by pregnancy-associated maternal morbidity and HIV (World Bank 2003). While overall STI disease burden is most prominent in adolescents and young adults, the most serious adverse health consequences, including adverse pregnancy outcomes and STI-associated cancers, are borne primarily by women and infants. For nations with high STI prevalence, prevention and control of these infections is a critical and cost-effective investment in preventing many of the most important long-term health consequences (World Health Organization 2007).

Since the licensure of the first STI vaccine, against hepatitis B virus (HBV) 25 years ago, a number of important advances have occurred in the field of STI. First, safe and effective vaccines are now available for two STI, including HPV as well as HBV (World Health Organization 2007; Munoz *et al.* 2003; Szmuness *et al.* 1980; Villa *et al.* 2005; CDC 2007; Koutsky *et al.* 2002; Harper *et al.* 2004; Schmiedeskamp & Kockler 2006; CDC 2006). Thus, an opportunity now exists to prevent the two viruses that account for most of the world's STI-related cancer burden (Pisani *et al.* 1999), although widespread programmatic implementation of HBV vaccine for infants is still limited in many countries and discussions about best ways to roll out HPV vaccines in pre-adolescents are just beginning for HPV vaccines (World Health Organization 2007). Second, since the early 1990s, with the World Health Organization's (WHO) recommendation that low-income countries use locally validated syndromic approaches for STI diagnosis and treatment, the prevalence of bacterial causes of genital ulcer disease and neonatal conjunctivitis have been observed to decline markedly in several low-income settings in Africa (World Health Organization 2007). Third, with the adoption of national screening policies for asymptomatic STI with serious adverse sequelae (e.g. antenatal syphilis screening, gonorrhoea and chlamydia screening for young women, cervical cancer screening) many nations have substantially reduced associated morbidity and mortality (World Health Organization 2007; Berman & Kamb 2007). Fourth, several fairly effective behaviour change approaches have been identified and effectively implemented among high-risk populations in health facilities and community settings (Greenberg *et al.* 1998; Kamb *et al.* 1998; Manhart & Holmes 2005; Fenton & Bloom 2007; McFarlane & Bull 2007; Vega & Ghanem 2007), although, again, these have not been widely implemented in most areas. Fifth, improved methods for contacting, counselling, and treating sex partners have been proven to reduce re-infections (Golden *et al.* 2005; Du *et al.* 2006; White *et al.* 2005; Passin *et al.* 2006; Brewer 2005; Hogben *et al.* 2007; Trelle *et al.* 2007). Sixth, better and more acceptable targeted interventions have been developed for highly affected, hard-to-reach populations who—through an improved understanding of STI transmission dynamics—are recognized in certain settings to contribute importantly to spread of infection into the general community (Dallabetta *et al.* 2007; World Health Organization 2007; Berman & Kamb 2007; Greenberg *et al.* 1998; Manhart & Holmes 2005; Fenton & Bloom 2007; Sanchez *et al.* 2003; Levine *et al.* 1998; Laga *et al.* 1994; Fleming & Wasserheit 1999; CDC 2001). Finally, aside from the interventions themselves, more efficient and affordable methods have been identified to assess STI health burden, implement STI prevention and control programmes and to evaluate their effects (World Bank 2003; Hassig *et al.* 1996).

Table 9.12.1 Sexually transmitted pathogens and associated diseases or syndromes

Pathogen	Associated disease or syndrome
Bacteria	
Neisseria gonorrhoeae	Cervicitis, urethritis, proctitis, pharyngitis, Bartholinitis, endometritis, pelvic inflammatory disease (PID), infertility, chronic pelvic pain, orchitis, epididymitis, urethral stricture, prostatitis, perihepatitis, disseminated infection, Reiter's syndrome; enhanced HIV risk; asymptomatic in up to 2/3 (women) and 1/3 (men) of cases. *Maternal:* Ectopic pregnancy, maternal death, preterm rupture of membranes; *Infant:* Neonatal conjunctivitis, corneal scarring, blindness, premature birth, low birth weight
Chlamydia trachomatis	Cervicitis, urethritis, proctitis, pharyngitis, Bartholinitis, endometritis, PID, infertility, chronic pelvic pain, orchitis, epididymitis, urethral stricture, prostatitis, perihepatitis, disseminated infection, Reiter's syndrome; lymphogranuloma venereum (LGV)—anogenital ulcer or inguinal swelling; enhanced HIV risk; asymptomatic in up to 2/3 (women) and 1/3 (men) of cases *Maternal:* Ectopic pregnancy, maternal death, preterm rupture of membranes; *Infant:* Neonatal conjunctivitus, pneumonia, premature birth, low birth weight
Mycoplasma hominis	Postpartum fever, PID
Mycoplasma genitalium	Urethritis, cervicitis; PID, enhanced HIV risk
Ureaplasma urealyticum	Urethritis, chorioamnionitis, premature delivery
Treponema pallidum (syphilis)	Genital ulcer (chancre), local adenopathy, skin rashes, condyloma lata, hepatitis, arthritis, enhanced HIV risk; bone, cardiovascular (e.g. aortic disease) and central nervous system disease (e.g. aseptic meningitis, cerebrovascular accidents, cranial nerve abnormalities, optic atrophy, tabes dorsalis, general paresis) *Maternal:* Spontaneous abortion, stillbirth, preterm delivery, low infant birth weight *Infant:* congenital syphilis
Gardnerella vaginalis (in association with other bacteria)	Bacterial vaginosis, PID, enhanced HIV risk, urethral discharge *Maternal:* Chorioamniotis, prematurity, low birth weight
Haemophilus ducreyi (chancroid)	Genital ulcers, inguinal adenitis, disfiguring lesions, tissue destruction, enhanced HIV risk
Calymmatobacterium granulomatis (granuloma inguinale, Donovanosis)	Nodular swellings and ulcerative lesions of inguinal and anogenital areas
Shigella spp.	Shigellosis in homosexual men
Salmonella spp.	Enteritis, proctocolitis in homosexual men
Campylobacter spp.	Enteritis, proctocolitis in homosexual men
Viruses	
Human immunodeficiency virus, types 1 and 2	HIV-related disease, opportunistic infections, lymphomas, AIDS *Maternal:* Vertical transmission to infants *Infant:* HIV infection
Herpes simplex virus types 1 and 2	Anogenital vesicular lesions and ulcerations, recurrent genital ulcers, cold sores cervicitis, urethritis, pharyngitis, proctitis, chronic pain, arthritis, aseptic meningitis, hepatitis, meningitis, enhanced HIV risk. *Maternal:* Vertical transmission to infants *Infants:* Ulcerations of skin, eye, mucous membranes; encephalitis, disseminated infection with hepatitis, pneumonitis, encephalitis; long-term neurologic abnormalities
Human papilloma virus (more than 30 genital genotypes identified)	Anogenital and oral warts; intraepithelial neoplasia of the cervix, penis, vulva, vagina, anus; carcinoma of the cervix, penis, vulva, vagina, anus; recurrent respiratory papillomatosis, oropharyngeal cancer *Maternal:* Vertical transmission to infant *Infants:* Recurrent respiratory papillomatosis
Hepatitis B virus	Acute hepatitis, liver cirrhosis, end-stage liver disease, hepatocellular cancer *Maternal:* Vertical transmission to infants; *Infants:* Cirrhosis, end stage liver disease, primary liver cancer
Hepatitis A virus	Acute hepatitis A
Hepatitis C virus	Acute hepatitis C, liver cirrhosis, end-stage liver disease, hepatocellular cancer
Cytomegalovirus (CMV)	Heterophil-negative infectious mononucleosis, hepatitis *Infant:* Primary infection of the newborn, hepatitis, sepsis, deafness, mental retardation
Molluscum contagiosum virus	Genital molluscum contagiosum,
Human T-lymphotrophic retrovirus, type 1	Human T-cell leukemia or lymphoma
Human herpesvirus 8 (HHV-8)	Kaposi's sarcoma, primary effusion lymphoma, Castleman's disease

Protozoa	
Trichomonas vaginalis	Vaginitis, cervicitis, urethretis, endometritis, salpingitis, probably enhanced HIV risk *Maternal:* Chorioamniotis, preterm delivery, low birth weight *Infants:* Pneumonitis, fever, vaginal discharge in female infants
Entamoeba histolytica	Amebiasis in men who have sex with men
Giardia lamblia	Giardiasis in men who have sex with men
Fungi	
Candida albicans	Vulvovaginitis, balanitis
Ectoparasites	
Phthirus pubis	Pubic lice infestation
Sarcoptes scabiei	Scabies, Norwegian (disseminated) scabies *Infants:* Norwegian (disseminated) scabies

Global burden of STI

WHO estimates that each year more than 340 million new curable STI (i.e. gonorrhoea, chlamydia, trichomoniasis, and syphilis) occur in reproductive-aged men and women (Fig. 9.12.1) (World Health Organization 2007). This estimate does not include the many millions of new viral STI that occur each year. Genital HPV infection is believed to be the highest incidence STI worldwide, infecting an estimated 50–70 per cent of sexually active persons and accounting for an estimated 5 million new infections each year in the United States alone (Baseman & Koutsky 2005; Weinstock *et al.* 2004). HSV-2 is also extremely common, with reported population prevalences among nations ranging from 20 per cent to 40 per cent even higher, and is now recognized to be the most common cause of genital ulcer disease worldwide (Paz-Bailey *et al.* 2007). Although not always transmitted sexually, HBV accounts for an estimated 360 million chronic infections globally; and additionally 3 per cent of the world's population is believed to be infected with hepatitis C virus (HCV), including an estimated 170 million people with severe liver disease (Global Burden of Hepatitis C Working Group 2004; Goldstein *et al.* 2005). Additionally, there are approximately 33 million new cases of HIV in adults each year, most of them transmitted sexually (World Health Organization 2007). Viral STI generally cannot be cured and result in either latent infection or active disease that can be transmitted to sex partners. Long-term infection with viral STI may lead to chronic conditions with serious

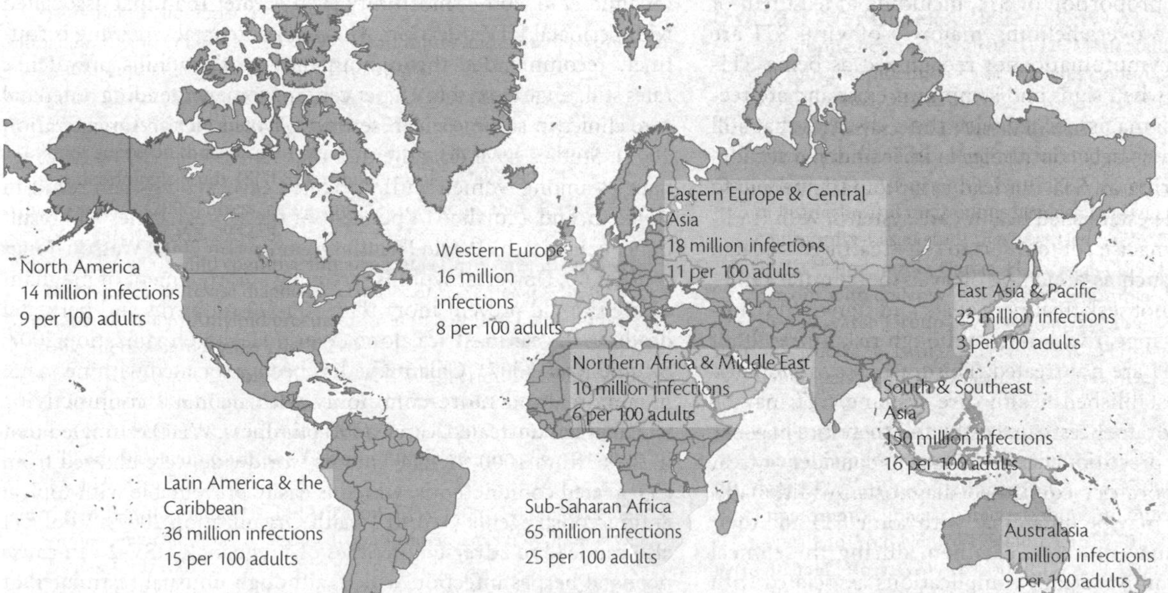

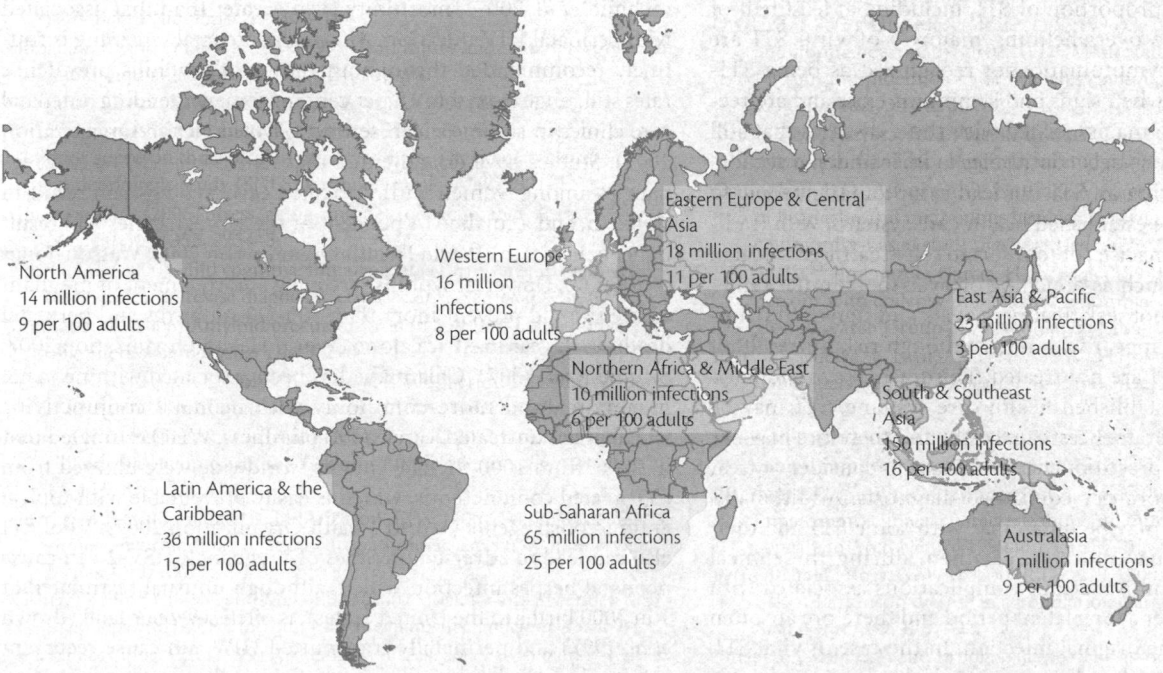

Fig. 9.12.1 Estimated annual numbers and incidence per 100 adults of curable STIs among men and women aged 15–44 years, globally and by region (2001). Each year, an estimated 340 million cases of curable STIs are due to gonorrhoea, chlamydia, syphilis, and trichomoniasis.
Source: World Health Organization (WHO), An Overview of Selected Curable Sexually Transmitted Diseases, Geneva: WHO, Global Programme on AIDS. 2001.

consequences, such as anogenital cancers associated with HPV and hepatocellular carcinomas and end-stage liver disease associated with HBV and HCV.

Most high- and moderate-income nations that have established national STI control programmes have seen marked declines in bacterial infections, notably gonorrhoea and syphilis (Berman & Kamb 2007). Consequently, 80–90 per cent of the global burden of curable STI currently occurs in developing countries, with incidence and prevalence rates up to 20 times higher than in industrialized nations (World Health Organization 2007; Adler 1996). The highest curable STI prevalence rates occur in sub-Saharan African nations, followed by Latin America and the Caribbean, and South and Southeast Asia (Fig. 9.12.1). For a variety of biologic, behavioural, and socioeconomic reasons, curable STI are most common in young adults and adolescents, particularly those under age 24. Although highest STI prevalence occurs in low-income settings in Africa, the largest overall numbers of curable STI occur in Asian nations with large populations under age 40. Viral STI are remarkably common both in industrialized and in developing countries. National population-based surveys in the United States indicate that 17 per cent of reproductive-aged adults are HSV-2 infected, and that prevalence increases with age (from 1.6 per cent in 14–19-year-olds to 26.3 per cent in 40–49-year-olds), and that prevalence varies considerably by racial/ethnic group (Xu *et al.* 2006). Conversely, because of the synergy between HIV and HSV-2, in which each virus enhances shedding of the other, countries with high HIV prevalence generally see increasingly higher HSV-2 prevalence, resulting in a continuing vicious cycle (Paz-Bailey *et al.* 2007). Some of these situations could change in the future. For example, widespread implementation of primary HPV prevention through newly available vaccines could reduce HPV incidence and prevalence in succeeding generations.

STI are greatly under-recognized and under-treated for several reasons. First, a large proportion of STI, including at least half of bacterial STI and the overwhelming majority of viral STI are asymptomatic or, if symptomatic, not recognized as being STI-related. Second, even when signs and symptoms exist and are recognized, the social stigma associated with these diseases that still exists in virtually every society contributes to their under-detection. Shame around acquiring an STI can lead symptomatic people to seek treatment outside established health care systems, with traditional healers or pharmacists, or to resort to self-treatment through inadequate methods such as douching or over-the-counter remedies. Many people do not seek treatment at all, and signs and symptoms will typically disappear with time, although risk for resultant sequelae persists if STI are not treated. Third, when symptomatic patients present to established health care systems, STI may be missed. Many STI laboratory tests are costly, and therefore may not be ordered, and often practitioners are hesitant to consider or treat an STI without a laboratory-confirmed diagnosis. Additionally, health care providers may be unfamiliar with some STI and their manifestations and may not consider them during the clinical work-up. Finally, the most serious complications associated with STI typically occur after a long latent period and therefore are often not associated with the original infection. In the case of viral STI, the sequelae of AIDS and malignancies typically do not occur for many years or decades after the initial exposure.

If left untreated, STI can cause a vast array of health consequences, ranging from relatively minor discomfort or cosmetic concerns to death (Table 9.12.1). The most important health consequences fall under the general categories of (1) reproductive morbidity and mortality including adverse pregnancy outcomes and infertility; (2) STI-associated cancers; and (3) enhanced transmission and acquisition of HIV. The most common of the serious STI consequences are adverse reproductive outcomes, particularly infertility, generally caused by chlamydia or gonorrhoea. As noted earlier, chlamydia and gonorrhoea are highly prevalent infections, and 10–40 per cent of women with untreated infection may develop pelvic inflammatory disease (PID), up to 25 per cent of which can result in infertility (World Health Organization 2007). These infections also can lead to ectopic pregnancy, which is associated with maternal morbidity and mortality as well as pregnancy loss. Women who have had PID are 6–10 times more likely than women without PID to develop a subsequent ectopic pregnancy, with an estimated 40–50 per cent of all ectopic pregnancies attributed to PID (World Health Organization 2007). Although mortality associated with ectopic pregnancy has declined markedly in industrialized nations (Ebrahim *et al.* 1997), hospital-based studies in some low-income nations have reported from 1 per cent to 3 per cent fatality rates associated with ectopic pregnancy, which is about 10 times higher than fatality rates reported in higher-income nations (Goyaux *et al.* 2003). Limited other data suggest ectopic pregnancy may be the source of as much as 11 per cent of maternal mortality in some developing-world settings (Goyaux *et al.* 2003; Meheus 1992). Chlamydial and gonorrhoeal infections also can lead to the long-term morbidity of chronic pelvic pain in women.

Another large proportion of the reproductive morbidity associated with STI is related to adverse pregnancy outcomes for infants, including foetal loss or stillbirth, premature birth or low birth weight infant, blindness, or neonatal death. Maternal syphilis is the most important cause of adverse pregnancy outcome, accounting for an estimated 750 000 to 1.5 million deaths worldwide each year (Schmid *et al.* 2007), morbidity even greater than that associated with perinatal HIV infection. Although antenatal screening is routinely recommended throughout the world, syphilis prevalence rates still range from 4 to 15 per cent in women attending antenatal care clinics in some African settings (World Health Organization 2007). Studies have documented that 25–40 per cent of all pregnancies among women with untreated early syphilis will result in stillbirth, and a further 14 per cent of these pregnancies will result in neonatal death (World Health Organization 2007; Watson-Jones *et al.* 2007). Universal syphilis screening and treatment of pregnant women would prevent more than 500 000 stillbirths and perinatal deaths each year in Africa alone (World Health Organization 2007; Schmid *et al.* 2007). Chlamydia has been associated with neonatal pneumonia and more commonly with neonatal conjunctivitis which, if left untreated, can lead to blindness. WHO estimated that in 2006, from 1000 to 4000 infants worldwide were blinded from STI-related conjunctivitis, which is easily preventable with topical antimicrobial agents (World Health Organization 2007). Viral STI also can lead to adverse outcomes of pregnancy. HSV-2 can cause neonatal herpes infection which, although unusual (estimated at 1 in 3000 births in the United States), is often severe or fatal (Brown *et al.* 1997) and perinatally transmitted HPV can cause recurrent respiratory papillomatosis, a chronic condition often requiring recurrent surgical procedures. On the other hand, the majority of HBV and HCV infections in infants are asymptomatic, although perinatal HBV infection will often result in chronic infection and subsequent complications (CDC 2006).

The second important category of serious STI-related health consequences are malignancies, including anogenital cancers, hepatocellular cancers, lymphomas (e.g. those associated with HIV), and sarcomas (e.g. Kaposi's sarcoma associated with human herpes virus type 8 [HHV-8]). It is now firmly established that certain HPV subtypes are the causal agents of cervical cancer and likely of other anogenital cancers (e.g. vulvar, vaginal, penile, anal) as well (Zur Hausen 1996; Cogliano *et al.* 2005). Two carcinogenic HPV subtypes, 16 and 18, are responsible for an estimated 70 per cent of all cervical cancers and likely of 80–90 per cent of anal and penile cancers worldwide (Munoz *et al.* 2003; Daling *et al.* 2004, 2005). Cervical cancer is now the most common cancer in women worldwide, after breast cancer, and in developing world settings, it is the leading cause of cancer mortality in women, estimated to account for more than 200 000 deaths per year (World Health Organization 2007). The cellular changes associated with carcinogenic HPV types occur slowly, presenting first with dysplasia and later with localized (*in situ*) disease before proceeding to invasive cancer, a natural history which allows early detection and treatment through cervical screening programmes (i.e. Pap test or direct cervical visualization). The large disparity in cervical cancer morbidity and mortality between industrialized and developing nations is largely attributed to limited availability of cervical screening and treatment in the latter. In addition, a significant interaction exists between HPV and HIV which can accelerate HPV-related cellular changes and may further contribute to disparities between developed and industrialized settings, at least in high HIV prevalence nations. Routine periodic cervical screening with a Pap test is the standard of care in most high-income nations and in an increasing number of moderate-income nations, with more frequent screening intervals recommended for HIV-infected women. However, in developing-world settings many women have never had a Pap smear (Schmiedeskamp & Kockler 2006).

HBV is a highly prevalent infection in developing-world settings, which is typically related to vertical transmission from mother-to-child. HBV also is commonly transmitted parenterally through tainted blood products, organs, or medical or illicit drug injection equipment. This virus also can be transmitted sexually, and in industrialized nations such as the United States where vertical transmission is unusual, sexual transmission now accounts for a majority of HBV infections, and is especially common among men who have sex with men (MSM). HBV is associated with several serious, long-term complications, including cirrhosis and end-stage liver disease and hepatocellular cancer (primary liver cancer). Hepatocellular cancer is the fifth leading cause of cancer deaths in adults worldwide but ranks third in developing-world settings, accounting for 415 000–500 000 deaths per year, of which 80 per cent occur in Asia and sub-Saharan Africa (Pisani *et al.* 1999; McGlynn & London 2005). Just over half of hepatocellular carcinomas globally are attributed to chronic HBV infection, with regional estimates varying greatly, ranging from 16 per cent in North America, 47 per cent each in Africa and Southeast Asia, 59 per cent in Eastern Mediterranean countries, and 65 per cent in East Asia (Perz *et al.* 2006). About 25 per cent of hepatocellular cancers are caused by HCV (which is sexually transmitted in about 20 per cent of cases) (Perz *et al.* 2006). In addition to malignancies, HBV and HCV also are major contributors to cirrhosis globally (causing 30 per cent and 27 per cent of all cases, respectively) (Perz *et al.* 2006).

The third important category of adverse STI-associated outcomes is related to HIV transmission and acquisition. Persons co-infected with HIV and certain STI, particularly those causing genital ulcers, have higher levels of HIV shedding than HIV-infected persons without other STI; co-infected individuals are more likely to transmit HIV to an uninfected partner; and successful STD treatment has been documented to reduce viral shedding (Fleming & Wasserheit 1999). Additionally, HIV-uninfected people with certain STI—again particularly genital ulcers—are more susceptible to acquiring new HIV infections from HIV-infected sex partners, probably by disrupting mucosal integrity and by increasing the presence and activation of HIV-susceptible cells in the genital tract (Fleming & Wasserheit 1999). Intervention studies have demonstrated that routine STI clinical services and condom promotion can result in large reductions in HIV incidence or prevention of epidemic increases among high-risk persons such as commercial sex workers (CSW) (Levine *et al.* 1998; Laga *et al.* 1994; Plummer *et al.* 2005). Furthermore, a community randomized trial conducted in Mwanza, Tanzania, in the early 1990s documented that communities receiving an improved programme of management of symptomatic STI had reduced HIV incidence compared with communities with typical STI management programmes—supporting an HIV prevention benefit at the community level (Grosskurth *et al.* 2000). The lack of a similar effect in subsequent community level intervention trials (i.e. Rakai study of mass treatment; Wawer *et al.* 1999, and Masaka study of enhanced syndromic management; Korenromp *et al.* 2005) evaluating various STI control strategies indicates that a community-level HIV benefit is not likely to occur in all circumstances or for all populations but that such benefit may be particularly important in settings of early (non-generalized) epidemics with a high prevalence of bacterial GUD (White *et al.* 2004). Nonetheless, the individual-level benefit of STI treatment for HIV-infected persons co-infected with curable STI or for HIV susceptible persons with symptomatic STI is compelling. Even in advanced HIV epidemics where STI care has less population-level impact on HIV, it remains an effective intervention at the individual level and may be particularly important in preventing transmission from persons with HIV infection, underlining the importance of offering STI services to those in HIV care. The strong association of genital ulcer disease with HIV transmission, along with the above-noted observation that high HSV-2 prevalence often occurs in countries with high HIV prevalence, raises the question of whether treatment of genital HSV-2 might reduce the likelihood of HSV-2 or HIV shedding (or both) and thus prevent transmission or acquisition of new HIV infections (Paz-Bailey *et al.* 2007; Weiss 2004). This is of particular interest because some antiviral agents (e.g. acyclovir) that are effective against genital HSV-2 are now off-patent and therefore may be affordably priced even for low-income nations with high HIV prevalence. A recent trial has demonstrated that treatment of HSV-2 infections can reduce HIV shedding in HSV-2/HIV co-infected, asymptomatic persons (Nagot *et al.* 2007), and a rigorous evaluation involving several larger, multinational randomized controlled trials in various populations is expected to provide additional data about this potential HIV prevention strategy within the next few years.

Conceptual framework for STD prevention

Individual vs. population benefit

STI prevention programmes provide benefits both to individuals and to the larger population. Individual benefits derive from activities that prevent acquisition of infection, ameliorate symptoms, and reduce complications of initial infection, while the general population benefits from efforts that prevent continuing transmission and thus reduce overall prevalence of infection and complications in the population (Aral *et al.* 2005; Douglas & Fenton 2007). Since activities that prevent acquisition of infection (behaviour change, condom use, vaccines) or lead to diagnosis and treatment of curable infections (e.g. screening, clinical care, management) also prevent subsequent transmission, they provide population-level as well as individual-level effects. Alternatively, some interventions may have greater effects on transmission, and thus population benefit, than on personal health. One example is vaccination of males for HPV 16/18, where models indicate that there may be an effect on disease in women but limited benefit for men (Hughes *et al.* 2002). Another example is measures to prevent transmission from persons chronically infected with HSV-2 or HIV (e.g. suppressive antiviral treatment to prevent HSV-2 transmission between sexual partners; maternal antiretroviral treatment to prevent vertical transmission, promotion of condom use; etc.) (White *et al.* 2004). The relative importance of individual versus population benefit can vary by specific subpopulation. For example, substantial STI prevention efforts are focused on subpopulations important in continuing transmission, such as 'core groups' (groups who have high STI prevalence and also high rates of partner change, discussed in depth later). Interventions aimed at core groups have the potential to have greater population-level impact than those targeted at the broader, general population, and thus are often higher priorities for public health programmes (Douglas & Fenton 2007; Aral *et al.* 1996).

Determinants of transmission

An important concept in understanding STI epidemiology in populations and the possible impact of prevention strategies is the STI transmission dynamics model of May and Anderson (1987). The reproductive rate of an STI in a population (R_0), which is the average number of new infections generated by each infected person, is based on three factors: (1) the likelihood of transmission per sexual contact between an infected person and a susceptible partner (B); (2) the average number of new sexual partnerships formed over time between infected and susceptible persons (c); and (3) the average duration of infectiousness (D), where $R_0 = BcD$. Incidence and prevalence of a specific STI within a population will increase when R_0 exceeds 1 and decrease if R_0 falls below 1. Circumstances that reduce any of the three factors will reduce R_0 and population prevalence (Brunham 2005).

A primary focus of STI prevention programmes has been reduction in duration of infectiousness (D) by detecting and treating infected persons. Measures to accomplish this goal include enhancing access to and utilization of health care, improving case finding, and improving completion of treatment after clinical contact. Prevention strategies that reduce transmission efficiency (B) and number of sexual partnerships (c) can affect all STI but are particularly important for those that are not curable by antimicrobial therapy, such as HIV, HSV-2, and HPV. Most approaches to reduce transmission efficiency are behavioural (e.g. efforts to promote male and female condom use; efforts to reduce higher-risk practices such as needle sharing), but a growing number of biomedical approaches shows promise. For example, suppressive antiviral therapy of HSV-2 has been proven to reduce transmission within discordant sexual partnerships (Corey *et al.* 2005). In addition, male circumcision has been recently shown to reduce transmission of HIV and possibly other STI (Weiss 2007). Most importantly, effective vaccines markedly reduce susceptibility. Vaccination programmes have substantially reduced the incidence of HBV in developed countries (CDC 2006) and may have similar effects in the future on HPV (Goldie *et al.* 2004). Even low-efficacy vaccines or those that reduce viral load without completely preventing infection can have substantial effects at the population level (Anderson & Hanson 2005). Finally, strategies to reduce sexual partnerships between susceptible and infected partners can have the broadest effects, but may be difficult to implement and sustain. For example, although programmes to encourage abstinence by adolescents have been strongly encouraged in the United States, there is growing evidence that such programmes may have limited effectiveness (Santelli *et al.* 2006). Encouraging a reduction in the number of sex partners, particularly among people with frequent sex partner change (e.g. sex workers), may be a more plausible approach, based on experiences in several countries where HIV prevalence has fallen (Shelton *et al.* 2004).

Sexual networks and core groups

In addition to these factors' affecting transmission at the level of individuals and their partners, networks of sexual interaction within populations also influence likelihood of contact between susceptible and infected persons (Aral *et al.* 1996; Adimora & Schoenbach 2005). Sexual networks consist of groups or individuals who are directly or indirectly sexually connected, and the location of an individual in such networks can influence the likelihood of infection as much as or more than personal behaviour by influencing the prevalence of infection in their partners. Larger numbers of sexual linkages in a subpopulation can result in transmission of STI from core groups to the general population, especially if the sexual partnerships are formed concurrently rather than sequentially and involve dissassortative (like-with-unlike) mixing patterns (Aral *et al.* 1996, 2005). Sexual networks can be affected by a variety of contextual factors, such as community norms about sexual behaviour; migration and travel patterns; economic circumstances; and the societal disruptions induced by natural disasters, political conflict, and wars. As noted earlier, a related concept in STI prevention is that of the 'core group', persons with multiple partners at well-connected points in sexual networks who are responsible for continuing STI transmission. From the perspective of STI transmission determinants, they are defined as groups or individuals with sufficient rates of sex partner change to maintain $R_0 > 1$, and their characteristics will vary by their location in the sexual network and by specific STI depending on duration of infection and efficiency of transmission. Targeting core groups with STI prevention efforts such as screening and condom promotion can be more efficient and cost-effective than efforts targeted more broadly (Over & Piot 1996; Douglas & Fenton 2007). Programmes focusing on CSWs, persons living in geographic areas with a high prevalence of reported cases of STD, incarcerated persons, or those with repeat STI infection have used the core group approach (Leichliter *et al.* 2007; Williams & Kahn 2007).

STI prevention programmes

The previous section described why, for communicable diseases such as STI, effective diagnosis and treatment is an important prevention strategy. Prompt and effective treatment of curable STI minimizes their adverse outcomes in the individual patient, but also reduces further spread of STI into the community (making STI exposure less likely). However, clinical case management considered alone has limitations that are illustrated by a tuberculosis management model developed using actual data from rural women in one African nation (Ryan *et al.* 2007; Waaler & Piot 1969). Figure 9.12.2a describes STI prevalence in a community and a series of steps required to ensure effective STI treatment, focusing on the proportion of STI missed (not effectively treated) at each step. The model illustrates that most people with STI, even those with symptoms, are not effectively treated; and even fewer have sex partners effectively treated. These issues can be addressed, however. Figure 9.12.2b shows the potential benefits of (i) well-conducted clinic-based management (i.e. persons coming to health facilities obtain effective STI treatment); (ii) the incremental benefits that might be attained if symptomatic patients who do not come to health facilities could be identified and receive STI services (e.g. through asymptomatic screening, targeted outreach programmes, community-based educational efforts and effective partner management); and (iii) the incremental benefits that primary prevention might bring (e.g. through high coverage of an effective STI vaccine; or widespread community education around STI prevention, whether abstinence, delaying initiation of sex in adolescents, or promotion of safer sex practices such as correct and consistent condom use).

With this concept that STI clinical services cannot, by themselves, control STI in a community, STI prevention programmes are based on several essential components working together. These include STI surveillance, STI prevention interventions, and programme support components.

Surveillance

As for other public health programmes, accurate STI surveillance is critical for assessing the magnitude of the problem, trends over

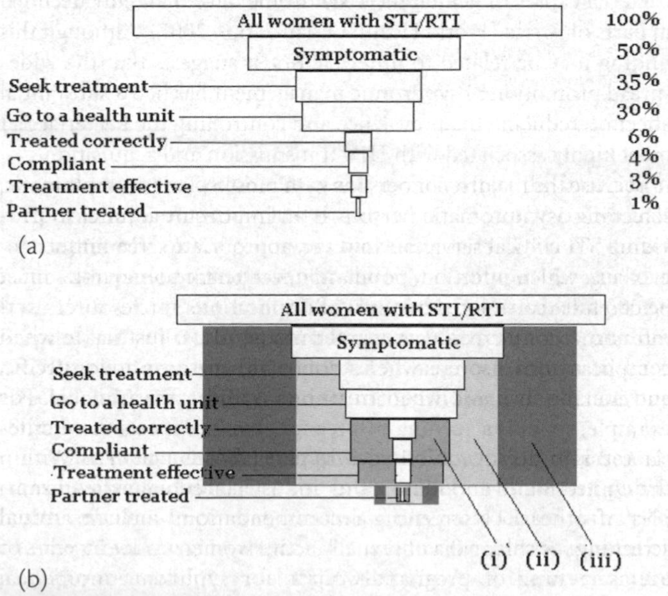

Fig. 9.12.2 (a) Piot–Fransen model of STI prevalence and typical STI case management. (b) Potential benefits of additional control strategies in concert with STI case management.

time, emergence of outbreaks or new problems, development of prevention strategies, prioritization of resources, and monitoring public health effects. There are several approaches to surveillance that can provide complementary information (World Health Organization 2007; Douglas & Fenton 2007). First, *case-reporting* provides a measure of new cases of STI or associated syndromes over a specified time interval and is the most common surveillance activity, especially in jurisdictions with functional reporting systems for notifiable infectious diseases. In industrialized countries, gonorrhoea, syphilis, and chlamydia are generally nationally reportable, with reports generated by clinicians, laboratories, or both. In developing countries where national reporting is more difficult, reporting from sentinel clinics can be useful. Second, *prevalence monitoring* can define the prevalence of STI or related syndromes in defined populations undergoing routine assessment (e.g. screening or diagnostic testing for infections, examination for syndromes) and can complement case-reporting in assessing the burden of infection or disease. For example, in the United States, while notifiable cases of chlamydia have continually climbed as screening has increased, prevalence monitoring in STI and family planning clinics has shown little change, indicating that the burden of infection is unlikely to be rising (CDC 2005, 2006). Third, *sentinel surveillance* generally refers to data collection from representative 'sentinel populations' for outcomes not routinely measured, such as antimicrobial resistance or infectious aetiology of various STI-related syndromes, and is often useful for generating broader guidance about appropriate treatment regimens and national lists of essential medications. Fourth, *population-based surveys*, involving collection of data such as prevalence of specific infections from persons considered representative of the general population are difficult to perform but provide the best assessment of population burden. In addition to these approaches for assessing morbidity, periodic surveillance of sexual behaviours or health services can be useful in monitoring the need for or responses to educational and health marketing efforts, and can also provide information on where prevention services are most needed (Douglas & Fenton 2007). Because of the large burden of disease and often limited resources for collection and analysis of STI surveillance data, conducting effective STI surveillance is challenging even in industrialized countries, and there is a critical need to enhance it in developing countries by improving laboratory facilities and surveillance personnel and strengthening reporting mechanisms (World Health Organization 2007).

STI prevention interventions

STI prevention interventions include clinical management, laboratory services, partner management strategies, and health education and behavioural interventions.

Clinical management

STI clinical management (i.e. diagnosis, treatment, and prevention services at a health facility) is generally considered the core intervention for STI prevention efforts. Effective clinical management can provide individual health benefits (e.g. ameliorating symptoms and preventing complications), but it can also provide overall population health benefits. From the perspective of transmission determinants, effective diagnosis and treatment reduce the duration of infection (D) and thus reduce efficiency of further transmission in the community. STI clinical services can be offered in virtually any type of clinical setting, ranging from specialty STI, HIV, and family planning clinics to primary care clinics and antenatal clinic services; additionally, STI screening is increasingly offered in non-clinical outreach settings. Because of the sensitive and often stigmatizing nature of STI, particular attention must be paid to offering services that are nonjudgmental and confidential.

The traditional approach to STI clinical management has been through dedicated specialty clinics classified as STI, genitourinary, or dermato-venereology clinics (Douglas & Fenton 2007). These are typically publicly funded clinics staffed by providers with greater clinical experience and who generally have greater access to comprehensive rapid and conventional diagnostic testing and treatment services than providers in other settings. Especially in wealthier countries, there is often heavy reliance on laboratory testing to establish aetiologic diagnoses that can enhance surveillance and partner services. Such clinics frequently offer a comprehensive range of sexual health services including HIV testing, risk-reduction counselling and condom provision, contraception, referral for other services (e.g. HIV and substance abuse care), Pap testing and immunizations (e.g. HBV vaccine). However, even in countries where such specialty clinic services are available, most STI management is provided in other types of health facilities. In the United States, for example, the majority of all reportable STI now originates from non-STI clinic sites (e.g. primary and secondary syphilis—67 per cent, gonorrhoea—65 per cent, chlamydia—76 per cent) (CDC 2006), with other important sites including family planning, correctional health care, and primary care clinics and specialty providers in both public and private sector settings. In developing countries, STI services are often provided by private providers, traditional healers, or pharmacists, and quality of management may be suboptimal (World Health Organization 2007; Douglas & Fenton 2007). The importance of integrating high quality, comprehensive STI management into a spectrum of other settings including private clinics, is particularly critical in developing countries in order to enhance coverage, access, and ultimately impact (World Health Organization 2007).

In an ideal world, STI clinical management would be guided by use of rapid, point-of-care diagnostic tests (done at the time of the initial clinic visit) that are affordable, easy to use, and highly sensitive and specific. Such rapid STI tests are generally not available, and tests that do exist are often costly and require several days for results. Given the limited availability of reliable, high-quality, or affordable diagnostic tests in most developing countries, WHO has recommended that settings with limited diagnostic infrastructure consider using locally validated syndromic management approaches for care of symptomatic STI and other reproductive tract infections (RTI) (Dallabetta *et al.* 2007; World Health Organization 2007; Ryan *et al.* 2007). Syndromic management is based on the identification of a 'syndrome', a constellation of easily elicited symptoms and recognizable clinical signs that are associated with a limited number of defined STI or RTI aetiologies. The approach is practical in that it can be carried out in almost any setting (Dallabetta *et al.* 2007). It does not require laboratory facilities, and patients are treated at the initial clinical visit, which allows prompt treatment and thus reduces chances for complications to develop or for further STI spread to sex partners. Costs are minimized because laboratory tests are avoided and drug regimens are simplified. The use of standardized algorithms covering all likely conditions reduces treatment failures, eliminating the need for repeated visits or referrals to higher level centres. Standardized regimens also help improve case-reporting for surveillance and, consequently, provide more information for programme management (Dallabetta *et al.* 2007; Ryan *et al.* 2007).

The syndromic approach also has important limitations (Dallabetta *et al.* 2007; World Health Organization 2007). The most critical is that it does not address asymptomatic patients, who account for the majority of curable STI. Asymptomatic women with cervical infections are at risk for serious adverse outcomes including tubal damage and infertility, but they are not covered by this approach. Furthermore, because many genitourinary symptoms are caused by other conditions or situations in the absence of an STI, the syndromic approach can lead to false positive diagnoses and thus to unnecessary drug use, additional costs and potential partner issues. Partner management is a particular issue, as many providers are hesitant to treat sex partners of individuals who are treated without a specific, laboratory-defined STI aetiology, even though re-infection of the patient would be very likely without treatment of a steady sex partner. Additionally, the most common presenting syndrome for women, vaginal discharge syndrome, is usually caused by non-STI related RTIs (e.g. bacterial vaginosis, candidiasis) or by other factors. Vaginitis can be complicated to treat, often requiring multiple visits and repeated presumptive treatment trials, which can be costly and may lead to side effects. Finally, some health care providers, particularly physicians, have been reluctant to adopt syndromic approaches because they have been trained in aetiologic diagnosis-based treatment and often view syndromic management as 'unscientific' (Dallabetta *et al.* 2007; Ryan *et al.* 2007).

Programmatic evaluations from a variety of settings indicate that syndromic management approaches are particularly effective for management of genital ulcer syndrome in men and women, urethritis or epididymitis in men, and neonatal conjunctivitis in infants (World Health Organization 2007). Over the past decade, repeated cross-sectional studies in several nations indicate that bacterial causes of genital ulcer syndrome have markedly declined in parts of Africa (World Health Organization 2007). Although this finding may be related to other factors, it suggests that the widespread promotion of syndromic management has had a substantial effect on reducing the prevalence and controlling the bacterial STI most highly associated with HIV transmission and acquisition.

Because the majority of persons with most STI are asymptomatic, screening asymptomatic persons is an important adjunct to providing STI clinical services. However, appropriate screening strategies (e.g. which infection, population, venue, frequency, etc.) must be carefully considered because of implications for resources and infrastructure. Screening programmes are most justifiable when complications are severe; when screening tests are sensitive, specific, and inexpensive; and when treatment options are available. For example, syphilis screening of pregnant women meets these criteria and is widely recommended as part of antenatal care. Within the United States and many other industrialized countries, examples of other STI screening recommendations include annual screening for chlamydia of sexually active women under 25 years of age; screening of pregnant women for syphilis, gonorrhoea, chlamydia, and HIV; annual screening of sexually active MSM for gonorrhoea, chlamydia, syphilis, and HIV; and routine Pap testing (every 1–3 years for women starting at age 21) (CDC 2006; Douglas & Fenton 2007).

Although not traditionally included in STI clinical services, the availability of safe and effective STI vaccines has increased interest in their provision in selected settings. Although HBV vaccine is a routine infant immunization in many countries, settings providing STI care or serving those at high STI risk have been recommended as additional venues for HBV immunization (CDC 2006; Douglas & Fenton 2007). The recent licensure of an HPV vaccine, now recommended in the United States for 11–12-year-old girls routinely and for young women from 13 to 26 years of age as a catch-up vaccine (CDC 2007), creates the possibility of linking a second vaccine to STI services to enhance population coverage. HPV vaccines are projected to be cost-effective even in settings with Pap test screening programmes (Elbasha *et al.* 2007), although they will have the greatest potential impact in developing countries with no organized cervical cancer prevention programmes. Possible ancillary benefit of an STI vaccine widely recommended for young women include the chance to establish vaccine platforms that are relevant to future HIV vaccines, and to destigmatize and normalize STI prevention services.

Laboratory services

Laboratory services are essential for effective surveillance and clinical services. In settings where diagnostic tests are available, they can provide accurate diagnosis of symptomatic persons and exposed sex partners and a means of screening asymptomatic high-risk populations. As noted earlier, for optimal utility, STI laboratory tests should be accurate, rapid, simple, and inexpensive. For curable STI, where administration of a short course of therapy can interrupt transmission as well as resolve symptoms and prevent complications, test sensitivity has traditionally been more important than specificity. However, in recent years, test specificity has been an increasing concern, owing to the growing importance of chronic viral STI (where a diagnosis can have lifelong implications), increased STI screening in asymptomatic populations (where low specificity can reduce positive predictive value and result in an unacceptable level of false positive diagnoses), and greater attention to partner services (where a false positive diagnosis can lead to unnecessary distress or relationship problems) (Cates & Holmes 1998).

In developing countries, insufficient resources and infrastructure limit the capacity of laboratory testing to affect clinical care of individuals. However, in these settings, laboratory services still play a critical role in validating and intermittently re-assessing the appropriateness of algorithms for syndromic case management. For example, as noted above, over the past 10 years, such assessments have pointed to the growing importance of HSV-2 in genital ulcer disease, leading to revised algorithms including empiric antiviral therapy. Laboratory services are also essential for monitoring trends in antimicrobial resistance, particularly for gonorrhoea. Because susceptibility testing for individual patients is impractical, national and regional surveillance systems have been important in detecting emerging gonococcal resistance and altering management guidelines (World Health Organization 2007).

Rapid, point-of-care laboratory tests are especially important for STI prevention for several reasons. In many settings, persons with STI may not return for follow-up visits. In addition, prompt diagnosis expedites the time to treatment and partner services, which can reduce spread of STI in the community. In settings with low rates of follow-up, use of rapid tests can result in more complete treatment of infected persons than can the use of more sensitive but slower conventional tests (Gift *et al.* 1999). Clinics specializing in STI care have emphasized rapid diagnosis in men by use of microscopy for diagnosis of gonorrhoea and urethritis by Gram stain, of trichomoniasis in women by wet mount examination, and of syphilis by darkfield examination. Rapid serologic tests for syphilis (e.g. RPR card tests) have been important in syphilis control, but can be difficult to use properly. Newer generation rapid tests that are simple enough to use in developing country settings offer great promise in screening pregnant women and preventing vertical transmission, and are one of the bases for new global efforts at elimination of congenital syphilis.

Partner management

Partner management has long been integral to STI control programmes, initiated in the first few decades of the twentieth century for syphilis control in many industrialized countries (Brewer 2005; Hogben *et al.* 2007). Its principal goal is notifying sex partners of persons with STI diagnoses of their exposure to enhance early diagnosis and treatment, providing health benefit at both the individual level (to index patients whose risk of re-infection is reduced and to partners, for whom early treatment may avoid complications) and the population level (by preventing continuing transmission). Additional benefits of partner management include fulfilment of an ethical duty to warn persons exposed to serious infections, as well as the opportunity to enhance understanding of sexual and drug-use networks in which STI transmission is occurring.

Two basic approaches are used for partner management services: Provider referral and patient referral (Brewer 2005; Hogben *et al.* 2007). The former involves the use of third parties, usually health care providers or public health workers, to interview the index patient to determine partner names and locating information, with subsequent confidential notification of partners about their exposure and their need for testing and treatment. In contrast, patient referral, which offers a less labour-intensive approach for the many settings with insufficient resources to conduct provider referral, relies upon the index patient to notify their partner(s), preferably assisted by written materials. A hybrid approach known as contract-referral begins with patient referral but is followed by provider referral if contacts have not been notified within a specified timeframe. The primary focus of partner management has been on the curable STI (e.g. syphilis, gonorrhoea, chlamydia, and trichomoniasis), although there is growing interest in partner services for persons with HIV infection, and, in some countries, for other viral STI such as genital HSV and HPV.

The efficacy of partner referral has been summarized in several recent reviews (Passin *et al.* 2006; Brewer 2005; Hogben *et al.* 2007). Provider referral has a similar yield for the curable STI of syphilis, chlamydia, and gonorrhoea, with a range of 0.22–0.25 infected partners identified and treated per index patient. Estimations of the effect of partner services on population transmission are limited, although several reports have described reductions in gonorrhoea incidence following increased partner management efforts (Du *et al.* 2006; Douglas & Fenton 2007; Han *et al.* 1999). Although there have been few direct comparisons, patient referral appears to have a lower yield than provider referral. However, even in industrialized countries, there are insufficient resources to offer provider services to more than a minority of patients. Therefore, novel approaches, such as expedited partner therapy, which relies on the delivery of therapy by patients to partners without a provider examination, are of increasing interest. This approach has been shown to increase partner treatment and to reduce index patient re-infection for both gonorrhoea and chlamydia, and modelling studies indicate that it may allow sufficiently increased population coverage to reduce population prevalence (Golden *et al.* 2005; White *et al.* 2005; Douglas & Fenton 2007). Increased operational research to better understand benefit and acceptability of different approaches, especially in developing countries, is an important STI prevention priority (World Health Organization 2007).

Health education and behavioural interventions

A mainstay of effective STI prevention programmes is the provision of health education and other strategies to promote healthful sexual behaviour. Basic educational messages should include primary prevention strategies such as the benefits of delaying initiation of sexual activity, reducing the number and concurrency of sex partners, and the benefit of the correct and consistent use of condoms in situations where partners are not known to be free of STI. They should also include information about the value of preventive interventions such as testing and immunizations, and the importance of seeking care for possible STI symptoms to facilitate early STI diagnosis and treatment and prevention of transmission to partners (World Health Organization 2007). In addition, for those in whom an STI is diagnosed, information on completing therapy, need for follow-up examinations or testing, notification of sex partners, and STI preventive measures in the future are all important.

Health education can be supplemented by behavioural intervention services that promote healthful sexual behaviour. Such interventions can be conducted at both individual and community levels. Individually focused interventions target behaviour change at the individual level by providing knowledge or strategies to modify attitudes, beliefs, motivation, or skills and such interventions include approaches such as risk-reduction counselling for adolescents, MSM and persons with an STI; outreach and counselling programmes for illicit drug users; and condom promotion and distribution programmes for high-risk individuals such as CSW. Such interventions are most efficiently delivered in settings where high-risk individuals can be easily accessed. Successful examples include risk-reduction counselling delivered in STI clinic settings (Kamb *et al.* 1998) and educational videos promoting safer behaviour in waiting room settings (Warner & Rietmeijer 2006), prevention counselling for persons with HIV infection in HIV care settings (CDC 2003), and street outreach projects targeting high-risk youth and injecting drug users (Greenberg *et al.* 1998). Such interventions may be particularly effective at 'teachable moments', when individuals first learn that they have an STI. In contrast, interventions targeted at the community level address individual risk in the broader context of their social networks and environments and attempt to modify social norms, influence social and sexual networks, and reduce community barriers to healthful sexual behaviour and health-care seeking behaviour (CDC 2001).

Health marketing, also known as social marketing, is an aspect of health communication directed at the community that is of emerging importance both in industrialized and in developing countries. It combines techniques from consumer marketing (e.g. consumer research and marketing) with theoretical models of behaviour change, creating a hybrid form of marketing whose goal is to change awareness, attitudes, beliefs, and behaviours, rather than selling a product (Vega & Ghanem 2007). With the realization that mass media are primary sources of health information for many consumers (Salmon 1989), health marketing campaigns can use a variety of mass media approaches (e.g. printed materials, broadcast media, and the Internet). Although public service announcements (PSAs) have usually been the primary broadcast media approach, these can be effectively complemented by messages conveyed by news reports and entertainment programming, also known as 'edu-tainment'. Recent efforts in the United States to respond to syphilis epidemics in MSM have successfully combined all of these approaches (Vega & Ghanem 2007). The interaction between perceived vulnerability, perceived severity of the health outcome, and efficacy of preventive behaviours is a central issue for development of effective messages. How much such campaigns should emphasize negative consequences has often been controversial, although it appears that appeals to fear can be effective if they are linked to specific protective recommendations and information about how to accomplish the recommendations, while fear appeals without a high-efficacy message can result in denial (Vega & Ghanem 2007; Witte & Allen 2000). STI prevention health marketing should emphasize positive outcomes of prevention (peace of mind, protecting personal and partner health) as well as the normative aspects of the recommended behaviour.

Programme support components

Several programme components are essential to support STI prevention and control interventions. These include leadership and advocacy around STI prevention, STI training for health providers and other public health specialists, monitoring and evaluation of existing programmes to ensure high quality and wide coverage of services, and STI research, including applied programme evaluations or primary research around intervention effectiveness.

Leadership and advocacy

Strong and effective programme leadership is essential for implementing and sustaining effective STI prevention programmes and for effectively integrating the other essential programme components. No matter how effective prevention technologies are, they cannot produce sustainable individual and population benefit without the leadership to develop political will and resources, and to ensure a supportive legal and policy environment for STI prevention and control. The need for effective leadership is especially critical for conditions such as STI because their associated stigma often makes public discussion and community involvement difficult (World Health Organization 2007). Important components of effective leadership include partnerships and collaboration, priority setting and planning, and policy development and implementation.

Given the magnitude of the STI burden, even in countries with dedicated STI prevention programmes and clinics, building effective partnerships and collaborations is increasingly recognized as critical to achieving population coverage and effect (World Health Organization 2007; Douglas & Fenton 2007). Such efforts can include professional organizations, academia, the pharmaceutical industry, the private health care sector, and community-based organizations. Professional organizations can be critical in providing endorsement of prevention activities and training. Regarding community-based organizations, while secular non-governmental organizations have generally been the primary source of partnerships, there has been recent emphasis on collaborations with faith-based organizations, which often have extensive networks including rural locations and which, because of their influence in shaping opinions and attitudes of their members, have great potential for reducing stigmatization (World Health Organization 2007).

To maximize effects and cost-effective use of limited resources, priority setting and planning is an equally important leadership activity. Most countries have developed broad, multisectoral responses to HIV prevention. However, many have not developed similar, comprehensive STI control strategies, and many nations have very limited engagement of private (and sometimes even the public) health sector in STI prevention and control efforts. Some examples of more comprehensive efforts exist, however, such as the national Infertility Prevention Program (CDC 2004) and Syphilis Elimination Plan (CDC 2006) in the United States and the National Strategy for Sexual Health and HIV in the UK (Department of Health 2007). Appropriate surveillance, monitoring, and evaluation are critical for effective priority setting and planning.

Finally, policy development creates an overarching structure for public health programmes and is the key determinant of long-term public health effects. It includes the broad planning efforts described above as well as attention to the legal and regulatory environment, the securing of financial resources, and advocacy for programme priorities. Examples of important legal issues affecting STI prevention include providing confidential (without parental consent) clinical services for young people, ability of non-physician providers to provide services or prescribe drugs, and the permissibility of expedited partner therapy (World Health Organization 2007; CDC 2006). Securing financial resources for STI prevention is a core function with a major effect on population coverage of services since in the private sector the cost of clinical services for low-income users is a major barrier to effective programmes (World Health Organization 2007). Finally, advocacy for and communication of prevention priorities to decision-makers is an increasingly critical policy priority, not only to raise political interest and will but also to mobilize resources. For developing countries, such efforts often involve attempts by multinational organizations such as WHO to work with leaders of possible donor countries.

Training

A well-trained workforce is critical for implementation of all other programme components. As public health and STI prevention have expanded from a largely biomedical focus to include other areas of expertise such as behavioural science, health communications, and informatics, the spectrum of training needs has likewise grown. In addition, with the increasing role of non-categorical STI clinics in providing services, the need to train providers in other sectors—especially primary care and HIV care providers—has increased. The development and dissemination of national guidelines can enhance the quality of care in all sectors (World Health Organization 2007). For example, in the United States, such efforts have included those focused specifically on STI programme operations as well as on more detailed STI management recommendations (CDC 2001, 2006).

Clinical training has historically been provided by health professional schools, but because inclusion of STI training is variable and often suboptimal, retraining of post-graduate staff through on-the-job training, continuing education efforts, and activities by professional organizations (e.g. conferences, journal articles, newsletters, etc.) is of primary importance (World Health Organization 2007). In addition, some countries have provided national training efforts (e.g. the clinical, behavioural, and partner services training provided by the US National Network of STD Prevention Training Centers; (World Health Organization 2007; CDC 2006) sexual health training provided in the UK through the Development Toolkit of the Department of Health). There is increasing interest in the use of the Internet as a low-cost and widely available training medium, particularly in its ability to provide 'just in time' training through rapid access to guidelines for non-specialist providers of STI care (Tietz *et al.* 2004). Retraining of post-graduates can aid in updating (e.g. on newer tests and therapies) and also introducing new approaches (e.g. on recent vaccines, risk-reduction counselling, expedited partner therapy).

All of these issues are compounded by challenges in workforce capacity both in industrialized and in developing countries which are not specific to STI programmes but which affect them. In the United States, the overall public health workforce is aging, with estimated retirement rates over the next several years of more than 40 per cent and chronic shortages in professional areas such as nursing, epidemiology and laboratory science (ASTHO 2004). In the developing world, there are grave shortages of health care workers in all sectors related to limited resources for education of professionals, but compounded both by 'brain drain', when trained professionals leave to go to wealthier countries experiencing shortages, as well as by donor support for scaling up vertical programmes (e.g. HIV treatment and care), causing a shift in workforce from other health sectors.

Monitoring and evaluation

The purpose of monitoring and evaluation is to ensure high-quality, appropriate services (Hassig *et al.* 1996). Fundamentally, monitoring and evaluation are tools that allow documentation of the overall value and improvement of an STI prevention and control programme over time. While programme monitoring was once mainly conducted as a periodic activity to assure aspects of programme quality, with funding nowadays increasingly linked to attainment of a programme's targeted goals and objectives, monitoring and evaluation have blossomed into a science in their own right. For best results, monitoring and evaluation should be introduced as part of the design and development of any programme, not only in the implementation phases. A number of useful 'how to' tools have become available to help with this (Salabarria-Pena *et al.* 2007). When monitoring and evaluation are approached as an expected part of an overall programme, data collection procedures are more likely to be done well and less likely to be considered a burden by members of the staff (Hassig *et al.* 1996).

Monitoring refers to tracking data that measure the progress of a specific STI prevention or control programme in carrying out the steps that the programme is designed to achieve. The data collected should identify programme strengths and weaknesses, and thus serve to document programme progress, identify resource needs and allocation and make changes needed to improve programmes. Programme monitoring often involves measuring factors such as service delivery, staff performance, adequacy of staffing patterns, client satisfaction, or resource needs and allocation (Hassig *et al.* 1996). Collecting data on programme operating costs (e.g. staff salaries), commodities, and other resources expended is an important part of programme monitoring, and is also important in the evaluation phase of a programme to measure cost-effectiveness. Examples of indicators monitoring service delivery include the hours of operation of a specific clinical facility, the number of patient encounters that took place during a specified time interval, the numbers of specific STI or disease syndromes diagnosed over a time interval, the numbers of commodities (e.g. condoms, drugs, syringes) dispensed during that interval, average patient waiting time, the number (or type, or training) of staff at the facility, and adequacy of water, lighting and cleanliness.

Ensuring 'good service' is not easy, as adequacy of service is seldom entirely objective. Important first steps for any STI programme are ensuring that expectations are clearly documented in programme procedures manuals, and that staff members receive training on specific programme expectations. Given clear programme expectations, managers have employed a variety of tools to try to measure quality of service delivery. One of these is periodic on-site observation of services by supervisors, using a predetermined checklist of events (e.g. provider treated patient with respect). Ideally, such observation would be followed by constructive feedback to providers while the specifics of a situation were still fresh in the mind. Several peer monitoring techniques have also been employed, such as periodic case conferences where providers are asked to share particularly satisfying or difficult patient interactions, with a chance for colleagues to offer feedback. The use of simulated patients who go through services and report back on how services were delivered has been used by programmes in many nations. Patient satisfaction surveys may also be useful, although they tend to provide fewer data on service quality than other techniques when patients are not aware of the quality of service that they ought to expect. Because providers tend to focus on the services for which they are judged, the focus should be on a small number of indicators that are vitally important to the programme. Ideally, these should be factors that can be easily collected; otherwise data collection may get interfere with service provision (Hassig *et al.* 1996). Some examples of helpful prevention indicators are the two developed by the WHO Global Programme on AIDS: (1) the proportion of clients presenting for STI diagnosis and treatment who are treated according to national guidelines (PI-6), and (2) the proportion of clients presenting for STI diagnosis and treatment who receive appropriate prevention-related services (PI-7). Both involve a combination of routine data collection and direct observation to assess quality of STI service delivery (World Health Organization 1994; Franco *et al.* 1997).

Evaluation measures a programme's impact, whether on intermediate-term goals (e.g. reducing chlamydia prevalence in a defined population) or longer-term goals (e.g. preventing chlamydia-related sequelae in a defined population). Evaluation measures may focus on specific disease pathogens, the burden of STI overall, longer-term sequelae, or cost-effectiveness of programmes (e.g. cost per case averted). Sometimes referred to as 'data for decision making', evaluation data are important in determining whether an STI programme is worth continuing, and convincing policy makers about the value of a specific programme. Because programme goals will vary among interested parties, many experts recommend that programme goals and objectives ought to be developed collaboratively by the major stakeholders involved (rather than imposed by outside evaluators); this approach is also likely to increase compliance in data collection (Salabarria-Pena *et al.* 2007). Some common ways to collect impact data are through evaluation of STI surveillance data (whether case-reports or population-based surveys), STI-related morbidity indicators collected from non-STI service sites, results of special studies conducted by the STI control programme itself, or by other means (e.g. Demographic and Health Surveys) (Hassig *et al.* 1996).

Ultimately, the value of findings identified in monitoring and evaluation systems is to modify, strengthen, and improve the programme. This is more likely to take place if simple feedback mechanisms are established to ensure that programme staff members are aware of problems and can make needed changes. Feedback mechanisms may range from simple procedures, such as routine monthly communication from a supervisor or manager to the clinic staff to sophisticated annual reports on all aspects of programme performance (Hassig *et al.* 1996).

Research

Research helps in identifying more effective ways to conduct current prevention activities and in developing effective approaches to emerging problems. Most of the advances in STI prevention programmes and policy over the past decade were stimulated by research findings in the areas of epidemiology, clinical manifestations, and natural history of infection, diagnostics, therapeutics, and primary prevention approaches such as behavioural strategies, barrier contraceptives, and vaccines. Research is typically not conducted by STI prevention programmes; however, it is increasingly apparent that programme involvement is important, if not essential, for successful research translation. Programme involvement helps ensure that programme-relevant research questions are identified and that appropriate approaches to prevention research are used to evaluate intervention effectiveness, whether at the individual or population level (Aral *et al.* 2007).

There are many research priorities facing the field of STI prevention. Some are the development of better diagnostic tests (e.g. more accurate, faster, and cheaper); improved therapies, especially for those STI for which antimicrobial resistance is a concern; new vaccines, especially for viral STI; enhanced approaches for partner services; use of new communications technologies for prevention (e.g. Internet, social networking websites); practical use of sexual network analysis to reduce STI transmission; effective strategies for reducing HIV transmission through STI control; and determining the best combinations of interventions to enhance STI control. These efforts will require the involvement of a variety of sectors, including the pharmaceutical industry, academia, government, research networks, and involved communities (Douglas & Fenton 2007).

Special issues for STI prevention

Access to care

Effective STI management requires symptomatic individuals to have access to appropriate quality health services. That is a deceptively simple statement, however, as gaining access to STI care is a remarkably complex transaction in almost all societies. In addition to the general issues surrounding availability, affordability, and acceptability of health services, seeking health care for an STI is a function of attitudes about disease and sex (Dallabetta *et al.* 2007). In virtually every society, STI are associated with substantial stigmatization and prejudice, and tend to be viewed as 'social diseases' that are dirty, shameful, and somehow deserved. This may be the general norm even in the situation that occurs for many women (and all infants), whose STI exposure may be related to a partner's risk rather their own. Access to STI services requires that services be available; that involves factors such as easy-to-reach locations, convenient hours of operation, and providers trained in effective STI management. Access to effective STI management also requires affordability of the services. In some communities, public clinics may exist which are free of charge, but individuals may be required to pay for drugs prescribed. A recent review found that STI drug treatment (excluding STI management) in low- and middle-income countries cost approximately US$3 for acute, bacterial STI (range US$0.05–35.23); this exceeds the average daily income for low-income nations (Terris-Prestholt *et al.* 2006). In some settings, individuals must cover all costs of the services, making it less likely that poor or vulnerable populations will have access to the services. Whether or not available STI services are acceptable can also be complicated. Perceived empathy and acceptance by service providers has been observed to have a profoundly positive effect on patients' opinions of services, and perceived judgmental or scolding attitudes have been observed to lead to equally negative opinions of the services, even if they are of otherwise high quality (Dallabetta *et al.* 2007). Other factors related to acceptability include real and perceived privacy of the setting and confidentiality of services. Adolescents and stigmatized or marginalized groups (e.g. CSW, MSM) are often the least likely to find services in official settings to be acceptable. This situation must be addressed because of the contribution of such groups to STI transmission dynamics in a community.

Antimicrobial resistance

Resistance to previously effective antimicrobial therapies has developed for several STI including gonorrhoea, chancroid, trichomoniasis, syphilis, and HSV-2. Evolving resistance of gonorrhoea to various antimicrobial agents has had the greatest effect, and the emergence of highly resistant strains of gonorrhoea has been deemed by some public health experts to be 'one of the major health care disasters of the twentieth century' (World Health Organization 2007). Gonorrhoea resistance has been increasingly observed throughout the world over the past 30 years. Penicillinase-producing strains were first isolated in South East Asia as early as the 1970s, and subsequently penicillin-resistant gonorrhoea has spread widely throughout the world (WHO 2007). Resistance to other first-line therapies such as spectinomycin and tetracycline emerged in Asia in the 1980s. Fluoroquinolone-resistant gonorrhoea strains were found in several Asian countries in the 1990s, and high levels of fluoroquinolone resistance subsequently spread throughout Asia and other parts of the world (Lawung & Buatiang 2005) including the United States, in which treatment guidelines have recently been revised to no longer recommend the use of fluoroquinolones for treatment against gonorrhoea (CDC 2006; WHO 2007). Globally, WHO no longer recommends a single, first-line treatment for gonorrhoea, and national experts must decide, based on the local resistance data, what drugs to recommend (WHO 2007). That is a problematic situation because many countries cannot afford surveillance and must rely on data from other areas. With loss of fluoroquinolones, at present only a single class of antibiotics—third generation cephalosporins—remains uniformly effective against gonorrhoea. This situation will be seriously compounded if resistance to available cephalosporins develops, and therefore the development of effective alternative treatment regimens is a high STI-control priority. Antimicrobial resistance is also emerging for *H. ducreyi*, the causative agent of chancroid, although oral antibiotic therapies are still effective against this disease (CDC 2006). Azithromicin resistance in syphilis has been reported in a few settings (Lukehart *et al.* 2004), although the geographic distribution of resistant strains has not been well established, and *T. pallidum* remains exquisitely sensitive to penicillin, the first-line recommended therapy against syphilis. Resistance of trichomoniasis to standard treatment with single dose metronidazole occurs occasionally, requiring lengthier drug regimens or alternative treatments (CDC 2006). Additionally, while resistance of HSV-2 to acyclovir and related antiviral regimens is uncommon in immunocompetent patients, it has been observed to occur in up to 5 of HIV-infected patients (Reyes *et al.* 2003).

Essential drugs

Effective treatment and cure of bacterial STI requires the availability of appropriate drugs, preferably those with minimal side effects, and for which antimicrobial resistance is unlikely to develop. Also, such drugs ideally should not be contraindicated in pregnant or lactating women, and should lend themselves to single-dose, oral administration (World Health Organization 2007). A continual problem for many nations is that the most desirable drugs may not be included on national essential drug formularies, and therefore are generally not available to clients who attend public clinics. Although availability of particular STI drugs is dependant on numerous factors, the most immediate issue for most developing nations is affordability. Local availability also depends on intact and efficient national distribution systems to ensure that STI drugs (as well as other needed commodities such as condoms and syringes) are provided to all levels of the health care system before product expiration dates. Effective treatment requires that health care practitioners provide or prescribe appropriate drugs. Chances of this increase when national or local STI management guidelines are provided and disseminated, when STI training is included in professional school curricula or when refresher training courses are part of licensure or recertification of public and private providers, and when alternative practitioners (such as pharmacists) are included in STI management courses. Correct choice of drugs by providers has been observed to increase when countries adopt national syndromic algorithms, because management then becomes locally validated and standardized (Dallabetta *et al.* 2007). Some alternative strategies, such as pre-packaged STI drug kits, may also increase the likelihood that effective STI drugs will be provided to clients (Crabbe *et al.* 1998).

Targeted interventions for high-risk populations

As noted earlier, core groups can contribute significantly to disease burden and to further sustaining or perpetuating STI spread. In many communities, the core groups are CSW or other sex traders (individuals who trade sex for commodities other than money, such as food or drugs), men with highly mobile occupations that take them away from their homes and families (e.g. miners, seafarers, truck drivers) and MSM. Other populations, particularly adolescents, may also be viewed as 'high risk' given their high vulnerability to STI and their adverse consequences, even if the subgroup does not contribute disproportionately to disease transmission in the community. In most settings, the high-risk populations noted here have minimal or reduced access to official health care services either because of stigma, lack of financial resources, lack of time or convenient hours of operation, or because the official services are unacceptable to them. Given the situation of high-frequency transmitters who may have limited access to effective STI management, and often, limited resources, there is growing interest in the use of specialized, highly accessible interventions that are particularly targeted toward core groups or other vulnerable populations (Dallabetta *et al.* 2007; World Health Organization 2007). In the context of STI control, several such targeted interventions have been proven effective in selective community settings (Table 9.12.2). Current research indicates that the utility of any particular intervention is likely highly contextual, and that what works in one community may not work in others. Additionally, effective implementation of even a good, community-specific targeted intervention can be challenging since core groups are often difficult to identify or access, or both (Dallabetta *et al.* 2007). Additionally, the intervention or the persons applying it must not be perceived as stigmatizing or discriminatory toward the targeted group since acceptability of a specific intervention is generally determined by what happens at the first visit.

New opportunities for prevention

New initiatives

In May 2006, WHO announced a new *Global Strategy for Prevention and Control of STI: 2006–2015* and has begun work in supporting development of an Action Plan that could be adapted by nations around the world (World Health Organization 2007). The strategy emphasizes the importance of scaling up STI prevention activities globally and better integrating STI prevention with other prevention programmes. The strategy also highlights specific priority prevention activities for implementation (Table 9.12.3). In addition to scaling up syndromic management for STI in developing settings (which has been a continuing focus since the 1990s), areas that are given particularly high priority in the Global Strategy are the elimination of congenital syphilis as a public health problem; scaling up STI prevention strategies and programmes for HIV-infected persons; increasing STI surveillance within the context of second generation HIV surveillance programmes; and the elimination of bacterial causes of genital ulcer disease.

The Global Strategy's continuing focus on STI diagnosis and treatment illustrates the fundamental importance of high quality STI management in preventing adverse STI-related health outcomes in individuals, and also preventing further disease spread in the community. In contrast, the Global Strategy's priority ranking of congenital syphilis represents a renewed emphasis on the serious, adverse pregnancy outcomes related to syphilis that is timely for several reasons. First, syphilis screening tests and treatment are now readily available, and national policies in most countries support universal syphilis screening for pregnant women. Furthermore, several new opportunities exist, including availability of new rapid diagnostic tests that allow point-of-care screening (and if positive, treatment) at increasingly affordable prices (discussed below); greater attention on improved health care for women and infants as a result of the new Millennium Development Goals (MDGs) of the United Nations; and the global re-interest in advancing and supporting integrated antenatal care services.

The Global Strategy's third priority, an emphasis on STI screening and prevention in HIV-infected persons, is related to an increasing understanding that, even as more and more HIV-infected persons are able to access effective HIV treatments, new cases of HIV continue to occur at an alarming rate. Targeting HIV prevention efforts, including STI screening and treatment, for persons already in care is recognized as an early (and relatively easy) step in primary HIV prevention, even in countries with limited resources. The Strategy's fourth priority aimed at upgrading STI surveillance illustrates a need for countries to define their STI burden and to understand the population groups and settings where STI are most likely to occur. Many HIV programmes have already developed population-level behavioural and risk surveys, or sentinel surveillance surveys. For many of these, linking STI testing to existing surveillance systems can provide information that is important for both HIV and STI programmes. Control and elimination of bacterial causes of genital ulcer disease is the fifth priority area of the Global Strategy. Although increasingly unusual in many parts of the world, bacterially-caused genital ulcers remain problematic in parts of Africa and the Americas. Of all STI syndromes, genital ulcer disease has been most associated with enhanced HIV acquisition and transmission, with ulcerogenic STI estimated to account for 5–11 per cent of new HIV infections in some settings (Wasserheit 1992). Data from syndromic management validation studies indicate that both syphilis and chancroid have decreased in many settings in Africa and the Caribbean over the past 20 years. Although their decline is likely multifactorial, the promotion by WHO of syndromic management approaches and of regular availability of sufficient and effective antibiotics is playing an important role in this effort.

Rapid diagnostic tests

As noted earlier, rapid diagnostic tests (e.g. point-of-care) facilitate screening and treatment of STI in asymptomatic persons (e.g. chlamydial infections, syphilis infections in pregnant women) in settings where it may be difficult for patients to learn of results and get prompt treatment if test results are positive (e.g. remote, hard-to-reach settings where reference laboratories are limited or have reduced capacity). Rapid tests may also be useful for symptomatic patients where more sensitive and specific diagnostic tests are unaffordable. Although syndromic treatment algorithms are used in many parts of the world for symptomatic patients, the use of appropriate diagnostic tests could greatly increase the specificity of the algorithms and thus reduce unnecessary treatment (e.g. for women with vaginitis). Recognizing the need for simple, affordable diagnostic tests for STI that can be performed during a clinic visit so as to allow immediate treatment, WHO's Sexually Transmitted Disease Diagnostic Initiative (SDI) is dedicated to the development, evaluation and application of rapid diagnostic tests for STI that are appropriate for use in primary health care settings in developing countries (Sexually Transmitted Diseases Diagnostics Initiative 2007). The SDI focus is on tests that meet the 'ASSURED' criteria—*a*ffordable, *s*ensitive, *s*pecific, *u*ser-friendly (simple to perform in only a few steps and with minimal training), *r*apid and *r*obust (to enable treatment at first visit, and not requiring refrigeration), *e*quipment-free (i.e. easy, non-invasive way to collect specimens), and *d*elivered to end users (Sexually Transmitted Diseases Diagnostics Initiative 2007).

To date, the SDI has prioritized evaluation of rapid tests for syphilis, gonorrhoea and chlamydia, as these are the STI most associated with substantial adverse health outcomes in developed settings and for which curative therapy is widely available. Rapid tests for syphilis have been particularly successful, and there are more than a dozen with good performance relative to the reference standard. Also, they are easy to use and often quite affordable (e.g. substantially

Table 9.12.2 Some targeted interventions for high-risk populations that have been found effective in reducing STI in selected community settings

Female sex workers	
Specialized sex worker clinics	STI clinical services, condoms and preventive education and counselling provided by specially trained staff, available at convenient locations and during hours that do not interfere with women's work. Ideally, such clinics can be easily accessed using public transport as many women work in neighbourhoods far from their homes and prefer treatment close to the work site and away from their homes (Dallabetta *et al.* 2007)
Ambulatory clinic vans	Mobile vans that travel from community to community and allow women to come in for routine STI clinical care and other health services. Integrating additional health services helps reduce stigma
Clinics at the work site	CSW establishment owners contract with private practitioners to provide routine on-site STI clinical evaluations and treatment (Dallabetta *et al.* 2007)
Brothel-based 100 per cent condom use programs	Structural intervention whereby brothel managers require clients and women to use condoms with every sexual encounter. Was particularly effective in Thailand
Periodic presumptive therapy	Single empiric mass treatment of sex workers has been found to reduce STI prevalence in some settings, however levels eventually rose again. Periodic empiric mass treatment appears to lower bacterial STI and particularly syphilis (Berman & Kamb 2007)
Men away from home	
Pharmacy-based interventions	Pharmacists trained in syndromic management can provide effective treatment to men with urethritis and GUD who may be unwilling to wait in primary health clinics. Use of prepackaged STI 'treatment kits' that include specific STI drugs, partner referral cards, and condoms has been found to increase rates of effective treatment in some communities and may be particularly useful in pharmacies (Ryan *et al.* 2007)
Clinics at the work-site	Many companies (e.g. shipping companies, mining operations, agricultural estates) provide STI clinical care, condoms and health education to employees. Services seem to be most acceptable if it is perceived that care is not related to employment (e.g. HIV testing may have low uptake if perceived related to employment)
Men who have sex with men	
Specialized clinics or services	Accessible, acceptable clinical services with specialized providers promotes trust and increases likelihood men will come promptly for treatment and refer partners (Peterman *et al.* 2005)
Venue-based interventions	Providing information or clinical services (or referral to services) at bars, bath houses or other venues where MSM are likely to congregate has been effective in some communities. Provision of integrated health services may be more acceptable and less stigmatizing (Blank *et al.* 2005; Ciesielski *et al.* 2005)
Network-based interventions	Internet or local gay press may be ways to provide preventive health information or information about where clinical services can be safely obtained without stigma (McFarlane *et al.* 2005)
Adolescents	
Specialized youth centres	Services catering toward youth and their issues, with specialized counselling. Special care units may be integrated within existing care facilities (e.g. within family planning services, within primary care with special days for youth) or in store-fronts in places easily accessible to youth (World Health Organization 2007)
Internet and mobile telephone interventions	Health education messages or referrals to specialized clinical services may be increasingly used as more adolescents have access to new technologies (Kachur 2007)

less than US$1 in many cases). Many syphilis tests can use whole blood and do not require refrigeration. Thus far, however, all of the licensed rapid syphilis tests have been treponemal tests, recognizing syphilis infection but unable to distinguish between new and prior (treated) infection, which has been the function of the non-treponemal tests (e.g. VDRL, RPR) that are typically used for screening and to quantify disease activity. Use of treponemal tests alone carries the potential for over-treatment, which may be substantial in settings with prior STI control activities, as many of these positive tests will simply indicate prior infection rather than active disease. Therefore, development of a simple, rapid, two-antigen test, including non-treponemal as well as treponemal tests, is an important priority.

Evaluations for rapid gonorrhoea and chlamydia tests are continuing, and some promising candidates are being evaluated now or are to be evaluated in the near future (Lee 2007). The tests developed thus far have had less than ideal sensitivity and specificity, although mathematical models indicate that in certain settings with relatively high STI prevalence even tests with lower than optimal sensitivity and specificity might have a significant effect on disease burden when asymptomatic people who would otherwise not be treated can be reached for screening and treatment (Peeling *et al.* 2006). The SDI notes that recent advances in the understanding about the pathogenesis of STI, and the availability of complete genome sequences for the pathogens causing specific STI syndromes, are likely to support the development of raid tests in upcoming years (Peeling *et al.* 2006).

Table 9.12.3 WHO global strategy for prevention and control of STI 2006–2015: prevention activities for priority implementation in resource-limited settings*

Priority 1 activities	**Indicators**	**National-level targets (to be reached by 2010* or 2015)**
1. Scale up STI diagnosis and treatment, using syndromic management where diagnostic resources are limited	◆ Per cent of primary care sites providing comprehensive case management for symptomatic STI ◆ Per cent of STI patients at selected health facilities who are diagnosed, treated and counselled per national guidelines	◆ 90 per cent of primary care sites provide comprehensive STI care ◆ 90 per cent of women and men with STI at health-care facilities are appropriately diagnosed, treated and counselled
2. Control congenital syphilis as a step towards elimination	◆ Per cent of 15–24-year-old pregnant women attending antenatal clinics with a positive serology for syphilis who are treated per national guidelines	◆ 90 per cent of first time 15–24-year-old antenatal care attendees screened for syphilis ◆ 90 per cent of syphilis sero-positive women are treated adequately
3. Scale up STI prevention strategies and programmes for HIV-positive persons	◆ Per cent of HIV-positive patients with STI who receive comprehensive STI care, including advice on condom use and partner notification	◆ Strategies and guidelines for HIV positive persons with STI interventions in place* ◆ 90 per cent of primary point-of-care sites provide effective STI care for HIV infected persons
4. Upgrade STI surveillance within the context of second generation HIV surveillance	◆ Number of STI prevalence studies regularly conducted (at sentinel sites or in sentinel populations) every three to five years ◆ Annual incidence of reported STI (syndromic or etiologic)	◆ At least two rounds of prevalence surveys conducted ◆ Routine STI reporting established and sustained over at least 5 consecutive years
5. Control bacterial genital ulcer disease (GUD)	◆ Per cent of confirmed bacterial GUD cases in patients with genital ulcerative diseases ◆ Per cent of 15–24-year-old pregnant women attending antenatal clinics with a positive serology for syphilis	◆ Zero cases of chancroid identified in GUD patients ◆ Reduction to below 2 per cent of positive syphilis serology among 15–24-year-old antenatal care attendees
Priority 2 activities	**Indicators**	**National-level targets (to be reached by 2010* or 2015)**
6. Implement targeted interventions for high-risk and vulnerable populations	◆ Health needs identified/ national plans developed and implemented for STI/HIV control for key high-risk and vulnerable populations ◆ Per cent of people aged 15-24 years with STI that are detected during diagnostic STI testing	◆ Health needs, policies, legislation and regulations reviewed; plans in place and country-specific targeted interventions implemented* ◆ At least two rounds of prevalence surveys done among groups with high-risk behaviour and among young people
7. Implement age-appropriate comprehensive sexual health education and services	◆ Per cent of schools with at least one teacher who can provide life-skills-based STI/HIV prevention education	◆ Review of policies, development of age-appropriate training and information material for schools completed (by 2007) ◆ Increased number of teachers trained in participatory life-skills-based STI/HIV education
8. Promote partner treatment and prevention of reinfection	◆ Per cent of patients with STI whose partner(s) are referred for treatment	◆ Plans/support materials for partner notification developed; and health-care provider training in place* ◆ Double the proportion of patients who bring in or provide treatment to their partner(s)
9. Roll out of effective vaccines (HBV, HPV and eventually HSV)	◆ Policy and plans for universal vaccination for hepatitis B ◆ Plans and policy reviews and strategies for implementation of HPV and potential HSV-2 vaccines.	◆ Plans in place regarding vaccination for hepatitis B and HPV (by 2008) ◆ Pilot vaccination programmes initiated and scaling up in progress*
10. Universal opt-out HIV voluntary counselling and testing in STI patients	◆ Per cent of STI patients who are routinely counselled and offered confidential HIV testing	◆ HIV testing and counselling available in all settings providing care for STI ◆ Double the proportion of STI patients who receive voluntary counselling and testing for HIV

STI, sexually transmitted infections; HIV, human immunodeficiency virus; GUD, genital ulcer disease; HBV, hepatitis B virus; HPV, human papillomavirus; HSV, herpes simplex virus.
Priority 1: Should be implemented in all nations
Priority 2: Should be implemented if resources exist
* Adapted from World Health Organization. (2007). *Global Strategy for the prevention and Control of Sexually Transmitted Infections 2006–2015*. Geneva, WHO.

Integration of services

Over the past century, the fashions around integrated public health programmes that focus on prevention as well as curative aspects of STD control, versus a more vertical approach that focuses on STI diagnosis and cure, have waxed and waned. With the MDGs clearly addressing women, infants and adolescents, the potential advantages of integrated programmes for some areas of STI control are important considerations. Antenatal service visits and delivery offer the opportunity to integrate a package of preventive services, including maternal syphilis screening and HIV testing (both preferably early in pregnancy), prophylactic treatment for conjunctivitis (at delivery), and neonatal HBV (postnatal period) in appropriate settings where vertical HBV transmission is high (e.g. parts of Asia). In settings where prevention of mother-to-child HIV transmission functions as a separate (often parallel) programme alongside antenatal services, introduction of syphilis testing has the potential both to reduce congenital syphilis infections and to enhance uptake of HIV testing, which can be more stigmatizing than syphilis testing. For reproductive-aged women, family planning services offer an opportunity for STI education and screening that target sexually active women who may be at risk for particular STI. In this setting, consideration must be given to encouraging condoms as a disease-prevention strategy that should be considered in conjunction with (rather than instead of) more effective contraceptive practices such as hormonal contraceptives. For men, on the other hand, opportunities for integrating STI care into other health services have not been particularly effective thus far, as many men do not use traditional public health clinics. Recently, the results of three African clinical trials found a substantial protective effect of adult male circumcision against new HIV infection, and strategies around safe and affordable circumcision may offer an opportunity for integrating STI services for men in those settings (World Health Organization 2007; WHO/UNAIDS Technical Consultation 2007). Many nations with high HIV prevalence are already grappling with best practices of providing circumcision to interested adult males, and public health experts have recognized that additional services around HIV/STI prevention education and counselling, HIV testing, condom promotion and screening for certain STI associated with HIV may be an efficient and cost-effective part of the package.

Conclusion

At the outset of the twenty-first century, STI continue to be a major global health problem, accounting for substantial reproductive, perinatal, and cancer-related morbidity and mortality—in addition to their contributions to HIV transmission. This chapter has outlined a number of successes that have occurred and several upcoming opportunities that exist in the field of STI control both in industrialized countries with established STI control programmes and in developing countries. For example, the use of syndromic case management in developing settings appears to have markedly reduced the burden of curable STI and their sequelae in many nations. Additionally, although viral STI remain highly prevalent in all countries, new tools for their control (e.g. vaccines, suppressive antiviral therapy) offer great promise. However, many challenges remain. In an era of increasingly available and affordable interventions, some very basic STI control programmes (e.g. universal syphilis screening of pregnant women) have not been well-adopted, especially in developing-world settings. New problems are also emerging, such as antimicrobial resistance and social disruption leading to gaps in health care and altered sexual networks, both of which enhance transmission. Because STI are stigmatizing conditions that have their greatest effect in vulnerable or marginalized populations, mobilizing societal and political support for their prevention and control remains challenging in all countries. However, in spite of this challenge, given the societal costs associated with STI and the new approaches available to prevent them, efforts to sustain and scale up effective STI control programmes must remain important global health priorities.

References

Adimora A.A., Schoenbach V.J. (2005). Social context, sexual networks, and racial disparities in rates of sexually transmitted infections. *J Infect Dis* 191 Suppl 1:S115–S122.

Adler M.W. (1996). Sexually transmitted diseases control in developing countries. *Genitourin Med* 72(2):83–88.

Anderson R., Hanson M. (2005). Potential public health impact of imperfect HIV type 1 vaccines. *J Infect Dis* 191 Suppl 1:S85–S96.

Aral S.O., Holmes K.K., Padian N.S. *et al.* (1996). Overview: individual and population approaches to the epidemiology and prevention of sexually transmitted diseases and human immunodeficiency virus infection. *J Infect Dis* 174 Suppl 2:S127–S133.

Aral S.O., Lipshutz J.A., Douglas J.M. (2007). Introduction. In Aral, S.O.; Douglas, J.M.; Lipshutz, J.A. eds., *Behavioral Interventions for Prevention and Control of Sexually Transmitted Diseases*: New York, Springer Science and Business Media, LLC. 60–101.

Aral S.O., Padian N.S., Holmes K.K. (2005). Advances in multilevel approaches to understanding the epidemiology and prevention of sexually transmitted infections and HIV: an overview. *J Infect Dis* 191 Suppl 1:S1–S6.

ASTHO. (2004). State Public Health Employee Shortage Report: A Civil Service Recruitment and Retention Crisis.

Baseman J.G., Koutsky L.A. (2005). The epidemiology of human papillomavirus infections. *J Clin Virol* 32 Suppl 1:S16–S24.

Berman S., Kamb M. (2007). Biomedical Interventions. In Aral, S.O.; Douglas, J.M.; Lipshutz, J.A. eds., *Behavioral Interventions for Prevention and Control of Sexually Transmitted Diseases*: New York, Springer Science and Business Media, LLC. 60–101.

Blank S., Gallagher K., Washburn K. *et al.* (2005). Reaching out to boys at bars: utilizing community partnerships to employ a wellness strategy for syphilis control among men who have sex with men in New York City. *Sex Transm Dis* 32(10 Suppl):S65–S72.

Brewer D.D. (2005). Case-finding effectiveness of partner notification and cluster investigation for sexually transmitted diseases/HIV. *Sex Transm Dis* 32(2):78–83.

Brown Z.A., Selke S., Zeh J. *et al.* (1997). The acquisition of herpes simplex virus during pregnancy. *N Engl J Med* 337(8):509–515.

Brunham R.C. (2005). Parran Award Lecture: insights into the epidemiology of sexually transmitted diseases from Ro = betacD. *Sex Transm Dis* 32(12):722–724.

Cates W. Jr., Holmes K.K. (1998). Public Health and Preventive Medicine. Wallace R, editor. *Sexually Transmitted Diseases,* 14th Edition, 137–155.

CDC. (2001). Community and individual behavior change interventions. Program Operations Guidelines for STD Prevention:1–24.

CDC. (2001). Guidelines for STD Prevention. Program Operations Guidelines for STD Prevention:1–27.

CDC. (2001). Overview. Program Operations Guidelines for STD Prevention:1–26.

CDC. (2003). Incorporating HIV prevention into the medical care of persons living with HIV. MMWR 52(RR-12):1–24.

CDC. (2004). Infertility and Prevention of Sexually Transmitted Diseases. Report to Congress. (Accessed on February 8, 2007, at http://www.cdc.gov/std/infertility/ReportCongressInfertility.pdf).

CDC. (2005). Sexually Transmitted Disease Surveillance. Atlanta, GA. U.S. Department of Health and Services.

CDC. (2006). Expedited partner therapy in the management of sexually transmitted diseases. Atlanta, GA: U S Department of Health and Human Services.

CDC. (2006). Hepatitis B Virus Infection: A comprehensive immunization strategy to eliminate transmission in the United States, Part II immunization of adults. MMWR:1–79.

CDC. (2006). Sexually Transmitted Disease Treatment Guidelines. MMWR 55(RR-11):1–94.

CDC. (2006). The National Plan to Eliminate Syphilis from the United States. Division of STD Prevention.

CDC. (2007). Quadrivalent human papillomavirus vaccine – recommendations of the Advisory Committee on Immunization Practices (ACIP). MMWR:1–24.

CDC. National Network of STD Prevention Training Center (NNPTC) (Accessed January 12, 2006, at http://www.cdc.gov/std/training/courses.htm).

Ciesielski C., Kahn R.H., Taylor M. *et al.* (2005). Control of syphilis outbreaks in men who have sex with men: the role of screening in nonmedical settings. *Sex Transm Dis* 32(10 Suppl):S37–S42.

Cogliano V., Baan R., Straif K. *et al.* (2005). Carcinogenicity of human papillomaviruses. *Lancet Oncol* 6(4):204.

Corey L., Huang ML., Selke S. *et al.* (2005). Differentiation of herpes simplex virus types 1 and 2 in clinical samples by a real-time taqman PCR assay. *J Med Virol* 76(3):350–355.

Crabbe F., Tchupo J.P., Manchester T. *et al.* (1998). Prepackaged therapy for urethritis: the 'MSTOP' experience in Cameroon. *Sex Transm Infect* 74(4):249–252.

Daling J.R., Madeleine M.M., Johnson L.G. *et al.* (2004). Human papillomavirus, smoking, and sexual practices in the etiology of anal cancer. *Cancer* 101(2):270–280.

Daling J.R., Madeleine M.M., Johnson L.G. *et al.* (2005). Penile cancer: importance of circumcision, human papillomavirus and smoking in in situ and invasive disease. *Int J Cancer* 116(4):606–616.

Dallabetta G., Field M., Lage M. *et al.* (2007). STDs: Global Burden and Challenges for Control. In G. Dallabetta, M. Laga, and Lamptey P. eds. 'Control of Sexually Transmitted Diseases: A handbook for the design and management of programs,' Durham, North Carolina; Family Health International/The AIDS Control and Prevention Project (AIDSCAP). 23–52.

Department of Health. Better prevention, better services, better sexual health - The national strategy for sexual health and HIV. Crown Copyright. July 2001. Accessed January 7, 2007 at http://www.dh.gov.uk/PublicationsAndStatistics/Publications/PublicationsPolicyAndGuidance/PublicationsPolicyAndGuidanceArticle/fs/en?CONTENT_ID=4003133&chk=/iTv%2BN).

Douglas J.M., Fenton K. (2007). STD/HIV Prevention Programs in Developed Countries. In: *Sexually Transmitted Disease*. Holmes KK. eds, Fourth edition. McGraw-Hill: New York (in press).

Du P., Coles F.B., Gerber T. *et al.* (2006). Effects of partner notification on reducing gonorrhea incidence rate. *Sex Transm Dis*:189–194.

Ebrahim S.H., Peterman T.A., Zaidi A.A. *et al.* (1997). Mortality related to sexually transmitted diseases in US women, 1973 through 1992. *Am J Public Health* 87(6):938–944.

Elbasha E.H., Dasbach E.J., Insinga R.P. (2007). Model for assessing human papillomavirus vaccination strategies. *Emerg Infect Dis* 13(1):28–41.

Fenton K., Bloom F. (2007). STD Prevention with Men Who Have Sex with Men in the United States. In: *Behavioral Interventions for Prevention and Control of Sexually Transmitted Diseases*. Aral S, Douglas J, eds. New York: Springer SBM, LLC.

Fleming D.T., Wasserheit J.N. (1999). From epidemiological synergy to public health policy and practice: the contribution of other sexually transmitted diseases to sexual transmission of HIV infection. *Sex Transm Infect* 75(1):3–17.

Franco L.M., Daly C.C., Chilongozi D. *et al.* (1997). Quality of case management of sexually transmitted diseases: comparison of the methods for assessing the performance of providers. *Bull World Health Organ* 75(6):523–532.

Gift T.L., Pate M.S., Hook E.W., III. *et al.* (1999). The rapid test paradox: when fewer cases detected lead to more cases treated: a decision analysis of tests for Chlamydia trachomatis. *Sex Transm Dis* 26(4): 232–240.

Global Burden of Hepatitis C Working Group. Accesed on August 17, 2007 at http://jcp.sagepub.com/misc/terms.shtml. (2004). *J Clin Phar* 44:20–29.

Golden M.R., Whittington W.L., Handsfield H.H. *et al.* (2005). Effect of expedited treatment of sex partners on recurrent or persistent gonorrhea or chlamydial infection. *N Engl J Med* 352(7):676–685.

Goldie S.J., Kohli M., Grima D. *et al.* (2004). Projected clinical benefits and cost-effectiveness of a human papillomavirus 16/18 vaccine. *J Natl Cancer Inst* 96(8):604–615.

Goldstein S.T., Zhou F., Hadler S.C. *et al.* (2005). A mathematical model to estimate global hepatitis B disease burden and vaccination impact. *Int J Epidemiol* 34(6):1329–1339.

Goyaux N., Leke R., Keita N. *et al.* (2003). Ectopic pregnancy in African developing countries. *Acta Obstet Gynecol Scand* 82(4):305–312.

Greenberg J.B., MacGowan R., Neumann M. *et al.* (1998). Linking injection drug users to medical services: role of street outreach referrals. *Health Soc Work* 23(4):298–309.

Grosskurth H., Gray R., Hayes R. *et al.* (2000). Control of sexually transmitted diseases for HIV-1 prevention: understanding the implications of the Mwanza and Rakai trials. *Lancet* 355(9219): 1981–1987.

Han Y., Coles F.B., Muse A. *et al.* (1999). Assessment of a geographically targeted field intervention on gonorrhea incidence in two New York State counties. *Sex Transm Dis* 26(5):296–302.

Harper D.M., Franco E.L., Wheeler C. *et al.* (2004). Efficacy of a bivalent L1 virus-like particle vaccine in prevention of infection with human papillomavirus types 16 and 18 in young women: a randomised controlled trial. *Lancet* 364(9447):1757–1765.

Hassig S., Hoffman I., Hamilton H. (1996). STD Monitoring and Evaluation, In: *Control of Sexually Transmitted Diseases; A Handbook for the Design and Management of Programs*, eds. Dallabetta, G.; Laga, M.; Lamptey, P.; Family Health International, AIDS Control and Prevention Project. 275–289.

Hogben M., Brewer D.D., Golden M.R. (2007). Partner Notification and Management Interventions. In: *Behavioral Interventions for Prevention and Control of Sexually Transmitted Diseases*. Aral S., Douglas J., eds. New York: Springer SBM, LLC.

Hughes J.P., Garnett G.P., Koutsky L. (2002). The theoretical population-level impact of a prophylactic human papilloma virus vaccine. *Epidemiology* 13(6):631–639.

Kamb M.L., Fishbein M., Douglas J.M., Jr. *et al.* (1998). Efficacy of risk-reduction counseling to prevent human immunodeficiency virus and sexually transmitted diseases: a randomized controlled trial. Project RESPECT Study Group. *JAMA* 280(13):1161–1167.

Korenromp E.L., White R.G., Orroth K.K. *et al.* (2005). Determinants of the impact of sexually transmitted infection treatment on prevention of HIV infection: a synthesis of evidence from the Mwanza, Rakai, and Masaka intervention trials. *J Infect Dis* 191 Suppl 1:S168–S178.

Koutsky L.A., Ault K.A., Wheeler C.M. *et al.* (2002). A controlled trial of a human papillomavirus type 16 vaccine. *N Engl J Med* 347(21): 1645–1651.

Laga M., Alary M., Nzila N. *et al.* (1994). Condom promotion, sexually transmitted diseases treatment, and declining incidence of HIV-1 infection in female Zairian sex workers. *Lancet* 344(8917):246–248.

Lawung R., Buatiang A. *et al.* (2005). Increasing trend of multiple resistance and genomic mobility of Neisseria gonorrhoeae to penicillin and quinolone. *EXCLI Journal* 4, 130–140.

Lee H. (2007). A new chlamydia rapid test using non-invasive samples. 17th International Society for STD Research, Seattle, Washington.

Leichliter J., Ellen J., Gunn R. (2007). STD Repeaters: Implications for the Individuals and STD Transmission in a Population In: *Behavioral Interventions for Prevention and Control of Sexually Transmitted Diseases*. Aral S, Douglas J, eds. New York: Springer SBM, LLC.

Levine W.C., Revollo R., Kaune V. *et al.* (1998). Decline in sexually transmitted disease prevalence in female Bolivian sex workers: impact of an HIV prevention project. *AIDS* 12(14):1899–1906.

Lukehart S.A., Godornes C., Molini B.J. *et al.* (2004). Macrolide resistance in Treponema pallidum in the United States and Ireland. *N Engl J Med* 351(2):154–158.

Manhart L.E., Holmes K.K. (2005). Randomized controlled trials of individual-level, population-level, and multilevel interventions for preventing sexually transmitted infections: what has worked? *J Infect Dis* 191 Suppl 1:S7–24.

May R.M., Anderson R.M. (1987). Transmission dynamics of HIV infection. *Nature* 326(6109):137–142.

McFarlane M., Bull S.S. (2007). Use of the Interest in STD/HIV Prevention. In: *Behavioral Interventions for Prevention and Control of Sexually Transmitted Diseases*. Aral S, Douglas J, eds. New York: Springer SBM, LLC. 214–231.

McFarlane M., Kachur R., Klausner J.D. *et al.* (2005). Internet-based health promotion and disease control in the 8 cities: successes, barriers, and future plans. *Sex Transm Dis* 32(10 Suppl):S60–S64.

McGlynn K.A., London W.T. (2005). Epidemiology and natural history of hepatocellular carcinoma. *Best Pract Res Clin Gastroenterol* 19(1): 3–23.

Meheus A. (1992). Women's health: importance of reproductive tract infections, pelvic inflammatory disease and cervical cancer, in A. Germain, K.K. Holmes, P. Piot, and J.N. Wasserheit eds., *Reproductive Tract Infections: Global Impact and Priorities for Women's Reproductive Health*: New York, Plenum Press, p. 61–91.

Munoz N., Bosch F.X., de S.S. *et al.* (2003). Epidemiologic classification of human papillomavirus types associated with cervical cancer. *N Engl J Med* 348(6):518–527.

Nagot N., Ouedraogo A., Foulongne V. *et al.* (2007). Reduction of HIV-1 RNA levels with therapy to suppress herpes simplex virus. *N Engl J Med* 356(8):790–799.

Over M., Piot P. (1993). HIV infection and sexually transmitted diseases. In D.T. Jameson, Mosley W.H., Measham A.R., Babadilla J.L., eds. *Disease Control Priorities in Developing Countries*, New York; Oxford University Press. 445–529.

Over M., Piot P. (1996). Human immunodeficiency virus infection and other sexually transmitted diseases in developing countries: public health importance and priorities for resource allocation. *J Infect Dis* 174(Suppl. 2):S162–S175.

Passin W.F., Kim A.S., Hutchinson A.B. *et al.* (2006). A systematic review of HIV partner counseling and referral services: client and provider attitudes, preferences, practices, and experiences. *Sex Transm Dis* 33(5):320–328.

Paz-Bailey G., Ramaswamy M., Hawkes S.J. *et al.* (2007). Herpes simplex virus type 2: epidemiology and management options in developing countries. *Sex Transm Infect* 83(1):16–22.

Peeling R.W., Mabey D., Herring A. *et al.* (2006). Why do we need quality-assured diagnostic tests for sexually transmitted infections? *Nat Rev Microbiol* 4(12):909–921.

Perz J.F., Armstrong G.L., Farrington L.A. *et al.* (2006). The contributions of hepatitis B virus and hepatitis C virus infections to cirrhosis and primary liver cancer worldwide. *J Hepatol* 45(4):529–538.

Peterman T.A., Collins D.E., Aral S.O. (2005). Responding to the epidemics of syphilis among men who have sex with men: introduction to the special issue. *Sex Transm Dis* 32(10 Suppl):S1–S3.

Pisani P., Parkin D.M., Bray F. *et al.* (1999). Estimates of the worldwide mortality from 25 cancers in 1990. *Int J Cancer* 83(1):18–29.

Plummer F.A., Countinho R.A., Ngugi E.N. *et al.* (2005). Sex workers and their clients in the epidemiology and control of sexually transmitted diseases. *Sexually Transmitted Diseases*, Third Edition. [10], 143–150.

Reyes M., Shaik N.S., Graber J.M. *et al.* (2003). Acyclovir-resistant genital herpes among persons attending sexually transmitted disease and human immunodeficiency virus clinics. *Arch Intern Med* 163(1):76–80.

Ryan C., Kamb M., Holmes K. (2007). STI Care Management. In: *Sexually Transmitted Disease*. Holmes K.K. eds, Fourth edition. McGraw-Hill: New York.

Salabarria-Pena Y., Pat B.S., Walsh C.M. (2007). Practical Use of Program Evaluation among Sexually Transmitted disease (STD) Programs, Atlanta (GA): Centers for Disease Control and Prevention.

Salmon, C.T. (1989)ed., *Information Campaigns: Balancing Social Values and Social Change*, Newbury Park, CA Sage.

Sanchez J., Campos P.E., Courtois B. *et al.* (2003). Prevention of sexually transmitted diseases (STDs) in female sex workers: prospective evaluation of condom promotion and strengthened STD services. *Sex Transm Dis* 30(4):273–279.

Santelli J., Ott M.A., Lyon M. *et al.* (2006). Abstinence-only education policies and programs: a position paper of the Society for Adolescent Medicine. *J Adolesc Health* 38(1):83–87.

Schmid G.P., Stoner B.P., Hawkes S. *et al.* (2007). The need and plan for global elimination of congenital syphilis. *Sex Transm Dis* 34(7 Suppl):S5–10.

Schmiedeskamp M.R., Kockler D.R. (2006). Human papillomavirus vaccines. *Ann Pharmacother* 40(7–8):1344–1352.

Sexually Transmitted Diseases Diagnostics Initiative website accessed on April 11, 2007 at http://www.who.int/std_diagnostics/.

Shelton J.D., Halperin D.T., Nantulya V. *et al.* (2004). Partner reduction is crucial for balanced 'ABC' approach to HIV prevention. *BMJ* 328(7444):891–893.

Szmuness W., Stevens C.E., Harley E.J. *et al.* (1980). Hepatitis B vaccine: demonstration of efficacy in a controlled clinical trial in a high-risk population in the United States. *N Engl J Med* 303(15):833–841.

Terris-Prestholt F., Vyas S., Kumaranayake L. *et al.* (2006). The costs of treating curable sexually transmitted infections in low- and middle-income countries: a systematic review. *Sex Transm Dis* 33(10 Suppl): S153–S166.

Tietz A., Davies S.C., Moran J.S. (2004). Guide to sexually transmitted disease resources on the Internet. *Clin Infect Dis* 38(9):1304–1310.

Trelle S., Shang A., Nartey L. *et al.* (2007). Improved effectiveness of partner notification for patients with sexually transmitted infections: systematic review. *BMJ* 334(7589):354.

Vega M.Y., Ghanem K.G. (2007). STD Prevention Communication: Using Social Marketing Techniques with an Eye on Behavioral Change. In Aral, S.O.; Douglas, J.M.; Lipshutz, J.A. eds., *Behavioral Interventions for Prevention and Control of Sexually Transmitted Diseases*: New York, Springer Science and Business Media, LLC, pp. 142–169.

Villa L.L., Costa R.L., Petta C.A. *et al.* (2005). Prophylactic quadrivalent human papillomavirus (types 6, 11, 16, and 18) L1 virus-like particle vaccine in young women: a randomised double-blind placebo-controlled multicentre phase II efficacy trial. *Lancet Oncol* 6(5):271–278.

Waaler H.T., Piot M.A. (1969). The use of an epidemiological model for estimating the effectiveness of tuberculosis control measures. Sensitivity of the effectiveness of tuberculosis control measures to the coverage of the population. *Bull World Health Organ* 41(1):75–93.

Warner L., Rietmeijer C. *et al.* (2006). A brief waiting room video intervention reduces incident sexually transmitted infections among STD clinic patients. 2006 National STD Prevention Conference, Jacksonville, FL, May 8–11.

Wasserheit J.N. (1992). Epidemiological synergy. Interrelationships between human immunodeficiency virus infection and other sexually transmitted diseases. *Sex Transm Dis* 19(2):61–77.

Watson-Jones D., Weiss H.A., Changalucha J.M. *et al.* (2007). Adverse birth outcomes in United Republic of Tanzania—impact and prevention of maternal risk factors. *Bull World Health Organ* 85(1):9–18.

Wawer M.J., Sewankambo N.K., Serwadda D. *et al.* (1999). Control of sexually transmitted diseases for AIDS prevention in Uganda: a randomised community trial. Rakai Project Study Group. *Lancet* 353(9152):525–535.

Weinstock H., Berman S., Cates W. Jr. (2004). Sexually transmitted diseases among American youth: incidence and prevalence estimates, 2000. *Perspect Sex Reprod Health* 36(1):6–10.

Weiss H. (2004). Epidemiology of herpes simplex virus type 2 infection in the developing world. *Herpes* 11 Suppl 1:24A-35A.

Weiss H.A. (2007). Male circumcision as a preventive measure against HIV and other sexually transmitted diseases. *Curr Opin Infect Dis* 20(1):66–72.

White P.J., Golden M.R. Thurner K.M.E. *et.al.* (2005). Patient-delivered partner therapy: when and where should it be used? predicting its impact in the USA and U.K. 16th International Society for STD Research, Amsterdam, Netherlands.

White R.G., Orroth K.K., Korenromp E.L. *et al.* (2004). Can population differences explain the contrasting results of the Mwanza, Rakai, and Masaka HIV/sexually transmitted disease intervention trials?: A modeling study. *J Acquir Immune Defic Syndr* 37(4):1500–1513.

WHO Report on Infectious Diseases 2000, Overcoming Antimicrobial Resistance. (Accessed August 18, 2007 at http://www.who.int/infectious-disease-report/2000/.

WHO/UNAIDS Technical Consultation. Male circumcision and HIV prevention: Research implications for policy and programming. Montreaux, 6–8 March, 2007; Conclusions and Recommendations (www.who.int/hiv/mediacentre/MCrecommendations_en.pdf).

Williams S.P., Kahn R.H. (2007). Looking Inside and Affecting the Outside: Corrections-based Interventions for STD Prevention. In: *Behavioral Interventions for Prevention and Control of Sexually Transmitted Diseases*. Aral S, Douglas J, eds. New York: Springer SBM, LLC. 374–396.

Witte K., Allen M. (2000). A Meta-analysis of Fear Appeals: Implications for Effective Public Health Campaigns. *Health Education and Behavior*, 27:591–615.

World Bank (2003). World Bank World Development Report 2004: New York, Oxford University Press.

World Health Organization. (1994). Evaluation of a national programme: a methods package 1. Prevention of HIV infection. Geneva.

World Health Organization. (2007). Global Strategy for the Prevention and Control of Sexually Transmitted Infections 2006–2015. Geneva, World Health Organization.

World Health Organization. Revised Global Burden of Disease 2002 Estimates, Accessed on April 11, 2007 at http://www.who.int/healthinfo/bodgbd2002revised/en/index.html.

Xu F., Sternberg M.R., Kottiri B.J. *et al.* (2006). Trends in herpes simplex virus type 1 and type 2 seroprevalence in the United States. *JAMA* 296(8):964–973.

Zur Hausen H. (1996). Papillomavirus infections--a major cause of human cancers. *Biochim Biophys Acta* 1288(2):F55–F78.

9.13

Acquired immunodeficiency syndrome

Salim S. Abdool Karim,
Quarraisha Abdool Karim, and
Roger Detels

Abstract

In the 25 years since the first reported cases of acquired immunodeficiency syndrome (AIDS), more than 70 million people have been infected with the human immunodeficiency virus (HIV). HIV is a retrovirus that is spread from mother to child, through blood contamination and through sex. Antiretroviral drugs administered to HIV-infected pregnant women and the newborn child, together with exclusive or no breastfeeding, have drastically reduced mother-to-child transmission. Screening of blood supplies, universal safety precautions in medical settings, and needle exchange programmes for intravenous drug users are effective in avoiding bloodborne spread. Reduction in sexual transmission is achievable through sexual abstinence, monogamy, condoms, treatment of concurrent sexually transmitted infections, male circumcision, and HIV counselling and testing.

When spread, HIV specifically infects and replicates in CD4+ cells, leading to the systematic destruction of CD4+ cells over a period of years. The drop in CD4+ T-cell numbers to low levels leads to individuals developing symptoms including weight loss, low-grade fevers, night sweats, frequent fungal infections, and eventually various opportunistic infections and malignancies, which signal the onset of AIDS. Until then, individuals who have been asymptomatic with HIV infection over several years have been infectious, thereby creating the conditions for the efficient spread of this virus. HIV infection is readily diagnosed by assays detecting antibodies, viral components, and the viral genome. More than 25 antiretroviral drugs are known to be effective against HIV. Combinations of these drugs, referred to as highly active antiretroviral therapy, are effective in treating HIV infection.

Globally, it has proven to be a substantial challenge to extend HIV prevention programmes and provide treatment to those who most need it, as a disproportionately large burden of this disease is in poor countries. This pandemic has created many ethical, social, human rights, and political challenges. The estimated 25 million people that have already died from AIDS far exceeds the total killed in all the major wars of the twentieth century. AIDS is the world's most devastating epidemic and the deadliest in the history of humankind.

History of AIDS

First reported cases of AIDS

AIDS was first reported in 1981 by a young physician from the University of California Los Angeles School of Medicine who described the occurrence, without identifiable cause, of *Pneumocystis carinii* pneumonia (PCP) in four gay men in Los Angeles (Gottlieb *et al.* 1981). This new disease was also reported to and published by the US Centers for Disease Control and Prevention (CDC) in June 1981 and marked the beginning of awareness of the epidemic potential of AIDS in the United States. In 1982, the disease was given the name 'acquired immunodeficiency syndrome (AIDS)'. At this time, very little was known about the epidemiology and transmission of AIDS, and initially it was thought that only homosexuals and injecting drug users were affected but reports soon emerged that the disease was also occurring in haemophiliacs and Haitian immigrants in the United States.

A greater understanding of the mode of transmission of AIDS was gained following the reported death, from infections related to AIDS, of a young child who had previously received multiple blood transfusions, causing worldwide concerns about the safety of the blood supply, and the first cases of possible mother-to-child transmission of AIDS. By the time reports emerged that the disease was also transmitted heterosexually, it was apparent that the world was facing a disease of epidemic proportions.

Discovery of HIV as the cause of AIDS

The discovery that HIV caused AIDS was not a simple or direct path and required a substantial collaboration among different groups of scientists and clinicians. Only after the discovery of the human T leukaemia virus types 1 and 2 (HTLV-1 and HTLV-2) in the 1980s, did the scientific community accept that it was possible for retroviruses to infect humans. The marked decline in CD4 cells and possible mode of transmission led scientists to believe that AIDS was possibly caused by a retrovirus. In 1983, a virus was isolated from a patient with lymphadenopathy, which was later named lymphadenopathy-associated virus (LAV). In the same year, two distinct viruses were isolated from an AIDS patient in Haiti, one which cross-reacted with antibodies to HTLV, while the other virus killed target T-cells. It proved to be challenging to make the link between the virus and the clinical disease, AIDS, because the clinical signs of disease develop several years after the infection. However, through persistent isolation of the virus from patients with AIDS, the linkage was made possible (Gallo 2002; Gallo & Montagnier 2003). A series of important papers describing isolates of the new retrovirus, methods for its continuous production, and analyses of its proteins, were published in *Science* and *Lancet* in 1984 and provided the scientific evidence that HIV is the cause of AIDS.

Viral structure and genetic diversity

Viral structure and replication

HIV belongs to the family Retroviridae and the genus *Lentivirus*: Lenti meaning slow due to the long time from infection to disease. HIV, being a retrovirus, encodes the enzyme, reverse-transcriptase, which makes DNA from viral RNA. HIV genetic material, as proviral DNA in the nucleus of infected cells, is able to persist in long-lived reservoirs such as resting T-cells, thwarting efforts to clear HIV from the body.

Viral particles are spherical, about 100 nm in diameter. HIV has two major structural components—the core and the envelope. The core comprises the Gag (*g*roup-associated *a*ntigens) proteins, including the matrix protein (p17), which lies just beneath the envelope, and the capsid protein (p24) which encloses the viral RNA. The envelope, a lipid membrane, consists of two 'Env' glycoproteins, gp120 and gp41. These proteins exist as trimers on the viral surface facilitating binding and entry to the host cell. Besides reverse transcriptase, two other enzymes, integrase and protease, collectively known as polymerases, are carried inside the viral particle and are encoded by the 'Pol' gene of HIV. In addition to the major structural proteins, a number of regulatory and accessory proteins are also produced, including: Tat and Rev, which enhance levels of gene expression, and Vif, Vpr, Vpu, and Nef, which function to increase viral production and infectivity. Regulatory and accessory proteins are usually only produced once the virus infects cells and are not present inside the viral particles (Morris & Cilliers 2005).

HIV can attach to any cell that has a CD4+ receptor. Although these receptors are found primarily on the CD4+ lymphocytes,

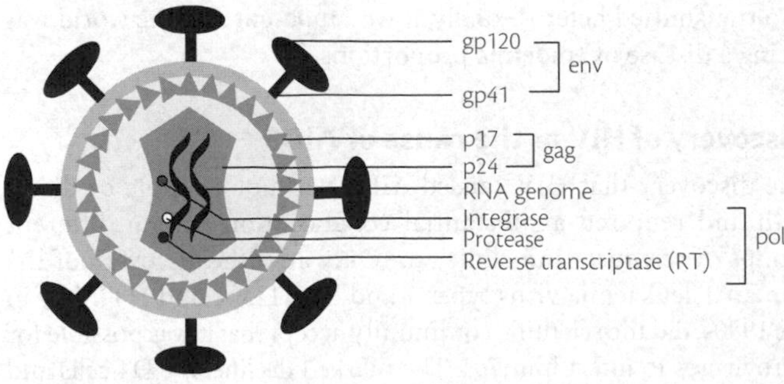

Fig. 9.13.1 Schematic diagram of HIV showing the constituent proteins and enzymes.
Source: Adapted from Morris & Cilliers (2005), with permission from Cambridge University Press.

they are also found on a range of mononuclear cells including macrophages, B cells, mature CD8+ cells, and cells in the central nervous system. The process of HIV replication begins when gp120 binds to surface CD4+ and a co-receptor molecule, either CCR5 or CXCR4 (Moore & Doms 2003). Once HIV has successfully attached to the cell, a conformational change occurs allowing gp41 to insert itself into the host cell membrane. The capsid is then intruded into the cytoplasm of the cell where the viral RNA is reverse-transcribed to DNA and transported to the nucleus where, with the aid of the viral enzyme integrase, it is incorporated into human DNA. The transcription process, however, is imperfect, and mutations are common occurrences during replication. The 'errors' in this step are a major reason why HIV is able to escape the immune system and persist (Weiss 2001).

After the viral DNA has been incorporated into the host DNA, it is indistinguishable from the host DNA and is referred to as the 'provirus'. Each time the cell divides, the viral DNA will be passed on to the progeny cells. Proviral DNA can remain quiescent for extended periods of time or become transcriptionally active, particularly in cases where there is inflammation (Simon & Ho 2003).

The virus makes use of the host cell machinery to replicate itself. Messenger RNA directs the production of viral proteins. After cleavage by viral proteases to generate individual proteins, structural proteins aggregate just beneath the plasma membrane surface for inclusion into the new virions. Envelope glycoproteins insert themselves into the cell membrane and mature viral particles are formed when the virus buds through the membrane. Full-length unspliced genomic RNA is transported to the plasma membrane to be incorporated into the viral progeny. As the new HIV is extruded from the host cell, lipid from the cell wall is incorporated onto the virus and forms the envelope of the progeny virus. A single CD4+ cell is capable of producing hundreds of new HIV progeny.

Genetic diversity

There are two HIV types, HIV-1 and HIV-2. HIV-2 is less pathogenic than HIV-1 and largely restricted to West Africa, with limited spread to other countries and is genetically more closely related to SIV than to HIV-1. Numerous HIV-1 subtypes and circulating recombinant forms (CRF) make up the complex mosaic of the global HIV-1 pandemic (McCutchan 2006). Specifically, HIV has been classified into three groups, M, N, and O. The Major Group (Group M) comprises the viruses that are currently dominating the global AIDS epidemic. The Outlier Group (Group O) and the non-M non-O group (Group N) are much less common. Based on their phylogenetic relatedness, the Group M viruses have been further subdivided into nine subtypes or clades; A, B, C, D, F, G, H, J, and K. Two of these, subtypes A and F have been further subdivided into sub-subtypes (referred to as A1, A2 and F1, F2, respectively).

An analysis of 23 874 HIV samples from 70 countries shows that, in terms of viral diversity, subtype C viruses dominate and account for half of all HIV-1 infections worldwide while subtypes A, B, D and G account for 12, 10, 3, and 6 per cent, respectively. Circulating recombinant forms are responsible for 18 per cent of infections worldwide. Subtype C is dominant in Africa and Asia, while subtype B is the commonest subtype in Europe and the Americas (Hemelaar *et al.* 2006).

HIV diversity is generated either through mutations introduced into viral genomes during replication or during the recombination of viral genomes. Mutations are introduced into the viral genome primarily due to the error-prone nature of the viral replication enzyme, reverse transcriptase. HIV has an average mutation rate of 5×10^{-6} mutations per nucleotide per cycle of virus replication (Smith *et al.* 2005). As a consequence, no two viruses are identical within an infected individual, allowing for rapid adaptation to fluctuating selection pressures such as immune responses and antiretroviral drugs.

Natural history of HIV infection

Following the introduction of HIV into the human body, there is replication in local CD4+ cells before spread to the gut-associated lymphoid tissue, where there is high-level HIV replication leading to virus levels in blood which can exceed ten million viral particles per ml. During viral replication in the gut-associated lymphoid tissue, there is a rapid decline in the numbers of CD4+ T lymphocytes, with the CD4+ cell count dropping by up to 50 per cent within weeks post-infection.

Within a few weeks of the onset of HIV infection, the host immune response curtails viral replication resulting in a decline in the viral load and a slow increase in CD4+ T-cell numbers for a few months before starting its slow progressive decline (Fig. 9.13.2). At the time of the immune response, many infected individuals experience influenza-like symptoms characterized by chills, malaise, and weakness for a few weeks.

Within 6–12 months following the onset of HIV, viral replication reaches a level which is referred to as the 'set point'. The level of the set point correlates with the rate of disease progression. Most individuals remain clinically well (asymptomatic) for an average of 8–9 years although the asymptomatic interval may vary widely. For reasons that are not fully understood, some individuals never develop control over viral replication and progress to AIDS within 1–2 years of infection (rapid progressors) while others have remained disease-free for up to 20 years, often with undetectable viral loads (long-term non-progressors).

Kinetic studies have shown that during the asymptomatic period up to a billion HIV particles and two billion CD4+ T-cells are destroyed and produced each day. Thus, while individuals may be clinically well, the virus continues to replicate, particularly in the lymph nodes, causing a gradual decline in CD4+ T-cell numbers. The drop in CD4+ T-cell numbers to low levels leads to individuals developing AIDS symptoms. With the deterioration of immune function, the viral load increases and, in the absence of treatment, death usually occurs within 6 months to 2 years after an AIDS diagnosis (Burger & Poles 2003). Treatment with Highly Active Antiretroviral Therapy (HAART) significantly extends the time period between AIDS diagnosis and death. There is accumulating evidence that the onset of AIDS may be about 1–2 years shorter following onset of HIV infection, in Africa compared to the developed world (Jaffar *et al.* 2004).

Laboratory assays

The isolation of HIV in 1984 and the establishment of its causal relationship with AIDS led to the development of the first commercially available HIV serological tests by 1985. Subsequently, there has been a rapid evolution in HIV diagnostic technology that has matched the rapidly evolving understanding of the natural history of HIV disease. Currently, a wide range of assays are available for adult and paediatric diagnosis, monitoring disease progression and therapeutic success, as well as for research and surveillance. These assays can be performed on a range of biological tissues such as serum, plasma, saliva, whole blood, urine, seminal fluid, and cervico-vaginal specimens.

Antibody detection

Detection of antibodies using serological tests such as a standard enzyme immunoassay (EIA) is most often used for screening or diagnosis of HIV infection. A major advance has been the availability of rapid HIV antibody tests. The two limitations of these serological tests are, firstly, detection of infection during primary infection when antibody levels are low or absent and secondly, determination of whether a reactive EIA or positive rapid HIV test in newborns is due to infection in the baby or due to passively

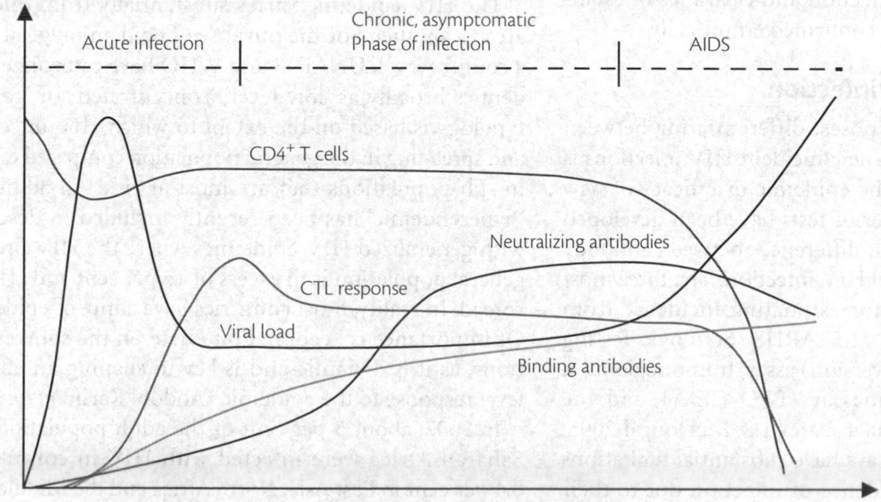

Fig. 9.13.2 Schematic diagram showing the natural history of HIV infection.
Source: Adapted from Morris & Cilliers (2005) with permission from Cambridge University Press.

transferred maternal antibodies. In these instances, the use of polymerase chain reaction technology for detection of viral RNA is helpful.

Antigen detection

Standard EIA tests are available for p24 antigen, which is often the earliest antigen that can be detected in acute HIV infection before the presence of antibodies is detectable. It is therefore used to identify the presence of HIV infection during the window period, the period between onset of HIV infection and the detection of HIV antibodies.

Nucleic acid detection

Plasma viral load is a marker of viral replication and is used to monitor therapeutic success in patients on antiretroviral treatment. A number of commercially available tests provide sensitive quantification as low as 50 copies of HIV RNA per ml (Berger *et al.* 2005). There are also tests for cell-associated HIV which measure branched DNA levels.

CD4+ cell counts

The number of CD4+ T-cells reveals the degree of immunodeficiency and is therefore a key criterion for initiating antiretroviral treatment. At present, flow cytometry analysis is the standard method for quantification of CD4+ cells. Where CD4+ quantification is not readily available, total white cell counts are sometimes used as a proxy marker (Spacek *et al.* 2006).

T-cell immune response detection

Various assays have been developed to assess the presence of a cellular immune response to HIV antigens. The earlier approaches like the Chromium release assay and the tetramer assay have now largely been superseded by the Elispot assay and the Intracellular cytokine stain assay. The latter two assays depend on the release of certain cytokines, such an interferon-gamma, when T-cells from the patient recognize HIV antigens used in the test. These assays are very sensitive and can sometimes be positive in the absence of any other markers of HIV infection—suggesting that the patient has previously encountered and can recognize HIV antigens, perhaps through a previous HIV exposure or aborted HIV infection. The hypotheses of aborted HIV infection and clearance of established HIV infection have not been confirmed empirically.

Assays to identify recent HIV infection

For research and surveillance purposes, differentiating between established/prevalent infection and new/incident HIV infections is critical for monitoring trends in the epidemic or efficacy of new interventions under trial. A number of tests have been developed for this purpose; most are based on differences between antibody responses in early versus established HIV infection. The three most commonly used serologic assays for estimating incidence from prevalent studies are the 'detuned' or STARHS (Serologic Testing Algorithm for Recent HIV Seroconversion) assay, Immunoglobulin G Capture BED-enzyme immunoassay (BED-CEIA), and the Avidity Index (AI) (Dobbs *et al.* 2004, Parekh & McDougal 2005; Janssen *et al.* 1998). All of these assays have substantial limitations and tend to over-estimate the incidence of infection due to their high false-positive rates.

STARHS consists of a less sensitive, first-generation ELISA followed by a later-generation ELISA with increased sensitivity. Recent infection (within the last 129 days, depending on viral sub-type) is indicated if the first-generation ELISA is negative and the second-generation ELISA is positive.

The *BED-CEIA* attempts to identify recent HIV infection by measuring increasing levels of anti-IgG as a proportion of overall IgG. Recent infection (within the last 153 days) is indicated by a ratio of HIV-specific IgG/total IgG less than 0.8.

The *AI* attempts to identify the weak antibody-antigen interaction present early in HIV infection compared to later stages where this interaction is stronger and more difficult to disrupt. Recent infection (within 120 days) is indicated by an Avidity Index less than 80 per cent.

Other assays in development are the Affinity assay, IgG3 isotype assay and anti-HIV p31 assay.

Global epidemiology of HIV

Since the first reported cases of AIDS in 1982, an estimated 70 million HIV infections and about 25 million AIDS-related deaths have occurred globally (UNAIDS 2006). In 2007, UNAIDS estimated that globally there were 33.2 million (upper and lower bound of estimate: 30.6–36.1 million) adults and children living with HIV infection. Furthermore, globally a total of 2.5 million (1.8–4.1 million) new infections occurred and 2.1 million (1.9–2.4 million) people died from AIDS in 2007 (UNAIDS 2007).

Differences in the time of introduction of HIV and rates of HIV transmission in specific countries and populations have resulted in a complex mosaic of epidemics (Abdool Karim *et al.* 2007). In most countries, HIV continues to spread and in countries with limited access to antiretroviral treatment, morbidity and mortality rates are on the rise.

A distinctive feature of the pandemic in the twenty-first century is its increasing burden in women. Women now comprise about 42 per cent of those infected globally, over 70 per cent of whom live in sub-Saharan Africa. Of significance is that a quarter of all new HIV infections occur in young adults under 25 years of age (UNAIDS 2003). Notably, where HIV transmission is predominantly sexual, HIV infection rates are 3–6-fold higher in adolescent girls compared to boys in the same age group (Pettifor *et al.* 2005; UNAIDS 2006).

The HIV epidemic varies substantially from one geographical area to another. For the purpose of epidemiological surveillance at a country level, UNAIDS and WHO have categorized the HIV epidemics broadly as 'low level', 'concentrated', or 'generalized'. The typology is based on the extent to which HIV infection is present and spreading in the general population compared to spread of HIV in sub-populations that are most at risk. An additional scenario 'hyperendemic' has been recently included to describe countries with generalized HIV epidemics where the HIV prevalence in the general population is in excess of 15 per cent and HIV continues to spread. In reality, most countries have a mix of epidemic scenarios. Of importance is keeping up to date on the sources of new infections, as it is dynamic and is key to shaping an effective country level response to the epidemic (Abdool Karim *et al.* 2007).

In 2007, about 5 per cent of the adult population living in sub-Saharan Africa were infected with HIV in contrast to less than 0.4 per cent in East Asia, North Africa and the Middle East, West and Central Europe, and Oceania (UNAIDS 2006). Sub-Saharan Africa is severely affected by HIV and accounts for 67.8 per cent [22.5 million (20.9 million–24.3 million)] of global infections (Fig. 9.13.3) (UNAIDS 2007). It is estimated that 1.7 million (1.4 million–2.4 million) people in this region became newly infected in 2007, while 1.6 million (1.5–2 million) died from AIDS in this period. The majority of infections in sub-Saharan Africa occur through heterosexual contact, where women have about 2–3 times more HIV infection compared to men (Abdool Karim & Abdool Karim 1999).

Southern Africa epitomizes a 'hyper-endemic' scenario and remains at the epicentre of the pandemic (Abdool Karim 2006a). HIV prevalence is >15 per cent in the general adult population fuelled by extensive heterosexual spread, widespread concurrent sexual partnerships, and transmission in discordant stable couples.

Several countries in sub-Saharan Africa have shown a decline in HIV prevalence in recent years, including Kenya, urban areas in Rwanda, Zimbabwe, and urban areas in Burkino Faso (Hallett *et al.* 2006; Kayirangwa *et al.* 2006; UNAIDS 2005, 2006). In contrast, while Uganda has for years been an excellent role-model for successfully impacting the HIV epidemic, more recent data demonstrate an increase in HIV infection in young women (Shafer *et al.* 2006).

HIV prevalence in the Middle East and North Africa is low, and the national HIV prevalence has not exceeded 0.3 per cent, with the exception of Sudan, where national prevalence in 2005 was estimated at 1.6 per cent. A total of 380 000 (270 000–500 000) people were living with HIV in this region in 2007. The main modes of transmission in this region are unprotected sexual contact (including commercial sex and sex between men) and injecting drugs using contaminated equipment. In some countries in North Africa and the Middle East, a significant number of infections still result from contaminated blood products, blood transfusions or lack of infection control measures in healthcare settings although the extent of this has decreased significantly over the last decade.

The HIV epidemics in Latin America and the Caribbean are associated mainly with unsafe sex (both heterosexual and men who have sex with men) and use of contaminated drug injecting equipment, especially among the poor and unemployed. In Latin America, an estimated 1.6 million (1.4–1.9 million) people were living with HIV in 2007. In most Latin American countries, HIV prevalence is highest among men who have sex with men.

In North America, and Western and Central Europe, HIV prevalence has remained below 1 per cent and AIDS mortality has been low because of the widespread availability of antiretroviral therapy. A total of 2.1 million people infected with HIV live in these regions (Fig. 9.13.3), of whom about 1.3 million live in the United States. A total of 77 000 people were newly infected in these regions in 2007 (UNAIDS 2007). Unsafe sexual practices between men and the use of contaminated drug injecting equipment are the most important routes of transmission of HIV in these regions. However, in recent years there has been an increase in heterosexual transmission and more women and members of minority ethnic groups have become infected through unsafe sex.

Epidemic patterns have also been changing in Eastern Europe and Central Asia in recent years, where an increasing number of women are being infected, many of whom acquire HIV infection from their male partners who became infected through injecting drugs using shared, contaminated injecting equipment. The epidemics in this region are continuing to grow. The total number of people living with HIV increased by about 36 per cent from 2003 to 2005 (UNAIDS 2006). UNAIDS estimates that, of the 1.6 million (1.2–2.1 million) people living with HIV in this region, 150 000 (70 000–290 000) were newly infected with the virus in 2007. The Russian Federation and Ukraine account for the majority of infections in this region; most are infected through injecting drugs using contaminated equipment.

In South and Southeast Asia, it is estimated that there were 4 million (3.3 million–5.1 million) people living with HIV at the end of 2007; 340 000 (180 000– 740 000) became newly infected with HIV; and 270 000 (230 000–380 000) died from AIDS during 2007 (UNAIDS 2007). About 69 per cent of all people infected with HIV in this region live in India. However, with a total population of

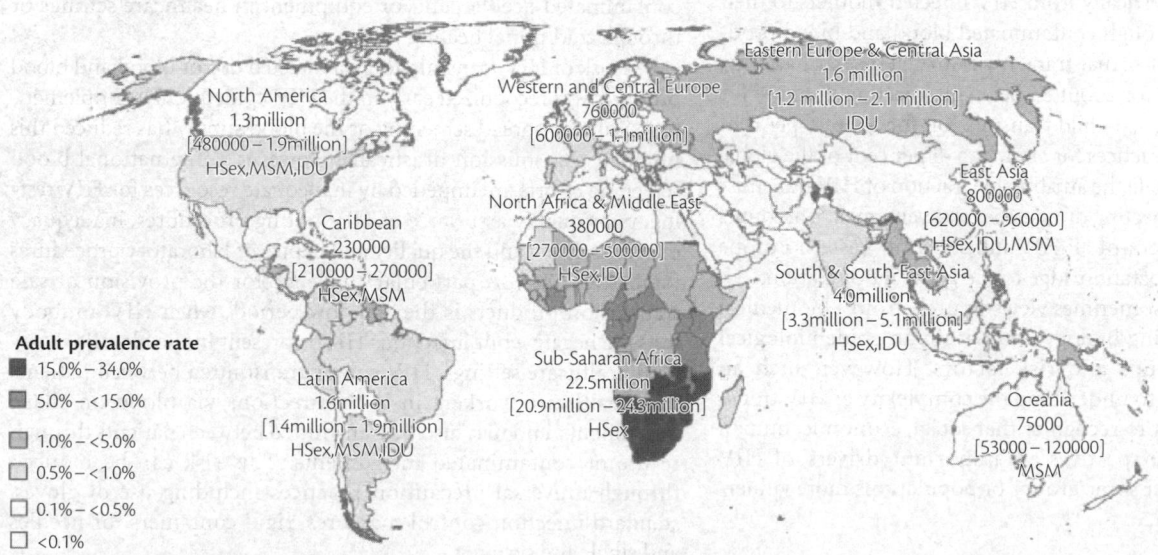

Fig. 9.13.3 Global distribution of people (adults and children) living with HIV in 2005 (33.2 million (30.6–36.1 million)). Major modes of HIV transmission are abbreviated as follows: MSM = men who have sex with men, HSex = heterosexual, and IDU = injection drug use (Adapted from: UNAIDS (UNAIDS 2007)).

over 1 billion people, the adult prevalence in India is still below 1 per cent (NACO 2006). In India, HIV transmission is primarily heterosexual, with female sex workers and their clients being the main drivers of HIV transmission (Mawar *et al.* 2005).

In East Asia (including China, Japan, Mongolia, Republic of Korea, and Democratic People's Republic of Korea) adult prevalence remains low and has not yet reached 0.1 per cent. In most of the rest of the countries in Asia, HIV prevalence remains low; only Cambodia, Thailand, and Myanmar had adult HIV prevalence rates above 1 per cent (1.6 per cent, 1.4 per cent, and 1.3 per cent, respectively) in 2005 (UNAIDS 2006).

Thailand provides an example of the dynamic nature of the evolving epidemic at a country level. The main routes of transmission in the late 1980s and early 1990s were through the use of non-sterile equipment in injecting drug users and through unsafe sexual behaviours. While the 100 per cent condom use policy in brothels made a major impact on preventing sexual spread of HIV to the general population, Thailand's more conservative policy on needle exchange and methadone treatment has enabled HIV to spread rapidly to injecting drug users, who are potentially an important bridge to the general population. In 2005, it was estimated that about 43 per cent of all new infections in Thailand occurred in the low-risk heterosexual population, while 21 per cent of new infections occurred among men who have sex with men (Gouws *et al.* 2006).

Of 75 000 (53 000–120 000) people infected with HIV in Oceania, it is estimated that over 70 per cent are living in Papua New Guinea, where the epidemic started recently, but is growing rapidly. The number of cases of HIV in Papua New Guinea has increased by about 30 per cent per year since 1997 (UNAIDS 2006), reaching an adult prevalence of 2.4 per cent in 2007, with the main mode of transmission being unsafe sex. HIV prevalence in other countries in this region (including Australia, New Zealand, and Fiji) has remained low at about 0.1 per cent (UNAIDS 2006) and is mainly concentrated in men who have sex with men and intravenous drug users.

Transmission of HIV

HIV spreads sexually, vertically from HIV infected mothers to their unborn infants, and through contaminated blood and blood products. It is estimated that sexual transmission (heterosexual and sex between men) accounts for about 84 per cent, injecting drug use for about 7 per cent, mother-to-child transmission for about 6 per cent and unsafe healthcare practices for about 2.5–5 per cent of the global HIV burden in 2006. While the attributable fraction of HIV transmission globally through injecting drug use is relatively small, it accounts for more than 80 per cent of all HIV infections in Eastern Europe and Asia and is an important bridge to the general population.

HIV transmission is sometimes viewed purely from a biomedical perspective of underlying biology and within an epidemiological paradigm of risk groups and risk factors. However, such an approach is inadequate to understand the complexity of HIV transmission. It is important to recognize that social, economic, human rights, and political perspectives are important 'drivers' of HIV transmission that render some groups or populations more vulnerable to HIV acquisition.

Sexual transmission

While the probability of HIV transmission through a single coital act is very low, this risk increases with repeated exposure, co-infection with sexually transmitted infection(s) especially genital ulcers, genital immaturity, receptive anal sex, circumcision status of male sexual partner, higher viral load in the HIV infected person, and the susceptibility of the exposed individual (Vernazza *et al.* 1999). The risk of HIV infection is 3 per 10 000 contacts for the male partner compared to 20 per 10 000 contacts for the female partner in peno-vaginal sex. Hence, on average, women are seven times more likely to become infected. This ratio rises in peno-anal sex, where the risk ratio for the receptive compared to insertive partner exceeds 20:1, highlighting the importance of receptive anal sex as an important factor not only for men but for women as well.

The underlying biological mechanisms of sexual transmission of HIV are poorly understood. Studies have shown that both semen and vaginal secretions have both cell-free virus and T-cells and macrophages which contain HIV. CD4+ positive cells are present both in the male urethra and female vagina—but it remains unclear whether CD4+ cells in the lumen or in the mucosa are involved in the infectious process.

High viral load is associated with more efficient transmission of HIV (Quinn *et al.* 2000). Viral load varies according to the stage of HIV infection, and is elevated during early infection, as well as during advancing HIV disease and progression to AIDS as immunity diminishes. Viral load is also higher during periods where there are other co-infections including herpes simplex virus type 2, malaria, tuberculosis and intestinal parasites. Ulcerative and non-ulcerative sexually transmitted infections contribute to higher HIV transmission and acquisition risk.

The various biological factors that influence the risk of HIV acquisition and transmission occur in a milieu of social, behavioural, and cultural situations which also impact on the spread of HIV. These include poverty, gender-based economic and power differentials, gender-based violence, migrant labour, sex work, and alcohol abuse.

Transmission through blood

Transmission through blood and blood products includes the sharing of needles and syringes during illicit drug use, inadequately screened or unscreened transfusion of blood and blood products, contaminated needles, and/or equipment in healthcare settings or through traditional healing practices.

The risk of HIV transmission via infected donor blood and blood products was recognized early in the HIV epidemic. The implementation of widespread screening of the blood supply has reduced this mode of transmission drastically. However, some national blood screening efforts are impeded by inadequate resources for HIV testing, poor quality assurance of HIV testing procedures, inadequacy of staff training and the quality and choice of laboratory procedures (UNAIDS 2006). A particular challenge for the provision of safe transfusion products is the 'window period', when HIV antibody tests are negative but infectious HIV is present in the blood.

In healthcare settings, HIV can be transmitted between patients and healthcare workers in both directions via blood on sharp instruments, and may also be transmitted between patients through re-use of contaminated instruments. This risk can be reduced through universal precaution practices including use of gloves, standard infection control measures, rigid containers for needles and single use syringes.

The sharing of needles and syringes among injecting drug users is a high-risk practice for HIV transmission. Sterile needle exchange programmes are effective in reducing HIV transmission among injecting drug users. The illicit nature of injection drug use and associated social stigma have compromised efforts to reduce HIV transmission in injecting drug users resulting in continuing high rates of transmission in these populations with bridging transmission to the general population in some instances.

Mother-to-child transmission

HIV is transmitted *in utero* (pre-partum), during the process of childbirth (intra-partum) and post-partum through breastfeeding. In the absence of any intervention, the mother-to-child transmission rate is between 20 per cent and 40 per cent. Most transmission from mother-to-child occurs during childbirth where mother's infected blood in the birth canal infects the baby, resulting in 10–20 per cent of babies becoming infected. About 5 per cent of babies become infected *in utero*. Breastfeeding accounts for 5–20 per cent of babies becoming infected, depending on length and type of breastfeeding. The risk of perinatal HIV transmission is influenced by the severity of HIV disease in the mother (high RNA viral load and low CD4+ count), the route of delivery (Caesarean section versus vaginal delivery), and the type of breastfeeding practices (exclusive breastfeeding or mixed feeding) and duration of breastfeeding. Notable advances have been made in reducing mother-to-child transmission of HIV to very low levels through the use of antiretroviral drugs, obstetric practices including Caesarean delivery, and management of breastfeeding.

As availability of antiretroviral therapy to reduce mother-to-child transmission during childbirth increases, breastfeeding is assuming a proportionately greater role as a source of HIV spread to newborn babies in settings where formula-feeding is not an affordable option.

Breastfeeding, particularly in poor countries, can account for one-third to one-half of all mother-to-child transmissions. This risk is reduced substantially if the mother exclusively breastfeeds her baby since mixed feeding (breastmilk plus formula milk or any other feeds, including water) increases the risk of HIV transmission to the baby. Duration of breastfeeding affects the rate of transmission. A meta-analysis (Coutsoudis *et al.* 2004) of breastfeeding studies from sub-Saharan Africa estimated the cumulative probability of acquiring HIV infection to be 3 per cent at 3 months, 5 per cent at 6 months, 9 per cent at 12 months, and 15 per cent at 18 months.

Obstetric practices, such as vaginal delivery (compared to Caesarean section) and prolonged rupture of membranes (>4 h), increase mother-to-child HIV transmission. Invasive procedures during labour and delivery, such as foetal scalp monitoring, amniocentesis, foetal scalp electrodes, episiotomy, and instrumental delivery, may also increase the risk of transmission. Circulating HIV variants in the mother are selected through immune pressure which is HLA dependent. Where the father has a substantially different HLA profile from the mother, the risk of transmission and/or the viral load in the baby is lower.

HIV prevention strategies

HIV prevention focuses, on the one hand, on reducing the likelihood of and vulnerability to infection in those who are currently uninfected and, on the other hand, on reducing the risk of transmission from those who are currently infected with HIV. The latter is an important new opportunity for enhancing prevention efforts through integration of prevention programmes into the health services which are scaling up AIDS treatment and the prevention of mother-to-child transmission. Knowledge of HIV status is an important gateway for targeted prevention and care efforts. It creates an opportunity to address prevention efforts along a continuum that includes those uninfected who are at high risk of getting infected, those recently infected, those with established infection but asymptomatic and those who have advancing HIV disease and those on antiretroviral treatment. Within this context, groups that are particularly vulnerable can be targeted and their particular needs addressed. Proven interventions are available for preventing HIV through any of its transmission modalities (Table 9.13.1).

Reducing sexual transmission

Globally, the incidence rate of new HIV infections continues to exceed AIDS mortality rates. Reducing sexual transmission, especially heterosexual transmission, of HIV is critical to altering the current epidemic trajectory in many parts of the world. Prevention of sexual transmission can be achieved through reduction in the number of discordant sexual acts and/or reduction of the probability of HIV transmission in discordant sexual acts (Fig. 9.13.4).

There is no risk of HIV infection among those who practice sexual abstinence or lifelong mutual monogamy. Serial monogamy, where there are multiple sequential individual short-lived monogamous partnerships, is associated with an increased risk of HIV, but not to the same extent as the substantial increase in risk of transmission emanating from multiple concurrent sexual partnerships (Morris & Kretzschmar 1997). Reduction in the number of concurrent sexual partnerships and the use of condoms are key components of HIV prevention messages, widely promoted as part of 'ABC' campaigns promoting *A*bstinence, *Be* faithful and *C*ondomize.

Male condoms

Condoms are a pivotal part of the fight against HIV/AIDS. They are inexpensive and relatively easy to use and provide protection against acquisition and transmission of HIV, a wide range of other sexually transmitted infections as well as pregnancy. When used correctly and consistently, the latex male condom is highly effective in preventing the sexual transmission of HIV. The strongest evidence for the role of condoms in preventing the transmission of HIV comes from sero-discordant couple studies, which uniformly show that increased condom use is associated with a substantially reduced risk of HIV transmission. However, there are still important questions regarding whether inconsistent condom use (that is, condom use in less than 100 per cent of sexual contacts) is protective. While some studies have suggested that inconsistent condom use may offer more protection than no condom use whatsoever, others have demonstrated that the transmission of HIV among irregular condom users is similar to that of individuals who do not use condoms (Ahmed *et al.* 2001).

To be effective as a prevention option to impact on the growth of the epidemic, access to condoms needs to be drastically scaled up. In 2001, it was reported, that the overall provision of condoms to sub-Saharan Africa was 4.6 per man per year. An estimated 1.9 billion additional condoms would be needed to raise all countries to the average procurement level (about 17 condoms per man per year) of the six African countries that use the most condoms (Shelton & Johnson 2001). It would cost an estimated US$47.5 million a year to fill the 1.9 billion condom gap excluding service delivery costs and production. However, based on data on condoms procured in public sector health facilities across South Africa, the estimated unmet need for condoms is probably closer to 13 billion (Myer *et al.* 2001).

Table 9.13.1 Biomedical technologies for prevention for each mode of HIV transmission

Mode	Technology	Intervention
Blood and blood products	◆ HIV screening for both virus and antibodies	◆ Selection of donors based on lower HIV risk profile ◆ Screening of all blood supplies with best available technology for viral detection during the window period of infection
Occupational exposure in health care settings	◆ Barrier nursing—gloves, goggles, gowns as appropriate ◆ Universal Infection control practices ◆ Proper sharps and other biohazards disposal systems ◆ Post-exposure prophylaxis	◆ Guidelines for universal precautions ◆ Trained health care workers ◆ Availability of post-exposure prophylaxis ◆ Availability of barrier nursing paraphernalia ◆ Availability of disposal systems for sharps and other biohazardous materials
Exposure to infected blood through traditional skin cutting and blood-letting practices	◆ Infection control practices ◆ Barrier nursing	◆ Guidelines for universal precautions ◆ Adequate training of traditional healers ◆ Information to public raising awareness of HIV risk through traditional practices
Injecting drug use	◆ Detoxification centres ◆ Sterile needles and syringes ◆ Maintenance therapy; e.g. buponorphine	◆ Treatment/rehabilitation centres ◆ Free needle exchange programmes
Mother-to-child transmission	◆ Determine mother and/or father's HIV status ◆ Antiretroviral drugs ◆ Alternative baby feeding options ◆ Non-invasive intra-partum procedures ◆ Caesarian section	◆ Implementation of a comprehensive prevention of mother-to-child transmission (PMTCT) programme
Sexual transmission		◆ Abstinence ◆ Delay age of sexual debut ◆ Mutually faithful monogamous relationship between concordant couples ◆ Zero-grazing', i.e. no concurrent multiple partnerships
Consensual sex	◆ Male condoms ◆ Female condoms ◆ HIV testing ◆ Sexually transmitted infection treatment ◆ Male medical circumcision	◆ Implementation of services for condom distribution, HIV education and counselling, HIV testing, sexually transmitted infection treatment, and circumcision services
Non-consensual/coerced sex	◆ Post-exposure prophylaxis ◆ Emergency contraception ◆ Sexually transmitted infection treatment	◆ Availability of health services for post-exposure prophylaxis, sexually transmitted infection treatment and emergency contraception
Experimental prevention tools to reduce sexual transmission (unproven)	◆ Antiretroviral drugs as pre-exposure prophylaxis for HIV uninfected persons ◆ Early antiretroviral therapy for HIV-infected persons ◆ Microbicides ◆ Vaccines	

Notwithstanding the challenges to condom access, a wide range of factors have been implicated as barriers to condom use; the most common being the widespread perception that condoms reduce sexual pleasure and that suggesting the use of condoms represents self-acknowledgement of HIV infection or a lack of trust in the partner. In the context of a marital relationship or stable partnership where pregnancy is desired, or where subordination of women limits their ability to negotiate safer sex practices, attempts to introduce or promote condom use have had limited success.

Several studies have demonstrated that alcohol consumption is associated with inconsistent condom use; this phenomenon is particularly problematic because many individuals meet high-risk sexual

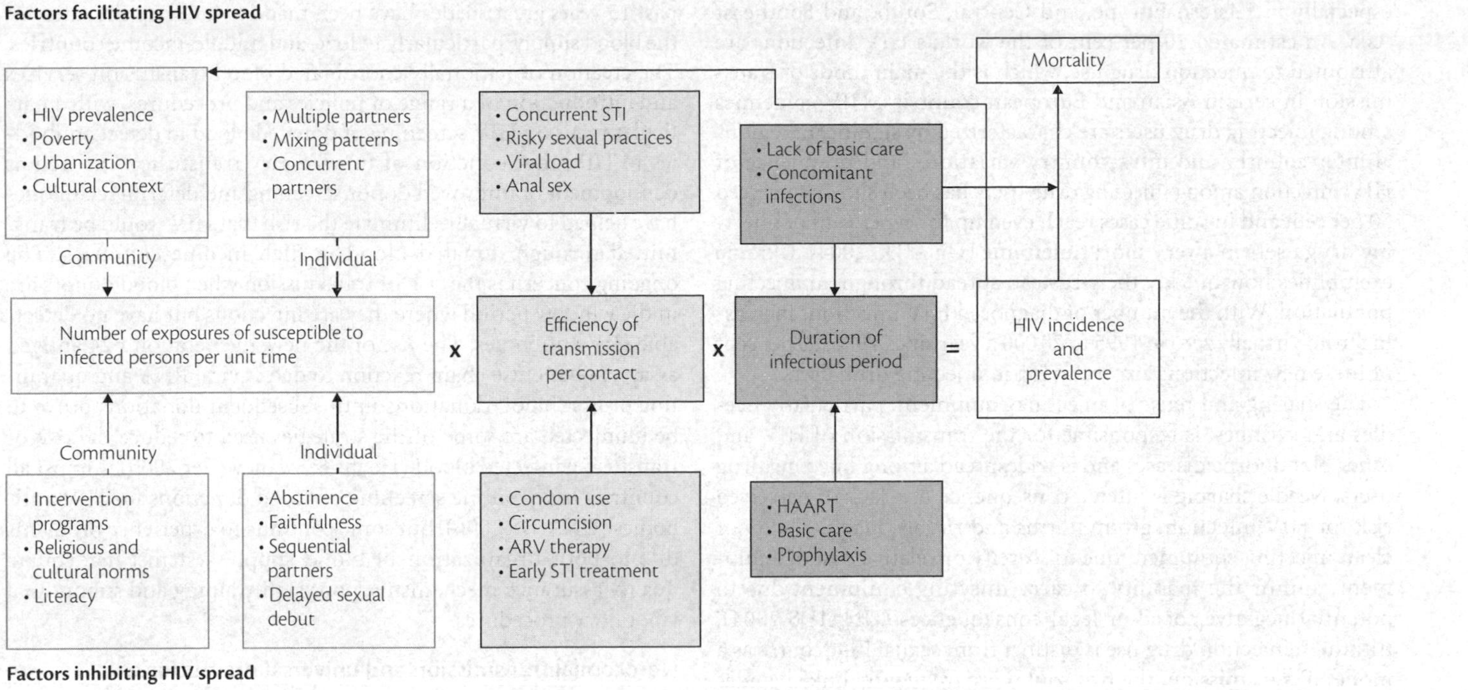

Fig. 9.13.4 Interplay between factors influencing sexual transmission of HIV infection.
Source: Department of Health, South Africa (2007).

partners in social settings where alcohol is available. Condoms use is lower in partnerships where an effective form of contraception is being used. This points to the need for interventions that promote dual method use (the simultaneous use of condoms with another form of contraception) among high-risk women. An important predictor of condom use is previous experience using condoms; individuals who have used condoms previously are more likely to use them in the future.

Female condoms

It is generally accepted that the efficacy of the female condom, when used correctly, is at least comparable to that of male condoms. While there are less data on the efficacy of the female condom, it protects essentially the same mucosal surface area as the male condom, and the polyurethane used in the construction of the female condom is stronger and less permeable than the latex used in most male condoms. Furthermore, female condoms do not degrade appreciably after several washings and, if they are cleaned appropriately, can be reused (unlike the male condom) though this practice is not widely recommended.

Sexually transmitted infections

HIV transmission and acquisition during heterosexual intercourse is enhanced in the presence of sexually transmitted infections, particularly ulcerative infections such as syphilis, chancroid, and herpes simplex virus type 2 virus infection. Genital ulceration or inflammation caused by sexually transmitted infections increase the infectiousness of HIV-positive individuals and the susceptibility of HIV negative individuals.

The incidence of curable sexually transmitted infections is highest in sub-Saharan Africa, with 69 million new cases per year in a population of 269 million adults aged 15–49 (WHO 2001). This is an important factor in accelerating the spread of HIV in this region. In rural South Africa, nearly 9 per cent of adults have syphilis, and almost one in 20 has gonorrhea (Colvin *et al.* 1998). The prevalence of HIV infection in sexually transmitted disease clinic patients has exceeded 70 per cent in Zimbabwe (WHO 2001) and exceeded 50 per cent in Swaziland (UNAIDS 2002). It is estimated that only 14 per cent of those in Africa in need of sexually transmitted disease services are able to access them.

Male circumcision

In 2006/2007, three randomized control trials conducted in Africa consistently demonstrated that medical male circumcision reduces the risk of female to male transmission of HIV by 50–60 per cent (Auvert *et al.* 2005; Bailey *et al.* 2007; Gray *et al.* 2007). There may be an increased risk of HIV infection in men who engage in sex before complete healing of the circumcision wound. It is unclear as to whether male circumcision has any impact on the risk of male to female HIV transmission or on male to male HIV transmission. Mathematical modelling of the introduction of male circumcision suggests that 2–3 million HIV infections could be averted in sub-Saharan Africa. If integrated into a comprehensive package of male sexual and reproductive health services it could mark a critical milestone in increasing male involvement in HIV prevention.

Reducing transmission through blood

Transmission of HIV through exposure to infected blood can occur through transfusion of blood and blood products, through sharing of needles and syringes among injecting drug users and through inadvertent nosocomial transmission (e.g. through needlestick injuries) in healthcare settings.

Injection drug use

Of the estimated 13.2 million injecting drug users worldwide, 78 per cent of them reside in low- and middle-income countries, especially in Eastern Europe, and Central, South, and Southeast Asia. An estimated 10 per cent of the world's HIV infections are attributed to injection drug use, which is the main mode of transmission in certain Asian and European countries. HIV epidemics among injecting drug users are characterized by significant regional inter-country and intra-country variations, and prevalence of HIV infection among injecting drug users has been shown to exceed 50 per cent and in some cases reach even up to 90 per cent of injecting drug users in a very short timeframe (UNAIDS 2004). Ukraine exemplifies how quickly the virus can spread through an injecting population: With the number of diagnosed HIV infections increasing from virtually zero in 1995 to 20 000 a year since 1996; 80 per cent of these new infections are occurring in injecting drug users.

The sharing and reuse of injecting equipment, particularly needles and syringes, is responsible for the transmission of HIV and other bloodborne diseases and is widespread among injecting drug users. Needle sharing is often a consequence of a lack of perceived risk for HIV infection, group norms and rituals, inaccessibility of clean injecting equipment due to scarcity or relative cost of equipment, and/or the inability to carry injecting equipment due to potential negative social or legal consequences (UNAIDS 2004). Although injection drug use is distinct from sexual intercourse as a mode of transmission, the two routes are frequently linked epidemiologically. Injection drug users are often young and sexually active, potentially exposing their sexual partners, children and foetuses to the virus. In addition, injection drug use is common in the commercial sex industry.

Over the past 20 years, research among injecting drug users and the experience from numerous programmes and projects indicate that the HIV epidemics among injecting drug users can be prevented, stabilized and even reversed. Effective programmes typically include; drug dependence treatment, including substitution treatment (e.g. methadone programmes), outreach to injecting drug users to promote safer sex and injecting practices, clean needles and syringes, condoms, voluntary counselling and HIV testing, treatment of sexually transmitted infections, and interventions for special populations-at-risk such as prisoners and sex workers who inject drugs (UNAIDS 2004).

'Needle exchange' or 'syringe exchange' programmes, when part of a comprehensive harm-reduction approach, have been shown to reduce the risk of transmission without contributing to an increase in drug use (Des Jarlais *et al.* 1996; Vlahov & Junge 1998). Early implementation of needle exchange, community outreach, and access to sterile injection equipment have been critical factors in helping several cities avoid a serious HIV outbreak among injecting drug users (Des Jarlais *et al.* 1995). An analysis of 81 cities around the world showed that HIV prevalence decreased 5.8 per cent in 29 cities with needle exchange projects compared to a 5.9 per cent increase in HIV prevalence in 52 cities without such programmes (Hurley *et al.* 1997).

Blood transfusions

The transfusion of HIV-infected blood or blood products is probably responsible for 5–10 per cent of cumulative infections worldwide (UNAIDS 2006), translating to an estimated 160 000 cases of HIV being transmitted every year (WHO 2005a).

In the 1980s and early 1990s, the majority of HIV infections through blood and blood products were in haemophiliacs. In the past 15 years great strides have been made to build up the safety of the blood supply, particularly in low- and middle-income countries. The creation of nationally coordinated blood transfusion services and introduction of a range of policies and procedures, with a particular focus on HIV screening of donated blood to detect antibodies to HIV, the reduction of unnecessary transfusions as well as development of improved donor screening and deferral techniques have helped to virtually eliminate the risk that HIV would be transmitted through donated blood in high-income countries. The ongoing concern is the risk of transmission when blood donors are in the window period where they are infectious but have no detectable HIV antibodies. The use of the newer generation p24 antigen assays, polymerase chain reaction to detect viral RNA and quarantine of first blood donations until subsequent donations prove to be uninfected are some of the strategies used to reduce the risk of transfusing infected blood (Heyns & Swanevelder 2005). Almost all countries have routine screening of blood donations for HIV antibodies (UNAIDS 2006), but some continue to experience problems due to poor organization of blood supply systems, inadequate quality assurance mechanisms, poor staff training and suboptimal laboratory procedures.

Nosocomial transmission and universal precautions

Healthcare workers exposed to blood and body fluids have a low but measurable risk of occupational infection with HIV. In a review of transmission probability estimates, infectivity following a needlestick exposure was estimated to range from 0.00 per cent to 2.38 per cent (weighted mean = 0.23 per cent) (Baggaley *et al.* 2006). While international guidelines recommend the use of relatively inexpensive auto-disable syringes as the 'equipment of choice' to help prevent HIV transmission in healthcare settings, only 62 per cent of low- and middle-income countries were using such syringes in their national vaccine programmes in 2004 (WHO 2005b). Risk of exposure to blood or other body fluids can be significantly lowered through workers' adherence to 'universal precautions', which involves the routine use of gloves and other protective gear to prevent occupational exposures, safe disposal of sharps, and timely administration of a 4-week prophylactic course of antiretroviral prophylaxis if a worker does get exposed.

Preventing mother-to-child transmission

Over 4 million HIV-infected children under the age of 15 have been born to HIV-infected mothers; in 2005 alone, an estimated 700 000 children became newly infected. With few exceptions, most children acquire their HIV infection from their mothers. Mother-to-child-transmission (MTCT) of HIV occurs in the intrauterine period, during labour and delivery, and postnatally through breastfeeding. Africa bears 70 per cent of the global burden of HIV in all age groups, but has at least 90 per cent of all the HIV-infected children in the world resulting in a reversal of decades of steady progress in child survival.

Substantial progress has been made in preventing MTCT. Before medical interventions became available, approximately one-third of babies of HIV positive mothers became infected with HIV. With a combination of antiretroviral drugs, changes in obstetric practices and alternatives to breastfeeding, MTCT rates below 1 per cent can be attained and MTCT has been virtually eliminated in high-income countries.

The first research breakthrough in MTCT occurred in 1994 when the Paediatric AIDS Clinical Trials Group 076 trial showed that HIV transmission from mother-to-child can be reduced from 25.5 per cent to 8.3 per cent using AZT. This efficacious regimen of AZT from about 12 weeks gestation and through labour and delivery in the infected mother and for a week post-birth to the infant has been widely implemented in industrialized countries. For resource-constrained settings, cheaper interventions using AZT or nevirapine are available. The Thai short course AZT regimen administered to mothers from 36 weeks gestation through the intra-partum period and the HIVNET 012-single dose nevirapine regimen (a dose to the mother at onset of labour and a dose to the infant within 72 h of birth) are preferred in resource-constrained settings. The main advantage of single-dose nevirapine is the ease of administration and low cost; the chief drawback is concern about drug resistance in the mother. Concerns about drug resistant viral strains have led to several trials using combination treatments to reduce transmission during the intra-partum period.

Breastfeeding is not recommended for HIV-positive mothers since this is associated with an increased risk of HIV transmission. However, lack of access to clean running water in resource-constrained settings has precluded the use of formula feeding. While exclusive breast feeding with abrupt weaning is one proven option of reducing breastfeeding risk in these settings, other options are under investigation (Coovadia *et al.* 2007), including studies of whether antiretrovirals given to baby (and mother) during breastfeeding may reduce MTCT.

Despite single-dose nevirapine being a readily implementable effective HIV prevention strategy to reduce MTCT in almost any country, only 9 per cent of pregnant women in low- and middle-income countries were offered services to prevent transmission to their newborns in 2005 (Global HIV Prevention Working Group 2006). A lot more still needs to be done to expand interventions to reduce MTCT.

Voluntary counselling and testing

Knowledge of HIV status is not only a vital entrée to treatment, it is also essential for prevention of MTCT, prevention of transmission through blood transfusions and reducing sexual transmission of HIV infection. Voluntary counselling and testing (VCT) has been shown to be both efficacious in reducing risky sexual behaviours (The VCT efficacy study group 2000) and cost-effective as a prevention intervention. In a large multi-centre study ($n = 4293$), both men and women randomized to receive VCT significantly reduced unprotected intercourse with their primary partners than those receiving only health information (The VCT efficacy study group 2000). In this VCT trial, the centres in Kenya and Tanzania averted an estimated 1104 and 895 HIV infections and this translated into a cost-saving of US$249 and US$346 per HIV infection averted in Kenya and Tanzania, respectively (Sweat *et al.* 2000).

Large numbers of HIV infected people, particularly in low- and middle-income countries, do not know their HIV status and are diagnosed too late (Shisana *et al.* 2005). While the aim is to put all those eligible for antiretroviral therapy (often defined as CD4 <200 cells/ml) on treatment, it is primarily those who are symptomatic and seeking care who are learning their HIV status and accessing care. VCT has traditionally been offered as an out-patient or ambulatory service based at primary care providers or specialized VCT centres. However, stigma, which is a common experience of those infected and affected by HIV, is a major obstacle to HIV testing and acknowledgement of individual risk of infection.

The traditional form of VCT was developed in the pre-ART era in response to human rights and ethical concerns about HIV testing that centred on the need to ensure autonomy and minimize harms for the client (Fylkesnes 1999). At that stage, VCT was mainly for prevention purposes. Unfortunately, this form of VCT has become a major obstacle to care due to the lack of capacity of health services to provide this time-consuming approach to VCT.

In an attempt to overcome this limitation, a number of different models to promote HIV testing have started to emerge, each designed to meet different goals, including:

a. Individual pre- and post-test counselling, which is the classic model that is client initiated and is typical of most free-standing VCT sites

b. Group information opt-in individual pre- and post-test counselling, which is widely used in high-prevalence settings

c. Group information opt-out individual testing with individual post-test counselling for sero-positives, which is widely used during routine medical screening, e.g. antenatal clinics

d. Group information opt-in couple/family pre-test counselling with individual post-test counselling

e. No specific pre-test information and testing is an opt-out option with individual post-test counselling, e.g. antenatal and sexually transmitted disease clinics

Routine opt-out testing, with a right to decline, was pioneered in Botswana in 2004. A population-based study on attitudes, practices, and human rights concerns showed that of 1268 adults interviewed, 81–93 per cent were in favour of opt-out HIV testing as it enhanced access to treatment. Barriers to testing included fear of learning one's status (49 per cent), lack of perceived HIV risk (43 per cent), and fear of having to change sexual practices with a positive HIV test (33 per cent) (Weiser *et al.* 2006). In the United States, routine opt-out testing in healthcare settings has been recommended since 2006.

While alternate models of VCT have engendered some concern about coercion of clients to participate in HIV testing, most of these concerns are readily remedied. Some have argued for a move away from the 'HIV exceptionalism' approach to a 'HIV normalization' approach wherein HIV is treated as any other infectious disease. In this context VCT is essential for both HIV prevention and early diagnosis for timely access to treatment (De Cock & Johnson 1998).

Community interventions for HIV prevention

Community intervention strategies can be categorized according to three approaches: Mass media (e.g. television, radio, newspapers/magazines, posters); community mobilization, through which the community becomes a participant in the design of the intervention; and interpersonal communication involving direct, face-to-face approaches such as counselling.

A common theoretical model used in developing behavioural interventions (Bertrand *et al.* 2006) requires the direct impact of the intervention to increase knowledge, change attitudes, and enhance self-efficacy, leading to a reduction in risk behaviours, greater utilization of health services and, ultimately, a reduction in HIV prevalence. An overall approach to the way interventions are designed and implemented suggests that for an intervention to be successful, it needs to be based on behavioural theory, designed to change specific risk behaviours, delivered by health professionals, delivered in an intensive manner, delivered to individuals, delivered as part of routine health services; and should incorporate skill-building (Crepaz *et al.* 2006).

The mass media approach targets the general population, regardless of level of HIV risk. Thus, the message that is delivered through the mass media must carefully consider the impact of the content and approach of their messages. In the early 1980s in the United States, mass media messages tended to emphasize the severity of the disease and the fatal outcome. The unexpected outcome of that approach was to induce fear and cause many people to shun individuals in high-risk groups and persons with AIDS, resulting in stigmatization. Stigmatization is now one of the major barriers to effective control of the epidemic, and has compromised efforts to promote HIV testing.

A systematic review (Bertrand *et al.* 2006) of interventions using the mass media in low- and middle-countries found that only two of the desired outcomes were achieved in 50 per cent or more of the trials: Knowledge of HIV transmission and reduction of high-risk activities (multiple partners, visiting sex workers, etc.). Few of the mass media intervention studies resulted in an increase in reported use of condoms.

A review (Eke *et al.* 2006) of community-based programmes, suggested that success was dependent on the interventions being tailored to respond to the unique contexts in which risk behaviours occur (e.g. in Thailand and Cambodia, a high proportion of sexual risk behaviour occurs in brothels, which then become a logical target for intervention), addressing contextual variables and practices such as sociocultural norms (e.g. acceptance that extra-marital sex is to be expected), and the provision of adequate resources with which to implement the intervention.

A successful example of a community mobilization strategy (Wu *et al.* 2002), aimed at new drug users in southern Yunnan Province in China, produced a two-thirds reduction in HIV incidence within one year. Another successful example of an intervention targeting a specific community is the Sonagachi Project, which organized commercial sex workers in Kolkata, India, to promote safer sex, better working conditions, better health-seeking behaviours, and better access to healthcare (Jana *et al.* 2004).

Community intervention strategies, like the successful examples above, can prevent HIV infection, but they must be carefully designed, and should mobilize the target population to participate in the intervention design and implementation.

Post-exposure prophylaxis

HIV infection is thought to initially established within the dendritic cells of the skin and mucosa before spreading through lymphatic vessels and developing into a systemic infection. Thus, there is a 'window of opportunity' following exposure for the use of antiretroviral therapy to prevent systemic infection.

There are several groups who could benefit from post-exposure prophylaxis (PEP). These include health workers, laboratory personnel, and individuals with likely exposure to HIV through sexual contact (including rape) or breast milk. The success of PEP in preventing established infection depends on a number of factors, including route and dose of exposure, efficacy of drug(s) used, interval between exposure and initiation of drug(s), and level of adherence to the drug. The dose of exposure depends primarily on the route of infection and the stage of infection of the source. Thus, receptive anal intercourse and deep accidental needle sticks carry the highest risk of exposure and the greatest challenge for effective PEP. People who are in the acute or terminal stages of HIV disease will also have the highest levels of HIV, and thus present the highest risk to those exposed to them.

It is unlikely that placebo-controlled double-blinded clinical trials of PEP will ever be conducted for logistical and ethical reasons. A case–control study of PEP following occupational exposures (Cardo *et al.* 1997) showed 81 per cent protection against HIV infection. A study of PEP following sexual exposure, primarily through anal intercourse, also showed a protective effect (Roland *et al.* 2005).

An important issue in implementing PEP is whether it will lead to behavioural disinhibition, i.e. individuals believing, because of PEP, they can safely engage in high-risk activities. Thus, counselling on the need for reduction of risk exposures should be an integral part of any PEP programme.

The US Centers for Disease Control and Prevention has issued guidelines for management of occupational, sexual, and other exposures to HIV (Panlilio *et al.* 2005). The current consensus is that combination antiretroviral therapy should be initiated as soon as possible after exposure, and continued for at least 4 weeks.

Scaling up prevention interventions

Despite substantial increases in knowledge of what works in preventing HIV infection, and resources for their implementation, the virus continues to spread. The inability to curb the epidemic in many settings is due to the inability to implement proven HIV prevention strategies at the necessary scale and magnitude to those who need it most, and not recognizing the link between HIV prevention and broader development needs especially in resource-constrained settings.

In 2006, the gap between HIV prevention needs and provision of prevention programmes was substantial. A significant constraint to prevention efforts has been the inability to integrate HIV prevention: (i) within a comprehensive AIDS strategy, including prevention integrated with AIDS treatment; (ii) within other national development programmes; (iii) into poverty reduction strategies; iv) into education programmes; (v) into health services, especially sexual and reproductive health services; (vi) into programmes aimed at reducing gender inequalities; and (vii) into initiatives to enhance economic and political opportunities for women and girls.

Prevention efforts have generally targeted whole communities or those who are HIV negative. There is a steady shift in prevention efforts from a narrow focus on HIV uninfected persons to a more effective continuum of prevention that includes those who are uninfected, recently infected, infected but asymptomatic as well as those with advancing HIV disease and on antiretroviral therapy.

To improve the impact of known effective HIV prevention interventions, implementation needs to be done to scale, targeting the key populations in the epidemic with integrated approaches that recognize that prevention planning and implementation needs to take the context into account.

New HIV prevention technologies under investigation

Several trials of new HIV prevention technologies are currently underway. Antiretroviral prophylaxis, microbicides, and vaccines are being tested and may have great potential in the future.

Pre-exposure prophylaxis

Certain groups are repeatedly exposed to possible infection by HIV. These include health workers, laboratory personnel, sex workers, injection drug users, and both homosexual and heterosexual individuals who have multiple partners and are unwilling to take precautions (as well as their spouses and/or regular partners). The concept of pre-exposure prophylaxis is not new, but has now gained considerable popularity as a possible strategy for reducing the risk of infection among high-risk groups.

However, there are many issues inherent in long-term prophylaxis with any drug. These include the need for inexpensive drugs, the potential for serious toxic side effects, development of viral resistance to the drug with repeated use, the potential impact on behavioural disinhibition (i.e. increasing risky behaviour and decreasing condom use), the possible need for multiple drug combinations, and assuring an acceptable cost:benefit ratio.

Several studies of the antiretroviral drug, tenofovir, were initiated to assess its effectiveness as pre-exposure prophylaxis (Liu *et al.* 2006). Results from one pre-exposure trial conducted in Ghana, Cameroon, and Nigeria (Peterson *et al.* 2007) showed no increased risk of drug-associated toxicity from oral tenofovir, and did not observe any increase in high-risk behaviour.

Whether pre-exposure prophylaxis becomes a widely implemented, acceptable prevention strategy will depend on the results of these trials evaluating efficacy/effectiveness, toxicity and behavioural disinhibition. If pre-exposure prophylaxis is shown to be safe and effective, implementation programmes of this potential prevention strategy will need to emphasize the concomitant use of other prevention strategies such as condoms.

Microbicides

Topical microbicides, products designed to prevent the sexual transmission of HIV and other sexually transmitted pathogens, are one of the most promising prevention tools currently under development that women can use to protect themselves from HIV (Stone 2002). Potentially, they can be applied vaginally to prevent both male-to-female and female-to-male transmission.

Currently in the research pipeline are over 60 substances that are being studied as possible microbicides. Some 50 of these substances are in pre-clinical development, and 11 have entered various stages of human clinical testing.

Microbicides in human trials have one of four mechanisms of action:

a. Surfactants, e.g. nonoxynol-9 and C31G (Savvy), which act by disrupting cell membranes
b. Vaginal defence enhancers, which boost the body's natural defences against infection by maintaining the naturally acidic environment of the vagina by increasing lactobacilli or by rapidly acidifying alkaline ejaculate, e.g. BufferGel
c. Attachment and fusion inhibitors, which bind to pathogens or to receptors on healthy human cells thereby preventing attachment, e.g. Carraguard, PRO2000, and Cellulose Sulphate
d. Replication inhibitors, or antiretroviral agents, which act locally in the reproductive tract mucosa at various steps in the HIV replication cycle and therefore have a narrow spectrum of activity, e.g. Tenofovir gel, Dapivirine, and UC781

Early studies of the spermicide, nonxynol-9, showed this product, which acts by disrupting cell membranes, to be harmful as it caused lesions in the genital tract and increased the risk of HIV infection. Subsequent studies of Savvy, another product in the same class, were halted due to low HIV incidence rates in the trial sites. Trials of Cellulose Sulphate, were stopped in 2007 due to safety concerns. Gel formulations of inhibitors of the chemokine receptor, CCR5 have shown promise in animal models and are currently being developed for early human studies.

There are significant challenges in conducting microbicide effectiveness trials, including the ethical need to promote condoms thereby undermining the ability to show the effect of the microbicide, low HIV incidence rates in some trial populations, poor adherence to study products and high rates of pregnancy as study products are discontinued during pregnancy.

Vaccines

A safe, protective and inexpensive vaccine would be the most efficient, effective, and possibly the only way to control the HIV pandemic. Despite intensive research, development of such a candidate vaccine remains elusive. Safety concerns prohibit the use of whole killed HIV or live attenuated virus as immunogens (Sheppard 2005). Many different approaches using recombinant technologies have been pursued over the past two decades. Initially, efforts were focused on generating neutralizing antibodies using recombinant monomeric envelope gp120 (AIDSVAX) as immunogen. This vaccine did not induce neutralizing antibodies and the phase III trials failed to show protection against HIV acquisition. Antibody-mediated HIV neutralization is complicated by the high genetic diversity of the variable Env regions, epitopes masked by a carbohydrate shield (glycosylation) and conformational rearrangements (Garber *et al.* 2004).

Since CD8+ T-cell responses have been shown to control viral replication *in vivo*, recent vaccine development has focused on eliciting cellular immune responses. Unfortunately, safety and immunogenicity studies of adenovirus vector-based T-cell vaccine have failed to show a protective effect and may be associated with an increased risk of HIV infection.

Vaccine development is severely hampered by the lack of any immune correlate which has been shown to prevent viral infection or clear initial viral infection. The human immune system generally fails to spontaneously clear HIV infection and so there is no natural immune process for the vaccine candidates to mimic. It is, however, believed that approaches aimed at eliciting both humoral and cell mediated immunity are most promising to prevent or at least control retroviral infection (Ho & Huang 2002).

Most of the efforts to produce a vaccine have concentrated on looking at components of the virus that may stimulate protective immunity and substrates that may enhance the immune response. While natural immunity has not been observed in HIV/AIDS, several researchers (Clerici *et al.* 1992; Detels *et al.* 1994; Detels *et al.* 1996) have identified groups of men who have sex with men and female sex workers who have been repeatedly exposed to HIV and have not become infected. Some of these individuals were shown to lack the CCR-5 receptor on CD4+ cells to which the HIV attaches (Dean *et al.* 1996). However, these individuals comprise only a subset of 'resistant' individuals. If the factors that allow these individuals to resist infection can be identified, it might be possible to confer the 'resistance factor' on individuals lacking it, thus artificially providing them some measure of protection against HIV infection. This approach would represent an alternative approach to the traditional strategies of vaccine development and might overcome the apparent lack of natural immunity to HIV.

The spectrum of clinical manifestations of AIDS

Opportunistic infections, which seldom cause serious disease in immunocompetent people, are common in HIV-infected individuals. Indeed, most of the morbidity and mortality associated with HIV infection is almost always as a consequence of opportunistic diseases or malignancies that occur when immunity is impaired, usually corresponding with a CD4+ count below 200 cells/ml. Infections caused by more virulent pathogens, such as *Mycobacterium tuberculosis* or *Streptococcus pneumoniae*, often occur with lesser degrees of immune suppression. Over 100 opportunistic infections by viruses, bacteria, fungi, and protozoa have been associated with AIDS. The spectrum of clinical manifestations includes:

Dermatological manifestations

Cutaneous abnormalities are common and some of the conditions are unique and virtually pathognomonic for HIV disease, e.g. Kaposi's sarcoma.

Neurological manifestations

Apart from dementia, HIV-infected patients are at risk for a wide range of neurologic diseases. Global cerebral disease can present with altered mental status or generalized seizures, whereas focal disease often produces hemiparesis, hemisensory loss, visual field cuts, or disturbances in language use. Fungal, viral, and mycobacterial meningoencephalitis are the most common causes of global cerebral dysfunction, and progressive multifocal leukoencephalopathy (PML), primary CNS lymphoma, and toxoplasmosis account for the majority of focal presentations.

Pulmonary manifestations

HIV-associated pulmonary conditions include both opportunistic infections and neoplasms. The opportunistic infections include bacterial, mycobacterial, fungal, viral, and parasitic pathogens. Some of the more common respiratory infections associated with HIV patients include: Pneumonia, tuberculosis, and pulmonary Kaposi's sarcoma.

Endocrine manifestations

A number of endocrine abnormalities develop in patients with HIV infection; some due to infiltration of endocrine glands by tumour or infection.

HIV wasting

This condition was first recognized as an AIDS-defining illness by the US Centers for Disease Control and Prevention in 1987. The 'wasting syndrome' is defined as a weight loss of at least 10 per cent in the presence of diarrhoea or chronic weakness and documented fever for at least 30 days that is not attributable to a concurrent condition other than HIV infection itself.

Haematologic manifestations

Clinically significant haematologic abnormalities are common in persons with HIV infection. Impaired haematopoiesis, immune-mediated cytopaenias, and altered coagulation mechanisms have all been described in HIV-infected individuals.

Renal manifestations

Renal disorders during HIV infection range from fluid and electrolyte imbalances commonly seen in hospitalized HIV-infected patients, to HIV-associated nephropathy, which can progress rapidly to end-stage renal disease.

Gastrointestinal manifestations

Common gastrointestinal disorders include diarrhoea, dysphagia and odynophagia, nausea, vomiting, weight loss, abdominal pain, anorectal disease, jaundice and hepatomegaly, gastrointestinal bleeding, interactions of HIV and hepatotropic viruses, and gastrointestinal tumours (Kaposi's sarcoma and non-Hodgkin's lymphoma).

Ophthalmic manifestations of HIV

Numerous ophthalmic manifestations of HIV infection may involve the eye including tumours of the periocular tissues, a variety of external infections, HIV-associated retinopathy, and a number of opportunistic infections of the retina and choroid.

Otolaryngologic manifestations

HIV disease is associated with a variety of problems in the head and neck region; as many as 70 per cent of HIV-infected patients eventually develop such conditions.

Oral manifestations

Oral manifestations of HIV disease are common and include oral lesions and novel presentations of previously known opportunistic diseases. Some are caused by fungal infections, e.g. candidiasis; while others are due to viral infections, e.g. herpes simplex, herpes zoster, human papillomavirus, cytomegalovirus, hairy leukoplakia, and Epstein–Barr virus. Other oral complications include periodontal disease, neoplastic lesions, and lymphomas.

Rheumatologic and musculoskeletal manifestations

Musculoskeletal syndromes that occur in HIV-infected patients include manifestations of drug toxicity, reactive arthritis, Reiter's syndrome, infectious arthritis, and myositis.

Tuberculosis and HIV

In resource-constrained settings, the most common presenting illness of AIDS is tuberculosis (TB). TB is a global public health problem that has been exacerbated by the HIV epidemic. In 2003 an estimated 8.8 million new cases of TB were diagnosed and 1.7 million people died from the disease. The most severely affected region has been sub-Saharan Africa, where TB notifications have, on average, trebled since the mid-1980s, and death rates on treatment have reached 20 per cent compared with the 5 per cent that can be achieved by good TB-control programmes without HIV (WHO 2005c).

AIDS has changed the profile of TB patients globally; from a disease of the malnourished, elderly and men to a disease of young people, predominantly women. Extra-pulmonary TB is common in

AIDS patients; together with other reasons for smear-negative TB, this has created a major diagnostic problem. The result is large numbers of patients being treated for TB without microbiological confirmation of infection. The rapid growth of the HIV epidemic has resulted in a rapidly growing TB epidemic. Rising TB incidence rates in those who are HIV infected has had a spillover effect of rising TB incidence rates even among those who do not have HIV infection.

In much of sub-Saharan Africa, the strain of growing TB and HIV epidemics has led to the emergence of extensively drug resistance TB. Global increases in multidrug-resistant (MDR-TB) and extensively drug-resistant (XDR-TB), are threatening both TB and HIV treatment programmes worldwide. The former is defined as resistance to both isoniazid and rifampin, whereas the newly defined XDR-TB consists of MDR and resistance to a fluroquinolone and at least one injectable second-line TB drug (kanamycin, amikacin, or capreomycin). Together, they raise concerns of a global epidemic of untreatable TB and pose a huge threat to TB control. In high-prevalence TB and HIV areas of the developing world, the current DOTS (Directly Observed Treatment, Short Course) strategy is proving ineffective because available resources are being outstripped by the large number of patients in need of treatment. As a consequence TB treatment and outcomes are sub-optimal and MDR and XDR TB are on the rise.

Treatment

Antiretroviral therapy (ART)

The ART era started in 1987 with the approval of AZT (also known as zidovudine), a thymidine nucleoside analogue that interrupts the transcription of viral RNA to viral DNA by blocking the action of the reverse transcriptase enzymes. During the late 1980s additional nucleoside reverse transcriptase inhibitors (NRTIs) were developed. As more antiretroviral drugs of different classes became available, triple combination therapy was shown to have greater and more durable benefits than either mono- or dual therapy. The big treatment breakthrough occurred in 1996 with the introduction of protease inhibitors (PIs) that are capable of blocking the assembly of the progeny HIV within the CD4+ cell, marking the beginning of the era of highly active antiretroviral therapy (HAART). A third class of antiretrovirals, the non-nucleoside reverse transcriptase inhibitors (NNRTIs) was developed soon after the first PIs became available.

Combinations of drugs from these three classes of antiretrovirals are widely used as the 'standard of care' (Wood 2005). The currently recommended regimens for adults that demonstrate the most potent virologic and immunologic efficacy are those composed of two NRTIs together with either a NNRTI or a PI (DHHS Panel on Antiretroviral Guidelines for Adults and Adolescents 2006b). Although HAART is not a cure, it has dramatically improved rates of mortality and morbidity, improved quality of life, revitalized communities and transformed perceptions of AIDS from a plague to a manageable, chronic illness.

Several international HIV treatment guidelines exist to guide clinicians in the management of HIV-infected individuals and are based on a combination of evidence from randomized clinical trials, observational cohorts and expert opinion.

Since the advent of HAART in 1996, most guidelines have evolved to keep up with new evidence. For example, the United States Department of Health and Human Services (US DHHS) guidelines initially advocated a more aggressive therapy but have subsequently moved towards a more conservative approach. The 2006 DHHS guidelines (DHHS Panel on Antiretroviral Guidelines for Adults and Adolescents 2006b) recommend initiation of treatment in all asymptomatic patients with <200 CD4+ cells/ml and allowing clinical judgement to be exercised at earlier stages of disease.

The WHO recommendations for expanded access in low- and middle-income countries (WHO 2004) take into account the lack of medical and laboratory infrastructure in many countries that have a high AIDS burden. The WHO guidelines emphasize treatment of patients with significant symptomatic disease and those with CD4+ cell count <200 cells/ml. A substitute for the CD4+ cell count criterion in resource-constrained settings where a CD4+ cell count is not available is a total lymphocyte count <1200 cell/ml. All of the guidelines emphasize initiation of ART for symptomatic patients with HIV-related symptoms (WHO stages 3 & 4), while the decision to initiate treatment of asymptomatic patients is more complex and is based on the patient's readiness to adhere to long-term therapy, together with an assessment of the level of existing immunodeficiency, the risk of disease progression and the risks and costs of therapy. In resource-constrained settings, the threshold for entry into an ART programmatic will also need to take cognizance of the resultant numbers to be treated, available financial and medical infrastructure and the resources necessary to identify treatment beneficiaries.

The dynamics of HIV in paediatric patients is distinct from that of adults. Most children infected with HIV have contracted the disease through vertical transmission from their mothers. The mean survival of vertically HIV infected children ranges from 75–90 months and only a fraction of the HIV-infected children survive to around 10 years of age without ART. In countries where it has been successfully introduced, ART has substantially changed the face of HIV infection in children, with many HIV-infected infants and children now surviving to adolescence and adulthood. Guidelines for treatment of HIV-infected children are also continually evolving. The decision to start therapy and what drugs to choose for children is complex (DHHS Panel on Antiretroviral Guidelines for Adults and Adolescents 2006a). While HIV-infected children suffering from impaired growth and development may benefit from earlier initiation of HAART, the criteria for treatment initiation is based on CD4+ percentage, viral load and clinical condition.

Prophylaxis and treatment of co-morbidities

The best way to prevent opportunistic infections is to prevent exposure to the infectious agent. However, this is not possible for all opportunistic infections because several are thought to be caused by a reactivation of latent infection, e.g. tuberculosis, herpes simplex virus, cytomegalovirus, and toxoplasmosis.

Improvement in immune function following the initiation of HAART can significantly lessen the morbidity of opportunistic infections. Furthermore, the incidence of a number of opportunistic infections and associated mortality can also be reduced through the use of prophylactic agents like cotrimoxazole.

Specifically targeted interventions like preventive therapy for tuberculosis in high-risk patients, chemoprophylaxis for malaria for HIV infected pregnant women in malaria endemic areas, and vaccinations against pneumococcal infections and influenza in HIV infected adults can be used to lessen the morbidity and mortality from opportunistic infections. Although not generally regarded as an opportunistic infection, vaccinations against hepatitis B should be considered in selected patients who are shown to be non-immune because of the effect that HIV has on the natural history of hepatitis B (Maartens 2005).

Challenges in ART provision

Since 2000, the collective efforts of activists, researchers, service providers, pharmaceutical companies, policy makers, and international agencies have generated real momentum in scaling up AIDS treatment and prevention across the globe, particularly in low- and middle-income countries. Coverage of ART in the developing world has more than doubled—increasing from 400 000 in 2003 to approximately 1 million by June 2005 (WHO 2006). While still short of the WHO goal of '3 by 5', the momentum in expanding treatment access is a remarkable achievement despite the initial challenges in implementing AIDS treatment programmes, especially in Africa where the burden is largest. The scale of ART provision was guided by what WHO refers to as the 'Public health approach to AIDS treatment'. This involved standardizing first and second line ART regimens, creating algorithms for determining who was eligible for ART, and how to manage patients on ART. This standardization enabled healthcare workers who are not physicians to become involved in AIDS care. Indeed, in much of Africa, nurse practitioners or intermediate-level clinicians are the main providers of ART. However, many challenges with respect to the scale up and sustained provision of treatment remain. These include constraints in scaling up VCT, stigma and discrimination, challenges in achieving high levels of treatment adherence, and side effects and toxicity such as hyperlipidaemia, insulin resistance, frank diabetes mellitus, acute life-threatening lactic acidosis, asymptomatic lactic acidaemia, chronic myopathy, peripheral neuropathy, and gastrointestinal intolerance.

While these challenges are being resolved, new challenges are emerging in scaling up the treatment and sustaining the ART provision in resource-constrained settings. While the various practical and political challenges in ART provision have changed since 2000, three over-arching challenges—under-developed, overburdened healthcare services, the persistence of stigma, and the failure to integrate prevention into care–continue to hamper the effort to maximize the benefits of ART implementation (Abdool Karim 2006b).

Impact of AIDS

Impact of AIDS on mortality

Globally, AIDS has joined the leading causes of premature death among both women and men 15–59 years of age (Piot 2006). In the worst affected countries like South Africa, AIDS is the single largest contributor to premature loss of life and accounts for about half of the disability adjusted life years lost. In Africa, one important feature of AIDS related mortality is its age and gender frequency distribution. While the overall AIDS related mortality rates are highest in the 20–40-year age group, women experience higher AIDS mortality rates at younger ages in Africa.

The introduction of ART has helped slow the rising mortality due to AIDS. In high-income countries the introduction of HAART led to significant declines in AIDS mortality rates (Palella *et al.* 1998; Detels *et al.* 1998) (See http://www.cdc.gov/hiv/topics/surveillance/resources/slides/trends/index.htm). Unfortunately, this trend has not yet become evident in most poor countries, where mortality rates due to AIDS continue to climb. However, as ART becomes more widely available in poor countries, it is hoped that mortality will start to fall.

Impact of AIDS on society

The social impact of AIDS is more pronounced in generalized epidemics and in settings where heterosexual transmission is dominant. For example, the AIDS epidemic in sub-Saharan Africa has had widespread impact on many sectors of society, impacting beyond the individual, to the family structure and society at large. High death rates in the socially and economically most active sectors of society are impacting dramatically on economic activity, financial wellbeing and social progress. Indeed, AIDS has become the biggest threat to the continent's development for the current generation of young adults as well as the next generation. UNAIDS estimates that AIDS is reducing the per capita growth rate by 0.5–1.2 per cent annually in sub-Saharan Africa. Life expectancy has halved in some countries and millions of adults are dying in their economically productive years, thereby impacting on the economic dependency ratio. Many families are losing their income earners and the families of those who die have to find money to pay for their funerals.

As the epidemic progresses, social cohesion in already fragile communities is being further eroded. An increasing number of households are either grandmother or child-headed. Children who are orphaned struggle to survive without parental care and frequently cease attending school because they cannot afford school fees and uniforms or have to look after younger siblings (Johnson 2001). A decline in school enrolment is one of the most visible effects of the HIV/AIDS epidemic on education in Africa.

Private industry and companies of all types face higher costs of training, insurance, benefits, absenteeism and illness. A number of skilled personnel in important areas of public management and core social services are being lost to AIDS. Essential services are being depleted and scarce resources are put under greater strain. As the epidemic matures, the health sector suffers the additional pressures of caring for those with AIDS. Not only has health utilization increased, but other illnesses that deserve attention (such as diabetes, malaria, hypertension, etc.) are being crowded out by the increasing morbidity that AIDS brings.

The worst of the epidemic impact has yet to come. In the absence of massively expanded prevention, treatment and care efforts, the AIDS death toll on the continent of Africa is expected to continue rising before peaking around the end of this decade.

Ethical and human rights issues

Human rights challenges in AIDS treatment provision

The continued spread of HIV globally and the immense and growing burden of AIDS places a moral, scientific and ethical imperative on individuals and societies to mobilize political will and resources to respond to the pandemic. This imperative extends to the urgent need to conduct research to find new ways of preventing and treating AIDS. The immediacy of the challenge and need for solutions has redefined the way medical practitioners, governments, and health service providers, amongst others, respond to an infectious disease and the way in which researchers conduct research and clinical trials.

During the early days of the epidemic, AIDS was identified with already socially and/or legally marginalized or stigmatized groups, such as men who have sex with men, injecting drug users, racial minorities, and sex workers. The uncertainty of the cause of the new disease and how it is spread created conflict between human rights activists and public health practitioners. Classical infectious diseases approaches of 'isolate and contain', as practised in the sanitoria of Cuba, the closure of bath-houses in San Francisco, and restrictions on entry of HIV infected persons to the United States were at odds with the ongoing campaigns in the gay community to secure their rights. As knowledge of natural history of infection grew, levels of social stigma and discrimination did not diminish but an uneasy balance was struck between respect of the right of the infected person and public good. A phrase coined by Bayer (Bayer & Fairchild 2006), 'HIV exceptionalism', captures the outcome of this balance between the rights of those infected with broader rights of society to be protected from an incurable infectious disease.

In the pre-HAART era, the manifestation of protection of the rights of the individual infected person was most apparent in HIV testing policies. All HIV testing had to be voluntary, client-initiated, and done in the context of pre- and post-test counselling by a trained person. In contrast to management of other health conditions where the clinician made decisions about what diagnostic tests are undertaken, HIV set new standards of patient autonomy to make this decision in an informed manner. Furthermore, disclosure was the prerogative of the infected person. Several precedent-setting judgements in the courts of law reinforced this right in several countries (Jonsen 1990; Kirp 1989; Kirp & Bayer 1992). Prohibitions on pre-employment HIV testing in the workplace are another of the human rights achievements in response to workplace-based discriminatory policies against those with AIDS.

Research showing the substantial benefit of AZT in reducing mother-to-child transmission of HIV re-opened some of the early HIV testing debates in industrialized countries, focusing now on whether HIV testing should be compulsory for all pregnant women in light of potential benefit to the unborn baby. These debates were echoed in poor countries as single-dose nevirapine became available for prevention of mother-to-child transmission of HIV. Despite the high HIV prevalence in pre-natal settings, many women choose not to test because of real or perceived fear of testing positive, fear emanating from the social consequences of having HIV infection. The status of women in these settings, as well as fear of violence and discrimination, impact a number of decisions infected mothers make—whether to have an HIV test, take their intra-partum dose of medication, ensure their babies receive nevirapine, or breastfeed their babies.

The introduction of HAART in industrialized countries in the late 1990s highlighted the economic disparities between north and south. Global activism, spurred on by social movements of people living with AIDS, community groups, professional organizations and advocacy groups, resulted in major reductions in drug prices. Importantly, it also led to the establishment of International Assistance Funds to help countries provide these life-saving drugs; the Global Fund against AIDS, Tuberculosis and Malaria and the US President's Emergency Plan for AIDS Relief (PEPfAR).

These initiatives have set important precedents for how the global community responds to public health crises. Other long-standing public health challenges are benefiting, such as maternal and child health, reproductive health services, tuberculosis and malaria. Importantly, these funds are supporting efforts to increase access to ART, expand training of healthcare workers, strengthen healthcare services, and build new facilities including laboratory infrastructure and drug distribution systems in resource-constrained settings. While these efforts cannot undo the historical inequities between north and south, they demonstrate the importance of global commitment and joint action.

Ethical challenges in AIDS research

The disparities between north and south in the context of HIV prevention trials have led to substantial debate on research ethics. In the mid-1990s, a prominent medical journal questioned the ethics of conducting placebo-controlled trials for the prevention of MTCT in Africa and Thailand. The argument was that PACTG 076 regimen of AZT, which has been shown to be effective in reducing MTCT in the United States, should be the control intervention in all subsequent MTCT trials. The counter-arguments were that the PATCG 076 regimen of AZT was not implementable in resource-constrained settings and hence the need to assess the efficacy of short implementable courses of antiretrovirals against the existing standard of care in the countries hosting the trials. The centrepiece of these debates is whether placebo-controlled trials were justifiable when an intervention exists regardless of whether the intervention was not affordable or feasible in the host country, as was the case with the AZT regimen emanating from the PACTG 076 trial. A certain level of paternalism dominated these debates—issues of exploitation, duties of sponsors, and questions about the voluntariness of the informed consent process in poor and low-literate populations. This debate led to the revision of several international ethical guidelines to clarify when placebo controlled trials are ethically justifiable.

New standards in HIV prevention and treatment research have emerged that pay particular attention to community engagement and participation through formalized structures such as Community Advisory Boards; assessments of comprehension of the informed consent process prior to enrolling volunteers into trials; upfront provision for post-trial access and provision of ancillary care. In contrast to non-HIV research, additional responsibilities are placed on HIV researchers to provide therapies unrelated to the study interventions, e.g. provision of HAART for HIV vaccine trial participants who become infected. In some instances, the pendulum has swung too far across and researchers have become over-protectionist and risk averse in the conduct of HIV prevention research in these settings.

Conclusion

The last 25 years has seen the emergence of a completely new pathogen and its devastating consequences. The magnitude of the global HIV epidemic also spurred the scientific community to develop several interventions that are proven to prevent HIV infection and over 25 new drugs that are effective in treating AIDS. For each of the three main modes of HIV transmission, there are effective strategies to prevent HIV infection using existing technologies (like circumcision and male condoms) or new technologies like antiretrovirals to prevent MTCT, female condoms, and new HIV tests to protect the blood supply. The challenge has been to implement these interventions to scale given the historical under-development of public health systems in the countries worst affected by AIDS.

While medical research has made enormous strides in the prevention of MTCT and bloodborne spread, changing sexual behaviour to reduce HIV risk has proved more challenging. However, there are notable exceptions. Thailand reversed its HIV epidemic through its 100 per cent condom programme in brothels, and Uganda has been able to alter the course of its epidemic through political will for programmes that reduced high-risk behaviours. Vaccines have been key to infectious disease control and, in some instances, eradication. Developing an HIV vaccine has proven to be elusive, due mainly to the absence of identifiable natural immunity against HIV infection in humans. The enormity of this vaccine development challenge led to the creation of the AIDS vaccine enterprise, which is a global collaboration amongst scientists to work towards the common goal of a safe and effective AIDS vaccine.

AIDS has redefined the way in which doctors relate to their patients, the way in which research is conducted and the way in which activism has forced redress in global inequities to life-saving medical care. The experiences of the AIDS epidemic over almost three decades has illustrated that AIDS is more than a medical problem; it is also a social and development problem with profound consequences on the very fabric of society. It is impacting on security, social cohesion, and economic growth, and is even reversing some of the health gains of the last century.

References

Abdool Karim Q. and Abdool Karim S.S. (1999). Epidemiology of HIV infection in South Africa. *AIDS*, **13**, S4-S7.

Abdool Karim S.S. (2006a). The African Experience. In Mayer K. and Pizer H.F., ed. *The AIDS Pandemic: Impact on science and society*, pp. 351–73. Elsevier Academic Press, San Diego, California.

Abdool Karim S.S. (2006b). Durban 2000 to Toronto 2006: The evolving challenges in implementing AIDS treatment in Africa. *AIDS*, **20**, N7–N9.

Abdool Karim S.S., Abdool Karim Q., Gouws E. *et al.* (2007). Global Epidemiology of HIV. *Infectious Disease Clinics of North America*, **21**, 1–18.

Ahmed S.T., Lutalo T., Wawer M. *et al.* (2001). HIV incidence and sexually transmitted disease prevalence associated with condom use: a population study in Rakai, Uganda. *AIDS*, **15**, 2171–9.

Auvert B., Taljaard, D., Lagarde E. *et al.* (2005). Randomized, controlled intervention trial of male circumcision for reduction of HIV infection risk: the ANRS 1265 Trial. *PLoS Med*, **2**, e298.

Baggaley R.F., Boily M.C., White R.G. *et al.* (2006). Risk of HIV-1 transmission for parenteral exposure and blood transfusion: a systematic review and meta-analysis. *AIDS*, **20**, 805–12.

Bailey R.C., Moses S., Parker C.B. *et al.* (2007). Male circumcision for HIV prevention in young men in Kisumu, Kenya: a randomised controlled trial. *Lancet*, **369**, 643–56.

Bayer R. and Fairchild A.L. (2006). Changing the Paradigm for HIV Testing—The End of Exceptionalism. *N Engl J Med*, **355**, 647–9.

Berger A., Scherzed L., Sturmer M. *et al.* (2005). Comparative evaluation of the Cobas Amplicor HIV-1 Monitor Ultrasensitive Test, the new Cobas AmpliPrep/Cobas Amplicor HIV-1 Monitor Ultrasensitive Test and the Versant HIV RNA 3.0 assays for quantitation of HIV-1 RNA in plasma samples. *J Clin Virol*, **33**, 43–51.

Bertrand J.T., O'Reilly K., Denison J. *et al.* (2006). Systematic review of the effectiveness of mass communication programs to change HIV/AIDS-related behaviors in developing countries. *Health Educ Res*, **21**, 567–97.

Burger S. and Poles M.A. (2003). Natural history and pathogenesis of human immunodeficiency virus infection. *Semin Liver Dis*, **23**, 115–24.

Cardo D.M., Culver D.H., Ciesielski C.A. *et al.* (1997). A case-control study of HIV seroconversion in health care workers after percutaneous exposure. Centers for Disease Control and Prevention Needlestick Surveillance Group. *N Engl J Med*, **337**, 1485–90.

Clerici M., Giorgi J.V., Chou C.C. *et al.* (1992). Cell-mediated immune response to human immunodeficiency virus (HIV) type 1 in seronegative homosexual men with recent sexual exposure to HIV-1. *J Infect Dis*, **165**, 1012–9.

Colvin M., Abdool Karim S.S., Connolly C. *et al.* (1998). HIV infection and asymptomatic sexually transmitted infections in a rural South African community. *Int J STD & AIDS*, **9**, 548–50.

Coovadia H.M., Rollins N.C., Bland R.M. *et al.* (2007). Mother-to-child transmission of HIV-1 infection during exclusive breastfeeding in the first 6 months of life: an intervention cohort study. *Lancet*, **369**, 1107–16.

Coutsoudis A., Dabis F., Fawzi W. *et al.* (2004). Late postnatal transmission of HIV-1 in breast-fed children: an individual patient data meta-analysis. *J Infect Dis*, **189**, 2154–66.

Crepaz N., Lyles C.M., Wolitski R.J. *et al.* (2006). Do prevention interventions reduce HIV risk behaviours among people living with HIV? A meta-analytic review of controlled trials. *AIDS*, **20**, 143–57.

De Cock K.M. and Johnson A.M. (1998). From exceptionalism to normalisation: a reappraisal of attitudes and practice around HIV testing. *BMJ*, **316**(7127), 290–3.

Dean M., Carrington M., Winkler C. *et al.* (1996). Genetic restriction of HIV-1 infection and progression to AIDS by a deletion allele of the CKR5 structural gene. Hemophilia Growth and Development Study, Multicenter AIDS Cohort Study, Multicenter Hemophilia Cohort Study, San Francisco City Cohort, ALIVE Study. *Science*, **273**, 1856–62.

Department of Health. (2007). HIV and AIDs and STI Strategic Plan for South Africa, 2007-2011. Department of Health, Pretoria. Available online at http://www.doh.gov.za/docs/misc/stratplan-f.html Accessed 30 January 2008.

Des Jarlais D.C., Hagan H., Friedman S.R. *et al.* (1995). Maintaining low HIV seroprevalence in populations of injecting drug users. *JAMA*, **274**, 1226–31.

Des Jarlais D.C., Marmor M., Paone D. *et al.* (1996). HIV incidence among injecting drug users in New York City syringe-exchange programmes. *Lancet*, **348**(9033), 987–91.

Detels R., Liu Z., Carrington M. *et al.* (1994). Resistance to HIV-1 infection. Multicenter AIDS Cohort Study. *Journal of Acquired Immune Deficiency Syndrome*, **7**, 1263–9.

Detels R., Mann D., Carrington M. *et al.* (1996). Persistently seronegative men from whom HIV-1 has been isolated are genetically and immunologically distinct. *Immunol Lett*, **51**, 29–33.

Detels R., Munoz A., McFarlane G. *et al.* (1998). Effectiveness of potent antiretroviral therapy on time to AIDS and death in men with known HIV infection duration. Multicenter AIDS Cohort Study Investigators. *JAMA*, **280**, 1497–503.

DHHS Panel on Antiretroviral Guidelines for Adults and Adolescents (2006). *Guidelines for the Use of Antiretroviral Agents in HIV-1-Infected Adults and Adolescents*. Available online at http://aidsinfo.nih.gov/ Accessed (8 March 2007), Office of AIDS Research Advisory Council (OARAC), National Institutes of Health.

DHHS Panel on Antiretroviral Guidelines for Adults and Adolescents (2006). *Guidelines for the Use of Antiretroviral Agents in Pediatric HIV Infection*. Available online at http://aidsinfo.nih.gov/ Accessed (8 March 2007), Office of AIDS Research Advisory Council (OARAC), National Institutes of Health.

Dobbs T., Kennedy S., Pau C.P. *et al.* (2004). Performance characteristics of the immunoglobulin G-capture BED-enzyme immunoassay, an assay to detect recent human immunodeficiency virus type 1 seroconversion. *J Clin Microbiol*, **42**, 2623–8.

Eke A.N., Mezoff J.S., Duncan T. *et al.* (2006). Reputationally strong HIV prevention programs: lessons from the front line. *AIDS Educ Prev*, **18**, 163–75.

Fylkesnes K., Haworth, A., Rosenvard, C. *et al.* (1999) HIV counseling and testing: overemphasizing high acceptance rates threat to confidentiality and the right not to know. *AIDS*, **13**:2469–74

Gallo R.C. (2002). Historical essay. The early years of HIV/AIDS. *Science*, **298**,1728–30.

Gallo R.C. and Montagnier L. (2003). The discovery of HIV as the cause of AIDS. *N Engl J Med*, **349,** 2283–5.

Garber D.A., Silvestri G. and Feinberg M.B. (2004). Prospects for an AIDS vaccine: three big questions, no easy answers. *Lancet Infect Dis*, **4**, 397–413.

Global HIV Prevention Working Group (2006). New approaches to HIV prevention—accelerating research and ensuring future access. Available from www.gatesfoundation.org and www.kff.org Accessed 18 January 2008.

Gottlieb M.S., Schroff R., Schanker H.M. *et al.* (1981). Pneumocystis carinii pneumonia and mucosal candidiasis in previously healthy homosexual men: evidence of a new acquired cellular immunodeficiency. *N Engl J Med*, **305**, 1425–31.

Gouws E., White P.J. Stover J. *et al.* (2006). Short term estimates of adult HIV incidence by mode of transmission: Kenya and Thailand as examples. *Sex Transm Infect*, **82**(Suppl 3), iii51–55.

Gray R.H., Kigozi G., Serwadda D. *et al.* (2007). Male circumcision for HIV prevention in men in Rakai, Uganda: a randomised trial. *Lancet*, **369**, 657–66.

Hallett T.B., Aberle-Grasse J., Bello G. *et al.* (2006). Declines in HIV prevalence can be associated with changing sexual behaviour in Uganda, urban Kenya, Zimbabwe, and urban Haiti. *Sex Transm Infect*, **82**(Suppl 1), i1–8.

Hemelaar J., Gouws E., Ghys P.D. *et al.* (2006). Global and regional distribution of HIV-1 genetic subtypes and recombinants in 2004. *AIDS*, **20**, W13–23.

Heyns A. and Swanevelder J.P. (2005). Safe Blood Services. In Abdool Karim SS and Abdool Karim Q, ed. *HIV/AIDS in South Africa*. pp. 203–16. Cambridge University Press, Cape Town.

Ho D.D. and Huang Y. (2002). The HIV-1 vaccine race. *Cell*, **110**, 135–8.

Hurley S.F., Jolley D.J. and Kaldor J.M. (1997). Effectiveness of needle-exchange programmes for prevention of HIV infection. *Lancet*, **349**, 1797–800.

Jaffar S., Grant A.D., Whitworth J., Smith P.G. and Whittle H. (2004). The natural history of HIV-1 and HIV-2 infections in adults in Africa: a literature review. *Bull World Health Organ*, **82**, 462–9.

Jana S., Basu I., Rotheram-Borus M.J. *et al.* (2004). The Sonagachi Project: a sustainable community intervention program. *AIDS Educ Prev*, **16**, 405–14.

Janssen R.S., Satten G.A., Stramer S.L. *et al.* (1998). New testing strategy to detect early HIV-1 infection for use in incidence estimates and for clinical and prevention purposes. *JAMA*, **280**, 42–8.

Johnson L. and Dorrington R. (2001). The Impact of AIDS on orphanhood in South Africa: A Quantitative Analysis: Monograph No.4. University of Cape Town: Centre for Actuarial Research.

Jonsen A.R. (1990). The Duty to Treat Patients with AIDS and HIV Infection. In Gostin LO ed. *AIDS and the Health care System*, pp. 155–68, 270–1. Yale University Press, New Haven.

Kayirangwa E., Hanson J., Munyakazi L. *et al.* (2006). Current trends in Rwanda's HIV/AIDS epidemic. *Sex Transm Infect*, **82**(Suppl 1), 127–31.

Kirp D.L. (1989). *Learning by Heart: AIDS and Schoolchildren in America's Communities*. Rutgers University Press, New Brunswick, New Jersey.

Kirp D.L. and Bayer R. (1992). *AIDS in the Industrialized Democracies. American Civil Liberties Union Epidemic of Fear: A Survey of AIDS Discrimination in the 1980s and Policy Recommendations for the 1990s (ACLU AIDS Project,1990) for other economically advanced democracies*. Rutgers University Press, New Brunswick New Jersey.

Liu A.Y., Grant R.M. and Buchbinder S.P. (2006). Preexposure prophylaxis for HIV: unproven promise and potential pitfalls. *JAMA*, **296**, 863–5.

Maartens G. (2005). Prevention of opportunistic infections in adults. In Abdool Karim SS and Abdool Karim Q (eds.) *HIV/AIDS in South Africa*, pp. 454–462 Cambridge University Press, Cape Town.

Mawar N., Saha S., Pandit A. *et al.* (2005). The third phase of HIV pandemic: social consequences of HIV/AIDS stigma & discrimination & future needs. *Indian J Med Res*, **122**, 471–84.

McCutchan F.E. (2006). Global epidemiology of HIV. *J Med Virol*, **78** (Suppl 1), S7-S12.

Moore J.P. and Doms R.W. (2003). The entry of entry inhibitors: a fusion of science and medicine. *Proc Natl Acad Sci USA*, **100**, 10598–602.

Morris L. and Cilliers T. (2005). Chapter 5: Viral structure, replication, tropism, pathogenesis and natural history. In Abdool Karim SS and Abdool Karim Q. *HIV/AIDS in South Africa.* pp 79–88. Cambridge University Press, Cape Town.

Morris M. and Kretzschmar M. (1997). Concurrent partnerships and the spread of HIV. *AIDS*, **11**, 641–8.

Myer L., Mathews C., Little F. (2001). Condom gap in Africa is wider than study suggests. *BMJ*, **323**, 937.

NACO (2006). HIV/AIDS epidemiological Surveillance & Estimation report for the year 2005. Delhi, National AIDS Control Organization, Ministry of Health & Family welfare, Government of India (Available at www.nacoonline.org Last accessed 22 January 2008).

Needle R.H., Coyle S.L., Normand J. *et al.* (1998). HIV prevention with drug-using populations - current status and future prospects: introduction and overview. *Public Health Reports,* **113**(Supp 1), 4–18.

Palella F.J., Delaney K.M., Moorman A.C. *et al.* (1998). Declining morbidity and mortality among patients with advanced human immunodeficiency virus infection. *N Engl J Med*, **338**, 853–60.

Panlilio A.L., Cardo D.M., Grohskopf L.A. *et al.* (2005). Updated U.S. Public Health Service guidelines for the management of occupational exposures to HIV and recommendations for postexposure prophylaxis. *MMWR Recomm Rep*, **54**(RR-9), 1–17.

Parekh B.S. and McDougal J.S. (2005). Application of laboratory methods for estimation of HIV-1 incidence. *Indian Journal for Medical Research,* **121**, 510–518.

Peterson L., Taylor D., Roddy R. *et al.* (2007). Tenofovir disoproxil fumarate for prevention of HIV infection in women: a phase 2, double-blind, randomized, placebo-controlled trial. *PLoS Clin Trials* **2**, e27.

Pettifor A.E., Rees H.V., Kleinschimidt I. *et al.* (2005). Young people's sexual health in South Africa: HIV prevalence and sexual behaviors from a nationally representative household survey. *AIDS*, **19**, 1525–34.

Piot P. (2006). AIDS: from crisis management to sustained strategic response. *Lancet*, **368**, 526–30.

Quinn T.C., Wawer M.J., Sewankambo N. *et al.* (2000). Viral load and heterosexual transmission of human immunodeficiency virus type 1. *N Engl J Med*, **342**, 921–9.

Roland M.E., Neilands T.B., Krone M.R. *et al.* (2005). Seroconversion following nonoccupational postexposure prophylaxis against HIV. *Clin Infect Dis*, **41**, 1507–13.

Shafer L.A., Biraro S., Kamali A. *et al.* (2006). *HIV prevalence and incidence are no longer falling in Uganda—a case for renewed prevention efforts: evidence from a rural population cohort 1989–2005, and from ANC surveillance [Abstract: THLB0108]*. XVI International AIDS Conference, Toronto, Canada.

Shelton J.D. and Johnson B. (2001). Condom gap in Africa: evidence from donor agencies and key informants. *BMJ*, **323**, 139.

Sheppard H.W. (2005). Inactivated- or killed-virus HIV/AIDS vaccines. *Curr Drug Targets Infect Disord*, **5**, 131–41.

Shisana O., Rehle T., Simbayi L.C. *et al.* (2005). South African National HIV prevalence, HIV incidence, behaviour and communication survey. Cape Town, Human Sciences Research Council Press.

Simon V. and Ho D.D. (2003). HIV-1 dynamics in vivo: implications for therapy. *Nat Rev Microbiol*, **1**, 181–90.

Smith R.A., Loeb L.A. and Preston B.D. (2005). Lethal mutagenesis of HIV. *Virus Res*, **107**, 215–28.

Spacek L.A., Shihab H.M., Lutwama F. *et al.* (2006). Evaluation of a low-cost method, the Guava Easy CD4 assay, to enumerate CD4-positive lymphocyte counts in HIV-infected patients in the United States and Uganda. *J Acquir Immune Defic Syndr*, **41**, 607–10.

Stone A. (2002). Microbicides: a new approach to preventing HIV and other sexually transmitted infections. *Nature Reviews*, **1**, 977–85.

Sweat M., Gregorich S., Sangiwa G., Furlonge C., Balmer D., Kamenga C. *et al.* (2000). Cost-effectiveness of voluntary HIV-1 counselling and testing in reducing sexual transmission of HIV-1 IN Kenya and Tanzania. *Lancet*, **356**, 113–21.

The Voluntary HIV-1 counseling and testing efficacy study group (2000). Efficacy of voluntary HIV-1 counseling and testing in individuals and couples in Kenya, Tanzania, and Trinidad: a randomised trial. *Lancet*, **356**, 103–12.

UNAIDS (2002). *Report on the global HIV/AIDS*. Geneva, Switzerland, UNAIDS.

UNAIDS (2003). *AIDS epidemic update December 2003*. Geneva, UNAIDS and WHO.

UNAIDS (2004). Chapter 1: The World Drug Problem: a status report. In UNAIDS *World Drug Report includes latest trends, analysis and statistics*, pp. 47–51. United Nations Office on Drugs and Crime (UNODC), Geneva, Switzerland.

UNAIDS (2005). *Evidence for HIV decline in Zimbabwe: a comprehensive review of the epidemiological data*. Joint United Nations Programme on HIV/AIDS. Geneva, Switzerland.

UNAIDS (2006). *2006 Report of the global AIDS epidemic*. Joint United Nations Programme on HIV/AIDS (Available at www.unaids.org). Geneva, Switzerland.

UNAIDS (2007). *2007 AIDS Epidemic Update*. http://data.unaids.org/pub/ EpiSlides/2007/2007 EpiUpdate_en.pdf (Accessed 27 November 2007). Joint United Nations Programme on HIV/AIDS. Geneva, Switzerland.

Vernazza P.L., Eron J.J., Fiscus S.A. *et al.* (1999). Sexual transmission of HIV: infectiousness and prevention. *AIDS*, **13**, 155–66.

Vlahov D. and Junge B. (1998). The role of needle exchange programs in HIV prevention. *Public Health Rep*, **113**(Suppl 1), 75–80.

Weiser S.D., Heisler M., Leiter K. *et al.* (2006). Routine HIV Testing in Botswana: A Population-Based Study on Attitudes, Practices, and Human Rights Concerns. *PLoS Med*, **3**, e261.

Weiss R.A. (2001). Gulliver's travels in HIVland. *Nature*, **410**, 963–7.

World Health Organization (WHO) (2001). Global Prevalence and incidence of selected curable sexually transmitted infections. Overview and estimates, World Health Organisation, Geneva, Switzerland.

WHO (2006). Progress on Global Access to HIV Antiretroviral Therapy: A report on 3 by 5 and Beyond. Geneva, World Health Organisation and United Nations Programme on HIV/AIDS.

WHO (2004). Scaling up antiretroviral therapy in resource-limited settings: Treatment guidelines for a public health approach. A revision. World Health Organisation, Geneva, Switzerland.

WHO (2005). The safety of immunization practices improves over last five years, but challenges remain. World health Organisation, Geneva, Switzerland.

WHO (2005). World alliance for patient safety: Global patient safety challenge, World Health Organisation, Geneva, Switzerland.

WHO (2005). Global tuberculosis control: surveillance, planning, financing. Geneva, Switzerland, World Health Organisation, Geneva, Switzerland.

Wu Z., Detels R., Zhang J., Li V. *et al.* (2002). Community-based trial to prevent drug use among youths in Yunnan, China. *Am J Public Health*, **92**, 1952–7.

9.14

Tuberculosis

Dermot Maher, Marcos Espinal, and Mario Raviglione

Abstract

We begin the chapter by describing the natural history of *Mycobacterium tuberculosis* infection. This underpins our understanding of tuberculosis epidemiology and the principles of tuberculosis control, for which the main stratagems are then briefly discussed. We continue with an historical account of the global tuberculosis epidemic as the necessary background to a description of the current burden of tuberculosis and recent trends. A brief account of tuberculosis control in the era of anti-tuberculosis chemotherapy serves as the backdrop to the development and implementation of the World Health Organization (WHO) strategy for tuberculosis control known as DOTS (a brand name derived from Directly Observed Treatment, Short-Course) and its adaptations. The next section reviews the basic principles in tuberculosis care which underpin the public health approach to tuberculosis control. We provide an assessment of the progress made towards the international targets for tuberculosis control for 2005, and then outline recent events in the evolving international response to the challenge of tuberculosis, including the development of the Stop TB Strategy and the Global Plan to implement it. We conclude with an assessment of the prospects for tuberculosis control in the future, looking forward to 2015 (the target year for the United Nations' Millennium Development Goals) and then beyond to 2050 (the target year for the elimination of tuberculosis as a global public health problem).

Introduction

Tuberculosis still represents a threat and a challenge to humanity today as it has done throughout history. There were an estimated 1.6 million tuberculosis deaths and 8.8 million new tuberculosis cases worldwide in 2005 (WHO 2007a), of which about 1 million cases (11 per cent) occur in children aged less than 15 years. Low- and middle-income countries suffer the brunt of the tuberculosis epidemic. Overall, it is estimated that 95 per cent of the world's tuberculosis cases and 98 per cent of the tuberculosis deaths occur in the developing world (Raviglione *et al.* 1995). Tuberculosis was the third leading cause of death (after HIV/AIDS and ischaemic heart disease) in adults aged 15–59 years in low- and middle-income countries in 2001 (Lopez *et al.* 2006).

The paradox is that tuberculosis continues to pose a great threat at a time when we are potentially well equipped to respond to the challenge. The explanation to the paradox lies in collective neglect. We have not yet dedicated enough effort and resources firstly, in technological innovation to replace the current generally old technologies for tuberculosis prevention and control; and secondly, in public health practice to ensure worldwide equitable access to the benefits of our understanding of the disease and of the means to control it.

The natural history of tuberculosis

In the practice of public health regarding tuberculosis prevention and control, the natural history of *M. tuberculosis* infection and tuberculosis disease underpins our understanding of tuberculosis epidemiology and the principles of tuberculosis control. A description of the contagious nature of pulmonary tuberculosis dates back to the tenth-century book *Qanun fi'l-Tibb* (The Canon of Medicine) by Avicenna (also known as Ibn Sina) (http://www.ummah.net/history/scholars/ibn_sina). Koch confirmed Avicenna's description 900 years later, by identifying the tubercle bacillus and its causative role in tuberculosis. Bacelli observed in 1882 that the tubercle bacillus is a necessary, but not a sufficient, cause of tuberculosis: '*Il bacillo non é ancora tutta la tubercolosi*' (The bacillus is not yet all there is to tuberculosis.) (quoted by Bloom 1994). Tuberculosis can only occur following infection with *M. tuberculosis*, but occurs in a small minority of those infected. The risk of *M. tuberculosis* infection is largely exogenous in nature, determined by the characteristics of the source case, environment and duration of exposure. In contrast, the risk of tuberculosis following *M. tuberculosis* infection is largely endogenous, determined mainly by the individual's immune status. Although tubercle bacilli may vary in virulence, the influence of the genetic diversity of the infecting organisms on the course of infection is not very well understood. The natural history of tuberculosis comprises the sequence of events following exposure to an infectious case: Transmission of *M. tuberculosis* infection, the process of becoming infected, the development of tuberculosis as one of the consequences of infection, and the completion of the disease cycle by transmission of *M. tuberculosis* by new or recurrent infectious cases.

Exposure to infection with *M. tuberculosis* and transmission of infection

The transmission of *M. tuberculosis* is almost exclusively airborne. The patient with pulmonary tuberculosis who is coughing (or talking, sneezing, spitting, or singing) produces droplets that may contain tubercle bacilli (Loudon & Roberts 1966). As the droplets expelled into the air evaporate, some form droplet nuclei (i.e. infectious particles of respiratory secretions usually less than 5 μm in diameter containing one or a few tubercle bacilli). A single cough can produce 3000 droplet nuclei which can remain suspended in the air for several hours. Whereas larger particles either fall to the ground or, if inhaled, are trapped either in the nose or in the mucociliary system of the tracheobronchial tree, droplet nuclei are so small that they avoid the defences of the bronchi and penetrate into the terminal alveoli of the lungs where infection begins. The particles containing tubercle bacilli on the clothing, bed-covers, or belongings of a tuberculosis patient cannot be dispersed in aerosols, so do not play a significant part in transmission of infection.

Those people with respiratory tract tuberculosis who produce the most tubercle bacilli are the most infectious. The number of tubercle bacilli found in sputum specimens reflects infectiousness (Frieden 2004). The most potent sources of infection are patients with sputum smear-positive pulmonary tuberculosis. This was demonstrated by the higher risk of tuberculosis found among contacts of sputum smear-positive than among contacts of smear-negative index cases in special studies and in classical contact tracing (Liippo *et al.* 1993). More recently, the use of molecular fingerprinting techniques has shown that the relative transmission rate from sputum smear-negative compared with sputum smear-positive source cases was 0.22 (Behr *et al.* 1999). Patients with extrapulmonary tuberculosis do not generally constitute a source of infection.

Risk of infection

Risk of infection depends on the extent of an individual's exposure to droplet nuclei and on susceptibility to infection.

Exposure to droplet nuclei

The two factors that determine an individual's risk of exposure are the concentration of droplet nuclei in contaminated air and the length of time spent breathing that air. The extent of an individual's exposure to droplet nuclei is determined by the proximity and duration of contact with an infectious source case.

The concentration of droplet nuclei depends on the number of infectious droplets expelled and the volume of air into which they are expelled. Risk of exposure is therefore much greater indoors than outdoors. Ventilation dramatically dilutes the concentration of droplet nuclei, and so is the most important environmental measure to decrease risk of infection among exposed persons. The simplest and least expensive way of ventilating a room or hospital ward is to maximize natural ventilation through open windows (WHO 1999a). Transmission generally occurs indoors since the concentration of droplet nuclei in contaminated air falls very quickly outdoors, and direct sunlight kills tubercle bacilli in 5 minutes.

A susceptible individual's risk of infection is therefore high with close, prolonged, indoor exposure to a person with sputum smear-positive pulmonary tuberculosis (generally considered 'close contact'). A contact tracing study in the Netherlands that cast the contact tracing 'net' very widely showed that the closer the contact of a susceptible individual to an infectious source case, the greater the chance of infection (Veen 1992). The number of cases of infection in a particular exposure group (defined by closeness to the source case) is the product of the risk and the number of people in the group. Thus, more cases of infection occur in a large group of distant, low-risk contacts than in a small group of close, high-risk contacts—an example of the Rose axiom (Rose 1985). Conventional contact tracing generally identifies the close, high-risk contacts and therefore identifies a minority of the contacts infected by a source case. The extent of an individual's exposure to infection determines not only risk of infection but also affects the risk of disease, since those with greater intensity of exposure are at greater risk of developing disease (Houk *et al.* 1968).

Susceptibility to infection

It has been difficult to separate the influence of the genetic and exogenous (socioeconomic and environmental) factors that determine susceptibility to infection. The role of genetic factors in determining susceptibility was suggested by a study in the United States of nursing home residents with apparently the same risk of exposure which found a higher risk of infection among black than white residents (Stead *et al.* 1990). Susceptibility to infection is affected by the ability of macrophages to phagocytose and destroy the bacilli that reach the terminal alveoli and begin the process of implantation and infection (Schluger & Rom 1998). Since several genes are involved in this process, the study of human genomics has the potential to increase our understanding of differences between individuals and populations in their susceptibility to infection (Davies & Grange 2001).

Some exogenous factors may cause increased susceptibility to infection by impairing the local immune response in the respiratory tract, e.g. silicosis and inhalation of smoke from cooking fires and industrial pollution, or by damaging the respiratory endothelium and mucociliary stairway, e.g. cigarette smoking (Aubry *et al.* 2000). In practice it has been difficult to separate the possible influence of these exogenous factors on susceptibility to infection versus progression of infection to disease. HIV may increase susceptibility to infection with *M. tuberculosis*. The evidence for this mainly depends on comparisons in hospital outbreaks of the outcome of exposure to source cases of tuberculosis, with higher rates of development of tuberculosis in HIV-positive than HIV-negative patients exposed. Assuming that the secondary cases have primary tuberculosis, the higher rates of tuberculosis in HIV-positive people reflect higher rates of *M. tuberculosis* infection and therefore increased susceptibility to infection with *M. tuberculosis*.

Primary infection and its outcomes

Primary infection occurs in persons without previous exposure to tubercle bacilli. When droplet nuclei are inhaled into the lungs, those small enough to avoid the mucociliary defences of the bronchi are ingested by alveolar macrophages. Bacilli virulent enough to withstand the proteolytic enzymes in the macrophage phagolysosomes multiply and initiate infection. About 2–4 weeks after infection, cell-mediated immunity results in the formation of granulomas, which usually constrain the spread of the bacilli. The initial focus of infection in the lungs (the Ghon focus) together with the related hilar lymphadenopathy comprise the primary complex, which develops without symptoms. The development of the immune response (delayed hypersensitivity and cellular immunity) about 4–6 weeks after the primary infection is indicated by a positive tuberculin skin test and occasionally by clinical hypersensitivity reactions.

The balance between host immunity and bacillary multiplication determines the outcome of infection. The immune response in most cases stops bacillary multiplication, but in a few cases is insufficient to prevent bacillary multiplication, and progression from infection to disease occurs within a few months. Young children are at increased risk of primary tuberculosis since the immune system may not be mature enough to contain the initial infection. Primary tuberculosis results from local bacillary multiplication and spread in the lung or spread in the blood from the primary complex throughout the body, with seeding of bacilli in various tissues and organs. In some cases dormant bacilli may persist and cause disease on later reactivation. The possible outcomes of primary infection with *M. tuberculosis* are therefore: (1) latent infection (with a positive tuberculin skin test and no clinical disease)—the usual outcome in 90 per cent of cases or more; (2) hypersensitivity reactions; (3) pulmonary and pleural complications; and (4) disseminated disease.

Progression of *M. tuberculosis* infection to disease

Once infected with *M. tuberculosis*, a person remains infected for many years, probably for life. The vast majority (90 per cent) of people without HIV infection who are infected with *M. tuberculosis* do not develop tuberculosis (Sutherland 1976). In contrast to the risk of *M. tuberculosis* infection that is largely determined by exogenous factors, the risk of tuberculosis following *M. tuberculosis* infection is largely endogenous, determined by the individual's immune status. Why some people with latent *M. tuberculosis* infection develop tuberculosis and others do not is still an unanswered question.

The 5–10 per cent of people infected with *M. tuberculosis* who develop tuberculosis in their lifetime do so mostly within 5 years of infection (Comstock & Cauthen 1993). The chance of developing disease is greatest shortly after initial infection and then steadily lessens over time. Various conditions or emotional stresses may trigger progression of infection to disease. The most important trigger is weakening of immune resistance, especially by HIV infection, but also by immunosuppressive therapies. The medical conditions that increase risk of progression to disease include diabetes mellitus, malnutrition, substance abuse, silicosis, malignancies, malabsorption, and chronic renal failure (Rieder 1999).

Impact of HIV co-infection on progression of *M. tuberculosis* infection

HIV increases the risk of progression to active tuberculosis both in people with recently acquired (DiPerri *et al.* 1989) and with latent (Selwyn *et al.* 1989) *M. tuberculosis* infection (for which HIV is the most powerful known risk factor for reactivation). This risk increases with increasing immunosuppression (Antonucci *et al.* 1995). As HIV infection progresses, CD4+ T-lymphocytes steadily decline in number and function, with a concomitant decreased ability to restrict tubercle bacilli to a few infected macrophages.

The impact of HIV on the outcome of primary infection is an increased risk and speed of progression to primary tuberculosis through local and disseminated bacillary spread. The tuberculin skin reaction is also suppressed. HIV increases not only the risk but also the speed of progression of latent *M. tuberculosis* infection to disease. Overall, compared to an individual who is not infected with HIV, an individual with untreated HIV infection has a 10 times increased risk of developing tuberculosis (Selwyn *et al.* 1989).

First episode (primary or post-primary) or recurrent tuberculosis

First episode of tuberculosis

A first episode of tuberculosis may be primary, i.e. occurring through progression of primary infection, or post-primary, i.e. occurring after a latent period of months or years after primary infection.

Primary tuberculosis

Primary tuberculosis mainly occurs in childhood since this is when most *M. tuberculosis* infections occur. Since HIV dramatically increases the risk of rapid progression of *M. tuberculosis* infection to disease, adults with HIV infection who become infected with *M. tuberculosis* often develop primary tuberculosis. The incidence of primary tuberculosis is therefore increased in countries with high HIV prevalence. The manifestations of primary tuberculosis mainly result from pulmonary and pleural complications and dissemination of primary infection.

Post-primary tuberculosis

Post-primary tuberculosis may occur either by reactivation of the dormant tubercle bacilli that have persisted in tissues for months or years after primary infection or by re-infection. The patient's immune response results in a characteristically localized pathological lesion, often with extensive tissue destruction and cavitation. Post-primary tuberculosis usually affects the lungs but can involve any part of the body. Patients with post-primary pulmonary tuberculosis often have extensive lung destruction with cavitation and positive sputum smear on microscopy, and are the main transmitters of infection in the community. People with latent *M. tuberculosis* infection who become infected with HIV are at increased risk of progression of infection to disease. The clinical picture depends on the degree of immunodeficiency, with disease dissemination more likely as immunodeficiency progresses.

Recurrent tuberculosis

A recurrent episode of tuberculosis is one that occurs after a previous episode has been considered cured, and may be due to relapse (reactivation of the same strain causing the original disease) or reinfection (indicating the lack of effectiveness of acquired immunity) (Lambert 2003). HIV increases the rate of recurrent tuberculosis (Korenromp *et al.* 2003), with increased likelihood of reinfection in settings of intense *M. tuberculosis* transmission.

Natural history of untreated tuberculosis (in the absence of HIV infection)

Studying the natural history of untreated tuberculosis would nowadays be unethical. However, in South India during the 1960s a study of untreated patients with sputum smear-positive pulmonary tuberculosis in a rural population found that five out of ten died within 5 years, three self-cured, and two remained ill with chronic, infectious tuberculosis (National Tuberculosis Institute, Bangalore 1974). As a rule of thumb in tuberculosis epidemiology (Styblo 1991), this finding is embodied in practically every conceptual model—qualitative or quantitative—of the way tuberculosis affects populations (Dye 2006a).

The disease cycle

In the absence of HIV infection, up to 10 per cent of people infected with *M. tuberculosis* will develop active tuberculosis (whether from progression of recent infection or from reactivation), of whom about one half will be infectious (usually with sputum smear-positive pulmonary disease) (Sutherland 1976). Thus, only one in 20 people infected with *M. tuberculosis* develops infectious tuberculosis, and each infectious case in turn needs to infect about 20 people in order to generate one further infectious case. This is the situation of stable tuberculosis incidence (i.e. the case reproduction number is one). Key determinants of the case reproduction number are the number of people infected by an infectious case, and the proportion of people infected with *M. tuberculosis* who develop active tuberculosis. Any factors that increase the number of people infected by an infectious case (e.g. lack of or inadequate anti-tuberculosis treatment) or that increase the proportion of people infected with *M. tuberculosis* who develop active tuberculosis will push the case reproduction number above one, with consequent increasing tuberculosis incidence.

Stratagems for tuberculosis control

The primary stratagem of tuberculosis control is to reduce the average number of people infected by each infectious case so that the case reproduction number is less than one. This can be achieved by prompt diagnosis and effective treatment, which lie at the heart of the approaches to tuberculosis control developed in the era of anti-tuberculosis chemotherapy (see 'The development of the approach to tuberculosis control in the chemotherapy era'). Other stratagems target individuals at risk of developing tuberculosis and are aimed at decreasing risk of primary infection with *M. tuberculosis*, risk of progression of *M. tuberculosis* infection to a first episode of disease, or risk of a recurrent episode of disease (whether due to relapse or reinfection).

Prompt diagnosis and effective treatment

The correct application of anti-tuberculosis drugs can cure over 90 per cent of new smear-positive tuberculosis patients who have neither tuberculosis resistance to first-line drugs nor HIV infection. Before the spread of HIV, countries that met the two international targets of at least 70 per cent case detection (among incident cases of sputum smear-positive pulmonary tuberculosis) and at least 85 per cent treatment success of those detected could expect to see a decline in tuberculosis incidence rates of 5–10 per cent per year or more (Dye *et al.* 1998). This expected epidemiological impact has been demonstrated in, for example, Peru (Suarez *et al.* 2001), and has been supported by observed reductions in prevalence, for example in the areas of China that have implemented the DOTS strategy (China Tuberculosis Control Collaboration 2004).

BCG immunization

A tuberculosis vaccine could potentially interrupt the disease cycle by decreasing risk of infection with *M. tuberculosis* or risk of progression of *M. tuberculosis* infection to disease. BCG provides protection against tuberculosis by decreasing risk of progression of *M. tuberculosis* infection to disease. Since BCG has a protective efficacy of 70–80 per cent against disseminated and severe forms of tuberculosis (e.g. meningeal and miliary tuberculosis) in children, WHO in 1996 recommended BCG vaccination for all neonates in countries with high tuberculosis incidence. Most of the infants vaccinated with BCG worldwide are therefore protected to a large extent against disseminated and severe tuberculosis for the first few years of their lives (WHO 1995). Although a meta-analysis of the published literature on efficacy of BCG in the prevention of tuberculosis found that, on average, BCG reduced the risk of tuberculosis by 50 per cent (Colditz *et al.* 1994), protective efficacy varies considerably in different populations (Fine & Rodrigues 1990). Most people who are vaccinated as children in countries with high tuberculosis incidence will not be protected against pulmonary tuberculosis as adults because the vaccine is unlikely to protect for longer than 15 years and, in many populations, often has low efficacy against adult pulmonary disease. BCG is therefore not expected to have any significant global impact in reducing *M. tuberculosis* transmission and tuberculosis incidence.

Preventive treatment

Preventive treatment can be aimed at decreasing risk of primary infection with *M. tuberculosis*, risk of progression of *M. tuberculosis* infection to a first episode of disease, or risk of a recurrent episode of disease (whether due to relapse or reinfection). The most common example of preventive treatment aimed at decreasing risk of primary infection with *M. tuberculosis* is the administration of isoniazid to an infant born to a mother with sputum smear-positive pulmonary tuberculosis and therefore at high risk of becoming infected. Most individuals who receive preventive treatment are those who are infected with *M. tuberculosis* and at high risk of developing tuberculosis, i.e. they receive treatment for latent *M. tuberculosis* infection. Isoniazid preventive treatment (IPT) for 6 months is recommended for such high-risk individuals, including children who are household contacts of an infectious case of tuberculosis and who, after screening, are found not to have active tuberculosis themselves (WHO 2006a) and people infected with HIV, since up to 15 per cent of tuberculin-positive, HIV-positive adults will develop tuberculosis each year (WHO 1999b). Preventive treatment is also of benefit in decreasing the risk of tuberculosis recurrence after successful treatment of a first tuberculosis episode in people who are HIV-infected (Fitzgerald *et al.* 2000).

Although cheap, IPT is at present used mostly for the protection of individuals, rather than to prevent transmission. This is because children rarely develop infectious tuberculosis, and because of the difficulties in large-scale administration of IPT to healthy adults. Since at least 6 months' daily consumption of isoniazid is difficult for health services and patients alike, many people who could benefit from treatment drop out before completion. The proportion of HIV-infected people who do complete a course of IPT is typically small (Aisu *et al.* 1994). For IPT to be effective in preventing a large number of tuberculosis cases, ways need to be found to maximize the detection of people infected with *M. tuberculosis* and at high risk of tuberculosis, and minimize the IPT dropout rate. For tuberculosis associated with HIV, maximizing the detection of people infected with *M. tuberculosis* depends on expanded provision of voluntary counselling services for HIV-positive patients (Hawken & Muhindi 1999).

Physical measures to decrease transmission

Removal of tuberculosis patients from their homes and their isolation in sanatoria may well have played a role in decreasing the transmission of *M. tuberculosis* in the pre-chemotherapy era. In the early years of chemotherapy, the usual policy for administration of treatment

anti-HBs positivity is related to the antibody peak level achieved after primary vaccination (Jilg *et al.* 1984, 1988). Follow-up of successfully vaccinated people has shown that the antibody concentrations usually decline over time, but clinically significant breakthrough infections are rare. Those who have lost antibody over time after a successful vaccination usually show a rapid anamnestic response when boosted with an additional dose of vaccine given several years after the primary course of vaccination or when exposed to the HBV. This means that the immunological memory for HBsAg can outlast the anti-HBs antibody detection, providing long-term protection against acute disease and the development of the HBsAg carrier state (West & Calandra 1996; Banatvala & Van Damme 2003). Hence, for immunocompetent children and adults the routine administration of booster doses of vaccine does not appear necessary to sustain long-term protection (European Consensus Group 2000). Such conclusions are based on data collected during the first 10–20 years of vaccination in countries of both high and low endemicity (Kao & Chen 2005; Zanetti *et al.* 2006).

Since the availability of hepatitis B vaccines in industrialized countries, strategies for HBV control have stressed immunization of high-risk groups (e.g. homosexual men, healthcare workers, patients in sexually transmitted infection clinics, sex workers, drug users, people with multiple sex partners, household contacts with chronically infected persons, some categories of patients) and the screening of pregnant women. As observed and reported in many countries, and though it is certainly desirable to immunize these persons, it is unlikely that such a programme limited to high-risk groups will control HBV infection in the community.

In 1991, the World Health Organization (WHO) called for all children to receive the HBV vaccine. Substantial progress has been made in implementing this WHO recommendation: By the end of 2006, 168 countries had implemented or were planning to implement a universal HBV immunization programme for newborns, infants and/or adolescents. Of these, 119 (62 per cent) countries reported HBV infant vaccination coverage over 80 per cent after the third dose; these countries are mainly situated in Europe, North and South America, Northern Africa, and Australia (WHO 2006).

High coverage with the primary vaccine series among infants has the greatest overall impact on the prevalence of chronic HBV infection in children (WHO 2004a). According to model-based predictions, universal HBV infant immunization (without administration of a birth dose of vaccine to prevent perinatal HBV infection), would prevent up to 75 per cent of global deaths from HBV-related causes, depending on the vaccination coverage for the complete series. Adding the birth dose would increase the proportion of deaths prevented up to 84 per cent (Goldstein *et al.* 2005).

In countries with high or intermediate disease endemicity, the most effective strategy is to incorporate the vaccine into the routine infant immunization schedule or to start immunization at birth (<24 h). Countries with lower prevalence may consider immunization of children or adolescents as an addition or an alternative to infant immunization (WHO 2004a, 2006).

Indeed, the effectiveness of hepatitis B newborn and infant immunization programmes has already been demonstrated in a variety of countries and settings (André & Zuckerman 1994; Lee 1997; WHO 2001). The results of effective implementation of universal hepatitis B programmes have become apparent in terms of reduction not only in the incidence of acute hepatitis B infections, but also in the carrier rate in immunized cohorts and in hepatitis-B-related mortality—two ways to measure the impact of a hepatitis B vaccination programme (Coursaget *et al.* 1994).

In Taiwan, the HBsAg prevalence in children under 15 years of age decreased from 9.8 per cent in 1984 to 0.7 per cent in 1999 (Chan *et al.* 2004). The average annual incidence of HCC among children aged 6–14 years was 0.7/100 000 for the period 1981–1986, and declined to 0.36/100 000 in 1990–1994 (Chang *et al.* 1997). In the Gambia, childhood HBsAg prevalence decreased from 10 per cent to 0.6 per cent since the introduction of the universal infant immunization programme (Whittle *et al.* 1995; Viviani *et al.* 1999). In Malaysia, HBsAg seroprevalence in children aged 7–12 years went down from 1.6 per cent in 1997 to 0.3 per cent in 2003 since the implementation of a universal infant programme in 1990 (Ng 2005). Recent data in Hawaii show a 97 per cent reduction in the prevalence of HBsAg since the start of the infant hepatitis B vaccination programme in 1991. The incidence of new acute hepatitis B infections in children and adults was reduced from 4.5/100 000 in 1990 to 0 in the period 2002–2004 (Perz *et al.* 2006b). In Bristol Bay, Alaska, 3.2 per cent of children were HBsAg positive before universal hepatitis B immunization; 10 years later, no child under 10 years of age was HBsAg positive (Wainwright *et al.* 1997). Finally, surveillance data from Italy, where a universal programme was started in 1991 in infants as well as in adolescents, have shown a clear overall decline in the incidence of acute hepatitis B cases from 11/100 000 in 1987 to 3/100 000 in 2000 (Romano *et al.* 2004).

Hepatitis C

Aetiological agent

HCV is classified in the family *Flavivridae*. Like other flaviviruses, HCV is an enveloped RNA virus with an inner nucleoprotein core. Its envelope contains two glycoproteins, E1 and E2, which form heterodimers (to form a functional subunit) at the surface of the virion. Efforts to isolate the virus by standard immunologic and virologic techniques were unsuccessful and HCV was finally identified by direct cloning and sequencing of its genome. Although the virus was identified 15 years ago, its pathogenesis and replication are still not fully understood. An important feature of HCV is that the viral genomes display extensive genetic heterogeneity at the local as well as the global level. Even within a host, the HCV genome population circulates as a 'quasi-species' of closely related sequences. Worldwide, a high degree of genetic variation exists, resulting in at least six major genotypes and more than 100 distantly related subtypes (Forns & Bukh 1999). It has been reported that virus pathogenicity and sensitivity to current standards of treatment appear to vary with different subtypes (genotypes 2 and 3, responding better than genotype 1). These characteristics of HCV, much like HIV, make it a moving target for vaccine design.

Epidemiology

HCV is a major cause of acute hepatitis and chronic liver disease, including cirrhosis and HCC. Globally, an estimated 170 million persons are chronically infected with HCV and 3–4 million persons are newly infected each year (Alter 2007). The worldwide prevalence of HCV ranges from 1 per cent in high-income countries to around 10 per cent in low- and middle-income countries (Fig. 9.16.2). Table 9.16.1 summarizes the global prevalence and mortality of HCV versus the observed prevalence and mortality of HBV and HIV/AIDS.

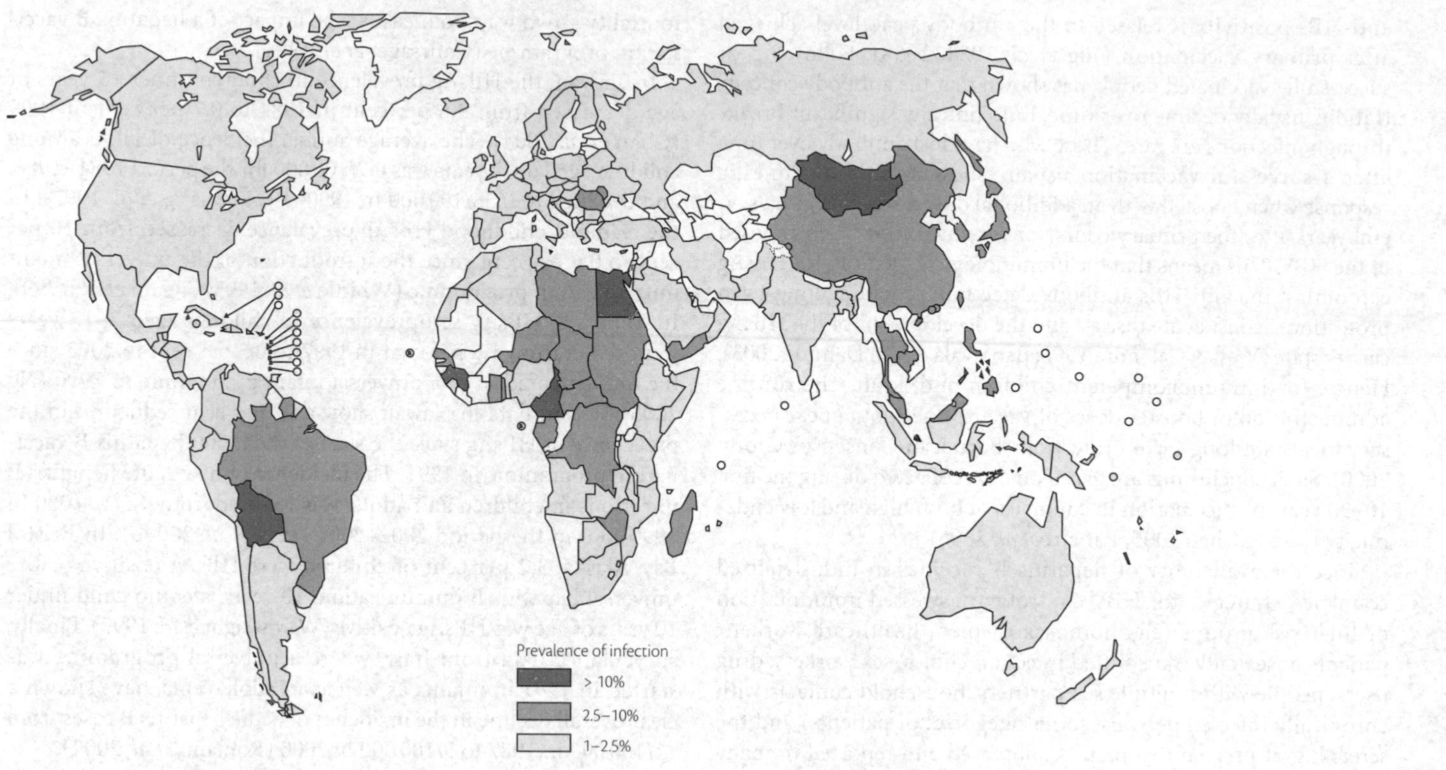

Fig. 9.16.2 Map representing countries with low (1–2.5%), moderate (2.5–10%), and high (>10%) hepatitis C virus prevalence.
Source: http://www.who.int/ith/maps/hepatitisc2007.jpg.

The reported seroprevalence in the Nile delta ranges from 19 per cent in the 10–19-year-old age group to ~60 per cent in the 30-year-old age group, and is associated with a high prevalence of liver cirrhosis in Egypt. The higher prevalence in the Nile delta is reported to be linked to parenteral anti-schistosomiasis therapy, which was carried out with inadequately sterilized injection material (Frank *et al.* 2000). Current estimates in the United States are that 3.9 million Americans are chronically infected with HCV, with prevalence rates as high as 8–10 per cent in African Americans. Haemodialysis patients, haemophiliacs, drug addicts, and people transfused with blood before 1990 are particularly affected by the disease. Despite infection control precautions, healthcare providers remain at risk for acquiring bloodborne viral infections due to accidental exposure. Therapeutic injections are reported as accounting for 2 million new HCV infections each year. Many of these injections are performed in less than ideal conditions, often with reuse of needles or multi-dose vials and mainly, but not exclusively, in low- and middle-income countries. The residual risk of transmitting HCV through blood transfusion is very low in industrialized countries but safety of blood supply remains a major source of public concern in low- and middle-income countries.

In Europe, up to 60–70 per cent of intravenous drug users living in urban areas are seropositive for HCV antibodies. The rate of infection depends on the length of drug use, with 25 per cent of infections occurring during the first year of addiction, 50 per cent after 5 years and up to 90 per cent for more than 5 years of intravenous drug use.

Transmission

The global epidemic of HCV infection emerged in the second half of the twentieth century and has been attributed, at least in part, to the increasing use of parenteral therapies and blood transfusion during that period. In high-income countries, the rapid improvement of healthcare conditions and the introduction of anti-HCV screening for blood donors have led to a sharp decrease in the incidence of iatrogenic HCV (Prati 2006). Injectable drug use remains the main route of transmission, accounting for nearly 90 per cent of new HCV infections. Mother-to-child transmission has been widely documented. The risk of perinatal infection ranges from 3 per cent to 10 per cent in different populations. Transmission is believed to occur *in utero*, as a consequence of a high viral load in the mother (in particular, from mothers who are HIV-co-infected) (Kato *et al.* 1994). Sexual transmission is thought to be relatively infrequent; however, an epidemiological review of current literature shows that, in many cases, no recognizable transmission factor or route is identified (Memon & Memon 2002).

It appears that HCV is inefficiently transmitted sexually; however, the large reservoir of HCV carriers provides multiple opportunities for exposure to potentially infected partners. Individuals with multiple sexual partners, prostitutes and their clients, patients with common sexually transmitted infections, and partners of HCV and HIV co-infected persons are at the highest risk of acquiring HCV sexually.

Clinical manifestations

The incubation period for hepatitis C before the onset of clinical symptoms ranges from six to seven weeks on average. In acute infections, the most common symptoms are fatigue and jaundice; however, the majority of cases (between 60 and 70 per cent), even those who develop chronic infection, are asymptomatic for years. Fulminant hepatitis C forms are rarely observed. While most patients with acute HCV infection have mild symptoms or no symptoms, 50–85 per cent of those infected develop chronic disease.

Chronic disease is difficult to recognize because symptoms are mild and infection passes silently and insidiously from the acute to the chronic phase. In fact, the vast majority of those affected are symptom free for at least 20 years. Serological diagnosis of acute HCV infection is based upon the detection of HCV RNA. Persistence of HCV infection is diagnosed by the presence of HCV RNA in the blood for at least 6 months.

The mechanisms of HCV persistence are currently unknown, although it is known that HCV chronicity develops despite humoral and cellular responses to HCV proteins. Factors associated with development of chronic disease appear to include older age at the time of infection, male gender, and an immunosuppressed state such as HIV infection (Lauer *et al.* 2001).

Treatment

The primary goals for treatment of HCV infection are to reduce morbidity and mortality through complete clearance of HCV and normalisation of liver enzymes, reducing disease progression, improving quality of life and reducing the reservoir of chronic carriers, thereby controlling further transmission. Treatment is recommended for patients with an increased risk of developing cirrhosis; most of these patients (but not all) have persistently elevated liver enzymes and high levels of HCV RNA (>60 IU/ml). Effective sustained virological response has been obtained in about 50 per cent of HCV patients with genotype 1 and 80 per cent of patients with genotype 2 and 3 who had received combined pegylated interferon-based treatment with ribavirin for 48 weeks (Chevalier & Pawlotsky 2007; Tan & Lok 2007). As with HBV treatment, therapy for chronic HCV is often too costly for most patients in low- and middle-income countries to afford.

Public health impact

HCV has been compared to a 'viral time bomb'. The WHO estimates that about 170 million people, some 3 per cent of the world's population, are infected with HCV, 130 million of whom are chronic HCV carriers at risk of developing liver cirrhosis and/or HCC. It is estimated that 3–4 million persons are newly infected each year and that 20 per cent of those infected with HCV progress to cirrhosis within the first 10 years after infection (Gerberding & Henderson 1992; Alter 2007). Furthermore, chronic HCV disease is the primary cause of liver transplantation in industrialized countries.

Prevention

There is no vaccine against HCV. Research is in progress, but the high mutability of the HCV genome complicates vaccine development. Although 20 per cent of patients with acute HCV infection clear the virus spontaneously, lack of knowledge of any protective immune response following HCV infection impedes vaccine research. Although some studies have shown the presence of virus-neutralizing antibodies, it is not fully clear whether and how the immune system is able to eliminate the virus. Thus, from a global perspective, the greatest impact on HCV disease burden will likely be achieved by focusing efforts on reducing the risk of HCV transmission from nosocomial exposures (e.g. screening of blood, rigorous implementation of infection control, reducing unsafe injection practices) and high-risk behaviours (e.g. injection drug use).

Adherence to fundamental infection control principles, including safe injection practices and appropriate aseptic techniques, is essential to prevent transmission of bloodborne viruses in health-care settings. Educational programmes aimed at the prevention of drug use and, for those already addicted, aimed at the prevention of shared needles and other equipment can decrease this source of infection. Some countries have established syringe exchange programmes that provide easy access to sterile syringes, accompanied by counselling and health education and instructions on the safe disposal of used syringes.

Alcoholic liver disease

Alcoholic beverages have been used in human societies since the beginning of recorded history. It has long been known that alcohol consumption is responsible for increased illness and death. Alcohol has been shown to be related to more than 60 different medical conditions (Room *et al.* 2005). Worldwide, alcohol causes 1.8 million deaths (3.2 per cent of total) and 58.3 million (4 per cent of total) of Disability Adjusted Life Years (World Health Organization 2004b). The burden is not equally distributed among the countries. The highest disease load attributable to alcohol is found in the heavy-drinking former socialist countries of Eastern Europe and in Latin America (Fig. 9.16.3). For most diseases there is a dose–response relation to volume of alcohol consumption, with the risk of the disease increasing with higher volume. Thirty-two per cent of all cases of cirrhosis worldwide are estimated to be attributable to alcohol (Room *et al.* 2005).

Alcoholic liver disease, resulting from the chronic and excessive consumption of alcoholic beverages, represents a considerable burden for the practising clinician, constituting the commonest reason for admitting patients with liver disease to hospital. Alcoholic liver disease is currently the second leading indication for liver transplantation in Europe and the United States after chronic hepatitis C, representing 17–33 per cent of transplants (European Liver Transplant Registry 2007) (Fig. 9.16.4).

The costs to society from alcohol abuse cannot be overemphasized. In 1998, overall costs in the United States amounted to US$186.6 billion, out of which healthcare costs accounted for US$26.5 billion, and hospital-related costs US$600 million to US$1.8 billion (Harwood 2000). In the United Kingdom, alcohol costs the country approximately £20 billion per year (Pincock 2003). Despite this burden, surprisingly little consensus exists on disease pathogenesis and on the factors that determine susceptibility.

Worldwide patterns of alcoholic intake and burden of disease in general and alcoholic liver disease in particular

Patterns of alcohol intake are constantly evolving as well as prevalence and incidence of alcoholic liver disease. The average volume of drinking was highest in established market economies in Western Europe and North America, and in the former Socialist economies in Eastern Europe, and lowest in the Eastern Mediterranean region and parts of Southeast Asia including India (Rehm 2003).

Overall, 4 per cent of the global burden of disease is attributable to alcohol. This is as much as the burden of disease from tobacco (4.1 per cent) (Room *et al.* 2005). Internationally, the highest disease load attributable to alcohol is found in the heavy-drinking former socialist countries in Eastern Europe, where 12.1 per cent of disease burden is related to alcohol. North America, Western Europe, Japan, and Australasia have a 6.8 per cent disease burden (Room *et al.* 2005). In most low- and middle-income countries,

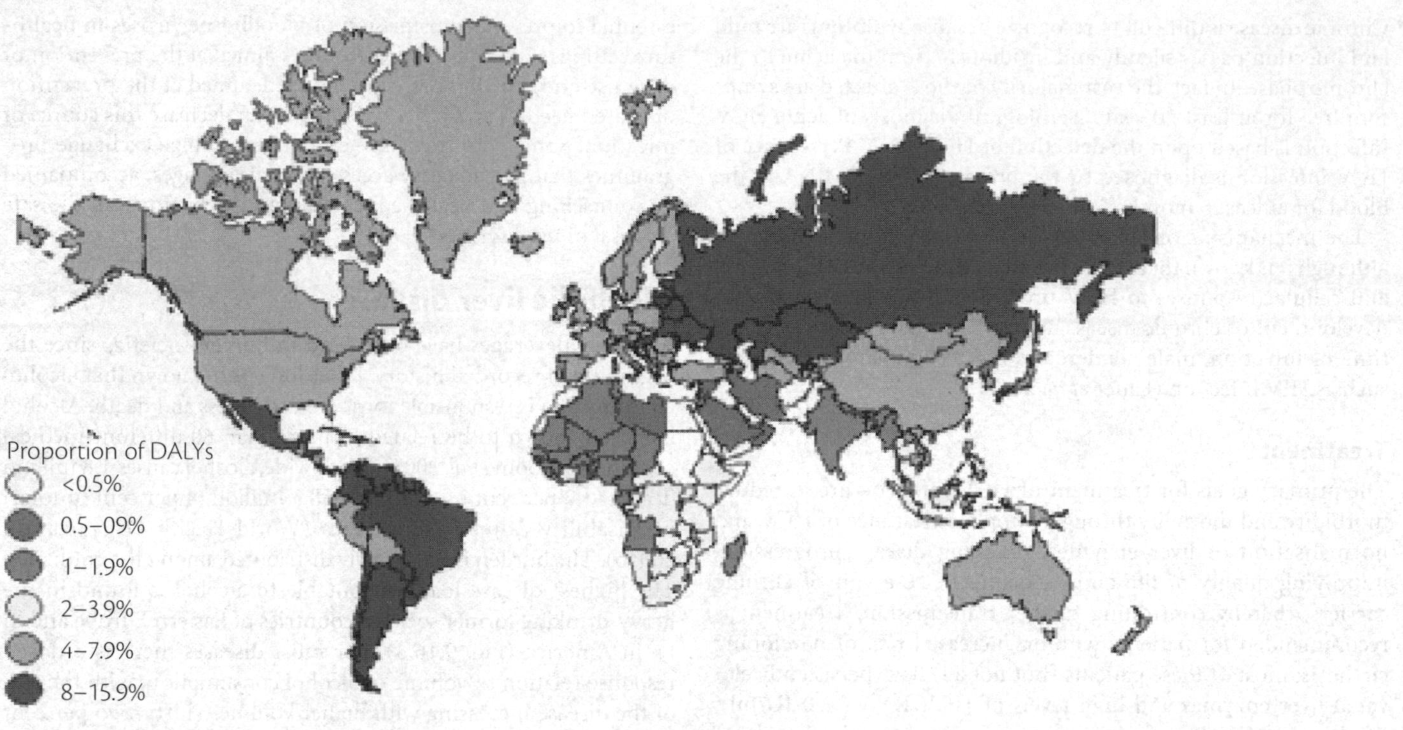

Fig. 9.16.3 Distribution of burden of disease attributable to alcohol in the world, expressed as disability adjusted life years (DALYs) (World Health Organization 2004b: http://www.who.int/topics/alcohol_drinking).

alcohol consumption is still relatively low, with a 1.3 per cent of the burden of disease in the Islamic Middle East and Indian subcontinent, and 2 per cent in the poorest countries of Africa and America (Room *et al.* 2005).

Given the relationship between alcohol consumption and cirrhosis, it would be expected that there is a lag period between changes in per capita alcohol consumption and cirrhosis-related mortality. Data regarding this lag effect have been conflicting. In fact, a long latency time is not observed, and the usual lag period is only one year or less (Kerr *et al.* 2000).

In Europe, 20–30 per cent of the population is estimated to consume excessive amounts of alcohol (Corrao *et al.* 1997). There was an increase in alcohol consumption until the late 1970s, followed by a period of stabilization. Along with this, there has been a pattern of stabilization to decline in cirrhosis mortality since the 1970s (Corrao *et al.* 1997; Ramstedt 2001).

In the United States, per capita consumption of all alcoholic beverages increased between 1962 and the early 1980s, and then decreased until 1998. Since then, there has a slight but persistent increase (Roizen *et al.* 1999). The cirrhosis mortality rate in the United States declined sharply in the early and mid-1970s in spite of the increase of overall per capita consumption till the early 1980s. The factors responsible for the discordance between US alcohol consumption and mortality rates have included better alcoholic liver disease treatments, increased 'Alcoholics Anonymous' memberships, and improved nutrition.

Despite a reduction of alcohol consumption in Europe in the 1970s, mortality rates for alcoholic liver disease decreased only in Western and Southern Europe, but did not change in Eastern and Northern Europe (Corrao *et al.* 1997). Studies in Australia (Saunders & Latt 1993) and Canada (Halliday *et al.* 1991) showed that cirrhosis-related mortality rates declined at almost the same time as the decrease per capita alcohol consumption. A similar pattern of almost simultaneous decrease in cirrhosis mortality and per capita alcohol consumption occurred in Europe during World Wars I and II, as well as in the United States during the Prohibition from 1919 to 1932 (Corrao *et al.* 1997; Saunders & Latt 1993).

In Japan alcohol consumption and all-type cirrhosis mortality increased for the past 50 years (Hasumura & Takeuchi 1991). The proportion of alcohol-induced liver disease increased to 5.1 per cent in 1968 to 10.7 per cent in 1977 and 14.1 per cent of cases in 1986. On the other hand, the Eastern Mediterranean Region—mostly countries with majority Muslim populations—displays a steady low alcohol consumption over a period of almost 40 years (World Health Organization 2004b).

In other parts of the world, including the most populous parts of the world, the trends have been alarming, showing increasing alcohol consumption, especially in the form of spirits, along with a tendency toward unhealthy patterns of alcohol intake (Campollo *et al.* 2001). This is the case in the Southeast Asian Region and the Western Pacific Region, driven by economic growth and aggressive marketing (Fig. 9.16.5) (World Health Organization 2004b; Pearson 2004). Without intervention, experts predict a future wave of alcohol-related problems in these countries. Korea has undergone dramatic socioeconomic transformation in the last 35 years. The per capita alcohol consumption rose from 1 l in 1970 to 7 l per year in 1980. There is also heavier consumption of distilled beverages. The proportion of patients in Korea with alcohol as aetiology of

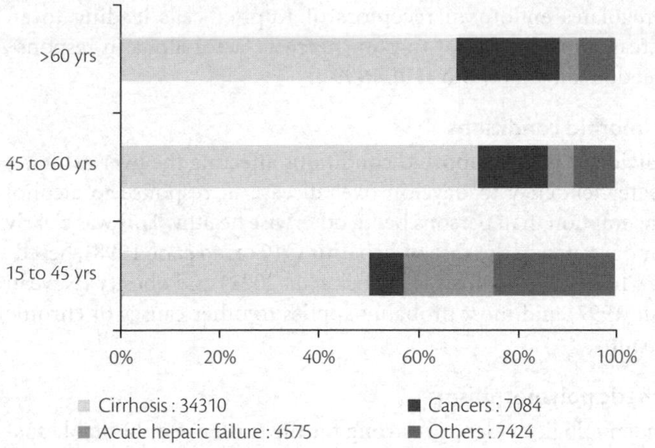

Fig. 9.16.4 Primary indications of liver transplantation in adult recipients (January 1988 to June 2006).
(*Source*: European Liver Transplant Registry, http://www.eltr.org/publi/IMG/gif/DIA8-2.gif).

liver disease increased from 1.5 per cent in 1980 to 24 per cent in 1993 (Park *et al.* 1998).

Morphology and natural history of alcoholic liver disease

Fatty liver (steatosis)

The first and most predictable hepatic change attributable to alcohol is the development of large droplet (macrovesicular) steatosis. This disorder usually resolves within two weeks if alcohol consumption is discontinued (Diehl 1997). In the past, it was assumed that alcoholic fatty liver was a benign process. However, it is now assumed that 5–15 per cent of patients will develop cirrhosis during a 10-year follow-up period (Sorensen *et al.* 1984).

Alcoholic steatohepatitis

The spectrum of alcoholic steatohepatitis includes fatty infiltration of hepatocytes associated with hepatocellular injury including: Ballooning degeneration, Mallory bodies inflammation with neutrophils and/or lymphocytes, and fibrosis with a perivenular, perisinusoidal, and pericellular disposition. These changes are present in 10–35 per cent of all alcoholics. It is not a benign process. Some patients will develop fatal decompensation. In addition, the risk of developing cirrhosis is increased. It is estimated that the probability of developing cirrhosis is ~10–20 per cent per year and ~70 per cent of patients with alcoholic hepatitis will eventually develop cirrhosis (Diehl 1997).

Cirrhosis

Worldwide, cirrhosis kills nearly 150 000 people each year (Corrao *et al.* 1997). Alcoholic cirrhosis accounts for ~38–50 per cent of all cirrhosis-related deaths (Stinson *et al.* 2001; Bellentani *et al.* 1997). The long-term prognosis of alcoholic cirrhosis improves with abstinence. The 5-year survival in compensated cirrhosis patients who continue to drink is <70 per cent, but can be as high as 90 per cent if they abstain from further alcohol intake. In patients with decompensated cirrhosis, the 5-year survival drops to <30 per cent in individuals who continue to drink, but is 60 per cent in those who stay abstinent (Diehl 1997; Alexander *et al.* 1971).

Hepatocellular carcinoma

Alcohol can be considered both as a primary cause of HCC and as a co-factor for the development of HCC. Most of the studies on incidence of HCC in alcoholic cirrhosis date from before the identification of the hepatitis C virus. As hepatitis C is relatively frequent in alcoholics, most of the reported HCC incidence rates in earlier studies are likely to be overestimated. Although the exact incidence rate of HCC in alcoholic cirrhosis is unknown, it is estimated to be over 1.5 per cent, making it worthwhile to offer patients surveillance (Bruix & Sherman 2005).

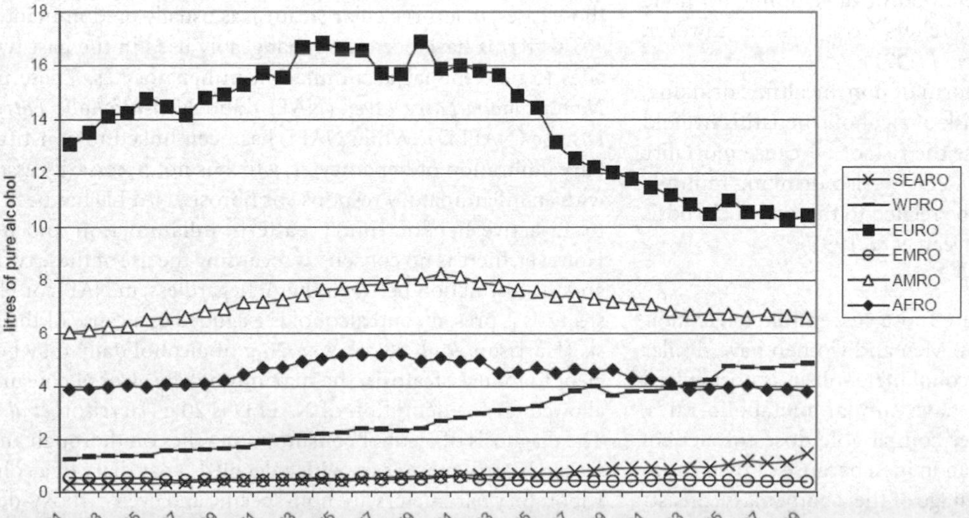

Fig. 9.16.5 Population-weighted means of the recorded adult per capita alcohol consumption in the WHO Regions 1961–1999 (World Health Organization 2004b: http://www.who.int/topics/alcohol_drinking)

Factors influencing the risk of alcoholic liver disease

Alcohol consumption can lead to steatohepatitis and cirrhosis. Most authors agree that persons who drink heavily (50–60 g of ethanol daily) represent a population at increased risk of developing liver disease (Becker *et al.* 2002). However, the absolute risk of acquiring alcoholic hepatitis or cirrhosis is relatively low (6.9 per cent in the two above-mentioned studies). This suggests that genetic factors and/or environment play a role in disease risk. Many studies that address the risk factors refer to their effect on 'alcoholic liver disease' in general rather than any specific aspect of alcoholic liver disease such as steatohepatitis.

Amount of alcohol

There is a general agreement that excessive alcohol consumption is associated with an increased risk of cirrhosis. However, the exact dose or a specific dose–response relationship for cirrhosis has not been agreed on. Measuring alcohol use in an individual or country has limitations. Most studies rely on interviews with patients and their families to estimate the amount, frequency and duration of alcohol consumption. Patients may not accurately report the quantity of alcohol they consume. The definition of a 'standard drink' varies from country to country: 8 g ethanol in the United Kingdom, 14 g in the United States, 19.75 g in Japan (Pearson 2004). The easiest would be to consider a standard drink containing 10 g of ethanol.

Evidence suggests that there is an increased risk for alcoholic liver disease with the ingestion of >60–80 g/day of alcohol in men and >20 g/day in women (Day 2000). 'Safe' limits of alcohol consumption for the liver are up to two drinks per day for women, and up to four drinks per day for men, with at least three alcohol-free days per week (Michielsen & Sprengers 2003).

Drinking behaviour

Researchers from Denmark showed in a large survey of 30 630 persons that beer or spirits are more likely to promote liver disease than wine (Becker *et al.* 2002). At present, it is uncertain whether wine *per se* is responsible for this reduced risk of liver disease compared to the other alcoholic beverages, or whether it represents a surrogate for other healthy behaviours such as increased consumption of fruits/vegetables (Everhart *et al.* 2003).

According to a Chinese study, drinking outside of mealtimes is a habit that might increase the likelihood of developing alcoholic liver disease (Lu *et al.* 2004). Researchers from France, however, found no such evidence (Pelletier *et al.* 2001).

Binge-drinking, an exaggerated form of non-mealtime drinking, has been reported to increase the risk of alcoholic hepatitis fivefold (Barrio *et al.* 2005), and to increase the risk of all-cause mortality in men and women (Tolstrup *et al.* 2004). Also drinking multiple types of drinks has been shown to be related to the risk of cirrhosis and non-cirrhotic liver disease (Naveau *et al.* 1997).

Gender

It is well recognized that women are more susceptible to alcohol-induced health disorders than men. Men and women have similar sized livers and when the rate of alcohol metabolism is normalized to liver mass, men and women have similar metabolic rates. However, blood alcohol levels after comparable doses of alcohol will usually be higher in women than in men because of their lower body volume and the higher percentage of their body mass consisting of fat. Evidence from animal models has suggested that oestrogen increases the gut permeability to endotoxin and accordingly upregulates endotoxin receptors of Kupffer cells leading to an increased production of tumour necrosis factor alpha in response to endotoxin (Enomoto *et al.* 1999).

Co-morbid conditions

Individuals with co-morbid conditions affecting the liver exhibit a greater tendency to develop liver disease in response to alcohol consumption than persons being otherwise healthy. This was clearly demonstrated in the case of hepatitis C (Corrao *et al.* 1998), hereditary haemochromatosis (Fletcher *et al.* 2002) and obesity (Naveau *et al.* 1997) and most probably applies to other causes of chronic hepatitis.

Genetic polymorphisms

Epidemiologic evidence is strong for the existence of heritable susceptibility to alcoholic liver disease. This appears related to several gene polymorphisms, some of which impact alcohol metabolism and others that influence hepatic immune responses.

Non-alcoholic fatty liver disease (NAFLD) and non-alcoholic steatohepatitis (NASH)

Definitions

Steatosis is defined as the accumulation of fat in the liver parenchymal cells or hepatocytes. A distinction is made between macrovesicular and microvesicular steatosis. Macrovesicular steatosis implies the presence of large fat vacuoles, containing predominantly triglycerides, and occupying a large part of the cell cytoplasm, displacing the nucleus towards the cell border. The hepatocytes may be enlarged by the presence of these fat vacuoles. Macrovesicular steatosis is graded according to the percentage of hepatocytes containing fat vacuoles: <5 per cent is minimal or no steatosis; >5 and ≤30 is mild steatosis; >30 and ≤60 is moderate; and >60 per cent is considered to be severe macrovesicular steatosis (D'Allessandro *et al.* 1991). In microvesicular steatosis, bipolar lipids are forming micelles, which are spread over the cytoplasm, and which do not displace the nucleus. The cells usually have normal dimensions. Grading is less complex: >45 per cent is considered to be severe microvesicular steatosis (Sheiner *et al.* 1995). In many patients, both types of steatosis are present, called mixed type steatosis. In those cases, macrovesicular steatosis is usually predominant.

Two terms have been interchangeably used in the past two decades to describe fat accumulation in hepatocytes. These include *Non-alcoholic Fatty Liver* (NAFL) and *Non-alcoholic Fatty Liver Disease* (NAFLD). While NAFL has been linked to constitutional fatty infiltration of hepatocytes, which is not necessarily associated with an inflammatory response or fibrosis, NAFLD has been linked to an active hepatic injury pattern, inflammation and fibrosis. However, there is no consensus regarding the use of these two terms and the distinction between them. Regardless, in NAFL or NAFLD, steatosis is present, and alcohol is excluded as a cause of the steatosis (Harrison *et al.* 2004). As >20 g of alcohol daily may be sufficient to induce steatosis, the maximum daily alcohol consumption allowed for the definition of NAFLD is 20 g (Harrison *et al.* 2004). The diagnosis of alcohol consumption relies on thorough anamnesis and hetero-anamnesis, with a detailed 7-day diary of alcohol use. Laboratory parameters are non-specific and even carboxy-deficient transferrin measurement is not very accurate in excluding significant alcohol consumption. In addition, the differential diagnosis cannot be made histologically, as the histological features of alcoholic and non-alcoholic liver disease seem to be identical. The diagnosis of the aspect of 'non-alcoholic' therefore constitutes a first problem in the interpretation of any data on the prevalence and natural history of NAFLD.

Non-alcoholic steatohepatitis (NASH) is a subgroup of NAFLD, in which liver steatosis is accompanied by signs of liver cell damage (especially ballooning of hepatocytes) and/or inflammation. In these patients, fibrous tissue may be generated, and patients can evolve to cirrhosis and its complications, including HCC. Although still debated, it is generally believed that pure steatosis does not lead to fibrogenesis and that only the NASH patients may present progressive liver disease (Angulo 2002).

Although not reflected by the name, NAFLD also implies the exclusion of other chronic liver diseases, including chronic viral hepatitis, toxic hepatitis (due to industrial toxins or solvents or to pharmacological agents), autoimmune liver disease, haemochromatosis, Wilson's disease, and some rare metabolic disorders. Hepatitis C, especially genotype 3, and Wilson's disease are two classical examples of liver diseases accompanied by steatosis, but they are not NAFLD. As will be discussed further, steatosis is no longer regarded as an innocent bystander, therefore the term NAFLD is preferred over NAFL.

Diagnosis

As already mentioned, a first problem is the diagnosis of the aspect 'non-alcoholic'. Laboratory tests, including elevation of AST (aspartate transaminase) more than ALT (alanine transaminase), elevation of γGT (gamma-glutamyl transpeptidase) or CDT (carboxy-deficient transferrin) measurement may be helpful, but are inaccurate. Thorough anamnesis and hetero-anamnesis is the cornerstone of the diagnosis, which therefore may always remain questionable.

A second problem is the diagnosis of steatosis and steatohepatitis. Abdominal ultrasound has a sensitivity of 70–75 per cent and a specificity of 60–70 per cent in diagnosing moderate to severe steatosis (Bellentani *et al.* 2000). CT scan and MRI are equally specific (100 per cent) and sensitive (75 per cent) in making the same distinction (Rinella *et al.* 2001). These non-invasive tools are thus not very sensitive, not able to accurately grade the steatosis, and not able to diagnose the presence of inflammation or fibrosis, and hence do not distinguish between NAFLD and NASH. Magnetic Resonance Spectroscopy can accurately quantify the fat content of a liver sample, but the need for specific software and practical considerations limits its use to specific research centres. Scores based on laboratory parameters are not validated for the diagnosis of steatosis (Miele *et al.* 2007). The gold standard for the diagnosis is still liver biopsy. The invasive character of that procedure, however, limits its use on a larger scale.

The diagnosis of steatohepatitis is even more complicated. Laboratory tests, especially the elevation of aminotransferase levels, are inaccurate, although frequently regarded as a sign of liver cell damage and hence inflammation, as patients with elevated liver tests may have pure steatosis without inflammation on liver biopsy, and 50 per cent of the patients with biopsy-proven steatohepatitis have normal transaminases (Prati *et al.* 2002). The cut-off values for normal aminotransferase levels have recently been questioned, and lowering the upper limit of normal to ≤30 U/l in males and ≤19 U/l in females increases the sensitivity for the diagnosis of NASH from 42 per cent to 80 per cent, but specificity decreases from 80 per cent to 42 per cent (Kunde *et al.* 2005). Scoring systems based on laboratory parameters are unvalidated to date. Imaging cannot distinguish steatosis from steatohepatitis. Again liver biopsy is the gold standard. This also holds true for the diagnosis of fibrosis. Laboratory parameters are not useful, except for a stage of cirrhosis, where more specific laboratory features can be present. Scoring systems based on laboratory parameters can distinguish between no or mild fibrosis versus advanced fibrosis and cirrhosis in hepatitis C (Rosenberg *et al.* 2004), but have not been validated in NASH. Imaging is not useful for the staging of fibrosis, and is only of value if signs of cirrhosis indicate advanced liver disease. Elastography, an ultrasound-based technique measuring liver stiffness (Ganne-Carrie *et al.* 2006), has been validated in hepatitis C, but not in NASH, and, like the laboratory scoring systems, only roughly distinguishes between no or mild versus severe fibrosis and cirrhosis. Also for fibrosis, liver histology is still the gold, or at least the best, standard (Miele *et al.* 2007).

Prevalence of steatosis, NAFLD, and NASH

As already mentioned, the difficulty in diagnosing of non-alcoholic steatosis, and the lack of accuracy of the tools for the diagnosis of steatosis, constitute two major problems in the acquisition of precise epidemiological data. Sample selection constitutes a third problem, as some categories of patients are more at risk. This will be discussed in the next section.

In screening studies with ultrasound, prevalence varies between 16 per cent and 23 per cent (Bellentani *et al.* 2000). In an autopsy series of traffic accidents, steatosis was histologically diagnosed in 24 per cent of cases. The prevalence was clearly age-related: In those aged <20 years the prevalence was 1 per cent, while in those >60 years the prevalence rose to 39 per cent (Hilden *et al.* 1997). In a series of cadaveric donor livers, 17.5 per cent were steatotic (Crowley *et al.* 2000). If specific lipid stainings are used, prevalence up to 50 per cent can be noted (Urena *et al.* 1998). Based on these figures, and making the distinction with alcoholic steatosis, the prevalence of non-alcoholic steatosis is estimated at 15–20 per cent in the general adult population (Angulo 2002). Exact data on the prevalence of NASH in the general population are scarce. In an autopsy series, a prevalence of 6.3 per cent was reported. The prevalence is usually estimated at 2 per cent, but this highly depends on sample selection. As a number of risk factors can be identified (see below), prevalence rates may vary geographically (Neuschwander-Tetri *et al.* 2003).

NAFLD and NASH and the metabolic syndrome

The metabolic syndrome, associating visceral overweight, dyslipidaemia, hyperinsulinaemia or diabetes mellitus, and arterial hypertension, as defined by the Third Report of the National Cholesterol Education Expert Panel on Detection, Evaluation, and Treatment of High Blood Cholesterol in Adults (Adult Treatment Panel-ATP III) (Expert Panel 2001), seems to be closely related with NAFLD and NASH. Some authors consider NAFLD and NASH as the hepatic manifestation of the metabolic syndrome. Many epidemiological data are at least in favour of a close relationship between the two entities.

In patients with NAFLD, the metabolic syndrome, according to the criteria of the ATP III, is fully present in 30 per cent of males and 60 per cent of females. Visceral adiposity is present in 40 per cent and 65 per cent of males and females, respectively, and diabetes in

10 per cent and 30 per cent, respectively. These prevalence rates are significantly higher than in the control population. The metabolic syndrome is significantly more prevalent in patients with NASH compared to patients with simple steatosis (38 per cent vs. 14 per cent, $p = 0.004$) (Marchesini *et al.* 2003).

In patients with obesity, steatosis is present in 60–95 per cent, according to the selection of patients and the way of diagnosis (e.g. ultrasound or histology in a series of patients undergoing bariatric surgery). The body mass index is an independent predictive factor for the accumulation of fat in the liver (Marchesini *et al.* 2003). Liver steatosis is more specifically associated with visceral obesity. Increasing obesity is also associated with an increased risk of NASH. Patients with NASH have visceral obesity in 48 per cent of cases versus 31 per cent of patients with pure steatosis ($p = 0.005$) (Marchesini *et al.* 2003). In morbid obese patients undergoing bariatric surgery, the prevalence of NASH is 15–25 per cent (compared to 2 per cent in the general population) (Kunde *et al.* 2005). In obesity, the relative risk of morbidity and mortality related to terminal liver failure is 4 (Ioannou *et al.* 2003), and the known increased risk for malignancy is largely related to the increased risk for developing HCC.

In patients with type 2 diabetes, cirrhosis and its complications are the second cause of disease-specific mortality (de Marco *et al.* 1999). NAFLD, as diagnosed by liver ultrasound, is present in 69.5 per cent, in an age-dependent manner (65.4 per cent in patients aged 40–59 years and 74.6 per cent in those aged ≥ 60 years) (Angulo 2002). Diabetes mellitus is a major risk factor for NASH: 15 per cent of patients with diabetes have simple steatosis, but 56 per cent have NASH. Among patients with NAFLD and diabetes, 23.9 per cent develop cirrhosis and 19 per cent experience liver-related death in 19 per cent, compared to 10.6 per cent and 2 per cent in NAFLD patients without diabetes, respectively (Abrams *et al.* 2004).

The close association between NAFLD/NASH and the metabolic syndrome and its components explains the variance in prevalence data according to the patient selection. The prevalence of NAFLD/NASH is therefore high in the Western population, and will increase, parallel with the increasing prevalence of the components of the metabolic syndrome. The prevalence of obesity is 31 per cent in the adult US population and is projected to be 45 per cent in 2025 (Mokdad *et al.* 2003). In Belgium, 15 per cent of the adult population is obese (Moreau *et al.* 2004). In Africa and Asia, the prevalence of overweight is <10 per cent (Kosti *et al.* 2006). The increase of the prevalence of overweight in children and adolescents is of particular concern. The prevalence of diabetes is also increasing, and is currently estimated at 5–6 per cent worldwide (Adeghate *et al.* 2006). In the United States, 22 per cent of the adult population fulfils the criteria of the metabolic syndrome (Lin *et al.* 2007).

The natural history of NAFLD/NASH

Data on the natural history of NAFLD and NASH have the same three problems as outlined for the prevalence data. In patients with NASH, 45 per cent will exhibit fibrosis progression and 19 per cent will ultimately develop cirrhosis (Fassio *et al.* 2004). In patients with NAFLD, lifetime progression to cirrhosis is estimated at 2–5 per cent (Dam-Larsen *et al.* 2004; Ekstedt *et al.* 2006).

It is not clear whether only NASH patients will progress, or if pure steatosis may also lead to progressive fibrosis and ultimately cirrhosis. A recent long-term follow-up study (mean follow-up of 13.7 years) showed no increase in mortality in patients with elevated liver enzymes and pure steatosis on an initial biopsy. Patients with biopsy-proven NASH, on the other hand, had a higher risk of dying from cardiovascular disease (15.5 per cent vs. 7.5 per cent, $p = 0.04$) and from liver-related causes (2.8 per cent vs. 0.2 per cent, $p = 0.04$). Disease progression was, however, noted: 41 per cent had fibrosis progression and 5.4 per cent of patients developed cirrhosis, and this did not depend on features of inflammation on the initial biopsy (Ekstedt *et al.* 2006).

In patients with cryptogenic cirrhosis, >60 per cent have features that might have been associated with NASH and in these patients cirrhosis is believed to be an end stage of NASH (Ekstedt *et al.* 2006). Actually cryptogenic cirrhosis accounts for 8 per cent of the indications for liver transplantation in Europe (European Liver Transplant Registry). NASH may recur after liver transplantation, further enforcing the concept of NASH as an aetiology of cryptogenic cirrhosis (Maheshwari *et al.* 2006).

HCC has been reported in patients with NASH-associated cirrhosis. Data on prevalence and risk, however, are scarce. In the Ekstedt series (Ekstedt *et al.* 2006), 2.3 per cent developed HCC or 43 per cent of those with documented cirrhosis. It is thus not clear whether the risk is comparable to the 10 per cent cumulative risk usually reported in cirrhosis of any aetiology, but it might be higher (Smedile *et al.* 2005). HCC has not been reported without cirrhosis or extensive fibrosis.

Risk factors reported to be associated with an increased risk of fibrosis are: Age (>40 or >50 years of age), the presence of diabetes, BMI > 25 or > 28 or > 30, hypertriglyceridaemia, elevated transaminases >2 times the upper limit of normal, and AST/ALT >1 (Angulo *et al.* 1999; Adams *et al.* 2005). As already mentioned, patients with NAFLD and diabetes have a higher probability of cirrhosis and liver-related death, compared to NAFLD patients without diabetes (Abrams *et al.* 2004). In the Ekstedt series (Ekstedt *et al.* 2006), the 41 per cent progression of fibrosis was associated with higher levels of ALT, a higher weight gain during follow-up, more severe insulin resistance and more pronounced fatty infiltration. As stated previously, patients with NASH more frequently meet the criteria of the metabolic syndrome and are more likely to have visceral obesity compared to patients with simple steatosis. As it is believed that NASH is a subgroup of NAFLD at risk for progressive fibrosis, the metabolic syndrome and its components clearly constitute a risk factor for fibrosis and cirrhosis, which will be a major burden of disease in view of the epidemic of obesity and diabetes and their related conditions.

HCC may also be the ultimate result of NAFLD-related cirrhosis, as stated earlier. A significant proportion of HCC (7–30 per cent) develops in patients with cryptogenic cirrhosis, suggesting that the risk of developing a HCC is higher than from other aetiologies of cirrhosis. Diabetes also seems to be a major risk factor for developing HCC (Bugianesi 2005).

Overall conclusion

In spite of the availability of safe and effective vaccines and their proven effectiveness in reducing the chronic consequences of HBV infections, the current burden of disease associated with hepatitis B remains substantial. To finally achieve the WHO goal of HBV elimination, continuous efforts will be required to keep prevention of hepatitis B on the agenda of public health officers worldwide, and to continue to improve treatment options for those already suffering chronic hepatitis B.

Even if the present burden of disease caused by hepatitis C is somewhat less impressive, the lack of an effective vaccine despite major efforts in its development, and the limited success of treatment pose a substantial future threat to public health.

Alcoholic liver disease remains a major cause of morbidity and mortality worldwide. There is concern that, worldwide, alcoholic liver disease may increase in the next several decades. Recent data indicate that alcohol consumption is increasing in low- and middle-income countries. In addition, rates of excessive alcohol intake appear to be rising in women. Although alcohol-related cirrhosis mortality rates decreased in many countries during the past 30 years, rates are no longer declining in several countries and are actually increasing in low- and middle-income countries.

Although data on the prevalence and natural history of NAFLD/NASH are scarce and suffer from multiple methodological problems, it is clear that, because of its association with the metabolic syndrome and its components, which tend to take epidemic proportions in the Western population, NAFLD and NASH will constitute a major health problem in the near future.

Key points

- Liver cirrhosis and primary liver cancer are important public health problems worldwide.
- Viral hepatitis B and C, and alcoholic as well as non-alcoholic fatty liver disease, represent the major causes for these chronic liver diseases.
- Despite the availability and widespread use of effective hepatitis B vaccines, efforts will be required to keep the immunization programmes on the political and donor agenda.
- As the development of a hepatitis C vaccine has not yet resulted in success, prevention and control measures will form a major challenge to all those involved in public health.
- In low- and middle-income countries experts predict a future wave of alcohol-related liver diseases.
- Fatty liver disease and steatohepatitis, chronic liver diseases associated with the metabolic syndrome, tend to take epidemic proportions in the near future in Western populations.

References

Abrams G.A., Kunde S.S., Lazenby A.J. *et al.* (2004). Portal fibrosis and hepatic steatosis in morbidly obese subjects: a spectrum of non-alcoholic fatty liver disease. *Hepatology*, **40**, 475–83.

Adams L.A., Lymp J.F., St Sauver J. *et al.* (2005). The natural history of nonalcoholic fatty liver disease: a population-based cohort study. *Gastroenterology*, **129**, 113–21.

Adeghate E., Schatter P., and Dunn E. (2006). An update on the etiology and epidemiology of diabetes mellitus. *Ann N Y Acad Sci*, **1084**, 1–29.

Alexander J.F., Lischner M.W., Galambos J.T. (1971). Natural history of alcoholic hepatitis. II. The long-term prognosis. *The American Journal of Gastroenterology*, **56**, 515–25.

Alter M.J. (2007). Epidemiology of hepatitis C virus infection. *World Journal of Gastroenterology*, **13**, 2436–41.

André F.E. and Zuckerman A.J. (1994). Review: protective efficacy of hepatitis B vaccines in neonates. *J Med Virol*, **44**, 144–51.

Angulo P., Keach J.C., Batts K.P. *et al.* (1999). Independent predictors of liver fibrosis in patients with steatohepatitis. *Hepatology*, **30**, 1356–62.

Angulo P. (2002). Nonalcoholic fatty liver disease. *N Engl J Med*, **346**, 1221–31.

Banatvala J.E., Van Damme P. (2003). Hepatitis B vaccine—do we need boosters? *J Hepatol* **10**, 1–6.

Barrio E., Tome S., Rodriguez I. *et al.* (2005). Liver disease in heavy drinkers with and without alcohol withdrawal syndrome. *Alcoholism, Clinical and Experimental Research*, **28**, 131–6.

Becker U., Gronbaek M., Johansen D. *et al.* (2002). Lower risk for alcohol-induced cirrhosis in wine drinkers. *Hepatology*, **35**, 868–75.

Bellentani S., Saccoccio G., Masutti F. *et al.* (2000). Prevalence of and risk factors for hepatic steatosis in northern Italy. *Ann Intern Med*, **132**, 112–17.

Bruix J. and Sherman M. (2005). AASLD Practice Guideline. Management of hepatocellular carcinoma. *Hepatology*, **42**, 1208–36.

Bugianesi E. (2005). Review article: steatosis, the metabolic syndrome and cancer. *Aliment Pharmacol Ther*, **22**(Suppl 2): 40–3.

Campollo O., Martinez M.D., Valencia J.J. *et al.* (2001). Drinking patterns and beverage preferences of liver cirrhosis patients in Mexico. *Substance Use & Misuse*, **36**, 387–98.

Centers for Disease Control and Prevention (1987). Recommendations of the Immunization Practices Advisory Committee. Update on hepatitis B prevention. *Morbid Mortal Wkly Rep*, **36**, 353–60.

Chan C.Y., Lee S.D., Lo K.J. (2004). Legend of hepatitis B vaccination: the Taiwanese experience. *J Gastroenterol Hepatol*, **19**, 121–6.

Chang M.H., Chen C.J., Lai M.S., *et al.* (1997). Universal hepatitis B vaccination in Taiwan and the incidence of hepatocellular carcinoma in children. Taiwan Childhood Hepatoma Study Group. *N Engl J Med*, **336**, 1855–9.

Chen C.J., Yang H.I., Su J. *et al.* (2006). Risk of HCC across a biological gradient of serum HBV-DNA levels. *JAMA*, **295**, 65–73.

Chevalier S. and Pawlotsky J.M. (2007). Hepatitis C virus: virology, diagnosis and management of antiviral therapy. *World J Gastroenterol*, **7**, 2461–6. Review.

Corrao G. and Arico S. (1998). Independent and combined action of hepatitis C virus infection and alcohol consumption on the risk of symptomatic liver cirrhosis. *Hepatology*, **27**, 914–9.

Corrao G., Ferrari P., Zambon A. *et al.* (1997). Are the recent trends in liver cirrhosis mortality affected by the changes in alcohol consumption? Analysis of the latency period in European countries. *Journal of Studies on Alcohol*, **57**, 486–94.

Coursaget P., Leboulleux D., Soumare M. *et al.* (1994). Twelve-year follow-up study of hepatitis B immunisation of Senegalese infants. *J Hepatol*, **21**, 250–4.

Crowley H., Lewis D., Gordon F. *et al.* (2000). Steatosis in donor and transplant liver biopsies. *Human Pathology*, **31**, 1209–13.

D'Allessandro A., Kalayoglu M., Sollinger H. *et al.* (1991). The predictive value of donor liver biopsies for the development of primary non-function after orthotopic liver transplantation. *Transplantation*, **51**, 157–63.

Dam-Larsen S., Franzmann M., Andersen I.B. *et al.* (2004). Long term prognosis of fatty liver: risk of chronic liver disease and death. *Gut*, **53**, 750–55.

Day C.P. (2000). Who gets alcoholic liver disease: nature or nurture? *Journal of the Royal College of Physicians of London*, **34**, 557–62.

de Marco R., Locatelli F., Zoppini G. *et al.* (1999). Cause-specific mortality in type 2 diabetes. The Verona Diabetes Study. *Diabetes Care*, **22**, 756–61.

Diehl A.M. (1997). Alcoholic liver disease: natural history. *Liver Transplantation and Surgery*, **3**, 206–11.

Dienstag J.L., Werner B.G., Polk B.F. *et al.* (1984). Hepatitis B vaccine in health care personnel: safety, immunogenicity, and indicators of efficacy. *Ann Intern Med*, **82**, 8168–72.

Duclos P. (2003). Safety of immunization and adverse events following vaccination against hepatitis B. *J Hepatol*, **39**, S83–S88.

Ekstedt M., Franzen L.E., Mathiesen U.L. *et al.* (2006). Long-term follow-up of patients with NAFLD and elevated liver enzymes. *Hepatology*, **44**, 865–73.

El Serag H.B. (2005). Epidemiology of hepatocellular carcinoma. *Clin Liver Dis*, **5**, 87–107.

Enomoto N., Yamashina S., Schemmer P. *et al.* (1999). Estriolsensitizes rat Kupffer cells via gut-derived endotoxin. *American Journal of Physiology*, **277**, G671–7.

European Consensus Group on Hepatitis B immunity (2000). Are booster immunisations needed for lifelong hepatitis B immunity? *Lancet*, **355**, 561–65.

European Liver Transplant Registry (2007). Available at: http://www.eltr.org/publi/IMG/gif/DIA8-2.gif Accessed 15 September 2007.

Everhart J.E. (2003). In vino veritas? *Journal of Hepatology*, **38**, 411–9.

Expert Panel on Detection, Evaluation and Treatment of High Blood Cholesterol in Adults (2001). Executive Summary of The Third Report of The National Cholesterol Education Program (NCEP) Expert Panel on Detection, Evaluation and Treatment of High Blood Cholesterol in Adults (Adult Treatment Panel III). *JAMA*, **285**, 2486–97.

Fletcher L.M., Dixon J.L., Purdie D.M. *et al.* (2002). Excess alcohol greatly increases the prevalence of cirrhosis in hereditary hemochromatosis. *Gastroenterology*, **122**, 281–9.

Forns X. and Bukh J. (1999). The molecular biology of hepatitis C virus. Genotypes and quasispecies. *Clin Liver Dis*, **3**, 693–716.

Frank C., Mohamed M.K., Strickland G.T. *et al.* (2000). The role of parenteral antischistosomal therapy in the spread of hepatitis C virus in Egypt. *Lancet*, **355**, 887–91.

Ganne-Carrie N., Ziol M., de Ledighen V. *et al.* (2006). Accuracy of liver stiffness measurements for the diagnosis of cirrhosis in patients with chronic liver diseases. *Hepatology*, **44**, 1511–17.

Gerberding J.L. and Henderson D.K. (1992). Management of occupational exposures to bloodborne pathogens: hepatitis B virus, hepatitis C virus, and human immunodeficiency virus. *Clin Infect Dis*, **14**, 1179–85.

Goldstein S.T., Zhou F., Hadler S.C. *et al.* (2005). A mathematical model to estimate global hepatitis B disease burden and vaccination impact. *Int J Epidemiol*, **34**, 1329-39. Available at: http://aim.path.org/en/vaccines/hepb/assessBurden/model/index.html Accessed on 18 December 2007.

Hadler S.C. and Margolis H.S. (1992). Hepatitis B immunization: vaccine types, efficacy, and indications for immunization. In: Remington J.S., Swartz M.N., eds. Current Topics In Infectious Diseases (vol. 12), pp. 282–308. Boston, Blackwell Scientific Publications.

Halliday M.L., Coates R.A. and Rankin J.G. (1991). Changing trends of cirrhosis mortality in Ontario, Canada, 1911–1986. *International Journal of Epidemiology*, **20**, 199–208.

Harrison S.A. and Neuschwander-Tetri B.A. (2004). Nonalcoholic fatty liver disease and non-alcoholic steatohepatitis. *Clinics in Liver Disease*, **8**, 861–79.

Harwood H. (2000). Updating estimates of the economic costs of alcohol abuse in the United States: estimates, update, methods and data. *National Institute on Alcohol Abuse and Alcoholism, Bethesda, MD.*

Hasumura Y. and Takeuchi J. (1991). Alcoholic liver disease in Japanese patients: a comparison with Caucasians. *Journal of Gastroenterology and Hepatology*, **6**, 520–7.

Hilden M., Christoffersen P., Juhl E. *et al.* (1997). Liver histology in a "normal" population-examination of 503 consecutive fatal traffic casualties. *Scand J Gastroenterol*, **12**, 593–98.

Hollinger F.B. (1989). Factors influencing the immune response to hepatitis B vaccine, booster dose guidelines and vaccine protocol recommendations. *Am J Med*, **87**(suppl3A), 36–40.

Hoofnagle J.H., Doo E., Liang T.J. *et al.* (2007). Management of hepatitis B: summary of a clinical research workshop. *Hepatology*, **45**, 1056–75. Review.

Ioannou G.N., Weiss N.S., Kowdley K.V. *et al.* (2003). Is obesity a risk factor for cirrhosis-related death or hospitalization? A population-based cohort study. *Gastroenterology*, **125**, 1053–59.

Jilg W., Schmidt M., Zachoval R. *et al.* (1984). Hepatitis B vaccination: how long does protection last? *Lancet*, **2**, 458.

Jilg W., Schmidt M. and Deinhardt F. (1988). Persistence of specific antibodies after hepatitis B vaccination. *J Hepatol*, **6**, 201–7.

Kato N., Ootsuyama Y., Nakazawa T. *et al.* (1994). Genetic drift in hypervariable region I of the viral genome in persistent hepatitis C virus infection. *J Virol*, **68**, 4776–84.

Kao J-H and Chen D.S. (2005). Hepatitis B vaccination: to boost or not to boost? *Lancet*, **366**, 1337–38.

Keating G.M. and Noble S. (2003). Recombinant hepatitis B vaccine (Engerix-B): a review of its immunogenicity and protective efficacy against hepatitis B. *Drugs*, **2003**, 63:1021–51.

Kerr W.C., Fillmore K.M. and Marvy P. (2000). Beverage-specific alcohol consumption and cirrhosis mortality in a group of English-speaking beer-drinking countries. *Addiction*, **95**, 339–46.

Kosti R.I. and Panagiotakos D.B. (2006). The epidemic of obesity in children and adolescents in the world. *Cent Eur J Public Health*, **14**, 151–9.

Kunde S.S., Lazenby A.J., Clements R.H. *et al.* (2005). Spectrum of NAFLD and diagnostic implications of the proposed new normal range for serum ALT in obese women. *Hepatology*, **42**, 650–6.

Lauer G.M. and Walker B.D. (2001). Hepatitis C virus infection. *N Engl J Med*, **345**, 41–52.

Lavanchy D. (2004). Hepatitis B virus epidemiology, disease burden, treatment, and current and emerging prevention and control measures. *J Viral Hep*, **11**, 97–107.

Lavanchy D. (2005). Worldwide epidemiology of HBV infection, disease burden, and vaccine prevention. *J Clin Virol*, **34** (**Suppl 1**), S1–3.

Lee W.M. (1997). Hepatitis B virus infection. *N Engl J Med*, **337**, 1733–45.

Lin S.X. and Pi-Sunyer E.X. (2007). Prevalence of the metabolic syndrome among US middle-aged and older adults with and without diabetes: a preliminary analysis of the NHANES 1999-2002 data. *Ethn Dis*, **17**, 35–9.

Lok A.S. and McMahon J. (2007) Chronic hepatitis B: AASLD Practice Guidelines. *Hepatology*, **45**, 507–39.

Lu X.L., Luo J.Y., Tao M. *et al.* (2004). Risk factors for alcoholic liver disease in China. *World Journal of Gastroenterology*, **10**, 2423–6.

Maheshwari A. and Thuluvath P.J. (2006). Cryptogenic cirrhosis and NAFLD: are they related? *Am J Gastroenterol*, **101**, 664–8.

Marchesini G., Bugianesi E., Forlani G. *et al.* (2003). Nonalcoholic fatty liver, steatohepatitis, and the metabolic syndrome. *Hepatology*, **37**, 917–23.

Memon M.I. and Memon M.A. (2002). Hepatitis C: an epidemiological review. *J Viral Hepat*, **9**, 84–100.

Michielsen P.P. and Sprengers D. (2003). Who gets alcoholic liver disease: nature or nurture? (summary of the discussion). *Acta Gastroenterologica Belgica*, **66**, 292–3.

Michielsen P.P., Francque S.M. and van Dongen J.L. (2005). Viral hepatitis and hepatocellular carcinoma. *World J Surg Oncol*, **20**, 3: 27.

Miele L., Forgione A., Gasbarrini G. *et al.* (2007). Noninvasive assessment of liver fibrosis in non-alcoholic fatty liver disease (NAFLD) and non-alcoholic steatohepatitis (NASH). *Transl Res*, **149**, 114–25.

Mokdad A.H., Ford E.S., Bowman B.A. *et al.* (2003). Prevalence of obesity, diabetes and obesity-related health risk factors. *JAMA*, **289**, 76–9.

Moreau M., Valente F., Mak R. *et al.* (2004). Obesity, body fat distribution and incidence of sick leave in the Belgian workforce: the Belstress study. *Int J Obes Relat Metab Disord*, **28**, 574–82.

Naveau S., Giraud V., Borotto E. *et al.* (1997). Excess weight risk factor for alcoholic liver disease. *Hepatology*, **25**, 108–11.

Neuschwander-Tetri B.A. and Caldwell S.H. (2003). Nonalcoholic fatty liver disease: summary of an AASLD Single Topic Conference. *Hepatology*, **37**, 1202–19.

Ng K.P., Saw T.L., Baki A. *et al.* (2005). Impact of expanded programme on immunization against hepatitis B infection in school children in Malaysia. *Med Microbiol Immunol*, **194**, 163–8.

Niu M.T. (1996). Review of 12 million doses shows hepatitis B vaccine safe. *Vaccine Weekly*, **4**, 13–5.

Park S.C., Oh S.I. and Lee M.S. (1998). Korean status of alcoholics and alcohol-related health problems. *Alcoholism, Clinical and Experimental Research*, **22**, 170S–172S.

Pearson H. (2004). Public health: The demon drink. *Nature*, **428**, 598–600.

Pelletier S., Vaucher E., Aider R. *et al.* (2002). Wine consumption is not associated with a decreased risk of alcoholic cirrhosis in heavy drinkers. *Alcohol and Alcoholism*, **37**, 618–22.

Perz J.F., Armstrong G.L., Farrington L.A. *et al.* (2006a). The contributions of hepatitis B virus and hepatitis C virus infections to cirrhosis and primary liver cancer worldwide. *J of Hepatol*, **45**, 529–38.

Perz J.F., Elm JL J.R., Fiore A.E. *et al.* (2006b). Near elimination of hepatitis B infections among Hawaii elementary school children universal infant hepatitis B vaccination. *Pediatrics*, **118**, 1403–8.

Pincock S. (2003). Binge drinking on the rise in UK and elsewhere. Government report shows increases in alcohol consumption, cirrhosis, and premature deaths. *Lancet*, **362**, 1126–7.

Prati D., Taioli E., Zanella A. *et al.* (2002). Updated definitions of healthy ranges for serum alanine aminotransferase levels. *Ann Intern Med*, **137**, 1–10.

Prati D. (2006). Transmission of hepatitis C virus by blood transfusions and other medical procedures: a global review. *J Hepatol*, **45**, 607–16.

Ramstedt M. (2001). Per capita alcohol consumption and liver cirrhosis mortality in 14 European countries. *Addiction*, **96** (Suppl 1), S19–33.

Raza S.A., Clifford G.M., Franceschi S. (2007). Worldwide variation in the relative importance of hepatitis B and hepatitis C viruses in hepatocellular carcinoma: a systematic review. *British Journal of Cancer*, **96**, 1127–34.

Rehm J., Rehn N., Room R. *et al.* (2003). The global distribution of average volume of alcohol consumption and patterns of drinking. *European Addiction Research*, **9**, 147–56.

Rendi-Wagner P., Shouval D., Genton B. *et al.* (2006). Comparative immunogenicity of a PreS/S hepatitis B vaccine in non- and low responders to conventional vaccine. *Vaccine*, **24**,2781–2789.

Rinella M., Alonso E., Rao S. *et al.* (2001). Body mass index as a predictor of hepatic steatosis in living liver donors. *Liver Transplant*, **7**, 409–13.

Roizen R., Kerr W.C., Fillmore K.M. (1999). Cirrhosis mortality and per capita consumption of distilled spirits, United States, 1949-1994: trend analysis. *The Western Journal of Medicine*, **171**, 83–7.

Romano L., Mele A., Pariani E. *et al.* (2004). Update in the universal vaccination against hepatitis B in Italy: 12 years after its implementation. *Eur J Public Health*, **14(Suppl)**, S19.

Room R., Babor T. and Rehm J. (2005). Alcohol and public health. *Lancet*, **365**, 519–30.

Rosenberg W.M.C., Voelker M., Thiel R. *et al.* on behalf of the European Liver Fibrosis Group (2004). Serum markers detect the presence of liver fibrosis: a cohort study. *Gastroenterology*, **127**, 1704–13.

Safary A. and André F. (1999). Over a decade of experience with the yeast recombinant hepatitis B vaccine. *Vaccine*, **18**, 57.

Saunders J.B. and Latt N. (1993). Epidemiology of alcoholic liver disease. *Ballières Clinics in Gastroenterology*, **7**, 555–79.

Sheiner P., Emre S., Cubukcu O. *et al.* (1995). Use of donor livers with moderate-to-severe macrovesicular fat. *Hepatology*, **22**, 205A.

Sherlock S. (1993). Clinical features of hepatitis. In Zuckerman A.J., Thomas H.S., eds. *Viral Hepatitis*, pp. 1–11. Churchill Livingstone, London.

Shouval D., Ilan Y., Adler R. *et al. (1994)*. Improved immunogenicity in mice of a mammalian cell-derived recombinant hepatitis B vaccine containing pre-S_1 and pre-S_2 antigens as compared with conventional yeast-derived vaccines. *Vaccine*, **12**, 1453–1459.

Smedile A. and Bugianesi E. (2005). Steatosis and hepatocellular carcinoma risk. *Eur Rev Med Pharmacol Sci*, **9**, 291–293.

Sorensen T.I., Orholm M., Bentsen K.D. *et al.* (1984). Prospective evaluation of alcohol abuse and alcoholic liver injury in men as predictors of development of cirrhosis. *Lancet*, **2**, 241–44.

Stinson F.S., Grant B.F. and Dufour M.C. (2001). The critical dimensions of ethnicity in liver cirrhosis mortality statistics. Alcoholism, *Clinical and Experimental Research*, **25**, 1181–7.

Szmuness W., Stevens C.E., Zang E.A. *et al.* (1981). A controlled clinical trial of the efficacy of the hepatitis B vaccine (Hepatavax B): a final report. *Hepatology* **5**, 377–85.

Tan J. and Lok A. (2007). Update on viral hepatitis: 2006. *Gastroenterology*, **23**, 263–267.

Tandon B.N. and Tandon A. (1997). Epidemiological trends of viral hepatitis in Asia. In Rizzetto M., Purcell R.H., Gerin J.L., Verme G., eds. *Viral Hepatitis and Liver Disease*, pp. 559–561. Edizioni Minerva Medica, Turin.

Tolstrup J.S., Jensen M.K., Tjonneland A. *et al.* (2004). Drinking pattern and mortality in middle-aged men and women. *Addiction*, **99**, 323–30.

Urena M., Ruiz-Delgado F., Moreno Gonzalez E. *et al.* (1998). Hepatic steatosis in liver transplant donors: common feature of donor population? *World J Surg*, **22**, 837–44.

Venters C., Graham W. and Cassidy W. (2004). Recombivax-HB: perspectives past, present and future. *Expert Rev Vaccines*, **3**, 119–29.

Viviani S., Jack A., Hall A.J. *et al.* (1999). Hepatitis B vaccination in infancy in the Gambia: protection against carriage at 9 years of age. *Vaccine*, **17**, 2946–50.

Wainwright R., Bulkow L.R., Parkinson A.J. *et al.* (1997). Protection provided by hepatitis B vaccine in a Yupik Eskimo Population: results of a 10 year study. *J Infect Dis*, **175**, 674–7.

West D.J. and Calandra G.B. (1996). Vaccine induced immunologic memory for hepatitis B surface antigen: implications for policy on booster vaccination. *Vaccine*, **14**, 1019–27.

Whittle H.C., Maine N., Pilkington J. *et al.* (1995). Long-term efficacy of continuing hepatitis B vaccination in infancy in two Gambian villages. *Lancet*, **345**, 1089–92.

World Health Onganization (2001). Expanded Programme on Immunization. Introduction of hepatitis B vaccination into childhood immunization services: management guidelines, including information for health workers and parents (WHO/V&B/01.31). Geneva, World Health Organization, 2001. Available at http://www.who.int/vaccines-documents/DocsPDF01/www613.pdf (accessed 12 December 2006).

World Health Organization (2004a). Hepatitis B vaccines (WHO position paper). *Weekly Epidemiol Rec*, **79**, 255–63.

World Health Organization (2004b). Global Status Report on Alcohol 2004. Available at http://www.who.int/topics/alcohol_drinking Accessed 20 December 2007

World Health Organization (2006). Vaccines and Biologicals. WHO vaccine preventable disease monitoring system. Global summary 2006 (data up to 2005). Available at http://www.who.int/vaccines-documents/GlobalSummary.pdf Accessed on 15 September 2007.

Worman H.J. (1999). Acute versus chronic disease. In: The Liver Disorders Sourcebook, pp. 12–15. Lowell House, Chicago, Illinois.

Zanetti A.R., Mariano A., Romanò L. *et al.* (2005). Long-term immunogenicity of hepatitis B vaccination and policy for booster: an Italian multicentre study. *Lancet* **366**, 1379–84.

9.17

Emerging and re-emerging infections

David L. Heymann

Introduction

The microbial world is complex, dynamic and constantly evolving. Infectious agents reproduce rapidly, mutate frequently, cross the species barrier between animal hosts and humans, and adapt with relative ease to their new environments. Because of these traits, infectious agents are able to alter their epidemiology, their virulence, and their susceptibility to anti-infective drugs.

When disease is caused by a microbe that is newly identified and not known previously to infect humans, it is commonly called an emerging infectious disease, or simply an emerging infection. When disease is caused by an infectious agent previously known to infect humans that has re-entered human populations or changed in epidemiology or susceptibility to anti-infective drugs, it is called a re-emerging infection. A report published by the United States Institute of Medicine in 1992 first called attention to emerging and re-emerging infectious diseases as evidence that the fight against infectious diseases was far from won, despite great advances in the development of antimicrobials and vaccines (Lederberg *et al.* 1992).

All forms of infectious agents—bacteria, viruses, parasites, and prions—are able to emerge or re-emerge in human populations, and it is estimated that 70 per cent or more of all emerging infections have a source in animals. When a new infectious agent enters human populations there are several potential outcomes. In some instances, infected humans become ill, while in others, infections are asymptomatic. Once humans are infected, human-to-human transmission may or may not occur. If it occurs, it may be limited to one, two, or more generations, or it may be sustained indefinitely. Among those infectious agents that cause disease, some maintain their virulence, while others attenuate over time. Changes in the epidemiological characteristics of infectious agents may occur gradually, or they may occur abruptly as the result of a sudden genetic change during reproduction and/or replication.

Epidemiology of emerging and re-emerging infections

Rabies and variant Creutzfeldt–Jakob disease are clear examples of human infections that cause illness but cannot transmit from human to human unless there is an iatrogenic cause of transmission through non-sterile medical procedures, blood transfusion, or organ transplant. In several instances, corneal transplantation from a person who died undiagnosed with rabies-infection has caused rabies in transplant recipients. The recent identification of several humans with vCJD associated with blood transfusion demonstrates its potential to spread iatrogenically within the human population.

Human monkeypox provides a clear example of an infectious agent that can infect humans but not sustain transmissibility. Thought to have a rodent reservoir in the sub-Saharan rain forest, the monkeypox virus infects humans who come in contact with an infected animal. Transmission is sustained through one or two generations and then ceases. In the first generation of cases, the case fatality rate can approach 10 per cent, but with passage through human populations the virulence and case fatality of human monkeypox decreases as its transmissibility declines.

The human immunodeficiency virus (HIV) is an example of an infectious agent that has been able to infect humans, maintain virulence and sustain transmission. A long incubation period for HIV has ensured sustained transmission resulting in endemnicity worldwide, causing an estimated 2 million deaths in 2007 alone. It is hypothesized that HIV entered human populations from a non-human primate sometime in the early twentieth century. It escaped detection in the late 1970s when human-to-human transmission was being amplified on the African continent, in island nations of the Caribbean, and in North America. By the time it was first identified in the early 1980s, it had spread widely throughout the world.

The short incubation period in persons infected with the Ebola virus, and the high case fatality rates are less compatible with long-term human-to-human transmission. Ebola endemnicity in humans has not developed, though frequent re-emergence and localized outbreaks with human-to-human transmission continue to be documented. The potential for attenuation of the Ebola virus with passage is unknown, though in its present form it is unlikely that it will be able to become endemic in human populations because of its short incubation period and rapid progression to death in the majority of those infected.

The RNA virus that causes seasonal influenza is highly unstable genetically and mutates frequently during replication, requiring annual antigenic modifications in seasonal influenza vaccines to ensure protection. Avian influenza viruses are likewise unstable and at times infect humans and cause sickness and death. Occasionally, avian influenza viruses cause human influenza pandemics. The trigger virus for the influenza pandemic of 1918 is thought to have been an avian influenza virus. One hypotheses of its origin is that over time it circulated among birds and possibly some mammals, and through adaptive mutation, the virus gradually assumed a form that could infect humans and easily transmit.

Two other influenza pandemics of the twentieth century, in 1957 and 1968, are thought to have been caused by more abrupt genetic reassortment during the intracellular replication process in an animal dually infected with a human and an avian influenza virus. Risk factors for emergence of influenza viruses in humans are thought to be highest in areas such as South China and Southeast Asia where there are large populations of aquatic birds (the hosts of many different types of avian influenza viruses) and where humans live in close proximity to animals that may be infected by these aquatic birds.

Currently, H5N1, an avian influenza virus that was first identified as the cause of human illness in 1997, continues to cause occasional severe infections in humans but remains a zoonotic human infection and does not transmit easily from human to human. Most scientists agree that this virus, like many other avian influenza viruses, has the potential to mutate and gain the epidemiological characteristics that would permit it to spread easily from human to human and cause a pandemic.

Susceptibility of infectious agents to anti-infective drugs

Bacteria, viruses, and parasites can develop resistance to anti-infective drugs through spontaneous mutation and natural selection, or through the exchange of genetic material between strains and species. They then transmit from human to human, replacing more susceptible organisms with resistant strains. Soon after development of the first antibiotics, warning signs of microbial resilience began to appear. By the end of the 1940s, resistance of hospital strains of *Staphylococcus aureus* to penicillin emerged in the United Kingdom with resistance levels as high as 14 per cent, and by the end of the 1990s, levels had risen to of 95 per cent or greater (Fig. 9.17.1).

In addition to acquiring genes encoding resistance to all penicillins—including methicillin and other narrow-spectrum β-lactamase-resistant antibiotics—*S. aureus* has developed resistance to methicillin. Methicillin-resistant *S. aureus* (MRSA) first identified in the United Kingdom in 1961, is now widespread in hospitals throughout the world.

By 1976, chloroquine-resistant *Plasmodium falciparum* malaria was highly prevalent in Southeast Asia and 10 years later was found worldwide, as was high-level resistance to two second-line drugs, sulphadoxine-pyrimethamine and mefloquine. Today combination therapy with two antimalarial drugs with different targets is required to ensure effective treatment, as is surveillance to measure the continuing evolution of antimalarial drug resistance.

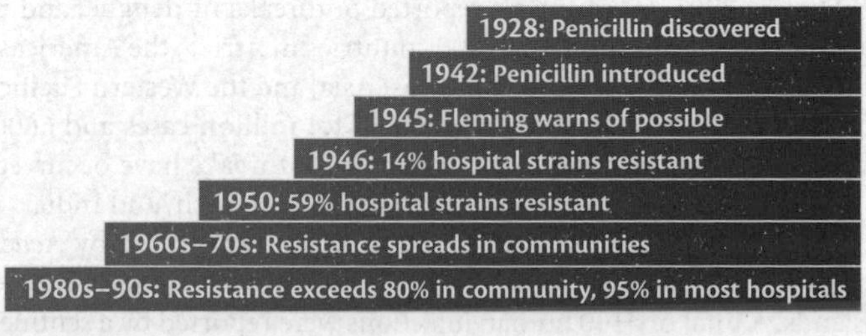

Fig. 9.17.1 Evolution of penicillin resistance in *Staphylococcus aureus*.

The bacterial and viral infections that contribute most to human disease are also those in which antimicrobial resistance is rapidly emerging: Diarrhoeal diseases such as dysentery; respiratory tract infections, including pneumococcal pneumonia and tuberculosis; sexually transmitted infections such as gonorrhoea and HIV; and infectious agents that have now accumulated resistance genes to virtually all currently available anti-infective drugs such as MRSA and extremely resistant tuberculosis (XDR-TB).

Geographic distribution of emerging and re-emerging infections

Emerging infections have the potential to occur in every country and on every continent (Fig. 9.17.2). Though the term emerging infections was newly introduced in the early 1990s, the previous 30 years had seen panoply of newly identified infections in humans on every continent. The year 1976 was especially illustrative of this phenomenon with the identification of the swine flu virus (H1N1), thought to be a direct descendant of the virus that caused the pandemic of 1918, at a military base in the Fort Dix (United States); the identification of *Legionella pneumophila* as the cause of an outbreak of severe respiratory illness among a group of veterans staying at a hotel in downtown Philadelphia (United States), initially feared to be a human outbreak of swine influenza (H1N1); and the identification of the Ebola virus as the cause of simultaneous outbreaks of haemorrhagic fever in Sudan and the Democratic Republic of Congo (then called Zaire).

Nine years earlier, in 1967, the Marburg virus had been identified in an outbreak in Germany that caused 25 primary infections and seven deaths among laboratory workers who were infected by handling monkeys from Uganda, and six secondary cases in health workers who took care of primary cases, with subsequent spread to family members. A member of the same filovirus family as Ebola, the Marburg virus has caused sporadic small outbreaks in Africa during the 1970s and 1980s, and larger outbreaks in 1998 in the Democratic Republic of Congo and 2005 in Angola. Since the Marburg virus was first identified in 1967 there have been over 40 other newly identified infectious agents in humans, an average of one per year.

Health workers and emerging/re-emerging infections

As clearly recorded during the Marburg outbreak of 1967, laboratory and health workers are at especially high risk of emerging and re-emerging infections. Outbreaks of Marburg, Ebola, and recently of severe acute respiratory syndrome (SARS), provide clear examples of the potential for health workers to become infected, and in some instances to sustain and amplify transmission in hospitals, and through their patients and family members, to the community. In the 1995 outbreak of Ebola haemorrhagic fever in Kikwit (Democratic Republic of Congo), almost one third of those infected were health workers, and in the 2003 SARS outbreak in Singapore, 10 health workers were thought to have been infected while treating an infected health worker colleague who is also thought to have infected her husband, three other patients and seven visitors to the hospital. Laboratory workers are also at risk of infection: The last human case of smallpox was caused by a laboratory accident in the United Kingdom, and the last-known human cases of SARS occurred in laboratory accidents in Singapore and China.

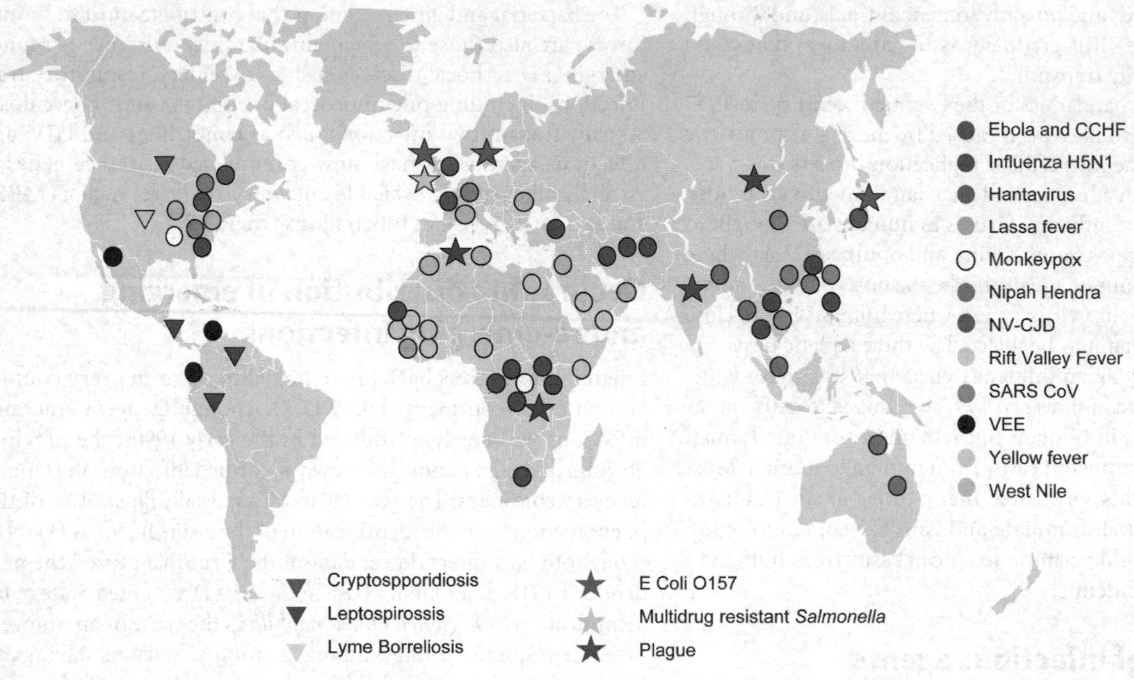

Fig. 9.17.2 Selected emerging and re-emerging infectious diseases: 1996–2004.

Economic impact of emerging and re-emerging infections

Outbreaks caused by emerging and re-emerging infections are costly (Fig. 9.17.3). They consume health-care resources and divert them from endemic disease problems, result in productivity loss, and decrease trade and tourism revenue. At times they economically devastate entire sectors. This has occurred after major outbreaks of emerging or re-emerging infections during the past 20 years, with economic losses ranging from an estimated US$39 million after the reemergence of cholera in Tanzania in 1998, to approximately US$39 billion after the emergence of bovine spongiform encephalopathy in the United Kingdom during the period 1990–1998.

SARS was likewise responsible for sizeable economic losses and insecurity in financial markets across Asia and worldwide. With fewer than 9000 cases, the outbreak was estimated by the Asian Development Bank to have cost Asian countries an estimated US$20 billion in gross domestic product (GDP) terms for 2003, and up to US$60 billion of gross expenditure and business losses.

The main drivers of the economic impact of outbreaks caused by emerging and re-emerging infections are travel, tourism, trade and consumer confidence. Fear of transmission causes international tourists to choose alternative holiday locations, and local population to avoid any perceived source of infection such as restaurants and other public leisure venues—sectors of the economy that are significant contributors to the GDP of many countries.

Factors influencing emergence and re-emergence

Many external factors provide opportunities for enhanced emergence or re-emergence of infectious diseases. They range from weakened public health infrastructure and failure of safety procedures/regulations to increases in population; anthropogenic activities or natural variances in climate; civil disturbance/human displacement; and human behaviour that varies from occupation and misperceptions about the use of anti-infective drugs to the safety of public health interventions and the desire to deliberately cause terror and harm.

Weakened public health infrastructure

Weakening of public health infrastructure resulted in part from decreased investment in public health during the second half of the twentieth century. *Aedes aegypti* has now become well established in many large cities worldwide following the deterioration of mosquito control campaigns during the 1970s. The resurgence of the *Aedes* species has been confounded by the adoption of modern consumer habits in urban areas where discarded household appliances, tyres, plastic food containers, and jars create abundant artificial mosquito breeding sites.

Along with the increase in *Aedes* species there has been an increased risk of outbreaks of dengue. Prior to 1970, nine countries, mainly in Latin America, reported outbreaks of dengue. Thirteen years later, during 1983, 13 countries in Latin America and Asia reported dengue outbreaks, and by 1998, 1.2 million cases were reported from 56 countries.

During 2001, 69 countries reported outbreaks of dengue, and it is now endemic in more than 100 countries in Africa, the Americas, the Eastern Mediterranean, Southeast Asia, and the Western Pacific. During 2003 there were approximately 1.4 million cases and 6600 deaths reported to WHO. Major dengue outbreaks have occurred in Brazil, Indonesia, Thailand, Viet Nam, Bangladesh, and India.

In 2005, the Chikungunya virus, likewise transmitted by *Aedes aegypti*, emerged and spread throughout several southern Pacific islands. A total of 3100 human infections were reported by a sentinel network on La Réunion within the first 6 months of the outbreak,

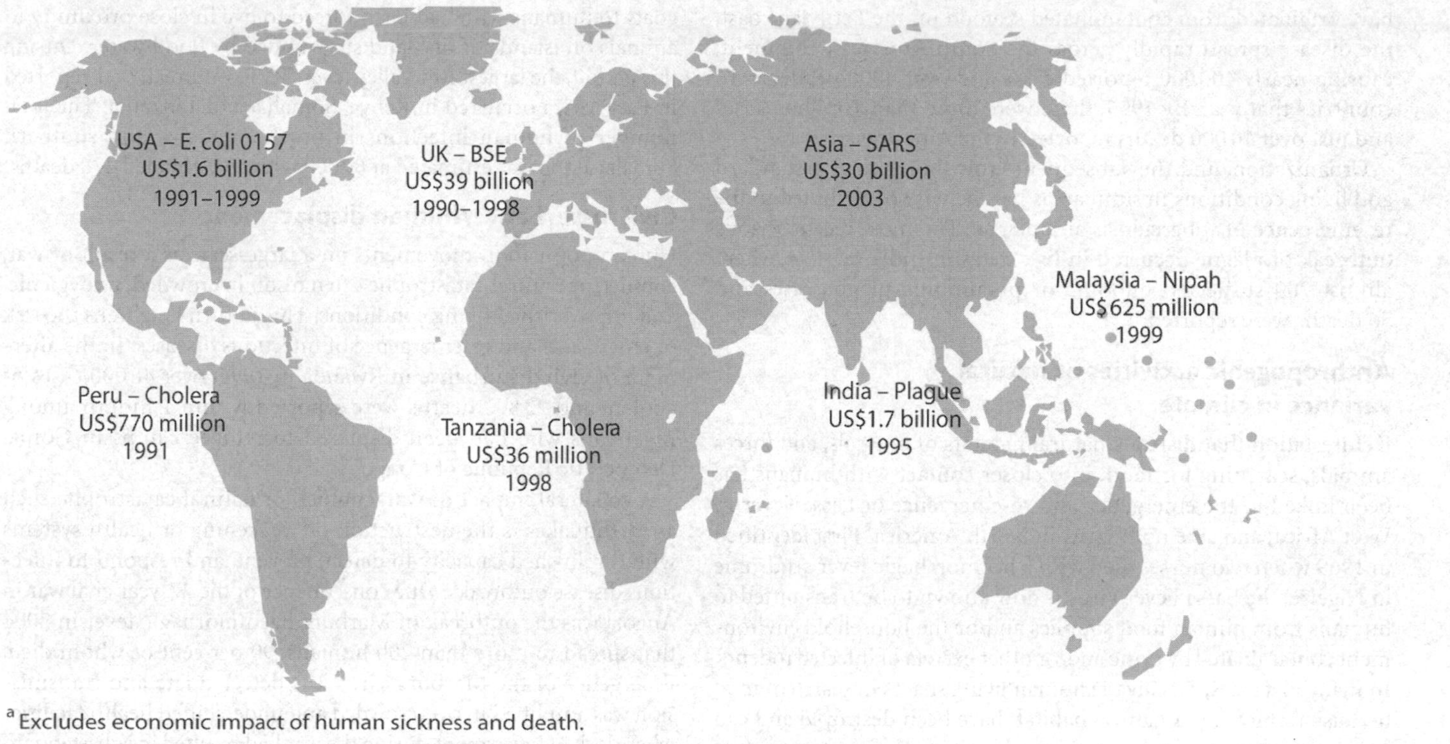

Fig. 9.17.3 Direct economic impact of selected infectious disease outbreaks, 1990–2003[a].

leading to an estimate of over 204 000 human infections by March 2006. In 2007, the Chikungunya virus spread north to Europe, where it caused an outbreak in northern Italy.

Lapses in childhood immunization coverage due to weakened childhood immunization programmes in Russia in the early 1990s resulted in the re-emergence of diphtheria, with major epidemics in the early 1990s. Reported cases of diphtheria in the Russian Federation increased from just over 1200 in 1990 to 3897 in 1992 to over 5000 in 1993. Likewise, lapses in yellow fever vaccination programmes in sub-Saharan Africa since the 1950s have left large susceptible populations in both rural and urban areas of sub-Saharan Africa, with sporadic urban outbreaks in cities in Côte d'Ivoire (2001), Senegal and Guinea (2002), and Burkina Faso (2004).

Most epidemiologists recognize that it was in part because of weak surveillance systems in developing countries that HIV rapidly spread during the late 1970s, and was not detected until it was first identified when it began to transmit in the United States.

Failure of safety procedures/regulations

Sub-standard universal precautions and hospital regulations during the 1980s led to breaches in sterile injection practices and nosocomial infections of HIV in the former USSR and Romania, together infecting over 250 children, accompanied by high levels of hepatitis B in both patients and health workers. Likewise sub-standard universal precautions led to nosocomial outbreaks of Ebola haemorrhagic Fever in the Democratic republic of Congo in 1976 and 1995, where syringes and/or failed barrier nursing amplified the transmission to patients, health workers, and the community. Lapses in universal precautions led to nosocomial transmission of SARS in hospitals in China and Hong Kong, Singapore, Vietnam, and Canada, where outbreaks then spread from hospitals to communities.

Changes in the process of rendering the carcasses of ruminant animals for the preparation of bone meal fed to other ruminant animals are thought to have been the cause of the outbreak of borine spongiform encephalopathy (BSE) in cattle that also led, in May 1995, to the death of a 19-year male in the United Kingdom, the first human death from what is now known to be variant Creutzfeldt–Jakob Disease (vCJD) or human Bovine Spongiform Encephalopathy (hBSE). The BSE and hBSE outbreaks demonstrate the health consequences of regulations for rendering that had changed over a 10-year period prior to 1995, inadvertently permitting rendered parts of cattle infected with the BSE-causing prion to contaminate bone meal made from rendered carcasses and used for livestock feed. The most likely source of human infection is thought to be through the consumption of contaminated meat. The BSE outbreak led to the recognition of the need for stronger government intervention along the entire 'feed to food' continuum to ensure the safety of foodstuffs for human consumption.

Population increase

The world's population more than doubled in the second half of the twentieth century, accelerating most rapidly in the developing countries of the tropics and sub-tropics. Rural–urban migration has resulted in inadequacy of water and sanitation systems, crowded living conditions and other basic infrastructure associated with population growth. In 1950, there were two urban areas in the world with populations greater than 7 million; by 1990, this number had risen to 23, and by 2005 to 30.

Population increases in Latin America resulted in breakdowns in sanitation and water systems in large coastal cities. In 1991, when cholera re-emerged in Peru after having been quiescent for approximately 100 years, it rapidly spread throughout Latin America. Thought to have originated from contaminated seafood on the Peruvian coast, the disease spread rapidly across the South American continent, causing nearly 400 000 reported cases and over 4000 deaths in 16 countries that year. By 1995, there were more than 1 million cases and just over 10 000 deaths reported in the Americas.

Urbanization, and the subsequent crowding with sub-standard and living conditions in slum areas has likewise contributed to the re-emergence of tuberculosis and plague. The most recent serious outbreak of plague occurred in five states in India in 1994, where almost 700 suspected bubonic or pneumonic plague cases and 56 deaths were reported.

Anthropogenic activities or natural variance in climate

Deforestation that disrupts natural habitats of animals, and forces animals, searching for food, into closer contact with humans has been linked to the emergence and re-emergence of Lassa Fever in West Africa, and sine nom virus in North America. First identified in 1969 when two nurses died with a haemorrhagic fever syndrome in Nigeria, the Lassa Fever virus is now known to be transmitted to humans from human food supplies and/or the household environment contaminated by urine and/or other excreta of infected rodents. In many instances, rats invade human living spaces in search of food because rainforests, a natural habitat, have been destroyed and can no longer support their needs. Sin nombre virus is a hantavirus, first identified in an outbreak in the southwestern part of the United States in 1993. It is now known to spread from infected rodents to humans through aerosolized excreta found in dust of homes that have been invaded by rodents as they scavenge for food.

In Latin America, Chagas disease re-emerged as an important human disease after mismanagement of deforested land caused triatomine populations to move from their wild natural hosts to involve humans and domestic animals in the transmission cycle, eventually transforming the disease into an urban infection that can be transmitted by blood transfusion. Other emerging infections influenced by changing habitats of animals include Lyme borreliosis in Europe and North America, transmitted to humans who come into contact with ticks that normally feed on rodents and deer, the reservoir of *Borrelia burgdorfi* in nature.

The narrow band of desert in sub-Saharan Arica, in which epidemic *Neisseria meningitides* infections traditionally occur, has enlarged as drought spread south so that Uganda and Tanzania experience epidemic meningitis. Climate extremes, whether involving excessive rainfall or drought, can likewise displace animal species and bring them into closer contact with human settlements, or increase vector breeding sites. A 1998 outbreak of Japanese encephalitis in Papua New Guinea has been linked to extensive drought, which led to increased breeding sites for the *culex* mosquito as rivers dried into stagnant pools. Mosquitoes then transmitted the Japanese encephalitis virus from infected pigs and or wild birds to humans. The Japanese encephalitis virus is now widespread in Southern Asia from India and Thailand to Malaysia, and as far north as Korea and Japan.

Above-normal rainfall associated with the occurrence of the warm phase of the El Niño Southern Oscillation phenomenon is thought to have caused extensive flooding in East Africa from December 1997 to March 1998, increasing the number of pooled-water breeding sites of *aedes* mosquitoes. Mosquitoes then facilitated the transfer of the Rift Valley Fever virus from infected cattle, sheep, and/or goats to humans who had been forced to live in close proximity to animals on islands of dry land surrounded by flood water. During this period, the largest Rift Valley fever (RVF) outbreak ever reported in East Africa occurred in Kenya, Somalia, and Tanzania. The total number of human infections in northern Kenya and southern Somalia alone was estimated at 89 000 with an estimated 478 deaths.

Civil disturbance/human displacement

Human population movements on a large-scale as a result of war, conflict, or natural catastrophe often result in crowded, unhygienic, and impoverished living conditions. This in turn heightens the risk of emergence and re-emergence of infectious diseases. In the aftermath of civil disturbance in Rwanda in 1994, over 48 000 cases of cholera and 23 800 deaths were reported within 1 month among Rwandans who had been displaced to refugee camps in Goma, Democratic Republic of Congo.

A collateral impact of war, conflict, or natural catastrophe such as earthquakes is the destruction or weakening of health systems with diminished capacity to detect, prevent, and respond to infectious disease outbreaks. One consequence of the 27-year civil war in Angola was the outbreak of Marburg haemmorhagic fever in 2004 that spread to more than 200 humans, 90 per cent of whom died. Emergence of the Marburg virus was detected late and transmission was amplified in overcrowded and understaffed health facilities where lack of investment during the war had resulted in sub-standard infection control.

Another large outbreak of Marburg virus infection was identified in late 1998 in the Democratic Republic of Congo, also a conflict-ravaged country. This emergence resulted in sporadic cases with small chains of transmission over a 2-year period in a remote area where civil war had interrupted supply lines and communication to health facilities in the region.

Human behaviour

Occupation

Throughout history, human occupations have been associated with infectious diseases. Anthrax, for example, has been called wool-sorters disease because of transmission of anthrax spores from infected animals to humans who sheer sheep and other wool-producing animals. It has also been associated with butchers who come into contact with infected animals at the time of slaughter or during preparation of meat for markets. Anthrax spores infect humans either intra-dermally, causing cutaneous anthrax, or by inhalation, causing pulmonary or inhalation anthrax.

Though intensive research has failed to confirm the origins of Ebola fever outbreaks, infection is thought to occur as humans encounter animal sources, possibly infected bats and/or non human primates, somewhere in the transmission cycle. An outbreak of Ebola haemorrhagic fever in humans in 1995 was linked to a woodsman, who worked deep within the tropical rainforest making charcoal, and who is somehow thought to have become infected with the Ebola virus that he then carried back to his home village and family members. A Swiss researcher infected with the Ebola virus while searching for the cause of a major die-out of chimpanzees in a forest reserve in West Africa is thought to have become infected while conducting chimpanzee autopsies in search of the cause of death.

In 2003, a veterinarian in the Netherlands became infected with the influenza A (H7N7) virus during an investigation of influenza outbreaks in poultry and later died in acute respiratory failure. A total of 89 humans, including the veterinarian, were confirmed to have H7N7 influenza virus infection associated with this poultry outbreak and no further deaths occurred. The majority of human infections are thought to have occurred as a result of direct contact with infected poultry; but there were three possible instances of transmission of infection from poultry workers to family members.

Mistrust and misinformation

During 2003, unsubstantiated rumours circulated in northern Nigeria that the oral polio vaccine (OPV) was unsafe and could cause infertility by vaccination of young children. Mistrust and misinformation that followed led to the government-ordered suspension of polio immunization in two northern states and substantial reductions in polio immunization coverage in those states, and a large number of others. The result was a polio outbreak across northern Nigeria that then spread to previously polio-free areas in sub-Saharan Africa. Over 70 per cent of all children worldwide who were paralyzed by polio during the following year, 2004, were living in Nigeria—or in other parts of sub-Saharan Africa that had been re-infected by polio virus genetically linked to viruses that had a Nigerian origin.

Misinformation about the safety of vaccines against pertussis, measles, and hepatitis B has likewise led to decreases in vaccine uptake among children, and in some instances industrialized country outbreaks of pertussis and measles.

Anti-infective drug prescription and use

Behaviours such as over- or under-prescribing of antibiotics by health workers, and excessive demand for antibiotics by the general population, have had a remarkable impact on the selection and survival of resistant microbes, rapidly increasing levels of microbial resistance.

The selection and spread of resistant infectious agents is paradoxically facilitated by either over or under-prescribing of drugs, and/or poor compliance to their use and unregulated sale that makes them available to any who have the ability to purchase them. In Thailand, among 307 hospitalized patients in the late 1990s, 36 per cent who were treated with anti-infective drugs did not have an infectious disease. Over-prescribing of anti-infective drugs occurs in most other countries as well. In Canada, it has been estimated of the more than 26 million people treated with anti-infective drugs, up to 50 per cent were treated inappropriately. Findings from community surveys of *Escherichia coli* in the stool samples of healthy children in China, Venezuela, and the United States suggest that although multi-resistant strains were present in each country, they were more widespread in Venezuela and China, countries where less control is maintained over antibiotic prescribing and sales.

Animal husbandry and agriculture use large amounts of anti-infective drugs, sometimes indiscriminately, resulting in the selection of resistant bacterial strains. Antibiotics are used as growth-promoting agents in animal feed in some countries, and for spraying of fruit trees, rice paddies, and flowers to avoid bacterial blights. Some of the infectious agents that infect animals freely circulate between animals and humans, providing opportunities for swapping or exchanging resistant genes, increasing the speed with which anti-infective resistance evolves in both agriculture and human populations.

From January 2005 to March 2006, 44 of 53 patients with multi-drug resistance to tuberculosis (MDR-TB) were further diagnosed with extreme drug resistant tuberculosis (XDR-TB). All were found to be HIV-positive as well. Widespread infection with HIV provides fertile ground for the transmission of all forms of TB, including XDR-TB, facilitated by inappropriate prescribing behaviour of health workers and poor adherence to treatment regimes by patients.

Deliberate use to cause terror and harm

The potential of organisms used as weapons of biological warfare or bioterrorism was graphically illustrated in 1979 in an accident involving anthrax in Sverdlovsk, 1400 km east of Moscow, in the then Soviet Union. Attributed at first by government officials to the consumption of contaminated meat, it was later shown to have been caused by the unintentional release of anthrax spores from a Soviet military microbiology facility. It is estimated that up to 358 humans were infected and that between 45 and 199 died.

In the United States in late September 2001, the deliberate dissemination of potentially lethal anthrax spores in four known letters sent through the United States Postal Service caused massive disruption of postal services in the United States and many other countries around the world. The anthrax letters—dated 11 September 2001, and postmarked 7 days later—caused huge public alarm and prompted a massive public health response. A total of 22 persons are thought to have been infected by anthrax spores sent through the postal system; 11 developed cutaneous anthrax and the remaining 11 developed inhalation anthrax, of whom five died. Twenty of the 22 patients were exposed to work sites that were found to be contaminated with anthrax spores. Nine of them had worked in mail processing facilities through which the anthrax letters had passed.

Other bacteria, viruses, mycotic agents, and biological toxins are also considered to have the potential for deliberate use to cause harm to humans. Great concern has been expressed by many countries about the potential health consequences that could be caused by the deliberate introduction of infectious agents such as the variola virus into a human population where smallpox vaccination is no longer practised, or the plague bacillus that could potentially cause an outbreak of pneumonic plague.

Public health security: Globalization and emerging/re-emerging infectious disease agents

Emerging and re-emerging infections enter a world of increased human mobility and interdependence that facilitates the transfer of infectious agents from country to country, and from continent to continent. Infectious agents efficiently travel in humans, insects, food and animals, and can spread around the globe and emerge in new geographic areas with ease and speed. Some are transported by the flights of migratory birds. Others, such as disease-carrying mosquitoes, travel in the passenger cabin or luggage hold of jets, to cause tropical infections in temperate countries when they bite airport workers or those who live nearby. They thus threaten public health security—our collective vulnerability to acute infectious disease outbreaks (Heymann 2003).

In 2000, among 312 athletes participating in an international triathlon held in Malaysia, 33 became infected with leptospirosis and returned to their home countries during the incubation period. While leptospirosis lacks human transmissibility and therefore did not set up local foci or transmission, another event in 2003—the outbreak of SARS, clearly demonstrates the full potential of emerging infectious agents for international spread. From a medical doctor who was infected by patients that he was treating in the Guangdong Province of China, and then unknowingly carried the newly emerged infectious agent to a Hong Kong hotel, SARS spread in individual chains of transmission form infected hotel guests to 8422 persons reported infected in North and South America, the Middle East, Europe, and Asia with a case-fatality rate of approximately 11 per cent.

During the years 1969–2003, 18 instances of airport malaria were reported to WHO—malaria infections in workers at airports or in persons who live nearby who had not travelled to malaria-endemic countries. Their infection originated from malaria-infected *anopheles* mosquitoes that had travelled from countries with endemic malaria and took a blood meal from airport workers or other persons upon landing, clearly demonstrating that insects, like humans, can transport infectious agents around the world to emerge in places where they are not endemic.

Livestock, animal products, and food can also carry infectious agents that emerge or re-emerge in non-endemic countries. Rift Valley Fever emerged in humans in Yemen and Saudi Arabia in 2000, 2 years after a major outbreak of Rift Valley Fever in East Africa. Infection has since become endemic in livestock in the Arabian Peninsula, and is thought to have been imported from East Africa in livestock traded across the Red Sea. In 1996, imported raspberries contaminated with *Cyclospora* caused an outbreak in the United States. It is hypothesized that the raspberries imported from Guatemala were contaminated when surface water was used to spray them with fungicide before harvest.

Concern about the international spread of emerging and re-emerging infections and the need for strong public health security are not new. By the fourteenth century, governments recognized the capacity for international disease transmission and legislated preventive measures, as reflected in the establishment of quarantine in the city state of Venice. Arriving ships were not permitted to dock for 40 days, in order to attempt to keep plague from entering by sea.

Many European leaders of the mid-nineteenth century, worried by the cholera pandemic of the time; threats of plague; and the weakness of quarantine measures, began to recognize that controlling the spread of infectious diseases from one nation to another required cooperation between those nations. International conventions were organized and draft covenants signed, almost all of which related to some type of quarantine regulations.

From 1851 to 1897, 10 international sanitary conferences were held among a group of 12 European countries, focusing exclusively on the containment of epidemics in their territories. The inaugural 1851 conference in Paris lasted 6 months and was followed in 1892 by the first International Sanitary Convention that dealt with cholera. Five years later, at the 10th International Sanitary Conference, a similar convention that focused on plague was signed.

New policies then emerged in the late nineteenth century, such as the obligatory telegraphic notification of first cases of cholera and plague, a model that a small group of South American nations followed when they signed the first set of international public health agreements in the Americas during the 1880s. In addition to cholera and plague, often carried by immigrants arriving from Europe, the agreements in the Americas covered yellow fever that was endemic in much of the American region at that time, and that from time to time caused major urban epidemics.

During the following decade, 12 countries attended the First International Sanitary Convention of the American Republics in Washington, DC, leading to the creation of the Pan American Sanitary Bureau (now called the Pan American Health Organization) in 1902. Its counterpart in Europe was the Office International d'Hygiène Publique (OIHP), established in 1907, and based in Paris.

In 1951, 3 years after its founding, WHO adopted a revised version of the International Sanitary Regulations (1892) that remained focused on the control of cholera, plague and yellow fever and rooted firmly in the preceding agreements of nineteenth and twentieth centuries.

The international health regulations

In 1969 the Member States of the World Health Organization agreed to new set of regulations—the International Health Regulations (IHR)—aimed at better ensuring public health security with minimal interruption in travel and trade. In addition to requiring reporting of four infectious diseases—cholera, plague, yellow fever, and smallpox—the IHR (1969) were aimed at stopping the spread of disease by pre-established control measures at international borders. They included requirements such as yellow fever and smallpox vaccination for passengers arriving from countries where yellow fever or smallpox outbreaks had been reported, and thus provided a legal framework for global surveillance and response, with the potential to decrease the world's vulnerability to four infectious diseases that were know to cross international borders.

By 1996, it had become clear, however, that the IHR (1969) were not able to ensure public health security as had been envisioned—countries reported the occurrence of cholera, plague and yellow fever late or not at all because of fear of stigmatization and economic repercussions (smallpox had been removed from the list when it was certified eradicated in 1980). At the same time it was realized that the IHR (1969) did not meet the challenges caused by emerging and re-emerging infectious diseases and the rapid global transit of these infections, sometimes still in the incubation period, by humans, insects, animals, and goods. From 1996 until 2005, the Member States of WHO therefore undertook a process to examine and revise the IHR (1969).

The result—the IHR (2005)—provide a more up-to-date legal framework requiring reporting of any public health emergency of international concern (PHEIC), and the use of real-time evidence to recommend measures to stop their international spread. A PHEIC is defined as an extraordinary event that could spread internationally or might require a coordinated international response (World Health Organization).

Under the IHR (2005) an event is evaluated for its potential to become a PHEIC by the country in which it is occurring, using a decision tree instrument developed for this purpose (Fig. 9.17.4). If the criteria for a PHEIC are met, an official notification must be provided to WHO. Notification is also required for even a single occurrence of a disease that would always threaten global public health security—smallpox, poliomyelitis caused by a wild-type poliovirus, human influenza caused by a new virus subtype, and SARS. In addition, there is a second list that includes diseases of documented—but not inevitable—international impact. An event involving a disease on this second list, which includes cholera, pneumonic plague, yellow fever, Ebola, and the other haemorrhagic fevers, still requires the use of the decision tree instrument to determine if it is a PHEIC. Thus, two

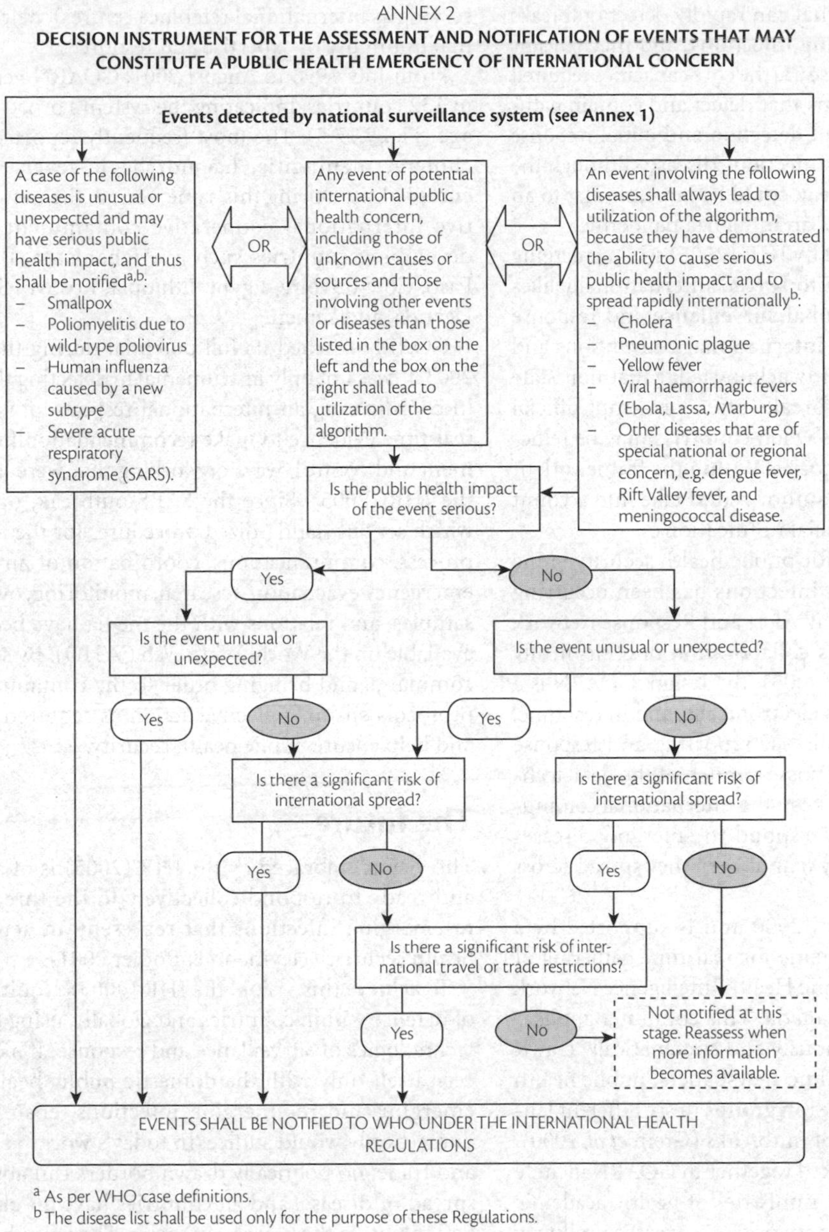

Fig. 9.17.4 Decision tree for assessment of a potential public health event of international concern.

safeguards create a baseline of public health security by requiring countries to respond, in designated ways, to well-known threats.

In contrast to previous regulations, the IHR (2005) introduced a set of core capacity requirements for surveillance and response. All countries must meet these requirements during the first 5 years of implementation of the IHR (2005) in order to detect, assess, notify, report, and contain the events covered by the regulations so that their potential for international spread and negative economic impact are minimized. The IHR (2005) likewise require collective action by all WHO Member States in the event that an emerging or re-emerging infectious disease threatens to spread internationally, and the free-sharing of information pertaining to this threat. They thus provide a safety net against the international spread of emerging or re-emerging infections, requiring collaboration between all states to ensure the timely availability of surveillance information and technical resources that better guarantee international public health security.

Other international frameworks have also been developed to contain and curtail the international spread of emerging infections. Among them are the WHO global strategy for containment of antimicrobial resistance (World Health Organization 2001). Though not legally binding, this framework calls on countries to work across the human health, animal health, and agricultural sectors to ensure more rational use of anti-infective drugs in order to limit the factors that accelerate the selection and proliferation of anti-infective-drug-resistant microbes.

National and international surveillance and response

For emerging and re-emerging infections that are able to transmit from person to person, the window of opportunity for effective intervention often closes quickly. The most important defence against their international spread is highly sensitive national surveillance systems, public health laboratories that can rapidly detect outbreaks caused by emerging and re-emerging infections, and mechanisms that permit timely containment. These are the core capacities required by the IHR (2005). The same systems that detect and contain naturally occurring outbreaks also permit detection and initial response to deliberately caused outbreaks of infectious disease, although the scale of a deliberately caused outbreak could be large, similar to an outbreak caused by an event such as an influenza pandemic.

The collaborative action required by IHR (2005) when emerging or re-emerging infections threaten to spread internationally likewise provides a framework for global surveillance and response that is a departure from previous international conventions and regulations. The IHR (2005) explicitly acknowledge that non-state sources of information about outbreaks often pre-empt official notification, especially in situations when countries may be reluctant to reveal an event in their territories. Within the framework of the IHR (2005), WHO is therefore authorized to take into account information sources other than official notifications.

Collaboration among countries for public health security in the face of emerging and re-emerging infections has been occurring since 1997 when the Global Outbreak Alert and Response Network (GOARN) was first envisaged. This collaboration now sits firmly within the framework of the HIR (2005). By design, GOARN is a network of networks that interlinks electronically, and in real time, over 140 existing laboratory and disease reporting and response networks. Together, these networks possess much of the data, technical expertise, and skills needed to keep the international community constantly alert and ready to respond to emerging diseases within countries and internationally if and when they spread across national borders.

GOARN was formalized in April 2000 and is supported by a customized artificial intelligence engine for real-time gathering of disease information, the Global Public Health Intelligence Network (GPHIN) maintained by Health Canada. This computer application heightens vigilance by continuously and systematically crawling web sites, news wires, local online newspapers, public health email services, and electronic discussion groups in six different languages in order to identify reports of outbreaks (Grein *et al.* 2000).

Other sources of information linked together in GOARN include government and university centres, ministries of health, academic institutions, other UN agencies, networks of overseas military laboratories, and nongovernmental organizations having a strong presence in epidemic-prone countries such as Medecins sans Frontières and the International Federation of Red Cross and Red Crescent Societies. Information from all these sources is assessed and verified on a daily basis by WHO and its partners in GOARN, and validated information is made public on the WHO web site.

If an outbreak of emerging or re-emerging infectious disease occurs in a country that requires international assistance to help in containment activities, as agreed upon in confidential pro-active consultation with the affected country and with experts in the network, electronic communications are used to describe the technical expertise required and to then provide prompt assistance and support. To this end, global databases of professionals with expertise in specific diseases or epidemiological techniques are maintained, together with nongovernmental organizations present in countries and in a position to reach remote areas. Such mechanisms, which are further supported by the WHO network of Collaborating Centres (national laboratories and institutes throughout the world serving as international reference centres), help the world make the maximum use of expertise and resources.

From July 1998 to August 2001, GOARN verified 578 outbreaks in 132 countries, indicating the system's broad geographical coverage (Fig. 9.17.5). The most frequently reported outbreaks were of cholera, meningitis, haemorrhagic fever, anthrax, and viral encephalitis. During this same period, the network launched effective international cooperative containment activities in many developing countries such as Afghanistan, Bangladesh, Burkina Faso, Côte d'Ivoire, Egypt, Ethiopia, Kosovo, Sierra Leone, Sudan, Uganda, and Yemen.

GOARN reached its full potential during the SARS outbreak in 2003. It was not only instrumental in detecting the outbreak, but also in coordinating an international response for the first time using real-time evidence to make recommendation for epidemic containment and control, ways of working that were later incorporated in the IHR (2005). Since the SARS outbreak, operational protocols which set out standardized procedures for the alert and verification process, communications, coordination of an epidemic response, emergency evacuation, research, monitoring, ownership of data and samples, and relations with the media have been finalized and are available on the World Wide Web (WHO). By setting out a chain of command, and bringing order to the containment response, such protocols ensure collective action as required by the IHR (2005) and help ensure public health security.

The future

The vision embraced by the IHR (2005) is of a world on the alert and ready to respond collectively to the threat of emerging and re-emerging infections that represent an acute threat to public health security (Heymann & Rodier 2001).

To achieve this vision, the IHR (2005) requires an unbroken line of defence within countries and globally, using the most up-to-date technologies of surveillance and response. If a country had to concern itself only with the domestic public health issues caused by emerging and re-emerging infections, ensuring core capacities domestically would suffice. In today's world of international travel and trade, no politically drawn borders can absolutely prevent the spread of disease, and all countries have an obligation to develop and maintain these core capacities. They also have an obligation to be part of an interconnected system engaged in risk management activities that collectively reduce international vulnerability to threats to public health security.

Adherence to the IHR (2005) requires adherence to new norms and standards for reporting and responding to emerging and re-emerging infections despite the economic consequences that may result. Their full achievement will provide the highest level of public health security possible. National core capacities as described in the IHR (2005) must be put in place within the national public health system that can detect, investigate, communicate, and contain events that threaten public health security as soon as they appear. An interconnected system must be operating at the national and international levels, engaged in specific threat and risk assessment and management activities that minimize collective vulnerability to public health events.

These two goals are interdependent and must be sustained. They involve measures that the international community must continually invest in, strive to achieve, and assess for progress. In today's mobile,

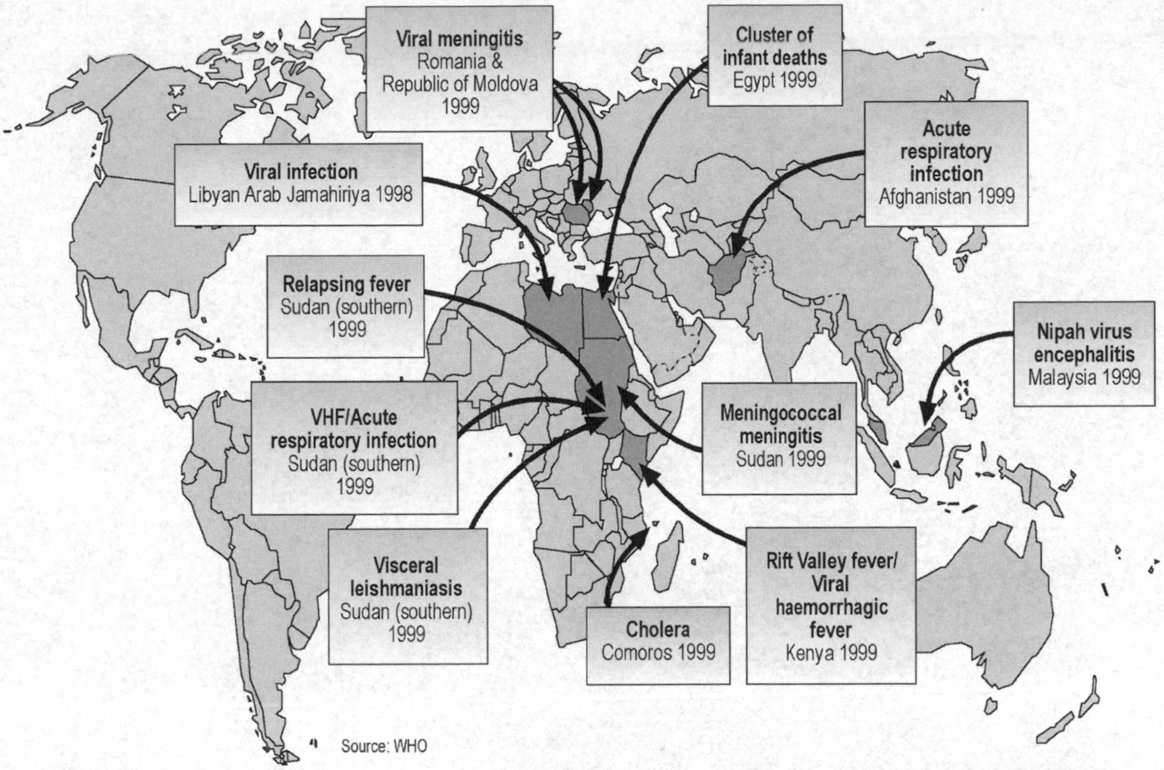

Fig. 9.17.5 Sample of international epidemic response missions during the first 12 months, Global Outbreak Alert and Response Network, 1998–1999.

interdependent, and interconnected world, threats arising from emerging and epidemic-prone diseases affect all countries. Such threats reinforce the need for shared responsibility and collective action in the face of universal vulnerability, in sectors that go well beyond health.

References

Grein T., Kamara K.B.O., Rodier G. *et al.* (2000) Rumours of disease in the global village: outbreak verification. *Emerging Infectious Diseases*, **6**, 97–102.

Heymann D.L. (2003) The evolving infectious disease threat: implications for national and global security. *Harvard University/Commission on Human Security for Global Health, Journal of Human Development*, **4**, 191–207.

Heymann D.L. and Rodier G. (2001) Hot spots in a wired world: Who surveillance of emerging and re-emerging infectiou diseases. *Lancet*, **1**, 345–53.

Lederberg J., Shope R.E., Oaks S.C. Jr., eds. *Emerging infections: microbial threats to health in the United States*, Washington DC: National Academy Press, 1992.

World Health Organization. International Health Regulations (2005), Geneva. Available at: http://www.who.int/gb/ebwha/pdf_files/WHA58/WHA58_3-en.pdf

World Health Organization. (2001) *WHO Global Strategy for Containment of Antimicrobial Resistance*. Geneva. Available at: http://www.who.int/drugresistance/WHO%20Global%20Strategy%20-%20Executive%20Summary%20-%20English%20version.pdf

SECTION 10

Prevention and control of public health hazards

10.1

Tobacco

Samira Asma, Douglas W. Bettcher,[1] Jonathan Samet, Krishna M. Palipudi, Gary Giovino, Stella Bialous, Katherine DeLand,[1] June Leung, Daniel Ferrante,[1] Gemma Vestal,[1] Gonghuan Yang, and Derek Yach

Abstract

Tobacco use is the single-most preventable cause of death and is unique in terms of its current and projected future impacts on global mortality. If current trends of tobacco use continue, the number of people killed by tobacco will reach 8.3 million annually by the year 2030. Tobacco is also the only legal consumer product that can harm everyone exposed to it, and it kills up to half of those who use it as intended. Despite the crises, there is also an opportunity. The current national and global momentum to promote smoke-free societies offers opportunity to apply proven strategies. The World Health Organization (WHO) Framework Convention on Tobacco Control, a multilateral legal framework, presents a blueprint for countries to reduce both supply and demand for tobacco. In addition, the WHO MPOWER package offers recommendations for countries to implement the most proven strategies. This chapter examines the history of tobacco use and dependence, and the current and projected pattern of the tobacco epidemic, reviews the structure, conduct, and strategies of the tobacco industry, and proposes proven tobacco control strategies, which may have relevance throughout the world.

Introduction

Today, tobacco use is the single-most preventable cause of death and is unique in terms of its current and projected future impacts on global mortality. If current trends of tobacco use continue, the number of people killed by tobacco will reach 8.3 million annually by the year 2030 (Mathers & Loncar 2006). Tobacco is also the only legal consumer product that harms every user, killing up to half of those who use it as intended. Tobacco use is widespread due to insufficient public awareness about its dangers, aggressive marketing and promotion of the products, and lack of strong, countering public health policies.

Nonetheless, there are substantial opportunities to slow the epidemic. After decades of implementing, evaluating, and fine-tuning tobacco control programmes, there is now a substantial evidence base identifying and supporting those policies that can be expected to have the greatest positive effect. Promisingly, this evidence base has not been neglected; in the face of the unprecedented toll caused by tobacco use and the worrying projections for the future, the global health community has taken strong steps toward reducing and eventually eliminating the morbidity and mortality caused by the tobacco epidemic; most notably, in the negotiation and implementation of the WHO Framework Convention on Tobacco Control (WHO FCTC).

The WHO FCTC is a multilateral evidence-based treaty, providing the legal framework for countries to reduce both supply and demand for tobacco. With over 160 Parties, the WHO FCTC is one of the most universal treaties in UN history. Over the next several years, its substantial impact should be felt in Parties and, insofar as tobacco is a transnational concern, also in non-Party jurisdictions. Building on this momentum, WHO launched an implementation strategy for the WHO FCTC as part of the WHO Report on the Global Tobacco Epidemic, 2008. The MPOWER technical assistance package contains a set of six proven strategies, each of which reflects one or more provisions of the WHO FCTC.

In addition to these two major global initiatives, the very way in which the tobacco debate is perceived has shifted with the multiple disclosures of internal industry documents revealing the tactics of the tobacco industry. Thus armed, the tobacco control community has expanded inroads for vigilant monitoring of the industry as it seeks to maintain and expand its markets, particularly in less-developed countries and among women.

The purpose of this chapter is to explore the opportunities to limit the epidemic by (a) examining the history of tobacco use and its dependence, and the current and projected pattern of the tobacco epidemic, (b) reviewing the structure, conduct, and strategies of the tobacco industry, and (c) encouraging the use of already proven tobacco control strategies, which have relevance throughout the world.

The tobacco epidemic

In this section, we review the history of tobacco use and dependence, the epidemiological model, and the characteristics of the

[1] The author is a staff member of the World Health Organization. The author alone is responsible for the views expressed in this publication and they do not necessarily represent the decisions or the stated policy of the World Health Organization.

tobacco epidemic. The characteristics of the epidemic include production of tobacco, patterns of tobacco use, smoking cessation and nicotine dependence, exposure to second-hand smoke (SHS), and the pattern and burden of tobacco-related diseases.

The history of tobacco use and dependence

The tobacco plant (*Nicotiana tabacum*) originates from South America, where tobacco was used for ceremonial and shamanistic purposes long before Columbus arrived; however, it was not consumed regularly. By the arrival of Columbus in 1492, tobacco was being chewed, smoked, or snuffed in many areas of both North and South America. In the 1700s and the early 1800s, large quantities of tobacco were being snuffed by the aristocracy of Europe and chewed by the American settlers. By the middle of the 1800s, the technology for making cigarettes in large quantities with a machine and the flue-curing of tobacco had been developed, and the chewing of tobacco was beginning to be considered unhygienic. The converging development of several technologies between the late-nineteenth and early-twentieth centuries made the modern cigarette possible. New tobacco blends and curing processes were developed, which produced a tobacco product that, when burned, could be inhaled. Machinery for manufacturing cigarettes cheaply was perfected, the safety match was invented, and advertising and promotion techniques promoted the products of the tobacco industry. By the start of the twentieth century, the mass production of cigarettes had begun and smoking among men in industrial countries began to rise dramatically. Cigarette smoking became increasingly accepted among women in industrial countries, starting about the time of World War II. At this time, smoking also began to rise in men in developing countries. Today, tobacco is cultivated commercially in more than 100 countries. The major producers are China, Brazil, India, the United States, Angola, Indonesia, Turkey, Greece, Italy, and Pakistan. Tobacco is consumed in all countries of the world (FAO 2006).

The epidemiological model

The epidemiological triad of agent, host, vector, and environment long used for infectious diseases also facilitates the understanding of factors that influence patterns, determinants, and consequences of tobacco use (Orleans & Slade 1993). An agent is traditionally defined as a factor whose presence is essential for the occurrence of disease (Last 1995). In this model, the myriad components of tobacco and tobacco smoke-cause disease. Tobacco and tobacco smoke contain over 3500 chemicals, including hundreds that are toxic or carcinogenic (USDHHS 1989, 2006; Hecht 1999). Tobacco also contains nicotine, an addictive compound that serves to maintain people's use of the agent even when they want to quit (USDHHS 1988; Giovino *et al.* 1995; FDA 1996). The bioavailability of nicotine can be increased by raising the pH of the product (FDA 1996; Fant *et al.* 1999). Many tobacco products (e.g. so-called 'low tar' cigarettes) may appear to be less dangerous than others on the basis of 'tar' and 'nicotine' ratings derived from a smoking machine. However, such products are rated by a machine testing system that does not represent smokers' intake of the toxic components of the cigarette, the way that smokers compensate for reduced nicotine yield, and their availability may undermine smokers' motivations to quit (USDHSS 1996; Kozlowski *et al.* 1998a,b).

The host in this model is the person who uses the product, i.e. one who smokes tobacco (through a cigarette, cigar, pipe, or other smoking device), chews or dips oral tobacco, or inhales snuff. Host factors found to be determinants of smoking include demographic characteristics, knowledge, attitudes, and behaviours, tobacco use by friends and family members, and genetic susceptibility to addiction and disease (USDHHS 2006). One significant challenge to tobacco control lies in understanding why some people who experiment with smoking easily discontinue, whereas others progress to become regular dependent users. Host factors can influence why some dependent smokers quit and others continue, and why some lifelong smokers develop smoking-attributable diseases while others do not.

Because SHS, also known as environmental tobacco smoke (ETS),[2] which is the combination of sidestream smoke and exhaled mainstream smoke inhaled by non-smokers causes disease in many exposed persons who do not consume tobacco products (SCOTH 1998; Samet & Wang 2000; California Environmental Protection Agency 2005; USDHHS 2006), the complete disease model also includes involuntary smokers as incidental hosts (DiFranza & Lew 1995; USDHHS 2006). The vector serves to transport the agent to susceptible individuals (Last 1995). Just as we understand, e.g. the role of the rat in the spread of the plague or the mosquito in the spread of malaria, we need to understand that tobacco has a vector—tobacco products' manufacturers. Thus, in the development of nicotine addiction and tobacco-attributable disease, tobacco products' manufacturers produce the agent and distribute it in ways that make the product appealing to both users and non-users. The industry uses packaging, advertising, and promotion to reach and influence as many people as possible to use their products. The price of the product (the lower the price, the more will be sold) and the ease with which it can be obtained (from vending machines, over-the-counter displays, and sales by street vendors) are also key distribution factors. In the case of tobacco, the vector also serves to undermine public health attempts to limit use by denying for decades the health consequences of use, and resisting many health-promoting programmes and policies (Hilts 1996; Kluger 1996; Jamieson 1998) in order to maintain the product affordable, to maintain the ability to market the product and to maintain the social acceptability of tobacco use. This vector actively markets products that tacitly claim to be less hazardous and engages in sophisticated public relations campaigns to promote itself as a responsible corporation, and while in some cases admitting the harmful effects of tobacco use (while continuing to deny the health impact of SHS), continues to deny any responsibility over the individual harm caused to smokers and the social harms caused by marketing (Hirschhorn 2004; Lee & Bialous 2006; McDaniel *et al.* 2006, 2008). Additionally, for decades, the vector has manipulated the product in ways that have made it more addictive and potentially more harmful. For example, by the manipulation of pH, manufacturers have enhanced the bioavailability of nicotine to the smoker (Ferris Wayne *et al.* 2006; Hammond *et al.* 2006).

---

[2] Several alternative terms are commonly used to describe the smoke emitted from the burning end of a cigarette or from other tobacco products usually in combination with the smoke exhaled by the smoker. The term 'second-hand smoke' is the preferred term used in the guidelines adopted by the Conference of the Parties for implementation of the WHO Framework Convention on Tobacco Control (WHO 2007a), and thus will be used in this chapter thereafter. Other terms such as 'passive smoking' or 'involuntary exposure to tobacco smoke' are best avoided as the tobacco industry may use these terms to support a position that 'voluntary exposure' is acceptable.

The environment includes diverse cultural, historical, economic, and political factors. In many countries, tobacco growing and tobacco product manufacturing have been, for decades, respected and lucrative businesses that wielded tremendous economic and political influence (World Bank 1999). When the health effects became known, and more recently when the industry's malfeasant activities became apparent, attitudes towards the industry changed precipitously. Nevertheless, the powerful effects of pro-tobacco forces have influenced many political decisions (Francey & Chapman 2000; Saloogee & Dagli 2000; Muggli *et al.* 2001; Neuman *et al.* 2002; McDaniel *et al.* 2008). In addition, the industry often attempts to gain cultural and political favour by sponsoring cultural events and promoting smoking prevention campaigns (Dewhirst & Hunter 2002; Barbeau *et al.* 2004; Anderson *et al.* 2006; Brandt 2007).

Economic and cultural influences in regions where tobacco is grown and/or where tobacco products are produced often result in reduced support for tobacco control activities, in comparison with areas that not affected by tobacco industry activities. Environmental factors also include efforts by the tobacco control community, whether governmental or non-governmental, to counter pro-tobacco influences.

This epidemiological model has proved useful for both research and intervention. Past and ongoing research addresses each of the components of this model, as well as the interactions among its elements. Most research has focused on host factors, although more recent attention has also turned to policy factors. With the widespread dissemination of industry documents, our understanding of the vector has increased and led to legal and regulatory strategies to better control it.

Interventions address different levels in a continuum that extends from the individual smoker to the national and international levels. Some attempt to influence host factors, e.g. by educating people about the dangers of tobacco use, how to quit, and ways to resist pro-tobacco influences from the peers and the media. Recent activities attempt to influence the environment, e.g. by promoting policy changes and mass media interventions. The industry is changing the agent, e.g. by developing nicotine-delivery products that heat (as opposed to burn) tobacco. Regulatory efforts strive to control both the agent and the activities of the vector; a global initiative has been launched with the advent of the World Health Organization's Framework Convention on Tobacco Control (WHO FCTC).

Characteristics of the tobacco epidemic

In this section, we provide an overview of the characteristics of the global tobacco epidemic, which will include tobacco production and its patterns of use. It will also describe smoking cessation and nicotine dependence, and discuss the exposure to SHS. Finally, we will conclude by reviewing the literature on the patterns and burden of tobacco-related diseases.

Tobacco production

In this section, we classify and describe the various tobacco products available, tobacco growing, and the world market in manufactured tobacco products.

Types of tobacco products

There are two main forms of tobacco in common use: Smoking tobacco and smokeless tobacco. Smoking tobacco includes manufactured cigarettes (filter and unfiltered) and 'roll-your-own' cigarettes. *Kretek* (clove-flavoured cigarettes), from Indonesia, are sticks made from a local variety of sun-cured tobacco known as *brus* and wrapped in cigarette paper. These are indigenous to Indonesia, but are also available in the United States (WHO 2006). *Bidis* (small hand-rolled cigarettes consisting of sun-dried tobacco wrapped in a *tendu* leaf) are smoked throughout Southeast Asia, particularly in India (Stratton *et al.* 2001). They are also becoming increasingly popular among teenagers in the United States (Malson & Pickworth 2002). Cigars are made of air-cured and fermented tobacco with a tobacco leaf wrapper, and come in many shapes and sizes, from cigarette-sized to 10-g double coronas. Pipes are used predominantly in Europe, America, and Southeast Asia; e.g. clay pipes known as *sulpa*, *chilum*, and *hookli* are common in Asia. *Chutta* is an Indian home-made cigar. Reverse smoking of *chutta* (with burning

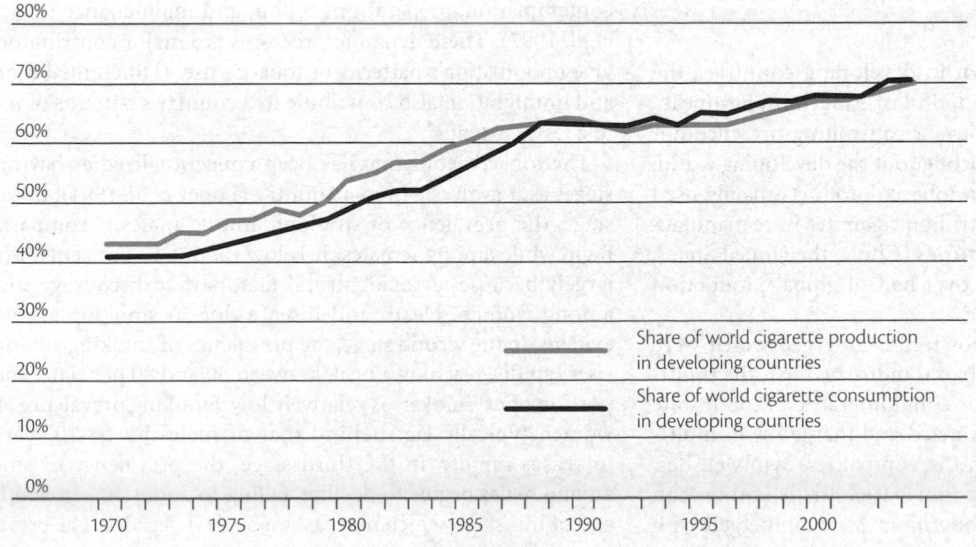

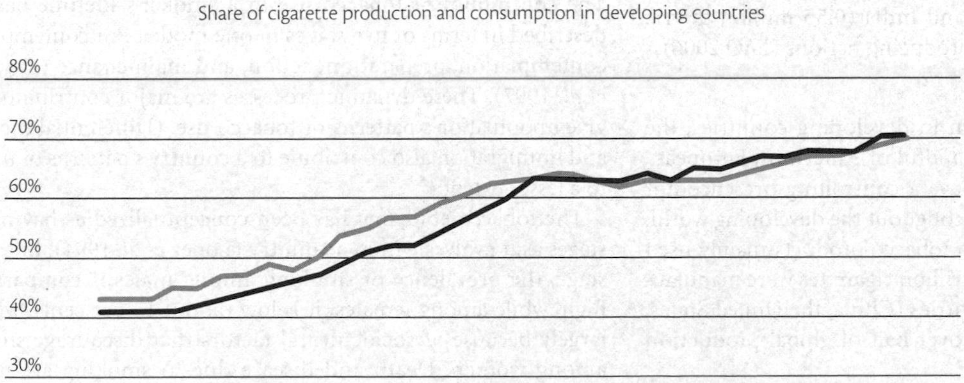

Fig. 10.1.1 Shifting epidemic (the tobacco industry reaches new markets in developing countries).
Source: Based on data from Food and Agriculture Organization FAOSTAT, United Nation Commodity Trade Statistic Database, United Nation Common Database, United States Department of Agriculture Economic Research Service, World Health Organization Statistics Information System, and ERC Group Plc's World Cigarettes Report (2005).

end inside the mouth) is prevalent among women in the rural communities of Andhra Pradesh (Van der Eb *et al.* 1993). Water pipes, also known as *hookah*, *gaza*, *narghile*, hubble-bubble, and *shisha*, are in common use in Eastern Mediterranean region, parts of Asia and North Africa.

Smokeless tobacco products, consisting of tobacco leaf and a wide variety of flavouring and other ingredients, are used either orally or nasally. Smokeless tobacco includes chewing tobacco and snuff (dry and moist varieties), used in South Asia, Western Europe and North America and parts of Africa. Chewing tobacco is produced by shredding tobacco leaf. The leaf can be consumed loosely, or by pressing into bricks (plugs), or by drying and forming twist. Snuff, which may be sniffed or placed in the mouth, has a much finer consistency than chewing tobacco and is made from powdered or finely cut tobacco leaves. Moist snuff taken orally has been used for many years in Sweden, where it is known as snus, and in the United States. Smokeless tobacco is being actively marketed as a popular form of tobacco among children and adolescents in the United States and Scandinavia (Tomar 2007). About 40 per cent of total tobacco consumption in India is in the form of smokeless or chewing tobacco (Reddy & Gupta 2004; WHO 2008).

Tobacco growing

Tobacco is grown in more than 115 countries on almost 4 million hectares of land, a third of which is in China (FAO 2006). In 1970, 4.7 million tons of tobacco were produced worldwide, by 1997 leaf production had peaked to almost 9 million tons and by 2006 had fallen to 6.7 million tons (FAO 2006). China is the world's leading producer of tobacco, with production increasing from 0.81 million tons in 1970 (17 per cent of total world output) to 2.75 million tons in 2006 (41 per cent of total world output). In 2006, the other nine leading producers were Brazil, India, the United States, Angola, Indonesia, Turkey, Greece, Italy, and Pakistan.

The pattern of production has shifted significantly in recent decades. Whereas exports from the United States have fallen slightly, those from Brazil, China and Zimbabwe have increased significantly (FAO 2006). According to the Food and Agricultural Organization (FAO) projections, developing countries will account for 87 per cent of world tobacco by 2010. FAO estimates revealed that China is projected to remain the largest producer of tobacco in the world. Brazil (0.91 million metric tons) and India (0.55 million metric tons) are also among top tobacco-producing nations (FAO 2006).

Manufactured tobacco products

Although tobacco is mainly grown in developing countries, the world market is dominated by a handful of American, European, and Japanese companies, which have a controlling presence not only in all Western countries but throughout the developing world. China is an exception, with its own tobacco products mainly used in the domestic market. About 5.5 trillion cigarettes were manufactured worldwide in 2004; four countries (China, the United States, Russia, and Japan) accounted for over half of global production (USDA 2004).

During the late 1990s, two major trends emerged which were significant for the future of the tobacco industry. First, the multinationals merged into a few major conglomerates. Second, state monopolies were increasingly privatized and merged with multinationals. For example, as seen in the companies' own websites, in the past decade, United Kingdom-based British American Tobacco acquired Cigarrera La Moderna in Mexico, merged with Rothmans in Canada, gained control of Peru's Tabacalera Nacional, Italy's ETI, and Serbia's Duvanska Industrija Vranje. It also combined the business of United States-based Brown and Williamson with RJ Reynolds Tobacco Company to form Reynolds American, where BAT has a 42 per cent share. Japan Tobacco International was established in 1999 as a separate division of Japan Tobacco group after the acquisition of RJ Reynolds International division, and recently, of United Kingdom-based Gallaher. Altadis, created from the merge of France's Seita with Spain's Tabacalera has recently acquired Morocco's Regie de Tabacs and United Kingdom's Imperial. Philip Morris International (PMI), similarly, has in the past decade acquired interests in tobacco companies in Greece, Serbia, Colombia, Pakistan and acquired Sampoerna Tobacco in Indonesia and in 2006 announced an agreement with the China National Tobacco Company for the licensed production of Marlboro in China. In March 2008, the parent corporation, Altria, finalized the spin-off of PMI, which becomes a separate tobacco company.

In some countries, state-owned tobacco companies continue to dominate within their own market; the most notable of these is the China National Tobacco Company, which is the largest tobacco company in the world in terms of number of cigarettes sold (WHO 2008). Increasingly, however, the multinationals are moving into countries formerly controlled by state monopolies and introducing aggressive marketing programmes (Szilagyi & Chapman 2003; Lawrence & Collin 2004; Gilmore *et al.* 2005, 2007; Lee K *et al.* 2008). For example, in the 1980s, the American tobacco companies relied upon the United States government, and the threat of trade sanctions, to open the cigarette markets in Japan, Taiwan, South Korea, and Thailand (Chaloupka & Corbett 1998). The shift in focus of the multinationals also comes at a time when they are under increasing attack in their home bases as new disclosures become public, detailing how the tobacco industry built and maintained its markets through decades of improper conduct. These disclosures, in addition to shedding important historical light on the tobacco industry, also provide sobering and relevant insight as the tobacco industry expands to conquer new markets.

Patterns of tobacco use

The continuum of tobacco use in a smoker's lifetime has been described in terms of five stages in one model: Pre-contemplation, contemplation, preparation, action, and maintenance (Prochaska *et al.* 1997). These dynamic processes are major contributors to a given population's patterns of tobacco use. (Differential mortality and immigration also contribute to a country's patterns of use, but to a lesser extent.)

The tobacco epidemic has been conceptualized as having four stages as it evolves within a country (Lopez *et al.* 1994). In the first stage, the prevalence of smoking among males is comparatively high, while among females, it is low (about 15 per cent), which is largely because of sociocultural factors that discourage smoking among women. Death and disease due to smoking are not yet evident. In the second stage, the prevalence of smoking among men rises rapidly, reaching a peak between 50 and 80 per cent. The proportion of ex-smokers is relatively low. Smoking prevalence among women typically lags behind that of males by 10–20 years, but increases rapidly. In the third stage, the prevalence of smoking among males begins to decline, falling to about 40 per cent by the end of this stage, which may last for several decades. The prevalence

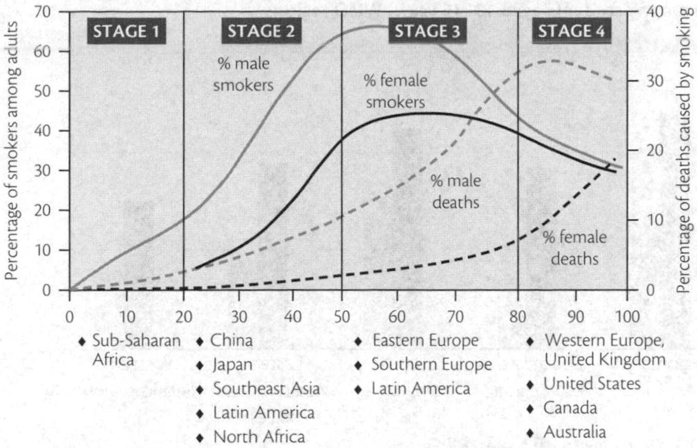

Fig. 10.1.2 Four-stage tobacco epidemic.
Source: Lopez *et al.* (1994).

tends to be lower among middle-aged and older men, many of whom have become ex-smokers. Most importantly, the end of the third stage is characterized by an initial decline in smoking among females. There is also likely to be a marked age gradient in prevalence among women, with about 40–50 per cent of all young women being regular smokers but with relatively few smokers (about 10 per cent) among women above 55–60 years of age. Another characteristic of this period is the rapid increase in smoking-attributable mortality, which rises from about 10 per cent of all deaths in males to about 25–30 per cent within three decades. In middle age (35–69 years), the proportionate mortality of males due to tobacco is even higher (about one in three deaths). The tobacco-related death rate among women is still comparatively low (about 5 per cent of all deaths) but rising. In the fourth stage, smoking prevalence for both sexes continues to decline more or less in parallel, but only slowly, 20–40 years after reaching its peak.

Although the prevalence of smoking has decreased and quitting rates have increased in some developed countries in recent decades, the overall global pattern of tobacco consumption is of major public health concern. Approximately 70 per cent of the world's smokers live in low- and middle-income countries. Nearly two-thirds of the world's smokers live in 10 countries, namely China, India, Indonesia, Russian Federation, the United States, Japan, Brazil, Bangladesh, Germany, and Turkey (WHO 2008).

The current smoking rate for the world's population is 25.3 per cent: 41.2 per cent among males and 9.3 per cent among females. In developed countries, the prevalence of smoking for males and females is 39.8 and 21.7 per cent, respectively. In developing countries, the gender difference in smoking prevalence is larger, with 41.6 per cent of males and 5.7 per cent of females smoking (unpublished data from WHO Tobacco Free Initiative).[3]

Trends in the consumption of tobacco

Trends in cigarette consumption rates have varied worldwide and also across WHO regions (WHO 2004, 2008). Overall, the world has seen an average annual increase of approximately 1 per cent in adult per capita consumption over the last two decades. The most rapid declines have been in countries such as Canada and the United Kingdom, where average annual decreases of 1.8 and 1.6 per cent, respectively, have been recorded since the early 1970s. These have not been matched by equivalent declines in prevalence.

In contrast, over the same time period, there have been dramatic average annual increases in per capita consumption in China (8 per cent), Indonesia (6.8 per cent), Syria (5.5 per cent), and Bangladesh (4.7 per cent). These high rates of increase are occurring from a low starting base, but China and Syria have already reached the per capita consumption levels of the United Kingdom; and in both countries, the rates of smoking among women remain low. There is a growing concern about the efforts of the tobacco industry to increase smoking rates among women in developing countries (WHO 1997a, 2008).

In many countries, people begin smoking at young ages, with the median age of initiation usually being under 15 years. The prevalence of smoking in youth continues to increase in both developed and developing countries, even where the overall prevalence of tobacco use is declining (WHO 1997b, 2008). Between 2000 and 2007, data for Global Youth Tobacco Survey (GYTS) were obtained

[3] The global and income aggregates represent adjusted prevalence estimates. Crude estimates received from WHO Member States are adjusted to obtain nationally representative prevalence estimates for current smokers of tobacco for the same year and age groups. These estimates are not age-standardised (i.e. do not remove the effects of the underlying age structures across countries) and should be used with caution when making comparisons of smoking prevalence across regions/income groups. For this reason, these estimates differ to those published in WHS (2008).

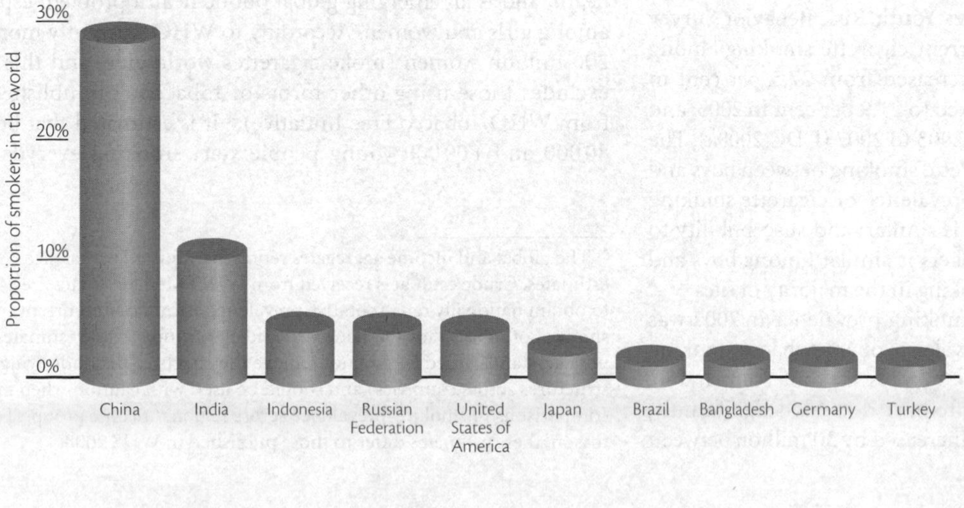

Fig. 10.1.3 Nearly two-thirds of the world's smokers live in 10 countries.
Sources: WHO (2008a).

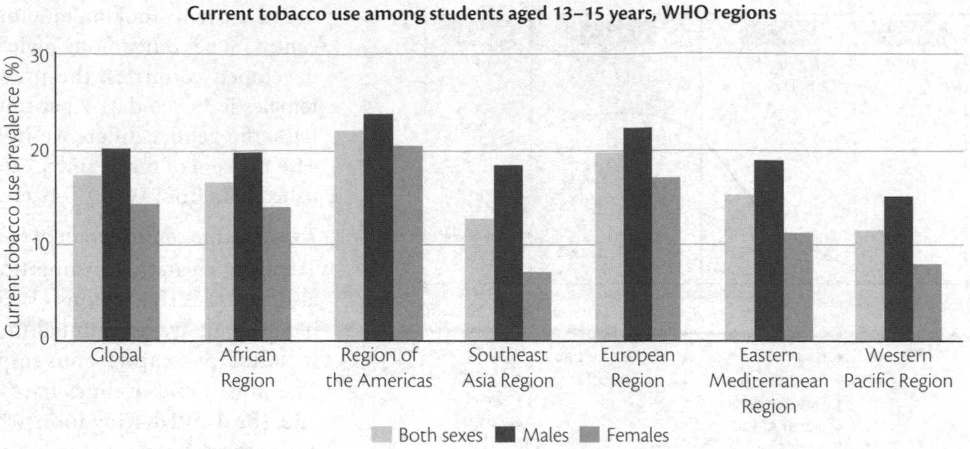

Fig. 10.1.4 Risk factor transition: High prevalence of tobacco use, youth worldwide.
Source: Worren *et al.* (2008a).

over 140 WHO Member States, six territories (American Samoa, British Virgin Islands, Guam, Monserrat, Puerto Rico, and the US Virgin Island), two geographic regions (Gaza Strip and West Bank), one United Nations administered province (Kosovo), one special administrative region (Macau) and one Commonwealth region (northern Mariana Islands). Among the students (aged 13–15 years) who were surveyed, it was revealed that overall 9 per cent of students currently smoke cigarettes. The rates were the highest in the European Region (19.2 per cent) and lowest in the Eastern Mediterranean Region (4.9 per cent). One in 10 (10.1 per cent) students currently used tobacco products other than cigarettes (e.g. pipes, water pipes, smokeless tobacco, and bidis), with the highest prevalence in the East Mediterranean Region (12 per cent) and lowest in the Western Pacific Region (6.6 per cent). Among students who had never smoked cigarettes, 19.1 per cent indicated they were susceptible to initiate smoking during the next year. The rate was highest in the European Union (29.8 per cent) and lowest in the Western Pacific Region (13.4 per cent). Cigarette smoking rates were significantly higher than other tobacco-use rates in the Americas, European Region, and Western Pacific Region; while other tobacco use was significantly more prevalent than cigarette smoking in the East Mediterranean Region and South East Asia Region. There was no difference between cigarette and other tobacco-use rates in the African Region or across all sites. Susceptibility rates were significantly higher than current cigarette smoking rates overall and in every region, except the Western Pacific Region, where no difference was reported (Warren *et al.* 2006; CDC 2008b).

Data from the 2005 United States Youth Risk Behavior Survey indicate that the prevalence of current cigarette smoking among American high-school students increased from 27.5 per cent in 1991 to 36.4 per cent in 1997, declined to 21.9 per cent in 2003, and remained stable (23 per cent) from 2003 to 2007 (CDC 2008a). The GYTS showed that the level of cigarette smoking between boys and girls is similar in many sites; the prevalence of cigarette smoking and use of other tobacco products is similar; and susceptibility to initiate smoking among never smokers is similar among boys and girls and is higher than cigarette smoking in the majority of sites.

In China, the current cigarette smoking prevalence in 2002 was 31.4 per cent, while in 1996, the prevalence of any tobacco smoking was 35.3 per cent. Although both surveys are not comparable, smoking prevalence did not appear to have decreased significantly, and the number of smokers in fact increased by 30 million between 1996 and 2002 (Yang *et al.* 2002). In the Kurdistan region of Iraq, among students aged 13–15, approximately 1 in every 10 ever-smokers of both sexes initiated smoking before 10 years of age. The initiation rates are slightly higher for girls than for boys (CDC 2006).

Many studies have shown that sociodemographic, environmental, behavioural, and personal factors are associated with the onset of tobacco use. Environmental factors include availability and advertising of cigarettes, the perception that tobacco use is the norm, peer and sibling attitudes, and lack of parental support during adolescence (Reid *et al.* 1995). Ease of acquiring cigarettes is another environmental factor that can have an impact on smoking among adolescents. Parental attitudes towards smoking, in particular towards their own children's smoking, has been shown to be related to adolescent smoking. Also important are school performance and psychosocial factors, including low academic achievement, rebelliousness, low self-esteem, alienation from school, and lack of skills to resist offers of cigarettes (Tyas & Pederson 1998). These findings are mainly from Western countries (Conrad *et al.* 1992; Tyas & Pederson 1998); although several studies from developing countries such as China have shown similar results (Wang *et al.* 1994b; Zhu *et al.* 1996). Additionally, data indicate that daily tobacco smoking is most prevalent among the lowest-income households in developing economies—that is, among the poorest of the poor (WHO 2007h).

Tobacco use by women

Tobacco use is one of the major causes of premature disease and death, and is an emerging global public health problem especially among girls and women. According to WHO, currently more than 200 million women smoke cigarettes worldwide, and this figure excludes those using other forms of tobacco (Unpublished data from WHO Tobacco Free Initiative).[4] It is estimated that between 80 000 and 100 000 young people start smoking everyday, and

[4] The global and income aggregates represent adjusted prevalence estimates. Crude estimates received from WHO Member States are adjusted to obtain nationally representative prevalence estimates for current smokers of tobacco for the same year and age groups. These estimates are not age-standardised (i.e. do not remove the effects of the underlying age structures across countries) and should be used with caution when making comparisons of smoking prevalence across regions/income groups. For this reason, these estimates differ to those published in WHS 2008.

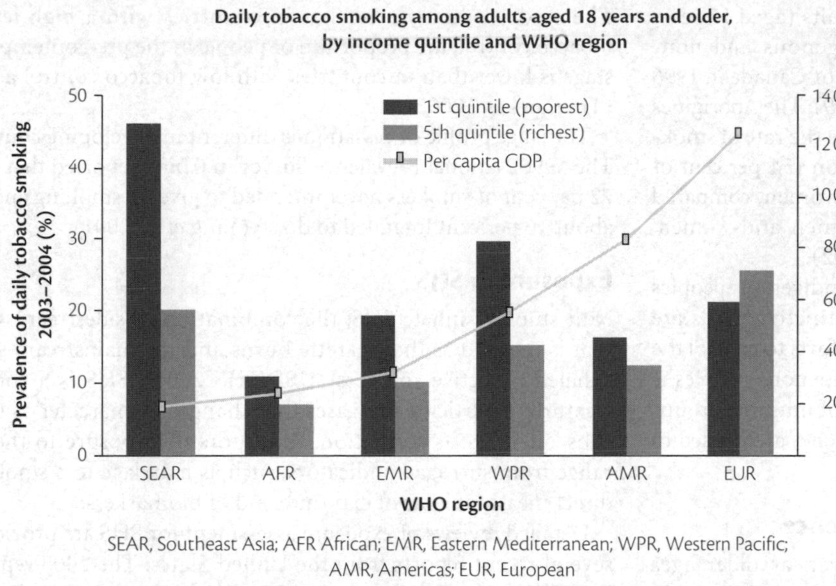

Fig. 10.1.5 Tobacco use and poverty: High prevalence among the world's poorest.
Source: WHO (2007h).

many of these are girls. An estimated 9.3 per cent of women smoke globally; about 21.7 per cent of women smoke in developed countries, while 5.7 per cent of women smoke in developing countries (estimates for adult population ≥15 years old for 2005, unpublished data from WHO Tobacco Free Initiative[4]). Again, these statistics do not include forms of tobacco use other than cigarettes. For example, in India, 30.8 per cent of men and only 2.8 per cent of women currently smoke (WHO 2008). On the other hand, the prevalence of other forms of tobacco use, i.e. chewing tobacco, is about 9.9 per cent (IIPS and Macro International 2007). Historically, smoking has been more common among men than among women in the majority of countries. In countries for which reliable data are available for assessing trends in smoking (primarily industrialized countries), peak prevalence among women occurred some years after it did so for men (Garfinkel 1997). While there are minor gender differences in smoking rates in some industrialized countries (such as the United States, New Zealand, and Australia), disparities between male and female current smoking rates in Asia are striking, specifically in Japan (43.3 per cent of men and 12 per cent of women), Korea (52.8 per cent of men and 5.8 per cent of women), and China (57.4 per cent of men and 2.6 per cent of women) (WHO 2008).

At the same time, smoking rates are rising among young women in many countries in Asia and the Pacific regions, where smoking is sometimes perceived as a symbol of women's liberation from traditional gender roles. There is an even greater cause for alarm here as statistics on cigarette consumption do not reflect the widespread use of smokeless tobacco among women in South Asia. For example, in Kerala, India, 22 per cent of rural women chew tobacco in a betel leaf. In the Bihar region and parts of Punjab and Haryana, women also smoke *bidis* and *hookahs*, while rural Indian women in the state of Goa rub and plug burnt powdered tobacco inside their mouths (Aghi *et al.* 2001). A major setback in public health would result if more women in developing countries began to smoke, similar to the trend observed in developed countries, and continued to use other forms of tobacco.

A contributing factor to this rising epidemic of tobacco use among women is the proliferation of seductive tobacco advertising worldwide, which may lead women and girls to believe that smoking is socially desirable. Typically, women's brands in developing countries feature false images of slimness, sophistication, emancipation, and modernity. To sell such images, tobacco companies are producing a range of brands aimed at women and feminized cigarettes which are long, extra slim, low-tar, light-coloured, or menthol.

The Kobe Declaration adopted in 1999 by women and youth leaders, scientists and policy-makers 'demanded a global ban on direct and indirect advertising, promotion and sponsorship by the tobacco industry across all media and in all forms of entertainment; and demanded public funding for counter-advertising that disconnects women's liberation and tobacco use and that reaches women and girls in all cultural contexts' (WHO 1999a, 2000a). WHO also recommends that gender issues be incorporated into the planning and implementation of tobacco control measures, in order to address the specific needs of women and men more effectively (WHO 2007g).

Tobacco use by indigenous people

Tobacco use is an important factor that impacts negatively on the health of indigenous peoples who have the highest rates of tobacco use in the world. It is not unusual for the rates of smoking of indigenous peoples to be twice that of the general population of the country in which they live. A survey among the Inuit of Greenland found that currently 82 per cent of Inuit men and 78 per cent of Inuit women are smokers. Furthermore, in the area of Disko Bay, approximately 65 per cent of pregnant women are smokers (AMAP 1998). Therefore, it is not surprising that the incidence and mortality of tobacco-related cancers are very high among the Inuit of Greenland (AMAP 1998). Similar patterns of smoking and smoking-related disease are evident among other groups of indigenous peoples, including the Maori of New Zealand, the First Nations and Inuit peoples of Canada, and the Aborigines and Torres Strait Islanders of Australia (Durie 1998). By 2006/2007, the rate of smoking among the Maori of New Zealand (42.2 per cent of Maori aged 15 years and over) was twice the rate of non-Maori New Zealanders. After adjusting for age, Maori women were more than twice as likely to be current smokers than women in the total population (Ministry of Health, New Zealand 2008). In 1997, 62 per cent of

First Nations and Labrador Inuit of Canada adults (aged 15 years and over) were smokers. The ratio for indigenous and non-indigenous peoples of the Northwest Territories of Canada in 1996 was similar (S. Gauthier, unpublished report, 1999). The Aborigines and Torres Strait Islanders of Australia have twice the rate of smoking of the non-indigenous Australian population (54 per cent of indigenous men and 46 per cent of indigenous women, compared with 28 and 22 per cent of non-indigenous men and women, respectively) (Australian Bureau of Statistics 2002).

Given the high level of tobacco use by many indigenous peoples around the world, it is essential that their distinctive needs are addressed in national and global public health efforts to control the tobacco epidemic. Tobacco control among indigenous peoples is not adequately addressed within the framework of minority groups or vulnerable populations; more specific approaches are needed to address their distinctive tobacco control needs.

Smoking cessation and nicotine dependence

Smoking cessation decreases health risks, even at older ages (USDHHS 2004). However, many smokers try to quit but fail. Nicotine dependence is the major reason for relapse after quitting. Nicotine, an alkaloid, is a constituent of all tobacco products and a drug that leads to addiction (USDHHS 1988). Nicotine administration can lead to tolerance and physiological dependence. Tolerance is indicated by the diminished response to repeated doses of nicotine. Nicotine-induced physiological dependence and withdrawal are specific to the administration or removal of nicotine itself. Cessation from tobacco following chronic use results in withdrawal symptoms, including a craving for nicotine, impaired ability to concentrate, disrupted cognitive performance, mood changes, and impaired brain function (Hatsukami *et al.* 1985).

Cessation of smoking is a dynamic process with a cyclical nature. Over the course of time, many people alternate between smoking and non-smoking. Smoking cessation is not a discrete process but rather a complex process involving several stages. As mentioned previously, the trans-theoretical model, which uses stages of change to integrate processes and principles of change on people's behaviour, conceives behavioural change as a process involving five stages: Pre-contemplation, contemplation, preparation, action, and maintenance (Prochaska *et al.* 1997). Pre-contemplation is defined as a stage in which current smokers have no intention to give up smoking within the next 6 months. During contemplation, current smokers intend to give up smoking within the next 6 months. Current smokers in the preparation stage are seriously preparing to give up smoking within the next 30 days and take some steps in this direction, such as reading relevant materials. The action stage is defined as the first 6 months after smokers stop smoking. Lastly, maintenance continues from 6 months after stopping smoking until the person is a confirmed non-smoker without relapse.

There may be different stage profiles of smoking cessation across different countries and population groups. Understanding the various stage profiles might help public health officials to target messages and projects more appropriately. Tobacco control efforts or other forms of support aimed at smokers who are less ready to quit may promote their intention to quit. For example, results from a 2006 survey of 1750 smokers, aged 16–59, from five different European countries showed that the majority of smokers (73.5 per cent) wanted to stop smoking, and between 62.6 and 77.7 per cent of smokers can be categorized in the pre-contemplation stage. The study demonstrated that in countries with a high level of tobacco control, the proportion of people in the pre-contemplation stage is lower than in countries with low tobacco control activity (Thyrian *et al.* 2008).

The stage profile of cessation is different in developing countries. The 1996 National Prevalence Survey in China reported that about 72 per cent of smokers never intended to give up smoking and only about 16 per cent intended to do so (Yang *et al.* 2001).

Exposure to SHS

Non-smokers inhale SHS, the combination of sidestream smoke that is released as the cigarette burns and the mainstream smoke exhaled by active smokers (USDHHS 2006). SHS is a complex mixture of particles and gases that changes in character as it ages subsequent to its formation. Indicators of exposure to the SHS range from surrogate indicators, such as marriage to a smoker, to direct measurements of exposure and of biomarkers.

Detailed reviews of exposure assessment for SHS are provided in several recent reports from the United States: The 2005 report of the California Environmental Protection Agency and the 2006 report of the US Surgeon General (California Environmental Protection Agency 2005; USDHHS 2006). Questionnaires have proved effective for epidemiological research as have biomarkers; the extent of misclassification associated with questionnaires has been characterized in a number of populations, using biomarkers or other 'gold standards'.

In some countries, in which male smoking prevalence exceeds female smoking prevalence, one useful index at the national level is the husband's smoking status as an estimate of SHS exposure for wives. This index is potentially incomplete because it does not capture smoking by other family members or exposure outside of the home (Wang *et al.* 1994). Indirect measures used for research and surveillance include self-reported exposure and description of the source of SHS in relevant microenvironments, most often the home and workplace, obtained by using standardized questionnaires.

Nicotine and its metabolite cotinine have long been used as measures of tobacco smoke intake, whether from active smoking or inhaling SHS. The concentrations of serum and urinary cotinine in non-smokers increase significantly with the reported number of cigarettes smoked by their spouses; cotinine can be used to identify second-hand smokers and is sensitive to the extent of tobacco smoke exposure (California Environmental Protection Agency 2005; USDHHS 2006). However, cotinine with a half-life of about 20 h in nonsmokers provides a measurement of exposure within the last few days and does not reflect the long-term exposure to second-hand smoking.

Second-hand smoking exposure of a non-smoker is influenced by the number of smokers in the indoor environment, the intensity of their smoking, the duration of exposure, the volume of the indoor environment, and its ventilation characteristics (USDHHS 2006). The doses of SHS components reaching the respiratory tract further depend on one's breathing pattern and activity level. Homes, workplaces, and public places can all be loci of exposure to SHS, particularly the home for women and children in many societies (Wipfli *et al.* 2008). The prevalence of SHS exposure remains high, particularly in countries where the prevalence of smoking is high among men and low among women. For example, in a 2002 survey in China, 53 per cent of non-smokers reported that they were exposed to SHS (Yang *et al.* 2002). The prevalence rate of SHS exposure in females (54.6 per cent) was higher than that in males (49.1 per cent). The highest exposure to SHS (up to 60 per cent) was in middle-aged women. The majority of second-hand smokers were exposed every day, with 82 per cent reporting exposure at home, 35 per cent reporting exposure in their work environments, and 67 per cent being exposed in public places (Yang personal communication).

Studies document substantial exposures of younger children to SHS as well. Children's exposure to SHS is involuntary, arising from smoking, mainly by adults, in the places where they live, work, and play. WHO estimates that about 700 million, or almost half, of the world's children breathe air polluted by tobacco smoke, particularly at home (WHO 1999b). The GYTS data show that approximately 4 in 10 students (42.5 per cent) were exposed to smoke in their home, approximately half (55.1 per cent) of all students were exposed to SHS in public places during the week preceding the survey and more than three-fourths (78.3 per cent) of students in all WHO regions thought smoking should be banned in all public places (CDC 2008). In Hong Kong, China, from data on 8327 newborns in April and May 1997, 41.2 per cent were exposed to SHS at home, mainly from smoking by the father (Leung *et al.* 2004). For older children, the proportion of SHS exposure at home ranges from 42.1 to 47 per cent, and SHS exposure outside their homes from 35.2 to 67.3 per cent (WHO 2008). In a recent 31-country study, Wipfli and colleagues (2008) measured air nicotine in homes with and without smokers as well as nicotine concentration in the hair of women and children living in the homes. Having a smoking parent was associated with a doubling of the hair nicotine concentration. Air concentrations were substantially higher if smokers lived in the home. Importantly, in only a few percentage of homes was a policy in force with regard to smoking in the home.

Patterns and burden of tobacco-related diseases

Toxicology of tobacco smoke

Tobacco smoke is generated by the burning of a complex organic material, tobacco, together with various additives and paper at a high temperature, reaching several thousand degrees Celsius in the tip during puffing. The resulting smoke, comprising numerous gases and particles, contains many toxic components that can cause injury through inflammation and irritation, asphyxiation, carcinogenesis, and other mechanisms. Active smokers inhale mainstream smoke, i.e. the smoke that is drawn directly through the end of the cigarette. Passive smokers inhale SHS, as noted earlier. Concentrations of SHS are far below the levels of mainstream smoke inhaled by the active smoker, but there are qualitative similarities between SHS and mainstream smoke, as SHS comes predominantly from mainstream smoke (USDHHS 2006).

Both active and second-hand smokers absorb tobacco smoke components through the lung's airways and alveoli, and many of these components, such as the gas carbon monoxide, enter into the circulation and are distributed throughout the body. There is also uptake of some components, such as benzo[*a*]pyrene, directly into the cells that line the upper airways and the lung's airways. Some of the carcinogens undergo metabolic transformation into their active forms. The genitourinary system is exposed to toxins in tobacco smoke through the excretion of these compounds in the urine. The gastrointestinal tract is exposed through direct deposition of smoke in the upper airways and the clearance of smoke-containing mucus from the trachea through the glottis into the oesophagus. Not surprisingly, tobacco smoking has proved to be a cause of disease in almost all organs of the body in addition to diminishing health generally (USDHHS 2004).

There is a vast bank of scientific literature on the mechanisms by which tobacco smoking causes disease, disability, and death (USDHHS 1989, 2004; WHO 2004d). This literature includes characterization of many of the toxic components in smoke, which include well-known toxins such as hydrogen cyanide, carbon monoxide, and nitrogen oxides. The toxicity of smoke has been studied by exposing animals to tobacco smoke, in cellular and other laboratory toxicity assays, and by assessing smokers for evidence of injury by tobacco smoke using biomarkers such as tissue changes and levels of damaging enzymes and cytokines. The data from these studies amply document the powerful toxicity of tobacco smoke. For example, young smokers in their twenties already show evidence of permanent damage to the small airways of the lung (Niewoehner *et al.* 1974; PDAY Research Group 1990), and lavage of the lungs of smokers shows increased numbers of inflammatory cells and higher levels of markers of injury compared with non-smokers (USDHHS 1990). The new tools of molecular and cellular biology have provided evidence of tobacco-induced changes at the molecular level as well. For example, an activated tobacco-smoke carcinogen has been shown as binding to the same codon in the p53 gene where mutations are found in smokers with lung cancer (Denissenko *et al.* 1996). A variety of genetic changes are also found in epithelial cells in smokers' lungs (Wistuba *et al.* 1997).

WHO and the International Union Against Tuberculosis and Lung Disease have recently confirmed an association between active smoking and tuberculosis mortality through a qualitative systematic review (WHO 2007f), which examined five studies investigating the role of active smoking and tuberculosis mortality. All the studies showed strong effects of smoking on tuberculosis mortality, with the risk ratio ranging from 1.02 to 6.62. This effect appears to be independent of the effects of alcohol use, socioeconomic status, and a large number of other potential confounders.

The most useful epidemiological studies for assessing the health risks of tobacco were the cohort studies initiated in the 1950s, 1960s, and 1970s, together with the follow-up mortality analyses pertaining to this period (Lopez 1999). All are limited to the study of mortality, and give quantitatively similar results for the relative risks of smoking for various diseases (and all causes of death), despite the fact that the cohorts were recruited from countries as diverse as the United States, Sweden, Japan, Canada, and the United Kingdom. These findings have complemented the results of numerous case–control studies, some including thousands of cases (USDHHS 1989, 1997, 2001, 2006).

In the United States, the United Kingdom, and Canada, where men had been smoking in large numbers for decades before these studies were carried out, smoking was typically associated with 70–80 per cent excess mortality from all causes (Peto *et al.* 1996). The relative risks varied substantially by disease, and were largest for cancers of the lung and upper aerodigestive tract (mouth, pharynx, larynx and oesophagus), and lowest for vascular diseases that have complex multicausal aetiologies. Typically, lung cancer death rates were 10–12 times higher in smokers than in non-smokers, with the notable exception of Japanese men and American women for whom the excess risks were three to four times that of non-smokers. Similarly, the all-cause mortality ratios (relative risks) were substantially lower in these two studies, reflecting the fact that tobacco use in the two populations had been much lower than in other cohorts.

Relative risks of lung cancer for American women smokers versus lifelong non-smokers increased from 2.7 in 1959–1965 to 11.9 in 1982–1986, reflecting the dominant role of duration of exposure in determining lung cancer hazards (USDHHS 1989, 2006).

Two large cohort studies have produced evidence on health hazards from smoking, which have emphasized the increasing hazards of smoking with longer duration of use. These two studies are the 50-year follow-up of the 1951 British doctors cohort (Doll *et al.* 2004) and the second American Cancer Society Cancer Prevention Study (CPS-II) cohort of over 1.2 million adults monitored since 1982, for which comparisons can be made with CPS-I, initiated 20 years earlier (Thun *et al.* 1997).

The alarming size of the hazards observable in populations that have been smoking for many decades is now apparent. In the first 20 years of follow-up of the British doctors cohort (1951–1971), smokers had, on an average, about a 1.5–2-fold higher death rate at each age, similar to the excess reported in other studies around that time (Doll *et al.* 1994, 2004). With a longer duration of smoking, the death rates of smokers increased substantially, so that during the second period of follow-up (1971–1991), the death rate of middle-aged smokers was three times higher than that of non-smokers (Doll *et al.* 1994, 2004). A similar excess mortality ratio was found in the CPS-II cohort based on follow-up in the latter half of the 1980s. These relative risks suggest that, on an average, a smoker who begins smoking in young adult life and continues to smoke has at least a 50 per cent chance of eventually being killed by tobacco in either middle or old age (Peto *et al.* 1994).

The evidence from these two studies of the disease-specific risks associated with smoking is similar (Lopez 1999). Current smokers have about a 20-fold higher death rate from lung cancer than never-smokers, among whom lung cancer death rates have remained low and constant. There is epidemiological evidence to suggest that this is also the case in other populations. For example, based on the two American Cancer Society studies with follow-up to 1959–1965 and 1982–1986, respectively, lung cancer death rates among lifelong non-smokers were remarkably constant at 15.4 and 14.7 per 1 00 000 (age-standardized) for men, and 9.6 and 12 for women; the rates for current smokers were 187.1 and 341.3 for men, and 26.1 and 154.6 for women (Thun *et al.* 1997). A more recent study on the CPS-II cohort showed that relative risks of colorectal cancer mortality ranged from 1.32 in male to 1.41 in female smokers when compared with never smokers (Chao *et al.* 2000). Smokers also incur a 10–20-fold excess mortality from chronic obstructive lung disease (primarily chronic bronchitis and emphysema), and a risk of death from major vascular diseases that is about twice that of non-smokers.

The excess mortality of smokers from vascular disease is particularly noteworthy. Vascular disease death rates are typically much higher than those for cancer or other causes associated with smoking. Therefore, cardiovascular diseases (especially ischaemic heart disease and stroke) contribute more to smoking-attributable deaths at a population level than other causes, including lung cancer for which the relative risk is much higher, although this pattern will change as cardiovascular disease mortality declines. Finally, it is worth noting that the all-age excess mortality ratio of about two from cardiovascular diseases masks a very significant age gradient in relative risks. At younger ages (<50 years), smokers have a 5–6-times higher death rate than non-smokers, with the relative excess declining with age. These data suggest that if a smoker dies from vascular disease before the age of about 50 years, there is a 70–80 per cent chance that death was caused by smoking, and that vascular disease is the chief mechanism through which smoking causes a threefold excess mortality rate in middle age (Parish *et al.* 1995). However, cigarette smoking is only one of several causative factors of cardiovascular disease. This is especially true for ischaemic heart disease, where smoking interacts synergistically with other factors such as hypercholesterolemia and hypertension to increase risk of heart disease substantially. Evidence suggests that the independent risk attributable to smoking is comparable with that of other major risk factors (USDHHS 2004). The interaction with dietary parameters probably explains the historically lower proportions of ischaemic heart disease attributable to smoking in populations such as China where low-fat diets have predominated (Liu *et al.* 1998).

Smoking by women adversely affects reproduction. Smoking during pregnancy reduces birth weight by approximately 200 g on an average (USDHHS 1990); and the degree of reduction is dose-related. With successful cessation by the third trimester, much of the weight reduction can be avoided. Smoking also increases rates of spontaneous abortion, placenta praevia and perinatal mortality, and smoking during pregnancy is now considered to be a cause of sudden infant death syndrome. There is more limited evidence suggesting that smoking may increase childhood cancer incidence and congenital defects (Charlton 1996; SCOTH 1998).

Cigarettes have changed substantially over the last 50 years (USDHHS 1997). Filtered cigarettes now dominate the market, and tar and nicotine yields, as assessed by smoking machines, have declined substantially. Although tar and nicotine deliveries to smokers have little relationship to machine-measured levels (USDHHS 1997), early epidemiological evidence comparing switchers to filtered cigarettes with continued use of non-filtered cigarettes showed some reduction in lung cancer risk. Subsequent epidemiological evidence on cancer risk in relation to yield of tar has shown little indication of reduced risk for lung cancer; in fact, comparisons of risks of lung cancer in smokers over time show an increase in relative risk, compared with never smokers (USDHHS 2001, 2004). A reduction has not been observed for cardiovascular disease in association with lower yield, as measured by a machine (USDHHS 2001, 2004). Although rising relative risks of smoking have been documented across recent decades when the lower-delivery products came into widespread usage (Doll *et al.* 1994), this is due to a longer duration of exposure and not to a change in the hazard.

Evidence on health risks of SHS

Evidence on the health risks of SHS comes from epidemiological studies which have directly assessed the associations of SHS exposure with disease outcomes and also from knowledge of the components of SHS and their toxicities. Judgements as to the causality of association between SHS exposure and health outcomes are based not only on this epidemiological evidence, but also on the extensive evidence derived from epidemiological and toxicological investigation of active smoking. The evidence is clear: Exposure to SHS causes illness and death. As US Surgeon General Richard Carmona commented in releasing his 2006 report on SHS, the scientific community has reached consensus on this point (USDHHS 2006).

In the United States, it is estimated to cause as many as 50 000 premature deaths each year, making it the third leading preventable cause of death (California Environmental Protection Agency 2005).

Additionally, studies using biomarkers of exposure and dose, including the nicotine metabolite cotinine and white cell adducts, document the absorption of SHS components by exposed non-smokers, adding to the plausibility of the observed associations of SHS with adverse effects.

Second-hand smoke exposure of the infant and child has adverse effects on respiratory health, including increased risk for more severe lower respiratory infections, middle-ear disease, chronic respiratory symptoms, and asthma, as well as a reduction in the rate of lung function growth during childhood. Maternal smoking during gestation and subsequent SHS exposure increase risk for sudden infant death syndrome (California Environmental Protection Agency 2005; USDHHS 2006). There is more limited evidence suggesting that SHS exposure of the mother reduces birth weight (Zhang & Ratcliffe 1993) and that child development and behaviour are adversely affected by parental smoking (Eskenazi & Castorina 1999; WHO 1999b). There is no strong evidence at present that SHS exposure increases childhood cancer risk (WHO 2004d; USDHHS 2006).

In adults, SHS exposure has been causally associated with lung cancer and may also increase the risk of ischaemic heart disease. In 1986, the conclusion was reached by a number of agencies that SHS caused lung cancer, including the United States Surgeon General (USDHHS 1986), and the US National Research Council (NRC 1986). The International Agency for Research on Cancer (IARC) also concluded that SHS must give rise to some risk of cancer. Arguments that the association of SHS exposure with lung cancer risk in never-smokers could reflect confounding or information bias were considered and set aside in these and subsequent reports. Since 1986, other expert groups have also found SHS to be a cause of lung cancer in non-smokers (EPA 1992; Australian National Health and Medical Research Council 1997; California Environmental Protection Agency 1997, 2005; SCOTH 1998; WHO 2004d; USDHHS 2006).

The risk has been quantified in several meta-analyses, beginning with the 1986 US National Research Council report (NRC 1986). The risk associated with marriage to a smoker has been around 20–30 per cent; a meta-analysis by IARC (WHO 2004d) of 46 studies and 6257 cases yielded a point estimate of 24 per cent (95% CI: 14–34 per cent). Several other recent meta-analyses further quantify the association between SHS and lung cancer. Stayner *et al.* performed a meta-analysis of 22 studies published through 2003 on workplace SHS exposure and lung cancer, in which the pooled relative risk was found to be 1.24 (95% CI: 1.18–1.29). Among highly exposed workers, the relative risk was 2.01 (95% CI: 1.33–2.60) (Stayner *et al.* 2007). Taylor *et al.* performed a meta-analysis to calculate a pooled estimate of relative risk of lung cancer associated with exposure to SHS in never-smoking women exposed to smoking spouses. Using 55 studies (7 cohort, 25 population-based case–control, and 23 non-population-based case–control studies) published through 2006, the authors found a pooled relative risk for lung cancer of 1.27 (95% CI: 1.17–1.37) (Taylor *et al.* 2007).

Coronary heart disease has also been causally associated with SHS exposure on the basis of observational and experimental evidence (Barnoya & Glantz 2005; California Environmental Protection Agency 2005; USDHHS 2006). Exposure to SHS has been shown to unfavourably affect blood clotting parameters and endothelial cell function. The meta-analysis prepared for the 2006 US Surgeon General's Report estimated the pooled excess risk for coronary heart disease from SHS exposure from marriage to a smoker as 27 per cent (95% CI: 19–36 per cent) (USDHHS 2006). There is also evidence linking SHS to other adverse effects in adults, including stroke (Bonita *et al.* 1999), exacerbation of asthma, reduced lung function and respiratory symptoms (USDHHS 2006).

Summarizing the health risks of SHS, the 2006 US Surgeon General Report examined the topics of toxicology of SHS, assessment and prevalence of exposure to SHS, reproductive and developmental health effects, respiratory effects of exposure to SHS in children and adults, cancer among adults, cardiovascular diseases, and the control of SHS exposure (USDHHS 2006). This report included six overall conclusions which are provided below.

'The scientific evidence with regard to the involuntary exposure of nonsmokers to tobacco smoke, supports the following major conclusions:

- Second-hand smoke causes premature death and disease in children and in adults who do not smoke.
- Children exposed to SHS are at an increased risk for sudden infant death syndrome, acute respiratory infections, ear problems, and more severe asthma. Smoking by parents causes respiratory symptoms and slows lung growth in their children.
- Exposure of adults to SHS has immediate adverse effects on the cardiovascular system and causes coronary heart disease and lung cancer.
- The scientific evidence indicates that there is no risk-free level of exposure to SHS.
- Many millions of Americans, both children and adults, are still exposed to SHS in their homes and workplaces despite substantial progress in tobacco control.
- Eliminating smoking in indoor spaces fully protects non-smokers from exposure to SHS. Separating smokers from non-smokers, cleaning the air, and ventilating buildings cannot eliminate exposures of non-smokers to SHS'.

Burden of tobacco-related diseases

In 1953, Levin proposed an epidemiological statistic, now referred to as the population attributable risk, for estimating the burden of disease caused by a particular factor in a population (Levin 1953). He was motivated to do so by the emerging information on the association of lung cancer with smoking and the consequent need to understand the related burden of disease. His basic approach has now been widely applied. The global and regional projections of mortality and burden of disease by cause had been published by Murray and Lopez in 1997, and were based on data from 1990. In 2006, Mathers and Loncar updated the projection using more recent data (Mathers & Loncar 2006). They applied the same method applied in the original Global Burden of Disease Study. In relation to tobacco-related deaths, the smoking impact ratios (SIR) were used as an indirect indicator of accumulated smoking risk based on excess lung cancer mortality. Smoking impact ratio measures the absolute excess lung cancer mortality due to smoking in the study population, relative to the excess lung cancer mortality in lifelong smokers of the reference population. Estimated tobacco attributable deaths were 5.4 million in 2005, 6.4 million in 2015 and 8.3 million in 2030. Tobacco attributable deaths are expected to decline in developed countries (9 per cent decrease between

2002 and 2030), but double in low- and middle-income countries (from 3.4 to 6.8 million). By 2015, smoking is expected to cause 50 per cent more deaths than HIV/AIDS, and will be responsible for 10 per cent of all deaths.

Certain countries have contributed to a significant proportion of the world's burden of disease and deaths attributed to tobacco. In China, tobacco killed 1 million smokers by 2000, and by 2020, 2 million will die if the number of smokers continues to grow at present rate (Gan *et al.* 2007). In India, in a national-and population-based case–control study that included 1.1 million households, prevalence of smoking was compared in 74 000 deceased subjects with 78 000 living unmatched subjects. The authors estimated that smoking was associated with higher risk of death in women (risk ratio 2) and in men (risk ratio 1.7). Smoking was associated with a reduction in life expectancy of 8 years in women and 6 years in men. By 2010, if the actual smoking prevalence remains unchanged, almost 1 million deaths will be attributed to tobacco, with 70 per cent of them occurring in middle-aged people (Jha *et al.* 2008).

The tobacco industry

A distinguishing feature of the tobacco epidemic has been the role of major corporations—some of the largest in the world—in promoting tobacco use and, as a consequence, death and disease. This presents a unique challenge for the public health community. The adversary is not only disease or natural forces. It also includes powerful corporations whose actions are antithetical to public health as discussed earlier in the chapter.

As the 21st century begins, the transnational tobacco companies are increasing their presence in global markets. While total consumption of cigarettes is falling in several high-income countries, consumption in low- and middle-income countries is increasing (WHO 2008).

Given the growing influence of the multinationals, an understanding of their history, conduct, and behaviour is essential to help guide strategies for tobacco control. In the mid- to late-1990s, the public health community gained an unprecedented view of the tobacco industry through the release of millions of pages of previously secret internal tobacco company documents (Bero 2003). These documents were obtained primarily through court proceedings in lawsuits against tobacco companies in the United States.

The global corporate actors

While tobacco in diverse forms has been used since antiquity, the modern cigarette did not become a popular phenomenon until the twentieth century, with the invention of the mechanical cigarette rolling machine. With a dramatically increased production capacity, the modern tobacco industry was born (Detels *et al.* 2002). Currently, much of the world's cigarette market is dominated by a few transnational tobacco companies, as articulated earlier in this chapter.

Decades of deceit

Starting in the mid-to-late 1990s, millions of pages of previously secret internal documents from mostly United States-based tobacco companies or companies doing business in the United States, were publicly released in the country secondary to a series of court cases against tobacco companies (WHO 2000b, 2004; Hirschhorn 2005). Analyses of these documents paint a damning picture of an industry which for decades suppressed scientific research and information on the health hazards and addictiveness of smoking, manipulated the amount and/or form of nicotine to exploit the addictive potential of tobacco, and targeted marketing campaigns at youth (Detels *et al.* 2002; Bero 2003). Recently, other sources of information about the tobacco companies' behaviour are also being used in the development of reports to guide policy-making in tobacco control (Hiilamo & Hirschhorn 2006).[5] One of the most comprehensive analyses of the tobacco companies' deceptive practices can be found in the final report of the United States Department of Justice case against the tobacco companies operating within the country (US Department of Justice 2004, 2006); while dozens of papers and reports have been published looking at the information contained in the tobacco companies' internal documents.[6]

The above documents make clear that many transnational tobacco companies, often in collaboration with each other, have engaged in a decades-long campaign to publicly deny the harmful effects of tobacco use and the addictive powers of nicotine, while these companies' internal research confirmed what was being said by academics and public health professionals. At the same time, these tobacco companies had developed technology in the production of cigarettes to enhance their addictive powers and had manipulated the cigarette development process so as to attract a larger number of consumers across different groups, such as women and ethnic minorities (Wayne & Connolly 2002; Cook *et al.* 2003; Ferris Wayne *et al.* 2006; Hammond *et al.* 2006; Lewis & Wackowski 2006; Milberger *et al.* 2006). The companies have also engaged in joint programmes to deny the harmful effects of SHS exposure, which is yet to be clearly accepted by tobacco companies, and developed sophisticated public relations and political campaigns to stop or deter public policies promoting smoking bans in public places (Ong & Glantz 2000; Drope & Chapman 2001; Samet & Burke 2001; Dearlove *et al.* 2002; Assunta *et al.* 2004). It is also clear how tobacco companies have used funding to subvert the scientific process, igniting the debate of the role of tobacco companies' funding in science and research and calls for such funding to be banned (Malone & Bero 2003; Parascandola 2003; Bero 2005; Chapman 2005; Thomson & Signal 2005; Hirschhorn *et al.* 2006).

In many instances, the tobacco companies indirectly exert their influence on tobacco control policy-making through the funding or creation of front groups and alliances, in order to avoid any negative publicity that might be associated with a tobacco company (Chapman 2003; Smith & Malone 2006; Apollonio & Bero 2007). Additionally, the internal documents show how the tobacco companies work in the political sphere at the local, national, and international levels to stop effective tobacco control policies from moving forward, including strategies to monitor and influence the development of the WHO FCTC and tobacco control advocacy efforts (Francey & Champman 2000; Jamrozik 2000; Saloojee & Dagli 2000; Bialous & Yach 2001; Carter 2002; Gilmore & McKee

---

5 These documents can be found online at: http://legacy.library.ucsf.edu/ and http://bat.library.ucsf.edu/.

6 A list of these publications can be found online at: http://www.library.ucsf.edu/tobacco/docsbiblio.html#mar.

2004; MacKenzie *et al.* 2007; Tong & Glantz 2004; McDaniel *et al.* 2006, 2008; Gilmore *et al.* 2007). Awareness of these strategies could better prepare policy-makers and public health officials to counter the industry efforts of derailing tobacco control (Ling & Glantz 2002; Thomson & Wilson 2005; Chapman 2006).

In the area of advertising and promotion, the tobacco companies have developed target marketing campaigns, including sponsorship of cultural and sports events, have worked to circumvent marketing restrictions when attempts to prevent or modify marketing restrictions had failed and have developed new products to continue to appeal to young people (Dewhirst & Hunter 2002; Pollay & Dewhirst 2002; Neuman *et al.* 2002; Wakefield *et al.* 2002; Assunta & Chapman 2004; Barbeau *et al.* 2004; Smith & Malone 2004; Anderson *et al.* 2005; Carpenter *et al.* 2005; LeGresley *et al.* 2006; MacKenzie *et al.* 2007). There is also an evidence of the tobacco companies' involvement, or at least, awareness of contraband of its products in several regions of the world (Joosens & Raw 2002; WHO 2003a; Collin *et al.* 2004; Lee & Collin 2006).

More recently, several transnational tobacco companies have engaged in efforts to present themselves as socially responsible corporations, when analysis of the industry documents demonstrate that these efforts are no more than public relations campaigns in response to increasing litigation against the industry, as well as increasing public perception of the tobacco companies as untrustworthy (Hirschhorn 2004; McDaniel & Malone 2005; Palazzo & Richter 2005; Szczypka *et al.* 2007).

As the multinational tobacco companies shift their attention to emerging markets, an understanding of the structure and behaviour of the tobacco industry becomes imperative as public health professionals attempt to fashion strategies to deal with a growing epidemic. These strategies cannot be formed and implemented in a vacuum. The tobacco industry is the vector, and only by knowing its history and conduct, monitoring its current behaviour, and regulating and restricting the environment in which the industry operates, can public health strategies be effective.

Tobacco control

The preventive potential for tobacco control to reverse the given forecast of a global tobacco epidemic is still high in many countries. We now have an improved understanding of the complexity of the tobacco epidemic, which will assist us to improve and activate interventions. The main focus of any strategy should be to prevent initiation of tobacco use, to promote quitting among the young and adults and to eliminate non-smokers' exposure to tobacco smoke. Cost-effective strategies are available and have already been proven to make a positive impact in many countries. To build on those successes, a comprehensive tobacco control strategy can provide a road map for national and global action. In this section, we explore the key components of a comprehensive tobacco control strategy that is applicable locally, regionally, and globally. A multifaceted strategy is needed to assure success of global tobacco control. The components of such a strategy will broadly include education and information, legislative measures, economic measures, cessation efforts, crop substitution and diversification, advocacy, litigation, and administration and management. Appropriate monitoring, evaluation, and surveillance are essential to assess the effectiveness of specific interventions. Strong political commitment on both national and global levels is essential for sustaining success.

The following sections will first provide the background and status of the WHO FCTC, followed by an outline of the MPOWER package as essential components of a comprehensive, WHO FCTC-based tobacco control strategy. Additionally, these sections will highlight other important measures such as product regulation, youth access, crop substitution and diversification, and litigation. Finally, the role of management and administration in establishing a sustained strategy will also be discussed.

The WHO framework convention on tobacco control

In May 1999, the WHO Member States unanimously paved the way for negotiations to begin on the WHO FCTC, a multilateral treaty addressing the tobacco epidemic, and possible related protocol agreements. Under Article 19 of its Constitution, WHO has the legal authority to serve as a platform for the development of binding treaties on health-relevant issues, which includes potentially all aspects of tobacco control, national and transnational. Major tobacco growers and exporters, as well as several countries in the developing and developed world that face the brunt of the tobacco industry's marketing and promotion, strongly supported the need for an international treaty to address the tobacco control epidemic.

The framework convention protocol approach has been used to address a wide range of international concerns, including environmental, arms control, and human rights issues. The term 'framework convention' does not have a particular technical meaning in international law. It is used to describe a variety of legal agreements which establish a general system of governance for an issue area, such as global tobacco control. Framework conventions, unlike more comprehensive forms of treaties, do not attempt to resolve all significant issues in a single document. Rather, they divide the negotiation of separate issues into separate agreements. States first adopt a framework convention, which creates an institutional forum in which states can co-operate and negotiate for the conclusion of separate implementing protocols containing detailed obligations or added institutional commitments. The framework convention/protocol approach is a dynamic and incremental process of global law-making that allows the political will of states, as signatories to international legal agreements, to be titrated gradually into legally binding commitments. The WHO FCTC is open for ratification, acceptance, approval, formal confirmation and accession indefinitely for States and eligible regional economic integration organizations wishing to become parties to it (WHO 2008). As of 1 February 2009, there were a total of 168 signatories and 162 Parties (WHO 2008).

The WHO FCTC entered into force on 27 February 2005, and WHO convened the first session of the COP, the treaty's governing body, in Geneva from 6 to 17 February 2006, in accordance with the Convention's Article 23 *Conference of the Parties*. During that first session, the Parties agreed on a number of procedural and substantive matters, formalized as decisions. They adopted Rules of Procedure to guide their interactions and a budget, funded exclusively by voluntary assessed contributions from Parties, and Financial Rules and Regulations to provide the necessary monetary structure for the work of the Convention. Additionally, the Conference established the Convention Secretariat in decision FCTC/COP1(10), which was confirmed and adopted by reference by the Health Assembly in May 2006. The Convention Secretariat is part of the WHO structure, reporting to the COP on technical and treaty matters and to the WHO Director General on administrative and certain technical matters. The Convention Secretariat is mandated to work closely and synergistically with TFI to provide the necessary support to implement the WHO FCTC.

At its first session, the COP also established two kinds of intersessional groups to move the work of the treaty forward. Working groups, composed of interested Parties and invited experts from civil society were formed to develop guidelines for the implementation of Article 8 *Protection from exposure to tobacco smoke* and Articles 9 and 10 *Regulations of the contents of tobacco products* and *Regulation of tobacco product disclosures*, respectively. Expert groups, comprising of four experts from each of the six WHO regions and invited experts from civil society, were established to draft templates for protocols on advertising, promotion and sponsorship of tobacco products and the illicit trade in tobacco products. The reports of the Working Groups and the Expert Groups were submitted to the Parties for their consideration at the second session of the COP, held in Bangkok, 30 June–6 July 2007.

At its second session, the Conference made important strides forward in the efforts to control tobacco use globally. Among the decisions taken in Bangkok, the Parties adopted guidelines for the implementation of Article 8 *Protection from exposure to tobacco smoke* that include strong language regarding the need for areas to be entirely smoke free. The work of the Articles 9 and 10 Working Group was continued and three new guideline development working groups were created, one each for Articles 5.3 *General Obligations*, Article 11 *Packaging and labelling of tobacco products*, Article 12 *Education, communication, training and public awareness* and Article 13 *Tobacco advertising, promotion and sponsorship*. At its third session, held in Durban, 17-22 November 2008, the Conference adopted guidelines for implementation of Articles 5.3, 11, and 13 and established two new working groups to develop guidelines, one each for Article 12 *Education, communication, training and public awareness* and Article 14 *Demand reduction measures concerning tobacco dependence and cessation*. Additionally, the Parties decided to enter into negotiation of a protocol on illicit trade in tobacco products. As such, the Conference established an intergovernmental negotiating body (INB), a subsidiary body of the Conference, mandated to negotiate the text of the protocol, using the template developed by the expert group as the basis for initiating its work. The INB has met twice in Geneva, the first time from 11 to 16 February 2008 and the second time from 20 to 25 October 2008. A Chairperson's text was submitted to the INB for its consideration at its second session; a revised Chairperson's text will be submitted for consideration at the third session, scheduled to take place from 28 June to 5 July 2009, in Geneva.

As noted in the chapter on International Public Health Instruments, the WHO FCTC provides an effective instrument for counteracting the globalization of the tobacco pandemic by serving as a platform for multilateral commitment, co-operation, and action to address the rise and spread of tobacco consumption. The globalization of the tobacco epidemic restricts the capacity of countries to control tobacco unilaterally within their sovereign borders (Bettcher & Yach 1998). All transnational tobacco control issues, including trade, smuggling, advertising and sponsorship, prices and taxes, control of toxic substances, and tobacco package design and labelling, require multilateral cooperation and effective action at the global level. It is clear that national and transnational dimensions of tobacco control must be addressed in tandem; in the absence of effective international co-operation even the most comprehensive national control programmes can be unravelled (Bettcher *et al.* 2000).

The adoption and entry into force of the WHO FCTC was the start of a unique new chapter in global public health. WHO's ongoing

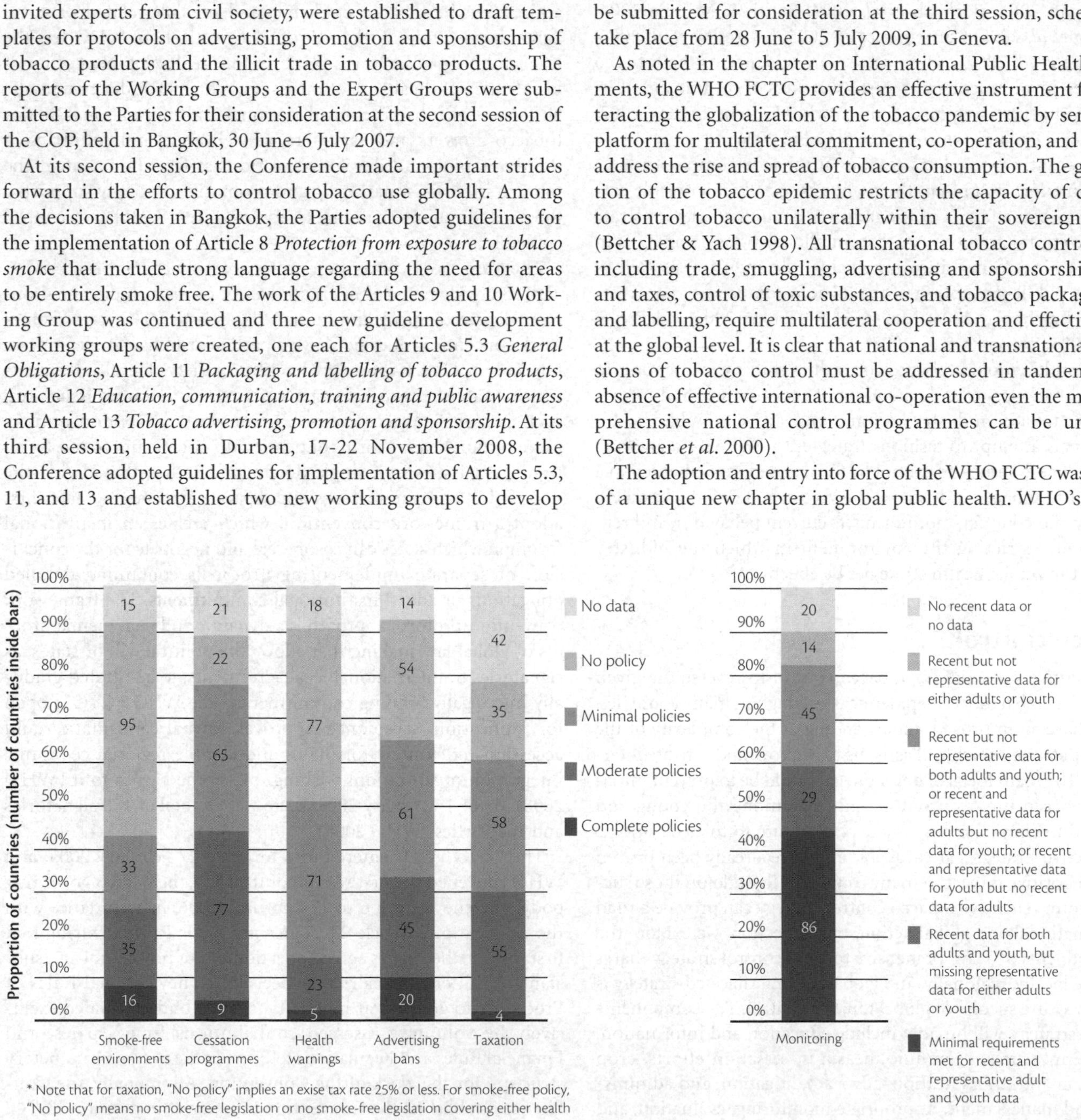

* Note that for taxation, "No policy" implies an exise tax rate 25% or less. For smoke-free policy, "No policy" means no smoke-free legislation or no smoke-free legislation covering either health care or educational facilities.

Fig. 10.1.6 The state of tobacco control policies in the world.
Source: WHO (2008a).

commitment to the WHO FCTC and global tobacco control implementation has been supported by its selection as a partner in the Bloomberg Initiative to Reduce Tobacco Use. The WHO FCTC and the MPOWER implementation strategy combine an overwhelming scientific evidence base with an evolving global social movement. This work links science and international relations at the global level as a vehicle for addressing a totally preventable man-made epidemic.

MPOWER

The WHO FCTC provides the foundation and context for effective global tobacco control policy intervention. As WHO's technical assistance package for the WHO FCTC, WHO released the MPOWER package of six cost-effective mechanisms proven to reduce tobacco use, each of which reflects at least one provision of the WHO FCTC (WHO 2008). Each of the elements of MPOWER reflects one or more provisions of the WHO FCTC. The six proven strategies of MPOWER are:

- Monitor tobacco use and prevention policies (Articles 20 and 21 of the WHO FCTC)
- Protect people from tobacco smoke (Article 8 of the WHO FCTC)
- Offer help to quit tobacco use (Article 14 of the WHO FCTC)
- Warn about the dangers of tobacco (Articles 11 and 12 of the WHO FCTC)
- Enforce bans on tobacco advertising, promotion and sponsorship (Article 13 of the WHO FCTC)
- Raise taxes on tobacco (Article 6 of the WHO FCTC)

Although there has been progress in recent years, no government is fully implementing all of these key interventions.

This translates to only a small portion—not more than 5 per cent in any circumstance—of the world's population being covered by comprehensive tobacco control policies (WHO 2008a).

Monitoring, surveillance and evaluation

Countries need accurate measures of tobacco use to effectively plan, implement, and evaluate tobacco control strategies. An effective national or international monitoring system must track several indicators, which include prevalence of tobacco use; impact of policy interventions; and tobacco industry marketing, promotion, and lobbying (WHO 2008). Comprehensive monitoring informs leaders of governments and civil society about the extent of the tobacco epidemic in their countries, helps them allocate tobacco control resources accordingly and shows them how effective the existing policies are.

Surveillance refers to the systematic and ongoing process of collection, collation, and analysis of data at national, regional, and global levels, as well as the timely dissemination of this information. Surveillance of tobacco use can guide policy decisions, research initiatives, and the development and evaluation of intervention programmes (Giovino 2000; WHO 2008). An ideal surveillance system would monitor variables contained in the traditional epidemiological model of agent, host, vector, and environment (Orleans & Slade 1993). Surveillance of agent factors (i.e. various tobacco products) may include monitoring of toxic constituents, pH, and additives. Most surveillance work monitors host factors (i.e. smoker/user or potential smoker/user) and the measures may include: Patterns of initiation, susceptibility of tobacco use, indicators of dependence, quitting patterns and methods, receipt of advice to quit from physicians and dentists, mental health indicators, use of behaviours, sources of tobacco, prices paid for cigarettes, usual brand, receptivity to marketing, awareness of tobacco control programmes and opinions about tobacco control policies. Surveillance of vector (i.e. tobacco product manufacturers) includes chronicling tobacco industry public relations, lobbying, and marketing activities. Environmental surveillance (economic, cultural, political, and historical) includes national tobacco control legislation and programmes, exposure to health messages; and tobacco promotions, prices, and placements (Giovino 2000).

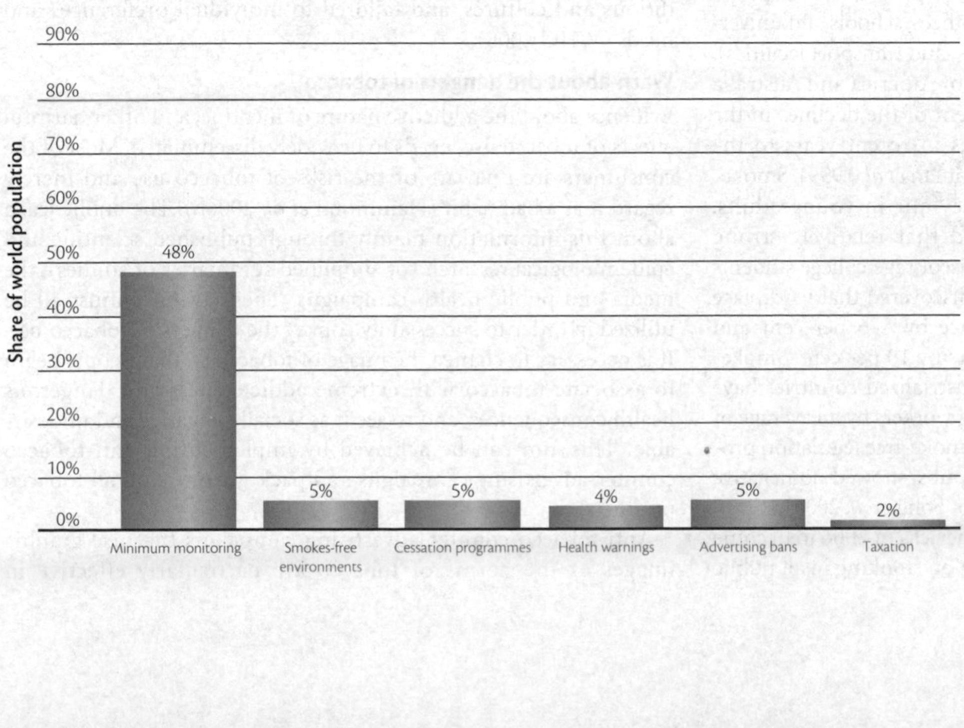

Fig. 10.1.7 Share of the world population covered by tobacco control policies.
Source: WHO (2008a).

For instance, the WHO Global Tobacco Surveillance System (GTSS) includes the collection of standard and comparable data through four surveys: Global Youth Tobacco Survey (GYTS), Global School Personal Survey (GSPS), Global Health Professions Students Survey (GHPSS) and Global Adult Tobacco Survey (GATS). The purpose of the GTSS is to enhance the capacity of countries to design, implement, and evaluate their national comprehensive tobacco action plan (GTSS Collaborative Group 2005). The GYTS focuses on youth aged 13–15 and collects information in schools. The GSPS surveys teachers and administrators from the same schools who participate in the GYTS. The GHPSS focuses on third-year students pursuing degrees in dentistry, medicine, nursing, and pharmacology. The GATS, a household survey, monitors tobacco use among adults aged 15 and above. The surveys cover a wide range of topics related to tobacco, including tobacco use prevalence (smoking and other tobacco products); exposure to SHS; cessation; risk perceptions; knowledge and attitudes; exposure to media; price and taxation on tobacco products; and sociodemographic characteristics.

Surveillance is also a crucial part of evaluation research. In order to ensure that the utility of both surveillance and evaluation research are maximized, programme evaluations should be built upon and complement tobacco-related surveillance systems. However, it is also important that specific evaluation surveys and data collection systems are implemented to evaluate individual programme activities. Ensuring that surveillance and evaluation are used in concert will serve to link programmes at national, regional, and global levels to facilitate progress towards intermediate and primary outcome objectives in tobacco control. It must also be highlighted that findings from the surveillance system must be effectively disseminated and used, especially in the policy-making process.

Protect people from tobacco smoke

Smoke-free environments are becoming increasingly popular, and such policies are important because they protect non-smokers from exposure to tobacco smoke, reduce smoker's consumption of cigarettes and induce some smokers to quit (Brownson *et al.* 1997; Chapman *et al.* 1999). Many countries are enacting comprehensive smoke-free legislation in all enclosed public spaces and workplaces (such as healthcare facilities, government offices, schools and universities, restaurants and bars, day-care centres, and transport facilities).

Studies conducted in the United States of America and Australia have attributed between 13 and 22 per cent of the declines in the tobacco consumption in these countries in recent years to the impact of smoke-free environments (Chapman *et al.* 1999). Smoke-free policies also alter tobacco use behaviour in young adults. Chaloupka and Wechsler (1997) found that relatively strong restrictions on smoking in public places discourage college students from smoking; while Evans *et al.* (1999) discovered that workplace smoking bans reduce smoking prevalence by 4–6 per cent and average daily consumption among smokers by 10 per cent. Smoke-free policies in workplaces in several industrialized countries have reduced total tobacco consumption among workers by an average of 29 per cent (Fichtenberg & Glantz 2002). Smoke-free legislation proposed in Ireland in 2006, which included pubs, showed no negative impact on business or profits (Howell 2005; Fong *et al.* 2006).

Uruguay was the first country in the Americas in 2006 to become 100 per cent smoke-free by enacting a ban on smoking in all public spaces and workplaces, including bars, restaurants and casinos. About half of all Americans and 90 per cent of Canadians live in areas where public spaces and workplaces are smoke-free (PAHO 2007). It is clear that there is growing support from countries to enact comprehensive smoke-free legislation. In this regard, WHO recommends a step by step approach to creating and enforcing smoke-free environments (WHO 2004a).

Offer help to quit tobacco use

Integrating tobacco cessation within primary healthcare systems and available healthcare services can be effective. Programmes that assist young and adult smokers to stop smoking can produce quicker public health benefits through incorporating cessation services in primary care, offering quit lines, providing affordable pharmacological treatment options and government support. Smokers who quit before the age of 50 halve their risk of dying in the next 15 years (USDHHS 1990). In addition, the cost savings from reduced tobacco use resulting from the implementation of moderately priced and effective smoking cessation interventions would more than pay for these interventions within 3–4 years (Wagner *et al.* 1995).

Evidence shows that advice from healthcare practitioners can increase cessation rates (Fiore *et al.* 2000). Quit lines linked to counselling and treatment are also effective, and if well-designed and managed, can be accessible widely.

On the other hand, pharmacological therapy such as nicotine replacement therapies (NRT) are generally expensive, considered to be less cost-effective than physicians' advice and quit lines and more difficult to obtain in many countries. However, NRT have been demonstrated to double or triple quit rates (Tobacco Advisory Group 2000; Silagy *et al.* 2004), and could increase demand for and effectiveness of cessation efforts (Fiore *et al.* 2000). Over-the-counter forms of NRT include nicotine patches, gum, nasal spray, inhaled nicotine and sublingual nicotine. Prescription drugs such as Bupropion and Varenicline have also proven to be effective. Access to low-cost pharmacological therapy is helpful to tobacco users who want to quit.

It is important for governments to provide support for tobacco users to quit in the context of robust public policies. Furthermore, treatment for tobacco dependence should be adapted to local conditions and cultures, and tailored to individual preferences and needs (WHO 2008).

Warn about the dangers of tobacco

Evidence about the addictive nature of nicotine, and other harmful effects of tobacco use, needs to be widely disseminated. Most of the consumers are unaware of the risks of tobacco use and merely regard it as a bad habit (Hammond *et al.* 2006b). The public learn about this information mainly through published scientific and epidemiological research (or simplified summaries of studies), the media and public health campaigns. These avenues must all be utilized in order to successfully convey the dangers of tobacco use. It is necessary to change the image of tobacco so that people begin to associate tobacco with extreme addictiveness and dangerous health consequences, and to see it as socially negative and undesirable. This aim can be achieved by implementing anti-tobacco counter-advertising campaigns and pack warnings on all tobacco products.

Anti-tobacco counter-advertising campaigns that use graphic images of the harms of tobacco are particularly effective in promoting users to quit (Siahpush *et al.* 2006). They should also be professionally designed and produced, relevant to the context of the country and strategically placed in all forms of media. By publicizing the full extent of tobacco's dangers, these campaigns have the potential to prevent use, promote quitting and expose the tobacco industry tactics, while promoting a tobacco-free society. The downside to counter-advertising is that effective campaigns can be expensive. The United States Centers for Disease Control and Prevention recommend that governments spend about 15–20 per cent of total tobacco control programme costs on counter-advertising campaigns (USDHHS 2007). In addition to paid advertising, 'earned media' in the form of television and radio coverage, news stories in print, broadcast and online media and letters to the editor and opinion articles can be a highly effective and inexpensive way to communicate the harms of tobacco, increase attention on tobacco control initiatives and counter tobacco industry misinformation.

Warnings on the packaging of tobacco products also play a pivotal role in conveying the health risks of tobacco to its users. Health warnings increase smokers' awareness of their risk (Hammond *et al.* 2006b), and their ultimate goal is to cause cessation. Evidence shows that the effectiveness of these warnings increases with their prominence—larger warnings with pictures have more impact compared to smaller, text-only health warnings. WHO also recommends that packaging of tobacco products should not contain deceptive terms such as 'low tar', 'light', or 'mild'—all of which create the false impression that a particular product is less harmful than others, but do not actually signify any reduction in health risk (WHO 2006).

Enforce bans on tobacco advertising, promotion and sponsorship

Tobacco marketing is a strong impediment to tobacco control efforts. It has the potential to 'normalize' tobacco, encourage potential users, mislead the consumer with false information and strengthen industry influence over the media. Tobacco advertising and promotion activities stimulate adult consumption and increase the risk of youth initiation (USDHHS 1994). Children buy the most heavily advertised brands (USDHHS 1994) and are three times more susceptible to advertising than are adults (Pollay *et al.* 1996).

The success of the Marlboro cigarettes advertising campaign highlights the obstacles in altering consumer behaviour (Elliot 1995). By projecting the image of a free-spirited, masculine cowboy, the Marlboro Man falsely associates smoking with independence, enjoyment, relaxation, and 'being cool'. Deceptive marketing strategies such as this make it difficult for the public to understand the hazards of smoking. In light of these ubiquitous and sustained pro-tobacco use messages, counter-marketing efforts of comparable intensity are needed to alter the environmental context of tobacco use.

Since 1972, the most high-income countries have introduced stronger restrictions on advertising and promotion of tobacco products across more media and on various forms of sponsorship. A study of 22 high-income countries based on data from 1970 to 1992 concluded that comprehensive bans on cigarette advertising and promotion can reduce smoking, while more limited partial bans have little or no effect. The study concluded that if the most comprehensive restrictions were in place, tobacco consumption would fall by more than 6 per cent in high-income countries (World Bank 1999). Another study of 100 countries compared consumption trends over time in those with relatively complete bans on advertising and promotion and those with no such bans. In the countries with nearly complete bans, the downward trend in consumption was much steeper (World Bank 1999).

There are reasons to believe that young people are more receptive to advertising than are adults (Pierce *et al.* 1991; McCann 1992); hence a comprehensive advertising ban may prevent potential users, mostly young people, from trying tobacco and consequently becoming long-term users. There is also growing evidence that the tobacco industry is directing increasing shares of its advertising and promotion activity towards markets where there is judged to be growth or potential for growth, including some youth markets and specific minority groups among whom tobacco use has been uncommon until recently (USDHHS 1998).

It must be emphasized that advertising, promotion, and sponsorship bans should be complete and apply to all marketing and promotional categories in order to be effective (WHO 2004a). Partial bans enable the tobacco industry to retain their marketing power, particularly towards young people who are potential users and adults who want to quit. If only certain marketing channels are blocked, e.g. television and radio, the tobacco industry will shift its budgets to other avenues such as magazines, newspapers, billboards, and the Internet. If only these traditional advertising channels are blocked, the industry can then replace advertising with sponsorship of events that are particularly attractive to young people. There is also a growing need for international bans as more tobacco companies are advertising and selling their products through the Internet. Comprehensive marketing bans must be regularly amended so as to keep up with the innovations in industry tactics and media technology (WHO 2008).

Raise taxes on tobacco

Evidence from several countries shows that increases in price on tobacco products are highly cost-effective in reducing demand. Higher taxes induce some smokers to quit and prevent others from starting. They also reduce the number of ex-smokers who return to cigarettes and reduce consumption among continuing smokers. On an average, a price rise of 10 per cent on a pack of cigarettes would be expected to reduce demand for cigarettes by about 4 per cent in high-income countries and by about 8 per cent in low- and middle-income countries (World Bank 1999). Evidence also shows that a 70 per cent increase in the price of tobacco could prevent up to a quarter of all smoking-related deaths worldwide (Jha *et al.* 2006). Children and adolescents are more responsive to price rises than older adults, and so this intervention would have a significant impact on them. Currently, four-fifths of high-income countries tax tobacco at more than 50 per cent of retail price while less than a quarter of low and middle income countries tax tobacco at 50 per cent or more of the retail price (WHO report 2008).

Several myths exist in the economics of tobacco control. First, it is often believed that smokers always bear the costs of their consumption choices. The reality is that smokers do impose certain costs on non-smokers. These costs include health damage, nuisance, and irritation from exposure to SHS. In addition, smokers can impose financial costs on others (e.g. treatment of diseases caused by exposure to second-hand smoke and bearing a portion of smokers' excess healthcare costs). In high-income countries, smokers' healthcare costs on an average exceed those of non-smokers in any given year (Warner 2000). Second, it is often argued that tobacco control will result in permanent job losses for an economy.

In actuality, tobacco control policies will lead to only a slow decline in global tobacco use so that the transition will be phased over several decades. Furthermore, money not spent on tobacco will be spent on other goods, generating alternative employment. Third, many believe that governments will lose revenues if they increase cigarette taxes, because people will buy fewer cigarettes. The reality is at complete variance with this claim. The evidence is clear: Calculations show that even substantial cigarette tax increases will still reduce consumption and increase tax revenues. This is in part because the proportionate reduction in demand does not match the proportionate size of the tax increase. Historically, raising tobacco taxes has led to increases in cigarette tax revenues. Fourth, it is often claimed that cigarette taxes have a disproportionate impact on the poor. Although less-wealthy individuals tend to smoke more, it does not necessarily follow that the poor pay a greater share of their income in tobacco taxes. This reasoning ignores the effect that tax increases have on the prevalence and initiation of tobacco use, and also ignores the benefits of cessation; it ignores the evidence that shows that the young and the poor are more responsive to price increases. It is also instrumental to note that the main concern of policy-makers should be the distributional impact of the entire tax and expenditure system, and not particular taxes in isolation. Finally, contrary to claims by the tobacco industry, tax increases do not necessarily promote smuggling. Other factors contribute to smuggling such as corruption, weak policies to tackle smuggling, and porous borders, among others. An interesting example is Spain, which for years had lower tobacco taxes and more smuggling than most other European countries. When the Spanish government raised tobacco taxes and stepped up law enforcement in the 1990s, tobacco revenues increased by 25 per cent while smuggling took a dramatic decline (WHO 2003b).

In summary, it is important to note that higher tax increases government revenues and effectively decreases consumption, in particular among the young and the poor. Smuggling, on the other hand, can only effectively be tackled through strict customs policies and law enforcement. Given the importance of controlling smuggling, the Parties to the WHO FCTC are currently negotiating a legally binding protocol on illicit trade that will counter smuggling and counterfeiting. This protocol should markedly increase international cooperation on this critical issue.

Other measures

Product regulation

As WHO seeks to minimize the impacts of tobacco on morbidity and mortality, it must create and endorse public health policies that rest on firm scientific foundation. In the area of tobacco product regulation, which is defined by WHO as the governmental oversight and enforcement of how tobacco products are manufactured (ingredients and emissions), distributed, packaged, and labelled in order to promote public health protection, the regulation of tobacco products is encompassed within a set of provisions contained in Articles 9, 10, and 11 of the Framework Convention that are targeted at the regulation of the manufacture and distribution of tobacco products. The scientific basis for the principles guiding the implementation of Articles 9 and 10 establishes the rationale for the principles guiding the implementation of Article 11. For this reason, and in order to achieve the synergistic effect of these provisions, all three articles should be treated as a single set of interrelated and mutually reinforcing regulations.

To assist countries in improving their capacity to regulate tobacco products, WHO has created an expert Study Group, working groups, and a global network of tobacco testing and measuring laboratories in order to increase capacity to inform policymakers as they make decisions at the international, regional, and national level. The work of these groups addresses the effects of nicotine, tobacco contents and emissions, smokeless tobacco, harm reduction products, and other tobacco product regulation issues, in accordance with Article 9, which provides for the adoption of guidelines on the testing and measuring of contents and emissions of tobacco products, and for the regulation of such contents and emissions, and Article 10, which sets forth requirements for product disclosures (WHO 2005).

Research and scientific evidence informed the negotiation of Articles 9, 10, and 11 of the WHO FCTC (WHO 2006), which govern tobacco product regulation. To help establish the content of Articles 9–11, WHO created an *ad hoc* Scientific Advisory Committee on Tobacco Product Regulation (SACTob), which held its first meeting in October 2000 (WHO 2004c). SACTob provided sound scientific information on tobacco product regulation, which eventually 'served as the basis for negotiations and subsequent consensus reached on the language of these three articles of the Convention' (WHO 2007e). In November 2003, recognizing the continuing critical importance of tobacco product regulation, the WHO Director-General changed the status of the SACTob from an *ad hoc* committee to a formal study group, the WHO Study Group on Tobacco Product Regulation (TobReg). TobReg is composed of experts on product regulation, tobacco-dependence treatment, and the laboratory analysis of tobacco ingredients and emissions. Its work is based on cutting edge research on tobacco product issues and recommends research and testing in order to fill in the regulatory gaps of tobacco control (WHO 2007b).

As mentioned earlier, to implement Articles 9, 10, and 11, government regulatory authorities require some degree of laboratory capacity and global uniformity to guide and validate tobacco product testing (WHO 2004b). Responding to this need, and to a TobReg recommendation, WHO Tobacco Free Initiative created the WHO Tobacco Laboratory Network (TobLabNet). TobLabNet is a global network of government, academic, and independent laboratories that furthers the objectives of Article 9 by addressing tobacco product testing and research on product contents and emissions on a global level. TobLabNet is unique in its scientific treatment of tobacco and in its consideration of the fact that 'temporal and geographical variations are important sources of product variability that should be included in any examination of the differences within and across products' (WHO 2005). Thus, TobLabNet strengthens national and regional capacity for the research and verification testing of the contents and emissions of tobacco products. Once capacity is established, TobLabNet will be a main source of laboratory support, methods development and validation, and scientific information for tobacco testing and research, allowing national governments to meet the requirements prescribed by the WHO FCTC (WHO 2007d).

The WHO Tobacco Free Initiative currently serves as the Secretariat and coordinating body for both TobReg and TobLabNet (WHO 2007d). In recognition of the valuable work of TobReg and TobLabNet and to avoid redundancy, the Conference of the Parties (COP) to the WHO FCTC at its first session in February 2006 (WHO 2007c) decided to set up a working group of Parties to develop guidelines for the implementation of Articles 9 and 10 of the WHO FCTC, referring to the work of TobReg and TobLabNet. The working group provided a progress report to the COP at its second session in July 2006 and another progress report at its third session in November 2008. The progress report provides an outline for future work that will take several years to accomplish. Therefore, the efforts by the working group are ongoing and TobReg and TobLabNet continue to provide expert and technical advice as needed (WHO 2007b). For example, and further to the work on the guidelines development for product regulation, TobLabNet is currently preparing to perform international validation of test methods for three contents (nicotine, ammonia, and humectants) and emissions (tobacco-specific nitrosamines, benzo[a]pyrene, aldehydes, and volatile organic compounds).

WHO looks forward to a day when tobacco, a product that kills half of its consumers when used as intended by manufacturers, is forced to operate under a heavily regulated environment such that regulatory agencies will have the information and resources to collaborate with other regulatory agencies (such as, trend data and product characteristic and design features linked to exposure and harm biomarkers) and to act to prevent further harm to the public.

Some current WHO recommendations related to product regulation are as follows:

- Ban the use of misleading terms such as 'light', 'mild', and other words or imagery (including certain brand names), which have the aim or effect of implying a reduced health risk attributable to low tar or nicotine measurements on tobacco products and in advertising/promotional material.
- Remove tar and nicotine measures derived from International Organization for Standardization methods from packages. Warning labels should emphasize the addictiveness of tobacco products.
- Require tobacco manufacturers to disclose the contents, purpose, and effects of constituents in all their products at regular intervals.
- Develop and implement a comprehensive long-term communication programme to accompany all the above actions that stresses that there is no safe cigarette and that nicotine addiction is a major public health concern.
- In order to reduce the addictiveness of tobacco products, research is urgently needed to evaluate the benefits and/or hazards of reducing nicotine and other possible addictive constituents in tobacco products over time. Particular attention should be given in research to determining whether a threshold exists for addictiveness.
- Determine whether countries should forbid addition of all new additives and explicitly address the possibility of reducing the use of additives that make tobacco products more attractive and/or taste better.

These recommendations are likely to be implemented in some form over the next few decades by many countries and represent a significant new focus of tobacco control efforts.

Youth access laws

As recognized in Article 16 of the WHO FCTC, youth access laws limit the supply of tobacco products to youths who are too young to comprehend the risks of consuming tobacco products. Youth access laws are designed to limit the availability of tobacco to minors from commercial sources (stores, pharmacies, vending machines, samples from distributors). The rationale for governments enacting youth access restrictions rests primarily on the fact that minors should be protected from the inherent dangers of tobacco as they do not know how to access or accurately appreciate the risks of becoming addicted to nicotine (USDHHS 1994). Jurisdiction attempts to prohibit the sale of cigarettes to minors by establishing minimum age-at-sale laws, banning self-service displays, limiting vending machines to adult-only locations or banning them completely, banning the sale of loose cigarettes, and outlawing the distribution of free samples to minors. Additionally, some jurisdictions require retail vendors to be licensed to sell tobacco products, and some laws include revocation of the license if retailers repeatedly violate minimum age-at-sale laws. In general, youth restrictions are difficult to enforce, because youths often obtain cigarettes from their older peers and sometimes from their parents. There have been several unsuccessful attempts to impose restrictions on the sale of cigarettes to teenagers in many developed countries. In many developing countries where tobacco consumption is rising, the infrastructure and resources needed to implement and enforce such restrictions are not available.

The literature provides mixed evidence on the effectiveness of youth access laws in reducing youth smoking prevalence. Retailer compliance with laws prohibiting sales to minors can be increased through active enforcement (DiFranza & Brown 1992; Cummings *et al.* 1998; Forster & Wolfson 1998), educational interventions (Altman *et al.* 1991; Feighery *et al.* 1991; Gemson *et al.* 1998), and community involvement (Forster *et al.* 1998). Forster and Wolfson (1998) summarize workable policies to restrict youth access to tobacco. Strong youth access intervention programmes should enforce one or all of the following means of restricting supply:

- Complete restrictions on distribution, such as bans on free samples and coupons
- Regulation of the means of sale through bans or locks on vending machines, placement of tobacco products behind service counters to limit self-service, and prohibitions on the single/loose cigarettes
- Regulation of the seller through tobacco products licensing requirements, which includes possible revocation and the passage of minimum age-at-sale laws whose violation results in stiff penalties and fines

Even successful efforts to reduce sales in stores can be undermined in two ways. First, young people can often locate the small percentage of stores that continue to sell to minors. Additionally, young people often can find an older (or older appearing) friend or acquaintance who will purchase tobacco for them.

Crop substitution and diversification

Historically, tobacco is a highly attractive crop to the farmers, providing a higher net income yield per unit of land than most cash crops and substantially more than food crops. In the best tobacco-growing areas of Zimbabwe, tobacco is approximately 6.5 times more profitable than the next best alternative crop. Farmers also find tobacco an attractive crop for more practical reasons because the global price of tobacco is relatively stable, the tobacco industry provides in-kind supports and loans to the farmers, tobacco is less perishable than many other crops, and the industry assists with delivery or collection (World Bank 1999).

There have been a number of experimental schemes to substitute other crops for tobacco. For example, in developing countries, a number of alternative crops have been identified, which include cassava in Brazil, sugarcane in Kenya, and chillies, soya beans, cotton, and mustard in India (Reddy & Gupta 2004). However, there is no hard evidence, except in Canada, that these schemes succeed, where a tobacco diversification plan provided incentives to stop growing tobacco and develop alternatives to assist the orderly downsizing the tobacco industry (PAHO 1992).

An important development in this area has been the establishment of the study group on economically sustainable alternatives to tobacco growing by the COP at its first session in February 2006. The aims of the study group include summarizing the uptake of existing economically viable alternatives for tobacco-related workers, growers and, as the case may be, individual sellers; recommending to the COP mechanisms to assess the impact over time of the tobacco companies practices; reporting on initiatives that are being taken at national level in accordance with Article 17; and recommending cost-effective diversification initiatives. The study group met for the first time in February 2007 in Brasilia, Brazil. Background documentation prepared for the meeting intended to summarize existing literature and research on the issues related to tobacco growing and crop substitution. One of the key conclusions of the meeting was that there was insufficient research on health, environmental and socioeconomic impacts of tobacco growing and that there was a need for deeper analysis of financial factors of crop substitution, particularly targeting at the case of small farmers. The second meeting of the study group was convened in June 2008 in Mexico and aimed particularly to expand the scope of work by updating experiences from the first study group meeting (current progress of case studies, focusing on challenges and lessons learned), and introducing additional relevant cases. Another objective is to review cross-national analysis in selected topics: Drawing common aspects, understanding different contexts, and identifying best practices.

Litigation

The WHO FCTC acknowledges that litigation can be an effective public health intervention in the area of tobacco control. This has been demonstrated most dramatically by recent events in the United States. In the mid- and late-1990s, there was a new wave of litigation against the tobacco industry in the United States. There were a variety of forms of litigation, including lawsuits filed by individual smokers, class action lawsuits by large groups of smokers, and lawsuits filed by victims of SHS. To date, the most successful litigation against the tobacco industry in the United States has been a series of actions brought by the Attorneys General of individual states.

The lawsuits brought by the Attorneys General focused on the conduct of the tobacco industry, not merely the product *per se*. Among other things, these lawsuits sought to recover the enormous sums of money that the states spent in healthcare costs for persons with smoking-related disease. These lawsuits alleged that the tobacco industry had misrepresented and concealed the health risks and addictiveness of smoking, manipulated the form and/or amount of nicotine in cigarettes to ensure their addictive potential, conspired to suppress health research, and targeted youth in their advertising and marketing campaigns. Thus, the legal bases for these lawsuits generally focused on consumer protection and antitrust statutes (JAMA 1995).

The Attorneys General lawsuits were all successfully resolved by settlement with the tobacco industry in 1997 and 1998. The settlement agreements resulted in the payment of billions of dollars to the states. While the ultimate disposition of this money is not entirely resolved, and in some cases is the subject of fierce political battles, some of the funds have been dedicated to tobacco control efforts, infusing the tobacco control community with unprecedented levels of funding. In addition, beyond the monetary terms, the settlements provided for a variety of injunctive relief, including the prohibition of marketing to children, the banning of certain types of advertising and promotion (i.e. billboards and movie placements), and the dissolution of two of the tobacco industry's longtime trade groups, the Tobacco Institute and the Council for Tobacco Research. The Attorneys General litigation and settlements also resulted in the release of millions of pages of previously secret documents from the files of the tobacco industry. These documents paint a damning picture of the tobacco industry's conduct for decades, and contain a wealth of information that can help guide public health activities for years to come.

The US Department of Justice filed a landmark lawsuit under the civil racketeering (RICO) law on 22 September 1999, to hold Philip Morris International legally accountable for decades of illegal and harmful practices. The trial in the case lasted from 21 September 2004 to 9 June 2005. It was recommended that the tobacco company be required to pay US$130 billion to fund cessation and prevention programmes, however in the end no financial remedies were given. The company was found guilty of decades of deception and fraud and was banned from making future deceptive statements, eliminating misleading descriptor words such as 'light' and 'mild', improving health warnings, and making all internal documents open to the government and public.

Class action lawsuits have also been successful. In Florida, a group of flight attendants filed a lawsuit on behalf of non-smoking flight attendants exposed to SHS. The case was settled in October 1997 in exchange for a US$300 million fund to research the diagnosis and treatment of diseases caused by SHS.

The litigation was successful in the United States in large part because new successful alliances forged between attorneys and the public health community. The American Medical Association, in an unusual step, recommended in 1995 that 'all avenues of individual and collective redress should be pursued through the legal system' (JAMA 1995). Prominent public health professionals provided invaluable assistance in the litigation by serving as expert witnesses.

Litigation against the tobacco industry is now being pursued in a number of countries, including Canada, France, India, Israel, Ireland, Germany, Australia, Poland, South Korea, Nigeria, and the Marshall Islands. In many countries, this type of litigation is unusual, and it is still too early to anticipate how the various actions will play out. The risks and challenges of litigation against the tobacco industry (which fiercely opposes lawsuits with virtually unlimited resources) are very large. In the United States, e.g. litigation against the tobacco industry began in 1954, and for more than 40 years (until the breakthroughs in the 1990s), the tobacco industry won every single case. Thus, the prospect of litigation needs to be carefully evaluated before any decisions to proceed are undertaken. However, the potential rewards in terms of public health objectives can be enormous. In some jurisdictions, where there are promising theories of liability and sufficient resources, litigation may be one way to achieve tobacco control objectives in a forum—the courts—which may not be subject to the same political influences as legislative bodies.

Administration and management

An effective global tobacco control requires a well-designed and efficient management structure to facilitate co-ordination of programme components at the country, regional, and global levels. Experience from other successful public health programmes such as smallpox, tuberculosis, and poliomyelitis has demonstrated the importance of an organized administrative and management systems. Because a comprehensive programme involves multiple partners, programme management and co-ordination is a challenging task. Furthermore, co-ordinating efforts require adequate resources, training and communication systems. Administration and management activities include (a) recruiting and training qualified, technical, programme, and administrative staff, (b) coordinating implementation across programme areas and assessing programme performance, (c) creating an effective communication system, and (d) developing a sound fiscal management and reporting systems.

Acknowledgements

The authors would like to acknowledge the following people for their contributions towards the chapter: A.D. Lopez, Derek Yach, Anne-Marie Perucic, Ayda Yurekli, Dongbo Fu, and Daniel Ferrante.

References

Aghi, M., Asma, S., Yeong, C.C., Vaithinathan, R. (2001). Initiation and maintenance of tobacco use among girls and women. In J.M. Samet and S.Y. Yoon, eds. *Women and the tobacco epidemic: Challenges for the 21st century*. WHO, Geneva.

Altman, D.G., Rasenick-Douss, L., Foster, V., Tye, J.B. (1991). Sustained effects of an educational program to reduce sales of cigarettes to minors. *American Journal of Public Health*, **81**, 891–3.

AMAP (Arctic Monitoring and Assessment Programme) (1998). *AMAP assessment report: Arctic pollution issues*. AMAP, Oslo.

Anderson, S.J., Glantz, S.A., Ling, P.M. (2005). Emotions for sale: Cigarette advertising and women's psychosocial needs. *Tobacco Control*, **14**, 127–35.

Anderson, S.J., Dewhirst, T., Ling, P.M. (2006). Every document and picture tells a story: Using internal corporate document reviews, semiotics, and content analysis to assess tobacco advertising. *Tobacco Control*, **15**(3), 254–61.

Apollonio, D.E., Bero, L.A. (2007). The creation of industry front groups: The tobacco industry and "Get Government off our Back". *American Journal of Public Health*, **97**(3), 419–27.

Assunta, M., Chapman, S. (2004). 'The world's most hostile environment': How the tobacco industry circumvented Singapore's advertising ban. *Tobacco Control*, **13**(2), ii51–7.

Assunta, M., Fields, N., Knight, J., Chapman, S. (2004). Care and feeding: The Asian environmental tobacco smoke (ETS) consultants programme. *Tobacco Control*, **13**(2), ii4–12.

Australian Bureau of Statistics (2002). *National aboriginal and torres strait islander social survey*, p. 13. ABS, Canberra.

Australian National Health and Medical Research Council (1997). *The health effects of passive smoking. A scientific information paper*. Australian Government Publishing Service, Canberra.

Barbeau, E., Leavy-Sperounis, A., Balbach, E. (2004). Smoking, social class, and gender: What can public health learn from the tobacco industry about disparities in smoking? *Tobacco Control*, **13**, 110–20.

Barnoya, J., Glantz, S.A. (2005). Cardiovascular effects of secondhand smoke: Nearly as large as smoking. *Circulation*, **111**, 2684–98.

Bero, L.A. (2003). Implications of the tobacco industry documents for public health and policy. *Annual Review of Public Health* **24**, 267–88.

Bero, L.A. (2005). Tobacco industry manipulation of research. *Public Health Reports*, **120**, 200–8.

Bettcher, D., Yach, D. (1998). The globalization of public health II: The convergence of self-interest and altruism. *American Journal of Public Health*, **88**, 839.

Bettcher, D., Yach, D., Guindon, G.E. (2000). Global trade and health: Key linkages and future challenges. *Bulletin of the World Health Organization*, **78**, 521–34.

Bialous, S., Yach, D. (2001). Whose standard is it anyway? How the tobacco industry determines the International Organization for Standardization (ISO) standards for tobacco and tobacco products. *Tobacco Control*, **10**, 96–104.

Bonita, R., Duncan, J., Truelsen, T., Jackson, R.T., Beaglehole, R. (1999). Passive smoking as well as active smoking increases the risk of acute stroke. *Tobacco Control*, **8**, 156–60.

Brandt, A.M. (2007). *The cigarette century: The rise, fall and deadly persistence of the product that defined America*. Basic Books, New York.

Brownson, R.C., Eriksen, M.P., Davis, R.M., Warner, K.E. (1997). Environmental tobacco smoke: Health effects and policies to reduce exposure. *Annual Review of Public Health*, **18**, 163–85.

California Environmental Protection Agency (1997). *Health effects of exposure to environmental tobacco smoke: Fnal report*. California Environmental Protection Agency, Office of Environmental Health Hazard Assessment, Sacramento, CA.

California Environmental Protection Agency (2005). *Proposed identification of environmental tobacco smoke as a toxic air contaminant*. California Environmental Protection Agency, Office of Environmental Health Hazard Assessment, Sacramento, CA.

Carpenter, C.M., Wayne, G.F., Pauly, J.L., Koh, H.K., Connolly, G.N. (2005). New cigarette brands with flavours that appeal to youth: Tobacco marketing strategies. *Health Affairs*, **24**, 1601–10.

Carter, S.M. (2002). Mongoven, Biscoe & Duchin: Destroying tobacco control activism from the inside. *Tobacco Control*, **11**, 112–8.

CDC (Centers for Disease Control and Prevention) (2008a). Youth Risk Behavior Surveillance United States 2005. Surveillance Summaries, *Morbidity and Mortality Weekly Report* 2008, **57** (No. 25).

CDC (Centers for Disease Control and Prevention) (2008b). Global youth tobacco surveillance, 2000–2007. Surveillance summaries. *Morbidity and Mortality Weekly Report 2008*, **55** (No. SS-1).

Chaloupka, F.J., Wechsler, H. (1997). Price, tobacco control policies and smoking among young adults. *Journal of Health Economics*, **16**, 359–73.

Chaloupka, F.J., Corbett, M. (1998). Trade policy and tobacco: Towards an optimal policy mix. In I. Abedian, ed. *The economics of tobacco control*, pp. 129–45. Applied Fiscal Research Center, University of Cape Town. Cape Town, South Africa.

Chao, A., Thun, M.J., Jacobs, E.J., Henley, S.J., Rodriguez, C., Calle, E.E. (2000). Cigarette smoking and colorectal cancer mortality in the Cancer Prevention Study II. *Journal of the National Cancer Institute*, **92**(23), 1888–96.

Chapman, S., Borland, R., Scotto, M., Brownson, R.C., Dominetto, A., Woodward, S. (1999). Impact of smoke-free workplaces on declining cigarette consumption in Australia and United States. *American Journal of Public Health*, **89**, 1018–23.

Chapman, S. (2003). 'We are anxious to remain anonymous': The use of third party scientific and medical consultants by the Australian tobacco industry, 1969 to 1979. *Tobacco Control*, **12**(3), 31–7.

Chapman, S. (2005). Research from tobacco industry affiliated authors: Need for particular vigilance. *Tobacco Control*, **14**, 217–9.

Chapman, S. (2006). Regulating the global vector for lung cancer. *Lancet*, **367**, 706–8.

Charlton, A. (1996). Children and smoking: The family circle. *British Medical Bulletin*, **52**, 90–107.

Collin, J., LeGresley, E., MacKenzie, R., Lawrence, S., Lee, K. (2004). Complicity in contraband: British American Tobacco and cigarette smuggling in Asia. *Tobacco Control*, **13**(2), ii104–11.

Conrad, K.M., Flay, B.R., Hill, D. (1992). Why children start smoking cigarettes: Predictors of onset. *British Journal of Addiction*, **87**, 1711–24.

Cook, B., Wayne, G., Keithly, L., Connolly, G. (2003). One size does not fit all: How the tobacco industry has altered cigarette design to target consumer groups with specific psychological and psychosocial needs. *Addiction*, **98**, 1047–61.

Cummings, K.M., Hyland, A., Saunders-Martin, T., Perla, J., Coppola, P.R., Pechacek, T.F. (1998). Evaluation of an enforcement program to reduce tobacco sales to minors. *American Journal of Public Health*, **88**, 932–6.

Dearlove, J., Bialous, S., Glantz, S.A. (2002). Tobacco industry manipulation of the hospitality industry to maintain smoking in public places. *Tobacco Control*, **11**, 94–104.

Denissenko, M.F., Pao, A., Tang, M., Pfeifer, G.P. (1996). Preferential formation of benzo[*a*]pyrene adducts at lung cancer mutational hotspots in P53. *Science*, **274**, 430–2.

Detels, R., McEwen, J., Beaglehole, R., Tanaka, H., eds (2002). *Oxford textbook of public health, 4th ed.* Oxford University Press, New York.

Dewhirst, T., Hunter, A. (2002). Tobacco sponsorship of Formula One and CART auto racing: Tobacco brand exposure and enhanced symbolic imagery through co-sponsors' third party advertising. *Tobacco Control*, **11**, 146–50.

DiFranza, J.R., Brown, L.J. (1992). The Tobacco Institute's 'It's the Law' campaign. Has it halted illegal sales of tobacco to children? *American Journal of Public Health*, **82**, 1271–3.

DiFranza, J.R., Lew, R.A. (1995). Effect of maternal cigarette on pregnancy complications and sudden death infant syndrome. *Journal of Family Practice*, **40**, 385–94.

Doll, R., Peto, R., Wheatley, K., Gray, R., Sutherland, I. (1994). Mortality in relation to smoking: 40 years observations on male British doctors. *British Medical Journal*, **309**, 901–11.

Doll, R., Peto, R., Boreham, J., Sutherland, I. (2004). Mortality in relation to smoking: 50 years' observations on male British doctors. *British Medical Journal*, **328**, 1519.

Drope, J., Chapman, S. (2001). Tobacco industry efforts at discrediting scientific knowledge of environmental tobacco smoke: A review of internal industry documents. *Journal of Epidemiology and Community Health*, **55**, 588–94.

Durie, M.H. (1998). *Whaiora–Maori health development*. Oxford University Press, Auckland.

Elliot, S. (1995). Uncle Sam is no match for the Marlboro Man. *The New York Times*, 27 August, C1.

EPA (Environmental Protection Agency) (1992). *Respiratory health effects of passive smoking: Lung cancer and other disorders.* EPA/600/006F. US Government Printing Office, Washington, DC.

Eskenazi, B., Castorina, R. (1999). Association of prenatal maternal or postnatal child environmental tobacco smoke exposure and neurodevelopmental and behavioral problems in children. *Environmental Health Perspectives*, **107**, 991–1000.

Evans, W.N., Farrelly, M.C., Montogomery, E. (1999). Do workplace smoking bans reduce smoking? *American Economic Review*, **89**, 728–47.

Fant, R.V., Henningfield, J.E., Nelson, R.A., Pickworth, W.B. (1999). Pharmacokinetics and pharmacodynamics of moist snuff in humans. *Tobacco Control*, **8**, 387–92.

FAO (Food and Agricultural Organization) (2006). *FAOSTAT database.* [Online]. Available at: http://faostat.fao.org/site/567/DesktopDefault.aspx?PageID=567.

FDA (Food and Drug Administration) (1996). Regulations restricting the sale and distribution of cigarettes and smokeless tobacco to children and adolescents: final rule. *Federal Register*, **61**, 44395–618.

Feighery, E., Altman, D.G., Shaffer, G. (1991). The effects of combining education and enforcement to reduce tobacco sales to minors. *Journal of the American Medical Association*, **266**, 3168–71.

Ferris Wayne, G., Connolly, G.N., Henningfield, J.E. (2006). Brand differences of free-base nicotine delivery in cigarette smoke: The view of the tobacco industry documents. *Tobacco Control*, **15**(3), 189–98.

Fichtenberg, C.M., Glantz, S.A. (2002). Effect of smoke-fee workplaces on smoking behaviour: Systematic review. *British Medical Journal*, **325**(7357), 188.

Fiore, M.C., Hyland, A., Borland, R. *et al.* (2000). Treating tobacco use and dependence: A public health service clinical guidelines. US Department of Health and Human Services, Rockville, MD, press briefing.

Fong, G.T., Bailey, W.C., Cohen, S.J. *et al.* (2006). Reductions in tobacco smoke pollution and increase in support for smoke-free public places following the implementation of comprehensive smoke-free workplace legislation in the Republic of Ireland: Findings from the International Tobacco Control (ITC) Ireland, UK Survey. *Tobacco Control*, **15** (Suppl. 3), iii51–8.

Forster, J.L., Wolfson, M. (1998). Youth access to tobacco: Policies and politics. *Annual Review of Public Health*, **19**, 203–35.

Forster, J.L., Murray, D.M., Wolfson, M., Blaine, T.M., Wagenaar, A.C., Hennrikus, D.J. (1998). The effects of community policies to reduce youth access to tobacco. *American Journal of Public Health*, **88**, 1193–8.

Francey, N., Chapman, S. (2000). Operation Berkshire: The international tobacco companies' conspiracy. *British Medical Journal*, **321**, 371–4.

Gan, Q., Smith, K.R., Hammond, S.K., Hu, T.W. (2007). Disease burden of adult lung cancer and ischaemic heart disease from passive tobacco smoking in China. *Tobacco Control*, **16**, 417–22.

Garfinkel, L. (1997). Trends in cigarette smoking in the United States. *Preventive Medicine*, **26**, 447–50.

Gemson, D.H., Moats, H.L., Watkins, B.X., Ganz, M.L., Robinson, S., Healton, E. (1998). Laying down the law: Reducing illegal tobacco sales to minors in central Harlem. *American Journal of Public Health*, **88**, 936–9.

Gilmore, A.B., McKee, M. (2004). Moving east: How the transnational tobacco companies gained entry to the emerging markets of the former Soviet Union. Part I: Establishing cigarette imports. *Tobacco Control*, **13**, 43–100.

Gilmore, A., Radu-Loghin, C., Zatushevski, I., McKee, M. (2005). Pushing up smoking incidence: Plans for a privatised tobacco industry in Moldova. *Lancet*, **365**, 1354–9.

Gilmore, A., Collin, J., Townsend, J. (2007). Transnational tobacco company influence on taxation policy during privatization: The case of BAT in Uzbekistan. *American Journal of Public Health*, **97**, 2001–9.

Giovino, G.A., Henningfield, J., Tomar, S.L., Escobedo, L.E., Slade, J. (1995). Epidemiology of tobacco use and dependence. *Epidemiologic Reviews*, **17**, 48–65.

Giovino, G.A. (2000). World's best practice in tobacco control. Surveillance of patterns and consequences of tobacco use: USA. *Tobacco Control*, **9**, 232.

GTSS (Global Tobacco Surveillance System Collaborating Group) (2005). Global Tobacco Surveillance System: Purpose, production, and potential. *Journal of School Health*, **75**, 15–24.

Hatsukami, D., Hughes, J.R., Pickens, R. (1985). Characterization of tobacco withdrawal: Physiological and subjective effects. In J. Grabowski and S.M. Hall, eds. *Pharmacological adjuncts in smoking cessation*, pp. 56–67. DHHS Publication (ADM) 85–1333. US Department of Health and Human Services, Public Health Service, Alcohol and Drug Abuse and Mental Health Administration, Washington, DC.

Hammond, D., Collishaw, N., Callard, C. (2006a). Tobacco industry research on smoking behaviour and product design. *Lancet*, **367**, 781–7.

Hammond, D., Fong, G.T., McNeill, A., Borland, R., Cummings, K.M. (2006b). Effectiveness of cigarette warning labels from informing smokers about the risk of smoking: Findings from the international Tobacco Control (ITC) Four Country Survey. *Tobacco Control*, **15** (Suppl. 3), iii19–25.

Hecht, S.S. (1999). Tobacco smoke carcinogens and lung cancer. *Journal of the National Cancer Institute*, **91**, 1194–210.

Hiilamo, H., Hirschhorn, N. (2006). Tobacco industry documents from outside sources: New perspectives on industry strategies on local levels. *Central European Journal of Public Health*, **14**(4), 175–9.

Hilts, P.J. (1996). *Smoke screen. The truth behind the tobacco industry cover-up*. Addison-Wesley, New York.

Hirschhorn, N. (2004). Corporate social responsibility and the tobacco industry: Hope or hype? *Tobacco Control*, **13**(4), 447–53.

Hirschhorn, N. (2005). *The tobacco industry documents. What they are, what they tell us, and how to search them. A practical manual. 2nd ed.* [Online]. Available at: http://www.who.int/tobacco/communications/TI_manual_content.pdf

Hirschhorn, N., Bialous, S., Shatenstein, S. (2006). The Philip Morris external research program: Results from the first round of projects. *Tobacco Control*, **15**(3), 267–9.

Howell, R. (2005). Smoke-free bars in Ireland: A runaway success. *Tobacco Control*, **14**(2), 73–4.

International Institute for Population Sciences (IIPS) and Macro International (2007). *National Family Health Survey (NFHS-3), 2005–2006: India: Volume, I.* IIPS, Mumbai.

JAMA (1995). The Brown and Williamson documents. Where do we go from here? *Journal of the American Medical Association*, **274**, 256–7.

Jamieson, K.H. (1998). *'Tax and spend' vs. 'little kids': Advocacy and accuracy in the tobacco settlement ads of 1997–1998*. Annenberg Public Policy Center, University of Pennsylvania, Philadelphia, PA.

Jamrozik, K. (2000). Barbarians inside the gate: How the tobacco industry penetrated the World Health Organization: Report of the Committee of Experts on Tobacco Industry Documents. Tobacco company strategies to undermine tobacco control activities at the World Health Organization. Geneva: World Health Organization, 2000, pp. 247. *International Journal of Epidemiology*, **30**, 633–4.

Jha, P., Chaloupka, F., Moore, J. *et al.* (2006). Tobacco Addiction. In D.T. Jamison, J.G. Breman, A.R. Measham. *et al.*, eds. *Disease control priorities in developing countries, 2nd ed*, pp. 869–85. Oxford University Press, New York and World Bank, Washington, DC.

Jha, P., Jacob, B., Gajalakshmi, V. *et al.* (2008). A nationally representative case–control study of smoking and death in India. *New England Journal of Medicine*, **13**, **358**(11), 1137–47.

Joosens, L., Raw, M. (2002). *Turning off the tap: An update on cigarette smuggling in the UK and Sweden, with recommendations to control smuggling.* [Online]. Cancer Research UK and National Institute of Public Health, Sweden. Available at: http://old.ash.org.uk/luk/lukdocs/turningoffthetap.pdf.

Kluger, R. (1996). *Ashes to ashes. America's hundred-year cigarette war, the public health, and the unabashed triumph of Philip Morris*. Alfred, A. Knopf, New York.

Kozlowski, L.T., Pillitteri, J.L., Ahern, F.M. (1998a). Advertising fails to inform smokers of official tar yields of cigarettes. *Journal of Applied Biobehavioral Research*, **3**, 55–64.

Kozlowski, L.T., Goldberg, M.E., Yost, B.A., White, E.L., Sweeney, C.T., Pillitteri, J.L. (1998b). Smokers' perceptions of light and ultra-light cigarettes may keep them smoking. *American Journal of Preventive Medicine*, **15**, 9–16.

Last, J.M., ed. (1995). *A dictionary of epidemiology, 3rd ed.* Oxford University Press, New York.

Lawrence, S., Collin, J. (2004). Competing with kreteks: Transnational tobacco companies, globalisation and Indonesia. *Tobacco Control*, **13**(2), ii96–103.

Lee, K., Bialous, S.A. (2006). Corporate social responsibility: Serious cause for concern. *Tobacco Control*, **15**(6), 419.

Lee, K., Collin, J. (2006). "Key to the Future": British American Tobacco and cigarette smuggling in China. *PLoS Med*, **3**(7), e228.

Lee, K., Kinh, H., MacKenzie, R., Gilmore, A., Minh, N., Collin, J. (2008). Gaining access to Vietnam's cigarette market: British American Tobacco's strategy to enter 'a huge market which will become enormous.' *Global Public Health*, **3**(1), 1–25.

LeGresley, E., Muggli, M.E., Hurt, R.D. (2006). Movie moguls: British American Tobacco's covert strategy to promote cigarettes in Eastern Europe. *The European Journal of Public Health*, **16**(5), 505–8.

Leung, G.M., Ho, L.M., Lam, T.H. (2004). Secondhand smoke exposure, smoking hygiene, and hospitalization in the first 18 months of life. *Archives of Paediatric and Adolescent Medicine*, **158**(7), 687–93.

Levin, M.L. (1953). The occurrence of lung cancer in man. *Acta Union International Contra Cancer*, **9**, 531–41.

Lewis, M.J., Wackowski, D. (2006). Dealing with an innovative industry: A look at flavoured cigarettes promoted by mainstream brands. *American Journal of Public Health*, **96**(2), 244–51.

Ling, P.M., Glantz, S. (2002). Using tobacco-industry marketing research to design more effective tobacco-control campaigns. *Journal of the American Medical Association*, **287**, 2983–9.

Liu, B.Q., Peto, R., Chen, Z.M. *et al.* (1998). Emerging tobacco hazards in China: Retrospective proportional mortality study of one million deaths. *British Medical Journal*, **317**, 1411–22.

Lopez, A.D. (1999). Measuring the health hazards of tobacco. *Bulletin of the World Health Organization*, **77**, 82–3.

Lopez, A.D., Collishaw, N.E., Piha, T. (1994). A descriptive model of the cigarette epidemic in developed countries. *Tobacco Control*, **3**, 242–7.

MacKenzie, R., Collin, J., Sriwongcharoen. K. (2007). Thailand – lighting up a dark market: British American Tobacco, sports sponsorship and the circumvention of legislation. *Journal of Epidemiology and Community Health*, **61**(1), 28–33.

MacKenzie R, Collin J, Sriwongcharoen K, Muggli ME. 'If we can just "stall" new unfriendly legislations, the scoreboard is already in our favour': transnational tobacco companies and ingredients disclosure in Thailand. *Tobacco Control*. 2004 Dec;**13** Suppl 2:79–87.

Mathers, C., Loncar, D. (2006). Projections of Global Mortality and burden of Disease from 2002 to 2030. *PLoS Medicine*, **3**(11:e442), 2011–30.

Malone, R.E., Bero, L.A. (2003). Chasing the dollar: Why scientists should decline tobacco industry funding. *Journal of Epidemiology and Community Health*, **57**, 546–8.

Malson, J.L., Pickworth, W.B. (2002). Bidis – Hand-rolled, Indian cigarettes: Effects on physiological, biochemical and subjective measures. *Pharmacology Biochemistry and Behaviour*, **72**, 443–7.

McCann, J. (1992). Tobacco logo recognition. *Journal of Family Practice*, **34**, 681–4.

McDaniel, P.A., Malone, R.E. (2005). Understanding Philip Morris's pursuit of US government regulation of tobacco. *Tobacco Control*, **14**, 193–200.

McDaniel, P.A., Smith, E.A., Malone, R.E. (2006). Philip Morris's Project Sunrise: Weakening tobacco control by working with it. *Tobacco Control*, **15**(3), 215–23.

McDaniel, P.A., Intinarelli, G., Malone, R.E. (2008). Tobacco industry issues management organizations: Creating a global corporate network to undermine public health. *Global Health*, **4**, 2.

Milberger, S., Davis, R., Douglas, C. *et al.* (2006). Tobacco manufacturers' defense against plaintiffs' claims of cancer causation: Throwing mud at the wall and hoping some of it will stick. *Tobacco Control*, **15**(4), iv17–26.

Ministry of Health, New Zealand (2001). *Inhaling inequality – tobacco's contribution to health inequality in New Zealand.* Available at: http://www.moh.govt.nz/moh.nsf/0/eb38a31c067f8776cc256af0000f6f1e/$FILE/InhalingInequality.pdf

Ministry of Health, New Zealand (2008) Tobacco Use In: A portrait of health - Key results of the 2006/07 New Zealand Health Survey. Available at: http://www.moh.govt.nz/moh.nsf/pagesmh/7440/$File/second-hand-smoke-and-tobacco-use-nz-health-survey-jun08.pdf.

Muggli, M., Forster, J., Hurt, R., Repace, J. (2001). The smoke you don't see: Uncovering tobacco industry strategies aimed against environmental tobacco smoke. *American Journal of Public Health*, **91**, 1419–23.

Murray, C.J.L., Lopez, A.D. (1997a). Global mortality, disability, and the contribution of risk factors: Global burden of disease study. *Lancet*, **349**, 1436–42.

Murray, C.J.L., Lopez, A.D. (1997b). Alternative projections of mortality and disability by cause, 1990–2020: Global burden of disease study. *Lancet*, **349**, 1498–504.

National Research Council (NRC) (1986). *Environmental tobacco smoke: Measuring exposures and assessing health effects*. National Academy Press, Washington, DC.

Neuman, M., Bitton, A., Glantz, S. (2002). Tobacco industry strategies for influencing European Community tobacco advertising legislation. *Lancet*, **359**, 1323–30.

Niewoehner, D.E., Kleinerman, J., Rice, D.B. (1974). Pathologic changes in the peripheral airways of young cigarette smokers. *New England Journal of Medicine*, **291**, 755–8.

Ong, E., Glantz, S. (2000). Tobacco industry efforts subverting the International Agency for Research on Cancer's second-hand smoke study. *Lancet*, **355**, 1253–9.

Orleans, C.T., Slade, J. (1993). Preface. In C.T. Orleans and J. Slade, eds. *Nicotine addiction. Principles and management*. Oxford University Press, New York.

PAHO (Pan American Health Organization) (1992). *Tobacco or Health: Status in the Americas*. Scientific Publication Number 536. PAHO, Washington, DC.

PAHO (Pan American Health Organization) (2007). *Smoke free inside*. PAHO, Washington, DC.

Palazzo, G., Richter, U. (2005). CSR business as usual? The case of the tobacco industry. *Journal of Business Ethics*, **61**, 387–401.

Parascandola, M. (2003). Hazardous effects of tobacco industry funding. *Journal of Epidemiology and Community Health*, **57**, 548–9.

Parish, S., Collins, R., Peto, R. *et al.* (1995). Cigarette smoking, tar yields, and non-fatal myocardial infarction: 14 000 cases and 32 000 controls in the United Kingdom. *British Medical Journal*, **311**, 471–7.

PDAY Research Group (1990). Relationship of atherosclerosis in young men to serum lipoprotein cholesterol concentrations and smoking. A preliminary report from the Pathological Determinants in Youth (PDAY) Research Group. *Journal of the American Medical Association*, **263**, 3018–24.

Peto, R., Lopez, A.D., Boreham, J., Thun, M., Heath, C. (1994). *Mortality from smoking in developed countries, 1950–2000*. Oxford University Press, Oxford.

Peto, R., Lopez, A.D., Boreham, J., Thun, M., Heath, C., Doll, R. (1996). Mortality from smoking worldwide. *British Medical Bulletin*, **52**, 12–21.

Pierce, J.P., Gilpin, E., Burns, D.M. *et al.* (1991) Does tobacco advertising target young people to start smoking? Evidence from California. *Journal of the American Medical Association*, **266**(22):3154–8.

Pollay, R.W., Siddarth, S., Siegel, M. *et al.* (1996). The last straw? Cigarette advertising and realized market shares among youths and adults, 1979–1993. *Journal of Marketing for Professions*, **60**, 1–16.

Pollay, R.W., Dewhirst, T. (2002). The dark side of marketing seemingly "light" cigarettes: Successful images and failed fact. *Tobacco Control*, **11**(1), i18–31.

Prochaska, J.O., Redding, C.A., Evers, K.E. (1997). The trans-theoretical model and stages of change. In K. Glantz, F.M. Lewis and B.K. Rimer, eds. *Health behaviour and health education, theory, research, and practice*. Jossey-Bass, San Francisco, CA.

Reddy, S.K., Gupta, P.C., eds. (2004). *Report on Tobacco Control in India*. Ministry of Health and Family Welfare, Government of India, New Delhi.

Reid, D.J., McNeill, A., Glynn, T.J. (1995). Reducing the prevalence of smoking in youth in Western countries: An international review. *Tobacco Control*, **4**, 266–77.

Saloojee, Y., Dagli, E. (2000). Tobacco industry tactics for resisting public policy on health. *Bulletin of the World Health Organization*, **78**, 911–2.

Samet, J.M., Wang, S.S. (2000). Environmental tobacco smoke. In M Lippmann, ed. *Environmental toxicants: Human exposures and their health effect. 2nd ed.* Wiley, New York.

Samet, J.M., Burke, T.A. (2001). Turning science into junk; the tobacco industry and passive smoking. *American Journal of Public Health*, **91**, 1742–4.

SCOTH (Scientific Committee on Tobacco and Health) (1998). *Report of the Scientific Committee on Tobacco and Health*. HMSO, London.

Siahpush, M., McNeill, A., Hammond, D., Fong, G.T. (2006). Socioeconomic and country variations in knowledge of health risks of tobacco smoking and toxic constituents of smoke: Results from the 2002 International Tobacco Control (ITC) Four Country Survey. *Tobacco Control*, **15**(3), iii65–70.

Silagy, C., Lancaster, T., Stead, L., Mant, D., Fower, G. (2004). Nicotine Replacement therapy for smoking cessation. *Cochrane Database Systematic Review*, **3**, C000146.

Smith, E.A., Malone, R.E. (2004). "Creative Solutions": Selling cigarettes in a smoke-free world. *Tobacco Control*, **13**, 57–63.

Smith, E.A., Malone, R.E. (2006). 'We will speak as the smoker': The tobacco industry's smokers' rights groups. *European Journal of Public Health*, **17**(3), 306–13.

Stayner, L., Bena, J., Sasco, A.J. *et al.* (2007). Lung cancer risk and workplace exposure to environmental tobacco smoke. *Americal Journal of Public Health*, **97**(3), 545–51.

Stratton, K., Shetty, P., Wallace, R., Bondurant, S., eds. (2001). Products for tobacco exposure reduction. In *Clearing the smoke. Assessing the science base for tobacco harm reduction*, pp. 78–98. National Academy Press, Washington, DC.

Szczypka, G., Wakefield, M., Emery, S., Terry-McElrath, Y., Flay, B., Chaloupka, F. (2007). Working to make an image: An analysis of three Philip Morris corporate image media campaigns. *Tobacco Control*, **16**(5), 344–50.

Szilagyi, T., Chapman, S. (2003). Hungry for Hungary: Examples of tobacco industry's expansionism. *Central Europe Journal of Public Health*, **11**, 38–43.

Taylor, R., Najafi, F., Dobson, A. (2007). Meta-analysis of studies of passive smoking and lung cancer: Effects of study type and continent. *International Journal of Epidemiology*, **36**(5), 1048–59.

Thomson, G., Signal, L. (2005). Associations between universities and the tobacco industry: What institutional policies limit these associations? *Social Policy Journal of New Zealand*, **26**, 186–204.

Thomson, G., Wilson, N. (2005). Directly eroding tobacco industry power as a tobacco control strategy. *New Zealand Medical Journal*, **118**, U1683.

Thun, M.J., Day-Lally, C., Myers, D.G. *et al.* (1997). Trends in tobacco smoking and mortality from cigarette use in Cancer Prevention Studies I (1959–1965) and II (1982–1988). In *Changes in cigarette-related disease risks and their implication for prevention and control, smoking and tobacco control monograph 8*, pp. 305–82. US Department of Health and Human Services, Public Health Service, National Institutes of Health, Bethesda, MD.

Thyrian, J.R., Panagiotakos, D.B., Polychronopoulos, E., West, R., Zatonski, W., John, U. (2008). The relationship between smokers' motivation to quit and intensity of tobacco control at the population level: A comparison of five European countries. *BMC Public Health*, **8**, 2.

Tomar, S.L. (2007). Epidemiologic perspectives on smokeless tobacco marketing and population harm. *American Journal of Preventive Medicine*, **33**(6), S387–97.

Tong, E.K., Glantz, S.A. (2004). ARTIST (Asian Regional Tobacco Industry Scientist Team): Philip Morris' attempt to exert a scientific and regulatory agenda on Asia. *Tobacco Control*, **13**(2), ii118–24.

Tyas, S.L., Pederson, L.L. (1998). Psychosocial factors related to adolescent smoking: A critical review of the literature. *Tobacco Control*, **7**, 409–20.

Tobacco Advisory Group of the Royal College of Physicians (2000). *Nicotine addiction in Britain; a report of the Tobacco Advisory Group of the Royal College of Physicians*. Royal College of Physicians of London, London.

USDA (US Department of Agriculture) (2004). *Global cigarette production, distribution and supply 2000–2004*. [Online]. Available at: http://www.fas.usda.gov/tobacco/circular/2004/092004/CIGARETTE2004.PDF

USDHHS (US Department of Health and Human Services) (1986). *The health consequences of involuntary smoking: A report of the Surgeon General*. DHHS Publication 87–8398. US Department of Health and Human Services, Centers for Disease Control, Center for Health Promotion and Education, Office on Smoking and Health, Rockville, MD.

USDHHS (US Department of Health and Human Services) (1988). *The health consequences of smoking: Nicotine addiction. A report of the Surgeon General*. DHHS Publication 88–8406. US Department of Health and Human Services, Public Health Service, Centers for Disease Control, Center for Health Promotion and Education, Office on Smoking and Health, Rockville, MD.

USDHHS (US Department of Health and Human Services) (1989). *Reducing the health consequences of smoking: 25 years of progress. A report of the Surgeon General*. DHHS Publication 89–8411. US Department of Health and Human Services, Public Health Service, Centers for Disease Control, Center for Chronic Disease Prevention and Health Promotion, Office on Smoking and Health, Rockville, MD.

USDHHS (US Department of Health and Human Services) (1990). *The health benefits of smoking cessation. A report of the Surgeon General*. DHHS Publication 90-8416. US Department of Health and Human Services, Public Health Service, National Centre for Chronic Disease Prevention and Health Promotion (Centers for Disease Control and Prevention), Office on Smoking and Health, Rockville, MD.

USDHHS (US Department of Health and Human Services) (1994). *Preventing tobacco use among young people. A report of the Surgeon General*. DHHS Publication 017-001-00491-0. US Department of Health and Human Services, Centers for Disease Control and Prevention, National Center for Chronic Disease Prevention and Health Promotion, Office on Smoking and Health, Atlanta, GA.

USDHHS (US Department of Health and Human Services) (1996). The FTC cigarette test method for determining tar, nicotine, and carbon monoxide yields of US cigarettes. Report of the National Cancer Institute Expert Committee. NIH Publication 96-4028. US Department of Health and Human Services, Public Health Service, National Institutes of Health, National Cancer Institute, Bethesda, MD.

USDHHS (US Department of Health and Human Services) (1997). *Smoking and tobacco control monograph 8: Changes in cigarette-related disease risks and their implication for prevention and control*. NIH Publication 97-1213, US Department of Health and Human Services, Public Health Service, National Institutes of Health, Bethesda, MD.

USDHHS (US Department of Health and Human Services) (1998). *Tobacco use among US racial/ethnic minority groups—African Americans, American Indians and Alaska Natives, Asian Americans and Pacific Islanders, and Hispanic. A report of the Surgeon General*. US Department of Health and Human Services, Centers for Disease Control and Prevention, National Center for Chronic Disease Prevention and Health Promotion, Office on Smoking and Health, Atlanta, GA.

USDHHS (US Department of Health and Human Services) (2001). *Smoking and tobacco control monograph 13: Risks associated with smoking cigarettes with low tar machine-measured yields of tar and nicotine*. National Cancer Institute, National Institutes of Health, Rockville, MD.

USDHHS (US Department of Health and Human Services) (2004). *The Health Consequences of Smoking: A report of the Surgeon General*. US Department of Health and Human Services, Centers for Disease Control and Prevention, National Center for Chronic Disease Prevention and Health Promotion, Office on Smoking and Health. Washington, DC.

USDHHS (US Department of Health and Human Services) (2006). *The Health Consequences of Involuntary Exposure to Tobacco Smoke: A report of the Surgeon General*. NIH Publication 97-1241, US Department of Health and Human Services, Public Health Service, National Institutes of Health, Bethesda, MD.

USDHHS (US Department of Health and Human Services) (2007). *CDC recommended annual per capita funding levels for state programs*. US Department of Health and Human Services, Centers for Disease Control and Prevention, Atlanta, GA.

United States Department of Justice (2004). United States of America, plaintiff v. Philip Morris *et al.* defendants. United States' Final Proposed Findings of Fact. United States District Court for the District of Columbia, Civil Action No. 99-CV-02496 (GK). Available at: http://www.usdoj.gov/civil/cases/tobacco2

United States Department of Justice (2006). United States of America, plaintiff v. Philip Morris. *et al.* defendants. Final Opinion. United States District Court for the District of Columbia, Civil Action No. 99-CV-02496 (GK). Available at: http://www.library.ucsf.edu/tobacco/litigation/uspm.html

Van der Eb, M.M., Leyten, E.M., Gavarasana, S., Vandenbroucke, J.P., Kahn, P.M., Cleton, F.J. (1993). Reverse smoking as a risk factor for palatal cancer: A cross sectional study in rural Andhra Pradesh, India. *International Journal of Cancer*, **54**, 754–8.

Wagner, E.H., Curry, S.J., Grothaus, L., Saunders, K.W., McBride, C.M. (1995). The impact of smoking and quitting on health care use. *Archives of Internal Medicine*, **155**, 1789–95.

Wakefield, M., Morley, C., Horan, J., Cummings, K. (2002). The cigarette pack as image: New evidence from tobacco industry documents. *Tobacco Control*, **11**(1), i73–80.

Wang, F.L., Love, E.J., Liu, N., Dai, X.D. (1994a). Childhood and adolescent passive smoking and the risk of female lung cancer. *International Journal of Epidemiology*, **23**, 223–30.

Wang, S.Q., Yu, J.J., Zhu, B.P., Liu, M., He, G.Q. (1994b). Cigarette smoking and its risk factors among senior high school students in Beijing, China, 1988. *Tobacco Control*, **3**, 107–14.

Warner, K.E. (2000). The economics of tobacco: Myths and realities. *Tobacco Control*, **9**, 78–89.

Warren, C.W., Jones, N.R., Eriksen, M.P., Asma, S., Global Tobacco Surveillance System (GTSS) collaborative group (2006). Patterns of global tobacco use in young people and implications for future chronic disease burden in adults. *Lancet*, **367**(9512), 749–53.

Wayne, G., Connolly, G. (2002). How cigarette design can affect youth initiation into smoking: Camel cigarettes 1983–1993. *Tobacco Control*, **11**(1), i32–9.

WHO (World Health Organization) (1997a). *Tobacco or health: A global status report*. WHO, Geneva.

WHO (World Health Organization) (1997b). *Smoking, drinking and drug taking in the European region*. WHO Regional Office for Europe, Copenhagen.

WHO (World Health Organization) (1999a). *World health report 1999*. WHO, Geneva.

WHO (World Health Organization) (1999b). *Tobacco free initiative consultation report, international consultation on environmental tobacco smoke (ETS) and child health*. WHO/TFI/99.10, WHO, Geneva.

WHO (World Health Organization) (2000a). *Kobe Declaration*. Tobacco Free Initiative Report. WHO, Geneva.

WHO (World Health Organization) (2000b). *Tobacco company strategies to undermine Tobacco Control activities at the World Health Organization*. Report of the Committee of Experts on Tobacco Industry Documents. WHO, Geneva.

WHO (World Health Organization) (2003a). *The cigarette "transit road" to the Islamic Republic of Iran and Iraq. Illicit tobacco trade in the Middle East*. WHO Regional Office for the Eastern Mediterranean, Cairo.

WHO (World Health Organization) (2003b). *Report on smuggling control in Spain.* WHO, Geneva. Available at: http://www.who.int/tobacco/training/success_stories/en/best_practices_spain_smuggling_control.pdf

WHO (World Health Organization) (2004a). Tobacco Free Initiative. *Building blocks for tobacco control: A handbook.* WHO, Geneva.

WHO (World Health Organization) (2004b). *Recommendation 6: Guiding principles for the development of tobacco product research and proposed protocols for the initiation of tobacco product testing.* [Online]. WHO Study Group on Tobacco Product Regulation. Available at: http://repositories.cdlib.org/context/tc/article/1172/type/pdf/viewcontent/

WHO (World Health Organization) (2004c). *Scientific advisory committee on tobacco product regulation.* [Online]. Tobacco Free Initiative. Available at: http://www.who.int/tobacco/sactob/en/ [Accessed on 3 November 2007].

WHO (World Health Organization) (2004d). *IARC monographs on the evaluation of carcinogenic risks to humans: Tobacco smoke and involuntary smoking, Vol.83*, pp. 53–119. International Agency for Research on Cancer, WHO, France.

WHO (World Health Organization) (2005). *The first meeting of the WHO Tobacco Laboratory Network (TobLabNet) on 28 & 29 April 2005 in the Hague, the Netherlands.* [Online]. Tobacco Free Initiative. Available at: http://www.who.int/tobacco/global_interaction/tobreg/laboratory/en/ [Accessed on 23 April 2008].

WHO (World Health Organization) (2006). *Tobacco: Deadly in any form or disguise.* WHO, Geneva.

WHO (World Health Organization) (2007a). *Elaboration of guidelines for implementation of the Convention (decision FCTC/COP1(15)) – Article 8: Protection from exposure to tobacco smoke.* [Online]. The Second Session of Conference of the parties to the WHO Framework Convention on Tobacco Control. Available at: http://www.who.int/gb/fctc/PDF/cop2/FCTC_COP2_7-en.pdf

WHO (World Health Organization) (2007b). *Elaboration of guidelines for implementation of the Convention (decision FCTC/COP1(15)) – Article 9: Product regulation.* [Online]. The Second Session of Conference of the parties to the WHO Framework Convention on Tobacco Control. Available at: http://www.who.int/gb/fctc/PDF/cop2/FCTC_COP2_8-en.pdf

WHO (World Health Organization) (2007c). *The first session of the Conference of the Parties to the WHO Framework Convention on Tobacco Control.* [Online]. Tobacco Free Initiative. Available at: http://www.who.int/tobacco/fctc/cop/en/index.html [Accessed on 3 November 2007].

WHO (World Health Organization) (2007d). *WHO Tobacco Laboratory Network (TobLabNet).* [Online]. Tobacco Free Initiative. Available at: http://www.who.int/tobacco/global_interaction/toblabnet/history/en/index.html [Accessed on 3 November 2007].

WHO (World Health Organization) (2007e). *The scientific basis of tobacco product regulation.* WHO Technical Report Series 945. WHO, Geneva.

WHO (World Health Organization) (2007f). *A WHO/The Union monograph on TB and tobacco control: Joining efforts to control two related global epidemics.* WHO, Geneva. Available at: http://whqlibdoc.who.int/publications/2007/9789241596220_eng.pdf

WHO (World Health Organization) (2007g). Gender and tobacco control: A policy brief. WHO, Geneva. Available at: http://www.who.int/tobacco/resources/publications/general/policy_brief.pdf.

WHO (World Health Organization) (2007h). World health statistics 2007. WHO, France; 15.

WHO (World Health Organization) (2008a). *WHO Report on the Global Tobacco Epidemic, 2008: The MPOWER package.* WHO, Geneva.

WHO (World Health Organization) (2008b). World health statistics 2008. WHO, Geneva; 66–75.

Wipfli, H., Avila-Tang, E., Navas-Acien, A. *et al.* (2008). Secondhand smoke exposure among women and children: Evidence from 31 countries. *American Journal of Public Health*, **98**(4), 672–9.

Wistuba, I.I., Lam, S., Behrens, C. *et al.* (1997). Molecular damage in the bronchial epithelium of current and former smokers. *Journal of the National Cancer Institute*, **89**, 1366–73.

World Bank (1999). *Curbing the epidemic: Governments and the economics of tobacco control.* World Bank, Washington, DC.

Yang, G., Ma, J., Chen, A. *et al.* (2001). Smoking cesation in China: Findings from the 1996 national prevalence survey. *Tobacco Control*, **10**(2), 170–4.

Yang, G.H., Ma, J.M., Liu, N., Zhou, L.N. (2005). Smoking and passive smoking in Chinese, 2002. [Article in Chinese]. *Zhonghua Liu Xing Bing Xue Za Zhi*, **26**(2), 77–83.

Zhang, J., Ratcliffe, J.M. (1993). Paternal smoking and birthweight in Shanghai. *American Journal of Public Health*, **83**, 207–10.

Zhu, B.P., Liu, M., Shelton, D., Liu, S., Giovino, G.A. (1996). Cigarette smoking and its risk factors among elementary school students in Beijing. *American Journal of Public Health*, **86**, 368–75.

10.2

Drug abuse

Don C. Des Jarlais and Robert L. Hubbard

Abstract

Abuse and dependence on alcohol and other drugs is a particularly complex and very important public health problem. Drug dependence disorders involve biomedical, pharmacological, psychological, and social factors. Drug abuse often involves multiple pharmacological agents used within a complex social environment in which some substances are legal and others illegal. The consequences of drug abuse are many and varied. Over the last 40 years, there have been major advances in prevention and treatment of drug abuse, but given present worldwide trends, the problems associated with psychoactive drug use are likely to continue increasing. Human immunodeficiency virus (HIV), the virus that causes acquired immunodeficiency syndrome (AIDS) has emerged as the most dramatic adverse consequence of drug use. HIV is not transmitted through drug use *per se*, but through the sharing of equipment to inject drugs and through unsafe sexual activities that are often facilitated by drug use. Sharing of injection equipment can lead to extremely rapid transmission of HIV, with half or more of a local drug user population becoming infected over a period of a few years. Conversely, programmes such as community outreach and syringe exchange can be highly effective in reducing injection-related HIV transmission. It is possible to prevent epidemics of HIV among injecting drug users. The main problems have been not implementing programmes to prevent HIV among injecting drug users at all, but waiting until after an epidemic has already occurred to implement programmes, or implementing programmes on an inadequate scale. The HIV/AIDS crisis has spurred development of the 'harm reduction' perspective towards the problems of psychoactive drug use. This perspective is based in a human rights approach to drug users—drug users should be treated with dignity and respect—and a pragmatic, public health perspective on drug related problems. It is not likely that the problems associated with drug use can be eliminated, so public health policy should focus on the many different ways in which those problems can be minimized.

Abuse and dependence on alcohol and other drugs is a particularly complex public health problem. The complexity of alcohol and other drug abuse is a function of its diverse nature. Dependence disorders involve biomedical, pharmacological, psychological, and social factors. Substance abuse often involves multiple pharmacological agents used within a complex social environment in which some substances are legal and others illegal. Furthermore, the distinctions among use, abuse, and dependence are often blurred. The consequences of substance abuse are many and varied. Some are acute and put an individual at immediate risk, such as driving while intoxicated. Use of addictive substances by biologically vulnerable individuals may result in long-term consequences such as criminal behaviour and loss of employment. Sharing of injection equipment by intravenous drug users immediately increases their risk of exposure to HIV and, once exposed, their life-styles compromise health and may lead to accelerated development of AIDS. Thus, simple definitions, explanations, or solutions for substance abuse are inadequate, inefficient, and potentially counterproductive. The evolution of research on the individuals using drugs, prevention, and treatment was summarized in a 2006 conference reflecting on 40 years of substance abuse research (Sloboda 2008). This chapter indicates some of the broad concepts necessary to understand substance abuse and dependence disorders, their consequences, and potential solutions.

The focus in the first section of the chapter is dependence on drugs other than alcohol, which is discussed in another chapter. While recognizing that problems of alcohol and drug abuse occur worldwide and across diverse cultures (Babor 1986), this discussion is limited by both space and data to the United States. In the United States, the problem is most profound. The history and current conditions in the United States illustrate many of the issues that exist or can be expected to emerge in many countries in the future. The abuse of alcohol (Aaron & Musto 1981) and other drugs (Brecher *et al.* 1972) has persisted for centuries. Since 1900, attention to alcohol and other drug abuse has waxed and waned in the United States (Jaffe 1979). Some of the foremost reasons for renewed attention on alcohol and drug abuse in the 1980s and the 1990s are the increasing costs for treatment for dependence, the violent crime associated with cocaine distribution, and the role of intravenous drug use in the transmission of HIV. Intravenous drug use is now the second most common risk behaviour associated with AIDS. It is also the major contributing factor to paediatric and heterosexual AIDS cases in the United States (Turner *et al.* 1989). In the last 5 years, rates are rapidly escalating among minorities and underserved populations in rural communities outside traditional epicentres (Reif *et al.* 2006).

This first section describes the definition, epidemiology, aetiology, and consequences of alcohol and drug abuse. The major efforts made in the United States to prevent and treat alcohol and other drug abuse are reviewed and their effectiveness documented. The chapter concludes with a discussion of the critical role of intravenous drug use in the HIV/AIDS epidemic. The last section incorporates a broader worldwide view. Within each section, a broad array of perspectives on these problems are presented. These perspectives range from the biomedical search for genetic markers to legal attempts to control alcohol and other drug use. A full discussion of all perspectives is beyond the scope of one particular presentation. Because of the orientation of the authors, this presentation necessarily has a social/psychological orientation. This is not to suggest that the other approaches are not important to consider, only that the authors of this chapter are most qualified to deal with the research literature in their own discipline.

Definition of dependence on drugs

Various approaches have been used to characterize the use, abuse, and dependence on drugs. Numerous personal interviews and self-report inventories have been developed to obtain a comprehensive history of use as well as assessments of current use patterns, dependence, and drug- and alcohol-related problems (Skinner & Horn 1984; Babor *et al.* 1988). No single measure has yet been accepted as fully characterizing use, abuse, or dependence. From an epidemiological perspective, frequency of use, and total number of times used in a lifetime are often the principal measures. Abuse refers to usage levels that have short-term acute personal or social consequences. Psychiatric diagnosis of dependence requires evidence of consequences over an extended period of time. The clinical definition of dependence, which is now undergoing careful review, has evolved over the past decade to include psychological as well as physiological components.

Assessment of alcohol dependence and problems has received more attention than diagnosis of drug abuse problems or dependence. Research on alcohol dependence has fostered interest in the measurement of drug dependence syndromes, using similar diagnostic criteria (Edwards *et al.* 1981). Many of the assessments that were used to measure alcohol abuse have been modified for drug abuse research. A factor analytical study (Skinner & Horn 1984) identified a general cluster resembling the alcohol dependence syndrome postulated by Edwards *et al.* (1976). The salient markers of this factor include loss of behavioural control over drinking, withdrawal symptoms, and obsessive-compulsive drinking style. Early validation research (Skinner & Horn 1984) indicates that the drug dependence symptoms correlate in predictable ways with clinic attendance, physical symptoms, and psychosocial problems.

Perhaps the most ambitious and theoretically sound approach to assessing dependence has been taken by Rounsaville *et al.* (1986) on the structured clinical interview for the revised edition of the Diagnostic and Statistical Manual of Mental Disorders (DSM-III-R). The structured clinical interview is designed to determine diagnoses and symptoms of substance use disorder according to the American Psychiatric Association's revised Diagnostic and Statistical Manual of Mental Disorders (Spitzer & Williams 1987). The structured clinical interview provides a more comprehensive assessment of alcohol and drug dependence symptoms than the substance use disorders section of the Diagnostic Interview Schedule, and provides diagnoses that can be applied to both the third edition and the third revised edition of the Diagnostic and Statistical Manual of Mental Disorders.

The criteria have been substantially revised (Rounsaville *et al.* 1986) and are designed to reflect aspects of the dependence syndrome (Edwards *et al.* 1981). Symptoms include: (1) more use than intended; (2) inability to reduce use; (3) amount of time seeking substance; (4) physical effects of use; (5) use replaces other activities; (6) continued use in spite of problems; (7) tolerance; (8) withdrawal symptoms; or (9) use to avoid withdrawal symptoms. Dependence severity is assessed by considering the number of symptoms reported and the extent of impairment, and the indication of level of dependence (mild, moderate, severe, partial remission, full remission) rather than simply the presence or absence of dependence or abuse. Abuse is defined as sporadic non-dependent patterns of use in spite of problems or physical hazards. Rounsaville (2002) reviewed the two emergent systems, International Classification of Diseases 10 (WHO 1992) and Diagnostic and Statistical Manual of Disease IV (APA 2000), and identified needs for consistency across the two systems, a consistency that may be achieved more easily for dependence.

Initial attempts to define alcohol and drug dependence have been confounded by increased multiple use of various drugs during the 1970s and 1980s (Clayton 1985; Hubbard *et al.* 1986) and the rise of cocaine use during the 1980s. A very complex typology is needed to capture the full extent of alcohol and other drug use. In fact, many individuals who use alcohol heavily also report the use of marijuana and, increasingly, the use of cocaine. Among those using marijuana, almost all will have used alcohol. At another extreme, most intravenous heroin users have used alcohol, cocaine, and marijuana (Hubbard *et al.* 1986). To address this problem, Spitzer and Williams (1987) introduce a general category of polydrug dependence to include dependence on three or more specific psychoactive substances or dependence on psychoactive substances in general. These emerging approaches to definition within and across the complex array of usage patterns offer the promise of a more comprehensive understanding of abuse and dependence (Cacciola & Woody 2005).

Epidemiology

Since the 1960s in the United States, national attention has been focused on the rapidly expanding problem of drug abuse. In particular, the concern was the involvement of adolescents with alcohol and other drugs. To trace these high levels of use, three series of national probability sample surveys have been conducted in the United States. Each year since 1974, a national sample of high school senior students has completed self-administered questionnaires on alcohol and drug use (Johnston *et al.* 1989). In the years 1972, 1974, 1975, 1979, 1982, 1985, and 1988, and annually since 1991, personal interviews on drug use have been conducted with a national sample of American household residents, stratified by ages 12–17, 18–25, and 26 years or older (National Institute on Drug Abuse 1989). These surveys have documented relative stability in alcohol use, but a rapid escalation from 1972 to 1979 in lifetime and current use of other drugs, particularly marijuana and cocaine. After 1979, the use of marijuana and, since 1985, cocaine, dropped rapidly (Table 10.2.1). For youth, the rates of marijuana use then began to increase in the mid-1990s, but since 2000, a gradual decline has been noted (Johnston *et al.* 2005).

Table 10.2.1 Trends in prevalence of self-reported use of marijuana, cocaine, and alcohol in the National Household Survey on Drug Abuse in the United States, 1974–2005

Year of survey	1974	1979	1985	1991	1995	2000	2005
Lifetime prevalence for youths aged 12–17							
Marijuana	23%	26.7%	20.1%	11.1%	16.2%	18.3%	17.4%
Cocaine	3.6%	5.5%	4.7%	2.4%	2%	2.4%	2.3%
Alcohol	54%	70.8%	56.1%	46.9%	40.6%	41.7%	40.6%
Past year prevalence for young adults aged 18–25							
Marijuana	34.2%	44.2%	34%	22.9%	21.8%	23.7%	28%
Cocaine	8.1%	17%	13.6%	6.7%	4.3%	4.4%	6.9%
Alcohol	77.1%	84.6%	84.2%	80.7%	76.5%	74.5%	77.9%
Past year prevalence for older adults aged 26–34							
Marijuana	3.8%	20.5%	20.2%	11.6%	11.8%	5%	6.9%
Cocaine	–	5.7%	10.5%	4.4%	3.1%	1%	1.5%
Alcohol	62.7%	81.7%	81.9%	79.1%	77%	63.7%	69%

The spectrum of problems associated with drug use persists, and now includes the crucial role of intravenous heroin and cocaine use in the transmission of HIV infection. The large-scale household or school-based surveys do not provide useful information on the relatively rare and hidden populations of intravenous drug users. Estimates of the size and usage patterns of this population are derived largely from studies of convenience samples, statistical models, and informed guesses.

Youth and young adults

While alcohol and other drug abuse occur at all income levels and in virtually all age groups, the high levels of abuse among youths and young adults causes the most concern. In the United States, approximately 70 per cent of all youth have at least experimented with illegal drugs by the time they leave high school (Johnston *et al.* 1999), and one in three senior students report current heavy drinking (five or more drinks in a row in the past 2 weeks). A survey of 7500 youth aged 11–14 years has shown that initiation of alcohol and drug abuse rises exponentially through the years of early adolescence (Hubbard *et al.* 1988). By the age of 14, two of five adolescents have at one time consumed two or more drinks or reported trying drugs for non-medical reasons. The patterns of use have also varied greatly since the first national surveys were conducted in 1972.

The trends in the use of drugs by youth showed a levelling off from the mid-1970s to the early 1980s, a rapid decline in the late 1980s, an increase in the mid-1990s, and fairly consistent rates through 2005 (Table 10.2.1). Percentages of youth who had ever tried marijuana, 26.7 per cent in 1979, had fallen to 20.1 per cent in 1985 and to 9.9 per cent in 1993, before beginning an annual increase to 17 per cent in 1998, where the figure has remained. Cocaine use rose rapidly from 1.5 per cent in 1972 to 5.5 per cent in 1979 to 6.1 per cent in 1982, but fell to 2.4 per cent in 1991 and to 1.1 per cent by 1993, then climbed to 2.2 per cent by 1998, where it has remained through 2005. Although the percentages of youths aged 12–17 years who used drugs in 2005 are lower than the 1979 figures, rates have fluctuated, but now appear to have been relatively stable from 2000 through 2005 (Substance Abuse and Mental Health Services Administration 1999, 2007).

The levels and trends for youth in the household surveys have paralleled those for high-school senior students, which show a downward trend in the use of marijuana and other illicit drugs from 1979 to 1993, with rates increasing through 1998 (Johnston *et al.* 1999). Beginning in 2000, a gradual trend in decreasing rates has been observed (Johnston *et al.* 2006). Cocaine use was an exception to this rapid downward trend, having stabilized through 1986 at the levels attained in the late 1970s. Rates decreased from 1986 through 1993 before beginning to climb again through 1998. By 1986, about one of every six high-school senior students reported trying cocaine, and one in 20 reported use in the 30 days prior to the survey. By 1998, about one of every 10 high-school senior students reported trying cocaine, and only one in 40 reported use in the last 30 days. Between 1983 and 1986, the proportion of seniors reporting daily cocaine use in the month before the survey and the proportion who had been unable to stop using in the prior year had both doubled. Between 1986 and 1998, the proportion of seniors reporting daily cocaine use in the month before the survey had fallen to the 1983 level. The proportion who had smoked crack cocaine, a more dangerous and effective route of administration, had also doubled from 1983 to 1986, but rapidly declined from 5.7 per cent (1986 level) to 1.5 per cent by 1991. In 1986, only half of the senior students thought there was much risk associated with occasional cocaine use. The 1988 survey, however, shows a marked decline in cocaine use coupled with a heightened perception of risk. One in eight report lifetime use, and one in 30 reported use in the past 30 days. About 7 in 10 high-school senior students viewed occasional cocaine use as harmful. By 1993, rates of lifetime use of cocaine had decreased to 6 per cent, and less than 2 per cent of high school senior students used cocaine in the 30 days prior to the survey. The 1993 data also reported an increased number of drugs used and less negative attitudes towards drugs. By 2005, only 8 per cent of high school seniors reported ever using cocaine, and in 2007, only 3 per cent of 8th graders reported ever using cocaine.

Although use among young adults also declined during the 1980s, many continue to use various types of drugs. The National Household Survey on Drug Abuse conducted in 1979 showed that 44.2 per cent of persons aged 18–25 years had used marijuana in the year before the survey (Table 10.2.1). There was a general downward trend until the mid-1990s (21.8 per cent in 1995), with an increase to 24.1 per cent in 1998. Cocaine use decreased from a high of 17 per cent in 1979 to 4.3 per cent in 1995, before rising slightly to 4.7 per cent in 1998. Self-reports of any illicit drug in the year before the survey fell from a high of 45.5 per cent in 1979 to around 25 per cent through 1998. Lifetime cocaine use prevalence for 19–28-year-olds was 32 per cent in 1986, but had dropped steadily to 12.3 per cent by 1998 (Johnston *et al.* 1999). The 2005 data from the national household survey shows a troubling increase in the rate of use in the past year to 28 per cent for marijuana and 6.9 per cent for cocaine, trends that parallel the trend for alcohol use (Substance Abuse and Mental Health Administration 2007).

Adults

Levels of drug use for adults (aged 26–34 years old) have not fluctuated as dramatically as those for youth and young adults. About 9 in 10 of older adults reported some experience with alcohol. Lifetime rates of marijuana (45 per cent in 1979, to 54.9 per cent in 1993, to 47.9 per cent in 1998) and cocaine use (13.4 per cent in 1979 to 25.4 per cent in 1993 to 17.1 per cent in 1998) have shown the same trends as youth and young adults. Use of all drugs in the past year remained relatively low (around 10 per cent for marijuana and under 5 per cent for cocaine) throughout the years of the household survey (Table 10.2.1).

More detailed and reliable data on dependence are available from a consortium of community epidemiological studies conducted from 1980 to 1982. In three American cities, lifetime rates between 11.5 and 15.7 per cent for alcohol abuse/dependence disorders and between 5.5 and 5.8 per cent for drug abuse/dependence were found for the adult residents interviewed in households (Robins *et al.* 1984). Current 6-month prevalence rates for men ranged between 8.2 and 10.4 per cent for alcohol dependence and 2.5 and 3.0 per cent for drug dependence (Myers *et al.* 1984). Rates for females were between 4.5 and 5.7 per cent for alcohol abuse/dependence and 1.8 and 2.2 per cent for drug abuse/dependence. Both of these data sets indicate that a substantial proportion of individuals in the United States have self-recognized problems with alcohol and drugs, and many meet the third edition criteria for dependence of the Diagnostic and Statistical Manual of Mental Disorders. Observations from community-based observers in 22 geographically dispersed communities have tracked trends from various data sources (e.g. emergency rooms, law enforcement, treatment) since the 1970s (Community Epidemiology Work Group 2007). They have reported geographically disparate rates of use of methamphetamine and prescription opioids, which cannot be easily accessed through household or school-based survey methodology.

Intravenous drug users

Estimating the number of intravenous drug users is an imprecise art. The problem of estimation is further hampered by differing definitions of past and current behaviour that qualifies an individual as an intravenous drug user. Spencer (1989) reviewed the variety of indirect estimates (derived from statistical models of indicators such as emergency room and medical examiner reports), direct estimates (based on surveys of convenience samples, back extrapolation, and capture-recapture estimates) or informed guesses. Considering all sources, Turner *et al.* (1989) conclude that a reasonable guess of the number of intravenous drug users in the United States is between 500 000 and 2 million. In the latest NSDUH, a likely underestimate, 3.8 million Americans, were projected to have used heroin, and 338 000 were projected to have used in the past month (SAMHSA 2007).

Consequences

Drug abuse costs were US$47 billion in 1980 (Harwood *et al.* 1984). The major contributors to these costs are lost productivity and treatment costs. Lost productivity attributed to drug abuse was estimated to be US$26 billion. Treatment services related to drug abuse were just over US$1 billion. This represents direct health services provided to victims, including long- and short-term hospitalization, services from physicians, and other sources. The overall costs also include the economic costs of crime, and violent crime due to drug abuse, premature mortality resulting from drug overdoses, liver disease, suicide, homicide, motor vehicle crashes, and other causes. Drug abuse costs US$2 billion for accidental overdoses. Drug addiction cost society approximately US$9 billion because of the addicts' pursuit of non-productive and criminal careers, another US$6 billion for criminal justice expenses, and US$1.5 billion for incarceration. These costs alone place drug abuse as one of the main contributors to the social cost of health-related problems in the United States. The costs were estimated to rise about 5 per cent a year, reaching US$181 billion in 2002 (Office of National Drug Control Policy 2004).

With the emergence of the AIDS epidemic in the 1980s, every drug abuser who contracts AIDS adds another US$80 000 in medical care costs to the equation (Scitovsky & Rice 1987). As described below, intravenous drug users play an important role in the AIDS epidemic, as they are second only to male homosexuals in the ranking of high-risk groups for AIDS in the United States (Turner *et al.* 1989). Intravenous drug use is also a major factor in cases involving children, heterosexuals, blacks, and Hispanics (Day *et al.* 1988; Des Jarlais & Friedman 1988). Regardless of sexual orientation, past or present intravenous drug users represent over one-quarter of reported AIDS cases in the United States, and the proportion continues to increase. Tests for HIV have shown that 10–58 per cent of sampled intravenous drug users are seropositive (Robert-Guroff *et al.* 1986; Chaisson *et al.* 1987; Des Jarlais *et al.* 1989). This increased risk of infection resulted in estimates of costs of US$2.5 to US$3.5 billion in the mid-1990s, with potentially greater costs due to the increased number of HIV/AIDS patients being treated (Office of National Drug Control Policy 2004).

Aetiology

The goal of efforts to deal with alcohol and drug abuse involves identifying those at risk and intervening to prevent or treat the problem. Information on risk factors to help target prevention, treatment, and rehabilitation efforts is largely limited to youth and young adults. Research is moving closer to uncovering basic biological and psychosocial mechanisms in alcohol and other drug use, but it does not appear likely that any simple explanation will be found. Being the child of a substance abuser has been found to be a consistent predictor of abuse. Both genetic and family environmental factors have been cited as influential agents (Kandel *et al.* 1978; Schuckit 1980; Cloninger *et al.* 1981; Goodwin 1985; Petrakis 1985).

Delinquent behaviour, including alcohol and drug abuse, often occur together (Jessor *et al.* 1980; Robins 1980). Many of the studies conclude that involvement in delinquent behaviour precedes drug use (Bachman *et al.* 1978; Elliott *et al.* 1985; Kandel *et al.* 1986), and that both behaviours have the same aetiological sources (Elliott *et al.* 1985; Hawkins *et al.* 1985). Early delinquent behaviour, usually before the age of 10, has also been linked to earlier initiation (Kandel *et al.* 1986) and frequent drug use (Kandel *et al.* 1978; Johnston *et al.* 1978; Kellam & Brown 1982; Rachal *et al.* 1982; Robins & Przybeck 1985; Kaplan *et al.* 1986). Other social factors such as low socio-economic status of parents, social isolation, and poor living conditions have also been found to be related to chronic delinquency and drug use (Farrington 1985; Hawkins *et al.* 1987). Studies have identified an association of alcohol and drug abuse with depression, low self-esteem, and psychological distress (Kandel *et al.* 1978; Kaplan *et al.* 1982; Aneshensel & Huba 1983).

One of the areas that has received relatively little attention in aetiological research is the examination of factors leading to cessation. Kandel and Raveis (1989) found that health and social factors discouraging use among young adults were predictive of cessation and a more extensive degree of previous involvement in drug use was predictive of continuation. Interpretation of these correlates of the likelihood of stopping use will require a more comprehensive understanding of use, abuse, and dependence (Meyer 1989), including the relative role of pharmacological, social, and physiological factors combined with the level and nature of involvement.

Another area where data is lacking is the dynamics of the initiation into intravenous drug use. Des Jarlais *et al.* (1986) suggest that initiation is often an unanticipated behaviour. Turner *et al.* (1989) conclude that some of the same factors contributing to initiation of other types of illicit use (such as peer groups) also predict initiation of intravenous use and continuation of usage. The uncertainty surrounding initiation, particularly in the face of the AIDS epidemic, dictates the need for more extensive and intensive research on initiation, development, maintenance, and cessation of intravenous drug use. More recent research has focused on the cessation rather that initiation of substance use. Laudet (2007) identified recovery as a multifaceted concept. The Betty Ford Institute Consensus Panel (2007) defined recovery as 'a voluntarily maintained lifestyle characterized by sobriety, personal health and citizenship'.

Prevention

Identifying youth at risk for alcohol/drug initiation and continued use is a potentially efficient and effective means for targeting prevention efforts. In the United States, however, youth in general are at risk for drug initiation (Hubbard *et al.* 1988). Surveys of high school students have shown that non-medical drug use begins in the early teens, peaks in early adulthood, and declines sharply thereafter (Kandel 1980). Initiation to marijuana is almost completed by the age of 20, and to psychedelic drugs by the age of 21 (Kandel & Logan 1984). More than half of inhalant, phencyclidine, and barbiturate users initiate use before tenth grade (15–16 years old). Prior to the crack epidemic, most cocaine users initiated use in the last 2 years of high school (Johnston *et al.* 1984).

Drug use prevention programmes should ideally first reach youth prior to adolescence, then reinforce the message throughout adolescence. Research findings suggest that prevention efforts oriented towards delaying the age of onset of initiation may prevent the initiation of other perhaps more dangerous drugs (Kandel 1982), a greater frequency of use (Rachal *et al.* 1982), and the involvement in other delinquent acts (Brunswick & Boyle 1979).

Prevention strategies seek to prevent substance abuse by informing, educating, and training individuals so that they have the necessary information, skills, and confidence to choose not to abuse alcohol or other drugs. Environmental approaches seek to restrict the opportunity for exposure to alcohol and other drugs. Prevention programmes and organizations offering prevention services often adopt one or more strategies (Tobler 1986):

1. Information activities are designed to provide accurate and timely information about alcohol and other drugs and their effects on the individual, family, and community.
2. Education activities use a structured process to assist individuals in learning and improving basic life skills (decision-making, problem-solving, community, and peer/social resistance skills).
3. Alternatives programmes provide challenging positive growth experiences in which individuals can develop the self-discipline, confidence, personal awareness, self-reliance, and independence they need to become socially mature individuals by offering positive alternatives to alcohol and other drug-using behaviours.
4. Intervention services identify individuals with early substance abuse problems, help them assess their problems and take action to resolve them, and provide emotional support and practical guidance during the early stages of recovery.
5. Environmental controls include efforts to make alcohol and other drugs less accessible by raising drinking ages, increasing enforcement, or otherwise reducing access to alcohol and other drugs.

Most of the drug education programmes are based on a knowledge/attitude, value/decision-making, or social competency theoretical approach (Moskowitz 1983). The knowledge/attitude approach has been used most widely, although empirical support for the assumed causal links between knowledge of the consequences of drug use, attitudes concerning use, and use behaviour is limited (Hanson 1980; Kinder *et al.* 1980; Goodstadt 1981). The effectiveness of the value/decision-making approach (Huba *et al.* 1980; Goodstadt 1981), which assumes that logical weighing of the costs and benefits of drug use takes place, is also not well supported. Studies measuring the effects of the teaching of social skills on drug use prevention among adolescents show promising results. Pentz (1983) concluded that teaching skills such as assertiveness, initiating/maintaining conversation, non-verbal expression, expressing feelings/empathy, decision-making, expressing an opinion or request, self-control, praise, and responding to criticism reduces drug use and related behaviours among adolescents. Similarly, Botvin (1983), after instituting a prevention programme teaching life skills to adolescents, found a 50 per cent reduction in new cigarette smoking 1 year after the programme.

Prevention efforts have been implemented and developed primarily in three social realms—the school, the family, and the community.

Educational programmes presented in schools are the most frequently employed approach to drug abuse prevention. Evaluative studies (Schaps *et al.* 1984) and reviews (Goodstadt 1980; Schaps *et al.* 1981), however, provide little support for the effectiveness of school-based programmes. Goodstadt (1980), in a review of several drug education programmes, observed that most had mixed results; i.e. they produced negative results on some attitudinal and behavioural dimensions and positive results on others. He concluded that although education programmes do not appear to be as harmful or counterproductive as some detractors claim, their results are not as strongly positive as one would like. While these educational programmes have reported some positive results, both the programmes and the evaluations of them have been criticized because of an inadequate theoretical base. They assume, albeit implicitly, that attitudes are strongly related to behaviours, and that a single exposure will have enduring effects throughout the adolescent years. Attitudes are usually not good predictors of behaviour (Fishbein & Ajzen 1975), and most programmes do not consider the complex development stages of adolescence (Greenspan 1985).

Many theories have addressed the importance of involving parents in any type of intervention. Bry (1983) notes the significance of modelling and the necessity for communication skills to teach young people how to say 'no' when dealing with the pressures of substance abuse behaviours and other negative behaviours. McAlister (1983) points specifically to the significance of prevention programmes that address low self-esteem, poor skills for coping with stress, and alienation from school and family. He addresses the significance of self-image being more related to family relationships than to school relationships. These theories give credence to involving parents with their children in a family approach to prevention.

Descriptions of community action programmes in alcohol (Hewitt & Blane 1984) and drug abuse (Flay & Sobel 1983) have generally focused on media campaigns. Project STAR (Students Taught Awareness and Resistance), a community-based drug and alcohol abuse prevention programme in Kansas City, MO, however, is a comprehensive approach that works through a liaison between the programme implementers and researchers (Pentz *et al.* 1986). Programme components are implemented, and progress is observed and tested for any effect on drug use. The component is then refined according to the evaluation results before the initiation of the next programme component. Data from the delayed implementation of this multicommunity trial (Pentz *et al.* 1989) indicate the potential effectiveness of comprehensive intervention. The interventions included a combination of mass media, school-based programmes, parental involvement, and community support. Prevalence of alcohol, tobacco, and marijuana was lower in the sites where the intervention had been implemented compared to control sites where the intervention had been delayed, 17 versus 24 per cent for cigarettes, 11 versus 16 per cent for alcohol, and 7 versus 10 per cent for marijuana. The rate of increase in usage was also lower in the sites where the intervention had been implemented.

Based on the success of public information campaigns to reduce smoking and the results of prevention research, a media effort to reduce drug use among youth was launched throughout the United States in 1998 (Westat 2003). While exposure to (70–80 per cent) and recall of (58–76 per cent) of the messages were high for both youth and parents, the effects were weak or absent. Parents did seem to be more likely to talk to youth about drugs and engaged in more activities. Although believing monitoring was important, those exposed to messages did not increase their monitoring behaviour. There was 'little evidence of direct favourable campaign effects on youths' beliefs, intentions or behaviour'. Delayed effect analyses have been planned, but are not yet available.

Treatment

Treatment in one form or another for both alcohol and drug abuse have been available since the turn of the century. It is, however, only in the late 1960s and early 1970s that both alcohol and drug abuse treatment have become major parts of the public health system in the United States. The administration of the public treatment system in America shifted from the federal government to states under the Omnibus Reconciliation Act of 1981. Treatment systems rapidly evolved to meet the demands of cost containment in the 1990s. In the next millennium, the evolution of treatment programmes and the system that supports them has continued. There is a major transformation to fee for service and evidence-based practice (Lewin Group 2005; Roman *et al.* 2006).

Approaches

The alcohol treatment system emerged from an effort in the late 1960s to establish community-based alcohol treatment centres throughout many parts of the United States. Combined with this public approach was the availability of proprietary inpatient programmes based on the Minnesota model treatment protocol (Laundergan 1982; Cook 1988). These short-term inpatient regimens help guide alcohol abusers through the first phases of the 12 steps of the Alcoholics Anonymous recovery programme.

The rapid escalation of heroin addiction in communities in the late 1960s, coupled with the high rates of addiction among returning Vietnam veterans, led to the establishment of a national system of drug abuse treatment programmes to deal with the increasing rates of addiction and associated crime (Jaffe 1979). Since these early years, there have been far-reaching changes in the drug abuse treatment system. The three major modalities or types of treatment developed and currently being administered under public funding in the United States are outpatient methadone clinics, therapeutic communities, and outpatient drug-free programmes. Outpatient methadone programmes treat opioid abusers, most of whom use heroin intravenously. After stabilization with medically prescribed doses of methadone, clients receive a variety of counselling and other services to help them resume productive lives. Therapeutic communities use group counselling with all types of drug abusers over long stays in a 24-h community environment. Outpatient drug-free programmes tend to be oriented towards non-opioid users, emphasizing counselling, often in community mental health centre settings. Among the three modalities, there are great variations in programme size, structure, therapeutic approach, services, and funding. Treatment for drug abuse, particularly cocaine, began to be provided in chemical dependency programmes originally designed for alcoholism in the late 1980s.

The treatment system in the United States now includes a broad array of public and private programme types. The proportion of privately funded alcohol and drug abuse treatment programmes increased during the 1980s. By the 1990s, drug abuse treatment was delivered in a wider variety of settings, including chemical dependency programmes (formerly exclusive alcohol treatment programmes), community mental health centres, as well as treatment programmes designed primarily for alcohol. The distinction between publicly funded and private treatment has become blurred. With the movement to a fee for service structure, substance abuse treatment clients may receive services from an even broader array of providers. Despite the multiple service need and the availability of community resources, the treatment of many clients in the traditional public treatment modalities has seldom been supported by public funds at a level that parallels annual inflation.

Effectiveness

The effectiveness of both alcohol and drug abuse treatment has been continually questioned. One of the major reasons for this is the difficulty of conducting broad-based epidemiological outcome studies or controlled clinical trials of sufficient scope to answer some of the major questions about treatment. In the United States, only one national study of alcohol treatment and three of drug abuse treatment have been successfully mounted in the past 30 years. Clinical trials based on unblinded random assignment have often failed because of limited compliance (Fuller *et al.* 1986) and retention (Bale *et al.* 1980) for sufficiently long periods of time to demonstrate the efficacy of any particular treatment approach.

Epidemiological outcome studies do indicate positive effects. The major clinical epidemiological study of alcohol treatment was conducted in the early 1970s with a sample of 593 clients followed 18 and 48 months after treatment (Armor *et al.* 1978; Polich *et al.* 1981). After 4 years, 21 per cent were abstinent for at least 1 year before the follow-up. A positive correlation was reported between those clients receiving five or more outpatient visits and those with more than 7 days worth of inpatient visits. Using a cost-offset framework in an analysis of health insurance data, Holder and Blose (1986) attributed substantial savings to alcohol treatment in health-care costs. Other follow-up studies of proprietary programmes reviewed by the Institute of Medicine (Committee to Identify Research Effectiveness in the Prevention and Treatment of Alcohol-Related Problems 1989) find abstinence rates between 40 and 60 per cent in the first year after treatment. Similar results were found in studies of state programmes (Hubbard *et al.* 1988) and proprietary programmes (Hoffman & Harrison 1987). Because of the often low rates of response to follow-up, the method of obtaining reports, imprecise measurement of treatment process, including continuing care and other methodological considerations, these rates of abstinence likely exaggerate the positive effects of treatment.

In contrast to these findings and those for drug abuse treatment reported below, the Institute of Medicine panel found little evidence supporting longer term treatment for alcohol abuse Reviews (Saxe *et al.* 1983; Annis 1986; Miller & Hester 1986), and a series of random assignment studies have found neither length of treatment nor intensity (inpatient versus outpatient) influenced outcome. In such unblinded research, however, the levels of severity of client problems likely interact with selection bias from compliance and attrition to confound the interpretation of results. Further, most alcohol treatment protocols tested, typically less than 3 months, may not be of sufficient duration or intensity to produce demonstrable effects. Controlled studies of alcohol treatment may need to focus more on comparison of different continuums of care to examine how inpatient and outpatient programmes can contribute to long-term compliance with aftercare and relapse prevention.

Such an approach has been implemented in a national multisite trial of three outpatient protocols for alcohol abuse based on 12-step, cognitive-behavioural, or motivational enhancement approaches (Project MATCH Research Group 1993). These studies demonstrated that in all three approaches, clients did achieve reductions in alcohol.

A series of studies conducted primarily over the past four decades has demonstrated the effectiveness of the publicly funded methadone maintenance and therapeutic community approaches (Tims 1981; Tims & Ludford 1984; Hubbard *et al.* 2008). Use of most drugs declines during and after treatment (Sells & Simpson 1976; Smart 1976; Sells 1979; Holland 1982; DeLeon 1984). Criminal activity is reduced among programme clients, particularly during treatment (Gorsuch *et al.* 1976; Nash 1976; McGlothlin *et al.* 1977; Dole & Joseph 1978).

In the late 1970s, a clinical epidemiological study of drug abuse treatments assessed outcomes for 10 000 methadone, residential, and outpatient drug-free clients up to 5 years after treatment (Hubbard *et al.* 1989). Substantial decreases in regular heroin, cocaine, and psychotherapeutic drug abuse, and diminished overall severity of drug abuse were apparent during and after treatment for clients treated over a period of at least 3 months. The prevalence of regular heroin use for methadone clients in the first year after treatment (17 per cent) was one-quarter of the pretreatment rate. For residential clients, the post-treatment prevalence of regular heroin (12 per cent) was one-third of the rate prior to treatment, and non-medical psychotherapeutic drug use (9 per cent) was one-fifth of the rate prior to treatment; regular use of cocaine declined by half to 16 per cent in the post-treatment period. In the case of outpatient drug-free clients, prevalence of non-medical psychotherapeutic drug use was half the pretreatment rate. In any given year of follow-up, less than 20 per cent of former clients in any modality were regular users of drugs other than marijuana or alcohol. Reductions in criminal activity were maintained up to 5 years after leaving treatment.

All types of treatment did achieve statistically and clinically significant reductions for the drug usage they were designed to treat if a client stayed in a programme long enough. In multivariate analysis controlling for a variety of factors, including demographics, drug use patterns, prior treatment, and reason for seeking treatment, the risk of relapse was reduced three- to four-fold for those clients who stayed in treatment for 6 months or more, compared to those who left earlier. The authors conclude that although treatment does have a demonstrable effect, substantial improvement is needed. Programmes only attract a relatively low proportion of individuals who might benefit from treatment. Retention rates have been low, particularly for long-term treatment or continuum of care necessary. The increasingly complex problems of multiple drug usage and impairment require more trained and committed staff. Further, recovering addicts and abusers must also have access to an array of relapse prevention rehabilitation, habilitation, and support services in the community.

This research was replicated in the Drug Abuse Treatment Outcome Studies (DATOS) for a sample of 10 000 adults entering treatment between 1991 and 1993 (Flynn *et al.* 1997). The DATOS research in community-based treatment has replicated a number of major findings that have been consistently found in other studies. In addition to replication of major findings, the DATOS studies also found positive effects of treatment for adolescents (Hser *et al.* 2001) and for cocaine abusers (Simpson *et al.* 1999). The changes in behaviour and the influence of time in treatment were confirmed 5 years after termination of treatment (Hubbard *et al.* 2003), even after taking into account the characteristics of the persons and a variety of intervening events over the 5 years.

Another set of findings requires further examination, as studies have included a broader variety of programmes in complex, changing health care, social service, and criminal justice environments. There has been a broad array of programmes designed to meet the needs of substance abusers, including therapeutic community or long-term residential, outpatient drug-free, methadone, and short-term inpatient programmes. The range of options, however, appears to be diminishing, including the elimination of short-term inpatient rehabilitation and longer-term stays in therapeutic communities (Etheridge *et al.* 1997). Clients select and are selected for different modalities of treatment based on the type of drug use, the severity of related problems, and the resources to pay for treatment. Few clients are referred to methadone treatment by the criminal justice system, and increasing proportions of clients in other modalities are referred by the criminal justice system. The source of referral can result in longer stays (Joe *et al.* 1999).

The diverse modality and programme approaches to treatment can be described by the nature of core therapy for substance abuse and the comprehensive services for related problems. Over the decades of the 1970s and 1980s, core services have improved, particularly the integration of 12-step components, while comprehensive services have declined and are less likely to meet the needs of clients (Etheridge *et al.* 1997).

Treatment has been effective for the type of drug use for which it has been targeted; opioids in the 1960s and 1970s, multiple drug use in the 1980s, and cocaine in the 1990s. Stays of 90 days significantly reduce the probabilities of relapse to drug use within the first year following treatment. Involvement in self-help at least twice a week is related to further decreases in the probability of relapse to cocaine for those who stayed in treatment more than 90 days (Etheridge *et al.* 1999).

The effects of treatment (particularly time in treatment) on related problems are not as consistent, and appear to be diminishing with the erosion of comprehensive services. A 1-year stay in a therapeutic community has been consistently related to increases in the probability of post-treatment employment and decreases in the probability of illegal activity. However, the effects of treatment duration on illegal activity for methadone and outpatient drug-free clients in the follow-up year found in the 1970s–1980s have not been consistently replicated in more recent studies (Hubbard *et al.* 1997).

Economic analyses of benefits and costs consistently show that treatments in therapeutic communities, methadone, and outpatient drug-free treatment generate benefits in crime reduction during and after treatment that more than pay for the costs of treatments (Flynn *et al.* 1999). Clients in therapeutic communities, who have the highest crime rates, generate the greatest reduction in crime costs after treatment.

The NIDA Clinical Trial Network was implemented as a response to the concerns that clinical research did not address the gaps in knowledge in actual practice. A series of over 20 trials of pharmacological and psychosocial interventions have been undertaken. The major studies to date have demonstrated efficacy of the buprenorphine detoxification regimen (Amass *et al.* 2004) in community settings, identified a feasible approach to using incentives to encourage abstinence for stimulant users (Petry *et al.* 2005), determined that manual guided motivational interviewing led to greater retention (Carroll *et al.* 2006), and determined that post-residential programme discharge phone contact with patients increased the likelihood of subsequent attendance at community-based treatment (Hubbard *et al.* 2007). The trials have also focused on interventions for injecting drug users at risk for HIV/AIDS.

HIV/AIDS among injecting drug users

Over the last several decades, HIV infection among injecting drug users (IDUs) has become a worldwide public health problem. According to the most recent estimate, there are now 13 million IDUs in the world (Aceijas *et al.* 2006), of whom over 10 million live in developing and transitional countries. HIV has been spreading rapidly among IDUs in Eastern Europe and Asia. Approximately 10 per cent of all new HIV infections worldwide are among IDUs, and approximately 30 per cent of all new HIV infections outside of sub-Saharan Africa are among IDUs (UNAIDS/WHO 2006). HIV/AIDS clearly become the most dramatic example of the many health and social problems associated with illicit drug use.

Injection of illicit psychoactive drugs does not in itself transmit HIV; rather, it is the micro-transfusions of HIV-infected blood that transmit the virus when two or more persons use the same injection equipment. It is thus possible to reduce HIV transmission among IDUs not only by reducing illicit drug injection itself, but also by reducing the instances in which two or more IDUs use the same injection equipment. The urgent need to control HIV transmission among IDUs and the possibility that HIV can be prevented in persons who continue to inject illicit drugs have led to a number of programmes that would not have been considered prior to the emergence of HIV/AIDS, and to a new public health-oriented perspective on the problems of drug misuse.

The first HIV epidemic among IDUs almost occurred in New York City during the mid-1970s (Des Jarlais *et al.* 1994). During the 1980s, HIV then spread among IDUs in the rest of the United States and in Western Europe and Australia (Ball *et al.* 1998). During the late 1980s, HIV spread to IDUs in Asia, most notably in Thailand (Des Jarlais *et al.* 1992b), and also in Latin America. The spread of HIV among IDUs continued during the 1990s, particularly in Asia, and from the mid-1990s, onwards in Russia and Eastern Europe (Ball *et al.* 1998). Given the development of this pandemic of HIV transmission among IDUs, public health officials need to plan on continued diffusion of HIV among IDUs throughout the world.

In many areas, HIV has spread extremely rapidly among IDUs, with the HIV seroprevalence rate (the percentage of IDUs infected with HIV) increasing from less than 10–50 per cent or greater within a period of 1–2 years (Des Jarlais *et al.* 1992a; Stimson *et al.* 1998). Several factors have been associated with extremely rapid transmission of HIV among IDUs. First, a lack of awareness of HIV/AIDS as a local threat can contribute to rapid spread. Without an awareness of AIDS as a local threat, IDUs are likely to use each other's equipment very frequently. Indeed, prior to an awareness of HIV/AIDS, providing previously used equipment to another IDU is likely to be seen as an act of solidarity among IDUs, or as a service for which one may legitimately charge a small fee.

Second, situations that promote 'rapid partner change' among persons who share needles and syringes contribute to rapid transmission.

Not all types of sharing of injection equipment will lead to rapid transmission of HIV within population of IDUs. Rapid transmission requires sharing within settings that permit IDUs to share with large numbers of other IDUs within short time periods (rapid risk partner change). 'Shooting galleries' (places where IDUs can rent injection equipment, which is then returned to the gallery owner for rental to other IDUs) and 'dealer's works' (injection equipment kept by a drug seller, which can be lent to successive drug purchasers) are examples of situations that provide rapid, efficient mixing within an IDU population. 'Hit doctors', who administer injections to IDUs who have trouble injecting themselves, may use the same needle and syringe for many different clients. In these situations, many different IDUs may share the same needle and syringe within a short time period. Sharing in these types of settings can spread HIV across potential social boundaries, such as friendship groups, which otherwise might have served to limit transmission.

Third, persons who are recently infected with HIV ('acute HIV infection') also tend to be highly infectious (Wawer *et al.* 2005). This increases the possibility of extremely rapid HIV transmission if the virus should enter an IDU population structured to produce rapid partner change syringe sharing.

At present, there is no vaccine to prevent HIV infection. There is effective treatment to manage HIV infection, but this treatment is expensive, does not cure infection, and drug resistance frequently develops. Thus, while it is very important to provide treatment for HIV-infected IDUs, public health efforts to reduce morbidity and mortality related to HIV among IDUs must focus on modifying the risk behaviour of IDUs. We will review current knowledge of HIV prevention programmes for IDUs. In doing so, it will be useful to provide some historical context on the evolution of these efforts.

Early risk reduction among IDUs

The first evidence that IDUs would change their risk behaviour in response to information about AIDS came from several studies in New York City (Des Jarlais *et al.* 1985; Friedman *et al.* 1987; Selwyn *et al.* 1987). This risk reduction occurred due to the implementation of formal HIV prevention programmes for IDUs in the city. In all of these studies, the majority of drug users reported that they knew about AIDS, that they knew that it was transmitted through the sharing of needles and syringes, and that they had already made at least some changes in their injection behaviour (e.g. reduced sharing of injection equipment).

IDUs in New York had learned about AIDS through the mass media and through their own oral communication networks. Because of the relatively large number of cases of AIDS among IDUs in New York City, even in the early 1980s, there had been a considerable amount of mass media coverage. The relatively large number of cases of AIDS among IDUs in New York also meant that a substantial number of IDUs either knew someone first-hand who had developed AIDS, or knew someone who knew someone who had developed AIDS. An additional potentially important factor in this early behaviour change/risk reduction was the expansion of the illicit market in sterile injection equipment (Des Jarlais *et al.* 1985).

While early studies indicated that IDUs would learn about AIDS from the mass media and through oral communication networks, it became clear by the mid-1980s that there would be many additional advantages to having health workers provide face-to-face AIDS education for IDUs. Face-to-face education would permit transmitting more detailed information, using culturally appropriate terminology (that might not have been possible in mass media), answering any questions that the drug users might have, and adopting an emotional tone responsive to the IDUs participating in the immediate communication.

It is possible to provide AIDS education for drug users in drug abuse treatment programmes, and many treatment programmes did develop AIDS education efforts (Des Jarlais *et al.* 1992c). With the great majority of drug users, however, various types of 'community outreach' programmes were developed to provide AIDS education to active drug users. The earliest programmes were in New Jersey (Jackson & Rotkiewicz 1987) and San Francisco (Watters 1994). Outreach programmes have since become a primary method for preventing HIV transmission among IDUs in most countries throughout the world. Outreach programmes have become increasingly sophisticated in terms of the theories utilized to lead to risk reduction, the use of former or current drug users as health outreach workers, and provision of the means for behaviour change (sterile needles and syringes for safer drug injection and condoms for safer sexual behaviour).

Using psychological theories of health-related behaviour to prevent HIV among IDUs

While the earliest studies did show an effect of providing 'education' about AIDS in changing HIV risk behaviour among IDUs, it was also clear that simple 'information-only' prevention programmes were not likely to be very strong in producing long-term behaviour change. Knowledge of possible adverse consequences is rarely sufficient to change behaviour in the health field.

Various theories of health-related behaviour, including the Health Belief model (Becker & Joseph 1988), social learning theory (Bandura 1977), and the theory of reasoned action (Fishbein & Ajzen 1975) have been utilized in programmes. While there are differences among these theories, there are also more important similarities. All include elements of expectancy-value decision-making analyses. Thus, these theories tend to emphasize perceived probabilities (of getting or avoiding AIDS, of being able to successfully perform new behaviours) and subjective valuations of different outcomes (the seriousness of developing AIDS, social costs of performing new behaviours if one's injecting or sexual partners are resistant). With some variation in explicitness, these theories also consider social factors (role models, perceived social norms) and various 'barriers' to changing HIV risk behaviours.

Utilizing these psychological theories of health behaviour required more than the one-way communication possible in mass-media approaches and more than the usually brief conversations that occur between outreach programme workers and IDUs encountered in the streets. The National AIDS Demonstration Research/AIDS Targeted Outreach Model programme began in the United States in 1987, and eventually included 41 projects in nearly 50 different cities (Brown & Beschner 1993). In all of the cities, the NADR/ATOM project involved street outreach to IDUs not in treatment programmes. The eligibility requirements for subjects to be enrolled in the research component of the NADR/ATOM projects required that the person must have injected illicit drugs in the previous 6 months and must not have been in drug abuse treatment in the preceding month. Approximately 40 per cent of the more than 30 000 subjects enrolled in the NADR/ATOM projects reported that they had never been in drug abuse treatment. Many of the NADR/ATOM projects used experimental designs to test psychological theories of health behaviour change. All subjects were provided with a 'standard' intervention to reduce HIV risk behaviour, which included information about HIV and AIDS, a baseline risk assessment, and the option of HIV counselling and testing. Some of these subjects were then randomly assigned to an 'enhanced' condition that typically involved several additional hours of counselling/education/skills-training that incorporated components of the psychological theories of health behaviour. Subjects were followed at 6-month intervals to assess changes in HIV risk behaviours and the incidence of new HIV infections.

The NADR/ATOM projects provided a wealth of data about HIV risk behaviours among IDUs not in drug treatment programmes. With respect to changes in HIV risk behaviours, there were two strong and very consistent findings. First, almost all of the NADR/ATOM projects showed substantial reductions in injection risk behaviour from the baseline assessment to the follow-up interviews. For example, those reporting sharing needles declined from 54 to 23 per cent (Stephens *et al.* 1993).

The second consistent finding was that almost none of the different projects showed significant differences in risk reduction between the 'standard' intervention and the 'enhanced' interview. The general lack of differences between the 'standard' and the 'enhanced' interventions should not be interpreted as meaning that the psychological theories of health behaviour are not relevant to HIV risk reduction among IDUs; rather, these results suggest two other possible explanations. First, after provision of basic information about AIDS (as in the standard intervention), 2–8 h of additional education and counselling does little to further 'strengthen' anti-AIDS attitudes, perceptions and intentions.

A second explanation is that risk reduction among IDUs—again, after basic HIV/AIDS education—is primarily a function of social processes rather than the characteristics of individual IDUs.

Using social network theories to prevent HIV among IDUs

There is increasing evidence that social network processes, particularly peer influences, are important in HIV risk reduction among IDUs (Des Jarlais *et al.* 1994; Neaigus *et al.* 1994; Latkin *et al.* 1996). Almost all injection risk behaviours (sharing of injection equipment) and all sexual risk behaviours occur within social settings. Initiating and maintaining safer injection and sexual behaviours may require changes in the social relationships among IDUs and their sexual partners.

In an analysis of factors associated with risk reduction among IDUs in four of the cities (Bangkok, Glasgow, Rio de Janeiro, and New York City) participating in the World Health Organization's Multi-Centre Study of AIDS and Drug Injection, 'talking with drug-using friends' was significantly associated with risk reduction in all four cities (Des Jarlais *et al.* 1993a). Despite the substantial variation in the drugs injected in these cities (heroin in Bangkok, heroin and buprenorphine in Glasgow, cocaine in Rio de Janeiro, and heroin and cocaine in New York) and the obvious cultural differences among IDUs in these cities, peer influence appeared to be an important component of risk reduction in all four cities.

Several of the NADR/ATOM models explicitly focused on peer influence and social change processes. The Chicago project (Wiebel *et al.* 1996) had its origins in the long tradition of ethnography, community research, and outreach to drug users by researchers at the University of Chicago. In this particular project, ex-addicts, under the supervision of trained ethnographers, conducted outreach for IDUs not in treatment. Specific efforts were made to enrol influential persons (indigenous leaders) within drug use networks into the project and have them act to influence other IDUs to practice safer injection. This project thus utilized the naturally occurring network structure among IDUs to change HIV risk behaviours. A cohort research design was used, with subjects followed for 5 years. The subjects reported dramatic reductions in injection risk behaviour. At the start of the project, 95 per cent of subjects reported engaging in injection risk behaviour, and this declined to only 15 per cent of the subjects reporting injection risk behaviour in the 5th year of the study. There was also a significantly lower HIV incidence among the IDUs who received the indigenous leader prevention compared to HIV incidence among IDUs who lived in a different neighbourhood and did not receive the intervention (Wiebel 1993).

One of the New York City NADR projects involved 'self-organization' among IDUs (Friedman *et al.* 1992, 1993). The Dutch 'Junkie Bonds'—one of which had initiated the first syringe-exchange programme in Holland—served as a model for how IDUs can act together to further their own health interests. In the New York City project, outreach workers recruited IDUs and assisted them in developing self-help groups to address HIV transmission and other issues of importance to them. In particular, the subgroup of commercial sex workers among IDUs had a number of common interests. Regular group meetings were held to discuss how the participants could change peer norms of injection and sexual risk behaviours. Attending the meetings was strongly associated with both the subjects' own risk reduction and efforts to change the behaviour of other IDUs (Friedman *et al.* 1993).

Broadhead and colleagues (1998) developed a 'peer-driven' outreach programme for IDUs. Individual IDUs are recruited into the study and provided with AIDS education. These initial subjects are then asked to recruit other IDUs into the study, and paid modest stipends for their recruiting efforts. The initial subjects are asked not only to recruit new subjects, but also to provide AIDS education to the new subjects. An AIDS information test is given to each of the peer-recruited subjects, and if the newly recruited subject passes the test, the original subject who did the recruiting and educating receives an increased stipend.

Latkin and colleagues (1996) developed an AIDS risk reduction programme that utilizes naturally occurring peer networks of IDUs. Existing peer networks or single network members are brought in for multiple sessions that not only provide information about HIV and AIDS, but also attempt to develop new social norms within the peer groups. These new norms emphasize practising safer injection and safer sex. These efforts have led to substantial reductions in risk behaviours.

Social network theories do not necessarily replace 'AIDS education' and psychological theories of health-related behaviour. Knowledge of HIV infection and AIDS and how to practice safer sex and safer injection are still important, as are perceptions of risk and a sense of efficacy in practising safer behaviours. Given the continuing developments in HIV/AIDS research (such as new therapies), AIDS education must also be done on a continuing basis.

Social network theories offer important additional power for reducing HIV risk behaviours, however. Influencing others to adopt new behaviours can also serve to strengthen the intentions of prevention programme participants to change their own risk behaviours. If social norms of injection and sexual behaviour can be changed, then it will be possible to change the behaviour of IDUs who do not directly participate in the prevention programme. Finally, the peer approval that comes with following the new norms can itself serve to reinforce safer injection and safer sex practices among IDUs.

Using social structural theory to prevent HIV among IDUs

Much recent theoretical work on HIV prevention for IDUs has centred on social structural interventions (Blankenship *et al.* 2000; Des Jarlais 2000; Sumartojo & Laga 2000). Structural invention theory often includes individual and social network components, but represents a major change in the focus for interventions. The focus in structural interventions is not on changing the individual IDU (increasing knowledge, motivation, skills) or changing social networks (changing social norms), but on changing the 'risk environment' in which drug injection occurs. The main problem to be addressed is not lack of knowledge or motivation among individual IDUs or inappropriate social norms among IDUs, but rather the many societal factors make it very difficult for IDUs to practice safer behaviours. There are a number of central ideas within the broad concept of structural interventions to reduce HIV transmission among IDUs, including: (1) providing the means for safer behaviours; (2) removing barriers to practising safer behaviours; (3) 'comprehensive' interventions; and (4) the amount of 'coverage' required.

1. Providing the means for behaviour change

While knowledge, motivation, skills, and social support are all important, having access to sterile needles and syringes is necessary for practising safer injection. Syringe exchange has become the prototype programme for HIV prevention for IDUs. As the name suggests, these programmes exchange new, sterile needles and syringes for used needles and syringes. Such exchange both provides IDUs with sterile injection equipment and removes the potentially HIV-contaminated needles and syringes from the community.

The first syringe exchange was set up in the city of Amsterdam in 1984. The exchange was implemented after a large pharmacy in the city centre stopped selling needles and syringes to drug users. The exchange was actually established to prevent hepatitis B, not HIV, transmission among IDUs in the city. In 1985, the HIV antibody test became available, and it became clear that many IDUs in the city (over 30 per cent) were already infected with HIV. This led to a rapid expansion of syringe exchange in Amsterdam and implementation of syringe exchanges in many other Dutch cities (Buning *et al.* 1988). In 1987, the United Kingdom implemented a nationwide system of syringe-exchange programmes (Stimson *et al.* 1988). In 1987, France repealed its laws requiring prescriptions for the sale of sterile injection equipment and set up a programme for encouraging pharmacists to sell injection equipment to IDUs (Espinoza *et al.* 1988; Ingold & Ingold 1989). Australia repealed its prescription requirement laws in 1984, then established a system of syringe-exchange programmes (Wodak 1995). In many European countries, such as Italy, Germany and Spain, there were no legal restrictions on the sale and possession of injection equipment, and education programmes were implemented to educate and encourage IDUs to inject with sterile equipment. Almost all of these countries have since established syringe exchange programmes as a means for providing sterile needles and syringes to IDUs (Lurie *et al.* 1993).

In the United States, there was also some early consideration of providing legal access to sterile injection equipment as a method for reducing HIV transmission among IDUs (Des Jarlais & Hopkins 1985). Early exchanges were implemented by activists in the northeast and by community-based organizations in the northwest (see Lurie *et al.* 1993; Normand *et al.* 1995 for histories of early syringe exchange efforts in the United States). There were many impediments to providing legal access to sterile injection equipment for IDUs in the United States (Des Jarlais & Friedman 1992a; Lurie *et al.* 1993; Normand *et al.* 1995; Gostin 1998). The states with large numbers of IDUs (e.g. New York, California, Illinois) had laws requiring prescriptions for the sale of injection equipment, and almost all states had laws criminalizing the possession of equipment for injecting illicit drugs.

Efforts to increase access by IDUs to sterile injection equipment, either through changing laws and/or by implementing 'underground' syringe exchanges in defiance of existing statutes, often generated intense controversy over whether this would increase illicit drug use and/or represent official 'condoning' of illicit drug use (Lurie *et al.* 1993; Normand *et al.* 1995). In some areas, racial/ethnic group antagonisms compounded the controversies (Anderson 1991). In 1989, federal legislation was enacted that prohibited the use of any federal funds to support syringe exchanges or other distribution of sterile injection equipment to persons who inject illicit drugs, and this prohibition remains in effect. Despite lack of federal funds, syringe exchange has expanded in the United States from 68 programmes in 1994 to 185 programmes in 2005 (McKnight *et al.* 2007). This expansion has occurred with funding from state, county, and local governments and from private sources.

There are now a moderately large number of studies that have used HIV infection (either incidence or trends in prevalence) as an outcome measure for assessing syringe exchange programmes. Almost all studies have shown low HIV incidence associated with syringe exchange programmes, including studies in Tacoma, WA (Hagan *et al.* 1995); Lund, Sweden (Ljungberg *et al.* 1991); Glasgow, Scotland (Frischer *et al.* 1993), the United Kingdom (Stimson *et al.* 1991; Stimson 1995), Portland, OR (Oliver *et al.* 1994); New York, NY (Des Jarlais *et al.* 1996, 2005), Seattle (Hagan & Thiede 2000), Australia (Wodak 1996), and France (Emmanuelli & Desenclos 2005; Des Jarlais *et al.* 2007). Although it is not possible to draw a direct causal connection, the expansion of syringe exchange programmes in the United States has been followed by reductions in HIV incidence among IDUs. HIV incidence is currently approximately 1/100 person-years at risk. Injecting drug use may be the only transmission category for which HIV incidence has declined over the last decade in the United States (Des Jarlais *et al.* 2005).

While the great majority of the studies of syringe exchange programmes have shown low HIV incidence associated with the programmes, there are also several studies of syringe exchange programmes that clearly did not provide sufficient protection against HIV infection for either their participants or for other IDUs in the community. In both Montreal (Bruneau *et al.* 1994) and Vancouver (Strathdee *et al.* 1997), HIV incidence exceeded 10/100 person-years at risk among syringe exchange participants. The factors that most probably led to the very high HIV incidence in Montreal and Vancouver included the exchanges attracting very high-risk drug injectors and that the supplies of sterile injection equipment were not sufficient to protect against HIV transmission within the context of very frequent cocaine injection. In response to the outbreaks of HIV among IDUs in Montreal and Vancouver, the syringe exchanges were expanded, and HIV incidence did then decline (Tyndall *et al.* 2001, 2002).

There have been a series of summary evaluations of syringe exchange programmes, including ones conducted by the United States National Commission on AIDS (1991), the United States Government Accounting Office (1993), the University of California (Lurie *et al.* 1993), and the National Academy of Science (Normand *et al.* 1995) (Gibson *et al.* 2002; Ksobiech 2003; Committee on the Prevention of HIV Infection 2006). All of these evaluations have concluded that syringe exchange programmes do lead to reductions in injection risk behaviour and do not lead to increases in illicit drug use.

2. Removing barriers to practising safer behaviours: Reducing stigmatization

Effective structural interventions require not only implementing programmes for IDUs, but removing barriers to IDUs participating in the programmes. Stigmatization of persons with (or at risk for) HIV is a critical aspect of the social environment of HIV transmission. Stigmatization can have multiple adverse consequences. First, stigmatization clearly increases the suffering of persons with HIV and AIDS. Second, stigmatization of groups at risk for or with HIV/AIDS can reduce public support for both prevention and treatment services. Third, fear of stigmatization may lead persons at risk for HIV/AIDS to avoid using the programmes that have been implemented, leading to increased transmission of HIV. Finally, members of ethnic/racial minority groups are at higher risk for HIV/AIDS in the United States and in many other countries. Stigmatization of HIV/AIDS can thus be compounded with stigmatization based on racial/ethnic minority status, increasing the multiple adverse consequences.

Stigmatization of HIV/AIDS, of illicit drug use, and of racial/ethnic minority status can all be difficult to change. However, there are important steps that can be taken. Civil rights laws clearly do not end stigmatization of racial/ethnic minorities, but such laws can reduce harmful actions based on stigmatization. The Americans with Disabilities Act (ADA) similarly prohibits discrimination based on AIDS and a history of drug use. (The ADA does not prohibit discrimination based on current drug use.) It is also possible and important to work with specific groups to reduce stigmatization of IDUs at risk for HIV/AIDS. There have been a number of projects that have worked with pharmacists to increase sales of sterile injection equipment to IDUs (Emmanuelli & Desenclos 2005; Fuller *et al.* 2007). It is also possible to work with local law enforcement agencies to reduce potential police interference with IDUs participating in HIV prevention programmes (Hammett *et al.* 2007).

3. Comprehensive programming to prevent HIV among IDUs

Structural analyses also include consideration of multiple prevention services rather than a single programme for all IDUs. Any IDU population is likely to have considerable diversity in terms of frequency of injection, frequency of needle sharing, and frequency of sexual risk behaviour. Different IDUs will also have different other issues, such as lack of stable housing, unemployment, and psychiatric problems, which may need to be addressed in order to consistently practice HIV risk reduction. Thus, no single programme is likely to be able to meet all of the needs within an IDU population. Over time, syringe exchange programmes have become multi-service organizations. In the United States and in other industrialized countries, syringe exchange programmes often provide services such as condom distribution, HIV and hepatitis C virus counselling and testing, and sexually transmitted disease screening on-site. Additional services are often provided through referrals. One critical aspect of syringe exchanges is that the great majority of the programmes provide referrals to drug abuse treatment programmes. Thus, rather than syringe exchange programmes keeping drug users from entering treatment, syringe exchange programmes have become an important linkage into drug abuse treatment (McKnight *et al.* 2007).

The most recent review of HIV prevention for IDUs emphasizes provision of sterile injection equipment within 'comprehensive programming' (Committee on the Prevention of HIV Infection 2006). This reflects both practical aspects of HIV prevention; many drug users require more than access to sterile injection equipment in order to avoid HIV infection. It also reflects a basic ethical position—that societies have an ethical obligation to address needs of drug users beyond HIV prevention; in particular, societies have an ethical obligation to provide effective treatment to reduce drug abuse.

4. The amount of 'coverage' required

Pilot programmes do not stop HIV epidemics. A critical aspect of structural interventions is having interventions that are large enough to control HIV transmission in a population of IDUs. Knowing what level of 'coverage' is needed to control HIV transmission is of obvious importance in areas with limited resources for HIV prevention. Studying the amount of 'coverage' needed, however, is difficult, and consensus among expert opinions and mathematical modelling are the two most frequently used methods of estimating coverage requirements. Coverage of sterile injection equipment for the number of injections in IDU populations has received the greatest amount of attention. The 'ideal' for HIV prevention is that each drug user would use a new, sterile needle and syringe for each injection (Des Jarlais *et al.* 1995a). Depending upon sharing patterns (sharing limited within small groups is much less likely to lead to widespread HIV transmission than sharing in large groups of IDUs) and the number of times IDUs re-use their own needles and syringes (which can lead to bacterial infections, but does not transmit HIV), the current estimate/opinion is that syringe distribution should cover about 25 per cent of injections (Vickerman *et al.* 2006).

High coverage to reduce unsafe injections does not require extremely large numbers of IDUs personally attending syringe exchange programmes or personally purchasing sterile needles and syringes at pharmacies. Rather, individual IDUs may exchange for peers ('secondary exchange') or purchase for peers who do not want to attend exchanges or purchase from pharmacies, usually because of concerns over confidentiality. Effective structural interventions need to provide for secondary exchange and purchasing for peers, and avoid artificial limits on the numbers of syringes that can be exchanged or purchased at a single visit (Des Jarlais *et al.* 1995b).

The low incidence rates in areas with syringe exchange programmes may occur through both direct and indirect effects of syringe exchanges. Participants in the exchanges receive both supplies of sterile injection equipment and counselling and information about HIV. Since syringe exchanges tend to attract IDUs who would otherwise be at very high risk for HIV infection, reducing risk behaviour among the IDUs who come to syringe exchanges can have a partial 'herd immunity' effect that protects the local IDU population as a whole. Sterile injection equipment, information about HIV, and new social norms against sharing injection equipment may also diffuse outwards from IDUs who directly participate in syringe exchange programmes to other IDUs in the community. Thus, large-scale syringe exchange programmes should probably be considered as community-level interventions whose protective effect extends beyond the IDUs who participate directly in the programmes.

New challenges

As discussed earlier, HIV prevention has been quite successful overall in industrialized countries, with incidence rates of 1/100 person-years or less in most of the countries. Certainly implementation of public health scale prevention programmes for IDUs could have been accomplished much earlier, and this would have averted thousands of HIV infections (Lurie & Drucker 1997). But injecting-related HIV transmission can now be considered under public health control in industrialized countries. The current challenges in industrialized countries concern hepatitis C virus and sexual transmission of HIV among injecting and non-injecting drug users. Hepatitis C virus (HCV) is hyperendemic among IDUs in both industrialized and developing/transitional countries, with prevalence rates of 60 to 90+ per cent (Hagan *et al.* 2007). HCV is also much more easily transmitted than HIV, and thus programmes that dramatically reduce HIV transmission may or may not be effective in controlling HCV transmission. Reduction in needle-borne HIV transmission has led to emergence of sexual transmission as the leading cause of new HIV infections among IDUs in some areas (Kral *et al.* 2001; Strathdee *et al.* 2001; Strathdee & Sherman 2003).

As noted above, however, the current predominant issue is rapid transmission of HIV among IDUs in many developing and transitional countries. An estimated one-third of incident HIV infections outside of sub-Saharan Africa are occurring among IDUs, particularly in parts of Eastern Europe and Central and Southeast Asia (UNAIDS/WHO 2006).

Harm reduction

The emergence of HIV/AIDS among IDUs has been a profound challenge to public health systems. In some areas, there was a rapid response and potential HIV epidemics among IDUs were averted. In other areas, HIV epidemics occurred before effective public health responses, but the responses eventually brought the epidemics under control, and in still other areas, HIV epidemics are occurring among IDUs without any effective public health responses. The HIV/AIDS crisis has furthered the development of a policy framework that provides a new perspective on the use of psychoactive drugs (both licit and illicit). This perspective has generally come to be known as 'harm reduction' (Berridge 1999; Buning 1991; see *Journal of Harm Reduction*).

It may be best to present Harm Reduction in the words of its practitioners (Harm Reduction Coalition 2007 [http://www.harmreduction.org/]).

Harm reduction is a set of practical strategies that reduce negative consequences of drug use, incorporating a spectrum of strategies from safer use to managed use to abstinence. Harm reduction strategies meet drug users 'where they're at', addressing conditions of use along with the use itself.

Because harm reduction demands that interventions and policies designed to serve drug users reflect specific individual and community needs, there is no universal definition of or formula for implementing harm reduction. However, HRC considers the following principles central to harm reduction practice.

- Accepts, for better and for worse, that licit and illicit drug use is part of our world, and chooses to work to minimize its harmful effects rather than simply ignore or condemn them.
- Understands drug use as a complex, multi-faceted phenomenon that encompasses a continuum of behaviours from severe abuse to total abstinence, and acknowledges that some ways of using drugs are clearly safer than others.
- Establishes quality of individual and community life and well-being—not necessarily cessation of all drug use—as the criteria for successful interventions and policies.
- Calls for non-judgmental, non-coercive provision of services and resources to people who use drugs and the communities in which they live in order to assist them in reducing attendant harm.
- Ensures that drug users and those with a history of drug use routinely have a real voice in the creation of programmes and policies designed to serve them.
- Affirms drugs users themselves as the primary agents of reducing the harms of their drug use, and seeks to empower users to share information and support each other in strategies that meet their actual conditions of use.
- Recognizes that the realities of poverty, class, racism, social isolation, past trauma, sex-based discrimination, and other social inequalities affect both people's vulnerability to and capacity for effectively dealing with drug-related harm.
- Does not attempt to minimize or ignore the real and tragic harm and danger associated with licit and illicit drug use.

The two basic components of harm reduction are respecting the civil rights of drug users (Gilmore 1996; Elliott 2004; Wolfe & Malinowska-Sempruch 2004) and pragmatism—doing what works. Harm reduction is thus a particularly appropriate policy framework for incorporating scientific data into public health practice (Des Jarlais 1995).

References

Aaron, P. and Musto, D. (1981). Temperance and prohibition in America: a private historical overview. In *Alcohol and public policy: beyond the shadow of prohibition* (eds. M.H. Moore and D.R. Gerstein). National Academy Press, Washington, DC.

Aceijas, C., Friedman, S.R., Cooper, H.L.F., Wiessing, L., Stimson, G.V., and Hickman, M. (2006). Estimates of injecting drug users at the national and local level in developing and transitional countries, and gender and age distribution. *Sexually Transmitted Infections*, **82** (Suppl III), iii10–7.

Amass, L., Ling, W. *et al.* (2004). Bringing buprenorphine-nalozone detoxification to community treatment providers: the NIDA clinical trials network field experience. *American Journal of Addictions*, **13** (Suppl 1), S42–66.

American Psychiatric Association. (1994). *Diagnostic and statistical manual of mental disorders*, 4th edn. (DSM-IV). American Psychiatric Association, Washington, DC.

Anderson, W. (1991). The New York needle trial: the politics of public health in the age of AIDS. *American Journal of Public Health*, **81**, 1506–17.

Aneshensel, C.S. and Huba, G.J. (1983). Depression, alcohol use, and smoking over one year: a four-wave longitudinal causal model. *Journal of Abnormal Psychology*, **92**, 134–50.

Annis, H.M. (1986). Is inpatient rehabilitation of the alcoholic cost effective, Con position. *Advances in Alcohol and Substance Abuse*, **5**, 175–90.

Armor, D.J., Polich, J.M., and Stambul, H.B. (1978). *Alcoholism and treatment*. Wiley, New York.

Babor, T.E. (ed.) (1986). *Alcohol and culture: comparative perspectives from Europe and America*. New York Academy of Sciences, New York.

Babor, T., Cooney, N., Hubbard, R. *et al.* (1988). The syndrome concept of alcohol and drug dependence: results of the secondary analysis project. In *Problems of drug dependence, 1987. Proceedings of the 49th Annual Scientific Meeting, The Committee on Problems of Drug Dependence, Inc.* Research Monograph Series 81 (ed. L.S. Harris). National Institute on Drug Abuse, Rockville.

Bachman, J.G., O'Malley, P.M., and Johnston, L.D. (1978). *Youth in transition Vol. VI: adolescence to adulthood—change and stability in the lives of young men*. Institute for Social Research, University of Michigan, Ann Arbor.

Bale, R.N., Van Stone, W., Kuldau, J.M., Engelsing, T.M.J., Elashoff, R.M., and Zarcone, V.P. (1980). Therapeutic communities vs. methadone maintenance. *Archives of General Psychiatry*, **37**, 179–93.

Ball, A.L., Rana, S. *et al.* (1998). HIV prevention among injecting drug users: responses in developing and transitional countries. *Public Health Reports*, **113** (Suppl 1), 170–181.

Bandura, A. (1977). *Social learning theory*. Englewood; Prentice-Hall, Englewood Cliffs.

Becker, M.H. and Joseph, J.K. (1988). AIDS and behavioral change to reduce risk: a review. *American Journal of Public Health*, **78**, 394–410.

Berridge, V. (1992). *Harm reduction: an historical perspective*. 3rd International Conference on Reduction of Drug-Related Harm, Melbourne.

Berridge, V. (1999). Histories of harm reduction: illicit drugs, tobacco, and nicotine. *Substance Use & Misuse*, **34**, 35–47.

The Betty Ford Institute Consensus Panel (2007). What is recovery? A working definition from the Betty Ford Institute. *Journal of Substance Treatment*, **33**, 221–8.

Blankenship, K., Bray, S., and Merson, M. (2000). Structural interventions in public health. *AIDS*, **14**, S11–21.

Botvin, G.J. (1983). Prevention of adolescent substance abuse through the development of personal and social competence. In *Preventing adolescent drug abuse: intervention strategies* (eds. T.J. Glynn, C.G. Leukefeld, and J.P. Ludford), pp. 115–40. Research Monograph 47. National Institute on Drug Abuse, Rockville.

Brecher, E.M. and the Editors of Consumer Reports (1972). *Licit and illicit drugs: the Consumers Union report on narcotics, stimulants, depressants, inhalants, hallucinogens, and marijuana—including caffeine, nicotine, and alcohol*. Consumers Union, Mount Vernon.

Broadhead, R.S., Heckathorn, D.D. *et al.* (1998). Harnessing peer networks as an instrument for AIDS prevention: results from a peer driven intervention. *Public Health Reports*, **113** (Suppl 1), 42–57.

Brown, B.S. and Beschner, G.M. (eds.) (1993). *Handbook on risk of AIDS: injection drug users and sexual partners*. Greenwood Press, Wesport.

Bruneau, J., Lamothe, E, Lachance, N., Soto, J., and Vincelette, J. (1994). *HIV prevalence and incidence in a cohort of IDUs in Montreal, according to their needle exchange attendance, Abstract PD0496*. Presented at the Tenth International Conference on AIDS, Yokohama.

Brunswick, A.F. and Boyle, J.M. (1979). Patterns of drug involvement: developmental and secular influences on age at initiation. *Youth and Society*, **2**, 139–62.

Bry, B.H. (1983). Empirical foundations of family-based approaches to adolescent substance abuse. In *Preventing adolescent drug abuse: intervention strategies* (eds. T.J. Glynn, C.G. Leukefeld, and J.P. Ludford), pp. 154–71. Research Monograph 47, National Institute on Drug Abuse, Rockville.

Buning, E.C. (1991). Effects of Amsterdam needle and syringe exchange. *International Journal of Addictions*, **26**, 1303–11.

Buning, E.C., van Brussel, G.H.A. *et al.* (eds.) (1988). *Amsterdam's drug policy and its implications for controlling needle sharing. Needle sharing among intravenous drug abusers: national and international drug perspectives*. Research Monograph, National Institute on Drug Abuse, Rockville.

Cacciola, J. and Woody, G.E. (2005). Evaluation and early treatment. In *Substance abuse: a comprehensive textbook* (eds. J.H. Lowinson, P.Ruiz, R.B. Millman, and J.G. Langrod), pp. 559–63. Lippincott Williams & Wilkins, Philadelphia.

Carroll, K.M., Ball, S.A., Nich, C. *et al.* (2006). Motivational interviewing to improve treatment engagement and outcome in individuals seeking treatment for substance abuse: a multisite effectiveness study. *Drug and Alcohol Dependence*, **81**, 301–12.

Chaisson, R.E., Osmond, D., Moss, A.R., Feldman, H.W., and Biernacki, P. (1987). HIV, bleach and needle sharing (letter). *Lancet*, **1**, 1430.

Clayton, R.R. (1985). Cocaine use in the United States: in a blizzard or just being snowed? In *Cocaine use in America: epidemiologic and clinical perspectives* (eds. N.J. Kozel and E.H. Adams), pp. 8–34. Research Monograph Series 61, National Institute on Drug Abuse, Rockville.

Cloninger, R., Bohman, M., and Sigvardsson, S. (1981). Inheritance of alcohol abuse. *Archives of General Psychiatry*, **38**, 861–8.

Committee on the Prevention of HIV Infection among Injecting Drug Users in High Risk Countries. (2006). *Preventing HIV infection among injecting drug users in high risk countries: an assessment of the evidence*. Institute of Medicine, Washington, DC.

Community Epidemiology Work Group. (2007). *Proceedings of the Community Epidemiology Work Group, January 2007*. National Institute on Drug Abuse, Rockville.

Cook, C.C.H. (1988). The Minnesota model in the management of drug and alcohol dependency: miracle, method, or myth? Part I. The philosophy and the programme. *British Journal of Addiction*, **83**, 625–34.

Day, N.A., Houston-Hamilton, A., Deslondes, J., and Nelson, M. (1988). Potential for HIV dissemination by a cohort of black intravenous drug users. *Journal of Psychoactive Drugs*, 179–226.

DeLeon, G. (1984). *The therapeutic community: study of effectiveness*. National Institute on Drug Abuse, Rockville.

Des Jarlais, D.C. (1997). *Fifteen years of research on HIV and injecting drug use*. Fourth Science Forum: Research Synthesis Symposium on the Prevention of HIV in Drug Abusers., Flagstaff.

Des Jarlais, D.C. (2000). Structural Interventions to reduce HIV transmission among injecting drug users. *AIDS*, **14**, S41–6.

Des Jarlais, D.C. and Hopkins, W. (1985). "Free" needles for intravenous drug users at risk for AIDS: current developments in New York City. *New England Journal of Medicine*, **313**(23), 1476.

Des Jarlais, D.C. and Friedman, S.R. (1988). HIV infection among persons who inject illicit drugs: problems and prospects. *Journal of Acquired Immune Deficiency Syndromes*, **1**, 267–73.

Des Jarlais, D.C. and Friedman, S.R. (1992a). The AIDS epidemic and legal access to sterile equipment for injecting illicit drugs. *Annals of the American Academy of Political and Social Science*, **521**, 42–65.

Des Jarlais, D.C. and Friedman, S.R. (1992b). AIDS prevention programs for intravenous drug users. In *AIDS and other manifestations of HIV infection*. (ed. G.P. Wormser) (2nd edn), pp. 645–j8. Raven Press, New York.

Des Jarlais, D.C., Friedman, S.R. *et al.* (1985). Risk reduction for the acquired immunodeficiency syndrome among intravenous drug users. *Annals of Internal Medicine*, **103**, 755–9.

Des Jarlais, D.C., Friedman, S.R., and Strug, D. (1986). AIDS and needle sharing within the intravenous drug use subculture. In *The social dimensions of AIDS: methods and theory* (eds. D. Feldman and T. Johnson), pp. 111–25. Praeger, New York.

Des Jarlais, D.C., Friedman, S.R., Novick, D. *et al.* (1989). HIV-1 infection among intravenous drug users in Manhattan. *Journal of the American Medical Association*, **261**, 1008–12.

Des Jarlais, D.C., Choopanya, K. *et al.* (1992a). Risk reduction and stabilization of HIV seroprevalence among drug injectors in New York City and Bangkok, Thailand. In *Science challenging AIDS*. (eds. G.B. Rossi, E. Beth-Giraldo, L. Chieco-Bianchi *et al.*), pp. 207–13. Karger, Basel.

Des Jarlais, D.C., Friedman, S.R. *et al.* (1992b). International epidemiology of HIV and AIDS among injecting drug users. *AIDS*, **6**, 1053–68.

Des Jarlais, D.C., Friedman, S.R., and Sotheran, J.L. (1992c). The first city: HIV among intravenous drug users in New York City. In *AIDS: the making of a chronic disease*. (eds. E. Fee and D. M. Fox), pp. 279–95. University of California Press, Berkeley.

Des Jarlais, D.C., Choopanya, K. *et al.* (1993a). Cross-cultural similarities in AIDS risk reduction among injecting drug users. 9th International Conference on AIDS, Berlin.

Des Jarlais, D.C., Friedman, S.R. *et al.* (1993b). Harm reduction: a public health response to the AIDS epidemic among injecting drug users. *Annual Review of Public Health*, **14**, 413–50.

Des Jarlais, D.C., Friedman, S.R. *et al.* (1994). Continuity and change within an HIV epidemic: injecting drug users in New York City, 1984 through 1992. *Journal of the American Medical Association*, **271**(2), 121–7.

Des Jarlais, D.C., Hagan, H.H., Friedman, S.R. *et al.* (1995a). Maintaining low HIV seroprevalence in populations of injecting drug users. *Journal of the American Medical Association*, **274**, 1226–31.

Des Jarlais, D.C., Paone, D., Friedman, S.R., Peyser, N., and Newman, R.G. (1995b). Regulating controversial programs for unpopular people: methadone maintenance and syringe exchange programs. *American Journal of Public Health*, **85**, 1577–84.

Des Jarlais, D.C., Marmor, M. *et al.* (1996). HIV incidence among injecting drug users in New York City syringe-exchange programmes. *The Lancet*, **348**, 987–91.

Des Jarlais, D.C., Perlis,T.P., Arasteh, K. *et al.* (2005). HIV incidence among injection drug users in New York City, 1990 to 2002: use of serologic test algorithm to assess expansion of HIV prevention services. *American Journal of Public Health*, **95**, 1439–44.

Des Jarlais, D.C., Kling, R., Hammett, T.M., Ngu, D., Liu, W., Chen, Y., Thanh Binh, K., and Friedmann, P. (2007). Reducing HIV infection among new injecting drug users in the China-Vietnam Cross Border Project. *AIDS*, **21** (Suppl 8), S109–14.

Dole, V.P. and Joseph, H. (1978). Long-term outcome of patients treated with methadone maintenance. *Annals of the New York Academy of Sciences*, **311**, 181–9.

Edwards, G., Gross, M.M., Keller, M., and Moser, J. (1976). Alcohol-related problems in the disability perspective. *Journal of Studies on Alcohol*, **37**, 1360.

Edwards, G., Arif, A., and Hodgson, R. (1981). Nomenclature and classification of drug and alcohol related problems: a WHO memorandum. *Bulletin of the World Health Organization*, **59**, 225.

Elliott, R. (2004). Drug control, human rights, and harm reduction in the age of AIDS. *HIV/AIDS Policy & Law Review*, **9**, 86–90.

Elliott, D.S., Huizinga, D., and Ageton, S.S. (1985). *Explaining delinquency and drug use*. Sage, Beverly Hills.

Emmanuelli, J. and Desenclos, J.C. (2005). Harm reduction interventions, behaviours and associated health outcomes in France, 1996–2003. *Addiction*, **100**(11), 1690–700.

Espinoza, P., Bouchard, I., Ballian, P., and Polo DeVoto, J. (1988). *Has the open sale of syringes modified the syringe exchanging habits of drug addicts*. Abstract 8522. Presented at the Fourth International Conference on AIDS. 12–16 June, Stockholm, Sweden.

Etheridge, R.M., Hubbard, R.L., Anderson, J., Craddock, S.G., and Flynn, P.M. (1997). Treatment structure and program services in the Drug Abuse Treatment Outcome Study (DATOS). *Psychology of Addictive Behaviors*, **11**(4), 244–60.

Etheridge, R.M., Craddock, S.G., Hubbard, R.L., and Rounds-Bryant, J.L. (1999). The relationship of counseling and self-help participation to patient outcomes in DATOS. *Drug and Alcohol Dependence*, **57**, 99–112.

Farrington, D.P. (1985). Predicting self-reported and official delinquency. In *Prediction in criminology* (eds. D.P. Farrington and R. Tarling), pp. 150–73. State University of New York Press, Albany.

Fishbein, M. and Ajzen, I. (1975). *Belief, attitude, intention and behavior*. Addison-Wesley, Reading.

Flay, B.R. and Sobel, J.L. (1983). The role of mass media in preventing adolescent substance abuse. In *Preventing adolescent drug abuse: intervention strategies*. (eds. T.J. G1ynn, C.G. Leukefeld, and J.P. Ludford), pp. 535. Research Monograph 47, National Institute on Drug Abuse, Rockville.

Flynn, P.M., Craddock, S.G., Hubbard, R.L., Anderson, J., and Etheridge, R.M. (1997). Methodological overview and research design for the Drug Abuse Treatment Outcome Study (DATOS). *Psychology of Addictive Behaviors*, **11**, 230–47.

Flynn, P.M., Kristiansen, P.L., Porto, J.V., and Hubbard, R.L. (1999). Costs and benefits of treatment for cocaine addiction in DATOS. *Drug and Alcohol Dependence*, **57**, 167–74.

Friedman, S.R., Des Jarlais, D.C., Sotheran, J.L., Garbar, J., Cohen, G., and Smith, D. (1987). AIDS and self-organization among intravenous drug users. *International Journal of Addictions*, **22**, 201–9.

Friedman, S.R., Des Jarlais, D.C. *et al.* (1992). Organizing drug injectors against AIDS: preliminary data on behavioral outcomes. *Psychology of Addictive Behaviors*, **6**(2), 100–6.

Friedman, S.R., de Jong, W. *et al.* (1993). Community development as a response to HIV among drug injectors. *AIDS*, S263–9.

Friedman, S.R., Jose, B., Deren, S., Des Jarlais, D.C., Neaigus, A., and the National AIDS Research Consortium (1995). Risk factors for HIV seroconversion among out-of treatment drug injector in high and low seroprevalence cities. *American Journal of Epidemiology*, **142**, 864–74.

Frischer, M., Des Jarlais, D.C. *et al.* (1993). Modeling AIDS awareness and behavior change among IDUs in Glasgow and New York. 9th International Conference on AIDS, Berlin.

Fuller, R.K., Branchey, L., Brightwell, D.R. *et al.* (1986). Disulfiram treatment of alcoholism. *Journal of the American Medical Association*, **245**, 1449–55.

Fuller, C.M., Galea, S., Caceres, W., Blaney, S., Sisco, S., and Vlahov, D. (2007). Multilevel community-based intervention to increase access to sterile syringes among injection drug users through pharmacy sales in New York City. *American Journal of Public Health*, **97**, 117–24.

Gibson, D.R., Brand, B., Anderson, K., Kahn, J.G., Perales, D., and Guydish, J. (2002). Two- to sixfold decreased odds HIV risk behavior associated with use of syringe programs. *Journal of Acquired Immune Deficiency Syndromes*, **31**, 237–42.

Gilmore, N. (1996). Drug use and human rights: privacy, vulnerability, disability, and human rights infringements. *Journal of Drug Policy*, **14**, 155–69.

Goodstadt, M.S. (1980). Drug education—a turn on or a turn off? *Journal of Drug Education*, **10**, 89–93.

Goodstadt, M.S. (1981). Planning and evaluation of alcohol education programs. *Journal of Alcohol and Drug Education*, **26**, 1–10.

Goodwin, D.W. (1985). Alcoholism and genetics: the sins of the fathers. *Archives of General Psychiatry*, **6**, 171–4.

Gorsuch, R.L., Abbamonte, M., and Sells, S.B. (1976). Evaluation of treatments for drug users in the DARP: 1971–1972 admissions. In *The effectiveness of drug abuse treatment, Vol. 4. Evaluation of treatment outcomes for the 1971-1972 Admission Cohort* (eds. S.B. Sells and D.D. Simpson). Ballinger, Cambridge.

Gostin, L. (1998). The legal environment impeding access to sterile syringes and needles: the conflict between law enforcement and public health. *Journal of Acquired Immune Deficiency Syndromes and Human Retrovirology*, **18**(1), S60–70.

Grant, B.E., Harford, T.C., Chou, P. *et al.* (1991). Epidemiologic Bulletin No. 27: prevalence of DSM-III-R alcohol abuse and dependence: United States, 1988. *Alcohol Health Research*, **15**(1), 91–6.

Greenspan, S.I. (1985). Research strategies to identify developmental vulnerabilities for drug abuse. In *Etiology of drug abuse: implication for prevention* (eds. C.L. Jones and R.J. Battles). National Institute on Drug Abuse, Rockville.

Hagan, H., Des Jarlais, D.C. *et al.* (1995). Reduced risk of hepatitis B and hepatitis C among injecting drug users participating in the Tacoma syringe exchange program. *American Journal of Public Health*, **85**(11), 1531–7.

Hagan, H., McGough, J. *et al.* (1999). Syringe exchange and risk of infection with hepatitis B and C viruses. *American Journal of Epidemiology*, **49**(3), 203–13.

Hagan, H. and Thiede, H. (2000). Changes in injection risk behavior associated with participation in the Seattle needle-exchange program. *Journal of Urban Health*, **77**, 369–82.

Hagan, H., Des Jarlais, D.C., Stern, R., Lelutiu-Weinberger, C., Scheinmann, R., Strauss, S., and Flom, P.L. (2007). HCV synthesis project: preliminary analyses of HCV prevalence in relation to age and duration of injection. *International Journal of Drug Policy*, **18**, 341–51.

Hammett, T.M., Wu, Z., Duc, T.T., Stephens, D., Sullivan, S., Liu, W., Chen, Y., Ngu, D., and Des Jarlais, D.C. (2007). 'Social Evils' and harm reduction: the evolving policy environment for human immunodeficiency virus prevention among injection drug users in China and Vietnam. *Addiction*, **103**, 137–45.

Hanson, D. (1980). Drug education: does it work? In *Drugs and the youth culture* (eds. E Scarpitti and S. Batesman). Sage, Beverly Hills.

Hanzo, C., Chatterjee, A. *et al.* (1997). Reaching out beyond the hills: HIV prevention among injecting drug users in Manipur, India. *Addiction*, **92**(7), 813–20.

Harm Reduction Coalition. (2007). *Harm Reduction Coalition Website*. Retrieved 2007 (http://www.harmreduction.org/).

Harwood, H.J., Napolitano, D.M., Kristiansen, P.L., and Collins, J.J. (1984). *Economic costs to society of alcohol and drug abuse and mental illness: 1980*. Research Triangle Institute, Research Triangle Park.

Hawkins, J.D., Lishner, D.M., and Catalano, R.F. (1985). Childhood predictors and the prevention of adolescent substance abuse. In *Etiology of drug abuse: implications for prevention. Research Monograph 56* (eds. C.L. Jones and R.J. Battjes). National Institute on Drug Abuse, Rockville.

Hawkins, J.D., Lishner, D.M., Jenson, J.M., and Catalano, R.F. (1987). Delinquents and drugs: what the evidence suggests about prevention and treatment programming. In *Youth at risk for substance abuse* (eds. B.S. Brown and A.R. Mills), pp. 81–133. National Institute on Drug Abuse, Rockville.

Heather, N., Wodak, A. *et al.* (eds.) (1993). *Psychoactive drugs and harm reduction: from faith to science*. Whurr, London.

Hewitt, L.E. and Blane, H.T. (1984). Prevention through mass media communication. In *Prevention of alcohol abuse* (eds. P.M. Miller and T.D. Nirenberg), pp. 281–323. Plenum Press, New York.

Hilton, M.E. and Clark, W.B. (1987). Changes in American drinking patterns and problems, 1967–1984. *Journal of Studies in Alcohol*, **48**, 515–22.

Hoffman, N.G. and Harrison, P.A. (1987). *Chemical abuse treatment outcome registry, 1986 report: findings two years after treatment*. Comprehensive Assessment and Treatment Outcome Research (CATOR), St Paul.

Holder, H.D. and Blose, J.O. (1986). Alcohol treatment and total health care utilization and costs. *Journal of the American Medical Association*, **256**, 1456–60.

Holland, S. (1982). *Residential drug-free programs for substance abusers: the effect of planned duration on treatment*. Gateway Houses, Chicago.

Hser, Y., Grella, C.E., Hubbard, R.L., Hsieh, S.C., Fletcher, B.W., Brown, B.S., and Anglin, M.D. (2001). An evaluation of drug treatment for adolescents in four U.S. cities. *Archives of General Psychiatry*, **58(7)**, 689–95.

Huba, G., Wingard, J., and Bentler, P. (1980). Applications of a theory of drug use to prevention programs. *Journal of Drug Education*, **10**, 25–38.

Hubbard, R.L., Bray, R.M., and Craddock, S.G. (1986). Issues in the assessment of multiple drug use among drug treatment clients. In *Strategies for research on drugs of abuse* (eds. M. Braude and H.M. Ginzburg), pp. 15–40. National Institute on Drug Abuse, Rockville.

Hubbard, R.L., Brownlee, R.F., and Anderson, R. (1988). Initiation of alcohol and drug abuse in the middle school years. *Elementary School and Guidance Counselling*, **23**, 118–23.

Hubbard, R.L., Marsden, M.E., Rachal, J.V., Harwood, H.J. Cavanaugh, E.R., and Ginzburg, H.M. (1989). *Drug abuse treatment: a national study of effectiveness*. UNC Press, Chapel Hill.

Hubbard, R.L., Craddock, S.G., Flynn, P.M., Anderson, J., and Etheridge, R.M. (1997). Overview of 1-year follow-up outcomes in the Drug Abuse Treatment Outcome Study (DATOS). *Psychology of Addictive Behaviors*, **11**(4), 261–78.

Hubbard, R.L., Craddock, S.G., and Anderson, J. (2003). Overview of 5-year follow-up outcomes in the Drug Abuse Treatment Outcome Studies (DATOS). *Journal of Substance Abuse Treatment*, **25(3)**, 125–34.

Hubbard, R.L., Simpson, D.D., and Woody, G. (2008). *Journal of Drug Issues: Special Issue.*

Ingold, E.R. and Ingold, S. (1989). The effects of the liberalization of syringe sales on the behavior of intravenous drug users in France. *Bulletin on Narcotics*, **41**, 67–81.

Institute of Medicine, Committee to Identify Research Effectiveness in the Prevention and Treatment of Alcohol Related Problems (1989). *Prevention and treatment of alcohol problems*. National Academy Press, Washington, DC.

Jackson, J. and Rotkiewicz, L. (1987). *A coupon program: AIDS education and drug treatment*. Third International Conference on AIDS, Washington, DC.

Jaffe, J.H. (1979). The swinging pendulum: the treatment of drug users in America. In *Handbook on drug abuse* (eds. R.L. DuPont, A. Goldstein, and J. O'Donnell), pp. 3–16. National Institute on Drug Abuse, Rockville.

Jessor, R., Chase, J.A., and Donovan, J.E. (1980). Psychosocial correlates of marijuana use and problem drinking in a national sample of adolescents. *American Journal of Public Health*, **70**, 604–13.

Joe, G.W., Simpson, D.D., and Broome, K.M. (1999). Retention and patient engagement models for different treatment modalities in DATOS. *Drug and Alcohol Dependence*, **57**, 113–25.

Johnston, L.D., O'Malley, P.M., and Eveland, L. (1978). Drugs and delinquency: a search for causal connections. In *Longitudinal research on drug use. Empirical findings and methodological issues* (ed. D. Kandel), pp. 137–56. Wiley, New York.

Johnston, L.D., O'Malley, P.M., and Bachman, J.G. (1984). *Highlights from drugs and American high school students 1975–1983*. National Institute on Drug Abuse, Rockville.

Johnston, L.D., O'Malley, P.M., and Bachman, J.G. (1989). *Drug use, drinking, and smoking: national survey of results from high school, college, and young adult populations.* National Institute on Drug Abuse, Rockville.

Johnston, L.D., O'Malley, P.M., and Bachman, J.G. (1999). *National survey results on drug use from the monitoring the future study, 1975–1998, Vol. I: secondary school students (NIH Publication No. 99-4660).* National Institute on Drug Abuse, Rockville.

Johnston, L.D., O'Malley, P.M., Bachman, J.G., and Schulenberg, J.E. (2005). *Monitoring the future national survey results on drug use, 1975–2004. Vol. 1: secondary school students (NIH Publication No. 05-5727).* National Institute on Drug Abuse, Bethesda.

Kandel, D.B. (1980). Drug and drinking behavior among youth. *Annual Review of Sociology*, **6**, 235–85.

Kandel, D.B. (1982). Epidemiological and psychosocial perspectives on adolescent drug use. *Journal of American Academy of Clinical Psychiatry*, **21**, 328–47.

Kandel, D.B. and Logan, J.A. (1984). Patterns of drug use from adolescence to young adulthood: I. Periods of risk for initiation, continued use, and discontinuation. *American Journal of Public Health*, **74**, 660–6.

Kandel, D.B. and Raveis, V.H. (1989). Cessation of illicit drug use in young adulthood. *Archives of General Psychiatry*, **46**, 109–16.

Kandel, D.B., Kessler, R., and Margulies, R. (1978). Antecedents of adolescents' initiation into stages of drug use: a developmental analysis. In *Longitudinal Research in drug use: empirical findings and methodological issues* (ed. D.B. Kandel), pp. 73–99. Hemisphere-Wiley, Washington, DC.

Kandel, D.B., Simcha-Fagan, O., and Davies, M. (1986). Risk factors for delinquency and illicit drug use from adolescence to young adulthood. *Journal of Drug Issues*, **60**, 67–90.

Kaplan, H.B., Martin, S.S., and Robbins, C.A. (1982). Applications of a general theory of deviant behavior: self derogation and adolescent drug use. *Journal of Health and Science Behavior*, **23**, 274–94.

Kaplan, H.B., Martin, S.S., Johnson, R.J., and Robbins, C.A. (1986). Escalation of marijuana use: application of a general theory of deviant behavior. *Journal of Health and Social Behavior*, **27**, 44–61.

Kellam, S.G. and Brown, H. (1982). *Social adaptational and psychological antecedents of adolescent psychopathology ten years later.* Johns Hopkins University, Baltimore.

Kral, A.H., Bluthenthal, R.N., Lorvick, J., Gee, L., Bacchetti, P., and Edlin, B.R. (2001). Sexual transmission of HIV-1 among injection drug users in San Francisco, USA: risk-factor analysis. *Lancet*, **357**, 1397–401.

Ksobiech, K. (2003). A meta-analysis of needle sharing, lending, and borrowing behaviors of needle exchange program attenders. *AIDS Education and Prevention*, **15**, 257–68.

Latkin, C.M.W.V.D., Oziemkowska, M., and Celentano, D. (1996). People and places: behavioral settings and personal network characteristics as correlates of needle sharing. *Journal of Acquired Immune Deficiency Syndromes and Human Retrovirology*, **30**, 273–80.

Laudet, A.B. (2007). What does recovery mean to you? Lessons from the recovery experience for research and practice. *Journal of Substance Abuse Treatment*, **33**, 243–56.

Laundergan, J.C. (1982). *Easy does it: alcoholism treatment outcomes, Hazelden and the Minnesota Model.* Hazelden Foundation, Duluth.

Lewin Group. (2005). Comparative evaluation of Pennsylvania's HealthChoices program and fee-for-service program. Report prepared for the Coalition of Medical Assistance Managed Care Organizations.

Ljungberg, B., Christensson, B. *et al.* (1991). HIV prevention among injecting drug users: three years of experience from a syringe exchange program in Sweden. *JAIDS*, **4**, 890–5.

Lurie, P. and Drucker, E. (1997). An opportunity lost: HIV infections associated with lack of a national needle-exchange programme in the USA. *Lancet*, **349,** 604–8.

Lurie, P., Reingold, A.L., and Bowser, B. (eds.) (1993). *The public health impact of needle-exchange programs in the United States and abroad, Vol. I.* Centers for Disease Control and Prevention, Atlanta.

McAlister, A.L. (1983). Social-psychological approaches. In *Preventing adolescent drug abuse: intervention strategies* (eds. T.J. Glynn, C.G. Leukefeld, and J.P. Ludford), pp. 36–50. Research Monograph 47, National Institute on Drug Abuse, Rockville.

McCoy, C.B., Rivers, J.E. *et al.* (1994). Compliance to bleach disinfection protocols among injection drug users in Miami. *Journal of the Acquired Immune Deficiency Syndrome*, **7**, 773.

McGlothlin, W., Anglin, M., and Wilson, B. (1977). *An evaluation of the California Civil Addict Program, DHEW Publication No. ADM 78-558.* National Institute on Drug Abuse, Rockville.

McKnight, C., Des Jarlais, D.C., Perlis, T. *et al.* (2007). Syringe exchange programs – United States, 2005. *Morb Mort Wkly Rep MMWR*, **56,** 1164–7.

Meyer, R.E. (1989). Who can say no to illicit drug use? *Archives of General Psychiatry*, **46**, 189–90.

Miller, W.R. and Hester, R.K. (1986). Inpatient alcoholism treatment: who benefits? *American Psychologist*, **41**, 794–805.

Moskowitz, J.M. (1983). Preventing adolescent substance abuse through education, In *Preventing adolescent drug abuse: intervention strategies* (eds. T.J. Glynn, C.G. Leukefeld, and J.P. Ludford), pp. 233–49. Research Monograph 47. National Institute on Drug Abuse, Rockville.

Myers, J.K., Weissman, M.M., Tischler, G.L. *et al.* (1984). Six-month prevalence of psychiatric disorders in three communities. *Archives of General Psychiatry*, **41**, 959–67.

Nash, G. (1976). An analysis of twelve studies of the impact of drug abuse treatment upon criminality. In *Drug use and crime: report of the panel on use and criminal behavior, Appendix.* Research Triangle Institute, Research Triangle Park.

National Institute on Drug Abuse (1989). *Highlights from the National Household Survey on Drug Abuse: 1988.* National Institute on Drug Abuse, Rockville.

National Institutes of Health, U. S. (1997). *Interventions to prevent HIV risk behaviors.* NIH Consensus Statement, National Institutes of Health.

Neaigus, A., Friedman, S.R., Curtis, R. *et al.* (1994). The relevance of drug injectors' social and risk networks for understanding and preventing HIV infection. *Social Science & Medicine*, **38**(1), 67–78.

Newmeyer, J.A., Feldman, H.W. *et al.* (1989). Preventing AIDS contagion among intravenous drug users. *Medical Anthropology*, **10**, 167–75.

Normand, J., Vlahov, D. *et al.* (eds.) (1995). *Preventing HIV transmission: the role of sterile needles and bleach.* National Academy Press/National Research Council/Institute of Medicine, Washington, DC.

Office of National Drug Control Policy (2004). *The economic costs of drug abuse in the United States, 1992–2002.* Executive Office of the President (Publication No. 207303), Washington, DC.

Oliver, K., Maynard, H., Friedman, S.R., and Des Jarlais, DC. (1994). Behavioral and community impact of the Portland syringe exchange program. In *Proceedings of the workshop on needle exchange and bleach distribution programs,* pp. 35–9. National Academy Press, Washington, DC.

Pentz, M.A. (1983). Prevention of adolescent substance abuse through social skill development, In *Preventing adolescent drug abuse: intervention strategies* (eds. T.J. Glynn, C.G. Leukefeld, and J.P. Ludford), pp. 195–232. Research Monograph 47. National Institute on Drug Abuse, Rockville.

Pentz, M.A., Cormack, C., Flay, B., Hansen, W.B., and Johnson, C.A. (1986). Balancing program and research integrity in community drug abuse prevention: project STAR approach. *Journal of School Health*, **56**, 389–93.

Pentz, M.A., Dwyer, J.H., MacKinnon, D.P. *et al.* (1989). A multi-community trial for primary prevention of adolescent drug abuse. *Journal of the American Medical Association*, **261**, 3259–66.

Petrakis, P.L. (1985). *Alcoholism: an inherited disease*. DHHS Publication No. ADM 85-1426. National Institute on Alcohol Abuse and Alcoholism, Rockville.

Petry, N.M., Peirce, J.M., Stitzer, M.L. *et al.* (2005). Effect of prize-based incentives on outcomes in stimulant abusers in outpatient psychosocial treatment programs. *Archives of General Psychiatry*, **62**, 1148–56.

Polich, J.M., Armor, D.J., and Braiker, H.B. (1981). *The course of alcoholism*. Wiley, New York.

Project MATCH Research Group. (1993). Project MATCH: rationale and methods for a multisite clinical trial matching patients to alcoholism treatment. *Alcoholism Clinical and Experimental Research*, **17**, 1130.

Rachal, J.V., Guess, L.L., Hubbard, R.L. *et al.* (1982). Facts for Planning No. 4: alcohol misuse by adolescents. *Alcohol Health and Research World*, **6**, 61–8.

Reif, S., Geonnotti, K., and Whetten, K. (2006). HIV infection and AIDS in the Deep South. *American Journal of Public Health*, **96**(6), 970–3.

Robert-Guroff, M., Weiss, S.H., Giron, J.A. *et al.* (1986). Prevalence of antibodies to HTLV-1, -2, and -3 in intravenous drug abusers from an AIDS endemic region. *Journal of the American Medical Association*, **255**, 3133–7.

Robins, L.N. (1980). The natural history of drug abuse. Evaluation of treatment of drug abusers. *Acta Psychiatrica Scandinavica*, **284** (Suppl 62), 7–20.

Robins, L.N. and Przybeck, T.R. (1985). Age of onset of drug use and other disorders. In *Etiology of drug abuse: implications for prevention. Research Monograph 56* (eds. C.L. Jones, R.J. Battjes *et al*). National Institute on Drug Abuse, Rockville.

Robins, L.N., Helzer, J.E., Weissman, M.M. *et al.* (1984). Lifetime prevalence of specific psychiatric disorders in three sites. *Archives of General Psychiatry*, **11**, 949–58.

Roman, P.M., Ducharme, L.J., and Knudsen, H.K. (2006). Patterns of organization and management in private and public substance abuse treatment programs. *Journal of Substance Abuse Treatment*, **31**(3), 235–43.

Rounsaville, B. (2002). Experience with ICD-10/*DSM-IV* substance use disorders. *Psychopathology*, **35**, 82–8.

Rounsaville, B.J., Spitzer, R.L., and Williams, J.B. (1986). Proposed changes in DSM-III substance use disorders: description and rationale. *American Journal of Psychiatry*, **143**, 463–8.

Saxe, L., Dougherty, D., Esty, K., and Fine, M. (1983). *The effectiveness and costs of alcoholism treatment, Health Technology Case Study No. 22.* US Congress, Office of Technology Assessment, Washington, DC.

Schaps, E., DiBartolo, R., Moskowitz, J., Palley, C.S., and Churgin, S. (1981). A review of 127 drug abuse prevention program evaluations. *Journal of Drug Issues*, **11**, 17–43.

Schaps, E., Moskowitz, J., Malvin, J., and Schaeffer, G. (1984). *The Napa drug abuse prevention project: research findings*, DHHS Publication No. ADM 84-1339. National Institute on Drug Abuse, Rockville.

Schuckit, M.A. (1980). Self-rating of alcohol intoxication by young men with and without family histories of alcoholism. *Journal of Studies in Alcohol*, **41**, 242–249.

Scitovsky, A. and Rice, D. (1987). Estimates of the direct and indirect costs of acquired immunodeficiency syndrome in the United States, 1985, 1986, 1990. *Public Health Reports*, **102**, 5–17.

Sells, S.B. (1979). Treatment effectiveness. In *Handbook on drug abuse* (eds. R.L. DuPont, A. Goldstein, and John O'Donnell). National Institute on Drug Abuse, Rockville.

Sells, S.B. and Simpson, D. (1976). *The effectiveness of drug abuse treatment, Vols. 1–5*. Ballinger, Cambridge.

Selwyn, P.A., Schoenbaum, E.E. *et al.* (1987). *Natural history of HIV infection in intravenous drug abusers (IVDAs)*. Third International Conference on AIDS, Washington, DC.

Skinner, H.A. and Horn, J.L. (1984). *Guidelines for using the Alcohol Dependence Scale (ADS)*. Addiction Research Foundation, Toronto.

Simpson, D.D., Joe, G.W., Fletcher, B.W., Hubbard, R.L., and Anglin, M.D. (1999). A national evaluation of treatment outcomes for cocaine dependence. *Archives of General Psychiatry*, **56**, 507–14.

Sloboda, Z. (2008). Reflections on 40 years of drug abuse research. *Journal of Drug Issues*.

Smart, R.G. (1976). Outcome studies of therapeutic community and halfway house treatment for addicts. *International Journal of Addiction*, **11**, 143–59.

Spencer, B.D. (1989). On the accuracy of estimates of numbers of intravenous drug users. In *AIDS: sexual behavior and intravenous drug use* (eds. C.F. Turner, H.G. Miller, and L.E. Moses). National Academy Press, Washington, DC.

Spitzer, R.L. and Williams, J.P. (1987). *Diagnostic and statistical manual of mental disorders (3rd edn. revised)*. American Psychiatric Association, Washington, DC.

Stephens, R.C., Simpson, D.D., Coyle, S.L., McCoy, C.B., and the National AIDS Research Consortium (1993). Comparative effectiveness of NADR interventions. In *Handbook on risk of AIDS* (eds. B.S. Brown and G.M. Beschner), pp. 519–56. Greenwood Press, Westport.

Stimson, G.V. (1995). AIDS and injecting drug use in the United Kingdom, 1987–1993: the policy response and the prevention of the epidemic. *Social Science and Medicine*, **41**(5), 699–716.

Stimson, G.V., Alldritt, L.J., Dolan, K.A., Donoghoe, M.S., and Lart, R.A. (1988). *Injecting equipment exchange schemes: final report*. Monitoring Research Group, Goldsmith's College, London.

Stimson, G.V., Keene, J. *et al.* (1991). *Evaluation of the syringe exchange programme Wales, 1990–1991*. Final Report to the Welsh Office, The Centre for Research on Drugs and Health Behavior, University of London.

Stimson, G.V., Des Jarlais, D.C., and Ball, A. (1998). Drug injecting and HIV infection: global dimensions and local responses. UCL Press, London.

Strathdee, S.A. and Sherman, S.G. (2003). The role of sexual transmission of HIV infection among injection and non-injection drug users. *Journal of Urban Health*, **90**(4 Suppl 3), iii 7–14.

Strathdee, S., Patrick, D. *et al.* (1997). Needle exchange is not enough: lessons from the Vancouver injection drug use study. *AIDS*, **11**, F59–65.

Strathdee, S.A., Galai, N., Safaeian, M., Celentano, D.D., Vlahov, D., Johnson, L., and Nelson, K.E. (2001). Sex differences in risk factors for HIV seroconversion among injection drug users: a 10-year perspective. *Archives Internal Medicine*, **161**, 1281–8.

Substance Abuse and Mental Health Services Administration (1999). *Summary findings from the 1998 National Household Survey on Drug Abuse*. Office of Applied Studies, Rockville.

Substance Abuse and Mental Health Services Administration (2007). Results from the 2006 National Household Survey on Drug Use and Health: National Findings.

Sumartojo, E. and Laga, M. (eds.). (2000). Structural factors in HIV prevention. *AIDS*, **14**, S1–73.

Tims, F.M. (1981). *Effectiveness of drug abuse treatment programs. Treatment Research Report DHHS Publication No. ADM 84-1143*. National Institute on Drug Abuse, Rockville.

Tims, F.M. and Ludford, J.P. (1984). Drug abuse treatment evaluation: strategies.

Titus, S., Marmor, M., Des Jarlais, D.C., Kim, M., Wolfe, H., and Beatrice, S. (1994). Bleach use and HIV seroconversion among New York City injection drug users. *Journal of Acquired Immune Deficiency Syndromes*, **7**, 700–4.

Tobler, N.S. (1986). Meta-analysis of 143 adolescent drug prevention programs: quantitative outcome results of program participants compared to a control or comparison group. *Journal of Drug Issues*, **16**, 537–67.

Turner, C.E, Miller, H.G., and Moses, L.E. (eds.) (1989). AIDS: sexual behavior and intravenous drug use. National Academy Press, Washington, DC.

Tyndall, M., Johnston, C., Craib, K. *et al.* (2001). HIV incidence and mortality among injection drug users in Vancouver – 1996–2000. *Canadian Journal of Infectious Diseases,* **12**, 69B.

Tyndall, M.W., Bruneau, J., Brogly, S., Spittal, P., O'Shaughnessy, M.V., and Schechter, M.T. (2002). Satellite needle distribution among injection drug users: policy and practice in two Canadian cities. *Journal of Acquired Immune Deficiency Syndromes,* **31**(1), 98–105.

UNAIDS/WHO. (2006). AIDS epidemic update: December 2006. Geneva: Joint United Nations Programme on HIV/AIDS (UNAIDS) and World Health Organization (WHO).

United States General Accounting Office (1993). *Needle exchange programs: research suggests promise as an AIDS prevention strategy.* Report to the Chairman, Select Committee on Narcotics Abuse and Control, House of Representatives. US House of Representatives, Washington, DC.

United States National Commission on AIDS (1991). *Twin epidemics of AIDS and substance abuse.* Government Report, Washington, DC.

Vickerman, P., Hickman, M., Rhodes, T., and Watts, C. (2006). Model projections on the required coverage of syringe distribution to prevent HIV epidemics among injecting drug users. *Journal of Acquired Immune Deficiency Syndromes,* **42**, 355–61.

Vlahov, D., Astemborski, J. *et al.* (1994). Field effectiveness of needle disinfection among injecting drug users. *Journal of the Acquired Immunodeficiency Syndromes,* **7**, 760–6.

Watters, J.K., Estilo, M.J., Clark, G.L., and Lorvick, J. (1994). Syringe and needle exchange as HIV/AIDS prevention for injection drug users. *Journal of the American Medical Association,* **271**(2), 115–20.

Wawer, M.J., Gray, R.H., Sewankambo, N.K. *et al.* (2005). Rates of HIV-1 transmission per coital act, by stage of HIV-1 infection, in Rakai, Uganda. *Journal of Infectious Diseases,* **191**(9), 1403–9.

Westat. (2003). *Evaluation of the national youth anti-drug media campaign: 2003 report of findings executive summary.* National Institute on Drug Abuse, Rockville.

Wiebel, W. (1993). *The indigenous leader outreach model: intervention manual.* National Institute on Drug Abuse, Rockville.

Wiebel, W.W., Jimenez, A. *et al.* (1996). Risk behavior and HIV seroincidence among out-of-treatment injection drug users: a four-year prospective study.

Wodak, A. (1995). Needle exchange and bleach distribution programmes: the Australian experience. *International Journal of Drug Policy,* **6**, 46–56.

Wolfe, D. and Malinowska-Sempruch, K. (2004). *Illicit drug policies and the Global HIV epidemic effects of UN and National Government approaches.* Open Society Institute, New York.

World Health Organization. (1992). *Tenth revision of the international classification of disease (ICD-10).* World Health Organization, Geneva.

10.3

Alcohol[1]

Robin Room

Abstract

This chapter begins with a discussion on alcohol, its uses, and its effects, both positive and negative, followed by a review of the recent research on its cumulative adverse effects on health. The history of alcohol as a public health issue is also briefly reviewed. The temperance movements of the nineteenth and early-twentieth centuries were succeeded by an impulse to deflate alcohol's adverse effects and, in turn, by a 'new public health' approach. Although this approach gained ground among researchers from the 1970s onwards, it has often been resisted in the policy process. Seven main strategies to prevent or control alcohol problems are described, and their effectiveness briefly assessed. The chapter concludes with an account of alcohol policy in a globalizing world. An international convention on alcohol control has been called for to counter the influence of trade agreements and the globalization of alcohol production, distribution, and promotion.

Alcohol and its effects

Alcoholic beverages have been consumed in most, if not all, human societies since the beginning of recorded history. Beverages containing ethanol (C_2H_5OH) can be fermented from a large number of organic materials that comprise carbohydrates, and in one part of the world or another, these products are prepared from fruits, berries, various grains, plants, honey, or milk. Under most circumstances, such fermented beverages can contain up to 14 per cent ethanol. The most widely commercialized fermented beverages are beer prepared from barley or other grains (usually 3–7 per cent ethanol), apple and other fruit ciders (usually 3–7 per cent ethanol), and grape wine (usually 8–14 per cent ethanol). Other fermented beverages are also common in particular cultures, often from home production or in commercial form: For example, sorghum or millet beers in Eastern and Southern Africa, palm wine toddy in West Africa and the Indian subcontinent, pulque (prepared from the maguey cactus) in Mexico, and rice wine (sake) in Eastern Asia.

Distilled beverages, in which ethanol is concentrated by evaporation and condensation from a fermented liquid, were a Chinese invention, which came to Europe *via* Arabia in the Middle Ages. In Europe, at first, their use was primarily medicinal, but by the 1600s, popular use as a social beverage spread rapidly. Distilled beverages can be made up of almost-pure ethanol, but those sold for drinking contain between 25 per cent and 50 per cent ethanol. Distilled alcohol is also added to wine, producing 'fortified wines' with about 20 per cent ethanol. Because distilled beverages and fortified wines do not readily spoil, they could be shipped over long distances, even before refrigeration and airtight packaging became available, and played a particularly important part in commerce and exploitation in the age of the European empires. Different cultures consume varying strengths of alcoholic beverages, often with water or a 'mixer' being added to distilled beverages and, in some cultures, also to wine and other fermented beverages.

Use-values of alcohol

Ethanol has many uses in human life. These include non-beverage uses as a fuel and as a solvent. Important beverage-related use-values include use as a medicine, as a religious sacrament, as a foodstuff, and as a thirst-quencher (Mäkelä 1983). But, alcoholic beverages have received special attention as a public health hazard because of their psychoactive properties. These properties carry with them another set of use-values: In terms of psychopharmacology, ethanol is a depressant, and alcoholic beverages have long been used to affect mood and feelings. With enough consumption, alcohol becomes an anodyne and, indeed, an anaesthetic; distilled spirits were used as an anaesthetic in surgical practice before the mid-nineteenth century. Many drinkers seek and appreciate the levels of intoxication, which lie between mild mood alteration at one end of the spectrum and being comatose at the other.

The decisions to drink and how much to drink are, however, often not made by the individual in isolation. Drinking is usually a social act, and the pace and level of drinking are frequently subject to collective influence, with drinking together being seen as an expression of solidarity and community. Although drunkenness may be sought to relieve misery or loneliness, it is more commonly associated with sociable celebration.

Adverse effects

Alcohol consumption can have a variety of adverse effects, some of which are acute effects associated with the particular drinking event.

[1] Author's note: Portions of this chapter have been adapted from 'Prevention of alcohol-related problems' in the *New Oxford Textbook of Psychiatry*. Oxford University Press.

Drinking progressively impairs physical coordination, cognition, and attention, resulting in an increased risk of accidents and injury. Above a threshold level, drinking can also affect intention and judgement, so intoxication potentially plays a causal role in violent behaviour and crime (Graham *et al.* 1998). This relation appears to be culturally mediated, because there is a substantial variation between cultures in the association of intoxication with violence and crime (MacAndrew & Edgerton 1969). A sufficient amount of alcohol may result in a potentially fatal overdose, by interrupting various autonomic bodily functions.

Other adverse effects of alcohol consumption are chronic effects related to a repeated pattern of drinking. Alcohol consumption can adversely affect nearly every organ of the body, although some effects are not common. Chronic conditions in which alcohol is implicated as an important cause include liver cirrhosis; cancers of the upper digestive tract, liver, and breast; cardiomyopathy; and gastritis and pancreatitis (Rehm *et al.* 2004). Through a variety of mechanisms, alcohol is also implicated in the incidence and course of infectious diseases (NIAAA 1997).

Repeated heavy drinking can also adversely affect mental health; specific neurological disorders are associated with sustained heavy drinking. More common concomitants include depression and affective disorders. Alcoholism—the experience of loss of control over drinking, along with other psychological and physical sequelae—has also been considered a mental disorder in modern times. In current nosologies, alcoholism has been replaced by the terms *alcohol dependence* (in *Diagnostic and Statistical Manual of Mental Disorders* [DSM-IV] terminology) and the *alcohol dependence syndrome* (in the *International Classification of Diseases* [ICD-10]).

The impairment of coordination and judgement produced by drinking potentially affects bystanders and the drinkers' acquaintances, friends, and family, as well as themselves: The effects can be through impairment of coordination or judgement during the drinking event, resulting in injury or distress, or through impairment of performance in family, friendship, work, and other social roles as a result of recurring drinking episodes. The actual and potential adverse effects on others have historically been the primary justification for alcohol controls and other societal responses to problematic drinking (Room 1996); the effects on the adult drinker's own health have been of much less importance in determining public policy on alcohol.

Positive effects

For the drinker, and sometimes for those around, alcohol consumption can have positive effects. We have already mentioned the different use-values of alcohol—which mean that drinkers are usually willing to pay more than just the cost of production and distribution of the beverage. Apart from its valued effects on mental state, alcohol use has some positive outcomes on health. By far, the most important of these, in terms of public health, is its potential for preventing cardiovascular disease (CVD). A fairly consistent finding in studies in several societies is that drinking at moderate levels protects against CVD (Klatsky 1999), although controversy about the existence and extent of this effect remains (e.g. Fillmore *et al.* 2006). The findings on the upper limit of drinking for such protection vary. Taken together, it appears that most of the protective effect can be gained with as little as one drink of an alcoholic beverage every second day (Maclure 1993). About half of this effect seems to come from inhibiting the build-up of plaque in arteries, whereas the other half seems to result from a relatively immediate effect of diminishing the likelihood of blood clots. To the extent this is true, irregular or occasional drinking is likely to have a less protective effect.

Although it has been argued that this protection comes primarily from red wine constituents (particularly resveratrol) rather than from the ethanol, the balance of evidence favours an ethanol effect (Klatsky 1999). However, relatively little is known about how this effect interacts with or overlaps other risk and protective factors for chronic heart disease (CHD), such as regular exercise, diet, or taking aspirin (acetyl salicylic acid [ASA]) or other pharmaceuticals (Criqui *et al.* 1998). The protective effect of alcohol appears to be higher for cigarette smokers than for non-smokers (Kozlowski *et al.* 1994).

Drinking is also often bad for the heart (Poikolainen 1999; Chadwick & Goode 1998). Studies have found that a pattern of intermittent heavy drinking, such as getting drunk every weekend, is associated with an elevated rate of coronary death (Kauhanen *et al.* 1997), probably through mechanisms such as heart arrhythmias (Kupari & Koskinen 1998; McKee & Britton 1998). Data from countries in the former Soviet Union, where a pattern of intermittent intoxication is common, support the strong adverse effect of binge drinking on heart disease mortality. During a period of deliberate restriction of alcohol supplies, the estimated per-capita consumption in Russia, including the illicit alcohol market, fell from 14.2 litres in 1984 to 10.7 litres in 1987 (Shkolnikov & Nemtsov 1997)—a fall of 25 per cent. The death rate from ischemic heart disease among males fell by 10 per cent in the same period (Leon *et al.* 1997). This rate rose again when the restrictions lapsed, although this time, unlike between 1985 and 1988, other risk factors also changed.

Research on cumulative effects of alcohol

Effects on the drinker's health

In most studies, the relationship between amount of drinking and overall mortality is a J-shaped curve, with abstainers, and often, very light drinkers showing a higher mortality than those drinking a little more. This may be because, in these findings, a substantial part of the study population were older adults, and thus were at risk of mortality from CVD. Studies limited to younger cohorts typically found a monotonic relationship between amount of drinking and mortality (Andréasson *et al.* 1991; Rehm & Sempos 1995). Such an association might also be expected in any population, such as in some developing countries, that has a low rate of CVD.

The pattern of drinking is also a potentially important factor in mortality due to alcohol. Although this has long been obvious in casualty deaths, there is growing recognition of its significance in other causes of death, as implied by the earlier-mentioned Russian data. However, until recently, there have been only few measurements of this pattern in studies on alcohol and overall mortality. Variations among cultures in drinking habits may partly explain why the J-curve relation of volume of drinking to mortality shows different low-points in different cultures.

The risks and potential benefits associated with a given level of drinking, thus, vary with the age and sex of the drinker, and possibly with other sociocultural characteristics, as well as with the pattern and circumstances related to drinking. This variation has posed a considerable challenge because of political demand in a number of countries for advice on 'low-risk drinking' or 'safe drinking' guidelines (Hawks 1994). Whereas earlier guidelines were inclined to be stated only in terms of the volume of drinking, in line with the measurement methods of medical epidemiology literature, more recent guidelines have also emphasized limits on the amount consumed on a given occasion or day (Bondy *et al.* 1999).

Current literature on the cumulative effects of drinking on health relies substantially on summations of prospective epidemiological literature, following the tradition set up by English *et al.* (1995). Using meta-analysis on studies of the relationship between volume of drinking and specific causes of death in which alcohol was either a risk or protective factor, the studies following this tradition derive attributable fractions for different levels of the volume of drinking and apply these fractions to segments of the population at each level in order to arrive at estimates on total lives and life-years lost and gained. In the WHO's estimation of the global burden of disease (GBD) for 2000, drinking patterns were also taken into account for injuries and heart disease, and the estimations were extended to cover all regions of the world (Rehm *et al.* 2004). In these estimates, the projected protective effects of alcohol are subtracted from the negative burden. In addition to life-years lost, the study's most comprehensive indicator, disability-adjusted life years (DALYs), includes a projection of the burden of disability attributable to alcohol.

According to GBD estimates, 4.0 per cent of the total burden of disease globally (as measured in DALYs) is attributable to alcohol (Ezzati *et al.* 2002). This compares with 4.1 per cent for tobacco and 0.8 per cent for illegal drugs. The alcohol share of the burden is highest in high-income societies, including Eastern Europe and Northern Asia, as well as in Latin America. The relative position of alcohol among risk factors is actually highest in middle-income countries, where it ranks first; although the alcohol share of all DALYs is lower in other developing regions, this fraction is calculated on the basis of a higher total burden of disease and disability in these countries.

Effects at the population level

So far, we have dealt with estimates of alcohol's effects at the individual level. The methodological difficulties in the studies underlying these estimates extend beyond those we have already discussed (Edwards *et al.* 1994). The estimates rely primarily on prospective epidemiological studies in which alcohol consumption is measured at one point in time; such a measurement is, at best, a poor surrogate for either of the main aspects of alcohol consumption as a risk factor—chronic effects of cumulated alcohol consumption or acute effects of intoxication at a specific event. In these studies, the effects of possible confounders are dealt with by statistically controlling for them in the analysis. But this can be problematic if drinking and the potential confounder are causally intertwined, as is true in the case of hypertension or tobacco smoking. Consider, for instance, a person who only smokes when under the influence of alcohol; controlling for that person's smoking behaviour potentially limits some of the alcohol effect.

From a public health perspective, it is the effects at the population level, rather than the individual level, that are the main concern. If drinking was entirely a matter of individual choice and behaviour, and if the effects of drinking happened only to the drinker, then effects at the population level would be a simple aggregation of the effects at the individual level. But neither of these conditions is applicable. Drinking is by and large a social activity, and the drinking behaviour of a person is likely to influence and be influenced by those around that person. In a given population, the amounts drunk by infrequent or light drinkers and by heavy drinkers tend to move up and down in concert. Thus, if there is some health gain when those at the lower end of the spectrum increase their consumption, there will also be health losses from an increase in consumption for those at the top end of the spectrum. In view of this, it has been argued that the level of per-drinker consumption where the balance of health benefits and losses is optimized in a population is likely to be considerably lower than the optimum level of consumption for the individual drinker (Skog 1996). For instance, Skog (1996) argued that the optimum level of alcohol consumption with respect to mortality was likely to be lower than the present-day per-capita consumption of any nation in western Europe. His argument is supported by findings of a generally positive relationship of the level of alcohol consumption with total mortality in time-series analysis of differenced data in a number of high-income countries (Norström & Ramstedt 2005).

By their design, the prospective studies typically used for investigations of alcohol's effects on mortality or morbidity do not measure the effects of drinking on others. Other types of individual-level studies, such as studies of the effects of drinking–driving (Perrine *et al.* 1989) or studies of homicide and other crimes (Wolfgang 1958), document the importance of such effects in terms of death or injury. But the strongest evidence of the magnitude of these effects comes from aggregate-level studies of the covariation of changes over time in a given society or place. Differenced time-series analyses in European societies have suggested that a 1 litre change in per capita alcohol consumption produces about a 1 per cent change in the overall mortality rate (Norström 1996; Her & Rehm 1998). Here again, however, drinking patterns and social circumstances are likely to make a difference. For instance, the drop in Russian total mortality during the alcohol restrictions of 1985–88 imply a decline of about 2.7 per cant in age-standardized mortality for each 1 litre drop in per capita consumption (calculated from Shkolnikov & Nemtsov 1997, and Leon *et al.* 1998). Even specifically for heart disease, any protective effects from changes in low-level drinking seem to be outbalanced in the population as a whole by negative effects from changes at high-consumption levels, levels of consumption typical in high-income societies. Thus, time-series analyses of differenced data on alcohol consumption and on CHD mortality in 14 European countries found no evidence of net protective effects and some evidence of net adverse effect (Hemström 2001; Ramstedt 2006).

Alcohol as an issue in public health

Shifting societal responses to problematic drinking

Efforts to control problematic drinking date back to the beginning of recorded history. These efforts have been many-sided, including informal responses in the family and community, as well as governmental controls. Religious teachings and movements have often been directed against drinking or intoxication: Moslems are forbidden by their faith to drink at all, and drinking is also discouraged or forbidden in at least some branches of all the major world religions.

In the last few centuries, European and Europe-derived societies have been hosts to conflicting trends in terms of alcohol issues. The production of alcoholic beverages became an important part of European economies and of imperial domination and trade in the age of European colonization. Alcohol production and exports took on political importance not only in the wine cultures of Southern Europe, but also in such countries as the Netherlands and Britain. In the British colonies as well as in America, in the late-eighteenth century, distilled spirits was the only profitable way to get grain to market (Rorabaugh 1979). In recent decades, alcohol beverage industries have become increasingly internationalized and concentrated (Jernigan 1997), and multinational companies, mostly based in Europe or North America, have pressed with considerable success to open up global markets for alcohol.

Starting in the early 1800s, there were substantial waves of popular, and eventually, governmental response to the problems that were resulting from the very heavy consumption of alcoholic beverages in English-speaking and Northern European societies (Blocker 1989; Levine 1991). As a culmination of decades of popular temperance movements, in the early-twentieth century, alcohol prohibition was adopted in several of these countries and stringent controls on the availability of alcohol in others. Although alcohol's impact on public order and morals and on family life were more central to the temperance movement thinking than the public health issues, mainstream thought in medicine and public health acknowledged the substantial adverse impacts of alcohol on health (Emerson 1932), and prohibition or an alternative, stringent controls on the availability of alcohol (Catlin 1931), were often identified with the public health interest.

In the United States, and other societies which had adopted alcohol prohibition, there was a strong reaction against it by the early 1930s, with middle-class youth in the lead (Room 1984a, 1984b). In this cultural–political context, as the new generation moved into professional and research positions, adverse effects of alcohol were downplayed or denied (Herd 1992; Katcher 1993), and alcohol issues almost disappeared from public health textbooks and discourse. Any problems with drinking were seen as attributable to a relatively small cadre of alcoholics, unable to control their drinking because of a mysterious predisposing factor. As late as 1968, the main emphasis of the American Public Health Association was on building treatment capacity for alcoholism (Cross 1968).

The 'new public health' approach

The last three decades of the twentieth century saw the rise of what has been termed in the alcohol literature the 'new public health' approach (Beauchamp 1976; Tigerstedt 1999) to alcohol issues. This approach brought together several strands of research and philosophy. In contrast to a concept in terms of 'alcoholism', the approach was premised on a disaggregated approach: There was a diversity of alcohol-related problems, fairly widely distributed among the drinking population (Knupfer 1967; World Health Organization, Expert Committee on Problems Related to Alcohol Consumption 1980). It was noted that for many problems, the heaviest drinkers accounted for only a minority, because there were so many more drinking at somewhat lower levels (Moore & Gerstein 1981); picking up Rose's (Rose 1981) phrase, Kreitman (Kreitman 1986) termed this the 'preventive paradox'. Attention was, therefore, paid not only to the heaviest drinkers, but also to the whole range of drinking levels, and indeed, to the distribution of consumption in the population (Ledermann 1956; De Lint 1968). What happens with moderate drinkers, it was argued, influences the social climate for heavy drinking, because drinking is largely a social activity, marked by mutual influences and norms of reciprocity (Bruun *et al.* 1975a; Skog 1985). In a given population, it was found that rates of alcohol-related problems tend to rise and fall with changes in the level of consumption (Seeley 1960). Controls on the availability of alcohol, including taxes, affect the level of consumption, and thus, also the rates of alcohol-related problems (Seeley 1960; Terris 1967; Popham *et al.* 1976). The level of alcohol consumption in a population, and controls on alcohol availability, is thus seen as a public health concern, and part of a society's overall 'alcohol policy' (Bruun *et al.* 1975a).

In enumerating the elements of the new public health approach, we have given references for early statements of each element. It will be seen that the strands of this approach were woven together gradually over a period of some years. A 1975 report by an international group of researchers (Bruun *et al.* 1975a) became a pivotal document for the approach. A few years later, the approach was given an authoritative endorsement in the United States by a committee of the National Academy of Sciences (Moore & Gerstein 1981). The most recent restatement of the approach by an international group of scholars appeared in 2003 (Babor *et al.* 2003), with a somewhat parallel analysis oriented to the developing world (Room *et al.* 2002).

The approach has had considerable influence on WHO programmes in the field of alcohol (Room 2005; World Health Organization 2007). At national levels, there has been a considerable variation in its influence on policy. In Sweden, where it is known as the Total Consumption Model, it attained dominance as the basis for official policy (Sutton 1998). However, policies based on this approach have been eroded as a consequence of Sweden's accession to the European Union (Holder *et al.* 1998). The approach also has had considerable backing in other Nordic countries.

In English-speaking countries, it has encountered substantial resistance in the cultural–political realm. Those allied with the alcoholic beverage industry have strongly attacked the approach, both in analyses and polemics (e.g. Mott 1991; Grant & Litvak 1998) and through direct political action to remove official proponents (Room 1984c). An approach that contemplates government regulation and influencing of private consumer choices is also unwelcome to those committed to consumer sovereignty and the primacy of individual choice (e.g. Peele 1987). Often, proponents of approaches seeking to 'domesticate' drinking—to reduce problems from drinking by integrating it into everyday life—have portrayed the new public health approach as antithetical to this (Olsson 1990), although some researchers have noted that there is no necessary antithesis (Whitehead 1979).

In terms of its influence on policy, the approach has undoubtedly had some effect in strengthening the defence of existing control structures and regulations. But efforts to get the approach adopted as the practical base for policy have met with resistance and failure in a number of countries (Baggott 1990; Hawks 1993). One response to this resistance has been some calls for an alternative approach (Stockwell *et al.* 1997), arguing that policy measures directed at heavy and problematic drinkers are more politically acceptable than measures directed at all drinkers.

The policy approach offered as an alternative is a focus on harm reduction, primarily by reducing instances of intoxication or insulating the drinkers from harm (Plant *et al.* 1997; Stimson *et al.* 2007). However, there is in fact usually no conflict between approaches aimed at total consumption and approaches aiming to reduce harm from heavy drinking. As Stockwell *et al.* (1997) noted, 'aggregate consumption levels are in fact likely to fall if effective (harm reduction) strategies are introduced'. Conversely, many measures that affect the whole drinking population—taxation being a good example—are especially hard on heavier drinkers. Nor are targeted harm reduction measures necessarily more politically acceptable than measures that affect all drinkers. Old systems of rationing and individual buyer surveillance (Järvinen 1991), which were directed specifically at restraining heavy drinking, are now politically unacceptable in any high-income society, although rationing, at least, was highly effective as a targeted prevention measure (Norström 1987).

Beyond its specific features, the controversy over the new public health approach replicates familiar patterns of controversy over public health approaches in general, particularly when those approaches impinge on familiar and valued patterns of behaviour, with substantial economic interests at stake. At the level of the knowledge base, the approach has had considerable success: The empirical evidence underlying the approach has considerably strengthened since the approach was first put forward. At a political level, however, the approach has had only limited success, and primarily in areas peripheral to its main focus—that is, in drinking–driving and minimum-age limits for drinkers.

Strategies of prevention and control and their effectiveness

Simplifying them, there are seven main strategies to minimize alcohol problems. One strategy is to educate or persuade people not to use alcohol or about ways to use it so as to limit harm. A second strategy, a kind of negative persuasion, is to deter drinking-related behaviour with the threat of penalties. A third strategy, in the positive direction, is to provide alternatives to drinking or to drink-related activities. A fourth strategy is in one way or another to insulate the user from harm. A fifth strategy is to regulate availability of alcohol or the conditions of its use; prohibition of supply may be regarded as a special case of such regulation. A sixth strategy is to work with social or religious movements oriented to reducing alcohol problems. And, a seventh strategy is to treat or otherwise help people who have in trouble with their drinking habits. We will consider, in turn, these strategies and the evidence on their effectiveness.

Education and persuasion

In principle, education can be offered to any segment of the population in a variety of venues, but it is usually education of youth in schools that first comes to mind in the prevention of alcohol problems. Community-based prevention programmes, which are often also directed at adults, also may include an educational component.

Education offers new information or ways of thinking and leaves it to the listener to draw conclusions concerning beliefs and behaviour. However, most alcohol education programmes go beyond this. Commonplace in North American evaluative literature on alcohol education is that 'knowledge-only' approaches do not result in changes in behaviour (Botvin 1995). School-based alcohol education has, thus, usually had a persuasional element, aiming to influence students in a particular direction.

Persuasion is directly concerned with changing beliefs or behaviours, and may or may not also offer information. Mass-media campaigns aimed at persuasion have been a very common component of prevention programmes for alcohol-related problems, but this can also be pursued through other media and modalities.

In most societies, public-health-oriented persuasion about alcohol must compete with a variety of other persuasive messages, including those intended to sell alcoholic beverages. The evidence that alcohol advertising influences teenagers and young adults towards increased drinking and problematic drinking is becoming stronger (Wyllie *et al.* 1998a, b; Casswell *et al.* 2002). Even where alcohol advertising is not allowed in the mass media, these messages are often conveyed to consumers and potential consumers in a variety of other ways.

Evidence on effectiveness

The literature on effectiveness of educational approaches is dominated by studies on school-based education from the United States. This means that alcohol education has usually been in the context of drug and tobacco education and that the emphasis has been on abstention (Beck 1998) or at least on delaying the start of drinking, in cultural circumstances where the median age of actually starting to drink is about 13 years although the minimum legal drinking age is 21 years. In general, despite the best efforts of a generation of researchers, this literature has had difficulty showing substantial and lasting effects (Foxcroft *et al.* 2003; Gorman *et al.* 2007). There is a good argument from general principles for alcohol education in the context of consumer and health, but there is little evidence from the formal evaluation literature at this point of its effectiveness beyond the short term.

Persuasive media campaigns have also been a favourite modality in many places in recent decades. In general, evaluations of such campaigns have been able to demonstrate impacts on knowledge and awareness about substance use problems, but show little success in affecting attitudes and behaviours (Babor *et al.* 2003). As with school education approaches, there are hints in literature that more success may come from influencing the community around the drinker—in terms of attitudes of significant others or popular support for alcohol policy measures—than from directly persuading the drinker himself or herself. Thus, media messages can be effective as agenda-setting mechanisms in the community, increasing or sustaining public support for other preventive strategies (Casswell *et al.* 1989).

Deterrence

In its broadest sense, deterrence means simply the threat of negative sanctions or disincentives for behaviour—a form of negative persuasion. Criminal laws deter in two ways: By general deterrence, which is the effect of the law in preventing a prohibited behaviour in the population as a whole; and specific deterrence, which is the effect of the law in discouraging those who have been caught from doing it again (Ross 1982). A law will have a greater preventive effect and be cheaper to administer to the extent it has a strong general deterrence effect.

Prohibitions on driving after drinking more than a specified amount are now in effect in most nations (World Health Organization 2004). In many societies, there have also been laws against public drunkenness (being in a public place while intoxicated) and against obnoxious behaviour while intoxicated. Other common prohibitions are concerned with producing or selling alcoholic beverages outside state-regulated channels and with aspects of drinking under a specified minimum age.

Evidence on effectiveness

Drinking–driving legislation, such as 'per-se' laws outlawing driving while at or above a defined blood-alcohol level, has been shown to be effective in changing behaviour and reducing rates of alcohol-related problems (Babor *et al.* 2003; Ross 1982; Hingson 1996). The effect is through both general and specific deterrence. The quickness and certainty of punishment as well as its severity are important in the deterrent value (too much severity tends to undercut the quickness and certainty). Drinking–driving is an ideal area for applying general deterrence, as the gains from breaking the law are limited and automobile drivers typically have something to lose by being caught.

Many English-speaking and Scandinavian countries have had a tradition of criminalizing drinking in public places or public drunkenness as such. The trend in the 1970s and following was to decriminalize public drunkenness, although in many places it remains illegal. In the 1990s and following, there has been some trend to criminalize drinking in specific public places (Edwards *et al.* 1994). Although there are few specific studies, criminalization of such behaviours has some effect in moving behaviour around, but is probably not very effective in changing the behaviour of marginalized heavy drinkers who have little to lose.

Providing and encouraging alternative activities

Another strategy, in principle involving positive incentives, is to provide and seek to encourage activities that are an alternative to drinking or to activities closely associated with drinking. This includes initiatives such as making soft drinks available as an alternative to alcoholic beverages, providing locations for sociability as an alternative to taverns, and providing and encouraging recreational activities as an alternative to leisure activities involving drinking. Job creation and skill development programmes are other examples.

Evidence on effectiveness

'Boredom' and 'because there's nothing else to do' are certainly among the reasons given by some for drinking. And, there are often good reasons of general social policy for providing and encouraging alternative activities. But as has been noted, the problem with alternatives to drinking is that drinking combines so well with many of them. Soft drinks are indeed an alternative to alcoholic beverages for quenching thirst, but they may also serve as a mixer in an alcoholic drink. Involvement in sports may go along with drinking as well as replace it. The few evaluation studies of providing alternative activities, again from a restricted number of societies, have generally not shown lasting effects on drinking behaviour (Moskowitz *et al.* 1983; Norman *et al.* 1997), although they undoubtedly often serve a general social purpose in broadening opportunities for the disadvantaged (Carmona & Stewart 1996).

Insulating use from harm

A major social strategy for reducing alcohol-related problems in many societies has been measures to separate the drinker, and particularly heavy drinkers, from potential harm. This separation can be physical (in terms of distance or walls), it can be temporal, or it can be cultural (e.g. defining the drinking occasion as 'time out' from normal responsibilities). These 'harm-reduction' strategies, as they are called in the context of illicit drugs, are often built into cultural arrangements around drinking, but can also be the object of purposive programmes and policies (Moore & Gerstein 1981), such as promotion of 'designated drivers', where one person in a social group is chosen to abstain and drive in the particular social situation (DeJong & Hingson 1998).

A variety of modifications to the driving environment positively affect casualties associated with drinking and driving, along with other casualties. These include mandatory use of seat belts, airbags, and improvements in the safety of vehicles and roads. Many other practical measures to separate intoxication episodes from casualties and other adverse consequences have been put into practice, although usually without formal evaluation.

Evidence on effectiveness

Drinking–driving countermeasures are a prime example of an approach in terms of insulating drinking behaviour from harm, as they seek to reduce alcohol-related traffic casualties without necessarily stopping or reducing alcohol use (Evans 1991). There is substantial evidence on the success of a range of such countermeasures, including environmental change approaches as well as deterrence (DeJong & Hingson 1998; Forsyth 1996). Some environmental measures that reduce traffic casualties in general—such as requiring the wearing of seat belts in cars or providing sidewalks separated from the road—may prevent casualties associated with intoxication even more than other casualties.

Regulating the availability and conditions of use

In terms of the substantial harm to health and public order they can cause, alcoholic beverages are not ordinary commodities. Governments have, thus, often actively intervened in the markets for such beverages, far beyond usual levels of state intervention in markets for commodities.

Total prohibition can be viewed as an extreme form of regulation of the market. In this circumstance, where no one is licensed to sell alcohol, the state has no formal control over the conditions of the sales that occur nevertheless and there are no legal sales interests, controlled through licensing, to cooperate with the state in market regulation.

With a general prohibition, typically, the consumption of alcohol does fall in the population, and there are also declines in the rates of the direct consequences of drinking such as cirrhosis or alcohol-related mental disorders (Moore & Gerstein 1981; Teasley 1992). But prohibition also brings with it characteristic negative consequences, including the emergence and growth of an illicit market and the crime associated with this. Partly for this reason, prohibition is now not a live option in any high-income society, although it still is in some other societies and local areas.

The features of alcohol control regimes that regulate the legal market in alcohol vary greatly. Special taxes on alcohol are very common, imposed often as much for revenue as for public health considerations. Many societies have minimum-age limits forbidding sales to underage customers and regulations forbidding sales to the already intoxicated. Often, the regulations include limiting the number of sales outlets, restricting hours and days of sale, and limiting sales to special stores or drinking places. Rationing of alcohol purchases—limiting the amount individuals can buy in a given time period—has also been used as a means of regulating availability. Regulations restricting or forbidding advertising of alcoholic beverages attempt to limit or channel efforts by private interests to increase demand for particular alcoholic beverages.

Such regulations potentially complement education and persuasion efforts. State monopolization on sales of some or all alcoholic beverages at the retail and/or wholesale level has also been commonly been used as a mechanism to minimize alcohol-related harm (Room 1993).

Effectiveness of specific types of regulation on availability

The decades since the 1970s have seen the development of a burgeoning literature on the effects of alcohol control measures. Reference guides for communities, summarizing the research evidence and attuned to particular national or regional conditions, are becoming available (e.g. Grover 1999; Neves *et al.* 1998). Specific types of regulation of the alcohol market, and the evidence on their effectiveness, are discussed as follows:

Minimum-age limits: A minimum-age limit is a partial prohibition, applied to one segment of the population. There is a strong evaluation literature showing the effectiveness of establishing and enforcing minimum-age limits in reducing alcohol-related problems (Babor *et al.* 2003). However, this literature is mostly based on North America, focusing mostly on youthful driving casualties and evaluating reduction from and increases to age 21 years as the limit, a minimum-age limit higher than in most societies. There is limited evidence on the applicability of the literature's findings in other societies and where youth cultures may be less automobile-focused (but see Møller 2002; Kypri *et al.* 2006).

Taxes and other price increases: Generally, consumers show some response on the price of alcoholic beverages, as on all other commodities. If the price goes up, the drinker will drink less; data from high-income societies suggests this is at least as true of the heavy drinker as of the occasional drinker (Babor *et al.* 2003). Studies have found that alcohol tax increases reduce the rates of traffic casualties, of cirrhosis mortality, and of incidents of violence (Cook 1981; Cook & Moore 1993).

Limiting sales outlets, and hours and conditions of sale: A substantial body of literature shows that levels and patterns of alcohol consumption, and rates of alcohol-related casualties and other problems, are influenced by such sales restrictions, which typically make the purchase of alcoholic beverages slightly inconvenient or influence the setting of and after drinking (Babor *et al.* 2003). Enforced rules influencing 'house policies' in drinking places on not serving intoxicated customers, for example, have also been shown to have some effect (Saltz 1997).

Monopolizing production or sale: Studies of the effects of privatizing retail alcohol monopolies have often shown some increase in levels of alcohol consumption and problems, in part because the number of outlets and hours of sale typically increase with privatization (Her *et al.* 1999) and partly also because the new private interests typically exert political influence for further increases in availability. From a public health perspective, it is the retail level that is important, although monopolization of the production or wholesale level may facilitate revenue collection and effective control of the market.

Rationing sales: Rationing the amount of alcohol sold to an individual potentially directly impacts on heavy drinkers and has been shown to reduce levels both of intoxication-related problems such as violence and of drinking-history-related problems such as cirrhosis mortality (Norström 1987; Schechter 1986). But, although a form of rationing—the medical prescription system—is well accepted in most societies for psychoactive medications, it has proved politically unacceptable nowadays for alcoholic beverages in high-income societies.

Advertising and promotion restrictions: Many societies have regulations on advertising and other promotion of sales of alcoholic beverages (World Health Organization 2004). Although it is well accepted that advertising can strongly affect consumer choices on products in the market, it has proved difficult to measure the effects of advertising on demand for alcoholic beverages as a whole, partly because the effects are likely to be cumulative and long-term, making them difficult to measure. However, the evidence on the effects of advertising and promotion on overall demand has become somewhat stronger in recent literature (Casswel 1995; Saffer 1998; Casswell & Zhang 1998).

Social and religious movements and community action

Substantial reductions in alcohol-related problems have often been the result of spontaneous social and religious movements, which put a major emphasis on quitting intoxication or drinking. In recent decades, efforts have also been made to form partnerships between state organizations and non-governmental groups to work on alcohol problems, often at the level of the local community. There has been an active tradition of community action projects on alcohol problems, often using a range of prevention strategies (Giesbrecht *et al.* 1990; Greenfield & Zimmerman 1993; Holmila 1997; Holder 1998). School-based prevention efforts have also moved increasingly to try to involve the community, in line with general perceptions that such multifaceted strategies will be more effective (Paglia & Room 1999).

Although some of the biggest historical reductions in alcohol problem rates have resulted from spontaneous and autonomous social or religious movements, support or collaboration from a government can easily be perceived as official co-optation or manipulation (Room 1997). Thus, there is considerable question about the extent to which such movements can or should become an instrument of government prevention policies.

Evidence on effectiveness

In the short term, movements of religious or cultural revival can be highly effective in reducing levels of drinking and of alcohol-related problems. Alcohol consumption in the United States fell by about half in the first flush of temperance enthusiasm in 1830–45 (Moore & Gerstein 1981). Rates of serious crime are reported to have fallen for a while to a fraction of their previous level in Ireland in the wake of Father Mathew's temperance crusade (Room 1983). The enthusiasm that sustains such movements tends to decay over time, although they often leave behind new customs and institutions of much longer duration. For instance, although the days when the historic temperance movement in English-speaking societies was strong are long gone, the movement had the long-lasting effect of largely removing drinking from the workplace in these societies.

Particularly in the developing world, religious or cultural renewal movements oriented to reducing or prohibiting drinking are often a strong avenue of preventive action (Room *et al.* 2002). A reform movement among poor indigenous people in a region of Ecuador touched off in 1987 by religious renewal movements and an earthquake appears to have had lasting effects on popular sobriety (Butler 2006).

Treatment and other help

Providing effective treatment or other help for drinkers who find they cannot control their drinking can be regarded as an obligation of a just and humane society. The help can take several forms: A specific treatment system for alcohol problems, professional help in general health or welfare systems, or non-professional assistance in mutual-help movements. To the extent such help is effective, it is also a means of preventing or reducing future alcohol-related problems in the person helped, although less clearly on a population basis.

Treatments for alcohol problems need not be complex or expensive. The evaluation literature suggests that brief outpatient interventions aimed at changing cognitions and behaviour around drinking are as effective in most circumstances as longer and more intensive treatment (Finney & Monahan 1998; Long *et al.* 1998). Positive results from such interventions in primary health-care settings were shown in a WHO study that included a number of countries (Babor & Grant 1994).

Evidence on effectiveness

In terms of the effects of treatment on those who come for it, there is good evidence on the effectiveness of treatment for alcohol problem. Typically, the improvement rate from a single episode of treatment is about 20 per cent higher than the no-treatment condition: Further treatment episodes are often needed. Brief treatment interventions or mutual-help approaches usually result in net savings in social and health costs associated with the heavy drinker (at least where health care is not self-paid), as well as improving the quality of life (Holder *et al.* 1992; Holder & Cunningham 1992).

The effectiveness of providing treatment as a strategy for reducing rates of alcohol problems in a society is more equivocal. In a North American context, it has been argued that the steep increase in alcohol problems treatment provision and mutual-help group membership in recent decades has contributed to reducing alcohol problems rates (Smart & Mann 1990). But the strength of the evidence for this contention is disputed (Holder 1997; Smart & Mann 1997). A treatment system for alcohol problems is an important part of an integrated national alcohol policy, but as an instrument of prevention—of reducing societal rates of alcohol problems—it is probably not very cost-effective.

Building integrated alcohol policies

Alcohol policy at a community or societal level

Often, the different strategies for preventing alcohol problems appear to be synergic in their effects (DeJong & Hingson 1998). For instance, controls on availability are more likely to be adopted, continued, and respected when the public has been successfully persuaded of their effects and effectiveness. But strategies can also work at cross-purposes: A prohibition policy, for instance, makes it difficult to pursue measures that insulate drinking from harm.

In a society where alcohol is a regular item of consumption, in view of the resulting rates of alcohol-related social and health problems, there is a strong justification for adopting a comprehensive policy concerning alcohol, taking into account production, marketing, and consumption, and the prevention and treatment of alcohol-related problems. In recent years, the idea that there should be an integrated alcohol policy at community or national levels, reaching across the many sectors of government and civil society that deal with alcohol issues, has become a common public health aim, although accomplishing this has often proved difficult (Smart & Mann 1997; Crombie *et al.* 2007).

In terms of strategies we have reviewed for managing and reducing the rates of alcohol problems in the society, there is a clear evidence for effectiveness and cost-effectiveness of measures regulating the availability and conditions of use, and measures which insulate use from harm. With respect to some aspects of alcohol problems, notably drinking–driving, deterrence measures also fall in the same category. Despite their perennial popularity, evidence of the effectiveness of education or persuasion and treatment strategies in reducing societal rates of problems is limited at best. Education and treatment are good things for a society and a government to be doing about alcohol problems, but they do not constitute in themselves a public health policy on alcohol. These strategies will nevertheless be pursued in most societies, and they can best pursued with attention to using cost-effective methods, and to integrating targets and messages with other aspects of alcohol policy.

Alcohol policy in a global perspective

Apart from agreements made a century ago among the European colonial powers about control of the spirits trade in Africa (Bruun *et al.* 1975b), there is little tradition of collaboration on alcohol policy at the international level. It has been largely up to each nation to cope on its own with the serious social and health problems associated with drinking. Although alcohol smuggling has a long history, the nation-state could usually rely on distances and traditional trade barriers to keep alcohol issues largely a matter within its borders, in terms of the supply as well as of the problems.

Since the 1980s, an accelerated rate of economic globalization has been seen, which has increasingly rendered obsolete the assumption that alcohol issues are local issues. This globalization affects alcohol issues in three main ways. The first of these is the influence of a global ideology of free markets. In its sweep, this ideology has caught up and dismantled a variety of market arrangements that served to hold down and to structure alcohol consumption. State and provincial alcohol monopolies in North America were weakened or dismantled (Her *et al.* 1999). In Eastern Europe and the countries in transition, alcohol monopolies were swept away along with most other governmental intrusions in the market (Moskalewicz 1993). Many of the municipally-run beer halls in Southern African countries were privatized (Jernigan 1997). In line with the general ideology, privatization of alcohol production and distribution has been often suggested, abetted or imposed on developing countries by international development agencies (White & Batia 1998).

Secondly, trade agreements, trade dispute mechanisms, and the growth of new sales media have effectively reduced the ability of national and subnational governments to control their local alcohol markets. The influence of trade agreements and trade dispute decisions in breaking down alcohol controls, including control of price through taxation, has been most fully documented for North America (Room *et al.* 2006) and Europe (Holder *et al.* 1998; Tigerstedt 1990), but these mechanisms also operate in the developing world. For instance, average taxes on alcoholic beverages in South Korea were lowered in 2000 as a result of complaints to the World Trade Organization by the European Union and the United States (Kim 2000). Sales of alcoholic beverages through the Internet have become a fast-growing threat to national or local control of alcohol markets (Apple 1999).

Third, alcohol production, distribution, and marketing became increasingly globalized (Jernigan 1997; Room *et al.* 2002). Transnational alcohol companies expanded rapidly into the developing world and the countries in transition in search of new markets, benefiting from weak policy environments and the sweeping tide of market liberalization. Alhough most alcoholic beverages are still produced in the country in which they are sold, industrially produced beverages were increasingly produced in plants owned, co-owned, or licensed by multinational firms. To promote increased sales, these firms have been able to transform and step up the marketing techniques used in the national market, bringing forth all the marketing resources and expertise they have developed in other markets.

In light of these converging trends, there is a growing need for mechanisms to express public health interests in alcohol issues at the international level, both in trade agreements and settlements of trade disputes, and in creating mutual obligations for one nation to back up rather than subvert the alcohol regulations and policies of another. There are growing calls for a framework convention on alcohol control to be negotiated under the WHO auspices or otherwise, on the model of the tobacco convention (Room 2006; A framework convention on alcohol control 2007).

Conclusion

The comparative risk analysis in the WHO's estimation of the global burden of disease has underlined the substantial role of alcohol in death and disability, particularly in high-income and middle-income countries. Over the last 30 years, sufficient literature has emerged, which allows a differentiation of prevention strategies and policies in terms of their effectiveness. Some strategies—for example, school education, public information campaigns, and provision of alternatives—are often politically popular but have limited or no effect. A few strategies that have proved effective—notably, drinking–driving countermeasures—have been applied in a number of countries. Other effective strategies—especially, controls on price and availability—have been widely resisted in the political process. In a globalized world, control of the alcohol market in the interest of public health is needed not only at the local and national level, but also internationally. This need has led to calls for a framework convention on alcohol control, which would also provide an impetus and template for actions at national and subnational levels.

References

A framework convention on alcohol control [editorial]. *Lancet* 2007 Sep 29;**370**(9593):1102.

Andréasson S., Romelsjö A., Allebeck P. Alcohol, social factors, and mortality among young men. *British Journal of Addiction* 1991;**86**:877–87.

Apple R.W. Zinfandel by mail? New York Times 1999 May 19.

Babor T., Caetano R., Casswell S. *et al. Alcohol: no ordinary commodity – research and public policy*. Oxford: Oxford University Press; 2003.

Babor T.F., Grant M. *et al.* Randomized clinical trial of brief interventions in primary health care: summary of a WHO project (with commentaries and a response). Addiction 1994;**89**:657–78.

Baggott R. *Alcohol, politics, and social policy*. Aldershot, UK: Avebury; 1990.

Beauchamp D. Exploring new ethics for public health: developing a fair alcohol policy. *Journal of Health Politics, Policy, and Law* 1976; **1**:338–54.

Beck J. 100 years of 'just say no' versus 'just say know'. *Evaluation Review* 1998;**22**:15–45.

Blocker J. *American temperance movements: cycles of reform*. Boston (MA): Twayne Publishers; 1989.

Bondy S.J., Rehm J., Ashley M.J. *et al.* Low-risk drinking guidelines: the scientific evidence. *Canadian Journal of Public Health* 1999;**90**:272–6.

Botvin G.J. Principles of prevention. In: Coombs RH, Ziedonis D, editors. *Handbook on drug abuse prevention: a comprehensive strategy to prevent the abuse of alcohol and other drugs*. Boston (MA): Allyn and Bacon; 1995. p. 19–44.

Bruun K., Edwards G., Lumio M. *et al. Alcohol control policies in public health perspective*. Helsinki: Finnish Foundation for Alcohol Studies; 1975a. FFAS Vol. 25.

Bruun K., Rexed I., Pan L. The gentlemen's club. Chicago (IL): University of Chicago Press; 1975b.

Butler B.Y. Holy intoxication to drunken dissipation: alcohol among Quichua speakers in Otavalo, Ecuador. Albuquerque (NM): University of New Mexico Press; 2006.

Carmona M., Stewart K. *Review of alternative activities and alternatives programs in youth-oriented prevention*. Rockville (MD): Center for Substance Abuse Prevention; 1996. CSAP Technical Report 13.

Casswell S. Does alcohol advertising have an impact on public health? *Drug and Alcohol Review*. 1995;14:395–404.

Casswell S., Gilmore L., Maguire V. *et al.* Changes in public support for alcohol policies following a community-based campaign. *British Journal of Addiction* 1989;**84**:515–22.

Casswell S., Pledger M., Pratap S. Trajectories of drinking from 18 to 26 years: identification and prediction. *Addiction* 2002;**97**(11): 1427–37.

Casswell S., Zhang J.F. Impact of liking for advertising and brand allegiance on drinking and alcohol-related aggression: a longitudinal study. *Addiction* 1998;**93**:1209–17.

Catlin G.E.G. *Liquor control*. London: Thornton Butterworth; 1931.

Chadwick D.J., Goode J.A., editors. Alcohol and cardiovascular diseases. Chichester, UK: John Wiley & Sons; 1998.

Cook P. Effect of liquor taxes on drinking, cirrhosis, and auto accidents. In: Moore M.H., Gerstein D.R., editors. *Alcohol and public policy: beyond the shadow of prohibition*. Washington (DC): National Academy Press; 1981. p. 255–85

Cook P.J., Moore M.H. Violence reduction through restrictions on alcohol availability. *Alcohol Health and Research World* 1993;**17**:151–6.

Criqui M. *et al.* Discussion. In: Chadwick D.J., Goode J.A., editors. *Alcohol and cardiovascular diseases*. Chichester, UK: John Wiley & Sons; 1998. p. 122–4.

Crombie I.K., Irvine L., Elliott L. *et al.* How do public health policies tackle alcohol-related harm? A review of 12 developed countries. *Alcohol and Alcoholism* 2007;**42**(**5**):492–9.

Cross J.N. *Guide to the community control of alcoholism*. New York (NY): American Public Health Association; 1968.

De Lint J., Schmidt W. The distribution of alcohol consumption in Ontario. *Quarterly Journal of Studies on Alcohol* 1968;**29**:968–73.

DeJong W., Hingson R. Strategies to reduce driving under the influence of alcohol. *Annual Review of Public Health* 1998;**19**:359–78.

Edwards G., Anderson P., Babor T.F. *et al. Alcohol policy and the public good*. Oxford: Oxford University Press; 1994.

Emerson H., editor. *Alcohol and man: the effects of alcohol on man in health and disease*. New York (NY): Macmillan; 1932.

English D.R., Holman C.D.J., Milne E. *et al. The quantification of drug caused morbidity and mortality in Australia* (2 vol.). Canberra: Australian Government Publishing Service; 1995.

Evans L. *Traffic safety and the driver*. New York (NY): Van Nostrand Reinhold; 1991.

Ezzati M., Lopez A.D., Rodgers A. *et al.* and the Comparative Risk Assessment Collaborating Group. Selected major risk factors and global and regional burden of disease. *Lancet* 2002;**360**(9343):1347–60.

Fillmore K.M., Kerr W.C., Stockwell T. *et al.* Moderate alcohol use and reduced mortality risk: systematic error in prospective studies. *Addiction Research and Theory* 2006;**14**(2):101–32.

Finney J.W., Monahan S.C. Cost-effectiveness of treatment for alcoholism: a second approximation. *Journal of Studies on Alcohol* 1998;**57**:229–43.

Forsyth I. Alcohol and drugs: the role of insurance in promoting effective countermeasures. In Proceedings of the Conference on Road Safety in Europe and Strategic Highway Research Program (SHRP). Linköping, Sweden: Swedish National Road and Transport Safety Institute; 1996. VTI Conferens No. 4A. Part 3. p. 45–63.

Foxcroft D.R., Ireland D., Lister-Sharp F.J. *et al.* Longer-term primary prevention for alcohol misuse in young people: a systematic review. *Addiction* 2003;**98** Suppl 4:397–411.

Giesbrecht N., Conley P., Denniston R. *et al.* editors. *Research, action and the community: experiences in the prevention of alcohol and other drug problems.* Rockville (MD): Office of Substance Abuse Prevention; 1990. DHHS Publication No. (ADM) 89–1651.

Gorman D.M., Conde E., Huber Jr. J.C. The creation of evidence in 'evidence-based' drug prevention: a critique of the Strengthening Families Program Plus Life Skills Training evaluation. *Drug and Alcohol Review* 2007;**26**(6):585–93.

Graham K., Leonard K.E., Room R. *et al.* Current directions in research on understanding and preventing intoxicated aggression. *Addiction* 1998;**93**:659–76.

Grant M., Litvak J. Introduction: beyond per capita consumption. In: Grant M, Litvak J, editors. *Drinking patterns and their consequences.* Washington (DC): Taylor and Francis; 1998. p. 1–4.

Greenfield T., Zimmerman R., editors. *Experiences with community action projects: new research in the prevention of alcohol and other drug problems.* Rockville (MD): Center for Substance Abuse Prevention; 1993. DHHS Publication No. (ADM) 93–1976.

Grover P.T., editor. *Preventing problems related to alcohol availability—environmental approaches: reference guide.* Washington (DC): Center for Substance Abuse Prevention; 1999. DHHS Publication No. SMA 99–3298. Available from: http://text.nlm.nih.gov/ftrs/dbaccess/csap

Hawks D. A review of current guidelines on moderate drinking for individual consumers. *Contemporary Drug Problems* 1994;**21**:223–37.

Hawks D. The formulation of Australia's National Health Policy on Alcohol. *Addiction* 1993;**88** Supplement:19S–26S.

Hemström Ö. Per capita alcohol consumption and ischaemic heart disease mortality. *Addiction* 2001;**96** Suppl 1:93–112.

Her M., Giesbrecht N., Room R. *et al.* Privatizing alcohol sales and alcohol consumption: evidence and implications. *Addiction* 1999;**94**:1125–39.

Her M., Rehm J. Alcohol and all-cause mortality in Europe 1982–1990: a pooled cross-section time-series analysis. *Addiction* 1998;**93**:1335–40.

Herd D. Ideology, history, and changing models of liver cirrhosis epidemiology. *British Journal of Addiction* 1992;**87**:179–92.

Hingson R. Prevention of drinking and driving. *Alcohol Health and Research World.* 1996;20;219–26.

Holder H.D. *Alcohol and the community: a systems approach to prevention.* Cambridge, UK: Cambridge University Press; 1998.

Holder H. Can individually directed interventions reduce population-level alcohol-involved problems?. *Addiction* 1997;**92**:5–7.

Holder H.D., Cunningham D.W. Alcoholism treatment for employees and family members: its effect on health care costs. *Alcohol Health and Research World* 1992;**16**:149–53.

Holder H.D., Kühlhorn E., Nordlund S. *et al. European integration and Nordic alcohol policies.* Aldershot, UK: Ashgate; 1998.

Holder H.D., Lennox R.D.L., Blose J.O. Economic benefits of alcoholism treatment: a summary of twenty years of research. *Journal of Employee Assistance Research* 1992;**1**:63–82.

Holmila M., editor. *Community Prevention of Alcohol Problems.* Basingstoke, UK: Macmillan; 1997.

Järvinen M. The controlled controllers: women, men, and alcohol. *Contemporary Drug Problems* 1991;**18**:389–406.

Jernigan D.H. *Thirsting for markets: the global impact of corporate alcohol.* San Rafael (CA): Marin Institute for the Prevention of Alcohol and Other Drug Problems; 1997.

Katcher B.S. The post-repeal eclipse in knowledge about the harmful effects of alcohol. *Addiction* 1993;**88**:729–44.

Kauhanen J., Kaplan G.A., Goldberg D.E. *et al.* Beer bingeing and mortality: results from the Kuopio ischaemic heart disease risk factor study, a prospective population-based study. *British Medical Journal* 1997;**315**:846–51.

Kim H-R. Revised liquor taxes leave soju makers in lurch. Korea Herald 2000 Mar 13.

Klatsky A.L. Moderate drinking and reduced risk of heart disease. *Alcohol Research and Health* 1999;**23**(1):15–23.

Knupfer G. The epidemiology of problem drinking. *American Journal of Public Health* 1967;**57**:973–86.

Kozlowski L.T., Heller D.A., Pillitteri J.L. *et al.* Tobacco use, the health effects of moderate alcohol drinking, and the assessment of their interaction. *Contemporary Drug Problems* 1994;**21**:81–9.

Kreitman N. Alcohol consumption and the preventive paradox. *British Journal of Addiction* 1986;**81**:353–63.

Kupari M., Koskinen P. Alcohol, cardiac arrhythmias and sudden death. In: Chadwick DJ, Goode JA, editors. *Alcohol and Cardiovascular Diseases.* Chichester, UK: John Wiley & Sons; 1998. p. 68–79.

Kypri K., Voas R.B., Langley J.D. *et al.* Minimum purchasing age for alcohol and traffic crash injuries among 15- to 19-year-olds in New Zealand. *American Journal of Public Health* 2006;**96**(**1**):126–31.

Ledermann S. *Alcool, Alcoolisme, Alcoolisation.* Paris: Presses Universitaires de France. INED Cahier No. 29; 1956.

Leon D.A., Chenet L., Shkolnikov V.M. *et al.* Huge variation in Russian mortality rates 1984–94: artefact, alcohol, or what?. *Lancet* 1997;**350**:383–8.

Levine H.G. Temperance cultures: concern about alcohol problems in Nordic and English-speaking cultures. In: Lader M, Edwards G, Drummond DC, editors. *The nature of alcohol and drug related problems.* Oxford: Oxford University Press; 1991. p. 15–36.

Long C.G., Williams M., Hollin C.R. (1998) Treating alcohol problems: a study of program effectiveness and cost-effectiveness according to length and delivery of treatment. *Addiction*;**93**:561–71.

MacAndrew C., Edgerton R.E. *Drunken Comportment.* Chicago (IL): Aldine; 1969.

Maclure M. Demonstration of deductive meta-analysis: ethanol intake and risk of myocardial infarction. *Epidemiologic Reviews* 1993;**15**:328–51.

Mäkelä K. The uses of alcohol and their cultural regulation. *Acta Sociologica* 1983;**26**:21–31.

McKee M., Britton A. The positive relationship between alcohol and heart disease in Eastern Europe: potential physiological mechanisms. *Journal of the Royal Society of Medicine* 1998;**91**:402–7.

Møller L. Legal restrictions resulted in a reduction of alcohol consumption among young people in Denmark. In: Room R, editor. *The effects of Nordic alcohol policies: what happens to drinking when alcohol controls change?* Helsinki: Nordic Council for Alcohol and Drug Research; 2002. NAD Publication 42 p. 93–100. Available from: http://www.nad.fi/pdf/NAD_42.pdf

Moore M.H., Gerstein D.R. (1981) (eds) *Alcohol and Public Policy: Beyond the Shadow of Prohibition.* Washington (DC): National Academy Press; 1981.

Moskalewicz J. Privatization of the alcohol arena in Poland. *Contemporary Drug Problems* 1993;**20**:63–275.

Moskowitz J.M., Mailvin J., Schaeffer G.A. *et al.* Evaluation of a junior high school primary prevention program. *Addictive Behaviors* 1983;**8**: 393–401.

Mott G. The anti-alcohol network. *Moderation Reader* 1991;**5**(5):6–20.

Neves P., de Pape D., Giesbrecht N. *et al.* (1998) Communities take action! A practical guide for municipalities, enforcement agencies, community groups, and others concerned about the impact of alcohol on public health and safety. Toronto: Addiction Research Foundation.

NIAAA. *Alcohol and the Immune System*. In the 9th special report to the US Congress on alcohol and health. Rockville (MD): National Institute on Alcohol Abuse and Alcoholism; 1997. p. 163–9. NIH Publication No. 97–4017.

Norman E., Turner S., Zunz S.J. *et al.* Prevention programs reviewed: what works? In: Norman E, editor. *Drug-free Youth: A Compendium for Prevention Specialists.* New York (NY): Garland Publishing; 1997. p. 22–45.

Norström T. Abolition of the Swedish rationing system: effects on consumption distribution and cirrhosis mortality. *British Journal of Addiction* 1987;**82**:633–41.

Norström T. Per capita consumption and total mortality: an analysis of historical data. *Addiction* 1996;**91**:339–44.

Norström T., Ramstedt M. Mortality and population drinking: a review of the literature. *Drug and Alcohol Review* 2005;**24**(**6**)**537–47**. Available from: http://www.informaworld.com.ezproxy.lib.unimelb.edu.au/smpp/title~content=t713412284~db=all~tab=issueslist~branches=24 - v24

Olsson B. Alkoholpolitik och alkoholens fenomenologi: uppfattningar som artikulerats i pressen [Alcohol policy and the phenomenology of alcohol: concepts articulated in the press]. *Alkoholpolitik* 1990;**7**: 184–95.

Paglia A., Room R. Preventing substance use problems among youth: a literature review and recommendations. *Journal of Primary Prevention* 1999;**20**:3–50.

Peele S. The limitations of control-of-supply models for explaining and preventing alcoholism and drug addiction. *Journal of Studies on Alcohol* 1987;**48**:61–77.

Perrine M.W., Peck R.C., Fell J.C. Epidemiologic perspectives on drunk driving. In: *Surgeon General's Workshop on Drunk Driving: Background Papers*. Washington (DC): US Department of Health and Human Services; 1989. p. 35–76.

Plant M., Single E., Stockwell T., editors. *Alcohol: Minimizing the Harm—What Works?* London and New York (NY): Free Association Books; 1997.

Poikolainen K. It can be bad for the heart, too—drinking patterns and coronary heart disease. *Addiction* 1999;**93**:1757–9.

Popham R., Schmidt W., de Lint J. The effects of legal restraint on drinking. In: Kissin B., Begleiter H., editors. *The Biology of Alcoholism: vol. 4. Social Aspects of Alcoholism*. New York (NY) and London: Plenum; 1976. p. 579–625.

Ramstedt M. Is alcohol good or bad for Canadian hearts? A time-series analysis of the link between alcohol consumption and IHD mortality. *Drug and Alcohol Review* 2006;**25**(**4**):315–20.

Rehm J., Room R., Monteiro M. *et al.* Alcohol use. In: Ezzati M., Lopez D., Rodgers A., Murray C.J.L., editors. *Comparative quantification of health risks. Global and regional burden of disease attributable to selected major risk factors: volume 1*. Geneva: World Health Organization; 2004. p. 959–1108.

Rehm J., Sempos C.T. Alcohol consumption and all-cause mortality. *Addiction* 1995;**90**:471–80.

Room R. A 'reverence for strong drink': the lost generation and the elevation of alcohol in American culture. *Journal of Studies on Alcohol* 1984b;**45**:540–6.

Room R. Alcohol and crime: behavioral aspects. In: Kadish S, editor. *Encyclopedia of crime and justice*. Vol. 1. New York (NY): Free Press; 1983. p. 35–44.

Room R. Alcohol and the World Health Organization: the ups and downs of two decades. *Nordisk Alkohol- & Narkotikatidskrift* 2005;**22** (English suppl):146–162.

Room R. Alcohol consumption and social harm—conceptual issues and historical perspectives. *Contemporary Drug Problems* 1996; **23**:373–88.

Room R. Alcohol control and public health. *Annual Review of Public Health* 1984a;**5**:293–317.

Room R. Former NIAAA directors look back: policy makers on the role of research. *Drinking and Drug Practices Surveyor* 1984c;**19**:38–42.

Room R. International control of alcohol: alternative paths forward. *Drug and Alcohol Review* 2006;**25**:581–95.

Room R. The evolution of alcohol monopolies and their relevance for public health. *Contemporary Drug Problems* 1993;**20**:169–87.

Room R. The idea of alcohol policy. *Nordic Studies on Alcohol and Drugs* 1999;**16** (English Suppl):7–20.

Room R. Voluntary organizations and the state in the prevention of alcohol problems. *Drugs and Society* 1997;**11**:11–23.

Room R., Giesbrecht N., Stoduto G. Trade agreements and disputes. In: Giesbrecht N, Demers A, Ogborne A *et al.* editors. *Sober reflections: commerce, public health, and the evolution of alcohol policy in Canada, 1980–2000*. Montreal and Kingston: McGill-Queen's University Press; 2006. p. 74–96.

Room R., Jernigan D., Carlini-Marlatt B. *et al. Alcohol and developing societies: a public health approach*. Helsinki: Finnish Foundation for Alcohol Studies; 2002.

Rorabaugh W.J. *The alcoholic republic*. New York (NY): Oxford University Press; 1979.

Rose G. Strategy of prevention: lessons from cardiovascular disease. *British Medical Journal* 1981;**282**:1847–51.

Ross H.L. Deterring the drinking driver: legal policy and social control. Lexington (MA): Lexington Books; 1982.

Saffer H. Economic issues in cigarette and alcohol advertising. *Journal of Drug Issues* 1998;**28**:781–93.

Saltz R.F. Prevention where alcohol is sold and consumed: server intervention and responsible beverage service. In: Plant M., Single E., Stockwell T., editors. *Alcohol: minimizing the harm—what works?* New York (NY): Free Association Books; 1997. p. 72–84.

Schechter E.J. Alcohol rationing and control systems in Greenland. *Contemporary Drug Problems* 1986;**13**:587–620.

Seeley J.R. Death by liver cirrhosis and the price of beverage alcohol. *Canadian Medical Association Journal* 1960;**83**:1361–6.

Shkolnikov V.M., Nemtsov A. The anti-alcohol campaign and variations in Russian mortality. In: Bobadilla J.L., Costello C.A., Mitchell F., editors. *Premature death in the new independent states.* Washington (DC): National Academy Press; 1997. p. 239–61.

Skog O-J. The collectivity of drinking cultures: a theory of the distribution of alcohol consumption. *British Journal of Addiction* 1985;**80**:83–99.

Skog O-J. Public health consequences of the J-curve hypothesis of alcohol problems. *Addiction* 1996;**91**:325–37.

Smart R.G., Mann R.E. Are increased levels of treatment and Alcoholics Anonymous large enough to create the recent reduction in liver cirrhosis?. *British Journal of Addiction* 1990;**85**:1385–7.

Smart R.G., Mann R.E. Interventions into alcohol problems: what works? *Addiction* 1997;**92**:9–13.

Stimson G., Grant M., Choquet M. *et al.* editors. *Drinking in context: patterns, interventions, and partnerships*. New York (NY) and Abingdon, Oxfordshire: Routledge; 2007.

Stockwell T., Single E., Hawks D. *et al.* Sharpening the focus of alcohol policy from aggregate consumption to harm and risk reduction. *Addiction Research* 1997;**5**:1–9.

Sutton C. Swedish alcohol discourse: constructions of a social problem. *Acta Universitatis Upsaliensis, Studia Sociologica Upsaliensia*. 1998;45.

Teasley D.L. Drug legalization and the 'lessons' of Prohibition. *Contemporary Drug Problems* 1992;**19**:27–52.

Terris M. Epidemiology of cirrhosis of the liver: national mortality data. *American Journal of Public Health* 1967;**57**:2076–88.

Tigerstedt C. Alcohol policy, public health, and Kettil Bruun. *Contemporary Drug Problems* 1999;**26**:209–35.

Tigerstedt C. The European Community and the alcohol policy dimension. *Contemporary Drug Problems* 1990;**17**:461–79.

White O.C., Batia A. *Privatization in Africa*. Washington (DC): World Bank; 1998.

Whitehead P.C. Prevention of alcoholism. In: Robinson D, editor. *Alcohol problems*. New York (NY): Holmes and Meier; 1979.

Wolfgang M.E. *Patterns in criminal homicide*. Philadelphia (PA): University of Pennsylvania Press; 1958.

World Health Organization, Expert Committee on Problems Related to Alcohol Consumption. Problems related to alcohol consumption. Geneva: World Health Organization; 1980. Technical Report Series 650.

World Health Organization, Expert Committee on Problems Related to Alcohol Consumption. Second Report. Geneva: World Health Organization; 2007. Technical Report Series 944. Available from: http://www.who.int/substance_abuse/activities/expert_comm_alcohol_2nd_report.pdf

World Health Organization. *Global status report: alcohol policy*. Geneva: World Health Organization; 2004.

Wyllie A., Zhang J.F., Casswell S. Positive responses to televised beer advertisements associated with drinking and problems reported by 18- to 29-year-olds. *Addiction* 1998a;**93**:749–60.

Wyllie A., Zhang J.F., Casswell S. Responses to televised advertisement associated with drinking behaviour of 10–17-year-olds. *Addiction* 1998b;**93**:361–71.

10.4

Injury prevention and control: The public health approach

Corinne Peek-Asa and Adnan A. Hyder

Abstract

Injuries are among the leading causes of death and disability throughout the world, and injury rates are highest among middle- and low-income countries. Efforts in injury prevention have high potential gain for society because they disproportionately reduce death and disability to the young. Many opportunities to implement injury prevention strategies exist, and a systematic approach to injury prevention can help identify the most effective and efficient approaches. Building capacity for injury prevention activities in low- and middle-income countries is an important public health priority.

Introduction

Injuries are a leading contributor to the disease burden worldwide. They contribute significantly to premature life lost and years lived with disability for all countries, all regions of the world, and all age groups. Injuries cause over 5 million deaths per year, with approximately 1.2 million of these due to road traffic injuries (Krug *et al.* 2000; Peden *et al.* 2002; World Health Organization 2004). For children under 14 years of age, road traffic crashes, drowning, fires, poisoning, interpersonal violence, and war are all in the leading 10 causes of death. Deaths represent just a small proportion of the many injuries that cause serious injury and potentially life-long disability, and injuries also cause significant psychological trauma and financial loss. The burden of traumatic injuries necessitates that injury prevention be considered an international public health priority.

Because the majority of us will suffer multiple minor injuries throughout our lives, most of which cause only minor discomfort or inconvenience, we may be lulled into believing that injuries are just part of life. However, a serious injury or the traumatic death of a loved one can completely change the course of the lives of those affected. Many of these severe and fatal injuries can be prevented, and global investment in traumatic injury prevention will have significant long-term health and financial benefits.

For developed countries, progress has been made in reducing the toll of traumatic injuries. In the United States, for example, road traffic crashes per million vehicle miles travelled decreased nearly 90 per cent from the 1930s into the twenty-first century (Institute of Medicine 1999). Mortality rates have decreased for deaths from drowning, residential fires, homicide, poisoning, among others. However, these rates remain unacceptably high knowing that many effective prevention strategies have not yet been widely implemented.

The burden of traumatic injury worldwide is disproportionately concentrated in lower-income countries (Hofman *et al.* 2005; Ameratunga *et al.* 2006). The World Health Organization (WHO) anticipates that, if current trends continue, road traffic injuries, interpersonal violence, war, and self-inflicted injuries will all be among the leading 15 causes of disability-adjusted life years lost by the year 2020. Road traffic crashes, which in 1990 ranked as the ninth leading cause of disability-adjusted life years lost, is predicted to reach the rank of three in 2020 (Peden *et al.* 2002). Operations of war will rise from the rank of 16 in 1990 to 8 by 2020, and interpersonal violence will rise from rank 19 to 12. Despite some successes in many areas of injury prevention, new risks, changing environments, and increasing population size constantly challenge injury control efforts.

Effective injury prevention strategies will require organization of the public health response and increased integration of professionals from many backgrounds. Modern injury control research combines ideas and skills from public health, biomechanics, engineering, behavioural sciences, law, law enforcement, medicine, and urban planning, among others. Research that identifies how effective interventions in high-income countries can be translated in low- and middle-income settings is a priority, but injury prevention strategies will need to be appropriate for local environments. Injury prevention activities that integrate multiple approaches within an organized public health response have a stronger chance of success.

This chapter will present the current state of knowledge regarding the burden of injuries and will introduce the basic concepts of building injury prevention infrastructure and capacity.

Causal model of injuries

Injuries are generally divided into the two broad categories of intentional and unintentional. Intentional injuries are those in which there was an intent to commit harm, either to oneself or someone else. Unintentional injuries occur without a direct intent to commit harm, even if gross negligence was involved. For example, a motor vehicle occupant death caused by a drunk driver would be considered an unintentional injury even though in many countries the driver could be prosecuted for a crime.

Injuries are further classified by their cause, such as motor vehicle occupant injuries, drowning, suicide/attempted suicide, homicide/assault, or residential fire injuries. Until the late 1990s, cause and intent were coded together, so that, for example, a poisoning death would not be distinguished as intentional or unintentional. In the 1990s, a collaboration between the US Centers for Disease Control and Prevention and the American Public Health Association recommended that cause and intent be considered as separate components of describing an injury, and most data are now coded accordingly (Centers for Disease Control and Prevention 1997). Through this collaboration, a matrix to code injuries by intent and cause using the International Classification of Diseases, 9th revision, was developed. This matrix served as a template to create codes for injury cause and intent that are now included in the 10th revision of this coding system.

Injury causes are very broad and represent a diverse range of physical harm. What, therefore, is the uniting feature that defines an injury? The traditional epidemiologic model for infectious diseases provides a framework for the epidemiologic study of traumatic injury (Fig. 10.4.1). At the centre of the causal pathway for injuries is the agent-host interaction. The agent, which in the case of injuries is energy, is absorbed by the host to cause injury. Energy can take many forms, such as mechanical, electrical, chemical, radiation, and thermal. An example of an agent-host relationship is a motor vehicle crash, in which the energy exerted on the individual is mechanical. The reservoir is the place in the environment where the agent is found. The potential for energy transfer exists everywhere, but its potential to cause injury is limited to specific conditions. For instance, the potential energy in a motor vehicle exists only when the car is being driven, and causes injury only when the vehicle crashes.

Vehicles and vectors are mechanisms which transport energy from the reservoir to the host. A vehicle is an inanimate object, such as a motor vehicle; a vector is animate, such as a dog biting a child. For many injury causes, vehicles and vectors are both involved in energy transfer, such as when one individual (vector) stabs another with a knife (vehicle). The injury outcome is the trauma or injury sustained by the individual, and is influenced by host responses to the energy. Only energy transmitted beyond a host's tolerance causes an injury, and therefore not all exposures to energy result in noticeable injury. A human has some resistance to energy which can be increased through exercise or protective devices, or reduced through changes in intrinsic factors such as existing medical conditions or age and through extrinsic factors such as fatigue and alcohol.

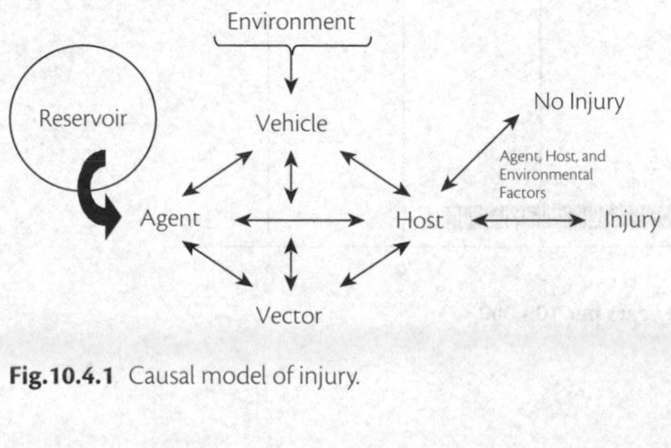

Fig.10.4.1 Causal model of injury.

This causal model is important when considering injury prevention strategies. Injury prevention aims to prevent energy transfer or to reduce the amount of energy that is transferred. Prevention activities can focus on the host, on the environment, on vehicles or vectors, or combine all of these components. A theoretical approach to injury prevention based on this model is presented later in this chapter.

Data sources

Data that describe injury events and that provide information related to injuries can be found from a wide variety of sources, both within and outside of the health sector (Hyder & Morrow 2006). Data sources within the health sector include some that capture a wide range of health conditions, such as health information systems, vital registration systems and hospital discharge data. Other sources are specific to injuries, such as emergency medical services data and trauma registries. Sources outside the health sector cover a wide spectrum, including data from police, the transportation sector, legal records, and insurance company claims. Sources such as newspaper articles and consumer reports have also been used to describe injury incidence and risk. This diversity of data sources makes the field of injuries and violence unique in terms of the inter-sectoral nature of the information (Norton *et al.* 2006).

In many instances, data sources need to be linked together to provide a complete description of the injury. Motor vehicle crash injuries, for example, often require data from traffic enforcement to describe the cause and nature of the crash and data from the health sector to describe the injuries and their severity. Linking these data sources can be impeded by issues of privacy and access to identifying information for linkage, as well as data quality issues. In low- and middle-income countries these data systems, if they exist at all, are often not computerized and have never been evaluated for quality, making such linkages even more challenging. However, information from multiple sources is often necessary to examine causal hypotheses about injuries.

The Global Burden of Disease study attempted to collect consistent and internationally comparable data (Murray & Lopez 1996; WHO 2002). This global data has several limitations in regard to injuries. For example, burn data include deaths from fire-related burns only, and exclude scalds, and drowning deaths exclude drowning deaths due to floods. However, this data is the most comprehensive source for describing the global burden of injuries, especially in relation to other health conditions, and it is thus very useful for public health purposes.

Generally, mortality data has the highest quality, and most high- and middle-income countries have some vital statistics systems that capture the majority of deaths and their causes. Population-based data that describe the causes and types of non-fatal injuries and their outcomes are more challenging to collect and far less available, especially in the developing world. The public health infrastructure and routine collection of health information in the developing world has been fragile, especially in regions such as sub-Saharan Africa and South Asia. It is thus not surprising that there has been little tradition of developing specific information sources for injuries. Population-based studies from low- and middle-income countries, though, consistently conclude that the injury burden is higher than reported in national official statistics and that injuries are significantly underreported in these regions.

One of the important developments over the past decades in the field of health information systems has been the development of summary measures of population health (Hyder & Morrow 2006). The sentinel work of the Ghana Health Assessment Team in the development of the days of life lost indicator evolved into the launch of the disability adjusted life year (DALY) by the World Bank and WHO (WDR 1993; Hyder *et al.* 1998). The DALY combines the loss of healthy life from premature mortality and that lost from life lived with disability in the uni-dimensional measure of time (Murray & Lopez 1996). This allows deaths, morbidity, disability—both fatal and non fatal health outcomes—from a disease to be measured (Fig. 10.4.2). The combination of years of life lost (premature deaths) and years lived with disability in summary measures of population health (like DALY) is important for injuries which cause both types of health outcomes. Technical details of the DALY and other measures are available elsewhere (Murray and Lopez 1996; www.who.int).

Global burden of injury

Over 5 million deaths occur from all injuries worldwide each year (Table 10.4.1), of which nearly 85 per cent are in low–middle income countries (LMIC) (World Health Organization 2002). Nearly 25 per cent of these deaths are caused by road traffic injuries, with self-inflicted injuries and violence comprising a further 17 and 11 per cent of deaths respectively (Fig. 10.4.3). Injury death rates are highest for road traffic injuries, followed by 'other' unintentional injuries, self-inflicted injuries and violence; similar patterns are observed for non-fatal health outcomes using DALY rates (Table 10.4.2).

Road traffic injuries (RTIs) alone kill over 1 million people every year, qualifying these types of injuries as the tenth leading cause of death worldwide (World Health Organization 1999). According to the Global Burden of Disease study, death and disability from road traffic injuries are projected to rise substantially in future years to become the third leading cause of disability-adjusted life years lost worldwide by 2020 (Murray & Lopez 1996). Globally, the majority of those killed are from low- or middle-income countries. The absolute number of fatalities and the mortality rate resulting from road traffic injuries vary considerably across countries, and although all age groups are affected young adults, particularly males, are most at risk of loss of life. Since this age group corresponds to the most economically productive segment of the population, road traffic injuries have serious implications for national economies.

The WHO estimates that there are over 3 million cases of acute poisoning resulting in over 300 000 deaths each year. More males die from poisoning and over 90 per cent of these events occur in LMIC. Non-fatal, unintentional poisoning resulted in a loss of over 7.5 million DALYs globally. Falls cause more than 350 000 deaths worldwide with a mortality rate of 6 per 100 000 globally. They result in more than 15 million DALYs lost per year (2 DALYs per 1000 population)—signifying the important contribution of morbidity and disability from falls. The global burden from falls is also disproportionately high in low- and middle-income countries. Over 300 000 deaths are caused by fire burns resulting in more than 10 million DALYs lost; however, unlike other injuries, more females than males died from fires (male to female ratio of 0.6:1.00). Causing an estimated 400 000 deaths each year, drowning is the second leading cause of unintentional injury death globally, with 97 per cent of these deaths in low- and middle-income countries. (These data include only 'accidental drowning and submersion and exclude drowning due to floods [cataclysms], boating and water transport'.) One-third of drowning occurs in the Western Pacific Region, though Africa has the highest drowning fatality rate. Overall, the male rate of drowning is more than twice that for females.

Self-inflicted injuries, including suicides, attempted suicide, self-destructive behaviours and self-mutilation, cause the deaths of over 850 000 people globally, resulting in more than 20 million DALYs lost. Interpersonal violence disproportionately affects low- and middle-income countries with an estimated rate of 32 per 100 000 people, compared to 14.4 per 100 000 in high-income countries

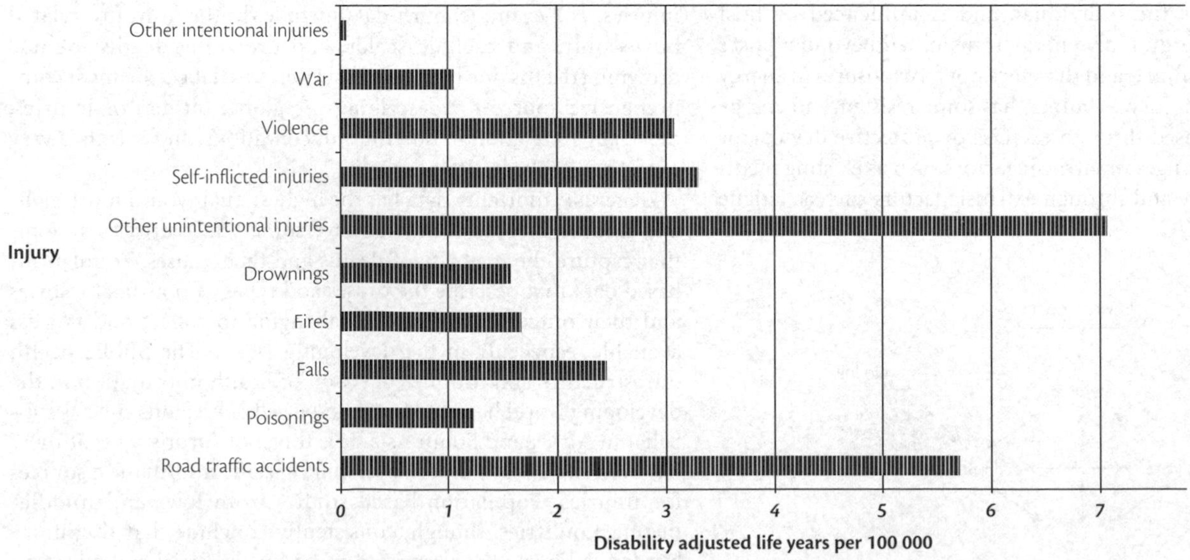

Fig. 10.4.2 Worldwide burden of injury by cause (2001).

Table 10.4.1 Deaths from injuries worldwide, 2001

	Total	Males	Females
All injuries	5 185 745	3 482 854	1 702 891
Unintentional injuries	3 534 562	2 296 318	1 238 244
Road traffic accidents	1 189 417	866 871	322 547
Poisonings	349 460	225 797	123 664
Falls	387 477	233 661	153 816
Fires	309 740	118 583	191 157
Drowning	384 666	263 145	121 521
Other unintentional injuries	913 802	588 262	325 539
Intentional injuries	1 651 183	1 186 536	464 647
Self-inflicted injuries	874 533	547 017	327 516
Violence	556 272	442 137	114 136
War	207 589	187 128	20 461
Other intentional injuries	12 788	10 253	2 534

(Krug *et al.* 2002). Surveys indicate that up to 8 per cent of women (over 16 years) report experiencing sexual violence within the past 5 years, while up to 27 per cent report experiencing sexual violence from an intimate partner in the past year (Krug *et al.* 2002). An estimated 200 000 youth homicides are committed globally varying from 1 in high-income countries to 36 per 100 000 in Latin America. It is estimated that for every youth homicide, there are up to 40 victims of non-fatal youth violence receiving hospital treatment (Krug *et al.* 2002).

Surprisingly, the burden of homicide is found in children under 5 years of age as well; the rate of homicides are 2.2 per 100 000 for boys and 1.8 per 100 000 for girls in high-, and 6.1 and 5.1 per 100 000 for boys and girls, respectively, in low-income countries (Krug *et al.* 2002). Abuse of the elderly occurs in the home and institutions and there is a lack of global data on this issue; however,

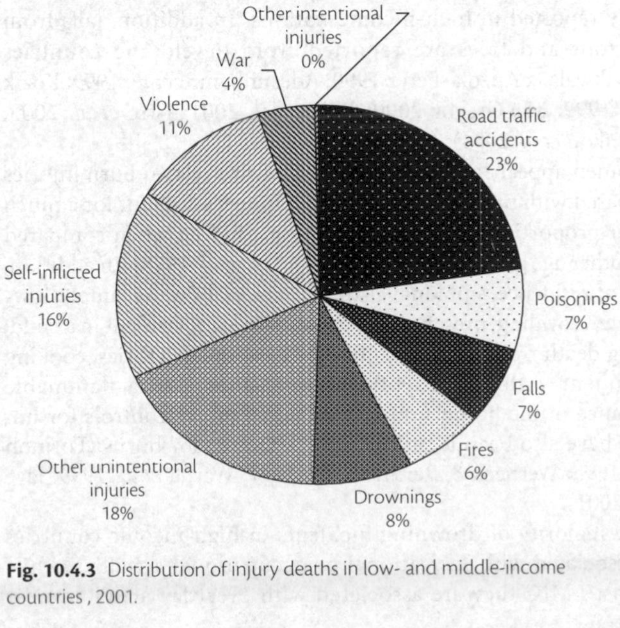

Fig. 10.4.3 Distribution of injury deaths in low- and middle-income countries, 2001.

surveys in the developed world indicate a prevalence of 4–6 per cent of abuse of older persons (Krug *et al.* 2002). War is also an important form of collective violence and was estimated by WHO to cause more than 200 000 direct deaths worldwide in 2001.

Disparity in injury morbidity and mortality

South Africa reported drowning as the 2nd leading cause of injury mortality for children less than 15 years (Kibel *et al.* 1990) and demonstrated an increasing trend in drowning deaths for all ethnic groups in the 1980s and 1990s (Cywes *et al.* 1990; Kibel *et al.* 1990). A review of more than 300 paediatric deaths (0–14 years) in the United Arab Emirates revealed that drowning was the 2nd leading cause of death for both genders (Bener *et al.* 1998). Drowning is also the second leading cause of death for the 10–19 year age group in Taiwan; while it remains the number one cause for males aged 10–14 years (Lu *et al.* 1998). China and India—the world's most populous nations—contribute 43 per cent of the world drowning deaths and 41 per cent of the total DALYS attributed to drowning globally (World Health Organization 2003).

Recent work from South Asia explores police data in Pakistan, and provides a unique picture of trends in suicides over 15 years (1985–1999). During this period, there were 2568 reported suicides, 71 per cent in men and 39 per cent in women. While firearms are the leading method of suicide in the United States, in Pakistan, the leading method was organophosphates followed by hanging (Khan & Hyder 2006).

The true extent of intimate partner violence is largely unknown but surveys in Paraguay and the Philippines reveal that 10 per cent of women surveyed reported being assaulted by an intimate partner compared to 22 per cent in the United States, 29 per cent in Canada, and 34 per cent in Egypt (Krug *et al.* 2002). Other studies show that 3 per cent of women in Australia, the United States and Canada had been assaulted by a partner in the previous 12 months, compared to 27 per cent in Nicaragua, 38 per cent in South Korea, and 53 per cent in West Bank and Gaza (Krug *et al.* 2002). Country comparisons are difficult because data is sparse and because of varying definitions of what constitutes abuse. Furthermore, cultural norms may lead to very different reporting tendencies. Women in countries who have conducted programmes to screen and respond to intimate partner violence, including victim's assistance programmes and social marketing campaigns against intimate partner violence, may be less inhibited to divulge their experiences with violence.

Economic and societal burden

The average annual cost of road crashes has been estimated at about 1 per cent of the gross national product in developing countries, 1.5 per cent in countries in economic transition, and 2 per cent in highly motorized countries. The annual economic cost of road traffic injuries globally is about US$518 billion. In low- and middle-income countries, the annual cost of road traffic crashes is about US$65 billion, exceeding the total annual amount received by these countries in development assistance (Jacobs 2000). Studies exploring the economic and social costs of road traffic injuries in low-income countries show that males who provided the majority of the household income in India and Bangladesh were the most common victims of road traffic fatalities; and the consequences included reduced household income and reduced food consumption for the victim's family

Table 10.4.2 The Haddon matrix for motor vehicle safety (illustrative)

Phases	Factors			
	Human	**Vehicle**	**Physical environment**	**Sociocultural environment**
Pre-injury	Reduce alcohol intoxication, programmes to increase defensive driving and decrease road rage	Increase vehicle stability, increased visibility	Improvements in road structure and traffic controls, traffic calming measures	Support safety programmes and increase consumer awareness of safety issues
Injury	Use of seat belts and car seats, proper placement of car seats, booster seats	Increase energy absorbed by the vehicle frame, safety features such as air bags, head rests, shatterproof windshields, and collapsible steering columns	Install energy-absorbing guard rails	Programmes to provide car seats, educational programmes about car seat installation and placement
Post-injury	Stabilize serious injuries, reduce bleeding and other complications	Design for easier extrication	Enhanced emergency medical systems and field care	Support infrastructure of trauma care, including 911 system, emergency and trauma care, and rehabilitation services

(Aeron-Thomas *et al.* 2004). In addition, the poor were found to spend a much greater proportion of their income on funeral and/or medical costs than the non-poor (Aeron-Thomas *et al.* 2004).

Estimates of the cost of violence the United States reach over 3 per cent of the gross domestic product. In England and Wales, the total costs from violence amount to an estimated US$40 billion annually. The economic effects of interpersonal violence are expected to be more severe in poorer countries, and yet, there is a scarcity of studies on the costs of violence in low- and middle-income countries (Waters *et al.* 2004). However, estimates from low- and middle-income countries indicate that the overall costs of violence are substantial, ranging up to 25 per cent of annual gross domestic product. Comparisons with high-income countries are complicated by the fact that economic losses related to productivity tend to be undervalued in lower-income countries. Child abuse results in US$94 billion in annual costs to the US economy (1 per cent of GDP) and intimate partner violence costs the US economy nearly US$13 billion (0.1 per cent of GDP); this can be compared to 1.6 per cent of GDP in Nicaragua and 2 per cent of GDP in Chile. The cost of gun violence also has been calculated at US$155 billion annually in the United States.

Risk factors for injuries

Motorization rates rise with income (Kopits & Cropper 2003), and in a growing number of LMIC where economies are experiencing growth, there has been a corresponding increase in the numbers of motor vehicles (Ghaffar *et al.* 1999). Data obtained from routinely collected police reports in a number of LMIC show that speed is a leading causal factor in road traffic crashes (Afukaar 2003; Odero 2003; Wang *et al.* 2003), accounting for up to 50 per cent of all crashes. Alcohol is associated with an increased risk of road crashes (Peden *et al.* 2004) and in studies conducted in LMIC alcohol has been shown to be present in up to 69 per cent of fatally-injured drivers (Odero & Zwi 1995). A study from China showed a two-fold increased risk of car crash associated with driver chronic sleepiness (Liu *et al.* 2003); while surveys of commercial road transport in African countries have shown that drivers often work unduly long hours and go to work when exhausted (Mock *et al.* 1999; Nafukho & Khayesi 2002). A significant risk factor for increased injury severity is non-use or inappropriate use of safety devices such as motorcycle helmets (Kulanthayan *et al.* 2000; Liu *et al.* 2004), and seat belts (Peden *et al.* 2004).

Risk factors for falls in older people include: Low bone density; poor nutritional status; low body mass index; low calcium intake; co-morbid conditions (hypertension, diabetes); poor performance in activities of daily living; poor cognitive function; poor vision; environmental factors affecting balance; family history of hip fracture; and alcohol consumption (Cummings *et al.* 1995; Dargent-Molina *et al.* 1996; Clark *et al.* 1998; Boonyaratavej *et al.* 2001). A study in Thailand suggested that features associated with poor socioeconomic status may also be risk factors, for example, lack of electricity in the house and living in Thai huts (Jitapunkul *et al.* 2001). In younger ages, falls from balconies, apartment windows, beds, nursery equipment, and playground equipment are commonly reported in high-income nations. In addition, falls from roof tops and trees are reported from developing countries (Bangdiwala & Anzola-Perez 1990; Adesunkanmi *et al.* 1999; Kozik *et al.* 1999; MacGregor 2000; Raja *et al.* 2001; Istre *et al.* 2003; Dedoukou *et al.* 2004).

Women appear to be at greater risk of fire-related burn injuries compared with men, and burn-related injuries account for a much higher proportion of injuries in young children when compared with other age groups (Jie & Ren 1992; Liu *et al.* 1998). In addition, place of residence, smoking, alcohol use, lack of water supply, low-income, crowding, presence of a pre-existing impairment in a child, sibling death from a burn, clothing of manmade fabrics, cooking equipment within reach of children, storage of a flammable substance in the home, and lack of temperature controls for hot water have also been identified as risk factors for burns (Forjuoh *et al.* 1995; Werneck & Reichenheim 1997; Warda *et al.* 1999; Jaye *et al.* 2001).

The majority of drowning incidents in high-income countries are associated with recreational or occupational activities, while in most LMIC they are associated with everyday activities near natural bodies of water (Celis 1997; Kobusingye *et al.* 2001; Brenner 2003; Hyder *et al.* 2003). Children aged 1–4 years, males, those living in rural areas, alcohol use, number of children in the family, presence of a well in the home, and lack of child supervision are additional risk factors for drowning (Kibel *et al.* 1990; Celis 1997; Ahmed *et al.* 1999; Kozik *et al.* 1999; Carlini-Cotrim & da Matta Chasin 2000; Kobusingye *et al.* 2001; Brenner 2003; Driscoll *et al.* 2004). Several studies have shown that young age, residential mobility, limited adult supervision of children, previous poisoning, the use of non-standard containers for storage (e.g. Coca-Cola bottles); and the storage of poisons at ground level are risk factors for childhood poisoning (Azizi *et al.* 1993; Chatsantiprapa *et al.* 2001; Soori 2001). Access to prescription drugs is also a frequent cause of poisoning.

A number of factors have been associated with an increased risk of suicide. Depression, schizophrenia, anxiety disorders and alcohol and drug abuse play a significant role in increasing risk (Krug *et al.* 2002). In addition, a previous suicidal attempt, family history of suicide, painful current illness, personal loss, interpersonal conflict, social isolation, place of residence (rural), unemployment, immigration status, religious affiliation, and poor economic conditions have been shown to pose a higher risk for suicide (Krug *et al.* 2002; Khan & Hyder 2006). Risk factors for violence, in general, have been identified in various studies including being male and young, abuse of alcohol and drugs, being a victim of child abuse, low socio-economic status, marital discord, parental conflict, and low access to medical care (Krug *et al.* 2002). In addition, macro-risk factors for violence in the literature include rapid social change, economic inequality, poverty, weak economic safety nets, corruption, gender inequalities, and high firearm availability. Previous victimization, having many sexual partners, and involvement in sex work have also been shown to be associated with increased levels of sexual violence in particular.

Theoretical basis for injury prevention

The causal model for injuries allows the injury process to be categorized into distinct phases which are important for prevention (Haddon 1970, 1972). The *pre-injury* phase is the period prior to the energy transfer, the *injury* phase is the often millisecond period in which the energy is transferred to the host, and the *post-injury* phase is the period of recovery and rehabilitation. Prevention approaches affect the injury process in one of these three injury phases.

Primary injury prevention includes prevention strategies that aim to prevent the transfer of injury to the host, and thus act in the pre-injury phase. Examples of successful primary prevention strategies include roadway designs that reduce motor vehicle collisions (Graham 1993), child-resistant caps on medication bottles to prevent ingestion and poisoning (Poison Prevention Technical Advisory Committee 1971), and pool fences to prevent submersion and drowning (Thompson & Rivara 2007).

Secondary injury prevention includes strategies that reduce the amount of energy that is transferred to the host. While these strategies are often put in place long before the injury event, their function acts to reduce energy transferred during the injury phase. Examples of secondary prevention strategies include seat belts and air bags (Evans 1995), motorcycle and bicycle helmets (US General Accounting Office 1991; Thomas *et al.* 1994). Seat belts and helmets do not prevent the crash itself, but they reduce the amount of energy transmitted to the host during the crash. Secondary prevention strategies might not prevent injury completely. For example, lower extremity injuries are not prevented by either seat belts or helmets. However, studies have consistently shown that when these devices are present, the risk for mortal injury is much less and injury severity is reduced.

Tertiary prevention strategies act in the post-injury phase to help with recovery and rehabilitation once an injury has occurred. One example is the development of trauma systems, which help with triage and transport of an injured individual to reduce the time between injury and definitive medical care (Mann *et al.* 1999; Nathens *et al.* 2000). Optimizing resources to enable recovery and rehabilitation does not prevent the injury or reduce the amount of energy transfer, but tertiary prevention strategies can have enormous impact on improving survival, function and quality of life following an injury.

The Haddon Matrix is a framework that combines these injury phases with the major components of the injury causal model to help identify prevention approaches (Fig. 10.4.1). This matrix, developed by Dr. William Haddon in the United States, was the foundation for the study of motor vehicle crashes and countermeasures for highway safety and continues to be an applicable theoretical framework for injury prevention (Haddon 1972). Using the three injury phases, Haddon categorized prevention approaches into those that affect the host, vehicles and vectors, the physical environment, and the socio-cultural environment. An example of the Haddon Matrix with examples from motor vehicle occupant protection is included in Table 10.4.2.

The Haddon Matrix provides a framework for identifying individual approaches to injury prevention. However, one single intervention strategy is unlikely to be highly effective. Multiple collaborative approaches need to be combined to maximize success. For example, the success of seat belt use in reducing motor vehicle occupant fatalities in the United States required a combination of engineering, education, policy, and enforcement that led to the current use rate of 80 per cent (National Highway Traffic Safety Administration 2007). Although seat belts were developed and available from the early 1900s, they were not required to be a standard feature on passenger cars in the United States until 1968. The steps to getting seat belts installed as a regular feature in passenger cars required considerable advocacy and policy initiatives. However, once the seat belts were installed, use rates without any occupant incentive or education were about 11 per cent. Efforts in the areas of legislation, enforcement, and public education were necessary to achieve the high use rates currently observed. Stricter legislation, for example, is associated with higher use, as evidenced by the higher use rates consistently observed among states with primary (not wearing a seat belt is by itself a citable offence) compared with secondary (not wearing a seat belt can be cited only along with another citation) laws in the United States (National Highway Traffic Safety Administration 2007).

Successful injury prevention strategies

It cannot be emphasized strongly enough that success in reducing injuries will depend on multi-faceted and comprehensive efforts. As demonstrated through the Haddon Matrix, injuries occur as a complex interplay between individuals and their physical and socio-cultural environments. Injury rates have very clear patterns within both individuals and geographic areas. Understanding these patterns within the context of the environment is essential to reducing the global burden of injuries. Below are some examples of successful injury prevention efforts.

Trends in road traffic injuries throughout the world provide a case study of how an integrated approach can lead to successful prevention. Over the last several decades, developed countries have experienced decreases in motor vehicle occupant death rates, even while the total miles driven, and thus exposure to the roadway, have dramatically increased. In contrast, developing countries have experienced large increases in the rate of road traffic fatality rates. For example, developed countries experienced a cumulative decrease in the number of road traffic fatalities of nearly 40 per cent between 1968 and 1985, while Asian countries experienced an increase of over 150 per cent and African countries an increase of over 300 per cent (Transport and Road Research Laboratory 1991; WHO 2004). Nearly 90 per cent of road traffic deaths now occur in low- or middle-income countries (WHO 2004).

The main reason for success in developed countries has been a comprehensive approach to intervention which has included environmental, engineering, legislative, and educational approaches. In the United States, The National Highway Traffic Safety Administration and the Federal Highway Safety Administration estimate that 243 000 lives were saved between 1966 and 1990 as a result of highway, traffic, and motor vehicle safety programmes (Institute of Medicine 1999). Road modifications mandated by the Federal Highway Traffic Safety Act of 1966 led to a shift from two-lane rural roads to interstate freeways. Although vehicle volume and speed are highest on interstate highways, the number of crashes per mile travelled on interstate highways is the lowest of all roadway types. Safety features built into interstate roads are numerous, and include: Divided highways that separate traffic flow in different directions, avoiding lane crossings and decreasing the risk for head-on crashes; graded curves; crash-absorbing barriers that reduce the risk of cars running off the road, especially in areas where roadside hazards exist; skid-resistant surfaces that reduce loss of traction while braking; and, lighted signage to increase visibility and reduce distraction (Graham 1993).

At the same time, changes to the motor vehicle itself increased the likelihood of survival in a crash. In addition to the implementation of seat belts and then air bags, legislation required modifications that improved vehicle crash worthiness. Some examples of these modifications include shatter-resistant windshields, collapsible steering columns, crash-friendly dashboard surfaces, frames that are resistant to passenger space intrusion, increased strength of the vehicle frame, seat, and doors, lap and shoulder belts, and airbags (Haddon & Baker 1981). Studies have found that these safety improvements to the motor vehicle led to a 24–40 per cent decrease in fatal crashes and saved over 9000 lives each year (Robertson 1981; Institute of Medicine 1999).

Most of these changes were due in part to legislative efforts, and these efforts were themselves collaborative in nature. For example, the successful modification of the roadway and vehicle environments was facilitated by the establishment of the National Highway Traffic Safety Administration (NHTSA) through the Federal Highway Act of 1966. NHTSA was established as the lead United States federal agency to identify and respond to road traffic hazards, and its establishment was due largely to advocacy efforts that educated the general public and legislators about the scope and potential to prevent roadway fatalities.

Additional legislative approaches that have contributed to motor vehicle occupant safety include laws to require seat belt use, driver training, speed limits, and laws that aim to reduce drunk driving. These laws were all introduced because of successful education of legislators. However, their effectiveness varies dramatically. For example, most countries have laws against drinking and driving, yet countries have wide variation in the rate of alcohol-involved crashes as well as the number of drinking drivers, drivers cited for drinking and driving, and punished for drinking and driving. While this variation has much to do with factors associated with patterns of alcohol consumption, access to transportation, and the driving culture, this variation is also due to factors associated with the laws themselves. The effectiveness of legislative approaches depends on the level of enforcement that accompanies them and on the perception that the legislated consequences will actually occur (Mann *et al.* 2003). The effectiveness of drinking and driving laws is influenced by the level of enforcement, the ability of courts to impose penalties, and that the nature of the penalties serves as a deterrent.

Historically, many developed countries have focused much of their efforts on protecting vehicle occupants, and these efforts have shown many successes. However, the focus on motor vehicle occupants without concomitant integration of urban planning, sustainable transportation, and pedestrian and bicycle safety may be problematic in the long run. More recently, countries throughout Europe as well as Australia and the United States have introduced an approach called 'traffic calming' that aims to control motor vehicle traffic and speed in neighbourhoods, and thus increase safety and walkability in communities (Ewing 1999; Richter *et al.* 2006). The concept of traffic calming dates back to the Dutch city of Delft in the 1960s, when residents angry with fast-moving cars cutting through their local streets blocked them with gardens, social areas, and play grounds (Ewing 1999). Modern traffic calming involves a variety of approaches to reduce traffic volume and speed in residential areas using visually appealing strategies.

Success in reducing road traffic deaths has depended on the development of an infrastructure that can identify and respond to road hazards, and a wide variety of approaches to address these hazards. In some developed and many developing countries, the car culture is growing without concomitant safety efforts (Bishai *et al.* 2003). Highway design standards are often outdated or translated too directly from an industrialized country, and insufficient resources for roadway maintenance are available (Transport and Road Research Laboratory 1991). Poorly designed and maintained roadways are even further stressed by an ever-increased number and variety of vehicles. In addition to a growing number of passenger cars and a high proportion of commercial vehicles and buses, developing countries' roadways include animal-powered vehicles, small engine vehicles (such as scooters and motorcycles) that carry multiple people, bicycles, human-powered transport vehicles (such as a rickshaw), and pedestrians. This complex mix of vehicles contributes to increased deaths on the road.

In order to avert the growing toll of road traffic deaths, the WHO has called for a 'systems approach' in which the interaction between vehicles, roads, road users and their physical, social, and economic environments form the basis for a multi-sectoral response (WHO 2004).

Road traffic crashes provide one example of the potential for injury prevention success, the necessity for an integrated approach, and the need for building capacity for injury prevention. Throughout the world, general capacity for conducted injury prevention activities is limited. Growing awareness of the burden of traumatic injury coupled with a growing evidence base of successful injury prevention approaches bode well for increasing injury prevention activities in many countries.

Resources to identify successful injury prevention programmes

In addition to information to measure the scope, burden, and cost of injuries, several good resources are available to identify evidence-based injury prevention approaches. Two international collaborative efforts provide structured and systematic reviews of existing literature.

The Cochrane Collaboration provides scientific evidence-based reviews of health care interventions through the Cochrane Library (Bero & Rennie 1995; Alderson *et al.* 2004). The library has more than 100 reviews on the prevention, treatment, and rehabilitation of traumatic injuries, including topics such as fall-related injuries to older persons, pool fencing to prevent drowning in children, and interventions for promoting smoke alarm ownership and function. Abstracts are available free of charge (http://www.cochrane.org/reviews/index.htm) and full reviews are available by subscription, with most major libraries holding subscriptions. Cochrane reviews are highly weighted towards evidence from randomized controlled trials, which excludes many of the observational evaluations conducted for injury interventions. The search strategy protocol requires inclusion of international findings as well as unpublished data, and when sufficient data are present meta-analyses are conducted. Thus, these reviews are meant to be applicable to an international audience.

The Campbell Collaboration, begun in 1999, includes systematic reviews of social service programmes, divided into the categories of education, crime and justice, and social welfare (Davies & Boruch 2001). The goal of the collaboration is to provide evidence for policy decisions regarding social issues. While the majority of injury prevention-related reviews are found within the crime and justice reviews, many reviews in the other categories are strongly related to injury and violence prevention. The Campbell Collaboration includes evidence from all types of study designs, and has methods groups to ensure systematic interpretation of findings. Methods groups include experimental methods, quasi-experimental methods, and process and quantitative methods. Campbell reviews can be accessed free of charge (http://www.campbellcollaboration.org/frontend.asp).

Another source of recommendations for injury prevention strategies is *The Guide to Community Preventive Services: Systematic Reviews and Evidence–Based Recommendations* (the *Guide*). This system was developed by the Task Force on Community Preventive Services, established by the United States Centers for Disease Control and Prevention (Pappaioanou & Evans 1998). The *Guide's* recommendations are primarily based on evidence of effectiveness, including the suitability of the study design, but they also assess the applicability of the intervention to other populations or settings, the economic impact, barriers observed in implementing the interventions, and if the intervention had other beneficial or harmful effects (Briss *et al.* 2000). The *Guide* then provides a recommendation as to whether the approach is 'strongly recommended', 'recommended', has 'insufficient evidence' or is 'discouraged'. The Guide has injury-related reviews in the categories of alcohol, motor vehicle, physical activity, substance abuse, worksite, mental health, social environment, and violence. Reviews are available free of charge at http://www.thecommunityguide.org/default.htm.

In addition there are more global sources of information that provide help and guidance on a variety of injury issues. The Department of Violence and Injuries Prevention of the WHO (www.who.int) offers a diversity of guidelines and manuals that provide assistance in implementing programmes or conducting research. Examples include guidelines for establishing injury surveillance systems, conducting community based surveys and evaluating pre-hospital care. International non-governmental organizations also offer a variety of assistance and expert members on specific issues. Examples include the International Society for Child and Adolescent Injury Prevention (www.iscaip.net), the Road Traffic Injuries Research Network (www.rtirn.net), and the International Society for Violence and Injury Prevention (www.isvip.org).

Another source of recent estimates of the burden of injuries and cost-effectiveness of interventions is the Disease Control Priorities for Developing Countries Project (www.dcp2.org). This project worked on both intentional and unintentional injuries as well as emergency care to present a consistent set of estimates for the global burden of injuries and their impact in low- and middle-income countries. In addition, using a consistent set of guidelines, the project worked out the cost-effectiveness of interventions to reduce the burden of injuries across the world.

Building capacity for injury prevention

In order to implement the comprehensive strategies for injury prevention that are most effective, countries, states, and local communities need to develop the infrastructure and capacity to conduct the essential activities needed for an injury prevention programme. Infrastructure includes the identification of agencies to oversee essential injury control activities and the integration of these activities. Capacity includes the availability of human, financial, relational, and structural resources.

Most important of these is the development of a critical mass of trained injury professionals in a country to understand the local environment, develop, implement, and evaluate prevention programmes. Because there is a lack of trained injury prevention professionals in low- and middle-income countries, capacity development should focus on the developing world. In order to facilitate training of injury prevention professionals, the WHO developed a training programme called Teach Violence and Injury Prevention—TeachVIP (http://www.who.int/violence_injury_prevention/capacitybuilding/teachvip/en/print.html)This programme provides teaching materials to introduce the major topics of the field of injury and violence prevention, and is an important tool for trainers. The WHO has also identified priorities for global reduction in the two leading causes of injury death: Motor vehicle injuries and violence. These priorities are listed in Box 10.4.1. Capacity-building efforts are best organized around the public health framework of surveillance, prevention/evaluation, and treatment.

Box 10.4.1 WHO's priorities for the future of injury prevention

Continued success in the prevention and control of injuries will depend on systematic and organized efforts. Worldwide, much progress has been made, and it is important to find efficient methods to share and adapt successful approaches. The World Health Organization has developed reports on two of the leading causes of injury mortality and morbidity: Road traffic injuries and violence. Below, the priorities that were identified in these reports are summarized.

Priorities from the World Report on Road Traffic Injury Prevention:[a]

1. Identify a lead agency in government to guide national road traffic safety efforts
2. Assess the problems, policies, institutional settings and capacity relating to road traffic injury
3. Prepare a national road traffic safety strategy and plan for action
4. Allocate financial and human resources to address the problem
5. Implement specific actions to prevent road traffic crashes, minimize injuries and their consequences, and evaluate these efforts
6. Support the development of national capacity and international collaboration

Priorities from the World Report on Violence and Health:[b]

1. Create, implement, and monitor a national action plan for violence prevention
2. Enhance capacity for collection of data on violence
3. Define priorities for, and support research on, the causes, consequences, costs and prevention of violence
4. Promote primary prevention responses
5. Strengthen responses for victims of violence
6. Integrate violence prevention into social and educational policies, and thereby promote gender and social equality
7. Increase collaboration and exchange of information on violence prevention
8. Promote and monitor adherence to international treaties, laws, and other mechanisms to protect human rights
9. Seek practical, internationally agreed responses to the global drug trade and the global arms trade

Sources:

[a] World Health Organization. *World Report on Road Traffic Injury Prevention.* (http://www.who.int/violence_injury_prevention/publications/road_traffic/world_report/en/index.html)

[b] World Health Organization. *World Report on Violence and Health.* (http://www.who.int/violence_injury_prevention/violence/world_report/en/index.html)

Surveillance

One of the most important priorities for injury prevention worldwide is the development of dependable local injury surveillance systems. These systems are necessary to identify and explain the nature of the injury problem, and also to track changes over time as interventions are implemented and new risks emerge. Surveillance efforts need to focus on two priorities: Enhanced data quality and the establishment of registry systems to track injury trends.

Several efforts to collect international injury mortality data have found that differences in death certification systems, methods of data collection, and definitions of variables severely challenge international comparisons (Krug *et al.* 2000; Fingerhut 2004; Hofman *et al.* 2005; Polinder *et al.* 2007). As mentioned in the previous section on data sources, many countries have an insufficient infrastructure to accurately enumerate and code traumatic injury deaths. The International Collaborative Effort on Injury Statistics, undertaken by the US National Center for Health Statistics as a multi-country exercise, was the first effort to compare international mortality rates (Fingerhut 2004). This collaboration has undertaken several projects to improve data compatibility between countries, such as the Barell injury diagnosis matrix that provides guidance for coding injury diagnoses by body region and nature of injury. Other efforts have been undertaken by the WHO and the European Union, among others (Krug *et al.* 2000; Polinder *et al.* 2007). These efforts consistently identify data quality as a major impediment.

The burden of traumatic injury is disproportionately born by low- and middle-income countries, and these countries are also the least likely to have established surveillance systems to monitor injury trends (Hofman *et al.* 2005). Surveillance systems are needed to identify and track trends in injuries for research and prevention efforts, and are also necessary to attract the attention of policymakers and community leaders. Data registries need to be developed using methods that are not highly resource-intensive, such as adding injuries to existing medical reporting systems for conditions such as infectious diseases. In order to be effective, minimum data elements with standard definitions need to be employed. If possible, surveillance should be developed to provide some benefit to the agencies responsible for collecting the data. One method of accomplishing this is to integrate measurable quality indicators into the data collection so that agencies can use the data systems to monitor their own performance.

Investment in data infrastructures will be critical to the long-term sustainability of injury prevention efforts. Data will be necessary to monitor changes over time, to evaluate new efforts, and to continue to engage new partners in injury control efforts. Guidelines for injury surveillance and surveys have been released by the WHO (www.who.int).

Prevention and evaluation

Effective and cost-beneficial injury prevention programmes are needed worldwide. In developed countries, a growing number of programmes are emerging, but far too many are not evaluated. Among approaches that are evaluated and found to be effective and adaptable to wider populations, few are the subject of wide-spread dissemination.

The wide-spread dissemination of injury prevention programmes takes concerted effort. For example, smoke alarms have been shown to reduce the risk of dying in a house fire by half (Hall 1994). When smoke alarms were first introduced, few homes had them, and currently, the majority of homes do not install them effectively (Harvey *et al.* 1998; Peek-Asa *et al.* 2005). In order to increase the number of homes with operational smoke alarms, several agencies in the United States, such as the National Fire Protection Agency and the Centers for Disease Control and Prevention, initiated national campaigns to educate consumers about smoke alarms, to change building codes to require smoke alarms, and to engage public health agencies in the dissemination and installation of alarms (Ballesteros *et al.* 2005). These efforts appear to be effective, and currently, nearly 90 per cent of US homes have at least one operational smoke alarm (Harvey *et al.* 1998).

Although a number of successful strategies for injury prevention have been identified, these have primarily been developed in high-income countries. Existing strategies will have varying success in different environments. For example, random breath alcohol screening for drivers has been an effective policy/enforcement method to reduce drinking and driving in Australia, especially when combined with social marketing campaigns raising awareness of the risks of drinking and driving, and bringing attention to the likelihood and penalties of being caught. However, random driver screening is not adaptable to the United States because law enforcement lacks the authority to randomly stop drivers without cause (Peek-Asa *et al.* 1999). Policy efforts need to work within the authorities of the local agencies as well as the local economic, political, and cultural environments. Without an understanding of the local environment, it is unlikely that translation of existing strategies will be effective.

Thus, injury prevention efforts can occur at multiple levels (national, regional, and local), but are most effective when integrated within the local environments. When developing a new approach to an injury problem, it is important to identify the scope of the problem, the populations that are at highest risk, the causal mechanisms of the injury, and the environment in which the injuries occur. For example, one could propose to address a high incidence of dog bites to children through an educational campaign focused on dog owners and veterinarians. However, if most of the bites are caused by feral dogs that have no owner and are unlikely to see a veterinarian, this educational campaign is unlikely to make any difference.

Priority should be placed on adapting proven interventions from high-income countries to low- and middle-income countries (Peden *et al.* 2004). Growing evidence supports this approach. Data from a controlled study undertaken in South Africa has shown that the free distribution of child resistant containers appears to be a highly effective means of preventing poisoning in children (Krug *et al.* 1994). Increased supervision of children around bodies of water, and use of barriers have also been proposed as measures that might reduce drowning in developing countries (Hyder *et al.* 2003).

There are many factors to consider when either developing a new strategy or adapting an existing strategy to a new community. Some of these factors are obvious, such as the cost of the programme, the existence of an agency or group of individuals to conduct the work, and good evidence that the strategy is effective when implemented correctly. Other considerations are equally important but less obvious. These include issues such as acceptance of the strategy by the community, equity or perceived equity, and the potential to stigmatize the affected community (Runyan 1998).

An international panel assembled by the Fogarty Center of the US National Institutes of Health recognized that, in addition to lack of data, the trained workforce to develop injury prevention programmes was lacking in most low- and middle-income countries (Hofman *et al.* 2005). In particular, the proportion of the trained public health workforce that focuses on injury prevention and safety issues is relatively small when compared to health conditions of equal magnitude. And, ironically, many health care professionals cannot mobilize to conduct prevention activities because they are overwhelmed in treating the injuries and illnesses of the individuals who are in need of the prevention services. In addition to a paucity of trained injury prevention professionals, funding to conduct injury prevention activities is scarce, if existent at all. Although resources are scarce, the potential of pooling resources among multiple agencies offers promise. Building sufficient infrastructure to bring the necessary stakeholders together will help identify better uses of existing resources, while also increasing the number of individuals who can move programmes forward. This, in turn, will help leverage increased resources to sustain efforts that can be proven effective.

Treatment

Many injuries lead to death because of inadequate emergency and trauma care, although an organized trauma response system can dramatically reduce deaths from injuries (Mann *et al.* 1999; Hofman *et al.* 2005). For example, one study reported up to 58 per cent pre-hospital mortality for intentional injuries in Pakistan (Chotani 2002), while in a comparative study trauma mortality was 65 per cent in resource poor settings compared with 55 per cent and 35 per cent in moderate and good resource settings (Mock 1998).

However, many countries lack trained medical personnel, equipment, and infrastructure (Kobusingye 2005). An evaluation of trauma care capabilities in Mexico, Vietnam, India, and Ghana indicated that even when a sufficient number of health care professionals were trained, 'brain drain' from rural to urban and from low- to higher-income communities led to widespread provider shortages (Mock *et al.* 2006). In order to develop a stronger trauma response system, improvements must be made in the areas of increased human resources, physical resources, security for health care personnel, transportation systems to get patients to definitive treatment, and administrative infrastructure (Kobusingye 2005; Mock *et al.* 2006).

Although many of these improvements require new resources, system-wide changes are possible through effective planning even in the absence of significantly increased resources. For example, several low-cost trauma training programmes have been developed and used effectively in low-income countries, and these have contributed to decreased injury mortality (Kobusingye 2005). Administrative changes, such as making necessary diagnostic equipment available for critical trauma cases, are also low-cost. However, identifying and implementing low-cost strategies cycles back to the need for data. Finding the low-cost strategies that will work in a health care facility will be enhanced by data systems that can track trends in patient treatment and be used for quality assurance. These systems are lacking in many health care organizations throughout the world.

Improving emergency medical systems and trauma treatment capacity could greatly reduce injury mortality worldwide, and also reduce the physical, emotional, and financial consequences of severe injuries. These efforts need to be in collaboration with general worldwide efforts to improve access to public health and medical services. Over the past few years, WHO has released guidelines for pre-hospital and trauma care with a special focus on low- and middle-income countries (www.who.int). In addition, an evaluation of interventions for emergency care has been evaluated and checklists developed to identify potentially useful approaches in the developing world (Kobusingye *et al.* 2006).

Necessary elements to sustainable injury programmes

Resources are the biggest challenge to implementing needed surveillance, prevention, and treatment components; although these needed resources come in a variety of forms. A review of the Swedish Safe Communities programme concluded that no single type of resource or programme component is sufficient to sustain injury prevention efforts (Nilsen *et al.* 2005). The Swedish Safe Communities model, adopted in many variations throughout the world, encourages communities to establish grassroots efforts to address local safety and injury prevention issues. Each local community identifies its own priorities, methods to address the priorities, and methods to integrate with regional and national safety efforts. The evaluation identified financial resources as necessary but not sufficient for sustainability, and, furthermore, that reliance on several key individuals was not predictive of sustainability. Sustainable efforts required financial, human, relational, and structural resources that bring together people with many different skills and capabilities to work together. This is a challenge in any community, but particularly challenging in a community with already limited public health and medical resources.

Conclusion

Despite the high burden of injuries throughout the world, investment in safety and injury prevention infrastructure has been low. In low-income countries such as Pakistan and Uganda, approximately US$0.07 per capita was devoted to safety. In every country, the amount invested in prevention is far surpassed by the amount spent on the treatment of traumatic injuries, and thus studies that focus on cost-benefits are badly needed. International assistance has also not prioritized safety or injury prevention. External assistance to the health sectors of low income countries was US$2–3 per DALY lost to infectious diseases, but only US$0.06 per DALY lost to injuries (Mock *et al.* 2004).

Since 90 per cent of the world's population lives in low- and middle-income countries, and the burden of injuries is predicted to increase in these countries, it is imperative that future research and development activities focus especially on their needs. Basic research to describe the existing burden, causes, and distribution of injuries is still needed in LMIC. Trials of injury interventions have largely not been conducted in LMIC, and there is a great need to modify, adapt and test existing, as well as new interventions in these specific settings (Peden *et al.* 2004). More work is also required to assess barriers to implementation of such interventions globally.

The role of international organizations (such as WHO and the World Bank) and national agencies (such as ministries of health or medical research councils) needs to be emphasized in moving ahead the injury prevention agenda. The international movements currently underway for violence prevention and road traffic injuries prevention as promulgated through the two World Reports are examples of how joint global-national partnerships are needed for making change.

Progress will also be supported if a growing number of professionals become advocates for safety. Professionals from public health, medicine, engineering, social services, urban planning, law and law enforcement, among others, can all have a strong voice in raising awareness for safety programmes and to encourage individuals to make safe choices.

Key points

- Injuries and violence are a leading cause of mortality and morbidity worldwide.
- Injuries disproportionately affect young and vulnerable populations, and injury rates are disproportionately high among low- and middle-income countries.
- Prevention of injuries is very feasible and works best with a multidisciplinary and integrated approach.
- Building capacity for injury prevention should be a priority for all countries, but is an urgent need for low- and middle-income countries.
- Improvement in global injury prevention efforts would be aided by increased capacity in data systems, building an evidence base for successful approaches, trauma care delivery, and trained injury prevention professionals.

References

Adesunkanmi, A. R., Oseni, S. A., & Badru, O. S. 1999, 'Severity and outcome of falls in children', *West African Journal of Medicine*, vol. 18, no. 4, pp. 281–5.

Aeron-Thomas, A., Jacobs, G. D., Stexon, B., Gururaj, G., & Rahmann, F. 2004, 'The involvement and impact of road crashes on the poor: Bangladesh and India case studies', *Published Project Report PRP 010*. Crowthorne: Transport Research Laboratory LTD.

Afukaar, F. K. 2003, 'Speed control in LMICs: Issues, challenges and opportunities in reducing road traffic injuries', *Injury Control and Safety Promotion*, vol. 10, no. 1–2, pp. 77–81.

Ahmed, M. K., Rahman, M., & van Ginneken, J. 1999, 'Epidemiology of child deaths due to drowning in Matlab, Bangladesh', *International Journal of Epidemiology*, vol. 28, no. 2, pp. 306–11.

Alderson, P., Green, S., & Higgins, J. P. T. (eds.) 2004, *Cochrane Reviewers Handbook 4.2.2*. Retrieved 3/07 from http://www.cochrane.org/resources/handbook/hbook.htm.

Ameratunga, S., Hijar, M., & Norton, R. 2006, 'Road traffic injuries: Confronting disparities to address a global health problem', *Lancet*, vol. 367, pp. 1533–40.

Anonymous. Bulletin of the Clearinghouse National Poison Control Centers Poisoning Prevention Technical Advisory Committee, 1971, *Poisoning Prevention Packaging Act of 1970*, May–June, 1–2.

Azizi, B. H., Zulkifli, H. I., & Kasim, M. S. 1993, 'Risk factors for accidental poisoning in urban Malaysian children', *Annals of Tropical Paediatrics*, vol. 13, no. 2, pp. 183–8.

Ballesteros, M., Jackson, M., & Martin, M. W. 2005, 'Working towards the elimination of residential fire deaths: CDC's Smoke Alarm Installation and Fire Safety Education (SAIFE) Program', *Journal of Burn Care and Rehabilitation*, vol. 26, no. 5, pp. 434–9.

Bangdiwala, S. I., & Anzola-Perez, E. 1990, 'The incidence of injuries in young people: II. log-linear multivariable models for risk factors in a collaborative study in Brazil, Chile, Cuba and Venezuela', *International Journal of Epidemiology*, vol. 19, no. 1, pp. 125–32.

Bener, A. K., Al-Salman, M., & Pugh, R. N. H. 1998, 'Injury mortality and morbidity among children in the United Arab Emirates', *European Journal of Epidemiology*, vol. 14, pp. 175–8.

Bero, L., & Rennie, D. 1995, 'The Cochrane Collaboration. Preparing, maintaining, and disseminating systematic reviews of the effects of health care', *Journal of the American Medical Association*, vol. 274, pp. 1935–8.

Bishai, D., Hyder, A. A., Ghaffar, A., Morrow, R. H., & Kobusingye, O. 2003, 'Rates of public investment for road safety in developing countries: Case studies of Uganda and Pakistan', *Health Policy and Planning*, vol. 18, no. 2, pp. 232–5.

Boonyaratavej, N., Suriyawongpaisal, P., Takkinsatien, A., Wanvarie, S., Rajatanavin, R., & Apiyasawat, P. 2001, 'Physical activity and risk factors for hip fractures in Thai women', *Osteoporosis International*, vol. 12, no. 3, pp. 244–8.

Brenner, R. A. 2003, 'Prevention of drowning in infants, children and adolescents', *Pediatrics*, vol. 112, no. 2, pp. 440–5.

Briss, P. A., Zaza, S., Pappaioanou, M. *et al.* 2000, 'Developing an evidence-based guide to community preventive services-methods', *American Journal of Preventive Medicine*, vol. 19, no. 1S, pp. 35–43.

Carlini-Cotrim, B., & da Matta Chasin, A. A. 2000, 'Blood alcohol content and death from fatal injury: A study in metropolitan area of Sao Paulo, Brazil', *Journal of Psychoactive Drugs*, vol. 32, no. 3, pp. 269–75.

Celis, A. 1997, 'Home drowning among preschool age Mexican children', *Injury Prevention*, vol. 3, no. 4, pp. 252–6.

Centers for Disease Control and Prevention and the Injury Control and Emergency Health Services Section of the American Public Health Association. 1997, 'Recommended framework for presenting injury mortality data', *MMWR Recomm Rep*., vol. 46, no. RR-14, pp. 1–30. http://www.cdc.gov/mmwr/preview/mmwrhtml/00049162.htm

Chatsantiprapa, K., Chokkanapitak, J., & Pinpradit, N. 2001. 'Host and environment factors for exposure to poisons: A case control study of preschool children in Thailand', *Injury Prevention*, vol. 7, no. 3, pp. 214–7.

Clark, P., de la Pena, F., Gomez Garcia, F., Orozco, J. A., & Tugwell, P. 1998, 'Risk factors for osteoporotic hip fractures in Mexicans', *Archives of Medical Research*, vol. 29, no. 3, pp. 253–7.

Cummings, S. R., Nevitt, M. C., Browner, W. S. *et al.* 1995, 'Risk factors for hip fracture in white women', *New England Journal of Medicine*, vol. 332, 12, pp. 767–73.

Cywes, S., Kibel, S. M., Bass, D. H., Rode, H., Millar, A. J. W. & De Wet, J. 1990, 'Paediatric trauma care', *South African Medical Journal*, vol. 78, pp. 413–8.

Dargent-Molina, Favier, P. F., Grandjean, H. *et al.* 1996, 'Fall-related factors and risk of hip fracture: The EPIDOS Prospective Study', *Lancet*, vol. 348, no. 9021, pp.145–9.

Davies, P., & Boruch, R. 2001, 'The Campbell Collaboration does for public policy what Cochrane does for health', *British Medical Journal*, vol. 323, no. 7308, pp. 294–5.

Dedoukou, X., Spyridopoulos, T., Kedikoglou, S., Alexe, D. M., Dessypris, N., & Petridou, E. 2004, 'Incidence and risk factors of fall injuries among infants: A study in Greece', *Archives of Pediatric and Adolescent Medicine*, vol. 158, no. 10, pp. 1002–6.

Driscoll, T. R., Harrison, J. A., & Steenkamp, M. 2004, 'Review of the role of alcohol in drowning associated with recreational aquatic activity', *Injury Prevention*, vol. 10, no. 2, pp. 107–13.

Evans, L. 1995, 'Restraint effectiveness, occupant ejection from cars, and fatality reductions', *Accident Analysis and Prevention*, vol. 22, pp. 167–75.

Ewing, R. H. 1999, 'Traffic calming: State of the practice', *Federal Highway Administration* FHWA-RD-99-135. Washington D.C., (http://www.ite.org/traffic/tcstate.htm#tcsop).

Fingerhut, L. A. 2004, 'International collaborative effort on injury statistics: 10 year review', *Injury Prevention*, vol. 10, pp. 264–7.

Forjuoh, S. N., Guyer, B., Strobino, D. M., Keyl, P. M., Diener-West, M., & Smith, G. S. 1995, 'Risk factors for childhood burns: A case-control study of Ghanaian children', *Journal of Epidemiology and Community Health*, vol. 49, no. 2, pp. 189–93.

Ghaffar, A., Hyder, A. A., Mastoor, M. I., & Shaikh, I. 1999, 'Injuries in Pakistan: Directions for future health policy', *Health Policy and Planning*, vol. 14, no. 1, pp. 11–17.

Graham, J. D. 1993, 'Injuries from traffic crashes: Meeting the challenge', *Annual Review of Public Health*, vol. 14, pp. 515–43.

Haddon, W., Jr. 1970, 'On the escape of tigers: An ecologic note', *American Journal of Public Health*, vol. 60, pp. 2229–34.

Haddon, W., Jr. 1972, 'A logical framework for categorizing highway safety phenomena and activity', *Journal of Trauma*, vol. 12, pp. 193–207.

Haddon, W., & Baker, S. P. 1981, *Injury Control*, eds. D. W. Clark & B. McMahaon, Preventive and Community Medicine, 2nd edn, pp. 109–40, Little, Brown, and Company, Boston, Massachusetts.

Hall, J. R., Jr. 1994, 'The U.S. experience with smoke detectors: Who has them? How well do they work? When don't they work?' *National Fire Protection Association Journal*, pp. 36–46.

Harvey, P. A., Sacks, J. J., Ryan, G. W., & Bender, P. F. 1998, 'Residential smoke alarms and fire escape plans', *Public Health Report*, vol. 113, pp. 459–464.

Hofman. K., Primack, A., Keusch, G., & Hrynkow, S. 2005, 'Addressing the growing burden of trauma and injury in low- and middle-income countries', *American Journal of Public Health*, vol. 95, pp. 13–17.

Hyder, A. A., Arifeen, S., Begum, N., Fishman, S., Wali, S., & Baqui, A. H. 2003, 'Death from drowning: Defining a new challenge for child survival in Bangladesh', *Injury Control and Safety Promotion*, vol. 10, no. 4, pp. 205–10.

Hyder, A. A., & Morrow, R. H. 2006, *Measures of Health and Disease in Populations*, eds. R. B. Black, M. Merson & A. Mills, International Public Health: Diseases, Programs, Systems and Policies, 2nd edn, Jones & Bartlett Publishers, Boston, MA.

Hyder, A. A., Rotllant, G., & Morrow, R. H. 1998, 'Measuring the burden of disease: Healthy life years', *American Journal of Public Health*, vol. 88, no. 2, pp. 196–202.

Institute of Medicine 1999, *Reducing the Burden of Injury: Advancing Prevention and Treatment*. Bonney, R. J., Fulco, C. E., & Liverman, C. T., eds, Washington, D.C. National Academy Press.

Istre, G. R., McCoy, M. A., Stowe, M. *et al.* 2003, 'Childhood injuries due to falls from apartment balconies and windows', *Injury Prevention*, vol. 9, no. 4, pp. 349–52.

Jaye, C., Simpson, J. C., & Langley, J. D. 2001, 'Barriers to safe hot tap water: Results from a National Study of New Zealand Plumbers', *Injury Prevention*, vol. 7, pp. 302–6.

Jie, X., & Ren, C. B. 1992, 'Burn injuries in the Dong Bei area of China: A study of 12,606 cases', *Burns*, vol. 18, no. 3, pp. 228–32.

Jitapunkul, S., Yuktananandana, P., & Parkpian, V. 2001, 'Risk factors of hip fracture among Thai female patients', *Journal of the Medical Association of Thailand*, vol. 84, no. 11, pp. 1576–81.

Khan, M. M., & Hyder, A. A. 2006, 'Suicides in the developing world: Case study from Pakistan', *Suicide & Life Threatening Behavior*, vol. 36, no. 1, pp. 76–81.

Kibel, S. M., Joubert, G., & Bradshaw, D. 1990, 'Injury-related mortality in South African children, 1981–1985', *South African Medical Journal*, vol. 78, no. 7, pp. 398–403.

Kobusingye, O. C. 2005, 'Emergency medical systems in low- and middle-income countries: Recommendations for action', *Bull World Health Organisation*, vol. 83, no. 8, pp. 626–31.

Kobusingye, O., Guwatudde, D., & Lett, R. 2001, 'Injury patterns in rural and urban Uganda', *Injury Prevention*, vol. 7, no. 1, pp. 46–50.

Kobusingye, O. C., Hyder, A. A., Bishai, D., Joshipura, M., Hicks, E. R., & Mock, C. 2006. Emergency Medical Services. *Disease Control Priorities in Developing Countries*, 2nd edn, Jamison, D. *et al*., eds., Disease Control Priorities in Developing Countries, 1261–9.Oxford University Press and the World Bank, New York, NY.

Kopits, E., & Cropper, M. 2003, *Traffic Fatalities and Economic Growth*, Policy Research Working Paper 3035, World Bank, Washington, DC.

Kozik, C. A., Suntayakorn, S., Vaughn, D. W., Suntayakorn, C., Snitbhan, R., & Innis B. L. 1999, 'Causes of death and unintentional injury among schoolchildren in Thailand', Southeast Asian *Journal of Tropical Medicine and Public Health*, vol. 30, no. 1, pp. 129–35.

Krug, E. G., Dahlberg, K. L., Mercy, J. A., Zwi, A. B., & Lozano, R, (eds.) 2002, *World Report on Violence and Health*, Geneva, World Health Organisation.

Krug, A., Ellis, J. B., Hay, I. T., Mokgabudi, N. F., & Robertson, J. 1994, 'The impact of child-resistant containers on the incidence of paraffin (kerosene) ingestion in children', *South African Medical Journal*, vol. 84, no. 11, pp. 730–4.

Krug, E. G., Sharma, G. K., & Lozano, R. 2000, 'The global burden of injuries', *American Journal of Public Health*, vol. 90, pp. 523–6.

Kulanthayan, S., Umar, R. S., Hariza, H. A., Nasir, M. T., & Harwant, S. 2000, 'Compliance of proper safety helmet usage in motorcyclists', *Medical Journal of Malaysia*, vol. 55, no. 1, pp. 40–4.

Liu, G. F., Han, S., Liang, D. H. *et al.* 2003, 'Driver sleepiness and risk of car crashes in Shenyang, a Chinese Northeastern city: Population-based case-control study', *Biomedical and Environmental Sciences*, vol. 16, no. 3, pp. 219–26.

Liu, B., Ivers, R., Norton, R., Blows, S., & Lo, S. K. 2004, 'Helmets for preventing injury in motorcycle riders', *Cochrane Database of Systematic Reviews*, vol. 4, CD004333.

Liu, E. H., Khatri, B., Shakya,Y. M., & Richard, B. M. 1998, 'A 3 year prospective audit of burn patients treated at the Western Regional Hospital of Nepal', *Burns*, vol. 24, no. 2, pp. 129–33.

Lu, T. H., Lee, M. C., & Chou, M. C.1998, 'Trends in injury mortality among adolescents in Taiwan, 1965–94', *Injury Prevention*, vol. 4, pp. 111–5.

MacGregor, D. M. 2000, 'Injuries associated with falls from beds', *Injury Prevention*, vol. 6, no. 4, pp. 291–2.

Mann, N., Mullins, R, MacKenzie, E. *et al.* 1999, 'A systematic review of published evidence regarding trauma system effectiveness', *Journal of Trauma*, vol. 47, pp. S25–33.

Mann, R. E., Smart, R. G., Stoduto, G. *et al.* 2003, 'The effects of drinking-driving laws: A test of the differential deterrence hypothesis', *Addiction*, vol. 98, no. 11, pp. 1531–6.

Mock, C., Amegashi, J., & Darteh, K. 1999, 'Role of commercial drivers in motor vehicle related injuries in Ghana', *Injury Prevention*, vol. 5, no. 4, pp. 268–71.

Mock, C., Nguyen, S., Quansah, R., Arreola-Risa, C., Viradia, R., & Joshipura, M. 2006, 'Evaluation of trauma care capabilities in four countries using the WHO-IATSIC Guidelines for Essential Trauma Care', *World Journal of Surgery*, vol. 30, pp. 946–56.

Mock, C., Quansah, R., Krishnan, R., Arreola-Risa C., & Rivara, F. 2004, Strengthening the prevention and care of injuries worldwide, *Lancet*, vol. 363, pp. 2172–9.

Murray, C., & Lopez, A. 1996, *Global Burden of Disease and Injuries*, Harvard University Press, Cambridge, MA.

Nafukho, F. M., & Khayesi, M. 2002, 'Livelihood, conditions of work, regulation, and road Safety in the small-scale public transport sector: A case of the Matatu mode of transport in Kenya', in Urban Mobility for All, ed X. Godard and I. Fatonzoun, pp. 241–5, Proceedings of the Tenth International CODATU Conference, Lome, Togo, 12–15 November 2002, Lisse, The Netherlands.

Nathens, A., Jurkovich, G., Cummings, P., Rivara, F., & Maier, R. 2000, 'The effect of organised systems of trauma care on motor vehicle crash mortality', *The Journal of the American Medical Association*, vol. 283, pp. 1990–4.

National Highway Traffic Safety Administration. 2007, 'Seat belt use in 2006 – Use rates in states and territories', *Traffic Safety Facts*. DOT-HS-810-960. January, 2007. (http://www-nrd.nhtsa.dot.gov/pdf/nrd-30/NCSA/RNotes/2007/810690.pdf).

Nilsen, P., Timpka, T., Nordenfelt, L., & Lindqvist, K. 2005, 'Towards improved understanding of injury prevention program sustainability', *Safety Science*, vol. 43, pp. 815–33.

Norton, R., Hyder, A. A., & Gururaj, G. 2006, *Unintentional Injuries and Violence*, R. B. Black, M. Merson, A. Mills, eds., International Public Health: Diseases, Programs, Systems and Policies, 2nd edn., Jones & Bartlett Publishers, Silver Boston, Massachusetts.

Odero, W. O., & Zwi, A. B. 1995, *Alcohol-Related Traffic Injuries and Fatalities in LMICs: A Critical Review of Literature*, C. N. Kloeden & A. J. McLean, eds., In Proceedings of the 13th International Conference on Alcohol, Drugs and Traffic Safety, pp. 713–20. Road Accident Research Unit, Adelaide.

Peden, M., McGee, K., & Sharma, G. 2002, *The Injury Chart Book: A Graphical Overview of the Global Burden of Injuries*, World Health Organisation, Geneva.

Peden, M., Scurfield, R., Sleet, D. *et al.* (eds.) 2004, *World Report on Road Traffic Injury Prevention*, World Health Organisation, Geneva.

Peek-Asa, C., Allareddy, V., Yang, J., Taylor, C., Lundell, J., & Zwerling, C. 2005, 'When one is not enough: Prevalence and characteristics of homes not adequately protected by smoke alarms', *Injury Prevention*, vol. 11, no. 6, pp. 364–8.

Polinder, S., Meerding, W. J., Mulder, S. *et al.* 2007, *Assessing the Burden of Injury in Six European Countries, Bulletin of the World Health Organisation* vol. 85, no. 1, pp. 27–34.

Pappaioanou, M., & Evans, C., Jr. 1998, 'Development of the Guide to Community Preventive Services: A U.S. Public Health Service initiative', *Journal of Public Health Management & Practice*, vol. 4, no. S2, pp. 48–54.

Raja, I. A.,Vohra, A. H., & Ahmed, M. 2001, 'Neurotrauma in Pakistan', *World Journal of Surgery*, vol. 25, no. 9, pp. 1230–7.

Richter, E. D., Friedman, L. S., Berman, T., & Rivkind, A. 2006, 'Death and injury from motor vehicle crashes: A tale of two countries', *American Journal of Preventive Medicine*, vol. 30, no. 5, pp. 440–9.

Robertson, L. S. 1981, 'Automobile safety regulations and death reductions in the United States', *American Journal of Public Health*, vol. 71, no. 8, pp. 818–22.

Runyan, C. W. 1998, 'Using the Haddon Matrix: Introducing the third dimension', *Injury Prevention*, vol. 4, pp. 302–7.

Soori, H. 2001, 'Developmental risk factors for unintentional childhood poisoning', *Saudi Medical Journal*, vol. 22, no. 3, pp. 227–30.

Thomas, S., Acton, C., Nixon, J., Battistutta, D., Pitt, W. R., & Clark, R. 1994, 'Effectiveness of bicycle helmets in preventing head injury in children: Case-control study', *British Medical Journal*, vol. 308, pp. 173–7.

Thompson, D. C., & Rivara, F. P. 2007, *Pool Fencing for Preventing Drowning in Children*, The Cochrane Database of Systematic Reviews, Issue 1.

Transport and Road Research Laboratory. 1991, *Towards Safer Roads in Developing Countries: A Guide for Engineers and Planners*, Overseas Development Administration, ISBN 1-851221-176-5, Berkshire, England.

U.S. General Accounting Office. 1991, *Motorcycle Helmet Laws Save Lives and Reduce Costs to Society*, Washington, DC: U.S. General Accounting Office, GAO/RCED-91-170.

Wang, S., Chi, G. B., Jing, C. X., Dong, X. M., Wu, C. P., & Li, L. P. 2003, 'Trends in road traffic crashes and associated injury and fatality in the People's Republic of China, 1951–1999', *Injury Control and Safety Promotion*, vol. 10, no. 1–2, pp. 83–7.

Warda, L., Tennebein, M., & Moffatt, M. E. K. 1999, 'House fire injury prevention update, Part I: A review of risk factors for fatal and non-fatal house fire injury', *Injury Prevention, vol.* 5, no. 3, pp. 145–50.

Waters, H., Hyder, A. A., & Rajkotia, Y. Basu, S., Rehwinkel, J. A., & Buchchart, A. 2004, *The Economic Dimensions of Interpersonal Violence*, World Health Organisation, Geneva.

Werneck, G. L., & Reichenheim, M. E. 1997, 'Pediatric burns and associated risk factors in Rio de Janeiro, Brazil', *Burns*, vol. 23, no. 6, pp. 478–83.

World Bank. 1993, *World Development Report 1993: Investing in Health*, 1993 World Health Organisation, Oxford University Press, New York. Available at www.who.int.

World Health Organisation. 2002, *The World Health Report 2002: Reducing Risks, Promoting Health Life*, World Health Organisation, Geneva.

World Health Organisation. 1999, *Injury: A Leading Cause of the Global Burden of Disease*, World Health Organisation, Geneva.

World Health Organisation. 2003, *Drowning Fact Sheet*, World Health Organisation, Geneva.

10.5

Interpersonal violence prevention: A recent public health mandate

Deborah Prothrow-Stith

Introduction

This chapter on public health presents approaches to prevent interpersonal violence in response to the epidemic of adolescent and young adult homicide in the United States, and the growing international attention and concerns about this problem. The chapter provides a short history of the efforts within public health to address violence, a definition and description of the problem, and a discussion of examples of public health approaches to violence prevention. While several types of violence are briefly discussed, the focus of the chapter is youth violence and the increase in youth homicide in the United States. The 1987 United States homicide rate for 15–24-year-old men of 22 per 100 000 was the highest among industrialized countries not at war in 1986/1987 (Fig. 10.5.1). By 1991, it had increased to 37 per 100 000, but declined to 20 per 100 000 in 2004, still the highest among industrialized nations. While high homicide rates also plagued South Africa at the same time, the political instability and violent freedom struggle make it an exception. For further details on international issues, we recommend the 2003 WHO report, *World Report on Violence and Health* (Krug 2002) and the WHO website, http://www.who.int/violence_injury_prevention/en/ (WHO).

The public's demand for solutions to violence in the United States has generated increased multidisciplinary attention, expanding the traditional criminal justice responses of punishment and deterrence to include public health and other health and human service disciplines. In the past 25 years, we have witnessed a dramatic effort by public health professionals to prevent violence in the United States. National leadership has emerged from the Centers for Disease Control (CDC) and the US Surgeon General's office. In addition, many state and local health department leaders have embraced the issue, creating offices of violence prevention within their departments. There are several international meetings, initially geared towards discussion of peace and ending war, which have included interpersonal violence prevention on their conference agendas.

The Centers for Disease Control and Prevention established the Violence Epidemiology Branch in 1983, for the study of homicide and suicide, and the early data fuelled the violence prevention efforts in public health. Initial Morbidity and Mortality Weekly Reports revealed that homicide is the leading cause of death for black men between 15 and 24 and 25 to 44 years, and that for all adolescents, homicide is the second leading cause of death (CDC 1982; CDC 1983; CDC 2007a). Additional information concerning the characteristics of homicides was published for public health audiences, indicating that 58 per cent of the victims knew their assailants, 47 per cent were precipitated by an argument, and only 15 per cent were as a result of another felony (burglary, drug trafficking, etc.) (CDC 1983). The application of basic epidemiology and reporting techniques became the impetus for public health professionals across the country to confront the issue.

In October 1985, C. Everett Koop convened an invitational meeting, the Surgeon General's Workshop on Violence and Public Health, in Leesburg, Virginia, in the United States. The interdisciplinary meeting focused on assault and homicide, child abuse, rape and sexual assault, domestic violence, elder abuse, and suicide. The disproportionate impact of homicide among young black men in the United States was addressed at the workshop, and a classroom-based violence prevention education programme designed for that population was presented (Prothrow-Stith 1985). The workshop and published proceedings continue to fuel public health professionals' efforts to frame violence as a mainstream public health problem. Over the next decade, the dramatic increase in public health attention to the problem that followed the Surgeon General's conference led to the establishment of the National Center for Injury Prevention and Control at the CDC in 1994. Every Surgeon General since Koop has encouraged the public health community to use its strategies to better understand and prevent violence. Into the new millennium, public health professionals' endeavours to understand and prevent violence have continued to grow with increasingly more programmes, publications, and presentations.

Public health efforts to prevent violence utilizing standard epidemiology, community outreach, screening, community-based programmes, health education, behaviour modification, public

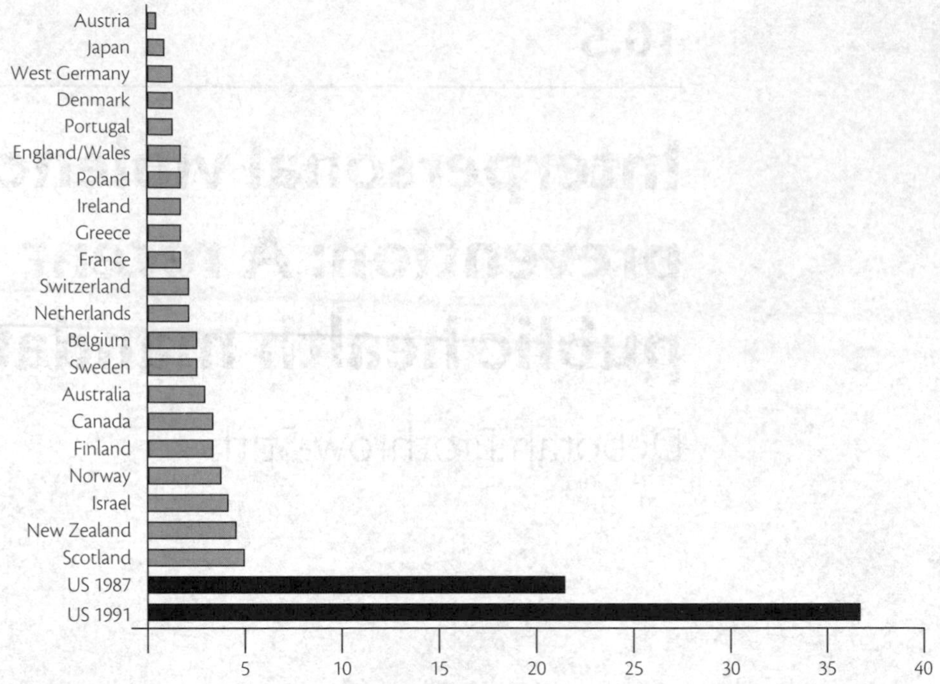

Fig. 10.5.1 International comparisons of homicide rates per 100 000 population (males, aged 15–24) in the years 1986 or 1987.

awareness, and education campaigns continue to involve every aspect of the United States Public Health Service. These efforts are based upon similar multidisciplinary efforts to prevent lung cancer deaths, heart disease, and fatal car crashes.

Consisting of thousands of local programmes scattered across the country, the dramatic increase in interpersonal violence prevention activities has the potential for the same level of success that public health professionals have had with reducing smoking and drunk-driving in the United States. The analogy between violence prevention and other public health problems is not flawless, yet over two decades of experience employing comparable techniques and strategies indicates enough similarity for success. In addition, a number of efforts to train health and public health professionals have been developed and disseminated (Sege & Hoffman 2005).

Definition and classification

The National Center for Injury Prevention and Control at the US Centers for Disease Control classifies both unintentional injuries (accidents) and intentional injuries (violence) as public health problems, as illustrated in Fig. 10.5.2. Intentional injuries are divided into self-directed violence (suicides and suicide attempts) and interpersonal violence (assaults and homicides) (Fig. 10.5.3). Violence is defined by the CDC, as 'the threatened or actual use of physical force or power against another person, against oneself, or against a group or community that either results or is likely to result in injury, death, or deprivation'.

Suicide, a more traditional problem for health and public health professionals, has several commonalities with interpersonal violence. Both often it involves alcohol and other drugs, and the risk for both increases with the presence of a firearm. Media and entertainment values appear to have an impact on both. Adolescent suicide and homicide rates rose dramatically during the early 1980s. While suicide remains an important public health concern, recent efforts using public health strategies to address interpersonal violence have proliferated.

There are at least four reasons why interpersonal violence became an important concern for public health professionals in the United States: (1) the magnitude and persistence of the problem; (2) the characteristics of and contributing risk factors for violence; (3) the contact health professionals and other professionals in the field of public health have with the victims and perpetrators of violence; and (4) the applicability of public health strategies to both understanding and preventing violence.

Public health professionals have offered a unique comprehensive and prevention-oriented approach to violence that has yielded significant contributions and offers further promise.

Violence is preventable

Perhaps not all of the violence is preventable, but it is clear from the literature and from history that much of it is. The United States and other countries that have similar youth violence problems have a preventable problem; a problem they do not have to have. Evidence that violence is a preventable problem comes from many sources. The comparisons of homicide rates for young men in industrialized countries published by the WHO demonstrate a 5–70-fold difference in rates. If homicide were a genetic or inevitable part of the human condition, one would expect rates from country to country to be fairly similar. The wide discrepancy in rates illustrated in Fig. 10.5.1 indicates a preventable problem. In addition, the changes and variability within US rates among different groups and at different times suggest a preventable problem. For example, the recent increases in the arrest rates for girls in the United States indicate that change is possible. What goes up can come down. In Boston, the significant reduction from 1996 to 2000 in the murder of children 16 or younger illustrated in Fig. 10.5.4 is further indication that violence is preventable. The Boston reduction was celebrated by many and some called it 'the Boston Miracle'. Boston, along with

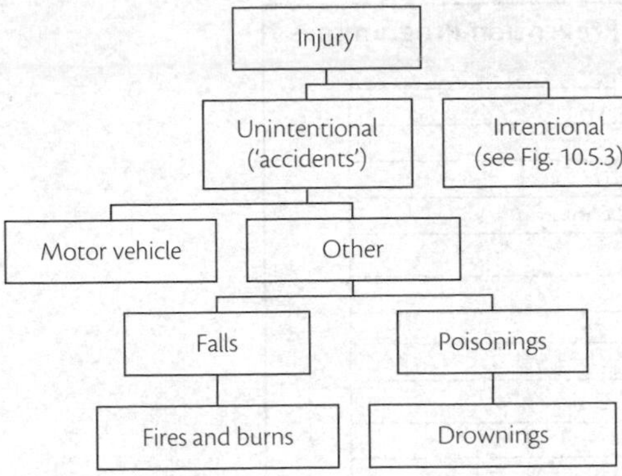

Fig. 10.5.2 Classifications of injury in public health.

most US urban settings, has experienced a recent increase in youth homicide. What goes down can go back up. An inverse relationship between youth homicide rates and resources appears to emerge. In Boston (Fig. 10.5.4), declines in youth homicide appear to be associated with increases in resources and programmes, and the recent increases with a retreat of resources. This appears to also hold true for the success of prevention efforts on a national scale.

The end of a former, rather ubiquitous, practice of duelling (often to the death) among elite white gentlemen of the 1800s in the United States (and many European countries for that matter) is further indication that violence is preventable. Peaking in the United States around 1850, duelling claimed the lives of many, including politicians, journalists, and even physicians, who were recorded as duelling over the proper treatment for a patient. Though illegal, this practice often drew crowds and became a public event. Harriet Martineau, a New Orleans-based journalist, wrote that there were 2–3 duels a day, and as many as 15 on the weekend in New Orleans. Women were advised not to marry a man unless he had proven himself with the blade. Duelling pistols were created to allow 'fairness' in the duels. The Code Duello (originally written in Ireland) was revised and published in 1838 in the United States by a former governor of South Carolina, John Lyde Wilson. Alexander Hamilton, signer of the US Constitution and the first Secretary of the Treasury in the United States, was killed in a duel in 1804. His son, Phillip Hamilton, was killed in a duel 3 years prior. Alexander Hamilton kept a diary, and the entry the night before he was killed in a duel with Aaron Burr is a powerful reminder of the role culture and social norms play in human behaviour (Fig. 10.5.5).

In the case of duelling, culture trumped laws for nearly 100 years. Today, in the United States, we are up against similar cultural forces that encourage children to fight and indicate that it is the strong superhero who justifies a wrong with violence. The extent to which the entertainment media propagate these messages corresponds to the extent to which the US exports them to a broader international community.

Data sources

There are several sources of data on violence in America which are accessible to the public or through community partnerships with academic institutions. The National Center for Education Statistics (NECS) and the Bureau of Justice Statistics (BJS) are the primary federal entities for collecting, analysing, and reporting data related to education and crime, respectively, in the United States and other nations. The Department of the Treasury, Bureau of Alcohol, Tobacco and Firearms (ATF) publication, *Commerce in Firearms in the United States*, is an annual report of activities relating to the regulation of firearms. The Youth Crime Interdiction Initiative (YCGII), *Crime Gun Trace Analysis Reports: The Illegal Youth Firearms Market in 27 Communities*, brings together federal, state, and local law enforcement officials to improve information about the illegal sources of guns recovered from juveniles and adult criminals.

The Uniform Crime Reports (UCR), published by the Federal Bureau of Investigation, is the most frequently cited source of national information on violent crime. These annual reports date back to 1930. The UCR use police data that are submitted to the FBI and which are aggregated into a national data source. Homicides are manditorily reported in these data sets, but other crimes (including non-fatal violent assaults) are reported voluntarily and therefore inconsistently. The reports give cursory information on homicides and assaults, including victim and perpetrator relationship, weapons used, location of the violent episode, and races of victim and perpetrator.

More recently, the National Violent Death Reporting System was established by the US Centers for Disease Control and Prevention (CDC) in 2002 and seeks to provide detailed information concerning each violent death in the United States. The system is organized and run on the state level, and includes data from vital statistics, medical, and criminal justice sources. Although the programme is planned to include the entire country, as of this writing, 17 states are contributing data.

Since 1991, behavioural risk factors reported by high school students in the United States have been measured every other year to the present in the YRBSS (Youth Risk Behavioral Surveillance System).

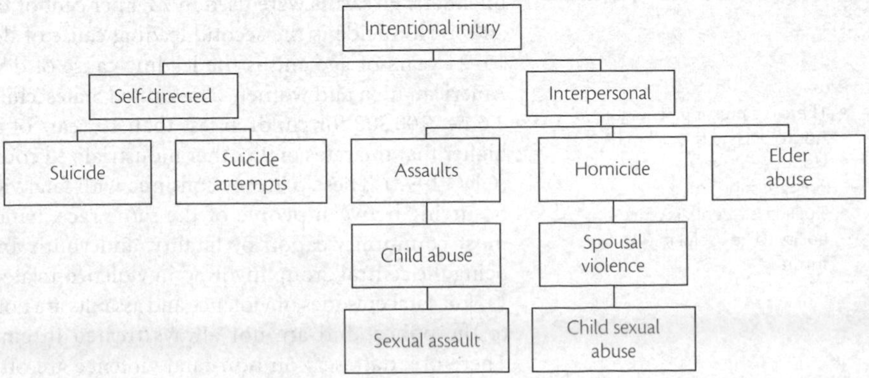

Fig. 10.5.3 Classifications of intentional injury.

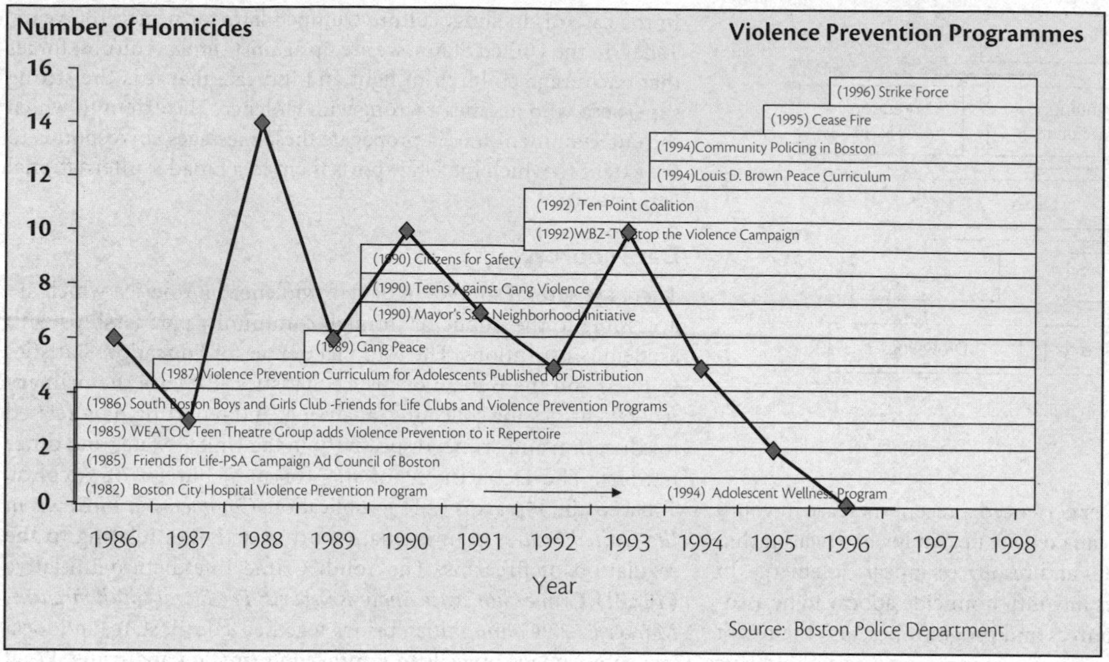

Fig. 10.5.4 Boston Violence Prevention Movement. The number of children under 17 murdered with guns and violence prevention programme examples by start date in Boston 1986–1996.

These data are collected nationally, with local- and state-enhanced collection where contracted. Violent behaviour, weapon carrying, and exposure to violence are measured along with many other health risk factors (drug use, smoking, exercise, etc.). YRBSS data are available on-line on a user-friendly website that facilitates several levels of analysis. In addition to being a site for researchers, the website has generated youth-run research activities. A similar survey of adults, the BRFSS (Behavioral Risk Factor Surveillance System), is on-line accessible as well. Both the YRBSS and the BRFSS are conducted by CDC.

The magnitude of the problem

The United States Federal Bureau of Investigation estimates that 1.8 million Americans are victims of violence each year. Adolescents are more likely than any other age group to be victims of violence, mostly from their peers (same race, from the same neighbourhood). A complete representation of the magnitude of violence is unavailable because of the unreliable and inconsistent measures of non-fatal episodes of violence. Homicides, the tip of the iceberg, are most accurately measured, as reporting is mandatory, as noted above. Other countries have made their homicide rates available through the World Health Organization.

Cons

- I have a wife and children whom I love.
- I am deeply in debt and should not leave this burden to my family.
- I have no ill-will for Burr.
- Dueling is illegal in NY.
- Dueling is condemned by Christianity, my religion.

Pros

- There is a pressing necessity not to decline the call.
- Not dueling will cost me political support.
- Dueling is essential to my ability to be useful in the future.

Fig. 10.5.5 Hamilton's pros and cons.

The magnitude of the problem of homicide in the United States was mind-boggling when compared to that of other industrialized nations not at war. Not only was the United States homicide rate 10–25 times higher than most industrialized nations, but the homicide rates rivalled some less-developed countries facing war or considerable social, political, and economic turmoil (Wolfgang 1986). An international study of 1985 homicide rates in industrialized countries showed that the United States rate for both sexes, ages 1–19, was more than three times that of the next highest rate, Canada (Williams & Kotch 1990). Little has changed with respect to these international comparisons over the past several decades.

In 2006, of the 14 990 murder victims, 50 per cent were black and 47 per cent were white. In 45 per cent of the murders, the relationships between the victim and perpetrator were not known; in 30 per cent, they were friends or acquaintances, in 13 per cent, they were in the same family, and in 12 per cent, they were strangers. In addition, 93.2 per cent of black victims were killed by black offenders and 82.9 per cent of white murder victims were killed by white offenders. Firearms were used in 73.4 per cent of the murders (FBI 2007). Homicide is the second leading cause of death for persons 15–24 years of age and is the leading cause of death for African–American men and women. The United States' child homicide rate, 2.6 per 100 000 for children less than 15 years of age, is five times higher that the rates of 25 other industrialized countries combined (CDC 1997). These patterns continue with fatal violence primarily occurring between people of the same race, handguns being the most common weapon of fatality, and youth and young adults being the central group involved in violence-related fatalities.

Non-fatal episodes of violence and assaults are not always reported to the police, and are not always treated in emergency rooms. Therefore, data sets on non-fatal violence are often inconsistent.

Police are often unaware of numerous, sometimes serious violent injuries and events. Emergency rooms capture a much larger number of the assaults. In 2004, 5292 youth aged 10 years were murdered, while an estimated 721 000 were treated in hospital emergency departments for violence-related injury—a ratio of approximately 120:1 (CDC 2007b). This ratio is a comparable to that in the Northeast Ohio Trauma Study, in which for each single homicide, there were 20 assaults reported to the police and 100 reported to the emergency rooms in one standard metropolitan statistical area in northeast Ohio. Furthermore, many episodes of violence, particularly those occurring among friends and family, are not reported to either the police or the emergency rooms.

The epidemic of youth violence in the United States is not limited to homicide. Arrest rates reported by police reveal an increase in nonfatal episodes of adolescent violence, despite the limitations of the data set. The decade of 1980–1990 saw the juvenile violent crime arrest rate for black adolescents increase by 19 per cent; for white adolescents, it increased 44 per cent, while the other race categories, despite a large increase in Asian youth, declined 53 per cent (FBI 1992). Although minors accounted for less than 14 per cent of the US population, in 1995, 37 per cent of homicide arrests, 28 per cent of rape arrests, and 51 per cent of robbery arrests were committed by minors. In 1982, 390 youth aged 13–15 were arrested for homicide. By 1992, this figure had nearly doubled. Although these rates dropped between 1994 and early 2000, they are starting to increase in most urban areas in the United States. The escalation of adolescent violent crime rates in the last several decades cuts across race, class, and geographic location, despite a common misconception that it is an urban black problem. More recently, the United States has experienced dramatic increases in violent crime rates involving girls as both perpetrators and victims, reflecting a growing involvement of girls in the epidemic of violence.

Adolescent violence

Violence involving youth has persisted at alarming levels in the United States. In 2003, the National Center for Health Statistics reported that homicide was the second leading cause of death for the 15–19-year age group (second only to motor vehicle accidents), at almost twice the rate of the overall United States population (CDC 2006). In 1997, 6146 people aged 15–24 years were victims of homicide. This amounts to an average of 17 youth homicide victims per day in the United States. Since then, the rate of youth homicide has dropped to 14 deaths per day (5085 total deaths). Homicide has remained the second leading cause of death for persons (men and women) 15–24 years of age (crude rate 12.8/100 000 for the period 1999–2007) and the leading cause of death for African–Americans, with 2004 rates still astronomically high: 77.2 per 100 000 for males, 8.8 for females.

Furthermore, adolescent mortality rate trends indicate that although overall death rates and death rates due to motor vehicle crashes both decreased for persons aged 10–24 years from 1979 to 1988, death rates for homicide increased by 6.7 per cent. In eight US states, firearm-related deaths surpassed automobile crashes as the leading cause of death for this age group (Centers for Disease Control and Prevention 1994). Since the peak in the late 1990s, these same rates have seen a modest decline of 5.6 per cent in the period 1999–2004.

Even for non-fatal violent victimizations, the 1990 National Crime Survey found that age was one of the most important single predictors of an individual's risk, which peaks at age 16–19 for both men (95 per 1000) and women (54 per 1000) (Bureau of Justice Statistics 1992, 1993). This was a dramatic change from several decades earlier, when the mean age of victims of violence was approximately 10 years older. Clearly, our nation's youth are at high risk for experiencing violence.

Dating violence is a form of adolescent and young adult violence that is often overlooked, even within discussions of domestic violence. Very little research has been done, and the general awareness of the problem of dating violence is relatively recent. A survey within a college population found that 21 per cent of the students admitted being in violent relationships and 62 per cent personally knew of someone affected by a violent relationship (Makepeace 1981). Several studies since then have indicated that between 12 and 19 per cent of high school students are involved in dating violence, either as a victim or as a perpetrator. As with domestic violence, women are more often the victims.

School violence

School suspension data offer another measure of the violence occurring, yet there are several limitations. Suspension numbers may vary within a school depending upon the persons responsible for collecting the data. There are not standard criteria within or between school systems as to what behaviour results in student suspension. There are also disincentives to reporting incidents of violence in schools, as this information may lead to negative consequences for school personnel themselves.

Violence in schools is not new, but it has become more severe and occasionally lethal. In the 2005 YRBSS, amongst students in the 9th to 12th grade in the 50 states, including the District of Columbia and Virgin Islands, 18.5 per cent reported carrying a weapon 30 days prior to the survey, and 5.4 per cent reported that they had carried a gun. Among students nationwide, 25.9 per cent had been in a physical fight one or more times during the 12 months preceding the survey (CDC 2007), and 3.6 per cent had required medical treatment for fighting-related injuries.

The CDC survey also revealed that 6 per cent of the students said that they missed at least 1 day of school in a month before because they felt unsafe at school (CDC 2007). In 1989, the United States Department of Justice found that 6 per cent of students report having to avoid certain places in school or on the way to or from school because they were afraid of being attacked. A poll conducted by Metropolitan Life showed that only 23 per cent of the students said they never saw violent incidents at school. A Louis Harris Associates Poll of youth and guns conducted in 1993 of 2500 students in the 6th to 12th grades showed that 15 per cent carried a handgun to school in the past year. Fifty-nine per cent said they could get a handgun if they wanted one. The addition of weapons to the typical school brawl has contributed significantly to the greater severity and mortality of school fights.

The CDC, the United States Department of Education, and the National School Safety Center conducted a study of actual deaths in schools. Data show that 105 school-associated violent deaths occurred in the school years 1992–1993 and 1993–1994, including 81 homicides, 19 suicides, and 5 unintentional firearm-related deaths. Sixty-six per cent of these occurred on school property and 75 per cent were committed with a firearm (Satcher 1985).

While the arrest rates for overall crime and violent crime are significantly lower for young women than young men, recent increases in girls' arrests have narrowed the gap. From 1981 to 1995, there was a 129 per cent increase in the violent crime arrest rate for young women when compared to a 56 per cent increase over the same time period for young men. Currently, girls account for over 25 per cent of juvenile arrests for violent crime, unheard of two decades ago. More girls are entering the juvenile justice system and doing so at younger ages; there has been a 10 per cent increase in the numbers of 13- and 14-year olds coming into juvenile court.

Some experts, including Meda Chesney-Lind (1998) at the University of Hawaii, believe that there really has not been a significant increase in the proportion of young women committing crimes. Rather, 'we're criminalizing a lot of schoolyard scuffles where, in the past, we'd call it a cat fight, we'd giggle and keep walking. Now we're calling the cops'.

Chesney-Lind and others also point to changes and biases within the juvenile justice system that they believe explain the increased number of girls arrested. For example, girls are twice as likely as boys to be detained, with the detention period lasting five times longer for girls than their male counterparts. Girls are more likely than boys to be charged with status offences, which if committed by an adult, would not be considered a crime (e.g. running away from home, truancy, incorrigibility), and are more likely to be incarcerated for these offences than males.

However, it is important to note that more recent increases in arrests for girls involve violent crimes, not status offences. Furthermore, these increases are occurring at the same time that arrest rates for boys for various categories of violent crime are either declining or barely increasing. With severely limited juvenile facilities and detention spaces for girls, police actually have a disincentive to arrest girls, as there is no place to take them.

Suicide

Historically, suicide in the United States was viewed as primarily a problem of older adult white men with clinical depression or other mental disorders; thus, suicide prevention involved identifying and treating mental illness. A steady rise in the adolescent and young adult (15–24-year old) suicide rates from 4.5 per 100 000 in 1950 to 10.1 per 100 000 in 1999–2004 created the need for new prevention strategies (CDC 1998). The rise was alarming, particularly as research indicated that only one out of three of those who committed suicide fit the criteria for clinical depression or other mental illness (Shaffer *et al.* 1988).

Race and gender disparities in suicide rates are striking. The rates for adolescent girls and women have remained relatively stable over the last 30 years, and the rates for white men have levelled since 1988. However, there has been a dramatic rise in the suicide rates for young black males (15–24-year old) since 1986 (Shaffer *et al.* 1994). While the suicide rates for white males remain higher than those for black males in each age cohort, the rates among black males increased at a faster rate than any other group. Male rates of completed suicide reflect their choice of rapidly lethal means (firearms and hanging), compared to females who more commonly choose ingestions resulting in high rates of non-lethal suicide attempts.

The CDC convened a panel of experts and conducted a study of youth suicide prevention programmes. The study reviewed the existing programmes and delineated eight suicide prevention strategies:

1. School gatekeeper training. This type of programme is directed at school staff to help them identify and defer students at risk of suicide and to organize the response in case of a suicide.
2. Community gatekeeper training. This type of programme provides the same service to community staff, clergy, police, merchants, etc.
3. General suicide education. These programmes are school-based education on suicide, often incorporating self-esteem building or social competency exercises.
4. Screening programmes. Screening involves administering an instrument to identify high-risk youth in order to provide services.
5. Peer support programmes. School- or community-based programmes to help adolescents develop competency in relationships and to help each other.
6. Crisis centres and hotlines. These programmes provide 24-h emergency counselling.
7. Means restriction. Strategies to restrict access to firearms, drugs, or other means of committing suicide.
8. Intervention after a suicide. Commonly called postvention, these programmes are designed to help survivors and prevent suicide clusters.

Miller and colleagues have published compelling evidence demonstrating the tragic role of firearms availability in youth suicide rates (Miller *et al.* 2006). As a result, suicide prevention recommendations now strongly support controlling access to firearms, as well as improved identification of depression and access to mental health services (AAP 2007).

Domestic violence

Domestic violence or partner violence is defined as violence between those involved in an intimate relationship. According to Department of Justice, approximately 4.8 million women and 2.9 million men were victims of intimate partner violence (Tjaden 2000). It involves physical abuse, sexual assault, threats of violence, and emotional abuse. Coercive control through degradation, malicious enforcement of petty rules, intermittent rewards and isolations are examples of the methods employed to demonstrate and maintain power.

However, in family situations, children under 12 years of age represent 62 per cent of all victims. Juveniles aged 12–17 comprise 30 per cent of the victims in overall offences, and 23 per cent in family occurrences. Females are most frequently the victims of family and overall offences, comprising 74–76 per cent of the victims of family and overall offences, respectively (Uniform Crime Reports 1998).

In 1998, 27 per cent of victims of family-related violence were reported to have been related to one or more of their offenders. A higher percentage of victims of family violence are over the age of 18 than the victims of overall crimes of violence (80 vs. 76 per cent). Additionally, victims of family violence are overwhelmingly female (71 per cent for family violence and 58 per cent for overall violence) (Uniform Crime Reports 1998).

Rape and sexual assault

The Federal Bureau of Investigation in the 1993 Uniform Crime Reports recorded 104 806 rapes in 1993, with a national rate of 79 per 100 000. The National Crime Victimization Survey indicates women report approximately 133 000 rapes each year, with half saying they reported them to the police and 55 per cent indicating that they knew the assailant.

Rape accounts for slightly less than 1 per cent of all violent offences. In particular, children under 12 years of age comprise a larger proportion of victims of family rape than all victims of rape (36 vs. 12 per cent) (FBI 1998).

Additional information is available from a national sample, the National Women's Study (Kilpatrick *et al.* 1992), suggesting a higher incidence and prevalence. According to this study, an estimated 683 000 women are raped each year, with 60 per cent being younger than 18 years old. The perpetrator was a stranger in only 22 per cent of the cases. This study estimates that 12.1 million American women are raped at some point in their lives. Only 16 per cent of them report the rape to the police.

Economic costs

In 2000, the total economic cost of violence in the United States from non-fatal injuries and death were over US$70 billion (Corso *et al.* 2007). Each year, US citizens pay about US$53.5 billion for criminal justice interventions for violence, and an additional US$158 billion for cost of lifetime care for victims of violence (medical treatment, rehabilitation, and lost productivity). These figures reflect only the monetary costs of violence, not the pain, suffering, and lost quality of life for victims. They do not reflect the cost for safety measures—the inability of children and adults to walk or play in their own neighbourhood, the cost of guard dogs and guns for 'protection', and an immeasurable sense of fear of crime victimization. In considering the impact of violence on society, it is also important to note the costs of violent crimes.

A framework model developed by Miller and colleagues (1993) was used to quantify costs of violent crime; it incorporated direct losses other than property losses (medical, mental health, and emergency services, insurance administration), productivity losses (wages, fringe benefits, housework), and non-monetary losses (pain, suffering, lost quality of life). Costs to victims of crimes resulting in injury were estimated to be US$110 000 for rape survivors, and US$23 000 for assault survivors (in 1993 dollars). Moreover, the lifetime costs of criminal victimizations for a person aged 12 and older was estimated to be US$10 billion for rape, US$96 billion for assault, and US$48 billion for murder (Miller *et al.* 1993).

Furthermore, these figures do not include property losses incurred during violent acts, nor the mammoth costs incurred by collective society's reactive response to violence, including law enforcement, adjudication, victim services, and correctional expenditures.

In 1993, the cost of direct medical spending, emergency services, and claims processed for the victims of gun violence nationwide totalled approximately US$3 billion. Average hospital charges for treating one child wounded by gunfire were more than US$14 000.

Taxpayers pay for gun violence. The average cost (including medical treatment and the prosecution and incarceration of the shooter) of one gunshot wound patient (all age groups) can be up to US$1.79 million (Lengel 1997). Approximately 80 per cent of patients who suffer from violence are uninsured and/or eligible for government medical care assistance. A study of all direct and indirect costs of gun violence, including medical, lost wages, and security costs, estimates that gun violence costs the nation US$100 billion a year (Cook 2000). The average total cost of one gun crime can be as high as US$1.79 million, including medical treatment and the prosecution and imprisonment of the shooter (Rice 1993). At least 80 per cent of the economic costs of treating firearm injuries are paid by taxpayer dollars (Wintemute 1992).

The characteristics of violence

Contrary to the stereotype of violence as predominantly stranger-related or occurring in the context of criminal behaviour such as racial harassment, robbery, or drug-dealing, much of the violence experienced in the United States is intimate and occurs in the context of personal relationships (FBI 2006). A typical homicide involves two people who know each other, who are under the influence of alcohol and get into an argument that escalates in the presence of a gun. Only 15 per cent of homicides occur in the course of committing a crime, as compared with over 50 per cent that stem from arguments among acquaintances (CDC 1982). This 50 per cent takes place in family relationships (e.g. child abuse, elder abuse, spouse abuse) or friends (interpersonal peer violence). In the remaining 35 per cent, the relationship between victim and perpetrator is unknown.

The perpetrators and victims of violence share many traits. They are likely to be young and male and of the same race. They are likely to be poor and to have been exposed to violence in the past, especially family violence. They may be depressed and use alcohol and/or other drugs (Prothrow-Stith & Weissman 1991). This incongruity between public perception and actual circumstances has resulted in demands for resources and solutions that address only part—possibly the smaller part—of the problem. While certainly not discarding established anti-crime and anti-violence strategies, we must recognize the diversity of violent circumstances that exist and must build a broader base of efforts that not only responds to violent events, but also focuses on preventive services as well.

A closer look at the demographic characteristics reveals certain noteworthy factors contributing to a complex picture of adolescent violence. Breaking down the 10–24 years of age spectrum further, 1997 homicide rates (deaths per 100 000) were considerably higher among 20–24-year-olds (19) and 15–19-year-olds (11.7) compared with 10–14-year-olds (1.7)—yet, it is still important to note that the rates increased among all three groups from 1979 to 1988 (CDC 1998). In terms of gender, males greatly exceed females in the number of violent victimizations, with the exception of sexual assault and are also more likely to be violent offenders and witnesses to violence.

Contact that health professionals have with victims and perpetrators

The regular contact physicians and nurses have with victims of violence, particularly in emergency departments, has caused many to begin to address this problem. The American College of Emergency Physicians has included violence prevention on the agenda of their annual meetings. The Journal of the American Medical Association has dedicated two special issues to the topic of violence, concurrent with the American Medical Associations publication of manuals for health providers on domestic violence, child abuse, and rape and sexual assault.

The Northeast Ohio Trauma Study illustrates the need for greater data from emergency departments in showing that five times the number of assaults reported to the police was reported to hospital emergency departments. Not only are non-fatal violent episodes inadequately measured with police data, but the greater contact health providers have with victims provides an opportunity to offer public health prevention and intervention strategies in the emergency department. Such programmes have been started at Boston City Hospital (now the Boston Medical Center and no longer a government hospital), Cook County Hospital in Chicago, Harborview Hospital in Seattle, and the Washington and Grady Memorial Hospital in Atlanta, Georgia, in the United States.

There is a substantial body of research which suggests that crime rates reflect 'community social disorganization'. The social disorganization theory was originally developed by the Chicago School researchers, Clifford Shaw and Henry McKay, in their classic work, *Juvenile Delinquency and Urban Areas* (1942). Shaw and McKay demonstrated that the same socioeconomically disadvantaged areas in 21 US cities continued to exhibit high delinquency rates over a span of several decades, despite changes in their racial and ethnic composition, indicating the persistent contextual effects of these communities on crime rates, regardless of what populations experienced them. This observation led them to reject individualistic explanations of delinquency and to focus instead on community processes such as disruption of local community organization and weak social controls, which lead to the apparent trans-generational transmission of criminal behaviour. In general, social disorganization is defined as the 'inability of a community structure to realize the common values of its residents and maintain effective social controls' (Sampson & Groves 1989). The social organizational approach views local communities and neighbourhoods as complex systems of friendship, kinship, and acquaintanceship networks, as well as formal and informal associational ties rooted in family life and ongoing socialization processes (Sampson 1995). From the perspective of crime control, a major dimension of social disorganization is the ability of a community to supervise and control teenage peer groups, especially gangs. Thus, Shaw and McKay (1942) argued that residents of cohesive communities were better able to control the youth behaviours that set the context for gang violence. Examples of such controls include 'supervision of leisure-time youth activities, intervention in street-corner congregation, and challenging youth who seem to be up to no good'. Socially disorganized communities with extensive street-corner peer groups are also expected to have higher rates of adult violence, especially among younger adults who still have ties to youth gangs' (Sampson 1995).

Application of public health strategies

Public health professionals have applied traditional public health strategies to violence prevention. They have brought a different perspective and orientation to bear on the problem. Applying public health techniques and strategies complements and strengthens the criminal justice approach.

Public health brings an analytic approach to problems by concentrating on identifying risk factors as well as factors that influence resiliency that could become the focus of preventive interventions. It also brings a record of accomplishment in controlling 'accidental' (unintentional) injuries through both environmental manipulations (for example, seat belts and childproof caps on medicines) and behavioural change (for example, laws and educational campaigns to reduce drunk-driving).

Identification of risk factors

Public health strategies have added to the literature on the understanding of violence and its risk factors. In combination with the work from other disciplines, major risk factors for youth violence have been identified. These factors can be broadly categorized into environmental and psychological risk factors. The major environmental risk factors include firearms, alcohol and other drugs, and cultural factors; being a victim of child abuse, witnessing family violence, exposure to media violence, and exposure to high levels of peer and community violence. A consistent and strong environmental risk factor for homicide is poverty. The mechanism for this interaction is not completely understood, but may include: (1) the anger and frustration associated with not having money and essential commodities; (2) the experience of classism; (3) the likely absence of adult male role models; (4) the scarcity of recreational, extracurricular, and after-school activities; and (5) more time spent watching television.

Corporal punishment is a controversial environmental factor that may be related to risk for violence. Certainly, in its extreme form, abuse, there is an evidence to suggest that it increases the risk of delinquency. Efforts to improve parenting and to reduce child abuse often focus on alternative disciplinary strategies. Other environmental risk factors for adolescents include peer pressure, the crack cocaine epidemic, and policing practices.

Race and poverty

There appear to be extremely large racial differences in violence rates among young Americans. In 1991, homicide was the number one cause of death for black youth aged between 15 and 24; the homicide rate for black youth (both sexes) was eight times the rate for white youth aged between 15 and 24 (90 per 100 000 vs. 10.8 per 100 000, respectively). National statistics concerning other ethnic minority groups, such as Latin Americans, Asian–Americans, and Native Americans, are scant.

The racial data are not indicative of any biological or genetic factor, because they are confounded by socioeconomic status, urban living, gun availability, and racism. Using family income as the primary indicator of socioeconomic status, the National Crime Survey found an inverse relationship between income and the risk of violent vicitmization (Bureau of Justice Statistics 1992). In 1988, the risk of victimization was found to be 2.5 times higher for people in low-income families (under US$7500 per year) when compared to high-income families (US$50 000 per year).

It is important to note, however, that the relationship of violence and social factors is complex and still unclear. For example, multivariate studies have shown a complicated interaction between race and socioeconomic status. That is to say, at low socioeconomic levels, black individuals have a higher risk of homicide compared to white individuals. At higher socioeconomic levels, however, the difference disappears. William Julius Wilson's work on neighbourhood poverty offers a possible explanation. Poor black people are much more likely than poor white people to live in neighbourhoods, where the majority of the people are poor. Although it appears that race is a significant social predictor in certain studies, multivariate studies show a more complex situation.

Other studies have suggested that, in fact, socioeconomic status is the major predictor, and race is merely a marker. One study that used several markers for poverty, including number of people per square foot of housing, disaggregated the race and socioeconomic variables. In this study, overcrowded white people had the same high domestic homicide rates as overcrowded black people.

Less-crowded members of both groups had the same lower rates (Centerwall 1984, 1993). In 1987, the homicide rate for young black men in the military was 1/12th of their national rate, strongly indicating the influence of social, structural, cultural, and economic factors.

Child neglect and abuse

Child abuse and neglect are general terms used to encompass many harmful behaviours toward children. Verbal, emotional, and sexual abuse are included, as well as failure to meet a child's needs, and outright physical violence. Child sexual abuse is most often considered separately, yet each state has its own definition and guidelines for protective custody.

Because child abuse has been a reportable crime for many years, better statistics are available. An annual 50-state survey estimated two million reports of child abuse and neglect in 1986. Over the decade of the 1980s, the number of reports increased by 184 per cent (Daro & Mitchel 1987). The number of child sexual abuse reports increased dramatically as well, a 12-fold increase within the decade. It is obvious that researchers have the same problem documenting both child abuse and child sexual abuse as they do documenting other forms of violence—unreliable data sources, under-reporting by victims, inconsistent definitions, and failure to recognize an event as precipitated by violence.

With child abuse, reporting biases work in both directions, both to inflate or deflate the numbers. Episodes of child abuse occurring in families of middle-class and professional parents are less likely to be reported, even with mandatory reporting laws, which diminish prevalence estimates. Yet, greater awareness and sensitivity to child abuse and the advent of mandatory reporting no doubt increase the numbers. There is a struggle among child health and human service professionals to determine the way to maintain mandatory reporting and improve the effectiveness of the state protective services. An over-reliance on foster care without adequate attention to family preservation seems to have been the rule in the past.

The cycle of violence

The relationship between child abuse, neglect, and witnessing violence to adolescent and adult violence has been demonstrated in several studies. Existing studies suggest that there is a greater likelihood of abuse by parents if they were abused as children. Estimates of the percentages of abusive parents who were abused as children ranged from 7 per cent (Gil 1973) to 70 per cent (Egeland & Jacobvitz 1984). Among adults who were abused, up to one-third of them abuse their children (Straus & Gelles 1990).

A retrospective look at violent juvenile delinquents compared with non-violent juvenile delinquents showed a significantly higher rate of physical child abuse. Both interviews with the delinquents and medical chart reviews yielded evidence of greater victimization, skull fractures, emergency trauma visits, and other physical injuries.

A cohort study of abused or neglected children demonstrated a greater risk for delinquency, adult criminal behaviour, and violent criminal behaviour, even though the majority of such children do not demonstrate these behaviours. The abused children had a number of offences, and began delinquent behaviour at earlier ages, regardless of race and gender (Widom 1989).

For black adolescents aged 11–19 living in or around an urban housing project, the self-reported use of violence was associated with exposure to violence and personal victimization, hopelessness, depression, family conflict, and previous corporal punishment. Those with a higher sense of purpose in life and less depression were better able to handle the exposure to violence in the home and community (Durant *et al.* 1994).

Children and exposure to media violence

The association between childhood exposure to media violence and subsequent aggressive behaviour has been firmly established over the past four decades. The American Psychological Association collected these data and decided unequivocally to pronounce the negative influence of entertainment media violence on children in a report (American Psychological Association Commission on Violence and Youth 1993). They expected the report to have an impact on parents and policy makers. Other reviews of the literature have been done with similar conclusions (Dietz & Strasburger 1991; Sege & Dietz 1994).

Pre-school children exposed to violent activity in a controlled setting were observed to imitate and repeat the violent behaviours (Bandura *et al.* 1963). It involved an actor appearing on screen attacking a Bobo-the-clown doll. Following this attack, in three separate video sequences, the actor was praised, ignored, or punished. The pre-school-aged viewers who saw the violent behaviour rewarded onscreen were more likely than the other two groups to repeat the violent actions when shown a Bobo-the-clown doll themselves. This experiment demonstrated that children can learn violent behaviours from television, and are especially likely to do so when these activities are depicted as socially acceptable.

Older children's behaviour is also heavily influenced by exposure to media violence. Meta-analysis of a series of experiences demonstrates conclusively that school-aged boys have more fights in the days following exposure to violent mainstream movies that they do in the days following exposure to less-violent movies (Turner *et al.* 1986; Wood *et al.* 1991).

In a landmark cohort study involving children raised in Pennsylvania, Huesmann and Eromn showed that preference for violent television programmes at age eight, as well as total hours of television viewing, predicted the severity of violent criminal convictions by age 30 (Huesmann *et al.* 1984). This effect should, however, be modified by parental interventions (Huesmann *et al.* 1983; Liebert 1988; Austin *et al.* 1990; Weaver & Barbour 1992; Sang *et al.* 1993).

Centerwall has shown that in three different countries (the United States, Canada, and South Africa), homicide rates doubled approximately 10–12 years after the introduction of English-language television (Centerwall 1992). In the United States, homicide rates doubled first among those portions of the population exposed to television first (white urban dwellers), and only later among those segments of the population who received television later. He attributes approximately 10 000 deaths annually in the United States as the results of exposure to media violence.

Taken together, we believe that these studies meet most of the criteria for causality set forth in the Surgeon General's 1964 report on smoking and health (United States Department of Health, Education, and Welfare 1964), and established that exposure to media violence places children at risk for subsequent violence.

Public debate flourishes concerning the roles of video games and violence-oriented musical lyrics in encouraging violence. Currently, however, no definitive data are available on these issues.

Firearms

The United States has more firearms than any other industrialized nation not at war, and the following facts, extracted from the well-referenced 2007 website of the Brady Campaign to Prevent Gun Violence, are astounding:

- There are approximately 192 million privately owned firearms in the United States—65 million of which are handguns.
- Currently, an estimated 39 per cent of US households have a gun, while 24 per cent have a handgun.
- In 1998 alone, licensed firearms dealers sold an estimated 4.4 million guns, 1.7 million of which were handguns. Additionally, it is estimated that one to three million guns change hands in the secondary market each year, and many of these sales are not regulated.
- In 2004, 29 569 people in the United States died from firearm-related deaths—11 624 (39 per cent) of those were murdered, 16 750 (57 per cent) were suicides, 649 (2.2 per cent) were accidents, and for 235 (0.8 per cent), the intent was unknown. In comparison, 33 651 Americans were killed in the Korean War and 58 193 Americans were killed in the Vietnam War.
- In 2004, firearms were used to murder 56 people in Australia, 184 people in Canada, 73 people in England and Wales, 5 people in New Zealand, and 37 people in Sweden. In comparison, firearms were used to murder 11 344 people in the United States.
- In 2005, there were only 143 justifiable homicides by private citizens using handguns in the United States.
- In 2004, nearly eight children and teenagers aged 19 and under were killed with guns each day.
- In 2004, firearm homicide was the second leading cause of injury death for men and women 10–24 years of age, second only to motor vehicle crashes.
- In 2004, firearm homicide was the leading cause of death for black males aged 15–34 years.
- From 1999 through 2004, an average of 916 children and teenagers took their own lives with guns each year.
- For each time a gun is used in a home in a legally justifiable shooting, there are 22 criminal, unintentional, and suicide-related shootings.
- The presence of a gun in the home triples the risk of homicide in the home.
- The presence of a gun in the home increases the risk of suicide five-fold. A gun in the home is 43 times more likely to kill a family member or friend than it is to be used in self-defence.
- In the United States, in 2006, firearms were used in 67.9 per cent of murders, 42.2 per cent of robbery offences, and 21.9 per cent of aggravated assaults.
- In 2002, 1830 children in the United States under the age of 19 years died from gunshot wounds; 167 of these children were shot accidentally.

Teenage and young adult homicides are uniquely American problems. This high rate of youth homicide in the United States has been attributed to the much higher rate of gun ownership in the United States. An international study of gun ownership and homicide found positive correlations between the rates of household gun ownership and the national rates and proportions of gun-related homicide (Lester 1988; Killias 1993).

Handgun availability appears to be playing an increasingly important role in youth homicides. As an example, the increasing trend seen in the total homicide rate among 15–19-year-olds from 1979 to 1989 is solely attributable to the increase in firearm homicides; the firearm-related homicide rate increased 61 per cent (6.9–11.1 per 100 000), while, at the same time, the non-firearm-related homicide rates actually decreased by 29 per cent (3.4–2.4 per 100 000) (Fingerhut *et al.* 1992). From 1980 to 1989, over 65 per cent of the 11 000 homicides committed by high-school aged youth were firearm-related.

Handguns are widely accessible to adolescents in the United States. The national 2005 Youth Risk Behavior Survey found that about 5.4 per cent of high school students had carried a firearm at least once in the 30 days preceding the survey. The incidence was higher among males, 9.9 per cent (Centers for Disease Control and Prevention 2006). In another study of inner-city youths, as many as 35 per cent of males carried a gun outside of school (Sheley *et al.* 1992).

Firearms contribute to both the violent victimization of youth and to the violent offences committed by youth. The presence of a weapon in the home is associated with a three-fold increase in the likelihood of homicide, compared with matched controls drawn from the neighbourhood surrounding the victim (Kellerman *et al.* 1993).

Comparisons of two cities (Seattle and Vancouver) with similar demographic characteristics showed that Seattle's excess homicide rate is entirely attributable to firearm homicides (Sloan *et al.* 1988) (Fig. 10.5.6). Another study designed to look at the effect of implementation of gun control legislation showed a positive effect of the enactment of tougher gun control laws in the District of Columbia compared with both neighbouring states (Loftin *et al.* 1991).

All of these studies demonstrate that availability of firearms is strongly correlated with increased homicide rates. Logically, this result coincides with the earlier observation that most homicides result from conflicts among people who know each other well, including friends and acquaintances, as well as relatives and spouses.

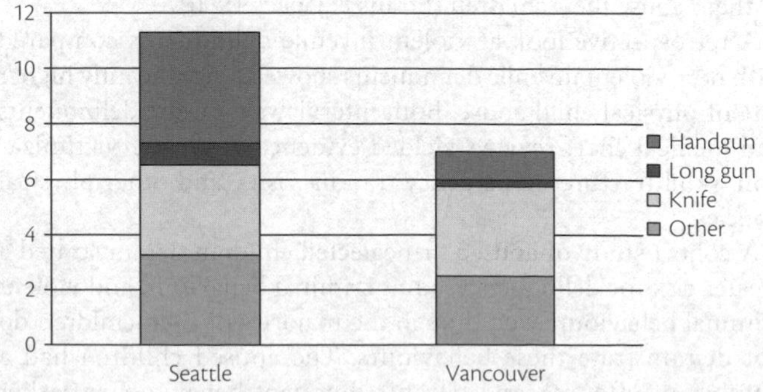

Fig. 10.5.6 Comparison of homicide rates in cities of similar demographics.

In a situation of passionate conflict, handgun availability appears to increase the likelihood of serious injury or death.

Psychological and behavioural factors

In pioneering studies conducted in the late 1980s, Slaby and Guerra (1988) demonstrated that adolescents involved in violence have habits of thought that lead them into violent confrontations. They examined the responses of three groups of teenaged boys to a specific scenario. One group of boys were in custody for the commission of violent crimes, a second group was identified by their teachers as being violence-prone, and a third group was identified by their teachers as not being violence-prone. Each boy was presented with the same scenario: They were going after school to work on their batting so that they could make the baseball team. As a boy arrived, another boy took the last bat. In understanding this scenario, the more violence-prone boys were more likely to assign malicious intent to the boy who took the bat than the less-violent boys. In imagining ways to resolve this scenario, these boys could envisage fewer alternative means towards resolution.

Slaby and Guerra concluded from this study that the more violence-prone boys got into more fights because they were more likely to see harmful intent in a given situation, and, having seen such intent, were less likely to come up with a peaceful way to resolve the situation. These results have been confirmed with a larger-scale study conducted in the New York City schools (Center for Disease Control and Prevention 1993). Boys who reported having been in serious fights were more likely to suggest that carrying a weapon or threatening to use a weapon were good ways to stay out of fights than the general school population; they were also far less likely to say that one could avoid fighting by apologizing compared with the overall population.

Witnessing violence

In addition to the young people directly injured by violence, increasing attention is being given to the scores more young people who are affected indirectly as witnesses to violent acts or by exposure to chronic violent environments (Groves *et al.* 1993). Pynoos and colleagues (1987) examined the appearance of post-traumatic stress disorder (PTSD) symptoms in children who experienced a fatal sniper attack on their elementary school, and reported a correlation between the type and number of post-traumatic stress disorder symptoms and proximity to the violent incident, as well as more severe symptoms in children who knew the deceased child.

In addition to acute incidents, other studies relate findings of correlations between exposure to chronic violence and distress symptoms (Fitzpatrick & Boldizar 1993; Freeman *et al.* 1993; Lorion & Saltzman 1993; Martinez & Richters 1993; Osofsky *et al.* 1993). In addition, Lorion and Saltzman (1993) described anecdotal reports from their research participants, including reports from teachers and administrators about children who lived in violent settings arriving at school in distress, who were unable to concentrate or maintain appropriate behaviour in class, and who hid in the classroom and were afraid to return home or take the bus. Clearly, there is a need to address not only the physical threat of violence, but also the potential for psychopathological and/or emotional disturbances in both victims and bystanders (Emde 1993; Durant *et al.* 1994).

Approaches to violence prevention and control

Historically, society has relied almost exclusively on the criminal justice system both to respond to and prevent violence. This tactic is rooted in the beliefs that violence is criminal, that those who commit violence should be punished, and that the threat of punishment is a potential deterrent to violent acts. A large, elaborate set of institutions has been developed to achieve these goals, which includes police, prosecutors, public defenders, judges, probation officers, and prison guards. It is principally designed to respond to crimes after they have been committed by identifying, apprehending, prosecuting, punishing, and controlling the violent offender. It is guided not only by the practical goals of reducing crimes of all types (including violence), but also by the normative goal of assuring justice to victims and the accused.

The public health and criminal justice systems historically have been separate in their conceptualization of approaches to violence and the development of activities to reduce or prevent violence. The public health field has approached the issue through efforts to identify the risk factors related to violent behaviour. The field comes to this issue in reaction to the magnitude of intentional injuries that are present in health care settings. The criminal justice system has approached the issue through efforts to identify and assign blame for criminal behaviour, maintain public safety, and remove violent offenders from the community.

Viewed from the perspective of those interested in reducing violence, the criminal justice system's responses have had only limited success. Part of the reason is inherent limitations in the overall approach of the criminal justice system. First, it is more reactive than preventive in its basic orientation. True, deterrence may produce some preventive results. True too, the criminal justice system has sought to rehabilitate offenders through special programmes in prisons, and to prevent children from becoming violent offenders through the development of the juvenile justice system, whose most fundamental goal is to prevent future criminal activity by children. Nonetheless, the criminal justice system comes into play only after a crime episode occurs.

Second, the criminal justice system, and particularly the police, is focused primarily on the predatory violence that occurs among strangers on the street. The violence that emerges from nagging frustrations and festering disputes and takes place in intimate settings is far more difficult for the criminal justice system to deal with than stranger-inflicted violence that arises from greed or desperate need, and takes place in the open. Robbery and burglary and their associated violence are more traditional and central to the criminal justice system's business (and consciousness) than aggravated assaults that spring up among friends in bars, lovers in bedrooms, or teenagers at dances.

Public health and criminal justice: Interdisciplinary challenges

Unfortunately, the collaboration of public health and criminal justice in the area of violence prevention has not reached its full potential. This may partially arise from a basic failure in effectively reducing the problem of violence that has put both disciplines on the defensive—criminal justice for its failure to bring the problem under control and meet societal expectations, and public health for the slowness with which it has recognized and taken on the problem. However, much of this tension probably comes from the divergence of perspective of the two disciplines and the fact that there are inadequate resources directed to addressing violence, which has forced the disciplines to compete rather than collaborate.

Public health is primarily focused on identifying causality (or its approximation) and intervening to control or reduce the risk factors; it has little interest in assigning blame or meting out punishment and does not discriminate between victim and offender. The public health community may agree that justice must be done, but is not professionally committed to the process. The criminal justice system, on the other hand, is deeply and morally rooted in 'justice' and criminal offenders being properly identified and punished. In this field, there is less emphasis on the precursors or factors that may have led to the violent event. The criminal justice system is less likely to consider external factors that might have motivated the offender to engage in violence, because it sees these issues as largely irrelevant to judgement of guilt and innocence. At worst, the claim that these other factors were causally important in the particular instance seems like a rationalization or an apology for what was a criminal deed. This rift is further exacerbated by the fact that the criminal justice profession continues to develop preventive agendas, such as first offender programmes and community policing initiatives, and probably feels that their 'thunder' and leadership are in jeopardy of being stolen by the entry of another professional player onto their turf.

This tension is clearly unproductive. It threatens effective collaboration and frustrates the opportunity to pool resources and expertise at a time when resources are seriously inadequate and the problem is increasing. Healing this rift requires a more collaborative spirit from both disciplines. The public health 'purists' must get beyond their science and recognize the invaluable contributions and practical experiences of the criminal justice professionals. The criminal justice 'moralists' must in turn recognize the limitations of a primary agenda of assigning blame and assuring justice is done.

If we are to get past these initial reactions and successfully exploit the complementary qualities of these two approaches to violence, it is essential to put aside professional jealousies. More importantly, we must better define the perspective, roles, and expertise both groups bring to the issue. This will not only lead to a more creative process, but will also establish productive working relationships.

Primary, secondary, and tertiary prevention

A conceptual framework that can alleviate professional tension, facilitate definitions of roles in addressing the problem, and assist in developing a broader perspective on programmatic strategies involves breaking the spectrum of violence into levels that reflect different points of intervention (Fig. 10.5.7). This framework, used frequently in public health circles, structures approaches to problems into three stages: Primary prevention, secondary prevention (or early intervention), and tertiary prevention (or treatment/rehabilitation). More recently, in public health, these levels have been labelled universal (primary), selected (secondary), and targeted (tertiary) (Prothrow-Stith & Weissman 1991; Guterman 2004). However, the most user-friendly label emerged from a group of young people working on the Blueprint for a Safer Philadelphia: Up-Front (primary), In-the-Thick (secondary), and After-the-Fact (tertiary). Labels aside, these three levels have proven to be valuable

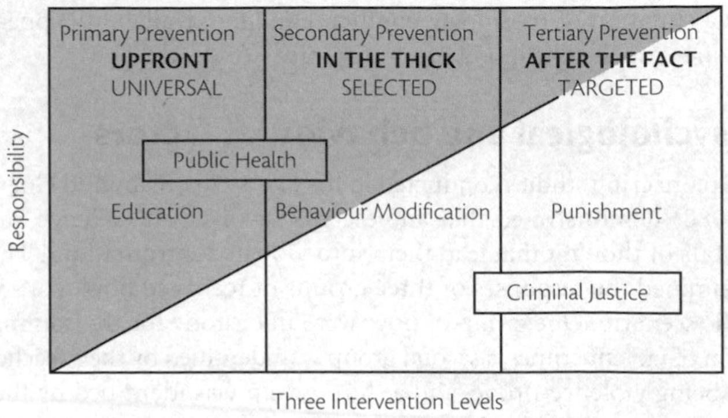

Fig. 10.5.7 Three levels of violence prevention: Public health and criminal justice.

in understanding a spectrum of intervention efforts. Their boundaries are not rigid or discrete; the same prevention activity for an adolescent or young adult 'in-the-thick' might actually be 'up-front' for a younger brother/sister or son/daughter. Tertiary prevention is distinguished from secondary and primary prevention in which it lies on the opposite side of the violent event than the other two. Its focus is on trying to reduce the negative consequences of a particular event after it has occurred, or on trying to find ways to use the event to reduce the likelihood of similar incidents occurring in the future. Thus, one might think of improved trauma care on the one hand, and increased efforts to rehabilitate or incapacitate violent offenders on the other hand, as tertiary prevention instruments in the control of or the response to violence.

Primary prevention, which by definition addresses the broadest level of the general public, might seek to reduce the level of violence that is shown on television or to promote gun control. This would be an effort directed towards dealing with the public values and attitudes that may promote or encourage the use of violence.

Secondary prevention is distinguished from primary prevention in that it identifies relatively narrowly defined subgroups or circumstances that are at high risk for being involved in or occasioning violence, and focuses its attention on them. Thus, secondary prevention efforts might focus on poor urban young men who are at particularly high risk for engaging in or being victimized by violence, and educating them in non-violent methods of resolving disputes or displaying competence and power.

The relative risk level of groups or circumstances is a continuum, with some people and circumstances at very high risk (a person who has been victimized by violence in his or her own home, also surrounded by violence in school, entering a bar in which members of a rival gang are drinking), and others at relatively low-risk (e.g. a happily married professor who owns no weapon more lethal than a screwdriver, writing on her computer at home). Moreover, it is generally true that the higher risk groups are smaller than the lower risk groups.

Primary prevention instruments are those that can affect larger and larger populations, ideally at relatively low cost. Indeed, the need to reach very large populations requires primary prevention efforts to be low cost per individual reached. Thus, primary prevention instruments tend to be those providing information and education on the problem of violence through the popular media; for example, the recruitment of Bill Cosby to the cause of using the media to prevent adolescent violence, or Sarah Brady's efforts to advocate for gun control laws and educate the public about the risks of handguns, rather than providing non-violence training to the entire population. There are, of course, the ultimate long-term primary prevention goals that have to do with eliminating some of the root causes of violence, such as social injustice and discrimination.

This public health model can be very useful when applied specifically to the issue of interpersonal violence. In the past, the criminal justice system has addressed each of the three points of intervention to varying degrees as represented, yet the bulk of the efforts have focused on the response to serious violent behaviour, with moderate attention to early identification and intervention and limited efforts in the area of primary prevention.

The major activities of the criminal justice system have historically involved the roles of the police, the courts, and the prison system in responding to criminal or violent events. Most resources have been directed to investigating and punishing criminal behaviour. Tertiary prevention has generally involved incarceration. In the area of secondary prevention, the police have focused efforts on 'situated' crime prevention, and the juvenile justice system has made attempts at early intervention with youthful offenders, although youth were frequently ignored by the courts and probation system until their criminal behaviour reached a relatively high level of concern. Primary prevention efforts have focused on elementary school drug and violence prevention education by the police, as well as on controlling 'criminogenic' commodities such as drugs, guns, and alcohol.

With the more recent involvement of the public health system, attention has been broadened, with enhanced efforts in the prevention arena. The public health agenda has focused primarily on prevention and early intervention, playing only a small role in the treatment of individuals with serious violence-related problems. The roles and activities of the public health system are newer, less extensive, and therefore less evolved than that of the criminal justice system.

Traditionally, public health responded by treating the violence-related injury in the emergency setting. Today, a new generation of committed health practitioners, community violence-prevention practitioners, social workers, and community activists have devised numerous intervention programmes to serve medium- to high-risk adolescents. At the primary prevention level, efforts have focused on gun control and safety, and enhanced public awareness of risk factors and the true characteristics of most violence to dispel myths and modify societal values around the use of violence. Additionally, some educational interventions (e.g. violence prevention curricula) have been applied to broader, less high-risk settings. Again, much of this work is relatively recent, and therefore has not yet established a long track record to fully assess its effects. Finally, public health has applied its analytical expertise to greatly enhance the understanding of risk factors, allowing for a broader vision in the planning and development of preventive approaches (Prothrow-Stith & Spivak 2004).

Recently published information regarding the effectiveness of school-based primary prevention (universal) programmes was encouraging for practitioners (Hahn *et al.* 2007; Prothrow-Stith 2007). Robert Hahn and colleagues, in a meta-analysis, demonstrated an average of 15 per cent reduction in fighting in those schools employing a universal programme, regardless of the grade level of the school, the socioeconomic status of students, or other related factors. One can conclude from these data that every US school should have an 'up-front' violence prevention programme for all students.

In the area of secondary prevention, public health has been involved in the development of educational interventions specifically focused on behaviour modification of high-risk individuals, particularly children and youth. A number of curricula are currently in use addressing both the risks of violence in solving problems and conflict resolution techniques (Prothrow-Stith & Spivak 2004).

It is important to note that the criminal justice system has more recently increased its involvement with primary and secondary prevention efforts. For example, some criminal justice professionals have become increasingly involved in gun control initiatives. In 1974, the Juvenile Justice and Delinquency Prevention Act was passed and it gave a primary responsibility to the Justice Department for delinquency prevention programmes. The Office of Juvenile Justice and Delinquency Prevention was designed in part to encourage the development of model delinquency prevention programmes. One such programme is the Boys Clubs of America Targeting Programs for Delinquency Intervention. Other community groups refer at-risk boys to the programme, who are then recruited. Early evaluations of these programmes seem promising. Data indicate that 39 per cent of the boys did better in school and 93 per cent of those who completed the programme have not been re-involved with the juvenile system (Boys Clubs of America 1986). These types of interventions reflect an important interface between the criminal justice and public health professions. With further attention and the dedication of resources of the public health system to this issue and the broadening vision of criminal justice, a more reasonable balance between prevention and treatment can be achieved in the future. Efforts can be broadened to reflect more fully the range of efforts needed to reduce both the extent of violent behaviour and respond to the violence that does occur. The emphasis of the public health system will be on prevention, with the criminal justice system prioritizing the response to violence, but with both disciplines working together across the spectrum.

Cigarette smoking reduction: A model for intervention

To illustrate the advantages of this approach, it is useful to the review how it has worked successfully in other areas. One example, which on the surface appears to be a considerable stretch from violence, is the multidisciplinary approach that has been developed to deal with tobacco use. It is important to note that while this example illustrates a collaboration between public health and the medical care system, it represents a useful analogy to the possible collaboration between public health and criminal justice.

Smoking is a major contributing factor to death and disability in the United States. Significant inroads have been made in turning the tide on this major health threat. What was once a valued, sexy, and socially acceptable behaviour is now viewed as a disgusting, unhealthy, and socially unacceptable behaviour. Heroes in the media used to smoke all the time; now they rarely do. Nationally, the number of people who smoke has declined dramatically, although smoking was and still is a learned behaviour; one that can be unpleasant or distasteful when starting, but is extremely difficult to stop.

The strategy to deal with smoking involved a three-pronged approach: Primary prevention for those not yet smoking to teach the reasons for not starting and to support the decision not to start; secondary prevention to encourage stopping or reducing use for those who had already started smoking (often this involves helping individuals to identify alternative behaviours to replace the smoking behaviour); and treatment in the form of surgery or chemotherapy and other medical interventions for those smokers who have developed cancer or other health consequences of their behaviour. Broad public initiatives to alter the societal values that encouraged smoking were also established to support the above efforts. This has been done through legislation (package labelling, advertising constraints, restrictions on sales to minors, establishment of smoke-free environments), public education, and pressure on media to change images and role models. Although, as stated earlier, this is an example of a public health/medical care interface, it represents an important success that has value in looking at the possibilities of a public health and criminal justice collaboration in addressing violence.

A similar approach could and should be taken with respect to violence. Primary prevention strategies and more targeted secondary prevention efforts need to be applied that proactively value and teach non-violent behaviours in response to anger and conflict. This is particularly important when the growing evidence that violence is a learned behaviour is given (Bandura *et al.* 1963; Liebert *et al.* 1973; Slaby & Quarfoth 1980; Allen 1981; Eron & Huesmann 1984; Straus 1991; Vissing *et al.* 1991; Prothrow-Stith & Spivak 2004; Prothrow-Stith & Spivak 2005). Well-child health visits in neighbourhood health centres provide an ideal window of opportunity for early intervention. Peter Stringham, a paediatrician at the East Boston Neighborhood Health Center, incorporates a violence prevention protocol for families, from newborn visits through the teenage years. Social skills are as important to teach our children as the academic subjects which we now emphasize in our society. This will in no way eliminate the underlying societal stresses that influence violent behaviour, but can affect and direct responses to these stresses toward a pro-social and productive outcome. Curricula that place emphasis on decision-making, non-violent conflict resolution, and self-esteem development currently exist, but are terribly under-utilized and viewed as an 'add on' in academic settings rather than a basic component. A move to place more emphasis on the use of such curricula, with enhanced investment in social and support services for families and youth, will be an important step in countering the learned use of violence by our youth. Such a move would also require that the education, human services, and public health institutions play major roles in effecting these changes in our communities.

Indeed, the recognition that education designed to teach non-violent behaviours might be an important part of a combined public health/criminal justice response to the problem of violence helps to remind us that the modern view of how the law operates on behaviour in the society has become far more narrow that it once was. In our modern conceptions of the law, we imagine it operating on individual behaviour primarily through its incentive effects—the promise of punishment for misconduct made concrete and credible through individual prosecutions.

In the classic writings on laws, however, a great deal of attention was devoted not only to the passage of laws and to their application to individual cases, but also to their promulgation throughout society (Friedman 1975). Extensive efforts to explain and educate citizens as to why the laws were necessary helped to ensure both their justice and their efficacy. Unless citizens knew about the law—its spirit as well as its letter—they could not reasonably be held accountable for failures to obey it. If the purpose of the law is not made clear, voluntary compliance—which is crucial to the law's effect—could not be counted upon.

The public health community's interest in non-violence education can be viewed as the modern rediscovery of the importance of explaining to and educating the public about violence, as well as simply having laws and applying them. It also incorporates an important modern discovery about the promulgation of obligations; it is often far easier to persuade people to comply with an important obligation when one can show individuals that it is in their best interests to do so, and when one can help them comply with the law. Persuasion and assistance are often more effective tools than accusation and blame. Still, it often helps in persuading and assisting if there is a broad social rule against violence that becomes part of the context for the education. Thus, behavioural change may depend on a combination of education and laws that were previously known as promulgation.

Gun control legislation efforts represent an important example of the interconnection between education and laws. Although there is growing support for increased handgun ownership restrictions as a primary prevention strategy, legislation alone is unlikely to create great change in violent injury rates in the foreseeable future. With over 60 million handguns in circulation in the United States (Bureau of Alcohol, Tobacco & Firearms 1991), understanding and acceptance of the risks of handgun ownership and carrying is as important as legislative restrictions to reduce intentional handgun injuries.

Secondary level strategies require a more targeted effort. They require early identification of individuals at high risk for or already beginning to exhibit violent behaviour and the development of treatment services for these individuals. This area represents an important interface between the human services and the criminal justice systems, because early identification of individuals at high risk for violence requires considerable collaboration. Points of early identification occur in schools, health facilities, police departments, courts, and a variety of other community institutions. Professional training in early identification and appropriate evaluation and treatment is necessary. This is not an easy process. Professional definitions and institutional boundaries have been established that encourage limited one-dimensional approaches.

Treatment interventions (tertiary prevention) for the most seriously affected individuals represent a key focal point for the criminal justice system. Violent behaviour cannot be condoned; punishment is an appropriate response to violent crimes or episodes, and some individuals with serious pathology are not able to live in the general society. While it is essential that we understand how violent behaviour evolves, we must deal with it firmly to maintain safety within communities.

Although tertiary prevention falls most extensively into the criminal justice realm, with incarceration as the major strategy, public health needs to work along with the prison system in the area of rehabilitation. Without increased attention to rehabilitative efforts, including supportive services for those returning from prison to the community, most of them will continue to leave the prison system without the skills to avoid violence in the future. Public health must advocate for and support drug and alcohol treatment services, job training efforts, conflict resolution and violence prevention skills, as well as the development of more extensive behavioural change interventions. To date, successful rehabilitative efforts are limited, further reinforcing the need for more attention focused on this area as well.

Promising prevention programmes using public health strategies

Researchers Joy G. Dryfoos and Lisbeth Schorr both agree that the most effective programmes must be comprehensive, family- and community-oriented, and collaborative in nature. Some schools, communities, social agencies, and politicians around the country have incorporated this formula for success and have developed strategies to help children and their families prevent or cope with violence. These programmes offer the opportunity to learn from their successes and failures.

Peace zone: An elementary school programme for emotional intelligence

Peace Zone is an elementary school-based programme (ages 4–11 years) that is designed to increase students' ability to make positive decisions, avoid risk-taking behaviour, and heal from trauma and loss. A secondary goal of the PZ programme is to assure that the adults are able to reinforce the core concepts with children, both at home and in school. 'Two Approaches to Violence Prevention' are integrated into Peace Zone. The programme combines classroom activities that build social skills with those that promote healing from trauma, grief, and loss. Psychomotor expressive activities (visual arts, music, dance, etc.) and community service shape the key healing activities. The programme includes a School Climate Change Module and six classroom-based units:

- The Louis D. Brown Story
- Pledge for Peace
- Trying Your Best
- Self-Control
- Thinking and Problem Solving
- Cooperation

Each unit contains four 30-min lessons and takes approximately 1 week to complete. The last lesson of each unit links the topic to a community service activity. The entire programme can be presented in 6 weeks; however, it should be continued and reinforced throughout the school year with supplemental booster activities. Full implementation of the programme includes lead teachers at each grade level, a half-time school counsellor to support both classroom- and school-wide activities, and a commitment to consistent utilization of the common Peace Zone language throughout the school.

A strong theoretical foundation supports the Peace Zone programme, which was created by an experienced, diverse, academic-practitioner partnership (comprised of Harvard Youth Violence Prevention Center, the Lesson One Company, the Louis D. Brown Peace Institute, and the Boston Public Schools). The programme is based upon social cognitive theory and the research of Howard Gardner (*Frames of Mind*), who advances the concept of developing 'emotional intelligence' to enhance a child's ability for personal adjustment and resiliency throughout life.

Positive evaluation data and a substantial developmental process underlie the efforts to adapt and disseminate Peace Zone. In 1998, the partners received a multi-million dollar competitive grant from the US Department of Education to create Peace Zone. The programme qualified for the maximum full 5 years of funding by demonstrating positive impact data. Pre- and post-surveys were conducted in grades 3–5 in experimental and comparison schools. Paired *t*-tests were conducted to assess changes in outcomes relevant to the programme in three intervention schools. Both boys and girls reported significant reductions in being victimized by other children at school. Boys reported a decrease in perpetration of violence, and there were remarkable reductions in mild to severe depression reported by both boys and girls.

Resolving Conflict Creatively Program—school-based conflict resolution programme in New York, California, and Alaska

The 'Resolving Conflict Creatively Program', a holistic school-based conflict resolution programme, works with the entire school structure to create safe schools. The K-12 curriculum, developed and refined since 1986, requires support from school administration, although it does not mandate that every teacher should be trained. Each of the 32 school districts in New York City that use the curriculum maintains a certain autonomy, leaving decision-making to the school community. After an intense 40-h training on the curriculum, teachers incorporate the methods into their classrooms.

The programme invites and encourages the participation of parents in training. Both teachers and administrators in these schools document fewer fights and a sense of peace. Students become peer mediators and receive special training to negotiate and mediate arguments that break out during school hours.

The programme provides a win–win situation. Not only do students develop leadership skills and a sense of responsibility for peace and respect, but teachers and administrators find practical use for conflict resolution skills in their lives. The programme also offers regular advanced training sessions in such topics as helping students deal with death and grief.

A walk through the hallways of the Satellite Academy High School in the Bronx gives the sense that despite unsafe surroundings, the school offers an oasis of safety, a place of mutual respect—a place where learning takes place. Programme evaluations show that both teachers and students notice a positive change in the schools. A more comprehensive programme evaluation was recently funded through a grant from the Centers for Disease Control and Prevention.

Louis D. Brown Peace Institute (LDBPI) and survivors of violence for prevention

The Louis D. Brown Peace Institute was founded in 1994 to continue the peacemaking legacy of a 15-year-old youth leader named Louis D. Brown. The following seven principles are the core of this work: Love, unity, faith, hope, courage, justice, and forgiveness. The LDBPI is a unique organization in the City of Boston and in the nation. Founded to assist and support the families of homicide victims, the LDBPI rapidly grew into a model agency offering shelter and services to families in the most difficult times of their lives and a model for nonviolence to the city that Louis D. Brown called home.

The LDBPI has now developed a fully integrated curriculum for all elementary, middle- and high-school students that prepares them to deal with trauma and grief, build nonviolence and conflict resolution skills, and commit themselves to peace work in their families and their communities. These skills are also taught in workshops for community-based groups throughout the Commonwealth.

Policy advocacy is an ongoing effort of the Peace Institute. The LDBPI has successfully advocated for a state-wide calendar of events related to violence prevention, and worked with the state legislators to establish a Survivors of Homicide Victims Awareness Month, from November 20 to December 20 every year. The LDBPI staff and volunteers have also testified against the death penalty. The LDBPI is committed to restorative justice and building sustainable peace in our home communities. To perform this, the LDPBI works hand-in-hand with young men who have been defined as 'the problem' to build peace block by block in the communities of Dorchester. Following the lead of these young men, mothers who have lost their sons to murder or to prison have reached out to each other to form the Massachusetts Mothers on the Move (Memo's).

The LDBPI works to create and promote an environment where families can live in peace and unity. It is committed to restorative justice practices and struggles together with the members of our communities to create and promote an environment, where young people and their families are valued for their peacemaking efforts. The goals are to develop programmes and activities that teach and instil the values of peace and enrich the lives of young people; to assist/empower survivors of homicide victims with tools that not only rebuild their lives but also their communities through education, collaboration, and policy advocacy; and to inform and educate the public about the causes and the consequences of violence on the individual, the family and the community, while transforming the community.

School-based management—Comer method schools

More than 300 schools from around the country have adopted an educational model designed by Yale University's James P. Comer. Comer, a psychiatrist, began his school-based work in one of New Haven's most troubled schools in 1968. He designed a multidisciplinary approach to school management. The programme stresses that a partnership between educators and parents is critical to a school's success. Its philosophy is based on the premise that each child is special and that schools should be places of learning.

Comer's model is also based on the premise that the initial relationship between schools and disadvantaged parents is too often wrought with mistrust and alienation. Comer schools require parental representation on all levels, including the school's management team. These parents also work to increase the involvement of other parents in the school's mission to educate all children.

Blueprint for a safer Philadelphia

In 2006, State Representative Dwight Evans of Philadelphia, Pennsylvania, in the United States, culminated several years of community organizing and partnership building activities by kicking off a 10-year initiative to end youth violence in Philadelphia, The Blueprint for a Safer Philadelphia. The Blueprint's mission is to use proven, research-based public health methods to develop and implement a long-term strategy to help reduce gun violence and end youth homicides in Philadelphia by the year 2016. The multi-tiered Blueprint for a Safer Philadelphia Initiative includes influencing attitudes and changing community norms surrounding youth violence, and uses social, cultural, and educational programmes as a way to prevent violence before it begins.

The *Blueprint* Campaign has more than 400 community partners citywide that have pledged their support. Community partners, including community-based organizations, schools, churches, recreation centres, clinics, etc., receive information and updates about various Blueprint events, meetings, and activities.

Created to stop rising gun and youth violence, the Blueprint for a Safer Philadelphia Initiative is a unique and innovative approach that augments the traditional criminal justice response with a public health prevention model.

The public health initiative is disseminating pro-social messages to both youth and adults through a variety of traditional and non-traditional communications channels. All elements of the violence prevention campaign are culturally relevant, street-credible, and audience-tested.

Over the next decade, the Blueprint Initiative will work to:

- Heighten public awareness of alternatives to violence.
- Provide youth and their families with access to support and resources, along with options for changing their lives.
- Empower local community-based organizations to address the root needs of the area youth.

Harvard Youth Violence Prevention Center (HYVPC)

The Harvard Youth Violence Prevention Center (HYVPC) is a multidisciplinary violence prevention centre dedicated to *working collaboratively to build community capacity for youth violence prevention in Boston*. Located at the Harvard School of Public Health, the Center activities are based on the premise that effective prevention evolves from mutually respectful, reciprocal relationships between community members, researchers, and policy-makers. HYVPC has an outstanding multidisciplinary staff with expertise in survey research, programme evaluation, youth violence prevention, social capital, and interactive collaborations with community agencies and organizations. Other important, inter-related issues addressed by the centre include injury and suicide prevention, collective efficacy and community capacity-building, safety for children and youth, and youth development.

HYVPC collaborates with 11 Grassroots Community Partners in Boston, as well as with the Boston Mayor's Office, Boston Centers for Youth and Families, Boston Public Schools, Boston After School and Beyond, Boston Redevelopment Authority, Boston Police Department, and the Boston Foundation. HYVPC's primary goals are to work collaboratively across multiple levels of community to: (1) define the problem of youth exposure to, victimization by, and perpetration of violence; (2) identify risk and protective factors for youth experiences with violence; (3) develop and test youth violence prevention strategies; and (4) assure widespread adoption of strategies shown to be effective. Central to this effort, HYVPC is creating a multi-layered data gathering and analysis system for youth violence in Boston that includes: (1) a comprehensive representative biennial survey of public and private high-school and middle-school students; (2) a concurrent biennial community-based telephone survey of adults in Boston households conducted in parallel with the youth survey; (3) GIS integration and mapping of city, state, and federal data on neighbourhood characteristics, city trends, and initiatives that affect youth and communities; and (4) an Emergency Department Surveillance System on violence-related injuries to youth serious enough to result in hospital visits. These data will be used to determine individual and community risk and resiliency factors, track the changing needs of Boston's youth and communities, supporting HYPV's Community Partners, develop evidence-based prevention programmes and track their effectiveness, and evaluate the impact of city and community policies on youth violence and well-being.

The Youth Violence Prevention Center also works with Boston's Office of Community Partnerships on the Annual Youth Development Symposium, and conducts a biannual Boston Peace Party to honour community members who have made significant contributions in violence reduction. Finally, the Center recognizes that research and programmatic support must be supplemented by training. The Center provides Community Partner agencies and community members with training in programme evaluation and works with Center Partners to create local- and city-wide community action plans to reduce violence. The Center also provides formal training to graduate students, residents, and other physicians, community leaders, and injury control personnel in State Health Departments. Through its emphasis on research, practice, and collaboration, the HYVPC is continuing the Boston tradition of developing, implementing, and evaluating cutting-edge violence prevention strategies.

A programme for students who exhibit emotional disturbances—Montgomery County, MD, public schools

A 20-member committee that included principals, teachers, and support services representatives in Montgomery County, Maryland, in the United States, developed an interagency plan to serve students who exhibit violent behaviour. The cooperating agencies include public schools, departments of social services, the juvenile justice system, police, family resource services, recreation departments, drug, alcohol and mental health services, the state's attorney office, and the Office of Management and Budget.

The school district, mandated to serve students under the age of 16, has traditionally placed violent students in home instruction and provided 6 h of instruction per week. The new plan includes creating centres that have school days longer than 8 h and a half-day Saturday session. The longer school days, coupled with the mandated Saturday sessions, are meant to encourage students to return to public school.

The programme employs a case management approach. First, an assessment team evaluates the student to determine individual and family needs. The intense interagency programme is then implemented according to each student's identified needs. The school instructional day includes science and mathematics, life-skills-building, physical education, group counselling, and English and social studies. The day also includes meetings with students, teachers, case managers, and counsellors. By coordinating existing resources and redirecting existing funds, the programme requires only a moderate budget increase.

'Overcoming Obstacles'

The Los Angeles-based 'Overcoming Obstacles' is an education, jobs, and entrepreneurship programme that teaches young people the skills needed to: (1) succeed in education; (2) find jobs; (3) develop entrepreneurial skills; and (4) involve themselves in the community. It is an example of business partnering with a community programme to give students a chance to succeed.

This three-phased programme includes course work to:

- Improve self-esteem
- Develop a sense of personal responsibility
- Instil a sense of pride in community
- Set realistic goals
- Develop communications and conflict resolution skills
- Gain employment-seeking and retention skills

An evaluation demonstrated positive behaviour change in successful students during the school year and after graduation.

After the first educational phase, high-school students move to a job placement phase. Through a network, part-time and summer employment is secured for students, while full-time employment is offered for programme graduates. One example is a special programme with ARCO Product Company/Prestige Stations, Inc. Students working for this company receive a salary subject to increases and bonuses based on performance and have the opportunity to attend college paid for by ARCO.

Phase three encourages students to learn to become managers and owners of a business. Presently, funding has been provided for several businesses designed and managed by graduates of Overcoming Obstacles.

Survivors for Violence Prevention, Inc. (SVP)

The Harvard School of Public Health (HSPH) convened the first SVP Inc. forum, with a gathering of approximately 150 parents and family members who had loved ones killed or injured as a result of violence. Participants recognized the need for the creation of a survivor-led initiative. The organizational goals became increasing education and effecting public policy regarding survivorship. SVP Inc. was created to provide extensive information dissemination, communication, training, and technical assistance around survivorship issues. Advisory board members were identified and came together the following year. Advisory board members included practitioners who typically provide services to survivors and victims at both individuals- and community-based organizations, located in the cities of Boston, Atlanta, Rochester, Detroit, Columbus, Minneapolis, San Diego, Seattle, and Orange County, CA. From 1998 through 2004, SVP Inc. convened six annual conferences in partnership with the HSPH, violence practitioners and survivors, along with community activists and committed systems change advocates supportive of survivor and victim services.

The mission of SVP Inc. is to provide a powerful, united voice for survivors of victims of a violent crime and homicide. SVP Inc. informs thought and encourages debate regarding national public policy for the purpose of reducing violence in the United States.

Urban Networks to Increase Thriving Youth Through Violence Prevention (UNITY)

Urban Networks to increase Thriving Youth Through Violence Prevention is a CDC-funded cooperative agreement awarded in 2005 to a partnership comprised of the Prevention Institute, Deborah Prothrow-Stith of the Harvard School of Public Health, and Billie Weiss from the University of California at Los Angeles Southern California Injury Prevention Research Center.

The goal of UNITY is to strengthen urban youth violence prevention, build national support for necessary resources and policies, and develop tools and framing to ensure long-term sustainability of youth violence prevention efforts. To accomplish this, UNITY aims to engage youth and representatives of the 45 largest cities, along with national violence prevention advocates and leaders, in a National Consortium to shape the US strategy for urban youth violence prevention. UNITY will provide tools, training, and technical assistance to help cities to be more effective in preventing youth violence.

Development of this programme is supported by the Centers for Disease Control and Prevention (CDC). Its contents are solely the responsibility of the authors and do not necessarily represent the official views of the US Department of Health and Human Services or the Centers for Disease Control and Prevention (CDC).

Co-coordinating coalitions

The Contra Costa County California Health Department is widely known for its efforts to develop comprehensive programmes harnessing existing resources to alleviate poor health outcomes. Rather than designing and implementing their own stand-alone projects, Contra Costa County Program, CCCP, coordinates and develops existing programmes to meet identified community needs. It serves as a lead agency for a number of health-related issues, including violence prevention. Some CCCP premises are that coalitions:

- Offer more resources for less money
- Can reach more people than a single organization
- Provide greater credibility than single organizations
- Offer more political clout
- Serve a community networking function
- Offer more diverse opinions and talents

The CCCP defines eight steps to building effective coalitions. An initial planning group should: (1) analyse programme objectives and decide if a coalition is needed; (2) recruit relevant and effective organizations/community representatives; (3) develop preliminary objectives and activities; and (4) convene the group. By using the input from the planning group, the coalitions should: (5) develop a budget and structure; (6) maintain coalition vitality (communications, public relations); (7) evaluate programmes; and (8) based on evaluation offer recommendations to improve programmes. A guide further defining the eight-step process is available from the Contra Costa County Health Department.

A school-based planning model: Pittsburgh safe schools project

The Safe Schools Project of the Pittsburgh Public Schools is a model for multidisciplinary violence prevention coalition. Members of the Pittsburgh Public Schools, the Jewish Healthier Foundation, the Western Psychiatric Institute and Clinic, the Center for Injury Research and Control at the University of Pittsburgh, and the Boys and Girls Club of Western Pennsylvania formed a working group that produced a Blueprint for Violence Reduction in Pittsburgh Public Schools. It is an action plan based on sound theoretical framework, data collection and analysis, a commitment to understand the causes of violence and an analysis of state-of-the-art school violence prevention programmes.

The blueprint contains a review of the project's components and discusses each step in a thorough manner which lends itself to replication in other school districts. The blueprint also includes a set of valuable guiding principles for school-based programme implementation:

- Violence prevention must be a long-term priority for the school district.
- Adequate resources should be focused on very young children, particularly those at risk for developing aggressive lifestyles.
- Developmentally appropriate programmes should be integrated in a comprehensive approach for all grade levels.
- Students, teachers, and parents should participate in planning and assessing violence prevention activities.
- Activities should be culturally and racially appropriate.
- Prevention efforts should include home, school and community coordination.
- Programme evaluation measures should be integrated into the programme design.
- New programmes should be built upon successful existing programmes.

Conclusions

The contributions made by public health professionals towards efforts to prevent violence have been tremendous. The continued application of public health strategies to the understanding and prevention of violence assures success. The public health campaign to reduce smoking took 30 years after the first Surgeon Generals' report to reduce smoking. Violence reduction can be expected to take at least as long and require as many, if not more diverse strategies.

References

Allen, N.H., (1981). Homicide prevention and intervention. *Suicide and Life Threatening Behavior*, **11**, 167.

American Academy of Pediatrics (2007). Suicide and suicide attempts in adolescents. *Pediatrics*, **120**, 669–76.

American Psychological Association Commission on Violence and Youth (1993). *Violence and Youth: Psychology's Response*.

Austin, E.W., Roberts D.F., and Nass, C.I. (1990). Influences of family communication on children's television-interpretation processes. *Communication Research*, **4**, 545–65.

Bandura, A., Ross, D., and Ross, S.A. (1963a). Imitation of film-mediated aggressive models. *Journal of Abnormal Social Psychology*, 3–11.

Bandura, A., Ross, D., and Ross, S.A. (1963b). Vicarious reinforcement and imitative learning. *Journal of Abnormal Psychology*, **63**, 601–7.

Blueprint for a Safer Philadelphia. Campaign information on website: http://www.phillyblueprint.com/ Last checked December 2007.

Boys Clubs of America (1988). *Targeted Outreach Newsletter*, Vol. II-1.

Brady Campaign to Prevent Gun Violence. Firearms Facts on the website: http://www.bradycampaign.org/facts/factsheets/pdf/firearm_facts.pdf Last checked December 2007.

Bureau of Alcohol, Tobacco and Firearms (1991). *Firearm Census Report*. U.S. Treasury Department, Washington, DC.

Bureau of Justice Statistics (1992). *Criminal victimization in the United States, 1991*. U.S. Department of Justice, Washington, DC.

Bureau of Justice Statistics (1993). *Highlights from 20 Years of surveying crime victims: The national crime victimization survey, 1972–1992*. U.S. Department of Justice, Washington, DC.

Bureau of Justice Statistics (1994). *Violence between inmates*. NCJ-149259. Office of Justice Programs, U.S. Department of Justice, Washington, DC.

CDC (Centers for Disease Control) (1982a). Homicide. *Morbidity and Mortality Weekly Report*, November 12, **31**, 594.

CDC (Centers for Disease Control) (1982b). Homicide – United States. *Morbidity and Mortality Weekly Report*, **31**, 599–602.

CDC (Centers for Disease Control) (1983a). Violent deaths among persons 15–24 years of age – United States, 1970–1978. *Morbidity and Mortality Weekly Report*, September 9, **32**, 453.

CDC (Centers for Disease Control) (1983b). *Homicide surveillance, high risk racial and ethnic groups – Blacks and Hispanics, 1970–1983*. U.S. Department of Health and Human Services, Public Health Service, Washington, DC.

CDC (Centers for Disease Control) (1990). Homicide among black males – United States, 1978–1987. *Morbidity and Mortality Weekly Report*, **39**, 869–72.

CDC (Centers for Disease Control) (1992). *Youth suicide prevention program: A resource guide*. Department of Health and Human Services, Public Health Service, Centers for Disease Control, National Center for Injury Prevention and Control, Atlanta.

CDC (Centers for Disease Control) (1993). *Advance report of final mortality statistics, 1991, Monthly vital statistics report*. August, Atlanta.

CDC. (1997). Rates of homicide, suicide, and firearm related deaths among children–26 industrialized countries. *Morbidity & Mortality Weekly Report*, **46**, 101–5.

CDC, National Center for Injury Prevention and Control, Office of Statistics and Programming. Web-based Injury Statistics Query and Reporting System (WISQARS). Online at http://www.cdc.gov/ncipc/wisqars/ Accessed September 2007a.

CDC. *Facts at a glance: Youth violence*. Summer 2007. Online at http://www.cdc.gov/ncipc/dvp/YV_DataSheet.pdf Accessed December 2007b.

Centers for Disease Control and Prevention (1991). Weapon carrying among high school students – United States, 1990. *Morbidity and Mortality Weekly Report*, **40**, 681–4.

Centers for Disease Control and Prevention (1993). Violence-related attitudes and behaviors of high school students – New York City, 1991. *Morbidity and Mortality Weekly Report*, **40**, 773–7.

Centers for Disease Control and Prevention (1994). Deaths resulting from firearm- and motor-vehicle-related injuries – United States, 1968–1991. *Morbidity and Mortality Weekly Report*, **3**, 37–42.

Centers for Disease Control and Prevention (CDC) (2006). Youth risk behavior surveillance—United States, 2005. *Morbidity & Mortality Weekly Report*, **55** (SS-05), 1–108.

Centerwall, B.S. (1984). Race, socio-economic status, and domestic homicide, Atlanta, 1971–1972. *American Journal of Public Health*, **8**, 813–15.

Centerwall, B.S. (1992). Television and violence: The scale of the problem and where to go from here. *Journal of the American Medical Association*, 3059–63.

Centerwall, B.S. (1993). Race, socio-economic status, and domestic homicide in New Orleans. The Second World Conference on Injury Control.

Cook, P.J., and Ludwig, J. (2000). *Gun violence: The real costs*. Oxford University Press, New York.

Corso, P.S., Mercy, J.A., Simon, T.R., Finkelstein, E.A., and Miller, T.R. (2007). Medical costs and productivity losses due to interpersonal violence and self-directed violence. *American Journal of Preventive Medicine*, **32**(6), 474–82.

Daro, D., and Mitchel, L. (1987). *Deaths due to maltreatment soar: The results of the 1986 annual fifty state survey*. National Center on Child Abuse Prevention Research, National Committee for Prevention of Child Abuse, Chicago.

Dietz, W.H., and Strasburger, V.C. (1991). Children, adolescents and television. *Current Problems in Pediatrics*, **1**, 8–31.

Durant, R. Pendergast, R., and Cadenhead, C. (1994). Exposure to violence victimization and fighting behavior by urban black adolescents. *Journal of Adolescent Health*, **4**, 311–8.

Egeland, B., and Jacobvitz, D. (1984). *Intergenerational continuity of parental abuse: Cases and consequences*, presented at the conference on the Bio Social Perspectives on Abuse and Neglect, New York.

Emde, R.N. (1983). The horror! The horror! Reflection on our culture of violence and its implication for early development and morality. *Psychiatry*, **1**, 119–23.

Eron, L., and Huesman, L.R. (1984). Television violence and aggressive behavior. In *Advances in clinical child psychology* (eds. B. Lahey and A. Kardin). Plenum Press, New York.

FBI (Federal Bureau of Investigation) (2006). *Uniform crime report: Crime in the United States*. U.S. Department of Justice, Washington, DC. Online at http://www.fbi.gov/ucr/cius2006/offenses/expanded_information/homicide.html.

Fingerhut, L.A., and Kleinman, J.C. (1990). International and interstate comparisons of homicide among young males. *Journal of the American Medical Association*, **24**, 3292–4.

Fingerhut, L.A., Ingram, D.D., and Feldman, J.J. (1992). Firearm and non-firearm homicide among persons 15 through 19 years of age. *Journal of the American Medical Association*, **22**, 3048–53.

Fitzpatrick, K.M., and Boldizar, J.P. (1993). The prevalence and consequences of exposure to violence among African-American youth. *Journal of the American Academy of Child and Adolescent Psychiatry*, **2**, 424–30.

Freeman, L., Mokros, H., and Poznanski, E. (1993). Violent events reported by normal urban school-aged children: Characteristics and depression correlates. *Journal of the American Academy of Child and Adolescent Psychiatry*, **2**, 419–23.

Friedman, L.M. (1975). *The legal system: A social science perspective*, pp. 56–66. Russell Sage Foundation, New York City.

Gil, D. (1973). *Violence against children: Physical child abuse in the United States*. Harvard University Press, Cambridge.

Groves, B.M. *et al.* (1993). Silent victims: Children who witness violence. *Journal of the American Medical Association*, **2**, 262–4.

Guterman, N.B. (2004). Advancing prevention research on child abuse, youth violence and domestic violence: Emerging strategies and issues. *Journal of Interpersonal Violence*, **19**(3), 299–321.

Hemenway, D. (2005). Private guns, public health. Insert Publisher.

Huesmann, L.R. *et al.* (1983). Mitigating the imitation of aggressive behaviors by changing children's attitudes about media violence. *Journal of Personality and Social Psychology*, 899–910.

Huesmann, L.R. *et al.* (1984). Stability of aggression over time and generations. *Developmental Psychology*, 1120–34.

Kellerman, A.L. *et al.* (1993). Gun ownership as a risk factor for homicide in the home. *New England Journal of Medicine*, **15**, 1084–91.

Kellermann, A.L. *et al.* (1998). Injuries and deaths due to firearms in the home. *The Journal of Trauma*, **45**, 263–7.

Killias, M. (1993). International correlations between gun ownership and rates of homicide and suicide. *Canadian Medical Association*, **10**, 1721–5.

Kilpatrick, D.G., Edmunds, C.N., and Seymour, A.K. (1992). *Rape in America: A report to the Nation*. National Victim Center, Arlington.

Krug, E.G. *et al.*, eds. (2002). *World report on violence and health*. World Health Organization, Geneva.

Wintemute, G.J., and Wright, M.A. (1992). Initial and subsequent hospital costs of firearm injuries. *The Journal of Trauma*, **34**, 556–60.

Lester, D. (1988). Firearm availability and the incidence of suicide and homicide. *Acta Psychiatrica*, 387–93.

Liebert, R.M. (1988). *Early window: The effects of television on children and youth*, 6th edition. Allyn and Bacon, Needham.

Liebert, R., Neale, J., and Davidson, E. (1973). *Early window: The effects of television on children and youth*. Pergamon Press, New York.

Loftin, C. *et al.* (1991). Effects of restrictive licensing of handguns on homicide and suicide in the District of Columbia. *The New England Journal of Medicine*, **23**, 1615–20, 1647–9.

Lorion, R.P., and Saltzman, W. (1993). Children's exposure to community violence: Following a path from concern to research to action. *Psychiatry*, **1**, 55–65.

Makepeace, J.M. (1981). Courtship violence among college students. *Family Relations*, **30**, 97–102.

Martinez, P., and Richters, J. (1993). The NIMH community violence project: II. Children's distress symptoms associated with violence exposure. *Psychiatry*, February, 22–35.

Miller, T.R., Cohen, M.A., and Rossman, S.B. (1993). Datawatch: Victim cost of violent crime resulting injuries. *Health Affairs*, Winter, 187–97.

Miller *et al.* (1996). *Victim costs and consequences: A new look*. National Institute of Justice, U.S. Department of Justice, Washington, DC. Online at http://www.ncjrs.org/pdffiles/victcost.pdf.

Miller, M., Azrael, D., Hepburn, L., Hemenway, D., and Lippmann, S.J. (2006). The association between changes in household firearm ownership and rates of suicide in the United States, 1981–2002. *Injury Prevention*, **12**, 178–82.

Osofsky, J. *et al.* (1993). Chronic community violence: What is happening to our children? *Psychiatry*, February, 36–45.

Prothrow-Stith, D. (1985). *Prevention of interpersonal violence and homicide in black youth*. Report of the Surgeon General's Workshop on Violence and Public Health, Leesburg, October 27–29. *Public Health Reports* No. HRS-D-MC 86-1, 35–43. U.S. Government Printing Office, Washington, DC.

Prothrow-Stith, D., and Weissman, M. (1991). *Deadly consequences: How violence is destroying our teenage population and a plan to begin solving the problem*, pp 1–203. Harper Collins Publishers, New York.

Pynoos, R.S. *et al.* (1987). *Life threat and post traumatic stress in school-age children. Archives of General Psychiatry*, December, 1057–63.

Rice, M. (1993). Shooting in the dark: Estimating the cost of firearm injuries. *Health Affairs*, **12**, 171–85.

Sang, F., Schmitz, B., and Tasche, K. (1993). Developmental trends in television coviewing of parent-child dyads. *Journal of Youth and Adolescence*, **5**, 531–43.

Satcher, D. (1985). *The Public Health Approach to Violence*. National Education Association National Conference, Los Angeles, California, April 8.

Sege, R., and Dietz, W. (1994). Television viewing and violence in children: The pediatrician as agent for change. *Pediatrics*.

Sege, R., and Hoffman, J. (2005). Training health professionals in youth violence prevention. *American Journal of Preventive Medicine (supplement)*, **29**(5S2), 175–81.

Shaffer, D., Garland, A., Gould, M., Fisher, P., and Trautman, P. (1988). Preventing teenage suicide: A critical review. *Journal of the American Academy of Child and Adolescent Psychiatry*, **27**, 673–87.

Shaffer, D., Garland, M., and Hicks, R. (1994). Worsening suicide rate in black teenagers, Brief Reports. *American Journal of Psychiatry*, **151**, 12.

Sheley, J., McGee, Z., and Wright, J. (1992). Gun-related violence in and around inner-city schools. *Journal of Diseases of Childhood*, June 677–82.

Slaby, R.G., and Guerra, N.G. (1988). Cognitive mediators of aggression in adolescent offenders: 1. Assessment. *Developmental Psychology*, **4**, 580–8.

Slaby, R., and Quarfoth, G. (1980). Effects of television on the developing child. *Advanced Behavioral Pediatrics*, **1**, 225–66.

Sloan, J.H. *et al.* (1988). *Handgun regulations, crime, assaults, and homicide: A tale of two cities. New England Journal of Medicine*, **19**, 1256–62.

Spivak, H., Prothrow-Stith, D., and Hausman, A. (1988). Dying is no accident: Adolescents, violence, and intentional injury. *Pediatric Clinics of North America*, **35**, 1339–47.

Straus, M. (1991). Discipline and deviance: Physical punishment of children and violence and other crime in adulthood. *Social Problems*, **38**, 137–54.

Straus, M., and Gelles, R. (1990). How violent are American families? Estimates from the National Family Violence Resurvey and other studies. In *Physical violence in American families: Risk factors and adaptations to violence in American families: Risk factors and adaptations to violence in 8,145 families* (eds. M. Straus and R. Gelles). Transaction, New Brunswick.

Tjaden, P., and Thoennes, N. (2000). Extent, nature, and consequences of intimate partner violence: Findings from the National Violence Against Women Survey. U.S. Department of Justice, Washington DC. Publication number 181867.

Turner, C.W., Hesse, B.W., and Peterson-Lewis, S. (1986). *Naturalistic studies of the long-term effects of television violence. Journal of Social Issues*, 51–73.

United States Department of Health, Education, and Welfare (1964). *Smoking and health*. Report of the Advisory Committee to the Surgeon General, Public Health Service, Washington, DC.

Vissing, Y., Straus, M., Gelles, R., and Harrop, J. (1991). Verbal aggression by parents and psychological problems of children. *Child Abuse and Neglect*, **15**, 223–38.

Weaver, B., and Barbour, N. (1992). Mediation of children's televiewing. Families in Society. *The Journal of Contemporary Human Services*, **4**, 236–43.

Widom, C.S. (1989). The cycle of violence. *Science*, April 14, **244**, 160–6.

Williams, B.C., and Kotch, B.J. (1990). Excess injury mortality among children in the United States: Comparison of recent international statistics. *Pediatrics* (Supplement), 1067–73.

Wolfgang, M. (1986). Homicide in other industrialized countries. *Bulletin of the New York Academy of Medicine*, **62**, 400.

Wood, W., Wong, F.Y., and Chachere, J.G. (1991). Effects of media violence on viewer's aggression in unconstrained social interaction. *Psychological Bulletin*, 3371–83.

World Health Organization (2007). Online at http://www.who.int/violence_injury_prevention/en/ Last checked August 18, 2007.

10.6

Collective violence: War

Victor W. Sidel and Barry S. Levy

Abstract

Three types of violence—self-directed, interpersonal, and collective—have been defined by the World Health Organization (WHO) in its efforts to urge public health workers to consider violence prevention as an important public health issue. This chapter deals with collective violence, which includes war, terrorism, and their health consequences, and suggests public health approaches to prevention of collective violence and promotion of justice and peace. These approaches include the following: Conducting research on the health and environmental consequences of collective violence; educating public health workers, the public, and decision makers on the impact of collective violence on health and environment; intervening to prevent collective violence or to end it; and advocating for changes in attitudes and policies on the public health aspects of collective violence.

Public health workers have a responsibility to promote four levels of prevention of collective violence as well as to promote peace and justice. Pre-primary prevention consists of alleviating the underlying causes of armed conflict. Primary prevention consists of preventing specific conflicts from turning into collective violence. Secondary prevention is minimizing the health consequences of collective violence and ending the violence. Tertiary prevention is the rehabilitation and reintegration of victims of the violence into society, the remediation of the physical, social, cultural, and economic damage, and the prevention of recurrence of the collective violence.

Collective violence as threat to public health

In 1966, the World Health Assembly declared violence 'a major and growing public health problem across the world' (World Health Assembly 1996). The World Report on Violence and Health, published by WHO in 2002, was the first comprehensive report by WHO on violence as a public health problem (Krug 2002). The WHO report presents a typology of violence that defines three broad categories based on the characteristics of those committing the violent acts: Self-directed violence, interpersonal violence, and collective violence. Other chapters in the textbook cover the first two categories of violence, and this chapter will deal primarily with war, an important component of collective violence.

Collective violence has been characterized as 'the instrumental use of violence by people who identify themselves as members of a group—whether this group is transitory or has a more permanent identity—against another group or set of individuals in order to achieve political, economic, ideological, or social objectives'. Collective violence includes armed conflict (such as war and genocide), state-sponsored violence (such as genocide, repression, disappearances, and torture), and organized violent crime (such as gang warfare and banditry).

The Report gives examples of collective violence: 'Violent conflicts between nations and groups, state and group terrorism, rape as a weapon of war, the movement of large numbers of people displaced from their homes, and gang warfare'. As the Report notes, 'all of these occur on a daily basis in many parts if the world' and 'the effects of these different types of events on health in terms of deaths, physical illness, disabilities, and mental anguish are vast'. Also included in this chapter is limited information on what has been termed *terrorism* and the *war on terror*, as Chapter 10.8 covers *bioterrorism*. This chapter will not cover the topic of *gang warfare*, which is covered in Chapter 10.5 ('Interpersonal violence prevention: A recent public health mandate').

The health impacts of collective violence

Direct consequences of war and military operations

Armed conflicts in the twenty-first century largely consist of the civil wars (conflicts within countries, to which other countries sometimes contribute military troops) that continue to rage in many parts of the world. For example, at the beginning of 2007, it was reported that there were 15 significant armed conflicts (1000 or more reported deaths) and another 21 'hot spots' that could slide into or revert to war (Smith 2007). During the post-Cold War period of 1990–2001, there were 57 major armed conflicts in 45 locations—all but three of which were civil wars (Stockholm International Peace Research Institute 2002).

Some of the impacts of war on public health are obvious, whereas others are not. The direct impact of war on mortality and morbidity is apparent. Many people, including an increasing percentage of civilians, are killed or injured during war. An estimated 191 million people died directly or indirectly as a result of conflict during the twentieth century, more than half of whom were civilians (Rummel 1994). The exact figures are unknowable because of the generally poor record keeping in many countries and its disruption in time of conflict.

War has direct, immediate, and deadly impact on human life and health. The 'body counts' and the data on those with war-caused injuries and disabilities, both physical and psychological, although woefully incomplete, document the many people tragically killed and wounded as a direct result of military activities. Through the early twentieth century up to the start of World War II, the vast preponderance of the direct casualties of war were uniformed combatants, usually members of national armed forces. Although non-combatants suffered social, economic, and environmental consequences of war and may have been the victims of what is now termed *collateral damage* of military operations, 'civilians' were generally not directly targeted and were largely spared direct death and disability resulting from war (Levy & Sidel 2008).

However, since 1937, when Nazi forces bombed the city of Guernica, a non-military target in the Basque region of Spain, military operations have increasingly killed and maimed civilians through purposeful targeting of non-military targets. The use of 'carpet bombing' and the collateral damage of heavy attacks on military targets have caused many civilian casualties. The percentage of civilian deaths as a proportion of all deaths directly caused by war has therefore increased dramatically. Many of these civilian deaths may have been indirectly rather than directly caused by war.

Since September 11, 2001, there has been increasing concern in the United States and other countries about violence conducted by individuals and groups to create fear and advance a political agenda—a form of violence commonly called *terrorism*. We believe that there needs to be a balanced approach to strengthening systems and protecting people in response to the threat of terrorism, an approach that strengthens a broad range of public health capacities and preserves civil liberties (Levy & Sidel 2007). Terrorism is often defined in a partisan fashion: Those called *terrorists* by one side in a conflict may be viewed as 'patriots', 'freedom fighters', or 'servants of God' by the other. We have defined terrorism as, 'politically motivated violence or the threat of violence, especially against civilians, with the intent to instil fear'. This definition includes violent acts conducted by nation-states against civilians with the intent to instil fear as well as acts committed by individuals and subnational groups. The term *terrorism* has considerable overlap with the term *war* and many actions conducted during war fit our definition of terrorism. The initiation of a 'war on terror', in contrast to use of education, law enforcement, economic aid, and other methods to prevent such acts, has led some analysts to include this war on terror as an example of collective violence.

Indirect effects of war and other military activities

Along with the direct impacts of war and other military activities on health, collective violence may also cause serious health consequences through its impact on the physical, economic, social, and biologic environments in which people live. The environmental damage may affect people not only in nations directly engaged in collective violence but also in all nations. Much of the morbidity and mortality during war, especially among civilians, has been the result of devastation of societal infrastructure, including destruction of food and water supply systems, health-care facilities and public health services, sewage disposal systems, power plants and electrical grids, and transportation and communication systems. Destruction of infrastructure has led to food shortages and resultant malnutrition, contamination of food and of drinking water and the resultant foodborne and waterborne illness, and health-care and public health deficiencies and resultant disease (Levy & Sidel 2008).

Preparation for war also can adversely affect human health. Some of the impacts are direct, such as injuries and deaths during training exercises, and others are indirect. As with war itself, preparation for war can divert human, financial, and other resources that otherwise might be used for health and human services.

Damage to the physical environment—water, land, air, and space—and use of non-renewable resources may be the result of preparation for war as well as war itself. Lakes, rivers, streams and aquifers, land masses, and the atmosphere may be polluted through testing and use of weapons. Outer space could be damaged by placement of weapons. Non-renewable resources may be used in weapons production, testing, and use.

The economic environment may also be adversely affected by the diversion of resources from education, housing, nutrition, and other human and health services to military activities and through an increase in national debt and/or taxation. These economic impacts affect both developed and developing countries.

Governmental and societal preoccupation with preparation for wars—often known as *militarism*—may lead to massive diversion and subversion of efforts to promote human welfare. This preoccupation may lead to policies that promote 'pre-emptive war' (when an attack is allegedly imminent) and to 'preventive war' (when an attack may be feared sometime in the future). Diversion of resources to war is a problem worldwide, but is especially important in developing countries. Many developing countries spend substantially more on military expenditures than on health-related expenditures; for example, in 1990, Ethiopia spent US$16 per capita for military expenditures and only US$1 per capita for health, and Sudan spent US$25 per capita for military expenditures and only $1 per capita for health.

The social environment may be affected by increasing militarism, by encouragement of violence as a means for settling disputes, and by infringement on civil rights and civil liberties. In addition, preparation for war, like war itself, can promote violence as a means for settling disputes.

Another indirect impact of war is the creation of many refugees and internally displaced persons: Many of the world's 12 million refugees have left their native countries as a result of war. Refugees often flee to neighbouring less-developed countries, which often face significant challenges in addressing the public health needs of their own populations. In addition, the vast majority of the 22–25 million internally displaced persons worldwide have left their homes to escape war. These internally displaced persons are often worse off than refugees who have left their countries because they frequently do not have easy access to food, safe water, health care, shelter, and other necessities. Approximately 8 million of these internally displaced persons live in the Democratic Republic of Congo, Uganda, and Sudan—all in Africa. In West Darfur, Sudan, more than 700 000 people have been internally displaced and more than 250 000 people have fled to refugee camps in neighbouring Chad as a result of bitter ethnic conflict. Refugees and internally displaced persons experience much higher rates of mortality and morbidity, much of it due to malnutrition and infectious diseases.

The vast majority of refugees and internally displaced persons as a result of war are women, children, and elderly people who may be highly vulnerable not only to disease and malnutrition, but also to threats of their security.

The environment may be disrupted during war or the preparation for war. Conventional weapons may damage the environment such that the health-supporting infrastructure—systems of food and water supply, sewage disposal, medical care, transportation, and communication—is severely disrupted or destroyed. Malnutrition of the affected population may increase the frequency and severity of infectious diseases. The biological environment may also be disrupted by the production, testing, and use of biological weapons. Ionizing radiation from the production, testing, use, and disposal of nuclear weapons and radioactive materials, such as depleted uranium, may also disrupt and damage the environment. So may toxic substances by the release of hazardous substances from damaged industrial facilities or from the production, testing, use, and disposal of chemical weapons.

Hazardous wastes from military operations represent potential contaminants of air, water, and soil. For example, groundwater was contaminated with trichloroethylene (TCE), a probable human carcinogen, and other toxins at the Otis Air Force Base in Massachusetts; 125 chemicals were dumped over a period of 30 years at the Rocky Mountain Arsenal in Colorado; and benzene, a definite human carcinogen, was found in extremely high concentrations at the McChord Air Force Base in the State of Washington (Renner 2000).

Both during war and the preparation for war, military forces consume huge amounts of fossil fuels and other non-renewable materials. Energy consumption by military equipment can be substantial. For example, an armoured division of 348 battle tanks operating for one day consumes more than 2.2 million L of fuel and a carrier battle group operating for one day consumes more than 1.5 million L of fuel. In the late 1980s, the US military annually consumed 18.6 million tons of fuel (more than 44 per cent of the world's total) and emitted 381 000 tons of carbon monoxide, 157 000 tons of oxides of nitrogen, 78 000 tons of hydrocarbons, and 17 900 tons of sulphur dioxide (Renner 2000).

Weapons systems

Conventional weapons

Conventional weapons consist of explosives, incendiaries, and weapons of various sizes, ranging from 'small arms and light weapons' to heavy artillery and bombs. Small arms and light weapons (SALW), which include pistols, rifles, machine guns, and other hand-held or easily transportable weapons, are the weapons most often used in wars. Although some restrictions have been placed on their use in war, such as the outlawing of the use of 'dum-dum bullets' (which cause extensive injuries when striking a human), there has been little effective effort to outlaw their use. In the Millennium Report of the UN Secretary-General to the General Assembly, Kofi Annan stated that small arms could be described as weapons of mass destruction (WMD) because the fatalities they produce 'dwarf that of all other weapons systems—and in most years greatly exceed the toll of the atomic bombs that devastated Hiroshima and Nagasaki'.

Conventional weapons have accounted for the overwhelming majority of adverse environmental consequences due to war. During World War II, for example, extensive carpet bombing of cities in Europe and Japan accounted not only for many deaths and injuries, but also for widespread devastation of urban environments. During the Persian Gulf War, the more than 600 oil fires in Kuwait accounted for widespread environmental devastation as well as for acute, and possibly chronic, respiratory ailments among people who were exposed to the smoke from these fires. The bombing of mangrove forests during the Vietnam War led to destruction of these forests, and the resultant bomb craters remain several decades afterward, often filling with stagnant water that serves as a breeding ground for mosquitoes transmitting malaria and other mosquito-borne diseases.

Nuclear weapons

Nuclear weapons have been increasingly widespread since their development in the 1940s. There are now an estimated 20 000 nuclear warheads in at least eight nations—the United States, Russia, the United Kingdom, France, China, Israel, India, and Pakistan—and possibly also in North Korea (Sutton & Gould 2007). The historic high in the explosive capacity of the world nuclear weapons stockpiles was reached in 1960 with an explosive capacity equivalent to 20 000 megatons (20 billion tons or 40 trillion pounds) of trinitrotoulene (TNT), equivalent to that of 1.4 million of the nuclear bombs dropped on Hiroshima (Yokoro & Kamada 2000). In the United States in 1967, the nuclear stockpile had reached approximately 32 000 nuclear warheads of 30 different types. In 2003, the US stockpile was about 10 400 warheads, totalling about 2000 megatons—equivalent to 140 000 Hiroshima-size bombs. Five thousand of the nuclear weapons in the United States, Russia, and possibly other countries are on 'hair-trigger' alert, ready to fire on a few minutes notice.

The detonation of nuclear bombs over Hiroshima and Nagasaki in August 1945 during World War II led to the immediate deaths of approximately 200 000 people, primarily civilians, as well as to lasting injury and later death of many others, with massive devastation—and widespread radioactive contamination—of the environment in these two cities (Yokoro & Kamada 2000). Atmospheric testing of nuclear weapons by the United States, the Soviet Union, and other countries has also led to environmental contamination, with increased rates of leukaemia and other cancers among populations who were downwind from these tests. The effects of exposure to iodine-131 (a radioactive isotope of iodine produced by the testing) on children has been well-documented (Institute of Medicine, National Research Council 1999). In addition to the potential for use of nuclear weapons by national armed forces, such as that described in the recent US Nuclear Posture Review, which threatened use of nuclear weapons under a wider range of circumstances, there is an increasing threat of their use by individuals and groups.

From 1945 to 1990, the United States produced approximately 70 000 nuclear weapons; other nations also produced many of these weapons. Production of nuclear weapons has led to major environmental contamination (Levy & Sidel 2005). For example, the area around Chelyabinsk in Russia has been heavily contaminated with radioactive materials from the nuclear weapons production facility in that area. The level of ambient radiation in and near the Techa River in the area has been documented to be as high as 28 times the normal background radiation level (Burmistrov *et al.* 2006). Another example is the leakage of radioactive materials from the storage of wastes from nuclear weapons production at Hanford, along the Columbia River in Washington State, leading to extensive radioactive contamination (Renner 2000).

The dismantling and disposal of nuclear weapons has also led to environmental contamination. The primary site for the disassembly of US nuclear weapons is the Pantex Plant, located 17 miles northeast of Amarillo in the Texas panhandle (Levy & Sidel 2005). Overall, the United States has dismantled about 60 000 nuclear warheads since the 1940s; during the 1990s, 11 751 warheads were dismantled. More than 12 000 plutonium pits (hollow shells of plutonium encased in steel or another metal that are essential components of nuclear weapons) are stored in containers at Pantex (Levy & Sidel 2005). Plutonium, an element first produced in the Manhattan Project in 1942, has a half-life of 24 000 years. Plans are underway to produce as many as 80 new pits annually at Los Alamos National Laboratory, and the Bush administration advocates building a modern pit facility capable of producing 250–900 pits annually by 2018 (Levy & Sidel 2005).

Radiologic weapons

'Dirty bombs', consisting of conventional explosive devices mixed with radioactive materials, or attacks on nuclear power plants with explosive weapons could widely scatter highly radioactive materials. Another example of a radioactive substance used in weapons is depleted uranium (DU), uranium from which the uranium isotope usable for nuclear weapons or as fuel rods for nuclear power plants has been removed (Depleted Uranium Education Project 1997). DU is used militarily as a casing for armour-penetrating shells. An extremely dense material, uranium used as a casing increases the ability of the shell to penetrate the armour of tanks; uranium is also pyrophoric and bursts into flames on impact. DU-encased shells were used by the United States during the Persian Gulf War and the Iraq War as well as the war in Kosovo; similar shells were used by the United Kingdom in the Iraq War. DU, which is both radioactive and extremely toxic, has been demonstrated to cause contamination of the soil and groundwater. Use of DU is considered legal by the nations using it, but its use is considered by others to be illegal under the Geneva Conventions and other international treaties.

Chemicals

A variety of chemical weapons and related materials have the potential for direct health effects during collective violence and also for contaminating the physical environment during war and the preparation for war. The potential for exposure exists not only for military and civilian populations, who may be exposed during the use of chemical weapons in wartime, but also for workers involved in the development, production, transport, and storage of these weapons and for community residents living near facilities where these weapons are developed, produced, transported, and stored. In addition, disposal of these weapons, including their disassembly and incineration, can be hazardous.

During the Vietnam War, the US military used defoliants on mangrove forests and other vegetation, which not only defoliated and killed trees and other plants, but may also have led to excessive numbers of birth defects and cases of cancer among nearby residents (Levy & Sidel 2005). In addition, development and production of conventional weapons involve the use of many chemicals that are toxic and can contaminate the environment. Furthermore, there is now a plausible threat of non-state agents using chemical weapons; a Japanese cult, Aum Shinrikyo, used sarin in the subway system of two Japanese cities in the mid 1990s, accounting for the death of 19 people and injuries to thousands (Spanjaard & Khabib 2007).

The Chemical Weapons Convention (CWC), which came into force in 1997, prohibits all development, production, acquisition, stockpiling, transfer, and use of chemical weapons. It requires each state party to destroy its chemical weapons and chemical weapons production facilities, as well as any chemical weapons it may have abandoned on the territory of another state party. The verification provisions of the CWC affect not only the military sector but also the civilian chemical industry worldwide through certain restrictions and obligations regarding the production, processing, and consumption of chemicals that are considered relevant to the objectives of the convention. These provisions are to be verified through a combination of reporting requirements, routine onsite inspection of declared sites, and short-notice challenge inspections. The Organization for the Prohibition of Chemical Weapons (OPCW) in The Hague, established by the CWC, ensures implementation of the provisions of the CWC. The disposal of chemical weapons required by the CWC has raised controversy about the safety of two different methods of disposal: Incineration and chemical neutralization. The controversy about safety and protection of the environment has delayed completion of the disposal by the date required by the CWC.

Biological agents

These consist of bacteria, viruses, other microorganisms, and their toxins, which can not only directly produce illness in humans, but can also be used against other animals or plants, thereby adversely affecting human food supplies or agricultural resources and indirectly affecting human health. Biological agents have been used relatively infrequently during warfare, but there has long been a potential for their use. These agents have been used as weapons, albeit sporadically, since ancient times. In the sixth century BC, Persia, Greece, and Rome tried to contaminate drinking water sources with diseased corpses. In AD 1346, Mongols besieging the Crimean seaport of Kaffa placed cadavers of plague victims on hurling machines and threw them into Kaffa. In the mid-eighteenth century, during the French and Indian War, a British commander sent blankets infected with smallpox to Native Americans. During World War I, Germany dropped bombs containing plague bacteria over British positions and used cholera in Italy. During the 1930s, Japan contaminated the food and water supplies of several cities and sprayed the cities with cultures of microorganisms.

Gruinard Island, off the coast of Scotland, was contaminated in 1942 by a test use of anthrax spores by the United Kingdom and the United States (Harris & Paxman 1962). During the 1950s and 1960s, secret large-scale open-air tests at the US Army Dugway Proving Ground may have introduced the microorganisms that cause Q fever and Venezuelan equine encephalitis into the deserts of Western Utah (Cole 1988). In 1979, the accidental release of anthrax spores near Sverdlovsk in the Soviet Union resulted in at least 77 cases of inhalation anthrax and at least 66 deaths (Meselson 1994).

There is concern that biological agents could be used as terrorist weapons. In the fall of 2001, anthrax spores were disseminated through the US mail, causing 23 cases of inhalational and skin anthrax, 5 of which were fatal. The Centers for Disease Control and

Prevention has identified three categories of diseases caused by biological agents, according to its level of concern that they may be used as terrorist weapons. Category A consists of the agents that cause anthrax, botulism, plague, smallpox, tularaemia, and several viral haemorrhagic fevers. Category B consists of the agents that cause brucellosis, glanders, melioidosis, psittacosis, Q fever, and food safety threats (such as salmonella and shigella species, and *Escherichia coli* O157:H7), as well as epsilon toxin of *Clostridium perfringens*, ricin toxin from castor beans, and staphylococcyl enterotoxin B. Category C consists of the agents that cause emerging infectious diseases such as Nipah virus and hantavirus (Centers for Disease Control and Prevention 2007).

Antipersonnel landmines

Approximately 80 million landmines are still deployed worldwide in at least 78 countries. These landmines have been termed 'weapons of mass destruction, one person at a time'. They have mostly been placed in rural areas, posing a threat to residents of these areas and often disrupting farming and other activities. Civilians are the most likely to be injured or killed by landmines, which continue to injure and kill 15 000–20 000 people annually; more than 90 per cent of landmine victims are civilians, primarily poor people living in rural areas. One-fourth of landmine victims are children, putting landmines among the six most preventable major causes of death to children throughout the world. It is estimated that half of all landmine victims die of their injuries before they reach appropriate medical care. Although a mine may cost as little as US$3 to produce, it may cost as much as a US$1000 to remove and its adverse economic impact on human health and well-being is substantially higher. Mines, in addition to maiming and killing people, also make large areas of land uninhabitable. Remaining in place for many years, they pose long-term threats to people, including refugees and internally displaced persons returning to their homes after long periods of war. Since the entry into force of the Anti-Personnel Landmine Convention in 1997, production of landmines has been markedly reduced and a number of those that had been implanted in the ground have been removed (International Campaign to Ban Landmines 2006). Many of the mines are still buried and additional resources will be required to continue unearthing and destroying them, tasks that pose inherent risks to demining personnel (Sirkin *et al.* 2008).

Weapons in space

The deployment of weapons in space represents another risk of weapons systems igniting armed conflict or adding to its potential health consequences. Attempts by the 65-member United Nations Conference on Disarmament in Geneva to limit weapons in space have failed. UN Secretary-General Ban Ki-moon opened the 2008 session of the Conference by urging progress. In early 2008, the Russian and Chinese delegates to the Conference presented a draft treaty banning weapons in space, but the United States opposed such a treaty. The risk of an arms race of weapons in space continues.

The role of public health in addressing war

War and the preparation for war have enormous adverse impact on humans and their environment. Public health has an important part to play in response to war. As the World Health Assembly declared in 1981, 'the role of health workers in promoting and preserving peace is a significant factor for achieving health for all' (World Health Assembly 1981).

Prevention of war

The health and environmental problems created by collective violence can appear to be overwhelming. However, standard public health principles and implementation measures can be successfully applied in addressing these problems. The following subsection of this chapter highlights three standard public health approaches that can be developed and implemented in addressing these environmental problems: (a) surveillance and documentation, (b) education and raising awareness, and (c) advocacy for sound policies and programmes.

Surveillance and documentation

Much can be accomplished by undertaking surveillance and other activities to document the problems caused by war. Although the numbers of deaths, injuries, and diseases among uniformed combatants are generally well-documented, deaths, injuries, and diseases among civilians are more difficult to document. Household cluster surveys have been used during the Iraq War to estimate the civilian casualties. Technical approaches to surveillance can include environmental monitoring as well as biological monitoring, the latter to document and assess the human burden of environmental contaminants and their adverse health consequences. Non-technical approaches can include information from physician reports, reports in the mass media, and assessments by government agencies.

Education and raising awareness

Much can also be accomplished by educating and raising the awareness of health professionals, policy makers, and the general public about the problems caused by war. A multifaceted approach that incorporates publications by citizens' groups and professional organizations, communications of the mass media, and personal communication is often valuable. In addition, efforts should be made to assist people in distinguishing between accurate and inaccurate information and in setting priorities.

Advocacy for sound policies and programmes

Finally, much can also be accomplished by advocating for improved policies and programmes that help prevent collective violence and minimize its public health impact.

Levels of prevention

Those concerned with the promotion and protection of health classify preventive measures into four basic categories: Primordial prevention (a recent addition, which in this chapter will be called *pre-primary prevention*), primary prevention, secondary prevention, and tertiary prevention. Pre-primary prevention consists of measures to prevent adverse health consequences by removing the conditions that lead to them. Primary prevention consists of measures to prevent the health consequences of a specific illness or injury by preventing its occurrence in a specific individual or among a specific group. Secondary prevention consists of measures to prevent or limit the health consequences of an illness or injury, or to limit the spread of an infectious disease to others, after the disease process has begun. Tertiary prevention consists of efforts to rehabilitate those injured and to reintegrate them into society or, in the case of prevention of collective violence, to prevent the resumption of violence.

Prevention of scurvy may be used as an example. Policies that assure that a population has information about and access to an adequate diet that includes vitamin C are examples of pre-primary prevention. Provision of foods containing vitamin C to ensure an adequate intake of this vitamin among a group that does not otherwise have access to it is an example of primary prevention; James Lind, a pioneer of public health in the 1700s, provided limes to sailors on British warships to prevent scurvy (Lind 2006). To use prevention of smallpox as another example, elimination of smallpox virus in the ecosphere is pre-primary prevention and vaccination against smallpox before exposure is primary prevention. Vaccination may also be used after exposure to smallpox has occurred to prevent the disease and its spread to others, an example of secondary prevention.

Pre-primary prevention

In general, pre-primary prevention requires political and social will. Pre-primary and primary prevention may be difficult to accomplish because the causes of the disease or injury may be unknown and, when they are known, the preventive methods may be difficult to implement technically or politically. As measures for pre-primary or primary prevention are usually more effective and rarely have negative consequences, they are generally considered preferable to secondary prevention even when implementation is difficult or expensive. Secondary prevention is usually easier to implement politically and technically but, because such methods are often ineffective or only partially effective, they may create a false sense of security and encourage risk taking, can be more expensive than primary prevention, and more likely than pre-primary or primary prevention methods to have adverse consequences. The health consequences of war and the aftermath of war can be prevented or reduced through primordial prevention. This generally requires cooperation among civil society (non-governmental) organizations, governmental agencies, and organizations of health professionals.

The underlying causes of collective violence include poverty, social inequities, adverse effects of globalization, and shame and humiliation. Some of the underlying causes of war and militarism are becoming more prevalent or worsening.

Persistence of socioeconomic disparities and other forms of social injustice are among the leading underlying causes of war. The rich–poor divide is growing. In 1960, in the 20 richest countries, the per-capita gross domestic product (GDP) was 18 times that of the 20 poorest countries; by 1995, this gap had increased to 37 times. Between 1980 and the late 1990s, inequality increased in 48 of the 73 countries for which there are reliable data, including China, Russia, and the United States (Marmot & Bell 2006). Inequality is not restricted to personal income, but includes other important areas of life, such as health status, access to health care, education, and employment opportunities. In addition, abundant national resources, such as oil, minerals, metals, gemstones, drug crops, and timber, have fuelled many wars in developing countries.

Globalization is similarly a two-edged sword. Insofar as globalization leads to good relations among nation-states and reductions in poverty and disparities within and among nations, it may play a powerful role in prevention of collective violence. Conversely, if globalization leads to exploitation of people, of the environment, and of other resources, it may be among the causes of war.

The Carnegie Commission on Preventing Deadly Conflict has identified the following factors that put nations at risk of violent conflict, including:

- Lack of democratic processes and unequal access to power, particularly in situations where power arises from religious or ethnic identity and leaders are repressive or abusive of human rights.
- Social inequality characterized by markedly unequal distribution of resources and access to these resources, especially where the economy is in decline and there is, as a result, more social inequality and more competition for resources.
- Control by one group of valuable natural resources, such as oil, timber, drugs, or gems.
- Demographic changes that are so rapid that they outstrip the capability of a nation to provide basic necessary services and opportunities for employment.

The United States and other nations must increase funding for humanitarian and sustainable development programmes that address the root causes of collective violence, such as hunger, illiteracy, and unemployment.

Promoting multilateralism

Since its founding in 1946, the UN has attempted to live up to the goal stated in its charter: 'To save succeeding generations from the scourge of war'. Its mandate, along with preventing war, includes protecting human rights, promoting international justice, and helping the people of the world to achieve a sustainable standard of living. Its affiliated programmes and specialized agencies include, among many others, the United Nations Children's Fund (UNICEF), the World Health Organization (WHO), the Food and Agriculture Organization (FAO), the International Labour Organization (ILO), the United Nations Development Programme (UNDP), and the Office of the UN High Commissioner for Refugees (UNHCR). These UN-related organizations, and the UN itself, have made an enormous difference in the lives of people.

The resources allocated to the UN by its member states are grossly inadequate. The annual budget for the core functions—the Secretariat operations in New York, Geneva, Nairobi, Vienna, and five required commissions—is far less than New York City's annual budget and far less than annual worldwide military expenditures. Indeed, the world's military expenditures for one year would pay for the annual core functions of the United Nations for close to a century. This is about 4 per cent of New York City's annual budget—and nearly a billion dollars less than the yearly cost of Tokyo's Fire Department. The entire UN system (excluding the World Bank and International Monetary Fund) spends US$12 billion a year. By comparison, annual world military expenditures—$1 trillion—would pay for the entire UN system for more than 65 years.

The UN has no army and no police. It relies on the voluntary contribution of troops and other personnel to halt conflicts that threaten peace and security. The United States and other member states on the Security Council decide when and where to deploy peacekeeping troops. Long-term conflicts, such as those in the Sudan and Kashmir and the Israeli–Palestinian conflict, fester while conflicting national priorities deadlock the UN's ability to act. In fact, if stymied by the veto, the organization has little power beyond the bully pulpit. The United States and the United Kingdom have severely weakened the UN by their unauthorized and illegal invasion of Iraq in 2003. The United States also failed to support the International War Crimes Tribunal through signature and ratification of the Statute of the International Criminal Court.

Ending poverty and social injustice

Poverty and other manifestations of social injustice contribute to conditions that lead to collective violence. Growing socioeconomic and other disparities between the rich and the poor within countries, and between rich and poor nations, also contribute to the likelihood of armed conflict. By addressing these underlying conditions through policies and programmes that redistribute wealth within nations and among nations, and by providing financial and technical assistance to less-developed nations, countries such as the United States can minimize poverty and other forms of social injustice that lead to collective violence.

Creating a culture of peace

Workers in the health and environment sectors can do much to promote a culture of peace, in which non-violent means are utilized to settle conflicts. A culture of peace is based on the values, attitudes, and behaviours that form the deep roots of peace. They are in some ways the opposite of the values, attitudes, and behaviours that reflect and inspire collective violence, but should not be equated with just the absence of war. A culture of peace can exist at the level of the family, workplace, school, and community as well as at the level of the state and in international relations. Health and environment professionals and others can play important roles in encouraging the development of a culture of peace at all these levels.

The Hague Appeal for Peace Civil Society Conference was held in 1999 on the 100th anniversary of the 1899 Hague Peace Conference. The 1899 conference, attended by governmental representatives, was devoted to finding methods for making war more humane. The 1999 conference, attended by 1 000 individuals and representatives of civil society organizations, was devoted to finding methods to prevent war and to establish a 'culture of peace'. The document adopted at the 1999 conference, the Hague Appeal for Peace and Justice for the 21st Century, has been translated by the United Nations into all its official languages and distributed widely around the world. Its ten-point action agenda addressed education for peace, human rights, and democracy; the adverse effects of globalization; sustainable and equitable use of environmental resources; elimination of racial, ethnic, religious, and gender intolerance; protection of children; reduction of violence; and other issues.

Primary prevention

Primary prevention includes preventing specific elements of collective violence and sharply reducing preparation for war, as follows.

Strengthening of nuclear weapons treaties

Unlike the implementation of treaties banning chemical weapons and biological weapons, there is no comprehensive treaty banning the use or mandating the destruction of nuclear weapons. Instead, a series of overlapping incomplete treaties have been negotiated. The Partial Test Ban Treaty (PTBT) of 1963, promoted in part by concerns about radioactive environmental contamination, banned nuclear tests in the atmosphere, under water, and in outer space. The expansion of the PTBT, the Comprehensive Nuclear Test Ban Treaty (CTBT), a key step towards nuclear disarmament and preventing proliferation, was opened for signature in 1996 but has not yet received sufficient signatures or ratifications to enter into force. It bans nuclear explosions, for either military or civilian purposes, but does not ban computer simulations and subcritical tests, which some nations rely on to maintain the option of developing new nuclear weapons. As of early 2008, the CTBT had been signed by 178 nations and ratified by 144. Entry into force requires ratification by the 44 nuclear-capable nations, of which 35 had ratified it by early 2008. The United States has not yet ratified the CTBT.

The Treaty on the Non-Proliferation of Nuclear Weapons (the 'Nuclear Non-Proliferation Treaty', or NPT) was opened for signature in 1968 and entered into force in 1970. By early 2008, a total of 189 states parties (nations) had ratified the treaty. The five nuclear weapon states recognized under the NPT—China, France, Russia, the United Kingdom, and the United States—are parties to the treaty. The NPT attempts to prevent the spread of nuclear weapons by restricting transfer of certain technologies. It relies on a control system carried out by the International Atomic Energy Agency (IAEA), which also promotes nuclear energy. In exchange for the non-nuclear weapons states' commitment not to develop or otherwise acquire nuclear weapons, the NPT commits the nuclear weapon states to good-faith negotiations on nuclear disarmament. Every five years since 1970 the states parties have held a review conference to assess implementation of the treaty. The review conference in 2000 identified and approved practical steps towards the total elimination of nuclear arsenals. The International Court of Justice (the World Court) in 1996 in an advisory opinion urged that the nations possessing nuclear weapons move expeditiously toward nuclear disarmament, as is required by Article VI of the NPT.

The Anti-Ballistic Missile (ABM) Treaty between the United States and the Soviet Union was signed and entered into force in 1972. The ABM Treaty, by limiting defensive systems that would otherwise spur an offensive arms race, has been seen as the foundation for the strategic nuclear arms reduction treaties. In late 2001, President Bush announced that the United States would withdraw from the ABM Treaty within six months and gave formal notice, stating that it 'hinders our government's ability to develop ways to protect our people from future terrorist or rogue-state missile attacks'. The United States in 2007 announced plans to establish a ballistic missile defence system in Eastern Europe, which led Russia to threaten to increase its arsenal of nuclear weapons.

The United States should help stop the spread of nuclear weapons by actively supporting and adhering to these treaties, and by setting an example for the rest of the world by renouncing the first use of nuclear weapons and the development of new nuclear weapons. It should work with Russia to dismantle nuclear warheads and increase funding for programmes to secure nuclear materials so that they will not fall into the hands of individuals and groups.

Increasing attention is being focused on the elimination of nuclear weapons. Policy makers, such as former US Secretaries of State Henry Kissinger and George Shultz and former military leaders, have called for measures towards the elimination of these weapons (Shultz *et al.* 2007). One measure that may accomplish this is a nuclear weapons convention comparable to the Chemical Weapons Convention, the Biological and Toxin Weapons Convention, and the Anti-Personnel Landmine Convention. A model nuclear weapons convention has been drafted by an international coalition of civil society and professional organizations, and has been presented by Costa Rica to the United Nations.

Strengthening the chemical weapons convention

The Chemical Weapons Convention (CWC) is the strongest of the arms control treaties outlawing a single class of weapons. Inspection and verification of compliance with its provisions lies in the hands of the Organization for the Prohibition of Chemical Weapons (OPCW) in The Hague, established by the CWC (Spanjaard & Khabib 2003). Controversies about safety and protection of the environment during the disposal of chemical weapons required by the CWC have delayed completion of the disposal, and large stockpiles still remain in a number of the world's nations that pose a continuing threat to health and to the environment. The United States has failed to fully support the OPCW in its difficult tasks of inspection and in urging nations to comply with the CWC.

Strengthening the biological and toxin weapons convention

Although the development, production, transfer, or use of biological weapons was prohibited by the 1975 Biological and Toxin Weapons Convention (BWC), several nations are believed to retain stockpiles of such weapons. The verification measures included in the BWC are weak and attempts to strengthen them have been unsuccessful. During 2002, the United States blocked attempts to strengthen the verification measures of the BWC, announcing that such measures might lead to exposure of US industrial or military secrets. The United States must be urged to reverse its rejection of the international community's attempts to develop strong inspection and verification protocols for the BWC. Efforts must be made to convince all nations to support strengthening of the BWC and all nations must refrain from secret activities, often termed *defensive*, that may fuel a biological arms race.

Perhaps even more important, global public health capacity to deal with all infectious disease must be strengthened. The best individual and collective efforts at diagnosing and treating disease outbreaks can be overwhelmed by any natural or intentionally induced epidemic. Consequently, support for strong global preventive public health capabilities provides the best ultimate defence against ever-evolving threats. The significant vulnerabilities to persistent global reservoirs of endemic illness in impoverished and underserved populations can provide the source of future pandemics. For example, in India during 1999, there were 2 million new cases of tuberculosis, causing about 450 000 deaths. An investment of $30 million annually over a few years, compared to the current US contribution to India of US$1 million for this purpose, could virtually wipe out the disease. In addition, the United Nations has estimated that US$10 billion invested in safe water supplies could cut by up to one-third the current 4 billion cases of diarrhoea worldwide that result in 2.2 million annual deaths.

Promoting the support of the Anti-Personnel Landmine Convention

As of April 2008, a total of 158 nations had signed or acceded to the 1997 Land Mines Convention. Of these, 156 nations had formally ratified. Regrettably, 37 nations had neither signed nor ratified, including China, India, Iran, Iraq, Israel, Russia, and the United States. Resources are desperately needed to clear the landmines currently deployed. All the nations of the world must be urged to contribute more resources to this task.

Secondary prevention

The consequences of collective violence can also be prevented or diminished by secondary prevention if war occurs, by preventing casualties among military personnel and civilians, by preventing environmental destruction, and by seeking an end to the war. Secondary prevention methods include strengthening adherence to the Geneva Conventions and other treaties that lessen the effects of war; reducing military activities, including preparation for war; and negotiating effective treaties to lessen environmental damage.

Tertiary prevention

Efforts after the end of an armed conflict to rehabilitate and reintegrate those living with disabilities due to the conflict, to repair the damage to the physical, social, cultural and economic environments, and thereby to prevent new conflicts and new collective violence are extremely important. Tertiary prevention methods include programmes for physical and social rehabilitation for individuals, groups and communities; provision of appropriate aid to communities and nations damaged by collective violence, such as the Marshall Plan after World War II; assurance of environmental remediation after the armed violence has ended; and the establishment of truth and reconciliation commissions, such as the highly successful commission set up in South Africa by President Nelson Mandela.

The role of non-governmental organizations

Important roles for public health workers in the prevention and alleviation of the consequences of collective violence lie in work with non-governmental organizations (NGOs). These organizations are increasingly being called *civil society organizations*, and focus on war from a medical and public health perspective in a variety of ways:

- Intervening to mitigate the consequences of armed conflict
- Researching the effects of war
- Educating the public and decision makers about its impact on health and the environment
- Advocating for changes in global attitudes and policies towards war and the most dangerous weapons and practices of war (Loretz 2008)

Other non-governmental organizations provide direct humanitarian assistance to the victims of collective violence. These organizations generally participate in secondary and tertiary prevention but some, such as the International Committee of the Red Cross, have also in recent years begun to play a role in primary prevention. Humanitarian assistance organizations may also play a role in primary prevention of specific acts of violence and atrocities. They may be strong advocates on behalf of civilian populations among whom they live and for whom they provide humanitarian assistance (Waldman 2008).

Acknowledgement

Parts of this chapter are modified from a background paper on 'Collective Violence: Health Impact and Prevention' for the Workshop on Violence Prevention in Low- and Middle-Income Countries conducted by the Institute of Medicine in 2007, which was published as an appendix in the Workshop Summary (Sidel & Levy 2008).

References

Burmistrov D., Kossenko M., Wilson R. *Radioactive contamination of the Techa River and its effects.* Cambridge (MA): Harvard University; 2006.

Available from: http://phys4.harvard.edu/~wilson/publications/pp747/techa_cor.htm. [Accessed 2006 Mar 8].

Centers for Disease Control and Prevention. Bioterrorism agents/diseases. Centers for Disease Control and Prevention; 2007. Available from: http://www.bt.cdc.gov/agent/agentlist-category.asp. [Accessed 2007 Jun 9].

Cole L.A. Clouds of secrecy: the Army's germ warfare tests over populated areas. Totowa (NJ): Rowman & Littlefield; 1988.

Depleted Uranium Education Project. *Metal of dishonor: depleted uranium*. New York (NY): International Action Center; 1997.

Harris R., Paxman J. A higher form of killing: the secret story of chemical and biological weapons. New York (NY): Hill and Wang; 1962.

Institute of Medicine, National Research Council. Exposure of the American people to iodine-131 from Nevada nuclear-test: review of the National Cancer Institute report and public health implications. Washington (DC): National Academy Press; 1999. p. 193.

International Campaign to Ban Landmines [Online]. Available from: www.icbl.org. [Accessed 2008 July 29].

Krug E.G. *et al.*, editors. 2002 *world report on violence and health*. Geneva: World Health Organization. Available from: http://www.who.int/violence_injury_prevention/violence/world_report/en/full_en.pdf

Levy B.S., Sidel V.W., editors. Terrorism and public health: a balanced approach to strengthening systems and protecting people. Updated ed. New York (NY): Oxford University Press; 2007.

Levy B.S., Sidel V.W., editors. *War and public health*. 2nd ed. New York (NY): Oxford University Press; 2008.

Levy B.S., Sidel V.W. War. In: Frumkin H, editor. *Environmental health: from local to global*. New York (NY): Jossey-Bass; 2005. p. 269–87.

Loretz J. The role of nongovernmental organizations. In: Levy B.S., Sidel V.W., editors. *War and public health*. 2nd ed. New York (NY): Oxford University Press; 2008. p. 381–92.

Marmot M., Bell R. The socioeconomically disadvantaged. In: Levy B.S., Sidel V.W., editors. *Social injustice and public health*. New York (NY): Oxford University Press; 2006. p. 25–45.

Meselson M., Guillemin J., Hugh-Jones M. *et al.* The Sverdlovsk anthrax outbreak of 1979. *Science* 1994;**266**:1202–8.

Renner M. Environmental and health effects of weapons production, testing, and maintenance. In: Levy B.S., Sidel V.W., editors. *War and public health*. Updated ed. Washington (DC): American Public Health Association; 2000. p. 117–36.

Rummel R.J. *Death by government: genocide and mass murder since 1900*. New Brunswick (NJ), London: Transaction Publications; 1994.

Securing our survival: the case for a nuclear weapons convention. Cambridge (MA): International Physicians for the Prevention of Nuclear War; 2007.

Shultz G.P., Perry W.J., Kissinger H.A. *et al.* A world free of nuclear weapons. Wall Street Journal 2007 Jan 4;Sect. A:15.

Sidel V.W., Levy B.S. Collective violence: health impact and prevention. In: Institute of Medicine (IOM). *Violence prevention in low- and middle-income countries*. Washington (DC): National Academies Press; 2008. p. 171–99.

Sirkin S., Cobey J.C., Stover E. Landmines. In: Levy B.S., Sidel V.W., editors. *War and public health*. 2nd ed. New York (NY): Oxford University Press; 2008. p. 102–16.

Smith D. World at war. *The Defense Monitor* 2007;**36**(1):1–9.

Spanjaard H., Khabib O. Chemical Weapons. In: Levy B.S., Sidel V.W., editors. *Terrorism and public health: a balanced approach to strengthening systems and protecting people*. Updated ed. New York (NY): Oxford University Press; 2007. p. 199–219.

Stockholm International Peace Research Institute. *SIPRI yearbook 2002: armaments, disarmament, and international security*. New York (NY): Oxford University Press; 2002.

Sutton P.M., Gould R.M. Nuclear, radiological, and related weapons. In: Levy B.S., Sidel V.W., editors. *Terrorism and public health: a balanced approach to strengthening systems and protecting people*. Updated ed. New York (NY): Oxford University Press; 2007. p. 220–42.

Waldman R. The roles of humanitarian assistance. In: Levy B.S., Sidel V.W., editors. *War and public health*. 2nd ed. New York (NY): Oxford University Press; 2008. p. 369–80.

World Health Assembly. Resolution WHA34.38 Geneva: World Health Organization; 1981.

World Health Assembly. Resolution WHA49.25 on prevention of violence: a public health priority. Geneva: World Health Organization; 1996.

Yokoro K, Kamada N. The health effects of the use of nuclear weapons. In: Levy BS, Sidel VW, editors. *War and public health*. Updated ed. Washington (DC): American Public Health Association; 2000. p. 65–83.

10.7

Urban health in low- and middle-income countries

Mark R. Montgomery

Abstract

Over the next 30 years, low- and middle-income countries will cross an historic threshold, becoming for the first time more urban than rural. This chapter explores the implications for urban public health. To date, health research and policy discussions have been overly concerned with urban–rural differences in health, which generally favour urban areas except for human immunodeficiency virus (HIV)/acquired immunodeficiency syndrome (AIDS), and insufficient attention has been paid to the wide disparities in health that exist within urban areas. Empirical studies show clearly that the urban poor—especially those who live in slums, without adequate drinking water, sanitation, and housing—face health risks that are similar to and sometimes markedly worse than the risks facing rural villagers.

The private sector is a more prominent element of the urban than the rural health system, and the monetary costs of care often cause the urban poor to delay or forgo needed treatment. In addition, although high-quality health care is in principle available in large cities, the quality of the basic health-care services accessible to the urban poor can be abysmally low. It is not so much the physical distance to services that matter for them, but the social, informational, and economic costs of access. A number of urban health risks warrant more attention: Women's mental health, which is doubtless a key determinant of self-efficacy and thus health-seeking behaviour; the incidence of intimate-partner violence and the risks of crime faced by the urban poor; injuries and deaths due to motor vehicles, typically ranking near the top of the urban burden of disease; tuberculosis and malaria (in sub-Saharan Africa and parts of Southeast Asia); the health threats posed by indoor and outdoor air pollution; and the risks that climate change will present for the cities of low- and middle-income countries, which are likely to experience increases in extreme weather in the coming decades. As national governments and health systems continue to decentralize, the health needs of smaller, secondary cities cannot continue to be neglected—it is in these smaller cities where the majority of urbanites live in most countries. To meet the health challenges of an urban era, the public health sector must engage in what Harpham (2007) terms 'joined-up government', forging partnerships with other urban agencies and sectors at the municipal and regional as well as the national level.

Introduction

Sometime in the next 30 years, if United Nations (UN) projections prove to be on the mark, the populations of poor countries will cross an historic threshold, becoming for the first time more urban than rural (United Nations 2005). In public health, as in other fields, the full implications of this urban transition are only beginning to be appreciated. Part of the difficulty is that the term *urban* refers to a bewildering variety of environments. The health circumstances of small cities and towns differ in many ways from those of larger cities. Within any given city, some residents live in secure, gated communities having all the amenities of Europe or the United States, whereas others—especially those who live in slums—exist in grim Dickensian settings lacking the most basic of human needs such as water supply, sanitation, and housing. The health systems of cities in low- and middle-income countries are also astonishingly varied.

An urban system will often present the full array of health providers, ranging from traditional healers, purveyors of drugs in street markets, ill-equipped pharmacists and chemists operating from ramshackle storefronts, and so on up the scale to the most highly-trained surgeons. Among all urban providers, a high percentage is likely to be engaged in private practice, whether on a full- or part-time basis, and for this reason, urban health care is more monetized than rural care. In urban areas, unlike rural, it is not so much the distance to services that presents a barrier to their use, but rather the social, informational, and economic costs of access.

To be sure, the urban–rural contrast should not be overdrawn. Many residents of the developing world live on the peripheries of cities in locations that are arguably neither urban nor rural; circular migration and other social linkages have long connected the two sectors, and the multiplicity of contacts provides opportunities for communicable diseases to pass between them. Although urban health cannot be separated out and studied apart from rural, it may nevertheless be useful to consider the features of urban health environments and behaviour that have a distinctive quality.

To convey the scale of the urban health challenge that lies ahead, we first provide a sketch of the demographic forces that are reshaping the landscape of low- and middle-income countries. The next section then summarizes the urban health differentials that can be identified in data from internationally comparable sample surveys.

Here, we begin by documenting urban–rural differences and proceed to give closer attention to the within-urban inequalities in health. Next, we draw out the salient features of the supply side of urban health, with particular emphasis on the money costs and quality of health care. Following this, we turn to a description of urban health risks that have not been sufficiently appreciated, or which, to be effectively addressed, would require an expansive conception of the role of the public health system. Finally, we provide a conclusion.

The demographic context

The urban population of the developing world, estimated by the United Nations Population Division to have been 1.97 billion persons in the year 2000, is projected to increase to 3.90 billion by 2030 and to 5.26 billion by 2050 (United Nations 2005). These additions to the cities and towns of poor countries will account for nearly 90 per cent of all world population growth over this period. By 2050, according to the projections, fully two-thirds of the inhabitants of poor countries will live in urban areas, with the number of large cities in these countries reaching historically unprecedented levels.

In 1950, there were only two metropolitan areas in the world—the Tokyo and the New York–Newark agglomerations—with populations of 10 million or more. (Cities of this size are commonly called megacities.) By 2025, according to the UN forecasts, the low- and middle-income countries alone will contain 21 cities of this size. Even more striking is the number of cities in the 1–5 million range. In 1950, only 33 such cities were found in the developing world, whereas by 2025, the UN projects a total of no fewer than 431 cities in this range.

Forecasts such as these seem to have fostered the impression that most urban-dwellers in poor countries live in huge urban agglomerations. This is simply not the case. As Fig. 10.7.1 shows, among all developing-country urbanites in cities of 100 000 and above, only 12 per cent live in megacities—about 1 in 8 of these urban residents. Twice as many people live in the small cities ranging from 100 000 to a half-million in size. As the Panel on Urban Population Dynamics (2003) has argued, such smaller cities warrant much more attention than they have been given.

These cities are generally less well-provisioned than larger places with basic services such as improved sanitation and adequate supplies of drinking water. Rates of malnutrition and the risks of infant and child mortality in small cities differs only little from what is seen in the countryside. Yet, the municipal governments of such cities seldom possess the range of health expertise and managerial talent that can be found in the governments of larger places. As low- and middle-income countries continue to decentralize their political and administrative systems—transferring more responsibilities for service delivery and revenue-raising from national governments and health ministries to the local tiers of government and the local ministry offices—the thinner resources and weaker capabilities of smaller cities will need careful attention (Panel on Urban Population Dynamics 2003). The preoccupation with the largest of developing-country cities in health-policy discussions, and the general neglect of small cities, has left unaddressed a wide array of important health concerns.

The urban burden of disease: Overview

Because very few low- and middle-income countries maintain reliable vital statistics systems, sample surveys provide much of what is known of urban health in these countries.[1] The two major ongoing survey programmes are the Demographic and Health Survey (DHS), which has fielded and put into the public domain over 150 surveys

[1] See the WHO report (*World health statistics* 2007. Geneva: World Health Organization 2007c), which indicates that, of the 115 countries reporting to the WHO on the quality of cause-of-death statistics, only 29 (representing a mere 13 per cent of world population) were judged to have adequate records.

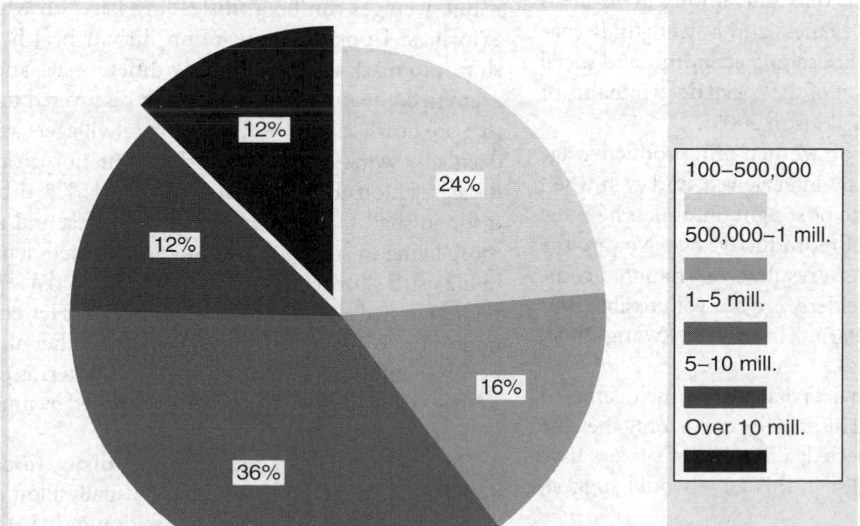

Fig. 10.7.1 Distribution of urban population by city size, population of 100 000 or more, in low- and middle-income countries in 2000.
Source: United Nations. *World urbanization prospects: the 2005 revision population database.* New York [NY]: Department of Economic and Social Affairs, Population Division, United Nations (2005).

Table 10.7.1 Health data routinely collected in the Demographic and Health Surveys (DHSs) and the Multiple Indicator Cluster Surveys (MICSs)

Demographic group	Health data	Gaps
Infants and children	Survival, approximate age at death Vaccination status Recent experience of fever, cough, diarrhoea Height and weight for age (in many surveys)	No reliable cause-of-death information No detailed account of health-seeking behaviour
Adolescents and women of reproductive age	Knowledge of reproduction, contraception, HIV/AIDS, and sources of contraception and health care Detailed data on use of contraception For recent births, nature and timing of prenatal care, place of delivery and attendance	Induced abortion and aftermath not studied Maternal mortality examined indirectly via 'sisterhood' methods No exploration of asymptomatic health conditions unless biomarkers are collected
Sources of care	Knowledge of sources of contraception and health care in some cases supplemented with an urban 'community questionnaire'	No systematic inventory of health providers Not obvious whether geographic boundaries effectively define urban accessible care

since the mid-1980s, and the Multiple Indicator Cluster Survey (MICS), for which some 50 surveys are now available.[2] The DHS and MICS are nationally representative, and are designed to provide reliable estimates for the urban sector as a whole. However, the sample sizes are too small to yield reliable health estimates at the level of individual cities. These programmes have broad data collection agendas in which health is only one among many areas of inquiry. This breadth is both a weakness and a strength: It enables health measures to be linked to household economic and social variables, allowing some investigation of the social determinants of health (Marmot 2005; Marmot & Wilkinson 2005).

The surveys have focused mainly on women of reproductive age and their children. Men are not always interviewed, and even when they are, it is uncommon for a man to be sought out unless he is the partner of an interviewed woman of reproductive age. Nor are the elderly eligible to be interviewed. As a result, cross-national comparisons of the health of the urban elderly are not yet possible (but see Wong *et al.* 2006; Hu *et al.* 2007; Zimmer & Kwong 2004; Kaneda *et al.* 2005; and WHO 2007a).

Table 10.7.1 summarizes the health data that are routinely gathered in the course of a DHS and MICS. This table presents only the core measures that are almost always collected; a number of surveys have been far more ambitious than the list in this table would suggest.

[2] For more information, see http://www.measuredhs.com/aboutdhs for the DHS and http://www.childinfo.org/index.htm for the MICS.

There are well-known limits on what can be learned about health in a survey interview. When they are led through their reproductive histories by a skilled interviewer, women can supply reliable information on infant and child survival, but they are unlikely to give medically meaningful accounts of the causes of death. Adult mortality also presents difficulties for the DHS and MICS instruments, given that the women who are the primary respondents are generally no older than 50 years of age themselves. (Ingenious attempts have been made to measure maternal mortality via the 'sisterhood' method (Graham *et al.* 1989), and the DHS and MICS could, in theory, do more along these lines.)

Obviously, asymptomatic conditions cannot be identified in the course of an interview unless blood or tissue samples are collected or the interviewee undergoes a physical examination. (Collection of biomarker data is becoming more common in the DHS programme, but is not yet the norm.) Even reports on symptomatic morbidities and conditions may be clouded by local understandings of what constitutes a disease. The measurement of health-seeking behaviour is also difficult via general-purpose surveys. Although instruments can be designed to retrace the steps leading from problem recognition to treatment, relatively few such surveys of this type have been fielded.

Averages and inequalities

It is commonly believed that in modern-day populations, rural levels of health are worse than urban, and this belief is supported by good scientific evidence. In its analysis of 90 surveys from the DHS programme, the Panel on Urban Population Dynamics (2003) found that, on average, the urban populations of poor countries exhibit lower levels of child mortality than rural populations, and similar urban–rural differences were evident across a range of health indicators. HIV/AIDS presents the large exception to the general rule of urban health advantage. As will be discussed, although the epidemic is penetrating rural areas and may be driving up incidence rates there, prevalence continues to be higher in urban areas, often substantially so. Apart from HIV/AIDS, however, in most low- and middle-income countries, the urban advantage in terms of average health levels is too well-documented to dispute.

But averages can be a misleading basis on which to set health priorities. Upon disaggregation, urban health averages can be shown to mask wide within-city differentials, and when these are examined, the urban poor are often discovered to face health risks that are nearly as bad as those of rural villagers and are sometimes decidedly worse. To see the urban situation clearly, two types of disaggregation are needed at a minimum: The urban poor must be distinguished from other urban residents; and among the poor, those living in communities of concentrated deprivation—slums, in the usual shorthand—need to be considered separately from the poor who live elsewhere (Montgomery & Hewett 2005). It is also important to distinguish cities from each other on the basis of their health institutions and personnel, and in terms of the strength of oversight and management that is exercised by municipal and other tiers of government.

The data needed to explore these distinctions are not always available. Demographic surveys will usually allow a country's urban poor to be studied as a group, but seldom provide reliable estimates of health among the poor in any given city, to say nothing of the subgroup of poor residents who live in a city's slums. Although there is good reason to expect deficiencies of health personnel and services in the smaller and less-advantaged cities, the empirical evidence on this point is still very thin. The comprehensive review provided by Dussault and Franceschini (2006) emphasizes urban–rural imbalances in health personnel, but does not differentiate among types of urban areas.

The urban poor

Intra-urban health inequalities—which are all too often overlooked by health and development agencies—are clearly apparent in household survey data. Using the 90 DHSs mentioned earlier, the Panel on Urban Population Dynamics (2003) estimated all-cause infant mortality for the urban poor, other urban households, and all rural households. The results are summarized in Table 10.7.2. As can be seen, the urban poor face significantly greater mortality risks than other urban residents, although as a rule, rural-dwellers face even higher levels of risk. In a survey-by-survey comparison of the poor urban and rural infants, this study found that the risks facing the urban poor were significantly lower in about two-thirds of the surveys. However, in 29 per cent of the surveys, poor urban infants faced significantly higher mortality risks than their rural counterparts. (In the remaining surveys, there was no significant difference between poor urban and rural infants.) Even the generalization that urban infant mortality is lower than rural needs to be carefully qualified; much depends on whether the urban poor are separated out in the urban–rural comparisons.

The evidence available does not yet permit broad pronouncements to be made about the relative risks of the urban poor and rural-dwellers that apply irrespective of health measure. The National Research Council study analysed children's height for age—an indicator that summarizes a child's history of nutrition and disease—obtaining the results shown in Table 10.7.3 for children in the age range of 3–36 months. (The table's entries are Z-scores, with a value of −100 indicating that a child is one standard deviation shorter, given its age and sex, than the median height of an international reference population.) The urban poor are again seen to exhibit worse health than other urban children. When the heights of poor urban and rural children were compared, in almost all surveys (60 of the 67 examined) the poor urban children were found to be significantly taller for their age than were rural children.

Table 10.7.2 Infant mortality estimates for urban poor, urban non-poor, and rural, by region

DHSs (in region)		Urban	
	Rural	**Poor**	**Non-poor**
North Africa	81	60	43
Sub-Saharan Africa	103	89	74
Southeast Asia	59	53	27
South, Central, West Asia	74	69	49
Latin America	69	62	39
Total	86	75	56

Rates expressed per 1000 births.
Source: Panel on Urban Population Dynamics. In: Montgomery MR *et al.*, editors. *Cities transformed: demographic change and its implications in the developing world.* Washington (DC): National Academies Press (2003).

Table 10.7.3 Height-for-age **Z**-scores among children 3–36 months of age, by residence and poverty status

DHSs		Urban	
(in region)	**All rural**	**Poor**	**Non-poor**
North Africa	−155.00	−122.35	−86.53
Sub-Saharan Africa	−184.60	−153.64	−125.86
Southeast Asia	−139.01	−106.46	−48.18
South, Central, West Asia	−176.78	−157.95	−120.31
Latin America	−157.09	−130.28	−80.61
Total	−173.51	−145.43	−109.37

Values are Z-scores, with a value of −100, indicating that a child is 1 SD shorter for its age and sex than the median height of an international reference population.
Source: Panel on Urban Population Dynamics. In: Montgomery MR *et al*, editors. *Cities transformed: demographic change and its implications in the developing world.* Washington (DC): National Academies Press ;(2003).

In the height-for-age measure, evidence of an urban advantage persists even for the urban poor.

As is well known, poor urban-dwellers are exposed to substantial risks when their neighbourhoods lack the public health infrastructure needed to safeguard water supply and assure sanitary disposal of waste (UN-Habitat 2003a, 2003b) The WHO (WHO 2002) estimates that in 2001, diarrhoeal diseases accounted for some 2 million deaths, almost all of which took place in low- and middle-income countries, with unsafe water, inadequate sanitation, and poor hygiene implicated as the possible causes in a large percentage of these. In its examination of data from the DHSs, the Panel on Urban Population Dynamics (2003) showed that urban poverty is associated with a lack of access to piped drinking water and with inadequate sanitation. Table 10.7.4 presents selected findings from this study, again comparing poor urban households with other urban and also rural households. As the table shows, the urban poor are markedly ill-served in comparison with other urban households. Rural households receive even less than poor urban households by way of water and sanitation services, although they benefit to an extent from lower population densities, which offer a form of natural protection against some communicable diseases.

Investments in public health infrastructure require the mobilization of substantial financial sums, and although public health authorities can help publicize needs and exert pressure, the key decision makers are generally located elsewhere in the political–bureaucratic system.[3] There are, however, complementary initiatives that lie squarely within the purview of public health. As McGranahan (2007) argues, citing Cairncross and Valdmanis (2006) among others, the literature on water and sanitation has tended to give too little attention to the hygienic and storage behaviours that cause

3 See Evans (Evans B. Understanding the urban poor's vulnerabilities in sanitation and water supply. Paper presented at *Innovations for an Urban World*, the Rockefeller Foundation's *Urban Summit*; 2007; Bellagio, Italy) on recent innovations in financing improvements in urban water supply, sanitation, and housing.

Table 10.7.4 Percentages of poor urban households with access to services, compared with rural households and the urban non-poor

DHSs (in region)		Piped water on premises	Water in neigh-bourhood	Flush toilet	Pit toilet
North Africa	Rural	41.6	37.3	41.3	17.5
	Urban poor	67.3	27.8	83.7	8.5
	Urban non-poor	90.8	7.8	96.3	2.6
Sub-Saharan Africa	Rural	7.8	55.7	1.1	47.6
	Urban poor	26.9	61.6	13.0	65.9
	Urban non-poor	47.6	45.8	27.4	67.2
Southeast Asia	Rural	18.6	53.7	55.5	24.3
	Urban poor	34.0	53.7	61.8	22.9
	Urban non-poor	55.8	40.1	89.0	9.4
South, Central, West Asia	Rural	28.1	53.6	4.3	55.4
	Urban poor	58.0	36.3	39.8	34.1
	Urban non-poor	80.2	17.7	64.0	23.2
Latin America	Rural	31.4	36.4	12.6	44.0
	Urban poor	58.7	35.2	33.6	47.0
	Urban non-poor	72.7	24.9	63.7	31.6
Total	Rural	18.5	50.7	7.5	46.6
	Urban poor	41.5	49.4	28.3	51.7
	Urban non-poor	61.5	34.0	48.4	46.5

Source: Panel on Urban Population Dynamics. In: Montgomery MR *et al.*, editors. Cities *transformed: demographic change and its implications in the developing world.* Washington (DC): National Academies Press (2003).

water to be contaminated after it has been drawn from the pipes. Important faecal–oral routes for contamination can be addressed through domestic hygiene interventions, including an emphasis on hand-washing especially after defecation, control of flies, and encouragement of safer practices in food preparation and water storage. Cairncross and Valdmanis (2006) assembled evidence showing that behavioural interventions in these areas can achieve substantial reductions in diarrhoeal diseases.

Other important health risks also arise in or near the homes of the poor, with the risks presented by indoor air pollution being increasingly recognized. Recent estimates suggest that, worldwide, more than 2 billion people rely on solid fuels, traditional stoves, and open fires for their cooking, lighting, and heating needs (Larson & Rosen 2002). These fuels generate hazardous pollutants—including suspended particulate matter, carbon monoxide, nitrogen dioxide, and other harmful gases—that are believed to substantially raise the risks of acute respiratory infections and chronic obstructive pulmonary disorders. Such fuels are often used by the urban poor, who must cook in enclosed or inadequately ventilated spaces. The health burdens associated with indoor air pollution are likely to fall heavily upon women, who spend much of their time cooking and tending fires, and also afflict the children who accompany them.

The spatially concentrated urban poor

It is not surprising that when poor city-dwellers live in close proximity to each other without the benefit of safe drinking water and adequate sanitation, they face elevated risks from water-, air-, and food-borne diseases. This much has been known since the eighteenth century in the West, well before the mechanisms of transmission were understood (Woods 2003). It remains difficult, however, to divide the overall risks facing slum-dwellers into the risks attributable to household poverty, and the additional risks produced by the spatial concentration of poverty in slum neighbourhoods and communities.

Although not definitive on this score, Fig. 10.7.2 is suggestive of the impact of concentrated poverty on child mortality in Nairobi, Kenya. In the slums of Nairobi, child mortality rates, at 150 per 1000 births, are substantially above the rates seen elsewhere in that city; slum mortality rates are high enough even to exceed rural Kenyan mortality. The addition to risk evident in these slums may be due to multiple factors: The poor quality and quantity of water and sanitation in these communities; inadequate hygienic practices; poor ventilation and dependence on hazardous cooking fuels; the city's highly monetized health system, which for the poor delays or prevents access to modern health services; and the transmission of disease among densely settled slum-dwellers.

There are additional factors of a social epidemiological character that are worth considering. Facing health threats from their unprotected physical environments—with the lack of services being a constant reminder of social exclusion—and lacking the incomes needed to counteract these daily threats, the urban poor may well feel unable to take effective action to safeguard their health. Poor individuals and families may thus lack the sense of self-efficacy needed to energize their health-seeking behaviour in such difficult environments. Poor communities may be reminded by the absence of basic services that the community as a whole is socially excluded and lacks the political voice needed to bring attention to its plight. At the individual and family level, as we will discuss, social exclusion combined with the daily stresses of poverty may bring on paralyzing fatigue, anxiety, low-level depression, and other expressions of mental ill-health. At the community level, the symptoms may be expressed in the weaknesses and fragilities of local community organizations; that is, in the lack of what has been termed 'bonding' social capital.

The urban health system

The concept of 'health system' is a very broad one and bringing definition to it is especially difficult in urban areas, within which a disparate set of health providers serves what is typically a highly diverse population, with core health needs arising in part from the many ways in which the population's subgroups come into contact. The urban health system is itself situated within larger political–economic frames at the country level. In the structural adjustment era of the 1980s and early 1990s, a number of low- and middle-income countries introduced user fees into public-sector care as they undertook broad health sector reforms (Harpham 2007). As discussed earlier, in many of these countries, the process of decentralization—a transformation of governance that accelerated in the mid-1990s, and which is in its way as profound as the urban transformation—is reshaping relationships between national, regional, and local governments, with important implications for health service planning, finance, and service delivery. These developments provide the context for our discussion of urban health systems.

A distinguishing feature of urban health systems is the prominence of the private sector. Not surprisingly, given the higher average

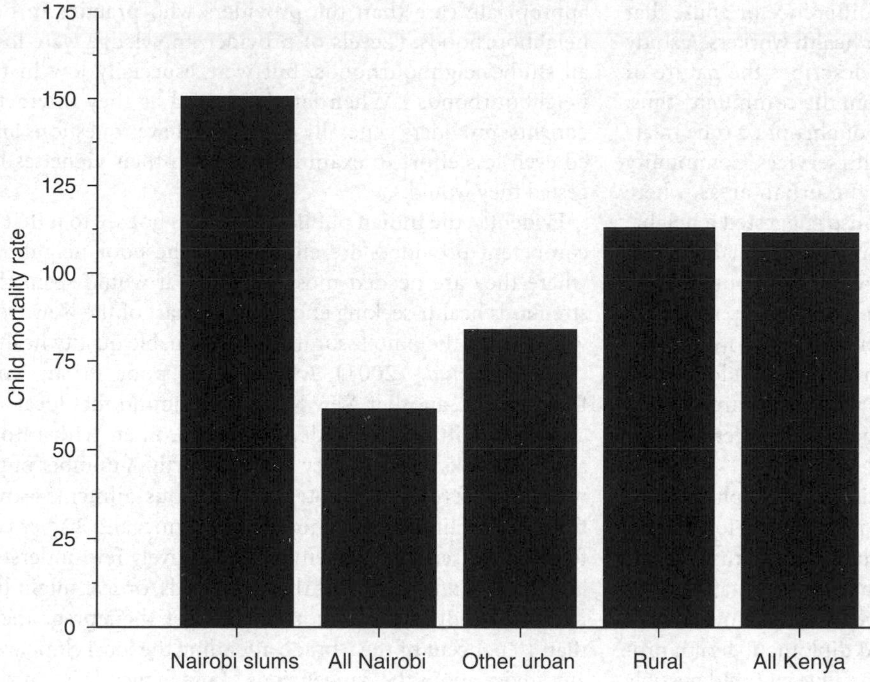

Fig. 10.7.2 Comparison of child mortality rates ($_5q_0$) in the Nairobi slums sample with rates for Nairobi, other cities, rural areas, and Kenya as a whole.
Source: African Population and Health Research Center. *Population and health dynamics in Nairobi's informal settlements: report of the Nairobi cross-sectional slums survey [NCSS] 2000*. Nairobi: African Population and Health Research Center (2002).

levels of income in urban populations and the income diversity that establishes market niches, private services tend to be much more developed in cities than in rural areas, especially in the larger cities (Dussault & Franceschini 2006). Fee-for-service arrangements are generally characteristic of urban health care, whereas rural services are often ostensibly provided free of cost (or made available for nominal fees) at public health posts and clinics.[4]

In the more monetized urban economy, the urban poor without cash on hand can find themselves unable to gain entry to the modern system of hospitals, clinics, and well-trained providers. They may then seek care in other niches of the urban system where less-trained providers make drugs and diagnoses available for affordable fees, and may also pursue traditional practitioners, who can adjust the level and type of payment to the needs of their poor clients.

As the Islam *et al.* (2006) study has documented for Manila and Indore, India, urban health providers are well aware of the effects of monetization on the health-seeking behaviour of the poor. They see poor clients who, having endured their illnesses until care cannot be put off any longer, finally present themselves in a more debilitated condition than they would otherwise have been. Health providers realize that the poor are likely to abandon courses of prescribed medication to save on the costs of purchasing medicines, or may economize by buying less than what was prescribed. They are not really surprised when the poor fail to return as requested for follow-ups and assessments of progress.

In only very few low- and middle-income countries is it possible for the urban poor to receive subsidized care from for-profit private providers, and generally such subsidies are available only through the private non-profit and public-sector clinics and hospitals. Manila's public-sector subsidy programme provides one instructive example. In this health system, subsidies are made available for the purchase of medicines but supplies are not similarly covered. As one physician said in exasperation: 'Sometimes, they say they can ask for discounts or even for free medicines, depending on the [income] class. But in supplies, they cannot. So, for instance, they get antibiotics for free [but] if you do not have syringe, how can you provide it? We still ask them to buy syringe to provide the vaccines'.

As this quotation suggests, stockouts of medicines and basic supplies such as syringes occur frequently in Manila's public-sector facilities. When they occur, it is left to the patient to find the funds to seek out prescribed medicines and supplies at private pharmacies or other sources. In Manila, the lowest tier of the public health system—the barangay health centre—is a vital component of the system for the poor because, for various reasons, the barangay centres are more likely to hold small stocks of some of the subsidized medicines.

As the Manila example illustrates, subsidies for the urban poor often depend on an unsystematic set of arrangements, requiring poor patients and their families to spend time searching and negotiating with what must be a bewildering variety of personnel at scattered locations. As they engage in this form of health-seeking behaviour, the poor can be discouraged by the difficulties of finding affordable transport, inconvenient hours of operation at clinics or health centres, the frequent absence of key staff, and long waits to receive care. In effect, the poor are being asked to substitute the costs of their time for the prospect of reduced costs of medicines. In a full-cost sense, a subsidy for the poor that exists in theory may prove to be no subsidy at all.

We have emphasized the monetary costs of health care, which clearly discourage the urban poor, but they can also be driven away

[4] Even in Latin America, where health-insurance systems are more inclusive than in other low- and middle-income regions, only 20 per cent of the urban poor are covered by insurance. (Fay M, editor. *The urban poor in Latin America*. Washington [DC]: The World Bank; 2005.)

from the modern health system by the indifference or abuse that they anticipate at the hands of formal sector health workers. A study of urban Zimbabwe (Bassett *et al.* 1997) describes the nature of interactions between nurses and women from the community thus:

'To community women, the expectation of abrupt or rude treatment was the main complaint about the health services. Community complaints were voiced most strongly in the urban areas, where accusations of patient neglect and even abuse suggested a heightened hostility between the clinic and community in the urban setting. Several explanations for nurse behaviour were put forward, chief among them was elitism . . . it is in urban areas that class differentiation is most advanced. [The perspective of nurses differed. For them] overwork and low pay promote the adoption of the attitude of an industrial worker—to do what is required and no more. Most nurses work more than one job, not to get rich but to survive'.

As this quotation suggests, much of the literature emphasizes the social distance between providers and their patients, the formal language that providers can use to reinforce their own status, and the possibilities for rude or abusive behaviour on part of the staff towards poor patients. But the literature has not much stressed how difficult it is, even for the most well-intentioned and diplomatic health provider, to get basic information across to poor, illiterate, and possibly intimidated patients. As a Manila obstetrician–gynaecologist explained (Islam *et al.* 2006):

'I guess, for 90 per cent of our patients, it is us who tell them things. Although there are some who are really inquisitive, especially those who have had some education. [But among the urban poor?] They just accept everything we tell them. They rarely ask questions. And sometimes it is difficult to relate to them. They have a hard time understanding what we are saying, even if we use the most basic words or terms. Like for instance, sometimes, we tell them, this is the right way to take the medicine; to make sure that they understand us, we ask them to demonstrate. [Are they receptive to that?] Some, yes. But the others just don't care. They don't know anything, they don't even know when was their last period, family history, nothing. It's really frustrating'.

When the poor do succeed in receiving formal health care, is that care likely to be of sufficient quality to make an effective difference to their health? A recent urban quality-of-care study in New Delhi raises serious doubts on this score (Das & Hammer 2007a, 2007b). The study was set in both slum and non-slum neighbourhoods, covering a range of income levels. A full inventory was made of the health providers who serve these neighbourhoods; it revealed that a 15-minute walk would bring a typical neighbourhood resident within reach of 70 health providers of some sort. Even for the poor, access in the sense of geographic distance was not the problem in this case; and if anything, the Delhi poor tended to seek care for illness at least as often as the non-poor. The study assessed the quality of health-care provision in two ways: Via a series of vignettes measuring provider knowledge of the steps to take in making a diagnosis and prescribing treatment or referral (rating the provider responses in relation to examination protocols); and by a follow-up in which many of the same providers were observed as they interacted with patients.

The study found that the quality of care available in the poor neighbourhoods was so low that the authors could fairly describe it as 'money for nothing'. Both public-sector and private providers serve the poor neighbourhoods of Delhi, and both know less about appropriate care than the providers who practice in better-off neighbourhoods. (Levels of provider knowledge were low across all study neighbourhoods, but were especially low in the poor neighbourhoods.) When later observed as they interacted with patients, providers generally asked even fewer questions and exerted even less effort in examinations than their vignettes had suggested they would.

Evidently, the Indian public sector does not see to it that its more competent providers are allocated to the poor neighbourhoods where they are needed most. In short, it would seem that even strenuous health-seeking efforts on the part of the New Delhi poor would bring them no assurance of reasonable quality health care.

Mayank *et al.* (2001), who studied poor urban women in Dakshinpuri, another New Delhi slum, found that local antenatal clinics did little to provide pregnant women with information about the risks of pregnancy and childbirth. A number of pregnant women suffered from potentially serious ailments—over two-thirds were clinically diagnosed as anaemic, and 12 per cent were found to be seriously anaemic. Yet, relatively few understood that high fevers and swelling of the face, hands, or feet might be symptoms of conditions that could endanger their pregnancy. Fewer than 10 per cent of the women attending the local clinic were given any advice about the danger signs of pregnancy. It is not altogether surprising that the maternal mortality rate in this urban sample was estimated at 645 deaths per 100 000, a rate not much different from that prevailing in rural India.

Figure 10.7.3 shows that low quality of care is generally characteristic of urban India (Fig. 10.7.3a) and is also a concern in the urban areas of the Philippines (Fig. 10.7.3b). The figure depicts the percentage of women who, in one or more prenatal care visits, were warned of the complications of pregnancy. Among poor urban Indian women, not even 40 per cent are told during prenatal visits of the danger signs of pregnancy. Although the percentages are somewhat higher in urban Philippines, less than half of the poor women are informed of the risks and fewer still are told where to seek care if signs of danger surface.

Urban health risks and risk factors

In this subsection, we turn attention to specific urban risks and causes of mortality and morbidity. Several themes unite this material. First among them is the importance of disaggregation of urban health conditions and risk factors by poverty and place. A second and closely-related theme is that of urban social epidemiology, with emphasis on the concepts of individual and collective efficacy in health seeking. A third theme in the discussion concerns health conditions or risks that are sometimes overlooked, or which are not as well-integrated as they might be in urban public health policies. Mental health is perhaps the leading example of such a condition. It is closely associated with poverty and with the health threats that arise from violence and alcohol abuse, which place disproportionate burdens on women. Other examples include the burdens of illness and death stemming from road traffic accidents and outdoor air pollution. In many countries, HIV/AIDS already occupies a prominent place on the urban health agenda, whereas urban tuberculosis and malaria receive less attention. Only the most expansive public health programmes in low- and middle-income countries have conceived of the field of action in such broad terms as to encompass all these areas.

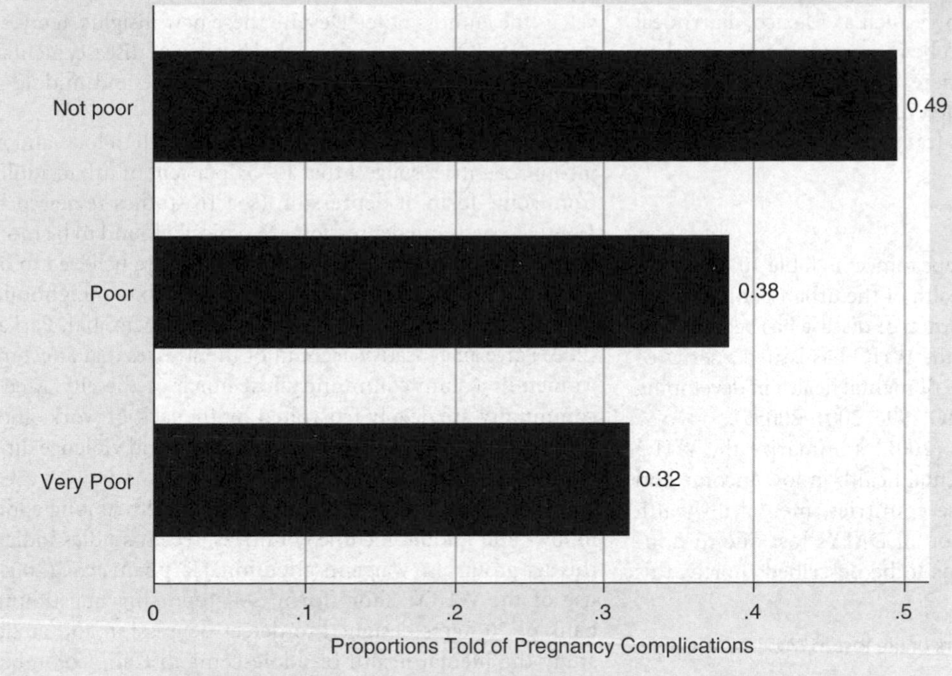

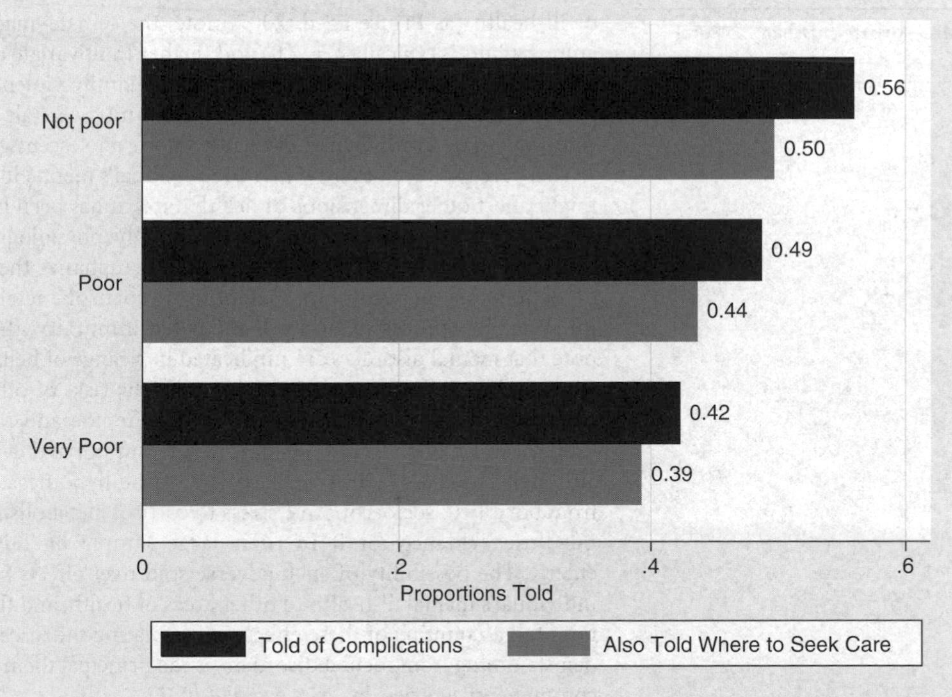

Fig. 10.7.3 Information on pregnancy complications given during prenatal care, by relative poverty, women with one or more visits, in urban India and urban Philippines:
(a) Women informed of complications and their danger signs during pregnancy, urban India; (b) Women informed of complications and danger signs during pregnancy, and told where to seek care if these appear, urban Philippines.
Source: Islam M, Montgomery MR, Taneja S. *Urban health and care-seeking behavior: a case study of slums in India and the Philippines.* Bethesda [MD]: PHRPlus Program, Abt Associates (2006).

To bring some order to a wide-ranging discussion, we begin with an overview of urban causes of death and disability, drawing upon data from Mexico, one of the few low- and middle-income countries that can provide reliable information. With this as background, we then present a series of remarks on the specific features of urban health that warrant closer study.

The urban burden of disease

Table 10.7.5 shows the 15 leading causes of disability-adjusted life years (DALYs) lost in rural and urban areas for Mexico. Several lessons can be extracted from this table. First, urban areas do not necessarily present health profiles that are wholly distinct from those of rural areas. In Mexico, the causes of DALYs lost are much the same in urban and rural areas, although they follow a different rank order. Of the top five causes in Mexico's urban areas, three (deaths related to motor vehicles, homicide and violence, and cirrhosis) are also found among the top five in rural areas. Second, interventions to address two of the most important causes of death and disability in urban Mexico—those related to violence, and to traffic-related deaths and injuries—would in many countries be considered outside the scope of the public health system. Third, the table reminds us that even in a middle-income country such as Mexico, diarrhoeal disease and pneumonia continue to be important causes of urban death and disability—here as elsewhere, an epidemiological transition is underway whereby the burden of disease is tilting towards non-communicable causes, but this transition is evidently far from being complete.

Mental health

Mental health, as such, makes no appearance in Table 10.7.5, but it is arguably a central factor in the health of the urban poor, and one whose contribution to the urban burden of disease has been underappreciated. Over the past decade, the WHO has issued a series of reports emphasizing the importance of mental health in developing as well as developed countries (WHO 1996, 2001, 2005a).

In a recent review, Prince *et al.* (2007) summarize the WHO burden-of-disease estimates for mental health in low-income and middle-income countries. In these countries, mental ill-health accounts for roughly 24 per cent of all DALYs lost due to non-communicable diseases. For reasons to be described shortly, this figure is likely to understate the full impacts of mental health. And yet, as the authors note, 'Despite these new insights, ten years after the first WHO report on the global burden of disease, mental health remains a low priority in most low-income and middle-income countries'.

Table 10.7.5 Disability-adjusted years of life lost in Mexico, by cause and area of residence

Cause	Rural	Rural rank	Urban	Urban rank	Rural urban
Diarrhoea	12.0	1	2.8	9	4.28
Pneumonia	9.3	2	3.9	7	2.39
Homicide and violence	9.2	3	7.4	2	1.23
Motor vehicle-related deaths	7.9	4	8.3	1	0.95
Cirrhosis	7.5	5	6.3	4	1.19
Anaemia and malnutrition	6.8	6	2.4	11	2.86
Road traffic accidents	5.5	7	6.8	3	0.81
Ischaemic heart disease	5.1	8	5.3	6	0.96
Diseases of the digestive system	4.7	9	1.7	15	2.74
Diabetes mellitus	4.1	10	5.7	5	0.72
Cerebrovascular disease	3.0	11	3.0	8	1.02
Alcohol dependence	3.0	11	1.9	13	1.56
Accidents (falls)	2.8	13	2.6	10	1.09
Chronic lung disease	2.6	14	1.9	13	1.39
Nephritis	2.2	15	2.2	12	1.01

1991 estimates, expressed per 1000 population.

Source: Lozano R, Murray C, Frenk J. El peso de las enfermedades en Mexico. In: Hill K, Morelos JB, Wong R, editors. *Las consecuencias de las transiciones demografica y epidemiological en América Latina.* Mexico City: El Colegio de México (1999).

Community-based studies of mental health in low- and middle-income countries suggest that 12–51 per cent of urban adults suffer from some form of depression (see 16 studies reviewed by Blue 1999). Anxiety and depression are typically found to be more prevalent among urban women than men and are believed to be more prevalent in poor than in non-poor urban neighbourhoods (Almeida-Filho *et al.* 2004). In a study of Mumbai, Parkar *et al.* (2003) give an evocative account of the stresses that affect men and women in a slum community just north of the city. Men in this community are deeply frustrated by the lack of work, and this is reflected in a high incidence of alcoholism and violence directed at their wives.

Although less is known about mental health among adolescents in low- and middle-income countries, recent studies indicate that this age group also warrants attention. Harpham *et al.* (2004) made use of the WHO's short-form, self-reporting questionnaire—a bank of 20 items designed to detect depression and anxiety—to study the mental health of adolescents in Cali, Colombia. Girls were found to be three times more likely than boys to exhibit signs of ill-health (as Prince *et al.* 2007, note, the female–male ratio among adults is typically 1.5–2.0) and further multivariate analysis showed that low levels of schooling, within-family violence, and perceptions that violence afflicts the community were all significantly associated with mental ill-health among adolescents.

There are two avenues by which an individual's mental ill-health might affect other dimensions of health. First, it has been hypothesized that socioeconomic stress undermines the physiological systems that sustain health. Prince *et al.* (2007) emphasize the effects of depression on serotonin metabolism, cortisol metabolism, inflammatory processes, and cell-mediated immunity; they also note that mental disorders are implicated in a range of behaviours (e.g. smoking, poor diet, obesity) that raise the risks of other diseases. Boardman (2004), McEwen (1998), Steptoe and Marmot (2002), and Cohen *et al.* (2006) provide supportive evidence, although Hu *et al.* (2007) are sceptical of the hypothesized link from poverty to socioeconomic stress to cortisol metabolism, finding little evidence for it in their large sample of Taiwanese elderly. The possibility of such adverse spill-over effects from an individual's mental ill-health to other areas of health, and the need for a full accounting of these effects in calculating the disease burden stemming from mental disorders, is the principal theme of the comprehensive review by Prince *et al.* (2007).

The second avenue needing exploration also involves spill-over effects, but in this case the posited linkage would connect women's mental health to the health-seeking energies they can deploy on behalf of their children and other family members. To judge from the review by Prince *et al.* (2007), very little research has been conducted on how mental health affects women's health-seeking behaviour. A few studies have linked mental ill-health to the difficulties that individuals face in adhering to their own treatment regimens, especially the demanding protocols required in antiretroviral therapies for HIV/AIDS and directly observed short-course treatments for tuberculosis. A bit more attention has been given to the associations between a woman's mental health and her reproductive health, and between the health status of pregnant women and their children's birth weight, with the latter possibly involving health-seeking behaviour. But almost nothing seems to have been written on whether and how mental ill-health undermines the sense of self-efficacy that motivates a woman to seek health-care for others in her family. This is a surprising gap in the literature, especially in view of the well-documented role that women play in protecting the health of their families and the equally common finding that mental ill-health is more common among women than men.[5]

Intimate-partner violence and alcohol abuse

Violence in urban areas takes a variety of forms, ranging from political and extra-judicial violence to gang violence, local violent crime, and abuse taking place within the home. Moser (2004) develops a framework within which these complex forms of violence can be analysed and describes the points of intervention within the judicial, public health, and other urban systems (also see Winton 2004). Garrett and Ahmed (2004) have developed a module for measuring aspects of crime, violence, and physical insecurity that could be adapted for use in surveys, so that these problems can be better documented than they are at present. Our discussion is mainly concerned with intimate-partner violence and its links to alcohol abuse and women's mental health.

Heise *et al.* (1994) reviewed community-based data for eight urban areas from different regions of the developing world, finding that mental and physical abuse of women by their partners was common, with damaging consequences for women's physical and psychological well-being. Using data collected from a module included in several DHSs, Kishor and Johnson (2004) examined whether women had ever been beaten by a spouse or partner. In Cambodia, 18 per cent of women had been beaten, and the percentages in the other study countries were also high: Colombia (44 per cent), Dominican Republic (22 per cent), Egypt (34 per cent), Haiti (29 per cent), India (19 per cent), Nicaragua (30 per cent), Peru (42 per cent), and Zambia (48 per cent). In seeking to understand why women who were the victims of violence did not seek help from the authorities or others outside the home, this study found that embarrassment was a major reason given by women, as well as the belief that it would be futile to seek care or that partner violence was simply a part of life. In some countries (but not in all), poor women were more likely than other women to have experienced violence at the hands of their spouses or partners. Where the connection could be explored, strong links were also found between spousal alcohol abuse and violence.

These findings were echoed in the WHO (2005b) study, summarized in Fig. 10.7.4, which covered both urban and rural study sites. The WHO analysis also documented a close association between the experience of violence and women's mental health. As Fig. 10.7.5 shows, among the women who had been abused by their partner in this study's Bangladeshi urban site (left-most bars), some 21 per cent had had thoughts of suicide, against only 7 per cent of the women who had not been abused. In all but one of the sites in the study, the difference in this measure of mental health was statistically significant, and as can be seen in the figure, the ratios are on the order of 2:1 or higher.

Other forms of urban violence also merit attention. Crime is particularly prevalent in Latin America's large cities, where it disproportionately victimizes men living in low-income neighbourhoods (Barata *et al.* 1998; Grant 1999; Heinemann & Verner 2006). Data collected between 1991 and 1993 in São Paulo suggested that men aged 15–24 years in low-income areas were over five times likelier to fall victim to homicide than were men of the same age in

[5] See Montgomery & Ezeh (2005b) for further discussion with attention to social capital and collective efficacy.

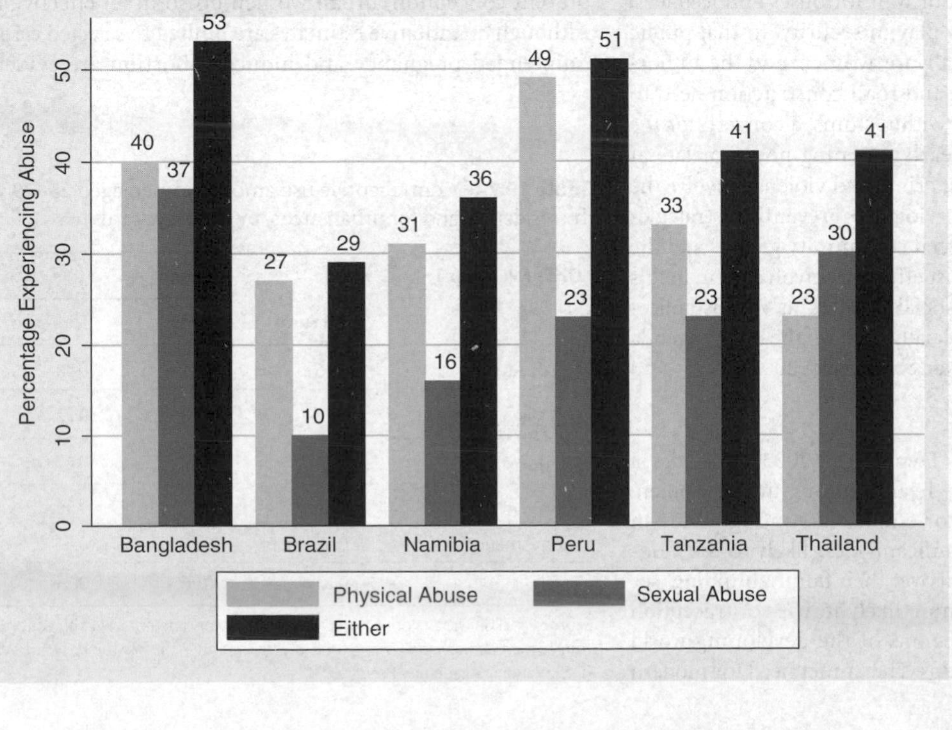

Fig. 10.7.4 Experience of physical or sexual violence by an intimate partner since age 15, among ever-partnered urban women.
Source: WHO. *WHO multi-country study on women's health and domestic violence against women: summary report of initial results on prevalence, health outcomes and women's responses.* Geneva: World Health Organization (2005b).

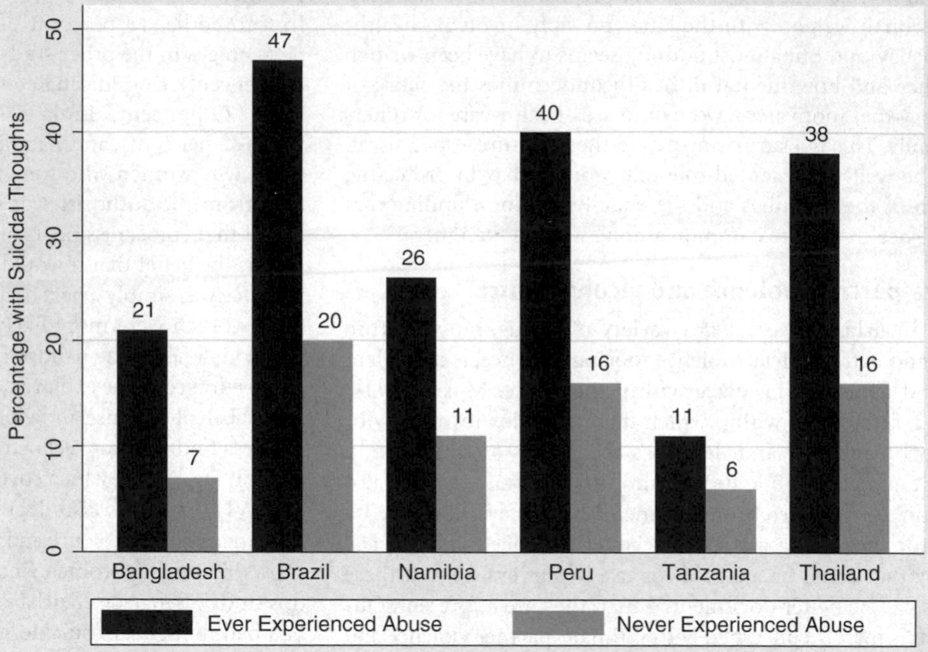

Fig. 10.7.5 Percentage of ever-partnered urban women reporting suicidal thoughts, according to their experience of physical or sexual violence, or both, by an intimate partner.
Source: WHO. *WHO multi-country study on women's health and domestic violence against women: summary report of initial results on prevalence, health outcomes and women's responses.* Geneva: World Health Organization (2005b).

higher-income areas (Soares *et al.* cited in Grant 1999). South African cities also exhibit extraordinarily high rates of violent crime (Stone 2006).

A need exists for systems that can provide women and the poor with some protection from the varied forms of urban violence to which they are vulnerable within and outside the home. To create such systems will require new partnerships linking agencies across urban sectors. In the transport sector, for example, there is a need to make safe the areas where the poor wait for buses and jeepneys; the health sector also has a role to play in security, in that public latrines can be places of risk especially for women; and the authorities responsible for electrification and road construction need to attend to the unlit paths and lanes within slums, a concern for the poor who must commute in the early morning hours or late at night. Effective partnerships against crime and violence involve the formulation of community-driven violence-prevention strategies and the initiation of dialogue between community groups and the police. (The police may initially resist efforts to involve them in this way, complaining of having to be 'social workers' as well as policemen.) Creation of safe spaces is especially high on the policy agenda for adolescent girls and boys (Erulkar & Matheka 2007).

Reproductive health

The Panel on Urban Population Dynamics (2003) provides a lengthy discussion of reproductive health among urban women; here, we select only a few points for emphasis. Among all urban women, those who are poor are significantly less likely to use modern contraception to achieve control over their family-building (see Table 10.7.6). They are generally more likely to use contraception than rural women, but in some regions of the developing world there is little to separate the two groups. The unmet need for modern contraception—this is measured by the proportion of women in a reproductive union who say that they want to prevent or delay their next birth, believe themselves to be capable of conceiving, and yet do not make use of modern contraception to achieve their stated aims—is markedly higher among poor urban than other urban women.

As the Panel on Urban Population Dynamics (2003) discusses, it is not clear that even when they use modern contraception to prevent conception, urban women do so in an effective manner. Although quantitative estimates are limited to selected case studies, unintended pregnancy and induced abortion are evidently not

Table 10.7.6 Contraceptive use among women aged 25–29 years, by residence, and for urban areas, by poverty status

DHSs (by region)		Urban	
	All rural	Poor	Non-poor
North Africa	0.26	0.37	0.48
Sub-Saharan Africa	0.08	0.13	0.22
Southeast Asia	0.44	0.40	0.47
South, Central, West Asia	0.33	0.35	0.44
Latin America	0.32	0.37	0.47
Total	0.22	0.26	0.35

Source: Panel on Urban Population Dynamics. In: Montgomery MR *et al.*, editors. *Cities transformed: demographic change and its implications in the developing world.* Washington (DC): National Academies Press (2003).

uncommon for urban women.[6] To cite a few examples: Women in three squatter settlements in Karachi, Pakistan, were estimated to have a lifetime rate of 3.6 abortions per woman (Jamil & Fikree 2002). Another study found abortion to be widespread in Abidjan, Côte d'Ivoire, where abortion is illegal yet nearly one-third of the women surveyed who had ever been pregnant had had one (Desgrées du Loû *et al.* 2000). A recent study of Ouagadougou, Burkina Faso by Rossier (2007) estimated an annual abortion rate of 4 per cent among women aged 15–49 years, suggesting that over a reproductive lifetime, a woman would have 1.4 abortions on average. Calvés (2002) studied women in their twenties living in Yaoundé, Cameroon; of these young women, 21 per cent reported having had an abortion, with just over 8 per cent having had more than one. Once again, the fact that modern contraceptive services are available in urban areas does not imply that women, especially poor women, have the knowledge and the social and economic wherewithal to make effective use of the methods.

Maternal mortality risks offer another revealing view of urban reproductive health. Because it is difficult to predict whether life-threatening problems will emerge in the course of a woman's pregnancy, delivery, and the aftermath, the prevention of maternal mortality depends crucially on fast access to emergency care. It might be thought that cities, which offer many more transport options than do rural areas, would exhibit much lower levels of maternal mortality. The cases in which the expected urban advantage does not emerge are therefore instructive about the circumstances of the urban poor.

Fikree *et al.* (1997) compared maternal mortality rates in the low-income communities of Karachi with rates in six rural districts elsewhere in Pakistan. Estimates of maternal mortality ratios (MMRs), together with their confidence bands, are shown in Fig. 10.7.6. Although the MMR estimate for Karachi is the lowest among all these sites, the rural estimates are significantly higher than Karachi's only for the remote districts of Loralai and Khuzdar. It appears that Karachi's poor suffer from maternal health disadvantages not unlike those that afflict Pakistan's rural-dwellers.

Why did the urban health advantage not prove greater in this case? In the poor communities of Karachi, some 68 per cent of the births are delivered at home and 59 per cent are attended by traditional birth attendants (TBAs). Yet, rural women are even more likely to deliver at home and to have family members or TBAs in attendance. Another study of Karachi slums (Fikree *et al.* 1994) identified the core of the problem: When acute pregnancy and delivery complications arise in these communities, there can be critical delays in locating male decision makers and obtaining their consent to hospital care. (It has not been customary for husbands or other men to be present at the time of childbirth.) Delays in initiating the search for care are compounded by the tendency for poor Karachi families to pursue local care first, going from place to place in the neighbourhood before making an effort to reach the modern health facilities located outside the neighbourhood. Fikree *et al.* (2004) have illustrated similar care-seeking patterns in a study of postpartum morbidities in the Karachi slums.

6 The Alan Guttmacher Institute (AGI. *Sharing responsibility: women, society, and abortion worldwide.* New York [NY]: Alan Guttmacher Institute; 1999) provides an excellent overview of induced abortion, a generally hidden and difficult-to-study area of health. See *International Family Planning Perspectives*, which is a good source of information on this topic; available from: http://www.guttmacher.org/pubs. The journal *Studies in Family Planning* is another helpful source; available from: http://www.blackwell-synergy.com/loi/sifp.

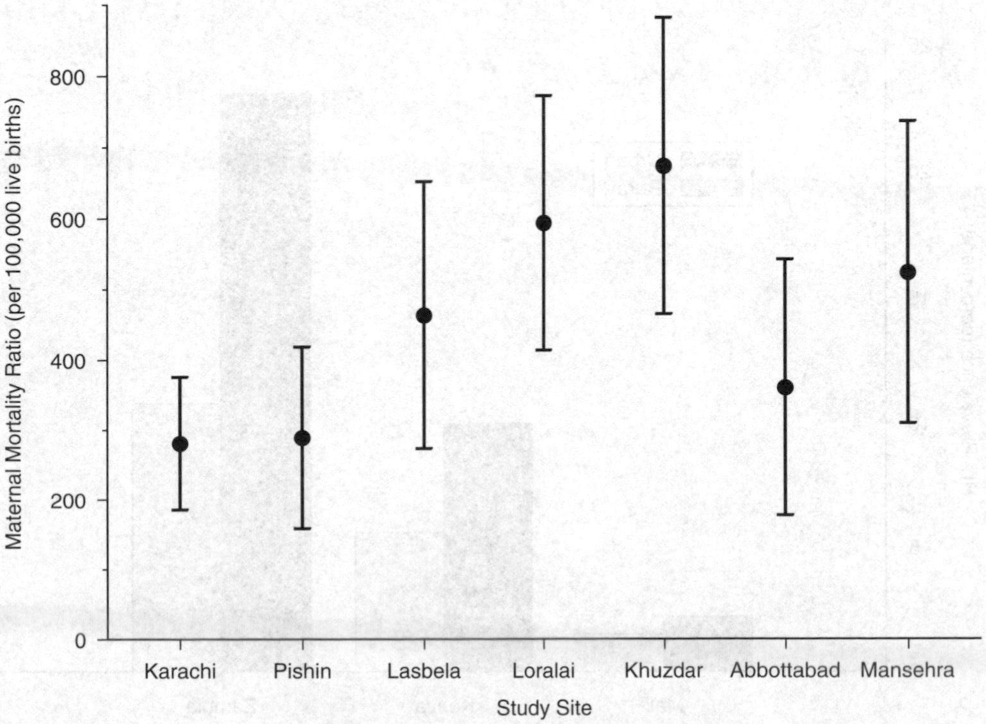

Fig. 10.7.6 Maternal mortality ratios in Karachi, Pakistan, and six rural sites. *Source:* Fikree FF, Midhet F, Sadruddin S *et al.* Maternal mortality in different Pakistani sites: ratios, clinical causes, and determinants. *Acta Obstetricia et Gynecologica Scandinavica* 1997;**76**:637–45.

HIV/AIDS

An enormous literature is now available on the social epidemiology of HIV/AIDS in both developing and developed countries. Despite the quantities of research underway on HIV/AIDS, much remains to be learned about its social components. Indeed, although HIV/AIDS is commonly thought to be more prevalent in urban than rural areas, until recently the scientific basis for this belief has been thin (UNAIDS 2004). In only a few low- and middle-income countries are community-based studies of prevalence now available that can quantify the urban–rural differences.[7]

Figure 10.7.7 presents findings from several nationally representative community-based studies in which prevalence is estimated from blood samples taken in connection with a DHS. In these three cases—Mali, Kenya, and Zambia—urban prevalence rates are clearly much higher than rural rates. Where HIV/AIDS is concerned, there is little evidence of the 'urban advantage' that is seen in other domains of health. However, circular and urban-to-rural migration is contributing to the spread of disease in rural areas (UNAIDS 2004), and many observers foresee an era of rising rural incidence and prevalence.

Because the community-based studies are relatively recent, the role played by urban poverty in the risks of HIV/AIDS in low- and middle-income countries is only beginning to be studied. Using the community surveys conducted under the DHS programme, Mishra *et al.* (2007) found that contrary to expectation, HIV prevalence is higher among the better-off families. These families were more likely to live in urban areas, which accounts for a part of the association, and other risk factors (including sexual risk-taking, use of condoms, and male circumcision) tended to mask the association between living standards and prevalence. Even with statistical controls for such factors in place, a positive association between living standards and HIV prevalence persisted.

In studies of urban adolescents and other selected socioeconomic groups, however, poverty has been linked to higher HIV prevalence as well as to a number of contributing risk factors, including earlier sexual initiation and more reported forced or traded sex, which would seem to place poor women at higher risk of contracting the virus (Hallman 2004). In short, the association with living standards is still a matter of dispute.

Tuberculosis

Tuberculosis is even today among the leading causes of death for adults in low- and middle-income countries, killing an estimated 1.6 million people worldwide in 2005 (WHO 2007b). As in the nineteenth century, urban crowding increases the risk of contracting tuberculosis (van Rie *et al.* 1999), and high-density low-income urban communities may face elevated levels of risk. The interactions between HIV/AIDS and tuberculosis, and the spread of multi-drug-resistant strains of the disease, have generated fears of a global resurgence of tuberculosis and have caused WHO to expand its programme beyond DOTS as such.

The concept of urban collective efficacy is directly relevant to the DOTS strategy, the core of WHO's treatment strategy. In a study of tuberculosis in urban Ethiopia, Sagbakken *et al.* (2003) showed how the local social resources of urban communities (organized in 'TB clubs') can be marshalled to reduce the stigma associated with

[7] See Dyson (Dyson T. HIV/AIDS and urbanization. *Population and Development Review* 2003;**29**:427–42.) Country profiles are available from http://www.census.gov/ipc/www/hivaidsn.html, but these profiles are worked up from the reports of selected clinics and various sentinel sites, which do not necessarily yield statistically representative portraits for urban or rural populations.

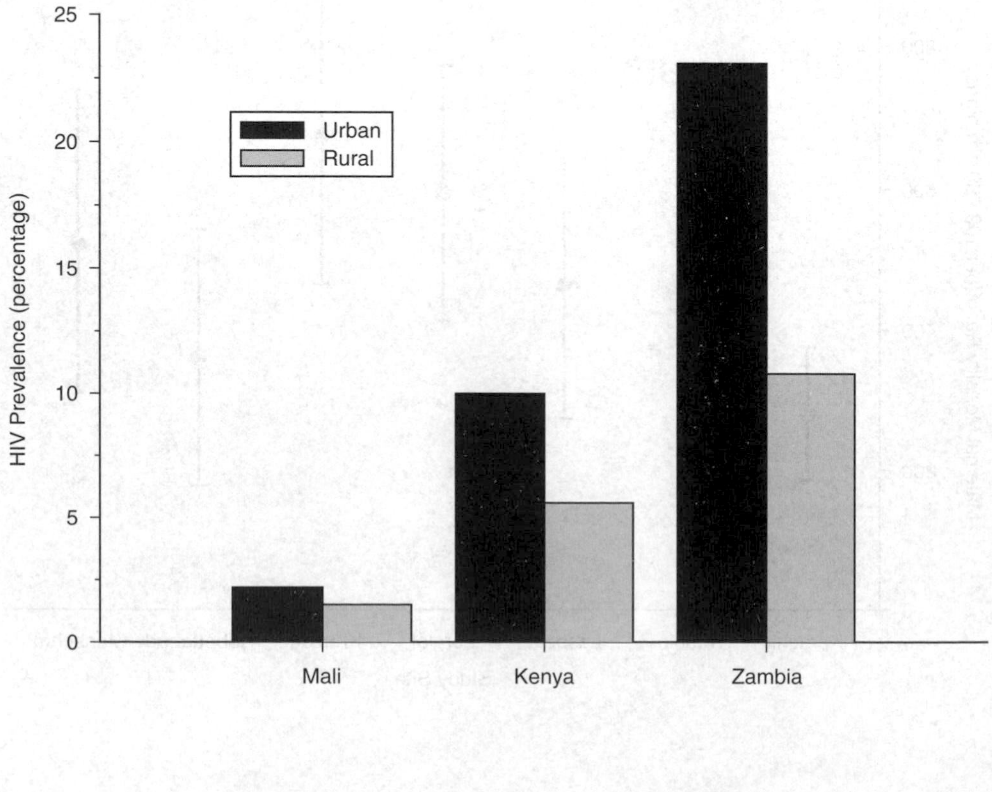

Fig. 10.7.7 Estimates of urban and rural prevalence of HIV from the Demographic and Health Surveys in Mali, 2001; Kenya, 2003; and Zambia, 2001–2002.
Source: Mali Ministère de la Santé. *Enquête Démographique et de Santé Mali 2001.* Mali; Calverton [MD]: Ministère de la Santé, ORC Macro; 2002; Kenya Central Bureau of Statistics. *Kenya Demographic and Health Survey 2003: preliminary report.* Nairobi, Kenya: Central Bureau of Statistics; 2003; Zambia Central Statistical Office. *Zambia Demographic and Health Survey 2001–2002.* Zambia; Calverton [MD]: Central Statistical Office, Central Board of Health; ORC Macro (2003).

the disease and encourage patients to adhere to the demanding short-course regimen of treatment. Similar interventions have been fielded in urban India, as described by Barua and Singh (2003), using community health volunteers to identify local residents with symptoms of tuberculosis and refer them to hospitals for diagnosis; local health workers attached to the hospitals then provide follow-up care and lend support during treatment.

An elaborate system of care, involving multiple urban community and health-service associations in Lima, Peru, is described in Shin *et al.* (2004) As reported in a WHO (2007b) report, Bangladesh has made urban DOTS a focus in a programme that links non-governmental organizations, private practitioners, medical colleges, and the corporate sector. As the country profiles presented in this report make clear, a number of countries have yet to reach WHO's treatment success rate target of 85 per cent of identified patients, and although data are scarce, it is very likely that detection rates of tuberculosis among the urban poor are well below rates for other urban residents.

Urban malaria

Although malaria has often been regarded as a problem afflicting rural populations, and rural rates of transmission are known to be markedly higher than urban rates, there is clear evidence that malaria vectors have adapted to urban conditions in sub-Saharan Africa (Modiano *et al.* 1999), and some evidence suggestive of urban risks has emerged for parts of Asia as well. As Hay *et al.* (2004) argue, urban population growth in Southeast Asia, as well as sub-Saharan Africa, may be contributing substantially to the global burden of malaria morbidity.

Keiser *et al.* (2004) calculate that in urban sub-Saharan Africa, some 200 million city-dwellers face appreciable risks of malaria, and they estimate that 25–100 million clinical episodes of the disease occur annually in this region's cities and towns. Indirect estimates suggest wide variations in prevalence by site, even within small geographic areas, with higher prevalence in the suburbs and city peripheries (especially when these are adjacent to wetlands) than in city centres.[8]

Pictet *et al.* (2004) describe a recent urban intervention programme mounted in Ouagadougou, Burkina Faso's capital, which aimed to make use of the social resources of urban communities to provide care in uncomplicated cases of child malaria. Inspired by a rural programme that yielded good results, this urban programme enlisted local community residents ('health agents'), gave them training in the recognition of malarial symptoms in young children, and supplied the agents with packets of chloroquine and paracetamol in age-appropriate doses. (In Ouagadougou, a high fraction of malaria cases still respond to chloroquine, although the parasite's resistance is evidently growing.)

In cases of childhood fevers, it has been common practice for residents of the Ouagadougou slums to buy chloroquine tablets (or drugs that have a similar appearance) in local markets, using these to medicate their ill children. Preliminary research showed, however, that the residents had little knowledge of the dosages or lengths of treatment appropriate for children. Hence, when judged against the medication practices that were already prevalent in these communities, the programme intervention was expected to improve the standard of malaria care.

When pilot-tested in two communities in Ouagadougou, the malaria intervention showed the expected positive results in the lower-income community, which was located on the fringes of the city and somewhat isolated from sources of modern health care. Of the two study communities, this was the more homogeneous in social and economic terms, and it exhibited evidence of greater 'neighbourliness' and other forms of social interaction through which information about the intervention might have circulated. In the other pilot community, however, easier access was already available to modern health clinics and reputable pharmacies, and more residents could afford to pay for their own care. In this middle-income site it proved difficult to sustain community interest in the intervention. As this Ouagadougou example shows, urban health interventions can be designed so as to tap the social energies and social organization of local neighbourhoods and communities, but the design may need to be tailored to fit the specific circumstances of each such community.

Traffic-related injuries and deaths

We now broaden the discussion to encompass sectors that have not always been linked to or carefully integrated with urban public health programmes, yet which have significant implications for health; injuries and deaths from traffic accidents are a case in point. Table 10.7.5 for Mexico showed just how important these are among all-urban causes of death and disability, but the great range of factors involved—touching on engineering concerns, and urban planning and land-use policies, as well as individual behaviour—seem in many countries to have inhibited the public health sector from taking action. The scale of this public health problem is enormous: The WHO (2004) estimates that road traffic injuries lead to 1.2 million deaths annually and an additional 20–50 million non-fatal injuries, the majority of which occur in low- and middle-income countries.

To elucidate the factors involved, Híjar *et al.* (2003) conducted a detailed analysis of pedestrian injuries in Mexico City, where pedestrian death rates are estimated at three times those of Los Angeles. Using a mix of spatially coded quantitative data and qualitative methods, these authors developed portraits of drivers and victims that underscore the importance of several mutually reinforcing risk factors: Poverty; a lack of understanding of how drivers are apt to react to pedestrians; inattention by drivers and pedestrians alike to risky conditions; insufficient public investment in traffic lights and road lighting; and dangerous mixes of industrial, commercial, and private traffic. Bartlett (2002) draws on hospital- and community-based studies to show how poverty and gender affect the risks, and how the time pressures on urban parents limit the effort they can devote to closely supervising their children.

In seeking to raise the public health profile of these important causes, the WHO (2004, 2007d) has given particular emphasis to the risks that are faced by adolescents and young adults, among whom road traffic injuries rank (worldwide) in the top three causes of death in the ages of 5–25 years. In the WHO's Africa region, it is pedestrians (especially children 5–9 years old) who face the greatest

[8] A detailed, time-series study of Dar es Salaam, Tanzania (see Caldas de Castro M, Yamagata Y, Mtasiwa D *et al.* Working paper on integrated urban malaria control: a case study in Dar es Salaam, Tanzania. Office of Population Research, Princeton University; 2004), which relies on an unusual combination of high-resolution aerial photography and extensive ground validation, depicts the micro-zones of high malaria risk within this city.

risks, whereas in Southeast Asia, the deaths occur disproportionately among riders of bicycles and motorized two-wheelers, who are aged 15–24 years.

Figure 10.7.8 shows how in poor countries of Asia, it is the vulnerable road users—pedestrians, bicyclists, and operators of motorized two-wheelers—who bear a greater share of the injury burden than the occupants of cars, vans, and buses. Among adolescents, young adults, and children, males face greater risks than females.

The full package of interventions known to be effective in high-income countries has typically not been implemented in low-income countries. The interventions include behavioural interventions—the promotion through media campaigns and other public-health communication outlets of seat belt use for adolescents and adults, appropriate restraints for infant and child passengers, and encouragement for bicycle and motorcycle riders to wear helmets—as well as traffic engineering concerns, such as the need to remove 'unforgiving' roadside objects, properly maintain existing roads, and situate new ones so that high-speed traffic is not routed through densely settled communities or placed near busy markets, schools, and children's play spaces.

In many low- and middle-income countries, only meagre resources are allotted to traffic control and enforcement of speed and road safety laws. Public health planners will also need to assess the priority that has been given to emergency rescue services (which may involve connections between the health system and the police) and the availability of pre-hospital care and in-hospital trauma centres.

Outdoor air pollution

Traffic and vehicular regulation are also key factors in outdoor air pollution. The Latin-American literature is especially rich in scientific analyses of outdoor urban air pollution and its effects on respiratory illness via the intake of airborne particulates and other pollutants emitted by industry and vehicles. Ribeiro and Alves Cardoso (2003) provide a thorough review of such studies for São Paulo; for Mexico City, Santos-Burgoa and Riojas-Rodríguez (2000) have assembled and reviewed a great range of studies.

There is increasing interest in the problem in India, China, and other rapidly developing countries of Asia, where the effects of economic growth are readily apparent in the levels and severity of outdoor air pollution.[9] In Delhi, a crucial public health intervention was recently made by the Supreme Court in a decision that mandated conversion to compressed natural gas (CNG) for bus, taxi, and other fleets of vehicles. There is reason to think that on a per-vehicle basis, this intervention has been effective; however, because the total volume of traffic has increased in Delhi, it is not yet obvious that the total volume of particulates and other pollutants has decreased (Kumar 2007; Narain & Krupnick 2007).

Future risks from climate change

Although much remains to be done to clarify the health implications of climate change, enough is already known to sketch the core

[9] For an overview of air pollution issues in Asia, see http://www.healtheffects.org/Asia/papasan-overview.htm.

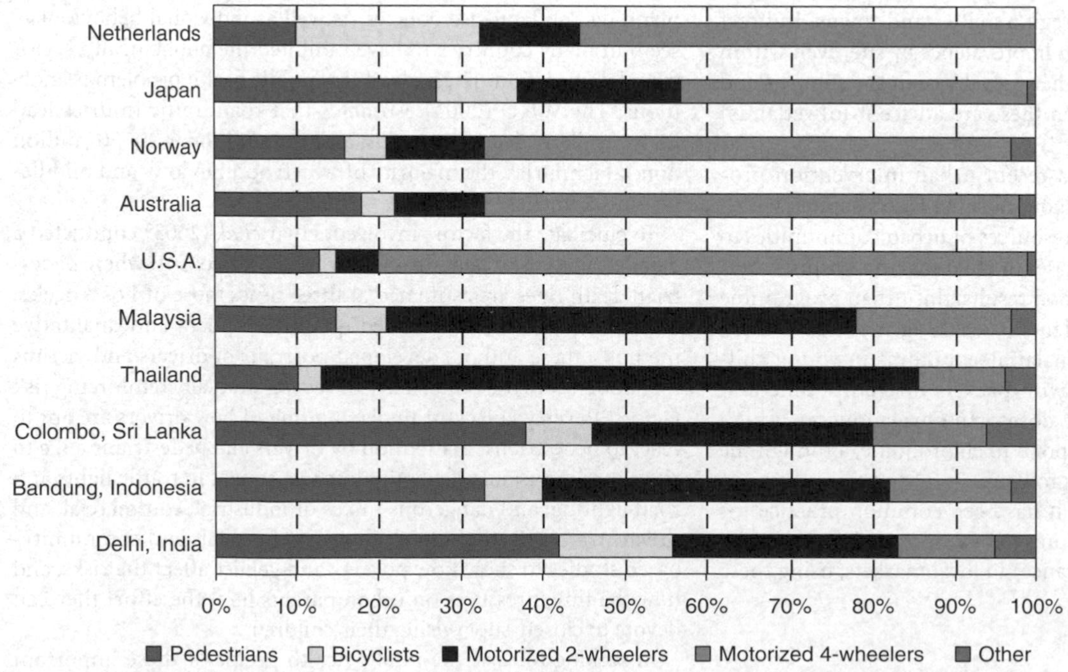

Fig. 10.7.8 Composition of road traffic injuries, by type, in selected high-income countries and Asian low- and middle-income countries.

Source: WHO. World report on road traffic injury prevention: main messages and recommendations. Geneva: World Health Organization; 2004. Available from: http://www.who.int/violence_injury_prevention/publications/road_traffic%'/world_report/whd_presentation.pdf elements of an urban adaptation strategy for low- and middle-income countries (Huq *et al.* 2007; McGranahan *et al.* 2007; Satterthwaite *et al.* 2007). According to current estimates, gradual increases in sea level are now all but inevitable over the coming decades, and this will place large coastal urban populations under threat. Alley *et al.* (2007) forecast rises in sea level of between 0.2 m and 0.6 m by 2100, which will be accompanied by periods of exceptionally high precipitation, more intense typhoons and hurricanes, and episodes of severe thermal stress. (The health effects of heat waves have not been much studied in the low- and middle-income countries, but the effects in Europe and the United States have been well-documented.)

In Asia, many of the region's largest cities are located in the flood plains of major rivers (the Ganges–Brahmaputra, Mekong, and Yangtze rivers) and in coastal areas that have long been cyclone-prone. Mumbai saw massive floods in 2005, as did Karachi in 2007. Flooding and storm surges also present a threat in coastal African cities (e.g. Port Harcourt, Nigeria, and Mombasa, Kenya) and in Latin America (e.g. Caracas, Venezuela). Figure 10.7.9 depicts one of the major low-elevation coastal zones of China near Shanghai and Tianjin, two of the world's fastest-developing economic regions, in which increasing numbers of urban dwellers will be placed at risk.

Urban flooding risks in poor countries stem from a number of factors: The predominance of impermeable surfaces that cause water run-off; the general scarcity of parks and other green spaces to absorb these flows; rudimentary drainage systems that are often clogged by waste and which in any case are quickly overloaded with

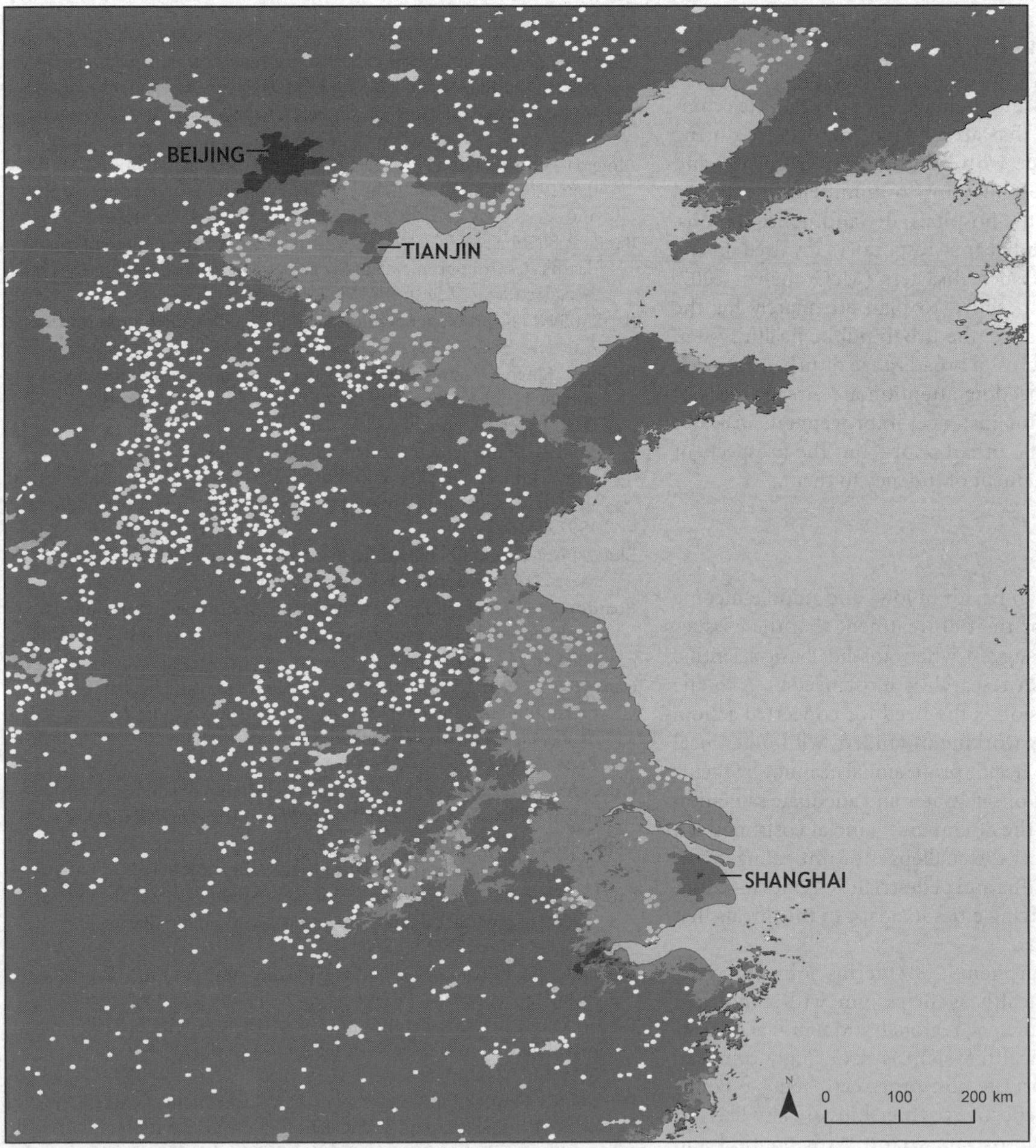

Fig. 10.7.9 Yellow Sea region of China, areas within 10 m of sea level.
Source: McGranahan G, Balk D, Anderson B. The rising tide: assessing the risks of climate change to human settlements in low-elevation coastal zones. *Environment and Urbanization* 2007;**19**:17–37.

water; and the ill-advised development of marshlands and other natural buffers. When urban flooding takes place, faecal and other hazardous materials contaminate flood waters and spill into open wells, elevating the risks of water-borne disease. The urban poor are often more exposed to these environmental hazards than others, because the housing they can afford tends to be located in the riskier areas.

As Revi (2008) discusses in a detailed analysis of urban adaptation needs in India, governments from the local to national levels and their public health systems will need to anticipate increases in extreme-weather events. The Indian Ocean tsunami of 2005 heightened attention to coastal zone management in India and the region, but to judge from Revi's account, the responsibilities for urban adaptation and disaster management have been strewn across the bureaucratic landscape and are not yet organized in any coherent manner.

He puts special emphasis on what is termed the 'lifeline' infrastructure needed to cope with extreme events: The roads, bridges and other transport systems; water, sewer, and gas pipelines; infrastructure for coastal defences and drainage; the power and telecommunications infrastructure that are of vital importance during disasters; arrangements made with local non-governmental and relief agencies for alerting populations to imminent threats and responding to disaster; and the hospitals, fire and police stations, schools, military forces and other first-responders involved during the onset and aftermath of such disasters (McGranahan 2007; Satterthwaite *et al.* 2007). In short, to plan adequately for the upcoming era of climate change, the urban public health system must engage with partners across a broad range of urban agencies. Many of the priority areas needing attention are already areas of concern on other counts—for instance, improvements in water and sanitation systems for the urban poor—but the prospects of climate change adds a new element of urgency to them.

Conclusions

The preceding sketch of urban health in low- and middle-income countries is no substitute for the full treatment that these issues deserve, but it may at least suggest where further basic scientific and programme intervention research is most needed. A theme running through the discussion is the need for concerted action, with the public health sector working in tandem with other local government agencies. Public health professionals cannot by themselves mandate the provision of safe water and adequate sanitation for the urban poor, with all the attendant financial costs; nor can they, acting alone, rise to meet the challenges of mitigating urban air pollution, reorganizing traffic and pedestrian activities to reduce deaths and injuries, and readying cities to adapt to the threats that will be posed by climate change.

What is needed is what Harpham (2007) terms 'joined-up government', whereby public health agencies join with concerned actors in other sectors of municipal, regional, and national governments. Because the urban health system is dauntingly complex, with private for-profit and private non-profit care being a significant presence in most cities, effective partnerships are also likely to require engagement with the private sector. With political and administrative decentralization now well underway in many low- and middle-income countries, the arena in which creative partnerships are forged will increasingly be the local and municipal level. Much remains to be learned about how health expertise, which is now situated in national ministries of health, and the international funding and technical assistance that has also been directed to national ministries, can be redeployed effectively to meet the many health needs of cities and their neighbourhoods.

Author's note: To draw out the distinctions of urban health environments and behaviour with proper care and nuance would, of course, require a book-length treatment. For those seeking more comprehensive accounts of urban health than can be provided in this chapter, I would like to direct attention to the recent US National Research Council report (Panel on Urban Population Dynamics 2003), to documents by Montgomery and Ezeh (2005a, 2005b), and especially, to papers by Harpham (2007), Mercado *et al.* (2007), and McGranahan (2007) for up-to-date reviews.

References

Alley R.B., Bertsen T., Bindoff N.L. *et al.* Summary for policymakers: contribution of Working Group I to the Fourth Assessment Report. Intergovernmental Panel on Climate Change; 2007. Available from: http://www.ipcc.ch [accessed 2007 Nov 7]

Almeida-Filho N., Lessa I., Magalhães L. *et al.* Social inequality and depressive disorders in Bahia, Brazil: Interactions of gender, ethnicity, and social class. *Social Science and Medicine* 2004;**59**:1339–53.

Barata R.B., Ribeiro M.C., Guedes M.B. *et al.* Intra-urban differentials in death rates from homicide in the city of São Paulo, Brazil, 1988–1994. *Social Science and Medicine* 1998;**47**:19–23.

Bartlett S.N. The problem of children's injuries in low-income countries: A review. *Health Policy and Planning* 2002;**17**:1–13.

Barua N., Singh S. Representation for the marginalized—linking the poor and the health-care system. Lessons from case studies in urban India. Draft paper, New Delhi. World Bank; 2003.

Bassett M.T., Bijlmakers L., Sanders D.M. Professionalism, patient satisfaction, and quality of health care: Experience during Zimbabwe's structural adjustment programme. *Social Science and Medicine* 1997;**45**:1845–52.

Blue I. Intra-urban differentials in mental health in São Paulo, Brazil. Ph.D. thesis. London: South Bank University; 1999.

Boardman J.D. Stress and physical health: the role of neighborhoods as mediating and moderating mechanisms. *Social Science and Medicine* 2004;**58**:2473–83.

Cairncross S., Valdmanis V. Water supply, sanitation, and hygiene promotion. In: Jamison D.T. *et al.* editors. *Disease control priorities in developing countries.* Washington (DC): World Bank; Oxford University Press; 2006. 2nd ed. p. 771–92.

Calvés A.E. Abortion risk and decision-making among young people in urban Cameroon. *Studies in Family Planning* 2002;**33**:249–60.

Cohen S., Doyle W.J., Baum A. Socio-economic status is associated with stress hormones. *Psychosomatic Medicine* 2006;**68**:414–20.

Das J., Hammer J. Location, location, location: residence, wealth, and the quality of medical care in Delhi, India. *Health Affairs* 2007a; **26**:w338–51.

Das J., Hammer J. Money for nothing: the dire straits of medical practice in Delhi, India. *Journal of Development Economics* 2007b;**83**:1–36.

Desgrées du Loû A., Msellati P., Viho I. *et al.* The use of induced abortion in Abidjan: a possible cause of the fertility decline. *Population* 2000;**12**:197–214.

Dussault G., Franceschini M.C. Not enough there, too many here: understanding geographic imbalances in the distribution of the health workforce. *Human Resources for Health* 2006;**4**:1–16. Available from: http://www.human-resources-health.com

Erulkar A.S., Matheka J.K. Adolescence in the Kibera slums of Nairobi, Kenya. New York (NY); Nairobi: Population Council; 2007.

Fikree F.F., Gray R.H., Berendes H.W. *et al.* A community-based nested case-control study of maternal mortality. *International Journal of Gynecology & Obstetrics* 1994;**47**:247–55.

Fikree F.F., Midhet F., Sadruddin S. *et al.* Maternal mortality in different Pakistani sites: ratios, clinical causes, and determinants. *Acta Obstetricia et Gynecologica Scandinavica* 1997;**76**:637–45.

Fikree F.F., Ali T., Durocher J.M. *et al.* Health service utilization for perceived postpartum morbidity among poor women living in Karachi. *Social Science and Medicine* 2004;**59**:681–94.

Garrett J., Ahmed A. Incorporating crime in household surveys: a research note. *Environment and Urbanization* 2004;**16**:139–52.

Graham W., Brass W., Snow R.W. Estimating maternal mortality: the sisterhood method. *Studies in Family Planning* 1989;**20**:125–35.

Grant E. State of the art of urban health in Latin America. European Commission funded concerted action: 'Health and human settlements in Latin America'. London: South Bank University; 1999.

Hallman K. Socio-economic disadvantage and unsafe sexual behaviors among young women and men in South Africa. New York (NY): Population Council; 2004. Policy Research Division Working Papers, No. 190.

Harpham T., Grant E., Rodriguez C. Mental health and social capital in Cali, Colombia. *Social Science and Medicine* 2004;**58**:2267–77.

Harpham T. Background paper on improving urban population health. Paper presented at Innovations for an Urban World, the Rockefeller Foundation's Urban Summit; 2007; Bellagio, Italy.

Hay S.I., Guerra C.A., Tatem A.J. *et al.* The global distribution and population at risk of malaria: past, present, and future. *The Lancet. Infectious Diseases* 2004;**4**:327–36.

Heinemann A., Verner D. Crime and violence in development: a literature review of Latin America and the Caribbean. Washington (DC): World Bank; 2006. World Bank Policy Research working paper no. 4041.

Heise L.L., Raikes A., Watts C.H. *et al.* Violence against women: a neglected public health issue in less developed countries. *Social Science and Medicine* 1994;**39**:1165–79.

Híjar M., Trostle J., Bronfman M. Pedestrian injuries in Mexico: A multi-method approach. *Social Science and Medicine* 2003;**57**:2149–59.

Hu P., Wagle N., Goldman N. *et al.* The associations between socio-economic status, allostatic load, and measures of health in older Taiwanese persons: Taiwan Social Environment and Biomarkers of Aging study. *Journal of Biosocial Science* 2007;**39**:545–56.

Huq S., Kovats S., Reid H. *et al.* Reducing risks to cities from climate change: an environmental or a development agenda? *Environment and Urbanization* 2007: Brief no. 15.

Islam M., Montgomery M.R., Taneja S. Urban health and care-seeking behavior: a case study of slums in India and the Philippines. Bethesda (MD): PHRPlus Program, Abt Associates; 2006.

Jamil S., Fikree F.F. Determinants of unsafe abortion in three squatter settlements of Karachi. Karachi, Pakistan: Department of Community Health Sciences, Aga Khan University; 2002.

Kaneda T., Zimmer Z., Tang Z. Socio-economic status differentials in life and active life expectancy among older adults in Beijing. *Disability and Rehabilitation* 2005;**27**:241–51.

Keiser J., Utzinger J., Caldas de Castro M. *et al.* Urbanization in sub-Saharan Africa and implications for malaria control. Working paper. Office of Population Research, Princeton University, Swiss Tropical Institute; 2004.

Kishor S., Johnson K. Profiling domestic violence: a multi-country study. Measure DHS+. Calverton (MD): ORC Macro; 2004.

Kumar N. Spatial sampling for demography and health survey. Paper presented at the 2007 Annual Meetings of the Population Association of America. New York (NY): Department of Geography, University of Iowa; 2007.

Larson B.A., Rosen S. Understanding household demand for indoor air pollution control in developing countries. *Social Science and Medicine* 2002;**55**:571–84.

Marmot M.G., Wilkinson R.G., editors. *Social Determinants of Health*. London: Oxford University Press; 2005. 2nd ed.

Marmot M.G. Social determinants of health inequalities. *Lancet* 2005;**365**:1099–104.

Mayank S., Bahl R., Rattan A. *et al.* Prevalence and correlates of morbidity in pregnant women in an urban slum of New Delhi. *Asia-Pacific Population Journal* 2001;**16**:29–44.

McEwen B.S. Protecting and damaging effects of stress mediators. *New England Journal of Medicine* 1998;**338**:171–9.

McGranahan G., Balk D., Anderson B. The rising tide: assessing the risks of climate change to human settlements in low-elevation coastal zones. *Environment and Urbanization* 2007;**19**:17–37.

McGranahan G. Evolving urban health risks in low- and middle-income countries: from housing, water, and sanitation to cities and climate change. Paper presented at Innovations for an Urban World, the Rockefeller Foundation's Urban Summit; 2007; Bellagio, Italy.

Mercado S., Havemann K., Nakamura K. *et al.* Responding to the health vulnerabilities of the urban poor in the 'new urban settings' of Asia. WHO Centre for Health Development, Alliance for Healthy Cities, and Southeast Asian Press Alliance. Paper presented at Innovations for an Urban World, the Rockefeller Foundation's Urban Summit; 2007; Bellagio, Italy.

Mishra V., Bignami S., Greener R. *et al.* A study of the association of HIV infection and wealth in sub-Saharan Africa. Calverton (MD): Macro International; 2007. DHS Working Papers, No. 31.

Modiano D., Sirima B., Sawadogo A. *et al.* Severe malaria in Burkina Faso: urban and rural environment. *Parassitologia* 1999;**41**:251–4.

Montgomery M.R., Ezeh A.C. The health of urban populations in developing countries: an overview. In: Galea S., Vlahov D., editors. *Handbook of Urban Health: Populations, Methods, and Practice.* New York (NY): Springer; 2005a.

Montgomery M.R., Ezeh A.C. Urban health in developing countries: insights from demographic theory and practice. In: Galea S., Vlahov D., editors. *Handbook of Urban Health: Populations, Methods, and Practice.* New York (NY): Springer: 2005b.

Montgomery M.R., Hewett P.C. Urban poverty and health in developing countries: household and neighborhood effects. *Demography* 2005;**42**:397–425.

Moser C. Urban violence and insecurity: an introductory roadmap. *Environment and Urbanization* 2004;**16**:3–16.

Narain U., Krupnick A. The impact of Delhi's CNG program on air quality. Washington (DC): Resources for the Future; 2007. Discussion Paper 07–08.

Panel on Urban Population Dynamics. In: Montgomery M.R. *et al.*, editors. *Cities Transformed: Demographic Change and its Implications in the Developing World.* Washington (DC): National Academies Press; 2003.

Parkar S.R., Fernandes J., Weiss M.G. Contextualizing mental health: gendered experiences in a Mumbai slum. *Anthropology and Medicine* 2003;**10**:291–308.

Pictet G., Kouanda S., Sirima S. *et al.* Struggling with population heterogeneity in African cities: the urban health and equity puzzle. Paper presented to the 2004 Annual Meetings of the Population Association of America; 2004; Boston (MA).

Prince M., Patel V., Saxena S. *et al.* No health without mental health. *Lancet* 2007;**370**:859–77.

Revi A. Climate change risk: an adaptation and mitigation agenda for Indian cities. *Environment and Urbanization* 2008;**20**:207–229.

Ribeiro H., Alves Cardoso M.R. Air pollution and children's health in São Paulo (1986–1998). *Social Science and Medicine* 2003;**57**:2013–22.

Rossier C. Attitudes towards abortion and contraception in rural and urban Burkina Faso. Paris: Institut National d'Etudes Démographique; 2007.

Sagbakken M., Bjune G., Frich J. *et al.* From the user's perspective—a qualitative study of factors influencing patients' adherence to medical treatment in an urban community, Ethiopia. Paper presented at the conference 'Urban Poverty and Health in Sub-Saharan Africa', African Population and Health Research Centre, Nairobi. Norway: Faculty of Medicine, University of Oslo; 2003.

Santos-Burgoa C., Riojas-Rodríguez H. Health and pollution in Mexico City Metropolitan Area: a general overview of air pollution exposure and health studies. Presentation to the Panel on Urban Population Dynamics, U.S. National Research Council; 2000; Mexico City.

Satterthwaite D., Huq S., Pelling M. *et al.* Building climate change resilience in urban areas and among urban populations in low- and middle-income nations. Paper prepared for Innovations for an Urban World, the Rockefeller Foundation's Urban Summit; 2007; Bellagio, Italy.

Shin S., Furin J., Bayona J. *et al.* Community-based treatment of multi-drug-resistant tuberculosis in Lima, Peru: 7 years of experience. *Social Science and Medicine* 2004;**59**:1529–39.

Steptoe A., Marmot M. The role of psychobiological pathways in socio-economic inequalities in cardiovascular disease risk. *European Heart Journal* 2002;**23**:13–25.

Stone C. Crime, justice, and growth in South Africa: toward a plausible contribution from criminal justice to economic growth. Cambridge (MA): Harvard University; 2006. Center for International Development working paper no. 131.

UNAIDS. 2004 report on the global AIDS epidemic. New York (NY): UNAIDS; 2004.

UN-Habitat. *The Challenge of Slums: Global Report on Human Settlements 2003*. London: Earthscan; 2003a.

UN-Habitat. *Water and Sanitation in the World's Cities: Local Action for Global Goals*. London: Earthscan; 2003b.

United Nations. World urbanization prospects: the 2005 revision population database. New York (NY): Department of Economic and Social Affairs, Population Division, United Nations; 2005.

van Rie A., Beyers N., Gie R.P. *et al.* Childhood tuberculosis in an urban population in South Africa: burden and risk factor. *Archives of Disability in Children* 1999;**80**:433–7.

WHO. Global age-friendly cities: a guide. Geneva: World Health Organization; 2007a.

WHO. Global tuberculosis control: surveillance, planning, financing. Geneva: World Health Organization; 2007b.

WHO. Investing in health research and development: report of the ad hoc committee on health research relating to future intervention options. Geneva: World Health Organization; 1996.

WHO. Mental health: facing the challenges, building solutions. Report from the WHO European Ministerial Conference; Copenhagen, Denmark. World Health Organization Regional Office for Europe; 2005a.

WHO. *The World Health Report 2001. Mental Health: New Understanding, New Hope*. Geneva: World Health Organization; 2001.

WHO. *The World Health Report 2002. Reducing Risk, Promoting Healthy Life*. Geneva: World Health Organization; 2002.

WHO. WHO multi-country study on women's health and domestic violence against women: summary report of initial results on prevalence, health outcomes and women's responses. Geneva: World Health Organization; 2005b.

WHO. World report on road traffic injury prevention: main messages and recommendations. Geneva: World Health Organization; 2004. Available from: http://www.who.int/violence_injury_prevention/publications/road_traffic%'/world_report/whd_presentation.pdf

WHO. Youth and road safety. Geneva: World Health Organization; 2007d.

Winton A. Urban violence: a guide to the literature. *Environment and Urbanization* 2004;**16**:165–84.

Wong R., Peláez M., Palloni A. *et al.* Survey data for the study of aging in Latin America and the Caribbean. *Journal of Aging and Health* 2006;**18**:157–79.

Woods R. Urban-rural mortality differentials: an unresolved debate. *Population and Development Review* 2003;**29**:29–46.

Zimmer Z, Kwong J. Socio-economic status and health among older adults in urban and rural China. *Journal of Aging and Health* 2004;**16**:44–70.

10.8

Public health aspects of bioterrorism

Manfred S. Green

Introduction

Biological warfare

While deliberate infliction of injury, other than in self-defence, runs contrary to almost all social norms, there is a special kind of abhorrence and dread associated with the use of biological agents. Many possible reasons for this can be suggested. The agents are 'invisible', they can cause injury indiscriminately and not only to those targeted and they can inflict disease and death in numbers quite out of proportion to the resources expended. Furthermore, their effects may only be experienced long after exposure and they may cause large outbreaks through person-to-person spread. Prior to the twentieth century, there were documented instances of crude attempts to use biological agents as weapons of war. For example, there are several reports of bodies of plague victims being hurled into the enemy ranks in order to infect their forces. There is also some evidence to suggest that European colonists in the Americas either actually used, or intended to use, 'smallpox' infected blankets to infect the native populations, who were previously unexposed (Patterson & Runge 2002).

Early in the twentieth century, rapid progress in the field of microbiology was accompanied by an increased interest in the use of biological weapons. This became evident during World War I, when German agents used glanders bacteria (*Burkholderia pseudomallei*) to infect horses, mules, and cattle being sent from the United States to the allied forces in Europe. As a result, several hundred soldiers became ill (Centers for Disease Control 2006). In 1918, the modern version of biological warfare became institutionalized when the Japanese established a biological weapons unit in their army. Due to growing concern about the potential military use of biological agents, in 1925 an international agreement to prohibit the use of biological weapons was signed by 132 countries. This agreement, 'the Geneva Protocol', did not limit development or production of such weapons. Despite the agreement, in 1931, the Japanese army began to experiment with biological weapons in Manchuria, including exposing prisoners to aerosolized anthrax spores. During World War II, other major powers, such as Germany, the United States, the Soviet Union, and the United Kingdom, initiated bioweapons programmes as part of their strategies to stockpile weapons of mass destruction.

In 1969, President Nixon ended the United States offensive bioweapons programme. Three years later, the 'Biological Weapons Convention' was signed by 171 countries. Article 1 of the convention states that 'each party to this convention undertakes never in any circumstances to develop, produce, stockpile or otherwise acquire or retain microbial or other biological agents, or toxins whatever their origin or method of production, of types and in quantities that have no justification for prophylactic, protective or other peaceful purposes'. The document also specifies a ban on the production of weapons, equipment or means of delivery designed to use such agents or toxins for hostile purposes or in armed conflict.

In 1985, the 'Australia Group' was formed to address the regulations governing exportation of materials necessary to manufacture chemical and biological weapons. It now has a membership of 40 countries plus the European Commission. The 'Wassenaar Arrangement', which regulates the control of exports of 'dual-use technologies' which could be applied to weapons of mass destruction, was confirmed in 1994 by more than 40 countries.

The emergence of bioterrorism

One of the earliest instances of the use of the term 'terrorism' in a political context, was during the French revolution (1789–1799). During the 1960s, cross-border terrorism became a major international issue. In general, terrorist objectives are considered to include the desire 'to promote nationalist or separatist objectives, to retaliate or take revenge for a real or perceived injury or to protest government policies' (Tucker 1999). While terrorism may be state-sponsored, terrorist groups usually commit their acts outside of formal government agencies and in most countries terrorism is defined as a criminal act. Terrorist groups tend to claim that they resort to illegal or illegitimate methods to achieve political or social change, because they have been excluded from, or frustrated by regular legal and diplomatic processes (Hoffman 2007).

Initially, conventional thinking held that biological weapons were so morally unacceptable and the means of production and dissemination so complex, that they would not be included in the armaments of terrorist groups. In the late 1990s, warnings began to appear in the professional literature about the potential use of biological agents by terrorist groups and the term 'bioterrorism' was coined (Franz *et al.* 1997; Henderson 1998). Several major events brought into focus the potential emergence of bioterrorism as a major threat to public security and health.

In the 1990s, it became evident that the Soviet Union had failed to adhere to the Biological Weapons Convention, and continued to develop biological weapons. In the early 1990s, investigations revealed that in 1979, anthrax spores were accidentally released from a military facility in Sverdlovsk (now Yekaterinburg), Russia, resulting in an outbreak of respiratory anthrax, with at least 70 deaths (Meselson *et al.* 1994). There was also evidence that a major facility in Novosibirsk, Siberia, housed a large programme to weaponize agents such as the smallpox and viral haemorrhagic fever viruses and anthrax spores (Henderson 1998). The breakup of the former Soviet Union increased concern that the biological agents that had been weaponized and the expertise acquired by the scientists, would fall into the hands of terrorist groups. There was also evidence that other countries were continuing to develop biological weapons (Zilinskas 1997).

Weaponizing biological agents is not trivial and generally requires a high level of technology and skill. However, state-sponsored biological weapons programmes could supply the necessary technology to terrorist groups. In 2001, the terrorist attacks on the Twin Towers in New York and the Pentagon in Washington renewed concern that international terrorist groups would attempt to expand their armaments to biological weapons.

A bioterrorist attack has been defined by the United States Centers for Disease Control (CDC) as 'the deliberate release of viruses, bacteria, or other germs (agents) used to cause illness or death in people, animals, or plants' (Centers for Disease Control 2006). This definition relates primarily to the physical impact of the attack. However, others have stressed the psychological impact, and defined bioterrorism as 'the use, or threatened use, of biological agents to promote or spread fear or intimidation upon an individual, a specific group, or the population as a whole for religious, political, ideological, financial, or personal purposes'. (Arizona Department of Health Services 2005). Since contagious agents are invisible, the threat of infection may be perceived to be ubiquitous with almost no way of avoiding it. Thus, while the potential physical impact is of major concern, the psychological impact may be much broader and longer-lasting than physical injury.

Four factors have been delineated as the basis for the assessment of the bioterrorism threat. They are the intent of the groups or individuals and willingness to use weapons of mass destruction, the technical capabilities of the groups, the attributes of the pathogens/toxins, and the range of possible targets for an attack (Zilinskas *et al.* 2004).

Contemporary incidents of bioterrorism and biocrimes

Until 2001, the only modern instance of bioterrorism recognized in the United States by the Federal Bureau of Investigation, occurred in 1984. The Bhagwan Shree Rajneesh sect deliberately contaminated salads with *Salmonella typhimurium* in salad bars in Oregon, with the intention of disrupting local elections and several hundred people became ill (Torok 1997). Bioterrorism attempts have been documented in other countries. For example, in 1980, a group called the Red Army Faction was reported to have used botulinum toxin against government officials in West Germany. In 1995, a Japanese cult, Aum Shinrikyo, produced quantities of anthrax spores, Q fever bacteria, botulinum toxin, and Ebola viruses and attempted to disseminate them (Sugishima 2003). Fortunately, there were no casualties.

Despite the paucity of actual events, there have been a number of bioterrorism threats. Among the most prominent occurred in the early 1970s when an extremist group in the United States, the 'Weather Underground', threatened to contaminate the urban water supplies with biological agents. In addition, there have been a number of so-called 'biocrimes' where biological agents have been used against individuals without a defined ideological motive. For example, in 1997, a disgruntled worker deliberately used *Shigella dysenteriae* type 2 bacteria to contaminate food served to co-workers (Kolavic *et al.* 1997).

The 'anthrax letters' incident in the United States, in 2001, dramatically demonstrated the potential for bioterrorism. During approximately three months, six envelopes contaminated with anthrax spores in powder form were identified in the regular mail and 22 people were infected. Half suffered from inhalation anthrax and the others from the cutaneous form (Jernigan *et al.* 2002). Recently, the United States Federal Bureau of Investigation announced that they had evidence to suggest that a scientist from a United States Army Medical Research laboratory may have been responsible for sending the letters (Federal Bureau of Investigation 2008). Since no clear motive has been established, this incident may be an example of either bioterrorism or a biocrime. There was major disruption of government offices and the mail services. Thousands of workers received prophylactic therapy, and there was a large-scale programme to decontaminate affected buildings. The cost of managing the incident may have exceeded one billion dollars. In addition, other countries also instituted safety measures and many suspected cases were investigated.

Confronting the threat of bioterrorism

Bioterrorism may be viewed from the perspective of the biological agents that pose the greatest danger, the potential impact on society and the likelihood that biological agents would be employed as terrorist weapons. Preparedness for a bioterrorism attack is multifaceted and includes prevention, detection, diagnosis, treatment, pre- and post-exposure prophylaxis, and risk communication. Prevention ranges from attempting to address the root causes of terrorism, implementation of deterrence measures and control of access to potentially dangerous pathogens to protection of food supplies and drinking water. Early detection of an incident will depend on effective human, environmental, and animal surveillance, rapid and accurate diagnoses, and comprehensive epidemiological investigations.

In order to deal effectively with an actual incident, countries will need to allocate substantial resources to develop contingency plans and training programmes. They will have to expand their infrastructure to ensure prompt diagnosis and treatment of patients and implement pre- and post-exposure prophylactic measures for both contagious and non-contagious diseases. Preparedness measures include stockpiling of medications, vaccines, and special protective equipment, and developing plans for non-pharmacological interventions in order to reduce spread of the disease. The possible need for decontamination of the environment following the incident will require prior investment in specialized equipment and supplies. Methods for risk communication and education of both health professional and the public will have to be tailored to the threat of bioterrorism. In addition, the special legal and ethical aspects must be resolved. This chapter addresses the above issues.

Biological weapons

General characteristics of bioterrorism agents

Biological weapons have features which make them particularly attractive for terrorist acts. They can be extremely difficult to detect in the environment and their effects are not felt for several hours to days. Both the agents and hardware for their production and dissemination are relatively easy to conceal. Thus, the perpetrators could produce and disseminate the agents and escape during the incubation or latent period before any illness is detected.

While the biological agents could be disseminated through food, human carriers or infected insects, aerosol spread will maximize the number of people exposed and produce the most damage. Since most of the potential agents do not transmit naturally as aerosols, their use in bioterrorism attacks may produce disease with shorter incubation periods and different manifestations of clinical disease. Furthermore, surreptitious and simultaneous aerosol dissemination of a contagious agent could produce an inordinately large number of second- and later-generation cases. The effects of each agent are likely to depend on the exposure dose and host factors such as age, sex, underlying illnesses, and immune status.

Classification of potential bioterrorism agents

Almost all potential bioterrorism agents occur naturally as known pathogens, although many are zoonoses that do not normally infect humans. The genetic composition of the biological agents may be modified to make them more virulent and increase their resistance to medications or vaccines.

In 1999, the United States CDC classified the potential agents for bioterrorism into three categories, A, B, and C (Tables 10.8.1 and 10.8.2), depending on how easily they can be spread, the severity of illness they might cause and the death rates that may result (Rotz *et al.* 2002). The highest priority is given to the category A agents which are considered the greatest risk to the public and national security. These agents can be classified into three types: Those that are both infectious and contagious, those that are infectious but not usually contagious and toxins. Category B includes diseases that are considered an intermediate risk to the public, since the causative agents are moderately easy to spread and the diseases result in moderately high death rates. Category C agents include emerging pathogens which have the potential to be engineered to spread and cause high rates of morbidity and mortality.

Table 10.8.1 CDC categorization of biological agents that may be used as weapons (http://www.bt.cdc.gov/agent/agentlist-category.asp)

Category A

High-priority agents include organisms and toxins that pose the highest risk to the public and national security

- They can be easily disseminated or transmitted from person to person.
- They result in high death rates and have the potential for major public health impact.
- They are likely to cause public panic and social disruption.
- They require special action for public health preparedness.

Category B

Second-highest-priority agents

- They are moderately easy to spread.
- They result in moderate illness rates and low death rates.
- They require specific enhancements of laboratory capacity and enhanced disease monitoring.

Category C

Third-highest-priority agents include emerging pathogens that could be engineered for mass spread in the future

- They are easily available.
- They are easily produced and spread.
- They have potential for high morbidity and mortality rates and major health impact.

Table 10.8.2 Examples of bioterrorism agents by category (http://www.bt.cdc.gov/agent/agentlist-category.asp)

Category A

Infectious and contagious diseases

- Smallpox (variola major)
- Plague (*Yersinia pestis*)
- Viral haemorrhagic fevers (filoviruses [e.g. Ebola, Marburg] and arenaviruses [e.g. Lassa, Machupo])

Infectious but not contagious diseases

- Anthrax (*Bacillus anthracis*)
- Tularaemia (*Francisella tularensis*)

Toxins

- Botulism (*Clostridium botulinum* toxin)

Category B

- Brucellosis (*Brucella* species)
- Epsilon toxin of *Clostridium perfringens*
- Food safety threats (*Salmonella* species, *Escherichia coli* 0157, *Shigella*)
- Glanders (*Burkholderia mallei*)
- Meliodosis (*Burkholderia pseudomallei*)
- Psittacosis (*Chlamidia psittaci*)
- Q fever (*Coxiella burnetii*)
- Ricin toxin from *Ricinus communis* (castor beans)
- Staphylococcal enterotoxin B
- Typhus fever (*Rickettsia prowazekii*)
- Viral encephalitis (alphavirus—e.g. Venezuelan equine encephalitis, eastern equine encephalitis, western equine encephalitis)
- Water safety threats (e.g. *Vibrio cholerae, Cryptosporidium parvum*)

Category C

- Emerging infectious diseases such as Nipah virus and hantavirus

Characteristics of category A bioterrorist agents

Since the category A biological agents are of greatest concern, they will be described in some detail.

Diseases which are both infectious and contagious

Smallpox (Henderson et al. 1999)

Smallpox is a severe, systemic illness caused by a large, brick-shaped, DNA virus from the orthopoxvirus genus. Prior to its eradication in 1978, it was endemic in many countries. The case-fatality rate for variola major in unvaccinated subjects was estimated at around 30 per cent. The infectious dose is unknown but may be as low as a few virions. There is evidence that smallpox may have been weaponized by the Soviet Union during the 1980s (Henderson 1998). The long period since cessation of universal vaccination, combined with the severity of the disease, has made smallpox one of the most feared potential bioterrorist agents.

After the virus enters the respiratory tract, it multiplies in the lymph nodes, and three to four days later produces an asymptomatic viremia. On about the eighth day, there is a second viremia accompanied by fever and toxemia. The virus then localizes in small blood vessels of the dermis and beneath the oral and pharyngeal mucosa. In addition to fever, the patient suffers from symptoms such as malaise, headache, backache, occasional abdominal pain, and delirium.

Macular-papular lesions appear on the mucosa of the mouth and oro-pharynx and the patient becomes infectious. Later the rash appears on the face, forearms, and legs and the lesions become vesicular, round, rubbery, and pustular. Scabs begin to form around the eighth day of the rash and following their separation, the person is no longer infectious. Overall, the patient may be infectious for an average of 16 days. The haemorrhagic and flat types of smallpox are less common, but more severe, with case-fatality rates approaching 80–90 per cent. The haemorrhagic type has a shorter incubation period and is more difficult to diagnose clinically. Pregnant women are particularly susceptible to these forms (Kiang & Krathwohl 2003).

Following the initial cases arising from the aerosolized virus, secondary cases may occur through droplet spread, usually over a distance of less than two meters, or through contact with the virus from the skin lesions or body fluids (Kiang & Krathwohl 2003). There are rare reports of apparent airborne transmission, such as in an outbreak in Germany in 1970. A single hospitalized patient, with severe cough, infected seventeen other patients on three floors in the hospital, probably through the ventilation system (Wehrle *et al.* 1970).

The spread of smallpox is likely to be slower than for diseases such as chickenpox and measles and pandemic influenza, since the reproduction number is smaller and the generation time longer. In addition, transmission of the disease only occurs after onset of the rash, at which stage patients are seriously ill and tend to remain at home or in healthcare facilities. Thus, family members and healthcare workers are at greatest risk.

Plague (Prentice & Rahalison 2007)

Plague is caused by a Gram-negative bacillus, *Yersinia pestis*, which is an enzootic infection of rodents and is transmitted by infected fleas. The natural disease begins as a blood-borne infection of the lymph nodes resulting in 'bubonic plague'. If the patient develops pneumonia, the disease is termed 'pneumonic plague' and can be transmitted by droplets. Weaponization of the plague bacillus was attempted during the United States programme and probably accomplished by Soviet scientists (Ingelsby *et al.* 2002).

Inhaled, aerosolized plague bacilli cause primary pneumonic plague. The incubation period may be as short as 24 h, but symptoms usually occur two to four days after exposure. The disease presents with fever, cough, and dyspnoea, sometimes with bloody, watery or purulent sputum. Occasionally there may be gastrointestinal symptoms including nausea, vomiting, abdominal pain, and diarrhoea. The subsequent clinical picture of primary pneumonic plague is similar to any type of severe, rapidly progressive pneumonia.

Untreated pneumonic plague has a case-fatality rate approaching 100 per cent, and the time from exposure to death has been found to be around 2–6 days. Since pneumonic plague can spread from person-to-person through droplets, several generations of the disease can occur. Appropriate isolative precautions are effective in preventing transmission. The epidemic curve for a simulated, point-source outbreak of pneumonic plague is shown for illustrative purposes in Fig. 10.8.1, where diagnosis is established at day four. The initial cases are due to exposure at source and treated appropriately once the cause is known. The second wave is due to secondary spread prior to control of the epidemic.

Viral haemorrhagic fevers (Borio et al. 2002)

The viral haemorrhagic fevers are illnesses associated with fever and bleeding diathesis caused by small RNA viruses belonging to the families, Filovioridiae, Arenaviridae, Bunyaviridae, and Flaviviridae. The filoviruses and arenaviruses have been weaponized by the former Soviet Union, Russia, and the United States. In particular, the Soviet Union is reported to have produced quantities of Marburg, Lassa, Ebola, Junin and Machupo viruses.

The incubation period varies from 2 to 21 days. Clinical manifestations include fever, myalgias, rash, and encephalitis. Patients display a non-specific prodrome of high fever, headache, malaise, arthralgias, myalgias, nausea, abdominal pain, and non-bloody diarrhoea, which may last about a week. Most have cutaneous flushing or a skin rash. Later patients show signs of haemorrhagic disease. Second and later generations of disease can occur through direct contact with body fluids of the patients, which are highly infectious. Healthcare workers are at the greatest risk.

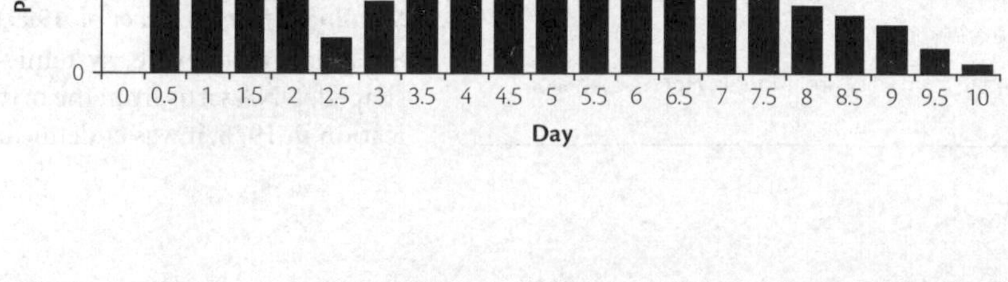

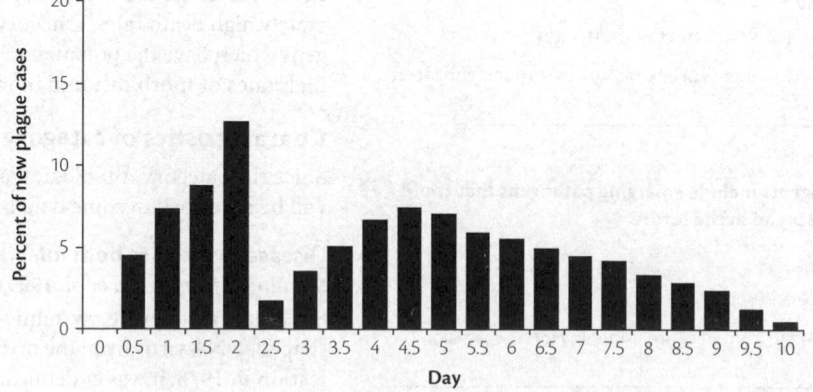

Fig. 10.8.1 Epidemic curve for a simulated point-source outbreak of pneumonic plague, with diagnosis on day four after exposure and appropriate treatment given to cases. *Source*: Scheulen, J., Latimer, C., and Brown, J. (2006). Electronic Mass Casualty Assessment and Planning Scenarios (EMCAPS). Johns Hopkins University. Available at: http://www.hopkins-cepar.org/EMCAPS/EMCAPS. Accessed July 14, 2007.

Diseases that are infectious but not contagious

Anthrax (Ingelsby et al. 2002)

Anthrax is caused by Gram-positive, aerobic, spore-forming, rod-shaped bacteria (*Bacillus anthracis*). It was one of the leading agents in the biological weapons programmes due to its stability and virulence. The vegetative spores are easily disseminated, resistant to drying and highly infectious. In addition, since the disease is not contagious, its effects can be restricted to the target population. There are three clinical manifestations of the disease: Cutaneous, gastrointestinal, and inhalation. The cutaneous form is not uncommon in nature, mainly among people occupationally exposed while handling domestic animals. Gastrointestinal anthrax is much less common and occurs as a result of the consumption of contaminated meat. Inhalation anthrax is exceedingly rare and has been reported mainly among woolsorters and workers exposed to contaminated animal hides and bones.

Aerosol dissemination of the spores, which is the likely scenario in a bioterrorist attack, causes inhalation anthrax (Ingelsby *et al.* 2002). Anthrax spores are about 1 μm in size and in order to enter the lung alveoli, the spore-bearing particles must be in the range of 1–5 μm. Thus, in order to weaponize the organism, the spore-bearing particles must be of the appropriate size and remain suspended in the air long enough to be inhaled. Once the spores penetrate the lung alveoli, they are ingested by macrophages, enter the lymphatic system and settle in the mediastinal lymph nodes, where they germinate. They cause disease by producing three factors called protective antigen, oedema factor and lethal factor. These combine to form two toxins, lethal toxin and oedema toxin. Protective antigen allows the binding of lethal and oedema factors to the cell membrane and facilitates their transport across it. To achieve full virulence, the bacteria must have an intact capsule together with the three toxin components.

The initial symptoms include fever, chills, sweats, fatigue, malaise, cough, nausea, and dyspnoea. This stage lasts from hours to a few days and is often accompanied by a brief period of recovery. The second stage is characterized by sudden fever, dyspnoea, dyaphoresis and shock. Cyanosis and hypotension progress rapidly, followed by death in a few hours. The disease is a sepsis syndrome with a haemorrhagic mediastinitis and many patients develop haemorrhagic meningitis. Alveolar pneumonia is not a major clinical feature. Untreated, the case-fatality rate is essentially 100 per cent.

Mathematical models based on the Sverdlovsk accident have been used to predict the incubation period and the dose-response of inhalation anthrax (Brookmeyer *et al.* 2001). The incubation period is estimated at 1–6 days but can be longer than 40 days, and is probably related to the exposure dose. For illustrative purposes, a possible epidemic curve for a simulated point-source outbreak of inhalation anthrax is shown in Fig. 10.8.2.

In fatal cases, the time between onset of symptoms and death in untreated cases has been found to be an average of three days (Ingelsby *et al.* 2002). The severity of the disease appears to be related to the exposure dose and it is possible that this is age-dependent. The spores can survive in the environment for many years, although once they are on the ground, they will tend to produce cutaneous anthrax.

Tularemia (Dennis et al. 2001)

Tularemia is a febrile illness caused by a small, non-motile, aerobic, Gram-negative, spore-forming coccobacillus, *Francisella tularensis*. It was initially identified in rodents and subsequently in humans exposed to infected animals. The agent has the potential for causing waterborne outbreaks and early on was described as a hazard for laboratory workers. Tularemia has been weaponised in biowarfare programmes.

The onset of the disease is usually abrupt with fever (38–40°C), headache, chills, rigors, generalized body aches, coryza, and sore throat. A pulse-temperature disassociation has been noted in many patients. There is often a dry or slightly productive cough. Inhalation tularaemia causes haemorrhagic inflammation of the airways early on in the course of the disease, which may progress to bronchopneumonia. Untreated, the fatality rates could be between 30–60 per cent. There is no secondary person-to-person spread.

Toxins

Botulism (Arnon et al. 2001)

Botulism is caused by a 150 Kd toxin which is produced by *Clostridium botulinum*, a spore-forming, obligate, anaerobic bacteria. Sporadic cases occur naturally such as through consumption of improperly canned foods. It is one of the most potent neurotoxins known and has been weaponized in biowarfare programmes. In a bioterrorist incident, it could be disseminated either through food or by aerosol.

After ingestion or inhalation of the toxin, an endopeptidase blocks acetylcholine-containing vesicles from fusing with the terminal membrane of the motor neurons. The incubation period for inhalational botulism is unknown for humans, but in animal experiments it was between 12 and 80 h. The main clinical manifestation is an acute, afebrile, symmetric, descending flaccid paralysis which

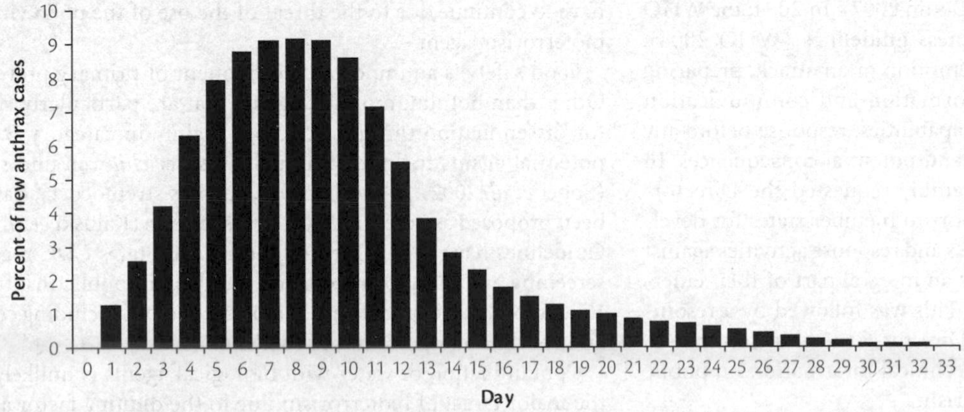

Fig. 10.8.2 Epidemic curve for a simulated point-source outbreak of inhalation anthrax, without intervention.
Source: Scheulen, J., Latimer, C., and Brown, J. (2006). Electronic Mass Casualty Assessment and Planning Scenarios (EMCAPS). Johns Hopkins University. Available at: http://www.hopkins-cepar.org/EMCAPS/EMCAPS. Accessed July 14, 2007.

begins in the bulbar musculature. The main presenting symptoms are difficulty in seeing, speaking, and swallowing with neurological signs such as ptosis, diplopia, blurred vision, enlarged or slow reacting pupils, dysarthria, dysphonia, and dysphagia. There are no significant sensory changes. In untreated cases, death occurs due to airway obstruction and inadequate tidal volume.

The patient is not contagious at any stage of the disease. Since aerosol spread of botulinum toxin does not occur in nature, the lethal dose is not known, but has been estimated at 0.70–0.90 μg.

Estimating the extent of a bioterrorist incident

Contagious diseases

The three major epidemiological factors affecting the spread of a contagious disease are the number of people initially exposed, the secondary reproduction rate and the generation time. The reproduction rate is defined by R_0, which is a measure of the average number of people who will be infected by each sick person. If it is less than one, transmission is not sustainable. The reproduction rate is not static and can change with the progression of the epidemic. $R(t)$ is the reproduction rate at a certain point in time t and is likely to drop following the introduction of control measures. For pneumonic plague, R_0 has been estimated at around 1.3 (Gani & Leach 2004). The R_0 for smallpox is larger and has been estimated as between 5 and 10, although it is likely to be closer to 5 (Leach 2007).

Estimates have been made of the extent of a smallpox incident under various bioterrorism scenarios, where the virus is disseminated by human vectors, in a building and in an airport (Bozzette *et al.* 2003). Since the number of initial cases will vary from tens to thousands, the total number of cases could be small or reach hundreds of thousands. Clearly, if vaccination is instituted early, the numbers could be reduced accordingly.

Infectious but not contagious diseases

Estimates have been made of the potential size of inhalation anthrax outbreaks under varying circumstances of the population exposed and the timing of antibiotic prophylaxis (Walden & Kaplan 2004). Since the disease is not contagious, the final total number of cases will only be a proportion of the number initially exposed. There could be some secondary cases of inhalation anthrax from reaerosolization of spores. However, most of the secondary cases are likely to be cutaneous anthrax.

Preparedness—general guidelines

During the 1990s, many countries began to actively prepare for the possibility of a bioterrorist event (Bonin 2007). In 2004, the WHO published bioterrorism preparedness guidelines (WHO 2004). They include threat analysis, pre-emption of an attack, preparing to respond, preparing public information and communication packages, validation of response capabilities, response before any overt release of biological agents, and potential consequences. In 2001, the 54th World Health Assembly requested the Director-General 'to provide technical support to member states for developing or strengthening preparedness and response activities against risks posed by biological agents, as an integral part of their emergency management programmes'. This was followed by a resolution in 2002, which requested the Director-General to continue to issue international guidance and technical information on public health measures related to bioterrorism.

In 2000, the United States CDC published a strategic plan for preparedness and response to biological and chemical terrorism (Khan *et al.* 2000). The strategic plan focused on five areas: Preparedness and prevention, detection and surveillance, diagnosis and characterization of biological and chemical agents, response and communication. In the preparedness area, the United States CDC undertook to provide public health guidelines and technical support to local and state public health agencies.

Prevention

The public health approach to the prevention of bioterrorism includes identifying the causes of terrorism and evaluating appropriate preventive strategies at the most basic level. The causes are likely to be multi-factorial. Political elements frequently dominate and the distinction between terrorist and 'freedom-fighter' is often blurred. There is no generic cause of terrorism. Poverty and deprivation can provide fertile ground for recruiting members to a terrorist organization. In addition to reducing ethnic and religious tensions, an international goal should be to ensure that there are adequate processes for non-violent resolution of differences. At a government level, there needs to be a clear, universal condemnation of terrorism as a means of achieving change. Rather emphasis should be placed on searching for common ground between groups.

Currently, the prevention of bioterrorism incidents remains largely in the hands of the security forces and intelligence agencies. At the international level, Interpol has established a special training programme to combat cross-border bioterrorism. Since bioterrorism will impact primarily on the health of the population, it is now considered to be an important public health issue. Coordination between professionals from various disciplines is needed to prepare for and manage an incident. They include specialists in epidemiology, infectious diseases, microbiology, vaccinology, general public health, medical informatics, emergency medicine, environmental health, food safety, veterinary medicine, health law, risk communication and management of health services.

Primary prevention of a bioterrorist incident is the first priority. This should be based on close cooperation between security authorities and international collaboration. The incentive for bioterrorism can be reduced if there are effective means to deal with a possible attack. Abuse of biological agents can be reduced by restricting access and good intelligence. The threat of bioterrorism has called into question some of the dogmas related to programmes to eradicate diseases such as poliomyelitis and measles. For example, if polio is successfully eradicated, universal vaccination may have to continue due to the threat of the use of the polio virus as a bioterrorism agent.

Food safety is an important component of primary prevention. Other than botulinum toxin, agents that are particularly suitable for dissemination through food are mainly in category B. Some potential agents include salmonella, *Escherichia coli* and *shigella* (Sobel *et al.* 2002). Other bacteria, such as streptococci, have also been proposed as potential bioterrorist agents (Kaluski *et al.* 2006). Guidelines have been issued by the United States CDC regarding screening and monitoring of food handlers in public institutions. Vulnerability assessments need to be carried out including controls and checks on importation of foods.

Contamination of water with biological agents is unlikely to be the major target of bioterrorism due to the diluting factor and the need for large quantities of the agent in order to cause significant outbreaks. Nevertheless, the cryptosporisium outbreak in Milwaukee, United States, in 1993, is an example of the large number of people that can be affected by a waterborne outbreak. Thus, the potential threat exists and should not be underestimated (Meinhardt 2005). In the United States, the Environmental Protection Agency addresses water security in three areas: Vulnerability assessments, emergency/incident planning and security enhancements.

Secondary prevention can be achieved by detection of the bioterrorist event in the early stages, in order to institute appropriate measures such as post-exposure pharmacological and non-pharmacological prophylaxis. Thus, comprehensive surveillance will be a cornerstone of secondary prevention. Tertiary prevention will include early treatment and rehabilitation of those people who contract the disease and public information campaigns to reduce the long-term psychological impacts of the incident.

Surveillance and early detection

The purpose of surveillance

The objectives of surveillance for bioterrorism incidents are twofold. The first is early detection of cases in order to facilitate prompt treatment of people already ill, identification of the exposure source and rapid introduction of prophylaxis for those who have been exposed or are at risk of exposure. If the disease is contagious, early detection will assist in limiting spread of the disease by ensuring isolation of cases and enforcing quarantine, where necessary. The second objective is monitoring the progress of the outbreak to assist the authorities in deciding to upgrade and redistribute health services and provide reliable and timely information for the media.

There are four main limitations of traditional surveillance systems for the detection and monitoring of bioterrorism incidents. Firstly, diagnosis of the early cases may be missed due to a failure to suspect or report unusual diseases. Secondly, there may be a considerable delay in reporting due to the lag time between clinical diagnosis and laboratory confirmation. Thirdly, since the flow of information in traditional surveillance systems tends to be relatively slow, there may be a substantial delay in alerting public health authorities. Finally, access to timely, processed information during the epidemic may be seriously limited.

Syndromic surveillance

Principles of syndromic surveillance

Most infectious diseases have prodromal periods characterized by non-specific symptoms and signs. As a result, surveillance of symptoms and signs of disease, or 'syndromic surveillance', was proposed as a more sensitive method for early detection and monitoring of an outbreak. Although syndromic surveillance is a relatively new term, surveillance for 'influenza-like illness' (ILI) is well-established for monitoring the incidence of influenza itself. Any system based on non-specific signs and symptoms will require balancing of sensitivity, specificity, and positive predictive value. Systems that are highly sensitive will tend to have low specificity and positive predictive value, with many false alarms.

The roles of syndromic surveillance

There are basically three potential roles for syndromic surveillance. These are detection of the first cases of the outbreak, detection of the outbreak at an early stage and management of the outbreak. Theoretically, syndromic surveillance could be successful in detecting the first cases of a slowly evolving outbreak. However, for bioterrorist scenarios, it is probably more realistic to describe the role of syndromic surveillance as detection of cases at an early stage of the outbreak. This would complement the reporting of the first cases clinically diagnosed by individual physicians. The system could be used to confirm the outbreak and help estimate its location. For this purpose, the syndromic surveillance system needs to be maintained and analysed periodically. In the event of a report of a suspicious or confirmed case, focused analysis of the data base could determine whether there are changes in the pattern of non-specific disease rates, relevant to the diagnosed cases reported.

Syndromic surveillance can also play a major role in the management and control of the outbreak. During large infectious disease outbreaks, occurring under emergency conditions, laboratory diagnosis of individual cases is likely to be limited and often not done at all. In addition, the transmission of information on diagnosed cases will often be delayed. Thus, once an outbreak has been confirmed, syndromic surveillance systems would provide timely and detailed data on the location and evolution of the outbreak. The system can also provide important, current information on general disease patterns in the total population so as to place the outbreak in perspective.

Sources of data

Syndromic surveillance has been facilitated by electronic reporting and the Internet. The sources of the data include visits to primary care physicians and emergency rooms, occasionally supplemented by medication prescription data. Since not all patients will visit a physician, surrogates of symptoms such as sales of the over-the-counter medications could also be used. In addition, other more crude indices of increased disease incidence could include hospital bed occupancy, mortality rates and the numbers of blood cultures requested. Syndromic surveillance could be complemented by special reporting systems such as PulseNet and FoodNet, which were established to monitor food-borne diseases. International data sharing will be essential for detecting cross-border bioterrorism.

Syndromic surveilance systems usually have statistical computing capabilities to determine whether there are unusual changes in either time or space or both (Kaufman *et al.* 2007; Rolka *et al.* 2007). Analytic tools, such as time series analysis and the cusum method, can be used to detect temporal changes in disease patterns. Detection of clusters, both in time and place, can be facilitated by the use of Geographic Information Systems (GIS), combined with statistical analysis tools. If a bioterrorist attack occurs in a public place, home addresses of the patients will not be helpful in detecting the location of the exposure. Clusters may be identified when only residential addresses are available if the communities surrounding a public place are overrepresented among people gathering at a public place (Green & Kaufman 2005). Other approaches that could be useful include searching for clusters in families or in age distributions. Once the outbreak has been identified, the syndromic surveillance data source should include a question on the location of the patient at the time of the attack.

Responding to alarms

A syndromic surveillance system must be accompanied by a response mechanism. It should include procedures to be followed in the event that an incident is suspected. In traditional surveillance, when a notifiable disease or obvious outbreak is diagnosed or suspected, the procedure to be followed is usually well-defined. For syndromic surveillance, it may not be clear which irregularities should be reported and investigated. This should include who should receive the report and what kind of investigation should be pursued. Since many of the systems use anonymized data, the investigation will need to be carried out together with those supplying the source data. Privacy issues should also be addressed. Unless there is a very large deviation from the expected incidence rates, each investigation is likely to be complex and time-consuming.

Syndromic surveillance systems

Guidelines for developing syndromic surveillance systems have been published by the United States CDC. They require that the goals of the system be detailed and include specifications of the kind of information that is expected. Syndromic surveillance systems are currently operating in a number of centres, mainly in the United States (Bravata *et al.* 2004a). One of the earliest systems was developed in the New York City Department of Health. Since 1999, they have been actively monitoring hotline calls on a daily basis to identify temporal or geographic increases in respiratory illnesses that might represent a potential bioterrorist event (Heffernan *et al.* 2004). The Health Department also developed systems to monitor community-based gastrointestinal outbreaks. The United States CDC is developing a national surveillance system called Biosense (Bradley *et al.* 2005).

Evaluation of syndromic surveillance systems

The surveillance system must be evaluated for each biological agent separately. The factors most likely to determine the success of the system have been listed as simplicity, flexibility, data quality, acceptability, sensitivity, predictive value, representativeness, timeliness, and stability (Centers for Disease Control 2001). Technical factors that should be considered include methods of collecting data, amount of follow-up, method of managing the data, methods for analysing and disseminating the data, staff training and time spent on maintaining the system.

Since there are essentially no actual bioterrorist events, evaluations of surveillance systems must be based on simulations. There is evidence that syndromic surveillance will identify influenza outbreaks earlier than sentinel surveillance based on laboratory isolates. However, since a bioterrorism incident is likely to be a point-source outbreak, it is questionable whether the efficacy of a system for detecting influenza outbreaks can be extrapolated to bioterrorism scenarios.

Benefits of syndromic surveillance

An appropriate surveillance system serves as the cornerstone of the information base at all stages of the outbreak. The benefits of electronic syndromic surveillance are primarily in the reduction in the lag time between early symptoms and clinical and laboratory, timeliness of the reports and reduced reliance on individual physicians to complete forms. This is of particular relevance in emergency situations. The system can provide current, updated information to decision-makers at the national or regional disease control centre. This information will be critical for confirming the outbreak, guiding decisions on intervention and monitoring the impact of control measures.

Limitations of syndromic surveillance

Despite the widespread implementation of syndromic surveillance systems, primarily in the United States, their contribution to the early detection of bioterrorism events has been questioned (Reingold 2003). There are two main criticisms. The first is the contention that early cases with clear clinical signs are likely to be detected in hospital emergency rooms earlier or at the same time as the outbreak is detected by syndromic surveillance. The second, and perhaps more dominant criticism, is that there is a real danger that an abundance of false reports could desensitize and paralyse the system. Thus, it is not at all clear whether these surveillance systems will play a significant role in early detection, and whether they can function efficiently in the long term, without overburdening the public health services.

The role of animals as sentinels

Where they have an enhanced sensitivity to the disease, illness in both domestic and wild animals could provide early warnings of exposure to biological agents (Rabinowitz *et al.* 2006). This could be relevant for anthrax, plague and tularaemia. Sheep and cattle could be sentinels for anthrax due to their sensitivity to the organism and the fact that they are largely outdoors. They may become ill quicker and at lower doses. For example, in the Sverdlovsk outbreak, sheep and cows began to die three days after the release of the aerosol, up to 50-km downwind from the point of release (Meselson *et al.* 1994). The incubation period for plague in cats may be as short as 1–2 days, compared with 1–6 days in humans. Rodents are sensitive to tularaemia and may become ill before humans. It is not known whether animals will be affected by aerosols of the haemorrhagic fevers. While the botulinum toxin type that would affect humans does not generally affect animals when transmitted by food, this does not exclude possible toxic effects if exposure is through the respiratory system.

Environmental and food surveillance

Bravata *et al.* (2004b) reviewed systems for environmental detection of biological agents and found that in many cases, the sensitivity and specificity of the systems had not been evaluated. The detection systems included particulate counters or biomass indicators that detect an increase in particles in aerosol samples, systems designed to rapidly detect biological agents collected from environmental, human, animal or agricultural samples and systems that integrate the collection, identification, and communication of the results. Autonomous detection systems for detecting anthrax spores are being developed particularly for use in the workplace (Meehan *et al.* 2004). Wherever any system installed, there should be detailed response plans in the event of a positive signal.

Current status of surveillance for bioterrorist incidents

Despite the increased sophistication of the surveillance systems, early identification of deliberately caused diseases will depend largely on the ability of primary care and emergency room physicians to identify and immediately report typical cases. The diagnosis of uncommon diseases may be missed by physicians who have rarely or never seen cases of the disease. Thus, medical personnel, particularly in hospital emergency rooms, should be updated regularly on the clinical manifestations of diseases which may result from bioterrorism.

The epidemiological investigation

In many respects, the epidemiological investigation of a bioterrorist incident is similar to any outbreak investigation. The main objectives are to identify and characterize the outbreak and predict its course.

For bioterrorism, the investigators should have specialized knowledge of the possible biological agents and the natural history of the diseases they produce. This will require a multi-disciplinary team led by specialists in infectious disease epidemiology. It will also require close cooperation with law enforcement authorities, risk communicators and the media. Where appropriate, those interviewing patients will need personal protective equipment (PPE).

There are likely to be three distinct phases of the investigation. The first is when an outbreak is suspected without a definitive diagnosis, the second is when the diagnosis has been confirmed and the third is when it is concluded that the outbreak was intentional. Clear, operational protocols for all phases, including agreed upon definitions of cases and contacts, and appropriate questionnaires, should be available for all potential agents. Data should be meticulously collected on each patient, including the date and time of onset of symptoms, the nature of the signs and symptoms, a history of all public places visited during a period compatible with the incubation periods of the suspected agents, details of personal acquaintances or knowledge of other patients with similar symptoms and contacts since the onset of symptoms. All relevant results of the medical examination should be recorded, including treatment received prior to presentation at a health care facility and that prescribed by the treating physician. The natural history of the disease should be described, including changes in the condition of the patient. A detailed history of previous vaccinations should be recorded. All relevant contacts of the patients need to be identified and interviewed.

Diagnosis in bioterrorist outbreaks

Most of the biological agents can be easily grown and diagnosed with high accuracy in hospital laboratories. However, some may require more specialized laboratories and there is a need for international collaboration. New technologies, especially those based on DNA technology, are being developed to speed up the pathogen recognition process. Concern for the safety of laboratory workers requires investment in safety equipment.

The clinical diagnosis of smallpox is based on the course of the disease and the typical rash (Henderson *et al.* 1999). The diagnosis is confirmed by electron microscopy. Recently, a real-time PCR method was described to identify the variola virus (Scaramozzino *et al.* 2007). The clinical diagnosis of anthrax is classically based on symptoms and chest X-ray findings which are usually abnormal, but can be confused with pneumonic plague (Ingelsby *et al.* 2002). There are not usually signs of classical bronchopneumonia, but later there is evidence of a widened mediastinum, pleural effusions, air bronchograms, necrotizing pneumonic lesions, and consolidation. The basic diagnostic tests for B anthracis are available in hospital laboratories and rapid tests are being developed. The confirmatory tests such as immuno-histochemical staining, gamma phage, and PCR assays are carried out in special reference laboratories.

The clinical diagnosis of plague is based on a finding of severe pneumonia and sepsis (Ingelsby *et al.* 2002; Prentice & Rahalison 2007). The index of suspicion is likely to be low unless there is a cluster of patients with fever, cough, shortness of breath, chest pain and a fulminant course. Gram stain may reveal Gram-negative bacilli or cocco-bacilli. A Wright, Giemsa or Wayson stain will often show bipolar staining and direct fluorescent antibody testing could be positive. Cultures of sputum, blood or lymph node aspirate should demonstrate growth approximately 24–48 h after inoculation. Up to 72 h may be required to identify the organism.

Since inhalation tularaemia presents with acute, non-specific, respiratory symptoms, the clinical diagnosis is difficult and usually, only a cluster of cases is likely to arouse suspicion (Dennis *et al.* 2001). The X-ray findings include atypical pneumonia, pleuritis and hilar lymphadenopathy, and routine microbiological tests may not be successful in identifying the bacteria. Diagnosis is made using direct examination of secretions, exudates and biopsy specimens using direct fluorescent antibody or immunohistological stains or blood cultures. Tests results can be obtained from reference laboratories within a few hours.

Botulism presents classically with a symmetric descending paralysis (Arnon *et al.* 2001). The electromyogram can sometimes help in the diagnosis. The CSF is unchanged in botulism. Laboratory testing for botulism is only obtainable at selected laboratories. The laboratory test is based on a mouse bioassay using serum, faeces, gastric aspirate. For food-transmitted botulism, vomitus and suspected foods can be tested. Suspected contaminated food should be refrigerated until tested. The mouse bioassay yields results within one to two days.

The clinical presentation of the viral haemorrhagic fevers varies widely and requires a high index of suspicion (Borio *et al.* 2002). Only specialized laboratories can currently make rapid diagnoses. The laboratory methods include antigen and antibody capture ELISA, RT-PCR, and viral isolation. Virus isolation requires a BSL-4 facility. Although a rise in antibody titre is diagnostic, antibodies appear late in the disease and are of limited value for early diagnosis.

Treatment of patients in bioterrorist incidents

Preparedness for bioterrorism will require an infrastructure that is capable of dealing with a variety of biological agents and clinical surge capacity. For contagious diseases such as smallpox, plague, and haemorrhagic fever, special precautions, such as patient isolation, will be necessary. Guidelines for isolation precautions for patients in healthcare facilities, have recently been published by the United States CDC (Siegel *et al.* 2007). The needs of special groups such as the paediatric population, pregnant women, and people with immunological disorders will need to be addressed.

For smallpox, standard, contact, and airborne precautions must be instituted. Therapy comprises supportive therapy and antibiotics for secondary infections. No drug has been found to be effective in modifying the course of the disease. There is some evidence of the potential efficacy of the thiosemicarbazones, but this is still under study. Patients with pneumonic plague must be managed using standard and droplet precautions. Streptomycin and gentamicin have been found to be effective in treatment. There is some evidence of the development of multiple, antimicrobial resistance in plague (Welch *et al.* 2007). For tularaemia, isolation of the patients is not necessary and standard precautions should be employed. The antibiotics, streptomycin, and gentamicin have been found to be effective. For the haemorrhagic fevers, initially standard, contact, and airborne precautions should be implemented until diagnosis has been confirmed. Subsequently, droplet can be used in place of airborne precautions. The treatment consists of supportive care and treatment of secondary infections. No drug has been found effective in modifying the course of the disease. There are no anti-viral drugs approved, although ribavirin may be effective.

Patients with inhalation anthrax need to be treated early (Ingelsby *et al.* 2002). Protective respirators (N95) and clothing should be used by healthcare personnel. Clothing of patients should undergo decontamination and thorough handwashing procedures should be enforced. Following the appearance of respiratory signs, the prognosis is very poor, even with treatment. In addition to supportive therapy, antibiotics such as ciprofloxacin, doxycycline, and ampicillin have been found to be effective. However, since the bacteria may have been engineered to be resistant to some of the antibiotics, the actual treatment regimen (Meselson *et al.* 1994) will dependent on the results of sensitivity testing. For symptomatic patients, antibiotics are given intravenously until the patient is stable, followed by oral therapy. In the event of a large number of casualties, intravenous therapy may not be feasible and only oral therapy will be used.

Patients with botulism do not need to be isolated and standard precautions should be maintained. Therapy includes supportive care and passive immunization with equine antitoxin. The licensed antitoxin contains types A, B, and C. There is also an investigational heptavalent (ABCDEFG) antitoxin held by the United States army. The dose is a single vial by slow intravenous infusion. Hypersensitivity reactions may occur. The rates of serum sickness or urticaria appear to be about 2 per cent and milder signs occur at rates as high as 18 per cent.

Handling of dead patients and burial procedures

The handling of dead patients should be carried out with the same barrier precautions as for live patients, according to the biological agent involved. Usually, post-mortem examinations should be kept to a minimum and should be carried out by staff appropriately protected and where necessary, given medications and/or vaccines. The burial procedures also have to be carried out using protective clothing which must be disposed in biohazard bags. At all times, the religions and traditions of the community involved should be respected.

For diseases such as smallpox, other than valuables, clothing and disposable medical equipment should be buried with the body. The body should be double-wrapped in sealed polyethylene bags. Some have proposed that quicklime should be added both inside the wrapping and in the grave itself. Care should be taken to bury the dead at places that are not near underground water sources, residential areas, agricultural sites or concentrations of animals.

Pharmacologic prophylaxis

Pre- and post-exposure prophylaxis

There are basically two modes of pharmacalogical prophylaxis, depending on the biological agent. Pre-exposure prophylaxis is given prior to the incident to people at increased risk of exposure. Post-exposure prophylaxis is given after known or suspected exposure to the biological agent. The first mode is generally confined to vaccines, whereas the second mode may combine the use of both antibiotics and vaccines. Antivirals and immunoglobulins are currently considered only for treatment and not for prophylaxis.

The role of vaccines

As part of primary prevention of bioterrorism, vaccines are one of the most effective means of protecting the public. Improved preparedness for bioterrorism will be heavily dependent on the development of new vaccines. Currently, vaccines are only relevant for smallpox and anthrax. If adverse events associated with these vaccines can be reduced to negligible levels, it is conceivable that some countries may consider including them in the infant vaccination schedules. For some of the other potential bioterrorist agents, vaccines are in various stages of development.

Smallpox

As a result of a world-wide campaign by the WHO, global eradication of smallpox was achieved in 1978 (Henderson *et al.* 1999). Since 1972, routine vaccination has been phased out and in most countries, more than 50 per cent of the population has never been vaccinated. Antibody titres have been shown to decline markedly after 5–10 years, although there is some evidence that residual immunity persists for many years (Eichner 2003). In such cases, even if the disease is not prevented, it is likely to be much milder. On the one hand this may reduce transmission (Nishiura & Eichner 2006), but on the other hand, milder cases may circulate in the community increasing the risk of spread (Kerrod *et al.* 2005).

The current vaccine is based on the established live, attenuated form of the vaccinia virus (Henderson *et al.* 1999). Some of the current vaccine stocks in the United States were produced during the 1970s using the New York City Board of Health (NHYBH) strain. Other types of smallpox vaccines include the Lister strains in the United States, LC16m8 in Japan and the modified Ankara strain (MVA) in Germany. Some 200 million doses of a cell-line vaccine are currently held by the United States government. New smallpox vaccines are currently being developed (Wiser *et al.* 2007).

The potential adverse effects of vaccination with vaccinia include post-vaccinial encephalitis, vaccinia necrosum, eczema vaccinatum, generalized vaccinia and accidental infection. The rates of life-threatening complications of post-vaccinia encephalitis and vaccinia necrosum in primary vaccinees are estimated as at least 3 and 1 per million, respectively (Aragon *et al.* 2003), although adverse effects may be higher for some strains. Rare, adverse effects on the cardiovascular system have been reported. The rates of adverse events may be substantially higher in areas where immunodeficiency is common.

Vaccinia immune globulin (VIG) is hyperimmune globulin produced from sera of previously vaccinated subjects. It is used under two circumstances. When a patient with relative contraindications to the vaccine is at high risk of contracting the disease, the smallpox vaccine is given together with VIG. In the event that a vaccinee experiences a severe adverse event, VIG is given intravenously and if the response is inadequate, it can be repeated after 72 h.

Smallpox pre-exposure prophylaxis

Most pre-exposure prophylaxis strategies call for vaccinating subgroups such as the military, healthcare workers, ambulance crews and police. Opinions vary on how large the portion of the population should be encouraged to be vaccinated. Healthcare workers have shown some resistance to vaccination due to concern about adverse effects and the perception that there is a low risk of a bioterrorist incident using smallpox.

Smallpox post-exposure prophylaxis

The method of post-exposure prophylaxis has been debated widely. There are data from the beginning of the twentieth century suggesting that vaccination within several days of exposure provides protection against clinical disease (Mortimer 2003). Since the incubation period for smallpox is around seven to fourteen days, if the identification of the first cases is the earliest indication of exposure, post-exposure vaccination will be too late to influence the outcome of those exposed at the site of the incident. It will therefore be relevant only for contacts.

Two approaches have been proposed for post-exposure prophylaxis. 'Ring vaccination', entails intensive tracing and vaccination of all primary contacts immediately following diagnosis of a case. This is followed by vaccination of the secondary contacts in the second ring. This approach was used successfully in the eradication of naturally occurring smallpox (Henderson *et al.* 1999). An alternative approach is to carry out mass vaccination of the population, following diagnosis of the first cases. Using mathematical modelling, some have favoured ring vaccination (Riley & Ferguson 2006) whereas others have found that rapid mass vaccination of the population is most effective (Kaplan *et al.* 2002). Ring vaccination accompanied by mass vaccination of affected regions (Hall *et al.* 2007), followed by countrywide mass vaccination, appear to be the most practical approach.

Anthrax

In the United States, the current vaccine is made from the cell-free filtrate of a non-encapsulated attenuated strain of *Bacillus anthracis*. It was licensed in 1970 to be given in a series of six doses. The United Kingdom produces a vaccine based on the same principles, where the protective antigen is the most important immunogen. Live spore vaccines from an attenuated strain have been produced in Russia and China. Pre-exposure prophylactic vaccination with the United States vaccine was shown to be protective in animal challenge studies. In a follow-up of vaccines, no unexpected local or systemic events were reported (Martin *et al.* 2005). Compliance may be a problem, due to factors such as concern about the safety of the vaccine. For post-exposure prophylaxis, the vaccine series, initiated together with antibiotics, has been shown to be the most cost-effective strategy (Fowler *et al.* 2005).

Vaccines for other category A agents

There are essentially no effective vaccines available for use in bioterrorist incidents for the other category A agents. The previous licensed, formalin-inactivated, whole bacilli, plague vaccine was not effective against primary pneumonic plague. Research continues in this area. A live, attenuated vaccine against tularaemia for high risk military personnel is held as an investigational new drug by the United States military. The vaccine has not been used widely for pre-exposure prophylaxis and does not appear to have any place in post-exposure prophylaxis.

A multivalent vaccine for some of the types of botulism is available at the CDC, but it is impractical to use in a bioterrorist incident. In the United States, an investigational pentavalent (ABCDE), botulinum toxoid is provided by the CDC for laboratory workers at high risk of exposure to botulinum toxin and by the military for protection against attack. Botulinum toxoid takes several months to produce immunity and has no value for post-exposure prophylaxis. New botulism vaccines are under development. As regards viral haemorrhagic fevers, with the exception of the yellow fever live attenuated 17D vaccine and Hunin virus vaccine, there are no licensed vaccines. Some progress appears to have been made in developing a vaccine for post-exposure prophylaxis of Ebola infection (Feldmann *et al.* 2007).

The role of medications in post-exposure prophylaxis

Antibiotics have a role in post-exposure prophylaxis mainly for anthrax and plague. Ciprofloxacin, doxycycline, and ampicillin should be effective against anthrax, depending on the sensitivity of the organism, and are recommended for a period of up to 60 days. Mild adverse events may be common, but serious reactions and hospitalizations are rare (Shephard *et al.* 2002). Since the response to antibiotics deteriorates rapidly following the onset of symptoms, prophylactic therapy should be provided as soon as possible to those who have been exposed. Due to the need to take the medications for a long period, compliance becomes a major problem. It may be possible to shorten the duration of antibiotic therapy, if vaccine is given concurrently.

Post-exposure prophylaxis for plague should be provided using appropriate antibiotics for a shorter period than required for anthrax. There is currently no effective vaccine for use under these circumstances.

It has been shown that antivirals, such as cidofovir or a related acyclic nucleoside phosphonate analogue, are more effective than post-exposure smallpox vaccine in preventing mortality, in monkeys experimentally infected with monkeypox virus (Stittelaar *et al.* 2006). This suggests that antivirals may have an important place in planning for a smallpox outbreak. For viral haemorrhagic fevers, ribavirin may have some efficacy in post-exposure prophylaxis.

National and international stockpiles of vaccines and medications

A number of countries have established national stockpiles of pharmaceuticals and vaccines, for use in the event of biological or chemical attacks or for serious diseases that may achieve epidemic proportions. The United States maintains the Strategic National Stockpile (SNS) of antibiotics, chemical antidotes, antitoxins, vaccines, life-supporting medications and emergency medical equipment. The operation of the SNS, in the event of an emergency, is based on 'push packages' that can be deployed to the designated sites within 12 h. The model is based on the 'Dispensing/Vaccination Centers' (DVCs). Either medications and vaccines will be taken directly to people's homes, or individuals will attend DVCs to receive medications or be vaccinated. The stocks in the SNS programme are rotated and kept within potency shelf-life limits.

NATO has initiated a programme to develop a deployable laboratory and biological defence stockpiles. In 2005, at least 40 countries had stockpiles of smallpox vaccine, varying from amounts sufficient to vaccinate the whole population to enough for only a proportion of the population (Arita 2005). The global inventory reported at that time was in excess of 800 million doses with a total global production potential of more than 400 million doses. Since some of the vaccines can be diluted at least one to five without losing potency (Couch *et al.* 2007), globally, the total number of doses potentially available in the event of an emergency may be in excess of three billion, with a production capacity in excess of two billion doses annually. International stockpiles of smallpox vaccine are held by the WHO with about 200 million doses being held under agreement by selected donor states, to be supplied to countries in need, in the event of an outbreak.

National vaccination programmes

Some countries have carried out active vaccination programmes against smallpox in the military and 'first-responders'. Since 2001, in the United States, more than half a million military personnel and about 40 000 healthcare workers have been vaccinated (Arita 2005). In addition, United States military personnel are now routinely vaccinated against anthrax and in the United Kingdom, the vaccine is offered to military personnel.

Non-pharmaceutical prophylaxis

Non-pharmacological prophylaxis is an important means of reducing the spread of the contagious diseases, smallpox, plague and the haemorrhagic fevers. These include strict isolation and barrier nursing procedures when treating patients, and public actions such as quarantine, social distancing, and the use of face masks, to reduce exposure in the community.

Isolation of sick patients

The first action to reduce propagation of contagious diseases, is to isolate sick patients. Isolation is defined as 'the separation and confinement of individuals known or suspected to be infected with a contagious disease to prevent them from transmitting the disease to others' (Barbera *et al.* 2001). This includes the transfer of patients to healthcare facilities. Once hospitalized, the highest level of isolation comprises special units with appropriate negative pressure air filtration. Simpler isolation with strict barrier nursing would represent a lower level of isolation. If the number of cases is large and overwhelms isolation facilities in hospitals, it may be necessary to establish isolation facilities at alternative locations. In addition, a policy of voluntary isolation could be implemented, where sick patients are encouraged to be treated at home.

Quarantine (curfews)

A second measure to limit spread of contagious diseases, is to quarantine those who may have been exposed. The definition of quarantine is: 'compulsory physical separation, including restriction of movement of populations or groups of healthy people who have been potentially exposed to a contagious disease, or to efforts to segregate them within specified geographical areas' (Barbera *et al.* 2001). The term 'cordon sanitaire' applies to restriction of movement of people and materials, and community-wide intervention strategies. The enforcement of quarantine is generally in the hands of the law-enforcement authorities. Since the quarantined population contains both people who have been exposed but are not yet ill, and others who were suspected of having been exposed but in fact were not, there is increased risk of disease transmission in the quarantined population.

Factors that contribute to imposing quarantine include the size of the exposed population and the severity and contagiousness of the disease (Barbera *et al.* 2001). Decisions have to be made regarding who should be quarantined and for how long. Border closure is a sensitive issue and will need special attention, according to the disease in question. The commercial consequences need to be recognized. Good risk communication is likely to improve compliance.

Social distancing

Social distancing has been proposed as an important non-pharmacological means of reducing the spread of transmissible diseases such as influenza. It includes measures such as closing of schools, limiting crowding in workplaces and other public places and reducing use of public transport. The possible impact on diseases caused by bioterrorism agents is less clear. Using mathematical modelling, there is evidence that social distancing could reduce the spread of smallpox (Kress 2005).

Masks and personal protective equipment (PPE)

There are clear, agent-specific, guidelines for the use of masks and PPE by healthcare personnel and the public health and emergency workers coming into contact with sick patients or moving in contaminated areas. The issue of whether the public should be encouraged to use masks during an outbreak of a contagious disease is less clear. The efficacy of the masks remains questionable and the type of masks to be used is not clear. Surgical masks may be adequate for droplet spread, but N95 type masks would be necessary to protect against aerosols. The N95 mask is more expensive, more complicated to use, requires special fitting and is uncomfortable to use for long periods of time.

Public education and risk communication

The goal of the terrorist has been described as 'an attempt to produce fear, magnified by an exaggerated sense of risk . . . and perpetuated by misinformation and rumors' (Shine 2001). The novel and largely unpredictable characteristics of biological weapons are likely to increase the uncertainty surrounding a bioterrorism incident. This uncertainty can reduce public trust in the ability of the authorities to control the incident. Public education and effective risk communication are essential in order to bolster public confidence and improve cooperation with the authorities.

Structured education programmes should be directed at healthcare personnel, other first responders and the general public. Clinicians and public health personnel should have access to up-to-date emergency information, which requires a solid infrastructure for rapid and reliable communication (Khan *et al.* 2000). The general public needs to have access to non-technical descriptions of the potential diseases that may be encountered and simple instructions on how to act in an emergency situation.

Risk communication plays a critical role in mitigating public panic responses and encouraging rational behaviour during an emergency. While there is a considerable literature on risk communication, relatively little has dealt with bioterrorism (Covello *et al.* 2001). Nevertheless, the general approaches that have been developed are relevant for a bioterrorism incident. Since the public's perception of risk may be somewhat different from the true risk, this is a critical component of risk communication (Slovic 1987). There are frequently misconceptions about what information should and should not be presented to the public. One approach is to encourage open discussion of the risk.

Due to the inherent uncertainty in a bioterrorism incident, the authorities may possess very little factual information. The impression may be that information is being withheld and the public may respond with hostility towards the authorities. In such situations, Sandman (2003) has proposed that 'one should not over-reassure, acknowledge uncertainty and share dilemmas'. Over-reaction or panic should be anticipated when new information about the risk is made public, although this is often complicated when rumours of ineffective and expensive solutions are propagated (Taig 1999).

As a convenient conceptual and operational framework, risk communication associated with a bioterrorist event may be divided into five stages—prior to the event, on suspicion of an event, on confirmation of the event, during the event and following the event. At each stage, the public is likely to ask questions relevant to that stage.

The main questions that are likely to be raised prior to a bioterrorist incident are whether in fact it can occur, and are the authorities well-prepared. On suspicion of an event, the public will want to know how likely it is that a bioterrorist incident has occurred. On confirmation of an incident, people will want to know where is it located, when did it start, is it contagious, are they at risk and is there a cure. During the event, there will be questions about the efficacy of the treatment, whether the disease is spreading, who is at risk and when will the event end. The questions after the event focus on whether the event has really ended and is there still a risk of exposure. The ability of the authorities to respond adequately to these questions depends on their access to good information. Timely and reliable surveillance data will be an important resource.

Problems that may be encountered during an outbreak

During an outbreak, the epidemiological investigation team should anticipate the numerous problems that may arise. These include atypical presentation of cases and varying responses to treatment. Unexpected laboratory difficulties are often more the rule than the exception and unexpectedly high percentages of false positive and negative diagnoses may be encountered. There are likely to be reports of side-effects of the medications and vaccines. In addition, there may be instances of vaccine or medication prophylaxis failure, which will reduce the trust of the public in the intervention procedures recommended.

Reports of the appearance of suspected new exposure foci are likely. A sense of mistrust may occur when disease is reported in apparently unexposed people. There may be incidences of inadequate isolation of patients and a breakdown of the implementation of quarantine regulations. It is possible that untried, new treatments will be proposed, often by professionals or lay persons not included among those handling the outbreak. Finally, unexpected changes in established policy may occur.

International cooperation (Bonin 2007)

The International Health Regulations (IHR) were first initiated in 1969 to 'prevent, protect against, control and provide a public health response to the international spread of disease in ways that are commensurate with and restricted to public health risks, and which avoid unnecessary interference with international traffic and trade'. The regulations were updated in 2005 and taken into account the increased threat of bioterrorism. They took effect in June 2007.

The WHO has established the Global Outbreak Alert and Response Network (GOARN) for international collaboration for the identification, confirmation and response to outbreaks with international implications. The Epidemic and Pandemic Alert and Response (EPR) component supports member states in epidemic preparedness in the context of the IHR. It includes training for preparedness and response, developing standardized approaches for readiness and response to major epidemic diseases, strengthening biosafety, biosecurity, and preparedness for outbreaks of diseases caused by dangerous pathogens and developing a global platform to support outbreak response.

The European Union also has a programme to improve cooperation between member states on preparedness and response to biological and chemical agent attacks (BICHAT). They operate the Early Warning and Response System (EWRS) for outbreaks of communicable diseases. A number of research activities are funded within the European Framework programmes and NATO funds activities such as Advanced Research Workshops where one of the major programme areas is bioterrorism preparedness.

Tabletop exercises

Tabletop exercises have been carried out, largely in the United States, to test the preparedness of the authorities in dealing with a bioterrorist attack. The 'Dark Winter' exercise in 2001, simulated a covert smallpox attack on the United States (O'Toole *et al.* 2002) and the TOPOFF exercise in 2000 simulated a simultaneous radiological, chemical and biological attack with *Yersinia pestis* (Ingelsby *et al.* 2001), They revealed serious deficiencies in the management of such incidents and provided impetus to the improvement of bioterrorism preparedness programmes. In 2005, the 'New Watchman' exercise, initiated by the European Commission, was conducted to evaluate European preparedness for a deliberate smallpox outbreak (Health Protection Agency 2007). Serious limitations were revealed in communications between member states, compatibility of response plans, countermeasures and adequacy of resources. In addition to recommendations on measures to overcome these limitations, it was stressed that similar exercises should be carried out as part of a routine programme.

Post-incident actions

Decontamination

Decontamination issues are relevant, mainly for anthrax and smallpox, in the general environment of an aerosol attack and places where patients were treated. This should including bedding, clothing and equipment. Methodologies for decontamination of the general environment from anthrax have been evaluated (Canter *et al.* 2005). Formaldehyde solution was effective in inactivating anthrax spores on the island of Gruinard, contaminated experimentally during the British biowarfare programme (Manchee *et al.* 1994). Hypochlorite solution is also effective.

Low humidity and temperature prolong survival of the smallpox virus in the environment (Kiang & Krathwohl 2003). Viruses on scab material can remain viable for as long as 12 weeks (Huq 1976). There are detailed procedures for sterilizing bedding and clothing and disinfecting the immediate environment of the patients.

Long-term consequences of bioterrorism incidents

Following a bioterrorist incident, residual public fear and anxiety is likely to persist. In a five-year follow-up of victims of the terrorist incident in the Tokyo subway attack, post-traumatic stress disorder symptoms were observed (Ohtani *et al.* 2004). There will inevitably be questions about the extent to which the authorities were able to control the incident, criticism of actions taken or not taken, and general recriminations. Part of the preparedness planning should include public education of the public on lessons learned from the incident and actions taken to address deficiencies.

Legal and ethical aspects

Bioterrorism preparedness requires the necessary legislation to enable the public health authorities to carry out measures with adequate legal backing. Laws that are of particular importance relate to closing buildings, taking over hospitals and ordering isolation and quarantine. Other issues that require regulation are active surveillance of presumed infected individuals and their contacts.

The authorities may have to exercise unusual powers to control the outbreak, which will require information campaigns. Civil liberties may be compromised. Questions that frequently arise relate to who enforces a quarantine, who detains an infected or exposed person and how civil liberties are protected. There will be a need for ethical review of surveillance procedures, but there is also 'an ethical mandate to undertake surveillance that enhances the well-being of the population' (Fairchild & Bayer 2004).

Agroterrorism

Agroterrorism includes the deliberate infection of livestock or crops with biological agents (Cupp *et al.* 2004). A number of countries, including the United States and the Soviet Union, had agricultural bioweapons programmes during the twentieth century. As previously noted, glanders was used against horses and mules in World War I, and it is alleged that Japan considered use of anthrax and rinderpest in World War II. The potential deliberate damage to crops or livestock will require special vigilance.

Conclusions

Bioterrorism falls into the category of low risk but high impact public health emergencies. Deterrence remains the prime goal, and delegitimization of the use of biological agents as weapons should be carried out at every level. The BioWeapons Prevention Project (BWPP) is an initiative based in Geneva with the objective of strengthening the opposition to the use of biological weapons. In addition, good preparedness for a bioterrorist incident both serves the goal of deterrence and ensures that the public health system and the society will deal effectively with the incident.

Questions have been raised about the justification for investing considerable resources in what is perceived to be a low risk event, possibly at the expense of the general public health services (Cohen *et al.* 2004). The United States CDC has defined 'ten essential services for public health' to respond to bioterrorism (CDC 2006). In summary, they recommend developing greater capacity to monitor health status and rapidly detect, diagnose, and investigate infectious disease and environmental health problems. The means to inform and educate people about health threats should be improved. Partnerships should be mobilized and policies and plans developed to respond to public health emergencies and enforce laws and regulations that protect health. Finally there is a need to develop a competent and trained public health workforce, evaluate the effectiveness, accessibility and quality of health services for emergencies and promote research for new and innovative solutions to health problems.

All these actions will serve public health in general, stressing the dual-benefit concept. An excellent example of such dual-benefit is the role played by of the United States military in developing new vaccines to protect the troops (Artenstein *et al.* 2005). This has resulted in vaccines for diseases affecting the general public, such as yellow fever, pneumococcal disease, hepatitis A and B and Japanese encephalitis. Preparedness for bioterrorism will benefit preparedness for disease outbreaks in general and other public health emergencies.

References

Aragon, T.J., Ulrich, S., Fernyak, S., and Rutherford, G.W. (2003). Risks of serious complications and death from smallpox vaccination: a systematic review of the United States experience, 1963–1968. *BMC Public Health*, **3**, 26–37.

Arita, I. (2005). Smallpox vaccine and its stockpile in 2005. *Lancet Infectious Diseases*, **5**, 647–52.

Arizona Department of Health Services. (2005). Bureau of Emergency Preparedness and Response. Bioterrorism. Available at: http://www.azdhs.gov/phs/edc/edrp/es/bthistor1.htm. Accessed July 1, 2007.

Arnon, S.S., Schechter, R., Ingelsby, T.V. *et al.* (2001). Botulism toxin as a biological weapon. Medical and public health management. *Journal of the American Medical Association*, **285**, 1059–70.

Artenstein, A.W., Opal, J.M., Opal, S.M., Tramont, E.C., Peter, G., Russell, P.K. (2005). *Military Medicine* **170**(4 Suppl):3–11.

Barbera, J., Macintyre, A., Gostin, L. *et al.* (2001). Large-scale quarantine following biological terrorism in the United States: scientific examination, logistic and legal limits, and possible consequences. *Journal of the American Medical Association*, **286**, 2711–8.

Bonin, S. (2007). In *International Biodefense Handbook. An inventory of national and international biodefense practices and policies* (series eds. A. Wegner, V. Mauer, and M. Dunn). *Center for Security Studies at ETH, Zurich.*

Borio, L., Ingelsby, T., Peters C.J. *et al.* (2002). Hemorrhagic fever viruses as biological weapons. *Journal of the American Medical Association*, **287**, 2391–405.

Bozzette S.A., Boer, R., Bhatnagar, V. *et al.* (2003). A model for a smallpox vaccination policy. *New England Journal Medicine*, **348**, 416–25.

Bradley C.A., Rolka, H., Walker, D., and Loonsk, J. (2005). BioSense: implementation of a national early event detection and situational awareness system. *Morbidity and Mortality Weekly Report*, **54**(Suppl), 11–9.

Bravata D.M., McDonald K.M., Smith W.M. *et al.* (2004a). Systematic review: surveillance systems for early detection of bioterrorism-related diseases. *Annals of Internal Medicine*, **140**, 910–22.

Bravata D.M., Sundaram, V., McDonald K.M. *et al.* (2004b). Evaluating detection and diagnostic decision support systems for bioterrorism response. *Emerging Infectious Diseases*, **10**, 100–8.

Brookmeyer, R., Blades, N., Hugh-Jones, M., and Henderson D.A. (2001). The statistical analysis of truncated data: application to the Sverdlovsk anthrax outbreak. *Biostatistics*, **2**, 233–47.

Canter D.A., Gunning, D., Rodgers, P., O'connor, L., Traunero, C., and Kempter C.J. (2005). Remediation of *Bacillus anthracis* contamination in the U.S. Department of Justice mail facility. *Biosecurity and Bioterrorism*, **3**, 119–27.

Centers for Disease Control and Prevention. (2001). Updated guidelines for evaluating public health surveillance systems. *Morbidity and Mortality Weekly Report*, **50**(RR13), 1–35.

Centers for Disease Control and Prevention. (2006). Bioterrorism overview. February 28, 2006. Available at: www.bt.cdc.gov/bioterrorism. Accessed July 1, 2007.

Cohen H.W., Gould R.M., and Sidel V.W. (2004). The pitfalls of bioterrorism preparedness: the anthrax and smallpox experiences. *American Journal of Public Health*, **94**, 1667–71.

Couch R.B., Winokur, P., Edwards K.M. *et al.* (2007). Reducing the dose of smallpox vaccine reduces vaccine-associated morbidity without reducing vaccination success rates or immune responses. *Journal of Infectious Diseases*, **195**, 826–32.

Covello V.T., Peters R.G., Wojtecki J.G., and Hyde R.C. (2001). Risk communication, the West Nile virus epidemic, and bioterrorism: responding to the communication challenges posed by the intentional or unintentional release of a pathogen in an urban setting. *Journal of Urban Health*, **78**, 382–91.

Cupp OS, Walker DE 2nd, Hillison J. Agroterrorism in the U.S.: key security challenge for the 21st century. (2004). *Biosecurity and Bioterrorism* **2**:97–105.

Dennis D.T., Ingelsby T.V., Henderson D.A. *et al.* (2001). Tularemia as a biological weapon. Medical and public health management. *Journal of the American Association*, **285**, 2763–73.

Eichner, M. (2003). Analysis of historical data suggests long-lasting protective effects of smallpox vaccination. *American Journal of Epidemiology*, **158**, 717–23.

Fairchild A.L., and Bayer, R. (2004). Public health. Ethics and the conduct of public health surveillance. *Science*, **303**, 631–2.

Federal Bureau of Investigation. Headline Archives. Anthrax investigation. Closing a chapter. Available at: http://www.fbi.gov/page2/august08/amerithtrax080608.html. Accessed October 1, 2008.

Feldmann, H., Jones S.M., Daddario-DiCaprio K.M. *et al.* (2007). Effective post-exposure treatment of Ebola infection. *PLOoS Pathogens*, **3**, 54–60.

Fowler R.A., Sanders G.D., Bravata D.M. *et al.* (2005). Cost-effectiveness of defending against bioterrorism: a comparison of vaccination and antibiotic prophylaxis against anthrax. *Annals of Internal Medicine*, **142**, 601–10.

Franz D.R., Jahrling P.B., Friedlander A.M. *et al.* (1997). Clinical recognition and management of patients exposed to biological warfare agents. *Journal of the American Medical Association*, **278**, 399–411.

Gani, R. and Leach, S. Epidemiologic determinants for modeling pneumonic plague outbreaks. (2004). *Emerging Infectious Diseases* **10**:608–614.

Green M.S. and Kaufman, Z. (2005). Syndromic surveillance for early location of terrorist incidents outside of residential areas. Morbidity and Mortality Weekly, **54** (Suppl), 189. Available at http://www.cdc.gov/mmwr/preview/mmwrhtml/su5401a35.htm. Accessed July 14, 2007.

Hall I.M., Egan J.R., Barrass, I., Gani, R., and Leach, S. (2007). Comparison of smallpox outbreak control strategies using a spatial metapopulation model. *Epidemiology and Infection*, **135**, 1133–44.

Health Protection Agency. Exercise New Watchman. A Smallpox exercise for the European Union. Serial 5.1. Final Report, March 2006. Available at: http://ec.europa.eu/health/ph_threats/com/watchman.pdf. Accessed October 6, 2007.

Heffernan, R., Mostashari, F., Das, D., Karpati, A., Kulldorff, M., and Weiss, D. (2004). Syndromic surveillance in public health practice, New York City. *Emerging Infectious Diseases*, **10**, 858–64.

Henderson D.A. (1998). Bioterrorism as a public health threat. *Emerging Infectious Diseases*, **4**, 488–92.

Henderson D.A., Ingelsby T.V., Bartlett J.G. *et al.* (1999). Smallpox as a biological weapon. Medical and public health management. *Journal of the American Medical Association*, **281**, 2127–37.

Hoffman, B. (2007). In "Terrorism". Microsoft Encarta Online Encyclopedia. Available at: http://encarta.msn.com. Accessed July 14, 2007.

Huq, F. (1976). Effect of temperature and relative humidity on variola virus in crusts. *Bulletin of the World Health Organisation*, **54**, 710–2.

Ingelsby T.V., Grossman, R., and O'Toole, T. (2001). A plague on your city: observations from TOPOFF. *Clinical Infectious Diseases*, **32**, 436–45.

Ingelsby T.V., O'Toole, T., Henderson D.A. *et al.* (2002). Anthrax as a biological weapon, 2002. Updated recommendations for management. *Journal of the American Medical Association*, **287**, 2236–52.

Jernigan D.B., Raghunathan, P.l., Bell B.P. *et al.* (2002). Investigation of bioterrorism-related anthrax, United States, 2001: epidemiologic findings. *Emerging Infectious Diseases*, **8**, 1019–28.

Kaluski D.N., Barak, E., Kaufman, Z. *et al.* (2006). A large food-borne outbreak of group A streptoccocal pharyngitis in an industrial plant: potential for deliberate contamination. *Israel Medical Association Journal*, **8**, 824.

Kaplan E.H., Craft D.L., and Wein L.M. (2002). Emergency response to a smallpox attack: the case for mass vaccination. *Proceedings of the National Academy of Sciences USA*, **99**, 10935–40.

Kaufman, Z., Wong W.K., Peled-Leviathan, T. *et al.* (2007). Evaluation of a syndromic surveillance system using the WSARE algorithm for early detection of an unusual, localized summer outbreak of influenza. Implications for bioterrorism surveillance. *Israel Medical Association Journal*, **9**, 3–7.

Kerrod, E., Geddes A.M., Regan, M., and Leach, S. (2005). Surveillance and control measures during smallpox outbreaks. *Emerging Infectious Diseases*, **11**, 291–7.

Khan A.S., Morse, S., and Lillibridge, S. (2000). Public-health preparedness for biological terrorism in the USA. *Lancet*, **356**, 1179–82.

Kiang K.M., and Krathwohl M.D. (2003). Rates and risks of transmission of smallpox and mechanisms of prevention. *Journal of Laboratory Clinical Medicine*, **142**, 229–38.

Kolavic S.A., Kimura, A., Simons S.L., Slutsker, L., Barth, S., and Haley C.E. (1997). An outbreak of Shigella dysenteriae type 2 among laboratory workers due to intentional food contamination. *Journal of the American Medical Association*, **278**, 396–8.

Kress, M. (2005). The effect of social mixing controls on the spread of smallpox—a two-level model. *Health Care Management Science*, **8**, 277–89.

Leach, S. (2007). Some public health perspectives on quantitative risk assessments for bioterrorism. In *Risk assessment and risk communication strategies in bioterrorism preparedness* (eds. M.S. Green, J. Zenilman, D. Cohen, I. Wiser, and R.D. Balicer). *NATO Security through Science Series – A: Chemistry and Biology. Springer, The Netherlands.*

Manchee R.J., Broster M.G., Stagg A.J., and Hibbs S.E. (1994). Formaldehyde solution effectively inactivates spores of Bacillus anthracis on the Scottish island of Gruinard. *Applied Environmental Microbiology*, **60**, 4167–71.

Martin S.W., Tierney B.C., Aranas, A. *et al.* (2005). An overview of adverse events reported by participants in CDC's anthrax vaccine and antimicrobial availability program. *Pharmacoepidemiology and Drug Safety*, **14**, 393–401.

Meehan P.J., Rosenstein N.E., Gillen, M. *et al.* (2004). Responding to detection of aerosolized Bacillus anthracis by autonomous detection systems in the workplace. *Morbidity and Mortality Weekly Report*, **53**(RR07),1–12.

Meinhardt, P.L. (2005). Water and bioterrorism: preparing for the potential threat to U.S. water supplies and public health. *Annual Reviews of Public Health*, **26**, 213–37.

Meselson, M., Guillemin, J., Hugh-Jones, M. *et al.* (1994). The Sverdlovsk anthrax outbreak of 1979. *Science*, **266**, 1202–8.

Mortimer, P.P. (2003). Can postexposure vaccination against smallpox succeed? *Clinical Infectious Diseases*, **36**, 622–8.

Nishiura, H., and Eichner, M. (2006). Estimation of the duration of vaccine-induced residual protection against severe and fatal smallpox based on secondary vaccination failure. *Infection*, **34**, 239–40.

Ohtani, T., Iwanami, A., Kasai, K., Yamasue, H., Kato, T., Sasaki, T., and Kato, N. (2004). Post-traumatic stress disorder symptoms in victims of Tokyo subway attack: a 5-year follow-up study. *Psychiatry Clinical Neuroscience*, **58**, 624–9.

O'Toole, T., Mair, M., and Inglesby T.V. (2002). Shining light on "Dark Winter". *Clinical Infectious Diseases*, **34**, 972–83.

Patterson K.B., and Runge, T. (2002). Smallpox and the native American. *American Journal of Medical Sciences*, **323**, 216–22.

Prentice M.B., and Rahalison, L. (2007). Plague. *Lancet*, **369**, 1196–207.

Rabinowitz, P., Gordon, Z., Chudnov, D. *et al.* (2006). Animals as sentinels of bioterrorist agents. *Emerging Infectious Diseases*, **12**, 647–52.

Reingold, A. (2003). If syndromic surveillance is the answer, what is the question? *Biosecurity and Bioterrorism*, **1**, 1–5.

Riley, S., and Ferguson N.M. (2006). Smallpox transmission and control: spatial dynamics in Great Britain. *Proceedings of the National Academy of Sciences*, **103**, 12637–42.

Rolka, H., Burkom, H., Cooper G.F., Kulldorff, M., Madigan, D., and Wong, W.-K. (2007). Issues in applied statistics for public health bioterrorism surveillance using multiple data streams: research needs. *Statistics in Medicine*, **26**, 1834–56.

Rotz L.D., Khan A.S., Lillibridge S.R., Ostroff S.M., and Highes J.M. (2002). Public health assessment of potential biological terrorism agents. *Emerging Infectious Diseases*, **8**, 225–230.

Sandman, P.M. (2003). Bioterrorism risk communication policy. *Journal of Health Communication*, **8** (Suppl 1), 146–7; discussion 148–51.

Scaramozzino, N., Ferrier-Rembert, A., Favier A.L. *et al.* (2007). Real-time PCR to identify variola virus or other human pathogenic orthopox viruses. *Clinical Chemistry*, **53**, 606–13.

Shephard C.W., Soriano-Gabarro, M., Zell E.R. *et al.* (2002). CDC adverse events working group. Antimicrobial post-exposure prophylaxis for anthrax: adverse events and adherence. *Emerging Infectious Diseases*, **8**, 1124–32.

Shine, K. (2001). "For a Hearing on Risk Communication: National Security and Public Health" (testimony presented to the Subcommittee on National Security, Veterans Affairs, and International Relations, House Committee on Government Reform, Washington, D.C.: November 29, 2001). Available at: http://www7.nationalacademies.org/ocga/testimony/Risk_Communication_Natl_Security_Public_Health.asp. Accessed July 1, 2007.

Siegel J.D., Rhinehart, E., Jackson, M., Chiarello, L. and the Healthcare Infection Control Practices Advisory Committee. (2007). Guideline for isolation precautions: preventing transmission of infectious agents in healthcare settings. pp. 119–24. Available at: http://www.cdc.gov/ncidod/dhqp/pdf/isolation2007.pdf. Accessed July 22, 2007.

Slovic, P. (1987). Perception of risk. *Science*, **236**, 280–5.

Sobel, J., Khan A.S., and Swerdlow D.L. (2002). Threat of a biological terrorist attack on the US food supply: the CDC perspective. *Lancet*, **359**, 874–80.

Stittelaar K.J., Neyts, J., Naesens, L. *et al.* (2006). Antiviral treatment is more effective than smallpox vaccine in monkeypox virus infection. *Nature*, **439**, 745–48.

Sugishima, M. (2003). Aum Shinrikyo and the Japanese law on bioterrorism. *Prehospital Disaster Medicine*, **18**, 179–83.

Taig, T, (1999). Benchmarking in government: case studies and principles. In *Risk Communication and Public Health* (eds. P. Bennett and K. Calman), pp. 117–32. Oxford University Press, Oxford.

Torok, T., Tauxe R.V., Wise R.P. *et al.* (1997). A large community outbreak of Salmonella caused by intentional contamination of restaurant salad bars. *Journal of the American Medical Association*, **278**, 389–95.

Tucker, J.B. (1999). Historical trends related to bioterrorism: an empirical analysis. *Emerging Infectious Diseases*, **5**, 498–504.

Walden, J., and Kaplan E.H. (2004). Estimating time and size of bioterror attack. *Emerging Infectious Diseases*, **10**, 1202–5.

Wehrle, P., Posch, J., Richter, K., and Henderson, D, (1970). An airborne outbreak of smallpox in a German hospital and its significance with respect to other recent outbreaks in Europe. *Bulletin of the World Health Organisation*, **43**, 669–79.

Welch, T.J., Fricke, W.F., McDermott, P.F. *et al.* (2007). Multiple antimicrobial resistance in plague: an emerging public health risk. *PloS ONE*, 2(3), e309. doi:10.1371/journal.pone.0000309.

Wiser, I., Balicer, R.D., and Cohen, D. (2007). An update on smallpox vaccine candidates and their role in bioterrorism related vaccination strategies. *Vaccine*, **25**, 976–84.

World Health Organization. (2004). Public health response to biological and chemical weapons: WHO guidance. Available at: http://www.who.int/csr/delibepidemics/biochemguide/en/print.html. Accessed July 1, 2007.

Zilinskas, R.A. (1997). Iraq's biological weapons. *Journal of the American Medical Association*, **278**, 418–24.

Zilinskas, R.A., Hope, B., North, D.W. (2004). A discussion of findings and their possible implications from a workshop on bioterrorism threat assessment and risk management. *Risk Analysis*, **24**, 901–8.

SECTION 11

Public health needs of population groups

11.1

The changing family

Julien O. Teitler

Abstract

Families are dynamic, heterogeneous entities that vary by size and age, gender, and generational compositions, and in political, social, and technological contexts. Thus, families can affect the health of its members in complex, indirect, and potentially overlapping ways. This chapter presents a broad overview of the micro- and macro-level processes by which families affect the health of individuals and highlights issues that are likely to be salient over the next several decades.

Introduction

How families affect health is a very broad area of inquiry, for several reasons: Families are dynamic, heterogeneous entities that vary by size and have different age, gender, and generational compositions. The political, social, and technological contexts that influence family structure and processes vary across place and over time. Families can affect health in a myriad of complex, indirect, and potentially overlapping pathways. Health itself is a broad construct that encompasses a variety of physical and mental health conditions, with varying degrees of severity. This chapter presents a broad overview of the micro- and macro-level processes by which families affect the health of individuals. It paints with broad strokes, emphasizing breadth over depth and offering salient examples rather than a detailed review of the complex pathways by which families can affect health.

The first section focuses on how processes within families affect health. The second section describes macro-level contexts that have influenced, and have been influenced by, family processes that are related to health. There is considerable overlap between these two sections, as the multidimensional topic of how families affect health cannot be divided neatly into categories. The third section will highlight issues related to family and health that will likely be at the forefront of future policy, legal, and ethical debates.

Within-family (micro) processes

Resource distribution

Perhaps the most central manner in which families affect health is through the distribution of resources. Families, as institutions, allocate resources both within and across generations. Family resources are usually fixed in quantity, so allocating them to one member of the family comes at the expense of another. Within-family resource allocation decisions can affect health directly through nutrition and healthcare. Parents' investments of resources in their children can also affect their children's health indirectly—through the children's educational attainment and future income, both of which are strongly associated with health and mortality.

Kinship systems and gender roles in societies define authority relationships within families, which determine who makes decisions of resource allocation and how they are made. Individuals whose status in the family is relatively low (typically based on sex, age, or birth order) tend to receive fewer resources. Examples of how expenditures, care, and food allocation to family members vary by status within the family abound. To give just a few examples: In the United States, parents allocate fewer resources to step-children than to their biological children (Case *et al.* 1999). In eighteenth and nineteenth century Bosnia, maternal mortality rates were higher among women married to husbands who were junior among brothers than among those married to oldest brothers (Hammel & Gullickson 2004). In China, where there are strong preferences for male children, infant mortality is higher among girls than boys and selective abortion favouring males is high (Coale & Banister 1994). In Egypt, where son preference is also present, infant mortality is higher among girls than boys, and girls receive lower-quality healthcare (Yount 2003). At the extreme, sex preferences can lead to infanticide or abandonment. Although this practice is uncommon today, studies continue to uncover differences in resource allocation by gender, even in the most economically advanced countries.

The health consequences of inequalities within families may not always benefit those who have higher status. For example, patriarchy appears to be associated not only with higher female mortality, but also with higher male mortality (Stanistreet *et al.* 2005). One explanation is that constructions of masculinity in patriarchal societies encourage males to engage in unhealthy behaviours (Courtenay 2000).

Resources may not always be directed disproportionately to family members who are healthy. While some parents may invest disproportionately in their healthy children, whom they may consider to have the best chance of achievement, others may invest more in children who are in poor health because of their greater needs, diverting resources away from healthy children.

Socialization

Families can affect children's health by modelling behaviours. Parents can shape tastes and health habits—including eating habits and food preferences, levels of physical activity, and standards of hygiene.

Some of the preferences and health behaviours that are transmitted to children have cultural origins. As such, families act as agents of socialization in ways that can have profound health consequences (positive and negative) that can reproduce across generations. For example, women of Mexican descent in the United States have birth outcomes on par with those of non-Hispanic whites despite being much poorer on average. Some have hypothesized that the Mexican-origin advantage is due to cultural factors, such as healthful diets and low rates of substance use.

Family gender roles determine whether and how much time women spend working in the paid labour force versus on childrearing and housework. Changes in women's social and economic status in many countries have had complicated implications for resource allocation and health. The greater earnings and increased status of women have given them more control over resources, but they also have contributed to large increases in the divorce rate from 1960 to 1980 in most industrialized countries as well as to increases in rates of non-marital childbearing. Both of these trends have resulted in increased poverty among women and children. Also, despite working more outside, the home than in the past, women continue to bear most of the childrearing and housework responsibilities (Hochschild & Machung 1989). Having dual responsibilities can result in overburden and role strain, taking a toll on women's physical and mental health and potentially having ripple effects on other members of the family. Of course, the net effects of female labour force participation depend on the family's unique circumstances and the characteristics of the individuals within those families.

Cultural variations (intra and cross-nationally, as well as over time) also shape gender norms, which affect health practices. One area in which gender norms play an important role is reproductive behaviour: Fertility decisions, contraception, and protection from sexually transmitted infections. In places with high levels of gender inequality, rates of contraception and condom use tend to be relatively low and fertility tends to be relatively high, though there are many exceptions to this pattern (McDonald 2000). Moreover, women often find ways to control their fertility even in regions with low levels of gender equality. Finally, changes in fertility over time, in turn, can affect gender equality and gender relations (Behrman *et al.* 2002).

Increases in gender equality may affect relationships and risks associated with sexual activity, even at very early ages. One illustrative example involves the timing of sexual initiation across European countries. As female labour force participation increased and the gender wage gap diminished during the second-half of the twentieth century, boys' and girls' age at sexual initiation converged (the age for boys decreased only slightly while that for girls decreased dramatically), teen fertility rates decreased, and condom use increased (Bozon & Kontula 1998; Teitler 2002).

Marriage may socialize health behaviours. Being married is associated with better health compared to not being married (Waite & Gallagher 2000). This 'marriage advantage' may reflect behavioural changes (i.e. refraining from engaging in risky behaviours) induced by social expectations of married individuals. It could also result from a more stable lifestyle with lower levels of stress. Or, it may simply reflect the people who get married (i.e. those who are healthier may be more likely to choose to get married). Despite numerous attempts to ascertain the reasons for the marriage advantage in health, the reasons remain very much an open question.

Social support

Families, including extended kin, can be a source of financial, social, and emotional support to the individuals within them. Support of these types can mitigate the negative effects of adverse shocks in life circumstances, which can be financial in nature (such as losing a job) or health-related (such as having an accident or experiencing a major illness). The more wealth a family has, the greater its ability to assist members through difficult times. In addition to the direct and immediate benefits that family and extended kin may offer in times of crisis, the security of having a resource buffer may make individuals more inclined to invest in education or training. Both the peace of mind that comes from social support and the accumulated wealth that may result from human capital investment that it affords can translate into improved immediate and longer-term physical and mental health.

There is a potential downside to having strong family or social support, which is that its obligations are usually reciprocal. Being on the receiving end of family support provides advantages, but at a cost to those providing the support—especially if family resources are relatively scarce. The fewer financially secure members in the family, the more taxing within-family support obligations will be to those members. Reciprocal obligations among family members may be particularly strong among low-income populations, which could explain why, in the United States, the returns to investments in education and training are smaller among African–Americans (who are more likely to be first-generation middle class with connections to large numbers of low-income kin) than Whites (whose families are more homogeneously middle class). In sum, more extensive family ties in disadvantaged communities can play very important safety net roles, but may also burden economically mobile members when public assistance programmes do not offset demands of their kin.

Kin obligations are likely to increase as family composition in the United States and some other countries further diversifies due to increased rates of union dissolution, re-partnering, and other changes in family structure described later. Recent studies are just beginning to examine the competing resource demands in complex families and their consequences for family members' well-being, but at the present time, very little about this topic is known.

Reciprocal effects

Not only can families affect individuals' health, but the health of individuals can also impact their families. Ill family members can draw resources away from others, and because care giving responsibilities can interfere with regular work hours, limit their ability to maintain stable employment. For example, stress from hardships associated with the care of ill or disabled children can lead to relationship strains and, in extreme cases, to parental separation or divorce (Reichman *et al.* 2004).

Macro-level processes

Demographic factors

Fertility and mortality

An indirect way that resources become allocated across family members is by parents regulating their fertility. The more children parents have, the fewer the resources available to each child. When total resources are limited, additional births can impact nutrition by reducing the per-person availability of food. The same is true for resources allocated to healthcare (both preventive care and treatments) and education. Larger families can affect children negatively for this reason, but can benefit parents later in life if they depend on their children for financial or emotional support. Support from children is particularly important in societies that do not have institutionalized income redistributive programmes (e.g. public retirement programmes) and among low-income families who are unable to accumulate sufficient financial reserves to achieve self-sufficiency later in life.

Two demographic changes have had large effects on fertility. One is the decline in infant and child mortality that began in the mid-1800s in industrialized countries and in the late 1900s in developing countries. The expectation that children would survive into adulthood increased their value to parents. As the perceived value of children increased for individual sets of parents, so too did the collective valuation of children by society at large—leading to greater investments on the part of social welfare institutions and expansions of legislative protections, including the enactment of child labour and compulsory education laws (Zelizer 1994). The lower child mortality rates and increased perceived value of children led to a reduction in the average number of children per family, which in turn increased the resources available to individual family members.

In sum, the shift from high mortality and high fertility to low mortality and low fertility, often referred to as the 'first demographic transition', profoundly reduced the size of families and increased the value of children, which in turn increased family and institutional investments in children, further benefiting their health.

Patterns of fertility declines, both caused by and positively affecting health, were observed throughout the nineteenth and most of the twentieth century (Coale & Watkins 1986). However, declines beyond replacement levels (approximately 2.1 children per woman) have the potential to negatively affect the health of both children and adult family members. Again, the reasons have to do with the supply and allocation of resources. Fertility declines below replacement level cause the population to age, meaning that the proportion of old people relative to young people increases. When fertility declines are accompanied by increases in longevity and delays in entry into the labour force, as was the case in many Western European countries during the latter part of the twentieth century, the ageing of the population can be highly consequential. One reason is that the healthcare costs for the elderly are high relative to those for other age groups because the elderly disproportionately have chronic expensive-to-treat health problems. Another is that the fraction of the population paying into programmes that support the elderly (e.g. health insurance and pensions) decreases.

Italy exemplifies how low fertility rates can burden the working-aged population. The total fertility rate in that country declined from 2.7 children per woman in 1965 to 1.2 children per woman in 2000. As a result, the working-aged population is expected to decline from 39 million in 1995 to 22 million in 2050. Life expectancy also increased in the latter half of the twentieth century and young adults have remained in school longer, delaying entry into the labour force and remaining financially dependent on their parents until later ages. Two indicators—the old age dependency ratio and the ratio of pensioners to workers—indicate the extent to which the burden placed on workers has increased and will continue to increase. The old age dependence ratio is the number of people over 65 divided by the number of people aged 15–64. In Italy, this ratio has been increasing rapidly and is projected to triple by 2050. The ratio of pensioners to workers is currently 0.8 and is projected to increase to 1.6 in 2050 (Bongaarts 2004), meaning that, in 2050, there will be 1.6 times more people drawing on pensions than there are workers paying into them. Italy is not the only extreme example and the ageing of the population is not unique to the West. Old age dependence ratio projections for Japan are similar to those for Italy.

Divorce and non-marital childbearing

Since the 1960s, most of the industrialized countries have experienced a series of demographic changes that have had profound impacts on family structure and the well-being of individuals within families. These changes include delays in marriage and childbearing, increases in non-marital cohabitation, increases in divorce, and increases in non-marital childbearing. These relatively recent trends are not confined to industrialized countries; Age at marriage and age at first birth have increased in much of the world in the past 50 years. In the United States, age at marriage rose from means of about 20 years for women and 23 years for men in 1950 to 25 years for women and 27 years for men in 2000. It rose about 3 years in Indonesia over the same period. Even African countries, which typically have very early ages at marriage, have experienced significant increases over the last decade.

Among Western industrialized countries, the proportion of marriages ending in divorce more than doubled between 1960 and 1980, reaching about 1 in 2, and has since stabilized. Divorce rates rose to similar levels in Russia and Cuba. And, though overall rates are comparatively low in Asia, the rates of increase in divorce in many Asian countries have been higher than in Western countries. For example, the divorce rate in China tripled between 1980 and 2000. Marriage delays and increased divorce rates have resulted in adults and children spending an increasing amount of time outside marital unions and in reconstituted families.

The impact of divorce (and family disruption more generally) on health can be direct or indirect. Parental separation, parental conflict, and changes in living environments and schools that often ensue can lead to emotional, behavioural, and academic problems among children, though, for most children, the effects are short-term (Hetherington 2002). In some instances, parental separation can have positive effects on the health of spouses and children if it ends physical or emotional abuse. Separation generally reduces material resources available to women and children (whose economic well-being tends to decline more than that of men after family disruption), which can negatively impact educational and occupational trajectories.

Rates of non-marital fertility have increased dramatically in all Western industrialized countries. In the United States, the proportion of births born to unmarried mothers increased from 5 per cent in 1960 to one-third in 2000. And the United States is not an outlier in this regard as shown in Fig. 11.1.1. Non-marital childbearing is now more common in the United Kingdom, France, Iceland, and Scandinavian countries than in the United States. About half of all births in Scandinavian countries and about two-thirds of births in Iceland are to unmarried parents. In the United States and United Kingdom, non-marital fertility is strongly associated with poverty, whereas elsewhere (e.g. France, the Netherlands, and Scandinavian countries), it crosses social strata,

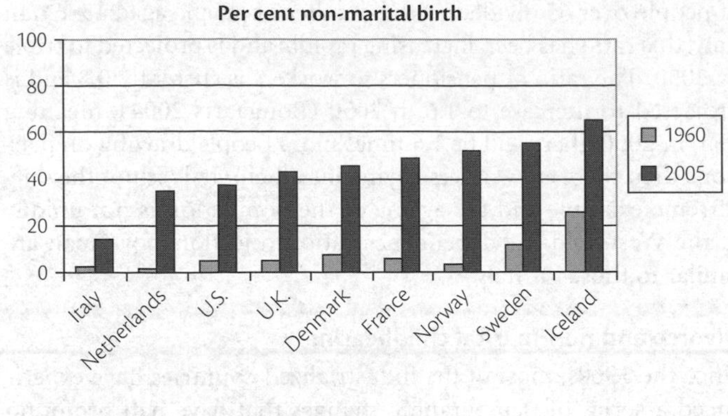

Fig. 11.1.1 Per cent non-marital birth.
Sources: NCHS Vital Statistics Reports, **48**(16). NCHD Births: Preliminary Data for 2005. Eurostat demographic trends 2005.

is not associated with single parenthood or poor child outcomes, and often leads to marriage of the biological parents.

Increases in cohabitation, divorce, and non-marital childbearing have resulted in large increases in multi-partner fertility (women bearing children with different fathers and men fathering children with more than one woman). One recent study estimates that close to one-third of low-income mothers in the United States had children with more than one partner, and over one-third of fathers had children with more than one partner (Meyer *et al.* 2005). The complexity of family structures and parental obligations that multi-partner fertility creates can increase resource strains.

The impact of the changes in family structure described above has not been uniform across country or socioeconomic status. Among highly educated women, delays in childbearing and expanded labour market opportunities have increased resources available for themselves and their children. Among less-educated women, rising rates of union dissolution and non-marital childbearing have led to increased poverty. The divergent trends have increased socioeconomic disparities in the conditions of children, particularly in the United States (McLanahan 2004). In most European countries, where cohabiting unions are more stable and family support policies provide greater supports to children than in the United States, increases in non-marital fertility are likely to be less consequential in terms of health-related resources available to children.

Maternal age

The age at which women give birth impacts their health and that of their children. In terms of children's health, there is a U-shaped association between maternal age and infant health as measured by birth weight (a risk factor for long term health and developmental outcomes). Rates of low birth weight are highest at very young and older ages. Since childbearing tends to begin earliest among low-income populations, the already higher risks of low birth weight for those groups may be compounded by early fertility.

Teen childbearing has costs for mothers as well as children. Women who have children before age 18 often interrupt their schooling. Though many eventually return to school or obtain high school equivalency diplomas, their academic achievement and attainment, on an average, suffers. The strong associations between socioeconomic status, income, and health—within and across generations—underscores the importance of fertility decisions on the health of parents and their dependents.

Rates of teen childbearing in most industrialized countries have decreased substantially since the 1960s, as shown in Fig. 11.1.2. The decline in teen pregnancy has been accompanied by an increase in the mean age of childbearing. In the United States, the mean age at first birth increased from 22 years in the 1950s to 25 years in 2000. In the Netherlands, the mean age increased from about 23 to 29 years over the same period. More recently, childbearing ages have been increasing in less-developed countries as well. The trend towards later childbearing may have positive implications for the health of children and their families.

The decoupling of sex and marriage

Across all social classes and most countries, the age of sexual initiation has been decreasing since 1960 as the age of marriage has been increasing. Consequently, men and women now spend many more years in short-term relationships than they did 50 years ago and have a greater number of sexual partners, both of which are associated with increased risks of sexually transmitted infections.

The middle generation squeeze

Increases in longevity, which were discussed earlier in terms of their impact on population-level resource allocation, also have consequences at the family level. As life expectancy increases, individuals experience more years of their adult lives with living parents, whose caretaking and financial needs may divert resources from other family members.

At the earlier end of the life cycle, transitions to adulthood are lengthening. Young adults are delaying marriage and childbearing, spending more years in school, and relying on parental support for longer periods of time (Settersten *et al.* 2005). Increasing delays in leaving the parental home have been observed in the most-developed countries (Fernández Cordon 1997; Corijn & Klijzing 2001), with Italian men representing an extreme example—leaving home at age 27, on an average (Billari *et al.* 2001).

Over the past 30 years, as longevity has increased, the period of schooling has lengthened, and the transition to adulthood has occurred at older ages, the costs of raising children have risen

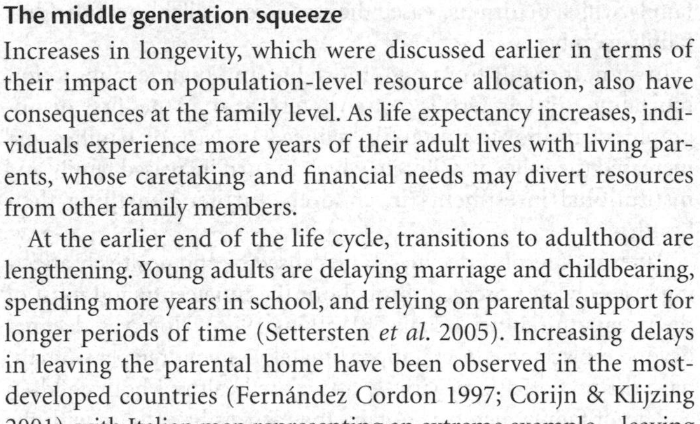

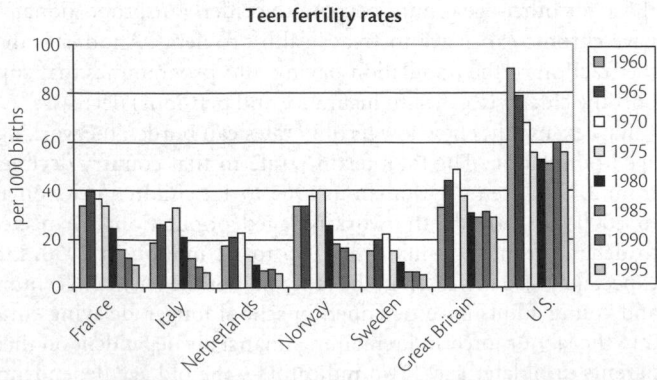

Fig. 11.1.2 Teen fertility rates.
Sources: Eurostat and US Vital Statistics Reports.

considerably (Schoeni & Ross 2004). Institutional supports have not kept pace with these changes. Consequently, many working age adults have been burdened with the support of both younger and older generations. Little is known about the extent to which the time, emotional, and financial costs of caring for both their parents and children have affected the allocation of resources or health in 'sandwich generation' families.

Technological factors

Contraception

Fertility regulation has been facilitated by modern, effective contraception. Most notably, the birth control pill has been available since the early 1960s. More recently, contraceptive patches, implants, and hormone shots offer protection for weeks or months at a time, making dose compliance much easier than in the past. These improvements in contraceptive technology have greatly reduced unplanned pregnancies. Additionally, newly available 'emergency contraception' provides women with the ability to end pregnancies up to 72 h after having sex. The increased efficacy of condoms has also improved fertility planning, while providing protection against sexually transmitted infections.

Neonatal care

Recent advances in neonatal care technology have led to the survival of infants born very preterm, who only decades ago would not have survived their first year (Reichman 2005). The tremendous benefits of saving lives are undisputable, but this progress has come with a big price tag because the technology is expensive and because modern medicine has lagged in terms of preventing chronic and disabling health conditions that arise from being born with an underdeveloped biological systems. Substantial costs are borne by healthcare systems, third-party payers, and families. Coping with the long-term needs of these 'new survivors' can create substantial financial and emotional hardships for families, which could take a toll on all family members' health.

Assisted reproduction

The benefits of assisted reproductive technology are clear. Medical advances over the past 20 years have allowed many couples, who would not have been able to do so in the past, to have children. These new opportunities, however, come with health related costs as well. One is an ageing parent population since the new technologies offset natural declines in women's ability to bear children. Another is an increase in the rate of multiple births. Because multiples are much more likely than singleton infants to be born low birth weight, assisted reproductive technology may be increasing chronic health problems among children.

Prenatal care

Advances in prenatal care technology provide information about the health and gender of foetuses (through genetic testing, ultrasound technology, or amniocentesis), creating opportunities for parents to selectively abort foetuses with unwanted traits. For example, parents can choose to terminate pregnancies if there are indications that the child will have Down Syndrome, abnormally developed organs, or be of the undesired sex. The ability to selectively abort can reduce hardships for family members, reduce the number of children with chronic health problems, and increase the proportion of 'wanted' children. However, selective abortions raise a host of complex ethical considerations that do not have easy answers.

Economic and political factors

Female labour force participation

Increases in female labour force participation, as discussed earlier, have had profound effects on organization of families. Mothers spending more time outside the home means that childcare is more likely to be delegated to others (childcare centres, relatives, children, and, less frequently, fathers). Housework, too, is either contracted out or reduced. Increased employment among women and entry into higher status occupations has obvious advantages for families in terms of household income. However, the health consequences of this change are not clear. For example, evidence of maternal employment on children's cognitive development is mixed (Waldfogel 2006).

Abortion laws

The criminalization of abortion in many countries can affect fertility control, the wantedness of children, and the health (and sometimes the life) of women who seek illegal and unregulated abortions. Worldwide, abortions are very common regardless of legality. The estimated number of abortions, in 1995 was 46 million. Abortion rates are no lower in places where they are restricted by law. 20 million of the 46 million abortions that took place in 1995 were illegal (Henshaw *et al.* 1999). Though some countries have at times increased restrictions on abortions, the overall trend has been toward liberalization. Most industrialized countries, Eastern European countries, China, and India legalized abortion between the 1950s and 1980s. Developing countries, overall, have been slower to legalize abortion, but many do not actively treat it as a crime (Henshaw 1994).

Gay marriage and civil unions

A few countries recognize unmarried same and opposite sex couples who are living together as families and confer legal rights to partners. It is not known whether legal recognition of alternative family forms will dissuade partners from marrying or encourage same sex unions or what effect either would have on individual well-being. While most research finds that many gay parent families are similar to heterosexual parents in terms of parenting, it is difficult to generalize from existing studies because of methodological limitations (Meezan & Rauch 2005). Evidence on domestic partnerships and civil unions is stronger and suggests that parents who cohabit are more likely to separate than those who are married (Manning *et al.* 2004). However, differences in dissolution rates by type of union vary by country, with smaller differences in countries where cohabitation is more prevalent (Liefbroer & Dourleijn 2006). Additionally, because individuals who enter different types of unions may be different in any number of ways, it is difficult to draw conclusive causal inferences about the effects of alternative family forms on individuals' health and well-being.

Future challenges

Across the world, families are becoming smaller, older, more complex, and more diverse. All of these changes have consequences for individuals' well-being and are likely to lead to important health related issues and ethical challenges in years to come. Several key issues at the nexus of family and health that will be at the forefront of ethical, legal, and policy debates are highlighted below:

- Legislation redefining parental rights and the acceptable scope of scientific research will need to be drafted as science increasingly makes it possible to screen foetuses for genetic predispositions to health and physical traits and to clone living organisms.
- In countries where non-marital fertility is both increasing and strongly associated with single-mother households, such as the United States and United Kingdom, social policies will need to adapt to declines in economic and social support that mothers and children receive from fathers.
- Legal definitions of family for the purposes of property and inheritance rights, child guardianship, and health insurance coverage will need to be revised. This will become increasingly necessary as complexities in family structure evolve. Some European countries provide legal status to non-marital domestic partnerships, but with only very specific and limited rights. In the United States, same-sex domestic partnerships are sometimes recognized for health insurance eligibility.
- Retirement systems will need to be adapted to an ageing population. This is a pressing challenge for developed countries. Either contributions into pension systems will have to increase (by increasing premiums or easing immigration restrictions) or disbursements will have to decrease (by reducing pension payments or delaying the retirement age). The interests of working and retired constituents will compete.
- End of life issues that arise because of advancing medical technologies will need to be debated. As families become more complex, the question of whose right and responsibility it is to make end of life decisions will become a particularly salient issue.

Acknowledgement

I am grateful to Nancy Reichman for her many helpful substantive and editorial comments.

References

Behrman, J.R., Kohler, H.-P., and Watkins, S.C. (2002). Social networks and changes in contraceptive use over time: evidence from a longitudinal study in rural Kenya. *Demography*, **39**(4), 713–38.

Billari, F.C., Philipov, D., and Baizán, P. (2001). Leaving home in Europe: the experience of cohorts born around 1960. *International Journal of Population Geography*, **7**(5), 339–56.

Bongaarts, J. (2004). Population aging and the rising cost of public pensions. *Population Council Working Paper* no. 185.

Bozon, M. and Kontula, O. (1998). Sexual initiation and gender in Europe. In *Sexual behavior and HIV/AIDS in Europe* (eds. M. Hubert, N. Bajos, and T. Sandfort), pp. 37–67. UCL Press, London.

Case, A., Lin, I., and McLanahan, S. (1999). Household resource allocation in stepfamilies: Darwin reflects on the plight of Cinderella. *The American Economic Review*, **89**(2), 234–8.

Coale, A.J. and Watkins, S.C. eds. (1986). *The decline of fertility in Europe*. Princeton University Press, Princeton.

Coale, A.J. and Banister, J. (1994). Five decades of missing females in China. *Demography*, **31**(3), 459–79.

Corijn, M. and Klijzing, E. (Eds.). (2001). *Transitions to Adulthood in Europe*. Kluwer Academic Publishers: Dordrecht.

Courtenay, W.H. (2000). Constructions of masculinity and their influence on men's well-being: a theory of gender and health. *Social Science & Medicine*, **50**, 1385–401.

Fernández Cordon, J.A. (1997). Youth residential independence and autonomy: a comparative study. *Journal of Family Issues*, **16**(6), 567–607.

Hammel, E.A. and Gullickson, A. (2004). Kinship structures and survival: maternal mortality on the Croatian-Bosnian border 1750–898. *Population Studies - A Journal of Demography*, **58**(2), 145–59.

Henshaw, S.K. (1994). Recent trends in the legal status of induced abortion. *Journal of Public Health Policy*, **15**(2), 165–72.

Henshaw, S.K., Singh, S., and Haas, T. (1999). The incidence of abortion worldwide. *International Family Planning Perspectives*, **25**, S30–8.

Hetherington, E.M. (2002). *For better or for worse: divorce reconsidered*. W.W. Norton & Co., New York.

Hochschild, A. and Machung, A. (1989). *The second shift: working parents and the revolution at home*. Viking Penguin, New York.

Liefbroer, A.C. and Dourleijn, E. (2006). Unmarried cohabitation and union stability: testing the role of diffusion using data from 16 European countries. *Demography*, **43**(2), 203–21.

Manning, W., Smock, P., and Majumdar, D. (2004). The relative stability of cohabitating and marital unions for children. *Population Research and Policy Review*, **23**(2), 135–59.

McDonald, P. (2000). Gender equity in theories of fertility transition. *Population and Development Review*, **26**(3), 427–39.

McLanahan, S. (2004). Diverging destinies: how children are faring under the second demographic transition. *Demography*, **41**(4), 607–27.

Meezan, W. and Rauch, J. (2005). Gay marriage, same-sex parenting, and America's children. *The Future of Children*, **15**(2), 97–115.

Meyer, D.R., Cancian, M., and Cook, S.T. (2005). Multiple-partner fertility: incidence and implications for child support policy. *Social Service Review*, **79**(5), 577–601.

Reichman, N.E. (2005). Low birth weight and school readiness. *The Future of Children*, **15**(1), 91–116.

Reichman, N.E., Corman, H., and Noonan, K. (2004). Effects of child health on parents' relationship status. *Demography*, **41**(3), 569–84.

Schoeni, R. and Ross, K. (2005). Material assistance received from families during the transitions to adulthood. In *On the frontier of adulthood: theory, research and public policy* (eds. R.A. Settersten, F.F. Furstenburg, and R.G. Rumbaut). The University of Chicago Press, Chicago.

Settersten, R.A., Furstenburg, F.F., and Rumbaut, R.G., eds. (2005). *On the frontier of adulthood: theory, research and public policy*. The University of Chicago Press, Chicago.

Stanistreet, D., Bambra, C., and Scott-Samuel, A. (2005). Is patriarchy the source of men's higher mortality? *Journal of Epidemiology and Community Health*, **59**, 873–6.

Teitler, J.O. (2002). Trends in youth sexual initiation and fertility in developed countries: 1960–1995. *The Annals of the American Academy of Political and Social Science*, **580**, 134–52.

Waite, L.J. and Gallagher, M. (2000). *The case for marriage: why married people are happier, healthier, and better off financially*. Doubleday, New York.

Waldfogel, J. (2006). *What children need*. Harvard University Press, Cambridge.

Yount, K.M. (2003). Gender bias in the allocation of curative health care in Minia, Egypt. *Population Research and Policy Review*, **22**(3), 267–99.

Zelizer, V.A. (1994). *Pricing the priceless child: the changing social value of children*. Princeton University Press, Princeton.

11.2

Women, men, and health

Sarah Payne and Lesley Doyal

Abstract

This chapter explores the ways in which sex and gender influence health. Figures for mortality and life expectancy reveal important differences between men and women in their risk of death and in the causes of death. In virtually every country around the world, men have a lower life expectancy than women, although the gap in life expectancy is narrower in low-income countries. Similarly, women and men have different patterns of ill health, and again, the gap varies between countries. Both sex and gender play a part in these variations. Sex, or biological factors, influences women's and men's risks of different diseases and health conditions, including reproductive disorders and diseases affected by the immune system and genetic factors, as well as survival following diagnosis. However, socially constructed gender-linked factors are also important. Gender affects behaviours such as smoking and alcohol use, which increase the risk of certain conditions, and also affects exposure to social and environmental risk factors, including paid and unpaid work, caring responsibilities, poverty and poor environmental conditions, and the risk of sexual and physical violence.

Introduction

This chapter explores the ways in which sex and gender influence health. It discusses variations in health between women and men across the life course, examines differences in male and female patterns of illness and premature death, and explores related differences in experiences of health care. It asks how far we can explain these differences with reference to biological sex and socially constructed gender.

Although the main determinants of health for a woman agricultural worker in rural China may be the same as those for a female office worker in New York or Sydney, the impact of different determinants will vary. Both women will be affected to some extent by their sex—by biological factors which increase or reduce the risk of particular health problems, including those associated with reproduction. However, social factors such as gender also play an important part in shaping morbidity and mortality. Key influences on the health of each woman may include whether or not she has children, the paid and unpaid work she performs, her access to material resources and to health care, and the levels of social support she receives.

But the impact of these influences on her health is also related to each woman's particular circumstances, which are in turn shaped by geographical, social, and cultural factors. The rural farm worker in China will have great difficulty accessing health care, particularly specialist services; she may have more access to familial support but experience greater stress from family relationships; and she may have little money in her own right and little say over the work she does, either inside the house or outside it. The office worker in New York, on the other hand, may have easier access to health care, depending on her insurance status and level of income, and she will almost certainly live closer to these services. She may have less family support, especially if she has moved to New York to find employment, but may have better sources of support from close friends. She may have money in her own right. In her employment, although she too may have little control over her work and it may offer little in terms of satisfaction, she will be less at risk from some forms of accidental injury and less exposed to noxious chemicals than the woman in agricultural work.

Both these women will be affected by their diet and by behaviours which impact on health, but again the effects are likely to be very different. The Chinese woman may be undernourished through lack of an adequate food supply combined with heavy physical work, whereas the woman in New York may be obese due to lack of exercise and overconsumption of a highly calorific diet. The two women will also probably show significant differences in their use of substances such as tobacco and alcohol.

If we compare the influences on men in the same location as these women, the main determinants of their health will again be the same for both men—the nature of work and paid employment, access to material resources, physical hazards encountered in daily life, health behaviour, and social support for example. But, as with the women, the relative importance and impact of these influences will vary between rural China and New York. And if we then compare the factors affecting the health of the man and woman in each location, there will be further differences between them reflecting gendered distributions of power, resources, and role expectations, associated with cultural and socioeconomic factors. This suggests that the roles of sex and gender in the health of men and women are complex and relational, reflecting various factors which come into play in different ways, with various intensities, and at different points in time.

In the following subsections, we will explore in detail some of the explanations for these differences between women and men in their experiences of health and health care, and their likelihood of developing specific diseases. We begin with an overview of the key differences between male and female mortality and morbidity, before turning to look at the part played by sex and gender in shaping these variations. The model of causality that will emerge from this exploration is not one by which the simple differences between women and men can provide a total explanation of variations in health outcomes. The next subsection will, therefore, look in more detail at the complex links between sex and gender and other determinants of heath such as geographical location, poverty, and socioeconomic status. This will be done by examining specific conditions, including coronary heart disease and HIV and AIDS. We finish this chapter with a discussion of the way gender differentials impact on the appropriateness and availability of health care.

Men, women, and mortality

Mortality data are widely available and relatively reliable, especially when looking at overall rates. These figures suggest that women have an advantage over men in terms of life expectancy and can expect to live longer than their male counterparts in virtually every country in the world. In 2004, for example, male life expectancy at birth was higher than female life expectancy in only 5 out of the 192 countries covered in the World Health Organization's (WHO) Annual Health Report (World Health Organization 2006). There were five countries where men and women had the same life expectancy. In all of the others—182 countries—women could expect to live longer than men.

The countries showing the narrowest gap between women and men are those in which life expectancy is low overall. These are also countries which are among the poorest in the world, notably those in the sub-Saharan region of Africa. For example, in Cameroon, women had only one year's advantage over men, whereas in Somalia and South Africa, women's life expectancy was two years higher than that of men. A number of influences are involved in creating health chances for women and men, but it is especially significant that in these countries where there is only a narrow gap there has been a reversal in both male and female life expectancy in recent years as a result of the increasing burden of HIV and AIDS together with persistent poverty.

Countries with gaps in life expectancy between women and men of five or more years are more diverse in terms of economic status, level of development, and culture: For example, Australia, Finland, Sri Lanka, and Cambodia (World Health Organization 2006). However, the countries showing the greatest divergence between male and female life expectancy are clustered in Eastern Europe, notably those countries which were formerly part of the Soviet Union. In the Russian Federation, for example, women might expect to live up to 13 years longer than men.

In these Eastern European countries, the gap between women and men in life expectancy has widened in recent years following the rapid rise in poverty and deprivation in the post-communist era, combined with high levels of unemployment and changing patterns of alcohol and substance use. This highlights not only the importance of socioeconomic factors in health experience but also the vulnerability of health gains to adverse conditions. In addition, it illustrates gender differences in the impact of socioeconomic change, as the widening gap between women and men reflects a dramatic reduction in life expectancy particularly for men in these countries (Macintyre 2001).

These variations in the gap between women and men across different cultures, time periods, locations, and levels of development suggest that the underlying reasons for such differences do not simply reflect economic factors or specific cultural factors but are explained by more complex influences involving both biological and social causes.

An alternative way of exploring the gap in mortality is through deaths in early childhood. Males and females have different risks of dying before their fifth birthday, and slightly fewer countries show a female advantage. There are 12 countries where girls under five have a higher mortality risk than boys, including China, India, Niger, Somalia, and Nepal, whereas in the majority of countries,

Table 11.2.1 Differences in male and female life expectancy, 2004—selected countries

Country	Male life expectancy at birth (2004)	Female life expectancy at birth (2004)	Difference
Russian Federation	59	72	−13
Estonia	66	78	−12
Republic of Korea	73	81	− 8
Cambodia	51	58	−7
Sri Lanka	68	75	−7
Finland	75	82	−7
Czech Republic	73	79	−6
Cote D'Ivoire	41	47	−6
United States of America	75	80	−5
Australia	78	83	−5
United Kingdom	76	81	−5
China	70	74	−4
Egypt	66	70	−4
Angola	38	42	−4
Iceland	79	83	−4
Samoa	66	70	−4
Sierra Leone	37	40	−3
India	61	63	−2
Somalia	43	45	−2
South Africa	47	49	−2
Pakistan	62	63	−1
Cameroon	50	51	−1
Nepal	61	61	0
Niger	42	41	+1
Kenya	51	50	+1

Source: WHO. *World health report 2006: working together for health*. Geneva: WHO; 2006. World Health Report Annex 1. Reproduced with permission from WHO.

Table 11.2.2 Under-5 male and female mortality rates, 2004—selected countries

Country	Male under-5 mortality rate per 1000 population (2004)	Female under-5 mortality rate per 1000 population (2004)	Male: female ratio (male rate as proportion of female)
Republic of Korea	5	7	0.7
China	27	36	0.8
India	81	89	0.9
Nepal	75	79	0.9
Somalia	222	228	1.0
Niger	256	262	1.0
Egypt	36	36	1.0
Pakistan	102	100	1.0
Angola	276	243	1.1
Sierra Leone	296	269	1.1
Cameroon	156	143	1.1
United States of America	8	7	1.1
Australia	6	5	1.2
Cambodia	154	127	1.2
South Africa	72	62	1.2
Kenya	129	110	1.2
United Kingdom	6	5	1.2
Czech Republic	5	4	1.2
Russian Federation	18	14	1.3
Sri Lanka	16	12	1.3
Cote D'Ivoire	225	162	1.4
Iceland	3	2	1.5
Finland	5	3	1.7
Estonia	10	6	1.7
Samoa	42	17	2.5

Source: WHO. *World health report 2006: working together for health*. Geneva: WHO; 2006. World Health Report Annex 1. Reproduced with permission from WHO.

more boys under five die than girls, including Angola and Cote D'Ivoire where male children have an especially high risk of such early death (World Health Organization 2006).

These differences between countries are explained by a mixture of social, cultural, and biological influences, including gender differences, which affect the treatment of girl and boy children. For example, the male advantage in some countries is partly explained by cultural factors including the practice of breastfeeding male children for longer, and giving boys more food and better access to health care in comparison with girls (Ravindran 2000).

It is also important to consider differences between women and men in causes of death. Overall, men and women have very similar patterns. Globally, around one-third of both men and women die from communicable diseases such as respiratory infections, tuberculosis, or HIV and AIDS (World Health Organization 2004b); similarly, around 60 per cent of both men and women die from non-communicable diseases, including cardiovascular disease and cancer. If we look in more detail at the major causes of death, there is a degree of consistency in this pattern: The top three causes of male deaths worldwide are ischaemic heart disease (13 per cent of total male deaths), cerebrovascular disease (8 per cent), and accidental injury (8 per cent) (World Health Organization 2004b). For women, the top two causes of death are the same as those for men—ischaemic heart disease (12 per cent of female deaths) and cerebrovascular disease (11 per cent)—but fewer women die from accidental injury, whereas deaths from lower respiratory infections are the third most common cause of female deaths (7 per cent).

However, although the key causes of death for women and men are similar, a main difference between them for the major mortality causes is age at death. Women tend to be older than men when they die of cardiovascular disease and cancer, and this reflects both biological and gendered differences, as we shall see.

One important cause of female deaths in many countries is maternal mortality. Although this accounts for less than 2 per cent of all female deaths worldwide, it is a relatively modifiable cause of death, in that improved health care before conception, during pregnancy, and in childbirth can dramatically reduce the risk of death. As such, maternal mortality figures are also important in explanations of the ways in which the ratio of male to female deaths varies over time and between countries.

Overall, more than half a million women die each year as a result of complications following pregnancy and childbirth, including problems arising from miscarriage and terminations (World Health Organization 2005a). Maternal mortality figures also include deaths among women that follow from a reduced immunity to some diseases during pregnancy or in which they suffer a deterioration in pre-existing illness as a result of pregnancy or childbirth.

The risk of such death varies widely, with very low rates in high-income countries and very high rates in low-income countries. For example, in 2000, the maternal mortality rate in Sierra Leone was 2000 deaths per 100 000 live births, compared with 6 in Australia and 11 in the United Kingdom (World Health Organization 2005a).

The relative risk of maternal mortality in different countries reflects social and economic differences rather than biological ones and is particularly associated with the availability of care, as well as maternal age and the number of previous pregnancies. In Sierra Leone, three-fifths of births are not attended by skilled health personnel; similarly, in Niger, a country with a maternal mortality rate of 1600 per 100 000 live births in 2000, only 11 per cent of women received skilled health care during childbirth.

A second major difference between women and men in terms of mortality risk is the higher male mortality rate for both accidental and non-accidental injury. For example, in the Russian Federation, four times many men as women die from injury, and in Thailand, male mortality from such causes is around three and a half times as high as female mortality.

More men than women die each year as a result of homicide, especially among younger age groups. In 2000, for example, global figures show that men aged 15–44 years were five times as likely to be the victims of homicide as women (World Health Organization 2003c). There are also gender differences in the perpetrators of such violence: Women are more at risk of being killed by close family, notably partners, whereas more men are killed by people outside their circle of family and acquaintances (Hemenway *et al.* 2002).

Men are similarly much more likely than women to die or be injured as a result of conflict, with more than 90 per cent of deaths in conflicts among men (World Health Organization 2004b). This reflects the ratio of men to women both in formal military organizations and in informal or paramilitary organizations, as well as the roles played by them in such organizations. However, conflicts also increase the risk of poor health for women, as a result of causes such as infectious diseases, accidental death, and sexual violence (World Health Organization 2003c). In addition, displacement among civilian populations due to conflict combined with the loss of employment, land, or source of income creates economic insecurity and poverty, leading to high risks of poor mental health and malnutrition among such people, a majority of whom are female.

Overall, women have longer life expectancies than men, although the gap varies between countries and there are differences between women and men for some causes of death. The following subsection explores an alternative indicator of the differences between women and men, focusing on measures of morbidity or illness.

Men, women, and morbidity

Figures for death are useful for broad comparisons between women and men but they also have limitations. Most importantly, they do not accurately capture health experience across the life course. Some causes of death are not usually associated with a period of ill health beforehand—for example, accidental injury. Other causes of death may have produced relatively short periods of illness, and still others may be associated with poor health and low quality of life for some years before death occurs. These considerations are important when exploring health differences between women and men as it is possible that excess male mortality does not equate to a similar disadvantage in terms of health enjoyed during a lifetime.

An alternative measure of health is morbidity, which refers to illness, both short-term acute periods of ill health and also longer-term or chronic illness. It has long been assumed that women experience poorer health during their lives in comparison with men—the suggestion that 'women get sicker but men die quicker' (Lorber 1997). But the true picture of the gap between women and men is more complex. The health of women and men varies across the life course and the gap widens or narrows reflecting different age-related patterns of health. Similarly, although women report more of some conditions (such as arthritis), men are more at risk of others, including respiratory diseases. There are also other variations in health status—for example, between socioeconomic groups and different ethnic groups—that may affect the health gap between women and men.

One of the reasons why there is no simple story to tell in terms of the burden of ill health among women and men is that morbidity can be measured in a number of ways, and each measure is potentially different in terms of how well it captures the experiences of men and women. The main indicators include self-reported health, which is based on individuals' judgements of their own health as either 'poor', 'good', or 'excellent'; data based on use of health-care services, including inpatient and community-based services; and composite indicators of health at population level, including measures of healthy life expectancy (HALE) and measures of disability-adjusted life years (DALYs). With each of these measures, there is a range of differences between women and men which varies across the life course, between different demographic groups, and also, between countries.

Self-reported health

In most countries, women report their health to be poorer, in comparison with men. In the WHO's *World Health Survey 2005*, for example, figures from China, France, India, Malawi, the Russian Federation, Pakistan, and Portugal all revealed that more women reported their health as either bad or very bad, whereas more men reported their health as either good or very good (World Health Organization 2005).

The gap between women and men in these countries also varies. One of the widest differences in self-reported health is found in the Russian Federation where nearly a quarter of women reported their health as either bad or very bad, compared with 13 per cent of men (World Health Organization 2005). When this finding is compared with the low male life expectancy in Russia discussed earlier, the data support the argument that in this country at least women report more illness while men have less chance of a long life.

However, women do not always report poorer health than men. In Australia, for example, national survey data for 2004–2005 show that slightly more women than men to say their health is either very good or excellent and, that in every age group other than young adults, more women than men report their health as either very good or excellent (ABS 2006). In the United Kingdom, similar numbers of men and women report their health as bad and although in the United States more men than women report good health, the gap between them is very narrow (ONS 2006; Schiller & Bernadel 2004).

These differences are difficult to interpret. They might reflect variations in the wording of survey questions and some are also influenced by whether or not the data are age-standardized. They might also reflect class or income differences as poorer health is reported by those in lower-income groups, which may include a greater proportion of women in some countries.

As these differences are based on a subjective measure, the findings specifically tell us about how men and women perceive themselves, rather than their objective health status. Variations among countries in terms of whether it is men or women who are more likely to report ill health might also suggest that cultural differences are important in shaping perceptions of health status.

However, the variations, particularly the relatively narrow gap between women and men in richer countries compared with the wider gap found in poorer countries, might also reflect the fact that men in some societies do enjoy better health than women.

One indication of the extent to which these self-reported measures reflect more objective indicators of health comes from evidence in the United States that men who report poor health more often die prematurely than those reporting themselves as being in good health (Benjamins *et al.* 2004). However, there is less evidence of such an association for women, which may mean that self-report surveys are measuring different things for women and men. One factor that affects self-reported health is the extent to which individuals make this judgement not only on any symptoms of illness, but also on the basis of their knowledge about their own behaviours (such as smoking, alcohol use, and diet) that might affect health risks.

Given the difficulties presented by self-report data on morbidity, especially in the context of whether there are gender differences in the measures used, we need to also look at other measures of health experience in order to understand the gap between women and men.

Use of health services

Another way in which health differences between women and men have been measured is through data on consultation with health professionals. Again, these figures are likely to be influenced by more than health status and symptoms alone. A number of issues affect the use of health care, including economic factors such as whether an individual has health insurance or the means to pay user fees in countries where access to health care requires payment; the ability to take time off from either paid employment or caring responsibilities to visit health facilities; and the availability of appropriate services and transport to reach them.

Of course these factors are themselves influenced by gender. For example, women are more often responsible for the care of children and vulnerable dependents, and this can limit their ability to seek help when faced with health symptoms. They are also less likely to be able to finance health consultations—for example, if they do not have command over household expenditure or when they earn less than men and are less able to afford user fees and charges. In some countries, women also need to be accompanied when using services and are therefore dependent on someone being available and willing to take them (Baghadi 2005).

Data from the *World Health Survey 2005* (World Health Organization 2005) shows that there are differences between women and men in their use of health-care services, with the pattern varying among countries and for different kinds of care. For example, in France, India, the Russian Federation, and China, more men than women reported using ambulatory services in the past 12 months, including primary care from general practitioners, community services, and outpatient care. In the United Kingdom and Portugal, similar percentages of men and women used this kind of care. More women than men reported receiving inpatient treatment in Portugal, Malawi, and China, but in France and the United Kingdom, more men reported such treatment. However, in all of these countries, more men than women reported not using any form of health care in the previous twelve months.

National survey data from the United Kingdom reveal that women consult more often than men throughout the health-care system and also take more prescribed medication. Similar gendered patterns of consultation are also found in the United States and Australia (Payne 2006).

There are further differences between women and men in terms of what they are treated for. For example, in general practice in the United Kingdom, more women than men are treated for hypertension, depression, and anxiety, whereas their male compatriots are more often treated for coronary heart disease and diabetes (ONS 2000). The difference in treatment for depression is particularly wide, with more than twice as many women receiving such a diagnosis in general practice.

Overall, data on consultation suggests that women do consult more often than men and are more likely to use health care, although patterns vary between countries and also in response to other factors including age. However, gender-linked influences, including financial or cultural constraints, limit their use of services in some countries and may help explain variations in the gap between women and men.

Composite health indicators

The third way in which we can assess the health gap between women and men is through composite indicators of health at population level. One of the best known of these is the estimate of healthy life expectancy (HALE) produced by the WHO. HALE is a measure that begins with life expectancy at birth and is then adjusted downwards to reflect an estimate of time spent during the life course in poor health (World Health Organization 2004b). This estimate is carried out for each of the WHO's member countries, using a range of survey statistics and other measures to calculate the adjustment separately for men and women.

HALE figures for 2002 revealed that, in 14 out of 192 countries, males had either the same or a better HALE than females. In the remaining 178 countries, women could expect to live a longer time in full health (World Health Organization 2004b). However, as with mortality and life expectancy, the extent of female advantage varies. In the Russian Federation, for example, female HALE was over 11 years greater than male HALE. In France, Spain, and Portugal, females had more than 5 years advantage, whereas in the United Kingdom, the advantage shrank to under three years. Again, it is useful to compare these figures with self-reported health—especially those which show that in the Russian Federation less women than men describe themselves as having good health.

However, if we look not at years spent in healthy life but at the proportion of overall life expectancy that is lost due to poor health, women appear to do rather less well. For the same 192 countries, there were only 4 countries in 2002 where men lost a greater proportion of their life expectancy to illness and disability; in the remaining countries, the proportion of life expectancy lost due to ill health was higher for women (World Health Organization 2004b).

An alternative measure of health, using disability-adjusted life years (DALYs), highlights the distribution of the burden of disease and combines data on death with data on poor health and disability. DALYs are based on calculations of the value of years of disability-free life that are lost as a result of either premature death or the onset of disability (Lopez *et al.* 2006). DALYs can be used in relation to specific conditions as well as to overall health and may also be used to indicate the value of particular interventions which reduce mortality or disability. For example, the number of DALYs gained through reductions in disease following health promotion or clean water policies can be measured. Worldwide, an estimated 1.5 billion DALYs are lost annually due to various health conditions (World Health Organization 2004b). Nearly 25 per cent of these are because of infectious and parasitic diseases, including HIV and AIDS (which accounts for almost 6 per cent of the total), and diarrhoeal diseases (which account for 4 per cent) (World Health Organization 2004b). Mental health problems account for between 12 and 15 per cent of the total number of DALYs lost each year, injuries account for 12 per cent, and heart disease contributes nearly 10 per cent.

Overall, there is only a narrow gap between women and men in their experience of morbidity using this measure: Men comprise 52 per cent of total DALYs lost per annum and women comprise the remaining 48 per cent (World Health Organization 2004b). However, men are much more likely than women to suffer illness or disability as a consequence of accidental and non-accidental injury, as well as from heart disease, alcohol-use disorders, and some cancers. Males also have higher risks of perinatal disabilities. Healthy years lost by women are most likely to result from complications of pregnancy and childbirth, depression, sensory disorders such as cataracts, and sexually transmitted infections.

For example, reproductive conditions including maternal deaths, disability arising from pregnancy and childbirth, sexually transmitted infections, and cancers of the reproductive organs account for between 5 and 15 per cent of all DALYs worldwide. There is a wide gap between men and women in the burden of disease associated with reproductive health and these conditions account for only 3 per cent of the male burden of disease compared with 22 per cent of female DALYs (Dejong 2006).

However, DALYs only measure a limited number of illnesses and health problems relating to reproduction and almost certainly undercount the poor health experienced by women due to various reproductive disorders. For example, infections of the reproductive tract that are not sexually transmitted—such as candidiasis—are not included, neither are menstrual disorders and psychosocial problems associated with difficulties conceiving or with sexuality (AbouZahr & Vaughan 2000). Similarly, mental health aspects of rape and sexual violence are not counted by the DALYs approach. Overall, the failure to include a range of health difficulties suggests that the burden of disease in relation to reproductive health is underestimated for women.

DALYs have also been criticized for their focus on economic rather than social costs of disease and poor health—the loss of income or the costs of care rather than suffering, stigma, and individual well-being (Sen & Bonita 2000). In addition, some have argued that because the severity of the impact of a disease was estimated by experts in the field rather than individuals with the condition, DALYs fail to measure the full burden of a disease, especially those illnesses with wider social costs affecting quality of life (Dejong 2006). This needs to be borne in mind when using DALYs to assess the gender gap in health, as there may well be variations between women and men in the social impact of different diseases.

For example, obstetric fistulae are highly debilitating conditions, which arise as a result of prolonged or obstructed labour, often in women who have undergone female genital mutilation (FGM). There are a number of serious health consequences for the women who are affected, including infection, ulcers, and incontinence. Fistulae are also highly stigmatizing and create enormous social problems for the women involved including, for some women, loss of home and economic security following marital breakdown. But this stigma and the consequences are not counted as part of the burden of DALYs, leaving the social and functional disabilities facing many women undercounted (Dejong 2006).

Summary—differences between women and men in morbidity

Taken together, the various ways of counting morbidity or ill health between women and men suggest that there is a complex relationship between sex, gender, and health, which is mediated by age. Other factors, including socioeconomic status and ethnicity, will also play a part. Although the picture for mortality is relatively straightforward, with most countries showing poorer life expectancy and higher death rates among men, morbidity data suggest that patterns of ill health vary for men and women around the world. On the whole, women report poorer health, use services more, particularly where health care is relatively accessible, and experience more of some conditions, notably those associated with chronic ill health. However, men experience higher levels of illness and disability from those conditions which also contribute to their higher mortality rates.

Sex and gender influences on health are central to explanations of these differences. First we need to define these terms and explore the ways in which each might affect health and health outcomes before going on to consider how sex and gender contribute to specific diseases.

Sex, gender, and health

In order to understand the ways in which sex- and gender-linked factors might influence health, it is important to clarify what is meant by these terms and particularly the differences between them. Despite increasing recognition of the various ways in which sex and gender can impact on the health of men and women, the terms are still sometimes used wrongly. Specifically, although the term *gender* is found more often than in the past in biomedical literature, it is often used interchangeably for *sex* rather than as a distinct concept with a very different meaning (Krieger 2003; Doyal 2001).

Sex and health

Sex refers to biological influences including not only differences between women and men based on the reproductive system, but also those reflecting genetic and hormonal factors. For many years reproductive differences between women and men were seen as the most significant sex-linked influence on health. However, more recent studies have widened our understanding of the complexity of sex-linked factors on men's and women's health.

The Committee on Understanding the Biology of Sex and Gender Differences, set up by the Institute of Medicine in the United States in 1999, produced an important review of the evidence relating to biological factors and their effects on health. The final report concluded that 'sex matters' (Wizeman & Pardue 2001). That is, the health of men and women is influenced in important ways by 'genetic, biochemical, physiological, and physical' elements, as well as those which are social in origin (Wizeman & Pardue 2001). Although hormonal and reproductive factors play a part in patterns of health and vulnerability to different conditions, this review also highlighted the significance of genetic and molecular factors, and important differences between men and women in gene expression. The report concluded with a number of recommendations for further research in the field stressing that genetic factors are not fully understood as yet.

The range of sex-linked influences on health

Sex-linked factors play a key part in human health throughout the life course. Males are more vulnerable to mortality than females at every age, from conception onwards (Waldron 1985). For example, studies of foetal mortality—deaths in the womb at any gestational age—reveal higher rates of mortality among males than females (MacDorman *et al.* 2007). Indeed, the higher rate of male deaths before birth is an important indication of the part played by biological factors in male excess mortality.

Hormones play a key role in differences in health experience between women and men. Female sex hormones appear to protect women against a range of conditions including ischaemic heart disease (Waldron 1985; Kane 1991). One explanation for this advantage is that oestrogen increases the flexibility of the female circulatory system, and that high blood pressure is less damaging for premenopausal women (Bird & Rieker 1999). Also, oestrogen affects cholesterol, increasing HDL cholesterol levels and decreasing LDL cholesterol, and improves the functioning of the heart (Wizeman & Pardue 2001).

Hormones are also implicated in irritable bowel syndrome, another condition demonstrating a female excess. Women are up to four times as likely to suffer from this chronic painful condition. Although this reflects gender-linked factors such as stress and anxiety, there is also evidence that men may receive protection from testosterone whereas female hormones may increase the severity of the symptoms experienced (Heitkemper *et al.* 2003).

Hormonal changes across the menstrual cycle also appear to affect health outcomes for women in the context of interventions as diverse as smoking cessation and surgery for breast cancer (Wizeman & Pardue 2001). Further evidence of biological influences comes from research on alcohol-related damage. Women and men have different patterns of risk from alcohol consumption. Women suffer the adverse effects of alcohol in terms of brain and liver damage more quickly than men do and are more likely to suffer health damage at the same level of consumption as men. These differences are partly due to differences in metabolism and hormonal factors, which means that women's bodies process alcohol differently (Redgrave *et al.* 2003).

There are also differences in male and female immune systems, which in turn are related to reproductive factors, especially the capacity of women to conceive and carry a child. These differences mean that women's immune systems are more at risk from autoimmune disorders (Bird & Rieker 1999). Changes in the immune system of pregnant women, particularly, put them at higher risk of some communicable diseases ranging from measles to malaria (Wizeman & Pardue 2001). However, other pregnancy-related changes such as the tendency for autoimmune diseases (such as rheumatoid arthritis) to go into remission highlight the complexity of the relationship between sex and the immune system.

Recent research has also suggested important sex differences in gene expression, contributing to women's higher risks for some forms of cancer. For example, among smokers, women appear to be more at risk of lung cancer than men at the same level of smoking, and lung cancer is also more common among non-smoking women than non-smoking men (Keohavong *et al.* 2003). This has been related to gene expression. Expression of genes related to lung cancer may be greater among women than men due to the location of the expressed gene on the X chromosome, leading to an increased risk of this cancer as well as shaping the type of lung cancer which women develop (Haugen 2002; Shields 2002; Payne 2001).

In addition, there is increasing evidence of sex differences in the way the brain is organized, including the use of language and verbal abilities. For example, women tend to recover more language ability than men following a left-hemisphere stroke (Wizeman & Pardue 2001). There are also differences between women and men in the way the brain responds to noxious stimuli, which in turn affect experiences of symptoms such as pain. Women have higher prevalence rates for what are often described as 'pain conditions', including headache, abdominal, and facial pain (Bradley & Alarcon 1999; LeResche 1999). Although this reflects the fact that the expression of pain is culturally more sanctioned for women than men, biological factors also play a part, especially differences between women and men, in particular certain neurological pathways (Yunus 2002).

However, we must be wary of attributing too much to biology. For example research on the relationship between parity and some health conditions, notably non-reproductive carcinomas such as colorectal cancer, has suggested that there might be a relationship in women between pregnancy and subsequent health risks. But recent studies have also revealed a similar relationship between parity and cancer for men, implying that social factors such as stress, access to resources, and expectations associated with having children may be more significant than biological factors in this association (Kravdal 1995).

Wizeman and Pardue (Wizeman & Pardue 2001) point out the limitations in this area of knowledge. Despite many years of research on the ways in which biology impacts on health, conclusive evidence and clear understanding of the pathways concerned remain scarce. There are various reasons for this, including a lack of research which is disaggregated for men and women and the fact that negative research findings which fail to find a difference between women and men are often not published, despite the fact that such results also advance our understanding.

What remains clear, however, is that biology or sex-linked factors interact with environmental factors, including gender, and the health of women and men is also shaped in a number of ways by socially constructed gender differences.

Gender and health

Gender refers to socially constructed differences between women and men; that is, the conventions, roles, and expectations of men and women that are culturally ascribed (Krieger 2003). Gendered influences on health include access to health promoting resources, exposure to health damaging and health promoting factors in daily life, and different expectations of behaviour such as drinking alcohol, risk taking, and the use of health care. In addition, gender impacts on health through the ways in which health services are organized and delivered, especially when such services operate in gender-insensitive ways.

One of the key differences between sex and gender is the extent to which they are fixed, or can change over time. Sex—male or female—is assigned to a child at birth on the basis of external genitalia and is fixed, other than for a minority of people undergoing medical sex reassignment. Gender is generally ascribed on the basis of biological sex, although what is meant in any one society or culture by gender may vary over the years and between social or other groupings. Thus, a child is identified at birth as either male or female and this in turn leads to the categorizations embedded in masculinity or femininity in that society.

Gender is an important influence on the health of men and women, both alone and in the interaction between gender and biology. Krieger and Zierler (Krieger & Zierler 1995) describe such interactions in terms of *the biologic expression of gender* and the *gendered expression of biology.* The biologic expression of gender refers to the ways in which gender becomes embodied. For example, in many societies, gender is constructed to mean that women see themselves, and are seen by others, as weaker than men. This in turn may result in women taking less exercise or choosing less strenuous forms of activity, which in turn affect the female body. The gendered expression of biology refers to the ways in which biological understandings of women and men lead to gendered differentiations, which often take the form of discrimination. So, for example, women's reproductive capacity is used to justify their exclusion from some forms of paid work on the basis that it is unsafe. Similarly, their exclusion from medical research is said to be justified on the basis that it may cause harm to an unborn child. This exclusion, in turn, strengthens social constructions of gender in which women are seen as less able to undertake some forms of paid work, or less vulnerable to some forms of disease.

For many writers, gender is seen as something that is 'performed' in various ways, in exchange with other people. That is, we 'do' gender in our daily lives—in our paid work, in relationships, in leisure activities, and so on (Courtenay 2000). This view of gender allows us to see how it changes over time and across societies, and also how individuals might 'do' gender differently at different times and in different settings. In addition, it highlights the fact that what is appropriate gendered behaviour for one group may not be so for another—for example, gender roles vary according to class and ethnicity. Finally, it allows for the possibility that individuals might choose to adopt gender roles that are not commensurable with their biological sex. But, although various gender roles may be available, it is also the case that in all societies some forms of masculinity and femininity are more sanctioned than others and this may impact on health in negative or positive ways.

Many writers have observed that in most (if not all) cultures, masculinity is privileged over femininity, but it is also true that all men are not equally advantaged. The term *hegemonic masculinity* has been used to refer to the most privileged form of masculinity, typically occupied by white middle-class men (Connell & Messerschmidt 2005). Men occupying different class positions may experience masculinity in a range of ways, with associated health benefits and/or risks. Similarly, women can experience gender in a number of ways, again with varying impacts on their health.

Gender affects the health of both men and women in numerous interlocking ways. Firstly, gender mediates the effect of physical and psychological risks encountered in daily life. There is substantial evidence, for example, that material factors such as poverty and social exclusion, socioeconomic status, poor housing and environmental disadvantage, and occupation and unpaid work all impact on health in varying ways and to varying degrees (Leon & Walt 2001; Krieger & Higgins 2002). And, men and women may face differential risks of experiencing these adverse effects, because of their gender. Secondly, gender roles and expectations are closely associated with individual behaviour, which in turn may impact on the health of women and men.

Socioeconomic determinants of health and gender

Material factors influence the health of women and men in complex ways through aspects of daily life such as paid work and employment status, household work and domestic labour, income, caring responsibilities, living arrangements, and experiences of conflict, stress, and violence. The extent to which men and women are exposed to these risk factors, and how they impact on their health, varies in relation to geographical location, socioeconomic status, and cultural differences.

Paid employment exerts numerous effects on health. There are a range of hazards associated with particular jobs, including exposure to unsafe chemicals, hazardous work environments, and dangers inherent in the nature of the work itself. The gender division of labour, which sees men more often employed in certain sectors and in certain occupations within sectors, creates a gendered division of occupational risk. Men typically work in industries and in jobs with a higher mortality risk, including construction, transport, and the emergency services.

However, in recent years, the occupational injury gap between women and men has narrowed, following a rise in the numbers of women in the labour force, and there has been a corresponding increase in some forms of injury-related mortality among women (Waldron *et al.* 2005). Other work-related hazards affect the risk of poor health, such as repetitive strain injury (RSI) from keyboard work and some production processes in manufacturing. Such injuries are more common among women partly as a result of the jobs they occupy and partly because the design of workstations is often based on male rather than female physiology (De Zwart *et al.* 2001; Lacerda *et al.* 2005).

Gender differences in occupational risk are compounded by differences outside the workplace and particularly by gender differences in domestic work. Women still carry out most household chores. For example, in the United Kingdom, despite their increasing participation in paid work, women still spend on average twice as many hours per day as men in housework and childcare (ONS 2003). In addition, even where men take on some of the work, women retain overall responsibility for domestic labour—for planning, organizing, and ensuring it is done (Hunt & Annandale 1993). Domestic labour carries further implications for health, including the stress of managing responsibilities combined with lack of reward, loneliness, and isolation, as well as lack of an independent income and low status for those women who are not also employed. Women working at home are notably vulnerable to mental health problems in comparison with those who have paid work, but the strain of juggling two roles and the dual burden of paid work and domestic labour also puts women who enter the labour market at risk of poor mental health (Doyal 1995).

Daily life brings pronounced health risks when either men or women are living in poverty or social exclusion. However, there are gender differences in the risk of such poverty, with women in most parts of the world being more likely to be poor. This is due to lower wages, reduced access to paid work as a result of caring responsibilities, and (in some countries) cultural restrictions, and also reflects the fact that women may not always share equally in household resources. Poverty is often especially severe among older women whose health is already frail (World Health Organization 2003a).

Exposure to violence creates further risks including poor mental health, post-traumatic stress disorders, and physical injuries. Violence is one of the most important causes of death for younger age groups (World Health Organization 2002c), but there are marked gender differences not only in the level of risk from violence but also in the source. Although both women and men are at risk from interpersonal violence, violence against men is more common in the public domain and they are more at risk from strangers. On the other hand, women are more often exposed to violence in the home, from partners and members of their family (World Health Organization 2002c). Women are at particular risk from sexual violence both in the home and elsewhere, and the consequences for their health can include pregnancy and sexually transmitted infections as well as mental health problems. Although sexual violence against men is less common, it may be especially damaging for their mental health due to feelings of stigma and shame (Ganju *et al.* 2004).

Taken together, these material aspects of daily life can create particular health stresses, which are often different for men and women.

To these health risks, we can add those associated with 'doing gender'—the ways in which social constructions of masculinity and femininity are associated with the increased risk of particular behaviours, which further impact on health.

'Doing gender'—masculinity, femininity, and health

Behaviour has long been seen as the leading gendered explanation for men's poorer health and premature mortality. In the seventeenth century, John Gaunt (quoted in Ciocco [1940]) suggested that women lived longer than men despite their experiences of illness because, 'Men, being more intemperate than women, die as much by reason of their vices, as women do by the infirmity of their sex'. There are still important differences between women and men in behaviours such as smoking, alcohol and substance use, physical activity, diet, risk taking, and the use of health-care services including preventive care and screening. These differences taken together are a key part of the explanation for men's higher mortality; a number of writers in this area have highlighted the extent to which masculinity accounts for the greater mortality risks experienced by men across a range of cultural settings (Courtenay 2000).

One of the most damaging behaviours—smoking and tobacco use—has a strongly gendered history. More men than women die each year from smoking-related diseases; lung cancer, for example, killed twice as many men as women worldwide in 2002 (World Health Organization 2004b). This reflects the gender ratio in smokers: Throughout the world more men than women smoke, and in countries where the epidemic is relatively new, the great majority of those using tobacco are male (World Health Organization 2002b). In Malaysia, for example, 53 per cent of men smoke compared with less than 3 per cent of women; in Malawi, 25 per cent of men and 6 per cent of women smoke; and in India, the comparable figures are 42 per cent and 9 per cent.

However, more developed regions where smoking has a longer history have seen increasing numbers of women beginning to use tobacco, to the point where in some countries similar proportions of women and men are smokers, such as in Norway and Sweden (World Health Organization 2002b). In the United States, 23 per cent of men and 19 per cent of women smoke, compared with 27 per cent of men and 24 per cent of women in the United Kingdom (Schiller & Bernadel 2004; GHS 2004). However, in the United Kingdom, female smokers have outnumbered males in recent years in younger age groups and there are also more women smokers than men in some minority ethnic groups, particularly those described as mixed race (GHS 2004).

Alcohol and substance use also have gendered profiles. Excessive consumption of alcohol on a regular basis is associated with an increased risk of a number of diseases, including liver cirrhosis and other liver disease, some forms of coronary heart disease, and oral cancers (World Health Organization 2004a). Other forms of alcohol consumption, including what is sometimes referred to as 'binge drinking' in which high levels of alcohol are consumed over a short period of time, also lead to an increased risk of violence and accidental injury, as well as self-harm and suicide (World Health Organization 2004a).

In surveys of national and international data, more women than men are described as 'abstainers', that is, as non-drinkers. The extent of the gender gap varies: In the Philippines, for example, women are seven times more likely than men to be abstainers, whereas in Iceland, the ratio of female to male abstainers is nearly equal (World Health Organization 2004a).

In many countries, more men than women are defined as heavy drinkers; that is, they consume a high number of units of alcohol on a weekly basis and/or have a high daily intake. Figures for Argentina, for example, show that over 11 per cent of male drinkers compared with 2 per cent of women are defined as consuming high levels of alcohol on a daily basis; similarly, 52 per cent of male drinkers in Colombia compared with 21 per cent of female drinkers are defined as heavy consumers; and 23 per cent of male drinkers in Japan compared with only 5 per cent of female drinkers are defined as having a problematic intake (World Health Organization 2004a). However, in some countries (including Australia, Nigeria, and the United Kingdom), more women than men are defined as drinking over recommended daily limits.

If we look at binge drinking rather than daily consumption, this remains much more common among men than women around the world, despite fears in some countries that such behaviour is increasing among younger women. Such drinking is highest among males in Finland where nearly half of male drinkers report very high consumption on single occasions compared with 14 per cent of women, although there are also high levels of binge drinking among men in Mexico, Nigeria, and Iceland. In Nigeria, nearly 40 per cent of female drinkers reported binge drinking at least once a month (World Health Organization 2004a).

Diet is also an important, modifiable contributor to health risks. The influence of diet on health is becoming increasingly clear, with growing evidence suggesting that a diet which is rich in fruit, vegetables, and fibre and low in fat may reduce the risk of various health problems including cancer and heart disease (Thune & Furberg 2001). Gender differences in what we eat may therefore play an important role in explaining different patterns of health for men and women. Men are more likely than women to die from colorectal cancer, for example, and part of the explanation for this seems to stem from differences in diet (Steinemetz & Potter 1991).

On the whole, men's diets are less healthy than those of women, especially in high-income countries, where men more often consume inadequate amounts of vegetables and fruit and also eat higher than recommended amounts of red meat (Payne 2006; Courtenay 2000). However, in low- and middle-income countries, notably those where food is scarce, women and girls are less likely than men to be eating adequate levels of fruit and vegetables. For example, in Malawi, 42 per cent of women and 37 per cent of men have diets with less than the recommended amount of fruit and vegetables. In other low-income countries (such as in Pakistan, India, Swaziland, and Kenya), a large majority of both men and women report diets insufficient in fruit and vegetables, and the differences between them are slight (World Health Organization 2006). In these countries, where there is a high risk of food insecurity, there are important gender differences in the distribution of food within households, in expectations about what men and women will eat, and also in what will be given to male and female children.

However, food intake and diet also need to be set against energy requirements, and again there are important gender differences both in levels of physical activity and in kinds of activity.

In high-income countries, lack of physical activity is a health concern that has increased in prominence in recent years. Physical activity can have a positive effect on health: It helps to protect against heart disease and may play a part in reducing vulnerability to other conditions, including some cancers and mental health problems (Thune & Furberg 2001). WHO estimate that around 2 million deaths and 19 million DALYs each year are associated with insufficient physical activity (World Health Organization 2002a). Physical activity levels in most communities are different for men and women, although the size of the gap varies in relation to other factors including employment-related activity levels and available leisure time.

Data on activity levels are complex and not always comparable. Some surveys refer to total physical activity including that associated with work and travel (e.g. cycling and walking) as well as leisure activities such as sport. One of the problems with this data is that physical domestic work, mainly carried out by women, is often not included in such measures (O'Brien 2005). This means that some figures (based on total activity), principally those from low- and middle-income countries, overestimate the extent to which women are leading sedentary lives. Data based on leisure activities alone, however, might also miss out some activities that are more frequent among women, such as dancing (O'Brien 2005).

Data from the West often focus on leisure activity rather than total activity, making it difficult to compare findings with poorer countries. However, in high-income countries, there is a gap between men and women in time spent in physical activity, with men tending to be more active. Figures from the United States, for example, show that a higher proportion of men participate regularly in physical activity (Schiller & Bernadel 2004). Similarly, in England, more men than women take part in such activity, with the widest gap among young adults between 16 and 24 years of age (NatCen 2003).

Figures for total physical activity in low- and middle-income countries suggest that men might be more likely than women to have active lifestyles, although this possibly reflects a failure to count some aspects of women's activities. In Kenya, for example, although less than 10 per cent of adults report physical activity levels that are too low (in terms of health benefit), slightly more women than men report insufficient time spent in physical activity (World Health Organization 2006). Similarly, in Malawi, few people have low levels of activity, but activity levels are lower among women than men. Activity levels are slightly lower in Pakistan, where women are twice as likely as men to report insufficient activity; and in India and China, fewer women than men report sufficient levels of activity.

However, in these countries it is also important to consider activity, or energy expenditure, alongside diet and calorie intake. In the poorest countries, women experience health risks because of activity levels that are high in the context of too little food. These problems are especially severe for pregnant and breastfeeding women, and carry long-term implications both for their health and that of their child. Jackson and Palmer-Jones (Jackson & Palmer-Jones 1998) talk of an 'energy trap' resulting from development policies that aim to increase various kinds of work in order to reduce poverty but which fail to take account of the increased need for food created by increased levels of activity. Gender differences in food allocation and access to calories, as well as in work carried out, mean this is an acute problem for women (Jackson & Palmer-Jones 1998; Standing 2002).

Diet and activity levels in high-income countries are also connected to a further measure of health risk: Obesity. Obesity is associated with various diseases including coronary heart disease, some forms of cancer, and diabetes. Obesity, defined as a body mass index (BMI) over 30, is more common among women than men although this varies between countries, whereas more men than women are defined as overweight (with a BMI of between 25 and 30) (Zaninotto *et al.* 2006; ASSO 2005). In older age groups and in lower-income groups in particular, women are more likely than men to be defined as obese (World Health Organization 2003a; NatCen 2003).

A final aspect of behaviour that is gendered and which affects health and mortality risk is the use of preventive services and health care. We have earlier discussed gender differences in consultation as a measure of morbidity, and economic factors play a part in the use of health care, but it is also important to consider the ways in which men and women differ in help-seeking behaviour. A number of studies have suggested that men are reluctant to seek medical help and attend services less readily than women. As one man put it, 'I don't go to the doctor unless something scares the hell out of me' (Stibbe 2004:36). Men describe themselves as unwilling to make a fuss or waste the time of health professionals (O'Brien *et al.* 2005). Although there are a number of variations in data on health-service use, such as those reflecting differences in age, in socioeconomic status, and for specific symptoms, men do appear less willing to see themselves as in need of health care. Similarly, men are more difficult to engage in health-promotion activities including screening, leading some health-care providers to devise various gender-sensitive strategies to increase take-up among men, such as placing clinics and information points in workplaces and bars (Alt 2002; Malterud & Okkes 1998). Overall, gender differences in roles, expectations, and behaviour combine to increase the risk of premature mortality for men and the risk of chronic health problems for women. Masculinity, insofar as it involves risk taking and unhealthy behaviours, increases risks of accidental and non-accidental injury, and of non-communicable diseases associated with smoking, alcohol, and substance use. Masculine practices also increase some health risks for women, notably the risks associated with male violence and sexually-transmitted infections.

Female gender roles and expectations may lead to reduced risks for some conditions because of lower rates of smoking, alcohol, and substance use, better diets, and less risk-taking, although the lower rates of physical activity more common among women will also affect their health risks. In poorer countries, however, women have different problems associated with insufficient food for the work they are expected to carry out. There are also pressures on both men and women arising from the stress of gender role expectations, especially in relation to failure to meet these expectations.

In order to illustrate these different influences and the complex associations between sex and gender, we now look at specific health problems: Cardiovascular diseases, cancer, HIV and AIDS, mental health difficulties, and malaria.

The impact of sex and gender on specific health problems

Cardiovascular diseases

Cardiovascular diseases include coronary heart disease (CHD) and stroke. Taken together, cardiovascular diseases account for around one-tenth of the global burden of disease, with more men than women affected. CHD is the major contributor to this burden, particularly among men, whereas strokes account for similar levels of illness among men and women. These conditions are also important in overall mortality: More men than women die as a result of CHD but more women die from a stroke (World Health Organization 2004b). One of the key differences between women and men in these illnesses is the age at which risk increases: Men are more likely than women to die prematurely from CHD and the male to female ratio is greatest in mid-life. On average, women with CHD die ten years later than men (Wizeman & Pardue 2001). In the United Kingdom, the male mortality rate for CHD is around five times the female rate between 45 and 54 years, whereas the male–female ratio has reduced to 1.4 to 1 by the age of 80 (Khaw 2006). Although trends in CHD have changed over time, men worldwide experience the greater risk of premature death and illness associated with this condition (Khaw 2006).

Why do men than women have higher risks for CHD at an early stage in the life course? In the aetiology of CHD, raised blood pressure and blood cholesterol are significant risk factors, and behaviours that are more common among men than women—notably poor diet and smoking—are important underlying explanations. Although women gain protection from heart disease due to female hormones, men increase their risks through the adoption of risky behaviours. The later age at which women appear to be at risk of CHD has led to speculation that until menopause female hormones might offer women some degree of protection. However, most recent research has failed to support this suggestion. For example, women's CHD risk does not increase immediately following menopause but some years later, suggesting that other factors may be important instead of, or alongside, female hormones. In addition, hormone replacement therapy does not appear to offer women protection from CHD (Khaw 2006).

However, there are also concerns over possible differences between women and men in the recognition and treatment of CHD. Because heart disease is seen as primarily a male condition, women may be less likely to have their illness diagnosed or to be offered appropriate treatment (Lockyer & Bury 2002). This topic is dealt with in a later subsection.

Cancer

Overall mortality from cancer is higher among men, and although both men and women are vulnerable to reproductive-related cancers, more men than women also die from cancers related to lifestyle and behaviours associated with an increased risk of cancer. Although cancers of the reproductive organs lead to more deaths among women than among men, the difference does not compensate for the male excess cancer mortality stemming from factors such as tobacco use, poor diet, and alcohol consumption.

Lung cancer, for example, accounts for more than twice as many deaths among men as among women, as well as for a large proportion of illnesses (World Health Organization 2004b). The main cause of lung cancer for both men and women is tobacco use, and in countries where tobacco use remains a predominantly male habit, the male–female ratio is especially high. In Thailand, for example, the ratio of men to women for lung cancer mortality is around 2.3:1, whereas in Denmark, where equal numbers of men and women now smoke, the ratio has reduced to 1.4 to 1 in recent years (World Health Organization).

However, research suggests that the risk of lung cancer is different for women and men irrespective of absolute levels of tobacco use. These differences stem from gendered differences in patterns of tobacco use—such as the type of cigarettes smoked and the depth of inhalation—and from biological factors. Women have a greater biological vulnerability to lung cancer due to genetic factors and their higher use of low-tar cigarettes leads to an increased risk of one form of lung cancer—adenocarcinoma. However, although lung cancer is a particularly fatal form of cancer with very low one-year and five-year survival rates, women appear to have better prospects for survival in comparison with men, which is also related to biological differences between women and men.

Thus, sex- and gender-linked factors interact to produce different risks of cancer for women and men, reflecting hormonal and genetic influences and the impact of certain behaviours.

Mental health and illness

Among chronic and debilitating conditions, the most significant in terms of numbers affected and the impact on daily living are those associated with mental illness. Mental health problems, including depression, anxiety, substance use, and schizophrenia, account for around 12 per cent of the global burden of disease (World Health Organization 2003b). Around 450 million people worldwide experience mental illness of one kind or another at any one time. There are important differences between women and men in their risks of different kinds of mental health problems or disorders. More women are diagnosed as suffering from depression and anxiety-related conditions, and in community-based surveys, more women are found to be suffering from symptoms of these illnesses (Payne 2006). This gender gap is found throughout the world: The *World Health Survey* (World Health Organization 2005) for 2005 found that in countries as diverse as Malawi, India, Portugal, Pakistan, and the Russian Federation more women than men were diagnosed with depression. It is estimated that worldwide women are almost twice as likely as men to experience an episode of depression in a twelve-month period (World Health Organization 2003b).

Men, on the other hand, are more frequently treated for mental health difficulties associated with alcohol and substance use, including harmful use, dependence, and psychosis (Payne 2006). Men are also more likely to commit suicide than women in every country in the world apart from China. In contrast, more women than men are involved in acts of deliberate self-harm.

Although there is some evidence that biological influences play a part in shaping mental health—especially in relation to specific conditions such as postnatal depression—most research suggests that gendered factors play the more significant role. These include stress-linked factors such as those associated with poverty, parenting, employment, exposure to the threat of violence, and gendered expectations, as well as the extent to which gender stereotyping in mental health services affects the delivery of care by increasing diagnoses of depression among women (Blair-West *et al.* 1999).

HIV and AIDS

In many parts of the world, HIV/AIDS is one of the most significant threats to the health of women and men. More than 39 million people worldwide were living with HIV in 2006, with over 4 million new infections and nearly 3 million deaths (UNAIDS 2006). Most of those who are HIV positive (nearly 25 million) live in sub-Saharan Africa, and most of the world's AIDS deaths occur in this region. Not surprisingly, HIV/AIDS accounts for a large proportion of illness worldwide and was the fourth largest contributor to the global burden of disease in 2001 (Lopez *et al.* 2006).

One of the main features of the pandemic is the increasing numbers of women affected in parts of the world where prevalence is highest. For example, in sub-Saharan Africa, women comprise nearly 60 per cent of adults living with HIV, compared with 26 per cent in North America (UNAIDS 2006). Increasing numbers of women are also being infected in Asia, Eastern Europe, and South American countries, with the proportion likely to rise in future years. In the Russian Federation, women now comprise 40 per cent of new infections (UNAIDS 2006).

Women are vulnerable to HIV/AIDS due to a mixture of biological and gender-linked factors. In unprotected vaginal intercourse, women are at greater risk than men because the absorbent vaginal wall is exposed to seminal fluid and because semen carries a higher viral load than other bodily fluids. However, women are also less able to negotiate sexual relationships—such as to demand protection—and may be forced or coerced into unprotected sex. Female sex workers in particular are at risk, especially when sex without condoms offers the opportunity for more money. Women in insecure situations, such as forced migrants, may also be pressurized into unsafe sex in order to gain protection or resources. For example, a recent study of HIV infection rates among displaced persons in North Uganda found that women living outside protected camps had higher risks of infection than those living inside such camps (UNAIDS 2006).

HIV and AIDS have severe consequences for the health of both women and men. For both, there is an increased risk of opportunistic infection, and levels of malaria, tuberculosis, and some forms of cancer are higher among people living with HIV and AIDS. Both also experience reduced fertility. However, although all of those living with HIV and AIDS are at risk of premature mortality without access to essential medicines, women are at risk of pelvic inflammatory disease, recurrent yeast infections, cervical cancer, and problems in pregnancy and childbirth, all of which complicate treatment (National Institute of Allergy and Infectious Diseases 2004). Men also have increased risks of some associated diseases, particularly Kaposi's sarcoma (a type of skin cancer), which can lead to weight loss, fever, and painful swelling especially in the legs, groin area, or skin around the eyes.

Thus, sex and gender again intertwine, both in terms of men's and women's vulnerability to infection and in the consequences of the disease.

Malaria

Between 350 and 500 million people become ill each year with malaria, and over 1 million people (mainly children) die from this disease (World Health Organization 2005b). The vast majority of those affected live in sub-Saharan Africa. The global impact of malaria on the burden of illness has been calculated at more than 46 million DALYs per annum (World Health Organization 2004b).

Reduction of the incidence of malaria has been included in the eight Millennium Development Goals (MDGs) and has been a key focus of the WHO's work in recent years. Incidence of malaria has been growing over the past decade for a variety of reasons, including increasing resistance to the drugs used to treat the disease and resistance to the insecticides used to prevent transmission. In addition, the disease burden has worsened due to an increase in the lack of access to necessary medicine and preventive measures, notably among those in poorer countries, and due to deforestation in some areas creating wider vectors of transmission.

There is an important difference between women and men in the risk of malaria, with more women being infected and dying from this disease. Biology plays a key part in this difference, as women have a much greater risk of contracting malaria when pregnant due to temporary changes in their immune system brought about by the pregnancy. However, gender factors also increase their risks of malaria. In many parts of the world (including those where malaria is rife), women have less access than men to preventive measures such as bed nets treated with insecticide, because of the household division of resources. In addition, women's responsibility for work, such as water collection and some agricultural labour, increases their exposure to mosquitoes and the risk of being bitten. Further, studies have found women to be less well-informed than men about the risks of malaria and the means of protection, and are less able to access health care when infected because of less control over household resources and, in many cultures, the need to be chaperoned when attending health services (Tanner & Vlassoff 1998). When they do seek help, research has also suggested that they are often blamed by health professionals for not attending earlier, and they feel poorly treated by such professionals and by being stigmatized in their communities (Tanner & Vlassoff 1998).

Gender and the delivery of health care

The final way in which gender impacts on health is through the delivery of health care. In addition to material circumstances and behaviour, the health of both men and women is also associated with the way in which health care is provided and we need to ask if health services are equally available for both, if they are accessible, and if they are appropriate.

Gender differences in availability and accessibility

Gender affects access to health in a number of ways. Most importantly perhaps, it affects the resources that are necessary in order to use health services. Around the world, women earn less than men, and, where health insurance is related to paid work, are more often in jobs without insurance cover (Collins *et al.* 1999).

In many low- and middle-income countries, although both men and women experience difficulty in obtaining health care due to the location of services and the need to meet the costs of user fees, women are more disadvantaged because of a lack of independent income or a say in how household resources are used (Ravindran 2000; Benjamins *et al.* 2004).

In addition to access, there may be further differences in availability. Where services are only open during the day, they are less available to those with paid work who cannot take time off or to those whose caring responsibilities prevent attendance. Although more men are prevented from using daytime services due to employment, they are also more often in jobs where time off for medical appointments is sanctioned. For women juggling full-time or part-time work with childcare, seeking medical help may be especially difficult.

Similarly, some cultures require women to consult with female health professionals, who may not always be available. Even where it is not culturally prescribed, more women report a preference for a female clinician, particularly when consulting about intimate health problems. For example, women are more likely to prefer a female colonoscopist when being screened for bowel cancer, but the lack of women in this profession means that their preferences are often not met, potentially delaying detection of bowel cancer among women (Menees *et al.* 2005).

Gender differences in the quality of care

The second way in which gender impinges on health care is through differences in the quality of care offered to men and women. One important factor affecting this is medical knowledge. Medical research has for some time been criticized for failing to disaggregate findings for women and men, and also for failing to include women in studies of health problems affecting both sexes (Doyal 1998). This focus on male subjects is problematic when it is assumed that findings can be extended to female populations as though there is no difference. Both symptom recognition and treatment based on men may fail women—for example, women metabolize pharmaceuticals differently to men and prescribed drugs may be more or less effective, or carry different risks for women if the research was conducted only on men (Wizeman & Pardue 2001). Similarly, risk factors affecting women's health tend to have been less intensively studied: The mental and physical risks associated with housework, for example, are relatively unexplored compared with some traditionally male occupations (Ruiz & Verbrugge 1997).

In the United States, the National Institutes of Health have required (since 1994) research funded by them to include sufficient numbers of men and women, and members of minority ethnic groups, as well as to provide separate analyses and reporting of results. Despite this, some evidence shows that a number of studies still either focus on men alone or fail to disaggregate findings for men and women (Vidaver *et al.* 2000). In countries without such guidelines, the bias is even greater.

Studies have also explored the different ways in which services respond to the health needs of women and men. For example, women are less likely to have heart conditions recognized by their primary physician because they often present with atypical symptoms including fatigue, shortness of breath, and cold sweats. Men, on the other hand, are seen as candidates for heart complaints by themselves, by their families, and by health care workers, and the symptoms they typically present with have become the norm (Lockyer & Bury 2002). In addition, chest pain, a key symptom of heart disease, will often have other causes for women and this also leads to an underdiagnosis of heart disease. Not surprisingly, women are less often referred for tests and for treatment, and tend to be at a more advanced stage of illness when they are treated, with more severe symptoms and the risk this implies (Lockyer & Bury 2002).

Equally, men are less likely than women to have mental health problems such as depression recognized (Blair-West *et al.* 1999). Underdiagnosis and undertreatment of depression in men contribute to higher rates of male suicide mortality; where there have been increases in prescriptions of antidepressants among men, suicide rates have fallen (Gunnell *et al.* 2003).

In addition, health care may not be sensitive to more subtle gender differences in health needs. Some services are gender-blind and unknowingly discriminate against men or women by failing to identify their specific needs. For example, most smoking cessation interventions do not highlight gender differences in successful strategies, including the fact that women and men appear to smoke for different reasons and may take up smoking again in response to different stress factors (Samet & Yoon 2001). In addition, women metabolize nicotine differently to men and have more adverse reactions to withdrawal compared with men (Perkins 2001). Women and men also may need different kinds of support, both from friends or family and from health services (Gritz *et al.* 1996).

Conclusion

What we have seen in this chapter is that both sex and gender play an important part in shaping the health of men and women, alongside other forms of diversity. Sex, or biology, is more than reproduction. The health of both men and women is also affected by hormonal differences, and by genetic factors, which impact on their vulnerability to different diseases as well as the chances of recovery and survival.

Gender, or socially constructed difference, also affects health—by increasing the chances of exposure to specific risk factors, such as poverty, or by helping to shape the behavioural choices made by men and women—the way we 'do' masculinity or femininity. Gender is also important in the way health services are delivered—from how research is conducted and how medical knowledge is constructed and disseminated to health policy and planning, which shape the availability of medical care, access to care, and how appropriately it meets the needs of men and women. All of these factors combine at the level of the individual to shape their health experience and their need for care, and that care itself needs to be planned and delivered in such a way that both men and women are able to benefit.

Key points

- Both sex and gender play a part in women's and men's health.
- Sex or biological factors affect incidence, and also, survival for various diseases.
- Gender is socially constructed and affects exposure to risk factors, as well as influencing health behaviours.
- Gender also affects the delivery of health care, access to care, and how well this care meets the needs of women and men.

References

AbouZahr C., Vaughan J.P. Assessing the burden of sexual and reproductive ill-health: questions regarding the use of disability-adjusted life years [online]. *Bulletin of the World Health Organization* 2000;**78**(**5**):655–66.

Alt R. Where the boys are not: a brief overview of male preventive health. *Wisconsin Medical Journal* 2002;**287**:337–43.

Australian Bureau of Statistics (ABS). *National health survey 2004–5*. Canberra: Australian Bureau of Statistics; 2006.

Australian Society for the Study of Obesity (ASSO). *Obesity in Australian adults: prevalence data*. Sydney: Australian Society for the Study of Obesity; 2005.

Baghadi G. Gender and medicines: an international public health perspective. *Journal of Women's Health* 2005;**14**:82–6.

Benjamins M., Hummer R., Eberstein I. *et al.* Self-reported health and adult mortality risk. *Social Science and Medicine* 2004;**59**:1297–306.

Bird C.E., Rieker P.P. Gender matters: an integrated model for understanding men's and women's health. *Social Science and Medicine* 1999;**48**:745–55.

Blair-West G.W., Cantor C.H., Mellsop G.W. *et al.* Lifetime suicide risk in major depression: sex and age determinants. *Journal of Affective Disorder* 1999;**55**:171–8.

Bradley L., Alarcon G. Sex-related influences in fibromyalgia. In: Fillingham B.D., editor. *Sex, gender, and pain*. Seattle (WA): IASP Press; 1999. p. 281–307.

Ciocco A. Sex differences in morbidity and mortality. *The Quarterly Review of Biology* 1940;**15**:59–73.

Connell R., Messerschmidt J.W. Hegemonic masculinity: rethinking the concept. *Gender and Society* 2005;**19**:829–59.

Courtenay W. Constructions of masculinity and their influence on men's well-being: a theory of gender and health. *Social Science and Medicine* 2000;**50**:1385–401.

De Zwart B., Frings-Dressen M., Kilbom A. Gender differences in upper extremity musculoskeletal complaints in the working population. *International Archives of Occupational and Environmental Health* 2001;**74**:21–30.

Dejong J. Capabilities, reproductive health, and well-being. *The Journal of Development Studies* 2006;**42**:1158–79.

Division for the Advancement of Women (DAW). *Gender equality, development, and peace for the twenty-first century: the feminization of poverty.* New York (NY): Division for the Advancement of Women, United Nations; 2000. Available from: http://www.un.org/womenwatch/daw/followup/session/presskit/fs1.htm [Accessed 24 April 2007].

Doyal L. *Gender and health technical paper*. Geneva: World Health Organization; 1998. WHO/FRH/WHD/98.16.

Doyal L. Sex, gender, and health: the need for a new approach. *British Medical Journal* 2001;**323**:1061–3.

Doyal L. What makes women sick? Gender and the political economy of health. Basingstoke, UK: Macmillan; 1995.

Ganju D., Jejeebhoy S., Nidadavoluand V. *et al. Sexual coercion: young men's experiences as victims and perpetrators*. New Delhi: Population Council; 2004.

General Household Survey (GHS). *Living in Britain: results from the 2002 general household survey*. London: The Stationery Office; 2004.

Gritz E.R., Nielsen I.R., Brooks L.A. Smoking cessation and gender: the influence of physiological, psychological, and behavioural factors. *Journal of American Medical Women's Association* 1996;**51**:35–42.

Gunnell D., Middleton N., Whitley E. *et al.* Why are suicide rates rising in young men but falling in the elderly? A time-series analysis of trends in England and Wales, 1950–1998. *Social Science and Medicine* 2003;**57**:595–611.

Haugen A. Women who smoke: are women more susceptible to tobacco-induced lung cancer? *Carcinogenesis* 2002;**23**:227–9.

Heitkemper M., Jarrett M., Bond E. *et al.* Impact of sex and gender on irritable bowel syndrome. *Biological Research for Nursing* 2003; **5**:56–65.

Hemenway D., Shinoda-Tagawa T., Miller M. Firearm availability and female homicide victimization rates among 25 populous high-income countries. *Journal of American Women's Medical Association* 2002;**57**:100–4.

Hunt K., Annandale E. Just the job? Is the relationship between health and domestic and paid work gender-specific? *Sociology of Health and Illness* 1993;**15**:632–64.

Jackson C., Palmer-Jones R. *Work intensity, gender, and well-being*. United Nations Research Institute for Social Development; 1998 Oct. Discussion Paper Number 96.

Kane P. *Women's health from womb to tomb*. London: St Martins Press; 1991.

Keohavong P., Lan Q., Gao W.M. *et al.* K-ras mutations in lung carcinomas from nonsmoking women exposed to unvented coal smoke in China. *Lung Cancer* 2003;**41**:21–7.

Khaw K-T. Epidemiology of coronary heart disease in women. *Heart* 2006;**92**:2–4.

Kravdal O. Is the relationship between childbearing and cancer incidence due to biology or lifestyle? Examples of importance of using data on men. *International Journal of Epidemiology* 1995;**24**:477–84.

Krieger J., Higgins D. Housing and health: time again for public health action. *American Journal of Public Health* 2002;**92**:758–68.

Krieger N., Zierler S. Accounting for the health of women. *Current Issues in Public Health* 1995;**1**:251–6.

Krieger N. Genders, sexes, and health: what are the connections—and why does it matter? *International Journal of Epidemiology* 2003;**32**:652–7.

Lacerda E., Nacul L., da S Augusto L. *et al.* Prevalence and associations of symptoms of upper extremities, repetitive strain injuries (RSI), and 'RSI-like condition': a cross-sectional study of bank workers in Northeast Brazil. *BMC Public Health* 2005;**5**:107.

Leon D., Walt G., editors. *Poverty, inequality, and health: an international perspective.* Oxford: Oxford University Press; 2001.

LeResche L. Epidemiological perspectives on sex differences in pain. In: Fillingham B.D, editor. *Sex, gender, and pain*. Seattle (WA): IASP Press; 1999. p. 233–49.

Lockyer L., Bury M. The construction of a modern epidemic: the implications for women of the gendering of coronary heart disease. *Journal of Advanced Nursing* 2002;**39**:432–40.

Lopez A.D., Mathers C.D., Ezzati M. *et al.* Measuring the global burden of disease and risk factors, 1990–2001. In: Lopez AD, Mathers CD, Ezzati M, Jamison DT, Murray CJH, editors. *Global burden of disease and risk factors*. New York (NY): World Bank; Oxford: Oxford University Press; 2006. p. 1–13.

Lorber J. Gender and the construction of illness. London: Sage; 1997.

MacDorman M., Hoyert D., Martin J. *et al.* Fetal and perinatal mortality, United States, 2003. *National Vital Statistics Reports* 2007;**55**(**6**):1–18.

Macintyre S. Inequalities in health: is research gender blind? In: Leon D., Walt G., editors. *Poverty, inequality, and health: an international perspective.* Oxford: Oxford University Press; 2001.

Malterud K., Okkes I. Gender differences in general practice consultations: methodological challenges in epidemiological research. *Family Practice* 1998;**15**:404–10.

Menees S.B., Inadomi J.M., Korsnes S. *et al.* Women patients' preference for women physicians is a barrier to colon cancer screening. *Gastrointestinal Endoscopy* 2005;**62**(**2**):219–23.

National Centre for Social Research (NatCen). *Health survey for England 2003: summary of key findings*. London: National Centre for Social Research; 2003.

National Institute of Allergy and Infectious Diseases. *HIV infection in women*. Rockville (MD): National Institute of Allergy and Infectious Diseases; 2004.

O'Brien Cousins S., Gillis M.M. 'Just do it … before you talk yourself out of it': the self-talk of adults thinking about physical activity. *Psychology of Sport and Exercise* 2005;**6**:313–34.

O'Brien R., Hunt K., Hart G. 'It's caveman stuff, but that is to a certain extent how guys still operate': men's accounts of masculinity and help seeking. *Social Science and Medicine* 2005;**61**:503–16.

Office for National Statistics (ONS). *2001 census data: focus on health*. London: Office for National Statistics; 2006. Available from: http://www.statistics.gov.uk/cci/nugget.asp?id=1325

Office for National Statistics (ONS). *Key health statistics from general practice 1998*. London: Office for National Statistics; 2000.

Office for National Statistics (ONS). *UK 2000 time use survey*. London: Office for National Statistics; 2003.

Payne S. Smoke like a man, die like a man? A review of the relationship between sex, gender, and lung cancer. *Social Science and Medicine* 2001;**53**:1067–80.

Payne S. *The health of men and women*. Cambridge: Polity; 2006.

Perkins K. Smoking cessation in women: special considerations. *CNS Drugs* 2001;**15**:391–411.

Ravindran T.K.S. Engendering health. Seminar 489: *Unhealthy trends (a symposium on the state of our public health system)*; 2000 May. Available from: http://www.india-seminar.com/2000/489/489%20ravindran.htm

Redgrave G.W., Swartz K.L., Romanoski A.J. Alcohol misuse by women. *International Review of Psychiatry* 2003;**15**:256–68.

Ruiz M.T., Verbrugge L.M. A two-way view of gender bias in medicine. *Epidemiology and Community Health* 1997;**51**:106–9.

Samet J., Yoon S-Y. Women and the tobacco epidemic: challenges for the 21st century. Geneva: World Health Organization; 2001.

Schiller J., Bernadel L. *Summary health statistics for the US population: national health interview survey*. Washington (DC): National Centre for Health Statistics; 2004. Washington Vital Health Stat Series 10 Number 22.

Sen K., Bonita R. Global health status: two steps forward, one step back. *Lancet* 2000;**356**:577–82.

Shields P. Molecular epidemiology of smoking and lung cancer. *Oncogene* 2002;**21**:6870–6.

Standing H. Understanding the links between energy, poverty, and gender. *Boiling Point* 2002;**48**:11. Available from: http://practicalaction.org/docs/energy/docs48/bp48_pp11.pdf

Steinemetz K.A., Potter J.D. Vegetables, fruit, and cancer. I. Epidemiology. *Cancer Causes and Control* 1991;**2**:325–57.

Stibbe A. Health and the social construction of masculinity in men's health magazine. *Men and Masculinities* 2004;**7**:31–51.

Tanner M., Vlassoff C. Treatment-seeking behaviour for malaria: a typology based on endemicity and gender. *Social Science and Medicine* 1998;**46**:523–32.

Thune I., Furberg A. Physical activity and cancer risk: dose-response and cancer, all sites and site-specific. *Medicine and Science in Sports and Exercise* 2001;**33**:S530–50.

UNAIDS. *AIDS epidemic update*. Geneva: World Health Organization, UNAIDS; 2006.

Vidaver R., Lafleur B., Tong C. *et al.* Women subjects in NIH-funded clinical research literature: lack of progress in both representation and analysis by sex. *Journal of Women's Health and Gender-based Medicine* 2000;**9**:495–504.

Waldron I., McCloskey C., Earle I. Trends in gender differences in accidents mortality. *Demographic Research* 2005;**13**:415–54.

Waldron I. What do we know about the causes of sex differences in mortality? *Population Bulletin of United Nations* 1985;**18**:59–76.

Wizeman T., Pardue M. *Exploring the biological contributions to health: does sex matter?* Washington (DC): National Academy Press; 2001.

World Health Organisation *WHOSIS World Health Organisation Health Statistics and Information System* Geneva at: http://www.who.int/whosis/database/core/core_select.cfm

World Health Organization. *Gender, health, and ageing*. Geneva: World Health Organization; 2003a.

World Health Organization. *Global status report on alcohol*. Geneva: World Health Organization; 2004a.

World Health Organization. *Investing in mental health*. Geneva: World Health Organization; 2003b.

World Health Organization. *Myths about physical activity*. Geneva: World Health Organization; 2002a.

World Health Organization. *Tobacco atlas*. Geneva: World Health Organization; 2002b.

World Health Organization. *World health report 2004: changing history*. Geneva: World Health Organization; 2004b.

World Health Organization. *World health report 2005: make every mother and child count*. Geneva: World Health Organization; 2005b.

World Health Organization. *World health report 2006: working together for health*. Geneva: World Health Organization; 2006.

World Health Organization. *World health survey 2005.* Geneva: World Health Organization; 2005. Available from: http://www.who.int/healthinfo/survey/en

World Health Organization. *World malaria report 2005*. Geneva: World Health Organization; 2005a.

World Health Organization. *World mortality database: tables*. Geneva: World Health Organization. Available from: http://www.who.int/healthinfo/morttables/en/index.html

World Health Organization. *World report on violence and health*. Geneva: World Health Organization; 2003c.

World Health Organization. *World report on violence and health*. Geneva: World Health Organization; 2002c.

Yunus M. Gender differences in fibromyalgia and other related syndromes. *Journal of Gender Specific Medicine* 2002;**5**:42–7.

Zaninotto P., Wardle H., Stamatakis E. *et al. Forecasting obesity to 2010*. London: Department of Health; 2006.

11.3

Child health

Elizabeth Mason, Olivier Fontaine, Bernadette Daelmans, Rajiv Bahl, Cynthia Boschi-Pinto, and Jose Martines

Abstract

This chapter focuses on the health status of children, particularly those less than five years of age—the main health risks faced by this age group and the interventions that promote their survival, growth, and development.

The under-five mortality rate (U5MR) is one of the most sensitive indicators of the socioeconomic status and well-being of a society, and has been chosen to monitor the global and national achievements of the Millennium Development Goal (MDG) 4 of reducing, between 1990 and 2015, the under-five mortality rate by two-thirds. The Global U5MR burden remains unacceptably high. Moreover, progress in reducing under-five mortality is not equally distributed across countries and regions. Poverty and its consequences are directly or indirectly associated with most of the poor outcomes in child health.

Most children suffer and die from a small number of conditions—the main causes of morbidity being highly correlated with the major causes of death. Likewise, child growth, nutritional status, and development are intertwined. Strikingly, even in the poorest settings, a significant proportion of these outcomes could be prevented with a few interventions that are well-known, feasible, deliverable without complex technology, and affordable. These interventions are in the following areas: Essential newborn care and case management of newborn illness, infant and young child feeding and case management of malnutrition, and the prevention and management of diarrhoea, pneumonia, malaria and HIV infection.

Strengthening the health system and integrating the interventions into packages of care that can be delivered at all levels during pregnancy, childbirth, neonatal period, and childhood—from home to hospital—will be key to increasing the coverage of health interventions. Achievement of the MDG of reducing child mortality will require significant acceleration in investments on child survival.

The situation of children in the world

The Convention of the Rights of the Child defines children as, 'all persons below the age of 18 years, unless under the law applicable to the child, majority is attained earlier'. The life-course approach to health care recognizes the continuum from birth through childhood, adolescence, and adulthood, reflecting the principle that care provided to children at birth, or even before it occurs, will affect their immediate well-being and will also have an impact on their health and development in later years (Fig. 11.3.1).

In the life-course approach, the period of life before attaining adulthood is divided into three age subgroups based on epidemiology and health-care needs: The first five years (under-five children), the next five years (older children), and the second decade of life (adolescents). The first five years of life are further subdivided into neonatal period, infancy, and preschool years.

This chapter focuses on the health of under-five children and touches upon the health of older children. Chapter 11.4 deals with adolescent health. The most important indicators of the health status of the under five relate to their mortality, morbidity, growth, and development.

Mortality in under-five children

The U5MR and infant mortality rate are broadly recognized as two of the most sensitive indicators of a country's socioeconomic situation and quality of life. The 1980s saw an acceleration of large-scale health programmes focused on immunization, control of diarrhoeal diseases, acute respiratory infections (ARIs), and nutrition in low- and middle-income countries, with an associated decline in U5MR. However, the progress has slowed down since the 1990s. During the first five years of the twenty-first century, the decline in U5MR was 17 per cent, from 94 per 1000 live births in the year 2000 to 78 per 1000 live births in 2004 (analysis based on the WHO mortality database (World Health Organization), available on request). The result is that about 9.7 million children less than five years of age continue to die in a year (World Health Organization 2005b). This figure corresponds to more than two-fold the number of all individuals dying in the same period from HIV infection or AIDS and tuberculosis combined.

When are under-five deaths occurring?

The risk of death is the highest closest to birth and then decreases over the subsequent days, months, and years. Almost 4 million of the 9.7 million under-five deaths occur in the first 28 days after birth, 3.3 million deaths occur in the following 11 months, and roughly the same number happen over the next four years (World Health Organization 2005b). Analysis of data from 39 demographic and health surveys (DHSs) shows that within the first month of life, about

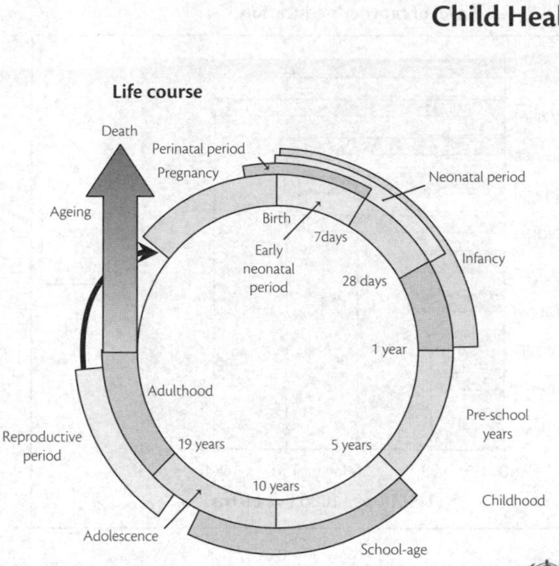

Age subgroups as defined by the World Health Organization

Terminology	Definition/Interval*
Under-five	***0–4 years***
Neonatal period	0–27 days
Early neonatal period	0–6 days
Post-neonatal period	28 days to 11 months
Infancy	0–11 months
Preschool	1–4 years
Older child	***5–9 years***
Adolescent	***10–19 years***

** The upper limit of the interval refers to completed days, months, or years.*

World Health Organization

Fig. 11.3.1 The life course and respective age subgroups.
Source: Adapted from World Health Organization. *Strategic directions for improving the health and development of children and adolescents.* Geneva: World Health Organization; 2002. WHO/FCH/CAH/02.21. Available from: http://www.who.int/child-adolescent-health/publications/OVERVIEW/CAH_Strategy.htm.

27 per cent of deaths occur on the day of birth, 45 per cent during days 0 and 1, and more than 70 per cent in the first week of life.

Where and why are under-five deaths occurring?

About three-quarters of all under-five deaths are clustered in just two regions of the world: Africa and Southeast Asia (Fig. 11.3.2). Although Africa has only about 20 per cent of the world's population, it accounts for 45 per cent of the global under-five deaths; in contrast, only 2 per cent of under-five deaths take place in the European region and 4 per cent in the region of the Americas. Similarly, most neonatal deaths occur in Africa and Southeast Asia, with about 30 per cent of all neonatal deaths in the African region and about 35 per cent in the Southeast Asian region. It is noteworthy that 90 per cent of the under-five deaths take place in just 40 countries, and even more striking is the fact that 50 per cent of all these deaths are concentrated in six countries: India, Nigeria, China, Democratic Republic of Congo (DRC), Ethiopia, and Pakistan.

Although the absolute number of deaths provides important information regarding the global magnitude of the problem, it does not take into account the size of the population at risk, and hence, it does not reflect the risk of death. For instance, although China is ranked third in the absolute number of under-five deaths, its under-five mortality rate is about 30 per 1000 live births, compared with several countries that have rates above 200 per 1000 (Afghanistan, Angola, Burkina Faso, DRC, Guinea-Bissau, Liberia, Mali, Niger, Sierra Leone, and Somalia).

Beyond inter-country inequities, further critical inequities are present within countries, where children from the poorest families living in rural areas and whose mothers are less educated are those more likely to die. Data from the DHSs, nationally representative household surveys with large sample sizes (usually between 5000 and 30 000 households), have been used in Fig. 11.3.3 to illustrate these important equity differentials within countries.

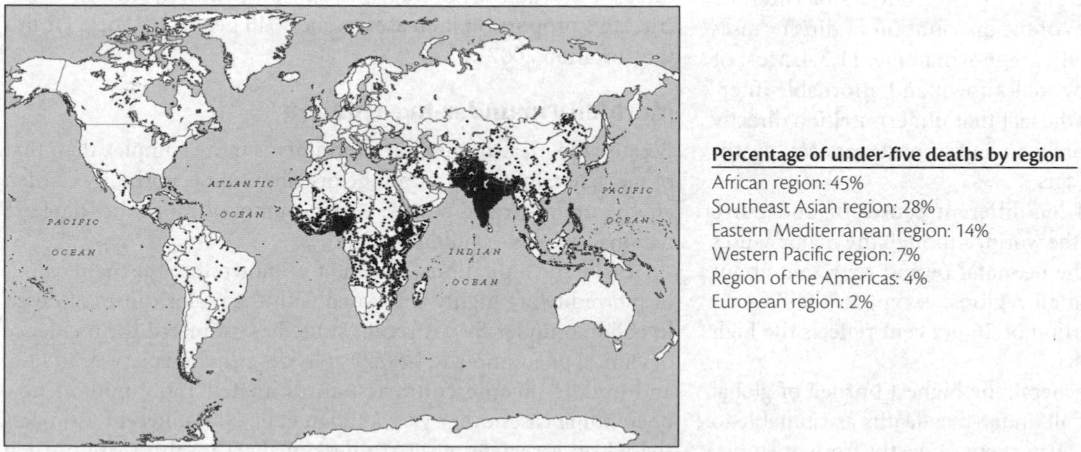

Fig. 11.3.2 World distribution of under-five deaths—each dot represents 5000 deaths. (From Black RE, Morris SS, Bryce J. Where and why are 10 million children dying every year? *Lancet* 2003;**361**:2226–34. Reprinted with permission from Elsevier.)

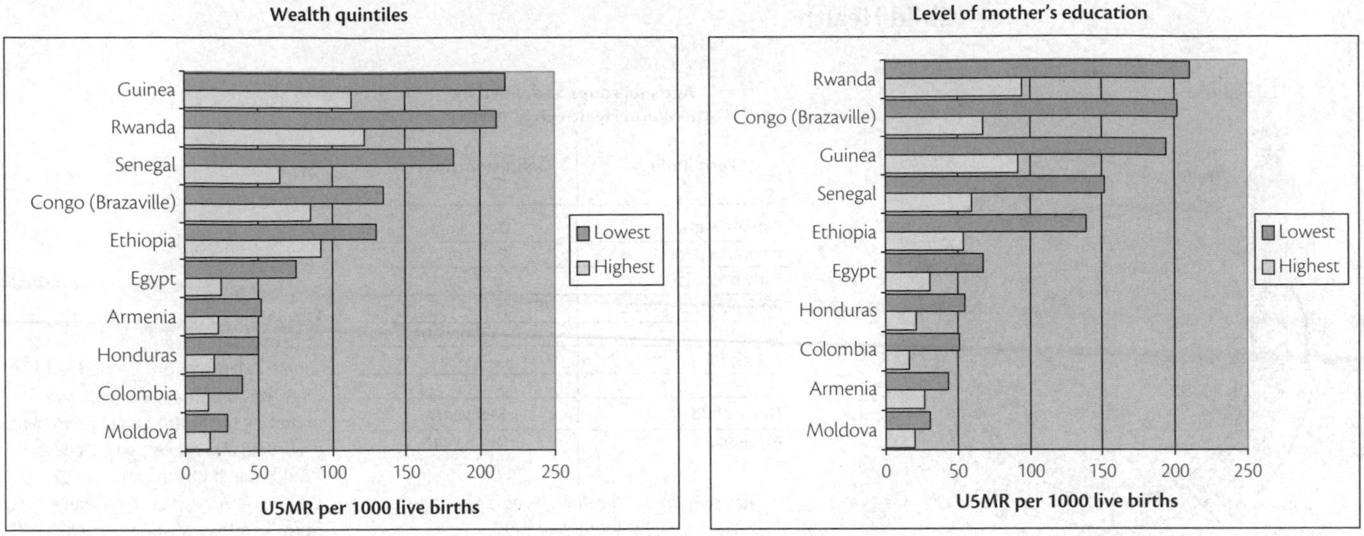

Fig. 11.3.3 Inequities in under-five mortality according to wealth and level of mother's education.
Source: Institut National de la Statistique du Rwanda (INSR), ORC Macro. *Rwanda demographic and health survey 2005.* Calverton (MD): Institut National de la Statistique du Rwanda, ORC Macro; 2006; Ndiaye S, Mohamed A. *Enquête Démographique et de Santé au Sénégal 2005.* Calverton (MD): Sénégal Centre de Recherche pour le Développement Humain, ORC Macro; 2006; National Institute of Public Health, National Institute of Statistics, ORC Macro. *Cambodia demographic and health survey 2005.* Phnom Penh, Cambodia, Calverton (MD): National Institute of Public Health, National Institute of Statistics, ORC Macro; 2006; National Institute of Population Research and Training (NIPORT), Mitra and Associates, ORC Macro. *Bangladesh demographic and health survey 2004.* Dhaka, Bangladesh: National Institute of Population Research and Training; 2005; Moroc Ministère de la Santé, ORC Macro, Ligue des États Arabes. *Enquête sur la population et la santé familiale (EPSF) 2003-4.* Calverton (MD): Ministère de la Santé, ORC Macro; 2005; Badan Pusat Statistik-Statistics Indonesia (BPS), ORC Macro. *Indonesia demographic and health survey 2002-3.* Calverton (MD): Badan Pusat Statistik-Statistics Indonesia (BPS), ORC Macro; 2003; El-Zanaty F, Way A. *Egypt demographic and health survey 2005.* Cairo, Egypt: Ministry of Health and Population, National Population Council, El-Zanaty and Associates, ORC Macro; 2006; National Statistics Office (NSO), ORC Macro. *National demographic and health survey 2003.* Calverton (MD): National Statistics Office (Philippines), ORC Macro; 2004; National Statistical Service, Ministry of Health, ORC Macro. *Armenia demographic and health survey 2005.* Calverton (MD): National Statistical Service, Armenian Ministry of Health, ORC Macro; 2006; Secretaría de Salud (SS), Instituto Nacional de Estadística (INE), Macro Internacional. *Encuesta nacional de salud y demografía 2005-6.* Tegucigalpa, Honduras, Calverton (MD): Secretaría de Salud, Instituto Nacional de Estadística, Macro International; 2006; National Scientific and Applied Center for Preventive Medicine (NCPM), ORC Macro. *Moldova demographic and health survey 2005.* Calverton (MD): National Scientific and Applied Center for Preventive Medicine, Moldova Ministry of Health and Social Protection, ORC Macro; 2006.

What are neonates and children dying from?

Poverty, low levels of maternal education, and poor quality health care are underlying determinants of most under-five deaths. However, most neonates and children eventually die from only a small number of disease conditions. Estimates of the distribution of direct causes of neonatal and under-five deaths are shown in Fig. 11.3.4. Most of these deaths are preventable by well-known and affordable interventions. Equally important is the fact that undernutrition directly or indirectly contributes to more than half of post-neonatal deaths in children under five years of age.

The relative importance of the different causes of under-five deaths varies across regions of the world, although the major causes remain the same. Deaths in the neonatal period represent about 45 per cent of child deaths in all regions, except in the African region where the lower proportion of 26 per cent reflects the high number of post-neonatal deaths.

The African region has, in general, the highest burden of global child mortality: 90 per cent of all under-five deaths attributable to malaria and to HIV and AIDS, 50 per cent of deaths from pneumonia, and 40 per cent of deaths from diarrhoea (World Health Organization 2005b). However, within the African region, the distribution of the burden of mortality attributable to HIV and to malaria differs substantially across countries. For example, in East African countries, HIV and AIDS contribute to 15 per cent of the under-five deaths on average, whereas in Southern African countries, this proportion increases to about 40 per cent (World Health Organization 2007).

Morbidity in under-five children

Because the measurement of morbidity is more complex than that of mortality, information on the distribution of morbidity burden among under-fives is scarce. Usual sources of morbidity data are national surveys or published studies.

Despite the limitations of data, it is known that the main causes of morbidity are highly correlated with the major causes of death in children under five. A recent study has estimated the incidence of clinical pneumonia to be 0.29 episodes per child per year in low- and middle-income countries, an estimated 150.7 million new pneumonia cases every year (Rudan *et al.* 2004). Recent estimates (based on a review of 27 studies) of diarrhoeal disease burden show a median of 3.2 episodes per child per year, with the highest incidence recorded in the African region (Kosek *et al.* 2003).

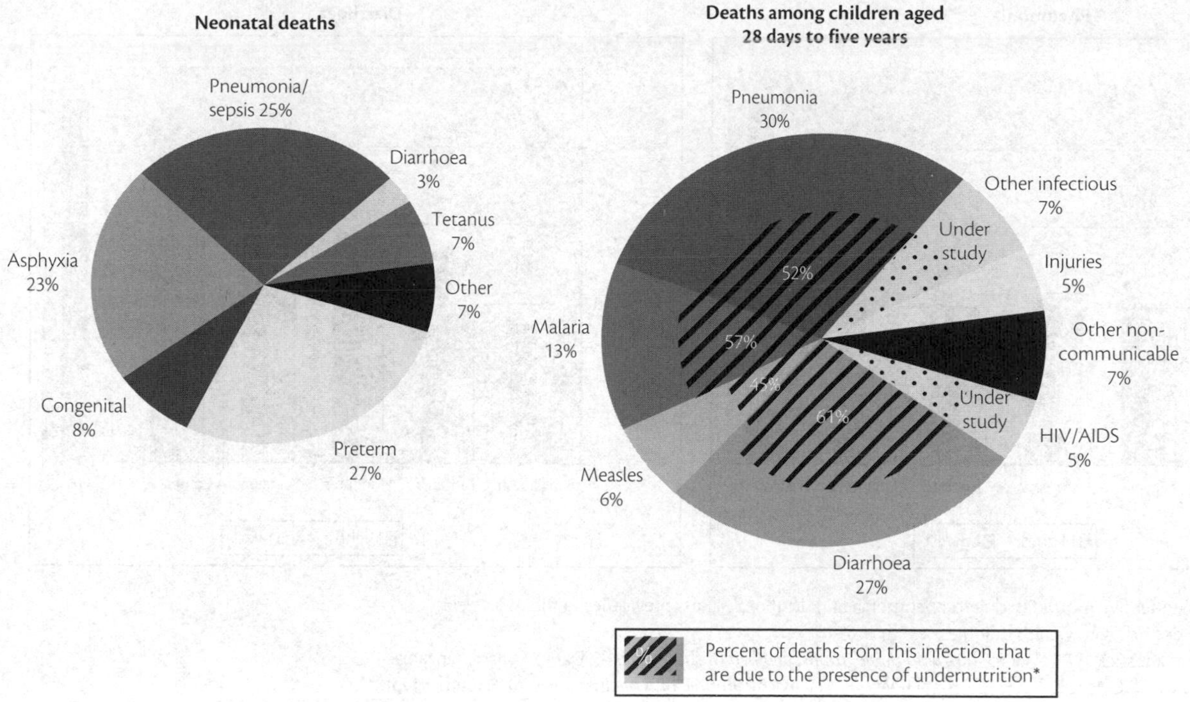

Fig. 11.3.4 Distribution of the main causes of death among neonates and children aged 28 days to 5 years in the year 2000.
Sources: World Health Organization (WHO 2005b), Caulfield *et al.* (2003).
* Recent estimates published by Black *et al.* (2008) indicate that nutrition-related factors are responsible for about 35% of all under-five deaths, but recent estimates of nutrition-related deaths by cause are not yet available.

An important consequence of persistently high rates of diarrhoea morbidity is a negative effect on child growth and development.

For both pneumonia and diarrhoeal diseases, morbidity rates are consistently higher in the first year of life, gradually decreasing from the second to the fifth year. The prevalence of pneumonia and diarrhoea can be more than twice as high among the poorest children as among the richest ones. Poor children are usually more exposed to health risks and less resistant to disease. Differences within and between countries are illustrated in Fig. 11.3.5.

Nutritional status of under-five children

Low weight at birth can be either the result of a birth that occurred too early (before 37 weeks of gestation) or of restricted growth during gestation. Low birth weight (LBW) is closely associated with increased risks of neonatal morbidity and mortality, cognitive problems, and chronic diseases during later periods in life. Every year, more than 20 million babies are born with LBW worldwide, the largest number of them in Africa and Southeast Asia (United Nations Children's Fund, World Health Organization 2004).

The nutritional status of under-five children is usually assessed through three standard indicators: Stunting, wasting, and underweight. A stunted child is a child who is too short for his or her age. Stunting is usually a result of chronic undernutrition or nutritional deprivation over a lengthy period of time. A child is considered wasted when the weight is too little for the child's height. Wasting usually reflects an acute nutritional deficiency, because of reduced food consumption or acute weight loss during an illness. Finally, a child is said to be underweight if his or her weight is too low for his or her age. This can be a result of stunting, wasting, or both.

It is estimated that 30 per cent of under-five children in the world are moderately or severely stunted, 9 per cent are moderately or severely wasted, and 25 per cent are underweight. In sub-Saharan Africa, these proportions are 37 per cent, 9 per cent, and 28 per cent, respectively (United Nations Children's Fund 2006). Poor nutritional status of a child is strongly correlated to his or her vulnerability to diseases, to delayed physical and mental development, and to an increased risk of mortality. As described for morbidity and mortality, underweight is usually associated with fewer years of mother's education and low levels in other indicators of well-being.

Development status of under-five children

The same biomedical risk factors, such as malnutrition and exposure to infectious diseases and to environmental contaminants, that threaten the survival of young children living in poverty in low- and middle-income countries also threaten their cognitive, motor, and socio-emotional development.

Currently, no global data on the status of early child development are available. Given the strong association of poor development with chronic growth retardation and poverty, to estimate the number of young children who are at risk for deficits in early development, country-level data on childhood chronic growth retardation (stunting, defined as length-for-age $< -2SD$) and living in absolute poverty (family income of less than US$1 per day) have been used to estimate the number of young who are at risk for deficits in early development (Grantham-McGregor *et al.* 2007). This estimate indicates that there are over 219 million, or 39 per cent of all children under five years of age, who are not fulfilling their developmental potential. Most of these children (89 million) live in South Asia. Ten countries (Bangladesh, China, DRC, Ethiopia,

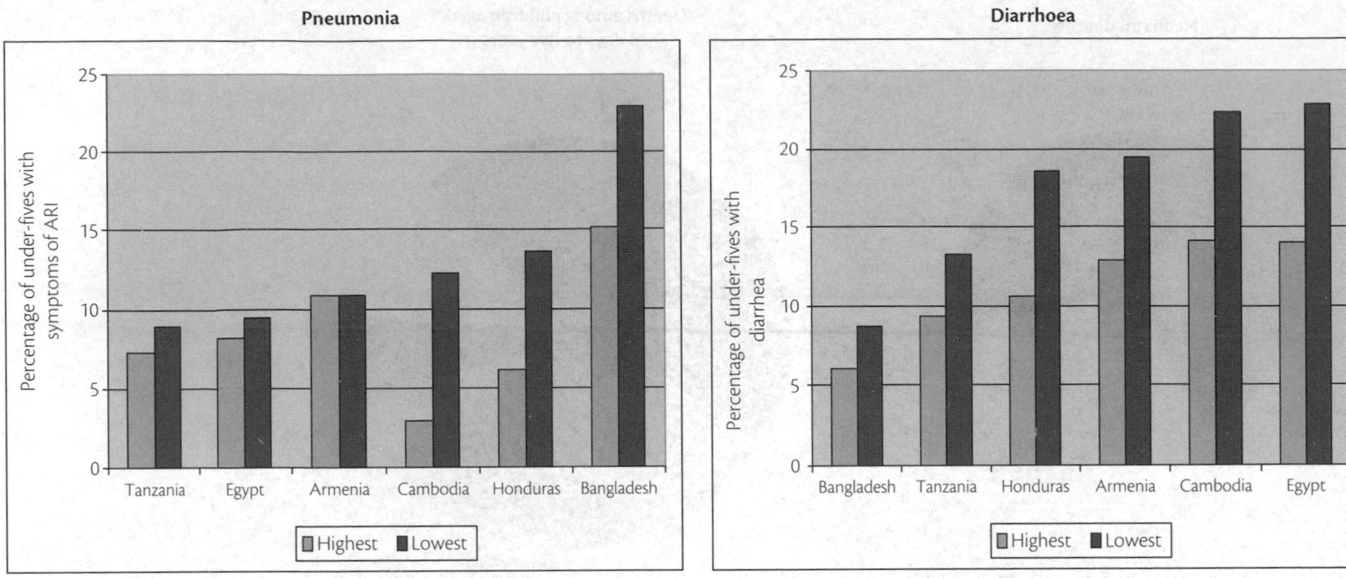

Fig. 11.3.5 Inequities in under-five morbidity due to pneumonia and diarrhoea (illness prevalence in the two weeks preceding the interview), according to wealth quintiles.
Source: National Bureau of Statistics, ORC Macro. *Tanzania demographic and health survey 2004-5*. Dar es Salaam, Tanzania: National Bureau of Statistics, ORC Macro; 2005; El-Zanaty F, Way A. *Egypt demographic and health survey 2005*. Cairo, Egypt: Ministry of Health and Population, National Population Council, El-Zanaty and Associates, ORC Macro; 2006; National Statistical Service, Ministry of Health, ORC Macro. *Armenia demographic and health survey 2005*. Calverton (MD): National Statistical Service, Armenian Ministry of Health, ORC Macro; 2006; National Institute of Public Health, National Institute of Statistics, ORC Macro. Cambodia demographic and health survey 2005. Phnom Penh, Cambodia, Calverton (MD): National Institute of Public Health, National Institute of Statistics, ORC Macro; 2006; Secretaría de Salud (SS), Instituto Nacional de Estadística (INE), Macro Internacional. *Encuesta nacional de salud y demografía 2005-6*. Tegucigalpa, Honduras, Calverton (MD): Secretaría de Salud, Instituto Nacional de Estadística, Macro International; 2006; National Institute of Population Research and Training (NIPORT), Mitra and Associates, ORC Macro. *Bangladesh demographic and health survey 2004*. Dhaka, Bangladesh: National Institute of Population Research and Training; 2005.

India, Indonesia, Nigeria, Pakistan, Tanzania, and Uganda) account for 145 million (66 per cent) of these 219 million disadvantaged children in the developing world (Grantham-McGregor *et al.* 2007).

Health status of the older child (children 5–9 years)

There is a considerably greater gap in knowledge of the epidemiology of health conditions and evidence for interventions for this age group as compared to under-five children. Although these children have survived the critical period of 0–59 months, when most deaths occur, many carry with them the consequences of a number of conditions suffered during their earlier years. Moreover, they are still exposed to additional health hazards during the 5–9 year period. Some of the main health problems related to this age group are as follows:

Poor growth and nutrition: Although the risk of acute clinical malnutrition is lower at this age, the accumulated consequences of poor diet and growth may significantly affect the school performance of these children.

Communicable diseases: Communicable diseases lead to considerable morbidity in this age group and, in some cases, to long-term disability. Major diseases that contribute to mortality and disability at this age are ARIs, diarrhoea, malaria, and tuberculosis, as well as nutritional deficiencies, particularly iron-deficiency anaemia.

Accidents, injuries, and violence: The older child has a higher risk of accidents, injuries, and violence than younger age groups. Children 5–9 years of age are primarily affected by poisoning, drowning, burns, and maltreatment by caregivers. Intentional injuries resulting from child maltreatment are associated with physical and cognitive deficits. Poor children, who commonly live in unsafe environments, are exposed to risks that increase their likelihood of being injured. Subgroups particularly at risk include those suffering abuse, exploitive labour, and also, street and orphaned children. Injury rates and patterns differ from country to country and from urban to rural areas. For example, in rural areas, injuries are related mainly to farming activities, pesticide poisoning, and drowning. In urban areas, most injuries in small children are traffic-related, linked to gadgets and electrical appliances, or to falls or poisonings resulting from the ingestion of household chemicals and pharmaceuticals.

Other conditions: Other main issues and conditions related to this age group are blood disorders, cardiac and respiratory diseases such as asthma and rheumatic cardiac disease, skin problems, and sensory and neurological diseases or impairment.

Child health in higher-income countries

The World Bank classifies countries into income group according to their growth national income (GNI) per capita. High-income countries (HIC) are those with a GNI per capita of US$10 726 or more (World Bank 2007), and account for approximately 10 per cent of the world under-five population and to less than 1 per cent of under-five deaths. In general, children living in the 56 countries in this group have the lowest U5MR (average of 7 per 1000 live births) and benefit from better health and development than children elsewhere.

Upper-to-middle-income economies include 40 countries that have a GNI per capita between US$3466 and US$10 725 (World Bank 2007). These countries have been experiencing a transition in child health epidemiology—transformation of the patterns of diseases and/or causes of death. These changes require prompt adjustments in national programmes and strategies to conform to the emerging new epidemiological profile.

Main challenges

The so-called 'epidemiological transition' has a complex and dynamic course and reflects the changes in various domains such as demographic, socioeconomic, cultural, biological, technological, and environmental factors. A major recent factor that has caused important changes in child health and survival patterns in high- and upper-middle-income economies was the emergence of HIV infection.

The beginning of HIV epidemics in Western European countries resulted in a threateningly large number of paediatric infections. Once interventions to prevent mother-to-child transmission became available, there was an impressive reduction in the transmission rates, which decreased from an initial level of 15–20 per cent to 2 per cent or less in more recent years. Nowadays, the HIV epidemics among infants in Western Europe can be considered mostly controlled, with only 149 reported cases of new infections among infants and young children in 2002 (World Health Organization 2004d).

However, Eastern Europe witnessed a dramatically growing rate of HIV infection over the same period. Following the collapse of the USSR, there was a large increase in injectable drug use and in the number of new HIV infections. Although there was an average decrease of more than 45 per cent in mother-to-child transmission in Western and Central European countries from 2002 to 2005, Eastern European countries faced an increase of 453 per cent during the same period. In the Russian Federation, for example, the number of infants born to HIV-positive mothers increased from 81 in 1998 to 2777 in 2002 (Euro HIV 2006).

Another example of the changing profile is illustrated by the increasing prevalence of overweight or obesity in high- and low-income countries. The number of children affected by these disorders continues to rise at an alarming rate. The current prevalence of childhood obesity is ten times higher than it was in the 1970s. In several countries of Western Europe, such as Greece, Malta, Spain, Sweden, and the United Kingdom, the prevalence of overweight children reached more than 15 per cent in 2002. Childhood obesity is associated with the premature burden of non-communicable diseases such as diabetes and cardiovascular disorder (World Health Organization 2005a).

The major challenge that wealthier nations face is the increasing socioeconomic inequities within their societies. Income inequalities are associated with poorer health and higher child mortality, regardless of the country's level of development. Gaps between and within countries have been widening in the last decade. Sometimes, differences between subgroups of the population within countries are so remarkable that these differences can constitute a contributory factor to social instability (United Nations Children's Fund 2005).

In a recent study, Collison *et al.* (2007) investigated the relationship between under-five mortality and income inequalities among the 24 countries that comprise the Organization for Economic Co-operation and Development (OECD). Most of these countries have achieved near-universal basic health care and education for children. Nevertheless, the investigators found a strongly significant association between the two variables examined. A recent review found an increase in the percentage of children living in relative poverty (households with income below 50 per cent of the national median income) in these same OECD countries in the last decade (United Nations Children's Fund 2005). According to this review, the proportion of children living below national poverty lines was lowest in the Scandinavian countries (2–4 per cent), ranged between 10 and 15 per cent in Australia, Austria, Canada, Greece, Germany, Japan, Netherlands, Spain, and the United Kingdom, and was as high as 22 per cent in the United States.

The impact of such inequities goes beyond child mortality and is likely to affect every stage of childhood development. For example, (1) overweight is more prevalent in children from lower income settings of industrialized countries than in those from higher income groups; (2) children from poor families are more likely to suffer injuries from road accidents or in the home than those from better-off families; (3) poor growth patterns are present in lower income groups in the United Kingdom; (4) poverty is closely associated with harmful environmental factors such as exposure to lead, poor housing, poor air quality, and undernutrition; and (5) there is strong evidence that poor diet, smoking, alcohol use, and lack of physical activity are all associated with lower socioeconomic conditions (World Health Organization 2004d).

Effective interventions for addressing major causes of child deaths

It is estimated that more than 60 per cent of under-five deaths can be prevented with universal coverage of a small set of known, effective interventions that do not require expensive technology (Jones *et al.* 2003). These interventions are reviewed in the following text for each of the major causes of under-five mortality and summarized in Table 11.3.1.

Newborn conditions

Improving newborn health and survival requires a continuum of care (World Health Organization 2005b) from pregnancy, childbirth, and the newborn period, into childhood and adolescence. Newborn health interventions can be classified into those relevant for all mothers and newborns, and those relevant only for newborns with conditions that require additional care.

Care for all mothers and newborns

The health and well-being of women and their children are closely associated with the education, nutrition, and health care they receive throughout the life cycle. Newborn health and survival requires empowerment (particularly of girls and women) and health promotion throughout life, which includes nutrition and education, prevention of harmful practices such as female genital mutilation, delay in sexual debut, prevention and treatment of sexually transmitted infections, and support for optimal timing and spacing of pregnancies.

Table 11.3.1 Summary of key interventions to address major causes of child deaths

Important causes of under-five mortality	Preventive interventions	Case management interventions
Newborn conditions	◆ Antenatal care ◆ Skilled care during labour and birth ◆ Care at the time of birth (warmth, resuscitation, cord care, and early initiation of breastfeeding) ◆ Care during the first days and weeks after birth (exclusive breastfeeding, warmth, hygienic skin and cord care, and prompt care-seeking for illness)	◆ Additional care of LBW infants (particularly feeding and warmth) ◆ Treatment of local eye, skin, and umbilical infections ◆ Treatment of neonatal sepsis
Diarrhoea	◆ Exclusive breastfeeding up to 6 months; continued breastfeeding with safe and appropriate complementary feeding at least up to 2 years ◆ Immunization against measles, rotavirus (candidates being evaluated in efficacy trials), and shigella (under development) ◆ Water and sanitation, hand washing	◆ Oral rehydration therapy, including use of the new low-osmolarity ORS ◆ Zinc for 10–14 days during diarrhoea ◆ Antibiotics for dysentery and cholera ◆ Continued feeding during diarrhoea
Pneumonia	◆ Immunization against measles, diphtheria, tetanus, and pertussis, *Haemophilus influenzae*, and pneumococcus ◆ Exclusive breastfeeding up to 6 months; continued breastfeeding with safe and appropriate complementary feeding at least up to 2 years ◆ *Pneumocystis jiroveci* pneumonia prophylaxis in HIV-exposed and HIV-infected infants ◆ Reduction in environmental risk factors—e.g. indoor air pollution	◆ Treatment of non-severe pneumonia with oral co-trimoxazole or amoxicillin ◆ Treatment of severe pneumonia with parenteral antibiotics, and oxygen and other supportive treatment
Malaria	◆ Vector control ◆ Use of ITNs	◆ Treatment of non-severe malaria with an oral antimalarial recommended for the area ◆ Treatment of severe malaria
HIV/AIDS	◆ Primary prevention of HIV and of unintended pregnancies in HIV-infected women ◆ Antiretrovirals—treatment of pregnant women when indicated, prophylaxis for others ◆ Safer infant feeding options—exclusive breastfeeding for 6 months if replacement feeding is not acceptable, feasible, affordable, sustainable, and safe; otherwise replacement feeding	◆ Co-trimoxazole prophylaxis for HIV-exposed and HIV-infected children ◆ ART for children who are eligible for it
Malnutrition	◆ Early initiation of breastfeeding ◆ Exclusive breastfeeding up to 6 months of age ◆ Continued breastfeeding with safe and appropriate complementary foods up to at least 2 years ◆ Preventing vitamin A, iron, iodine, and zinc deficiency through supplementation, food fortification, or dietary diversification	◆ Community-based management of children with severe malnutrition without complications ◆ Hospital management of children with severe malnutrition with complications

Care during pregnancy is important for newborn survival. Antenatal care provides a platform to promote healthy lifestyles, including hygiene, nutrition, and family planning, and for integrating programmes that address malnutrition, HIV and AIDS, sexually transmitted infections, malaria, and tuberculosis. Interventions of proven benefit for newborn health provided during antenatal care include tetanus immunization, screening for and treatment of syphilis and HIV, and prevention and treatment of malaria. Antenatal care provides the basis for continued care during and after childbirth by planning for birth with a skilled attendant and preparing for unforeseen complications, and by helping the family prepare for good mother and newborn care practices, such as early initiation of and exclusive breastfeeding.

Box 11.3.1 Basic newborn care at the time of birth and in the days and weeks after birth

Care at the time of birth

- Birth in a warm room
- Resuscitation, if required
- Drying the baby thoroughly immediately after birth
- Keeping the baby in skin-to-skin contact with the mother
- Hygienic cord care
- Eye care
- Early initiation of breastfeeding as soon as the mother and the baby are ready (usually within the first hour of birth)

Care during the first days and weeks

- Initiation of breastfeeding, if not already initiated
- Exclusive breastfeeding
- Keeping the newborn warm
- Hygienic cord and eye care
- Vaccination
- Prompt recognition of danger signs (not feeding well, reduced activity, fast or difficult breathing, fever or low body temperature, or convulsions) and care seeking by the family

Skilled care at childbirth is needed for all women and babies without exception because the complications that may occur during and immediately following childbirth (for both mothers and babies) cannot be predicted and may very rapidly become fatal. This means that skilled childbirth care in first-level health facilities, with the backup of a hospital that can manage complications, should be available 24 hours a day, every day. For a home birth, it is crucial to have access to a skilled attendant and a companion who can stay with the mother and baby for the first 12–24 hours. For a woman and her family who cannot have access to a skilled attendant in a home birth, it is essential to ensure that they have knowledge of maternal and newborn danger signs (*see* Box 11.3.1), and a plan for a clean delivery and early care-seeking if problems arise.

Care for all newborns at the time of birth and during the days and weeks that follow includes several relatively simple and effective interventions that do not require advanced technology (Box 11.3.1). The most critical time to deliver these interventions is immediately after birth. Also important are the first 12–24 hours after birth, the period during which a large proportion of maternal and neonatal deaths occur (World Health Organization 2006c). Thereafter, at least one additional contact with a health provider within the first week, preferably on the second or third day of life, is required.

Management and care of newborn conditions

Additional care of LBW infants is critical for improving newborn survival because 60–80 per cent of neonatal deaths occur in these infants. Identification of LBW infants within the first hours after birth should be a part of the basic newborn-care package. In settings where birth weight measurement is not feasible, such as for home births, all newborns perceived to be 'small' should receive additional care.

In addition to basic newborn care, LBW infants need more attention for warmth, feeding, hygiene, early detection of infections, and growth monitoring. Kangaroo mother care or skin-to-skin care is the best way to keep them warm and to encourage breastfeeding. Mothers who cannot breastfeed directly should be taught to express breast milk and to feed from a cup. Much of this additional care can be provided at home and in first-level health facilities. However, care for babies weighing less than 1500 g, who may not be able to feed, or for a baby with any danger sign is best provided in a hospital. It is recommended that LBW infants have more contacts with health providers than envisaged for newborns who are not LBW. These may include one additional contact in the first week and weekly contacts thereafter until the infant is feeding and growing well.

Management of newborn illness in a prompt and appropriate manner can reduce neonatal mortality by about half. Community- and health-facility-based activities to support families in identifying the danger signs and seeking timely and appropriate care are therefore very important. The first step in the WHO Integrated Management of Childhood Illness (IMCI) for 0–2 month old infants is the assessment and classification for severe disease (World Health Organization 2006b). The next step is the assessment and treatment of eye, skin, and umbilical infections, diarrhoea, and feeding problems. The last step is giving advice on home care for sick newborns, including advice on feeding, keeping the young infant warm, and when to return. Newborns with severe disease (including those who have suffered from severe birth asphyxia, are very premature or have very LBW, or who have a severe infection), who require referral, should receive intravenous fluids or alternative feeding methods and other supportive therapy such as oxygen and parenteral antibiotics in a hospital.

Diarrhoea

Diarrhoea remains a leading cause of death in under-five children in low- and middle-income countries. Strategies for the control of diarrhoeal diseases have remained substantially unchanged since the initiation of the Diarrhoeal Diseases Control Programme in the early 1980s (Jamison *et al.* 2006).

Prevention

Exclusive breastfeeding, which means that no food or drink (not even water) other than breast milk (with the exception of vitamin and mineral supplements or necessary medicines), is recommended for the first six months of life. A review of studies shows that breastfed children under six months of age are 6.1 times less likely to die of diarrhoea than non-breastfed infants (World Health Organization 2004b). Exclusive breastfeeding protects infants from diarrhoeal disease because breast milk contains both immune and non-immune antimicrobial factors, and because exclusive breastfeeding eliminates the intake of potentially contaminated food and water.

Sequential diarrhoeal disease leads to a vicious cycle of increasing nutritional deterioration, impaired immune function, and greater susceptibility to infection. The cycle may be broken by interventions to decrease infection or by improving nutritional status. Safe and appropriate complementary foods introduced at six months of age and continued breastfeeding for at least up to two years can improve nutritional status of infants and young children.

Almost all infants acquire rotavirus diarrhoea early in life. Rotavirus accounts for at least one-third of severe and potentially fatal watery diarrhoea episodes, primarily in low- and middle-income countries, where an estimated 440 000 vaccine-preventable rotavirus deaths per year occur. Two licensed rotavirus vaccines, derived from human or bovine rotavirus, are being marketed in a few countries (85 per cent protective efficacy against severe diarrhoea), and other candidate vaccines are undergoing field trials in low- and middle-income countries.

For cholera, the two oral vaccines licensed offer reasonable protection, but for only a limited period of time (60–65 per cent protective efficacy for about six months). There are no licensed vaccines against shigella. Although scientific interest in a cholera vaccine remains high, its public health priority is less than a vaccine for rotavirus or shigella. Measles is known to predispose to diarrhoeal disease secondary to measles-induced immunodeficiency; thus, measles vaccine also protects against post-measles diarrhoea.

Human faeces are the primary source of diarrhoeal pathogens. Poor sanitation, lack of accessible clean water, and inadequate personal and domestic hygiene are responsible for an estimated 90 per cent of childhood diarrhoeal cases. Hand-washing promotion reduces incidence of diarrhoea by an average of 33 per cent, and is best when part of a package of behaviour-change interventions. However, the required behaviour change is complex and significant resources are needed, the most important of which is access to water.

Case management

Most deaths from diarrhoea occur because of dehydration associated with acute diarrhoea, and because of dysentery (bloody diarrhoea). Management of diarrhoea includes:

- Treating dehydration with oral rehydration salts (ORS) solution, or with an intravenous electrolyte solution in cases of severe dehydration
- Continuing or increasing breastfeeding during and increasing feeding after the diarrhoeal episode
- Providing children with 20 mg per day of zinc for 10–14 days
- Using antibiotics only when appropriate (i.e. bloody diarrhoea) and not administering antidiarrhoeal drugs
- Advising mothers of the need to increase fluids and continue feeding during future episodes

Two recent advances are noteworthy in managing acute diarrhoea: Newly formulated ORS containing lower concentrations of glucose and salts, and zinc supplementation.

The ORS formulation recommended by UNICEF and WHO has proved safe and effective in the prevention and treatment of dehydration. However, mothers' and health workers' acceptance of standard ORS has been suboptimal because watery stools persist and the duration of diarrhoea is not reduced. Efforts over the past 20 years have led to the development of a new ORS formulation. Compared with standard ORS, this lower sodium and glucose ORS reduces stool output, vomiting, and the need for intravenous fluids (Hanh *et al.* 2001). The new ORS is safe and effective in both non-cholera diarrhoea and cholera in children and adults. WHO and UNICEF now recommend the use of ORS containing 75 meq of sodium and 75 mmol of glucose per litre (total osmolarity of 245 milliosmols per litre) everywhere (World Health Organization and United Nations Children's Fund 2004).

A review of all relevant clinical trials indicates that zinc supplements given during an episode of acute diarrhoea reduces both the duration and severity, and could prevent 300 000 deaths in children each year (Fontaine 2001). WHO and UNICEF now jointly recommend that all children with acute diarrhoea be given zinc in some form for 10–14 days during and after diarrhoea (10 mg per day for infants younger than six months of age and 20 mg per day for those over six months). Pilot studies in several countries show that including zinc routinely in the management of acute diarrhoea has two programmatically important effects: (1) use-rates of ORS increase and (2) use of antidiarrhoeals and antimicrobials decreases significantly.

The primary treatment for shigellosis—the most common and severe cause of bloody diarrhoea—is the use of antimicrobials. The choice of effective, safe, oral, and inexpensive drugs for use in low- and middle-income countries has, however, become problematic because of the increasing prevalence of antimicrobial drug resistance to several commonly used antibiotics. Because of its effectiveness, safety, ease of administration by the oral route, short course, and low cost (US$0.10 for a 3-day course for a 15-kg child), ciprofloxacin is the current drug of choice for shigellosis; however, ciprofloxacin-resistant strains are already appearing. Increasing antimicrobial resistance has made development of a vaccine for shigella a high priority.

ARIs

ARIs, particularly pneumonia, are a major cause of under-five child mortality in low- and middle-income countries. Interventions to control ARIs can be divided into preventive interventions such as immunization against specific pathogens, improvements in nutrition, and safer environments, and case management interventions (Jamison *et al.* 2006).

Prevention

Widespread use of vaccines against measles, diphtheria, pertussis, *Haemophilus influenzae* (Hib), pneumococcus, and influenza has the potential to substantially reduce the incidence of ARIs in children in low- and middle-income countries. Two particularly important vaccines are those against Hib and pneumococcus, pathogens responsible for about half of all cases of pneumonia.

The use of Hib conjugate vaccines in developed countries has resulted in the virtual elimination of invasive Hib disease (meningitis and bacteraemic pneumonia) because of immunity in vaccinated children and a herd effect in those not vaccinated. Studies in Bangladesh, Brazil, Chile, and the Gambia have shown that Hib vaccine reduced the incidence of radiological pneumonia by 20–30 per cent, but the results of a large study in Indonesia were inconclusive with regard to the effect of this vaccine on pneumonia. Several Hib conjugate vaccines are available; all are effective when given in early infancy and have virtually no side effects except occasional temporary redness or swelling at the injection site. To reduce the number of injections, Hib vaccine is sometimes given in combination with other vaccines, such as DTP and hepatitis B. Two to three doses are recommended depending on the manufacturer. The three-dose schedule is delivered at 6, 10, and 14 weeks of age.

Two types of pneumococcal vaccines are currently licensed for use: A polysaccharide vaccine effective against 23 different strains of pneumococcus and protein-conjugated vaccines effective against 7 strains. The polysaccharide vaccine is not recommended for use in children aged less than two years. A randomized controlled trial in the Gambia found a protein-conjugated vaccine with 9 strains to have a 77 per cent efficacy against vaccine-type pneumococcal invasive disease, 35 per cent reduction in radiologically confirmed pneumonia, and 16 per cent reduction in all-cause mortality. A similar study in South Africa showed that this vaccine was efficacious against vaccine-type invasive pneumococcal disease in both HIV-negative and HIV-positive children. One of the problems with the currently licensed protein-conjugated vaccine is that the serotypes included cover only 65–80 per cent of serotypes associated with pneumococcal disease among young children in Western industrialized countries, and this proportion may be lower in many low- and middle-income countries. Other pneumococcal conjugate vaccines with wider serotype coverage are in late stages of development.

Interventions that reduce the prevalence of LBW, malnutrition, and non-breastfeeding can reduce the incidence of pneumonia. Exclusive breastfeeding in the first six months of life and continued breastfeeding with complementary feeding up to at least two years of age reduce the incidence and severity of ARIs (Victora *et al.* 1999).

In a recently completed trial in Guatemala, environmental interventions to reduce exposure to indoor air pollution have been shown to reduce the incidence of severe respiratory infections in children. Therefore, wide use of interventions such as non-smoke stoves has the potential to substantially reduce pneumonia disease burden.

Case management

The simplification and standardization of ARI case management have enabled first-level health workers to provide effective treatment to millions of children in low- and middle-income countries. WHO clinical guidelines for ARI case management, which are part of IMCI, rely on two simple clinical signs: Fast breathing to identify children with ARI who need antibiotic therapy and lower chest wall in-drawing to identify children with severe pneumonia (World Health Organization 2006b). The latter sign requires referral and treatment in a hospital with parenteral antibiotics. Additionally, presence of audible stridor when calm and any of the general danger signs such as lethargy or unconsciousness, inability to feed and drink, or convulsions are also indications for referral to a hospital.

Fast breathing, defined by WHO as a respiratory rate of 60 or more for infants younger than 2 months, 50 or more for infants of 2–11 months, and 40 or more for children 1–4 years of age, detects about 85 per cent of pneumonia patients. The specificity of fast breathing is 70–80 per cent, which means that 20–30 per cent of children with ARI who do not need antibiotics will receive them. However, the use of this sign makes decision making by first-level health workers simple and, therefore, has increased the proportion of children with pneumonia who receive antibiotics. Children with fast breathing should be given an oral antibiotic (e.g. co-trimoxazole or amoxicillin) twice daily. It has been shown that oral antibiotic therapy for three days is as effective as that for five days (Qazi 2005).

Chest in-drawing is the inward movement of the lower chest wall when a child breathes in. WHO currently recommends that children with chest wall in-drawing should be referred to a hospital and treated with parenteral antibiotics. WHO also recommends the use of oxygen for children who are unable to feed or drink, or have cyanosis, respiratory rate of 70 or more, or severe chest wall in-drawing. Recent evidence shows that children with chest wall in-drawing who do not have any of the danger signs can be successfully treated with oral amoxicillin (Addo-Yobo *et al.* 2004). The safety and effectiveness of this approach is now being further evaluated. If confirmed, this could result in a substantially lower number of hospitalizations.

In HIV-positive children, who should be on oral co-trimoxazole prophylaxis, oral amoxicillin is recommended as the first-line treatment of non-severe pneumonia. Children older than 2 months who have severe pneumonia should receive therapy for *Pneumocystis jiroveci* in addition to the standard injectable antibiotics.

Malaria

Malaria kills more than a million people annually, 90 per cent of them in sub-Saharan Africa and the majority of whom are children under five. Chapter 9.15 on malaria describes malaria interventions in greater detail (Morrow & Moss 2008).

Prevention

Vector control remains the most generally effective measure to prevent malaria transmission in all ages. Insecticide-treated nets (ITNs) are a form of effective vector control and have been shown to be particularly effective in reducing mortality in young children (Lengeler 2004).

Case management

The two diagnostic approaches currently used are based on clinical diagnosis and detection of the causative parasite or its products. The IMCI strategy has practical algorithms for management of the sick child presenting with fever where there are no facilities for laboratory diagnosis. The additional use of parasitological diagnosis, either by light microscopy or by rapid diagnostic tests (RDTs), is becoming particularly important with the introduction of the more expensive artemisinin-based combinations in national malaria and IMCI treatment guidelines of many countries.

Once diagnosed as malaria, either on a clinical or parasitological basis, the child should be treated early with a safe and effective antimalarial medicine because a delay in treatment could result in progression to severe disease, which is associated with a high case-fatality rate. Malaria case management has been greatly affected by the emergence and spread of chloroquine and sulfadoxine-pyrimethamine (SP) resistance, which have been replaced by artemisinin-based combinations in many countries (World Health Organization 2006a). In areas with poor access to health facilities, early recognition and prompt and appropriate treatment of malaria in children requires treatment in the home or community.

HIV and AIDS

Currently, an estimated 2.3 million children under the age of 15 are living with HIV, and every day more than 1400 are newly infected. Without interventions, over half of the infected children die before their second birthday. Chapter 9.13 on HIV and AIDS describes HIV and AIDS interventions in greater detail (Karim *et al.* 2008).

Prevention

Over 90 per cent of HIV-infected children are infected through mother-to-child transmission (MTCT), which occurs during pregnancy, during birth, or through breastfeeding. Without any interventions, the risk of transmission is between 20 and 45 per cent, but this can be reduced to less than 2 per cent with a package of evidence-based interventions (World Health Organization 2004c).

Antiretroviral therapy (ART) for all pregnant women who are eligible for treatment is the most effective method of preventing MTCT. Pregnant women with HIV who do not yet require ART should be offered prophylactic regimens (World Health Organization 2004a).

The most effective way of eliminating the risk of HIV transmission through breastfeeding is by avoiding it altogether. However, exclusive breastfeeding for the first six months of life is the most effective preventive measure available for reducing child mortality in low- and middle-income countries. UN agencies have developed recommendations that recognize this dilemma and help in balancing the risks, considering the HIV-infected mother's individual circumstances and health services, counselling, and support available to her (World Health Organization 2006d):

- Exclusive breastfeeding is recommended for HIV-infected women for the first six months of life unless replacement feeding is acceptable, feasible, affordable, sustainable, and safe for them and their infants before that time; it has been shown that exclusive breastfeeding carries a lower risk of HIV transmission than mixed feeding (i.e. breastfeeding while also giving other fluids or foods).
- When replacement feeding is acceptable, feasible, affordable, sustainable, and safe, avoidance of all breastfeeding by HIV-infected women is recommended.
- Breastfeeding mothers of infants and young children who are known to be HIV-infected should be strongly encouraged to continue breastfeeding.

Management and care of HIV-exposed and HIV-infected children

All children born to HIV-infected mothers are considered to be HIV-exposed, whereas those in whom HIV has been transmitted from the mother are HIV-infected. Diagnosis of HIV-infection in children is based on demonstrating the presence of HIV (PCR-virological test) at age less than 18 months and on the presence of antibodies to HIV (ELISA) beyond this age. This is because maternal antibodies to HIV can pass through the placenta and will be present in HIV-exposed children until the age of 18 months.

HIV-exposed or HIV-infected children may acquire a serious life-threatening form of pneumonia caused by an organism called *Pneumocystis jirovecii* (previously *carinii*), which often occurs before their HIV status has been confirmed. Regular prophylaxis with trimethoprim-sulfamethoxazole (co-trimoxazole) provides a simple, inexpensive, and effective strategy to prevent this illness, and has been shown to reduce mortality of HIV-infected children by up to 40 per cent even in the absence of ART (Chintu *et al.* 2004).

HIV-exposed and HIV-infected children should receive all vaccines as early in life as possible, except BCG and yellow fever vaccines. In asymptomatic children, the decision to give late BCG should be based on the local risk of tuberculosis. Infants with symptomatic HIV infection should not receive yellow fever vaccines.

ART, which means antiretroviral drugs given in the correct way and with adherence, can substantially improve survival of HIV-infected children.

Malnutrition

Malnutrition contributes to more than half of all under-five deaths globally. Malnourished children, particularly those who are severely malnourished, have substantially higher risks of death from common childhood illness such as diarrhoea, pneumonia, and malaria.

Prevention

Interventions to prevent malnutrition include promotion of optimal feeding of infants and young children, prevention and treatment of illness, and amelioration of micronutrient deficiencies in the diet.

Early initiation of breastfeeding, ideally within the first hour after birth, has been shown to be associated with a reduced risk of neonatal mortality (Edmond *et al.* 2006). Exclusive breastfeeding during the first six months of life is associated with about a tenfold lower risk of death due to any cause than not breastfeeding at all, and a two- to threefold lower risk of death than partial breastfeeding (Bahl *et al.* 2003). Continued breastfeeding into the second year of life has also been shown to reduce the risk of child mortality and malnutrition (World Health Organization Collaborative Study team 2001). WHO, therefore, recommends early initiation of breastfeeding, exclusive breastfeeding up to six months of age, and continued breastfeeding along with complementary foods up to at least two years of age. Multiple approaches exist to promote breastfeeding through health facility and community programmes, including health education, professional support, lay support, and mass media campaigns.

Safe and appropriate complementary feeding started at six months of age can reduce the prevalence of malnutrition and contribute to reduced mortality. Promotion of safe and appropriate complementary feeding has been shown to improve weight-for-age and height-for-age gains by 0.24–0.87 SD in pilot studies (World Health Organization 1998). Effects of this magnitude if reproduced on a large scale could translate into tangible reductions in rates of malnutrition and the mortality attributable to it.

Prevention and prompt case management of common childhood illness, as discussed in the earlier subsections, can reduce the nutritional adverse effects of illness and, thereby, help break the vicious cycle of malnutrition–infections–malnutrition.

Common micronutrient deficiencies such as that of vitamin A, iron, iodine, and zinc, both at clinical and subclinical levels, contribute to illness and mortality in children. Approaches to prevent these deficiencies include supplementation, food fortification, and dietary diversification.

Case management of severe malnutrition

Children with severe malnutrition are usually identified by the weight-for-height criterion (< 70 per cent or < −3 SD of WHO reference median) and/or the presence of bilateral oedema. An additional independent criterion that can be used is mid-upper arm circumference (MUAC) of < 110 mm in children 6–59 months of age. For infants < 6 months of age, 'visible severe wasting' can be used to identify severe malnutrition in addition to the weight-for-height criteria (Prudhon *et al.* 2006).

Severely malnourished children without any complications can be managed in the community, whereas those with complications should be admitted to a hospital for treatment. These complications include anorexia, severe oedema, or both severe wasting and mild or moderate oedema.

In communities with limited access to proper local diets for nutritional rehabilitation, ready-to-use therapeutic foods (RUTFs) have been shown to be highly effective in the treatment of severe malnutrition in children 6–59 months of age without complications

(Collins *et al.* 2006). When families have access to nutrient-rich foods, children with severe malnutrition without complications can be managed in the community (without RUTFs) by carefully designed diets using low-cost family foods, provided appropriate minerals and vitamins are given. Children under six months, however, should not receive RUTFs or any solid family foods. They need milk-based diets and should be managed in a hospital, where their mothers can obtain support to re-establish breastfeeding.

Children with severe malnutrition who have complications should be admitted in a hospital. They need careful evaluation and treatment of infections, electrolyte imbalance, hypoglycaemia, and hypothermia. They should be fed carefully during the acute phase and should be given micronutrient supplements but no iron during the acute or stabilization phase. Subsequent rehabilitation, when appetite has returned and there is no severe oedema, can be done at home using RUTFs or nutrient-dense family foods, along with micronutrient supplements (World Health Organization 1999).

Integrated delivery of interventions

Despite the fact that effective interventions exist against all major conditions from which children die, the coverage of these interventions remains low in general. The key to achievement of substantial mortality reduction in children is universal coverage of the interventions described in the previous subsection.

Before the mid-90s, child health programmes in low- and middle-income countries focused on immunization, control of diarrhoeal diseases, ARIs, and nutrition. Their implementation led to reduction in under-five mortality in many countries, but this approach also encountered limitations. The narrow focus on single interventions has failed to consider the child in a holistic manner, leading to many missed opportunities for care in contacts with a health practitioner. Also, it was difficult to resolve upstream health-system constraints such as management or human resource policies by using this approach.

Solving these problems involves ensuring access to an integrated package of interventions that are organized around a 'continuum of care' from pregnancy, birth, neonatal period, infancy, childhood, and adolescence into adulthood. It also means that care should span across the home, community, health centre, and hospital. Trying to do so has profound consequences for the way programmes are organized. It requires realigning the scope of programme activities, specifying the packages, establishing benchmarks, and integrating delivery strategies. It also means adapting programme management procedures to reflect integration and to embed them within health-system development processes.

Packaging interventions for health-system delivery

The advantages of delivering interventions as packages include the following:

1. Many interventions go naturally together because they are delivered by the same person at the same time; for example, keeping the baby warm immediately after birth and initiation of breastfeeding within one hour.
2. Packaging is more cost-effective in terms of training, implementation, and supervision; for example, it is more efficient to run a course for IMCI than four separate courses on management of diarrhoea, pneumonia, malaria, and infant and young child feeding.
3. Packaging meets the needs of the individual caregiver and the child much better than isolated and uncoordinated single-intervention delivery, thus reinforcing the continuum of care.

Individual interventions should, therefore, be packaged and, if new interventions become available, they should be integrated within the existing packages and current strategies for their delivery. The delivery levels at which the programmes will focus for each of the packages should be decided, with the aim of achieving high and equitable coverage. The following is a suggested list of packages, which could be adapted to the country situation:

1. Care before pregnancy—reproductive health package, including family planning
2. Care during pregnancy—antenatal care package, including birth preparedness, syphilis screening, intermittent preventive treatment for malaria during pregnancy, HIV and AIDS counselling, nutrition counselling, and micronutrient supplementation
3. Care during labour, birth, and immediate 1–2 hours after birth—skilled birth attendant, basic and comprehensive emergency obstetric and neonatal care package (Basic and Comprehensive EmONC)
4. Care during postnatal period—postnatal or neonatal care package, including warmth, early initiation of exclusive breastfeeding, hygienic eye and cord care, and early recognition of and timely care seeking for signs of illness
5. Management of childhood illness—integrated management of newborn and childhood illnesses, based on assessment and classification of signs that are highly sensitive and specific, and that can be completed by a health practitioner with minimal equipment
6. Community-based promotion of optimal newborn and child care practices which have an impact on survival and health of infant and young children

Potential obstacles to packaging of interventions should also be considered. This may include those related to policy, programmes, and the organizational structure of ministries and health services. For example, managers responsible for single issue-focused programmes such as EPI, malaria, or HIV may feel that packaging their interventions with other maternal and child health services might make their delivery less efficient. Another concern about packaging interventions is that vulnerable groups may not get any of the interventions if enough attention is not given to equitable delivery of the package.

To overcome the gaps in access to care, which is a barrier to improved health in many countries with a high burden of newborn and child mortality, governments increasingly invest in strengthening provision and quality of care that can be provided by community health workers. For example, in Pakistan, a cadre of lady health workers now acts as the first line of contact in many villages. In India, the government is complementing the role of the village-based *anganwadi* worker with that of an *ayah*, both of whom are responsible for delivering health promotion, nutrition counselling, and basic medical care for the mother and child. The Government of Ethiopia has recently adapted a new policy that will put in place over 30 000 health extension workers. Where such effectors are undertaken, it remains critical to invest in strengthening other levels of care simultaneously in order to ensure functional referral pathways and care, as well as adequate supervision and other health-system supports.

Integrated management of childhood illness as a key strategy for improving child survival

IMCI was developed as an integrated primary health-care approach to child health based on the principles of primary health care as set out in the Alma Ata Declaration. This approach includes strengthening health workers' skills at the first level of the health system for appropriate treatment of common diseases, promotion of proper nutrition, and reduction of missed opportunities for immunization. Further, it includes strengthening the provision of essential drugs and supplies, supervision, and referral links. Finally, the promotion of key family and community practices contributes to the remaining components of PHC as related to children.

The IMCI approach to managing common childhood diseases is practical and scientifically sound. It focuses on the child as a whole, including his or her nutrition and immunization status, and not just a particular disease. IMCI addresses the major global causes of mortality and morbidity (malnutrition, newborn conditions, pneumonia, diarrhoea, malaria, measles, and HIV) (Bryce *et al.* 2005). It can be adapted to include or exclude conditions based on the national- and subnational-level epidemiological data. The key family and community practices to promote are also based on scientific evidence.

Where it has been implemented well, IMCI has been shown to improve health-worker performance (Gouws *et al.* 2004), drug availability, rational use of drugs, organization of work at health facilities, use of referral notes, and maintenance of records at district level, and to increase health facility utilization (Arifeen *et al.* 2004).

Strengthening of child health services

It will not be possible to scale-up child health interventions effectively without dealing with the challenges that affect health systems in many low-income countries. In order to translate knowledge of effective interventions into practical action, programme management is a key function at all levels of the health system (e.g. national, subnational, district, and community levels). Many countries have established a national programme that is responsible for child health, bringing together diarrhoea and ARI control programmes, in addition to a national immunization programme. However, considering the range of interventions that impact on the health of children, the inputs of other programmes are also required to ensure that a complete package is delivered with the desired level of coverage. In this context, programme management involves specific tasks of:

- Strategic planning—required periodically (every five years or so) to identify or reformulate the main strategic directions to improve child health, which is based on priority needs and resource availability, and with a view to building a continuum of care. This should promote harmonization of inputs across various programme areas (such as IMCI, nutrition, EPI, malaria, HIV and AIDS, maternal and newborn health) and among partners.
- Operational planning—required more frequently (often annually) to identify the concrete activities that will be implemented based on the strategic plan. Operational planning can involve activities in the areas of policies, guidelines, training, supervision, provision of drugs and supplies, health management information, monitoring, and evaluation.
- Implementation—the application of the operational plan in conducting activities. It requires programme managers to have skills of organization, facilitation, negotiation, and supportive supervision, among others.

Programme management for child health will also need to consider the broader context of health-systems development. In many countries, health-sector reforms that will affect the way child health programmes are planned and implemented are in progress. If covered by the definition of an essential health package, it is important that child health interventions are well reflected therein. Sector-wide approaches promote pooling of finances to address wider health-sector needs and are often accompanied by decentralization. It may not always be easy to harmonize the specific interests of child health programmes and the needs of the health sector as a whole; hence the need for programme managers who have a good understanding of health policy and planning. In this regard, human resources and health financing are two areas that are of specific relevance for scaling-up the implementation of interventions in order to achieve high population coverage (World Health Organization 2005b).

Economic hardship and financial crises have eroded the health sector in many countries over the past two decades. Many national health systems are in disarray, with a deteriorating infrastructure and a public health sector subject to the resource restrictions consequent to structural adjustment and macroeconomic ceilings. As a result, human resources working in the health sector have been destabilized and undermined. Low density of health workers, poor motivation, and drainage of the most qualified staff to urban centres and abroad have left rural population and even the urban population in some low-income countries deprived of the much needed human resources to provide adequate health care.

It is estimated that there is a global shortage of more than 4 million health professionals worldwide (World Health Organization 2006e). A global assessment of the shortfall has suggested that, on average, countries with fewer than 2.5 health workers per 1000 population failed to achieve 80 per cent coverage rates for deliveries by skilled attendants or for measles immunization. For child health services specifically as well to increase access among deprived populations, the deployment of an equivalent of 100 000 full-time multipurpose professionals backed up by many more community health workers is required. Governments in various countries are responding to this challenge by instituting a new cadre of community health workers or upgrading the skills of existing community resource persons, to deliver an essential package of health services that include child health interventions.

Ensuring universal access to child health services, however, is not merely a question of increasing the supply of services. Financial barriers to access have to be reduced or eliminated as well. In many countries, households spend considerable amounts on health care and out-of-pocket expenditures for health services can be between two and three times greater than the total health expenditure by governments and donors. User fees refer to the payment of out-of-pocket charges at the time of use of health care and constitute the largest share of out-of-pocket payments.

The higher the proportion of user payments in the total mix of financing for health, the greater is the relative share of the financing burden falling on poor people. The poorest population groups often forgo the care they need because it is unaffordable. When people do use available services, the costs incurred can force them to miss out on other necessities such as food, clothing, or children's education. Household expenditure surveys suggest that more than 150 million individuals globally face severe financial hardship each year because of health-care costs. Rather than relying on user fees and out-of-pocket payments, systems of prepayment can be used to promote fair access to health services.

Prepayment systems involve advance collection of funds through tax-based insurance or social health insurance schemes. Both provide financial risk protection and promote equity through prepayment of health-care costs and pooling of health risks. WHO recommends that out-of-pocket expenditures should be gradually converted into prepayment schemes, including community finance programmes. Unfortunately, to move from a situation of limited supply of health services, high out-of-pocket expenditures, and exclusion of the poor to a situation of universal access and financial protection can take many years.

Monitoring child health programmes

The phrase 'what gets measured gets done' summarizes the importance of monitoring and evaluation in programme planning and implementation.

Health status indicators

Health status of children is usually measured in terms of mortality, morbidity or disability, growth, and development. Changes in health status are influenced by social, economic, behavioural, and environmental determinants of health, as well as by the health system. Some examples of frequently used health status indicators relevant for child health programmes are:

- Under-five mortality rate
- Neonatal mortality rate
- Proportion of infants infected by HIV
- Proportion of wasted, stunted, or underweight children

The following methods are used to collect data on health status indicators:

- Large, nationally representative household surveys—large sample-size surveys are used to calculate health status indicators such as under-five, infant, and neonatal mortality rates.
- Vital registration—it is the best source of information related to the number and causes of death. However, many low- and middle-income countries have low coverage of vital registration.
- Qualitative research studies—research that uses focus groups, in-depth interviews, participatory approaches, and observations is conducted to get information on local beliefs, attitudes, terms, and cultural practices.
- Quantitative studies—these research studies are used to evaluate the effectiveness of different intervention delivery approaches.

Outcome indicators

Outcomes are the changes in the coverage of selected effective interventions produced as a result of programme activities. Improved coverage is expected to contribute to improved health status. Changes in outcome measures usually cannot occur unless programme outputs have changed. Some examples of outcome indicators used in child health programmes are:

- Proportion of children with diarrhoea who received oral rehydration treatment
- Proportion of children with pneumonia treated with antibiotics
- Proportion of HIV-exposed infants on co-trimoxazole prophylaxis
- Proportion of newborns who receive at least one postnatal care visit within 2 days of birth
- Proportion of infants less than 6 months who are exclusively breastfed
- Proportion of HIV-exposed infants less than 6 months who receive either replacement feeding or exclusive breastfeeding

Methods that can be used to collect data on outcome indicators are as follows:

- Large, nationally representative household surveys—commonly conducted large household surveys include the DHS and the UNICEF Multi Intercountry Cluster Survey (MICS).
- Small-sample household surveys, such as 30 cluster household surveys.

Reports from health facilities—routine reports from health facilities are sometimes used to estimate coverage of an intervention.

Inputs and output indicators

Inputs are the financial, material, and human resources that must be mobilized and made available to carry out programme activities. These include supportive laws and policies, human resources to carry out planned activities, health financing that supports universal access to health care, and efficient organization of services.

Some examples of input indicators are as follows:

- Countries or districts have a strategy and costed implementation plan for improving newborn and child survival.
- Countries or districts are implementing IMCI.
- Countries have adopted a policy promoting the new WHO/UNICEF recommendations on the management of diarrhoea.
- Countries have adopted a policy of community management of pneumonia for areas with low access to facilities.
- Countries have adopted a national policy on IYCF, including national targets.

Outputs are immediate results that are produced by a combination of making inputs available and conducting the planned activities. For example, the proportion of training courses or supervisory visits that have been completed as planned and according to an acceptable level of quality, and the proportion of trainees who had been trained and who are competent at the end of training. Some other examples of output indicators are:

- Proportion of first-level health facilities with at least 60 per cent of health workers who care for children trained in IMCI
- Proportion of first-level health facilities that have all the essential drugs for IMCI available
- Proportion of mothers who received early and exclusive breastfeeding advice during pregnancy or the first day of the infant's life

Methods which can be used to collect data on input and output indicators are listed as follows:

- Small-sample household surveys (output indicators)—these provide the best data related to knowledge and practices of caretakers for the prevention and treatment of illness in children and newborns.

- Health facility or provider surveys (output indicators)—these provide the best data on case-management practices and on the availability of facility supports.
- Reports from health facilities (output indicators)—almost all health facilities prepare and send routine reports to higher levels, usually the district health managers, providing information on patient treatment and availability of supplies.
- Supervisory visits (input and output indicators)—during supervisory visits, one can frequently also obtain information on human resources, and on material and drug supplies.
- Health facility auditing (input and output indicators)—the process of auditing allows comparison of the provision of a selected intervention or service with the standard set by the country.
- National or district programme records (input indicators)—details of availability of health workers, training activities, purchase of drugs and supplies and their distribution, and monitoring visits are usually available with programme managers.

International goals to accelerate progress in child survival

At the United Nations Millennium Summit in September 2000, 189 national leaders endorsed 'The Millennium Declaration' with an aim to promote the achievement of poverty elimination, which includes the development of education, promotion of and respect for human rights and equality, and improvement of the environment. As a roadmap to accomplish these aims, a commitment to attain eight specific goals by 2015 was made. Although all the Millennium Development Goals (MDGs) are relevant to child health, MDGs 1, 4, 5, and 6 are directly related to child survival (*see* Box 11.3.2). The fourth MDG has the explicit target of 'reducing by two-thirds, between 1990 and 2015, the under-five mortality rate'.

The global target (based on an U5MR of 94 per 1000 live births in 1990) is, therefore, to reach a mortality rate of 31 per 1000 live births by 2015. However, if recent trends (2000–2005) continue unchanged, the global U5MR is likely to be still more than twofold higher than the target for 2015. Even more worrisome are the facts that progress has been slowing down in recent years and it is not equally distributed across countries and regions (Fig. 11.3.6).

Box 11.3.2 The millennium development goals

Goal 1 Eradicate extreme poverty and hunger

Goal 2 Achieve universal primary education

Goal 3 Promote gender equality and empower women

Goal 4 Reduce child mortality

Goal 5 Improve maternal health

Goal 6 Combat HIV/AIDS, malaria and other diseases

Goal 7 Ensure environmental sustainability

Goal 8 Develop a global partnership for development

In May 2002, the UN Special Session on Children (UNGASS) adopted a declaration and plan of action set out in a document 'A World Fit for Children'. The document committed governments to a time-bound set of goals for children and young people, with particular focus on (a) promoting healthy lives; (b) providing quality education; (c) protecting children against abuse, exploitation, and violence; and (d) combating the HIV/AIDS epidemic. The UNGASS goals and targets provide an intermediate framework for assessing progress towards the MDGs, with many targets set for 2010, and a periodic review process agreed on as part of the UN General Assembly that takes places every year.

The Millennium Declaration and the Roadmap towards its implementation, as well as the UNGASS Declaration, stress the need for placing human rights at the centre of peace, security, and development programmes. As emphasized in the Roadmap, a rights-based approach to development should be the basis for equality and equity, both in the distribution of developmental gains and in the level of participation in the developmental process. From a child health perspective, therefore, integration of human rights norms and standards into country and United Nations system policies, programmes, and strategies is a crucial contribution towards achieving more equitable child health outcomes.

In this context, the United Nations Convention on the Rights of the Child (CRC) provides an important, holistic, legal, and normative framework for addressing child health, and for tackling the prevailing equity gaps within countries. It provides guidance for identifying and clarifying the legal obligations of governments and other actors to address and improve child health, and enhances accountability at the national and international levels. It requires a systematic and in-depth assessment of the possible impact that child health policies and programmes may have on the health and development of all children within a country.

Measuring progress towards MDGs

In 2005, the 'Countdown to 2015: Tracking progress in child survival' initiative was launched This initiative biennially measures and publishes the progress made in improving coverage of essential health interventions and in mortality reduction in the 60 countries that suffer the highest burden of child deaths. The second Countdown report 2008 showed that 16 countries were on track to achieving MDG 4, 26 were judged to have made insufficient progress in reducing child mortality, and 26 countries had made no progress at all (UNICEF, WHO, UNFPA and partners 2008).

The neonatal period stands out as one in which too few children are reached by effective care, and data on postnatal visits are yet to be systematically collected and reported. Given the important contribution of newborn mortality to under-five mortality, it is expected that in most countries, newborn mortality needs to be halved in order to achieve the MDG 4. To achieve MDG 4, efforts are also necessary to achieve MDGs 5 and 6, as they contribute to improved newborn survival and reduction in incidence and case fatality of malaria and HIV/AIDS, respectively.

Emphasis on children's early development is also needed given that two of the major United Nations 2000 MDGs are to reduce poverty and to ensure that all children complete primary schooling. These goals will not be achieved in countries where a large proportion of children live in poverty, suffer from poor nutrition and health, or lack psychosocial care.

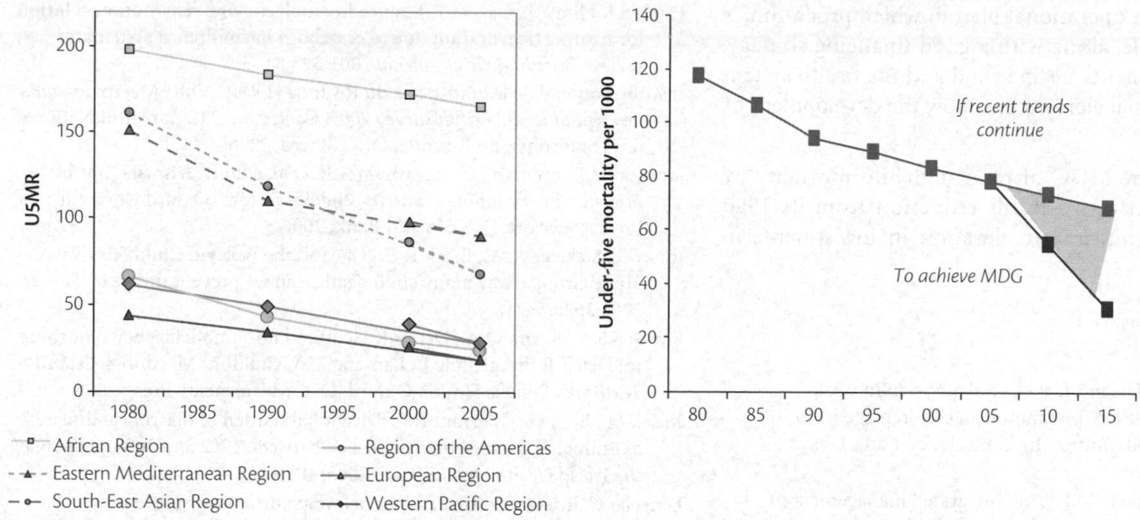

Fig. 11.3.6 Global and regional under-five mortality trend, 1980–2015.
Source: WHO mortality database. Data available on request from WHO-CAH Department.

Mobilizing resources for children

To achieve improved health outcomes for all children, development strategies and programmes need to increase the investments on building the capacity of families and communities in order to provide for and protect the physical, emotional, and cognitive development of children. It is important to ensure universal access to good-quality basic health, clean water, sanitation, and other social sector services such as education. This also includes creating the national legal, policy, and budget frameworks to promote the realization of children's rights to these services.

WHO and UNICEF support programmes to improve health and advocate protecting the rights of children across the world, along with other UN and external partners. The responsibility of success of child health programmes lies ultimately with governments. Only a fraction of resources for health in low- and middle-income countries originates in the international system, most of the resources being national. Scaling-up delivery of child health interventions will require additional investments in commodities, equipment, and human resources, as well as strengthening of the operational health system. This has cost implications. It has been estimated by WHO that universal coverage with known child health interventions will require an additional US$50 billion in the ten years from 2005 to 2015. At country level, financial needs for child survival will depend on the current situation as well as the targets set and the strategies employed for reaching those targets. Undertaking a cost assessment for child survival can help bring national programmes together to address priority needs, set joint targets, and plan complementary activities.

Once a multiyear budgeted child survival plan is available, it can be inserted into insurance plans, sector-wide approaches, poverty reduction strategy papers, and medium-term expenditure frameworks, allowing financing options to be discussed concretely with actors both inside and outside the health sector.

The additional financial resources will have to be mobilized by increasing both the national health budgets and the amount of official development assistance for health. In addition to these increased resources, greater efficiency and equity are required for their allocation and use.

Conclusion

Almost 10 million children under five die each year, 4 million of them dying in the neonatal period. Most neonatal deaths are due to three causes: Infections, prematurity, and birth asphyxia. ARIs, diarrhoea, malaria, measles, and HIV are the main causes of death in children aged 28 days to 5 years. Undernutrition is associated with over 35 per cent of these deaths. Child deaths are unequally distributed in the world. Three-quarters of child death occur in Africa and Southeast Asia; half of the child deaths take place in 6 countries. Within countries, child mortality tends to be higher in the rural areas and within the poorer and least educated families.

Key points

- Approximately two-thirds of under-five deaths could be prevented by universal coverage with a small set of existing interventions that do not require expensive technology. Among these interventions, the promotion of breastfeeding, management and prevention of diarrhoea, ARIs, malaria, and HIV infection, in addition to improved feeding practices to prevent malnutrition have the highest impact in reducing child mortality.
- Coverage with the earlier-mentioned interventions remains low. Integrating the interventions into packages of care that are organized along a continuum from pregnancy, birth, neonatal period, and childhood, and delivered at all levels—from the home and community through the first-level facility and hospital—would contribute to improved efficiency in intervention delivery and to the achievement of high coverage.
- Strengthening the health system will be key for increasing the coverage of health interventions. This requires improved programme management, with attention to strategic and implementation planning, implementation, monitoring, and evaluation.

- The development of an operational plan to which programmes can be held accountable, along with a good financing strategy, will yield long-term benefits for the child and the health system at large and is an essential element to follow the development of a child survival strategy.
- The achievement of the MDG of reducing child mortality by 2015—with a target of a two-thirds reduction from its 1990 level—will require significant acceleration in investments in child survival.

References

Addo-Yobo E., Chisaka N., Hassan M. *et al.* Oral amoxicillin *versus* injectable penicillin for severe pneumonia in children aged 3 to 59 months: a randomised multicentre equivalency study. *Lancet* 2004;**364**(9440):1141–8.

Arifeen S.E., Blum L.S., Hoque D.M.E. *et al.* Integrated management of childhood illness (IMCI) in Bangladesh: early findings from a cluster randomized study. *Lancet* 2004;**364**:1595–602.

Badan Pusat Statistik-Statistics Indonesia (BPS), ORC Macro. *Indonesia demographic and health survey 2002–3*. Calverton (MD): Badan Pusat Statistik-Statistics Indonesia, ORC Macro; 2003.

Bahl R., Frost C., Kirkwood B.R. *et al.* Infant feeding patterns and risks of death and hospitalization in the first half of infancy: multicentre cohort study. *Bulletin of the World Health Organization* 2003;**83**: 418–26.

Black R.E., Morris S.S., Bryce J. Where and why are 10 million children dying every year? *Lancet* 2003;**361**:2226–34.

Bryce J., Boschi-Pinto C., Shibuya K. *et al.* and the Child Health Epidemiology Reference Group. WHO estimates of the causes of death in children. *Lancet* 2005;**365**:1147–57.

Caulfield L.E., de Onis M., Blössner M. *et al.* Undernutrition as an underlying cause of child deaths associated with diarrhoea, pneumonia, malaria, and measles. *American Journal of Clinical Nutrition* 2004;**80**:193–8.

Chintu C., Bhat G.J., Walker A.S. *et al.* Co-trimoxazole as prophylaxis against opportunistic infections in HIV-infected Zambian children (CHAP): a double-blind randomized placebo-controlled trial. *Lancet* 2004;**364**:1865–71.

Collins S., Dent N., Binns P. *et al.* Management of severe acute malnutrition in children. *Lancet* 2006;**368**:1992–2000.

Collison D., Dey C., Hannah G. *et al.* Income inequality and child mortality in wealthy nations [e-pub ahead of print]. *Journal of Public Health (Oxford)* 2007 Mar 13.

DfID, UNICEF, USAID, WHO. The analytic review of the integrated management of childhood illness strategy. Geneva: World Health Organization; 2003.

Edmond K.M., Zandoh C., Quigley M.A. *et al.* Delayed breastfeeding initiation increases risk of neonatal mortality. *Paediatrics* 2006;**117**:380–6.

El-Zanaty F., Way A. *Egypt demographic and health survey 2005*. Cairo, Egypt: Ministry of Health and Population, National Population Council, El-Zanaty and Associates, ORC Macro; 2006.

Euro HIV. *HIV/AIDS surveillance in Europe: end-year report 2005*. Saint-Maurice, France: Institut de Veille Sanitaire; 2006. Number 73.

Fontaine O. Effect of zinc supplementation on clinical course of acute diarrhoea. Report of a meeting held in New Delhi, India; 2001 May 7–9. *Journal of Health, Population, and Nutrition* 2001;**19**:338–46.

Gouws E., Bryce J., Habicht J.P. *et al.* Improving antimicrobial use among health workers in first-level facilities: results from the multicountry evaluation of the integrated management of childhood illness strategy. *Bulletin of the World Health Organization* 2004;**82**:509–15.

Grantham-McGregor S., Cheung Y.B., Cueto S. *et al.* (on behalf of the International Child Development Steering Group). Developmental potential in the first 5 years for children in developing countries. *Lancet* 2007;**369**:60–70.

Hanh S.K., Jim Y.J., Garner P. Reduced-osmolarity oral rehydration solution for treating dehydration due to diarrhoea in children: a systematic review. *British Medical Journal* 2001;**323**:81–5.

Institut National de la Statistique du Rwanda (INSR), ORC Macro. *Rwanda demographic and health survey 2005*. Calverton (MD): Institut National de la Statistique du Rwanda, ORC Macro; 2006.

Jamison D.T., Breman J.G., Measham A.R. *et al.* editors. *Diseases control priorities in developing countries*. 2nd ed. Oxford: Oxford University Press; New York (NY): World Bank; 2006.

Jones G., Steketee R.W., Black R.E. *et al.* and the Bellagio Child Survival Study Group. How many child deaths can we prevent this year? *Lancet* 2003;**362**:65–71.

Karim S.S.A., Karim Q.A., Detels R. Acquired immunodeficiency syndrome. In: Detels R, Beaglehole R, Lansang MA, Gulliford M, editors. *Oxford Textbook of Public Health*. Oxford: Oxford University Press; 2008.

Kosek M., Bern C., Guerrant R.L. The global burden of diarrhoeal disease, as estimated from studies published between 1992 and 2000. *Bulletin of the World Health Organization* 2003;**81**:197–204.

Lengeler C. Insecticide-treated bed nets and curtains for preventing malaria. [Cochrane review]. Cochrane Database Syst. Review 2004;(2). CD000363.

Maroc Ministère de la Santé, ORC Macro, Ligue des États Arabes. *Enquête sur la population et la santé familiale (EPSF) 2003–4*. Calverton (MD): Ministère de la Santé, ORC Macro; 2005

Morrow R., Moss W. Malaria. In: Detels R., Beaglehole R., Lansang M.A., Gulliford M, editors. *Oxford Textbook of Public Health*. Oxford: Oxford University Press; 2008.

National Bureau of Statistics, ORC Macro. *Tanzania demographic and health survey 2004–5*. Dar es Salaam, Tanzania: National Bureau of Statistics, ORC Macro; 2005.

National Institute of Population Research and Training (NIPORT), Mitra and Associates, ORC Macro. *Bangladesh demographic and health survey 2004*. Dhaka, Bangladesh: National Institute of Population Research and Training; 2005.

National Institute of Public Health, National Institute of Statistics, ORC Macro. *Cambodia demographic and health survey 2005*. Phnom Penh, Cambodia, Calverton (MD): National Institute of Public Health, National Institute of Statistics, ORC Macro; 2006.

National Scientific and Applied Center for Preventive Medicine (NCPM), ORC Macro. *Moldova demographic and health survey 2005*. Calverton (MD): National Scientific and Applied Center for Preventive Medicine, Moldova Ministry of Health and Social Protection, ORC Macro; 2006.

National Statistical Service, Ministry of Health, ORC Macro. *Armenia demographic and health survey 2005*. Calverton (MD): National Statistical Service, Armenian Ministry of Health, ORC Macro; 2006.

National Statistics Office (NSO), ORC Macro. *National demographic and health survey 2003*. Calverton (MD): National Statistics Office (Philippines), ORC Macro; 2004.

Ndiaye S., Mohamed A. *Enquête Démographique et de Santé au Sénégal 2005*. Calverton (MD): Sénégal Centre de Recherche pour le Développement Humain, ORC Macro; 2006.

Prudhon C., Briend A., Weise Prinzo Z. *et al.* guest editors. WHO, UNICEF, and SCN informal consultation on community-based management of severe malnutrition in children. *Food and Nutrition Bulletin* [supplement] 2006;**27**. SCN Nutrition Policy Paper Number 21.

Qazi S. Short-course therapy for community-acquired pneumonia in paediatric patients. *Drugs* 2005;**65**:1179–92.

Rudan I., Tomaskovic L., Boschi-Pinto C. *et al.* and the WHO Child Health Epidemiology Reference Group. Global estimate of the incidence of clinical pneumonia among children under five years of age. *Bulletin of the World Health Organization* 2004;**82**:895–903.

Secretaría de Salud (SS), Instituto Nacional de Estadística (INE), Macro Internacional. *Encuesta nacional de salud y demografía 2005–6*. Tegucigalpa, Honduras, Calverton (MD): Secretaría de Salud, Instituto Nacional de Estadística, Macro International; 2006.

UNICEF, WHO, UNFPA and partners: Countdown to 2015: Tracking progress in maternal, newborn and child survival. The 2008 Report. New York: UNICEF, 2008. www.Countdown2015MNCH.org).

United Nations Children's Fund, World Health Organization. *Low birth weight: country, regional, and global estimates*. New York (NY): UNICEF; 2004.

United Nations Children's Fund. *Child poverty in rich countries*. Florence, Italy: UNICEF Innocenti Research Centre; 2005. Innocenti Report Card Number 6. Available from: http://www.unicef.org/brazil/repcard6e.pdf [Accessed 2007 Oct 1].

United Nations Children's Fund. The state of the world's children 2007. Women and children: the double dividend of gender equality. New York (NY): UNICEF; 2006.

Victora C.G., Kirkwood B.R., Ashworth A. *et al.* Potential interventions for the prevention of childhood pneumonia in developing countries: improving nutrition. *American Journal of Clinical Nutrition* 1999;**70**:309–20.

World Bank. *Data and statistics*. Washington (DC): World Bank; 2007. Available from: http://www.worldbank.org/ [Accessed 2007 May 14].

World Health Organization and United Nations Children's Fund. *Joint statement: clinical management of acute diarrhoea*. Geneva: World Health Organization; New York (NY): UNICEF; 2004.

World Health Organization Collaborative Study team on the Role of Breastfeeding on the Prevention of Infant Mortality. Effect of breastfeeding on infant and child mortality due to infectious diseases in less developed countries: a pooled analysis. *Lancet* 2001;**355**:451–5.

World Health Organization. Antiretroviral drugs for treating pregnant women and preventing HIV infection in infants: guidelines on care, treatment, and support for women living with HIV/AIDS and their children in resource-constrained settings. Geneva: World Health Organization; 2004a.

World Health Organization. Complementary feeding of young children in developing countries: a review of current scientific knowledge. Geneva: World Health Organization; 1998. WHO/NUT/98.1.

World Health Organization. Family and community practices that promote child survival, growth, development—a review of the evidence. Geneva: World Health Organization; 2004b.

World Health Organization. *Guidelines for the treatment of malaria*. Geneva: World Health Organization; 2006a.

World Health Organization. *HIV transmission through breastfeeding—a review of available evidence*. Geneva: World Health Organization; 2004c. WHO/UNICEF/UNFPA/UNAIDS

World Health Organization. Integrated management of childhood illness: complementary course on HIV/AIDS. Geneva: World Health Organization; 2006b.

World Health Organization. *Management of severe malnutrition: a manual for physicians and other senior health workers*. Geneva: World Health Organization; 1999. ISBN 92 4 154511 9 (NLM Classification: WD 101).

World Health Organization. Pregnancy, childbirth, postpartum, and newborn care: a guide for essential practice. 2nd ed. Geneva: World Health Organization; 2006c.

World Health Organization. *Strategic directions for improving the health and development of children and adolescents*. Geneva: World Health Organization; 2002. WHO/FCH/CAH/02.21 Available from: http://www.who.int/child-adolescent-health/publications/OVERVIEW/CAH_Strategy.htm [Accessed 2007 Oct 1].

World Health Organization. *Strategic framework for the prevention of HIV infection in infants in Europe*. Copenhagen, Denmark: Regional Office for Europe of the World Health Organization; 2004d. Available from: http://www.who.int/hiv/mtct/PMTCTEURO.pdf and http://www.unicef.org/ceecis/Strategic_framework_for_the_prevention_of_HIV.pdf [Accessed 2007 Oct 1].

World Health Organization. *The European health report 2005: public health action for healthier children and populations*. Copenhagen, Denmark: Regional Office for Europe of the World Health Organization; 2005a.

World Health Organization. *The world health report 2005: make every mother and child count*. Geneva: World Health Organization; 2005b.

World Health Organization. *WHO HIV and infant feeding technical consultation consensus statement*. Held on behalf of the interagency task team (IATT) on prevention of HIV infections in pregnant women, mothers, and their infants; 2006 Oct 25–7. Geneva: World Health Organization; 2006d. Available from: http://www.who.int/child-adolescent-health/publications/NUTRITION/consensus_statement.htm [Accessed 2007 Oct 1].

World Health Organization. WHO mortality database

World Health Organization. *World health report 2006: working together for health*. Geneva: World Health Organization; 2006e.

World Health Organization. *World health statistics 2007*. Geneva: World Health Organization; 2007. Available from: http://www.who.int/whosis/whostat2007.pdf [Accessed 2007 Oct 1].

11.4

Adolescent health

Pierre-André Michaud,
Venkatraman Chandra-Mouli,
and George C. Patton

Abstract

Around 30% of the world's population is aged 10–24 years, and close to 90% of these young people live in low- and middle-income countries. In recent decades, there have been marked shifts in the health problems affecting this age group. Infectious diseases, including HIV and TB, have become prominent and are major causes of death in Africa and South Asia. Accidents and injuries have also become common and are a greater cause of mortality and morbidity in this age group than others. Chronic illnesses, including mental and behavioural disorders, are the leading cause of disability in the age group. There are emerging problems with obesity in many parts of the world, but undernutrition also remains important in lower-income countries.

Various strategies are likely to be useful in responding to the health problems of young people. The health care system should offer 'youth-friendly' services that take into account the social context, developmental stage, and emerging autonomy of their young patients. The school setting can be used in many countries to implement and sustain broader health promotion initiatives in the age group. Ideally, young people, their parents, and the broader community in which young people live and work should be engaged in the implementation of preventive health programs.

At a broader level, policies that promote easy access to health care and contraception, traffic safety, limitation of access to licit and illicit drugs as well as weapons, and better access to health foods are likely to have a great effect on the health of this age group. Some of the most effective health interventions are likely to be around ongoing engagement in education and promoting a smooth transition into the workforce.

Adolescence and youth: A bio-psychosocial developmental concept

The WHO defines 'adolescence' as the age group of 10–19 years and 'youth' as the age group of 15–24 years. These two overlapping age groups are combined in the category of 'young people', covering the age range of 10–24 years. In this chapter, we will interchangeably use the words 'adolescents' and 'young people', as the categories are arbitrary and the health problems faced are similar. Indeed, adolescence is better viewed as a flexible life phase rather than a fixed time period. In most cultures and in individuals, it begins with the appearance of puberty and ends with a transition to greater emotional and social autonomy. This stage of transition between childhood and adulthood is largely shaped by biological and socioeconomic factors.

There is considerable variation in the onset of adolescence. At an individual level, there is a 4–5 year variation in the age of onset of puberty among healthy individuals, which is a physiological peculiarity of man and is observed even where living conditions are similar for all members of a group. At a population level, there are variations in the timing of puberty across races and across time periods. In Western countries, since around 150 years, pubertal timing has decreased by 4–5 years: The mean age for menarche is now 12–13 years in most high-income countries, whereas it used to occur between 16 and 17 years some centuries ago (Ong *et al.* 2006).

This biological trend is accompanied by an increasing duration of education and training, with a later acquisition of professional capabilities that are the hallmarks of an adult status (Patton & Viner 2007). In pre-industrial societies, the adolescent transition from puberty to adult roles, as defined by the onset of sexual activity, marriage, and parenthood, ranged from around two years in girls to four years in boys. In today's developed economies, longer periods of education, increased affluence, and the availability of effective contraception mean that adolescence commonly persists for well over a decade. Current concepts of adolescence typically encompass a biological onset at puberty and highly variable social transitions that mark its completion. The biological processes initiated at puberty interact with the social context to affect an individual's emotional and social development.

A modern pattern for reproductive capacity, as well as sexual activity, to precede (by more than a decade) role transitions into parenthood and marriage has been accompanied by a rise in the number of sexual partners before marriage and higher rates of sexually transmitted diseases. Similarly, the delay in taking on mature social roles and responsibilities in marriage, parenthood, and employment, associated with earlier initiation of substance use, has been linked to rises in substance use and mental health problems among young people. This phenomenon was limited to high-income countries for many years, but is increasingly being observed in low- and middle-income countries (Lloyd 2005).

Recent neuroscience research has shown that many brain changes continue to take place until the end of the third decade of life. Some changes precede and initiate puberty; others continue well beyond puberty. The possibility that behavioural problems arise because of a mismatch between the emotional reactions and cognitive capacities of young adolescents has long interested clinicians. The importance of this biological gap might be accentuated for those adolescents who mature earlier than their counterparts. Indeed, it has been repeatedly shown that early maturers, both boys and girls, engage in health-compromising behaviours at a higher rate than normal or late maturers and as such may represent a subgroup of adolescents with special vulnerability (Michaud *et al.* 2006).

This gap between the biological maturation of the brain and the acquisition of an adult status within society has important implications, as it creates a period of psychosocial vulnerability: Young people are offered tools and opportunities that they cannot master in terms of their cognitive abilities (Steinberg 2004). For instance, the use of fast motorized vehicles requires anticipation skills that are not necessarily acquired in middle adolescence. Therefore, public health professionals, as we will review later in this chapter, should not expect too much from purely educational strategies and need to place as much emphasis as they can on developing safe environments for adolescents.

Adolescents are a heterogeneous group (Steinberg & Morris 2001). There are great differences between a 12-year-old girl struggling to come to terms with a new body and the emergence of her menstrual periods, and a 19-year-old young woman who is pregnant and engaged to be married. For these reasons, adolescence has been divided into three phases:

- Early adolescence is marked by puberty and a rapid physical growth, with a raised interest in one's self image.
- Middle adolescence is characterized by a period of experimentation with potentially risky behaviours such as unprotected sexual intercourse, and the use of legal and illegal psychoactive substances. Many health-risk behaviours are transitory, but some can have harmful long-term consequences, such as unsafe sex resulting in an HIV infection.
- Late adolescence is a period of progressive stabilization during which young people tend to form more stable relationships and acquire long-term perspectives, a developmental process that extends into early adulthood.

In low- and middle-income countries (mainly in Africa and South Asia), young people currently represent 1.3 billion individuals, a number that will continue to increase up to 1.5 billion by the middle of the century. This is largely due to the improved child survival initiatives implemented over the last three decades. However, in the rest of the world, the proportion of young people within the total population will slowly decrease over the next few decades; that is, the relative size of the youth population will fall. This is largely due to the growing number of people who remain alive at older ages. Another demographic factor that impacts on the health of young people is the increasing age of marriage. Postponing marriage allows young female adolescents to access better education. It also alleviates some of the harmful consequences of very early childbearing.

Also, over the last 20 years, a steadily growing number of low- and middle-income countries have placed emphasis on education (Lloyd 2005; United Nations 2005; World Bank 2007). Learning gives the individual the knowledge and skills needed to master daily tasks and make decisions, including those that relate to health. In the poorest countries, efforts have been directed at ensuring that all children receive primary school education, and in many middle-income countries, authorities have invested in the development of post-primary education. The rate of achievement still varies a great deal across countries: Whereas the retention rate in Thailand up to the ninth grade is around 80 per cent, it drops to 20–40 per cent in countries such as Nicaragua or Senegal, with a large discrepancy between pupils from low and high socioeconomic groups.

The level of education attained should be looked at as one of the main determinants of health. Health literacy is closely linked with the learning process: Adolescents from poor families who drop out of school do much worse than those from wealthier families who have greater access to education and employment (World Bank 2007). With the emergence of new electronic media, young people around the world have access to information that was not previously available. The Internet and other information and communications technologies have created new means of socialization in which young people can reach out without geographic limits. Media use can be considered as potentially harmful in some instances (e.g. depriving physical activity or promoting violent behaviour among vulnerable youngsters), but it should also be viewed as an effective way to disseminate information, especially information on health that could potentially have a positive influence on young people's behaviour.

Adolescence can be viewed as a period of great opportunity and also of vulnerability during which public health interventions can greatly affect current and future health. According to the WHO (World Health Organization 2002a), there are at least three reasons for investing in the health and development of adolescents:

1. Reduction in the burden of morbidity and mortality in later life, because healthy behaviours and practices adopted during adolescence tend to last a lifetime.
2. From an economic perspective, gains in national productivity when healthy and well-educated adolescents enter the workforce.
3. Lastly, adolescent health is a basic human right. The UN Convention on the Rights of the Child (CRC) declares that, 'children and adolescents have a right to life, development, and to benefit from the highest attainable standard of health'.

The health of adolescents and young people: An overview

The health of young people is determined by influences within and outside the health system. Epidemiological research has highlighted the role of these risk and protective factors in shaping the health of young people at an individual and collective level. Figure 11.4.1, adapted from a recent publication (Blum *et al.* 2002), summarizes some of the biological, psychological, and socioenvironmental determinants that have been found to affect adolescent health.

Preventive intervention should address these determinants in the environment, in addition to interventions that are addressed to young people directly. For example, in injury prevention, strategies aimed at improving the environment have been shown to be more effective in reducing injuries than those attempting to directly modify the behaviour of young people (Toroyan & Preden 2007).

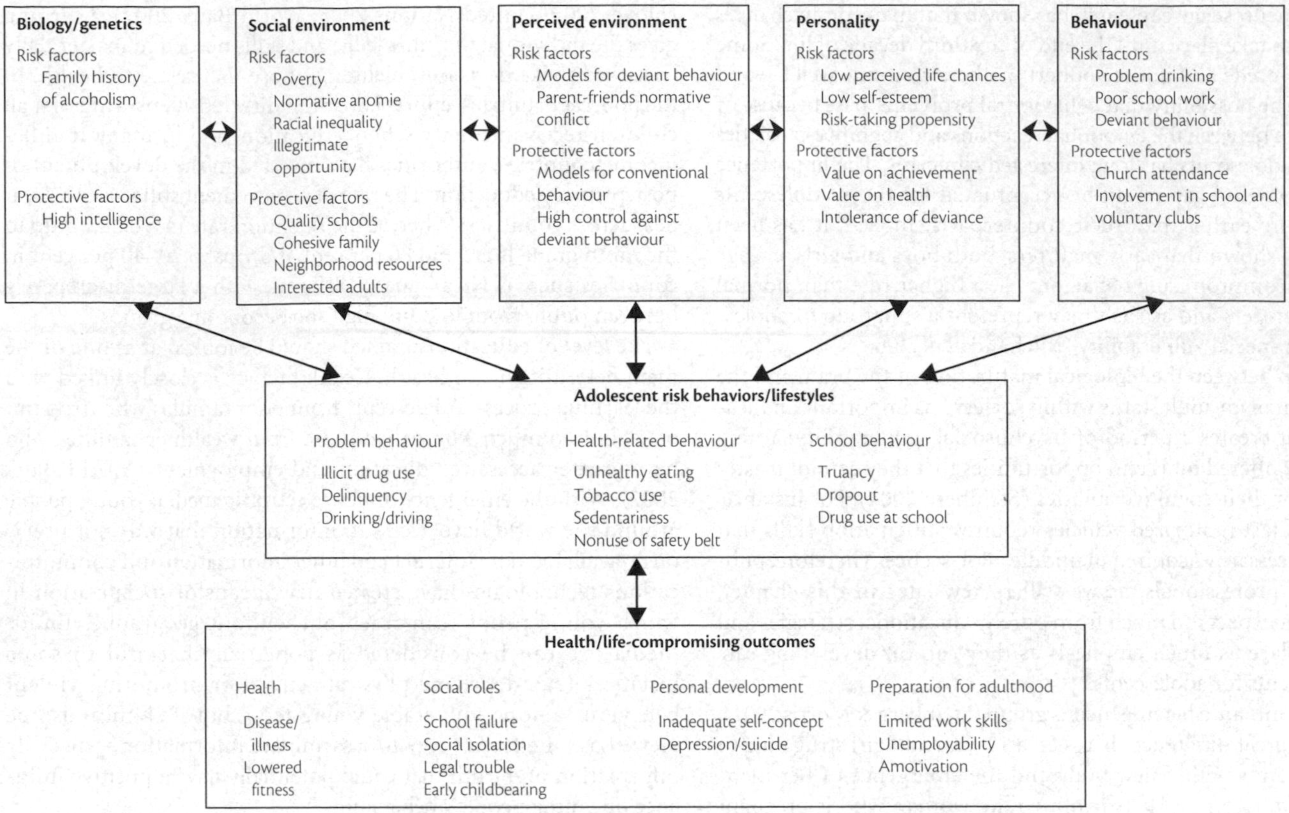

Fig. 11.4.1 Risk and protective factors that impact on the health of adolescents at the individual, family, community, and environmental levels. (Adapted from Blum RW, McNeely C, Nonnemaker J. Vulnerability, risk, and protection. *The Journal Adolescent Health* 2002;**31** Suppl 1:28–39.)

Although the scope and magnitude of health problems among youth vary greatly from one continent and country to another, the profile of problems and burdens found around the world is quite similar. The main current fatalities, diseases or burden of disease, and future threats to health can be observed in both rich and poor countries—such as malnutrition; self-inflicted violence and violence directed at others; HIV, sexually transmitted infections (STIs), and unplanned pregnancies; health problems resulting from substance use; mental health problems; and health and social problems arising from chronic conditions.

Overall, the health of young people has improved over the last decade. Between the 1970s and 1990s, life expectancy at birth increased in low- and middle-income countries more than in high-income countries (Lloyd 2005). This is largely due to the decline in infant mortality and a decrease in the rate of infectious diseases. A notable exception is the epidemic of HIV/AIDS in Africa, particularly in sub-Saharan Africa, where around 60 per cent of deaths among 15–29 year old individuals is attributed to the epidemic. The situation is far less dramatic in Middle East and Asia, but could deteriorate in the future.

In most countries, rich or poor, the overall mortality rate of young people is low in comparison with that of infants, adults, and older people, but the likelihood of premature death is much higher in poor countries. The average 15 year old boy has a 90 per cent chance of surviving to the age of 60 in Western Europe or North America, but only a 50 per cent chance in sub-Saharan Africa, primarily because of communicable diseases such as AIDS. In most parts of the world, with the exception of sub-Saharan Africa and South America, the main cause of premature deaths among young people is injuries, as exemplified in Table 11.4.1.

The second highest cause of death is suicide, which represents but one consequence of the burden of mental health problems and disorders among young people. Homicides are a notable cause of deaths among young people: Although it is often the result of crimes due to a violent environment in some US suburbs and in South America, it should not be forgotten that in other parts of the world, notably in Africa, it is the result of war and armed conflict. In 2003, more than 70 countries were considered as 'unstable' (UNAIDS 2006), and UNICEF estimates that there are approximately 300 000 young people under the age of 18 enrolled as soldiers, many of them forcibly recruited (United Nations 2005). Finally, in Africa, Southeast Asia, and to some extent in Eastern Mediterranean countries, other infectious diseases constitute an important cause of mortality and morbidity (Blum 1991).

The data on the global burden of disease estimated by Lopez *et al.* (2006) represent another view of the top-priority health concerns among young people. Health habits and lifestyles acquired during adolescence will impact on the future state of health and the global burden of disease. Among the top ten conditions that affect the global burden of disease worldwide, at least five are directly linked with health behaviours largely developed during the adolescent period: Unsafe sex, legal and illegal use of psychoactive

Table 11.4.1 Five leading causes of mortality in 15–29-year-olds[a]

World regions	Leading causes of death[b] Unintentional injuries	AIDS	Other infectious causes	Homicide/war/other intentional injuries	Suicide/self-inflicted injuries
All world regions	**1** (531 000)	**2** (326 000)	**3** (229 000)	**4** (227 000)	**5** (124 000)
South America/Caribbean	**2** (64 000)	**5** (11 000)	**4** (12 000)	**1** (72 000)	**3** (14 000)
Africa	**4** (56 000)	**1** (225 000)	**2** (104 000)	**3** (66 000)	**5** (6000)
Southeast Asia	**1** (178 000)	**3** (72 000)	**2** (81 000)	**5** (33 000)	**4** (37 000)
Western Pacific	**1** (119 000)	**5** (8000)	**3** (19 000)	**4** (17 000)	**2** (32 000)
Eastern Mediterranean	**1** (40 000)	**4** (7000)	**2** (21 000)	**3** (15 000)	**5** (5000)
Europe	**1** (74 000)	**5** (2000)	**4** (10 000)	**3** (23 000)	**2** (30 000)
North America[c]	**1**	**6**	**5**	**3**	**2**

[a] Between brackets: Number of deaths worldwide.
[b] Data on maternal mortality among 15–29-year-olds not available.
[c] In North America, cancer is the fourth leading cause of death in the adolescent/young adult years.
Source: Blum RW, Nelson-Mmari K. The health of young people in a global context. *The Journal of Adolescent Health* 2004:**35** 402–16.

substances and of tobacco, physical inactivity, and high body mass index (BMI).

Injuries and other forms of violence inflicted against and among adolescents

Injuries among young people are mainly due to traffic accidents, interpersonal violence, war, and suicide, and account for substantial mortality and morbidity. Apart from sub-Saharan Africa, where HIV accounts for a large proportion of deaths, in the rest of the world, violent deaths make up half of the mortality. A recent review run by the Department of Injuries and Violence Prevention of the WHO (World Health Organization 2002b) gives a good overview of the importance of injuries to the health of young people. In 2002, worldwide, among males aged 15–29 years, road traffic injuries accounted for approximately 285 000 deaths per year and for 12.4 billions disability-adjusted life years (DALYs), whereas the figures for females were 70 000 deaths and 2.7 billions DALYs. As motorized transportation grows, it is expected that the number of deaths linked with traffic accidents will also grow.

Overall, the profile of deaths by injuries varies greatly between males and females: Males experience more than twice the rate of fatalities than females do. Whereas road traffic injuries are the most common injuries among males, self-inflicted injuries (suicide) are the most common among females. Among males, interpersonal violence is the second most common cause of violent deaths: In some regions of the world (e.g. in South America), it is the most frequent cause of death as well as the leading cause of DALYs among both males and females. In Africa, the leading cause of death and of DALYs is war; in 2000, an estimated 53 856 young people aged 15–29 years lost their lives as a result of armed conflict. These deaths are not only those of young people enrolled in the army, but also of barbaric acts perpetrated among young people, especially among females.

The problem of violence affecting young people is not only reflected by high rates of mortality, but also of various injuries and handicaps. Severe traffic injuries often result in permanent brain or limb damage. The same applies to young people who are victims of anti-personnel mines. It is in the Americas that one observes the highest rates of homicide among young people. In many countries of this region, homicides account for one-third of the deaths among young people. Homicide is the second highest cause of death among young people in half of the South American countries and accounts for high rates of death in the United States as well (McAlister 2006).

Violence prevention needs to address risk factors at the individual, family, community, and societal levels (Dahlberg & Potter 2001; World Health Organization 2004c). Evidence shows that life-skills and social development programmes for children and adolescents aged 6–19 years are effective, as are mentoring programmes to develop attachments between at-risk youth and caring adults (Tremblay 2006). Visiting and supporting parents of young children at home and building their skills in problem solving and non-violent disciplining have also been shown to be effective in reducing parental violence. Preschool enrichment programmes (for children aged 3–5 years), and life-skills and social development programmes (for children and adolescents aged 6–19 years) have been shown to be effective in reducing violent behaviour later in life.

Several school-based violence prevention programmes have been implemented with a special focus on dating violence prevention and the promotion of healthy relationships. Those which have been proven effective have usually involved the surrounding community. A good example of such a programme is the Seattle Social Development Project, a theory-guided preventive intervention that strengthened teaching and parenting practices, and taught children interpersonal skills during the elementary grades, as well as showed wide-ranging beneficial effects on functioning in early adulthood, including better mental functioning and reduced crime and substance abuse (Hawkins *et al.* 2005).

Reducing the availability of alcohol and other legal substances, and decreasing the demand for and access to lethal weapons are effective ways of reducing violence. Actions to make health systems more responsive and to build the empathy and competence of health workers can help ensure that adolescents who experience violence, including sexual violence, get effective and sensitive care and treatment. Also, the provision of ongoing psychological and social support can help adolescents deal with the long-term psychological effects of violence, and reduce the likelihood of their becoming perpetuators of violence in the future. Finally, it should be stressed that reducing poverty, economic inequality, and social exclusion, which strongly impact on the occurrence of violence, is probably among the most effective strategies. However, outcome evaluation research to test all these strategies in low- and middle-income countries is urgently needed.

Road traffic accidents are increasing alarmingly in some low- and middle-income countries. This is due to the growth of motorized transport, a rise in the number of vehicles, and perhaps, a lack of education in driving skills. Four main types of strategies can be developed to address traffic injuries: Modifying the road environment, increasing the safeness of vehicles, providing guidance and support, and reducing the exposure of young people to traffic (Munro *et al.* 1995). Traffic calming measures and enforcing speed limits have proven particularly effective. Another environmental measure tested in high-income countries is preventing driving while under the influence of alcohol by providing alternative means of transportation for young people during late hours of the night. The use of seat belts and helmets is another very effective way to diminish the potential health impact of accidents.

Mental health

In nearly all countries, mental disorders account for an important, and often underestimated, part of the burden of disease. Five of the ten leading causes of DALYs in people aged 15–44 years are mental disorders: Unipolar depressive disorders, alcohol use disorders, self-inflicted injuries, schizophrenia, and bipolar affective disorders (Patel *et al.* 2007). One of the reasons for this is that several mental disorders start during adolescence (Michaud & Fombonne 2005). Mental health problems during adolescence constitute a heavy burden at the individual as well as the societal level, because they are not only a significant source of suffering for the adolescent and his or her family, but also often negatively influence the future of life course emotionally, socially, and professionally. Also, suicide, which frequently is a result of a mental disorder, represents one of the leading causes of deaths in many countries.

It is not easy to distinguish mental health problems from true disorders. Mental disorders are defined as situations characterized by lasting behavioural or psychological burden accompanied by a concomitant distress and/or a raised risk of death, or an important loss of freedom, involving an unexpected cultural response to any situation (Michaud & Fombonne 2005). Over the last few decades, it has been estimated that the rate of adolescents suffering from mental health problems and disorders is on the rise (Rutter & Smith 1995). In industrialized countries, the most prominent increase has been observed in the area of substance use, eating disorders, and conduct disorders (antisocial behaviour).

Many adolescents suffer from several mental health problems that tend to cluster. For example, psychoactive substance use disorder (PSUD) is often associated with depression and suicide attempts. The WHO estimates that this trend will continue and that there will be a 50 per cent increase in the percentage of young people suffering from mental disorders worldwide (World Health Organization 2003). One important problem linked with mental health disorders is that adolescents are often reluctant to seek help or to express their mental health problem in a way that is readily identifiable by family members, teachers, peers, or even health practitioners.

Public health interventions must tackle both risk and protective factors for mental health. Promoting mental health, preventing mental health problems, and responding to them if and when they arise requires a continuum of responses ranging from the community level, through health services at the primary level, to specialist health and social services at the referral level (Patel *et al.* 2007). The fact that mental health problems are very often correlated with other health problems (e.g. substance abuse and violence) must be taken into account. By identifying and treating individuals with attention-deficit hyperactivity disorder, psychoses, mood disorders, and anxiety disorders, one may well decrease the number of adolescents who will engage in violent behaviour, delinquency, or substance abuse.

A growing body of evidence suggests that effective interventions could reduce risk factors and enhance protective factors at the level of the child or adolescent, the family, and the community. These interventions include enhancing social skills, problem-solving skills, and self-confidence, and can address all the children in a community (universal interventions) or those at particular risk (selective interventions). They have been shown to help prevent specific mental health problems such as conduct disorders, anxiety, depression, and eating disorders, as well as other risk behaviours, including those that relate to sexual behaviour, substance use behaviour, and violent behaviour (World Health Organization 2004b).

There is some evidence that broad school-based approaches can have a beneficial midterm effect on the behaviour and mental health of pupils (Patton *et al.* 2006), as will be discussed later. These measures are particularly effective for young people who are at risk of developing mental health problems because of their family or social environment. Another complementary approach is to integrate mental health interventions with other existing youth programmes. For example, mental health prevention can be coupled with programmes focusing on sexual and reproductive health or programmes directed at the reduction of violent behaviours.

Also, another important area of intervention is to provide adolescents with mental health problems and disorders with better access to adequate treatment. Health workers at the primary level need to have the competencies to relate to young people, to detect mental health problems early, and to provide appropriate treatment, which includes counselling, cognitive-behavioural therapy and, where appropriate, psychotropic medication. However, these workers should be backed by specialist services at the referral level (Patel *et al.* 2007).

Worldwide, it is estimated that between 100 000 and 200 000 young people commit suicide every year. In industrialized countries, it is the first or second most common cause of death among young people, and also accounts for a large proportion of deaths in other countries (Wasserman *et al.* 2005). In 26 countries for which data were available for the period 1965–99, a rising trend of suicide in young males was observed, which was marked in the years before 1980 and in countries outside Europe. The determinants of suicide are multiple and complex, and include both personal vulnerability factors as well as family and psychosocial characteristics (Beautrais *et al.* 2006). Dysfunctional social networks, such as being disconnected from community and family ties, seem to play a predominant role.

Several countries have engaged in large, population-based, effective suicide prevention programmes (Wilson 2004), which include a sensitization of the whole population as well as training of target groups of professionals such as health workers, clergymen, policemen, teachers, and educators. Some countries have implemented formal teaching sessions addressing the issue of suicidal behaviours within the school setting. Most workers point out that such universal approaches show no evidence of a beneficial effect on suicide attempts and suicide. Ploed *et al.* (1996) suggest that more broadly based comprehensive school health programmes should be developed, addressing the determinants of adolescent risk behaviour. A promising more selective approach is the identification by lay professionals, such as teachers and social workers, of potentially suicidal adolescents who can then be referred to their doctor or to mental health facilities (Hawton & James 2005).

Substance use, misuse, and abuse

Psychotropic substances ('drugs') include both legal and illegal drugs such as, among others, tobacco, alcohol, psychoactive medication, cannabis, synthetic substances, cocaine, and heroin. Tobacco currently represents a major cause of death among adults in the world (Lopez & Mathers 2006): Nearly 5 million persons die every year from tobacco-related illnesses, with disproportionately higher mortality occurring in low- and middle-income countries. For instance, chronic obstructive lung diseases cause almost as many deaths as HIV/AIDS (2.7 million). Among those people who smoke, nearly a quarter had smoked their first cigarette before they reached the age of ten.

The Global Youth Tobacco Survey (GYTS), initiated in 1999 by WHO, the Centers for Disease Control, and the Canadian Public Health Association, is a school-based survey that provides self-reported data on the prevalence of cigarette and other tobacco products use within each of the six WHO regions (Centers for Disease Control 2007). The GYTS data indicate that nearly 2 of every 10 students report currently using a tobacco product (smoking: 8.9 per cent; other tobacco use: 11.2 per cent). Use of any tobacco products is highest in the American and European regions (22.2 per cent and 19.8 per cent, respectively) and lowest in the Southeast Asian and Western Pacific regions (12.9 per cent and 11.4 per cent, respectively). Boys are significantly more likely than girls to use any tobacco products in the Eastern Mediterranean, Southeast Asian, and Western Pacific regions, and significantly more likely than girls to smoke cigarettes in the African, Southeast Asian, and Western Pacific regions. Deterring young people from starting tobacco use is one of the big public health challenges health policy makers currently face.

The use of alcohol is heavily linked with cultural and religious contexts, which explains why its use varies considerably across countries. Although no evidence exists of significant health benefits from moderate alcohol consumption for young adults, it is essentially the hazardous use of alcohol (also named 'alcohol misuse' or 'problematic alcohol use') that represents a serious problem during adolescence because of its short- and long-term consequences, such as violence, unprotected sex, and injuries while driving under the influence of alcohol, or developing alcohol dependence once they enter adulthood (Bonomo *et al.* 2004). In Western countries, especially in Europe, the rate of adolescents reporting hazardous use of alcohol (on a more or less regular basis) has increased over the last two decades (Zaborskis *et al.* 2006). In Africa and South America, alcohol use and hazardous use are also on the rise, because of societal changes.

Besides alcohol, cannabis is the most frequently used illicit drug worldwide. The lifetime prevalence of cannabis use, however, differs greatly from one country to another. The available data suggest that lifetime prevalence rates of cannabis use, misuse (problematic use), and abuse are increasing in many countries. According to the Global Youth Network of the UN Commission on Narcotic Drugs (CND) (United Nations Economic and Social Council, Commission on Narcotic Drugs 1991), the percentage of young people having ever used cannabis varies between 1 per cent in poor countries such as Romania and 40–45 per cent in countries with high prevalence such as Canada, the United States, and Switzerland, with several countries such as those in Asia displaying intermediate figures (~5 per cent). A much lower but still substantial percentage of young people have access to other illicit drugs such as ecstasy, cocaine, and heroin, especially in high-income countries.

Young people initiate substance use for a range of reasons that may include curiosity and some peer pressure. Perceptions of prevailing norms on substance use are relevant to the extent that young people commonly conform to such norms in defining their identity (Hawkins *et al.* 1991). Influences on continuing and escalating use include vulnerability related to mental health, family difficulties, school failure, and unemployment, but the cultural, economic, and legal contexts in which adolescent development takes place also influence patterns of initiation and progression of substance use (Kodjo & Klein 2002). Several countries are currently debating whether the penalties for possessing small amounts of cannabis should be reduced: Reducing penalties for cannabis use does not necessarily lead to widespread use in the young. In the Netherlands, where cannabis use is not a criminal offence, the lifetime prevalence of cannabis use is lower than in the United States, which has some of the toughest cannabis laws in the Western world (Korf 2002).

Public health responses to adolescent substance use may take a variety of forms (Toumbourou *et al.* 2007). As mentioned before, regulatory interventions seek to limit the availability of substances through taxation and legislation. Legislation includes regulation of sales through age restrictions on purchase as well as regulation at points of sale, on hours of sale, and on quantities that can be sold. Regulation extends to limiting use in public spaces, a strategy that has been the cornerstone of tobacco control, although with less success in young people than in adults. Developmental interventions seek to reduce demand for substances by promoting healthy development and tackling risks that arise in the course of development.

Improving the social climate of secondary schools and/or implementing a life-skills approach among pupils could contribute to decreasing the likelihood of engagement in both licit and illicit substance use (Tobler 2000). Screening of young people and brief psychological interventions may be effective in reducing substance abuse (McCambridge & Strang 2004). Family interventions also appear very relevant and effective for the younger adolescent substance abuser (Kumpfer & Alvarado 2005). Finally, harm-reduction interventions are important in an overall public health response to substance abuse (Toumbourou *et al.* 2007). In those with harmful use, abuse, and dependence, these interventions seek to reduce the likelihood of negative outcomes without necessarily affecting the level of substance use. For example, needle and syringe exchange programmes have been shown to be effective in preventing HIV transmission without encouraging an increase in substance use through injection or other routes.

Nutritional problems and obesity

Chronic malnutrition in earlier years is responsible for widespread stunting and adverse health and social consequences throughout the life span. This is best prevented in childhood, but actions to improve access to food could benefit adolescents as well. Anaemia is one of the key nutritional problems in adolescent girls. Preventing too-early pregnancy and improving the nutritional status of girls before they enter pregnancy could reduce maternal and infant mortality, and contribute to breaking the cycle of intergenerational malnutrition. This will involve improving access to nutritious food and to micronutrient supplementation and, in many places, preventing infections as well. Adolescence is a timely period to shape healthy eating and exercise habits that can contribute to physical and psychological benefits during the adolescent period and to reducing the likelihood of nutrition-related chronic diseases in adulthood.

Over the past decade, WHO has recognized that overweight and obesity represent a major public health challenge, reaching pandemic proportions among adults as well as among children and adolescents. This pandemic was first observed and is still prominent in high-income countries such as the United States and those in Western Europe (Ogden *et al.* 2003), but has also occurred in Eastern Europe (Musaiger 2004), South America, and East Asia (Wang *et al.* 2002). The prevalence of overweight and obesity has increased markedly in the last two decades in most high- and middle-income countries (Wang *et al.* 2002). For instance, in the European Union, the number of overweight children is increasing by at least 400 000 every year, of which 85 000 are obese (Lobstein & Frelut 2003). This trend has arisen as a result of obesogenic environments, more sedentary time, diminished physical activity, and increasing calorie consumption. Urbanization encourages the use of automobiles and other motorized vehicles; in high-income countries, suburbs lack stores, entertainment, or other destinations within walking distance. Also, outside Northern European countries, infrastructure that supports walking and cycling has been neglected.

Linked with the area of obesity is an upward trend in the incidence of eating disorders in high- and middle-income countries. Anorexia nervosa is a condition that typically affects adolescents (0.5–1 per cent of the female population below 20 years), whereas bulimia nervosa tends to affect young adult females (3–5 per cent of this population). Increasingly, more girls (and even boys) suffer from typical and atypical eating disorders (so-called EDNOS for 'eating disorder not otherwise specified'), which are conditions only partially fulfilling the criteria for anorexia or bulimia, but are the source of much suffering, and often, of an overuse of health care (Chamay-Weber *et al.* 2005).

Most public health strategies addressing the area of overweight and obesity of young people have focused on the school setting. Several recent meta-analyses have reviewed the factors that contribute to the success of interventions in the field (Flodmark *et al.* 2006). In general, long-lasting programmes with a sound conceptual framework appear successful. Multifaceted interventions addressing intake as well as energy expenditure appear to be the most effective. An example of this approach is the CATCH intervention (Coordinated Approach to Child Health) run in 24 schools of the San Diego County in the United States, and directed at elementary and middle-school children. The intervention was designed to modify the pupils' environment by increasing the number and intensity of physical education sessions and modifying available food within the school. These principles apply to interventions targeting specifically obese adolescents as well.

Although encouraging youngsters to engage in physical activity has only a modest effect on their weight, it has a significant effect on health-compromising correlates of obesity such as glucose metabolism and cardiovascular fitness. The prevention of obesity should be progressively achieved through environmental measures set up in close collaboration with the food industry, such as political and economic measures, and large media campaigns. Physical and sports activities should be encouraged by increasing opportunities and facilities both within and outside the school. For instance, the European community set up the European Childhood Obesity Group, which has developed a comprehensive programme in cooperation with the food industry, advertisement agencies, and associations of consumers, and puts a strong emphasis on environmental measures (Widhalm & Fussenegger 2005).

Sexual and reproductive health

There is no area that has been more influenced by the biological and societal shifts reviewed at the beginning of this chapter as has the sexual and reproductive health of young people. Both societal transformation and behavioural patterns create a situation of unique vulnerabilities and expose young people to heightened risks for poor health outcomes, such as unplanned (early) pregnancy, STIs including HIV/AIDS, and sexual coercion and abuse (Bearinger *et al.* 2007). Biological as well as psychosocial factors contribute to this vulnerability: For example, young girls are at increased risk for acquiring an STI or facing difficulty in childbirth because of the immaturity of their reproductive and immune systems. The psychological vulnerability of adolescents, both girls and boys, also places them at greater risk of sexual exploitation, and in several countries, adolescents who are compelled to become sex workers are at heightened risk of STIs, pregnancy, and violence.

Sexual behaviour, contraception, and safe sex

Several surveys conducted among young people in high-income countries show that they tend to engage in premarital sexual activity in a progressive way; that is, from kissing to petting,and then, non-penetrative and penetrative intercourse (Brown *et al.* 2001), but this may not apply to some low-income countries where sexual activity starts with marriage, at least among women. Indeed, cultural and contextual factors do play an important role in the sequencing of these events. For instance, in the United States, which has promoted 'abstinence-only programmes', young people tend to replace penetrative vaginal intercourse with oral sex, which has raised a number of controversies in that country about the adequacy of this strategy (Brown *et al.* 2001).

The age at which young people tend to engage in sexual experiences varies, depending on contextual and cultural factors (Bearinger *et al.* 2007). In Africa, the percentage of young people aged 15–24 years reporting being sexually experienced varies between 30 and 60 per cent among males, and between 7 and 60 per cent among females. In Eastern Europe and Central Asia, the percentages among females and males are lower. In Latin America, they are between 40 and 60 per cent among males, and between 10 and 25 per cent among females ; whereas in high-income countries, the rates vary between 45 and 60 per cent, and are fairly similar among males and females.

In high-income as well as in many low- and middle-income countries, the gap between the first sexual intercourse and marriage is widening, which means that most early sexual experiences occur among unmarried young women and men. However, it has to be recognized that, in some places, many adolescent girls (an estimate of 100 million within the next 10 years) have their first sexual intercourse while married, with the consequence that they often do not use any contraception or protection and could be at high risk of acquiring STIs (Wellings *et al.* 2006).

The use of effective contraception and protection among young people has increased considerably over the last decades; around 1990, the reported rates were as low as 2–4 per cent in Africa and South America and between 10–30 per cent in the Middle East and Asia (Lloyd 2005). According to the most recent data available, in Africa and Latin America, it is around 20 per cent in the Middle East and around 50 per cent in Asia. As can be seen, the rates vary substantially from one region to another: In Western Europe, in the year 2000, 70–80 per cent of young people reported to have used effective contraception at first intercourse (Bajos & Guillaume 2003).

The most readily available contraceptive device is the condom, which also protects against STIs. It is thus very important to assess to what extent young people are informed on the issues of both contraception and infection protection, and are provided easy access to condoms. Many countries have embarked on information campaigns, resulting in increased condom usage among sexually active young people. Unfortunately, even in regions with high rates of HIV/AIDS, a substantial proportion of young people still do not use condoms: For example, the rates of males aged 15–24 years using condoms vary between 20 (e.g. in Mali, Haiti, and Malawi) and 40 per cent in many low-income countries.

Early childbearing and abortion

The average birth rate for young people varies considerably across regions (World Health Organization 2004a). In countries in sub-Saharan Africa, it ranges from 40–230 per 1000 adolescents; in North Africa, the Middle East, and Central and South Asia, the figures are lower (~7–120 per 1000). In Europe, the rates vary between a low of 5 per 1000 in Switzerland and a high of 40 per 1000 in Bulgaria. In South America, the figures vary roughly between 50 and 150 per 1000. The United States has a high rate of birth of around 40 per 1000, one of the highest among high-income countries, whereas Canada's rate is much lower at around 15 per 1000.

As a result of their biological immaturity and psychosocial vulnerability, adolescents who are pregnant face higher risks of medical complications and death. Indeed, maternal mortality and morbidity related to pregnancy constitute a significant threat to the health of many young women in low- and middle-income countries, especially among adolescents younger than 14 or 15 years of age. Worldwide, the death rates vary between around 6 per 100 000 in East Asia and 25 per 100 000 in North Africa and the Middle East (WHO 2001b). The gap between high-income countries and low- and middle-income countries is impressive: The lifetime risk of dying from maternal causes is 1 in 2800 in wealthy countries whereas it reaches 1 in 61 in sub-Saharan African countries (Lloyd 2005). Besides death, childbearing at a younger age has a greater likelihood of complications such as infection, haemorrhage, eclampsia, obstructed labour, and vesicovaginal fistula. Many of these adverse consequences are linked with absence of services, poor access to adequate medical care, and lack of confidentiality, and may thus be addressed in the future by more adequate coverage of the specific needs of pregnant adolescents.

Faced with an unplanned pregnancy, girls may choose to have the baby or elect to have an abortion. Such decisions are not only dependent on personal and family factors, but are heavily linked to environmental and cultural factors as well. The number of abortions taking place outside the formal or legal health-care system or taking place in countries in which it is considered illegal is obviously difficult to estimate. Performed in adequate conditions, with up-to-date methods, abortion is safe and carries little health risks.

However, every year, about 19–20 million abortions are performed by individuals without adequate skills and in unsafe environments; 97 per cent of these are in low- and middle-income countries (Grimes *et al.* 2006). Young women aged 15–24 years account for about 25 per cent of these unsafe abortions in Africa, whereas the percentages are lower in Asia and Latin America. A recent comparison of birth and abortion rates among 46 countries showed that the adolescent birth rate has declined in the majority of industrialized countries over the past 25 years and that pregnancy rates in 12 of the 18 countries with accurate abortion reporting showed declines (Lloyd 2005).

Sexual coercion and violence, female genital mutilation

Sexual coercion can be defined as an act of forcing, or attempting to force, an individual to engage in sexual behaviour against his or her will, using violence, threats, verbal insistence, and deception. The consequences of such sexual violence both among females and males are important, including intense mental suffering, depression, post-traumatic stress disorder, and even suicide. Moreover, some young people may engage in casual and unsafe sex as a result of having experienced forced sex. Young female and young male adolescents with homosexual orientation are at high risk for such events because of their inexperience and because of the age gap with the perpetrator.

For social and cultural reasons, female genital mutilation (FGM) remains common in many countries, including African countries where over 136 million women have been 'multilated' despite persistent and consistent efforts by various governments (Magoha & Magoha 2000). Besides measures such as repression through legislation, which can be set up in these countries, proper education of young girls, and above all, sensitization of families and communities to change social norms in this area should be set up. Moreover, health professionals should be sensitized to this issue: Even Western high-income countries should consider the risk of FGM when caring for migrant adolescents from countries where these operations still take place.

STIs and HIV

The WHO (World Health Organization 2001a) estimated that there were 340 million new cases of syphilis, gonorrhoea, chlamydia, and trichomoniasis worldwide in 1999 in men and women aged 15–49 years, whereas in 1990, the figure was around 250 million new cases. Within and between countries, the prevalence and incidence of STIs vary greatly due to many factors such as differences between urban and rural environments, levels of knowledge, and availability of protection. STIs tend to occur at a younger age in females than in males, which may be explained by differences in patterns of sexual activity and in the relative rates of transmission from one sex to the other (World Health Organization 2001a). Data in this field must be interpreted with caution, because the surveillance of STI spread is a neglected field in many countries worldwide.

An estimated 38.6 million people worldwide were living with HIV in 2005. Every year, around 4.1 million become newly infected with HIV and around 2.8 million lose their lives to HIV-related illnesses. Globally, an estimated 10.3 million young people aged 15–24 years are living with HIV/AIDS, and half of all new infections—over 6000 daily—are occurring among young people. About two-thirds of young people aged 15–24 years with an HIV infection live in sub-Saharan African countries (Bearinger *et al.* 2007). Many young people are vulnerable to HIV because of unsafe sexual behaviour, substance use, and their lack of access to HIV information and prevention services.

Young people who are marginalized and homeless, injecting drugs, or working in the sex industry have the highest risks. The UN estimates that there are more than 150 million street children worldwide injecting drugs using non-sterile needles and syringes, accounting for an estimated 10 per cent of all new HIV infections. Intravenous drug use (IDU) is often initiated at a young age and, in some places, the injecting trend among young people is increasing. Moreover, it is estimated that only 16 per cent of HIV-positive youth know their serological status, which means that the vast majority of young people who are HIV-positive do not know that they are living with HIV. Moreover, few young people engaging in sex know the HIV status of their partners.

Primary prevention is the cornerstone of HIV/AIDS prevention and does actually also address the transmission of other STIs. A recent publication of the WHO (World Health Organization 2006) provides a comprehensive review of evidence-based strategies to reach this objective. A second important area of intervention is secondary prevention: Public health programmes should focus on offering HIV testing to young people to identify those who are already HIV-positive and to help them access the services that will keep them healthy and teach them the skills needed to protect their sex partners. Moreover, testing and identifying young people who are HIV-negative helps them to stay negative as long as they are provided counselling sessions along with the test itself.

Although the search for an effective vaccine against HIV is still on its way, the recent introduction of the human papilloma virus (HPV) vaccine gives a good example of future avenues to control the spread of some STIs. Worldwide, HPV infections are responsible for approximately 493 000 cervical cancer cases annually, about half of which result death each year (Bosch & de Sanjose 2003). It remains to be shown that, given the price of the vaccine and the logistics required to vaccinate young people, this vaccine will represent an effective means to prevent cervical cancer, especially in low- and middle-income countries.

Services, community health, and policies

The continuum-of-care approach is one that has been applied to maternal and child health and which is also applicable to adolescent health, in which interventions commonly aim to affect more than one health outcome (Mahler 1986). In this subsection, we describe approaches at three levels of care: Hospital care, ambulatory or primary-level care, and the scope for health promotion.

Youth-friendly health services

The WHO, in collaboration with UNICEF, developed the concept of adolescent- or youth-friendly health services (YFHS) (McInthyre 2003). This approach stressed the need for a holistic and developmental approach to ambulatory care for young people. Factors contributing to adolescent-friendly service delivery are outlined in Table 11.4.2. The principles of YFHS have initially been conceptualized and implemented in specialized ambulatory youth clinics. They are, however, relevant to other health-care settings such as inpatient hospital care.

There is growing evidence that younger patients experience better quality of care in adolescent wards compared to child or adult wards (Viner 2007), but this seems particularly relevant in high-income countries. A recent review concluded that: 'Enough is known to recommend that each country, state, and locality has a policy and support to encourage provision of innovative and well-assessed youth-friendly health services' (Tylee *et al.* 2007). The principles of adolescent-friendly health services are not only appropriate for creating specific youth clinics, but they also apply to existing school health centres, primary-care clinics, private practice, and outreach facilities.

Indeed, primary-care physicians play a role in promoting adolescent health through a strategy of providing health guidance

Table 11.4.2 Basic principles of youth-/adolescent-friendly services

Policies	◆ Fulfil the right of adolescents ◆ Address the special needs of vulnerable adolescents ◆ No stigmatization (ethnicity, social status, *etc.*) ◆ Confidentiality guaranteed ◆ Affordability of services
Procedures	◆ Easy access ◆ Easy registration ◆ Short waiting time
Healthcare providers	◆ Technically competent ◆ Communication skills ◆ Adequate time ◆ Provide information and support ◆ Evidence-based approach
Environment	◆ Convenient location ◆ Convenient opening hours ◆ Outreach activities ◆ Link with the community
Youth participation	◆ Young people consulted/youth council ◆ Young people's satisfaction surveyed ◆ Young people disseminating information

Source: McInthyre P. *Adolescent-friendly health services.* Geneva: World Health Organization; 2003.

to adolescents and parents, screening, and encouraging immunizations; the rationale is that many aspects of lifestyle relevant to health are adopted in adolescence (Elster & Levenberg 1997). Goldenring and Rosen (Goldenring & Rosen 2004) proposed a simple mnemonic tool, HEEADSSS, to define the main areas to be covered in screening: Home, Education, Eating, Activities, Drugs, Sexuality, Suicide, and Security.

School-based preventive strategies

Adolescents, up to the age of 15–18 years, spend just under half their waking hours in school. Thus, schools remain one of the most important settings for health promotion and preventive interventions for young people, which include the following:

- Programmes aimed at increasing physical activity, often with a nutrition component: As in other instances, the available evidence suggests that programmes extending outside the school zone and involving the parents are more effective than those targeting the pupils only (Van Sluijs *et al.* 2007).
- Drug education, such as programmes promoting the adoption of life and social skills: Some evidence from efficacy trials shows that modest sustained effects in reducing uptake of licit and illicit drugs can take place with such programmes, but there are few models of effective, sustained, and system-wide implementation (Tobler 2000). Interventions involving parents and the community are more effective than those involving the students only (Kumpfer & Alvarado 2005).
- Sexuality education programmes: The issue of sexual education is a hotly debated one; carefully designed interventions such as those based on sound theoretical frameworks have had positive effects on the adoption of safe sex behaviours, without increasing the percentage of young people engaging in active sexual life (World Health Organization 2006).

The extension of health education to health promotion led the WHO to develop the concept of a health promoting school (HPS). The network of HPSs currently involves more than 35 countries. Schools commit to establishing a healthy physical and social environment. Youth participation such as setting up pupils' councils, or mediation sessions in case of conflict, and the use of life-skills interventions are encouraged. Some evidence supports key components of the HPS programme, namely that the programmes should be sustained, multifaceted, and have the commitment of the head of the school to provide appropriate training to the staff and to work in a holistic way (World Health Organization 2006). An excellent example of this approach was the Gatehouse project (Patton *et al.* 2006), a multilevel systemic programme focusing on promoting social inclusion of students with a view to promoting mental health and diminishing health-risk behaviours. Reductions in health-risk behaviours over a period of four years ranged from around 25 per cent for substance use and socially disruptive behaviours to around 50 per cent for levels of very early sexually activity. These are substantially greater than the effects obtained from health education alone and, given that they are largely based on changes in the schools' environment, offer a better prospect for sustainable system change.

Community health and policies

Other promising community strategies to promote the health of young people include media campaigns, the adoption of policies outside the health sector, and interventions within the community. In the field of smoking prevention, a recent review has shown some superiority of programmes involving the whole community over traditional approaches targeting young people only (Sowden *et al.* 2003). Community-based preventive interventions have shown an effect on youth substance use (Wu *et al.* 2002), suicide (Omar 2005), harmful drinking (Stafstrom *et al.* 2006), and rates of teen pregnancy (Cassell *et al.* 2005).

The International Policy Context around Adolescent Health and Development has received considerable attention in the past five years with a range of initiatives affecting the way in which health and other systems address young people and their development. Several of these initiatives have frameworks that extend beyond a health focus, a concept referred to as the 'new public health'. The World Bank Report on (Adolescent) Development and the Next Generation (World Bank 2007) dealt with the potential for interventions around young people to have a impact on the health and development of the next generation. The report took important steps in outlining a comprehensive framework for youth health and development. It focused on investments in five areas: Reducing health risks, promoting education, ensuring transition into employment, promoting citizenship, and family formation. The report stressed the value of a broad policy framework in that education and the transition to employment affect health risks.

Another broad initiative with a potential impact on the health of young people is the Millennium Development Goals (MDGs) which was adopted by the UN General Assembly in 2000. They have provided a framework for cooperation across the UN agencies. The MDGs grew out of an overall aim of reducing extreme poverty. As far as adolescent health is concerned, they focus on HIV prevention and the prevention of mortality in young mothers.

As already mentioned, all the available evidence accumulated in these reports show that, besides the quality of the health-care system and the preventive strategies set up, in most if not all countries, the level of education attained should be looked at as one of the main determinants of health. Adolescents from poor families who drop out of school do much worse than those from wealthier families who have greater access to education and employment (World Bank 2007). Thus, improving health literacy and the level of education of the adolescent population as well as providing young people with a perspective of their professional future and role in the society is probably one of the single most effective ways to improve their health and well-being.

Future directions

The advances in developing policy frameworks and recommendations outlined earlier raise questions about how to measure the progress made as well as the functioning of service systems. Several groups have proposed indicators ranging from health measures to sociodemographic determinants and health-system indicators (Harris *et al.* 2006). Currently, most agencies do not provide numbers by five-year strata, even for such basic data as mortality. Because indicators are essential for the monitoring of public health policies as well as for advocacy, it is important to achieve a fair consensus in this area in the future. Also, although we have more and more data showing evidence of what works (Evidence for Policy and Practice Information and Co-ordinating Centre 2002; Health Evidence Network, World Health Organization 2006), such information remains limited by the paucity of available evidence-based evaluations conducted outside high-income countries. Some of the approaches that have been validated in specific settings and ethnic backgrounds may not be as effective for young people and communities outside the cultural mainstream. Still another limitation is that most of the 'evidence-based' approaches that are available have emerged from randomized controlled trials (RCTs), which may limit their broad application in the public health context. Several authors have proposed more feasible and valid alternatives to RCTs, insisting on the importance of taking into account the context of the research and the interest of measuring trends over time (Victora *et al.* 2004).

Another more strategic issue is whether to put emphasis on the prevention of specific health problems or to use a more holistic health-promotion approach. Both strategies work, and may need to be used in judiciously in combination. 'New public health' has called for an approach to adolescent health that cuts across traditional fields such as social welfare, education, environment, and the health sectors. In many countries, basic public health engineering has been achieved, such as immunization, but new factors including psychological, social, and economic, and are becoming increasingly relevant as determinants of health and causes of illness, such as access to higher education and reduction of socioeconomic disparities.

Conceptual approaches targeting the whole population (and not only adolescents) may indeed positively impact on the health of young people. It requires better sensitization of politicians and policy makers to the health consequences of decisions and policies developed outside the field of health. An example of such a strategy comes from the Swedish Parliament, which in 2003 adopted a policy aimed to create social conditions that would ensure good health for the entire population, identifying the contribution of other sectors in creating safe environments and products, including the participation of the society (Hogstedt *et al.* 2004).

Conclusion

Young people aged 10–24 years represent a large part of the population, especially in low- and middle-income countries, where they will constitute about 1.5 billion people by 2050. Important epidemiological shifts have occurred and are still occurring in terms of the main health problems affecting young people. We have reviewed several types of strategies that can potentially address these important issues, which are as follows:

- The health-care system has to develop specific responses, taking into account the bio-psychosocial and developmental specificities of adolescents and their struggle for autonomy. Health-care settings and staff have to become more accessible and user-friendly to young people.
- We now have good evidence that the school setting can implement and sustain effective programmes to address specific problems as well as, more globally, the well-being of pupils. Implementing sound information provision and life skills building approaches as well as fostering a climate of confidence and trust among pupils and between pupils and teachers has a positive impact in terms of healthy habits as well as mental health.
- Young people as well as their parents and the community members should participate in the conceptualizing and implementing of preventive programmes. Young people represent an enormous resource that has proven extremely useful when used appropriately by health professionals, educators, or even policy makers.
- At a global level, there is substantial evidence showing that legislative and environmental policies—such as easy access to health care and contraception, improvement of traffic conditions, limitation of access to legal drugs or to lethal weapons, control of the quality of foods served in school or provided in shopping areas, and better access to sports areas—impact positively on the health of young people.
- Improving the socioeconomic conditions in which deprived families live positively affects the health of young people as well as the other segments of the population.
- Above all, improving health literacy and the level of education of adolescents as well as providing them with a perspective of their role in society is probably one of the single most effective ways to improve their health and well-being.

References

Bajos N., Guillaume A.K.O., editors. *Reproductive health behaviour of young Europeans*. Strasbourg, France: Council of Europe; 2003.

Bearinger L.H., Sieving R.E., Ferguson J. *et al.* Global perspectives on the sexual and reproductive health of adolescents: patterns, prevention, and potential. *Lancet* 2007;**369**:1220–31.

Beautrais A.L., Wells J.E., McGee M.A. *et al.* Suicidal behaviour in Te Rau Hinengaro: the New Zealand Mental Health Survey. *The Australian and New Zealand Journal of Psychiatry* 2006;**40**:896–904.

Blum R. Global trends in adolescent health. *Journal of the American Medical Association* 1991;**265**:2711–9.

Blum R.W., McNeely C., Nonnemaker J. Vulnerability, risk, and protection. *The Journal Adolescent Health* 2002;**31** Suppl 1:28–39.

Blum R.W., Nelson-Mmari K. The health of young people in a global context. *The Journal of Adolescent Health* 2004;**35**:402–18.

Bonomo Y.A., Bowes G., Coffey C. *et al.* Teenage drinking and the onset of alcohol dependence: a cohort study over seven years. *Addiction* 2004;**99**:1520–8.

Bosch F.X., de Sanjose S. Human papilloma virus and cervical cancer – burden and assessment of causality. *Journal of the National Cancer Institute (Monographs)* 2003;**31**:3–13.

Brown A.D., Jejeebhoy S., Shah I. *et al.*, editors. Sexual relations among young people in developing countries: evidence from WHO case studies. Geneva: World Health Organization; 2001.

Cassell C., Santelli J., Gilbert B.C. *et al.* Mobilizing communities: an overview of the Community Coalition Partnership Programs for the Prevention of Teen Pregnancy. *The Journal of Adolescent Health* 2005; **37** Suppl 3:S3–10.

Centers for Disease Control. Use of cigarettes and other tobacco products among students aged 13–15 years worldwide, 1999–2005. *Morbidity and Mortality Weekly Report* 2007;**55**:553–6.

Chamay-Weber C., Narring F., Michaud P.A. Partial eating disorders among adolescents: a review. *The Journal of Adolescent Health* 2005;**37**:417–27.

Dahlberg L.L., Potter L.B. Youth violence. Developmental pathways and prevention challenges. *American Journal of Preventive Medicine* 2001; **20** Suppl 1:3–14.

Elster A.B., Levenberg P. Integrating comprehensive adolescent preventive services into routine medicine care. *Rationale and approaches. Pediatric Clinics of North America* 1997;**44**:1365–77.

Evidence for Policy and Practice Information and Co-ordinating (EPPI) Centre. Barriers to and facilitators of the health of young people: a systematic review of evidence on young people's views and on interventions in mental health, physical activity, and healthy eating.

London: Evidence for Policy and Practice Information and Co-ordinating Centre; 2002.

Flodmark C.E., Marcus C., Britton M. Interventions to prevent obesity in children and adolescents: a systematic literature review. *International Journal of Obesity (2005)* 2006;**30**:579–89.

Goldenring J., Rosen D. Getting into adolescent heads: an essential update. *Contemporary Pediatrics* 2004;**21**:64–90.

Grimes D.A., Benson J., Singh S. *et al.* Unsafe abortion: the preventable pandemic. *Lancet* 2006;**368**:1908–19.

Harris K.M., Gordon-Larsen P., Chantala K. *et al.* Longitudinal trends in race/ethnic disparities in leading health indicators from adolescence to young adulthood. *Archives of Pediatrics and Adolescent Medicine* 2006;**160**:74–81.

Hawkins J.D., Abbott R., Catalano R.F. *et al.* Assessing effectiveness of drug abuse prevention: implementation issues relevant to long-term effects and replication. *NIDA Research Monograph* 1991;**107**:195–212.

Hawkins J.D., Kosterman R., Catalano R.F. *et al.* Promoting positive adult functioning through social development intervention in childhood: long-term effects from the Seattle Social Development Project. *Archives of Pediatrics and Adolescent Medicine* 2005;**159**:25–31.

Hawton K., James A. Suicide and deliberate self-harm in young people. *British Medical Journal* 2005;**330**:891–4.

Health Evidence Network, World Health Organization. *What is the evidence on school health promotion in improving health or preventing disease?* Geneva: World Health Organization; 2006.

Hogstedt C., Lundgren B., Moberg H. *et al.* The Swedish public health policy and the National Institute of Public Health. *Scandinavian Journal of Public Health (Supplement)* 2004;**64**:6–64.

Kodjo C.M., Klein J.D. Prevention and risk of adolescent substance abuse. The role of adolescents, families, and communities. *Pediatric Clinics of North America* 2002;**49**:257–68.

Korf D.J. Dutch coffee shops and trends in cannabis use. *Addictive Behaviors* 2002;**27**:851–66.

Kumpfer K.L., Alvarado R. Family-strengthening approaches for the prevention of youth problem behaviors. *The American Psychologist* 2005;**58**:457–65.

Lloyd C. *Growing up global: the changing transitions to adulthood in developing countries*. Washington (DC): National Research Council and Institute of Medicine, National Academies Press; 2005.

Lobstein T., Frelut M.L. Prevalence of overweight among children in Europe. *Obesity Reviews* 2003;**4**:195–200.

Lopez A.D., Mathers C.D. Measuring the global burden of disease and epidemiological transitions: 2002(2030. *Annals of Tropical Medicine and Parasitology* 2006;**100**:481–99.

Magoha G.A., Magoha O.B. Current global status of female genital mutilation: a review. *East African Medical Journal* 2000;**77**:268–72.

Mahler H. International Conference on Health Promotion in industrialized countries; 1986 Nov 17–21; Ottawa, Canada. *Canadian Journal of Public Health* 1986;**77**:387–92.

McAlister A.L. Acceptance of killing and homicide rates in nineteen nations. *European Journal of Public Health* 2006;**16**:260–6.

McCambridge J., Strang J. The efficacy of single-session motivational interviewing in reducing drug consumption and perceptions of drug-related risk and harm among young people: results from a multi-site cluster randomized trial. *Addiction* 2004;**99**:39–52.

McInthyre P. *Adolescent-friendly health services*. Geneva: World Health Organization; 2003.

Michaud P.A., Fombonne E. Common mental health problems. *British Medical Journal* 2005;**330**:835–8.

Michaud P.A., Suris J.C., Deppen A. Gender-related psychological and behavioural correlates of pubertal timing in a national sample of Swiss adolescents. *Molecular and Cellular Endocrinology* 2006;**254–255**:172–8.

Munro J., Coleman P., Nicholl J. *et al.* Can we prevent accidental injury to adolescents?. *A systematic review of the evidence. Injury Prevention* 1995;**1**:249–55.

Musaiger A.O. Overweight and obesity in the Eastern Mediterranean region: can we control it?. *Eastern Mediterranean Health Journal* 2004;**10**:789–93.

Ogden C.L., Carroll M.D., Flegal K.M. Epidemiologic trends in overweight and obesity. *Endocrinology and Metabolism Clinics of North America* 2003;**32**(vii):741–60.

Omar H.A. A model program for youth suicide prevention. *International Journal of Adolescent Medicne and Health* 2005;**17**:275–8.

Ong K.K., Ahmed M.L., Dunger D.B. Lessons from large population studies on timing and tempo of puberty (secular trends and relation to body size): the European trend. *Molecular and Cellular Endocrinology* 2006; **254–255**:8–12.

Patel V., Flisher A.J., Hetrick S. *et al.* Mental health of young people: a global public-health challenge. *Lancet* 2007;**369**:1302–13.

Patton G.C., Bond L., Carlin J.B. *et al.* Promoting social inclusion in schools: a group-randomized trial of effects on student health risk behaviour and well-being. *American Journal of Public Health* 2006;**96**:1582–7.

Patton G.C., Viner R. Pubertal transitions in health. *Lancet* 2007;**369**:1130–9.

Ploeg J., Ciliska D., Dobbins M. *et al.* A systematic overview of adolescent suicide prevention programs. *Canadian Journal of Public Health* 1996;**87**:319–24.

Rutter M., Smith D. Psychosocial disorders in young people. Time trends and their causes. New York (NY): Wiley; 1995.

Santelli J., Ott M.A., Lyon M. *et al.* Abstinence and abstinence-only education: a review of U.S. *policies and programs. The Journal of Adolescent Health* 2006;**38**:72–81.

Sowden A., Arblaster L., Stead L. Community interventions for preventing smoking in young people. [Online]. *Cochrane Database of Systematic Reviews* 2003;(1):CD001291.

Stafstrom M., Ostergren P.O., Larsson S. *et al.* A community action programme for reducing harmful drinking behaviour among adolescents: the Trelleborg Project. *Addiction* 2006;**101**:813–23.

Steinberg L., Morris A.S. Adolescent development. *Annual Review of Psychology* 2001;**52**:83–110.

Steinberg L. Risk taking in adolescence: what changes, and why?. *Annals of the New York Academy of Sciences* 2004;**1021**:51–8.

Tobler N. School-based adolescent drug prevention programs: 1998 meta-analysis. *The Journal of Primary Prevention* 2000;**20**:275–336.

Toroyan T., Preden M. *Youth and road safety*. Geneva: World Health Organization; 2007.

Toumbourou J.W., Stockwell T., Neighbors C. *et al.* Interventions to reduce harm associated with adolescent substance use. *Lancet* 2007;**369**: 1391–401.

Tremblay R.E. Prevention of youth violence: why not start at the beginning?. *Journal of Abnormal Child Psychology* 2006;**34**:481–7.

Tylee A., Haller D.M., Graham T. *et al.* Youth-friendly primary-care services: how are we doing and what more needs to be done?. *Lancet* 2007;**369**:1565–73.

UNAIDS. AIDS epidemic update: December 2006. Geneva: UNAIDS; 2006.

United Nations Economic and Social Council, Commission on Narcotic Drugs. Youth and drugs: a global overview. Report of the 42nd session of the Secretariat; 1991 Mar 16–25; Vienna. Available from: http://www.unodc.org/pdf/document_1999-01-11_2.pdf [Accessed on 2008 Feb 4].

United Nations. Millennium development goals. Available from: http://www.un.org/millenniumgoals/

United Nations. *World youth report*. New York (NY): United Nations; 2005. p. 148–60.

Van Sluijs E.M., McMinn A.M., Griffin S.J. Effectiveness of interventions to promote physical activity in children and adolescents: systematic review of controlled trials. *British Medical Journal* 2007;**335**:703.

Victora C., Habicht J., Bryce J. Evidence-based public health: moving beyond randomized trials. *American Journal of Public Health* 2004;**94**:400–5.

Viner R.M. Do adolescent inpatient wards make a difference? Findings from a national young patient survey. *Pediatrics* 2007;**120**:749–55.

Wang Y., Monteiro C., Popkin B.M. Trends of obesity and underweight in older children and adolescents in the United States, Brazil, China, and Russia. *The American Journal of Clinical Nutrition* 2002;**75**:971–7.

Wasserman D., Cheng Q., Jiang G.X. Global suicide rates among young people aged 15–19. *World Psychiatry* 2005;**4**:114–20.

Wellings K., Collumbien M., Slaymaker E. *et al.* Sexual behaviour in context: a global perspective. *Lancet* 2006;**368**:1706–28.

Widhalm K., Fussenegger D. Actions and programs of European countries to combat obesity in children and adolescents: a survey. *International Journal of Obesity (2005)* 2005;**29** Suppl 2:130–5.

Wilson J.F. Finland pioneers international suicide prevention. *Annals of Internal Medicine* 2004;**140**:853–6.

World Bank. World development report: development and the next generation. Washington (DC): World Bank; 2007.

World Health Organization. *Adolescent pregnancy: issues in adolescent health and development.* Geneva: World Health Organization; 2004a.

World Health Organization. *Caring for children and adolescents with mental disorders.* Geneva: World Health Organization; 2003.

World Health Organization. Global prevalence and incidence of selected curable sexually transmitted infections. Geneva: World Health Organization; 2001a.

World Health Organization. Growing in confidence: programming for adolescent health and development. Geneva: World Health Organization; 2002a.

World Health Organization. *Injury: a leading cause of the global burden of disease.* Geneva: World Health Organization; 2002b.

World Health Organization. Preventing HIV/AIDS in young people: a systematic review of the evidence from developing countries. Geneva: World Health Organization; 2006.

World Health Organization. Preventing violence: a guide to implementing the recommendations of the world report on violence and health. Geneva: World Health Organization; 2004c.

World Health Organization. *Prevention of mental disorders. Effective interventions and policy options.* A report of the WHO, Department of Mental Health and Substance Abuse in collaboration with the Prevention Research Unit of the Universities of Nijmegen and Maastricht. Geneva: World Health Organization; 2004b.

World Health Organization. *World health report. Mental health: new understanding, new hope.* Geneva: World Health Organization; 2001b.

Wu Z., Detels R., Zhang J. *et al.* Community-based trial to prevent drug use among youths in Yunnan, China. *American Journal of Public Health* 2002;**92**:1952–7.

Zaborskis A., Sumskas L., Maser M. *et al.* Trends in drinking habits among adolescents in the Baltic countries over the period of transition: HBSC survey results, 1993–2002. *BMC Public Health* 2006;**6**:67.

11.5

Ethnic minorities and indigenous peoples

Myfanwy Morgan, Martin Gulliford, and Ian Anderson

Abstract

This chapter considers the health of ethnic minorities and indigenous peoples. The term *ethnicity* is currently employed to refer to groupings of people defined according to shared characteristics including ancestral and geographical origins, cultural tradition, language, and religion. Ethnicity is a fluid, multifaceted construct whose characteristics are not fixed or easily measurable, with classification dependent on context. The concept of ethnicity has superseded the largely discredited biological notion of racial differences that emerged in the first half of the nineteenth century as the basis for differentiating groups in a population. The term *indigenous peoples* refers to groups who are descendants of populations that inhabited a country or geographical region at the time of conquest or colonization and who retain some or all of their own social, economic, cultural, and political institutions. Ethnic-minority and indigenous populations generally have younger age distributions than the majority of the population, and often show some degree of concentration into geographically distinct areas or communities. Where data are available, ethnic minorities and indigenous peoples may have increased mortality and diminished life expectancy compared with the majority, demonstrating an ethnic patterning of cause-specific mortality and morbidity. Determinants of health that are of particular relevance for explaining the ethnic patterning of health outcomes include genetics, culture and lifestyles, consequences of migration and discrimination, lack of access to services, and socioeconomic inequalities and poverty, all of which are interrelated. The significance of these determinants may vary for different health outcomes and in different contexts. More recent perspectives regard cultural beliefs and identities as flexible and shaped by the structural conditions of people's lives and experiences. The final section of the chapter considers policies at the societal level, including the question of self-determination for indigenous peoples, the assumptions and ideology of multiculturalism, and the critiques of this approach.

Introduction

This chapter analyses, from the standpoint of public health, the health of ethnic minorities and indigenous peoples. The health status of ethnic-minority groups and indigenous populations is important for several reasons. From the perspective of the 'right to the highest attainable level of health', the ethnic patterning of health outcomes observed in many populations may indicate that the right to health is not equally respected, protected, or fulfilled for all groups. Ethnic inequalities in health are particularly likely to be inequitable and unfair, stemming from wider social inequalities and the experience of deprivation across a range of social and environmental domains. Ethnic variation in health status may also be indicative of particular health needs that should be addressed through appropriate policies and services. Research into ethnicity and health may sometimes also provide insights into the causes of disease.

The first section of the chapter explores the concepts of ethnicity, race, and indigenous peoples. It also examines approaches to the classification of ethnic groups. The next section presents empirical data for several aspects of health status in relation to ethnic-minority or indigenous status. This is followed by an analysis of traditional approaches for explaining health risks and behaviour patterns of ethnic minorities and indigenous people in terms of distinct determinants, including economic disadvantage and cultural beliefs and behaviours. This is contrasted with more recent perspectives that regard cultural beliefs and identities as flexible and shaped by the structural conditions of people's lives and experiences, with examples of the significance of ethnicity and identity.

The concept of ethnicity

The concept of ethnicity is derived from the Greek word *ethnos*—meaning a nation, people, or tribe—and is currently employed to refer to groupings that people belong to, or are perceived to belong to, based on certain shared characteristics. These characteristics typically include ancestral and geographical origins, cultural tradition, language, and religion. Ethnicity is, thus, a multifaceted construct whose characteristics are not fixed or easily measurable. The concepts of ethnicity and ethnic groups have increasingly replaced the biological notion of racial differences that emerged in the first half of the nineteenth century as the basis for differentiating groups in the population.

Concept of race: Use and misuse

The historical notion of racial groups assumed that humankind could be differentiated into distinct subgroups based on physical characteristics, such as skin colour, hair type, eye colour, shape of head and face, and specific features such as the nose and lips. Underpinning this interest in racial types were questions of whether these biological differences were associated with indicators of social worth, particularly intelligence, and thus with the superiority and inferiority of different peoples. This notion of racial differences reflected the belief in a natural biological hierarchy, and led to the development of various crude classifications. These were based on continental groupings and trace their origin to Linnaeus (1806), a biologist who devised a biological classification of all living things (cited in Bhopal 2007). Linnaeus' grouping of humans had four categories: *Homo afer* (later synonyms: Black, African origin, Negro, Negroid), *Homo europaeus* (later synonyms: white, European origin, Caucasian, Caucasoid), *Homo asiaticus* (later synonyms: Mongoloid, Asian), and *Homo americanus* (later synonyms: American Indian, North American Indian, Native American). Variants of such classifications also have a grouping for the Aborigines (Australia).

From the 1930s, the concept of race was increasingly criticized for its use in justifying the unequal treatment of racial groups, involving economic exploitation, segregation, and genocide. This criticism was fuelled by the Nazi's abuse of the concept of race during World War II. Attempts to distinguish racial types have been shown to lack biological foundation and scientific legitimacy. This view was supported by evidence that 90–95 per cent of the genetic variation occurs within rather than among allegedly different races. Furthermore, only small differences in genotype are identified as being responsible for differences in facial and skin colour characteristics that form supposedly essential markers of racial difference (Cooper *et al.* 2003). Another conceptual distinction can be made based on much of contemporary thinking in population genetics, that the distribution of many gene frequencies is graduated across populations. Whereas a biological concept of race assumes a particular genetic structure within a racially defined population this does not hold for the socially based concept of ethnicity. However, the concept of ethnicity does not discount the role of genetic factors in some health conditions.

Concerns regarding both the biological basis and social misuse of racial categorizations has led to a shift from crude biological notions of race to the recognition that the variable of race measures some combination of social class, culture, and genes (Jones 2001). The concept of race, particularly the distinction between black and white racial groups, continues to be identified as a key social division in many countries. However, there is also increasing use of the concept of ethnicity to distinguish migrant groups, with the term *indigenous peoples* being used to refer to non-migrant minority groups, notably the Maoris (New Zealand), Native Americans, and the Inuit (Canada).

There are currently differing views regarding the importance of racial categories in the health field. Goldberg (1993), recognizing the contribution of genetic factors to disease, has argued for retention of the concept of races, while acknowledging that the use of this concept in modernity differs from the notions of superiority and inferiority that marked earlier usage and now merely identifies difference. Jones (2001), from a US perspective, similarly recommends the analysis of race-observed differences in health in order to eliminate them, with the important provisos that race is regarded as a social rather than a biological category, the diversity within racial groups is acknowledged, and the impacts of social class and racism are measured in explaining differences in health. A more critical view is to reject racial classifications altogether on the grounds that race-based research is inherently racist. Osborne and Feit (1992) take this approach, observing that explanations of differences between blacks and whites in stigmatized conditions such as sexually transmitted diseases and mental illness are frequently attributed to race rather than to socioeconomic status and other aspects of their conditions of life. This often reflects a general failure to move beyond associations between racial groups and disease, with the causal mechanisms such as poverty or lack of access to services remaining unknown and hidden from view.

Concept of ethnicity

Concerns about the misuse of racial categories has led to an increased emphasis on the concept of ethnicity in order to describe the social groupings that people identify based on common descent and shared culture or history. Sivanandan (1987) has argued that differentiating racial groups in terms of ethnicity can have the negative effect of dividing people who experience racism. He favoured expanding boundaries and using the political term 'black' as a social construct (as opposed to a biological construct) to signify the shared interests of peoples of African, African-Caribbean, and South Asian descent. However, as Modood (1994) noted, many members of minority groups reject inclusion in the political term 'black', as this does not acknowledge the substantial variations that exist in economic advantage with a consequent lack of shared class interests.

Classification of ethnicity

The development of acceptable and useful ethnic classifications has proved difficult and classifications currently vary between countries (see Bhopal 2007). This partly reflects the particular composition and characteristics of migrant groups arising from historical patterns of migration. For example, the group categorized as 'Asian' in the United States reflects particular patterns of migration to that country and comprises people of Chinese, Japanese, and Malayan descent, whereas in the United Kingdom the category of 'Asian' refers to people from the Indian subcontinent, reflecting the major migrations from India, Pakistan, and Bangladesh. Other differences are in the numbers of categories identified and variations in the marker of ethnicity employed (e.g. ethnic origin or self-identity).

The Canadian census uses one of the most detailed ethnic classifications and focuses on individuals' origins as the marker of ethnicity. The 2001 Canadian census identified 25 ethnic categories and sub-categories that included British Isles origins; Aboriginal origins; Caribbean origins; Latin American, Central American, and South American origins; African origins; Arab origins; West Indian origins; and South Asian origins. In the United States census, five major groups have been identified: black or African-American; white; Asian; native Hawaiian or other Pacific Islander; and American Indian or Alaska native. A distinction is also made between Hispanic and non-Hispanic ethnicity. In the United Kingdom, an ethnic classification that focused on self-perceived ethnicity as the marker was first introduced in the 1991 census, at a time when over half the black ethnic groups were born in the United Kingdom. Subsequently, a more comprehensive classification was included in the 2001 census. New features were to specifically identify Irish self-identity within the white population (although neglect of other white groups reflects the tendency to regard white ethnicity as invisible) and the introduction of categories that acknowledge the increasing numbers of people of mixed parentage and identity (14.6 per cent of the ethnic-minority population; Table 11.5.1).

Ethnic classifications lend themselves to subdivision, as with the distinction between black African and black Caribbean. White people may similarly perceive themselves as English, Turkish, Irish, Swedish, etc. However, individuals' self-perceived ethnicity may depend on context. For example, people who identify themselves as Nigerian in their country of origin may define themselves as black African or black British in the United Kingdom. Differences in self-perceived ethnicity also occur across generations. Migrants from the Caribbean to the United Kingdom in the 1950s and 1960s often identified themselves as coming from a particular island or from the West Indies, whereas today second- and third-generation migrants tend to perceive themselves as black British, black Caribbean, or African-Caribbean. Broad ethnic groupings also describe heterogeneous categories that may mask important variations by country of origin, religion, education, language, and diet. In the United Kingdom, people categorized as Asian were characterized by differences in language, religion, education, and place of origin, with the Indian group including Hindu (45 per cent), Sikh (29 per cent), and Muslim (13 per cent). People classified as black African come from a number of African countries with different cultural traditions, religions, and languages and include disproportionate numbers in the professional classes, and unemployed and semi-skilled workers. Neglect of such substantial within-group variations leads to dangers of stereotyped assumptions.

Examples of ethnicity in different contexts

Table 11.5.1 provides data on the ethnic composition of three countries: Trinidad and Tobago, England and Wales, and the United States of America. In these countries, both the classification of ethnicity and the ethnic distributions of populations reflect the differing histories and cultures of the three countries.

In Trinidad and Tobago, before the first arrival of Europeans, there was an indigenous population of 30 000–40 000; however, this population declined rapidly after European colonization and is no longer distinguishable. The largest groups are now formed of well-established populations of African or Indian-subcontinent descent who migrated to the islands, under varying degrees of coercion, as agricultural workers mostly in the period between 1783 and 1919 (Brereton 1981). There is an increasing group of 'mixed ethnicity', as well as small but economically significant

Table 11.5.1 Distribution of population by ethnic group in three countries

Trinidad and Tobago (2000)		England and Wales (2001)		United States (2000)	
Ethnic group	**Per cent population**	**Ethnic group**	**Per cent population**	**Ethnic group**	**Per cent population**
African descent	37.5	White:		White	75.1
Indian descent	40.0	British	87.0	Black/African American	12.3
White	0.6	Irish	1.3	American Indian/Alaska native	0.9
Chinese	0.3	Other	2.7	Asian:	3.6
Mixed	20.5	Mixed:		Asian Indian	0.6
Other	0.3	White and black Caribbean	0.5	Chinese	0.9
Not stated	0.8	White and black African	0.2	Filipino	0.7
		White and Asian	0.4	Japanese	0.3
		Other	0.3	Korean	0.4
		Asian/Asian British:		Vietnamese	0.4
		Indian	2.1	Other Asian	0.5
		Pakistani	1.4	Native Hawaiian and Other	
		Bangladeshi	0.6	Pacific Islander	0.1
		Other Asian	0.5	Some other race	5.5
		Black/black British:		Two or more races	2.4
		Caribbean	1.1		
		African	1.0		
		Other	0.2		
		Chinese	0.4		
		Other	0.4		

Source: Trinidad and Tobago Central Statistical Office. *Statistical pocket digest*. Port of Spain: Central Statistical Office; 2004; Office for National Statistics. *Census 2001: ethnicity and religion in England and Wales*. London: Office for National Statistics; 2007; United States Census Bureau. *Overview of race and Hispanic origin*. Washington (DC): United States Census Bureau Population Division; 2007.

groups of Chinese, Portuguese, and Lebanese or Syrian origin. In Fenton's (1999) classification, Trinidad and Tobago provides an example of ethnic groups in a plural society.

In England, the white population remains the largest ethnic group, but there are significant populations of Indian-subcontinent and African descent who migrated to England in the period after 1945. The group of African descent can be separated into earlier migrants from the Caribbean islands and more recent arrivals from various African countries. The Indian-subcontinent-origin population in England includes groups that are diverse with respect to language, religion, culture, and national origin, including people from India, Pakistan, and Bangladesh, as well as migrants from Indian-origin communities in East Africa and elsewhere. There are a wide range of smaller ethnic groups, including significant numbers from Southern Europe, and a growing population of migrants from Eastern Europe. England exemplifies the typology of ethnic groups as urban minorities derived from migrant worker populations (Fenton 1999).

In the United States, indigenous populations now represent a small minority. The largest ethnic grouping is formed from the descendants of settler migrants who travelled from Western Europe between the seventeenth and twentieth centuries. However, there is a significant African-American population mostly descending from involuntary migrants from West African countries between the seventeenth and nineteenth centuries. There is also a significant 'Asian' grouping in the United States, but this is more diverse in origin than in the United Kingdom. In the United States, ethnic minorities represent three distinct typologies including an indigenous minority, a post-slavery minority, and an urban-migrant minority group (Fenton 1999).

These data from three countries in the Western hemisphere illustrate how the ethnic composition of contemporary populations is generally formed through the interaction between the indigenous population and migrant groups that have moved to a country at different times in history. Migration is driven by social, political, and economic forces that are, to a greater or lesser extent, unique to a given national context. These influences also determine the experience of immigrant populations. In the United States, the African-American population was for a long time the subject of systematic segregation, discrimination, and denial of civil rights. These problems have only begun to be addressed in recent decades. In Trinidad and Tobago, a somewhat similar state of affairs existed during the colonial era but, in contrast to the United States, this experience generally applied to each of the major population groups and was ended as the country became independent (Brereton 1981). In England, large-scale immigration is a more recent phenomenon and, although difficulties with discrimination exist, the civil rights of ethnic minorities as well as their access to services are officially protected and promoted. These formative influences have implications for the determinants of health experienced by ethnic groups and influence the comparative age distribution of different ethnic groupings, their socioeconomic position, and geographical concentration.

Age distribution

Table 11.5.2 shows the proportion of the population in different age groups for the three countries. In Trinidad and Tobago, the population has a young age distribution, consistent with its status as a middle-income country. However, the age distribution of the population is similar in each ethnic group, which reflects the fact that the majority of the population have been established in the country over several generations. In the United Kingdom, in contrast, ethnic-minority populations are generally more youthful, with a higher proportion of children and a much smaller proportion of old people. This is a consistent finding across all the ethnic groups. There is also a different age distribution between older first-generation migrants and younger second-generation immigrants who were born in Britain. Data for the United States are between those obtained from the other two countries.

Table 11.5.2 Age-distribution in relation to ethnicity in three countries

Country and ethnic group	Age group (years)	
	< 15	≥ 65
Trinidad and Tobago (1990)		
African descent	33	8
East Indian	31	4
Mixed	41	6
United Kingdom (2001)[a]		
White British	19	16
Indian	22	6
Pakistani	35	4
Bangladeshi	38	3
Other Asian	22	4
Black Caribbean	25	9
Black African	33	2
Mixed	55	2
United States (2000)		
White	19	14
African-American	26	8
Asian	20	8

Figures are percentages of the total.

[a] Data are for <16 years.

Source: Trinidad and Tobago Central Statistical Office. *Statistical pocket digest*. Port of Spain: Central Statistical Office; 2004; Office for National Statistics. *Annual local area labour force survey*. London: Office for National Statistics; 2002; United States Census Bureau. *Overview of race and Hispanic origin*. Washington (DC): United States Census Bureau Population Division; 2007.

Geographical concentration and deprivation

Ethnic-minority groups are typically unevenly distributed geographically forming, to a greater or lesser extent, defined communities characterized by concentration according to ethnic group. In Trinidad at the 1990 census, African and Indian groups each contributed about 40 per cent of the total population, but people of Indian descent only comprised 11 per cent of the population of the capital Port of Spain; in contrast, in the town of Chaguanas in Central Trinidad, 65 per cent of the population were of Indian descent (Republic of Trinidad and Tobago, Central Statistical Office 1994). This distribution reflects local employment patterns; the immigrant Indian population was initially employed in agriculture and is still now more heavily concentrated in the former sugar-producing areas of the country.

In the United Kingdom, there is also significant spatial concentration of minority ethnic groups, in this case towards the inner cities. At the 1991 census, 35 per cent of the total UK population was located in nine metropolitan areas compared with 81.1 per cent for black Caribbeans, 86.5 per cent for black Africans, 67.8 per cent for Indians, 71.1 per cent for Pakistanis, and 77.6 per cent for Bangladeshis (Peach 1996). This concentration was still present at the 2001 census but there was evidence of ethnic minorities migrating out from these areas of concentration, leading to increasing diversity in other areas (Rees & Butt 2004). Data for the 2001 census in England have been analysed in relation to a small-area Index of Multiple Deprivation (IMD 2004), which summarizes measures of deprivation across seven domains (including income, employment, education, health and disability, housing, living environment, and crime). In the most deprived decile of areas, people of Bangladeshi and Pakistani origin made up a four-times higher proportion of the population than they did for England as a whole, whereas people of black Caribbean and black African descent represented a two and half times higher proportion of the population than they did for England as a whole. The distribution of the Indian-origin population varied in different regions. In London, Indians lived in areas with intermediate deprivation scores, whereas in the West Midlands they were more heavily concentrated in the most deprived areas.

In the United States, there is also a high degree of segregation of ethnic-minority groups by neighbourhood. Polednak (1997) used an index of residential dissimilarity to evaluate the segregation of African-Americans. The index gives an indication of the per cent of African-Americans that would have to move in order to achieve an even distribution. Across 38 metropolitan areas in 1990, the index gave values of 89 in Detroit, 87 in Chicago, 86 in Cleveland, and 84 in Milwaukee and Buffalo, with only two out of 38 metropolitan areas having values less than 50. Recently, African-American segregation has shown a modest decrease but segregation has increased for US 'Asians' and 'Hispanics' (Logan *et al.* 2004).

The geographical separation of minorities often provides a context in which the processes of social exclusion may be enacted (Peace 2001). The quality of housing, employment opportunities, and access to education and health services are characteristic of particular areas. The geographical context may therefore be associated with the social, economic, and health outcomes achieved by ethnic minorities. In the United States, for example, black:white mortality differentials at area level are strongly associated with indicators of segregation (Polednak 1997). These processes of social exclusion are particularly relevant to the experience of indigenous peoples.

The concept of indigenous peoples

On 13 September 2007, the United Nations General Assembly adopted a Declaration on the Rights of Indigenous Peoples (hereafter the Declaration). There had been over two decades of negotiations between representatives of indigenous peoples and governments within the United Nations system. The international political movement that led to this result provoked considerable—at times apparently intransigent—debate on the definition of indigenous peoples and the rights that were consequent to this. There was, for example, an ongoing dispute between indigenous delegates and states about whether the appropriate terminology should be indigenous peoples, indigenous people, or indigenous populations (Niezen 2003). Some governments resisted the use of the first construct—on the basis that the other terms inferred that indigenous people had collective rights, such as self-determination (Niezen 2003; Feiring & Partners 2003). Others governments denied that there were indigenous peoples within their jurisdiction notwithstanding the contrary claims of representatives of those peoples.

In 1972, a United Nations study proposed the following 'working definition':

> *Indigenous communities, peoples, and nations are those having a historical continuity with pre-invasion and pre-colonial societies that developed on their territories, consider themselves distinct from other sectors of the societies now prevailing in those territories, or parts of them* (Coates 2004: p. 6).

In 1989, The International Labour Organization (2007), an agency of the United Nations that deals with labour issues, defined indigenous peoples in its convention on Indigenous and Tribal Peoples as follows:

> *Peoples in independent countries who are regarded as indigenous on account of their descent from the populations which inhabited the country, or a geographical region to which the country belongs, at the time of conquest or colonization or the establishment of present State boundaries and who, irrespective of their legal status, retain some or all of their own social, economic, cultural, and political institutions* (Office of the High Commission for Human Rights 2007).

These formulations continue to be influential within the United Nations system. However, the representatives of indigenous organizations who were involved in the negotiation of the Declaration rejected the idea of a formal definition of indigenous peoples that would be adopted by States. This view was supported by governmental delegations for whom it was 'neither desirable nor necessary to elaborate a universal definition of indigenous peoples (Department of Economic and Social Affairs 2004: p. 3). Indigenous delegates resisted the inclusion of formal definitions on the basis that they did not wish to exclude groups from participating in debates on the basis of a technicality. This also reflected the emphasis placed by many indigenous delegates on the right to self-definition, a view that was preserved in the final version of the Declaration in Article 33 clause 1, which states:

> *Indigenous peoples have the right to determine their own identity or membership in accordance with their customs and traditions. This does not impair the right of indigenous individuals to obtain citizenship of the States in which they live* (United Nations General Assembly 2007).

Many contemporary commentators, when surveying the application of the concept of indigeniety internationally, have commented on the difficulty in developing definitions that satisfactorily embrace the full range of this diversity (Niezen 2003; Coates 2004; Barsch 1989; Stamatopoulou 1994; Kingsbury 1998; Stephens & Nettleton 2006). Indigenous identities are also contested within and between indigenous communities (Weaver 2001). These debates between indigenous peoples do have considerable social significance, but they are not unusual in their own right, as is attested to by many other similar disputes among people who belong to communities of religion, language, or ethnicity.

When the medical journal, *The Lancet*, put out a call for papers on indigenous health as part of a series that it intended to run on these issues (Stephens & Nettleton 2006), one anthropologist felt so troubled by the use of the term *indigenous* that he wrote to the journal arguing that the word 'is commonly used as a euphemism for primitive' when in fact those contemporary indigenous peoples who are hunters and who are seen as 'the contemporary heirs to the Upper Paleolithic way of life [when] the relation between contemporary and Upper Paleolithic hunting is very distant indeed' (Kuper 2006: p. 983). Kuper argues that peoples such as the Kalahari Bushmen (the San) and Central African pygmies have been interacting with African farming communities for centuries, whereas other hunting peoples such as the Inuit in Northern Canada have been integrated within a global trade network for a similar period of time. As a consequence of these definitional problems and the difficulties in identifying 'genuine' indigenous people, Kuper argues that:

> *The category of indigenous peoples is so problematic, it is unwise for The Lancet to devote a series of papers to their supposedly special health problems* (Kuper 2006: p. 983).

Despite the misgivings of Kuper and others, the concept persists and it has growing currency in global political processes. Further, given the entanglement with this idea and rights, there are compelling reasons to intellectually engage with this agenda. The various attempts to define indigenous peoples have resulted in two distinct, but related, definitional strategies: Culturist and political (Coates 2004).

The culturalist framework emphasizes the cultural characteristics of indigenous communities, placing particular emphasis on cultural difference relative to urban capitalist societies. Classically, the cultural and social organization of indigenous communities are characterized as small-scale societies which are generally a society of a few dozen to several thousand people who live by foraging wild foods, herding domesticated animals, or non-intensive horticulture on the village level. Such societies lack cities as well as complex economies and governments. Kinship relationships are usually highly important in comparison to the common pattern of large-scale societies (O'Neil 2007).

Indigenous communities that might be candidates in this regard include the Aborigines living in remote areas; the Yanomami of the Amazon River basin; and the San, who live a mobile lifestyle in the Kalahari Desert. However, this approach tends to fix indigenous peoples at a particular point in history, and ignores the impact of colonialism and globalization on even the most traditional of indigenous communities. Four-wheel-drive vehicles, Coca-Cola, and welfare payments are as characteristic of contemporary indigenous lifestyles in many remote regions of the globe as are classificatory kinship structure and hunting or foraging. Furthermore, during the twentieth century, many indigenous populations have became increasingly urbanized and integrated within capitalist economies—even though they many have continued to maintain traditional economic practices and occupy a relatively marginal position within the broader economy. Although many indigenous peoples were historically mobile peoples, the demography of indigenous peoples has changed within the context of colonial history. However, not all pre-colonial societies were mobile; many, such as in Central America, had long histories of urbanization.

Although it is not possible to identify a cultural archetype for indigenous society, indigenous peoples may respond to social trends and cultural change in a way that is distinct from the dominant society. Some change may be resisted for a range of complex reasons, even though indigenous peoples may also embrace some forms of development. Although it is not possible to predict responses to mining or the incursion of other economic modes of production (such as agriculture) into indigenous territories, the fault lines for these conflicts do re-inscribe the social and political relations between indigenous communities and dominant societies. In that respect, many indigenous peoples retain the desire to maintain a distinct identity and cultural practices in the face of a history of dispossession and social marginalization; they continue to maintain an understanding and sense of connection to a pre-colonial past, often passed on through oral testimony, ceremonies, and cultural activities, which serve to preserve the understanding of history.

Political definitions of indigenous people emphasize the relationship between indigenous people and states in which ethnic settler majorities dominate. Indigenous peoples are commonly political minorities in nation states dominated by settler societies or other ethnic majorities. Their contemporary political circumstance has been historically shaped by colonization in which they have been dispossessed from their traditional lands and natural resources, and subsequently incorporated within the institutional and political structures of the settler state. The management of indigenous peoples by the settler state has often involved the development of administrative structures and programmes. The rights of indigenous peoples and those of the settler majority are frequently differentiated. This pattern of political disempowerment is reflected in other forms of social and cultural marginalization. Increasingly, and perhaps most significantly, indigenous peoples, in the face of ongoing social and political incorporation into the state-centric structures, have increasingly over the last forty years formed political alliances with other indigenous peoples. These alliances are a response to globalizing processes and in working through the United Nations system have attempted to transcend the local politics of exclusion and marginalization.

The development of a globally applicable terminology that is sufficiently flexible for all contexts is clearly a challenge. However, this problem may have greater significance for jurists and legal scholars than the public-health practitioner. The anthropologist Ronald Neizen (2003), who spent some time observing the political machinations of the United Nations processes in the negotiations that led to the Declaration on the Rights of Indigenous Peoples, took the view that the ongoing debate about definitions were valuable in that they continued to draw attention to the different social and political contexts in which this idea has currency. The concept of indigeniety provides a conceptual lens through which we can frame our understanding of the health and social status of distinct populations. It directs our analytical gaze towards the historically unfolding relationships of power within the context of colonial relationships and it also focuses our attention on the role of the state in the production of social inequalities. The diversity of indigenous experience and context should keep our analytical attention on the particular histories and social relations of the peoples in question.

Indigenous peoples in a global context

People who either describe themselves as indigenous or who are defined as such by others are found around the world in widely varying social, cultural, political, and geographical contexts. This includes those peoples who are descended from the 'aboriginal' populations of Australia, New Zealand, North America, and most of Latin America where the history of European colonialism has produced and maintained the social distinction between native peoples and European-settler colonial societies (Stephens *et al.* 2006). The Aborigines inhabited the continent of Australia and the island of Tasmania for up to 60 000 years. Most were hunter–gatherers and there were up to 500 distinct language groups at the time of British colonization in 1788 (Anderson *et al.* 2006). The Maoris of New Zealand are descendants of Pacific Polynesian peoples and share an older cultural and linguistic heritage with many indigenous peoples in the Pacific including Native Hawaiians (Anderson *et al.* 2006). Despite the much longer history of European colonization in the Caribbean and Latin America, indigeniety here is also 'most clearly defined as those who pre-dated European conquistadores' (Montenegro & Stephens 2006: p. 1859). There is considerable linguistic and cultural diversity between indigenous peoples across this region. This includes the present-day descendents of the pre-Columbian complex societies of Central America such as the Maya and the many diverse cultures of the Amazon basin. It is estimated that there are nearly 400 different indigenous languages across the region (Montenegro & Stephens 2006). Indigenous peoples in this region also vary considerably in the extent to which they constitute the population of various nation states—from 71 per cent of the population of Bolivia and 66 per cent of the population of Guatemala to 0.2 per cent of the population of Brazil and 0.03 per cent of the population of Uruguay (Montenegro & Stephens 2006). Although the link between indigenous identities and colonial histories might lend an appearance of definitional clarity for these particular contexts, in other regions of the world—such as in Asia, the Middle East, and Africa—the history of colonialism is more complex and layered. In these contexts, 'colonization took place between ethnic groups within and between countries, and in some case native populations were almost entirely eradicated' (Stephens *et al.* 2006).

A number of Asian minority groups were involved in the global political processes that led to the adoption of the Declaration. These include tribal peoples from India, Taiwanese aboriginal groups, the Ainu, West Papuans, the Hmong peoples from Southeast Asia, and indigenous groups from the Philippines and the Republic of South Mollucas. In India, social hierarchy such as the caste system has created social categories in which social position is established at birth with some groups recognized as indigenous or tribal on a sociocultural basis (Stephens *et al.* 2006). Here, there are about 532 scheduled tribes, speaking over 100 different languages, each with its own ethnic or cultural identity (FAO Investment Centre 2006). Historically, these communities were characterized on the basis of their distinct non-agrarian lifestyles. Their forest-based subsistence economy used a combination of cultivation, hunting, and foraging strategies. British colonial rule had a significant impact on these communities through both the appropriation of forests and the loss of access to their traditional modes of economic production (FAO Investment Centre 2006).

By contrast, the Ainu people of Japan are a small proportion of the total Japanese population, found mainly on the island of Hokkaido. In 1999, there were approximately 23 767 Ainu people living in Hokkadio and 5000 in the Kanto area (Cheung 2003). Over the last four centuries, they have retained a distinct cultural identity—although in the contemporary world very few speak the Ainu language or practice a traditional way of life. They have over this period of time been subject to different political and legislative interventions such as the 1899 Law for the Protection of Native Hokkaido Aborigines, which attempted to impose a policy of assimilation on the Ainu (Cheung 2003).

Benedict Kingsbury (1998) documented some of the political controversy that followed the recognition of some Asian peoples as indigenous peoples. One group of delegates petitioned a meeting of the United Nations Working Group on Indigenous Populations in 1991:

> *First and foremost, we want to bring to your attention the denial of some Asian governments of the existence of indigenous peoples in our part of the world. This denial presents a significant obstacle to the participation of many indigenous peoples from our region in the Working Group's deliberations. The denial also seeks to withhold the benefits of the Declaration from the indigenous, tribal, and aboriginal peoples of Asia. We hereby urgently request that peoples who are denied the rights to govern themselves, and are called tribal, and/or aboriginal in our region, be recognized, for the purpose of this Declaration, and in accordance with [International Labor Organization] practice, as equivalent to indigenous peoples* (Kingsbury 1998: p. 417).

In 1995, the People's Republic of China put the following position to a working group of the UN Commission on Human Rights:

> *The Chinese Government believes that the question of indigenous peoples is the product of European countries' recent pursuit of colonial policies in other parts of the world. As in the majority of Asian countries, the various nationalities in China have all lived for aeons on Chinese territory. Although there is no indigenous peoples' question in China, the Chinese Government and people have every sympathy with indigenous peoples' historical woes and historical plight. China believes it absolutely essential to draft an international instrument to protect their rights and interests. The special historical misfortunes of indigenous peoples set them apart from minority nationalities and ethnic groups in the ordinary sense. For this reason, the draft declaration must clearly define what indigenous peoples are, in order to guarantee that the special rights it establishes are accurately targeted at genuine communities of indigenous people and are not distorted, arbitrarily extended, or muddled* (Kingsbury 1998: p. 417–418).

Within Africa, the recognition of some minorities as indigenous is even more highly contested. Many of these critics would claim to the contrary that all Africans are indigenous in relation to European colonization (Stephens *et al.* 2006; Ohenjo & Willis 2006). According to Ohenjo *et al.* (2006), there are 14.2 million people in Africa who identify as indigenous; these people can be historically grouped into three major categories: Hunter–gatherers (such as the Pygmy peoples of Central Africa and the San of Southern Africa); fisher peoples; and pastoralists (such as the Masai of Kenya and Tanzania, pastoral communities in Ethiopia and Sudan, the Taureg of West and Northern Africa, and the Himba of Namibia). One of the problems in the African context is that within this longer history, which pre-dates European colonial expansion in the continent, the patterns of settlement and political relations between various groups are contested. This situation is rendered more complex in the political context of the era following European colonization, when negotiation of post-colonial borders disrupted many existing cultural and political alliances. Ohenjo *et al.* (2006) take the view that being indigenous is related to the relation between peoples and the state and its dominant and economic and political structures. To that end, they point out that the national identity movements that emerged in the twentieth century sought to disregard internal ethnic differences with numerically dominant populations such as the Twana in Botswana being established as culturally normative and politically dominant with respect to the indigenous populations, such as the San peoples, who were now spliced within and between the political boundaries of a post-colonial Africa.

Health and social outcomes for indigenous peoples

Health status of indigenous peoples

The social circumstance of indigenous peoples across the globe varies considerably; in part, this reflects their different histories and location in resource-poor or resource-rich nations. However, it is the social inequalities experienced by indigenous peoples that have provided the political momentum for the increasing focus on indigenous issues in the international arena. These inequalities are evident in the measurement of health and social outcomes. There are a few instances in which some health indicators match that of benchmark populations. Patterns of disease also reflect the broader social context of the indigenous people in question, with patterns of disease varying between those peoples who live in resource-rich and resource-poor nations.

Despite the increasing global attention on the question of indigenous health, specific and accurate information concerning their health status is fragmented and incomplete. This quality of health data varies considerably, and in part reflects the capacity or political will of various nations to develop health-information systems that enable the disaggregation of data according to indigenous status. In resource-poor countries, the capacity to develop health-information systems more generally impacts on the collection of indigenous health data. For example, the US-associated Micronesia, where indigenous peoples constitute a majority of the population, does not have the capacity to support a sophisticated health-information system (Anderson *et al.* 2006). Not all nations record indigenous status in health data collections. Even in those that do, the quality of the data collected and recorded is variable. In Australia, for example, good-quality mortality data are available for only 60 per cent of the indigenous population (Anderson *et al.* 2006). Factors that compound some of these difficulties include the extent to which health services can systematically record indigenous status, when indigenous people may be a relatively invisible minority. There are also different approaches to how indigenous status is defined. Some communities cross international and other jurisdictional boundaries—making it even more difficult to get an accurate picture of health and social status (Stephens & Porter 2006).

Life expectancy

In general, indigenous populations experience lower life expectancies relative to other benchmark populations. The life expectancy among the Maya of Guatemala is 17 years shorter than that for non-Indigenous (Feiring & Partners 2003). The life expectancy for indigenous Australians for the years 1996–2000 was 59.4 years for men (compared with 76.6 years for non-Aboriginal men) and 64.8 years for women (compared with 82 years for non-Aboriginal women) (Anderson *et al.* 2006). The Maoris, in 1996–1999, had a life expectancy of 66.3 years for men and 71 years for women compared with 75.7 years and 80.8 years, respectively, for the non-Maori, non-Pacific population (Anderson *et al.* 2006). For the peoples of the Federated States of Micronesia (FSM), life expectancy was 68 years for men and 71 years for women compared with US benchmarks (Anderson *et al.* 2006). In 2001, the differences between the Mexican indigenous population were 67.6 years for men (72.4 years in the total population) and 71.5 years for women (78.1 years for the total population) (Feiring & Partner 2006).

Infant mortality

Measures of infant mortality rates also provide a useful insight in the differences between health outcomes for indigenous and non-indigenous peoples. The infant mortality rate among indigenous peoples of Mexico is almost double that of its non-indigenous population. In Australia and the FSM, indigenous infant mortality rates are approximately three times that of their benchmark populations (Freemantle & Read 2006). In New Zealand, Maori infants had twice the mortality rate (Anderson *et al.* 2006). Native Hawaiians have a similar rate of infant mortality with the non-native population of Hawaii (Anderson *et al.* 2006). Tribal peoples in the Indian state of Bihar had approximately three times the infant mortality rate, with over half of the children of this group experiencing malnutrition (FAO Investment Centre 2006). There are also documented differences in the prevalence of low birth weight. In Australia, 12.9 per cent of the total indigenous births were under 2500 g (compared with 6.1 per cent for the total Australian population), and in New Zealand, 7.9 per cent of Maori births were low birth weight compared with 6.1 per cent of the non-Maori non-Pacific population. However, the figures for native Hawaiians and non-native Hawaiians were very similar in 2001 at 8 and 8.1 per cent, respectively (Anderson *et al.* 2007).

Morbidity

It is difficult to make global generalization with respect to patterns of morbidity. In part, this reflects differences in the global pattern of disease. Many indigenous populations have higher incidences of chronic diseases such as diabetes, mental disorders, and cancers. In wealthy countries, diseases that are now relatively rare, such as tuberculosis and rheumatic fever, are significantly over-represented in indigenous populations.

Disability is often more frequent; for instance, 31 per cent of First Nations people in Canada report some form of disability linked to high accident rates, poor housing, substance abuse, or chronic disease. Alaskan Natives report unintentional-injury death rates more than three times the national average (Beavon & Cooke 2003). The suicide rate among indigenous Hawaiians is more than 150 per cent greater than that of non-Indigenous Hawaiians.

Indigenous health inequalities are reflected in broader social inequalities (Anderson *et al.* 2006). For example, in Peru, the rate of poverty among indigenous populations is 150 per cent that of the non-indigenous (Feiring & Partners 2003). Ninety-one per cent of the indigenous people in Guatemala lived in extreme poverty in 1989, compared to 45 per cent of the non-indigenous. In Ecuador, 76 per cent of the indigenous children live in poverty. The impact of poverty is clear from figures found in Honduras where an estimated 95 per cent of indigenous children under the age of 14 are malnourished (Feiring & Partners 2003).

Social determinants of indigenous health

There are a range of different explanatory frameworks that have been used to account for the persistent health and social disparities experienced by indigenous peoples. These include racial or genetic models; health behaviours; socioeconomic models and approaches, which have drawn upon the social and historical analysis of colonialism and the social relations that this has produced. With the exception of the latter, there is in fact a considerable degree of overlap with some of the approaches taken to theoretical and research agenda in ethnic health disparities (e.g. Dressler *et al.* 2005).

In contemporary analysis, there is a growing interest in the application of thinking drawn from the work on the social determinants of health of indigenous populations (e.g. Anderson *et al.* 2007; Carson *et al.* 2007). The convergence of thinking in indigenous health with this broader agenda in public health recognizes that many of those social processes which have been demonstrated to play a role in the production of health outcomes in other populations—such as economic circumstances, access the health and social services, experiences of racism and other forms of discrimination—are likely to play a role in the production of health inequalities for indigenous peoples. Nonetheless, it is also possible that there are particular social processes, or more likely a particular sociohistorical configuration of social processes, that conceptually distinguishes indigenous social determinants of health. To date, most of this analysis in indigenous health has been at the more theoretical end of the spectrum—with a relatively smaller body of research that empirically investigates the relationship between social processes and health outcomes.

The World Health Organization's Commission on the Social Determinants of Health (CSDH) decided to establish a process at its meeting in Nairobi in June 2006 to inquire into the role of the social determinants in the health of indigenous peoples. As a consequence, an International Review of Social Determinants of Indigenous Health was established to synthesize existing knowledge and expertise in this field (Mowbray 2007). This review included a commissioned international situational analysis and an international call for case studies, both of which formed the background papers for an International Symposium on the Social Determinants of Indigenous Health, which was convened by the CSDH in Adelaide, Australia, in April 2007, and attended by seventy-four participants from Australia, Belize, Cambodia, Canada, Chile, China, Ecuador, Guatemala, New Zealand, the Philippines, and the United Kingdom. The workshop subsequently covered a number of themes that were consistent with the analysis emerging from the document review. They included issues such as the following:

- The politics of indigenous self-determination
- The health consequences of ecological and environmental change
- Economic factors such as poverty or prosperity, fairness, and equity
- The development of indigenous leadership and capacity building in indigenous communities
- The impact of racism, political dominance, and imperialism
- Healing the access to health services, systems, and structures
- Cultural sustainability, protection, stewardship
- Land tenure, territorial integrity, and human rights

These ideas and themes had remained remarkably consistent through the entire process, in both the written material and workshop process. Despite the differences in the social and political contexts of indigenous peoples worldwide, there was a high degree of concordance throughout this process in the collective understanding about the role played by social processes in the development of disparities in indigenous health. However, it was also clear, particularly through the more detailed local case studies, that these broad ideas need to be critically interpreted within particular historical and social environments. In this sense, local research is required to identify how these more broadly defined processes might impact on local lives and realities.

Another significant finding was the understanding that, although the influence of social determinants on health can be identified in all populations, there is a specific cluster of factors and relationships that can be identified in the indigenous context. The role of work and other economic relationships is likely to be different within the context of the Aborigines, where the realm of social life is distinctly organized relative to other Australians. The historical processes of colonialism, and the ongoing processes of social marginalization, have effects on the health of indigenous Australians that require the development of a particular approach to the analysis of social relationships critical to health outcomes. These challenges are pivotal to the future development of research in this field.

Health status of ethnic minorities

A sizeable literature has described differences in health status and health outcomes between ethnic groups at different stages in the life course that are comparable to those described for indigenous peoples. The description of such variations is dependent on the collection of data for ethnicity in systems for vital registration, as well as population censuses and special surveys. These types of data may not be available in some countries and less satisfactory measures, such as the country of birth, may sometimes be collected instead of ethnic group. Systems for classification may also differ for health events as numerators as compared with population data as denominators. Much attention has focused on relative differences between ethnic groups, but evaluation of absolute risks will also be relevant for developing appropriate policy responses. For example, people of African descent in Europe are characterized as having a high risk of stroke and a low risk of coronary heart disease compared with white Europeans, but the absolute risk of coronary heart disease in the African group is generally higher than for stroke, as it is in most populations.

Mortality and life expectancy

Differences in mortality in relation to ethnic group or race are well documented in the United States (Tables 11.5.3 and 11.5.4). Infant mortality is twice as high in African-Americans and is 50 per cent higher in Native Americans, when compared to whites. In the Hispanic and Latino group, overall infant mortality is similar to that in whites, but the rate for Puerto Ricans (8.3 per 1000) is close to that for Native Americans. All-cause mortality is increased in African-Americans; life expectancy at birth in 2004 was 73.1 years

Table 11.5.3 Infant mortality rate by ethnic group in the United States, 2001–2003

Ethnic group	Infant mortality per 1000 live births
White	5.7
African American	13.6
Hispanic/Latino	5.6
Asian/Pacific Islander	4.8
American Indian/Alaskan Native	8.9

Source: United States Department of Health and Human Services. Health United States, 2006. Washington (DC): US Department of Health and Human Services; 2006.

for African-Americans compared with 78.3 for whites. There is considerable variation in the relative increase for different causes of death. African-American mortality shows greatest relative increases for HIV, homicide, diabetes, and cerebrovascular disease with no increase observed for unintentional injuries, chronic liver disease and cirrhosis, and chronic lower respiratory disease (Table 11.5.4).

In the United Kingdom, mortality has been analysed according to country of birth since 1981 (Balarajan 1995; Wild & Mckeigue 1997; Harding *et al.* 2008). These analyses are derived from the collection of data for country of birth in the national census and in death certification. Increased mortality from coronary heart disease in Indian-subcontinent-origin populations is a consistent finding, especially at younger ages. In the population under 65 years, mortality from coronary heart disease in people born in the Indian subcontinent is 1.5–1.7 times higher than in people born in England and Wales, and mortality for stroke is 1.8–2.5 times higher. For people born in Africa or the Caribbean, relative mortality is higher for stroke and lower for coronary heart disease. For migrants born in Europe, the evidence is conflicting; migrants from Ireland have increased mortality from both coronary heart disease and stroke, whereas mortality for both outcomes is lower among those born in continental Europe. Recent analyses by Harding *et al.* (2008) have shown that this ethnic patterning of mortality has been consistent over the three decades from 1979 to 2003, but mortality relative to those born in England and Wales has increased as mortality rates declined more rapidly in the England- and Wales-born population. Elevated mortality from coronary heart disease has been observed in Indian-subcontinent-origin populations in a number of countries including Trinidad and Tobago (Miller *et al.* 1988).

Diabetes, hypertension, and metabolic syndrome

A number of studies have shown that ethnic patterning of mortality is associated with variation in risk-factor profiles. The prevalence of type 2 diabetes is generally higher among people of African or Indian-subcontinent descent when compared with white Europeans (Chaturvedi *et al.* 1994; Simmons *et al.* 1992). The prevalence of hypertension, and mean blood pressure levels, are also higher among people of African descent (Chaturvedi *et al.* 1993). There is also variation in lipid profiles and anthropometric measures, including the prevalence of obesity and abdominal fatness, among ethnic groups that are also patterned by gender (Chaturvedi *et al.* 1994).

These observations have been used to raise questions concerning whether anthropometric reference standards should be developed for different groups; most present reference data having been obtained from white European-origin populations. One illustration is provided by the ethnic-group-specific criteria suggested for the definition of metabolic syndrome, a clustering of risk factors that is associated with increased risk of diabetes and vascular

Table 11.5.4 Age-adjusted mortality rates by ethnic group and cause in the United States, 2004

Cause of death	Age-adjusted mortality rate per 100 000		Rate ratio
	White	African American	
All causes	786.3	1027.3	1.31
Ischaemic heart disease	149.2	179.8	1.21
Cerebrovascular disease	48.0	69.9	1.46
Lung cancer	53.6	59.8	1.12
Breast cancer	23.9	32.2	1.35
Chronic lower respiratory disease	43.2	28.2	0.65
Chronic liver disease and cirrhosis	9.2	7.9	0.86
Diabetes	22.3	48.0	2.15
HIV	2.3	20.4	8.87
Unintentional injuries	38.8	36.3	0.94
Homicide	3.6	20.1	5.58

Source: United States Department of Health and Human Services. Health United States, 2006. Washington (DC): US Department of Health and Human Services; 2006.

disease (Okosun *et al.* 2000; Alberti *et al.* 2005). Lower cut-points for the definition of abdominal obesity have been proposed for men of Indian subcontinent or Chinese origin because diabetes is generally more frequent at lower values for waist circumference in these groups (Alberti *et al.* 2005). However, the significance of this observation is unclear (see Chapter 9.5 on obesity for further discussion).

Results from multi-site international studies make it clear that environmental influences are important in conditioning health outcomes within groups. For example, the International Collaborative Study on Hypertension in Blacks included population surveys in rural and urban populations in West Africa, in several Caribbean islands, and in Maywood, Illinois (Kaufman *et al.* 1996). The prevalence of obesity ranged from 5 per cent in rural African men to 36 per cent in African-American women in the United States. The prevalence of hypertension, with blood pressure ≥ 140/90 mm Hg or treated, ranged from 12 per cent in rural African men to 35 per cent in African-American women (Kaufman *et al.* 1996). These results draw attention to the potential importance of environmental determinants on supposed 'ethnic differences' and raise questions concerning how these differences may be explained.

Determinants of health among ethnic groups

As for indigenous peoples, a number of determinants of health are considered to have particular relevance to the ethnic patterning of health outcomes. These include variations in gene frequencies between populations; culture and lifestyles; migration, including selection effects and the consequences of migration; discrimination; lack of access to services; and socioeconomic influences, including poverty and deprivation in terms of income, education, and housing. The significance of these explanations varies for different health outcomes and different contexts. As we shall see, these explanations are not separate but closely interconnected and dependent.

Gene frequencies

Single gene defects

Inherited disorders of haemoglobin, including sickle cell disease and thalassaemias, are the most frequent diseases associated with single gene defects, with up to 7 per cent of the world population being carriers and up to half a million severely affected births each year (Weatherall *et al.* 2007). Disorders of haemoglobin vary greatly in frequency between ethnic groups in high-income countries. This is because the genes associated with these conditions are only present at low frequency in Northern European populations but in other regions—including Africa, South Europe, the Middle East, and South and Southeast Asia—up to 40 per cent or more of the population may be carriers. As a result of migration, there are significant numbers of affected births among minority ethnic groups in countries whose populations are primarily of Northern European origin. There is important morbidity, including transfusion dependency in thalassaemia or painful crises and increased risk of stroke in children with sickle cell disease, leading to increased health-care utilization.

As a policy response, neonatal screening programmes have been introduced to facilitate earlier detection and treatment of affected infants together with antenatal screening to facilitate prenatal diagnosis, so as to provide parents with an opportunity for informed choice concerning reproductive outcomes. An important question in the implementation of these programmes concerns whether screening should be universal, covering all pregnancies and births, or whether a selective strategy should be introduced to target minority ethnic groups. In the United Kingdom, universal antinatal screening is implemented in high-prevalence areas whereas a selective strategy is employed in low-prevalence areas. In the selective strategy, a preliminary screening question is used to identify individuals who, because of their ethnicity or family origin, may be more likely to be carriers of inherited haemoglobin disorders. This screening question asks 'What are your family origins?', with responses classified by geographical region, and does not depend on self-assigned ethnicity (Aspinall *et al.* 2003; Dyson *et al.* 2006). Screening is thus performed according to the restricted criterion of parental family origin in a region of the world where the population has a high gene-carrier frequency, rather than according to the broader, self-assigned concept of ethnicity.

Complex traits

The genetic evaluation of complex traits and their associations with ethnicity has generally been intractable. Interest in the genetic determinants of ethnic variation in complex traits has been stimulated recently by the development of pharmacogenomics, the study of the effect of genetic variation on responses to drug therapy. This raises the commercially attractive possibility that drugs may be tailored to the expected responses of patients in different groups. For example, it has been proposed that selection of antihypertensive drug therapy should be guided by assessment of ethnicity (Brown 2006). Those interested in the genetic evaluation of ethnic variations in complex traits must be sensitive to the antecedent history of research into race and health (Bhopal 1997). One example of a research study is provided by a case–control study in Trinidad that evaluated genetic markers of West African ancestry as risk factors for systemic lupus erythematosus (SLE) (Molokhia *et al.* 2003). The authors proposed that their results were consistent with a genetic basis for the difference in risk of SLE between West Africans and Europeans.

Culture and lifestyle

The term *culture* has several different meanings. It was defined by the United Nations Educational, Scientific, and Cultural Organization (UNESCO 2007) as 'the set of distinctive spiritual, material, intellectual, and emotional features of society or a social group that encompasses, in addition to art and literature, lifestyles, ways of living together, value systems, traditions, and beliefs'. The contribution of culture to ethnic variation in health status may derive from the distinct traditions and beliefs of communities that contribute to different lifestyles and ways of living which are associated with risk of illness and disease. Differences between communities are graded. On the one hand, there is usually substantial within-group variation in the degree of conformity with cultural norms; on the other hand, differences between groups are non-specific. There is cultural regulation or modulation of the uptake of the main lifestyle risk factors for diseases. Different cultures also vary in their social construction of illness and appropriate responses in terms of help-seeking behaviour.

An example of a culturally specific behavioural norm is provided by the requirement for women in some Muslim communities to be covered by clothing when outdoors. There is a concern that this might contribute to low vitamin D production in the skin with potential risks to women's bone health and the potential for development of rickets in children who are breastfed. A study in Turkey found that women who were habitually veiled had substantially lower serum 25-hydroxy vitamin D concentrations than women who usually wore western clothes (Guzel *et al.* 2001). In England, early clinical reports of rickets, osteomalacia, and vitamin D deficiency in people of Indian-subcontinent-origin led to the introduction of local strategies for vitamin D supplementation (Dunnigan *et al.* 1981). Recently, there has been a re-emergence of vitamin D deficiency among second-generation immigrants, leading to renewed calls for vitamin D supplementation in pregnancy to prevent foetal and maternal vitamin D deficiency (Shaw & Pal 2002). However, the causes for this vitamin D deficiency are unclear. Both men and women of Indian origin have been found to have low serum vitamin D concentrations (Shaunak *et al.* 1985), and this deficiency is not confined to particular religious groups (Jonnalagadda & Diwan 2002). Low vitamin D levels have also been found among African-Americans in the United States and in other minority groups (Dawson-Hughes 2004). Dietary deficiency and lack of vitamin D supplementation appear to be the more important causes of this increased susceptibility to vitamin D deficiency (Dawson-Hughes 2004).

Analysis of data for other lifestyle determinants of health reveal important differences between groups (Sproston & Mindell 2006). Smoking cigarettes and drinking alcohol are generally less frequent among ethnic minorities than in the general population. In particular, Indian, Pakistani, Bangladeshi, and Chinese women in England generally do not smoke. Alcohol is generally not used by men and women from Pakistan and Bangladesh. The proportion of men and women of Indian-subcontinent origin achieving recommended levels of physical activity is considerably lower than in the general population, more so among women. Crude dietary indicators such as consumption of fruit and vegetables generally reveal less variation between groups, but these crude measures conceal substantial differences between groups in the types of foods consumed, with further differences between first- and second-generation immigrants (Landman & Cruickshank 2001).

Data such as these are important in contributing to the development of strategies to promote health and prevent disease. They inform, for example, strategies to promote physical activity in women of Indian subcontinent origin (Carroll *et al.* 2002). Culturally-appropriate interventions are required that address the needs of groups in the context of their particular cultural traditions, beliefs and norms.

Migration and discrimination

The experience of migration is generally key to the formation of ethnic-minority groups in the high-income countries; these countries have a need to attract skilled as well as less-skilled workers and may offer a destination for asylum-seekers and refugees. Migrants are often in better general health than the populations from which they are drawn, contributing to the 'healthy migrant effect'. However, migration may itself have significant negative consequences for health and this is well illustrated with respect to mental health problems (Bhugra & Minas 2007).

Much research has addressed the question of differing frequency of schizophrenia and other psychoses among ethnic groups. In England, there is a well-documented excess of new diagnoses of schizophrenia in African-Caribbean populations. The AESOP study (Fearon *et al.* 2006) evaluated the incidence of schizophrenia and other psychoses among different ethnic groups in three areas of England with a combined population of just over 1 million. The results (Table 11.5.5) show a 6.7-fold increase in risk of new-onset psychosis in African-Caribbean men and women, a 4.1-fold excess risk in Africans, with more modest elevations in risk in other ethnic groups. This has led to suggestions that genetic predisposition or experiences of migration and racial discrimination may contribute to the increased risk of schizophrenia in people of African descent.

Studies in Trinidad (Bhugra *et al.* 1996), Jamaica (Hickling & Rodgers-Johnson 1995), and Barbados (Mahy *et al.* 1999) have evaluated the incidence of new-onset schizophrenia in Caribbean populations. These studies show that the incidence of schizophrenia in the Caribbean is similar to that observed in other regions, including the white British population in England, and much lower than those observed in Caribbean-origin populations in England. These studies provide strong evidence that environmental factors are responsible for the increased incidence of schizophrenia among ethnic minorities in England.

In the AESOP study (Fearon *et al.* 2006), the absence of a major elevation in risk in 'Asians' was viewed as diminishing a potential role for racial discrimination in the aetiology of schizophrenia, as the Asian group may be equally exposed to problems of racial discrimination as black Caribbean and Africans. A modest elevation in risk of psychosis among non-British whites was also regarded as important, as this group is exposed to the stresses of migration and acculturation. This is consistent with the findings of a systematic review, which found that both first- and second-generation migrants has an increased relative risk of schizophrenia compared with non-migrants in the same population (Cantor-Graae & Selten 2005).

Bhugra and Minas (2007) discuss four interrelated reasons why migration may represent a significant stressor with respect to mental health. First, migration generally occurs between communities with different cultural orientations. Immigrants are often derived from poor communities which have a collectivist or 'sociocentric' outlook, but the destination country will often be more affluent

Table 11.5.5 Age-adjusted incidence rate ratios (95 per cent confidence intervals) for all psychosis using the white British group as reference

Ethnic group	Relative risk of all psychosis (95 per cent confidence interval)
White British	1.0
African-Caribbean	6.7 (5.4–8.3)
Black African	4.1 (3.2–5.3)
Asian	1.5 (0.9–2.4)
Other	2.6 (1.7–3.9)
White other	1.6 (1.1–2.2)

Source: Fearon P, Kirkbride JB, Morgan C *et al.* AESOP Study Group. Incidence of schizophrenia and other psychoses in ethnic minority groups: results from the MRC AESOP Study. *Psychological Medicine* 2006; **36**: 1541–50.

and have a more individualistic or 'egocentric' culture. The resulting tensions may lead to mental distress (Bhugra & Minas 2007). Second, removing an individual from his or her familiar context including family and social support, together with the problems encountered in settling into a new environment, may increase the risk of mental illness. Third, experiences of racial discrimination may have significant impacts on mental well-being. These may result from individual-level interactions or from institutional racism, which may be more difficult to confront. Institutional racism is a term attributed to Stokely Carmichael and is defined as 'the collective failure of an organization to provide an appropriate and professional service to people because of their colour, culture, or ethnic origin' (Wikipedia 2007). Accusations of institutional racism have been specifically levelled at mental health services with the suggestion that methods for diagnosing and managing ethnic-minority patients with serious mental illness may be discriminatory (Singh & Burns 2006). However, these suggestions have not generally been supported by epidemiological studies in the United Kingdom (Singh & Burns 2006; Morgan *et al.* 2004). Fourth, the dominant majorities in countries that receive migrants may not embrace the prospect of increasing cultural pluralism and may not develop adequate responses to linguistic and ethnic diversity (Bhugra & Minas 2007). Questions of cultural sensitivity may be of most immediate concern in the delivery of health services used by ethnic-minority groups.

Access to services

The access that ethnic-minority groups have to health services is a significant source of concern, but the extent to which equity of access is achieved depends on the health-system context. In countries such as England and Trinidad and Tobago, which offer universal eligibility to health services, all groups may be said to have access to services, but there may be significant barriers to utilization that prevent particular groups from gaining access on an equitable basis. In other settings which, such as the United States, do not offer services with universal coverage, there are generally greater threats to achieving equity of access.

In Trinidad and Tobago, successive governments have adopted a strongly egalitarian approach to the provision of services. Findings from ad hoc surveys suggest that a fair degree of equity may be achieved in respect of ethnicity (Gulliford *et al.* 2002). In health-care services, the main threat to equity comes from the expanding private sector with access dependent on ability to pay, regardless of ethnic group.

In England, ethnic minorities are more concentrated in deprived areas that generally have less well-developed primary-care services consistent with the 'inverse-care law'. However, a number of studies have found that, after allowing for differences in needs, ethnic-minority groups are generally higher users of primary-care consultations then the white English population (Smaje & LeGrand 1997). Analysis of utilization of preventive medical care reveals a mixed picture. Local studies have shown increased uptake of immunization among ethnic minorities, especially those of Indian-subcontinent origin (Mixer *et al.* 2007; Deshpande 2004), but lower uptake of breast- and cervical-cancer screening (Webb *et al.* 2004; Atri *et al.* 1996). Some studies suggest that there is evidence of inequitable uptake of specialist services by people from ethnic minorities, especially with respect to the management of coronary heart disease (Feder *et al.* 2002), but this has not been confirmed in other studies (Britton *et al.* 2004). Significantly, there do not appear to be important differences in health-care-seeking behaviour with respect to chest pain between different ethnic groups (Adamson *et al.* 2003). Although these studies suggest that a fair degree of equity of access is achieved overall, local studies show that difficulties may be encountered when services do not deliver services that are sufficiently tailored to the needs of specific groups. The concepts of 'linguistic competence' and 'cultural competence' have been developed to describe organizations' ability to communicate effectively with minority groups and deliver services that are sensitive to cultural concerns which may influence the acceptability, uptake, and outcomes of services (Szczepura 2004).

In the US health system, there is strong and consistent evidence of inequitable treatment of ethnic minorities, especially African-Americans. The evidence was summarized most authoritatively in the US Institute of Medicine (Institute of Medicine 2003) report 'Unequal Treatment'. This report found that, even when difficulties of accessing health care because of financial barriers or lack of insurance coverage were excluded, there were significant racial or ethnic inequalities in the delivery of care that were sufficient to impact negatively on health outcomes. The report identified persistence of racial and ethnic discrimination at the societal, health-service, and practitioner levels as significant causes of these inequalities. In particular, bias and prejudice on the part of health-care providers were identified as significant causes of the lower-quality care received by ethnic minorities (Institute of Medicine 2003; Betancourt & King 2003). One example of the impact of such inequalities in access and delivery of care is provided by an analysis of black:white mortality differentials from human immunodeficiency virus (HIV) in the United States before and after the introduction of highly active antiretroviral therapy (HAART) (Levine *et al.* 2007). In men aged 25–34 years, the black:white mortality rate ratio for HIV was 3.1 in the period 1990–1995, but this ratio increased to 6.36 in the period 1997–2002 after the introduction of HAART. In women of the same age, the mortality rate ratio was 8.25 in the pre-HAART period and 13.24 after the introduction of HAART (Levine *et al.* 2007).

Socioeconomic position and deprivation

Deprivation and poverty are key determinants of the health of ethnic minorities. In a plural society such as Trinidad and Tobago, the social stratifiers of education, income, and wealth generally have similar significance for all ethnic and cultural groups (Ryan 1991). In other settings, ethnic minorities—or significant portions of minority populations—may, to a greater or lesser extent, be at risk of marginalization or social exclusion with ethnicity contributing tacitly to social stratification.

The concept of social exclusion is hard to define but has found wide application to social policy in recent years (Peace 2001). In a narrow sense, social exclusion refers to income poverty, encompassing groups that are not included in the labour market or who are confined to low-paid work. In this sense, the concept of social exclusion is often applicable to urban minorities. In a wider sense, social exclusion refers to a combination of lack of resources and denial of social rights that contributes to deprivation across multiple domains, in turn leading to a breakdown in social ties and a loss of sense of purpose (Peace 2001).

Evaluation of individual measures of socioeconomic position in England reveals a complex picture (Sproston & Mindell 2006).

Whereas African-Caribbean, Pakistani, and Bangladeshi men are less likely to have educational qualifications, black African and Indian men are more likely than the general population to be educated to degree level. Pakistani and Bangladeshi women have particularly low educational qualifications, but Chinese and African women in England are better-educated than the general population. In terms of occupational social class, ethnic-minority groups are more likely to be classified into routine or semi-routine occupations, but people of Indian-subcontinent origin as well as the Chinese are more likely than the general population to be small employers or working on their own account. It is an oversimplification to characterize ethnic-minority groups as invariably associated with lower socioeconomic position and social exclusion. There is considerable diversity both within and between groups, the effect of gender varies between groups, with inconsistency among indicators of socioeconomic position. In spite of this complexity, there are recognizable vulnerable groups within ethnic-minority populations that are excluded through lack of access to education and employment or because of poor health.

Nazroo (2003) and Smith (2002) have analysed the complexity of the interrelationship between ethnicity and socioeconomic position. Analyses have usually focused on the average socioeconomic position of different ethnic groups, but within ethnic groups, there is gradation of socioeconomic circumstances with some households having more, or less, advantaged status leading to socioeconomic inequalities within groups. Thus, in England, poor self-rated health in Bangladeshis is observed among lower-income groups and not in the top-income tertile. The overall poor health of the Bangladeshi group may be 'explained' by poverty and not ethnicity (Nazroo 2003).

The significance of indicators of socioeconomic status may vary between groups as, for example, if the income achieved for a given level of occupational social class is not the same between groups (Nazroo 2003). This is a methodologically important point because in conventional multiple regression analyses, adjustment for indicators of socioeconomic position, such as occupational social class, may not fully account for socioeconomic differences between groups. Proposed ethnic differences may in reality be explained by residual confounding with socioeconomic position (Nazroo 2003; Smith 2002). The same social indicator may sometimes have different associations with health measures in different ethnic groups. For example, in white European families, children's height diminishes as the number of children in the family increases, but this association is generally less apparent in children of African or Indian-subcontinent descent (Gulliford *et al.* 1991), perhaps because of the differing cultural significance of family size across ethnic groups.

At the societal level, segregation and discrimination may be important in restricting social and economic freedoms, contributing to the lower socioeconomic status of minority ethnic groups (Nazroo 2003). This is particularly evident in the situation of African-Americans in the United States. Furthermore, in a system in which there are significant financial barriers to accessing health care, lack of access to good-quality care and effective treatment may compromise outcomes in treatable conditions such as HIV infection. The low socioeconomic status of poorly educated migrant workers is often associated with poverty and poor overall health status, as is evident in some migrant groups in England. However, although cigarette smoking is a significant contributor to social inequalities in health in the general population, a lower cultural acceptance of smoking makes this a less significant hazard in African- and Indian-origin ethnic-minority groups, in whom there is a relatively low incidence of lung cancer (Wild & Mckeigue 1997).

Ethnicity and identity

Whereas cultural factors have traditionally been viewed as major but fairly static influences on the beliefs and health-related practices of ethnic minorities, increasingly the cultural beliefs and identities of minority ethnic groups are viewed as flexible and shaped by the structural conditions of people's lives and experiences, including those of racism and disadvantage. As Bhopal *et al.* (1991: p. 244) observed:

> *Far from being immutable categories, the labels to which ethnicity give rise vary in time and space, and according to social and political context.*

Ethnicity has thus been described as a 'hybrid' identity that is influenced by internal and external factors, including a group's history, prevailing circumstances, and the responses of the wider society. For example, the finding that smoking rates are strongly related to age on migration to the United Kingdom, with those migrating at younger ages or born in the United Kingdom having higher rates of smoking, may reflect the differing circumstances and experiences of different age groups (Nazroo 2003). Similarly, differences may arise from an ethnic groups varying experience of the wider society in terms of acceptance or discrimination, and from the extent to which traditional beliefs and practices conform or differ from those of the dominant culture. Ethnic categories are, therefore, shaped by their particular experiences as members of a group, rather than global categories for whom findings can be generalized from one context or group to another. Ethnicity, although a key dimension of identity, is also only one aspect of individuals' identity that includes socioeconomic position, gender, and age, with differing aspects of identity varying in importance between different peoples and in different contexts. Where race and ethnicity tend to be the organizing principle of people's lives, this has been described as 'thick' identity, and is contrasted with 'thin' ethnic identity that occurs where there are less frequent and less dense ethnic interactions, and where other dimensions of social life (including class and occupation) tend to be more powerful shapers of daily life and experiences (Cornell & Hartman 1998).

Recent research has aimed to move beyond the mere identification of differences in patterns of behaviour between ethnic groups to explain these behaviours in terms of the meanings and significance of ethnic identity in people's lives. For example, there is concern about low levels of participation by some marginalized groups in local-community consultation exercises and activist networks, including those focusing on the provision of facilities for children, women's issues, health issues, neighbourhood safety, policing, and leisure and entertainment facilities, which limits their access to community resources. This has traditionally been explained in terms of lack of knowledge or awareness and motivation. However, in-depth interviews conducted with a sample of African-Caribbean residents in a deprived multi-ethnic area in the United Kingdom indicated that such non-participation partly arose from experiences of racism and exclusion at school and work, which led to feelings of being an 'outsider' (Campbell & McLean 2002).

In addition, African-Caribbean residents' collective identity as a group was identified as weak and thus failed to unite people at the local-community level beyond particular face-to-face networks. This lack of solidarity was attributed to a number of factors including the relatively low numbers of African-Caribbean residents in the area relative to other groups, their partial integration into mainstream culture, and life and decline of black consciousness, together with the divisions that existed within the African-Caribbean community associated with social class and their particular island identity as 'Jamaican', 'Trinidadian', etc.

The authors concluded that policy recommendations which simply advocate grassroots participation in community networks as a means of tackling health inequalities are likely to fail without acknowledging the obstacles to such participation that arise from a groups collective identity and experiences, and making recommendations for addressing these barriers. Similar barriers to participation among the African-Caribbean population in the United Kingdom were identified in a qualitative interview study to understand the reasons for their low-organ-donor registration (Morgan *et al.* 2008). This indicated that these respondents' low levels of trust in the medical profession and the process of organ donation reflected their feelings of a lack of 'belonging' to mainstream society and reported experiences of discrimination and exclusion in relation to major social institutions such as hospitals, the police, and schools. Respondents also placed considerable emphasis on their ideal of returning 'home' to the Caribbean for burial, thus reaffirming their ethnic identity at death, which was associated with a desire that their body should return home 'whole', or without organs removed. In contrast, studies with South Asian communities in the United Kingdom indicate that their major concerns about the body associated with a reluctance to donate arise from religious concerns. This includes requirements among Muslims for rapid burial and proper handling of the corpse (Alkhawar *et al.* 2005) and concerns among Sikh Asians about whether their body will be reincarnated if tampered with (Exeley *et al.* 1999). This identifies ways in which similar negative attitudes in terms of the survey responses of ethnic groups may reflect differing cultural and situational factors arising from collective and personal experiences as an ethnic minority (Morgan *et al.* 2006).

Policy responses

Indigenous peoples and self-determination

The Declaration on the Rights of Indigenous peoples was passed with an overwhelming majority of 143 votes in favour. Only four countries—Canada, Australia, New Zealand, and the United States—cast negative votes, and there were 11 abstentions (Morgan *et al.* 2006). The inclusion of the term *self-determination* in the declaration was the most significant cause of controversy in this debate. The idea of self-determination has a long genesis outside the indigenous arena and is generally seen as a universal right that protects all peoples from political tyranny. Those who are opposed to the idea of indigenous self-determination argue that this concept threatens the unity of nation states—even though there are relatively few examples, if any, of indigenous secessionists in recent global history. Niezen (2003) argues that indigenous peoples have not pursued a secessionist political strategy for a number of reasons which include the fact that this would discharge nation states from their treaty obligations and further result in the creation of relatively poor nations. Indigenous peoples have preferred to develop global political alliances rather than internal secessionist movements.

The political idea of self-determination has been manifest in a number of ways. At one end of the spectrum, some indigenous peoples have sought forms of regional autonomy; at the other end, they have insisted that governments consult with them on issues that impact of the development of policy, services, and indigenous social and economic development.

However, although most indigenous peoples have some form of self-determination in health policy, the range of policy responses have been quite diverse. These have included strategies to improve access to health services (particular primary-care services), address the social determinants of health, improve health data, and develop strategies that address the broad range of health inequalities in indigenous populations.

Ethnicity and health policy

Policies and provision for ethnic minorities in the health field are shaped by wider assumptions and policies that accord with either multicultural or assimilationist perspectives. *Multiculturalism* (or cultural pluralism) is an ideology advocating that society should allow and include distinct cultural and religious groups with equitable status, and is generally supported by the view that cultural diversity is a positive force for society and justified in terms of civil rights to equality of cultures. In contrast, assimilationist policies and practices encourage forms of acculturation to the norms and language of the dominant culture to achieve a monoculture.

In the United States, the mass immigrations of the early nineteenth century were associated with what was termed as the 'melting pot' concept, which emphasized the assimilation of each group of immigrants into American society at their own pace, although Federal and state governments now support many multiculturalist policies in the United States. Multiculturalism as an official national policy is regarded to have started in Canada, which in 1971 became a bilingual and bicultural country, and was followed by Australia in 1973. Multiculturalism has since been adopted by most member states of the European Union as the official policy. In the health-care field, this ideology has led to considerable emphasis on the provision of culturally sensitive services to respond to differences in language, religion, diet, and lifestyles through the provision of interpreter services, patient advocates and link workers, information provided in minority languages, and provision for women patients to be attended only by women staff where this is a cultural expectation (Kai 2003).

A number of governments have recently expressed concerns that multiculturalism is divisive, and several European countries have begun to reverse this policy and to emphasize the importance of acculturation, often accompanied by the provision of compulsory language and citizenship courses to achieve this goal. The emphasis on cultural sensitivity has also been criticized from an anti-racist perspective as focusing overwhelmingly on supposed 'problems' of ethnic-minority groups that are internally generated through inappropriate cultural, familial, and community traditions. This in turn leads to a benevolent model of health-service provision in which the solution to problems are essentially technical and professional rather than political, based on the assumption that services will be improved with greater knowledge of different cultures, with improved skills in cross-cultural communication, and through the creation of particular ethnic specialisms. In contrast, an anti-racist perspective takes racism rather than culture as the starting point, and views racism as a pervasive reality structuring interactions at the interpersonal, organisational or institutional, and the structural or societal levels (Stubbs 1993). Thus, rather than merely responding to differences in cultural beliefs and practices, key requirements are to address the relatively disadvantaged position occupied by many ethnic-minority groups that increases health risks and discourages participation, and in particular to achieve the goal of equity among ethnic groups in the provision of health services (Bhopal 2007).

References

Adamson J., Ben ShlomoY., Chaturvedi N. *et al.* (2003). Ethnicity, socio-economic position and gender—do they affect reported health-care-seeking behaviour?. *Social Science and Medicine*;**57**:895–904.

Alberti K.G.M., Zimmet P., Shaw J. (2005). The metabolic syndrome—a new worldwide definition. *Lancet*;**366**:1059–62.

Alkhawar F.S., Stimson G.V., Warrens A.N. (2005). Attitudes towards transplantation in UK Muslim Indo-Indians in West London. *American Journal of Transplantation*;**5**:1326–31.

Anderson I., Baum F. *et al.* (2007). *Beyond bandaids: exploring the underlying social determinants of Aboriginal health*. Papers from the Social Determinants of Aboriginal Health Workshop, Adelaide, 2004 Jul. Darwin, Australia: Cooperative Research Centre for Aboriginal Health.

Anderson I., Crengle S., Kamaka M.L. *et al.* (2006). Indigenous health Part 1: indigenous health in Australia, New Zealand and Pacific. *Lancet*;**367**:1775–6.

Aspinall P.J., Dyson S.M., Anionwu E.N. (2003). The feasibility of using ethnicity as a primary tool for antenatal selective screening for sickle cell disorders: pointers from the research evidence. *Social Science and Medicine*;**56**:285–97.

Atri J., Falshaw M., Livingstone A. *et al.* (1996). Fair shares in health care? Ethnic and socioeconomic influences on recording of preventive care in selected inner London general practices: Healthy Eastenders Project. *British Medical Journal*;**312**:614–7.

Balarajan R. (1995). Ethnicity and variations in the nation's health. *Health Trends*;**27**:114–9.

Barsch R.L. (1989). United Nations seminar on indigenous peoples and states. *American Journal of International Law*; **833**:599–604.

Beavon D., Cooke M. (2003). An application of the United Nations human development index to registered Indians in Canada, 1996. In: White JP, Maxim PS, Beavon D, editors. *Aboriginal conditions: research as a foundation for public policy*. Vancouver, Canada: University of British Columbia Press.

Betancourt J.R., King R.K. (2003). Unequal treatment: the Institute of Medicine report and its public health implications. *Public Health Reports*;**118**:287–92.

Bhopal R. (1997). Is research into ethnicity and health racist, unsound, or important science? *British Medical Journal*;**314**:1751.

Bhopal R.S., Phillimore P., Kohli H.S. (1991). Inappropriate use of the term 'Asian': an obstacle to ethnicity and health research. *Journal of Public Health Medicine*;**13**:244–6.

Bhopal R.S. (2007). Ethnicity, race, and health in multicultural societies. Oxford: Oxford University Press.

Bhugra D., Hilwig M., Hossein B. *et al.* (1996). First-contact incidence rates of schizophrenia in Trinidad and one-year follow-up. *British Journal of Psychiatry*;**169**:587–92.

Bhugra D., Minas I.H. (2007). Mental health and global movement of people. *Lancet*;**370**:1109–11.

Brereton B. (1981). *A history of modern Trinidad 1783 to 1962*. Oxford: Heinemann International.

Britton A., Shipley M., Marmot M. *et al.* (2004). Does access to cardiac investigation and treatment contribute to social and ethnic differences in coronary heart disease? The Whitehall II prospective cohort study. *British Medical Journal*;**329**:318.

Brown M.J. (2006). Hypertension and ethnic group. *British Medical Journal*;**332**:833–6.

Campbell C., McLean C. (2002). Ethnic identities, social capital and health inequalities: factors shaping African-Caribbean participation in local community networks in the UK. *Social Science and Medicine*; **55**:643–57.

Cantor-Graae E., Selten J.P. (2005). Schizophrenia and migration: a meta-analysis and review. *American Journal of Psychiatry*; **162**:12–24.

Carroll R., Ali N., Azam N. (2002). Promoting physical activity in South Asian Muslim women through 'exercise on prescription'. *Health Technology Assessment*;**6**:1–101.

Carson B., Dunbar T. *et al.* (2007). *Social determinants of indigenous health*. Crows Nest, NSW: Allen and Unwin.

Chaturvedi N., McKeigue P.M., Marmot M.G. (1994). Relationship of glucose intolerance to coronary risk in Afro-Caribbeans compared with Europeans. *Diabetologia*;**37**:765–72.

Chaturvedi N., McKeigue P.M., Marmot M.G. (1993). Resting and ambulatory blood pressure differences in Afro-Caribbeans and Europeans. *Hypertension*;**22**:90–6.

Cheung S.C.H. (2003). Ainu culture in transition. *Futures*;**35**:951–9.

Coates K.S. (2004). A global history of indigenous peoples struggle and survival. New York (NY): Palgrave Macmillan.

Cooper R.S., Kaufman J.S., Ward R. (2003). Race and genomics. *New England Journal of Medicine*;**348**:1166–70.

Cornell S., Hartman D. (1998). Ethnicity and race: making identities in a changing world. London: Pine Forge Press.

Dawson-Hughes B. (2004). Racial/ethnic considerations in making recommendations for vitamin D for adult and elderly men and women. *American Journal of Clinical Nutrition*;**80**:S763–6.

Department of Economic and Social Affairs (2004). The concept of indigenous peoples: workshop on data collection and dissagregation for indigenous peoples. New York (NY): United Nations.

Deshpande S.A. (2004). Ethnic differences in the rates of BCG vaccination. *Archives of Disease in Childhood*;**89**:48–9.

Dressler W.W., Orths K.S. *et al.* (2005). Race and ethnicity in public health research: models to explain health disparities. *Annual Review of Anthropology*;**34**:231–52.

Dunnigan M.G., McIntosh W.B., Sutherland G.R. *et al.* (1981). Policy for prevention of Asian rickets in Britain: a preliminary assessment of the Glasgow rickets campaign. *British Medical Journal*;**282**:357–60.

Dyson S.M., Culley L., Gill C. *et al.* (2006). Ethnicity questions and antenatal screening for sickle cell/thalassaemia [EQUANS] in England: a randomised controlled trial of two questionnaires. *Ethnicity and Health*;**11**:169–89.

Exeley C., Sim J., Reid N. *et al.* (1999). Attitudes and beliefs within the Sikh community regarding organ donation: a pilot study. *Social Science and Medicine*;**43**:23–8.

FAO Investment Centre (2006). Overview of socio-economic situation of the tribal communities and livelihoods in Madhya Pradesh and Bihar. Rome: FAO Investment Centre.

Fearon P., Kirkbride J.B., Morgan C. *et al.* (2006). AESOP Study Group. Incidence of schizophrenia and other psychoses in ethnic minority groups: results from the MRC AESOP Study. *Psychological Medicine*;**36**:1541–50.

Feder G., Grook A.M., Magee P. *et al.* (2002). Ethnic differences in invasive management of coronary disease: prospective cohort study of patients undergoing angiography. *British Medical Journal*;**324**:511–6.

Feiring B., Partners M. (2003). Indigenous peoples and poverty: the cases of Bolivia, Guatemala, Honduras and Nicaragua. London: Minority Rights Group International.

Fenton S. (1999). *Ethnicity: racism, class and culture*. Basingstoke: Macmillan.

Freemantle C.J., Read A.W. *et al.* (2006). Patterns, trends, and increasing disparities in mortality for Aboriginal and non-Aboriginal infants born in Western Australia, 1980–2001: population database study. *Lancet*;367.

Goldberg D. (1993). Racist culture: philosophy and the politics of meaning. Oxford: Blackwell.

Gulliford M.C., Chinn S., Rona R.J. (1991). Social environment and height: England and Scotland 1987 and 1988. *Archives of Disease in Childhood*;**66**:235–40.

Gulliford M.C., Mahabir D., Rocke B.C. *et al.* (2002). Free school meals and children's social and nutritional status in Trinidad and Tobago. *Public Health Nutrition*;**5**:625–30.

Guzel R., Kozanoglu E., Guler-Uysal F. *et al.* (2001). Vitamin D status and bone mineral density of veiled and unveiled Turkish women. *Journal of Women's Health and Gender-Based Medicine*;**10**:765–70.

Harding S., Rosato M., Teyhan A. (2008). Trends for coronary heart disease and stroke mortality among migrants in England and Wales, 1979–2003: slow declines notable for some groups. Heart **94**, 463–70.

Hickling F.W., Rodgers-Johnson P. (1995). The incidence of first-contact schizophrenia in Jamaica. *British Journal of Psychiatry*;**167**:193–6.

Institute of Medicine (2003). Unequal treatment: what healthcare providers need to know about racial and ethnic disparities in healthcare. Washington (DC): Institute of Medicine.

International Labour Organization (2007). International Labour Organization 1996–2007. [Online]. Available from: http://www.ilo.org/global/lang--en/index.htm [retrieved 2007 Nov 6]

International Work Group for Indigenous Affairs (2007). Declaration on the rights of indigenous peoples 2007. [Online]. Available from: http://www.iwgia.org/sw248.asp [retrieved 2007 Oct 19]

Jones C.P. (2001). Invited commentary: 'Race', racism and the practice of epidemiology. *American Journal of Epidemiology*;**154**:299–304.

Jonnalagadda S.S., Diwan S. (2002). Nutrient intake of first-generation Gujarati Asian Indian immigrants in the US. *Journal of the American College of Nutrition*;**21**:372–80.

Kai J., editor (2003). *Ethnicity, health, and primary care*. Oxford: Oxford University Press.

Kaufman J.S., Durazo-Arvizu R.A., Rotimi C.N. *et al.* (1996). Obesity and hypertension prevalence in populations of African origin. *Epidemiology*;**7**:398–405.

Kingsbury B. (1998). 'Indigenous peoples' in international law: a constructivist approach to the Asian controversy. *American Journal of International Law*;**92**:414–57.

Kuper A. (2006). Indigenous people: an unhealthy category. *Lancet*;**366**:983.

Landman J., Cruickshank J.K. (2001). A review of ethnicity, health and nutrition-related diseases in relation to migration in the United Kingdom. *Public Health Nutrition*;**4**:647–57.

Levine R.S., Brigs N.C., Kilbourne B.S. *et al.* (2007). Black–White mortality from HIV in the United States before and after introduction of highly active antiretroviral therapy in 1996. *American Journal of Public Health*;**97**:1884–92.

Linnaeus C. (1806). A general system of nature through the three grand kingdoms of animals, vegetables and minerals: Systems Naturae. London: Lackington Allen and Co.

Logan J.R., Stults B.J., Farley R. (2004). Segregation of minorities in the metropolis: two decades of change. *Demography*;**41**:1–22.

Mahy G.E., Mallett R., Leff J. *et al.* (1999). First-contact incidence rate of schizophrenia in Barbados. *British Journal of Psychiatry*;**175**:28–33.

Miller G.J., Kirkwood B.R., Beckles G.L. *et al.* (1988). Adult male all-cause, cardiovascular and cerebrovascular mortality in relation to ethnic group, systolic blood pressure and blood glucose concentration in Trinidad, West Indies. *International Journal of Epidemiology*;**17**:62–9.

Mixer R.E., Jamrozik K., Newsom D. (2007). Ethnicity as a correlate of the uptake of the first dose of mumps, measles and rubella vaccine. *Journal of Epidemiology and Community Health*;**61**:797–801.

Modood T. (1994). Political blackness and British Asians. *Sociology*; **28**:859–76.

Molokhia M., Hoggart C., Patrick A.L. *et al.* (2003). Relation of risk of systemic lupus erythematosus to West African admixture in a Caribbean population. *Human Genetics*;**112**:310–8.

Montenegro R.A., Stephens C. (2006). Indigenous health in Latin America and the Caribbean. *Lancet*;**367**:1859–69.

Morgan C., Mallett R., Hutchinson G. *et al.* (2004). Negative pathways to psychiatric care and ethnicity: the bridge between social science and psychiatry. *Social Science and Medicine*;**58**:739–52.

Morgan M., Hooper R., Mayblin M. *et al.* (2006). Attitudes to kidney donation and registering as a donor among ethnic groups in the UK. *Journal of Public Health*;**28**:226–34.

Morgan M., Mayblin M., Jones R. (2008). Ethnicity and registration as a kidney donor: the significance of identity and belonging. *Social Science and Medicine*;**66**:147–58.

Mowbray M. (2007). The social determinants of indigenous health. The international experience and its policy implications. Adelaide: Commission on Social Determinants of Health.

Nazroo J.Y. (2003). The structuring of ethnic inequalities in health: economic position, racial discrimination, and racism. *American Journal of Public Health*;**93**:277–284.

Niezen R. (2003). The origins of indigenism. Human rights and the politics of identity. Berkeley (CA): University of California Press.

O'Neil D. (2007). Social organisation: glossary of terms, 2005. [Online]. Available from: http://anthro.palomar.edu/status/glossary.htm [retrieved 2007 Oct 25]

Office for National Statistics (2007). *Annual local area labour force survey*. London: Office for National Statistics; 2002. Available from: http://www.statistics.gov.uk/StatBase/Expodata/Spreadsheets/D6300.xls [accessed 2007 Dec 3]

Office for National Statistics (2007). Census 2001: ethnicity and religion in England and Wales. London: Office for National Statistics; 2007. Available from: http://www.statistics.gov.uk/pdfdir/ethnicity0203.pdf [accessed 2007 Dec 3]

Office of the High Commission for Human Rights (2007). Convention concerning indigenous and tribal peoples in independent countries No.169 [Online].Available from: http://www.unhchr.ch/html/menu3/b/62.htm [retrieved 2007 Aug 10]

Ohenjo N.O., Willis R. *et al.* (2006). The health of indigenous people in Africa. *Lancet*;**367**:1937–46.

Okosun I.S., Rotimi C.N., Forester T.E. *et al.* (2000). Predictive value of abdominal obesity cut-off points for hypertension in Blacks from West African and Caribbean island nations. *International Journal of Obesity*;**24**:180–6.

Osborne N.G., Feit M.D. (1992). The use of race in medical research. *Journal of American Medical Association*;**267**:275–9.

Peace R. (2001). Social exclusion: a concept in need of definition? *Social Policy Journal of New Zealand*;**16**:1172–438.

Peach C. (1996). The ethnic minority populations of Great Britain. In: *Ethnicity in the 1991 census;* vol. 2. London: Office for National Statistics.

Polednak A.P. (1997). Segregation, poverty and mortality in urban African Americans. New York (NY): Oxford University Press.

Rees P., Butt F. (2004). Ethnic change and diversity in England 1981 to 2001. *Area*;**36**:174–86.

Republic of Trinidad and Tobago, Central Statistical Office (1994). Age structure, religion, ethnic group, education. In: *Population and housing census 1990;* vol. 2. Port of Spain: Office of the Prime Minister, Central Statistical Office.

Ryan S. (1991). *Social and occupational stratification in contemporary Trinidad and Tobago*. St Augustine: Institute of Social and Economic Research, University of the West Indies.

Shaunak S., Colston K., Ang L. *et al.* (1985). Vitamin D deficiency in adult British Hindu Asians: a family disorder. *British Medical Journal*;**291**:1166–8.

Shaw N.J., Pal B.R. (2002). Vitamin D deficiency in UK Asian families: activating a new concern. *Archives of Disease in Childhood*;**86**:147–9.

Simmons D., Williams D.R., Powell M.J. (1992). Prevalence of diabetes in different regional and religious South Asian communities in Coventry. *Diabetic Medicine*;**9**:428–31.

Singh S.P., Burns T. (2006). Race and mental health: there is more to race than racism. *British Medical Journal*;**333**:648–51.

Sivanandan A. (1987). RAT and the degradation of the black struggle. In: *Racism awareness training: a critique*. London: Strategic Policy Unit; p. 54–87.

Smaje C., Le Grand J. (1997). Ethnicity, equity and the use of health services in the British NHS. *Social Science and Medicine*;**45**:485–96.

Smith D.G. (2002). Learning to live with complexity: ethnicity, socioeconomic position, and health in Britain and the United States. *American Journal of Public Health*;**90**:1694–8.

Sproston K., Mindell J. (2006). *Health survey for England 2004*. The health of minority ethnic groups. Leeds: The Information Centre.

Stamatopoulou E. (1994). Indigenous peoples and the United Nations: human rights as a developing dynamic. *Human Rights Quarterly*;**16**(1):58–81.

Stephens C., Nettleton C. *et al.* (2006). Indigenous peoples' health—why are they behind everyone, everywhere? *Lancet*;**366**:10–13.

Stephens C., Porter J. *et al.* (2006). Disappearing, displaced, and undervalued: a call to action for indigenous health worldwide. *Lancet*; **367**:2019–28.

Stubbs P. (1993). 'Ethnically sensitive' or 'anti-racist'? Models for health research and service delivery. In: Ahmad W.I.U., editor. *'Race' and health in contemporary Britain*. Buckingham: Open University Press; p. 34–50.

Szczepura A. (2004). Access to health care for ethnic minority populations. *Postgraduate Medical Journal*;**81**:141–7.

Trinidad and Tobago Central Statistical Office (2007). *Statistical pocket digest*. Port of Spain: Central Statistical Office; 2004. Available from: http://cso.gov.tt/files/cms/Pocket%20Digest%202004.pdf [accessed 2007 Dec 3.

UNESCO (2007). Universal declaration on cultural diversity, 2001. [Online]. Available from: http://unesdoc.unesco.org/images/0012/001271/127160m.pdf [accessed 2007 Nov 29]

United Nations General Assembly (2007). United Nations declaration on the rights of indigenous peoples. United Nations General Assembly; A/RES/61/295.

United States Census Bureau (2007). Overview of race and Hispanic origin. Washington (DC): United States Census Bureau Population Division; 2007. Available from: http://www.census.gov/population/www/cen2000/briefs.html [accessed 2007 Dec 3].

United States Department of Health and Human Services (2006). Health United States, 2006. Washington (DC): US Department of Health and Human Services.

Weatherall D., Akinyanju O., Fucharoen S. *et al.* (2007). Inherited disorders of haemoglobin. In: Jamison D.T. *et al*, editors. *Disease control priorities in developing countries*. 2nd ed. Washington (DC): World Bank Publications; 2007. Available from: http://files.dcp2.org/pdf/DCP/DCP34.pdf [accessed 2007 Nov 29]

Weaver H.N. (2001). Indigenous identity: what is it, and who really has it. *American Indian Quarterly*;**25**:240–55.

Webb R., Richardson J., Esmail A. *et al.* (2004). Uptake for cervical screening by ethnicity and place-of-birth: a population-based cross-sectional study. *Journal of Public Health*;**26**:293–6.

Wikipedia (2007). Stokely Carmichael. [Online]. Available from: http://en.wikipedia.org/wiki/Stokely_Carmichael [accessed 2007 Nov 29]

Wild S., Mckeigue P. (1997). Cross-sectional analysis of mortality by country of birth in England and Wales, 1970–92. *British Medical Journal*;**314**:705.

11.6

People with disabilities

Donald Lollar

Abstract

Disability is traditionally associated with morbidity and mortality as the negative public health outcomes. Primary prevention activities addressing birth defects, developmental disabilities, injuries, and chronic illnesses associated with disabling conditions are seminal to public health. There are, however, always going to be people in the population who fall through the primary prevention net and live with disabling conditions. Public health is beginning to acknowledge the potential role it plays in promoting the health and well-being of this population. This chapter addresses the emerging field of public health and disability.

The essential public health functions of assessment, policy development, and assurance are outlined for this population across countries and age groups. The World Health Organization's *International Classification of Functioning, Disability and Health* provides the framework for the conceptual and scientific issues. Clarifying definitions of 'disability' for purposes of public health surveillance and epidemiology, as well as research, are major emphases, including child disability measurement and caregiving or carers. Policy development emerges from the national and international conventions and activities, including the recently adopted UN Convention on the Rights of People with Disabilities, and supports the notion that the public health and disability communities have mutual responsibility for improving the health and well-being of this population. Assurance begins by asserting the relationship between poverty and disability, and includes discussion on interventions such as clinical preventive services, along with community-based rehabilitation activities.

Finally, the chapter outlines directions for public health and disability to develop more fully. Recommendations are made for improving communication, cooperation, and coordination of activities between the public health and disability communities. Curricula are coming available for the education and training of public health professionals in disability. Use of these curricula is strongly encouraged so that people with disabilities are included in public health science, programmes, and policy activities.

Introduction

Disability has traditionally been placed alongside morbidity and mortality as the negative public health outcomes. Preventing disabilities, therefore, has been a goal of public health activities. The activities to prevent disabling conditions are, indeed, a crucial aspect of public health work in the areas of birth defects, injuries, chronic illnesses, and even aging. However, this primary prevention emphasis begs the question: 'What happens to those who become disabled in spite of our best primary prevention efforts?' Individuals who fall through the public health prevention net by experiencing disabling conditions have been regarded as best served by medical and rehabilitation systems and services, and thus are seemingly outside the purview of public health. Medical and rehabilitative services are, indeed, crucial to those living with disabilities, but in fact do not take the place of public health.

In recent years, public health practitioners have begun to rethink this traditional stance, acknowledging that people with disabilities as a population are at greater risk for additional health and health-related problems, and therefore, are worthy of appropriate public health intervention. The most basic premise of this chapter, however, is that people with disabilities can experience and should experience a health status comparable to their peers without disabling conditions. People with disabilities can live healthy lives.

Public health emphasizes prevention. In the public health field of disability, this would include preventing secondary conditions among those with existing disabling conditions, in addition to promoting health and well-being. In some countries, medical care and rehabilitation are equated with disability; however, these services are rarely identified with public health. This chapter will describe current issues surrounding the inclusion of disability as an evolving concept and people with disabilities as an emerging population in public health. The three core public health functions—assessment, policy development, and assurance—will be applied to this population (Institute of Medicine 1988). Dimensions of disability, crossing the lifespan, international comparisons, and the role of environmental factors, will be described as they interact with these three public health functions. This chapter is meant to redefine disability and its conceptual and scientific relationship to public health.

As a preface, however, recent history must be invoked to provide a context for how public health and disability are evolving towards each other. Public health, although concerned with the population as a whole, has become progressively more concerned about certain populations at greater risk for disease, injury, and other aetiologic agents. This trend has focused primarily on ethnic minorities and other excluded groups who are more susceptible to diseases by virtue of being poor and marginalized with less access to health care. Simultaneously, a civil rights movement has been emerging among people with disabilities over the past 25 years, culminating in the UN's adoption of a Convention on the Rights of Persons with Disabilities in 2006 (United Nations 2006a). Although public health has evolved naturally from a medical approach to disability conditions, the disability rights movement has focused on disability as a social construct. Although these two models have vastly different emphases, there is growing awareness among public health professionals that people with disabilities can be viewed as a large minority population who are more vulnerable to various co-morbid conditions or secondary conditions, those that are more probable due to a primary disabling condition. Table 11.6.1 provides an overview of basic differences between the perspectives. The World Health Organization (WHO) has developed a framework for viewing disability that accounts for both models, and is becoming both the conceptual and scientific framework for integrating public health and disability.

Over the past 40 years, several paradigms of disability have developed. Disability models are currently best represented by the WHO's *International Classification of Functioning, Disability and Health* (ICF) (World Health Organization 2001). The ICF was approved by the World Health Assembly in 2001, and it is becoming the global standard both conceptually and scientifically. The ICF combines the medical and social models into what is described as a bio-psychosocial model of disability. Figure 11.6.1 depicts the ICF model.

The WHO began work to revise a previous disability classification in the early 1990s. Over the course of almost a decade, over 800 individuals, including individuals living with disabling conditions, representing more than 60 countries participated in the revision process. The resultant product emerged as a member of the WHO family of international classifications, the most notable member being the *International Classification of Diseases* (ICD) (World Health Organization 1992). The ICF took a different conceptual approach, addressing components of health rather than consequences of disease—the focus of the earlier rendition. In addition, a most crucial conceptual and coding component was added to the ICF—environmental factors. The importance of the environment as it interacts with health and functioning is explicit in this system. Environmental elements for the ICF interact with every other component.

The ICF does not address causes or aetiologies, but rather addresses function and health. From the beginning, the emphasis has been to provide a complement to the ICD. In addition, the purpose of the classification is to provide a foundation for the scientific study of function, health, and disability, as well as to provide a common language to be used across populations, sectors, ages, and users. The coding system outlined in the ICF allows public health professionals to collect data for population use, in addition to its use in clinical work to assess individual needs, plan interventions, and assess outcomes.

Table 11.6.1 Differences between the medical and social model perspectives

Area of concern	Medical model	Social model
Locus of problem	Individual	Society
Focus of change	Individual behaviour	Societal attitudes/culture
Changes needed	Personal adjustment	Environmental changes
Intervention strategy	Individual treatment	Social action
Policy issues	Medical/health care	Human rights/access to care

The components of the framework illustrated in Fig. 11.6.1 include functioning across all spheres—body structures and functions, personal activities, and societal participation. Body functions and structures refer to the physiological functions of body systems and the anatomical parts of the body, respectively. A problem with body functions or structures is referred to as *impairment*. A personal task or action undertaken by an individual is termed as an *activity*, and a difficulty in this area is called an *activity limitation*. Likewise, functioning in society in a life situation is termed as *participation*, with a problem in this functioning being called a *participation restriction*. Finally, an *environmental factor* includes any physical, social or attitudinal, and systemic element that affects the functioning of the individual, potentially in all components of body, person, and society (World Health Organization 2001). Figure 11.6.2 provides an outline of the one-level two-character codes for each of the components of the ICF. The full coding system allows coding up to six characters, permitting functional descriptions at both broad and specific levels. The functional codes can be used in both public health surveillance and in epidemiologic studies. Of particular importance for epidemiologic studies is the inclusion of qualifier codes that can be attached after the functional dimension. Qualifiers range from zero to four for severity and encompass a spectrum from 'no problem' to 'complete problem'. In addition, qualifiers can be used clinically to show changes in limitation and participation because of interventions and can be used to monitor change over time (World Health Organization 2001).

This framework provides the most plausible system for common understanding of disability concepts, definitions, and specific functional codes across countries, ages, and sectors, which are relevant for public health purposes related to assessment, policy development, and assurance.

Assessment

Public health assessment is defined as the regular, systematic collection and analysis of information on the health of a community or population. It should include data on health status, health needs of the population, and epidemiologic and other studies of health difficulties. Assessment begins with a most basic tenet—a definition of which health issue is to be assessed. Case definitions are crucial to appropriate identification and are the basis for surveillance, epidemiology, and potential intervention strategies.

Historically, definitions of disability and identification of those experiencing disability have varied greatly in those public health or other sector activities in which this population was included. Definitions for the purpose of identification of individuals with disabilities fall into one of several categories. Traditional approaches to defining disability for public health have focused on equating a particular diagnosis with disability: An individual with a diagnosis of cerebral palsy or blindness, for example, would be assumed to have a disability. A second approach has been to focus on the

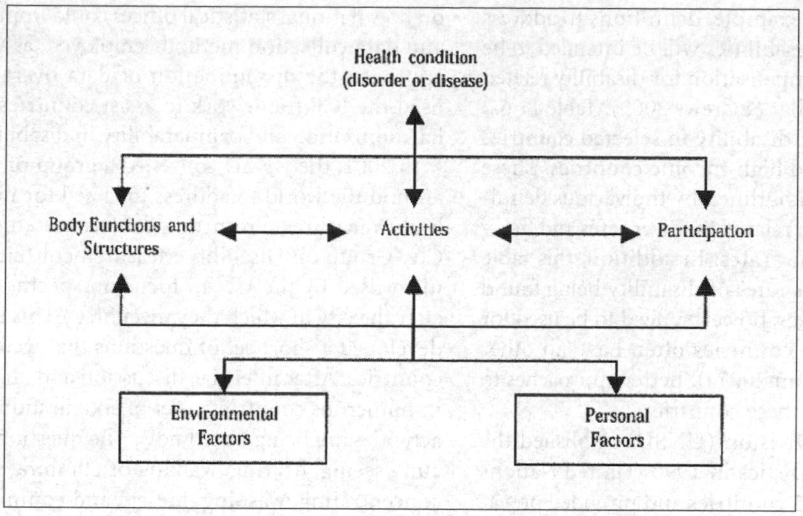

Fig. 11.6.1 Interactions among the *International Classification of Functioning, Disability and Health* components.
Source: Reprinted with permission of the World Health Organization.

impairment—that is, if someone cannot hear in one ear or has an intellectual or learning difficulty, he or she would be considered to have a disability. Third, limitations in particular activities, such as self-care or moving around, have been defined as disabilities. Another approach has been to identify those with problems in working or going to school because of a health problem as having a disability. Yet another approach is to identify those who need special programmes, such as special education or vocational rehabilitation, or special therapies such as physical, occupational, or speech therapy as having a disability. Further, another approach is to ask the individuals themselves if they or others would identify them as someone with a disability (self-identification).

Using these different definitions will produce different prevalence rates. For example, countries using a question such as 'Is anyone in the household deaf, blind, or mute?' as a disability identifier usually will find a prevalence of disability in the 1–2 per cent range. On the other hand, for an activity-oriented question or set of questions—such as, 'Does anyone in your household have difficulty seeing a friend across the street?' or 'Does anyone in your household have difficulty taking care of themselves in eating, drinking, toileting, or dressing?'—the prevalence of disability reaches double digits, and in some countries might approach 20 per cent (United Nations 1990). In more developed countries, several of the approaches to defining disability can be used according to the government agency

Body functions

- b1 Mental functions
- b2 Sensory functions and pain
- b3 Voice and speech functions
- b4 Cardiovascular, haematological, immunological, and respiratory
- b5 Digestive, metabolic, and endocrine functions
- b6 Genitourinary and reproductive functions
- b7 Neuromusculoskeletal and movement-related functions
- b8 Functions of the skin and related functions

Body structures

- s1 The nervous system
- s2 Eye, ear, and related structures
- s3 Structures for voice and speech
- s4 Cardiovascular, immunological, and respiratory structures
- s5 Digestive, metabolic, and endocrine structures
- s6 Genitourinary and reproductive structures
- s7 Structures related to movement
- s8 Skin and related structures

Activities and participation

- d1 Learning and applying knowledge
- d2 General tasks and demands
- d3 Communication
- d4 Mobility
- d5 Self-care
- d6 Domestic life
- d7 Interpersonal interactions and relationships
- d8 Major life areas
- d9 Community, social, and civic life

Environmental factors

- e1 Products and technology
- e2 Natural environment and human-made changes to environment
- e3 Support and relationships
- e4 Attitudes
- e5 Services, systems, and policies

Fig. 11.6.2 Outline of the one-level two-character codes for each of the *International Classification of Functioning, Disability and Health* components.

or purpose for the definition. For example, definitions to address civil rights issues for people with disabilities will be intended to be broad, whereas those providing compensation for disability related to work will be more stringent (Lollar & Crews 2003). Table 11.6.2 provides data on the prevalence of disability in selected countries by source, across low-, middle-, and high-income countries. These figures highlight the different rates outlined by the various definitions described—self-identification related to lower rates and functional approaches producing higher rates. In addition, this table highlights the trend towards higher rates of disability being found in surveys than in censuses. Censuses, however, need to be used for comparisons because low-income countries often have no other mechanism for data collection (Mont 2007a). Better approaches to question formation are needed for these countries.

The United Nations Statistics Division (UNSD) published the first compendium of disability statistics in 1990 (United Nations 1990), which included data from 55 countries and provided prevalence figures and differing case definitions. A major goal of the volume was to begin to develop international standards for disability statistics. Since that initial effort, the UNSD has published the *Guidelines and Principles for the Development of Disability Statistics* (United Nations 2001). This document provided clearer guidelines on how national statistical offices could improve the questions used and data collection methods employed, as well as how they could approach the dissemination of data overall. The UN guidelines used the ICF framework to assist countries as they work towards harmonization and comparability in disability data.

Table 11.6.2 Prevalence of disability in selected countries, by source.*

Censuses			**Surveys**		
Country	*Year*	*Per cent with disability*	*Country*	*Year*	*Per cent with disability*
United States	2000	19.4	New Zealand	1996	20.0
Canada	2001	18.5	Australia	2000	20.0
Brazil	2000	14.5	Uruguay	1992	16.0
United Kingdom	1991	12.2	Spain	1986	15.0
Poland	1988	10.0	Austria	1986	14.4
Ethiopia	1984	3.8	Zambia	2006	13.1
Uganda	2001	3.5	Sweden	1988	12.1
Mali	1987	2.7	Ecuador	2005	12.1
Mexico	2000	2.3	Netherlands	1986	11.6
Botswana	1991	2.2	Nicaragua	2003	10.3
Chile	1992	2.2	Germany	1992	8.4
India	2001	2.1	China	1987	5.0
Colombia	1993	1.8	Italy	1994	5.0
Bangladesh	1982	0.8	Egypt	1996	4.4
Kenya	1987	0.7			

Note: Rates vary according to type of disability-identifier questions used, and are explained in the text.

* Statistics complied using data from UNSD, IBGR (Brazil), INEC (Nicaragua), INEC (Ecuador), INEGI (Mexico), Statistics New Zealand, INE (Spain), Census of India 2001, and SINTEF Health Research 2006 (Zambia).

Source: Reprinted with permission of the World Bank. SP Discussion Paper No. 0706 by Mont D; 2007 Mar.

In 2001, the UNSD convened a group of disability experts from around the world to address the need for more standardized disability measures. From this conference emerged the Washington City Group on Disability Measurement (city groups are a mechanism used by the UN to focus on specific topics and are named after the city in which they meet first.) This international group has developed a short set of questions that were field-tested in several countries. After intensive discussion and analysis of questions used in numerous countries, a set of six questions focusing on personal activities are being tested now. The questions currently cover difficulty seeing, hearing, walking or climbing stairs, remembering or concentrating, washing oneself, and communicating (Centers for Disease Control and Prevention 2006a). The conclusion has been that, in surveys and censuses, respondents can report person-level activities more reliably and validly than they can diagnoses or impairments. Therefore, across settings and countries, comparable data on disabilities can be generated. There is continuing discussion about how to ensure the inclusion of those with cognitive or mental health problems in short sets of disability questions.

As definitions are clarified, there are several kinds of questions that can be further asked by public health about a subpopulation, such as: 'What characterizes this group beyond its disability status?', 'Which conditions are most associated with disability?', and 'Are there disparities between this group and the general population?'

In a recent publication from the United States, data on chronic health conditions contributing to a limitation of activity (disability) indicated that arthritis and other musculoskeletal conditions were most frequently associated with limitations among working-age adults, aged 18–44 years. Mental illness was the second condition most associated with activity limitation, followed by fractures or joint injuries. With increasing age (45–64 years), arthritis was still the most frequently cited condition associated with activity limitation, but was followed by heart and circulatory conditions. Mental illness and diabetes were also mentioned often. The same conditions were associated with activity limitation in the 65–74 age group, but in the 75 years and over age group, senility and vision or hearing problems substantially increased. Throughout all age groups, however, arthritis and heart problems were most related to causing activity limitations (Centers for Disease Control and Prevention 2006b).

In Australia, data have indicated that 20 per cent of the people are living with a disability, also defined as limitation of activity but including impairments and participation restrictions. Among the population, 6.3 per cent have experienced a profound or severe core activity limitation, indicating a need for help with self-care, mobility, or communication. Australia uses a four-factor approach to the kind of disability reported—physical or diverse, sensory or speech, psychiatric, and intellectual or learning. Fifteen per cent of the population have reported physical or diverse category as the disability most affecting their everyday lives. Approximately 2 per cent of the population reported the psychiatric and sensory or speech categories, whereas the intellectual category contributed just less than 1 per cent. As with the United States, older age groups experience more disabling conditions, but the prevalence of severe disability is rather stable (Australian Institute of Health and Welfare 2006).

The Canadian Participation and Activity Limitation Survey from 2001 indicated that 12.4 per cent of individuals reported some degree of disability, defined as limitations in daily living due to a physical, psychological, or health condition. Among adults, the most common limitation was mobility, defined as having problems walking, climbing stairs, or moving from one room to another. Working-age adults reported that the next most common form of disability was from pain (69.5 per cent) (Statistics Canada 2002).

Data from the United Kingdom used 'limiting long-term illness' as the disability approach, and reported 16 per cent of the population in that category. Similar to the Canadian data, the most common limitation was mobility, followed by lifting, carrying, and dexterity. Musculoskeletal problems were most commonly reported as the cause of limitations, then heart and circulatory difficulties, followed by respiratory disorders (Department of Health 1991).

All of these high-income countries have the ability to collect disability data from several sources, such as censuses and varied surveys, and use several definitions of disability—from reported impairments, activity limitations, and participation restrictions. Population-based interventions can be better tailored to a particular group when the characteristics of the population are more clearly understood. Low-income countries, on the other hand, are usually able to collect disability data only during a decennial census and, thus, have substantially less information for the purpose of policy development or assurance of services.

An example of characterizing those identified as having a disability, regardless of the definition, is the data from the United States. The public health agenda for the country has been established every 10 years since the 1980s. The current *Healthy People 2010* includes 'disability status' as a demographic variable for many of the health objectives. For example, one objective is to reduce the number of adults with disabilities who feel sad, depressed, or unhappy; the disparity between those with and those without disabilities in the general population at baseline was 21 per cent (28 per cent adults with disabilities *versus* 7 per cent of the general population). Likewise, a 9 per cent disparity was reported on life satisfaction between adults with and those without disabilities (United States Department of Health and Human Services 2000). In the United States, people with disabilities report obesity at a rate of 31.2 per cent, whereas those without disability reported a 19.6 per cent rate. Physical inactivity was also twice as prevalent among people with disabilities as those without disabilities (22.4 per cent *versus* 11.9 per cent) (Centers for Disease Control and Prevention 2006c).

In a report from the Special Rapporteur on Disability of the UN Commission for Social Development in 2006, results of a UN survey were presented. The survey included questions related to national monitoring of disability. Of the 73 countries responding, about 50 per cent had adopted an official definition of disability and 48 per cent had worked on collecting disability data. In terms of the range of data, 43 per cent were collecting data on the prevalence of disability, and 55 per cent included the types of disabilities. Fifty-six percent reported using data to develop policy (United Nations 2006b).

Using the ICF framework, and given the importance of the environment on the health and well-being of individuals with disabilities, assessment of environmental factors is also emerging. Satariano (1997) noted the importance of environment in the aging process and indicated that public health professionals need to understand and conceptualize the role of the physical environment so as to enhance the independence and mobility of this population. Altman *et al.* (2003), using data from the National Health Interview Survey in the United States, concluded that people with disabilities are more likely to report environmental barriers to their participation in everyday life. The type of functional or activity limitation appears to be related to which barriers are most reported, and respondents in this survey emphasized physical barriers rather than attitudinal or policy barriers. This element of assessment is continuing to develop.

Child disability measurement

Assessing children and youth can be just as or more difficult than assessing adults. First, a child or youth is not usually asked to respond to questions, rather a parent or other proxy. Second, if activity limitation is the approach used to assess disability, at early ages the inability to complete the tasks is developmentally appropriate—that is, the child is not supposed to be able to complete a task, such as dressing or toileting. Also, developmental stages make interpretation of limitations more problematic. Because of these differences, the WHO empowered a working group of international consultants in childhood disability to revise the ICF so that unique aspects of child and youth development and function would be captured (Lollar & Simeonsson 2005). The ICF-CY (Children and Youth) was approved by the WHO in 2006, and published in 2007 (World Health Organization 2007b).

In a 2006 report from the Australian Institute of Health and Welfare, 8.3 per cent of Australian children were reported to have a disability. The report indicated that the most prevalent disabling conditions related to intellectual or learning (4.3 per cent) and physical or diverse (4.2 per cent). Sensory or speech accounted for 3.4 per cent, and psychiatric conditions were reported for 1.2 per cent of the children and youth.

A 2003 study from the United States used the ICF as a framework and the National Health Interview Survey Disability Supplement from 1994–95 to show limitations in activities among children and youth (Fedeyko & Lollar 2003); a prevalence rate of 12 per cent was found using this approach. Learning limitations were more than twice as prevalent as the next highest contributors—communication and social or emotional difficulties. Sensory (vision and hearing) disability was a distant fourth. The *Chart Book on Trends in the Health of Americans* (Centers for Disease Control and Prevention 2006b) indicated that, according to age, different health conditions undermine function more often. Preschoolers have a higher prevalence of speech problems, breathing difficulties related to asthma, and learning or other developmental problems. Learning problems and attention-deficit hyperactivity disorder were the major contributors to activity limitations among school-age children. Older children added emotional and behavioural problems as important aetiologies. Stein and Silver (2002) compared four different definitions of chronic conditions and disabilities among children; the children and youth ranged in age from birth to 17 years. Using a common data set, the National Health Interview Survey from the United States, operational definitions identified between 13.7 and 17 per cent of the population of children with chronic conditions or disabilities. Differing definitions included those using specific diagnoses associated with developmental disabilities and those using consequences of conditions, such as limitations, need for therapies or medication, and the use of compensatory equipment or assistive technology. They concluded that there was significant overlap in the characteristics and prevalence rates, even using different conceptual definitions.

Durkin *et al.* (1995) employed an activity limitation approach to develop a screener of 10 questions for childhood disability. It has been used in several countries, including Bangladesh, Jamaica, and Pakistan where 15.6 per cent, 14.7 per cent, and 8.2 per cent, respectively, of children were identified as having disabilities (Durkin *et al.* 1994). The method used to identify the children was different, however, in that the studies are not usually population-based. The positive aspect is that children identified by the screener can be evaluated more thoroughly, if resources are available; intervention is then possible. The US National Survey of Children with Special Health Care Needs uses a similar activity-oriented approach, which more explicitly follows the ICF-CY model: It includes 13 questions, some of which are related to social and emotional limitations (Maternal and Child Health Bureau 2005). Analysis will allow a substantially greater understanding of both functioning and service use and satisfaction than has been previously possible.

Carers, caregivers, and personal assistance services (PAS)

Beyond obtaining the data to determine the prevalence of people with disabilities, public health should also address the health and well-being of those who provide assistance or care to individuals with disabilities. Most often, this involves family members but also includes paid caregivers or carers. Carers UK suggests that approximately 3 million carers work in the United Kingdom, and that 60 per cent of people will be a carer at some point in their life (ACE National Action for Carers and Employment 2007; Carers UK 2007). Australian data (Australian Institute of Health and Welfare 2006) indicates that 202 000 persons are the primary carers of individuals under 65 of age and live with the person for whom they care. These carers are primarily parents caring for a child or persons caring for a spouse or partner. It was reported that respite care was limited for these carers. Data from Canada indicate that parents of children with disabling conditions report substantial tension as a result of trying to coordinate work, family, and child-care duties, compromising the quality of life (Canadian Institute of Child Health 2000). In the United States, approximately 53 million people are caregivers, providing unpaid services estimated at US$257–389 billion (Arno *et al.* 1999). The persons providing the most intense level of care reported poor health more often than those providing moderate levels of care (Talley & Crews 2007). The numbers and economic impact of caregiving are substantial. Public health associations in high-income countries are only beginning to address this subject, and low-income countries are even less able to address this important health issue.

Measures of health and disability

As more data and sophisticated methods of data analysis are becoming available in many countries, attempts have been made to generate statistics that can better inform public health. Some statistics particularly focused on evaluating the relative effectiveness of public health interventions, among which are the years of healthy life (YHL), quality-adjusted life years (QALYs), and disability-adjusted life years (DALYs). The DALYs indicator was developed with support from the World Bank (Murray & Lopez 1996), and has been used in numerous reports to assess public health priorities and to set a future public health agenda. Because DALYs use the term disability, and because it is being employed so frequently to set public health priorities, it is important that public health professionals understand the relationship between DALYs and the 'current' definitions of disability.

DALYs are based on a definition of disability that correlates with individual disease states. This emphasis on disease assumes that all disease states translate into similar activity limitations and participation restrictions, and assumes no influence of, equal influence of, or only random influence of environmental factors. Over several years, public health professionals, economists, and the disability community have questioned several of the core terms, methods, and implications of the use of DALYs, including using the term disability to describe the statistics. Chamie (1995) suggested that DALYs misrepresent the concept of disability, and it would be better using a term such as *morbidity-adjusted* or *illness-adjusted*, given the method used to generate the measure.

The method requires health professionals to assess the burden of 22 disease-related conditions using preference weighting—the Person Trade-off (PTO) Method. Personal preferences, not population-based data, are used to characterize disability. The methodology used to generate DALYs, the lack of a functional definition of disability in most countries to identify people with disabilities, and the exclusion of people with disabilities in the development process makes the outcomes of this utility suspect (Grosse *et al.* 2009). Mont (2007b) suggested that DALYs were a poor indicator of how public health interventions affect or improve the lives of people with disabilities. He reported that the primary objective in the development of this indicator was to implement a metric that could help national policy makers in allocating resources to reduce poor health. Given the competing needs of people and the minimal resources available, governments have to make difficult decisions regarding public health improvement. Mont concluded that 'an indicator that does not properly embody the intended goals can build in systematic bias against achieving them' (Mont 2007b). The use of DALYs to inform public health policy is questionable, and methods incorporating increased levels of participation by people with disabilities compared to people without disabilities should be developed. Mont and Loeb (2008) have developed a protocol for addressing impact of activity limitations and impairments on participation using population-based data from Zambia. This approach provides a more scientific and generalizable approach to measuring the impact of disabling conditions on people with disabilities. In addition, it allows monitoring of changes in participation across the population and for comparisons across populations.

In summary, whatever the source (e.g. survey, census, or administrative data), public health data should be both periodic and predictable in timing. It is important that disability definitions be separated from outcomes so that analyses can compare groups with and without disabilities. When possible, environmental factors affecting outcomes should also be included in surveys, if not in censuses. Finally, if disability data are to be accepted for the purpose of policy development, people with disabilities should be included at each point in the development, collection, and analysis of data. The disability community dictum of 'nothing about us without us' is particularly important as public health assesses, characterizes, and compares this population with the general population.

Policy development

Data obtained about persons with disabilities alone do not make a difference in public health or in their own lives. Policy development addresses the need for public health policies to use scientific knowledge in decision making, as public health policy is best formulated on the foundation of strong data. Integral to the development of a more consistent approach to public health data collection on disability is the application of this data. Since 1982, when the World Programme of Action was adopted by the United Nations General Assembly, disability policy has been a global mandate (United Nations 1982). The Standard Rules on the Equalization of Opportunities for Persons with Disabilities (United Nations 1993) were developed by the UN to operationalize the Programme, and have been the basis for policy directions globally. Disability data allow countries to evaluate themselves, or have others evaluate them, as to how people with disabilities fare in relation with the general population.

The Standard Rules are divided into three groups—preconditions for equal participation (Rules 1–4), target areas for equal participation (Rules 5–12), and implementation measures (Rules 13–22). Figure 11.6.3 provides an outline of the rules. The end product of these rules is that people with disabilities have an opportunity to participate in society as equals to people without disabilities. It is a step beyond traditional public health and moves further than the emphasis on preventing disease, injury, and disability to embrace the higher-order outcome of participation. This move made when the WHO adopted as its mission 'to improve health and well-being' around the globe. This broader interpretation is the result of an ongoing interaction between public health professionals and the disability community.

It is noteworthy that Rules 2 and 3—medical care and rehabilitation—are the traditional roles acknowledged by public health. The emphasis in Rule 2 (medical care) is on early detection, assessment, and treatment of *impairment*, which can 'prevent, reduce, or eliminate disabling effects'. Also, states are encouraged to provide regular treatment and medication that is needed for people with disabilities to maintain or improve functioning. Rule 3 recommends that national rehabilitation programmes for all people with disabilities be developed. Programmes should focus on the daily needs of these individuals with the goal of full participation and equality. Recommendations are that individuals be involved in their own rehabilitation, that services be available in the local community, and that advocacy groups be included in national programme planning.

Implementation measures are, in fact, the processes that must be in place for the preconditions and target areas to be addressed. Most of the target areas are really the specific outcome areas in which opportunities should arise—for example, education, employment, recreation and sports, culture, and religion. Throughout the Document, the term *health* is rarely found. The concept of health promotion is also absent, and can only be found by an extensive reading of the early detection, assessment, and treatment of impairment or the provision of health care and related services to all people in order to reduce or prevent the 'disability effects of impairment' (United Nations 1993). An emerging area for public health intervention focuses specifically on promoting health and preventing secondary conditions often associated with primary disabilities—such as decubitus ulcers or skin sores among persons with spinal injuries. Physical activity and nutrition, smoking, and alcohol abuse, for example, are clear areas for public health policy and assurance in many countries. However, people with disabilities are often not seen as a vulnerable population for public health messages. Formulation of policy addressing not only rehabilitation and medical services but also health promotion and secondary condition prevention are important areas to be addressed among people with disabilities.

South Africa has provided arguably the most complete national strategy interpreting the UN Standard Rules (Office of the Deputy President 1997). The White Paper on an Integrated National Disability Strategy comprises policy guidelines for the major areas

Major areas

Preconditions		*Target areas*	
Rule 1	Awareness raising	Rule 5	Accessibility
Rule 2	Medical care	Rule 6	Education
Rule 3	Rehabilitation	Rule 7	Employment
Rule 4	Support services	Rule 8	Income maintenance/social security
		Rule 9	Family life and personal integrity
		Rule 10	Culture
		Rule 11	Recreation and sports
		Rule 12	Religion

Implementation measures

Rule 13	Information and research	Rule 18	Organizations of persons with disabilities
Rule 14	Policy making and planning	Rule 19	Personnel training
Rule 15	Legislation	Rule 20	National monitoring/evaluation of disability programmes
Rule 16	Economic policies	Rule 21	Technical and economic cooperation
Rule 17	Coordination of work	Rule 22	International cooperation

Fig. 11.6.3 Adapted from outline of the standard rules on the equalization of opportunities for persons with disabilities.
Source: United Nations. *Standard rules on equalization of opportunities for disabled persons*. New York [NY]: United Nations; 1993.

of the Standard Rules, including prevention, health care, and rehabilitation. Secondary prevention is included and suggests that the targets might be the prevention of complications, such as contractures for those with cerebral palsy. Inclusion of secondary prevention is a critical element in health policy related to disability. A national data base is being developed to provide an array of medical- and disability-related services, as well as to collect information on health-related needs and incidence of impairments. The policy objectives for data and research focus on the gaps between physical and mental conditions and their causes, including the environmental factors influencing them.

In 2007, countries began to sign the first UN convention of the new century—a convention establishing the rights of people with disabilities. This convention provides a roadmap to end discrimination and marginalization of people with physical or mental conditions and has a goal to eliminate exploitation and abuse. Its premise is that people with disabilities have an inherent right to life equal to that of people without disabilities and should receive equal protection and rights, including control of their own financial affairs and the right to privacy. Health is addressed in Article 25, and addresses access to health care, financing, and health professionals' training. Provision of population-based health programmes equivalent to the general population is included—for the first time. Implicit, though not explicitly stated, is the notion that people with disabilities can live healthily.

Although public health professionals can be faulted for not including people with disabilities in health messages for the population, and not recognizing their unique characteristics of vulnerability (for example, the difficulty of balancing nutrition and exercise among those using wheelchairs), the disability community must also recognize its complicity in this omission. In many policy debates surrounding the rights of people with disabilities, there has been an ambivalence to include health. For many people living with disabilities, health is equated with medical intervention and contact. At times, if not often, both medical care and rehabilitation are a source of (1) painful physical experiences, even for treatment; (2) difficulty accessing services; and (3) negative attitudes from medical staff. Therefore, when issues such as civil rights emerge, there is emphasis on employment, education, accessibility to public accommodations, transportation, and so forth, but little acknowledgment of the importance of health as one of the foundations for use of these other rights.

Countries have begun formulating public health policy by setting national health goals. *The Health of the Nation* was published by the Department of Health in the United Kingdom in 1991 (Department of Health 1991). Key areas were selected for attention, which included causes of substantial mortality such as cancer, causes of substantial ill health such as diabetes and mental health, factors contributing to mortality and morbidity such as smoking and diet, areas having potential for great harm (e.g. HIV/AIDS), and areas in which there was clear scope for improvement. This final area included rehabilitation services for people with a physical disability. Emphasis is placed on raising the awareness of medical professionals about care of individuals with chronic physical conditions by raising expectations for people with disabilities. Employing doctors with training in rehabilitation is seen as a step towards better service and higher expectation for function. The assumption is that better rehabilitation services will reduce pressure sores, contractures, and incontinence. Tailored health messages for wheelchair users or relating smoking to elevated skin breakdown associated with decubitus ulcers, however, are not considered as a possible broader public health awareness approach.

Healthy People 2010 (HP 2010) is the national public health agenda for the United States. The inclusion of a chapter in this volume that focuses on improving the health and well-being of people with disabilities is a major step forwards for public health policy in the United States. Addressing four basic misconceptions is at the core of the HP2010 chapter on disability and secondary conditions. First, there is a misconception that people with disabilities are, by definition, in poor health by virtue of living with a disabling condition; it follows, then, that people living with disabilities cannot be healthy. Second, public health has no responsibility for promoting the health of people with disabilities and is responsible only for preventing disabling conditions. Third, there is no need, therefore, to create or develop a case definition for 'people with disabilities'. Fourth, there is a misconception that the environment is unrelated to disability and that any disabling condition lies within the person. The 13 HP 2010 objectives address these misconceptions most clearly by setting targets that match those for the general population. For example, Objective 6-3 has the goal of reducing the proportion of adults with disabilities who are depressed to a level that has parity with all adults aged 18 years and older without disabilities in the United States. Objective 6-13 addresses the goal of having data and programmes for people with disabilities and caregivers in all 50 states by 2010. Figure 11.6.4 outlines the HP2010 objectives for Chapter 6: Disability and Secondary Conditions (United States Department of Health and Human Services 2000).

Regional reports from countries selected in Asia and the Americas have been completed by the International Disability Rights Monitor (Center for International Rehabilitation 2003; Center for International Rehabilitation 2004; Center for International Rehabilitation 2005). These reports include information from 33 countries and reflect policy data on disability measures, as well as on health, rehabilitation, and medical issues.

Child disability policy

As with public health assessment, policy issues are different for children with disabling conditions. The 1989 UN Convention on the Rights of the Child specifically addresses children with disabilities in Article 23 (United Nations 1989). It is committed to the view that these children should enjoy a full life under conditions that allow them to live with dignity, self-determination, and participation in the life of their community. It indicates the right to special care and assistance for them and their families or caregivers. Finally, any such help should come without cost and should include education, training, health care, rehabilitation, and services with the goal of individual development and social integration. This convention has been signed by virtually all countries in the world, and provides the foundation for national policies addressing the needs of children with disabilities. As noted, health care and rehabilitation are included in those rights.

Assessment can identify the magnitude of problem and the population to be targeted. Policies that provide special attention to those needing it can be developed. The final core function of public health, however, is most crucial to those individuals living with a disability—assurance.

Goal: Promote the health of people with disabilities, prevent secondary conditions, and eliminate disparities between people with and without disabilities in the US population.

Number	Objective short title
6-1	Standard definition of people with disabilities in data sets
6-2	Feelings and depression among children with disabilities
6-3	Feelings and depression interfering with activities among adults with disabilities
6-4	Social participation among adults with disabilities
6-5	Sufficient emotional support among adults with disabilities
6-6	Satisfaction with life among adults with disabilities
6-7	Congregate care of children and adults with disabilities
6-8	Employment parity
6-9	Inclusion of children and youth with disabilities in regular education programmes
6-10	Accessibility of health and wellness programmes
6-11	Assistive devices and technology
6-12	Environmental barriers affecting participation in activities
6-13	Surveillance and health-promotion programmes

Fig. 11.6.4 Outline of the *Healthy People 2010* objectives for Chapter 6: Disability and Secondary Conditions. *Source:* United States Department of Health and Human Service, 2000.

Assurance

Assurance focuses on the certitude that needed services will be provided to individuals and communities so that health goals can be reached. Assurance also suggests that services must not only be present but also maintained so that goals can be met. Implicit in these assertions is the notion that there are challenges or barriers to the provision and use of services that must be addressed. Assurance advises that the use of authority may be required to ensure that services will be provided and will not be too costly to access (IOM 1988).

Assurance of services includes not only the presence of services but also the access to those services. Access includes physical proximity or reasonable transport to travel to the services, physical accessibility to the services, policies and systems that allow financial access, and attitudes that encourage participation in the services. The services include clinical preventive services usually set as a baseline for everyone in any particular country, health promotion activities, and prevention of secondary conditions, in addition to basic medical care and rehabilitation.

A basic barrier to assurance of public health services and attention is poverty. Poverty not only contributes to disability but the presence of a disability contributes to poverty, particularly in low-income countries. This applies to any country or group, and it is applicable to people with disabilities because employment rates among them are substantially lower (in the United States, 75 per cent *versus* 37 per cent for individuals with and without disabilities, respectively) (United States Department of Health and Human Services 2000).

In public health, primary prevention programmes are extremely important across the life span. However, even with intense efforts to prevent birth defects, developmental disabilities, injuries, and chronic illnesses, for the foreseeable future, children and adults will continue to live with disabling conditions. They will be affected by poor nutrition, prenatal exposures and events, poorly controlled diseases, conflicts, and environmental factors. A recent Canadian report reflects that 'among those experiencing the worst income inequity are children with disabilities or children with parents who have disabilities' (Canadian Institute of Child Health 2000).

The relationship between poverty and disability has long been established, alongside the general relationship between health status and poverty (Fujiura & Kiyoshi 2000; United Kingdom Public Health Association 2007; Park *et al.* 2002). Yeo and Moore (2003), in discussing the relationship between poverty and disability, concluded that people with disabilities are among the poorest of the poor and are not represented in international development organizations and activities.

Often, people with disabilities, for reasons such as stigma, few resources, or transport, are unable to access appropriate health, medical, or rehabilitation services. In many countries, public health activities are difficult to implement for any of the general population. It is important, however, to remember that societies are judged by the way they relate to the most vulnerable of their citizens. In 2004, the World Bank held a conference on development and disability. James D. Wolfensohn, the World Bank Group President at that time, reported that the Millennium Development Goals set by the UN and the World Bank could not be achieved without the inclusion of people with disabilities (Wolfensohn 2004). Increasing development and improving economic standards cannot be successful without all populations being included.

Public health services

Primary prevention messages can be of equal importance for all segments of a population, including persons with disabilities. For example, people with disabilities might be just as vulnerable, or more so, to heart problems as the general population. Public health messages are often not tailored to ensure that those living with disabilities feel included. Sometimes, people with disabilities are even shown in messages to demonstrate the outcome of inappropriate behaviour, such as showing someone in a wheelchair in a message to promote safe driving. It is important, therefore, that prevention messages be developed so as to acknowledge that people with disabilities can be affected by the same images as the general population. At times, messages should be customized to reach individuals with disabilities. For example, people who have limited mobility are at greater risk for weight gain than the general population because of reduced physical activity (United States Department of

Health and Human Services 2006). However, some in the disability community might interpret primary prevention activities related to injuries or screening for birth defects as inimical to their being alive, and thus, might be suspicious, if not angry, about such activities. Communication between public health professionals and the disability community is critical so that important public health education can be delivered with appropriate input from people having disabilities, but without losing the impact of poignant messages.

Perhaps, the most important public health message for individuals with disabilities is consistent with that for the general population. Encouraging children, youth, and adults to be responsible for their own health is a powerful message that is particularly cogent for people with disabilities. For anyone who experiences multiple medical interventions, a sense of losing control over one's body can develop, which can further be equated with a loss of control over one's health as well. Both at the individual and population level, self-efficacy—a belief in one's ability to have control over one's life and health—is an important mediating factor for positive health outcomes.

Beyond public health education are the clinical services that all countries, whether well-developed or less-developed, attempt to provide for their citizens (US Preventive Services Task Force 1996). These services include immunizations, cancer screenings for both men and women, health guidance regarding nutrition and physical activity, sexuality and pregnancy education, drug use education including alcohol and smoking, and other important health information. In more-developed countries, medical care and rehabilitation are emphasized, whereas clinical preventive services are not. Often, rehabilitation becomes equated with medical rehabilitation and providers focus on the disabling condition and its medical complications. Primary care is not emphasized, with the assumption that medical-care generalists will provide the immunizations, health screenings, education, and other primary-care activities. Also, specialists might not be familiar with or sensitive to the need for these services in this population. Many individuals with disabilities, if they have specialized care, do not use primary care, and therefore, might not receive appropriate services. Jones and Kerr (1997) reported that individuals with cognitive impairments did not receive annual health screenings. Austin (2003) found that people with disabilities, in the US state of Oregon, using services funded through public mechanisms are at greater risk of developing smoking-related cancers, are more likely to be diagnosed at a later stage of cancer, and therefore, not receive timely screening for it. In addition, treatment was more often delayed among this population. A public health responsibility is to ensure that people with disabilities are not lost to the provision of clinical preventive services.

Secondary conditions prevention

The term *secondary conditions* is new and is evolving in the vocabulary and objectives of public health. Introduced in the early 1990s into public health in the United States, the term has come to denote those conditions that are preventable but are present because of a pre-established primary disabling condition. A secondary condition is one to which an individual is more susceptible by virtue of living with a disability. 'Secondary' does not reflect the level of importance but rather means that it comes after the primary condition (Lollar 1999). 'Conditions' was chosen to indicate that this secondary problem could have characteristics beyond the medical or even physical ones. Thus, depression could be a primary disabling condition, but could also be a secondary condition associated with a physical impairment. Social isolation is another common secondary condition not physical in nature, but certainly related to the presence of and vulnerability associated with a disabling condition. Of course, more common examples are physical fatigue from the exertion of moving a wheelchair or urinary tract infections associated with but not a required co-morbid diagnosis of spinal cord injury or spina bifida.

To reiterate, an important characteristic of a secondary condition is that it can be prevented. Thus, medical, rehabilitative, and public health professionals are involved with activities to prevent secondary conditions at the individual and the population level. Given that Disabled Persons International has affiliates in more than 120 countries (Disabled Persons International 2007), it is clear that people live with disabilities around the globe. The health of people with disabilities, however, should not be assumed to be poor by virtue of having a disabling condition. Health is also a right for people with disabilities.

Ravesloot *et al.* (1997) completed a study on adults with disabilities across several diagnostic categories. They indicated that the results were surprising because they had assumed that each diagnostic group would report different secondary conditions. Instead, the results indicated common secondary conditions across all diagnoses. Traci *et al.* (2002) used a survey of common secondary conditions in a study on individuals with developmental disabilities. Physical fitness and conditioning problems were the most prevalent (590/1000), followed by communication and mobility difficulties (573/1000 and 509/1000, respectively). Low frustration tolerance and weight problems were next in prevalence. They concluded that these difficulties included major behavioural and lifestyle limitations, whereas more medically oriented conditions, such as bowel problems or respiratory difficulties, were substantially less reported.

This topic is not complete without a mention of the 'secondary benefits'. Disabling conditions usually challenge the individual and family's functioning and participation, and often lead to secondary conditions. There are, however, benefits that may come as a result of living with a disability or being a family member of such an individual. Benefits often include openness to and acceptance of differences in other human beings and seeing the humanity beyond the difference. Creative problem solving is also frequently required in adapting to a world that is often not accommodating. Strength of will is more developed due to increased physical and emotional energy required to complete tasks (Lollar 2006). Friendships based on the shared experience of disability provide both social and emotional support, and the identifications created are often long lasting. These benefits may become protective factors in future adjustment and participation for both children and adults, and should be included in public health evaluation, policy, and assurance. Prevention of secondary conditions should be an integral part of any nation's public health agenda for people with disabilities, regardless of the health-care financing system.

Public health interventions

Interventions must be provided at both an individual and a population level. Using a self-efficacy conceptual model, several programmes have been developed to improve the health and well-being of people with disabilities. Seekins *et al.* (1991) developed an eight-session workshop, Living Well with a Disability, co-led by people with disabilities and a professional who helps participants learn to set health goals and find ways to meet them. This approach has reduced secondary conditions and medical visits among the participants. Fifteen US states have implemented the programme. In addition, state programmes that educate health-care providers about how to make their physical office space and medical staff attitudes more accessible to those with disabilities have also been instituted (North Carolina Office on Disability and Health 1999).

Many low-resource countries have medical and rehabilitation services—usually proportionate to their overall level of resources. These services, however, are not equivalent to public health. This translation of medicine and rehabilitation into public health is a necessary, but not sufficient, approach to improving the health and well-being of people with disabilities. Medical care is important, even critical, for all citizens regardless of disability status. Rehabilitation services, whether medical, educational, vocational, or social, are specific services focused on outcomes related to the designated area—for example, work or school. The experiences of individuals with disabilities are much broader than just medicine or rehabilitation, even defined broadly. Public health must encompass these services, but must also include those services discussed in previous subsections—health education, preventive services, prevention of secondary conditions, and environmental facilitators of health and well-being.

Towards this end, community-based rehabilitation (CBR) activities have been developed in more than 90 countries and strive to provide comprehensive strategies to include people with disabilities in the life of their communities (World Health Organization 2007a). This emphasis, sponsored by the WHO, focuses on providing equal access to medical and rehabilitation services, but also to education, employment, and numerous other community activities. Public health professionals, in conjunction with CBR staff, can collaborate to provide the expertise from both public health and the disability community to improve the health of people with disabilities.

Major directions

Communication, cooperation, coordination

The most pressing need is for public health and disability communities to acknowledge their respective perspectives of the other. Public health professionals do not easily acknowledge that people with disabilities are a legitimate population—a minority population, even—who deserve public health attention. The disability community must accept that health is a core issue for all, and particularly, for themselves because they are often more vulnerable to additional health problems. The public health community can be a strong partner towards improving health and well-being among people with disabilities. Likewise, the disability community can assist the public health community in achieving these goals.

There is a growing interaction between public health professionals and members of the disability community. A prime example of this cooperation was a leader from Disabled Persons International (DPI) co-chairing the WHO Environmental Task Force to complete the ICF. On the DPI website, there is support for use of the ICF to conceptualize disability and to collect data using ICF definitions. In the United Kingdom, a report on The Life Chances of Disabled People has been completed by disability researchers and addresses inclusion of people with disabilities. The Office on Disability Issues has created an advisory body of 23 people with disabilities called Equality 2025, whose responsibility is to advise the Government on disability issues, including health and well-being. Likewise, in 2006, the UN Department of Social and Economic Affairs commissioned an audit to evaluate the accessibility of the Internet for people with disabilities (Nomensa 2006). Five sectors from the Convention on the Rights of Persons with Disabilities were selected for assessment—travel, finance, media, politics, and retail. Interestingly, health was again not included. The evaluation concluded that only 3 sites, among the 100 audited from 20 countries, achieved appropriate accessibility ratings and that there was a failure around the world to provide basic levels of Internet accessibility for those living with disabilities.

In 2001 and 2002, the UN sponsored two workshops on measuring disability. The groups were composed equally of disability advocates and national statistical office representatives from the same countries. Representatives of English-speaking countries from Eastern Africa met in Kampala, Uganda in 2001 and those from the ESCWAR region, including Arab-speaking countries and Israel, met in Cairo, Egypt in 2002 (United Nations Statistics Division 2001, 2002). During each of the 2 weeks, the groups interacted to come to a better understanding of how disability statistics and disability policy were connected; the advocates and statisticians developed pilot questions to be used in censuses or surveys in their countries. These activities have not, until now, been the norm, but should become part of every nation's public health efforts to achieve valid disability data and pragmatic disability policy.

Disability framework and measurement

The WHO disability framework approved in 2001 along with the children's version approved in 2006 provide the foundation for public health functions to be achieved. The ICF is finding more traction in countries around the world. Clinical use of ICF codes can be found, in Germany, in the work of Stucki *et al.* (2002a, 2002b) Physicians throughout Italy are being trained to use ICF coding alongside ICD codes in clinical work (Disability Italian Network 2005). The Measuring Health and Disability in Europe (MHADIE) project of the European Union is implementing an ICF approach in addressing a standardized method to data collection on disability in its 25 member states (Measuring Health and Disability in Europe 2005).

Surveys have been incorporating the ICF framework in Qatar (Simeonsson RJ, Evaluation of children with activity limitations in Qatar schools, personal communication; 2007) and in the United States (Maternal and Child Health Bureau 2005). The Washington Group on Disability Measurement included 75 countries in its early efforts to develop a short set of ICF-based functional questions in order to identify people living with some of the most prevalent activity limitations associated with disability (Centers for Disease Control and Prevention 2006a). There is still the challenge of identifying individuals with mental health problems or with cognitive impairments, but the process has begun. Because the process for revision of both the ICD and the ICF are under the auspices of the Committee on Family of International Classifications (WHO-FIC), there will be growing congruence in the use of these complementary classifications in both clinical and public health settings.

Public health education and training

Public health education is expanding around the world. A study by Tanehaus *et al.* (2000) indicated that schools of public health in the United States are beginning to include disability-related course work. They recommend the inclusion of dedicated courses addressing disability issues, as well as integration of disability issues into courses across the public health curricula. As an outgrowth of this study, two products have been developed. A course dedicated to disability and public health has been developed by the Oregon Office on Disability and Health (Drum *et al.* 2004). In addition, a handbook of disability and public health has been completed. This volume encompasses all major public health core areas—epidemiology, health services, global health, environmental health, and ethics. Public health experts in these fields have contributed chapters that provide a link between public health and disability in their particular specialty and provide references and case studies for each area. Using this approach, any discipline within public health could integrate disability into its courses (Allen & Garberson 2009).

Conclusions

People living with disabilities have traditionally not been included in public health activities. As more people with disabilities live longer because of better nutrition, medical interventions, and public health interventions such as immunizations, there is a greater need for this population to be included in public health interventions, to be a target for specific public health messages, and to be acknowledged as a population worthy of attention when public health planning is being instituted. This 'epidemic of survival' provides an opportunity for public health to address a minority population around the world.

People with disabilities need to be encouraged to take responsibility for their health behaviours, but also to challenge the systems that undermine progress towards health and well-being. Both groups can address environmental barriers to health, including non-health issues such as access to health care and education, societal attitudes towards those with disabling conditions, and policies and systems. Training of public health professionals in disability issues is emerging, and this education of young people can lead to long-term changes in public health perceptions and practice.

References

ACE National Action for Carers and Employment. Work and Families Act 2006 [Online]. 2007. Available from: www.acecarers.org.uk

Allen D., Garberson W., editors. *One in Five: Public Health Perspectives on Disability*. 2009. New York: Springer Publishing Co.

Altman B., Lollar D.J., Rasche E. The experience of environmental barriers among persons with disabilities. Presentation to the American Sociological Association; 2003.

Arnesen T., Nord E. The value of DALY life: problems with ethics and validity of disability-adjusted life years. *British Journal of Medicine* 1999;**319**:1423–5.

Arno P.S., Levine C., Memmott M.M. The economic value of informal caregiving. *Health Affairs* 1999;**18**(2):182–8.

Austin D. Disabilities are risk factors for late stage or poor prognosis cancers. Paper presentation on Changing Concepts of Health and Disability at the Science and Policy Conference. Portland (OR): Oregon Health and Science University; 2003.

Australian Institute of Health and Welfare. Disability and disability services in Australia. Canberra: Australian Institute of Health and Welfare; 2006.

Canadian Institute of Child Health. *The health of Canada's children*. Ottawa: Canadian Institute of Child Health; 2000.

Carers UK. The voice of carers [Online]. 2007. Available from: www.carersuk.org

Center for International Rehabilitation. *International disability rights compendium*. Washington (DC): Center for International Rehabilitation; 2003.

Center for International Rehabilitation. *International disability rights monitor: regional report of the Americas 2004*. Chicago (IL): International Disability Network; 2004.

Center for International Rehabilitation. *International disability rights monitor: regional report of Asia 2005*. Chicago (IL): International Disability Network; 2005.

Centers for Disease Control and Prevention. *Chart book on trends in the health of Americans*. Washington (DC): Centers for Disease Control and Prevention; 2006b.

Centers for Disease Control and Prevention. *Disability and health state chart book*. Atlanta (GA): Centers for Disease Control and Prevention; 2006c.

Centers for Disease Control and Prevention. Washington City group report on disability measurement. Washington (DC): Centers for Disease Control and Prevention; 2006a.

Chamie M. What does morbidity have to do with disability? *Disability and Rehabilitation* 1995;**17**(7):323–7.

Department of Health. *The health of the nation*. London: Her Majesty's Stationery Office; 1991.

Disability Italian Network. *ICF: basic and advanced course*. Gardolo, Italy: Disability Italian Network; 2005.

Disabled Persons International [Online]. Available from: http://v1.dpi.org/lang-en/index

Drum C.E., Krahn G.L., Ritacco B.A. *et al.*, editors. *Disability and public health curriculum outline*. Portland (OR): Oregon Office on Disability and Health; 2004.

Durkin M.S., Islam S., Hasan Z.M. *et al.* Measures of socioeconomic status for child health research: comparative results from Bangladesh and Pakistan. *Social Science and Medicine* 1994;**38**(9):1289–97.

Durkin M.S., Wang W., Shrout P.E. *et al.* Evaluating a ten-questions screen for childhood disability: reliability and internal structure in different cultures. *Journal of Clinical Epidemiology* 1995;**48**(5):657–66.

Fedeyko H.J., Lollar D.J. Classifying disability data. In: Barnarrt S, Altman B, Hendershot G *et al.*, editors. *Using survey data to study disability: results from the national health interview survey on disability*. Research in Social Science and Disability. Vol. 3. Oxford: Elsevier; 2003. p. 55–72.

Fujiura G.T., Kiyoshi Y. Trends in demography of childhood poverty and disability. *Exceptional Children* 2000;**66**(2):187–99.

Grosse S., Lollar D.J., Campbell V.A., and Chamie M. (2009) Disability and disability-adjusted life years (DALYs): not the same. *Public Health Reports,* accepted for publication.

Institute of Medicine. *The future of public health*. Washington (DC): National Academy Press; 1988.

Jones R.G., Kerr M.P. A randomized control trial of an opportunistic health screening tool in primary care for people with intellectual disability. *Journal of Intellectual Disability Research* 1997;**41**:409–15.

Lollar D.J., Crews J.E. Redefining the role of public health in disability. *Annual Review of Public Health* 2003;**24**:195–208.

Lollar D.J., Simeonsson R.J. Diagnosis to function: classification for children and youths. *Developmental and Behavioral Pediatrics* 2005;**26**(4): 323–30.

Lollar D.J. Clinical dimensions of secondary conditions. In: Simeonsson RJ, McDevitt LN, editors. *Issues in disability and health: the role of secondary conditions and quality of life*. Chapel Hill (NC): University of North Carolina; 1999. p. 41–50.

Lollar D.J. Preventing secondary conditions and promoting health. In: Rubin IL, Crocker AC, editors. *Medical care for children and adults with developmental disabilities*. Baltimore (MD): Paul H Brookes Publishing; 2006. p. 33–42.

Maternal and Child Health Bureau. Survey of children with special health care needs. Washington (DC): Maternal and Child Health Bureau; 2005.

Measuring Health and Disability in Europe. MHADIE Press Release 2005 [Online]. Available from: http://www.mhadie.it/aboutus.aspx

Mont D. and Loeb M. (2008). *Beyond DALYs: Developing Indicators to Assess the Impact of Public Health Interventions on the Lives of People with Disabilities.* SP 0185. World Bank: Washington, DC.

Mont D. Measuring disability prevalence. *Social protection discussion paper.* New York (NY): World Bank; 2007a.

Mont D. Measuring health and disability. *Lancet* 2007b;**369**:1658–63.

Murray C.J.L., Lopez A.D., editors. The global burden of disease: a comprehensive assessment of mortality and disability from diseases, injuries and risk factors in 1990 and projected to 2000. Cambridge (MA): Harvard University Press; 1996.

Nomensa. United Nations global audit of web accessibility [Online]. 2006. Available from: http://www.nomensa.com/resources/research/united-nations-global-audit-of-accessibility.html

North Carolina Office on Disability and Health. Removing barriers: tips and strategies to promote accessibility. Chapel Hill (NC): North Carolina Office on Disability and Health; 1999.

Office of the Deputy President. Integrated national disability strategy: a white paper. Ndabeni, South Africa: Office of the Deputy President; 1997.

Park J., Turnbull A.P., Turnbull H.R. Impacts of poverty on quality of life in families of children with disabilities. *Exceptional Children* 2002;**68**(2):151–70.

Ravesloot C., Seekins T., Walsh J. A structural analysis of secondary conditions experienced by people with physical disabilities. *Rehabilitation Psychology* 1997;**42**(1):3–16.

Satariano W.E. The disabilities of aging—looking to the physical environment. *American Journal of Public Health* 1997;**87**(3):331–2.

Seekins T., Clay J., Kirchmyer S. *et al.* Developing and implementing a program for preventing and managing secondary conditions experienced by adults with physical disabilities. Missoula (MT): Research and Training Center on Rural Rehabilitation; 1991.

Statistics Canada. Participation and activity limitation survey: a profile of disability in Canada. Ottawa: Statistics Canada; 2002.

Stein R.E.K., Silver E.J. Comparing different definitions of chronic conditions in a national data set. *Ambulatory Pediatrics* 2002;**2**:63–70.

Stucki G., Cieza A., Ewert T. *et al.* Application of the international classification of functioning, disability and health in clinical practice. *Disability and Rehabilitation* 2002a;**24**:281–2.

Stucki G., Ewert T., Cieza A. Value and application of the ICF in rehabilitation medicine. *Disability and Rehabilitation* 2002b;**24**:932–8.

Talley R.C., Crews J.E. Framing the public health of caregiving. *American Journal of Public Health* 2007;**97**(2):224–8.

Tanehaus R.H., Meyers A.R., Harbsion L.A. Disability and the curriculum in US graduate schools of public health. *American Journal of Public Health* 2000;**90**:1315.

Tracy M.I., Seekins T., Szalda-Petree A. *et al.* Assessing secondary conditions among adults with developmental disabilities: a preliminary study. *Mental Retardation* 2002;**40**(2):119–31.

United Kingdom Public Health Association. The state of Britain's health: poverty and inequality [Online]. Available from: http://www.ukpha.org.uk/default.asp?action=article&ID=71&KeyWords=poverty%2Cand%2Cinequality

United Nations Statistics Division. *Workshop report on disability statistics for Africa.* 2001 Sept 10–14; Kampala, Uganda.

United Nations Statistics Division. *Workshop report on disability measurement for ESCWA countries.* 2002 Jun 1–5; Cairo, Egypt.

United Nations. Convention on the Rights of Persons with Disabilities; 2006 Aug 25. New York (NY): United Nations; 2006a.

United Nations. *Convention on the rights of the child.* New York: United Nations; 1989.

United Nations. *Disability statistics compendium.* New York (NY): United Nations; 1990.

United Nations. Global survey on government action on the implementation of the standard rules on the equalization of opportunities for persons with disabilities. New York (NY): United Nations; 2006b.

United Nations. Guidelines and principles for the development of disability statistics. New York (NY): United Nations; 2001. Series Y, No. 10.

United Nations. Standard rules on equalization of opportunities for disabled persons. New York (NY): United Nations; 1993.

United Nations. *World programme of action.* New York (NY): United Nations; 1982. Resolution 37/52.

United States Department of Health and Human Services. Disability and secondary conditions. In: *Healthy people 2010.* Washington (DC): Department of Health and Human Services; 2000.

United States Department of Health and Human Services. *Midcourse review on healthy people 2010: disability and secondary conditions.* Washington (DC): Department of Health and Human Services; 2006.

US Preventive Services Task Force. *Guide to clinical preventive services.* 2nd ed. Alexandria (VA): International Medical Publishing; 1996.

Wolfensohn J.D. Disability and inclusive development. Keynote presentation at the World Bank Conference; 2004 Dec 1; Washington (DC).

World Health Organization. Disability and rehabilitation team [Online]. 2007a. Available from: www.who.int/disabilities/cbr/en.

World Health Organization. *International classification of diseases.* 10th revision. Geneva: World Health Organization; 1992.

World Health Organization. *International classification of functioning, disability and health.* Geneva: World Health Organization; 2001. pp. 29–30.

World Health Organization. International classification of functioning, disability and health—children and youth. Geneva: World Health Organization; 2007b.

Yeo R., Moore K. Including disabled people in poverty reduction work: 'nothing about us without us'. *World Development 2003* Mar;**31**(3):571–90.

11.7

Health of older people

Shah Ebrahim and Julie E. Byles

Abstract

Declines in death rates and fertility have resulted in population ageing and an associated epidemiologic transition from infectious to chronic diseases. Dramatic improvements in life expectancy have occurred, although these have not been equally distributed among socioeconomic groups or seen in politically or economically unstable countries. Ageing is associated with increased health- and social-care needs, not only due to increased risk of chronic diseases but also due to multiple pathologies, and ironically, greater risk of iatrogenic problems associated with polypharmacy. Measures of functioning and disability provide a comprehensive and pragmatic means of assessing older people's needs and evaluating the effects of interventions. Older people are capable of benefiting from a wide range of preventive interventions that reduce mortality and morbidity in middle age—such as cardiovascular disease (CVD) risk factor reduction, increased physical activity, and a healthy diet. Specific preventive interventions—such as falls-prevention schemes and screening or anticipatory care—are probably of less value than was thought, which may reflect the increased access and acceptability of high-quality health services for older people in many high-income countries. These include disease-specific services—such as stroke units, orthogeriatric units, and psychogeriatric units—and general services such as assessment and rehabilitation units, day hospitals, and long-term care. Many countries, particularly low- and middle-income ones, have yet to establish these essential requirements for meeting older people's needs. Informal family support remains the backbone of care for older people in all countries, and without these contributions, statutory formal health- and social-care sectors would be inundated. The costs of care are wrongly considered to increase with age; in reality, costs are more strongly concentrated in the short period before death. Long-term care in institutions is expensive, and reducing the need for such care by increasing home care and avoiding the use of acute-sector institutions are both important measures for reducing costs. Considerable debate is required in order to develop new policies on societal and individual responsibilities for meeting the costs of long-term care. Public health has responsibilities for monitoring trends and transition in risk factors, disease, and disability in ageing populations. In addition, it has roles in encouraging effective health-promotion practices and in setting policy for the equitable and efficient use of health-care resources for the growing population of older people.

Introduction

This chapter considers the phenomenon of population ageing and the public health implications. The case for considering older people as a special-needs group is discussed, together with the health problems they face. The available evidence on the efficacy of preventive intervention, primary care and hospital services, and long-term care and social support is reviewed.

Concepts of ageing vary across societies and settings, over time, and from person to person. Even the definition of 'old age' is imprecise, and varies with the situation and purpose. In the past, the United Nations and other international agencies defined 'the elderly' as 60 years and over, but more recently, there is a growing consensus that it be defined as 65 years and over. However, people over this age are not one homogenous group. Indeed, older people are a very heterogeneous group comprising those who are actively pursuing careers in industry or politics, enjoying healthy retirement, or caring for frail and dependent relatives or friends, and others who are themselves very frail and dependent. Such diverse people are frequently grouped together as 'the elderly', as if they have similar needs and would respond uniformly to interventions. It is essential to recognize this heterogeneity when defining needs, assessing effects and relevance of intervention, and planning for the future.

It is common to categorize older people as the 'young old'—aged 60–69 years, the 'old old'—aged 70–79 years, and the 'oldest old'—aged 80 years and over. Further, as more and more people reach older ages, there is increasing interest in studying the needs and characteristics of centenarians and 'super-centenarians' (110 years and over). However, ageing is a biological and social process that affects individuals at different rates and which is related to but not synonymous with chronological age. Characteristics, apart from age, also contributing to the differences between older people include gender, geographic location, and socioeconomic and ethnic background. At any age, there is great variance in experience, capacity, and health status between individuals. The process of ageing is universal but not uniform.

Demographics and projections

Over the last century, the world has undergone an extraordinary demographic transition. The proportion of people aged 65 years is expected to increase from around 1 per cent of the world's population 100 years ago to an estimated 20 per cent by the middle of the twenty-first century (United Nations 2002). Currently, the world population is around 6.5 billion, of whom an estimated 485 million (7.4 per cent) were aged 65 and over in 2006 (United States Census Bureau 2007). The relative size of the population aged 65 years and over is expected to increase to more than 9 per cent in 2020 and to almost 17 per cent by 2050.

Figure 11.7.1 shows the age and sex structure of the world's population in 2000 and the projected structure in 2050. Figure 11.7.2 shows the proportions of people aged 65 years and over in various world regions in 2002.

More affluent countries tend to have older average population ages than lower-income regions. In affluent countries, ageing involves a large cohort of people born out of post-World War II prosperity. A majority of these people are health conscious, educated, and resourceful, and have access to a wide range of technologies. They also have relatively low levels of disability and have the health capacity to remain productive well into their old age. However, the majority of the world's older people live in low-income countries. In low-income countries, ageing is occurring rapidly against a background of prevailing poverty, immense social and cultural change, changes in family structure, vast urban–rural differences, the existing endemic diseases (e.g. malaria), and newer epidemic diseases (e.g. AIDS and obesity).

Moreover, the pace of population ageing in many low-income countries is more rapid than in high-income countries (see Fig. 11.7.3). In low-income countries, the annual population growth of people aged 65 years and over is almost 3 per cent per year, whereas in high-income countries, the growth has fallen to less than 2 per cent per year (Kinsella 1996). Belgium took over 100 years to double the proportion of its 60-plus population from 9 to 18 per cent. China will take 34 years to undergo the same transition, and Singapore will take only 20 years.

In high-income countries, the proportion of the 'oldest old' is growing more rapidly than any other age group. In the United States, the proportion of persons aged 85 years and over increased by 274 per cent from 1960 to 1994, compared with 100 per cent for persons aged 65 years and 45 per cent for the total population (United States Census Bureau 2007). It is these oldest old who tend to present major challenges for health and social services in these regions. Figure 11.7.4 illustrates the numbers of people aged 80 years or over projected to 2050.

Projections of population ageing are important for planning services, but are subject to error. These are particularly sensitive to assumptions about mortality rates at older ages and tend to underestimate the true numbers of older people. Population projections are also sensitive to phenomena such as changes in fertility rates, mass migrations, wars, and pandemics. The AIDS pandemic has had a major impact on the age and sex structure of many countries (most particularly those in sub-Saharan Africa), and the full effects are yet to be seen. The other population phenomenon of current interest is the post-war 'baby boom', which has created a bulge in the mid-aged populations of many high-income countries. Maintenance of the health and productivity of these people as they age is of particular importance for the sustainability of health services and welfare systems.

Determinants of population ageing

Population ageing is not only due to greater numbers of people living longer, but also due to lower fertility rates resulting in fewer

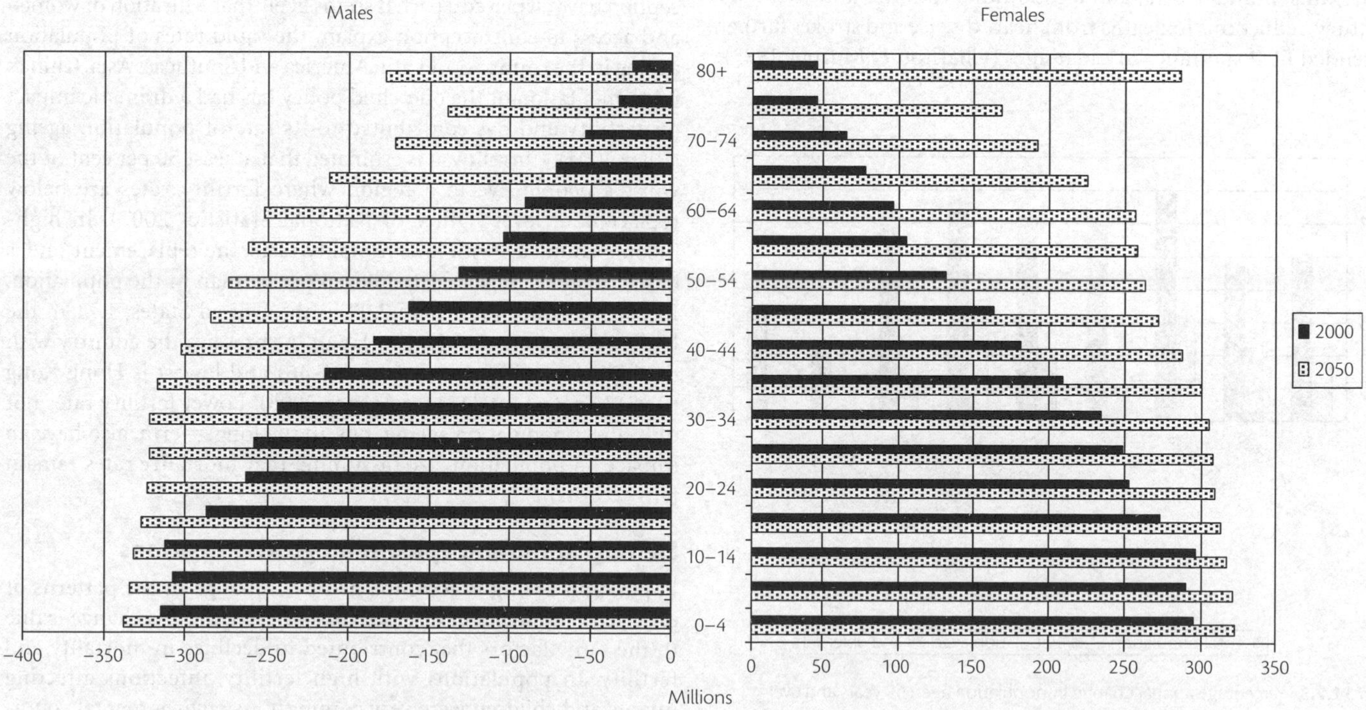

Fig. 11.7.1 World population pyramids, showing age and sex structure, in 2000 and the 2050 projection.
Source: United States Census Bureau (Online). Available from: http://www.census.gov/

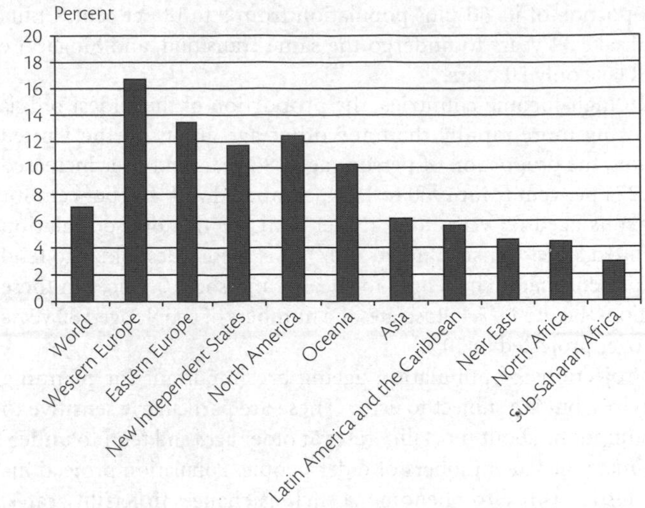

Fig. 11.7.2 Population aged 65 years and over in 2002 represented as a percentage of the total population, by region.
Source: United States Census Bureau. Global population profile 2002 (Online). Available from: http://www.census.gov/

young people entering the population. Therefore, although improvements in medical care have contributed to population ageing, the major drivers are declines in fertility and childhood mortality. In the United Kingdom, the drop in infant and childhood mortality began in the nineteenth century, pre-dating the era of modern effective medical care by many decades. In the twentieth century, population ageing was accelerated by lower infant and child mortality, initially because of improved living conditions and sanitation, and then as a result of better nutrition, immunization, antitoxins, immune sera, and antibiotics. From the mid-twentieth century, reductions in deaths from heart disease and strokes further extended life expectancy at older ages (Charlton & Murphy 1997).

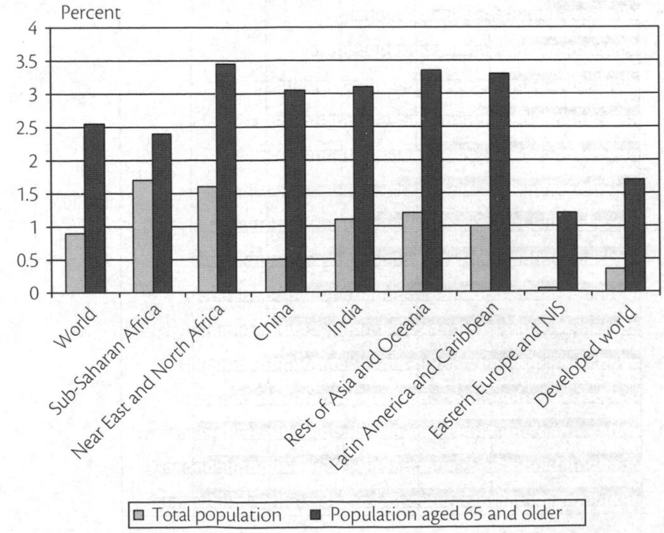

Fig. 11.7.3 Percentage annual change in population aged 65 years and over compared with the total population, by region, 2002–2025.
Source: Adapted from United States Census Bureau (Online). Available from: http://www.census.gov/

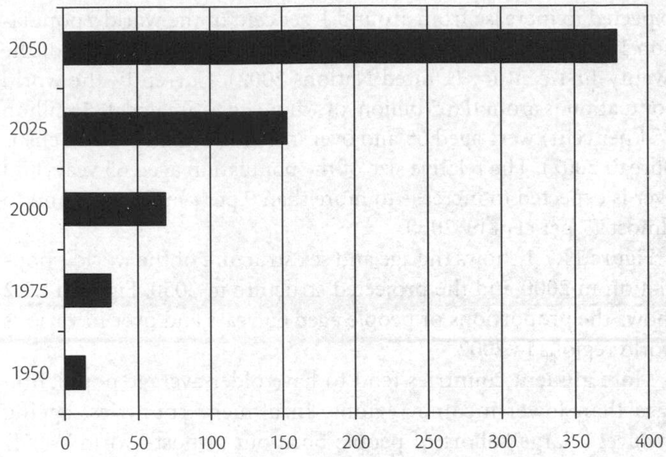

Fig. 11.7.4 World population aged 80 years or over, 1950–2050.
Source: Adapted from Department of Economic and Social Affairs. New York (NY): Population Division, United Nations; 2001. Available from: www.un.org.au

However, even recently in the United Kingdom, mortality declines have only been experienced by the better-off, demonstrating the continuing influence of social and economic factors (Drever & Whitehead 1997). In low-income countries, the successful infant and child health programmes (such as growth-chart monitoring, oral rehydration for diarrhoea, breastfeeding, and immunization for common infections) are probably responsible for the rapid rates of mortality decline at younger ages.

Declines in fertility are attributed to urbanization, industrialization, and social mobility, which have all had an influence on family structures. In addition, the emancipation of women, their greater chances for education, later age at marriage, and access to contraception have all played a part. It seems likely that education of women and access to contraception explain the rapid rates of population ageing in the countries of Latin America and Southeast Asia. China's implementation of the one-child policy has had a dramatic impact on fertility and has contributed to its rate of population ageing (Riley 2004). Currently, it is estimated that at least 50 per cent of the world's people live in a region where fertility rates are below replacement level (Office of National Statistics 2007). In high-income countries with low mortality rates, the replacement rate is based on an average of 2.1 children per woman in the population. In 2003, fertility rates were 2.07 in the United States, 1.71 in the United Kingdom, and 2.91 in Japan. At present, the country with the highest fertility rate is Niger (7.46) and lowest is Hong Kong (0.95) (Central Intelligence Agency 2006). Lower fertility rates not only affect population ageing, but, in the longer term, also have an impact on population size (assuming that mortality rates remain fairly constant).

Demographic and epidemiological transitions

Population ageing is accompanied by a change in the patterns of prevalent and incident diseases. To some extent, this change is due to the same factors that contributed to declines in mortality and fertility. In populations with high fertility, infections affecting infants and children were very common. As environmental conditions contributing to risk of infections improved, and as nutritional patterns changed from periods of famine to a more plentiful food supply throughout the year, so were the seeds of chronic and degenerative diseases sown. These epidemiological transitions have been defined as the age of pestilence and famine, the age of receding pandemics, and the age of degenerative and man-made diseases (Omran 1971). However, rapidly ageing low-income countries are experiencing high levels of infectious diseases that take their toll on infants and children, and also, emerging burdens of smoking- and diet-related diseases, particularly cardiovascular diseases, cancers, and diabetes mellitus. An additional 'age' has been defined to accommodate the populations experiencing reversals in longevity due to economic and political instability (Yusuf *et al.* 2001).

Mortality rates and life expectancy

Mortality rates tend to increase at older ages; however, in recent decades, the rate of death has slowed at all ages. Also, at advanced ages (after age 70 or 80), 'old-age mortality deceleration' takes place. The mortality rates of a population can be summarized in a 'life table', which can be used to calculate life expectancy of people at different ages. Table 11.7.1 shows the life expectancy at birth and at age 65 years for men and women in England and Wales. Note that for people who achieve 'old age', their life expectancy is greater than life expectancy at birth. A male born in 1841 could be expected to survive to 40.2 years, but another male who had already survived childhood and reached 65 years could expect to live a further 10.9 years. The difference between the situation in 1841 and now is that far fewer people actually survived the hazards of early life then.

Over recent decades, there has been a substantial increase in life expectancy at birth. Global life expectancy was around 46 years in 1950 and increased to 66 years in 1998. Even in the two decades since 1978, life expectancy increased by 5 years for men (reaching 65 years in 1998) and by 6 years for women (reaching 69 years in 1998) (World Health Organization 1999). Gains in life expectancy have been most pronounced at younger ages, but even at older ages increases have occurred due to falling death rates. Life expectancy gains have mainly benefited the better-off.

Life expectancy shows great variation between countries and even within countries. The country with the highest life expectancy at birth is Andorra, where a child born in 2006 can be expected to live 83.5 years. The lowest life expectancy is found in Swaziland, where the life expectancy at birth is only 32.6 years. Even among the most developed countries, there is substantial variation, with Australia at 80.5, Canada at 80.2, Great Britain at 78.5, and the United States at 77.8 years (Central Intelligence Agency 2006). Many of the countries with the lowest life expectancies have very high rates of HIV infection or AIDS. In sub-Saharan Africa, life expectancy in several countries has been reduced by 15–20 years following increases in the prevalence of HIV, and is now as low as 30 years (Mathers *et al.* 2001).

Other factors can also have a dramatic influence on life expectancy. Life expectancy for men in the former Soviet Union and Eastern European countries has declined following political reforms (Chenet *et al.* 1998; Leon *et al.* 1997). The reason for this trend is unclear, but sudden deaths due to binge alcohol drinking, increased risks of violent death, and suicide play a part (Chenet *et al.* 1996; Shkolnikov *et al.* 2001). The reunification of the former East Germany with West Germany shows a different picture; in the decade since the removal of the Berlin Wall in 1989, mortality rates in the East have fallen towards those in the West among women but not men (Haussler *et al.* 1995) These 'natural experiments' of the effects of social and economic engineering provide examples of how public health is influenced by political change. It also reinforces the importance of social and economic factors as major forces in determining life expectancy.

Differences in life expectancy between groups within countries have been long recognized. William Farr calculated average life expectancies in 1841 for Liverpool, Surrey, and London, which were 26, 45, and 37, respectively. By 1992, although the rank order by place of residence was much the same, life expectancy over the age of 65 years showed even greater variation than it did in 1841. Similarly, life expectancy shows a marked social-class gradient. As shown in Fig. 11.7.5, the difference in life expectancy for men in England and Wales at age 65 years between social class I (professional) and V (unskilled manual) has increased from 3.4 years in 1972–76 to 5 years in 1997–2001: Similar gradients exist for women. Analysis of health inequalities indicate that the cause of these gradients is more complex than simply poverty, but that relative deprivation is also important (Marmot 2001).

Table 11.7.1 Life expectancy at different ages in England and Wales, 1841–2005.

Year	Birth		65 years	
	Male	Female	Male	Female
1841	40.2	42.2	10.9	11.5
1901–10	48.5	52.4	10.8	12.0
1930–32	58.7	62.9	11.3	13.1
1960–62	68.1	74.0	12.0	15.3
1990–92	73.4	79.0	14.3	18.1
1993–95	74.1	79.3	14.6	18.2
1998–2000	75.3	80.1	15.5	18.8
2003–05	76.9	81.2	16.8	19.6

Source: Charlton J, Murphy M. *The health of adult Britain 1841-1994*. London: Her Majesty's Stationery Office; 1997.
Office of National Statistics [Online]. Available from: www.statistics.gov.uk

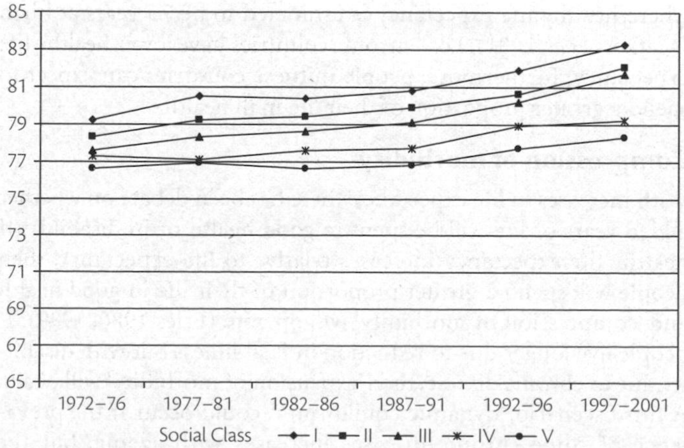

Fig. 11.7.5 Life expectancy for men at age 65, by social class, in England and Wales. *Source:* Office of National Statistics (Online). Available from: www.statistics.gov.uk/downloads~Life_Expect_Social_Class_1972-2001.pdf (accessed 9 February 2007).

Within the United States, African-American men have a life expectancy at birth of up to 20 years less than white men (Murray *et al.* 1998), and the difference in life expectancy is increasing. Levine *et al.* (2001) reported a 29-year lag in age-adjusted all-cause mortality, with the value for African-Americans in 1998 (6.9 per 100 000) equalling the value for white people in 1969. The age-adjusted all-cause mortality rate for African-Americans in 1965 showed a lag of 27 years compared with the rate for white persons (Levine *et al.* 2001). Interestingly, beyond the age of 80 years, African-Americans have better life expectancy than white populations—perhaps suggesting survival of the fittest (Manton 1980).

Similar differences in life expectancy exist between indigenous and non-indigenous populations in many countries, including New Zealand, Australia, Canada, and the United States. Within these developed, 'rich' countries, indigenous people regularly suffer from poorer levels of general health, and have an excess of early mortality and lower life expectancy when compared with the non-indigenous population. A study by Bramley *et al.* (2004) found that indigenous male life expectancy was highest in New Zealand (69 years) and indigenous female life expectancy was highest in Canada (76.6 years). The lowest life expectancy for indigenous people, males (56 years) and females (63 years), was in Australia. According to the Australian Bureau of Statistics (2000), 53 per cent of Aboriginal male deaths occur at ages less than 50 years.

Life expectancy is different from the maximum lifespan, which is the longest an individual member of a species or group has survived. Animals in the wild seldom achieve their maximum lifespan; in captivity, they are capable of reaching much older ages because major risks of predation, starvation, and accidents have largely been eliminated (Kirkwood 1999). Although the maximum lifespan that humans can achieve is widely debated, it is unlikely that we have reached it yet.

Other measures of ageing and health

Health-adjusted life expectancy provides an index of the equivalent years of full health that a person can expect to live at any given age, taking account of prevalent health states in the population and the value placed on ill health.

Figure 11.7.6 presents the inequalities in life expectancy (LE) and health-adjusted life expectancy (HALE) at birth across regions. The best HALE is seen in low-mortality countries such as Japan, where healthy life expectancy is estimated to be 75 years at birth (Mathers *et al.* 2001). Low-income countries have lower healthy life expectancy; furthermore, people in these countries can expect to spend a greater proportion of their life in ill health.

Compression of morbidity

With increases in life expectancy, there has been debate on whether added years of life will be spent in good health or in disability. If healthy life expectancy increases relative to life expectancy, then people will spend a greater proportion of their life in good health and 'compression of morbidity' will operate (Fries 1980, 1989). If people live longer due to reduction in fatal illness but with disability due to chronic disease, then 'expansion of morbidity' will occur. A third scenario, 'dynamic equilibrium', could occur if the prevalence of some chronic diseases increases with ageing, but the progression of some degenerative diseases reduces. In this scenario, people might suffer chronic illness for a longer period, but with less serious effects (Andrews 2001). This steady state could also be

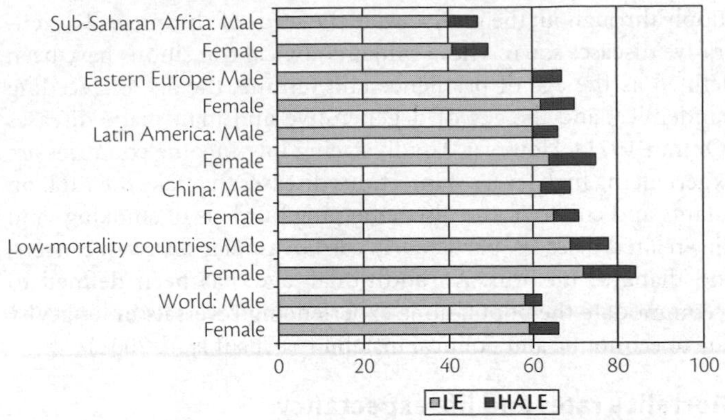

Fig. 11.7.6 Inequalities in years of life expectancy (LE) and healthy life expectancy (HALE) at birth, by gender and region, in 2002.
Source: Adapted from Mathers CD, Iburg KM, Salomon JA *et al.* Global patterns of healthy life expectancy in the year 2002. *BMC Public Health* 2004;**4**:66.

achieved if there are parallel declines in both disease incidence and total mortality (Manton 1982).

Fries (2005) argues that compression of morbidity may be prevailing in some populations. However, data to test this hypothesis are difficult to find and hard to interpret. Very few countries are capable of making reliable assessments over time, between geographic regions, or between socioeconomic groups. Investment in research infrastructure is required to ensure that regular health and disability surveys using comparable methodology are established. The US Health and Retirement Study has found that successive cohorts of people aged 51–56 years are in relatively poorer health, reporting more difficulty with daily tasks, more pain, more chronic conditions, more psychiatric problems, and higher use of alcohol (Soldo *et al.* 2006). Similar findings have also been reported for people in the United Kingdom (Banks *et al.* 2006).

Evidence of compression of morbidity is mostly seen among higher socioeconomic status people, particularly those with low levels of risk factors for chronic disease. In the United States, not only are disability rates higher among African-Americans than white people, but also the trends between 1990 and 1996 show that white people have enjoyed a reduction in disability whereas African-Americans people have suffered an increase (National Center for Health Statistics 1999). Among university alumni followed prospectively, those with high-risk health behaviours (i.e. smoking, high body mass index [BMI], and lack of physical exercise) suffered twice the cumulative incidence of disability, with the onset of disability postponed by an average of 5 years in those with low-risk health behaviours (Vita *et al.* 1998). If compression of morbidity is to occur at a population level, greater health-promotion and risk-reduction activities will be needed for disadvantaged groups who have high levels of health risks. Moreover, even if preventive activities were highly successful in reducing or postponing disability, increasing numbers of people living to very old ages mean that there will also be greater numbers of people with disabling conditions. At a population level, even if compression of morbidity dominates, there will be increasing needs for health and other care as the population ages.

Ageing in specific populations

Ageing in rural areas

The experience of ageing, need for care, and service availability vary greatly between people living in large cities and those living in rural and remote areas. Living in rural areas is also generally associated with economic hardship and poorer quality housing. Not only are incomes lower in rural areas, but prices of commodities such as fuel and food are higher as well.

The special circumstances of ageing in rural communities have not received much attention. However, the majority of the world's elderly live in rural and remote areas. Even in highly urbanized countries, a significant minority of the elderly live in rural and remote parts. Moreover, as younger people leave rural areas to work in cities, the proportion of older people in the rural population increases; so, rural and remote populations are ageing at a faster rate than urban populations. This effect is magnified when rural communities become popular places to live in retirement. Migration of young adults away from rural areas diminishes opportunities for family support, which is particularly important in rural areas, where societies tend to be more traditional and there is greater reliance on family structures.

The UN Madrid International Plan of Action on Aging considers the need to improve living conditions and infrastructure in rural areas, and to alleviate the marginalization of rural-dwelling older persons, particularly in low-income countries. Environmental factors, including lack of safe drinking water and poor sanitation, inadequate housing and absence of electricity, and poor roads and transport make life increasingly difficult for elderly people in rural areas. Further, in times of stress, such as during drought or other natural disasters (or war), rural elderly are likely to be particularly vulnerable (Mitka 2000).

Ethnic minority elders

Immigrations associated with trade, the colonial past, wars, and famine have produced complex multicultural societies in many countries. Different countries will have experienced immigration at different times and the contexts that will affect how ethnic minorities are viewed, their place in society, and their absolute and relative numbers will differ. Australia, for instance, has had a long history of immigration, from the early settlers and convicts, to the wave of immigrants from Europe following the Second World War, to more recent immigrants from Southeast Asia and other countries. The population is drawn from 200 countries, and 23 per cent of the population were born overseas (Australian Bureau of Statistics 2001). Ethnic minority populations that emigrated from other countries are now ageing rapidly and are often at a disadvantage due to poor health, poor economic circumstances and reliance on public services, as well as cultural and racial discrimination (Villa & Wallace 2007).

Data from United States indicate that immigrants such as Latinos and Asians, as well as African-American elders, are more likely to live in poverty and have lower median incomes than the general population. Further, many of these people are in poor health. African-Americans, for instance, have higher rates of disease and disability as compared to the rest of the population, and also appear to be more vulnerable to the impacts of disease (Villa & Wallace 2007).

Census information from the United Kingdom also shows older people from major ethnic minority groups, with the exception of the Chinese, to have more long-standing disability than the Anglo-Saxon majority. Explanations for excess morbidity may be found in poverty, poor housing and diet, and limited physical activity, all of which are likely to contribute to higher rates of CVD, diabetes, and other chronic health problems. The aetiology of ethnic minority health problems may be classified as 'home' country influences, influences of the new adopted country, selection of who migrates, and processes of adaptation and adjustment to migration (Marmot *et al.* 1984). However, once people from ethnic minorities reach old age, the selective 'healthy migrant' factors attenuate and they become prey to the common causes of chronic ill health in the wider population. Moreover, relocation and adaptation to a new country is a major lifetime stress that may have negative effects on health at later ages (Noh & Kaspar 2003). People who emigrate at older ages are particularly vulnerable; not only do they have poor health associated with ageing and disadvantage, but they also have more difficulty adjusting to a new culture and language than younger people, and they may also be less likely to use health care than others with similar needs.

Subtle barriers to referral, investigation, and treatment may also affect the care received by ethnic minority elders (Ebrahim 1996). People from ethnic minorities are less likely to receive social-support services, although given their need, they should be represented in greater proportion. In Australia, older people from non-English speaking backgrounds comprise around 25 per cent of the population aged 65 years and over, but only represent 16 per cent of the home-care clients and 7 per cent of the residential aged-care clients (Australian Institute of Health and Welfare 2002). Much more work is required to develop and evaluate appropriate services for ethnic minority elders.

Age and gender

Although the main conditions that affect people at older ages are similar among men and women (except for breast cancer and reproductive cancers), there are differences in the incidence of these conditions and the peak age of onset. For instance, men experience peak incidence of coronary artery disease earlier than women do. Lung cancer is more common among men who have had higher rates of smoking, although lung cancer is now the second most common cancer among women, reflecting their increasing smoking habits. There are also gender differences in terms of social roles and human rights, and these will have significant effects on the experience of ageing. Although there are few differences in self-rated health and long-standing illness, older women have higher rates of functional disability than men. Women also tend to live longer than men do, and so are more likely to experience disease and disability associated with advanced age.

Women's longevity also means that they are more likely to experience the death of their spouse and to spend a proportion of their older age widowed. Single older men, however, are more likely to be admitted to residential care than single older women, and married men are more likely to remain living in the community than married women (Arber & Cooper 1999).

Older women are especially vulnerable in the event of crises such as war, natural disaster, and famine, partly because they generally control fewer economic resources than older men do and because much of the care of children and other vulnerable people falls to older women.

Gender differentials in health and ageing have been poorly studied, but are important because of the gender imbalance in the population at older age due to women's longer life expectancy. In 2002 healthy life expectancy at the global level was 57.8 years for women, 2 years higher than that for men at 55.8 years. In Russia, healthy life expectancy was 66.4 years for women, 3 years below the European average, but just 56.1 years for men, 7 years below the European average (Mathers *et al.* 2004).

Health needs of older people

As people age, they have increased risk of disease and disability, and often, increasing health needs. Many conditions become more common at older ages, partly because of physiological changes associated with ageing, accumulated exposure to adverse health behaviours and risk factors across the life course, toxins and injury, and simple 'wear and tear'. Older people also tend to experience more than one health problem at any given time, and these problems are frequently under-reported and under-treated. In many cases, social circumstances add to the difficulties that people face as they age, making it harder for them to manage their health problems, and requiring a given broad and special consideration for the health needs of older people.

Physiological and functional changes

Physiological changes that occur with ageing affect all body systems. These normal changes limit bodily reserves, reduce the ability to maintain homeostasis, and increase the potential for illness. Obvious external signs of ageing appear on the skin, but along with these cosmetic changes skin also loses some of its function with age. The dermis becomes thinner and more fragile, and there are fewer and slower dividing keratinocytes—which means slower healing and less efficient production of vitamin D. Other changes in skin function include increased vulnerability to extremes of temperature and reduced sensitivity to touch. Muscle and bone mass decline with age, tendons become shorter, and cartilages become stiffer. Diseases such as osteoporosis and osteoarthritis exacerbate these losses and effects.

Changes to the cardiovascular system include stiffening of arteries (even among those with normal blood pressure), slowed electrical activity, postural hypotension, and reduced right ventricular function. The lungs become stiffer, alveoli enlarge, bronchioles collapse, and the chest muscles weaken, reducing respiratory capacity. Also, the cough reflex is reduced, leading to increased susceptibility to infection. The digestive system becomes less efficient at absorbing nutrients (especially vitamins), leaving older people vulnerable to nutritional deficiencies, particularly folate-deficiency anaemia. Changes in smooth muscle function can predispose to constipation. The liver reduces in size and becomes less efficient at synthesizing proteins and metabolizing toxins (increasing the risk of drug toxicity). Likewise, there is a decrease in kidney mass and renal function. Older people find it harder to maintain fluid and electrolyte balance, and are vulnerable to dehydration. Bladder capacity is reduced and bladder muscles may become weak and unstable (increasing the risk of incontinence), and in men, the prostate enlarges (increasing the risk of obstruction).

Physiological changes in body function are not due to disease (just as menopause is the loss of reproductive function but is not a disease). However, certain diseases and states can accelerate the onset of disability and shorten life. A number of longitudinal studies have been conducted in an attempt to disentangle the effects of ageing and disease on health and well-being (see United States National Institute of Ageing 2007). For example, the MacArthur Study of Successful Aging followed 1189 relatively healthy people aged between 70 and 79 years, for a period of seven years, to investigate factors that influence physical and cognitive functioning. They found that 'successful ageing' was associated with exercise, social engagement, and a positive mental attitude, including feelings of being useful to others (Seeman & Chen 2002; Gruenewald *et al.* 2007).

Common conditions affecting older people

Causes of death and disability

Some conditions are particularly strongly associated with age. These include conditions that are rapidly fatal (such as lung cancer) and which contribute greatly to years of life lost (YLL), and those that are chronic and associated with years of life lost to disability (YLD).

The most common recorded causes of death among people aged 60 years and over are diseases of the circulatory system, diseases of the respiratory system, and malignant neoplasms (see Box 11.7.1).

Worldwide, ischaemic heart disease and cerebrovascular disease are the leading causes of disability and death among people aged 60 years and over, measured by disability-adjusted life years (DALYs), (see Box 11.7.2).

Other major causes of DALYs include chronic obstructive lung disease, dementias, and cataract (and other vision disorders). Older people are also particularly susceptible to respiratory infections such as pneumonia. In regions where TB is endemic, older people are particularly vulnerable.

Musculoskeletal conditions (such as osteoarthritis and osteoporosis) are also common among older people, although they tend to contribute to disability more than death. In high-income countries, more than one in four women will have sustained at least one osteoporotic fracture by the age of 70. In 1990, a worldwide estimate of 1.7 million hip fractures occurred as a result of

Box 11.7.1 Mortality—adults aged 60 years and over

Rank	Cause	Deaths (1000)
1	Ischaemic heart disease	5825
2	Cerebrovascular disease	4689
3	Chronic obstructive pulmonary disease	2399
4	Lower respiratory infections	1396
5	Trachea, bronchus, lung cancers	928
6	Diabetes mellitus	754
7	Hypertensive heart disease	735
8	Stomach cancer	605
9	Tuberculosis	495
10	Colon and rectum cancers	477

Source: World Health Organization. *World health report 2003: shaping the future*. Geneva: World Health Organization; 2003.

Box 11.7.2 Disease burden—adults aged 60 years and over

Rank	Cause	DALYs (1000)
1	Ischaemic heart disease	31 481
2	Cerebrovascular disease	29 595
3	Chronic obstructive pulmonary disease	14 380
4	Alzheimer and other dementias	8569
5	Cataracts	7384
6	Lower respiratory infections	6597
7	Hearing loss, adult onset	6548
8	Trachea, bronchus, lung cancers	5952
9	Diabetes mellitus	5882
10	Vision disorders, age-related, and other	4766

Source: World Health Organization. *World health report 2003: shaping the future*. Geneva: World Health Organization; 2003.

osteoporosis; this number is expected to exceed 6 million by 2050 (World Health Organization 2001).

These common conditions are associated with a range of functional limitations such as cognitive impairment, mobility restrictions, and urinary incontinence. Urinary incontinence affects 10–30 per cent of older people, and women are affected twice as often as men (Chiarelli *et al.* 2005). Under-nutrition is another problem that commonly underlies and exacerbates many conditions affecting older people, even in countries where food supplies are generally reliable and plentiful.

Multiple pathology

Most older adults have a range of active health problems that interact with one another and complicate approaches to treatments. Figures vary from study to study, but at least 80 per cent of the people older than 65 years have one chronic condition or more, and 65 per cent have multiple chronic conditions (Wolff *et al.* 2002). For example, in one Australian study of men and women aged 70 years and over, the median number of conditions per person was 7 (Byles *et al.* 2005). This state (called multi-morbidity or co-morbidity) is important because it is associated with many important health outcomes such as quality of life, activities of daily living, health-service utilization, and mortality (Byles *et al.* 2005).

Population statistics often do not recognize the prevalence of co-morbidity among older people. For instance, deaths are enumerated according to the underlying cause and contributing causes are often not counted. However, although the recorded cause of death may be quite specific, the reality is that a number of co-morbid conditions could have caused or contributed to the person's death. In other cases, deaths among older people are attributed to 'senility' or to 'ill-known and undefined causes'. These cases represent the notion of multiple system failure, which accompanies old age, but again they do not provide information on those conditions that contribute most to morbidity and mortality.

Iatrogenic disease

Iatrogenic disease is common in older people, particularly in those taking multiple medications. Although medications can be beneficial in the management of multiple health problems of older people, they also have the potential to cause serious adverse effects. Older people have a reduced volume of distribution for drugs, and slower rates of drug metabolism and elimination, and so are vulnerable to overdose. Reduced physiological reserve renders older people more susceptible to drug toxicity. Also, multiple medications increase the risk of drug–drug interaction. Multiple medicines also increase medication complexity, which can increase risk of medication error and reduce adherence. In high-income countries, an estimated 60–90 per cent of community dwelling people aged 65 years and over take medications. Over 50 per cent use at least one drug on a regular basis, with the average number of medications used ranging from two to five (Byles *et al.* 2003). Adverse reactions are estimated to account for up to 22 per cent of hospital admissions, 35 per cent of unplanned readmissions, and almost half of nursing home admissions (Schmader *et al.* 1997). It is estimated that up to half of these adverse reactions could be prevented (Simonson & Feinberg 2005).

Functioning, disability, and health

The International Classification of Functioning, Disability and Health (known as the ICF) recognizes that functioning and disability occur in personal, environmental, and social contexts (World Health Organization 2007). This new classification scheme replaces the original International Classification of Impairment, Disability and Handicap.

The ICF has two parts: Part 1—Functioning and Disability (Body Functions and Structures, and Activities and Participation) and Part 2—Contextual Factors (Environmental Factors and Personal Factors). Any significant problem in body function or structure is classified as 'impairment'. Depending on the amount of impairment and on personal and environmental factors, impairments can result in activity limitations and restrictions on an individual's involvement in everyday life. A person can have impairment without having any limitation (e.g. disfigurement), but a person may also have activity limitations without obvious impairment (e.g. incontinence). The interaction with environmental and personal factors means that a person may have capacity limitations without assistance, but no performance restrictions when provided with a supportive social and physical environment.

People who work in aged care and in rehabilitation use the terms *activities of daily living* (ADL) and *instrumental activities of daily living* (IADL) to describe the functional limitations of many of the people they care for and to evaluate the effects of rehabilitation. ADLs are the basic functions of being able to walk, wash, dress, eat, groom, and go to the toilet. IADLs are higher-order activities that are needed to function independently in modern life, including using the telephone, going shopping, cooking meals and housekeeping, doing the laundry, using transport, using medications, and managing finances.

Frailty and geriatric syndromes

Although *frailty* is a term that is commonly used to describe older people, it is poorly defined and not well understood. Fried *et al.* (2001) have developed an operational definition of frailty that includes decreased resiliency and reserve, cycles of decline across multiple systems, negative energy balance, sarcopenia, and decreased strength and exercise tolerance. The symptoms and signs include exhaustion, weight loss, weak grip strength, slow walking pace, and low energy expenditure.

The common coexistence of disease in older people has led some to describe certain combinations of conditions as 'geriatric syndrome'. As with frailty, this term is not well defined and various usages are made. Common combinations associated with this term include falls, dementia, and incontinence.

Health-related quality of life

With longer lifespans, importance is placed not only on the quantity of life but also the quality of life. Quality of life is a subjective element that relates to the adequacy of people's circumstances and to their feelings about these circumstances. In terms of health, relevant aspects of the quality of life range from negatively valued aspects such as pain and disability to more positively valued aspects such as role function or happiness. Recently, there has been great attention given to quantification of quality of life as a measure of general health status, and for comparing outcomes of different treatments.

Health-related quality of life in older age is affected not only by disease but also by symptoms, which may not be associated with specific pathology, and by social circumstances. Common symptoms include joint stiffness, constipation, incontinence, and memory complaints. However, despite the presence of symptoms, medical conditions, and disability, older people often report their health as good or better and record high quality of life scores. This is a 'disability paradox' (Albrecht & Devlieger 1999), and was explored quantitatively in a national sample of British women, where it was found that one-fifth reported 'fairly' to 'very severe' levels of difficulty with daily living activities, but 62 per cent of these women rated their quality of life as 'good' or better. Multivariable analysis indicated that worse-perceived health, chronic diseases, and sociopsychological resources, including perceived control over life, distinguished between those who perceived their quality of life to be good in the face of functional difficulties (Bowling *et al.* 2007).

Trajectories of ageing and functional decline

The Established Populations for Epidemiologic Studies of the Elderly (EPESE) analysed four classical trajectories of functional decline by comparing activity of daily living scores for 4190 people who died in the first six years of follow-up (Lunney *et al.* 2003). Of the people studied, 15 per cent experienced sudden death, 21 per cent had a primary diagnosis of cancer and demonstrated a rapid decline to death, 20 per cent had congestive heart failure or chronic lung disease and exhibited a fluctuating level of function due to organ failure, and 20 per cent with none of these diseases had been in a nursing home in the year before death and had a prolonged steady decline in function, probably attributable to a dementia syndrome. The remaining 24 per cent were classified as 'other', and died outside of a nursing home. The different modes of death were associated with age (people dying of cancer were generally younger, people dying in nursing homes were generally older), gender (those dying of following a steady decline were more likely to be women), and race (those experiencing sudden death were more likely to be non-white). Importantly, only deaths from cancer had a predictable terminal period, which is important information for elderly people, their relatives, and those planning and funding palliative aged care.

Health and social care for older people

Health-care policy makers and planners are often challenged by concerns about the rising costs of health care in the face of an ageing population. The argument is that increasing numbers of older people will result in an explosion of costs and an unsustainable demand on services. People aged 65 years and over tend to have more admissions to hospital than younger people, and they have longer lengths of hospital stay. They also have more visits to doctors and use more medications. However, people aged 65 years and older contribute only modestly to time trends in per-capita costs of health care compared with the rest of the population. It has also been noted that the proportion of health-care expenditure that is allocated to older people is actually decreasing as the population ages. Rather, it is terminal illness that is expensive, not age as such, and the costs of health care increase with proximity to death (Normand 1998; Dixon *et al.* 2004). Also, very old people have lower health-care costs than young people with the same survival prospects (Himsworth & Goldacre 1999). The notion that we should restrict expensive acute- and tertiary-level services for older people overlooks the important benefits that even very old people can gain from both acute and technologically innovative health care.

Health promotion for old age

Three stages in promoting healthy old age have been described (see Fig 11.7.7). The first is increasing capacity for health in early life, which includes good maternal nutrition, and optimizing the development of vital organs such as brain, muscle, bone and blood vessels during childhood and early adulthood to build resources that may affect later capacity (such as increasing peak bone density to protect against osteoporosis). The second stage occurs in adult life and involves strategies to reduce damage (such as avoiding smoking), to protect against damage (a balanced fruit- and vegetable-focused diet), or to prevent loss through lack of use (such as physical activity). The third stage is in late life and involves minimizing the progression of disease and disability, protecting against increased environmental demands or stresses, and compensating for lost capacity. Examples of these approaches to health promotion include secondary prevention of stroke, rehabilitation, exercise and strength training, social support, correction of deficits in vision and hearing, and modifications to domestic and outdoor environments.

Several key health behaviours are associated with diseases that are common in older age. These associations would suggest that primary-prevention approaches are likely to be effective in reducing the incidence of disease at older ages. However, randomized

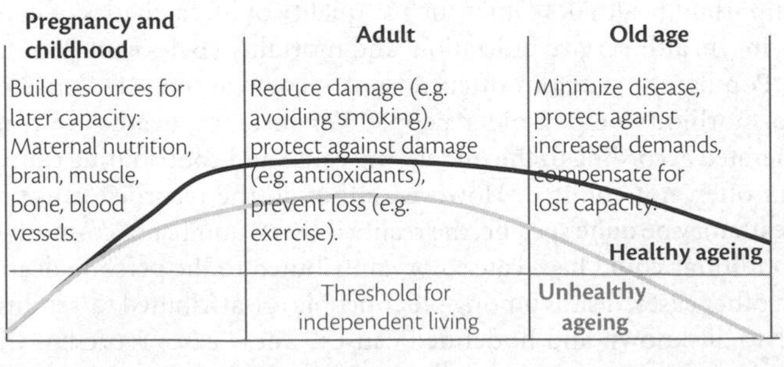

Fig. 11.7.7 Health promotion for old age.
Source: Adapted from Alexandre Kalache World Health Organization, personal communication 2008.

controlled trials have frequently failed to show that behavioural interventions addressing these risk factors are effective. For example, large-scale randomized controlled trials of dietary advice, smoking cessation advice, and exercise did not demonstrate a reduction in disease incidence (Ebrahim & Davey Smith 1997). This does not mean that reducing these risk factors is not important, rather that standard approaches to health promotion are not sufficiently effective. Strategies that take a more holistic approach, that involve the whole community (not just individuals), and that address environmental and cultural determinants of ill health are more important.

Social inequity is one of the major determinants of ill health at all ages (Marmot 2005). Poor circumstances have their first impact during pregnancy, when deficiencies in nutrition, maternal stress, smoking, and misuse of drugs and alcohol, insufficient exercise, and inadequate prenatal care can inhibit optimal foetal development. As seen in the life-course approach to health promotion, poor foetal development is a risk for health in later life. The impact of disadvantage continues throughout childhood and adult life, and is manifest in terms of psychosocial stress (which can have both physical and mental health impacts), poor education, poor nutrition, social exclusion, underemployment and poor job security, and work-related stress and injury. Smoking, alcohol, and drug use are higher among people in disadvantaged circumstances. Disadvantaged people also tend to live in poorer neighbourhoods with high rates of violence and crime, in overcrowded circumstances, and in areas with high levels of environmental hazards. Thus, although it is useful to highlight behaviours of individuals as risk factors for ill health at later ages, addressing these problems requires that the social circumstances that underpin these behaviours are also understood and improved where possible.

Smoking is a risk factor for CVD, stroke, respiratory disease, and many cancers, and smoking prevention is important in reducing the incidence of these conditions, even at older ages. The British Doctor's Study shows that over seven years of life expectancy are gained by avoiding smoking after the age of 35 years (Doll *et al.* 2004). Quitting smoking is also important in reducing up to 36 per cent of future coronary events. Systematic reviews of many trials show that brief advice and nicotine supplements do help people to stop smoking (Lancaster & Stead 2005a, 2005b).

Physical activity is strongly associated with lower rates of CVD, depression, and osteoporosis in many observational studies, and some small trials have demonstrated short-term health benefits among older participants. However, older people may find it difficult to maintain high levels of exercise, and the encouragement of exercise requires attention to physical environments as well as education of the individual. Neighbourhood factors such as the availability of transport, housing density, pedestrian-oriented urban design, and diversity of land use can increase physical activity (Handy *et al.* 2002; Saelens *et al.* 2003).

Observational studies suggest a clear association between nutrition and health at older ages. For example, the Baltimore Study of Ageing found that men who consumed at least five servings of fruits and vegetables per day and who obtained 12 per cent energy or less from saturated fat had 31 per cent lower all-cause mortality ($P < 0.05$), and were 76 per cent less likely to die from coronary heart disease (CHD; $P < 0.001$) than other men in the study (Tucker *et al.* 2005). However, dietary intervention studies and studies of vitamin supplementation have not demonstrated significant health benefits (Bengmark 2006; Davey Smith & Ebrahim 2005).

Obesity and overweight are increasing in prevalence and are associated with increased risk of stroke, coronary artery disease (CAD), diabetes, arthritis, and some cancers (World Health Organization 2000). There is currently little evidence from well-designed randomized controlled trials of the effectiveness of weight reduction on reducing longer-term morbidity.

A number of studies have demonstrated an association between social support and improved survival, reduced disability and health-care use, and improved quality of life (Berkman & Syme 1979; Bowling & Browne 1991; Steinbach 1992; Mendes de Leon *et al.* 1999). It is thought that these health effects are mediated through the influence of social support on health behaviour, improved access to care, and possibly through physiological pathways. A systematic review of 30 studies of social-support interventions for older people identified some evidence that educational- and social-activity group interventions that target specific groups can alleviate social isolation and loneliness among older people (Cattan *et al.* 2005). However the methods and generalizability of the reported studies varied, and more work is required to develop both theoretically sound social-support interventions and better methods for evaluating the outcomes of these approaches.

Prevention of specific conditions affecting older people

CVDs and diabetes

Many clinical trials provide evidence in support of the effectiveness of drug therapy in primary and secondary prevention of CVDs. It has been estimated that six preventative drugs in combination (three low-dose anti-hypertensives, a statin to lower cholesterol, aspirin, and folic acid) could prevent up to 88 per cent of CHDs and 80 per cent of strokes (Wald & Law 2003). This therapy has been proposed for all people over the age of 55 years regardless of CVD risk, but may be more beneficial among older people and people with pre-existing disease among whom the risk–benefit ratio is greater. However, there are many cost and safety issues to consider before universal multi-chemoprophylaxis becomes common practice. Furthermore, recent randomized trials of folate supplementation have not demonstrated the anticipated reductions in CVD risk, suggesting that this component of any combination treatment will not be useful.

Hormone replacement therapy (HRT) was thought to be cardioprotective (Stampfer & Colditz 1991), but large trials have demonstrated an increase in CHD among women on long-term HRT (Lawlor *et al.* 2004). However, a recent re-analysis of the Women's Health Initiative trials has shown that among women started on HRT shortly after the menopause, there was no evidence of an increased risk of CHD, a finding that has rekindled the HRT debate (Rossouw *et al.* 2007).

When treating diabetes in elderly patients, one must consider not only the importance of glucose control, but also other health risks and priorities as well as patient preferences. Life expectancy should also be considered. Control of other risk factors such as lipids and hypertension, as well as glucose control, is also important and may have considerable short-term advantages. For people with shorter life expectancy, long-term control of hyperglycaemia may be less important than for younger patients (Durso 2006). As with many conditions affecting older people, randomized controlled trial evidence is lacking. Observational evidence suggests that intensive control of diabetes mellitus can have favourable effects on microangiopathy (Katakura *et al.* 2007). Trials among people with impaired glucose tolerance have revealed that physical activity reduces the likelihood of developing diabetes (Toumilehto & Lindstrom 2003; Bethel & Califf 2007).

Mental health

Depression is the most common psychiatric disorder in the elderly, and is commonly under-diagnosed and under-treated. Once detected, however, it responds well to pharmacotherapy and/or psychotherapy (Wilson *et al.* 2001).

Dementia is a major cause of years of life lost to disability (Mathers *et al.* 2000). At this stage, there is no evidence that any treatment will prevent or slow the progression of dementia. However, many dementias appear to be partially attributable to CVD risk factors such as hypertension and control of these risk factors may reduce the incidence of dementia.

Falls and fractures

Numerous modifiable risk factors for falls and osteoporosis have been identified. However, reduction of fall-related injury at a population level requires that preventive activities become embedded within everyday social functions and physical structures (McClure *et al.* 2005). A number of interventions have been shown to reduce the risk of falls, including health and environment risk factor screening or intervention programmes, muscle strengthening and balance retraining, and home hazard assessment and modification (Gillespie *et al.* 2003). Multifactorial fall-prevention programmes have been shown to be effective in reducing falls among community-dwelling older people, OR 0.73 (0.63 to 0.86), and for older people with a history of falling, OR 0.79 (0.67 to 0.94) (Tinetti *et al.* 1994). Increased calcium and vitamin D as well as physical activity may also protect against osteoporosis (Boonen *et al.* 2006), although recent large-scale randomized trials of calcium and vitamin D supplementation in community-dwelling people did not demonstrate reductions in the risk of fracture (Porthouse *et al.* 2005; Jackson *et al.* 2006; The RECORD Trial Group 2005). A recent Cochrane review concluded that vitamin D has a significant effect in preventing fractures (including hip fracture) among people living in institutional care (Avenell *et al.* 2001). Evidence shows that bisphosphonates improve bone density and reduce osteoporotic fractures (Cranney *et al.* 2002). HRT may also reduce fractures; however, recent studies show increased risk of CVD and breast cancer, so HRT is not currently recommended for fracture prevention (Writing Group for the Women's Health Initiative Investigators 2002).

Osteoarthritis

Little attention has been paid to the prevention of osteoarthritis. Weight loss and prevention of obesity may have a role in prevention, and in the relief of symptoms and maintenance of activities of daily living for those with established disease (Bliddal & Christensen 2006). Established arthritis may also respond to exercise, orthotics, pharmacological therapies, and joint replacement.

Gains in healthy life expectancy due to the elimination of disease

The elimination of some diseases (such as CVD and cancer in men) would result in an increase in life expectancy, but with expansion of morbidity. Compression of morbidity is predicted with the elimination of musculoskeletal disorders and mental conditions; endocrine, nutritional, and metabolic disorders; respiratory and digestive disorders in men; and neoplasms in women (Mathers 1999). Population effects of preventing a condition such as arthritis would be considerable, as so many individuals are affected. Also, in addition to the direct effects of pain and stiffness, arthritis has indirect effects by limiting physical activity and thereby increasing risk of other conditions.

Preventive activities in primary care

Immunization

Vaccination of community-dwelling older people may be a cost-effective way to prevent hospitalization for influenza or pneumonia and to prevent deaths. However, much of the evidence on vaccination in the elderly comes from observational studies and may reflect other differences between vaccinated and non-vaccinated groups (Rivetti *et al.* 2006). In the United States, the Centers for Disease Control are aiming to achieve influenza vaccination coverage of 90 per cent for persons aged 65 years and over by 2010. Influenza vaccination levels have increased from 33 per cent in 1989 to 66 per cent in 1999 for people in this age group. However, vaccination rates are lower among certain groups (such as African-Americans and Hispanics) and among people in residential care, who are at greater risk and for whom there is also greater benefit (Centers for Disease Control 2006).

Medication review

Some studies have shown medication review to be beneficial for older people living in the community (e.g. Zermansky *et al.* 2002), but other studies did not find any effect of medication review on the use of medicines (e.g. Allard *et al.* 2001; Sellors *et al.* 2003). One large Australian randomized controlled trial demonstrated a positive effect on medication use and a reduced incidence of falls 12 months after the medication review (Pit *et al.* 2007).

Health assessments, case finding, and screening

Multiple problems: Reviews of the evidence on prevention-based assessment programmes for older people have come to varying conclusions: That the assessments have positive effects (Stuck *et al.* 2002), no effect (Cole 1998), or small mixed effects (Van Haastregt *et al.* 2000; Byles 2000; Elkan *et al.* 2001). These reviews also found differences between studies in content and duration of assessments and the length of follow-up. The effectiveness of assessments may depend on multiple follow-ups, and benefits may be most pronounced for the 'young old' (under 78 years) and for those with a low risk of death (Stuck *et al.* 2002). Further randomized controlled trials of health assessments have been published in the last four years (Byles *et al.* 2004; Fletcher *et al.* 2004), which demonstrated only limited health benefits associated with health assessments.

Cancer screening: Many cancer screening programmes for younger people are not promoted for older people; for instance, breast cancer screening is encouraged for women aged 40–70 years (United States Preventive Services Task Force 2006). Evidence for ceasing screening after age 70 is not clear because few mammography screening controlled trials enrolled women older than 69 years and no trials enrolled women older than 74 years. The incidence of breast cancer increases with age, but the benefits of screening may be outweighed by competing morbidities among older women. Screening for cervical cancer is not recommended for women over the age of 70 years if they have had three normal

Pap smears in the past ten years (United States Preventive Services Task Force 2006): The incidence of cervical cancer decreases at older ages, and so screening older women has low yield. Also, in Western countries, many women have had a hysterectomy and do not require cervical screening. Screening for colorectal cancer is recommended for adults over the age of 50 years and up to the age of 80 years depending on the person's health and co-morbidities (United States Preventive Services Task Force 2006). As for breast cancer, few trials enrolled older patients. Although there is limited evidence of the benefit of screening for oral cancer, assessment of the mouth, teeth, and gums is helpful for older people with cognitive impairment and who may have conditions that limit chewing, swallowing, and communication (Research Dissemination Core 2002). Box 11.7.3 lists some recommended screening procedures for older adults.

Cardiovascular diseases: Treatment of high blood pressure as a means for preventing stroke among relatively fit people up to the age of 80 years is supported by strong evidence from randomized controlled trials (Insua *et al.* 1994; Mulrow *et al.* 1994). Treatment of people over the age of 80 years has been examined in a subgroup analysis of seven randomized controlled trials of drug treatments. Reductions in non-fatal cardiovascular events were found with no overall reduction in total mortality (Gueyffier *et al.* 1999). However, increased efforts to screen for high blood pressure, either by case finding or screening, have not shown improvements in population coverage, adherence to treatment, or blood pressure control (Ebrahim 1998). Screening for lipid disorders is not considered to be important for older people because lipid levels are less likely to increase after age 65 years (United States Preventive Services Task Force 2006).

Osteoporosis: Although there is no direct evidence that screening for osteoporosis prevents fractures, the prevalence of osteoporosis and fractures increase with age, and the short-term risk of fracture can be estimated by bone measurement tests and risk-factor assessment. Treatment may reduce fracture risk among women with low bone density (Nelson *et al.* 2002).

Vision and hearing: Annual screening for vision and hearing problems is recommended for adults after the age of 65 years (Mouton & Espino 1999). However, screening for visual problems has not been associated with improvements in visual impairment (Smeeth & Iliffe 2003).

Mental health: Screening for depression may improve the recognition and treatment of this condition as well as quality of life or mood. A meta-analysis of screening for depression among adults showed screening to be associated with a 13 per cent reduction in relative risk and a nine-percentage-point absolute reduction in the proportion of patients with persistent depression (Pignone *et al.* 2002). Available evidence is insufficient to recommend for or against routine screening for dementia in older adults (United States Preventive Services Task Force 2006).

Box 11.7.3 Screening procedures for older adults

	US Preventive Services Task Force	UK National Screening Committee
Breast cancer (women)	◆ Up to age 70 years	◆ Age 50–70 years
Cervical cancer (women)	◆ Up to age 70 years	◆ Age 25–64 years
Colorectal cancer	◆ Up to age 80 years (depending on co-morbidities)	◆ Age 50–75 years
Blood pressure	◆ No age limit	◆ All adults
Lipids	◆ Up to age 65	◆ Relatives of people with familial hypercholesterolaemia
Diabetes	◆ Screening recommended for adults with hypertension or hyperlipidaemia	◆ General population screening not recommended
Osteoporosis	◆ Women aged 65 years and older, women 60 years and older with increased risk for osteoporotic fractures	◆ Screening not recommended
Dementia	◆ Insufficient evidence to recommend for or against	
Depression	◆ Recommended if appropriate systems for follow-up	◆ Screening not recommended
Smoking	◆ Screening and advice to quit recommended for all adults	
Glaucoma	◆ Insufficient evidence	◆ Screening not recommended
Elder abuse	◆ Insufficient evidence	

Sources: United States Preventive Services task Force. *The guide to clinical preventive services, 2006.* Rockville (MD): Agency for Healthcare Research and Quality; 2006. UK National Screening Committee. Policy positions. 2006 Jul. Available from: http://www.nsc.nhs.uk/pdfs/policy position chart july06%5B1%5D.pdf. Last accessed 2007, Feb 09.

Elder abuse: There is little evidence to make recommendations about screening for elder abuse (United States Preventive Services Task Force 2006). Elder abuse, however, is common and health workers should remain alert. Factors associated with the abuse of older adults include increasing age, low-income status, functional impairment, cognitive disability, substance use, poor emotional state, low self-esteem, cohabitation, and lack of social support.

In summary, efforts to improve disability and to prevent disease through health assessments and systematic case finding are not well supported by currently available evidence. It is likely that the failure to achieve benefits is due to inadequately specified actions to be taken in the light of problems detected by case finding. Further work in this area needs to ensure that interventions are better planned and should evaluate how well the processes of care operate, in addition to examining outcomes. Also, the trials of preventive approaches are subject to many methodological problems; of these problems, small sample sizes and loss to follow-up are the most common. Reliance on trials performed in diverse health-care systems is unwise owing to the very different barriers to care, expectations of people, and differences in need. More data are required to guide policy on the application of trial evidence for the prevention of morbidity and disability among elderly people.

Systems of care

There are many strategies that enable people to successfully manage existing specific conditions and live a normal life. Quality care for chronic diseases to prevent complications and to compensate for functional impairment is essential in order to optimize health and quality of life for older people.

Primary care

Primary care is considered to be of great importance in reducing health-care inequalities and in improving the quality and outcomes of health care among older people. However, training in health care for older people is not a high priority in undergraduate curricula in many medical and health schools. It is essential that the needs of the growing numbers of older people are reflected in health-care education. The first step is to examine the common health problems among older people seen in primary care and to match training to meeting these needs. Without appropriate training, it is likely that older people will simply receive an increasing number of pills for each of their symptoms, running the risk of iatrogenesis, and potentially diagnosable and treatable problems will be missed.

Hospital services

People are more likely to use hospital services as they age and occupy hospital beds for longer (McCallum *et al.* 2003). It is, therefore, expected that older people will consume an increasing proportion of the available hospital resources in the future. Older people presenting to hospital tend to be sicker, with more urgent conditions, and have more co-morbid diseases and medications than young people (Bridges *et al.* 2005). Cardiopulmonary disorders are among the most common medical reasons for presentation, and fall-related injury is the most common surgical emergency among older people presenting to emergency departments. Adverse drug-related events (unfavourable medical events related to medication use or misuse) account for around 10 per cent of emergency department visits, the most frequently implicated medications being non-steroidal anti-inflammatory drugs (NSAIDs), antibiotics, anticoagulants, diuretics, hypoglycaemics, β-blockers, calcium-channel blockers, and chemotherapeutic agents.

Older patients tend to have complex health problems, with longer length of stay; the discipline of geriatric medicine has evolved to meet these needs, and specialist geriatric units now exist within major hospitals. A systematic review shows positive effects of hospital geriatric evaluation and management units on mortality, place of discharge, and change in functional status (Stuck *et al.* 1993). Although these results support current working methods, there is a possibility that these results are affected by publication bias. Also, better characterization of the process of care in trials of complex interventions is essential for the interpretation and implementation of findings.

Disease-specific services

Specialist services for patients suffering strokes have been evaluated in several small randomized controlled trials and appear to reduce mortality, disability, and institutionalization by about 20 per cent at 12 months. A meta-analysis of these studies concluded that the outcome appeared to be better in stroke units based in a discrete ward (Stroke Unit Trialists' Collaboration 2001). Similar models have also been applied for the management of diabetes, respiratory disease, and CVD (Gentles & Potter 2001). Specialist services for fractured neck-of-femur patients (orthogeriatric services) have also been examined in systematic reviews of small randomized controlled trials; pooled effects show a non-significant trend towards improved survival and less dependence. However, the trials are very heterogeneous in terms of the interventions used and do not provide secure evidence for or against such services (Cameron *et al.* 2001).

Health services for elderly people suffering from functional mental illnesses (largely, depressive illness) and organic brain syndromes (largely, dementia) have followed the general trend of moving out of psychiatric hospitals and into the community. The specialty of geriatric psychiatry has developed to meet the needs of an ageing population with an increased burden of dementia (Arie & Jolley 1998). As with hospital services for physically ill people, convincing evidence to support particular styles of psychogeriatric practice in terms of costs and outcomes is not available.

Hospital-at-home and day services, rehabilitation, and transitional care

Various 'hospital-at-home' and early-discharge schemes have been promoted in efforts to reduce demand on acute hospital services. A review of 22 trials evaluating early-discharge and hospital-at-home schemes found little evidence of benefits or costs savings. However, early-discharge schemes for older patients may reduce the pressure on acute hospital beds (Shepperd & Iliffe 2001).

There is an increasing demand for rehabilitation for older people. Traditionally, this process has occurred in hospital or other institutional settings, but more recently community-based rehabilitation options have been explored. In countries lacking investment in hospital services for elderly people, community-based rehabilitation offers an alternative model, but requires evaluation. Many studies have been undertaken to evaluate this approach to rehabilitation, but these studies have not been considered adequate to provide evidence of its effectiveness (Ward *et al.* 2003).

Specific issues that need further study are the role of families in the process of rehabilitation, local low-cost production of disability aids and appliances, and education and training in rehabilitation for primary-care teams.

Long-term care

A common approach to population ageing has been to establish institutional care, despite its costs and very limited accessibility for a majority of elderly people. In Egypt, for example, the number of aged-care institutions has more than doubled over the past 20 years (Boggatz & Dassen 2005).

At any one time, the majority of older people will not live in institutions, but many will require some form of long-term care during the course of their life. In high-income countries, there is a trend towards care being increasingly provided in community settings. Care in the community is now the preferred and most common care arrangement, and there has been a reduction in the numbers of people in institutional care, despite the ageing of the population.

Future need for long-term care will be determined by demographic trends, the strong relationship between age and disability, the extent to which community care permits people to stay at home, and the willingness of relatives to provide continued unpaid help. Most of these factors will tend to result in more rather than less need for long-term institutional care. In many countries, current levels of provision will be inadequate to meet future needs. Ignoring the problem is likely to have predictable consequences for waiting lists and admission of acutely ill elderly people as beds become 'blocked' with people waiting for some alternative to an acute hospital bed.

Informal care and social support, community and social care

In the United Kingdom, almost three million people provide care for someone over the age of 75 years, and informal care is recognized as an essential component of aged care and support (Department of Health 1999). Many people providing care for older people are themselves old.

The move to community care relies on the availability of informal carers, and there is increasing concern about who will care for older people in need. Not only will there be more people in need of care, but also the demands of modern society reduce people's ability to provide adequate care for their friends and families. For example, the increased emphasis on community care has come at the same time as a massive increase in the numbers of women who work in paid jobs.

Although both caregivers and care recipients generally regard home-based care as preferable to institutionalization, there is a lot of evidence that care giving can be physically and emotionally taxing (e.g. Schulz & Martire 2004; Lee 2001). Lee and Porteous (2002) found that mid-age women who have never had a role in providing care were more likely to be in full-time employment, and had better physical and mental health as well as lower levels of stress than carers. They were more likely to be within a healthy weight range, were less likely to use medications for sleeping difficulty or depression, and had higher life satisfaction scores and lower depression scores. When women gave up their caring roles, they reported fewer general-practice visits and less use of medications for nerves than current caregivers. In many cases, people who took on caring were already in poor health themselves. The demands of being in or taking on caring roles are frequently overlooked by health professionals, who may actually trade on the emotional ties between daughters and parents to achieve community care for very dependent patients.

The tradition of family support for older people is changing in many countries as a result of economic and political conditions, and where diseases such as AIDS have affected mid-aged adults leaving older people and children without support. In China, where filial piety is a traditional value, family responsibility for older people is made explicit in policy and is incorporated into the marriage contract (Zavoretti 2006). Even so, economic development, urbanization, and demographic transition are having an impact on intergenerational support.

Costs of care

There is much concern about costs associated with an ageing population. However, many analysts predict that the cost implications will be small in relation to the overall economies of most high-income countries. Across countries belonging to the Organization for Economic Cooperation and Development (OECD), population ageing is not associated with health expenditure as a proportion of gross domestic product (GDP). For example, 17.3 per cent of the Swedish population were aged 65 years or older in 2001, and 8.6 per cent of the Swedish GDP was spent on health. In contrast, around 12.7 per cent of the Australian population were aged 65 years and over, but 9.3 per cent of the GDP was spent on health (Coory 2004). Other analyses suggest that the greatest proportion of lifetime health-care costs are incurred in the last two years of life, and are more closely associated with the proximity to death than with chronological age (Dixon *et al.* 2004).

The major increases in costs associated with ageing occur in association with community and residential aged care. Nursing home costs in the United States have grown at a far faster rate since the 1960s than other sectors of health-care spending (National Center for Health Statistics 1999). British long-term care costs also dominate the overall projections over a period of decades, far outstripping primary-care and hospital-sector costs (Laing *et al.* 1991). Hotel 'board and lodging' costs make up a high proportion of long-term care costs and individual payment for these costs is generally acceptable (Royal Commission on Long-Term Care 1999; Fitzgerald 2000).

A number of studies have compared the relative costs of residential and community care. A study in British Columbia found that, although people receiving community care spent more days in hospital than people in residential care, the overall costs of community care were half to three-quarters the cost of residential care. However, much of this cost difference is contributed by families (Chappell *et al.* 2004). Variation in costs of care depend on levels of dependency, the number of residents and number of short-stay admissions, qualified nursing staff and supervisory staff, and building standards (Fitzgerald 2000). However, although the relationship between severity of dependency and cost of care is relatively flat for institutional care, costs for care at home increase exponentially with increasing dependency (Evans 1993). Anyone can be looked after at home if sufficient resources are available.

The issue of who pays for long-term care is important, as 'protection' of health- and social-services budgets coming from different sources may not result in the optimal use of resources or good standards of care. A move towards private funding also raises concerns regarding equity of access to care, especially for people with the greatest need. Older people who would benefit from specific interventions (e.g. coronary revascularization) are less likely to receive them (Bowling 1991). Ironically, acute hospital beds are used by older patients waiting for transfer to a social-care sector, either their own homes or institutional accommodation.

Increasing the barriers to gaining entry into secondary care for older people is an obvious but misplaced response because it exacerbates inequity for some. Ensuring that both health- and social-care costs are considered in economic appraisals, rather than just the costs of one or other system, should guarantee that the balance of care is of net benefit to society and not simply to one payer. The role of family and community in reducing costs of care need to be recognized as being of fundamental importance.

Unfortunately, much of urban planning has ignored the needs of older people, is designed inappropriately (e.g. high-rise public housing), and is suited to small nuclear families rather than larger extended families. Also, although promoting care at home is a desirable policy, the practice may be unaffordable for poor families.

Rationing of care

Rationing of care for older people may result from paternalistic ageism or from (often incorrect) assumptions and value judgments that older people are less likely to benefit from treatments than younger people. In many circumstances, the old, who have the greatest need for care and the greatest potential to benefit, are least likely to receive care. Moreover, there is often a dearth of evidence on which to base decisions about what care is most appropriate and effective for older people.

How much should be spent on care for older people can only be determined by reference to ethical principles. If no value is placed on life once economic productivity ceases, then an argument to not waste resources on health services for elderly people will prevail. But if quality of life in older age is seen to have its own value, then there is an argument for providing care. The amount that one generation should spend on supporting earlier generations remains to be decided. The 'fair innings' argument—after so many years, old people should not expect any more—is used by health economists to argue for transfers from old to young rather than vice versa (Williams & Evans 1997). An obvious flaw in such arguments is the notion that we only get sick and in need of health and social care when we get old ; the 'fair innings' does not relate to health status or to the ability to benefit from health care, only to years lived.

An alternative economic argument can also be made, that older people have contributed to society for their whole lives and are denied the support of society at the point in their lives when they need it most. Of importance in this debate is a consideration that most health care for older people is not about prolonging life but about ensuring that their old age is as comfortable and humane as possible. For the most part, it is not health care at older age that contributes to longevity, but rather survival from health risks at younger ages. Furthermore, provision of timely and appropriate health care for older people may potentially offset other costs.

The ethics of state provision of a health service is based on utilitarianism—the greatest good for the greatest number. Health-care policy generally aims at targeting resources to where they will do the most good, rather than issue them in response to the distribution of disease. This approach appears appropriate at one level, but may have unintended consequences if the ability to gain health benefits are not distributed equitably across the population in need (Aldrich *et al.* 2003). Targeting also requires relevant information on service inputs and health outcomes. In the face of inadequate information on costs and benefits, it seems inevitable that doing the best for the patient regardless of cost should gain hold over utilitarianism. With stronger evidence on the effects of pharmacological interventions, it is also inevitable that conflicts between groups holding different ethical precepts (and with different financial incentives) will emerge. Older people will stand to lose on two counts: First, evidence is weakest and hardest to obtain for complex non-pharmacological interventions from which they may benefit, and second, the inherent ageism of society will ensure that elderly people will lose in an individual or collectivist fight for resources. Without better and wider evidence on the benefits of innovative patterns of care for elderly people, more resources will not necessarily mean better care.

Public health implications of population ageing

As seen in this chapter, population ageing is a global phenomenon that will have a major impact on disease and disability patterns, and on health-service use. A coordinated and appropriate public health response is essential if this phenomenon is to translate into an opportunity for longevity and healthy ageing, rather than a threat to global health and resources. Public health is important in monitoring trends and transitions in risk factors, disease, and disability, in encouraging effective health-promotion practices, and in setting policy for equitable and efficient use of health-care resources for this growing population. Health promotion for older age begins in early life and continues throughout life to the oldest age. Much more knowledge is needed as to how we can optimize the conditions and experiences of ageing. The recognition of contributions made by older people themselves to their families and communities as well as to national wealth is also of fundamental importance in meeting the challenges of an ageing population and in meeting the health needs of increasing numbers of older people.

Key points

- Ageing is occurring at far greater rates in low- and middle-income countries than it does in high-income countries, which will place considerable strain on the health- and social-care sectors.
- Increased longevity has not been experienced uniformly across socioeconomic groups or in different countries.
- Severe disability is becoming less common in successive cohorts of elderly people, indicating that a compression of morbidity and disability is occurring.
- Health services for older people have had dramatic effects in improving survival and reducing disability associated with the inevitable increases in chronic diseases at older ages.
- In all countries, families provide a major part of the care needed by older people, but require the knowledge and support of formal health and social services.
- Public health has major roles in surveillance, prevention, and development of services for older people.

References

Albrecht G.L., Devlieger P.J. The disability paradox: high quality of life against all odds. *Social Science and Medicine* 1999;**48**:977–88.

Aldrich R., Kemp L., Williams J.S. *et al.* Using socio-economic evidence in clinical practice guidelines. *British Medical Journal* 2003;**327**(7426):1283–5.

Allard J., Hebert R., Rioux M. *et al.* Efficacy of a clinical medication review on the number of potentially inappropriate prescriptions prescribed for community-dwelling elderly people. *Canadian Medical Association Journal* 2001;**164**(9):1291–6.

Andrews G.R. Care of older people: promoting health and function in an ageing population. *British Medical Journal* 2001;**322**:728–9.

Arber S., Cooper H. Gender differences in health in later life: the new paradox. *Social Science and Medicine* 1999;**48**:61–76.

Arie T., Jolley D. Psychogeriatric services. In: Tallis R.C., Fillit H.M., Brocklehurst J.C., editors. *Brocklehurst's textbook of geriatric medicine and gerontology*. 5th ed. Edinburgh: Churchill Livingstone; 1998.

Australian Bureau of Statistics. Australia demographic statistics. Canberra: Australian Bureau of Statistics; 2001. Cat. No. 3101.

Australian Bureau of Statistics. Mortality of Aboriginal and Torres Strait islanders. Canberra: Australian Bureau of Statistics; 2000. Occasional paper 3315.0.

Australian Institute of Health and Welfare. Australia's health 2002. Canberra: Australian Institute of Health and Welfare; 2002.

Avenell A., Gillespie W.J., Gillespie L.D. *et al.* Vitamin D and vitamin D analogues for preventing fractures associated with involutional and post-menopausal osteoporosis. [Online]. Cochrane Database Systematic Reviews 2001;1:CD000227.

Banks J., Marmot M., Oldfield Z. *et al.* Disease and disadvantage in the United States and in England. *Journal of the American Medical Association* 2006;**295**(17):2037–45.

Bengmark S. Impact of nutrition on ageing and disease. *Current Opinion in Clinical Nutrition and Metabolic Care* 2006;**9**(1):2–7.

Berkman L.F., Syme S.L. Social networks, host resistance and mortality: A nine year follow-up study of Alameda County residents. *American Journal of Epidemiology* 1979;**109**:186–204.

Bethel M.A., Califf R.M. Role of lifestyle and oral anti-diabetic agents to prevent type 2 diabetes mellitus and cardiovascular disease. *American Journal of Cardiology* 2007;**99**:726–31.

Bliddal H., Christensen R. The management of osteoarthritis in the obese patient: practical considerations and guidelines for therapy. *Obesity Reviews* 2006;**7**(4):323–31.

Boggatz T., Dassen T. Ageing, care dependency, and care for older people in Egypt: a review of the literature. *International Journal of Older People Nursing* 2005;**14**:56–63.

Boonen S., Vanderschueren D., Haentjens P. *et al.* Calcium and vitamin D in the prevention and treatment of osteoporosis—a clinical update. *Journal of Internal Medicine* 2006;**259**(6):539–52.

Bowling A., Browne P.D. Social networks, health, and emotional well-being among the oldest old in London. *Journal of Gerontology* 1991;**46**(1): S20–32.

Bowling A., Seetai S., Morris R. *et al.* Quality of life among older people with poor functioning. *The influence of perceived control over life. Age and Ageing Advance Access* 2007;**36**(3):310–5.

Bowling A. Ageism in cardiology. *British Medical Journal* 1991;**319**: 1353–5.

Bramley D., Hebert P., Jackson R. *et al.* Indigenous disparities in disease-specific mortality, a cross-country comparison: New Zealand, Australia, Canada, and the United States. *New Zealand Medical Journal* 2004;**117**:1207.

Bridges J., Meyer J., Dethic L. *et al.* Older people in accident and emergency: implications for UK policy and practice. *Reviews in Clinical Gerontology* 2005;**14**:15–24.

Byles J., Heinze R., Nair K. *et al.* Medication use among older Australian veterans and war widows. *Internal Medicine Journal* 2003;**33**:388–91.

Byles J.E., D'Este K., O'Connel R. *et al.* Single index of multi-morbidity did not predict multiple outcomes. *Journal of Clinical Epidemiology* 2005;**58**(10):997–1005.

Byles J.E., Tavener M., Nair K. *et al.* A randomized controlled trial of health assessments for older Australian veterans and war widows. *Medical Journal of Australia* 2004;**181**:186–90.

Byles J.E. A thorough going over: evidence for health assessments for older persons. *Australian and New Zealand Journal of Public Health* 2000;**24**:117–23.

Cameron I.D., Handoll H.H.G., Finnegan T.P. *et al.* Co-ordinated multidisciplinary approaches for inpatient rehabilitation of older patients with proximal femoral fractures. [Online]. Cochrane Database of Systematic Reviews 2001;(3):CD000106.

Cattan M., White M., Bond J. *et al.* Preventing social isolation and loneliness among older people: a systematic review of health promotion interventions. *Ageing and Society* 2005;**25**:41–67.

Centers for Disease Control. Prevention and control of influenza: recommendations of the Advisory Committee on Immunization Practices. *Morbidity and Mortality Weekly Report* 2006;**55**:1–42.

Central Intelligence Agency [Online]. 2006. Available from: www.cia.gov [accessed 2007 Feb 9].

Chappell N.L., Haven B., Hollander M.J. *et al.* Comparative costs of home care and residential care. *Gerontologist* 2004;**44**:389–400.

Charlton J., Murphy M. The health of adult Britain 1841–1994. London: Her Majesty's Stationery Office; 1997.

Chenet L., Mckee M., Fulop N. *et al.* Changing life expectancy in central Europe: is there a single reason? Journal of Public Health Medicine 1996;18:329–36.

Chenet L., McKee M., Leon D. *et al.* Alcohol and cardiovascular mortality in Moscow; new evidence of a causal association. *Journal of Epidemiology and Community Health* 1998;**52**:772–4.

Chiarelli P., Bower W., Wilson A. *et al.* Estimating the prevalence of urinary and faecal incontinence in Australia: systematic review. *Australasian Journal on Ageing* 2005;**24**(1):19–27.

Cole M.G. Impact of geriatric home screening services on mental state: a systematic review. *International Psychogeriatrics* 1998; **10**:97–102.

Coory M.D. Ageing and healthcare costs in Australia: a case of policy-based evidence? Medical Journal of Australia 2004;**180**:581–3.

Cranney A., Guyatt G., Griffith L. *et al.* the Osteoporosis Methodology Group, the Osteoporosis Research Advisory Group. Meta-analyses of therapies for postmenopausal osteoporosis. *IX: Summary of meta-analyses of therapies for postmenopausal osteoporosis. Endocrine Reviews* 2002;**23**(4):570–8.

Davey Smith G., Ebrahim S. Folate supplementation and cardiovascular disease. *Lancet* 2005;**366**:1679–81.

Department of Health. Caring about carers: a national strategy for carers. London: Her Majesty's Stationery Office; 1999.

Dixon T., Shaw M., Frankel S. *et al.* Hospital admissions, age and death—'the cost of ageing' or 'the cost of dying'? A retrospective cohort study. *British Medical Journal* 2004;**328**:1288.

Doll R., Peto R., Boreham J. *et al.* Mortality in relation to smoking: 50 years observations on male British doctors. *British Medical Journal* 2004;**328**:1519.

Drever F., Whitehead M. Health inequalities. London: Office for National Statistics, Her Majesty's Stationery Office; 1997. DS No. 15.

Durso S. Using clinical guidelines designed for older adults with diabetes mellitus and complex health status. *Journal of the American Medical Association* 2006;**295**:1935–40.

Ebrahim S., Davey Smith G. Systematic review of randomized controlled trials of multiple risk factor interventions for preventing coronary heart disease and stroke. *British Medical Journal* 1997;**319**:1358–60.

Ebrahim S. Detection, adherence and control of hypertension for the prevention of stroke: a systematic review. *Health Technology Assessment* 1998;**2**:1–78.

Ebrahim S. Ethnic elders. *British Medical Journal* 1996;**313**:610–3.

Elkan R., Kendrick D., Dewey M. *et al.* Effectiveness of home based support for older people: systematic review and meta-analysis. *British Medical Journal* 2001;**323**:719.

Evans J.G. Institutional care and elderly people. *British Medical Journal* 1993;**306**:806–7.

Fitzgerald V. Financial implications of caring for the aged. Melbourne: Myer Foundation; 2000.

Fletcher A., Price G., Ng E. *et al.* Population-based multidimensional assessment of older people in UK general practice: a cluster-randomized factorial trial. *Lancet* 2004;**364**(9446):1667–77.

Fried L.P., Tangen C.M., Walston J. *et al.* Frailty in older adults: evidence for a phenotype. *The Journal of Gerontology Series A: Biological Sciences and Medical Sciences* 2001;**56**:146–57.

Fries J.F. Aging, natural death, and the compression morbidity. *New England Journal of Medicine* 1980;**303**:130–5.

Fries J.F. Frailty, heart disease, and stroke: the compression of morbidity paradigm. American Journal of Preventive Medicine 2005;**29** (5 Suppl 1):164–8.

Fries J.F. The compression of morbidity: near or far? The Milbank Quarterly 1989;67:208–32.

Gentles H., Potter J. Alternatives to acute hospital care. *Reviews in Clinical Gerontology* 2001;**11**(4):373–8.

Gillespie L.D., Gillespie W.J., Robertson M.C. *et al.* Interventions for preventing falls in elderly people. [Online]. Cochrane Database Systematic Review 2003;(4):CD000340.

Gruenewald T.L., Karlamangla A.S., Greendale G.A. *et al.* Feelings of usefulness to others, disability, and mortality in older adults: the MacArthur Study of Successful Aging. *Journals of Gerontology Series B: Psychological Sciences and Social Sciences* 2007;**62**:28–37.

Gueyffier F., Bulpitt C.J., Boissel J.P. *et al.* the INDIANA Group. Antihypertensive drugs in very old people: a sub-group meta-analysis of randomized controlled trials. *Lancet* 1999;**353**:793–6.

Handy S.L., Boarnet M.G., Ewing R. *et al.* How the built environment affects physical activity: views from urban planning. *American Journal of Preventive Medicine* 2002;**23**:64–73.

Haussler B., Hempel E., Reschke P. Changes in life expectancy and mortality in East Germany after reunification (1989–1992). *Gesundheitswesen* 1995;**57**:365–72.

Himsworth R.L., Goldacre M.J. Does time spent in hospital in the final 15 years of life increase with age at death? A population based study. *British Medical Journal* 1999;**319**:1338–9.

Insua J.T., Sacks H.S., Lau T.S. *et al.* Drug treatment of hypertension in the elderly: a meta-analysis. *Annals of Internal Medicine* 1994;**121**:355–62.

Jackson R.D., LaCroix A.Z., Gass M. *et al.* Calcium plus vitamin D supplementation and the risk of fractures. *New England Journal of Medicine* 2006;**354**:669–83.

Katakura M., Naka M., Kondo T. *et al.* Development, worsening, and improvement of diabetic microangiopathy in older people: six-year prospective study of patients under intensive diabetes control. *Journal of the American Geriatrics Society* 2007;**55**:541–7.

Kinsella K. Demographic aspects. In: Ebrahim S, Kalache A, editors. Epidemiology in old age. London: BMJ Publishing; 1996. p. 32–40.

Kirkwood T. The time of our lives: the science of human ageing. London: Weidenfield and Nicolson; 1999.

Laing W., Hall M., Lumley P. Agenda for health. The challenges of ageing. London: Association of the British Pharmaceutical Industry; 1991.

Lancaster T., Stead L.F. Individual behavioural counselling for smoking cessation. [Update of Cochrane Database Syst Rev. 2002;(3):CD001292; PMID:12137623]. Cochrane Database of Systematic Reviews 2005b;(2): CD001292.

Lancaster T., Stead L.F. Self-help interventions for smoking cessation. [Update of Cochrane Database Syst Rev. 2002;(3):CD001118; PMID:12137618]. Cochrane Database of Systematic Reviews 2005a;(3): CD001118.

Lawlor D.A., Davey Smith G., Ebrahim S. Commentary: The hormone replacement–coronary heart disease conundrum: is this the death of observational epidemiology?. *International Journal of Epidemiology* 2004;**33**:464–7.

Lee C., Porteous J. Experiences of family caregiving among middle-aged Australian women. *Feminism and Psychology* 2002;**12**(1):79–96.

Lee C. Experiences of family caregiving among older Australian women. *Journal of Health Psychology* 2001;**6**:393–404.

Leon D.A., Chenet L., Shkolnikov V.M. *et al.* Huge variation in Russian mortality rates 1984–94: artefact, alcohol or what? Lancet 1997;**350**:383–8.

Levine R.S., Foster J.E., Fullilove R.E. *et al.* Black–white inequalities in mortality and life expectancy, 1933–1999: implications for healthy people 2010. *Public Health Reports* 2001;**116**:474–83.

Lunney J.R., Lynn J., Foley D.J. *et al.* Patterns of functional decline at end of life. *Journal of the American Medical Association* 2003;**289**(18): 2387–92.

Manton K.G. Changing concepts of morbidity and mortality in the elderly population. *Milbank Memorial Fund Quarterly – Health and Society* 1982;**60**:183–244.

Manton K.G. Sex and race specific mortality differentials in multiple causes of death data. *Gerontologist* 1980;**20**:480–93.

Marmot M., Adelstein A.M., Bulusu L. Lessons from the study of immigrant mortality. Lancet 1984;**1**(8392):1455–7.

Marmot M. Inequalities in health. *New England Journal of Medicine* 2001;**345**(2):134–6.

Marmot M. Social determinants of health inequalities. *Lancet* 2005;**365**(9464):1099–104.

Mathers C. Health differentials among older Australians. Canberra: AGPS ; 1999. Health Monitoring Series No. 2.

Mathers C.D., Iburg K.M., Salomon J.A. *et al.* Global patterns of healthy life expectancy in the year 2002. *BMC Public Health* 2004;**4**:66.

Mathers C.D., Sadana R., Salomon J.A. *et al.* Healthy life expectancy in 191 countries, 1999. *Lancet* 2001;**357**(9269):1685–91.

Mathers C.D., Vos E.T., Stevenson C.E. *et al.* The Australian Burden of Disease Study: measuring the loss of health from diseases, injuries and risk factors. *Medical Journal of Australia* 2000;**172**:592–6.

McCallum J., Simons L., Simons J. The Dubbo Study of the Health of the Elderly 1988–2002. Sydney: University of Sydney; 2003.

McClure R., Turner C., Peel N. *et al.* Population-based interventions for the prevention of fall-related injuries in older people. [Online]. Cochrane Database Systematic Review 2005;(1):CD004441.

Mendes de Leon C.P., Glass T.A., Beckett L.A. *et al.* Social networks and disability transitions across eight intervals of yearly data in the New Haven EPESE. *Journal of Gerontology SeriesB: Psychological Sciences and Social Sciences* 1999;**54**:S62–72.

Mitka M. International conference considers health needs of the rural elderly. *Journal of the American Medical Association* 2000;**284**(4): 423–34.

Mouton C.P., Espino D.V. Problem-oriented diagnosis: health screening in older women. *American Family Physician* 1999;**59**(7):1835–42.

Mulrow C.D., Cornell J.A., Herrera C.R. *et al.* Hypertension in the elderly. Implications and generalizability of randomized trials. *Journal of the American Medical Association* 1994;**272**:1932–8.

Murray C.J.L., Michaud C.M., McKenna M.T. *et al.* US patterns of mortality by county and race: 1965–1994. Cambridge (MA): Harvard School of Public Health; Atlanta (GA): Centers for Disease Control and Prevention; 1998.

National Center for Health Statistics. Health, United States 1999. Hyattsville (MD): National Center for Health Statistics; 1999.

Nelson H.D., Helfand M., Woolf S.H. *et al.* Screening for postmenopausal osteoporosis: a review of the evidence for the US Preventive Services Task Force. *Annals of Internal Medicine* 2002;**137**:529–41.

Noh S., Kaspar V. Perceived discrimination and depression: moderating effects of coping acculturation, and ethnic support. *American Journal of Public Health* 2003;**93**(30):232–8.

Normand C. Ten popular health economic fallacies. *Journal of Public Health Medicine* 1998;**20**:129–32.

Office of National Statistics. Population trends 119 [Online]. Spring 2005. Available from: http://www.statistics.gov.uk/downloads/theme_population/PT119v2.pdf [accessed 2007 Feb 9].

Omran A.R. The epidemiologic transition: a theory of the epidemiology of population change. *Milbank Memorial Fund Quarterly* 1971;**49**(4): 509–38.

Pignone M.P., Gaynes B.N., Rushton J.K. *et al.* Screening for depression in adults: a summary of the evidence for the US Preventive Services Task Force. *Annals of Internal Medicine* 2002;**136**:765–76.

Pit S.W., Byles J.E., Henry D.A., Holt L., Hansen V., Bowman D.A. A Quality Use of Medicines program for general practitioners and older people: a cluster randomised controlled trial *Medical Journal of Australia* 2007; **187**(1):23–30.

Porthouse J., Cockayne S., King C. *et al.* Randomized controlled trial of calcium and supplementation with cholecalciferol (vitamin D3) for prevention of fractures in primary care. *British Medical Journal* 2005;**330**:1003–8.

Research Dissemination Core. Oral hygiene care for functionally dependent and cognitively impaired older adults. Iowa City (IA): University of Iowa Gerontological Nursing Interventions Research Center; 2002.

Riley N.E. China's population: new trends and challenges. *Population Bulletin* 2004;**59**:3–35.

Rivetti D., Jefferson T., Thomas R. *et al.* Vaccines for preventing influenza in the elderly. [Online]. Cochrane Database of Systematic Reviews 2006;(2):CD004876.

Rossouw J.E., Prentice R.L., Manson J.E. *et al.* Postmenopausal hormone therapy and risk of cardiovascular disease by age and years since menopause. *Journal of the American Medical Association* 2007;**297**:1465–77.

Royal Commission on Long-Term Care. With respect to old age: long-term care— rights and responsibilities. London: Her Majesty's Stationery Office; 1999.

Saelens B.E., Sallis J.F., Frank L.D. Environmental correlates of walking and cycling: findings from the transportation, urban design, and planning literatures. *Annals of Behavioral Medicine* 2003;**25**:80–91.

Schmader K.E., Hanlon J.T., Landsman P.B. *et al.* Inappropriate prescribing and health outcomes in elderly veteran outpatients. *Annals of Pharmacotherapy* 1997;**31**(5):529–33.

Schulz R., Martire L. Family caregiving of persons with dementia: prevalence, health effects, and support. *American Journal of Geriatric Psychiatry* 2004;**12**:240–9.

Seeman T., Chen X. Risk and protective factors for physical functioning in older adults with and without chronic conditions: MacArthur Studies of Successful Aging. *Journals of Gerontology Series B: Psychological Sciences and Social Sciences* 2002;**57**:S135–44.

Sellors J., Kaczorowski J., Sellors C. *et al.* A randomized controlled trial of a pharmacist consultation program for family physicians and their elderly patients. *Canadian Medical Association Journal* 2003;**169**(1):17–22.

Shepperd S., Iliffe S. Hospital at home versus in-patient hospital care. [Online].Cochrane Database of Systematic Reviews 2001;(3): CD000356 [last update 2005 May].

Shkolnikov V., McKee M., Leon D.A. Changes in life expectancy in Russia in the mid-1990s. *Lancet* 2001;**357**:917–21.

Simonson W., Feinberg J.L. Medication-related problems in the elderly: defining the issues and identifying solutions. *Drugs Aging* 2005;**22**(7):559–69.

Smeeth L., Iliffe S. Community screening for visual impairment in the elderly. [Online]. Cochrane Database Systematic Reviews 2003;(4): CD001054.

Soldo B.J., Mitchell O.S., Tfaily R. *et al. Cross-cohort differences in health on the verge of retirement.* Cambridge (MA): National Bureau of Economic Research; 2006. Working paper 12762.

Stampfer M.J., Colditz G.A. Estrogen replacement therapy and coronary heart disease: a quantitative assessment of the epidemiologic evidence. *Preventative Medicine* 1991;**20**:47–63.

Steinbach U. Social networks, institutionalization, and mortality among elderly people in the United States. *Journal of Gerontology* 1992; **47**:S183–90.

Stroke Unit Trialists' Collaboration. Organized inpatient (stroke unit) care for stroke. In: The Cochrane Library. Issue 3. [Online]. Oxford: Update Software; 2001.

Stuck A.E., Siu A.L., Wieland G.D. *et al.* Comprehensive geriatric assessment: a meta-analysis of controlled trials. *Lancet* 1993;**342**(8878): 1032–6.

Stuck A.Q., Egger M., Hammer A. *et al.* Home visits to prevent nursing home admission and functional decline in elderly people. *Journal of the American Medical Association* 2002;**287**:1022–8.

The RECORD Trial Group. Oral vitamin D3 and calcium for secondary prevention of low-trauma fractures in elderly people (Randomized Evaluation of Calcium Or vitamin D, RECORD): a randomized placebo-controlled trial. *Lancet* 2005;**365**:1621–8.

Tinetti M., Baker C., McAvay G. *et al.* A multifactorial intervention to reduce the risk of falling among elderly people living in the community. *New England Journal of Medicine* 1994;**331**:821–7.

Toumilehto J., Lindstrom J. The major diabetes prevention trials. *Current Diabetes Report* 2003;**3**:115–22.

Tucker K.L., Hallfrisch J., Qiao N. *et al.* The combination of high fruit and vegetable and low saturated fat intakes is more protective against mortality in aging men than is either alone: the Baltimore Longitudinal Study of Aging. *Journal of Nutrition* 2005;**135**:556–61.

United Nations. World Population Ageing 1950–2050. New York (NY): Population Division, United Nations; 2002. Available from: http://www.un.org/esa/population/publications/worldageing19502050/[accessed 2007 May 8].

United States Census Bureau [Online]. Available from: http://www.census.gov/[accessed 2007 Feb 6].

United States National Institute of Ageing [Online]. Available from: http://www.nia.nih.gov/[accessed 2007 May 8].

United States Preventive Services Task Force. The guide to clinical preventive services, 2006. Rockville (MD): Agency for Healthcare Research and Quality; 2006.

Van Haastregt J.C.M., Diederiks J.P.M., van Rossum E. *et al.* Effects of preventive home visits to elderly people living in the community: systematic review. *British Medical Journal* 2000;**320**:754–8.

Villa V.M., Wallace S.P. Diversity and ageing: implications for aging policy. In: Carmel S., Morse C.A., Torres-Gil F.M., editors. Lessons of ageing from three nations. Volume I: The art of ageing well. New York (NY): Baywood Publishing Company Inc; 2007.

Vita A.J., Terry R.B., Hubert H.B. *et al.* Aging, health risks and cumulative disability. *New England Journal of Medicine* 1998;**338**:1035–41.

Wald N.J., Law M.R. A strategy to reduce cardiovascular disease by more than 80%. *British Medical Journal* 2003;**326**:1419–24.

Ward D., Severs M., Dean T. *et al.* Care home versus hospital and own home environments for rehabilitation of older people. In: The Cochrane Library. Issue 2. [Online]. Oxford: Update Software; 2003.

Williams A., Evans J.G. The rationing debate. *Rationing health care by age. British Medical Journal* 1997;**314**:820–5.

Wilson K., Mottram P., Sivanranthan A. *et al.* Antidepressants versus placebo for the depressed elderly. [Online]. Cochrane Database Systematic Review 2001:CD000561.

Wolff J.L., Starfield B., Anderson G. Prevalence, expenditures, and complications of multiple chronic conditions in the elderly. *Archives of Internal Medicine* 2002;**162**:2269–76.

World Health Organization. International Classification of Functioning, Disability and Health. Geneva: World Health Organization. Available from: www.who.int/icf [accessed 2007 May 8].

World Health Organization. Obesity: preventing and managing the global epidemic. Report of a WHO consultation. Geneva: World Health Organization; 2000. Technical Report Series 894.

World Health Organization. The bone and joint decade. Geneva: World Health Organization; 2001.

World Health Organization. World health report 1999: making a difference. Geneva: World Health Organization; 1999.

Writing Group for the Women's Health Initiative Investigators. Risks and benefits of estrogen plus progestin in healthy postmenopausal women: principal results from the Women's Health Initiative Randomized Control Trial. *Journal of the American Medical Association* 2002;**288**:321–33.

Yusuf S., Reddy S., Ounpuu S. *et al*. Global burden of cardiovascular diseases—Part II: variations in cardiovascular disease by specific ethnic groups and geographic regions and prevention strategies. *Circulation* 2001;**104**(23):2855–64.

Zavoretti R. Family-based care for China's ageing population. *Asia Europe Journal* 2006;**4**:211–8.

Zermansky A.G., Petty D.R., Raynor D.K. *et al*. Clinical medication review by a pharmacist of patients on repeat prescriptions in general practice: a randomized controlled trial. *Health Technology Assessment* 2002;**6**(20):1–86.

11.8

Forced migrants and other displaced populations

Catherine R. Bateman and Anthony B. Zwi

Abstract

This chapter provides an overview of the global health dimensions of forced migration and the associated public health challenges. The chapter begins by identifying different categories of forced migrants including refugees, internally displaced persons, asylum seekers, trafficked or smuggled persons, as well as environment and development displacees. The causes must be viewed in global context in which globalization is simultaneously a force for greater integration while at the same time contributing to forced migration. Global influences include economic inequalities, armed conflicts, human rights abuses, environmental degradation, and natural disasters among others. The problem of forced migration is difficult to quantify, and statistics are contested. In 2006, the United Nations High Commissioner for Refugees (UNHCR) recognized 32.9 million 'persons of concern' including 9.9 million refugees and 12.8 million internally displaced persons. Legal frameworks, including the 1951 UN Convention on Refugees and its successors, identify formal protections to which refugees and other groups of forced migrants are entitled. Nevertheless, the public health situation of forced migrants are varied and often poor. They may form distinct populations or be dispersed amongst host populations; they may be displaced within their own country, to a nearby country, or to a more distant country of asylum; and they may dwell in a developing country experiencing conflict, a more peaceful but poverty-stricken developing country, or a wealthy developed nation. The health of each forced migrant population will be shaped by these contextual factors, but also by prior health and social conditions, the journeys they have had to take, the social structures within which they now live, including access to services, and the stability of these new structures. The role of public health professionals in developing a comprehensive understanding of these dynamics, advocating for forced migrant health, and enabling forced migrants to speak and be heard, aiding them in transforming their own health outcome is discussed.

Introduction

This chapter provides a global overview of forced migration and the public health challenges facing populations forced to move from their usual homes. It begins by presenting a brief history of forced migration and the legal definition of 'refugee'. We describe the emergence of categories of forced migrants that do not meet the legal definition of 'refugee', describe how these groups are treated by states, and the implications for peoples' lives and health. The chapter then explores the social and political factors that have influenced the treatment of refugees by states. We lay out some of the major health issues that refugees face in both developing and developed countries. The wide variety of actors involved in both protecting forced migrants and providing health services is presented, along with a discussion of the contextual conditions that have an impact, often detrimental, on the health of forced migrants. As well as describing the structural factors that create and limit health outcomes, this analysis seeks to highlight the agency and voice of forced migrants, exploring the importance of understanding and projecting these, and of appreciating the rationales for how forced migrants may act in the often chaotic situations in which they find themselves. We consider how interactions with other actors, within the complex social, political, and legal context of forced migration, may lead to seemingly unhealthy choices, and at times, barriers to engaging with services. Yet, forced migrants make choices, when possible, seeking to protect their well-being and fight for better, and healthier, outcomes.

Categories of forced migrants

Definitions of forced migration have been debated for more than 50 years, dating back to the first UN Convention on Refugees in 1951. The legal framework that emerged under the Convention centred on 'refugees' as a specially defined group and is based upon the 1951 Convention and a subsequent 1967 protocol. According to these, a refugee is a person who:

> *owing to a well-founded fear of being persecuted for reasons of race, religion, nationality, membership of a particular social group, or political opinion, is outside the country of his nationality, and is unable to or, owing to such fear, is unwilling to avail himself of the protection of that country* (UNHCR 2007).

This definition has been modified by regional instruments in Africa and Latin America, as described in a later section.

The International Association for the Study of Forced Migration (IASFM), however, defines forced migration much more widely as:

> *a general term that refers to the movements of refugees and internally displaced people (those displaced by conflicts) as well as people displaced by natural or environmental disasters, chemical or nuclear disasters, famine, or development projects* (FMO 2008).

This definition encompasses a wide range of forced migrants, and these can be distinguished into several distinct groups (Box 11.8.1).

The definitions of other forced migrant groups, and their sources, are outlined below. They highlight the increased attention devoted to both describing, and defining, the many forms of forced migration that exist. The discourse and narratives presented have a marked impact on how people see, and respond, to those forced to leave their usual homes and livelihoods.

Internally displaced persons (IDPs)

Unlike refugees, there is no legal definition of an IDP. It is generally accepted that if a person meets the definition of a refugee, but their displacement does not take them across an international border, then they are internally displaced. The Secretary General of the United Nations has appointed a representative to deal with IDPs and the Office of the United Nations High Commissioner for Human Rights (OHCHR) has produced a set of Guiding Principles to address the specific needs of IDPs who are described as:

> *persons or groups of persons who have been forced or obliged to flee or to leave their homes or places of habitual residence, in particular as a result of, or in order to, avoid the effects of armed conflict, situations of generalized violence, violations of human rights or natural or human-made disasters, and who have not crossed an internationally recognized State border* (Deng 1998).

Asylum seekers

Asylum seekers are those who are fleeing persecution and are seeking refugee status in another country. According to UNHCR, an asylum seeker:

> *is a person who has left their country of origin, has applied for recognition as a refugee in another country, and is awaiting a decision on their application* (UNHCR 2007).

The application referred to relates to being recognized under the 1951 Convention as a refugee and therefore entitled to the protection and support stipulated by the Convention. They may or may not arrive in a country with authorization, nevertheless, they have a legal right to claim asylum and are therefore not 'illegal'.

Trafficked persons

The 2003 Protocol to Prevent, Suppress and Punish Trafficking in Persons, especially Women and Children, describes trafficking as:

> *recruitment, transportation, transfer, harbouring, or receipt of persons, by means of the threat or use of force or other forms of coercion, of abduction, of fraud, of deception, of the abuse or power or of a position of vulnerability or of the giving or receiving*

Box 11.8.1 Categories of forced migrants

Refugee	A person who 'owing to a well-founded fear of being persecuted for reasons of race, religion, nationality, membership of a particular social group, or political opinion, is outside the country of his nationality, and is unable to or, owing to such fear, is unwilling to avail himself of the protection of that country' (UNHCR 2008).
Internally displaced persons	'Persons or groups of persons who have been forced or obliged to flee or to leave their homes or places of habitual residence, in particular as a result of, or in order to, avoid the effects of armed conflict, situa tions of generalized violence, violations of human rights or natural or human-made disasters, and who have not crossed an internationally recognized State border' (Deng 1998).
Asylum seeker	'A person who has left their country of origin, has applied for recognition as a refugee in another country, and is awaiting a decision on their application' (UNHCR 2007).
Trafficking in persons	'Recruitment, transportation, transfer, harbouring or receipt of persons, by means of the threat or use of force or other forms of coercion, of abduction, of fraud, of deception, of the abuse for power or of a position of vulnerability or of the giving or receiving of payments or benefits to achieve the consent of a person having control over another person, for the purpose of exploitation' (United Nations 2003).
Smuggling in persons	'The procurement, in order to obtain, directly or indirectly, a financial or other material benefit, of illegal entry of a person into a state, party of which the person is not a national or permanent resident' (United Nations 2000) [Article 3 (a)].
Environmentally displaced person	'A person displaced owing to environmental causes, notably land loss and degradation, and natural disaster' (United Nations 1997).
Development displacees	"People who are compelled to move as a result of policies and projects implemented to supposedly enhance 'development'" (Forced Migration Online 2008).

of payments or benefits to achieve the consent of a person having control over another person, for the purpose of exploitation. Exploitation shall include, at a minimum, the exploitation of the prostitution of others or other forms of sexual exploitation, forced labour or services, slavery or practices similar to slavery, servitude or the removal of organs (United Nations 2003).

Smuggled persons

Smuggling of aliens or 'illegal migrant smuggling' is defined by the UN 2000 Protocol Against Smuggling of Migrants by Land, Sea and Air, which supplemented the UN Convention Against Transnational Organized Crime, to mean:

the procurement, in order to obtain, directly or indirectly, a financial or other material benefit, of illegal entry of a person into a state, party of which the person is not a national or permanent resident (United Nations 2000) [Article 3 (a)].

Environmentally displaced persons

The OECD glossary of statistical terms 2001 describes an environmental refugee as 'a person displaced owing to environmental causes, notably land loss and degradation, and natural disaster' (United Nations 1997). However, the term was first described by Essam El-Hinnawi (1985), a researcher from United Nations Environment Program (UNEP) in 1985, who defined environmental refugees as:

those people who have been forced to leave their traditional habitat, temporarily or permanently, because of a marked environmental disruption (natural and/or triggered by people) that jeopardized their existence and/or seriously affected the quality of their life.

'Environmental disruption' in this definition is taken to mean any physical, chemical, and/or biological changes in the ecosystem (or resource base) that render it, temporarily or permanently, unsuitable to support human life. The validity of the term 'environmental refugees' has been debated greatly since that time. Actors emerge from a realm of perspectives including environmentalists, economists, and refugee advocates, each with a different interpretation of the term. Some prefer to use the term 'environmental migrant' or 'environmental displacee'; different terms establish different implications for both the individuals and states involved.

Development displacees

There is no legal definition for development displaces; however, Forced Migration Online (http://www.forcedmigration.org) suggests they are:

people who are compelled to move as a result of policies and projects implemented to supposedly enhance 'development'. These include large-scale infrastructure projects such as dams, roads, ports, airports; urban clearance initiatives; mining and deforestation; and the introduction of conservation parks/reserves and biosphere projects. Affected people usually remain within the borders of their country. People displaced in this way are sometimes also referred to as 'oustees', 'involuntarily displaced' or 'involuntarily resettled' (Forced_Migration_Online 2008).

Interestingly, large-scale agricultural projects do not seem to be specifically mentioned.

Causes of displacement

The global context

Forced migration cannot be fully understood without considering the global context and the shifting global forces that shape the form and patterns of migration. Globalization and its role in shaping the dynamics of forced migration need to be considered. Although globalization is a contested concept with disputed definitions, most people accept it as a global process of integration which affects sociocultural, economic, and political domains (see Chapter 2.1).

There is a polarized debate over the affects of globalization on health. Some commentators argue, like Feachem (2001), that the forces of economic globalization can be beneficial to the poor, increasing wealth and therefore health; while others (Baum 2001; MacDonald 2007) highlight the poor health situation in many developing countries and the vast inequities present, and suggest that globalization plays a part in generating these conditions. The latter argue that globalization cannot be separated from economic policies that serve the interests of the wealthy, reinforcing or exacerbating inequalities, fuelling conflicts and contributing to public health crises in developing countries. This analysis suggests that the only way to improve health is to seriously restructure the dominant international financial institutions. Taking the middle ground, Lee (2004) suggests that rigorous, ongoing analysis is required to assess the positive and negative impacts on health within the overall conceptual domain of globalization. Zwi and Alvarez-Castillo (2003) argue that globalization has often led to poor health outcomes for vast populations and that this in turn is responsible for fuelling forced migration. Regardless of our standpoint on globalization, what it is, how it impacts on health, and its influence, what is clear is that global health inequities exist and are dramatic, producing some of the major contributors to forced migration, whether or not associated with violence.

Castles' (2004) analysis suggests that the global context should be carefully examined when considering forced migration dynamics. He argues that the current perception of a global 'asylum crisis' should be seen more as a crisis of North–South relationships, within which 'asylum' is but one aspect. The current picture of forced migration, he argues, is a result of disparities between North and South. While these disparities exist and people search for a better life, or simply for survival, forced migration will continue. The disparity is also reflected in how the effects of forced migration are absorbed globally, further deepening the crisis in North–South relations. He shows that while there has repeatedly been a perception of impending asylum crises ever since the 1800s, which largely do not fully emerge as feared, there are some new features. He cites the increase in endemic violence and human rights violations as a feature that has increased the volume of forced migration in recent times. Castles (2004) shows, however, that for the North, there is no significant economic or social crisis resulting from forced migration and contrary to popular belief, the North has not had to absorb large influxes of people. The situation is nonetheless construed by those in the North as a crisis because it highlights the 'erosion of nation-state sovereignty'. The South, however, has absorbed the vast majority of forced migrants from neighbouring countries (Allotey & Reidpath 2003). This combined with increasingly restrictive policies of wealthy countries that seek to limit refugee absorption from the South, leads to a tension in North–South relations, and opens space for people smuggling and trafficking, further threatening the sense of control over borders that the North is seeking to maintain, and therefore deepening the sense of crisis perceived by the North. Hence the burden has been left largely with the South, while in the North, incomplete pictures of fear that exclude vulnerable people have been painted and promoted (Grove & Zwi 2006). In their review of globalization, forced migration, and health, Zwi and Alvarez Castillo (2003) suggest that public health professionals have a responsibility to examine the context and whole picture, and in so doing, to advocate for a more humane globalization that has a chance of decreasing forced migration and the associated poor health outcomes.

Immediate causes of displacement

There is general agreement on the range of factors that contribute to displacement and forced migration. However, the importance of particular factors, and the linkages between them, varies in different contexts. Identification of specific causes has implications for both the states involved and the migrants themselves, given that the perceived cause of displacement has an impact on the international response, the level of funding support provided and the attitudes of host populations to those seeking protection. The health consequences of forced migration will be shaped by not only the causes of displacement, but by the perceptions of all actors regarding these causes and their relationship to them. In this respect, the terms and context within which forced migrants are described and 'presented' greatly affects the societal response and opportunities, or constraints, operating.

Forced migration has traditionally been associated with war and violence. The conception of a refugee as defined by the UN Convention, fleeing from persecution to a place of safety in another country, was clear-cut and well understood. As Moore and Shellman (2004) describe, the central model was one of:

Violence in = Forced migration out

However, whilst the main causes of involuntary displacement remain armed conflict, repression and war, other factors such as natural disaster and development projects are also important, as are the more complex set of economic, social, and political circumstances that may lead to trafficking and people smuggling.

Martin (2002) focuses attention on natural and man-made disasters and border changes leading to statelessness, as factors which lead to forced migration, alongside the well recognized factors related to persecution, human rights violations, repression, and conflict. Environmental factors, such as rising sea levels and extreme weather conditions, are also increasingly recognized as important. Some argue that these causes may, over time, supercede conflict as a primary cause of forced migration (Myers & Kent 1995). Resource constraints, including depleted access to land and water, and conflict over precious minerals, are likely to become increasingly important, especially as the global population increases from around six billion people at present to nearly nine billion by 2050.

While all these factors are important, quantifying their effects is difficult. Data are available regarding numbers of 'Convention' refugees and also, more recently, regarding IDPs. These data may give some indication of the level of displacement produced by conflicts and violence, alongside immediate natural disasters such as tsunami and earthquakes. However, more insidious environmental and economic effects are far harder to quantify.

The increased complexity of recent times in describing and understanding factors that cause displacement rise new concerns that go beyond the simple 'violence = migration' model therefore calls for new approaches. Major challenges include an increased focus on economic migrants and those who are forced to move as a result of environmental and climate changes; there is also a rise in 'mixed migration', a term which recognizes that many migrants fall somewhere on the spectrum between forced and voluntary migration and are hard to categorize as one or the other.

Particularly important is a call for a shift in policies of protection for host countries to developing policies which address the root causes within countries from which people are forced to migrate; and a growing understanding that understanding causes may allow predictions of impending displacement as well as the identification of the means to avert large-scale displacement.

Some analyses continue to support the primacy of violent conflict, or threat of conflict as the major predictor of populations leaving their homes. Moore and Shellman (2004) analysed a global sample of 40 countries and using a model that incorporated a wide range of indicators (government threat, dissident threat, government-dissent interaction, ethnic or non-ethnic civil wars, war on territory, income opportunity, political freedom and the rule of law, and cultural and family ties), they found that the first three were the primary determinants of forced migration flows. These were more important than other factors such as size of economy or type of political institution. Apodaca (1998) analysed a variety of models developed to predict forced migration and concluded that human rights violations are one of the most important predictors.

Economic migration has often been portrayed in the media as freely chosen migration that should not confer a responsibility to protect on accepting states. However, analysts such as Castles (2003) argue that forced migration is linked to economic migration and that the two are 'closely related (and indeed often indistinguishable) forms of expression of global inequalities and societal crises'. These inequities have intensified since the end of the Cold War. He argues that studies of the causes of forced migration have neglected the over-arching economic and social structures which should be seen in relation to 'US political and military domination, economic globalization, North–South inequality and transnationalism'.

Debates regarding causes of displacement have particular salience in relation to the protection offered to forced migrants. As subsequent sections of the chapter describe, the nature and extent of protection is often determined by perceived cause. Therefore, understanding these debates is crucial as they may have effects on what and how protection, if any, is offered to forced migrant populations.

Forced migration statistics

Assessing the volume of global flows of forced migrants is valuable in identifying trends, and the patterns of distribution with respect to where the burden for providing assistance and care lies. In specific countries and contexts, where people are forced to migrate from their place of origin, the first step in addressing public health and other more general concerns is often to define the size of the population at risk. Donors, governments, aid agencies, and community organizations require basic demographic and related data to inform planning and service delivery. The collection of data is complicated and surrounded by controversy, having the potential to immediately reframe what looks like a technical issue into a political one.

The two main sources of statistics on forced migrants are the United Nations High Commissioner for Refugees (UNHCR) and the US Committee for Refugees and Immigrants (USCRI). These organizations produce differing estimates for different types of forced migrants in different geographical contexts. The logistic difficulties of collecting reliable data from shifting forced migrant populations leaves space for political interests to enter, and seek to shape, the field. This is compounded by disagreement over definitions of forced migrants and which groups to include in which categories, as mentioned earlier, with significant implications for the rights and entitlements of such groups, as well as for who bears the responsibilities for addressing their needs. Despite contested data, available sources provide valuable information on trends and distribution.

UNHCR provides data based on 'persons of concern', an increasingly wide-ranging term. 'Persons of concern' includes refugees (as defined by the 1951 Convention or the 1969 Organisation of African Unity (OAU) Convention); persons granted complementary protection (alternative forms of protection for those that fall outside of the terms of the 1951 Convention) and those with forms of temporary protection; asylum seekers who in the year of data collection are still pending a final decision on an application for protection; stateless persons; refugees who returned to their country of origin in the year of data collection; and IDPs. For the purposes of UNHCR the latter are limited to conflict-generated IDPs to whom UNHCR protection or assistance is extended, but does not include all IDPs.

The changes seen between 2005 and 2006 in the UNHCR estimates (Tables 11.8.1 and 11.8.2) illustrate how dramatically statistics may fluctuate due to real, methodological, and political influences on data.

The number of 'persons of concern' to UNHCR increased substantially in 2006. Although 2006 saw a real increase in refugee numbers as a result of 1.2 million Iraqis seeking refuge in Syria and Jordan, there were other factors that led to the increased numbers (Tables 11.8.1 and 11.8.2). The UNHCR became involved at this point as a player in the cluster approach, through which UN agencies have been seeking to enhance their efficiency, and consequently extended its activities to include a larger number of IDPs. Methodological changes in collecting data also contributed to the increase partly as a result of moves to better reflect individual refugee registration in UNHCR operations, but also due to a review of the caseload of countries such as the United States.

Table 11.8.1 'Persons of concern' to United Nations High Commissioner of Refugees (UNHCR, April 2007, December 2007)

	2005	2006
Refugees	8.7 million	9.9 million
Asylum seekers	773 500	744 000
IDPs	6.6 million	12.8 million
Stateless	2.4 million	5.8 million
Returnees	1.6 million	2.6 million
Resettlement	80 000	71 700
Others of concern	960 400	1 million
Total	20.8 million	32.9 million

Table 11.8.2 World Refugee Survey (USCRI 2006, 2007)

	2005[a]	2006[b]
Refugees and asylum seekers	12 million	13.9 million
New refugees and asylum seekers	1.04 million	1.1 million
IDPs	21 million	–
New IDPs	2.1 million	–

[a] World Refugee Survey (2006) reports data from 2005.
[b] IDP data not available in World Refugee Survey (2007).

It is important to note that 4.3 million Palestinian refugees falling under the mandate of the United Nations Relief and Works Agency for Palestinian Refugees in the Near East (UNRWA) are not included in these UNHCR figures. The Palestinian community has been one of the largest groups of refugees that has remained without being fully resettled or absorbed into host-nations; a reflection of how community members on the ground suffer while local, national, regional, and global powers resolve, or fail to resolve, higher-level strategic and political issues.

Given the importance of these numbers, they are invariably contested and debated; with key actors seeking to shape what data are collected and presented, who are counted, and what the implications are for future activities. Indeed each 'player' in the system, whether they be a UN or non-governmental agency, a recipient or state of origin, a local community or professional group, and many others, has their own rationale for inflating or deflating the numbers of people whether they be refugees or IDPs, in or outside of camps, dependant or free of other major influences.

Legal framework

Refugees

The 1951 Convention, which forms the basis of all international refugee law, was drafted in the aftermath of World War II in response to the large numbers of displaced people caused by the war. The Convention included restrictions on who would be classified as a 'refugee' based on geographical and temporal factors that were specific to the European context. As a result, the 1967 Protocol relating to the Status of Refugees was adopted which removed these restrictions and allowed for more general application of the Convention. The Convention and Protocol laid out not only the definition of a refugee but also the scope of protection to which refugees were entitled. The most fundamental of these is *non-refoulement*, the right to remain rather than be returned to a place where their lives or freedoms would be at risk. Debate has raged over the continuing relevance of the Convention definition, given that it excludes large numbers of people in need of international protection, notably internally displaced persons and those that have migrated as a result of generalized (as opposed to individualized) violence, civil war, and widespread human rights abuses.

Africa and Latin America responded to the limitations of the Convention and Protocol by adopting their own regional laws and standards. The Organisation of African Unity (now known as the African Union) adopted the 1967 Convention Governing the Specific Aspects of Refugee Problems in Africa (Barnett 2002).

This is the only legally binding regional instrument and has a refugee definition similar to that of the convention but includes those who flee due to 'external aggression, occupation, foreign domination or events seriously disturbing public order in either part or the whole of his country of origin or nationality' (OAU 1969).

In Latin America, the Cartagena Declaration, adopted in 1984, included a definition of refugee similar to that of the OAU Convention but which also included reference to 'massive violation of human rights' (Cartagena Declaration 1984). The latter is not legally binding but has been adopted by many states and incorporated into some national legislation in the region.

Persons who have participated in war crimes and violations of humanitarian and human rights law, including the crime of terrorism are specifically excluded from the convention and cannot be recognized as refugees.

The UNHCR has been given a mandate to provide international protection to refugees and seek permanent solutions to their problems through its Statute, adopted by the UN General Assembly (UNGA) in December 1950. Over the years, the UNGA has allowed UNHCR to extend its responsibilities and is increasingly focused not only on refugee protection but also on managing refugees in the field.

IDPs

Whilst IDPs do not have the same legal framework of protection, they have become included in UNHCRs 'people of concern' and are therefore often covered by its mandate. The United Nations Office for Coordination of Humanitarian Affairs (OCHA) has produced a set of Guiding Principles to address the specific needs of internally displaced persons (OCHA 1998). The guidelines identify rights and guarantees that should be afforded to IDPs although they are not legally binding.

Asylum seekers

The Declaration of Territorial Asylum (DTA) adopted by the UN General Assembly in 1967 is based on article 14 of the Universal Declaration of Human Rights, which declares that 'everyone has the right to seek and to enjoy in other countries asylum from persecution'. The principles of the DTA are that all States recognize asylum granted by one State, that States themselves evaluate the grounds for asylum, and that no one seeking asylum should be rejected at borders or if already within a country should not be compulsorily returned to any State in which they may be subject to persecution. Exceptions can only be made in situations of national security or for asylum seekers that have committed a crime against humanity, against peace or a war crime.

Asylum may be granted by States on the basis of the 1951 Refugee Convention, in which an individual has been deemed a 'refugee' as defined by the Convention. However, given the restrictions of this definition and the increasing numbers of people who are seeking protection but do not fit the Convention definition, alternative forms of protection have developed. Often termed 'complementary' or 'subsidiary' protection, McAdam (2006) describes the plethora of alternative forms of protection for 'non-Convention refugees' that previously had been treated much the same as Convention refugees by states.

'Non-Convention' refugees, such as those fleeing widespread violence rather than targeted individual persecution, have to look to instruments of human rights law, rather than refugee law, for protection. However, human rights instruments do not attach the same clear rights and standards as the Refugee Convention and it has also been argued that human rights law can be weak on implementation (McAdam 2006). This has led many to argue that complementary protection is a lesser form of protection, and there is a danger of States using these forms of protection to decrease the numbers of Convention refugees and therefore their level of commitment. Debate continues as to whether expanding the current Convention definition, or expanding systems of complementary protection, will weaken or broaden protection to those seeking asylum.

Trafficking and smuggled persons

Although the reasons for a person to be trafficked or smuggled are very similar, international agreements and national laws treat them quite differently. Unlike trafficking, which may occur internally in a country, smuggling always involves the illegal crossing of an international boundary. Smuggling is seen as a crime against a *state* whereas trafficking is a crime against an *individual*. Consequently persons that are trafficked or smuggled are likely to be treated quite differently. The UN Convention on Trafficking mandates states to consider granting victims permanent or temporary resident status, whereas the Smuggling of Migrants Protocol calls on states to facilitate the return of smuggled persons to the country from which they came.

Environmental and developmental displacees

The concept of environmental refugees or displacees is particularly contentious and the subject of much current debate. There is little agreement on the whether environmental factors can be seen as primary causes of displacement and equally no consensus on a definition for those displaced from their homes by these factors. As a result the legal protection available is marginal. The current legal regime has no specific mandate to protect environmental displaces, if they are displaced across international borders, however, 'natural or human-made disasters' are covered by the Guiding Principles on Internal Displacement. These place the primary duty for protection with the national authority, however, no duty is placed on other states to recognize the need for protection. A growing body of opinion has begun calling for a system of global governance that recognizes environmental factors as a cause of displacement and for the displacees to be protected under international law (Courtland Robinson 2003; Biermann & Boas 2007).

Similarly developmental displacees do not have frameworks of protection of their own but are covered by the Guiding Principles on Internal Displacement. There is a need to recognize the needs of this group and for research on displacement not to fall into a dichotomy that separates conflict-related displacement from development-related displacement (Cernea 2007).

Evolving rights of protection

Protection based on a definition of refugees fleeing from the effects of violent conflict has been the prevailing paradigm, and whilst the centrality of conflict-related displacement has been debated, conflict and violence clearly remain significant causes of forced migration and suffering. Analysis reflecting the increasingly complex drivers of forced migration, including economic and environmental concerns, whilst vital, should be careful not to compromise existing rights of protection. These rights of protection, based on conflict as the central tenet, should not be further eroded by the recognition that there are other causes of forced migration that need to be seriously considered.

Political interests and control

Harrell-Bond (1992), the doyen of analysts examining forced migration, along with other key commentators such as Crisp (1999), and Bakewell (2008), demonstrate how resources to deal with forced migration are structured by broader ideological, political, and economic decisions. Harrell-Bond (1992) argues that refugee camps and many of the structures and organizations set up are part of a system of control of those in need. She argues that the allocation of resources (whether aid, political or military resources), is a 'central component in an ideology of control'. The granting of aid often legitimizes a group and their struggles; politics influences the status and visibility accorded to different groups. Even where humanitarian and development assistance are well targeted at forced migrants in need, the impact of services, systems, and funds, may be both positive and negative. While the forced migrants in great need may be able to access resources, these are not distributed equitably, and local populations, which often bear the brunt of providing for such community members, frequently are marginalized and unable to access new resources or services.

A valuable compilation of insights (Essed *et al.* 2004) highlights how forced migrants interact with agencies and the implications for ethics, policies, and politics. A case study by Turner (2004) in the same volume, for example, demonstrates how UNHCR effectively displaces older men as providers in their families and in so doing creates new dependencies. UNHCR becomes 'a better husband'—at the same time undermining and transforming traditional household and family relationships.

Public health situation of forced migrants

Forced migrants live in a range of different social, political, and geographical conditions. They may form distinct populations or be dispersed amongst host populations; they may be displaced within their own country, to a nearby or distant country of asylum; and may dwell anywhere from a developing country experiencing conflict, to a more peaceful but poverty-stricken developing country, to a wealthy developed nation. The health of each forced migrant population, and each individual within the group, will be shaped by these factors, as well as their prior health and social condition, the journeys they have had to take, the stability and security present in their new environments, the social structures within which they live, and the access they have to services and social support.

Gushulak and MacPherson (2000) describe migration health in terms of 'three distinct but interdependent undertakings: The predeparture phase, the migratory journey itself, and the arrival at destination', each of which influences health. Factors such as social networks, assets, language, knowledge, information or access to services, food security issues, poor shelter, sanitation, and availability of safe water will influence health outcomes.

In this section we describe the major health challenges facing forced migrant populations. This is followed by an overview of the public health responses and an indication of where more detailed technical advice may be found.

Refugees in developing countries

Developing countries continue to absorb the vast majority of forced migrants, in particular as developed nations have become more restrictive. Within developing countries, people who are forcibly displaced either within or across borders may find themselves in a variety of possible contexts, settling short or long term either in a camp situation or dispersed within a host population. Each presents threats and opportunities.

The type of settlement formed has implications for health and well-being. The typical refugee camp setting has presented a range of problems, although improvements in public health knowledge and experience, and informing policy and practice with evidence, have led to better outcomes.

The impact of forced migration falls heavily on developing nations, and within these countries, on host populations. This is particularly so where forced migrants reside in non-camp situations.

Camps and non-camp settlements

Camps, whilst constructed with the intention of providing protection, safety and access to services, may also pose risks. Poorly planned refugee settlements may have inadequate infrastructure, may pose risks to safety, or set up new inequalities. The combination of overcrowding, poor hygiene and sanitation, lack of water, poor nutrition, and inadequate shelter provides conditions for spread of many diseases, particularly communicable disease. Refugees may arrive in a poor condition, suffering from malnutrition, and with poor immunity, reflecting limited access to immunization services. Disrupted social structures decrease the capacity to deal with sickness. Communicable disease spreads quickly and may be particularly severe. Psychological distress is also a major issue due to the insecure, restricted environment and lack of resources.

Debates over the utility of camps are highlighted by Harrell-Bond (2000) who argues that as a concept they have failed. Originally based on modernization theory, the premise was that camp settlements would become new agricultural centres and eventually be integrated with host populations to the benefit of all. However, this was abandoned as the theory became discredited and was replaced by a view that refugees should be seen as temporary. Harrell-Bond suggests that those in camps are in 'prison-like' settlements with poor conditions, increased vulnerability to disease and often poor nutrition. She also argues that camps do not help host populations, as large sums of money are diverted to camps which may be demolished if refugees do move on, as well as diverting scarce human and material resources from the host population. She suggests that it would be far more appropriate and cheaper to help integrate refugees into host populations and invest in the country and strengthening existing social structures, as a whole.

In many situations of forced migration, for example, when the Kosovar Albanians fled from Kosovo over the border into Albania, integration with host populations there was the norm. Following political instability and violence in Timor-Leste in 2006, 4 years after independence, makeshift camps were established within Dili, the capital city, for IDPs, while many also fled and were integrated with host communities in the districts. The latter necessarily absorbed a portion of the social and economic costs associated with accommodating those who fled.

However, Salama *et al.* (2004) show that, despite the problems associated with camps, there are also benefits. The increased knowledge base and co-ordination of humanitarian interventions have led to improvements in health, with better nutrition, sanitation, and health services. The burden of ill-health may shift from displaced populations who are relatively well serviced, especially if they cross international borders and become refugees, relative to host populations and IDPs whose needs may be greater and who have less access to assistance.

Mortality

Crude mortality rates are often used as an indicator of the immediate impact of complex emergencies. Toole and Waldman (1990) proposed a definition of the acute phase of a complex emergency as greater than one death per 10 000 people per day, based on a doubling of the baseline mortality rate in sub-Saharan African countries. Surveillance systems to monitor the impact of emergencies have been established in the past 15 years based on this definition. In recent decades, it has not been unusual to see CMRs in refugee populations of 30 times the baseline in the country of origin (Toole & Waldman 1997); some of the highest recorded were amongst Rwandan refugees who flooded into North Kivu in 1994 where average crude mortality rates were 20–35 deaths per 10 000 (Salama *et al.* 2004). In refugee camps, CMRs of 2 per 10 000 are now rarely seen, however, the situation in non-camp situations has deteriorated (Salama *et al.* 2004). Refugees are usually at greatest risk in early days of displacement, with mortality rates subsequently diminishing. The highest risk group is young children with most deaths occurring in the under-5 age group, demonstrated dramatically in one Somali camp in which 70 per cent of children under 5 appear to have died over an 8-month period (Moore *et al.* 1993; cited in Toole & Waldman 1997).

Causes of death

The main causes of death in developing country refugee situations are similar to those of developing country populations in general. The most common causes of death in Africa are diarrhoeal disease, measles, acute respiratory infections, and malaria (where endemic), exacerbated by a high prevalence of acute malnutrition (Toole & Waldman 1997). These diseases typically account for the vast majority of reported deaths in refugee populations, at times up to 95 per cent thereof. This is in contrast to European countries affected by war, where the most common causes of death are injuries, as well as communicable diseases, neonatal problems, and nutritional deficiencies. Recent analyses suggest that chronic diseases require attention, given the ageing population, and violence, instability, and forced migration in populations in which communicable diseases have been relatively well controlled and chronic diseases have emerged as problems (Chan & Sondorp 2007).

The conditions affecting refugees may have been brought with them from the country of origin, may be acquired in the host country (with refugees susceptible due to lack of sufficient immunity), or may result from the camp conditions themselves.

Diarrhoeal disease

Possibly the greatest threat to life amongst refugees is diarrhoeal disease. The main pathogens of concern are usually cholera and shigella. In some refugee camps, more than 40 per cent of deaths in the acute phase of an emergency can be attributed to diarrhoeal disease, and over 80 per cent of these deaths are in children under the age of 2 years (Salama *et al.* 2004). Outbreaks are exacerbated by factors such as the sharing and contamination of water sources and food, the scarcity of soap, and inadequate sanitation.

Amongst Rwandan refugees in camps in North Kivu, 85 per cent of the 50 000 deaths amongst the 800 000 people that flooded into the area early July 1994 were caused by diarrhoea, with 40 per cent from shigella dysentery and 60 per cent from cholera (Salama *et al.* 2004). The primary drinking source, which was lake water, became rapidly contaminated, and as water was also scarce, infection spread swiftly through the refugees. Deaths in Goma were associated with a number of preventable causes (Siddique *et al.* 1995). Among Kurdish refugees, 70 per cent of deaths were a result of diarrhoea (Toole & Waldman 1997). In the elderly and young children, dysentery case-fatality rates can be as high as 10 per cent. Important public health interventions include the need to supply sufficient water, control excreta and hygiene, and increase public awareness of basic rules of hygiene. Evidence-informed case management is necessary to avoid unnecessary deaths.

Measles

Another of the most feared diseases in camps is measles—a particularly large problem in refugee situations in the 1970s and 1980s until it was recognized that vaccination should be accorded priority. The risk of death from measles is exacerbated in the presence of malnutrition, a common occurrence amongst refugee populations, as are secondary complications. Globally, measles kills approximately 450 000 people each year. While it is less of a problem in previously well-vaccinated populations, in developing countries, measles death rates can range from 1–5 per cent, and in refugee settings among malnourished children, the death rate may reach 10–30 per cent.

In 1985, 53 and 42 per cent of refugee deaths in eastern Sudan and Somalia, respectively, were caused by measles (Salama *et al.* 2004). The situation has improved in refugee camps due to mass vaccination, but IDPs still suffer as they have less access to vaccinations and, since 1990, it is more common to find high rates of measles in IDPs than in refugees. Measles is included in the Expanded Program on Immunisation but there is often low coverage in young children especially where human resources for health are limited or conflict affects normal service delivery. Increasing attention is being devoted to ensuring that services can continue to be supplied in fragile states.

Malaria

In areas where malaria is endemic, it can cause high rates of mortality and morbidity amongst refugees. This is particularly the case when people are displaced from an area of low endemicity to one of high endemicity. Drug resistance also plays a large part with chloroquine resistance and more recent resistance to fansidar reported in Rwandan refugees in Zaire. Local communities in low endemic areas may be placed at risk by refugees arriving from high endemic areas, especially if local conditions favour the mosquito. In Africa, 30 per cent of annual malarial deaths occur in complex emergency settings. This is because in complex emergencies (CEs) overcrowding increases the frequency of bites and also delays intervention thereby increasing the time that the parasite is in the blood (Salama *et al.* 2004). An example is Burundi which had a major epidemic in 2000–2001 when the population of 7 million reported 2.8 million cases of malaria, the war in 1993 caused control efforts to break down, populations were moving and there was widespread resistance to chloroquine.

Acute respiratory infections (ARIs)

Refugee camp conditions facilitate the spread of ARIs and rank amongst the leading causes of death in displaced populations. The lack of shelter, overcrowding with poor ventilation, and exposure that characterize the refugee existence contribute to the susceptibility to ARIs with poor outcomes. Young children are particularly affected. In Kabul, in 1993, 30 per cent under-five deaths and 23 per cent of deaths in displaced persons were a result of ARIs (Salama *et al.* 2004). Vaccinations against malaria, diphtheria, and pertussis have led to decreased mortality from ARIs. It is not just that these pathogens cause ARIs but they also render hosts less able to defend themselves from bacterial infection.

Tuberculosis (TB)

Tuberculosis is becoming increasingly important in complex emergencies and situations of forced migration—in part as a result of disrupted therapy (Connolly *et al.* 2004). TB can become a major problem, leading to a large numbers of deaths. Poor nutrition and over-crowding exacerbate the risk of TB, as may underlying HIV in some populations. A recent study of instability and internal displacement in Timor-Leste revealed a number of problems in maintaining continuity of treatment for those with TB. As a result many may have incomplete or inadequate treatment.

Meningococcal meningitis

Meningococcal meningitis is a potentially major problem for refugees when they are in overcrowded settlements in an endemic area, such as the 'meningitis belt' of sub-Saharan Africa that stretches from Senegal to Ethiopia. In Africa, a threshold incidence of 15 cases per 100 000 population per week is used to define the presence of an 'epidemic'. In CEs, large epidemics have also been reported outside the traditional malaria belt. Democratic Republic of the Congo had six epidemics in 6 months in 2002 and epidemics have also occurred in Uganda, Rwanda, Tanzania (Salama *et al.* 2004). Immunization has proved to be an effective control measure but is only effective in epidemics, routine immunization is not effective as the current vaccines only produce immunity for 3–5 years and may not be used in children under two. Therefore, WHO only recommends mass immunization in areas where epidemic proportions have been reached, and they estimate that this can reduce deaths by up to 70 per cent.

Hepatitis

Outbreaks of hepatitis E have occurred in African refugee camps. It is transmitted by the entero-faecal route, and therefore water supplies are often involved. Case-fatality rates vary from 1–4 per cent but there have been particularly high attack rates and case-fatality rates (up to 20 per cent) reported amongst pregnant women. The high level of previous exposure to hepatitis A and B in developing countries makes it likely that any hepatitis epidemic with high attack rates in adults is likely to be caused by hepatitis E.

HIV/AIDS and other sexually transmitted diseases (STIs)

The pattern of HIV/AIDS and STIs amongst refugee populations in developing countries will depend on many factors, including the level of infection prior to displacement (Dualeh & Shears 2002). Spiegel (2004), working at the UNHCR, has highlighted the key preventive and other responses to HIV/AIDS. Conflict situations and camp conditions have often been thought to exacerbate the spread of sexually transmitted infections, due to breakdown of social structures, behavioural change, sexual violence, and lack of access to services and testing (Zwi & Cabral 1991). However, Spiegel (2004) describes other factors inherent in refugee situations that may retard the spread of these diseases, such as decreased mobility, and the possibility of a host country having increased services in comparison to the country from which people have fled. He argues that each situation should be examined independently and that the spread of sexually transmitted infections are most likely to be determined by the complex interactions between a number of groups: Refugees and their hosts, the original conflict-affected population, IDP populations in the country of origin and host communities in country of origin. He argues for public health responses to be broad and focus not only on camps but the entire situation, including host populations.

Other communicable diseases

Outbreaks of other less common communicable diseases have been reported in some refugee camps, as highlighted by Dualeh and Shears (2002). Typhoid fever is endemic in many tropical areas and may occur sporadically in refugee situations. Leishmaniasis and Trypanosomiasis have also been reported in epidemic proportions amongst displaced populations in Uganda and Sudan. Viral haemorrhagic fevers occur in selected areas and may place refugee communities at risk. Rift valley fever has been documented among Somali refugees in Kenya, Yellow fever occurred amongst displaced populations from Ethiopia to Sudan, and Dengue affect refugees in endemic areas of Southeast Asia.

Connolly *et al.* (2004) provide an excellent overview of the literature on communicable diseases and complex emergencies.

Malnutrition—protein energy deficiencies

Moderate to severe acute malnutrition is a common occurrence in refugee settings. Children are particularly affected, with some deteriorating in terms of nutritional status after arrival in camps, due to inadequate nutrition or diarrhoeal disease. Surveys undertaken between 1988–1995 documented a range of 11–81 per cent of children under 5 years suffering acute malnutrition in conflict affected populations (Toole & Waldman 1990). Acute malnutrition can be both the cause and effect of other illnesses, and contributes to mortality both directly and indirectly. Malnutrition and measles are particularly linked with malnutrition exacerbating measles, and measles itself contributing to high malnutrition rates in those that survive it (Toole & Waldman 1990). This 'synergistic relationship' that malnutrition has with communicable disease requires an integrated response aimed at improving nutrition combined with efforts to improve public health services.

Micronutrient deficiencies

As a result of inadequate food rations micronutrient deficiencies occur frequently in refugee populations. The most common diseases seen are iron and vitamin A deficiencies but other diseases include scurvy (vitamin C deficiency), pellagra (niacin and/or trytophan deficiency), and beriberi (thiamine deficiency). As Prinzo and Benoist (2002) discuss, the solutions are not simple and each setting may require a different approach, including providing fortified blended cereal and finding ways to exchange rations for locally produced fresh fruit and vegetables.

Food and nutritional interventions need to be responsive to cultural as well as economic issues.

Reproductive health

The reproductive health needs of refugees have gained recognition since the mid-1990s. The burden is undeniably greater for women as a result of insecurity in their social situations and gender-based violence.

Women lack basic necessities such as sanitary napkins and condoms, and pregnancy itself can be a serious health threat in settings in which services are lacking or overwhelmed (Krause *et al.* 2000). Referral services are often non-existent and birthing or abortion may be undertaken in unsafe situations. Women may have no, or limited, access or means to carry out family planning, rape and sexual coercion are typically increased, and pressures on women to rebuild the population. Female genital mutilation may occur and sexually transmitted infections, including HIV, may be relatively common (Krause *et al.* 2000). A particularly important set of risks relate to sexual and other forms of gender-based violence, common in all societies and increased where societal norms are less able to be enforced or reinforced, and in which men with guns can demand whatever they like in return for precious resources such as safety, food, and onward passage. Intense efforts have focused on improving all aspects of reproductive health for women affected by complex emergencies and forced migration—and a Minimum Initial Services Package has been produced to address these needs. A study by Hynes *et al.* (2002) showed that due to the strength of the response there have actually now been better reproductive health outcomes in refugee camps than in host population or origin countries. However, the lessons learned require expansion across settings.

Mental health and psychosocial needs

Mental health problems are recognized as an important source of morbidity globally (Prince *et al.* 2007) and are likely to be even greater amongst displaced populations. Epidemiological assessments have documented high rates of mental illness in these populations. Studies have tended to focus on trauma-related conditions, although low prevalence conditions such as psychosis have also proven significant in post-conflict and refugee setting. There is much debate about the validity of western-derived measurement and about the trauma focus, with further development of relevant culturally valid ways to measure psychiatric morbidity still required. Despite the measurement debate, there is clearly a substantial burden of mental distress in these settings, and support for vulnerable people is vital in situations of social breakdown, especially where usual systems of social support and healing are disrupted (Silove *et al.* 2000). It may be of value to identify and respond to the needs of three different groups of people who experience psychosocial and mental distress in these situations: Those who are mentally ill, who need treatment; those who have had particularly horrific experiences and need care and support in order to recover; and the vast majority who need a more stable social and political environment in which they can resume their normal day-to-day activities necessary to promote mental health.

IDPs

While IDPs in developing countries have very similar health problems to refugees, they also have particular vulnerabilities. Some of these result from falling through gaps in a system geared to protect a particular group of forced migrants (i.e. 'Convention refugees'). Particularly in developing countries, but also in more developed states, the limited data available suggest higher morbidity and mortality in IDPs compared with refugees (Salama *et al.* 2001). With limited protection granted by the international community, the responsibility for protection and assistance often lies with their own governments. Yet, it is these governments themselves that have often contributed to the displacement experienced. Governments may not even officially recognize the existence of IDPs for fear of international scrutiny or interference. A growing number of countries have developed laws and policies to govern responses to IDP populations but not all make concerted attempts to implement these policies, and even when there is political will the states involved are often the poorest countries of the world limiting their ability to respond. There is no mandated international body although UNHCR may include them amongst their persons of concern and they are increasingly supported by agencies which follow the UN's Guiding Principles on Internal Displacement.

IDP populations rarely experience access to health services at the same standard as offered to other citizens and are likely to be markedly poorer than those available to refugees. Recent efforts to improve quality and responsiveness of interventions in humanitarian crises and complex emergencies have contributed to better health outcomes. IDPs, however, have poor access to these improved systems of protection and assistance.

Collection of data is more difficult amongst IDP populations and relatively few studies focus specifically on IDPs. However, the IDP-specific health data that are available suggest that access to health care for IDPs is often extremely limited. Salama *et al.* (2001) show how some of highest mortality rates in humanitarian emergencies have been found in IDP populations; Sudan and Somali, for example, reached 8 per 10 000/day and 17 per 10 000/day (Salama *et al.*, quoting Toole & Waldman 1993). In Ethiopia and DRC, delays in vaccinations led to measles outbreaks. In Ajiep (southern Sudan), severe acute malnutrition amongst IDPS reached 36 per cent during a famine in 1998.

Although international humanitarian law applies to all civilians affected by armed conflict and therefore IDPs should be afforded the same protection and assistance as the un-displaced host population, they may be multiple reasons why IDPs face discrimination and therefore do not receive the help they need.

Even in developed countries IDPs may have poor health outcomes. They are often subject to the discrimination and exclusion experienced by their developing country counterparts. The Internal Displacement Monitoring Centre (IDMC) describe the situation for a number of IDP groups in developed nations; 'While IDPs in the Balkans generally have satisfactory access to water, sanitation and health care, they are more likely than the local population to suffer from trauma-related problems. Roma IDPs usually live in informal settlements with very poor sanitary conditions. IDPs in Azerbaijan and the Russian Federation access health care less easily than the local population in some areas, due to administrative inconsistencies, lack of health care facilities and the demand for informal payments for medical treatment' (Internal Displacement Monitoring Centre 2008).

IDPs, whether in developing or developed countries, are clearly living with a higher burden of illness and mortality than many other forced migrant groups. Initiatives are emerging that aim to support this extremely vulnerable population, but they are yet to be supported by any legal framework.

Refugees and asylum seekers in developed countries

Refugees and asylum seekers often reach destinations in developed countries after long, precarious journeys. Prior to the journey, they will have faced many of the routine health problems that present themselves in disrupted developing country settings. The journey itself will have produced health challenges; people may have been detained at points along the way or experienced significant anxiety and distress through difficult and dangerous journeys and experiences. On arrival, the range of situations they find themselves in will further shape their health condition. Those who have applied for refugee status prior to arrival may have undergone health checks already in the country of origin, as is the practice of many developed countries; therefore, certain health conditions may have been picked up. Depending on the country they arrive in, they will then have a different range of options available to address their health problems. However, those applying for refugee status on arrival have an even more complicated journey; they may be detained for short or long periods, they may have extensive periods on temporary visas or they may find themselves living illegally without authorization from the host country. Typically asylum seekers are often isolated with difficulty in communication, in a situation of poverty, discrimination and a lack of social structure, causing many to suffer from trauma-related problems and many general health problems, exacerbated by poor provision of health information and barriers to accessing to services.

Biggs and Skull (2003) discuss the specific medical conditions that may be present amongst refugees in developed countries. These include communicable disease such as TB, HIV, STIs, hepatitis B and C, and parasitic diseases, all compounded by incomplete immunization. In addition, nutritional deficiencies (vitamin D in particular), mental health problems, and other non-communicable diseases such as diabetes and reproductive health issues are common.

Screening for health problems among newly 'arrived' refugees, or prior to arrival for those applying for refugee status overseas, is common practice. Biggs and Skull (2003) point out that there is little evidence demonstrating that screening has proved effective as many people have limited contact with services and many are lost to follow up. Refugees seeking asylum in the United States are screened before arrival to identify 'inadmissible conditions' such as HIV, TB, and leprosy. They may also be screened for diseases that are known to be prevalent and targets of public health intervention. For example, Somali refugees were mass treated for malaria and intestinal parasites. The types of health problems sought and treated in newly arrived immigrants also reflect particular areas of concern for asylum seekers, including infectious disease, gynaecological health (rape, genital surgery, STIs), and mental health (torture, trauma) (Adams *et al.* 2007).

Burnett and Peel (2001) evaluated the health needs of asylum seekers and refugees in Britain. They point out that these groups are subject to 'poverty, dependence, and lack of cohesive social support' as well as racial discrimination. They consider a range of studies examining the health status of refugees and found, for example, that 21 per cent of migrants to Spain from sub-Saharan Africa were chronic carriers of hepatitis B, and 3.4 per cent of refugees arriving in the United States in 1988 had tuberculosis. They highlight the lack of screening programmes available and how the focus has tended to be on protecting hosts rather than a responsibility to provide health care to all.

One specific refugee and asylum health condition that has been investigated somewhat more extensively than other health issues is mental health (see Chapter 9.7). Gerritsen *et al.* (2004) describe how early research focused on those who used services, or victims of trauma, followed by early population-based studies in Western settings which have tended to focus on psychiatric disorders such as post traumatic stress disorder (PTSD), anxiety, and depression. In a review of the literature, Fazel *et al.* (2005) show documented rates of PTSD from 4–70 per cent, depression 3–88 per cent, and anxiety 2–80 per cent. Their meta-analysis suggests that 1 in 10 refugees in Western countries have PTSD, 1 in 20 has major depression, 1 in 25 has a generalized anxiety disorder. Although lower than some estimates, this is still 10 times higher than rates of PTSD in the general population in the United States. Data for asylum seekers alone is sparse but there are reasons to believe even they have even higher rates due to their vulnerability because of disruption, separation from family members, increased levels of torture and trauma, lack of language skills and the often hostile reception from host population fuelled by media perceptions. The current trend towards detention, and temporary rather than permanent protection have added extra stress, as evidenced by studies of asylum seekers in detention centres and on temporary protection visas showing very high rates of mental illness (Silove *et al.* 2000, 2007).

Problems that asylum seekers in particular face, rather than refugees, relate to issues of having a temporary and often contested legal status, and in some cases actually being considered illegal, with implications (real or perceived) for access to health services. Many countries such as the United Kingdom and Australia have fluctuating policies with regards to what asylum seekers, of differing categories, may be entitled to in terms of health care. This can act as a barrier to health for many asylum seekers. The increased use of detention for asylum seekers, whilst claims are processed, has been challenged heavily by health professionals as a result of evidence that it is detrimental to health. The other popular policy of extending only temporary protection to some asylum seekers, therefore also causing confusion with regards to health entitlements, and long-term insecurity with associated health risks, has also caused concern to health professionals (Silove *et al.* 2000). Health care for asylum seekers may be difficult to access on many levels; policies of active deterrent of asylum seekers may mean they are not entitled to care, or there may be lack of prioritizing refugees, health professionals often misunderstand what the policies are and may refuse to register asylum seekers, they also fear the burden of vulnerable groups, those that do offer treatment may lack of understanding of the refugee health situation, temporary registration with GPs may be offered rather than permanent (limiting access to immunizations and screening), language problems are also a great barrier, with many practitioners having inadequate access to interpreting services.

Harris and Telfer (2001) estimated that in 1999–2000 there were over 10 000 asylum seekers living in the community in Australia. Many had to survive for many months or years with no right to work and no medical cover through the national Medicare scheme, resulting in untreated medical conditions. A study in Sydney suggested that most presenting to a Asylum Seeker Centre (ASC) providing health services had fairly serious psychological or physical symptoms. Some related to trauma and torture, others were infectious diseases, musculoskeletal complaints, and gynaecological problems. Up to 40 per cent of the asylum seekers were denied Medicare. A few are picked up by Asylum Seeker Assistance Scheme (ASAS) and the Red Cross assists others. Hospital fees are particularly high and case studies have shown that some are denied hospital treatment until assurance of payment is provided.

Trafficked and smuggled people

People that are trafficked or smuggled are not an entirely distinct group from other types of forced migrants already described.

Trafficked people have been coerced or tricked into allowing another person to organize their passage to another country; also smuggled across borders are those who 'voluntarily' migrate for a vast range of reasons but feel unable to do so through legal channels. Although these groups may appear distinct from refugee populations they may include convention refugees and others whose circumstances are very close to those of refugees. Resorting to illegal and clandestine methods of migrating to another country, either through being coerced and misled or through having such limited choices as to choose this route, is often a result of many of the factors behind the forced migration of refugees and internally displaced people.

Gushulak and MacPherson (2000) describe some of the reasons why people may fall into a trafficking situation. Poverty, exposure to violence, restrictive barriers—e.g. screening for certain diseases or security barriers, slow processing of routine immigration application which may cause delay to family reunification—all may encourage people to take alternative routes—especially when traffickers may offer what appear to be attractive possibilities. They state that the reasons why someone is more likely to migrate through these illegal methods are also reasons that place a person at higher risk of having poor health prior to migration. The journeys faced by trafficked and smuggled people are often extremely precarious, with high levels of morbidity and mortality attached as a result. Un-seaworthy and over crowded boats on long journeys, stowed in containers, attached to carriers, attempts to cross inhospitable land with extremes of temperature, drowning from swimming attempts, violence from traffickers, illegal activities such as smuggling drugs with people. On arrival people are then subject to many of the difficulties already outlined that face asylum seekers. Some trafficked and smuggled people may seek asylum and depending on the policies of the countries may incur some health benefits, however, many will be forced into illegal employment and be either too scared or prevented from approaching health services. Disease prevention and control in this population will be extremely poor—leading to increased prevalence of disease in the trafficked community as a whole.

Busza *et al.* (2004) examine the need for careful understanding of trafficking situations and to unravel the local dynamics. They state that even when intermediaries are involved, and even when they are taking people into exploitative arenas such as sex work, these situations remain a complex mixture of voluntary and forced migration. Whilst economic disadvantage may fuel the choice, there is still a choice being made in some contexts and organizations seeking to stem the flow or break up these systems may compromise the health or the individuals involved more than it helps. Attempts to 'save' people may make them even more vulnerable—e.g. the raiding of brothels and other such moves can force vulnerable people to go underground making engagement with health services difficult.

The health of trafficked and smuggled people is affected by fact they cannot easily be separated out from each other or from other types of 'voluntary' migration that are not truly voluntary but have strong forces pushing people on. The policies developed by states towards any of these groups are likely to impact on the capacity of other groups to access health care. Displaced people are more vulnerable to trafficking and may in desperation turn to smugglers. This should be kept in mind by health professionals to avoid vulnerable people missing out on essential services and support.

Public health solutions and interventions

Forced migration, as described above, clearly has major impacts on public health. Specific solutions and interventions need to be sensitive to culture and context.

Key actors and organizations in refugee health

There is an extensive range of organizations involved in addressing forced migration. The United Nations has designated the United Nations High Commissioner for Refugees as the key multilateral agency for identifying and dealing with refugee issues. More recently, the mandate of UNHCR, as described earlier, has been extended to include other 'people of concern' including IDPs and asylum seekers. Other agencies with a specific mandate for dealing with forced migrants include the International Organisation on Migration, the International Centre for Migration and Health, the American Refugee Committee International, the US Committee on Refugees, and the Global IDP Project.

A wide range of multilateral agencies including the World Health Organization (WHO), UN Population Fund (UNFPA), UNICEF, International Committee of the Red Cross (ICRC), International Federation of Red Cross and Red Crescent Societies (IFRC), and UNAIDS have some concern with forced migrants. Key non-governmental organizations (NGOs) include Merlin, Medicines sans Frontieres (MSF), International Medical Corps (IMC), International Rescue Committee (IRC), OXFAM, Save the Children Fund, CARE, Caritas, CONCERN, and the Norwegian Refugee Council. Academic bodies include the Oxford University Refugee Studies Program, the Centers for Disease Control (CDC), and the Refugee Studies Program in Cairo. A number of important journals, notably the *Journal of Refugee Studies, Disasters, Conflict and Health*, and *Forced Migration Online*, provide avenues for academic debate.

Developing countries and complex emergency settings

The principles of public health and epidemiology only began to be systematically applied to complex emergency situations from the early 1970s (Salama *et al.* 2004). Since then, new academic and practitioner fields have developed, including emergency public health and public health nutrition. With the introduction of an indicator to measure the impact of a complex emergency through crude mortality rates (CMRs), alongside the development of simplified measurements of malnutrition, and threshold rates for epidemics, it has become increasingly possible to draw meaningful inferences from data collected.

An understanding of the dynamics of disease and related mortality in CEs has grown, and practice improved on the basis of experience and research evidence. Guidelines and technical manuals have been produced and efforts enhanced to promote organizational learning and enhanced service delivery, building on a growing evidence-base. The call for evidence with which to inform policy and practice (Banatvala & Zwi 2000) reinforced what was already happening in the field where practitioners and academics were drawing lessons from experiences and enhancing the quality of their responses.

Mortality rates are now much lower than previously seen, malnutrition declining in many settings, and measles, a major killer in the past, less catastrophic following efforts to ensure early immunization of children. Enhanced understanding of risks of communicable diseases has decreased risks, although failures to apply evidence, such as in Goma following the Rwandan genocide, still lead to tens of thousands of preventable deaths. Epidemics of some communicable diseases are better controlled and may be less serious and last for shorter periods given improved surveillance and earlier detection of outbreaks. The pattern seen is often similar to the baseline in developing countries, in terms of the major killers. However, the shift has been to seeing many of the highest mortality rates outside of camps, where the public health response has not been as well developed.

Toole and Waldman (1997) describe the need for primary, secondary, and tertiary prevention. In primary prevention, they argue that political and diplomatic mechanisms should be developed to prevent conflicts evolving to the point of mass displacement, and that epidemiology may be able to add value in studying some of the dynamics that indicate conflict developing on a large scale. Secondary prevention comprises early detection of population movements, contingency planning so that relevant actors are prepared for the scale and nature of likely public health crises, having well trained personnel with knowledge and experience in dealing with the health problems associated with refugee situations and able to rapidly assess and intervene in partnership with local organizations, along with the capacity to monitor and evaluate programmes swiftly and effectively. Tertiary prevention involves channelling resources into combating the sources of morbidity and mortality already outlined. This involves providing shelter and protection, adequate food rations, adequate clean water and sanitation facilities, programmes for preventing specific communicable diseases, preparing for epidemics, specific programmes such as maternal and child health or mental health, managing diarrhoeal disease, and setting up health information systems.

The social, cultural, and political challenges of instituting these levels of prevention, alongside the practical implications of working in such settings, are substantial. Salama *et al.* (2004) describe how the field has been growing over 30 years, with increasing attention by humanitarian actors since the 1990s to codify technical guidelines. In the early 1990s, there was a growing disappointment and recognition amongst the actors attempting to engage with these complexities, and provide emergency assistance to refugees, that the field was uncoordinated and lacking in technical direction. Research, adverse publicity, and heightened calls for accountability around standards of service delivery and to the supposed beneficiaries of humanitarian interventions, all pointed to the need for significant improvements.

Initiatives were beginning to emerge that were investigating ways to address these issues, but the field was ultimately galvanized by events in 1994 in Goma, Zaire. The unprecedented rapid influx of refugees and the resulting massive cholera epidemic, producing one of the highest mortality rates recorded, led to a serious reappraisal of humanitarian work in these settings. The Joint Evaluation of Emergency Assistance to Rwanda was an impressive, multi-agency, multi-donor-funded initiative, paving the way to a deep review of the humanitarian and relief field and the standards of care and conduct.

In terms of future public health directions, Salama *et al.* (2004) describe the need to move beyond the current refugee and IDP paradigms, as non-camp populations affected by conflict are now often greater in number and burden, and mechanisms to deliver services to such populations are less clear. There is a need for enhanced coverage in all settings of known effective public health interventions, and for the more upstream causes of CEs to be addressed. The technical needs identified include the development of more context-specific methods for assessing mortality rates as an indicator based on surrounding baseline CMRs, and considering which other indicators may point to a deteriorating situation such as fluctuations in disease incidence, levels of displacement, and decreasing food security. They suggest that implementation of control measures should be early, not when mortality and malnutrition are already high, and that whilst communicable disease control should continue to be prioritized along with nutrition and food security, that enhanced efforts at addressing mental health, reproductive health, and neonatal health should also be incorporated. Important policy issues include better means of determining direction and co-ordination of public health interventions, early identification of a lead agency, and greater effort to support fledgling governments to take the lead with the support of a coherent international system. They suggest that the skills of relief workers should be strengthened and broadened to include knowledge of assessment and prevention of disease, monitoring and evaluation, and international systems, policies, and regulatory bodies.

Ensuring equity in the response and equity in access to services and resources made available remains a considerable and under-emphasized challenge.

Developed countries

In developed countries, the complex political arena and the increasingly restrictive views of host populations towards asylum seekers and refugees complicates the task of addressing the public health of forced migrants. Whilst an array of motivated and effective actors plays a number of different roles in this field, there are few central bodies charged with overseeing the public health of forced migrants as a whole. The policies of the host nations themselves are likely to shape the public health landscape and in situations where these policies seem to be detrimental to the health of this population, public health professionals may find themselves having to take increasingly political roles to fulfil their public health duties.

Advocacy groups and health professional organizations have set up refugee and asylum seeker health networks and centres through which to provide services and support and advocate for more inclusive social and health policies.

The Health of London Project established a health centre in 1999 to provide access to good-quality primary care for forced migrants. The service aims to provide a thorough initial health assessment, along with effective responses to issues such as mental health problems and communicable diseases. In Europe, Medecins du Monde, an NGO, has stepped in to provide care for groups with restricted access to healthcare, particularly failed asylum seekers.

The best way in which to organize health care for resettled refugees, and for asylum seekers, remains contentious. A key issue point of debate is whether they should be integrated within mainstream services, or offered separately through distinct services for these marginalized groups (Finney Lamb & Cunningham 2003). Such centres are often voluntarily run and unable to cover the full extent of need. Hull and Boomla (2006) discuss the implications of such NGO provision, including some of the unanticipated negative aspects.

Another potential theoretical divide that can emerge with health approaches to asylum seekers and refugees is that between public health and human rights frameworks. Governments are more responsive to public health arguments whereby health problems of forced migrant populations may be addressed for the benefit of the wider population, often highlighting the risk brought with incoming refugees and forced migrants of communicable diseases. However, these approaches focus more on protecting the host than the forced migrants' right to receive health care (Burnett & Peel 2001) and may reinforce discrimination and marginalization of the migrants who are seen as posing a risk to the general community and demanding excessive use of public services (Grove & Zwi 2006). Tarantola *et al.* (2008) argue for much closer links between public health, human rights and development—all equally relevant to forced migration.

Hull and Boola (2006) describe recent UK government proposals to deny GPs the discretion of registering overseas visitors including failed asylum seekers, and to provide care to them. They highlight the possibility that such a policy will inadvertently increase costs through more emergency admissions, and they stress that such a policy is a breach of human rights, ethically unsupportable, and may place clinicians in conflict with their professional duties.

Ashcroft (2005) describes the language of the UK and Australian governments as 'Orwellian' in an overview of their approaches to asylum seekers and health. In discussing the UK government's move to make failed asylum seekers pay for all non-emergency care, despite not having the right to work, he states that the treatment of asylum seekers is an ethical issue and that denial of medical treatment should not be used as a lever to exclude people or get them to leave the country. In some cases, the presence of HIV seropositivity has been used to exclude refugees from the opportunity to resettle in a third country; this is of particular concern given the heightened risk of violence and infection that may characterize the lives of many refugees. Using this against such vulnerable community members is a double victimization.

As Silove et al. (2000) stated 'the medical profession has a legitimate role in commenting on the general and mental health risks of imposing restrictive and discriminatory measures on asylum seekers, especially when some of these administrative procedures threaten one of the fundamental principles underpinning the practice of medicine: primum non nocere' (do no harm).

Further study to document the patterns of disease, the links to the asylum experience and impact of policies, not only on forced migrant health but also the implications for host populations are required. Given the more restrictive policy environment, health professionals require a strong evidence base from which to lobby for improved access to services as a first step in improving the health of refugees and asylum seekers in developed countries.

Emerging issues for public health professionals

Many of the issues raised above have a technical focus, even if their links with broader sociopolitical issues have been acknowledged. In this concluding section of the chapter, we highlight some of the many issues which challenge professionals and societies, not only on a technical level, but in terms of the values underpinning how we, individually and collectively, whether as citizens or professionals, see and respond to others, especially those who have been forced to flee.

This section seeks to highlight, briefly, a number of key themes: Globalization and poverty, quality and accountability, ethics and researching with forced migrants, voice, visibility, and agency. They are central to understanding the context within which forced migration arises and health needs should be understood and addressed.

Globalization and poverty

There is increasing evidence of widening gaps in income and basic needs between the well-off and the impoverished in many settings. Labonte and Schrecker (2005) identify the key links between current patterns of globalization and the influence these have on the social determinants of health. The challenges are evident in the failure to address the Millennium Development Goal (MDG) targets, while extreme wealth continues to be generated and monopolized by small fractions of the world's population. Resource constraints are likely to increase; countries engaging actively with global economic and political opportunities may do well but not all their citizens will necessarily benefit.

Evidence of gaps are widespread; and it is apparent that the MDGs, a major driving force at present in international development, do not adequately address issues of equity (Attaran 2005). Such concerns are likely to be amplified in relation to especially vulnerable and socially excluded communities such as forced migrants, data on whom may be unavailable and systems of response to which will be fragmented, uncoordinated, and inadequately monitored. Colson (2007) argues cogently that much greater emphasis should be placed on understanding the 'factors that provide the impetus to leave' and not focusing only on the aftermath of such forced migrations.

Quality and accountability

A key challenge in engaging with situations of violence, social exclusion, and disempowerment is in ensuring that work undertaken to assist those affected does no harm, or at least strives to limit the potential harm and maximize the potential value. The international community, through the United Nations, other multilateral and bilateral agencies, international NGOs, all ostensibly seek to assist those forced to flee or migrate.

One way in which evidence improvements are underway is in relation to enhancing and seeking to assure the quality of humanitarian and relief work. Major Quality and Accountability initiatives such as SPHERE, the Humanitarian Code of Conduct, the Humanitarian Accountability Partnership, and many others contribute to enhanced practice. There remains a need to facilitate self-reflection and open review, transparency of difficulties limitations and failures, and promotion and funding for the search to do better.

The vast majority of incentives currently in place, however, encourage the hiding, rather than the declaration, of weaknesses, so as to elicit the next tranche of funding. This is counter-productive when seeking to reflect and improve services and their responsiveness to need. New thinking is required: How do we develop systems of trust and collegiality, mutual support between affected communities, services providers, and agencies, to ensure that all incentives operate to maximize the gain for those at greatest risk?

New initiatives in the humanitarian and relief areas of activity seek to enhance practice and open out debate and public scrutiny. In so doing, weaknesses are identified, guidelines and lessons for better practice formulated, and processes which seek to engage and creatively respond to problems, developed. Taking forward such action requires promoting an ability to report and record limitations and inadequacies, and to carefully and systematically document strengths and limitations, weaknesses and potentials, to address real problems. Services are never ideal and always have constraints and limits; it is crucial to establish ways of examining them such that opportunities to change, to experiment, to creatively engage with solving problems are established.

New and enhanced knowledge management systems would be most valuable if they assisted in finding innovative means of conceptualizing problems, sharing information and insights of what works in different contexts, and develop systems to ensure accountability to the intended beneficiaries, the forced migrants themselves.

Ethics and researching with forced migrants

Ethical issues require considerable attention especially given the power imbalances present and in relation to research. Forced migrants may be especially vulnerable and risk being abused, either through their stories and survival strategies being exposed and used by their opponents to undermine them; the very practice of talking with an outsider or sharing information may heighten risk, vulnerability, and the attention of those seeking further to undermine and disempower. Real risks may result from security lapses, confidentiality lapses, exposure of coping strategies and adaptations; as well as stigma and reinforcement of difference and of 'otherness'.

A major challenge in research with refugees and other forced migrants is to assist them in documenting their experiences of forced migration (Mackenzie *et al.* 2007). In so doing, the locus of power in the research relationship has the potential to shift from the researcher him or herself, to the communities being researched. The project may shift from research *on* refugees to research *with* refugees and research *by* refugees for action and change.

While this may be conceptually and morally attractive, the practicalities of achieving this are impeded at multiple levels, not least of which is establishing a trusting relationship between the researcher and the communities with whom they research. Engaging with forced migrants is itself a major challenge: Such communities are often highly dependent on others, and may be reliant on outside agencies with expertise and resources and/or on local power-brokers in control of the basic necessities of life and survival—food, water, shelter, and security.

Zwi *et al.* (2006) have highlighted the importance of reconceptualizing such research to consider the potential to ensure benefit and reciprocity for the subjects of research and to shift the locus of decision-making in their direction. They offer a model to describe this process, while Mackenzie *et al.* (2007) present a case study of applying many of these considerations to work with forced migrants on the Thai–Burmese border. Of note is the transfer of power to community organizations, with women's groups from the Thai–Burmese border having control over the stories and narratives collected from them and academics being required to obtain permission from them to publish and distribute and write up such material.

Innovative approaches to research are emerging and warrant support. Youth-focused research highlights the importance of young people in exploring and documenting their own lives and experiences. Young people play a central role in refining and redefining the issues, identifying the challenges and the potential approaches to solving them through new models of participatory action research. Such collaboration needs to build skills, resilience, and opportunities to shape the future.

Voice, visibility, and agency

There is increasing recognition of the importance of hearing from those most affected by any public health condition and ensuring that their voices are heard; empowering them to help shape the proposed solutions. Black (2003) emphasizes the importance of advocacy as a central component of work with marginalized and disempowered groups and reinforces the centrality of ensuring that the voices of those affected, and of the range of stakeholders engaged, is heard.

The voices of forced migrants may be silenced while those of powerful agencies and governments are privileged in shaping our understanding both of the problems and of the solutions which surround forced migration (Harrell-Bond & Voutira 2007). Power imbalances, vulnerability, and cultural and linguistic differences are among the many barriers to creating an environment in which refugees and IDPs are able to take an active part in shaping solutions. As with the youth, truly participatory models of action and research require sensitivity to the challenges of the context and understanding of the conditions that usually deny refugees a voice.

It is crucial that we hear the voices of those most affected by forced migration if we are to recognize the range of experiences, and the positive and negative change and transformation which results. As Eastmond (2007) states eloquently: 'while transformation and change are part of the refugee experience, not all change is perceived as loss or defined as problematic or unwelcome by all individuals involved. Nor are refugees necessarily helpless victims, but rather likely to be people with agency and voice'. Learning and recognizing how agency, transformation, resilience, adaptation and change are shaped, notably, but not only, in relation to gender and power, would not be possible without hearing from and learning with, those most affected.

Concluding remarks

Forced migrant populations frequently suffer vast health challenges. Their experiences need to be understood within the context of accelerating globalization, with its positive and negative features transforming the lives of millions of people.

The role of public health professionals in working alongside forced migrants to bring about improvements in their health is demanding and complex. A comprehensive understanding of the dynamics of forced migration and sensitivity to the constraints placed on individuals and populations is vital to gain trust and provide opportunities for transforming health outcomes. Particularly, given the increasingly restrictive environments that forced migrants find themselves in, public health professionals can have a crucial role in advocating for forced migrant health, enabling forced migrants to speak and be heard, and to bring about improvements in their own health.

Improving knowledge and understanding is central to affirming the rights and the agency of those affected. Public health can play an important role, and indeed has done so, in improving technical quality of service delivery. Key gaps remain, however, in understanding, appreciating, and responding to the varied ways in which those forced to move seek to shape, transform, and better their own lives and experiences.

Further reading

The following manuals give technical advice in managing public health aspects of forced migration.

Médecins Sans Frontières (MSF)(1997) *Refugee health: an approach to emergency situations.* London: Macmillan. Available at http://www.refbooks.msf.org/msf_docs/en/Refugee_Health/RH1.pdf accessed 28th May 2008.

World Health Organization (2006). Communicable disease control in emergencies. A field manual. Available at http://www.who.int/infectious-disease-news/IDdocs/whocds200527/whocds200527chapters/ accessed 28th May 2008.

Relevant websites

Forced Migration Online—http://www.forcedmigration.org/

The Humanitarian Accountability Partnership—http://www.hapinternational.org/

SPHERE—www.sphereproject.org

ALNAP—'learning, accountability, performance in humanitarian action' www.alnap.org

United Nations High Commission for Refugees—www.unhcr.org

References

Adams, K., Gardiner, L., and Assefi, N. (2007). Healthcare challenges from the developing world: post-immigration refugee medicine. *British Medical Journal*, **328**, 1548–52.

Allotey, P.A. and Reidpath, D.D. (2003). Refugee intake: reflections on inequality. *Australian and New Zealand Journal of Public Health*, **27**, 12–6.

Apodaca, C. (1998). Human rights abuses: precursor to refugee flight? *Journal of Refugee Studies*, **11**, 80–93.

Ashcroft, R. (2005). Standing up for the medical rights of asylum seekers. *Journal of Medical Ethics*, **31**, 125–6.

Attaran, A. (2005). An immeasurable crisis? a criticism of the millennium development goals and why they cannot be measured. *PLoS Medicine*, **2**(10): e318 doi:10.1371/journal.pmed.0020318.

Bakewell, O. (2008). Can we ever rely on refugee statistics? Radical statistics. Available at http://www.radstats.org.uk/no072/article1.htm accessed 25th May 2008.

Banatvala, N. and Zwi, A.B. (2000). Public health and humanitarian interventions: developing the evidence base. *British Medical Journal*, **321**, 101–5.

Barnett, L. (2002) Global governance and the evolution of the international refugee regime. *International Journal Refugee Law*, **14**, 238–262.

Baum, F. (2001). Health equity justice and globalisation: some lessons from the People's Health Assembly. *Journal of Epidemiology and Community Health*, **55**, 613–6.

Biermann, F. and Boas, I. (2008). Preparing for a warmer world – towards a global governance system to protect climate refugees. Available at http://www.glogov.org/images/doc/WP33.pdf accessed 27th May 2008.

Biggs, B. and Skull, S. (2003). Refugee health: clinical issues. In *The health of refugees: public health perspectives from crisis to settlement* (ed. P. Allotey), pp. 54–67. Oxford University Press, Melbourne.

Black, R. (2003). Ethical codes in humanitarian emergencies: from practice to research? *Disasters*, **27**(2), 95–108.

Burnett, A. and Peel, M. (2001). Asylum seekers and refugees in Britain: health needs of asylum seekers and refugees. *British Medical Journal*, **322**, 544–7.

Busza, J., Castle, S. and Diarra, A. (2004). Trafficking and health. *British Medical Journal*, **328**, 1369–71.

Cartagena Declaration on Refugees. (1984). Colloquium on the International Protection of Refugees in Central America, Mexico and Panama. Available at http://www.unhcr.org/cgi-bin/texis/vtx/research/opendoc.htm?tbl=RSDLEGAL&id=3ae6b36ec accessed 27th May 2008.

Castles, S. (2003). Toward a sociology of Forced Migration and Social Transformation. *Sociology*, **37**, 13–34.

Castles, S. (2004). Confronting the realities of forced migration. Available at http://www.migrationinformation.org/Feature/print.cfm?ID=222 accessed 27th May 2008.

Cernea, M. (2007). Development-induced and conflict-induced IDPs: bridging the research divide. *Forced Migration Review*, March, 25–7.

Chan, E.Y. and Sondorp, E. (2007). Medical interventions following natural disasters: missing out on chronic medical needs. *Asia Pacific Journal of Public Health*, **19**(Special Issue), 45–51.

Colson, E. (2007). Linkage methodology: no man is an island. *Journal of Refugee Studies*, **20**, 321–33.

Connolly, M.A., Gayer, M., Ryan, M.J. *et al.* (2004). Communicable diseases in complex emergencies: impact and challenges. *The Lancet*, **364**, 1974–83.

Crisp, J. (1999). *'Who has counted the refugees?' UNHCR and the politics of numbers*. UNHCR, Geneva.

Courtland Robinson, W. (2003). Risks and rights: the causes, consequences, and challenges of development-induced displacement: The Brookings Institution-SAIS Project on Internal Displacement. Available at http://www.brookings.edu/~/media/Files/rc/reports/2003/05humanrights_robinson/didreport.pdf accessed 27th May 2008.

Deng, F. (1998). The guiding principles on internal displacement. United Nations, New York, February 11.

Dualeh, M. and Shears, P. (2002). *Refugees and other displaced populations.* In *Oxford Textbook of Public Health* (eds. R. Detels, J. McEwen, R. Beaglehole, H. Tanaka). Oxford University Press, Oxford.

Eastmond, M. (2007). Stories as lived experience: narratives in forced migration research. *Journal of Refugee Studies*, **20**, 248–64.

El-Hinnawi, E. (1985). *Environmental refugees.* United Nations Environment Programme, Nairobi.

Essed, P., Frerks, G. and Schrijvers, J. (eds.) (2004). *Refugees and the transformation of societies. Agency, policies, ethics and politics*. Berghahn Books, New York and Oxford.

Fazel, M., Wheeler, J. and Danesh, J. (2005). Prevalence of serious mental disorder in 7000 refugees resettled in western countries: a systematic review. *Lancet*, **365**, 1309–14.

Feachem, R. (2001). Globalisation is good for your health, mostly. *British Medical Journal*, **323**, 504–6.

Finney Lamb, C., Cunningham, M. (2003). Dichotomy or decision-making: specialization and mainstreaming in health service design for refugees. In: Allotey P, ed. *The Health of Refugees. Public Health Perspectives from Crisis to Settlement.* Melbourne: Oxford University Press. pp. 156–168.

Forced_Migration Online. (2008). *What is Forced Migration?* Available at http://www.forcedmigration.org/whatisfm.htm accessed 25th May 2008.

Gerritsen, A., Bramsen, I., Deville, W., van Willigen, L., Hovens, J. and van derPloeg, H. (2004). Health and health care utilisation among asylum seekers and refugees in the Netherlands: design of a study. *BMC Public Health*, **4**, 1–10.

Grove, N. and Zwi, A.B. (2006). Our health and theirs: forced migration,othering and public health. *Social Science and Medicine*, **62**, 1931–42.

Gushulak, B. and MacPherson, D. (2000). Health issues associated with the smuggling and trafficking of migrants. *Journal of Immigrant Health*, **2**, 67–78.

Harrell-Bond, B. (2000). 'Are refugee camps good for children?' UNHCR, Geneva. Available at http://www.jha.ac/articles/u029.htm accessed 28th May 2008.

Harrell-Bond, B. and Voutira, E. (2007). In search of 'invisible actors': barriers to access in refugee research. *Journal of Refugee Studies*, **20**, 282–98.

Harrell-Bond, B., Voutira, E., and Leopold, M. (1992). Counting the refugees: gifts, givers, patrons and clients. *Journal of Refugee Studies*, **5**, 205–25.

Harris, M.F. and Telfer, B.L. (2001). The health needs of asylum seekers living in the community. *Medical Journal of Australia*, **175**, 589–92.

Hull, S. and Boomla, K. (2006). Primary care for refugees and asylum seekers. *British Medical Journal*, **332**, 62–3.

Hynes, M., Sheik, M., Wilson, H.G. and Spiegel, P. (2002). Reproductive health indicators and outcomes among refugee and internally displaced persons in postemergency phase camps. *Journal of the American Medical Association*, **288**, 595–603.

Internal Displacement Monitoring Centre (2008). Health and IDPs. Accessed 27th May 2008. http://www.internal-displacement.org/8025708F004D404D/(httpPages)/61944755DF644EE1C12570C9005BAC3A?OpenDocument

Krause, S.K., Jones, R.K., and Purdin, S.J. (2000). Programmatic Responses to Refugees' Reproductive Health Needs. *International Family Planning Perspectives*, **26**, 181–7.

Labonte, R. and Schrecker, T. (2005). Globalization and social determinants of health: promoting health equity in global governance (part 3 of 3). *Globalization and Health*, **3**, 7.

Lee, K. (2004). Globalisation: what is it and how does it affect health? *Medical Journal of Australia*, **180**, 156–8.

MacDonald, T.H. (2007). *The Global Human Right to Health – dream or possibility?* Radcliffe Publishing, Oxford, New York.

Mackenzie, C., McDowell, C., and Pittaway, E. (2007). Beyond 'Do No Harm': The Challenge of Constructing Ethical Relationships in Refugee Research. *Journal of Refugee Studies*, **20**, 299–319.

Martin, S. (2002). Averting forced migration in countries in transition. *International Migration*, **40**, 25–40.

McAdam, J. (2006). The Refugee Convention as a rights blueprint for persons in need of international protection. UNHCR, Geneva.

Moore, W. and Shellman, S. (2004). Fear of persecution: forced migration 1952–1995. *Journal of Conflict Resolution*, **48**, 723–45.

Moore, P.S., Marfin, A.A., Quenemoen, L.E., Gessner, B.D., Ayub, Y.S. and Sullivan, K.M. (1993). Mortality rates in displaced and resident populations of Central Somalia during the famine of 1992. *Lancet*, **341**, 935–8.

Myers, N. (1993). Environmental refugees in a globally warmed world. *BioScience*, **43**, 752–61.

Myers, N. and Kent, J. (1995). *Environmental Exodus: An Emergent Crisis in the Global Arena*. Climate Institute, Washington DC.

Organisation of African Unity (1969). *OAU Convention Governing the Specific Aspects of the Refugee Problems in Africa*. Addis-Ababa. Available at http://www.unhcr.org/basics/BASICS/45dc1a682.pdf accessed 28th May 2008.

Office for the Coordination of Humanitarian Affairs (1998). *Guiding Principles on Internal Displacement*. Available at http://www.reliefweb.int/ocha_ol/pub/idp_gp/idp.html accessed 28th May 2008.

Prince, M., Patel, V., Saxena, S. *et al.* (2007). No health without mental health. *Lancet*, **370**, 859–77.

Prinzo, W.Z. and Benoist, B. (2002). Meeting the challenges of micronutrient deficiencies in emergency affected populations. *Proceedings of the Nutrition Society*, **61**, 251–7.

Salama, P., Spiegel, P., and Brennan, R. (2001). No less vulnerable: the internally displaced in humanitarian emergencies. *Lancet*, **357**, 1430–2.

Salama, P., Spiegel, P., Talley, L., and Waldman, R. (2004). Lessons learned from complex emergencies over past decade. *Lancet*, **364**, 1801–13.

Siddique, A.K., Salam, A., Islam, M.S., Akram, K., Majumdar, R.N., Zaman, K., Fronczak, N., and Laston, S. (1995). Why treatment centres failed to prevent cholera deaths among Rwandan refugees in Goma, Zaire. *The Lancet*, **345**, 359(3).

Silove, D., Steel, Z., and Watters, C. (2000). Policies of deterrence and the mental health of asylum seekers. *Journal of the American Medical Association*, **284**, 604–11.

Silove D., Ekblad S., Mollica R. (2000). The rights of the severely mentally ill in post-conflict societies. *Lancet*. Vol **355**, issue 9214, 1548–1549.

Silove, D., Austin, P., and Steel, Z. (2007). No refuge from terror: The impact of detention on the mental health of trauma-affected refugees seeking asylum in Australia. *Transcultural Psychiatry*, **44**, 359–93.

Spiegel, P. (2004). HIV/AIDS among conflict-affected and displaced populations: dispelling myths and taking action. *Disasters*, **28**, 322–39.

Stanley, J. (2008). *Development induced displacement and resettlement – global overview*. Forced Migration Online. Available at http://www.forcedmigration.org/guides/fmo022/ accessed 28th May 2008.

Tarantola D., Byrnes A., Johnson M., Kemp L., Zwi A.B., Gruskin S. (2008). Human rights, health and development. *Australian Journal of Human Rights*, **13**, 2.

Toole, M. and Waldman, R. (1990). Preventing excess mortality in refugee and displaced populations in developing countries. *Journal of the American Medical Association*, **263**, 3296–302.

Toole, M. and Waldman, R. (1997). The public health aspects of complex emergencies and refugee situations. *Annual Review of Public Health*, **18**, 283–312.

Turner, S. (2004). New opportunities: angry young men in a Tanzanian refugee camp. In *Refugees and the transformation of societies. Agency, policies, ethics and politics* (eds. P. Essed, G. Frerks and J. Schrijvers) pp. 94–105. Berghahn Books, New York and Oxford.

United Nations General Assembly (2003). *Protocol to Prevent, Suppress and Punish Trafficking in Persons, Especially Women and Children, Supplementing the United Nations Convention Against Transnational Organized Crime*, G.A. Res. 25, Annex II, U.N. GAOR, 55th Sess. UN; 2003. p. Supp. No. 49, at 60.

United Nations (2000). *Protocol against the smuggling of migrants by land, sea and air*. United Nations, New York.

United Nations (1997). *Glossary of environment statistics, studies in methods*. United Nations, New York. Available at http://stats.oecd.org/glossary/detail.asp?ID=839 accessed 28th May 2008.

United Nations High Commissioner for Refugees (2005). *Statistical Yearbook 2005 – trends in displacement, protection and solutions*. UNHCR, Geneva. Available at http://www.unhcr.org/cgi-bin/texis/vtx/home/opendoc.pdf?id=464049e80&tbl=STATISTICS accessed 28th May 2008.

United Nations High Commissioner for Refugees (2006). *Statistical Yearbook 2006 – trends in displacement, protection and solutions*. UNHCR, Geneva. Available at http://www.unhcr.org/cgi-bin/texis/vtx/home/opendoc.pdf?id=478ce2e62&tbl=STATISTICS accessed 28th May 2008.

United Nations High Commissioner for Refugees (2007). *Definitions and obligations*. Available at http://www.unhcr.org.au/basicdef.shtml accessed 28th May 2008.

US Commitee for Refugees and Immigrants (2006). *World Refugee Survey 2006*. Available at http://www.refugees.org/article.aspx?id=1565&subm=19&ssm=29&area=Investigate& accessed 28th May 2008.

US Commitee for Refugees and Immigrants (2007). *World Refugee Survey 2007*. Available at http://www.refugees.org/article.aspx?id=1941&subm=19&ssm=29&area=Investigate accessed 28th May 2008.

Zwi, A.B. and Cabral, A.J. (1991). Identifying "high risk situations" for preventing AIDS. *British Medical Journal*, **303**, 1527–9.

Zwi, A.B. and Alvarez-Castillo, F. (2003). *Forced migration globalization and public health: getting the big picture into focus*. In *The health of refugees* (ed. P. Allotey), pp. 14–34. Oxford University Press, Melbourne.

ZWI, A.B. *et al.* (2006) Placing ethics in the centre: Negotiating new spaces for ethical research in conflict situations. *Global Public Health*, **1**(3): 264–277.

SECTION 12

Public health functions

12.1

Need: What is it and how do we measure it?

Di McIntyre, Gavin Mooney, and Stephen Jan

Abstract

The concept of need is interpreted in different ways. The principle adopted in this chapter is that need is defined by the notion of 'capacity of benefit'. This means that need derives its meaning from the various pathways in which it can contribute to the achievement of a particular objective, i.e. it is 'instrumental'. Here we focus on need in relation to healthcare; a need for healthcare can be seen to be instrumental to the achievement of the objective of health. As a consequence, the type of healthcare that is needed in any given circumstance is a function of factors such as the level of prevailing resources, the availability and effectiveness of healthcare, and the perspective and values of whomsoever is making the assessment.

Need is a critical concept in the pursuit of efficient healthcare, in terms of maximizing health benefits, given the limited resources. There are a number of tools such as programme budgeting and marginal analysis and quality-adjusted life years (QALY) league tables which enable decision makers to systematically allocate resources efficiently according to need. Recent policy initiatives such as the Oregon Health Plan, the World Bank's essential package concept, and the Commission for Macroeconomics and Health have also incorporated cost-effectiveness as a basis for determining need to ensure best use of limited resources.

Need is also useful in planning for the equitable allocation of resources as it provides a measure by which policy makers may pursue objectives such as 'equal access for equal need' or 'equal use for equal need'. The application of these principles in practice can be seen most readily in health needs assessment exercises such as those carried out in the United Kingdom in the 1990s and the various needs-based resource allocation formulae that have been employed over recent decades in the United Kingdom, Australia, and recently in a number of low- and middle-income countries. One of the challenges in implementing these policies is in ensuring that any measure of need takes into account social values, absorptive capacity constraints, and is sensitive to variations in mortality and morbidity. These are issues that provide a focus for future research on this topic.

There is a beguiling simplicity about the proposition that healthcare services should be designed to meet the needs of the community. Indeed, the healthcare policies of a great many countries have as a key goal meeting the needs of the population. Faced with the obvious appetite for healthcare exhibited by virtually all communities exposed to it, it is traditional to distinguish between wants and needs: Wants, by implication, being less rational, possibly even related to greed. Needs, by contrast, are seen as objective states, things that can be measured and agreed upon by rational people often on behalf of those who have them, as deserving attention.

The purpose of this chapter is first to explore the concept of need and its relevance within a public health framework. The purposes for which need might be measured—for action in the clinical and population settings and for planning—are then reviewed. Some currently available measures of need are then examined and some conclusions are drawn. Given the elusive nature of the concept of need, a glossary of relevant terms used in this chapter is provided in Box 12.1.1 as a reference point for readers.

The concept of need within the context of public health

Need as an instrumental concept

The starting point for exploring the concept of need is to address the question of the need for what? If we are focusing on the health sector, there is general agreement that we are concerned with the need for healthcare—it is this need for healthcare that is the focus of this chapter. However, the need is not for healthcare as an end in itself; instead, healthcare is instrumental to achieving improved health, which is the ultimate objective. It is evident that there are instruments other than healthcare that are able to promote health, such as good housing and sanitation services, but we restrict ourselves mainly to health sector services in this chapter, even though many interventions outside the health sector are of relevance from the public health perspective (Culyer 1991; Culyer & Wagstaff 1993).

There is often a tendency to refer to healthcare needs in very general terms, usually with an implication that all needs ought to be addressed. However it is important to recognize that any given form of healthcare can be one of a number of instruments to achieving health benefit. For example, it would be helpful to indicate that a particular person with arthritis needs a hip-replacement *in order that* they are able to walk more easily and suffer less pain. This allows for critical assessment of whether a hip-replacement is

Box 12.1.1 Glossary of terms

Capacity to benefit	The notion that health care need is measured by the extent to which individuals or populations are able to benefit from care. One implication of using this criterion is that need is directly associated with the effectiveness and cost-effectiveness of health care.
Need as an instrumental concept	Health care is seen to have no intrinsic value; it is valued only insofar as it contributes to health or health related benefits such as information and autonomy. Therefore the need for health care is seen as instrumental in achieving these outcomes.
Need as a subjective concept	Need is seen to be a function of individual and community perception and therefore may vary across individuals and communities.
Equal health as a health care objective	The view that the objective of health care systems is the achievement of equal health across individuals
Equal access for equal need	The view that the objective of health care systems is the achievement of equal access to health services for individuals with the same level of need. It says nothing about how individuals with different needs should be treated relative to one another.
Equal use for equal need	The view that the objective of health care systems is the achievement of equal use of health services for individuals with the same level of need. The difference between this objective and the previous one is that 'equal access' implies a tolerance for inequalities in the use of services based on differing preferences, i.e. some individuals may choose not to use services whilst others in the same position do use them.
Absorptive capacity	This relates to the ability of a community or organization to utilize fully the resources which it has been allocated. It is a problem with resource allocation formulae, particularly in low income settings, where the policy of shifting resources to poorer regions is undermined by the inability of those regions to transform such investment into additional services.

really necessary, based on whether this intervention is appropriate for achieving the specified health improvement goal and whether or not there are other interventions that may be more effective and more cost-effective in achieving that goal. These sorts of critical assessments assist in deciding which needs should be addressed and to what extent, given that there is a scarcity of resources.

The instrumental nature of healthcare highlights firstly that effectiveness is closely associated with need; a need can only exist for effective healthcare. Thus, it is necessary to ask whether specific health services will actually prolong life, improve quality of life (e.g. improved mobility, relief of pain) or at least prevent further deterioration in quality of life. Secondly, it also underlines that need has a forward-looking perspective. Need is not equivalent to a person's or a group's existing health or illness status but focuses on how healthcare could lead to improved health.

Need as capacity to benefit

A useful concept that encapsulates this perspective is that of capacity to benefit from healthcare, in that there should be the potential for health to be improved relative to what it would be in the absence of the healthcare intervention. Culyer and Wagstaff (1993) define need as 'the minimum resources required to exhaust an individual's capacity to benefit from healthcare'. Defining need in this way not only points to the instrumental nature of healthcare but also places a limit on the amount of healthcare needed.

Whose perspective?

While the above ideas seem to provide quite clear guidance on the issue of need, they are quite difficult to implement in practice. They also fail to recognize that need can be viewed from different perspectives. A community experiencing high levels of infant mortality due to tetanus might be seen by a preventivist as one in need of the development of an effective maternal education programme focusing on hygiene at the time of cutting the umbilical cord, and maternal immunization. Conversely, an intensive care physician may see the same phenomena and compute them in terms of needs for neonatal intensive care beds to effect rescue of the young victims. The individuals involved—the parents of the children affected—may have a third interpretation of what they need, which may have little to do with healthcare.

These constructs of need—which is what they are, melding essentially the same 'facts' into different shapes—each have their legitimacy. Unless health is to be seen as something occupying a quiet biological space, independent of culture and society, then these different constructs should be accepted. Each derives from the fact that any relevant concept of need is subjective. Definitions of need vary depending on whose perception, interpretation and values are in play. As it is most unlikely that some universally valid construct of need can be adopted that will be apposite in all circumstances, the question arises of whose values ought to come into play and in which circumstances. Thus, another key issue is who should determine that a need exists and what the value is of meeting it in part or full.

Need is most frequently seen as being formed or perceived in the eyes of another, a third party. Thus, Liss (1990) wrote 'A need for healthcare exists when an assessor believes that healthcare ought to be provided'. With this conceptualization of need it is not the patient who is doing the assessing but someone else, an agent (often a medical doctor), on behalf of the patient. (While it would be possible to deduce from the quote from Liss (1990) that need might be self-assessed, it is clear elsewhere in his and in much other literature in this area that is not what he intends).

Such third-party assessment requires, for the assessment to have legitimacy, that wider concerns are at play. If a doctor, for example, assesses a patient's needs, this is only of interest if that assessment leads to rights for the patient or clarification or quantification of rights which then provide the patient with access to services which might be of assistance in addressing the problems identified by the doctor. It is not the assessment by the doctor that provides the needs with their rights base, with their element of 'social legitimacy'. That can only come from the concept of a social contract. When it is claimed that individuals have a right to certain basic necessities, that is the language of a social contract. As Loewy (1990) stated 'Social contract consists of those things which "go without saying" and which we consider to be the legitimate expectations we have of others and of our community'.

Tension arises with respect to what sort of community it is in which we are trying to assess needs. As Loewy (1990) reminded us, according to the Aristotelian dictum 'justice consists of giving everyone their due'. He continues, however:

> *What is and what is not someone's due . . . is another matter. Minimalist communities which . . . accept freedom as an absolute condition of the moral life will see what is due quite differently than will more generously based communities. What is due in minimalist communities is doing to each other no harm; what is due in broader-based communities is a far more difficult matter and one which will ultimately be determined by an ongoing dialectic between communal values and individual interests.*

Needs and wants

It immediately follows that the separation of wants and needs, which for some seems so simple, in practice is far from simple. There is an astonishing lack of research into individuals or communities as to what they actually want from their healthcare services and so the pejorative view of wants as little more than expressions of greed by the ignorant is particularly unfortunate. Paternalistic professionalism has blocked progress in understanding how the community views health and healthcare and where they place them in the context of other things that they also want for their lives.

Distinctions between needs and wants are made still more difficult by the fact that different disciplines also use different definitions. A potentially useful set of constructs is provided by the discipline of economics. Wants are the preferences of individuals on behalf of themselves but do not have to be expressed through taking action to have the wants 'fulfilled'. 'Demands' are based on wants, that is on an individual's own preferences, by some action on the part of the individual in seeking to have the wants addressed. Thus, a want for better health can be expressed as a demand for healthcare if the individual visits a general practitioner. A need for healthcare would arise if the general practitioner were to agree that some relevant and effective action could be taken by the healthcare services on behalf of the patient. It is clear that need could exist without want or demand, demand could exist without need but not without want, and want could exist without demand or need.

This distinction between need on the one side and wants and demands on the other emphasizes still further the value-laden nature of these phenomena. Such emphasis is merited. While wants and demands are normally readily recognized as being subjective in this way, this is less commonly the case with the conceptualization of need.

Need over time

Need is also likely to be dynamic over time. The need for care today, for example, is very different from the need for care 20 years ago. Partly, it is that the incidence and prevalence of diseases have changed. Also, expectations and values of both the population and the health professional have changed. Technological change and changing availability of services have also altered the extent and pattern of needs. Similarly, needs are likely to vary in moving from one culture or one society to another.

Need within the paradigms of public health

Policy and research in public health have not often adopted a multidisciplinary approach to the understanding of either wants or needs for healthcare. A great deal of ignorance thus lies undisturbed and the strengths and limits of the various public health sciences and discourses are thrown into relief when each comes to examine the nature of need. Epidemiology, with its reductionist roots, can provide a count of cases, deaths, and denominators, and can also provide insights into some of the causal pathways that manifest as these health states that we declare as needs. The social sciences can provide an interpretation of needs in terms of how society views departures from health—ranging from their perception as religious events through to secular phenomena that require government intervention that reinforces social values such as equity and efficiency. As indicated above, health economists can contribute to the understanding of healthcare needs by setting them within the context of what demands individuals and society place upon the resources available to them, in terms of their individual and corporate happiness and satisfaction. For example, where do healthcare needs fit in the total spectrum of needs, alongside the basic ones in the lower orders of the Maslow hierarchy (food, shelter, etc.) and in relation to the more sophisticated ones for education, justice, and freedom of speech (Maslow 1943)?

Any simple interpretation of need must therefore be suspect. The reductionist quality of measures of need should be understood if we are to avoid making useless extrapolations from them. Nevertheless, reductionist measures of need share with much reductionist science a remarkable capacity to get the job done, things improved, wars won, and health status elevated. The major issue confronting those involved in public health, therefore, is not so much to search endlessly for an all-embracing definition of need, but to be willing to live with pared-down versions of need that may be useful within a particular context, whilst recognizing their limitations. The debate about measuring need therefore shares much with the debate about measuring the quality of life.

What is not to be applauded, however, are those interpretations of need which are driven by data availability rather than the purpose for which the need measure is required. There are too many examples in the literature of needs estimation based on inappropriate grasping at available numbers without due consideration as to whether in ordinal or cardinal terms the interpretation of the numbers does reflect the construct of need which is claimed implicitly or explicitly.

The purpose of measuring need

If we accept that the generic notion of need is complex and elusive, we can proceed to identify different settings in which different measures of need, each with their limitations, may prove useful.

Need in the clinical setting

Within clinical practice, the measurement of need is an integral part of the daily routine. While it is a necessary and accepted part of such practice, it is not always judged explicitly.

The relevance of need and its usefulness in clinical decision-making are obvious and seemingly unchallenged and unchallengeable. Yet a challenge does arise from the extent to which there are substantial variations in clinical practice for similar or even identical health conditions. At this level, seemingly similar problems—identified perhaps with respect to reduced health status—are interpreted quite differently by different clinicians in terms of what is needed to deal with them. Manifestations of such apparent variations in interpretation can be a function not only of a diversity in respect of need but also of availability of resources to treat particular problems.

However, variations in the rates of performing various surgical procedures exist to a very great extent, even after allowing for or controlling for variations in the supply of resources and the characteristics of the populations being served. There is little doubt that this is a function of differences in perception and/or interpretation of needs at a clinical level across different clinicians.

In the face of a value-laden concept of need, the 'medical model'—if A, then B—can appear somewhat mechanistic. Neither A (the diagnosis) nor B (the choice of therapy) is devoid of value judgements on the part of the clinician. Yet historically it was possible to read into the concept of need in clinical medicine something that appeared concrete, objective, and largely value free. At the very heart of clinical medicine lies an increasing recognition of the extent to which medicine is about values, including the assessment and interpretation of needs.

At a clinical level there will be variations in interpretation of need across similar conditions but in different contexts. This can very clearly be influenced by the nature and structure of incentive systems (and not just financial incentives), which emphasizes still more the subjective nature of need. It is not possible to interpret the results of various studies on changes in remuneration systems in any other way. Need at a clinical level is a function, among other things, of how doctors are paid. As a consequence, care is sometimes provided that may not be 'needed' as viewed by a third party.

To point this out is not to criticize or to express regret about such a phenomenon. More importantly it is to recognize that there is potentially a useful tool for influencing clinical practice, in terms of not only the effectiveness of that practice but also its efficiency and its contribution to concerns for equity. Given the central place of need in clinical decision making, the fact that need can be perceived differently within different remuneration systems (Krasnik *et al.* 1990) has to be an important consideration for policy-makers. Yet the potential for using the remuneration system for policy purposes has been underexploited to date although recent initiatives in the United States and United Kingdom highlight growing interest in this area (Institute of Medicine 2001; Berwick *et al.* 2003; Mason *et al.* 2005).

Need at the level of the population

Although need may be considered in absolute terms, it is principally in relative terms that it finds its place in contemporary health service development and appraisal. Thus, 'standardized mortality ratios', that is mortality rates standardized to some common population, are compared from one region or country to another and implications are drawn about need. A community that has a 10 per cent higher mortality rate from ischaemic heart disease than the national average is seen, in particular by the popular press, as being 'in need'—of more coronary care beds, or more preventive programmes, or more ambulances fitted with defibrillators, etc.

Need is defined in these settings as some correlate of mortality, in no small part because mortality statistics despite all their weaknesses are, like democracy, pretty good compared with anything else. However, there is a particular problem in low- and middle-income countries in that many deaths are unreported and, hence, mortality statistics are very unreliable. What is of particular concern is that death reporting is especially poor in rural areas and, although residents of these areas in reality often bear the greatest burden of ill-health, this is not reflected in official mortality data. This is to some extent being addressed by the practice in a great many low- and middle-income countries of regularly conducting Demographic and Health Surveys (DHS), which provide data on infant, child and maternal mortality that are more reliable than official statistics.

Where there is a problem with mortality measures is with respect to answering the question: 'need for what?' Other things being equal, a higher level of mortality implies a higher level of need in some general rather unspecific sense—but greater need for what? It might be for health services but perhaps also for many other goods, services or activities. We believe that in the continuing tension between, on the one hand, treatment services for meeting healthcare needs and, on the other hand, public health services, one of the reasons why the latter may 'lose out' in resource allocation is the failure to specify needs adequately in terms of instrumentation. Instruments or interventions in treatment services tend to be of a much more specific and identifiable nature than is the case with public health measures. The former are also drawn from a defined set of healthcare services whereas public health interventions can be present in very many areas of the economy—transport, housing, the environment, food policy, etc.

Doctors working in the acute hospital sector always have seductively simple and clear instruments at hand. In the battle for meeting needs at that level as opposed to the public health level, they have the imperative of current sickness to provide still more weight to their claims over a still greater share of society's scarce resources. The latter is difficult to push aside and there are arguments that in the context of rescue, there is no reason to push them aside. It is important, however, to decide the extent of influence since it cannot be the case that treating current sickness can be seen as an absolute, or at least ought not to be. An important issue to draw into such considerations is that of effectiveness of alternative interventions, in that even though current sickness exists, there may not be the 'capacity to benefit' from currently available interventions.

Need from a planning perspective

The discussion in this section is framed largely within the context of tax funded health systems. However, many of the same issues apply to planning in health systems that are funded primarily through social or national health insurance. There are two places where need impacts upon planning. The first is in relation to what economists refer to as 'allocative efficiency'. This involves first an acceptance that resources are scarce, and second that the over-riding goal is to maximize benefits with the available resources. In terms of needs, this translates as maximizing the needs met or the value of the needs met with the resources available.

The second place where need and planning converge is in the pursuit of equity. In relation to equity, issues of distribution are often set in terms of 'equal use for equal need' or 'equal access for equal need'.

Allocative efficiency issues

For allocative efficiency, the health service planner approaches needs as but one ingredient in a complex equation which he or she is expected to solve. In this context, the planner may identify 'need' as being those margins of existing programmes for which additional resources might achieve more than similar sized investments in other programmes. An implication of this is that there may be situations for which resources might be withdrawn and devoted elsewhere with greater well-being than is currently derived from the system.

The following statement might be made: The returns to health of monies spent here, on this programme, in this location, on this group of patients, on this effort on prevention, are not high enough—the money would be better spent over there on that other programme, on that other group of patients. If it is possible to take US$100 000 from the treatment of cancer patients and do still more good in treating the elderly for, perhaps, chronic arthritis, then it should be done. If the reverse is true then the direction of the resource shift should be reversed.

It is not enough to be able to say that resources which are scarce are being well spent; the issue is rather, could they be better spent? Are there more needs or more highly valued needs that resources could be used to address?

The idea of shifting resources to where they can meet the greatest need (or more correctly where they will do most good)—what economists call marginal analysis—is not difficult to grasp. If more good can be done than is being done, if more needs can be met with the same resources, then the argument is that that is what should be done.

It is here that the necessity for measurement of need becomes paramount, as judgements have to be made about where resources will meet the greatest need. If, with the same amount of resources, pain, suffering and death can be reduced still more, then let us do so. That is the simple notion of economic efficiency.

The concept of need incorporated into this planning framework is that of capacity to benefit (Culyer 1991), outlined earlier. This concept is a somewhat different type of need as compared with that which is used frequently at the population level, which is interpreted in terms simply of the extent of illness and death in a population (as described above). Even if a health problem exists, if there is no capacity to benefit, such as where no effective treatment exists for that particular health problem, under this definition there is no need.

Programme budgeting and marginal analysis

This planning framework stands to benefit if we can obtain a picture of how resources are currently being spent and linked in an appropriate way to what the objectives and priorities are. This picture is what is known as a set of 'programme budgets'.

Most commonly in healthcare, expenditure data are available categorized by inputs, for example, expenditure on doctors, nurses, pharmaceuticals, and linen. In programme budgeting the interest is in categorization of sets of needs that we seek to alleviate or meet—the needs of the elderly, children, cancer patients, etc. The link is thus between expenditure and health objectives for relevant social or disease groupings.

Therefore, prior to proceeding with the marginal analysis or shifting resources, it is relevant to find out what is being spent on these groupings or 'programmes'. The two keys to designating programmes are first that the programmes together are comprehensive in that, first, all the health services—hospital, general practitioner, and community—are included, and second, the programmes are output or outcome orientated and not input orientated as is the case with most forms of budgeting.

This approach—programme budgeting plus marginal analysis—is what economists recommend for use in pursuing the meeting of needs at a planning level (*Health Policy* 1995). With respect to the marginal analysis part of the approach, trying to form a judgement about whether US$1 million is better spent on maternity care rather than on care of the elderly is difficult. There are major measurement problems here and greater effort needs to be invested in developing appropriate measures to enable these comparisons to be made.

A recent example of the use of programme budgeting and marginal analysis (PBMA) is that undertaken by two of the regional health authorities in New Zealand to inform their purchasing of health services (Bohmer *et al.* 2001). This PBMA initiative focused on identifying the optimal allocation of resources between existing and potential respiratory disease interventions. Respiratory diseases are seen as important given that they account for up to 16 per cent of deaths in these two regions. The establishment of an advisory group for the PBMA process allowed for the inputs of all concerned groups, including community representatives. As a result of the PBMA, both regions prioritized additional or new investment in smoking cessation programmes and educating health professionals and communities in respiratory disease issues including appropriate antibiotic use, amongst others, and prioritized disinvestment in lung transplants and relatively ineffective treatments such as the use of cough syrups and bronchodilators. Although decision-makers viewed the process as having been of considerable value and the results were being implemented, it was noted that PBMA can be very data and resource intensive (Bohmer *et al.* 2001).

Quality-adjusted life years (QALYs) league tables

QALY league tables may be seen as a form of marginal analysis. Such tables allow comparisons to be made between conditions according to the impact they have on the quantity and quality of life of sufferers. As discussed in more detail below, the QALY, which weights chronological survival according to the quality of life, has also been used as an output currency to compare what is attainable for investment in various healthcare procedures. Thus, for US$10 000 spent on treatment for one condition one may purchase 300 QALYs, compared with 700 QALYs for the same price if one is treating a different condition. Yet QALY league tables have limited applicability in resource allocation contexts for several reasons (Gerard & Mooney 1993). For example, different studies will often be based on different comparators for the intervention being assessed. There are difficulties in making meaningful QALY league tables if the comparators do not reflect current standard practice.

Recent initiatives

The moves in, for example, the United States (through the Patient Outcome Research Team programme etc.), the United Kingdom (through health needs assessment—see later section), New Zealand, and New South Wales in Australia, to plan health services with the focus on health outcomes or health gain, place emphasis on efficiency and equity in the context of needs. Such an emphasis demands that objectives be more precisely and explicitly stated and needs identified more carefully and then quantified. It is to the quantification of needs that we will turn shortly.

Attempts to reallocate limited Medicaid dollars to a wider pool of recipients in Oregon attracted great attention, in no small part because need, effective therapy and cost were subject to public scrutiny in determining a pattern of resource expenditure for healthcare (Dixon & Welch 1991; Kitzhaber 1993). In 1991, after extensive consultation, a proposal was put forward that Medicaid coverage for the poor in Oregon should cease to cover everything possible for the poorest 200 000 recipients of aid and instead provide for 709 disease categories and paired treatments for an additional 100 000 recipients. The plan was approved by President Clinton on 19 March 1993.

Teng (1996) argues that compromises which led to the development of the list of services to be covered meant that the original objective of cost-effectiveness was largely undermined. Regardless of how the list was devised, however, it is doubtful whether cost-effectiveness is compatible, in general, with an approach to funding that partitions services above and below a fixed line. Its main limitation is that it takes no account of differences across individuals in terms of their capacity to benefit from the same treatment.

Despite this, the Oregon Health Plan was successful in one of its major objectives; increasing healthcare coverage across the state (Oregon Health Plan 1997; Jacobs *et al.* 1999). Conversely, it has been less successful in reducing overall healthcare expenditure and has relied to a large extent on funding from increases in tobacco taxes (Jacobs *et al.* 1999).

On the basis of the success of the Oregon Health Plan, which achieved its goal of providing cover to an additional 100 000 people, in 2002 the State decided to pursue a further extension to an additional 46 000 low income Oregon residents. The proposal was to move the cut-off point on the service priority list up, i.e. reduce the services covered in order to reallocate funds to cover new enrolees. As expressed by a senior Oregon health department official: 'It comes down to an old issue. Is it better for everybody to have something than for some to have a lot and others to have nothing?' (Oberlander 2007). Co-payments, both for premiums and at the point of service use, were also introduced. These changes were introduced in early 2003, with unexpectedly negative consequences. While there were 104 000 'additional' enrollees from the original Oregon Health Plan by January 2003, this had declined to 49 000 by December 2003 and even further to 24 000 by 2006. Instead of achieving a 50 per cent increase in enrolment for the Oregon Health Plan, the changes resulted in a 75 per cent decrease in enrolment. This decline has been attributed largely to the introduction of cost-sharing. In thinking about how to resuscitate the Oregon Health Plan, policy makers wanted to reorder the list of priorities, emphasizing chronic care and preventive services, with an emphasis on reducing costs of the services covered (Oberlander 2007).

Another initiative to prioritize among interventions which has received considerable attention is the World Bank's efforts to promote the development of 'essential packages' in low- and middle-income countries. The essential package concept was linked to the 1993 World Development Report, in which it was argued that governments should only finance those public health services which have *substantial* externalities and a defined package of essential clinical services (World Bank 1993). It was recommended that the essential package should include the most cost-effective health services which address the major health problems within that country (determined in terms of the 'burden of disease' measured as disability-adjusted life years or DALYs—discussed in more detail in 'DALYs'). A key component of this reform measure was the creation of an enabling environment for the private health sector to grow and to finance and provide all services outside of this essential package. Another World Bank (1994) publication that followed shortly thereafter, designed an 'essential package' that was seen to be appropriate for a wide range of low- and middle-income countries. Countries could determine which elements of the package to include based on their major diseases and available funds. Although the World Development Report suggested that each country should undertake its own burden of disease study and cost per DALY calculations in order to develop a country-specific essential package, the package defined in a wide range of African countries is almost identical to the package proposed in the World Bank's 'Better Health in Africa' report (World Bank 1994). The fact that the relative cost-effectiveness of specific interventions may vary considerably in different country contexts was not acknowledged by the World Bank.

The Commission on Macroeconomics and Health recommended an almost identical approach stating that low- and middle-income countries should identify essential interventions that are the most cost-effective and address the main contributors to the burden of disease (World Health Organization 2001). The main differences are that the Commission recommended that 'the needs of the poor should be stressed', estimated that the essential package would cost about US$35 per person per year, compared to the World Bank's previous estimate of US$13 per person per year and called for greater national and international investment in health. A veritable 'industry' has arisen around these suggestions, with each African country being encouraged to set up a National Commission on Macroeconomics and Health (see, for example, http://www.afro.who.int/cmh/index.html). The practice of identifying need in relation to measures such as DALYs and defining limited service packages in relation to these 'needs', is firmly entrenched in many African countries as well as some other low- and middle-income countries.

The dilemma of deciding which health services can be provided to meet the needs of the population best is not unique to tax funded health systems. Indeed, this challenge is even more evident in insurance funded systems; while tax funded systems often avoid making explicit decisions about service rationing and effectively leave these decisions to clinicians, health insurance schemes (whether voluntary private or mandatory social health insurance) have to specify the benefit package to which their members will be entitled.

Equity issues

The second consideration that planners will be interested in concerns equity. One of the most problematical aspects of this is that there is so much confusion in healthcare policy circles as to what this word means. The chief contenders are 'equal health', 'equal use for equal need', and 'equal access for equal need'. Clearly the last two of these incorporate some view of need within them. Here our concern is restricted to the relationship between equity and need and, within that, the issue of resource allocation formulas.

The international industry of needs-based (or weighted capitation) resource allocation formulas began with the Resource Allocation Working Party (RAWP) in England whose report was published in 1976 (DHSS 1976). The approach has been used in several other places since (e.g. New South Wales in Australia, New Zealand, Portugal, as well as several African and Latin American countries such as Ghana, Tanzania, Zambia, Brazil, Chile, Colombia and Mexico).

What the original RAWP sought was a formula for allocating resources fairly to the 14 geographical regions of England based on the principle of equal access for equal need (although in practice it did not go beyond equal expenditure for equal need). The RAWP formula (and the various versions it has spawned) emphasized horizontal equity, i.e. equity that ensures that individuals with similar characteristics are treated equally. Vertical equity—the unequal, yet equitable, treatment of unequals—is not included directly in the formulation except in so far as different needs are weighted by the cost of dealing with each.

In the last decade, some attention has been devoted to Mooney's (1998) argument that there may be a case for developing the notion of 'communitarian claims' to replace needs or at least to complement them. It is normally the case that need is conceptualized in terms of purely health and that in meeting need, all nominally equal health gains (such as QALYs) be weighted equally. Communitarian claims, it is suggested, allow for other considerations (e.g. information or respect for patient dignity) to enter and for health gains to some recipients (e.g. those in particularly poor health) to be weighted more highly than others. A further claimed advantage is that it is the community who determine first what constitutes a claim, and second the differential strengths of different claims. These would determine what healthcare resources were to be made available to different groups in society. These claims are communitarian not only in the sense that the responsibility to arbitrate over them lies with the community but also that it is beneficial to the community that they do so. For example, in Australia the overall community may feel better as a result of knowing that it has contributed to the betterment of the health of its Indigenous peoples.

Measuring need—available instruments and their application

Needs-based formulas

In several countries measures of need have been constructed to guide the allocation of healthcare resources. The methods vary from allocating resources to geographical areas on the basis of prevailing patterns of mortality and social class, through to case-mix payment to hospitals on the basis of the need (in terms of diagnosis and severity) of patients admitted to their care.

The approach adopted in the RAWP formula (see above) aimed at measuring relative (and not absolute) need for healthcare in different regions. Such healthcare was divided into seven categories: Non-psychiatric inpatient services, all day-patient and outpatient services, mental illness inpatient services, mental handicap inpatient services, community services, ambulance services, and administration of general practitioner services but not these services *per se*.

The relative need for each of these services in each region was calculated on the basis of a formula which weighted the population according to a number of factors. For example, the factors relevant to non-psychiatric inpatient services were size of population, age/sex composition, morbidity (although in practice this was actually the standardized mortality rate), cost, patient cross-boundary flows, medical education and capital investment. Relative need was calculated for each of the services listed and then weighted according to the national proportion of the total spending on that service. These were then summed to give an overall regional weight. Thus, if a region with a population of, say, 5 million was above average in terms of need, for example to the extent of 10 per cent, then it would receive funding which assumed a weighted population of 5.5 million. In a later revision of the RAWP formula (DHSS 1986), the regional population was also weighted by a deprivation index (i.e. a composite index of socioeconomic indicators). This was in response to criticisms that standardized mortality rates do not account for regional variations in the need for health services arising from differences in socioeconomic conditions. Subjective indicators of health, in the form of self-rated health in household surveys, have also been used in the United Kingdom, although concerns exist about their validity given their high variability and low statistical association with mortality (O'Reilly 2005).

As indicated earlier, the idea of needs-based formulas to guide resource allocation has been taken up by a wide range of high-, middle- and even low-income countries. This is probably due to the success that RAWP had in effecting a relative redistribution of healthcare resources between regions in England. The difference in expenditure per capita (of weighted population) between the poorest and wealthiest regions was approximately 30 per cent when the RAWP report was published; this gap had virtually been eliminated one and a half decades later.

Box 12.1.2 provides an overview of the indicators of 'need' included in resource allocation formulas in a range of low- and middle-income countries. These countries face particular challenges in that there is limited access to data on many indicators. While all formulas have a common starting point, namely population size, and many adjust for the age and sex composition of the population, low- and middle-income countries tend to use infant or child mortality instead of standardized mortality ratios. Many also include some measure of socioeconomic status (poverty or a broader deprivation index) and adjust for the differential cost of providing services (particularly in rural or low-density areas). A factor that was not relevant in the English context, but is critical in many low- and middle-income countries is that of funds that may accrue at district or regional level other than central government tax funding. Given that different areas have different abilities to attract donor funding or to generate their own revenue (e.g. through local government rates and taxes or user fees charged at health facilities), it is necessary to take such revenue into account in order to promote equity in the overall funding envelope but at the same time, avoid undermining incentives to raise revenue locally.

What these formulas assume is that the total relative need in a region and across regions is a meaningful entity. That is open to challenge, however, if total need for healthcare is seen as in part a function of supply. Thus total relative need cannot be defined in the absence of some budget constraint which makes the argument for using total relative need as a measure for allocating a budget between different regions somewhat circular. It further assumes that the relative total need can be measured sufficiently accurately by just a few factors. Thirdly, it assumes that using standardized mortality rates (or infant or child mortality) as a measure of relative morbidity is a valid measure (again a doubtful assumption).

Box 12.1.2 Examples of low- and middle-income countries using a needs-based resource allocation formula

Africa

Ghana

Since 2004, Ghana has been allocating its tax funded and donor pooled fund health budget between regions using a formula which includes the regional population size, weighted for deprivation (measured as the population below the poverty line) and under 5 mortality.

Tanzania

The Tanzanian formula for the allocation of 'basket' (donor-pooled) funds to districts includes population size, under-five mortality as a proxy for disease burden, poverty level and adjusts for the differential cost of providing health services in rural and low population density areas.

Uganda

The primary health care budget is allocated between districts using a formula based on population size, the inverse of the Human Development Index (HDI), the inverse of per capita donor and NGO spending and a supplement for districts with a difficult security situation and those with no district hospital. In this formula, the HDI component includes measures of both socio-economic status and ill-health. Taking account of donor and NGO funding ensures that the full resource envelope for each district is taken into account when determining the allocation of government funds.

Zambia

Initially, a simple per capita formula was used in Zambia because of the scarcity of accurate data on other needs-based indicators. However, weightings for remoteness and disease patterns have been recently included in the formula.

Latin America

Chile

Resources for primary health care are allocated from central government to municipalities on the basis of population size, with an adjustment for rurality and municipal poverty level.

Colombia

Central government in Colombia allocates general funds to municipalities on the basis of a formula that includes the size of the municipal population, adjusted for poverty level, unmet basic needs, quality of life indicators and locally-generated revenue. A portion of these funds is explicitly earmarked for health services. Thus, they use a needs-based formula to determine an overall allocation for all municipal services but limit municipal autonomy in deciding on the distribution of these funds between types of services by protecting part of the grant for health (and similarly for education). This approach has dramatically promoted equity in the distribution of health care resources between municipalities.

Mexico

The Mexican Ministry of Health quite recently introduced a resource allocation formula which includes population size, child mortality rate and a 'marginalization index'. The last is a composite index of socio-economic status which includes educational status, access to potable water and to sanitation and overcrowding.

Source: Bossert *et al.* (2003); Pearson (2002); Rocha *et al.* (2004)

Finally, it assumes that differences in need are proportional to the resources required to address them. For example, if a particular region is judged to have needs that are on average 10 per cent greater than the national average, they are allocated 10 per cent more resources than they would have received based purely on their population size. In effect, this procedure for allocating resources is not consistent with the concept of allocating resources according to capacity to benefit *at the margin*.

We would not want to appear overcritical of this process, as these formulas have been instrumental in breaking historical inertia in resource allocation patterns and contributing to considerable resource redistribution in some countries. What we would emphasize is the desirability in many instances of trying to fund health services on an equitable basis and that using some concept of need is the way to follow. It remains the case, however, that the assumptions typically used in needs-based formulas and the problems of measurement are such that we are less than convinced that this is the best way to proceed. In particular, we would submit that not weighting different needs according to social values remains problematical.

Weighting need to reflect social values

In order to weight needs on the basis of social values, some form of survey needs to be carried out to determine such weights. Various methods have been posited in the literature including both surveys and citizen jury-based approaches—typically entailing scenario-based allocations across hypothetical populations differing with respect to various characteristics such as socioeconomic status, age and sex. For examples of such approaches, see Mooney *et al.* (1995), Nord *et al.* (1995), Wiseman *et al.* (2003), and Mooney and Blackwell (2004).

Similar efforts to elicit social views on the relative weights that should be accorded to different needs have been undertaken in low- and middle-income countries such as Zambia and Namibia. In Namibia, 101 people were interviewed, with two-thirds being elected representatives at national, regional or local level (MHSS & WHO 2005). The vast majority were in favour of adopting a vertical equity approach and weighting the needs of certain groups more highly than others (e.g. rural residents and the poor).

Absorptive capacity issues

When efforts are made to reallocate resources to promote equity in meeting the needs of the population, it is important to ensure that communities benefiting from additional allocations are able to 'absorb' and benefit from these resources. There are too many examples of substantial budgetary resource redistribution occurring where historically under-funded areas are unable to utilize all the funds allocated to them while historically well-resourced areas struggle to cope with budget cuts. This was experienced in South Africa, for example, shortly after its first democratic elections, where an overly ambitious initiative to achieve equal per capita spending in each province within 5 years (the term of government) encountered major absorptive capacity problems (Gilson *et al.* 1999). In this instance, this was clearly a problem of too rapid a pace of change, which the original RAWP had avoided by setting explicit 'floors and ceilings' which limited the annual percentage decrease or increase in any region's budget. There are, however, other issues that are important to take into account in relation to absorptive capacity, and it may be necessary to explicitly invest in developing such capacity.

It has been proposed that this be done through the building of 'MESH' infrastructure (where MESH is management, economic, social and human) (Mooney & Houston 2004). The idea is simple. The capacity to benefit from any set of resources allocated to improving health will in practice be realized only to the extent that there is an adequate infrastructure available to use the resources in an efficient way. If in some jurisdiction there is a lack of leadership and other skills to operate programs successfully to the benefit of their communities, then the capacity to benefit will not be realized as fully as it otherwise might be. The policy response should then be to build MESH. This governance issue is one that internationally is increasingly recognized as important in Indigenous affairs (Cornell *et al.* 2004) but the ideas are applicable in any population. (see, for example, Thomas, Mooney and Mbatsha 2007 in relation to South Africa).

Thus, different jurisdictions and communities may differ in terms of their capacities to produce benefits for the people they serve. This can be for three reasons: (i) some populations already have relatively good health, so the capacity to benefit further is limited compared with others; (ii) even where the health levels of two populations are similar, one population's health problems can be more amenable to health service interventions, i.e. its capacity to benefit from healthcare interventions is greater; and (iii) even where both the health levels and the health problems are similar, one health service may be better placed or better equipped to deliver benefit to its population than the other. In the case of (iii), the capacity to benefit is inhibited because the service lacks the necessary MESH infrastructure to deliver health benefits to its population.

The basis of the approach to resource allocation outlined here takes as its starting point the issue of governance. If progress is to be made in improving the health of any population, it must be through the preferences and the wishes of the people concerned. Insofar as there are variations in the abilities of different communities and health services with respect to MESH infrastructure, this can result in uneven implementation of health service interventions and consequent inequities and inefficiencies for the relevant populations.

It is thus necessary to address this problem of variation through providing support to those jurisdictions that are deficient in these abilities. The building of MESH infrastructure can be seen as a major plank in any equity strategy, as it may well be those jurisdictions with the greatest healthcare need that are most often lacking in MESH. The lack of MESH in these communities will then exacerbate the inequities in healthcare need between communities.

Needs-based formulas in insurance-funded systems

While the needs-based resource allocation formulas discussed above refer largely to the allocation of nationally collected general tax funds to provinces, regions, districts or similar geographical localities, a similar approach is also used in the case of what is termed 'risk-equalization' between different health insurance schemes (van Vliet & van de Ven 1992; Beck *et al.* 2003). 'Risk' in actuarial terms has a similar meaning to need as discussed in this chapter. Risk-equalization has both equity and efficiency objectives. It particularly aims to respond to 'cream-skimming' (or risk selection) by competing health insurance schemes, whereby they seek to attract young, healthy members leaving other schemes with a large share of older and less healthy members. The risk profile of individual schemes is assessed, particularly using demographic variables such as age and gender but may also include the number of members with particular chronic diseases. Schemes with a high proportion of low-risk members are required to pay into a 'risk-equalization fund' while those with a high proportion of high-risk members will receive payments from the fund. This applies pressure on schemes to operate efficiently and promotes risk cross-subsidies (the healthy subsidising the costs of the ill), which are seen as a key component of promoting equity in health service benefits, between schemes. This risk equalization process thus seeks to promote equal expenditure for equal need.

Risk-equalization or risk-adjustment between competing health insurance schemes exists in many high-income countries with a mandatory requirement for the population to purchase health insurance cover, such as the Netherlands, Switzerland, and Ireland. However, in many cases, the risk-equalization is based purely on demographic variables (age and gender), with these variables only being able to predict a small proportion of the variance in health expenditure, thus allowing for schemes to continue to 'cream-skim' (van Vliet & van de Ven 1992; Beck *et al.* 2003). Interestingly, it is a middle-income country, South Africa, that has developed one of the more comprehensive risk-equalization methodologies. This includes age, a maternity or delivery indicator, the number of people with any of the 25 most prevalent chronic conditions, the number of people with multiple chronic conditions and the number of people with HIV on anti-retroviral therapy (McLeod 2004). At the time of writing (March 2007), the risk-equalization methodology has been finalized, all health insurance schemes have submitted information of these variables and the process will be fully implemented within the next year or two.

Health needs assessment

Health needs assessment (HNA) has been described as 'a systematic method for reviewing the health issues facing a population, leading to agreed priorities and resource allocation that will improve health and reduce inequalities' (Cavanagh & Chadwick 2005). The HNA approach was developed to assist in the 'commissioning' of services in the United Kingdom after the separation of purchaser and provider functions within the National Health Service in the early 1990s. Its growing importance as a planning instrument has been promoted by the trend towards evidence-informed decision making in the health sector. In recent years, considerable emphasis has been placed on HNA as a mechanism for ensuring that community views are taken into account in the planning process.

HNA is described as a five-step planning process:

1. Preliminary activities, including: The identification of the population to be considered (particularly from an equity perspective such as a group or area which suffers from multiple deprivation); and establishing clear objectives
2. Identifying health priorities, including: Gathering general information on the target population; identifying how the population perceives its own needs; identifying the health conditions and underlying factors that have a significant impact (in terms of size and severity) on health status in this population (using a broad health determinants framework) and whose health is most at risk from these priority conditions; which priority conditions or factors influencing these conditions can effectively be improved; and shortlisting priorities for action
3. Assessing a health priority for action, including: Identifying effective interventions for the health priority; defining the specific target population; identifying the changes required; confirming that the proposed changes will help reduce health inequalities; identifying the most acceptable interventions; and assessing the resource feasibility of the interventions including a marginal analysis of whether resources can be shifted from their current use to more cost effective interventions
4. Planning for change which focuses on detailed programming of the necessary actions and tasks to implement the identified interventions
5. Monitoring and review, particularly to assess if the planned impact is being achieved and ways of improving impact

There are a number of ways in which HNA is an advance on previous efforts to measure needs within a planning context. Firstly, it recognizes the instrumental nature of need for healthcare, as the explicit goal is the improvement of health, and it focuses on areas where effective interventions exist. Throughout the HNA process, decision-makers are required to consider two criteria in the selection of priorities: 'impact' and 'changeability' (Cavanagh & Chadwick 2005). In terms of 'impact', one is required to evaluate whether the specific health problem being considered has a significant impact on the health functioning of the population, both in relation to severity and size of the impact. The criterion of 'changeability' requires explicit assessment of the extent to which the health problem can be addressed *effectively* within the local context and by the groups involved.

Secondly, HNA also ensures that resource scarcity is explicitly taken into consideration and is designed as a marginal analysis. In the third step of the HNA process, decision-makers have to estimate the resources required to implement a priority intervention and to address questions such as: 'Can existing resources be used differently?'; 'What resources might be released if existing ineffective interventions are stopped?'; and 'Which actions will achieve the greatest impact on health for the resources used?' (Cavanagh & Chadwick 2005). In effect, a marginal analysis is required to identify existing interventions that are less cost-effective and should be de-prioritized.

Third, equity is an explicit objective and a vertical equity approach is used in that there is an emphasis on identifying particularly deprived populations and assessing whether interventions identified as priorities will achieve a reduction in health inequalities. In the first step, the population to be prioritized is identified on the basis of answering the questions 'Does this population have significantly worse health than others locally' and do they suffer from 'significant health inequalities'? (Cavanagh & Chadwick 2005). In addition, groups that suffer not only worse health status but also social and material deprivation are given priority. There is also explicit consideration of whether an intervention will reduce inequalities, before it is included on the priority list.

Finally, the community is extensively involved in identifying priority interventions. Community involvement is required at various stages of the HNA, including to contribute to identifying the key health issues affecting that community, the interventions regarded as most acceptable, and prioritizing the target population, health conditions and potential interventions. Particular emphasis is placed on ensuring that marginalized communities are reached and that their perspectives and preferences are taken into account (Cavanagh & Chadwick 2005).

Measuring instruments

Measuring needs, as indicated above, is likely to be problematical for the various reasons already stated. Whatever process is adopted, it involves establishing a measure of some shortfall in health status from some ideal, some norm, from some achievable health status, or some measure of 'capacity to benefit'.

There are many ways of trying to measure needs which are severely deficient and reflect more the availability of data than any real attempt to grapple seriously with the conceptualization of needs as spelt out so far in this chapter. Various activity measures—number of admissions, visits to general practitioners, vaccinations carried out, etc.—are sometimes used to measure need. Yet, it is readily apparent that such indicators reflect not only need (although visits to general practitioners may perhaps be designated a measure of consumer demand, in particular first visits during a specific episode) but also supply-side considerations such as availability and appropriateness of services.

Certainly, there are a number of vehicles that can be adopted to allow measurement of need to take place. Most common here would be epidemiological and social surveys. The question then is how to measure needs within any such survey. The emphasis around the world is on identifying measures of need that combine indicators of length of life (mortality) and quality of life or health (morbidity). We first consider some of these aggregate quantity and quality of life measures and then consider in more detail specific instruments frequently used to measure health-related quality of life.

QALYs

The QALY, and its later 'stable mate' the healthy year equivalent (HYE), have been developed largely by economists (Williams 1985;

Torrance 1986; Mehrez & Gafni 1989) to allow health status to be measured in various circumstances. Both are based on the concept of health-related utility which recognizes that health, as an output of health services and of other activities that promote health, is a function of both quantity of health and quality of health—or mortality and morbidity.

The QALY allows individuals, groups, or societies to 'trade-off' quantity of life against quality of life arguing, for example, that according to people's preferences, 10 years living with a chronic condition which results in the individual being confined to his or her own home is equivalent to 8 years of full health. The implication is that the 'quality adjustment' for the chronic condition is 0.8. Furthermore, it is implied that intervening to cure the chronic condition would result in an improvement in quality of life of 0.2 per annum which over 10 years means 2 QALYs.

While there are various criticisms that can be made of QALYs (Loomes & McKenzie 1989), they do have considerable merit over the more conventional measures of health status and of need such as mortality rates or standardized mortality rates in that they do endeavour to combine both quantity of life and quality of health. The development of QALYs has helped to gain greater acceptance for the point that health status, and in turn need, have large subjective elements (Sculpher 2006). In practice, to date QALYs have been used to measure need, essentially marginal-met need, in the context of priority setting through QALY league tables, as discussed above.

DALYs

The DALY is a variant of the QALY. DALYs were first introduced by the World Bank in the early 1990s (World Bank 1993) as a means of calculating the burden of different diseases. The approach involves the measurement of health status (strictly lost health status) into a universal index of mortality and morbidity.

Specifically, the DALYs for a given condition or disease are the sum of years of life lost due to premature mortality and the number of years of life lived with disability, adjusted for the severity of the disability (Murray & Lopez 1997). In terms of the disability severity weights, these were originally based on the opinions of experts in international health and fell into six classes of severity ranging from 0 (for perfect health) to 1 (for death) but, more recently, social values have been incorporated in DALYs (Murray & Lopez 1997*a*).

DALYs and their use as an aggregate measure of health status in the monitoring of population health, in the establishment of priorities between interventions, and as a guide to research priorities have been criticized by a number of authors (Ugalde & Jackson 1995; Anand & Hanson 1997; Paalman *et al.* 1998). One of the most controversial aspects of the DALY calculation is the differential age weighting applied to life years lost (Barendregt *et al.* 1996). Murray (1994), a key designer of DALYs, argues that it is valid to weight life years lost for working age adults more highly than for young children and the elderly, given that 'because of social roles the social value of that time may be greater' and that it is purely 'an attempt to capture different social roles at different ages'. Anand and Hanson (1997) highlight the extent of age discrimination by noting that 'in the construction of a DALY, a year lived at age 2 counts for only 20 per cent of a year lived at age 25 where the age-weighting function is at a maximum, while that lived at age 70 counts for 46 per cent of the maximum'. The effect of this age weighting is that if two people have the same illness and can be treated effectively for the same cost, preference would be given to treating a young adult rather than an older person or a child. A number of authors have argued that the age weights should be considered 'inequitable in principle' (Paalman *et al.* 1998; Anand & Hanson 1997). Others have commented that DALYs inadequately reflect social preferences for health, that the assumed or posited goals of healthcare systems are not validated, that such goals are assumed to be constant across all societies, and that using DALYs, as is advocated, to measure the burden of disease to assist with priority setting is at best a misuse of analytical resources and at worst potentially misleading (Mooney & Creese 1993; Sayers & Fliedner 1997; Wiseman & Mooney 1998; Williams 1999).

More recently, Murray and colleagues have developed variations of DALYs, namely disability-free life expectancy (DFLE) and disability-adjusted life expectancy (DALE) (Murray & Lopez 1997*b*). For these measures, they developed seven categories of disability and associated weights ranging from 0 (for minimal disability) to 1 (for very severe disability). The weights were based on preferences for different health states according to nine groups of people from 25 countries. A single set of disability weights was developed, which the authors regard as applicable across the world.

This reflects one of the key challenges with measures such as QALYs, HYEs, DALYs, and DALEs. It is unlikely that a single set of social values can be developed that is universally applicable, or that a set of values developed in one country would be applicable or reflect social values in a very different country. Values of health, trade-offs between quantity and quality of life, and the influence of spirituality on health are all likely to vary from culture to culture. Even the very construct of health can be culturally specific. For example, the construct of Australian Aboriginal health is holistic in a way not recognized in Western biomedical definitions. It also includes elements of reciprocity, mutuality, and obligation (Houston 2004).

It is of concern that little work has been undertaken in low- and middle-income countries to develop quality of life or disability weights that are relevant within specific country contexts, although more work has been undertaken in this regard in recent years. Low- and middle-income countries most frequently take an existing instrument for measuring health-related quality of life, which usually has been developed in the United States or in a European context, translate it into the local language and collect data to estimate locally relevant valuation of different health states (Bowden & Fox-Rushby 2003). Nevertheless, the emphasis appears to be placed more on ensuring that the quality of life measures are equivalent to that in other countries than on ensuring that the measures are appropriate for assessing need within the individual country contexts. The preoccupation with being able to perform cross-country comparisons appears to take precedence over appropriately informing local decision-making.

Measuring quality of life

What are some of these generic health-related quality of life instruments that are used around the world? The two most widely used instruments are 'SF-36' (or Short Form 36) and EuroQol (European Quality of Life) EQ-5D. The SF-36 was developed by the RAND Corporation in the United States for use in the Health Insurance Study Experiment/ Medical Outcomes Study (Ware *et al.* 1993). It is a concise 36-item health status questionnaire and has become one of the most widely used measures of subjective health status (Ware *et al.* 1993; Jenkinson *et al.* 1996).

The SF-36 contains 36 items which measure eight dimensions: Physical functioning (ten items), role limitations due to physical problems (four items), role limitations due to emotional problems (three items), mental health (five items), energy/vitality (four items), social functioning (two items), pain (two items), and general health perception (five items). There is also a single item about perceptions of health changes over the past 12 months.

The validity and reliability of the SF-36 in patient populations has been confirmed in the United States (McHorney *et al.* 1992, 1993). For example, patients with chronic heart failure reporting oedema, orthopnoea, or dyspnoea on exertion were classified as having a serious medical condition. The SF-36 could detect difference in health status among these patient groups across all eight scales. Garratt *et al.* (1993) claim on the basis of their own empirical work in the United Kingdom that the SF-36 seems 'acceptable to patients, internally consistent, and a valid measure of the health status of a wide range of patients'.

However, not all studies have been favourable to the SF-36. For instance, it has been criticized for failing to detect low levels of morbidity in some patient groups (Bowling 1997). Kurtin *et al.* (1992) reported 'floor' effects in the role of functioning scales in severely ill patients, where 25 to 50 per cent of patients obtained the lowest score possible, the implication being that deterioration in condition will not be detected by the scale. Other studies have revealed that it has little discriminatory power among women receiving different treatments for stage II breast cancer (Levine *et al.* 1988; Guyatt *et al.* 1989). Detailed reviews of the instrument are given by Anderson *et al.* (1993) and Bowling (1997).

More recently, an abbreviated version of the SF-36, the SF-12, has been developed (Ware *et al.* 1996). The SF-12 health survey generates the physical and mental component summary scores of the SF-36 'with considerable accuracy, while imposing less burden on the respondents' (Jenkinson & Layte 1997). However, there do appear to be trade-offs in terms of reliability. For example, Jenkinson and Layte (1997) warn that 'the questionnaire contains a number of areas of health tapped with only a single item . . . consequently the SF-36 will provide a more reliable profile of scores across the eight domains than could be gained using the SF-12'.

Both the SF-36 and SF-12 can now be used to estimate QALYs through the SF-6D algorithm. This provides a single summary measure of quality of life based on preference-based weights (Brazier *et al.* 2002; Brazier & Roberts 2004). Likewise, the EQ-5D, provides a simple summary measure of quality of life based on five questions (The EuroQol Group 1990).

Recently there has also been the development of the World Health Organization's Quality of Life Measure (WHOQOL) which seeks to assess inter alia the relevance of spirituality, religion and personal beliefs to health (WHOQOL SRPB Group 2006). These factors are likely to vary, sometimes markedly, from one culture to another, as will their influence on health. This measure is thus particularly important in acknowledging the diversity of cultures and the fact that the construct of health is a cultural phenomenon.

The measurement of both need and health status is thus constantly undergoing improvement and development. That will undoubtedly continue in the future.

Which measure is to be preferred in measuring need is not only a function of why need is being assessed but also the context or environment in which it is being assessed. Many normative factors influence health perceptions including the health of others in the individual's community or group, the nature and severity of the illness, demographic characteristics, and social class (Festinger 1954; Sen 1987; Crawford 1994; Olsen & Dahl 2007). While many measurement efforts are mathematically sophisticated and some are reliable in the sense that they can reproduce the same results from one application to another, they tend to be of questionable validity in so far as they fail to recognize the importance of these normative factors. Currently, most health status indices do not take account of the variation in criteria that individuals or groups use to make judgements about their own health status.

The consistent underperception of ill health observed in many disadvantaged and marginalized groups has 'obvious implications for the design and implementation of public health programs particularly if these programs aim to bring treatment to those most in need of such help' (Wiseman 1999). Secondly, resource allocation decision-making which relies on potentially different subjective measures of health may provide a misleading picture of the resource requirements of some groups in society. This will have implications for estimating healthcare priorities and the funding and planning of health services. There is a need to learn more about the criteria of health which are relevant in judging the well being of these groups and to investigate alternative elicitation procedures which would allow for a more accurate reflection of the preferences of such groups.

Conclusion

The concept of need is elusive but useful. In confronting the notion of need, we acknowledge the value-laden quality of the community's expectation of health services, whether these be for the relief and treatment of illness or the preservation and maintenance of good health. Need derives its meaning from the instrumental pathways we can follow in meeting it and inevitably involves third parties in its definition. Key issues identified in this chapter include:

- The focus of the need for healthcare is on the outcome of such care, namely improved health. This implies that there must be a capacity to benefit from healthcare and that a need can only exist for effective healthcare.
- In determining how to meet need in a setting of limited resources, the allocation of resources must take account of the likely health gain and the cost of that achievement. Moving resources at the margins of our principal programmes of care and health development, according to estimates or measurement of the cost and outcome, offers ways in which we can move in the direction of the wisest use of those resources in meeting need.
- Needs-based formulas have been important in pursuing equitable resource allocation in many countries, generally in relation to promoting equal expenditure for equal need. More emphasis should be placed on incorporating social values in this process, to identify whose needs should be given relatively greater weight in the allocation of limited resources.
- Measuring needs involves assessing the shortfall in health status from some achievable norm, generally using a measure that combines indicators of length of life (mortality) and quality of life (morbidity). There are a few instruments, developed in the United States and Europe, for measuring health-related quality of life that are regarded as valid and reliable. However, further

work is required to assess the appropriateness of these instruments in different cultural contexts and how to account for normative factors that influence health perceptions in need measures.

- Despite the considerable outstanding agenda of work in refining concepts and measures of need, disappointingly little published work has been forthcoming over the past few years. If we are to progress in addressing health sector efficiency and equity, this trend should be reversed.

Acknowledgement

We are grateful to Steve Leeder and Virginia Wiseman for allowing us to use materials contained in previous versions of this chapter, which they co-authored with Gavin Mooney, and the latter also with Stephen Jan.

References

Anand S. and Hanson K. (1997). Disability-adjusted life years: a critical review. *Journal of Health Economics*, **16**, 685–702.

Anderson R., Aaronson N., and Wilkin D. (1993). Critical review of the international assessments if health-related quality of life. *Quality of Life Research*, **2**, 369–95.

Barendregt J.J., Bonneux L., and Van der Maas P.J. (1996). DALYs: the age-weights on balance. *Bulletin of the World Health Organization*, **74**(4), 439–46.

Beck K., Spycher S., Holly A. *et al.* (2003). Risk adjustment in Switzerland. *Health Policy*, **65**, 63–74.

Berwick D.M., DeParle N.A., Eddy D.M. *et al.* (2003). Paying for performance: Medicare should lead. *Health Affairs (Millwood)*, **22**, 8–10.

Bohmer P., Pain C., Watt A. *et al.* (2001). Maximising health gain within available resources in the New Zealand public health system. *Health Policy*, **55**, 37–50.

Bossert T., Larranaga S., Giedion U. *et al.* (2003). Decentralization and equity of resource allocation: evidence from Colombia and Chile. *Bulletin of the World Health Organization*, **81**, 95–100.

Bowden A. and Fox-Rushby J.A. (2003). A systematic and critical review of the process of translation and adaptation of generic health related quality of life measures in Africa, Asia, Eastern Europe, the Middle East, South America. *Social Science and Medicine*, **57**, 1289–306.

Bowling A. (1997). *Measuring health. A review of quality of life measurement scales* (2nd edn). Open University Press, Milton Keynes.

Brazier J.E. and Roberts J. (2004). Estimating a preference-based index from the SF-12. *Medical Care*, **42**(9), 851–9.

Brazier J.E., Roberts J., and Deverill M (2002). The estimation of a preference-based measure of health from the SF-36. *Journal of Health Economics*, **21**, 271–92.

Cavanagh S. and Chadwick K. (2005). *Health needs assessment: A practical guide*. Health Development Agency (now National Institute for Health and Clinical Excellence), London.

Cornell S., Curtis C. and Jorgensen M. (2004). *Joint Occasional Paper on Native Affairs No 2004–02: The concept of governance and is implications for First Nations*. The Harvard Project on American Indian Economic Development, Boston.mhttp://www.jopna.net/pubs/jopna_2004-02_Governance.pdf

Crawford R. (1994). The boundaries of the self and the unhealthy other: reflections on health, culture and AIDS. *Social Science and Medicine*, **38**, 1347–65.

Culyer A.J. (1991). *Equity in health care policy.* Paper presented to the Ontario Premier's Council on Health, Well-Being and Social Justice. University of Toronto, Toronto.

Culyer A.J. and Wagstaff A. (1993). Equity and equality in health and health care. *Journal of Health Economics*. **12**, 431–57.

DHSS (Department of Health and Social Security) (1976). *Report of the Resource Allocation Working Party (RAWP)*. HMSO, London.

DHSS (Department of Health and Social Security) (1986). *Review of the Resource Allocation Working Party Formula.* Report by the NHS Management Board. DHSS, London.

Dixon J. and Welch H.G. (1991). Priority setting: Lessons from Oregon. *Lancet*, **337**, 912–6.

The EuroQol Group (1990). EuroQol: A new facility for the measurement of health-related quality of life. *Health Policy*, 16, 199–208.

Festinger L. (1954). A theory of social comparison processes. *Human Relations*, **7**, 117–40.

Garratt A., Ruta D., Abdalla M. *et al.* (1993). The SF36 Health survey Questionnaire: an outcome measure suitable for routine use within the NHS? *British Medical Journal*, **306**, 1440–4.

Gerard K. and Mooney G. (1993). QALY league tables: handle with care. *Health Economics*, **2**, 59–64.

Gilson L., Doherty J., McIntyre D. *et al.* (1999). *The Dynamics of Policy Change: Health Care Financing in South Africa 1994–99. Monograph No. 66.* Centre for Health Policy and Health Economics Unit, Johannesburg.

Guyatt G., Nogradi S., Halcrow S. *et al.* (1989). Development and testing of a new measure of health status for clinical trials in health failure. *Journal of General Internal Medicine*, **4**, 101–7.

Health Policy (1995). Special issue on programme budgeting and marginal analysis. *Health Policy*, **33**.

Houston S. (2004). *Aboriginal Health Policy: The Past, the Present, the Future.* PhD Thesis. Curtin University, Perth.

Institute of Medicine (2001). *Crossing the quality chasm: a new health system for the 21st century*. National Academy Press, Washington, D.C.

Jacobs L., Marmor T., and Oberlander J. (1999). The Oregon Health Plan and the political paradox of rationing: what advocates and critics have claimed and what Oregon did. *Journal of Health Politics, Policy and Law*, **24**, 161–80.

Jenkinson C. and Layte R. (1997). Development and testing of the UK SF-12. *Journal of Health Services Research and Policy*, **2**, 14–8.

Jenkinson C., Layte R., Wright L. *et al.* (1996). *The UK SF-36: an analysis and interpretation manual*. Health Services Research Unit, Oxford.

Kitzhaber J.A. (1993). Prioritizing health services in an era of limits: the Oregon experiment. *British Medical Journal*, **307**, 373–7.

Krasnik A., Groenewegen P., Pedersen P.A. *et al.* (1990). Changing remuneration systems: effects on activity in general practice. *British Medical Journal*, **300**, 1698–701.

Kurtin P., Davies A., Meyer K. *et al.* (1992). Patient-based health status measurements in outpatient dialysis: early experiences in developing an outcomes assessment program. *Medical Care*, **30** (Supplement 5), MS136–49.

Levine M., Guyatt G., Gent M. *et al.* (1988). Quality of life in stage II breast cancer: an instrument for clinical trials. *Journal of Clinical Oncology*, **6**, 1798–810.

Liss P.E. (1990). *Health care need: meaning and measurement.* Linkoping University, Linkoping.

Loewy E.H. (1990). Commodities, needs and health care: a communal perspective. In: *Changing values in medical and health care decision making* (ed. J.J. Jensen and G. Mooney), pp. 17–31. Wiley, Chichester.

Loomes G. and McKenzie I. (1989). The scope and limitations of QALY measures. *Social Science and Medicine*, **28**, 299–308.

McLeod H. (2004). *Social Health Insurance: An introduction for practitioners.* University of Pretoria, Pretoria.

McHorney C., Ware J., Rogers W. *et al.* (1992). The validity and relative precision of MOS short- and long-form health status scales and Dartmouth COOP charts: results from the medical outcomes study. *Medical Care*, **30** (Supplement 5), MS253–65.

McHorney C., Ware J., and Raczek A. (1993). The MOS 36-item short form health survey. II: Psychometric and clinical tests of validity in measuring physical and mental health constructs. *Medical Care*, **31**, 247–63.

Maslow A.H. (1943). A theory of human motivation. *Psychological Review*, **50**, 370–396

Mason A.R., Drummond M.F., Hunter J.A. *et al.* (2005). Prescribing incentive schemes: a useful approach? *Applied Health Economics and Health Policy*, **4**(2), 111–117

Mehrez A. and Gafni A. (1989). Quality adjusted life years, utility theory and healthy year equivalents. *Medical Decision Making*, **9**, 142–9.

MHSS (Ministry of Health and Social Services) and WHO (World Health Organization), Namibia (2005). *Equity in health care in Namibia: Towards needs-based allocation formula.* Regional Network for Equity in Health in Southern Africa (EQUINET), Harare. (http://www.equinetafrica.org/bibl/docs/DIS26finNamibia.pdf)

Mooney G. (1998). 'Communitarian claims' as an ethical basis for allocating health care resources. *Social Science and Medicine*, **47**, 1171–80.

Mooney G.H. and Blackwell S.H. (2004) Whose health service is it anyway? Community values in healthcare. *Medical Journal of Australia*, **180**, 76–8.

Mooney G. and Creese A. (1993). Priority setting for health service efficiency: the role of measurement of burden of illness. In *Disease control priorities in developing countries* (ed. D. Jamison, W. Mosely, A. Measham and J. Bobadilla). Oxford University Press, New York.

Mooney G. and Houston S. (2004). An alternative approach to resource allocation: weighted capacity to benefit plus MESH infrastructure. *Applied Health Economics and Health Policy*, **3**(1), 29–33.

Mooney G., Jan S., and Wiseman V. (1995). Examining preferences for allocating health gains. *Health Care Analysis*, **3**, 261–5.

Murray C.J.L. (1994). Quantifying the burden of disease: the technical basis for disability-adjusted life years. *Bulletin of the World Health Organization*, **72**(3), 429–45.

Murray C. and Lopez A. (1997a). The utility of DALYs for public health policy and research: a reply. *Bulletin of the World Health Organization*, **75**, 377–81.

Murray C.J.L. and Lopez A.D. (1997b). Regional patterns of disability-free life expectancy and disability-adjusted life expectancy: Global Burden of Disease Study. *The Lancet*, **349**, 1347–52.

Nord E., Richardson J., Street A. *et al.* (1995). Maximising health benefits versus egalitarianism: an Australian survey of health issues. *Social Science and Medicine*, **41**(10),1429–37.

Oberlander J. (2007). Health reform interrupted: The unravelling of the Oregon Health Plan. *Health Affairs*, **26**(1), 96–105.

Olsen K.M. and Dahl S.A. (2007). Health differences between European countries. *Social Science and Medicine* (in press).

Oregon Health Plan (1997). *The uninsured in Oregon 1977.* Office for Oregon Health Plan Research, Salem.

O'Reilly D., Rosato M., and Patterson C. (2005) Self reported health and mortality: ecological analysis based on electoral wards across the United Kingdom. *British Medical Journal*, **331**(7522), 938–939.

Paalman M., Bekedam H., Hawken L. *et al.* (1998). A critical review of priority setting in the health sector: the methodology of the 1993 World Development Report. *Health Policy and Planning*, **13**(1), 13–31.

Pearson M. (2002). *Allocating Public Resources for Health: Developing Pro-poor Approaches.* DFID Health Systems Resource Centre, London.

Rocha G., Martinez A., Rios E. *et al.* (2004) Resource allocation equity in northeastern Mexico. *Health Policy*, **70**, 271–9.

Sayers B.M. and Fliedner T.M. (1997). The critique of DALYs: a counter-reply. *Bulletin of the World Health Organization*, **75**, 383–4.

Sculpher M. (2006) The use of quality-adjusted life-years in cost-effectiveness studies. *Allergy*, **61**(5), 527–30.

Sen A. (1987). *On ethics and economics.* Basil Blackwell, Oxford.

Teng T.O. (1996). An evaluation of Oregon's Medicaid rationing algorithms. *Health Economics*, **5**, 171–81.

Thomas S., Mooney G., and Mbatsha S. (2007). The MESH approach: strengthening public health systems for the MDGs. *Health Policy*, **83**(2-3), 180–5.

Torrance G.W. (1986). Measurement of health state utilities for economic appraisal. *Journal of Health Economics*, **5**, 1–30.

Ugalde A. and Jackson J.T. (1995). The World Bank and international health policy: A critical review. *Journal of International Development*, **7**(3), 525–41.

van Vliet R.C.J.A. and van de Ven P.M.M. (1992). Towards a capitation formula for competing health insurers: An empirical analysis. *Social Science and Medicine*, **34**(9), 1035–48.

Ware J., Kosinski M., and Keller S. (1996). A 12-item short-form health survey: construction of scales and preliminary tests of reliability and validity. *Medical Care*, **34**, 220–33.

Ware J., Snow K., Kosinski M. *et al.* (1993). *SF-36 survey manual and interpretation guide.* Health Institute, New England Medical Center, Boston, MA.

WHOQOL SRPB Group (2006). A cross cultural study of spirituality, religion, and personal beliefs as components of quality of life. *Social Science and Medicine*, **62**(6), 1486–97.

Williams A. (1985). Economic of coronary artery bypass grafting. *British Medical Journal*, **49**, 825–31.

Williams A. (1999). Calculating the global burden of disease: time for a strategic reappraisal? *Health Economics*, **8**, 1–8.

Wiseman V. (1999). Culture, self-rated health and resource allocation decision-making. *Health Care Analysis*, **7**, 207–23.

Wiseman V. and Mooney G. (1998). Burden of illness estimates for priority setting: a debate revisited. *Health Policy*, **43**, 243–51.

Wiseman V., Mooney G., Berry G. *et al.* (2003). Involving the general public in priority setting: experiences from Australia. *Social Science and Medicine*, **56**, 1001–12.

World Bank (1993). *World Development Report 1993: Investing in Health.* Oxford University Press for The World Bank, New York.

World Bank (1994). *Better Health in Africa: Experience and Lessons Learned.* The World Bank, Washington, D.C.

World Health Organization (2001). *Macroeonomics and Health: Investing in Health for Economic Development. Report of the Commission on Macroeconomics and Health.* World Health Organization, Geneva.

12.2

Needs assessment: A practical approach

Aileen Clarke, John Powell, and Mary Ann Lansang[1]

Abstract

Needs assessment is an essential part of planning for health care and public health. This chapter describes a practical approach to needs assessment, building on the previous chapter on need and its measurement (McIntyre *et al.* 2009). Needs assessment aims to ensure a population-based, epidemiological, and public health approach to the planning of health interventions. It is of particular importance in publicly funded systems but is also of value in other systems. A needs assessment should provide a specific plan for meeting the needs of a specific population, with a specified health condition or set of conditions, taking questions of effectiveness, affordability, allocative efficiency, equity, and access into account and independent of competing clinical or commercial interests. A conventional needs assessment includes epidemiological, comparative, and corporate components although this chapter also considers rapid needs assessment and participatory community appraisal techniques. In the past, needs assessment has been seen as failing to contribute expected benefits; however, needs assessment has great potential to contribute valuable practical public health inputs to any health organization's activities.

Introduction

Need for needs assessment

In any health system, decisions must be made about the introduction of new services, the closure of old services, and the re-organization of others. How should such decision be taken? While there is often an underlying emphasis on financial considerations, health and health improvement have to be key considerations.

Health planning often follows an incremental approach, with a varying ability of planners and managers to respond rationally to changes in demography, the epidemiology of disease or the availability of new pharmaceuticals or technologies (Buse *et al.* 2007). Needs assessment can provide a rational, systematic, and analytical approach to planning health care as part of a cycle of planning, execution, or implementation of change, management, and review (Fig. 12.2.1).

Definitions and issues of definition in needs assessment

Needs assessment is the process of identifying need for health interventions and its distribution in a population. Need has been defined as 'the capacity to benefit' (McIntyre *et al.* 2009), but it is important to consider definitions of both 'capacity' and 'benefit'. Capacity is defined here as the ability to make use of a needed intervention. Benefit is defined as a reduction in disease or disability or an improvement in health. However, need is a value-laden and contested concept as McIntyre, Mooney, and Jan demonstrate (McIntyre *et al.* 2009). This raises questions concerning whose view of capacity should be taken into account? And whose estimate of the extent of a reduction in disease or disability should be considered as representing a legitimate benefit?

It is also important to distinguish 'need' from 'demand or want' and from 'utilization' or 'supply' (Fig. 12.2.2). Need has sometimes

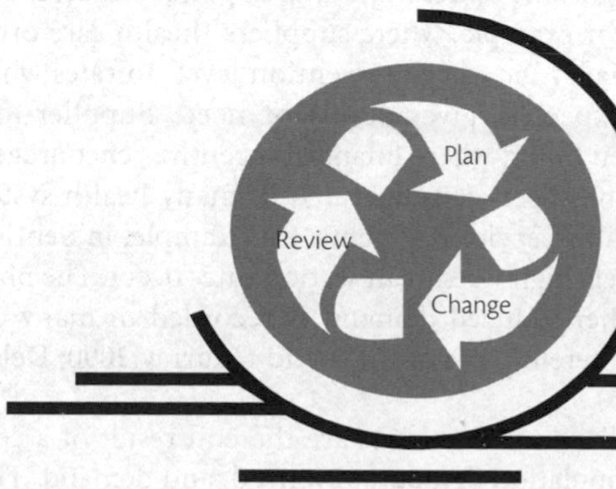

Fig. 12.2.1 Forward rolling cycle of management planning, implementing change, and review.

[1] M. A. Lansang, chapter co-author, currently works at The Global Fund to Fight AIDS, Tuberculosis and Malaria. The views expressed in this chapter are those of the named authors and do not necessarily reflect the decisions or stated policy of The Global Fund.

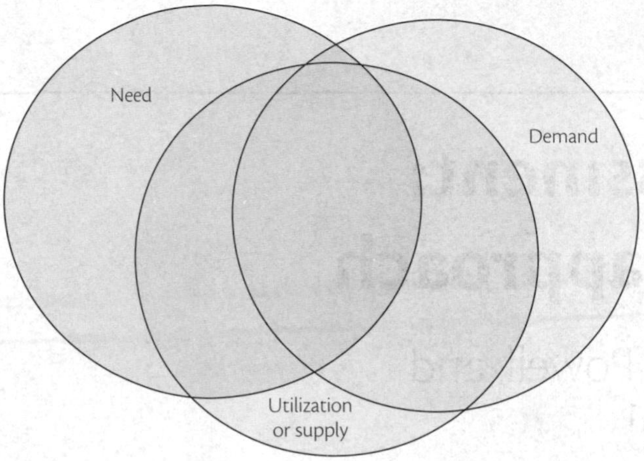

Fig. 12.2.2 Overlapping circles of need, demand, and utilization. (For most conditions there is little empirical evidence for the extent to which these circles overlap.)

been defined as the professional view of capacity to benefit; if the clinical professional view is that those with a certain level of severity of a condition will benefit from a specific intervention, then they are considered to have a 'need'. If a person believes that they have a capacity to benefit from an intervention that is considered a 'want'. The want can be translated into a demand by a request for that intervention. Need and demand can of course co-exist or exist separately. When professionally-defined need is not addressed by services, there is said to be 'unmet need'.

Utilization (or use or supply) of health services can exist in the absence of need. As an example, some would say that high rates of upper gastrointestinal endoscopy may represent utilization without need (NICE 2007). It is much rarer for utilization to occur without demand. Usually if a person takes up a service or intervention, it can be assumed that it is demanded (although compulsory psychiatric intervention could be seen as utilization without demand).

It is also important to be aware that supplier-induced demand can occur, as for example, where suppliers (health care organizations or clinicians) increase intervention levels to rates which are higher than expected, given levels of need. Supplier-induced demand is often found where financial incentives encourage intervention. This has been demonstrated in many health systems in relation to fee-for-service payments, for example, in dentistry, or where excessively high Caesarean section rates occur. The phenomenon of supplier-induced demand is recorded in many clinical areas and in different parts of the world (Murray 2000; Delattre & Dormont 2003).

Rates of utilization of services are the end result of a complex interplay of population demography, need, and demand. They are related to the extent of unmet need, supplier-induced demand, and the availability of services, as well as a population's ability to access them (McKee & Clarke 1995). In some rare urgent and emergency cases, for example severe head injury due to road accidents (Williams *et al.* 1997), utilization rates may come close to reflecting the actual level of need within a population, but in most cases, utilization rates used in this way will not give an accurate estimate of need.

Levels of needs assessment

It is important to be aware that needs assessment as defined may be undertaken at a number of different levels. Needs assessment can be undertaken for:

a) A whole population

b) A subgroup of the population (McNeil *et al.* 2006; Wright & Tomkins 2006)

c) A subgroup of the population suffering from a specific condition, e.g. stroke (Mant *et al.* 2004) or drug misuse (Marsden *et al.* 2004) or for specific interventions, e.g. hip replacement (Dawson *et al.* 2004), carotid endarterectomy (Ferris *et al.* 1998), or emergency obstetric care (Orinda *et al.* 2005)

d) For a population using a particular service, e.g. psychology and counselling services, rural primary care services, accident and emergency services (Williams *et al.* 1997); and prison health service (Cresswell *et al.* 2005)

e) For an individual person or family. Need for healthcare, housing, food, sanitation, safety, etc., can be gauged for individuals and a service or treatment plan put in action

This chapter will focus mainly on needs assessment at levels c and d in the above classification (subgroups of the population either suffering from a specific condition or in need of a specific intervention, and assessment of need for a particular health service). Level e will not be considered further because in this chapter concentrates on needs assessment at the population level. The principles of needs assessment for levels a and b are similar to those for c and d, although this sort of needs assessment can sometimes be important (McNeil *et al.* 2006). The process of starting from a zero base to work out the whole health care needs of a population is rarely undertaken except in emergency situations (McNeil *et al.* 2006). Thinking further about levels c and d, it is also possible to undertake needs assessment either for a service, e.g. blood transfusion services or smoking prevention services or for a recognized disease or problem, e.g. alcohol misuse (Cook 2004). Needs assessment can be undertaken for different types of health intervention, e.g. for health protection and infectious disease control; for health education, health promotion and disease prevention; for screening and immunization; for diagnostics; for acute treatments and ongoing treatment for chronic disease, for rehabilitation, and for terminal and palliative care. A public health approach would normally include health education, health promotion, and disease prevention as part of the range of interventions for any condition.

Timing of needs assessment

When should a needs assessment be undertaken? Ideally, a needs assessment should be undertaken whenever a major change in a health services or programme is anticipated or occurs. Of course, a needs assessment should be undertaken in advance of a planned change in order to inform that change. A needs assessment should not be undertaken simply to provide a post hoc justification for a change that has already been agreed.

When does a needs assessment end? This is not a spurious question since many models of needs assessment discuss the process of implementing change. This chapter will cover the process of needs assessment until a recommended, evidence-based, and costed plan for change has been produced, but many would suggest that the needs assessment does not end here and that the management processes for implementing change are also part of the needs assessment.

The definitions and distinctions outlined in this section are important because they impact on methods for undertaking needs assessments. Often in needs assessments, normative judgements of need are used, demands are not always included or viewed as legitimate, unmet need is considered too difficult to measure, and utilization rates are used as a proxy for need. However, needs assessment should distinguish between demand and need and evaluate met and unmet needs taking into account the contextual and value-laden nature of the definition of need. This may be of particular importance if either the health care intervention under consideration or proposed changes are controversial. Community participatory techniques and rapid assessment procedures (RAP), which are discussed later in the chapter, both tackle some of these issues directly.

Undertaking a needs assessment

The aim of needs assessment is to deliver practical information to change public health and health services. One useful definition is; 'to maximize the appropriate delivery of effective health interventions or care and to minimize both the provision of ineffective health intervention or care and the existence of unmet need for healthcare in an evidence-based way', and to 'maximize equity' (Powell 2006). This definition gives the overall aim of a needs assessment and in the following section we will break down the practicalities of needs assessment into a series of steps. In practice these will require adaptation to local circumstances.

A needs assessment is highly dependent on data. Variations occur in the availability, extent, reliability, and validity of data sources both for the evidence of effectiveness and for the underlying demography of the population of interest. One of the recurring themes in needs assessment is to what extent can, or should, new data be gathered? We would suggest that for a practical needs assessment to be of value in usual health management timescales, new data collection should be kept to an absolute minimum, but that pragmatism should prevail. In some low- and middle-income countries, there are often no alternatives to the collection of new data as many routine health statistics are incomplete, unreliable, and inaccurate. In emergency situations, *ad hoc* data collection is the rule. Rapid Appraisal Procedures are of particular value in this context.

A number of models for undertaking a needs assessment have been proposed including those of Cavanagh and Chadwick (2005) and Stevens and Raftery (2004), and we draw on both of these in the following sections. In particular, we will draw on an 'epidemiological, corporate and comparative' model (Stevens & Raftery 2004) in the following plan of action for a needs assessment.

Problem definition

As with any project, planning is required in the early stages to clarify aims and objectives and the reasons for undertaking a needs assessment. It is important to clarify who the 'customer' or commissioner of the needs assessment is, what they hope to achieve from the needs assessment, how much resource they can offer for the needs assessment to be undertaken, their role within the health or public health system and their relationships with other stakeholders. Needs assessments can present those managing health services with hard choices and difficult decisions, and it is important that those undertaking a needs assessment are aware of this from the outset. Certain questions should be asked, and answered, at this stage before a needs assessment can proceed, and these are shown in Box 12.2.1.

Box 12.2.1 Seven questions to be asked before undertaking a needs assessment

1. Why is this needs assessment needed now?
2. Who will be affected?
3. What would be the consequences of doing nothing?
4. How much time is available? There may be pivotal decision points within the organization for which the results of the needs assessment will be needed.
5. How can the results and recommendations of the needs assessment be produced and presented to facilitate informed action?
6. Are sufficient resources available? This includes managerial support at the appropriate level for implementation
7. How will the needs assessment itself be assessed and evaluated?

Stakeholder advisory group

A number of stakeholders will need to give their view on the definition of the problem and the issues which will need to be included. Ideally at the earliest stage, a stakeholder advisory group should be set up. The group should include the commissioner of the needs assessment, and other key stakeholders. These would usually include clinical or health experts in the field (current providers of services either may or may not be included); and may also include methodological experts; members of local communities, users of services and their representatives; voluntary sector, religious and charity representatives, and representatives of other concerned organizations (e.g. local councils or local or district authorities) or individuals. While it is very important to be clear about the advisory nature of these stakeholders' roles, is also important to be inclusive at this stage, in order to offer the needs assessment the optimal chance of legitimacy and implementation. Community participatory needs assessments tend to afford greater emphasis to engagement of members of the community at this stage. Box 12.2.2 shows an example of stakeholder involvement.

Project plan

The next phase of the needs assessment is to develop a formal costed project plan. The work should be broken down into manageable steps. For each step, an estimate of how long it will take, and how much it will cost should be made, and tasks should be allocated so that is clear who will undertake the work and how dependencies in timings between different project components will be managed. Production of a project plan may seem either a luxury or a nuisance; however, this planning stage is invaluable in developing a proper understanding of the work. The project plan can be used to monitor progress and can be amplified and modified as a working document which can be built on to produce the report of the work.

Box 12.2.2 Stakeholders in a needs assessment for male circumcision for HIV/AIDS prevention and control

Recent evidence from three randomized controlled trials in Africa shows reduction of HIV/AIDS by more than half among males who were circumcised (see detailed discussion of the evidence in Chapter 6.11, this volume). Male circumcision has been hailed by many international health organizations as an important intervention for HIV/AIDS prevention, particularly in high-burden areas like sub-Saharan Africa, India, and China.

But Sawires *et al.* (2007) have identified at least 13 issues that need to be considered for effective implementation, for example, acceptability among men and women, and among different ethnic and religious groups; perceptions of benefits and risks; timing of circumcision; safety and complications; and health system requirements.

For a needs assessment for services to increase the use of male circumcision for HIV/AIDS prevention, stakeholders will include:

- Experts: HIV/AIDS, epidemiology, behavioural sciences, mathematical modelling, health economics, communications, bioethics
- Policy makers: Local, regional, and national
- Health service payers and providers
- NGOs
- Religious and rights-based groups
- Community representatives especially for young people, and people living with AIDS

Box 12.2.3 Stages of a needs assessment

A. *Epidemiological needs assessment*—which answers the questions: How many people 'need' care for this condition in the local population and what effective interventions should be available for them?

B. *Comparative needs assessment*—which answers the question: How do others provide services for this condition?

C. *Corporate or local needs assessment*—which answers a series of questions. How are services currently provided locally? How does this compare with expected provision given evidence on incidence and prevalence? How do current treatments and interventions compare with the evidence of effectiveness? How do local services compare with those in other places? How do local treatments and services compare with what others consider should be done? (e.g. patient groups, government departments insurers, payers, etc.). What are the gaps? What are the options for improvement? What changes are required and how much will they cost?

Models of needs assessment

Drawing on Stevens and Raftery (2004) we are going to describe a detailed plan for how to undertake a needs assessment using epidemiological, corporate, and comparative approaches. Box 12.2.3 shows these stages of the Stevens and Raftery model. After describing this approach we will describe Rapid Assessment Procedures which are useful to provide information where data sources are limited and/or when the needs assessment is required urgently.

Epidemiological needs assessment: The population of interest

How many people 'need' care for this condition in the local population and what effective interventions are available for them?

The first phase of the actual work is to begin to understand the underlying characteristics of the population of interest from whom the population of those with a need for the service/s under consideration is drawn. As mentioned in the introductory section, the local population may be defined geographically, or by a particular insurance plan, or as a particular subgroup of a community. The demography of the local population, including age and sex structure and mortality, needs to be understood, along with any information available on broader health, welfare, and public health issues, health status, inequalities, and socioeconomic status, demand for health care, and underlying relevant risk factors.

Gathering data on the local or denominator population will be important for two reasons. First, it is important to be able to locate a needs assessment properly within an understanding of competing priorities for both the organization and for the population itself. This can only be done by developing an understanding of the population of interest. Secondly, much of the available epidemiological evidence for particular conditions is available, using age- and sex-standardized rates per hundred thousand population. In order to derive local estimates and to understand need (absolute numbers of those requiring interventions), the age and sex structure and characteristics of the local population need to be understood.

Many organizations publish demographic data which are relatively easily accessible for geographic areas and for appropriate reference populations. In many countries, routine data collection and manipulation, including censuses, death certification statistics and population projections, and estimates together allow for a picture of the structure of a population to be built up (National Statistics 2007). Insurance companies keep their own enrollees' demographic data (Young *et al.* 1991). Exceptions exist in poor countries or countries where breakdown in civil structures has occurred, during war, for example, where censuses are non-existent or unreliable, where special surveys may have to be undertaken to provide estimates of the relevant population structure. For some countries, where national information systems are weak, there have been efforts over the past 30 years to establish health and demographic surveillance systems to provide longitudinal, population-based data on important health and vital events for specific geographic areas or sentinel sites (Adazu *et al.* 2005). The INDEPTH Network (an International Network of field sites with continuous Demographic Evaluation of Populations and Their Health in developing countries) has 37 demographic surveillance sites in 19 countries. Problems can also arise in attempting to undertake a needs assessment for a subgroup of a community where no reliable population data exist and the issue of whether such data should be collected *de novo* arises.

Information on the structure of the local population may be relatively easy to access in many countries, but information on broader health and welfare, inequalities, socioeconomic status, and health status and demand for health care, and underlying relevant risk factors, may be much more difficult to obtain. In many countries, data on mortality by cause are collected which have been used as a measure of demand for health care, although there are drawbacks to this use of mortality data in needs assessments, as McIntyre, Mooney, and Jan point out (McIntyre *et al.* 2009). In the United Kingdom, the Health Survey for England (DH Health Survey 2007) provides data on levels of smoking or obesity, or health status but these rates are derived from relatively small samples of the overall UK population and are not always valid for smaller population groups. However, many local public health organizations undertake local health surveys, which document demography, health determinants (e.g. health risks and health behaviours), and health status, and these can be extremely valuable. Community participation can also be valuable here, where communities themselves can participate in local data collection. This is discussed again later in this chapter.

Epidemiological needs assessment: Conditions and levels of severity

The next step is to consider the conditions or diseases for which the needs assessment is being undertaken and, in particular, to consider known levels of severity, since need for intervention will vary with levels of severity. The main sources of information include published research literature, grey literature, policy documents, guidelines, and textbooks, but in some countries there will be morbidity surveys, or disease registries, for example, cancer registry data, which can be used. It may also be the case that others have already undertaken a needs assessment in the area and already listed relevant categories of severity. Literature searching techniques are not covered in detail in this chapter, but for this stage of a practical needs assessment, literature searching in order to understand categories of severity does not have to be exhaustive and governed by the same strict rules as for systematic reviews. It does, however, need to be systematic in its coverage of the important information and reasonably up-to-date since methods of categorizing diseases change.

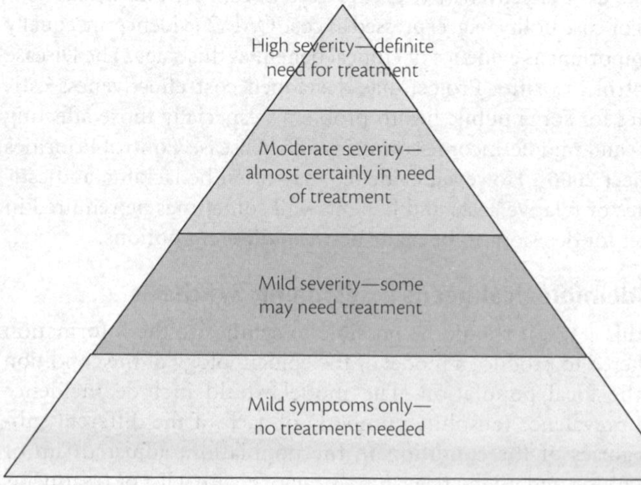

Fig. 12.2.3 Subcategories and levels of need in a population.

For some conditions and diseases, reliable and valid methods for measuring grades of severity are well documented. Examples include the American Urologists Association (AUA) categorization for prostatic hypertrophy (Barry *et al.* 1992), the international TNM (tumour, node, metastasis) systems for the classification of cancers (UICC and TNM 2007), the Oxford hip score (Dawson *et al.* 2001), and many more. Figure 12.2.3 gives a diagrammatic representation of the information to be collected on levels of severity.

A common scenario is that it is only possible to obtain estimates of incidence and prevalence for those in the most severe category of illness. However, a 'public health' approach, means that all those in each relevant category including those in the general population eligible for screening or primary prevention should also be estimated.

Epidemiological needs assessment: Risk factors

While it is very important to know the likely numbers of people in each grade of severity, it is also important to understand these differential risk subgroups in the population of interest who may experience a different rate of the disease under consideration. They may be either unequally exposed to an important determinant or unequally susceptible to the exposure and the likelihood of disease. There may be specific risk factors for the condition under consideration which need taking into account. One example would be in needs for diabetes services where the levels of people in any particular severity category are related to characteristics of the underlying population, e.g. levels of diet and physical activity (Chowdhury *et al.* 2005). For example, in hepatic cirrhosis, levels of alcohol consumption in the population will need to be measured or estimated.

Epidemiological needs assessment: Numbers affected by conditions and levels of severity within the reference population

Information on the population of interest and information on the diseases or conditions under consideration should be combined to estimate the absolute numbers of people suffering from the condition both overall and within each category of severity. It is important at this stage to be clear about absolute numbers in each level of severity and not to confuse absolute and relative measures of risk. Ideally, it would be possible to obtain incidence and prevalence values directly for the local population itself, but the possibilities either of data being available or for them to be collected within the time available for a needs assessment are low. There are often gaps in the evidence, and it is almost always necessary to extrapolate from other populations from epidemiological surveys or from health needs assessments elsewhere.

Given this extrapolation it is important for assumptions made to be made explicit. For example, one might assume that epidemiology of cataracts of the eye might be comparable between different cities in the same country (Wadud *et al.* 2006), or that rates of severe ankle sprain in children and young people apply equally in two different European cities. These are testable assumptions and contestable if clearly stated in the needs assessment. Figure 12.2.4 gives an example of an epidemiological study where information might be used in a needs assessment. Figure 12.2.4 shows World Health Organization (WHO) estimated numbers of new TB cases in different countries in the world in 2005. This map illustrates variations in numbers, and the complete lack of data from some countries. Of course, for a local or regional needs assessment it is very important to have more detailed data on absolute numbers of

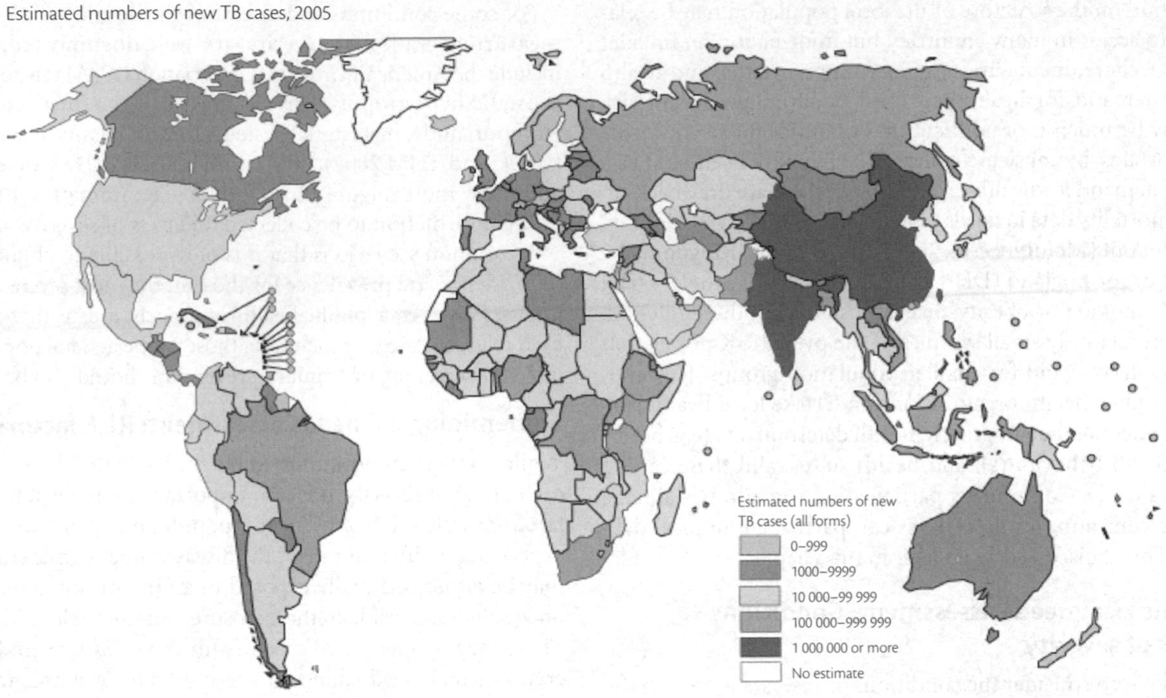

Fig. 12.2.4 Estimated numbers of new cases of TB by country in 2005.
Source: WHO Report 2007. Global Tuberculosis Control. Surveillance, Planning and Financing http://www.who.int/tb/publications/global_report/2007/pdf/full.pdf

those affected. An ideal approach is to have estimates of both incidence and prevalence. Need for services varies with stages in the trajectory of illness, but service use is often highly concentrated around the time of diagnosis, and assessment of needs is enhanced if absolute numbers of both incident cases per year and prevalent cases can be estimated. A significant problem in this part of a needs assessment is that often there is very little evidence relating to the natural history of disease. Little is known about what happens in the absence of treatment. However, natural history is important when 'unmet need' is being considered. Evidence may be sparse or lacking in this area, and discussion with clinicians may provide the most fruitful information. Another problem is attempting to understand factors affecting demand. This may not be an easy task although there is some literature which is published on this topic for different disease areas (e.g. reluctance to attend for screening appointments (Chan *et al.* 2002), but the relationship between need and demand is under-researched, and there may be little evidence to find.

Epidemiological needs assessment: The evidence on effectiveness and costs

The next stage of the needs assessment is to find and appraise evidence of the clinical and cost-effectiveness of interventions for the condition and for its different subcategories. This part of the needs assessment again requires searching of the research literature, grey literature, and policy documents to find the range of interventions available and estimates of their effectiveness. Interventions can act at a number of different levels and may include methods for screening or prevention as well as pharmaceutical or surgical interventions, rehabilitation services, etc. It is customary to take as much account of the hierarchy of evidence as possible in deriving the evidence base in a needs assessment. Therefore, for example, evidence consisting of systematic reviews of large number of large randomized controlled trials (RCTs) should clearly be given more weight than single RCTs which should themselves be given more weight than observational designs and other evidence further down the hierarchy. However, it is often hard to find evidence to support the use of a particular well-known intervention which is believed to be beneficial. It is important to document these evidence gaps, and many needs assessments include recommendations for further research, recognizing a need for more and better evidence for common interventions. It is important at this stage not to be constrained by an awareness of the health services that are already currently provided to the population for the conditions under consideration but to approach the evidence in a spirit of inquiry. Sometimes radically different combinations of treatments or specific interventions can be shown to be more beneficial than those which are currently provided. Cost-effectiveness (e.g. expressed as cost per unit health benefit) or cost-utility (e.g. expressed as cost/QALY) evidence are equally as important as evidence of clinical benefit at this stage. The Disease Control Priorities Project, has developed cost-effectiveness estimates for some public health problems, especially those affecting low- and middle-income countries (The Disease Control Priorities Project 2006). However, evidence may often be lacking, and estimates of relative costs and benefits will sometimes be required in order for decisions to be made between different options.

Epidemiological needs assessment: Synthesis

At this stage, it should be possible to synthesize the information gathered to produce a model of the epidemiology of the condition in the local population. The model would include incidence and prevalence (absolute numbers) of each of the different subcategories of the condition in the population, adjusted (up or down) for underlying relevant risk factors; with a list of treatments and interventions ranked according to evidence of effectiveness and evidence relating to costs effectiveness and estimated actual likely costs where available. Often, the information estimated will be incomplete and imprecise, but this summary is the basis on which the next stages can be built.

Comparative needs assessment

How do others provide services for this condition?

Armed with the evidence of clinical and cost-effectiveness and an understanding of the local populations' needs, the aim of this phase of the needs assessment is to investigate how others approach meeting need and organizing services for the condition under consideration.

Comparative needs assessment: Models of care in practice

The research and grey literatures may be helpful in investigating others' approaches to organizing services and care pathways and patterns. It will be important to identify similar populations, systems, and services to the one under study and to meet those providing those services, to investigate what they do and the problems and issues that they face. This phase does not have to be restricted by country, and other countries may offer useful insights into how to provide care for particular conditions.

This phase may also simply be about opening a dialogue with other health service or health care providers to find out how they plan and offer services for this condition. It may help to be reasonably systematic about data gathering especially if a number of providers are being consulted at this stage, in order to ensure that all important items are covered. This part of the needs assessment should result in a list of models of care including patient care patterns and pathways and their relative strengths in practice.

Comparative needs assessment: The existence of variation

The existence of variation in intervention rates presents a problem for comparative needs assessment. Internationally, substantial variation in health care provision and utilization has been described, much of it not explained by known factors such as the apparent level of morbidity or 'need' within a population (Weinstein 2004). Therefore, it should be recognized that chosen comparators may be outliers, either under- or over-providing services for patients with a particular condition. Figure 12.2.5 illustrates this graphically. Women living in different districts in England had a varying likelihood of undergoing hysterectomy within the NHS between 1999 and 2003. Age-standardized rates can be seen to vary dramatically (Goldacre *et al.* 2005). Although the best comparators from a population point of view should be chosen, the possibility should also be considered that these chosen comparators may not be representative.

These figures show that quantitative, comparative needs assessment can be useful for highlighting variation and raising questions about that variation. However, comparative needs assessment may be most useful for providing a list of organizational models and patterns of care.

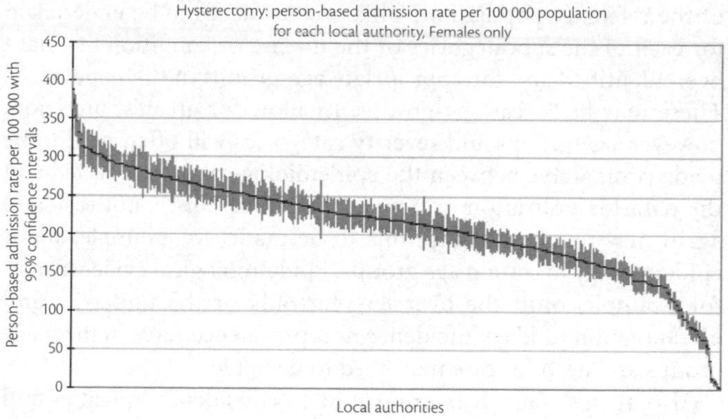

Fig. 12.2.5 Standardized admission rates (SARs) for hysterectomy per 100 000 women for a 3-year period (1998–1999 to 2002–2003), by local authority area with 95% confidence intervals.

Source: Unit for Health care Epidemiology, University of Oxford. (Each dot shows the rate for women in a single local authority and the border shows 95% confidence intervals.)

Corporate needs assessment

How are services currently provided locally? How does this compare with expected provision given evidence on incidence and prevalence? How do current treatments and interventions compare with the evidence of effectiveness? How do local services compare with those in other places? How do local treatments and services compare with what others consider should be done (e.g. patient groups, government departments insurers, payers, etc.)? What are the gaps? What are the options for improvement? What changes are required, and how much will they cost?

Corporate needs assessment: Current model of care

The corporate needs assessment is the stage where ongoing input from the stakeholder group will be most useful. For the first task of the corporate needs assessment, it is necessary to understand current service provision and utilization statistics. The best approach to this phase is a thorough and systematic data gathering process where all providers, and all relevant service users and members of the public are identified. Utilization data should be collected for all aspects of the care pathway, to organize data into a current working model of care used in practice. Routine data should, if possible, be gathered from primary or first contact care, from secondary and tertiary care, and from community and local government providers. There will be a problem in many regions and countries of missing, incomplete, or out-of-date data. Some commercial providers are unwilling to release data on patient flows through specific care pathways, and in some countries such data are not collected at all and often best estimates of current provision need to be made. At this stage, it is important to attempt to gather information in the same subcategories of disease that were developed earlier. However, information is not always collected in this way and again a pragmatic approach may be needed.

Corporate needs assessment: Comparison of current model of care with epidemiological needs assessment

Next a comparison needs to be made between the current model of care, 'the observed model', and the 'expected model' based on evidence derived from the epidemiological needs assessment. Is the pattern and level of provision equivalent to expected levels, given the known epidemiology, the evidence base, and the local demography of the reference population? This process needs to be undertaken for each of the subcategories of the disease or condition that have been identified and for appropriate age-groups in the population. These may be 5-year age-groups, to allow for greatest precision, however, age-groups and severity categories will often need to be made comparable between the epidemiological data collected and the data for utilization or actual provision. This is not easy and again may require assumptions to be made, for example, about epidemiology in certain age groups. Epidemiological evidence may, for example, omit the over 85-year-olds or the under-5s, and extrapolation of likely incidence and prevalence rates in these age groups and need for care may need to be made.

Also at this stage, it is important to consider inequalities and equity. The needs of otherwise underserved groups need special consideration. People such as the very elderly, those with social or language barriers to accessing services (the homeless, refugees, etc.), and those who are very poor, will almost certainly need special consideration. There may or may not be relevant evidence to cover the needs of these groups, but best efforts should be made to ensure that the model being constructed of care pathways is inclusive of the relevant social and care groups.

However, the idea here is not to build up the perfect definitive picture of expected provision versus observed utilization—but to derive practical working estimates of the discrepancies between the two, whilst acknowledging assumptions which have had to be made on the way.

At this stage, the issue of 'use-for-need' needs consideration. Although observed and expected levels of treatment for a particular condition may be consistent, it is possible that both unmet and over-met needs exist. Figure 12.2.6 illustrates this point.

This model, referred to previously in Fig. 12.2.3, can also be used to consider the problem of unmet need. There is a small group at the top of the pyramid who have a clear and definite need for the intervention(s) under consideration. At lower levels, there are more people in each layer but their need for intervention is less. If we assume that everybody above line B 'needs' intervention but that most services are provided along line C, then some people who need services do not receive it, whilst others who do not need it receive it. Needs assessment should be able to help make line B more horizontal, reducing 'unmet' and also 'over-met' needs. This diagram can also be used to consider equity and inequalities. Perhaps some of those inappropriately above line C are more vociferous and demanding, and some of those who are below the line do not come forward even though they 'need' services. It is important to consider how current treatments and interventions compare with the evidence of effectiveness that has been compiled. Which interventions are commonly used for our population under consideration, and what is the evidence in favour of them? As we mentioned previously, for some areas of care there is very little good evidence. But if relevant evidence is already being used in providing care it is important to understand this.

Corporate needs assessment: Consultation with stakeholders

This is the stage where the input of the different pressure groups and interest group views can formally be taken into account. Systematic qualitative data collection should be undertaken to understand the views of the stakeholders and interest groups about what should be changed and why. It is valuable at this stage to include patient groups and providers as well as those involved in strategic planning for the service. Stakeholders will include patient and community groups, professional bodies, government departments, insurers, and payers, clinicians, auditors, and managers and others. Information on stakeholders' views of what currently works badly and what works well will also help with planning for change. At this stage, it is important to remember that some 'corporate' contributors may have their own strong agenda to bring to the table, and it will be important to consider the best strategy for dealing with these stakeholders, especially where there may be vested interests. There may also be national governmental or regional or local imperatives related to legislation or guidance. In many countries 'evidence-based' clinical practice guidelines or treatment guidelines have been adopted by national disease control programmes, which should be taken into account.

Community participation in needs assessment

Community participation can be included at many different stages of a needs assessment. Community participation might be thought of as part of the 'corporate' phase of a needs assessment where

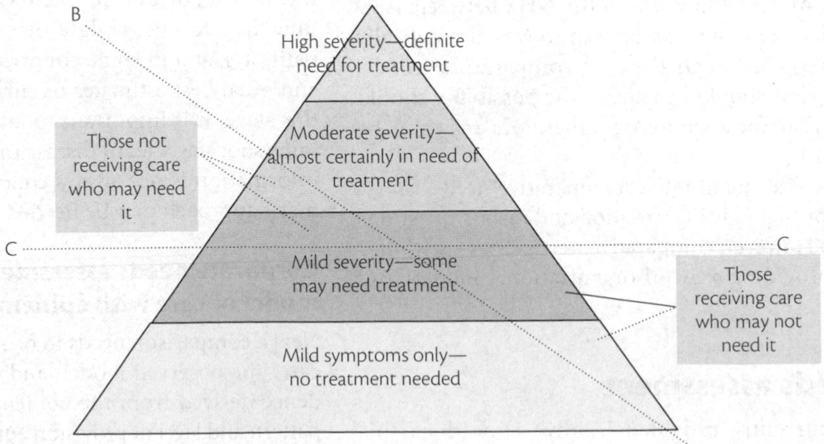

Fig. 12.2.6 Levels of need in a population. Line B represents the 'line of treatment or utilization'. Line C represents the 'line of need'.

stakeholders are consulted, but communities can play an important role in many different stages of a needs assessment in data collection; in understanding and making informed choices; in determining collective needs and priorities; and in reconciling these priorities to externally driven programme objectives. Through community participation, a sense of empowerment and ownership can be engendered among local stakeholders, increasing the chances of success of programme implementation and optimizing the use of local resources. This is in contrast to more superficial models of 'participation', which can range from passive participation, participation in information giving, participation in consultation and participation for material incentives.

Box 12.2.4 gives some examples of community participation.

Rapid assessment procedures (RAP)

Rapid assessment procedures cover a shorter period of systematic data collection than in the usual needs assessment, to provide information on health needs and status of a given community for planning and programming purposes. RAP has also been labelled as rapid ethnographic studies (RES) or rapid ethnographic procedures (REP). A related approach that allows clients and the community some control over some needs assessment tools has been labelled participatory rural appraisal (PRA). Uses include:

- Where health statistics and information are very limited or unreliable: For example, to assess needs among highly mobile such as urban slum dwellers (Rifkin *et al.* 1992) or refugees.
- During disease outbreaks, health emergencies, and disasters where health statistics and information may have broken down, to determine needs and plan interventions rapidly (McNeil *et al.* 2006).

The steps of RAP basically follow the general methodology of health needs assessment, as described earlier in this chapter. RAP, as its name suggests, is quick and generally uses less resources and RAP studies often have small samples of key informants or other respondents. As a result RAP is often the less rigorous option—although it may be the only option available in some cases.

Methods of RAP are both quantitative and qualitative. RAP is often more participatory, partly as a pragmatic necessity. The range of qualitative research methods used in RAP and PRA are varied. They include: In-depth interviews, formal and informal observation, participant observation, focus group discussions, community mapping, case studies, community assemblies and discussions, and other cognitive or ethnographic techniques. A detailed description of some of the most commonly used ethnographic methods are provided in Chapter 7.1 of this Textbook (Morgan *et al.* 2009). Quantitative methods such as quick surveys are used in RAP to supplement or validate qualitative findings.

Box 12.2.4 Some examples of community participation in needs assessment

A. *Epidemiological needs assessment:* This was a health needs assessment using a thirty-cluster survey method in three urban areas in Dublin where there were inadequate health information systems, weak planning data and a history of inadequate recipient involvement in health service planning. Local community members, local general practitioners and other healthcare providers were trained and participated as data collectors in the surveys while the local health boards and NGOs were involved in the planning that ensured from the needs assessment (Smith *et al.* 2005)

B. *Epidemiological and 'corporate' needs assessment:* In Bangladesh communities with arsenic contamination of the water supply, a public participatory geographical information system and focus groups resulted in the development of community priorities for spatial planning of deep tubewell water for reducing arsenic contamination (Hassan 2005).

C. *Epidemiological and 'corporate' needs assessment*: Community members and local leaders in an area affected by conflict were involved in data collection and in in-depth discussions on their values and priorities for a reproductive health care needs assessment in southern Sudan. Findings revealed clear needs in reproductive health; a mismatch between the views of service providers and the community; variation in perception of need according to age, sex and whether the community was settled or displaced; lack of supplies and other barriers to accessing services (Palmer 1991).

Synthesis and constructing the case for change

All the information gathered must be synthesized to construct the 'case for change'. It is important to be aware of how the many possible models now available—(what is *currently* in place—'the observed model'; what the evidence and epidemiology tell us *ought* to be done—'the expected model'; what the stakeholders and community *believe* should be done or *want* done—the 'hoped for' model) compare with each other. Gaps in treatments and services need to be identified, along with options for improvement, the likely changes required and the costs of such changes. Sometimes the gaps will be relatively minimal or require reorganization and changed patient care pathways within a service, but occasionally whole services will need providing. It is also important at this stage to continue to bear in mind inequalities, equity, and access to services.

Costed options are essential to allow for decision makers to understand the overall strengths and weaknesses of possible courses of action and to select between them. It is at this stage also that questions of allocative efficiency come in. How does investment in the area covered by the needs assessment compare with investment in other areas? How can the efficiency of the organization of the whole be maximized? Formal decision-making tools may be employed at this stage in order to make explicit the values, assumptions, and evidence that are being taken into consideration.

Discussion: Value and potential contribution of needs assessment

Value of needs assessments

Two evaluations of needs assessment have been undertaken (Hensher & Fulop 1999; Jordan *et al.* 2002) in the United Kingdom, and a critique has also been produced by the Department of Health in England and Wales (South Eastern Public Health Observatory 2007). Critiques suggest a lack of focus by needs assessments on population health and health outcomes, rather than on health care services; a lack of focus on prevention rather than treatment; a failure of some needs assessment to involve patients and the public; and the lack of actual use of needs assessments to change services in the 'real world'. Although important health-related costs and benefits have been identified in needs assessments, these have not necessarily been used in decision-making in the same way as purely financial considerations. It is unfortunate that evaluations paint a somewhat negative picture, and this research may need further investigation. The redesignation in 2006–2007 by the Department of Health for England and Wales as 'strategic' needs assessment suggests that needs assessments should be better tied into the needs and values of the organizations they are designed to help (South Eastern Public Health Observatory 2007).

However, it is always worth being reflective in public health practice. What went well? What went badly? What are the important research needs? Table 12.2.1 shows some of the strengths and weaknesses of the different elements of needs assessments. Later, for evaluation and audit, questions such as whether and how the needs assessment was valuable should be asked.

Boxes 12.2.5 and 12.2.6 show examples of successful needs assessments in different countries. The stages are not necessarily ordered in the same way as in this chapter but are nevertheless identifiable.

Needs assessment can be thought of as essential 'public health action' designed to tailor health programmes not to demand, or to unthinking cost restrictions, but to objectively assessed need. It has huge potential to allow for a rational approach to changing health care. As such it should be recognized as a key component of any health organization's planning framework.

The aim of needs assessment is to deliver practically useful information to change health services; to maximize the appropriate delivery of effective healthcare and to minimize the provision of ineffective care and the existence of unmet need for healthcare in an evidence-based way; and to maximize equity (Powell 2006). In this chapter, we have seen how many of the basic skills of public health, including epidemiology, statistics, and ethnographic skills, provide useful information for a needs assessment. The main steps of a needs assessment were shown to be: Understanding the rationale for the needs assessment; developing a good project plan; involving stakeholders; constructing a model of the problem in the population using the best evidence and information available (epidemiological needs assessment); comparing the model with practice in other areas (comparative needs assessment); understanding current practice and consulting widely on the problem and possible plans for change within the organization (corporate needs

Table 12.2.1 Some of the strengths and weaknesses of the different elements of needs assessments

Needs assessment	Strengths	Weaknesses
Epidemiological	◆ Rigorous ◆ Valid ◆ Reliable ◆ Uses best available evidence ◆ Gives absolute numbers ◆ Potentially less biased ◆ Potentially allows for clear understanding of 'the ideal model'	◆ Statistical expertise required ◆ Time-consuming ◆ More costly ◆ May require primary data collection ◆ Adaptation for local factors ◆ Data may not be available
Comparative	◆ Face validity ◆ Improved communications with colleagues, other stakeholders ◆ Can use routine data if available ◆ Provides comparators and benchmarks ◆ Good for identifying models used in practice	◆ Variation in service provision and organization and in health systems may make comparisons problematic ◆ Other may not be acting on the best evidence ◆ Requires adaptation for local factors
Corporate or local	◆ Essential basis on which to plan change ◆ Can use routine data if available ◆ Improved communications with decision makers and other stakeholders—allows for understanding of 'the hoped-for model' ◆ Potentially allows for clear understanding of 'what we do now—the observed model'	◆ May be swayed by local stakeholders with strong vested interests
Rapid assessment procedures	◆ Good use of limited resources ◆ Useful in an emergency situation ◆ Potentially allows for strengthened community involvement and partnerships ◆ Possibility of deeper understanding of community health needs and resources ◆ Potential for development of working hypotheses for future research or explanatory models for quantitative findings	◆ May require primary data collection ◆ Restricted generalizability of findings beyond the community studied ◆ Potential for 'bias' owing to small numbers of participants or respondents ◆ Potential for subjectivity in interpretation of qualitative data and of cultural differences in perceptions of different respondents

Box 12.2.5 Example of needs assessment for severe (morbid) obesity

The need

A local health board serving a population of 450 000 adults identified an increasing number of referrals of patients to specialist centres for the treatment of severe (morbid) obesity. There was no systematic approach to these referrals, and patients were sent to a variety of centres for a range of treatments such as various bariatric surgery procedures, with or without other interventions such as psychological assessment, and modifications to diet or physical activity The health board needed a consistent strategy for the future management of this population who have high health needs due to the associated morbidity.

Epidemiological approach

An epidemiological approach was used to estimate the numbers of adults in the local population likely to fit the clinical criteria for severe (morbid) obesity. This approach combined local population statistics with results from a health and lifestyle survey undertaken in the same region. This gave a prevalence figure for severe obesity (BMI $> 40 kg/m^2$) of 0.80 per cent (95% confidence interval 0.61–0.99%), implying a local population prevalence of 3 600 adults with severe obesity (95% confidence interval 2 750 to 4 460). Secondly, a systematic review was undertaken to determine the effectiveness and cost-effectiveness of the five main interventions for severe (morbid) obesity, namely diet, physical activity, psychological treatments, drug therapy, and surgery.

Corporate approach

A variety of local and national stakeholders were interviewed to capture their views on future service provision. Interviews were held with user representatives (including a voluntary organization for people with severe obesity), local clinical managers, local commissioners, local finance managers, national policymakers, and national experts on obesity treatment. A search was undertaken for relevant local or national guidelines. Finally routine activity data were examined to determine the current level of service provision. This showed that very few people with severe obesity were receiving effective interventions from the health service.

Comparative approach

Local health boards with similar populations were contacted to compare current policies and levels of service provision. Routine data collected nationally were also used to compare local provision with national averages. This data showed that the local level of need, and the local level of provision, was very similar to neighbouring areas.

Problems faced

Some of the problems faced in this needs assessment included:

- Difficulty ensuring involvement of a representative range of stakeholders
- Difficulty finding the evidence and in ensuring adequate time and skill available to synthesize it
- Difficulty with not having direct population statistics and therefore relying on extrapolation
- difficulty in incorporating new treatments (especially drugs) as they are being developed and introduced all the time with insufficient (cost)effectiveness data.

The conclusion

Nevertheless, through using the three approaches it was possible to identify and quantify significant unmet treatment needs for the local population with severe (morbid) obesity. Recommendations were made regarding future service provision, based on epidemiology, evidence of effectiveness and cost-effectiveness, expert opinion, and practice in neighbouring areas. These included increasing local provision of psychological assessment, dietary and physical activity advice. In addition local guidelines for the prescribing of obesity drugs and for the referral of patients for bariatric surgery were drawn up, to provide consistency in the future management of individuals. The prior involvement of stakeholders in the corporate element was important in ensuring implementation of the recommendations.

Source: Personal communication

Box 12.2.6 Example of needs assessment for services for mobile populations at high risk for HIV/AIDS along selected border towns in southern Africa

The need

The 'Corridors of Hope' Initiative, focused on mobile populations at high risk for HIV/AIDS along selected border towns in southern Africa. Overall, the plan was to develop 'a standard participatory methodology for evaluating HIV risk, identifying prevention opportunities and designing grounded, coordinated regional prevention initiatives'. To achieve this, a needs assessment was done from July to November 1999 in four border towns in 3 southern African countries, namely: Messina in northern South Africa, Beitbridge in southern Zimbabwe, Chirundu in northern Zimbabwe and Chirundu in southern Zambia. Specific objectives relating to these border towns were: (1) to identify STI/HIV risk factors and STI/HIV prevention opportunities at the Beitbridge–Messina and Chirundu highway and borders; and (2) to develop an implementation plan for priority STI/HIV prevention initiatives at these sites.

Epidemiological approach

Literature searches and reviews were undertaken, focusing on: Socioeconomic and health status, and morbidity and mortality data on STI and HIV/AIDS.

Corporate and comparative approaches

Policy documents and programme reports relating to STI/HIV/AIDS were reviewed.

As part of the stakeholder consultations on policy and programme priorities, the seven-member needs assessment team interviewed regional, national and provincial policymakers in the three southern African countries, including donor representatives, health employees, AIDS programme staff, NGO staff, and experts in various aspects of STI/HIV/AIDS health service delivery and education/communication.

Box 12.2.6 Example of needs assessment for services for mobile populations at high risk for HIV/AIDS along selected border towns in southern Africa *(continued)*

Rapid appraisal procedures approach

The field research in the selected sites employed a wide range of community participatory approaches, e.g. site inventories, mapping, behavioural surveys of sex workers, in-depth interviews, focus group discussions, ethnographic observations, and participatory learning appraisals. The field research focused on migrant men and women, including truckers, informal traders, and sex workers, but additional information on educational institutions and health services for STI.

Conclusions

The needs assessment found 'exceptional HIV vulnerability' at each border post, particularly among truckers and traders. While there were some interventions directed at sex workers, there was a notable lack of interventions for truckers as well as members of the permanent border communities who had migrant sexual partners. The needs assessment team recommended the following to the sponsoring agency and its government partners:

- A comprehensive prevention programme, with the following core services: Strengthened STI services, targeted interventions to protect truckers and their partners, workplace interventions; youth interventions; condom social marketing and targeted communication interventions for behavior change.
- Improved STI care for both sex workers and clients, including innovative strategies to reach truckers who may not avail of public health services, and regular screening for sex workers.
- Establishment of simple but effective project evaluation and quality assurance systems.

Acknowledgement: This regional assessment is part of the 'Corridors for Hope' Initiative funded by the United States Agency for International Development, in partnership with southern African governments and organizations. It was conducted under the auspices of Family Health International, which manages the Implementing AIDS Prevention and Care (IMPACT) Project, USAID's flagship effort for addressing the global HIV/AIDS pandemic (http://www.fhi.org/en/HIVAIDS/Projects/res_IMPACT±main±page.htm).

Source: Implementing AIDS Prevention and Care (IMPACT) Project (2007). Corridors of hope in southern Africa: HIV prevention needs and opportunities in four border towns. Family Health International and the United States Agency for International Development. Also available at: http://www.fhi.org/en/HIVAIDS/pub/guide/corrhope/correg.htm Last accessed on 5 May 2007

assessment); and developing a realistic, evidence-based, costed plan for change. We have described different methods of needs assessment including rapid appraisal techniques and their strengths and weaknesses and the special role of stakeholder, particularly community, involvement and participation. We have seen how important data are for needs assessment but how data systems and availability are likely to vary.

The next step is to act on the health needs assessment. At the beginning of the chapter we described the importance of locating a needs assessment within the planning and management cycles of the responsible organization (Box 12.2.1). We described a series of questions that should be asked before a needs assessment is undertaken. They relate to the timing of the needs assessment and its role. Perhaps the most important question of all to ask at the beginning is 'How can the results and recommendations of the needs assessment be produced and presented to best inform action?' If the needs assessment has been undertaken with care, using the best data available, and this question has been properly answered, then the likelihood of the needs assessment informing action is high.

References

Barry M.J., Fowler F.J. Jr., O'Leary M.P. *et al.* (1992). The American Urological Association symptom index for benign prostatic hyperplasia. *Journal of Urology*, **148**:1549–57.

Buse K., Walt G., Mays N. (2005) *Making Health Policy*. Open University Press, Maidenhead. England.

Busse J.W., Mills E., Dennis R. *et al.* (2009). Clinical epidemiology. In: Detels R., Beaglehole R., Lansang M.A., Gulliford M., eds. *Oxford Textbook of Public Health, 5th ed.* Oxford University Press, Oxford.

Cavanagh S., Chadwick K. (2005) *Health needs assessment: A practical guide.* UK National Institute for Health and Clinical Excellence (NICE). Available at http://www.nice.org.uk.

Chan C., Ho S.C., Chan S.G. *et al.* (2002) Factors affecting uptake of cervical and breast cancer screening among perimenopausal women in Hong Kong. *Hong Kong Medical Journal*, **8**(5):334–41.

Chowdhury P.P., Balluz L., Murphy W. *et al.* (2007) Centers for Disease Control and Prevention (CDC) (2007). Surveillance of certain health behaviours among states and selected local areas—United States, 2005. *MMWR Surveillance Summaries*, **56**(4):1–160.

Cook C. (2004) *Alcohol Misuse needs assessment.* Health Care Needs Assessment. First Series. Second Edition. Volume 1 Radcliffe Medical Press, Oxford.

Cresswell P., Learmonth A., Chappel D. (2005) *The Health Needs of Prisoners.* North East Public Health Observatory. Occasional Paper 16. Available at http://www.nepho.org.uk.

Dawson J., Fitzpatrick R., Frost S., *et al.* (2001) Evidence for the validity of a patient-based instrument for assessment of outcome after revision hip replacement. *Journal of Bone and Joint Surgery (British Volume)*, **83**(8):1125–9.

Dawson J., Fitzpatrick R., Fletcher J. *et al.* (2004) *Osteoarthritis affecting the hip and knee. Health Care Needs Assessment. First Series. Second Edition.* Volume 1 Radcliffe Medical Press, Oxford.

DH Health Survey for England (2007). Available at http://www.dh.gov.uk/en/Publicationsandstatistics/PublishedSurvey/HealthSurveyForEngland. Accessed 21 June, 2007.

Delattre E., Dormont B. (2003) Fixed fees and physician-induced demand: A panel data study on French physicians *Health Economics*, **12**(9):741–754.

Disease Control Priorities Project: Cost-Effective Interventions (2006). Available at http://www.dcp2.org.

Ferris G., Roderick P., Smithies A. *et al.* (1998) An epidemiological needs assessment of carotid endarterectomy in an English health region. Is the need being met? *British Medical Journal*, **317**:447–451.

Goldacre M., Yeates D., Gill L., *et al.* (2005) *A geographical profile of hospital admissions.* Published by Unit of Health-Care Epidemiology, Oxford University, and South East England Public Health Observatory.

Hassan M.M. (2005). Arsenic poisoning in Bangladesh: spatial mitigation planning with GIS and public participation. *Health Policy*, **74**, 247–60.

Hensher M., Fulop N. (1999) The influence of health needs assessment on health care decision-making in London health authorities. *Journal of Health Services Research & Policy*, **4**(2):90–5.

INDEPTH Network (2005) INDEPTH Demographic Surveillance Sites. Available at http://www.indepth-network.org/dss_site_profiles/dss_sites.htm.

International Union against Cancer (UICC) TNM (Tumour Node Metastasis) system. Available at http://www.uicc.org/index.php?id=508. Accessed 21 June 2007.

Jordan J., Wright J., Ayres P. *et al.* (2002) Health needs assessment and needs-led health service change: a survey of projects involving public health doctors. *Journal of Health Services Research & Policy*, **7**: 71–80.

Marsden J., Strang J. *et al.* (2004) Drug misuse needs assessment. *Health Care Needs Assessment. First Series. Second Edition*. Volume 2 Radcliffe Medical Press, Oxford.

Mant J., Wade D., Winner S. (2004) Stroke needs assessment. *Health Care Needs Assessment. First Series. Second Edition*. Volume 1 Radcliffe Medical Press, Oxford.

McIntyre D., Mooney G., Jan S. (2009) Need: What is it and how do we measure it? In: Detels R., Beaglehole R., Lansang M.A., Gulliford M., eds. *Oxford Textbook of Public Health, 5th ed.* Oxford University Press, Oxford.

McKee M., Clarke A. (1995) Guidelines, enthusiasms, uncertainty and the limits to purchasing. *British Medical Journal*, **310**;101–4.

McNeil M., Goddard J. *et al.* (2006) Rapid Community Needs Assessment After Hurricane Katrina—Hancock County, Mississippi. Centers for Disease Control (CDC) *MMWR*, **55**(09);234–236.

Morgan M., Reid M., Ogden J. (2009). Sociology and psychology in public health. In: Detels R., Beaglehole R., Lansang M.A., Gulliford M., eds. *Oxford Textbook of Public Health, 5th ed.* Oxford University Press, Oxford.

Murray S. (2000) Relation between private health insurance and high rates of Caesarean section in Chile: qualitative and quantitative study. *British Medical Journal*, **321**:1501–1505.

National Statistics. Available at http://www.statistics.gov.uk/StatBase/Product.asp. Accessed 21 June 2007.

Mortality Statistics: Cause (Series DH2).

National Institute for Clinical Excellence (2007) Determining local service levels for upper GI endoscopy: Assumptions used in estimating a population benchmark. Available at http://www.nice.org.uk. Accessed 13 June 2007.

Orinda V., Kakande H., Kabarangira J. *et al.* (2005) A sector wide approach to emergency obstetric care in Uganda. *International Journal of Genecology and Obstetrics*, **91**(3):285–291.

Palmer C.A. (1999). Rapid appraisal of needs in reproductive health care in southern Sudan: Qualitative study. *British Medical Journal*, **319**, 743–8.

Powell J. (2006) Health Needs Assessment: A systematic approach. National Library for Health; Health Management Specialist Library. Available at http://www.library.nhs.uk/healthmanagement/ViewResource.aspx?resID=29549.

Rifkin S., Annett H., Tabibzadeh I. (1992). Rapid appraisal to assess community health needs: A focus on the urban poor. In: Scrimshaw N.S. and Gleason G.R. (eds.). *Rapid assessment procedures: Qualitative methodologies for planning and evaluation of health related programs*, pp. 357–63. International Nutrition Foundation for Developing Countries, Boston, MA, USA.

Smith S.M., Long J., Deady J. *et al.* (2005). Adapting developing country epidemiological assessment techniques to improve the quality of health needs assessments in developed countries. *BMC Health Services Research* 5, 1472-6963-5-32. Available at http://www.biomedcentral.com/1472-6963/5/32.

South Eastern Public Health Observatory (SEPHO) 2007 Joint Strategic needs assessment. Available at http://www.sepho.org.uk/ViewResource.aspx?id=10769.

Stevens A., Raftery J. (2004) Health Care Needs Assessment. First Series. Second Edition. Volume 1 Radcliffe Medical Press, Oxford.

Young T.K., Roos N.P., Hammerstrand K.M. (1991) Estimated burden of diabetes mellitus in Manitoba according to health insurance claims: A pilot study. *Canadian Medical Association Journal*, **144**(3): 318–324.

Wadud Z., Kuper H., Polack S. *et al.* (2006) Rapid assessment of avoidable blindness and needs assessment of cataract surgical services in Satkhira District, Bangladesh. *British Journal of Ophthalmology*, **90**(10):1225–9.

Weinstein J.N., Bronner K.K., Morgan T.S. *et al.* (2004) Trends and geographic variations in major surgery for degenerative diseases of the hip, knee, and spine. *Health Affairs,* Suppl Web Exclusives:VAR81–9.

Williams B. Nicholl J. Brazier J. (1997) Accident and emergency departments. *Health Care Needs Assessment. Second Series*. Radcliffe Medical Press, Oxford.

Wright N., Tomkins C. (2006) How can health services effectively meet the health needs of homeless people? *British Journal of General Practice*, **56**(525):286–293.

12.3

Socioeconomic inequalities in health in high-income countries: The facts and the options

Johan P. Mackenbach

Abstract

Socioeconomic inequalities in health have been studied extensively in past decades. In all high-income countries with available data, mortality and morbidity rates are higher among those in less advantaged socioeconomic positions, and as a result differences in health expectancy between socioeconomic groups typically amount to 10 years or more. Good progress has been made in unravelling the determinants of health inequalities, and a number of specific determinants (particularly material, psychosocial and lifestyle factors) have been identified which probably contribute to explaining health inequalities in many high-income countries. Although further research is necessary, our understanding of what causes health inequalities has progressed to a stage when rational approaches to reduce health inequalities are becoming feasible. Although different countries are in widely different phases of awareness of, and willingness to take action on, health inequalities, several European countries have endeavoured to develop comprehensive policy programmes to tackle health inequalities.

Introduction

Socioeconomic inequalities in health have been studied extensively around the world in past decades. Inequalities in health have been documented from the United States (Davey Smith *et al.* 1996) to Russia (Shkolnikov *et al.* 2006), from Sweden (Ljung *et al.* 2005) and the Netherlands (Mackenbach & Stronks 2002) to Japan (Fukuda *et al.* 2007) and Korea (Khang *et al.* 2004), and from New Zealand (Shaw *et al.* 2005) to Canada (Lasser *et al.* 2006). At the start of the twenty-first century, all high-income countries are faced with substantial inequalities in health within their populations. People with a lower level of education, a lower occupational class, or a lower level of income tend to die at a younger age, and to have, within their shorter lives, a higher prevalence of all kinds of health problems. This leads to truly tremendous differences between socioeconomic groups in the number of years that people can expect to live in good health ('health expectancy'). In countries with available data, differences in health expectancy typically amount to 10 years or more, counted from birth. According to widely accepted principles, such differences in health are unjust (Whitehead 1990) and represent one of the greatest challenges for public health in these countries.

Historical notes

Historical evidence suggests that socioeconomic inequalities in health is not a recent phenomenon. However, it was only during the nineteenth century that socioeconomic inequalities in health were 'discovered'. Before that time, health inequalities simply went unrecognized due to lack of information. In the nineteenth century great figures in public health, such as Villermé in France, Chadwick in England, and Virchow in Germany, devoted a large part of their scientific work to this issue (Ackerknecht 1953; Coleman 1982; Chave 1984). This was facilitated by national population statistics, which permitted the calculation of mortality rates by occupation or by city district. Louis René Villermé (1782–1863), for example, analysed inequalities in mortality between 'arrondissements' in Paris in 1817–21. He showed that districts with a lower socioeconomic level, as indicated by the proportion of houses for which no tax was levied over the rents, tended to have systematically higher mortality rates than more well-to-do neighbourhoods. He concluded that life and death are not primarily biological phenomena, but are closely linked to social circumstances (Coleman 1982). Rudolf Virchow (1821–1902) went even further in his famous statement that 'medicine is a social science, and politics nothing but medicine at a larger scale' (Ackerknecht 1953).

Since the nineteenth century, the magnitude of socioeconomic inequalities in health has probably declined in absolute terms in developed countries. There has been a marked decline in the average mortality rate in the population, leading to a doubling of life expectancy at birth. This was largely due to improvements in living standards and public health. As a result, the absolute difference in mortality rates and in life expectancy at birth between people with a high and a low socioeconomic position has probably become smaller, as suggested by the limited historical evidence which has been uncovered in a few European countries (Pamuk 1985). It is less clear, however, whether inequalities in mortality have also declined in relative terms, i.e. in terms of the percentage excess death rates in lower as compared to higher socioeconomic groups. In the long run, the relative risks of dying for those with a low as compared to those with a high socioeconomic position seem to have remained very stable, and have even unexpectedly increased during the last decades of the twentieth century in many developed countries (Pamuk 1985; Mackenbach *et al.* 2003a). Particularly in Western Europe, with its high levels of prosperity and highly developed social security, public health, and health care systems, this was a disturbing finding. These developments have contributed to a heightened awareness of health inequalities, and of the challenge they pose to public health policy, around the world.

The start of the resurgence of an active interest in health inequalities in Europe can be linked to the publication of the Black Report in England in 1980 (Townsend & Davidson 1992), which first highlighted the widening of health inequalities despite the rise of the welfare state in the decades after World War II. The Black Report contributed to heightened awareness of health inequalities all around Europe as well as in developed countries in other parts of the world. As a result, an enormous amount of descriptive data has been collected and analysed in many countries, testifying to the existence of substantial inequalities in health in all countries with good data.

While all these descriptive studies were going on, the emphasis of academic research in this area has shifted from description to explanation, not only to satisfy scientific curiosities but also to find entry-points for policies and interventions to reduce health inequalities (Marmot & Wilkinson 2006; Mackenbach & Bakker 2002). This was greatly facilitated by increased research funding, both from national research programmes (e.g. in England, the Netherlands, and Finland), and by international agencies (e.g. the European Commission and the European Science Foundation) (Siegrist & Marmot 2006). As a result, our understanding of the causes of socioeconomic inequalities in health has expanded tremendously, and has allowed interested policy makers to start searching for strategies to reduce these inequalities. Countries are in widely different stages of policy development in this area, but in some countries (e.g. England) political windows of opportunity have arisen which have led to large-scale implementation of policies to tackle health inequalities.

The purpose of this chapter

This chapter aims to review the available evidence on the description and explanation of socioeconomic inequalities in health in high-income countries, and to present the current (2007) state of the art with regard to the available options for reducing health inequalities.

For the purpose of this chapter, socioeconomic inequalities in health will be defined as systematic differences in morbidity or mortality rates between people of higher and lower socioeconomic status, as indicated by, e.g. level of education, occupational class, or income level. Where possible, we will draw upon international overviews, such as comparative studies, in order to avoid biases related to the selective experiences of single countries. We will, however, mainly draw upon the European experience, which has become very well documented in the past two decades.

The facts: Description

Mortality

Although no individual can escape death, important differences in mortality *rates* are typically found between men and women, city dwellers and inhabitants of rural areas, native people and immigrants, and population groups classified according to many other characteristics. Some of the largest inequalities are found when individuals are classified according to their socioeconomic position. In all high-income countries with available data, mortality rates are higher among those in less advantaged socioeconomic positions, regardless of whether socioeconomic position is indicated by educational level, occupational class, or income level (Mackenbach 2006).

Levels and trends

Table 12.3.1 summarizes these inequalities for a wide range of European countries. The overall picture is extremely clear: The mortality rates are consistently higher in lower, than in higher socioeconomic groups. Many of the figures given in Table 12.3.1 apply to middle-aged adults, and this implies that differences in mortality rates can be interpreted as differences in the risks of dying prematurely. From studies that have included women, it has become clear that inequalities in mortality exist among women as they do among men, but that inequalities are smaller among women than among men (Mackenbach *et al.* 1999).

Not only is the size of these inequalities often substantial, in the order of an excess relative risk of dying in the lowest socioeconomic groups of 25–50 per cent. But inequalities in mortality have also risen substantially in the past decades, without much evidence that the widening of the mortality gap will stop in the near future. To the surprise of many, mortality differences between socioeconomic groups have widened in many Western European countries during the last three decades of the twentieth century. This has continued into the 1990s, and has led to considerable increases of the relative excess risk of dying in the lowest socioeconomic groups (Fig. 12.3.1) (Mackenbach *et al.* 2003a).

The explanation of this disturbing phenomenon is only partly known. One aspect which should certainly be taken into account, however, is that this widening of the relative gap in death rates is generally the result of a difference between socioeconomic groups in the speed of mortality *decline*. While mortality declined in all socioeconomic groups, the decline has been proportionally faster in the higher socioeconomic groups than in the lower. The faster mortality declines in higher socioeconomic groups were in their turn mostly due to faster mortality declines for cardiovascular diseases (Mackenbach *et al.* 2003a). In many developed countries, the 1980s and 1990s have been decades with substantial improvements in cardiovascular disease mortality. These have been due to improvements in health-related behaviours (less smoking, modest improvements in diet, more physical exercise, etc.), and to the introduction of effective health care interventions (hypertension detection and treatment, surgical interventions, thrombolytic therapy, etc.). Apparently, while these improvements have to some extent been taken up by all socioeconomic groups, the higher socioeconomic groups have tended to benefit more.

Table 12.3.1 Inequalities in mortality by socioeconomic position in 21 European countries[a]

Country	Indicator of socioeconomic position	Period	Age-group	Rate ratio[b]		Source
				Men	Women	
Austria	Education	1991–1992	45+	1.43*	1.32*	National census-linked mortality follow-up
Belgium	Education	1991–1995	45+	1.34*	1.29*	National census-linked mortality follow-up
	Housing tenure	1991–1995	60–69	1.44*	1.43*	
Czech Republic	Education	End 1990s	20–64	1.66*	1.09*	Unlinked cross-sectional study
Denmark	Education	1991–1995	60–69	1.28*	1.26*	National census-linked mortality follow-up
	Housing tenure	1991–1995	60–69	1.64*	1.47*	
	Occupation	1981–1990	45–59	1.33*	n.a.	National census-linked mortality follow-up
England/Wales	Education	1991–1996	45+	1.35*	1.22*	National census-linked mortality follow-up
	Housing tenure	1991–1996	60–69	1.65*	1.58*	
	Occupation	1981–1989	45–59	1.61*	n.a.	National census-linked mortality follow-up; representative sample
Estonia	Education	2000	20+	2.38*	2.23*	National cross-sectional study
	Education	1988	20–74	1.50*	1.31*	National cross-sectional study
Finland	Education	1991–1995	45+	1.33*	1.24*	National census-linked mortality follow-up
	Housing tenure	1991–1995	60–69	1.90*	1.73*	
France	Education	1990–1994	60–69	1.31*	1.14	National census-linked mortality follow-up
	Housing tenure	1990–1994	60–69	1.27*	1.25*	
	Occupation	1980–1989	45–59	2.15*	n.a.	National census-linked mortality follow-up; representative sample
	Occupation	1984–1985	45–64	1.61	1.33	National cross-sectional study
Ireland	Occupation	1980–1982	45–59	1.38*		National cross-sectional study
Italy	Education	1991–1996	45+	1.22*	1.20*	Urban census-linked mortality follow-up (Turin)
	Housing tenure	1991–1996	60–69	1.37*	1.33*	
	Education	1981–1982	18–54	1.85*	n.a.	National census-linked mortality follow-up
	Occupation	1981–1982	45–59	1.35*	n.a.	National census-linked mortality follow-up
Latvia	Education	1988–1989		1.50	1.20	National cross-sectional study
Lithuania	Education	2001	25+	2.40*	2.90*	Unlinked cross-sectional analysis
Netherlands	Education	1991–1997	25–74	1.92*	1.28	GLOBE Longitudinal study (Eindhoven)
Norway	Education	1990–1995	45+	1.36*	1.27*	National census-linked mortality follow-up
	Housing tenure	1990–1995	60–69	1.44*	1.36*	
	Occupation	1980–1990	45–59	1.47*		National census-linked mortality follow-up
Poland	Education	1988–1989	50–64	2.24	1.78	National cross-sectional study
Portugal	Occupation	1980–1982	45–59	1.36*	n.a.	National cross-sectional study
Slovenia	Education	1991 & 2002	25–64	2.44	2.66	Unlinked cross-sectional study
Spain	Education	1992–1996	45+	1.24*	1.27*	Urban and regional census-linked mortality follow-up (Barcelona & Madrid)
	Occupation	1980–1982	45–59	1.37*	n.a.	National cross-sectional study
Sweden	Occupation	1980–1986	45–59	1.59*		National census-linked mortality follow-up
Switzerland	Education	1991–1995	45+	1.33*	1.27*	National census-linked mortality follow-up
	Occupation	1979–1982	45–59	1.37*		National cross-sectional study

[a] Because of differences in data collection and classification, the magnitude of inequalities in health cannot always directly be compared between countries.

[b] Rate ratio: Ratio of mortality rate in lower socioeconomic groups as compared to that in higher socioeconomic groups. Asterisk(*) indicates that difference in mortality between socioeconomic groups is statistically significant. n.a. indicates 'not available'.

Source: Mackenbach 2006.

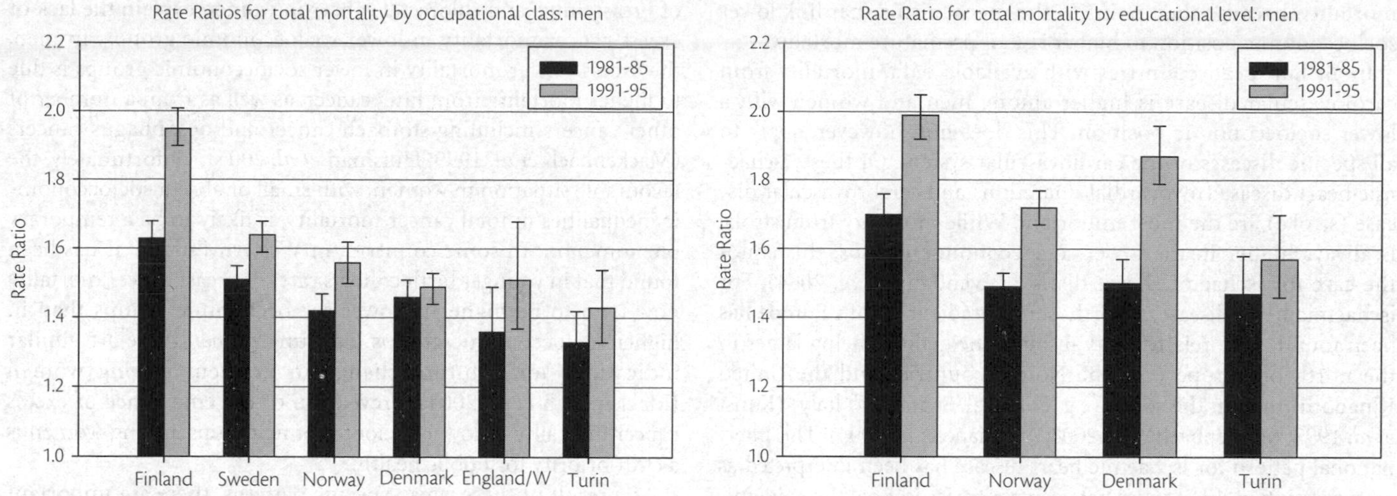

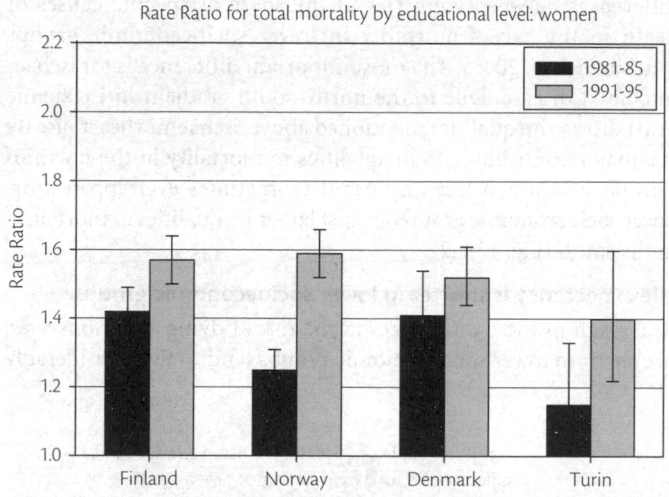

Fig. 12.3.1 Inequalities in mortality by educational level and occupational class, 1981–1985 and 1991–1995. Finland, Sweden, Norway, Denmark, England/Wales, Turin.
Source: Mackenbach et al. (2003).

Differences between countries

Some comparative studies have tried to assess whether the magnitude of inequalities in mortality differs systematically between countries. The most extensive of these studies have been performed in Europe (Mackenbach *et al.* 1997; Kunst *et al.* 1998, 1999; Huisman *et al.* 2004, 2005a) and have found that the range of between-country variation in relative inequalities is rather small within Western Europe. Due to the fact that countries differ substantially in average mortality rates for the population as a whole, absolute differences in mortality between socioeconomic groups usually do show clear between-country variations, in contrast to relative inequalities which tend to be more similar. For example, because of its low average death rates, Sweden has rather small absolute differences in mortality between socioeconomic groups, although relative differences are not clearly smaller than elsewhere (Mackenbach *et al.* 1997).

This is not to say that systematic differences between countries in the magnitude of relative inequalities in mortality do not exist: Relative inequalities in mortality are larger than elsewhere in some Eastern European countries, perhaps as a result of the economic and social developments following the political changes around 1990 (Mackenbach 2006). Since these transitions, mortality rates have changed dramatically in many countries in Eastern Europe, sometimes to the better (e.g. in the Czech Republic) but often to the worse, at least temporarily (e.g. in Hungary and Estonia), particularly among men. This is probably due to a combination of (interlinked) factors: A rise in economic insecurity and poverty; a breakdown of protective social, public health, and health care institutions; and a rise in excessive drinking and other risk factors for premature mortality. The available evidence clearly shows that these changes in mortality have not been equally shared between socioeconomic groups: In the countries with available data, mortality rates have generally improved less, or deteriorated more, in the lower socioeconomic groups. Apparently, people with higher levels of education have been able to protect themselves better against increased health risks, and/or have been able to benefit more from new opportunities for health gains. Evidence from several Eastern European countries (Estonia, Hungary, Russia) suggests a substantial widening of the gap in death rates (Leinsalu *et al.* 2003; Shkolnikov *et al.* 2006).

Cause-specific mortality

Variations in patterns of cause of death between socioeconomic groups provide valuable clues for the explanation of disparities in mortality, because they point to the mechanisms that link lower socioeconomic position to higher risk of premature mortality.

In all European countries with available data, mortality from cardiovascular disease is higher among men and women with a lower socioeconomic position. This does not, however, apply to all specific diseases of the cardiovascular system. Of these, ischaemic heart disease (myocardial infarction) and cerebrovascular disease (stroke) are the most important. While mortality from stroke is always higher in the lower socioeconomic groups, this is not the case for ischaemic heart disease (Avendano *et al.* 2004). For ischaemic heart disease, a north–south gradient within Europe has been found, with relative and absolute inequalities being larger in the north of Europe (e.g. the Nordic countries and the United Kingdom) than in the south (e.g. Portugal, Spain, and Italy) (Kunst *et al.* 1999; Mackenbach *et al.* 2000; Avendano *et al.* 2004). This international pattern for ischaemic heart disease has been interpreted as an expression of differences between countries in how the epidemiology of this disease has developed. In many countries, particularly in the north of Europe, mortality from ischaemic heart disease increased substantially after the World War II, probably as a result of changes in health-related behaviours, such as smoking, diet, and physical exercise. During the 1970s, however, a decline set in, and is still continuing. During this epidemiological development, important changes occurred in the association between socioeconomic position and ischaemic heart disease mortality. In the north of Europe, during the 1950s and 1960s ischaemic heart disease mortality was higher in the higher socioeconomic groups, leading to the notion of ischaemic heart disease being a 'manager's disease'. It was only during the 1970s, coinciding with the start of the decline of ischaemic heart disease mortality in the population as a whole, that a reversal occurred, and the current association emerged (Marmot & McDowell 1986). This is due to differences between socioeconomic groups in both the timing and the speed of decline of ischaemic heart disease mortality. As we have seen above, the widening of the gap in ischaemic heart disease mortality was still continuing in the 1990s. In the south of Europe, a similar 'epidemic' of ischaemic heart disease mortality has not occurred, and inequalities in ischaemic heart disease mortality have not undergone such clear-cut changes as in the north of Europe. It is possible that the lack of clear inequalities in ischaemic heart disease mortality in some southern European populations represents an earlier stage of epidemiological development, and will turn out to be a temporary phenomenon, because the protection of southern European populations against ischaemic heart disease which their traditional living habits offered, is gradually eroding.

Inequalities in cancer mortality tend to be smaller than those for cardiovascular disease mortality (Mackenbach *et al.* 1999; Huisman *et al.* 2005a). Among women, inequalities in mortality from all cancers combined are even negligible in magnitude in many countries. Among men, however, the usual pattern of higher mortality in lower socioeconomic groups applies to cancer as it does to most other diseases. These patterns for all cancers combined are the net result of strongly diverging patterns for specific forms of cancer. For some cancers, 'reverse' patterns (with higher death rates in the upper socioeconomic groups) are seen in some countries. Examples include prostate cancer among men, and breast and lung cancer in women. For colorectal cancer, another important cause of death, inequalities in mortality tend to be small everywhere. The 'reverse' or absent gradients *and* large contributions to cancer mortality of breast, lung, and colorectal cancer in women explain the lack of excess cancer mortality in lower socioeconomic groups. In men, the excess cancer mortality in lower socioeconomic groups is due to higher mortality from lung cancer, as well as from a number of other cancers including stomach cancer and oesophagus cancers (Mackenbach *et al.* 1999; Huisman *et al.* 2005). Unfortunately, the favourable situation in women, with small or absent socioeconomic inequalities in total cancer mortality, is likely to be a temporary phenomenon. In some countries in Western Europe, it has been found that in younger birth cohorts rates of breast cancer mortality now tend to be higher in lower socioeconomic groups than in higher socioeconomic groups. For lung cancer, there are similar indications for a future change in gradient among women (Mackenbach *et al.* 2004). Prevention of the emergence of excess cancer mortality in lower socioeconomic groups among women is a clear priority for public health.

As a result of these cause-specific patterns, there are important differences between countries in the share of specific causes of death in the excess mortality in lower socioeconomic groups (Huisman *et al.* 2005). The most important difference is for ischaemic heart disease: Due to the north–south gradient in ischaemic heart disease inequalities mentioned above, ischaemic heart disease is a major contributor to inequalities in mortality in the north of Europe, and much less important (sometimes even 'protecting' lower socioeconomic groups against larger inequalities in mortality) in the south (Fig. 12.3.2).

Life expectancy is shorter in lower socioeconomic groups

As a result of these differences in the risk of dying at various ages, people from lower socioeconomic groups tend to live considerably

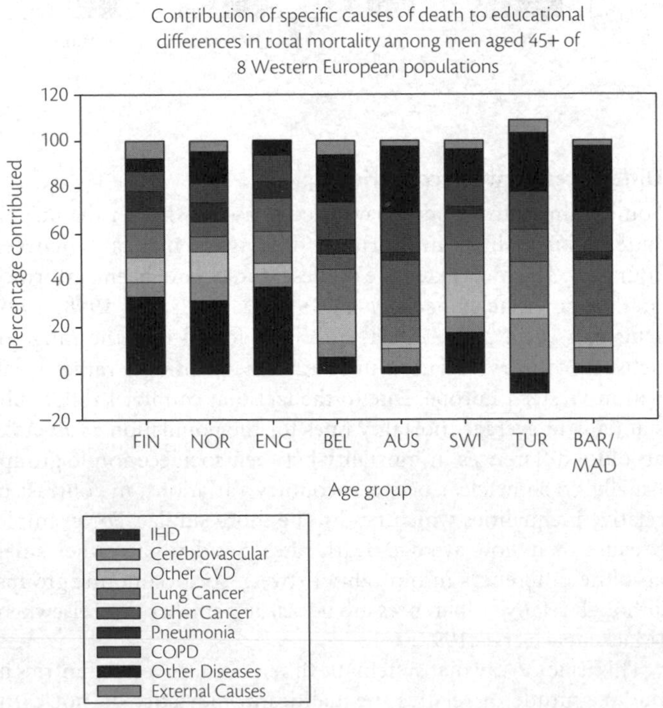

Fig. 12.3.2 Contribution (%) of specific causes of death to difference between low and high educational groups in total mortality in eight European populations, men and women aged 45 years and over, 1990s.
Source: Huisman *et al.* (2005).

shorter lives than those with more advantaged social positions. Differences in life expectancy at birth between the lowest and highest socioeconomic groups (e.g. manual versus professional occupations, or primary school versus postsecondary education) are typically in the order of 4–6 years among men, and 2–4 years among women, but sometimes larger differences have been observed (Mackenbach 2006). In England and Wales, for example, inequalities in life expectancy at birth among men have increased from 5.4 years in the 1970s to more than 8 years in the 1990s (Department of health 2004). A similarly strong increase has been observed in Finland (Martikainen *et al.* 2001).

Morbidity

Many countries have nationally representative surveys with questions on both socioeconomic status and self-reported morbidity (e.g. self-assessed health, chronic conditions, disability). Inequalities in the latter are substantial everywhere, and practically always in the same direction: Persons with a lower socioeconomic status have higher morbidity rates.

Inequalities in generic health indicators

For one indicator, self-assessed health (measured with a single question on an individual's perception of his or her own health), the availability of these data is almost as great as that for inequalities in mortality (Table 12.3.2). The overall pattern is clear again: Prevalence rates of less-than-'good' self-assessed health are higher in lower socioeconomic groups. No clear patterns have emerged in the magnitude of socioeconomic inequalities in self-assessed health between European countries (Mackenbach 2006).

These inequalities in self-reported morbidity persist into old-age. Beyond early adulthood, socioeconomic differences in self-reported morbidity have been found in all European countries where this has been examined (Cavelaars *et al.* 1998; Dalstra *et al.* 2005). For children and adolescents, however, the picture is more mixed. Some studies have suggested that in adolescence, the period between childhood and adulthood, there is a genuine narrowing of health inequalities, perhaps as a result of the transition between socioeconomic position of family of origin and own socioeconomic position. Among children the picture is more consistent: Many studies find that parents in lower socioeconomic groups report more ill-health for their children than parents in higher socioeconomic groups (Haldorsson *et al.* 2000).

Respondents to health interview surveys are unlikely to be perfect reporters of their health problems, and there may also be differences between socioeconomic groups in the accuracy of reporting health problems. Where more objective data have been available for comparison, however, similar pictures of higher incidence and prevalence of health problems have been obtained. Although height is partly genetically determined, it is also strongly influenced by childhood living conditions, such as nutrition, occurrence of disease, psychosocial stress, and housing conditions. It is often used as a summary indicator of health during childhood and adolescence, and shows consistent differences between socioeconomic groups. In all countries there are clear differences in average adult height between socioeconomic groups: The higher educated are 1–3 cm taller (Table 12.3.3) (Cavelaars *et al.* 2000a).

Inequalities in diseases and disabilities

Socioeconomic inequalities have not only been found for general health indicators, which are usually measured on the basis of self-reports, but can also be found for many specific indicators, including objective measurements of the incidence or prevalence of diseases and disabilities. In the large majority of these studies, higher incidences or prevalences of health problems have been found in the lower socioeconomic groups (Huisman *et al.* 2003; Dalstra *et al.* 2005).

No socioeconomic inequalities in the prevalence of cancer are usually found, while many epidemiological studies have found an increased incidence of many cancers in lower socio-economic groups. Among men, lung, larynx, oropharyngeal, oesophageal, and stomach cancers are among those with usually higher incidences in lower socioeconomic groups. Among women, this applies to oesophageal, stomach, and cervical cancer. Interestingly, some cancers have a higher incidence in higher socioeconomic groups: Colon and brain cancer and skin melanoma in men, and colon, breast, and ovary cancer and skin melanoma in women. We already saw similar patterns on the basis of cancer mortality (see 'Mortality') (Dalstra *et al.* 2005).

The fact that cancer prevalence is not higher in lower socioeconomic groups can perhaps be explained by differences in cancer survival. Put simply, incident ('new') cases of cancer can either die or stay alive, and only those who stay alive contribute to the number of prevalent ('current') cases. There is extensive evidence for socioeconomic inequalities in cancer survival: Most studies show a survival advantage for patients with a higher socioeconomic position. The lower survival rates of cancer patients in lower socioeconomic groups may to some extent numerically 'compensate' the higher incidence rates, and contribute to the lack of an excess prevalence of cancer in lower socioeconomic groups. These data for cancer are illustrative for many other potentially fatal conditions: Patients from higher socio-economic groups are usually likely to have better survival, because of more favourable prognostic factors (e.g. less comorbidity, better psychosocial profiles, etc.), because of better treatment (better access, higher quality treatments, better compliance, etc.), or both. Although inequalities in health care utilization are not among the most important contributors to the explanation of socioeconomic inequalities in health, at least not in Western Europe, these data suggest that improvements in the health care system could still be of some help in tackling health inequalities.

Mortality data by cause of death show that suicide tends to occur more frequently in lower socioeconomic groups, particularly among men (Lorant *et al.* 2005). One of the underlying risk factors, mental ill-health, also tends to be more prevalent in lower socioeconomic groups. The higher prevalence of mental illness in lower socioeconomic groups is likely to have a complex explanation. In psychiatric epidemiology, there is a long tradition of looking at the possible effects of mental health problems on downward social mobility. This 'drift hypothesis' has indeed found some support, for example in the case of schizophrenia, whose onset usually occurs in adolescence and young adulthood, and which may consequently interfere with school and early work careers. On the other hand, incidence studies have also found higher rates of many mental health problems among those who are currently in a lower socioeconomic position. It seems likely that this at least partly reflects a causal effect, perhaps through a higher exposure to psychosocial stressors and/or a lack of coping resources.

As a result of the higher frequency of physical and mental health problems in lower socioeconomic groups, the prevalence of limitations in functioning and various forms of disability also tends to

Table 12.3.2 Inequalities in self-assessed health by socioeconomic position in 18 countries[a]

Country	Indicator of socioeconomic position	Period	Age	Odds ratio[b] Men	Odds ratio[b] Women	Source
Austria	Education	1991	25–69	3.22*	2.67*	Mikrozensus Fragen zur Gesundheit
Belgium	Education	1997	25–74	2.55*	2.36	Belgium Health Interview Survey
Bulgaria	Education	1997	18+	2.19*	2.84*	National representative survey of the population of Bulgaria
	Income			1.86	1.50	
Denmark	Education	1994	25–69	2.16*	3.00*	Danish Health and Morbidity Survey
	Occupation	1986–1987	25–69	2.19*	n.a.	Danish Health and Morbidity Survey
Estonia	Education	1996	25–79	3.11*	3.59*	Estonian Health Interview Survey
	Income			2.37*	1.66*	
Finland	Education	1994	25–69	2.99*	3.29*	Finnish Survey on Living Conditions
	Income			3.09*	2.43*	
France	Occupation	1991–1992	25–69	2.24*		Enquête sur la Santé et les Soins Médicaux
Germany (West)	Education	1990–1991	25–69	1.76*	1.91*	National Health Survey
	Income			2.05*	2.40*	
	Occupation			1.63*		
Great Britain	Income	1996	25–69	3.88*	3.92*	British General Household Survey
	Occupation	1991	25–69	2.32*	n.a.	General Household Survey
England	Education	1995	25–69	3.08*	2.66*	Health Survey for England
Italy	Education	1994	25–69	2.94*	2.55*	Health Interview Survey
Latvia	Education	1999	25–70	2.21*	2.48*	Norbalt-II Living Conditions Survey
	Income			5.10*	3.26*	
The Netherlands	Education	1997–1999	25–69	2.81*	2.12*	Permanent Survey on Living Conditions
	Income			4.50*	3.01*	
	Occupation	1991–1992	25–69	2.40*		Health Survey
Norway	Education	1995	25–69	2.30*	2.84*	Health Survey
Poland	Education	1993	35–64	1.27	1.72	Household Survey Pol-MONICA survey (Warsaw)
Poland	Education	1993	35–64	2.08	0.93	Household Survey Pol-MONICA survey (Tarnobrzeg)
Spain	Education	1997	25–69	2.58*	3.10*	Spanish Health Survey
Sweden	Education	1997	25–69	2.37*	3.06*	Swedish Survey on Living Conditions
	Income			4.11*	2.80*	
	Occupation	1991	25–69	2.79*	n.a.	Swedish Level of Living Survey
Switzerland	Occupation	1992–1993	25–69	2.12*	n.a.	

[a] Because of differences in data collection and classification, the magnitude of inequalities in health cannot always directly be compared between countries.

[b] Odds ratio: Ratio of odds (a measure of risk) of less-than-'good' self-assessed health in lower socioeconomic groups as compared to that in higher socioeconomic groups. Asterisk (*) indicates that difference in mortality between socioeconomic groups is statistically significant. n.a. indicates 'not available'.

Source: Mackenbach (2006).

Table 12.3.3 Differences in average height (cm) between higher and lower educational groups in 10 European countries, around 1990

	Men differences (95% CI)	Women differences (95% CI)
Norway	1.8 (0.7–3.0)	1.2 (0.1–2.2)
Sweden	2.5 (1.8–3.1)	1.5 (0.9–2.0)
Finland	1.6 (1.0–2.2)	1.5 (0.9–2.0)
Denmark	2.8 (2.0–3.7)	1.8 (1.0–2.6)
Netherlands	2.5 (2.1–3.0)	1.6 (1.2–1.9)
Germany	2.2 (1.7–2.6)	2.2 (1.8–2.6)
Switzerland	2.9 (2.4–3.4)	2.2 (1.8–2.6)
France	2.6 (2.2–3.0)	1.6 (1.2–2.0)
Italy	2.5 (2.2–2.7)	1.3 (1.1–1.5)
Spain	3.0 (2.7–3.3)	1.3 (1.0–1.7)

This table shows people with higher educational level to be 1–3 cm taller.
Source: Cavelaars *et al.* (2000).

be higher. This applies to many aspects of functioning (mobility, sensory functioning, grip strength, walking speed, etc.) and is particularly evident among the elderly (Avendano *et al.* 2005). These inequalities in functioning translate into inequalities in limitations with activities of daily living such as dressing and bathing (ADL), and limitations with instrumental activities of daily living such as preparing hot meals and making telephone calls (IADL). This illustrates the high burden of physical limitations among those with a lower socioeconomic position, and is likely to contribute to substantially higher professional care needs, including institutionalized care (e.g. nursing homes). As suggested by the results for objective measures of grip strength and walking speed, inequalities in self-reported disability are real, and not a matter of reporting bias.

'Healthy life expectancy' is shorter in lower socioeconomic groups

We have seen above that the higher mortality rates in lower socioeconomic groups lead to substantial inequalities in life expectancy: People in lower socioeconomic groups tend to live between 2 and 8 years less than people in higher socioeconomic groups. The fact that morbidity rates (among those who are still alive) are higher too, contributes to even larger inequalities in 'healthy life expectancy' (the number of years which people can expect to live in good health). Inequalities in the number of years lived in good health are often seen of more than 10 years (Sihvonen *et al.* 1998; Mackenbach 2006).

The facts: Explanation

'Selection' versus 'causation'

During the past decade, great progress has been made in unravelling the determinants of health inequalities, and although further research is certainly necessary, our understanding of what causes health inequalities has progressed to a stage when rational approaches to reduce health inequalities are becoming feasible.

Early debates about the explanation of socioeconomic inequalities in health focused on the question whether 'causation' or 'selection' was the more important mechanism (Townsend & Davidson 1992; Macintyre 1997). Social selection explanations imply that health determines socioeconomic position, instead of socioeconomic position determining health. The term 'selection' here refers to the process of social mobility (changes in socioeconomic position), during which a selection occurs on health or health-related characteristics.

The occurrence of health-related selection as such is undisputed: During social mobility, some degree of selection on (ill-)health does indeed occur, with people who are in poor health being more likely to move 'downward' (e.g. get a lower status job, or lose income) and less likely to move 'upward' (e.g. finish a high-level education, or obtain a highly paid job), than people who are in good health. It is less clear, however, what the contribution of health-related selection to the explanation of socioeconomic inequalities in health is. The few studies which have investigated this, have concluded that this contribution is likely to be small (Bartley & Plewis 1997; Van de Mheen *et al.* 1999).

Furthermore, longitudinal studies in which socioeconomic status has been measured before health problems are present, and in which the incidence of health problems has been measured during follow-up, show clearly higher risks of developing health problems in the lower socioeconomic groups. These studies have demonstrated clearly that 'causation' instead of 'selection' is the main explanation for socioeconomic inequalities in health (Marmot *et al.* 1991; Marmot & Wilkinson 2006).

The unspoken assumption in debates about the role of selection versus causation often was that social selection is less of a problem for public policy than social causation. This assumption was incorrect, however, because limiting the social consequences of health problems is one of the classical objectives of social security and public health policies in many developed countries.

Specific determinants

The 'causal' effect of socioeconomic status on health is likely to be largely indirect: Through a number of more specific health determinants which are differentially distributed across socioeconomic groups (Fig. 12.3.3). Many risk factors for morbidity and mortality are more prevalent in lower socioeconomic groups, and it is these inequalities in exposure to specific health determinants which should be seen as the main explanation of health inequalities.

There is no doubt that 'material' factors, i.e. exposure to low income and to health risks in the physical environment, are part of

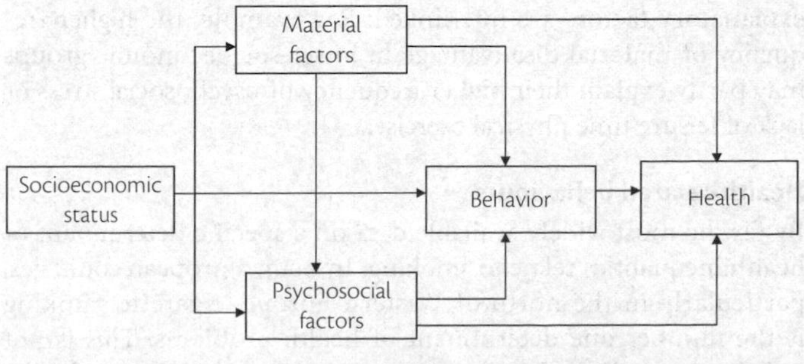

Fig. 12.3.3 Simple explanatory diagram: Factors which have been shown to 'mediate' between low socioeconomic position and risk of ill-health.

the explanation. All European countries have large inequalities in income. According to Eurostat, the 20 per cent of the population with the highest income in the European Union (EU-25) received 4.5 times more than the 20 per cent of the population with the lowest income in 2001. The proportion of the population who is at risk of poverty (defined as having an income less than 60 per cent of the national average) was 15 per cent in the EU as a whole. Although income inequality and poverty rates differ between countries, partly as a result of differences in income taxation and social security benefit schemes, it is quite likely that inequalities in financial disadvantage play an important role in the explanation of health inequalities in all developed countries. Financial disadvantage may affect health through various mechanisms: Psychosocial stress and subsequent risk-taking behaviours (smoking, excessive alcohol consumption, etc.), reduced access to health-promoting facilities and products (fruits and vegetables, sports, preventive health care services), etc. Occupational health risks (exposure to chemicals, accident risks, physically strenuous work, etc.) and health risks related to housing (crowding, dampness, accident risks, etc.) are other examples of 'material' factors which have been shown to make important contributions to the explanation of some health inequalities (Marmot & Wilkinson 2006; Siegrist & Marmot 2006).

The second group of specific determinants which contribute to the explanation of health inequalities are psychosocial factors. Those who are in a low socioeconomic position on average experience more psychosocial stress, in the form of negative life events (loss of beloved ones, financial difficulties, etc.), daily hassles, 'effort-reward imbalance' (high levels of effort without appropriate material and immaterial rewards), and a combination of high demands and low control. These forms of psychosocial stress can in their turn lead to ill-health, either through biological pathways (e.g. by affecting the endocrine or immune systems) or through behavioural pathways (e.g. by inducing risk-taking behaviours). Psychosocial factors related to work organization, such as job strain, have been shown to play an important role in the explanation of socioeconomic inequalities in cardiovascular health (Marmot & Wilkinson 2006; Siegrist & Marmot 2006).

The third group of contributory factors are health-related behaviours, such as smoking, inadequate diet, excessive alcohol consumption, and lack of physical exercise. In many developed countries, one or more of these 'lifestyle' factors are more prevalent in the lower socioeconomic groups, as will be discussed in the next section of this report. As we have seen above, many of the disease-specific patterns of health inequalities also suggest a substantial contribution of health-related behaviours to inequalities in mortality.

It is important to be aware of the fact that the three groups of explanatory factors are interlinked: For example, the higher frequency of material disadvantage in lower socioeconomic groups may partly explain their higher frequency of psychosocial stress or lack of leisure time physical exercise.

Health-related behaviours

By far the most widely available data on a specific determinant of health inequalities relate to smoking. In many European countries, particularly in the north of Western Europe, cigarette smoking is the number one determinant of health problems. This is not only because of its role in lung cancer and some other specific diseases, for which smoking is the main cause, but also because of its role in (premature) mortality in general, less-than-'good' self-assessed health and disability, for which smoking is an important contributory factor. The prevalence of smoking differs strongly between socioeconomic groups in many European countries, so one can safely assume that it plays an important role in generating health inequalities (Cavelaars *et al.* 2000b; Huisman *et al.* 2005).

In general, the prevalence of smoking is higher in the lower socioeconomic groups, but there are important differences between countries in the magnitude, and sometimes even the direction, of these inequalities. A number of comparative studies within Europe have demonstrated a north–south gradient, with larger inequalities in current smoking in the north of Europe and smaller (sometimes even 'reverse') gradients in the south (Fig. 12.3.4) (Cavelaars *et al.* 2000b; Huismand *et al.* 2005). This is particularly clear in the case of women: Higher educated women smoke less in the north of Europe (represented by the Nordic countries, Great Britain, the Netherlands, Belgium, etc.), but they smoke more than lower educated women in the south of Europe (represented by Italy, Spain, Greece, Portugal, etc.). Current rates of smoking are the result of trends which have played out over the past decades: The habit of cigarette smoking started early in the twentieth century with the advent of industrially produced cigarettes, and in many European countries it was only after the World War II that smoking became highly prevalent, first among men

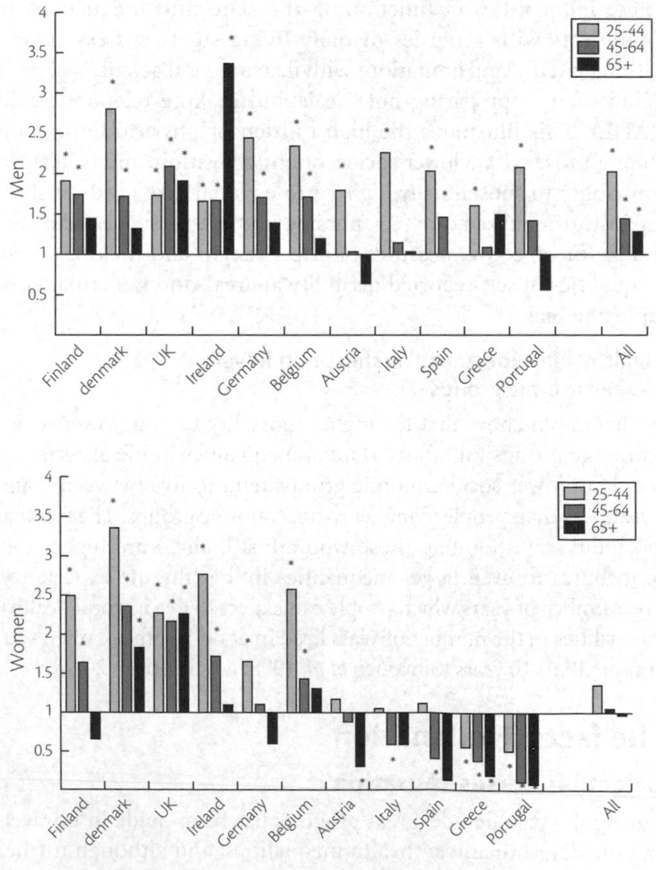

Fig. 12.3.4 Inequalities in current daily smoking by level of education in 11 European countries, 1998.
Source: Huisman, Kunst, and Mackenbach (2005).

(with rates of up to 90% smokers), then among women. In many countries, smoking prevalence has declined over the past decades, at least among men, as a result of health education efforts and other anti-tobacco measures such as raising excise taxes and bans on smoking in public places. This decline in smoking is still continuing, but there have been, and still are, clear socio-economic differences in this decline.

While smoking is clearly bad for health, alcohol is a more complex risk factor: Both abstinence and excessive alcohol consumption are bad for health (as compared to moderate drinking). Abstinence usually is more common in the lower socioeconomic groups, both among men and among women, but the pattern for excessive alcohol consumption is more variable. Many studies report a higher prevalence in lower socioeconomic groups, particularly among men, but the results for women are far from consistent (Droomers *et al.* 1999). These inconsistencies may well be due to real differences between countries in the social patterning of excessive alcohol consumption. In some countries, such as the Nordic countries (e.g. Finland) and several Eastern European countries, 'binge drinking' (drinking more than, say, 8 units on a single occasion) is a more serious source of health problems than regular overconsumption of alcohol. In these countries, binge drinking tends to be more common in lower socioeconomic groups, and is likely to contribute to the explanation of health inequalities, e.g. through a higher rate of ischaemic heart disease, stroke, and injury mortality (Makela *et al.* 1997).

Comparable data on dietary behaviour by socioeconomic status are even more difficult to obtain. The measurement of diet is notoriously difficult, and collecting nationally representative data on diet by socioeconomic position from a range of countries a costly exercise. Only a few comparative studies have been conducted, and these show that men and women in lower socioeconomic groups tend to eat fresh vegetables less frequently, particularly in the north of Europe. Differences in fresh vegetable consumption are smallest in the south of Europe, perhaps because of the larger availability and affordability of fruits and vegetables in Mediterranean countries. A similar north–south gradient has been found for the consumption of fruits (Cavelaars *et al.* 1997). Literature reviews have shown that it is likely that many other aspects of diet, such as consumption of meat, dairy products, and various fats and oils, also are socially patterned in many European countries, and that these social patterns differ between countries (Lopez-Azpiazu *et al.* 2003).

Lack of leisure-time physical activity tends to be more common in the lower socioeconomic groups, and so do overweight and obesity. Interestingly, this is one of the very few health aspects where patterns of social variation are clearer for women than for men. Among women, overweight and obesity are more prevalent in lower socioeconomic groups in all countries with available data, whereas the patterns are more variable among men (Fig. 12.3.5) (Sobal & Stunkard 1989; Cavelaars *et al.* 1997).

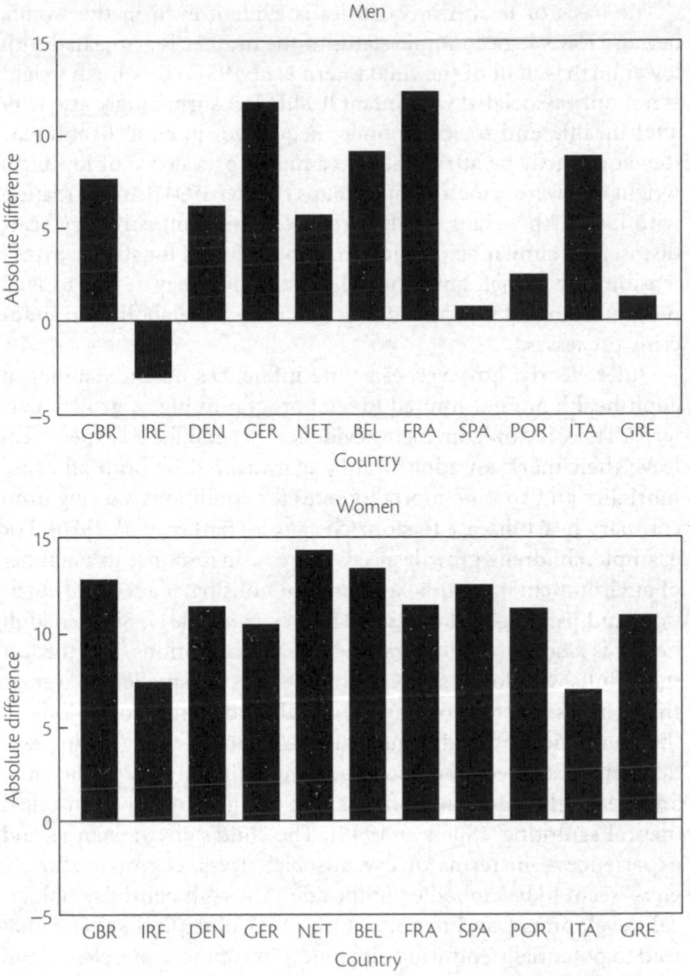

Fig. 12.3.5 Educational differences in overweight (% of individuals with body mass index higher than or equal to 25 kg/m^2) in 10 European countries, men and women aged 20–74 years, ca. 1990.
Source: Cavelaars et *al.* (1997).

Additional perspectives

During the 1990s, substantial progress has been made in understanding the mechanisms and factors involved in generating these variations in health. What has emerged from recent research efforts is a rather complex picture of how individuals in the lower socioeconomic strata are exposed over their lifetime to a wide variety of unfavourable and interacting material, cultural and psychological conditions, and how these exposures lead to ill-health—either directly, or indirectly through unhealthy behaviours or psychosocial stress. This research has opened a number of new perspectives which we review here: Life-course perspectives (dealing with the clustering of advantage and disadvantage over an individual's lifetime), and macrosocial perspectives (dealing with the effect of the wider social, economic, and political environment).

Life-course perspective

One of the interesting new perspectives on health inequalities has come from developmental research. The life-course perspective postulates that inequalities in the structure of society shape individuals' 'life chances'. Advantages and disadvantages not only cluster cross-sectionally, but also longitudinally (Davey Smith *et al.* 1997; Power & Matthews 1997). Interestingly, a life-course perspective also resolves the 'selection' versus 'causation' debate, because a material disadvantage in one stage of the life-course may translate into a health disadvantage in the next, which may then in turn lead to a material disadvantage 5 years later (Davey Smith *et al.* 1994).

The basis of health inequalities is evident even in the womb, because low socioeconomic status of the mother is associated with lower birth weight of the child (Stern *et al.* 1987). Low birth weight is not only associated with infant health, but surprisingly also with adult health, and socioeconomic inequalities in adult health may therefore partly be attributable to a higher prevalence of low birth weight in lower socioeconomic groups (Barker 1994). An association with low birth weight was first reported for adult coronary heart disease, but similar associations have been found for stroke, hypertension, and diabetes mellitus. The association may be due to 'fetal programming' of growth patterns and related metabolic and endocrine processes.

Quite clearly, however, early life influences on inequalities in adult health are not limited to fetal programming of growth patterns. There is now convincing evidence that childhood experiences leave their mark on adult health, as measured by both all-cause mortality and specific mortality rates for conditions varying from coronary heart disease to stomach cancer (Barker *et al.* 1990). For example, children's growth speeds decrease in response to a number of environmental hazards, such as poor housing, inadequate nutrition, and psychosocial stressors (Berney *et al.* 2001). Shorter adult height is associated with a range of health conditions, and the fact that adults with lower socioeconomic status are smaller on average thus suggests a role of adverse childhood living conditions in the generation of health inequalities. There is also growing evidence that socioeconomic circumstances literally shape the child and hence the adult in a process that has graphically been called 'neural sculpting' (Spencer 1996). The child's circumstances and experiences—in terms of psychosocial stress, cognitive stimuli, etc.—seem to be embodied in the adult through neuropsychological development and its impact on other biological systems that lead to potentially enduring differences in coping, competence, and health (Keating & Hertzman 1999). Circumstances in early life also set up a pattern of social learning, which may generate a sense of powerlessness reinforced by others in the social network who have been similarly disadvantaged and socially excluded, sometimes over generations (Keating & Hertzman 1999). The consequence of all this would be that observed socioeconomic differences in health in older people can plausibly be seen as the biological correlates of socially structured, differential exposure to health hazards over an entire lifetime (Berney *et al.* 2001). This view implies cumulative effects of adverse childhood living conditions, instead of latent effects.

Macrosocial perspectives

At the other end of the scale from biological factors is the macrosocial environment. Recent evidence suggests that factors such as 'social capital' and neighbourhood deprivation are independent determinants of health and may also play a part in generating health inequalities.

Partly spurred by studies suggesting that areas with more unequal income distribution have higher mortality rates, and that this may be due to less investments for the public good (Kaplan *et al.* 1996), there has been increased attention to the possible role of a lack of 'social capital' in generating health inequalities. Social capital can be depleted by high residential mobility, fear of strangers and by street crime that possibly inhibits people going to meetings and supporting their neighbours. There is some evidence that low social capital has an effect on overall levels of health, at ward and state levels in the United States and elsewhere (Kawachi *et al.* 1999; Subramanian *et al.* 2001). While social capital is usually defined as the voluntary organizations that can bridge different social groups and whose activities can benefit members as well as those outside the membership, the concept remains contentious and has been employed quite differently by different schools of researchers.

In many countries, indices have been developed of socioeconomic deprivation of neighbourhoods and other geographical areas. These indices combine various factors known to be disadvantageous to health, such as being unemployed, part of a sole-parent household, or on a welfare benefit, and having no car or renting rather than owning a home. In recent years, a number of studies have consistently shown that even after taking account of individual circumstances, living in a deprived area is associated with ill-health both in subjective and objective terms (Diez-Roux *et al.* 2001). Pathways are likely to involve lack of access to amenities that are necessary to maintain or restore good health (such as sports facilities, stores with affordable fresh fruit and vegetables, health care), psychosocial effects (such as psychosocial stress, feelings of hopelessness, experiences of being disrespected by others), as well as depletion of social capital (Lynch *et al.* 2000; Marmot & Wilkinson 2001).

The options: How to build a strategy to reduce inequalities in health?

Policy developments vis-à-vis health inequalities

Different countries are in widely different phases of awareness of, and willingness to take action on, socioeconomic inequalities in health. Figure 12.3.6 illustrates these differences for nine countries from various parts of Europe (Mackenbach *et al.* 2003b). Four common

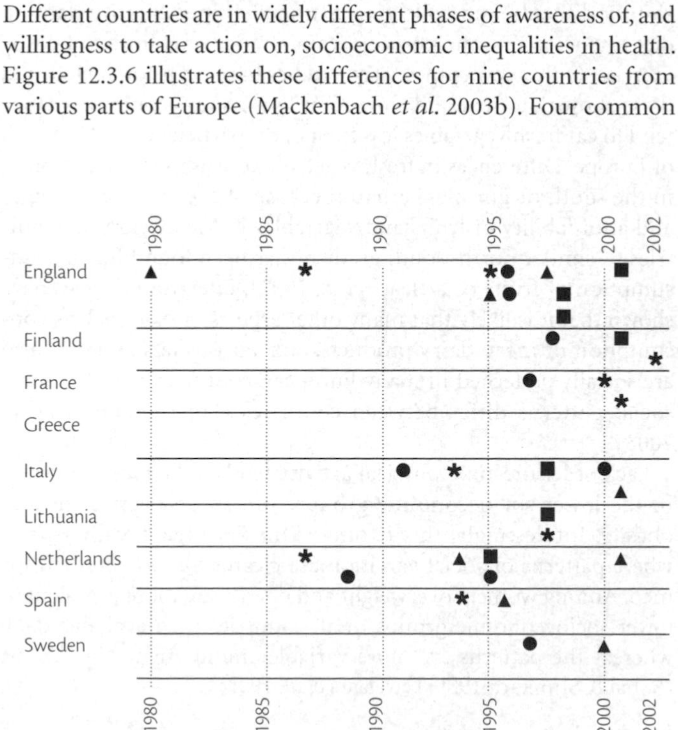

★ High-profile independent report recommending policy action on health inequalities
● Start of national research program on health inequalities
▲ Report of government advisory commission focusing on health inequalities reduction
■ Government policy document focusing on health inequalities reduction

Fig. 12.3.6 Time-lines representing concurrent policy development in nine European countries.
Source: Mackenbach and Bakker (2003).

milestones in policy development have been distinguished: High-profile independent reports recommending research or policy on health inequalities; national research programmes on health inequalities; government advisory committees recommending policies to reduce health inequalities; and coordinated government action to reduce health inequalities.

The first event included that is shown in Fig. 12.3.6 is the publication of the Black Report in 1980 in Britain (Townsend & Davidson 1992)—which has spurred research in Britain and increased awareness of health inequalities in the rest of Europe. It took more than a decade before further action was taken in Britain, first in the form of national research programmes and important government and non-government reports, then culminating in the Independent Inquiry published in 1998 (Acheson 1998). National governments in several other countries responded earlier, probably because of differences in political climate. In the Netherlands (late 1980s) and Italy (early 1990s), heightened awareness of health inequalities, partly generated by the Black Report, led to government-sponsored research programmes in this field. In Finland (mid-1980s) and Sweden (early 1990s), inequalities in health were addressed in major government policy documents on public health generally (not shown in Fig. 12.3.6) (Mackenbach *et al.* 2003b).

Whitehead has proposed a schematic 'action spectrum' to characterize the stage of diffusion of ideas on socioeconomic inequalities in health (Whitehead 1998). Starting with a primordial stage in which socioeconomic inequalities in health are not even measured, the spectrum covers the stages of 'measurement', 'recognition', 'awareness', 'denial/indifference', 'concern', 'will to take action', 'isolated initiatives', 'more structured developments', and 'comprehensive coordinated policy'. Among the countries included in the analysis shown in Fig. 12.3.6, which was carried out in 2002, Greece is the only one that found itself still in a pre-measurement stage. Data on socioeconomic inequalities in health were almost completely lacking, and awareness of the issue was limited to a small number of academics who do not have structural research funding for studies in this area. Spain, after a period with heightened awareness due to the publication of a Spanish 'Black Report', found itself in a 'denial/indifference' stage, largely because of a change in political colour of the national government. France and Italy both were in a 'concern' stage: Important reports on socioeconomic inequalities in health had been published, and policy-makers were increasingly paying attention to the issue. Lithuania, after the fall of the Soviet empire, has rapidly reached a 'will to take action' stage, as evidenced by parliamentary resolutions and reports from government advisory councils. The Netherlands and Sweden were in a 'more structured developments' stage, with national research programmes as well as high-level advisory committees that have recently issued comprehensive policy advice on how to reduce socioeconomic inequalities in health (see 'Blueprints for comprehensive strategies') (Mackenbach *et al.* 2003b).

The international comparison suggests that Britain, after a period of lagging behind other European countries, now is ahead of continental Europe in developing and implementing policies to reduce socioeconomic inequalities in health. It is the only country where policy advice has led to a significant number of new government initiatives specifically addressing health inequalities. Since the introduction of devolution in 1999, there have been a growing number of differences in health and other public policies between different parts of the United Kingdom, and it has therefore become difficult to make general statements. England seems to have entered a 'comprehensive coordinated policy' stage. Many recommendations from the Independent Inquiry have been accepted by the government in major policy documents (Department of Health 1999, 2001, 2004), and a series of new policies have been implemented ranging from neighbourhood renewal programmes to a fuel poverty strategy and from a national school fruit scheme to a child tax credit. Although from a European perspective some of these policies could be seen as a form of 'catching up' (similar programmes have been adopted long ago in other countries), the level of official government commitment was certainly unique at this point in time.

Innovative approaches

A number of innovative approaches to reduce health inequalities have been developed, some of which have been listed in Box 12.3.1.

Box 12.3.1 Innovative approaches for tackling socioeconomic inequalities in health developed during the 1990s in various European countries

Policy steering mechanisms
- Quantitative policy targets
  - Reduction of inequalities in 11 intermediate outcomes (poverty, smoking, working conditions, etc.)—the Netherlands
- Health inequalities impact assessment
  - Qualitative assessment of impact on health inequalities of EC agricultural policy—Sweden

Labour market and working conditions
- Universal approaches
  - Strong employment protection and active labour market policies for chronically ill citizens—Sweden
  - Occupational health services offering annual check-ups and preventive interventions to all employees—France

Targeted approaches
  - Reduction in retirement age for manual workers—Italy
  - Job rotation among dustmen—the Netherlands

Health-related behaviours
- Universal approaches
  - Serve low-fat food products through mass catering in schools and workplaces—Finland
- Targeted approaches
  - Multi-method intervention to reduce smoking among low-income women—Britain

Health care
- Improving quality of care
  - Nurse practitioners to support GPs working in deprived areas—the Netherlands
- Working with other agencies
  - Community strategies led by local government agencies, but integrating care across all the local public sector services, including health—England

Territorial approaches
- Comprehensive health strategies for deprived areas
  - Health Action Zones—England
  - Municipal health policy towards Ciutat Vella, Barcelona—Spain

Source: Mackenbach and Bakker (2003).

For each of the innovations (with the exception of policy steering mechanisms), there is at least some empirical evidence suggesting that they can help to reduce health inequalities (Mackenbach & Bakker 2002). Here, we will only highlight a few examples in the areas of 'labour market and working conditions', 'health-related behaviour', and 'health care'.

Health inequalities are partly due to labour market and working conditions. Swedish labour market policies enforce strong employment protection and active promotion of labour market participation for citizens with chronic illness. A comparison with England suggests that these policies have been effective in protecting vulnerable groups from labour market exclusion during the recession of the 1990s (Burström *et al.* 2000). In France, occupational health services are mandatory and include an annual health check for every employee. This provides a good setting for introducing preventive activities for those who otherwise have few medical contacts, particularly those in manual occupations. Randomized controlled trials within this setting have shown that interventions aimed at detection and treatment of hypertension and smoking cessation were successful (Lang *et al.* 1995, 2000). In Italy, a financial crisis in the early 1990s led to a reform of the pension scheme and a postponement of retirement age. Trade unions called attention to socioeconomic inequalities in life expectancy, and negotiated a 1-year reduction in retirement age for manual workers (Costa *et al.* 2002). Improvements of working conditions have made important contributions to reducing health inequalities in the past, but a lot remains to be done. In the Netherlands, a recent intervention study suggests that task rotation among garbage collectors reduces sickness absenteeism. Rotation of tasks (truck driving and mini-container loading) reduces physical load and possibly also increases job control (Kuijer *et al.* 1999).

Health-related behaviours like food consumption, smoking, and physical exercise also contribute to socioeconomic inequalities in health. Finnish nutrition policies have followed the Nordic welfare ideology where universalism has been the general principle. School children, students, and employees in Finland receive free or subsidized meals at school or workplace, and special dietary guidelines have been implemented ensuring the use of low-fat food products. This has probably contributed to the favourable trend of narrowing socioeconomic inequalities in use of butter and high-fat milk in Finland (Prättälä *et al.* 1992). In many countries, smoking is increasingly concentrated in lower socioeconomic groups, and reviews show that a variety of policies and interventions is effective in reducing smoking in these groups. While the price weapon (raising excise taxes) is very effective, its regressive impact on the poorest smokers who cannot stop should be counteracted by active promotion of the use of nicotine replacement therapy and other cessation support. Low-income women are a group where it is particularly difficult to change smoking behaviour, and a promising Scottish initiative therefore combined various approaches (community development, drama and poetry, fitness, cessation services, social support) (Gaunt-Richardson *et al.* 1999).

Universal access to effective health care, regardless of income or other forms of social disadvantage, is another important factor. Unequal access to health care services (according to need) may aggravate socioeconomic inequalities in health or even cause them. In addition, health care can contribute to reducing health inequalities by offering dedicated services to lower socioeconomic groups and by taking the lead in working with other agencies. In England, recent health service reforms gave local health authorities the lead responsibility for working with other agencies to improve health and reduce inequalities. The key integrating device is the production of a 3-year rolling plan for health, which feeds into a wider community strategy, committing all the local public sector services to a programme to improve the economic, social and environmental well-being of each area (Department of Health 2001).

Blueprints for comprehensive strategies

As it is unlikely that any single policy or intervention will significantly reduce socioeconomic inequalities in health, 'packages' of policies and interventions of a more comprehensive nature have been devised by government advisory committees in Great Britain, Sweden, and the Netherlands (Box 12.3.2).

Box 12.3.2 Comparison of three blueprints for comprehensive packages of policies and interventions to reduce inequalities in health

British Independent Inquiry into inequalities in health (1998)

39 main recommendations (123 with sub-clauses)

Seven overarching policy areas reviewed, corresponding to the major departments of state:

- Taxation and social security
- Education
- Employment
- Housing and environment
- Mobility, transport, and pollution
- Nutrition and the common agricultural policy
- National Health Service

Demographic factors over the life course considered, including:

- Mothers, children, and families
- Young people and adults of working age
- Older people
- Ethnicity
- Gender

Three priority areas are emphasized as crucial to addressing inequalities:

1. Health inequalities impact assessment
2. A high priority for the health of families with children
3. Reduction in income inequalities and improvement of living standards of poor households

The Dutch program committee on socioeconomic inequalities in health (2001)

26 recommendations

Four specific strategies:

1. Reduction of inequalities in education, income and other socioeconomic factors, e.g. no increase in income inequalities; anti-poverty measures; benefits to counter health effects of poverty

2. Reduction of the negative effects of health problems on socioeconomic position, e.g. decent benefits for work-incapacity; improved labour market participation of chronically ill
3. Reduction of the negative effects of socioeconomic position on health, e.g. reduction of smoking, overweight, physical and psychosocial work load in lower socioeconomic groups
4. Improve access and quality of healthcare for lower socioeconomic groups, e.g. preserve equal access; strengthen primary care in deprived neighbourhoods

Eleven quantitative targets relating to intermediate outcomes.

In general, strong emphasis on continuation of research, development, monitoring, and evaluation.

Swedish National Public Health Commission (2000)

18 health policy objectives
Six overarching themes:

1. Strengthening social capital, e.g. reduce poverty; reduce segregation in housing; reduced isolation and loneliness
2 Growing up in a satisfactory environment, e.g. secure parent-child bond; schools that strengthen pupils' self-confidence
3. Improving conditions at work, e.g. low unemployment; adapt physical and mental work demands; reduced overtime
4. Creating a satisfactory physical environment, e.g. green areas and playgrounds; high standards of building; safe traffic environment
5. Stimulating health-promoting life habits, e.g. more physical exercise; reduce overweight; reduce unwanted pregnancies
6. Developing a satisfactory infrastructure for health, e.g. strengthening prevention; coordination of public health efforts; intensified research

Development of 'indicators for achievement' recommended.

Source: Mackenbach and Bakker (2003).

Great Britain

The Black Report, mentioned above, contained the first example of such a comprehensive strategy (Townsend & Davidson 1992), but was received coolly and largely ignored by the Conservative government that was in power when it was issued in 1980. Further high-profile reports, such as The Health Divide (Whitehead 1992), stimulated widespread debate in the late 1980s, but were rejected by the government of the day. By the mid-1990s, however, the political climate had softened, and the King's Fund revisited the area and made a systematic attempt to review the scientific evidence for effective policies and interventions to reduce socioeconomic inequalities in health (Benzeval *et al.* 1995). The King's Fund report paved the way for the Independent Inquiry into Inequalities in Health, held by the Acheson Committee. The committee came up with 39 recommendations (123 in total, counting sub-clauses) (Acheson 1998). Without a doubt, this is the most comprehensive set of recommendations ever prepared. It has consequently been criticized for its lack of clear priorities, although three areas were singled out as priorities in the report, as detailed in Box 12.3.2. There is a certain emphasis on addressing 'upstream' factors like income, education, and employment, while recommendations on 'downstream' factors, like health-related behaviour, are presented as part of more general strategies directed towards groups defined in terms of age, gender, and ethnicity. The role of the National Health Service in reducing health inequalities is presented under a separate heading, probably to emphasize that even though deficiencies in health services are not a major cause of inequalities in health status, the health sector has an important part to play in any strategy to address observed health inequalities. Since the publication of the report, important progress has been made in implementing a number if its recommendations (Department of Health 1999, 2001, 2004).

The Netherlands and Sweden

Two recent reports from the Netherlands and Sweden provide an interesting contrast. In the Netherlands, a national 'Program Committee on Socioeconomic Inequalities in Health' has issued a set of 26 specific recommendations (Mackenbach & Stronks 2002). The committee is commonly called after its chairman, Albeda, a former Christian-Democrat Minister of Social Affairs. The committee had an equal representation of scientists and policy-makers, the latter representing different political parties. The recommendations were partly based on a series of intervention studies in which 12 different interventions addressing inequalities in health were subjected to, mostly quasi-experimental, process or outcome evaluations. A consultation exercise involving policy-makers and practitioners in various fields was part of the exercise (Stronks & Hulshof 2001). The recommendations were grouped in four strategies to address four different entry-points: Reduction of inequalities in socioeconomic factors; reduction of the negative effect of health on socioeconomic position; reduction of the negative effect of socioeconomic disadvantage on health (through reduced exposure to specific risk factors); and improved access and quality of health care. These entry points were derived from a simple and pragmatic model that was devised to help policy-makers understand how socioeconomic inequalities in health are generated. Examples of recommendations include 'no further increase in income inequality', 'no cuts in disability benefits', 'increase labour participation of the chronically ill', 'reduce physically demanding work', 'increase tobacco taxation', 'implement school health policies', and 'strengthen primary care in deprived areas' (Mackenbach & Stronks 2002). Due to recent political instabilities in the Netherlands, the national government has only recently started to implement some of the recommendations of the Albeda committee. At the local and regional level, however, many new initiatives have been taken to tackle health inequalities (Mackenbach & Stronks 2004).

In Sweden, the National Public Health Commission, a committee consisting of representatives of all political parties, scientific experts and advisers from governmental and non-governmental organizations, has recently developed a new national health policy with a strong focus on reducing health inequalities. The commission used a conceptual model resembling the Dutch model, but with contextual factors and the social consequences of disease added. Although the exercise involved a review of scientific evidence, like in the Independent Inquiry this review focused on explanations of inequalities in health, not on the evaluation of policies and interventions. It further involved extensive consultation of numerous organizations, and the proposal itself includes action by a wide range of actors in society. The commission formulated

18 health policy objectives grouped in six large areas: Strengthening social capital; growing up in a satisfactory environment; improving conditions at work; creating a satisfactory physical environment; stimulating health-promoting life habits; and developing a satisfactory infrastructure for health. Specific factors addressed by the strategy range from contextual factors such as social cohesion and housing segregation (with effects on children's educational opportunities) to work organization (with effects on job strain) and tobacco and alcohol consumption. The commission recommended to develop quantitative targets related to each of these policy objectives, but although specific targets were presented in draft versions of the strategy, these were withdrawn as the process progressed (Ministry of Health and Social Affairs, Stockholm 2000).

Towards evidence-based policy-making to tackle socioeconomic inequalities in health

The role of evidence

Within high-income countries, there is considerable diversity in the way scientific evidence has been used to underpin policies to reduce health inequalities. This is illustrated by the way the three comprehensive blueprints mentioned above were developed. The Acheson Committee commissioned 18 reviews of the evidence covering seven overarching policy areas, together with major sociodemographic factors over the life-course. Much of the evidence in the commissioned reviews related to the contribution of specific factors to the explanation of health inequalities, not to the effectiveness of policies and interventions tackling them (Macintyre *et al.* 2001). In contrast, the Dutch strategy was developed at the end of a 6-year research programme in which 12 studies were carried out to assess the effectiveness of various intervention options. The results of these studies were then discussed with experts and policy-makers, to see how these fitted into the existing evidence-base and in current policy (Stronks & Hulshof 2001). Although the approach proved only partly successful, because some entry-points for policy were not covered by evaluation studies, and some evaluation studies failed while others had design weaknesses, in the end a sizable fraction of policy recommendations was related to specific results of the programme (Mackenbach & Stronks 2002). In the Swedish case, the emphasis again was strongly on evidence relating to the explanation of health inequalities. The process was one of consultation with practitioners and policy-makers that ensured their commitment with the final recommendations. Evidence demonstrating that the strategies will actually work in terms of reducing health inequalities was not provided (Ministry of Health and Social Affairs, Stockholm 2000).

This diversity is also seen in the opinions of different researchers on what type of evidence is needed to underpin policies and interventions in this field. There are those who argue that in view of the urgency of starting to tackle health inequalities ('doing nothing is not an option') (Petticrew *et al.* 2004), one should be prepared to start intervening on the basis of plausibility. Political 'windows of opportunity' are usually short, e.g. 4 years at most, and they may be closed before careful evaluation studies have been conducted (Whitehead *et al.* 2004). A parallel has been drawn with nineteenth-century public health interventions for which controlled intervention studies have never been done, but which were implemented on the basis of plausibility and have proven to be highly successful (Davey Smith *et al.* 2001). Under the pressure of politicians wanting to see rapid results, the best that can be achieved in terms of scientific evaluation may then be large-scale implementation accompanied by a 'real time' evaluation study of the intervention, concurrent with its implementation, using some quasi-experimental design (before-after study, interrupted time-series study, etc.) (Macintyre 2003).

On the other hand, there are those who argue that this is a strategy with serious risks. Like in other areas of social and health policy, the actual results of policies and interventions to reduce health inequalities could easily be counterintuitive. There are many historical examples of 'plausible' interventions and policies that did not work, or actually had adverse effects (Macintyre *et al.* 2001). The fact that there are no systematic differences between countries in the magnitude of health inequalities, despite large differences in health, social and economic policies, should also warn us against optimism about the effects of policies and interventions that seem plausible. Shouldn't one expect the magnitude of health inequalities in the Nordic countries, with their long histories of egalitarian economic, social, and health care policies, to be smaller than in other Western European countries? The fact that this is not the case, suggests that policies which could plausibly be seen as conducive to reducing health inequalities, may actually not be of much help, or at the very least far from sufficient. Several explanations have been suggested, including that the generous 'welfare state regimes' in the Nordic countries may actually have enabled people in lower socioeconomic groups to participate in an affluent life-style, including smoking, lack of physical exercise, overeating, and excessive alcohol consumption (Dahl *et al.* 2006). In addition to that, one could argue that any investment in reducing health inequalities should be justified on the basis of a comparison of its cost-effectiveness with that of other possible investments in health and well-being, and that producing credible evidence is therefore essential (Oliver 2001). A plea could therefore be made for more systematically collecting evidence on the (cost-)effectiveness of interventions and policies to reduce health inequalities (Macintyre *et al.* 2001).

What types and levels of evidence are needed?

Despite the disagreements on what types and levels of evidence are needed before policies and interventions to reduce health inequalities, there is a general consensus that collection of such evidence is needed. The next question then is what types and levels of evidence should be collected. Schematically, the evidence-base underpinning decisions to implement a policy or intervention to tackle health inequalities could be built up in the following sequence:

- Creating a theoretical rationale for the intervention or policy: Identifying factors which make a substantial, independent contribution to the explanation of health inequalities.
- Developing an intervention or policy which could target these factors: Adapting existing, or creating new, interventions or policies which are likely to do more good than harm, which will differentially benefit lower socioeconomic groups, and which can be implemented on a sufficiently large scale to have an impact on health inequalities at the population level.
- Demonstrating the (cost-)effectiveness of this intervention or policy: Showing empirically that the policy or intervention reduces health inequalities in settings similar to that in which it will be implemented, taking into account any harmful side-effects, and to an extent that justifies its cost.

For the first step, one must rely on evidence from carefully designed observational studies, such as longitudinal (or prospective cohort) studies in which exposure to low socioeconomic status and specific health determinants has been measured at base-line, and health outcomes are measured during follow-up. A number of such longitudinal studies have been set up over the past decades in some Western European countries, and have contributed importantly to the evidence-base (Marmot *et al.* 1991; Mackenbach *et al.* 1994). A variety of factors has been shown to make important contributions to the explanation of health inequalities, particularly inequalities in mortality or incidence of cardiovascular disease. Evidence on other outcomes is much more scarce. Because of the complexity of the explanation of health inequalities, in which chains of interconnected factors are thought to be operating over the life-course, one must be careful in interpreting the results of these studies. It is not necessarily the case that factors which have been identified by conventionally designed cohort studies, indeed make an 'independent' contribution to the explanation of health inequalities, in the sense that if this particular factor would be removed, the magnitude of health inequalities can be assumed to be reduced by its contribution as measured in multivariate analyses. It is important to be aware of the fact that the explanation of health inequalities, in terms of specific 'downstream' factors, is likely to be substantially different between Western European countries, and that theoretical rationales constructed for one country may have limited generalizability to other countries. This was illustrated above with the example of smoking.

Generally speaking, it is unlikely that suitable policies or interventions which effectively target factors identified in the first step are already available. Many of the factors known to be involved in the explanation of health inequalities, such as working and housing conditions, health-related behaviours, or psychosocial stressors, have been known to be health determinants for a long time, and many of them have been addressed by health or intersectoral policies. The fact that they still make important contributions to the explanation of health inequalities implies that current policies to address these factors are insufficiently effective in lower socioeconomic groups. More powerful and/or tailored approaches will therefore have to be developed, and carefully assessed, e.g. with regard to the balance between benefits and harms. In this stage of development, powerful evaluation designs are usually not necessary, just as in the case of drugs development where so-called phase I and II studies are usually small and uncontrolled (Thomson *et al.* 2004). Because of the scale of the problem of health inequalities, which requires changing the 'gradient' of health problems in whole populations, it is crucial that policies and interventions are developed which can effectively reach large sections of the population.

After the development stage, 'promising' new approaches will need to be evaluated for their effectiveness under 'real-life' circumstances. Clearly, randomized controlled trials will not always be feasible, particularly for the evaluation of policies and interventions that are applied on a population-wide scale. Sometimes, Community Intervention Trials, in which groups of people (school classes, neighbourhoods, etc.) instead of individuals are allocated to the intervention and control condition, will then be a good alternative. But in many circumstances one will have to rely on quasi-experimental or even observational designs to inform policy-makers on the effectiveness of new approaches. Controlled before-after studies or interrupted time-series designs could then be used, or observational studies of 'natural experiments', e.g. by making comparisons between countries (Thomson *et al.* 2004). A complicating factor in evaluating the effectiveness of policies and interventions to reduce health inequalities is that this effectiveness should be measured in terms of favourably changing the distribution of health problems in the population, not of reducing the rate of health problems in a particular group. A 'full' study-design therefore requires the measurement, in one or more experimental populations and one or more control populations, of changes over time in the magnitude of health inequalities. Any other design, such as an experimental study of changes over time in the rate of health problems in lower socioeconomic groups only, requires rather strong assumptions to be made, in this case on the absence of health effects in higher socioeconomic groups (Mackenbach & Gunning-Schepers 1997). Fulfilling this requirement is rather difficult in experimental study designs, which is an additional argument for accepting quasi-experimental and observational evidence in this area.

Conclusions

Whether it will actually be possible to substantially reduce socioeconomic inequalities in health remains an open question. Western European trends in inequalities in mortality during the last decades of the twentieth century have generally shown a widening of the gap in relative terms, and at best a stable situation in absolute terms (Mackenbach *et al.* 2003a). This was despite the WHO equity target for the period 1985–2000 (WHO 1985), but as previous analyses have shown, despite good intentions in some countries, scale and intensity of efforts aiming to reduce health inequalities have been very modest, at least until 1998 (Mackenbach *et al.* 2003b). It was only towards the end of the 1990s that a few countries reached a stage of policy development in which serious efforts can be, and sometimes are, considered.

There is a lot of good news too, however. First, in Western Europe, during the 1990s, there has been enormous progress in explanatory research, and this has identified a large number of targets for policies and interventions to tackle health inequalities. Second, there has also been a beginning of research and development for effective interventions and policies to tackle health inequalities. While this is still a modest beginning, it does put us in a better position to reduce socioeconomic inequalities in health in the coming decades. A number of innovative approaches have been developed for which there is at least some evidence of effectiveness. Blueprints of comprehensive packages have been developed in several countries that have a sound theoretical basis and clear inspirational value, and that have been taken or are being taken seriously by policy-makers. Progress in research and increased awareness among policy-makers have created an enormous 'window of opportunity' that should be used for moving policy forward.

Developing effective strategies to reduce health inequalities is a daunting task. No single country has the capacity to contribute more than a fraction of the necessary knowledge. This is a matter not only of restricted manpower or financial resources for research, but also of restricted opportunities for implementing and evaluating policies and interventions. Some policies can be implemented and evaluated in some countries and not in others, either because they have already been implemented or because they are politically infeasible. International exchange is therefore necessary to increase learning speed. Such international exchange should be supported strongly by international agencies such as the World Health Organization, the European Union, and the Cochrane and Campbell Collaborations.

References

Acheson, D. (1998) *Independent Inquiry into Inequalities in Health Report*. London: The Stationery Office.

Ackerknecht, E.H. (1953) Rudolf Virchow. Doctor, statesman, anthropologist. University of Wisconsin Press, Madison, WI.

Avendano, M., Kunst, A.E., Huisman, M. *et al.* (2004) Educational level and stroke mortality: a comparison of 10 European populations during the 1990s. *Stroke*, **35**, 432–7.

Avendano, M., Aro, A.R., Mackenbach, J.P. (2005). Socio-economic disparities in physical health in 10 European countries. In *Health, ageing and retirement in Europe. First results from the survey of health, ageing and retirement in Europe* (eds. A. Börsch-Supan, A. Brugiavini, H. Jürges, J.P. Mackenbach, J. Siegrist, G. Weber). Strauss GmbH, Morlenbach, pp. 89–94.

Barker, D.J.P. (1994) *Mothers, babies and health in later life*, 2nd ed. Churchill, Livingstone, Edinburgh.

Barker, D.J.P., Coggon, D., Osmond, C., Wickham, C. (1990) Poor housing in childhood and high rates of stomach cancer in England and Wales. *British Journal of Cancer*, **61**, 575–8.

Bartley, M., Plewis, I. (1997) Does health-selective mobility account for socioeconomic differences in health? Evidence from Engeland and Wales, 1971 to 1991. *Journal of Health Social Behaviour*, **38**, 376–86.

Benzeval, M., Judge, K., Whitehead, M. (1995) Tackling inequalities in health: An agenda for action. King's Fund, London.

Berney, L., Blane, D., Davey Smith, G. *et al.* (2001) Lifecourse influences on health in early old age. In *Understanding health inequalities* (ed. H. Graham), pp. 79–95. Open Univ. Press, Buckingham.

Burström, B., Whitehead, M., Lindholm, C. *et al.* (2000) Inequality in the social consequences of illness: how well do people with long-term illness fare in the British and Swedish labor markets? *International Journal of Health Services*, **30**, 435–51.

Cavelaars, A.E.J.M., Kunst, A.E., Mackenbach, J.P. (1997) Socio-economic differences in risk-factors for morbidity and mortality in the European Community. An international comparison. *Journal of Health Psychology*, **2**, 353–72.

Cavelaars, A.E.J.M., Kunst, A.E., Geurts, J.J.M. *et al.* (1998) Morbidity differences by occupational class among men in seven European countries: an application of the Erikson Goldthorpe social class scheme. *International Journal of Epidemiology*, **27**, 222–30.

Cavelaars, A.E.J.M., Kunst, A.E., Geurts, J.J.M. *et al.* (2000b) Educational differences in smoking: international comparison. *British Medical Journal*, **320**, 1102–7.

Cavelaars, A.E.J.M., Kunst, A.E., Geurts, J.J.M. *et al.* (2000a) Persistent variations in average height between countries and between socio-economic groups: an overview of 10 European countries. *Annals of Human Biology*, **27**, 407–21.

Chave, S.P.W. (1984) The origins and development of public health. In *Oxford Textbook of Public Health* (ed. W.W. Holland, R. Detels, G. Knox). Oxford University Press, Oxford.

Coleman, W. (1982). Death is a social disease; public health and political economy in early industrial France. University of Wisconsin, Madison, WI.

Dalstra, J.A.A., Kunst, A.E., Borrell, C. *et al.* (2005) Socio-economic differences in the prevalence of common chronic diseases: an overview of eight European countries. *International Journal of Epidemiology*, 34, 316–26.

Davey Smith, G., Neaton, J.D., Wentworth, D. *et al.* (1996). Socioeconomic differentials in mortality risk among men screened in the Multiple Risk Factor Intervention Trial: I: White men. *American Journal of Public Health*, **86**, 486–96.

Davey Smith, G., Blane, D., Bartley, M. (1994) Explanations for socioeconomic differentials in mortality. Evidence from Britain and elsewhere. *European Journal of Public Health*, **4**, 131–44.

Davey Smith, G., Hart, C., Blane, D. *et al.* (1997). Lifetime socio-economic position and mortality: Prospective observational study. *British Medical Journal*, **314**, 547–52.

Davey Smith, G., Ebrahim, S., Frankel, S. (2001) How policy informs the evidence. *British Medical Journal*, **322**, 184–5.

Department of Health (1999) *Reducing health inequalities: an action report*. Stationery Office, London.

Department of Health (2001) *From vision to reality. Stationery Office*, London.

Department of Health (2004) *Choosing health: making healthy choices easier*. Stationery Office, London.

Diez Roux, A.V., Merking, S.S., Arnett, D. *et al.* (2001) Neighborhood of residence and incidence of coronary heart disease. *New England Journal of Medicine*, **345**, 99–106.

Dahl, E., Fritzell, J., Lahelma, E. *et al.* (2006) Welfare state regimes and health inequalities. In *Health inequalities in Europe* (eds. J. Siegrist and M. Marmot). Oxford University Press, Oxford.

Dromers, M., Schrijvers, C.T., Stronks, K. *et al.* (1999) Educational differences in excessive alcohol consumption: the role of psychosocial and material stressors. *Preventive Medicine*, **29**, 1–10.

Fukuda, Y., Nakamura, K., Takano, T. (2007) Higher mortality in areas of lower socioeconomic position measured by a single index of deprivation in Japan. *Public Health*, **121**, 163–73.

Gaunt-Richardson, P., Amos, A., Howie, G. *et al.* (1999) Women, low income and smoking – breaking down the barriers. ASH Scotland/Health Education Board for Scotland, Edinburgh.

Halldórsson, M., Kunst, A.E., Köhler, L. *et al.* (2000) Socioeconomic inequalities in the health of children and adolescents. A comparative study of the five Nordic countries. *European Journal of Public Health*, **10**, 281–8.

Huisman, M., Kunst, A.E., Andersen, O. *et al.* (2004) Socioeconomic inequalities in mortality among elderly people in 11 European populations. *Journal of Epidemiology and Community Health*, **58**, 468–75.

Huisman, M., Kunst, A.E., Bopp, M. *et al.* (2005a) Educational inequalities in cause-specific mortality in middle-aged and older men and women in eight Western European populations. *The Lancet*, **365**, 493–500.

Huisman, M., Kunst, A.E., Mackenbach, J.P. (2005) Educational inequalities in smoking among men and women aged 16 years and older in 11 European countries. *Tobacco Control*, **14**, 106–13.

Kaplan, G.A., Pamuk, E.R., Lynch, J.W. *et al.* (1996). Inequality in income and mortality in the United States: Analysis of mortality and potential pathways. *British Medical Journal*, **312**, 999–1003. Published erratum appears in *British Medical Journal*, **312**, 1253.

Kawachi, I.B.P., Kennedy, Glass, R. (1999) Social capital and self-rated health: A contextual analysis. *American Journal of Public Health*, **89**, 1187–93.

Keating, D.P., Hertzman, C. eds. (1999). *Developmental health and the wealth of nations: Social, biological and educational dynamics*. Guilford, New York.

Khang, Y.H., Lynch, J.W., Yun, S. *et al.* (2004) Trends in socioeconomic health inequalities in Korea: use of mortality and morbidity measures. *Journal of Epidemiology and Community Health*, **58**, 308–14.

Kuijer, P.P., Visser, B., Kemper, H.C. (1999) Job rotation as a factor in reducing physical workload at a refuse collecting department. *Ergonomics*, **42**, 1167–78.

Kunst, A.E., Groenhof, F., Mackenbach, J.P. and the EU Working Group on Socioeconomic Inequalities in Health (1998). Occupational class and cause-specific mortality in middle aged men in 11 European countries: a comparison of population based studies. *British Medical Journal*, **316**, 1636–41.

Kunst, A.E., Groenhof, F., Andersen, O. *et al.* (1999) Occupational class and ischemic heart disease mortality in the United States and 11 European countries. *American Journal of Public Health*, **89**, 47–53.

Lasser, K.E., Himmelstein, D.U., Woolhandler, S. (2006) Access to care, health status, and health disparities in the United States and Canada: results of a cross-national population-based survey. *American Journal of Public Health*, **96**, 1300–7.

Lang, T., Nicaud, V., Darne, B. *et al.* (1995) Improving hypertension control among excessive alcohol drinkers: a randomised controlled trial in France. The WALPA Group. *Journal of Epidemiology and Community Health*, **49**, 610–16.

Lang, T., Nicaud, V., Slama, K. *et al.* (2000) Smoking cessation at the workplace. Results of a randomised controlled intervention study. Worksite physicians from the AIREL group. *Journal of Epidemiology and Community Health*, **54**, 349–54.

Leinsalu, M., Vagero, D., Kunst, A.E. (2003) Estonia 1989-2000: enormous increase in mortality differences by education. *International Journal of Epidemiology*, **32**, 1081–7.

Ljung, R., Peterson, S., Hallqvist, J. *et al.* (2005) Socioeconomic differences in the burden of disease in Sweden. *Bulletin of the World Health Organisation*, **83**, 92–9.

López-Azpiazu, I., Sánchex-Villegas, A., Johansson, L. *et al.* (2003) FAIR-97-3096 Project. *Journal of Human Nutrition and Dietics*, **16**, 349–64.

Lorant, V., Kunst, A.E., Huisman, M. *et al.* (2005) Socio-economic inequalities in suicide: an European comparative study. *British Journal of Psychiatry*, **187**, 49–54.

Lynch, J.W., Davey Smith, G., Kaplan, G.A. *et al.* (2000) Income inequality and mortality: importance to health of individual income, psychosocial environment, or material conditions. *British Medical Journal*, **320**, 1200–4.

Macintyre, S. (1997) The Black Report and beyond: what are the issues? *Social Science and Medicine*, **44**, 723–45.

MacIntyre, S., Chalmers, I., Horton, R. *et al.* (2001) *Using evidence to inform health policy: case study. British Medical Journal*, **322**, 222–5.

Macintyre, S. (2003) Evidence based policy making. *British Medical Journal*, **326**, 5–6.

Mackenbach, J.P. (1994) Socioeconomic inequalities in health in the Netherlands: impact of a five year research programme. *British Medical Journal*, **309**, 1487–91.

Mackenbach, J.P., van de Mheen, H., Stronks, K. (1994) A prospective cohort study investigating the explanation of socioeconomic inequalities in health in The Netherlands. *Social Science of Medicine*, **38**, 299–308.

Mackenbach, J.P., Gunning-Schepers, L.J. (1997) How should interventions to reduce inequalities in health be evaluated? *Journal of Epidemiology and Community Health*, **51**, 359–64.

Mackenbach, J.P., Kunst, A.E., Cavelaars, A.E.J.M. *et al.* and the EU Working Group on Socioeconomic Inequalities in Health (1997) Socioeconomic inequalities in morbidity and mortality in Western Europe. *Lancet*, **349**, 1655–9.

Mackenbach, J.P., Kunst, A.E., Groenhof, F. *et al.* (1999) Socioeconomic inequalities in mortality among women and among men: an international study. *American Journal of Public Health*, **89**, 1800–6.

Mackenbach, J.P., Cavelaars, A.E.J.M., Kunst, A.E. *et al.* and the EU Working Group on Socioeconomic Inequalities in Health (2000) Socioeconomic inequalities in cardiovascular disease mortality: an international study. *European Heart Journal*, **21**, 1141–51.

Mackenbach, J.P., Bakker, M.J. (eds.) (2002). *Reducing inequalities in health: a European perspective.* Routledge, London.

Mackenbach, J.P., Stronks, K. (2002) A strategy for tackling health inequalities in the Netherlands. *British Medical Journal*, **325**, 1029–32.

Mackenbach, J.P., Bakker, M.J. and the European Network on Interventions and Policies to Reduce Inequalities in Health (2003b) Tackling socioeconomic inequalities in health: an analysis of recent European experiences. *Lancet*, **362**, 1409–14.

Mackenbach, J.P., Bos, V., Andersen, O. *et al.* (2003a) Widening socioeconomic inequalities in mortality in six Western European countries. *International Journal of Epidemiology*, **32**, 830–7.

Mackenbach, J.P., Stronks, K. (2004) The development of a strategy for tackling health inequalities in the Netherlands. *International Journal for Equity in Health*, **3**, 11.

Mackenbach, J.P., Huisman, M., Andersen, O. *et al.* (2004) Inequalities in lung cancer mortality by the educational level in 10 European populations. *European Journal of Cancer*, **40**, 126–35.

Mackenbach, J.P. (2006) *Health inequalities: Europe in profile.* Presidency of the EU, London, UK.

Mäkelä, P., Valkonen, T., Martelin, T. (1997) Contribution of deaths related to alcohol use of socioeconomic variation in mortality: register based follow up study. *British Medical Journal*, **315**, 211–6.

Marmot, M.G., McDowall, M.E. (1986). Mortality decline and widening social inequalities. *Lancet*, **2**, 274–76.

Marmot, M.G. *et al.* (1991) Health inequalities among British civil servants: The Whitehall II study. *Lancet*, **337**, 1387–93.

Marmot, M.G., Wilkinson, R.G. (2001). Psychosocial and material pathways in the relation between income and health. *British Medical Journal*, **322**, 1233–36.

Marmot, M., Wilkinson, R.G. (2006) *Social determinants of health.* Second Edition. Oxford University Press, Oxford.

Martikainen, P., Valkonen, T., Martelin, T. (2001) Change in male and female life expectancy by social class: decomposition by age and cause of death in Finland 1971-95. *Journal of Epidemiology and Community Health*, **55**, 494–9.

Mheen, H. van de, Stronks, K., Schrijvers, C.T.M. *et al.* (1999)The influence of adult ill health on occupational class mobility and mobility out of and into employment in The Netherlands. Results from a longitudinal study. *Social Science of Medicine*, **49**, 509–18.

Ministry of Health and Social Affairs. Hälsa på lika villkor – nationella mål för folkhälsan. Slutbetänkande av nationella folkhälsokommittén (Health on equal terms – final proposal on national targets for public health). (2000) Ministry of Health and Social Affairs, Stockholm (SOU 2000:91).

Oliver, A. (2001) Health inequalities policy: do we need evidence on effectiveness? [letter to the editor]. (rapid responses to: Davey Smith G, Ebrahim S, Frankel S. How policy informs the evidence.) *British Medical Journal*, **322**, 184–5.

Pamuk, E. (1985) Social class inequality in mortality from 1921 to 1972 in England and Wales. *Population Studies*, **39**, 17–31.

Petticrew, M., Whitehead, M., Macintyre, S.J. *et al.* (2004) Evidence for public health policy on inequalities I: The reality according to policymakers. *Journal of Epidemiology and Community Health*, **58**, 811–6.

Power, C., Mathews, S. (1997). Origins of health inequalities in a national population sample. *Lancet*, **350**, 1584–9.

Prättälä, R., Berg, M.A., Puska, P. (1992) Diminishing or increasing contrasts? Social class variation in Finnish food consumption patterns 1979-1990. *European Journal of Clinical Nutrition*, **42**(suppl), 16–20.

Shaw, C., Blakely, T., Crampton, P. *et al.* (2005) The contribution of causes of death to socioeconomic inequalities in child mortality: New Zealand 1981-1999. *New Zealand Medical Journal*, **16**, 118.

Shkolnikov, V., Andreev, E.M., Jasilionis, D. *et al.* (2006) The changing relation between education and life expectancy in central and Eastern Europe in the 1990s. *Journal of Epidemiology and Community Health*, **60**, 875–81.

Siegrist, J., Marmot, M. (eds.) (2006) *Health inequalities in Europe.* Oxford University Press, Oxford.

Sihvonen, A.-P., Kunst, A.E., Lahelma, E. *et al.* (1998) Socioeconomic inequalities in health expectancy in Finland and Norway in the late 1980s. *Social Science of Medicine*, **47**, 303–15.

Stern A. *et al.* (1987). Social adversity, low birth weight, and pre-term delivery. *British Medical Journal*, **295**, 291–3.

Stronks, K., Hulshof, J. (red.). (2001) *De kloof verkleinen.* Assen: Van Gorcum.

Subramanian, S.V., Kawachi, I., Kennedy, B.P. (2001). Does the state you live in make a difference? Multilevel analysis of self-rated health in the US. *Social Science and Medicine*, **53**, 9–19.

Thomson, H., Hoskins, R., Petticrew, M. *et al.* (2004) Evaluating the health effects of social interventions. *British Medical Journal*, **328**, 282–5.

Townsend, P., Davidson, N. (1992) The Black Report 1982. In *Inequalities in health: The Black Report and the health divide* (eds. Townsend, P., Whitehead, M., Davidson, N.), pp. 29–213. Penguin Books, London.

Whitehead, M. (1990) *The concepts and principles of equity and health.* World Health Organization, Copenhagen.

Whitehead, M. (1992) The Health Divide. In *Inequalities in health: The Black Report and the health divide* (eds. Townsend, P., Whitehead, M., Davidson, N.), pp. 215–450. Penguin Books, London.

Whitehead, M. (1998) Diffusion of ideas on social inequalities in health: a European perspective. *Millbank Quarterly*, **76**, 469–92.

Whitehead, M., Petticrew, M., Graham, H. *et al.* (2004) Evidence for public health policy on inequalities II: Assembling the evidence jigsaw. *Journal of Epidemiology and Community Health*, **58**, 817–21.

World Health Organization (1985) *Targets Health for All.* WHO, Copenhagen.

12.4

Reducing health inequalities in developing countries

Davidson R. Gwatkin

Abstract

This chapter provides a review of current thinking about health inequalities in developing countries and how to reduce them. The chapter initially discusses the relationship between three related indicators that describe distributional aspects of health status: The health of the poor, health inequality and health inequity. A concern for the health of poor flows from a broader concern for disadvantaged population groups. The definition of poverty may concern 'absolute poverty', with poverty defined in terms of a given level of income or consumption which is equally relevant for people wherever they may be. The concept of 'relative poverty' is more country-specific and attempts to define the poverty line in terms of relevance for a specific society. An alternative approach is to focus more on reducing inequalities, both in general and with respect to health in particular. Such a focus has traditionally occupied a particularly important place in thinking about international health issues and it is rare for a prominent international health statement not to give significant weight to inequality reduction. Poverty and inequality are both primarily empirical concepts. Equity, by contrast, is a normative concept, closely associated with the concept of social justice. One of the most widely cited definitions of health inequity is that it 'refers to differences in health which . . . are considered unfair and unjust'. At present, the greatest amount of attention in the overall economic development field is being paid to reducing absolute poverty, rather than to lessening relative poverty or decreasing inequality or inequity. This orientation is reflected most prominently in Millennium Development Goals (MDGs), a set of objectives that currently guide the strategy of most international and bilateral donor agencies. The second section of the chapter summarizes what is known about the dimensions and magnitude of health inequalities. The discussion focuses first on differences in life-expectancy and under-5 mortality between countries, and then describes variations in the distribution of health status and health service use within countries. The third section of the chapter presents a summary of current thought about how best to reduce inequalities and improve the health of the poor. This focuses on two, complementary issues. One is on reducing the social and economic inequalities that underlie the health inequalities described. The second is on reaching the poor more effectively with health and related services that are relevant to the principal health conditions from which they suffer. The chapter closes with a brief conclusion.

This is a review of current thinking about health inequalities in developing countries and how to reduce them. It is in three parts. The first is a discussion of the concept of health inequalities, and of the similarities and differences between other distributional concepts in current use. The second summarizes what is known about the dimensions and magnitude of health inequalities. The third presents a comparable summary of current thought about how best to reduce inequalities and improve the health of the poor. The review closes with a brief conclusion.

Concepts: The health of the poor, health inequality, health inequity

While the title of this chapter refers to health inequalities, it is important to recognize that such inequalities constitute only one of the several related indicators of interest to those dealing with the distributional aspects of health status and service use. Two others are health equity and the health of the poor.

These three indicators or concepts are similar in some ways, different in others. Those concerned with different ones of them all share a recognition that in health, as in many other fields, societal averages typically disguise as much as they reveal. Their interest is thus not in health conditions that prevail in society as a whole, but in the condition of different socioeconomic groups within society—especially in that of the lowest or most disadvantaged groups.

But within this shared concern lie a number of distinctions. Those interested with the health of the poor are typically concerned primarily with improving the health of that group alone, rather than with reducing differences between poor and rich. For those oriented towards equality, the principal objective is the reduction of poor–rich health differences. Those concerned with health inequities are concerned with righting the injustice represented by inequalities or poor health conditions among the disadvantaged.

These similarities and differences can most easily be understood by considering each the three indicators and concepts in turn, and then reviewing the practical implications of thinking in terms of one or the other:

The health of the poor

A concern for the health of poor flows from a broader concern of disadvantaged population groups that has occupied a central role in established thinking about overall socioeconomic development for over two decades. This concern emerged in the late 1960s and early 1970s in reaction to the then-dominant emphasis on countries' overall *per capita* income growth rates. At the time, a concern for distribution was thought likely to detract from the overall economic growth that was considered a necessary condition for the long-term alleviation of poverty. Concentrate first on overall growth, was the prevailing view. The result might be a rise in inequality over the short term. But, eventually, the benefits would trickle down to the poor and, over the long run, the poor would end up better off than under a development strategy oriented towards their immediate needs.

The 'trickle-up' and 'basic human needs' schools of thought, which emerged to counter the view just presented, advocated dealing directly with the poor as the best means of producing sustainable growth. The many discussions about how best to define the poor population groups of concern produced two approaches:

- *Absolute poverty*. The first, based on what is often called 'absolute poverty', takes a universal perspective and defines poverty in terms of a given level of income or consumption which is equally relevant for people wherever they may be. This is usually done by defining a 'poverty line' as the lowest amount of money sufficient to purchase the amount of food necessary for a minimally adequate diet (and still have enough left over to buy other essentials).
- *Relative poverty*. The second approach, more country-specific, deals with what is frequently referred to as 'relative poverty'. The practice here is to define the poverty line in terms of relevance for a specific society. This is typically done in one of three ways. One way, analogous to the international approach just described, is to determine how much income one needs to live decently according to some locally established definition of decency. The second approach is simply to define the national poverty line as some proportion—often arbitrarily determined—of a society's average per capita income or expenditure. The third is to define a certain percentage of a society's population, again usually arbitrarily established, as being poor.

Traditionally, advocates of absolute or relative approaches have both defined poverty in primarily in economic terms, with the poor seen as those suffering from inadequate incomes or purchasing power. However, the strictly materialistic view of this outlook has recently been increasingly challenged. Leading the charge has been the Nobel Laureate economist Amartya Sen, who has gained many adherents to his 'capabilities' approach, which defines poverty as a limited capability of an individual to realize his or her life aspiration (Sen 1999). Defined in this way, poverty becomes a much broader concept, since economic constraints constitute but one of the many obstacles that the poor must overcome. Other important ones include inadequate education, characteristics like race or religion that attract prejudice—and, of special interest for present purposes—poor health.

As of this writing, there is general agreement among those concerned with the health of the poor, and also with health inequalities as discussed in the next section, that poverty is a multi-dimensional phenomenon involving far more than economic status. There is less agreement on just which of poverty's many non-economic dimensions deserve highest priority, but many have been attracted to the dimensions included on what might be called 'the progress list'. In this case, 'progress' is an acronym, with each letter referring to a dimension of poverty thought to be important: Place of residence, religion, occupation, gender, religion, education, socio-economic status, and social capital (Evans & Brown 2002). Yet another approach might be called 'pure' health inequality—that is, the ordering of people on the basis of their health status, from most to least healthy regardless of income or any other attribute, for the purpose of measuring health diversity in a society (Gakidou *et al.* 2000).

Health inequality

An alternative approach is to focus more on reducing inequalities, both in general and with respect to health in particular. Such a focus has traditionally occupied a particularly important place in thinking about international health issues. To be sure, it is possible to cite expressions of concern for poverty in prominent international health documents from at least the time of the 1978 Declaration of Alma-Ata onwards. But it is rare for a prominent international health statement not to give at least equal, if not more, weight to inequality reduction. For example, at the same time as the Declaration of Alma-Ata professed its concern for the unacceptable health conditions found among the hundreds of millions among the world's poor, it also advocated primary health care because of its potential 'to close the gap between the "haves" and the "have-nots"', i.e. to lessen health inequalities (World Health Organization 1978). Similarly, health inequalities have played a central role in a long European tradition of concern. Thus, for instance, well-known 1980 Black Report in the United Kingdom was titled *Inequalities in health* (Department of Health and Social Security 1980), as was the exercise that produced its successor, the 1998 Acheson Report (Independent Inquiry 1998). In the same vein, the 1984 targets of the WHO Regional Office for Europe (EURO) were expressed in terms of reducing poor–rich disparities. 'By the year 2000', said the WHO document in which these targets were presented, 'the actual differences in health status between countries and between groups within countries should be reduced by at least 25 per cent, by improving the health of disadvantaged nations and groups' (Whitehead 1990).

However, just as there are different approaches to poverty alleviation, so too are there various views about the most appropriate strategies for the reduction of inequalities. One, referred to in the previous section, concerns which dimension of health inequalities—economic, gender, ethnic, health status or some other—deserve highest priority. Other issues include:

- *How inequality is to be measured*. There are almost as many statistical definitions of inequality as there are statisticians; and the different definitions can produce very different interpretations of the same situation or trend. This is particularly true of measures of relative and of absolute inequality (e.g. a relative measure like the ratio of some death rate in the highest group under review relative to the rate in the lowest rate, or an absolute measure like the difference between the two rates). The measure that is currently in widest use is a relative one known as the concentration index. As in the case of the Gini coefficient for income distribution from which it is derived, the value of the concentration index can range from –1.0 (if all infant or under-5 deaths, for instance, occur in the poorest population group to +1.0 (if all deaths are in the richest group) (Wagstaff *et al.* 1991).
- *What aspects of inequality are most important*. Some would argue for considering inequality in health status as the outcome that

counts, especially when poor health is seen as an important limitation to an individual's capability to realize his or her lifetime aspirations. Others favour focusing on health services, of any of several reasons. One is that health status can be determined by many factors, like diet and exercise practices, which are volitional; and thus, from a libertarian perspective, lie outside the realm of appropriate public policy. Another, more pragmatic reason for a health services focus is that health service access and coverage are the determinants of health status which health professionals can most easily influence.

Within each of these two streams of thought are further distinctions. Health status, for example, can be determined either through a physical examination or through self-assessment. (The two approaches can produce quite different results, in that people found to be relatively unhealthy through a physical examination do not always consider themselves to be less healthy than people whose health was determined by examination to be considerably better.) With respect to health services, there are distinctions between inequalities in service use and financing; among public, private non-profit and private for-profit services; and between preventive and curative services. People who come out ahead in one of these dimensions may lag from another perspective.

- *Whether the focus should be local or global.* A great deal of media and policy attention has been given to global inequalities, especially between wealthy regions like Western Europe and North America and particularly poor ones like sub-Saharan Africa, As will be discussed further below, this global outlook has recently been supplemented by the concern for inequalities among groups within countries that constitutes the principal focus of this review.

Health equity

Poverty and inequality, as described above, are both primarily empirical concepts. Equity, by contrast, is a normative one—a question of values, and closely associated with the concept of social justice. When applied to health, equity has traditionally been most often linked to the reduction of inequalities. Thus, one of the most widely cited definitions of health inequity is that it 'refers to differences in health which . . . are considered unfair and unjust'. In a similar vein, the above-cited WHO/EURO document on health equity indicated that 'equity requires reducing unfair disparities . . .' and that 'pursuing equity in health and health care development means trying to reduce unfair and unnecessary social gaps in health and health care . . .' (Whitehead 1990).

However, equity need not be exclusively a matter of reducing inequalities. It can also be associated with poverty, since one could argue that it is unjust to allow people to continue living in poverty when adequate resources are available within the society at large to lift them out of it. A particularly well-known example of poverty-oriented general thought about equity is the 'maximin' principle of distributive justice posited by John Rawls. That principle and others like it call for resources to be distributed in a way that the worst-off people in society (i.e. those occupying the 'minimum' position) get the maximum possible amount of gain. What happens to the better-off through such a pattern of resource distribution is extraneous to the maximin principle (Rawls 1971).

While not many equality-oriented advocates of health equity seem prepared to go this far, almost all incorporate at least traces of such a poverty-oriented equity definition in their statements. The traces are to be seen most clearly in the tendency of equality-oriented discussions to disavow interest in one of the arguably more effective potential ways of reducing poor–rich health inequalities: Elimination of the rich. Rather, the focus of all known inequality-oriented health equity proposals is on lessening poor–rich differences through special efforts to improve the health of the poor.

However, regardless of whether one considers health equity to be related more to equality or poverty, the introduction of normative or social justice considerations also raises questions. For example:

- *When is an inequality unfair?* Not always, certainly. It is quite possible to imagine a situation marked by health inequalities that are not necessarily inequitable. One example is an inequality that is irremediable (Whitehead 1990). Another might be two population groups with similar incomes but marked differences in life expectancy attributable to different lifestyles. If the less healthy group adopts its lifestyle in full awareness of the risks involved, the resulting differences in life expectancy might be said to be simply a reflection of differences in the social preferences of the two groups, rather than any fundamental inequity. Or, to illustrate the same point by a more general example: If two individuals are in fact unequal in capacity, equal treatment would be unfair to the more capable of the two. In such a case, equity might well call for unequal treatment. In other words, equity and equality are by no means synonymous and need to be carefully distinguished from one another.
- *On what basis can one decide when the resources in a society are adequate to alleviate poverty?* 'Adequacy' is not a binary concept, such that there is one level of resource availability above which availability is totally adequate, and below which it is completely inadequate. Rather, there is a spectrum running from a total lack to infinite availability of resources, often with no obvious cut-off point along the way. Also, perceptions can differ: Resources that seem adequate to one person may not be so to another.

The policy and programme implications of the poverty-inequality-equity distinction

At present, the greatest amount of attention in the overall economic development field is being paid to reducing absolute poverty, rather than to lessening relative poverty or decreasing inequality or inequity. This orientation is reflected most prominently in MDGs, a set of objectives that currently guides the strategy of most, possibly all, international and bilateral donor agencies. The MDGs, which are contained in a declaration adopted unanimously in September 2000 by members of the United Nations drew together and enlarged a set of development objectives that had been agreed to during a set of global conferences over the preceding decade. As subsequently published (http://www.un.org/millenniumgoals/; http://www.undp.org/mdg/basics.shtml), they consist of eight specific aims. The overall tone of the MDGs is set by the by the first and most prominent of the eight is 'to eradicate extreme poverty and hunger'. This goal is accompanied by two targets that are unambiguously stated in terms of absolute poverty reduction. They are to halve, by 2015, the proportion of people with daily incomes of less that US$1.00, and suffering from hunger in 1990.

The three of the eight goals devoted explicitly with health are rather more ambiguously framed, in that all refer to improvements in national averages, without reference to how these improvements are to be distributed across groups within the nations concerned.

Goal four, on reducing child mortality, calls for reducing the under-5 mortality rate by two-thirds; goal five, to improve maternal mortality, sets a target of a three-quarters decline in the maternal mortality ration; goal six, on combating HIV/AIDS, malaria, and other diseases, says simply that the spread and incidence of these diseases should be halted and reversed.

While the ambiguity of these health goals leaves room for different interpretations, their association with goal one's unambiguous focus on the alleviation of absolute poverty implies at least to some degree that they, too, share this orientation. To the extent this is the case, they display less concern for lessening relative poverty, intergroup inequalities, or inequity than for improving the health of the people below the US$1.00 per day, who numbered just under one billion in 2004, representing around 18 per cent of the developing world's population in that year (World Bank 2007).

Whether the (apparent) adoption of this absolute poverty approach rather than some other has significant programme or policy approaches is a matter of debate. On the one hand, as has been noted, even those who seem furthest apart—those giving highest priority to reductions in poor–rich health inequalities in the name of equity, and those concerned with improving the health of the absolute poor—end up sounding rather similar once one realizes that the approach preferred by advocates of inequality reduction looks primarily to improvements in the health of the disadvantaged.

This is the approach taken in this article: Namely, that the most legitimate approach to reducing health inequalities is through improving the health of the poor, making the three terms close to synonymous In practice. However, it should be noted that there are at least some circumstances where an interest in improving the health of the poor can imply a different approach from that resulting from a concern for inequality reduction. An example concerns inter-regional resource allocations by international agencies:

- *An absolute poverty approach.* According to the World Bank figures cited earlier, nearly 80 per cent of the world's people living below the poverty line are in Asia and Africa (World Bank 2007). This being the case, an international agency guided by an absolute poverty objective would wish to put virtually all of its health resources into those regions. There would be much less justification for working in Latin America; and practically none at all for health activity in the Middle East or in Eastern Europe, where hardly anyone is so poor as to lie below the international poverty line.
- *A relative poverty approach.* Relative poverty exists in every country. From this perspective, there could thus be as strong a justification for supporting pro-poor health activities in one region of the world as in any other.
- *An equality approach.* Assuming that most of the existing health inequalities observed in the developing world are also inequitable and that inequality reduction interventions are equally effective, an equity approach would imply a particularly high priority to countries where health inequalities are greatest. Recent research points to the existence of large country-to-country differences in the degree of health inequality, which in turn suggests that some countries deserve much more attention than others from an equity perspective. According to the data presented in one recent review (Gwatkin *et al.* 2007a), intra-country economic inequalities in health (with regard to under-5 mortality) are highest in East Asia and the Pacific, and in Latin America so that these regions would deserve highest priority according to an equality criterion. Countries in sub-Saharan Africa, where intra-country economic inequalities in health are lower, would receive less attention.

Evidence: The dimensions of the problem

Since space limitations prevent adequate coverage of the full range of health inequalities that might be considered, the discussion deals primarily, albeit not exclusively, on inequalities by economic status. It first covers global inequalities: Inequalities among regions and countries. It then turns to inequalities within countries.

A global perspective

To begin with what is perhaps obvious, the health of people in low-income regions is quite poor, much worse than in better-off countries. The situation is particularly deficient in sub-Saharan Africa.

Table 12.4.1 presents summary figures, drawn from the World Bank's *World Development Indicators*. In 2005, the latest year for which data are available:

- Life expectancy at birth in the low-income countries was around 59 years, 20 years or 25 per cent lower than the 79 years recorded in high-income countries. The worst conditions were in sub-Saharan Africa, where life expectance was only 47 years, more than ten years (20 per cent) below the low-income country average, more than thirty years (40 per cent) under the high-income country average.
- Under-5 mortality rates show the same pattern. In the low-income countries, 114 of all children born could be expected to die during the first 5 years of her or his life. This is nearly 100 (over 15 times) more than the seven who would die in the high-income countries. In sub-Saharan Africa, the 163 deaths would be almost 50 (30 per cent) higher than in the typical low-income country, over 150 (more than 23 times) above the average high-income one.

A comparison between the Table 12.4.1 figures for 2005 and 1980 provides an idea of how much the situation has changed in the past quarter-century. In brief:

- Life expectancy has improved significantly in almost all areas, rich and poor. But there are two exceptions: Eastern Europe, where the increase has been only one year, and in sub-Saharan Africa, where there has been a 1-year decline.
- Under-5 mortality has decreased in every region with available data, but the size of the increase has varied widely. Measured in absolute terms, the decrease has been largest in South Asia (97 deaths per thousand live births), lowest in the high-income countries (eight deaths per thousand live births). The percentage changes show quite a different picture, with under-5 mortality declining on the order of 50–60 per cent in all areas except sub-Saharan Africa, where a reduction of less than 15 per cent was recorded.

Any effort to summarize these trends is difficult, since the outcome varies widely with the trend and mortality measure used. All in all, however, it seems reasonable to conclude that overall conditions have improved significantly in most areas of the world, especially the middle-income countries. The major exceptions have been sub-Saharan Africa, which as clearly lagged behind the other regions; and Eastern Europe and Central Asia, where conditions appear to be improving only slowly at best.

Table 12.4.1 Global disparities in life expectancy at birth and in under-5 mortality, 1980 and 2005

Region	Life expectancy at birth (years)				Under-5 mortality (per 1000)			
	Levels in 1980, 2005		1980–2005 change		Levels in 1980, 2005		1980–2005 change	
	1980	2005	Absolute	Percentage	1980	2005	Absolute	Percentage
Low-income countries	53	59	+6	+11.3	177	114	−63	−35.6
Mid-income countries	60	70	+10	+16.7	79	37	−42	−53.2
High-income countries	74	79	+5	+6.8	15	7	−8	−53.3
East Asia, Pacific	65	71	+6	+9.2	82	33	−49	−59.8
East Europe, Central Asia	68	69	+1	+1.5	NA	32	NA	NA
Latin America, Caribbean	65	72	+7	+10.8	80	31	−49	−61.3
Middle East, North Africa	59	70	+11	+18.6	136	53	−83	−61.0
South Asia	54	63	+9	+16.7	180	83	−97	−53.9
Sub-Saharan Africa	48	47	−1	−2.1	189	163	−26	−13.8
High-income countries	74	79	+5	+6.8	15	7	−8	−53.3
World	63	68	+5	+7.9	123	75	−48	−39.0

Source: World Bank 2001, 2007

A country perspective

A concern for conditions among disadvantaged groups within developing countries is more recent than the attention given to the global situation outlined in the preceding section. To at least some degree, this resulted from the absence of standardized, comparable data that lent itself to easy review. However, this situation has changed greatly over the past few years, as international organizations have begun to provide increasing amounts of distributional information in the reports issued from comparable, multi-country household survey programmes that they have sponsored. The most readily available of these tables appear in programmes sponsored by the Demographic and Health Survey (DHS) Program, the World Bank in cooperation with the DHS Program, UNICEF, and the World Health Organization. Each has its strengths and limitations. To describe each briefly for the benefit of readers wishing to explore health equity issues more fully than is possible on the basis of information here:

- The DHS Program has conducted similar household surveys, focused on fertility and maternal/child health, in some 75 poor and middle-income countries. In many countries, there have been multiple surveys at different points in time. Many of the core tables in each country survey report (available at www.measuredhs.com/countries) have included data disaggregated according to such dimensions of poverty or inequality as gender, place of residence, and educational level. Since 2003, many tables have also provided information according to economic status.
- The World Bank, in cooperation with the DHS Program secretariat, has recently prepared a set of 56 country health and poverty reports based on information from 95 DHS surveys undertaken between 1990 and 2005. (Gwatkin *et al.* 2007a). While the reports contain information disaggregated by gender and place of residence, the principal focus is on economic disparities.
- UNICEF has sponsored a set of Multiple-Indicator Cluster (household) Surveys (MICS), which are generally similar to the DHS programme but cover a somewhat different set of countries and indicators. (Available at: www.childinfo.org/mics.) Like the DHS reports, those produced by MICS include data disaggregated by several dimensions of poverty.
- In 2002, the World Health Organization organized a World Health Survey, a set of comparable household surveys undertaken in some seventy developed and developing countries. (Available at www.who.int/healthinfo/survey/en/index.html.) These cover a considerably broader range of indicators than the mother/child-focused DHS and MICS: Self-assessed adult health status, for example; interventions against adult chronic diseases; household health expenditures; etc.

A flavour of what the massive amount of data available from these sources show can be gained from the contents of Table 12.4.2, based on DHS data. The figures presented there refer to the unweighted country averages for each of nine illustrative indicators, from as many of the 56 countries as had data available (ranging in number from 49 to 56). The average date of the surveys producing the data was around 2000. Among other things, they suggest that, overall:

- Economically disadvantaged groups are notably worse off with respect to almost all indicators of health status and health service use, and also with respect to almost underlying factors. For instance under-5 mortality and fertility in the lowest 20 per cent of the population is nearly twice as high as in the highest 20 per cent (135.4 vs. 73.5 for infant/child mortality, 5.7 vs. 3.0 for fertility); almost three times as high for severe malnutrition (18.0 per cent vs. 6.2 per cent). Coverage of basic health services is 50–200 per cent higher among the population's top 20 per cent as in its lowest 20 per cent, with attended deliveries being particularly skewed

Table 12.4.2 Distribution of health status, health service use in 56 low-and middle-income countries, ca. 2000

	Economic		Place of residence		Gender	
	Lowest 20%	**Highest 20%**	**Rural**	**Urban**	**Females**	**Males**
Health status						
Infant/child mortality	135.4	73.5	125.9	89.3	109.8	120.5
Severe malnutrition	18.0	6.2	15.0	8.6	12.6	13.5
Fertility	5.7	3.0	5.1	3.5	NA	NA
Health service use						
Immunization	40.7	64.0	46.6	59.3	50.9	50.7
Attended delivery	35.8	85.0	44.6	78.1	NA	NA
Contraceptive use	17.6	36.4	23.8	35.7	28.7	23.5
Underlying factors						
Breastfeeding	38.4	32.9	37.2	35.2	NA	NA
School completion	37.8	8.15	49.2	74.2	53.7	64.6
HIV/AIDS knowledge	64.3	88.2	69.9	83.3	69.7	83.9

Source: Gwatkin *et al.* 2007a. *Definitions:* Under-5 mortality for infant/child mortality (per 1000); third-degree stunting for severe malnutrition (%); total fertility rate for fertility (births/woman); full basic coverage for immunization (%); attendance by any medically trained person for attended deliveries (%); use of any modern contraceptive method for contraceptive use (%); exclusive breastfeeding up to six months for Breastfeeding (%); completion of five or more years of education for school completion (%); knowledge that HIV/AIDS is sexually transmitted for HIV/AIDS knowledge (%).

Note: Figures are unweighted averages for 49–56 low- and middle-income countries according to the indicator presented.

toward the best off. The only exception is breastfeeding, generally considered an important health-promoting behaviour, which tends to be somewhat higher in low economic groups.

- Rural-urban differences tend to parallel economic differences, presumably because of the fairly close relationship between place of residence and prevalence of economic poverty.
- Gender differences are quite mixed. For some indicators, there appears to be little difference among females and males, albeit with possibly higher rates among males. Examples include infant/child mortality (109.8 females, 120.5 males), severe malnutrition (12.6 per cent females, 13.5 per cent males), and immunization (50.9 per cent females, 50.7 per cent males). In some other respects, however, women seem clearly worse-off than males. School completion (53.7 per cent females, 64.7 per cent males) and HIV/AIDS knowledge (69.7 per cent females, 83.9 per cent males) are illustrations. There are yet other indicators where women seem to do better than men—as in contraceptive use (28.7 per cent female, 23.5 per cent male).

Averages, however, tell only part of the story, since there are large variations among regions and countries with respect to inequalities. A noteworthy example concerns female–male disparities with respect to infant/child mortality. Male infant/child mortality is higher than female in 50 of the countries covered; but it is lower is six. One of those six is India, which has one of the largest disparities in favour of males (female, 105.1; male 97.8). Since India is by far the most populous of the countries covered, an average figure weighted for population size—rather than unweighted as shown in Table 12.4.2—would probably show female mortality to be higher than male.

Further information on health services indicate clearly that government services, while less regressive on average that private services, almost always deliver more benefits to the better-off than to the poor. This can be seen from Table 12.4.3, which indicates the amount of subsidy from government health expenditures accruing to the lowest and highest 20 per cent of the population in 21 countries (or large areas within countries). The highest 20 per cent of the population gained on average over 25 per cent of total financial subsidies provided through government health expenditures, compared with just over 15 per cent in the lowest 20 per cent of the population. Only four of these countries—all in Latin America—show a progressive pattern of subsidies through government services. But, in that region, government-provided services are usually accompanied by a large, highly regressive, government-sponsored social security system that provides services to formal sector employees and their families.

Benefits from government primary care expenditures seem much less inequitably distributed than those from total government health expenditures, with only about 20 per cent of primary care benefits going to the highest 20 per cent of the population, compared with 19 per cent of benefits going to the population's lowest 20 per cent. This is line with data for attended deliveries from the World Bank–DHS data exercise referred to above (but not presented here), strongly suggesting that coverage of lower-level services tends to notably less inequitable than that of higher-level ones.

The record with regards to trends in this pattern of intra-country inequalities has been limited largely to changes in economic disparities with regard to under-5 mortality. A notable exception has been the study of gender inequalities of infant and child mortality in Bangladesh, which shows a sharp decline in differences between boys and girls, which had disappeared by 2004 (Gwatkin *et al.* 2007b). The two known studies of this issue suggest that the picture has been mixed at best. This is the general conclusion from

Table 12.4.3 Subsidies from government health services accruing to top and bottom 20 per cent of a country/region's population

Subsidy from	Percentage of total subsidy to		Number of countries/regions where subsidy to bottom 20% of population is		
	Bottom 20% of population	Top 20% of population	Less than subsidy to top 20%	Same as subsidy to top 20%	More than subsidy to top 20%
All health expenditures	15.9%	26.4%	15	2	4
Primary health care expenditures only	18.8%	19.7%	12	0	9

Source: Filmer (2004).

a review, based on DHS data from the World Bank–DHS exercise. It found that among the 13 countries with a trend of decline in overall mortality, relative disparities had declined in only four, and had increased in five (Moser *et al.* 2005). The other study, by UNICEF researchers, relied on separate tabulations of DHS data. In the 24 countries covered, differentials were reduced in two, remained constant in a few others, but worsened in the majority (Minujin & Delamonica 2003).

The significance of these intra-country inequalities can be seen by considering the degree to which the total global health gap, in terms of potentially avoidable mortality, can be reduced by alleviating them. Around the year 2000, the global gap in child mortality stood at around 5 000 000 deaths, in the sense this is the number of deaths among infants and children under 5 years in the 56 countries covered by the World Bank–DHS exercise that would be eliminated by reducing mortality in those countries to the levels currently enjoyed in high-income societies. If instead, mortality levels in all economic groups within those 56 countries were reduced to the levels then experienced by the economically top 10 per cent in those same countries, slightly over 3 000 000 child deaths—representing about 60 per cent of the total global gap—would be averted. The crude nature of such estimates argues against drawing too firm a conclusion from them, but they are sufficient to suggest that intra-country disparities contribute at least as much to global health inequality as do differences among countries (Gwatkin 2007).

Evidence: Ways of remedying the problem

Current thought about how to reduce the inequalities discussed in the preceding sections focuses on two, complementary issues. One is on reducing the social and economic inequalities that underlie the health inequalities just described. The second is on reaching the poor more effectively with health and related services that are relevant to the principal health conditions from which they suffer.

Social and economic approaches

The rationale behind focusing on social and economic approaches is two-fold. The first is that social and economic improvement is in itself an important end—arguably the most important end—of development. From this perspective, while reducing health disparities between, say, economic groups is well worth doing, if one leaves the pre-existing economic inequalities unchanged, then the accomplishment is far smaller than achieving the broader goal of reducing both health and economic disparities. The second element of the rationale is based on the argument that social and economic inequalities are the principal causes of health disparities, and only by tackling those underlying inequalities can one make significant progress toward reducing disparities in health.

Current efforts to reduce health inequalities through social and economic approaches can best be illustrated with reference to two active initiatives. One is the drive to achieve the MDGs, referred to earlier. The second is the work of a WHO Commission on the Social Determinants of Health (CSDH).

As noted previously, the MDGs consist of a set of development objectives adopted by the United Nations in 2000 that deal with a wide range issues related to human well-being: Income, hunger, education, health and others. While some of the indicators for progress toward the health MDGs refer to the coverage of health services (such as measles immunizations for reducing infant mortality and attended deliveries for improving maternal health), the goals themselves are stated in terms of health outcomes like mortality and disease prevalence levels that are influenced by far more than health services alone. Furthermore, the MDG health components are but one part of a broad, multi-pronged approach to development that focuses primarily on many other dimensions of economic and social improvement that affect health conditions.

The CSDH is a group of prominent international health professionals that began its 3-year programme of work in March 2005. The vision guiding this programme, as stated in the Commission's recent interim statement, is that 'strengthening health equity . . . means going beyond contemporary concentration on the immediate causes of disease . . . [and focusing on] the "causes of the causes"—the fundamental structures of socially determined conditions these structures crate in which people grow, live, and age—the social determinants of health'. (http://www.who.int/social_determinants/resources/ interim_statement/en/index.html) The Commission's principal aim is 'to set solid foundations for its vision: The societal relations and factors that influence health and health systems will be visible, understood and recognized as important . . . Success will be achieved if institutions working in health . . . will be using this knowledge to set and implement relevant public policy affecting health' (Marmot 2005).

At the heart of this work is the idea of a 'social gradient' in health, whereby health outcomes become worse as one descends the socio-economic ladder. This means that not only do the poor have worse health than the rich, but the middle classes have worse health than the rich as well. While this is itself far from startling, the idea incorporates two other points that are much less intuitively obvious and that greatly increase its significance. One is the finding that these gradients exist not just in poor countries, but also in better-off ones where living conditions among even the lowest groups studied are far above any meaningful absolute poverty line. From this, it is pretty clear that there are causes of ill health that lie well outside the nexus of poor nutrition, inadequate education, unfavourable environmental surroundings, and the like that is normally blamed for particularly high rates of illness and death among the poor. The second is the identification of psychological factors—degree of control over one's work environment, for example—that appear to be responsible for these high rates, and the delineation of the biological channels through which such psychological and other factors work.

Such findings lead toward an emphasis on social and economic policies, more than on health services, as the most promising approaches to the reduction of socioeconomic health inequalities. One of the several examples that could be cited involves unemployment, which has been shown to affect health not only through loss of income, but also through the anxiety that it causes. Government moves to smooth the business cycle, and to ensure reasonable unemployment benefits illustrate ways of countering ill health and the other effects of this factor. Another illustration concerns transport, where government policies focusing on cycling, walking and the use of public transport can promote health by providing exercise, reducing fatal accidents, increasing social contact, and reducing air pollution (Wilkinson & Marmot 2003).

Thus far, most work on the social gradients of health has dealt with Northern, developed countries, particularly in Europe. If the Commission is successful, the same approach will be applied increasingly to health equity research and policy development in middle and lower income countries over the years ahead.

Health service approaches

For some, the case for reforming health services in order to reduce disparities rests on the view that the equal availability of social services is a desirable equity end in itself, regardless of how important or unimportant those services may be for reaching some other desired objective like improved health services. Recently, however, this rationale is becoming less common, and is being replaced by three others. All three acknowledge that improved health status is the desired end; that health service coverage constitutes only one of the many means to that end; and that its contribution to improved health status improvement may well be considerably less than that of broader social and economic progress. The first of the three rationales is that while health service coverage may well be a relatively minor contributor to better health, it is easier to influence than overall social and economic development. This is not to argue that even health service coverage and universal access are easy to achieve, just that it is not so difficult as the truly Herculean efforts require to increase, say, the incomes of poor people. Thus, when judged from a cost-benefit perspective, expanding health service coverage among the poor might compare quite favourably with other, social or economic approaches that might be considered. The second, closely related rationale is that with nearly US$400 billion being spent each year on health services in low- and middle-income countries, the sector is large and important enough to justify an effort to ensure that funds allocated to it are equitably spent as one component of an overall drive to improve health equity. The third rationale, also closely related to the other two, is that health professionals have a far greater expertise in the health sector than in the other sectors related to social and economic development. Thus, while they no doubt have a potentially valuable supporting role to play in advocating and initiating change in these other sectors, the most direct contribution they can make is with respect to the health services whose provision they dominate. Some would add a moral dimension to this rationale, arguing that the first responsibility of health professionals to get their own house in order, before they try telling people in other sectors what they should be doing.

Among those working to improve health service coverage among the poor, there are two schools of thought about how to proceed. One would emphasize focusing on a few services of particular importance of health for the poor—basic immunization and attended deliveries, for example—and working to achieve universal coverage with respect to them. That is, the objective is to achieve 100 per cent coverage among all groups, better-off as well as poor. The other school prefers more targeted approaches—approaches that seek to identify the poor through one of the many methods described below—and focus on delivering services to them.

In cases where achievement of universal coverage can be realistically expected within an acceptably short period of time, the universal coverage approach would probably be generally accepted as the one of choice. When universal coverage is achieved, it provides 100 per cent coverage for the poor; and it is inherently egalitarian, in that the poor receive the same type and quality of the services concerned as do the better-off. This avoids the potential stigma, as well as the possibility of lower-quality services, that are present when special programmes are developed for disadvantaged groups. It also has the advantage of simplicity, in that it obviates the need for often-difficult and expensive mechanisms required to identify the poor and ensure that they are the ones who receive services. Also, when starting from a base of high initial overall coverage, a universal coverage approach is inherently targeted, in the sense that those not already covered are likely to be concentrated in disadvantaged groups.

There are a number of cases where universal care strategies can be shown to have largely achieved their objectives. Examples include the poor republics of the former Soviet Union, which have achieved high immunization coverage rates that are close to equal across economic classes, and even higher and well-distributed delivery attendance. Even here, however, there are notable class differences by type of delivery attendance with most deliveries in lower income groups handled by nurses or midwives, and most upper-income deliveries attended by doctors (Gwatkin *et al.* 2007a). Several Asian countries/areas with universal care strategies—Hong Kong, Malaysia, Sri Lanka, Thailand—have achieved government health service expenditure patterns that provides larger subsidies to the lowest than to the highest economic groups (O'Donnell *et al.* 2005).

The advantages of universal care strategies become considerably less obvious in settings where initial overall coverage is low, and where the prospects for achieving universal service availability in the foreseeable future are limited. Here, large numbers of people at all levels remain unserved. In such a situation is possible and tempting to increase national average rates by serving first the better-off uncovered groups, which are often the easiest to reach, and deferring expansion of coverage to the poor until some later stage of programme development. In the least unfavourable scenario, coverage of the poor can be delayed for an extended period marked by increased inequality as coverage rises among the better-off. In cases where the drive for coverage expansion slows or stalls before the achievement of universality, then this situation of heightened inequality could be extended indefinitely.

In these and other settings, an alternative is to use some 'targeted' approach. The expression 'targeting' refers to a set of techniques used to increase the percentage of benefits from a particular intervention that flow to the poor. There are many different targeting techniques available, and many ways of categorizing them. One of the more common categorization approaches features a distinction between 'individual', 'direct', or 'narrow' targeting on the one hand; and 'indicator/characteristic', 'indirect', or 'broad' targeting on the other.

The former type refers to efforts to identify poor individuals and see that as much of the service concerned reaches as many of them as possible. The objective is come as close as possible to the goal of 100 per cent coverage with 0 per cent leakage—that is, the goal of seeing that all of the poor are served and that all of those served are poor. The latter type of targeting deals with attributes rather than individuals. Rather than trying to identify individuals who are poor, for instance, it might feature the provision of services in slum areas in anticipation that the great majority of recipients will be poor. In doing so, it recognizes that it will not be able to reach all of the poor (some of whom live outside slums), and that at least some of those receiving services will not be poor (since not everyone living in a poor area is her/himself poor). But it accepts these limitations as prices worth paying in order to attain two important advantages. One is administrative practicality or efficiency, through avoidance of the considerable effort typically required to distinguish between poor and non-poor individuals with even a modest degree of precision. The second is political: The belief that poverty-oriented service programmes are much more likely to gain the political support needed for survival if members of the middle and upper classes gain enough from them to have an incentive to defend their continuation.

There are many specific targeting techniques available, each with unique features, strengths, and weakness. Three can serve to illustrate the different options. The three are individual targeting, and two forms of categorical targeting: Geographic and disease/age:

- *Individual targeting*. Recently, a great deal of attention has been given to the identification of poor individuals in order to exempt them from users' fees introduced in developing country government health facilities during health sector reforms. This is done with varying degrees of formality. At one end of the spectrum is the highly statistical 'proxy means test'. Under this approach, household possessions are taken as a proxy for income or consumption, the preferred measures of economic status; households are surveyed to determine what their residents possess; the results are amalgamated into a single index, using various statistical techniques to weight the different possessions; households are scored on the basis of this index; and those receiving below some specified score are deemed eligible for benefits. At the spectrum's other, least formal end are participatory approaches that leave it largely to village residents to determine what household characteristics best characterize poverty, and which households are poorest in terms of those characteristics.
- *Geographic targeting*. The idea behind geographic targeting is straightforward: The poorer the area to which resources are allocated, the greater the likelihood that the individuals who benefit from those resources will be poor. Geographic targeting can be applied with widely varying degrees of precision. Perhaps the simplest, least precise form of geographic targeting is the emphasis often placed on rural areas, where the available information about suggests that poverty is in general considerably more prevalent than it is in the cities. Other, more precise forms of targeting involve a focus on poor states or provinces, or subdivisions within each. Typically, these are identified on the basis of data for per capita income or output produced by government statistical offices. Several countries, particularly in Latin America, have sought to be even more precise by using census data on things like house construction and educational levels to identify villages or other small communities that are especially poor. Recently, there has been experimentation with techniques to for identifying small areas on the basis of measures more obviously and directly related to consumption, traditionally the indicator preferred by economists concerned with poverty. The techniques concerned involve combining data from in-depth sample surveys, which ask many questions from a relatively small number of households, and from national censuses, which ask a few questions about all the households in a country. The basic idea is to identify those questions on the household survey instruments that: (1) are also included in the national census; and (2) best predict the consumption levels of the households covered. Then, average values for the questions thus identified can be calculated for individual villages covered by the census data in order to predict the average consumption levels prevailing in those villages; and the poorest villages can be selected on this basis. The amount of improved accuracy resulting from such increases in precision will depend upon the spatial distribution of poverty in the society concerned.
- *Targeting by disease and age*. While the poor generally suffer more at all ages and from all diseases than the better-off, the gaps tend to be considerably larger among young people suffering from communicable diseases. Also, because fertility is much higher among the poor, children tend to cluster in lower-income groups. For reasons like these, poverty-oriented health service programmes often focus on them through agencies like UNICEF and drives to deal with malaria, diarrhoea, immunization-preventable diseases, and acute respiratory infections. (However, as seen in the immunization figures of Table 12.4.2, many of the programmes that employ disease/age targeting end up achieving much lower coverage among the poor than among the better-off, indicating that this type of targeting alone is not necessarily sufficient to reach the poor children who suffer from the communicable diseases in question.)

These different targeting methods are not mutually exclusive and are often used in combination. Nor are they specific to health: They are also widely employed in determining the provision of other social services and benefits, and in public works programmes. There is no known instance of their achieving or even approaching perfection, when perfection is defined is full coverage of the poor, and all programme benefits flowing to them. However, there is considerable evidence that they often significantly increase the percentage of programme benefits flowing to disadvantaged groups.

A recent review of over 120 projects dealing with a wide range of development issues in nearly 50 low- and middle-income countries

(Coady *et al.* 2004) found that, on average, targeted programmes transferred around 25 per cent more to poor beneficiaries than they would have received under universal allocation. However, the range of experiences was wide, with a quarter of the interventions delivering more to the better-off. Some methods—proxy means testing and geographic means testing—seemed to work better than others. But the range of outcomes within each of the particular targeting approaches covered was very wide, suggesting that implementation effectiveness was more important in achieving success than was the targeting method selected.

Further evidence, specific to health, comes from a recent World Bank effort to identify programmes with reliable evidence concerning their record in reaching economically poor population groups (World Bank 2005). Of the 27 programmes it found, two-thirds delivered more than 20 per cent of their benefits to the population's poorest 20 per cent; in nearly a quarter of these cases, more than 40 per cent of the programme benefits went to the poorest quintile. Over half of these programmes also achieved coverage rates of over 50 per cent in the areas where they operated.

Illustrations of these programmes include:

- *Mexico's 'Progresa/Opportunidades' initiative* that pays rather than charges poor families for clinic and school attendance. The programme serves of 20 million people, and provides 20 per cent of the income to participating families. Almost 60 per cent of the people reached belong to the poorest 20 per cent of Mexico's population; 80 per cent of beneficiaries are in the poorest 40 per cent.
- *Colombia's use of a refined individual targeting technique* to provide subsidized health insurance to the disadvantaged. This raised insurance coverage in the poorest quintile of the population from well under 10 per cent in the early 1990s to nearly 50 per cent four years later. 35 per cent of the total programme subsidy went to the poorest 20 per cent of the population; 65 per cent to the poorest 40 per cent.
- *Cambodia's experiment in contracting with non-governmental organizations* to operate governmental rural primary health services, under contracts calling for attainment of specified coverage levels among the poor. During a 4-year experiment, the coverage among the poorest 20 per cent of the population of eight basic services rose from an average of below 15 per cent to over 40 per cent in two experimental districts with a total population of around 200 000. This increase was nearly two and one-half times as large as that experienced in two control districts that continued to receive standard government services.
- *Distribution of insecticide-treated bednets through measles immunization campaigns in Ghana and Zambia*. In Ghana, the Red Cross and the Government Health Service raised, from 3 per cent to nearly 60 per cent, the rate of treated bednet use among children in the poorest 20 per cent of people in a Northern district with a population of around 90 000. A similar programme in Zambia produced comparable results: An increase in ITN coverage from 18 per cent to 82 per cent in the poorest 20 per cent of the population in five rural districts with a total population of 450 000.
- *Marketing of insecticide-treated bednets in Tanzania*. In two southern districts, with a total population of about 60 000, the Ifakara Health Research and Development Centre developed and implemented a social marketing programme that raised the ownership of bednets in the poorest 20 per cent of households from 20 per cent to 73 per cent. As in Ghana and Zambia, the increase in bednet use/ownership was higher among the poor than among the better-off.

As can be seen, the range of techniques featured in the apparently successful projects and programmes was wide (and included techniques that are believed not to have worked very well in other settings). Among the techniques were: Improved means of identifying poor individuals (Colombia, Mexico), cash payments for use of services (Mexico); services provided by NGOs working under contracts with carefully specified pro-poor performance indicators (Cambodia); mass campaigns (Ghana, Zambia); and social marketing (Tanzania). This is in line with the Coady-Grosh-Hoddinot finding reported above that differences in the effectiveness with which targeted programmes are administered, and in the care with which programme designs are fitted to the settings where they operate, are more important than the type of targeting approach used in determining success.

Conclusion

The conventional way to end a review of this kind is with a statement that further research is needed. Such a conclusion would no doubt be as valid with respect to health inequalities as with any of the other topics covered in this volume. Yet in the case of health inequalities, it would be difficult to argue that the need for further research is the highest priority. For, while much remains to be determined, a great deal is already understood, both about the magnitude and principal features of the problem that inequalities represent, and about approaches that can be taken to reduce them. As a result, much more is known than is being acted upon, and the principal constraints to progress are the many factors that prevent the translation of research findings into effective actions. Principal among these factors are the political ones that explain how societies determine which issues deserve their greatest attention. In other words: Political will.

References

Coady, D., Grosh, M., and Hoddinot, J. (2004). *Targeting of transfers in developing countries: review of lessons and experience*. World Bank: Washington.

Evans, T. and Brown, H. (2002). *Opportunities for action: applying an equity lens to global health initiatives*. Presentation at the National Press Club, Washington.

Evans, T. and Brown, H. (2002). *Applying an equity lens to the safe motherhood initiative*. Presentation to the Safe Motherhood Interagency Group, London.

Filmer, D. (2004). *The incidence of public expenditures in health and education*. Available at http://econ.worldbank.org/wdr/wdr2004/library/doc?id=29478.

Gakidou, E., Murray, C., and Frenk, J. (2000). Defining and measuring health inequality: an approach based on the distribution of health expectancy. *Bulletin of the World Health Organization*, **78**, 42–54.

Gwatkin, D., Rutstein, S., Johnson K. *et al.*(2007a). *Socio-economic differences in health, nutrition, and population within developing countries*. World Bank, Washington.

Gwatkin, D., Rutstein, S., Johnson K. *et al.* (2007b). *Socio-economic differences in health, nutrition, and population within in Bangladesh*. World Bank, Washington.

Gwatkin, D. (2007). *Health coverage for the poor*. Presentation at the Johns Hopkins University Bloomberg School of Public Health, Baltimore.

Marmot, M. (2005). Social determinants of health inequalities. *The Lancet*, **365**, 1099.

Minujin, A. and Delamonica, E. (2003) Mind the gap! widening child mortality disparities. *Journal of Human Development*, **4**, 397–418.

Moser, K., Leon, D., and Gwatkin, D. (2005) How does progress toward the child mortality millennium development goal affect inequalities between the poorest and least poor? Analysis of Demographic and Health Survey data. *British Medical Journal*, **331**, 2280–2.

O'Donnell, O. *et al.* (2005). *Who benefits from public spending on healthcare in Asia?* Equitap Working Paper No. 3. Institute for Health Policy, Colombo.

Sen, A. (1999). *Development as freedom*. Oxford University Press, Oxford.

Wagstaff, A., Paci, P., and van Doorslaer, E. (1991). On the measurement of inequalities in health. *Social Science and Medicine*, **33**, 545–s57.

Whitehead, M. (1990),*The concepts and principles of equity and health*. Document EUR/ICP/RPD/414. World Health Regional Office for Europe, Copenhagen.

Wilkinson, R. and Marmot, M. eds. (2003*). Social determinants of health: the solid facts*, 2nd ed., Healthy Cities 21st Century, and the International Centre for Health and Society. World Health Organization Regional Office for Europe, Copenhagen.

World Bank (2001). *2001 world development indicators*. World Bank, Washington.

World Bank (2005). *Reaching the poor with health, nutrition, and population services: what works, what doesn't and why*. Available at http://siteresources.worldbank.org/INTPAH/ Resources/Reaching-the-Poor/summary.pdf

World Bank (2007). *2007 world development indicators*. World Bank, Washington.

12.5

Prevention and control of chronic, non-communicable diseases[1]

Jørn Olsen, Virasakdi Chongsuvivatwong, and Robert Beaglehole

Abstract

Chronic, non-communicable diseases have reached epidemic proportions worldwide. These diseases include cardiovascular diseases, mainly heart disease and stroke; several important cancers; chronic respiratory conditions; and type-2 diabetes. They affect people of all ages, nationalities, and classes. Over the coming decades, the burden of chronic diseases is projected to rise particularly fast in low- and middle-income countries. Unfortunately, the prevention of disability and death from chronic diseases gets little attention worldwide. Fortunately, the main causes of these conditions are known and are similar in all regions of the world. Various strategies and interventions are available to prevent and control chronic diseases at relatively modest costs. Urgent action is required by multiple agencies to ensure that this knowledge is translated into action.

Introduction

Chronic, non-communicable diseases have reached epidemic proportions worldwide (WHO 2005). These diseases include cardiovascular diseases, mainly heart disease and stroke; several important cancers; chronic respiratory conditions; and type-2 diabetes; they affect people of all ages, nationalities, and classes. Over the coming decades the burden of chronic diseases is projected to rise particularly fast in low- and middle-income countries. Unfortunately, the prevention of disability and death from chronic diseases gets little attention worldwide, at least in part because of the persistence of myths and half-truths about them (WHO 2005). In poor sub-Saharan African countries, it is understandable that governments, donors, and research funding agencies have channelled most resources into infectious diseases. In most other richer countries, the focus of biomedical research on chronic diseases has been on treatment rather than prevention (Daar *et al.* 2007).

In response to the rising burden of chronic diseases, the World Health Assembly has adopted many resolutions—the first in 1956—calling for increased action to be taken to prevent and control the growing burden of chronic diseases. Most recently, the World Health Assembly has adopted a series of related resolutions which amplify WHO's mandate in the area of chronic diseases: Resolution WHA56.1 on the WHO framework convention on tobacco control; resolution WHA57.16 on health promotion and healthy lifestyles; resolution WHA57.17 on the global strategy on diet, physical activity and health; resolution WHA58.22 on cancer prevention and control; resolution WHA58.26 on public-health problems caused by harmful use of alcohol; and WHA 60.23 on prevention and control of non-communicable diseases: Implementation of the global strategy.

This chapter reviews the current and projected health and economic impacts of chronic diseases and strategies for their prevention and control with emphasis on low- and middle-income countries. Other chapters review the specifics of the major chronic diseases including mental disorders and their common risk factors.

The global burden of chronic diseases

Approximately 58 million deaths occurred in 2005. Around 17 million deaths, approximately 30 per cent, were due to infectious diseases (including HIV/AIDS, tuberculosis, and malaria), maternal and perinatal conditions, and nutritional deficiencies combined. An additional 5 million deaths, 9 per cent of the total, resulted from violence and injuries (WHO 2005; Abegunde *et al.* 2007).

Chronic diseases cause 60 per cent of all deaths. Cardiovascular diseases (mainly heart disease and stroke) are the leading cause of death, responsible for 30 per cent of all deaths (Fig. 12.5.1). Cancer and chronic respiratory diseases are the other leading causes of chronic disease deaths. The contribution of diabetes is underestimated because, although people may live for years with diabetes, their deaths are usually recorded as being caused by heart disease or kidney failure. About 80 per cent of all chronic disease deaths occur in low- and middle-income countries.

[1] The term 'chronic diseases' is preferred to 'noncommunicable diseases'.

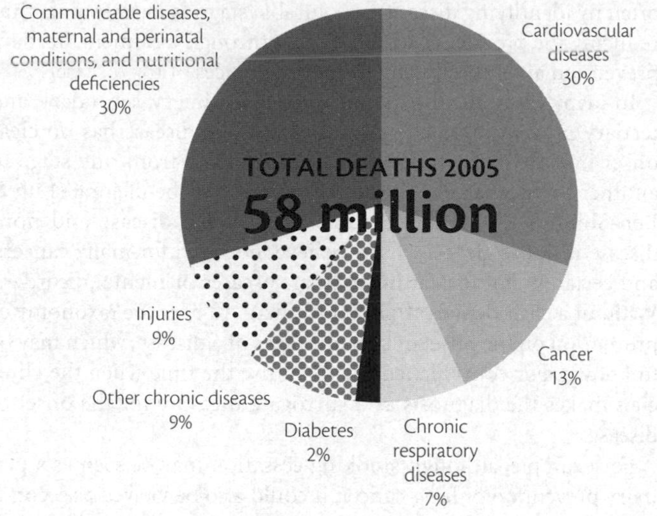

Fig. 12.5.1 Projected main causes of death, worldwide, all ages, 2005.

The number of deaths is similar in males and females. It is often assumed that chronic disease deaths are restricted to older people, but this is not the case. Moreover, chronic disease deaths occur at earlier ages in low- and middle-income countries than in high-income countries. The death rates for all chronic diseases rise with increasing age, but almost 45 per cent of chronic disease deaths occur under the age of 70 years.

Along with a high death toll, chronic diseases also cause disability, often for decades of a person's life. The most widely used summary measure of the burden of disease is the disability-adjusted life year (or DALY), which combines the number of years of healthy life lost to premature death with time spent in less than full health. One DALY can be thought of, under a number of conditions, as one lost healthy year of life (Murray & Lopez 1996). It focuses upon the health aspect of quality of life, and is based upon a number of assumptions; it is a concept that is population and time specific.

The projected global burden of disease for all ages, as measured by DALYs, is shown in Fig. 12.5.2, along with the burden of the leading chronic diseases. Approximately half of the burden of disease is caused by chronic diseases, 13 per cent by injuries, and 39 per cent by communicable diseases, maternal and perinatal conditions, and nutritional deficiencies combined. Cardiovascular diseases are the leading contributor, among the chronic diseases, to the global burden of disease. The number of DALYs caused by chronic disease is greatest in adults aged 30–59 years, and the rates increase with age. Overall, the burden of disease is similar in men and women. Approximately 86 per cent of the burden of chronic disease occurs in people under the age of 70 years.

Chronic disease is the leading cause of death in males and females in all WHO regions except Africa, as shown in Fig. 12.5.3 for males.

Chronic diseases are the leading cause of the burden of disease in all regions except Africa; HIV/AIDS is a major contributor in Africa (Fig. 12.5.4).

The challenges of prevention

Although, in principle it is known how to prevent many of the most important chronic diseases, it is not often known how best to implement this knowledge. The common major risk factors for chronic diseases are the same for men and women in all regions of the world: Unhealthy diet, physical inactivity, and tobacco and excessive alcohol use. These risks, which are expressed through raised blood pressure, raised glucose concentrations in blood, abnormal concentrations of lipids in blood, overweight, obesity, and consequences of harmful use of tobacco and alcohol, are mainly driven by underlying social, economic, and environmental determinants of health (see Chapter 2.2). About 80 per cent of premature heart disease and stroke, 80 per cent of type-2 diabetes, and 40 per cent of cancers are probably preventable (WHO 2005).

Prevention aims to avoid diseases at a premature stage, not necessarily to prevent the diseases from occurring at the later stages of life. In fact, the occurrence of chronic diseases will increase with

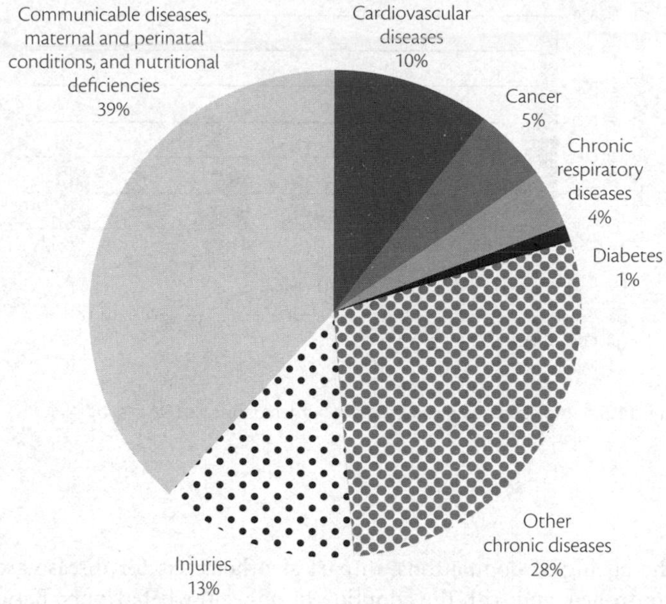

Fig. 12.5.2 Projected main causes of global burden of disease (DALYS), worldwide, all ages, 2005.

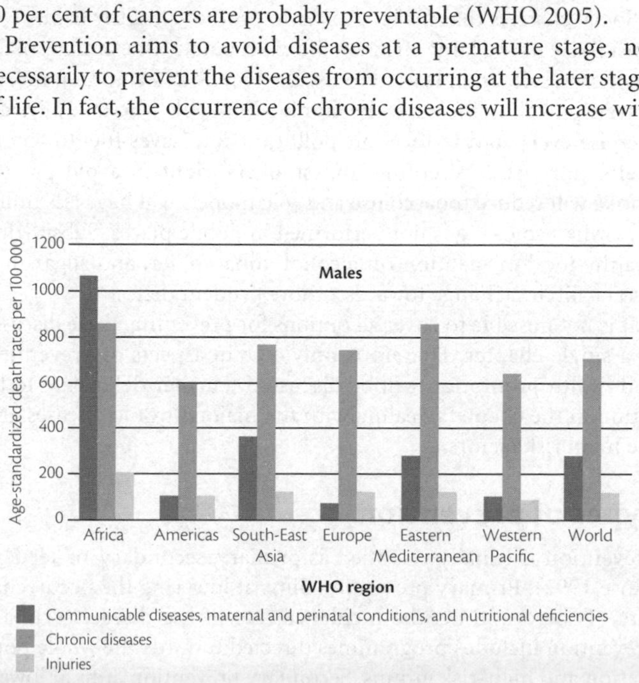

Fig. 12.5.3 Projected main causes of death by WHO region all ages, 2005—males.

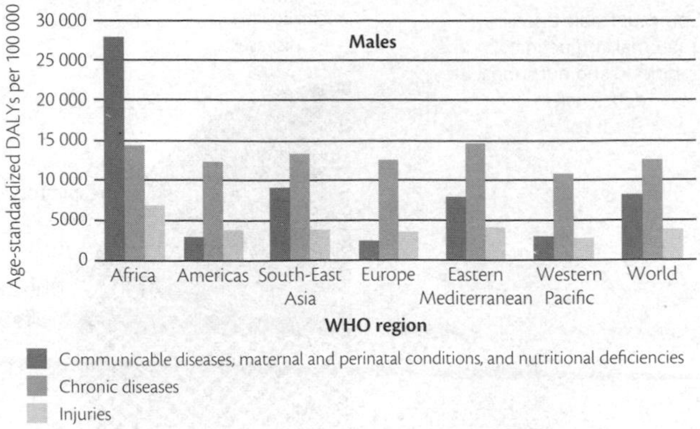

Fig. 12.5.4 Projected main causes of the burden of disease (DALYs) by WHO region, all ages, 2005, males.

the ageing of populations, in part as other risks for disease are controlled, and with the adoption of unhealthy behaviours. Basic health care will also lead to good-quality treatment of infections, and implementation of vaccination programmes will increase life expectancy; therefore, the lifelong occurrence of many chronic diseases will increase. The shift from communicable to chronic diseases in many low- and middle-income countries is in some respects a positive achievement. The challenges lie in reducing the avoidable deaths and disabilities related to chronic diseases at the same time as maintaining a focus on the remaining infectious diseases.

Although wealthy countries spend 90 per cent of world health resources on 10 per cent of world health problems, history clearly shows that expenditure of health resources on treatment alone has not been a very efficient way of reducing the number of non-communicable diseases. However, an increasing number of effective and cost-effective interventions are now available, including for chronic diseases (Jamison *et al.* 2006; Gaziano *et al.* 2007).

Social changes that make it easier to promote healthy habits will most likely have a large effect on life expectancy. For example, making it easy, safe, and pleasant to use the bicycle as a common means of transportation increases the number of people who take physical exercise every day, reduces air pollution, and saves fuel for more useful purposes. Accepting non-smokers' right to avoid passive smoke will reduce tobacco use and role models will have less influence when smoking is not performed in public places. Subsidizing healthy food or taxation on alcohol, tobacco, fat, and sugar may also facilitate a change towards a more prudent diet.

It is not possible to cover all options for preventing these diseases in a single chapter. Therefore, only certain aspects of prevention and health promotion will be discussed. Further details are to be found in the chapters dealing with the major chronic diseases and the main risk factors.

Types of prevention

Prevention is usually classified as primary, secondary, or tertiary (Rose 1992). Primary prevention aims at lowering the occurrence rate of the event, i.e. the incidence rate of the disease. Primary prevention includes programmes directed towards the whole population and high-risk groups. Secondary prevention aims at lowering the occurrence of later and more severe stages of the disease, often by identifying diseases at a curable stage as in screening, thus reducing the prevalence of the disease through treatment. Tertiary prevention aims at reducing the consequences of the disease.

In many cases, the distinction between primary, secondary, and tertiary prevention is not clear, because the disease has no clear onset in time or a precise transmission time from one stage to another but is a result of processes which may be lifelong (Kuh & Ben-Shlomo 1997). The distinction between disease and non-disease is not as clear as many believe, not even for many cancers, and certainly not for cardiovascular diseases or mental disorders. Without a clear demarcation, it is difficult to base the taxonomy of prevention on the onset of certain stages of a disease, which may be unknown. For convenience, we often use the time when the clinician makes the diagnosis as a surrogate measure for the onset of disease.

For example, although smoking cessation may be seen as a primary prevention of lung cancer, it could also be viewed as secondary prevention if lung cancer is seen as a disease that starts with a first-stage transformation in a multistage carcinogenic process. A screening programme would aim at diagnosing lung cancer at a stage where treatment is possible and thereby removing the patient from the pool of prevalent cases (most attempts to do this have not been promising), but spiral CT screening may be an option (The International Early Lung Cancer Action Program Investigators 2006). Tertiary prevention would aim at securing work and income as long as possible and then to provide aid to reduce the losses following the disease, or to rehabilitate the patient to make it possible for him or her to work at a reduced physical or mental capacity.

The periconceptual intake of folic acid to prevent neural tube defects is primary prevention (Berry *et al.* 1999). Prenatal screening for neural tube defects by ultrasound examination is secondary prevention if a finding leads to an induced abortion, which removes the child from the pool of prevalent cases at birth. High-quality surgical treatment followed by extensive physical and social training is tertiary prevention, aimed at reducing the social consequences for the affected child and the family. Fortification of bread or flour with folic acid is primary prevention on a large scale and requires further knowledge about its consequences other than just its effects on the unborn child. Recent findings indicate that this vitamin (as well as other vitamins given in excess) may have unwanted side effects (Cole *et al.* 2007).

Screening

Screening is usually considered to be secondary prevention as it aims at identifying those with diseases at a time when they will still benefit from early detection and treatment (see Chapter 12.7). Thus, those with diseases are identified before reaching the critical point where only palliative treatment is available. Screening consists of a programme, not just the application of a screening test, and it must be evaluated as a programme. Even in situations where a well-accepted screening test is available, a health benefit is expected, and the necessary health-care facilities are available, a screening programme must be carefully evaluated before it is implemented; the screening programme takes up resources that could be spent in other areas, and also a screening activity often has severe side-effects for some of the participants. When a screening test is applied to people without symptoms, it aims at identifying the diseased before the disease has reached a non-reversible stage.

Table 12.5.1 Illustration of the outcome of a screening test

Test result	Diseased	Not diseased
Positive	True positive	False positive
Negative	False negative	True negative

An illustration of the simplest possible outcome after using a screening test on a population without symptoms shows how participants fall into four groups (Table 12.5.1).

The *true positives* benefit from the screening if they are diagnosed at a curable stage. Those who are diagnosed late may be harmed by the screening in some cases. The *true negatives* often benefit as they do not have the disease and are reassured by the testing. The false negatives may have the normal diagnostic routines delayed as the test was negative, and the false positives may have to go through unpleasant and perhaps even risky diagnostic routines due to the screening result. Therefore, the validity of the screening test is a key parameter for the success of a screening programme. It is usually measured as sensitivity, i.e. the probability of being tested positive given that you have the disease, and as specificity, i.e. the probability of being tested negative given that you do not have the disease. Screening tests often have a sensitivity ranging from 30 to 95 per cent and a specificity ranging from 80 to 95 per cent. When such a test is applied to a population with a low prevalence of the disease to be screened, many false-positive results are obtained, and not all with the disease are identified. Screening for a rare disease with a test that has low specificity will produce an unfavourable ratio between true and false positives (low predictive value; the number of true positives divided by all positives).

Randomized control trials have shown a reduction in cause-specific mortality after screening for breast cancer and colorectal cancer (Weitz *et al.* 2005). It is also generally believed that screening for cervical cancer is useful in affluent societies (WHO 2006). Identification of the subtypes of HPV that causes cervical cancer and the development of appropriate vaccines is one of the major success stories in preventive medicine and primary prevention may replace screening for cervical cancer in two to three generations (Muñoz *et al.* 2003, 2004). It is expected that more useful screening programmes will be available in cancer prevention in the future, but it would be dangerous to rely upon screening only in the fight against cancer.

Causation

The search for the causes of chronic diseases usually addresses proximal determinants of a disease because the cause must make a difference for at least some of the exposed. For example, tobacco smoking, asbestos, and some other exposures cause lung cancer, and by using counterfactual reasoning it is assumed that if these causes are removed some of the expected cases will not occur. Very few of the proximal determinants are in themselves sufficient or necessary causes. Most of the necessary causes are made necessary by including the cause in the definition of the disease (Olsen 1993). However, the component causal model presents a framework for causal thinking that matches actual evidence (Rothman & Greenland 1998). In many situations, prevention may, however, fail if it is not taken into consideration that causes also have causes and more proximal causes may be more efficient. Poverty is probably a cause of many risk factors, and without eliminating poverty many preventive programmes will fail, especially in the most disadvantaged population groups.

WHO (2002) estimated that the five most important risk factors worldwide are malnutrition (underweight), unsafe sex, elevated blood pressure, tobacco, and alcohol misuse (in that order), with variations by level of development. Prevention should, if possible, aim at these proximal determinants directly, but in practice we may be more successful if we try to modify the determinants of, say, malnutrition or smoking. The first of these risk factors is to a large extent associated with poverty, and the tobacco, for example, is to some extent associated with ignorance and powerful marketing in some countries. Although it is known that specific subtypes of human papilloma virus are necessary causes of cervical cancer, dealing with more distal risk factors, such as reducing the number of sexual partners or encouraging condom use, may be the only way of preventing cervical cancers while we wait for an affordable vaccine to be available for the public in poor countries. Whether we should move upstream or downstream in the search for public health determinants remains an important topic for discussion.

Health promotion

Health promotion (see Chapter 7.3) includes activities that aim at improving health rather than preventing specific diseases. A prudent diet, physical exercise, better social networks, and a stimulating work environment will improve well-being and lower the risk of several diseases (see other chapters for details). Preventing chronic diseases will, with our present technology, rest upon encouraging healthy habits such as non-smoking, more physical exercise, a better diet low in fat and rich in fruit and vegetables, and better stress control by, for example, improving social networks. However, poverty-related problems such as homelessness, drug and alcohol abuse, and physical violence have not yet been eliminated, even in the most affluent societies. Basic needs concerning housing and food for all have not yet been secured, which makes health promotion meaningless for many people. A reduction in environmental exposures from pesticides, heavy metals, radon exposure, and other chemical and physical exposures are important, but at present these risk factors have a much smaller role than unhealthy lifestyle factors (WHO 2002). As many chronic diseases develop over the entire lifespan, prevention may be seen as a lifelong investment (Galobardes *et al.* 2006). The importance of taking a life course approach to disease prevention is perhaps best illustrated for obesity. Different growth curves at different age intervals correlate strongly with long-term obesity in a way we do not fully understand (Drake *et al.* 2007).

Changing behavioural risk factors is more difficult and perhaps also more expensive than changing environmental factors. Not all are willing to accept responsibility for their own health. Many people prefer, reasonably, to blame their bad health on some external factor—the environment in general, work conditions, or lack of social or personal support. Or they like to believe that medical treatment will solve all the problems that they may have in the future, perhaps not with the present technology but when they become patients in 10–20 years. The health-care industry has in many ways promised more than it could deliver. How much influence these promises have on health promotion and disease prevention is not known, but the detrimental effect could be substantial and it will continue since the health industry thrives on hope.

It is possible to change behaviour, and many private enterprises achieve this through repeated advertising. Usually large budgets are required as it is often necessary to create a perceived need and then to maintain it. Some health-related changes may benefit from being linked to profit-making enterprises. Commercial interest in selling smoking cessation tools may also be more efficient in reducing smoking habits than traditional anti-smoking campaigns. Recognition of the effectiveness of commercial methods has led to the development and application of the concept of 'social marketing', which aims to use marketing techniques to promote behaviour change for social good rather than commercial benefit.

Setting up systems that provided safe drinking water needed financial resources and political leadership in Europe in the nineteenth century (Holland & Stewart 1998). The same is true for organizing a well-functioning health-care system with a strong emphasis on health promotion. Strong political leadership is necessary to improve health behaviour. Health insurance companies, public health activities, private and public health care, pharmaceutical companies, strong medical professions, etc., do not have the same interests or goals, and they are powerful players in the health field and difficult to co-ordinate. Countries with a publicly funded health care system are often willing to provide the health care that is supported by evidence but rarely evidence-based prevention.

Building on the Ottawa Charter, the Bangkok Charter for Health Promotion (Tang *et al.* 2006) adds value to health promotion practice worldwide. Four new commitments were identified: To make the promotion of health central to the global development agenda, a core responsibility for all of government, a key focus of communities and civil society and a requirement for good corporate practices.

Prevention and healthcare

Usually only a small fraction of the overall budget for healthcare is spent on prevention, and most of the money is spent on screening and regular health examinations. Most experts agree that only changes in the most important lifestyle factors will succeed in substantially improving global health indicators in developed countries, and improving social conditions, reducing family size and providing safe water in developing countries. Still, it is difficult to see how the balance between treatment and prevention could change. Treatment deals with named patients in need. Prevention is about anonymous individuals who are at present healthy and who, in general, will not know whether or not they will benefit from the preventive action.

Convincing circumstantial evidence indicates that changing the sleeping position in early childhood from a prone to a supine position has saved thousands of children from sudden infant death syndrome (Gilbert *et al.* 2005), but there are no grateful parents who donate money to research or tell their member of parliament that prevention is an important activity to support. Prevention may be better than cure. Still, prevention will never be able to compete with cure on resources for many reasons, some of which are reasonable. A utilitarian approach to health care would allocate more resources to disease prevention, but a strictly utilitarian approach is not acceptable for ethical reasons and will be in conflict with the aim of equity in treatment (Jensen & Mooney 1990). In like manner it will not be acceptable to shift resources from necessary and efficient treatments to prevention. On the other hand, many treatments have little or no scientific justification and in these situations money is much better spent on evidence-based prevention. However, it may often be more difficult to obtain high-level evidence for preventive strategies than for clinical interventions.

A healthcare system needs to be organized towards well-defined health goals to make any difference in the priority setting. This message was probably the most important result of the WHO Health for All policy. Still, day-to-day problem solving and short-term goals, where the media's treatment of case stories plays an important part, drives most healthcare policy systems. WHO has proposed a global goal, additional to the Millennium Development Goals, which aims to reduce chronic disease death rates by an additional 2 per cent per year over current trends. The goal, if reached, would avert approximately 36 million chronic disease deaths by 2015 and would result in substantial economic savings (Abegunde *et al.* 2007). This goal is achievable even at our present level of knowledge. A small number of interventions directed towards the whole population and high-risk people will readily achieve the goal in 23 low- and middle-income countries at a relatively modest cost (Asaria *et al.* 2007; Lim *et al.* 2007).

Although prevention may be better than cure, few people act according to this precept. It is unlikely that this will change substantially in the near future, which is why every opportunity should be taken to discuss and change unhealthy habits. One such opportunity is illness. Stopping smoking after a myocardial infarction is late—too late in some cases, but not in all. Involving all healthcare workers in prevention carries an important potential for lowering the disease burden. In most countries, this potential resource has not been used to any large extent.

Social determinants of health

It is expected that disease and death would be closely correlated to poverty. It is disappointing that social inequalities in health are strong even in welfare states that have eradicated poverty in a materialistic sense for almost everyone in their societies and provided access to health care for all (see Chapter 2.2). It is perhaps difficult to avoid the fact that chronic disease can lead to unemployment and loss of income, but it should be within our reach to limit the inequalities in health that follow differences in social status. This has been one of the key targets in the WHO plan for Health for All by the Year 2000. However, in many countries, the trend has been the opposite. Reasons for social inequalities could be genetic, due to differences in access to health care, or due to differences in exposures to health hazards in the working environment or in personal life. Poor social conditions may also lead to greater exposure to stress and more changes in social conditions and other life events. In some of the East European states, there has been a substantial decline in life expectancy in males over the past 15–20 years (Eberstadt 2006).

Changes in the social classification system may explain some of the changes in social inequalities over time. If the population is classified into, say, quintiles according to a given social indicator, selection bias hardly explains changes in social inequalities. However, if the social classification system is based on educational levels, those who remain in the lower social groups need not be comparable with those from the same level in the past. This type of selection bias is expected to be present in many societies where social grouping is based on, for example, educational levels or the skill required to hold certain jobs (Cavelaars *et al.* 1998).

Social indicators are usually developed within social research. Although there are many possible ways that social factors may impair health (Marmot 2007), further knowledge is required on how best to classify social conditions in relation to health. Income, housing and working conditions, health behaviour, and access to health care may be related to health through very different mechanisms that may change over time and be different in different societies. How all these factors should be included in a social classification system that relates to health issues is not well understood.

It is likely that mandatory public health programmes, or programmes offered to all, such as vaccination programmes, free school meals, or control of work exposures help to reduce social inequalities in health. Health campaigns and voluntary screening programmes may, on the other hand, be better accepted by the best educated. Health-care workers have an important task in providing information to be used in primary or secondary prevention in a way that is understood by all. This potential for health improvements in patients with lifestyle-related diseases has not been widely used in most countries.

Genetic and molecular epidemiology

The mapping of the human genome provides new tools and new challenges in epidemiology. For most of the chronic diseases, the genetic risk factors will probably be complex and their individual contributions may be small. Stratifying the participants on genetic factors will sometimes make it easier to identify environmental and preventable causes of diseases, as has been shown for the Leiden V mutation and oral contraception (Appleby & Olds 1997). However, other gene–environment interactions may be much more difficult to detect. Important genetic determinants of breast cancer, colorectal cancer, cardiovascular diseases, obesity, and many other diseases have been identified (Frayling *et al.* 2007), but the importance of these findings in primary prevention is still not clear. The use of new genetic technologies has been most successful in identifying better treatment options by providing a better understanding of the causal pathways in disease progression. Although research may show that obesity to a large extent is a genetic disease this will not explain why obesity has an epidemic development in many countries. Even lung cancer would appear to be a predominantly genetic disorder in a population where all smoked 20 cigarettes per day. Epidemiology has had a strong link to public health. New research methods incorporating molecular biology have the potential to enhance the ability of epidemiologists to study disease processes; however, it is important for those epidemiologists using these new molecular tools to use them to help elucidate public health issues (Olsen *et al.* 1999). The development of diseases over time cannot be understood outside a social context. Diseases have causes and many of these causes are man-made and, therefore, often avoidable. Although these causes interact with genetic factors to produce their effect, it seems more appropriate to target or prevent these causes rather than change susceptibility, which may have unknown side-effects.

Environmental risk factors

Since Ramazzini published his book *De Morbis Artificium* about occupational diseases in the eighteenth century, many diseases have been accepted as having an occupational or environmental aetiology. Percival Pott was the first to identify an occupational cancer in 1775 when he recognized soot from chimney sweeping as the cause of scrotal cancer. Much later the culprit was identified as one of the polycyclic hydrocarbons. Now it is known that 4-aminophenyl, arsenic, asbestos, benzene, benzidine, chromium, polyclorinated biphenyls, vinyl chloride, and other compounds cause cancer but the fraction of cancers attributable to specific occupations is probably small in most affluent countries. Most countries have been successful in finding substitutes for some of the carcinogens or in reducing exposure levels to very low levels, but heavy metals and pesticides with very long biological half-lives are of concern, especially if they accumulate in human food chains. Asbestos exposure and exposure to radon daughter elements are still widespread and constitute important public health problems.

Environmental diseases have to be identified and their determinants located. Some diseases are so closely related to their causes that the task may be easy, such as cancer of the nose in furniture workers or liver cell angiosarcoma in people exposed to vinyl chloride. Most other diseases have environmental as well as non-environmental causes and thus are more difficult to detect despite the fact that they are much more frequent. Weak associations between exposure to high levels of electromagnetic fields and childhood leukaemia (UK Childhood Cancer Study Investigators 1999) or cell phone use and brain cancer have been difficult to interpret, as weak associations indicate that other causes of the disease are not included in the statistical model used.

In countries with very poor occupational standards, education may be the most cost-effective way of reducing exposures. Reducing environmental exposures need not be very expensive if the exposure levels are high. Exposure to, say, organic solvents may often be greatly reduced by minor rearrangements at the work site. Knowing what to do is often the first step to getting it done, but many newly industrialized countries lack the knowledge or the infrastructure to implement the knowledge.

A life-course approach to disease prevention

A growing body of evidence indicates that there may be new avenues of disease prevention in the future. The early phase of life from conception into early childhood may 'program' disease susceptibility, even for disease with an onset much later in life. As the field of life-course epidemiology evolves, it may lead to research results that can be translated into prevention (Gluckman & Hanson 2006).

It is well known that, for example, neurotoxic exposures in early life may permanently impair brain functioning, as is the case in fetal alcohol syndrome (Abel 1998). Infections may also cause damage that is not detected clinically within a short follow-up period, but could cause chronic disease in adulthood. Cardiovascular diseases, type-2 diabetes, and cancer have been seen as diseases that were the result of high-fat intake, smoking, and lack of physical exercise in adult life for genetically susceptible people. This susceptibility need not only be a function of genetic factors, but also a result of exposures that took place early in life (Gluckman & Hanson 2006). It is known from animal experiments that the functioning of some organs may be permanently altered if the diet is poor in nutritional components such as proteins, and this alteration is called 'programming'. The first human evidence came from

Forsdahl's (1977) studies in Norway showing that middle-aged males who were born in regions of high infant mortality at the time of their birth had a high mortality 50 years later, mainly due to cardiovascular diseases. Men born in regions with low infant mortality had a low risk of dying from cardiovascular diseases in middle age. A similar ecological correlation was found to be present for serum cholesterol (Bakketeig *et al.* 1991). Barker (1995) and Barker *et al.* (2005) followed up these ideas and established a link between birth weight and chronic diseases at the individual level. The mechanisms could operate via epigenetic changes where the fetus tries to adapt to the intrauterine environment. If this adoption does not match environmental conditions later it may have negative health consequences.

It is also believed that some cancers have a fetal aetiology, especially childhood cancers and cancer of the testis, but also breast cancers, ovarian cancers, and perhaps cancer of the prostate (Adami *et al.* 1998; Ekbom 1998). The intrauterine hormonal level may be of importance for these cancers, especially oestrogen or the balance between oestrogen and progesterone. Stress and nutrition are prenatal exposures with possible long-term effects (Ozanne & Hales 2004; St Clair *et al.* 2005).

The number of Sertoli cells at birth partly determines sperm production, and male fecundity may similarly be affected by external or internal disrupters of the hormonal balance acting during the time period of organogenesis (Sharpe & Skakkebæk 1993). New data indicates prenatal smoking may even be more important (Ramlau-Hansen *et al.* 2007). It is not known whether some types of medication have a programming effect or not but more than half of all pregnant women use medication during pregnancy.

However, whether or not these hypotheses are true is not crucial to the life-course approach in preventing chronic diseases. Arteriosclerosis is a process that starts very early in life, and dietary habits and the tendency to abuse alcohol, tobacco, or drugs depend on social and psychological factors in early life. Obesity in childhood is strongly associated with obesity in adult life. Given these conditions, health promotion as well as disease management must focus on the longitudinal track of a given disease process on the health status of individuals as well as populations. Antenatal care is only the first process in a lifelong health promotion and disease prevention endeavour and needs to take into consideration not only diseases that surface to clinical detection shortly after the onset of the programme but also health in the long run. A healthcare system strongly specialized within certain time periods of the lifespan or certain organ systems will not be well suited to meet the challenges raised by life-course research. Health promotion and diseases prevention must start early in life and should be an ongoing process like what is seen for many dental health plans.

Integrated prevention and control

Taking action

Creative solutions are necessary to address the escalating demands of reducing the frequency of chronic diseases and their common risk factors in countries with limited or stressed health systems where annual health expenditures are very low. With this limited funding, many countries must contend with a high prevalence of chronic malnutrition of children, relatively high maternal and neonatal mortality, an unfinished agenda around infectious diseases, and a steady increase in cardiovascular diseases, cancer, and other chronic diseases. Within contexts such as these, ministries of health are faced with a seemingly daunting task: To rally support for chronic disease prevention and control; to provide a unifying vision and action plan to ensure that intersectoral action is emphasized at all stages of policy formulation and implementation; and to make certain that actions at all levels and by all sectors are mutually supportive. Additionally, actions need to be prioritized in keeping with the specific population needs for chronic disease prevention and control, range of possible interventions, and availability of human and financial resources to implement them.

Stepwise framework for preventing chronic diseases

The WHO stepwise framework offers a flexible and practical approach to assist ministries of health in balancing diverse needs and priorities while implementing evidence-based interventions (Epping-Jordan *et al.* 2005). The framework is guided by a set of principles based on a public health approach to chronic disease prevention and control:

- The national level of government provides the unifying framework for chronic disease prevention and control, so that actions at all levels and by all stakeholders are mutually supportive.
- Intersectoral action is necessary at all stages of policy formulation and implementation because major determinants of the chronic disease burden lie outside the health sector.
- Policies and plans focus on the common risk factors and cut across specific diseases.
- As part of comprehensive public-health action, population-wide and individual interventions are combined.
- In recognition that most countries will not have the resources to immediately do everything implied by the overall policy, activities that are immediately feasible and likely to have the greatest impact for the investment are selected first for implementation. This principle is the heart of the stepwise approach.
- Locally relevant and explicit milestones are set for each step and at each level of intervention with a particular focus on reducing health inequalities.

Figure 12.5.5 outlines the framework, which includes three main planning steps and three main implementation steps. The first planning step is to assess the current risk factor profile and burden of chronic diseases of a country or subpopulation. The distribution of risk factors among the population is the key information required by countries in their planning of prevention and control programmes, and can be assessed using WHO's stepwise surveillance approach (WHO 2003). This information must then be synthesized and disseminated in a way that successfully argues the case for the adoption of relevant policies. This is a key aspect of making the case for action.

The second planning step is to formulate and adopt a chronic disease policy that sets out the vision for prevention and control of the major chronic diseases and provides the basis for action in the next 5–10 years. In all countries, a national policy is essential to give chronic diseases appropriate priority and to organize resources efficiently. For example, China's Ministry of Health, with the support of WHO and the cooperation of relevant sectors, has been developing a national plan for chronic disease prevention and control that focuses on cardiovascular diseases, stroke, cancer, chronic

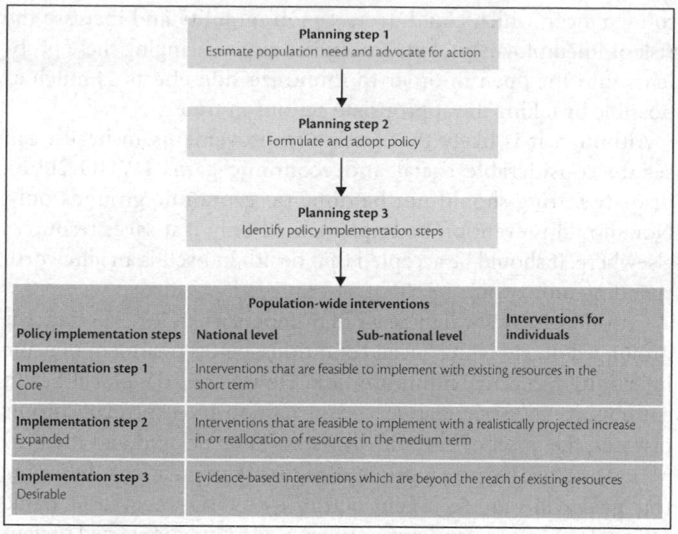

Fig. 12.5.5 Stepwise framework for prevention.

obstructive pulmonary disease, and diabetes. It will include an action plan for 3–5 years (Wang *et al.* 2005). Depending on the configuration of each country's governance, complementary policies can also be developed at the state, province, district, or municipal levels. In these cases, it is vital that subnational policies are fully integrated and aligned with national policies.

The third planning step is to identify the most effective means of implementing the adopted policies. The comprehensive approach requires a range of interventions to be implemented in a stepwise manner, depending on their feasibility and likely impact in the local conditions, and taking into account potential constraints and barriers to action. Some of the selected interventions might be primarily under the control of the health ministry, such as realigning health systems for chronic disease prevention and control. Others might be primarily the responsibility of other government sectors or the legislative branch, such as health financing, laws, and regulations, and improving the built environment. In these cases, the ministry of health must ensure coordination and cooperation with all government partners, civil society, and the private sector.

Planning is followed by a series of implementation steps: Core, expanded, and desirable. The chosen combination of interventions for core implementation forms the starting point and the foundation for further action. Each country must consider a range of factors in deciding the package of interventions that constitute the first, core implementation step, including capacity for implementation, likely impact, acceptability, and political support. Selecting a smaller number of activities and doing them well is likely to have more effect than tackling a large number haphazardly (Asaria *et al.* 2007; Lim *et al.* 2007). Countries should also try to ensure that any new activities complement those already underway locally, provincially or nationally.

Putting the framework into action

A number of countries, such as Vietnam and Tonga, have successfully used the stepwise framework for policy formulation and implementation (WHO 2005). They show how the stepwise approach has general applicability to solving chronic disease problems without sacrificing specificity for any given country.

Across these and other countries, the following factors have been associated with successful implementation:

- A high-level political mandate to develop a national policy framework
- A committed group of advocates who are often involved with estimating need, advocating for action, and developing the national policy and plan
- International collaboration providing political and technical support
- Wide consultation in the process of drafting, consulting, reviewing and re-drafting the policy until endorsement is achieved
- Development and implementation of a consistent and compelling communication strategy for all stages of the process
- Clarity of vision on a small set of outcome-oriented objectives

Involvement of civil society and the private sector

Any single organization or group is unlikely to have enough resources to address the complex public health issues related to the prevention and management of chronic diseases. The stepwise framework initiated by governments allows all health and non-health sectors to see how their role is an integral part of an overall framework. It becomes quickly apparent that it can be best implemented by working with the private sector, civil society, and international organizations. In the Philippines, for example, the Department of Health has assumed a coordination and advocacy role in the development of a response to chronic disease, marshalling the multiple inputs of local governments, non-governmental associations, and the Philippine Health Insurance Corporation. Using the stepwise framework as a basis for planning, a Philippine Coalition for the Prevention of Noncommunicable Diseases has been formed and a Memorandum of Understanding for action between these parties was signed in 2004 (Philippine Coalition for the Prevention of Noncommunicable Disease. Memorandum of understanding. April 14, 2004). The relations between government, civil society, and the private sector also apply at the international level, where WHO collaborates with a range of partners on chronic disease prevention and control.

The future of chronic diseases

'It is difficult to make predictions, especially for the future' was a statement made by the Danish writer Storm P., with which most people will agree. On the other hand, all preventive activities try to change undesirable expected future events and therefore are, or should be, based on predictions for the future. Not even the obesity epidemic was well predicted, although most of the risk factors were well known and monitored over time.

Most preventive activities address elimination or reduction of known risk factors, but often without giving much consideration to other consequences of behavioural or environmental changes. Most of the present predictions are based on what we know about the long-term consequences of present risk factors or long-term trends in, for example, life expectancy. Based on information of this type, we expect most populations to age in developed as well as in many developing countries and we expect chronic disease morbidity to increase from 28 million deaths worldwide in 1990 to 50 million in 2020. In 2020, the five leading causes of DALYs worldwide are expected to be ischaemic heart diseases, unipolar major depression, road traffic accidents, cerebrovascular diseases, and chronic obstructive pulmonary diseases (Murray & Lopez 1997). Although it is known how some of these diseases may be prevented, it is not in general known how to implement this knowledge. Predicting future trends rests upon many assumptions, guesses, and intuition that call for the use of many different sources of information coming from experts as well as non-experts. These methods include Delphi techniques, brainstorming, and simulation games, as well as quantitative approaches in time-series analyses, use of Markov chains, and many other related techniques (Garrett 1999; Kirchhoff *et al.* 1999).

The future will partly reflect the past (be predictable) but also partly reflect unpredictable opportunities and problems. Changes in climate, living conditions, wars, and behaviours will generate new diseases and provide new opportunities in new areas for existing diseases. Global warming may not only lead to mass migration from areas that will be flooded but will also lead to migration of diseases like malaria into areas where they do not exist at present. New infectious diseases may also emerge when conditions are right. Huge investments are being made in the hope that new technology may produce better predictions of pandemics and shorten the time for preventive measures like vaccines to be available.

A better understanding of diseases at the genetic and molecular level will change clinical medicine. It is less obvious it will change public health practice to the same extent but it has impact on public health research and large-scale studies are beginning to find results on genetic risk factors that are replicable in other studies as a better understanding of molecular pathways to diseases may reveal new hypotheses on gene–environment interaction which may advance a research area that focuses upon the avoidable causes of diseases.

Future research is a risky matter, as time will show if the prediction were accurate. It is necessary because it emphasizes the need to imagine what will happen with or without the preventive activity we want to implement. It is important to try to capture all consequences of preventive activities by focusing upon the larger picture rather than just single outcomes. For example, it is a noble aim to reduce childhood accidents in day-care centres, but as accidents are an unavoidable part of the way in which children explore and learn about the environment, they should not be reduced at all costs. Eradication of serious disease is extremely important for diseases such as smallpox, even though this makes the smallpox virus a frightening biological weapon. Elimination of measles will also be valuable if the virus is not replaced with other more harmful infectious agents, or if the disease or vaccination against it has no beneficial effect on the immune system in general.

Screening programmes may replace primary prevention if it is believed that the health problem can be solved by early treatment. However, if a screening programme is followed by increased risk behaviour at work or in personal life, the net benefit may be less than expected and could even be negative. If priorities were set entirely upon how much health a unit of cost would produce, the healthcare system would look very different from what we have at present. Few people would welcome such a radical approach as many other aspects have to be taken into consideration.

Setting higher standards for automobile safety equipment leads to more expensive cars and may make it impossible for poor people to own a car, which could decrease job mobility and increase the risk of unemployment. Futures studies aim at bringing these problems into the open in order to minimize side-effects as much as possible by taking the appropriate actions in time.

Although it is likely that lasting improvements in health can secure considerable social and economic gains (WHO 2001), priority setting should not be done on economic grounds only. Nor should prevention be implemented only if it saves resources elsewhere. It should be accepted that health in itself is an aim worth spending money on.

Chronic diseases will increase in numbers when life expectancy is prolonged due to better social conditions, better treatment of acute infections and active immunization. However, if the global health community gets serious about the prevention and control of chronic diseases, the onset of chronic diseases will be delayed and the time period of active life prolonged in all high-risk populations. Achieving this goal will require urgent action by WHO, the World Bank, regional banks and development agencies, foundations, civil society, non-governmental organizations, the private sector including the pharmaceutical industry, and academics (Beaglehole *et al.* 2007).

Key points

- Chronic diseases, principally cardiovascular diseases, cancer, chronic respiratory diseases, and diabetes, are leading causes of death and disability but grossly neglected on the global health agenda.
- Achievement of the global goal for chronic disease prevention and control would avert 36 million deaths by 2015 and would have major economic benefits.
- An integrated and stepwise approach to the prevention and control of chronic diseases will be the most efficient approach.
- Urgent action is required by WHO, the World Bank, regional banks and development agencies, foundations, civil society, non-governmental organizations, the private sector including the pharmaceutical industry, and academics.

References

Abegunde, D.O., Mathers, C.D., Adam, T. *et al.* (2007) The burden and costs of chronic diseases in low-income and middle-income countries. *Lancet*, **370**, 1929–38.

Abel, E.L. (1998) Prevention of alcohol abuse-related birth effects. II: Targeting and pricing. *Alcohol and Alcoholism*, **33**, 417–20.

Adami, H.O., Signorello, L.B., and Trichopoulos, D. (1998). Towards an understanding of breast cancer etiology. *Seminars in Cancer Biology*, **8**, 255–62.

Appleby, R.D. and Olds, R.J. (1997). The inherited basis of venous thrombosis. *Pathology*, **29**, 341–7.

Asaria, P., Chisholm, D., Mathers, C. *et al.* (2007) Chronic disease prevention: health effects and financial costs of strategies to reduce salt intake an control tobacco use. *Lancet*, **370**, 2044–53.

Bakketeig, L.S., Magnus, P., and Sundet, J.M. (1991). In *Problems and methods in longitudinal research* (ed. D. Magnusson, L.R. Bergman, G. Rudinger, *et al.*). Cambridge University Press, Cambridge.

Barker, D.J. (1995). Fetal origins of coronary heart disease. *British Medical Journal*, **311**, 171–4.

Barker, D.J., Osmond, C., Forsén, T.J. *et al.* (2005). Trajectories of growth among children who have coronary events as adults. *New England Journal of Medicine*, **353**, 1802–9.

Beaglehole, R., Ebrahim, S., Voute, J. *et al.* (2007) Prevention of chronic disease: a call to action. *Lancet*, **370**, 2152–7.

Berry, R.J., Li, Z., Erickson, J.D. *et al.* (1999). Prevention of neural-tube defects with folic acid in China. *New England Journal of Medicine*, **341**, 1485–90.

Cavelaars, A.E.J.M., Kunst, A.E., Geurts, J.J. *et al.* (1998). Differences in self reported morbidity by educational level: a comparison of 11 Western European countries. *Journal of Epidemiology and Community Health*, **52**, 219–27.

Cole, B.F., Baron, J.A., Sandler, R.S. *et al* (2007). Folic acid for the prevention of colorectal adenomas. *JAMA*, **297**, 2351–9.

Daar, A.S., Singer, P.A., Persad, D.L. *et al.* (2007). Grand challenges in chronic noncommunicable diseases. *Nature*, **450**, 494–6.

Drake, A.J., Tang, J.I., Nyirenda, M.J. (2007). Mechanisms underlying the role of glucocorticoids in the early life programming of adult disease. *Clinical Science*, **113**, 219–32.

Eberstadt, N. (2006). Commentary: reflections on "The Health Crisis in the USSR". *International Journal of Epidemiology*, **35**, 1394–7.

Ekbom, A. (1998). Growing evidence that several human cancers may originate in utero. *Seminars in Cancer Biology*, **8**, 237–44.

Epping-Jordan, J.E., Galea, G., Tukuitonga, C. *et al.* (2005). Preventing chronic diseases: taking stepwise action. *Lancet*, **366**, 1667–71.

Forsdahl, A. (1977). Are poor living conditions in childhood and adolescence an important risk factor for arteriosclerotic heart disease? *British Journal of Preventive and Social Medicine*, **31**, 91–5.

Frayling, T.M., Timpson, N.J., Weedon, M.N. *et al.* (2007). A common variant in the FTO gene is associated with body mass index and predisposes to childhood and adult obesity. *Science*, **316**, 889–94.

Garrett, M.J. (1999). *Health Futures*. WHO, Geneva.

Galobardes, B., Smith, G.D., Lynch, J.W. (2006). Systematic review of the influence of childhood socioeconomic circumstances on risk for cardiovascular disease in adult childhood. *Annals of Epidemiology*, **16**, 91–104.

Gaziano, T.A., Galea, G., Reddy, K.S. (2007) Scaling up interventions for chronic disease prevention: the evidence. *Lancet*, **370**, 1939–46.

Gilbert, R., Salanti, G., Hareden, M. *et al.* (2005). Infants sleeping position and the sudden infant death syndrome: systematic review of observational studies and historical review of recommendations from 1940 to 2002. *International Journal of Epidemiology*, **34**, 874–87.

Gluckman, P. and Hanson, M. (2006). *Developmental origins of health and disease*. Cambridge University Press.

Gotzsche, P.C. and Olsen, O. (2000). Is screening for breast cancer with mammography justifiable? *Lancet*, **355**, 129–34.

Holland, W.W. and Stewart, S. (1998). *Public health. The vision and the challenge*. Nuffield Trust, London.

Jamison, D., Breman, J., Measham, A. *et al.* (eds) (2006). *Disease control priorities in developing countries. 2nd ed.* New York, NY—Washington, DC: Oxford University Press; World Bank.

Jensen, U.J. and Mooney, G. (1990). *Changing values in medical and health care decision making*. Wiley, Chichester.

Kirchhoff, M., Davidsen, M., Bronnun-Hansen, H. *et al.* (1999). Incidence of myocardial infarction in the Danish MONICA population 1982– 1991. *International Journal of Epidemiology*, **28**, 211–18.

Kuh, D. and Ben-Shlomo, B. (eds) (1997). *A life course approach to chronic disease epidemiology. Tracing the origins of ill-health from early to adult life*. Oxford University Press, Oxford.

Lim, S.S., Gaziano, T.A., Gakidou, E. *et al.* (2007) Prevention of cardiovascular disease in high-risk individuals in low-income and middle-income countries: health effects and costs. *Lancet*, **370**, 2054–62.

Marmot, M. (2007) Achieving health equity: from root causes to fair outcomes. *Lancet*, **370**, 1153–63.

Muñoz, N., Bosch, F.X., de Sanjosé, S. *et al.* International Agency for Research on Cancer Multicenter Cervical Cancer Study Group. (2003) Epidemiologic classification of human papillomavirus types associated with cervical cancer. *New England Journal of Medicine*, **348**, 518–27.

Muñoz, N., Bosch, F.X., Castellagué, X. *et al.* (2004) Against which human papillomavirus types shall we vaccinate and screen? The international perspective. *International Journal of Cancer*, **111**, 278–85.

Murray, C.J.L. and Lopez, A.D. (1996). *The global burden of disease: A comprehensive assessment of mortality and disability from diseases, injuries, and risk factors in 1990 and projected to 2020.* Cambridge: Harvard University Press.

Murray, C.J.L. and Lopez, A.D. (1997). Global mortality, disability, and the contribution of risk factors: Global Burden of Disease Study. *Lancet*, **349**, 1436–42.

Olsen, J. (1993). Some consequences of adopting a conditional deterministic causal model in epidemiology. *European Journal of Public Health*, **3**, 204–9.

Olsen, J., Andersen, P.K., Sørensen, T.I.A. *et al.* (1999). The future of epidemiology. *International Journal of Epidemiology*, **28**, S996.

Ozanne, S.E. and Hales, C.N. (2004). Lifespan: catch-up growth and obesity in male mice. *Nature*, **427**, 411–2.

Ramlau-Hansen, C.H., Thulstrup, A.M., Storgaard, L. *et al.* (2007). Is prenatal exposure to tobacco smoking a cause of poor semen quality? A follow-up study. *American Journal of Epidemiology*, **165**, 1372–9.

Rose, G. (1992). *The strategy of preventive medicine*. Oxford University Press, Oxford.

Rothman, K.J. and Greenland, S. (1998) *Modern epidemiology. 2nd edn.* Philadelphia: Lippincott-Raven.

St. Clair, D., Xu, M., Wang, P. *et al.* (2005). Rates of adult schizophrenia following prenatal exposure to the Chinese famine of 1959-1961. *JAMA*, **294**, 557–62.

Sharpe, R.M. and Skakkebæk, N.E. (1993). Are oestrogens involved in falling sperm counts and disorders of the male reproductive tract. *Lancet*, **341**, 1392–5.

Tang, K.C., Beaglehole, R., Pettersson, B. (2006). Implementation of the Bangkok Charter on Health Promotion in a Globalized World: experience and challenges of selected high income countries in Europe. *Sozial- und Präventivmedizin*, **51**, 1–3.

The International Early Lung Cancer Action Program Investigators (2006). Survival of Patients with Stage I Lung Cancer Detected on CT Screening. *New Engl Journal of Medicine*, **355**, 1763–71.

UK Childhood Cancer Study Investigators (1999). Exposure to powerfrequency magnetic fields and the risk of childhood cancer. *Lancet*, **354**, 1925–31.

Wang, L., Kong, L., Wu, F. *et al.* (2005). Preventing chronic diseases in China. *Lancet*, **366**, 1821–4.

Weitz, J., Koch, M., Debus, J. *et al.* (2005). Colorectal cancer. *Lancet*, **365**, 153–65.

WHO (2001). *Macroeconomics and health: investing in health for economic development*. Geneva, Switzerland.

WHO (2002). *The world health report 2002. Reducing Risks, Promoting Healthy Life*. WHO, Geneva.

WHO (2003). *STEPS: A framework for surveillance*. WHO, Geneva.

WHO (2005). *Preventing chronic diseases: A vital investment*. WHO, Geneva.

WHO (2006). Comprehensive cervical cancer control. A guide to essential practice. WHO, Geneva.

12.6

Principles of infectious disease control

Robert J. Kim-Farley

Abstract

This chapter provides a global and comprehensive view of the principles of infectious disease control through examination of the magnitude of disease burden, the chain of infection (agent, transmission, and host) of infectious diseases, the varied approaches to their prevention and control (measures applied to the host, vectors, infected humans, animals, environment, and agents), and the factors conducive to their eradication as well as emergence and re-emergence.

Introduction and overview

Ingenuity, knowledge, and organization alter but cannot cancel humanity's vulnerability to invasion by parasitic forms of life. Infectious disease which antedated the emergence of humankind will last as long as humanity itself, and will surely remain, as it has been hitherto, one of the fundamental parameters and determinants of human history. (William H. McNeill 1976)

Infectious diseases remain a leading cause of morbidity, disability, and mortality worldwide. Their control is a constant challenge that faces health workers and public health officials in both industrialized and developing countries. Only one infectious disease, smallpox, was eradicated and stands as a landmark in the history of the control of infectious diseases. The international community is now well down the path towards eradication of poliomyelitis and dracunculiasis (guinea-worm infection). Other infectious diseases, like malaria and tuberculosis, foiled eradication attempts or control efforts and are re-emerging as increasing threats in many countries. Some infectious diseases, such as tetanus, will always be a threat if control measures are not maintained. Newer infectious diseases, like AIDS, demonstrate the truth of McNeill's statement that infectious disease will remain 'one of the fundamental parameters and determinants of human history'. The history of infectious diseases is an exciting story in itself, and readers interested in the subject are referred to McNeill (1976) or the comprehensive work on the history of human diseases (Kiple 1993).

This chapter provides many examples of infectious diseases that illustrate modes of transmission and approaches to infectious disease control; however, it does not attempt to be comprehensive in listing all infectious diseases. Detailed recommendations on control measures for any specific disease are outlined periodically in the updated reports of the American Public Health Association, *Control of Communicable Diseases Manual* (Heymann 2004), the comprehensive two-volume work *Mandell, Douglas and Bennett's Principles and Practice of Infectious Diseases* (Mandell *et al.* 2005), and the textbook *Infectious Diseases* (Gorbach *et al.* 2004). For readers specifically interested in paediatric infectious diseases, there is the comprehensive two-volume *Textbook of Pediatric Infectious Diseases* (Feigin *et al.* 2004); for infectious diseases in emergency medicine settings, there is the textbook on *Infectious Disease in Emergency Medicine* (Brillman & Quenzer 1998); and for tropical infectious diseases, there is *Tropical Infectious Diseases: Principles, Pathogens, and Practice* (Guerrant *et al.* 2006). A comprehensive treatment of the worldwide distribution and diagnosis of infectious diseases is provided in *A World Guide to Infections: Diseases, Distribution, Diagnosis* (Wilson 1991). The Centers for Disease Control and Prevention (CDC) publishes up-to-date disease surveillance information for the United States and recommendations for control measures in the *Morbidity and Mortality Weekly Reports* and provides annual summaries of notifiable infectious diseases in the *Summary of Notifiable Diseases, United States* (CDC 2008). Many other countries have similar types of publications. The World Health Organization (WHO) publishes worldwide surveillance information and recommendations for control measures in the *Weekly Epidemiological Record*. A more detailed background on infectious agents as determinants of health and disease is provided in Volume 1, Chapters 2.7, and Volume 3, Chapters 9.11–9.15, and 9.17.

Definitions of infectious diseases and their control

Infection occurs when an infectious agent enters a body and develops or multiplies. *Infectious agents* are organisms capable of producing inapparent infection or clinically manifest disease and include bacteria, rickettsia, chlamydiae, fungi, parasites, viruses, and prions. An *infectious disease*, or communicable disease, is an infection that results in a clinically manifest disease. Infectious disease may also be due to the toxic product of an infectious agent, such as the toxin produced by *Clostridium botulinum* causing classical botulism. As this is a textbook of public health, the infectious diseases considered are those that manifest in human hosts and are a result of the interaction of people, animals, and their environment. Infectious diseases may be due to infectious agents exclusively found in human hosts such as rubella virus, in the environment such as *Legionella pneumophila*, or primarily in animals such as *Brucella abortus*.

Control of infectious diseases refers to the actions and programmes directed toward reducing disease incidence (new infections), reducing disease prevalence (infections in the community at any given point in time), or completely eradicating the disease. Control aimed at reducing the incidence of infectious disease can be considered as *primary prevention* of infectious disease. Primary prevention protects health through individual and community-wide measures, including such actions as maintaining good nutritional status, keeping physically fit, immunizing against infectious diseases, providing safe water, and ensuring the proper disposal of faeces.

Control aimed at reducing the prevalence by shortening the duration of infectious disease can be considered as *secondary prevention* of infectious disease. Secondary prevention corrects departures from good health through individual and community-wide measures, including such actions as early detection of disease, prompt antibiotic treatment and ensuring adequate nutrition. It should be noted that such control efforts in secondary prevention in a group of infected individuals may also result in primary prevention in uninfected persons. For example, prompt and specific drug therapy for tuberculosis patients resulting in sputum conversion to culture negative status renders them no longer a source of infection to others.

Control aimed at reducing or even eliminating long-term impairments of infectious disease can be considered as *tertiary prevention* of infectious disease. Tertiary prevention reduces or eliminates disabilities, minimizes suffering, and promotes adjustment to permanent disabilities through such actions as providing orthopedic appliances, counselling and vocational training, and prevention of opportunistic infections. For example, the prevention of opportunistic infections in HIV infection can be considered as tertiary prevention (Osterholm *et al.* 2005).

Global burden of infectious diseases

A World Health Organization (WHO) analysis of the global burden of disease estimates that infectious diseases caused 14.9 million deaths, accounting for 26 per cent of total global mortality of 57.0 million deaths in 2002 (WHO 2004a). Five diseases, respiratory infections, AIDS, diarrhoeal diseases, tuberculosis and, malaria, account for some 77 per cent of the total infectious disease burden. Most infectious disease (some 95 per cent, or 14.1 million) deaths occur in the economically developing group of countries where approximately one in three deaths (14.1 out of 43.6 million) are due to an infectious cause. However, infectious diseases are also of importance in more developed countries. In the United States, for example, AIDS rose to become the leading cause of death in persons aged 25–44 years in the late 1980s and early 1990s, and still ranks as an important cause of death in this age group.

The current magnitude of morbidity and mortality due to infectious diseases worldwide is highlighted by the WHO as follows (WHO 2004a):

- *Acute respiratory infections*, including pneumonia and influenza, cause some 451 million episodes of illness each year and result in 4 million deaths annually. These infections are the highest cause of infant and child mortality in developing countries.
- *HIV* newly infects about 2 million people each year and causes an estimated 2.7 million AIDS-related deaths annually. There are now about 33 million people living with HIV as of the end of 2007 (UNAIDS 2007).
- *Diarrhoeal diseases* are also a major cause of morbidity and mortality in infants and children in developing countries. Each year there are some 4.5 billion episodes with 1.8 million deaths due to diarrhoeal disease, of which the vast majority are among children under five years of age.
- *Tuberculosis*, caused by *Mycobacterium tuberculosis*, infects about one-third of the world's population. It is estimated that there are approximately 7.6 million people who develop clinical disease and 1.6 million who die of tuberculosis each year.
- *Malaria* is estimated to cause some 408 million cases of acute illness. An estimated 1.3 million deaths per year worldwide are attributable to malaria, mainly in children under the age of five years.
- *Influenza* epidemics, caused by influenza A and B viruses, are estimated to kill from 500 000 to 1 million people worldwide each year. Influenza pandemics, of which there were three in the last century, have killed as many as 40–50 million people (as occurred during the 1918–1919 'Spanish flu' pandemic) and, as with the current concerns regarding avian influenza (H5N1), continue to threaten to re-emerge as a major public health emergency.

Chain of infection: Agent, transmission, and host

The chain of infection is the relationship between an infectious agent, its routes of transmission, and a susceptible host. The prevention and control of infectious diseases depend on the interaction of these three factors that may result in the human host clinically manifesting disease.

Agent

The infectious agent is the first link in the chain of infection and is any micro-organism whose presence or excessive presence is essential for the occurrence of an infectious disease. Examples of infectious agents include the following:

- *Bacteria:* For example, spirochetes such as *Treponema pallidum* causing syphilis, curved bacteria such as *Borrelia burgdorferi* causing lyme disease, Gram-negative rods such as *Yersinia pestis* causing plague, Gram-positive cocci such as *Streptococcus pyogenes*, group A causing erysipelas, and Gram-positive rods such as *Mycobacterium tuberculosis* causing tuberculosis
- *Rickettsiae:* For example, *Rickettsia ricketsii* causing Rocky Mountain spotted fever, and *Rickettsia prowazekii* causing epidemic louse-borne typhus fever
- *Chlamydiae:* For example, *Chlamydia psittaci* causing psittacosis, and *Chlamydia trachomatis* causing trachoma and genital infections
- *Fungi*: For example, *Trichophyton schoenleinii* and *Microsporum canis* causing tinea capitis, and *Trichophyton rubrum*, *Trichophyton mentagrophytes* and *Epidermophyton floccosum* causing tinea pedis
- *Parasites:* For example, helminths such as *Trichinella spiralis* causing trichinosis, filaria such as *Brugia malayi* causing filariasis, nematodes such as *Enterobius vermicularis* causing enterobiasis (pinworm disease), trematodes such as *Clonorchis sinensis* causing clonorchiasis (oriental liver fluke disease), cestodes such as

Taenia solium causing taeniasis (beef tapeworm disease), and protozoa such as *Trypanosoma cruzi* causing American trypanosomiasis (Chagas' disease)

- *Viruses:* For example, Paramyxoviridae such as measles virus which causes measles, Togaviridae such as rubella virus which causes rubella, and arthropod-borne viruses (arboviruses) such as dengue viruses which cause dengue fever
- *Prions:* Small proteinaceous infectious particles which cause such diseases as kuru, Creutzféldt–Jakob disease (and its variant associated with exposure of humans to the bovine spongiform encephalopathy, or 'mad cow', agent), and the Gerstmann–Straussler–Scheinker syndrome (see Volume 3, Chapter 9.11)

There is increasing evidence that some infectious agents, often with cofactors, are associated with human tumours. Examples include *Shistosoma haematobium* with bladder cancer, *Shistosoma japonicum* with colorectal cancer, *Clonorchis sinensis* with cholangiocarcinoma, hepatitis B and C viruses with hepatocellular carcinoma, *Helicobacter pylori* with gastric cancer, and human papillomaviruses with cervical cancer. Cancers attributed by the International Agency for Research on Cancer (IARC) to infectious agents are considered to account for some 26 per cent and 8 per cent of the total number of cancers in the developing world and industrialized world, respectively (WHO 2003).

Agents can be described by their ability to cause disease (pathogenicity) as well as their ability to cause serious disease (virulence). The *pathogenicity* of an infectious agent is the extent to which clinically manifest disease is produced in an infected population and is measured by the ratio of the number of persons developing clinical illness to the total number infected. Examples of highly pathogenic infectious agents are the measles virus and the human (α) herpesvirus 3 (varicella-zoster), causing measles and chickenpox, respectively, in which most infected susceptible persons will manifest disease.

The *virulence* of an infectious agent is the extent to which severe disease is produced in a population with clinically manifest disease. It is the ratio of the number of persons with severe and fatal disease to the total number of persons with disease. An example of a highly virulent infectious agent is HIV whereby nearly all untreated persons with AIDS will die.

Characteristics of infectious agents that effect pathogenicity include their ability to invade tissues (invasiveness), produce toxins (intoxication), cause damaging hypersensitivity (allergic) reactions, undergo antigenic variation, and develop antibiotic resistance. An example of an infectious agent with high *invasiveness* is the *Shigella* organism which can invade the submucosal tissue of the intestine and cause clinically manifest shigellosis (bacillary dysentery). An example of an infectious agent that has a high degree of ability to *produce toxins* is the *Clostridium botulinum* organism which can elaborate toxins in inadequately prepared food and cause classical botulism. An example of an infectious agent that is highly *allergenic* is the *Mycobacterium tuberculosis* organism which can cause tuberculosis. An example of an infectious agent that has a high degree of *antigenic variation* is the type A influenza virus which frequently experiences minor antigenic changes—antigenic 'drift'. Influenza A viruses, on an irregular basis, may also undergo a major antigenic change creating an entirely new subtype—antigenic 'shift'. Antigenic shifts that have the characteristic of high transmissibility between persons may result in an influenza pandemic when large numbers of individuals are exposed to the new subtype for which they have no prior immunity. An example of an infectious agent that can develop *antibiotic resistance* that challenges control efforts is *Neisseria gonorrhoeae* that has both chromosomally mediated and resistance transfer plasmid mediated genetic factors for antibiotic resistance.

The *infective dose* of an infectious agent is the number of organisms needed to cause an infection. The infective dose may vary depending on the route of transmission and host susceptibility. An example of an infectious agent that need only a very low infective dose (as few as 10 organisms) is *Escherichia coli* O157:H7 which causes enterohaemorrhagic diarrhoea.

Control measures for infectious diseases directed at inactivating the agent are designed according to the type of agent and its reservoirs and sources. For example, an agent like *Vibrio cholerae* can be inactivated through adequate chlorination of the water supply. This is a chemical method for provision of safe water to control cholera. An agent like hepatitis B virus can be inactivated through adequate autoclaving of injection and surgical equipment. This is a sterilization method to control hepatitis B. Details of these and other methods of control directed at the agent are provided in the sections in this chapter on control measures applied to the agent and the environment.

Routes of transmission

Control efforts are often designed to break the routes of transmission, the mechanisms by which infectious agents are spread from reservoirs or sources to human hosts. A *reservoir* of an infectious agent is any person, other living organism, or inanimate material in which the infectious agent normally lives and grows. The *source* of infection for a host is the person, other living organism or inanimate material from which the infectious agent came. *Horizontal transmission* refers to transmission between individuals whereas *vertical transmission* refers to the specific situation of transmission between parent to offspring (for example, transplacentally *in utero*, during passage through the birth canal, or through breast milk). The routes of transmission have been summarized in the *Control of Communicable Diseases Manual* (Heymann 2004) as follows:

Direct transmission

Direct and essentially immediate transfer of infectious agents to a receptive portal of entry through which human or animal infection may take place. This may be by direct contact as touching, biting, kissing, or sexual intercourse, or by the direct projection (droplet spread) of droplet spray onto the conjunctiva or onto the mucous membranes of the eye, nose or mouth during sneezing, coughing, spitting, singing or talking (usually limited to a distance of about 1 m or less). It may also occur through direct exposure of susceptible tissue to an agent in soil or through the bite of an animal, or transplacentally.

Indirect transmission

Vehicle-borne

Contaminated inanimate materials or objects (fomites) such as (a) toys, handkerchiefs, soiled clothes, bedding, cooking or eating utensils, surgical instruments or dressings; (b) water, food, milk, and biological products including blood, serum, plasma, tissues, or organs; or (c) any substance serving as an intermediate means by which an infectious agent is transported and introduced into a susceptible host though a suitable portal of entry. The agent may or may not have multiplied or developed in or on the vehicle before being transmitted.

Vector-borne

Mechanical: Includes simple mechanical carriage by a crawling or flying insect through soiling of its feet or proboscis, or by passage of organisms through its gastrointestinal tract. This does not require multiplication or development of the organism.

Biological: Propagation (multiplication), cyclic development, or a combination of these (cyclopropagative) is required before the arthropod can transmit the infective form of the agent to humans. An incubation period (extrinsic) is required following infection before the arthropod becomes infective. Maintenance of infectious agents may occur within vectors through transovarian or transstadial transmission. In transovarian transmission, the infectious agent is passed vertically to succeeding generations (for example, an important mechanism for maintaining *Rickettsia rickettsii* in nature is the through infected eggs passed by an infected adult female tick which will hatch into infected larvae). In transstadial transmission the infectious agent is maintained in the vector as the vector passages from one stage of its lifecycle to another (for example, ticks infected with *Rickettsia rickettsii* can remain infected with this agent as they passage from nymph to adult stages). Transmission may be by injection of salivary gland fluid during biting, or by regurgitation or deposition on the skin of faeces or other material capable of penetrating through the bite wound or through an area of trauma from scratching or rubbing. This transmission is by an infected non-vertebrate host and not simple mechanical carriage by a vector as a vehicle. However, an arthropod in either role is termed a vector.

Airborne transmission

It is the dissemination of microbial aerosols to a suitable portal of entry, usually the respiratory tract. Microbial aerosols are suspensions of particles in the air consisting partially or wholly of microorganisms. They may remain suspended in the air for long periods of time, some retaining and others losing infectivity or virulence. Particles in the 1–5 μm range are easily drawn into the alveoli of the lungs and may be retained there. Microbial transmission through droplets and other large particles that promptly settle out of the air is considered as direct, not airborne, transmission.

Droplet nuclei: Usually the small residues which result from evaporation of fluid from droplets emitted by an infected host. They also may be created purposely by a variety of atomizing devices, or accidentally as in microbiology laboratories or in abattoirs, rendering plants or autopsy rooms. They usually remain suspended in the air for long periods.

Dust: The small particles of widely varying size which may arise from soil (for example, fungus spores), clothes, bedding, or contaminated floors.

Control measures for infectious diseases directed at interrupting transmission are designed according to the type of transmission for the agent. Direct transmission of an agent like *Neisseria gonorrhoeae*, for example, can be reduced by using condoms as a barrier method of control of gonorrhoea. Vector-borne transmission of an agent like *Plasmodium falciparum* can be reduced by using a residual insecticide against *Anopheles* mosquitoes as a chemical vector control method for malaria. Airborne transmission of an agent like *Mycobacterium tuberculosis* from sputum-positive pulmonary tuberculosis patients in hospital can be reduced by the use of special ventilation in the patient's room as an environmental method of control of tuberculosis. It should be recognized that some infectious agents may have more than one route of transmission. Poliovirus, for example, can be spread via direct transmission through the faecal–oral route and pharyngeal spread, or indirect transmission through contaminated food or other materials. Details of these and other methods of control directed at interrupting transmission are provided in the sections on control measures in this chapter.

Host

The human host is the final link in the chain of infection. The infectious agent may enter the host through the following portals of entry.

- *Respiratory tract:* Infectious agents can be inhaled into the respiratory tract and will be deposited at different levels of the pulmonary tree according to the size of the aerosol, droplet nuclei or dust particles. For example, *Mycobacterium tuberculosis* in airborne droplet nuclei, 1–5 μm in diameter, may be inhaled into the alveoli of the lungs of a vulnerable host and result in tuberculosis.
- *Intact skin:* Some infectious agents, such as *Necator americanus* which causes hookworm disease, can penetrate the intact skin.
- *Gastrointestinal tract:* An infectious agent, such as *Vibrio cholerae* which causes cholera, may enter via the gastrointestinal tract. Persons who have a compromised gastric function, such as gastric achlorhydria, may be at increased risk of disease.
- *Mucous membranes:* Infectious agents, such as measles viruses, may be deposited on mucous membranes, including the conjunctiva of the eye, by droplet spread or by direct contact with infected persons or contaminated objects.
- *Urinary tract:* Some infectious agents, such as *Escherichia coli* which causes urinary tract infections, can enter the urinary tract via an ascending route from the urethra colonized with the organism. Structural abnormalities of the urinary tract and procedures such as urinary catheterization may predispose the host to disease.
- *Placenta:* Certain infectious agents, such as rubella virus which causes congenital rubella syndrome, can cross the placenta resulting in transplacental transmission, a direct route of transmission from the mother to the fetus that is a form of vertical transmission.

Infectious agents also enter the host though mechanisms that get past the body's natural barriers, including wounds that break the integrity of the skin or mucous membranes; invasive procedures, parenteral injections, parenteral infusions, blood transfusions, or organ transplants that may introduce an agent into the body; or insect vectors that may inject agents through the skin.

The most important host factors regarding developing clinically manifest disease and the severity of disease are immune status and age. Infants, young children, and the elderly are at generally higher risk from more severe disease due to immaturity or deterioration of their immune systems, respectively.

Many host defence mechanisms help prevent infection or disease. *Non-specific* host defence mechanisms include the intact skin, nasal cilia, tears, saliva, mucus, and gastric acid. *Specific* host defence mechanisms include naturally acquired immunity from previous infection, tranplacentally acquired passive immunity in the newborn from the mother, artificially acquired active immunity from immunization, and artificially acquired passive immunity from immunoglobulins and antitoxins.

Host responses to infection that prevent or reduce the severity of infectious disease include (a) polymorphonuclear leukocytosis stimulated by some bacterial infections that increases the number of phagocytic white blood cells, (b) fever that may slow the multiplication of some infectious agents, (c) antibody production that may neutralize some infectious agents or their toxins, (d) interferon production that may block intracellular replication of viruses, and (e) cytotoxic immune cell responses that kill cells infected with viruses.

The *manifestation of infection* in the host may vary from inapparent (subclinical) infection to severe disease that may even result in death. The interaction between an infectious agent, routes of transmission, and host factors determines the spectrum of signs and symptoms. Sometimes the host may become an asymptomatic carrier of the infectious agent and be a source of infection for others.

Control measures for infectious diseases directed at the host are designed according to the immune status of the host and the likelihood of host exposure to certain infectious agents. For example, measles disease can be prevented by active immunization with measles vaccine to develop host immunity. Pneumonic plague can be prevented in those in close contact with patients with plague pneumonia by chemoprophylaxis using tetracycline or sulphonamide. Details of these and other methods of control directed at the host are provided in the section on control measures applied to the host in this chapter.

Tools for control of infectious diseases

The primary concern of infectious disease control in public health, whether in developing or industrialized countries, is the reduction, elimination or even eradication of infectious disease. This is accomplished by directing control measures to the agent, the routes of transmission, or the host. Such control measures include: (a) identifying and then reducing or eliminating infectious agents at their sources and reservoirs, (b) breaking or interfering with the routes of transmission of infectious agents, and (c) identifying susceptible populations and then reducing or eliminating their susceptibility.

The tools for control of infectious diseases are related to recognition and evaluation of the patterns of diseases and the results of interventions to control them. In infectious disease control, the most important tool for recognition and evaluation is *surveillance* of disease defined as:

> *the process of systematic collection, orderly consolidation, analysis, and evaluation of pertinent data with prompt dissemination of the results to those who need to know, particularly those who are in a position to take action. It includes the systematic collection and evaluation of: (a) morbidity and mortality reports; (b) special reports of field investigations of epidemics and of individual cases; (c) isolation and identification of infectious agents by laboratories; (d) data concerning the availability, use, and untoward effects of vaccines and toxoids, immune globulins, insecticides, and other substances used in control; (e) information regarding immunity levels in segments of the population; and (f) other relevant epidemiologic data. A report summarizing the above data should be prepared and distributed to all cooperating persons and others with a need to know the results of the surveillance activities. The procedure applies to all jurisdictional levels of public health from local to international* (Heymann 2004).

Surveillance, therefore, is 'information for action'. More detailed information on surveillance or on field investigations is given in Volume 2, Chapters 6.4, 6.17, and 8.3.

Tools for control related to *interventions* include:

- *Control measures applied to the host:* Active immunization, passive immunization, chemoprophylaxis, behavioural change, reverse isolation, barriers, and improving host resistance.
- *Control measures applied to vectors:* Chemical, environmental, and biological.
- *Control measures applied to infected humans:* Chemotherapy, isolation, quarantine, restriction of activities, and behavioural change.
- *Control measures applied to animals:* Active immunization, isolation, quarantine, restriction or reduction, chemoprophylaxis, and chemotherapy.
- *Control measures applied to the environment:* Provision of safe water, proper disposal of faeces, food and milk sanitation, and design of facilities and equipment.
- *Control measures applied to infectious agents:* Cleaning, cooling, pasteurization, disinfection, and sterilization.

Achieving maximum impact on control of a specific infectious disease may involve more than one of these interventions. For example, the control of hepatitis A infection can be achieved through interventions that may include: Active immunization, passive immunization, food preparation and handwashing behaviours, provision of safe water, food sanitation, and proper disposal of faeces.

The tools for control can also be considered according to the level at which they are applied: Individual, institutional, or community-based. At the *individual level*, control measures, usually initiated by a clinician, are directed toward the specific infectious disease threats to the particular individual. Examples include chemoprophylaxis to prevent wound infection, pre-exposure prophylactic immunization against rabies for a veterinarian, and use of diphtheria antitoxin in a patient with diphtheria.

At the *institutional level*, control measures, usually initiated by the officials of the institution, are directed to a group of people who are in close contact with each other, such as persons in daycare centres, schools, military barracks, hospital wards, nursing homes, and correctional facilities. Examples include (a) administering amantadine hydrochloride or rimantadine for chemoprophylaxis or chemotherapy of influenza A in a high-risk institutional population; (b) quarantining institutionalized young children during a measles outbreak; and (c) hepatitis B immunization of staff and clients of institutions for the developmentally disabled.

At the *community level*, control measures, usually initiated by local, state or national public health agencies, are directed to the community at large. Examples include childhood immunization programmes, provision of safe water, regulation of food supplies, and recall of contaminated food products.

It should be noted that some control measures, such as immunization, may take place at all levels while others, such as the provision of safe water to a community, are more specifically applied at a particular level.

The tools for the control of infectious diseases and their relationship to the chain of infection are the main focus of the remainder of this chapter.

Control measures applied to the host

Control measures applied to the host range from relatively easily administered immunization to behavioural changes that may be extremely difficult for an individual to accept and practice. This section details the types of control measures applied to susceptible hosts and gives examples of their application in the control of selected infectious diseases.

Active immunization

One of the most efficient control measures applied to a host is one that renders the host immune from infectious disease by an infectious agent. Active immunization is a cornerstone of public health measures for the control of many infectious diseases and is considered one of the most cost-effective methods of individual, institutional and community protection for vaccine-preventable infectious diseases. The most powerful example of the potential impact of active immunization against an infectious disease is that of smallpox vaccination. Mobilization of political will on a worldwide basis, coupled with full application of the strategies of active surveillance and containment immunization against smallpox, ultimately resulted in the complete global eradication of the disease and cessation of transmission of the infectious agent, variola virus.

Active immunization is usually considered synonymous with the term vaccination, and is the process of administration of an antigen that can induce a specific immune response that protects a susceptible host from an infectious disease. Some draw a distinction between the two terms. Narrowly defined, *vaccination* is the process of administration of an antigen and *immunization* is the development of a specific immune response. Administering an antigen without evoking an immune response is possible, since no vaccine is 100 per cent effective. Conversely, someone can become immunized even if they were not administered an antigen. For example, the live, attenuated oral polio vaccine viruses can be transmitted from the recipient to other close contacts.

Active immunization can be accomplished through different types of antigens, including the following:

- *Inactivated toxins:* Diphtheria toxoid is an example of a formaldehyde-inactivated preparation of diphtheria toxin that protects against clinically manifest disease, although the immunized person may still become infected with toxin-producing strains of *Corynebacterium diphtheria*. Tetanus toxoid and *Clostridium perfringens* toxoid (pig bel vaccine) are other examples of inactivated toxin preparations.
- *Inactivated complex antigens:* Whole-cell pertussis vaccine is an example of a heat or chemically treated preparation of killed whole pertussis bacteria that protects against clinically manifest disease, although the immunized person may still become infected with *Bordetella pertussis*. Inactivated polio vaccine and inactivated influenza vaccine are other examples of inactivated vaccines.
- *Purified antigens:* Acellular pertussis vaccine is an example of a vaccine composed of isolated and purified immunogenic pertussis antigens. Other vaccines with purified components include polyvalent capsular polysaccharide pneumococcal, polysaccharide meningococcal, protein–polysaccharide conjugate *Haemophilus influenzae* type b, and plasma-derived hepatitis B vaccines.
- *Recombinant antigens:* Hepatitis B recombinant vaccine is an example of a vaccine composed of hepatitis B surface antigen sub-units made through recombinant DNA technology. Human Papilloma Virus vaccine is another example of a DNA recombinant vaccine.
- *Live, attenuated vaccines:* Measles vaccine is an example of a vaccine containing live infectious agents that are of reduced virulence, but induce protective antibodies against measles viruses. Other live, attenuated vaccines include oral polio, mumps, rubella, yellow fever, and bacille Calmette–Guérin (BCG) vaccines.

Protective *antibody responses* usually take 7–21 days to develop. Although most vaccines must be given before exposure to be effective, some vaccines may protect even if administered after exposure to an infectious agent. For example, measles vaccine may provide protection against measles disease if given within 72 h of exposure. This occurs since the percutaneous route of administration of the antigen evokes an immune response faster than the measles virus results in disease through the respiratory route of natural exposure.

Duration of protection varies from only months, such as with killed whole-cell cholera vaccine, to years or even life with some live attenuated vaccines, such as measles vaccine. Some inactivated toxoids and vaccines, such as tetanus toxoid, may require a priming series of doses to be optimally effective and additional booster doses to maintain protective antibodies. Many new technologies are being explored that may increase the number and efficacy of vaccines available against infectious disease, including immune stimulating complexes, live viral or bacterial vector vaccines, and timed-release vaccines.

It should be recognized that vaccines vary in their efficacy and that no vaccine is 100 per cent effective. *Vaccine efficacies* vary with type of vaccine, manufacturing techniques, storage and handling conditions, skill of administration, age of vaccination, and other host factors. Vaccines for routine use are safe. However, no vaccine is 100 per cent safe. Potential vaccinees, or their parents or guardians, should be screened for contraindications and be informed of potential side-effects.

Immunization schedules for the routine control of infectious diseases preventable by immunization vary between countries and are usually based on expert advice to governments and physicians. For example, recommended policies for immunization in the United States are provided by the Advisory Committee on Immunization Practices (ACIP) and are published in the *Morbidity and Mortality Weekly Report* (ACIP 2006). In addition, the American Academy of Pediatrics periodically publishes comprehensive immunization recommendations in its *Report of the Committee on Infectious Diseases* (Committee on Infectious Diseases 2006). At the global level, the WHO publishes recommended immunization schedules and control strategies for vaccine-preventable diseases that are periodically updated by expert advisory groups in the WHO *Weekly Epidemiological Record*.

In *outbreak settings*, immunization schedules may be modified. For example, the age of immunization for measles may be lowered to

6 months of age during an outbreak. In such situations, persons receiving vaccine before the routinely recommended age of immunization should be immunized again at the recommended age since immunization at the earlier age may not have been optimally effective.

Immunization programmes include vaccines for routine child, routine adult, travel, selected high risk populations, and occupational settings. For example, tetanus toxoid is universally recommended; yellow fever vaccine is only recommended in geographic areas of epidemiologic risk; typhoid fever vaccine is only recommended for individuals subject to unusual exposure to typhoid, including persons living in the same household as known carriers; and anthrax vaccine is only recommended for veterinarians and persons occupationally exposed to possibly contaminated industrial raw materials.

Beyond protection of the individual, vaccination may also provide a degree of community protection. This phenomenon is known as herd immunity. *Herd immunity* is the relative protection of a population group achieved by reducing or breaking the chains of transmission of an infectious agent because most of the population is resistant to infection through immunization or prior natural infection. Herd immunity is a complex phenomenon and varies according to the infectious agent, its routes of transmission, the degree to which immunization protects against infection versus only clinically manifest disease, and the distribution of immunization in the population (for example, groups of persons with low vaccination coverage vulnerable to disease introduction may exist within populations with high average levels of vaccination coverage). The mechanisms of herd immunity are several, including 'direct protection of vaccinees against disease or transmissible infection and indirect protection of nonrecipients by virtue of surreptitious vaccination, passive antibody, or just reduced sources of transmission and, hence, risks of infection in the community' (Fine 1993).

A particularly difficult problem for vaccine-preventable infectious disease control programmes is complacency by the population that can result from the very successes of the programmes. Low rates of vaccine-preventable infectious disease may mistakenly lead parents to consider that vaccination is no longer important for maintaining their children's health and may result in political leaders reducing funding for immunization programmes. Low disease rates may also focus undo attention on the relatively rare serious side-effects of vaccination in relation to current rates of disease. Such side-effects should only be compared in relation to rates of disease and its complications that would occur without immunization programmes.

A comprehensive treatment of active immunization is given by Plotkin and Orenstein (2004).

Passive immunization

Passive immunization is a temporary immunity in a host due to the protection afforded by antibody produced in another host. Passive immunity may be acquired either naturally or artificially.

Naturally acquired passive immunity is achieved through transfer of maternal antibodies via the placenta. It is the way that newborn infants are provided with a temporary immunity against many infectious diseases for which the mother is immune. This immunity wanes over time and eventually leaves the infant susceptible to these diseases.

An important use of transplacental immunity as a control measure is in the prevention of tetanus neonatorum (neonatal tetanus) by immunization of women before or during pregnancy with tetanus toxoid. The disease typically occurs when the umbilical cord is cut with an unclean instrument contaminated with tetanus spores or when substances contaminated with tetanus spores are placed on the umbilical stump after delivery. Control by active immunization of the infant cannot be achieved in sufficient time since the average incubation period is only 6 days (with a range from 3 to 28 days). An adequately immunized mother, however, will usually effectively transfer maternal antibodies against tetanus across the placenta to her newborn and prevent tetanus neonatorum.

Another example of naturally acquired passive immunity is the relative protection against measles disease in a young infant born to a mother who previously had the disease. Typically, such infants are immune for approximately 6–9 months or more after birth, depending upon how much residual maternal antibodies are present at the time of pregnancy. Other diseases for which there is usually an effective transplacental immunity in infants, for variable amounts of time, include diphtheria, mumps, poliomyelitis, rubella, and varicella (chickenpox). It should be noted that if the mother is not immune, or if residual maternal antibodies have significantly waned, then the infant may be susceptible to disease.

Research is ongoing as to other infectious diseases that may be preventable in the neonate or infant though immunization of the mother before or during pregnancy. Examples include *Haemophilus influenzae* type b, group B streptococcal and meningococcal diseases (Insel *et al.* 1994). Many diseases, however, are not prevented by transplacental immunity.

Breastfeeding is a form of naturally acquired passive antibody transfer to neonates and infants. Breast milk and colostrum contain secretory immunoglobin A (IgA) antibodies that may play a protective role in the prevention of infections with such agents as respiratory syncytial virus, rotavirus and *Haemophilus influenzae* type b.

Artificially acquired passive immunity is acquired through administration of an antibody-containing preparation, antiserum, or immune globulin. It has a place in the control of certain infectious diseases in special situations. This immunity also wanes over a relatively short period of time.

Examples of the use of artificially acquired passive immunity to control infectious disease include the following:

- *Rabies:* Natural immunity to rabies in humans does not exist. Susceptible individuals bitten by an animal known or suspected to be rabid should receive rabies immune globulin to neutralize the rabies virus in the wound. It should be noted that, besides passive immunization with rabies immune globulin, such individuals should also receive active immunization with rabies vaccine.
- *Hepatitis A:* In areas where sanitation is poor, hepatitis A infection commonly occurs at an early age and therefore most adults in developing countries are already immune. However, epidemics may occur in industrialized countries. Passive immunization with immune globulin may be given to: (a) all household and sexual contacts of patients with hepatitis A; (b) other food handlers in an establishment where hepatitis A has occurred in a food handler; (c) all individuals in an institution where a focal outbreak of hepatitis A has occurred; and (d) persons from industrialized countries travelling to highly endemic areas. It should be noted that vaccines for active immunization for hepatitis A are available.

- *Diphtheria:* Treatment of this disease is an example of the use of an antibody containing product (diphtheria antitoxin) produced in an animal (only diphtheria antitoxin from horses is available) administered as part of the treatment regimen for secondary prevention of disease. In suspected cases of diphtheria, the antitoxin must be given as soon as possible because it is only effective in neutralizing diphtheria toxins not yet bound to cells.
- *Other important infectious diseases, including hepatitis B, measles, tetanus, varicella:* Depending upon the circumstances of exposure, susceptibility of the host, and status of the host's general immune system there are circumstances under which hepatitis B immune globulin, tetanus immune globulin, varicella-zoster immune globulin, or immune globulin may be warranted.

Chemoprophylaxis

Chemoprophylaxis is the prevention of infection or its progression to clinically manifest disease through the administration of chemical substances, including antibiotics. Chemoprophylaxis can also consist of the treatment of a disease to prevent complications of that disease (Solomon *et al.* 2004). Chemoprophylaxis may be specifically directed against a particular infectious agent or it may be non-specifically directed against many infectious agents. The use of antibiotics before surgical procedures is an example of non-specific chemoprophylaxis to prevent wound infections in the postoperative period. Examples of specific chemoprophylaxis are given below.

The use of chemoprophylaxis to *prevent development of infection* is illustrated by using chloroquine to prevent malarial parasitemia caused by *Plasmodium vivax, Plasmodium ovale, Plasmodium malariae* and chloroquine-sensitive strains of *Plasmodium falciparum*. For some chloroquine resistant strains of *Plasmodium falciparum*, alternative regimes include mefloquine alone, doxycycline alone, primaquine alone, or an atovaquone/proguanil combination. Primaquine may be given to reduce the risk of a relapse from intrahepatic forms of *Plasmodium vivax* and *Plasmodium ovale* after discontinuation of chemoprophylaxis with any chemosuppresive drugs other than primaquine. Determination of a specific malaria chemoprophylactic regimen is complex. It must take into account the geographic area, the possibility of pregnancy, the weight of an individual (dose size for children is determined by body weight), and the risks of adverse reactions to the chemoprophylactic regimen.

Other examples of prevention of development of infection include the following:

- The use of silver nitrate, erythromycin or tetracycline instilled into the eyes of a newborn to prevent gonococcal ophthalmia by transmission of *Neisseria gonorrhoeae* from an infected mother during birth
- The use of tetracycline, sulphonamides (including sulphadiazine and trimethoprim-sulphamethoxazole), chloramphenicol or streptomycin in close contacts of confirmed or suspected cases of plague pneumonia to prevent plague pneumonia by transmission of *Yersinia pestis*
- The use of benzathine penicillin in those in sexual contact with confirmed cases of early syphilis to prevent syphilis by transmission of *Treponema pallidum*

An example of the use of chemoprophylaxis to 'prevent the progression of an infection to active manifest disease' is the use of isoniazid (INH) to prevent the progression of latent infection with *Mycobacterium tuberculosis* to clinical tuberculosis. Persons less than 35 years of age who are tuberculosis test positive should receive isoniazid to prevent clinical tuberculosis. The decision to use isoniazid, especially in individuals more than 35 years of age, must be determined based on such information as length of infection, closeness of association with a current case, status of the immune system, presence of acute liver disease, possibilities of pregnancy and risks of adverse reactions.

Other examples of prevention of progression of an infection to active manifest disease through the use of chemoprophylaxis include the following:

- Co-trimoxazole or pentamidine to prevent subclinical latent infection with *Pneumocystis carinii* from progressing to clinically manifest pneumocystis pneumonia in immunosuppressed persons such as HIV-infected individuals
- Mebendazole, albendazole, or pyrantel pamoate to prevent infection with *Necator americanus, Ancylostoma duodenale*, and *Ancylostoma Ceylanicum* from progressing to the clinically manifest anaemia of hookworm disease
- Pyrimethamine combined with sulphadiazine and folinic acid (to avoid possible bone marrow depression) to prevent asymptomatic infants congenitally infected with *Toxoplasma gondii* from progressing to clinically manifest chorioretinitis and other sequelae of congenital toxoplasmosis

In some situations, establishing *screening* programmes to detect and treat asymptomatic or unrecognized infections in defined populations is useful. An example is the screening for *Chlamydia trachomatis* in sexual partners of persons infected with *Chlamydia Trachomatis*, women with mucopurulent cervicitis, sexually active women 25 years of age or younger, and women older than 25 years of age with risk factors for chlamydia. A more detailed background on screening as a public health function is given in Volume 3, Chapter 12.7.

An example of the use of chemoprophylaxis to 'treat an infectious disease to prevent complications of the disease' is the use of penicillin (or erythromycin in penicillin-sensitive patients) to treat streptococcal sore throats caused by *Streptococcus pyogenes* group A to prevent acute rheumatic fever.

Other examples of prevention of complications of an infectious disease through the use of chemoprophylaxis include the following:

- Tetracycline for adults, or penicillin for children, for treatment of lyme disease caused by *Borrelia burgdorferi* in the erythema chronicum migrans stage to prevent or reduce the severity of late cardiac, arthritic or neurologic complications
- Benzathine penicillin for treatment of syphilis in its primary, secondary, or early latency period to prevent late manifestations of the disease such as cardiovascular syphilis
- Ketoconazole for treatment of blastomycosis caused by *Blastomyces dermatitidis* in its early stages to prevent progression of chronic pulmonary or disseminated blastomycosis that may lead to death

Potential problems with the use of chemoprophylaxis may include compromise of the host's own non-specific defence mechanisms, other replacement infectious agents causing disease by growing in the place of the infectious agent affected by the specific chemoprophylactic regimen, and emergence of resistant strains of the infectious agent. The development of antibiotic resistance can be reduced by using antibiotics only when needed, selecting the proper antibiotic (or, in some situations, the appropriate multidrug therapy) for the infectious agent, and ensuring compliance with the appropriate regimen for the duration of treatment.

Behavioural change

Perhaps the most challenging tool for the control of infectious diseases, and sometimes one of the most powerful and cost-effective, is behaviour change in the host that reduces or eliminates risk of exposure to an agent. Everyone has developed habits of living (lifestyles) that are not easily changed. Some of these behaviours are protective against infectious diseases. Others render the individual at higher risk of infection.

Examples of higher risk of exposure to infectious agents through behaviour, and behaviour changes that can have an impact on the chain of transmission, include the following.

Sexual behaviour

Many infectious agents are transmitted by the direct transmission route through sexual contact, including *Chlamydia trachomatis* causing chlamydial genital infections, *Neisseria gonorrhoeae* causing gonorrhoea, *Treponema pallidum* causing venereal syphilis, *Calymmatobacterium granulomatis* causing granuloma inguinale, *Heamophilus ducreyi* causing chancroid, herpes simplex virus causing herpes simplex, *Trichomonas vaginalis* causing trichomoniasis, human papillomaviruses causing condyloma acuminate, and HIV causing AIDS.

Abstinence behaviour, i.e. refraining from sexual activity with other persons, eliminates the risk of transmission of these agents through sexual contact. The delaying of age of first sexual activity avoids the risk of transmission of these agents at an early age. Restricting sexual contact to only between two uninfected persons who do not have sexual activity with any other persons virtually eliminates the risk of transmission of these agents through sexual behaviours. The exceptions are due to other routes of transmission of some of these agents (for example, HIV acquired through intravenous drug use in one partner being transmitted through sexual contact to the other partner). Limiting the number of sexual partners, and limiting those sexual partners to persons who also have few sexual partners, reduces the risk of exposure. However, at the individual level, if one of these sexual partners has an infectious agent transmissible by sexual contact, the risk of transmission may still be high. Finally, condom use during sexual activity in high risk situations will markedly reduce, but not eliminate, transmission. A more detailed background on sexually transmitted diseases is provided in Volume 3, Chapters 9.12 and 9.13.

Intravenous drug use behaviour

Injection of drugs using non-sterile needles or syringes previously used by other intravenous drug users may transmit infectious agents in blood through the vehicle-borne route of indirect transmission, including HIV causing AIDS; hepatitis B virus causing viral hepatitis B; and *Plasmodium vivax, Plasmodium malariae*, and *Plasmodium ovale* causing malaria.

Abstinence behaviour, i.e. refraining from intravenous drug use, eliminates the risk of transmission of such agents through contaminated needles and syringes. Using a sterile needle and sterile syringe for intravenous drug use will break the chain of transmission of these infectious agents through this route. Some community public health programmes, in addition to promoting drug abstinence and drug rehabilitation, conduct needle and syringe exchanges and education regarding methods of decontamination to help promote the use of sterile injection equipment among intravenous drug users (see Volume 3, Chapter 10.2).

Eating behaviour

Eating certain foods may result in exposure to infectious agents through the vehicle-borne route of indirect transmission. These behaviours include consuming raw molluscs by which an infectious agent like the hepatitis A virus can cause viral hepatitis A, eating raw eggs by which an infectious agent like a *Salmonella* serotype can cause salmonellosis, and consuming raw beef by which an infectious agent like *Taenia saginata* can cause beef tapeworm infection.

Although food and diet are strongly ingrained behaviours, modification of dietary patterns is possible. Cooking foods like beef, pork, and eggs can markedly reduce risk of transmission of infectious agents. In addition, reducing risks by elimination of infectious agents from the food may be possible (see the section on control methods applied to the environment). Handwashing before eating also reduces risk of transmission of many infectious agents that are spread through direct or indirect routes of faecal–oral transmission, such as *Shigella dysenteriae, Shigella flexneri, Shigella boydii*, and *Shigella sonnei* which may cause shigellosis (bacillary dysentery).

Working behaviour

In certain occupations, many behaviours may result in exposure to infectious agents and should be targets for control programmes in occupational safety and health settings. Specific examples include the following:

- Dental workers performing procedures with bare hands may result in exposure to hepatitis B viruses from infected patients.
- Health workers improperly handling used needles may result in needle-stick injuries leading to exposure to HIV from infected patients.
- Hospital laboratory workers improperly processing specimens containing infectious agents without appropriate glove or eyewear protection may result in exposure to these agents.
- Veterinarians who do not properly handle animals may result in brucellosis (undulant fever) due to exposure to *Brucella abortus, Brucella melitensis, Brucella suis*, or *Brucella canis*.

Occupational hazards related to non-infectious materials may predispose an individual to increased risk of infectious diseases. For example, working conditions and behaviours in industrial plants and mines that lead to silicosis due to long-term inhalation of free crystalline silica dust will greatly increase the risk of developing tuberculosis.

Working behaviours appropriate for the particular occupational setting may include wearing protective clothing, eyewear and gloves; handwashing and changing clothes after work; meticulous adherence to needle disposal and equipment sterilization procedures; and using hooded laboratory benches when handling highly infectious specimens.

Other behaviours

Other behaviours that may reduce the transmission of infectious agents include the following:

- Scheduling outdoor activities at periods of low vector activity, applying insect repellents and sleeping under bednets reduce the indirect transmission of vector-borne agents of infectious diseases like malaria

- Searching oneself for attached ticks every 3–4 h when playing or working in tick-infested areas reduces the indirect transmission of vector-borne agents of infectious diseases like Rocky Mountain spotted fever
- Avoiding sharing of utensils, cups, toothbrushes, or towels reduces the indirect transmission of vehicle-borne agents of infectious diseases like mononucleosis
- Wearing of shoes reduces the direct transmission of infectious agents like those causing hookworm disease
- Frequently bathing and regular washing of clothes in hot soapy water controls body lice
- Breastfeeding reduces diarrhoeal diseases in the infant, although it may transmit HIV from HIV-infected mothers
- Handwashing after defecation or touching potentially contaminated surfaces, persons, or animals prior to preparing food or touching ones own eyes, mucus membranes, or mouth reduces the risk of direct or indirect transmission of a wide variety of infectious agents
- Large family sizes and crowding may facilitate airborne transmission of infectious agents in droplet nuclei for infectious diseases like tuberculosis

Some of these other behaviours, like crowding, are conditioned by circumstances such as poverty that are not easily or directly amenable to programmes promoting behavioural change.

Reverse isolation

Certain rare circumstances exist where a means of avoiding transmission of an infectious disease to a highly susceptible host is to provide reverse, or protective, isolation. Such isolation attempts to protect infection-prone patients from potentially harmful infectious agents. Reverse isolation procedures range from provision of a private room with the use of masks, gloves and gowns by all persons entering the room, to elaborate facilities with laminar airflow rooms and sterilization of all food. Protective isolation is usually conducted for a limited time until the normal immune system recovers, a regimen of passive immunization is begun, or a bone marrow transplant is successful.

Examples of persons who may need periods of reverse isolation include those who have such diseases as X-linked agammaglobulinemia, DiGeorge's syndrome, and severe combined immunodeficiency; or those who have received therapies, such as some forms of cancer chemotherapy, that have severely compromised the person's immune system.

Barriers

One tool of control that can be applied to the host is the use of barriers between the host and the infectious agent. The effectiveness of such barriers, however, may be dependent on the behaviour of the host to use them consistently. Examples of barriers include the following:

- Screens, bednets (including bednets impregnated with pyrethroid insecticides such as permethrin), long-sleeved shirts and trousers (with the cuffs tucked into boots as a mechanical barrier), and repellents (such as *N*,*N*-diethyl-meta-toluamide known as DEET) to prevent transmission of malaria through the bite of infected female *Anopheles* mosquitoes or West Nile virus through *Culix* mosquitoes
- Condoms to prevent transmission of HIV and other sexually transmitted infectious agents through sexual intercourse
- Masks (air-purifying respirators) to prevent transmission of tuberculosis through airborne droplet nuclei from patients with sputum-positive pulmonary tuberculosis

General improvement in host resistance

Improving host resistance though general improvement of the immune system is a non-specific approach, but may be important in certain settings. Kwashiorkor, marasmus, and other forms of malnutrition debilitate the host's immune system and may make an individual more susceptible to infectious diseases. Moreover, persons who are malnourished and succumb to an infectious disease are at higher risk of the disease being of greater severity and leading to other complications.

Malnutrition also encompasses micronutrient deficiencies. Vitamin A deficiency, for example, has been linked to higher rates of mortality associated with measles disease. Correcting vitamin A deficiency, through programmes of supplementation, fortification, and dietary modification in high-risk populations, can reduce mortality rates due to measles.

A complex interaction exists between infectious diseases, such as diarrhoeal diseases and malnutrition. A downward spiral of infection may lead to malnutrition that, in turn, leads to more infections, and so on. If unchecked, especially in developing countries, this downward spiral can ultimately result in death.

International travel

The special situation of international travel combines many control measures applied to the host already mentioned. The increase in the numbers of travellers, the speed of travel, and the ability to reach areas previously infrequently visited have reduced the effectiveness of surveillance for infectious diseases at ports of arrival and increased infectious disease risks. Advice for prevention against infectious diseases must be both general and specific.

General advice includes such issues as avoidance of eating and drinking potentially contaminated food or drink (including ice) and swimming or bathing in polluted water. Specific advice must be provided based on information about the area to be visited and may include such measures as active immunization against yellow fever, active or passive immunization against hepatitis A, chemoprophylaxis against malaria, repellents against potentially infected mosquitoes, and not walking barefoot in areas of risk for infection with hookworms *Strongyloides stercoralis* and *Strongyloides fuelleborni*. A more detailed background on international travel and health is provided in the annually updated WHO publication on *International Travel and Health* (WHO 2008).

Control measures applied to vectors

Vector-borne transmission is the only or main route of transmission for many infectious diseases. There exist more than 100 arthropod-borne viruses that may produce clinically manifest diseases in humans. Control of vector-borne diseases includes measures to: (a) Change behaviour and create barriers to the susceptible host; (b) reduce or break the chain of transmission of the infectious agent from an infected host to the vector; and (c) directly control the vector population itself. Chemical, environmental, and biological controls are the primary means of directly controlling the vector population.

Chemical control

Chemicals used in the control of vectors include minerals, natural plant products (botannicals), chlorinated hydrocarbons, organophosphates, carbamates, and fumigants. Chemical control measures include the following public health interventions:

- Spraying chemical insecticides such as organochlorine insecticides (for example, dichlorodiphenyltrichlorothane, or DDT, and dieldrin), organophosphorus insecticides (for example, malathion and fenitrothion), and carbonate insecticides (for example, propoxur and carbaryl) to prevent malaria through control of mosquitoes
- Spraying chemical biodegradable insecticides such as temephos (Abate®) to prevent onchocerciasis through control of *Simulium* fly vectors
- Using traps impregnated with decamethrin to prevent African trypanosomiasis (sleeping sickness) through reduction of the population of infective species of *Glossina* (tsetse fly) vectors
- Treating snail breeding places with chemical molluscicides to prevent schistosomiasis due to the free-swimming cercariae (larval forms) of *Schistosoma mansoni, Schistosoma haematobium, and Schistosoma japonicum* that develop in snails
- Treating step-wells and ponds with chemical insecticides such as temephos (Abate®) to prevent dracunculiasis due to infected cyclops (a crustacean copepod)
- Suppressing rat populations by poisoning, preceded or accompanied by measures to control fleas, as an additional measure to supplement environmental sanitation to control rodent populations to prevent human plague

The use of spraying for control of mosquitoes is complicated due to concerns of environmental contamination by chemicals such as DDT and dieldrin which have lead to their being banned in many countries. In addition, the emergence of mosquito vectors resistant to the insecticides diminishes their effectiveness in many areas. New methods of application, such as ultra low-volume spraying of malathion, reduce the amounts of insecticide used.

Environmental control

Environmental control of vectors includes the following public health interventions:

- Eliminating breeding sites of mosquito larvae by filling and draining areas of stagnant water and removing objects around houses that may collect water
- Destroying the habitats of the tsetse fly vector
- Properly implementing landfill procedures, placing lids on rubbish bins, covering food for human consumption, screening privies, cleaning up spilled food, and appropriately storing food
- Placing roach and fly traps
- Constructing rat-proof houses
- Eliminating rodent habitats

It is also important to note that certain development projects may have an impact on the environment that facilitates the growth of vector or intermediate host populations and results in increased infectious diseases. Construction of artificial waterways may serve as breeding sites for *Simulium* fly vectors that can transmit *Onchocerca volvulus* resulting in onchocerciasis. Irrigation schemes can foster the growth of snail intermediate hosts required for the transmission of species of *Schistosoma* resulting in schistosomiasis. Carefully conducted environmental and health impact studies that consider the impact of a construction project on the vector and intermediate host populations, and ways to modify the project to reduce such populations, are important environmental control measures.

Biological control

Biological control of vectors includes the following public health interventions.

- *Introduction of predators and parasites:* The introductions of *Gambusia affinis*, a small fish that feeds on mosquito larvae, and of *Coelomomyces*, a fungal parasite, are examples of control measures that are effective against *Aëdes* mosquitoes.
- *Insect growth regulators*: The use of such regulators may result in death or sterility of vectors by interfering with normal insect development. An example is the use of methoprene (Altosid®) to control flood water mosquitoes.
- *Genetic modification:* Although still at an experimental phase, researchers have developed transgenic, or genetically modified, mosquitoes that are malaria resistant with higher survival rates that could eventually replace mosquitoes that carry malaria parasites.

Control measures applied to infected humans

Control measures may be applied to infected persons at the individual level, in the institutional or hospital setting, and at the community level.

Hospital infection control

The hospital setting is a unique situation that requires special efforts to prevent and control nosocomial infections, or healthcare-associated infections (HAIs), which are infections that originate or occur in a hospital or other healthcare setting. HAIs are a major problem world-wide. In the United States alone, some 2 million HAIs occur annually resulting in an estimated 90 000 deaths and US$4.5 billion in excess healthcare costs (McKibben 2005).

Infection control programmes for hospitals should ideally include the following elements:

- An infection control committee responsible for overall co-ordination of infection control activities
- One or more infection control practitioners responsible for nosocomial disease surveillance, analysis of data, consultation and training of hospital staff
- A hospital epidemiologist to supervise the infection control practitioners, oversee data collection and analysis, and implement any needed emergency infection control measures
- An engineer to direct engineering and preventive maintenance operations, especially ventilation equipment

- A sanitarian to develop procedures for proper disposal of liquid and solid wastes; and sanitation of water, ice, and food
- Effective guidelines for patient care practices
- Surveillance of patient care practices, patient infections, and environmental contamination by infectious agents
- Co-ordination with other departments (microbiology laboratory, central services, housekeeping, food service, and laundry)
- Vector control
- Thorough investigation of problems

Examples of specific control measures that may be applied to infected humans at the individual, institutional, and community levels are detailed in the next section.

Chemotherapy

Treatment of persons with infectious diseases or subclinical infections may be a control tool for some infectious diseases. Such treatment may or may not have an impact on disease progression in the patient. It should be noted that rapid case detection and prompt application of appropriate chemotherapeutic agents are needed to limit infectivity.

Some important examples of control by chemotherapy include the following:

- Treatment of patients with sputum-positive pulmonary *tuberculosis* with appropriate multi-drug therapy will usually result in sputum conversion rendering them non-infectious to others within a few weeks. Recommended treatment regimens include isoniazid (INH) combined with one or more of the following antibiotics: Rifampin, streptomycin, ethambutol, and pyrazinamide. The WHO has recommended that adherence to a complete course of multi-drug therapy be directly observed by another responsible person as part of the DOTS (directly observed treatment, short-course) global strategy for the control of tuberculosis.
- Patients with *leprosy* treated with appropriate multi-drug therapy are considered no longer infectious within 3 months of regular and continued treatment. Recommended treatment regimens for multibacillary leprosy include the following antibiotics: Rifampicin, dapsone and clofazimine.
- Treatment of patients with *streptococcal sore throats* with penicillin (or erythromycin for penicillin-sensitive patients) will usually render them no longer be infectious after 24 to 48 hours.
- Patients with *pertussis* treated with antibiotics such as erythromycin or trimethoprim-sulphamethoxazole, although they may not affect the patient's symptoms, will usually result in the patient no longer being infectious after 5–7 days.

Of special note is the situation of treatment of persons who are carriers. A *carrier* is

> *a person or animal that harbors a specific infectious agent without discernible clinical disease and serves as a potential source of infection. The carrier state may exist in an individual with an infection that is inapparent throughout its course (commonly known as* healthy *or* asymptomatic carrier*), or during the incubation period, convalescence, and post-convalescence of an individual with a clinically recognizable disease (commonly known as* incubatory carrier *or* convalescent carrier*). Under either circumstance the carrier state may be of short or long duration (*temporary *or* transient carrier*, or* chronic carrier*)* (Heymann 2004).

A chronic carrier of diphtheria, for example, may shed the infectious agent *Corynebacterium diphtheriae* for 6 months or more, but appropriate antibiotic therapy will usually promptly stop the carrier state. Another example is that of untreated patients with typhoid fever due to *Salmonella typhi*. Between 2 and 5 per cent of such patients will become permanent carriers. Treatment with appropriate antibiotics may be effective in ending the carrier state.

Antibiotic treatment may not always eliminate a carrier state for some infectious agents. For example, the treatment of persons with salmonellosis with an antibiotic may not terminate the period of communicability and can even result in emergence of antibiotic-resistant strains. However, antibiotic therapy may be still warranted under certain circumstances.

In some situations, establishing screening programmes in defined target populations for identification of asymptomatic or unrecognized infections that could be transmitted to others may be appropriate. Such screening should include the necessary follow-up with appropriate chemotherapy and counselling. An example would be screening close contacts of diphtheria patients with nose and throat cultures for the presence of *Corynebacterium diphtheriae*. Identified carriers with positive cultures should be treated with appropriate antibiotic therapy.

Isolation

Isolation is the 'separation, for the period of at least equal to the period of communicability, of infected persons or animals from others in such places and under such conditions as to prevent or limit the direct or indirect transmission of the infectious agent from those infected to those who are susceptible to infection or who may spread the agent to others' (Heymann 2004).

The Centers for Disease Control and Prevention (CDC), USA, and the Hospital Infection Control Practices Advisory Committee (HICPAC) have provided guidelines for isolation precautions in hospital settings (HICPAC 1996). There are two levels of isolation precautions, namely, (a) a standard precautions level designed for the care of all hospitalized patients, and (b) a transmission-based precautions level designed for the care of hospitalized patients that are suspected or confirmed to be infected by agents spread by contact, droplet, or airborne routes of transmission. These are summarized from HICPAC (1996) as follows.

Standard precautions are universally applied precautions designed to reduce the risk of transmission by infectious agents from blood; body fluids, secretions, and excretions; non-intact skin; and mucous membranes. The essential elements of standard precautions include handwashing; use of gloves; appropriate application of mask and eye protection or a face shield; utilization of gowns; proper handling of patient-care equipment; adequate environmental control measures for routine care, cleaning and disinfection of frequently touched surfaces; appropriate handling, transporting, and processing of used linen; proper handling and disposal of needles, scalpels, and other sharp instruments; and placement of patients who contaminate the environment in private rooms.

Airborne precautions are used, in addition to standard precautions, in settings where patients are suspected or confirmed to be infected by agents transmitted by airborne droplet nuclei.

The essential elements of airborne precautions include placement of patients in a private room that has monitored negative air pressure (if necessary, it is possible to use cohorting of patients with the same active infections); use of mask respirators (N-95 air-purifying respirators); and limiting patient movement and transport from the room (placing a surgical mask on the patient if they are being moved for an essential purpose). An example of an infectious disease for which patients are recommended to be placed under airborne precautions is a patient in hospital with measles through the fourth day of rash. Although isolation of patients with measles not in hospital is not practical in the general population, schoolchildren should remain out of school through at least the fourth day of rash.

Droplet precautions are used, in addition to standard precautions, in settings where patients are suspected or confirmed to be infected by agents transmitted by droplets. The essential elements of droplet precautions include placement of patients in a private room (if necessary, it is possible to use cohorting of patients with the same active infections or maintaining a spatial separation of at least 3 feet between the infected patient and other patients and visitors); use of a mask when working within 3 feet of the patient; and limiting patient movement and transport from the room (placing a surgical mask on the patient if they are being moved for an essential purpose). Examples of infectious diseases for which patients are recommended to be placed under droplet precautions include pharyngeal diphtheria caused by *Corynebacterium diphtheriae* and pneumonic plague caused by *Yersinia pestis*.

Contact precautions are used, in addition to standard precautions, in settings where patients are suspected or confirmed to be infected or colonized by agents transmitted by direct or indirect contact. The essential elements of contact precautions include placement of the patient in a private room (if necessary, it is possible to use cohorting of patients with the same active infections); use of gloves when entering the patient's room and removing them before leaving the room; wearing a gown when entering the patient's room and removing the gown before leaving the room; limiting patient movement and transport to essential purposes only; and, when possible, dedicate the use of patient-care equipment to a single patient (if necessary, it is possible to use such equipment on a cohort of patients with the same active or colonized infections). Examples of infectious diseases for which patients are recommended to be placed under contact isolation precautions include cutaneous diphtheria caused by *Corynebacterium diphtheriae*, rubella, and disseminated herpes simplex caused by herpes simplex virus.

Quarantine of potentially infected persons

Quarantine is the 'restriction of the activities of well persons or animals who have been exposed (or are considered to be at high risk of exposure) to a case of communicable disease during its period of communicability (i.e. contacts) to prevent disease transmission during the incubation period if infection should occur'. Two categories of quarantine are as follows (Heymann 2004):

- *Absolute* or *complete quarantine*. The limitation of freedom of movement of those exposed to a communicable disease for a period of time not longer than the longest usual incubation period of that disease, in such manner as to prevent effective contact with those not so exposed.
- *Modified quarantine*. A selective, partial limitation of freedom of movement of contacts, commonly on the basis of known or presumed differences in susceptibility and related to the assessed risk of disease transmission. It may be designed to accommodate particular situations. Examples are exclusion of children from school, exemption of immune persons from provisions applicable to susceptible persons, or restriction of military populations to the post or to quarters. Modified quarantine includes: *Personal surveillance*, the practice of close medical or other supervision of contacts to permit prompt recognition of infection or illness but without restricting their movements; and *segregation*, the separation of some part of a group of persons or domestic animals from the others for special consideration, control or observation; removal of susceptible children to homes of immune persons; or establishment of a sanitary boundary to protect uninfected from infected portions of a population (known as a *cordon sanitaire)*.

Examples of diseases where quarantine may be considered include the following:

- *Pneumonic plague:* Persons who have been in the same household or in face-to-face contact with patients with pneumonic plague and who do not accept chemoprophylaxis should be placed under *absolute quarantine* with strict isolation, including careful surveillance, for 7 days.
- *Measles:* Although absolute quarantine is impractical, a *modified quarantine* is recommended in settings where young children are living in dormitories, wards or institutions. When measles occurs in such institutional settings, strict *segregation* of infants is recommended.
- *Lassa fever:* Close *personal surveillance* of all close contacts is recommended. Such persons include those who live or are in close contact with lassa fever patients as well as laboratory personnel testing specimens from such patients.

Restriction of activities

Controlling infectious disease transmission by restriction of the activities of persons in the community who are potentially infectious to others may be appropriate in certain circumstances. Examples include the following:

- Individuals with a diarrhoeal disease should be excluded from handling food and caring for patients in hospital, children, and elderly persons.
- Known carriers of *Salmonella typhi* should be excluded from foodhandling and care of patients.
- Persons with staphylococcal disease should avoid contact with debilitated persons and infants.
- Persons with rubella should be excluded from school or work for seven days after the onset of rash and from contact with pregnant women.

Behavioural change

Behaviour change in an infected person to protect others may be difficult to accomplish. However, this should be considered in preventing the transmission of infectious agents in the following situations.

Sexual behaviour. Examples of infectious agents transmitted through sexual activities are discussed in the section above on control measures applied to the host and in more detail in Volume 3, Chapter 9.12. Individuals who suspect that they may have a sexually transmitted disease should be encouraged to have health-seeking behaviours. Persons with a sexually transmissible infectious agent should be treated and asked to co-operate with health officials to trace their sexual contacts. Patients with diseases such as lymphogranuloma venereum and syphilis, for example, should refrain from sexual contact until all lesions are healed. HIV-infected individuals should be counselled to treat genital ulcer disease promptly since such disease may increase transmissibility of HIV. Also, HIV-infected persons should avoid sexual intercourse with HIV-negative individuals. For a more detailed overview of HIV and AIDS see Volume 3, Chapter 9.13.

Intravenous drug use behaviour. In addition to counselling to abstain from intravenous drug use and establishing drug rehabilitation programmes to help individuals who wish to abstain, promoting behaviour change in the use of injection equipment is important. Discouraging the sharing of injection equipment and education on methods for the decontamination of needles and syringes for intravenous drug use reduce risks of transmission of infectious agents through contaminated injection equipment.

Food preparation behaviour. Individuals who should be restricted from handling food (for example, carriers of *Salmonella typhi*) should be counselled regarding their condition and potential to infect others if they handle food. Foodhandlers who have an infectious disease that is potentially transmissible through the vehicle-borne means of food should be discouraged from handling food for others. The importance of hand washing, especially after defecation and before handling food, should be stressed.

Other behaviours that may reduce risk of transmission of infectious agents to other persons include the following:

- *Cough and sneeze behaviour:* Patients with infectious diseases directly transmitted by droplet spread or airborne transmitted by droplet nuclei (for example, patients with sputum-positive tuberculosis) should cover their mouth and nose when coughing or sneezing;
- *Avoidance of contaminated drinking water:* Persons suffering from dracunculiasis should avoid entering a source of drinking water if they have an active ulcer or blister;
- *Avoidance of vector bites:* Patients with the vector-borne disease of African trypanosomiasis (sleeping sickness) with trypanosomes in their blood should prevent tsetse flies from biting; and
- *Avoidance of donating organs or bodily fluid by certain persons:* Individuals who are infected with HIV or who have sexual and other behaviours that have placed them at increased risk for HIV infection should not donate blood, plasma, tissues, cells, semen for artificial insemination, or organs for transplantation.

Control measures applied to animals

A zoonosis is any infectious agent or infectious disease that may be transmitted under natural conditions from vertebrate animals, both wild and domestic, to humans. A detailed approach to zoonoses is given in the comprehensive work *CRC handbook series in zoonoses* (Beran & Steele 1994). In the control of zoonoses many approaches are used that are applied to animals, including the following:

Active immunization

Active immunization, or vaccination, of selected animals may protect susceptible animal hosts from certain infectious diseases. This protection of animals, in turn, prevents susceptible humans from exposure to the infectious agent of those diseases from animals. An example of an infectious disease in animals in which some control can be achieved through immunization in selected animal populations is rabies. The reservoir of the rabies virus is varied and includes dogs, foxes, wolves, skunks, raccoons and bats. Preventive measures include efforts to vaccinate all dogs.

Other examples of immunization of animals under certain conditions include: (a) immunization of young goats and sheep using a live attenuated strain of *Brucella melitensis* and calves using a strain of *Brucella abortus* in areas of high endemicity for brucellosis; and (b) immunization of animals at risk for acquiring infection with *Bacillus anthracis* that could be transmitted to man causing anthrax.

Restriction or reduction

Restriction is the limiting of the movement of animals and includes isolation and quarantine. Reduction is the killing, known as culling, of selected animals. Selective use of restriction of animals or reduction of animal populations that are infected, or potentially infected, with a zoonotic infectious agent are methods used to decrease or eliminate the opportunity of exposure of susceptible humans, or other animals, to such animals.

The example of rabies can also be used to illustrate the use of restriction or reduction of an animal population to help control an infectious disease. Heymann (2004) recommends that a comprehensive rabies control programme include:

> *register, license, and immunize all dogs in enzootic countries; collect and sacrifice ownerless animals and strays; educate pet owners and the public on the importance of restrictions for dogs and cats (for example, pets must be leashed in congested areas when not confined on owner's premises; strange-acting or sick animals of any species, domestic or wild, should not be picked up/handled; reporting of such animals and animals that have bitten a person or another animal to the police/local health department; confinement and observation of such animals as a preventive measure; and wild animals should not be kept as pets). Immediately sacrifice unimmunized dogs or cats bitten by known rabid animals; if detention is elected, hold the animal in an approved secure pound or kennel for at least 6 months under veterinary supervision, and immunize against rabies 30 days before release. If previously immunized, reimmunize and detain (leashing and confinement) for at least 45 days. Cooperative programmes with wildlife conservation authorities to reduce fox, skunk, raccoon and other terrestrial wildlife hosts of sylvatic rabies may be used in circumscribed enzootic areas near campsites and areas of human habitation. If such focal depopulation is undertaken, it must be maintained to prevent repopulation from the periphery.*

In epizootic situations, 'in urban areas of industrialized countries, strict enforcement of regulations requiring collection, detention and killing of ownerless and stray dogs, and of non-immunized dogs found off owners' premises, and control of the dog population by castration, spaying or drugs have been effective in breaking transmission cycles' (Heymann 2004).

Other examples of restricting or reducing of animal populations include the following:

- Rat-proofing dwellings and reduction of the rat population to prevent rat bites that may transmit the infectious agents *Streptobacillus moniliformis* and *Spirillum minus* causing the rat-bite fevers of streptobacillosis and spirillosis, respectively
- Rat suppression by poisoning (after achieving flea control) in rodent populations with a high potential for epizootic plague
- Culling of domestic poultry flocks that are infected with highly pathogenic avian influenza, such as H5N1
- Elimination of animals infected with *Brucella abortus, Brucella melitensis, Brucella suis*, and *Brucella canis* by segregation or slaughter to prevent brucellosis
- Slaughtering dairy cattle that test positive for infection with *Mycobacterium bovis*, the infectious agent of bovine tuberculosis

Chemoprophylaxis and chemotherapy

Chemoprophylaxis of an animal is using chemical substances (e.g. antibiotics) that prevent infection or its progression to clinically manifest infectious disease in the animal. Chemotherapy of an animal is using these chemical substances to treat an infectious disease in an animal. Both chemoprophylaxis and chemotherapy are control measures that may be used to reduce or prevent the opportunity of an infectious agent from being transmitted from an animal to susceptible humans.

Psittacosis is an example of a zoonosis controlled by chemoprophylaxis or chemotherapy in selected animal populations. The infectious agent, *Chlamydia psittaci*, may be directly transmitted to humans from infected birds when the dried droppings, secretions, or dust from the feathers of such infected birds are inhaled. Imported psittacine species of birds should be placed under quarantine and receive an appropriate antibiotic chemotherapeutic regimen such as chlortetracycline administered in their feed for 30 days.

Another example is chemoprophylaxis in selected dogs at high risk of infection with *Echinococcus granulosus*. This infectious agent can be transmitted to humans through hand to mouth transmission of the tapeworm eggs from dog faeces causing echinococcosis due to *Echinoccus granulosus*, or cystic hydatid disease. Such high-risk dogs (for example, sled dogs) should periodically receive antihelminth treatment with a chemotherapeutic agent such as praziquantel (Biltricide®). Routine use of chemoprophylaxis in cattle, feed lots, and poultry farms, however, can promote serious drug-resistance problems.

Control measures applied to the environment

Control measures applied to the environment are designed to interrupt the routes of transmission by which an infectious agent may be spread through the environment. Just as the routes of transmission are varied, so, too, are the control methods that can be applied. Control measures that affect transmission that can be applied to the host, agents, vectors, infected humans and other animals are reviewed elsewhere in this chapter. Environmental factors may also have a direct impact on the host, agent, or vector. For example, low humidity may predispose to certain infections due to a greater permeability of mucus membranes in the host; cold, dry climates inhibit development of the infective larvae agent of hookworm disease; and higher altitudes and colder climates limit the mosquito vector.

The recognition of the relationship between disease and filth led to a sanitary revolution in industrialized countries that markedly reduced infectious diseases even before the arrival of the antibiotic era. Improved methods for storing and preserving food, better housing, and smaller families with a resultant decrease in the risk of infections at an early age all contributed to reductions in infant and child mortality rates.

This section focuses on general environmental control measures not mentioned elsewhere. Some of these methods, such as provision of safe water, have the potential to prevent several different infectious diseases and significantly reduce rates of disease in the community.

Provision of safe water

It has been estimated that about 1.3 billion people in the developing world lack access to clean and plentiful water (World Bank 1993). Contaminated drinking water, sometimes the result of poorly designed or maintained systems of sewerage, may lead to the water-borne indirect transmission of such infectious agents as *Giardia lamblia* causing giardiasis, pathogenic serotypes of *Salmonella* causing salmonellosis, and *Cryptosporidium* species causing cryptosporidosis.

Purification of water can occur though natural methods or human intervention. Examples of natural methods that contribute to water purification include the processes of evaporation and condensation, filtration through the earth, plant growth, aeration, and reduction and oxidation of organic material by bacteria. Purification of water for public consumption is conventionally done through such processes as coagulation of colloids by aluminium salts or with other techniques; filtration through such materials as coal, sand, or diatomaceous earth; and disinfection with such chemicals as chlorine derivatives. In special situations, boiling and distillation can be used for purification (Solomon *et al.* 2004).

Proper disposal of faeces

It has been estimated that nearly 2 billion people in the developing world do not have an adequate system for proper disposal of faeces (World Bank 1993). Infectious agents in faeces that may result in infectious diseases include poliovirus causing poliomyelitis; *Shigella dysenteriae, Shigella flexneri, Shigella boydii*, and *Shigella sonnei* causing shigellosis; and *Entamoeba histolytica* causing amebiasis.

Infectious agents in faeces may be transmitted by the direct transmission route (including the faecal–oral mode), the vehicle-borne route (including water as noted in the previous section) and the vector-borne route (including the simple mechanism of flies carrying infected faeces on their feet). Public health environmental control measures to interrupt these routes of transmission by ensuring the proper disposal of faeces include the following:

- Appropriate on-site disposal through such means as properly constructed sanitary privies in rural areas with no sewerage systems.
- On-site disposal of domestic wastewater (such as use of septic tanks or cesspools).

- Sewerage systems with treatment of wastewater. Such treatment may include preliminary treatment, sedimentation, chemical coagulation and flocculation, biological treatment (such as activated sludge units and trickling filters), stabilization ponds, sludge management, and disinfection (usually with chlorine) of effluents discharged into drinking, bathing, or shellfish-growing waters.

The importance of personal-health-promoting behaviours of using toilets, keeping toilets clean, and handwashing after defecation are a part of control efforts aimed at the proper disposal of faeces.

Food sanitation

Food-borne infectious diseases remain a problem in both industrialized and developing countries. In the United States alone, an estimated 76 million persons are affected each year, resulting in some 5000 deaths annually. Significant food-borne outbreaks and sporadic cases continue to occur due to such factors as the following:

- Contamination of meat, poultry and eggs with infectious agents, including pathogenic serotypes of *Salmonella, Yersinia pseudotuberculosis* and *Yersinia entercolitica*, and *Listeria monocytogenes*.
- Contamination of vegetables, especially lettuce and leafy green vegetables, with the infectious enterohaemorrhagic strain of *Escherichia coli* O157:H7. Other outbreaks in fruits, juices, and vegetables have been due to contamination with hepatitis A and pathogenic serotypes of salmonella.
- Problems in food storage, handling, and preparation in commercial eating places and in homes.
- Larger and more centralized production and processing facilities, coupled with increasingly extensive distribution networks, which may result in transmission of infectious agents to many persons if a commercial product becomes contaminated.

Industrialized countries have significantly reduced the transmission of some infectious agents through major public health programmes in food sanitation, including: (a) inspecting eating and drinking establishments; (b) inspecting meat and poultry; (c) improving shellfish sanitation; and (d) promoting adequate cooking, canning and refrigeration methods. Some cities and counties have instituted restaurant grading systems based on inspection reports, including required public display of the restaurant's grade as a guide for consumers.

Examples of vehicle-borne indirect transmission of infectious agents through food that can be controlled though a comprehensive public health food sanitation programme include the following:

- Pathogenic serotypes of *Salmonella* transmitted by ingesting food made from infected animals or contaminated by the infectious agent in faeces that may cause salmonellosis. Control is achieved through '(a) handwashing before, during and after food preparation; (b) refrigerating prepared foods in small containers; (c) thoroughly cooking all foodstuffs derived from animal sources, particularly poultry, pork, egg products and meat dishes; (d) avoiding recontamination within the kitchen after cooking is completed; and (e) maintaining a sanitary kitchen, protecting prepared foods against rodent and insect contamination. Inspect for sanitation and adequately supervise abattoirs, food-processing plants, feed-blending mills, egg-grading stations and butcher shops' (Heymann 2004).
- *Staphylococcus aureus* causing staphylococcal food intoxication by ingesting food containing the staphylococcal enterotoxin. Control is achieved through means to '(a) educate food handlers about strict food hygiene, sanitation and cleanliness of kitchens, proper temperature control, handwashing, cleaning of fingernails; (b) the danger of working with exposed skin, nose and eye infections and the need to cover wounds; (c) reduce food handling time (from initial preparation to service) to a minimum, with no more than 4 h at ambient temperature. If they are to be stored more than 2 h, keep perishable foods hot (above 60°C/140°F) or cold (below 7°C/45°F; best is below 4°C/39°F) in shallow containers and covered; and (d) temporarily exclude people with boils, abscesses and other purulent lesions of hands, face or nose from food handling' (Heymann 2004).
- *Trichinella spiralis* transmitted by ingesting raw or improperly cooked meat or meat products, mainly pork, containing infectious encysted larvae that may cause trichinosis. Control is achieved through means to '(a) educate the public on the need to cook all fresh pork and pork products and meat from wild animals at a temperature and for a time sufficient to allow all parts to reach at least 71°C/160°F, or until meat changes from pink to grey, which allows a sufficient margin of safety. This should be done unless it has been established that these meat products have been processed either by heating, curing, freezing or irradiation adequate to kill trichinae; (b) grind pork in a separate grinder or clean the grinder thoroughly before and after processing other meats; (c) adopt regulations to encourage commercial irradiation processing of pork products. Testing carcasses for infection with a digestion technique and immunodiagnosis of pigs with an approved ELISA test are both useful; (d) adopt and enforce regulations that allow only certified trichinea-free pork to be used in raw pork products that have a cooked appearance or in products that traditionally are not heated sufficiently to kill trichinea during final preparation; and (e) adopt laws and regulations to require and enforce the cooking of garbage and offal before feeding to swine' (Heymann 2004).

Milk sanitation

Milk may be a vehicle for indirect transmission of infectious agents like: *Mycobacterium bovis* causing tuberculosis, *Corynebacterium diphtheriae* causing diphtheria, *Listeria monocytogenes* causing listeriosis, and *Campylobacter jejuni* and *Campylobacter coli* causing campylobacter enteritis.

Public health control measures to break the chain of transmission of infectious agents through milk include:

- Mechanization and sanitization of milking processes
- Refrigeration of milk
- Pasteurization of milk through high-temperature short-time, batch, ultra-pasteurization, or ultra-high-temperature methods
- Monitoring milk quality by testing for bacteria using a standard bacterial plate count, by testing for density of coliform organisms, and by use of the phosphatase test to assay for pasteurization
- Periodic testing of cows for tuberculosis and brucellosis

The use of raw milk for human consumption as well as post-pasteurization contamination of milk may result in outbreaks of milk-borne diseases.

Design of facilities and equipment

The design and proper maintenance of buildings, rooms, and equipment can help break the chain of transmission of infectious agents. Laminar airflow hoods in laboratory workbenches, ventilation systems in hospitals, and disposable intravenous equipment are examples of systems designed to reduce risk of transmission. Routine maintenance needed to retain the original design standards for control of transmission of infectious agents include: (a) replacement of air filters; (b) cleaning of cooling towers; (c) monitoring of positive pressure rooms and airlocks; and (d) replacement of in-dwelling peripheral venous catheters.

Examples of infectious agents whose transmission can be reduced through proper design and maintenance include the following:

- *Legionella* species, the infectious agents responsible for legionellosis, are usually transmitted through airborne transmission via aerosol-production. Transmission of the agent from cooling towers can be reduced by periodically cleaning off any scale or sediment, routinely using biocides to kill slime-forming organisms, and draining such towers when not in use.
- *Staphylococcus aureaus*, the infectious agent responsible for staphylococcal disease in medical and surgical wards of hospitals, can be controlled by enforcing strict aseptic techniques, including procedures to change intravenous infusion sites at least every 48 h and replace indwelling peripheral venous catheters every 72 h.
- *Bacillus anthracis*, the infectious agent responsible for anthrax, can be transmitted, among other ways, through inhalation of anthrax spores. Proper design of industrial plants that handle raw animal fibres include providing facilities for adequate ventilation and control of dust, washing and changing clothes after work, and eating away from the places of work.

Other methods

In addition to the environmental methods of control of transmission of infectious agents already mentioned, the following are other methods, some specific and some general, that should also be noted.

- Improvement of housing conditions to *reduce crowding* (as measured by the number of persons per room and not total population density). Reduction in crowding is a general measure that can reduce the transmission of infectious agents, especially direct transmission from direct contact or direct projection (droplet spread).
- *Improvement in working conditions* can affect the risk of infectious disease. For example, control of particulate matter by proper ventilation in occupations such as textile mill workers, metal grinders, and pottery factory workers can reduce inflammation of the lungs and thus decrease the risk of developing tuberculosis. Excessive physical exertion and the stress of exhausting work can also increase the risk of tuberculosis.
- Improved *irrigation* and agricultural practices and *removing vegetation* or *draining* and *filling* of snail-breeding sites can reduce or eliminate the freshwater snail hosts of such infectious agents as *Schistosoma mansoni, Schistosoma haematobium*, and *Schistosoma japonicum* that cause schistosomiasis in humans.
- *Adequate screening* of blood, serum, plasma, tissues or organs can break the chain of vehicle-borne transmission from such biological products. Examples include screening for hepatitis B surface antigen and HIV antibodies in donated blood to prevent transmission of hepatitis B and HIV, respectively.
- Installation of *screened living* and *sleeping quarters* and the use of *bednets*, including bednets impregnated with a synthetic pyrethroid such as permethrin, can reduce exposure to mosquitoes infected with the infectious agents of malaria.

Control measures applied to the agent

Control of some infectious diseases can be achieved through means that remove the infectious agents from the environment or inactivate the agents. Physical measures (such as heat, cold, ultraviolet light, and ionizing radiation) and chemical measures (such as liquid disinfectants and antiseptics, gases, and chlorination) can be used. Examples of control measures applied to infectious agents include the following:

- *Cleaning* is the removing of infectious agents from surfaces through such physical actions as vacuum cleaning or washing and scrubbing using soap or detergent and hot water. Cleaning also helps remove organic materials that might support the growth or survival of infectious agents.
- *Cooling* may inhibit bacterial multiplication and some infectious agents, such as *Trichinella* cysts and *Taenia solium* larvae (cysticerci), which can be killed by freezing temperatures.
- *Pasteurization* is heating to a temperature of 75°C/167°F for 30 min to kill pathogenic vegetative bacteria. It does not inactivate bacterial spores. Pasteurization is a commonly used process to help ensure safety of milk and to prolong its storage quality.
- *Disinfection* is the reduction or killing of vegetative harmful bacterial infectious agents outside the body or on objects. Disinfection may not inactivate all bacterial spores and viruses. *Disinfectants* are used to eliminate pathogenic bacteria from the skin surface and from contaminated inanimate surfaces and include: (a) alcohols; (b) halogens such as iodine and chlorine; (c) surface active compounds such as the quaternary ammonium compound benzalkonium chloride; (d) phenolics; and (e) alkylating agents such as glutaraldehyde and formaldehyde. *Antiseptics* are a class of disinfectant that can be applied on body surfaces; they have a lower toxicity than environmental disinfectants and are usually less effective in killing micro-organisms.
- *Sterilization* is the complete removal or killing of all infectious agents in, or on, an object. Sterilization of equipment for surgery and wound dressings; parenteral administration of drugs, vaccines, or nutrients; catheterization; and dental work are all important means of controlling infectious diseases by killing infectious agents. Sterilization can be accomplished through use of fire, steam (such as in an autoclave), heated air, certain gases (such as ethylene oxide), ultraviolet light, ionizing radiation, liquid chemicals, and filtration. The method of sterilization chosen depends on the type of equipment to be sterilized.

The use of sterilized *disposable equipment*, such as disposable needles, syringes, and catheters, has the potential to reduce the risk of transmission of infectious agents. However, it must be assured that such equipment is disposed of properly and is not reused. For example, disposable syringes cannot be properly resterilized because the plastic from which they are made cannot withstand the heat necessary for sterilization. Technologies, such as the single-use disposable needle and syringe developed for immunization programmes, help assure such disposable equipment is not reused.

Control and prevention programmes

The preceding sections have considered the issues and given examples of control measures for infectious diseases at individual, institutional and community levels and the tools for control directed at the host, routes of transmission, and the agent. Control and prevention programmes using these tools must be developed according to a number of factors including: (a) the risk of disease; (b) the magnitude of disease burden (as measured by mortality, degree of disability, morbidity, and economic costs); (c) the feasibility of control strategies; (d) the cost of control measures; (e) the effectiveness of such measures (on current levels of disease and impact on future cases or outbreaks); (f) the adverse effects or complications of the control measures; and (g) the availability of resources. Public heath planning for the control of infectious diseases must consider these issues to design optimal, evidence-based control and prevention programmes.

The tools of disease surveillance for recognition and evaluation of the patterns of disease can provide the information on the risk and magnitude of disease burden to individuals, persons in institutions, subgroups of populations, and the community at large. Establishment and maintenance of the infrastructure for surveillance, including a system for the reporting of notifiable infectious diseases and unusual events, must be a high priority.

Feasibility of possible control and prevention strategies must be assessed through operational research, pilot projects, or from field experience. The fact that a particular measure can help control a disease does not mean it can be applied on a sufficient scale to have the desired impact. The cost of control activities (in both human and material resources) can be assessed through costing studies that can also provide the data needed to conduct more rigorous cost-benefit and cost-effectiveness analyses. A costly measure, even if it provides a high degree of control for an infectious disease, may not be affordable to the society or reasonable to apply in the light of other less expensive alternative strategies. Effectiveness of control measures may be assessed through epidemiologic studies to find out their impact on reduction in the incidence or prevalence of disease.

The availability of resources for prevention and control programmes forces public health planners to set priorities by taking into account all these factors and then designing programmes that have maximum impact within available resources. Planners have a responsibility to mobilize additional necessary resources by raising public awareness and generating political will. Effective communication of disease burden and the results achievable through well-managed and effective control programmes can be a powerful tool for advocacy. Ideally, communities or their representatives should actively participate in the planning, execution, and evaluation of public health programmes.

Prevention effectiveness is 'the measure of the impact on health (including effectiveness, safety and cost) of prevention policies, programmes, and practices. The assessment of prevention effectiveness is the ongoing process of applying evaluation tools to prevention practices' (CDC 1995). Recognizing that systems for assessing the effectiveness of prevention strategies (including prevention strategies for infectious diseases) are weak or non-existent in both developing and industrialized countries alike, the CDC has suggested the following objectives for prevention effectiveness activities: 'evaluate the impact of prevention, use results of evaluation research to establish programme priorities, and establish or apply standardized methods to compare the benefits and effectiveness of alternative prevention strategies' (CDC 1995).

The current situation of *international migration* of many people worldwide presents an additional complexity to the design of programmes for the control of infectious diseases. Pertinent issues include refugee camps, legal status of migrants in recipient countries, and temporary return migration. Public health officials must consider the most effective mix of combined control measures applied to the host, agent, and routes of transmission when designing suitable control and prevention programmes (Gellert 1993).

International commerce and transportation are important areas of concern for public health infectious disease control programmes, especially as the speed of travel has increased. The tools of control include such measures as:

- Spraying insecticides effective against mosquito vectors of malaria in aircraft before departure, in transit, or on arrival
- Rat-proofing or periodic fumigation to control rats on ships, docks, and warehouses to prevent plague

Specific international control measures relating to aircraft, ships, and land transportation for infectious diseases are detailed in the *International Health Regulations (2005)* (WHO 2005).

The challenge facing infectious disease control programmes is to design an optimal set of interventions at local, institutional, community, national, and international levels supported and accepted by the political leadership and the persons to whom these measures are applied.

Eradication

A unique endpoint in the control of infectious diseases is that of eradication. Eradication is the cessation of all transmission of an infectious agent by extermination of that agent. To date, only one infectious disease, *smallpox*, has been eradicated. The WHO World Health Assembly in May 1980 confirmed its global eradication some three years after the last naturally acquired case of smallpox in October 1977 (Fenner *et al.* 1988). The magnitude of this accomplishment is appreciated when one realizes that, in the early 1950s, it was estimated 50 million cases of smallpox still occurred each year in the world, some 150 years after Edward Jenner had performed the first vaccination and wrote: 'it now becomes too manifest to admit of controversy, that the annihilation of the Small Pox, the most dreadful scourge of the human species, must be the final result of this practice' (Fenner *et al.* 1988).

The goal of global eradication has been set by the World Health Assembly for two other infectious diseases, poliomyelitis caused by wild poliovirus and dracunculiasis (guinea-worm infection), the latter caused by the infectious agent *Dracunculus medinensis*. A high level of sustained political will, aggressively applied disease surveillance, and effective control measures are the required elements to achieve eradication of the infectious agents for these diseases.

Impressive progress has been made toward the global *eradication of poliomyelitis* since the 1988 World Health Assembly set the goal for its eradication. The entire region of the Americas succeeded in interrupting transmission of indigenous wild poliovirus since August 1991. The Western Pacific region succeeded in interrupting transmission since 1997. In other regions of the world, countries endemic for poliomyelitis are carrying out the necessary strategies to eradicate the poliovirus. Poliomyelitis control measures that will lead to eradication include the following:

- Achieving and maintaining high levels of routine coverage of infants with at least three doses of oral polio vaccine.
- Mass application of oral polio vaccine in countries where poliomyelitis is endemic through national immunization days, usually by providing oral polio vaccine to every child less than 5 years of age twice each year, separated by 4–6 weeks, and conducted during the low season of poliovirus transmission.
- 'Mopping-up' operations after the use of national immunization days has reduced transmission of disease to defined focal geographic areas, usually by providing oral polio vaccine house-to-house to all children less than 5 years of age on two occasions separated by 4–6 weeks.
- Aggressive action-oriented surveillance for acute flaccid paralysis. Such surveillance includes: (a) case investigation; (b) a laboratory network for isolation and characterization of polioviruses in suspect cases of poliomyelitis and people in close contact with them; and (c) limited outbreak response immunization providing one house-to-house round of oral polio vaccine to children less than 5 years of age living in the same village or neighborhood of the patient.

Significant strides in the *eradication of dracunculiasis* have also been made. Over the last decade the total number of dracunculiasis cases have declined by more than 95 per cent. The disease is now limited to only certain parts of some African countries in a band between the Sahara desert and the equator. India was certified as dracunculiasis free in the year 2000. Dracunculiasis control measures that are leading to its ultimate eradication include the following:

- Establishing a national programme office, conducting baseline surveys and preparing and refining a national plan of action.
- Educating the population in endemic areas that the source of guinea-worm comes from their drinking water.
- Ensuring that persons with blisters or emerging worms do not enter sources of drinking water through behaviour changes and by converting step-wells into draw-wells.
- Promoting the boiling or filtering of water through a fine mesh cloth to remove copepods. Treating drinking water with chlorine or iodine will also kill the copepods and infective larvae.
- Providing non-infected water through construction of wells or rainwater catchments.
- In selected endemic villages, controlling copepod populations with temephos (Abate®) insecticide placed in reservoirs, tanks, ponds, and step-wells.
- Implementing an intensified surveillance and aggressive case-containment strategy as programmes get close to achieving eradication.

The eradication of a disease requires a unique set of conditions, including the following: (a) a defined, accessible reservoir of the infectious agent; (b) affordable and effective control measures that can interrupt the chain of infection directed at the host, agent or route of transmission; and (c) a surveillance mechanism adequate to monitor and ultimately certify the disappearance of the infectious agent.

It is likely that measles may be targeted for global eradication in the future. Some countries and geographic regions have already targeted measles for elimination—a term sometimes used to describe the eradication of a disease from a large geographic area. Other diseases that may potentially be targeted for eradication in the future include: Mumps, rubella, hepatitis B, leprosy and diphtheria.

Emerging infectious diseases

New, emerging, and re-emerging infectious diseases have become a focus for the attention of public health prevention and control programmes in both industrialized and developing countries. Such infectious diseases have thwarted any expectation that infectious diseases will soon be eliminated as public health problems and resulted in a widening spectrum of diseases, many of which were once thought to be almost conquered. Krause has reflected on this as follows:

> *Microbes and vectors swim in the evolutionary stream, and they swim faster than we do. Bacteria reproduce every 30 min. For them, a millennium is compressed into a fortnight. They are fleet afoot, and the pace of our research must keep up with them, or they will overtake us. Microbes were here on earth 2 billion years before humans arrived, learning every trick for survival, and it is likely that they will be here 2 billion years after we depart.* (Krause 1998)

Many factors contribute to the emergence of new or re-emergence of those previously known (Lederberg *et al.* 1992; CDC 1994; Murphy 1994), including: Human demographic change; breakdowns of sanitary and other public health measures; economic development and changes in the use of land; climate change; other human behaviours (such as increased use of child-care facilities, sexual and drug use behaviours, and patterns of outdoor recreation); international travel and commerce; changes in food processing and handling; evolution of pathogenic infectious agents; development of resistance of infectious agents; resistance of the vectors of vector-borne infectious diseases to pesticides; imunosuppression of persons; and deterioration in surveillance systems for infectious diseases, including laboratory support, to detect new or emerging disease problems at an early stage.

An aggressive public health response to these new, emerging and re-emerging infectious disease threats must be made to characterize them better and to mount an effective response for their control. For example, the 1999 outbreak of West Nile fever in New York City and surrounding areas that, within a 4-year period, spread throughout the United States demonstrates how a viral encephalitis, initially classified as St. Louis encephalitis and later confirmed to be due to West Nile virus, can reach far beyond its normal setting.

The WHO has outlined the following high priority areas (WHO 1995):

- Strengthen global surveillance of infectious diseases
- Establish national and international infrastructures to recognize, report, and respond to new disease threats

- Further develop applied research on diagnosis, epidemiology, and control of emerging infectious diseases
- Strengthen the international capacity for infectious disease prevention and control

Emerging infectious diseases are addressed in detail in Volume 3, Chapter 9.17.

Bioterrorism: The deliberate use of biological agents to cause harm

Another unfortunate source of an infectious disease threat is the spectre of biological warfare or bioterrorism, especially in an age where terrorist acts are frequent events (Christopher *et al.* 1997). The 2002 World Health Assembly resolution urges member states 'to treat any deliberate use, including local, of biological and chemical agents and radionuclear attack to cause harm also as a global public health threat, and to respond to such a threat in other countries by sharing expertise, supplies and resources in order rapidly to contain the event and mitigate its effects' (WHO 2002).

The WHO recommends the following (WHO 2004b):

- Public health authorities, in close cooperation with other government bodies, should draw up contingency plans for dealing with a deliberate release of biological or chemical agents intended to harm civilian populations. These plans should be consistent or integral with existing plans for outbreaks of disease, natural disasters, large-scale industrial or transportation accidents, and terrorist incidents.
- Preparedness for deliberate releases of biological or chemical agents should be based on standard risk-analysis principles, starting with risk and threat assessment in order to determine the relative priority that should be accorded to such releases in comparison with other dangers to public health in the country concerned. Considerations for deliberate releases should be incorporated into existing public health infrastructures, rather than developing separate infrastructures.
- Preparedness for deliberate releases of biological or chemical agents can be markedly increased in most countries by strengthening the public health infrastructure, and particularly public health surveillance and response, and measures should be taken to this end.
- Managing the consequences of a deliberate release of biological or chemical agents may demand more resources than are available, and international assistance would then be essential.

Many countries are developing rapid response capability to deal with such contingencies, especially in the light of the 2001 bioterrorist attack using anthrax in the United States.

Conclusion

In summary, the aggressive application of the principles of infectious disease control outlined in this chapter (including the measures applied to the host, vectors, infected humans, animals, environment, and agents), is needed to control, eliminate, or even eradicate infectious diseases. The public's health is continually at risk for infectious disease and we must ensure that our guard against these diseases is not let down and, in fact, is continually raised as the factors that favour emerging infectious diseases result in new challenges for their control.

It is only through worldwide concerted action will the effort to control infectious disease be effective. We have now in an era where, as Nobel Laureate Dr. Joshua Lederberg has stated, 'The microbe that felled one child in a distant continent yesterday can reach yours today and seed a global pandemic tomorrow' (quoted in CDC 1994). As Hans Zinsser stated over 60 years ago:

> *Infectious disease is one of the few genuine adventures left in the world. The dragons are all dead and the lance grows rusty in the chimney corner . . . About the only sporting proposition that remains unimpaired by the relentless domestication of a once free-living human species is the war against those ferocious little fellow creatures, which lurk in the dark corners and stalk us in the bodies of rats, mice and all kinds of domestic animals; which fly and crawl with the insects, and waylay us in our food and drink and even in our love.* (Hans Zinsser 1934 quoted in Murphy 1994)

References

ACIP (Immunization Practices Advisory Committee) (2006). General recommendations on immunization. *Morbidity and Mortality Weekly Report*, **55**, RR 15.

Beran, G.W. and Steele, J.H. (ed) (1994). *Handbook series of zoonoses*. CRC Press, Boca Raton, FL.

Brillman, J.C. and Quenzer, R.W. (ed.) (1998). *Infectious disease in emergency medicine* (2nd ed). Lippincott-Raven, Philadelphia, PA.

CDC (Centers for Disease Control and Prevention) (1994). *Addressing emerging infectious disease threats: a prevention strategy for the United States*. CDC, Atlanta, GA.

CDC (Centers for Disease Control and Prevention) (1995). *Prevention effectiveness: making prevention a practical reality*. CDC, Atlanta, GA.

CDC (Centers for Disease Control and Prevention) (2008). Summary of notifiable diseases, United States, 2006. *Morbidity and mortality weekly report*, **55**(53), 2–94.

Cristopher, G.W., Cieslak, T.J., Pavlin, J.A. *et al.* (1997). Biological warfare: A historical perspective. *Journal of the American Medical Association*, **278**, 412–7.

Committee on Infectious Diseases (2006), *American Academy of Pediatrics: report of the committee on infectious diseases*, (25th ed). American Academy of Pediatrics, Elk Grove Village, IL.

Evans, A.S. and Kaslow, R.A. (ed.) (1997). *Viral infections of humans: Epidemiology and control*, (4th ed). Plenum Press, New York.

Evans, A.S. and Brachman, P.S. (ed.) (1998). *Bacterial infections of humans: epidemiology and control* (3rd ed). Plenum Press, New York.

Fenner, F., Henderson, D.A., Arita, I. *et al.* (1988). *Smallpox and its eradication*. World Health Organization, Geneva.

Feigin, R.D. *et al* (ed.) (2004). *Textbook of pediatric infectious diseases* (5th ed). W.B. Saunders, Philadelphia, PA.

Fine, P.E. (1993). Herd immunity: history, theory, practice. *Epidemiologic reviews*, **15**, 265–302.

Gellert, G.A. (1993). International migration and control of communicable diseases. *Social Science and Medicine*, **37**, 1489–99.

Gorbach, S.L., Bartlett, J.G., and Blacklow, N.R. (ed.) (2004). *Infectious diseases* (3rd ed). Lippincott Williams and Wilkins, Philadelphia, PA.

Guerrant, R.L., Walker, D.H., and Weller, P.F. (ed.) (2006). *Tropical infectious diseases: Principles, pathogens, and practice* (2nd ed). W.B. Saunders, Philadelphia, PA.

Heymann, D.L. (ed.) (2004). *Control of communicable diseases manual*, (18th ed). American Public Health Association, Washington.

HICPAC (Hospital Infection Control Practices Advisory Committee) (1996). Guideline for isolation precautions in hospitals part II. Recommendations for isolation precautions in hospitals. *Am J Infect Control*, **24**:32–52.

Insel, R.A., Amstey, M., Woodin, K. *et al.* (1994). Maternal immunization to prevent infectious diseases in the neonate or infant. *International Journal of Technology Assessment in Health Care*, **10**, 143–53.

Jamison, D.T. *et al.* (ed.) (2006). *Disease control priorities in developing countries* (2nd ed). Oxford University Press, New York.

Kiple, K.F. (ed.) (1993). *The Cambridge world history of human disease.* Cambridge University Press.

Krause, R.M. (ed.) (1998). *Emerging infections.* Biomedical Research Reports, Academic Press, New York.

Last, J.M. *et al.* (ed.) (2001). *A dictionary of epidemiology* (4th ed). International Epidemiological Association. Oxford University Press, New York.

Lederberg, J., Shope, R.E., and Oaks, S.C. Jr. (ed) (1992). *Emerging infections: microbial threats to health in the United States.* National Academy Press, Washington, D.C.

McKibben, L. *et al.* (2005). Guidance on public reporting of healthcare-associated infections: recommendations of the Hospital Infection Control Practices Advisory Committee). *Am J Infect Control*, **33**, 217–26.

McNeill, W.H. (1976). *Plagues and peoples.* Anchor Press/Doubleday, Garden City, New York.

Mandell, G.L., Bennett J.E., and Dolin, R. (ed.) (2005). *Mandell, Douglas and Bennett's principles and practice of infectious diseases* (6th ed). Elsevier Churchill Livingstone, New York.

Murphy, F.A. (1994). New, emerging, and reemerging infectious diseases. *Advances in Virus Research*, **43**, 1–52.

Osterholm, M.T. and Hedberg C.W. (2005). Epidemiolologic principles. In *Mandell, Douglas and Bennett's principles and practice of infectious diseases* (6th edn) (ed. G.L. Mandell, J.E. Bennett and R. Dolin), pp. 158–68. Elsevier Churchill Livingstone, New York.

Plotkin, S.A. and Orenstein, W.A. (ed) (2004). *Vaccines.* (4th ed.). W.B Saunders, Philadelphia.

Ryan, K.J. and Ray, C.G. (ed.) (2004). *Sherris Medical microbiology: an introduction to infectious diseases* (4th ed). McGraw-Hill, New York.

Solomon, S.L., Fraser, D.W., and Kaplan, S.L. (2004). Public health considerations. In *Textbook of pediatric infectious diseases*, (ed. R.D. Feigin *et al*) (5th edn), pp. 3221–44. W.B. Saunders, Philadelphia, PA.

UNAIDS (Joint United Nations Programme on HIV/AIDS) (2007). *UNAIDS/WHO AIDS epidemic update: December 2007.* UNAIDS, Geneva.

Wilson, M.E. (1991). *A world guide to infections: diseases, distribution, diagnosis.* Oxford University Press, New York.

World Bank (1993). *World Bank development report: investing in health.* World Bank, Washington.

WHO (World Health Organization) (1995). *Communicable disease prevention and control: new, emerging, and re-emerging infectious diseases*, No. A48/15. WHO, Geneva.

WHO (World Health Organization) (2002). Global public health response to natural occurrence, accidental release or deliberate use of biological and chemical agents or radionuclear material that affect health. World Health Assembly Resolution, WHA55.16, WHO, Geneva.

WHO (World Health Organization) (2003). *Communicable disease 2002: global defence against the infectious disease threat.* WHO/CDS/2003.15, WHO, Geneva.

WHO (World Health Organization) (2004a). *World health report 2004.* WHO, Geneva.

WHO (World Health Organization) (2004b). Public health response to biological and chemical weapons. WHO, Geneva.

WHO (World Health Organization) (2005). *International health regulations (2005).* WHO, Geneva.

WHO (World Health Organization) (2008). *International travel and health.* WHO, Geneva.

12.7

Population screening and public health

Allison Streetly and Walter W. Holland

Abstract

Screening is concerned with actively identifying disease or pre-disease conditions in individuals who presume themselves to be healthy but may benefit from early treatment. Population screening should be distinguished from the testing of individuals to facilitate case finding in clinical settings. The chapter begins by outlining the historical development of screening as a health intervention. It then discusses the properties of screening tests and the criteria that must be fulfilled before a screening programme is introduced. The initiation of a screening programme raises a number of ethical questions that must be addressed at the level of the health system and the screening programme, as well as at the level of the individual subject who may be offered a screening test. The meaning and limitations of informed choice are discussed. The practical problems that must be negotiated when organizing the delivery of a screening programme are outlined. Processes of quality assurance are described. The final section of the chapter summarizes recommendations for screening at different stages of life.

Introduction

The concept of screening, that is actively identifying a disease or pre-disease condition in individuals who presume themselves to be healthy but may benefit from early treatment, sounds easy and attractive. The presumption is that if this is done the clinical course of the disease will be altered and the prognosis will be improved for the person who has been screened. Unfortunately, the reality of screening is more difficult and screening programmes, like other healthcare interventions, may do harm (Raffle & Gray 2007). Unlike most other healthcare interventions, screening programmes are offered to individuals who consider themselves to be healthy and the harms caused by screening programmes are therefore particularly difficult to accept. Consequently, it is important to appreciate what screening can and cannot achieve, and the conditions required for a cost-effective programme. Public health scientists and practitioners contribute by providing and appraising evidence concerning the benefits and harms of screening, managing screening programmes, and informing the expectations of the public and other stakeholders. This chapter outlines the principles that underpin the development and implementation of screening programmes. It also provides a brief summary of screening applications at different stages of life.

History of screening

The benefits of screening were first demonstrated by the use of mass miniature radiography (MMR) for the identification of individuals with tuberculosis (TB). The use of MMR became common in many countries after the introduction of effective treatment for TB after 1946. With the reduction in the burden of tuberculosis, the application of screening to other chronic conditions began to be considered. This was particularly so in the United States, where a law on the control of chronic diseases and the availability of screening was passed in the late 1950s. Lester Breslow, head of the Division of Chronic Diseases in the California State Health Department (later its Commissioner for Health), was a particularly enthusiastic advocate. A Commission on Chronic Illness was founded in 1957 and a major review published in the Journal of Chronic Disease (Breslow & Roberts 1955). Raffle and Gray (2007) identified Horace Debell, a London physician, who promoted comprehensive periodical examinations in the nineteenth century and exhorted people to prevent disease. He suggested that physicians should give advice on living conditions and other necessary measures and thus prevent the progression of disease. While the concept of routine comprehensive periodic medical examinations was adopted most avidly in the United States, the use of routine medical examinations was also developed by industry, in order to identify those who already had a disease and should not be employed, and by insurance companies, in order to identify those with excess risk (Raffle & Gray 2007).

One of the first comprehensive reviews of screening was published by Thorner and Remein (1961) of the United States Public Health Service; much of this is still relevant. Morris Collen (1988), Medical Director of the Kaiser Permanente Health Maintenance Organization in Oakland, California, was also a great advocate of regular screening and comprehensive medical examinations of adults for chronic disease. Collen believed that regular screening could reduce healthcare costs and utilization of medical care. Screening was introduced as a component of subscribing to the Kaiser Permanente HMO. Unfortunately, no clear benefits to subscribers could be demonstrated.

In the United Kingdom, there was initially much less enthusiasm for the concept of screening. Nonetheless, the concept and belief in the benefits of screening was soon apparent, largely because of the growth of cervical cytology screening for the early identification of the precursors of cancer of the cervix. This was greatly promoted by the women's movement in the early 1960s. The ease of performing these smears meant that these were very popular; only Ahluwahlia and Doll (1968) and Knox (1982) raised critical comments concerning questions of effectiveness. As a result, pathology services were required to devote increasing resources to cervical cytology and rapidly became overwhelmed and other pathology services suffered.

The Ministry of Health in England recognized the importance of the growth of demand for screening as a component of preventive medical services. Dr J.M.G. Wilson was despatched to the United States to review the situation, and he and Jungner, a Swedish biochemist, developed their view and published under the auspices of the WHO, a landmark publication (Wilson & Jungner 1968) that outlined some of the criteria under which a screening programme might be adopted.

In the past 40 years, professional attitudes towards screening have changed. At the start of the period, health professionals were enthusiastic of the promise that early diagnosis could provide in the improvement of prevention and reduction of morbidity from chronic diseases. This enthusiasm has become much more tempered with the appreciation that screening also has disadvantages and should only be applied for certain defined conditions and in carefully controlled circumstances (Holland & Stewart 1990, 2005b).

By contrast, and in spite of widely quoted mishaps, screening has become much more popular with the general public. In recent years, the population has become much more health conscious and, with the growth of the Internet, knowledgeable about health matters. This has increased the demand for health interventions. A firm belief has developed that the earlier a diagnosis is made, the better will be the outcome. The parallel of the annual test for roadworthiness of motor vehicles (MOT) is often quoted. This belief in the efficacy of screening is fuelled through the advocacy of charities concerned with individual diseases, such as prostate cancer; by private clinics and private providers who may have good intentions but can see a way to make money; and by some doctors and politicians, who are anxious to publicize their belief in the importance and value of prevention. Screening has become a commercial enterprise, not only in terms of the promotion of procedures but also in terms of the supply of reagents and equipment. It has become a process driven by financial incentives of services, the promotion of unproven tests and the presence of booths or mobile screening units in supermarkets. Governments are often willing to 'invest' in screening services, even at relatively high cost and with relatively small benefits, as for example in screening for breast cancer, in order to show that they care. Critics who advocate caution in particular instances have been undermined or attacked (Holland & Stewart 1990, 2005b).

The concept of screening

Definitions of screening

McKeown (1968) defined screening as 'medical investigation which does not arise from a patient's request for advice for a specific complaint'. This definition of screening may encompass: (i) research for the validation of a procedure; or (ii) tests done for the promotion of the public health, for example, to identify a source of infection in a food outbreak; or (iii) as a direct contribution to the health of the individual. It is this last, prescriptive screening, which is now the most common objective.

There have been a number of modifications of this definition since 1968. The UK National Screening Committee (2000) defined screening as 'a public health service in which members of a defined population, who do not necessarily perceive that they are at risk of, or are already affected by, a disease or its complications are asked a question or offered a test to identify those individuals who are more likely to be helped than harmed by further tests or treatment to reduce the risk of disease or its complications'.

Clinical practitioners commonly use the term 'screening' when they systematically apply tests to their patients in order to detect evidence of elevated risks or early-stage complications as, for example, when diabetic patients are examined annually for signs of retinal disease or peripheral nerve damage. The term 'screening' is also used inappropriately when individuals are offered tests nonsystematically, as when they are tested for infectious diseases. However, these approaches are more correctly termed 'testing' (Gostin 2000) or 'opportunistic screening' or 'case finding'. The term 'screening' should only be used when populations, or groups of people who are thought to be at risk, are systematically offered screening tests as in national programmes for cancer of the breast and cervix.

Criteria for introducing a screening programme

The basic criteria to be fulfilled before the introduction of screening for a condition are fundamental to the screening process. The criteria proposed by Wilson and Jungner (1968) were widely accepted and quoted for many years and these provide the basis for a more elaborate set of the necessary criteria listed in the UK National Screening Committee's Second Report (2000) (Box 12.7.1). The condition sought should be an important health problem whose whole natural history should be understood. The condition must have a recognizable early or latent stage. The diagnosis should be made by a suitable acceptable test and there should be agreement as to whom to regard as a patient. There must be acceptable, effective treatment or intervention for individuals found to have the disease or pre-disease condition and facilities for this must be available. The cost of case finding (including diagnosis and treatment) should be economically balanced in relation to possible expenditure on medical care as a whole. As well as meeting the above criteria and principles there must be adequate, on-going evaluation and quality control.

Properties of screening tests

Screening tests must be applied to large numbers of healthy individuals most of whom will be identified as screen negative. This means that screening tests must be evaluated and judged in low-prevalence settings and not just in the high-prevalence settings, as in hospitals, where they are often developed. Cochrane and Holland (1971) listed some desirable characteristics of screening tests including the requirement that they should be acceptable to screened subjects, safe, rapidly and easily applied and not too costly.

A screening test is not a diagnostic test. Instead, screening tests separate individuals into groups who have either a low probability or a high probability of disease being present. This is commonly misunderstood by members of the public who assume that a positive

Box 12.7.1 UK National Screening Committee criteria for adopting a screening programme

Ideally, all the following criteria should be met before screening for a condition is initiated:

1. The condition should be an important health problem.
2. The epidemiology and natural history of the condition, including development from latent to declared disease, should be adequately understood, and there should be a detectable risk factor, disease marker, latent period, or early symptomatic stage.
3. All the cost-effective primary prevention interventions should have been implemented as far as practicable.
4. If the carriers of a mutation are identified as a result of screening, the natural history of people with this status should be understood, including the psychological implications.
5. There should be a simple, safe, precise, and validated screening test.
6. The distribution of test values in the target population should be known, and a suitable cut-off level defined and agreed.
7. The test should be acceptable to the population.
8. There should be an agreed policy on the further diagnostic investigation of individuals with a positive test result and on the choices available to those individuals.
9. If the test is for mutations, the criteria used to select the subset of mutations to be covered by screening, if all possible mutations are not being tested, should be clearly set out.

The treatment

10. There should be an effective treatment or intervention for patients identified through early detection, with evidence of early treatment leading to better outcomes than late treatment.
11. There should be agreed evidence based policies covering which individuals should be offered treatment and the appropriate treatment to be offered.
12. Clinical management of the condition and patient outcomes should be optimized in all healthcare providers prior to participation in a screening programme.

The screening programme

13. There should be evidence from high-quality randomized controlled trials that the screening programme is effective in reducing mortality or morbidity. Where screening is aimed solely at providing information to allow the person being screened to make an 'informed choice' (e.g. Down's syndrome, cystic fibrosis carrier screening), there must be evidence from high-quality trials that the test accurately measures risk. The information that is provided about the test and its outcome must be of value and readily understood by the individual being screened.
14. There should be evidence that the complete screening programme (test, diagnostic procedures, treatment/intervention) is clinically, socially, and ethically acceptable to health professionals and the public.
15. The benefit from the screening programme should outweigh the physical and psychological harm (caused by the test, diagnostic procedures, and treatment).
16. The opportunity cost of the screening programme (including testing, diagnosis and treatment, administration, training, and quality assurance) should be economically balanced in relation to expenditure on medical care as a whole (i.e. value for money).
17. There should be a plan for managing and monitoring the screening programme and an agreed set of quality assurance standards.
18. Adequate staffing and facilities for testing, diagnosis, treatment and programme management should be available prior to the commencement of the screening programme.
19. All other options for managing the condition should have been considered (e.g. improving treatment, providing other services), to ensure that no more cost effective intervention could be introduced or current interventions increased within the resources available.
20. Evidence-based information, explaining the consequences of testing, investigation, and treatment, should be made available to potential participants to assist them in making an informed choice.
21. Public pressure for widening the eligibility criteria for reducing the screening interval, and for increasing the sensitivity of the testing process, should be anticipated. Decisions about these parameters should be scientifically justifiable to the public.
22. If screening is for a mutation, the programme should be acceptable to people identified as carriers and to other family members.

Source: National Screening Committee (2000).

result is 'bad news' and a negative result is the 'all clear'. This can result in considerable anxiety for the individuals concerned if these perceptions are not addressed appropriately. A positive screening test result must usually be followed up by appropriate confirmatory tests to establish whether the screening result was a true positive, confirming the diagnosis and need for treatment, or more commonly that the result was a 'false positive' and the individual can be reassured.

The classification of individuals which results from a screening test result may be compared with true disease status obtained using a reference method or 'gold standard' (Fig. 12.7.1). Important characteristics to be assessed before any screening test can be considered for use in a screening programme include specificity and sensitivity. Specificity is defined as the proportion of disease-free subjects who are classified as true negatives by the test. Sensitivity is defined as the proportion of subjects with the condition of interest who are classified as true positives by the test. Ideally, both measures should be high. A common misperception among clinicians is that high sensitivity is more important than specificity, in other words, a case must not be 'missed'. In reality, all screening programmes will 'miss' some true positive cases and specificity is as, if not more, important for an effective and acceptable programme because a high rate of false positives can outweigh the benefits to the few true positives identified, with negative consequences for individuals who test false-positive. This is an important issue for programmes such as breast screening. It is generally more important if the prevalence of condition to be identified is low.

The positive predictive value of a test is the proportion of subjects with a positive test result who have the condition of interest. The positive predictive value is determined by the relative proportions of true positives and false positives and, with sensitivity and specificity remaining constant, the positive predictive value depends on the prevalence of the condition of interest. When the condition is common, true positives will be frequent but if the condition is rare, true positives will be infrequent. Conditions that are sought by screening programmes commonly have a prevalence lower than 1 per cent, consequently the positive predictive value of a screening test will be low unless both sensitivity and specificity are extremely high (Table 12.7.1). In practical terms, this means that false positive results may outnumber true positive results, and the impact of screening on those who do not have the condition of interest is an important concern.

As an example, a cut-point for mean cell haemoglobin (MCH) of 27 pg is used in the detection of beta thalassaemia. This has been shown to have a sensitivity of 100 per cent in a sample of 6314 results with 104 carriers from two London hospitals that serve a high-prevalence population (Wald and Leck 2000, p. 255). At this prevalence, the positive predictive value in this sample is approximately 77.4 per cent. In lower-prevalence areas, the predictive value of the same cut-point was estimated to range from 1.3 to 30 per cent (NHS Sickle Cell and Thalassaemia Screening Programme 2008). Using HbA2 estimation, in combination with the MCH result, to increase the specificity of the testing procedure, resulted in important reductions in the workload associated with follow-up of screen positives without compromising detection rate. In the detection of maternal alpha zero carriers, use of a MCH cut-point of 25 pg gives a predictive value, in a research setting with results validated against DNA analysis, of 1:424 with 100 per cent sensitivity. Use of the MCH cut-point in combination with a question about family origins to increase specificity gives an estimated predictive value of 1:3 [12/36] (Sorour *et al.* 2007). Applying this approach in practice reduces partner recall from 1:61 requiring follow up to 1:1497 requiring partner follow-up (a 96 per cent reduction in partner recall). These examples show how important the predictive value is as a measure of the impact of screening test on programme workload. These examples also demonstrate that when conditions are of low prevalence attending to the specificity of a test is extremely important if staff and public commitment to a programme are to be maintained.

When a screening test generates a quantitative measure, rather than a binary classification, the cut-point used to separate 'normal' from 'abnormal' may be varied. This is illustrated in Fig. 12.7.2 which presents data for prostate-specific antigen (PSA) in relation to later development of prostate cancer (Thompson *et al.* 2005). Sensitivity and specificity have been estimated and plotted for different PSA cut-points. A low cut-point will give a high sensitivity but low specificity, as the cut-point is increased the sensitivity decreases and the specificity increases. Thus, there is a reciprocal relationship between sensitivity and specificity. The area under the ROC curve is used as a summary measure of test performance. Note that, in this example, PSA test performance is better for detecting tumours that are Gleason grade 8 or higher, these are poorly differentiated tumours that are more likely to spread rapidly and be clinically and prognostically important. The authors of the study observed that lowering the PSA cut-point sufficiently to ensure detection of high-grade tumours would not only have the effect of increasing false positive diagnoses, but would also increase detection of tumours that might be of less clinical importance (Thompson *et al.* 2005).

In general, the performance of a screening procedure may be improved by modifications that increase both sensitivity and specificity. This can sometimes be achieved by combining several tests

	Disease present	Disease absent
Test positive	TP	FP
Test negative	FN	TN

$$\text{Positive predictive value (PPV)} = \frac{TP}{(TP + FP)}$$

$$\text{Negative predictive value (NPV)} = \frac{TN}{(TN + FN)}$$

$$\text{Sensitivity} = \frac{TP}{(TP + FN)} \qquad \text{Specificity} = \frac{TN}{(TN + FP)}$$

$$\text{Likelihood ratio } (+) = \frac{\text{sensitivity}}{(1 - \text{specificity})}$$

TP, True positive
FP, False positive
TN, True negative
FN, False negative

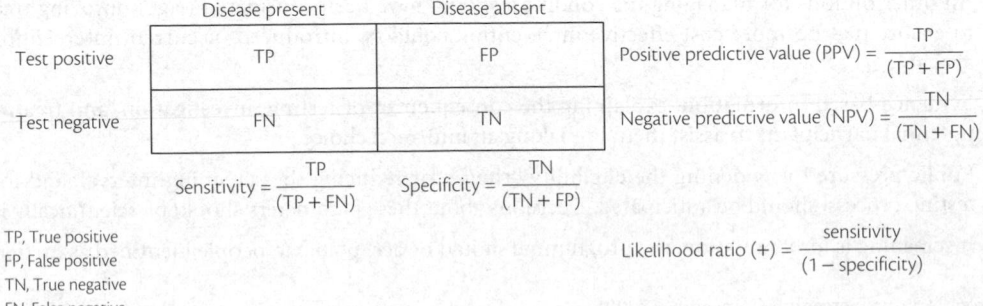

Fig. 12.7.1 Properties of a screening test.

Table 12.7.1 Positive predictive values (PPV) at different values for sensitivity and specificity and disease prevalence

Prevalence	PPV (%) if sensitivity = 75% and specificity = 75%	PPV (%) if sensitivity = 95% and specificity = 95%
10%	25.0	67.9
1%	2.94	16.1
0.1%	0.30	1.9
0.01%	0.03	0.2

together, as in the 'quadruple test' used in antenatal screening for Down syndrome. Wald *et al.* (2003) compared combinations of two, three, or four biochemical measures in the detection of Down's syndrome pregnancies. They reported that the 'double', 'triple', or 'quadruple' tests gave detection rates of 57, 62, and 70 per cent, respectively, while the odds of being affected given a positive result were 1:56, 1: 52, and 1:45, respectively.

The likelihood ratio of a positive test provides another measure for analysing measure of test performance. The post-test odds of disease are given by the product of the likelihood ratio of a positive test and the pre-test odds of disease. The likelihood ratio provides a measure of the relative increase in frequency of the disease in subjects who test positive compared with the untested population. The likelihood ratio of a positive test is given by sensitivity divided by (1 – specificity) (Fig. 12.7.1).

Benefits and disadvantages

As noted earlier, screening may cause harm to individuals and populations (Raffle & Gray 2007). It is therefore essential to be aware

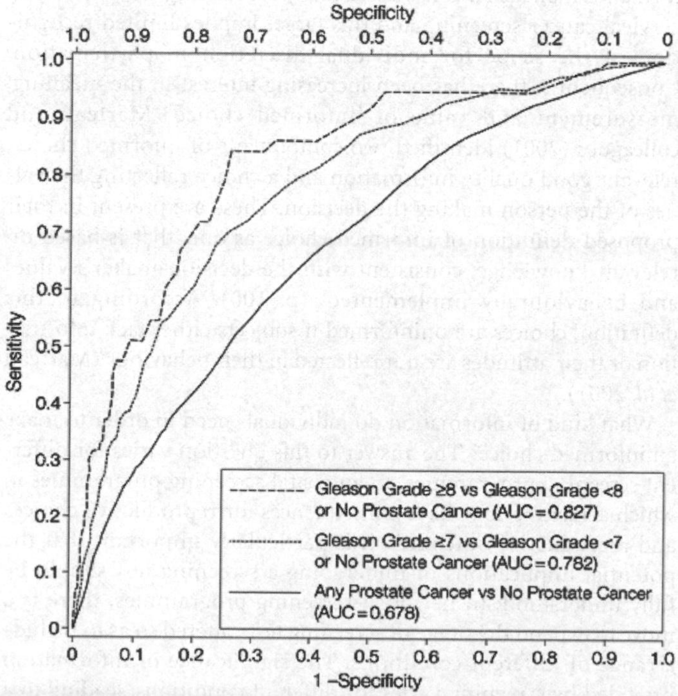

Fig. 12.7.2 Receiver-operating characteristic curve for prostate-specific antigen (PSA) and different grades of prostate cancer. AUC, area under curve.

Table 12.7.2 Potential benefits and disadvantages of screening programmes

Benefits	Disadvantages
Improved prognosis for some cases detected	Longer morbidity for cases whose prognosis is not altered
Less radical treatment which cures some early treated cases	Over-treatment of questionable abnormalities
Resource savings	Resource costs
Reassurance for those with negative test results	False reassurance for those with false negative results
	Anxiety and sometimes morbidity for those with false positive results
	Hazards of screening test itself

Source: Chamberlain (1984).

of both the benefits and possible harms of screening (Table 12.7.2) (Chamberlain 1984). Some of the problems of screening are not easy to communicate to the public. If thousands of tests are done, 'errors' are bound to occur. All programmes must be subject to continuing quality control to minimize such 'errors'. Yet, even under optimal conditions, some individuals will be labelled as positive and yet not have the condition sought and others labelled as negative and yet have the condition sought. Thus, individuals will be wrongly labelled, stigmatized, and may become anxious, while others are falsely reassured. There is thus a great need to appreciate the ethics of screening. Cochrane and Holland (1971) emphasized that screening differs from other forms of healthcare in that it is the healthcare provider who offers a test with the implicit promise that undergoing this test may provide benefit, in contrast to the normal situation, where the individual seeks the help of the provider. It is thus essential that screening services are only introduced if the necessary principles and criteria are met. In countries other than the United Kingdom, including the United States and Canada, national and professional bodies have published the tests and conditions for which screening must be justified, often with appropriate reviews. There is a national body in the United Kingdom, the National Screening Committee, responsible for the review and ongoing assessment of those screening tests that meet the necessary criteria and the responsibility for their introduction and use in the NHS that provides a model approach to these issues.

Ethics and screening

Lawrence Gostin (2000) observed that 'screening is far from a neutral scientific pursuit. Rather, screening is political . . . fraught with complex choices and weighing values—cost, efficiency, autonomy, and justice' (p. 201). This challenging perception shows that screening must be viewed within its social and ethical context. However, the ethical framework for screening can be considered at more than one level. The traditional biomedical ethical approach, which primarily considers the individual level, is arguably not the most relevant level at which to consider the ethics of screening. All relevant levels, including the level of the screening programme and the health system or society, must be considered to ensure that introduction of a screening programme is as consistent as possible, with a given society's values. This section of the chapter outlines some key ethical questions that must be negotiated if a screening programme is to be introduced.

At the *health system* or *societal* level, the implementation of screening raises questions concerning resource allocation and prioritization. Any screening programme is associated with an opportunity cost that represents the healthcare foregone through allocating resources to screening. The criteria used to justify screening programme implementation are generally oriented towards increasing efficiency, a utilitarian value of ensuring the greatest good for the greatest number given available resources. However, the valuation of different outcomes may present difficult problems. For example, in Down's syndrome screening, it may be feasible to estimate the cost per affected birth prevented but it is difficult, and in some societies unacceptable, to weigh this cost against the cost of treatment and care of affected individuals. This issue is discussed in more detail in a later section.

Allocation of resources to screening programmes also raises questions of equity because the proposed health benefits of screening may be differentially distributed to certain groups in the population. Some men's groups argue that since screening programmes are implemented to detect women's cancers, including breast and cervical cancer screening, fairness requires that screening programmes should also be implemented to detect cancers that affect men, including cancer of the prostate, even if considerations of efficiency do not support this. More generally, screening programmes may be differentially utilized by higher socio-economic groups, with lower-income groups and minorities showing lower uptake. Screening, thus, has the potential to increase inequalities in health while improving the overall health of the total population. Screening outcomes, and inequalities in outcomes, should be important measures for quality assurance of screening programmes.

At the level of the *screening programme*, the selection of population groups to be screened, the choice of screening procedures, the value attached to different screening outcomes and the nature of available treatment services might appear to be purely technical issues, but these processes also raise ethical questions. A screening programme may be either universal or targeted. If a targeted strategy is chosen, then there is a risk of stigmatizing the target population as being particularly associated with an undesirable health outcome, such as a sexually transmitted disease. If the target population is defined on grounds of age, as is done for breast cancer screening, then this raises questions concerning the 'right to health' of women who are either younger or older than the proposed age cut-points. While efficiency arguments may favour a more focused strategy, considerations of equity favour a more universal approach (Sassi *et al.* 2001).

As discussed earlier, screening tests often have low-positive predictive values and this means that there may be large numbers of subjects with false positive results and a smaller number of subjects with true positive results. Subjects with false positive results may be exposed to significant harm through the communication of anxiety producing information and through follow-up tests that may be risky and uncomfortable. Major benefits from screening are shared by a few true positives and these benefits must be balanced against potential harm to many false positives. As a minimum, this indicates an ethical requirement for adequate quality assurance to ensure the reliability and validity of testing procedures, the safety of diagnostic services, and the adequacy of information communication to screened subjects.

The selection of screening outcomes also requires careful consideration. This is especially true for screening processes that may impact on reproductive outcomes. The possibility of making diagnoses before birth and giving parents informed choice over reproductive outcomes appear to be positive developments. However, these processes may be related to the concept of 'eugenics'. The term 'eugenics' literally means 'well-born'. It is a social philosophy which advocates the improvement of human hereditary traits through various forms of intervention (Osborn 1937; Wikipedia 2008). Although, the notion of eugenics was introduced with good intentions, the concept of eugenics now has negative connotations that mainly date from the Nazi period from 1933 to 1945. Contemporary developments in genetics have increased the potential for genetic screening, but there is now a 'guarded attitude towards eugenics, which had become a watchword to be feared rather than embraced' (Wikipedia 2008).

Finally, it is ethically unjustified to initiate screening unless adequate treatment services are available to provide treatment and care for subjects identified through the screening programme. The resources required for treatment services may seldom be provided through a screening programme, and those advocating the programme must also advocate for investment in appropriate treatment services.

At the level of the *individual subject*, ethical issues are raised concerning the autonomy of the individual. Most screening programmes are voluntary and should be offered to individuals, enabling them to make an informed choice whether to participate in screening or not. In reality, as Gostin (2000) describes, voluntary population screening programmes are offered as routine interventions with limited opportunities for individuals to opt-out of participation. Family practices in the United Kingdom are performance managed against a nationally agreed target for uptake of cervical cancer screening and this target implies limited recognition of the scope for individual discretion in participation. Consequently, there has been increasing interest in the meaning, measurement and value of 'informed choice'. Marteau and colleagues (2001) identified two components of informed choice, relevant good quality information and a choice reflecting the values of the person making the decision. These are present in their proposed definition of informed choice as one 'that is based on relevant knowledge, consistent with the decision-maker's values and behaviourally implemented' (p. 100). According to this definition, choices are uninformed if subjects either lack information or their attitudes are not reflected in their behaviour (Marteau *et al.* 2001).

What kind of information do individuals need in order to make an informed choice? The answer to this question varies for different screening programmes. In antenatal screening programmes in which screening may have consequences for reproductive choices and reproductive outcomes, it is particularly important that the potential implications of undergoing a screening test should be fully understood. In newborn-screening programmes, there is a move to expand the range of screening tests offered so as to include a range of different conditions. The significance of information provided by screening varies for different conditions, leading to a situation in which the concept of informed choice becomes difficult and impractical (Nijsingh 2007).

In the context of cancer screening, potential benefit of screening may be communicated in terms of the 'number needed to screen', which is the inverse of the absolute risk reduction (Welch 2001). Rembold (1998) estimated that the 'number needed to screen' to prevent one death from colon cancer was 1374 over 5 years and for mammography, to prevent one death from breast cancer was 2451 over 5 years for women aged 50–59 years. From the individual's perspective, these statistics are not encouraging, however, understanding the limitations of screening and the potential for harm from screening are equally, if not more, important (Welch 2001). More aggressive cancers are most likely to be missed by screening programmes; these cancers are often diagnosed by clinical services as 'interval' cancers between screening rounds. Screening tests are not diagnostic tests and typically have a low-positive predictive value. This means that a positive screening test may lead on to more invasive procedures that may be associated with negative consequences. Screening may identify abnormalities that might never have caused clinical disease, leading to unnecessary treatment. This is exemplified by prostate cancer screening because sub-clinical prostate cancer is a frequent finding in older men. Histopathological definitions of cancer are unreliable contributing to incorrect diagnoses and unnecessary treatment in some cases or under-treatment in others (Welch 2001).

The information required to inform an individual's choice to participate in screening is technically complex and wide-ranging. Consequently, there may be limited opportunities for truly informed choice in routine screening programmes. In democratic societies, it may be legitimate for the state to make decisions on the implementation of screening programmes through what the Nuffield Council on Bioethics (2007) terms the state's 'stewardship' role. It is through the stewardship role that states discharge their obligation to protect and fulfil their citizens' right to health. However, this should also include promoting citizens' capacity to make informed choices through better public education about screening. Helping individuals, who may have little understanding of the issues, to make decisions at difficult times in their lives should not be the sole or even main approach (Nijsingh 2007). It may be more helpful to increase people's awareness of relevant issues from before they plan families or are offered screening tests. More needs to be done to develop an educated public which can benefit from screening programmes, whose focus should not be limited to technical issues while broader social perspectives are neglected.

Organizing and delivering screening programmes

Challenges in implementing screening programmes

Introducing and sustaining screening programmes

The first step in implementing a screening programme should be a formal review of the evidence to evaluate whether this supports the introduction of screening or not (Box 12.7.1). This step is sometimes omitted and screening may be initiated by enthusiasts with testing diffusing into routine practice without formal evaluation. This is particularly likely to occur with tests that are not costly and have broad public support. As noted earlier, this was exemplified by the introduction of the 'pap smear' for cervical screening. Even when there is good evidence to support such a programme, converting existing variable local practices into a standard programme across a region or country may be more difficult than introducing a new planned programme *de novo*.

The decision to introduce a programme must be viewed in the context of a particular time and place. This is illustrated by international differences in approach. For example, screening for toxoplasmosis in pregnancy is recommended in France but not in the United Kingdom. This difference may be attributed to the different prevalence and epidemiology of the condition in these two countries associated with different meat eating habits. A screening programme that is considered cost-effective in a high-income country may often be unaffordable in a middle- or low-income country.

Temporal variations in the need for screening are illustrated by the example of antenatal syphilis screening in the United Kingdom. Syphilis declined dramatically after World War II, following the introduction of antibiotics to treat the disease. By the 1990s, there were calls for the antenatal screening programme for syphilis to be stopped. However, a 1999 review argued against this because of recent outbreaks of the disease. On the basis of this review, the decision was made to continue screening and rates of syphilis have increased since that time, albeit mostly in men (Connor *et al.* 2000).

Clarifying aims and objectives of the programme

Clarifying the aims and objectives of the screening programme represents another important step. This is not merely a technical exercise but one that should involve professionals, users and the voluntary sector. A classic example of a well-meaning approach to introducing screening that miscarried was the US Sickle Cell Act of 1970. This was intended to help identify those with sickle cell disease and provide care for them. However, the programme was introduced without adequate public education or planning. As a result, carriers identified by the programme were stigmatized, sometimes being refused jobs or losing employment due to misunderstanding of the differences between the disease and carrier states. Ultimately, the public refused to be tested because of the negative impacts of testing (Anionwu 2001). An important lesson from this experience is that the public need to be well informed, educated and continuously engaged, if the implementation of screening programmes is to achieve the potential benefit and be well-accepted with sustained support.

Defining the scope of the programme

Defining the scope of a screening programme should be considered prior to more detailed planning because if this is not considered carefully and comprehensively, some aspects of required service development may be omitted, causing difficulties later. In the United Kingdom, the term 'screening programme' is defined as 'the whole system of activities needed to deliver high-quality screening. This encompasses identifying and informing those to be offered screening through to the treatment and follow-up of those found to have an abnormality, as well as support for those who develop disease despite screening' (National Screening Committee 2000). A key criterion for the introduction of a screening programme is that 'clinical management of the conditions and patient outcomes should be optimized by all healthcare providers prior to participation in a screening programme' (National Screening Committee 2000). For example, the introduction of a newborn hearing programme requires planning and development of a service of adequate capacity and quality in tertiary specialist centres if the programme is to be effective and achieve its goal of timely appropriate treatment of screen positive children. These aspirations have seldom been achieved by the time screening is introduced.

Planning implementation

Planning and implementing the programme should cover a range of aspects such as education and training and standardization of testing procedures. These processes require project planning skills and the overall co-ordination and sequencing of programme implementation is important. Clinical services may be overwhelmed if a screening programme were to suddenly start, placing significantly increased demands on their services. On the other hand, if services are set up and referrals do not occur relatively quickly, then there may be disillusionment and disinvestment. It may be optimal if services do experience some increase in demand early on to ensure that there is a recognition of the increased service need that will be forthcoming but without overwhelming them. Another area that requires sequencing and will take some time to implement is professional and public education. Professional education and training should be implemented before a screening programme undertakes public awareness campaigns in order to avoid difficulties for front-line professionals. The UK experience and approach to planning and implementation are discussed in detail by Raffle and Gray (2007).

Information systems

The importance of adequate information and information systems should not be neglected in the planning and budgeting for a screening programme. Information systems are needed to manage the process of screening. Information systems are also required to provide fail-safe systems and to monitor the outcomes of screening.

Information systems are an important part of ensuring that adequate fail-safe processes are in place to guarantee the benefits of the programme, follow-up those with positive screening tests and assure the safety and quality of the programme. A characteristic of an effectively delivered screening programme is that fail-safe systems operate independently of the individual practitioners who are responsible for patient care. These systems should ensure that all those eligible are offered screening, that those with inconclusive, missing or screen positive results are followed up and managed appropriately. Problems with these processes should be rapidly identified and addressed. In the cervical screening programme in the United Kingdom, a series of fail-safe actions are identified at the level of the call–recall system, the general practice, the cytology laboratory and the colposcopy clinic that follows up cases requiring further management (NHS Cancer Screening Programmes 2004). These fail-safe actions are intended to ensure that errors are minimized in calling women for screening, monitoring test uptake, repeating smears, referring women for colposcopy with the required degree of urgency and ensuring that necessary treatment is received. Screening programmes that do not operate such systems are unsafe and risk high-level failures of process with consequent disengagement of population support.

Data derived from information systems are also important in the quality assurance (QA) of programmes and in monitoring programmes' success against specified objectives and criteria in terms of population outcomes. Failures of process may be less visible in the early stages of the programme but may cause problems later on. In addition, without adequate information, it may be difficult to demonstrate the benefits of the programme and hence to maintain investment.

Quality assurance in screening programmes

Importance of quality assurance

Quality assurance and performance management should be an integral part of any organized screening programme. Screening offers the promise of benefiting individuals and populations by identifying health problems about which they are unaware, unlike the usual situation in which an individual presents for healthcare. Screening is also offered to, and taken up by, many individuals from large populations. Consequently, failures of systems or processes can cause harm to many individuals, and the promise of screening may not be fulfilled. The overall aim of quality assurance should be to ensure that a screening programme achieves the potential health benefits while minimizing associated risks and harms. The processes of quality assurance should include assessment of all relevant risks, particularly those that are most likely to have adverse effects on subjects who are screened.

The process of quality assurance

The term 'quality assurance' is used to refer to the process by which the quality of a screening programme, in all its key dimensions, can be evaluated and improved. Variations in quality should be identified and addressed, so as to correct problems or implement improvements. Quality assurance is not a passive process; therefore, it requires the potential to intervene so as to address any problem that may be identified. According to Donabedian (2003), a narrow definition of quality assurance requires the collection and interpretation of information, followed by making adjustments to the system. A wider definition includes processes of system design or redesign, linked to resource allocation so as to address problems, as well as including educational and motivational activities to modify the behaviour of health professionals. Quality assurance should be cyclical; moving from assessment of performance, to action, followed by review. Quality assurance has little meaning if it operates only as a monitoring and reporting cycle, in isolation from those able to make real changes and allocate resources to address problems. A well-developed quality management system should specify when and how any task is to be undertaken and by whom (Balmer *et al.* 2000). A named individual should be identified as responsible for the quality of each component of the screening process, with involvement of the whole organization to plan, deliver, and evaluate quality of services (Moullin 2002). Strong user involvement in the process is recommended. Service quality is dynamic and standards should be continually reviewed and tightened so that quality is maintained and progressively increased, particularly in response to rising expectations from patients. Communication is a key aspect of maintaining quality and good partnerships between service providers are required (Moullin 2002).

Dimensions of quality

The processes of quality assurance should address several dimensions of quality (Donabedian 2003). *Effectiveness* should be enhanced so as to optimize the benefits or health gains from screening. *Efficiency* is required to ensure that the maximal benefits are obtained from available resources. The *equity* of screening uptake and screening outcomes should be evaluated to ensure that screening is accessible to all eligible groups and benefits are fairly distributed. The *safety* of screening programmes is important to ensure that errors are avoided and harms are minimized. The *acceptability* of the screening programme to the public and service users should be ensured. Standards for any programme should encompass each relevant dimension of quality.

Measuring and monitoring quality: Developing criteria and standards

A first step for successfully measuring and monitoring the quality of a programme is determining what to monitor. Clarifying and agreeing the aims and objectives for a programme should be the first step, using the evidence that supports the introduction of the programme as a starting point. Following from this, key priorities for monitoring should be identified including structures, processes, and outcomes (National Screening Committee 2003).

Raffle and Gray (2007) recommend defining the objectives of a programme to encapsulate what a 'good' programme should look like. Box 12.7.2 gives an example from the sickle cell and thalassaemia screening programme in England. A similar approach has been used in the United Kingdom for other programmes including the breast screening and diabetic retinopathy programmes. Once objectives are defined, ways of measuring the achievements of these objectives need to be identified. This requires the development of criteria and standards to measure achievement of each objective; criteria and standards are the tools by which quality of care is measured. A criterion is defined 'as an attribute of structure, process, or outcome that is used to draw an inference about quality' (Donabedian 2003, p. 60). A standard is defined as 'a specified quantitative measure of magnitude or frequency that specified what is good or less so' (Donabedian 2003, p. 60). Criteria, therefore, should cover the key dimensions of quality to be assured. Standards then specify exactly what is to be expected for each dimension.

Setting standards for a screening programme should follow from a baseline assessment of performance where possible. Standards are then set using informed judgement of the level of performance that should be achieved. Standards may include both minimum standards, to be achieved by all, and achievable standards that might be reached by the top quartile of programmes. Minimum standards indicate an acceptable level of service below which services should not fall. Achievable or developmental standards target attainment in an environment of increasing expectations. The process of setting standards is iterative and continuous, requiring regular review, particularly in the early years following the development and implementation of a programme. Once standards have been set, it is necessary to identify the interventions required to meet the standards, to monitor service delivery against standards and aim for continuous improvement of services. Standards should also be based on an understanding of patients' requirements and expectations. Moullin (2002) recommends that standards should be realistic and achievable within available resources; service users should contribute to the development process with user involvement, an indicator of quality; and standards must be measurable and capable of being monitored.

The measurement of outcomes for screening programmes can be a particular challenge but is important in evaluating the extent to which a programme has achieved its aims. Measurement of outcomes of a programme may be treated as an overall national- or state-wide evaluation of the programme and not part of the quality assurance process which mostly deals with structural and process measures which are more useful for assessing the operation of a programme at a local or unit level. Table 12.7.3 gives an example of the outcome standards set for the newborn screening programme for sickle cell disease in England (NHS Sickle Cell and Thalassaemia Screening Programme 2006).

Box 12.7.2 Example of screening programme aims and objectives. (NHS Sickle Cell and Thalassaemia Screening Programme, 2006)

NHS newborn sickle cell screening programme

Programme aims

- To achieve the lowest possible childhood death rate and to minimize childhood morbidity from sickle cell disorders

Overall outcome to be achieved at national level

- Mortality rate in children with sickle cell disorders under 5 years of less than 4 per 1000 person years of life (2 deaths per 100 affected infants) by 2010
- To accurately diagnose infants born with specific conditions where early intervention is likely to be beneficial

Programme objectives

- To offer screening for sickle cell disorders to all infants
- To process tests in a timely manner
- To identify and arrange timely follow-up of infants identified as needing further investigation
- To ensure effective and acceptable follow-up, care and support for affected infants and their carers
- To offer treatment and start parental education in a timely manner
- To minimize the adverse effects of screening—including failure to follow-up screen positive infants, inaccurate or inadequate information, unnecessary investigation and follow-up, inappropriate disclosure of information and failure to communicate results to parents (normal and carrier)
- To ensure that responsibility, accountability, and performance management for all aspects of the programme are clear and that these link together from local to national level and between the newborn and antenatal programme

Different types of programmes present different challenges

The challenges of screening are typically presented in relation to screening for cancer, but this is not the only type of screening programme. Four different types of programme are considered, including infections, genetic conditions, vascular screening, and cancers.

Infections

Examples of screening for infection include pre-conception syphilis screening as recommended in the United States; Hepatitis B, rubella susceptibility and HIV screening in pregnancy in the United Kingdom; or toxoplasmosis screening in pregnancy in France. The purpose of screening should be clarified as, depending on the purpose, different actions may be required. Screening for infection may identify susceptibility, as in the case of rubella screening that may indicate a need for immunization to prevent infection in a future pregnancy. Screening may identify past infection and

Table 12.7.3 Outcome measures for a newborn sickle cell screening programme in England

Outcome	Criteria	Minimum standard	Achievable standard
Best possible survival for affected infants detected by the programme	Mortality rates expressed in person years	Mortality rate in children under 5 of less than four per 1000 person-years of life (two deaths per 100 affected children)	Mortality rate in children under 5 of less than two per 1000 person years of life (one death per 100 affected children)
Accurate detection of all infants born with major clinically significant abnormalities	Sensitivity of the screening programme	99% for HbSS 98% for HbSC 95% for other variants	99.5% for HbSS 99% for HbSC 97% for other variants

Source: NHS Sickle Cell and Thalassaemia Screening Programme (2006).

sero-conversion, as in the case of hepatitis B and HIV, with potential benefits of intervention for the infant (Hepatitis B) or both mother and infant (HIV) (Department of Health 1998). In pregnancy, there may be benefits either for the mother and/or the baby. Without clarity as to the purpose of screening, the potential benefits of the programme may not be realized. For example, while surveillance of infections is important, screening for this reason can be offered at any stage in pregnancy. Most of the benefits to the infant will be gained if infections, such as syphilis, are identified before pregnancy, as is the policy in the United States, rather than later in pregnancy, when the infection may already have affected the infant. If test information is only to be used for surveillance purposes, this point may be lost and result in a programme that does not deliver optimal benefit.

Another challenge for such programmes is ensuring that information identified as relating to the mother can be transferred to the infant's record to ensure that it receives appropriate care. For example, infants of HIV-infected mothers should receive anti-viral drugs and the mother should be counselled not to breast-feed. In the United Kingdom, well-intentioned data protection legislation has made the transfer of such information very difficult, on occasion effectively preventing the benefits of the screening programme being achieved.

A specific problem for screening programmes for infections, such as HIV in pregnancy, is that the screen performed only relates to a specific point in time and any non-immune individual can subsequently become infected at any point after this screen. This also relates, for example, to screening of migrants for tuberculosis when subsequent poor living conditions may provide an environment for acquiring and developing an active infection. Screening may also fail to detect very recently infected individuals if the screening test is for sero-conversion rather than acute infection. Screening may, if inappropriately applied as in the case of a meningitis outbreak, identify asymptomatic carriers of a particular organism.

Genetic testing and screening

Developments in genetics have opened up many new possibilities for the diagnosis of a variety of diseases, but it is important to note that the same principles apply as in other forms of screening. If genetic tests are offered to any individual, either there must be an effective intervention available for individuals found to be affected, or the information provided by the result must help the individual or other family members to make better decisions than if the information was not available. There are a number of instances where genetic testing and screening may be helpful. For example, a child known to have multiple endocrine neoplasia type 2 can be spared medullary carcinoma by undergoing prophylactic thyroidectomy or an adult with hereditary haemochromatosis can avoid cirrhosis by the early initiation of phlebotomy treatment. This section includes the application of genetic tests to individuals and populations, that is, testing and screening.

Uses of genetic tests

Genetic tests may be used in a variety of settings for a number of purposes, including diagnostic testing, to confirm or exclude a genetic disorder in an asymptomatic individual; and predictive testing in asymptomatic individuals who have a family history. This may be presymptomatic, when the gene mutation is present (e.g. Huntingdon's disease), or predispositional, when eventual development of symptoms is possible but not certain (e.g. cancer of the breast). It is important that adequate counselling services be available if predictive testing is used. Testing may be useful at different stages of the life course.

(a) Offering carrier testing or screening to allow identification of couples at risk. Tests can be offered at any time up to early pregnancy and in high-risk groups to enable individuals to make informed choices. Examples include testing for thalassaemia, Tay–Sachs, and sickle cell disease. For autosomal recessive conditions, if both partners are carriers, then there is a one-in-four risk in each pregnancy of an affected infant.

(b) Foetal testing in cases where there is thought to be an increased risk of an affected foetus. This is usually done by amniocentesis or chorionic villus sampling. These tests carry risks and may result in foetal loss. Non-invasive genetic tests of maternal blood are under development but not in routine practice at present (Free Foetal DNA testing).

(c) Pre-implantation genetic diagnosis in early embryos after *in vitro* fertilization to minimize the risk of genetic condition in couples at particular risk. This is the option of choice for some parents who have been identified pre-conception as being a couple at risk of a particular condition. This can be extended to the selection of 'saviour siblings' to allow for earlier bone marrow transplantation.

(d) Newborn screening to identify individuals as early a stage as possible in order to start treatment, where there is evidence of benefit or treatment available, e.g. cystic fibrosis, sickle cell disease.

Some of the tests employed are not strictly *genetic tests* but are biochemical tests used to identify genetic diseases.

(e) In a number of common conditions, preventive genetic testing may contribute to the identification of individuals at high risk; for example, BRCA1 and BRCA2 mutations, which can identify women at particular risk for developing breast cancer. However, positive findings are rare. For example, out of 10 000 women, 1000 will have a mother or a sister who has had breast cancer but only 15 will have a mutation that confers a high risk. Furthermore, it must be noted that it has been estimated that lifetime risk of breast cancer associated with a mutation ranges from 26 to 85 per cent. Testing for BRCA1 and BRCA2 do not meet the criteria for a screening programme.

Problems of genetic screening

Public expectations of genetic screening have been greatly magnified by the human genome project, but it is essential to appreciate the problems and difficulties of genetic screening. The Human Genome has several million single nucleotide polymorphisms, and thus, the 'number of possible genetic associations is limited only by the rate at which laboratories are able to type these polymorphisms' (Colhoun *et al.* 2003). These difficulties are often neglected and it must be realized that associations of a gene with a condition should be treated with the same degree of rigorous assessment as the findings of an environmental risk factor associated with a disease.

As with all screening tests, genetic screening may have psychological consequences, thus adequate counselling services must be provided. For common conditions, genetic screening is unlikely to be of great use in view of the complex interaction between environmental, behavioural, biological, and genetic factors. Its use is likely to be greatest in screening certain high-risk groups and populations for a few clearly defined conditions, e.g. to prevent thalassaemia in a high-risk population in Iran, where the costs of treatment for those affected are considered unaffordable to the society and in general, individuals wish to have the option of prenatal diagnosis and termination because of the economic consequences of having an affected child (Samavat & Modell 2004).

Particular problems arising with newborn screening programmes for both cystic fibrosis (to a lesser degree) and sickle cell disease (to a greater degree) are that the methods used by the programme which aims to detect those with disease but unavoidably also detects the carrier state. In the United Kingdom and the United States, this has resulted in a considerable debate as to the merits of revealing carrier status to parents of infants at a stage in life before a child can make such a decision. In both the United States and United Kingdom, the view that has prevailed is that 'carriers should be reported to parents and follow-up counselling is offered to ensure understanding of the difference between carrier state and disease and also the genetic significance of the carrier state' (Human Genetics Commission 2006; Lin & Barton 2007). The UK Human Genetics Commission (2006) emphasizes that such decisions must at their core reflect societal views and not the views of technical experts.

A second common problem, particularly relevant to newborn screening and carrier testing to identify couples at risk, relates to the potential of such programmes to identify non-paternity if counselling and information sharing is not handled sensitively. This emphasizes the importance of public education and awareness about such programmes.

Vascular screening programmes

Vascular programmes include risk assessments for cardiovascular disease, diabetic retinopathy screening and aortic aneurysm screening. Questions have been raised concerning whether some of these procedures should be identified as screening programmes. Cardiovascular risk assessment, it has been argued, is not a screening programme as all people in a given population are at risk of cardiovascular disease and screening cannot sort individuals into two groups. Diabetic retinopathy screening is not always considered to be a true screening programme as it calls a clinically identified population with diabetes. In other respects, this programme does operate as a population screening programme. Aortic aneurysm screening, followed by surgery for those at risk can result in mortality of screen identified cases through operative mortality. This raises ethical questions about the suitability of a programme that may lead directly to mortality. Overall, however, the life years saved by successful intervention outweigh the risks and, on this basis, the UK National Screening Committee has recommended a national programme which is currently being introduced.

Cancer screening

Cancer screening programmes represent the model in which much screening theory has been developed and which are most familiar to the public. Cancer screening is particularly relevant in high-income countries where cancer contributes most to total mortality. Mature breast and cervical programmes are in place in many European countries and North America. A particular problem with cancer programmes has been the difficulty in demonstrating the impact of screening because of the multiple influences on outcomes. In the case of breast cancer screening, there are changes in disease incidence associated with utilization of hormone replacement therapy as well as changes in case management that may be associated with improving prognosis.

Specific problems for cancer screening are 'length time' and 'lead time' biases. Length time bias refers to the fact that screening is most effective at detecting slow developing cancers which are less likely to be the cause of an individual's death but by detection can cause considerable anxiety. More aggressive tumours are likely to develop rapidly in the intervals between screening rounds. Lead time bias refers to the problem for evaluation of programmes that screening programmes detect cancers earlier than would have been the case with symptomatic screening and may thus appear to lengthen the time from diagnosis to survival when there is no true change in natural course or treatment may even shorten life expectancy.

Screening at different stages of life

This section provides a brief summary of debates concerning screening at different stages of life. Current recommendations from the United Kingdom are used for illustration.

Antenatal and newborn screening

One of the most comprehensive reviews on appropriate procedures in the antenatal and neonatal period is published by Wald

Table 12.7.4 Recommendations for antenatal screening tests to be offered routinely

Recommended	NOT recommended
Maternal anaemia	Bacterial vaginosis
Bacteriuria in pregnancy	Chlamydia
Blood group and RhD status	Cytomegalovirus
Down syndrome	Cystic fibrosis
Foetal anomalies (ultrasound)	Diabetes in pregnancy
Thalassaemia and sickle cell disease	Domestic violence
Haemolytic disease of newborn	Foetomaternal alloimmune thrombocytopaenia
Hepatitis B	Fragile X syndrome
HIV	Hepatitis C
Neural tube defects	Genital herpes
Pre-eclampsia	HTLV1
Placenta praevia	Streptococcus B
Psychiatric illness	Thrombophilia
Rubella immunity	Toxoplasmosis
Syphilis	Postnatal depression
Tay–Sachs disease	

Source: Holland and Stewart (2005).

and Leck (2000). It is at this period of life that screening has been shown to be of particular importance and has been used longest. Even so, there are still questions about certain tests and much still needs to be developed. The accepted recommendations in the United Kingdom are shown in Table 12.7.4. If one examines the recommendations of Wald and Leck (2000), differences of opinion can be seen.

It is important to realize that termination of pregnancy is the only effective intervention for some of the conditions listed in Table 12.7.4. This has implications on the need to provide a clear ethical framework for service availability and delivery and informed decision-making before any tests are done. It also means that timing of offer of tests is important and relevant to informed decision-making. Advice on these issues is often omitted or is of poor quality, and testing may be too late to allow informed decision making (Dormandy 2008).

Foetal ultrasound scanning has greatly increased in popularity and utilization. This test is not as uncomplicated as some obstetricians and mothers might imagine. It requires careful application at defined periods of gestation and skilled interpretation. The arguments about its utility are analysed by Holland and Stewart (2005).

The need to continuously review and appraise antenatal screening procedures is well illustrated by the case of Down syndrome. The diagnosis of this condition has been greatly improved by the use of combined serum tests and ultrasound so that the likelihood of detection is now of the order of 80 per cent (Wald & Leck 2000). Nonetheless, the only treatment is termination of the pregnancy and the necessary diagnostic amniocentesis or chorionic villus sampling carries a risk of foetal damage. Thus, the requirement of informed parental consent is paramount. The timing of testing is important. The quadruple test is offered in the second trimester, but first trimester screening with ultrasound and biochemical markers provides relevant information at an earlier stage of pregnancy, is therefore more acceptable to women, and is now recommended in the United Kingdom.

A further ethical concern has also arisen over time. Whereas 20–30 years ago the prognosis for Down syndrome children was very poor—few lived beyond puberty and almost all were not educable—now many such children live to early middle age, are able to participate in education and are able to pursue a simple occupation and become self-sufficient—hence the need for very careful balanced advice in every case before tests are done.

Newborn screening

Screening of newborn infants consists of routine biochemical tests on an infant's blood spot and physical examination including testing for hearing impairment (Table 12.7.5). Bloodspot screening should be done in the first week of life. In the United Kingdom, current recommendations are for testing for phenylketonuria, congenital hypothyroidism, cystic fibrosis, sickle cell disease and, Medium Chain Acyl-CoA Dehydrogenase deficiency (UK Newborn Screening Programme Centre 2005). Physical examination and testing for hearing loss are performed in the first year of life. It is important that methods of routine physical examination are properly standardized, that individuals performing them are trained in these methods and that the programme is kept under continuous review.

Table 12.7.5 Recommendations for newborn screening tests to be offered routinely in the United Kingdom

Condition	Comment
Blood spot for	
Phenylketonuria	
Congenital hypothyroidism	
Cystic fibrosis	
Sickle-cell disease	
Medium chain acyl-CoA dehydrogenase deficiency (MCADD)	In process of introduction for all newborns
Physical examination	
Congenital heart disease	Training programme in physical examination being developed
Congenital cataract	
Cryptorchidism	
Congenital dislocation/dysplasia of the hip	
Other tests	
Hearing impairment	Automated otoacoustic emission (AOAE) test used as first-line screening method in England
Under review	
Additional biochemical screening on the newborn blood spot for fatty acid disorder and amino acid metabolism defects introduced in the United States but currently not recommended in the United Kingdom	

Source: Adapted from Holland and Stewart (2005).

Examination is for signs of congenital heart disease, congenital cataract, cryptorchidism, congenital dislocation or developmental dysplasia of the hip, as well as other congenital malformations. Screening for congenital dislocation of the hip has been the subject of much controversy, but evidence of the effectiveness of ultrasound as a screening method is now accumulating. A national screening programme for hearing impairment has been implemented in the United Kingdom.

Screening in childhood

Screening in childhood is important, both to follow up findings from the neonatal period and to identify remediable defects or problems. A large number of bodies recommend a variety of procedures at different stages. Screening for hearing and visual impairment and congenital displacement of the hip is straightforward, but there is also a need to identify children from deprived and disadvantaged households in order to identify those children who are at particular risk to develop both physical and behavioural impairments—a matter often neglected.

Screening in adolescence

The major need at this stage of life is to build on the findings of the schoolchild examinations and to provide confidential accessible health services to aid the adolescent to confront and deal with such problems as fertility and sex, drugs and alcohol use. All opportunities should be taken to educate the adolescent in methods of healthy living, personal safety, nutrition, exercise, etc. The only opportunistic screening procedure that may be recommended is for chlamydia, a common, curable sexually transmitted disease which is often asymptomatic but can lead to life threatening ectopic pregnancy, pelvic inflammatory disease and infertility. However, evidence about the effectiveness of screening or the best way to deliver this service is limited.

Screening in adults

As we have already stated, screening in adults is big business. Media interest in health is insatiable and politicians have capitalized on public expectations and attitudes in the belief that 'prevention is better than cure'. This has been the mantra of many advocates, who carefully abstain from reminding people that death cannot be avoided. It is therefore essential to consider what screening procedures actually can do in all cases and to appreciate that there are also disadvantages in all the cases. In the United Kingdom, there is a National Screening Committee charged with the task of continuously reappraising the evidence and research to identify those procedures that meet the criteria we have enunciated and to monitor the application of these approved tests. In this chapter, most attention is given to those tests that meet the criteria and principles enunciated. It is essential to realize that these are not 'set in stone' but are subject to continuous research and evaluation. Recommendations are also context-dependent. It is also emphasized that all procedures must be subject to quality control, audit, and evaluation.

Cancer

As the second largest cause of mortality in the high-income countries, it is obviously a candidate for screening. Screening for cervical cancer was one of the main driving forces for the introduction of screening in healthcare. It is thus not surprising that cancer screening has been the subject of a great deal of attention.

Breast cancer

The major trials of breast cancer screening have been done in the United States (Shapiro *et al.* 1982) and Sweden (Taban *et al.* 1985, 1989). Other trials have been done in the United Kingdom, which before introducing a national scheme of breast cancer screening, had a major public enquiry (Forrest 1987). Screening for breast cancer is a highly emotive subject which has been the subject of very critical analysis (Gøtzsche & Olsen 2000). Under experimental conditions, as in the two original studies (Shapiro *et al.* 1982; Taban *et al.* 1985), there is a reduction in breast cancer mortality following mammographic screening. The reduction of total mortality in the test group is not so marked. The benefits in practice are smaller than in the experimental studies. There are arguments about which age range of women should be included in the scheme, the methods of mammography, the interval between repeat screening and the interpretation of mammograms. There is no doubt that for the scheme to be effective, there needs to be a good organization, careful quality control of both mammography and the subsequent breast biopsy as well as good expert-specialized treatment services including surgery, radiotherapy, and chemotherapy. The scheme, if properly executed, is costly, and critics suggest that the resources could be better used on clinical breast cancer treatment services. The major problems with the services are poor information to participants, increased anxiety in those screened, particularly the false positives, side effects from the biopsy and the risks of radiation exposure. Details of the pros and cons are summarized by Holland and Stewart (2005), who follow the UK National Screening Committee guidelines and accept screening 50–70-year-old women every 3 years as worthwhile. In view of the popularity of breast cancer screening, it would be a daring policy-maker who would suggest that the scheme should cease.

Cervical cancer

A programme of screening was first proposed in the mid-1960s. The original scheme was wasteful, including any woman attending any gynaecological service or family planning. In the United Kingdom, since 1998, the service has been re-launched on the basis of a call–recall system based on the GP patient register. Women are first invited at the age of 25 years and then recalled every 3 years until age 50 when the interval is increased to 5 years. About 80 per cent of the eligible women are screened, comparable to breast cancer screening coverage. Although mortality from cervical cancer has fallen considerably, it is worthwhile appreciating that an enormous effort is required. Raffle (2004), in an analysis of screening records of 348 419 women in Bristol, calculated that 1000 women need to be screened for 35 years to prevent one death, over 80 per cent of women with high-grade cervical intra-epithelial neoplasia will not develop invasive cancer, but all will need to be treated, and for each death that is prevented, over 150 women have an abnormal result, over 80 women are referred for investigation, and over 50 women receive treatment.

The method of cytological examination used is also subject to development. Straightforward cytological examination has been superseded by liquid-based cytological examination and now by human papilloma virus (HPV) culture. This is, of course, in order to automate the procedure. Cervical cancer prevention through screening may be superseded by the use of an HPV vaccine which is now being introduced for girls aged 13 years.

Colorectal cancer

A number of studies have shown that early detection by screening can reduce mortality (Hardcastle *et al.* 1996; Kronborg *et al.* 1996). As a result, screening for individuals aged more than 50 years is gradually being introduced in the United Kingdom (UK Colorectal Cancer Screening Pilot Group 2004). Individuals are mailed a filter paper which tests for faecal occult blood (FOBT). These filter papers are then returned to the centre. If the screening test is positive, then a colonoscopy and/or double contrast barium enema are done. The alternative advocated by some is flexible sigmoidoscopy. Followed if necessary by colonoscopy and/or double contrast barium enema. It is suggested that the screening tests are done at a five yearly intervals. Some authorities advocate screening by colonoscopy, however, it is important to note that this is found to be a very unpleasant procedure by many and carries a risk of bowel perforation of 0.5–5 per cent. It is important that the necessary surgical facilities and pathological and radiological facilities are available for those positives identified.

Prostate cancer

Although a biochemical screening test—prostate specific antigen (PSA) and digital rectal examination and transrectal ultrasound are available, confirmation by biopsy is essential.

Prostate cancer is one of the commonest cancers in men, particularly, the elderly. It has therefore become a 'cause celebre' in screening arguments. Many groups, particularly prostate charities, male advocacy groups and commerce are strong advocates. It has been the subject of intense argument and review. Although it is a very common cancer, many more men die with the cancer than of it (Martin 2007). Many studies have not shown any evidence that mortality is reduced or postponed if screening is undertaken in asymptomatic individuals. In our view, with present knowledge, there is no case for screening well individuals but those with prostate symptoms of frequency nocturia, inadequate voiding, etc. should be investigated.

Other cancers

Lung cancer is the commonest cancer in the United Kingdom. Unfortunately symptoms develop late. Trials of sputum cytology and chest x-ray have not shown any benefit with mortality of those screened compared with controls not improved. Diagnosis is too late. Major trials of spiral-computed tomography are ongoing and offer possible hope of an effective screening tool but the results are not yet available. Far more effective is to persuade smokers to give up smoking.

Ovarian cancer screening is the subject of at least three large randomized trials. Results are awaited before any recommendations can be given. Skin cancer and melanoma are a significant cause of morbidity. Theoretically, they seem a suitable condition for screening. However, no empirical evidence has yet been provided to suggest that benefits outweigh disadvantages. Protection from the sun and by suitable health education is preferable.

Coronary heart disease, stroke, and abdominal aortic aneurysm

Cardiovascular and related diseases are now the commonest causes of death in most developed Western countries and are rapidly catching up with infectious diseases as the main cause of death in developing countries. Since diabetes and cardiovascular diseases are closely related, it is worthwhile to consider them together.

The most effective preventive strategy for these conditions is not to smoke, improve the diet by reducing and maintaining cholesterol level of less than 4 mmol/l, increase the amount of physical exercise and reduce levels of blood pressure to 76-mm Hg diastolic or below. To achieve these goals, the most important changes that need to be made are to behaviour and attitude. As the important risk factor, exposures are so common in the general population, whole population screening programmes are unlikely to be an effective use of resources. Since, in all countries, most of the population has contact with the health services at least annually, it is essential that this contact should be used to reduce these risk factors. Populations with organized primary care systems can develop patient registers on which risk factor details should be noted. Any individual consulting should be advised and helped to stop smoking, have blood pressure measured and if necessary antihypertensive treatment instituted, have cholesterol and weight measured and if necessary given advice re-diet and anti-cholesterol drug treatment (statin) instituted. In addition, of course, appropriate public health measures should be taken to aid people in their decision to stop smoking; for example, by reducing cigarette advertising; banning smoking in public places; improving the provision and reducing the cost of healthy food particularly in deprived areas; providing and encouraging the use of public open spaces, cycling and running tracks, etc.; and labelling food so that people can make better informed choices.

Recent controlled trials and a systematic review have demonstrated the effectiveness of ultrasound screening of men aged 65–74 years for abdominal aortic aneurysm, linked with appropriate vascular surgical services (Cosford & Leng 2007). It is, however, important to note that the risk from surgery is high, and renal disease can result in a minority of cases.

Type 2 diabetes and diabetic retinopathy

Type 2 diabetes is not uncommon. There are divided views about the usefulness of screening for this condition. Wareham and Griffin (2001) do not advocate universal screening. This has also been the view of the National Screening Committee in the United Kingdom. We do not consider that population screening is worthwhile, but as stated above, those considered to be at risk should be tested, and treated if necessary. Spijkeman and colleagues (2002) used a simple validated questionnaire—the Cambridge risk score shows that these individuals are at high risk of mortality and suggests that direct public health interventions may be helpful.

Diabetic eye disease is the most common cause of preventable visual loss in the UK working population. Different methods of screening for diabetic retinopathy are available and have been evaluated by Squirrel and Talbot (2003). These use retinal photography and screening by optometrists. They are certainly worthwhile, but must be subject to stringent quality control and audit. They are quite difficult to establish satisfactorily although a successful programme has been implemented in the United Kingdom.

Mental illness

Depression is the third commonest reason for consultation in UK general practice. A variety of questionnaires have been proposed for screening for this condition. Unfortunately, none of them have met the criteria for an effective instrument. Arrol *et al.* (2003) in New Zealand found two questions: 'During the past month, have you often been bothered by feeling down depressed or hopeless?' and 'During the past month, have you often been bothered by little interest or pleasure in doing things?' detected most cases of depression.

There is a case for opportunistic screening for depression using such a simple questionnaire in general practice. There do not appear to be appropriate indications for screening for other mental conditions or personality disorders or alcohol misuse or domestic violence.

Occupational health

In view of the changes in the distribution of manufacturing and industry, there is now much less concern with the hazards of coal mining and steel production in high-income countries. Thus, in Western countries, most work-site screening is concerned with emphasis on lifestyles, etc., rather than pneumoconiosis or 'bent knees'. This continues to be of importance in areas where heavy industry is common. Thus, in work-site screening, the main concerns are to:

- Assess fitness for the task pre-employment or pre-placement for a specific task, e.g. food handler crane operators.
- Assess fitness during routine exposure to hazards, e.g. specific chemical, noise, radiation, vibration, etc.
- Assess general health risks from history or lifestyle, e.g. smoking, entry to a pension plan.
- Assess capability, e.g. taking drugs.
- Genetic screening—this is still in development and raises major ethical concerns but may be useful to 'screen out' individuals at particular risk for a specific hazard, e.g. chemical exposure.

Screening in the elderly

This is an important issue in view of the increasing proportion of elderly in many societies. There is little scientific evidence of the benefits of screening in this age group largely because of a lack of clear objectives.

In a randomized controlled trial over a period of 3 years in Denmark, Hendricksen *et al.* (1984 and 1989) showed reduced mortality resulting from a programme of home visits and three monthly intervals that led to an improvement in the provision of home helps, equipment, and modifications to the home. Although this incurred costs, they reckoned to have saved about twice as much because of the reduction in hospital nursing home care.

Since most elderly persons have most contact with primary care services than any other age group, these contacts should be used for opportunistic case finding. Obviously, search should be made for potentially treatable condition including hypertension, hearing loss, and visual impairment. It is also worthwhile considering symptomatic conditions such as bacteriuria and incontinence. In addition, a common condition which causes distress are foot problems. Behavioural concerns such as inappropriate medication, lack of physical exercise, depression, dementia, alcohol problems, and social isolation should be considered. Home visits to those aged over 75 years may make one aware not only of inappropriate housing, hazards in the home which may cause falls, but also social isolation under-nutrition and elder abuse. Thus, screening in this age group is concerned with case finding and improvement in quality of life.

Conclusion

The concept of screening for disease offers the possibility of bringing the benefits of health interventions to apparently healthy subjects, free from known disease. This chapter has discussed some of the difficulties associated with this approach. These problems must be analysed from several different disciplinary perspectives. The epidemiological approach is required to analyse problems of screening test performance, as well as questions of the effectiveness of intervention through screening. Applying screening techniques raises important ethical questions concerning the relationships between individuals, screening programmes, and the wider society. These reflect uncertainty and disagreement as to how the benefits and harms from intervening through screening should be valued and distributed. Developing a screening programme represents a complex technical challenge and sound planning and project management strategies should be employed for implementation. Ongoing screening programmes should be continuously improved through application of quality assurance and the implementation of systems to minimize errors and harm. Application of these principles to different screening programmes in the main areas of infections, genetic conditions, vascular disease, and cancer, and at different stages of life, requires detailed knowledge, and the reader is referred to specialist texts for further information.

Further reading

Holland, W.W. and Stewart, S. (1990). *Screening in healthcare*. The Nuffield Provincial Hospitals Trust, London.

Holland, W.W. and Stewart, S. (2005a). *Screening in Europe*. Copenhagen, European Observatory on Health Systems and Policy. World Health Organization.

Holland, W.W. and Stewart, S. (2005b). *Screening in disease prevention. What works?* Radcliffe Publishing, Oxford.

Raffle, A.E. and Muir Gray, J.A. (2007). *Screening: evidence and practice*. Oxford University Press, Oxford.

Wald, N. and Leck, I. (eds.) (2000). *Antenatal and neonatal screening (2e)*. Oxford University Press, Oxford.

References

Ahluwahlia, H.S. and Doll, R. (1968). Mortality from cancer of the cervix uteri in British Columbia and other parts of Canada. *British Journal of Preventive and Social Medicine*, **22**, 161–4.

Anionwu, E. (2001). *The politics of sickle cell and thalassaemia*. Open University Press, Milton Keynes.

Arrol, B., Khin, N., and Kerse, N. (2003). Screening for depression in primary care with two verbally asked questions. Cross sectional study. *British Medical Journal*, **327**, 1144–6.

Balmer, S., Bowens, A., Bruce, E., Farrar, H., Jenkins, C., and Williams, R. (2000). *Quality management for screening*. University of Leeds, Leeds. Available at http://www.leeds.ac.uk/hsphr/ nuffield_publications/ documents/screening.pdf. Accessed at http://www.nsc.nhs.uk/uk_nsc/ uk_nsc_ind.htm.

Breslow, L. and Roberts, D.W. (eds.) (1955). Screening for asymptomatic disease. *Journal of Chronic Disease*, **2**, 363–490.

Chamberlain, J.M. (1984). Which prescriptive screening programmes are worthwhile? *Journal of Epidemiology and Community Health*, **38**, 270–7.

Cochrane, A.L. and Holland, W.W. (1971). Validation of screening procedures. *British Medical Bulletin*, **27**, 3–8.

Colhoun, H.M., McKeigue, P.M., and Davey Smith, G. (2003). Problems of reporting genetic associations with complex outcomes. *The Lancet*, **361**, 865–72.

Collen, M.F. (1988). *History of the Kaiser Permanente Medical Care Programme*. An interview conducted with Sally Smith Hughes. Regional Oral History Office. Bancroft Library. University of California, Berkeley.

Connor, N., Roberts, J., and Nicoll, A. (2000). Strategic options for antenatal screening for syphilis in the United Kingdom: a cost effectiveness analysis. *Journal of Medical Screening*, **7**, 7–13.

Cosford, P.A. and Leng, G.C. (2007). Screening for abdominal aortic aneurysm. *Cochrane Database of Systematic Reviews* (2):CD002945.

Department of Health (1998). *Screening of pregnant women for hepatitis B and immunisation of babies at risk (Health Service Circular: HSC 1998/127)*. Department of Health, London.

Donabedian, A. (2003). *An introduction to quality assurance in healthcare*. Oxford University Press, Oxford.

Dormandy, E., Gulliford, M.C., Reid, E.P. *et al.* (2008) Delay between pregnancy confirmation and sickle cell and thalassaemia screening: a population-based cohort study, *British Journal of General Practice*, **58**, 154–9.

Forrest Report. (1987). *Breast cancer screening. Report to the Health Ministries of England Wales Scotland and Northern Ireland by a working group chaired by Sir Patrick Forrest*. HMSO, London.

Gostin, L.O. (2000). *Public health law. Power, duty, restraint*. University of California Press, Berkeley and Los Angeles.

Gøtzsche, P.C. and Olsen, O. (2000). Is screening for breast cancer with mammography justifiable? *The Lancet*, **355**, 129–34.

Hardcastle, J.D., Chamberlain, J.O., Robinson, M.H., Moss, S.M., Amar, S.S., Balfour, T.W., James, P.D., and Mangham, C.M. (1996). Randomised controlled trial of faecal-occult-blood screening for colorectal cancer. *The Lancet*, **348**, 1472–7.

Hendriksen, C., Lund, E., and Tromgaard, E. (1984). Consequences of assessment and intervention among elderly people a three year randomised controlled trial. *British Medical Journal*, **289**, 1522–4.

Hendricksen, C., Lund, E., and Stromgaard, E. (1989). Hospitalisation of elderly people a three year controlled trial. *Journal American Geriatric Society*, **37**, 119–22.

Human Genetics Commission (2006). *Making babies: reproductive decisions and genetic technologies*. Human Genetics Commission, London. Available at http://www.hgc.gov.uk/UploadDocs/DocPub/Document/Making%20Babies%20Report%20-%20final%20pdf.pdf accessed 13 April 2008.

Knox, E.G. (1982). *Cancer of the uterine cervix*. In Trends in cancer incidence (ed. J. Magnus). Hemisphere, Washington.

Kronborg, O., Fenger, C., Olsen, J., Jørgensen, O.D., and Søndergaard, O. (1996). Randomised study of screening for colorectal cancer with faecal-occult-blood test. *The Lancet*, **348**, 1467–71.

Lin, K. and Barton, M. (2007). Screening for haemoglobinopathies in newborns. Reaffirmation update for the US Preventive Services Taskforce. Evidence synthesis No. 52. Agency for Health Care Quality, Rockville. AHRQ Publication Number 07-05104-EF-1. Available at http://www.ahrq.gov/cliic/serfiles.htm#sicklecell accessed 13 April 2008.

Marteau, T.M., Dormandy, E., and Michie, S. (2001). A measure of informed choice. *Health Expectations*, **4**, 99–108.

Martin, R.M. (2007). Commentary: prostate cancer is omnipresent, but should we screen for it? *International Journal of Epidemiology*, **36**, 278–81.

McKeown, T. (ed.) (1968). *Screening in medical care: reviewing the evidence*. Oxford University Press for Nuffield Provincials Hospital Trust, Oxford.

Moullin, M. (2002). *Delivering excellence in health and social care*. Open University Press, Buckingham.

National Health Service Cancer Screening Programme (2004). *Guidelines on failsafe actions for the follow-up of cervical cytology reports*. NHS Cancer Screening Programmes, Sheffield.

National Health Service Sickle Cell and Thalassaemia Screening Programme (2006). *Standards for the linked antenatal and newborn screening programmes*. NHS Sickle Cell and Thalassaemia Screening Programme, London. Available at http://www.sickleandthal.org.uk/Documents/ProgrammeSTAN.pdf accessed 13 April 2008.

National Screening Committee (2000). Second Report of the National Screening Committee. Department of Health, London. Available at http://www.nsc.nhs.uk/pdfs/secondreport.pdf accessed 13 April 2008.

National Screening Committee (2003). *New world symphony – screening and quality management in the reorganised NHS in England*. Available at www.nsc.nhs.uk accessed 13 April 2008.

Nijsingh, N. (2007). Informed consent and the expansion of newborn screening. In *Ethics, prevention and public health* (eds. A. Dawson and M. Verweij). Oxford University Press, Oxford.

Nuffield Council on Bioethics (2007). *Public health: ethical issues*. Nuffield Council on Bioethics, London.

Osborn, F. (1937). Development of a Eugenic Philosophy. *American Sociological Review*, **2**, 389–97.

Raffle, A. (2004). Cervical screening. *British Medical Journal*, **328**, 1272–3.

Rembold, C.M. (1998). Number needed to screen: development of a statistic for disease screening. *BMJ*, **317**, 307–12.

Samavat, A. and Modell, B. (2004). Iranian national thalassaemia screening program. *British Medical Journal*, **329**, 1134–7.

Sassi, F., Le Grand, J., and Archard, L. (2001). Equity versus efficiency: a dilemma for the NHS. *British Medical Journal*, **323**, 762–3.

Shapiro, S., Venet, W., Strox, P. *et al.* (1982). Ten to fourteen year effect of screening on breast cancer mortality. *Journal of the National Cancer Institute*, **69**, 349–55.

Sorour, Y., Heppinstall, S., Porter, N., Wilson, G.A., Goodeve, A.C., Rees, D. and Wright, J. (2007). Is routine molecular screening for common a-thalassaemia deletions necessary as part of antenatal screening programme? *Journal of Medical Screening*, **14**, 60–1.

Spijkeman, A., Griffin, S., Dibben, J., Nijpels, G., and Wareham, N.J. (2002). What is the risk of mortality for people who are screen positive in a diabetes screening programme but who do not have diabetes on biochemical testing? Diabetes screening programmes from a public health perspective. *Journal of Medical Screening*, **9**, 187–90.

Squirrel, D.M. and Talbot, J.F. (2003). Screening for diabetic retinopathy. *Journal of the Royal Society of Medicine*, **96**, 273–6.

Streetly, A., Clarke, M., Downing, M. *et al.* (2008). Implementation of the newborn screening programme for sickle cell disease in England: results for 2003–2005. *Journal of Medical Screening*, **15**, 9–13.

Taban, L., Gad, A., Holmberg, L.H. *et al.* (1985). Reduction in mortality for breast cancer after mass screening with mammography. *The Lancet*, **ii**, 829–32.

Taban, L., Fagerberg, G., Gunman, D. *et al.* (1989). The Swedish two county Trial of mammographic screening for breast cancer: recent results and calculation of benefit. *Journal of Epidemiology and Community Health*, **43**, 107–14.

Thompson, I.M., Ankerst, D.P., Chi, C., Lucia, M.S., Goodman, P.J., Crowley, J.J., Parnes, H.L., and Coltman, C.A., Jr. (2005). Operating characteristics of prostate-specific antigen in men with an initial PSA level of 3.0 ng/mL or lower. *Journal of the American Medical Association*, **294**, 66–70.

Thorner, R.M. and Remein, Q.R. (1961). *Principles and procedures in the Evaluation of screening for disease*. PHS Publication No. 846. Public Health Monograph No. 67. Public Health Service, Washington DC.

UK Colorectal Cancer Screening Pilot Group (2004). Results of the first round of a demonstration pilot of screening for colorectal cancer in the United Kingdom. *British Medical Journal*, **329**, 133.

UK Newborn Screening Programme Centre (2005). Newborn blood spot screening in the UK Policies and Standards. Available at www.newbornscreening-bloodspot.org.uk. Accessed 13 April 2008

Wald, N.J., Huttly, W.J., and Hackshaw, A.K. (2003). Antenatal screening for Down's syndrome with the quadruple test. *The Lancet*, **361**, 835–6.

Wareham, N.J. and Griffin, S.J. (2001). Should we screen for type 2 diabetes? Evaluation against national screening committee criteria. *British Medical Journal*, **322**, 986–8.

Welch, H.G. (2001). Informed choice in cancer screening. *Journal of the American Medical Association*, **285**, 2776–8.

Wikipedia (2008). *Eugenics*. Available at http://en.wikipedia.org/wiki/Eugenics#_note-Osborn1937 accessed 13 April 2008.

Wilson, J.M.G. and Jungner, G. (1968). *Principles and practice of screening for disease*. Paper Number 34. World Health Organization, Geneva.

12.8

Environmental health practice

Lynn R. Goldman and Elma B. Torres

Abstract

Environmental health practice occurs within the context of physical, chemical, biological, social, and psychosocial processes in the environment that impact health, and actions to modify these factors to promote health for present and future generations. There are many professional disciplines and players in the environmental health practice arena, all of whom have important roles in the process. Environmental health practice is a three-phase process involving health impact assessment, policy development, and assurance that action is taken. Developing countries have a greater focus on prevention of infectious diseases and on efforts to reduce poverty, but their priorities are shifting along with economic transitions. Prevention of global environmental impacts is of increasing priority.

Several international policy goals have been adopted in principle, including sustainable development, the precautionary principle, and the concept of 'polluter pays'. Policy approaches include: Use of best available technology to control pollution, requirements for environmental impact reviews, consideration of economic impacts and equity (environmental justice), and ability to address issues across entire ecosystems. Assuring that policies are carried out largely depends on the strength of the rule of law in a country. Approaches include command and control, pollution prevention, and environmental monitoring. More recently, countries have increased the use of 'right-to-know' approaches. Environmental education plays an important role in strengthening the awareness and role of individuals. Increasingly, international agreements are being used to curb harmful environmental practices, for example, the Montreal Protocol to phase out ozone-depleting chemicals. Such global capacity building is occurring on a number of fronts, for example, control of greenhouse gases and management of chemical in commerce.

The rapid pace of global change, including, population growth, economic globalization, natural resource depletion, and climate change, is creating challenges for environmental health practice, even as economic transitions are creating new opportunities in developing countries.

Introduction

Environmental health practice can be best understood within an overall context of health. In 1993, the World Health Organization (WHO) stated that 'environmental health comprises those aspects of human health, including quality of life, that are determined by physical, chemical, biological, social, and psychosocial processes in the environment. It also refers to the theory and practice of assessing, correcting, controlling, and preventing those factors in the environment that can potentially affect adversely the health of present and future generations' (World Health Organization 1994). Thus, as defined, environmental health encompasses a wide array of determinants that can impact the health of the individual. Elsewhere in this textbook (Volume I, Chapter 2.5 'Water and sanitation', Chapter 2.6 'Food and nutrition', and Chapter 2.8 'The global environment'), chapters provide overviews of the environmental determinants of health. Also, Volume II, Chapter 8.1 ('Environmental health issues in public health') provides a general overview of environmental health issues.

This chapter will focus on the practice of environmental health with respect to non-occupational environmental exposures. It will also focus on those aspects of the environment that are largely not under the control of individuals, such as contaminants in food, drinking water, and indoor and outdoor air. It will not cover voluntary exposures like smoking nor will it cover injury prevention and control of radiation hazards, which are covered in other chapters. This chapter will not cover occupational health, which is discussed in Volume II, Chapter 8.5 ('Occupational health').

Many factors modify the relationship between environment and health. The practice of environmental health should take into account the variability in individual responses to the environment. Differences in age, gender, and individual genetic make-up influence both exposure and susceptibility to environmental agents. Gene–environment interactions are presented in Volume III, Chapter 9.1. A challenge in environmental health is the consideration of all age groups, as well as the very ill and the very healthy, in evaluation of hazards. Behaviour is also important and can have a major impact on exposure. In addition, social differences can affect exposure. For example, diets vary greatly across different cultural groups. People who live in poverty may experience multiple environmental threats, dietary inadequacies, and other factors that contribute to increased risk from environmental exposures.

The practice of environmental health is inextricably involved with the prevention of chronic diseases such as, cancers, asthma, and birth defects as well as acute illnesses such as viral gastroenteritis. The general state of knowledge about causation of many chronic diseases is less advanced than for communicable diseases so that while outbreaks or statistical excesses (so-called 'clusters') of chronic disease are often attributed by the public to environmental exposures, in many cases, the cause is unknown. Thus, practitioners of environmental health are often called upon to address not only known exposures and links to disease but also diseases of unknown aetiology and public concern about the potential for environmental links. How to investigate such issues is outlined in Volume II, Chapter 6.4 ('Principles of outbreak investigation'). In the United States, the Centers for Disease Control (CDC) National Center for Environmental Health and the Agency for Toxic Substances and Disease Registries (ATSDR), as well as state and local public health agencies, are often called upon to address such community outbreaks.

From the outset, it is important to emphasize that certain environmental health problems are much more serious in developing countries; for example, drinking water contamination with microorganisms and toxic substances is much more prevalent and consequent morbidity and mortality more serious. Indoor and outdoor air pollution are much more impacted by the burning of coal, wood, and other biomass fuel sources for cooking and heating homes. Air is much more polluted because many of the controls and technological changes that have been required in developed countries have not yet been applied. Chemical spills and plant accidents are more common and there are fewer means to protect nearby communities and passers-by. Not covered in this chapter, but very important worldwide, is disaster prevention and management. Worldwide there are large numbers of unnecessary deaths and injuries due to earthquakes, storms, and floods, which are completely preventable with appropriate environmental measures like construction standards for homes and buildings.

Environmental health practice in developing countries will follow a unique course according to traditions, culture, and legal structures. Because poverty is at the root of many environmental health problems, elimination of poverty is in itself a major component of environmental health policy-making. Thus, the eradication of extreme poverty and hunger by 2015 globally, a key target of the United Nations Millennium Development Goal, would be expected to result in a number of environmental health improvements (United Nations Millennium Summit 2000).

As developed countries successfully combated most, if not all, communicable diseases and a number of non-communicable diseases, the developing world is still coping with the control of both communicable and non-communicable diseases. This situation is further aggravated by global ecological changes affecting habitats of disease vectors such as those for malaria, Lyme disease, and tick-borne encephalitis (Yassi *et al.* 2001). Further, the global technological progress and ease of travel have likewise facilitated the occurrence and transmission of emerging diseases such as severe acute respiratory syndrome (SARS) and avian flu.

Control of non-communicable diseases is an even bigger hurdle for developing societies to surmount than communicable diseases. This is largely because non-communicable diseases lack a single aetiology and involve numerous factors including environmental exposures, individual behaviours, and other modifying factors, as described above. In developing countries, there is scarcity of information generated from local environmental epidemiological research, thus, making environmental health practice highly dependent on international standards. Although this approach has achieved progress in environmental health, it is open to criticism as to the appropriateness and relevance of using data from more developed countries with different cultures, climates and lifestyle, for assessing local exposures and health risks.

In 1965, Rene Dubos noted that indices of environmental health are 'expressions of the success or failure experienced by the (human) organism in its efforts to respond adaptively to environmental challenges' (Dubos 1965). This effort to respond adaptively to environmental challenges becomes ever more complex as the environment is changed by humans at a very rapid pace. Despite the difficulty of adapting to an environment that has been changed dramatically within just a few generations, there is evidence of remarkable success in this century. The sanitation movement of the 1800s resulted in enormous reductions in mortality due to infectious diseases and marked increases in life expectancy. This has resulted in much of the increase in life expectancy in the United States, from 47 years in 1900 to almost 77 in 1997.

In the last 30 years, in the industrialized nations, stronger environmental laws have resulted in cleaner air, safer drinking water, and recovery of some water bodies that in 1970 had unacceptable levels of pollution for fishing and recreation. In developing countries, on the other hand, economic development and the rapid pace of urbanization have resulted in opposite trends with alarming increases in pollution of air and water and in the generation of municipal and hazardous wastes.

The global trends in environmental health are more disturbing and indicative of a failure to adapt to a changing environment (McMichael *et al.* 2006). (This is further covered in Chapter 2.8 'The global environment'.) On a global basis, the trend for pollution of air and drinking water supplies is upward. Drinking water is under pressure both from pollution and from consumption and in many parts of the world, there are serious shortages of drinkable water today. Even in the United States, there are shortages of potable drinking water in many parts of the country, shortages which may become more chronic with the onset of global warming. Climate extremes associated with global warming are associated with increased risk of epidemics of heat related mortality, increased severity of major weather events and resultant impacts on human health and wellbeing and changes in ranges of vector borne diseases. In addition, over fishing and pollution of water bodies is posing an increasing threat to fish harvests. In most of the world, there is little control of chemicals and pesticides in commerce and chemical waste disposal, even while development is moving forward at a very rapid pace.

Even in developed nations, there are numerous challenges that remain. To a great extent, the easiest problems have been addressed, leaving environmental threats that are much more difficult to control and require more participation from a broader range of society. Often the problems that must be faced today involved multiple small sources of pollutants rather than a few large and visible ones. Many of these small sources are from sectors, like agriculture and small business, which are less familiar with environmental regulations and often resistant to change. Clearly, they will need to be involved; yet, they do not have the resources of large industries to address environmental issues. As automobile emissions become a larger component of air pollution, land use and transportation planning and urban sprawl are becoming greater concerns. Further, problems like non-point source pollution engage everyone in society from the farmer to the weekend car mechanic who needs to know how to properly dispose of used motor oil. All of this means that new tools for assessing and managing environmental hazards will be needed in order to continue to achieve gains in environmental health.

In 1988, the US Institute of Medicine published a report *The Future of Public Health*, which defined three major functions for the practice of public health practice: Assessment, policy development, and assurance (Institute of Medicine 1988). This chapter will take this approach in describing the practice of environmental health. The general principles underlying the practice of environmental health do not differ between developed and developing nations, however, the methods and tools distinctly vary according to the individual country's social, cultural and demographic attributes, economic development, trends in science and technology, management of natural resources, and by the institutional and policy framework that the country supports.

Environmental health assessment

Environmental health assessment is necessary in preventing diseases attributable to environmental exposures. The impact of environment on health is significant. In 2006, WHO estimated that 24 per cent of the global disease burden and 23 per cent of all deaths can be attributed to environmental factors and that developing regions carry a disproportionately heavy burden for communicable diseases and injuries (Pruss-Ustun & Corvalan 2006). Some developing countries have initiated efforts to estimate the burden of communicable diseases attributable to environmental factors using regularly collected national statistics (census, demographic, health, and environmental) and available epidemiological data. Whenever epidemiological and surveillance data are limited, expert opinions from the health and non-health sectors are sought particularly in setting exposure scenarios.

The weight of evidence approach employed in environmental health inevitably involves a multitude of disciplines. Toxicology is the study of how chemicals and pollutants can be hazardous to humans and other organisms. Environmental epidemiologists study and interpret the distributions and relationships among diseases and exposure in the environment. Exposure assessors and industrial hygienists have expertise in measuring and estimating human exposure to contaminants. Analytic chemical laboratories are important for measuring levels of pollutants whether in human blood and tissues or in environmental samples such as air, food, water and soil. Statistics and modelling experts contribute an understanding of how to utilize the often-immense quantity of data in order to inform decision-making. Many science disciplines, ranging from environmental and atmospheric chemistry to hydrogeology, which looks at the dynamics of flow of water in the environment, are needed to understand how pollutants move in the environment and the ultimate fate in terms of exposures to humans and ecosystems. There are many fields of engineering involved: Chemical engineers who can design processes to minimize, eliminate or treat wastes, sanitary engineers who can design treatment systems for wastewater, and so forth. Engineering may play a role not only in the management of environmental hazards but also in the development of standards, as described below.

Thus, environmental health assessment requires specialists from a range of science disciplines and branches of medicine, engineering, and chemistry as well as facilities such as chemical and analytical laboratories. However, many developing countries are constrained in undertaking human health risk assessments, environmental health monitoring and epidemiological studies due to shortage of trained environmental health professionals and practitioners. In addition, support infrastructures and equipment such as chemical analytical laboratories are not widely available and whenever available, are poorly managed and maintained. This problem becomes apparent particularly during reported 'outbreaks' of environmental diseases such as cholera and other gastroenteritis, malaria, paralytic shellfish poisoning, etc. and when community health concerns are raised during industrial 'disasters' such as chemical spills and leaks contaminating air, water and food sources. Developing countries often seek technical assistance from the international community in order to address and manage such situations, but, in the near term, need support to build such capacity.

Generally, the assessment of environmental health threats involves the identification of hazards that may lead to disease states, on the one hand and measurement or monitoring of exposures or doses to the population. *Hazard* is a measure of the intrinsic ability of the stressor to cause harm. *Dose* is the amount of the stressor delivered to the person, organism, or ecosystem. *Effect modifiers* are other factors that influence the relationship between exposure to a hazardous agent and health. These include biologic factors like age and gender, socioeconomic factors such as poverty, and exogenous agents such as exposure to other environmental agents, tobacco, alcohol, drugs, and pollutants.

The principles are those used in the evaluation of epidemiology, the nine Bradford Hill principles: Strength of association, consistency, specificity, temporality, biological gradient, biological plausibility, coherence of evidence, experimental evidence, and reasoning by analogy. A strong association between hazard and dose is one where the risk or odds of disease is relatively large. A consistent association is one that is demonstrated in different studies and perhaps using different methods. Specificity is the extent to which the effect is uniquely associated with a disease. For example, vinyl chloride is the only exposure known to cause a rare cancer, angiosarcoma of the liver. Temporality has to do with the relationship between time of exposure and time of disease. Some diseases like cancer may have long latency periods, as much as 10 or more years. Other diseases are caused by more immediate exposures, for example, pesticide poisoning from carbamates occurs within an hour of exposure. Biological gradient refers to the ability to demonstrate that there is a dose–response between the exposure and the disease. Biological plausibility is the extent to which the association is consistent with what is already known about the response to the exposure and/or the disease. Coherence of evidence has to do with the fit between the studies and what else is known that is relevant to the association and experimental evidence is evidence from controlled experiments that is relevant. Reasoning by analogy is the extent to which the observed pattern is similar to known exposure/disease relationships. For example, knowledge about how benzene causes cancer has been helpful in interpreting data for similar compounds, with similar results from animal studies, but which lack the epidemiologic information available for benzene.

Hazard identification

Hazard identification generally relies on two types of information, data from epidemiologic studies, and data from animal testing and other scientific studies of animals. There are many sources of hazard

Table 12.8.1 Sources of hazard information

Data	Observational studies	Controlled studies
Human	Epidemiology	Dosing studies
	Case reports	Clinical trials
	Surveillance	
	Disease	
	Exposure	
	Case control studies	
	Prospective studies	
Environmental/ animal	Incident reports	*In vitro* studies
	Emissions inventories	General toxicity
	Field studies	Specialized toxicity
	Environmental monitoring	
	Ecological impacts	

information (Table 12.8.1). *Environmental epidemiology* is defined as 'the study of the effect on human health of physical, biologic, and chemical factors in the external environment, broadly conceived. By examining specific populations or communities exposed to different ambient environments, it seeks to clarify the relationship between physical, biologic or chemical factors and human health' (National Research Council 1991).

Environmental health surveillance is an important tool for community environmental health; it is defined as the ongoing systematic collection, analysis, and interpretation of data on specific health events affecting a population (Thacker & Stroup 1994). Surveillance of hazards and exposures, as well as diseases, is critical to the practice of environmental health (Wegman 1992). By tracking exposures and diseases we can identify and respond to different kinds of public health problems. Surveillance and monitoring are also essential to the assurance function, that is, the follow-up to make sure that the treatment for the community is effective (Thacker *et al.* 1996). Examples of environmental health surveillance include air pollution monitoring, blood lead monitoring, poison centre surveillance for pesticide and chemical ingestions, pesticide illness reports, asthma surveillance and birth defects registries. All of these are tools for monitoring trends, and identifying opportunities to prevent and control environmental disease and exposures. Another form of surveillance is post-market monitoring for adverse effects. In the United States, there are provisions under both the pesticide and chemicals laws for reporting to the Environmental Protection Agency (EPA) of adverse health (as well as environmental) effects of toxic chemicals. This can be an important safety mechanism for chemicals approved as a result of animal testing alone since such limited testing cannot detect effects that are expected to occur in a small percentage of the population, especially idiosyncratic effects that are not completely dose-dependent.

It is important to recognize that environmental health monitoring is not the same as environmental quality monitoring. Although many of these data systems have other important uses for enforcement and administrative purposes as well as for assessment of ecological systems, it is clear that environmental health assessments need to be better informed by information about both exposure and disease rates in populations. There are examples of remarkable successes that have resulted in application of the public health model for surveillance in environmental health. The Centers for Disease Control and Prevention (CDC) surveillance of lead levels in children in the United States demonstrated the benefits of the US phase-out of lead in gasoline at a time when this was in doubt and there were efforts to overturn the decision. Despite this and other successes, the capacity for environmental surveillance at the federal, state, and local level is quite limited.

Environmental epidemiology suffers from some limitations. For one, it cannot detect risks of concern when there is little variation in exposure across the population. For example, dioxin exposures are difficult to evaluate in the general population because most people have dioxin body burdens within a narrow range. Second, epidemiology cannot be applied before approving the introduction into commerce of a chemical, product, or technology. Third, studies of environmental exposures often rely on measurements for the ambient environment as a whole rather than measurements of individual exposures. Such studies are known as *ecologic studies* and they are often the only feasible way to study exposures; air pollution is often studied this way. Generally, the larger the area over which exposures are averaged, the greater are the methodological limitations with these studies. The major limitation of ecologic studies is the *ecological fallacy*, which in some circumstances can result from making causal inferences based on ecological data (Morgenstern 1982). Issues related to use of ecological data in epidemiology are discussed in Section II, Chapter 6.2 ('Ecologic variables, ecologic studies, and multilevel studies in public health research').

Animal *toxicity testing* allows examination of a wide range of exposures, use of experimental controls to limit the possibility of confounding and pre-market prediction of hazards. In the practice of environmental health, governments have established regulatory standards or guidelines to ensure that any testing required by the law meets strict standards for quality of the data generated. The international standard that is available, and employed by most industrialized nations, is the set of internationally harmonized guidelines developed by the Organization for Economic Cooperation and Development (OECD). Test guidelines attempt to assay toxic properties of chemicals in a manner that is valid, reproducible, standardized between different laboratories, and is as humane to laboratory animals as possible. In countries, specific requirements for testing vary with the type of substance and the statute under which the substance is covered. In the United States, the most highly tested substances are food-use pesticides, for which numerous health tests are required including: Tests of acute and chronic toxicity, neurotoxicity tests, cancer bioassays, and multiple generation studies to assess reproductive and developmental toxicity. In addition, there are new requirements for tests of immunotoxicity, developmental neurotoxicity, and endocrine toxicity that are being implemented by the EPA. The OECD is currently developing new and enhanced assays for endocrine disruption for oestrogen, androgen, and thyroid effects. Because most chemicals and pesticides are marketed in many countries, the OECD has also established an agreement for Mutual Acceptance of Data to avoid unnecessary duplication of tests.

Toxicity testing is done under *good laboratory practices* (GLP), standards established by governments to eliminate extraneous factors, such as poor nutrition of animals, sloppy laboratory practices, or unclean environments, which would tend to bias or distort the results of laboratory tests. These practices also include record-keeping requirements that allow intensive peer review of studies to ensure their quality. There is an internationally agreed upon set of GLP for chemicals adopted by the OECD.

Despite efforts to carry out accurate toxicity tests, these tests have limitations. To be cost-effective and humane, they are designed with as few animals as statistically possible, while dosing animals at high levels. Outcome measures have been refined over the years but may be cruder than the measurements that can be taken in humans; for example, a mouse cannot report a headache. There can be phenomena that occur in the high-dose groups that are not relevant to human risk assessment. Thus, expert judgement is needed to interpret such data and it is important that scientists review all of the evidence before making a judgement. Unfortunately, there is a perception that animal testing is irrelevant. When we have both epidemiological and animal testing data, there is a striking concordance between the two with respect to relevance to risk assessment. Further, most chemicals that have been subjected to high-dose testing do not cause cancer, refuting the often-made assertion that 'everything causes cancer if you give a high enough dose'.

Despite the availability of accepted tests and practices to assess hazards, the truth is that we know very little about the chemicals in commerce worldwide. The industrialized nations belonging to the OECD have for years been collaborating on an effort to obtain at least screening information about such chemicals (Organization for Economic Co-operation and Development and Environment Directorate 1991).

Exposure assessment

Assessment of exposure involves numerous factors. Usually, in risk assessment, one does not have access to precise measurements of all of these exposure attributes, and yet they are all important in being able to calculate an average daily lifetime exposure. We would like to know the rate and duration of exposure and the amount absorbed, as well as the body weight. Issues related to assessment of human exposures are examined in Chapter 8.4 ('The science of human exposures to contaminants in the environment').

Almost never available to decision-makers are direct measurements of exposure to the human population. It is recognized that such direct measurements, in combination with better information about environmental sources and levels, would be a vast improvement over the current methods for modelling and estimating exposure. In the United States, the National Health Assessment and Nutrition Examination Survey (NHANES) has conducted some population monitoring of exposures and the CDC is beginning to publish data about trends (Centers for Disease Control and Prevention 2005).

As a practical matter, actual exposure measurements are often replaced by defaults. At the US EPA, the policy is to assess a *reasonable high-end exposure*—that is, an exposure at the upper 90th or 95th percentile. Summation of numerous high-end exposures can greatly overestimate exposure, however. Exposure to pesticides in food is a good example of this. Adding up the upper 90th percentile bound for all foods would result in a theoretical individual who eats 5000 calories/day—not exactly a reasonable high-end estimate of exposure. If there are data on distributions of food consumption and on pesticide levels in the food, it is possible to use *probabilistic modelling*, which incorporates those distributions for all foods to compute the distribution of exposure to pesticide residues in the food. Most frequently, this is done using Monte Carlo modelling techniques, not only for pesticide residues on food but also for other aggregate exposure situations. Monte Carlo and other probabilistic modelling techniques simulate the distributions of individual combinations of multiple exposures, to produce a theoretical distribution of an aggregate exposure to the population.

There is not currently a process underway for international harmonization of exposure assessment. This is probably because of the large differences—cultural, dietary, climatic, and others—which can lead to differences in exposures for different countries. For example, in a hot equatorial climate, there is more consumption of drinking water; in the Arctic among traditional societies there is more consumption of marine mammals.

Effect modification

Assessment of effect modification involves a number of considerations. Are there age or life stage 'windows of vulnerability' that need to be taken into consideration (as described below)? It is important to consider whether there are higher (or lower) exposures during these vulnerable times. Another factor is whether there are concurrent exposures or other situations in the population. For example, children exposed to lead may be more vulnerable if they also have iron or calcium deficiency. For another example, risk of cancer from exposure to asbestos is magnified by concurrent exposure to tobacco smoke. Such considerations are especially important in developing countries. Poverty, which by itself is a consequence of the country's economy and social structures, exerts tremendous consequences on health status of individuals. Malnutrition, poor access to water supply, sanitation and garbage disposal, exposures to pollution of air, water, soil and food are the major health concerns brought about by poverty. These factors often occur in combination.

Risk assessment

There are a number of tools used for integrating and summarizing information about environmental health hazards. Environmental health relies extensively on the use of *risk assessment* to evaluate environmental stressors. Use of risk assessment allows us to extrapolate either between human populations or from laboratory animals to humans. It involves weighing all of the evidence in order to develop estimates of the risks to populations who may be exposed. The current practice of risk assessment in environmental health is largely based on a set of principles developed by the National Research Council (1983). Risk is a function of hazard and dose. Four steps in risk assessment have been delineated: Hazard identification, dose–response evaluation, exposure assessment, and risk characterization (National Research Council 1983). These are laid out in detail in Volume II, Chapter 8.7 ('Toxicology and risk assessment in the analysis and management of environmental risk'). Some aspects of hazard and exposure assessment have been addressed above. The section below discusses some aspects of dose–response evaluation and risk characterization that are important to the practice of environmental health.

The practice of *dose–response assessment* differs significantly between a carcinogen and a non-carcinogen. *Cancer assessment* is one of the most established areas of risk assessment. There are several authoritative bodies, all of which conduct cancer risk assessment in a similar fashion. On the international level, there is the International Agency for Research in Cancer (IARC), which publishes monographs on assessments of individual carcinogens.

There are many bodies in the United States, but the most important is the National Toxicology Program, which in its *Biennial Report on Carcinogens* reviews the evidence and lists substances likely to be carcinogenic (US Department of Health and Human Services and National Toxicology Program 2005).

At the present time, hazard assessments for cancer are done in a roughly similar fashion worldwide. At the hazard assessment phase, all studies relevant to the assessment of cancer are reviewed. If there is definitive human evidence of cancer causation, all of these bodies rate the chemical as a human carcinogen. A substance can also be rated as a human carcinogen when the human evidence alone does not prove a causal relationship, but the weight of the evidence is convincing. (This is a change from the past, when only human data could be used to make this judgement.) When there is strong evidence, but not probative, of carcinogenicity to humans, the substance is considered to be a 'probable' human carcinogen. Most systems then have a category for 'possible' carcinogens, those with weaker evidence and non-carcinogens, chemicals that despite testing show no evidence for carcinogenicity.

At the dose–response assessment phase, the default assumption is that the dose–response curve is linear at low doses and starts at zero. This means that we assume that for every additional exposure there is additional cancer risk. In other words, we generally assume that if 20 out of 100 people exposed at 1 part per 1000 in air will get cancer, the risk for an exposure to a much lower level of 1 part per million would be 200 cancers for every 1 million people exposed. This relationship is assumed unless there is compelling evidence for a different dose–response relationship at low doses.

There are many mechanisms for carcinogenicity and it is believed that not all of these mechanisms have linear dose–response relationships at low doses. However, there are rigorous criteria for accepting arguments to depart from the low-dose linear model, and most carcinogens are still considered to have linearity at low doses. Whether from human or from animal data, the dose–response curve is modelled using statistical techniques that extrapolate the curve from the higher doses in the occupational or laboratory setting to the lower doses that are often of concern in environmental settings. Because of the uncertainties in extrapolating from high to low doses, and to account for the variability in the general human population, the dose–response curve is plotted with 95 percentile confidence limits and the upper 95th percentile bound is generally used for risk assessment. This estimate is combined with the exposure assessment to give a probabilistic estimate of risk, e.g. 10^{-3}, 10^{-5}, 10^{-6}.

Non-cancer risk assessment generally involves use of the *reference dose* (RfD) or *acceptable daily intake* (ADI) approach. It is important for decision-makers to understand that a reference dose is a dose considered safe with a margin of uncertainty rather than a bright line for toxicity. A chronic RfD is an estimate of a daily exposure to a population, which, over a 70-year life span, is likely to have no significant deleterious effects (Barnes & Dourson 1988). An acute RfD considers a 1-day exposure only. Generally, the RfD for an acute exposure may be much higher than the RfD for a chronic exposure, but this is very much dependent on the nature of the chemical and effects under study.

Susceptible populations

Children and other susceptible populations pose a special challenge for assessment of environmental hazards. Children are not just small adults. Children develop very rapidly in the first few years of life, their diets vary from those of adults, and they require more caloric intake, oxygen, and water for their body weights than adults. Children's metabolism changes over the first few years of life, affecting how their systems handle pharmaceuticals and toxic substances. Normal childhood behaviour includes intense exploration of the environment and hand-to-mouth activities that can lead to increased exposures to contaminants in soil and around the home. Children lack judgement and thus cannot avoid exposures unless adults ensure that their environments are safe (Rogan 1995).

These differences between children and adults influence toxicity and exposure assessments for children, as well as options for risk management. A National Research Council (NRC) committee in its 1993 report *Pesticides in the Diets of Infants and Children* concluded that the toxicity of, and exposures to, pesticides are frequently different for children and adults. It found that, despite a wealth of scientific information to warrant addressing risks to children, the EPA rarely did so in making regulatory decisions about pesticides. The committee advised EPA to incorporate information about dietary exposures to children in risk assessments, and augment pesticide testing with new assessments of neurotoxicity, developmental toxicity, endocrine effects, immunotoxicity, and developmental neurotoxicity. It recommended that the EPA include cumulative risks from pesticides that act via a common mechanism of action and aggregate risks from non-food exposures when developing a tolerance for a pesticide. Since that time, there has been a major undertaking by government to incorporate these recommendations into federal management of the use of pesticides (National Research Council 1993).

While this is good in theory, children in developing countries may have much more emergent environmental health risks that need to be addressed. A recent review identified unsafe drinking water, lack of sanitation, and household burning of fossil fuels as being responsible for huge number of completely preventable childhood deaths every year: 49 700 in Latin America and the Caribbean, 0.8 million in South Asia, and 1.47 million in sub-Saharan Africa (Gakidou *et al.* 2007).

There are other vulnerable populations as well, many of whom are not in the workplace. Those who live in poverty are very vulnerable because of the potential to multiple exposures, poorer diets, and lack of access to medical care (Institute of Medicine and Committee on Environmental Justice 1999). For example, children who are relatively deficient in iron or calcium absorb more lead per gram of intake than children who have adequate nutrition. The elderly population may be particularly susceptible to some environmental exposures and may have slower elimination of many toxicants. Those who have chronic illnesses are often more susceptible as well. For example, people who have human immunodeficiency virus (HIV) infections or are immunosuppressed as a result of cancer therapy are much more at risk for serious infections from pathogens in drinking water or food. Pregnant women are at risk not only from the perspective of exposure to the developing child but also because of altered physiology and metabolism of many toxic agents. For women, menopause may be another time of vulnerability. For example, there is evidence that at the time of menopause, blood lead levels increase because of liberation of stored lead from bones.

It is easy to conclude that the process of dose–response assessment has become ever more complex, given considerations of the increasing sophistication in understanding of mechanisms of toxicity as well as increased appreciation that there are some in the population that are more vulnerable. This is creating challenges for practitioners in environmental health in developing a language that can be used and understood by stakeholders as well as decision-makers to achieve the public involvement and transparency that are so important in environmental health practice.

Risk characterization

The *risk characterization* is the final step of the risk assessment process. No additional scientific information is added during this phase, which involves estimating the magnitude of the public health or environmental problem. Much judgement is needed in appropriate selection of populations and exposure levels for analysis. In addition, it is important that relevant statistical and biological uncertainties are made clear at this stage. This part of the risk assessment process is the largest nexus between risk assessment and risk managers, and it is important that risk managers receive a complete set of information to guide decisions. This is where the very complex interactions between scientists, decision-makers and the public occur and yet where some of the most difficult communication issues occur as well. Issues related to risk communication are described in Section II, Chapter 8.8 ('Risk perception and communication').

The International Program for Chemical Safety, which is a collaborative effort between the World Health Organization (WHO), the United Nations Environment Program (UNEP), the International Labor Organization (ILO), and the Food and Agriculture Organization (FAO), publishes Environmental Health Criteria documents which are intended to serve as international characterizations of risk for substances. In addition, there is information available in the ILO Chemical Safety Cards, in the WHO/FAO pesticide assessments and in summary form on the UNEP Global Information Network. Many nations make risk assessments widely available via the Internet and other means but it is important to emphasize that the exposure assessment may differ between countries, as mentioned above. While all of this information is helpful, it is also true that the best efforts to accurately characterize risk are hobbled by the great variability in risk among different populations, the uncertainties in our models for assessing risk, and the enormous knowledge gaps that remain even after the most thorough assessment.

Environmental health policy-making

For the most part, environmentally induced diseases and injuries are completely preventable, using pollution prevention, product design, engineering controls, personal protection, housing policies, consumer product safety, and education—all within the context of supportive policy environments including engagement of various industry sectors, government at all levels, as well as the general public, in active efforts to protect the environment. So much of environmental health practice falls outside the realm of traditional medicine because the focus is generally on primary prevention, preventing exposures before the development of disease. At the same time, other interventions flow directly from a physician encounter that diagnoses the health problem and forms a connection between that problem and an environmental exposure (for example, childhood lead poisoning, pesticide poisoning, and asthma exacerbation by air pollution). As with occupational disease, single or small numbers of diagnosed cases can be sentinels for more widespread population exposures and disease. However, environmental health requires a broad range of disciplinary approaches and the application of engineering, sanitation, public health nursing, education and communication, epidemiology, toxicology, statistics, laboratory, administration, enforcement and legal expertise as well as the expertise of public health generalists and physicians. This is therefore a complex web of scientific expertise and information and much of the science of environmental policy-making involves the job of weaving together information from multiple disciplines in order to define problems and develop alternative approaches to solving them.

Who makes environmental health policy? The players

Who makes environmental health policy? Nearly everyone at some level is involved with decisions related to the environment and health. At all the levels, decisions about planning of towns and cities, road building, and economic development all have an impact on environmental health. Much of the time, the policy-makers may not be aware of the environmental health implications of these decisions. Yet, there is a need for more input of public health assessment data into such decision-making processes at all levels. For example, health experts are rarely engaged in discussions about transportation planning in the United States. Involvement of 'stakeholders', literally those with a stake in the outcome of decision-making, is important in environmental health policy-making. In a sense, since everyone wants to be able to breathe clean air, drink safe drinking water and eat healthful food, all are stakeholders in environmental policy-making. Much of the art of environmental health practice is in not only informing but also involving stakeholders in all stages of the decision-making process, from problem definition through selection of alternative solutions to the problem at hand (The Presidential/Congressional Commission on Risk Assessment and Risk Management 1997). It also involves no small amount of political will to see solutions through since by its very nature environmental health protection inevitably involves either costs to taxpayers, costs to industry or both. At the same time, environmental health practice usually creates winners as well as losers and planning for transition from more to less polluting activities is at the heart of environmental health policy-making at its best.

The role of various players in environmental health policy-making is recognized by many nations. It has been promoted internationally as exemplified by the UNCED (United Nations Conference on Environment and Development) Principles of Sustainable Development in 1992 (United Nations Conference on Environment and Development 1992) the Health and Environment Linkages Initiative launched by the WHO and UNEP during the World Summit on Sustainable Development in Johannesburg, South Africa in 2002, and the UN Millennium Development Goals of 2000 (United Nations Millennium Summit 2000). These initiatives are global efforts to promote and facilitate inter-sectoral partnerships and networking in reducing environmental threats to human health in concert with support of sustainable development objectives.

For example, as a commitment to the UNCED principles, the Philippine government enacted a 1992 Executive Order that created the National Interagency Committee on Environmental Health to develop environmental health policies addressing those threats confronting the country (Office of the President and Republic of the Philippines 1992). The Committee is chaired by the Department of Health and vice-chaired by the Department of Environment and Natural Resources. Other sectors represented in the committee are agriculture, public works and highways, science and technology, trade and industry, transportation and communication, labour, economic development, and public information. A successful policy developed by the Committee and put into action is the reduction of paralytic shellfish poisoning morbidity and mortality. Participation of other sectors in the Committee such as non-governmental organizations, the industry sector, and the private sector are sought by the Committee whenever issues concern these sectors. To manage environmental health concerns of various administrative regions of the country, the Committee created the Regional Interagency Committee on Environmental Health; these address local environmental issues and thus support the national policy- and decision-making processes.

Environmental health policy principles adopted by governments

In 1992, more than 100 nations signed the United Nations Commission on Environment and Development (UNCED) treaty that formally adopted the goal of *sustainable development* and 27 principles of sustainable development (Table 12.8.2). Chief among these is principle 1, which states: 'Human beings are at the centre of concerns for sustainable development. They are entitled to a healthy and productive life in harmony with nature'. The second principle is also very fundamental; it describes a 'sovereign right' of states 'to exploit their own resources pursuant to their own environmental and developmental policies, and the responsibility to ensure that activities within their jurisdiction or control do not cause damage to the environment of other States or of areas beyond the limits of national jurisdiction' (United Nations Conference on Environment and Development 1992). The outcomes of UNCED were reviewed in the 2002 World Summit on Sustainable Development (WSSD) held in Johannesburg. The WSSD identified six major environmental treaties that flowed directly from UNCED: The Framework Convention on Climate Change with the Kyoto Protocol; the Convention on Biological Diversity with the Cartagena Protocol; the Convention to Combat Desertification; the Convention on Persistent Organic Pollutants; the Convention on Straddling and Highly Migratory Fish Stocks; and the Convention on the Prior Informed Consent (PIC) Procedure for Certain Hazardous Chemicals and Pesticides in International Trade. All of these directly or indirectly involve environmental health and some are discussed further. At the same time, fighting poverty was a major theme of the WSSD meeting and particularly the urgent need to strengthen the UN institutions working on sustainable development. The WSSD called for a focus on provision of safe drinking water and sanitation, more sustainable sources of energy, and addressing economic and social imbalances in world trade rules and the ecological impacts of the globalized economy in order to contribute to sustainable development (World Summit on Sustainable Development 2002). Thus, while in theory development leads to economic improvements that enhance health, there are enormous problems related to overconsumption, pollution, poverty and inequities that will continue to create challenges for generations to come.

The *precautionary principle* is another UNCED principle for environmental policy-making. As governments agreed in 1992: 'In order to protect the environment, the precautionary approach shall be widely applied by States according to their capabilities. Where there are threats of serious or irreversible damage, lack of full scientific certainty shall not be used as a reason for postponing cost-effective measures to prevent environmental degradation' (United Nations Conference on Environment and Development 1992). For example, the pesticide dichlorodiphenyltrichloroethane (DDT) was banned in the United States long before its precise mechanisms of action had been described by scientists. Despite the agreement to this principle at UNCED, there has been a great deal of disagreement on its applicability within other global contexts, none more evident than in the context of the disputes by the United States and Canada versus the European Union over Europe's ban of hormones fed to farm animals (Carlarne 2007).

Another important principle, adopted in many nations, is the principle of *polluter pays* (United Nations Conference on Environment and Development 1992). Put very simply, this means that those who profit from pollution should pay the price for cleaning it up. More recently, this has evolved to the concept of *economic instruments* such as pollutant trading systems that seek to shift the societal cost of pollution to the polluter, in order to ratchet down the overall levels of pollution. While these principles are important, it is obvious, from the trends that have been mentioned above, that they have not been put in place consistently and that, too often, it is possible to profit at the expense of the health of others as well as the degradation of resources that are needed for human well-being. Worldwide, the practice of environmental health involves not only the application of science but also policy approaches to shift the costs of pollution onto the shoulders of the polluter, because this is one of the most effective ways to prevent pollution.

Environmental health policy tools

There are a number of tools that are used in environmental policy-making. In some cases, an *economic analysis* of costs or feasibility in developing standards is an important driver in decision-making. Economic analyses can play a number of roles including attempting to weight costs and benefits of an action (so called cost-benefit analysis) weighing the relative *cost effectiveness* of alternative solutions to a problem and identification of economic inequities in impact that can inform decision-making.

Pollution and its consequences are not distributed equally in society, and thus it is important to consider *environmental justice* issues in assessment of hazard (Institute of Medicine and Committee on Environmental Justice 1999). Unfortunately, in the past there was a failure to do so, accounting for concentrations of polluting industries, sources of air pollution, and waste disposal operations in certain low income and minority communities. In addition, there are higher rates of many diseases in poor and minority communities globally, lending support to the notion of differential exposure and risk (Goldman & Tran 2002).

Another important tool at a community level is an *ecosystem-based* approach or a *community-based* approach to environmental protection. For air pollution control, it has long been recognized that, for many communities, it would not be possible to meet standards unless management is undertaken for an entire air shed. This approach is now being adopted for protection of large

Table 12.8.2 UNCED principles of sustainable development most relevant to environmental health

Principle 1	Human beings are at the centre of concerns for sustainable development. They are entitled to a healthy and productive life in harmony with nature.
Principle 2	States have, in accordance with the Charter of the United Nations and the principles of international law, the sovereign right to exploit their own resources pursuant to their own environmental and developmental policies, and the responsibility to ensure that activities within their jurisdiction or control do not cause damage to the environment of other States or of areas beyond the limits of national jurisdiction.
Principle 3	The right to development must be fulfilled so as to equitably meet developmental and environmental needs of present and future generations.
Principle 4	In order to achieve sustainable development, environmental protection shall constitute an integral part of the development process and cannot be considered in isolation from it.
Principle 5	All States and all people shall cooperate in the essential task of eradicating poverty as an indispensable requirement for sustainable development, in order to decrease the disparities in standards of living and better meet the needs of the majority of the people of the world.
Principle 10	Environmental issues are best handled with the participation of all concerned citizens, at the relevant level. At the national level, each individual shall have appropriate access to information concerning the environment that is held by public authorities, including information on hazardous materials and activities in their communities, and the opportunity to participate in decision-making processes. States shall facilitate and encourage public awareness and participation by making information widely available. Effective access to judicial and administrative proceedings, including redress and remedy, shall be provided.
Principle 11	States shall enact effective environmental legislation. Environmental standards, management objectives and priorities should reflect the environmental and developmental context to which they apply. Standards applied by some countries may be inappropriate and of unwarranted economic and social cost to other countries, in particular developing countries.
Principle 13	States shall develop national law regarding liability and compensation for the victims of pollution and other environmental damage. States shall also cooperate in an expeditious and more determined manner to develop further international law regarding liability and compensation for adverse effects of environmental damage caused by activities within their jurisdiction or control to areas beyond their jurisdiction.
Principle 14	States should effectively cooperate to discourage or prevent the relocation and transfer to other States of any activities and substances that cause severe environmental degradation or are found to be harmful to human health.
Principle 15	In order to protect the environment, the precautionary approach shall be widely applied by States according to their capabilities. Where there are threats of serious or irreversible damage, lack of full scientific certainty shall not be used as a reason for postponing cost-effective measures to prevent environmental degradation.
Principle 18	States shall immediately notify other States of any natural disasters or other emergencies that are likely to produce sudden harmful effects on the environment of those States. Every effort shall be made by the international community to help States so afflicted.
Principle 19	States shall provide prior and timely notification and relevant information to potentially affected States on activities that may have a significant adverse transboundary environmental effect and shall consult with those States at an early stage and in good faith.
Principle 22	Indigenous people and their communities and other local communities have a vital role in environmental management and development because of their knowledge and traditional practices. States should recognize and duly support their identity, culture and interests and enable their effective participation in the achievement of sustainable development.
Principle 24	Warfare is inherently destructive of sustainable development. States shall therefore respect international law providing protection for the environment in times of armed conflict and cooperate in its further development, as necessary.
Principle 25	Peace, development and environmental protection are interdependent and indivisible.

and complex watersheds both within countries and internationally. Increasingly, it is recognized that *non-point sources* of pollution to air and water—that is, sources that are diffuse rather than from large industrial incinerator stacks and water disposal outfalls—are important. Ecosystem-based approaches are more effective than individual permitting activities in controlling such sources. Across the world today of increasing concern is agricultural runoff from confined animal feeding operations, which can release harmful pathogens and nutrients to aquatic environments. Aquaculture, if not done properly, may directly pollute aquatic ecosystems with animal waste as well as antibiotics and nutrient loadings from feeds. The nutrients in turn have been associated with blooms of harmful organisms like toxic algal blooms and with the production of 'dead zones', areas of hypoxia which damages health by diminishing the productivity of fish and other seafood. Only watershed based management schemes can address this kind of pollution.

Global environmental health policy issues

The threats of large-scale changes to the *global environment*, such as destruction of the tropospheric ozone layer and global climate change, are encouraging nations to cooperate on environmental policy issues. For example, air pollutants can persist and travel long distances, creating environmental damage. Hazardous wastes can be transported across borders and into nations with little or no capacity to handle them. Pollution to large water bodies like the Great Lakes or the Baltic Ocean can affect the quantity and quality of food available to neighbouring nations. Clearly, when pollutants cross boundaries environmental decision-making must occur on an international basis.

Another international issue in environmental policy is the emergence of a global economy, and along with it, a global trading system that is more open than in the past. Although trading agreements have recognized past environmental agreements, there is always the possibility of trade taking precedence over future environmental actions. Environmental policy-making today must take into account not only national economic interests but international ones as well, while upholding the sovereign right of nations to establish their own health and environmental standards as agreed in UNCED.

Environmental health assurance

Environmental health assurance is a complex process that involves a multitude of players. In most nations, there are a number of governmental entities that carry out the process of providing environmental health protection. Generally, there is a national environmental ministry that carries out most national environmental regulatory responsibilities. In the United States, this function is divided between the Department of the Interior and the Environmental Protection Agency (EPA), but this is the exception rather than the rule. Generally, there are separate regulatory authorities for food safety that are either located in the health or agriculture ministry or, in the case of the United States, both. In addition, in many nations, the health or labour ministry also has some responsibility in the area of management of chemicals. There may be separate radiation safety and consumer products agencies as well. There may also be a justice agency (in the United States, the Department of Justice), with additional enforcement responsibilities.

In addition to agencies with direct responsibility for environmental health, there are many others who may become involved because of how regulations affect economic interests in society. Thus, in the United States, the Departments of Energy, Commerce, and Defense, the Office of Management and Budget, the Small Business Administration, and others all become involved where their interests may be affected by regulations. Therefore, at a national level, assurance of environmental health involves a complex web and much of the practice of environmental health involves learning how to coordinate and work effectively within this kind of complex environment.

In most nations, environmental regulation is delegated to state and local government levels. For example, municipal waste disposal is primarily a state and local function in the United States. At a local level in the United States, environmental assurance primarily is in the hands of environmental health divisions within local health agencies. However, there are many other players, including those as diverse as environmental agencies, fire departments, and agriculture departments. Whereas activities at a national level may focus on assuring that there is a minimum standard for clean air, drinking water and food, on a local level there are different responsibilities, such as, inspection of food preparation establishments, rat control, sanitation services, spill cleanups, lead poisoning prevention, and the like.

Command and control approaches to environmental health management

In most of the world, much environmental health assurance is via a *command and control* approach that involves the development and enforcement of *laws, regulations* and *standards*. For example, there may be rules against leaking septic tanks or creating cross connections between water and sewer lines in cities. In addition, for chemicals and pesticides there are licensing functions like new chemicals approvals and pesticide registrations. *Environmental impact assessments* allow the review of proposed projects to ensure compliance with environmental standards prior to the commitment of resources for new development and construction. *Permitting* of facilities for air emissions, water discharges, and waste disposal are essential to controlling point sources of pollution as is a strong environmental *enforcement* presence. Generally, enforcement is targeted to specific goals; hopefully goals that are informed by priorities for protection of health and ecosystems. Generally, the first line of responsibility for enforcement is with local and state health and environmental agencies. Command and control approaches require a strong infrastructure including adherence to rule of law, standards setting ability and authorities, and strong monitoring and enforcement capacities.

The *environmental impact assessment* is one of the best ways of achieving goals related to sustainable development. While the ultimate goal of economic development is the attainment of the highest possible level of well-being of its citizens, and while economic development has brought improvements to general health status, it has likewise brought an array of new and complex health problems. Thus, many countries, including developing countries, have enacted environmental laws related to economic development, environmental degradation and impact on human health. Such laws required environmental impact assessments (EIAs) before development projects are implemented. Impact on health is generally based on secondary health data sets which cover communicable diseases and only limited information on environmentally-induced chronic diseases. Often, a major focus of EIA in the developing world is the social acceptability to communities primarily impacted by the development project. As an example of EIAs in developing countries, in the Philippines, the Health Department developed a National Framework and Guidelines for Environmental Health Impact Assessment (EHIA) (DOH 1997) to strengthen EIAs. The EHIA is integrated into the EIA system and helps assure that human health is considered in economic development in the case of environmentally critical projects (resource extractive industries, power generation, heavy industries and infrastructure projects) and for projects in critical locations (national parks and watersheds, areas where indigenous cultural communities reside, and areas frequently hit by natural calamities such as earthquakes, volcanic activities and floods). The WHO Regional Office for Western Pacific (WPRO) has also commissioned a similar study to develop a regional EHIA framework and guidelines for reference of its member states where about 80 per cent are developing countries (WHO/WPR1997). It is too soon to evaluate these nascent efforts, however. They should provide significant benchmarks for later assessment of impacts of such projects as well as informing decisions about future projects.

Much of command and control regulation is premised on the establishment of environmental standards. Environmental standards may be *risk-based*, that is, wholly or in part based upon assessments of environmental or public health risks. Many environmental standards are *technology-based*. There are many examples of regulatory programs based on *best available technology*, such as the air toxics Maximum Achievable Control Technology (MACT) standards under the US Clean Air Act and similar Best Available Technology (BAT) standards in many European countries. Technology standards can be combined with risk based standards. For example, for hazardous air pollutants, the US EPA was directed by Congress to regulate using MACT standards and then to assess the 'residual risks' and tighten the regulations if necessary. While technology standards can speed the development of regulations they do not help with controlling substances in other media. For example, a MACT standard reducing air emissions of a chemical from a toy manufacturer will not reduce the amount of the chemical in the toys.

Environmental health management tools

There are a number of tools that are used in risk management. *Environmental engineering* has played a very important role in identifying alternative methods for pollution prevention and control.

Pollution prevention is an important tool for environmental management as well as for policy. Increasingly, it is understood that trying to address environmental problems one medium at a time can result in just moving pollutants from water to air to land to water, without a net reduction in risk. The rungs of the pollution prevention ladder go from the most preferable strategy, reduction of pollution at the source (source reduction), to waste minimization, reuse, recycling, emissions controls, and, least preferably, clean-up. It is generally less expensive to reduce pollution at the source and thus avoid costs of emissions controls and environmental cleanup. So called multimedia approaches look at all of the impacts of decisions. Pollution prevention can also be an important driver for decision-making. Often changes that involve source reduction occur over a longer production life cycle than more incremental changes. In the United States, pollution prevention is used in both regulatory and also voluntary approaches to environmental assurance. As an example of the latter in the United States, there is a Presidential Award called the Green Chemistry Challenge, a contest in which companies and universities compete to be recognized for innovative new chemistries that reduce waste and are safer for health and the environment.

Environmental monitoring is also an important tool for evaluating the success of efforts and for targeting future regulatory and enforcement actions. Monitoring can involve reporting by regulated entities or actual sampling and analysis of pollutants in the air, water, food, etc. Such monitoring can be enforcement driven or at random to reflect population exposure. While important for environmental health assurance, environmental monitoring that is directly relevant to human health can feed back into the assessment process and inform future environmental health practice.

Right to know and the power of information

Community right to know is a powerful driver for reducing pollution. It was first introduced at a national level in the United States with passage of the 1986 Emergency Preparedness and Community Right to know Act (EPCRA) and establishment of the Toxic Release Inventory (TRI), which initially required the manufacturing industry to report releases of some 300 chemicals to the public. In the rest of the world, such reporting systems are called *Pollutant Release and Transfer Registries (PRTRs)*. Like the material safety data sheets (MSDSs) in workplaces, community right to know is designed to empower citizens to make informed decisions either as individuals or as a community. Community right to know is a powerful tool not only to inform citizens but also workers within plants as well as plant and corporate managers. In the United States, the TRI helped industry recognize that it often was more cost-effective to prevent the pollution by better managing the flows of materials into, in, and through facilities. In the United States, the TRI was also the basis for a voluntary pollution reduction programme in which industry reduced TRI emissions of several toxic air contaminants by 33 per cent by 1992 and 50 per cent by 1995 from the TRI baseline year of 1988. Canada and Mexico have developed PRTRs that are similar to TRI and work is underway for a North American PRTR that would combine the data for the three countries. Other nations that have developed PRTRs include Australia and the United Kingdom (Kyesku 2003).

Today, with the increasing availability of information online, we will probably continue to see expanded availability of information. A challenge for environmental health professionals will be keeping up with the available information, and helping communities and individuals sift through it to understand what is important and relevant for their communities and how to place it into perspective. Keeping up with and understanding this information is a critical part of environmental health practice. Industry has long been concerned that provision of information is damaging to competitiveness. There are other concerns that information can be easily taken out of context and misunderstood by communities. Clearly, while there is an appropriate balance between providing information and other concerns, right to know has proven to be a useful tool for environmental health protection. Since it is here to stay, an important role of environmental health practitioners is to promote the right to understand as well as the right to know, that is, to provide the context for information so that communities can understand it as well as acquiring it.

Another powerful force in assuring environmental health is the private right of action. This varies with the legal system in countries but in the United States, the tort liability system sometimes has been a powerful driver toward prevention of exposures to environmental pollutants. In some instances, US environmental statutes give the public the right to sue the US EPA to enforce standards (called 'citizen suits' provisions). Completely unique in the United States is California's Proposition 65, which combined the right to know and the citizen suit approach. In a nutshell, companies must label products: (1) if they may cause more than a 1 in 100 000-lifetime cancer risk; or (2) if they may cause reproductive toxicity and have exposures at levels greater than 1000 times the level where no effects are seen (the 'no observed effect level'). Citizens can sue the companies if they fail to provide such warning. Proposition 65 has prompted numerous product reformulations inspired by a desire to avoid having to use the label.

Environmental education also plays an important role in the management of environmental hazards. In the United States, hazards like radon gas in homes and environmental tobacco smoke have largely been managed, on a federal level, by providing education to the public. Environmental educators can also play an important role in helping to translate complex hazard and prevention information so that it is better understood by the public.

International agreements and the emergence of international standards for chemicals

A number of international organizations are responsible for aspects of environmental health practice (Table 12.8.3). As is true for nations, this too is a complex web of activity. Already mentioned are the roles of international organizations in the assessment and policy-making functions of environmental health practice. There are global and regional agreements to prevent climate change,

Table 12.8.3 International organizations involved in environmental protection

Acronym	Organization	Environmental health scope
UNEP	United Nations (UN) Environment Program	Environmental agreements, chemical information systems, technical assistance, right to know
WHO	World Health Organization	Toxicology and epidemiology, IARC, technical assistance
UNCED	UN Commission for Environment and Development	Implementation of Agenda 21 treaty signed in 1992
UNDP	UN Development Program	Sustainable development, growth and population issues
FAO	Food and Agriculture Organization	Pesticides and other agricultural health issues. Food safety (Codex Alimentarius)
IMO	International Maritime Organization	Seafood safety and protection of the seas
OECD	Organization for Economic Cooperation and Development	Harmonization of chemicals testing and classification, good laboratory practices for chemicals, cooperation on waste disposal, climate and other issues
IPCC	International Program on Climate Change	Scientific assessment of climate change
IFCS	Intergovernmental Forum on Chemical Safety	Cooperation on global chemical safety issues
ILO	International Labor Organization	Workplace health and safety; chemicals labelling in the workplace (MSDSs)
SAICM	Strategic Approach to International Chemicals Management	Carries out Global Plan of Action for international management of chemicals
UNCTDG	UN Commission on Transport of Dangerous Goods	Harmonization of classification and labels for chemicals in transport

control emission of ozone-depleting chemicals and decrease acid rain. These include: The Montreal Protocol on Substances that Deplete the Ozone Layer (United Nations Environment Programme, Secretariat for The Vienna Convention for the Protection of the Ozone Layer, and The Montreal Protocol on Substances that Deplete the Ozone Layer 2000), the Rotterdam Convention on Prior Informed Consent, for import of certain toxic chemicals (United Nations Environment Programme 1998) and the Stockholm Convention on Persistent Organic Pollutants (United Nations Environment Programme 2001).

Given the reality of the extensive global trade in chemicals, an internationally-harmonized approach to classification and labelling, which was called 'Globally Harmonized System of Classification and Labeling of Chemicals (GHS)', has recently been adopted. The 2007 edition of the GHS is published at http://www.unece.org/trans/danger/publi/ghs/ghs_welcome_e.html. It is a voluntary system for hazard classification of chemicals. Implementation by nations will require several years but will be important for public health protection and right to know internationally.

Only in recent years have pollutant release and transfer registers begun to be established globally. Under the Aarhus Convention on Access to Information, Public Participation in Decision-making and Access to Justice in Environmental Matters of the UN Economic Commission for Europe (UNECE), there is a protocol for pollutant release and transfer registries that was adopted in 2003. It is not yet in force but is open for participation by all countries globally.

These developments are evidence of a gradual emergence of *international standards*. However, it is important to emphasize that all environmental agreements in existence today recognize the sovereign right and responsibility of nations to set their own standards and tend to get involved only with transboundary issues such as movement of pollutants, trade in hazardous goods and trade in hazardous wastes. For example, the Basel Convention on the Control of Transboundary Movements of Hazardous Wastes and their Disposal contains no provisions relevant to the proper handling and disposal of such wastes generated within a country. As another example, under the Rotterdam Convention on Prior Informed Consent, the covered chemicals may be manufactured and distributed within a country without any prior consent.

In the chemicals arena, the SAICM (Strategic Approach to International Chemicals Management) has developed an *overarching policy strategy* that established objectives for international chemicals risk reduction, knowledge and information, governance, capacity-building and technical cooperation and illegal international traffic, as well as underlying principles and financial and institutional arrangements. Coordinated by UNEP the SAICM Global Plan of Action, which sets out proposed 'work areas and activities' for implementation of the Strategic Approach (http://www.chem.unep.ch/saicm/). Additionally, the Intergovernmental Forum on Chemical Safety contributes to the implementation of the Strategic Approach to International Chemicals Management (SAICM) and the work of other chemicals-related international organizations and institutions by providing an open and inclusive forum where governments and nongovernmental organizations can bring forth new issues with regards to chemicals management (http://www.who.int/ifcs/en/).

Environmental management in developing countries

Environmental health policies and laws are the major driving forces in the prevention of environment-related diseases. Many developing countries are signatories to international treaties and agreements as to environmental protection, sustainable development and health protection and promotion. However, achieving the goals of these agreements is, in many instances, very difficult for these countries.

As primary prevention of disease, some developing countries have enacted and enforced environmental laws covering areas such as water resources, clean air, toxic chemicals, pesticides, hazardous waste management, and solid waste management. However, specific policy-making and environmental standard setting efforts are limited by the lack of relevant epidemiological data and control measures to underpin strategies for preventing the health effects of environmental pollution. For example, indoor air pollution has taken its toll on children's health in many developing countries. Indoor smoke from biomass cooking fuel and second-hand cigarette smoke are significant triggers for asthma attacks (Etzel 2003; Desai *et al.* 2004). The lack of local epidemiological and exposure data deters the development of environmental standards for indoor air pollutants, so that pollution abatement strategies are difficult if not impossible to implement.

Another example for developing countries is the lack of remediation goals for sites contaminated by chemicals. There are insufficient local epidemiological, exposure and environmental data to support development of environmental clean-up standards to reduce the contamination to practically reasonable levels by which health risks are minimized. Moreover, many contaminated sites—such as vacant lot or open spaces or rivers, where wastes have been dumped or buried—have no known legal 'owners' and there are no funds for the government to clean these sites.

Conclusions

In conclusion, the practice of environmental health has come a long way in the last several decades. Although there is still much to be learned about environmental health risks, today, we do possess not only a tremendous fund of knowledge but also a number of tools, and areas of expertise, that can be brought to bear to address the most hazardous environmental conditions. We can point to many achievements that have been gained over the years such as, improvements in sanitation, alleviation of some of the worst sorts of air pollution, prevention of lead poisoning and removal of some of the most hazardous substances from consumer and household products. At the same time, the job is not done and there is a tremendous need for strengthening the practice of environmental health on a global basis. Particularly, those living in poverty continue to be deprived of safe drinking water, food, air, housing and consumer products. The rapid pace of several factors involved with global change, including, population growth, economic globalization, natural resource depletion, and climate change, are likely to create even more challenges to assuring safe environments globally. At the same time, these same conditions are opening up new opportunities. As economies transition, there can be more opportunities to engage in efforts to improve environmental health, as well as to expand the opportunities for training environmental health professionals in developing countries. Likewise, the global nature of many of the challenges we face today are likely to promote further action to develop global governance systems for assuring environmental health (Carpenter 2003).

Key points

- Environmental health practice is best understood within a broader context of efforts to improve health of communities, but it involves a much broader range of interests and stakeholders than other areas of public health practice.
- A critical component of environmental health practice is assuring a healthy environment through environmental management efforts, which involve a broad range of disciplines (medical, engineering, public health) as well as approaches (based on engineering controls, risk-based standards setting, information-based efforts and pollution prevention).
- Environmental health impact assessment is an important tool for review of development projects in order to determine the likely environmental and health consequences before decisions are taken.
- Environmental health policy development occurs at all levels of government and, internationally; it is informed by scientific evidence, economic analyses, considerations of justice, and principles of sustainable development, such as, the precautionary principle and the polluter pays principle.
- Environmental health assessment and monitoring provide important feedback to practitioners in developing priorities for action and assessing the efficacy of past efforts; numerous data are relevant, including risk assessments, environmental health surveillance, and monitoring levels of pollutants in air, water, food, and products.

References

Barnes, D. and Dourson, M. (1988). Reference dose (RfD): description and use in health risk assessments. *Regulatory Toxicology and Pharmacology*, **8**, 471–86.

Carlarne, C. (2007). From the USA with love: sharing home-grown hormones, GMOs, and clones with a reluctant Europe. *Environmental Law*, **37**(Spring), 301–36.

Carpenter, D.O. (2003). The need for global environmental health policy. *New Solutions*, **13**(1), 53–9.

Centers for Disease Control and Prevention (2005). *Third National Report on human exposure to environmental chemicals*. CDC, Atlanta.

Desai, M., Mehta, S., and Smith, K. (2004). Indoor smoke from solid fuels: assessing the environmental burden of disease at national and local levels. *Environmental Burden of Disease Series*, (4). World Health Organization, Protection of the Human Environment, Geneva.

Dubos, R. (1965). *Man adapting*. Yale University Press, New Haven.

Etzel, R.A. (2003). How environmental exposures influence the development and exacerbation of asthma. *Pediatrics*, **112**(1 Pt 2), 233–9.

Gakidou, E., Oza, S., Vidal Fuertes, C. *et al.* (2007). Improving child survival through environmental and nutritional interventions: the importance of targeting interventions toward the poor. *JAMA*, **298**(16), 1876–87.

Goldman, L.R. and Tran, N. (2002). *Preventable tragedies: the impact of toxic substances on the poor in developing countries: a report to the World Bank*. The World Bank, Washington, DC.

Institute of Medicine (1988). *The future of public health*. National Academy Press, Washington, DC.

Institute of Medicine and Committee on Environmental Justice (1999). *Toward environmental justice: research, education and health policy issues*. National Academy Press, Washington, DC.

Kyesku, P. (2003). The evolution of the pollution inventory. *Environmental Information Bulletin*, **128**, 12–5.

McMichael, A.J., Woodruff, R.E., and Hales, S. (2006). Climate change and human health: present and future risks. *Lancet*, **367**(9513), 859–69.

Morgenstern, H. (1982). Uses of ecologic analysis in epidemiologic research. *American Journal of Public Health*, **72**(12), 1336–44.

National Research Council (1983). *Risk assessment in the federal government: managing the process*. National Academy Press, Washington, DC.

National Research Council (1991). *Environmental epidemiology: public health and hazardous wastes*. National Academy Press, Washington, DC.

National Research Council (1993). *Pesticides in the diets of infants and children*. National Academy Press, Washington, DC.

Office of the President and Republic of the Philippines (1992). *Executive Order No. 489. Institutionalizing the Inter-agency Committee on Environmental Health.*

Organisation for Economic Co-operation and Development and Environment Directorate (1991). *Decision-recommendation of the council on the co-operative investigation and risk reduction of existing chemicals C(90)163/final*. Organisation for Economic Co-operation and Development, Paris.

Pruss-Ustun, A. and Corvalan, C. (2006). *Preventing disease through healthy environments*. World Health Organization, Geneva.

Rogan, W.J. (1995). Environmental poisoning of children – lessons from the past. *Environmental Health Perspectives*, **103** (Suppl. 6), 19–23.

Thacker, S.B. and Stroup, D.F. (1994). Future directions for comprehensive public health surveillance and health information systems in the United States. *American Journal of Epidemiology*, **140**(5), 383–97.

Thacker, S.B., Stroup, D.F., Parrish, R.G., and Anderson, H.A. (1996). Surveillance in environmental public health: issues, systems, and sources [see comments] [published erratum appears in Am J Public Health 1996 Nov;86(11):1526]. *American Journal of Public Health*, **86**(5), 633–8.

The Presidential/Congressional Commission on Risk Assessment and Risk Management (1997). *Framework for Environmental Health Risk Management*, Washington, DC.

U.S. Department of Health and Human Services and National Toxicology Program (2005). *Report on carcinogens, Eleventh Edition*. U.S. Department of Health and Human Services, Public Health Service, Research Triangle Park.

United Nations Conference on Environment and Development (1992). *Rio declaration on environment and development*. United Nations, Rio de Janeiro.

United Nations Environment Programme (1998). *Convention on the prior informed consent procedure for certain hazardous chemicals and pesticides in international trade*. UNEP, Rotterdam.

United Nations Environment Programme (2001). *Convention on persistent organic pollutants*. UNEP, Stockholm.

United Nations Environment Programme, Secretariat for The Vienna Convention for the Protection of the Ozone Layer, and The Montreal Protocol on Substances that Deplete the Ozone Layer (2000). *The Montreal protocol on substances that deplete the ozone layer*. United Nations Environment Programme, Nairobi.

United Nations Millennium Summit (2000). *United Nations millennium declaration. Millennium development goals*. UN, New York.

Wegman, D. (1992). Hazard surveillance. In *Public health surveillance* (eds. W. Halperin and E.J. Baker), pp. 62–75. Van Nostrand Reinhold Co, New York.

World Health Organization (1994). Action plan for environmental health services in Eastern and Central Europe and the Newly Independent States: Report on a WHO Consultation, Sofia, Bulgaria, 19–22 October 1993. WHO Regional Office for Europe, Copenhagen.

World Health Organization.(1997). *EHIA Framework for the Western Pacific Region*.

World Summit on Sustainable Development (2002). *World summit declares 'fault line' between rich and poor threatens prosperity, adopts broad measures to alleviate poverty, protect environment (17th Plenary Meeting (PM) and Round-up) ENV/DEV/J/35*. UN Department of Public Information, Johannesburg; News and Media Services Division, New York.

Yassi, A., Kjellstrom, T., de Kok, T., and Guidotti, T. (2001). *Basic environmental health*. Oxford University Press, New York.

12.9

Structures and strategies for public health intervention

Don Nutbeam and Marilyn Wise

Abstract

The earlier chapters of this book confirm that the scientific basis for public health is well developed and evolving in response to emerging public health challenges. However, to achieve the goal of improving the health of populations and improving equity in health, this science must be applied both within the health sector and more broadly in society in ways that have an impact on the social determinants of health.

The application of the science of public health is dependent upon the existence of an infrastructure for public health action that provides strategic and technical public health leadership, and contributes directly to the development and implementation of policies and programmes that are necessary to deliver improvements in the health of populations. Such infrastructure must also include the capacity to form partnerships with communities and with organizations across different sectors that support the delivery of public health services and programmes, as well as the capacity to evaluate and report routinely on progress.

This chapter analyses and describes key elements of an infrastructure for public health that have been found to be effective in guiding national action, and the components of an infrastructure and delivery system required to design, deliver, and evaluate public health interventions. Public health intervention requires a complex mix of science, art (of practice), and politics. Four key challenges for the future emerge from this analysis: The need to address all determinants of health, the importance of gaining greater public visibility for public health, the need to increase our capacity to work across sectors to develop policy and plans to improve health, and the importance of working with all the people and organizations that have a role in improving or protecting the health of populations.

Introduction

Current and emerging public health problems require the application of existing knowledge and strategies within the health sector and more broadly in society in ways that have an impact on the key determinants of health such as environment, education and employment. The greatest contemporary public health challenge is to ensure that there is action to achieve equity—to eliminate the unjust gaps in life expectancy and health across the life span that have proven to be persistent within wealthy and poor nations and, of course, between nations.

The most explicit sign of a nation's commitment can be found in the extent to which public policy and investment are linked explicitly to achieving improved population health and reducing inequity. Examples of this type of commitment can be observed in countries such as Sweden, Canada, and the United Kingdom (Agren 2003; Public Health Agency of Canada 2007; Wanless 2004). But in addition to policy, action is needed. The translation of policy (and resources) into effective action is dependent upon the existence of an infrastructure for public health action that provides both strategic and technical public health leadership, and that contributes directly to the development and implementation of policies and programmes that are necessary to deliver improvements in the health of populations. Such infrastructure must also include the capacity to form partnerships with communities, and with organizations across different sectors that support the delivery of public health services and programmes, as well as the capacity to evaluate and report routinely on progress.

Figure 12.9.1 provides an overview of the essential elements of such a system, and provides the structure for this chapter. Based on analysis of experiences in several countries, the Figure traces the steps which link identification of the determinants of health, through definition of priorities and development of policy, to the infrastructure and delivery systems required by countries and regions to guide and implement effective public health action (International Union for Health Promotion and Education 1999; National Health and Medical Research Council 1997; Mittelmark *et al.* 2007).

Figure 12.9.1 describes an infrastructure and delivery system that enables countries or regions to apply public health science both to the identification and analysis of the determinants of public health problems, and to the design, delivery and evaluation of public health interventions. The infrastructure includes the capacity to link evidence of the effectiveness of these public health actions with regular review and re-definition of problems and priorities for public health and for related policy, and to a system of public accountability for progress (Australian Institute of Health and Welfare 2006a; NSW Health 2007).

Following the structure in Fig. 12.9.1, the chapter explores the need for an initial analysis of the determinants of public health problems—economic and social, alongside behavioural and environmental—and of their distribution across populations and communities. These analyses then provide the raw material for political, professional and community debate on the issues/problems to be given greatest priority, and to identify the most effective interventions to address their causes and health consequences. This will often include action with sectors other than the health sector in the development of public policy interventions.

Expanding the vision of national health policies beyond the provision of health care services has proved to be consistently challenging around the world. This is especially the case in attempting to develop 'health policies' that address the underlying determinants of health that are often outside of the scope and immediate influence of Health Ministries or Health Ministers. The chapter begins with examples of different initiatives taken to date by governments. It goes on to identify the explicit components of infrastructure and capacity needed by the health sector in particular (and government in general) to direct and guide action to achieve improved population health and reductions in inequity.

Policies and interventions to address the determinants of health in populations

Earlier chapters in this book describe the range of personal, social, economic and environmental factors that are related to increased risk of disease, and of adverse outcomes from disease. Analysis of the determinants of the health of populations is essential to clarify the relative importance of each, and to identify those that are modifiable through public health intervention.

These determinants include individual characteristics and behaviours, such as smoking, physical activity, hypertension or diet, which have been the focus for the majority of public health interventions in high-income countries to reduce the burden of non-communicable disease in the population over recent decades. Epidemiological analysis also reveals major differences in the disease experiences of different groups in populations with different social, economic and environmental circumstances. Although some of these differences can be explained by differences in individuals' health-related behaviours (such as tobacco use and food choices), more of the difference is explained by the different social, economic and environmental circumstances in which people live and work (Raphael 2007; Marmot & Wilkinson 1999).

For example, in the case of coronary heart disease Marmot's work in the United Kingdom has indicated that a high proportion of the variance in premature deaths between different social groups cannot be adequately explained by known behavioural and other personal risk factors. Other factors, related to differences in the social status and economic conditions of different groups within a population, clearly play a major role in determining the health status of populations. The distribution of these conditions is socially determined and is beyond the control of individuals, and is not amenable to change through health sector related activities alone.

However, it is increasingly clear that policies and interventions to modify these social, economic, and environmental conditions have

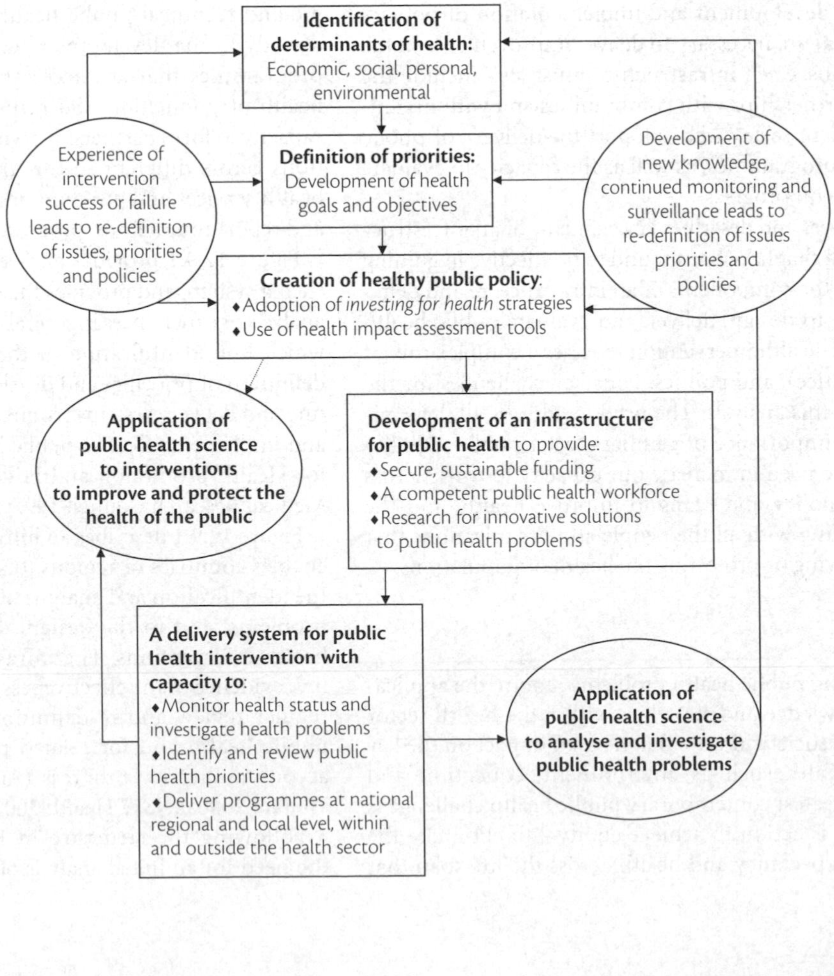

Fig. 12.9.1 Overview of an infrastructure for public health intervention.

the potential to produce even greater gains in health status than those attributed to changes in lifestyles and improved health care in many high-income countries in the past two decades.

This is not a new discovery. Creating supportive environments for health has been a major goal of public health policy and action for the past 150 years. Environmental interventions to provide clean water and waste disposal, safe food, and safe living and working conditions led to major improvements in public health in industrialized countries. Programmes to improve maternal and child health, and effective mass immunization programmes have been effective in reducing morbidity and mortality among children in most countries throughout the twentieth century.

However, over the course of the twentieth century the very success of public health policy, research and practice meant that it became 'invisible' in many countries. In industrialized countries, the public health policies, strategies and structures that had been so effective in reducing mortality and morbidity across their populations were in decline by the middle of the twentieth century. In most countries the great proportion of health sector investment has been (and remains) in biomedical intervention. In high-income countries, in particular, public health interventions have tended to become marginalized within the health sector, and rather narrowly focused on the identification of biological and behavioural risk factors for non-communicable diseases—followed by interventions that aimed to change individuals' lifestyles.

This has meant that progress toward improving the health of populations has been limited and that the benefits have been distributed unequally and unfairly. Limited public health interventions to address behavioural risks have had an impact on the lifestyles of those who are wealthier and better educated—those best placed to make personal changes in their lifestyles. But there is evidence that these interventions may also have had an unintended effect of exaggerating existing differences in health status between social groups.

The need to expand health policy to include explicit commitment to improving the health of populations (and not, simply, to responding to disease and injury), and to eliminating unjust inequalities in the distribution of health was identified more than 30 years ago by the World Health Organization (WHO). The concept of *Health for All* was adopted as the main social target of governments and the WHO at that time (World Health Organization 1980). This resolution represented a commitment to explore new avenues to solve public health problems and gave prominent attention to the need to reduce growing health inequalities between and within countries. *Health for All* provided a major focal point for a renaissance in public health action, and impetus for a long overdue examination of health policy, infrastructure, capacity and evidence.

However, even with the evidence and WHO leadership it has proven difficult for health sectors (and governments) in most countries to use this knowledge to design and implement the interventions necessary to achieve the goal of *Health for All*, and to build the infrastructure and capacity to deliver these effectively and efficiently.

Designing effective interventions

All health problems in any population have multiple causes or determinants. Finding ways of taking action that effectively address these represents a major challenge for governments and public health systems in all countries. In the 1980s, WHO led a series of processes designed to reinvigorate public health practice by bringing a wider range of disciplinary perspectives to public health interventions. These reforms were in response to changes in the disease profile in most high-income countries resulting from the emergence of health problems that have their origins in individual behaviours and social conditions. This 'new public health' methodology was referred to as *health promotion*. For many, a significant turning point in the conversion of this renewed interest and understanding into public health action came through the *Ottawa Charter for Health Promotion* (World Health Organization 1986). The Charter advocated a 'new' approach to public health, where public health intervention had come to be understood as action which is directed towards improving people's control over all modifiable determinants of health.

The late twentieth century saw the growth of evidence confirming that it is possible to act purposefully to improve the health of populations—to reduce the incidence of acute and chronic conditions, to reduce the prevalence of some conditions, and to reduce deaths associated with these (International Union for Health Promotion and Education 1999; Centers for Disease Control and Prevention 1999; Wanless 2004). Although progress has been achieved through interventions that are highly targeted to the needs of specific population groups, on its own, this is neither optimally effective nor efficient in achieving the shift in population risk first described by Geoffrey Rose (1992). Taking smoking as an example, although there are some good targeted interventions (e.g. for pregnant women) the greatest progress in reducing the prevalence of smoking in a population has been achieved by combining efforts to communicate to people the benefits of not smoking with a wider set of measures to reinforce and sustain this healthy lifestyle choice. This has meant taking action to reduce demand through restrictions on promotion and increases in price, to reduce supply by restrictions on access (especially to minors), and to reflect social unacceptability through environmental bans (Bonnie *et al.* 2007). Such a comprehensive approach addresses the underlying social and economic determinants of individuals' behavioural choices, and was recognized formally in the world's first international public health treaty—the Framework Convention on Tobacco Control (2003) that was adopted at the World Health Assembly in 2003.

This same comprehensive approach to implementing a complex array of actions to address public health problems is being highlighted in contemporary efforts to reduce or at least slow the advance of obesity in populations across the globe (Popkin 2007).

However, such actions, although successful in reducing the prevalence of some major diseases and behavioural risk factors across populations (on average), have not, as yet, proven to be effective in reducing the pre-existing inequities in the distribution of the social determinants of health within populations. The need to expand action to more overtly address these social determinants is now being recognized (Norwegian Ministry of Health and Care Services 2007). Evidence-based actions to address the impact of social determinants of health are gradually emerging (Raphael 2007; Whitehead 2007; World Bank Povertynet 2007; Cutler & Lleras-Muney 2007; Kawachi *et al.* 1999). More needs to be done to convert our understanding of the causes of inequalities into practical, politically manageable policies and actions. In 2003, the World Health Organization established a Commission on the Social Determinants of Health to focus more precisely on identifying actions to address the social determinants of health effectively, and to stimulate governments, the private sector and civil society to take these actions (World Health Organization 2006). The WHO Bangkok Charter (2005) affirmed that policies and partnerships to empower communities and to improve health and health equality should be at the centre of global and national development.

Determining directions and priorities for public health intervention

The 1980s saw the development of national health policy in several countries that incorporated, for the first time, national health goals and objectives—expressed as quantifiable, population-wide health outcomes. The US national health objectives (US Department of Health and Human Services 1980) and the World Health Organization European Region promoted health targets as a mechanism for defining the outcomes expected of nations' investment in 'health', as a mechanism for defining differences in health status between populations and as a mechanism for targeting reductions in these differences—the central tenet of *Health for All* (World Health Organization, Regional Office for Europe 1985, 1999). Several other nations followed these leads in the 1980s and 1990s (Nutbeam & Wise 1996).

The initial rationale for setting national health goals and targets was to link national health investment with improved population health outcomes. In specifying this link, it was intended that the role of public health interventions (in addition to the provision of health care services) would become more prominent—highlighting the need for interventions to prevent the onset of disease and occurrence of injury, in addition to the interventions to diagnose, treat, and rehabilitate people with symptoms or established illness. For the first time, nations were establishing *a priori* benchmarks against which to measure the effectiveness and efficiency of their investments in the health of populations. In itself, this shift in focus was a significant conceptual step for governments, for health professionals and populations—from a focus on the provision of health care services to a focus on the achievement of population health outcomes.

Although there are similarities in the rationale for setting national health goals and targets across nations, there has been considerable strategic and technical variation in their development, in their scope, and in their intended impact. It is useful to analyse some of these variations in order to identify the strengths and weaknesses of the different approaches, and to assess their implications for the future.

Developing national health goals and targets is a significant technical undertaking, and the process in most countries has revealed the need for expanded national health information systems to gather, analyse and report on the health of their populations over time. This has required clarity in understanding of the links between health outcomes and their determinants. It has also required the definition of indicators that measure health outcomes (mortality and morbidity, life expectancy and quality of life), as well as indicators of the social and behavioural determinants of the health of populations, and of the distribution of health in populations. These challenges in turn have highlighted strengths and weaknesses in national health data and in the data available from other sectors that impact on health determinants.

Setting health objectives and targets also requires some form of explicit prioritization—inevitably it involves identification of objectives and targets in relation to a relatively defined range of health issues, population groups or settings that would receive greatest attention and investment.

Australia's experience in setting national health goals and targets provides an example of these processes. Work on national targets began in 1987, resulting in a narrowly defined group of priority health issues and behavioural risk factors in 1988 (Health Targets and Implementation Committee 1988). But in 1993 a major revision expanded the scope of the targets beyond the limited range of the initial report (Nutbeam *et al.* 1993). This work saw the inclusion of two new categories of health targets concerned with *personal health literacy* and *healthy environments*, and a section focusing explicitly on the role of health services in achieving the overall goals and targets.

Figure 12.9.2 is derived from the report and provides an illustration of the framework for the targets, showing how each of three key determinants of health—health literacy, health behaviours, and healthy environments—is inextricably linked to the other. The report made a strong case for coordinated public health action to address all of the determinants, particularly by adding to existing efforts to promote health literacy and healthy lifestyles with matching attention to the creation of healthy environments.

The Australian experience provides an example of the ways in which health targets can be used to highlight and address the social, economic and environmental determinants of health status. The report was also structured partly to reflect the way in which government was organized into Ministries (e.g. housing, employment, environment), and partly to build upon existing working relations between the health sector and other sectors (e.g. health promoting schools). Such an approach was seen as important both in defining the respective roles of the different sectors, in establishing a workable model for monitoring progress, and determining accountability for the achievement of targets (Nutbeam *et al.* 1993).

More recently, other governments have been strong advocates of the use of targets in all sectors to set priorities, and to make explicit expectations for change over time. In England two 'headline' targets were set to reduce health inequalities over a 10-year period. These medium-term targets are backed by a set of 12 short-term indicators that were adopted as a way of assessing progress within 10 years through several ministries in addressing the underlying determinants of health across a range of sectors (Department of Health 2003). Table 12.9.1 lists the two headline targets and 12 national indicators.

A further distinction among the goals and targets set by different nations exists in the extent to which the process was used to identify the strategies (policies and programmes) that would be necessary to achieve them, and to allocate responsibility for action. In the United States for example, the implementation of policies and programmes to achieve the objectives was substantially a responsibility of each individual state (and not of the Federal government), and of organizations/agencies of civil society as well as the private sector that had contributed to setting the goals and targets, and to establishing priorities.

By contrast, the targets and indicators established in England have been developed following a Treasury review of spending by different ministries to assess the extent to which their respective policies and programmes contributed to the action necessary to reduce health inequalities. This review led to a cross-government strategy that specifies the actions and responsibilities of different

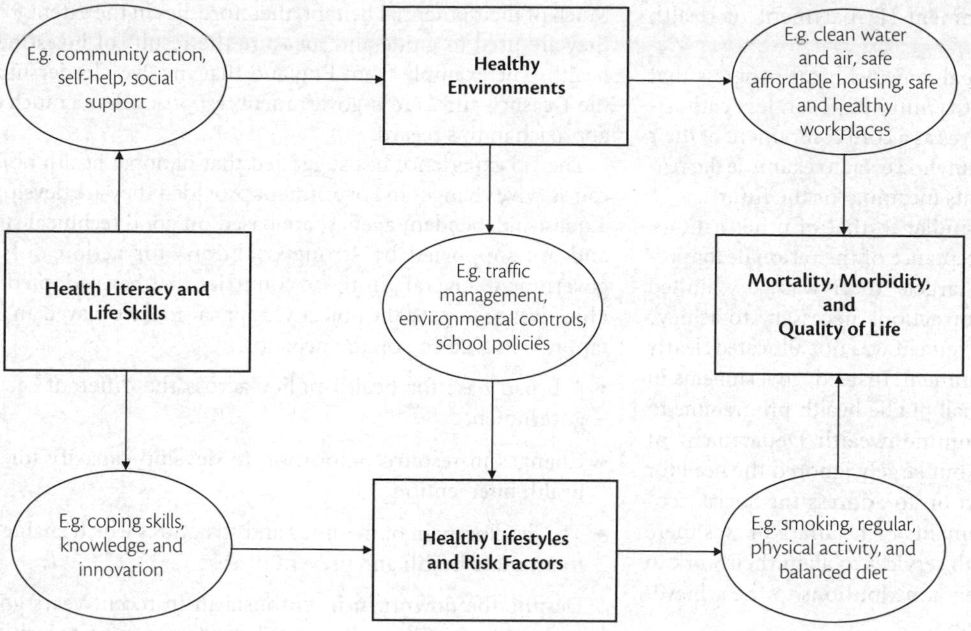

Fig. 12.9.2 The relationship between the four groups of health targets. Examples of targets are shown in oval boxes.
Source: Nutbeam *et al.* (1993).

Table 12.9.1 English health inequalities targets, and headline indicators

Health inequalities targets	
1. Infant mortality	A 10% reduction in the relative gap (i.e. percentage difference) in infant mortality rates between the 'routine and manual' socioeconomic group and England as a whole from the baseline year of 1998 (the average of 1997–1999) to the target year 2010 (the average of 2009–2011).
2. Life expectancy	A 10% reduction in the relative gap (i.e. percentage difference) in life expectancy at birth between the fifth of areas with the worst health and deprivation indicators and England as a whole.
Headline indicators	
1. Preventable deaths	Age-standardized death rates per 100 000 population for the major killer diseases (cancer, circulatory disease), ages under 75 (for the 20% of areas with the highest rates compared with the national average.
2. Teenage pregnancies	Rate of under-18 conceptions comparing differences by area of deprivation.
3. Road accident casualties	Road accident casualties comparing differences by area of deprivation.
4. Access to primary care	Number of primary care professionals per 100 000 population comparing differences by area of deprivation.
5. Uptake of flu vaccinations	Percentage uptake of flu vaccinations by older people (aged 65+) comparing differences by area of deprivation.
6a. Prevalence of smoking	Prevalence of smoking among people in manual social groups.
6b. Prevalence of smoking among pregnant woman	Prevalence of smoking among pregnant woman comparing differences by area of deprivation.
7. Educational attainment	Proportion of those aged 16 who get qualifications equivalent to five GCSEs at grades A to C comparing national average with schools in the most disadvantaged communities
8. Fruit consumption	Proportion of people consuming five or more portions of fruit and vegetables per day in the lowest quintile of household income distribution.
9. Housing quality	Proportion of households living in non-decent housing comparing private and social housing status.
10. Physical activity	Percentage of schoolchildren who spend a minimum of two hours each week on high-quality PE and school sport and beyond the curriculum comparing national average with schools in the most disadvantaged communities
11. Poverty	Proportion of children living in low-income households.
12. Homelessness	Number of homeless families with children in temporary accommodation

Source: Department of Health (2006). *Tackling health inequalities: Status report on the program for action 2006, Update on headline indicators*. London, DOH.

ministries and agencies of government (Department of Health 2002; Department of Health 2003).

Despite the significant conceptual and technical progress that has been achieved, the twenty-first century has seen less enthusiasm for the use of goals and objectives as a core component of their national health policy. It is important, however, to examine the reasons for this shift and to reflect on its meaning for the future.

The Australian experience was similar to that of other nations. Although there was widespread acceptance of the rationale for preparing national health goals and targets, there was very limited investment in the infrastructure or actions necessary to achieve them. Responsibility for their achievement was not allocated clearly in the ensuing health policy environment. Instead, governments in Australia invested in a relatively small public health programme to address some priority issues (Commonwealth Department of Human Services and Health 1994) but largely ignored the need for their own commitment to lead action to address the social, economic and environmental determinants of health. Nor was there any investment in reorienting health services to align their work to ensure that they accounted for their contributions to the achievement of population health outcomes.

Other nations' experiences mirrored these. Busse and Wismar (2002) highlighted the fact that in no country or region did the health goals and targets policy outline the scale and redistribution of health sector resources that would be necessary to achieve the health goals and targets. Nor did the policies identify the health service and public health infrastructure and capacity necessary to lead and deliver interventions, or to report on progress.

Reviewing experience in eight countries, Allin *et al.* (2004) concluded that, to date, health goals and targets remain political constructs that have been a source of inspiration rather than explicit benchmarks against which to account for progress in improving a nation's health. As with all political processes to set priorities for spending, changes in government, or even changes in Ministers, have led to reinterpretation of the nature and purposes of the targets, and substantial dislocation of any actions that had been previously committed to (Nutbeam & Wise 1996; Beaglehole & Davis 1992; Wismar 2002).

The processes of establishing goals and targets have contributed significantly to the technical development of public health. The conceptual frameworks, the indicator development, the evolution of national and local health information systems to report on social and economic determinants of health in addition to the biological and behavioural determinants, and the development of a much stronger body of research identifying and tracking inequalities in the health status of populations are all positive outcomes of the initiatives to establish national health goals and targets. So, too, is the growing body of evidence of effective interventions, and the routine public reporting on the health of populations that provides governments, organizations and communities with the information necessary to guide future investment. This applies not only at the national level but also at the state/province/regional level (NSW Health 2007). In the United States, the objectives offered a benchmark against which changes in population health status could be observed over time, and acted as a catalyst for response (US Department of Health and Human Services 1995, 2006).

Conceptually, health goals and targets are the proposed outcomes of a nation's entire investment in the health of its population. Much of their potential benefit, therefore, lies in the extent to which they are used to guide and measure the results of investments in health. The example from England that involved leadership from the Treasury, and a cross-government response offers a much clearer approach in this regard.

The US experience has suggested that national health objectives can survive changes in government provided they are developed by a quasi-independent agency, are based on good technical support, and are supported by strong coalitions for action outside of government. Overall, in those countries that have adopted health objectives or targets, the objectives appear to have played an important role in focusing on the need for:

- A broad base for health policy across the different sectors of government
- Changes in resource allocation to develop capacity for public health intervention
- The development of methods and structures which enable action to promote health and prevent disease

Despite the downturn in enthusiasm in recent years goal and target setting is still used as a tool for determining priorities, and achieving accountability for health outcomes. One example of great public health significance has been the commitment of countries and international organizations to the Millennium Development Goals (MDGs). The MDGs are intended to provide a mechanism through which to join public health initiatives to engage with the global organizations, industries and social movements that make global economic, social, environmental, and trade decisions, in particular (United Nations. 2000).

Developing public policy for health: Health in all policies

Whilst setting goals for improvement in the underlying determinants of health that are outside the health sector have provided a useful stimulus in some situations, other mechanisms need to be utilized as an alternative, or to complement and extend this approach. Actions to improve and protect the health of the public have to be grounded in a policy structure which is sensitive to the impact on health policy decisions across all government sectors, and which maximises opportunities for matching economic and social development goals with health development goals and objectives.

This logic is the basis for WHO's *Investment for Health* strategy which offers a model for achieving a 'whole of government' approach to improving public health. This strategy is described as:

> *a practical approach based on the rationale that resources are best applied in a way that not only addresses the main causes of ill-health in a credible, effective and ethical manner, but also furthers the achievement of goals for social and economic development.*

The key elements of the *Investment for Health* concept concern achieving a strong commitment to health in policy making across all government ministries, a commitment to intersectoral working, and a continued focus on equity (World Health Organization 2002). Health improvement will not always be the primary policy goal, but the strategy represents a commitment to assess the *population health impact* (both positive and negative) of public policy decisions, development strategies and investment decisions, particularly those with social and economic implications. Economic development becomes a means of improving both the social infrastructure and people's health. Tools for *health impact assessment* are essential to support this element of the strategy and there is a growing body of evidence on the use of formal health impact assessment and its impact on policy-making (Kemm 2006).

Though the rationale for the health sector to work with other sectors is strong, the experience with working in partnership with other sectors has highlighted the need for the health sector to avoid imposing its own priorities on the core business of other sectors and to ensure that all partners are able to identify the benefits that will flow from working in collaboration. Building on existing common ground between sectors, combined with transparency in purpose, and investment in building inter-organizational and interpersonal relationships appear to offer a basis for developing effective partnerships that are required to advance health and achieve greater equity in health by addressing its underlying determinants (Padgett *et al.* 2004). Where progress has been achieved it has, most often, been through bilateral partnerships between the health services and other sectors. In the latter case such action is most achievable where there is obvious mutual benefit, and where the roles and responsibilities of each sector and are clearly defined (Harris *et al.* 1996).

The WHO has revived its focus on equity through the work of the Commission on the Social Determinants of Health. The work of the commission is directed toward improving understanding of the social determinants of health and their unequal impact on health between and within populations, and between countries. Equity in this case implies that all people will have equal opportunity to develop and maintain their health through a fair distribution of the resources and opportunities that support health. A mix of programmes to address fundamental differences in opportunity and access to resources, as well as targeted programmes for disadvantaged individuals and communities, is required to support this element of the strategy.

Achieving such a substantial commitment to health is by no means an easy political task. The European Office of the WHO carried out national *Investment for Health* Appraisals in several countries including Slovenia, Hungary, Romania, and Malta (Ziglio *et al.* 2000). This involved external appraisal and reporting back to the Health Ministry and/or Parliament on:

- The strategy needed to improve the health status of the population
- The potential for investment for health in the country
- The infrastructure needed to build, support, and sustain *Investment for Health*

Each part of the appraisal identified the opportunities to promote health more effectively through key economic and social development policies. This strategy represented a sophisticated attempt to put into public health practice the logical consequences of contemporary analyses of what determines health in populations. Although the approach has been implemented for less than a decade, it illustrates the important challenge facing public health advocates and practitioners. This challenge is to engage government, civil society, and the private sector in dialogue about the health impact of policies and practices, and to consider the scope for a synergistic relationship between health, economic, and social development strategies.

Like health goals and targets, the *Investing in Health* strategy is not a substitute for investment in a public health infrastructure in countries. Rather, it is a mechanism that facilitates the dialogue needed to link investment for health with economic and social development, and support action across sectors to improve the health of the public. One recent example of this mechanism at work is that of the European Commission, which has taken action to ensure that there is a high level of human health protection in all Community activities, and has codified this as a central part of the Community's responsibilities (WHO European Office for Investment in Health and Development 2007; Stahl *et al.* 2006).

Developing infrastructure and delivery systems for public health interventions

To be effective, the science of public health must be 'applied'. The science, strategies, and tools used in public health are too often used only to describe and analyse public health problems, and to develop policy. To enjoy the fruits of this analysis, and of health-oriented public policy, it is essential that attention is also given to the development of the organizational capacity for effective public health intervention. This capacity is most often concentrated in the health sector but can be found in other sectors of government and in the non-government sector. The public health interventions include the health education and health promotion strategies described in previous chapters, as well as other forms of public health intervention required to assist people and communities *improve their control over the determinants of health.*

The limited shifts in government investment and action to support the achievement of their national health goals and priorities are both a cause and consequence of the frailty of the infrastructure for public health intervention in many countries. Although the last two decades have seen a rejuvenation of interest and investment in public health in many countries, it is still the case that much of that investment has been and continues to be *ad hoc*—in targeted programmes and services rather than in a well-resourced, sustained public health infrastructure that is capable of programme development and implementation and for routinely reporting on progress (Baker *et al.* 2005).

Creating a sustainable, specialized infrastructure for public health has proven to be a complex undertaking. Although there is strong evidence that the greatest improvements in the health of populations have arisen from social and economic developments that have an impact on health, modern health sectors have evolved to diagnose and treat diseases, their symptoms, and injuries. As a result, the 'health' debate and investment in most countries continues to centre on the accessibility and quality of health care services. The need for an effective public health service tends to be invisible both to governments and to the public except in times of crisis, and is often oriented towards the control of infectious diseases (such as the SARS epidemic). There is relatively limited public demand for a strong public health service (compared with demand for health care services) in all but exceptional circumstances (Grossman & Scala 1993). However, the evolution of health policy to include recognition of the social determinants of health and to commit governments to tackle non-communicable diseases has stimulated action by a number of countries to review and strengthen their infrastructure for public health.

Although there remain significant unanswered questions about the most effective systems or structures through which to design and deliver public health interventions, there are emerging models for defining priorities for action, for working across government to address determinants of health, and for establishing elements of an effective public health infrastructure.

The range of activities and sectors in which practitioners need to act, and the broad range of disciplines that can be said to make up the field of public health have made it challenging to define the 'core business' of public health. Several recent initiatives have sought to identify these 'core functions' (Population Health and Wellness 2005; Institute of Medicine 2003). Within these lists of core functions, essential services, and public health practices there is still a considerable lack of conceptual consistency. A mix of intended outcomes, interventions (or strategies), and principles for good practice is represented in all the lists. To help untangle these conceptual inconsistencies the distinction is made in Fig. 12.9.1 between the essential **infrastructure** required to lead the development of policy and interventions to achieve priority health goals and targets, and the **delivery system** required to develop and execute public health interventions.

Key elements of infrastructure for public health

The components of public health infrastructure are similar to those needed by all organizations to conduct their core business. In addition to the strategic direction and priority setting outlined in previous sections in this chapter, the infrastructure for public health is made up of material resources, a skilled workforce, and information from research and evaluation, that are then combined by organizations to develop and implement policies and to deliver services or interventions that promote, protect, and maintain the health of populations, and to account for progress (Baker & Koplan 2002).

Figure 12.9.1 highlights three essential components of an **infrastructure** for public health including secure and sustainable funding, a well-trained workforce, and supportive research.

Secure and sustainable funding

Aside from the *investing for health* strategy discussed earlier, secure, recurrent financial resources are required to support a public health infrastructure within the health sector. Without such investment in a dedicated infrastructure there is little chance to build a sustainable infrastructure, and even where one exists, experience has shown that the public health system can quickly lose capacity if investment declines (National Health and Medical Research Council 1997; US Department of Health and Human Services 1999).

Public health cannot work if left to market forces. Most countries have recognized the need to invest in a public health infrastructure as a 'public good'. These investments have provided capacity to analyse public health status, guide decision-making on priorities for action, and respond to public health threats, especially infectious disease outbreaks. This latter capacity has been tested considerably in past years with outbreaks of SARS and avian flu, and more general concern with preparedness for bio-terrorism. Despite these dramatic reminders, secure, sustainable funding for the design, delivery and evaluation of public health interventions directed to addressing non-communicable diseases, and to tackling the social determinants of health has proved more elusive.

This secure 'programme funding' necessary to tackle non-communicable diseases is especially vulnerable when interventions run counter to prevailing government policy or ideology, and especially when they contradict economic policy—such as in relation to the sale of alcohol or tobacco, or nutritional programmes which conflict with agricultural practices or with the food supplied by significant food industries. Providing a strong rationale for investing in public health interventions continues to be a major part of the role of public health professionals—requiring the use of science (to demonstrate effectiveness), political argument (to demonstrate professional and community concern) and practical demonstration in the form of case studies (Nutbeam 2003). Achieving sustainable funding may require more active communication and political advocacy. Baker and Koplan (2002) argue for the development of a new language to increase the public's understanding of public health, and the use of case reports and studies to sustain interest in and support for public health infrastructure.

Data on the proportion of national recurrent health sector expenditure that is accounted for by public health infrastructure and programmes in different countries indicate that it is very small, relative to expenditure on acute and chronic health care services. Furthermore, there has been little tangible progress in the last three decades in the proportion of health budgets invested in public health or health promotion. For example, in Australia, recently published data by the Australian Institute for Health and Welfare (2006b) indicates that expenditure on public health activities by Australian health departments in 2004–2005 was approximately 1.7 per cent of total recurrent health expenditure, or A$71 per person. The greatest proportion of public health expenditure (23.6%, or A$338.3 million) was on organized immunization, followed by selected health promotion (A$232.8 million) and communicable disease control (A$232.0 million). While this does not include all the funding invested in public health it provides some indication of the minimal level of public investment through the health sector that might be expected to support public health infrastructure and intervention programmes.

In many countries low levels of funding have meant that it has been necessary to find alternative sources of funding for public health interventions. A growing number of countries have established Health Promotion Foundations based, most commonly, on funding generated by taxation levied by government on the sale of tobacco products. This type of Foundation was first established in Australia as part of a strategy to replace lost income from tobacco company sponsorship of sports, arts, and cultural events. The model has been copied in several countries, both high- and middle-income countries, with general success. Foundations now engage in a diversified range of programmes and have been able to make a significant contribution to funding public health research as well as to actions to address social and environmental determinants of health (International Network of Health Promotion Foundations 2007).

The non-government and community sectors play significant roles in funding research and delivering interventions on issues such as cardiovascular disease prevention, tobacco control, or childhood injury prevention. Organizations such as Heart Foundations and Cancer Councils perform important roles in many countries, not only in raising money for research, but in conducting direct community interventions to promote health and prevent disease. There are limitations imposed by their focus on single issues and by the level of funding that they are able to raise directly from their constituencies (in addition to government support). But their high levels of credibility among health professionals and community members mean that they can also be attractive to partners in developing and implementing public health interventions.

The private sector, too, has begun to take an increasing interest in contributing to public health and social development. In many cases the benefits of partnership are obvious and mutual. For example, in several countries, the insurance industry has contributed significant levels of funding to specific programmes to reduce motor vehicle crashes, and the food industry has committed to a programme to improve consumers' recognition of healthier food options.

It is important to recognise that private sector contributions, in particular, are linked to the needs of business for community support and to assist marketing of specific goods and products. These needs do not automatically clash with public health goals, but the mutual benefit in partnerships with the private sector is not always as apparent as it could be. The WHO Jakarta Declaration provides some useful general guidance on this issue concerning the need for transparency in relationships and clearly defined mutual benefit (World Health Organization 1998). In negotiating partnership agreements with the private sector it is important to ensure that there is no potential conflict between the outcomes required by the company and the intended public health outcomes.

A well-trained, competent workforce, including capacity for leadership to guide and direct action within and outside the health sector

The delivery of essential public health services requires a skilled, competent workforce, often working in partnership with other organizations and the community (Gebbie *et al.* 2000; Gebbie and Turnock 2006; Joint Task Group on Public Health Human Resources 2005). In addition to a specifically trained public health workforce, professionals from many different sectors can be considered as part of the broad public health workforce. There is equal need to support education and professional development for both groups.

Most specialist public health training is provided at the postgraduate level through universities—usually through schools or departments of public health. In some countries medical qualifications have been a prerequisite for entry into public health training; in others a wide range of undergraduate qualifications is accepted. Many disciplines contribute to the body of knowledge that underpins the field, but there is growing agreement about the core competencies required of all members of the specialist public health workforce (Council on Linkages between Academia and Public Health Practice 2006; Joint Task Group on Public Health Human Resources 2005; Commonwealth Department of Health and Aged Care 2000). Within the field there are also several specialities that have developed advanced training programmes—epidemiology and biostatistics, health economics and health promotion being three of the more common speciality groupings. Specific competencies are also being developed in these disciplines within public health (Howat *et al.* 2000; McCracken-Rance 2000).

In some countries, governments have recognized the need to invest in training programmes to ensure that there are adequate numbers of trained public health professionals. In Australia, for example, the Public Health Education and Research Program (PHERP) was established by the Federal Department of Health and Aged Care in 1986 to fund universities to develop Master of Public Health programmes. Later, the PHERP was expanded to include funding to develop the quality and quantity of teaching and research in specific areas of special need, including environmental health, health promotion, mental health, health economics, and public health nutrition. More recently, the Program has funded innovation in developing the public health workforce necessary to meet emerging needs (such as bioterrorism, or SARS, as well as issues such as obesity), and it has expanded its focus on mechanisms to ensure that the public health workforce is 'judgement safe'. These initiatives have led to the expansion of the quality and effectiveness of the public health workforce in Australia—and to recognition of the need for regular review to ensure that the workforce is adequately prepared to meet current and emerging public health challenges (Durham & Plant 2005).

Professional associations, too, make a significant contribution to workforce development. Some of the global professional bodies with members in most countries include: Public Health Associations (linked through the World Federation of Public Health Associations [http://www.wfpha.org]), Epidemiological Associations (linked through the International Epidemiological Association [http://www.dundee.ac.uk/iea]), Health Promotion and Health Education Associations (linked through the International Union of Health Promotion and Education [http://www.iuhpe.org]). The conferences and journals produced by these organizations are essential components of workforce development infrastructure. Such associations are also important in the development of and advocacy for healthy public policy.

The opportunities for collaboration among institutions that are offered by the Internet have resulted in new possibilities to establish national and international programmes and standards of quality in public health workforce training. The Internet also offers students the opportunity to access a wider range of public health training—some of it across national borders (Davies *et al.* 2000).

Public health intervention requires special skills that are different to those required to analyse health problems in a population. Influencing health behaviour in populations, and influencing the structural and environmental determinants of health requires public health specialists to have substantial knowledge and skills in the behavioural, social and political sciences. This will require educational institutions to extend the range of current training in many cases (Institute of Medicine 2003).

This emphasis on intervention also highlights the need for a different style of leadership from senior public health practitioners. Earlier sections in this chapter have pointed to some of the difficulties inherent in collaboration across sectors. Leadership for public health intervention requires practitioners to work more closely with other sectors, to advocate effectively for the development and adoption of healthy public policy, and to create, with communities, a shared vision for the public's health. There are few programmes that explicitly address the need for advanced training for public health leadership. One example is a National Public Health Leadership Institute supported by the Centers for Disease Control and Prevention (CDC) in the United States, and based at the University of North Carolina at Chapel Hill (http://www.phli.org/aboutPHLI/index.htm).

The training of other health professionals is gradually being adapted to provide them with basic knowledge of public health. Professionals in the health sector (doctors, nurses, allied health professionals), and professionals in other sectors (such as teachers, social workers, architects and urban planners) are increasingly being involved in developing policies and programmes that contribute to improvements in the health of the population. This is a major challenge and significant area for development in public health education in the next decade.

The education systems responsible for providing workforce development lie, largely, outside the ambit of the health sector. It is necessary that there be strong links between academic institutions and agencies responsible for public health. Examples of efforts to achieve this can be seen in the United States, by the formation of the Council on Linkages between Academia and Public Health Practice, and in Australia by the Public Health Education and Research Programme.

Supportive research policy, funding, and training

Public health research and development is central to continuous improvement in the relevance, quality and impact of public health intervention. An effective system for public health research is dependent upon a national/organizational research policy that highlights the need for specific public health research—as distinct from biomedical research. It then depends upon the availability of funds specifically for public health research, and upon a strong system of peer review by qualified public health researchers. Furthermore, the strength of the research system depends on there being high-quality research training available to young researchers, and upon a career development path for public health researchers.

Research funding for public health can come from many sources. However, competition for health research funding is fierce, and public health research often competes poorly through institutions which are dominated by biomedical and health services research. Within public health research, there is also a strong bias towards descriptive/investigative epidemiological research at the cost of adequate investment in intervention research (Millward *et al.* 2003). It is important to ensure that research addresses priority health/structural issues, population groups and settings and that it also addresses the need for methodological development specific to public health intervention.

Although no single model has been identified to ensure the funding and conduct of policy-driven research that is necessary to supplement the investigator-driven research in public health, there has been growing recognition of the need for research funding bodies to ensure the balance between biomedical and public health research funding (Wanless 2004). Experience has shown that there is a continuous need for review of research funding criteria so that nations are able to develop the information they need to make effective, efficient decisions on health and medical policies and practices. But within this generic concern to find balance, strong advocacy for public health research, in particular, is required. The need for research on the systems needed to design and deliver optimal public health interventions and services to defined populations at different levels of jurisdiction has been identified (Institute of Medicine 2003). This is in addition to research on strengthening health systems more generically (Travis *et al.* 2004).

Even within the discipline of public health there has been tension between the twin intellectual approaches to public health practice—with many public health researchers focusing on the development of knowledge rather than on the actions required to solve public health problems (Hunter & Berman 1997). The most obvious manifestation of this can be seen in the overwhelming investments made in monitoring and surveillance, and in research focused on improving knowledge about public health problems and their causes, rather than on research that improves knowledge of effective action to resolve the problems (Millward *et al.* 2003). In reviewing the available information on research funding and publication in the public health literature, it is hard to escape the conclusion that the policies of research funding agencies need to give greater weight to 'intervention' and evaluation research, and ensuring that the peer review process includes reviewers with appropriate knowledge and skills in such research.

Because effective public health interventions include a complex set of actions to bring about widespread social change there is a need for the development of research and evaluation methods that better 'fit' the context of the intervention (Nutbeam & Bauman 2006; Rootman *et al.* 2001). Several efforts are being made to identify frameworks and criteria to ensure that the quality of evidence to guide public health interventions meets the highest possible standards of scientific rigour within this more complex environment (Weightman *et al.* 2005).

The infrastructure for public health is not, on its own, sufficient to ensure that effective public health interventions are developed, delivered and evaluated. The infrastructure must then work to develop organizational capacity within and beyond the health sector to create a *delivery system* for public health intervention referred to in Fig. 12.9.1. The components of the delivery system include population health surveillance, mechanisms for priority setting, programme delivery systems, and mechanisms for quality control, as discussed in the succeeding sections.

A system for population-wide health monitoring and surveillance

Understanding the complex and changing health status of the population is a cornerstone of public health. A national, comprehensive system for population-wide health monitoring and surveillance is an essential component of public health infrastructure. Such a system should facilitate on-going, systematic collection, analysis and interpretation of national or local population data relevant to the national public health effort. Such data need to be collected at national or more local levels repeatedly over time. This 'health intelligence' is needed to identify problems, to set priorities for action, and to monitor progress (National Health and Medical Research Council 1997). The US Centers for Disease Control and Prevention are a widely recognized example of an organization with this important function.

Health information in many countries is largely restricted to data on mortality, morbidity and health system use. This information is vitally important for epidemiological investigation, and to provide broad guidance on public health priorities and policy, but has limitations in its usefulness for planning and monitoring public health interventions (Nutbeam & Bauman 2006). For this a much wider range of information is needed, including information that is either national in coverage or has relevance nationally such as:

- Measures of health status in the population (including mortality and morbidity data)
- Measures of the determinants of the population's health, including those in the external environment (physical, biological, social, cultural and economic) and those internal to individuals (such as knowledge, behaviour, disease risk factors)
- Measures of the distribution of health in the population, and measures of the distribution of the determinants of a population's health

- Health interventions or health services, including interventions provided directly to individuals and those provided to communities, covering information on the nature of interventions, management, resourcing, accessibility, use, and effectiveness
- The relationships among these elements (National Health and Medical Research Council 1997)

Any type of health information system should enable analysis of the needs and progress of specific population sub-groups, with particular emphasis on disadvantaged groups. It must be capable of identifying inequities in health status and their determinants.

The system for monitoring and surveillance should also be responsible for reporting on the 'state of the health of the population'—on progress toward achieving health goals and targets, and on emerging issues or gaps. There are some useful examples of such reports being used effectively to highlight progress and the need for specific investment in action to address the needs of socially and economically marginalized populations. In the United Kingdom, the regular reports of the Chief Medical Officer (e.g. Department of Health 2005), and in the United States, Reports of the Surgeon General (http://www.surgeongeneral.gov/reportspublications.html) are practical examples of well-researched public health reports that are produced largely independent of the political administration

Examples of efforts to improve the relevance and range of health status indicators are beginning to emerge. To measure the influence of social, economic and environmental factors on the health of populations an expanded range of information is needed in national systems of monitoring and surveillance. The importance of developing a broader set of health indicators is strongly supported by the work of the WHO Commission on the Social Determinants of Health (2007), particularly through its Knowledge Networks.

A system for identifying national, regional, local priorities for action, and for regular review and redefinition of priorities

The identification of priorities for investment in public health interventions remains one of the most contentious issues in contemporary public health. The use of different criteria for establishing priorities leads to very different priorities for action (Nutbeam & Bauman 2006). Nationally determined priorities do not always resonate with local needs and perceptions of what actions are important to improve health.

Among the different approaches to priority development are those determined by epidemiological, economic, and community perspectives. Although not mutually exclusive, each of these perspectives places 'value' on different outcomes and processes.

To date, epidemiological analysis has dominated priority setting at national levels. The national health goals and targets identified by many nations and regions discussed earlier have given priority to leading causes of preventable deaths and morbidity. Criteria that have been used to identify priorities include: Analysis of the incidence, prevalence, costs to the health care system and to society associated with the disease/injury, and an assessment of the feasibility of acting to prevent or reduce the incidence or prevalence of the condition. Actions that are linked through epidemiological analysis to a reduction in disease are valued in such an analysis (Lopez 2003).

Increasingly, economic principles of efficiency are being proposed as a means of identifying priorities for public health intervention (Woodley 2001). Efficiency is used here to mean obtaining optimal gain from investment. However to use the concept of 'efficiency' as a criterion for identifying public health priorities, it is important to distinguish between two components of 'efficiency'. The first component has to do with ensuring that the services to address a particular issue or problem (e.g. cardiovascular disease) are organized and resourced. This means placing investment across the range of interventions (preventive, curative, palliative, or all three) for a particular condition to maximise individual and community health gain. It is called 'technical efficiency'. It means giving the greatest proportion of investment to the 'part' of the service that produces the greatest health gains—sometimes this will be prevention; sometimes it will be treatment. The evidence is also continually changing, and needs to be applied to readjust the balance of investment.

However, even if investment within a programme area (e.g. cardiovascular disease) is efficient, it is possible that investment across the range of health issues and population groups is not well-balanced. The second component of efficiency is 'allocative' efficiency. The analysis of the balance of investment based on assessment of allocative efficiency helps to identify priority issues or problems across the whole range of potential programme or service areas. At its most basic it is a tool for ensuring that a significant issue (such as mental illness) does receive adequate resources compared with other equally prevalent, severe issues. More sophisticated analyses will link investment in programme areas to predetermined population health outcomes, making decisions about the relative level of investment across different service/programme areas.

The third approach to priority setting reflects the growing evidence that the most effective and sustainable public health interventions have been characterized by high levels of community, organizational and political support. This is particularly true at the local level, which is also where national priorities are often seen to be remote from local concerns. Criteria for establishing priorities at local levels include: Extent of community concern about an issue, the capacity of the community to act to address the issue, and the capacity of local institutions, organizations, and people to contribute to action (Hancock & Minkler 1998). The process of participation in decision-making, and perceived responsiveness to local priorities are valued through such an analysis (Perrons & Skyler 2003).

These three perspectives on setting priorities are not mutually exclusive, and are best combined to achieve a sound basis for effective action that is nationally relevant, locally sensitive and financially sound.

Further, the development of priorities for public health intervention should not be considered a one-off event. The 'health intelligence' system established for defining priorities should also be capable of use in the review and redefinition of priorities. This is to ensure that there is capacity to redirect resources (as well as to increase the pool of resources) to address new priorities.

Programme delivery systems at national, regional, local levels of jurisdiction—within and outside the health sector

As indicated earlier, epidemiological analysis of priorities for intervention has generally led public health intervention towards reducing risk factors and behaviours in individuals. This in turn has led frequently to highly differentiated, vertical programmes within health sectors to tackle specific risks, such as tobacco use, or diseases such as coronary heart disease. Such programmes tend to have their own goals, resources, workforces, and research programmes (National Health and Medical Research Council 1997). As a consequence there is limited scope for integrated programmes to address the social, economic and physical environmental determinants of health. In contrast to disease/risk factor-specific programmes, such integrated programmes are more likely to focus on policy and institutional changes, in addition to public information, education and mobilization programmes.

Recently in Europe and in Australia there are examples of processes being implemented that, amongst other things, are intended to encourage the redefinition of priorities to include greater emphasis on the underlying factors and environments that are 'shared' across different causes of disease and injury. The significant burden of chronic disease being experienced by so many nations has led to the development of 'integrated' chronic disease-prevention programmes. The WHO has organized its work into chronic diseases and health promotion, together with a series of 'issue-specific' programmes. And, encouragingly, there is evidence of countries exploring initiatives to shift the focus of their public health programmes and funding away from vertical programmes to address the underlying determinants of health (Department of Health 2003). Again, WHO has established a structure on equity, poverty and social determinants of health to lead work on these 'cross-cutting' issues. Although vertical programmes continue to be the dominant organizational structure guiding public health investment and intervention, these new initiatives are interesting attempts to link funding with the more contemporary analysis of determinants of health and the need for explicit efforts to achieve equity.

The comprehensive programmes that are needed to bring about the wide-scale changes in the health of populations require public health infrastructure and action at national, regional and local levels of jurisdiction. Experience has demonstrated the need for clear role delineation and mechanisms for coordinating activity—particularly where the focus of the activity is change in legislation, policy, or programmes in sectors other than health. The exact nature of infrastructure needed at each level of jurisdiction has not been defined.

In most countries the greater part of the systems for programme delivery are devolved to state, regional, or local levels. A significant factor in improving the infrastructure for programme delivery in some countries, including the United Kingdom and Australia, has been the establishment of sub-regional administrative structures within the health sector that are responsible for protecting, promoting and maintaining the health of defined geographic populations. Within these structures, there have been initiatives to draw together the parts of the health care system that have the greatest 'affinity' with public health. This has been an effective means of ensuring an ongoing public health service at local and regional levels. However, it has been less effective in refocusing public health action to address inequalities in health and the determinants of health, and it has not been an effective mechanism through which to increase the proportion of health sector spending on public health action.

In addition to its specialist public health services, the health sector has many other opportunities to make significant contributions to improving the health of the population—through its hospitals, general practitioners, nursing homes, and early childhood services, for example. The sector also has a more direct role in public health—as a major employer, as a consumer of non-renewable resources, and as a physical and social setting that can influence the health of patients, staff, visitors and the community (Coote 2002; Swedish National Institute of Public Health 2006). Mobilizing this significantly untapped resource remains a major challenge for specialist public health practitioners.

As noted above, non-government, community and professional organizations also play significant roles in the design and delivery of public health interventions. Many of these are linked to specific health issues, e.g. sudden infant death syndrome, HIV/AIDS, or schizophrenia. Others focus on the needs of specific population groups, e.g. older people, immigrants, or indigenous people. Such organizations have specific knowledge, experience, and access to individuals and communities that is often difficult for government agencies to obtain.

Local government, too, has a key role in public health. The *Healthy Cities* movement is based, largely, on this level of government. Municipal public health planning has been found to be an effective mechanism to bring together local government, communities and key government agencies (including health) to define steps that each can take separately and together to improve the health of the population (Bagley *et al.* 2007; Lenihan 2005.) In the United Kingdom, a derivation of the healthy cities concept in the form of Health Action Zones represents a deliberate attempt to bring together the different agencies for public health at a local level (Barnes *et al.* 2005). It is through this type of organizational structure that other sectors can be more successfully engaged in public health action. The health sector's role in such relationships varies, depending on the context and the issue being addressed (Harris *et al.* 1996). However, a nation's public health infrastructure must include people with the knowledge, skills and resources (including power) to work effectively with other sectors. This is particularly important as the emphasis of public health action shifts from programmes developed and delivered by and within the health sector, to influencing public policy and organizations and programmes delivered by other sectors.

Systems for quality control, evaluation, promotion of best practice

Public health interventions need to be evaluated. The frameworks for assessing the quality of evidence to guide public health interventions referred to above are a component of an effective public health infrastructure. However, such frameworks have tended to focus on the quality of research design, and methods, rather than on the quality of the interventions (relevance, use of evidence and theory, practicality of implementation, etc.). There is a growing body of evidence that defines the characteristics of effective public health interventions (International Union for Health Promotion and Education 1999; McQueen & Jones 2007; Jackson & Waters 2005). It is a base from which to develop standards of quality for the design and implementation of public health interventions in relation to specific issues or population groups. The National Institute for Clinical Excellence (NICE) in the United Kingdom and the Centers for Disease Control and Prevention in the United States have developed standards for application to national and regional intervention programmes (Zaza *et al.* 2005). Use of such standards and guidelines in the development and implementation of public health interventions will be vitally important in improving the quality and impact of public health intervention in the future.

Concluding remarks: Key tasks to improve structures and strategies for public health intervention into the twenty-first century

This chapter has described key elements of health policy and strategy that have been found to be effective in guiding national public health action, and the components of an infrastructure and delivery system required to design, deliver and evaluate public health interventions. Public health intervention requires a complex mix of science, art (of practice), and politics. The emergence of high rates of non-communicable diseases in most high-income countries has required a radical re-appraisal of what determines health, and what public health responses are most appropriate and effective. In addition, many low- and middle-income countries are now experiencing both high rates of communicable and of non-communicable diseases. Four key challenges emerge from this chapter:

- **Addressing all determinants of health:** It is increasingly apparent that, in many cases, public health practitioners need to expand the range of research methods used to identify public health problems and their causes. As well as using the traditional public health tools of epidemiology and demography, it is necessary to use the social, behavioural and environmental sciences to obtain a more complete picture. More complex analysis of patterns of disease in populations, and of the determinants of disease will lead to better informed and potentially more effective interventions as a response.

  In addition, knowledge of current infrastructure and existing strengths in communities is a powerful platform from which to build effective public health interventions (Labonte 1999). Identifying this capacity within communities also requires the use of a wider range of research and consultation methods (McKnight & Kretzmann 1998). It also emphasises the key role of communities in defining and prioritizing problems and in developing solutions, and is particularly important when working with communities that are disadvantaged or socially excluded.

- **Gaining visibility for public health:** It is also clear from the analyses in this chapter that public health action often involves political processes. Public health practitioners need to better use health data to influence these political processes. Reporting on ever more sophisticated analyses of public health problems and their determinants will not, on its own, result in any action. However, this data is of great use in raising public and political awareness of health problems, and in highlighting the obligation of governments to develop policy that enables action to improve the health of the population. This includes engaging politicians in dialogue to identify priorities for efficient health sector investment, and when appropriate, advocating for action to support investment in public health interventions in the face of pressure for increased investment in health care services.

- **Influencing policy and plans for improving public health**: The range of determinants of health means that public health practitioners will be required increasingly to provide technical advice on the impact on health of policies and practices in sectors other than the health sector. *Health impact analysis* is a relatively new and underdeveloped tool to assist this process. Such technical advice will inevitably lead to conflict in some cases that will require the public health practitioner to act as an advocate for health in the face of competing pressures.

  More positively, as evidence grows of the effectiveness of public health interventions it will be necessary for public health practitioners to operate across different sectors of government at national, regional and local levels. Public health practitioners need skills in identifying the policy relevance of the evidence and in identifying the most effective ways to ensure the use of evidence in the development and implementation of public policy.

- **Working with people and organizations to improve health:** Public health practitioners need to be able to engage people and organizations in practical action to address the determinants of health. Such action will often occur at a local level. The capacity to develop and deliver interventions within local communities and through different settings (such as schools and worksites) is an essential public health skill. The chapter by Kickbusch and McQueen (and other chapters) provides practical guidance on the type of skills and strategies required of public health practitioners to achieve change for public health at this level.

The development of effective organizational structures through which to bring together the components of an effective public health infrastructure within the health sector (in particular) to provide the capacity to 'orchestrate' public health action is a major challenge for the twenty-first century. It is important, however, to reflect on the fact that having the technical capacity to develop and deliver effective interventions is not sufficient, on its own. Without political commitment, action to promote health is, at best, difficult—at worst, impossible. The national infrastructure for promoting health must include people and strategies aimed at building and maintaining political support both for public health in general as a key area of government activity, as well as for the specific actions that must be taken, if we are to succeed in improving the health of the population.

References

Agren G. (2003). *Sweden's new public health policy: national public health objectives for Sweden*. Stockholm: Swedish National Institute of Public Health.

Allin S., Mossialos E., McKee M., and Holland W. (2004). *Making decisions on public health: a review of 8 countries*. European Observatory on Health Systems and Policies. Copenhagen, Denmark: World Health Organization (on behalf of the European Observatory on Health Systems and Policies.

Australian Institute of Health and Welfare(2006a). *Australia's Health 2006. The tenth biennial health report of the Australian Institute of Health and Welfare*. Canberra: Australian Institute of Health and Welfare.

Australian Institute of Health and Welfare (2006b). *National public health expenditure report 2000–2001 to 2003 – 4*. Health and welfare expenditure series no. 26. Canberra: Australian Institute of Health and Welfare.

Bagley P., Lin V., Sainsbury P., Wise M., Keating T., and Roger K. (2007). In what ways does the mandatory nature of Victoria's municipal public health planning framework impact on the planning process and outcomes? *Australia and New Zealand Health Policy* **4**. Available at: www.anzhealthpolicy.com/content/4/1/4 (accessed on 1 July 2007).

Baker E., Potter M., Jones D., Mercer S., Cioffi J., Green L. *et al.* (2005). The public health infrastructure and our nation's health. *Annual Review of Public Health* **26**, 303–18.

Baker E. and Koplan J. (2002). Strengthening the nation's public health infrastructure: historic challenge, unprecedented opportunity. *Health Affairs* **21**, 15–27.

Barnes M., Baule L., Benzeval M., Judge K., MacKenzie M., and Sullivan H. (2005). *Building capacity for health equity*. London, Routledge.

Beaglehole R. and Davis P. (1992). Setting national health goals and targets in the context of a fiscal crisis: the politics of social choice in New Zealand. *International Journal of Health Services*, **22**, 417–28.

Bonnie R., Stratton K., Wallace R. (eds.) (2007). *Ending the tobacco problem: a blueprint for the nation*. Washington DC, The National Academies Press.

Busse R. and Wismar M. (2002). Health target programmes and health care services – any link? A conceptual and comparative study (Part 1). *Health Policy* **59**, 209–221.

Centers for Disease Control and Prevention (1999). *An ounce of prevention . . . what are the returns?* 2nd ed. revised. Atlanta, Centers for Disease Control and Prevention, US Department of Health and Human Services.

Commonwealth Department of Human Services and Health (1994). *Better health outcomes for Australians: national goals, targets and strategies for better health outcomes into the next century.* Canberra, Australian Government Publishing Service.

Commonwealth Department of Health and Aged Care (1999). *Independent review of the public health education and research program.* Report to the Commonwealth Department of Health and Aged Care. Canberra, Department of Health and Aged Care.

Commonwealth Department of Health and Aged Care (2000). *National Public Health Education Framework.* Public Health Education and Research Program. Canberra, Department of Health and Aged Care.

Coote A., ed. (2002). *Claiming the health dividend: unlocking the benefits of NHS spending*. London, King's Fund.

Cutler D., Lleras-Muney A. (2007). *Education and health: evaluating theories and evidence*. National Poverty Centre. Policy Brief 9. Gerald R. Ford School of Public Policy, University of Michigan. Available at: www.npc.umich.edu/publications/policy_briefs/brief9/policy_brief9/pdf (accessed 1 July 2007).

Davies J., Colomer C., Lindstrom B., Hospers H., Tountas Y., Modolo M., and Kannas L. (2000). The EUMAHP Project – the development of a European Masters programme in health promotion. *Promotion and Education*, **VII**, 15–18.

Department of Health (2002). *Tackling health inequalities – 2002 cross-cutting review 2002*. London, Department of Health.

Department of Health (2003). *Tackling health inequalities: a programme for action*. London, Department of Health.

Department of Health (2005). *The Chief Medical Officer on the state of public health. Annual Report 2006*. London, Department of Health.

Department of Health (2006). *Tackling health inequalities: Status report on the program for action 2006, Update on headline indicators*. London, DOH.

Health Inequalities Unit, Department of Health (2006). *Tackling health inequalities: status report on the programme for action – 2006 update of headline indicators*. London, Department of Health.

Durham G. and Plant A. (2005). *The Public Health Education and Research Program Review 2005: strengthening workforce capacity for public health.* Canberra, Commonwealth of Australia.

Gebbie K., Rosenstock L., and Hernandez L. (eds.) (2000). *Who will keep the public healthy? Educating public health professionals for the 21st century*. Washington D.C, The National Academies Press.

Gebbie K. and Turnock B. (2006). The public health workforce 2006: new challenges. *Health Affairs*, **25**, 923–933.

Grossman R. and Scala K. with the assistance of Untermarzoner D. (1993). *Health promotion and organizational development: developing settings for health.* European Health Promotion Series No. 2. Vienna, World Health Organization, Regional Office for Europe and IFF Health and Organizational Development.

Hancock T. and Minkler M. (1998). Community health assessment or healthy community assessment: whose community? whose health? whose assessment? In Minkler M. *Community organizing and community building for health*, pp. 139–156. New Jersey, Rutgers University Press.

Harris E., Wise M., Hawe P. *et al.* (1996). *Working together: intersectoral action for health.* Canberra/Sydney, National Centre for Health Promotion and Commonwealth Department of Human Services and Health.

Health Targets and Implementation Committee (1998). *Health for all Australians.* Report to the Australian Health Ministers' Advisory Council and the Australian Health Ministers' Conference. Canberra, Australian Government Publishing Service.

Howat P., Maycock B., Jackson L. *et al.* (2000). Development of competency-based university health promotion courses. *Promotion and Education*, **VII**, 33–38.

Hunter D., and Berman P. (1997). Public health management. Time for a new start? *European Journal of Public Health*, **7**, 345–349.

Institute of Medicine (2003). The governmental public health infrastructure. In: *The future of the public's health in the 21st century*. Washington DC, Institute of Medicine of the National Academies.

International Network for Health Promotion Foundations (2007). Available at: www.hp-foundations.net (accessed on 5 June 2007).

International Union for Health Promotion and Education (1999) *The evidence of health promotion effectiveness. Shaping public health in a new Europe. A report for the European Commission* (2nd edition). Brussels/ Luxembourg,The European Commission.

Jackson N. and Waters E. (2005). Criteria for the systematic review of health promotion and public health interventions. *Health Promotion International*, **20**, 367–374.

Joint Task Group on Public Health Human Resources (2005). *Building the public health workforce for the 21st century.* A Pan-Canadian framework for public health human resources planning. Ottawa, Advisory Committee on Health Delivery and Human Resources, Advisory Committee on Population Health and Health Security.

Kawachi I., Kennedy B. and Wilkinson R. (eds.) (1999). *Income inequality and health: a reader.* New York, New Press.

Kemm J. (2006) Health impact assessment and health in all policies. In Stahl T., Wismar M., Ollila E., Lahtinen E., Leppo K. (eds.) (2006). *Health in all policies: prospects and potentials*. Helsinki, Finnish Ministry of Social Affairs and Health.

Labonte R. (1999). Health promotion in the near future: remembrances of activism past. *Health Education Journal* **58**, 365–377.

Lenihan P. (2005). MAPP and the Evolution of Planning in Public Health Practice. *Journal of Public Health Management and Practice*, **11**, 381–386.

Lopez A. (2003). Evidence and information for health policy: a decade of change. *Medical Journal of Australia*, **179**, 396–7.

McCracken-Rance H. (2000). Developing competencies for health promotion training in Aotearoa-New Zealand. *Promotion and Education*, **VII**, 40–3.

McKnight J. and Kretzmann J. (1988). Mapping community capacity. In Minkler M. *Community organizing and community building for health*, pp. 157–174. Rutgers University Press, New Jersey.

McQueen D. (2000). Perspectives on health promotion: theory, evidence, practice and the emergence of complexity. *Health Promotion International*, **15**, 95–97.

McQueen D. and Jones C. (2007). *Global Perspectives on Health Promotion Effectiveness*. New York, Springer Science & Business Media.

Marmot M. and Wilkinson R. (eds.) (1999). *Social determinants of health*. Oxford, Oxford University Press.

Millward L., Kelly M. and Nutbeam D. (2003). *Public health intervention research – the evidence*. London, Health Development Agency.

Mittelmark M., Wise M., Nam E.W. *et al.* (2007). Mapping national capacity to engage in health promotion: overview of issues and approaches. *Health Promotion International*, **21** (S1).

National Health and Medical Research Council (1997). *Promoting the health of Australians: a review of infrastructure support for national health advancement*. Canberra, National Health and Medical Research Council.

NSW Department of Health (2007). *The health of the people of New South Wales*: Report of the Chief Health Officer 2006. Sydney, NSW Department of Health.

Norwegian Ministry of Health and Care Services (2007). *National strategy to reduce social inequalities in health*. Report No. 20 (2007–7) to the Storting. Oslo: Norwegian Ministry of Health and Care Services.

Nutbeam D., Wise M., Bauman A. *et al.* (1993). *Goals and targets for Australia's health in the year 2000 and beyond*. Canberra, Australian Government Publishing Service.

Nutbeam D. and Wise M. (1996). Planning for Health for All: international experience in setting health goals and targets. *Health Promotion International*, **11**, 219–226.

Nutbeam D. (1996). Achieving 'best practice' in health promotion: improving the fit between research and practice. *Health Education Research*, **11**, 317–325.

Nutbeam D. (1998). Evaluating health promotion – progress, problems and solutions. *Health Promotion International*, **13**, 27–44.

Nutbeam D. (2003). How does evidence influence public policy? Tackling health inequalities in England. *Health Promotion Journal of Australia*, **14**: 154–8.

Nutbeam D. and Bauman A. (2006). *Evaluation in a nutshell*. Sydney, McGraw Hill.

Padgett S., Bekemeier B. and Berkowitz B. (2004). Collaborative partnerships at the state level: promoting systems changes in public health infrastructure. *Journal of Public Health Management Practice*, **10**, 251–257.

Perrons D. and Skyers S. (2003). Empowerment through participation? Conceptual explorations and a case study. *International Journal of Urban and Regional Research*, **27**, 265–285.

Popkin B. (2007). Understanding global nutrition dynamics as a step towards controlling cancer incidence. *Nature*, **7**: 61–67.

Population Health and Wellness (2005). *A framework for core functions in public health. Resource Document*. Province of British Columbia, Canada, Population Health and Wellness, Ministry of Health Services.

Public Health Agency of Canada (2007). *About the Agency*. Available at: http://www.phac-aspc.gc.ca/about_apropos/index.html (accessed 3 July 2007).

Raphael D. (2007). *Poverty and policy in Canada: Implications for health and quality of life*. Toronto, Canadian Scholars' Press.

Rootman I., Goodstadt M., Hyndman B. *et al.* (2001). *Evaluation in health promotion: principles and perspectives*. Who Regional Publications, European Series No. 92. Denmark, World Health Organization.

Rose G. (1992). *The strategy of preventive medicine*. Oxford, New York, Tokyo, Oxford University Press.

Stahl T., Wismar M., Ollila E. *et al.* (eds.) (2006). *Health in all policies: prospects and potentials*. Helsinki, Finnish Ministry of Social Affairs and Health.

Swedish National Institute of Public Health (2006). *Towards a more health-promoting health service*. Stockholm, Swedish National Institute of Public Health.

Travis P., Bennett S., Haines A., Pang T., Bhutta Z., Hyder A. *et al.* (2004). Overcoming health-systems constraints to achieve the Millennium Development Goals. *The Lancet*, **364**, 900–906.

United Nations (2000) Millennium Development Goals. New York. Available at: http://www.un.org/millenniumgoals (accessed 7 August 2008).

US Council on Linkages (1999). *Competencies*. Available at: www.TrainingFinder.org/competencies (accessed 8 August 2007).

US Department of Health and Human Services (1980). *Promoting health/preventing disease: objectives for the nation*. Washington D.C, Department of Health and Human Services, Public Health Service.

US Department of Health and Human Services (1995). *Healthy people 2000. Midcourse review with 1995 revisions*. US Department of Health and Human Services, Public Health Service. Washington DC, US Government Printing Office.

US Department of Health and Human Services (1999). *The Public Health Functions Project*. Available at: http://www.healthypeople.gov/document/HTML/Volume2/23PHI.htm (accessed 9 August 2007).

US Department of Health and Human Services (2006). *Midcourse Review: Healthy people 2010*. Washington, DC: US Government Printing Office.

Wanless D. (2004). *Securing good health for the whole population. Final report*. HM Treasury. London: HMSO.

Weightman A., Ellis S., Cullum A. *et al.* (2005). *Grading evidence and recommendations for public health interventions: developing and piloting a framework*. Support Unit for Research Evidence, Information Services (Cardiff University) and Health Development Agency. London, Health Development Agency.

Whitehead M. (2007). A typology of actions to tackle social inequalities in health. *Journal of Epidemiology and Community Health*, **61**, 473–478.

Wismar M. and Busse R. (2002). Outcome-related health targets – political strategies for better health outcomes. A conceptual and comparative study (Part 2). *Health Policy*, **59**, 223–241.

Woodley P. (2004). *Health financing and population health*. Occasional papers. Health Financing Series Vol. 7. Canberra, Population Health Division, Commonwealth Department of Health and Aged Care.

World Bank Povertynet (2007). *Poverty and health*. Available at: http://web.worldbank.org/WBSITE/EXTERNAL/TOPICS/EXTPOVERTY (accessed 3 July 2007).

World Health Organization (1980). *Global strategy for Health for All*. Geneva, World Health Organization.

World Health Organization.(1985). *Targets for Health for All*. Copenhagen, World Health Organization, Regional Office for Europe,.

World Health Organization, Health and Welfare Canada, Canadian Public Health Association (1986). *Ottawa Charter for Health Promotion*. (Available through) Copenhagen, World Health Organization, Regional Office for Europe.

World Health Organization (2002). *Investment for health: a discussion of the role of economic and social determinants*. WHO Regional Office for Europe. Copenhagen, World Health Organization.

World Health Organization (1998). *Jakarta Declaration on leading health promotion into the 21st century*. Geneva,World Health Organization.

World Health Organization (1999). *Health 21 – health for all in the 21st century*. Copenhagen, World Health Organization.

World Health Organization (2003). *WHO Framework Convention on Tobacco Control*. Geneva, World Health Organization.

World Health Organization (2006). *Commission on the Social Determinants of Health*. Geneva, World Health Organization.

World Health Organization (2005). The Bangkok Charter for Health Promotion in a globalized world. *Health Promotion Journal of Australia*, **16**, 168–171.

WHO European Office for Investment in Health and Development (2007). http://www.euro.who.int/ihd (accessed 3 July 2007.)

World Health Organization (2007). *Knowledge Networks. How the knowledge networks work?* Commission on the Social Determinants of Health. Available at: www.who.int/social_determinants/knowledge_networks/how_kn_operate/en/index.html (accessed 3 July 2007).

Zasa S., Briss P. and Harris K. (2005). *The guide to community preventive services: what works to promote health*? Oxford, New York, Oxford University Press.

Ziglio E., Hagard S., McMahon L. *et al.* (2000). Principles, methodology and practices of investment for health. *Promotion and Education*, **VII**, 4–15.

12.10

Strategies for health services

Martin McKee, Ellen Nolte, and Josep Figueras

Abstract

This chapter starts from the premise that a health system should, fundamentally, seek to improve population health. It first reviews the evidence that modern healthcare can impact positively on population health. Employing the concept of avoidable mortality, which identifies deaths that should not occur in the presence of timely and effective care, it shows that modern healthcare does make an important contribution to health but it also notes that some care provided is either ineffective or even harmful. It continues by examining the many factors that are acting on health systems and to which they must respond. One factor is the changing economic situation, with increasing evidence that investment in health promotes economic growth. Another is the evolving burden of disease, characterized in particular by the growing number of people with multiple complex disorders. Others include changing beliefs about the relationship between the individual and the state, and greater knowledge and expectations among actual and potential users. It then examines what public health professionals can do to maximize the amount of effective care provided to those in need while minimizing what is ineffective or harmful. It identifies a series of strategies. One is priority setting, which should be based on evidence and underpinned by explicit values, including the pursuit of equity in healthcare funding and delivery. Another is optimal allocation of resources, based on the quest to maximize health gain, which includes assessment of need and intelligence-led purchasing of appropriate care. Another is defining models of service delivery, ensuring that care is provided in the most appropriate setting and in ways that achieve optimal outcomes. Finally, the chapter examines some of the ways in which health systems can provide a setting for prevention and health promotion. It concludes by arguing that public health professionals must engage in the debate about how healthcare is funded and delivered if they are to maximize population health.

Introduction

The inclusion of this chapter in a textbook of public health begs a question. Why should public health professionals be interested in health services? This seemingly naïve question brings to the fore a more fundamental question; what are health services for? The answer one gets will vary according to whom the question is addressed. A financial analyst on Wall Street, viewing with pleasure the return on capital of an American for-profit hospital chain will see the provision of healthcare as an economic activity like any other service industry, no different, fundamentally, from running chains of hotels, theme parks or even casinos. A regional development agency may view a healthcare facility as something that enhances the attraction of a run down post-industrial area, an essential element of infrastructure similar to a road network, an airport, and high-speed Internet links, a view endorsed by those responsible for the European Union's structural funds, which actively support investment in health infrastructure. A trade union representing healthcare workers may see it as a source of employment for its members.

From a public health perspective, however, this chapter draws on a framework set out initially in the seminal 2000 World Health Report (World Health Organization 2000) and used subsequently by other writers. In it, the key functions of a health system are to improve population health, to collect the necessary money in a way that is fair, thus protecting people from catastrophic expenditure when they fall ill, and to respond to their legitimate expectations about how a health service should be provided. Public health professionals have a crucial role in ensuring that health systems achieve these objectives, but especially the first of these. To do so, they must promote the equitable use of interventions that are effective and appropriate for the population in question, reduce interventions that are ineffective or harmful, and thus maximize the health gain obtained with the available resources.

Yet, they must do so within a changing environment. This brings both opportunities and threats for public health professionals. On the one hand, change offers the possibility to challenge existing arrangements and maximize the contribution of health services to population health. On the other hand, it brings threats as those responsible for health policy may seek to meet other objectives, such as the narrow pursuit of profit or the exclusion of those in need. Consequently, this chapter explores the changing nature of health services, the roles that public health professionals can play in these processes, and the strategies that they can pursue to enhance health gain and promote equity. It begins by assessing the contribution that health services make to population health.

Do health services affect population health?

There is little argument that some interventions, most obviously immunization against diseases such as smallpox, poliomyelitis and measles, but also some low-technology strategies such as integrated management of childhood illness, have been remarkably successful in reducing mortality in many parts of the world. However, there is much less agreement about many other elements of health services.

At the risk of simplification, the debate has become somewhat polarized. Thus, some have argued that healthcare contributes little to population health, a view that is associated most closely with the work of McKeown (1979). He argued that three-quarters of the decline in mortality in England and Wales between 1841 and 1971 had been due to a reduction in deaths from infectious disease, yet three-quarters of this reduction had preceded the widespread introduction of immunization or antibiotics. This, he contended, demonstrated that the main drivers of improvements in health had been nutrition, environment, and behaviour. A different, but related, perspective is offered by those who argue that it is unrealistic to expect healthcare to contribute significantly to population health because so little of it has been adequately evaluated and found to be effective (Chappell 1993).

To others, however, it is not just that healthcare has little impact on health. Instead, it may actually damage it. This view receives some support from studies that have related healthcare inputs to outputs. If anything, these have suggested that there is an inverse association, with greater healthcare resources leading to worse overall health (Cochrane *et al.* 1978). One explanation advanced for this observation is that scarce resources are being channelled into healthcare rather than sectors such as education where they might have a greater, albeit less immediately obvious, impact on health. Another is that healthcare has a direct and adverse effect on health, a view advanced by Illich (1976), who coined the term iatrogenesis to describe the adverse consequences of prescribed drugs, hospital-acquired infections, poorly performed surgery, and the harm done by following up spurious abnormalities found among the vastly increased number of laboratory investigations being undertaken.

These views have elicited a range of responses. Some physicians have simply dismissed them, arguing that they are completely at odds with the everyday experience of clinicians who see the results of the care that they provide. In contrast, others have argued that the existing level of healthcare provision in some countries is excessive (Lavis & Stoddart 1994) and that politicians should shift expenditure from healthcare to sectors such as education, housing, and employment.

This debate has considerable implications for the role of public health professionals. Thus, if the major determinants of health lie outside the healthcare sector, is the involvement of public health professionals in the delivery of healthcare at best an irrelevance and, at worst, a diversion from the more important roles of advocacy and mobilizing inter-sectoral action (Whitty & Jones 1992)? Or have public health professionals a role in ensuring that healthcare is provided effectively and efficiently, on the basis that this will maximize population health?

However, the debate has to be interpreted in the light of the context within which it was held. Thus, while Illich and McKeown may have been correct in the 1960s and 1970s when they were developing their arguments, the intervening period has seen major changes, with many formerly fatal conditions now amenable to treatment. Furthermore, many of the criticisms made by Illich concerning unnecessary and inappropriate investigations and treatment have now been addressed by the greater acceptance of evidence-based healthcare. In this scenario, healthcare is seen as an important determinant of health of a population. It is thus worthy of the attention of public health professionals, who have a role in enhancing access to effective care and reducing exposure to ineffective and dangerous care.

Quantifying the contribution of healthcare to population health

It is important to recall that healthcare has changed remarkably in a relatively short time. Many new treatments have been shown, in high-quality evaluative research, to be able to prolong life. Examples include effective treatment for hypertension and heart failure, secondary prevention following myocardial infarction and chemotherapy for many childhood cancers. There has also been, in many countries, a revolution in the approach to evidence in making treatment decisions. These changes are part of a long-term trend. Beeson (1980) showed how many treatments advocated in a 1927 edition of a major textbook of medicine were, at the time he was writing, known to be either ineffective or harmful. By the time that the 1975 edition was published there was a major shift to treatments that had been proven to be effective. However, the pace of change has accelerated during the 1980s and 1990s. There has been a much greater willingness to challenge professional judgement where it is not supported by evidence of effectiveness and to question whether clinical performance is optimal. This has led from early pioneers of the medical audit to the enormous expansion of evidence-based healthcare (see below). It encompasses a wide range of activities which together have helped to eliminate many interventions that do not work and have increased the uptake of those that are effective. Thus there is a case that if healthcare had made little contribution to population health during the period that McKeown was looking at, up to the mid-1960s, it may now be doing so. The following section asks whether this has actually happened.

Rutstein *et al.* (1976) asked an expert panel to identify a list of conditions from which death should not occur in the presence of timely and effective care. These deaths were deemed to be 'preventable' although subsequent writers have also used the terms 'avoidable' and 'amenable to medical care'; and were interpreted as a measure of the quality of the healthcare system. This concept was later applied empirically by other researchers, with publication of regional atlases permitting cross-national comparisons. A seminal study by Mackenbach *et al.* (1988) related changes in deaths from particular causes to the time that various interventions were introduced. By doing so, they were able to show that the impacts of specific treatments were observable as accelerating falls in mortality from the conditions they were intended to treat. They concluded that the healthcare interventions they examined added 2.9 years to life expectancy at birth for men and 3.9 years for women in the Netherlands between 1950 and 1984.

More recently, Nolte and McKee (2004) undertook a systematic review of the evidence that deaths from specific causes of death could be avoided. This enabled them to update the previous lists of 'avoidable' causes, taking account of advances in medical knowledge and technology, while extending the upper age limit to 75 years of age. Figure 12.10.1 shows the age standardized death rates in 2003 in a range of industrialized countries.

A comparison of trends over time in selected European countries showed that reductions in avoidable mortality contributed substantially to increasing life expectancy in Western European countries

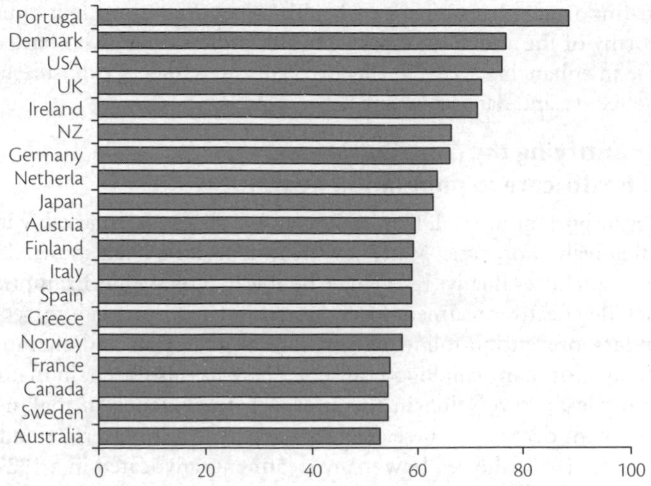

Fig. 12.10.1 Age-standardized death rates (0–74 years per 100 000) from conditions amenable to care (2003 or most recent year).
Source: Authors' calculations using data from the WHO mortality database.
Note: Denmark 2001, Italy, Sweden, United States 2002.

during the 1980s. They continued to do so during the 1990s, although by then the contribution was greater in southern European countries such as Italy and Spain, suggesting some catching up with their northern neighbours. In contrast, the then communist countries in central and eastern Europe saw little benefit from healthcare during the 1980s but this changed in the 1990s and has continued, with further substantial reductions in avoidable mortality in the first decade of the twenty-first century (Nolte *et al.* 2004). Finally, a comparison of Russia and the United Kingdom shows how the two countries had very similar rates of avoidable mortality in the mid-1960s, a time when there were relatively few modern pharmaceuticals available in either country. The rate in the United Kingdom then began to fall steadily while they remained steady in Russia, which during the Soviet era never managed to develop a modern pharmaceutical system and where the principles of evidence-based care were essentially unknown (Andreev *et al.* 2003).

Further evidence that healthcare can impact positively on population health comes from studies of particular causes of death. Beaglehole (1986) estimated that 42 per cent of the decline in deaths from cardiovascular disease in New Zealand between 1974 and 1981 could be attributed to advances in medical care. The long-term decline in mortality from coronary heart disease in the Netherlands between 1969 and 1993 accelerated significantly after 1987, coinciding with the wider availability of interventions such as coronary care units and thrombolysis (Bonneux *et al.* 1997).

Thus, while there is increasing evidence for a positive impact of healthcare on population health, it is also important not to dismiss Illich's views entirely. The thalidomide scandal in the 1960s, in which what was thought to be a safe sedative was found later to cause serious limb deformities in the children of mothers who took it while pregnant, confirmed the potential for an effective drug to cause harm to susceptible individuals. Subsequently other apparently safe drugs have been shown to have caused unanticipated long-term side effects. For example, the growing burden of multi-drug resistant tuberculosis is entirely a creation of healthcare, providing a classic example of iatrogenesis. In some countries, the 1990s have seen a marked increase in the rate of resistance among hospital-acquired infections. Rates vary markedly between countries, and there is compelling evidence that they are related to the approach taken to the prescribing of antibiotics. Thus, hospitals and other healthcare facilities in which prescribing is uncontrolled and haphazard represent a threat to the wider population, and not only in the country concerned. Unfortunately, surveillance systems are often weak, even in many industrialized countries. It is easy to forget that, until the early twentieth century, one's probability of dying was increased by coming into hospital because of the risk of infection and the growth of iatrogenic antibiotic resistance is perhaps one of the greatest challenges facing public health professionals today.

It is also important to recognize the accumulating evidence of patient harm resulting from medical errors, with one analysis suggesting this could account for as much as 44 000 deaths among Americans each year (Institute of Medicine 2000). Finally, it is salutary to recall that even well-established interventions may be ineffective or even harmful, as in the example of albumin, long given to patients with burns and multiple trauma on the basis, incorrectly, of an intuitive belief that it was likely to be beneficial (Alderson *et al.* 2004). In this context, it is necessary to consider the specific situation in the countries of the former Soviet Union. Its isolation from international developments during the Soviet era led to the widespread adoption of many entirely ineffective treatments based on various forms of electromagnetic and ionizing radiation, many of which remain in widespread use (McKee 2007).

Healthcare and health equity

The health impact of health services raises the important issue of equity. When healthcare had little measurable impact on health, socio-demographic inequalities in access to care may have been of little importance. Indeed, it is arguable that the wealthy, exposed at considerable personal expense to such painful and ineffective treatments as cupping and bleeding were actually disadvantaged compared with the poor who patiently waited for the inevitable death spared such indignities. The present situation is quite different. If healthcare does contribute materially to population health, then lack of access to it will exacerbate health inequalities (Arblaster *et al.* 1996).

There is considerable evidence from many countries that such inequalities exist and that they have an impact on health. This is intuitive in healthcare systems where there is not universal access to care, such as the United States. For example, American research has found that people living in deprived areas with poor access to care have high rates of hospital admission with chronic medical conditions, such as asthma, heart failure, and diabetes that, if detected and treated early should not require admission to hospital (Billings *et al.* 1996). Death rates from many chronic disorders responsive to healthcare are very much higher among African Americans than white Americans (Kunitz & Pesis-Katz 2005), with similar differences in survival from many cancers, reflecting both later presentation (itself a reflection of access to primary care) and lower rates on intervention once a diagnosis has been made (Morris *et al.* 2006).

Inequalities are, however, also seen in countries offering universal coverage. In the United Kingdom, women, people from minority ethnic populations, older people, and those living in deprived areas are all disadvantaged in access to surgical interventions for coronary artery disease.

Differential access is a factor in the observation that social class gradients are substantially greater for causes amenable to medical care than other causes of death (Marshall *et al.* 1993).

Inequitable access to care can disadvantage many groups of people other than those listed above (Healy & McKee 2004). Thus, those living in rural areas may be disadvantaged unless specific measures are taken to ensure their access to care. This will often require innovative delivery models, taking advantage of technological developments such as near-patient testing and telemedicine to compensate for the increasing pressure to centralize facilities. Prisoners in many countries receive poor quality care, while disabled people may face structural obstacles in accessing health facilities and obtaining services. At a global level there are enormous inequalities in access to basic, but essential, treatments such as immunization and life-sustaining drugs such as anti-retrovirals and insulin.

This section has highlighted how, unlike the situation prior to the 1970s, healthcare can make a substantial difference to population health. However, as the World Health Organization noted in the Ottawa Charter (World Health Organization 1986), health services are only one of the determinants of health, others being genetic predisposition, individual behaviour and lifestyle, and environmental circumstances (Lalonde 1974), whose importance are recognized in the creation by the World Health Organization, in March 2005, of a Commission on Social Determinants of Health.

Public health professionals must look at the wider picture and take into account these other determinants but it is important that, in taking a broad perspective, they do not lose sight of the contribution that healthcare can make to population health, ensuring that what care is provided is effective and is provided equitably. The remainder of this chapter explores the changing nature of health services, the impact that various policies have, and the role that public health professionals can play in maximizing the health gain that health services can provide.

Why are health systems changing?

Health systems face a range of pressures, from both within and outside. External factors include the macroeconomic climate and the evolving framework of values of the society within which the system is located. Internal factors include the changing pattern of health in the population being served, upward pressures on expenditures arising from ageing populations and technological change, a search for improvements in the quality of healthcare that is delivered, and the expansion of information technology. These will be considered in turn.

Macroeconomic factors

Health systems are influenced strongly by their economic environments. One is the nature of the market within which resources are procured. In general, the costs of some inputs into health services have tended to reflect local market conditions, such as salaries for healthcare professionals. Others, such as pharmaceuticals and technology, have tended to reflect world market prices although, in practice, the situation is not quite so simple. Thus, the cost of employing health professionals will reflect the market within which they function. Those in countries where few speak one of the major international languages may still be operating in what is essentially a national market, allowing salaries to remain low. Conversely, where most speak a language such as English, French, or Spanish, health workers operate increasingly in a global market, so that healthcare providers must pay high salaries if they are to retain them. The inability to do so has contributed to the emigration of vast numbers of health professionals from low-income countries. In the case of pharmaceuticals, the price paid in a low-income country may actually be several times higher than in a developed one because of the fragmentation of the purchasing function and multiple mark-ups along the supply chain (Mossialos *et al.* 2004). The different costs of inputs will shape the pattern of care that is provided.

A second consideration relates to the resources available for healthcare. There are two issues to be considered. The first is the overall state of the economy. The second is the share of the economy devoted to health.

Clearly, the healthcare system is likely to come under pressure during an economic crisis. Examples include events in some Latin American countries in the 1980s and 1990s, in the countries of the former Soviet Union in the years following 1991 or, in many low-income countries, in the face of externally imposed structural adjustment policies. The effects may be seen in death rates from treatable conditions. Thus, deaths from diabetes among young people increased many times in the former Soviet Union during the early 1990s (Telishevka *et al.* 2001) while child mortality has increased in countries facing structural adjustment.

These circumstances are, however, unusual and economic swings are typically much less severe. Yet, they still impact on the health system. An economic downturn, especially where it leads to long-term unemployment, will increase demand for many elements of healthcare at a time when financial resources are scarce, although, paradoxically, death rates from cardiovascular disease, traffic injuries, and cirrhosis increase during an economic boom.

The share of the economy devoted to healthcare is, inevitably, the result of the interplay between market forces and political choices. Regardless of the funding system in place, governments in all industrialized and middle-income countries play an important role in determining how much will be spent. This is easiest in countries where healthcare is financed from taxation but governments in countries with social insurance systems are usually partners to negotiations on contribution levels, salaries, or pharmaceutical prices, simply because of the important macroeconomic implications. Even in a country such as the United States, where the role of the government in healthcare is often considered to be minimal, almost 50 per cent of the population have their healthcare paid from government funds.

The way in which healthcare expenditure is viewed has changed over the past decade. During the 1980s and 1990s it was often regarded as a drain on the economy, with high social costs damaging national competitiveness. In particular, the cost of healthcare was sometimes cited as a reason for trans-national corporations to relocate production in a country where the costs were less (Stephens *et al.* 1999). This was exacerbated in some places by specific factors. In the mid-1990s, the countries of Southeast Asia suffered a major economic crisis. However, countries responded in different ways, providing a valuable natural public health experiment. Thailand and Indonesia followed advice from the World Bank to cut back on public expenditure while Malaysia did not (Hopkins 2006). There was a short- lived but detectable increase in mortality in the first two countries but not in Malaysia, highlighting the importance of maintaining social safety nets at times of economic crisis.

More recently, there are signs of a change of direction in the prevalent thinking. Research, initially in low-income countries (World Health Organization and Commission on Macroeconomics and Health 2001), but later confirmed in high-income countries (Suhrcke *et al.* 2006), has highlighted the contribution of good health to economic growth, with better health leading to greater wages, higher labour force participation, higher savings, and greater investment in one's own education.

Historical improvements in health and nutrition have contributed substantially to the favourable economic status of today's advanced industrialized countries (Fogel 1994). People who are healthy are more likely to remain in the workforce, where they are more productive. They are likely to save more, increasing the resources available for capital investment, and to invest in their own skills. Furthermore, there is a growing recognition that investment in timely care can reduce the frequency of complications, which are much more expensive to treat (Billings *et al.* 1996). One example of this new thinking is the Wanless Report (Wanless 2001), commissioned by the United Kingdom Treasury. This report showed how investment in better health now would lead to a substantial reduction in expenditure in the future.

While, in most cases, public health professionals must work within the constraints imposed by the macroeconomic context in which they find themselves, they also have a major role, as advocates for the public's health, in shaping the debate, arguing for sustained investment in health on the basis of its contribution to future economic growth.

Norms and beliefs

A second set of factors driving change in healthcare systems relate to the underlying norms and beliefs of the society within which the system is embedded (Contandriopoulos *et al.* 1998). Healthcare systems act as mirrors reflecting deeply rooted social and cultural expectations of the population that they serve. Although these norms and beliefs are generated outside the formal structure of the healthcare system, they play a major role in defining the system's overall characteristics.

The impact of different norms and beliefs is apparent when comparing the United States, where healthcare is generally seen as a commodity to be bought and sold, and Europe, where healthcare is seen predominantly as a social or collective good, in which citizens benefit when an individual receives effective care (McKee 2002).

Societies thus have dominant belief systems (Benson 1975). This does not imply that a single view is held by all members of that society; rather, the tension and negotiation that exist between various beliefs and values have some stability. A useful approach to understanding belief systems sees these tensions as grouped around four poles (Habermas 1987): Values, understanding of phenomena, definition of jurisdictions and allocation of resources, and logic of regulation. Values include tensions and trade-offs between equity, individual autonomy, and efficiency (Clark 1998). Understanding of phenomena relates to how concepts such as life, death, sickness, health, and pain are interpreted and thus viewed as relating to the objectives of a healthcare (Gillett 1995). Definition of jurisdictions and allocation of resources comprise the perceptions of the role and functions of those responsible for and working in the healthcare sector, as well as the allocation of resources between prevention and cure and between healthcare and broader determinants of health. The logic of regulation relates to how society chooses to regulate the delivery of healthcare (Contandriopoulos *et al.* 1998). This may be technocratic, with trained experts guiding the system on the basis of their knowledge and position within the hierarchy; professional self-regulatory, which has the physician, as the best agent of the patient, at the centre of the system; the market-based model, in which regulations reflect supply and demand in a competitive market; or the democratic model, in which the population, either directly or, more often, through elected or appointed representatives, is responsible for setting out the framework for delivery of healthcare.

Although dominant belief systems have some stability, they are in a state of constant tension as different classes and groups within society struggle for ascendancy, a phenomenon most clearly seen in the fluctuating electoral success of political parties. In some societies, the process of change will be evolutionary and incremental. In others, as exemplified by the countries in Central and Eastern Europe after the collapse of communism, it will be abrupt. An understanding of the dominant belief system in a society is important for public health professionals as it contributes to knowledge of why systems are as they are, how they have changed, and the objectives that individuals within the healthcare system are pursuing. It will also influence the choice of strategies that should be adopted to bring about change.

Changing burden of disease

Although it would be naive to think that the health needs of the population are the only factor driving the configuration of health services, they do play an important role. For example, the creation of public health services in many industrialized countries was a direct result of the global epidemics of cholera in the mid-nineteenth centuries. Recognition of the infectious nature of tuberculosis led, somewhat controversially, to the creation of sanatoria in rural areas. As the need for surgery for tuberculosis declined, thoracic surgeons turned first to undertaking mitral valvotomies for rheumatic heart disease, and then to more advanced forms of cardiac surgery, explaining why some world-famous cardiac surgical hospitals are currently situated on their own in open countryside. More recently, the discovery of the agent responsible for hepatitis B and, especially, the emergence of the HIV virus, have both had significant implications for the organization of systems designed to reduce cross-infection in healthcare facilities, and in the latter case, the approaches taken to issues of patient consent and confidentiality.

The burden of disease worldwide is dynamic (Mathers & Loncar 2006). One factor is the changing age structure of the population. In many populations, the number of old people, and especially the very old, is increasing. This is something to be celebrated, especially as there is growing evidence that it is associated with compression of morbidity, so that people are living even longer in good health. Yet, when coupled with the ability to maintain people with chronic diseases in good health, this is leading to a situation wherein there are many more people with multiple chronic diseases (McKee & Nolte 2004). This will be perhaps the greatest challenge to health systems in the twenty-first century. Yet traditionally, health services have been based on a model of individual self-limiting illnesses in which a patient is attended to by a single health professional. This model is inappropriate in a situation where a patient must navigate a complex maze of health facilities and health professionals. In such circumstances, the patient (or his or her carer, where the patient has cognitive impairment) may be the only person who has a comprehensive view of the total package of care.

Recognition of these challenges has led to the development of new models of care, especially in the United States where, as already noted, outcomes of chronic disease are poor. One of the best known, the Chronic Care Model, illustrates many of the issues related to these new models of care (Wagner *et al.* 1999). Most other models are variations on the same theme. The Chronic Care Model comprises four interacting system components: Self-management support, delivery system design, decision support and clinical information systems. Evaluations have linked individual components to improvements in some process or outcome measures, such as perceived quality of care, patient outcomes, pathways to care, and reduced cost (Tsai *et al.* 2005). However it is less clear whether this is a consequence of applying the model as a whole, or whether the same benefits can be achieved using only some of the components (Bodenheimer *et al.* 2002). The message to emerge from this body of work is that appropriate care for the growing number of people with multiple chronic disorders requires systems that empower patients and help them to navigate through a complex system, secure in the knowledge that the care available is co-ordinated and based on evidence of effectiveness.

There are, however, many other ways in which the burden of disease is changing that have implications for health services. To a considerable extent this reflects changing risk factors. It is increasingly likely that the epidemic of tobacco-related disease will be seen as a transient phenomenon of the twentieth and early twenty-first century, at least in industrialized countries. Other changes are a result of a general improvement in living conditions, such as the long-standing decline in stomach cancer, reflecting falling rates of infection with *Helicobacter pylori* in childhood. Still others are more complex. Death rates from cardiovascular disease have fallen by about 50 per cent in many industrialized countries over the past three decades, reflecting a combination of lower rates of smoking, improved diet (in part a result of global trade), and improved understanding of risk factors. Yet, not all changes are so encouraging. A combination of energy-rich diets and reduced levels of exercise are leading to a rapid increase in obesity in many countries, with an accompanying rise in the prevalence of type II diabetes. Finally, successes against some infectious diseases, such as measles, contrast with failures with others, exemplified by increasing rates of HIV infection and drug-resistant bacteria in many places.

The key message for public health professionals is that they have a central role in tracking and predicting these emerging trends, in designing mechanisms that address them, and in supporting the changes in service delivery that are required.

Upward pressure on healthcare expenditure

The debate on the future of health systems often seems to be dominated by discussion of the cost of providing care. This is an issue that is surrounded by a great deal of mythology. For example, the observation that healthcare costs increase with age is often used to support the argument that an ageing population will render the provision of universal healthcare unsustainable. However, it is now clear that age per se does not increase costs but rather proximity to death (McGrail *et al.* 2000). In fact, in the United States, Medicare data show that payments associated with an additional year of death fall as age at death increases (Lubitz *et al.* 1995) and that the most costly patients are those who die young, possibly because, for a variety of reasons, they are more intensively treated. An ageing population will, however, incur increased costs for social care, largely reflecting the effects of cognitive decline (Meerding *et al.* 1998). However, when looking to the future it is necessary to take account of evidence that tomorrow's elderly population is likely to be considerably healthier than today's, as they will have benefited from a lifetime of better nutrition and social conditions. This is known as compression of morbidity (Fries 2003). For these reasons, simplistic extrapolation of cross-sectional cost data to a future population with a longer life expectancy is flawed.

The changing composition of the population does, however, have one important consequence. In many countries ageing populations are coinciding with falling birth rates, leading to an increasing old-age dependency ratio (ratio of people 65 and over to those aged 15–64). These changes vary greatly between countries. Some countries, such as Germany and Japan, face substantial challenges while others, such as the United Kingdom, will be somewhat less affected, at least until the middle of the twenty-first century. This development, taken with the evidence of compression of morbidity noted above, is leading several countries to explore the possibility of raising the retirement age as a means of addressing what would otherwise be a shrinking share of the population in working ages. Projections indicate that a relatively small increase in retirement age, coupled with efforts to increase the participation in the workforce of people over 50, would overcome many of the anticipated problems.

Another area where there appears to be considerable misunderstanding relates to the oft-quoted statement that healthcare costs inevitably rise at a faster rate than the economy, or in economic terms, that healthcare is a luxury good. This is often linked to a view, usually implicit, that it is legitimate to restrict health expenditure because the additional expenditure is not yielding proportionate health gains. However, cost estimates are only as good as the underlying data and models used. Thus, Parkin and colleagues have shown it is possible to derive widely differing figures for the elasticity of health spending on national income in industrialized countries, depending on whether exchange rates or purchasing power parities are used and on how the model is specified (Parkin *et al.* 1987). Furthermore, analyses inside countries consistently indicate that healthcare is not a luxury good.

A third issue is the introduction of new pharmaceuticals and technology. The pace of change in healthcare is steadily accelerating. The growth of healthcare technology is widely held to have contributed substantially to the upward pressure on healthcare expenditure, for several reasons, although its precise contribution is controversial (Mossialos & Le Grand 1999). New technologies can be more expensive than the ones they replaced. Even where the actual technology is less expensive, it may lead to increased costs as other aspects of the service are reorganized to reflect changing patterns of treatment. The introduction of new treatments may lead to an expansion in the number of individuals with indications for treatment, either because a previously untreatable condition becomes treatable or, as side-effects or contraindications are reduced, the threshold for treatment falls. Finally, the diffusion of technology from tertiary centres, in some cases into primary care, can markedly reduce barriers to access and thus increase uptake. In response to the increasing use of expensive new technologies, many countries have established health technology assessment programmes and related systems to control introduction and diffusion. One example is the United Kingdom's National Institute for Health and Clinical Excellence, which looks beyond specific technologies to evaluate a wide range of health interventions. It assesses evidence of cost-effectiveness, typically recommending the adoption of interventions where the cost of an additional quality-adjusted life year gained is under about £30 000 (€44 000). It also identifies gaps in the available research. While some of its decisions not to recommend interventions or products have attracted considerable controversy, it has also been credited with increasing the uptake of innovations of proven effectiveness.

Fourth, consumers have increased their expectations about the services provided by the healthcare system, in some cases encouraged by governments. As noted above, the development of new and more expensive technologies coupled with the increased access to information via the Internet have led people to demand a wider range of services of high quality from healthcare providers, an issue dealt with in more detail below.

Each of these issues has implications for public health professionals. Public health professionals must contribute to the process of anticipating future health needs. This requires an understanding of the relationship over time between a change in exposure and its corresponding outcome. This may be very short, as was seen following the collapse of the USSR where rapid fluctuations in mortality were driven by large-scale changes in alcohol consumption (Shkolnikov *et al.* 2001). In contrast, there is a delay of many years between an increase in smoking in a population and the development of many tobacco-related diseases. It is, however, important to recognize that relationships may be asymmetrical, with reductions in exposure leading to rapid declines in disease or death.

Public health professionals must also contribute to discussions on how health services can be reconfigured to meet the increasingly complex needs of the elderly population with multiple disease processes, as well as how to invest effectively in prevention so as to extend the years that people live in good health. Discussions about new health technology require inputs from public health professionals, drawing on skills such as epidemiology and economics, to assess appropriateness and cost-effectiveness. However, it is also important to stress that attention to these issues may lead to a conclusion that there is a need for greater expenditure on healthcare, as was the case in the United Kingdom, where the Wanless Report demonstrated how the National Health Service was underperforming because of long-term underinvestment (Wanless 2001).

The quest for enhanced quality of care

Research undertaken in the 1970s and 1980s drew attention to widespread geographical variations in the use of common procedures (McPherson 1989) and led to a questioning of clinical judgements about the appropriateness of healthcare interventions. The International Cochrane Collaboration has played a major part in this process by highlighting the extent to which much care that was provided was ineffective, while effective interventions were not adopted widely (Chalmers & Altman 1995). Similar findings have emerged from the health technology assessment activities discussed above. More recently, there has been growing attention to patient safety, in the light of research showing unacceptably high levels of patient injury and death due to clinical errors (Institute of Medicine 2000).

These developments reflect a change in dominant belief systems, challenging traditional models based on clinical autonomy. They are contributing to a range of changes in healthcare systems that include not only the elimination of ineffective treatments and adoption of effective ones but also new organizational structures to bring about change. Again, public health professionals have key roles to play because of their skills in healthcare evaluation and the management of change. Strategies to ensure quality of care are discussed in more detail below.

The information society

The 1980s and 1990s have seen an unparalleled revolution in the pace and volume of communication. This brings both challenges and opportunities for health systems, discussed in more detail in Chapter 5.3 (Web-based public health information dissemination and evaluation).

Strategies for health services

Given these changing circumstances, coherent strategies are needed to enable health systems to respond appropriately. Four such strategies are considered here. The first includes those that address resource scarcity, which here includes the process of setting priorities for healthcare. The second relates to healthcare funding, focusing on the issue of equity and, specifically, the tension between competition and solidarity. The third includes those designed to achieve a more effective allocation of resources, here including assessment of healthcare need and purchasing healthcare. The final set includes strategies designed to achieve more cost-effective and higher-quality care.

Tackling scarcity of resources

Upward pressures on healthcare costs in the face of limited resources confront governments with two interconnected options. One is to increase the resources for healthcare by shifting funds from other areas of public sector expenditure or by increasing taxation, social insurance contributions, or direct payments. The second is to seek to control healthcare expenditure by pursuing strategies that influence either the demand for or the supply of healthcare. Strategies that act on supply of health services include reducing the number of healthcare professionals or facilities, setting global budgets for providers, giving professionals incentives to reduce the amount of care provided, and reducing access to care (Abel-Smith *et al.* 1995).

Strategies acting on demand include priority setting to ration access to certain services, the use of cost-sharing, incentives to encourage greater private expenditure, such as tax concessions, and the right to opt out of the statutory system.

Each of these measures seeks to reduce demand by shifting some portion of healthcare costs to the individual. They have all been discussed elsewhere (Mossialos & Le Grand 1999) and here only one approach, that of setting priorities, is considered as it is the one in which public health professionals have played the greatest role.

During the 1990s, many countries addressed the issue of explicit rationing of publicly funded healthcare. The debate has been lengthy and complex, with many different views. Perhaps the only issue where there is a degree of unanimity is that, in all healthcare systems, some form of rationing has always taken place although, in most cases, this was implicit, inextricably linked to clinical judgement. Beyond this, the consensus breaks down as illustrated by the situation in the United Kingdom where there was fundamental disagreement between politicians and others about even the choice of the terms 'rationing' or 'priority setting' as a means of describing the process.

In this debate, some commentators have argued that rationing should not be necessary if either sufficient funding was made available typically by redirecting it from other areas of public expenditure or raising taxes or by ensuring that available resources are used more efficiently. However, others have argued that the continuing upward pressure on healthcare costs has made explicit rationing of effective care necessary. For these commentators, the key issue is transparency.

Concerns about the affordability of healthcare have led, in several countries, to initiatives that examine priority setting on a more systematic and explicit basis. These processes have brought together a wide range of individuals, including public health professionals, managers, politicians, economists and philosophers.

Explicit setting of priorities involves making decisions at different levels within the healthcare system, ranging from the overall funders of healthcare to the treatments available to individual patients. If explicit priority setting is to be undertaken, a co-ordinated, strategic approach is most effective to integrate decision-making at these different levels.

Decisions may lead to blanket exclusions of intervention, or of condition–intervention combinations, as in the approach taken in Oregon in the United States, or production of guidelines, such as those developed by the National Institute of Health and Clinical Excellence in the United Kingdom. The experience of Oregon was especially interesting because of the technical and ethical issues it raised (Oregon Health Services Commission 1991). It was designed to create a list of condition intervention pairs, ranked on the basis of cost-benefit, with a cut-off point based on available resources below which combinations would not be funded. The idea was that this would maximize the return on resources invested in healthcare. However, the process was extremely problematic when it became clear that many of the data required were unavailable and some results were quite counterintuitive—for example, appendectomy was rated lower than cosmetic dentistry.

An alternative approach was used in the Netherlands. There the Dunning Committee (Dunning 1992) proposed four criteria that an intervention to be funded from social health insurance should meet. These were necessity, effectiveness, efficiency, and whether treating the condition should be a matter of individual rather than community responsibility. As a result of this process, it was recommended that services such as dentistry for adults, homeopathic treatment, *in vitro* fertilization and physiotherapy for sports injuries should be excluded.

This debate has created a recognition that the priority-setting process must include government, providers, the public and patients, as well as evidence on health needs and on the cost and effectiveness of available interventions (Ham 1993). Priority setting cannot be reduced to a technical exercise and should be combined with a thorough public debate about the values underpinning the choices to be made. This is seen in the approach taken in Sweden (McKee & Figueras 1996), which focused on the need to reach a shared view of the ethical basis on which priorities should be set. This rejected a narrow economic approach and gave priority to the treatment of life-threatening conditions. It also emphasized the importance of social solidarity.

Ultimately, while public health professionals have an important role in providing the evidence on which any debate on priority setting must be based and on examining the consequences of any decisions for equity, priority setting in a publicly funded system is the responsibility of politicians. Decision-making inevitably involves trade-offs between objectives as a balance is sought among universal coverage, comprehensiveness of services, equity, efficiency, cost-containment, and broader social values. However, it is also important to note that, despite enormous efforts being devoted to the setting of priorities, it has been extremely difficult for any health system ostensibly providing universal coverage to exclude any treatments except for a few on the margin, such as cosmetic surgery.

Equitable funding of health systems

Whitehead (1988) has shown how access to services is a key element of strategies designed to reduce health inequalities. Throughout the twentieth century the steady expansion of coverage in many countries has served to improve access to healthcare for those in greatest need, based on the principle of solidarity, in which individual financial contributions are related to ability to pay and are not dependent on the individual's health status.

At present, however, certain developments threaten to undermine the principle of solidarity. One is the pressure from advocates of market-based policies to establish competition among healthcare insurers. A second is the development of information technology and, increasingly, the use of genetic profiling, enabling individual risks to be predicted more accurately and permitting exclusion or higher premiums for those at greatest risk, although this is raising enormous technical and ethical issues. A third is the failure, by some governments, to collect sufficient taxes or social insurance contributions from the wealthy to fund the system. This has several causes. One is a neo-liberal agenda that argues that, for countries to attract inward investment and employment, they must reduce taxes. A second cause, which is especially problematic in, but not exclusive to, low- and middle-income countries, is widespread tax avoidance by the wealthy.

Each of these issues has important implications for equity and thus for public health professionals. The third is beyond the scope of this chapter, but the first and second, which are linked in that competitive insurers have a strong incentive to identify the risks attached to those they accept, are relevant as public health professionals may have to work with such competitive systems.

Competition between health insurers (whether private or public) tends to erode solidarity in healthcare financing, since health insurers seek to select good risks. In the absence of regulation, older people and those with pre-existing illness or even a strong family history of illness are either excluded from coverage or charged higher premiums. As noted above, advances in information technology and genetics are making this ever easier, although this is raising enormous ethical issues. For example, should an insurer be permitted to know an individual's genotype?

Two responses are open to policy-makers. One is mandatory open enrolment, so that insurers are unable to refuse coverage to an individual. This is typically linked to regulation of the level of contributions, such as community ratings. The second is the use of risk-adjustment schemes that redistribute the health insurance system's revenue among competing health insurers on the basis of the risk profile of those enrolling with each insurer.

While these responses might work in theory, they are much more problematic in practice. Apparently open enrolment can be distorted in many subtle ways by targeting promotional activities or manipulating access so that insurers tend to 'cream skim'. Risk pooling requires development of valid formulas, which have proved elusive, with several systems relying purely on crude measures such as age.

If politicians choose to introduce competitive markets in healthcare financing, despite a widespread consensus from health economists and others that such initiatives are fraught with danger, public health professionals have an important role in monitoring and responding to any effects on equity. Maintaining solidarity in healthcare financing while introducing competition among insurers is an ambitious and difficult undertaking. The 'safety-net' for solidarity has to be designed very carefully, and such an undertaking requires experienced supervision of healthcare markets. Moreover, several crucial questions have not yet been answered. Whether competition among insurers really leads to more efficient and more effective healthcare has yet to be demonstrated (Chinitz *et al.* 1998), not least because of the need for expensive regulatory and risk adjustment systems, as has the question of whether mechanisms seeking to combine solidarity with competition can succeed.

Optimal allocation of resources

Upward pressure on costs and an increasing willingness of politicians, managers and the public to challenge established patterns of care have placed an increased emphasis on the optimal allocation of scarce healthcare resources. Several interconnected strategies are available to health policy-makers. These include ensuring that the health services provided reflect the health needs of the population that they serve, enhance the efficiency with which services are delivered, and control the cost of key inputs such as pharmaceuticals and technology. Public health professionals can play an important role in both the assessment of health needs and, increasingly, in the process of intelligent purchasing of healthcare so as to maximize health gain for a given set of inputs.

Assessing need for healthcare

Assessment of healthcare needs has arisen from recognition that, left to itself, the pattern of health services will frequently reflect only partially the health needs of the population it is serving, and often those whose needs are greatest will receive least, a phenomenon described by Tudor Hart (1971) as the Inverse Care Law. Instead, other factors come into play, such as, the specialist interests of individual physicians, the structure of financial incentives, and the ease of interacting with different groups of patients. Three types of needs assessment have been described: Epidemiological, comparative, and corporate (Stevens & Gabbay 1991). These are examined in detail in Chapter 12.2 (Needs assessment: A practical approach). Public health professionals play a central role in assessment of need, drawing on the skills they possess, especially where there is a major epidemiological perspective.

Intelligent purchasing

In an increasing number of countries intelligent purchasing is seen as an instrument to implement health policy objectives, including ensuring that health services closely reflect the health needs of the population that they serve (Øvretveit 1995). Purchasing acts as a co-ordinating mechanism that offers an alternative to a traditional command-and-control approach. Its essential characteristic is that it separates purchasers from providers but binds each party by means of contracts to explicit commitments, with creation of the economic motivation to fulfil these commitments.

Contracts have always been a feature of those healthcare systems based on social insurance systems, with complex institutional structures developed to represent health insurers and physicians in negotiations over payment schedules. Governments have often played some role in these discussions, typically to ensure cost containment and preservation of solidarity. However, both insurers and governments are increasingly using contracts as a means of reorienting the focus of health services, to ensure that they reflect health needs and provide cost-effective care.

In contrast, in most tax-based systems, relationships between health authorities and providers have traditionally been based on hierarchies. This is also changing as policy-makers seek new ways of influencing provider behaviour, based on a clearer identification of the objectives of the health system.

In systems where private insurance plays an important role, similar changes are taking place. Instead of simply reimbursing costs incurred retrospectively, insurers are introducing what is described as managed care, in which entitlements are defined in advance and treatment patterns are closely scrutinized.

From a public health perspective, interest in purchasing relates to whether or not it can achieve health gain and promote equity. Whether it does so will depend on both the objectives being pursued and on the quality of the contracting process. Contracts bring many potential benefits but also some risks.

For purchasing to promote health gain it must be based on an assessment of health needs coupled with a strong focus on the cost-effectiveness of clinical interventions and the organizational context within which they are delivered. Conversely, if it is based primarily on cost-saving, it will reduce health gain.

Purchasing can support equity if, through needs assessment, they take explicit account of vulnerable and disadvantaged groups as well as under-served communities. From this perspective, purchasers represent the interests of their populations, allocating resources and purchasing services in accordance with their needs. However, purchasing also carries the risk of undermining equity if providers are able to underemphasize or phase out services that are less profitable. Purchasing also offers a means for enhancing participation by the population in the organization of healthcare, thus increasing the accountability of governments and the medical profession and making health policy more relevant to the needs and priorities of society.

In some countries, especially where public health professionals have played a central role in the contracting process, it has been possible to use contracts to develop intersectoral responses to health problems or to reorient healthcare providers so that they integrate prevention with curative care. The opportunities for doing so are discussed in more detail below.

Implementation of an intelligent purchasing system is a complex process requiring a high level of skills and well-developed information systems (Figueras *et al.* 2005). At a minimum, information is required on patient flow, cost, and utilization information across specialties or diagnostic groups, and demographic and risk groups. It is important that expectations of what can be achieved are realistic. Medical care is extremely complex. Diagnostic labels are often imprecise and clouded by a degree of legitimate uncertainty. Decisions on clinical management incorporate values and beliefs relating to factors such as attitude to risk and the utility placed on different health states. Contracts must incorporate sufficient flexibility and reflect the views of all those concerned if they are to retain any credibility.

Purchasing also involves transaction costs to cover activities such as needs assessment, performance analysis, negotiating, and monitoring. A substantial increase in quality and efficiency is required to justify these additional costs. If transaction costs can be minimized without compromising the pursuit of the objectives of equity and health gain, intelligent purchasing can provide a formidable instrument to promote population health.

Efficient and effective service delivery

The increasing use of intelligent purchasing is focusing the attention of public health professionals on the delivery of healthcare. Evaluative research has highlighted the extent of use of treatments that are unsupported by evidence of effectiveness and the importance of appropriate organizational structures and cultures in the provision of high-quality care. This section examines three areas in which public health professionals can play an important role: The design of systems that ensure that patients are managed at the level of the healthcare system that is most appropriate, the creation of mechanisms that identify and promote high-quality clinical care, and the reorientation of curative services towards prevention.

Shifting interfaces

Health services are typically organized on different levels, reflecting the need to balance two competing objectives. On the one hand, dispersion permits easy access to those facilities in which most people receive care and where they can obtain an initial contact with the system. On the other hand, concentration of specialized resources required by relatively small numbers of patients optimizes scarce resources, with potential gains in effectiveness and efficiency, although the relationships are complex and often counterintuitive (Ferguson *et al.* 1997). Movement between the various levels (primary, secondary, tertiary, and community care) typically involves passage across an interface that is governed by rules of varying degrees of formality. Examples include referral to hospital by a primary care physician or discharge from an acute hospital to a long-stay facility.

The nature of these interfaces is steadily changing in the face of the new circumstances discussed above. Upward pressure on costs is causing policy-makers to ensure that patients are treated in the most cost-effective settings. Changing patterns of disease, coupled with evolving patient beliefs about the nature of healthcare, are challenging established ways of delivering care. New technologies in fields such as imaging, diagnosis, surgery, pharmaceuticals, and information are having a substantial impact on clinical practice. Healthcare professionals are developing new and different sets of skills.

These changes involve a process of substitution, by which there has been a continual regrouping of resources across care settings to exploit the best available solutions. This can take many forms. One typology differentiates three kinds of substitution: Moving the location of care, introducing new technologies, and shifting the mix of staff and skills (Warner 1996).

From a public health perspective, substitution brings the potential of both benefits and risks. Benefits include increased patient satisfaction, improved clinical outcomes, greater efficiency, and more appropriate management of certain diseases. Risks include fragmentation of services, loss of specialized skills, increased costs, and wasteful duplication of expensive technology. Each case must be assessed on its merits as initiatives that have seemed intuitively better than what they replaced have often, on detailed evaluation, failed to live up to the initial expectations.

Effective substitution policies require co-ordination, with clear strategic objectives. A system-wide perspective is necessary to identify unintended consequences for other services. Too often substitution involves simply changing the location, without an appropriate shift in skills and technology or without a reallocation of resources. However, substitution offers a valuable tool to public health professionals to make services more accessible and appropriate to the population and to ensure that care is provided as cost-effectively as possible.

Improving outcomes

As noted above, former deference to medical judgement about how to deliver healthcare is giving way, in the face of wide variations, to how care is delivered (Institute of Medicine 2001). The view expressed by the editor of *The Lancet* in 1951, that central guidance on clinical care should be rejected because of the harm that it would do to the sense of personal responsibility of the physician (Fox 1951), is no longer tenable.

Variations in clinical practice have many causes, the most important being clinical uncertainty about the most appropriate treatment in any given circumstance. Studies of treatment patterns reveal both over-treatment, where patients receive treatments that are ineffective, and under-treatment, where those who would benefit are denied effective treatment. This has led to four related questions. Firstly, which treatments can be expected to produce improved health outcomes? Secondly, does a treatment that has been shown to be efficacious in evaluative research achieve the intended objective in routine clinical practice? Thirdly, why are treatments of known effectiveness not used in circumstances where they would achieve health improvement? Finally, how does one change professional behaviour so as to ensure that the most effective, efficient, and humane treatments are provided? Together, these questions contribute to the quest for what is termed 'evidence-based healthcare'.

Four aspects of quality assurance are relevant. The first is that it should be based on evidence, typically organized as guidelines or protocols. While these should take full account of local circumstances, there are a number of international collaborations seeking to achieve economies of effort. Second, it is a continuous process, involving repeated cycles of setting standards, introducing change to meet those standards, and review of the results of change. The third is that it is necessary to differentiate three types of quality measures (Donabedian 1966). Measures of structure relate to inputs such as facilities and the availability of trained staff. Measures of process include adherence to agreed good practice. Measures of outcome assess the extent to which the objectives of treatment are achieved. A fourth relates to the question of whether quality assurance should be internal or external.

Quality assurance activities often deal with structures and processes of care rather than outcomes. Ideally, the focus would be on outcomes, but outcomes are typically more difficult to measure and may only become apparent long after the intervention took place. Some outcomes may also be rare and the sample size required to detect a deviation from what is expected may be very large. For example, Mant and Hicks (1995) showed, on the basis of knowledge of effective treatment for myocardial infarction, that, in a comparison of two typical hospitals, it would take 73 years of data to detect a significant 3 per cent reduction in mortality. In contrast, a significant difference in process measures, here uptake of treatments, would emerge after only 4 months. Where process or structure measures are used there should be evidence that they correlate with a good outcome. Measures based on structure can be of some value, based on the assumption that high-quality care cannot be provided in the absence of basic prerequisites, such as adequately trained staff, but this is a necessary rather than a sufficient measure and should normally be supplemented by measures of either process or outcome.

Internal and external forms of quality assurance have quite different characteristics. In the former, the activity is conducted by those undertaking the clinical activities concerned, such as the physicians in a hospital. They are responsible for setting standards and implementing change. This has the advantage of fostering a sense of ownership and is less open to opportunistic manipulation of results. However, it does require a culture in which it is accepted that clinical practice should be open to examination by one's peers. Professional bodies have often played a major role in promoting this approach.

External quality assurance involves a body outside the healthcare facility examining measures of quality. This typically focuses on structure, largely because this is so much easier to measure than process or outcome. A typical example is hospital accreditation. Accreditation is especially important for countries seeking to establish a mix of private and public health services, as it offers a means of reassurance that all facilities meet an agreed minimum level of quality. In some countries there is growing pressure to make public assessments of the performance of individual health professionals and facilities yet there is now considerable evidence that comparisons can be highly misleading (Jacobson *et al.* 2003) and that they can create strong incentives for perverse behaviour (Green & Wintfeld 1995). Such behaviour includes imaginative use of disease coding to increase the apparent severity of patients' conditions, refusal to operate on patients at high risk, and even frank distortion of data.

Perhaps the greatest challenge facing those seeking to improve the quality of healthcare is how to change clinical behaviour. An increasing volume of research on this topic is being brought together by the work of the Cochrane Collaboration on Effective Practice and Organization of Care. This has examined behavioural, financial, and organizational approaches to changing practice. It has shown how many traditional approaches, such as conferences and short educational events, are of little value. Educational outreach visits have a small effect, and financial and organizational initiatives, such as the introduction of co-payments, tend to reduce appropriate and inappropriate care to a similar extent. The most successful strategies involve combing a range of behavioural approaches, such as audit and feedback, production of guidelines, and, where appropriate, computer-generated reminders (Grimshaw *et al.* 2006). However, the main conclusion of this research is that change is very difficult and requires carefully targeted sustained action.

Public health professionals have played a key role in the development of evidence-based healthcare, although its elements, from research through dissemination to implementation, are in place in only a few countries and health policy discussion often remains focused on issues of financing and organization.

Health services as a setting for promoting health

Public health professionals have a particularly important role in promoting the reorientation of health services to address the broader determinants of health. Health services are important settings in which it is possible actively to promote health through primary preventive strategies. Health professionals have an important role as opinion formers, both in individual patient encounters and, among the wider public, as respected advocates for healthy public policies (Chapman & Lupton 1994). Conversely, contradictory images, such as physicians and nurses smoking while they advise their patients to quit, can do much to undermine public health messages.

Relatively simple approaches, such as brief interventions by health professionals, can often be very effective. Yet it is not sufficient to assume that such approaches are always going to be effective, and, as with treatment interventions, each must be assessed individually. For example, while advising patients to take more exercise or eat more nutritious food may seem intuitively beneficial, there is little evidence that it is effective. There is no evidence that attempts to reduce the risk of coronary heart disease through multiple risk factor interventions have an impact on either total or coronary heart disease mortality (Ebrahim & Smith 1997), and fiscal and legislative measures seem more appropriate.

Many people come into contact with healthcare facilities, either as patients or staff. This provides an important opportunity to demonstrate support for health-promoting policies by means of an ethos based on healthy lifestyles. Most obviously, it is no longer acceptable for healthcare facilities to permit smoking on their premises (McKee *et al.* 2003). Ideally, smokers should be seen several weeks before admission and supported with advice and nicotine replacement therapy (Moller *et al.* 2002). In contrast, failure to ban smoking provides an implicit message that health promotion is simply not taken seriously and the obvious conflict between the culture of the organization and the advice given to patients will make behavioural change more difficult.

There is, however, much more that can be done to create a healthy environment. For example, patients and staff should be able to choose healthy diets. The provision of cycle parks, gyms, and showers will encourage staff to cycle to work. Many of these ideas have been brought together in the WHO's Health-Promoting Hospitals project, which seeks to increase participation in health-promoting activities by patients, staff, and others outside the hospital, as well as improving communication and reorienting hospitals towards health promotion.

Finally, the contribution that health services can make to health by employing people should not be ignored. The adverse health effects of unemployment are well recognized (Bartley 1994), in particular the impact of job insecurity and anticipation of unemployment (Ferrie *et al.* 1995). Health services have always been labour intensive. Healthcare reforms in many countries have led to substantial reductions in staff numbers, either through redundancy or, in some countries, transfers to private sector agencies where levels of pay and conditions of service are substantially worse. While reducing the direct costs to the health service, such policies often increase overall government expenditure through increased social costs. However, some governments are recognizing the role of health services as a source of employment, as illustrated by the use of the European Union's structural funds to support investment in healthcare infrastructure.

The contribution of public health to health services

This chapter began by showing how healthcare can no longer be regarded as peripheral to attempts to improve the health of populations. Notwithstanding the importance of tackling the wider determinants of health, modern medical care offers new opportunities to reduce mortality and improve quality of life. Healthcare is also taking on a greater importance as evidence emerges of how differential access can increase health inequalities.

Health services are changing, bringing new opportunities for public health to increase its impact on this process by reorienting health services towards the maximization of health gain. However, if public health professionals are to take full advantage of these new opportunities, they will need to have a thorough understanding of the pressures that are driving the health services change.

This chapter has highlighted the contributions that they can make to the response to the changing demands on healthcare systems. These various strategies can be summarized through a conceptual shorthand suggested by Saltman and Figueras (1998). This approach compresses activities into two traditional economic parameters: Policy interventions instituted on the demand side as against those instituted on the supply side of the healthcare system.

The demand side incorporates all strategies that influence funding of the healthcare system and more specifically the relationships between the consumer and the third-party payers. A number of health system strategies have concentrated on the demand side by introducing measures shifting costs to the patient, such as cost-sharing arrangements or limiting the public package of care, and by introducing market competition incentives among third-party insurers. Many of these have led to inequities. The role of public health here is twofold: First to ensure that solidarity in the health system is not harmed by these measures which tend to reduce access and coverage particularly for the most vulnerable groups in our society, and second to shift the policy-makers' agenda from these individual patient-based demand policies towards strategies dealing with aggregate population-based demand. Indeed, the latter is very much at the core of a public health role.

The introduction of effective health promotion and primary prevention strategies will ultimately reduce the total demand for healthcare services and healthcare costs. However, health promotion has not played a central role in the health reform agenda. Public health professionals need to strive to develop more and better ways to evaluate health promotion that satisfies the needs of policy-makers, managers and clinicians so the full potential of health promotion can be realized.

The supply side includes strategies forming a continuum that moves from the allocation of health resources to the delivery of health services. Some of the key strategies include the introduction of quality-oriented strategies, and the integration and substitution of services across the hospital and primary healthcare sectors. In many instances, these reforms have met with considerable success (Saltman & Figueras 1998), but the extent of their success will depend on the availability of a series of skills traditionally linked to the public health profession. These include assessing the health needs of the population, evaluating and monitoring interventions, assessing health outcomes, and reorienting healthcare delivery so that the focus is on prevention as well as cure.

Health services can make an important contribution to improving the health status of populations. This chapter has identified mechanisms through which public health can have a major role in maximizing the health gain obtained from health services, but much will depend on the ability of the public health profession to adapt and bring its portfolio of tools and skills to bear on rapidly changing health services.

Key points

- Modern healthcare has the potential to make a substantial contribution to population health and has been doing so in high-income countries for at least four decades.
- While much healthcare that is provided is effective in improving health, some is ineffective or even harmful.
- Healthcare systems must continually adapt to changing circumstances, including the economic situation, the burden of disease and scope for intervention, and public expectations.
- Expenditure on improved health should be seen not as a drain on the economy but as an investment in future growth.
- Public health professionals have a critical role to play in maximizing the health gain achieved by healthcare.

References

Abel-Smith, B., Figueras, J., Holland, W. *et al.* (1995). *Choices in health policy: An agenda for the European Union* Aldershot, Dartmouth Press/ Office for Official Publications of the European Communities.

Alderson, P., F. Bunn, C. Lefebvre. *et al.* (2004). Human albumin solution for resuscitation and volume expansion in critically ill patients. *Cochrane Database Syst Rev* (4): CD001208.

Andreev, E.M., E. Nolte, V.M. Shkolnikov. *et al.* (2003). The evolving pattern of avoidable mortality in Russia. *Int J Epidemiol* **32**, 437–46.

Arblaster, L., M. Lambert, V. Entwistle. *et al.* (1996). A systematic review of the effectiveness of health service interventions aimed at reducing inequalities in health. *J Health Serv Res Policy* **1**, 93–103.

Bartley, M. (1994). Unemployment and ill health: understanding the relationship. *J Epidemiol Community Health* **48**, 333–7.

Beaglehole, R. (1986). Medical management and the decline in mortality from coronary heart disease. *Br Med J (Clin Res Ed)* **292**, 33–5.

Beeson, P.B. (1980). Changes in medical therapy during the past half century. *Medicine* **59**, 79–99.

Benson, J.K. (1975). The interorganisational network as a political economy. *Administrative Science Quarterly* **20**, 229–49.

Billings, J., G.M. Anderson and L.S. Newman (1996). Recent findings on preventable hospitalizations. *Health Aff* **15**, 239–49.

Bodenheimer, T., E.H. Wagner and K. Grumbach (2002). Improving primary care for patients with chronic illness. *JAMA* **288**, 1775–9.

Bonneux, L., C.W. Looman, J. J. Barendregt. *et al.* (1997). Regression analysis of recent changes in cardiovascular morbidity and mortality in the Netherlands. *BMJ* **314**, 789–92.

Chalmers, I. and D.G. Altman (1995). *Systematic reviews*. London, BM Publications.

Chapman, S. and D. Lupton (1994). *The fight for public Health*. London, BMJ Publications.

Chappell, N.L. (1993). The future of health care in Canada. *Journal of Social Policy* **22**, 495.

Chinitz, D., Preker A., and Wasem J. (1998). Balancing competition and solidarity in health care financing. *Critical challenges for health care reform*. R.B. Saltman, J. Figueras and C. Sakellarides. Buckingham, Open University Press: xvi, p. 424.

Clark, D.G. (1998). Autonomy, personal empowerment and quality of life in long-term care. *Journal of Applied Gerontology* **7**, 279–97.

Cochrane, A.L., A.S. St Leger and F. Moore (1978). Health service 'input' and mortality 'output' in developed countries. *Journal of Epidemiology and Community Health* **32**, 200–5.

Contandriopoulos, A.P., M. Lauristin and E. Leibovich (1998). Values, norms and the reform of health care systems. *Critical challenges for health care reform*. R. B. Saltman, J. Figueras and C. Sakellarides. Buckingham, Open University Press: 339–62.

Donabedian, A. (1966). Evaluating the quality of medical care. *Milbank Mem Fund Q* **44**(3), Suppl,166–206.

Dunning, A. (1992). Choices in health care: a report by the Government Committee on Choices in health care. Rijkswijk, the Netherlands, Ministry of Welfare, Health and Culture.

Ebrahim, S. and G.D. Smith (1997). Systematic review of randomised controlled trials of multiple risk factor interventions for preventing coronary heart disease. *BMJ* **314**(7095), 1666–74.

Ferguson, B., T. Sheldon, and J. Posnett (1997). *Concentration and choice in health care*. Glasgow, Royal Society of Medicine Press.

Ferrie, J.E., M.J. Shipley, M.G. Marmot. *et al.* (1995). Health effects of anticipation of job change and non-employment: longitudinal data from the Whitehall II study. *Bmj* **311**(7015), 1264–9.

Figueras, J., R. Robinson, and E. Jakubowski (2005). *Purchasing to Improve Health Systems Performance*. European Observatory Series. Maidenhead. Open University Press. McGraw Hill Education.

Fogel, R.W. (1994). Economic Growth, Population Theory, and Physiology: the bearing of long-term process on the making of economic policy. *American Economic Review* **84(3)**, 369–395.

Fox, T.E. (1951). Professional freedom. *Lancet* **2**(3), 115–9.

Fries, J.F. (2003). Measuring and monitoring success in compressing morbidity. *Ann Intern Med* **139**(5 Pt 2), 455–9.

Gillett, G. (1995). Virtue and truth in clinical science. *J Med Philos* **20**(3), 285–98.

Green, J. and N. Wintfeld (1995). Report cards on cardiac surgeons. Assessing New York State's approach. *New England Journal of Medicine* **332**, 1229–32.

Grimshaw, J., M. Eccles, R. Thomas. *et al.* (2006). Toward evidence-based quality improvement. Evidence (and its limitations) of the effectiveness of guideline dissemination and implementation strategies 1966-1998. *J Gen Intern Med* **21 Suppl 2**, S14–20.

Habermas, J. (1987). *Theorie de l'agir communicationnel*. Paris, Fayard.

Ham, C. (1993). *Priority setting in the NHS: reports from six districts. Rationing the action*. London, BMJ Publications.

Healy, J. and M. McKee (2004). *Accessing healthcare: responding to diversity*. Oxford, Oxford University Press.

Hopkins, S. (2006). Economic stability and health status: evidence from East Asia before and after the 1990s economic crisis. *Health Policy* **75**(3), 347–57.

Illich, I. (1976). *Limits to medicine: medical nemesis, the expropriation of health*. London, Boyars.

Institute of Medicine (2000). *To err is human: building a safer health system*. Washington, D.C., Institute of Medicine.

Institute of Medicine (2001). *Crossing the quality chasm: a new health system for the 21st century*. Washington DC, Institute of Medicine.

Jacobson, B., J. Mindell and M. McKee (2003). Hospital mortality league tables. *British Medical Journal* **326**, 777–8.

Kunitz, S.J. and I. Pesis-Katz (2005). Mortality of white Americans, African Americans, and Canadians: the causes and consequences for health of welfare state institutions and policies. *Milbank Q* **83**(1), 5–39.

Lalonde, M. (1974). *A new perspective on the health of Canadians: a working document*. Ottawa, Department of Health and Welfare.

Lavis, J. and G.L. Stoddart (1994). Can we have too much health care? *Daedalus* **123**, 43–60.

Lubitz, J., J. Beebe, and C. Baker (1995). Longevity and medical care expenditures. *New England Journal of Medicine* **332**, 999–1003.

Mackenbach, J.P, C.W.M. Looman, A.E. Kunst. *et al.* (1988). Post-1950 mortality trends and medical care: gains in life expectancy due to declines in mortality from conditions amenable to medical interventions in the Netherlands. *Soc Sci Med*; 27, 889–94.

Mant, J. and N. Hicks (1995). Detecting differences in quality of care: the sensitivity of measures of process and outcome in treating acute myocardial infarction. *BMJ* **311**(7008), 793–6.

Marshall, S.W., I. Kawachi, N. Pearce. *et al.* (1993). Social class differences in mortality from diseases amenable to medical intervention in New Zealand. *Int J Epidemiol* **22**(2), 255–61.

Mathers, C.D. and D. Loncar (2006). Projections of global mortality and burden of disease from 2002 to 2030. *PLoS Med* **3**(11), e442.

McGrail, K., B. Green, M.L. Barer. *et al.* (2000). Age, costs of acute and long-term care and proximity to death: evidence for 1987-88 and 1994-95 in British Columbia. *Age Ageing* **29**(3), 249–53.

McKee, M. (2002). Values, beliefs and implications. *Health targets in Europe*. M. Marinker. London, BMJ Books: 181–205.

McKee, M. (2007). Cochrane on Communism: the influence of ideology on the search for evidence. *Int J Epidemiol* **36**(2):269–73.

McKee, M. and J. Figueras (1996). Setting priorities - can Britain learn from Sweden? *BMJ* **312**, 691–4.

McKee, M., A. Gilmore and T. Novotny (2003). Smoke-free hospitals. *BMJ* **326**, 941–2.

McKee, M. and E. Nolte (2004). Responding to the challenge of chronic diseases: ideas from Europe. *Clin Med* **4**(4), 336–42.

McKeown, T. (1979). *The role of medicine: drama, mirage or nemesis?* Oxford, Blackwell.

McPherson, K. (1989). International comparisons in medical care practices. *Health Care Financing Review* **Annual supplement**, 9–20.

Meerding, W. J., L. Bonneux, J. J. Polder. *et al.* (1998). Demographic and epidemiological determinants of healthcare costs in Netherlands: cost of illness study. *Bmj* **317**(7151), 111–5.

Moller, A. M., N. Villebro, T. Pedersen. *et al.* (2002). Effect of preoperative smoking intervention on postoperative complications: a randomised clinical trial. *Lancet* **359**(9301), 114–7.

Morris, A. M., Y. Wei, N. J. Birkmeyer and J. D. Birkmeyer (2006). Racial disparities in late survival after rectal cancer surgery. *J Am Coll Surg* **203**(6), 787–94.

Mossialos, E. and J. Le Grand (1999). Cost containment in the EU: An overview. *Health care and cost containment in the European Union*. E. Mossialos and J. Le Grand. Aldershot, Ashgate: 1–154.

Mossialos, E., M.F. Mrazek, and T. Walley (2004). *Regulating pharmaceuticals in Europe: striving for efficiency, equity and quality*. Maidenhead, Open University Press.

Nolte, E. and M. McKee (2004). *Does healthcare save lives? Avoidable mortality revisited*. London, The Nuffield Trust.

Nolte, E., V. Shkolnikov, R. Scholz. *et al.* (2004). Progress in health care, progress in health? Patterns of amenable mortality in central and eastern Europe before and after political transition. *Demographic Research* **Special Collection 2**, 139–162.

Oregon Health Services Commission (1991). Prioritization of health services. Salem, Or, Oregon Health Commission.

Øvretveit, J. (1995). *Purchasing for health: a multidisciplinary introduction to the theory and practice of health purchasing*. Buckingham, Open University Press.

Parkin, D., A. McGuire, and B. Yule (1987). Aggregate health care expenditures and national income. Is health care a luxury good? *J Health Econ* **6**(2), 109–27.

Rutstein, D. D., W. Berenberg, and T. C. Chalmers (1976). Measuring the quality of medical care: a clinical method. *New England Journal of Medicine* **294**, 582–8.

Saltman, R. B. and J. Figueras (1998). Analyzing the evidence on European health care reforms. *Health Aff (Millwood)* **17**(2), 85–108.

Shkolnikov, V., M. McKee, and D. A. Leon (2001). Changes in life expectancy in Russia in the 1990s. *Lancet* **357**, 917–21.

Stephens, C., G. Leonardi, S. Lewin. *et al.* (1999). The multilateral agreement on investment. Public health threat for the twenty-first century? *European Journal of Public Health* **9**(3–5).

Stevens, A. and J. Gabbay (1991). Needs assessment needs assessment. *Health Trends* **23**(1), 20–3.

Suhrcke, M., M. McKee, R. S. Arce. *et al.* (2006). Investment in health could be good for Europe's economies. *BMJ* **333**(7576), 1017–9.

Telishevka, M., L. Chenett and M. McKee (2001). Towards an understanding of the high death rate among young people with diabetes in Ukraine. *Diabet Med* **18**(1), 3–9.

Tsai, A. C., S. C. Morton, C. M. Mangione. *et al.* (2005). A meta-analysis of interventions to improve care for chronic illnesses. *Am J Manag Care* **11**(8), 478–88.

Tudor Hart, J. (1971). The inverse care law. *Lancet* **1**(7696), 405–12.

Wagner, E. H., C. Davis, J. Schaefer. *et al.* (1999). A survey of leading chronic disease management programs: are they consistent with the literature? *Manag Care Q* **7**(3), 56–66.

Wanless, D. (2001). Securing our future: taking a long-term view. An interim report, London, HM Treasury.

Warner, M. (1996). *Implementing health care reforms through substitution*. Cardiff, Welsh Institute for Health and Social Care.

Whitehead, M. (1988). *The health divide*. Harmondsworth, Penguin.

Whitty, P. and I. Jones (1992). Public health heresy: a challenge to the purchasing orthodoxy. *BMJ* **304**(6833), 1039–41.

World Health Organization (1986). *Ottawa Charter for Health Promotion: First International Conference on Health Promotion. WHO/HPR/HEP/95.1*. Geneva, World Health Organization.

World Health Organization (2000). *Health systems: improving performance*. Geneva, W.H.O.

World Health Organization and Commission on Macroeconomics and Health (2001). *Macroeconomics and health: investing in health for economic development*. Geneva, World Health Organization.

12.11

Public health workers

Suwit Wibulpolprasert and Piya Hanvoravongchai

Go to the people.
Live among them. Learn from them.
Plan with them. Work with them.
Start with what they know. Build on what they have.
Teach by showing. Learn by doing.
Not a showcase, but a pattern.
Not odds and ends, but a system.
Not piecemeal, but integrated approach.
Not to conform, but to transform.
Not relief, but release.

Dr Y.C. James Yen

The Constitution of the World Health Organization (WHO) defines 'health' as: 'A state of complete physical, mental, social well-being, and not merely the absence of diseases and infirmity'. This broad perspective of health underscores its multi-factorial nature. Health improvement depends much on the educational status (particularly of women), and other socioeconomic development, as well as on the development of healthcare systems (Roemer 1991; World Health Organization 1999) (Fig. 12.11.1).

'Health workers', as defined in the World Health Report (2006), includes 'all people engaged in actions whose primary intent is to enhance health'. According to the Joint Learning Initiative (2004) and the WHO (2006), health workers are a crucial component of the health sector because they manage all other financial and non-financial resources. Workers are also the key to improve performance of the health system in regards to quality, efficiency and accessibility of health services.

Moreover, spending on health workers accounts for a large share of public health spending in most countries (Joint Learning Initiative 2004). On an average, a country spends over 40 per cent of its public health budget on its health workforce (World Health Organization 2006). Many developing countries spend more than half of their public health funding on salaries and remuneration. For example, Ecuador in 1995 and the Dominican Republic in 1996 spent 72 per cent and 67 per cent, respectively, of their Ministries of Health's budget on health workforce salaries (Berman *et al.* 1999).

History has proved that health workers, especially public health workers, are essential for effective disease control programmes and increases in child survival (Beaglehole & Dal Poz 2003; Joint Learning Initiative 2004). Therefore, the current weakness of health workforce systems in many countries are major obstacles to the provision of necessary health services in order to achieve national health targets and internationally agreed upon health-related development goals (Chen *et al.* 2004; Haines & Cassels 2004; Kober & Van Damme 2004; Travis *et al.* 2004; World Health Organization 2006). In addition, many global health initiatives, such as the Global Fund to fight AIDS, tuberculosis, and malaria, and the Global Alliance on Vaccine and Immunization, are vertical programmes that have put tremendous pressure on the already weak health workforce and diverted limited resources from other important public health problems.

This chapter focuses on an important group of health workers, the public health workforce. They are at the core of the health system in delivering public health interventions to achieve health goals. This chapter is divided into four sections: (1) background on public health workers, including the definition, their roles and functions, and their importance to public health; (2) key management principles necessary for an effective, efficient, and equitable public health workforce system; (3) a specific case of frontline public health workers, namely, community health workers (CHWs); and (4) definition, history, and functions of CHWs, as well as the keys to successful and efficient management of this group. It concludes by addressing key challenges to public health workforce development.

Who are the public health workers and what are their roles?

Defining public health workers

The term 'public health worker' has been used in at least three different ways: (1) the *sector* in which a person works (public sector); (2) their *functions*, referring to all workers whose goal is to improve public health, but does not distinguish whether the workers are employed by public, private, or non-government agencies; and (3) the work *setting* where the workers are employed. In this case, all workers in the agencies that work primarily for public health would be defined as public health workers.

Sometimes 'public health workers' is limited to a group of workers based on their *credentials*. This would include all workers with a degree in public health. However, the term 'public health professional' is more frequently used. For example, the US Institute of

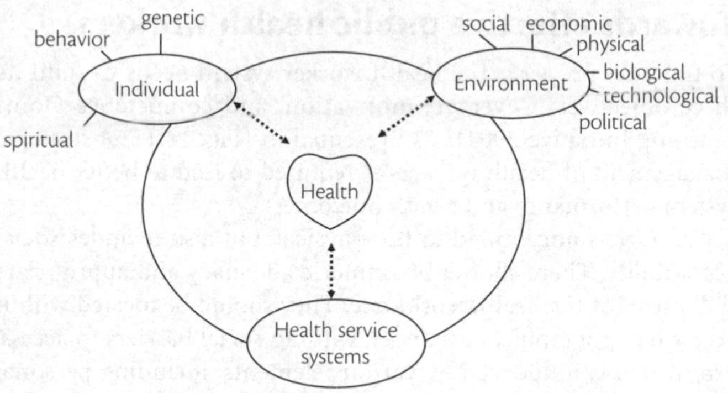

Fig. 12.11.1 Multifactorial relationship of health and its determinants.
Source: Wibulpolprasert (2006).

Medicine defines a public health professional as 'one educated in public health or related discipline who is employed to improve health through a population focus' (Gebbie *et al.* 2003).

The most commonly used operational definition of various agencies and among scholars is the one based on their functions; i.e. those whose work is primarily for public health (Box 12.11.1).

Public health workers' functions

Through broad definition, the public health workforce is a diverse and complex group of workers. Their education can range from primary level to graduate degrees. They could be from the professional sector, the popular sector, or the folk sector. Their occupational backgrounds could be as wide-ranging as farmers, teachers, social scientists and health professionals such as physicians, nurses, and laboratory technicians. What characterizes them as public health workers are their primary functions in public health (Box 12.11.2).

Another way to understand the scope of public health workers' functions is to look at the classification of public health workers. Based on the types and areas of work, public health workers can be classified into various categories (US Bureau of Labor Statistics 2007). A sample list includes the following:

- Health educators
- Community health workers, public health and community social workers
- Occupational safety technicians/technologists
- Environmental engineers/technicians/technologists/scientists/specialists
- Health services managers/administrators
- Public health policy analysts, health planners
- Public health administrative or clerical staff
- Health information systems specialists
- Biostatisticians/health economists/public health researchers
- Epidemiologists
- Public health physicians/nurses/dentists/dental workers/veterinarians/nutritionists
- Mental health and substance abuse social workers/counsellors

Box 12.11.1 Defining public health workers based on their functions

'A public health worker is one for whom a significant portion of work content advances or contributes to accomplishing one or more of the ten essential public health services identified by the Public Health System Performance Standards' (Tilson and Gebbie 2004).

'Public health workers are defined as all those responsible for providing the essential services of public health regardless of the organization in which they work' (US Department of Health and the US Department of Health and Human Services 1994; cited in Gebbie *et al.* 2002).

Box 12.11.2 US public health workers' functions

- Monitor health status to identify community health problems
- Diagnose and investigate health problems and health hazards in the community
- Inform, educate, and empower people about public health issues
- Mobilize community partnerships to identify and solve health issues
- Develop policies and plans that support individual and community health efforts
- Enforce laws and regulations that protect health and ensure safety
- Link people to needed personal health services and ensure the provision of health care when otherwise unavailable
- Ensure a competent public health and personal health care workforce
- Evaluate effectiveness, accessibility and quality of personal and population-based health services
- Conduct research for new insights and innovative solutions to health problems

Source: US Department of Health and Human Services (1994).

Roles of public health workers

Public health workers contribute to the improvement of population health worldwide. Smallpox eradication is an example that would not have been successful without active contributions by public health workers (Joint Learning Initiative 2004). When properly trained and provided with appropriate incentives and resources, non-professional public health workers and community health workers are capable of effectively delivering health interventions to reduce child mortality in developing countries (Bryce *et al.* 2003; Haines *et al.* 2007). For ongoing health efforts such as the eradication of polio or prevention and control of the burden of non-communicable diseases, public health workers have a major contributory role in their success.

The effectiveness of improving the population's health in Shasta Shabikas by community workers in Bangladesh, the Lady Health Workers in Pakistan, and the Brazilian Community Health Agents, is well documented (Joint Learning Initiative 2004). In Africa, community health workers from Gambia, South Africa, Tanzania, Zambia, Madagascar, and Ghana cost-effectively improved health programme performance at the community level (Gericke *et al.* 2003; Lehmann *et al.* 2004).

In addition, frontline workers such as community health workers and village health staff improved coverage and increased health equity. They are generally better distributed geographically (Berman *et al.* 1987; Chapman *et al.* 2005). They are also more accessible and acceptable to communities, resulting in an increase in health service utilization, especially among poorer households (Berman 1984). Extending services through community health workers is seen as a way to reduce inequity in child health (Victora *et al.* 2003; Masanja *et al.* 2005).

Public health workers can also contribute to strategic policy development, planning and regulation, and organization, delivery and evaluation of health.

Enumerating public health workers

Despite the importance of public health workers, information about numbers and dynamics of public health workers is very limited. The problem of limited data availability occurs in both poor and rich countries (Cioffi *et al.* 2004; World Health Organization 2006). Additionally, quantification of public health workers is not an easy task, given the diversity in occupational backgrounds, education and experience, as well as functions.

The World Health Report of 2006 provides the latest counts of the health workforce in member countries estimated from available surveys, censuses and other national statistics (World Health Organization 2006). The actual numbers of public health workers are estimated to be much higher than those reported, because they do not include public health workers from countries with no data and they are limited only to some cadres. In addition, some public health workers may have reported their occupations in different categories that were not captured as public health workers in the surveys or censuses. The information provided is mostly for key health professionals such as nurses, physicians, pharmacists and dentists. Data on the numbers of environmental and public health professionals are available for 70 countries, totalling 655 415 professionals. Similarly, data on numbers of community health workers are available in only 40 countries, totalling 563 348 community workers worldwide. This figure is definitely an underestimate, as village health volunteers in a country such as Thailand totalled more than 800 000 in 2007.

Even in a wealthy country such as the United States, information is limited, and mostly restricted to public health professionals. The latest information on US public health professionals employed to deliver public health services in the country, estimated from employer and employee surveys, is approximately 500 000 persons (US Health Resources and Services Administration 2000). It has been found that nurses are the largest professional group in public health (Gebbie *et al.* 2002). However, this figure does not include approximately 2.8 million volunteers who are engaged in unspecific public health activities (Gebbie & Merrill 2001). The total number of public health workers in the United States could therefore be over three million, or more than one per 100 population.

Towards effective public health workers

To function properly, the health worker system needs to fulfil its three objectives: Coverage, motivation, and competence (Joint Learning Initiative 2004). As presented in (Fig. 12.11.2) strategic management of health workers is required to lead to better health system performance and health outcomes.

Coverage is not limited to the physical, but also includes social accessibility. There should be numeric adequacy and appropriate skill mixes of the health workforce. They should be located within accessible geographical distances, with no social barriers to access. *Motivation* is influenced by various elements, including personal beliefs, financial and non-financial incentives, support provided by the system, and work environment. *Competency* is the result of education, training, and experience that can be fostered prior to their recruitment, as well as while they are in service in the field (Kennedy & Moore 2001; Joint Learning Initiative 2004; World Health Organization 2006). To achieve these three workforce objectives, the system requires active strategic management and health workforce development and concerted action.

Public health worker education and training

Health worker education and training is aimed at ensuring numeric adequacy of a well-qualified and appropriate mix of staff. A set of knowledge and skills that are recommended for public health workers is proposed, and transformed into the appropriate mode of recruitment, education and training. Appropriate policy interventions to empower and guide public health education and training are needed.

Public health worker competency

Competency of public health workers includes adequate *knowledge* and *skills* that are necessary for their functions.

Knowledge: Afifi and Breslow (1994) proposed that public health knowledge essential to public health functions is comprised of five major disciplines: Epidemiology, biostatistics, behavioural and social sciences, environmental health, and health services management. Recent advancement in science and technology means that additional knowledge in areas such as informatics and genomics would be beneficial to their work (Tilson & Gebbie 2004).

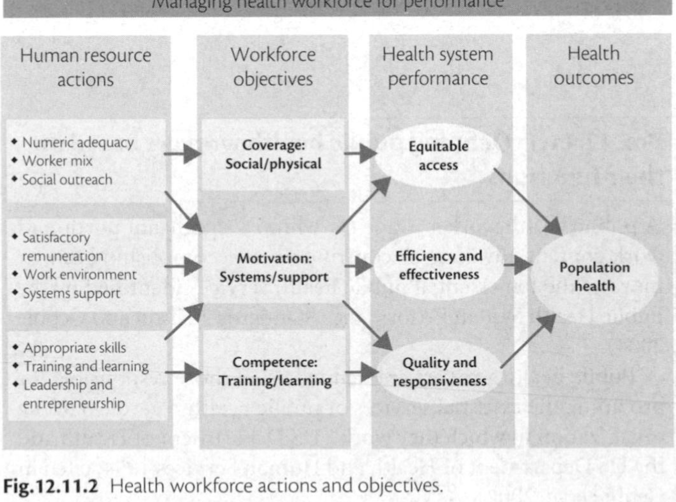

Fig.12.11.2 Health workforce actions and objectives.
Source: Joint Learning Initiative (2004).

Similarly, the increasing importance of social determinants of health requires that public health workers be knowledgeable in the areas of law and public policy. Global health is also an emerging area, with threats from emerging diseases.

Skills: A core set of public health workers' skills should encompass eight domains: (1) critical analysis and assessment; (2) policy development and programme planning; (3) communication; (4) cultural competency; (5) community dimensions of practice; (6) basic public health science; (7) financial planning and management; and (8) leadership and systems (Tilson & Gebbie 2004). For each of these eight domains, the level of proficiency required for frontline staff, senior level staff, and supervisory and management staff could vary from being aware, being knowledgeable and being proficient in that skill.

In addition to the core skill set, additional skills are required for each public health worker that differ by his/her function and responsibility. Moreover, each public health worker should have general work skills such as computer literacy, presentation skills and writing skills. These skill sets can be grouped or classified in several ways. An example is the competencies framework for public health workers as proposed by the US Center for Disease Control (Box 12.11.3).

Education for public health workers

Public health education can be carried out through various mechanisms and at different phases. The training could occur before recruitment (pre-service training) or after workers are already working (in-service training). It could be through formal public health degree programmes or through specific training courses for specific tasks.

Schools of public health

Schools of public health are a product of the twentieth century. Before having public health schools, most professional public health training occurred in medical schools through a department of preventive or community medicine. The emergence of schools of public health in many countries is the result of the demand for workforce training to support public health campaigns (World Health Organization 2006). In the United States, establishment of schools of public health was a result of a conference in 1914 that designed the educational system for the public health profession and was presented in the Welch-Rose Report on Schools of Public Health by the Rockefeller Foundation in 1915 (Fineberg *et al.* 1994). The number of public health schools then increased significantly thereafter. It is claimed that in the United States, 'the emergence of schools of public health was a major factor in the development of public health' (Gordon & McFarlane 1996).

The WHO estimated that there are 375 schools of public health globally (World Health Organization 2006). However, more than half of them are located in the Americas and Europe. In South Asia, with a major share of the global population and the burden of disease, there are less than 10 schools of public health. More than half of the countries in Africa also have no graduate training programme in public health (Joint Learning Initiative 2004).

Schools of public health are not the only source of training for professional public health practitioners. There are many public health programmes outside schools of public health (Gordon & McFarlane 1996; Tulchinsky & Bickford 2006). These programmes are offered in other health professional schools, such as medical and nursing schools, as well as by users, such as the health ministries.

Other modes of public health training

Since most schools of public health are usually under the control of education ministries or independent universities, their isolation from ministries of health and health providers is a major concern as a weakness of the system. Public health education through an institution-based model may be far from actual field experience, and the knowledge learned may be irrelevant to real-world practices and health problems in the community (Beaglehole & Dal Poz 2003). Additionally, the students or trainees may lack public health skills that could have been gained from public health programme implementation and practices.

One innovative project to address the weakness described above is by the Rockefeller Foundation, which initiated the Public Health Schools Without Walls Initiative in many developing countries (Beaglehole & Dal Poz 2003). It uses a broad-based, integrative and adaptive model, with focus on community-based services and practical health problems. The curricula incorporate a large proportion of field training, with close collaboration with the ministry of health. Students gain competence in key areas through actual work in the field, such as health problem investigation, health programme management and workplace communications.

Distance education in public health

Another mode of public health education that is increasingly popular is the use of distance education. Distance education occurs when teachers and the students are distant from each other (Keegan 1996; Knebel 2001). Distance could refer to geographical distance or time difference or both. The instructors use various form of media, such as printed materials, electronic devices, and audio and video to deliver pedagogical messages to the students.

The advantages of distance education for public health training are numerous. First, it expands the access of health education programmes to the prospective students who are unable to physically attend classes at schools or colleges. Second, most distance learning programmes allow for flexibility of times so it is more convenient for many, especially those who have full-time jobs. Third, good distance learning programmes for health workers can benefit from a closer link between training and actual field experiences for the students.

Box 12.11.3 US CDC key competency sets for public health workers

- Core: Basic public health skills (skills needed to perform the essential functions of public health)
- Function-specific: For example, leadership, management, supervisory, and support staff
- Discipline-specific: For example, community dentistry for public health dentists, other professionals or technical specialists
- Subject-specific (within a discipline): Maternal and child health, sexually transmitted diseases, vaccine preventable diseases, cancer, other chronic diseases
- Workplace basics: Required of all personnel, including literacy, writing, and presentation skills, and computer literacy

Source: Appendix E: Competencies for Public Health Workers: A Collection of Competency Sets for Public Health-Related Occupations and Professions (Institute of Medicine 2002).

Fourth, distance education programmes are generally less expensive for students, with savings on travel expenses and infrastructure (such as buildings). The cost to the educators also decreases with the number of students, as instructional media development costs are fixed. Availability of distance education is also compatible with the concept of life-long learning that is recommended for all public health workers.

The distance education approach also has its limitations. It is based on limited personal contact, with no active face-to-face interactions, so communication errors can occur. These could be complicated by cultural differences between the instructors and students in the case of cross-regional or cross-country programmes. The lack of personal interaction also means that the style of teaching will be more formal, which could be less stimulating to some students. Also, for distance education, teachers need to play additional roles as facilitators, coaches, and mentors. Their workload is generally greater than in traditional modes of education. More importantly, this method generally has lower graduation rates, as the programme relies heavily on the responsibility and motivation of the students.

Nevertheless, distance education is continually gaining in popularity in the public health sector. Since the first distance education programme in health in the 1960s, many public health training programmes have been offered through distance learning (Knebel 2001). In both developed and developing countries, distance education has been used for pre- and in-service education, for degree programmes, and for short courses. Several public health schools are now offering masters of public health programmes through distance education.

Numerous studies have shown that distance education programmes in health are equally effective as traditional training programmes, with lower costs and greater satisfaction of the students (Knebel 2001). However, pre-service training by distance education may be less attractive to some because of the lack of peer interaction and the lower prestige compared to traditional university education.

Policies on education of public health workers

There are several health workforce education policies that can be used to influence the performance of the health workforce system:

- First, there should be an adequate link between the public health education system and the healthcare system.
- Second, the policy on public health education, especially the number of trainees and their required mix of skills, should consider the current and future demand for the health workforce in the country.
- Third, public health education policy could contribute to improving equity in health service provision in several ways. The geographical location of training institutions could affect the practice location of the workforce once they are trained. Additionally, the recruitment policy based on the socioeconomic and geographical backgrounds of the students may also influence the population they will serve.
- Fourth, financing policy for public health education as well as its social ties after graduation may be effective tools to ensure better distribution and fairness of financial burden.
- Fifth, public health education should be expanded to other health and public policy professions. Professors and medical specialists, as well as other non-public-health persons, can serve as very strong advocates for public health if they are sensitized to it. Thus, building a 'public health mind' for non-public health individuals may be as important as training public health workers.

System for effective management of public health workers

A study in the United States shows that competency comprises about 2–20 per cent of service performance (Mayer 2003), which suggests that larger roles may be played by other factors, including individual, organizational and social influences. This section describes key factors of health workforce and health system management that can influence the effectiveness and performance of the health workforce. They are remuneration and financial incentives, non-financial incentives and system support, policy and regulation, and monitoring and evaluation.

Remuneration and financial incentives

Satisfactory remuneration is considered an important factor to promote workplace motivation. However, in some developing countries, the level of payment for public health workers is based on the civil service system, and is very low and may not be enough for living expenses. Inadequate or late payments may lead public health workers to pursue informal or unwanted economic activities that contribute to inefficiency and lower health service accessibility.

There are several forms of dubious coping strategies that public health workers have been known to use in such cases (McPake *et al.* 1999; Van Lerberghe *et al.* 2002; Muula & Maseko 2006). These include requesting informal payments or under-the-counter fees for services that are meant to be free, misusing or stealing drugs, overtime work at public facilities for private income, and treating private patients during official and non-official work hours. Ensuring a timely and adequate level of remuneration is therefore important.

Payment mechanisms to remunerate public health workers is another area for policy decision. Salaries provide a secure source of income, but may not create incentive for active service provision. Case-based payments could increase motivation and reflect workloads for which the workers are responsible but may lead to excessive provision of unnecessary services. The use of a mixed payment system, such as providing basic salary with top-up payments based on performance, could combine the benefit of both payment mechanisms.

Financial incentives could also be formulated to influence decisions on practice locations of the health workforce. There is a tendency for health workers, especially health professionals, to be concentrated in highly populated and affluent areas. Providing extra monetary incentives specifically for service in deprived areas or to those specialists in shortage has been used to recruit and maintain health workers in under-served areas or unpopular specialties (Wibulpolprasert & Pengpaibon 2003).

Non-financial incentives, work environment and system support

Social recognition, fairness of management and the opportunity to fulfil self-determination, as well as work environment and system support, play significant roles in the performance of the health workforce (World Health Organization 2006). Dieleman and colleagues indicated that the main motivating factors for health workers, in addition to stable jobs and income, are appreciation by managers, colleagues and the community, and availability of continued training (Dieleman *et al.* 2003).

Work environments can be improved in many ways. Good management and leadership in the health system are seen as a simple step to improve individual and organization performance. Since public health functions require teamwork, good team management is necessary. Having clear job descriptions and responsibilities can reduce tension and increase job satisfaction and compliance. In addition, the public health workforce should also be provided with an opportunity for continuous learning and training to be ready for changing public health demands.

The public health workforce's motivation and performance can also improve with better system support, such as an effective information and communication system. The availability of a functioning infrastructure, necessary supplies, and a safe workplace can promote the workforce's functions. In many cases, provision of support to the families of the workforce, such as safe housing for the family and good schooling for their children, is a very effective incentive for health workers to work and remain in underserved areas.

Roles of certification and credentials

One emerging issue in public health workforce management is certification and credentials of public health professionals. Certain members of the health sector, such as clinical scientists, doctors, nurses and technicians, are required to have certain certification or credentials before they can practice. However, in public health, this issue has only been recently raised in some countries. In the United States, only the state of New Jersey requires licensure of public health administrators employed to run a local health department, while the state of Illinois is moving to certify directors of local health departments.

Proponents of certification argue that it has several benefits (Akhter 2001; Tilson & Gebbie 2004). Certification can help identify professionals with adequate training experience and appropriate competency to deliver public health functions successfully. The establishment of national competency standards and certification could influence health workers to participate in lifelong learning activities to be qualified. It could also facilitate recognition and respect of the profession by the public, and could be used for job promotions or as one of the criteria for remuneration increases.

On the other hand, requiring credentials could mean rising costs of health professional employment. It may also limit the number of people willing to work in public health from a previously open arena. The majority of those practising public health do not have specific training or public health competency, but may have speciality training in other fields such as medicine or nursing.

There is also a practical difficulty in the public health certification process, as the scope of public health is very broad and entails several disciplines. The effort could also face political resistance from other professions perceiving certification as a threat to their scope of practice. In Thailand, there is an effort to legislate for the requirement of credentials of public health officers, but it faces strong resistance from eight professional groups, including medical and nursing councils. The bill introduced in 2007 was finally voted down in the parliament.

Health workforce system monitoring and evaluation

Health workforce system monitoring and evaluation is very important for public health workforce management. The current system is suffering from a lack of data and information for strategic decision-making. With increasing interest in outputs and outcomes of health investment, it is essential that there be more monitoring and evaluation of the health workforce system, especially performance measurement.

To measure performance, it is important to monitor inputs, processes, outputs and/or outcomes in a sound and effective way. The World Health Report of 2006 proposes four dimensions to monitor health workforce performance: Availability, competence, responsiveness, and productivity.

- *Availability* of the health workforce should be monitored in terms of space and time, covering both the distribution and attendance of existing workers.
- *Competence* includes the combination of technical knowledge, skills, and behaviours.
- *Responsiveness* measures how people are treated, regardless of who they are or how ill they are.
- *Productivity* refers to how effective health services and health outcomes are produced, given the existing stock of health workers.

Several methods of data collection are available for public health workforce system monitoring and evaluation. They include routine reporting systems, such as personnel records and health service reports; rapid appraisal methods, such as key informant interviews, focus group discussions, and direct observation; or formal surveys. In the case of performance measurement, it is recommended that all key stakeholders are involved in the planning process, so that the results of the monitoring and evaluation processes are accepted by all.

Planning for an effective public health workforce

Strategic planning for a public health workforce system should be done within the context of overall health workforce and health system planning, as the public health workforce is a part of the overall health system, which is complex and influenced by interactions between multiple players and stakeholders. Health workers are also employed in competitive labour market environments. Public health problems are influenced by demographic and epidemiological changes, changing patterns of public behaviours, and expectations. Innovative strategies and implementation plans are necessary to prepare the public health workforce with an evolving capacity in response to the changing needs of a modern health system. One common mistake in health workforce planning is that it usually focuses on the number and responses to adequate numbers of workers, which does not take into consideration the important issues of motivation, distribution and productivity.

The WHO and its partnerships propose that six interlinking thematic areas should be considered when dealing with public health workforce development and planning (Dal Poz *et al.* 2006). They are human resource management systems, policy, finance, education, partnership, and leadership (Fig. 12.11.3). These six areas should be considered concurrently in health workforce planning, as well as in situation analysis, implementation and monitoring and evaluation.

Specifically regarding public health personnel, Cioffi *et al.* (2004) proposed six strategic elements for public health workforce development, which include: (1) monitoring the workforce composition; (2) identifying competencies/developing curriculum; (3) designing integrated learning systems; (4) using incentives to

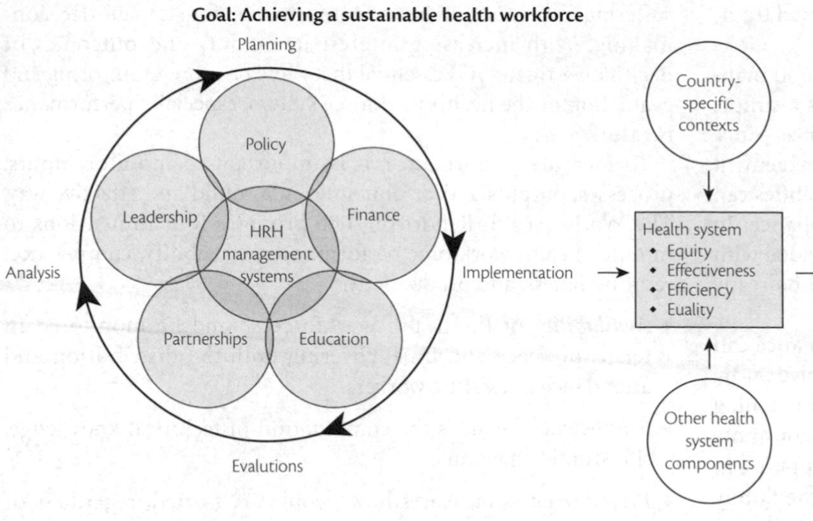

Fig. 12.11.3 Health Workforce Action Framework.
Source: Dal Poz *et al.* (2006).

assure competency; (5) conducting evaluation and research; and (6) assuring financial support.

In addition to the components of the public health workforce system and the strategic elements required, public health workforce planning should also take into account external factors that could affect its functions and roles over time. Since the health workforce is a component of health systems, it is almost always affected by changes in health systems. In many countries, the public health workforce is mostly in the public sector, which is therefore sensitive to any public sector or civil service reform, such as downsizing, decentralization or privatization.

The notion of public sector reform often receives lukewarm and sceptical responses by public health workers. They are generally seen as weakening workers' positions as professionals and undermining job security, which can lower workers' motivation (Kyaddondo & Whyte 2003). In Uganda and Bangladesh, decentralization of health services creates a change in the power structure, with a power struggle between various stakeholders (Ssengooba *et al.* 2004). It is perceived as jeopardizing job security, especially career structure and the opportunity for promotion. In the United States, privatization of public health agencies and the use of temporary workers (Keane *et al.* 2002) are seen by some managers as a cost–control measure, but it could mean a contract-based staff who may not closely adhere to public health principles and are less dedicated to the work and public health goals.

Community health workers (CHWs)

Community health workers comprise a major workforce for public health in many developing countries. Expansion of the roles of CHWs is seen as a model to alleviate the ongoing crisis due to a severe shortage of health workers in many sub-Saharan African countries. This sector uses CHWs as a case to demonstrate the development and effective management of one cadre of public health workers as part of the health system to achieve public health goals.

What is a CHW?

Accessibility to modern healthcare services depends not only on availability, but also on affordability, cultural acceptability, and effectiveness (Fig. 12.11.4) (World Health Organization 1984). Countries usually respond to the problem of inadequate physical access to professional services first by providing a lower level of health personnel. For example, auxiliary midwives and junior sanitarians have been produced in Thailand since 1953. In the United States and Canada, physician assistants and nurse practitioners have been produced since the mid-1960s (Jonas 1998). Nevertheless, even with the expanded services by these auxiliaries, basic health services are still not accessible by large numbers of rural villagers and poor people in urban slums.

The WHO (1978, p. 62; 1987, p. 10) defined CHWs as people with limited education trained in a short time to carry out either a wide range or restricted aspects of healthcare services. They include:

> *men and women chosen by the community, and trained to deal with the health problems of individuals and the community, and to work in close relationship with the health services.*

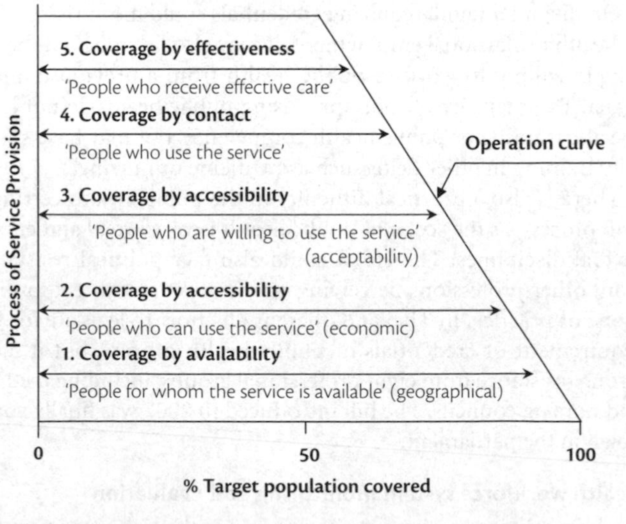

Fig. 12.11.4 Coverage of health services.
Source: Adapted from World Health Organization (1984).

Most CHWs are volunteers and receive short but systematic training. However, some CHWs receive longer-term training and even civil servant status; e.g. auxiliary midwives in Myanmar and community health aides in Jamaica. The WHO (1989) proposed that CHWs should be:

- Members of the communities where they work
- Selected by the communities
- Answerable to the communities for their activities
- Supported by the health system but not necessarily a part of its organization
- Have shorter training than professional workers

CHWs may go by different names in different countries and in different situations, and have different responsibilities. They may be called, for example, community health workers, village health volunteers (VHVs), village health communicators (VHCs), health guides (HGs), sanitation monitors, barefoot doctors, feldschers, health guides, lady health workers, etc. In addition, there may be more than one category of CHWs adopted by a country. Table 12.11.1 shows the various categories of CHWs and community financing schemes for nine elements of PHC in Thailand in 1988.

The origin of community health workers

Inadequate access to basic health services by a large portion of the population prompted many countries to start piloting the creation of systematically trained local CHWs. For example, in Thailand, the first pilot project to involve communities and to appoint CHWs for sanitation activities was started in 1960 (Vacharotai 1978). In DPR Korea, female sanitation monitors were recruited and trained in 1955. However, reliance on pilot or small-scale top-down projects not adapted to local conditions and lacking community participation, local support and resources resulted in disappointments and failures.

In the early 1970s, the health of the Chinese people improved dramatically, partly as a result of what is now called the nationwide primary healthcare approach. One of its guiding principles was the use of CHWs to extend health services to the places where the people live and work, support communities in identifying their own health needs, and helping people solve their own health problems. This new concept that communities should assume substantial responsibility for their own health brought a new dimension to the management of healthcare services. It opened up an opportunity to redraft and expand basic health services in many countries.

The Alma Ata International Conference on Primary Health Care (PHC) in 1978, organized jointly by the WHO and UNICEF, proposed the development of national CHW programmes as an important strategy for improving access to primary healthcare (World Health Organization 1978). Since then, CHW programmes have expanded to many developing countries,

Table 12.11.2 provides a summary of CHWs in nine countries of the WHO's South-East Asia Region.

After several decades of development, ample evidence has been published on the CHW role as a key agent in improving health. In Africa, the use of community health workers has evidently been found to improve health development (World Bank 1994; Gericke *et al.* 2003; Uta Lehmann 2004). Walt (1990) concluded that CHWs not only provide basic health services, but also promote the key principles of primary healthcare; i.e. equity, intersectoral collaboration, community involvement and use of appropriate technology. CHWs have shown that they can reduce mortality and improve other indices of health status. In certain communities, they can satisfy basic healthcare needs that cannot realistically be met by other means (World Health Organization 1989). They are also more accessible and acceptable to communities, resulting in an increase in health service utilization, especially among poorer households (Berman 1984; Berman *et al.* 1987). Extending services through

Table 12.11.1 Categories of CHWs and community financing schemes for nine elements of PHC, Thailand, 1988

Elements	CHWs[a]	Role	Financing schemes[b]
Health education	VHVs/VHCs	Village broadcasts/ education/motivation	–
Control of locally endemic diseases	Some VHVs/VHCs and malaria volunteers	Malaria surveillance, bleeding site control, provision of antimalarials	Mosquito Net Fund
Immunization (EPI)	VHVs/VHCs	Communication for immunization	Health Card Fund
Maternal and child health, family planning	VHVs/VHCs and trained traditional birth attendants	Advocate breast-feeding, supplementary diet, family planning, and maternal and child health; distribute oral pills and condoms	Health Card Fund
Nutrition	Model mother VHVs/VHCs	Nutritional surveillance, demonstration of supplementary diets	Nutrition Fund
Essential drugs and treatment of basic medical problems	VHVs/VHCs	Provision of essential drugs, first aid, and basic medical care	Village Drug Fund
Sanitation	Village sanitary craftsmen	Building latrines and water jars	Sanitation Fund
Dental health	VHVs/VHCs	Education and demonstration of regular and correct tooth brushing	Toothbrush and Toothpaste Fund

Note: VHV, village health volunteer; VHC, village health communicators.

[a] Only VHVs and malaria volunteers still existed in 1999.

[b] Most community financing schemes have diminished and been integrated into multipurpose village development funds.

Source: Adapted and updated from Wibulpolprasert (1991).

Table 12.11.2 Main categories of community health workers/volunteers in nine countries of the WHO's Southeast Asia Region, by country

Country	Category	Date initiated	CHW per number of population (pop) or households (hh)	Duration of training	Percentage of females	Numbers trained
Bangladesh	Village health volunteer	1988	1: 30 hh	4 days	80	38 262
Bhutan	Village health volunteer/worker	1978–1979	1:20–30 hh	12 days	10	1400
Democratic People's Republic of Korea	Sanitation monitor	1955	1:20–30 hh	5 days	100	NA
India	Village health guides	1977	1:1000 pop	3 months	25	416 724 (1985)
	Anganwadi worker	1975	1:1000 pop	3 months	100	NA
Indonesia	Health cadre	1978	1:10 hh	3 days	100	1.8 million (1991)
Myanmar	Community health worker	1977	1:1000 pop	4 weeks	5	36 358
	Auxiliary midwife	1977	1:2266 pop	6 months	100	17 856 (1994)
	Ten-household health worker	1987	1:10 hh	7 days	90	41 643 (1994)
Nepal	Female village health volunteer	1988–1989	1:400 (normal terrain) 1:250 (hill area) 1:150 (mountains)	12 days + 3 days refresher yearly	100	32 000
Sri Lanka	Volunteer health worker	1975–1977	Cluster of hh	6 hours (spread out)	66	40 000 (1996)
Thailand	Village health communicator	1979	1:10–15 hh	5 days	NA	598 908 (abolished in 1994)
	Village health volunteer	1979	1:80–150 hh	15 days	NA	642 532 (1998)
	Village sanitary craftsmen	1982	1:5–10 villages	15 days	NA	4132 (1990)
	Family health leaders	1996	1:1 hh	1 day	NA	1 177 464 (1998)

Notes:
[1] Many countries train traditional birth attendants as volunteer health workers; e.g. Thailand.
[2] Numbers of community health volunteers enlisted are mainly those selected and trained in the government health care system; figures from NGOs are not included.
[3] NA, not available.
Source: Adapted and updated from World Health Organization (1996).

CHWs is seen as a way to reduce inequity in child health (Victora *et al.* 2003; Masanja *et al.* 2005; Haines *et al.* 2007).

Responsibilities of CHWs

CHWs usually serve in roles as educators, communicators, problem detectors, problem-solvers, community organizers, and leaders for health. They serve as the link between the community and the healthcare system. They play an important role in galvanizing communities for action. They provide information that promotes individual and family self-care and responsibility as integral components of everyday life.

Some CHWs support delivery of general basic health services; e.g. village health volunteers in Bangladesh, Bhutan, and Thailand. Others play more specific roles; e.g. trained traditional birth attendants and village sanitary craftsmen in Thailand, and sanitation monitors in DPR Korea. The specific roles of CHWs are adapted to local situations and health demands. Nevertheless, their roles must be specifically defined. In Pakistan, the lady health workers are female workers recruited from the same community for which they serve, to provide reproductive health services and to promote positive health behaviours.

As a member (and leader) of the community, CHWs can integrate health issues into other community development activities, a role that is difficult for health professionals. In many countries, CHWs combine service and developmental functions that are not confined to the field of health. The relative importance of these two functions varies according to the socioeconomic situation and the availability and accessibility of local health services. The service function is less important where there is ready access to healthcare facilities. The developmental function is useful in all circumstances, and is crucial in less developed communities.

Table 12.11.3 shows the duties of CHWs in 11 different countries (World Health Organization 1987). Most CHWs play education and motivation roles, as well as delivering first aid treatment and dispensing basic medications. More specific or sophisticated service is provided only by CHWs in some countries. For example, CHWs in Columbia and Papua New Guinea also give injections, particularly for immunization. CHWs in Botswana, Sudan, and Yemen provide regular school health activities. CHWs in Botswana, Jamaica, China and Papua New Guinea assist in health centre clinic activities.

Community health workers: Conditions for success

Early evaluation of CHW programmes points to four necessary (but difficult) conditions for success; i.e. CHWs must be well trained, well supervised, provided with logistic support, and linked to functioning district health systems for referral when needed (World Bank 1993). These four conditions are relevant technical and managerial conditions, which require clear policy and leadership support. Experiences with many developing countries point to three necessary conditions for success of CHW programmes; namely, strong political support, intersectoral approaches and active community participation.

Strong political support

Initiating a CHW programme means accepting the health for all policy based on primary healthcare. It also means that the limitations of health professionals and the potential of the community are well accepted. This inevitably means a decision to put more resources into primary healthcare, which includes resources to support activities to establish and strengthen CHWs. It may also mean shifting resources from secondary and tertiary care in urban areas to support basic health services and primary healthcare in rural settings. Shifting of resources is a painful process that requires strong political leadership. Strong political support is also needed for CHW programmes to overcome resistance and win acceptance from health professionals.

The Alma-Ata declaration on health for all policy based on primary healthcare in 1978 provided very strong political support for CHW programmes in many developing countries. The Kenyan community-based healthcare project initiated in 1979 was a good example (Kaseje 1990). Political commitment for further and real decentralization of health services also allows more active participation by the community. At the local level, political leadership support from village leaders, religious leaders, teachers and other informal leaders are crucial to the success of CHW programmes.

Intersectoral approach

The priorities of most rural communities mainly focus on roads, water for agriculture, electricity, schools and employment, rather than on health. To attract higher priority and more community involvement, CHW programmes should be integrated into overall community development programmes. This approach complements the holistic, multifactorial nature and 'All for Health' concept of health.

This intersectoral concept, although not difficult to accept, is not easy to implement. In most developing countries, ministries usually have their own interests in maintaining a vertical bureaucracy. Vertical non-integrated activities are normal phenomena in different ministries or in different departments or divisions within one ministry. Thus, it is not uncommon to see health, education, rural development and agriculture ministries compete for the recruitment of volunteers in villages.

Active community participation

Sustainability of CHW programmes depends heavily upon acceptance by the communities, its relevance to their demands, and their participation. Active community participation should be included in all activities of CHW programmes, including community preparation, selection of CHWs, decisions on types and strategies of health development activities, and management of the programmes.

Active community participation is not easy to achieve in prevailing patron-client relationships between government officials and villagers of most rural communities. Reorientation of health personnel perspectives and the release of community potential are essential for its achievement. This requires not only community preparation, but also active preparation of health personnel. Socioeconomic and political reform of the country toward more decentralization and more participatory democracy is also conducive to its success.

One possibility to increase active community participation is to increase the flexibility of CHW programmes. Most developing countries implement CHW programmes based on a single rigid top-down primary healthcare model. This approach usually leaves little room for lower-level health personnel and the community to make adjustments to fit the local context. A single rigid top-down primary healthcare model implemented on a nationwide scale may yield rapid impressive results, but is usually short-lived.

Leaders in villages, formal or informal, are important resource persons who can actively participate in CHW programmes. Religious leaders, schoolteachers, youth leaders, and leaders of housewife groups are examples of local leaders conducive to CHW programmes. Local health personnel should contact these leaders and seek their opinions and support for the success and sustainability of CHW programmes.

Efficient management of CHW programmes

Even when the rationale for a CHW programme receives high political support and active community participation, managing the programme is not an easy task. Several factors in the programme management need to be addressed.

Preparation of health personnel

Preparation is one of the most crucial components of CHW programmes. Health personnel, particularly at the district level, are the prime (and closest) trainers and supporters of CHWs. Their attitudes and skills for working together with CHWs need to be developed and monitored.

In general, health personnel at the district level health infrastructures (e.g. district hospitals and health centres) are responsible for community preparation, selection and training, providing supervision and support, and direct communication with CHWs. They must be trained as trainers, primary healthcare supporters, and social advocates. Most important is their positive attitude towards CHWs, their respect for the community capacity, and their community skills. They should be able to build friendly relations with community leaders, CHWs and active members of the community.

Table 12.11.3 Duties of community health workers in different countries

Task summary	Benin	Botswana	Colombia	India	Jamaica	Liberia	Papua New Guinea	Philippines	Sudan	Thailand	Yemen
1. First aid, treat accidents and simple illness	/	/	/	/	/	/	/	/	/	/	/
2. Dispense drugs	/	/	/ (including injections)	/	/	/	/ (including injections)	/	/	/	/
3. Pre- and post-natal advice, motivation	/	/	/	/	/	/	/	/	/	/	/
4. Deliver babies	/	X	/	X	X	X	X	X	X	/ (trained TBA)	X
5. Child care advice, motivation	/	/	/	/	/	/	/	/	/	/	/
6. Nutrition motivation, demonstration	/	/	/	/	/	/	/	/	/	/	/
7. Nutrition action (W=weigh children, maintain chart; F=distribute food supplements)	F	W	W	X	W, F	X	W	W, F	F	W, F	X
8. Immunization motivation, assistance during clinics	/	/	/	/	/	/	/	/	/	/	/
9. Immunization—give injections	X	X	/	X	X	X	/	X	/	X	X
10. Family planning motivation	/	/	/	/	/	/	X	/	/	/	/
11. Family planning—distribute supplies	X	/	/	/	X	X	X	/	/	/	/
12. Environmental sanitation, personal hygiene, general health habit motivation	/	/	/	/	/	/	/	/	/	/	/
13. Communicable disease screening, referral, prevention, motivation	/	/	/	/	X	/	/	/	/	/	/
14. Communicable disease follow-up, motivation of confirmed cases	/	/	/	/	X	Sometimes	/	/	/	/	Sometimes
15. Communicable disease action (D=provide drug resupply; M=take malaria slides)	X	D	D, M	M	X	X	D, M	TB sputum smear	D	D, M (Malaria volunteers)	D
16. Assist health centre clinic activities (i.e. not in village)	Occasionally	/	Occasionally	X	/	X	/	X	Occasionally	Occasionally	X
17. Refer difficult cases to health centre or hospital	/	/	/	/	/	/	/	/	/	/	/
18. Perform school health activities regularly	X	/	X	X	X	X	X	X	/	X	/
19. Collect vital statistics	X	/	/	/	X	/	X	/	/	/	/
20. Maintain records, reports	/	/	/	/	/	/	/	/	/	/ (VHV only)	/
21. Visit homes on a regular basis	/	/	/	/	/	Sometimes	/	/	/	/	X
22. Perform tasks outside the health sector (e.g. agriculture)	/	/	X	/	X	/	X	/	/	/	/
23. Participate in community meetings	/	/	/	/	/	/	/	/	/	/	/

Note: /, task performed by CHWs; X, task not performed; VHV, village health volunteer; TBA, traditional birth attendant.

Source: Adapted from World Health Organization (1987).

These skills will enable them to be effective supporters of CHWs. Their preparation can be achieved through short courses, on-the-job-training of primary healthcare, CHW programmes, and training methodology.

Training materials and working guides for health personnel should be locally prepared. They may be adapted from the one provided by WHO (McMahon 1980). In addition, reorientation of basic medical education curricula to build understanding, positive attitudes and community skills for health professionals is also very important.

Financial incentives

Schemes based on financial incentives (e.g. Jamaica CHW programme) often collapse when the incentives are discontinued. In the case of needs for financial incentives, the community should be consulted and asked to decide on suitable recompense. For sustainability and acceptance, financial incentives should come more from the community than from the government.

The WHO Study Group (Rohde 1983) warned against a 'fee-for-service' arrangement, because of its tendency to concentrate on curative services for which CHWs can charge fees. However, fee-for-service for preventive and health promotion tasks may be allowed; e.g. fees for distribution of oral pills and condoms. Other additional incentives such as free medical care for CHWs and their family members, and nominal profit from sales of essential drugs may be given. If the time required to carry out the functions assigned is not a significant proportion of their time, direct financial remuneration could be counterproductive, and is therefore not recommended.

Continuing education

Some CHWs with an adequate level of education may be good candidates for recruitment into health personnel training colleges. They usually have better attitudes toward the community, as well as better community skills, than other students in these colleges. Nevertheless, providing this incentive may also have some detrimental effects, and must be carried out with great care and be highly selective. China's barefoot doctors are a good example.

China's barefoot doctors contributed greatly to the success of preventive health that had a proven effect on mortality and morbidity. In the late 1970s and 1980s, as a result of changes in economic policy and in the demand for medical care, they were offered the opportunity to become village doctors through training and qualifying exams. They then provided more sophisticated services and, in many provinces, moved to a fee-for-service financing system. Thus, a national CHW programme evolved to become a private practice model free from any governmental guidance resulting in a decline in preventive and promotion services (Zhu 1989; De Geyndt 1992; Ministry of Public Health 1999).

Resources and support

CHW programmes require initial investment, plus additional reinvestment in training, management, logistics, and supervision. Although the resource need is sizable, it is nevertheless usually a small fraction of the total national health budget.

In addition to public resources, other resources can be recruited from the community. Community financing schemes can be established to support various elements of primary healthcare, or to support integrated community health development activities. These additional resources may be used to provide incentives to CHWs. For example, in Thailand, the multipurpose village development fund pays the village sanitary craftsmen to build latrines and water jars. The dividend from these community-financing schemes, if sufficient, may also encourage active community participation.

Evaluation of CHW programmes

Evaluating any health programme is a complex and difficult exercise, beginning with the problem of methodology. Although there is some general agreement on the measurements in terms of reduction in morbidity and mortality, the methodology for evaluating social impact is more complex. Qualitative phenomena such as community participation, behaviour, and perceptions are difficult to measure. Some subjectivity and criticism are thus inevitable.

No matter how complex and difficult it is, a built-in system of monitoring and evaluating CHW programmes is needed, from formulation through to implementation. Evaluation is intended not only to measure progress and success, but also to yield necessary proposals for further development. Necessary relevant, valid, and reliable indicators need to be developed to measure the input, processes, and outcomes of the programme. In addition to the built-in system, some periodic external evaluations are helpful to guide further development of the CHW programme.

Information from the built-in monitoring and evaluation system of the Thai primary healthcare programme in 1986 revealed several constraints in the CHW programme; e.g. high drop-out rates, low levels of activity and low morale. This led to a systematic external evaluation in 1988, which resulted in abolishment of village health communicators, an increase in social and financial incentives, and more involvement of village headmen and village committees, as well as further strengthening of health service system support (Wibulpolprasert 1991).

Community management structures

CHWs should not be left alone in the community. Linkages to community infrastructures can gain more acceptability, and also allow CHWs to gain access to community resources conducive to health development. CHWs should be included as members in the community development committee. In Thailand, CHWs are now supported mainly by local administrative authorities rather than by the central government; they are therefore part of the local community.

Sometimes separate village health development committees have been set up. Top-down establishment of village health committees may be unsuccessful or even counterproductive. In the Saradidi project in Kenya, it was learned that reorganizing the community or setting up a new leadership system of the village health committee was not appropriate.

Certain community financing schemes may provide a good basis for the activities of the CHWs in the community development committee. They can also empower their community management skills. The resources generated can be used for further development of CHWs and the community. Figure 12.11.5 shows three important components for community health development; i.e. CHWs, management committees, and community financing schemes.

Conclusions

This chapter has provided an overview of the public health workforce and its roles, functions, and related factors that contribute to its effectiveness. An example of one public health workforce cadre,

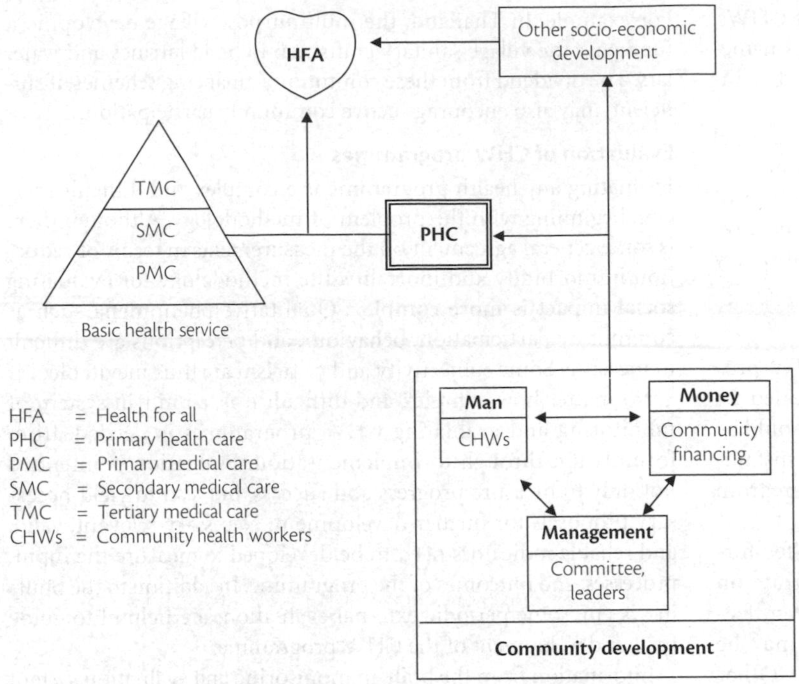

Fig. 12.11.5 Conceptual framework for community development in support of primary health and health for all.

community health workers, is discussed in detail to demonstrate the complexity of workforce development and management, as well as the support required by all factors.

One major challenge to the success of the public health workforce system is the lack of policy and political attention. In most developing countries, there has been a general neglect of both the public health workforce and its related infrastructure, as well as its long-term development. High-profile health professionals working in clinical care, such as doctors and nurses, are generally better organized, and their problems often get media attention more easily.

The Joint Learning Initiative, a global network of public health experts, called for increased attention to current failures in the health workforce system and the necessity to overcome the crisis (Joint Learning Initiative 2004). They indicated five main challenges, including shortages, skill-mix imbalance, geographical maldistribution, poor work environment, and a weak knowledge base. These problems are similarly shared by the public health workforce system, a major component of the overall health workforce, with a stronger intensity of problems in developing countries.

The Fifty-Seventh World Health Assembly in 2004 requested the WHO Director General to include human resources for health development as a top-priority programme area in the organization's General Programme of Work for 2006–2015 (World Health Organization 2004). Development of the public health workforce should be at the core of health workforce development for WHO, as well as all countries. Successful action requires active involvement of the public, communities and all stakeholders inside and outside health system. More importantly, there is a huge shortfall of rigorous research to provide the needed evidence base for policy decision-making regarding the public health workforce, similar to the problems in the public health field in general (Tilson & Gebbie 2004).

Only a strong public-health workforce will be able to respond to the global and national health challenges (Beaglehole *et al.* 2004).

Acknowledgements

The authors are thankful for research supported by Paichit Pengpaiboon and Sirianong Peyasuntiwong. The chapter also benefits from helpful comments and suggestions by the reviewers.

References

Afifi, A.A. and Breslow, L. (1994) The maturing paradigm of public health. *Annual Review of Public Health*, **15**, 223–35.

Akhter, M.N. (2001) Professionalizing the public health workforce: the case for certification. *Journal of Public Health Management Practice*, **7**, 46–9.

Beaglehole, R. and Dal poz, M. (2003) Public health workforce: challenges and policy issues. *Human Resources Health*, **1**, 4.

Berman, P.A. (1984) Village health workers in Java, Indonesia: coverage and equity. *Soc Sci Med*, **19**, 411–22.

Berman, P.A., Gwatkin, D.R., and Burger, S.E. (1987) Community-based health workers: head start or false start towards health for all? *Soc Sci Med*, **25**, 443–59.

Berman, P., Arellanes, L., Henderson, P., and Magnoli, A. (1999) Health care financing in Eight Latin American and the Caribbean Nations: the first regional national health accounts network. *Latin America and Caribbean Health Sector Reform Initiative.* Bethesda, MD, Partnerships for Health Reform Project, Abt Associates.

Bryce, J., EL Arifeen, S., Pariyo, G. *et al.* (2003) Reducing child mortality: can public health deliver? *Lancet*, **362**, 159–64.

Chapman, J., Congdon, P., Shaw, S. *et al.* (2005) The geographical distribution of specialists in public health in the United Kingdom: is capacity related to need? *Public Health*, **119**, 639–46.

Chen, L., Evans, T., Anand, S. *et al.* (2004) Human resources for health: overcoming the crisis. *Lancet*, **364**, 1984–1990.

Cioffi, J.P., Lichtveld, M.Y., and Tilson, H. (2004) A research agenda for public health workforce development. *J Public Health Management Practice*, **10**, 186–192.

Dal poz, M.R., Quain, E.E., O'neil, M. *et al.* (2006) Addressing the health workforce crisis: towards a common approach. *Human Resources Health*, **4**, 21.

De geyndt, W., Zhoa, X., Liu, S. (1992) From barefoot doctor to village doctor in rural China. World Bank Technical Paper, No.187. *World Bank Technical Paper.* Washington DC, World Bank.

Dieleman, M., Cuong, P., Anh, L. *et al.* (2003) Identifying factors for job motivation of rural health workers in North Viet Nam. *Human Resources Health*, **1**, 10.

Fineberg, H.V., Green, G.M., Ware, J.H. *et al.* (1994) Changing public health training needs: professional education and the paradigm of public health. *Annual Rev Public Health*, **15**, 237–257.

Gebbie, K.M., Merrill, J., and Tilson, H.H. (2002) The public health workforce. *Health Affairs (Project Hope)*, **21**, 57–67.

Gebbie, K.M. and Merrill, J. (2001) Enumeration of the public health workforce: developing a system. *J Public Health Management Practice*, **7**, 8–16.

Gebbie, K.M., Rosenstock, L., and Hernandez, L.M. (2003) *Who Will Keep the Public Healthy? Educating Public Health Professionals for the 21st Century,* Washington DC, National Academies Press.

Gericke, C., Kurowski, C., Ranson, M.K. *et al.* (2003) Feasibility of Scaling-up Interventions: The Role of Intervention Design. *Disease Control Priority Project Working Paper.*

Gordon, L.J. and Mcfarlane, D.R. (1996) Public health practitioner incubation plight: following the money trail. *J Public Health Policy*, **17**, 59–70.

Haines, A. and Cassels, A. (2004) Can the millennium development goals be attained? *Br Med Assoc*, **329**(7462), 394–397.

Haines, A., Sanders, D., Lehmann, U. *et al.* (2007) Achieving child survival goals: potential contribution of community health workers. *Lancet*, **369**(9579), 2121–2131.

Hongwiwatana, T., Sri-Ngernyuang, L. and Chuengsatiensap, K. (1988) *Alternatives to primary health care volunteers in Thailand,* Bangkok, Sangdad Publishing Co., Ltd.

Institute of Medicine (2002) *The Future of Public Health in the 21st Century,* Washington DC, National Academy Press.

Joint Learning Initiative (2004) *Human resources for health: Overcoming the crisis,* Cambridge, MA, Harvard University Press.

Jonas, S. (1998) *An introduction to the U.S. health care system.* New York, Springer Publishing Company.

Kaseje, D.C.O. (1990) Community-based health care: The Saradidi, Kenya experience. In Walsh, S.H.A.J. (Ed.) *Why Things Work.* Boston, Adams Publishing Group.

Keane, C., Marx, J., and Ricci, E. (2002) Public health privatization: proponents, resisters, and decision-makers. *J Public Health Policy*, **23**, 133–152.

Keegan, D. (1996) *Foundations of Distance Education*, Routledge.

Kennedy, V.C. and Moore, F.I. (2001) A systems approach to public health workforce development. *J Public Health Management Practice*, 7, 17–22.

Knebel, E. (2001) The use and effect of distance education in healthcare: What do we know? *Operations Research Issue Paper*, 2.

Kober, K. and Van damme, W. (2004) Scaling up access to antiretroviral treatment in southern Africa: who will do the job? *Lancet*, **364**, 103–107.

Kyaddondo, D. and Whyte, S.R. (2003) Working in a decentralized system: a threat to health workers' respect and survival in Uganda. *Int J Health Plan Management*, **18**, 329–42.

Lehman, U., Friedman, I., Sanders, D. (2004) Review of the Utilisation and Effectiveness of Community-Based Health Workers in Africa. *Joint Learning Initiative Working Paper.*

Masanja, H., Schellenberg, J.A., De savigny, D. *et al.* (2005) Impact of integrated management of childhood illness on inequalities in child health in rural Tanzania. *Health Policy Plan*, **20** Suppl 1, i77–i84.

Mayer, J.P. (2003) Are the public health workforce competencies predictive of essential service performance? A test at a large metropolitan local health department. *J Public Health Manag Pract*, **9**, 208–213.

Mcpake, B., Asiimwe, D., Mwesigye, F. *et al.* (1999) Informal economic activities of public health workers in Uganda: implications for quality and accessibility of care. *Soc Sci Med*, **49**, 849–65.

Ministry of Public Health (1999) *Health in Thailand 1997-1998,* Bangkok, The Veteran Press.

Muula, A.S. and Maseko, F.C. (2006) How are health professionals earning their living in Malawi? *BMC Health Services Res*, **6**, 97.

Roemer, M.I. (1991) *National Health System of the World*, New York, Oxford University Press.

Rohde, J. (1983) Health for All in China: principles and relevance for other countries. In D. Morley, J.R., G. Wiliams (Ed.) *Practising Health for All.* Oxford, Oxford University Press.

Ssengooba, F., Rahman, A., Hongoro, C. *et al.* (2004) The Impact of Health Sector Reforms on Human Resources in Health in Uganda and Bangladesh.

Tilson, H. and Gebbie, K.M. (2004) The public health workforce. *Annual Rev Public Hlth*, **25**, 341–356.

Travis, P., Bennett, S., Haines, A. *et al.* (2004) Overcoming health-systems constraints to achieve the Millennium Development Goals. *Lancet*, **364**, 900–906.

Tulchinsky, T.H. and Bickford, M.J. (2006) Are schools of public health needed to address public health workforce development in Canada for the 21st century? *Can J Public Health. Revue Canadienne De Sante Publique*, **97**, 248–250.

U.S. Bureau of Labor Statistics (2007) 2000 Standard Occupational Classification. Washington, DC, U.S. Bureau of Labor Statistics.

U.S. Department of Health and Human Services (1994) *The public health workforce: an agenda for the 21 century,* Washington DC, Government Printing Office.

U.S. Department of Health and Human Services, P. H. S., Public Health Functions Steering Committee (1994) *Public Health in America,* Washington, DC, Government Printing Office.

U.S. Health Resources and Services Administration (2000) *The public health workforce:enumeration 2000.,* Washington DC, Bureau of Health Professions, National Center for Health Workforce Analysis.

Vacharotai, S. (1978) *Lampang health development project: a Thai primary health care approach.,* Bangkok, Amarin Press.

Van lerberghe, W., Conceio, C., Van damme, W. *et al.* (2002) When staff is underpaid: dealing with the individual coping strategies of health personnel. *Bull WHO*, **80**, 581–584.

Victora, C.G., Wagstaff, A., Schellenberg, J.A. *et al.* (2003) Applying an equity lens to child health and mortality: more of the same is not enough. *Lancet*, **362**, 233–241.

Walt, G. (1990) *Community Health Workers in National Health Programmes. Just Another Pair of Hands?* Oxford University Press, Oxford.

Wibulpolprasert, S. (1991) Community financing: Thailand's experiences. *Health Policy Planning*, **4**, 354–360.

Wibulpolprasert, S. (2006) *Thailand Health Profile 2001-2004,* Nonthaburi, Bureau of Policy and Strategy, MOPH.

Wibulpolprasert, S. and Pengpaibon, P. (2003) Integrated strategies to tackle the inequitable distribution of doctors in Thailand: four decades of experience. *Human Resources Health*, **1**, 12.

World Bank (1993) *World Development Report 1993. Investing in Health*, Oxford University Press, Oxford.

World Bank (1994) *Better Health in Africa. Experiences and Lessons Learned.* Washington DC, World Bank.

World Health Organization (1978) *Primary Health Care.* Geneva, World Health Organization.

World Health Organization (1984) Evaluating primary health care in South East Asia. *WHO/SEARO technical publication.* World Health Organization, South-East Asia Regional Office, New Delhi.

World Health Organization (1987) *The Community Health Worker.* Geneva, World Health Organization.

World Health Organization (1989) *Strengthening the Performance of Community Health Workers in Primary Health Care.* Report of a WHO study group. *WHO Technical Report Series.* Geneva, World Health Organization.

World Health Organization (1996) *Role of Health Volunteers in Strengthening Action for Health*. Report of an intercountry consultation, Yangon, 20–24 February 1995. New Delhi, World Health Organization.

World Health Organization (1999) *The World Health Report 1999. Making a Difference.* Geneva, World Health Organization.

World Health Organization (2004) International migration of health personnel: a challenge for health systems in developing countries. In the *Proceedings of the 57th World Health Assembly.*

World Health Organization (2006) *The World Health Report 2006: Working Together for Health,* Geneva, World Health Organization.

Zhu, N. (1989) Factors associated with the decline of the Cooperative Medical System and barefoot doctors in rural China. *Bull WHO*, 431–441.

12.12

Planning for and responding to public health needs in emergencies and disasters

Khanchit Limpakarnjanarat and Roderico H. Ofrin

Abstract

Natural and man-made disasters have cause significant harm throughout history. However, the frequency and level of devastation caused by disasters appears to be increasing. Disasters not only cause loss of life and property, but also cause tremendous psychological damage, affecting the society and culture of the area as well. Poverty increases the impact of disasters, and developing countries tend to suffer more. The impact of disasters can be mitigated by disaster preparedness planning. To be effective, disaster planning must involve the entire community and must anticipate the range of disasters to which the community is vulnerable. In the modern world, disasters in one region often affect other regions. Thus, there is a need not only for local and national disaster preparedness, but also for international preparedness. The World Health Organization (WHO) has developed the International Health Regulations (IHR-2005), which has been approved by all Member States, and has established the Benchmarks for Emergency Preparedness and Response. The Benchmark provides a framework for systematic monitoring of health systems that comprise preparedness for natural and man-made disasters.

Synopsis

The importance of disasters as a major public health problem is widely recognized (Godschalk *et al.* 1999; Goel 2006). The sudden impact of natural disasters may cause many deaths, injuries, and illness. For example, the earthquake and tsunami in December 2004 resulted in approximately 280 000 deaths in Indonesia, Thailand, Sri Lanka, Southern India, Maldives, and Myanmar, and left 1 723 543 homeless (Kohl *et al.* 2005; World Health Organization 2005). The impact on the health system can also be drastic: Disaster can destroy health infrastructures, health staff may perish in the event, and funds must be re-allocated to support relief efforts. Surveillance systems need to be scaled up and public health interventions have to be re-prioritized quickly. Consequently, national healthcare goals may be set back for years (Noji 1997).

At the global level, the natural disasters continue to cause substantial loss of lives and property, despite scientific and material progress in disaster management. In 1989, the United Nations General Assembly declared the decade 1990–2000 as the International Decade for Natural Disaster Reduction with the objective to reduce loss of lives and property through international actions especially in developing countries (United Nations Department of Economic and Social Affairs 1996).

Human culture is also vulnerable to destruction. As a result of disasters, ancient structures and sometimes traditional customs can disappear due to the impact of an event or its related effects such as relocation and displacement (Cuny 1993).

The damage from natural and man-made disasters tends to be more severe if there is no proper preparedness in place (Lechat 1990). The goal of preparedness is to strengthen a public health system to be more efficient and effective at a time when special and immediate needs have to be addressed such as those in an emergency. This can be achieved if the approach is based on well-organized scientific principles of vulnerability and risk analyses. The approach can make prevention more effective, relief more relevant, and management more efficient at the local, national, and international levels. Overall, this will help save more lives and prevent avoidable morbidity (Armenian 1986).

The aim of public health disaster preparedness is prevention and control of unnecessary morbidity and mortality (Pan American Health Organization 1983). Therefore, application of effective prevention strategies can minimize the effects of disasters on public health. Preparedness can make a difference to minimize the destruction caused by natural disasters. As with all public health interventions, emergency preparedness and response requires involvement of many sectors. The involvement of sectors such as infrastructure, water and sanitation, finance, disease control, media and legal sectors can ensure that lives are saved.

In many instances, when city planning ignored building codes, communities were located in dangerous areas, warnings were not issued or followed, or a plan was not tested prior to the events, disasters caused more harm than necessary. Understanding the risks of people who died or were injured in disaster is a prerequisite for preventing and reducing deaths and injuries from future disasters (Guha-Sapir & Lechat 1986a). This chapter will review the basic concepts of disasters, provide a global review of the epidemiology of disasters, identify key public health problems in specific scenarios, and present the WHO strategic recommendations for emergency planning and response.

Classification of disasters

We can divide disasters into two broad categories: Natural and human generated (Rutherford *et al.* 1983).

- Natural events arise from hazards whose origin is from nature, such as earthquakes, volcanic eruptions, hurricanes, floods, fires, tornadoes, and extremes of temperature (Goel 2006).
- Man-made disasters fall into two categories (Pan American Health Organization 1982). The first are results from accidental destructive activity. Such events may be acute, as with aeroplane crashes, explosions, fires, and intoxications, or they may be chronic processes like deforestation and the contamination of the environment. Accidental man-made disasters, which usually pose little, if any, additional risk of communicable disease to the community, are beyond the scope of this chapter. The second category consists of man-made disasters caused by warfare, economic or social disruption and civil disturbances. Warfare is frequently subdivided into the conventional type, including siege and blockade, and the non-conventional type, including biological, chemical (toxic gas) and nuclear warfare. Experience with the effect of non-conventional warfare on communicable disease is limited. Public health handles biological agents capable of producing epidemics that incapacitate military or civilian populations (e.g. anthrax and plague) through taking the same measures as those used for naturally occurring outbreaks.

Other authors (Goel 2006) further specify these broad classifications as: (a) Complex emergencies usually involving situations in which civilian populations suffer casualties and loss of property, loss of basic services, and a means of livelihood as a result of war, civil unrest, or other political conflict. In many instances, people are forced to leave their homes temporarily or permanently, others become refugees in other countries; (b) technological disasters are those in which large numbers of people, property, infrastructure, or economic activity affected by major industrial accidents, severe pollution, unplanned nuclear release, major fires, or explosions from hazardous substances, e.g. fuel, chemicals, explosive, or nuclear materials; and (c) other disasters such as transportation (vehicular), material shortages resulting from energy embargoes, and dam breaks that are not caused by natural hazards but that occur in human settlements.

The distinction between natural and man-made disasters may not be clear-cut. A natural disaster may trigger secondary disasters—such as fires after an earthquake, hazardous air pollution may result from temperature inversion, or release of toxic chemicals into the environment in the aftermath of floods.

Natural disasters and those generated by people can be divided into acute- or sudden-impact events, such as earthquake and tropical cyclones, and those of chronic- or slow genesis, such as droughts leading to famine or chronic exposure to harmful chemicals from local industry or radiation from toxic disposal sites by community (Noji 1997).

Global overview of epidemiology of disasters

Trends show that events leading to emergencies and disasters are increasing as shown from data from the Center for Research on the Epidemiology of Disasters. Figure 12.12.1 shows the number of natural disasters at the country level during the past two decades has increased four- to fivefold worldwide.

The numbers of affected populations are also increasing. Natural disasters such as earthquakes, tropical cyclones, floods, and volcanic eruptions have claimed approximately 3 million lives worldwide during the past 20 years. They have adversely affected the lives of at least 800 million more displaced people. They have also caused more than US$50 billion in property damage.

The number of people killed in natural disasters in the past decade by continents is reflected in data from World Disaster Report 2006 (International Federation of the Red Cross and Crescent Societies 2006), which shows that disasters in the Asia Pacific region were responsible for 78 per cent of the total deaths globally (Fig. 12.12.2).

Many parts of the world experience major natural disasters which resulted in very high mortality (Table 12.12.1) (Advisory Committee on the International Decade for Natural Hazard Reduction 1987). Worldwide, a major disaster occurs almost daily, and natural disasters that require international assistance for affected populations occur weekly (Binder & Sanderson 1987).

From 1960 to 1990, floods were the most frequent type of natural disaster, accounting for more than one-third of all disasters. Windstorms (e.g. cyclones, hurricanes, and tornadoes) were the next most frequent disaster, contributing one-quarter of the total number. Earthquakes and cyclones caused the greatest devastation in terms of numbers of deaths and economic loss (Berz 1984) (Table 12.12.2). From 1965 to 1992, more than 90 per cent of all natural-disaster-affected persons lived in Asia and Africa. The following is the distribution for major natural disaster occurrences per year: Asia, 15; Latin America and Africa, 10; North America, Europe, and Australia, 1. Whether disasters in a region are measured by economic loss or by numbers of deaths and injuries, data show that Asia is the most natural-disaster-prone area of the world, Latin America and Africa are the second-most prone, and North America, Europe, and Australia are the least prone (IDNDR Promotion Office 1994).

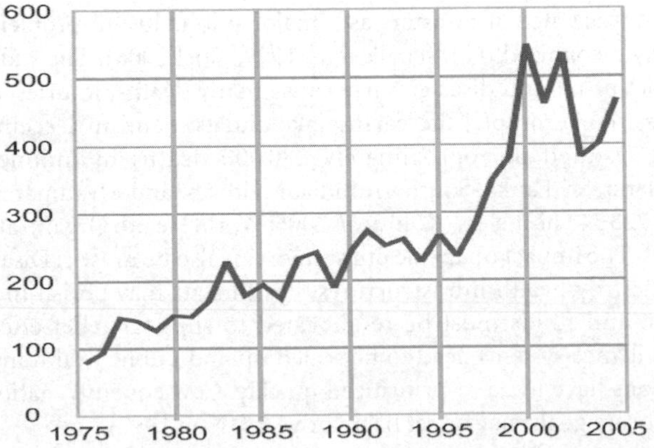

Fig. 12.12.1 Number of disasters from 1975 to 2005.
Source: Center for Research on the Epidemiology of Disasters (2007).

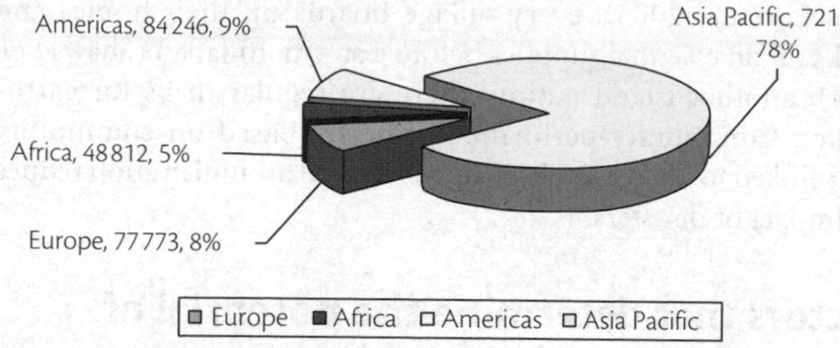

Fig. 12.12.2 Total number of people killed in natural disasters (1996–2005) Numbers.
Source: World Disaster Report (2006).

During the period 1947–1980, cumulative data gathered worldwide showed the top 10 major types of disasters ranked by the number of lives lost to be caused by heavy storms such as cyclones, hurricanes, or typhoons, with an almost equal number caused by earthquakes, followed by floods, thunderstorms and tornadoes, snowstorms, volcanoes, heat waves, avalanches, and landslides, respectively (Table 12.12.3).

Factors that may contribute to a disaster and the severity of its impact, particularly in developing countries, are human vulnerability resulting from poverty and social inequality, environmental degradation resulting from poor land use, lack of sophisticated health structures and disaster preparedness plans, and rapid population growth, especially among the poor. It has been estimated that 95 per cent of the deaths that are the result of natural disasters occur among 66 per cent of the world's population that lives in the poorest countries (Anderson 1991). For example, more than 3000 deaths per disaster occur in low-income countries compared with the average of 500 deaths per disaster that occur in high-income countries. The poor are most at risk because they are least able to afford housing that can withstand earthquake activity, often live

Table 12.12.1 The 10 worst natural disasters worldwide, 1945–2005.

Year	Location	Type of disaster	Number of deaths
1948	USSR	Earthquake	100 000
1949	China	Flood	57 000
1954	China	Flood	40 000
1965	Bangladesh	Cyclone	30 000
1968	Iran	Earthquake	30 000
1970	Peru	Earthquake	70 000
1970	Bangladesh	Cyclone	500 000
1971	India	Cyclone	30 000
1976	China	Earthquake	250 000
1990	Iran	Earthquake	40 000
2004	Indonesia, Sri Lanka, Maldives, India, Thailand, Myanmar, Somalia	Tsunami	280 000

Source: Office of US Foreign Disaster Assistance. (1995). *Disaster history: significant data on major disasters worldwide, 1900–present*; Agency for International Development, Washington DC.

Table 12.12.2 Crude disaster mortality by type of disaster, 1960–1969, 1970–1979, and 1980–1989 (Office of US Foreign Disaster Assistance 1995).

Disaster type	Deaths		
	1960–1969	1970–1979	1980–1989
Floods	28 700	46 800	38 598
Cyclones	107 500	343 600	14 482
Earthquakes	52 500	389 700	53 740
Hurricane			1263
Other disasters			1 011 777
Total			1 119 800

along coasts where storms or tidal waves strike, or live in floodplains subject to flooding. Their economic circumstances force them to live in substandard housing susceptible to landslides or are located near industrial sites. Furthermore, they are not educated about lifesaving behaviours. Risks and vulnerabilities are higher in poor countries and poorer subsets of the population because there is less investment in preparedness. Preparing for emergencies decreases mortality and morbidity from the impact of events. It prevents events from turning into emergencies, and emergencies into disasters (Guha-Sapir & Lechat 1986b).

Hazards, risks, and vulnerabilities

The basis of any preparedness planning is risk and vulnerability analysis. Understanding the dynamics of risks, hazards, vulnerability, and capacities provides essential information for proper prioritization of resources and actions. A definition of these three terminologies is essential (International Strategy for Disaster Reduction 2003).

Hazard A hazard is a potentially damaging physical event, phenomenon or human activity that may cause the loss of life or injury, property damage, social and economic disruption, or environmental degradation.

Table 12.12.3 Ten major types of disasters ranked by the number of lives lost worldwide during the period 1947–1980 (Shah 1983).

Type of disaster	Number of deaths
Tropical cyclones, hurricanes, typhoons	499 000
Earthquakes	450 000
Floods (other than those associated with hurricanes)	194 000
Thunderstorms and tornadoes	29 000
Snowstorms	10 000
Volcanoes	9000
Heat waves	7000
Avalanches	5000
Landslides	5000

Hazards can include latent conditions that may represent future threats and can have different origins: Natural (geological, hydro meteorological and biological) or induced by human processes (environmental degradation and technological hazards). Hazards can be single, sequential or combined in their origin and effects. Each hazard is characterized by its location, intensity, frequency and probability.

Vulnerability comprises the conditions determined by physical, social, economic, and environmental factors or processes that increase the susceptibility of a community to the impact of hazards.

The opposite of vulnerability is *capacity*. It is defined as a combination of all the strengths and resources available within a community, society or organization that can reduce the level of risk or the effects of a disaster. Capacity may include physical, institutional, social, or economic resources, as well as skilled personal or collective attributes such as leadership and management. Capacity may also be equivalent to capability.

Risk is defined as the probability of harmful consequences or expected losses (deaths, injuries, property, livelihoods, economic activity disrupted or environment damaged) resulting from interactions between natural or human-induced hazards and vulnerable conditions. Conventionally, risk is expressed by the notation: Risk = Hazards × Vulnerability.

Some disciplines also include the concept of exposure to refer particularly to the physical aspects of vulnerability.

Beyond expressing a possibility of physical harm, it is crucial to recognize that risks are inherent or can be created or exist within social systems. It is important to consider the social context in which risks occur, and that people do not necessarily share the same perceptions of risk and their underlying causes.

Taking these concepts together—hazards, risks, vulnerabilities, and capacities—will comprise the key information for planning. Knowing risks and vulnerabilities, one will be able to identify what to plan for and what to prioritize. Identifying existing capacities will also inform us of which gaps to fill and what to strengthen.

There are differences in health effects, depending on the hazards that cause an event (Goel 2006) (Table 12.12.4). Planning for disasters and emergencies should be based on analysis of risks, and vulnerabilities, *vis-à-vis* capacities that are in place in the areas where the planning is being conducted (e.g. national, subnational). It would be important to plan to examine all hazards, also known as the all-hazard approach, and developing scenarios around each possible event.

Specific examples

Islands are prone to extremely damaging natural disasters, such as hurricanes and tropical storms, volcanic eruptions, storm surges, landslides, extended droughts, and extensive floods. A recent study of the UN/DHA shows that at least 13 of the 25 most disaster-prone countries worldwide are small island developing country states. The impact of natural disasters is especially severe for islands because of their small size, dependence on agriculture and tourism, narrow resource base, and the pervasive impact of such events on their people, environment and economies, including loss of insurance coverage. For those affected by these natural disasters, these particular characteristics mean that the economic, social, and environmental consequences are long-lasting and the costs of rehabilitation are high. Island nations which are prepared and aware of the consequences they may face suffer less from such events. In Cuba (Mas Bermejo 2006), every village boards up their homes and stocks up on essential supplies before a storm. In Japan (Shaw *et al.* 2004), another island nation, there are regular drills for earthquakes. Community-performed exercises based on community plans linked to higher levels of authority and administration reduce the impact of disasters.

Factors that determine the potential of communicable disease transmission

One of the most common myths associated with disasters is that epidemics of communicable diseases are inevitable. This myth is often perpetuated by the media and by local politicians who demand mass vaccination campaigns immediately following natural disasters such as hurricanes, earthquakes, and floods. The public perception that disease outbreaks are imminent often derives from its exaggerated sense of the risk posed by dead bodies that remain exposed after an acute natural disaster. The truth is that communicable disease epidemics are relatively rare after rapid onset natural disasters unless large numbers of people are displaced from their homes and placed in crowded and unsanitary camps (Seaman *et al.* 1984; World Health Organization 1986). Six types of adverse changes influence the potential risk of communicable diseases after disasters (Noji 1997). These are changes in pre-existent levels of disease, changes in ecology that are the result of the disaster, changes due to population displacement, changes in population density, changes due to disruption of public utilities, and changes due to interruption of basic public health services.

Changes in pre-existent levels of disease

Usually the risk of a communicable disease in a community affected by a disaster is proportional to the endemic level. There is generally no risk of a given disease when the organism that causes it is not present beforehand. Developing countries frequently have poor systems for reporting communicable diseases; thus, their national authorities lack adequate information about levels of specific organisms. Political pressure nonetheless is sometimes exerted demanding public health measures against diseases such as smallpox, cholera, yellow fever, or other vector-borne diseases in geographic areas considered free of them by communicable disease specialists.

Relief workers can conceivably introduce communicable diseases into areas affected by disasters. Diseases potentially introduced include new strains of influenza, foot-and-mouth disease, and those borne by insect vectors, particularly by *Aedes aegypti*. In addition, non-immune relief workers may be susceptible to endemic diseases to which the local population is tolerant or immune, and may become ill.

Changes in ecology caused by disasters

Natural disasters, particularly droughts, floods, and hurricanes, frequently produce ecological changes in the environment that increase or reduce the risk of communicable diseases. Vector-borne and water-borne diseases are the most significantly affected. A hurricane with heavy rains that strikes the Caribbean coastal area of Central America may, for example, reduce the number of *Anopheles aquasalis* hatched, since the vectors prefer brackish tidal swamps, and increase *A. albimanus* and *A. darlingi*, which breed easily in

Table 12.12.4 Short-term effects of major disasters.

Effect	Earthquakes	High winds (without flooding)	Tidal waves/flash floods	Slow onset floods	Landslides	Volcanoes
Deaths*	Many	Few	Many	Few	Many	Many
Severe injuries requiring extensive treatment	Many	Moderate	Few	Few	Few	Few
Increased risk of communicable diseases	Potential risk following all major disasters (probability rising with overcrowding and deteriorating sanitation)					
Damage to health facilities	Severe (structure and equipment)	Severe	Severe but localized	Severe (equipment only)	Severe but localized	Severe (structure and equipment)
Damage to water systems	Severe	Light	Severe	Light	Severe but localized	Severe
Food shortage	Rare (may occur due to economic and logistic factors)	Rare (may occur due to economic and logistic factors)	Common	Common	Rare	Rare
Major population movement	Rare (may occur in heavily damaged areas)	Rare (may occur in heavily damaged areas)	Common (generally limited)	Common (generally limited)	Common (generally limited)	Common (generally limited)

*Potential lethal impact in absence of preventive measures.

Source: Goel (2006) *Encyclopedia of Disaster Management* (vol. 1—Disaster Management Policy and Administration)—page 6.

fresh, clear water and overflows. The net effect of the hurricane on human malaria, of which both mosquitoes are vectors, would be difficult to predict. Rain from such a hurricane would also cause flooding of streams and canals in rural areas that are often the source of drinking water. Under some circumstances, a water-borne zoonotic disease such as leptospirosis may become more widely disseminated via water-contact or drinking from contaminated sources. There is evidence that the short-term effect of diluting supplies of already contaminated drinking water with rain may reduce the level of disease (Rutherford *et al.* 1983). The population may avoid drinking water contaminated by flooding for a cultural/psychological reason such as the presence of animal carcasses.

Changes due to population displacement

Movement of populations away from the areas affected by a disaster can affect the relative risk for communicable diseases in three ways. If the population moves nearby, the existing facilities and services in the receiving community will be strained. When resettlement occurs at some distance, the chances increase that the displaced population will encounter diseases not prevalent in their own community, to which they are susceptible. For example, non-immunized, rural Andean populations brought together in camps after an earthquake may then be exposed to measles. Alternatively, displaced populations may bring the agents or vectors of communicable diseases with them. The latter concern frequently occurs when populations from low-lying coastal areas with malaria move further inland before a hurricane.

Changes in population density

Population density is a critical factor in the transmission of diseases spread by the respiratory route and through person-to-person contact. Because of the destruction of houses, natural disasters almost invariably contribute to increased population density. Survivors of severe disasters seek shelter, food, and water in less affected areas. When the damage is less severe, crowding may occur when people move in with other families and congregate in such public facilities as schools and churches. The resulting problems most commonly mentioned are acute respiratory illness, and include influenza and non-specific diarrhoeas.

Changes due to disruption of public utilities

Disasters may interrupt electricity, water, sewage disposal, and other public utilities. In situations with disruption of public utilities, there are promiscuous defecation habits and contaminated sources of water that promote communicable diseases. However, in economically more developed areas, the extended disruption of basic services increases the risks of food- and water-borne disease. Insufficient water for washing hands and bathing promotes the spread of diseases transmitted by contact.

Changes due to interruption of basic public health services

The interruption of basic public health services such as vaccination, ambulatory treatment of tuberculosis, and programmes for the control of malaria and vectors are frequent, but often overlooked factors increase the probability of disease transmission after disaster in a developing country. The risk of transmission increases proportionally to the extent and the duration of the disruption. An outbreak of communicable disease may occur months or years after a drought, famine, or civil disturbance. The interruption causing such an occurrence is usually the result of the diversion of staff and financial resources to the relief effort, beyond the critical period.

In addition or in conjunction with this, the failure to reestablish resources at sufficient levels contributes to the interruption.

Phases of a disaster and its link to sustainable development

The UN International Strategy for Disaster Reduction identifies the phase of a disaster as follows:

Preparedness	Activities and measures taken in advance to ensure effective response to the impact of hazards, including the issuance of timely and effective early warnings and the temporary evacuation of people and property from threatened locations.
Prevention	Activities to provide outright avoidance of the adverse impact of hazards and means to minimize related environmental, technological, and biological disasters. *Depending on social and technical feasibility and cost/benefit considerations, investing in preventive measures is justified in areas frequently affected by disasters. In the context of public awareness and education, related to disaster risk reduction changing attitudes and behaviour contribute to promoting a 'culture of prevention'.*
Recovery	Decisions and actions taken after a disaster with a view to restoring or improving the pre-disaster living conditions of the stricken community, while encouraging and facilitating necessary adjustments to reduce disaster risk. *Recovery (rehabilitation and reconstruction) affords an opportunity to develop and apply disaster risk reduction measures.*
Relief/ response	The provision of assistance or intervention during or immediately after a disaster to meet the life preservation and basic subsistence needs of those people affected. It can be of an immediate, short-term, or protracted duration.
Mitigation	Structural and non-structural measures undertaken to limit the adverse impact of natural hazards, environmental degradation, and technological hazards.

These phases can be better understood as a cycle:

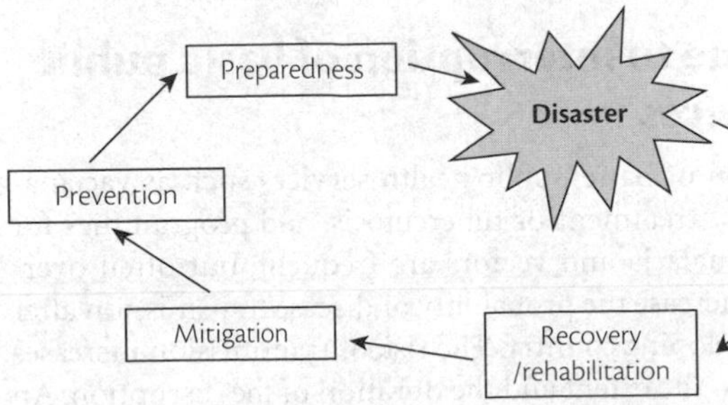

It is important to note that the cycle and its phases should be viewed in terms of managing risks. This cycle illustrates the process by which various stakeholders (e.g. governments, civil society, private sector) plan for, respond to, and conduct activities to reduce the impact of disasters even before they happen. With appropriate legislation, policies, regulations and activities in place at every point in the cycle, then the net effect is contribution to:

- Greater reduction of vulnerability of communities
- Increased capacities in preparedness
- Increased response capacity
- Increased resilience in recovery of communities

As the cycle recurs with every event, there is also the opportunity to improve the legislation, policies, regulations, and investments in mitigation, prevention, and preparedness. Events and emergencies will continue to help improve public policies that modify the causes of, or reduce the impacts of disasters on communities. All of which then ensure continuous development.

Indeed, the link between disasters and development becomes crucial as we view the cycle. Managing disasters is all about understanding and managing risks at all points of this cycle and the health sector has much to contribute in this. This being so, it is clear why the health sector plays a key role in disaster and emergency preparedness and response, and development of nations in general.

Sustainable development requires various approaches and among them is risk management of which a safer community is the main end goal. Managing risks goes hand in hand with developing capacity to adequately manage emergencies and disasters when they occur. There is a synergistic and cyclical relationship between disasters and development: The goal of disaster and emergency management is to reduce risks to create safer communities and to safeguard the existing as well as the potential gains of development. Conversely, development that is risk approach-oriented prevents and mitigates the deleterious effects of catastrophic events. A good example would be establishing good hospital systems and training health professionals to attend to affected populations of an earthquake. But then, in many cases, hospitals themselves cannot withstand tremors and earthquakes due to poor construction. It then becomes a case of development creating more risks and vulnerabilities; this should be prevented. This is an example from within the health sector. However, there are development issues impinging on wider areas, such as the environment, urban planning, and migration in which development may generate further risks and disasters if not addressed properly. The health sector does not only act to prepare and respond to disasters but needs to involve itself in other sustainable development issues. After all, a risk to health is a risk to achieving development, with the reverse being true as well. A holistic view of the various phases, how they link, and what are the appropriate interventions that can be done per phase can help in ensuring that health and development are protected.

Health sector functions in emergencies: Components for planning

The WHO categorizes its functions for emergencies described below. This framework can also apply to the health sector in its preparedness and responses for emergencies. The following are the four major areas:

1. *Capacity building for health responses in disasters*: The concept of capacity building covers a wide range of operational and

disciplinary factors. These can range from the capacity of the government military, civil society groups, and the community response to the capacity of laboratories for providing testing at the approved quality level. It also covers a wide range of activities from building systems and policies to training community members or health staff for specific skills. The goals of building capacity in the health sector are not different from those in other sectors; i.e. autonomy and self-reliance, local capacities, and sustainability:

- *Autonomy and self-reliance* is the primary goal for all communities at risk. In this context, building the capacity of local communities is the main strategy to accomplish this objective.
- *Local capacities* in the areas of relief and responses are most effective when people in local communities are well trained and the community is well prepared for disasters. Persons at the community level will reach the affected areas the quickest, and are most familiar with local conditions. Thus, the efficiency and effectiveness of the responses are enhanced greatly by improving the capacity of local health professionals. Experienced and skilled international relief workers are useful in disaster management, but require adjustment to the conditions and the customs and characteristics of the area in which the disaster occurs.
- Skilled, well-trained local personnel in place can ensure *sustainability*. When the relief efforts stop, these personnel will continue to provide the affected community with long-term recovery.

2. *Assessments*: Needs assessment is one of the most important aspects of disaster responses and relief planning. The main reason to conduct needs assessment is to inform decision-makers about what to do in relation to a given situation. The assessment will help answer five decision-making questions: (1) Should there be an intervention?; (2) What is the nature and scale of intervention needed?; (3) What are the priorities for the allocation of resources?; (4) What are the gaps that need to be filled?; and (5) What is the program design and what planning is required? Several problems can result from poor needs assessment, including unnecessary repetition, lack of coordination, inadequate determination of effectiveness, changes over time, inadequate dissemination, and need for standards.

   Assessments are keys in the event of various disasters. The accident at Chernobyl (Ukraine 1986) (World Health Organization 2007), the explosions in fireworks storage (The Netherlands, 2000) (Ruijten 2007), the AZF factory (France, 2001) (Verger *et al.* 2007), fuel explosion (The United Kingdom, 2005) (Russell & Saunders 2007), terrorist attacks on the Twin Towers (United States, 2001) (Herbert *et al.* 2006), the summer 2003 heat wave in Europe (Sardon 2007), the tsunami in Southeast Asia (2004) (World Health Organization 2005) and, most recently, hurricanes Katrina and Rita (United States, 2005) (Blendon *et al.* 2007) and the earthquake in Pakistan (2005) (Laverick *et al.* 2007) all had serious human health, social, and economic effects on human societies. However, no comprehensive strategy for investigating and learning more about health, social, and societal consequences of disasters has been defined at the international level. Health assessment involves exposure and health risk assessment, as well as epidemiologic surveillance and in-depth studies. Standardization and coordination of assessment activities require consensus at the international, national, and subnational levels.

   There is a role for health assessment after an event, as well as using epidemiology to anticipate catastrophes. These evaluations face many difficulties, including lack of pre-disaster health indicator information such as post-traumatic stress disorders (PTSD), availability of soil contamination data, lack of pre-exposure data, relevant demographic databases, loss of follow-up of subjects, etc. Post-disaster assessments and health information systems that are set up shortly after an emergency can provide decision-making support to manage health hazards, screening for specific health problems, and organization of medical follow-up and health surveillance. Public information about health risks must be transparent and available to the media, the public, affected populations, healthcare professionals, and various other stakeholders. Scientific knowledge resulting from research will increase knowledge and improve responses to any future event.

3. *Coordination*: The elements in emergencies that require coordination in the health sector include efforts by affected communities, national and local governments in the affected areas, donor governments (bilateral), multi-lateral agencies (UN and international financial institutions), national and international non-government organization (NGOs), academic institutions, the military, and the media. The national government, especially the Ministry of Health, should coordinate all health responses in emergencies in their respective countries. However, in areas that the national government has failed during the conflict, organizations such as World Health Organization may take a leadership role in health sector coordination to guarantee minimum standard healthcare for the affected populations. Roles of coordinating bodies responsible for medical care and public health functions are:
   - Working with all players to establish and agree to norms and standards
   - Leading in emergency preparedness and drills
   - Actively engaging other players within the sector, sharing information as it becomes available
   - Integrating health expertise and activities for maximum effectiveness and efficiency
   - Acknowledging the roles of all of actors

4. *Filling gaps in available services*: To identify gaps in available services, health authorities should consider these general points; i.e. uniqueness of the types of disasters, such as floods, tsunamis, earthquakes. Decision-makers require adequate and accurate needs assessment to generate information, and population data to determine the impact of the event. Gaps in the early phase of relief common to all sudden onset disasters are interventions relating to provision of food, supply of adequate safe water and sanitation facilities, construction of temporary shelters, and rapid restoration of preventive and curative healthcare services. The healthcare services that should be considered as high priority are field hospitals, mental health, and women's health.

New tools to address new challenges for health emergencies

- International Health Regulations (2005)
- Benchmarks for Emergency Preparedness and Response

Disaster response relies upon the concept of International Health Security. There is a need to reduce the vulnerability of people to the escalation of existing, new, acute, or rapidly spreading risks to health, particularly those that threaten to cross international borders. Health issues present new challenges that go far beyond national borders, and have an impact on the collective security of people around the world.

Globalization with its easy, frequent travel, as well as large-scale trade, offers ample opportunity for disease to spread across borders quickly and easily. Epidemic-prone diseases, both new and re-emerging, humanitarian emergencies, bioterrorism, climate change, and environmental degradation have the potential to become international public health emergencies.

No single institution or country has all the capacities needed to respond to international public health emergencies caused by epidemics, natural hazards, conflicts, or by epidemics of existing diseases, or new and emerging infectious diseases.

The earth's climate is changing. Temperatures are rising, tropical storms are increasing in frequency and intensity, and polar ice caps and permafrost regions are melting. The acute impact of climate change-related events may be local, but the cause is global. When floods contaminate international waters, when people migrate across borders to find food and shelter, when disease patterns change due to an altered climate, the impact is felt internationally. As a result, trends and predictions for changes in morbidity and mortality patterns all point to an increase.

Humanitarian emergencies arise from the effects of crises such as natural hazards, food and water shortages, and armed conflict. Just as these situations affect individuals, they also affect the already stressed health systems that people rely on for maintaining health security. The World Disasters Report 2006 (International Federation of the Red Cross and Crescent Societies 2006) indicates that approximately 58 per cent of the total number of people killed in natural disasters occurred in the Southeast Asia region during the decade of 1996–2005. In this decade, the Asian region had the highest number of natural disasters (1273 reported events) and technological disasters (1387 reported events). Disaster preparedness strategies and humanitarian response operations together can create a balanced approach to alleviating the negative impact of natural disasters. Both rely on planning, collaboration, and coordination of roles of the various sectors involved.

Considering all these elements of International Health Security, *vis-à-vis* risks and hazards in the region, it would be practical to focus on two key aspects: (1) international health regulations; and (2) systematic emergency preparedness and response.

The International Health Regulations (2005) (WHO 2006)

The revised International Health Regulations (IHR) (2005) unanimously adopted by the World Health Assembly of WHO came into force in June 2007. Their implementation will help build and strengthen effective mechanisms for alert and response for events of public health concern at national and international levels.

Member states will work towards the implementation of the IHR (2005) and towards greater collaboration across borders and between sectors to counter the negative influences on health posed by globalization, disasters, climate change, and existing and emerging diseases.

Key elements of the IHR (2005) are as follows:

- This legal framework seeks to protect against, control, and provide a mechanism to initiate a public health response to the threat of international spread of diseases of biological, chemical, or radionuclear origin.
- IHR (2005) is a major paradigm shift from IHR (1969), and focuses now on:
  - Containment at the source of a possible Public Health Emergency of International Concern (PHEIC) as opposed to only control at borders
  - All public health threats as opposed to a few diseases
  - Adapted responses as opposed to pre-set measures
  - Facilitates development of proactive systems as opposed to reactive ones

As a binding global legal framework, the adoption of the IHR (2005) requires certain requirements for Member States, including:

- Designation of a national IHR focal point
- Strengthening core capacity to detect, report, and respond rapidly to events that pose a threat to public health
- Assessing events occurring in their territory and notifying WHO within 24 h of all events that may constitute a PHEIC
- Providing routine inspection and control activities at international airports, ports and some ground crossings
- Building a legal and administrative framework in line with IHR (2005) requirements

In accordance with these needs, WHO will support the development of core capacities in health systems for IHR to be fully functional. This includes its own institutional readiness to support Member States with appropriate staffing, conducting global surveillance and health intelligence gathering, providing technical assistance and guidance to Member States, developing guidelines and measures for PHEIC, and updating the IHR (2005) as appropriate to maintain its scientific and regulatory validity.

WHO South-East Asia Region (SEAR) benchmarking framework for emergency preparedness and response (EPR)

The Benchmarks Framework is a response to the collective experiences of five Asian countries affected by the tsunami of 26 December 2004, the recurring emergencies in all SEAR member countries, and the global call for improved emergency preparedness.

Member States formulated the benchmarks to set standards for emergency preparedness through a participatory approach applicable to the specific situations in the countries of the region and other countries in the world. This gap in standards and benchmarks was a clearly identified need after many lessons learned from the tsunami experience.

The benchmarks are the product of a regional consultation in Bangkok in November 2005 (World Health Organization, Regional Office of South-East Asia 2006) involving all 11 SEAR member countries. In addition to Ministries of Health (MOH), a number of other stakeholders were present, notably from Ministries of Home Affairs, Foreign Affairs and Education, as well as UN agencies, the International Federation of Red Cross, International Non-Governmental Organizations (INGO), donors, and universities.

The consultation's main objective was to identify gaps in addressing response, preparedness, and recovery for health needs of affected and vulnerable populations. The 12 benchmarks address the key issues necessary to establish a disaster preparedness mechanism as identified by the participants at the consultation.

Following a regional consultation in Bali in June 2006 (World Health Organization, Regional Office for South-East Asia 2007a), the Benchmarks Framework was further refined to include standards and indicators to make planning, monitoring, and evaluation more accurate.

The following are the 12 benchmarks (World Health Organization, Regional Office for South-East Asia 2007b)

1. A legal framework and functioning coordination mechanisms and an organizational structure in place for health EPR at all levels involving all stakeholders.
2. Regularly updated disaster preparedness and emergency management planning for the health sector and standard operating procedures (SOP) (emergency directory, national coordination focal point) in place.
3. Emergency financial (including national budget), physical and regular human resource allocation and accountability procedures established.
4. Rules of engagement (including conduct) for external humanitarian agencies, based on needs established.
5. Community planning for mitigation, preparedness and response developed, based on risk identification and participatory vulnerability assessment, backed by a higher level of capacity.
6. Community-based response and preparedness capacity developed, and supported with training and regular simulation/mock drills.
7. A local capacity for emergency provision of essential services and supplies (shelters, safe drinking water, food, communication).
8. Advocacy and awareness developed through education, information management and communication, including media relations (pre-, during, and post-event).
9. The capacity to identify risks and assess vulnerability at all levels.
10. Human resource capabilities continuously updated and maintained.
11. Health facilities built/modified to withstand expected risks.
12. Early warning and surveillance systems for identifying health concerns.

Corresponding to each benchmark are standards, indicators and a question/checklist. All these complete the framework for identifying gaps and monitoring progress towards improved emergency preparedness and response.

Each benchmark has two or three standards, and each standard has one to four health sector indicators for which monitoring can take place. The standards denote the technical reference level of quality or attainment of the benchmark. The standards are qualitative, universal in nature, and applicable in any operating environment, as they specify the minimum level to be attained.

Each standard is equipped with tools to measure the progress towards achieving the standards; i.e. a set of indicators. The indicators provide a way to measure and determine progress in achieving the standards. As the indicators are formulated to be very specific to the standards, they can also be used to guide strategic thinking and planning.

The health sector indicators all refer to health-related issues that various partners have a mandate to ensure, including the Ministry of Health, district health authorities, hospitals, UN agencies, NGOs, and community partners,.

For each standard, a set of non-health sector or 'other sectors indicators' has been included. The other sectors indicators refer to essential preparedness issues that are not within the means of the health sector to achieve, but that nonetheless have a crucial impact on the overall preparedness levels of the country.

Although their implementation might not be the mandate of the health sector, they are important to consider when planning and evaluating the health sector emergency preparedness activities. Some of these indicators point to key areas of intersectoral coordination and collaboration, and highlight the importance of including public health concerns in areas such as national emergency planning, capacity building, and community disaster mitigation.

The last tool in the benchmarks framework is a checklist that consists of pertinent questions for each standard that can help guide analysis of the existing situation.

The questions predominantly relate to health sector issues, but also refer to important factors outside the health sector when the absence or presence of these is a potentially determining factor for the overall vulnerabilities and capacities of the national and local systems.

Use of the benchmarks

Other partners are increasingly looking to the SEAR benchmarks. In May 2007, Yale New Haven Center for Emergency Preparedness and Disaster Response (YNH-CEPDR), the Joint Commission, the Pan American Health Organization (PAHO), and the University of Wisconsin, Department of Surgery/World Association for Disaster and Emergency Medicine (WADEM) used six of the benchmarks as the basis for discussion during a workshop on 'The Safe and Resilient Hospitals: Preparing for the Next Disaster'.

The emergency preparedness and response programme in the WHO Regional Office for Europe is planning to introduce the benchmarks as part of the framework of upcoming country assessments of health security capacities. In the initial phase, assessments are planned for three countries (Armenia, Azerbaijan, and either Ukraine or Georgia).

The IHR and the SEAR benchmark frameworks are new tools to measure the progress in improving emergency preparedness and response in more complex contexts that we live in and in which emergencies occur.

References

Advisory Committee on the International Decade for Natural Hazard Reduction (1987). *Confronting natural disasters: an international decade for natural hazard reduction*. Washington DC: National Academy Press.

Anderson, M.B. (1991). Which costs more: prevention or recovery? In *Managing natural disasters and the environment* (eds. A. Kreimer and M. Munasinghe). World Bank, Washington DC.

Armenian, H.K. (1986). Wartime: options for epidemiology. *American Journal of Epidemiology*, July, **124**(1), 28–32.

Berz, G. (1984). Research and statistics on natural disasters in insurance and reinsurance companies. *The Geneva Papers on Risk and Insurance*, **9**, 135–57.

Binder, S. and Sanderson, L.M. (1987). The role of epidemiologist in natural disasters. *Annals of Emergency Medicine*, September, **16**(9), 1081–4.

Blendon, R.J., Benson J.M., DesRoches C.M., Lyon-Daniel K., Mitchell E.W., Pollard W.E. *et al.* (2007). The public's preparedness for hurricanes in four affected regions. *Public Health Reports*, March–April, **122**(2), 167–76.

Center for Research on the Epidemiology of Disasters (2007). *Report of CRED 2007*. Brussels.

Cuny, F.C. (1993). Introduction to disaster management. Lesson 5: technologies of disaster management. *Journal of Prehospital and Disaster Medicine*, **6**, 372–4.

Cuny, F.C., Abrams, S., and America, O. (1983). *Disasters and development*. Oxford University Press, New York.

Godschalk, D.R. *et al.* (1999). *Natural hazard mitigation: recasting disaster policy and planning*. Island Press, Washingon DC.

Goel, S.L. (2006). *Encyclopedia of disaster management*. Vol. 1 – Disaster management policy and administration). Deep and Deep Publications, New Delhi.

Guha-Sapir, D. and Lechat, M.F. (1986a). Information systems and needs assessment in natural disasters: an approach for better disaster relief management. *Disasters*, **10**(3), 232–7.

Guha-Sapir, D. and Lechat, M.F. (1986b). Reducing the impact of natural disasters: why aren't we better prepared? *Health Policy and Planning*, **1**(2), 118–26.

Herbert, R. *et al.* (2006). The World Trade Center disaster and the health of workers: five-year assessment of a unique medical screening program. *Environmental Health Perspectives*, December, **114**(12), 1853–8.

IDNDR Promotion Office (1994). *Natural disasters in the world: statistical trends on natural disasters*. National Land Agency, Tokyo.

International Federation of the Red Cross and Crescent Societies (2006). *World disasters report – focus on neglected crises*. International Federation of Red Cross and Red Crescent Societies. Geneva.

International Strategy for Disaster Reduction (2003). Glossary. Geneva. Availabale at http://www.unisdr.org/eng/public_aware/world_camp/2003/english/5_Glossary_eng.pdf, accessed 13 September 2007).

Kohl, P.A. *et al.* (2005). The Sumatra–Andaman Earthquake and Tsunami of 2004: the hazards, events, and damage. *Prehospital and Disaster Medicine*, November–December, **20**(6), 355–63.

Laverick, S. *et al.* (2007). Asian earthquake: report from the first volunteer British hospital team in Pakistan. *Emergency Medical Journal*, August, **24**(8), 543–6.

Lechat, M.F. (1990). Updates: the epidemiology of health effects of disasters. *Epidemiologic Reviews*, **12**(1), 192–7.

Mas Bermejo, P. (2006). Preparation and response in case of natural disasters: Cuban programs and experience. *Journal of Public Health Policy*, **27**(1), 13–21.

Noji, E.K. (1997). *The public health consequences of disasters*. Oxford University Press, New York.

Office of US Foreign Disaster Assistance (1995). *Disaster history: significant data on major disaster worldwide, 1900-present*. Agency for International Development, Washington DC.

Pan American Health Organization (1982). *Epidemiologic surveillance after natural disaster*. PAHO, Washington DC.

Pan American Health Organization (1983). *Health services organization in the event of disaster*. PAHO, Washington DC.

Ruijten, M. (2007). The Dutch experience with health impact assessment of disasters. *European Journal of Public Health*, February, **17**(1), 5–6.

Russell, D. and Saunders, P. (2007). The UK experience with Health Impact Assessment of disasters. *European Journal of Public Health*, February, **17**(1), 4–5.

Rutherford, W.H. *et al.* (1983). The definition and classification of disasters. *Injury*, July, **15**(1), 10–2.

Sardon, J.P. (2007). The 2003 heat wave. *Euro Surveillance*, March 1, **12**(3), 226.

Seaman, J. *et al.* (1984). *Epidemiology of natural disasters*. Karger, New York.

Shah, B.V. (1983). Is the environment becoming more hazardous? A Global survey 1947–1980. *Disasters*, **7**, 202–9.

Shaw, R. *et al.* (2004). From disaster to sustainable civil society: the Kobe experience. *Disasters*, March, **28**(1), 16–40.

United Nations Department of Economic and Social Affairs (1996). *International Decade for Natural Disaster Reduction*. Resolution 196/45 at 52nd plenary meeting, 26 July 1996. Available at http://www.un.org/documents/ecosoc/res/1996/eres1996-45.htm accessed 1 September 2007).

Verger, P. *et al.* (2007). French experiences with Health Impact Assessment of disasters. *European Journal of Public Health*, **17**(1), 3–4.

World Health Organization (1986). Communicable diseases after natural disasters. *Weekly Epidemiological Record*, **11**(14), 79–81.

World Health Organization (2005). *Communicable disease toolkit for tsunami affected areas: surveillance system for emergency phase*. Geneva.

World Health Organization (2006). *International health regulations (2005)*. Geneva.

World Health Organization (2007). *The world health report 2007: a safer future: global public health security in the 21st century*. Geneva.

World Health Organization, Regional Office for South-East Asia (2006). *Health Aspects of Emergency Preparedness and Response: Report of the Regional Meeting Bangkok, 21–23 November 2005*, New Delhi. Document SEA/EHA/13.

World Health Organization, Regional Office for South-East Asia (2007a). *Emergency preparedness and response: from lessons to action: report of the regional consultation, Bali, Indonesia, 27–29 June 2006*, New Delhi. Document SEA/Dis. Prep/3.

World Health Organization, Regional Office for South-East Asia (2007b). *Benchmarking emergency preparedness: Emergency & humanitarian action*, New Delhi: p. 8. Available at http://www.searo.who.int/LinkFiles/EHA_BenchmarkingEPP_Aug07.pdf accessed 1 September 2007).

12.13

Private support of public health

Roger Detels and Sheena G. Sullivan

Abstract

Although private funding of health initiatives has existed for some time, in recent years, private investment in health, particularly in developing countries, has increased considerably and has often resulted in improvements in health and alleviation of suffering. However, the donation of large sums of money to address one or a handful of health problems can have, and has occasionally had, unintended repercussions in developing nations. Left unchecked, cause-specific funding may undermine the public health systems of these countries, rather than improving them. The purpose of this chapter is to present the positive and negative aspects of private funding of public health and to make suggestions to minimize the harmful unintended negative impacts and to maximize positive outcomes of donor investments in public health.

History

The late twentieth and early twenty-first centuries have witnessed a huge influx of private support for public health as exemplified by generous gifts from the Bill and Melinda Gates Foundations, Warren Buffett, the William Clinton Foundation, the Carter Center, the Wellcome Trust, industry, professional and non-governmental organizations, and others. However, such generous giving, especially by Americans, actually dates back to the formation of the original foundations in the earliest years of the twentieth century. The earliest foundation in the United States was the Russell Sage Foundation founded in 1906, which had a limited focus on working women and social ills. The establishment of the large, broadly focused foundations began with the founding of the Carnegie Foundation by Andrew Carnegie in 1911 'to do real and permanent good in this world' (Carnegie Foundation 2007) followed by the founding of the Rockefeller Foundation in 1913 (Rockefeller Foundation 2007).

These early gifts had a significant impact on public health. The Rockefeller Foundation, for example, founded the International Health Commission in its first year. This was the first appropriation of funds by private sources for international public health activities and has helped 52 countries on 6 continents and 29 islands to improve their public health systems. In the same year, the Foundation began 20 years of support for the *Bureau of Social Hygiene* which focused on research and education on birth control, maternal health and sex education. Moreover, they played a key role in founding the world's first schools of public health, first at Johns Hopkins, then at Harvard and later in other parts of the United States, as well as in 21 foreign countries. Overseas, they helped to establish the London School of Tropical Medicine and Hygiene with a large gift in 1921, as well as the China Medical Board (1914) and the Peking Union Medical College (1921), both of the latter having played a significant role in the development of public health in China.

Since the establishment of these early foundations, the culture of donation to support public health has increased, particularly in recent years. Now, there are over 40 major foundations based in both the United States and abroad (see Table 12.13.1), as well as countless smaller ones. This increase can be attributed in part to at least two phenomena: The AIDS epidemic and the rise in public pressure for corporate social responsibility.

AIDS and the new culture of donation

With the discovery of therapy that could control the progression of HIV disease came the recognition, strongly expressed at the International AIDS Meeting in 1996, that millions of people, especially in developing countries, were being denied access to treatment because of the cost of the drugs. This realization spurred a tripling of funding for international projects to provide treatment for HIV/AIDS and to address the problems of malaria and tuberculosis, two of the major diseases responsible for loss of life and disability internationally. The increased funding was led by the Global Fund to Fight AIDS, Tuberculosis and Malaria (GFATM 2007) and the Bill and Melinda Gates Foundation (Bill and Melinda Gates Foundation 2007) which by 2006 had total assets of US$33.7 billion, more than the total budget of many developing countries. Every year, the Gates Foundation gives away approximately US$800 million approaching the total budget of the World Health Organization and equivalent to the budget for fighting infectious diseases given by the US Agency for International Development. The commitment of the Gates Foundation stimulated additional large donations by Warren Buffett and the William Clinton Foundation.

Corporate social responsibility (CSR) and public–private partnerships

Concurrent with these increases in funding for health has been the rise of CSR. Although corporations are required to abide by certain laws and regulations to reduce any adverse consequences of their

Table 12.13.1 Wealthiest foundations globally

	US$ (billion)
Canada	
The MasterCard Foundation of Toronto, Ontario	2.2
Denmark	
Realdania of Copenhagen	5.6
A.P. Møller og Hustru Chastine Mc-Kinney Møllers Fond til almene Formaal of Copenhagen ca	1.5
Carlsberg Foundation of Copenhagen	1.4
Germany	
Robert Bosch Foundation	6
Landesstiftung Baden-Württemberg	3.3
Volkswagen Foundation	2.7
Deutsche Bundesstiftung Umwelt	2.1
Liechtenstein	
Onassis Foundation of Vaduz, Liechtenstein	2.1
The Netherlands	
Stichting INGKA Foundation	>36
Norway	
Sparebankstiftelsen DnB NOR of Oslo	1.8
Institusjonen Fritt Ord of Oslo	0.4
Cultiva—Kristiansand Kommunes Energiverksstiftelse of Kristiansand	0.3
UNIFOR—Foundation of the University of Oslo of Oslo	0.2
Spain	
La Caixa	0.32
Sweden	
Knut and Alice Wallenberg Foundation of Stockholm	3.9
Nobel Foundation of Stockholm	0.4
United Kingdom (according to Charities Direct)	
Wellcome Trust of London	26.57
The Church Commissioners for England	8.32
Garfield Weston Foundation	6.94
The Leverhulme Trust	2.12
Esmée Fairbairn Foundation	1.82
The National Trust	1.66
Bridge House Trust	1.46
The Henry Smith Charity	1.4
Wolfson Foundation of London	1.32
Whitgift Foundation	0.51
Nuffield Foundation	0.5
Joseph Rowntree Foundation	0.48
United States (according to Foundation Center)	
Bill & Melinda Gates Foundation (WA)	33.12
The Ford Foundation (NY)	13.66
J. Paul Getty Trust (CA)	10.13
The Robert Wood Johnson Foundation (NJ)	10.09
The William and Flora Hewlett Foundation (CA)	8.52
W.K. Kellogg Foundation (MI)	8.40
Lilly Endowment Inc. (IN)	7.60
The David and Lucile Packard Foundation (CA)	6.35
John D. and Catherine T. MacArthur Foundation (IL)	6.18
The Andrew W. Mellon Foundation (NY)	6.13
Gordon and Betty Moore Foundation (CA)	5.84
The California Endowment (CA)	4.41
The Rockefeller Foundation (NY)	3.81
The Kresge Foundation (MI)	3.33
The Starr Foundation (NY)	3.30
The Annie E. Casey Foundation (MD)	3.27
The Duke Endowment (NC)	2.98
The Annenberg Foundation (PA)	2.68
Charles Stewart Mott Foundation (MI)	2.63
Carnegie Corporation of New York (NY)	2.53
Casey Family Programs (WA)	2.49
John S. and James L. Knight Foundation (FL)	2.34
The Harry and Jeanette Weinberg Foundation, Inc. (MD)	2.27
Tulsa Community Foundation (OK)	2.26
Robert W. Woodruff Foundation, Inc. (GA)	2.25
The McKnight Foundation (MN)	2.21
Richard King Mellon Foundation (PA)	2.08
Ewing Marion Kauffman Foundation (MO)	2.07
The New York Community Trust (NY)	2.04
Doris Duke Charitable Foundation (NY)	1.95
India	
Tata Trusts	

businesses, CSR takes this concept further to encourage corporations to take actions to improve the quality of life of their employees and their families, customers, stakeholders, and the community in general (WBCSD 2000). As part of the Millennium Development Goals (UN 2008), corporations, especially large multinationals, are encouraged to increase their awareness of their impact on the societies in which they operate. Many corporations have since established a CSR division to run social programmes. For example, the Standard Chartered Bank, recognizing the need to maintain a stable and healthy workforce, has an extensive HIV/AIDS programme to provide healthcare and support for staff and their families affected by HIV/AIDS in Africa (Standard Chartered 2006).

General CSR programmes may include production of healthful foods, design and manufacturing of low-emission vehicles with higher standards of safety, improvement of the work environment of workers, control of industrial waste, etc.

In addition, corporations, particularly pharmaceutical companies, have been increasingly signing public–private partnerships. These are generally joint ventures between private industry, government, or international agencies such as the WHO or UN agencies, and civil society including universities or NGOs to achieve a shared health objective (Widdus 2005). There were more than 90 international partnerships in health in 2004 (Nishtar 2004). The majority address infectious diseases, notably AIDS, TB, and malaria. Some involve individual governments or NGOs or both forming an alliance with the for-profit sector. For example, Sanofi-Aventis has an extensive international programme of humanitarian sponsorship, including a partnership with the Nelson Mandela Foundation and the South African Department of Health to provide free tuberculosis treatment in areas badly affected within South Africa (Sanofi-Aventis 2008). Other partnerships may involve many players. The most notable are the global health alliances, such as the Global Alliance for Vaccines and Immunizations, Roll Back Malaria, the Stop TB partnership, the Global Polio Eradication Program, and the International AIDS Vaccine Alliance. They may be principally driven by a company, be legally independent, or hosted by a civil society organization (Nishtar 2004). Stop TB, for example, comprises a network of more than 500 partners, including governments of both developed and developing countries, research and technical health institutes, multilateral organizations, civil society, pharmaceutical companies and other industry partners and is housed within the WHO (Stop TB 2007).

Examples of private support

Private support of public health, given by foundations, industry, pharmaceutical companies, and professional organizations has been directed towards disease control and treatment, poverty alleviation, education, training of health workers, infrastructure development, research, improved agricultural practices, health information dissemination, and sponsorship of the many global health alliances.

Specific examples include the provision of drugs and the reduction of drug prices for developing countries, the earliest example being the Metzican Donation Program by Merck & Co. Inc. for treatment for onchocerciasis (river blindness) in West Africa in 1988 (Mectizan 2008). In 1998, GlaxoSmithKline provided albendazole for treatment of lymphatic filiarisis as part of the Mectizan programme. To date, this ongoing programme has reached more than 40 million people (Mectizan 2008).

Another major contribution has been the establishment of special training programmes and scholarships/fellowships for training health personnel. Many foundations are set up for this purpose alone or as part of a broader portfolio. For example, the Robert Wood Johnson Foundation has a clinical scholars programme for US students (Robert Wood Johnson Foundation 2008). Additionally, foundations may provide gifts to schools, such as equipment or teaching resources.

Another important contribution of private agencies has been to research. The Hughes Medical Institute, for example, was established by Hughes Aviation to conduct research into human illness (HHMI 2008) (although the motivation for doing so has been attributed to tax evasion rather than philanthropy; Wikipedia 2008). The Gates Foundation currently supports a large number of research projects related to HIV prevention strategies including vaccine and microbicide development. There are also the very significant contributions made by pharmaceutical companies to the research and development of vaccines and treatments, both independently and in public–private partnerships. Increasingly, these efforts are focusing on the so-called 'neglected diseases' that disproportionately affect the world's poorest nations.

Industry is realizing that improving the health of the public is in their best interest in the long run. These generous gifts and actions have unquestionably had a very significant impact on the growth of public health in the twentieth century and played a significant role in shaping the character and missions of public health. For these significant contributions to 'promote the well-being of mankind throughout the world', they are to be commended (Rockefeller Foundation Charter 1913).

Unforeseen problems

Many of these very generous gifts have benefited the recipient countries enormously and have achieved goals which otherwise would have been impossible to achieve. There is no question that the recent surge in international giving, which shows no signs of slowing, is a positive step towards reducing the disparities between the rich and poor countries and benefiting all mankind. Why, then, have there been critics of this surge in generosity?

From the beginning, the foundations have determined their goals for giving based on the personal perspectives of their founders and subsequent leaders. Often, they did not consult public health leaders in determining these goals. This strategy has the risk of distorting the public health agenda with the influx of large sums of money, which often dwarfs the national budgets of the recipient countries and cannot be matched by the local government. This presents a myriad of problems for these countries.

First, their public health agenda is being determined by outside agencies. This agenda may not coincide with the country's needs, and may deplete existing resources, especially trained personnel. When a huge donor driven programme is established, it must rapidly acquire an infrastructure for its management. Programmes will often attract qualified personnel by providing higher salaries than can realistically be provided by local government agencies. Thus, much of the staff is drawn from the existing public health infrastructure, leaving fewer staff within government to work on other health priorities. The result—the goals of the donors are met, but at the expense of the country's health system resulting in deterioration of other important public health programmes and exacerbating the existing public health human resource crisis extant in most developing countries. For example, in Haiti, the dramatically improved HIV/AIDS situation has paralleled a decline in other measures of the population's health, including infant mortality (Farmer & Garrett 2006).

Second, the governments, in many developing countries, have invested little of their funds, often less than 5 per cent, in health. Large infusions of donor funds allow these countries to continue to underfund health. Kwame Ampomah, a Ghanaian with the UNAIDS programme in Gaborone, Botswana, asserts that 'you need a clear health system with equity that is not donor-driven' (Garrett 2007).

The influx of huge sum of money can also contribute to corruption, inflation, and destabilization of the economy. In countries with entrenched bureaucracies and rampant corruption, the donor funds may not all be used for implementation of public health programmes. In the absence of any evaluation to measure the benefits of a programme or any auditing to account for spending, donations may simply serve to exacerbate corruption and bureaucracy. In addition, increasing the salaries of some, especially government officials, can widen the rich–poor gap and generate inflation (Garrett 2007).

Further, programmes that appear acceptable to the Western intellect may not be culturally acceptable to people of other countries. For example, family-planning programmes, in order to be successful, had to demonstrate that smaller families meant increased survival for the children and an increased probability that parents would have a viable male to support them in their old age.

Sustainability

The donation of large sums of money to tackle specific health problems does not lend itself to a sustainable solution. For example, the Gates Foundation now provides 17 per cent of the global budget (US$86 million) to eradicate poliomyelitis and also supports vaccine programmes for HIV/AIDS, Japanese encephalitis, and other diseases, as well as research in HIV/AIDS, particularly towards development of female-controlled interventions. In an effort to assist women to become more independent, the foundation has given money to the Grameen Foundation, whose founder recently received the Nobel Peace Prize. With the Rockefeller Foundation, the Gates Foundation has also provided funds to support improved agricultural practices in developing countries. But, when Gates' and other donor monies are discontinued, are these programmes going to be sustained by the local governments which do not have the resources of these large donors?

Currently, massive funding is being injected to provide treatment for HIV/AIDS to those in need, but it is likely that other major health problems will occur in the future which will divert donors' attention away from HIV/AIDS. The countries now receiving these massive infusions of money for treatment programmes for HIV/AIDS patients will not be able to sustain them. Thus, it is unclear what the long-term impact of the huge influx of funds will be on HIV/AIDS. A larger investment in prevention may have a more long-lasting benefit, but currently the majority of donors have concentrated their funds on treatment with little allocated to prevention, in part because it is difficult to show immediate outcomes with prevention.

The implementation of demonstration/pilot projects needs to consider whether the projects can be sustained by the local government if they are demonstrated to be effective, and whether it will be feasible to upscale the project to the point where it will have a significant impact on the health of the country. Often, outside support to maintain a programme is provided without seeking in-country solutions to supply issues, and there is a focus on treatment rather than prevention. In the case of pharmaceuticals, for example, the solution is usually to help countries find cheap avenues for importing drugs, rather than helping them to establish their own pharmaceutical plants to manufacture generic medicines. By supporting development of local industries, donor money can have an impact that reaches far beyond health.

Reliance on imported pharmaceuticals has very real risks for disease control. Cessation of an externally funded programme, including the drug supply, can lead to the resurgence of disease, as was the case in Uganda when sleeping sickness quickly resurfaced once control had apparently been achieved and the project staff withdrew (Widdus 2005). Irregular supply or inadequate storage facilities, both common in developing countries, can lead to treatment failure and subsequent resistance to medications. Simple mismanagement of programmes has also had serious adverse consequences—such as the reckless provision of TB therapy without adequate medical supervision in KwaZulu Natal, which has led to the evolution of the most drug-resistant strains of the mycobacteria (Garrett 2007). Ironically, by providing quick fixes to a problem, some foundations are doing what medicine has long known as unsustainable—treating symptoms without preventing the cause!

Coordination

In some countries, there are so many donors, each targeting their own agendas, that the country's public health professionals are not aware of all the programmes being conducted in their country. Without this information for coordination, national programmes may be duplicating donor programmes while other urgent needs may be unmet. This lack of coordination is exacerbated in countries where the donors feel that the government is corrupt and therefore bypass it. In developed countries, governments that have played a central role in funding health have had better control over growth and may lead to a more efficient health service (Navarro 1985). Thus, external investment in a country's health should prioritize partnering with, improving and supporting existing public infrastructures, and should recognize that a country's elected government may be able to judge its health priorities better than an external organization based in a rich country (Widdus 2003). Donors may also bypass established health authorities who work closely with governments to determine priorities, such as the WHO, which undermines their role in international health and fractures the system further.

For HIV/AIDS, at least, UN agencies have overseen the development of the 'Three Ones' agreement: *One* agreed-upon HIV/AIDS action framework that provides the basis for coordinating the work of all partners; *one* national AIDS coordinating authority, with a broad based multi-sector mandate; and *one* consensus for country-level monitoring and evaluation system (WHO 2004). Similar agreements are needed for donor-supported health projects in general. China provides a unique example of how government authoritarianism has helped achieve this kind of coordination. Although it was motivated by a different purpose, China insists that large donor agencies have government approval before being allowed to work in-country, and thus, the relevant officials have been able to have a direct role in deciding where and how donor money should be channelled.

Dubious motives

Because of charitable tax deductions by the US government, the foundations are able to reduce their tax burden by as much as 25 per cent. The *New York Times* has estimated that charitable deductions cost the US government US$40 billion in lost tax revenue in 2006 (Strom 2007). Thus, to some extent, the foundations, not the US government, are determining where public health funds are spent. Recognizing this fact, Eli Broad, one of the major donors, has said that, 'What smart entrepreneurial philanthropists and their foundations do is get greater value for how they invest their money than if the government were doing it' (*The New York Times*, September 6, 2007). Not everyone would agree with him. Foundations often determine their targets and objectives on emotional grounds rather than an objective assessment of international and national need.

It is well to remember that the founders of many of these large foundations or organizations obtained their massive wealth though questionable business and labour practices—exploitation of the very public that these foundations strive to serve! Thus, it is not surprising that the motives of these organizations are viewed with suspicion (Reich 2000). Several of the large foundations have been criticized because they obtained their funds through questionable business practices and currently derive some of their income from investments that negatively impact the public and the environment (*Los Angeles Times*, January 7, 2007, January 8, 2007). Thus, they help the public with one hand while harming it with the other.

Recommendations

Clearly, the generous giving of the foundations, industry, and private donors has benefited public health greatly. Nonetheless, they have sometimes also had unintended negative consequences. How can the behaviour of the foundations and other donors be modified to maximize the positive impact and minimize the negative? Several changes, suggested below, may contribute to this goal:

- Careful objective assessment of the goals of the foundation *vis-a-vis* the needs of the proposed recipient countries
- Consultation with health leaders of the recipient countries and the World Health Organization on the health priorities/needs of the recipient countries
- Consideration of the impact that the infusion of money and the programme will have on the existing public health structure and economy of the country
- Strengthening the existing national and local public health infrastructures by incorporating foundation programmes into the existing public health system
- Periodic evaluation of the impact of the donor's programmes by an objective group not affiliated with the donors, but including local expertise
- Establishment of advisory committees that include both international and local public health experts from developing countries and targeted areas
- Introducing ethical evaluations, as many universities currently do, in determining in which companies, institutions and commodities to invest, so that investment practices are not counter to the charitable goals of the donor/foundation. Investments in companies, etc. that negatively impact the health and quality of life of the public to make money to do good do not make sense
- Implementation of projects that can be sustained by the local governments when funding is discontinued
- Partnering with countries to contribute to the programmes in an effort to encourage countries to increase their investment in health
- Investment in local businesses to reduce reliance on external sources of health consumables
- Development of clear governance mechanisms, as well as transparent policies and procedural frameworks that facilitate monitoring and evaluation

Many of these recommendations have already been incorporated by the Global Fund to Fight AIDS, Tuberculosis and Malaria and other private donors. Private funding of public health has contributed greatly to the goals of public health. Let us hope that foundations, industry, and other private donors/agencies will continue to generously support public health in ways that will strengthen the public health structures, stability, and well-being of the recipient countries.

References

Bill and Melinda Gates Foundation. (2007). Available at www.gatesfoundation.org/aboutus/, www.gatesfoundation.org/GlobalHealth/, accessed October 2007.

Carnegie Corporation of New York. (2007). Available at http://www.carnegie.org/, accessed October 2007.

Farmer, P., and Garrett, L. (2007). From "marvellous momentum" to health care for all: success is possible with the right programs. *Foreign Affairs*, March/April. Available at http://fullaccess.foreignaffairs.org/20070301faresponse86213/paul-farmer-laurie-garrett/from-marvelous-momentum-to-health-care-for-all-success-is-possible-with-the-right-programs.html, accessed October 2008.

Garrett, L. (2007). The challenge of global health. *Foreign Affairs*, January/February. Available at http://fullaccess.foreignaffairs.org/arp/to_fullaccess?u=%2F20070101faessay86103%2Flaurie-garrett%2Fthe-challenge-of-global-health.html, accessed October 2008.

Global Fund to Fight AIDS, Tuberculosis and Malaria. (2007). Available at www.theglobalfund.org/en/about/record, accessed October 2007.

HHMI: Howard Hughes Medical Institute. (2008). Available at http://www.hhmi.org/, accessed January 2008.

Mectizan Donation Program. (2008). Available at http://www.mectizan.org/, accessed January 2008.

Navarro, V. (1985). The public/private mix in the funding and delivery of health services: an international survey. *American Journal of Public Health*, **75**, 1318–20.

Nishtar, S. (2004). Public–private partnerships in health – a global call to action. *Health Research Policy and Systems*, **2**, 5.

Pillar, C. (2007). Money clashes with mission. *Los Angeles Times*, January 8; Business.

Pillar, C., Sanders, E., and Dixon, R. (2007). Dark clouds over good works of Gates Foundation. *Los Angeles Times*, January 7; National.

Reich, M.R. (2000). Public–private partnerships for public health. *Nature Medicine*, **6**, 617–20.

Robert Wood Johnson Foundation. (2008). Available at http://www.rwjf.org/applications/m accessed January 2008.

Rockefeller Foundation Charter. (1913). Available at http://www.rockfound.org/about_us/Rockefeller_Foundation_Charter.pdf, accessed March 2008.

Rockefeller Foundation. (2007). Available at http://www.rockfound.org/aboutus/aboutus.shtml, accessed October 2007.

Sanofi-Aventis. (2008). *Sanofi-Aventis joins the fight against tuberculosis in South Africa*. http://en.sanofi-aventis.com/ethics_responsibilities/humanitarian_sponsorship/humanitarian_sponsorship.asp, accessed October 2008.

Sanofi-Aventis. (2006). *Humanitarian sponsorship*. http://en.sanofi-aventis.com/group/sponsorship/sponsorship_developpementproject.asp, accessed December 2007.

Standard Chartered. (2006). *Sustainability review 2006 leading the way in Asia, Africa and the Middle East*. Available at http://www.standardchartered.com/_documents/2006-sustainability-review/sc_2006_sustainabilityReview.pdf, accessed December 2007.

Stop TB. (2007). *Partnership*. Available at http://www.stoptb.org/stop_tb_initiative/, accessed December 2007.

Strom, S. (2007). Big gifts, tax breaks and a debate on charity. *New York Times*, September 6; Business.

UN. (2008). *The millennium development goals*. Available at http://www.un.org/millenniumgoals/, accessed January 2008.

WBCSD. (2000). *Corporate social responsibility: making good business sense*. World Business Council for Sustainable Development. Available at http://www.wbcsd.org/web/publications/csr2000.pdf, accessed October 2008.

WHO. (2004). *"Three Ones" agreed by donors and developing countries*. Available at http://www.who.int/3by5/newsitem9/en/, accessed December 2007.

Widdus, R. (2003). Public–private partnerships for health require thoughtful evaluation. *Bulletin of the World Health Organization*, **81**, 235–6.

Widdus, R. (2005). Public–private partnerships: an overview. *Transactions of the Royal Society of Tropical Medicine and Hygiene*, **995**, S1–8.

Wikipedia. (2008). *Howard Hughes*. http://en.wikipedia.org/wiki/Howard_Hughes, accessed January 2008.

12.14

Global health agenda for the twenty-first century

Adrian Ong, Mary Kindhauser, Ian Smith, and Margaret Chan

Introduction

... the preservation of health is ... without doubt the first good and the foundation of all the other goods of this life.

(*René Descartes,* Discours de la méthode, *1637*)

The right to the highest attainable level of health is enshrined in the charter of the World Health Organization (WHO) (2002a) and many international treaties. It is this aspiration that spurs the work of the Organization and frames the broader global public health agenda for the twenty-first century. It is a tall order. But the right to health is more important today than ever before given the dramatic evolution in the architecture of global public health and the growing prominence of health within the human security, rights, and development agendas.

The past century had witnessed remarkable gains in health, rapid economic growth, and unprecedented scientific advances. These advances have led to major improvements in health care in which millions more lives are protected than ever before. Life expectancy at birth has continued to rise, by almost 8 years between 1950 and 1978, and 7 more years since (WHO 2007c). These transformations are unmatched in history.

Yet, in spite of this optimistic outlook, the international community faces a demanding health agenda. Many public health problems, both new and old, remain to be solved. Despite progress, nearly 2.6 billion people, especially in fragile states, remain in extreme poverty and live on less than US$2 a day. Nearly 10 million children die before their fifth birthday, with approximately four million of these deaths occurring during the neonatal period (UNICEF 2007). Nutrition is a major problem with one-third of all children in developing countries underweight or stunted; half the people in developing countries lack access to improved sanitation (World Bank 2007a). Health inequalities are growing wider between and within countries, between rich and poor, between men and women, and between different ethnic groups.

These stark numbers reinforce the urgent need for collective global action. The United Nations Millennium Declaration in 2000 committed states to a global partnership to reduce poverty, improve health and education, and promote peace, human rights, gender equality, and environmental sustainability by 2015 (UN 2000). These Millennium Development Goals (MDGs) establish health as a key driver of socioeconomic progress. In so doing, they elevate the status of health within the development agenda and recognize the two-way, though uneven, link between poverty and health. Poverty contributes to poor health, and poor health anchors large numbers of people in poverty. In all countries, poverty is associated with high childhood and maternal mortality, malnutrition, and increased exposure to infectious diseases as well as chronic diseases such as cardiovascular diseases, diabetes, and cancer.

Investments in health must thus work to reduce poverty, ensure the poor have access to health care, and prevent economic ruin as a result of high health expenditures. As the world around us is becoming progressively interconnected and complex, human health is contingent on the integrated outcome of ecological, sociocultural, economic, and institutional determinants. It is increasingly recognized, also in the Millennium Declaration, that broad intersectoral action in tackling these determinants of health is needed to achieve significant and more durable health gains, especially for the poor.

This chapter lays out, in three sections, a strategy and agenda for global public health by assessing the current context, challenges and opportunities in the global health landscape. Many of the issues highlighted are not new. The first section examines current global health problems and the challenges they present. It reviews the revolution in health spurred, in part, by demographic transitions in societies and by globalization and its related nutritional and behavioural transitions. The second section analyses the impediments to scaling up health service delivery and improving access to care. Building upon these lessons and issues, the final section outlines the fundamental principles and means by which health systems can meet the challenges of the twenty-first century.

The evolving global health landscape

The issues and actors in global health today are myriad and complex. Shaped by the potent forces of globalization, demographic changes and emergent diseases, the agenda for health has never been more challenging nor more pressing. This section surveys current trends and phenomena in international health that meaningfully impact the public health agenda for the new century.

Health within the larger human context

Health in its own right is of fundamental importance and, like education, is among the basic capabilities that give value to human life (Sen & Sen 1999). It is an intrinsic right as well as a central input to poverty reduction and socioeconomic development. Health-related human rights are core values within the United Nations and WHO, and are endorsed in numerous international and regional human rights instruments. They are intimately related to and dependent on the provision and realization of other social and economic human rights such as those of food, housing, work, and education. Appreciation of this defining value underscores all efforts to provide equitable health care for all.

Health is also a central element of human security. The WHO Constitution defines health as a state of complete physical, mental and social well-being and not merely the absence of disease or infirmity (2002a). Humanitarian emergencies, including natural and human-made disasters, outbreaks of epidemic-prone diseases, conflicts and complex emergencies, constitute what has traditionally been considered the main threat to health security worldwide. However, wider considerations of human security, with the individual as a focus, also encompass issues of safe food and water, adequate shelter, clean air, poverty-related threats, violence, and the adverse effects of climate change on health (Ogata & Sen 2003). Strengthening the capacity of health and related sectors and improving international coordination can effectively contribute to reducing avoidable morbidity and mortality resulting from these threats to health security.

The pace of global economic integration has accelerated over the past decade, dramatically transforming the world's economic and political landscape. Globalization, with its remarkable acceleration of trade, knowledge, and resource flows, offers unprecedented promise for improving human health. Many experts assumed that as economic conditions within a country improved, health would improve accordingly through income growth, poverty alleviation and the broader availability of health and other social services.

Yet, to date, globalization has had a complex influence on health and results have been uneven. Opinions differ with regard to the economic benefits of globalization and its impact on poverty and health. Some have argued that income inequality has not widened and that the higher growth rates that follow market integration in developing countries have benefited the poor (Ben-David 2000; Dollar 2001; Dollar & Kraay 2002). Others hold that the economic benefits of recent globalization have been largely asymmetrical, creating among countries and within populations, beneficiaries, losers, and growing inequalities between the two with consequent effects on health (Mazur 2000; Wade 2004; Globalization Knowledge Network 2007).

Globalization may thus create wealth but has no rules that guarantee its fair distribution. Economic growth per se does not ensure equitable health improvement for all. Rather, action within and between countries to mitigate and remove structural inequality is the necessary counterpart to worldwide growth itself and the policies that aim to support it (Marmot 2007). New governance policies structured around equity, distributive fairness, and social justice should be strengthened to minimize the negative externalities of global integration.

A changing world

Populations of the world are experiencing unprecedented demographic change. There are three billion more people today than there were in 1960. Another 2.5 billion will likely be added by 2050 based on mid-range population estimates (UN 2008).

Behind these numbers lie other important demographic trends common to many countries. Women are bearing fewer children, people are living longer and healthier lives, populations are aging, and increasing numbers of migrants are moving from villages to cities and from one country to another in search of better opportunities (UN 2008). A sharp contrast exists between the poorest nations with their rapidly growing and young populations, and the more demographically advanced and richer nations with near zero population growth and aging populations.

In populations with increasing life expectancy, the number and proportion of people reaching old age has risen throughout the world. Every month, one million people worldwide reach the age of 60 years. Of these, 80 per cent live in the developing world (WHO 2006c). Also with improved public health, more children are now surviving into adolescence and adulthood. One in every five people in the world is an adolescent. Out of 1.2 billion adolescents worldwide, about 85 per cent live in developing countries and the remainder live in the industrialized world (UN 2008).

This growth in human numbers is already leading to greater demand for food, water, energy and other natural resources. Importantly, the demographic heterogeneity and transition strongly impacts priorities and resources required to meet the shifting health needs of populations.

Each age category of persons faces a differing burden and nature of diseases. Many adolescents suffer premature deaths arising through accidents (including road crashes), suicide, violence, pregnancy-related complications, and other illnesses. They are exposed to tobacco-related diseases, harmful use of alcohol, substance abuse, sexually transmitted infections, unwanted pregnancy, and other health problems related to behaviour. Every year, an estimated 1.7 million young men and women between the ages of 10 and 19 lose their lives to preventable or treatable causes (WHO 2002b).

In many developing countries, the speed of modernization has outpaced the ability of governments to provide the necessary supporting infrastructures. Road traffic injuries are a growing public health issue, disproportionately affecting the poor and persons in the most economically productive age group. Such events kill an estimated 1.2 million people annually and injure as many as 5.2 million. Over 70 per cent of road traffic fatalities are under 45 years of age (Peden *et al.* 2004).

Maternal mortality has remained virtually unchanged for the past 20 years. Each year, more than half a million women die from complications of pregnancy and child-birth (Hill *et al.* 2008). Developing countries account for almost all of maternal deaths. The greatest burden is felt in sub-Saharan Africa, where more than half of all maternal deaths occur; in these countries, a woman is 100 times more likely to die from complications of pregnancy than a woman in the industrialized world. Underlying many of these deaths is the poor availability of health services. Seven in ten of all maternal deaths are estimated to arise from complications requiring emergency obstetric services. Yet, access to these services in many developing countries is limited, making improving health systems and access to assistance from trained attendants during birth imperative for reducing maternal mortality.

Addressing chronic diseases are another major challenge that now has global dimensions. Current demographic trends, together with deteriorating environmental conditions, unhealthy lifestyles and improper nutrition, has led to a rise in non-communicable or chronic diseases, including mental and substance abuse disorders, and a subsequent demand for long-term medical care in many societies (WHO 2006c). In developing countries, this has created a second burden of disease alongside the continuing struggle to control infectious diseases and the HIV/AIDS epidemic.

While the proportion of burden from chronic diseases, including mental disorders, in adults in developed countries remains stable at over 80 per cent, the proportion in middle-income countries has already exceeded 70 per cent. Almost 50 per cent of the adult disease burden in the high-mortality regions of the world is now attributable to chronic diseases (WHO 2003b). The health impact of this 'risk' transition affects all countries, though the effects may be more severe in the developing world, where health services and social support systems are often inadequate to meet the rising needs.

A few common risk factors are responsible for a considerable proportion of the burden of chronic diseases. Attributable causes include improper diet, inadequate exercise, smoking, and excessive alcohol consumption. An intervention that addresses one of these risk factors can possibly reduce the risk for several diseases, thus giving special impetus for health promotion and disease prevention efforts in controlling chronic diseases. The long time lag between the development of high population levels of risk and the emergence of non-communicable disease epidemics, testifies to the importance of intervening now to control the major risk factors, especially in poorer countries where they tend to be neglected in the face of competing priorities.

Tobacco addiction is a global epidemic and remains the second major cause of death in the world, being currently responsible for about one in ten adult deaths—nearly five million deaths each year. By 2030, unless urgent action is taken, tobacco's annual death toll will rise to more than eight million (Mathers & Loncar 2006). Today, almost one in three adults of the global population smoke. Of these, almost 80 per cent live in low- and middle-income countries (WHO 2008c). Due to the increase in the global adult population, coupled with expanded marketing by the tobacco industry, the total number of smokers is expected to reach about 1.6 billion by 2025, making the negative economic and health implications of tobacco use simply staggering. This growth is being driven largely by the rise in tobacco use in low-income countries and, more ominously, among young persons, especially females, in highly-populous countries (WHO 2008c).

Similar disturbing trends are occurring in the area of nutrition. Changes in global dietary patterns involve the increasing consumption of fats, energy-dense and highly processed foods. The world faces in many ways a double burden of nutrition—the co-existence, often in the same country, of under-nutrition and over-nutrition, with both as leading determinants of morbidity and mortality.

The next few decades will also see an unprecedented escalation of urban growth. About half of the world's population now lives in urban areas (UN 2008). In developing countries, 43 per cent of the urban population lives in slums, and in the least developed countries, 78 per cent of urban residents are slum-dwellers, with 30 per cent of families headed by women.

The flow of migrants from villages to cities is so rapid that the population growth in the rural areas of the developing world has virtually stopped. As a result, most of the 3 billion people expected to be added to the world population in the future are going to be added to urban centres and shantytowns in developing countries, further aggravating already overburdened infrastructure and public services (UNFPA 2007). More disturbingly, this urban population growth will be composed to a large extent, of poor people (Garau *et al.* 2005), the needs of whom are often overlooked in urban planning.

The contribution of human activities to changes in the climate system is irrefutable. Increases in global average air and ocean temperatures, widespread melting of snow and ice, and rising global average sea levels are phenomena associated with the ongoing and accelerating warming of the climate system (Climate Change 2007). Climate change—possibly the defining issue of the new millennium—poses a significant addition to the spectrum of environmental health hazards faced by humankind. The impacts of climate on human health will not be evenly distributed around the world, with the impoverished populations of the developing world being the first and hardest hit (Confalonieri *et al.* 2007). It will affect, in profoundly adverse ways, the most basic determinants of health—air, water, food, shelter, and freedom from disease—and could vastly increase the current huge imbalance in health outcomes. The implications of climate variability for human health and security are far-reaching, effecting death and disease through heat waves, floods, droughts, and other extreme weather events. Yet, the greatest health impact may not come from such acute shocks, but from the indirect pressure on the natural, economic, and social systems that sustain health, many of which are already under stress in much of the developing world (Parry *et al.* 2007).

In recent years, there has been a notable rise in the supply and trade of counterfeit and substandard medicines, including useless and, in some cases, even toxic products (WHO 2006b). This is a vast and under-reported problem that particularly affects countries where regulatory and legal oversight is weakest; it is an important cause of unnecessary morbidity, mortality, and negatively impacts public confidence in medicines and the effectiveness of health programmes (Dondorp *et al.* 2004). The drugs most commonly counterfeited include antibiotics, anti-malarials, hormones, and steroids. Yet, increasingly, more sophisticated and deceptive practices have seen even anticancer and antiviral drugs, including those used to treat HIV/AIDS, being faked. It has been estimated that some 10–30 per cent of medicines on sale in developing countries, especially those in sub-Saharan Africa, are counterfeit (Cockburn *et al.* 2005). The impact of this exploitive and poorly regulated trade on health outcomes has been enormous.

Similarly, widespread and inappropriate use of antimicrobials has created high levels of drug resistance and a growing crisis in health care management. Mainstay antimicrobials are now failing at a rate that outpaces the development of replacement drugs (Heymann *et al.* 2001). Hospital-acquired infections with drug resistant organisms are a serious and mounting complication of hospitalization, contributing significantly to morbidity, mortality and health care costs. Formerly curable diseases such as gonorrhoea and typhoid are rapidly becoming difficult to treat, while old killers such as tuberculosis and malaria are now growing increasingly resistant to mainstay therapy (Smith & Coast 2002). Ominously, the emergence of multi-drug resistant tuberculosis, which is 100 times more expensive to treat than susceptible tuberculosis, and extensively drug-resistant tuberculosis, which is virtually impossible to treat, is jeopardizing current control and elimination efforts (Raviglione & Smith 2007). Drug resistance is a deepening and complex problem accelerated by the overuse of antibiotics in developed nations and the paradoxical underuse of quality antimicrobials in developing nations owing to poverty, trade in counterfeit medicines and a dearth of effective health care.

Communicable diseases, crises, and epidemics

Armed conflicts, epidemics, famine, natural disasters, and other major emergencies have a significant impact on populations and their health. Each year, one in five countries experiences a crisis, often overwhelming national capacities to mitigate and manage such emergencies. These complex humanitarian crises often arise unpredictably and cause untold suffering, population displacement and death. The dislocation of large populations creates immense public health challenges with regard to food, water, sanitation, shelter the risk of epidemics in already vulnerable groups of persons, and the provision of routine immunizations, care, and essential medicines.

New infectious diseases have been emerging at the unprecedented rate of about one a year for the past three decades, a trend that is expected to continue (Smolinski *et al.* 2003). The shrinking of the world by technology and economic interdependence has allowed diseases to spread with great speed. The dissemination of HIV/AIDS and SARS are just two contemporary examples.

Constant evolution is the survival mechanism of the microbial world, and these organisms are well equipped to exploit opportunities to adapt and spread. The opportunities are numerous: Through increased population movements via tourism, migration or disasters; growth in international trade in food and biological products; social and environmental changes linked with urbanization, deforestation and alterations in climate; advancement in medical procedures; and changes in animal husbandry and food production methods (Ong & Heymann 2007).

The free movement of goods, capital, and labour in an increasingly interconnected world facilitates the transnational spread of diseases and places all countries at common risk. However, the same globalizing forces that create such rampant opportunities for pathogens can also provide mechanisms for innovative, global efforts to control infectious diseases. Recognition of shared vulnerability to these diseases, and their often considerable economic consequences, has brought a strong global commitment to make their detection, reporting, control, and prevention a collaborative effort (WHO 2007b).

Health actors and partners

Globalization is eroding traditional distinctions between domestic and foreign affairs. The health of populations largely depends on health and welfare policies of national governments. Yet, growing internationalization, migration, and macroeconomic considerations are, to greater extents, influencing the policy space of national governments and their ability to sustain health and welfare policies for their constituencies. Increasingly, health determinants have become more multifaceted, complex and shaped by factors outside the control of the health sector.

Indeed, the framework of international health is no longer dominated by a few organizations, and now involves numerous players. Health activities are now being pursued by more than 40 bilateral donors, 26 UN agencies, 20 global and regional funds, and 90 global health initiatives (Alexander 2007). An increasing number of non-governmental, faith-based and private sector organizations are delivering care and complement the efforts of national health systems. New philanthropists have emerged, and fast-growing economies have become aid givers and international investors. Governments acting alone, or in international partnerships, have initiated programmes and made available new funding. The number of innovative funding mechanisms continues to grow, as does the size of resources they provide. In quantity, aid for health has almost tripled over 10 years and nearly doubled in the last 5 years (OECD 2007).

Public–private partnerships in the area of research are increasingly important, as they often focus on health needs otherwise neglected by market-driven forces. Academic, industrial, government and non-governmental research continue to shape the directions and use of knowledge acquisition. Industry, trade and finance are powerful drivers of research and development and a massive force in producing and distributing goods. They can also influence decisions on health policy.

In just the past 7 years, more than 100 partnerships, focused on individual diseases, have formed. In addition, the formation of public–private partnerships, often involving large donations of medicines, has marked a watershed, by bringing new actors, resources, business models and a sense of urgency to bear on neglected diseases. Partnerships focused on product access have proven remarkably effective in supplying communities with free or reduced cost, quality-assured medicines and vaccines. The Mectizan Donation Program, The Stop TB Global Drug Facility, and the Global Alliance for Vaccines and Immunization (GAVI) provide three examples.

Globally, there has been a down-sizing of government and a marked trend towards privatization of many functions formerly within the public domain. To varying degrees, many countries have experienced a shift from centrally planned and regulated to market-dominated economies.

Health care policy in most developing countries has generally emphasized the development of government-owned health services, largely financed by government tax revenues. However present, evidence indicates that private health care supply is significant and growing rapidly in many countries (Preker *et al.* 2007). Despite public policies promoting universal access to subsidized public services, the majority of health care contacts in developing countries are with private providers on a fee-for-service basis. Private health care is typically dominant for ambulatory treatment of illness, which in developing countries accounts for the largest share of total health care spending. It is usually less dominant for inpatient treatments and limited for preventive and public health services.

The extensive private sector activity in the health sector has seen growing public–private linkages, such as the contracting-out of selected services or facilities, development of new purchasing arrangements, franchising and the introduction of vouchers. Selective contracting out of services to the private sector is often a component of national health policy, leveraging on these private resources in the service of the public sector and to improve the efficiency of publicly funded services (Mills *et al.* 2002). Contracts for primary care with private providers serve as a quick and simple solution to gaps in coverage, especially in areas where government provision is inadequate and there are private providers already practising. The private sector represents a resource that is available and used even in the poorest countries and among lower income groups (Berman 2000). For example, the majority of malaria episodes in sub-Saharan Africa are initially treated by private providers, mainly through the purchase of drugs from shops and peddlers (Goodman *et al.* 2007). For some diseases of high priority, e.g. malaria, tuberculosis and sexually-transmitted infections and where public infrastructure is limited, scaling up of prevention and treatment efforts in the many countries hinges on enhancing utilization of private sector services (WHO 2008a).

Challenges and gaps

Addressing discrimination, equity, and social justice

Inspection of health outcomes through an equity lens reveals that the impressive gains in health experienced in recent decades are unevenly distributed. Aggregate indicators, whether at the global, regional or national level, do not offer sufficient granularity and often hide striking variations in health outcomes between men and women, rich and poor, both across and within countries.

However, health inequities involve more than inequality—in health determinants or outcomes, or in access to the resources needed to improve and maintain health. They also represent a systematic failure to avoid or overcome social differences in health and opportunities for health and their causes (Whitehead 1992; WHO 2006a). Indigenous people, ethnic minorities, people in poor communities, people living with HIV/AIDS, people with disabilities, and migrants suffer most especially from avoidable discriminatory social, economic, and welfare policies and practices. Beyond this, many marginalized groups are also disenfranchised and voiceless in the economic and social policy-making process.

For example, the richest one-tenth of the population of Latin America and the Caribbean earn 48 per cent of total income, while the poorest tenth earn only 1.6 per cent (ECLAC 2005). This inequality in income distribution extends to unequal access to education, health, water and electricity, as well as huge disparities in voice, assets and opportunities (World Bank 2007b). In some countries of Latin America, greater that 97 per cent of the people in the highest income quintile have access to health care services as compared to less than 10 per cent in the lowest quintile. Not surprisingly, 40 per cent of child deaths in the region occur among those living in the poorest quintile whereas the highest quintile accounts for only 8 per cent (*Lancet* 2007). Further, the poorest quintile of the population showed 3–10 times the prevalence of stunted children than the richest quintile in nine countries (Belizan *et al.* 2007).

In the case of health, the disadvantaged position of women in many societies undermines their ability to protect and promote their own physical, mental and emotional health. Women's status and empowerment—as measured by education, employment, household decision-making, intimate partner violence, and reproductive health—strongly influences their effective use of health information and services (Gill *et al.* 2007). Independent of related factors, educated women are more likely than are uneducated women to use antenatal care, to use trained providers and to have safe deliveries (Grown *et al.* 2005). Similarly, education not only results in substantial improvements in a woman's own health as a mother, but also has positive intergenerational effects on the health and nutrition of her children and their households (Bloom *et al.* 2001). For a variety of reasons, health policies and programmes all too often fail to adequately address these issues around women's autonomy but instead perpetuate gender stereotypes.

The dimensions of inequities in health are also evident in the health status and access to health services of populations. The poor availability of drugs that can significantly reduce AIDS-related mortality in regions of the world most affected by AIDS is a case in point.

It is estimated that, globally, over 33 million people are living with HIV, with more than two out of three adults and nearly 90 per cent of children infected with HIV living in sub-Saharan Africa (UNAIDS 2007). Yet, this region still accounts for over 70 per cent of the global unmet antiretroviral treatment need. Worldwide, over 2 million people living with HIV were receiving treatment in resource-poor countries, representing less than a third of the estimated 7.1 million people in need (UNAIDS 2006).

Such stark disparities in health outcomes are not unique to any one country or region. They exist, to a greater or lesser extent, within all societies of all nations. In many societies, overconsumption and obesity coexist with hunger and malnutrition. Great differences in life expectancy can be seen between the social classes, different occupations, ethnic groups and between the sexes in many countries, including those of highly developed economies (Marmot 2005).

Addressing governance and coordination

In recent years, there has been a unprecedented profusion of new actors, partners and sectors involved in the work and delivery of health care. In the past, few global actors possessed the political or financial authority to influence global health agendas. Today, a rich diversity of new institutions is actively reshaping global health priorities for policy and investment. These new partnerships and initiatives have added significant resources for tackling diseases of the poor and benefiting the health of large populations.

At the same time, this crowed health landscape has created a new set of challenges. The multiplicity of actors has led to an increasingly fragmented, reactive, and disparate agenda for international health (Ruger & Yach 2005). Despite efforts towards better global health partnerships, global health governance has been criticized as being too fragmented, uncoordinated, and largely donor driven. Results on the ground have been mixed; lower-income countries are growing increasingly reliant on external assistance; aid frequently does not support health systems or countries' health priorities; and financing is unpredictable and unsynchronized among donors.

Partnerships are by their very nature, issue-specific and results focused; their interventions are not always congruous with recipient countries' national priorities nor do they efficiently leverage national system resources. Non-aligned international aid skews national priorities of recipient countries by imposing those of donor partners. To achieve their narrow issue-specific goals, there is often insufficient consideration of the impact of their activities on the wider health system, including distortion of local wage structures and health worker resources. The lack of harmonization across agencies has led to inefficiency and overlap in implementation; duplication in planning, project-specific monitoring and evaluation, missions and financial management, and parallel systems for health service delivery (e.g. drug procurement and distribution). This increases significantly the transaction costs of these ventures and jeopardizes sustainable health gains.

Historically, the locus of health governance has been at the national and subnational level as governments of individual countries have undertaken primary responsibility for the health of their domestic populations. However, a range of health determinants are increasingly affected by factors outside the remit of the health sector—trade and investment flows, conflict, illicit and criminal activity, environmental change, and communication technologies (Dodgson *et al.* 2002).

Similarly, the health of individuals suffers or benefits not just from the impact of their domestic environment or personal choices, but also from decisions made at national levels and outside their own countries. Yet, ministries of health and even nation states themselves may lack the power to effect change for health due to a range of developments: Decentralization to regional and local health authorities, decisions set by donors or by lending institutions, rules set by international agreements and regimes, and of course the wider forces of globalization.

Globalization has in many ways eroded the boundary between the determinants of public and individual health, and made health a global public good. Many public health goods can no longer be achieved through domestic policy action alone and depend on international cooperation. This has arisen from the international transfer of risk, intensification of cross-border flows of people, goods, services, and ideas and the increasing threat to common resources. Yet, policy-making is still largely organized on a country-by-country basis and there is no international equivalent of the state. As a result, global public goods are increasingly underprovided for and global public bads are increasingly overprovided.

This blurring of health and jurisdictional frontiers is most obvious in the case of communicable disease transmission and the spread of non-communicable disease risk factors.

For example, susceptibility to tobacco-related diseases, once strongly linked to, and blamed on the lifestyle choices of individuals, is also increasingly being attributable to a variety of complex factors with cross-border effects, including trade liberalization, direct foreign investment, global marketing, transnational tobacco advertising, and the international movement of contraband and counterfeit cigarettes (Chen *et al.* 1999; Bettcher *et al.* 2000). In response to this globalization of the tobacco epidemic, the WHO Framework Convention on Tobacco Control (FCTC) (WHO 2003a) was developed to provide both demand- and supply-side strategies for curbing global tobacco consumption. This includes restrictions on tobacco advertising, sponsorship and promotion; raising prices through tax increases; as well as strengthening legislation to clamp down on tobacco smuggling.

The issue of antimicrobial resistance is also illustrative. It is a global problem that must be addressed in all countries as no single nation, however effective it is at containing resistance within its borders, can protect itself from the importation of resistant pathogens through travel and trade. Poor prescribing practices in any country now threaten to undermine the potency of vital antimicrobials everywhere.

Gaps in health services

Health is the final common pathway, contingent on the good functioning of many other processes and sectors. In many cases, the power of global health interventions is not matched by the power of health systems to deliver them to those in greatest need, on an adequate scale or in time. Many low-income countries are facing a double crisis of devastating disease and failing health systems. There is growing awareness in international health groups that weak national health systems limit the gains and opportunities that can be made in many areas of health, including the health MDGs. Chronic under-investments have led to fragile and fragmented health systems that are especially lacking capabilities in key areas such as health financing, information systems, health workforce, and drug supply.

There has been an implicit assumption that through the implementation of narrow disease-specific interventions, broader health systems will be strengthened more generally. Yet, the evidence of benefit for these selective initiatives on national health system capacities has been mixed. Already weak systems may be further compromised by the over-concentration of resources in specific 'vertical' programmes, leaving many other areas further under-resourced. The establishment of many selective and disease-specific initiatives within countries have resulted in competing and overlapping subsystems within the broader health care system. This can lead to duplication of work processes, distortions of local salary and work norms, service disruptions in existing programmes, and distraction from core work activities (Travis *et al.* 2004).

Further, many groups and communities still do not have access to essential public health interventions even when these are known to be cost effective. This is largely due to inadequate allocation of resources to health and disproportionate allocation to curative and high technology services in urban settings. Also, the funds that are committed often do not benefit those who need them most, and remain underutilized. Equitable health systems need financing mechanisms which remove the barriers to health care, specially those confronting disadvantaged groups. Gaps in implementation include, in some cases, too much emphasis on pilot projects and islands of excellence, with inadequate plans and health system capacity to scale up (WHO 2006c).

The role of the private sector

New challenges have emerged with the commoditization of health care and the often unregulated delivery of health care in the non-government health sector. Private health care is expanding rapidly and is acknowledged as an important and often well-resourced provider of health care services in many countries. Yet, this important component of the health care system has received little policy attention. Increasingly, experience with the private sector has indicated a number of problems with the quality, price and distribution of private health services. This has led to a growing focus on the critical role of government in regulation and the orientation of the private sector with public health goals.

The effectiveness of private services is often very low. Poor treatment practices have been reported for diseases such as tuberculosis (Uplekar *et al.* 2001) and sexually transmitted infections (Chalker *et al.* 2000), with implications not only for the individuals treated but also for disease transmission and the development of drug resistance. For example, to improve affordability, partial doses of drugs may be sold as private services are priced to the purchasing power of the client. In Sierra Leone, for example, the price of purchased drugs was almost a third of the cost of treatment at a public health centre (Fabricant *et al.* 1999). The rise of chronic diseases in the developing world, often bringing with it a life-long need for medication, is expected to compound this problem considerably.

The use of the more expensive private services, or treatment for chronic conditions, can result in households being unable to afford other vital requirements or being driven into poverty through greater out of pocket expenditure. Moreover, rapidly growing private services compete with the public sector for trained human resources, further weakening public services (Mills *et al.* 2002).

A crisis in human resources for health

Human resources have been described as 'the heart of the health system in any country' (WHO 2006d). Yet, many national health systems are in crisis, with the shortage of workers severely compromising the delivery of essential health services and interventions. Abundant evidence demonstrates that progress in health in the poorest countries will not be possible without strong national health systems for which the work force is essential. The work force determines health outputs and outcomes and drives health systems performance.

Uneven distribution deprives many groups of access to life-saving services, a problem compounded by accelerating migration in open labour markets that draw skilled workers away from the poorest communities and countries. Health workers are leaving poorer areas for wealthier ones, and often leaving the countries that invested in their training to take up jobs abroad. Strikingly, for every Liberian physician working in Liberia, about two live abroad in developed countries; similarly for every Gambian professional nurse working in the Gambia, likewise about two live in a developed country overseas (Clemens & Pettersson 2008).

Many health services are consequently jeopardized by this trend, including childhood immunization, care during pregnancy and childbirth, and access to treatment for HIV/AIDS, tuberculosis, and malaria. The inadequacy of human resources for health significantly correlates with poorer maternal mortality, infant mortality, under five mortality rates (Anand & Barnighausen 2004), and childhood vaccination coverage (Anand & Barnighausen 2007). As the number of health workers declines, survival declines proportionately. Unless the workforce crisis is addressed, neither priority disease initiatives, including those aimed at achieving the health-related MDGS, nor health systems strengthening can succeed.

Sub-Saharan Africa faces the greatest crisis: This part of the world accounts for 11 per cent of the global population and 24 per cent of the global burden of disease, but has only 3 per cent of the world's health workforce (WHO 2006d). Shortages are widespread, with a gap of more than 1 million health workers estimated for Africa alone. Globally, WHO estimates that more than 4 million more health workers are required to achieve the health-related MDGs and has identified 57 countries with critical shortages of health workers—36 of these countries are in Africa.

The causes of these shortages are manifold. There is a limited production capacity in many developing countries as a result of years of underinvestment in health education institutions. Decades of economic and sectoral reform capped expenditures, froze recruitment and salaries, and restricted public budgets, depleting working environments of basic supplies, drugs, and facilities (Narasimhan *et al.* 2004). Moreover, the training output is poorly aligned with the health needs of the population. There are also 'push' and 'pull' factors that encourage health workers to leave their workplaces, mainly related to unsatisfactory working conditions, low salaries, political instability and poor career opportunities. Surveys among health workers intending to migrate or already migrated consistently cite issues of remuneration and living conditions as primary reasons for their departure (Vujicic *et al.* 2004). Other factors contributing to the shortage of health workers include growth of the global population as training of health workers stagnates, the rise in chronic diseases, and the ageing of populations, which increases the need for long-term care. The devastation of HIV/AIDS is also a major force assailing health workers in the hardest hit societies of sub-Saharan Africa, Asia, the Americas, and eastern Europe; it is a triple threat that is increasing workloads on health workers, exposing them to infection, and stressing their morale (Joint Learning Initiative 2004).

Undoubtedly, health workers have a clear human right to emigrate in search of a better life. Yet, people in source countries hard hit by an exodus of health workers also have the right to health in their own countries, and to see a return on their considerable investments in education and training (Robinson & Clark 2008). The space between these two fundamental rights is the area where a clear global framework for response and cooperation is needed. It will require working in partnership and across sectors in both source and recipient countries, to implement and monitor effective strategies to develop a well-performing health workforce (Global Health Workforce Alliance 2008).

Gaps in knowledge

There is growing recognition that research is critical in the fight against disease. Knowledge contributes to the policies, activities, and performance of health systems, and to the improvement of individuals' and populations' health.

However, gaps in research and the dissemination of knowledge and health information are growing ever more acute. International research efforts are poorly coordinated and fragmented. Spending on health research, when viewed from a global perspective, is grossly skewed and under-funded. The landmark findings of the Commission on Health Research for Development (1990) almost two decades ago, highlighted the discrepancy in research funding and priorities–that only 5 per cent of the total global research funds were spent on research addressing the problems of developing countries whose citizens bore greater than 90 per cent of the global burden of preventable conditions affecting health. The magnitude of this discrepancy is an issue of continuing concern (Global Forum for Health Research 2007).

Despite impressive advances in science, technology, and medicine, society has failed to allocate sufficient resources to fight the diseases that particularly affect the poor. There is a dearth of research and development into neglected diseases such as African trypanosomiasis, lymphatic filariasis, schistosomiasis, and Chagas disease, which account for a high burden of disease in disability-adjusted life years. Sex-disaggregated data is important for developing effective and gender-sensitive health services and policies, yet these data are seldom collected. Lack of access to information through modern communications technology in poor parts of the world is hampering the wider dissemination of best practices in diverse fields such as hygiene, injury prevention, tobacco and substance abuse.

The limited resources available can fund only a fraction of the promising research opportunities. Hence, prioritization is essential for health research in order to focus on areas of greatest need. Yet, the degree to which research funding should reflect the burden of disease has been the subject of extensive debate. Even where there is agreement on existing or new research priorities, the best way of financing the discovery, production and delivery of these pubic goods for health, and making them affordable by poor countries, is seldom clear.

Prescription for the new millennium

An agenda for health

As can be appreciated from the above discussion, the world is falling short in winning sustainable and equitable improvements for health. Aggregate global health indicators have improved substantially since the middle of the past century, but gross health inequalities persist. Indeed, the gaps are widening between the world's poorest people and those better placed to benefit from economic development and public health progress. This trend takes place within an evolving global health landscape characterized by a complex and challenging mixture of old and new health problems and greater pluralism in health actors, funding resources and opportunities.

An analysis of the past provides a starting point for defining an agenda for the future. From the gaps thus examined and our understanding of current key challenges and shortfalls in response, it is evident that greater global commitment and solidarity are needed to forge greater health gains. Lasting health progress, including attainment of the health-related MDGs, depends on strong political will, supported by sound, integrated and evidence-based policies and broad participation from actors both within and outside the health sector.

Global efforts to improve health are inseparable from medical science, but social, economic, environmental and political factors also determine health opportunities and outcomes. Although trends in some major determinants of health, such as demographic changes, are relatively predictable, many are not (WHO 2006c). Progress in public health is rarely linear. Health emergencies—whether climatic, seismic, or infectious in nature—illustrate how quickly situations can change and how precarious health can be. The fragility of health gains has repeatedly been shown in response, for example, to economic and social changes and civil disruption. As such, any global public health agenda has to plan for inherent unpredictability and volatility in the health of populations and societies.

The following outline of a global health agenda identifies seven priority areas. The broad agenda borrows from the eleventh general programme of work of the WHO, which was endorsed and adopted by its 193 Member States at the World Health Assembly in May 2006. It serves as a strategic framework and direction for the future work of the Organization and all it Member States in the new millennium. Of the seven areas, the first three frame the fundamental principles and concepts underlying health advancement: Investing in health to reduce poverty; building individual and global health security; and promoting universal coverage, gender equality and health-related human rights. The remaining four items focus on more strategic and explicit areas of endeavour: Tackling the determinants of health; strengthening health systems and equitable access; harnessing knowledge, science and technology; and strengthening governance, leadership, and accountability.

Establishing the role of health in development and poverty reduction

Elimination of poverty and extreme hunger is foremost among the MDGs. For the poor with few possessions, health is their main, if not their only, asset—if they do not have even that, they have nothing. For many of these people, being healthy means the possibility to work, earn a living and support their families. When the health of the main earner in poor families is compromised, the implications for economically dependent family members, particularly children, are particularly severe. By definition, poor people have few reserves and may be forced to sell what assets they have, including land and livestock, or borrow at high interest rates, to deal with the immediate crisis precipitated by illness. Each option leaves them more vulnerable, less able to recover, and in greater danger of moving down the poverty spiral (Braveman & Gruskin 2003). Poor people are thus caught in a vicious circle: Poverty breeds ill-health, ill-health maintains poverty.

Yet, the escape from poverty rests on more than just one pillar. Having a population that is healthy and educated enough to participate in the global economy is as important as enlightened economic reform. At the international level, priorities for improving public health are clear: Focus on health problems and diseases that affect the poor disproportionately. Health gains require directing programme benefits towards the poor and increasing the quality and availability of health services, especially where they are most scarce (World Bank 2007b).

Good health enables individuals to be active agents of change in the development process, both within and outside the health sector. The provision of health services is no longer viewed merely as a consumer of resources and an onerous obligation of governments. Health is also a producer of economic gains and integral to development in a broader sense. Beyond raising living standards through economic growth, health and development improve human capital through empowerment and enhancement of individual agency (Sen & Sen 1999). As such, health and poverty alleviation hold a prominent place in debates on priorities for development. Countries, at all levels of development, are realizing the need for sustained, equitable increases in health investment as a contribution to prosperity and social stability.

Our understanding of poverty has broadened from a narrow focus on income and consumption. Poverty is now known to encompass many other dimensions—lack of education, inadequate housing, social exclusion, unemployment, and environmental degradation. Each of these elements diminishes opportunity, limits choices and threatens health. Thus, poverty encompasses not just low income, but also lack of access to services, resources and skills; vulnerability; insecurity and powerlessness.

Poor countries, and poor people within countries, suffer from a multiplicity of deprivations that translate into high levels of ill-health. These wide differences in health status are considered unfair, or inequitable, because they correspond to differing societal, cultural, and system-wide constraints and opportunities. Further, these differences lie largely beyond the choice of the individual (Wagstaff 2002). Poverty-oriented health strategies require complementary policies in other sectors (WHO 2003b). These include improving access to education, enhancing the position of women and other marginalized groups, shaping development policies in agriculture and rural development, and promoting open and participatory governance.

Multidimensional poverty is a potent determinant of health risks, health seeking behaviour, health care access and health outcomes. Economic indicators focusing primarily on income alone offer a limited assessment of poverty, and a limited platform for attacking poverty. In contrast, health indicators provide a greater measure of the multi-faceted nature of poverty. For this reason health should be a key measure of the success or failure of development and of poverty reduction policies during this century (Haines *et al.* 2000).

Government expenditures on health are often designed to give everyone equal access to health care. Yet, in practice, equal access is usually elusive. Health improvements have not been shared equally and health inequalities among and within countries remain entrenched. Publicly financed health care fails to reach the poor in almost all developing countries. Most research conducted in developing countries in the last 20 years has confirmed that publicly financed health care benefits the well-off more than the poor (Devarajan 2003). If access to health services were distributed according to need, the poor would come first. However, in many cases, the 'inverse care law' unduly prevails and, as a result, the availability of good medical care tends to vary inversely with the need for it in the population served (Tudor Hart 1971).

Health services can fail poor people in many ways—in access, in quantity, in quality, and in costs. The striking differences in health status among different economic groups reflect inequalities in access to information, to facilities that provide decent standards of care, and to the means to pay for good care. In most instances, the poor are less educated than the rich and lack knowledge in areas of hygiene, nutrition and good health practices. Regressive patterns of health financing force greater out-of-pocket expenditure, and exacerbate poverty and ill health. For example, poor people often delay health care until a problem is advanced, more difficult or impossible to treat, and much more costly. This well-documented tendency becomes more of a problem with the rise of chronic diseases in low- and middle-income countries, as it jeopardizes early preventive and protective care.

If policy-makers want health to reduce poverty, they cannot allow the costs of health care to drive impoverished households even deeper into poverty. As noted above, the provision of effective and accessible health services helps protect the poor from spiralling into worsening economic problems. To achieve this, propagation of more equitable socioeconomic policies is paramount. Programmes can address barriers to health for the poor in many ways: Through better education and health promotion, better targeting of services to specific groups, improvements in quality of care, incentives for health providers, and financing mechanisms that make care affordable to those most in need (Mundial 2005). Fair health financing schemes promote the alignment of contribution with the ability to pay, and the use of services with the degree of need. An emphasis on prepayment for health care through taxes or insurance, with contribution tied to an individual's disbursement capacity, goes far in supporting the poor. The emphasis in conditional cash transfer programmes, such as those in Brazil and Mexico, on channelling resources through female household members, shows the importance policy places on supporting their role in protecting children's development and promoting family health (Marmot 2007).

Since demand for health care by poor people is price sensitive, any reduction in the price charged to the user will induce an increase in demand. Yet, access to ostensibly free health care is, for most users, far from free (Gwatkin *et al.* 2004). Indeed, use of this entitlement has associated participation costs, such as transportation, food expenditure, and loss of time. Ensuring that the poor access and participate in health services may therefore necessitate the employment of various schemes to reduce participation costs. Examples include the use of vouchers, fee waivers, social health insurance and reimbursement for transport and food.

In addition to supply-driven pro-poor schemes, several complementary approaches are being explored. These focus on creating an effective demand and pressure for relevant health services on the part of the poor, to offset the influence of better-off groups that traditionally shape priorities and programmes. Individuals should have the opportunity to participate in political and social decisions about public policies that affect them (Ruger 2003). This strengthens agency, a process that is central to the sustainability of effective health systems and the achievement of broader development goals; it also provides a foundation for cohesive societies. Participation and enablement allow people to hold service providers accountable, both directly and indirectly, through influence and feedback to policy-makers. Community-level programmes that involve beneficiaries in aspects of programme design, implementation and evaluation can achieve better health outcomes through empowerment and creating a greater sense of ownership. The recently introduced approach of community-led total sanitation, which offers no subsidies but relies on communities to make sanitation a priority and devise local solutions, provides a good example of the potential for rapid, community-wide, and sustainable results (Kar & Bongartz 2006).

In addition, models of social protection have been put forward to lessen the vulnerability of the poor to adverse health crises and catastrophic expenses. An array of social safety nets, social assistance programmes such as cash transfers, food-subsidy programmes, public works, and microfinancing schemes can be used to ameliorate adverse shocks and alleviate poverty. Such schemes, which can enhance social security, need to be targeted to reach poor and vulnerable populations.

Good policies and investments in health are not, in themselves, sufficient to ensure growth and poverty reduction. Institutions and governance are additional key determinants. Efforts to improve governance may aim to increase political accountability, strengthen civil society participation, create a competitive private sector, impose institutional restraints on power or improve public sector management. The role of government in all these processes is critical. Poverty reduction strategies, where they exist, also place national governments in a central role, making them responsible for the cross-sectoral implementation of policies specifically designed to tackle the causes and consequences of poverty in their country.

Promoting universal coverage, gender equity, and health-related human rights

Effective public health action needs an ethical position as well as technical competence. To shape a healthier future, public health must be clear about its values, as well as its scientific principles. As enshrined in the WHO constitution and many international instruments of law, the enjoyment of the highest attainable standard of health is one of the fundamental rights of every human being. Appreciation of this defining value underscores all efforts to provide good health for all. The foundation for realizing physical, mental and social well-being is inextricably linked to the protection and fulfilment of human rights. For example, the violation or neglect of human rights, as expressed by torture or violence against women, can lead to ill-health. Conversely, the fulfilment of human rights can reduce a person's vulnerability to ill-health (Mann *et al.* 1999).

The progressive realization of rights to health requires action and policies that make appropriate and affordable health care accessible to those in greatest need in the shortest possible time. The underlying determinants of health also need to be addressed: Access to safe and potable water, adequate sanitation, safe and nutritious food, and housing; healthy occupational and environment conditions; and access to health education and information, also in the area of sexual and reproductive health.

Health and development outcomes are greatly enhanced by employing human rights as an integral dimension in the design, implementation, monitoring and evaluation of health-related policies and programmes. Through this approach, substantive rights-based elements such as attention to vulnerable groups, safeguarding dignity, equality and freedom from discrimination, employing a gender perspective and ensuring accessible health systems, can be considered and addressed.

A pressing problem in many countries is the deficiency in access by poor and marginalized groups to essential health services. A commitment to universal coverage embraces the principle of fair distribution of opportunities for well-being based on people's needs, rather than their social privileges. It implies equitable health systems characterized by accessibility, affordability, quality and acceptability, and prioritized towards the needs of the marginalized and vulnerable population groups—children, women, indigenous and tribal populations; ethnic, religious and national minorities; immigrants, persons with disabilities and people living with HIV/AIDS. Indeed, some low-income countries with policies that emphasize equitable access to essential care have achieved greater life expectancies than wealthy countries with no such policy objective. These better health outcomes are achieved when equitable access to care is, at the outset, a categorical and unambiguous objective of policy-makers.

Inequities in health occur along several axes of social stratification, including sex, race, ethnic group, language, educational level, occupation, and residence. Whole classes of people whose health is compromised by economic or social disadvantages are beset by many other problems that make their lives miserable; yet their health plight is often invisible to policy-makers and poorly captured in statistics. To better unmask these variations in health, the employment of disaggregated health data that go beyond gross health statistics and national averages allows for a more profound appreciation of inter-group disparities. Such data go far in informing the redistribution of social and economic resources to those in greatest need and in bringing evidence to bear on political choices in health. Further, mitigation of these health inequities serves the dual goals of equity and efficiency for health services.

A rights-based approach to health also recognizes the need for empowerment and participation. All groups, including the vulnerable and marginalized, have the right to participate in the design, implementation and monitoring of health policies, programmes and legislation that can affect their health. However, a characteristic common to marginalized groups is their lack of power to influence their political, social and economic conditions. Thus, to be effective and sustainable, interventions that aim to redress inequities must typically go beyond remedying a particular health inequity. The broader aim is to help empower the target group through systemic changes, such as legislative reform or changes in economic or social relationships, and the reduction of stigma and discrimination.

In recent decades, great strides have been made in the health of women. Yet, in most societies, disadvantages for women persist. Women's health is compromised by the disproportionate prevalence among them of poverty, few prospects of employment beyond the home, the indignities of violence and rape, limited influence on their sexual and reproductive lives and limited power to influence decisions. Goal 3 of the MDGs—to achieve gender equality and empower women—seeks specifically to rectify those disadvantages through policies and programmes that build women's capabilities, improve their access to economic and political opportunities, and guarantee their safety. Complementary health interventions, such as expanding access to sexual and reproductive health care, health information and education, are also needed to ensure sustainable improvements in women's health. Moreover, policies and programmes designed with a gender perspective must explicitly aim to rectify inequalities and disadvantages faced by women. Ample evidence demonstrates that when women are given opportunities to develop their potential, health indicators for families and communities rapidly improve. As noted in the Millennium Declaration, the empowerment of women is an effective way to combat poverty, hunger and disease and to stimulate development that is truly sustainable.

Many countries are working to expand coverage of essential health services by renewing their systems of primary health care, an approach that is again being strongly supported by WHO. A commitment to the values, principles and approaches of primary health care encourages a focus on vulnerable and marginalized populations, promotes population-based and personal care services, emphasizes prevention as well as cure, and strengthens the referral system It also encourages intersectoral action to address the root causes of ill health and helps orient the private sector to public health goals (WHO 2006c).

Building individual and global health security

In recent years, health has been conceptualized as a security issue, both in terms of individual and community health security, expressed as access to the fundamental prerequisites for health, and global health security. Global health security seeks protection from risks and dangers to health that arise from the ways in which nations and their populations interact at the international level.

At the international level, the relationship between health and security faces many new challenges (and opportunities) in an increasingly globalized world characterized by the unprecedented speed and volume of international travel, the interdependence of businesses and financial markets, and the interconnectedness brought on by the revolution in information technology.

Acute threats to human health posed by conflicts, disease outbreaks, natural disasters and zoonoses have become a larger menace in a globalized society. The 2003 outbreak of severe acute respiratory syndrome (SARS)—the first severe new disease of the twenty-first century—demonstrated how much the world has changed in terms of its vulnerability to emerging diseases. SARS spread rapidly along the routes of international air travel and caused enormous economic losses and social disruption well beyond the outbreak zones. As the emergence of diseases is tied to fundamental changes in the way humanity inhabits the planet, more new diseases can be anticipated as this century progresses. In particular, the behaviour of emerging and epidemic-prone diseases has made all nations acutely aware of their shared vulnerability and their shared responsibility for mutual self-protection. Global public health security is thus both a collective aspiration and a mutual responsibility (WHO 2007d).

Public health emergencies throw into sharp relief the strengths and weaknesses of infrastructures designed to protect the public on a daily basis. To ensure global health security, two interrelated strategies are required: A significant strengthening of public health within both developed and developing countries and the establishment of mechanisms that facilitate the collaborative action of countries. The Global Outbreak Alert and Response Network (GOARN), which proved instrumental in the response to SARS, is one such mechanism. The revised International Health Regulations are another. These regulations, which came into force in 2007, are designed to minimize the international consequences of public health emergencies. For those caused by emerging and epidemic-prone diseases, the regulations follow a proactive approach to risk management that aims to stop an outbreak at source, before it has an opportunity to spread internationally. To do so, the regulations further recognize that all countries must posses a set of core capacities for outbreak surveillance and detection, laboratory diagnosis, and response. Meeting these core requirements, as set out in the regulations, would greatly strengthen collective global health security. Unfortunately, the necessary systems and infrastructures in many countries are lacking, making greater investment in capacity building an urgent priority.

The effectiveness of many collective agreements, including the International Health Regulations, depends on transparency and cooperation between national governments and the larger international community. Accordingly, the open and timely sharing of essential health information and knowledge is a central obligation under the revised Regulations that must be honoured by all countries as a prerequisite for collective security. In addition, given the multidimensional challenges to health security, governments must also foster greater cooperation between different sectors and stakeholders. For example, the engagement of sectors such as health, agriculture, trade and tourism is a key element in preparedness plans for a future influenza pandemic.

While conflicts and natural disasters are localized events, they can also take on international dimensions. During such events, routine health services are frequently disrupted; the health consequences can be compounded by breakdowns in water supply and sanitation or interruptions in the supply of essential medicines and equipment. The risk of epidemics increases dramatically when people are crowded together in temporary shelters. Most natural disasters and long-term conflicts will require assistance and cooperation from the international community. Ensuring the capacity for such swift global response reduces avoidable loss of lives and mitigates suffering.

At the level of the individual and the community, more proximal determinants, such as access to food, water, and shelter, healthy environments, and protection from violence, especially for women, are the focus of security concerns. Broader issues in human security, such as education, gender equality, poverty and globalization have consequential effects on health and require the continued action of governments in framing more equitable development and international policies. Climate change is a further contemporary challenge to collective security (CNA Corporation 2007) and demands urgent attention. Numerous adverse effects on health are projected. While the warming of the planet is expected to be gradual, the effects of extreme weather events—more storms, floods, heat waves, and droughts—will be abrupt and acutely felt. Both trends can have profoundly adverse effects on health. WHO has focused attention on five main health consequences of climate change: (1) Increases in malnutrition and in the severity of childhood infectious diseases; (2) increases in death, disease and injury due to extreme weather events; (3) increases in episodes of diarrhoeal disease; (4) increases in the frequency of cardiorespiratory diseases; and (5) altered distribution of vectors responsible for infectious diseases, most notably malaria and dengue (WHO 2008b). To address these challenges, Member States have called on WHO to promote research and pilot projects aimed at health protection, especially in vulnerable countries. While climate change is a global phenomenon, scientists predict that developing countries, especially in sub-Saharan Africa, will experience the earliest and most severe consequences, also for health.

Health systems strengthening and ensuring equitable access

Appropriately constituted and managed health systems provide a vehicle to improve people's lives, protecting them from the vulnerability of sickness, generating a sense of security, and building social cohesion within society; they can ensure that all groups benefit from socioeconomic development and they can generate the political support needed to sustain them.

Patterns of disease, care and treatment are not static. Health systems have to cope with a spectrum of competing health changes and challenges. Their capacity to respond is similarly impacted by many factors operating at different levels. On a more local level, services and programmes are challenged by the availability of resources, both financial and human, as well as government policies in relation to decentralization and the role of the private sector and civil society. With increasing globalization, issues such as migration, transnational spread of disease, and trade, including obligations under international treaties, are constraining the policy and fiscal space of national governments. In the face of multiple objectives and limited resources, governments have to reconcile the competing demands for access and efficiency against those of ensuring affordability and quality. Strategies for strengthening the health sector also need to be linked to broader processes of national development planning, such as civil service reform, public expenditure reviews and reform, decentralization, and poverty-reduction strategies.

As can be appreciated, strengthening health system performance is a wide-ranging subject, requiring action on many levels and management fronts. Given the contextual complexity, there is no one blueprint or single set of best practices that can be put forward as a model for improved performance. Yet, health systems across countries share commonalities in function, services and objectives; they also share some common experiences and face some similar difficulties. By addressing these challenges through a collaborative, coordinated way, driven by desired health outcomes, sustainable system-wide benefits can be achieved. To be most effective, this process must be country-led and based on priorities set out in comprehensive national health plans. It requires attention to the various functions of the health system to achieve the objectives of: Improved health and health equity through accessible, affordable, quality services to all who need them, greater social and financial risk protection, improved efficiency and responsiveness to health needs, and greater patient safety (WHO 2006c).

Strengthening health systems means addressing key constraints related to health worker staffing, governance, infrastructure, health commodities, logistics, tracking progress, and effective financing. Stronger leadership and governance helps ensure good oversight, accountability, attention to regulation and coalition building both within and outside the national health sector. Stewardship in government seeks innovative engagement with civil society and the private sector and to orient programmes and resources towards public health goals. Communities and individuals must be actively engaged to participate in the decision-making process of policies that affect their health. Policy-making needs to be more collaborative, better coordinated and better informed. A well-functioning health information system contributes to this by the generation, analysis and dissemination of timely and critical information on health determinants, status, and performance. Building up managerial skills at all levels and accommodating reform is critically important, as is the delivery of primary health care.

The contributions of primary health care to improvements in many aspects of population and individual health are well documented (Starfield *et al.* 2005). Evidence demonstrates that health systems oriented towards primary health care—with its underpinning values of universal access, equity, community participation, and intersectoral action—produce better outcomes, at lower costs, and with higher user satisfaction (Doherty & Govender 2004). Its emphasis on health promotion, continuity of care across levels of care and over the life course, use of appropriate technology and care that is 'close-to-client' is central to health policies in many countries. Equally important, especially as a contribution to efficiency, is the provision of as much care as possible at the first point of contact effectively supported by secondary level facilities through a fully functioning referral processes. Large gains in health outcomes have been seen in countries with a strong political commitment to aligning their health system to the principles of primary health care. Such an approach is relevant to both developing and developed countries alike.

The health workforce is central to managing and delivering health services in all countries. The effectiveness of health systems and the quality of the health services depend on a well-functioning workforce that is responsive, motivated and skilled. Yet, the current crisis of human resources, including shortages and mal-distribution, is jeopardizing the delivery of services in all countries, especially those in sub-Saharan Africa. This shortfall is aggravated by skewed distribution geographically between urban and rural areas and between the private and public sector. To address this crisis, governments must exercise leadership in developing holistic national strategic policies for workforce development, based on sound evidence and participatory feedback. Increased investments to improve performance and productivity are also essential through compensation adjustments, incentives, education, and the provision of safer working conditions. National and international efforts need to be aligned to address the issues of ethical hiring of health workers trained abroad and the negotiation of policies that shape migration and international labour markets (WHO 2006d).

To achieve sustainable funds for health and social protection, regressive patterns of financing need to be addressed. Reducing reliance on out-of-pocket payments where they are high, and by moving towards prepayment systems based on pooling of financial risk across population groups should be encouraged. Additionally, where needed, social protection schemes should be supported to ensure the poor and other vulnerable groups have access to services based on need, while ensuring that health care costs do not lead to financial catastrophe.

Tackling the determinants of health and promoting intersectoral participation

Modern concepts of health recognize that underlying conditions establish the foundation for realizing physical, mental, and social well-being. Health is a consequence of multiple interacting determinants operating in dynamic biological, behavioural, social, and economic contexts that change as a person develops. Health risks are created and maintained by social systems; the magnitude of those risks is largely a function of socioeconomic disparities and psychosocial gradients. Some social circumstances that affect health relate to social exclusion and other multidimensional disadvantages, such as education, gender, poverty, discrimination, and ethnicity. Beyond these, exposure risks such as working environments, living conditions, unsafe sex and the availability of food and water also contribute to health risks. Wider economic, political and environmental determinants include urbanization, intellectual property rights, trade and subsidies, globalization, air pollution, and climate change.

Accordingly, any effort to reduce health disparities cannot be confined to the provision of better access to care and resources alone but must also go beyond to address the underlying determinants. Such an approach supports the advancement of global health equity. Acting on the structural conditions in society affecting health offers a better hope for sustainable and equitable outcomes in health beyond just medical or social interventions alone. As a framework for this, a strategy of health promotion is needed that enables the fulfilment of health through the creation of supportive environments, healthy public policies, access to information, life skills and opportunities for making healthy choices (Charter 1986). Such policy options are expected to increase after the Commission on Social Determinants of Health publishes its findings (Marmot 2005). The work of the Commission will be instrumental for rendering the problem of health inequity real and actionable by institutional authorities and policy practitioners.

Given their aetiology, many of the attributable causes of chronic disease lend themselves to prevention or control. Physical inactivity, improper diets, tobacco use, and excessive alcohol consumption represent major modifiable risk factors. These factors are now recognized as being amenable to alleviation throughout life, even into old age. Just as the risk occurs at all ages, so all ages are part of the continuum of opportunity for prevention. This can be best applied through a life-course approach that includes maternal health, exclusive breastfeeding for six months, health promotion in schools, and in the work-place, sex education, a healthy diet, and regular physical activity from childhood into old age (WHO 2006c).

However, against a backdrop of globalization and changing health risks, the advocacy for change in individual behaviour alone is insufficient by itself. In many instances, the individual and even the health sector have little or no control over many of the powerful influences on health; many of these issues lie within the ambit of governments and commercial responsibilities. Action on these determinants requires the collaborative engagement of multiple stakeholders across many levels—from communities to governments, local to international and private to non-governmental. Cooperation and advocacy must necessarily push the boundaries of public health action to overcome such structural factors.

Governments, and ministries of health in particular, must play a leading role in intersectoral action to secure better public health policies and achieve some control over the transnational forces that affect the health of their populations. The widespread influence of globalization has increased the need for new frameworks of international collaboration, including conventional international law, to address and formulate policy responses to emerging opportunities for and threats to global health (Taylor 2002). International organizations, such as the WHO, play a pivotal role in contributing to the coherent development of greater global dialogue, building effective partnerships, and stimulating effective governmental and intergovernmental action on public health issues.

Multilateral collective strategies, especially the development of international standards and instruments, are central for protecting and promoting public health. Increasingly, international health legislation is proving an important tool for creating global health covenants in promoting cooperative action against shared health challenges. Agreements such as the revised International Health Regulations (2005) have demonstrated the power of multilateral cooperative arrangements to protect against the transnational spread of disease and pathogens. In the same way, governments must move to strengthen corresponding national regulatory and enforcement frameworks and capacities to support and advance many of these same themes.

Health damaging behaviours in particular, such as the use of tobacco, poor diet and sedentary lifestyles, have proven amenable to such collective action. On an international level, a strong model of cooperation and intersectoral action is provided by the WHO Framework Convention on Tobacco Control, an instrument that embraces a social determinants approach to tobacco control and demands broad intersectoral action on matters as diverse as trade, agriculture, education and the environment (Taylor & Bettcher 2000). Similarly, the WHO global strategy on diet, physical activity and health emphasizes community-based approaches and engagement with industry for action on the structural drivers of food availability, accessibility and acceptability at the global and national levels (Chopra *et al.* 2002).

Contemporary international cooperation efforts have also seen the linkage of health with other traditionally distinct but substantive issues become increasingly common. For example, the fundamental interdependence of sustainable development and health necessitates intersectoral coordination of economic, social, and environmental policies to promote population well-being. Other growing issue linkages to health have been elaborated in international processes on public health, innovation, and intellectual property, as well as conventions on biological diversity, climate change, and sustainable development. In all these, governments must display strong leadership and give equity and health a central place in their agendas.

Strengthening governance, leadership, and accountability

Good national governance, wise leadership, and strong political will are central societal structures underpinning economic growth and equitable development. The gaps between policies and their implementation are often huge. Governments need to bridge these gaps and address deeper sources of policy failure that can undermine health development. Enlightened policy-making brings coherence to the delivery of health services and outcomes. It is important that the health of populations feature as a principal concern of all governments. Experiences shows that as governance improves, fewer women die in childbirth, more physicians exist per population, there is better access to improved water, and life expectancy is longer. Such is its power and importance.

At the national level, ministries of health must exercise stewardship and advocacy to centre health in development planning and secure increased financial allocation to health in the national budget. This implies the ability to formulate strategic policy direction and clarify the roles and responsibilities of the different actors in health; clear policy priorities must be established while maintaining an overview of societal interests and reorienting policies towards pro-poor public health goals. It also implies ensuring good regulation and the tools for implementing it, and to provide the necessary intelligence on health system performance in order to ensure accountability and transparency.

Through intersectoral engagement, ministries must create a platform for coordination and consensus-building across mutually-reliant sectors—public, civil, and private. Such engagement needs to address cross-cutting issues such as civil service reform, social determinants of health, macroeconomic policy, gender equality, and health-related human rights. Where they exist, health targets must be in integrated into poverty reduction strategies, based on comprehensive and equity-based health sector investment plans.

Recent years have also seen greater expansion and commitment in external resources for health. Concomitantly, there has been an upsurge in the number of external agencies involved in the health sectors of developing countries with growing volumes of resources transferred to these health systems. Notwithstanding the beneficial impact of increased resources, recipients and donors must find greater efficiency in the aid policy process to deliver sustainable health development (Buse & Walt 1997).

In countries where there is significant health sector investment by international partners, there is an imperative to develop capacities and policies to coordinate and manage such cooperation. Substantive challenges regarding development assistance revolve around its possible distortion of country priorities, and the issues of volatile and unpredictable aid that impedes long term macroeconomic and sectoral policy formulation (WHO 2007a). In many developing countries, progress towards rationalizing the new flow and mechanisms of such aid has been limited by the lack of comprehensive national health strategies, and critical deficits in national absorptive and planning capacity.

It is recognized that for aid to become truly effective, stronger and more balanced accountability mechanisms are required at different levels. Aid is more effective when partner countries exercise ownership with strong and effective leadership over their development policies and strategies. This fundamental tenet underpins the

Paris Declaration (OECD 2005) and other multilateral initiatives that aim to increase the effectiveness of aid. To strengthen health systems, expand use and coverage of health services and help achieve the MDGs in developing countries, new initiatives such as the International Health Partnerships (IHP) have been successfully launched; an agreement between donors and developing countries, the IHP aims to put the Paris Declaration into practice in the health sector by setting out a process of mutual responsibility and accountability for the development and implementation of national health plans of developing countries (Alexander 2007). Above all, the IHP recognizes that successful and sustainable health initiatives must be country-led and country-owned.

Globalization and the liberalization of trade and services have materially transformed the capacity of governments to monitor and protect public health. As such, governments must effectively assess and respond to the risks and opportunities for population health presented by negotiated international agreements such as the Agreement on Trade Related Aspects of Intellectual Property Rights (TRIPS) and the General Agreement on Trade in Services (Blouin *et al.* 2006). Governments are challenged to remain informed and engaged in a wide range of issues—covering food, insurance, occupational and environmental health conditions, pharmaceuticals, and affordable access to medicines among others—and their deeper implications for health equity and public health.

Harnessing knowledge, science, and technology

Against a backdrop of unprecedented technological and economic resources for health, the stark reality of large inequities in health status looms ever larger. Across many developing countries, the health status of populations has declined, largely as a result of HIV/AIDS, but also because of enduring poverty, an inadequate tax base in many developing countries, a resurgence in infectious diseases, and a upsurge in non-communicable diseases. Indeed a key imperative for health research must be to bring a sharper focus on mitigating these inequities and the unacceptable gap between unprecedented knowledge about diseases and their control, and the implementation of that knowledge, especially in poor countries.

It is recognized that the creation and diffusion of knowledge is one of the major driving forces for health progress and improving health equity (Jamison *et al.* 2006). Evidence derived from scientific knowledge can help transform health, be it through new and better technologies, promoting better health practices, or the application of evidence in health policy formulation.

Gaps in essential health information prevent effective global and country responses to health challenges. Good health metrics and evaluation is vital. It allows comparative health-system research, building the evidence-base for policy, baseline monitoring and programme performance evaluation. Greater investments are needed to produce actionable learning that national leaders and development partners can use to improve health programmes and assess effectiveness.

Even though the greatest burden of ill health and premature mortality occurs in the developing world, only a small fraction of global research funding is devoted to communicable, maternal, perinatal, and nutritional disorders that constitute the major burden of disease in developing countries (WHO 2002b). As such, developing countries need greater investments to build stronger scientific and institutional capacity to address problems unique to their circumstances. Greater emphasis should be placed on research on the social, economic, and political determinants of ill health and how the structural barriers to application of existing technologies might be overcome. Advocacy for health systems and implementation research needs to be strengthened to bridge the gap between knowledge and action (Sanders & Haines 2006). This demands stronger capacity for indigenous and multidisciplinary health research, to deliver socially and culturally sensitive evidence to inform practical health systems development.

The opportunities created by advances in biomedical science need to be harnessed more effectively to develop new products. The agenda for research should be guided by national and internationally agreed priorities and biased towards the greatest unmet health needs. There is a strong necessity to continue to develop safe and affordable new products for such communicable diseases as AIDS, malaria and tuberculosis, and for other diseases disproportionately affecting developing countries. Insufficient research has been focused on interventions for the poor, such as treatment for neglected tropical diseases, antibiotic delivery mechanisms for children with pneumonia and access to perinatal care (WHO 2007a).

There has been considerable momentum in recent years by governments, industry, charitable foundations, and non-governmental organizations in funding initiatives to develop new products to fight diseases affecting developing countries, and to increase access to new ones. Strong advocacy must continue to sustain the political will and commitment for such initiatives, and the unprecedented opportunities for health they have created. Multilateral finance mechanisms such as the International Finance Facility for Immunization, the use of Advance Market Commitments to stimulate the development of new vaccines, the Global Fund, UNITAID, and the Global Alliance for Vaccines and Immunization provide long-term, sustainable and predictable funding needed to scale up access and reduce prices of drugs, vaccines, and diagnostics for the treatment of diseases disproportionably affecting developing countries.

The sharing of knowledge and research also serves to promote health through its effect on individual behaviour and better health practices. The dissemination of health information, especially through the use of media, on such issues as tobacco use, and sexual and reproductive health in adolescents and young adults, helps raise awareness, and enhance health promoting behaviour. Advances in the use of information and communication technology to provide health care in remote or hard to reach areas, data collection and research remains an expanding and valuable resource.

Conclusion

At the midpoint to 2015—the target year for the achievement of the MDGs at a global level—we are mindful of the significant gaps and challenges in health that still confront us. We cannot afford to fail. To attain these goals requires action on equity and the underlying social determinants that influence health. It also demands our attention to improving the performance of health systems and for better evidence in policy. The impact of our outputs will be measured by the real and qualitative improvement of the health of women and the people of Africa. Progress on these fronts necessitates unwavering political will and global participation. Only then can we hope to achieve true health for all.

References

Alexander, D. (2007). The international health partnership. *The Lancet*, **370**(9590), 803–4.

Anand, S. and Barnighausen, T. (2004). Human resources and health outcomes: cross-country econometric study. *The Lancet*, **364**(9445), 1603–9.

Anand, S. and Barnighausen, T. (2007). Health workers and vaccination coverage in developing countries: an econometric analysis. *The Lancet*, **369**(9569), 1277–85.

Belizan, J.M., Cafferata, M.L., Belizan, M., and Althabe, F. (2007). Health inequality in Latin America. *The Lancet*, **370**(9599), 1599–600.

Ben-David, D. (2000). *Trade, growth and disparity among nations*. WTO Geneva, WTO Secretariat Geneva.

Berman, P. (2000). Organization of ambulatory care provision: a critical determinant of health system performance in developing countries. *Bulletin of the World Health Organization*, **78**(6), 791–802.

Bettcher, D.W., Yach, D., and Guindon, G.E. (2000). Critical reflection global trade and health: key linkages and future challenges. *Bulletin of the World Health Organization*, **78**(4) 521–534.

Bloom, S.S., Wypij, D., and Das Gupta, M. (2001). Dimensions of women's autonomy and the influence on maternal health care utilization in a north Indian city. *Demography*, **38**(1), 67–78.

Blouin, C., Drager, N., and Smith, R. (2006). *International trade in health services and the gats: current issues and debates*. World Bank Publications, Washington D.C.

Braveman, P. and Gruskin, S. (2003). Poverty, equity, human rights and health. *Bulletin of the World Health Organization*, **81**(7), 539–45.

Buse, K. and Walt, G. (1997). An unruly melange? Coordinating external resources to the health sector: a review. *Social Science & Medicine*, **45**(3), 449–63.

Chalker, J., Chuc, N.T.K., Falkenberg, T., Do, N.T., and Tomson, G. (2000). STD management by private pharmacies in Hanoi: practice and knowledge of drug sellers. *British Medical Journal*, **76**(4), 299.

Charter, O. (1986). *Ottawa charter for health promotion*. Paper presented to First International Conference on Health Promotion, Ottawa, viewed 12 March 2008 <http://www.who.int/hpr/NPH/docs/ottawa_charter_hp.pdf>.

Chen, L.C., Evans, T.G., Cash, R.A., Kaul, I., Grunberg, I., and Stern, M. (1999). *Global public goods: International cooperation in the 21st century*. Oxford University Press, Oxford.

Chopra, M., Galbraith, S., and Darnton-Hill, I. (2002). A global response to a global problem: the epidemic of overnutrition. *Bulletin of the World Health Organization*, **80**(12), 952–8.

Clemens, M. and Pettersson, G. (2008). New data on African health professionals abroad. *Human Resources for Health*, **6**(1), 1.

Climate Change. (2007). *The physical science basis. Summary for policymakers. (Contribution of Working Group I to the Fourth Assessment Report of the Intergovernmental Panel on Climate Change)*, Intergovernmental Panel on Climate Change (IPCC), Geneva.

CNA Corporation. (2007). National security and the threat of climate change, viewed 20 April 2008, <http://securityandclimate.cna.org/>.

Cockburn, R., Newton, P.N., Agyarko, E.K., Akunyili, D., and White, NJ. (2005). The global threat of counterfeit drugs: why industry and governments must communicate the dangers. *PLoS Med*, **2**(4), e100.

Commission on Health Research for Development. (1990). *Health research: essential link to equity in development*. Oxford University Press, Oxford.

Confalonieri, U., Menne, B., Akhtar, R., Ebi, K.L., Hauengue, M., Kovats, R.S., Revich, B., and Woodward, A. (2007). Human health. In *Intergovernmental panel on climate change fourth assessment report: climate change impacts, adaptation, and vulnerability* (eds. M.L. Parry, O.F. Canziani, J.P. Palutikof, P.J. van der Linden and C.E. Hanson), pp. 391–431. Cambridge University Press, Cambridge.

Devarajan, S. (2003). *World Development Report 2004: making services work for poor people*. World Bank Publications, Washington DC.

Dodgson, R., Lee, K., and Drager, N. (2002). *Global health governance*.

Doherty, J. and Govender, R. (2004). The cost-effectiveness of primary care services in developing countries: a review of the international literature. *Background Paper: Disease Control Priorities Project*, World Bank, Washington DC, viewed 12 March 2008, <http://www.dcp2.org/file/49/wp37.pdf>.

Dollar, D. (2001). Is globalization good for your health? *Bulletin of the World Health Organization*, **79**(9), 827–33.

Dollar, D. and Kraay, A. (2002). Growth is Good for the Poor, *Journal of Economic Growth*, **7**(3), 195–225.

Dondorp, A.M., Newton, P.N., Mayxay, M., Van Damme, W., Smithuis, F.M., Yeung, S., Petit, A., Lynam, A.J., Johnson, A., Hien, T.T., McGready, R., Farrar, J.J., Looareesuwan, S., Day, N.P.J., Green, M.D., and White, N.J. (2004). Fake antimalarials in Southeast Asia are a major impediment to malaria control: multinational cross-sectional survey on the prevalence of fake antimalarials. *Tropical Medicine & International Health*, **9**(12), 1241–6.

ECLAC. (2005). *Social panorama of Latin America*. Economic Commission for Latin America and the Caribbean, viewed 12 March 2008, <www.eclac.org/publicaciones/xml/4/24054/PSI2005_Cap2_GastoSocial.pdf>.

Fabricant, S.J., Kamara, C.W., and Mills, A. (1999). Why the poor pay more: household curative expenditures in rural Sierra Leone. *The International Journal of Health Planning and Management*, **14**, 179–99.

Garau, P., Sclar, E., and Carolini, G.Y. (2005). *A home in the city: UN Millenium project. Task force on improving the lives of slum dwellers*. UNDP, James & James (Science Publishers) Ltd, London.

Gill, K., Pande, R., and Malhotra, A. (2007). Women deliver for development. *The Lancet*, **370**(9595), 1347–57.

Global Forum for Health Research. (2007). *Global forum update on research for health volume 4. Equitable access: research challenges for health in developing countries*. Pro-Book Publishing Limited, viewed 12 March 2008, <http://www.globalforumhealth.org/filesupld/global_update4/GlobalUpdate4Full.pdf>.

Global Health Workforce Alliance. (2008). *Health workers for all and all for health workers. The Kampala Declaration and agenda for global action*. Paper presented to First Global Forum on Human Resources for Health, Kampala, Uganda.

Globalization Knowledge Network. (2007). *Towards health-equitable globalisation: rights, regulation and redistribution*, viewed 12 March 2008 <http://www.who.int/social_determinants/resources/globlalization_kn_07_2007.pdf>.

Goodman, C., Brieger, W., Unwin, A., Mills, A., Meek, S., and Greer, G. (2007). Medicine sellers and malaria treatment in Sub-Saharan Africa: what do they do and how can their practice be improved? *The American Journal of Tropical Medicine and Hygiene*, **77**(6) (Suppl.), 203.

Grown, C., Gupta, G.R., and Pande, R. (2005). Taking action to improve women's health through gender equality and women's empowerment. *The Lancet*, **365**(9458), 541–3.

Gwatkin, D.R., Bhuiya, A., and Victora, C.G. (2004). Making health systems more equitable. *The Lancet*, **364**(9441), 1273–80.

Haines, A., Heath, I., and Smith, R. (2000). Joining together to combat poverty. *BMJ*, **320**(7226), 1–2.

Heymann, D. L. and Rodier, G. R. (2001). Hot spots in a wired world: WHO surveillance of emerging and re-emerging infectious diseases. *The Lancet Infectious Diseases*, **1**, 345–353.

Hill, K., Thomas, K., AbouZahr, C., Walker, N., Say, L., Inoue, M., and Suzuki, E. (2008). Estimates of maternal mortality worldwide between 1990 and 2005: an assessment of available data. *The Lancet*, **370**(9595), 1311–9.

Jamison, D.T., Mosley, W.H., Measham, A.R., and Bobadilla, J.L. (2006). *Disease control priorities in developing countries*. World Bank Group, Washington DC.

Joint Learning Initiative. (2004). *Human resources for health: overcoming the crisis*. Harvard University Press, Cambridge, viewed 12 March 2008, <www.who.int/hrh/documents/JLi_hrh_report.pdf>.

Kar, K. and Bongartz, P. (2006). *Update on Some Recent Developments in Community-Led Total Sanitation*, viewed 20 April 2008 <http://www.livelihoods.org/hot_topics/docs/CLTS_update06.pdf>.

Lancet. (2007). Editorial: progress and inequity in Latin America. *The Lancet*, **370**(9599), 1589.

Mann, J.M., Gostin, L., Gruskin, S., Brennan, T., Lazzatin, Z., and Fineberg, H. (1999). *Health and human rights health and human rights: a reader*, Routledge, New York.

Marmot, M. (2005). Social determinants of health inequalities. *The Lancet*, **365**(9464), 1099–104.

Marmot, M. (2007). Achieving health equity: from root causes to fair outcomes. *The Lancet*, **370**(9593), 1153–63.

Mathers, C.D. and Loncar, D. (2006). Projections of global mortality and burden of disease from 2002 to 2030. *PLoS Med*, **3**(11), e442.

Mazur, J. (2000). Labor's new internationalism. *Foreign Affairs*, **79**(1), 79–93.

Mills, A., Brugha, R., Hanson, K., and McPake, B. (2002). What can be done about the private health sector in low-income countries? *Bulletin of the World Health Organization*, **80**(4), 325–30.

Mundial, B. (2005). *World Development Report 2006: equity and development*. World Bank Publications, Washington DC.

Narasimhan, V., Brown, H., Pablos-Mendez, A., Adams, O., Dussault, G., Elzinga, G., Nordstrom, A., Habte, D., Jacobs, M., and Solimano, G. (2004). Responding to the global human resources crisis. *The Lancet*, **363**(9419), 1469–72.

OECD. (2005). *Paris declaration on aid effectiveness: ownership, harmonisation, alignment, results and mutual accountability, organization for economic co-operation and development*. OECD High-Level Forum, Paris.

OECD. (2007). *Reporting directives for the Creditor Reporting System*. Development Assistance Committee, Organisation for Economic Co-operation and Development, Paris.

Ogata, S. and Sen, A. (2003). *Human security now. protecting and empowering people*. United Commission on Human Security, Final Report, New York.

Ong, A.K. and Heymann, D.L. (2007). Microbes and humans: the long dance. *Bulletin of the World Health Organization*, **85**, 422–23.

Parry, M.L., Canziani, O.F., Palutikof, J.P., van der Linden, P.J., and Hanson, C.E. (2007). *Climate change 2007: impacts, adaptation and vulnerability*. Contribution of Working Group II to the Fourth Assessment Report of the Intergovernmental Panel on Climate Change.

Peden, M., Scurfield, R., Sleet, D., Mohan, D., Hyder, A.A., Jarawan, E., and Mathers, C. (2004). *World report on road traffic injury prevention*. World Health Organization, Geneva.

Preker, A.S., Liu, X., and Velenyi, E. (2007). *Public ends, private means: strategic purchasing of health services*. World Bank Publications, Washington DC.

Raviglione, M.C. and Smith, I.M. (2007). XDR tuberculosis – implications for global public health. *The New England Journal of Medicine*, **356**(7), 656–9.

Robinson, M. and Clark, P. (2008). Forging solutions to health worker migration. *The Lancet*, **371**(9613), 691–3.

Ruger, J.P. (2003). Health and development. *The Lancet*, **362**(9385), 678.

Ruger, J.P. and Yach, D. (2005). Global functions at the World Health Organization. *BMJ*, **330**(7500), 1099–100.

Sanders, D. and Haines, A. (2006). Implementation research is needed to achieve international health goals. *PLoS Med*, **3**(6), e186.

Sen, A.K. and Sen, A. (1999). *Development as freedom*. Oxford University Press, Oxford.

Smith, R.D. and Coast, J. (2002). Antimicrobial resistance: a global response. *Bulletin of the World Health Organization*, **80**(2), 126.

Smolinski, M.S., Margaret, A., and Lederberg, J. (2003). *Microbial threats to health emergence, detection, and response*. National Academies Press, Washington DC.

Starfield, B., Shi, L., and Macinko, J. (2005). Contribution of primary care to health systems and health. *The Milbank Quarterly*, **83**(3), 457–502.

Taylor, A.L. (2002). Global governance, international health law and WHO: looking towards the future. *Bulletin of the World Health Organization*, **80**(12), 975–80.

Taylor, A.L. and Bettcher, D.W. (2000). WHO Framework Convention on Tobacco Control: a global "good" for public health. *Bulletin of the World Health Organization*, **78**(7), 920–9.

Travis, P., Bennett, S., Haines, A., Pang, T., Bhutta, Z., Hyder, A.A., Pielemeier, N.R., Mills, A., and Evans, T. (2004). Overcoming health-systems constraints to achieve the Millennium Development Goals. *The Lancet*, **364**(9437), 900–6.

Tudor Hart, J. (1971). The inverse care law. *The Lancet*, **297**(7696), 405–12.

UN. (2000). *United Nations millennium declaration (United Nations General Assembly Resolution 55/2)*. United Nations, New York.

UN. (2008). *Department for economic and social affairs, population division. world urbanization prospects: the 2007 revision*. United Nations, New York.

UNAIDS. (2006). *UNAIDS Annual Report. Making the money work*. Joint United Nations Programme on HIV/AIDS (UNAIDS), Geneva.

UNAIDS. (2007). *AIDS epidemic update: December 2007*. Joint United Nations Programme on HIV/AIDS (UNAIDS) and World Health Organizations (WHO), Geneva.

UNFPA. (2007). *State of world population 2007. Unleashing the potential of urban growth*. United Nations Population Fund, New York.

UNICEF. (2007). *Progress for children. A world fit for children. Statistical Review Number 6*. United Nations Children's Fund, New York.

Uplekar, M., Pathania, V., and Raviglione, M. (2001). Private practitioners and public health: weak links in tuberculosis control. *The Lancet*, **358**(9285), 912–6.

Vujicic, M., Zurn, P., Diallo, K., Adams, O., and Dal Poz, M. (2004). The role of wages in the migration of health care professionals from developing countries. *Human Resources for Health*, **2**(1), 3.

Wade, R.H. (2004). Is globalization reducing poverty and inequality? *World Development*, **32**(4), 567–89.

Wagstaff, A. (2002). Poverty and health sector inequalities. *Bulletin of the World Health Organization*, **80**, 97–105.

Whitehead, M. (1992). The concepts and principles of equity and health. *International Journal of Health Services*, **22**(3), 429–45.

WHO. (2002a). Constitution of the World Health Organization. *Bulletin of the World Health Organization*, **80**, 983–4.

WHO. (2002b). *Global forum for health research: The 10/90 report on health research 2001–2002*. World Health Organization, Geneva.

WHO. (2003a). *WHO framework convention on tobacco control*. World Health Organization, Geneva.

WHO. (2003b). *The World Health Report 2003: shaping the future*. World Health Organization, Geneva.

WHO. (2006a). The commission on social determinants of health: tackling the social roots of health inequities. *PLoS Medicine*, **3**(6), e106.

WHO. (2006b). *Counterfeit medicine*. World Health Organization, viewed 12 March 2008 <http://www.who.int/mediacentre/factsheets/fs275/en/index.html>.

WHO. (2006c). *Engaging for health. Eleventh general programme of work 2006–2015. a global health agenda*. World Health Organization, Geneva.

WHO. (2006d). *World Health Report 2006: working together for health*. World Health Organization, Geneva.

WHO. (2007a). *Tough choices: investing in health for development: experiences from national follow-up to the Commission on Macroeconomics and Health*. World Health Organization, Geneva.

WHO. (2007b). *WHA 58.3 Revision of the International health regulations*. World Health Organization, viewed 12 March 2008 <http://www.who.int/gb/ebwha/pdf_files/WHA58/WHA58_3-en.pdf >.

WHO. (2007c). *WHO mortality database: tables [online database]*. World Health Organization, Geneva.

WHO. (2007d). *World Health Report 2007 – a safer future: global public health security in the 21st century*. World Health Organization, Geneva.

WHO. (2008a). *Global tuberculosis control: surveillance, planning, financing*. WHO Report 2008, Geneva.

WHO. (2008b). *Protecting health from climate change – World Health Day 2008*. World Health Organization, viewed 20 April 2008, <http://www.who.int/world-health-day/en/>.

WHO. (2008c). *WHO report on the global tobacco epidemic, 2008. The MPOWER package*, viewed 12 March 2008 <http://www.who.int/tobacco/mpower/en/index.html>.

World Bank. (2007a). *Global monitoring report 2007: confronting the challenges of gender equality and fragile states*. World Bank, Washington DC.

World Bank. (2007b). *World Development Indicators 2007*. Washington DC.

Index

Page numbers in **bold** refer to major sections of the text.

Since the major subject of this title is public health, entries under this keyword have been kept to a minimum, and readers are advised to seek more specific references.

Indexing style

Alphabetical order. This index is in letter-by-letter order, whereby hyphens, en-rules and spaces within index headings are ignored in the alphabetization. Terms in brackets are excluded from initial alphabetization.

Main abbreviations used

AIDS acquired immunodeficiency syndrome
ANOVA analysis of variance
BMI body mass index
CJD Creutzfeldt-Jakob disease
COPD chronic obstructive pulmonary disease
HIV human immunodeficiency virus
SARS sudden acute respiratory syndrome
STIs sexually transmitted infections.

Other abbreviations are defined in the index

H

M

Q

R